FUNDAMENTALS
of NURSING

ELEVENTH EDITION

A tailored education experience —
Sherpath book-organized collections

Sherpath is the digital teaching and learning technology designed specifically for healthcare education.

Sherpath book-organized collections offer:

Objective-based, digital lessons, mapped chapter-by-chapter to the textbook, that make it easy to find applicable digital assignment content.

Adaptive quizzing with personalized questions that correlate directly to textbook content.

Teaching materials that align to the text and are organized by chapter for quick and easy access to invaluable class activities and resources.

Elsevier ebooks that provide convenient access to textbook content, even offline.

VISIT
myevolve.us/sherpath
today to learn more!

ELEVENTH EDITION

FUNDAMENTALS of NURSING

Patricia A. Potter, RN, MSN, PhD, FAAN
Formerly, Director of Research
Patient Care Services
Barnes-Jewish Hospital
St. Louis, Missouri

Anne Griffin Perry, RN, MSN, EdD, FAAN
Professor Emerita
School of Nursing
Southern Illinois University—Edwardsville
Edwardsville, Illinois

Patricia A. Stockert, RN, BSN, MS, PhD
Formerly, President, College of Nursing
Saint Francis Medical Center College of Nursing
Peoria, Illinois

Amy M. Hall, RN, BSN, MS, PhD, CNE
Professor and Dean
School of Nursing
Franciscan Missionaries of Our Lady University
Baton Rouge, Louisiana

SECTION EDITOR:
Wendy R. Ostendorf, RN, MS, EdD, CNE
Contributing Faculty
Masters of Science in Nursing
Walden University
Minneapolis, Minnesota

ELSEVIER

Elsevier
3251 Riverport Lane
St. Louis, Missouri 63043

Notice

Practitioners and researchers must always rely on their own experience and knowledge in evaluating and using any information, methods, compounds or experiments described herein. Because of rapid advances in the medical sciences, in particular, independent verification of diagnoses and drug dosages should be made. To the fullest extent of the law, no responsibility is assumed by Elsevier, authors, editors or contributors for any injury and/or damage to persons or property as a matter of products liability, negligence or otherwise, or from any use or operation of any methods, products, instructions, or ideas contained in the material herein.

Previous editions copyrighted 2021, 2017, 2013, 2009, 2005, 2001, 1997, 1993, 1989, 1985.

Library of Congress Control Number: 2021936924

Director, Traditional Education: Tamara Myers
Senior Content Development Manager: Lisa P. Newton
Senior Content Development Specialist: Tina Kaemmerer
Publishing Services Manager: Julie Eddy
Senior Project Manager: Jodi Willard
Design Direction: Maggie Reid

Printed in India

Last digit is the print number: 9 8 7 6 5 4 3 2

Working together
to grow libraries in
developing countries

www.elsevier.com • www.bookaid.org

CONTRIBUTORS TO PREVIOUS EDITIONS

Jeanette Adams, PhD, MSN, APRN, CRNI

Michelle Aebersold, PhD, RN

Paulette M. Archer, RN, EdD

Myra. A. Aud, PhD, RN

Katherine N. Ayzengart, MSN, RN

Marjorie Baier, PhD, RN

Sylvia K. Baird, RN, BSN, MM

Karen Balakas, PhD, RN, CNE

Brenda Battle, RN, BSN, MBA

Kimberly Diane Baxter, DNP, APRN, FNP-BC

Sharon Ferguson Beasley, PhD, MSN, RN, CNE

Lois Bentler-Lampe, RN, MS

Janice Boundy, RN, PhD

Jessica L. Bower, DNP, MSN, RN

Karen Britt, DNP, RN-BC, CNE

Anna Brock, PhD, MSN, MEd, BSN

Sheryl Buckner, RN-BC, MS, CNE

Jeri Burger, PhD, RN

Linda Cason, MSN, RN-BC, NE-BC, CNRN

Pamela L. Cherry, RN, BSN, MSN, DNSc,

Janice C. Colwell, RN, MS, CWOCN, FAAN

Rhonda W. Comrie, PhD, RN, CNE, AE-C

Maureen F. Cooney, DNP, FNP-BC

Eileen Costantinou, MSN, RN

Cheryl A. Crowe, RN, MS

Ruth M. Curchoe, RN, MSN, CIC

Sarah Delgado, MSN, RN, ACNP

Marinetta DeMoss, RN, MSN

Bronwyn Doyle, PhD, RN, CNE

Alice E. Dupler, MSN, JD, RN, CNP, Esq.

Christine R. Durbin, PhD, JD, RN

Margaret Ecker, RN, MS

Martha Keene Elkin, RN, MS, IBCLC

Antoinette Falker, DNP, RN, CMSRN, CBN, GCNS-BC

Jane Fellows, MSN, CWOCN-AP

Linda Felver, PhD, RN

Susan Fetzer, BA, BSN, MSN, MBA, PhD

Victoria N. Folse, PhD, APRN, PMHCNS-BC, LCPC

Leah W. Frederick, MS, RN CIC

Kay Gaehle, PhD, MSN

Lorri A. Graham, DNP-L, RN

Carla Armstead Harmon, PhD (Curriculum & Instruction), MSN, BSN

Susan Hendricks, EdD, MSN, RN, CNE

Maureen Hermann, BSN, MSN, DNP, RN

Mimi Hirshberg, RN, MSN

Tara Hulsey, BSN, MSN, PhD

Lenetra Jefferson, PhD, MSN, BSN, LMT

Noël Marie Kerr, PhD

Steve Kilkus, RN, MSN

Judith Ann Kilpatrick, RN, DNSc

Shari Kist, PhD, RN, CNE

Lori Klingman, MSN, RN

Mary Koithan, PhD, MSN, BSN

Karen Korem, RN-BC, MA

Gayle L. Kruse, RN, ACHPN, GCNS-BC

Anahid Kulwicki, RN, DNS, FAAN

Jerrilee LaMar, PhD, RN, CNE

Joyce Larson, PhD, MS, RN

Kristine M. L'Ecuyer, RN, MSN, CCNS

Kathryn Lever, MSN, WHNP-BC

Ruth Ludwick, BSN, MSN, PhD, RNC

Annette G. Lueckenotte, MS, RN, BC, GNP GCNS

Frank Lyerla, PhD, RN

Deborah Marshall, MSN

Barbara Maxwell, RN, BSN, MS, MSN, CNS

Erin H. McCalley, RN, BSN, MS, CCRN, CCNS

Emily McClung, MSN, RN, PhD

Angela McConachie, FNP, DNP

Judith A. McCutchan, RN, ASN, BSN, MSN, PhD

Emily McKenna, APN, CNS

Theresa Miller, PhD, MSN, MHA, RN

Elaine K. Neel, RN, BSN, MSN

Patricia A. O'Connor, RN, MSN, CNE

Wendy Ostendorf, RN, MS, EdD, CNE

Dula Pacquiao, BSN, MA, EdD

Nancy C. Panthofer, RN, MSN

Jill Parsons, PhD, RN

Elaine U. Polan, RNC, BSN, MS

Beverly J. Reynolds, RN, EdD, CNE

Kristine Rose, BSN, MSN

Patsy L. Ruchala, DNSc, RN

Debbie Sanazaro, RN, MSN, GNP

Lynette Savage, BS, BSN, MS, PhD

Marilyn Schallom, RN, MSN, CCRN, CCNS

Carrie Sona, RN, MSN, CCRN, ACNS, CCNS

Matthew R. Sorenson, PhD, APN, ANP-C

Angela Renee Starkweather, PhD, ACNP-BC, FAAN

Marshelle Thobaben, RN, MS, PHN, APNP, FNP

Donna L. Thompson, MSN, CRNP, FNP-BC, CCCN-AP

Jelena Todic, MSW, LCSW

Ann B. Tritak, EdD, MA, BSN, RN

Shellye A. Vardaman, PhD

Janis Waite, RN, MSN, EdD

Mary Ann Wehmer, RN, MSN, CNOR

Pamela Becker Weilitz, RN, MSN(R), BC, ANP, M-SCNS

Joan Domigan Wentz, BSN, MSN

Katherine West, BSN, MSEd, CIC

Terry L. Wood, PhD, RN, CNE

Carolyn J. Wright Boon, MSN, BSN

Rita Wunderlich, PhD, RN

Valerie Yancey, PhD, RN

We would like to dedicate this 11th edition of *Fundamentals of Nursing* to three awe-inspiring groups of people—working nurses, nurse educators, and nursing students. Hardworking, caring nurses have provided and will continue to provide care to hundreds of thousands of patients hospitalized with COVID-19 during the pandemic. It has been a challenging time to deliver care for patients, and all of you have stepped up to the challenge and continued to provide safe, competent, high-quality care to all patients. You have provided patients with support and comfort during the hardest times in their lives. Nurse educators, you have been challenged during the pandemic to continue providing education to nursing students who often were not in your classroom. You have been thoughtful and creative in your approaches and have embraced online and nontraditional delivery of nursing content, determined to prepare future nurses entering the profession. Nursing students, you have embraced these nontraditional styles of learning and have continued to move forward with your education so that you can join the nursing workforce.

Thank you to all the nurses, nurse educators, and nursing students for continuing to excel and meet the unforeseen challenges of the COVID-19 pandemic. We are proud to be a part of the nursing profession with all of you!

Patricia A. Potter
Anne Griffin Perry
Patricia A. Stockert
Amy M. Hall
Wendy R. Ostendorf

PREFACE TO THE INSTRUCTOR

The nursing profession is always responding to dynamic change and continual challenges. Today, nurses need a broad knowledge base to know how to use sound clinical judgment by applying critical thinking and best evidence in practice to ensure the best outcomes for their patients. The role of the nurse includes assuming the lead in preserving nursing practice and demonstrating its contribution to the health care of our nation. Nurses of tomorrow, therefore, need to become competent clinicians using sound clinical judgment, critical thinkers, patient advocates, and patient educators within a broad spectrum of care services.

The eleventh edition of *Fundamentals of Nursing* was revised to prepare today's students for the challenges of tomorrow. This textbook is designed for beginning students in all types of professional nursing programs. The comprehensive coverage provides fundamental nursing concepts, skills, and techniques of nursing practice and a firm foundation for more advanced areas of study.

Fundamentals of Nursing provides a contemporary approach to nursing practice, discussing the entire scope of primary, acute, and restorative care. In an effort to continue to inform and build students' knowledge of the complexities of nursing practice, the authors have developed a new Critical Thinking and Clinical Judgment model that incorporates the major themes and constructs of the National Council of State Boards of Nursing Clinical Judgment Measurement Model (NCSBN-CJMM). The model has been integrated into all clinical chapters of the text along with case studies and more examples of clinical applications. The student is shown throughout the text how clinical judgment is unique to each patient and the patient's clinical condition.

This new edition continues to address a number of key practice issues, including an emphasis on patient-centered care, cultural sensitivity and diversity, evidence-based practice, and globalization of health care. Evidence-based practice is one of the most important initiatives in health care today. The increased focus on applying current evidence in patient care helps students understand how the latest research findings should guide their clinical decision making. Current evidence is reflected in each chapter's references.

KEY FEATURES

We have carefully developed this eleventh edition with the student in mind. We have designed this text to welcome the new student to nursing, communicate our own love for the profession, and promote learning and understanding. Key features of the text include the following:

- **Clinical examples** that assist students in understanding how clinical judgment is practiced.
- Students will appreciate the **clear, engaging writing style.** The narrative actually addresses the reader, making this textbook more of an active instructional tool than a passive reference. Students will find that even complex technical and theoretical concepts are presented in a language that is easy to understand.
- **Comprehensive** coverage and readability of all fundamental nursing content.
- The **attractive, functional design** will appeal to today's visual learner. The clear, readable type and boldface headings make the content easy to read and follow. Each special element is consistently color-keyed so students can readily identify important information.
- Hundreds of **large, clear, full-color photographs and drawings** reinforce and clarify key concepts and techniques.

- The **nursing process** format provides a consistent organizational framework for clinical chapters.
- **Learning aids** to help students identify, review, and apply important content in each chapter include Objectives, Key Terms, Key Points, QSEN activities, Next-Generation NCLEX®–based Reflective Learning Questions, and Review Questions.
- **Reflect Now** boxes interspersed throughout the chapters prompt students to consider a recent clinical experience based on the topic being discussed in the text.
- **Review Questions** have been updated in each chapter and include several alternate-item–type questions. Answers are provided at the end of the chapter, with rationales provided in the Evolve Student Resources.
- **Health promotion and acute and continuing care** are covered to address today's practice in various settings.
- A **health promotion/wellness** thread is used consistently throughout the text.
- **Cultural competence,** care of the **older adult,** and **patient teaching** are stressed throughout chapter narratives, as well as highlighted in special boxes.
- **Evidence-Based Practice** is consistently used within the chapters, including an Evidence-Based Practice box relevant to the content of the chapter. This box includes a brief summary of the evidence related to a PICOT question and appropriate nursing actions.
- **Procedural Guidelines** boxes provide more streamlined, step-by-step instructions for performing very basic skills.
- **Concept Maps** included in clinical chapters show you the association between multiple nursing diagnoses for a patient with a selected medical diagnosis and the relationships among nursing interventions.
- **Nursing Care Plans** guide students on how to conduct an assessment, analyze the defining characteristics in order to select nursing diagnoses, and then determine the expected outcomes of care. The plans include NIC and NOC classifications to familiarize students with this important nomenclature. The evaluation section of the plans shows students how to evaluate whether the identified outcomes of care were achieved.
- Information related to the **Quality and Safety Education for Nurses (QSEN)** initiative is highlighted by headings that coordinate with the key competencies. Building Competency scenarios in each chapter incorporate one of the six key competencies in QSEN. Answers to these activities can be found online in the Evolve Student Resources.
- **More than 55 nursing skills** are presented in a clear two-column format with steps and supporting rationales that are supported with current evidenced-based research.
- **Delegation Considerations** guide when it is appropriate to delegate tasks to assistive personnel.
- **Teach-back** is included in the evaluation section of each skill and in the Patient Teaching boxes.
- **Unexpected Outcomes and Related Interventions** are highlighted within nursing skills to help students anticipate and appropriately respond to possible problems faced while performing skills.
- **Evolve Resources** lists at the beginning of every chapter detail the electronic resources available for the student.
- **Video Icons** indicate video clips associated with specific skills that are available on the Evolve Student Resources.
- **Printed endpapers** on the inside back cover provide information on locating specific assets in the book, including Skills, Procedure Guidelines, Nursing Care Plans, and Concept Maps.

ix

NEW TO THIS EDITION

- Revised unit on Clinical Judgment in Nursing Practice. This unit integrates a model for Clinical Judgment that incorporates elements and constructs from the National Council of State Boards of Nursing Clinical Judgment Measurement Model (NCSBN-CJMM) and Next-Generation NCLEX® to prepare students to know how to make the right clinical decisions for their patients. The model provides a foundation for the nursing process chapters and is applied in all clinical chapters.
- New to the clinical chapters is the inclusion of an **evolving case study** throughout the chapter. Within the nursing process sections of the chapters, these case studies demonstrate how nursing assessment reveals relevant data cues and how the nurse analyzes the data to identify accurate and appropriate nursing diagnoses, identify and prioritize outcomes of care, and select individualized nursing interventions. Last, these case studies demonstrate how the nurse evaluates the outcomes of patient care.
- Increased emphasis on **delegation considerations**. The goal is to help the student understand the professional importance of correctly delegating a skill to the right assistive personnel and of completing any related nursing actions prior to or following delegation.
- **Clinical Judgment points** are included within the Skills and Procedural Guidelines boxes to alert the student to current research or appropriate patient-specific adaptations to a certain skill or technique.
- **Evidence-Based Practice** boxes in each chapter have been updated to reflect current research topics and trends.
- The **Reflective Learning** section uses the chapter case study to help students better understand and think about their clinical and simulation experiences as they progress through their first nursing courses.
- **Teach-Back** has been incorporated into the Evaluation section of the Patient Teaching boxes.

LEARNING SUPPLEMENTS FOR STUDENTS

- The **Evolve Student Resources** are available online at http://evolve.elsevier.com/Potter/fundamentals/ and include the following valuable learning aids organized by chapter:
  - Chapter Review Questions with Answers and Rationales
  - Answers and rationales to Building Competency scenario questions
  - Video clips highlight common skills
  - Concept Map Creator included in each clinical chapter
  - Conceptual Care Map included in each clinical chapter
  - Case Study with questions
  - Audio glossary
  - Fluids & Electrolytes Tutorial
  - Calculation Tutorial
  - Printable versions of chapter Key Points
  - Printable Skills Performance Checklists for each skill in the text
- A thorough *Study Guide* by Geralyn Ochs provides an ideal supplement to help students understand and apply the content of the text. Each chapter includes multiple sections:
  - Preliminary Reading includes a chapter assignment from the text.
  - Case Study includes related questions.
  - Comprehensive Understanding provides a variety of activities to reinforce the topics and main ideas from the text.
  - Review Questions include multiple-choice, matching, and fill-in-the-blank questions. Answers and rationales are provided in the answer key.

- Clinical chapters include a discussion of the Clinical Judgment Measurement Model that expands the case study from the chapter's Nursing Care Plan and asks students to develop a step in the synthesis model based on the nurse and patient in the scenario. This helps students learn to apply both content learned and the critical thinking synthesis model.
- Twenty chapters include a new Next-Generation NCLEX® question to help prepare students for practice.
- The handy *Clinical Companion* complements, rather than abbreviates, the textbook. Content is presented in tabular, list, and outline format that equips your students with a concise, portable guide to all the facts and figures they will need to know in their early clinical experiences.

TEACHING SUPPLEMENTS FOR INSTRUCTORS

The **Evolve Instructor Resources** (available online at http://evolve.elsevier.com/Potter/fundamentals) are a comprehensive collection of the most important tools instructors need, including the following:

- **TEACH for Nurses** ties together every chapter resource you need for the most effective class presentations, with sections dedicated to objectives, teaching focus, nursing curriculum standards (including QSEN, BSN Essentials, and Concepts), instructor chapter resources, student chapter resources, answers to chapter questions, and an in-class case study discussion. Teaching Strategies include relations between the textbook content and discussion items. Examples of student activities, online activities, new health promotion–focused activities, and large group activities are provided for more "hands-on" learning.
- The **Test Bank** contains 1100 questions with answers coded for the NCLEX® Client Needs category, nursing process, and cognitive level. The ExamView software allows instructors to create new tests; edit, add, and delete test questions; sort questions by NCLEX® category, cognitive level, nursing process step, and question type; and administer/grade online tests.
- Updated **PowerPoint Presentations** include over 1500 slides for use in lectures. Art is included within the slides and progressive case studies include discussion questions and answers.
- The **Image Collection** contains more than 1150 illustrations from the text for use in lectures.
- **Simulation Learning System** is an online toolkit that helps instructors and facilitators effectively incorporate medium- to high-fidelity simulation into their nursing curriculum. Detailed patient scenarios promote and enhance the clinical decision-making skills of students at all levels. The system provides detailed instructions for preparation and implementation of the simulation experience, debriefing questions that encourage critical thinking, and learning resources to reinforce student comprehension. Each scenario in *Simulation Learning System* complements the textbook content and helps bridge the gap between lectures and clinicals. This system provides the perfect environment for students to practice what they are learning in the text for a true-to-life, hands-on learning experience.

MULTIMEDIA SUPPLEMENTS FOR INSTRUCTORS AND STUDENTS

- **Nursing Skills Online 4.0** contains 19 modules rich with animations, videos, interactive activities, and exercises to help students prepare for their clinical lab experience. The instructionally designed lessons focus on topics that are difficult to master and pose a high risk to the patient if done incorrectly. Lesson quizzes allow students to check their learning curve and review as needed, and the module exams feed out to an instructor grade book. Modules cover Airway Management, Blood Therapy, Bowel Elimination/Ostomy Care, Cardiac Care, Cardiac Care, Closed Chest Drainage Systems, Enteral Nutrition, Infection Control, Maintenance of IV Fluid Therapy, IV Fluid Therapy, Administration of Parenteral Medications: Injections and IV Medications, Nonparenteral Medication Administration, Safe Medication Preparation, Safety, Specimen Collection, Urinary Catheterization, Caring for Central Vascular Access Devices (CVAD), Vital Signs, and Wound Care. Available alone or packaged with the text.

ACKNOWLEDGMENTS

The eleventh edition of *Fundamentals of Nursing* is one that we believe continues to prepare the nursing student to be able to practice in the challenging health care environment. Collaboration on this project allows us to be creative, visionary, and thoughtful regarding students' learning needs. Each edition is a new adventure for all of us on the author team as we try to create the very best textbook for beginning nurses. Each of us wishes to acknowledge the professionalism, support, and commitment to detail from the following individuals:

- To the editorial and production professionals at Elsevier, including:
    - Tamara Myers, Director, Traditional Education, for her vision, organization, professionalism, energy, and support in assisting us to develop a text that offers a state-of-the-art approach to the design, organization, and presentation of *Fundamentals of Nursing*. Her skill is in motivating and supporting a writing team so it can be creative and innovative while retaining the characteristics of a high-quality textbook.
    - Tina Kaemmerer as our Senior Content Development Specialist for *Fundamentals of Nursing* for her dedication to keeping the writing team organized and focused and for performing considerable behind-the-scenes work to ensure accuracy and consistency in how we present content within the textbook. She has limitless energy and is always willing to go the extra mile.
    - Jodi Willard, Senior Project Manager, for consistently performing miracles. She is an amazing and accomplished production editor who applies patience, humor, and attention to detail. It is an honor to work with Jodi because of her professionalism and ability to coordinate the multiple aspects of completing a well-designed finished product.
- To our contributors and clinician and educator reviewers, who share their expertise and knowledge about nursing practice and the trends within health care today, helping us to create informative, accurate, and current information. Their contributions allow us to develop a text that embodies high standards for professional nursing practice through the printed word.
- And special recognition to our professional colleagues at Barnes-Jewish Hospital, Southern Illinois University—Edwardsville, Saint Francis Medical Center College of Nursing, and Franciscan Missionaries of Our Lady University.

We believe that *Fundamentals of Nursing*, now in its eleventh edition, is a textbook that informs and helps to shape the standards for excellence in nursing practice. Nursing excellence belongs to all of us, and we are happy to have the opportunity to continue the work we love.

Patricia A. Potter
Anne Griffin Perry
Patricia A. Stockert
Amy M. Hall
Wendy R. Ostendorf

CONTENTS

Any updates to this textbook can be found in the Content Updates folder on Evolve at http://evolve.elsevier.com/Potter/fundamentals/.

1

Nursing Today

OBJECTIVES

- Explain how nursing standards affect nursing care.
- Discuss the development of professional nursing roles.
- Discuss the roles and career opportunities for professional nurses.
- Discuss the influence of social, historical, political, and economic changes on nursing practices.
- Discuss how advances in nursing science and evidence-based practice improve patient care.
- Compare and contrast the educational programs available for professional registered nurse (RN) education.
- Explain how professional nursing organizations affect both the profession and the standards of care.

KEY TERMS

Advanced practice registered nurse (APRN)
American Nurses Association (ANA)
Caregiver
Certified nurse-midwife (CNM)
Certified registered nurse anesthetist (CRNA)
Clinical nurse specialist (CNS)
Code of ethics

Continuing education
Genomics
In-service education
International Council of Nurses (ICN)
Nurse administrator
Nurse educator
Nurse practitioner (NP)

Nurse researcher
Nursing
Patient advocate
Professional organization
Quality and Safety Education for Nurses (QSEN)
Registered nurse (RN)

MEDIA RESOURCES

http://evolve.elsevier.com/Potter/fundamentals/
- Review Questions
- Audio Glossary

- Case Study with Questions
- Content Updates
- Answers to QSEN Activity and Review Questions

Nursing is an art and a science. As an art, nursing involves learning to deliver care with compassion, caring, and respect for each patient's dignity and individuality. It evolves as you gain more experience and witness how patients respond to your actions. As a science, nursing practice is based on a body of knowledge and evidence-based practices that are continually changing with new discoveries and innovations. Through integration of the art and science of nursing, the quality of care you provide meets the highest standards and benefits patients and their families. Your care reflects your patients' multidimensional needs as well as the needs and values of society and professional standards of care.

Nursing offers personal and professional rewards every day. This chapter presents a contemporary view of the evolution of nursing and nursing practice and the historical, practical, social, and political influences on the discipline of nursing.

NURSING AS A PROFESSION

The patient is the center of your practice. Depending on the setting and situation, your patients may include individuals, families, and/or communities. Patients have a wide variety of health care needs, knowledge, experiences, vulnerabilities, and expectations, but this is what makes nursing both challenging and rewarding. Making a difference in your patients' lives is fulfilling (e.g., helping a young mother learn parenting skills, finding ways for older adults to remain independent in their homes, assisting family care givers with end-of-life care and symptom management).

Nursing is not simply a collection of specific skills, and you are not simply a person trained to perform specific tasks. Nursing is a profession. No one factor absolutely differentiates a job from a profession, but the difference is important in terms of how you practice. To act

1

professionally, you will use critical thinking (see Chapter 15) to administer high-quality evidence-based patient-centered care in a safe, prudent, and knowledgeable manner. You are responsible and accountable to yourself, your patients, and your peers.

A variety of career opportunities are available in nursing, including clinical practice, education, research, management, administration, and even entrepreneurship. As a student it is important for you to understand the scope of professional nursing practice and how nursing influences the lives of your patients, their families, and their communities.

Health care advocacy groups recognize the importance of the role high-quality professional nursing plays in a nation's health care. One such program was the Robert Wood Johnson Foundation (RWJF) *Future of Nursing: Campaign for Action* (RWJF, 2014). This program was a multifaceted campaign to transform health care through nursing, and was a response to the Institute of Medicine (IOM) publication *The Future of Nursing* (IOM, 2010). A new RWJF (2017) initiative, *Catalysts for Change: Harnessing the Power of Nurses to Build Population Health in the 21st Century,* reinforces the fact that nurses are educated to consider health care issues within a broader context, and as a result nurses identify factors outside of health care that affect a person's level of health. These initiatives prepare a professional workforce to meet health promotion, illness prevention, and complex care needs of the population in a changing health care system.

Science and Art of Nursing Practice

Because nursing is both an art and a science, nursing practice requires a blend of current knowledge and practice standards with an insightful and compassionate approach to your patients' health care needs. Your care must reflect the needs and values of society and professional standards of care and performance, meet the needs of each patient, and integrate evidence-based findings to provide the highest level of care. For example, when caring for a patient with a pressure injury, you use evidence-based practice guidelines from professional organizations, such as the Wound, Ostomy, and Continence Nurses Society (WOCN) to individualize wound care interventions.

Clinical expertise takes time and commitment. According to Benner (1984), an expert nurse passes through five levels of proficiency when acquiring and developing generalist or specialized nursing skills (Box 1.1). Expert clinical nursing practice is a commitment to sound clinical judgment involving application of knowledge, ethics, evidence-based practices, and clinical experience. Your ability to interpret clinical situations and make complex decisions is the foundation for your nursing care and the basis for the advancement of nursing practice and the development of nursing science (Benner et al., 1997; Benner et al., 2010).

Critical thinking applied with clinical judgment helps you acquire and interpret scientific knowledge, integrate knowledge from clinical experiences, and become a lifelong learner (Chapter 15). Integrate the competencies of critical thinking in your practice. This includes incorporating knowledge from the basic sciences and nursing, applying knowledge from past and present experiences, considering environmental factors, applying critical thinking attitudes, and implementing intellectual and professional standards. When you provide well–thought-out care with compassion and caring, you provide each patient the best of the science and art of nursing care (see Chapter 7).

Scope and Standards of Practice

When giving care, it is essential to provide a specified service according to standards of practice and to follow a code of ethics. Professional practice includes knowledge from social and behavioral sciences, biological and physiological sciences, and nursing theories. In addition, nursing practice incorporates ethical and social values, professional autonomy, and a sense of commitment and community

---

BOX 1.1   Benner: From Novice to Expert

- **Novice:** Beginning nursing student or any nurse entering a situation in which there is no previous level of experience (e.g., an experienced operating room nurse chooses to now practice in home health). The learner learns via a specific set of rules or procedures, which are usually stepwise and linear.
- **Advanced Beginner:** A nurse who has had some level of experience with the situation. This experience may be only observational in nature, but the nurse is able to identify meaningful aspects or principles of nursing care.
- **Competent:** A nurse who has been in the same clinical position for 2 to 3 years. This nurse understands the organization and specific care required by the type of patients (e.g., surgical, oncology, or orthopedic patients). This nurse is a competent practitioner who is able to anticipate nursing care and establish long-range goals. In this phase the nurse has usually had experience with all types of psychomotor skills required by this specific group of patients.
- **Proficient:** A nurse with more than 2 to 3 years of experience in the same clinical position. This nurse perceives a patient's clinical situation as a whole, is able to assess an entire situation, and can readily transfer knowledge gained from multiple previous experiences to a situation. This nurse focuses on managing care as opposed to managing and performing skills.
- **Expert:** A nurse with diverse experience who has an intuitive grasp of an existing or potential clinical problem. This nurse is able to zero in on the problem and focus on multiple dimensions of the situation. This nurse is skilled at identifying both patient-centered problems and problems related to the health care system or perhaps the needs of the novice nurse.

Data from Benner P: *From novice to expert: excellence and power in clinical nursing practice,* Menlo Park, CA, 1984, Addison-Wesley.

(American Nurses Association [ANA], 2021). The following definition from the ANA illustrates the consistent commitment of nurses to provide care that promotes the well-being of their patients and communities (ANA, 2021):

> ***Nursing*** *incorporates the art and science of caring and focuses on the protection, promotion, and optimization of health and abilities; prevention of illness and injury; facilitation of healing; and alleviation of suffering through compassionate presence. Nursing is the diagnosis and treatment of human response, and advocacy in the care of individuals, families, groups, communities, and populations in recognition of the connection of all humanity.*

The **International Council of Nurses (ICN)** has another definition (ICN, 2021):

> *Nursing encompasses autonomous and collaborative care of individuals of all ages, families, groups, and communities, sick or well, and in all settings. Nursing includes the promotion of health; prevention of illness; and the care of ill, disabled, and dying people. Advocacy, promotion of a safe environment, research, participation in shaping health policy and in patient and health systems management, and education are also key nursing roles.*

Both of these definitions support the prominence and importance that nursing holds in providing safe, patient-centered health care to the global community.

The ANA develops, revises, and maintains the scope of practice statement and standards that apply to the practice of all professional nurses (ANA, 2021). It is important that you know and apply these

BOX 1.2 American Nurses Association (ANA) Standards of Nursing Practice

1. **Assessment:** The registered nurse collects pertinent data and information relative to the healthcare consumer's health or the situation.
2. **Diagnosis:** The registered nurse analyzes the assessment data to determine the actual or potential diagnoses, problems, and issues.
3. **Outcomes Identification:** The registered nurse identifies expected outcomes for a plan individualized to the healthcare consumer or the situation.
4. **Planning:** The registered nurse develops a plan encompassing strategies to achieve expected outcomes.
5. **Implementation:** The registered nurse implements the identified plan.
   5a. **Coordination of Care:** The registered nurse coordinates care delivery.
   5b. **Health Teaching and Health Promotion:** The registered nurse employs strategies to teach and promote health and wellness.
6. **Evaluation:** The registered nurse evaluates progress toward attainment of goals and outcomes.

Copyright © American Nurses Association: *Nursing scope and standards of practice*, ed 4, Silver Springs, MD, 2021, The Association. Reprinted with permission. All rights reserved.

BOX 1.3 American Nurses Association (ANA) Standards of Professional Performance

7. **Ethics:** The registered nurse integrates ethics in all aspect of practice.
8. **Advocacy:** The registered nurse demonstrates advocacy in all roles and settings.
9. **Respectful and Equitable Practice:** The registered nurse practices with cultural humility and inclusiveness.
10. **Communication:** The registered nurse communicates effectively in all areas of professional practice.
11. **Collaboration:** The registered nurse collaborates with health care consumers and other key stakeholders.
12. **Leadership:** The registered nurse leads within the professional practice setting and the profession.
13. **Education:** The registered nurse seeks knowledge and competence that reflects current nursing practice and promotes futuristic thinking.
14. **Scholarly Inquiry:** The registered nurse integrates scholarship, evidence, and research findings into practice.
15. **Quality of Practice:** The registered nurse contributes to quality nursing practice.
16. **Professional Practice Evaluation:** The registered nurse evaluates one's own and others' nursing practice.
17. **Resource Stewardship:** The registered nurse utilizes appropriate resources to plan, provide, and sustain evidence-based nursing services that are safe, effective, and fiscally responsible and avoid waste.
18. **Environmental Health:** The registered nurse practices in a manner that advances environmental safety and health.

Copyright © American Nurses Association: *Nursing scope and standards of practice*, ed 4, Silver Springs, MD, 2021, The Association. Reprinted with permission. All rights reserved.

standards in your practice (Box 1.2). Most schools of nursing and practice settings have published copies of the scope and standards of nursing practice. The scope and standards of practice guide nurses to make significant and visible contributions that improve the health and well-being of all individuals, communities, and populations (ANA, 2021).

Standards of Professional Nursing Practice. The Standards of Professional Nursing Practice contain authoritative statements of the duties that all registered nurses (RNs), regardless of role, population, specialty, setting, or APRN foci, are expected to competently perform (ANA, 2021). The Standards of Professional Nursing Practice describe a competent level of nursing care demonstrated by a critical thinking model known as the nursing process: assessment, diagnosis, outcomes identification and planning, implementation, and evaluation (ANA, 2021). The nursing process is the model for clinical decision making and includes all significant actions taken by nurses in providing care to patients (see Unit 3).

Standards of Professional Performance. The ANA Standards of Professional Performance (Box 1.3) describe a competent level of behavior in the professional nursing role. All RNs are expected to engage in professional role activities reflective of their education, experience, and position (ANA, 2021). The standards set a level of performance to assure patients that they are receiving high-quality care. This assumes that nurses know exactly what is necessary to provide nursing care. The standards are used as a measure to determine whether nursing care meets the standards.

Code of Ethics. The nursing code of ethics is a statement of philosophical ideals of right and wrong that define the principles you will use to provide care to your patients. It is important for you to also incorporate your own values and ethics into your practice. As you incorporate these values, explore what type of nurse you will be and how you will function within the discipline (ANA, 2021; Fowler, 2015). Ask yourself how your ethics, values, and practice compare with established standards. The ANA has a number of publications that address ethics and human rights in nursing. *The Code of Ethics for Nurses with Interpretive Statements* (ANA, 2015) lists the nine succinct provisions and interpretive statements that establish the ethical framework for RNs' practice

across all roles, levels, and settings. Chapter 22 provides a review of the nursing code of ethics and ethical principles for everyday practice.

Professional Responsibilities and Roles

Nurses provide care and comfort for patients in all health care settings. Their concern for meeting patients' needs remains the same whether care focuses on health promotion and illness prevention, disease and symptom management, family support, or end-of-life care. As a nurse, you are responsible for obtaining and maintaining specific knowledge and skills for a variety of professional roles and responsibilities.

Autonomy and Accountability. Autonomy is an essential element of professional nursing that involves the initiation of independent nursing interventions without medical orders. Although the nursing profession regulates accountability through nursing audits and standards of practice, you also need to develop a commitment to personal professional accountability. For example, you independently implement coughing and deep-breathing exercises to clear the lungs of secretions and promote oxygenation in a patient who recently had major surgery. As you continue to care for this patient, a complication arises. You note that the patient has a fever and the surgical wound has a yellow-green discharge. You collaborate with other health care professionals to develop the best treatment plan for this patient's surgical wound infection. With increased autonomy comes greater responsibility and accountability.

Accountability means that you are responsible professionally and legally for the type and quality of nursing care provided. This includes dependent, independent, and interdependent nursing actions (see Chapter 18). You must remain current and competent in nursing and scientific knowledge and technical skills.

Caregiver. As a caregiver you help patients maintain and regain health, manage disease and symptoms, and attain a maximal level of function and independence through the healing process. You provide evidence-based nursing care to promote healing through both physical and interpersonal skills. Healing involves more than achieving improved physical well-being. You support patients by providing measures that restore their emotional, spiritual, and social well-being. As a caregiver you help the patient and family set outcomes and assist them with meeting those outcomes with minimal financial cost, time, and energy.

Advocate. As a patient advocate you protect your patient's human and legal rights and provide assistance in asserting those rights if the need arises. As an advocate you act on behalf of your patient, such as safeguarding their care against errors, suggesting alternatives to care, securing your patient's health care rights, and facilitating personal and cultural preferences (Abbasinia et al., 2019; Kowalski, 2016). For example, you provide additional information to help a patient decide whether to accept a treatment, or you find an interpreter to help family members communicate their concerns. Sometimes you need to defend patients' rights to make health care decisions in a general way by speaking out against policies or actions that put patients in danger or conflict with their rights (Takenouchi, 2018). Furthermore, advocates ensure that patients' autonomy and self-determination are respected (Gerber, 2018). Patient advocacy is hard and often provides unique emotional challenges to health care providers, especially when providing high-quality palliative or end-of-life care or caring for patients with debilitating chronic illnesses (Takenouchi, 2018; O'Mahony et al., 2017). As an advocate, it is important to be mindful of your own personal stressors and to identify ways to cope with these stressors (see Chapter 37).

Educator. Your value as a patient educator is important to your patients' health and recovery. Your ability to teach effectively improves patients' knowledge, skills, self-care activities, and ability to make informed decisions (Flanders, 2018). As an educator you identify patients' willingness and ability to learn, explain concepts and facts about their health, describe the reason for care activities, demonstrate procedures such as self-care activities, reinforce learning or patient behavior, and evaluate the patient's progress in learning. Some of your patient teaching is unplanned and informal. For example, during a casual conversation you respond to questions about the reason for an intravenous infusion, a health issue such as smoking cessation, or necessary lifestyle changes. Other teaching activities are planned, more formal, and individualized, such as when you teach your patient how to self-administer insulin injections. Assess your patient's and family caregiver's learning styles and needs and develop a teaching plan that meets your patients' self-management objectives and includes teaching methods that match your patient's and family's needs (Pinchera et al., 2018) (see Chapter 25).

Communicator. An effective communicator is central to the nurse-patient relationship. It allows you to know your patients, including their preferences, strengths, weaknesses, and needs. High-quality communication is essential for all nursing roles and activities (see Chapter 24). You routinely communicate with patients and families, other nurses and health care professionals, resource people, and the community. Effective communication strategies are fundamental to providing high-quality care, coordinating and managing patient care, assisting patients in rehabilitation, advocating for patients, assisting patients and families in decision making, and providing patient education (Christian, 2017).

Manager. Today's health care environment is fast-paced and complex. Nurse managers direct groups of nurses by establishing an environment for collaborative patient-centered care and safe, evidence-based quality care with positive patient outcomes. A manager coordinates the activities of members of a nursing staff in delivering nursing care and has personnel, policy, and budgetary responsibility for a specific nursing unit or agency. A manager uses appropriate leadership styles to create a nursing environment for patients and staff that reflects the mission and values of the health care organization (see Chapter 21).

Career Development

Innovations in health care, expanding health care systems and practice settings, and the increasing needs of patients have created new nursing roles. Today the majority of nurses practice in hospital settings, followed by community-based care, ambulatory care, home care, and nursing homes/extended care settings.

Nursing provides an opportunity for you to commit to lifelong learning and career development. Because of increasing educational opportunities for nurses, the growth of nursing as a profession, and a greater concern for job enrichment, the nursing profession offers different career opportunities. Your career path is limitless. You will probably switch career roles more than once. Take advantage of the different clinical practice and professional opportunities. Examples of these career opportunities include advanced practice registered nurses (APRNs), nurse researchers, nurse risk managers, quality improvement nurses, consultants, and entrepreneurs.

Clinician. Most nurses provide direct (hands-on) patient care in acute care settings. However, as changes in health care services and reimbursement continue, there will be an increase in direct care activities provided in the home care setting and an increased need for community-based health promotion activities, restorative care, and end-of-life care.

In the hospital you may choose to practice in a medical-surgical setting or concentrate on a specific area of specialty practice such as pediatrics, critical care, or emergency care. Most specialty care areas require some experience as a medical-surgical nurse and additional continuing or in-service education. Many intensive care unit and emergency department nurses are required to have certification in advanced cardiac life support and critical care, emergency nursing, or trauma nursing. When developing as a clinician in acute care, you will learn a variety of hands-on technical procedures, the rationale for those procedures, and how to ensure safe implementation. Career advancement promotes a maturing of clinical skills and clinical decision making.

In community and home care settings, nurses' clinical abilities will include technical skills. However, because nurses in these settings usually have more contact with patients and family members over time, expertise in communication and assessment skills is crucial for clinical development. Community and home care nurses have an advantage of gaining a greater insight into how patients live and work daily and to thus apply clinical skills for promotion of long-term improvement in health.

Advanced Practice Registered Nurses. The advanced practice registered nurse (APRN) is the most independently functioning nurse. An APRN has a master's degree or Doctor of Nursing Practice (DNP) degree in nursing; advanced education in pathophysiology, pharmacology, and physical assessment; and certification and expertise in a specialized area of practice (American Association of Colleges of Nursing [AACN], 2021a). The APRN Consensus Model for APRN Regulation: Licensure, Accreditation, Certification and Education provides guidance for states to adopt uniformity in the regulation of APRN roles (National Council of State Boards of Nursing [NCSBN], 2021). The model addresses inconsistent standards in APRN education, regulation, and practice, which had limited APRN mobility from one state to another

(Doherty et al., 2018). The consensus model identified that the title of APRN is for nurses with advanced graduate-level knowledge prepared in one of four roles: clinical nurse specialist (CNS), nurse practitioner (NP), certified nurse-midwife (CNM), and certified registered nurse anesthetist (CRNA). The educational preparation for the four roles is in at least one of the following six populations: adult-gerontology, pediatrics, neonatology, women's health/gender related, family/individual across life span, and psychiatric mental health (NCSBN, 2021).

These advanced practice roles provide additional career opportunities for nurses and expand the professional health care opportunities for patients, many of whom are underserved. However, prior to progressing to an advanced practice role, it is important for the new graduate nurse to obtain solid bedside clinical practice. This clinical practice helps the new graduate increase knowledge about disease processes and how the body responds to illnesses. The nurse gains expertise and confidence in basic and complex skills. As a result, new graduates refine their critical thinking and have opportunities to make sound clinical judgments. The knowledge and skill acquisition, refinement of critical thinking, and opportunities for clinical judgment are essential preparation for the education and practice in an advanced role (Faraz, 2017).

Clinical nurse specialist. A **clinical nurse specialist (CNS)** is an APRN who has graduate preparation (master's degree or doctorate) in nursing and is an expert clinician in a specialized area of practice (National Association of Clinical Nurse Specialists [NACNS], 2019). The specialty may be identified by a population (e.g., geriatrics), setting (e.g., critical care), disease specialty (e.g., oncology, diabetes), type of care (e.g., rehabilitation), or type of problem (e.g., pain) (NACNS, 2019). Clinical nurse specialists provide diagnosis, treatment, and ongoing management of patients in all health care settings (Fig. 1.1). They also provide expertise and support to nurses caring for patients at the bedside, help drive practice changes throughout an organization, and ensure the use of evidence-based practices and evidence-based care to achieve the best possible patient outcomes (Wallace et al., 2019; NACNS, 2019).

Nurse practitioner. A **nurse practitioner (NP)** is an APRN who has graduate preparation (master's degree or doctorate) in nursing. NPs provide primary, acute, and specialty health care to patients of all ages and in all types of health care settings. This care includes assessment, diagnosis, planning, and treatment; monitoring ongoing health status; evaluation of therapies; and health education (American Association of Nurse Practitioners [AANP], 2021). Some NPs provide care to acutely ill patients in hospital settings, including critical care units.

Other NPs provide comprehensive care in outpatient settings, directly managing the nursing and medical care of patients who are healthy or who have chronic conditions. It is important to review state regulations for advanced practice. Some states require the NP to have a collaborative provider agreement with an agency or physician/physician group to treat a specific group of patients; other states do not.

Certified nurse-midwife. A **certified nurse-midwife (CNM)** is an APRN who has graduate preparation (master's degree or doctorate) in nursing, is also educated in midwifery, and is certified by the American College of Nurse-Midwives (ACNM). The scope of practice of nurse-midwifery has been defined by the ACNM (2012) as encompassing a full range of primary health care services for women from adolescence beyond menopause. These services include primary care; gynecological and family planning services; preconception care; care during pregnancy, childbirth, and the postpartum period; care of the normal newborn during the first 28 days of life; and treatment of male partners for sexually transmitted infections (ACNM, 2012). The nurse-midwife conducts physical examinations; prescribes medications, including controlled substances and contraceptive methods; admits, manages, and discharges patients; orders and interprets laboratory and diagnostic tests; and orders the use of medical devices.

Certified registered nurse anesthetist. A **certified registered nurse anesthetist (CRNA)** is an APRN with advanced education from an accredited nurse anesthesia program. Before applying to a nurse anesthesia program, a nurse must have at least 1 year of critical care or emergency experience. Nurse anesthetists practice both autonomously and in collaboration with a variety of health care providers on the interprofessional team to deliver high-quality, holistic, evidence-based anesthesia and pain care services (American Association of Nurse Anesthetists [AANA], 2020). CRNAs practice under the guidance and supervision of an anesthesiologist, a physician with advanced knowledge of surgical anesthesia.

Nurse Educator. A **nurse educator** works primarily in schools of nursing, staff development departments of health care agencies, and patient education departments. Nurse educators need experience in clinical practice to provide them with practical skills and theoretical knowledge.

A faculty member in a nursing program educates students to become professional nurses. Nursing faculty members are responsible for teaching current nursing practice; trends; theory; and necessary skills in classroom, laboratories, and clinical settings. Faculty development is essential to improve and maintain a faculty member's clinical skills in addition to preparing faculty to adapt to new teaching and learning methods (Monsivais and Robbins, 2020). Nursing faculty have graduate degrees such as a master's degree in nursing or an earned doctorate in nursing or a related field. In general, they have a specific clinical, administrative, or research specialty and advanced clinical experience.

Nurse educators in staff development departments of health care agencies provide educational programs for nurses within their agencies. These programs include orientation of new personnel, critical care nursing courses, assisting with clinical skill competency, safety training, and instruction about new equipment or procedures. These nursing educators often participate in the development of nursing policies and procedures.

The primary focus of the nurse educator in a patient education department of an agency such as a wound treatment clinic is to teach and coach patients and their families how to self-manage their illness or disability, make positive choices or change their behaviors to promote their health, and improve their health outcomes (Flanders, 2018). These nurse educators are usually specialized and hold a certification and see only a specific population of patients. One example is a certified diabetic nurse

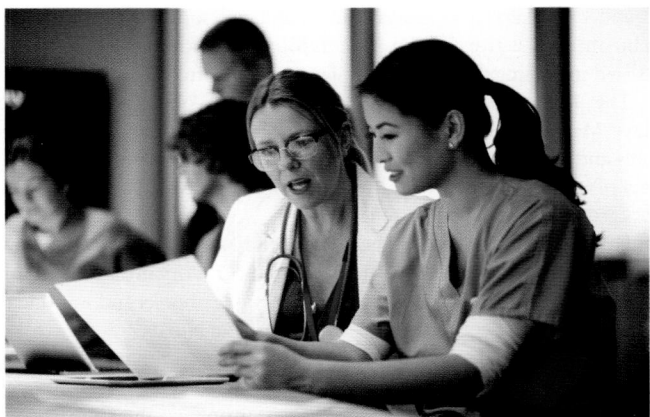

FIG. 1.1 Clinical nurse specialist consults on a complex patient case. (iStock.com/Sturti.)

educator (CDE), who partners with patients and their caregivers to improve diabetic self-management and reduce the rate of hospitalizations or disease-related complications (Wilson et al., 2019).

Nurse Administrator. A nurse administrator is responsible for management of the nursing staff in a health care agency. Nursing administration begins with positions such as clinical care coordinators and assistant nurse managers. Experience and additional education sometimes lead to a middle-management position such as nurse manager of a specific patient care area or house supervisor or to an administrative position such as an associate director or director of nursing services. The American Organization of Nurse Executives (AONE) (2015) has outlined five competencies detailing the skills, knowledge, and abilities that guide the practice of nurse leaders in administrative or executive practice. These include communication and relationship management; knowledge of the health care environment; leadership; professionalism; and business skills and principles.

Nurse manager positions usually require at least a bachelor's degree in nursing, and director and nurse executive positions generally require a master's degree. Requirements will vary by agency. Chief nurse executive and vice president positions in large health care organizations often require preparation at the doctoral level. Nurse administrators often have advanced degrees such as a master's degree in nursing administration, hospital administration (MHA), public health (MPH), or business administration (MBA).

In today's health care organizations, directors have responsibility for more than one nursing unit. They often manage a particular service or product line, such as medicine or cardiology. Vice presidents of nursing or chief nurse executives often have responsibilities for all clinical functions within the hospital (e.g., pharmacy, respiratory care, and rehabilitation). This may include all ancillary personnel who provide and support patient care services. The nurse administrator needs to be skilled in business and management and understand all aspects of nursing and patient care. Functions of administrators include budgeting, staffing, strategic planning of programs and services, employee evaluation, and employee development.

Nurse Researcher. The nurse researcher conducts evidence-based practice, performance improvement, and research to improve nursing care and further define and expand the scope of nursing practice (see Chapter 5). She or he often works in an academic setting, hospital, or independent professional or community service agency. Academic researchers generally pursue a specific area of research that they have identified and developed over the course of their experiences. Researchers for hospitals often pursue research on topics of priority or interest to the agency. Researchers within community service agencies conduct research based on the service focus of that agency. The preferred educational requirement is a doctoral degree, with at least a master's degree in nursing.

REFLECT NOW

In reviewing the roles and responsibilities of the professional nurse and career options, think about your personal academic and career goals. Design a plan that you can modify as you progress through your academic nursing program.

HISTORICAL INFLUENCES

Nurses have responded and will always respond to the needs of their patients. In times of war they have responded by meeting the needs of

the wounded in combat zones and military hospitals in the United States and abroad. When communities face health care crises such as natural disasters, disease outbreaks, or insufficient public health resources, nurses establish community-based immunization and screening programs, treatment clinics, and health promotion activities. Our patients are most vulnerable when they are injured, sick, or dying.

Today nurses are active in determining best practices in a variety of areas such as pressure injury prevention, wound care management, pain control, nutritional management, and care of individuals across the life span. Nurse researchers are leaders in expanding knowledge in nursing and other health care disciplines. Their work ensures that nurses have the best available evidence to support their practices (see Chapter 5).

Knowledge of the history of the nursing profession increases your understanding of the social and intellectual origins of the discipline. Although it is not practical to describe all the historical aspects of professional nursing, some of the more significant nursing leaders and milestones are described in the following paragraphs.

Florence Nightingale

In *Notes on Nursing: What It Is and What It Is Not,* Florence Nightingale established the first nursing philosophy based on health maintenance and restoration (Nightingale, 1860). She saw the role of nursing as having "charge of somebody's health" based on the knowledge of "how to put the body in such a state to be free of disease or to recover from disease" (Nightingale, 1860). During the same year she developed the first organized program for training nurses, the Nightingale Training School for Nurses at St. Thomas' Hospital in London.

Nightingale was the first practicing nurse epidemiologist. Her statistical analyses connected poor sanitation with the incidence of cholera and dysentery. She volunteered during the Crimean War in 1853 and traveled the battlefield hospitals at night, carrying her lamp; thus, she was known as the "lady with the lamp." The sanitary, nutritional, and basic conditions in the battlefield hospitals were poor, and she was asked to ensure the quality of sanitation facilities. As a result of her actions, the mortality rate at the Barracks Hospital in Scutari, Turkey, was reduced from 42.7% to 2.2% in 6 months (Donahue, 2011).

The Civil War to the Beginning of the Twentieth Century

The Civil War (1860–65) stimulated the growth of nursing in the United States. Clara Barton, founder of the American Red Cross, cared for soldiers on the battlefields, cleansing their wounds, meeting their basic needs, and comforting them at end of life. Dorothea Lynde Dix, Mary Ann Ball (Mother Bickerdyke), and Harriet Tubman also influenced nursing during the Civil War (Donahue, 2011). Dix and Bickerdyke organized hospitals and ambulances, appointed nurses, cared for the wounded soldiers, and oversaw and regulated supplies to the troops. Tubman was active in the Underground Railroad movement and assisted in leading more than 300 slaves to freedom (Donahue, 2011).

The first professionally educated African-American nurse was Mary Mahoney. She was concerned with relationships between cultures and races. As a noted nursing leader, she brought forth an awareness of cultural diversity and respect for the individual, regardless of background, race, color, or religion.

Isabel Hampton Robb helped found the Nurses' Associated Alumnae of the United States and Canada in 1896. This organization became the ANA in 1911. She authored many nursing textbooks and was one of the original founders of the *American Journal of Nursing*.

Nursing in hospitals expanded in the late nineteenth century. However, nursing in the community did not increase significantly until 1893, when Lillian Wald and Mary Brewster opened the Henry Street Settlement, which focused on the health needs of poor people who lived in tenements in New York City (Donahue, 2011).

Twentieth Century

In the early twentieth century a movement toward developing a scientific, research-based defined body of nursing knowledge and practice evolved. Nurses began to assume expanded roles. Mary Adelaide Nutting, who became the first nursing professor at Columbia Teachers College in 1906, was instrumental in moving nursing education into universities (Donahue, 2011).

The Magnet Recognition Program® designates organizations worldwide in which nursing leaders successfully align their nursing strategic goals to improve the organization's patient outcomes. The Magnet Recognition Program® provides a roadmap to nursing excellence, which benefits the whole of an organization. To nurses, Magnet Recognition means education and development through every career stage, which leads to greater autonomy at the bedside. To patients, it means the very best care, delivered by nurses who are supported to be the very best that they can be. In 1994 the University of Washington Medical Center in Seattle, Washington was the first American Nurses Credentialing Center (ANCC) Magnet®-designated organization (ANCC, n.d.).

As nursing education developed, nursing practice also expanded, and the Army and Navy Nurse Corps were established. By the 1920s nursing specialization started to develop. The last half of the century saw the creation of specialty-nursing organizations such as the American Association of Critical Care Nurses, Association of peri-Operating Room Nurses (AORN), Infusion Nurses Society (INS), and Emergency Nurses Association (ENA). In 1990 the ANA established the Center for Ethics and Human Rights, which provides a forum to address the complex ethical and human rights issues confronting nurses and designs activities and programs to increase ethical competence in nurses (Fowler, 2015).

Twenty-First Century

Today the profession faces multiple challenges. Nurses are revising nursing practice and school curricula to meet the ever-changing needs of society, including an aging population, cultural diversity, bioterrorism, emerging infections, and disaster management. Advances in technology and informatics (see Chapter 26), the high acuity level of care of hospitalized patients, and early discharge from health care institutions require nurses in all settings to have a strong and current knowledge base from which to practice. In addition, nursing and the RWJF are taking a leadership role in developing standards and policies for end-of-life care through the *Last Acts Campaign* (see Chapter 36). The End-of-Life Nursing Education Consortium (ELNEC) is a national and international education initiative to improve palliative care offered collaboratively by the AACN and the City of Hope Medical Center. The educational programs focus on end-of-life care and practices in nursing curricula and professional continuing education programs for practicing nurses (AACN, 2021b).

CONTEMPORARY INFLUENCES

Multiple external forces affect nursing, including the need for nurses' self-care, health care reform and rising health care costs, demographic changes of the population, human rights, and increasing numbers of the medically underserved.

Importance of Nurses' Self-Care

Nursing is a dynamic and gratifying career. However, it also has both physical and emotional demands and challenges. You cannot give fully engaged, compassionate care to others when you feel depleted or do not feel cared for yourself. You and your colleagues will have many self-care needs that must be met to function as healthy professionals.

In your educational experience and in your career, you will experience grief and loss. Many times, even before you have a chance to recover from an emotionally draining situation, you will encounter another difficult human story. Nurses in acute care settings frequently witness prolonged, concentrated suffering, leading to feelings of frustration, anger, guilt, sadness, or anxiety (Hairong et al., 2021). The 2020 outbreak of coronavirus disease 2019 (COVID-19) demonstrated the psychological stress experienced by nurses on the front lines. Nursing students are not immune. They report feeling initially hesitant and uncomfortable with their first encounters with a dying patient and identify feelings of sadness and anxiety.

Frequent, intense, or prolonged exposure to grief and loss places nurses at risk for developing compassion fatigue. *Compassion fatigue* is a term used to describe a state of burnout and secondary traumatic stress (Graystone, 2020; Potter et al., 2013a). It occurs without warning and often results from giving high levels of energy and compassion over a prolonged period to those who are suffering, often without experiencing improved patient outcomes (Hairong et al., 2021). *Secondary traumatic stress* is the trauma that health care providers experience when witnessing and caring for others suffering trauma. Examples include an oncology nurse who cares for patients undergoing surgery and chemotherapy over the long term for their cancer or a spouse who witnesses his wife deteriorating over the years from Alzheimer disease.

Burnout is the condition that occurs when perceived demands outweigh perceived resources (Graystone, 2020; Potter et al., 2013a; Potter et al., 2013b). It is a state of physical and mental exhaustion that often affects health care providers because of the nature of their work environment. Over time, giving of oneself in often intense caring environments sometimes results in emotional exhaustion, leaving a nurse feeling irritable, restless, and unable to focus and engage with patients. This often occurs in situations in which there is a lack of social support, organizational pressures influencing staffing, and the inability of the nurse to practice self-care.

Compassion fatigue typically results in feelings of hopelessness, a decrease in the ability to take pleasure from previously enjoyable activities, a state of hypervigilance, and anxiety. Compassion fatigue negatively affects the health and wellness of nurses and the quality of care provided to patients. It also affects health care agencies as nurses experience changes in job performance and in their personal lives; it can result in nurses' desire to leave the profession or their specialty. High nurse turnover can result. In addition, these factors affect patient satisfaction and an agency's ability to maintain a caring, competent staff (Graystone, 2020).

There is a need for health care agencies to identify programs for the early recognition of compassion fatigue and to develop interventions to help nurses manage it. Prompt interventions and creating work environments in which nurses feel supported by co-workers and management improve nurse retention and job satisfaction rates (Graystone, 2020.) Agency-based programs that provide opportunities for nurses to validate their experiences and to talk about the challenges of the type of care they give help nurses cope with compassion fatigue and its implications for professional nursing care (Wenzel and Brysiewicz, 2017).

Compassion fatigue may contribute to what is described as *lateral violence* (see Chapter 24). Lateral violence sometimes occurs in nurse-nurse interactions and includes behaviors such as withholding information, making snide remarks, and demonstrating nonverbal expressions of disapproval, such as raising eyebrows or making faces. New graduates and nurses new to a unit are most likely to face problems with lateral or horizontal violence (Sanner-Stiehr and Ward-Smith, 2017).

All nurses require resiliency skills to better manage the stressors that contribute to compassion fatigue and lateral violence. Managing stress and conflict, building connections with colleagues to share difficult stories, practicing self-care, and maintaining an appropriate work-life balance are helpful stress-management techniques in dealing with difficult situations and contribute to safe and effective care (see Chapter 37) (Cooper et al., 2020).

Health Care Reform and Costs

Health care reform affects not only how health care is paid for but also how it is delivered. There will be greater emphasis on health promotion, disease prevention, and illness management in the future. More services will be in community-based care settings. However, hospitals will continue to manage the care of very seriously ill patients. As a result, more nurses will be needed to practice in community care centers, patients' homes, schools, and senior centers. This will require nurses to be skilled at assessing for resources, service gaps, and how patients adapt to return to their communities. Nursing needs to respond to such changes by assessing for resources, improving staffing and management models in hospitals, changing nursing education, helping patients adapt to new health care delivery methods, and providing care to safely return patients to their homes.

Skyrocketing health care costs present challenges to the profession, the consumer, and the health care delivery system. As a nurse you are responsible for providing patients with the best-quality care in an efficient and economically sound manner, including following established protocols, exercising timely well-planned patient discharge from a care setting, and judiciously using supplies and equipment. The challenge is to use health care and patient resources wisely. Chapter 2 summarizes reasons for the rise in health care costs and its implications for nursing.

Demographic Changes

The U.S. Census Bureau (2015) predicts that the 2030s will be a transformative decade, with the population expected to grow at a slower pace, age considerably, and become more racially and ethnically diverse. These changes will require expanded health care resources. The U.S. Census Bureau's population projections predict that by 2030, all baby boomers will be older than 65 years of age. This will expand the size of the older population such that one of every five residents will be of retirement age. It is also predicted that by 2044 more than half of the U.S. population will be part of a minority group (U.S. Census Bureau, 2015). To effectively meet all the health care needs of the expanding minority and aging populations, changes need to occur as to how care is provided, especially in public health. The population is still shifting from rural areas to urban centers, and more people are living with chronic and long-term illnesses. Not only are outpatient settings expanding, but more and more people want to receive outpatient and community-based care and remain in their homes or community (see Chapters 2 and 3).

Medically Underserved

Nursing has a strong history in advocating for and meeting the needs of the medically underserved (Porter-O'Grady, 2018). Unemployment, underemployment and low-paying jobs, mental illness, homelessness, and rising health care costs all contribute to increases in the medically underserved population. Caring for this population is a global challenge; social, political, economic, and health literacy factors affect both access to care and access to health care–related resources (Kaphingst et al., 2016).

In addition, the number of underserved patients who require home-based palliative care services is increasing. This is a group of patients whose physical status does not improve and whose health care needs increase. People with low health literacy are less likely to participate in decision making regarding their care because they do not understand the medical information provided, nor do they understand the consequences of indecision (Seo et al., 2016).

TRENDS IN NURSING

Nursing is a dynamic profession that grows and evolves as society and lifestyles change, as health care priorities and technologies change, and as nurses themselves change. The current philosophies and definitions of nursing have a holistic focus, which addresses the needs of the whole person in all dimensions, in health and illness, and in interaction with the family and community. In addition, there continues to be an increasing awareness of patient safety in all care settings.

Evidence-Based Practice

A core responsibility of an RN is to make sound clinical judgments. This applies to acquiring a view of each patient (what you can learn about the patient), identifying the patient's health problems, and knowing what actions to take. Clinical judgment is influenced by the critical thinking element of knowledge (see Chapter 15). Knowledge helps shape clinical judgment. Evidence-based knowledge is a critical element of that knowledge.

Today the general public is more informed about their health care needs, the cost of health care, best practices, and the incidence of medical errors within health care institutions. Your current and future practice needs to be based on current evidence. This means you do not rely solely on information gained during your education, experiential knowledge, or policies and procedures of health care agencies (see Chapter 5). It means you always need to search for the best scientific evidence to apply to recurrent patient health care problems. Delivery of and reimbursement for evidence-based nursing care is essential (Melnyk and Gallagher-Ford, 2018). Health care agencies must show their commitment to each health care stakeholder (e.g., patients, insurance companies, and governmental agencies) to control health care costs, reduce health care errors, and improve patient safety by implementing evidence-based practices (National Quality Forum [NQF], 2021). In addition, many hospitals are achieving Magnet Recognition®, which is an extensive hospital certification program that recognizes excellence in nursing practice and the implementation and dissemination of successful evidence-based nursing practices and strategies (ANCC, n.d.).

Quality and Safety Education for Nurses

The overall goal of the Quality and Safety Education for Nurses (QSEN) project is to meet the challenge of preparing future nurses and advanced practice nurses to have the knowledge, skills, and attitudes (KSAs) necessary to continuously improve the quality and safety of the health care systems within which they work (QSEN, 2020a). To achieve this goal, the IOM and QSEN faculty defined quality and safety competencies for nurses and proposed targets for the KSAs developed for prelicensure programs (Table 1.1). For each competency there are targeted KSAs for prelicensure programs and graduate programs (QSEN, 2020a; QSEN, 2020b).

As you gain experience in clinical practice, you will face situations in which your critical thinking and knowledge will help you to make a difference in improving patient care. Whether that difference is to provide evidence for implementing care at the bedside, identify a safety issue, or study patient data to identify trends in outcomes, each of these situations requires competence in patient-centered care, safety, or informatics. Although it is not within the scope of this textbook to present the QSEN initiative in its entirety, subsequent clinical chapters will provide you an opportunity to address how to build competencies in one or more of these areas.

TABLE 1.1 Quality and Safety Education for Nurses

Competency	Definition With Examples
Patient-centered care	Recognize the patient or designee as the source of control and full partner in providing compassionate and coordinated care based on respect for patient's preferences, values, and needs. *Examples: Involve family and friends in care. Integrate an understanding of patient, family, community preferences, values. Provide patient-centered care with sensitivity and respect for the diversity of the human experience.*
Teamwork and collaboration	Function effectively within nursing and interprofessional teams, fostering open communication, mutual respect, and shared decision making to achieve high-quality patient care. *Examples: Recognize the contributions of other individuals and groups helping patient/family achieve health goals. Discuss effective strategies for communicating and resolving conflict. Participate in designing systems to support effective teamwork.*
Evidence-based practice	Integrate best current evidence with clinical expertise and patient/family preferences and values for delivery of optimal health care. *Examples: Demonstrate knowledge of basic scientific methods. Appreciate strengths and weaknesses of scientific bases for practice. Appreciate the importance of regularly reading relevant journals.*
Quality improvement	Use data to monitor the outcomes of care processes and use improvement methods to design and test changes to continuously improve the quality and safety of health care systems. *Examples: Use tools such as flow charts and diagrams to make process of care explicit. Appreciate how unwanted variation in outcomes affects care. Identify gaps between local and best practice.*
Safety	Minimize risk of harm to patients and providers through both system effectiveness and individual performance. *Examples: Examine human factors and other basic safety design principles as well as commonly used unsafe practices (such as work-arounds and dangerous abbreviations). Value own role in preventing errors.*
Informatics	Use information and technology to communicate, manage knowledge, mitigate error, and support decision making. *Examples: Navigate an electronic health record. Protect confidentiality of protected health information in electronic health records.*

Adapted from QSEN Institute: *QSEN competencies,* 2020a. https://qsen.org/competencies/pre-licensure-ksas/. Accessed April 2021.

QSEN Building Competency in Patient-Centered Care You are caring for Kitty, a 10-year-old with severe delayed development. Kitty, an only child, lives with her parents and goes to a school that is able to meet her needs. Her mom gives her seizure medicine each day, and her seizures are well controlled. Kitty has very little independent function. She needs assistance with all of her activities of daily living (e.g., bathing, toileting, eating, and hygiene). Up to now Kitty's parents have been able to provide all of her care and meet her needs. As a patient advocate, what do you need to know about Kitty's parents' goals for her future care? Think about how you can use this information to advocate for Kitty and her parents to achieve these goals.

Answers to QSEN Activities can be found on the Evolve website.

Impact of Emerging Information Technologies

Emerging information technologies directly affect nursing practice. These technologies provide more accurate, noninvasive assessment tools; help you to implement evidence-based practices automatically; collect and trend patient outcome data; and use clinical decision support systems. The electronic health record (EHR) is an efficient method for documenting and managing patient health care information (see Chapter 26.) Computerized physician/provider order entry (CPOE), allowing health care providers to directly enter medical orders, is a critical patient safety initiative especially in the area of medication ordering and administration (Crespo et al., 2018).

Emerging information technologies will help you to communicate with, provide care for, and build relationships with your patients. Telehealth, e-visits, and devices that allow your patients to phone in pertinent health information are examples of technology that open new venues for providing care. Learn how these electronic tools work so that you can teach patients how to use them. Evidence-based practice, clinical decision support systems, and case-based reasoning are all methods to increase information acquisition and distribution.

Technological innovations help family caregivers monitor and manage home environments of older adults, enable older adults to stay in their homes but stay connected to their support systems, and help with decision support and care coordination (Andruszkiewicz and Fike, 2015–2016). In addition, there is an increase in the availability and use of telehealth and telemedicine functions for providing patient-centered care to urban and rural populations, in all age-groups, to patients with acute and chronic illness, and to patients and families for end-of-life care and support (Smaradottir and Fensli, 2018).

Genomics

Genetics is the study of inheritance, or the way traits are passed down from one generation to another. Genes carry the instructions for making proteins, which in turn direct the activities of cells and functions of the body that influence traits such as hair and eye color, and susceptibility to disease. Genomics is a newer term that describes the study of all the genes in a person and interactions of these genes with one another and with that person's environment (Centers for Disease Control and Prevention [CDC], 2021). Genomic information combined with technology can potentially improve health outcomes, quality, and safety and reduce health care costs (McCormick and Calzone, 2016). This information allows health care providers to determine how genomic changes contribute to patient conditions and influence treatment decisions (Sharoff, 2016). For example, when a family member has colon cancer before the age of 50, it is likely that other family members are at risk for developing this cancer. Genomics counseling and testing can determine family status. Knowing this information is important for family members who will need a colonoscopy before the age of 50 and repeat colonoscopies more often than the patient who is not at risk. Nurses help to assess and interpret genomic test results, identify patients' risk factors, and counsel patients about what this genomic finding means to them personally and to their families. As you use and understand genomics, remember to use genomic test information in a confidential, ethical, and culturally appropriate manner to help health care providers and patients and their families make informed care decisions (Tluczek et al., 2019).

Public Perception of Nursing

Nursing is a pivotal health care profession. As frontline health care providers, nurses practice in all health care settings and constitute the largest number of health care professionals. They are essential to providing skilled, specialized, knowledgeable care; improving the health status of the public; and ensuring safe, effective, high-quality care (ANA, 2021).

Consumers of health care are more informed than ever; with the Internet, consumers have access to more health care and treatment information. For example, *Hospital Compare* is a consumer-oriented website that allows people to select multiple hospitals and directly compare performance measure information on specific diseases and procedures such as heart attack, heart failure, pneumonia, and surgery (Centers for Medicare and Medicaid Services [CMS], n.d.). This information can help consumers make informed decisions about health care.

Consumers can also access the *Hospital Consumer Assessment of Healthcare Providers and Systems* (HCAHPS) website to obtain information about patients' perspectives on hospital care. CMS and the Agency for Healthcare Research and Quality (AHRQ) developed the HCAHPS Survey, also known as Hospital CAHPS®, to provide a standardized survey instrument and data collection methodology for measuring patients' perspectives on hospital care (CMS, 2020). Most hospitals collect information on patient satisfaction; HCAHPS offers a survey that helps consumers obtain valid comparisons about patient perspectives across all hospitals. This information is intended to allow consumers to make "apples to apples" comparisons to support their choice (HCAHPS, 2021).

REFLECT NOW

A nurse is often the first health care professional a patient sees when in the emergency department or following admission to a hospital. Think about the type of impression you want to make in terms of compassion, competency, and professionalism.

Impact of Nursing on Politics and Health Policy

Political power or influence is the ability to influence or persuade an individual holding a governmental office to exert the power of that office to effect a desired outcome. Nurses' involvement in politics is receiving greater emphasis in nursing curricula, professional organizations, public health policy, and health care settings. Professional nursing organizations and State Boards of Nursing employ lobbyists to urge state legislatures and the U.S. Congress to pass legislation that will improve the quality of health care (Mason et al., 2020).

The ANA works for the improvement of health standards and the availability of health care services for all people, fosters high standards of nursing, stimulates and promotes the professional development of nurses, and advances their economic and general welfare. The ANA's purposes are unrestricted by considerations of nationality, race, creed, lifestyle, color, gender, or age.

You can influence policy decisions at all governmental levels. One way to get involved is by participating in local and national efforts (Mason et al., 2020). This effort is critical to exerting nurses' influence early in the political process. Nurses can help make the future bright by becoming serious students of social needs, activists in influencing policy to meet those needs, and generous contributors of time and money to nursing organizations and to candidates working for universal good health care (Mason et al., 2020).

PROFESSIONAL REGISTERED NURSE EDUCATION

A significant amount of formal education is necessary to become a professional RN. The issues of standardization of nursing education and entry into practice remain a major controversy, making it sometimes difficult for individuals to choose nursing programs. Various prelicensure educational programs are available for individuals intending to become an RN. In addition, graduate nurse education and continuing and in-service education are available for practicing nurses.

Prelicensure

Currently in the United States the most frequent way to become a registered nurse (RN) is through completion of either an associate or bachelor's degree program. Graduates of both types of programs are eligible to take the National Council Licensure Examination for Registered Nurses (NCLEX-RN®) to become RNs in the state in which they will practice.

The associate degree program in the United States is a 2-year program that is usually offered by a university or community college. This program focuses on the basic sciences and theoretical and clinical courses related to the practice of nursing. A nurse with an associate degree can later progress to earn a bachelor's degree. Each university determines the additional coursework, and an RN Bachelor of Science in Nursing (BSN) program may take 12 to 18 months depending on a student's associate degree transcript.

The bachelor's degree program usually includes 4 years of study in a college or university. It focuses on the basic sciences; theoretical and clinical courses; and courses in the social sciences, arts, and humanities to support nursing theory. In Canada the degree of Bachelor of Science in Nursing (BScN) or Bachelor in Nursing (BN) is equivalent to the degree of BSN in the United States. *The Essentials: Core Competencies for Professional Nursing Education* (AACN, 2021a) encompasses 10 Domains for the baccalaureate-prepared nurse and guides faculty on the structure and evaluation of the curriculum (Box 1.4). Standards published by nursing program accrediting organizations specify that core competencies for the professional nurse should be in the nursing curriculum. In addition, one of the IOM recommendations is that 80% of nurses be prepared with a bachelor's degree in nursing by 2020 (IOM, 2010) (see Chapter 2).

BOX 1.4   American Association of Colleges of Nursing (AACN) Essential Domains (2021)

Domain 1: Knowledge for Nursing Practice
Domain 2: Person-Centered Care
Domain 3: Population Health
Domain 4: Scholarship for Nursing Practice
Domain 5: Quality and Safety
Domain 6: Interprofessional Partnerships
Domain 7: Systems-Based Practice
Domain 8: Informatics and Healthcare Technologies
Domain 9: Professionalism
Domain 10: Personal, Professional, and Leadership Development

From American Association of Colleges of Nursing (AACN): *The essentials: core competencies for professional nursing education,* 2021a, https://www.aacnnursing.org/Education-Resources/AACN-Essentials. Accessed April 2021.

Graduate Education

After obtaining a bachelor's degree in nursing, you can pursue graduate education leading to a master's or doctoral degree in any number of graduate fields, including nursing. Other fields include public health, epidemiology, and informatics. *The Essentials: Core Competencies for Professional Nursing Education* (AACN, 2021a) provides direction for structure and evaluation of graduate nursing curricula, to include strong knowledge skills in nursing science and theory; advanced knowledge in the basic sciences; and research-based clinical practice. A master's degree in nursing is important for the roles of nurse educator, nurse administrator, and future nurse researcher, and it is a minimum requirement for an APRN.

Doctoral Preparation. Professional doctoral programs in nursing (Doctor of Nursing Science [DSN or DNSc] degree) prepare graduates to apply research findings to clinical nursing. Other doctoral programs prepare nurses for more rigorous research and theory development and award the research-oriented Doctor of Philosophy (PhD) in nursing. The DNP is the terminal practice degree and provides advanced preparation for APRNs. The DNP is a practice-focused doctorate. *The Essentials: Core Competencies for Professional Nursing Education* (AACN, 2021a) provides direction for structure and evaluation of DNP nursing curricula, to include skills in obtaining expanded knowledge through the formulation and interpretations of evidence-based practice.

The need for nurses with doctoral degrees is increasing. Expanding clinical roles and continuing demand for well-educated nursing faculty and administrators, nurse administrators, and APRNs in the clinical settings and new areas of nursing specialties such as nursing informatics are just a few reasons for increasing the number of doctoral-prepared nurses.

Continuing and In-Service Education

Nursing is a knowledge-based profession, and clinical decision making and technological expertise are qualities that health care consumers demand and expect. Continuing education updates your knowledge about the latest research and practice developments, helps you to specialize in a particular area of practice, and teaches you new skills and techniques, all of which are crucial factors to improving patient care (Wellings et al., 2017). Continuing education involves educational programs offered by universities, hospitals, state nurses' associations, professional nursing organizations, and educational and health care institutions. An example is a program on caring for older adults with dementia offered by a university or a program on safe medication practices offered by a hospital. Although many of these programs are conducted on-site as a lecture, seminar, or skills training, there is a growth in virtual learning and mobile simulation programs, especially for those nursing subspecialties, such as oncology, that require continuing nursing education or to meet the educational needs of nurses in rural areas (das Gracas Silva Matsubara and De Domenico, 2016; Smith et al., 2020). Many states require a set number of continuing education hours as part of license renewal. In some cases there are continuing education requirements for specific topics such as bioterrorism and pain management.

In-service education programs are instruction or training programs provided by a health care agency or institution. An in-service program is held in the institution and is designed to increase the knowledge, skills, and competencies of nurses and other health care professionals employed by the institution. Often in-service programs are focused on new technologies such as how to correctly use the newest safety syringes. Many in-service programs are designed to fulfill required competencies of an organization. For example, a hospital might offer an in-service program on safe principles for administering chemotherapy or a program on cultural sensitivity.

NURSING PRACTICE

You will have an opportunity to practice in a variety of settings, in many roles within those settings, and with caregivers in other related health professions. The ANA standards of practice, standards of performance, and code of ethics for nurses are part of the public recognition of the significance of nursing practice to health care and implications for nursing practice regarding trends in health care. State and provincial nurse practice acts (NPAs) establish specific legal regulations for practice, and professional organizations establish standards of practice as criteria for nursing care.

Nurse Practice Acts

In the United States each State Board of Nursing oversees its NPA. The NPA regulates the scope of nursing practice for the state and protects public health, safety, and welfare. This protection includes protecting the public from unqualified and unsafe nurses. Although each state has its own NPA that defines the scope of nursing practice, most NPAs are similar. The definition of nursing practice published by the ANA is representative of the scope of nursing practice as defined in most states. During the last decade, many states have revised their NPAs to reflect the growing autonomy of nursing, minimum education requirements, certification requirements, and the expanded roles and scope of practice of APRNs.

Licensure and Certification

Licensure. In the United States all boards of nursing require RN candidates to pass the NCLEX-RN®. Regardless of educational preparation, the examination for RN licensure is the same in every state in the United States. This provides a standardized minimum knowledge base for nurses. Other requirements for licensure such as criminal background checks vary from state to state.

Certification. After passing the NCLEX-RN®, a nurse may choose to work toward certification in a specific area of nursing practice. Minimum practice and/or educational requirements are set, based on specific certification. National nursing organizations such as the ANA have many types of certification to enhance your career, such as certification in medical-surgical or geriatric nursing. After passing the initial examination, you maintain your certification through ongoing continuing education and by maintaining a set number of hours in clinical or administrative practice.

PROFESSIONAL NURSING ORGANIZATIONS

A professional organization deals with issues of concern to those practicing in the profession. In addition to the educational organizations previously discussed, a variety of specialty nursing organizations exist. For example, some professional organizations focus on specific areas such as critical care, advanced practice, maternal-child nursing, oncology, and nursing research. These organizations seek to improve the standards of practice, expand nursing roles, and foster the welfare of nurses within the specialty areas. In addition, professional organizations present educational programs and publish journals.

As a student you need to take part in organizations such as the National Student Nurses' Association (NSNA) in the United States and the Canadian Nursing Students' Association (CNSA) in Canada. These organizations consider issues of importance to nursing students such as career development and preparation for licensing. The NSNA often cooperates in activities and programs with the professional organizations.

KEY POINTS

- Nursing standards provide the guidelines for implementing and evaluating nursing care.
- Changes in society, such as health care reform, changing demographic patterns, increases in the medically underserved population, and increased consumerism, affect the practice of nursing.
- A nurse may take multiple professional career paths, such as advanced practice, nurse educator, research, and administration, to advance within the discipline.
- Nurses are increasingly aware of the role of politics and its influence on the health care system. As a result, nurses are more aware of the profession's influence on health care policy and practice.
- Advances in nursing's scientific knowledge base and the application of evidence-based practice have improved patient care and patient outcomes.
- Although nursing programs are available for professional registered nurse (RN) education, all programs should adhere to educational standards established by a professional nursing organization.
- Professional nursing organizations have an impact on educational standards and certifications, specialty practice, consumerism, and patient advocacy.

REFLECTIVE LEARNING

- Thinking back on a recent clinical experience, which QSEN competencies in knowledge, skills, or attitudes did you use while providing care?
- What impact do evidence-based practice and emerging technologies have on high-quality patient-centered care?
- You are on the patient safety committee at your hospital. Your assignment is to identify two resources related to safety. One resource must relate to the individual nurse, and the second must relate to the practice and work environment.

REVIEW QUESTIONS

1. You are preparing a presentation for your classmates regarding the clinical care coordination conference for a patient with terminal cancer. As part of the preparation, you have your classmates read the Nursing Code of Ethics for Professional Registered Nurses. Your instructor asks the class why this document is important. Which statement best describes this code?
   1. Improves self–health care
   2. Protects the patient's confidentiality
   3. Ensures identical care to all patients
   4. Defines the principles of right and wrong to provide patient care
2. A nurse is caring for a patient with end-stage lung disease. The patient wants to go home on oxygen and be comfortable. The family wants the patient to have a new surgical procedure. The nurse explains the risk and benefits of the operation to the family and discusses the patient's wishes with them. The nurse is acting as the patient's:
   1. Educator
   2. Advocate
   3. Caregiver
   4. Communicator
3. The nurse spends time with a patient and family reviewing a dressing change procedure for the patient's wound. The patient's spouse demonstrates how to change the dressing. The nurse is acting in which professional role?
   1. Educator
   2. Advocate
   3. Caregiver
   4. Communicator
4. The examination for RN licensure is the same in every state in the United States. This examination:
   1. Guarantees safe nursing care for all patients
   2. Ensures standard nursing care for all patients
   3. Provides the minimal standard of knowledge for an RN in practice
   4. Guarantees standardized education across all prelicensure programs
5. Contemporary nursing requires that the nurse have knowledge and skills for a variety of professional roles and responsibilities. Which of the following are examples of these roles and responsibilities? (Select all that apply.)
   1. Caregiver
   2. Autonomy
   3. Patient advocate
   4. Health promotion
   5. Genetic counselor
6. Match the advanced practice nurse specialty with the statement about the role.

   1. Clinical nurse specialist
   2. Nurse anesthetist
   3. Nurse practitioner
   4. Nurse-midwife

   a. Provides independent care, including pregnancy and gynecological services
   b. Expert clinician in a specialized area of practice such as adult diabetes care
   c. Provides comprehensive care, usually in a primary care setting, directly managing the medical care of patients who are healthy or have chronic conditions
   d. Plans and delivers anesthesia and pain management to patients across the life span

7. Health care reform will bring changes in the emphasis of care. Which of these models is expected from health care reform?
   1. Moving from an acute illness to a health promotion, illness prevention model
   2. Moving from an illness prevention to a health promotion model
   3. Moving from hospital-based to community-based care
   4. Moving from an acute illness to a disease management model
8. The nurse manager meets with the registered nursing staff about an increase in urinary tract infections in patients with a Foley catheter. The staff work together to review the literature on catheter-associated urinary tract infections (CAUTIs), identifies at-risk patients, and establishes new catheter care practices. This is an example of which QSEN competency?
   1. Patient-centered care
   2. Safety
   3. Teamwork and collaboration
   4. Quality improvement
9. A critical care nurse is using a new research-based intervention to correctly position patients who are on ventilators to reduce pneumonia caused by accumulated respiratory secretions. This is an example of which QSEN competency?
   1. Patient-centered care
   2. Evidence-based practice
   3. Teamwork and collaboration
   4. Quality improvement

10. The nurses on an acute care medical floor notice an increase in pressure injury formation in their patients. A nurse consultant decides to compare two types of treatment. The first is the procedure currently used to assess for pressure injury risk. The second uses a new assessment instrument to identify at-risk patients. Given this information, the nurse consultant exemplifies which career?
 1. Clinical nurse specialist
 2. Nurse administrator
 3. Nurse educator
 4. Nurse researcher

Answers: 1. 4; **2.** 3; **1.** 4, 3; **5.** 1, 2, 3, 4; **6.** 1b, 2d, 3c, 4a; **7.** 1; **8.** 4; **9.** 2; **10.** 4.

Rationales for Review Questions can be found on the Evolve website.

REFERENCES

American Association of Colleges of Nursing (AACN): *The essentials: core competencies for professional nursing education,* 2021a, https://www.aacnnursing.org/Education-Resources/AACN-Essentials. Accessed April 2021.

American Association of Colleges of Nursing (AACN): *End-of-Life Education Consortium (ELNEC) Fact Sheet,* 2021b, https://www.aacnnursing.org/Portals/42/ELNEC/PDF/ELNEC-Fact-Sheet.pdf . Accessed April 2021.

American Association of Nurse Anesthetists (AANA): Scope of nurse anesthesia practice, 2020, https://www.aana.com/docs/default-source/practice-aana-com-web-documents-(all)/professional-practice-manual/scope-of-nurse-anesthesia-practice.pdf?sfvrsn=250049b1_6. Accessed April 2021.

American College of Nurse Midwives (ACNM): *Definition of Midwifery and scope of practice of certified nurse-midwives and certified midwives,* 2012, https://www.midwife.org/acnm/files/ACNMLibraryData/UPLOADFILENAME/000000000266/Definition%20of%20Midwifery%20and%20Scope%20of%20Practice%20of%20CNMs%20and%20CMs%20Feb%202012.pdf. Accessed April 2021.

American Association of Nurse Practitioners (AANP): *What is a Nurse Practitioner (NP)?* https://www.aanp.org/about/all-about-nps/whats-a-nurse-practitioner, 2021. Accessed April 2021.

American Nurses Association (ANA): *Code of ethics for nurses with interpretive statements,* Silver Spring, MD, 2015, The Association. Available at: https://www.nursingworld.org/practice-policy/nursing-excellence/ethics/code-of-ethics-for-nurses/coe-view-only/. Accessed April 2021.

American Nurses Association (ANA): *Nursing: Scope and Standards of Practice,* 4th edition. Silver Spring, MD, 2021, The Association.

American Nurses Credentialing Center (ANCC): *Facts about the magnet recognition program,* n.d., https://www.nursingworld.org/globalassets/organizational-programs/magnet/magnet-factsheet.pdf. Accessed April 2021.

American Organization of Nurse Executives. *AONE Nurse Executive Competencies.* Chicago, IL, 2015, Author. https://www.aonl.org/sites/default/files/aone/nec.pdf. Accessed April 2021.

Benner P: *From novice to expert: excellence and power in clinical nursing practice,* Menlo Park, CA, 1984, Addison-Wesley.

Benner P, et al: The social fabric of nursing knowledge, *Am J Nurs* 97(7):16, 1997.

Benner P, et al: *Educating nurses: a call for radical transformation,* Stanford, CA, 2010, Carnegie Foundation for the Advancement of Teaching.

Centers for Disease Control and Prevention (CDC): *Genomics and health topics,* 2021, https://www.cdc.gov/genomics/disease/genomic_diseases.htm. Accessed April 2021.

Centers for Medicare and Medicaid Services (CMS): *Find & compare nursing homes, hospitals & other providers near you,* n.d., https://www.medicare.gov/care-compare/?providerType=Hospital&redirect=true. Accessed April 2021.

Centers for Medicare and Medicaid Services (CMS): *Hospital CAHPS (HCAHPS),* 2020, https://www.cms.gov/Research-Statistics-Data-and-Systems/Research/CAHPS/HCAHPS1. Accessed April 2021.

Donahue MP: *Nursing: the finest art—an illustrated history,* ed 3, St Louis, 2011, Mosby.

Doherty CL et al: The consensus model: What current and future NPs need to know, *American Nurse Today* 13(12), 2018, https://www.americannursetoday.com/consensus-model-nps/. Accessed April 2021.

Flanders SA: Effective patient education: evidence and common sense, *MedSurg Nursing,* 27(1): 55, 2018.

Fowler DM: *Guide to the Code of Ethics for nurses with interpretive statements: development, interpretation and application, second edition,* Silver Spring, MD, 2015, The Association.

Gerber L: Understanding the nurse's role as a patient advocate. *Nursing* 2018, 48(4): 55, 2018.

Graystone R: Prevent compassion fatigue and burnout with a magnet culture, *JONA* 49(5): 231, 2020.

Hospital Consumer Assessment of Healthcare Providers and Systems (HCAHPS): *CAHPS® Hospital Survey,* 2021, https://hcahpsonline.org/. Accessed April 2021.

Institute of Medicine (IOM): *The future of nursing: leading change, advancing health,* Washington DC, 2010, National Academies Press.

International Council of Nurses (ICN): *Nursing definitions,* 2021, https://www.icn.ch/nursing-policy/nursing-definitions. Accessed April 2021.

Kowalski K: Professional behavior in nursing, *J Contin Educ Nurs* 47(4):158, 2016.

McCormick KA, Calzone KA: The impact of genomics on health outcomes, quality, and safety, *Nurs Manage* 47(4):23, 2016.

Mason DJ, et al: *Policy & politics in nursing and health care,* ed 8, St. Louis, 2020, Elsevier.

Monsivais DB, Robbins LK: Better together: faculty development for quality improvement in the nurse educator role, *Teach Learn Nurs,* 15(1): 7, 2020.

National Association of Clinical Nurse Specialists (NACNS): *Statement on CNS practice and education* ed 3, Reston, VA, 2019, The Association.

National Council of State Boards of Nursing (NCSBN): *APRN Consensus Model for APRN Regulation: Licensure, Accreditation, Certification and Education,* 2021, https://www.ncsbn.org/aprn-consensus.htm, accessed April 2021.

National Quality Forum (NQF): *A strategic plan for achieving the care we need,* 2021, https://www.qualityforum.org/A_Strategic_Plan_for_Achieving_The_Care_We_Need.aspx . Accessed April 2021.

Nightingale F: *Notes on nursing: what it is and what it is not,* London, 1860, Harrison and Sons.

Porter-O'Grady T: Bringing nursing to the homeless and underserved, *Nurs Admin Q,* 42(2): 115, 2018.

QSEN Institute: *QSEN Competencies,* 2020a, http://qsen.org/competencies/pre-licensure-ksas/. Accessed April 2021.

QSEN Institute: *Graduate QSEN Competencies,* 2020b, https://qsen.org/competencies/graduate-ksas/. Accessed April 2021.

Robert Wood Johnson Foundation (RWJF). *Catalysts for change: Harnessing the power of nurses to build population health in the 21st century,* 2017, https://www.rwjf.org/en/library/research/2017/09/catalysts-for-change--harnessing-the-power-of-nurses-to-build-population-health.html Accessed April 2021.

Robert Wood Johnson Foundation (RWJF). *Campaign for action is chalking up successes that will improve patient care,* 2014, https://www.rwjf.org/en/library/articles-and-news/2014/06/campaign-for-action-is-chalking-up-successes-that-will-improve-p.html Accessed April 2021.

Sanner-Stiehr, Ward-Smith P: Lateral violence in nursing: Implication and strategies for nurse educators, *J Prof Nurs,* 33(2): 113, 2017.

Sharoff L: Holistic nursing in the genetic/genomic era, *J Holist Nurs* 34(2):146, 2016.

Smith SD et al: Adapting a nurse-managed mobile simulation program to meet rural health nursing continuing education needs, *J Cont Educ Nurs,* 51(2): 82, 2020.

Takenouchi S: Empowering nursing through end-of-life nursing education in Asia: Nurses as advocates for patients' dignity, *Asia Pac J Oncol Nurs,* 5(1): 9, 2018.

Tluczek A et al: How American Nurses Association Code of Ethics informs genetic/genomic nursing, *Nursing Ethics,* 26(5): 1505, 2019.

U.S. Census Bureau, Population Division: *Projections of the size and composition of the US Population,* 2014-2060, released 2015, https://www.census.gov/library/publications/2015/demo/p25-1143.html. Accessed April 2021.

Wallace I et al: The impact of clinical nurse specialists in the decision making in cancer multidisciplinary team meetings: A qualitative study, *European J Onc Nurs,* 43:1, 2019.

Wilson M et al: Impact of nurse champion on quality of care and outcomes in type 2 diabetes patients, *Int J Evid Based HealthC,* 17(1): 3, 2019.

RESEARCH REFERENCES

Abbasinia M et al: Patient advocacy in nursing: a concept analysis, *Nursing Ethics* 27(1): 141, 2019.

Andruszkiewicz G, Fike K: Emerging technology trends and products: how tech innovations are easing the burden of family caregiving, *Generations* 39(4):64, 2015–2016.

Christian BJ: Translational research-effective communication and teaching strategies for improving the quality of pediatric nursing care for hospitalized children and their families, *J Ped Nurs,* 34: 90, 2017.

Cooper AL et al: Nurse resilience: a concept analysis, *Int J Mental Health Nurs,* 29:553, 2020, https://doi.org/10.1111/inm.12721.

Crespo A et al: Improving the safety and quality of systemic treatment regimens in computerized prescriber order entry systems. *J Oncol Pract,* 14(6): e393, 2018.

das Gracas Silva Malsubara M; De Domenico EBL: Virtual learning environment in continuing education in nursing in Oncology: an experimental study, *J of Cancer Education* 31(4): 804, 2016.

Faraz A: Novice nurse practitioner workforce transition and turnover intention in primary care. *J Am Assoc Nurs Pract,* 29:26, 2017.

Hairong Y et al: Predictors of compassion fatigue, burnout, and compassion satisfaction among emergency nurses: a cross-sectional survey. *International Emergency Nursing,* 55(2021):100961, 2021, Available at: https://www.sciencedirect.com/science/article/pii/S1755599X20301336, 2021. Accessed April 2021.

Kaphingst KA et al: Relationships between health literacy and genomics-related knowledge, self-efficacy, perceived importance, and communication in a medically underserved population, *J Health Comm* 21:58, 2016.

Melnyk BM, Gallagher-Ford L: Outcomes from the first Helene Fuld Health Trust National Institute for Evidence-Based Practice in Nursing and Health Care Invitational Expert Forum, *Worldviews Evid Based Nurs* 15(1): 5, 2018,

O'Mahony J et al: Hospice palliative care volunteers a program and patient/family advocates, *Am J Hosp Palliat Med,* 34(9): 844, 2017.

Pinchera B et al: Best practices for patient self-management: implications for nurse educators, patient educators, and program developers, *J Cont Ed Nurs,* 49(9): 432, 2018.

Potter PA, et al: Developing a systemic program for compassion fatigue, *Nurs Adm Q* 37(4):326, 2013a.

Potter PA, et al: Evaluation of a compassion fatigue resilience program for oncology nurses, *Oncol Nurs Forum* 40(2):180, 2013b.

Seo J, et al: Effect of health literacy on decision-making preferences among medically underserved patients, *Med Decis Making* 36:550, 2016.

Smaradottir B, Fensli R: Evaluation of a telemedicine service run with a patient-centered model, *Stud Health Technol Inform,* 251:297, 2018.

Wellings CA et al: Evaluating continuing nursing education: a qualitative study of intention to change practice and perceived barriers to knowledge translation, *J Nurs Prof Dev,*33(6): 281, 2017.

Wenzel D, Brysiewicz P: Integrative review of facility interventions to manage compassion fatigue in oncology nurses, *Oncol Nurs Forum,* 44(3): E124, 2017.

The Health Care Delivery System

OBJECTIVES

- Discuss the features of an integrated health care system.
- Summarize the scope of the six levels of health care.
- Discuss the role of nurses in various health care settings.
- Explain the relationship between levels of health care and levels of prevention.
- Examine the types of settings in which professionals provide primary, secondary, and tertiary health care.
- Discuss the factors that affect a person's access to health care.
- Summarize the importance of discharge planning.

- Identify barriers to effective discharge planning.
- Explain how the concept of "Pay for Value" is used to reward hospitals financially.
- Explain the approaches nurses can use to improve patient satisfaction.
- Discuss how the nursing shortage is affecting the nursing profession.
- Explain the concept of patient-centered care.
- Explain the effects of health disparities on the health of a community.

KEY TERMS

Acute care
Adult day care centers
Affordable Care Act
Assisted living
Diagnosis-related group (DRG)
Discharge planning
Extended care facility
Health care disparities
Health care equity

Home care
Hospice
Inpatient Prospective Payment System (IPPS)
Medicaid
Medicare
Minimum Data Set (MDS)
Nursing-sensitive outcomes
Palliative care

Patient-centered care
Primary health care
Rehabilitation
Respite care
Restorative care
Secondary health care
Skilled nursing facility
Telehealth
Tertiary health care

MEDIA RESOURCES

http://evolve.elsevier.com/Potter/fundamentals/
- Review Questions
- Audio Glossary

- Case Study with Questions
- Content Updates
- Answers to QSEN Activity and Review Questions

The U.S. health care system is complex and constantly changing. Over the past decade, efforts were focused on reducing the costs of health care while improving access to the health care system and ensuring high-quality outcomes. However, in the first 6 months of 2020, approximately 30 million Americans did not have health insurance (Assistant Secretary for Planning and Evaluation [ASPE], 2021). In 2018, health care expenditures in the United States totaled 17.7% of the gross domestic product, which averaged $11,172 per person (Centers for Medicare and Medicaid Services [CMS], 2019a). A variety of services are available from different disciplines of health care professionals, but gaining access to services is often difficult for those with limited health care insurance and other economic resources. Millions of Americans have health insurance but do not seek preventive or needed health care because of the high cost of shared expenses (Himmelstein et al., 2018). Patients who are uninsured or do not seek health care early present a challenge to health care providers because they are more likely to skip or delay treatment for acute and chronic illnesses and die prematurely (Young and Kroth, 2018).

You will better succeed in your career if you understand the functioning of the health care system and the roles nurses play. Nursing is a caring discipline. The profession's values are rooted in helping people to regain, maintain, or improve their health; prevent illness; and find comfort and dignity at the end of life.

The practice of nursing is changing. The American Nurses Association (ANA) states, "Nursing promotes the health, well-being, comfort, dignity, and humanity of all individuals, families, groups, communities, and populations. Nursing's focus on the healthcare consumer is enhanced by interprofessional collaboration, sharing knowledge, scientific discovery, integrative healthcare approaches, and social justice" (ANA, 2021, p. 5). Buerhaus et al. (2017) identified four challenges facing nursing in the upcoming years. The first is the aging baby boomer generation, which will have increased health care needs and thus require more health services and increasingly more complex nursing care. The second is the shortage and uneven distribution of physicians, particularly primary care physicians, which increases the health care that nurses will need to provide. The third is the accelerating rate of nurses' retirements due to an aging nursing workforce, which results in loss of experienced nurses' knowledge and skills in all areas of practice. The fourth is the uncertainty of health care reform with each new government administration that is elected, which results in changes in roles for nurses within the health care system. It is critical to prepare nurses to face these and other challenges in the health care system today and to work toward improving access and maintaining quality and safety, while working to lessen health care costs that create a barrier to optimal wellness. Developing clinical judgment through the use of critical thinking is important to deliver safe, high-quality patient care in a changing health care environment.

TRADITIONAL LEVEL OF HEALTH CARE

The U.S. health care system has six levels of care for which health care providers offer services: preventive, primary, secondary, tertiary, restorative, and continuing health care. Levels of care describe the scope of services and settings delivered by health care providers to patients in all stages of health and illness. It is important to understand how the health care industry organizes and delivers services for patients and families within these six levels of care (Box 2.1)

Each level of care presents different requirements and opportunities for a nurse. For example, in your role within a primary care setting, you will be extensively involved in patient assessment. You will be expected to identify changes in chronic conditions or the development of new acute conditions. You will educate patients on how to perform self-care activities (e.g., teaching new mothers how to care for their babies, or young adults how to use inhalers). In a continuing care setting, you will apply gerontological nursing principles to help patients adapt to permanent health changes so that they can remain active and engaged.

Levels of care are not the same as levels of prevention (see Chapter 6). Levels of prevention describe the focus of health-related activities in a care setting. These include health promotion and disease prevention (primary prevention), curing or managing disease (secondary prevention), and reducing complications (tertiary prevention). For example, in a tertiary level of care, such as an intensive care unit (ICU), a nurse practices primary prevention by preventing pneumonia through repositioning a patient frequently, secondary prevention by administering antibiotics on time to treat the pneumonia, and tertiary prevention by assessing the patient frequently for signs of antibiotic intolerance.

At every level of care, nurses and other health care providers offer a variety of prevention services. For example, a nurse working in a specialized acute care (secondary/tertiary) hospital setting monitors the recovery of a patient following open heart surgery while also providing health promotion information to the patient and family caregiver concerning diet and exercise.

Health care reform has led to changes unique to each level of care. For example, the health care industry now places greater emphasis on wellness. Thus, the industry directs more resources toward primary and preventive care. Wellness care focuses on the health of populations and their communities rather than simply curing an individual's disease. In wellness care, nurses can help lead communities and health care systems in coordinating resources to better serve their populations.

INTEGRATED HEALTH CARE DELIVERY

Integrated health care delivery (IHCD) came about as part of the U.S. health care reform movement in response to the fragmented, costly, and varying quality of health care found in the United States at the time. An IHCD system is a network of health care organizations that work together to provide a continuum of health services to a defined population with intended outcomes of better aligning resources, improving quality, and controlling costs (Al-Saddique, 2018). IHCDs were developed with a primary focus on improving health care quality and decreasing overall health care costs. The goal of focusing on population health is to decrease health care costs through effective management of patients with chronic health problems. An example of an IHCD is the Accountable Care Organizations (ACOs) that were developed in response to health care reform, with the intended goals of improving quality and decreasing costs of health care (McWilliams et al., 2016).

There is no single model for an integrated health care system. Basically, two types of IHCDs exist: an organizational structure that follows economic imperatives (such as combining financing with all providers, from hospitals, clinics, and physicians to home care and long-term care facilities) and a structure that supports an organized

---

BOX 2.1 Examples of Health Care Services

Preventive Care
- Adult screenings for blood pressure, cholesterol, tobacco use, and cancer
- Pediatric screenings for hearing, vision, autism, and developmental disorders
- HIV screening for adults at higher risk
- Wellness visits
- Immunizations
- Diet counseling
- Mental health counseling and crisis prevention
- Community legislation (seat belts, car seats for children, bike helmets)

Primary Care (Health Promotion)
- Diagnosis and treatment of common illnesses
- Ongoing management of chronic health problems
- Prenatal care
- Well-baby care
- Family planning
- Patient-centered medical home care

Secondary (Acute Care)
- Urgent care; hospital emergency care
- Acute medical-surgical care: ambulatory care, outpatient surgery, hospital
- Radiological procedures

Tertiary Care
- Highly specialized: intensive care, inpatient psychiatric facilities
- Specialty care (such as neurology, cardiology, rheumatology, dermatology, oncology)

Restorative Care
- Rehabilitation programs (such as cardiovascular, pulmonary, orthopedic)
- Sports medicine
- Spinal cord injury programs
- Home care

Continuing Care
- Long-term care: assisted living, nursing centers
- Psychiatric and older-adult day care

care delivery approach (coordinating care activities and services into seamless functioning) (Al-Saddique, 2018).

The Patient-Centered Medical Home model is an example of an IHCD. The Patient-Centered Medical Home strengthens the physician-patient relationship with coordinated, goal-oriented, individualized care. In this approach, a patient's primary health care provider is the coordinator/manager who enlists the skills and knowledge of health care professionals from various services. These professionals include nurses, medical assistants, nutritionists, social workers, pharmacists, hospice care providers, and other caregivers. Members of a Patient-Centered Medical Home care team are linked by information technology, electronic health records (EHRs), and system best practices to ensure that patients receive care how they want it and when and where they need it. Patient-centeredness is a unifying principle. It describes an ongoing, active partnership with a personal primary care physician or nurse practitioner who leads a team of professionals dedicated to providing proactive, preventive, and chronic care management through all stages of a patient's life (American Academy of Family Physicians, 2020.)

Primary and Preventive Health Care Services

Primary health care focuses on improved health outcomes for an entire population by promoting regular health care visits, health education, proper nutrition, maternal/child health care, family planning, immunizations, and control of diseases. The World Health Organization (WHO) (2021) notes that most of a person's health care needs in their lifetime can be met with primary care services. Primary health care requires collaboration among health professionals, health care leaders, and community members. In settings in which patients receive preventive and primary care, such as schools, physicians' offices, and occupational health clinics, health promotion is a major theme (Table 2.1). Health promotion programs are designed to reduce the incidence of disease, minimizing complications and the need to use more expensive health care resources. As a result, the overall costs of health care are also reduced. In contrast, preventive care is more disease oriented and focused on reducing and controlling risk factors for disease through activities such as immunization and occupational health programs. Chapter 3 provides a more comprehensive discussion of primary health care in the community.

Secondary and Tertiary Care

The traditional reason people use health care services (such as a hospital) is for diagnosis and treatment of illness. When the nature or severity of a condition makes primary care insufficient, secondary and tertiary care may become necessary. The difference between secondary and tertiary care arises from the complexity of a patient's medical needs. Secondary health care is provided by a specialist or agency on referral by a primary health care provider. It requires more specialized knowledge, skill, or equipment than the primary care physician or nurse practitioner can provide. For example, an individual sees a cardiologist because of increasing shortness of breath with activity.

Tertiary health care is specialized consultative care, usually provided on referral from secondary medical personnel. For example, the cardiac surgeon sees the patient referred from the cardiologist for possible cardiac bypass surgery. However, changes in medical cost reimbursement, improved technology, and less invasive treatments have often made secondary and tertiary care available at the primary care level. For example, more surgeons are performing simple surgeries in outpatient surgical centers or office suites. However, if a patient develops a problem that the surgeon or primary health care provider is not able to treat and/or if intensive nursing care is needed, the patient needs a medical specialist, often resulting in hospitalization. Secondary and tertiary care (also called acute care) typically are expensive, especially if the patient has waited to seek care until after symptoms have developed. Delays in treating or diagnosing chronic illness may cause disability, decreased quality of life, and increased health care costs (Young and Kroth, 2018).

Hospitals. Hospitals provide comprehensive secondary and tertiary health care to patients who are acutely ill. During 2018 more than 36 million patients were admitted to American Hospital Association (AHA)–registered hospitals (AHA, 2020a). Even allowing for the fact that some patients are admitted multiple times during a year, a large percentage of the U.S. population receives health care in a hospital each year.

Hospitals vary in the services they offer. Most small rural hospitals offer general inpatient services but have limited emergency and diagnostic services. The exception is Critical Access Hospitals (CAHs). In comparison, large urban medical centers offer comprehensive, state-of-the-art diagnostic services, trauma and emergency care, surgical intervention, ICUs, inpatient services, and rehabilitation centers. Larger hospitals hire professional staff from a variety of specialties, such as nursing, social services, respiratory therapy, physical and occupational therapy, and speech therapy. Most patients who require these services are having acute episodes of illness. Thinking critically and using clinical judgment are needed to assess patients' changing problems quickly and intervene safely and accurately. This is a challenge when you are assigned multiple patients. Using clinical judgment enables you to better organize patient care to deliver an array of nursing interventions safely and effectively, and recognize when the needs of your patients change and no longer match the level of health care where they are receiving treatment. You also must be able to plan and coordinate care with other health care providers quickly and competently.

Hospitals use evidence-based practice guidelines and clinical protocols (see Chapter 5) in the delivery of care to patients. Current evidence-based practices ensure safe, effective, state-of-the art care. Throughout the nursing process, clinical judgment requires the continual evaluation of whether patients achieve outcomes so plans of care can be revised as needed to meet patient needs.

According to the AHA (2020b), delivering the right care, at the right time, in the right setting is the core mission of hospitals across the country. To fulfill this mission, hospitals fully support quality and safety initiatives. An example of a quality initiative is patient satisfaction. Patient satisfaction is challenging to achieve in a stressful setting, such as an inpatient nursing unit. Patients expect to be treated courteously and respectfully and to be involved in daily care decisions (Santana et al., 2019). Hospitals are adopting models of patient-centered care that focus on care that is responsive to individual patient and family preferences, needs, and values and ensuring that patient values guide clinical decisions (Santana et al., 2019). In a patient-centered care model, nurses partner with patients and families early in the decision-making process to develop an individualized plan of care (Santana et al., 2019). As a nurse, you have a key role in learning patient needs and expectations early to form effective therapeutic partnerships. By treating the nurse-patient relationship with respect and dignity, nursing care delivery is improved, which enhances patient satisfaction.

Intensive Care. An ICU or critical care unit (CCU) is a hospital unit in which patients receive close monitoring and intensive medical and nursing care. The status of a patient who is critically ill can change by the minute, so health care providers must have specialized knowledge and skills. ICUs have advanced technologies such as computerized cardiac monitors and high-tech mechanical ventilators. Although many of these devices are on regular nursing units, patients hospitalized within ICUs are monitored and maintained on multiple devices. An ICU is the most expensive health care delivery site because each

TABLE 2.1   Preventive and Primary Care Services

Type of Service	Purpose	Available Programs and Services
School health	Comprehensive programs integrate health promotion principles into a school curriculum. Services emphasize program management, interprofessional collaboration, and community health principles. Research shows a link between the health outcomes of young people and their academic success (CDC, 2021).	Health education Physical education and physical activity Nutrition environment and services Health services Physical environment Social and emotional climate Counseling, psychological services, and social services Employee wellness Family engagement Community involvement
Occupational health	The workplace is an important setting for delivering comprehensive health protection, health promotion, and disease and accident prevention programs. Americans working full time spend an average of more than one-third of their day, 5 days a week, at the workplace (CDC, 2015). The goal is to increase worker productivity, reduce absenteeism, reduce health risks, and reduce the use of expensive medical care.	Environmental surveillance Create company policies that promote healthy behaviors such as a tobacco-free campus policy Work environment: offer healthy foods through vending machines or cafeterias Physical assessment and health screening Health education classes Communicable disease control Counseling
Physicians' offices	Provide primary health care and diagnose and treat acute and chronic illnesses. Practitioners are beginning to focus more on health promotion practices. Advanced nurse practitioners often partner with a physician in managing a patient population.	Routine physical examination Health screening and risk appraisal Diagnostics Disease management Prevention services: diabetes and osteoporosis screenings, smoking cessation programs, and immunizations Wellness counseling
Nurse-managed clinics	Nurse-managed clinics or centers deliver nursing services with a focus on health promotion and health education, chronic disease assessment and management, and support for self-care and caregivers. Clinics often are associated with a school, college, department of nursing, federally qualified health center, or independent nonprofit health care agency.	Day care Clinical education site for other health care providers in school Prevention services: diabetes screenings, smoking cessation programs, and immunizations Physical examinations, cardiovascular checks Health risk appraisal Wellness counseling Employment readiness Acute and chronic care management
Block and parish nursing	Nurses deliver health care services to patients (e.g., older adults or those unable to leave their homes) within their own religious communities. Provide services that are unavailable in traditional health care system.	Running errands/transportation Respite care Counseling Spiritual health: balancing body and mind health to achieve overall wellness
Community centers	Provide comprehensive and cost-effective primary care and supportive services that promote access to health care. Often deliver services to a specific patient population (such as well-baby care, mental health, patients with diabetes) within underserved communities. Sometimes affiliated with a hospital, medical school, church, or other community organization. The care offered by community centers is culturally appropriate and delivered in languages that many in these communities speak.	Physical assessment and health screening Nutrition education Translation services Dental care Mental health services Care coordination and case management Specialty care (such as orthopedic, cardiac, or podiatric care) Disease management Health education

nurse usually cares for only one or two patients at a time and because of all the treatments and procedures the patients in the ICU require.

Mental Health Facilities. According to the National Alliance on Mental Illness (NAMI) (2021), about one in five adults in the United States experience mental illness in a given year, with 1 in 20 adults experiencing a serious mental illness such as depression, schizophrenia, or bipolar disorder. Perhaps more concerning is the report that only 44.8% of adults in the United States with a mental health condition received mental health services in 2019 (NAMI, 2021). Patients who have emotional and behavioral problems such as depression, mood disorders, violent behavior, and eating disorders require special counseling and treatment in psychiatric facilities.

The massive cuts to non-Medicaid state mental health spending in 2011 resulted in states having to cut vital mental health services for tens of thousands of youth and adults living with the most serious mental illnesses. These services include community- and hospital-based psychiatric care, housing, and access to medications (NAMI, 2011). This reduction in mental health agencies and services continues to have consequences today, such as loss of income due to missed work, high suicide rates, and high education dropout rates (NAMI, 2021). Individuals with serious mental illness are more likely to suffer chronic disease and as a result die earlier than others, largely from treatable medical conditions (NAMI, 2021).

The psychiatric facilities that exist are located in hospitals, independent outpatient clinics, and private mental health hospitals. They offer inpatient and outpatient services, depending on the severity of a patient's problem. Patients enter mental health facilities voluntarily or involuntarily. In voluntary admission, the patient or guardian completes an application requesting admission to the mental health facility with the ability to request release at any time. Involuntary admission is made without patient consent if patients require psychiatric treatment, cannot meet their own basic needs, or are a danger to themselves or others. During an involuntary admission, patients retain their right to informed consent, right to refuse medications, and right to freedom from unreasonable restraint (Varcarolis and Fosbre, 2021). Patients who are hospitalized usually have short stays intended to stabilize them before transfer to outpatient treatment centers. Patients with mental illness receive a comprehensive interprofessional treatment plan that engages patients and their families. Medical, nursing, social work, and activity therapy providers collaborate to develop a plan of care that enables patients to become more functional within their communities. Patients usually receive referrals for follow-up care at clinics or with counselors during discharge from inpatient settings.

Rural Hospitals. Lack of access to health care in rural areas is a serious public health problem. Only about 13% of physicians practice in rural America, but nearly 20% of the U.S. population lives in these areas (National Rural Health Association [NRHA], 2020). Rural Americans face a unique combination of factors that create health care disparities that are not found in urban areas, including (1) economic factors (rural Americans are more likely to live below the poverty level), (2) cultural and social differences, (3) educational shortcomings, (4) lack of recognition by legislators, and (5) isolation from living in remote rural areas (NRHA, 2020).

Many rural hospitals have failed economically and closed. To address this problem, the Balanced Budget Act of 1997 changed the designation of some rural hospitals to Critical Access Hospital (CAH) when certain criteria were met (CMS Medical Learning Network [MLN], 2019). A CAH is located in a state that established a rural health plan as of February 2018, is in a rural area (35 miles from another hospital or CAH), provides 24/7 emergency services with no more than 25 inpatient beds, and reports 96 hours or less as an average length of stay (LOS) for temporary care for patients needing stabilization before transfer to a larger hospital. CAHs may operate a distinct rehabilitation and/or psychiatric care unit, each with up to 10 beds. Physicians, advanced practice nurses, or physician assistants staff a CAH. The CAH provides inpatient care to people who are acutely ill or injured before they are transferred to better-equipped health care centers. Basic radiological and laboratory services are also available. To improve care for patients residing in rural areas, rural hospitals are expected to (HealthIT.gov, 2017):

- Improve access to services, including urgent care services, and to meet unmet health needs in isolated rural communities.
- Engage rural communities in developing rural health care systems.

- Develop collaborative delivery systems in rural communities as the hubs of rural health care.
- Create protocols for coordinating care transition by aligning urban health care systems.
- Be the subject matter experts and coordinators for the health care environment of providers, patients, and staff.

Health care reform enabled urban health care systems to branch out and establish affiliations or mergers with rural hospitals. Rural hospitals and CAHs provide a referral base to the larger tertiary care medical centers. Nurses who work in rural hospitals or clinics often function independently without a physician. These nurses must be competent in physical assessment, clinical judgment and decision making, and emergency care. Advanced practice nurses (such as nurse practitioners and clinical nurse specialists) use medical protocols and establish collaborative agreements with staff physicians.

Health care payers, such as CMS and private insurers, expect patients who are hospitalized to be treated and discharged within a reasonably predictable time period. Reimbursements are affected by the quality and timeliness of care. Nurses must use resources efficiently and effectively to help patients recover and return home. For example, a nurse collaborates with members of the interprofessional health care team, such as case managers, advanced practice providers such as nurse practitioners, physical therapists, physicians, and social workers, to plan a quick yet realistic transition to another level of health care. This process is known as *discharge planning.*

Discharge Planning. Discharge planning is a coordinated, interprofessional process that develops a plan for continuing care after a patient leaves a health care agency. Studies have shown that patients tend to be discharged "quicker and sicker" from hospitals. This can result in adverse events during the immediate postdischarge period (Aicher et al., 2019; Meek et al., 2018). Such problems include medication prescribing errors, poor communication between hospital and primary care providers, readmission to health care agency, and lack of coordination with community health care services. The focus of discharge planning is to ensure that a patient transitions to the setting in which health care needs can be appropriately met.

With the emphasis on decreased LOS in hospitals, *discharge planning with coordination of services must begin the moment a patient is admitted to a hospital.* As a nurse you will play a large role in discharge planning by knowing a patient's plan of care (developed by the interprofessional team) as soon as possible, informing the patient and family of that plan, encouraging their participation, acting on the plan, and evaluating progress (Fig. 2.1). Discharge planning for patients and their caregivers involves these elements (CMS, 2019b):

- Determining the appropriate post-hospital destination for a patient. A case manager or social worker usually selects this setting based on a patient's health care needs, self-care capacity, insurance, and place of residence.
- Identifying a patient's needs for a smooth and safe transition from the acute care hospital/post–acute care agency to the patient's discharge destination. Nurses, therapists, health care providers, and dietitians usually identify these needs.
- Beginning the process of meeting a patient's needs while the patient is still hospitalized, with approaches such as early mobility protocols, health education, and new medication regimens.

With a well-developed discharge plan, a patient is less likely to have unavoidable complications or unrelated illnesses or injuries and will be able to continue progressing toward the goals of the plan of care after discharge (CMS, 2019b). As a nurse, participate in discharge planning by anticipating and identifying each patient's continuing needs before

FIG. 2.1 Providing discharge teaching to decrease hospital readmission. (Copyright © FatCamera/iStock/Getty Images.)

the actual time of discharge and coordinating efforts to achieve an appropriate discharge plan.

The CMS does not require discharge planning for outpatients, including those who present to an emergency department and are not admitted as hospital inpatients. At the same time, hospitals may help some outpatients (such as emergency department or same-day surgery patients) by providing some discharge planning services (CMS, 2019b). A nurse-driven discharge planning model that includes discharge teaching and follow-up after discharge can help reduce hospital readmission rates (Dizon and Reinking, 2017; Meek et al., 2018). Box 2.2

BOX 2.2   Discharge Planning Models

Coleman's "Care Transitions Program" (Coleman et al., 2006)

Emphasizes the role of a transition coach in managing/facilitating the discharge of a patient to home or to a rehabilitation center. Model is based on four pillars: (1) medication self-management, (2) patient-centered record, (3) follow-up, and (4) indicators of worsening medical condition. Each pillar has different interventions depending on the stage of the hospitalization.

Naylor's "Transitional Care Model" (Naylor et al., 2009)

Emphasizes comprehensive discharge planning and follow-up for older adults who are chronically ill. Model contains six key components: (1) in-hospital assessment and development of the discharge care plan by a transitional care nurse/advanced practice nurse/gerontological nurse; (2) discharge preparation by an interprofessional care team; (3) patient participation (communication between nursing staff and the patient) regarding the process, the decision making, the discharge planning, and the discharge education; (4) continuity of care and communication among health care providers; (5) predischarge assessment; and (6) postdischarge follow-up.

High-Intensity Care Model (GRACE Model)

The interprofessional team is headed by *both* a nurse practitioner *and* a social worker. Other team members include a pharmacist, geriatric specialist, and mental health provider. This team works in tandem to support the primary care physician and, following best practice protocols, to fully address a patient's health conditions. The focus is to help patients manage their health conditions, coordinate their health care, and achieve optimal health (Blue Cross Blue Shield of Michigan, n.d.; Center for Consumer Engagement in Health Innovation, 2018). This achieves a patient's goal from the convenience and security of the patient's own home (Counsell, 2015).

---

describes models of discharge planning that focus on the patient and family caregiver.

Some patients are more in need of discharge planning because of their health-related risks. For example, some patients have poor health literacy, limited financial resources, or limited family support; others have long-term disabilities or chronic illness; and older adults sometimes have cognitive and/or hearing impairments affecting their attention to discharge instruction. There are also barriers to effective discharge planning, including ineffective communication (health care provider to provider; health care provider to patient), lack of role clarity among health care team members (responsibility and follow-up), and lack of resources (e.g., rehab and nursing home beds) (Abu et al., 2018; Shinall et al., 2019). You can reduce barriers to discharge planning by clearly communicating about the plan of care with patients, families, and members of the health care team. Change-of-shift, hand-off reporting, and hourly bedside rounds are ways to keep all health care providers and patients informed (see Chapter 24). Communicate clearly both verbally and in the entries you make in the EHR (see Chapter 26). Clarify any role confusion to be sure that elements of the plan are completed.

Discharge instructions prepare patients for transition from a hospital to the next level of care (such as home, rehabilitation, or long-term care). Nurses offer useful and relevant information to prepare patients and their family caregivers for postdischarge care. To develop discharge instructions, you must understand the proper timing for discharge, engage the patient and family caregiver (when allowed by the patient) in the process, and know the health care team's plan of care. Patients cannot learn when they are having pain, nausea, confusion, or other disabling symptoms. Family caregivers can be excellent resources when the patient desires their help. Always involve patients and family caregivers in the decisions about the patient's discharge destination.

Provide discharge instruction as early as possible so that you and other health care team members can reinforce the information several times to improve learning. For example, when a patient is receiving care that follows a standard protocol, you can easily anticipate the treatment and the patient's estimated discharge date. When the patient has multiple complications, the plan of care and estimated discharge date might not be clear. Begin to explain discharge instruction as soon as you know the plan of care. The following are required discharge instruction topics (The Joint Commission [TJC], 2020): discharge medications, follow-up care (if needed), list of all medications changed and/or discontinued, dietary needs, and follow-up tests or procedures.

Some patients assume passive roles when they receive instructions. They might be satisfied when a nurse, physician, or therapist rushes through an explanation and finishes by simply inquiring, "Any questions?" This often leads the patient to automatically answer "no." This patient might never have been invited to actively participate in the health care plan. A patient-centered approach does more. For example, the health care provider *invites* the patient to participate: "I want to make sure that I've helped you understand everything you need to know about your illness. Patients usually have questions because their situations can be complicated. Could you tell me what you do not understand, and then I can help clarify?" or "Do you understand which medications were changed or discontinued?" The teach-back approach (see Chapter 25) helps to ensure that a patient understands instructions. Teach-back is an evidence-based health literacy intervention that promotes patient engagement, patient safety, adherence, and quality (Agency for Healthcare Research and Quality [AHRQ], 2020). Comprehensive discharge instruction ensures that patients know what to do when they get home, how to perform care activities, and what to do when problems develop.

Discharge planning often leads to referrals to other health care providers, especially when specific therapies are planned (such as physical therapy) (see Chapter 18). Some tips for making a successful referral include the following:

- Engage the patient and family caregiver in the referral process, including selecting the care provider. Explain the reason for the referral, the service to be provided, and how the service will be provided.
- Make the referral as soon as possible.
- Give the care provider receiving the referral as much information as possible about the patient. This can avoid unnecessary duplication of assessment (e.g., current vital signs or pain status) and omission of important information.
- The care provider, such as a physical therapist, social worker, dietitian, or radiologist, will make recommendations for the patient's care. Learn these recommendations and incorporate them into the treatment plan as soon as possible.

Restorative Care

Patients recovering from an acute or chronic illness or disability often require additional services in order to return to their previous level of function or to reach a new level of function limited by their illness or disability. The goals of restorative care are to help individuals regain maximal functional status and to enhance quality of life through promotion of independence and self-care. With the emphasis on early discharge from hospitals, patients usually require some level of restorative care. For example, some patients require ongoing wound care and activity and exercise management until they recover enough strength and/or function following surgery to independently resume normal activities of daily living.

The intensity of care has increased in a number of restorative care settings because patients are being discharged from hospitals earlier. Patients in a home or rehabilitation setting often still receive intravenous (IV) fluids (see Chapter 42), aggressive pain control (see Chapter 44), or enteral nutrition (see Chapter 45). The restorative health care team is interprofessional and includes the patient and family or significant others. In restorative settings, nurses recognize that success depends on effective and early collaboration with patients and their families. Patients and families require a clear understanding of goals for physical recovery, the rationale for any physical limitations, and the purpose and potential risks associated with therapies. Patients and families are more likely to follow treatment plans and achieve optimal functioning when they are engaged in their care.

Home Care. Home care is the provision of medically related professional and paraprofessional services and equipment to patients and families in their homes for health maintenance, education, illness prevention, diagnosis and treatment of disease, rehabilitation, and palliative care. This care consists of part-time, medically necessary skilled care (nursing, physical therapy, occupational therapy, and speech-language therapy) that is prescribed by a health care provider (CMS, 2020a). A home care service also coordinates the access to and delivery of home health equipment, or durable medical equipment, which is a medical product adapted for home use.

Home care nurses have their own patient caseloads and deliver highly individualized nursing care. They help patients adapt to many permanent or temporary physical limitations so that the patients can assume a daily home routine that is as normal as possible. Home care requires a strong knowledge base in many areas, such as family dynamics (see Chapter 10), cultural competence (see Chapter 9), spiritual values (see Chapter 35), and communication principles (see Chapter 24). Home health nurses must also have expertise in assessment (see Chapter 30). Nurses who work in Medicare-certified home care agencies conduct patient-specific comprehensive assessments at a patient's start of care, at 60-day follow-ups, at discharge, and before and after an inpatient stay

(Research Data Assistance Center [ResDac], 2020). This comprehensive assessment, OASIS (the Outcome and Assessment Information Set), includes a group of standardized core assessment items for an adult home care patient. OASIS forms the basis for measuring patient outcomes and improving home health care for the purposes of outcome-based quality. Data items within OASIS include sociodemographic information on the patient's home environment and informal caregivers, support system, health status, functional status, psychosocial status, and health service utilization (e.g., emergent care, hospital admissions) (ResDac, 2020). The OASIS assessment tool was designed to gather the data items needed to measure both outcomes and patient risk factors in the home setting.

Home health care focuses on the goal of helping patients and their family members achieve independence. Home care addresses the recovery from and stabilization of an illness. In addition, home care identifies problems related to lifestyle, safety, environment, family dynamics, and health care practices. Home care agencies provide skilled and intermittent professional services, such as wound care, administration of parenteral and enteral nutrition, administration of medications and blood therapy, and home care aide services. The frequency of these services is based on patient need and may range from a couple of times a week to once or twice a day as often as 7 days a week.

Approved home care agencies usually receive reimbursement for services from governmental programs (such as Medicare and Medicaid in the United States), private insurance, and private payers. The government strictly regulates reimbursement for home care services. An agency cannot simply charge whatever it wants for a service and expect to receive that amount. Governmental programs set the amount of reimbursement for most professional services.

Rehabilitation. The WHO defines rehabilitation as the process aimed at enabling people with disabilities to reach and maintain their optimal physical, sensory, intellectual, psychological, and social functional levels. Rehabilitation gives people with disabilities the tools they need to attain independence and self-determination (WHO, 2020). Patients require rehabilitation after a physical or mental illness, surgery affecting musculoskeletal function, injury, or chemical addiction. Rehabilitation was once offered mostly to patients with illnesses or injury to the nervous or musculoskeletal system, but the expanded scope of services now also includes cardiovascular, neurological, pulmonary, and mental health rehabilitation programs. The goal of these specialized rehabilitation services is to help patients and families adjust to necessary changes in lifestyle and learn to function with the limitations of their disease. For example, drug rehabilitation centers help patients become free from drug dependence and return to the community.

Rehabilitation services after acute care include physical, occupational, and speech therapy and social services. Ideally rehabilitation begins the moment a patient enters a health care setting for treatment. For example, some orthopedic programs now have patients perform physical therapy exercises before major joint repair to enhance their recovery after surgery. Initially rehabilitation usually focuses on preventing complications related to an illness or injury, such as promoting early mobility in patients after surgery. As the patient's condition stabilizes, rehabilitation helps to maximize functioning and level of independence, often by examining the need for assistive devices such as walkers or canes or adapting approaches for performing self-care.

Rehabilitation settings include rehabilitation units within acute care centers, freestanding outpatient settings, and the home. Patients who have severe disabilities may not be able to carry out the activities of daily living independently. An example would be a patient who has had a stroke or spinal cord injury. These patients may benefit from long-term rehabilitation to reach their maximum potential.

Patients who use rehabilitation services in an outpatient setting receive treatment at appointments during the week but live in their home. Sometimes, specific rehabilitation services are also used in the home to help the patient.

Extended Care Facilities. An extended care facility provides intermediate medical, nursing, or custodial care for patients recovering from acute illness or those with chronic illnesses or disabilities. Extended care facilities include intermediate care and skilled nursing facilities. Some include long-term care and assisted-living facilities. In the past, extended care facilities primarily cared for older adults; now, because of the focus on early discharge from hospitals, there is a greater need for intermediate care settings for patients of all ages. For example, health care providers transfer a young patient who has a traumatic brain injury resulting from a car accident to an extended care facility for rehabilitative or supportive care until discharge to the home becomes a realistic and safe option.

An intermediate care or skilled nursing facility offers skilled care from a licensed nursing staff. This often includes administration of IV fluids, wound care, long-term ventilator management, and physical rehabilitation. Patients receive extensive supportive care until they are able to move back into the community or into residential care. Extended care facilities provide around-the-clock nursing coverage. Nurses who work in a skilled nursing facility need nursing expertise similar to that of nurses working in acute care inpatient settings, along with a background in gerontological nursing principles (see Chapter 14).

Continuing Care

Continuing care describes a variety of health, personal, and social services provided over a prolonged period. These services are for people who have disabilities, who were never functionally independent, or who have a terminal disease. The need for continuing health care services is growing in the United States. People are living longer, and many of those with continuing health care needs have no immediate family members to care for them. A decline in the number of children that families choose to have, the aging of care providers, and the increasing rates of divorce and remarriage complicate this problem.

Continuing care is available within institutional settings (e.g., nursing centers or nursing homes, group homes, and retirement communities), communities (e.g., adult day care and senior centers), or the home (e.g., home care, home-delivered meals, and hospice) (Meiner and Yeager, 2019). Another alternative for the patient who does not need nursing care but needs some assistance to stay independent is elder care services. These services offer companionship, assistance with activities of daily living, and food preparation.

Nursing Centers or Facilities. The language of long-term care is confusing and constantly changing. *Nursing home* was formerly the name for the dominant setting for long-term care (Meiner and Yeager, 2019). With the 1987 Omnibus Budget Reconciliation Act, *nursing facility* became the term for nursing homes and other facilities that provided long-term care. Now *nursing center* is the most appropriate term. A nursing center typically provides 24-hour intermediate and custodial care such as nursing, rehabilitation, dietary, recreational, social, and religious services for residents of any age with chronic or debilitating illnesses. Nursing center services provided by Medicaid-certified nursing homes offer:
- Skilled nursing
- Rehabilitation
- Long-term care (Medicaid.gov, n.d.)

These three services include 24-hour licensed nursing, rehabilitation, medically related social services, and pharmaceutical services. In addition there are dietary services individualized to the needs of each resident, a professionally directed program of activities to meet the interests and needs for the well-being of each resident, emergency dental services, room and bed maintenance services, and routine personal hygiene items and services. A skilled nursing facility must care for its residents in a manner and in an environment that will promote maintenance or enhancement of the quality of life of each resident (Legal Information Institute, n.d.).

Most people living in nursing centers are older adults. A nursing center may be a resident's temporary or permanent home with surroundings made as homelike as possible. Residents receive a planned, systematic, and interprofessional approach to care to help them reach and maintain their highest level of function.

Nursing centers must comply with the Omnibus Budget Reconciliation Act of 1987 and its minimum requirements for nursing facilities to receive payment from Medicare and Medicaid. Government regulations require that staff members in nursing centers comprehensively assess each resident and that care planning decisions be made within a prescribed period. A resident's functional ability (such as the ability to perform activities of daily living and instrumental activities of daily living) and long-term physical and psychosocial well-being are the focus.

A nursing facility must complete the Resident Assessment Instrument (RAI) for each resident. The RAI helps nursing facility staff gather definitive information on a resident's strengths and needs, which must then be addressed in an individualized care plan (CMS, 2019). The RAI has three components: the Minimum Data Set (MDS) Version 3.0, the Care Area Assessment (CAA) process, and the RAI Utilization Guidelines (Box 2.3). The components of the RAI yield information about a resident's functional status, strengths, weaknesses, and preferences, as well as offering guidance on further assessment once problems have been identified (CMS, 2019). The MDS Version 3.0 is an initial overview of a resident's health care needs. It is a preliminary assessment to identify the resident's potential problems, strengths, and preferences. The CAAs are triggered by individual MDS item responses that reveal the need for additional assessment. These item responses identify problems, known as "triggered care areas," which form a critical link between the MDS and decisions about care planning. CAAs enable facilities to identify and use tools that are grounded in current clinical standards of practice, such as evidence-based or expert-endorsed research, clinical practice guidelines, and resources.

The information gathered using the RAI provides a national database for nursing facilities that enables policy makers to better understand the health care needs of the long-term care population. The MDS and CAAs are a rich resource for nurses in selecting interventions that best meet the health care needs of this growing population.

Assisted Living. Assisted living is one of the fastest-growing industries within the United States. There are almost 30,000 assisted-living facilities with nearly one million licensed beds that house more than 800,000 people in the United States (National Center for Assisted Living [NCAL], 2020). Assisted living offers an attractive long-term care setting with an environment more like home and greater resident autonomy. Residents require some assistance with activities of daily living but remain relatively independent within a partially protective setting. A group of residents live together, but residents have their own rooms and share dining and social activity areas. Usually people keep all of their personal possessions in their residences.

Assisted-living residences range from hotel-like buildings with hundreds of units to modest group homes that house a handful of seniors. Assisted living provides independence, security, and privacy all at the same time (Touhy and Jett, 2018). These settings promote physical and psychosocial health (Fig. 2.2). Services in an assisted-living center include laundry, assistance with meals and personal care, 24-hour oversight, and housekeeping (NCAL, 2020). Some centers provide assistance with medication administration. Nursing care services are not always

BOX 2.3   Components of the Resident Assessment Instrument (RAI)

Minimum Data Set (MDS)
A core set of screening, clinical, and functional status elements, including common definitions and coding categories, which forms the foundation of a comprehensive assessment for all residents of nursing homes that are Medicare or Medicaid certified. Elements include:

- Identification information
- Hearing, speech, and vision
- Cognitive patterns
- Mood
- Behavior
- Preferences for customary routine and activities
- Functional status
- Functional abilities and goals
- Bladder and bowel
- Active diagnoses
- Health conditions
- Swallowing/nutritional status
- Oral/dental status
- Skin conditions
- Medications
- Special treatments, procedures, and programs
- Restraints and alarms
- Participation in assessment and goal setting
- Care Area Assessment (CAA) Summary

Care Area Assessment (CAA) Process
This process is designed to assist the assessor to systematically interpret the information recorded on the MDS. Once a care area has been triggered, nursing home providers use current, evidence-based clinical resources to conduct an assessment of the potential problem and determine a plan of care for it. The CAA process helps the clinician to focus on key issues.

- Care Area Triggers (CATs) are specific resident responses for one or a combination of MDS elements. The triggers identify residents who have or are at risk for developing specific functional problems and require further assessment.
- Care Area Assessment is the further investigation of triggered areas, to determine if the CATs require interventions and care planning.
- CAA Summary provides a location for documentation of the care area(s) that have triggered from the MDS and the decisions made during the CAA process regarding whether to proceed to care planning.

Utilization Guidelines
The Utilization Guidelines provide instructions for when and how to use the RAI.

Adapted from Centers for Medicare and Medicaid Services (CMS): *Long-Term Care Facility Resident Assessment Instrument 3.0 User's Manual Version 1.17.1*, 2019. https://downloads.cms.gov/files/mds-3.0-rai-manual-v1.17.1_october_2019.pdf. Accessed July 2021.

directly available, although home care nurses can visit patients in assisted-living residences. Unfortunately, most residents of assisted-living residences pay privately. The national median monthly fee is $4000 for a private unit (NCAL, 2020). With no government fee caps and little regulation, assisted living is not always an option for individuals with limited financial resources.

Respite Care. Caring for family members within the home creates great physical and emotional burdens for adult caregivers. This is especially true when the family member who needs assistance is physically or cognitively limited. The caregiver is usually an adult who not only has the responsibility for providing care to a loved one (such as a spouse, parent, or sibling) but often maintains a full-time job, raises a family, and manages the routines of daily living as well.

FIG. 2.2 Providing nursing services in assisted-living facilities promotes physical and psychosocial health. (Copyright © DGLimages/iStock/Thinkstock.)

Respite care is a service that offers short-term relief by providing a new environment or time to relax for family caregivers who support the ill, disabled, or frail older adult (Alzheimer's Association, 2021). Recommend respite services to the family caregivers of your patient whenever indicated. Respite care can be provided at home by a friend, another family member, or a volunteer; by a paid service; or in a care setting such as adult day care or a residential center (Alzheimer's Association, 2021). Research has shown that family caregivers must have great trust in the respite care service and that they perceive that the major benefits for the recipients of care are social interaction and meaningful activity, with a resulting improvement in well-being (Whitmore and Snethen, 2018).

Adult Day Care Centers. Adult day care centers provide a variety of health and social services to specific patient populations who live alone or with family in the community. Services offered during the day allow family members to maintain their lifestyles and employment and still provide home care for their relatives (Meiner and Yeager, 2019). Day care centers are associated with a hospital or nursing home or exist as independent centers. Frequently the patients need continuous health care services but not hospitalization (e.g., physical therapy, meals, recreational activities, or counseling) while their families or support people work. Patients who typically use adult day care are physically frail, cognitively impaired, or both and require some supervision but not continuous care (Meiner and Yeager, 2019).

The centers usually operate weekdays during typical business hours and usually charge on a daily basis. Adult day care centers allow patients to retain more independence by living at home, thus potentially reducing the costs of health care by avoiding or delaying an older adult's admission to a nursing center. Nurses working in day care centers provide continuity between care delivered in the home and the center. For example, nurses ensure that patients continue to take prescribed medication and administer specific treatments. Knowledge of community needs and resources is essential in providing adequate patient support (Touhy and Jett, 2018).

Palliative and Hospice Care. Palliative care is a holistic, patient- and family-centered care approach with a goal of improving the quality of life of patients and families who are experiencing problems related to life-threatening illnesses. Palliative care is delivered through the continuum of illness with a focus on early identification and treatment of physical, psychosocial, and spiritual problems; relief of pain and suffering; continuity of care; and helping patients and families make informed decisions (National Hospice and Palliative Care Organization [NHPCO], 2021; Parola et al., 2018). Palliative care can be delivered in any health care setting. Some health care agencies have dedicated palliative care units to care for these patients with complex health problems. Key to palliative care delivery is the nurse-patient and nurse-family relationship. With the patient, the nurse develops a singular relationship, and with the family or a partner, a supportive relationship is formed (Parola et al., 2018).

A hospice is a system of family-centered care that allows patients to live with comfort, independence, and dignity while easing the pain of terminal illness. A patient entering into hospice care is in the terminal phase of illness, and the patient, family, and health care provider agree that no further treatment will reverse the disease process. Hospice care is provided in a setting that best meets the needs of each patient and family, such as in a patient's home or in nursing homes, assisted-living facilities, freestanding hospices, and hospitals. The focus of hospice care is supportive care, not curative treatment (see Chapter 36). Hospice benefits families and patients in the terminal phase of any disease, such as cardiomyopathy, multiple sclerosis, acquired immunodeficiency syndrome (AIDS), and cancer. Hospice team members are available 24 hours a day, 7 days a week to answer questions or visit anytime the need for support arises. Team members collaborate to provide care that ensures death with dignity. Services continue without interruption even if a patient's care setting changes.

Palliative and hospice care are similar in that both focus on symptom management and ensuring the patient's comfort. Both care delivery methods are managed by an interprofessional team that works together with the patient's primary health care provider to develop and maintain a patient-directed, individualized plan of care (Pawlow et al., 2018). An essential member of the interprofessional team is the advanced practice registered nurse (APRN). To meet the increasing need for APRNs in palliative and hospice care, integration of core competencies into APRN education, development of clinical education opportunities in palliative and hospice care, and provision of continuing education in palliative and hospice care for practicing APRNs need to occur (Pawlow et al., 2018).

ISSUES IN HEALTH CARE DELIVERY FOR NURSES

The climate in health care today influences both health care professionals and consumers. Because those who provide patient care are the most qualified to make changes in the health care delivery system, you need to participate fully and effectively within all aspects of health care. Health care agencies today are working hard to improve patient experience and engagement while delivering high-quality care, improving outcomes, and controlling costs (Considine, 2018). In today's health care system, the outcomes of patient satisfaction and quality care indicators such as infection rates are tied to health care payments (McCay et al., 2018). As you face challenges in maintaining health care quality while reducing costs, you need to develop clinical judgment, applying the nursing process and thinking critically as you make the clinical decisions needed in each patient situation. It is also more important than ever to collaborate with other health care professionals to design and deliver new approaches for patient care delivery.

Health Care Costs and Quality

It is impossible today to separate two initiatives facing health care institutions: managing costs and achieving high-quality patient care. Health care payers (Table 2.2) (such as Medicare, Medicaid, and private insurers) have been trying to manage and address health care costs for many years. The Social Security Act established a system of payment for the operating costs of acute care hospital inpatient stays under Medicare Part A (hospital insurance) based on prospectively set rates (CMS, 2020c). This payment system is referred to as the Inpatient Prospective Payment System (IPPS). Under the IPPS, each patient case is categorized into a diagnosis-related group (DRG). Each DRG has a payment weight assigned to it, based on the average resources used to treat Medicare patients in that DRG (CMS, 2020c). Regardless of the amount a hospital spends to care for a patient, the DRG-established payment is the amount the hospital receives. The DRG payment groups are still used, but many payers now demand that evidence-based standards of care be followed to further reduce the cost of health care.

The U.S. Congress created the CMS Innovation Center to test "innovative payment and service delivery models to reduce program expenditures . . . while preserving or enhancing the quality of care" for those who receive Medicare, Medicaid, or Children's Health Insurance Program (CHIP) benefits (CMS, 2021). The Innovation Center supports the following priorities: testing new payment and service delivery models, including Quality Payment Program Advanced Alternative Payment Models, evaluating results and advancing best practices, and engaging a broad range of stakeholders to develop additional models for testing. One example of an initiative supported by the Innovation Center is the creation of Medicare ACOs. The ACOs are groups of doctors, hospitals, and other health care providers who come together voluntarily to give coordinated high-quality care to their Medicare fee-for-service (FFS) beneficiaries and reduce unnecessary costs (CMS, 2020d). As of 2015, 424 ACOs participate in the CMS Shared Savings Program (CMS, 2020d).

The Affordable Care Act ties payment to organizations offering Medicare Advantage plans to the quality ratings of the coverage they offer. If hospitals perform poorly in quality scores, they receive lower payments for services. Quality outcome measures include patient satisfaction and more effective management of care by reducing complications and readmissions and improving care coordination. Examples of reforms that incent or "Pay for Value," designed to build a health care system that better serves the American population (CMS, 2015), include the following:

- *Hospital Value-Based Purchasing:* This program links a portion of hospitals' Medicare payments (1.5% of base operating DRG payment) for inpatient acute care to their performance in important quality measures. The Hospital Consumer Assessment of Healthcare Providers and Systems (HCAHPS) is the standardized survey instrument and data collection methodology that CMS requires for measuring patients' perceptions of hospital care. HCAHPS is a patient satisfaction measure that sets a national standard for collecting or publicly reporting patients' perceptions that enables users to make valid comparisons across all hospitals (HCAHPS, 2021). Research shows that when hospitals have a higher percentage of hospitalists providing care, services are linked and there is improved coordination of care, resulting in higher performance scores (Spaulding et al., 2018).
- *Hospital Readmissions Reduction Program:* This CMS program reduces Medicare payments to hospitals with excess patient readmissions within 30 days of hospital discharge. It is designed to encourage patient safety and care quality. Heart attack, heart failure, and pneumonia are conditions regulated under this program, and readmissions dropped from 18.4% to 17.5% (National Quality Forum, 2021a). Nurses are a vital part of interprofessional teams. These team

TABLE 2.2 Common Health Care Payers in the United States

Among the current health care payment models, quality is a key component. Most health care cost reimbursement arrangements tie the final payment to the achievement of key quality metrics.

Fee-for-service	• The most traditional health care payment model. • Requires patients or payers to reimburse the health care provider for each service performed. • No incentive to implement preventive care strategies, prevent hospitalization, or take any other cost-saving measures.
Pay for coordination	• Coordinates care between the primary care provider and specialists. • Coordinating care among multiple providers can help patients and their families manage a unified care plan and can help reduce redundancy in expensive tests and procedures.
Pay for performance (P4P)	• Same as value-based reimbursement. • Health care providers are compensated only if they meet certain metrics for quality and efficiency. • Quality benchmark metrics tie physicians' reimbursement directly to quality of care they provide.
Bundled payment or episode-of-care payment	• Reimburses health care providers for specific episodes of care, such as an inpatient hospital stay. • Encourages efficiency and quality of care because only a set amount of money will pay for the entire episode of care.
Upside shared savings programs (Centers for Medicare and Medicaid Services [CMS] or commercial)	• Provide incentives for providers treating specific patient populations. • A percentage of any net savings realized is given to the provider. • Upside-only shared savings is most common with Medicare Shared Savings Program (MSSP) Accountable Care Organizations, but all MSSP participants must move to a downside model after 3 years.
Downside shared savings programs (CMS or commercial)	• Includes both the gain share potential of an upside model, but also the downside risk of sharing the excess costs of health care delivery between provider and payer. • Because providers are taking on greater risk with this model, the upside opportunity potential is larger in most cases than in an all-upside program.
Partial or full capitation	• Patients are assigned a per-member per-month (PMPM) payment based on their age, race, sex, lifestyle, medical history, and benefit design. • Payment rates are tied to expected usage regardless of whether the patient visits more or less. • As with bundled payment models, health care providers have an incentive to help patients avoid expensive procedures and tests in order to maximize their compensation. • Only certain types or categories of services are paid on a capitation basis.

Data from American Academy of Pediatrics: *Getting paid: alternative payment models*, 2020. https://www.aap.org/en-us/professional-resources/practice-transformation/getting-paid/Pages/Payment-Models.aspx. Accessed June 2020; American Hospital Association: *Current and emerging payment models*, 2020. https://www.aha.org/advocacy/current-and-emerging-payment-models. Accessed June 2020; and Brookings: *The beginner's guide to new healthcare payment models*, 2014. https://www.brookings.edu/blog/usc-brookings-schaeffer-on-health-policy/2014/07/23/the-beginners-guide-to-new-health-care-payment-models/. Accessed June 2020.
CMS, Centers for Medicare and Medicaid Services; *MSSP*, Medicare Shared Savings Program.

members collaborate to design treatment and discharge instruction protocols to reduce unnecessary patient readmissions.

• *Bundled Payments for Care Improvements:* Certain health care organizations are testing whether bundled payments (single payment for all services performed to treat a patient) for a specific episode of care (inpatient stays in an acute care hospital) can better coordinate care for Medicare patients and reduce Medicare costs. A bundled payment includes payments for services such as medical, radiological, and therapeutic. This initiative focuses on improving care for specific conditions. Bundling payments for services, such as heart bypass surgery, is one way to encourage doctors and hospitals to better coordinate care during hospitalization and after discharge (CMS, 2020b). Health care institutions enter into payment arrangements that include financial and performance accountability for an episode of care

• *Hospital-Acquired Condition (HAC) Reduction Program:* This program was developed by CMS to encourage hospitals to improve health care quality and patient safety. As a component of this program, hospitals that have a high incidence of HACs in patients—such as pressure injury development, catheter-associated urinary tract infections (CAUTIs), central line–associated bloodstream infections (CLABSIs), surgical site infections, and *Clostridium difficile* infection (CDI)—received reduced or no funding from CMS for the treatment of these HACs. This program saves CMS approximately $350 million

annually (CMS, 2020e). Because of this reduced funding, hospitals have focused quality improvement efforts on reducing and preventing these HACs.

Patient Satisfaction. Patient satisfaction is the responsibility of all health care providers. It is more important than ever because patient satisfaction measures are linked to hospital reimbursement. Patient perceptions of the quality of their health care have been incorporated into quality assessment. As a result, health care organizations have made the patient experience and patient-centered care major components of their health care missions (Cody and Williams-Reed, 2018; Niederhauser and Wolf, 2018). Hospitals now report patient satisfaction scores for patient care units monthly. All health care staff members help identify satisfaction trends and determine ways to improve quality of care. Hospitals and other health care agencies use a variety of instruments to measure patient satisfaction (NEJM Catalyst, 2018). Instruments are provided by private vendors. They usually are not published, and their reliability and validity are unclear:

• Public and standardized instruments such as patient satisfaction questionnaires (e.g., PSQ-18) and consumer assessment health plans (e.g., HCAHPS) have the advantage of good reliability and validity; however, they have a limited scope of survey questions.

• Internally developed instruments are derived mainly from questions extracted from other instruments.

The HCAHPS is used widely by hospitals to collect and publicly report patient satisfaction data for comparison purposes (HCAHPS, 2021). The HCAHPS survey has 29 items, including 19 that encompass critical aspects of the hospital experience (e.g., communication with doctors, communication with nurses, responsiveness of hospital staff, pain management, communication about medicines, discharge information, cleanliness of the hospital environment, quietness of the hospital environment, transition of care, and willingness to recommend the hospital). The remaining 10 items forward patients to appropriate disease- and procedure-specific questions, adjust for the mix of patients across hospitals, and support congressionally mandated reports (HCAHPS, 2021).

Much research has been conducted to identify the factors that patients perceive affect their satisfaction, including relational communication techniques, hourly rounding, nurse staffing patterns, and bedside shift report (Cody et al., 2018; Persolja, 2018; Dilts Skaggs et al., 2018). One common factor among the studies is interpersonal skills, especially the courtesy and respect of health care providers. This is in addition to the communication skills of providing explanations and clear information, which are more influential in affecting patient perceptions than other technical skills (George et al., 2018; Pattison et al., 2017).

Nursing Shortage

The American Association of Colleges of Nursing (AACN) has warned of a shortage of registered nurses (RNs) that is expected to intensify as baby boomers age and the need for health care grows (AACN, 2020). The problem is complicated by the fact that nursing schools across the country are struggling to expand their capacity to meet the rising demand for RNs. In addition, aging nurses are retiring from the workforce. The AACN noted important shortage indicators:

- The Bureau of Labor Statistics (BLS) Employment Projections for 2018–28 show that RNs are among the top occupations in terms of job growth through 2028 (BLS, n.d.). The RN workforce is expected to grow 12% (increase of 371,500) by 2028. The Bureau also predicted the need for 203,700 replacement nurses in the workforce, bringing the total number of RN job openings to 3.4 million by 2026 (AACN, 2020).
- The Institute of Medicine (IOM) 2010 report *The Future of Nursing: Leading Change, Advancing Health* called for an increase in the percentage of nurses who attain a bachelor's degree to 80% and a doubling in the number of nurses with doctoral degrees. The current nursing workforce falls far short of these recommendations, with only 56% of RNs prepared at the bachelor's or graduate degree level (IOM, 2010; AACN, 2020).

The shortage affects all aspects of nursing, including patient care, administration, and nursing education, but it also represents challenges and opportunities for the profession. Many health care dollars are invested in strategies aimed at recruiting and retaining a well-educated, critically thinking, motivated, and dedicated nursing workforce. There is a positive correlation between direct patient care provided by an RN and positive patient outcomes, reduced complication rates, and a more rapid return of the patient to an optimal functional status (Box 2.4) (Aiken, 2017; Twigg et al., 2019). Research also correlates poor staffing with missed nursing assessments and missed nursing care. In postoperative patients whose status changes rapidly, these missed assessments and care result in poor patient outcomes (Ball et al., 2018).

Professional nursing organizations predict that the number of nurses will continue to diminish (AACN, 2020). With fewer available nurses, it is important for you to learn to use your patient contact time efficiently and professionally. Time management, therapeutic communication, patient education, and compassionate implementation of bedside skills are just a few of the essential skills you need. It is important for your

---

BOX 2.4 EVIDENCE-BASED PRACTICE

Impact of Nurse Staffing and Patient Outcomes

PICOT Question: What is the impact on patient outcomes in hospitals with adequate nurse staffing versus hospitals with lower nurse staffing?

Evidence Summary

There is a growing body of research that shows that nurse staffing affects patient outcomes, patient survival, and the occurrence of adverse events. A systematic quantitative review of the literature found that higher nurse staffing mixes were associated with better patient outcomes. Examples of the outcomes affected by staffing mix included length of stay (LOS), incidence of pressure ulcers, pneumonia, sepsis, catheter-associated urinary tract infections (CAUTIs), 30-day mortality rate, infection, and acute myocardial infarction (Twigg et al., 2019). Patients experiencing an in-hospital cardiac arrest were more likely to survive when there was a decreased patient-to-nurse ratio (Twigg et al., 2019). Combining higher nurse staffing with an evidence-based intervention such as a sepsis bundle results in improved patient outcomes, including decreased mortality and length of stay (Lasater et al., 2021).

Higher nurse staffing was also found to significantly correlate with nursing-sensitive outcomes, such as reduced falls and improved risk assessment for pressure injuries (Burnes Bolton et al., 2017; Brooks Carthon et al., 2018). When there is poor nurse staffing, resulting in larger numbers of patients assigned to a nurse, there is an increase in the occurrence of medication errors, missed care, pressure injury formation, and falls with injuries (ANA, 2019; Griffiths et al., 2018). Studies have found that a higher professional nurse staffing mix results in decreased inpatient mortality, decreased length of stay, decreased patient readmissions, and increased patient satisfaction (Aiken et al., 2021; McHugh et al., 2021). Studies demonstrating the positive impact that increased nurse-to-patient ratios have on outcomes provide nursing administrators with evidence to support the hiring of qualified professional nurses.

Application to Nursing Practice

- Consider the nurse-to-patient ratio and staffing mix when looking at a hospital or unit for employment (Aiken et al., 2017; Lasater et al., 2021).
- Adequate nursing levels help to improve the nursing work environment, resulting in improved patient safety and quality of care (AHRQ, 2019; McHugh et al., 2021; Sloane et al., 2018).
- Patient care units in which there is an increased risk for falls due to the patient population or diseases need increased nurse staffing (Burnes Bolton et al., 2017).
- Although research supports the economic impact of nurse staffing and improved nursing-sensitive outcomes and other patient outcomes, there needs to be continued research on the impact of nurse staffing ratios (Lasater et al., 2021; Twigg et al., 2019).

---

patients to leave the health care setting with a positive image of nursing and a feeling that they received high-quality care. Your patients should never feel that they received rushed or incomplete care. They need to feel that they are important and are involved in decisions and that their needs are met. If a certain aspect of patient care requires 15 minutes of contact, it takes you the same time to deliver organized and compassionate care as it does if you rush through your nursing care.

The nursing shortage opens great opportunities for every nurse. If you pursue further education and watch trends in health care, you will be able to find employment in any professional position you choose.

Competency

Health care practitioner competencies are an excellent tool for measuring how well a nurse practices nursing and serve as a guide for the development of a professional nursing career. The Quality and Safety

BOX 2.5 Registered Nurse Competencies

QSEN Competencies
- Patient-Centered Care
- Teamwork and Collaboration
- Evidence-Based Practice (EBP)
- Quality Improvement (QI)
- Safety
- Informatics

Massachusetts Nurse of the Future Nursing Core Competencies
- Patient-Centered Care
- Professionalism
- Leadership
- Systems-Based Practice
- Informatics and Technology
- Communication
- Teamwork and Collaboration
- Safety
- Quality Improvement
- Evidenced-Based Practice (EBP)

Data from Massachusetts Department of Higher Education Nursing Initiative (MDHENI): *Massachusetts Nurse of the Future Nursing Core Competencies© REGISTERED NURSE*, 2016. https://www.mass.edu/nahi/documents/NOFRNCompetencies_updated_March2016.pdf. Accessed April 2021; and Quality Safety Education for Nursing (QSEN): *QSEN competencies*, 2020. http://qsen.org/competencies/pre-licensure-ksas/. Accessed April 2021.

Education for Nurses (QSEN) project developed quality and safety competencies for nurses so that they would have the knowledge, skills, and attitudes to meet the challenges in today's health care settings (QSEN, 2020). The Massachusetts Nurse of the Future Nursing Core Competencies were developed by the Massachusetts Department of Higher Education and the Massachusetts Organization of Nurse Executives (now part of the Organization of Nurse Leaders) to identify knowledge, attitude, and skills for 10 competencies considered essential for the RN for the future (Box 2.5) (Massachusetts Department of Higher Education Nursing Initiative [MDHENI], 2016). A consumer of health care expects that the standards of nursing care and practice in any health care setting are appropriate, safe, and effective. Health care organizations ensure high-quality care by establishing policies, procedures, and protocols that are evidence based and follow national accrediting standards. Your responsibility is to follow policies and procedures and know the most current practice standards. Ongoing competency is your responsibility. You are also responsible for obtaining necessary continuing education, following an established code of ethics, and earning certifications in specialty areas.

Patient-Centered Care

In a landmark report, *Crossing the Quality Chasm,* the IOM defined patient-centered care as "care that is respectful of and responsive to individual patient preferences, needs, and values and [ensures] that patient values guide all clinical decisions" (IOM, 2001). Hospitals across the country have implemented patient-centered care strategies, specifically delivery of care models (see Chapter 21). Patient-centered care is a component of the total patient experience, which includes all interactions that a patient has in a health care setting. The overall patient experience is influenced by the culture of the health care setting and patient perceptions (Wolf, 2017).

Patient-centered care is much more than simply "individualizing" patient care. A critical component of patient-centered care is the partnering of the nurse, patient, and family caregiver to identify the patient's health care needs within the context of the patient's lifestyle and to coordinate the entire health care team so that patient and family are engaged in the care process and associated decisions. This is a major shift in how care is delivered, empowering the patient and family to participate in the plan of care and engaging patients and families in a dialogue about the patient experience (Niederhauser and Wolf, 2018). The following are the Picker Institute's eight principles of person-centered care (Picker, 2021), based on input from patients, families, and health care experts:

1. Fast access to reliable health care advice
2. Effective treatment delivered by trusted professionals
3. Continuity of care and smooth transitions
4. Involvement and support for family and carers
5. Clear information, communication, and support for self-care
6. Involvement in decisions and respect for preferences
7. Emotional support, empathy, and respect
8. Attention to physical and environmental needs

REFLECT NOW

After completing your assigned clinical experience, complete a self-assessment evaluating your use of the principles of patient-centered care. Identify areas that you can improve on for your next clinical assignment.

QSEN Building Competency in Patient-Centered Care Nathan, a new graduate nurse, is assigned to care for a patient who had surgery yesterday for cancer. The plan is for the patient to be discharged home in 2 days. Identify strategies that Nathan can use to meet his patient's expectations.

Answers to QSEN Activities can be found on the Evolve website.

Magnet Recognition Program®

The American Nurses Credentialing Center (ANCC) established the Magnet Recognition Program® to recognize health care organizations that achieve excellence in nursing practice (ANCC, 2020). Health care organizations that apply for Magnet® status must demonstrate high-quality patient care, nursing excellence, and innovations in professional practice. The professional work environment needs to allow nurses to practice with a sense of empowerment and autonomy to deliver high-quality nursing care. The Magnet® Model has five components affected by global issues that are challenging nursing today (ANCC, 2020). The five components are (1) Transformational Leadership, (2) Structural Empowerment, (3) Exemplary Professional Practice, (4) New Knowledge, Innovation, and Improvements, and (5) Empirical Quality Results (Box 2.6). In Magnet® hospitals, the organizational culture is focused on nurse engagement, use of evidence-based practices to provide high-quality care, commitment to quality improvement, clear strategic direction, shared governance, and trust in leadership (Fischer and Nichols, 2019; Lavenberg et al., 2019). Peer review is often used as a mechanism to improve accountability and foster professional growth (Roberts and Cronin, 2017). Magnet® status requires nurses to collect data on specific nursing-sensitive quality indicators or outcomes and compare their outcomes against a national, state, or regional database to demonstrate quality of care. Research shows that patient outcomes for nursing-sensitive indicators such as patient falls, CAUTIs, and CLABSIs are

BOX 2.6 Model and Forces of Magnetism

Magnet® Model Components	Forces of Magnetism
Transformational leadership—A vision for the future and the systems and resources to achieve the vision are created by nursing leaders.	• Quality of nursing leadership • Management style
Structural empowerment—Structures and processes provide an innovative environment in which staff are developed and empowered and professional practice flourishes.	• Organizational structure • Personnel policies and programs • Community and the health organization • Image of nursing • Professional development
Exemplary professional practice—Strong professional practice is established, and accomplishments of the practice are demonstrated.	• Professional models of care • Consultation and resources • Autonomy • Nurses as teachers • Interprofessional relationships
New knowledge, innovations, and improvements—Contributions are made to the profession in the form of new models of care, use of existing knowledge, generation of new knowledge, and contributions to the science of nursing.	• Quality improvement
Empirical quality results—Focus is on structure and processes and demonstration of positive clinical, workforce, and patient and organizational outcomes.	• Quality of care

Adapted from American Nurses Credentialing Center (ANCC): *Magnet Model—creating a magnet culture,* 2020. https://www.nursingworld.org/organizational-programs/magnet/magnet-model/. Accessed June 1, 2020.

significantly better in Magnet® organizations than in non-Magnet® organizations (Fischer and Nichols, 2019). One contributing factor to this may be the higher levels of transformational leadership found in nurse managers in Magnet® organizations (Fischer and Nichols, 2019).

Nursing-Sensitive Outcomes. Nursing-sensitive outcomes are patient outcomes and nursing workforce characteristics that are directly related to nursing care, such as changes in patients' symptom experiences, functional status, safety, psychological distress, RN job satisfaction, total nursing hours per patient day, and costs. As a nurse you assume accountability and responsibility for achieving and accepting the consequences of these outcomes. Measuring and monitoring nursing-sensitive outcomes reveal the interventions that improve patients' outcomes. Nurses and health care agencies use nursing-sensitive outcomes to improve nurses' workloads, enhance patient safety, and develop sound policies related to nursing practice and health care. The ANA developed the National Database of Nursing Quality Indicators (NDNQI) to measure and evaluate nursing-sensitive outcomes with the purpose of improving patient safety and quality care (NDNQI, n.d.). The NDNQI reports quarterly results on nursing outcomes at the nursing unit level. This provides a database for individual hospitals to compare their performance against national nursing performance. The evaluation of patient outcomes and nursing workforce characteristics remains important to nursing and the health care delivery system. Chapter 5 describes approaches for measuring outcomes.

Technology in Health Care

Technological advances continually affect health care organizations and change the ways in which nurses deliver evidence-based care to patients. Emerging technologies that will change how nurses practice include genetics and genomics, less invasive and more accurate tools for diagnosis and treatment, three-dimensional printing, robotics, biometrics, EHRs (see Chapter 26), and computerized physician/provider order entry and clinical decision support. Technology makes your work easier in many ways, but the technology does not replace your clinical judgment and clinical decision making. For example, when you manage an IV infusion smart pump, you must monitor the infusion to ensure that the device infuses on schedule and without complications despite its numerous automatic settings. An infusion device infuses at a constant rate, but you must confirm that the rate is calculated correctly. An infusion device sets off an alarm if the infusion slows but does not indicate why the infusion slowed. You must assess why the alarm sounded and use clinical judgment to determine the problem and how to resolve it. Technology never replaces a nurse's astute, critical eye and clinical judgment.

Robotics is an emerging technology that will greatly affect how nursing is practiced in the future. It is estimated that robotic use will grow because of workforce shortages, a growing elderly population, and a call for higher-quality care not subject to human limitations (Backonja et al., 2018; Hauser and Shaw, 2020). Most robotic applications are limited to food service, medication distribution, infection control, surgery, and even diagnosing patients. However, one area with huge potential for affecting nursing is the use of robots as direct care providers. Daily care robots provide support to older adults and people with disabilities in such activities as preparing and serving meals and in daily care tasks such as retrieving items (Kyarini et al., 2021; Sefcik et al., 2018). In addition, exoskeleton-powered robots are used to help patients who are paralyzed stand, with the goal of reducing morbidity and augmenting physical therapy for patients with impaired extremities (Kyarini et al., 2021). The implications for nursing are significant. Telenursing robots are a component of a telenursing system in which a robot is physically present with the patient and has an interlink to nurses or other health care providers who are at a different location (Hauser and Shaw, 2020). The telenursing robot provides two-way communication, is mobile to move between patients or rooms, is able to collect diagnostic and assessment data, provides accuracy and precision in data collection, and is able to use human- or robot-developed health care tools and instruments (Hauser and Shaw, 2020; Kyarini et al., 2021). The use of robots in health care and to perform nursing tasks presents challenges (Kyarini et al., 2021). The cost of robots is high for health care systems, and there is still concern about the maturity and readiness of the technology (Kyarini et al., 2021). Concerns for patient privacy have been voiced because of the cameras on the robots. There is also a question about how willing patients will be to accept care from robots (Kyarini et al., 2021). Nursing must be on the front line in deciding how robotics is used in order to advocate for patients and families and to ensure that professional standards of care are delivered.

Telemedicine is a technology that relies on interactive video; it uses medical information gathered and reviewed at one site (such as a hospital, home, clinic, or urgent care center) and transmits treatment recommendations to another site to improve a patient's clinical health status (American Telemedicine Association, 2020). There are a variety of applications and services using two-way video, smartphones, wireless tools, and other forms of telecommunications technology. The benefits of telemedicine include providing services that meet patient demand, increasing access to care, and decreasing cost (American Telemedicine Association, 2020). However, varying federal and state policies on telemedicine use and reimbursement pose an obstacle to wider adoption of this emerging practice (Young and Kroth, 2018).

Nurses need to play a role in evaluating and implementing new technological advances. You use technology to improve the effectiveness of nursing care, enhance safety, and improve patient outcomes. Most important, it is essential for you to remember that the focus of nursing care is not the machine or the technology; it is the patient. Therefore you need to constantly attend to and connect with your patients and ensure that their dignity and rights are preserved at all levels of care.

Health Care Disparities

Health care disparities are the differences in health care outcomes and dimensions of health care, including access, quality, and equity, among population groups (Almgren, 2018; Kneipp et al., 2018). Disparities can be related to many variables, such as race, ethnicity, gender, location, disability, or social determinants (Artiga et al., 2020). Social determinants greatly affect health disparities. They are the conditions in the environments in which people are born, live, learn, work, play, worship, and age that affect health, functioning, and quality-of-life outcomes and risks (ODPHP, n.d.). The *Healthy People 2030* initiative identifies five categories of social determinants: Economic Stability, Education Access and Quality, Health Care Access and Quality, Neighborhood and Built Environment, and Social and Community Context (Office of Disease Prevention and Health Promotion [ODPHP], n.d.). Disparities in health status, particularly in a community in which the majority have poor health, will affect the productivity and vulnerability of a population. The National Quality Forum (2021b) reported that health care disparities are linked to the following social determinants: inadequate resources, poor patient-provider communication, a lack of culturally competent care (see Chapter 9), and inadequate access to patient language services, among other factors (Box 2.7) (Fig. 2.3). The health care system and the many professionals who serve patients must address these factors and reduce their effect on patients' health so that all patients receive needed care. One strategy is to establish and support policies that positively influence social and economic conditions and support changes in individual behavior (such as pursuing healthful diets and adhering to medication regimens).

Healthy People 2030 (ODPHP, n.d.) aims to promote the nation's health and create a society in which all people throughout the life span can achieve their fullest potential for health and well-being. An important goal is to eliminate health disparities, achieve health care equity, and attain health literacy to improve the nation's health and well-being. Nurses practice in a wide variety of settings that require an awareness of the social determinants of health that contribute to health disparities (see Chapter 9). Social determinants of health impact a person's health, overall functioning, and quality of life (Kneipp et al., 2018). Nurses play a key role in promoting access to health care and in

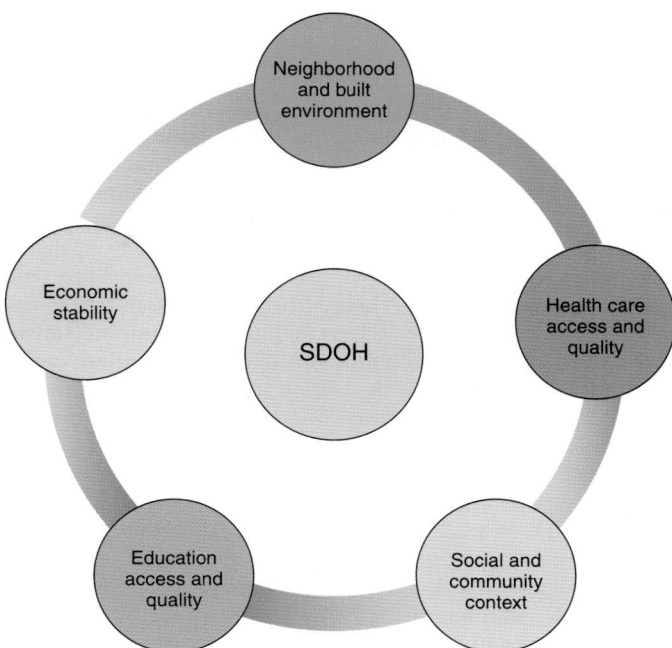

FIG. 2.3 Social determinants of health (SDOH). (From Office of Disease Prevention and Health Promotion [ODPHP]: Social determinants of health. *Healthy People 2030.* n.d., U.S. Department of Health and Human Services. https://www.healthypeople.gov/2020/topics-objectives/topic/social-determinants-of-health.)

providing appropriate education to patients and families to promote healthy development, healthy behaviors, and well-being to all individuals across the life span.

REFLECT NOW

Discuss with your clinical group the social determinants of health impacting the community where you are assigned to complete your clinical experiences. How have they created health disparities in the community?

THE FUTURE OF HEALTH CARE

A discussion of the health care delivery system today is incomplete without discussing the issue of change. The current system is in a constant state of change and reform, making it challenging to predict the future but also opening opportunities for improvement (Young and Kroth, 2018). The ultimate issue in redesigning and delivering health care is to ensure the health and welfare of the populations that health care institutions serve. It is predicted that the health care model of the future will have the consumer in the center (Batra et al., 2019). Young and Kroth (2018) reported that the U.S. health care system is a paradox—extreme successes and technological advances offset by limited access, high costs, and quality issues. One example of how the health care landscape is changing is the increasing emergence and reliance on technology and digital health (Batra et al., 2019; Larsen, 2020). Over the last few years, there has been increasing use of telehealth and digital care, with both expected to continue to grow over the next 5 years (Heller, 2019). Telehealth, sometimes called telemedicine—is the

BOX 2.7   Examples of Social Determinants of Health

- Safe housing, transportation, and neighborhoods
- Racism, discrimination, and violence
- Education, job opportunities, and income
- Access to nutritious foods and physical activity opportunities
- Polluted air and water
- Language and literacy skills

Adapted from Office of Disease Prevention and Health Promotion. Social determinants of health. *Healthy People 2030*, n.d., U.S. Department of Health and Human Services. https://health.gov/healthypeople/objectives-and-data/social-determinants-health. Accessed July 2021.

use of electronic information and telecommunication technologies (e.g., using cloud-based video conferencing tools) to provide care when a patient and health care provider are not in the same place at the same time (Telehealth.hhs.gov, 2021). All that is needed is access to the internet. Digital technology (e.g., computers and applications using the internet, video cameras, and mobile devices such as smartphones and electronic tablets) is providing patients the first access they will have into health care and with a health care provider, making a "digital front door" (Larsen, 2020). Using digital technology will decrease office visits as they occur today and streamline care for patients (Larsen, 2020). The use of technology will allow health care providers to continually monitor individuals with chronic or major health problems so that interventions can be implemented at the first indication of problems. Artificial intelligence (AI) will be used more to assist in the treatment of diseases through early detection and better understanding of disease progression (Batra et al., 2019). Technology will also help decrease cost of health care and remove the barrier of geography and access to services (Batra et al., 2019). Health care organizations are implementing new and improved technologies that are changing how they provide their services, reducing unnecessary costs, improving access to care, and improving the quality of patient care. Professional nursing is an important player in the future of health care delivery. The solutions necessary to improve the quality of health care depend largely on the active participation of nurses.

KEY POINTS

- An integrated health care system consists of a network of health care organizations that work together to provide a continuum of coordinated health care services to a defined group of people to improve quality of care and control health care costs.
- Each of the six levels of health care describe the types of services and different settings in which health care is delivered to patients in all stages of health and illness.
- Each level of care presents different requirements and opportunities for a nurse. In a primary care setting, nurses are extensively involved in patient assessment, whereas in restorative care settings, nurses know that success depends on their effective and early partnering with patients and their families in planning and care delivery.
- Levels of prevention are not the same as levels of care. Levels of prevention describe the focus of health-related activities in a care setting, such as health promotion and disease prevention (primary prevention) and curing or managing disease (secondary prevention)
- Health care professionals provide patient care in different settings. For example, primary care focuses on health promotion and tends to be provided in community settings, whereas hospitals provide comprehensive secondary and tertiary care to patients who are acutely ill.
- Health care access is influenced by access to hospitals, clinics, and physician offices; availability of transportation; ease in scheduling appointments; availability of appointments when needed; accessibility of specialty services when a referral is made; and clear instructions provided on when and how to get referrals.
- Rural Americans' access to health care is affected by economic factors (rural Americans are more likely to live below the poverty level), cultural and social differences, educational shortcomings, lack of recognition of the problem by legislators, and the isolation of living in remote rural areas.
- Discharge planning begins at admission to a health care agency, helps determine the best place for a patient to go after discharge

from the hospital, and creates a smooth transition of a patient's care from the acute care or post–acute care agency to the patient's next environment
- Barriers to effective discharge planning include ineffective communication, lack of role clarity among health care team members, and lack of resources.
- "Pay for Value" ties reimbursement to quality; if hospitals perform poorly in quality scores, they receive lower payments for services from CMS.
- Nurses promote patient satisfaction through providing patient- and family-centered care and applying good interpersonal skills, including courtesy, respect, and good communication skills.
- The nursing shortage is an issue in health care that affects all aspects of nursing (e.g., patient care, nursing administration, nursing education) and opens vast opportunities to nurses. Furthering education and following trends in health care open professional options for nurses.
- Patient-centered care is care that is focused on the patient's preferences, needs, and values and involves the patient in the clinical decision-making process. This type of care is based on the patient's lifestyle and is coordinated with the health care team so that the patient is engaged in the care process.
- Social determinants of health contribute to health disparities, creating differences in the health status of different groups of people in a community. Disparities in health status, particularly in a community in which the majority have poor health, will affect the productivity and vulnerability of a population.

REFLECTIVE LEARNING

- Investigate whether the clinical unit on which you are assigned displays its patient satisfaction data on the unit. If so, review the data and identify areas that, as students, you can work on to help improve patient satisfaction. Discuss with your clinical group.
- Select one of the RN competencies identified in Box 2.5. Develop a plan for improving your knowledge, skills, and attitudes for the competency during your upcoming clinical experience.
- Discuss with your clinical group changes in health care that have occurred in the last 5 years. How have these changes affected how you practice nursing today?

REVIEW QUESTIONS

1. Which activity performed by a nurse is related to maintaining competency in nursing practice?
   1. Asking another nurse about how to change the settings on a medication pump
   2. Regularly attending unit staff meetings
   3. Participating as a member of the professional nursing council
   4. Attending a review course in preparation for a certification examination
2. Which of the following are examples of a nurse participating in primary care activities? (Select all that apply.)
   1. Providing prenatal teaching on nutrition to a pregnant woman during the first trimester
   2. Assessing the nutritional status of older adults who come to the community center for lunch
   3. Working with patients in a cardiac rehabilitation program
   4. Providing home wound care to a patient
   5. Teaching a class to parents at the local elementary school about the importance of immunizations

3. Which of the following statements is true regarding Magnet® status recognition for a hospital?
   1. Nursing is run by a Magnet® manager who makes decisions for the nursing units.
   2. Nurses in Magnet® hospitals make all of the decisions on the clinical units.
   3. Magnet® is a term that is used to describe hospitals that are able to hire the nurses they need.
   4. Magnet® is a special designation for hospitals that achieve excellence in nursing practice.
4. The nurse is working in a tertiary care setting. Which activity does the nurse perform while providing tertiary care?
   1. Conducting blood pressure screenings at a local food bank
   2. Administering influenza vaccines for older adults at the local senior center
   3. Inserting an indwelling catheter for a patient on a medical-surgical unit
   4. Performing endotracheal suctioning for a patient on a ventilator in the medical ICU
5. A nurse is providing restorative care to a patient following an extended hospitalization for an acute illness. Which of the following is the most appropriate outcome for this patient's restorative care?
   1. Patient will be able to walk 200 feet without shortness of breath.
   2. Wound will heal without signs of infection.
   3. Patient will express concerns related to return to home.
   4. Patient will identify strategies to improve sleep habits.
6. Which of the following describe characteristics of an integrated health care system? (Select all that apply.)
   1. The focus is holistic.
   2. Participating hospitals follow the same model of health care delivery.
   3. The system coordinates a continuum of services.
   4. The focus of health care providers is finding a cure for patients.
   5. Members of the health care team link electronically to use the EHR to share the patient's health care record.
7. The school nurse has been following a 9-year-old student who has shown behavioral problems in class. The student acts out and does not follow teacher instructions. The nurse plans to meet with the student's family to learn more about social determinants of health that might be affecting the student. Which of the following potential social determinants should the nurse assess? (Select all that apply.)
   1. The student's seating placement in the classroom

2. The level of support parents offer when the student completes homework
   3. The level of violence in the family's neighborhood
   4. The age at which the child first began having behavioral problems
   5. The cultural values about education held by the family
8. A nurse is assigned to care for an 82-year-old patient who will be transferred from the hospital to a rehabilitation center. The patient and her husband have selected the rehabilitation center closest to their home. The nurse learns that the patient will be discharged in 3 days and decides to make the referral on the day of discharge. The nurse reviews the recommendations for physical therapy and applies the information to fall prevention strategies in the hospital. What discharge planning action by the nurse has not been addressed correctly?
   1. Patient and family involvement in referral
   2. Timing of referral
   3. Incorporation of referral discipline recommendations into plan of care
   4. Determination of discharge date
9. Which of the following are common barriers to effective discharge planning? (Select all that apply.)
   1. Ineffective communication among providers
   2. Lack of role clarity among health care team members
   3. Number of hospital beds to manage patient volume
   4. Patients' long-term disabilities
   5. The patient's cultural background
10. A nurse newly hired at a community hospital learns about intentional hourly rounding during orientation. Which of the following are known evidence-based outcomes from intentional rounding? (Select all that apply.)
   1. Reduction in nurse staffing requirements
   2. Improved patient satisfaction
   3. Reduction in patient falls
   4. Increased costs
   5. Reduction in patient use of nurse call system

Answers: 1.4; 2.1, 5; 3.4, 4; 4.4; 5.1; 6.1, 3, 5; 7.2, 3, 5; 8.2; 9.1, 2; 10.2, 3, 5

Rationales for Review Questions can be found on the Evolve website.

REFERENCES

Agency for Healthcare Research and Quality (AHRQ): *Nursing and patient safety,* 2019, https://www.psnet.ahrq.gov/primer/nursing-and-patient-safety. Accessed September 5, 2020.

Agency for Healthcare Research and Quality (AHRQ): *Teach-Back: Intervention. Quick Start Guide Full Page. March 2020.* Agency for Healthcare Research and Quality, Rockville, MD. https://www.ahrq.gov/health-literacy/quality-resources/tools/literacy-toolkit/healthlittoolkit2-tool5.html Accessed June 2020.

Almgren G: *Health career politics, policy, and services: a social justice analysis,* New York, 2018, Springer Publishing.

Al-Saddique A: Integrated delivery systems (IDSs) as a means of reducing costs and improving healthcare delivery, *J Healthcare Comm* 3(1):19, 2018.

Alzheimer's Association: *Alzheimer's and dementia caregiver center: respite care,* https://www.alz.org/care/

alzheimers-dementia-caregiver-respite.asp, 2021. Accessed April 2021.

American Academy of Family Physicians.: *The medical home,*. https://www.aafp.org/practice-management/transformation/pcmh.html, 2020. Accessed July 2020.

American Association of Colleges of Nursing (AACN): *Nursing shortage fact sheet*, https://www.aacnnursing.org/Portals/42/News/Factsheets/Nursing-Shortage-Factsheet.pdf 2020. Accessed April 2021.

American Hospital Association.: *Fast facts on US hospitals,* 2020, https://www.aha.org/statistics/fast-facts-us-hospitals, 2020a, accessed July 2020.

American Hospital Association.: *Quality and patient safety,* 2020b. https://www.aha.org/advocacy/quality-and-patient-safety. Accessed July 2020.

American Nurses Association (ANA): *Scope and standards of practice,* ed 4, Silver Spring, MD, 2021, American Nurses Association.

American Nurses Association: *Safe staffing literature review,* 2019, https://www.nursingworld.org/~49ebbb/globalassets/practiceandpolicy/work-environment/nurse-staffing/safe-staffing-literature-review.pdf. Accessed September 5, 2020.

American Nurses Credentialing Center (ANCC).: *Magnet model– creating a magnet culture,* https://www.nursingworld.org/organizational-programs/magnet/magnet-model/, 2020. Accessed June 1, 2020.

American Telemedicine Association: *Telehealth basics*: Telehealth: Defining 21st Century Care. https://www.americantelemed.org/resource/why-telemedicine/, 2021. Accessed April 2021.

Artiga S et al: *Disparities in health and health care: five key questions and answers,* Henry J. Kaiser Family Foundation, 2020. https://www.kff.org/disparities-policy/issue-brief/disparities-in-health-and-health-care-five-key-questions-and-answers/. Accessed July 2020.

Assistant Secretary for Planning and Evaluation (ASPE): *Trends in the U.S. uninsured population, 2010-2020, Issue Brief,* February 2021, https://aspe.hhs.gov/system/files/pdf/265041/trends-in-the-us-uninsured.pdf. Accessed April 10, 2021.

Batra N et al.: *Forces of change: the future of health,* 2019, https://www2.deloitte.com/us/en/insights/industry/health-care/forces-of-change-health-care.html. Accessed August 6, 2020.

Blue Cross Blue Shield of Michigan (BCBS): *High intensity care model,* n.d., https://micmt-cares.org/sites/default/files/2020-02/HICM%20Self-Study%20Module_v8.pdf, Accessed August 6, 2020.

Buerhaus PI et al.: Four challenges facing the nursing workforce in the United States, *J Nurse Regulation* 8(2):40, 2017.

Bureau of Labor Statistics: *Occupational outlook handbook: Registered nurses,* n.d., https://www.bls.gov/ooh/healthcare/registered-nurses.htm. Accessed May 2020.

Center for Community Engagement in Health Innovation: *Care That Works: Geriatric Resources for Assessment and Care of Elders (GRACE):* 2018, https://www.healthinnovation.org/resources/publications/document/Care-That-Works-GRACE_4_5_18.pdf?1522963914. Accessed August 6, 2020.

Centers for Disease Control and Prevention (CDC): *Workplace health promotion: health outcomes measures,* http://www.cdc.gov/workplacehealthpromotion/model/evaluation/outcomes.html, 2015. Accessed July 2020.

Centers for Disease Control and Prevention (CDC): *Whole school, whole community, whole child (WSCC).* http://www.cdc.gov/healthyschools/wscc/index.htm, 2021. Accessed April 2021.

Centers for Medicare and Medicaid Services (CMS): *Better care, smarter spending, healthier people: improving our health care delivery system,* 2015, https://www.cms.gov/newsroom/fact-sheets/better-care-smarter-spending-healthier-people-improving-our-health-care-delivery-system-0. Accessed September 5, 2020.

Centers for Medicare and Medicaid Services (CMS): *Long-term care facility Resident Assessment Instrument 3.0 user's manual version 1.17.1,* 2019. https://downloads.cms.gov/files/mds-3.0-rai-manual-v1.17.1_october_2019.pdf. Accessed July 2021.

Centers for Medicare and Medicaid Services (CMS): *National Health Expenditures 2018 Highlights,* 2019a, https://www.cms.gov/files/document/highlights.pdf. Accessed August 5, 2020.

Centers for Medicare and Medicaid Services (CMS): *Your discharge planning checklist,* https://www.medicare.gov/pubs/pdf/11376-discharge-planning-checklist.pdf, 2019b. Accessed June 2020 .

Centers for Medicare and Medicaid Services (CMS): *Home Health Quality Initiative,.* https://www.cms.gov/Medicare/Quality-Initiatives-Patient-Assessment-Instruments/HomeHealthQualityInits/index.html?redirect=/HomeHealthQualityInits/, 2020a. Accessed June 2020.

Centers for Medicare and Medicaid Services (CMS): *Bundled payments for care improvements: general information,* https://innovation.cms.gov/initiatives/bundled-payments/, 2020b. Accessed June 2020.

Centers for Medicare and Medicaid Services (CMS): *Acute inpatient PPS,* https://www.cms.gov/Medicare/Medicare-Fee-for-Service-Payment/AcuteInpatientPPS, 2020c. Accessed August 6, 2020.

Centers for Medicare and Medicaid Services (CMS): *Shared savings programs.* https://www.cms.gov/Medicare/Medicare-Fee-For-Service-Payment/sharedsavingsprogram/index.html, 2020d. Accessed August 6, 2020.

Centers for Medicare and Medicaid Services (CMS): *Hospital-acquired condition (HAC) reduction program,* https://www.cms.gov/Medicare/Quality-Initiatives-Patient-Assessment-Instruments/Value-Based-Programs/HAC/Hospital-Acquired-Conditions.html, 2020e. Accessed June 2020.

Centers for Medicare and Medicaid Services (CMS): *About the CMS Innovation Center,.* https://innovation.cms.gov/about/index.html, 2021. Accessed April 2021.

Centers for Medicare and Medicaid Services Medicare Learning Network (CMS MLN): *Critical access hospital,* https://www.cms.gov/Outreach-and-Education/Medicare-Learning-Network-MLN/MLNProducts/downloads/CritAccessHospfctsht.pdf, 2019. Accessed July 2020.

Considine J: *Better patient experience hinges on improving financial journey,* https://www.hcinnovationgroup.com/home/article/13010171/better-patient-experience-hinges-on-improving-financial-journey, 2018. Accessed August 6, 2020.

Counsell S: *10 key components of a post-discharge care model,.* http://www.beckershospitalreview.com/quality/10-key-components-of-a-post-discharge-care-model.html, 2015. Accessed April 2021.

George S et al.: Commit to sit to improve nurse communication. *Crit Care Nurse* 38(2):83, 2018.

Hauser K, Shaw R: *How medical robots will help treat patients in future outbreaks,* 2020, https://spectrum.ieee.org/automaton/robotics/medical-robots/medical-robots-future-outbreak-response. Accessed July 2021.

HealthIT.gov.: *Benefits for critical access hospitals and other small rural hospitals,* https://www.healthit.gov/topic/health-it-initiatives/benefits-critical-access-hospitals-and-other-small-rural-hospitals, 2017. Accessed June 2020.

Heller B: *The future of healthcare: 3 predictions for the next five years,* 2019, https://hitconsultant.net/2019/12/02/the-future-of-healthcare-3-predictions-for-the-next-five-years/. Accessed August 6, 2020.

Himmelstein DU et al.: The ongoing U.S. health care crisis: a data update, *Int J Health Serv* 48(2):209, 2018.

Hospital Consumer Assessment of Healthcare Providers and Systems (HCAHPS).: *HCAHPS Hospital Survey,* http://www.hcahpsonline.org, 2021. Accessed April 2021.

Institute of Medicine (IOM).: *Crossing the quality chasm: a new health system for the 21st century,* Washington DC, 2001, National Academies Press.

Institute of Medicine (IOM).: *The future of nursing: leading change, advancing health,* Washington DC, 2010, National Academies Press.

Larsen M: *The future of healthcare starts with a 'digital front door',* 2020, https://healthtechmagazine.net/article/2020/06/future-healthcare-starts-with-digital-front-door.* Accessed August 6, 2020.

Legal Information Institute.: *42 U.S. Code § 1395i–3. Requirements for, and assuring quality of care in, skilled nursing facilities,.* https://www.law.cornell.edu/uscode/text/42/1395i-3, n.d. Accessed June 2020.

Massachusetts Department of Higher Education Nursing Initiative (MDHENI): *Massachusetts nurse of the future nursing core competencies© registered nurse,* https://www.mass.edu/nahi/documents/NOFRNCompetencies_updated_March2016.pdf, 2016. Accessed June 2020.

Medicaid.gov.: *Nursing facilities,.* https://www.medicaid.gov/medicaid/ltss/institutional/nursing/index.html, n.d. Accessed June 2020.

Meek KL et al.: Outsourcing an effective postdischarge call program: a collaborative approach. *Nurs Admin Q* 42(2):175, 2018.

Meiner SE, Yeager JJ: *Gerontologic nursing,* ed 6, St Louis, 2019, Mosby.

National Alliance on Mental Illness (NAMI).: *Mental health by the numbers,* https://www.nami.org/mhstats. 2021. Accessed June 2021.

National Alliance on Mental Illness (NAMI).: *NAMI describes state mental health cuts in congressional briefing; comprehensive report expected soon,* https://www.nami.org/Press-Media/Press-Releases/2011/NAMI-Describes-State-Mental-Health-Cuts-in-Congres, 2011. Accessed June 2020.

National Center for Assisted Living (NCAL): *Facts and figures,* https://www.ahcancal.org/ncal/facts/Pages/default.aspx 2020. Accessed August 6, 2020.

National Database of Nursing Quality Indicators (NDNQI): *How is NDNQI used?* n.d., https://nursingandndnqi.weebly.com/how-is-ndnqi-used.html. Accessed August 6, 2020.

National Hospice and Palliative Care Organization (NHPCO): *An Explanation of Palliative Care,* 2021. shttps://www.nhpco.org/palliative-care-overview/explanation-of-palliative-care/. Accessed April 12, 2021.

National Quality Forum.: *Home vs. Hospital: national efforts to reduce readmissions are helping more patients heal at home,* 2021a. http://www.qualityforum.org/Readmissions_-_Home_vs_Hospitals.aspx. Accessed April 2021.

National Quality Forum; *Disparities,* 2021b. http://www.qualityforum.org/Topics/Disparities.aspx. Accessed April 2021.

National Rural Health Association (NRHA).: *About Rural Health Care,.* https://www.ruralhealthweb.org/about-nrha/about-rural-health-care, 2020. Accessed June 2020.

NEJM Catalyst: *Patient satisfaction surveys,* 2018, https://catalyst.nejm.org/doi/full/10.1056/CAT.18.0288. Accessed August 6, 2020.

Niederhauser V, Wolf J: Patient experience: a call to action for nurse leadership. *Nurs Adm Q* 42(3):211, 2018.

Office of Disease Prevention and Health Promotion (ODPHP): Social determinants of health, *Healthy People 2030.* n.d., U.S. Department of Health and Human Services. https://health.gov/healthypeople/objectives-and-data/social-determinants-health. Accessed April 2021.

Picker: *Principles of person centred care,* 2021, https://www.picker.org/about-us/picker-principles-of-person-centred-care/. Accessed July 2021.

Quality and Safety Education for Nurses (QSEN).: *QSEN competencies,.* http://qsen.org/competencies/pre-licensure-ksas/, 2020. Accessed June 2020.

Research Data Assistance Center.: *The home health outcome and assessment information set (OASIS),.* https://www.resdac.org/cms-data/files/oasis, 2020 . Accessed June 2020.

The Joint Commission (TJC): *2020 Comprehensive accreditation manual for hospitals,* Oakbrook Terrace, IL, 2020, The Commission.

Touhy TA, Jett K: *Ebersole & Hess' Gerontological nursing & healthy aging,* ed 5, St Louis, 2018, Elsevier.

Varcolis EM, Fosbre CD: *Essentials of psychiatric-mental health nursing: a communication approach to evidence-based care,* 4e, St. Louis, 2021, Elsevier.

Wolf JA: Critical considerations for the future of patient experience., *J Healthc Manag* 62(1):9, 2017.

World Health Organization (WHO): *Health topics: rehabilitation,.* https://www.who.int/health-topics/rehabilitation#tab=tab_1 2020. Accessed July 2020.

World Health Organization (WHO): *Primary health care,* 2021, https://www.who.int/health-topics/primary-health-care#tab=tab_1 2021. Accessed April 2021.

Young KM, Kroth PJ: *Sultz & Young's Health care USA: understanding its organization and delivery,* ed 9, Sudbury, 2018, Jones & Bartlett.

RESEARCH REFERENCES

Abu HO et al.: Are we "missing the big picture" in transitions of care? Perspectives of healthcare providers managing patients with unplanned hospitalization. *Appl Nurs Res* 44: 60, 2018.

Aicher BO et al.: Reduced length of stay and 30-day readmission rate on an inpatient vascular surgery service *J Vasc Nurs* 37(2):78, 2019.

Aiken LH et al.: Nursing skill mix in European hospitals: cross-sectional study of the association with mortality, patient ratings, and quality of care. *BMJ Qual Saf* 26:559, 2017.

Aiken LH et al.: Hospital nurse staffing and patient outcomes in Chile: a multilevel cross-sectional study, *Lancet Glob Health* published online July 2, 2021. http://dx.doi.org/10.1016/S2214-109X(21)00209-6.

Backonja U et al.: Comfort and attitudes towards robots among young, middle aged, and older adults: a cross-sectional study. *J Nurs Scholarsh* 50(6): 623, 2018.

Ball JE et al.: Post-operative mortality, missed care and nurse staffing in nine countries: a cross-sectional study. *Int J Nurs Stud* 78:10, 2018.

Brooks Carthon JM, et al: Association of nurse engagement and nurse staffing on patient safety. *Journal of Nurs Care Quality* 34(1):40, 2018.

Burnes Bolton L et al.: Mandated nurse staffing ratios in California: a comparison of staffing and nursing-sensitive outcomes pre- and post regulation, policy. *Polit Nurs Pract* 8(4):238, 2017.

Cody SE, et al.: Making a connection: family experiences with bedside rounds in the intensive care unit. *Crit Care Nurse* 38(3):18, 2018.

Cody R, Williams-Reed J: Intentional nurse manager rounding and patient satisfaction. *Nurs Manage* 49(4):16, 2018.

Coleman EA, et al.: The care transitions intervention: results of a randomized controlled trial. *Arch Intern Med* 166(17):1822–1828, 2006.

Dilts Skaggs MK, et al.: Using the evidence-based practice service nursing bundle to increase patient satisfaction. *J Emerg Nurs* 44(1):37, 2018.

Dizon ML, Reinking C: Reducing readmissions: nurse-driven interventions in the transition of care from the hospital. *Worldviews Evid Based Nurs* 14(6):432, 2017.

Fischer JP, Nichols C: Leadership practices and patient outcomes in Magnet® vs non-Magnet hospitals. *JONA* 49(10):S50, 2019.

Griffiths P, et al: The association between nurse staffing and omissions in nursing care: A systematic review. *Journal of Adv Nurs.* 74(7):1474, 2018.

Kneipp SM, et al.: Trends in health disparities, health inequity, and social determinants of health research: a 17-year analysis of NINR, NCI, NHLBI and NIMHD funding. *Nurs Res* 67(3):231, 2018.

Kyarini M et al.: A survey of robots in healthcare, *Technologies* 9(8):1, 2021.

Lasater KT et al.: Evaluation of hospital nurse-to-patient staffing ratios and sepsis bundles on patient outcomes, *Am J Inf Control* 49:868, 2021.

Lavenberg JG et al.: Impact of a hospital evidence-based practice center (EPC) on nursing policy and practice. *Worldviews Evid Based Nurs* 16(1): 4, 2019.

McCay R, et al.: Nurse leadership style, nurse satisfaction, and patient satisfaction: a systematic review. *J Nurs Care Qual* 33(4):361, 2018.

McHugh MD et al.: Effects of nurse-to-patient ratio legislation on nurse staffing and patient mortality, readmissions, and length of stay: a prospective study in a panel of hospitals. *Lancet* 397:1905, 2021.

McWilliams JM et al: Early performance of accountable care organizations in Medicare. *New Engl J Med* 374(24):2357, 2016.

Naylor MD, et al.: Translating research into practice: transitional care for older adults. *J Eval Clin Pract* 15(6):1164, 2009.

Parola V, et al.: Caring in palliative care: a phenomenological study of nurses' lived experiences. *J Hosp Palliat Nurs* 20(2):180, 2018.

Pattison KH, et al.: Patient perceptions of sitting versus standing for nurse leader rounding. *J Nurs Care Qual* 32(1):1, 2017.

Pawlow P, et al.: The hospice and palliative care advanced practice registered nurse workforce: results of a national study. *J Hosp Palliat Nurs* 20(4):349, 2018.

Persolja M: The effect of nurse staffing patterns on patient satisfaction and needs: a cross-sectional study. *J Nurs Manag* 26(7):858, 2018.

Roberts H, Cronin SN: A descriptive study of nursing peer-review programs in US Magnet® hospitals. *J Nurs Adm* 47(4):226, 2017.

Santana MJ et al: Measuring patient-centred system performance: a scoping review of patient-centred care quality indicators, *BMJ Open.* 2019;9:e023596. doi:10.1136/bmjopen-2018-023596, 2019.

Sefcik JS et al.: Stakeholders' perceptions sought to inform the development of a low-cost mobile robot for older adults: a qualitative descriptive study. *Clin Nurs Res* 27(1): 61, 2018.

Shinall MC et al: Facility placement as a barrier to hospice for older adult patients discharged from a palliative care unit. *Am J Hosp Palliat Care* 36(2): 93, 2019.

Sloane DM, et al.: Effect of changes in hospital nursing resources on improvements in patient safety and quality of care: a panel study. *Medical Care* 56(12): 1001, 2018.

Spaulding A, et al.: The impact of hospitalists on value-based purchasing program scores. *J Healthc Manag* 63(4):e43, 2018.

Telehealth.hhs.gov: What is telehealth? 2021, https://telehealth.hhs.gov/patients/understanding-telehealth/ Accessed April 12, 2021.

Twigg DE et al.: A quantitative systematic review of the association between nurse skill mix and nursing-sensitive patient outcomes in the acute care setting. *J Adv Nurs* 75:3404, 2019.

Whitmore KE, Snethen J: Respite care services for children with special healthcare needs: parental perceptions. *J Spec Pediatr Nurs* 23(3): e12217, 2018.

3

Community-Based Nursing Practice

OBJECTIVES

- Explain the relationship between public health and community health nursing.
- Contrast community-oriented nursing with community-based nursing.
- Discuss the role of the community health nurse.
- Discuss the role of the nurse in community-based practice.
- Identify characteristics of patients from vulnerable populations that influence the community-based nurse's approach to care.
- Explain the competencies important for success in community-based nursing practice.
- Discuss how global health impacts the health of a community.
- Identify elements of a community assessment.

KEY TERMS

Community-based nursing center
Community-based nursing
Community health nursing
Community-oriented nursing

Health disparities
Incident rates
Population
Public health nursing

Social determinants of health
Vulnerable populations

MEDIA RESOURCES

http://evolve.elsevier.com/Potter/fundamentals/
- Review Questions
- Case Study with Questions
- Audio Glossary
- Content Updates
- Answers to QSEN Activity and Review Questions

Community-based care focuses on health promotion, disease prevention, and restorative care. Some patients are discharged from acute care settings and require ongoing care outside traditional settings. Patients also require preventive care such as immunizations, screenings, lifestyle teaching, and counseling. Health care delivery has changed greatly over the past few decades, resulting in a growing need to provide health care services where people live, work, socialize, and learn. One way to achieve this goal is through a community-based health care model. Community-based health care is a collaborative, patient-centered approach to provide culturally appropriate health care within a community (Centers for Medicare & Medicaid Services [CMS], 2019). A healthy community includes elements that maintain a high quality of life and productivity, such as access to health services, preventive care, nutrition, safety, physical activity, oral health, and environmental quality (Office of Disease Prevention and Health Promotion [ODPHP], n.d.c). Including interventions that address both mental and physical health is essential for community health programs (CDC, 2018). Nurses directly influence the health and well-being of patients every day and can encourage lifestyle changes within communities (American Nurses Association [ANA], n.d.). As more community health care partnerships develop, nurses are in a strategic position to play an important role in health care delivery and to improve the health of the community.

The focus of health promotion and disease prevention continues to be essential for the holistic practice of professional nursing. Historically, nurses have established and met the public health needs of their patients. Within community health settings, nurses continue to be leaders in making the clinical judgments needed to provide patients public and community health services. Community health nursing and community-based nursing are components of a health care delivery system that improve the health of the general public.

COMMUNITY-BASED HEALTH CARE

Regardless of where you practice nursing, you need to understand the focus of community-based health care. Community-based health care is a model of care that reaches everyone in a community (including the poor and underinsured), focuses on primary rather than institutional or acute care, and provides knowledge about health and health promotion and models of care to the community. Community-based health care occurs outside traditional health care institutions such as hospitals. It provides services to individuals and families in nontraditional settings such as ambulatory care clinics, community hospice centers, senior centers, parishes, and schools. These settings allow those who would not be able to access care in other areas to receive the care they need. Providing necessary care to maintain and restore health decreases vulnerability in at-risk populations.

Today the challenges in community-based health care are numerous. Political policy, social determinants of health, increases in health disparities, and economics all influence public health problems and subsequent health care services. Some of these problems include a lack of adequate health insurance, chronic illnesses (e.g., heart disease and diabetes), substance abuse, an increase in sexually transmitted infections, and underimmunization of infants and children (ODPHP, n.d.c).

34

Today's leaders in the health care system must commit to reform and bring attention to health promotion and disease prevention and provide health care services to all communities. Many community health programs are trying to decrease disparity by addressing ways to improve quality of care, access to care, and cost (ODPHP, n.d.c).

Achieving Healthy Populations and Communities

The U.S. Department of Health and Human Services Public Health Service designed a program to improve the overall health status of people living in this country. The *Healthy People Initiative* was created to establish ongoing health care goals for the U.S. population (see Chapter 6) to meet the diverse public health needs and to seize opportunities to achieve its goals. Health of the nation is tracked, and goals are updated every 10 years based on data gathered during program evaluation and national health trends. *Healthy People* has become a broad-based public engagement initiative, with thousands of citizens helping to shape it at every step along the way. The overall goals of *Healthy People 2030* are to increase life expectancy and quality of life, attain health literacy, achieve health equity, and eliminate health disparities through improved delivery of health care services (ODPHP, n.d.b). Improved delivery of health care involves three key components: assessment, development and implementation of public health policies, and improved access to care.

Assessment of the health care needs of individuals, families, and communities is the first component. Assessment includes systematic data collection on the population, monitoring of the health status of the population, and accessing available information about the health of the community (Stanhope and Lancaster, 2018). An example of community assessment includes the gathering of information on **incident rates**, such as identifying and reporting new infections or diseases, such as rates for influenza or COVID-19, determining adolescent pregnancy rates, and reporting the number of motor vehicle accidents caused by teenage drivers. A comprehensive community assessment informs the development and maintenance of community health programs aimed at infection control, adolescent sex education, or ways to reduce distractions for teen drivers.

The second component of improved health care delivery is policy. Health professionals provide leadership in developing public policies to support the health of the population (Stanhope and Lancaster, 2018). Strong policies are driven by community assessment. For example, assessing the level of lead poisoning in young children often results in a lead cleanup program to reduce the incidence of lead poisoning. This is the case in Flint, Michigan. Nurses were instrumental as case managers for children exposed to lead but also led public health efforts to lobby for and educate about water filtration and successfully reduced the lead levels (Gomez et al., 2018). Nurses also play an important role in advocating and educating about the nation's opioid epidemic. Strict prescription monitoring programs, as well as referrals and the implementation of evidence-based substance abuse or pain relief treatments, can reduce the abuse of opioids (Becker and Starrels, 2020). Identifying evidence-based practices to help people manage chronic illnesses in the home and the community addresses the needs of nurses and their patients (Coffin, 2020; Croft et al., 2018).

The last component of improved health care delivery is access to care. Improved access to care ensures that essential community-wide health services are available and accessible to all members of a community (Stanhope and Lancaster, 2018). Insurance coverage, geographic availability of care, and the development of relationships with health care providers are essential in establishing access to community-wide health promotion and health maintenance activities (ODPHP, n.d.c). Examples include prenatal care programs and programs focusing on disease prevention, health protection, and health promotion. The five-level health services pyramid is an example of how to provide community-based

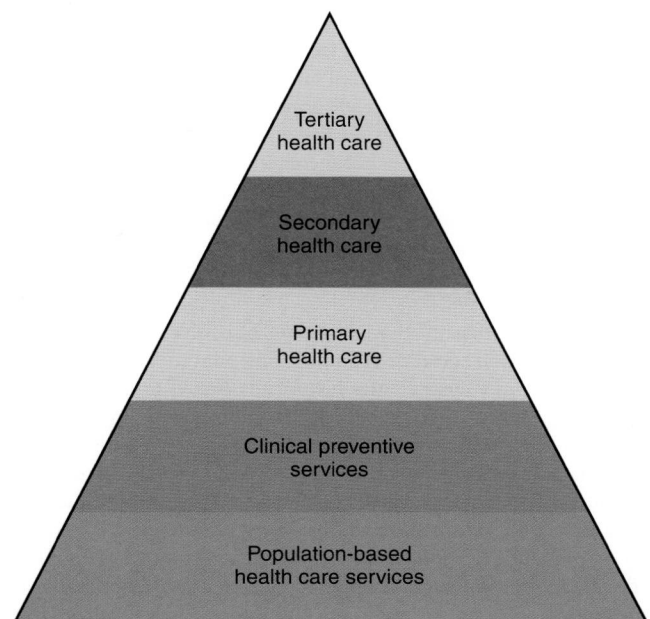

FIG. 3.1 Health services pyramid. (Courtesy U.S. Public Health Service: For a healthy nation: return on investments in public health, Washington DC, 2008, USDHHS.)

services within existing health care services in a community (Fig. 3.1). In this population-focused health care services model, the goals of disease prevention, health protection, and health promotion provide a foundation for primary, secondary, and tertiary health care services.

A rural community does not always have a hospital to meet the acute care needs of its citizens. However, the community may have the resources for providing childhood immunizations, flu vaccines, and primary preventive care services and is able to focus on child developmental problems and child safety. For example, a nurse completing a community assessment identifies services available to meet the needs of expectant mothers, reduce teenage smoking, and provide nutritional support for older adults. In addition, the nurse also identifies the health care gaps for the community. Community-based programs provide needed services and are effective in improving the health of the community by ensuring that members of the community are aware of the resources that are available.

Public health services aim at achieving a healthy environment for all individuals. Health care providers apply these principles for individuals, families, and the communities in which they live. Nursing plays a role in all levels of the health services pyramid. By using public health principles, you are better able to understand the types of environments in which patients live and the interventions necessary to help keep them healthy.

Social Determinants of Health

Our health is determined in part by access to social and economic opportunities. These include the resources and support systems available in our homes, neighborhoods, and communities; the quality of our schooling; the safety of our workplaces; the cleanliness of our water, food, and air; and the nature of our social interactions and relationships.

Health starts in our homes, schools, workplaces, neighborhoods, and communities. Research shows that taking care of ourselves by eating well and staying active, not smoking, getting recommended immunizations and screening tests, and seeing a health care provider when we are sick all influence our health. However, there are also social determinants of health. Social determinants of health are biological, socioeconomic, psychosocial, behavioral, or social factors that contribute to a person's current state of health (CDC, 2019a). *Healthy People 2030* lists five determinants of health that are grouped into five domains: economic stability; education access and quality; health care access and quality; neighborhood and built environment; and social and community context (ODPHP, n.d.d). Whether these factors affect a single family or the community, they impact the overall health and wellness of that community (see Chapter 2).

Health Disparities

Health disparities negatively affect groups of people who have systematically experienced social or economic obstacles to health. These obstacles stem from characteristics historically linked to discrimination or exclusion, such as race or ethnicity, religion, socioeconomic status, gender, mental health, sexual orientation, or geographic location. Other characteristics include cognitive, sensory, or physical disability.

Health disparities are preventable differences in a population's ability to achieve optimal health. Disparity exists if health outcomes vary by population. Populations can be disadvantaged by the burden of disease, injury, violence, or opportunities to achieve optimal health due to social, political, economic, or environmental resources (ODPHP, n.d.e). Disparity is multifactorial, including poverty, environmental threats, inadequate access to health care, individual and behavioral factors, and educational inequalities (ODPHP, n.d.e).

REFLECT NOW

Consider the community in which your nursing program is located. What are some health disparities that are present within your community?

COMMUNITY-ORIENTED NURSING

Frequently the terms *community health nursing* and *public health nursing* are used interchangeably and fall under the umbrella term *community-oriented nursing*. Community health nursing is nursing practice in the community, with the primary focus on the health care of individuals, families, and groups within their communities. The goal is to preserve, protect, promote, or maintain health (Stanhope and Lancaster, 2018). The emphasis of such nursing care is to improve the quality of health and life within a community. Public health nursing is a nursing specialty that requires understanding the needs of a population, or a collection of individuals who have one or more personal or environmental characteristics in common (Stanhope and Lancaster, 2020). Examples of populations include high-risk infants, older adults, or an ethnic group such as Native Americans. A public health nurse understands factors that influence health promotion and health maintenance, the trends and patterns influencing the incidence of disease within populations, environmental factors contributing to health and illness, and the political processes that affect public policy. For example, a public health nurse uses data on increased incidence of playground injuries to lobby for a policy to use shock-absorbing material rather than concrete for new public playgrounds.

The community health nurse may also provide direct care services to subpopulations within a community. These subpopulations often have a clinical focus in which the nurse has expertise. For example, a case manager follows older adults recovering from stroke and sees the need for community rehabilitation services, or a nurse practitioner gives immunizations to patients with the objective of managing communicable disease within the community. By focusing on subpopulations, a community health nurse cares for the community and considers an individual or family as only one member of a group at risk. In summary, the focus of community-oriented nursing is on health promotion, disease prevention, and improving quality of life of the population (Stanhope and Lancaster, 2018).

Public health nurses are sometimes required to have a baccalaureate degree in nursing educational preparation and clinical practice in public health nursing. A specialist in public health has a graduate-level education with a focus in the public health sciences (ANA, 2014). Competence as a community health nurse requires the ability to use interventions that include the broad social and political context of the community (Stanhope and Lancaster, 2020). The educational requirements for entry-level nurses practicing in community health nursing roles are not as clear as those for public health nurses. Not all hiring agencies require an advanced degree. However, nurses with a graduate degree in nursing who practice in community settings are considered community health nurse specialists, regardless of their public health experience (Stanhope and Lancaster, 2020).

Nursing Practice in Community Health

Community health nursing practice requires a unique set of skills and knowledge. In the health care delivery system, nurses who become experts in community health practice usually have advanced nursing degrees, yet the baccalaureate-prepared nurse generalist is also able to formulate and apply population-focused assessments and interventions. The expert community health nurse understands the needs of a population or community through experience with individual families or populations, which includes working through their social and health care issues. In this context, clinical judgment involves applying knowledge of public health principles, community health nursing, family theory, communication principles, and critical thinking to the best approaches to partner with families.

Successful community health nursing practice involves building relationships with the community and being responsive to changes within the community. For example, when there is an increase in the incidence of grandparents assuming child care responsibilities, a community health nurse becomes an active part of a community by establishing an educational program in cooperation with local schools to assist and support grandparents in this caregiving role. The nurse knows the community members, along with their needs and resources, and works in collaboration with community leaders to establish effective health promotion and disease prevention programs. This requires working with highly resistant systems (e.g., welfare system) and trying to encourage them to be more responsive to the needs of a population. Skills of patient advocacy, communicating people's concerns, and designing new systems in cooperation with existing systems help to make community nursing practice effective.

COMMUNITY-BASED NURSING

Community-based nursing care takes place in community settings such as a home or clinic, where nurses focus on the needs of an individual or family. It involves the safety needs and acute and chronic care of individuals and families, enhances their capacity for self-care, and promotes autonomy in decision making (Stanhope and Lancaster, 2018). Community-based nurses tend to provide illness care within the community setting (Stanhope and Lancaster, 2018). This type of nursing requires clinical judgment and decision making for the individual patient and family—assessing health status, critically applying knowledge, recognizing and analyzing cues, diagnosing health problems, planning care, implementing interventions, and evaluating outcomes of care. Because nurses provide direct care services where patients live,

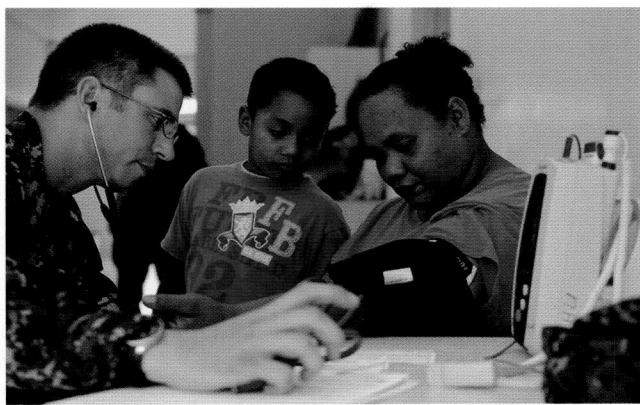

FIG. 3.2 Patient and family receiving care in a community-based care center. (Courtesy Mass Communication Specialist 2nd Class Daniel Viramontes.)

work, and play, it is important that they place the perspectives of the community members first and foremost when planning care (Stanhope and Lancaster, 2018). This is an example of population-focused care where community is the client.

Community-based nursing centers function as the first level of contact between members of a community and the health care delivery system (Fig. 3.2). Ideally health care services are provided near where patients live, work, and socialize. This approach helps to reduce the cost of health care for the patient and the stress associated with the financial burdens of care. In addition, these centers offer direct access to nurses and comprehensive patient-centered health services and readily incorporate the patient and the patient's family or friends into a plan of care. Community-based nursing centers often care for the most vulnerable of the population (Stanhope and Lancaster, 2018).

With the individual and family as the patients, the context of community-based nursing is family-centered care within the community. This focus requires a strong knowledge base in family theory (see Chapter 10), principles of communication (see Chapter 24), group dynamics, and cultural diversity (see Chapter 9). Nurses partner with their patients and families to enable them to ultimately assume responsibility for their health care decisions.

Impact of Global Health on Community Health

In the role of a community health nurse, consider the impact of global health on that community. Global health focuses on understanding health within an interprofessional and international context. Its aims are to improve health and health care equity for populations across the world (Torres-Alzate, 2019). The World Health Organization (WHO) works across the world to promote health and serve vulnerable populations (WHO, 2020). WHO was formed as an international organization in 1948 and is composed of members from 150 countries. The organization serves as the directing and coordinating authority on international health. The three focuses for WHO are universal health coverage, health emergencies, and health and well-being (WHO, 2020). The global health issues identified by WHO for the next decade impact your community. Examples of priorities in global health issues for WHO include: equitable access to safe and effective vaccines, air pollution and climate change, infectious diseases, health care equality, affordable and available medications for all, shortages of health care workers, the use of new technologies to disseminate accurate information, and clean water and sanitation (Brooks, 2020).

The health within a community in the United States can be impacted by events occurring anywhere in the world. Globally, there has been an increase in the incidence of heart disease, stroke, and diabetes, as well as infectious diseases, such as HIV, tuberculosis, viral hepatitis, and malaria (Brooks, 2020; ODPHP, n.d.a). An increase in international travel, an increase in the number of densely populated urban areas, and climate change have contributed to an increase in emerging infections and pandemics. Emerging infections are infections that were previously unknown or infectious diseases that are unable to be controlled (Johns Hopkins Medicine, 2020; ODPHP, n.d.a). Examples of emerging infections that have caused epidemics or pandemics impacting health worldwide include: Ebola virus, influenza (H1N1), severe acute respiratory syndrome (SARS), West Nile virus, Zika virus, dengue, and novel coronavirus (COVID-19) (Bloom and Cadarette, 2019; Johns Hopkins Medicine, 2020). These emerging infections not only affect the health of the community, but also threaten economic and social functions within the community. Emerging infections can result in economic and social disruption because of closure of schools, businesses, churches, and commercial and public services within a community to slow the spread of the illnesses (Stanhope and Lancaster, 2020). Health care systems are often overwhelmed with treating patients, there may be a shortage of medical supplies and medications, and there are increased costs to health care systems to deal with the infections (Stanhope and Lancaster, 2020). During a pandemic, you also see loss of income to individuals and businesses and increased mortality (Bloom and Cadarette, 2019). The financial losses and loss of life, along with the social isolation that could occur, can lead to increased mental health problems, such as depression, in individuals.

Nurses are at the forefront of both community and global health. During times of crisis, such as a pandemic, nurses play critical roles as patient caregivers, educators on sanitation measures (particularly hand hygiene) and disease prevention and spread, and managers of equipment and supplies for patient care and personal protection (Jordan, 2020). Nurses are also involved in the prevention and early detection of the disease and illness (Corless et al., 2018). During times of emerging infections and pandemics, nurses have an ethical responsibility to care for themselves as well as their patients (ANA, 2020). Nurses serve as liaisons between patients and the health care team in the treatment and the prevention of spread of illness during a pandemic (Anzalone, 2020). During a crisis, nurses, particularly public health nurses, are important members of the community teams serving to investigate cases, provide education using telehealth or home visits, and provide direct patient care within the community (Edmonds et al., 2020).

Vulnerable Populations

Nurses care for patients from diverse cultures and backgrounds and with various health conditions. Changes in the health care delivery system have made high-risk groups the principal patients. For example, you are unlikely to visit low-risk mothers and babies. Instead, you are more likely to visit adolescent mothers or mothers with drug addiction. Vulnerable populations are groups of patients who are more likely to develop health problems because of excess health risks, who are limited in their access to health care services, or who depend on others for care. Vulnerable populations include those living in poverty, older adults, the disabled, people who are homeless, immigrants, individuals in abusive relationships, people living with substance abuse, and people with mental illnesses. These vulnerabilities are often associated with the individual's/community's social determinants of health or individual health disparities.

Public and community health nursing and primary care providers share health care responsibility for health promotion, screening, and early detection and disease prevention for vulnerable populations. These patients have intense health care needs that are unmet or ignored or require more care than can be provided in outpatient or hospital settings. Individuals and their families who are vulnerable often belong to more than one of these groups. In addition, health care vulnerability affects all age-groups (Stanhope and Lancaster, 2020).

Patients who are vulnerable often come from various cultures, have different beliefs and values, face language and literacy barriers, or have few sources of social support. These diverse needs will be challenging as you care for patients with increasingly complex acute and chronic health conditions. To provide competent care for vulnerable populations, you need to assess these patients accurately (Box 3.1), including a patient's and family's cultural beliefs, values, and practices, to make decisions about their specific needs and the interventions that will be most successful in improving their state of health (see Chapter 9). It is important not to judge or evaluate your patient's

beliefs and values about health in terms of your own culture, beliefs, and values. Communication and caring practices are critical in learning patients' perceptions of their problems and then planning health care strategies that will be meaningful, culturally appropriate, and successful.

Barriers to access and use of services often lead to adverse health outcomes for vulnerable populations (ODPHP, n.d.e). Because of these poorer outcomes, vulnerable populations have shorter life spans and higher morbidity rates. Members of vulnerable groups frequently have multiple risk factors, resulting in cumulative effects of individual risk factors. It is essential for community-based nurses to assess members of vulnerable populations by considering the multiple stressors that affect their patients' lives. It is also important to learn patients' strengths and resources for coping with stressors. Complete assessment of vulnerable populations enables a community-based nurse to design interventions within the context of the patient's community (Stanhope and Lancaster, 2020).

Immigrant Population. The CDC (2016) predicts a continued increase in the immigrant population. This growth creates many social and health care needs. Social problems involved with immigration sometimes include poverty, acculturation, education, housing, and employment. Some immigrant populations face multiple diverse health issues that cities, counties, and states need to address. These health care needs pose significant legal and policy issues. For some immigrants, access to health care is limited because of language barriers and/or lack of benefits, resources, and transportation. Immigrant populations often have higher rates of hypertension, diabetes mellitus, and infectious diseases; decreased outcomes of care; and shorter life expectancies (Stanhope and Lancaster, 2018).

Frequently patients from immigrant populations practice nontraditional healing practices (see Chapter 9). Although many of these healing practices are effective and complement traditional therapies, it is important that you know how the therapies act physically and understand your patient's health beliefs about these healing practices.

Certain immigrant populations left their homes because of oppression, war, or natural disaster. You must be sensitive to these physical and psychological stressors and identify the appropriate resources to help your patients meet their health care needs (Stanhope and Lancaster, 2018).

Effects of Poverty and Homelessness. People who live in poverty are more likely to have health disparities because they are at a higher risk of living in hazardous environments, working at high-risk jobs, eating less nutritious diets, having multiple stressors in their lives, lacking adequate transportation, and being homeless. Patients who are experiencing homelessness have even fewer resources than people who are poor. They are often jobless, do not have the advantage of a permanent shelter, and must continually cope with finding food and a place to sleep at night. Chronic health problems tend to worsen because of poor nutrition and the inability to store nutritional foods. In addition, people who are experiencing homelessness usually have barriers to accessing health care, causing them to seek health care in emergency departments (American Public Health Association [APHA], 2017).

BOX 3.1   Guidelines for Assessing Members of Vulnerable Population Groups

Setting the Stage
- Create a comfortable, nonthreatening environment.
- Obtain information about a patient's culture so that you understand the practices, beliefs, and values that affect the patient's health care.
- If the patient speaks a different language, use a professional interpreter, and observe nonverbal behavior to complete a culturally competent assessment (see Chapter 9).
- Be sensitive to the fact that patients often have priorities other than their health care (e.g., financial, legal, or social issues). Ask patients to explore these issues with you. If a patient needs financial assistance, consult a social worker. If there are legal issues, provide the patient with a resource. Do not attempt to provide financial or legal advice yourself.

Nursing History of an Individual or Family
- Obtain an organized history of the patient's health condition and impact on daily living.
- Collect data that focus on the specific needs of the vulnerable population with whom you work. However, be flexible so as not to overlook important health information. For example, when with a mother who is an adolescent, obtain a nutritional history on both the mother and baby. Be aware of the developmental needs of the young mother, and listen to her social needs as well.
- Identify both developmental and health care needs. Remember, the goal is to collect enough information to provide family-centered care.
- Identify any risks to the patient's immune system. This is especially important for vulnerable patients who are homeless and sleep in shelters.

Physical Examination and Home Assessment
- Complete a thorough physical and/or home assessment. Only collect data that are relevant to providing care to the patient and family.
- Be alert for signs of physical abuse, substance abuse, or neglect (e.g., inadequately clothed, underweight).
- When assessing a patient's home, observe: Is there adequate water and plumbing? What is the status of the utilities? Are foods and perishables stored properly? Are there signs of insects or vermin? Is the paint peeling? Are the windows and doors adequate? Are there water stains on the ceiling, evidence of a leaky roof? What is the temperature? Is it comfortable? What does the outside environment look like: Are there vacant houses/lots nearby? Is there a busy intersection? What is the crime level?

Modified from Stanhope M, Lancaster J: *Public health nursing: population-centered health care in the community*, ed 10, St Louis, 2020, Elsevier.

REFLECT NOW

What health care resources are available to help the homeless and those living in poverty within your community? How can you participate in providing health care to these vulnerable groups?

Patients Who Are Abused. Physical, emotional, and sexual abuse and neglect are major public health problems that often affect older adults, women, and children. Risk factors for abusive relationships include mental health problems, substance abuse, socioeconomic stressors, lack of understanding of child development or parenting skills, and dysfunctional family relationships (CDC, 2020). One recent study showed a higher incidence and severity of physical intimate partner violence (IPV) during the COVID-19 pandemic compared with the previous 3 years (Gosangi et al., 2021). For some, risk factors may not be present. When dealing with patients at risk for or who have suffered abuse, it is important to provide protection. Interview a patient you suspect is abused at a time when the patient has privacy and the individual suspected of being the abuser is not present. Patients who are abused may fear retribution if they discuss their problems with a health care provider. Nurses use therapeutic communication techniques that reinforce that the abuse is not the victim's fault. Nurses are mandatory reporters for abuse involving elders over the age of 65, children under the age of 18, and individuals with disabilities.

Patients With Mental Illness. Patients with severe mental illness such as schizophrenia or bipolar disorder may experience multiple health and socioeconomic problems. Many patients with severe mental illnesses are homeless or live in poverty and lack the ability to remain employed or to care for themselves daily (SAMHSA, 2020). Patients who have a mental illness often require medication therapy, counseling, housing, and vocational assistance. In addition, they are at a greater risk for abuse and assault. Patients with mental illnesses are no longer routinely hospitalized in long-term psychiatric institutions. Instead, resources are offered within the community. Although comprehensive service networks may be available in the community, many patients still go untreated or undertreated because of an inability to navigate the health care system (Stanhope and Lancaster, 2018).

Older Adults. The older adult population is increasing, resulting in simultaneous increases in the number of patients suffering from chronic diseases and a greater demand for health care services. Take time to understand what health means to an older adult and which assessment findings to expect; view health promotion in the older adult within a broad context (see Chapter 14). Help older adults and their families understand which steps older adults need to take to maintain their health and improve their level of function through physical activity (CDC, 2019b). Design appropriate community-based interventions that provide an opportunity to improve the lifestyle and quality of life of older adults (Table 3.1).

Competency in Community-Based Nursing

A nurse in community-based practice needs a variety of skills and talents to be successful. In addition to assisting patients with their health care needs and developing relationships within the community, the community-based nurse needs skills in health promotion and disease prevention. Nurses use the nursing process and critical thinking (see Unit 3) to make the clinical judgments and decisions needed to ensure individualized nursing care. Students' clinical practice in a community-based care setting will probably be in partnership with a community nurse.

Caregiver. First and foremost, a nurse is a caregiver (see Chapter 1). In the community setting you manage and care for the health of patients and families in the community.

Use a critical thinking approach to apply the nursing process (see Unit 3) and ensure appropriate, individualized nursing care for your patients and their families. Historically, well-baby and child care was integral to community nursing practices. Community child care services

are increasing to address changes in the health care delivery system, changing economics, homelessness, and the increased number of people who are medically underinsured. Community nurses are undertaking more complex and expanded child health services for increasingly diverse patient populations (ODPHP, n.d.f).

In addition, the community nurse must individualize care within the context of a patient's community so that long-term success is more likely. Together with a patient and family you develop a caring partnership to recognize actual and potential health care needs and identify needed community resources. For example, if a patient is placed on an exercise program, you recommend a safe park or recreational area where the patient can exercise. Competent community-based practice builds healthy communities that are safe and include elements to enable people to achieve and maintain a high quality of life.

QSEN **Building Competency in Safety** Maria Perez is a 74-year-old widow with heart failure (HF) who has been referred to the Home Care Agency for services. Maria has been admitted to the hospital three times in the past two months. Two admissions were for HF exacerbation and the other was for a fractured wrist after falling in the bathroom. Maria lives alone in a senior housing apartment building that has an elevator. The hospitalist requests a home safety evaluation, along with assessment of medication management. What information does the nurse need to begin this assessment?

Answers to QSEN Activities can be found on the Evolve website.

Case Manager. In community-based practice, case management is an important competency (see Chapter 2). Case managers establish an appropriate plan of care based on assessment of patients and families and coordinate needed resources and services for a patient's well-being across a continuum of care. Generally, a community-based case manager assumes responsibility for the case management of multiple patients. The greatest challenge is to coordinate the activities of multiple providers and payers in different settings throughout a patient's continuum of care. An effective case manager eventually learns the obstacles, limits, and even the opportunities that exist within the community that influence the ability to find solutions for patients' health care needs.

Change Agent. A community-based nurse is also a change agent. This involves identifying and implementing new and more effective approaches to problems. You act as a change agent within a family system or as a mediator for problems within a patient's community. You identify any number of problems (e.g., quality of community childcare services, availability of older-adult day care services, or the status of neighborhood violence). As a change agent you empower individuals and their families to creatively solve problems or become instrumental in creating change within a health care agency. For example, if your patient has difficulty keeping regular health care visits, you determine why. Maybe the health clinic is too far and difficult to reach, or perhaps the hours of service are incompatible with a patient's transportation resources. You work with the patient to solve the problem and help identify an alternative site such as a nursing clinic that is closer and has more convenient hours.

To effect change, you gather and analyze facts before you implement programs to help people make changes to improve their health. This requires you to be very familiar with the community itself. Many communities resist change, preferring to provide services in the established manner. Before analyzing facts, it is often necessary to manage conflict among the health care providers, clarify their roles, and clearly identify the needs of the patients. If the community has a history of poor problem solving, you will have to focus on developing problem-solving capabilities (Stanhope and Lancaster, 2018).

TABLE 3.1 Major Health Problems in Older Adults and Community-Based Nursing Roles and Interventions

Problem	Community-Based Nursing Roles and Interventions
Hypertension	Monitor blood pressure and weight; educate about nutrition and antihypertensive drugs; teach stress-management techniques; promote a good balance between rest and activity; establish blood pressure screening programs; assess patient's current lifestyle and promote lifestyle changes; promote dietary modifications by using techniques such as a diet diary.
Cancer	Obtain health history; promote monthly breast self-examinations and recommended screening intervals for Papanicolaou (Pap) smears and mammograms for older women; promote colorectal screening; promote regular physical examinations; encourage smokers to stop smoking; correct misconceptions about processes of aging; provide emotional support and quality of care during diagnostic and treatment procedures.
Arthritis	Educate about management of activities, reducing stress on affected joints, availability of mechanical appliances, and adequate rest; promote stress management; counsel and assist the family to improve communication, role negotiation, and use of community resources.
Visual impairment (e.g., loss of visual acuity, eyelid disorders, opacity of the lens)	Provide support in a well-lighted, glare-free environment; use printed aids with large, well-spaced letters; help adult clean eyeglasses; help arrange for vision examinations and obtain necessary prostheses.
Hearing impairment (e.g., presbycusis)	Speak with clarity at a moderate volume and pace, and face audience when performing health teaching; help arrange a hearing examination and obtain necessary prostheses; teach how to care for hearing aids.
Cognitive impairment	Provide complete assessment; correct underlying causes of impairment (if possible); provide for a protective environment; promote activities that reinforce reality; help with personal hygiene, nutrition, and hydration; provide emotional support to the family; recommend applicable community resources such as adult day care, home care aides, and homemaker services.
Dementia	Maintain high-level functioning, protection, and safety; encourage human dignity; demonstrate to the primary family caregiver techniques to dress, feed, and toilet adult; provide frequent encouragement and emotional support to caregiver; act as an advocate for patient when dealing with respite care and support groups; protect the patient's rights; provide caregiver support to maintain family members' physical and mental health and to prevent caregiver role strain; maintain family stability; recommend financial services if needed.
Dental problems	Perform oral assessment and refer to dentist as necessary; emphasize regular brushing and flossing, proper nutrition, and dental examinations; encourage patients with dentures to wear and take care of them; calm fears about dentist; help provide access to financial services (if necessary) and dental care resources.
Substance and alcohol abuse	Get drug use history; educate about safe storage and risks for drug, drug-drug, drug-alcohol, and drug-food interactions; give general information about drug (e.g., drug name, purpose, side effects, dosage); instruct adult about presorting techniques (using small containers with one dose of drug that are labeled with specific times to take drug). Counsel adults about substance abuse; promote stress management to avoid need for drugs or alcohol and arrange for and monitor detoxification if appropriate. Provide community resources for substance abuse treatment.
Sexually transmitted infections	Perform a full sexual risk assessment, and bring awareness regarding risk factors and susceptibility to human immunodeficiency virus/acquired immunodeficiency syndrome (HIV/AIDS). Educate about safe sexual practices such as abstinence or use of condoms, and refer as necessary for HIV and other infection testing and HPV immunization.

Data from Centers for Disease Control and Prevention (CDC): Promoting health for older adults, https://www.cdc.gov/chronicdisease/resources/publications/factsheets/promoting-health-for-older-adults.htm, 2019b; Stanhope M, Lancaster J: *Public health nursing: population-centered health care in the community,* ed 10, St Louis, 2020, Elsevier; National Institute on Aging: Health information, n.d., https://www.nia.nih.gov/health. Accessed June 28, 2020.

Patient Advocate. Patient advocacy is important in community-based practice mainly because of the confusion surrounding access to health care services. Patients often need someone to help them walk through the system and identify where to go for services, how to reach individuals with the appropriate authority, which services to request, and how to follow through with the information they receive. As a patient advocate, you ensure patients have the information necessary to make informed decisions in choosing and using services appropriately. In addition, it is important for you to support and at times defend your patients' decisions.

Collaborator. Community-based nursing practice requires you to be competent in communicating and working with patients, their families, and other members of the health care team. Collaboration, or working in a combined effort with all those involved in care delivery, is necessary to develop a mutually acceptable plan that will achieve common goals (Stanhope and Lancaster, 2020). For example, when your patient is discharged home with terminal cancer, you collaborate with hospice staff, social workers, and pastoral care to initiate a plan to support interprofessional end-of-life care for the patient in the home and support the family. For collaboration to be effective, you need mutual trust and respect for each professional's roles, abilities, and contributions.

Counselor. To be an effective counselor, you need to be aware of a patient's community resources (e.g., mental health clinics, day care services, respite care). A counselor helps patients identify and clarify health problems as well as choose appropriate courses of action to solve those problems. Motivational interviewing is often very useful (see Chapter 24). For example, if you are a nurse in an employee-assistance program or a women's shelter, you will often assume the role of counselor with your patients. As a counselor, you are responsible for providing information; listening objectively; and being supportive, caring, and trustworthy. You do not make decisions but rather help your patients reach decisions that are best for them (Stanhope and Lancaster, 2020). Patients and families often require assistance in first identifying and clarifying health problems. For example, a patient who repeatedly reports a problem in following a prescribed diet is unable to afford nutritious foods or has family members who do not support healthy eating habits. You discuss with your patient factors that block or aid problem resolution, identify a range of solutions, and then discuss which solutions are most likely to be successful. You also encourage your patient to make decisions and express your confidence in the choice the patient makes.

Educator. Patient education is often a priority in community-based nursing. Become familiar with community service organizations that offer educational support to a wide range of individuals and patient groups. Prenatal classes, infant care, child safety, and cancer screening are just some of the health education programs provided in a community.

When the goal is to help your patients assume responsibility for their own health care, being an educator takes on greater importance (Stanhope and Lancaster, 2020). Patients and families need to gain skills and knowledge to care for themselves. Assess your patient's learning needs and readiness to learn within the context of the individual, the systems with which the individual interacts (e.g., family, business, and school), and the resources available for support. Adapt your teaching skills so you can instruct a patient within the home setting and make the learning process meaningful. Community-based nursing gives you the opportunity to follow patients over time. Planning for return demonstration of skills, using follow-up phone calls, and referring to community support and self-help groups give you an opportunity to provide continuity of instruction and reinforce important instructional topics and learned behaviors (see Chapter 25).

Epidemiologist. As a community-based nurse, you apply principles of epidemiology, the science dealing with the incidence, distribution, and possible control of diseases and other health problems. Your contacts with families, community groups such as schools and industries, and health care agencies place you in a unique position to initiate epidemiological activities, such as case finding, health teaching, and tracking incident rates of an illness. For example, a cafeteria worker in the local high school is diagnosed with active tuberculosis (TB). As a community health nurse, you help find where the exposure to TB may have occurred, such as within the worker's home, place of employment, or community.

Nurse epidemiologists are responsible for community surveillance (e.g., tracking incidence of elevated lead levels in children and identifying increased fetal and infant mortality rates, increases in adolescent pregnancy, presence of infectious and communicable diseases, and outbreaks of head lice). Nurse epidemiologists protect the level of health of the community, develop sensitivity to changes in the health status of the community, and help identify the cause of these changes.

COMMUNITY ASSESSMENT

When practicing in a community setting, you need to learn how to assess the community at large. Completing the community assessment requires clinical judgment and critical thinking to be able to analyze the multiple sources of data collected (Stanhope and Lancaster, 2020). Community assessment is the systematic data collection on the population, monitoring the health status of the population, and making information available about the health of the community (Stanhope and Lancaster, 2020). This is the environment in which patients live, work, play, and learn. Without an adequate understanding of that environment, any effort to promote a patient's health and bring about necessary change is unlikely to be successful. The community has three components: structure or locale, the people, and the social systems. To

---

BOX 3.2 Community Assessment

Structure
- Name of community or neighborhood
- Geographical boundaries
- Emergency services
- Water and sanitation
- Housing
- Economic status (e.g., average household income, number of residents on public assistance)
- Transportation
- Safety

Population
- Age distribution
- Sex distribution
- Growth trends
- Density
- Education level
- Predominant ethnic groups
- Predominant religious groups

Social System
- Educational system
- Government
- Communication system
- Welfare system
- Volunteer programs
- Health system

---

develop a complete community assessment, take a careful look at each of the three components to identify needs for health policy, health programs, and needed health services (Box 3.2).

When assessing the structure or locale, you travel around the neighborhood or community and observe its design, the location of services, and where residents meet. As you assess the physical environment, you look for possible environmental hazards in the air, water, or soil, as well as safety issues, such as abandoned buildings, a lack of sidewalks, or roads that are in poor repair. You obtain the demographics of the population by accessing statistics on the community from reliable websites, a local public health department, or public library. You acquire information about existing social systems such as schools or health care agencies by visiting various sites and learning about their services.

Once you have a good understanding of the community, you can perform all individual patient assessments against that background. For example, when assessing a patient's home for safety, you consider the following: Does the patient have secure locks on doors? Are windows secure and intact? Is lighting along walkways and entryways operational? As you conduct a patient assessment, it is important to know the level of community violence and the resources available when help is necessary. Always assess an individual in the context of the community.

REFLECT NOW

Complete a community assessment in the geographic area surrounding your nursing school. What are the demographics of the population? What social systems exist within the community?

CHANGING PATIENTS' HEALTH

In community-based practice, nurses care for patients from diverse backgrounds and in diverse settings. It is relatively easy over time to become familiar with the available resources within a community practice setting. Likewise, with practice you learn how to identify the unique needs of individual patients. Similarly, you bring together the resources necessary to improve a patient's continuity of care. When you collaborate with your patients and their health care providers, you provide patient-centered care and help reduce duplication of health care services. For example, when caring for a patient with a healing wound, you coordinate wound care services and help the patient and family locate cost-effective dressing materials.

You need to promote and protect a patient's health within the context of the community using an evidence-based practice approach when possible. For example, nurses can help reduce health disparities surrounding childhood obesity in racial/ethnic minority populations through community engagement (Frerichs et al., 2018; Luesse et al., 2018; Otterbach et al., 2018) (Box 3.3). Frerichs et al. (2018) investigated the effect of an evidence-based community approach to develop strategies to support reducing obesity risk factors among minority groups. Evidence showed that community involvement in collaborative initiatives has a high success rate in reducing obesity among racial/ethnic minority children.

When providing community-based nursing care, it is important to consider how well you understand your patients' lives. Begin by establishing strong, caring relationships with your patients and their families (see Chapter 7). As you gain experience and are accepted by a patient's family, you are able to advise, counsel, and teach effectively and understand what truly makes your patient unique. The day-to-day activities of family life are the variables that influence how you will adapt nursing interventions. The time of day a patient goes to work, the availability of the spouse and patient's parents to provide childcare, and the family values that shape views about health are just a few examples of the many factors you will consider in community-based practice. Once you acquire a picture of a patient's life, you then design patient-centered interventions to promote health and prevent disease within the community-based practice setting.

BOX 3.3   EVIDENCE-BASED PRACTICE

Promoting Community Involvement in Reducing Childhood Obesity in Racial/Ethnic Minority Population

PICOT Question: Do community-based interventions for families affect childhood obesity rates in diverse populations?

Evidence Summary

Obesity is more prevalent in children from ethnically diverse populations in the United States (Isong et al., 2018; Klish and Skelton, 2020). Research has found that there are genetic, epigenetic, biological, social, and environmental risk factors associated with obesity in children (Isong et al., 2018; Klish and Skelton, 2020). Current evidence shows links among childhood obesity and ethnicity, lack of physical activity, increased screen time from television and electronics, nutrition, sleep, and socioeconomic status, as well as maternal smoking and breastfeeding (Isong et al., 2018; Klish and Skelton, 2020). Childhood obesity has lifelong physical, mental, and social health consequences (Klish and Skelton, 2020; Otterbach et al., 2018).

Evidence shows that early interventions are most successful in decreasing racial/ethnic disparities related to childhood obesity (Isong et al., 2018). Adult perceptions of obesity must align with interventions for success (Perreault and Apovian, 2020). Evidence shows that when caregivers perceive interventions as useful, children have greater success in adhering to interventions to address obesity (Skelton, 2020). Asking children to adhere to lifestyle changes without adult support and role modeling will not result in positive outcomes (Skelton, 2020; Stanhope and Lancaster, 2018; Trude et al., 2018).

Community engagement in childhood obesity programs can include community workshops and media resources to gain attendance and community buy-in (Luesse et al., 2018). Collaborative initiatives with community involvement have high success rates in reducing obesity among children, especially those from a variety of racial and ethnic groups (Frerichs et al., 2018). Public policy must ensure that people from underserved communities have access to healthful food choices as well as improved socioenvironmental areas (Stanhope and Lancaster, 2018). It is important to ensure that families have access to the recommended food to ensure that healthy choices can be made (Frerichs et al., 2018; Luesse et al., 2018). Communities can also help address the socioenvironmental aspects associated with obesity such as underutilized parks (Frerichs et al., 2018). With collaborative community partnerships, childhood obesity in the racial/ethnic minority population can be reduced.

Application to Nursing Practice
- Understand the modifiable risk factors for obesity, and design effective interventions targeted at reducing the risk factors (Isong et al., 2018).
- Interventions need to include both diet and physical activity recommendations (Skelton, 2020). Nutritional information must include information pertaining to both the school and home environments (Luesse et al., 2018).
- Include culturally and linguistically appropriate interventions and communication, especially when providing care to patients who are from ethnically diverse populations (Luesse et al., 2018).
- Engaging youth from racial and ethnic minority communities as leaders through a curriculum on obesity prevention solutions is a potential strategy to mobilize support for addressing childhood obesity (Frerichs et al., 2018).

█ KEY POINTS

- The terms *community health nursing* and *public health nursing* are used interchangeably and fall under the umbrella term *community-oriented nursing.*
- The community-oriented nurse's focus is on health promotion, disease prevention, and improving quality of life of the population, while the focus of the community-based nurse is to provide direct illness care to individuals and families within the community setting.
- Nurses play a critical role in community health during a pandemic through identification of cases, prevention of disease/illness spread, education, direct patient care, and managing supplies and equipment.
- Vulnerable populations are groups of patients who are more likely to develop health problems as a result of excess health risks, who have limited access to health care services, or who depend on others for care. Individuals living in poverty, older adults, people who are homeless, immigrant populations, individuals in abusive relationships, people with substance abuse disorders, and people with severe mental illnesses are examples of vulnerable populations.
- The community-based nurse needs skills in health promotion, disease prevention, and relationship building to fill the role of caregiver, case manager, change agent, patient advocate, collaborator, counselor, educator, and epidemiologist.
- Community assessment is the systematic collection of data on the population, monitoring of the health status of the population, and making information available about the health of the community. Community assessment includes structure, population, and social system.

█ REFLECTIVE LEARNING

- What population in the community do you see most frequently in your clinical setting? What are some nursing assessments, skills, or tasks you can perform with this population?
- Using key information you gathered in doing a community assessment, evaluate your community's readiness and preparedness for a community health crisis. What are your community's strengths? What are the areas for improvement?
- Identify key information you learned in your clinical setting that you can take with you in your future nursing practice. How were you inspired to improve your nursing knowledge, practice, and skills by the people you worked with?

REVIEW QUESTIONS

1. The public health nurse is working with the local city/county health department during a pandemic that has created a crisis within the community. What are responsibilities of the public health nurse during the pandemic? (Select all that apply.)
   1. Educate the public on disease prevention
   2. Serve as liaison between patients and health care services and providers
   3. Investigate cases as they arise
   4. Monitor trends of the disease outbreak
   5. Assist with testing for identification of the disease

2. A community health nurse is working in a clinic with a focus on asthma and allergies. What is the primary focus of the community health nurse in this clinic setting? (Select all that apply.)
   1. Decrease the incidence of asthma attacks in the community
   2. Increase patients' ability to self-manage their asthma
   3. Treat acute asthma in the hospital
   4. Provide asthma education programs for the teachers in the local schools
   5. Provide scheduled immunizations to people who come to the clinic

3. The nurse caring for a refugee community identifies that the children are undervaccinated and the community is unaware of resources. The nurse assesses the community and determines that there is a health clinic within a 5-mile radius. The nurse meets with the community leaders and explains the need for immunizations, the location of the clinic, and the process of accessing health care resources. Which of the following practices is the nurse providing? (Select all that apply.)
   1. Raising awareness about community resources for the children
   2. Teaching the community about health promotion and illness prevention
   3. Promoting autonomy in decision making about health practices
   4. Improving the health care of the community's children
   5. Participating in professional development activities to maintain nursing competency

4. What factor results in vulnerable populations being more likely to develop health problems?
   1. The ability to use available resources to find housing
   2. Adequate transportation to the grocery store and community clinics
   3. Availability of others to help provide care
   4. Limited access to health care services

5. Many older homes in a neighborhood are undergoing a lot of restoration. Lead paint was used to paint the homes when they were built. The community clinic in the neighborhood is initiating a lead screening program. This activity is based on which social determinant of health?

6. A community health nurse conducts a community assessment focused on adolescent health behaviors. The nurse determines that a large number of adolescents smoke. Designing a smoking-cessation program at the youth community center is an example of which nursing role?
   1. Epidemiologist
   2. Counselor
   3. Collaborator
   4. Case manager

7. A nurse in a community health clinic reviews screening results from students in a local high school during the most recent academic year. The nurse discovers a 10% increase in the number of positive tuberculosis (TB) skin tests when comparing these numbers to the previous year. The nurse contacts the school nurse and the director of the health department. Together they begin to expand their assessment to all students and employees of the school district. The community nurse is acting in which nursing role(s)? (Select all that apply.)
   1. Epidemiologist
   2. Counselor
   3. Collaborator
   4. Case manager
   5. Caregiver

8. A nursing student is giving a presentation to a group of other nursing students about the needs of patients with mental illnesses in the community. Which statement by the student indicates that the nursing professor needs to provide further teaching?
   1. "Many patients with mental illness do not have a permanent home."
   2. "Unemployment is a common problem experienced by people with a mental illness."
   3. "The majority of patients with mental illnesses live in long-term care settings."
   4. "Patients with mental illnesses are often at a higher risk for abuse and assault."

9. The nurse in a new community-based clinic is requested to complete a community assessment. Order the steps for completing this assessment.
   1. Structure or locale
   2. Social systems
   3. Population

10. The public health nurse is working with the county health department on a task force to fully integrate the goals of *Healthy People 2030*. Most of the immigrant population do not have a primary care provider, nor do they participate in health promotion activities; the unemployment rate in the community is 25%. How does the nurse determine which goals need to be included or updated? (Select all that apply.)
    1. Assess the health care resources within the community.
    2. Assess the existing health care programs offered by the county health department.
    3. Compare existing resources and programs with *Healthy People 2030* goals.
    4. Initiate new programs to meet *Healthy People 2030* goals.
    5. Implement educational sessions in the schools to focus on nutritional needs of the children.

Answers: 1. 1, 2, 3, 4, 5; **2.** 1, 2, 4; **3.** 1, 2, 4, 4; **4.** 4; **5.** Physical environment; **6.** 2; **7.** 1, 3; **8.** 3; **9.** 1, 3, 2; **10.** 1, 2, 3.

Rationales for Review Questions can be found on the Evolve website.

REFERENCES

American Nurses' Association (ANA): *Nurses, ethics, and the response to the COVID-19 pandemic*, 2020, https://www.nursingworld.org/~495c6c/globalassets/practiceandpolicy/work-environment/healthsafety/coronavirus/nurses-ethics-and-the-response-to-the-covid-19-pandemic.pdf. Accessed May 16, 2020.

American Nurses Association (ANA): *Standards of public health nursing practice*, ed 2, Washington, DC, 2014, The Association.
American Nurses Association (ANA): *Public health nursing*, n.d. https://www.nursingworld.org/practice-policy/workforce/public-health-nursing/. Accessed June 28, 2020.

American Public Health Association (APHA): *APHA policy statement 20178: housing and homelessness as a public health issue*, 2017, https://www.apha.org/policies-and-advocacy/public-health-policy-statements/policy-database/2018/01/18/housing-and-homelessness-as-a-public-health-issue. Accessed June 28, 2020.

Anzalone C: *The role of nurses in the COVID-19 pandemic*, 2020, http://www.buffalo.edu/ubnow/stories/2020/04/qa-sands-nurses-covid.html. Accessed May 16, 2020.

Bloom DE, Cadarette D: *Infectious Disease Threats in the Twenty-First Century: Strengthening the Global Response, 2019*, https://www.frontiersin.org/articles/10.3389/fimmu.2019.00549/full. Accessed May 3, 2020.

Brooks M:*WHO Names Top 13 Global Health Challenges for the New Decade*, 2020, https://www.medscape.com/viewarticle/923799. Accessed May 3, 2020.

Centers for Disease Control and Prevention (CDC): *Child abuse and neglect: risk and protective factors.* https://www.cdc.gov/violenceprevention/childabuseandneglect/riskprotectivefactors.html, 2020. Accessed June 28, 2020.

Centers for Disease Control and Prevention (CDC): *Social determinants of health: know what affects health*, 2019a, http://www.cdc.gov/socialdeterminants/faqs/index.htm, 2019a. Accessed June 28, 2020.

Centers for Disease Control and Prevention (CDC): *Promoting health for older adults*, https://www.cdc.gov/chronicdisease/resources/publications/factsheets/promoting-health-for-older-adults.htm, 2019b. Accessed August 9, 2020.

Centers for Disease Control and Prevention (CDC): *Health-related quality of life*, 2018, https://www.cdc.gov/hrqol/wellbeing.htm. Accessed June 28, 2020.

Centers for Disease Control and Prevention (CDC): *Immigrant and refugee health*, 2016, https://www.cdc.gov/immigrantrefugeehealth/. Accessed June 28, 2020.

Centers for Medicare and Medicaid Services (CMS): Home- and community-based services. https://www.cms.gov/Outreach-and-Education/American-Indian-Alaska-Native/AIAN/LTSS-TA-Center/info/hcbs.html, 2019. Accessed June 28, 2020.

Corless IB et al.: Expanding nursing's role in responding to global pandemics 5/14/2018, *Nurs Outlook* 66:412, 2018.

Croft JB et al.: Urban-rural county and state differences in chronic obstructive pulmonary disease — United States. *MMWR* 67(7):205, February 23, 2018. https://www.cdc.gov/mmwr/volumes/67/wr/mm6707a1.htm?s_cid=mm6707a1_w/.

Edmonds JK et al.: A call to action for public health nurses during the COVID-19 pandemic, *Publ Hlth Nurs* 37:323, 2020.

Gomez H et al: Blood lead levels of children in Flint, Michigan: 2006-2016, *The Journal of Pediatrics* 197, 158-201, 2018.

Johns Hopkins Medicine: *Emerging Infectious Diseases, 2020*, https://www.hopkinsmedicine.org/health/conditions-and-diseases/emerging-infectious-diseases. Accessed May 3, 2020.

Jordan A: *On the front lines: the role of nurses during a pandemic*, 2020, https://www.provocollege.edu/blog/on-the-front-lines-the-role-of-nurses-during-a-pandemic/. Accessed May 16, 2020.

Office of Disease Prevention and Health Promotion (ODPHP): *Global health. n.d.a*, U.S. Department of Health and Human Services. https://health.gov/healthypeople/objectives-and-data/browse-objectives/global-health. Accessed April 11, 2021.

Office of Disease Prevention and Health Promotion (ODPHP): *Healthy People 2030 Framework. n.d.b*, U.S. Department of Health and Human Services. https://www.healthypeople.gov/2020/About-Healthy-People/Development-Healthy-People-2030/Framework. Accessed April 11, 2021.

Office of Disease Prevention and Health Promotion (ODPHP): Leading health indicators. *Healthy People 2030. n.d.c*, U.S. Department of Health and Human Services. https://health.gov/healthypeople/objectives-and-data/leading-health-indicators. Accessed April 11, 2021.

Office of Disease Prevention and Health Promotion (ODPHP): Social determinants of health. *Healthy People 2030. n.d.d*, U.S. Department of Health and Human Services. https://health.gov/healthypeople/objectives-and-data/social-determinants-health. Accessed April 11, 2021.

Office of Disease Prevention and Health Promotion (ODPHP): Health care access and quality. *Healthy People 2030. n.d.e*, U.S. Department of Health and Human Services. https://health.gov/healthypeople/objectives-and-data/browse-objectives/health-care-access-and-quality. Accessed April 11, 2021.

Office of Disease Prevention and Health Promotion (ODPHP): Children. *Healthy People 2030. n.d.f*, U.S. Department of Health and Human Services. https://health.gov/healthypeople/objectives-and-data/browse-objectives/children. Accessed April 11, 2021.

The Substance Abuse and Mental Health Services Administration (SAMHSA): Housing and shelter, https://www.samhsa.gov/homelessness-programs-resources/hpr-resources/housing-shelter, 2020.

Stanhope M, Lancaster J: *Foundations for population health in community/public health nursing*, ed 5, St Louis, 2018, Elsevier.

Stanhope M, Lancaster J: *Public health nursing: population-centered health care in the community*, ed 10, St. Louis, 2020, Elsevier.

World Health Organization (WHO): *What we do*, 2020, https://www.who.int/about/what-we-do. Accessed May 3, 2020.

RESEARCH REFERENCES

Becker W, Starrels J: Prescription drug misuse: Epidemiology, prevention, identification, and management, *UpToDate*, 2020, https://www.uptodate.com/contents/prescription-drug-misuse-epidemiology-prevention-identification-and-management. Accessed July 4, 2020.

Coffin P: Prevention of lethal opioid overdose in the community, *UpToDate*, 2020, https://www.uptodate.com/contents/prevention-of-lethal-opioid-overdose-in-the-community. Accessed July 4, 2020.

Frerichs L et al.: Development of a systems science curriculum to engage rural African American teens in understanding and addressing childhood obesity prevention, *Health Educ Behav* 45(3):423–434, 2018.

Gosangi B et al: Exacerbation of physical intimate partner violence during COVID-19 pandemic, *Radiology* Jan;298(1):E38–E45, 2021. Epub 2020 Aug 13.

Isong IA et al.: Racial and ethnic disparities in early childhood obesity, *Pediatrics* 141(1):1–11, 2018.

Klish W, Skelton J: Definition, epidemiology, and etiology of obesity in children and adolescents, *UpToDate*, 2020, https://www.uptodate.com/contents/definition-epidemiology-and-etiology-of-obesity-in-children-and-adolescents. Accessed July 4, 2020.

Luesse HB et al.: Challenges and facilitators to promoting a healthy food environment and communicating effectively with parents to improve food behaviors of school children, *Matern Child Health J* 22(7):958–967, 2018.

Otterbach L et al.: Community-based childhood obesity prevention intervention for parents improves health behaviors and food parenting practices among Hispanic, low-income parents, *BMC Obesity* 5:11, 2018.

Perreault L, Apovian C: Obesity in adults: Overview of management, *UpToDate*, 2020, https://www.uptodate.com/contents/obesity-in-adults-overview-of-management. Accessed July 4, 2020.

Skelton J: Management of childhood obesity in the primary care setting, *UpToDate*, 2020, https://www.uptodate.com/contents/management-of-childhood-obesity-in-the-primary-care-setting. Accessed July 4, 2020.

Torres-Alzate H: Nursing global health competencies framework, *Nursing Education Perspectives* 40(5): 295, 2019.

Trude ACB et al.: A youth-leader program in Baltimore City recreation centers: lessons learned and applications, *Health Promot Pract* 19(1):75–85, 2018.

Theoretical Foundations of Nursing Practice

OBJECTIVES

- Explain how theory is used in nursing practice.
- Analyze the components of a theory.
- Propose examples of the four concepts included in the nursing metaparadigm.
- Summarize the evolution of nursing theory.
- Discuss types of nursing theories.
- Describe theory-based nursing practice.
- Review selected shared theories from other disciplines.
- Determine how to apply different nursing theories in different patient situations.
- Apply the National Council of State Boards of Nursing Clinical Judgment Model (NCSBN-CJM) when making clinical judgments when providing nursing care.
- Elaborate on the use of theories in nursing research.

KEY TERMS

Assumptions

Conceptual framework

Concepts

Content

Descriptive theories

Domain

Environment/situation

Feedback

Grand theories

Health

Input

Metatheory

Middle-range theories

Nursing

Nursing metaparadigm

Nursing theory

Output

Paradigm

Person

Phenomenon

Practice theories

Prescriptive theories

Shared theory

Theory

MEDIA RESOURCES

http://evolve.elsevier.com/Potter/fundamentals/
- Review Questions
- Case Study with Questions

- Audio Glossary
- Content Updates
- Answers to QSEN Activity and Review Questions

Providing patient-centered nursing care is an expectation for all nurses. As you progress through your nursing program, you will learn to apply knowledge from nursing; social, physical, and biobehavioral sciences; ethics; and health policy. Theory-based nursing practice helps you design and implement evidence-based nursing interventions that address individual and family caregiver responses to health problems. Some nurses find nursing theory difficult to understand. However, as your knowledge about theories improves, you will find that nursing theories help to describe, explain, predict, and/or prescribe nursing care measures.

Common questions nurses have about theory include: What is theory? How are nursing theories created? Why is theory important to the nursing profession? This chapter will answer these questions and help you understand how to use theory in your nursing practice.

Imagine that you are building a house. You need to complete the foundation before you start building the walls. Without a strong foundation, the house will collapse. Such is the case with nursing practice. Theory serves as the foundation for nursing care. Nurses use theory every day but are not always aware of it. For example, when a nurse ensures that a patient's room is free of clutter, excess noise, and soiled linens, the nurse is using Florence Nightingale's environmental theory to promote healing and comfort. A nurse uses Imogene King's theory of goal attainment when encouraging patients to set outcomes for their recovery. Dorothea Orem's self-care deficit theory is used when feeding or bathing a patient until the patient can do this independently. Even though the term *theory* may sound intimidating, you will find that it is a standard part of everyday nursing practice.

The scientific work used to develop theories expands the scientific knowledge of the profession. Theories offer well-grounded rationales for how and why nurses perform specific interventions and for predicting patient behaviors and outcomes. Expertise in nursing is a result of knowledge, clinical experience, and clinical judgment. Nursing knowledge improves nursing practice by connecting theory and research. Theory, research, and practice are bound together in a continuous interactive relationship (Fig. 4.1). Nurses develop theories to explain the relationship among variables. Theories may be tested through critical reasoning, description of personal experiences, and use in practice. Throughout this process new information often comes to light that indicates the need to revise a theory, and the cycle repeats (Meleis, 2018). Throughout your nursing career you need to reflect and learn from your experiences to grow professionally and use well-developed theories as a basis for your approach to patient care.

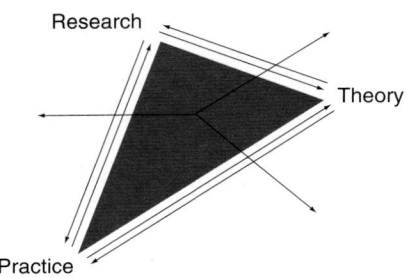

FIG. 4.1 Cyclical relationship among theory, research, and practice. (From LoBiondo-Wood G, Haber J: *Nursing research: methods for critical appraisal for evidence-based practice*, ed 9, St Louis, 2018, Elsevier.)

THEORY

What is theory? A **theory** helps explain an event by defining ideas or concepts, explaining relationships among the concepts, and predicting outcomes (McEwen and Wills, 2019). In the case of nursing, theories are designed to explain a phenomenon such as self-care or caring.

A **metatheory** is an area of study that looks at the relationships of various components that make up the knowledge of a discipline. These include philosophical, theoretical, and empirical components and provide a broad overview of discipline. Metatheory is used to derive theories and theoretical concepts (Reed and Shearer, 2018).

A **nursing theory** conceptualizes an aspect of nursing to describe, explain, predict, or prescribe nursing care (Meleis, 2018). Theories offer a framework for assessing your patients' situations. They also help you recognize and analyze cues that emerge from data. For example, if you use Orem's theory in practice, you assess and interpret data to determine patients' self-care needs, deficits, and abilities in the management of their disease. Orem's theory then guides your development of patient-centered nursing interventions.

Nursing is both a science and an art. The *science* of nursing is based on data from current research, whereas the *art* of nursing stems from a nurse's experience and the unique caring relationship that a nurse develops with a patient (Chinn and Kramer, 2018). A nursing theory helps to identify the focus, means, and goals of practice. Nursing theories enhance communication and accountability for patient care (Meleis, 2018).

Components of a Theory

A theory contains a set of concepts, definitions, and assumptions or propositions that explain a phenomenon. It explains how these elements are uniquely related to the phenomenon (Fig. 4.2). These components provide a foundation of knowledge for nurses to direct and

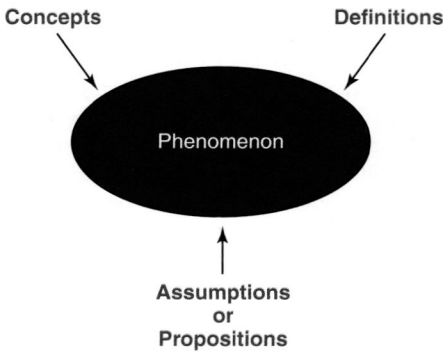

FIG. 4.2 Components of a nursing theory.

deliver caring nursing practices. Researchers test theories, and as a result they gain a clearer perspective and understanding of all parts of a phenomenon.

Phenomenon. Nursing theories focus on the phenomena of nursing and nursing care. A **phenomenon** is the term, description, or label given to describe an idea or responses about an event, a situation, a process, a group of events, or a group of situations (Meleis, 2018). Phenomena may be temporary or permanent. Examples of phenomena of nursing include caring, self-care, and patient responses to stress.

Concepts. A theory also consists of interrelated concepts that help describe or label phenomena. A concept is a thought or idea of reality that is put into words or phrases to help describe or explain a specific phenomenon (Smith and Liehr, 2018). **Concepts** can be abstract such as emotions or concrete such as physical objects (Chinn and Kramer, 2018). For example, in Meleis and colleagues' theory of transitions, abstract concepts include coping and adapting, while Nightingale described concrete concepts such as physical conditions and health care environments (Meleis, 2018). Theories use concepts to communicate meaning.

Definitions. Theorists use definitions to communicate the general meaning of the concepts of a theory. Definitions may be *theoretical/conceptual* or *operational*. Theoretical or conceptual definitions simply define a concept, much like what can be found in a dictionary, based on the theorist's perspective (Meleis, 2018; McEwen and Wills, 2019). Operational definitions state how concepts are measured (Chinn and Kramer, 2018). For example, a nursing concept *conceptually* defines pain as physical discomfort and *operationally* as a patient reporting a score of 3 or above on a pain scale of 0 to 10.

Assumptions. **Assumptions** are the "taken-for-granted" statements that explain the nature of the concepts, definitions, purpose, relationships, and structure of a theory. Assumptions are accepted as *truths* and are based on values and beliefs (Meleis, 2018). For example, Watson's transpersonal caring theory has the assumption that a conscious intention to care promotes healing and wholeness (Alligood, 2018).

The Domain of Nursing

The **domain** is the perspective or territory of a profession or discipline (Meleis, 2018). It provides the subject, central concepts, values and beliefs, phenomena of interest, and central problems of a discipline. The domain of nursing provides both a practical and a theoretical aspect of the discipline. It is the knowledge of nursing practice and nursing history, nursing theory, education, and research. The domain of nursing provides you with a comprehensive perspective that allows you to identify and treat patients' health care needs in all health care settings.

A **paradigm** is a pattern of beliefs used to describe the domain of a discipline. It links the concepts, theories, beliefs, values, and assumptions accepted and applied by the discipline (McEwen and Wills, 2019). The term **conceptual framework** is often used synonymously with paradigm. A conceptual framework provides a way to organize major concepts and visualize the relationship among phenomena. Different frameworks provide alternative ways to view the subject matter of a discipline and represent the perspective of the author. For example, the grand theorists all address similar concepts in their respective theories, but each theorist defines and describes the concepts in a different way based on the theorist's own ideas and experiences (Schmidt and Brown, 2019).

The **nursing metaparadigm** allows nurses to understand and explain what nursing *is*, what nursing *does*, and *why* nurses do what they do (Peterson and Bredow, 2017). The nursing metaparadigm includes the four concepts of person (or human beings), health, environment/situation, and nursing. **Person** is the recipient of nursing care and includes individual patients, groups, families, and communities. The person is central to the nursing care you provide. Because each person's needs are often complex, it is important to provide individualized patient-centered care. **Health** has different meanings for each patient, the clinical setting, and the health care profession (see Chapter 6). It is a state of being that people define in relation to their own values, personality, and lifestyle. It is dynamic and continuously changing. Your challenge as a nurse is to provide the best possible care based on a patient's level of health and health care needs at the time of care delivery.

Environment/situation includes all possible conditions affecting patients and the settings where they go for their health care. There is a continuous interaction between a patient and the environment. This interaction has positive and negative effects on a person's level of health and health care needs. Factors in the home, school, workplace, or community all influence the level of these needs. For example, an adolescent girl with type 1 diabetes mellitus needs to adapt her treatment plan to adjust for physical activities of school, the demands of a part-time job, and the timing of social events such as her prom.

Nursing includes "care of individuals of all ages, families, groups and communities, sick or well and in all settings. Nursing includes the promotion of health, prevention of illness, and the care of ill, disabled and dying people" (International Council of Nurses, 2021). The scope of nursing is broad. For example, a nurse does not medically diagnose a patient's health condition as heart failure. However, a nurse assesses a patient's response to the decrease in activity tolerance because of the disease and develops *nursing diagnoses* of fatigue, activity intolerance, and difficulty coping (see Chapter 17). From these nursing diagnoses the nurse creates an evidence-based patient-centered plan of care for each of the patient's health problems (see Chapter 18). Use critical thinking and clinical judgment to integrate knowledge, experience, attitudes, and standards into the individualized plan of care for each of your patients (see Chapter 15).

Evolution of Nursing Theory

How are theories created? Nursing theories often build on prior theories. Florence Nightingale is generally regarded as the first nursing theorist; her theory was founded on her belief that nursing could improve a patient's environment to facilitate recovery and prevent complications. In the Nightingale era, nurses were taught to observe each patient's condition and report changes to the physician, thus beginning the status of nursing as subservient to the physician—a sign of the Victorian era in which Nightingale lived (Chinn and Kramer, 2018).

Nursing began to transition from a vocation to a profession in the twentieth century, which prompted American nurses to standardize nursing education in diploma programs and encouraged more nurses to seek academic degrees. The first national gathering of nurses occurred at the World's Fair in Chicago in 1893, and the first edition of the *American Journal of Nursing* (AJN) was published in 1900. The "curriculum era" of nursing spanned the 1900s to the 1940s. During this period nursing education expanded beyond basic anatomy and physiology courses to include courses in the social sciences, pharmacology, and "nursing arts" that addressed nursing actions, skills, and procedures (Alligood, 2018).

The "research era" encompassed the 1950s, 1960s, and 1970s, during which nurses became increasingly involved in conducting studies and sharing their findings. The earliest research studies had a psychosocial, anthropological, or educational focus. Nurses studied their own attitudes, their relationships with other disciplines, and their functions in work and political settings. In the early years, nursing research did not explore clinical questions based on the medical model of research

because the discipline was attempting to show its uniqueness from medicine. At this same time, the "graduate education era" began, and early versions of nursing theories were developed that offered more structure to nursing research. The renowned theorists during this time included Johnson, King, Levine, Neuman, Orem, Rogers, and Roy (Alligood, 2018).

The *theory* era, which included the 1980s and 1990s, significantly contributed to knowledge development, and the nursing metaparadigm was proposed by Fawcett. This era resulted in the publication of several nursing journals, the development of nursing conferences, and the offering of more doctoral programs in nursing (Alligood, 2018).

The twenty-first century is considered the era of *theory utilization*. Today nurses strive to provide evidence-based practice (EBP), which stems from theory, research, and experience. The focus of EBP is safe, comprehensive, individualized, quality health care (see Chapter 5). The original *grand* theories served as springboards for the development of the more modern *middle-range* theories, which, through testing in research studies, provided "evidence" for EBP and promoted the translation of research into practice. Theory use is congruent with current national goals for quality health care (Alligood, 2018).

Nursing theories have changed over time in response to changes in society and the world. The environment of war was a primary factor in developing Nightingale's theory. At the other end of the nursing spectrum, Rogers' introduction of "energy fields" was developed during the 1980s when the advent of the space shuttle program brought an allure of space (Meleis, 2018).

Theorists developed their theories from their own experiences in nursing education and nursing practice and from knowledge gained from the disciplines of philosophy, sociology, psychology, and anthropology. Many nursing theorists revise their theories over time to remain current with health care changes. Such evolution shows that theories are not stagnant; rather they are dynamic and responsive to the changing environment in which we live (McEwen and Wills, 2019).

Types of Theory

The unique theories of a discipline help to distinguish the discipline from other professions. Before the development of nursing theories, nursing was considered a task-oriented occupation that functioned under the direction of the medical profession (McEwen and Wills, 2019). "The primary uses of theory are to provide insights about nursing practice situations and to guide research" and to provide a guideline or explanation of why nurses do what they do (Meleis, 2018, p. 35). Theories have different purposes and are sometimes classified by levels of abstraction (grand vs. middle-range vs. practice theories) or the goals of the theory (descriptive or prescriptive). For example, a descriptive theory describes a phenomenon such as grief or caring and identifies conditions or factors that predict when a phenomenon may occur. Prescriptive theory details nursing interventions for a specific phenomenon and the expected outcome of the interventions. Box 4.1 summarizes goals of theoretical nursing models.

BOX 4.1 Goals of Theoretical Nursing Models

- Identify domain and goals of nursing.
- Provide knowledge to improve nursing administration, practice, education, and research.
- Guide research to expand the knowledge base of nursing.
- Identify research techniques and tools used to validate nursing interventions.
- Develop curriculum plans for nursing education.
- Establish criteria for measuring quality of nursing care, education, and research.
- Guide development of a nursing care delivery system.
- Provide systematic structure and rationale for nursing activities.

Grand theories are abstract, broad in scope, and complex; therefore, they require further clarification through research so that they can be applied to nursing practice. A grand theory does not provide guidance for *specific* nursing interventions. Instead, it provides the structural framework for general, global ideas about nursing. Grand theories intend to answer the question "What is nursing?" and focus on the *whole* of nursing rather than on a *specific* type of nursing. The grand theorists developed their works based on their own experiences and the time in which they were living, which helps to explain why there is so much variation among the theories. Grand theories address the nursing metaparadigm components of person, nursing, health, and environment. For example, in Imogene King's theory of goal attainment, the focus of nursing is the interaction of human beings and the environment with an end goal of health (Meleis, 2018).

Middle-range theories are more limited in scope and less abstract. They address a specific phenomenon and reflect practice (administration, clinical, or teaching). While grand theories take a wide-angled lens perspective to nursing, middle-range theories expand on specific concepts or phenomena in a specific field of nursing such as uncertainty, incontinence, social support, quality of life, and caring (Peterson and Bredow, 2017; Smith and Liehr, 2018). For example, Kolcaba's theory of comfort encourages nurses to meet patients' needs for comfort in physical, psychospiritual, environmental, and sociocultural realms (Schmidt and Brown, 2019). Like many middle-range theories, Kolcaba's theory was based on the works of a grand theorist—in this case, Nightingale. Middle-range theories are also sometimes developed from research, nursing practice, or the theories of other disciplines (McEwen and Wills, 2019).

Practice theories, also known as situation-specific theories, bring theory to the bedside. Narrow in scope and focus, these theories guide the nursing care of a *specific* patient population at a *specific* time (Meleis, 2018). An example of a practice theory is a pain-management protocol for patients recovering from cardiac surgery. Practice theories are less abstract and are often easier to understand and apply than the grand and middle-range theories (Meleis, 2018). Fig. 4.3 demonstrates the level of abstraction for each of the grand, middle-range, and practice theory categories.

Descriptive theories are the first level of theory development. They describe phenomena and identify circumstances in which the phenomena occur (Meleis, 2018). For example, theories of growth and development describe the maturation processes of an individual at various ages (see Chapter 11). Descriptive theories do not direct specific nursing activities or attempt to produce change but rather help to explain patient assessments.

Prescriptive theories address nursing interventions for a phenomenon, guide practice change, and predict the consequences. Nurses use prescriptive theories to anticipate the outcomes of nursing interventions

(McEwen and Wills, 2019). Prescriptive theories direct nursing actions toward an explicit goal. Wiedenbach's prescriptive theory of the helping art of nursing conveys the purpose of nursing through three components: to motivate a patient, to facilitate efforts to overcome obstacles, and to develop nursing action based on the immediate situation (Meleis, 2018).

> **REFLECT NOW**
>
> Think about your most recent clinical day.
> Consider what type(s) of nursing theories you used when providing care to your patient.

Theory-Based Nursing Practice

Why is theory important to the nursing profession? Nursing knowledge is derived from basic and nursing sciences, experience, aesthetics, nurses' attitudes, and standards of practice. As nursing continues to grow as a practice-oriented profession, new knowledge is needed to prescribe specific interventions to improve patient outcomes. Nursing theories and related concepts continue to evolve. Florence Nightingale spoke with firm conviction about the "nature of nursing as a profession that requires knowledge distinct from medical knowledge" (Nightingale, 1860). The overall goal of nursing knowledge is to explain the practice of nursing as different and distinct from the practice of medicine, psychology, and other health care disciplines. Theory generates nursing knowledge for use in practice, thus supporting EBP (see Chapter 5). The integration of theory into practice leads to coordinated care delivery and therefore serves as the basis for nursing (McEwen and Wills, 2019).

The nursing process is used in clinical settings to determine individual patient needs (see Unit 3). Although the nursing process is central to nursing, it is not a theory. It provides a systematic process for the delivery of nursing care, not the knowledge component of the discipline. However, nurses use theory to provide direction in how to *use* the nursing process. For example, the theory of caring influences what nurses need to assess, how to determine patient needs, how to plan care, how to select individualized evidence-based nursing interventions, and how to evaluate patient outcomes.

SHARED THEORIES

To practice in today's health care systems, nurses need a strong scientific knowledge base from nursing and other disciplines such as the biomedical, sociological, and behavioral sciences. **Shared theory**, also known as a *borrowed* or *interdisciplinary* theory, explains a phenomenon specific to the discipline that developed the theory (McEwen and Wills, 2019). For example, Piaget's theory of cognitive development helps to explain how children think, reason, and perceive the world (see Chapter 11). Knowledge and use of this theory help pediatric nurses design appropriate therapeutic play interventions for toddlers or school-age children who are experiencing chronic illness. Knowles' adult learning theory helps a nurse plan and provide appropriate discharge teaching for a patient who is recovering from surgery.

Several nursing theories are based on systems theory. The nursing process is a system (Fig. 4.4). Like all systems, the nursing process has a specific purpose or goal (see Unit 3). The goal of the nursing process is to organize and deliver patient-centered care. As a system the nursing process has the following components: input, output, feedback, and content. **Input** for the nursing process is the data or information that comes from a patient's assessment. **Output** is the end product of a system; in the case of the nursing process, it is whether

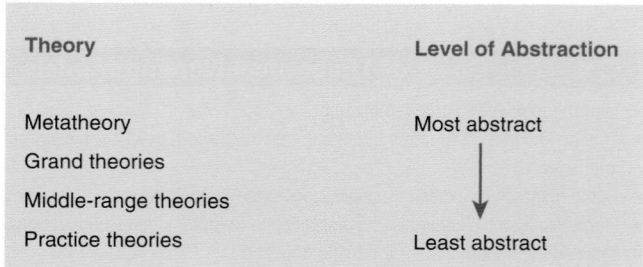

Theory	Level of Abstraction
Metatheory	Most abstract
Grand theories	
Middle-range theories	
Practice theories	Least abstract

FIG. 4.3 Correlation of theory category with level of abstraction. (From McEwen M, Wills EM: *Theoretical basis for nursing,* ed 5, Philadelphia, 2019, Wolters Kluwer Health.)

FIG. 4.4 The nursing process is a system.

the patient's health status improves, declines, or remains stable as a result of nursing care.

Feedback serves to inform a system about how it functions. For example, in the nursing process the outcomes reflect the patient's responses to nursing interventions. The outcomes are part of the feedback system to refine the plan of care. Other forms of feedback in the nursing process include responses from family members and consultation from other health care providers.

The content is the product and information obtained from the system. For example, patients with impaired bed mobility have common skin care needs and interventions (e.g., hygiene and scheduled positioning changes) that are successful in reducing the risk for pressure injuries. Table 4.1 provides an overview of additional select shared theories that are often used in nursing practice.

SELECT NURSING THEORIES

Definitions and theories of nursing can help you understand the practice of nursing. The following sections describe select theories and their concepts. See Table 4.2 for a review of additional grand and middle-range nursing theories.

Nightingale's Environmental Theory

Known as the founder of modern nursing, Florence Nightingale is credited with developing the first nursing theory. The focus of Nightingale's grand theory is a patient's environment, which Nightingale believed nurses should improve (e.g., ventilation, light, decreased noise, hygiene, nutrition) so that nature is able to restore a patient to health (McEwen and Wills, 2019). Through observation and data collection, she linked the patient's health status with environmental factors and initiated improved hygiene and sanitary conditions during the Crimean War. Nightingale taught and used the nursing process, noting that "vital observation [assessment] . . . is not for the sake of piling up miscellaneous information or curious facts, but for the sake of saving life and increasing health and comfort" (Nightingale, 1860).

Peplau's Interpersonal Theory

Hildegard Peplau is considered the mother of psychiatric nursing; the focus of her middle-range theory includes interpersonal relations among a nurse, a patient, and a patient's family and developing the nurse-patient relationship (McEwen and Wills, 2019). According to Peplau,

nurses help patients reduce anxiety by converting it into constructive actions (McEwen and Wills, 2019). Nurses develop therapeutic relationships with patients that are respectful, empathetic, and nonjudgmental (Hagerty et al., 2017). The following phases characterize the nurse-patient interpersonal relationship: preorientation (data gathering), orientation (defining issue), working phase (therapeutic activity), and resolution (termination of relationship). In developing a nurse-patient relationship, the nurse serves as a resource person, counselor, and surrogate. For example, when a patient seeks help, the nurse and patient first discuss the nature of any problems, and the nurse explains the services available. As the nurse-patient relationship develops, the nurse and patient mutually define the problems and potential solutions. When the patient's original needs are resolved, new needs sometimes emerge. This middle-range theory is useful in establishing effective nurse-patient communication when obtaining a nursing history, providing patient education, or counseling patients and their families (see Chapter 24).

Orem's Self-Care Deficit Nursing Theory

Dorothea Orem's Self-Care Deficit Nursing Theory is commonly used in nursing practice (Alligood, 2018). When applying this grand theory, a nurse continually assesses a patient's ability to perform self-care and intervenes as needed to ensure that patients meet physical, psychological, sociological, and developmental needs. According to Orem, people who participate in self-care activities are more likely to improve their health outcomes (Rutledge et al., 2019; Rezaeean et al., 2020). Nursing care becomes necessary when patients are unable to fulfill biological, psychological, developmental, or social needs. Nurses continually assess and determine why patients are unable to meet these needs, identify goals to help them, intervene to help them perform self-care, and evaluate how much self-care they can perform. For example, a patient may need a nurse to provide a bath or assist with feeding during acute illness, but as the patient's condition improves, the nurse encourages the patient to begin doing these activities independently.

> **REFLECT NOW**
>
> Consider Orem's Self-Care Deficit Nursing Theory. How can you apply this theory to promote recovery in your patient?

TABLE 4.1 Overview of Select Shared Theories

Theory Categories	Focus	Application To Nursing
Human needs	Need motivates human behavior. Maslow's hierarchy of basic human needs includes five levels of priority (e.g., physiological, safety and security, love and belonging, self-esteem, and self-actualization) (see Chapter 6; Fig. 6.3).	Basic physiological and safety needs are usually a patient's first priority, especially when the patient is dependent on others to meet these needs. When a patient has no emergent physical or safety needs, the nurse gives high priority to psychological, sociocultural, developmental, or spiritual needs. Patients entering the health care system generally have unmet needs. A patient in pain after surgery (basic need) is not ready for discharge teaching (higher-level need) until the pain is relieved. The hierarchy of needs is a way to plan for individualized patient care (McEwen and Wills, 2019).
Stress/adaptation	Humans respond to actual or perceived threats by adapting to maintain function and life.	Patients demonstrate a similar pattern of reacting to stress through physiological and psychological responses. Failure to adapt to stress can lead to exhaustion and decline in health. Nurses need to understand the reaction of body and mind to stress and intervene to help patients develop methods of coping/adapting to prevent or manage illness and disease (Alligood, 2018).
Developmental	Humans have a common pattern of growth and development.	Human growth and development are orderly, predictive processes that begin with conception and continue through death. Varieties of well-tested theories describe and predict behavior and development at various phases of the life continuum (McEwen and Wills, 2019).
Biomedical	Theory explains causes of disease; principles related to physiology.	Nurses must have knowledge of theories from the fields of biology, medicine, public health, physiology, and pharmacology to provide holistic patient care, promote health, and prevent illness (McEwen and Wills, 2019).
Psychosocial	Theory explains and/or predicts human responses within the physiological, psychological, sociocultural, developmental, and spiritual domains.	Nursing is a diverse discipline that strives to meet holistic needs of patients. Chapter 9 discusses models for understanding cultural diversity and implementing care to meet the diverse needs of the patient. Chapter 10 describes family theory and how to meet the needs of the family when the family is the patient or the caregiver. Chapter 36 discusses several models of grieving and demonstrates how to help patients through loss, death, and grief.
Educational	Theory explains the teaching-learning process by examining behavioral, cognitive, and adult learning principles.	Nurses provide education to patients, families, community groups, and members of the health care team. A basic understanding of various teaching-learning theories is critical for this aspect of the professional nursing role (Butts and Rich, 2018).
Leadership/management	Theory promotes organization, change, power/empowerment, motivation, conflict management, and decision making.	Nurses often assume leadership positions in the health care realm and as such are expected to effectively manage individuals and groups to promote change and improve quality care and outcomes (McEwen and Wills, 2019).

Leininger's Culture Care Theory

As early as the 1950s Madeleine Leininger recognized the need to focus on culture in nursing as she predicted that nursing and health care would become more global. She blended her background in anthropology with nursing to form her middle-range theory of cultural care diversity and universality (Alligood, 2018). Human caring varies among cultures in its expressions, processes, and patterns. Social structure factors such as a patient's politics, culture, and traditions are significant forces affecting care and influencing the patient's health and illness patterns. Think about the diversity of patients and their nursing care needs (see Chapter 9). The major concept of Leininger's theory is cultural diversity, and the goal of nursing care is to provide a patient with culturally specific nursing care (Alligood, 2018). To provide care to patients of unique cultures, nurses safely integrate their cultural traditions, values, and beliefs into a plan of care. Leininger's theory recognizes the importance of culture and its influence on everything that involves a patient, including health beliefs, the role of family and community, and dietary practices (Alligood, 2018). For example, some cultures believe that the leader of the community needs to be present during health care decisions. As a result, a health care team needs to reschedule when rounds occur to include the community leader. In addition, symptom expression also differs among cultures. One patient might be stoic and not complain about pain, whereas a person from a different culture might be very vocal about pain. In both cases a nurse needs to skillfully incorporate the patient's cultural practices in assessing the level of pain (e.g., asking, "Is the pain getting worse or remaining the same?").

QSEN **Building Competency in Patient-Centered Care** You are caring for a high school student who was in a motor vehicle accident on the way to spring break. The parents are not present. The patient has not previously been hospitalized and has never been away from home this long. How could you use *Peplau's interpersonal theory* when caring for this patient?

Answers to QSEN Activities can be found on the Evolve website.

TABLE 4.2   Overview of Select Grand and Middle-Range Nursing Theories

Theory Category	Theorist	Focus	Application
Grand theory	Henderson	Principles and practice of nursing	Nurses assist patients with 14 activities (e.g., breathing, eating/drinking, elimination, movement/positioning, sleep/rest, clothing, body temperature, hygiene, safety, communication, play, work, worship, learning) until patients can meet these needs for themselves or they help patients have a peaceful death (Butts and Rich, 2018; McEwen and Wills, 2019).
	Johnson	Behavioral system	Nurses perceive patients as being more important than their disease; a patient is viewed as a collection of subsystems that form an overall behavioral system focused on meeting basic drives of achievement, affiliation, aggression/protection, dependence, elimination, ingestion, sex, and restoration. The goal of nursing is to help the patient attain/maintain balance, function, and stability in each of the subsystems (Butts and Rich, 2018).
	Neuman	Systems	Nurses view a patient (physical, psychological, sociocultural, developmental, and spiritual) as being an open system that is in constant energy exchange with both internal and external environments. Nurses help a patient (individual, group, family, or community) cope with intrapersonal, interpersonal, and extrapersonal *stressors* that can break through the patient's line of defense and cause illness. The role of nursing is to stabilize a patient or situation, and the focus is on *wellness* and *prevention* of disease (McEwen and Wills, 2019).
	Abdellah	Patient-centered care	Nurses address 21 "nursing problems" to meet patients' physical, psychological, and social needs and should strive to *know* each patient. Nurses use knowledge constructed from previous experiences to determine a general plan of care and then personalize the plan to the patient to provide *patient-centered care*. A nurse also involves a patient's family in the plan of care when appropriate (McEwen and Wills, 2019).
	King	Goal attainment	Nurses view a patient as a unique personal system that is constantly interacting/transacting with other systems (e.g., nurse, family, friends); nurses help patients become active participants in their care by working *with* them to establish goals for attaining, restoring, or maintaining health (McEwen and Wills, 2019).
	Roy	Adaptation	Nurses help a patient cope with or adapt to changes in physiological, self-concept, role function, and interdependence domains (Alligood, 2018).
	Watson	Caring	Caring is a fundamental component of professional nursing practice and is based on 10 *carative factors* (see Chapter 7). The purpose of nursing is to understand the interrelationships among health, illness, and human behavior rather than focus on the disease-cure model. Caring occurs when a nurse and patient engage in a *transpersonal relationship* that facilitates the patient's ability for self-healing (Alligood, 2018).
	Rogers/Parse/Newman	Unitary beings/human becoming/ expanding consciousness	Nurses view a patient as a unique, dynamic energy field in constant energy exchange with the environment; nursing care focuses on helping patients use their *own* potential to identify and alter personal rhythms/patterns (e.g., eating, breathing, sleeping) to promote and maintain health. Nurses understand that patients are responsible for their own health and that health stems from how patients live their lives in accordance with their own values; the nurse's role is to be truly *present* with patients and accept their view of reality while providing guidance to them in making health-related choices in accordance with their belief system (McEwen and Wills, 2019).
Middle-range theory	Benner	Skill acquisition	Nurses progress through five stages of skill acquisition: novice, advanced beginner, competent, proficient, and expert (Butts and Rich, 2018).
	Kolcaba	Comfort	Nurses facilitate health-seeking behaviors in patients by striving to relieve physical, emotional, social, environmental, and/or spiritual distress (McEwen and Wills, 2019).
	Pender	Health promotion	Nurses understand that patients' personal characteristics, experiences, and beliefs affect motivation for adopting healthy behaviors (see Chapter 6) (McEwen and Wills, 2019).
	American Association of Critical-Care Nurses	Synergy	Matching nurse competencies to patient needs in the critical care environment improves patient outcomes (McEwen and Wills, 2019).
	Meleis, Sawyer, Im, Messias, and Schumacher	Transitions	Patients are more vulnerable during changes in health and illness. Nurses can facilitate healthy *transitions* through the development of nursing interventions specific to each patient—for example, a patient's transition from living at home to a nursing home due to declining health (Alligood, 2018).

The National Council of State Boards of Nursing Clinical Judgment Model

Nurses must use clinical judgment to make sound decisions when providing patient care. The National Council of State Boards of Nursing Clinical Judgment Model (NCSBN-CJM) was developed to help guide nursing educators in evaluating nursing students' abilities to make the clinical judgments necessary when providing competent nursing care (Dickison et al., 2019). Building upon other nursing theories related to critical thinking, clinical judgment, and decision making (see Chapter 6), the NCSBN-CJM is a model with multiple layers that help explain the cognitive process nurses use to make clinical judgments to guide their care (Fig. 4.5). Layers 3 and 4 describe the cognitive process that nurses use to make decisions for layer 2. If the patient does not respond positively to nursing care, the nurse moves through the cognitive processes in layers 3 and 4 again. Nursing clinical judgment in layer 1 impacts the nurse's clinical decisions made based on the patient's needs at layer 0. Nurses and nursing students repeat the six steps included in layer 3. Their competence improves over time as their level of nursing experience and clinical exposure increase. Layer 4 consists of individual and environmental factors that when combined with layer 3 inform a nurse's clinical judgment.

Nursing students can use this model to learn how to think like a nurse and make safe clinical decisions to positively influence patient care and patient outcomes. Nursing faculty can use this model to teach nursing students how to make complex decisions and provide safe care in an ever-changing health care environment. Additionally, the NCSBN plans to use this model to create the Next Generation NCLEX (NGN) exam, which all nursing graduates in the United States will need to pass to obtain a license to practice as a registered nurse (NCSBN, 2021).

LINKS AMONG THEORY AND KNOWLEDGE DEVELOPMENT AND RESEARCH IN NURSING

Nursing has its own body of knowledge that is both theoretical and experiential. You acquire nursing knowledge by learning from, thinking about, and reflecting on your clinical experiences. Experiential or clinical knowledge, often called the *art* of nursing, is formed from nurses' clinical experience. Theoretical knowledge stimulates deeper thinking and creates a broad understanding of nursing science and practice (Alligood, 2018). Both types of knowledge are needed to provide safe, comprehensive nursing care.

Nursing theories guide nursing practice (McEwen and Wills, 2019). When using theory-based nursing practice, you apply the principles of a theory in delivering nursing interventions. Grand theories help shape and define your practice, middle-range theories continue to advance nursing knowledge through nursing research, and practice theories help you provide specific care for individuals and groups of diverse populations and situations (Peterson and Bredow, 2017).

Research validates, refutes, supports, and/or modifies theory, while theory stimulates nurse scientists to explore significant issues in nursing

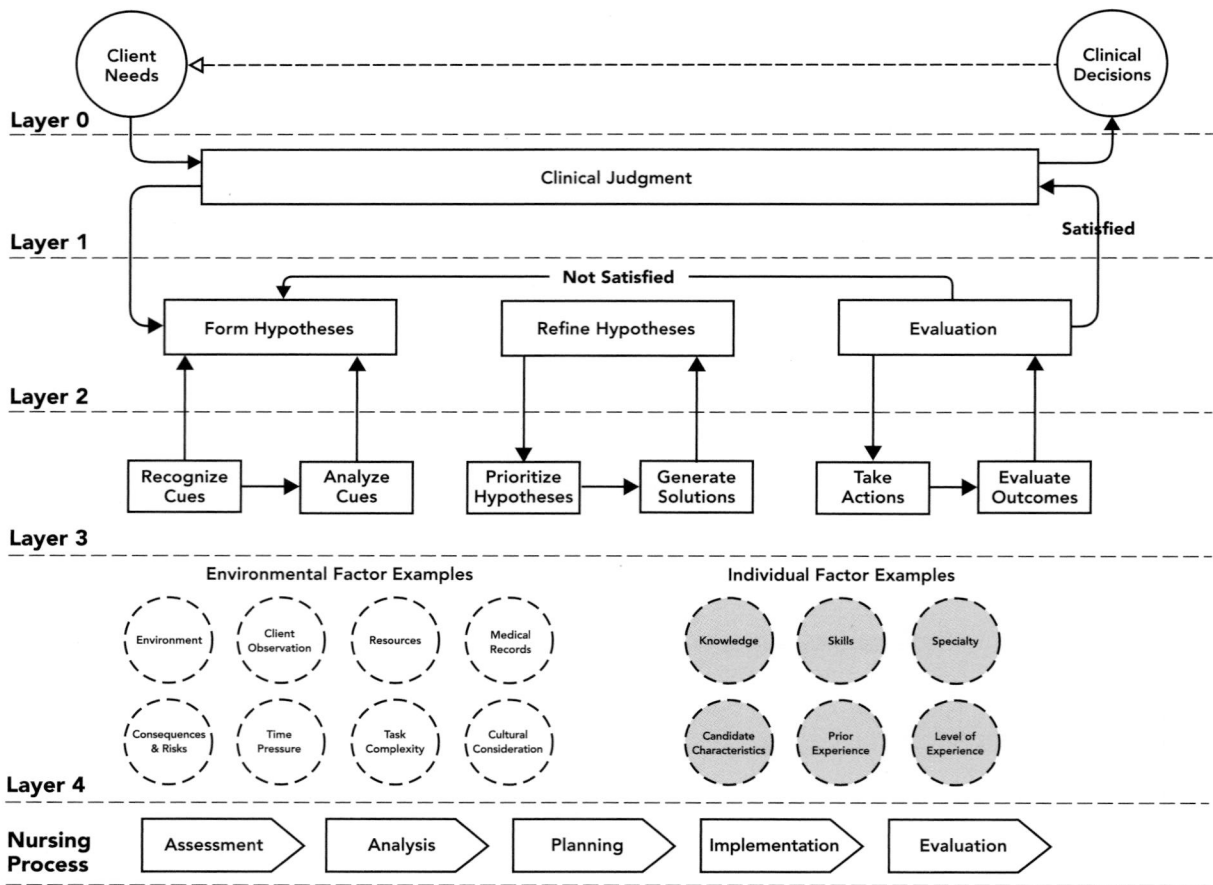

FIG. 4.5 The National Council of State Boards of Nursing Clinical Judgment Model (NCSBN-CJM). (From NCSBN: The NGN Clinical Judgment Measurement Model and Action Model, 2019, https://www.ncsbn.org/13444.htm. Accessed February 21, 2021.)

practice (McEwen and Wills, 2019; Meleis, 2018). The relationship between nursing theory and nursing research builds the scientific knowledge base of nursing, which is then applied to practice. Nurses better understand the appropriate use of a theory to improve patient care as more research is conducted. The relationships among the components of a theory often help identify research questions and determine the overall design of a study. For example, nurse researchers used Peplau's interpersonal theory as the framework for a project to improve the communication within a health care team. The aim of the project was to increase health care staff teamwork and communication (Holtmann, 2018). Table 4.3 provides some examples of how theories are used in nursing research. Nurses consider findings from theory-based research to determine whether the theory can be used in practice.

Sometimes research is used to develop new theories (Meleis, 2018). *Theory-generating* research uses logic to explore relationships among phenomena (McEwen and Wills, 2019). In theory-generating research an investigator makes observations (*without* any preconceived ideas) to view a phenomenon in a new way. Middle-range theories are often developed in this manner. For example, the middle-range theory of chronic sorrow stemmed from a researcher's initial observations of cyclic periods of sadness in parents of children with intellectual or developmental disabilities (Batchelor and Duke, 2019).

Theory-testing research determines how accurately a theory describes a nursing phenomenon. Testing develops the evidence for describing or predicting patient outcomes. A researcher has *some* preconceived idea as to how patients describe or respond to a phenomenon and generates research questions or hypotheses to test the assumptions of the theory. No one study tests *all* components of a theory; researchers test the theory through a variety of research activities. For example, nurse researchers studied Kolcaba's middle-range nursing theory of comfort when investigating how the perception of comfort experienced by older adults who lived in an extended care facility influenced their feelings of well-being (Gaibor et al., 2021).

Both theory-generating and theory-testing research refine the knowledge base of nursing. In turn, nurses incorporate research-based interventions into theory-based practice (Box 4.2). As research activities continue, not only do the knowledge and science of nursing increase, but patients receive high-quality evidence-based nursing care (see Chapter 5). As an art, nursing relies on knowledge gained from practice and reflection on past experiences. The "expert nurse" translates both the art and science of nursing into the realm of *creative caring*, which takes the extra step of individualizing care to the specific

TABLE 4.3 Theories Used in Nursing Practice and Research

Theory	Main Concepts Utilized in Research Example	Example of Use in Research
Kolcaba's theory of comfort	Enhanced comfort	Kolcaba's theory was used to better understand how older adults' perception of comfort is related to feelings of well-being (Gaibor et al., 2021).
AACN Synergy Model	Nurse competencies, environmental factors, patient characteristics	Clinical judgment and duration of transport were found to influence patient safety during critical care transport (Swickard et al., 2018).
Mishel's uncertainty in illness theory	Appraisal and management of uncertainty	Study results indicate that young adults with congenital heart disease are at risk for posttraumatic stress disorder (PTSD) and long-term stress due to chronic uncertainty (Moreland and Santacroce, 2018).
Meleis et al.'s transitions theory	Nursing therapeutics (assessment of readiness, preparation for transition, role supplementation), mindfulness	A mindfulness-based transition program was applied to mothers with premature rupture of membranes to measure acceptance of pregnancy, readiness to give birth, maternal attachment, and competency in the role of motherhood (Korukcu and Kukulu, 2017).

AACN, American Association of Critical-Care Nurses.

BOX 4.2 EVIDENCE-BASED PRACTICE

Theory-Based Practice in the Management of First-time Parents

PICOT Question: In patients experiencing their first pregnancy, how does application of Meleis' theory of transitions compared to no specific theory application influence a healthy transition to parenthood?

Evidence Summary

The transition to parenthood is a life-changing and often challenging time. Successful transitioning to the role of a parent can be accomplished by gaining confidence, planning for the birth, and developing a strong support system (Barimani et al., 2017; Korukcu and Kukulu, 2017). According to Meleis et al.'s theory of transitions, a transition is required when one's reality is interrupted, causing the need for a change and a new reality to be formed (Fitzpatrick and Tzouvara, 2019). Transitions theory can be applied to various types of transitions: developmental, health-illness, situational, and organizational. Nurses can assist expectant parents by providing professional support during the prenatal period. Expectant parents will require information regarding birth plans, feeding routines, maternal and child appointments, and routine testing before birth (Barimani et al., 2017). It is important for parents to be engaged in all decisions and for the nurse to understand and meet the parents' psychosocial needs, especially if they are experiencing a miscarriage or if their child is born with a serious health condition such as congenital heart disease (Elliott et al., 2021). Nursing actions based on Meleis et al.'s theory can assist patients in managing life's transitions (Elliott et al., 2021; Hua et al., 2021).

Application to Nursing Practice
- Ensure that expectant parents are knowledgeable about health care access in the prenatal period (Barimani et al., 2017).
- Help patients identify support groups in the community, allowing expectant parents to share knowledge and emotions with others (Barimani et al., 2017).
- Provide new-parent education that covers expectations, coping behaviors, and changes in relationships to facilitate successful transitions (Elliott et al., 2021).
- Recognize that a first-time parent's level of self-confidence may change during the pregnancy (Barimani et al., 2017; Korukcu and Kukulu, 2017).

needs of each patient. For example, a nurse provides creative caring when arranging for a patient who is in the hospital to visit with a beloved pet or in finding a way to honor a patient's wish to die at home.

Theory is the foundation of nursing; it defines our unique profession and sets it apart from other disciplines. Theory provides a basis for research and practice and serves as a guide in providing safe, comprehensive, individualized care, which is the hallmark of nursing. As you progress in your nursing education and practice, you will use theory in a variety of ways. Keep in mind that these theories apply not only to patient care but are useful in communicating with other members of the health care team.

> **REFLECT NOW**
>
> Analyze the nursing program you are enrolled in to determine what theories are reflected in the nursing program and nursing curriculum.

KEY POINTS

- Nurses use theory to describe, explain, predict, or prescribe nursing care.
- The components of a theory provide a foundation for knowledge for nurses to direct and deliver nursing care.
- The nursing metaparadigm includes the four concepts of person, health, environment/situation, and nursing, which allows nurses to understand what nursing is, what nursing does, and why nurses do what they do.
- Theories are dynamic and responsive to the changing environment in which we live.
- The types of nursing theories include grand theories, middle-range theories, practice theories, and descriptive and prescriptive theories.
- The integration of theory into practice leads to coordinated care delivery.
- Nurses need a strong scientific knowledge base from nursing and other disciplines, such as the biomedical, sociological, and behavioral sciences.
- Grand and middle-range nursing theories can help you understand the practice of nursing.
- The National Council of State Boards of Nursing Clinical Judgment Model (NCSBN-CJM) builds upon other nursing theories and can be used to guide your critical thinking, clinical judgment and decision making while planning and providing patient care.
- The relationship between theory and research builds the scientific knowledge base of nursing, which is then applied to practice.

REFLECTIVE LEARNING

- Reflect on a patient you recently were assigned to care for during a clinical or simulation experience. Describe how you did or could have applied Nightingale's environmental theory while you were caring for this patient.
- Reflect on a patient with a chronic health condition you were recently assigned to care for during a clinical or simulation experience. Explain how you would apply the National Council of State Boards of Nursing Clinical Judgment Model (NCSBN-CJM) to plan patient care, help this patient prevent complications, and promote disease management.

- Reflect on a patient you were assigned to care for in a recent clinical or simulation experience who required total patient care. Describe how you would apply Orem's self-care deficit theory for this patient.

REVIEW QUESTIONS

1. The components of the nursing metaparadigm include:
   1. Person, health, environment, and theory.
   2. Health, theory, concepts, and environment.
   3. Nurses, physicians, health, and patient needs.
   4. Person, health, environment, and nursing.
2. Theory is essential to nursing practice because it: (Select all that apply.)
   1. Contributes to nursing knowledge.
   2. Predicts patient behaviors in situations.
   3. Provides a means of assessing patient vital signs.
   4. Guides nursing practice.
   5. Formulates health care legislation.
   6. Explains relationships between concepts.
3. A nurse ensures that each patient's room is clean; well ventilated; and free from clutter, excessive noise, and extremes in temperature. Which theorist's work is the nurse practicing in this example?
   1. Henderson
   2. Orem
   3. King
   4. Nightingale
4. A nurse is caring for a patient admitted to the neurological unit with the diagnosis of a stroke and right-sided weakness. The nurse assumes responsibility for bathing and feeding the patient until the patient can begin performing these activities. The nurse in this situation is applying the theory developed by:
   1. Johnson.
   2. Orem.
   3. Roy.
   4. Peplau.
5. Match the following types of theory with the appropriate description.

   ____ 1. Middle-range theory   a. Very abstract; attempts to describe nursing in a global context

   ____ 2. Shared theory   b. Specific to a particular situation; brings theory to the bedside

   ____ 3. Grand theory

   ____ 4. Practice theory   c. Applies theory from other disciplines to nursing practice

      d. Addresses a specific phenomenon and reflects practice

6. Match the following descriptions with the appropriate grand theorist.

   ____ 1. King   a. Based on the theory that focuses on *wellness* and *prevention* of disease

   ____ 2. Henderson

   ____ 3. Orem   b. Based on the belief that people who participate in self-care activities are more likely to improve their health outcomes

   ____ 4. Neuman

      c. Based on 14 activities, the belief that the nurse should assist patients with meeting needs until they are able to do so independently

      d. Based on the belief that nurses should work with patients to develop goals for care

7. Which of the following statements related to theory-based nursing practice are correct? (Select all that apply.)
   1. Nursing theory differentiates nursing from other disciplines.
   2. Nursing theories are standardized and do not change over time.
   3. Integrating theory into practice promotes coordinated care delivery.
   4. Nursing knowledge is generated by theory.
   5. The theory of nursing process is used in planning patient care.
   6. Evidence-based practice results from theory-testing research.
8. A nurse is caring for a patient who recently lost a leg in a motor vehicle accident. The nurse best assists the patient to cope with this situation by applying which of the following theories?
   1. Roy
   2. Watson
   3. Johnson
   4. Benner
9. Using Maslow's hierarchy of needs, identify the priority for a patient who is experiencing chest pain and difficulty breathing.
   1. Self-actualization
   2. Air, water, and nutrition
   3. Safety
   4. Esteem and self-esteem needs
10. A nurse is analyzing data generated during a patient assessment to determine the best plan of care. Which layer of the NCSBN-CJM best describes the cognitive process being used by the nurse at this time?
    1. Layer 0
    2. Layer 1
    3. Layer 2
    4. Layer 3
    5. Layer 4

Answers: 1. 4; **2.** 1, 2, 4, 6; **3.** 4; **4.** 2; **5.** 1d, 2c, 3a, 4b; **6.** 1d, 2c, 3b, 4a; **7.** 1, 3, 4, 6; **8.** 1; **9.** 2; **10.** 4.

Rationales for Review Questions can be found on the Evolve website.

REFERENCES

Alligood MR: *Nursing theorists and their work*, ed 9, St Louis, 2018, Elsevier.

Batchelor LL, Duke, G: Chronic sorrow in parents with chronically ill children, *Pediatric Nursing*, 45(4), 163, 183, 2019.

Butts JB, Rich KL: *Philosophies and theories for advanced nursing practice*, ed 3, Burlington, MA, 2018, Jones & Bartlett Learning.

Chinn PL, Kramer MK: *Knowledge development in nursing: theory and process*, ed 10, St Louis, 2018, Elsevier.

Dickison P et al: Integrating the National Council of State Boards of Nursing Clinical Judgment Model into Nursing Educational Frameworks, *Journal of Nursing Education*, 58(2):72, 2019.

International Council of Nurses.: *Who we are: definition of nursing*, ©2018, International Council of Nurses, 2021. https://www.icn.ch/nursing-policy/nursing-definitions. Accessed February 21, 2021.

McEwen M, Wills EM: *Theoretical basis for nursing*, ed 5, Philadelphia,, 2019, Wolters Kluwer Health.

Meleis AI: *Theoretical nursing: development & progress*, ed 6, Philadelphia, 2018, Wolters Kluwer.

National Council of State Boards of Nursing (NCSBN): Next generation NCLEX project, 2021, https://www.ncsbn.org/next-generation-nclex.htm. Accessed February 21, 2021.

Nightingale F: *Notes on nursing: what it is and what it is not*, London, 1860, Harrison & Sons.

Peterson SJ, Bredow TS: *Middle range theories: application to nursing research and practice*, ed 4, Philadelphia, 2017, Wolters Kluwer.

Reed PG, Shearer NBC: *Nursing knowledge and theory innovation: advancing the science of practice*, ed 2, New York, 2018, Springer.

Schmidt NA, Brown JM: *Evidence-based practice for nurses: appraisal and application of research*, ed 4, Burlington, MA, 2019, Jones and Bartlett.

Smith MJ, Liehr PR: *Middle range theory for nursing*, ed 4, New York, 2018, Springer.

RESEARCH REFERENCES

Barimani M et al.: Facilitating and inhibiting factors in transition to parenthood – ways in which health professionals can support parents, *Scand J Caring Sci* 31(3):537, 2017.

Elliott M et al: Defining a new normal: a qualitative exploration of the parent experience during the single ventricle congenital heart disease interstage period, *J Adv Nurs* 77(5):2437, 2021.

Gaibor DM et al.: Stories of the elderly in relation to Katharine Kolcaba's Theory (Chillanes-Ecuador). *J Adv Pharm Edu Res* 11(1):48, 2021. Available at: https://japer.in/storage/models/article/JFVPzYs0La6s-VQLS38exY5cCA4siLPl7EbP8tlsBD2Shy0UbRYcuCw2mhlMV/stories-of-the-elderly-in-relation-to-katharine-kolcabas-theory.pdf. Accessed February 21, 2021.

Fitzpatrick JM, Tzouvara F: Facilitators and inhibitors of transition for older people who have relocated to a long-term care facility: a systematic review, *Health & Social Care in the Community* 27(3):e57, 2019.

Hagerty TA et al.: Peplau's theory of interpersonal relations: an alternative factor structure for patient experience data? *Nurs Sci Q* 30(2):160, 2017.

Holtmann M: Does the utilization of interactive learning during TeamSTEPPS SBAR, CUS, and debriefing tool sessions increase the perceptions of teamwork and communication in the hospital setting? (Doctoral project), Retrieved from *ProQuest Dissertations & Theses Global*, 2018 (Order No. 10792142).

Hua W et al.: Understanding preparation for preterm infant discharge from parents' and healthcare providers' perspectives: challenges and opportunities. *J Adv Nurs* 77(3):1379, 2021.

Korukcu O, Kukulu K: The effect of the mindfulness-based transition to motherhood program in pregnant women with preterm premature rupture of membranes, *Health Care for Women International* 38(7):765, 2017.

Moreland P, Santacroce SJ: Illness uncertainty and posttraumatic stress in young adults with congenital heart disease, *J Cardiovasc Nurs* 33(4):356, 2018.

Rezaeean S et al.: The effect of prenatal self-care based on Orem's theory on preterm birth occurrence in women at risk for preterm birth, *Iran J Nurs Midwifery Res* 25(3): 242, 2020. Available at: https://www.ncbi.nlm.nih.gov/pmc/articles/PMC7299423/. Accessed on February 21, 2021.

Rutledge P et al.: The relationship between family support, self-care, and health outcomes in selected African-American females with type 2 diabetes, *The Journal of the National Black Nurses Association*, 30(2):1, 2019. Available at: https://www.researchgate.net/profile/Zina-Mcgee/publication/342278555_The_Relationship_Between_Family_Support_Self-Care_and_Health_Outcomes_in_Selected_African-American_Females_with_Type_2_Diabetes/links/5eeb9c2292851ce9e7ed2a09/The-Relationship-Between-Family-Support-Self-Care-and-Health-Outcomes-in-Selected-African-American-Females-with-Type-2-Diabetes.pdf. Accessed February 21, 2021.

Swickard S et al.: Patient safety events during critical care transport, *Air Med J* 37(4):253, 2018.

Evidence-Based Practice

OBJECTIVES

- Discuss the benefits of evidence-based practice.
- Explain the relationship between evidence-based practice and clinical judgment.
- Explain the steps of evidence-based practice.
- Develop a PICOT question.
- Summarize the levels of evidence available in the literature.
- Discuss how nurses apply evidence in practice.
- Discuss the steps of the research process.
- Summarize the characteristics of quantitative research methods.
- Summarize the characteristics of qualitative research methods.
- Elaborate on how nursing research improves nursing practice.
- Explain the purpose of translation research in nursing.
- Discuss how performance improvement (PI) affects health care.
- Compare the similarities and differences among evidence-based practice, research, and performance improvement.

KEY TERMS

Active errors

Bias

Confidentiality

Empirical data

Evaluation research

Evidence-based practice (EBP)

Experimental study

Generalizability

Hypotheses

Inductive reasoning

Informed consent

Latent errors

Nursing research

Peer-reviewed

Performance improvement (PI)

PICOT question

Qualitative nursing research

Quantitative nursing research

Reliability

Sampling error

Scientific method

Sentinel event

Validity

Variables

MEDIA RESOURCES

http://evolve.elsevier.com/Potter/fundamentals/
- Review Questions
- Audio Glossary
- Case Study with Questions
- Content Updates
- Answers to QSEN Activity and Review Questions

Many nurses practice nursing according to what they learned in nursing school, their experiences in practice, and the policies and procedures (P&Ps) of their health care agency. These approaches to practice alone do not guarantee that nursing practice is always based on up-to-date scientific information. Sometimes P&Ps, for example, are based on tradition and not on current evidence. A wealth of new scientific information regarding nursing practice and the health care problems nurses encounter is being developed daily. Nursing practice is in an "age of accountability," in which nursing care affects the quality, safety, and cost of health care. People are more informed about their own health and the incidence of medical errors within health care agencies. Health care agencies are required to show their commitment to each health care stakeholder (e.g., patients, insurance companies, governmental agencies) to reduce health care errors and improve safety by putting into place evidence-based safe practices (National Quality Forum, 2020). The American Nurses Association's (ANA) *Nursing: Scope and Standards for Practice (2021)* state that nursing knowledge and scholarly inquiry occur on a continuum of scholarship to evidence-based practice to research. Standard 14 of professional performance states that the "registered nurse integrates scholarship, evidence and research findings into practice" (ANA, 2021, p. 100). Nurses and other health care providers can no longer accept traditional practices and practice the status quo. Nurses need to better understand the scientific reasoning behind why certain health care approaches are used, which ones work, and which ones do not. This involves the application of the most current and relevant scientific evidence available.

Research priorities identified by nurse administrators include nursing workforce and nursing workflow, communication, interprofessional collaboration, patient and family satisfaction, prevention of hospital-acquired infections, improving patient outcomes, and patient safety (Sun and Prufeta, 2019). Evidence-based practice (EBP) guides nurses' clinical judgments in making effective, timely, and appropriate clinical decisions.

Cathy and Tom are two nurses who work in the surgical intensive care unit (ICU). They are members of the interprofessional unit practice committee (UPC) that meets monthly to discuss practice issues and quality indicators for the unit. Cathy notes that the monthly quality report shows an increased incidence of central line–associated bloodstream infections (CLABSIs) over each of the past 3 months. Patients with central venous catheters (CVCs) that are used to deliver fluids and medications are becoming infected, but why? Tom questions whether the problem is related to the type of dressing placed over catheters or the way sites are cleansed before insertion. The occurrence of CLABSIs is considered a "hospital-acquired condition" (HAC), a condition that (1) is high cost or high volume or both, (b) results in the assignment of a case to a diagnosis- related group (DRG) that has a higher payment when present as a secondary diagnosis, and (c) could reasonably have been prevented through the application of evidence-based guidelines (Centers for Medicare and Medicaid Services [CMS], 2020a). All conditions classified as HACs are monitored by hospitals as quality measures because payments to hospitals that rank in the worst-performing 25% of all hospitals with respect to HAC quality measures are adjusted (CMS, 2020b). Thus because CLABSIs are considered an HAC, a hospital is reimbursed less by Medicare and other payers. It is important for the UPC to find ways to prevent CLABSIs from occurring. The UPC decides to explore these questions as part of its evidence-based practice (EBP) process. The first step is to develop a clinical question to efficiently search the scientific literature. Tom volunteers to do the search with the aid of the hospital librarian. The aim is to determine what evidence is available so that the committee can make an informed decision about standards needed to reduce CLABSIs in their patients.

THE NEED FOR EVIDENCE-BASED PRACTICE

Nursing practice involves the application of critical thinking in the making of clinical judgments that guides nurses' decision making (see Unit 3). Scientific knowledge is an integral element of critical thinking, as it guides how nurses interpret information about patients, identify problems, and select nursing interventions. **Evidence-based practice (EBP)** is a problem-solving approach to clinical practice that combines the deliberate and systematic use of best evidence in combination with a clinician's expertise, patient preferences and values, and available health care resources in making decisions about patient care (Fig. 5.1) (Melnyk and Fineout-Overholt, 2019). Put in simpler terms, EBP involves nurses addressing clinical problems by looking for the very best knowledge and scientific and clinical evidence that are available for treating or managing patient problems and implementing changes in

practice. Research studies show that EBP enhances the patient experience and patient satisfaction, decreases cost, empowers clinicians, and improves patient outcomes (Melnyk and Fineout-Overholt, 2019; Skaggs et al., 2018). Use of EBP competencies by nurses and advanced practice nurses further improves the quality and consistency of health care (Melnyk et al., 2017).

Nurses regularly face important clinical decisions when caring for patients (e.g., What further assessment information do I require? Why do I use the approach in this policy in providing patient care? Is a change in practice needed? Is there a way to improve patient outcomes?). Implementing health care processes or practices that are known to work (evidence based) in a reliable way is a feature of "quality care" and effective timely and appropriate clinical decisions (Chiwaula et al., 2018). Implementing new knowledge into nursing practice requires a systematic approach that applies evidence to improve clinical, educational, and administrative practices. EBP is one of the Quality and Safety Education for Nurses (QSEN) competencies. The overall goal of the QSEN initiative is to prepare nurses in prelicensure and graduate programs with the knowledge, skills, and attitudes (KSAs) necessary to continuously improve the quality and safety of the health care systems where they work (QSEN, 2020). Following this, Melnyk et al. (2017) developed and validated 12 EBP competencies considered essential for practicing registered nurses (RNs) and an additional 11 competencies essential for practicing advanced practice nurses. These EBP competencies are foundational for delivering high-quality care.

There are many sources of evidence-based knowledge. A textbook incorporates evidence into the information, practice guidelines, and procedures it includes. Articles from nursing and health care literature are available on almost any topic involving nursing practice in either journals or on the Internet. Although the scientific basis of nursing practice has grown, some nursing care practices do not have adequate research to guide practice decisions. The challenge is to obtain the very best, most relevant, current, and accurate information when you need it for patient care.

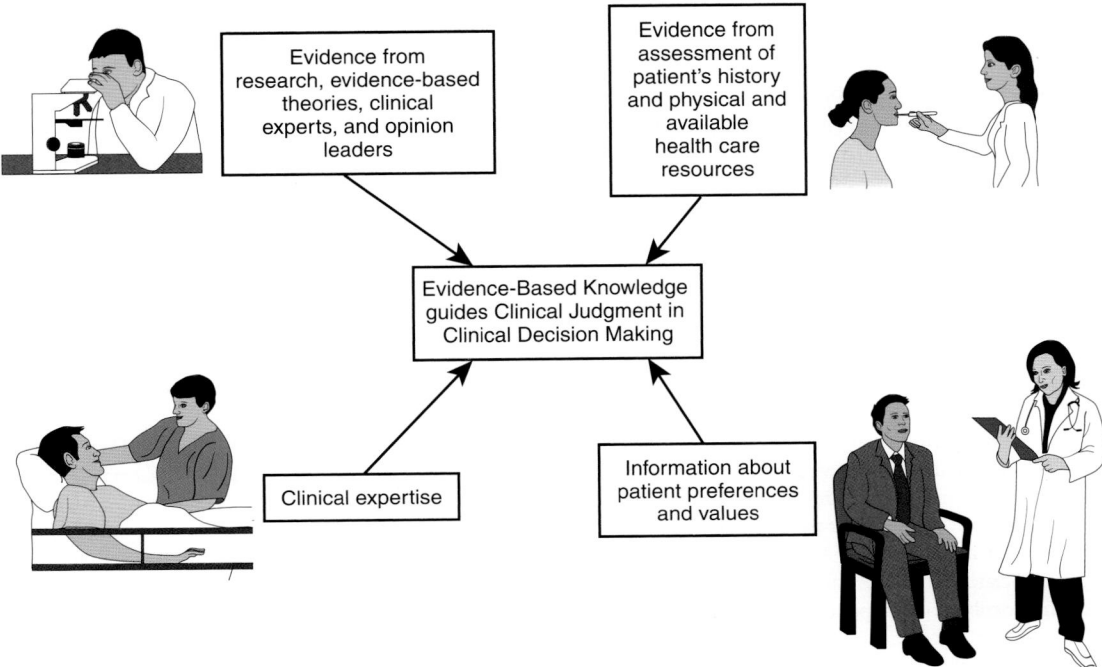

FIG. 5.1 Model for evidence-based clinical decision making.

The best scientific evidence comes from well-designed, systematically conducted research studies found in scientific, peer-reviewed journals. Researchers are usually able to conclude whether a new treatment or approach truly makes a difference at the completion of a research study. Unfortunately, much of that evidence never reaches the bedside. Although more health care settings have adopted EBP, there are still nurses who may not have easy access to databases for scientific literature. Instead, they often care for patients based on tradition or convenience.

Remember, knowledge derived from scientific evidence guides nurses' clinical judgments. Even when you use the best evidence available, application of the evidence and outcomes differs based on your patients' physical and psychological health, values and health beliefs, health care preferences, concerns, and/or expectations. The correct application of EBP also involves ethical and accountable professional nursing practice. As a nurse you use critical thinking to determine which evidence is appropriate and related to your patients' clinical situations (see Chapter 15). For example, a single research article involving adults shows that the use of therapeutic touch is effective in reducing patients' perceptions of abdominal pain after surgery. However, if your patients have cultural beliefs that discourage use of touch, you probably need to search for a different evidence-based therapy that your patients will accept. Using your clinical expertise and considering patients' values and preferences ensure that you apply the evidence available in practice both safely and appropriately.

Steps of Evidence-Based Practice

EBP is a systematic problem-solving process that facilitates achievement of best practices. Consistently following a step-by-step approach ensures that you will obtain the strongest available evidence to apply in patient care. There are seven steps of EBP, which are numbered from zero to six (Melnyk and Fineout-Overholt, 2019):

0. Cultivate a spirit of inquiry within an EBP culture and environment.
1. Ask a clinical question in PICOT format.
2. Search for the most relevant and best evidence.
3. Critically appraise the evidence you gather.
4. Integrate the best evidence with your clinical expertise and patient preferences and values to make the best clinical decision.
5. Evaluate the outcomes of practice changes based on evidence.
6. Communicate the outcomes of EBP decision or changes.

Cultivate a Spirit of Inquiry. Changes in health care are often made slowly because of multiple barriers that often prevent the implementation of EBP. To be an effective change agent and foster optimal patient care, you need to have a never-ending spirit of inquiry. Constantly questioning current practices and believing in the value of EBP lead to the consistent use of EBP in clinical nursing practice. For a health care agency to be successful at implementing and sustaining EBP changes, there must be a culture that promotes and supports a spirit of inquiry (Melnyk and Fineout-Overholt, 2019).

Health care agencies that promote and support EBP demonstrate a culture in which nurses are encouraged to question practice and identify EBP mentors to mentor other nurses in the process. These agencies have an infrastructure that supports inquiry and provides tools to support EBP, evidence-based P&Ps, nursing leaders who value EBP, integration of EBP competencies in performance evaluations and clinical ladders, and recognition programs for nurses for their work in EBP (Caramanica and Spiva, 2018; Melnyk et al., 2018a). As a nurse, you need to gain knowledge and skills associated with EBP and maintain a commitment to provide the best care possible to your patients and their families.

Ask a Clinical Question in PICOT Format. Always think about your practice when caring for patients. Question what does not make sense

to you and what needs to be clarified. Think about a problem or area of interest that is time-consuming, costly, or illogical. These thoughts are part of an ongoing spirit of inquiry into best practice. Nurses witness everyday events or situations that might be improved with better evidence.

There are different approaches for identifying problems requiring evidence-based solutions. A problem-focused trigger is one you face while caring for patients or a trend you see on a nursing unit. *For example, Cathy and Tom identified from the quality indicator report that the trend in CLABSIs increased over each of the previous 3 months.* Data gathered from a health care setting allows you to examine clinical trends and form questions. Most hospitals keep monthly records on key quality or performance indicators such as medication errors or infection rates. All Magnet®-designated hospitals maintain the National Database of Nursing Quality Indicators (NDNQI) (American Nurses Credentialing Center [ANCC], n.d.; NDNQI, n.d.). The database has information on falls, pressure injury incidence, and nurse satisfaction. Quality- and risk-management data do not give you evidence for finding a solution to a problem (Speroni et al., 2020). Rather, the data inform you about the nature or severity of problems, which then allows you to form practice questions. Other examples of problem-focused triggers include a patient injury following a fall or a patient who develops a Stage 3 pressure injury following surgery.

A knowledge-focused trigger is a question regarding new information available on a topic. For example, "What current evidence exists to improve pain management in patients with migraine headaches?" Important sources of this type of information are standards and practice guidelines available from national agencies such as the Agency for Healthcare Research and Quality (AHRQ), the American Pain Society (APS), or the American Association of Critical-Care Nurses (AACN). Other sources of knowledge-focused triggers include recent research publications and nurse experts within an organization.

Sometimes you use data gathered from a health care setting to examine clinical trends when developing clinical questions. For example, most hospitals keep monthly records on key quality indicators such as medication errors or infection rates. You use quality and risk-management data to help you understand the nature or severity of problems, which then allows you to form practice questions. The questions you ask eventually lead you to the evidence for an answer.

After you identify an area of interest, there are two types of questions you may ask: a background question or foreground question. A background question asks general information about a clinical issue and needs to be answered before a searchable and answerable foreground question can be posed (Melnyk and Fineout-Overholt, 2019). For example: What is the best way to reduce wandering in patients with dementia? The question might lead you to a variety of references, some that are even irrelevant, describing approaches for reducing wandering. But background information is often important to help you form a more specific foreground question. A foreground question focuses on specific knowledge that comes from a background question (Melnyk and Fineout-Overholt, 2019). For example, a foreground question might be: In patients with dementia, does the use of stress reduction techniques reduce wandering? Forming a foreground question using a PICOT format is very specific and assists you in finding the right evidence to answer the question with some certainty. When you ask a question and then go to the scientific literature, you do not want to read 100 articles to find the handful that are most helpful. You want to be able to read the best six articles that specifically address your practice question. Melnyk et al. (2017) suggest using a PICOT format to state a foreground question. Box 5.1 summarizes the five elements of a PICOT question. The more focused your question is, the easier it becomes to search for evidence in

BOX 5.1 Developing a PICOT Question

P = Patient population of interest
  Identify patients by age, gender, ethnicity, and disease or health problem.
I = Intervention or area of interest
  Which intervention is worthwhile to use in practice (e.g., a treatment, diagnostic test, prognostic factor)? What area of interest influences a desired outcome (e.g., complementary therapy, motivational interviewing)?
C = Comparison intervention or area of interest
  What is the usual standard of care or current intervention used now in practice?
O = Outcome
  What result do you wish to achieve or observe as a result of an intervention (e.g., change in patient behavior, physical finding, or patient perception)? Make an outcome statement nondirectional. For example: "Does use of chlorhexidine affect incidence of CLABSI?" instead of "Does the use of chlorhexidine reduce incidence of CLABSI?" A directional outcome may limit the articles in your search.
T = Time
  What amount of time is needed for an intervention to achieve an outcome (e.g., the amount of time needed to change quality of life or patient behavior)?

TABLE 5.1 Searchable Scientific Literature Databases and Sources

Databases	Sources
AHRQ	Agency for Healthcare Research and Quality; includes legacy clinical guidelines and evidence summaries. http://www.ahrq.gov The National Guideline Clearinghouse™ was taken down on July 16, 2018, because federal funding though AHRQ was no longer available to support it.
CINAHL	Cumulative Index to Nursing and Allied Health Literature; includes studies in nursing, allied health, and biomedicine. https://www.ebscohost.com/nursing/products/cinahl-databases/cinahl-complete
MEDLINE	Includes studies in medicine, nursing, dentistry, psychiatry, veterinary medicine, and allied health. https://www.nlm.nih.gov/bsd/medline.html
EMBASE	Biomedical and pharmaceutical studies http://www.embase.com
PsycINFO	Psychology and related health care disciplines http://www.apa.org/psycinfo/
Cochrane Database of Systematic Reviews	Full text of regularly updated systematic reviews prepared by the Cochrane Collaboration; includes completed reviews and protocols. https://www.cochrane.org/search/site/systematic%20reviews
PubMed	Health science library at the National Library of Medicine; offers free access to journal articles. https://www.ncbi.nlm.nih.gov/pubmed/
World Views on Evidence-Based Nursing	Electronic journal containing articles that provide a synthesis of research and an annotated bibliography for selected references

the scientific literature. *For example, Cathy and Tom first went to the literature with a general background question: "Which factors cause CLABSI in CVCs?" They were quickly frustrated when they found numerous articles about different factors that influence CLABSIs in CVCs. They screened the literature and decided to write two focused PICOT questions on one intervention found successful in reducing CVCs: (1) "Does the use of 2% chlorhexidine (I) compared with alcohol (C) for cleansing central catheter insertion sites in hospitalized patients (P) affect the incidence of CLABSI (O) within 6 months (T)?" and (2) "Does the use of sterile barrier techniques during catheter insertion (I) compared with sterile gloving only (C) affect the incidence of CLABSI (O) in patients who have had surgery (P) during their hospitalization (T)?"*

Proper question formatting allows you to identify key words to use when conducting your literature search. Note that a well-designed EBP question does not have to follow the sequence of *P, I, C, O,* and *T.* For example, a specific intervention (I), comparison (C), and time (T) are not used in every question. The aim is to ask a question that contains as many of the PICOT elements as possible. For example, here is a meaningful qualitative question that contains only a P and an O: How do patients with cystic fibrosis (P) perceive their quality of life (O)? The PICOT format allows you to ask questions that are intervention focused. For questions that are not intervention focused, the meaning of the letter I can be an area of interest instead of an intervention (Melnyk and Fineout-Overholt, 2019). For example, does the use of complementary therapies (I) compared with analgesics (C) affect pain (O) in patients with osteoarthritis (P)?

The questions you ask using as many elements as possible in a PICOT format help to identify knowledge gaps within a clinical situation. Asking well-thought-out questions allows you to identify evidence needed to guide clinical practice. Remember: Do not be satisfied with clinical routines. Always question and use critical thinking to consider better ways to provide patient care.

Search for the Best Evidence. Once you have a clear and concise PICOT question, you are ready to search for scientific evidence. A variety of sources will provide the evidence needed to answer your question, such as agency policy and procedure manuals, quality improvement data, existing clinical practice guidelines, and journal articles. Do not

hesitate to ask for help to find appropriate evidence. Key resources include nursing faculty, librarians, advanced practice nurses, staff educators, risk managers, and infection control nurses.

When using scientific literature for evidence, seek the assistance of a medical librarian who knows the various online databases available to you (Table 5.1). The databases contain large collections of published scientific studies, including peer-reviewed research. A **peer-reviewed** article is reviewed for accuracy, validity, and rigor and approved for publication by experts before it is published. MEDLINE and the Cumulative Index to Nursing and Allied Health Literature (CINAHL) are among the best-known online databases for scientific knowledge in health care (Melnyk and Fineout-Overholt, 2019). Some databases are available through vendors at a cost, some are free of charge, and some offer both options. Students typically have access provided by their schools. One of the more common vendors is OVID, which offers several different databases. Databases are also available on the Internet free of charge. The Cochrane Database of Systematic Reviews is a valuable source of high-quality evidence. It includes the full text of regularly updated systematic reviews and protocols for reviews currently under way. Collaborative review groups prepare and maintain the reviews. The protocols provide the background, objectives, and methods for reviews in progress (Melnyk and Fineout-Overholt, 2019).

Seek the help of a librarian to identify the databases and key words that will provide the best evidence to answer your PICOT question.

FIG. 5.2 Levels of evidence. (From LoBiondo-Wood G, Haber J: *Nursing research,* ed 10, St Louis, 2022, Elsevier.)

When conducting a search, you need to enter and manipulate different key words until you get the combination of terms that provides the best articles to help answer your question. It usually takes several searches to find the most appropriate articles. *For example, Cathy and Tom's first PICOT question includes the key words "catheter-associated bloodstream infection," "surgical patients," "chlorhexidine," and "alcohol."* The key words you select often have one meaning to one author and a very different meaning to another. Be patient and persistent and keep trying different words and combinations of words until you find the evidence you need.

It is important to use the hierarchy of evidence available as depicted in Fig. 5.2. The level of rigor or amount of confidence you can have in the evidence (e.g., findings from a study) decreases as you move down the pyramid. As a nursing student, you cannot be an expert on all aspects of the types of studies that comprise the first six levels of the pyramid. But you can learn enough about the types of studies to help you know which ones have the best scientific evidence. At the top of the pyramid are systematic reviews or meta-analyses, which are state-of-the-art summaries from an individual researcher or panel of experts. Meta-analyses and systematic reviews are the perfect answers to PICOT questions because they rigorously summarize current evidence about a specific topic or intervention.

During either a meta-analysis or a systematic review, a researcher asks a PICOT question, reviews the highest level of evidence available (e.g., randomized controlled trials [RCTs]) for a well-defined area of study, summarizes what is currently known about the area of study, and reports whether current evidence supports a change in practice or whether further study is needed. The main difference is that in a

meta-analysis the researcher uses statistics to show the effect of an intervention on an outcome. In a systematic review, no statistics are used to draw conclusions about the evidence. In the Cochrane Library, all entries include information on meta-analyses and systematic reviews. If you use MEDLINE or CINAHL, enter a text word such as *meta-analysis, systematic reviews,* or *evidence-based medicine* to obtain scientific reviews on your PICOT question.

An RCT is the highest level of experimental research. In an RCT a researcher tests an intervention (e.g., method for intravenous [IV] site care or patient education) against the usual standard of care. Researchers randomly assign subjects in an experiment to either a control or a treatment group. In other words, all of the subjects have an equal chance to be in either group. The treatment group receives the experimental intervention, and the control group receives the usual standard of care. The researchers measure both groups for the same outcomes and then perform statistical tests to see whether the experimental intervention made a significant difference. When an RCT is completed, the researcher has evidence showing whether the intervention leads to better outcomes than the standard of care.

A single RCT is not as conclusive as a review of several RCTs on the same question. However, a single RCT that tests the intervention included in your question yields useful evidence. If an RCT on your question is not available, use results from other research studies such as descriptive or qualitative studies to answer your PICOT question. The use of clinical experts may be at the bottom of the evidence pyramid, but do not consider clinical experts to be poor sources of evidence. Expert clinicians use evidence frequently as they build their own practices, and they are rich sources of information for clinical problems.

Critically Appraise the Evidence. With the help of the hospital librarian, *Tom searched three databases: PubMed, CINAHL, and the Cochrane Database of Systematic Reviews. He found a systematic review summary on central line dressings in the Cochrane Database. An article from the highly regarded* New England Journal of Medicine *reported on a research study that showed a reduction in CLABSIs after use of a bundling of several interventions (including use of chlorhexidine and barrier precautions). Cathy helped by searching the Centers for Disease Control and Prevention (CDC) website for clinical guidelines on central line catheters. Once they obtained the full text of all articles (not just the abstracts), Cathy and Tom distributed them to members of their UPC for critical review and evaluation.*

Critically reviewing and analyzing the available evidence requires a systematic approach. When evaluating the available evidence, you determine the value, feasibility, and usefulness of evidence for making a practice change (Mitchell and Freise, 2020). There are numerous critical appraisal guides available for nurses to use to evaluate the evidence using a structured format (Buccheri and Sharifi, 2017). Review each source of evidence (article, clinical guideline, expert summary) to determine its value, feasibility, and utility of evidence for making a practice change. This requires you to review each source of evidence carefully to determine its scientific worth and the strength of any study methods (when appropriate), to identify the level of evidence from each source, to summarize your findings, and to determine whether the evidence is conclusive regarding your practice question (Buccheri and Sharifi, 2017). *The ICU UPC committee reviews the evidence summaries for each of the articles and clinical guidelines on CLABSIs. The committee decides whether there is convincing evidence for the use of chlorhexidine instead of alcohol in cleansing catheter sites. The team also determines whether the use of barrier precautions during catheter insertion makes a difference in infection rates.*

It takes time to develop skills needed to critique the evidence like an expert. When you read an article, do not put it down and walk away because of the statistics and technical language. To determine its worth to practice, consider:

- What is the level of evidence?
- How well was the study (if research) conducted?
- How useful are the findings to practice?

Know the elements of an article when reviewing each one. Read each article carefully to decide how well the study was conducted. When reading through a scientific study, summarize key elements. Many EBP committees use critical appraisal guides or useful checklists for evaluating studies (Buccheri and Sharifi, 2017). A guide lists questions about essential elements of research (e.g., purpose, sample size, setting, method of study). It is important to know the elements of scientific articles to decide the value and relevance to your PICOT question (Buccheri and Sharifi, 2017). Evidence-based articles include the following elements:

- *Abstract.* An abstract is a summary that quickly tells you if the article is research or clinically based. An abstract summarizes the purpose of the article. It also includes the major themes or findings and the implications for nursing practice.
- *Introduction.* The introduction contains more information about the purpose of the article. There is usually brief supporting evidence

as to why the topic is important. Together the abstract and introduction help you decide if you want to continue to read the entire article. You will know if the topic of the article is similar to your PICOT question or related closely enough to provide useful information. If you decide that an article will most likely help answer your question, continue to read the next elements of the article.

- *Literature review or background.* A good author offers a detailed background of the level of science or clinical information about the topic of interest. The review involves reading, analyzing, and synthesizing scholarly articles about the research topic. It then offers an argument for what is known and what is not known, so as to provide an argument about what led the author to conduct a study or report on a clinical topic. This section of an article is valuable. Even if the article itself does not address your PICOT question the way you desire, the literature review overall may lead you to more useful articles and build your knowledge base in nursing. After reading a literature review, you should have a good idea of how past research led to the researcher's question. *For example, one article Tom found described a study designed to test the effects of aseptic practices on CLABSI. This study reviewed literature that describes the nature of CLABSI and the patients most at risk, the type of factors shown previously in the literature to contribute to CLABSI, and previous interventions used to prevent CLABSI.*
- *Manuscript narrative.* The "middle section," or narrative, of an article differs according to the type of evidence-based article it is (Melnyk and Fineout-Overholt, 2019). A clinical article describes a clinical topic, which often includes a description of a patient population, the nature of a certain disease or health alteration, how patients are affected, and the appropriate nursing therapies. An author sometimes writes a clinical article to explain how to use a therapy or new technology. A research article contains several subsections within the narrative, including the following:
  - *Purpose statement:* Explains the focus or intent of a study. It includes research questions or hypotheses—predictions made about the relationship or differences among study variables (concepts, characteristics, or traits that vary within or among subjects). *An example of a research question is: Does the use of chlorhexidine 2% compared with povidone-iodine reduce CLABSI in patients with CVCs? Within this question the author is studying the variables (independent) of chlorhexidine and povidone-iodine solutions as they affect the outcome (dependent variable) of CLABSI in patients. In contrast, a hypothesis might state: Chlorhexidine 2% for site care reduces the incidence of CLABSI in patients with CVCs.*
  - *Methods or design:* Explains how a research study was organized and conducted to answer the research question or test the hypothesis (a proposed explanation for a phenomenon that can be tested). This section explains the type of study that was conducted (e.g., RCT, case control study, or qualitative study) and the number of subjects or people who participated in the study. In health care research, subjects often include patients, family members, or health care staff. The methods section is sometimes confusing because it explains details about how the researcher designed the study to obtain the most accurate results possible. Use your faculty member as a resource to help interpret this section.
  - *Analysis:* Explains how the data collected in a study are analyzed. If quantitative data such as physical measurements and scores on surveys are collected, statistical results from the study are explained. Statistics can be confusing. Focus on learning whether the researcher found differences between groups or if an association was found between different variables. For example, if a researcher tests a new fall prevention strategy, did the strategy reduce falls

more than the standard approach to care? The researcher statistically reports a "*p* value." The *p* value (usually set at 0.05) is a probability level that tells you whether the difference between two groups was likely related to the intervention or if it was simply a difference by chance (Lobiondo-Wood and Haber, 2018). When the statistic shows that the value was less than the *p* value ($p < 0.05$), the result was likely the result of the intervention (less than 5% probability that it was caused by chance). If a study involved collection of qualitative information such as audiotaped interviews or open-ended surveys, the analysis describes the major themes reflected in the data. The analysis section helps to determine whether a study was conducted in a way that allows you to trust the results and use them to inform practice (Lobiondo-Wood and Haber, 2018).

- *Results or conclusions:* Clinical and research articles have a summary section. In a clinical article the author explains the clinical implications for the topic presented. In a research article the author details the results of the study and explains whether a hypothesis is supported or how a research question is answered. This section includes a statistical analysis if it is a quantitative research study. A qualitative study summarizes the descriptive themes and ideas that arose from the researcher's analysis of data. Do not let the statistical analysis in an article overwhelm you. Read carefully and ask these questions: Does the researcher describe the results? Were the results significant? An effective author also discusses limitations to a study in this section. The information on limitations is valuable in helping you decide if you want to use the evidence with your patients. Have a faculty member or an expert nurse help you interpret statistical results.
- *Clinical implications:* A research article includes a section that explains whether the findings from the study have clinical implications. The researcher explains the generalizability or how to apply findings in a practice setting for the type of subjects studied.

After you have critically reviewed each article for your PICOT question, combine the findings from all of the articles to determine the state of the evidence. If you used a critical appraisal guide for each article, summarize information in all of the forms into a final evaluation table. As you complete the evaluation table, use critical thinking to consider the scientific rigor or strength of the combined evidence and how well it answers your area of interest. Consider the evidence in light of your patients' concerns, values, preferences, and available health care resources. Your review of articles offers a snapshot conclusion of the combined evidence on your PICOT question. As a new nurse you learn to judge whether to use the evidence for a particular patient or group of patients who usually have complex health care situations (Melnyk and Fineout-Overholt, 2019). Ethically it is important to consider evidence that benefits patients and does no harm.

After appraising all articles, the UPC in the case study focuses on the systematic review, the research study, and CDC clinical guidelines as offering the most information about the use of chlorhexidine and other interventions for preventing CLABSI. The committee collaborates by discussing their conclusions, reviews the results of the final evaluation tables, and applies their clinical expertise. They consider the types of patients they see in the ICU and determine whether the evidence is strong enough for use in practice. The systematic review article (Level I evidence) did not address chlorhexidine use but concluded that there was no definitive advantage of transparent IV dressings over gauze for preventing CLABSI. Although they were Level VII evidence, the clinical guidelines from the CDC contained recommendations categorized on the basis of strength of existing scientific data and applicability. The CDC guidelines reported that research has shown no difference between transparent and gauze dressings in causing bloodstream infection

(BSI) and highly recommends use of chlorhexidine for IV site care and the use of sterile barriers during catheter insertion. The cohort study (Level IV evidence) showed a significant reduction in CLABSI in ICUs that used a bundle of interventions, including rigorous hand hygiene, chlorhexidine site care, and sterile barriers. The data from all studies were applicable to adult critically ill patients. The committee recommended adopting practice changes to include chlorhexidine site care, sterile barrier precautions for catheter insertion, and reinforcement of strict hand hygiene during all forms of central line site care.

Integrate the Evidence. If you decide that the evidence is strong and applicable to your patients and clinical situation, you begin to identify how to incorporate it into practice. When the evidence is of a qualitative nature or provides data on assessment guidelines, you identify ways that you can use the evidence to assess patient conditions. For example, the evidence available on the common causes for falls among older adults is integrated into most evidence-based fall risk assessment tools. If the evidence applies to an intervention, your first step is simply to apply the research in your plan of care for a patient (see Chapter 18). Use the evidence you find as a rationale for an intervention you plan to try. For instance, you learned about an approach to bathe older adults who are confused and decide to use the technique during your next clinical assignment. If you find that the bathing technique is successful with your own assigned patients, you may begin to work with a group of other students or nurses to revise the policy and procedure for bathing patients or develop a new clinical protocol.

When you work as a part of a hospital committee or task force, sometimes EBP change occurs on a larger scale. Engagement involves bringing all stakeholders (individuals who have an interest or concern in the practice change) together to explain why the evidence-based interventions are important. For example, administrators want to know if the practice change improves patient outcomes and lowers costs. Staff nurses want to know if the practice change improves patient outcomes and how it will affect the way they provide care. Health care providers also want to know how the practice change affects the way they provide care. Many agencies use EBP mentors who act as informal leaders to influence staff at a unit level (John Hopkins, 2018). A mentor should be someone within an organization who has the knowledge and skills to move an EBP initiative forward, can offer the best support, and has the most at stake to see that EBP is successful (John Hopkins, 2018). An example of an effective mentor is an advanced practice nurse or unit educator.

When integrating evidence it is important to consider the setting in which you want to apply the evidence and ask if stakeholders support the change. To integrate evidence into practice, education of all those involved in the practice change must occur. This requires approaches such as teaching seminars, informational newsletters, and ongoing discussions during staff and UPC meetings. The key to integrating evidence successfully is to increase buy-in by involving as many staff as possible to champion the EBP process by focusing on a problem that is important to them (John Hopkins, 2018).

The actual execution of a practice change requires planning, especially if it occurs on a large scale, involving more than one nursing unit or work area. The staff who are implementing a practice change must work closely with those who will be adopting the new practice to anticipate what will be needed to make a change successful. For example, new documentation forms, different types of supplies, or a change in the way information is communicated among disciplines may be needed. It is often best to test a new practice change by conducting a 3-month pilot before implementing on a large scale. A pilot study is a small-scale research study or one that includes a quality or performance improvement (PI) project. The results of the pilot tell you whether the practice change can be implemented easily and whether it results in desired outcomes. Nursing staff buy-in is important to the success of the pilot project and to sustaining the change. Nurses are more likely to use evidence-based practices if they perceive the practices to be useful and relevant and if their work environment is supportive and promotes communication (Jun et al., 2020; Mathieson et al., 2018).

A common approach used for integrating evidence into practice is to incorporate new evidence into P&Ps. A key feature of a practice environment that supports the use of best evidence is to require clinical practice P&Ps to be evidence based (Dols et al., 2017). Traditionally policies were reviewed annually or less often for updating. Today, policies and protocols are updated when new evidence justifies a revision (Dols et al., 2017). Updates are designed to share the most recent evidence and facilitate staff adherence to new practices Many agencies involve staff nurses and research-prepared advanced practice nurses to review scientific articles relevant to P&Ps and make appropriate revisions. P&Ps are important tools for supporting hospital-based nurses in using evidence in their everyday practice and promoting positive patient outcomes (Harvey et al., 2020).

After reviewing the evidence on CLABSI, the UPC committee decides to revise the P&P for central catheter insertion and maintenance. Cathy and Tom recommend that the committee conduct in-service sessions to educate all staff about the new P&P. A brief explanation about the change is also placed in the monthly newsletter of the unit. The bundle of interventions (hand hygiene, chlorhexidine use, and full barrier precautions) is implemented after the staff have the opportunity to ask questions about the new protocol in staff meetings. The ICU implements the new P&P with the UPC committee monitoring the monthly reports on CLABSI to determine whether infection rates change. In addition, the UPC audits staff practices to be sure that the new interventions are being followed consistently and that the change in practice is sustained.

Evaluate the Outcomes of the Practice Decision or Change. After applying evidence in your practice, your next step is to evaluate the outcome. How does the intervention work? How effective was the clinical decision for your patient or practice setting? Sometimes your evaluation is as simple as determining whether the expected outcomes you set for an intervention are met (see Chapters 18 and 20). For example, after the use of a transparent IV dressing, does the IV line dislodge, or does the patient develop the complication of phlebitis? When using a new approach to preoperative teaching, do patients learn what to expect after surgery?

When an EBP change occurs on a larger scale, an evaluation is more formal. *For example, evidence of factors that reduce the incidence of CLABSI leads the ICU to adopt the new P&P for central line catheter care. To evaluate the procedure, the members of the EBP committee track the outcome of incidence of CLABSI over a course of time before and after the practice change (e.g., 3–6 months). Measures from pre-intervention and postintervention are needed to determine change. In this case the CLABSI measure is collected by the hospital monthly. In addition, the staff collect data to describe both the patients who develop CLABSI and those who do not. This comparative information is valuable in determining the effects of the protocol and whether modifications are necessary.*

When evaluating an EBP change, determine whether the change was effective, whether modifications in the change are needed, or whether the change needs to be discontinued. Events or results that you do not expect may occur. *For example, the changes made in the protocol developed by Cathy and Tom might lead to an increase in CLABSIs. If this is not determined during evaluation, the practice would continue, and patients would suffer.* Never implement a practice change without evaluating its effects.

Communicate the Outcomes of the Evidence-Based Practice Decision. After implementing an EBP change, it is important to communicate the results. If you implement an evidence-based intervention with one patient, you and the patient determine the effectiveness of that intervention. When a practice change occurs on a nursing unit level, the first group to discuss the outcomes of the change is often the clinical staff on that unit. Unit huddles and visual management tools, such as a Gemba board to collect process issues, are effective strategies for communicating EBP changes and practices (Bourgault et al., 2018). To enhance professional development and promote positive patient outcomes beyond the unit level, share the results with various groups of nurses or other care providers such as the nursing practice council, EBP council, or research council (Carter and Rivera, 2018). Clinicians enjoy and appreciate seeing the results of a practice change. In addition, the practice change will more likely be sustainable and remain in place when staff are able to see the benefits of an EBP change. A good way to share this information on the nursing unit is through a poster presentation to the unit staff.

As a professional nurse it is critical to contribute to the growing knowledge of nursing practice. Nurses often communicate the outcomes of EBP changes during clinical grand rounds and at professional conferences and meetings. Being involved in professional organizations allows them to present EBP changes in scientific abstracts, poster presentations, or even podium presentations.

> **REFLECT NOW**
>
> On your assigned patient care clinical unit, discuss with two nurses the most effective strategies they use to communicate EBP changes to the nursing staff.

Sustain Knowledge Use. Sustaining change in practice as a result of the EBP process is a challenge. Health care agencies are bombarded by change from governmental and accrediting agencies, internal administrative initiatives, and the ongoing demands of delivering safe and effective patient care. For EBP to become fully adopted and integrated into an agency, the perception that changing practice will improve quality of care and make a difference in patients' lives must be felt by all staff (John Hopkins, 2018). When a new practice change is introduced, it is important that it be incorporated into the culture and practice environment of an organization. It is important for health care agencies to use targeted strategies to sustain use of EBP decisions and changes (Box 5.2). Often larger hospitals or health care systems will hire nurse researchers or nurse scientists to manage and further develop the EBP and nursing research programs within the agency (Carter and Rivera, 2018). Mentorship and modeling of EBP by advanced practice nurses facilitate implementation of EBP in clinical settings (Melnyk et al., 2018b). *After the ICU adopts the new P&P for central line catheter care, the committee posts the monthly CLABSI outcome measure on the conference room bulletin board for all staff to see. Members of the UPC conduct occasional audits to be sure that the processes of using chlorhexidine and sterile barriers are being followed by staff members. When the incidence of CLABSI starts to go back up, the UPC committee discusses the results and reviews the causes for each patient situation.* Translating new knowledge into practice requires transformational nursing leadership (see Chapter 21) that provides the resources to develop EBP education for nurses to increase EBP knowledge, such as a toolkit to standardize nursing practices, participation on interprofessional EBP teams, and role modeling of EBP behaviors (Harvey et al., 2020; Tucker and Melnyk, 2019).

BOX 5.2 EVIDENCE-BASED PRACTICE

Strategies to Sustain Nurses' Use of Evidence-Based Practice

PICOT Question: Does the use of targeted strategies result in nurses' implementation and sustained use of evidence-based practice (EBP)?

Evidence Summary

Nurses' implementation and sustained use of EBP continues to be a challenge. To be successful in implementing and sustaining EBP, units within health care agencies need to develop cultures focused on collaboration, human development, empowerment of staff, and promotion of interpersonal relationships (Jun et al., 2020; Yoo et al., 2019). It is essential that leaders in the institution have a clear vision, actively engage in and role model EBP behaviors, support staff efforts to use EBP, and provide mentorship to other nurses (Tucker and Melnyk, 2019). Nurses who work on units where the leaders have clear vision and use integrated strategies and EBP activities have higher levels of continued use of EBP practices (Caramanica and Spiva, 2018; Harvey et al., 2020). Forming a regional EBP Institute or a Clinical Research and Practice Collaborative as well as EBP work groups within nursing shared governance councils were found to be effective targeted strategies to engage nurses in EBP (Ecoff et al., 2020; Migliore et al., 2020). Nurses are more interested in and willing to adopt innovative practices when they have nursing leaders who provide ongoing communication related to research and EBP (Tucker and Melnyk, 2019). Research found that nurses who hold specialty certifications are more likely to use EBP when providing nursing care (Jun et al., 2020). Scholarly mentorships from nursing faculty through academic partnerships or from advanced practice nurses and participation in journal clubs helped nurses develop EBP skills (Carter and Rivera, 2018; Fritz, 2017). EBP fellowship programs increased nurses' EBP knowledge as well as EBP implementation (Friesen et al., 2017; Kim et al., 2017). Visual management tools, such as Gemba boards (visual board that includes a method for collecting process issues identified by nurses), and huddles foster an EBP culture (Bourgault et al., 2018). Targeted approaches help nurses engage in EBP in their practices.

Application to Nursing Practice

- Be familiar with the nursing leader's vision as it relates to strategies and activities for EBP in the health care agency (Melnyk et al., 2018a; Tucker and Melnyk, 2019).
- Form an EBP team or journal club with other nurses to help create a culture of inquiry in your agency (Fritz, 2017).
- Join with other nurses in the region to support each other in EBP (Ecoff et al., 2020).
- Consider becoming certified in a nursing specialty (Jun et al., 2020).
- Watch for strategic communication from leadership about research and EBP educational opportunities and improvements within your agency (Melnyk et al., 2018a; Yoo et al., 2019).
- Partner with a nursing professor or an advanced practice nurse who can mentor you as you develop your skills in EBP (Carter and Rivera, 2018; Melnyk et al., 2018b).
- As a student, partner with a nurse on the unit to search the literature to answer a practice improvement question and share your findings with the other nurses.

THE SCIENTIFIC METHOD

When there is no evidence for the support of a practice-related, educational, or administrative change, the next option is conducting research—the process of creating new knowledge. For example, when conducting EBP you may find a gap in knowledge that makes your PICOT question go unanswered. When this happens, the best way to answer your PICOT question is to conduct a research study.

The scientific method is the foundation of all research, an objective methodology for scientific investigation that results in unbiased interpretations of the phenomenon under study and refinement of knowledge. It is a process that, when done formally and rigorously, yields new knowledge critical to a science, be it nursing, psychology, or medicine. The scientific method is a systematic, step-by-step process. When performed correctly, you know whether a study supports the validity, reliability, and generalizability of a study's findings. In other words, when a nursing research study is performed correctly, you know if the findings apply to similar patients cared for (generalizability) and whether the same results will occur when the study is repeated under the same conditions (reliability). Valid findings exist when a study has followed all steps of the scientific method without bias.

Nurse researchers use the scientific method to understand, explain, predict, or control a nursing phenomenon (Lobiondo-Wood and Haber, 2018). Systematic, orderly procedures reduce the possibility for error. Although the possibility of error always exists, the scientific method minimizes the chance that a researcher's bias or opinion will influence the results of a study and thus the knowledge gained. Research using the scientific method includes the following steps:

1. *Make an observation.* The researcher identifies a problem area or area of interest to study.
2. *Ask questions about the observation and gather information.* The researcher conducts a thorough literature review of the area of interest.
3. *Analyze the literature and form a research question or hypothesis*—a proposed explanation for a phenomenon that can be tested, often involving a prediction based on that question or hypothesis.
4. *Conduct a study using scientific rigor.* Test the question or the hypothesis and prediction in an experiment (quantitative or qualitative) that can be reproduced. The type of study is driven by the research question. For example, "Does the use of chlorhexidine reduce incidence of CLABSI?" is a quantitative study involving statistical analysis. "What are nurses' perceptions of their own grieving when caring for COVID-19 patients?" is a research question best studied qualitatively. Researchers gather empirical data through the use of observations and assessments (e.g., surveys, physiological data, observation) and use the data to discover new knowledge.
5. *Analyze the data and draw conclusions.* Accept or reject the question/hypothesis or modify the hypothesis if necessary.

The goal of any study conducted by means of the scientific method is to apply the knowledge gained from a study to a broader group of patients. As you review the steps of the scientific method you will notice its similarity to the nursing process (Table 5.2). Understanding the scientific method enables you to understand how researchers perform research objectively, to gain and test knowledge. The method is useful in guiding research, but many of the elements of the scientific method also apply to how one conducts EBP projects: forming questions, searching the literature, and conducting pilot testing.

Types of Research Studies

A research question or hypothesis drives the method used by a researcher to answer the question. At the same time, a researcher must consider the population to be represented (e.g., cancer patients, undergrad nurses, patients with depression) in a study, access to the population, methods of data collection, and the setting where a study is to be performed. If the correct type of study is not selected, the results may be very limited or not useful at all. If there is little in the literature about a research question, a researcher will initially take an exploratory approach, and not be overly ambitious and attempt a formal experimental study. An example is research on fall prevention. Instead of prematurely testing a proposed intervention to reduce falls, early researchers first conducted studies to identify what factors are associated with falls. Once those factors were

Nursing Process	Research Process Using the Scientific Method
Assessment	Observe and ask questions. Identify area of interest or clinical problem. • Review literature. • Formulate theoretical framework. • Reflect on personal practice and/or discuss clinical issues with experts to better define the problem.
Diagnosis	Develop research question(s)/hypotheses.
Planning	Determine how study will be conducted: • Select research design/methodology. • Identify plan to recruit sample, taking into consideration population, number, and assignment to groups. • Identify study variables: specific interventions (independent variable) and outcomes (dependent variables). • Select data collection methods. • Select approach for measuring outcomes: questionnaires, surveys, physiological measures, interviews, observations. • Formulate plan to analyze data: statistical methods to answer research questions/hypotheses.
Implementation	Conduct the study: • Obtain necessary approvals. • Recruit and enroll subjects. • Implement the study protocol/collect data.
Evaluation	Analyze results of the study and form conclusion: • Continually analyze study methodology. Is study consistently carried out? Are all investigators following study protocol? • Interpret demographics of study population. • Analyze data to answer each research question/hypothesis. • Interpret results, including conclusions, limitations. Communicate the findings: • Formulate recommendations for further research. • Determine implications for nursing. • Disseminate the findings: presentations, publications, need for further study, how to apply findings in practice.

TABLE 5.2   Comparison of Steps of the Nursing Process With the Scientific Method Process

identified, new studies were developed to create fall risk assessment tools. Then researchers used the tools to identify high-risk patients and test interventions targeted at eliminating the risks. Choosing the right research method is critical to eventually revealing new, relevant knowledge (Box 5.3).

Quantitative Research. Quantitative nursing research relies on methods that precisely measure and quantify a study's variables. Two examples of quantitative research are (1) a study dealing with a new pain therapy that quantitatively measures participants' self-reported pain severity and (2) a study testing different forms of surgical dressings to measure the extent of wound healing. Quantitative research is the precise, systematic, objective examination of specific concepts. It focuses on numerical data, statistical analysis, and controls to eliminate bias in findings (Lobiondo-Wood and Haber, 2018). There are many quantitative methods. Some of the more commonly used quantitative methods include experimental, nonexperimental, survey, and evaluation research.

Experimental Research. An RCT is a true **experimental study** that tightly controls conditions to eliminate bias with the goal of generalizing the results of the study to similar groups of subjects. Researchers test an intervention (e.g., a new drug, therapy, or educational method) against the usual standard of care. They randomly assign similar subjects to either a control or a treatment group. When an RCT is completed, the researcher hopes to know whether the intervention leads to better outcomes than the standard of care.

Controlled trials without randomization test interventions, but researchers have not randomized the subjects into control (group with no intervention) or treatment (group receiving experimental intervention) groups. Thus there is bias in how the study is conducted. Some

BOX 5.3   Types of Research

- **Exploratory research:** Initial nonexperimental study designed to develop or refine the dimensions of phenomena (facts or events) or to develop or refine a hypothesis about the relationships among phenomena. Example: Pilot study testing the benefits of a new exercise program for older adults with dementia.
- **Evaluation research:** A form of quantitative research. Study that tests how well a program, practice, or policy is working. When programs are unsuccessful, evaluation research identifies problems with the program and opportunities for change or barriers to program implementation. Example: Study measuring the outcomes of an informational campaign designed to improve parents' ability to follow immunization schedules for their children.
- **Descriptive research:** Study that measures characteristics of people, situations, or groups and the frequency with which certain events or characteristics occur. Example: Study to examine RNs' biases toward caring for obese patients.
- **Historical research:** Descriptive research designed to establish facts and relationships concerning past events. Example: Study examining the societal factors that led to the acceptance of advanced practice nurses by patients.
- **Experimental research:** Study in which the investigator controls the study variable and randomly assigns subjects to different conditions to test the variable. Example: RCT comparing chlorhexidine with povidone-iodine in reducing the incidence of IV-site phlebitis.
- **Correlational research:** Nonexperimental study that explores the interrelationships among variables of interest without any active intervention by the researcher. Example: Study examining the relationship between RNs' educational levels and their satisfaction in the nursing role.

IV, Intravenous; *RCT,* randomized controlled trial; *RN,* registered nurse.

findings are distorted because of how the study was designed. A researcher wants to be as certain as possible when testing an intervention that the intervention is the reason for the desired outcomes. In a nonrandomized controlled trial, the way in which subjects fall into the control or treatment group sometimes influences the results. For example, consider a study in which there are more older adults who happen to fall into one group compared with another. This could influence outcomes. This suggests that the intervention tested was possibly not the only factor affecting the results of the study. Careful critique allows you to determine whether bias was present in a study and what effect, if any, the bias had on the results of the study.

Although RCTs investigate cause and effect and are excellent for testing drug therapies or medical treatments, this approach is not always the best for testing nursing interventions. The nature of nursing care causes nurse researchers to ask questions that are not always answered best by an RCT. For example, nurses help patients with problems such as knowledge deficits and symptom management. When researchers attempt to plan an RCT, ethical issues will often develop if the control group does not receive the new therapeutic intervention. Also, learning to understand how patients experience health problems cannot always be addressed through an RCT. Therefore, nonexperimental descriptive studies are often used in nursing research.

Nonexperimental Research. Nonexperimental descriptive studies describe, explain, or predict phenomena (an observable fact, event, or occurrence). Two examples include (1) a study examining factors that lead to adolescents' decisions to smoke cigarettes, and (2) a study determining factors that lead patients with dementia to fall in a hospital setting.

In a case control study, researchers study one group of subjects with a certain condition (e.g., asthma) at the same time as another group of subjects who do not have the condition. A case control study determines whether there is an association between one or more predictor variables and the condition (Melnyk and Fineout-Overholt, 2019). For example, is there an association between predictor variables such as family history or environmental exposure to dust and the incidence of asthma? Often a case control study is conducted retrospectively, or after the fact. Researchers look back in time and review available data about the two groups of subjects to understand which variables explain the condition. These studies involve a small number of subjects, creating a risk of bias. Sometimes the subjects in the two groups differ with regard to certain other variables (e.g., amount of stress or history of contact allergies) that also influence the incidence of the condition, more so than the variables being studied, which can make it difficult to interpret the results of the study.

Correlational studies describe the relationship between two variables (e.g., the age of the adolescents and whether the adolescents smoke). The researcher determines whether the two variables are correlated or associated with one another and to what extent.

Many times, researchers use findings from descriptive studies to develop studies that test interventions. For example, if a researcher determines that adolescents 15 years of age and older tend to smoke, the researcher might later test whether participation in a program about smoking for older adolescents is effective in helping adolescents stop smoking.

Surveys. Quantitative research often uses surveys or questionnaires to obtain information regarding the frequency, distribution, and interrelation of variables among subjects in the study (Lobiondo-Wood and Haber, 2018). An example is a survey designed to measure nurses' perceptions of physicians' willingness to collaborate in practice. Surveys obtain information about practices, perceptions, education, experience, opinions, and other characteristics of people. The most basic function of a survey is description. Surveys gather a large amount of data to describe

the population and the topic of study. It is important in survey research that the portion of the population sampled is large enough to keep sampling error (sample does not represent entire population under study) to a minimum.

Qualitative Research. Qualitative nursing research studies phenomena that are difficult to quantify or categorize, such as patients' perceptions of illness or quality of life. This research method describes information obtained in a nonnumeric form. Data are typically gathered during interviews via recording of each subject. Then the recordings are transcribed into written transcripts, serving as the data for interpretation. Qualitative researchers aim to understand patients' (and others') experiences with health problems and the contexts in which the experiences occur. Patients tell their stories and share their experiences in these studies. The findings have depth because patients are usually descriptive in what they choose to share. Examples of qualitative studies include (1) patients' perceptions of nurses' caring in a palliative care unit and (2) the perceptions of stress by family members of critically ill patients. Qualitative research may also involve nurses or other health care providers in an effort to understand their perceptions of issues affecting health care delivery.

Qualitative research involves inductive reasoning to develop generalizations or theories from specific observations or interviews (Lobiondo-Wood and Haber, 2018). For example, a nurse extensively interviews cancer survivors and then summarizes the common themes from the interviews to inductively determine the characteristics of cancer survivors' quality of life. Qualitative research involves the discovery and understanding of important behavioral characteristics or phenomena.

There are several different qualitative research methods, including ethnography, phenomenology, and grounded theory. Each is based on a different philosophical or methodological view of how to collect, summarize, and analyze qualitative data.

NURSING RESEARCH

The National Institute of Nursing Research (NINR) is the one nursing institute within the National Institutes of Health (NIH). The NINR supports the conduct of clinical and basic research and research training on health and illness, research that spans and integrates the behavioral and biological sciences, and research that develops the scientific basis for clinical practice (NIH, 2020). The institute had a 2020 budget of $92 million to fund research project grants (U.S. Department of Health and Human Services [USDHHS], 2020). The four areas of scientific research supported by the NINR include symptom science, wellness, self-management of chronic conditions, and end-of-life and palliative care. Many other professional nursing organizations have research priorities or agendas for directing the type of studies they support or conduct. For example, the Oncology Nursing Society (ONS) has three research priorities: (a) symptom science, (2) health disparities, and (3) palliative and psychosocial care in oncology. Whether a nurse is conducting a study in affiliation with a professional organization or more independently within a large health care center, nursing research targets some aspect of nursing's scope of practice (see Chapter 1). Nursing research addresses issues important to the discipline of nursing.

Nursing research improves the health and welfare of people who are underserved (NINR, n.d.). Nursing research is a way to identify new knowledge that can improve nursing practice, professional education and practice, and the use of nursing and health care resources effectively. Rigorous nursing research provides a scientific basis for nursing practice (clinical, educational, and administrative) and validates the effectiveness of nursing interventions. For example, nursing research with an educational focus can improve professional education and practice by revealing new educational approaches that improve learning outcomes. From an administrative perspective, nursing research can help nurses use resources more effectively (e.g., how to best use human resources by determining the best practice mix of nurses and assistive personnel on a nursing unit). The scientific knowledge base of nursing continues to grow, and it is this knowledge that guides clinical judgment when nurses enter a variety of practice experiences. Nursing research provides evidence that nurses can use to provide safe and effective patient care.

Translation Research

Translation research focuses on "testing implementation interventions to improve uptake and use of evidence to improve patient outcomes and population health" (Titler, 2018, p. 1). It is also called implementation science. The purpose of studies in translation research is to test implementation strategies in real-world settings to determine which strategies work best among diverse patient groups in various contexts to promote use of EBP (Titler, 2018; Naylor, 2018). In testing strategies, translation research helps to uncover which strategies work for whom, in what settings, and why. In conducting translation research, nurses can improve and sustain use of best evidence in everyday practice with the goal of improving patient care delivery, population health, and health outcomes (Titler, 2018). For example, Dr. Mary Naylor has done extensive research since 1994 in the development of the Transitional Care Model (Naylor et al., 1994). Despite the fact that numerous studies have shown its efficacy, health care agencies have not adopted the model on a broad scale (Naylor, 2018). The model is designed to prevent health complications and rehospitalizations of chronically ill, elderly hospital patients by providing them with comprehensive discharge planning and home follow-up, coordinated by a master's-level "Transitional Care Nurse" who is trained in the care of people with chronic conditions (Social Programs That Work, 2018). A translational research approach would test Naylor's model to determine how best to implement the model in the particular agency.

Translation research occurs along a dynamic continuum that moves through five phases from basic research to application of research findings in a variety of settings. The five phases include:
- Preclinical and animal studies—basic science research
- Phase 1 clinical trials—testing safety and efficacy in a small group of human subjects
- Phases 2 and 3 clinical trials—testing safety and efficacy in a larger group of human subjects and testing for comparison with standard treatment
- Phase 4 clinical trials and outcomes research—translation to practice
- Phase 5 population-level outcomes research—translation to community (Titler, 2018)

Translation research differs from EBP. In translation research, a research study tests the strategies that are used to implement and sustain EBP, whereas EBP focuses on the use of best evidence in practice and measuring outcomes. Translation research poses a research question or hypothesis. Then a variety of research designs and methods are used to answer the research question and test the hypothesis, revealing what is most effective in implementing evidence. Doctorally prepared nurses play a key role in conducting translation research to improve health outcomes (Trautman et al., 2018).

Outcomes Research

In today's health care delivery system, it is more important than ever to understand the results of health care practices. Outcomes research helps patients, health care providers, and those in health care policy make informed decisions based on current evidence (Patient-Centered Outcomes Research Institute [PCORI], 2020). Outcomes research typically focuses on the benefits, risks, costs, and holistic effects of a treatment on patients. For example, researchers are conducting outcomes research when they study the effects of managing Parkinson disease in patients using videoconferencing and telemedicine to increase access to health care.

Care delivery outcomes are the observable or measurable effects of health care interventions (Melnyk and Fineout-Overholt, 2019). Like the expected outcomes you develop in a plan of care (see Chapter 18), a care delivery outcome focuses on the recipients of service (e.g., patient, family, or community) and not the providers (e.g., nurse or physician). For example, an outcome of a diabetes education program is that patients are able to self-administer insulin, not the nurses' success in teaching patients who have diabetes to administer insulin.

Nurses sometimes experience difficulty in clearly defining or selecting measurable outcomes. Components of an outcome include the outcome itself, how it is observed (the indicator), its critical characteristics (how it is measured), and its range of parameters (Melnyk and Fineout-Overholt, 2019). For example, health care agencies commonly identify patient satisfaction as an outcome when introducing new services (e.g., new care delivery model or outpatient clinic). Patient satisfaction is often measured by patients' responses to a satisfaction instrument, which asks patients to rank their satisfaction with different aspects of their experience, such as nursing care, physician care, support services, and the care environment. Patients complete the instrument, responding to a scale (parameter) designed to measure their degree of satisfaction (e.g., scale of 1–5). The combined score on the instrument yields a measure of patient satisfaction, an outcome that the agency and health care team can track over time.

Nurse-sensitive indicators are outcomes that are directly influenced by nursing practice (Grove and Gray, 2019) (see Chapter 18). Although it is important to research the effects of nursing care on nurse-sensitive indicators, some researchers choose outcomes that do not measure a direct effect of nursing care, such as length of stay, mortality, quality of life, and patient satisfaction. Researchers need to select appropriate outcomes when designing their studies. For example, if a nurse researcher intends to measure the success of a nurse-initiated protocol to manage blood glucose levels in patients who are critically ill, the researcher will not likely measure mortality because it is too broad and susceptible to many factors outside the control of the nurse-initiated protocol (e.g., the selection of medical therapies, the patients' acuity of illness). Instead the nurse researcher will have a better idea of the effects of the protocol by measuring the outcome of patients' blood glucose ranges. The researcher obtains the blood glucose levels of patients placed on the protocol and compares them with a desired range that represents good blood glucose control.

The Conduct of Nursing Research

At this time in your career you will not be conducting formal research. However, you may observe nurses performing research within your health care agency. It is important for you to understand how the scientific method is used in the process of conducting a nursing research study and how it potentially generates new knowledge.

Nursing research allows you to study nursing questions and problems in greater depth within the context of nursing. Application of the scientific method in nursing research begins with making an observation. This will often occur within context of a nurse's practice. For example, a nurse observes that many surgical patients on a nursing unit have recently experienced more nausea and paralytic ileus shortly after colon surgery. The nurse may go to the literature to gather a broad view of the problem, or sometimes ideas about observations come from colleagues, such as after professional meetings. But a clear and concise research question is needed to proceed with research so that new knowledge can be identified. In the example, the nurse reviews the literature about studies designed to reduce postoperative ileus and nausea following colon surgery. She specifically looks for nursing interventions that have been used. After reading the available literature, two studies in particular interest her, so she asks the following research question: "Does chewing peppermint gum postoperatively reduce postoperative ileus in patients undergoing colon surgery?" Note that a well-formed research question assumes many characteristics of a PICOT question. The nurse consults with a nurse researcher in the nursing department, who recommends starting with a simple and realistically well-designed study. The nurse decides to conduct an experimental pilot study on the nursing unit to determine whether chewing peppermint gum following colon surgery reduces the incidence of postoperative ileus and nausea. The nurse will test a group of 30 patients who chew the gum versus 30 who are not given the gum. She will measure all 60 subjects for the incidence of nausea and paralytic ileus postoperatively. The nurse reviews the relevant literature to determine what is known about chewing peppermint gum and its effect on bowel mobility and nausea after abdominal surgery. Are there any risks to giving patients the gum? What is the best way to measure nausea and ileus? The nurse notes that although many patients report problems with nausea and return of bowel function, the two studies that she found do not form a conclusion as to the effects of chewing gum on these two outcomes.

Following identification of the research question and further review of the literature, the nurse forms a research team to design the study. The research team includes a nurse from the unit, a clinical nurse specialist, the hospital nurse researcher, a gastrointestinal surgeon, and a statistician. The study sample includes 60 patients who are having elective colon resections. Subjects are excluded if they need to have surgery because of an emergency situation. After obtaining approval from the hospital institutional review board (IRB), the research team approaches patients scheduled for surgery for their written consent. Those who agree to be in the study are then randomly assigned into one of the two groups (experimental or control), which means subjects have a 50-50 chance of being in each group. Sampling continues until 30 subjects are assigned to each group. The control group receives standard postoperative care. Subjects in the experimental or treatment group get standard postoperative care, and they chew gum for 5 minutes 3 times a day until discharge. The research team selects appropriate instruments to measure postoperative nausea (self-report rating scale). Patient assessment data including when nurses first hear bowel sounds and when patients first pass flatus and have their first bowel movement after surgery are gathered as outcomes for reducing ileus.

Before conducting any study with human subjects, a researcher obtains approvals from the human subjects committee or IRB of an agency. An IRB includes scientists and laypeople who review all studies conducted in the institution to ensure that ethical principles, including the rights of human subjects, are followed. **Informed consent** means that research subjects (1) are given full and complete information about the purpose of a study, procedures, data collection, potential harm and benefits, and alternative methods of treatment; (2) are capable of fully understanding the research and the implications of participation; (3) have the power of free choice to voluntarily consent or decline participation in the research; and (4) understand how the researcher maintains confidentiality or anonymity. **Confidentiality** guarantees that any information a subject provides will not be reported in any manner that identifies the subject and will not be accessible to people outside the research team.

Once the peppermint gum study begins, the nurses on the unit collect data as indicated in the study protocol. Once all data are collected from every patient in the study, the team analyzes the data from the nausea self-report instrument and the chart review about bowel function from the two groups studied. With the help of the statistician, analysis of the results determines whether patients who chewed peppermint gum experienced less nausea and a quicker return of bowel function than the patients who had standard nursing care. The nurse knows that results from this study may advance postoperative nursing care for the nursing unit.

Researchers always need to consider study limitations. Limitations are factors that affect study findings, such as a small sample of subjects, a unique setting where the study was conducted, or the failure of the study to include representative cultural groups or age-groups. The research team in this example conducted a pilot study because few data were available about the benefits of chewing gum following abdominal surgery. The sample size included only 30 patients in each group, and it was challenging to collect all the data from the patient charts because of inconsistencies in documentation. Therefore the results of the study have limited generalizability to other patients who are experiencing abdominal surgery. These limitations help the team decide how to refine or adapt the study for further investigation in the future.

A researcher also addresses the implications for nursing practice. This ultimately helps fellow researchers, clinicians, educators, and administrators apply findings from a study in practice. At the end of the chewing gum study, the research team recommends that patients who have elective colon resections be offered the opportunity to chew peppermint gum following surgery. The surgeons on the unit agree to the change in practice. The team decides to conduct another larger study to investigate this intervention with patients who have other types of abdominal operations to enhance the generalizability of the results. In addition, the team suggests ways to effectively introduce the use of chewing gum into other surgical units following surgery.

PERFORMANCE IMPROVEMENT

Performance improvement (PI) is a formal approach for the analysis of health care–related processes at a local level. *Local* means analysis of processes unique to a nursing unit, health care agency, or health care system. PI is not a process allowing for generalizability of findings to other settings. PI is one approach that organizations use to learn how processes (e.g., discharge process, medication delivery to patient care units, radiological procedure scheduling) can be altered to yield higher-quality care, better patient experience, and lower costs ("triple aim") (Song and Tucker, 2016).

PI does not involve introduction of new practices, as is the case with EBP, but instead involves review of how existing interventions within a process function. Health care organizations routinely promote efforts for improving patient care processes and outcomes, particularly with respect to reducing medical errors and enhancing patient safety. PI is the continuous and ongoing effort to achieve measurable improvements in the efficiency, effectiveness, performance, accountability, outcomes, and other indicators of quality services or processes (Green et al., 2018).

Every health care organization gathers and reports data on multiple performance and health outcome measures to determine its quality of care. When findings, such as monthly trending, suggest potential problems, an organization institutes a formal PI initiative. In many cases the same trending from PI data reveals problems that lead to EBP projects. PI projects usually occur more quickly than an EBP or research project. An organization analyzes and evaluates current performance data to solve system problems (e.g., supply delivery, appointment scheduling), people problems (e.g., staffing ratios, communication protocols), or clinical problems (e.g., surgical incision infection rates, patient injuries from falls). When interprofessional teams participate in PI activities,

TABLE 5.3 Examples of Performance Improvement Models

Performance Improvement Model	Summary Description
Balanced scorecard	A multidimensional framework for managing strategy by linking objectives, initiatives, targets, and performance measures across key organization perspectives.
Root cause analysis (RCA)	A structured method used to analyze serious adverse events. A central tenet of RCA is to identify underlying problems that increase the likelihood of errors while avoiding the trap of focusing on mistakes by individuals.
Six Sigma	A disciplined methodology for process improvement that deploys a wide set of tools based on rigorous data analysis to identify sources of variation in performance and ways of reducing them.
Plan-Do-Study-Act (PDSA)	An experiential learning method that involves analyzing a quality problem and testing a change by developing a plan to test the change (Plan), carrying out the test (Do), observing and learning from the consequences (Study), and determining which modifications should be made to the test (Act).

they may or may not use research findings to develop strategies; however, an evidenced-based approach is advised when dealing with clinical problems.

Performance Improvement Programs

A well-organized PI program focuses on processes or systems that significantly contribute to outcomes of a specific organization, and how to sustain measurable improvements over time. Agencies need an organization-wide, systematic approach to ensure that everyone supports a continuous PI philosophy. This begins with the organizational culture, in which all staff members understand their responsibility toward maintaining and improving quality (Connelly, 2018). Typically in health care many people are involved in single processes of care. For example, medication delivery involves the health care provider who prescribes medications, the secretary who communicates new orders being written, the pharmacist who prepares the dosage, the transporter who delivers medications, and the nurse who prepares and administers the drugs. When an agency identifies a need to improve the medication administration process, all professions involved in medication administration need to be engaged in the PI process. Because most health care processes are interprofessional, all members of the health care team collaborate in PI activities. As a member of the nursing team, you participate in recognizing trends in practice, identifying recurrent problems, and initiating opportunities to improve care.

The PI process begins at the staff level, where all disciplines become involved in identifying quality problems. This requires staff members to know the outcomes measured by the organization and the practice standards or guidelines that define quality. Unit PI committees review quality data and the activities or services considered to be most important in providing high-quality care to patients. One way to identify the greatest opportunity for improving quality is to consider activities that are high volume (greater than 50% of the activity of a unit); high risk (potential for trauma or death); and problem areas for patients, staff, or the institution. For example, on an orthopedic nursing unit hip surgery volume is high, adults older than 80 years have more postoperative complications, and family members are dissatisfied with patients' pain control. Any one of these factors could become the focus of a PI project.

Another approach to PI is to use The Joint Commission's (TJC's) annual patient safety goals (TJC, 2021), which provide an excellent focus for PI initiatives (see Chapter 27). Sometimes a problem is presented to a committee in the form of a sentinel event, an unexpected occurrence involving death or serious physical or psychological injury of a patient. After a sentinel event, the unit conducts a root cause analysis (RCA). The goal of the RCA is to review all information and identify how the event occurred through identification of active errors (i.e., the acts that personnel perform) and why it occurred through

identification and analysis of latent errors (i.e., the organization or steps of the process). Once a committee defines the problem, it applies a formal PI model for exploring and resolving quality concerns. There are several models for PI (Table 5.3). Health care organizations today are changing current organizational culture toward the concept of a "just culture." In a just culture, the organization values the reporting of errors and is focused on the processes that lead to the error. A just culture also values nurses' critical thinking and problem-solving skills and the nurses' work on improving patient care processes (Paradiso and Sweeney, 2019).

When findings from PI efforts are ultimately combined with EBP, this creates a foundation for excellent patient care and outcomes. Once a PI committee makes an EBP change, it is important to monitor the results and then communicate the results to staff from all appropriate departments. Practice changes are unlikely to last when PI committees fail to report findings and the results of interventions (Nilsen et al., 2017). Regular discussions of PI activities through staff meetings, newsletters, and memos are good communication strategies. Often a PI study reveals information that prompts organization-wide change. An organization must be responsible for responding to the problem with the appropriate resources. Revision of P&Ps, modification of standards of care, and implementation of new support services are examples of ways an organization responds.

QSEN Building Competency in Evidence-Based Practice The Nursing Practice Council notes that the incidence of falls with injuries has increased on all units in the agency over the past year. When checking its fall prevention protocol, the council notes it was last reviewed 4 years ago. The council knows that falls with injuries are a nursing-sensitive outcome (NDNQI) and establishes a goal to reduce the incidence of falls in the upcoming year. How should the Nursing Practice Council proceed?

Answers to QSEN Activities can be found on the Evolve website.

THE RELATIONSHIP AMONG EVIDENCE-BASED PRACTICE, RESEARCH, AND PERFORMANCE IMPROVEMENT

EBP, research, and PI are closely interrelated (Fig. 5.3) and exist along a continuum of clinical scholarship (Carter et al., 2017). All three processes require you to ultimately use the best evidence to provide the highest quality of patient care. As a nurse you are professionally accountable to know the differences and which process to select when facing clinical problems or when you desire to improve patient care.

FIG. 5.3 The overlapping relationship among research, evidence-based practice *(EBP),* and performance improvement.

Although you will use all of these processes in nursing practice, it is important to know the similarities and differences among them (Carter et al., 2017) (Table 5.4). When implementing an EBP project, it is important to first review evidence from appropriate research literature as well as PI data, when available. This information helps you better understand the extent of a problem in practice and within your organization. PI data inform you about how processes work within an organization and thus offer information about how to eventually make EBP changes. EBP and PI sometimes reveal problems that then create opportunities for research.

The following is an example of how the three processes merge to improve nursing practice:

A nursing unit has been experiencing a decrease in patient satisfaction with pain management over the last several months. PI data identify factors associated with pain management for patients on the unit (e.g., the types of pain medications typically ordered, patient reports of pain relief following administration of pain medications). A thorough analysis of PI data leads a unit-based PI team of nurses to conduct a literature review and implement the best evidence available to improve their pain-management protocol for the type of patients on the unit. The staff implement a revised pain-management protocol and evaluate its results. Despite the implementation of the revised pain-management protocol, patient satisfaction data continue to be lower than desired. Therefore staff decide to conduct a research study to further investigate this clinical problem and improve patient care. The study will focus on the factor that patients perceive as most likely influencing their perception of pain management.

■ KEY POINTS

- EBP guides nurses in addressing clinical problems by looking for the very best scientific and clinical evidence available for treating or managing the problems and implementing changes in practice.
- Use EBP and clinical judgment and consider the patient's values and preferences to ensure that you provide competent, safe, patient-centered care.
- The steps of EBP include cultivating a spirit of inquiry, asking a clinical question in PICOT format, searching for the most relevant

TABLE 5.4	**Similarities and Differences Among Evidence-Based Practice, Research, and Performance Improvement**		
	Evidence-Based Practice	**Research**	**Performance Improvement**
Purpose	Use of information from research, professional experts, personal experience, and patient preferences to determine safe and effective nursing interventions with the goal of improving patient outcomes.	Systematic inquiry answers questions, solves problems, and contributes to the generalizable knowledge base of nursing; it may or may not improve patient care.	Improves local work processes to improve patient outcomes and efficiency of health systems; results usually not generalizable.
Focus	Implementation of evidence already known into practice.	New knowledge is generated to find answers for questions that are not known about nursing practice.	Measures effects of practice and/or practice change on specific patient population.
Data sources	Multiple research studies, expert opinion, personal experience, patients	Subjects or participants have predefined characteristics that include or exclude them from a study; researcher collects and analyzes data from subjects.	Data from patient records or patients who are in a specific area such as on a patient care unit or admitted to a particular hospital.
Who conducts the activity?	Practicing nurses and possibly other members of the health care team	Researchers who may or may not be employed by the health care agency and usually are not a part of the clinical health care team	Employees of a health care agency such as nurses, physicians, pharmacists
Is activity part of regular clinical practice?	Yes	No	Yes
Is IRB approval needed?	Sometimes	Yes	Sometimes
Funding sources	Internal, from health care agency	Funding is usually external, such as a government grant. However, larger health care organizations often have internal grants available from their foundations.	Internal, from health care agency

IRB, Institutional review board.

and best evidence, critically appraising the evidence, integrating the best evidence, evaluating the outcomes of the practice change, and communicating results of the change.

- A well-developed PICOT question having the components of population (P), intervention (I), comparison (C), outcome (O), and time (T) will guide your search for evidence in the scientific literature.
- The systematic review or meta-analysis of RCTs and clinical practice guidelines based on systematic reviews provide the highest level of evidence to include when conducting a literature review; opinions are the lowest level of evidence to use in research literature review.
- Nurses apply evidence in practice through direct application or use of the evidence in patient care or by using the evidence to make a larger scale practice change for a health care agency.
- The research process is an orderly series of six steps that allow the researcher to move from problem identification to development of the research question, through study development with data collection and data analysis, to finding an answer to the research question and sharing the findings.
- Quantitative research methods include experimental, nonexperimental, survey, and evaluation research. These methods are similar in that these methods are systematic, objective methodologies that use numerical data and statistical analyses to examine a study's variables and answer the research question.
- Qualitative research methods include phenomenology, ethnography, and grounded theory research. These methods use nonnumerical data gathered through interviews or observation to understand patients' experiences with health problems and the contexts in which the experiences occur.
- Nursing research is a systematic process that asks and answers questions to generate knowledge and provide a scientific basis for nursing practice.
- Translation research in nursing is conducted to promote the use of evidence-based practice by testing implementation strategies in real-world settings to determine which strategies work best among diverse patient groups.
- Performance improvement (PI) is a formal approach used to study the processes or systems that contribute to the outcomes of an organization. PI also focuses on how to attain and sustain measurable improvements over time.
- EBP, research, and performance improvement (PI) are closely related but separate processes that use best evidence. EBP uses research literature and PI data when available to provide evidence for practice change, and EBP and PI can lead to opportunities for research.

REFLECTIVE LEARNING

- Reflect on the decisions you made during your clinical day. Describe you how used EBP to guide your clinical judgment in making one of the clinical decisions for your patient.
- Think about the nursing care that you provided to your patients on the clinical unit today. What questions came to your mind about the practices that you were doing? Formulate one of the questions in PICOT format.
- After asking a PICOT question, search the literature and find two or three research studies on the topic. What is the current state of the evidence related to your question?

REVIEW QUESTIONS

1. Match the components of PICO using the question "Does the use of guided imagery compared with standard care affect the postoperative pain in hospitalized adolescents?

_____ (P) Patient/population   A. Adolescents receiving standard care
_____ (I) Intervention   B. Postoperative pain
_____ (C) Comparison   C. Hospitalized adolescents
_____ (O) Outcome   D. Guided imagery

2. Place the steps of the EBP process in the appropriate order.
   1. Critically appraise the evidence you gather.
   2. Ask the clinical question in PICOT format.
   3. Evaluate the outcomes of the practice decision or change.
   4. Search for the most relevant and best evidence.
   5. Cultivate a spirit of inquiry.
   6. Integrate the evidence.
   7. Communicate the outcomes of the EBP change.

3. A nurse is reading a research article discussing a new practice to decrease the incidence of catheter-associated urinary tract infections. One section of the article describes who was studied and how the data were collected to answer the research questions and hypotheses. What section of the research article is currently being read?
   1. The literature review
   2. The data analysis
   3. The methods
   4. The implications for practice

4. A nurse implements an EBP change that teaches patients the importance of taking their diabetes medications correctly and regularly on time using videos streamed on the Internet. The nurse measures the patients' behavioral outcome from the practice change by using which type of measurement?
   1. Measuring the patients' weight
   2. Chart auditing teaching sessions
   3. Observing patients viewing the videos
   4. Checking patients' blood sugars

5. A patient in the ICU experiences a sentinel event related to central line catheter care that resulted in serious injury. What PI model should the unit use to identify errors that led to the sentinel event?
   1. Six Sigma
   2. Root cause analysis
   3. PDSA
   4. Balanced scorecard

6. The nurse identifies which of the following as outcomes measurements? (Select all that apply.)
   1. A nurse teaches a patient how to administer an injection and then watches the patient do a return demonstration.
   2. A nurse implements a new pain-management protocol and checks patients' charts to confirm whether interventions are being provided.
   3. A nursing unit adopts a set of strategies for reducing pressure injuries, and the UPC members use direct observation of the skin to measure incidence of pressure injuries.
   4. A nursing unit implements a new fall prevention protocol and checks the monthly performance data for incidence of falls on the unit.
   5. A nursing unit implements a patient rounding program, and the charge nurse watches the assistive personnel to see whether hourly rounding is being done on patients.

7. The nurses on a medical unit have seen an increase in the number of pressure injuries developing in their patients. The nurses decide to initiate a PI project using the PDSA model. Which of the following is an example of "Plan" from that model?
   1. Orienting patients to the unit's practice of hourly rounding on patients
   2. Reviewing the incidence of pressure injuries on patients cared for using the protocol

3. Based on findings from patients who developed injuries, implementing an evidence-based skin care protocol on all units
4. Meeting with all disciplines to develop a multidisciplinary approach for reducing pressure injuries

8. The nurse is using the QSEN competency of EBP when working with the unit council to initiate a change related to pain management. Which behaviors demonstrate that the nurse is practicing behaviors associated with EBP? (Select all that apply.)
   1. Initiating plan for self-development as a team member
   2. Reading original research related to pain management
   3. Demonstrating effective use of strategies to reduce risk of harm to self or others
   4. Valuing EBP as critical to the development of pain management guidelines for the unit
   5. Describing to the unit council reliable sources for locating clinical guidelines
   6. Applying technology and information management tools to support safe processes of care

9. Nurses in a community clinic are conducting an EBP project focused on improving the outcomes of children with asthma. The PICO question asked by the nurses is "In school-age children, does the use of an electronic gaming education module versus educational book affect the usage of inhalers?" In the question, what is the "O"?
   1. School-age children
   2. Educational book
   3. Use of inhalers
   4. Electronic gaming education

10. A nurse research investigator is explaining a research study to a patient. The patient is interested in participating in the research study. The nurse investigator reviews the informed consent with the patient. The patient asks the nurse why he must sign the consent to participate in the study. What is the nurse's best response(s) to the patient's question? (Select all that apply.)
   1. "The informed consent (IC) provides you with complete information on the research study."
   2. "By reviewing the consent with you, I can make sure that you understand the study and what it means for you to participate."
   3. "The informed consent provides details on the limitations of the study."
   4. "The informed consent provides your voluntary agreement to participate in the research study."
   5. "The informed consent explains how the data collected from you will be kept confidential during and after the study."

Answers: 1. C; D, A, B; 2. 5, 2, 4, 1, 6, 3; 7; 3. 3, 4, 5; 2, 6, 1, 3, 4; 7, 4; 8. 2, 4, 5; 9. 3; 10. 1, 2, 4, 5

Rationales for Review Questions can be found on the Evolve website.

REFERENCES

American Nurses Association (ANA). *Nursing: scope and standards of nursing practice*, ed 4, Washington, DC, 2021, American Nurses Publishing.

American Nurses Credentialing Center (ANCC): *Why become Magnet?* n.d., https://www.nursingworld.org/organizational-programs/magnet/about-magnet/why-become-magnet/. Accessed September 16, 2020.

Carter EJ et al: Clarifying the conundrum: evidence-based practice, quality improvement, or research? *J Nurs Adm* 47(5):266, 2017.

Centers for Medicare and Medicaid (CMS): *Hospital acquired conditions*, 2020a, https://www.cms.gov/Medicare/Medicare-Fee-for-Service-Payment/HospitalAcqCond/Hospital-Acquired_Conditions, Accessed September 17, 2020.

Centers for Medicare and Medicaid (CMS): *Hospital-Acquired Condition Reduction Program (HACRP)*, 2020b, https://www.cms.gov/Medicare/Medicare-Fee-for-Service-Payment/AcuteInpatientPPS/HAC-Reduction-Program" https://www.cms.gov/Medicare/Medicare-Fee-for-Service-Payment/AcuteInpatientPPS/HAC-Reduction-Program Accessed September 17, 2020.

Connelly LM: Overview of quality improvement, *Med Surg Nurs* 27(2):125, 2018.

Dols JD et al: Developing Policies and Protocols in the Age of Evidence-Based Practice, *J Contin Educ Nurs*, 48(2):87, 2017.

Green R et al.: The CFO's role in accelerating systemwide performance improvement: finance leaders can leverage their operational expertise to serve as catalysts for comprehensive performance improvement: a systematic approach to increasing overall value, *Healthc Financl Manage* 72(6):48, 2018.

Grove SK, Gray JR: *Understanding nursing research: building an evidence-based practice*, ed 7, St. Louis, 2019, Elsevier.

Johns Hopkins: *Johns Hopkins nursing evidence-based model & guidelines*, ed 3, Indianapolis, IN, 2018, Sigma Theta Tau International. https://sigma.nursingrepository.org/bitstream/handle/10755/623549/Free Download_JohnsHopkinsEBPModelGuidelines3rdEdition_DangDearholt.pdf;jsessionid=3148EA4AC5A18445D0C8EBBE7116A7A5?sequence=1. Accessed September 17, 2020.

Lobiondo-Wood G, Haber J: *Nursing research: methods and critical appraisal for evidence-based practice*, ed 9, St Louis, 2018, Elsevier.

Melnyk BM et al.: *Implementing the evidence-based practice competencies in healthcare: a practical guide for improving quality, safety, & outcomes*, Indianapolis, IN, 2017, Sigma Theta Tau International.

Melnyk BM, Fineout-Overholt E: *Evidence-based practice in nursing and healthcare: a guide to best practice*, ed 4, Philadelphia, 2019, Lippincott Williams & Wilkins.

Mitchell SA, Freise CR: *Decision rules for summative evaluation of a body of evidence*, 2020. https://www.ons.org/explore-resources/pep/decision-rules-summative-evaluation-body-evidence. Accessed September 17, 2020.

National Database of Nursing Quality Indicators (NDNQI): *Benefits of NDNQI: what is in it for you?* n.d., https://nursingandndnqi.weebly.com/benefits-of-ndnqi.html. Accessed September 16, 2020.

National Institutes of Health: *National Institute of Nursing research (NINR)*, 2020, https://www.nih.gov/about-nih/what-we-do/nih-almanac/national-institute-nursing-research-ninr#:~:text=It%20is%20organized%20around%20four,areas%20of%20NINR's%20research%20programs. Accessed September 17, 2020.

National Institute of Nursing Research (NINR): *The National Institute of Nursing Research,* n.d., http://www.ninr.nih.gov. Accessed September 17, 2020.

National Quality Forum (NQF): *NQF's strategic direction 2016-2019: lead, prioritize, and collaborate for better healthcare measurement*, http://www.qualityforum.org/NQF_Strategic_Direction_2016-2019.aspx, 2020. Accessed September 16, 2020.

Naylor, M.D.: Overview and Summary: Translational Research: From Knowledge to Practice. *OJIN: Online J Issues Nurs* 23(2), 2018.

Nilsen P et al.: Implementation of evidence-based practice from a learning perspective, *Worldviews Evid Based Nurs* 14(3):192, 2017.

Patient-Centered Outcomes Research Institute (PCORI): PCORI. 2020, http://www.pcori.org/. Accessed September 17, 2020.

Quality and Safety Education for Nurses (QSEN) Institute: *QSEN Competencies*, 2020, http://qsen.org/competencies/pre-licensure-ksas/. Accessed September 17, 2020.

Social Programs That Work: *Social Programs That Work Review—Evidence Summary for the Transitional Care Model, Laura and John Arnold Foundation*, 2017. https://evidencebasedprograms.org/document/the-transitional-care-model-evidence-summary/ Accessed September 17, 2020.

Song H, Tucker A: Performance Improvement in Health Care Organizations, *Foundations and Trends in Technology, Information and Operations Management*, 9(3-4): 153, 2016.

The Joint Commission (TJC): 2021 *National Patient Safety Goals*, Oakbrook Terrace, IL, 2021, The Commission. https://www.jointcommission.org/standards/national-patient-safety-goals/. Accessed April 14, 2021.

Titler MG: Translation research in practice: an introduction. *Online J Issues Nurs* 23(2):1, 2018.

Trautman DE et al.: Advancing scholarship through translational research: the role of PhD and DNP prepared nurses *Online J Issues Nurs* 23(2):1, 2018.

Tucker S, Melnyk BM: A leader's guide to implementing evidence-based practice: Lead the way to healthcare quality and safety, *American Nurse Today* 14 (6): 6, 2019.

U.S. Department of Health and Human Services: National Institutes of Health – NINR, 2020 budget, https://www.ninr.nih.gov/sites/files/docs/NINR-Budget-FY-2020-508c.pdf. Accessed September 17, 2020.

RESEARCH REFERENCES

Bourgault AM et al.: Using Gemba boards to facilitate evidence-based practice in critical care. *Crit Care Nurse* 38(3):e1, 2018.

Buccheri RK, Sharifi C: Critical appraisal tools and reporting guidelines for evidence-based practice. *Worldviews Evid-Based Nurs* 14(6):463, 2017.

Caramanica L, Spiva L: Exploring nurse manager support of evidence-based practice: clinical nurse perceptions. *JONA* 48(5):272, 2018.

Carter EJ, Rivera RR: Targeted interventions to advance a culture of inquiry at a large multicampus hospital among nurses. *JONA* 48(1):18, 2018.

Chiwaula CH et al.: Evidence-based practice: a concept analysis. *Health Syst Policy Res* 5(3): 75, 2018.

Ecoff L et al.: Design, implementation and evaluation of a regional evidence-based practice institute. *Applied Nursing Research* 55: 151300, 2020.

Friesen MA et al.: Findings from a pilot study: bringing evidence-based practice to the bedside. *Worldviews Evid Based Nurs* 14(1):22, 2017.

Fritz E: Interventions to increase use of evidence-based practice by ambulatory care nurses. *AAACN ViewPoint* 4, 2017. July/August.

Harvey G et al.: Leadership for evidence-based practice-enforcing or enabling implementation? *Collegian* 27:57, 2020.

Jun J et al.: Does unit culture matter? The association between unit culture and the use of evidence-based practice among hospital nurses. *Applied Nursing Research* 53: 151251, 2020.

Kim SC et al.: Benefits of a regional evidence-based practice fellowship program: a test of the ARCC model. *Worldviews Evid Based Nurs* 14(2):90, 2017.

Mathieson A et al.: Strategies, facilitators and barriers to implementation of evidence-based practice in community nursing: a systematic mixed-studies review and qualitative synthesis. *Primary Health Care Research & Development* 20(e6): 1, 2018.

Melnyk BM et al.: Outcomes from the first Helene Fuld Health Trust National Institute for Evidence-Based Practice in Nursing and Healthcare Invitational Expert Forum. *Worldviews Evid Based Nurs* 15(1):5, 2018a.

Melnyk BM et al.: The first U.S. study on nurses' evidence-based practice competencies indicates major deficits that threaten healthcare quality, safety, and patient outcomes. *Worldviews Evid Based Nurs* 15(1):16, 2018b.

Migliore L et al.: Clinical research and practice collaborative: an evidence-based nursing clinical inquiry expansion. *Military Medicine* 185(S2):35, 2020.

Naylor, MD., et al: Comprehensive Discharge Planning for the Hospitalized Elderly: A Randomized Clinical Trial. *Annals of Internal Medicine*, 120: 999, 1994.

Paradiso L, Sweeney N: Just culture: it's more than policy. *Nurs Manage* 50(6):38. 2019.

Skaggs MKD et al.: Using evidence-based practice service nursing bundle to increase patient satisfaction. *J Emerg Nurs* 44(1): 37, 2018.

Speroni KG et al.: Use of evidence-based practice models and research findings in Magnet-designated hospitals across the United States: national survey results. *Worldviews Evid Based Nurs* 17(2):98, 2020.

Sun C, Prufeta P: Using a Delphi Survey to develop clinical nursing research priorities among nursing management. *JONA* 49(3): 156, 2019.

Yoo JY et al: Clinical nurses' beliefs, knowledge, organizational readiness and level of implementation of evidence-based practice: The first step to creating an evidence-based practice culture. *PLoS ONE* 14(12): e0226742, 2019.

6

Health and Wellness

OBJECTIVES

- Explain how *Healthy People* guides public health goals for Americans.
- Discuss how individuals define health.
- Discuss the health belief, health promotion, basic human needs, and holistic health models to understand the relationship between patients' attitudes toward health and health practices.
- Identify variables influencing health, health beliefs, and health practices.
- Discuss health promotion, health education, and illness prevention activities.

- Compare the three levels of prevention.
- Compare and contrast nonmodifiable and modifiable risk factors that threaten health.
- Discuss the nurse's role in risk-factor modification and changing health behaviors.
- Analyze variables influencing illness behavior.
- Discuss the effect of illness on patients and families.

KEY TERMS

Acute disease
Chronic disease
Health
Health Belief Model
Health education

Health promotion
Holistic Health Model
Illness
Illness behavior
Illness prevention

Primary prevention
Risk factor
Secondary prevention
Tertiary prevention

MEDIA RESOURCES

http://evolve.elsevier.com/Potter/fundamentals/
- Review Questions
- Case Study with Questions

- Audio Glossary
- Content Updates
- Answers to QSEN Activity and Review Questions

Nurses function in the unique roles of caregiver, advocate, and educator to help individuals, families, communities, and populations achieve their highest level of health in all health care settings. Nurses use their knowledge, assessment skills, and clinical judgment to identify actual and potential risk factors that predispose individuals or groups to illness. In addition, nurses use strategies to help patients modify their risk factors to prevent or limit the effects of illness.

People react differently to their own illnesses or the illnesses of their family members. When nurses use clinical judgment to understand how patients react to illness, they can better help patients and their families maintain or return to the highest level of functioning, resulting in reduced health care costs. Thus, it is important that you analyze assessment data to identify how to help patients make changes to improve their health and wellness.

HEALTHY PEOPLE

The *Healthy People* initiative provides evidence-based, 10-year national objectives for promoting health and preventing disease. *Healthy People* sets objectives to help the United States increase its focus on health promotion and disease prevention (instead of illness care) and encourages cooperation among individuals, communities, and other public, private, and nonprofit organizations to improve health (Office of Disease Prevention and Health Promotion [ODPHP], n.d.). Widely cited by the media, in professional journals, and at health conferences, *Healthy People* emphasizes how the health of communities affects the overall health status of the nation. Because of its interprofessional approach, it has inspired health promotion programs throughout the country since its first publication in 1979.

The current publication, *Healthy People 2030,* promotes a society in which all people live long, healthy lives. *Healthy People 2030* identifies leading health indicators (LHIs) (e.g., household food insecurity and hunger; homicides; suicides; children and adolescents with obesity), which are high-priority health issues in the United States. Although the United States has made great progress on the LHIs, it falls behind other developed countries on key measures of health and well-being, including life expectancy, infant mortality, and obesity (ODPHP, n.d.). The *Healthy People 2030* website provides data about the LHIs to explain existing health disparities (ODPHP, n.d.).

DEFINITION OF HEALTH

The World Health Organization (WHO) defines health as a "state of complete physical, mental, and social well-being, not merely the absence of disease or infirmity" (WHO, 1947, 2021a). Health is a state of being that people define in relation to their own values, personality, and lifestyle. Each person has a personal concept of health. Health is the actualization of inherent and acquired human potential through goal-directed behavior, competent self-care, and satisfying relationships with others (Pender et al., 2015; Murdaugh et al., 2019). People adjust as needed to maintain structural integrity and harmony with the environment.

People who are free from disease are not necessarily healthy (Pender, 1996). Health is influenced by a person's culture and lifestyle (Murdaugh et al., 2019). Culture influences our values, how we define health, what we believe about illness, where we seek health care, and the treatments we prefer. Culture also influences the types of health promotion activities people practice. Sometimes people define their health by the circumstances surrounding their lives rather than by their physical condition. Life conditions can have positive or negative effects on health long before an illness is evident (Murdaugh et al., 2019). Life conditions include socioeconomic variables such as environment, diet, lifestyle practices or choices, and many other physiological and psychological variables.

Individual perceptions and definitions of health change with age and are affected by a person's health beliefs. For example, some older adults define health by the health practices they use regularly, while others define their health as the absence of disease and disability, the maintenance of physical and cognitive functioning, and having connections with others (Griffith et al., 2018). Thus, you need to consider the total person, including the environment, to individualize nursing care and enhance a patient's health.

MODELS OF HEALTH AND ILLNESS

Models help explain complex concepts or ideas, such as health and illness. Models help you understand the relationships between these concepts and a patient's attitudes toward health and health behaviors.

Health beliefs are a person's ideas, convictions, and attitudes about health and illness. They can be based on reality or false expectations, facts or misinformation, common sense or myths, or good or bad experiences. Because health beliefs influence health behavior, they can positively or negatively affect a patient's level of health. Positive health behaviors maintain, attain, or regain health and prevent illness. Common positive health behaviors include immunizations, scheduled screenings (e.g., colonoscopy, mammogram), proper sleep patterns, adequate exercise, stress management, and nutrition. Negative health behaviors include practices that are harmful to health, such as smoking, drug or alcohol abuse, risky sexual behaviors, poor diet, and refusing to take necessary medications.

Nurses use several health models to understand patients' unique attitudes and values about health and illness and to provide effective health care. These models allow you to understand and predict patients' health behaviors, including how they use health services and adhere to recommended therapy. Positive health models focus on an individual's strengths, resiliencies, resources, potential, and capabilities rather than on disease or pathology (Murdaugh et al., 2019).

Your clinical judgment will help you identify which model to use when creating individualized plans of care that will be effective in restoring or promoting a patient's health. Remember that each patient has a unique view of health and wellness. A person's individual belief system influences the ability to make lasting changes in health status. Do not make judgments when your patients have views and beliefs that differ from your own.

Health Belief Model

The Health Belief Model (Fig. 6.1) addresses the relationship between a person's beliefs and behaviors (Rosenstoch, 1974; Becker and Maiman, 1975). The first component of this model involves an individual's perception of susceptibility to an illness. For example, a patient whose family history includes one parent and two siblings who have died from a myocardial infarction (MI) recognizes the familial link for coronary artery disease and perceives a personal risk of heart disease.

The second component is an individual's perception of the seriousness of the illness. This perception is influenced and modified by demographic and sociopsychological variables, perceived threats of the illness, and cues to action (e.g., mass media campaigns and advice from family, friends, and medical professionals). For example, a patient may not perceive his or her heart disease to be serious, which may affect self-care.

The third component is the likelihood that a person will take preventive action. This component results from a person's perception of the benefits of and barriers to taking action. Preventive actions include lifestyle changes, increased adherence to medical therapies, or a search for medical advice or treatment. A patient's perception of susceptibility to disease and perception of the seriousness of an illness help to determine the likelihood that the patient will adopt healthy behaviors. Use of this model helps you understand factors influencing patients' perceptions, beliefs, and behaviors to plan care so that you can more effectively help patients maintain or restore health and prevent illness.

Health Promotion Model

The Health Promotion Model (HPM) (Pender, 1982; Murdaugh et al., 2019) defines health as a positive, dynamic state, not merely the absence of disease (Fig. 6.2). Health promotion increases a patient's level of well-being. The HPM describes the multidimensional nature of people as they interact within their environment to pursue health (Murdaugh et al., 2019). The model focuses on the following three areas: (1) individual characteristics and experiences; (2) behavior-specific cognitions and affect; and (3) behavioral outcome, in which the patient commits to or changes a behavior. Each person has unique personal characteristics and experiences that affect subsequent actions. The variables for behavioral-specific cognitions and affect influence a patient's motivation to change or adopt healthy behaviors. When applying this model, you help a patient modify these variables through nursing interventions. Health-promoting behaviors result in improved health, enhanced functional ability, and better quality of life at all stages of development (Murdaugh et al., 2019).

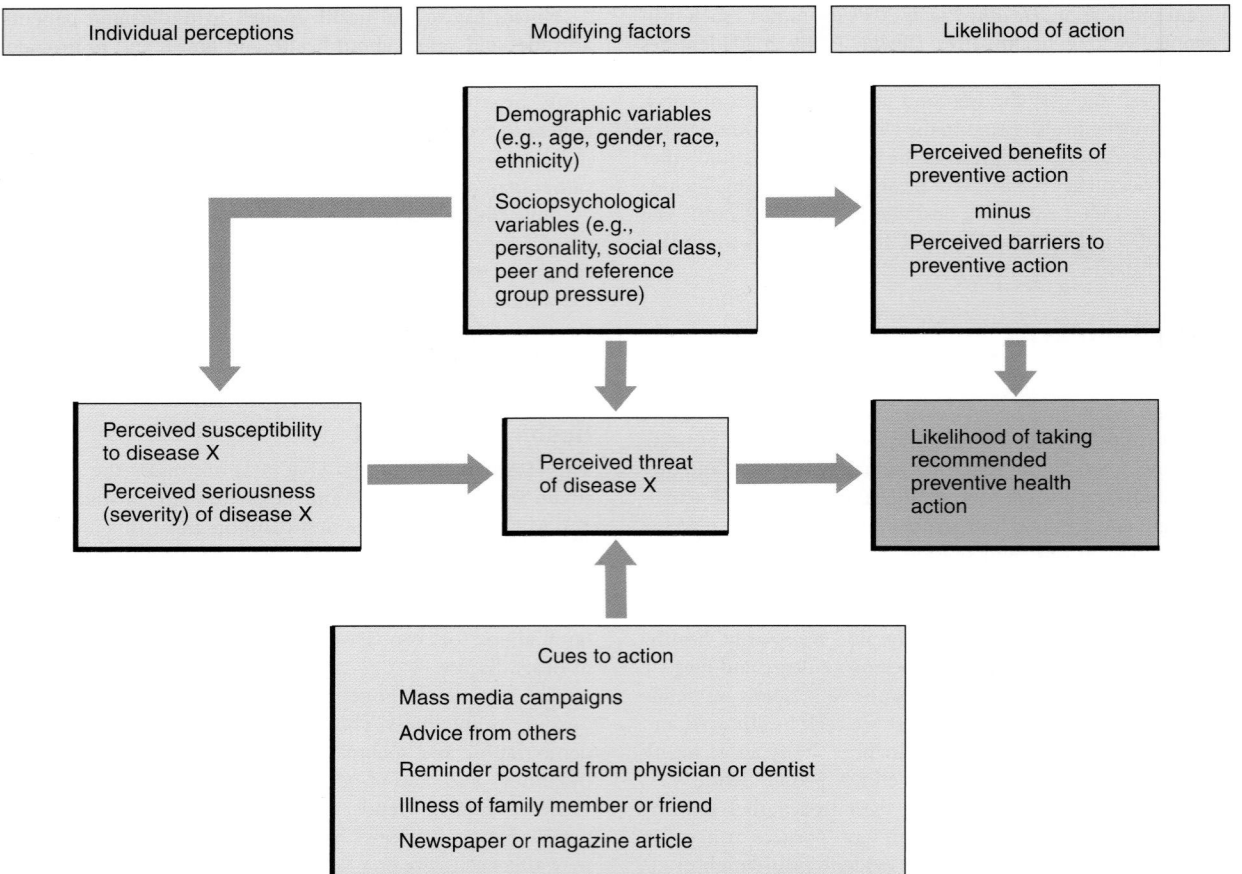

FIG. 6.1 Health Belief Model. (Data from Becker M, Maiman L: Sociobehavioral determinants of compliance with health and medical care recommendations, *Med Care* 13[1]:10, 1975.)

Maslow's Hierarchy of Needs

Nurses use Maslow's hierarchy of needs to understand the interrelationships of basic human needs (Fig. 6.3). Basic human needs (e.g., food, water, safety, and love) are necessary for human survival and health. Although each person has unique needs, all people share basic human needs, and the extent to which people meet their basic needs is a major factor in determining their level of health.

According to this model, certain human needs are more basic than others, and some needs must be met before other needs (e.g., fulfilling physiological needs before the needs of love and belonging). Self-actualization is the highest expression of one's individual potential and allows for continual self-discovery. Maslow's model considers individual experiences, which are always unique to that individual (Touhy and Jett, 2020).

Maslow's hierarchy provides a basis for nurses to care for patients of all ages in all health settings. However, when applying the model, focus your care on a patient's needs rather than on strict adherence to the hierarchy. It is unrealistic to always expect a patient's basic needs to occur in the fixed hierarchical order. In all cases an emergent physiological need takes precedence over a higher-level need. In other situations, a psychological or physical safety need takes priority. For example, in a house fire, fear of injury and death takes priority over self-esteem issues. As another example, while you are caring for a patient following a partial mastectomy, you anticipate her priority need will be pain control based on Maslow's hierarchy. However, after completing her assessment and analyzing her cues, you realize that while she needs pain control, her greatest need at this time is in the areas of love, belonging, and self-esteem. Although reflecting on your experience is important, do not assume a patient's needs just because other patients reacted in a certain way. Apply Maslow's hierarchy to each patient individually. To provide the most effective care, you need to understand the relationships among different needs and the factors that determine the priorities for each patient.

Holistic Health Model

The relationships among body, mind, and spirit affect a person's overall health. The Holistic Health Model of nursing promotes a patient's optimal level of health by considering the dynamic interactions among the emotional, spiritual, social, cultural, and physical aspects of an individual's wellness (LaVela et al., 2017). You put your patients at the center of their care and recognize your patients as the ultimate experts concerning their own health. A patient's subjective experience is relevant in maintaining health or assisting in healing. The Holistic Health Model empowers patients to engage in their own recovery and assume some responsibility for health maintenance (Edelman and Kudzma, 2018).

The Holistic Health Model supports how our choices powerfully affect our health. Some of the most widely used holistic interventions include meditation, music therapy, reminiscence, relaxation therapy, therapeutic touch, and guided imagery (see Chapter 32). These holistic strategies, which can be used in all stages of health and illness, are integral in the expanding role of nursing.

INDIVIDUAL
CHARACTERISTICS
AND EXPERIENCES

BEHAVIOR-SPECIFIC
COGNITIONS
AND AFFECT

BEHAVIORAL
OUTCOME

FIG. 6.2 Health Promotion Model (revised). (From Pender NJ, et al.: *Health promotion in nursing practice,* ed 5, Upper Saddle River, NJ, 2006, Prentice Hall.)

FIG. 6.3 Maslow's hierarchy of needs. (Redrawn from Maslow AH: *Motivation and personality,* ed 3, Upper Saddle River, NJ, 1970, Prentice Hall.)

Nurses use holistic therapies either alone or in conjunction with conventional medicine. For example, using reminiscence sometimes helps relieve anxiety for older patients dealing with memory loss. Meditation sometimes helps patients cope with the difficult side effects of chemotherapy. Helping your patients understand different holistic therapies allows them to make choices that may enhance their health.

VARIABLES INFLUENCING HEALTH AND HEALTH BELIEFS AND PRACTICES

Many variables influence a patient's health and health beliefs and practices. Internal and external variables influence how a person thinks and acts. Health beliefs usually influence health behaviors or health practices, which positively or negatively affect a patient's level of health. Understanding the effects of these variables, as well as your prior experiences, allows you to plan and deliver individualized care.

Internal Variables

Internal variables include a person's developmental stage, intellectual background, perception of functioning, and emotional and spiritual factors.

Developmental Stage. A person's perceptions of health, illness, and health behaviors change over time (see Chapter 11). Considering a patient's growth and developmental stage helps you predict a patient's response to an actual illness or the threat of a future illness. Fear and anxiety are common among children who are ill, especially if thoughts about illness, hospitalization, or procedures are based on lack of information or lack of clarity of information. Emotional development may also influence personal beliefs about health-related matters. For example, you use different techniques for teaching about the need to be physically active to an adolescent than you use for an adult. A person's developmental stage sometimes differs from the chronological age. Adapt your nursing care based on a patient's developmental stage and the ability to participate in self-care.

Intellectual Background. A person's beliefs about health are shaped in part by educational background, traditions, and past experiences, all of which influence knowledge or misinformation about body functions and illnesses. These variables influence how a patient thinks about health. In addition, cognitive abilities shape the way a person thinks, including the ability to understand factors involved in illness and apply knowledge of health and illness to personal health practices. Cognitive abilities also relate to a person's developmental stage. Consider your patient's intellectual background while providing patient teaching (Edelman and Kudzma, 2018).

Perception of Functioning. Perceptions of physical functioning affect people's health beliefs and practices. When you assess a patient's level of health, gather subjective data about the way a patient perceives physical functioning, such as level of fatigue, shortness of breath, or pain. Then obtain objective data about actual functioning such as blood pressure, height measurements, and lung sounds. Analyzing this information allows you to plan and implement individualized approaches to improve a person's ability to function (e.g., self-care, mobility) more successfully.

Emotional Factors. A patient's degree of stress, depression, or fear influences health beliefs and practices. How people handle stress throughout each phase of life influences their reaction to illness. A person who generally is very calm may have little emotional response during illness, whereas another individual may be unable to cope emotionally with the threat of illness and may overreact or deny the presence of symptoms and not take therapeutic action (see Chapter 37).

Spiritual Factors. Spirituality is reflected in how people live their lives. It affects an individual's values and beliefs, the relationships established with family and friends, and the ability to find hope and meaning in life. Spirituality serves as an integrating theme in people's lives and often provides motivation to participate in health promoting activities (Lindell et al., 2019; Dadipoor et al., 2020). Religious practices are one way that people exercise spirituality. Some religions restrict the use of certain forms of medical treatment. For example, there are some religions and faiths that discourage followers from having blood transfusions. You need to understand patients' spiritual beliefs to incorporate them effectively in nursing care (see Chapter 35).

External Variables

External variables influencing a person's health beliefs and practices include family practices, psychosocial and socioeconomic factors, and cultural background.

Family Role and Practices. The roles and organization of a family influence how each family member defines health and illness and values health practices. Families' perceptions of the seriousness of diseases and their history of preventive care behaviors (or lack of them) influence how patients think about health. For example, a child whose parents believe in the importance of physical activity and eating healthy foods may continue to practice these health beliefs, whereas parents who have misconceptions and unhealthy perceptions about diet quality often contribute to eating habits that lead to obesity in their children (Ontai et al., 2019; Russell et al., 2016).

Social Determinants of Health. Health is determined by a person's circumstances and environment. External factors such as where a person lives, the quality of the environment, income, educational level, and relationships with others have a considerable impact on a patient's health. Social determinants of health (SDOH) include a variety of social, commercial, cultural, economic, environmental, and political factors that affect health disparities. They refer to the conditions in which people are born, grow, live, work, and age (WHO, 2021b). There are five categories of SDOH: economic stability, education access and quality, health care access and quality, social and community context, and neighborhood and built environment (ODPHP, n.d.). Examples of SDOH include poverty, food insecurity, no primary health care in a community, culture, exposure to violence, and access to green spaces (Schroeder et al., 2018).

REFLECT NOW

What is food insecurity, and how does it affect the health of your community?

SDOH, especially those related to economic stability, often affect a patient's level of health by increasing the risk for disease, affecting the ability to find affordable and safe housing, and influencing how or at what point the patient enters the health care system (Schroeder et al., 2018). A person's adherence to a treatment designed to maintain or improve health is also affected by economic status. For example, a patient may give higher priority to food and shelter than to medications, treatments, and food for special diets if the patient has high utility bills, cares for a large family, and has a low income.

Culture. Culture, a social and community context, influences a patient's beliefs, values, and customs. It influences the approach to the health care systems, personal health practices, and the nurse-patient relationship. Cultural background also influences an individual's beliefs about causes of illness and remedies or practices to restore health (Box 6.1). If you are not aware of your own cultural patterns of behavior and language, you will have difficulty interacting with your patients and recognizing and understanding your patient's behaviors and beliefs. Effective nursing interventions incorporate cultural factors into a patient's, family's, or community's plan of care (Leh and Saoud, 2020; Schroeder et al., 2018) (see Chapter 9).

HEALTH PROMOTION, WELLNESS, AND ILLNESS PREVENTION

Public health focuses on health promotion, wellness, and illness prevention (see Chapter 3). Health education, legislation, and policy help individuals, groups, and communities improve their health, decrease the incidence of disease and disability, and improve their quality of life.

Health policies and laws affect all people in a community, state, or country, even if the people affected by the policies or laws are unaware of them. For example, because of the current opioid crisis, all 50 states

Cultural Health Beliefs

Cultural beliefs shape patients' views of health, how they treat and prevent illness, and preferences for care (Galbraith-Gyan et al., 2019). Health beliefs often vary within a cultural group; therefore, it is important to assess the health beliefs of each patient and not stereotype a patient based on cultural background (Gerend et al., 2021). Cultural health beliefs influence individuals' responses to health and illness, such as eye contact, response to pain and pain management, use of touch, perception and treatment of mental illness, and sick role behaviors (Giger and Haddad, 2021). Recognizing a patient's health beliefs helps you provide culturally competent nursing care that considers the physical, psychological, social, emotional, and spiritual needs of each patient.

Implications for Patient-Centered Care

- Be aware of the effect of culture on a patient's view and understanding of illness (Giger and Haddad, 2021).
- Understand a patient's traditions, values, and beliefs and how these dimensions may affect a patient's perceptions about illness prevention and treatment (Galbraith-Gyan et al., 2019).
- Do not stereotype patients based on their culture, and do not assume that they will adopt all cultural beliefs and practices (Giger and Haddad, 2021).
- Recognize your patient's unique cultural perceptions regarding the cause of an illness and attitudes and beliefs about disease prevention when providing patient education about illness and treatment options (Galbraith-Gyan et al., 2019).
- Be aware of your own cultural background and recognize prejudices that lead to stereotyping and discrimination (Giger and Haddad, 2021; Lekas et al., 2020).

have passed legislation that facilitates the availability and dispensation of naloxone, especially to certain people, such as first responders and caregivers of people who are addicted to opioids. Most states allow health care providers to order naloxone without examining the patient who needs it to allow qualified individuals the ability to administer naloxone in an emergency (The Network for Public Health Law, 2021). Other health promotion programs provide guidance in pain management and improve access to substance abuse treatment.

The concepts of health promotion, health education, and illness prevention are closely related and sometimes overlap. All are focused on the future; the differences among them involve motivations and goals. **Health promotion** helps individuals maintain or enhance their present health. It motivates people to engage in healthy activities such as routine exercise and good nutrition to reach more stable levels of health. **Health education** includes providing information on topics such as physical awareness, stress management, and self-responsibility to enable individuals to improve their health. Health education helps people develop a greater understanding of their health and how to better manage their health risks. **Illness prevention** activities such as immunization programs and blood pressure screenings protect people from actual or potential risks to health. They also help people avoid declines in their level of health or functional ability.

Health promotion activities are often classified as either passive or active. Individuals gain from passive strategies (the activities of others) without acting themselves. The fluoridation of municipal drinking water and the fortification of homogenized milk with vitamin D are examples of passive health promotion strategies. In contrast, individuals become personally involved with active strategies of health promotion. For example, weight-reduction and smoking-cessation programs require patients to be actively involved in measures to improve their present and future levels of wellness while decreasing the risk of disease.

Health promotion is a process of helping people gain control of and improve their health and focuses on a wide range of socioeconomic and environmental interventions (WHO, 2021c). An individual takes responsibility for health and wellness by making appropriate lifestyle choices. Lifestyle choices are important because they affect a person's quality of life and well-being. Making positive lifestyle choices and avoiding negative lifestyle choices also play a role in preventing illness.

Some health promotion programs help individuals change their lifestyles by developing more health-oriented habits that affect their overall health. Other programs are aimed at preventing specific health care problems. For example, support groups help people with human immunodeficiency virus (HIV) infection. Exercise programs encourage participants to exercise regularly to reduce their risk of cardiac disease. Stress-reduction programs teach participants to cope with stressors and reduce their risks for multiple illnesses, such as infections, gastrointestinal disease, and cardiac disease.

Illnesses, especially chronic illnesses, increase health care costs. Improving self-management and providing preventive services help to reduce health care needs and costs and improve overall health. Taking a holistic approach recognizes that many factors affect a person's health and helps improve well-being in all dimensions (Box 6.2).

Health Promotion Strategies

PICOT Question: Do holistic approaches used with vulnerable populations effectively promote adult health and assist individuals with lifestyle changes?

Evidence Summary

Nurses use a variety of holistic strategies to improve health promotion in individuals. Holistic strategies focus on a person's body, mind, and spirit and take a person's culture, spirituality, and faith into consideration. Research shows that using culturally appropriate approaches that include a person's faith or provide social support are effective when helping individuals make lifestyle changes (D'Alonzo et al., 2018; Brown et al., 2019).

For example, health promotion programs that include spiritual and social support within an African-American faith community are effective in helping people adopt healthy behaviors such as exercise and healthy food choices to reduce the risk of developing type 2 diabetes (Kitzman et al., 2021; Brown et al., 2019). Health promotion programs that use *promotoras*, trained Latino community leaders, to provide evidence-based health promotion interventions and education that is culturally appropriate and includes social support also improve health outcomes. One study found that using *promotoras* to provide tailored patient education to help Latino employees in service or manual labor jobs navigate the health system was very effective in improving screening rates for breast, cervical, and colorectal cancers (Warner et al., 2019). Another program used *promotoras* to promote obesity prevention activities such as healthy food choices and exercise for Hispanic women who lived in rural communities. The culturally sensitive patient education coupled with the emotional and social support of the *promotoras* resulted in the women adopting healthier lifestyles (Sanchez et al., 2021)

Application to Nursing Practice

- Use role models from similar cultures when possible to encourage individuals to make health promotion and lifestyle changes (D'Alonzo et al., 2018; Sanchez et al., 2021; Warner et al., 2019).
- Provide evidence-based interventions that include a person's faith and provide social support when helping individuals make lifestyle changes (Kitzman et al., 2021; Brown et al., 2019).
- Work with churches and other faith-based organizations when implementing community-based health promotion strategies (Kitzman et al., 2021; Brown et al., 2019).

Some health promotion, wellness education, and illness prevention programs are operated by health care agencies; others are operated independently. Many businesses have on-site health promotion activities for employees. Likewise, colleges and community centers offer health promotion and illness prevention programs. These programs often include nurses who provide direct care, act as consultants, or refer patients to them. The goal of these activities is to improve a patient's level of health through preventive health services, environmental protection, and health education.

Examples of the health topics and objectives as defined by *Healthy People 2030* include physical activity; adolescent health; tobacco use; substance abuse; sexually transmitted diseases; mental health and mental disorders; injury and violence prevention; environmental health, immunization and infectious disease; access to health services; and LGBTQ+ health (ODPHP, n.d.). A complete list of topics and objectives is available on the *Healthy People* website (https://health.gov/healthypeople). These objectives and topics show the importance of health promotion, wellness, and illness prevention and encourage all to participate in the improvement of health.

Three Levels of Prevention

Nursing care oriented to health promotion, wellness, and illness prevention is described in terms of health activities on primary, secondary, and tertiary levels (Table 6.1). As a nurse, you will care for patients in all three levels.

Primary Prevention. Primary prevention is true prevention. Its goal is to reduce the incidence of disease. Many primary prevention programs are supported by the government (e.g., federally funded immunization programs). Primary prevention includes health education programs, nutritional programs, and physical fitness activities. It includes all health promotion efforts and wellness education activities that focus on maintaining or improving the general health of individuals, families, and communities (Edelman and Kudzma, 2018). Examples of primary prevention include promoting hearing protection in occupational settings and providing education to reduce cardiac disease risk factors.

Secondary Prevention. Secondary prevention focuses on preventing the spread of disease, illness, or infection once it occurs. Activities are directed at diagnosis and prompt intervention, thereby reducing severity and enabling the patient to return to a normal level of health as early as possible (Edelman and Kudzma, 2018). Examples include identifying people who have a new case of a disease or following

people who have been exposed to a disease but do not have it yet. It includes screening techniques and treating early stages of disease to limit disability by averting or delaying the consequences of advanced disease. Screening activities may lead to primary prevention intervention. For example, a nurse screens a patient who is obese for diabetes mellitus. After gathering more information from the patient, the nurse provides health education about physical activity and preventing hypertension.

Tertiary Prevention. Tertiary prevention occurs when a defect or disability is permanent and irreversible. It involves minimizing the effects of long-term disease or disability by interventions directed at preventing complications and deterioration (Edelman and Kudzma, 2018). Activities are directed at rehabilitation rather than diagnosis and treatment. For example, a patient with a spinal cord injury undergoes rehabilitation to learn how to use a wheelchair and perform activities of daily living independently. Care at this level helps patients achieve as high a level of functioning as possible, despite the limitations caused by illness or impairment.

RISK FACTORS

A risk factor is any attribute, quality, environmental situation, or trait that increases the vulnerability of an individual or group to an illness or accident. Impaired gait, reduced vision, and lower extremity weakness are examples of risk factors for falls. Risk factors and behaviors, risk factor modification, and behavioral modification are integral components of health promotion, wellness, and illness prevention. Nurses in all areas of practice have opportunities to reduce patients' risk factors to promote health and decrease risks of illness or injury.

Risk factors do not cause diseases or accidents. Instead, they increase the chances that the individual, community, or population will experience a disease or dysfunction. Risk factors play a major role in how you identify a patient's health status. They also often influence health beliefs and practices if a person is aware of their presence. People can modify some of their risk factors, while other risk factors are unmodifiable.

Nonmodifiable Risk Factors

Nonmodifiable risk factors such as age, gender, genetics, and family history cannot be changed. You use your understanding of nonmodifiable risk factors along with your patient's assessment data and preferences (e.g., developmental stage, social networks, access to transportation, and motivation) to select appropriate secondary prevention strategies.

TABLE 6.1 Three Levels of Prevention

PRIMARY PREVENTION		SECONDARY PREVENTION		TERTIARY PREVENTION
Health Promotion	Specific Protection	Early Diagnosis and Prompt Treatment	Disability Limitations	Restoration and Rehabilitation
Health education	Providing immunizations	Individual and mass screening surveys	Adequate treatment to stop disease process and prevent further complications	Providing retraining and education to return to highest level of functioning
Good nutrition based on developmental stage	Attention to personal hygiene	Focused examinations to cure and prevent diseases, prevent spread of communicable diseases, prevent complications, limit disability, and prevent death	Provision of facilities to limit disability and prevent death	Helping people with disabilities find work and accommodating them in the workplace
Provision of adequate housing, recreation, and working conditions	Use of environmental sanitation			
	Protection from occupational hazards			
Marriage counseling, sex education, and genetic screening	Protection from accidents and carcinogens			

Modified from Edelman C, Kudzma E: *Health promotion throughout the life span,* ed 9, St Louis, 2018, Mosby.

For example, a person's age increases the susceptibility to certain illnesses and accidents. Premature infants and neonates are more susceptible to infections. Children are at risk for accidental deaths due to drowning and aspiration. As a person ages, the risk of heart disease and many types of cancers increases. Age risk factors are often closely associated with other risk factors such as family history and personal habits. Educate your patients about the importance of regularly scheduled screenings based on their age. Various professional organizations and federal agencies develop and update recommendations for health screenings, immunizations, and counseling. Box 6.3 discusses ways to support health promotion in older adults.

Sometimes gender affects a person's risk factors. For example, the risk for asthma is higher in males than females. However, after puberty, the number of women with asthma becomes more prevalent and severe (Fuseini and Newcomb, 2017). Men have a higher risk for cardiovascular disease (CVD) than premenopausal women. However, after menopause, the risk for CVD is similar between men and women (The North American Menopause Society, 2021).

Family history and genetics are other risk factors for some illnesses. Cancers such as breast, ovarian, and colon appear to have a genetic link. These patients can benefit from genetic counseling. A person with a family history of diabetes mellitus or CVD is at higher risk for developing these diseases. Sometimes it is difficult to determine whether the family link to illness is related to genetics, lifestyle choices, environmental exposure, or a combination of these factors. For example, you are caring for a patient who is obese and develops hypertension. Her parents have hypertension, and her husband smokes. It is difficult for you to determine which risk factor—lifestyle, genetics, or environmental toxins—contributed to her hypertension or whether it was a combination of all of these. In this example, you introduce health promotion strategies targeted at modifiable risk factors for obesity, such as nutrition counseling and exercise.

BOX 6.3   FOCUS ON OLDER ADULTS

Health Promotion

- Base health promotion for older adults on their common risk factors, chronic health conditions, and health promotion needs, including heart disease, cancer, chronic bronchitis, stroke, diabetes mellitus, dementia, caregiving, and injury prevention (https://health.gov/healthypeople/objectives-and-data/browse-objectives/older-adults/evidence-based-resources, ODPHP, n.d.).
- Consider an older adult's social environment and strengthen social support to promote health and provide access to resources (Touhy and Jett, 2020).
- Injury prevention is a key strategy to promote and improve health (Touhy and Jett, 2020).
- Assess for polypharmacy, which is common in older adults. Polypharmacy is associated with falls, confusion, adverse outcomes, and increased length of hospital stays (Mizokami et al., 2019).
- Promote holistic health promotion programs such as community-based exercise programs and programs that encourage creativity, such as creating art or improvised comedy to improve well-being, decrease social isolation, and increase independence (Cantu and Fleuriet, 2018; Morse et al., 2018; Seo and Chao, 2018).
- Carefully assess each older adult you care for to determine various factors that affect health. Every individual is unique. Current evidence shows factors such as an older adult's social networks, access to transportation, knowledge of local services, mobility, perceptions of age, personal motivation, and perceived confidence in the ability to make effective changes can influence health-promoting behaviors and quality of life (Frost et al., 2018; Hong et al., 2018).

Modifiable Risk Factors

Some risk factors such as lifestyle practices and behaviors can be modified. Modifiable behavioral risk factors include smoking, drinking alcohol, unhealthy diet, obesity, physical inactivity, and insufficient rest and sleep. These risk factors put people at risk for certain chronic illnesses, such as diabetes and heart disease (Ryan et al, 2020). There are risk factors that put a person at risk for developing specific diseases. For example, excessive sunbathing increases the risk of skin cancer, and smoking also increases the risk of lung diseases, including cancer.

Poor control of hypertension and elevated lipid and glucose levels are additional modifiable risks (CDC, 2021). Modifiable risk factors for people who are 10 to 24 years of age include behaviors that lead to unintentional injuries (e.g., bullying, texting while driving, driving under the influence of drugs or alcohol); carrying a weapon; the use of tobacco, smokeless tobacco products, alcohol, or other drugs; sexual behaviors leading to unintended pregnancy and sexually transmitted infections; unhealthy diet choices; and physical inactivity (Kann et al., 2018).

Lifestyle behavioral choices are also modifiable. Lifestyle choices can lead to health problems that cause a significant impact on our health care system, our economy, and our communities. Therefore, it is important to understand the effect of lifestyle behaviors on health status. For example, a teenager who makes nutritional choices that lead to obesity will most likely make similar nutritional choices as an adult. Lifestyle choices affect patients throughout the life span. Thus, it is important to understand the relationship between growth and development and lifestyle behaviors, and your patient's preferences and health status.

Stress is a lifestyle risk factor if it is severe or prolonged or if the person is unable to cope with life events adequately. Stress threatens both mental health (emotional stress) and physical well-being (physiological stress). Stress also interferes with health promotion activities and the ability to implement needed lifestyle modifications. Some emotional stressors result from life events, such as divorce, pregnancy, death of a spouse or family member, and financial instabilities. For example, job-related stressors overtax a person's cognitive skills and decision-making ability, leading to "mental overload" or "burnout" (see Chapters 1 and 37). Stress also threatens physical well-being and is associated with illnesses such as heart disease, cancer, and gastrointestinal disorders (Chiang et al., 2018). Always review life stressors as part of a patient's comprehensive risk factor analysis.

Environment

Where we live and the condition of that area (its air, water, and soil) determine how we live, what we eat, the disease agents to which we are exposed, our risk factors, our state of health, and our ability to adapt. The physical environment in which a person works or lives can increase the likelihood that certain illnesses will occur. For example, some kinds of cancer and other diseases are more likely to develop when people are exposed to certain chemicals at work or when people live near toxic waste disposal sites. Environmental exposure rarely occurs at one time, in one location, and from one source because we are constantly interacting with our environment (Edelman and Kudzma, 2018).

RISK-FACTOR IDENTIFICATION AND CHANGING HEALTH BEHAVIORS

Your patient interviewing and assessment skills will help identify your patients' modifiable and unmodifiable risk factors. Health risk appraisal forms help identify health threats based on the presence of

TABLE 6.2 Transtheoretical Model of Change: Stages of Health Behavior Change

Stage	Definition	Assessment Findings
Precontemplation	No intent to make changes within the next 6 months	Patient is unaware of, not interested in, or underestimates the problem. May be defensive. "There is nothing I really need to change."
Contemplation	Considering a change within the next 6 months	May be ambivalent about the change or is thinking about making a change. "I have a problem that I think I need to work on."
Preparation	Making small changes in preparation for a change in the next month	May have tried to make changes in the past but was unsuccessful. Patient believes that advantages outweigh disadvantages of behavior change. "I started running once, but I didn't keep it up. I think I might try again in a few weeks."
Action	Actively engaged in strategies to change behavior; lasts up to 6 months	Committed to change. Previous habits may become barriers to change. "I am really working hard to stop smoking."
Maintenance stage	Sustained change over time; begins 6 months after action has started and continues indefinitely	Changes integrated into the patient's lifestyle and behaviors adopted to prevent relapse. "I need to avoid people who smoke so I won't be tempted to start smoking again."

various risk factors (Edelman and Kudzma, 2018). Use data from a health risk appraisal tool to identify modifiable risks, and then apply knowledge of the patient's motivation and cultural preferences to design educational approaches. These approaches help your patients understand what they can modify, control, or even eliminate to improve their health. Identify community resources if a patient needs to make lifestyle changes to reduce health risks (Murdaugh et al., 2019).

Once you identify a patient's risk factors, you implement appropriate and relevant health education and counseling to help a person change or implement behaviors to maintain or improve health status (Edelman and Kudzma, 2018). Risk-factor modification, health promotion, illness prevention activities, or any program that attempts to change unhealthy lifestyle behaviors is a wellness strategy. Ask patients which changes they perceive they need to make or are willing to make. Patients typically will not change their behaviors unless they see a need and are motivated to change.

Sometimes patients need to stop health-damaging behaviors (e.g., tobacco use or alcohol misuse), while other times patients need to adopt healthy behaviors (e.g., healthy diet or exercise) (Murdaugh et al., 2019). Changing health behavior, especially long-term lifestyle habits, is difficult. Using a health promotion model to identify risky behaviors and implement the change process will help you motivate patients and facilitate health behavior changes (Edelman and Kudzma, 2018). Use evidence-based guidelines and recommendations when helping patients make health behavior changes.

You will be able to help your patients make difficult changes more effectively if you understand the process of change. Current evidence supports that many people go through a series of five stages when they make a change, described by the Transtheoretical Model of Change (Table 6.2) (pro-change Behavior Systems, Inc., 2018; Martinasek et al., 2021). These stages range from no intention to change (precontemplation) to maintaining a changed behavior (maintenance stage) (DiClemente and Prochaska, 1998). Change is not a linear process. People often relapse and cycle through the stages (pro-change Behavior Systems, Inc., 2018). When relapse occurs, a person will return to the contemplation or precontemplation stage before attempting the change again. Help your patients understand that relapse is a learning process; they can apply the lessons learned from relapse to their next attempt to change. It is important to understand what happens at the various stages of the change process to time the implementation of interventions (wellness strategies) adequately and provide appropriate assistance at each stage.

Once an individual identifies a stage of change, the change process facilitates movement through the stages. To be most effective, you

BOX 6.4 PATIENT TEACHING

Lifestyle Changes

Objective
- Patient will use behavioral change to reduce health risks by improving diet and exercising 150 minutes (2 hours and 30 minutes) to 300 minutes (5 hours) a week (moderate-intensity exercise).

Teaching Strategies
- Practice active listening and establish rapport with the patient.
- Begin with determining information that the patient knows regarding health risks related to poor lifestyle.
- Ask which barriers the patient perceives with diet modifications and exercising.
- Help the patient establish goals for change using a standard such as *The Physical Activity Guidelines for Americans* (U.S. Department of Health and Human Services, 2018).
- Collaborate with the patient to select safe areas to exercise and to establish timelines for modification of eating and exercise lifestyle habits.
- Reinforce the process of change.
- Have patient maintain a log of key behavioral changes (Chan et al., 2020).
- Ensure that educational materials are tailored to meet a patient's health needs, are easy to understand, and are culturally appropriate (Abboud et al., 2017; Bai et al., 2020).
- Include family members and significant others to support the lifestyle change (Khanom et al., 2020).

Evaluation
Use the principles of teach-back to evaluate patient/family caregiver learning:
- "Please tell me what you remember that we discussed last week regarding reducing risks and lifestyle changes" (O'Brien and Meyer, 2020).
- "Tell me how your log went this week. Show me what you tracked of your activity and diet" (Chan et al., 2020).
- "How many minutes did you exercise last week?"

choose nursing interventions that match the stage of change. Most behavior-change programs are designed for (and have a chance of success with) people ready to take action regarding their health behavior problems. Changes are maintained over time only if they are integrated into an individual's overall lifestyle (Box 6.4). Maintaining healthy lifestyles can prevent hospitalizations and potentially lower the cost of health care.

> **QSEN** **Building Competency in Safety** A nurse who works at a health center on a university campus notices that there are many students who smoke. The nurse partners with the local health department to implement a smoking-cessation program on campus. The program is based on the Transtheoretical Model of Change. In applying this model, which strategies does the nurse need to consider?
>
> Answers to QSEN Activities can be found on the Evolve website.

ILLNESS

Illness and disease are different concepts. A medical condition that causes distress for a person in the form of its symptoms is referred to as a *disease*. It is a generic term that includes all disorders, infections, disabilities, and deformities that can afflict human beings. **Illness** is a state in which a person's physical, emotional, intellectual, social, developmental, or spiritual functioning is diminished or impaired. It is a feeling of poor health. A person can feel ill in the presence or absence of a disease such as cancer or multiple sclerosis. A patient with leukemia continues to function as usual, whereas another patient with leukemia feels well physically but experiences great emotional and spiritual distress. A person can feel ill even when there is no underlying medical condition. In addition, many patients who have a disease feel healthy. Sometimes illness (i.e., feeling the impact of a disease) motivates people to adopt healthy behaviors. Although you need to be knowledgeable about different diseases, you also need to understand illness, which includes the holistic effects of diseases and treatments on your patient's functioning and well-being.

Acute and Chronic Diseases

Both acute and chronic diseases have the potential to affect many dimensions of functioning. An **acute disease** is usually reversible and has a short duration. The symptoms appear abruptly, are intense, and subside after a relatively short period. A **chronic disease** usually lasts more than 6 months, is irreversible, and affects functioning in one or more systems. Patients often fluctuate between maximal functioning and serious health relapses that may be life threatening. A person with a chronic disease is like a person with a disability in that both have varying degrees of functional limitations (Larsen, 2019).

Chronic diseases and disabilities remain a leading health problem in the United States. Coping and living with a chronic disease is usually complex and overwhelming. Half of the adults in the United States have one chronic disease, and one in four adults has two or more chronic health problems (CDC, 2021). Many chronic diseases are related to four modifiable health behaviors: physical inactivity, poor nutrition, tobacco use and secondhand smoke exposure, and excessive alcohol use (Ryan et al., 2020; CDC, 2021). A major role for nursing is to educate patients on how to manage their diseases or disabilities to help reduce the occurrence or improve the severity of symptoms.

Patients with chronic diseases and their families must continually adjust and adapt to the effects of their diseases. An individual's perceptions of a disease and its symptoms influence the type of coping responses that individual uses. In response to a chronic disease, an individual develops an illness career. The illness career is flexible and changes in response to changes in health, interactions with health professionals, psychological changes related to grief, and stress related to the disease (Larsen, 2019).

The nature of the disease, either acute or chronic, also affects a patient's illness behavior. Patients with acute diseases are likely to seek health care and adhere to therapy. On the other hand, a patient with a chronic disease in which symptoms are not cured but only partially relieved may not be motivated to adhere to the therapy plan. Some patients who have chronic diseases become less actively involved in their care, experience greater frustration, and adhere less readily to care. Because nurses often spend more time than other health care professionals with patients who are living with a chronic disease, they are in the unique position of being able to help these patients overcome problems related to illness behavior. A patient's coping skills and locus of control (the degree to which people believe they control what happens to them) are other internal variables that affect the way the patient behaves when ill (see Chapter 37).

Illness Behavior

People who are ill from a disease generally act in a way that medical sociologists call **illness behavior**. People often adopt cognitive, affective, and behavioral reactions to their diseases that are influenced by sociocultural and psychological factors. Classic work by Mechanic (1995) found that illness behaviors affect how people monitor their bodies, define and interpret their symptoms, take remedial actions, and use health care resources. Personal history, social situations, social norms, and past experiences affect illness behaviors (Larsen, 2019). How people react varies widely; illness behavior displayed in sickness is often used to manage life adversities (Mechanic, 1995). In other words, if people perceive themselves to be ill, illness behaviors become coping mechanisms. For example, illness behavior can result in a patient being released from roles, social expectations, or responsibilities.

The nature of the disease also affects a patient's illness behavior. Patients with acute diseases are likely to seek health care. On the other hand, patients with a chronic disease in which symptoms are only partly relieved may become less actively involved in their care, experience greater frustration, and have difficulty adhering to their treatment plan.

Variables Influencing Illness and Illness Behavior

Many variables influence a person's response to a disease and the resulting illness behaviors. Physical stressors such as a poor living environment, work stress, exposure to air pollution, and living in an unsafe environment affect health. Heredity and individual practices, such as poor eating habits or lack of regular exercise, also influence health and illness behaviors. The influences of emotional, intellectual, social, developmental, and spiritual factors often affect the likelihood of seeking health care, adherence to therapy, and health outcomes. Although patients' illness behaviors may seem unsafe or ineffective from your perspective as a nurse, your patients may perceive their illness behaviors to be helpful (Mathar et al., 2020). Plan individualized care based on an understanding of the variables that affect your patients and their behaviors to help patients cope with their illnesses at various stages. The goal is to promote optimal functioning in all dimensions throughout an illness.

Internal Variables. Internal variables are a patient's perceptions of symptoms and the nature of a disease. A patient's coping skills and locus of control (the degree to which people believe they control what happens to them) are other internal variables that affect the way a patient behaves when ill (see Chapter 37). If patients believe that the symptoms of their diseases disrupt their normal routine, they are more likely to seek health care assistance than if they do not perceive the symptoms to be disruptive. Patients are also more likely to seek assistance if they believe the symptoms are serious or life threatening (Gorbani et al., 2020). A patient awakened by crushing chest pain in the middle of the night who sees this symptom as serious and life threatening is motivated to seek assistance. However, such a perception also can have the opposite effect. Another patient with the same symptoms becomes fearful, reacts by denying it, and does not seek medical assistance.

External Variables. External variables influencing a patient's illness behavior include the visibility of symptoms, social group, cultural background, economic variables, accessibility of the health care system, and social support. The visibility of an individual's symptoms affects body image and illness behavior. A patient with a visible symptom (e.g., a high fever) is often more likely to seek assistance than a patient with no visible symptoms (e.g., symptoms associated with ovarian cancer such as fatigue and bloating).

Patients' social groups help them accept or deny the threat of their diseases. Families, friends, and co-workers all influence patients' illness behaviors. Patients often react positively to social support while practicing positive health behaviors. A person's family and cultural background teach the person how to be healthy, how to recognize disease, and how to be ill. For example, dietary practices, influenced by family and by spiritual, religious, and cultural beliefs, contribute to the development of a disease and disease maintenance (Giger and Haddad, 2021).

Economic variables are SDOH that influence the way a patient reacts to a disease. Financial difficulties often lead to delayed treatment and affect a patient's or family's ability to carry out prescribed treatments and therapies (Horner, 2020). Patients' access to the health care system is closely related to economic factors (Henderson et al., 2020). The health care system is a socioeconomic system that patients enter, interact within, and exit. For many patients, entry into the system is complex or confusing. Some patients seek nonemergency medical care in an emergency department because they do not know how to obtain health services in other ways or do not have access to care. The physical proximity of patients to a health care agency often influences how soon they enter the system after deciding to seek care.

Impact of Illness on the Patient and Family

Illness is never an isolated life event. A patient and family deal with changes resulting from disease, illness, and treatment. Each patient responds uniquely, requiring you to individualize nursing interventions. The patient and family commonly experience behavioral and emotional changes and changes in roles, body image and self-concept, and family dynamics.

Behavioral and Emotional Changes.
Short-term, non–life-threatening diseases usually require few changes in the functioning of a patient or family. For example, a father who has a cold lacks the energy and patience to spend time in family activities. He becomes irritable and prefers not to interact with his family. This is a behavioral change, but the change is subtle and does not last long. Some may even consider such a change a normal response.

Diseases that are life-threatening or chronic, such as ALS or emphysema, lead to a more extensive sense of illness, such as the emotional and behavioral changes of anxiety, shock, denial, anger, and withdrawal. The needs of patients and families, as well as the ways in which families function, change over time (Cox et al., 2020). Carefully assess a patient's and family's responses to the stress of disease and illness and analyze cues to develop interventions to help a patient and family cope with and adapt to their stress.

Impact on Body Image.
Body image is the subjective concept of physical appearance (see Chapter 33). Some diseases and illnesses (e.g., cancer and obesity) result in changes in physical appearance. Patient and family reactions differ and usually depend on the type of changes (e.g., loss of a limb or an organ), their adaptive capacity, the rate at which changes take place, and the support services available.

With a profound change in body image, such as after a leg amputation or mastectomy, the patient generally adjusts by experiencing phases of the grief process (see Chapter 36). Initially the patient is in shock because of the change or impending change. As the patient and family recognize the reality of the change, they become anxious and

often withdraw, refusing to discuss it. Withdrawal is an adaptive coping mechanism that helps the patient adjust. As a patient and family acknowledge the change, they gradually accept the loss. During rehabilitation, the patient becomes ready to learn how to adapt to the changed body image.

Impact on Self-Concept.
Self-concept is a mental self-image of all aspects of your personality. Self-concept depends in part on body image and roles but also includes other aspects of psychology and spirituality (see Chapters 33 and 35). The effect of a disease or illness on a patient's or family member's self-concept is usually more complex and less readily observed than role changes.

Self-concept is important in relationships with other family members. For example, a patient whose self-concept changes (e.g., feeling like a failure) because of illness may no longer meet family expectations, leading to tension or conflict. As a result, family members change their interactions with the patient. While providing care, you observe changes in a patient's self-concept (or in the self-concept of a family member) and develop a care plan to facilitate adjustment to the changes resulting from the illness.

Impact on Family Roles.
People have many roles in life, such as wage earner, decision maker, professional, child, sibling, or parent. Role reversal is common when a family member is diagnosed with a disease or becomes ill (see Chapter 10). If a parent becomes ill and cannot carry out usual activities, an adult child often assumes many of the parent's responsibilities and in essence becomes a parent to the parent. Such a reversal of the usual situation sometimes leads to stress, conflicting responsibilities for the adult child, or direct conflict over decision making (Guerrero and Mendez-Luck, 2019; Gelman and Rhames, 2020).

An individual and family generally adjust more easily to subtle, short-term changes. In most cases they know that the role change is temporary and will not require a prolonged adjustment. However, long-term changes require an adjustment process similar to the grief process (see Chapter 36). A patient and family often require specific counseling and guidance to help them cope with role changes.

REFLECT NOW

Think about a patient or family member who recently experienced a change in health status. How did this change affect the individual's family?

Impact on Family Dynamics.
Family dynamics is the process by which a family functions, makes decisions, gives support to individual members, and copes with everyday changes and challenges. Family dynamics often change because of the effects of diseases and illnesses (Agerskov et al., 2020; Gelman & Rhames, 2020). For example, a single parent experiences severe injury from a car accident. Her brother assumes some of her roles and responsibilities, such as getting the children to and from school. Although the patient and her brother are very close, the family experiences some tension as roles and responsibilities change. Include the whole family when appropriate to help patients and their families attain the maximal level of functioning and well-being (see Chapter 10).

CARING FOR YOURSELF

To be able to provide competent, quality, and safe care, nurses need to take care of themselves to ensure they remain healthy. Nurses are particularly susceptible to the development of compassion fatigue, which is a combination of secondary traumatic stress (STS) and burnout (BO) (see Chapter 1). STS develops because of the relationships that nurses develop with their patients and families, especially those in which nurses frequently witness suffering. Burnout stems from a chronic lack of resources (e.g., staffing, time) that results in conflicts or nurse job dissatisfaction within the work setting (Kelly and Lefton, 2017). Compassion fatigue frequently affects a nurse's health, often leading to a decline in health, changes in sleep and eating patterns, emotional exhaustion, irritability, restlessness, impaired ability to focus and engage with patients, feelings of hopelessness, inability to take pleasure from activities, and anxiety (Henson, 2017; Kurosaka and Payton, 2020). In the workplace the effects of compassion fatigue are often manifested by diminished performance, reduced ability to feel empathy, depersonalization of the patient, poor judgment, chronic absenteeism, high turnover rates, and conflict between nurses (Henson, 2017; Sullivan et al., 2019). It is important for nurses to engage in personal and professional strategies to help combat compassion fatigue and promote resiliency (Kurosaka and Payton, 2020).

Personal strategies focus on health-promoting behaviors and healthy lifestyle choices. To combat STS and burnout, you need to eat a nutritious diet, get adequate sleep regularly, engage in regular exercise and relaxation activities, establish a good work-family balance, and engage in regular nonwork activities (Kelly and Lefton, 2017; Mendes, 2017). Other strategies that can help you prevent or deal with STS and burnout include developing coping skills, allowing personal time for grieving the loss of patients, and focusing on your spiritual health (Kim and Yeom, 2018). Another strategy is to find a mentor or experienced nurse who understands the stress of the job and can help you identify coping strategies (Doré et al., 2017).

An increasing number of health care institutions and organizations offer educational programs and resources for nurses that are designed to help decrease compassion fatigue and increase resiliency (Kelly and Lefton, 2017; Sullivan et al., 2019). These programs educate nurses about compassion fatigue and its negative effects and provide resources and tools for nurses to use to prevent or cope with STS and burnout (Kurosaka and Payton, 2020). For example, participating in debriefing sessions or a compassion fatigue support group allows nurses to identify stressors and work as a group to develop healthy coping strategies (Schmidt and Haglund, 2017; Doré et al., 2017). Health care organizations need to also provide resources for nurses, such as a mental health professional to provide assistance in managing STS and burnout.

KEY POINTS

- *Healthy People* identifies leading health indicators that are high-priority health issues in the United States.
- Definitions of health vary among individuals based on a person's health beliefs, developmental age, and level of functioning.
- Multiple models of health in which people are active participants explain relationships among health beliefs, health behaviors, health promotion, and individual well-being.
- Internal variables, such as a person's developmental stage and spirituality, and external factors, such as family roles and SDOH, influence a person's health, health beliefs, and health practices.
- Health promotion activities help maintain or enhance health, health education helps people better understand their health and health risks, and illness prevention activities protect against health threats.
- Primary prevention reduces the incidence of disease, secondary prevention prevents the spread of disease when it occurs, and tertiary prevention minimizes the effects of disease or disability.
- You use your knowledge about different types of risk factors to select appropriate secondary prevention strategies for your patients.

- Nonmodifiable risk factors, such as age and family history, cannot be changed, while modifiable risk factors, such as smoking and activity levels, can be changed.
- Reducing risk factors and improving health usually require a change in health behaviors.
- Illness behaviors are different reactions people have when they become ill. Variables such as perceptions of the illness, the type of illness or disease, and the visibility of symptoms affect a person's illness behaviors.
- Illness has many effects on a patient and family, including changes in behavior and emotions, family roles and dynamics, body image, and self-concept.
- Using personal and professional strategies that focus on caring for oneself can help to decrease or prevent compassion fatigue.

REFLECTIVE LEARNING

- Understanding a person's risk factors helps you determine appropriate health education and health promotion interventions. Reflect on a patient you recently cared for or someone you know such as a friend or family member. What actual and/or potential health problems does this person have? What risk factors contribute to these health problems? Are the risk factors nonmodifiable or modifiable? What health education or health promotion interventions could you implement to limit the effect of these risk factors?
- Interview a patient or someone you know who is trying to make a health behavior change. What behavior change is the person trying to make? In what stage of change is this person currently based on the Transtheoretical Model of Change (see Table 6.2)? Once this person moves into the maintenance stage, what can you do to help this person prepare for potential relapses?
- Reflect on your own health as well as your beliefs and values. How do you define health? Do you consider yourself healthy? What health behaviors would you like to change or implement right now to improve your health? Develop a plan to make a change in your behavior to improve your health. What barriers might prevent you from implementing your plan? If you implemented this plan, how might your health improve? Remember to consider your health holistically as you reflect on your answers.

REVIEW QUESTIONS

1. A patient discharged a week ago following a stroke is currently participating in rehabilitation sessions provided by nurses, physical therapists, and registered dietitians in an outpatient setting. In what level of prevention is the patient participating?
   1. Primary prevention
   2. Secondary prevention
   3. Tertiary prevention
   4. Transtheoretical prevention
2. Based on the Transtheoretical Model of Change, what is the most appropriate response to a patient who states: "Me, stop smoking? I've been smoking since I was 16!"
   1. "That's fine. Some people who smoke live a long life."
   2. "OK. I want you to decrease the number of cigarettes you smoke by one each day, and I'll see you in 1 month."
   3. "What do you think is the greatest reason why stopping smoking would be challenging for you?"
   4. "I'd like you to attend a smoking-cessation class this week and use nicotine replacement patches as directed."
3. A nurse working on a medical patient care unit states, "I am having trouble sleeping, and I eat nonstop when I get home. All I can think of when I get to work is how I can't wait for my shift to be

over. I wish I felt happy again." What are the best responses from the nurse manager? (Select all that apply.)

1. "I'm sure this is just a phase you are going through. Hang in there. You'll feel better soon."
2. "I know several nurses who feel this way every now and then. Tell me about the patients you have cared for recently. Did you find it difficult to care for them?"
3. "You can take diphenhydramine over the counter to help you sleep at night."
4. "Describe for me what you do with your time when you are not working."
5. "The hospital just started a group where nurses get together to talk about their feelings. Would you like for me to e-mail the schedule to you?"

4. A patient has been laid off from his construction job and has many unpaid bills. He is going through a divorce from his marriage of 15 years and has been praying daily to help him through this difficult time. He does not have a primary health care provider because he has never really been sick, and his parents never took him to a physician when he was a child. Which external variables influence the patient's health practices? (Select all that apply.)

1. Difficulty paying his bills
2. Praying daily
3. Age of patient (46 years)
4. Stress from the divorce and the loss of a job
5. Family practice of not routinely seeing a health care provider

5. A nurse is conducting a home visit with a new mom and her three children. While in the home the nurse weighs each family member and reviews their 3-day food diary. She checks the mom's blood pressure and encourages the mom to take the children for a 30-minute walk every day. The nurse is addressing which level of need, according to Maslow's Hierarchy of Needs?

1. Physiological
2. Safety and security
3. Love and belonging
4. Self-actualization

6. When taking care of patients, a nurse routinely asks whether they take any vitamins or herbal medications, encourages family members to bring in music that the patients like to help the patients relax, and frequently prays with her patients if that is important to them. The nurse is practicing which model?

1. Holistic
2. Health belief
3. Transtheoretical
4. Health promotion

7. Using the Transtheoretical Model of Change, order the steps that a patient goes through to make a lifestyle change related to physical activity.

1. The individual recognizes that he is out of shape when his daughter asks him to walk with her after school.
2. Eight months after beginning walking, the individual participates with his wife in a local 5K race.
3. The individual becomes angry when the physician tells him that he needs to increase his activity to lose 30 pounds.
4. The individual walks 2 to 3 miles, 5 nights a week, with his wife.
5. The individual visits the local running store to purchase walking shoes and obtain advice on a walking plan.

8. Which of the following are symptoms of secondary traumatic stress and burnout that commonly affect nurses? (Select all that apply.)

1. Regular participation in a book club
2. Lack of interest in exercise
3. Difficulty falling asleep
4. Lack of desire to go to work
5. Anxiety while working

9. As part of a faith community nursing program in her church, a nurse is developing a health promotion program on breast self-examination for the women's group. Which statement made by one of the participants is related to the individual's accurate perception of susceptibility to an illness?

1. "I have a hanging tag on my bathroom door to remind me to do my breast self-examination monthly."
2. "Since my mother had breast cancer, I know that I am at increased risk for developing breast cancer."
3. "Since I am only 25 years of age, the risk of breast cancer for me is very low."
4. "I participate every year in our local walk/run to raise money for breast cancer research."

10. A nurse is assessing the risk factors for coronary artery disease (CAD) in a female patient. For each assessment finding (see below), indicate with an X whether the finding is modifiable, non-modifiable or unrelated to the risk for CAD.

Assessment Finding	Modifiable	Nonmodifiable	Unrelated
Patient is 67 years old			
B/P 146/88 mm Hg			
Father had type 2 diabetes mellitus			
Eats at fast food restaurants every day for lunch			
Patient treated with radiation to the chest 30 years ago to treat Hodgkin's disease			
Does not participate in regular activity			

Answers: 1. 3; 2. 3; 3. 2, 4, 5; 4. 1, 5; 5. 1; 6. 1; 7. 3, 1, 5, 4, 2; 8. 2, 3, 4, 5; 9. 2; 10. See Evolve.

Rationales for Review Questions can be found on the Evolve website.

REFERENCES

Becker M, Maiman L: Sociobehavioral determinants of compliance with health and medical care recommendations, *Med Care* 13(1):10, 1975.

Centers for Disease Control and Prevention (CDC): *National center for chronic disease prevention and health promotion,* https://www.cdc.gov/chronicdisease/, 2021. Accessed February 21, 2021.

DiClemente C, Prochaska J: Toward a comprehensive transtheoretical model of change. In Miller WR, Heather N, editors: *Treating addictive behaviors.* New York, 1998, Plenum Press.

Edelman C, Kudzma E: *Health promotion throughout the life span,* ed 9, St Louis, 2018, Mosby.

Fuseini H, Newcomb DC: Mechanisms driving gender differences in asthma, *Curr Allergy Asthma Rep* 17(3):19, 2017.

Giger JN, Haddad LG: *Transcultural nursing: assessment and intervention,* ed 8, St Louis, 2021, Mosby.

Henson JS: When compassion is lost, *Medsurg Nurs* 26(2):139, 2017.

Kurosaka A, Payton J: Prevention strategies to cope with nurse burnout in nephrology settings, *Nephrol Nurs J* 47(6):539-563, 2020.

Larsen PD: *Lubkin's chronic illness: impact and intervention,* ed 10, Boston, 2019, Jones & Bartlett.

Lekas HM et al.: Rethinking cultural competence: shifting to cultural humility, *Health Serv Insights* 13:1, 2020.

Lindell JM et al.: Developing healthy habits: a faith-based interdisciplinary action framework, *Nurse Leader* 17(6):498-504, 2019.

Mechanic D: Sociological dimensions of illness behavior, *Soc Sci Med* 41(9):1207, 1995.

Mendes A: How to address compassion fatigue in the community nurse, *Br J Community Nurs* 22(9):458, 2017.

Murdaugh CL et al.: *Health promotion in nursing practice,* ed 8, New York, 2019, Pearson.

Office of Disease Prevention and Health Promotion (ODPHP): *Healthy People 2030.* n.d., https://health.gov/healthypeople, n.d. U.S. Department of Health and Human Services. Accessed February 21, 2021.

Pender NJ: *Health promotion and nursing practice,* Norwalk, Conn, 1982, Appleton-Century-Crofts.

Pender NJ: Health promotion and nursing practice, ed 3, Stamford, C., 1996, Appleton & Lange.

Pender NJ et al.: *Health promotion in nursing practice,* ed 7, Upper Saddle River, NJ, 2015, Prentice Hall.

pro-change Behavior Systems: Inc.: the transtheoretical model, https://www.prochange.com/transtheoretical-model-of-behavior-change, 2018. Accessed February 22, 2021.

Rosenstoch I: Historical origin of the health belief model, *Health Educ Monogr* 2:334, 1974.

Schmidt M, Haglund K: Debrief in emergency departments to improve compassion fatigue and promote resiliency, *J Trauma Nurs* 24(5):317, 2017.

Schroeder K et al.: Addressing the social determinants of health: a call to action for school nurses, *J Sch Nurs* 34(3):182, 2018.

The Network for Public Health Law: *Drug overdose prevention and harm reduction,* 2021, https://www.networkforphl.org/resources/topics/substance-use-prevention-and-harm-reduction/#resources-5f0df313e5733. Accessed February 21, 2021.

The North American Menopause Society: *Keeping your heart healthy at menopause,* 2021, https://www.menopause.org/for-women/menopauseflashes/bone-health-and-heart-health/keeping-your-heart-healthy-at-menopause. Accessed February 21, 2021

Touhy TA, Jett K: *Ebersole and Hess' toward healthy aging: human needs and nursing response,* ed 10, St Louis, 2020, Mosby.

U.S. Department of Health and Human Services (USDHHS): *Physical activity guidelines for Americans,* ed 2, 2018 Office of Disease Prevention and Health Promotion.

World Health Organization Interim Commission (WHO): *Chronicle of WHO,* Geneva, 1947, The Organization.

World Health Organization (WHO): *Constitution,* http://www.who.int/about/mission/en/, 2021a. Accessed February 21, 2021.

World Health Organization (WHO): *Social determinants of health,* http://www.who.int/social_determinants/en/, 2021b. Accessed February 21, 2021.

World Health Organization (WHO): *Health promotion,* http://www.who.int/topics/health_promotion/en/, 2021c. Accessed February 21, 2021.

RESEARCH REFERENCES

Abboud S et al: Cervical cancer screening among Arab women in the United States: an integrative review. *ONF* 44(1):E20, 2017.

Agerskov H et al: The significance of relationships and dynamics in families with a child with end-stage kidney disease: a qualitative study, *J Clin Nurs* 29(5/6):987, 2020.

Bai Y et al.: Effectiveness of tailored communication intervention in increasing colonoscopy screening rates amongst first-degree relatives of individuals with colorectal cancer: a systematic review and meta-analysis, *Int J Nurs Stud* 101:103397, 2020. Doi: 10.1016/j.ijnurstu.2019.103397

Brown CW et al.: Perceptions and practices of diabetes prevention among African Americans participating in a faith-based community health program, *J Community Health,* 44(4): 694, 2019.

Cantu AG, Fleuriet KJ: "Making the ordinary more extraordinary": exploring creativity as a health promotion practice among older adults in a community-based professionally taught arts program, *J Holistic Nurs* 39(9):123, 2018.

Chan K et al.: A school-based programme promoting healthy eating, *Health Educ J* 79(3):277, 2020.

Chiang JJ et al.: Affective reactivity to daily stress and 20-year mortality risk in adults with chronic illness: findings from the national study of daily experiences, *Health Psychol* 37(2):170, 2018.

Cox ED et al: Reliability and validity of PROMIS® pediatric family relationships short form in children 8-17 years of age with chronic disease, *Qual Life Res* 29(1):191, 2020.

Dadipoor S et al.: Explaining the determinants of hookah smoking cessation among southern Iranian women: a qualitative study, *J Subst Use,* 25(5): 469, 2020.

D'Alonzo KT et al.: Outcomes of a culturally tailored partially randomized patient preference controlled trial to increase physical activity among low-income immigrant Latinas, *J Transcult Nurs* 29(4):335, 2018.

Doré C et al.: Perspectives on burnout and empowerment among hemodialysis nurses and the current burnout intervention trends: a literature review, *CANNT J* 27(4):16, 2017.

Frost R et al: Identifying acceptable components for home-based health promotion services for older people with mid frailty: a qualitative study, *Health Soc Care Community* 26(3):393, 2018.

Galbraith-Gyan KV et al.: HPV vaccine acceptance among African-American mothers and their daughters: an inquiry grounded in culture, *Ethn Health* 24(3): 323, 2019.

Gelman C, Rhames K: "I have to be both mother and father": the impact of young-onset dementia on the partner's parenting and the children's experience, *Dementia* 19(3):676, 2020.

Gerend M et al.: Acculturation and health beliefs: interactions between host and heritage culture underlie Latina/o caregivers' beliefs about HPV vaccination, *J Immigr Minor Health* 23(1):113, 2021.

Gorbani F et al.: Predictive performance of Pender's Health Promotion Model for hypertension control in Iranian patients, *Vasc Health Risk Manag* 16:299, 2020.

Griffith D et al.: "Health is the ability to manage yourself without help": how older African American men define health and successful aging, *J Gerontol B Psychol Sci Soc Sci* 73(2):240, 2018.

Guerrero LR & Mendez-Luck CA: Overcoming a bad day: a qualitative look into the dementia caregiving experiences of Mexican-origin women in East Los Angeles, *J Cross Cult Gerontol* 34(4):373, 2019.

Henderson LM Et al.: The role of social determinants of health in self-reported access to health care among women undergoing screening mammography, *J Womens Health* 29(11):1437, 2020.

Hong M et al.: Social networks, health promoting behavior and health related quality of life in older Korean adults, *Nurs Health Sci* 20(1):79, 2018.

Horner SD: Examining social determinants of health in childhood asthma management, *Clin Nurse Spec* 34(5):222, 2020.

Kelly LA, Lefton C: Effect of meaningful recognition on critical care nurses' compassion fatigue, *Am J Crit Care* 26(6):438, 2017.

Khanom A et al: Parent recommendations to support physical activity for families with young children: results of interviews in deprived and affluent communities in South Wales (United Kingdom), *Health Expect* 23(2):284, 2020.

Kann L et al.: Youth risk behavior surveillance—United States, 2017, *MMWR Surveill* 67(No. SS-8):1, 2018. https://www.cdc.gov/mmwr/volumes/67/ss/ss6708a1.htm#suggestedcitation. Accessed February 21, 2021.

Kim HS, Yeom H: The association between spiritual well-being and burnout in intensive care nurses: a descriptive study, *Intensive Crit Care Nurs* 46(92), 2018.

Kitzman H et al.: Better me within randomized trial: faith-based diabetes prevention program for weight loss in African American women, *Am J Health Promot* 35(2):202, 2021.

LaVela SL et al.: Relational empathy and holistic care in persons with spinal cord injuries, *J Spinal Cord Med* 40(1):30, 2017.

Leh SK, Saoud S: Using community-based participatory research to explore health care perceptions of a select group of Arab Americans, *J Transcult Nurs* 31(5):444, 2020.

Martinasek M et al: Predictors of vaping behavior change in young adults using the Transtheoretical Model: a multi-country study, *Tob Use Insights* 14:1, 2021.

Mathar H et al.: Self-reported illness behaviour related to chronic obstructive pulmonary disease and rehabilitation: a theory-guided qualitative study, *Scand J Caring Sci* 34(2):484, 2020.

Mizokami F et al: Clinical medication review type III of polypharmacy reduced unplanned hospitalizations in older adults: A meta-analysis of randomized clinical trials, *Geriatr Gerontol Int* 19: 1275, 2019.

Morse LA et al.: Humor doesn't retire: improvisation as a health-promoting intervention for older adult, *Arch Gerontol Geriatr* 75(1), 2018.

O'Brien T & Meyer, T: A feasibility study for teaching older kidney transplant recipients how to wear and use an activity tracker to promote daily physical activity, *Nephrol Nurs* 47(1):47–51, 2020, https://doi.org/10.37526/1526-744X.2020.47.1.47

Ontai LL et al.: Parent food-related behaviors and family-based dietary and activity environments: associations with BMI z-scores in low-income preschoolers, Child Obes, 2019, https://doi.org/10.1089/chi.2019.0105

Russell CG et al.: Effects of parent and child behaviours on overweight and obesity in infants and young children from disadvantaged backgrounds: systematic review with narrative synthesis, *BMC Public Health* 16(151), 2016, available at: https://bmcpublichealth.biomedcentral.com/articles/10.1186/s12889-016-2801-y. Accessed February 21, 2021.

Ryan N et al: Smoking, drinking, diet, and physical activity-modifiable lifestyle risk factors and their associations with age to first chronic disease, *Intl J Epidemiol* 49(1): 113, 2020.

Sanchez JI et al.: Eat Healthy, Be Active Community Workshops implemented with rural Hispanic women. *BMC Womens Health* 21(1): 1, 2021.

Seo JY, Chao YY: Effects of exercise interventions on depressive symptoms among community-dwelling older adults in the United States: a systematic review, *J Gerontol Nurs* 44(3):31, 2018.

Sullivan CE et al.: Reducing compassion fatigue in inpatient pediatric oncology nurses, *Oncol Nurs Forum* 46(3):338, 2019.

Warner EL et al.: A workplace-based intervention to improve awareness, knowledge, and utilization of breast, cervical, and colorectal cancer screenings among Latino service and manual labor employees in Utah, *J Community Health* 44(2): 256, 2019.

7

Caring in Nursing Practice

OBJECTIVES

- Analyze how caring affects the nurse-patient relationship.
- Compare and contrast theories on caring.
- Discuss the evidence about patients' perceptions of caring.
- Explain how an ethic of care influences nurses' clinical judgment.
- Discuss the role that caring plays in the nurse-patient relationship.
- Identify ways to express caring through presence and touch.
- Examine the therapeutic benefit of listening to patients.
- Explain the relationship between knowing a patient and clinical decision making.
- Explain the relationship of compassion to caring.

KEY TERMS

Caring
Comforting
Compassion

Ethic of care
Presence
Transcultural

Transformative

MEDIA RESOURCES

http://evolve.elsevier.com/Potter/fundamentals/
- Review Questions
- Case Study with Questions

- Audio Glossary
- Content Updates
- Answers to QSEN Activity and Review Questions

Caring principles are foundational to the nurse-patient relationship and nursing practice as nurses provide care for patients and families in both health and illness (Romero-Martin et al., 2019). Caring is a complex and multifaceted activity. It is more important in today's hectic, high-tech health care environment, where productivity and efficiency can interfere with nurses' capacity to be caring, compassionate professionals (Young et al., 2019; Letourneau et al., 2017). The environmental demands, pressure, and time constraints in the health care environment threaten nurses' opportunities to establish therapeutic relationships and interpersonal connections with patients and family caregivers (Percy and Richardson, 2018; Adams, 2016).

It is important to maintain a patient-centered approach to patient care for all aspects of clinical nursing, whether the care focuses on managing pain, teaching self-care, administering medications, or providing basic hygiene measures. Caring relationships require sincerity, listening, presence, respect, and acceptance. Despite the challenges in health care, patient-centered care is key to transforming health care delivery and improving patient outcomes (Grant et al., 2019; Ortiz, 2018). Professional organizations also stress the importance of caring in health care and of keeping the nurse engaged at a patient's bedside (RWJF, 2014). The American Organization of Nurse Executives (AONE, 2010) describes caring and knowledge as the core of nursing, with caring being a key component of what a nurse brings to a patient experience (Fig. 7.1).

Competent nursing practice values and embraces caring practices and expert knowledge (Grant et al., 2019; Benner et al., 2010). Your expertise in caring will come with experience in clinical practice. When you engage

patients in a caring and compassionate manner, the therapeutic gain in caring contributes greatly to your clinical judgment and the health and well-being of your patients. Your compassion creates an openness with patients who then choose to share more of their illness experiences with you. This knowledge then enables you to make better clinical judgments and decisions about patients' needs. Think about a time when you were ill or experienced a problem requiring health care intervention. Then consider the following two scenarios and select the situation that you believe most successfully demonstrates a sense of caring:

- A nurse enters a patient's room, greets the patient warmly while touching the patient lightly on the shoulder, makes eye contact, sits down for a few minutes and asks about the patient's thoughts and concerns, listens to the patient's story, looks at the intravenous (IV) solution hanging in the room, briefly examines the patient, and then checks the vital sign summary on the bedside computer screen before leaving the room.
- A second nurse enters the patient's room, looks at the IV solution hanging in the room, checks the vital sign summary sheet on the bedside computer screen, and acknowledges the patient but never sits down or touches the patient. The nurse makes eye contact from above while the patient is lying in bed, asks a few brief questions about the patient's symptoms, and leaves.

Both of these scenarios take about the same amount of a nurse's time, but they may be perceived differently by a patient and impact patient satisfaction. In times of illness or when a person seeks the professional guidance of a nurse, caring is essential in helping an individual achieve the best outcomes.

89

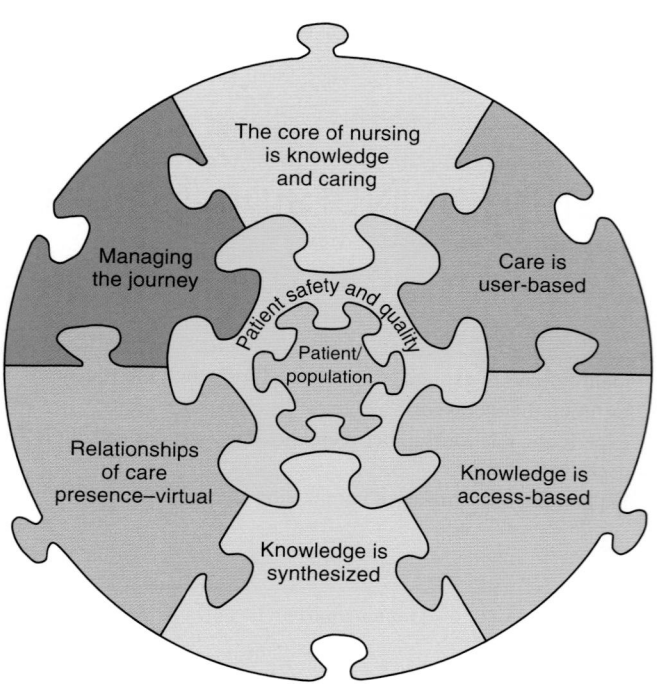

FIG. 7.1 AONE guiding principles for the role of the nurse in future patient care delivery. (Copyright© 2015 by the American Organization of Nurse Executives [AONE]. All rights reserved.)

 BOX 7.1 CULTURAL ASPECTS OF CARE

Nurse Caring Behaviors

Caring includes knowing your patient's cultural values and beliefs; respecting privacy, diversity, and individual needs; and interacting and listening to the patient and family (Colman, 2019). Having a sense of what it is like to live in a patient's world is critical. To provide culturally sensitive patient-centered care, you must understand and respect the impact of a patient's cultural beliefs and values on health condition, treatments, and self-care habits.

Implications for Patient-Centered Care

- Collect a culturally based nursing history by letting patients tell their stories and listening to them (Chapter 9).
- Know and clarify a patient's beliefs, attitudes, and cultural practices regarding health care, caring practices, and end-of-life-care (Zolnierek, 2014; Colman, 2019).
- Determine whether a member of a patient's family or cultural group is the best resource to guide the use of caring practices, such as providing presence or touching (Merritt et al., 2019; Marion et al., 2017).
- Encourage the patient and the family caregiver, if appropriate, to share the perspective of the personal impact of the patient's illness/trauma (Mohammadipour et al., 2017).
- Know the patient's cultural practices (such as touching, family involvement) or beliefs that impact the uncertainty related to diagnoses, treatments, and outcomes of care (Markey et al., 2018).

THEORETICAL VIEWS ON CARING

Caring is a universal phenomenon influencing the ways in which people think, feel, and behave in relation to one another. Since Florence Nightingale, nurses have studied caring from a variety of philosophical and ethical perspectives. Some nursing scholars developed theories on caring because of its importance to nursing practice. This chapter does not detail all of the theories, but it is designed to help you understand how caring enables a nurse to work with all patients in a respectful, therapeutic way.

Caring Is Primary

Dr. Patricia Benner offers nurses a rich, holistic understanding of nursing practice and caring through her research involving the interpretation of expert nurses' stories. After listening to nurses' stories and analyzing their meaning, she described caring as the essence of excellent nursing practice. The stories revealed the nurses' behaviors and decisions that expressed caring. Caring means that people, events, projects, and things matter to people (Benner and Wrubel, 1989; Benner et al., 2010). It is a word for being connected.

Caring underlies a wide range of interactions, from parental love to friendship, from caring for one's work to caring for one's pet, to caring for and about one's patients, and caring for one's self (Hines and Gaughan, 2017). "Caring creates possibility." Personal concern for another person, an event, or a thing provides motivation and direction for people to care. Through caring, nurses help patients recover in the face of illness, give meaning to their illness, and maintain or reestablish connection. Research shows that nursing students identify caring and **compassion** as interventions that are essential components of nursing care and that need to be taught and practiced early in nursing education and emphasized in all clinical practice settings (Atar and Asti, 2020; Labraque et al., 2017).

Patients are not all the same. Each person brings a unique background of experiences, values, and cultural perspectives to a health care encounter. Caring is specific and relational for each nurse-patient encounter. As nurses acquire more experience, they typically learn that caring helps them focus on their patients' needs. Caring improves a nurse's ability to know a patient, recognize a patient's problems, and find and implement individualized solutions (Romero-Martin et al., 2019; Young et al., 2019).

Because illness is the human experience of loss or dysfunction, any treatment or intervention given without consideration of its meaning to an individual is unlikely to be effective. Develop a caring relationship with your patients and listen to their stories to fully understand the meaning and impact of their conditions and to provide patient-centered care.

Leininger's Transcultural Caring

Madeleine Leininger (1991) offers a **transcultural** view of caring. She describes the concept of care as the domain that sets nursing apart from other health care disciplines (see Chapter 4). Care is an essential human need. Care, unlike cure, helps an individual or group improve a human condition. Acts of caring are nurturing and skillful activities, processes, and decisions that help people in empathetic, compassionate, and supportive ways. A caring act depends on the needs, problems, and values of a patient.

Nurses need to understand and apply cultural caring behaviors (Leininger, 1991). Even though human caring is a universal phenomenon, the expressions, processes, and patterns of caring vary among people of different cultures (Box 7.1). Caring is very personal; thus its expression differs for each patient. For caring to be effective, nurses need to learn culturally specific behaviors and words that reflect human caring in different cultures to identify and meet the needs of all patients (see Chapter 9). As nurses we care for patients from certain "subcultures" that have unique needs (e.g., people who are chronically ill, physically disabled, developmentally challenged, poor, or homeless).

TABLE 7.1 Watson's 10 Carative Factors

Carative Factor	Example in Practice
Forming a human-altruistic value system	Use loving kindness to extend yourself. Use self-disclosure appropriately to promote a therapeutic alliance with your patient (e.g., share a personal experience in common with your patient such as a child-rearing experience, an illness, or an experience with a parent who needs assistance).
Instilling faith-hope	Provide a connection with the patient that offers purpose and direction when trying to find the meaning of an illness.
Cultivating a sensitivity to one's self and to others	Learn to accept yourself and others for their full potential. A caring nurse matures into becoming a self-actualized nurse.
Developing a helping, trusting, human caring relationship	Learn to develop and sustain helping, trusting, authentic caring relationships through effective communication with your patients.
Promoting and expressing positive and negative feelings	Support and accept your patients' feelings. In connecting with your patients, you show a willingness to take risks in sharing in the relationship.
Using creative problem-solving, caring processes	Apply critical thinking in the nursing process to systematically make sound clinical judgments.
Promoting transpersonal teaching-learning	Learn together while educating the patient to acquire self-care skills. The patient assumes responsibility for learning.
Providing for a supportive, protective, and/or corrective mental, physical, societal, and spiritual environment	Create a healing environment at all levels, physical and nonphysical. This promotes wholeness, beauty, comfort, dignity, and peace.
Meeting human needs	Intentionally help patients meet basic needs with a caring consciousness.
Allowing for existential-phenomenological-spiritual forces	Allow spiritual forces to provide a better understanding of yourself and your patient.

Data from Watson J: *The philosophy and science of caring,* Boulder, CO, 2008, University Press of Colorado.

Watson's Transpersonal Caring

According to Jean Watson, caring is a central focus of nursing, and it is integral to maintain the ethical and philosophical roots of the profession (Dey, 2016). The changing health care delivery system, the increasing economic pressure for productivity, and the shortages of health care professionals increase the risk for dehumanized care. Patients and their families expect a high quality of human interaction from nurses; they need conversations with their nurses and caregivers that are meaningful and address their needs (da Rocha Rodrigues and Sechaud, 2019; Sitzman, 2017). Unfortunately, many conversations between patients and nurses are brief and disconnected. Many are not really "conversations" but rather simply the nurse reporting information to a patient and family. Watson's theory of caring is a holistic model that supports a nurse's conscious intention to care to promote healing and wholeness (Watson, 2008, 2010). It integrates the human caring process with healing environments, incorporating the life-generating and life-receiving processes of human caring and healing for nurses and their patients (Watson Caring Science Institute [WCSI], 2021). The theory describes a consciousness that allows nurses to raise new questions about what it means to be a nurse, to be ill, and to be caring and healing. The transpersonal caring theory rejects the disease orientation to health care and *places care before cure* (Watson, 2008). A nurse who focuses on transpersonal caring looks for deeper sources of inner healing to protect, enhance, and preserve a person's dignity, humanity, wholeness, and inner harmony.

Creating caring-healing environments in the current high-tech health care system is crucial to establishing and maintaining the nurse-patient relationship (Sitzman, 2017). Watson's model emphasizes the nurse-patient caring relationship with the focus on carative behaviors (Table 7.1). A nurse communicates caring-healing to a patient through the nurse's consciousness. This takes place during a single caring moment between nurse and patient when a connection forms. The model is transformative because the relationship influences both the nurse and the patient for better or for worse (Watson, 2008, 2010). Caring-healing

consciousness promotes healing. Application of Watson's caring model in practice enhances nurses' caring practices (Box 7.2).

Swanson's Theory of Caring

Kristen Swanson (1991) studied patients and professional caregivers to develop a theory of caring for nursing practice. This theory of caring was developed from three perinatal studies involving interviews with women who miscarried, parents and health care professionals in a newborn intensive care unit, and mothers who were socially at risk and received long-term public health intervention (Swanson, 1999). After analyzing the stories and descriptions of the three groups, Swanson developed a theory of caring, which includes five caring processes (Table 7.2). Swanson (1991) defines caring as a nurturing way of relating to an individual (i.e., when one feels a personal sense of commitment and responsibility). The theory guides nurses in developing caring interventions that improve patient satisfaction (Ray and Stargardt, 2020). In a study involving women giving birth, caring was shown as a central nursing phenomenon that was not unique to nursing practice; it improved patient satisfaction and outcomes (Ortega Barco and de Rodriguez, 2018). Teaching students and new nurses how to use Swanson's five caring processes helps new nurses gain confidence when providing patient-centered care (Moffa, 2015).

Summary of Theoretical Views

Caring theories translated into behaviors are valuable when nurses assess patient perceptions of being cared for in a multicultural environment. Research by Labraque et al. (2017) notes that there are commonalities, such as human interaction or communication, mutuality, appreciation of the uniqueness of individuals, and improvement in the welfare of patients and families. Caring is relational, and in a health care setting a nurse and patient enter into a relationship that is much more than one person simply doing tasks for another. In a caring relationship a mutual give-and-take develops as nurse and patient begin to know and care for each other (da Rocha Rodrigues and Sechaud, 2019; Su et al., 2020).

BOX 7.2   EVIDENCE-BASED PRACTICE

Enhancing Caring

PICOT Question: Do carative practices of nurses affect patient satisfaction among hospitalized and long-term care adult patients?

Evidence Summary

Researchers identify a strong, positive relationship between nurse caring behaviors and patient satisfaction. Patients feel that their care is individualized when nurses listen to their stories and concerns, and as a result they report greater satisfaction (Brewer and Watson, 2015). While the promotion of caring, compassionate, supportive, and therapeutic environments increases patient satisfaction, these factors also increase nurses' job satisfaction (Nightingale et al., 2018). Evidence shows that patient and family caregiver satisfaction improves when nurses demonstrate caring behaviors when including patients' specific requests into their care or communicating the reasons why these requests cannot be met immediately (Wyant et al., 2017). Caring nursing practices also help to improve patients' functional status, self-efficacy, coping, and self-care (Su et al., 2020; Ortiz, 2018). Finally, patient-centered care models emphasize that caring interventions promote patient advocacy and predict patient satisfaction (Compton et al., 2018).

Application to Nursing Practice

- Use the caring practices of listening, presence, and connectedness to partner with a patient and family through their illness. Use these practices with humility, love, kindness, and compassion (Nightingale et al., 2018).
- Ask patients whether they have questions about their illness, treatment, or home care needs (Compton et al., 2018).
- Knowing the patient enables you to partner with a patient and family caregiver to obtain vital health care information; understand the patient's health care priorities, expectations, and fears; explore the meaning of the illness; and when necessary help with end-of-life decision making (Murali, 2020; Compton et al., 2018).
- Being with and doing for a patient are components of presence, whether it is a dedicated one-on-one physical interaction or quietly sitting with a patient (Mohammadipour et al., 2017). Presence often helps elicit important health care information from a patient and reduces patient fear and anxiety.
- Caring nursing practices benefit nursing and nursing staff by reducing workplace stress and increasing job satisfaction (Wei et al., 2019; Nightingale et al., 2018).

TABLE 7.2   Swanson's Theory of Caring

Caring Process	Definition	Subdimensions
Knowing	Striving to understand an event as it has meaning in the life of the other	Avoiding assumptions Centering on the one cared for Assessing thoroughly Seeking clues to clarify the event Engaging the self or both
Being with	Being emotionally present to the other	Being there Conveying ability Sharing feelings Not burdening
Doing for	Doing for the other as one would do for self if it were at all possible	Comforting Anticipating Performing skillfully Protecting Preserving dignity
Enabling	Facilitating the other's passage through life transitions (e.g., birth, death) and unfamiliar events	Informing/explaining Supporting/allowing Focusing Generating alternatives Validating/giving feedback
Maintaining belief	Sustaining faith in the other's capacity to get through an event or transition and face a future with meaning	Believing in/holding in esteem Maintaining a hope-filled attitude Offering realistic optimism "Going the distance"

Data from Swanson KM: Empirical development of a middle-range theory of caring, *Nurs Res*, 40(3):161, 1991.

Caring is often invisible when a nurse and patient enter a relationship of mutual respect, concern, and support. A nurse's empathy and compassion become a natural part of every patient encounter. However, it is obvious when caring is absent. For example, a nurse who shows disinterest or chooses to avoid a patient's request for help quickly conveys an uncaring attitude. Benner and Wrubel (1989) relate the story of a clinical nurse specialist who learned from a patient what caring is all about: "I felt that I was teaching him a lot, but actually he taught me. One day he said to me (probably after I had delivered some well-meaning technical information about his disease), 'You're doing an OK job, but I can tell that every time you walk in that door you're walking out.'" In this nurse's story the patient perceived that the nurse was simply going through the motions of teaching and showed little caring toward the patient. Patients quickly know when nurses fail to relate to them.

As you gain clinical experience, continue to practice caring, and your patients and their family caregivers will sense your commitment and willingness to enter into a relationship that allows you to understand their experiences of illness (Monsen et al., 2017). In a study of patients with metastatic breast disease patients reported that a patient-centered approach was essential for their self-management of their cancer therapies. Patients also noted that a partnership with the nurse not only maintained adherence to the therapies but also improved patients' ability to manage symptoms and side effects (Komatsu et al., 2016; Yagasaki and Komatsu, 2013).

One aspect of caring is enabling—when a nurse and patient work together to identify alternatives in approaches to care and resources. The nurse becomes a patient advocate (see Chapter 1). Consider a nurse working with a patient recently diagnosed with diabetes mellitus. The nurse enables the patient by helping the patient identify lifestyle modifications that incorporate individualized strategies for diabetes self-management, such as timing medication administration, identifying exercises the patient can do, and recommending changes in diet that the patient is willing to make.

Another common theme of caring is understanding the context of a person's life and illness. It is difficult to show caring for another without understanding who the person is and the person's perception of the illness. Ask your patients the following questions to understand their perceptions: How was your illness first recognized? How do you feel about the illness? How does your illness affect what you do each day? Knowing the context of a patient's illness helps you choose and individualize patient-centered interventions that will actually help the patient. This approach is more successful than simply selecting interventions on the basis of your patient's symptoms or disease process.

PATIENTS' PERCEPTIONS OF CARING

Theories of caring help nurses understand the behaviors and processes that characterize caring. Researchers have explored nurse caring behaviors as perceived by patients (Table 7.3). Their findings emphasize what patients expect from their caregivers and thus provide useful guidelines for your practice. Patients continue to value nurses' effectiveness in performing tasks, but clearly patients value the affective dimension of nursing care, which reflects the art of nursing.

You need to understand patients' perceptions of caring and the association between these perceptions and their satisfaction of care (see Chapter 2). Health care consumers can search online for specific information about health care agencies with regard to their ratings by patients in various areas of performance. The Caring Assessment Tool (CAT) was developed to measure caring from a patient's perspective (Duffy et al., 2007). This tool and other caring assessments help you, as a beginning professional, to appreciate the types of behaviors that patients in the hospital identify as caring (Box 7.3). When patients sense that health care providers are sensitive, sympathetic, compassionate, and interested in them as people, they usually become active partners in the plan of care. Suliman et al. (2009) studied the impact of Watson's caring theory as an assessment framework in a multicultural environment. Patients in the study indicated that they did not perceive any cultural bias when they perceived nurses to be caring. As health care agencies strive to improve patient satisfaction, creating an environment of caring is a necessary and worthwhile goal. Patient satisfaction with nursing care is an important factor in a patient's decision to return to a specific health care agency.

As you begin clinical practice, determine how you practice caring behaviors, and consider the best approaches to provide care and how patients perceive caring. Assess what your patient expects. Build nurse-patient relationships to learn what caring behaviors are important to your patients (Ackerman, 2019). For example, you are caring for a patient who had breast cancer 2 years ago. She needs another breast biopsy, is fearful of the outcome, and has many questions. Instead of giving a lengthy description of why the procedure is necessary, you obtain assistance from an oncology nurse specialist. Knowing your patients helps you select caring approaches that are most appropriate to their needs.

BOX 7.3 Factors and Items Constituting the Caring Assessment Tool (CAT)

Each item begins with the stem: "Since I have been a patient here, the nurse(s)":

Mutual Problem Solving
- Help me understand how I am thinking.
- Ask me how I think treatment is going.
- Help me explore alternative ways of dealing.
- Ask me what I know.
- Help me figure out questions to ask.

Attentive Reassurance
- Are available.
- Seem interested.
- Support sense of hope.
- Help me believe in self.
- Anticipate my needs.

Human Respect
- Listen to me.
- Accept me.
- Treat me kindly.
- Respect me.
- Pay attention to me.

Encouraging Manner
- Support my beliefs.
- Encourage me to ask questions.
- Help me to see some good.
- Encourage me to go on.
- Help me deal with bad feelings.

Appreciation of Unique Meanings
- Are concerned with how I view things.
- Know what is important to me.
- Acknowledge my inner feelings.
- Show respect for things having meaning.

Healing Environment
- Check up on me.
- Pay attention to me when I am talking.
- Make me feel comfortable.
- Respect my privacy.
- Treat my body carefully.

Affiliation Needs
- Are responsive to my family.
- Talk openly with my family.
- Allow my family to be involved.

Basic Human Needs
- Make sure I get food.
- Help me with routine needs for sleep.
- Help me feel less worried.

Modified from Duffy JR, et al.: Dimensions of caring: psychometric evaluation of the Caring Assessment Tool, *Adv Nurs Sci* 30(3):235, 2007.

TABLE 7.3 Comparison of Research Studies Exploring Nurse Caring Behaviors (As Perceived by Patients)

Nurses' Caring Behaviors: The Perception of Patients With Cancer at the Time of Discharge After Surgery (Compton et al., 2018)	Learning the Patient's Stories (Ragan and Kanter, 2017; Engle, 2010; Frank, 1998)	The Need for a Nursing Presence in Self-Management of Metastatic Cancer (Komatsu et al., 2016; Yagasaki and Komatsu, 2013)
Used the Caring Assessment Tool (CAT, see Box 7.3) to determine patients' perceptions of nurse caring behaviors at the time of discharge. It was important to patients that nurses appreciated the unique impact of the illness on patient and family caregiver. Patients perceived that the nurses knew what was important to them. Caring behaviors, such as knowing, listening, and being present, contributed to patient satisfaction. Respecting the patient's values, beliefs, and health care choices, such as explaining choices, advocating for resources, and accepting patient decisions, was essential.	Learning and knowing the patient's story are essential elements of caring nursing practice. Listening and presence help nurses know patients. Understanding a patient's story establishes a nurse-patient relationship and maintains caring practice. To really hear a patient's story, start by refining listening skills and take the time to "sit and make eye contact" while listening. Knowing the patient and the story is critical to collecting clinical and personal information so that the nurse can better know and understand the patient's health care story and expectations for care, identify and correct missing information, and design patient-centered care.	Nursing presence contributes to knowing the patient. Illness and treatments often cause major changes in a patient's lifestyle. Nursing presence for helping patients manage their cancer therapies, including receiving oral chemotherapy, is as important as identifying those patients at risk for nonadherence. Nursing presence provides emotional and knowledge-based support for patients who are new to or receiving additional oral chemotherapy. As a result of this knowledge-based support, patients gain confidence in self-management and managing symptoms and treatment side effects (Komatsu et al., 2016).

ETHIC OF CARE

Caring is an interaction between a nurse and patient in an atmosphere of mutual respect and trust. In this collaborative environment, the nurse provides encouragement, hope, support, and compassion to help achieve desired outcomes. It is a professional, ethical covenant that nursing has with its public. It is also a standard applied in the critical thinking process for clinical judgment (see Chapter 15). Caring science provides a disciplinary foundation from which you deliver patient-centered care. Chapter 22 explores the importance of ethics in professional nursing. The term *ethic* refers to the ideals of right and wrong behavior. In any patient encounter a nurse needs to know what behavior is ethically appropriate. Nurses do not make professional decisions based solely on intellectual or analytical principles. Instead, an ethic of care places caring at the center of decision making.

An ethic of care is concerned with relationships between people and with a nurse's character and attitude toward others. Nurses who function from an ethic of care are sensitive to unequal relationships that lead to an abuse of one person's power over another—intentional or otherwise. In health care settings patients and families are often on unequal footing with professionals because of a patient's illness, lack of information, regression caused by pain and suffering, and unfamiliar circumstances. An ethic of care places the nurse as the patient's advocate, influences the nurse's clinical judgment, and helps guide clinical decision making regarding ethical dilemmas by attending to relationships and giving priority to each patient's unique personhood.

REFLECT NOW

A patient requires a lot of physical and emotional care and is frequently using the nurse call system. The health care providers alternate answering the nurse call system, stating "I just did it" or "It's your turn."
Think about how these comments and actions affect the ethic of care.
How would you convey your thoughts to the health care team?

CARING IN NURSING PRACTICE

It is impossible to determine when a nurse becomes a caring professional. As you encounter patients in various states of health and illness in your practice, you grow in your ability to care and to develop caring behaviors. We learn from our patients when we are willing to be open and to establish relationships that convey caring. Our patients tell us that a simple touch, a simple phrase (e.g., "I'm here"), or a promise to remain at the bedside represent caring and compassion (Engle, 2010).

Caring is one of those human behaviors that we can give and receive. As a nurse it is important to assess both your caring needs and your caring behaviors. Recognize the importance of nurses' self-care (see Chapters 1 and 6). You cannot give fully engaged, compassionate care when you feel depleted. Take time to recognize stressors and reach out to colleagues, family, and friends to help you cope. Use caring behavior to reach out to colleagues to care for them as well. For example, work among your colleagues to create a culture where they are supported when they express tension and stress related to increases in patient acuity levels, difficult working relationships, and end-of-life care (Frankenfield et al., 2018; Monsen et al., 2017). Whether you are giving or receiving care, the value of caring in your nursing practice benefits your patients, your colleagues, and your health care agency.

Providing Presence

Nursing practice and patient satisfaction improve when "nursing presence" is part of the health care culture (Mohammadipour et al., 2017; Yagasaki and Komatsu, 2013). Providing presence is a person-to-person encounter conveying a closeness and sense of caring. Presence involves "being there" and "being with." "Being there" is not only a physical presence; it also includes communication and understanding. A nurse who is present in a nurse-patient relationship is available and responsive to a patient's expressed needs. Nursing presence is the connectedness between a nurse and a patient (Hansbrough and Georges, 2019; Plessis, 2016).

Presence is an interpersonal process that is characterized by sensitivity, holism, intimacy, vulnerability, and adaptation to unique circumstances. It results in improved mental well-being for nurses and patients and improved physical well-being in patients. The interpersonal relationship of "being there" requires a nurse to be attentive to the perspectives of the patient and family caregiver. It translates into an actual caring art that affects the healing and well-being of both the nurse and patient (Mohammadipour et al., 2017). Nurses use presence in conjunction with other interventions, such as establishing the nurse-patient relationship, providing comfort measures, providing patient education, and listening (Plessis, 2016). The outcomes of nursing presence include the relief of suffering, a decrease in the sense of isolation and vulnerability, and personal growth.

Establishing presence strengthens your ability to provide effective patient-centered care. Presence is also valuable during patient- and family-centered rounds, during which nurses offer their presence to help patients achieve positive outcomes, diminish the intensity of unwanted feelings, promote reassurance, and guide family caregivers. As a result, patients often are more satisfied with the nursing care and the health care system in general (Hansbrough and Georges, 2019).

"Being with" involves a nurse giving of himself or herself, which means being available and at a patient's disposal. If a patient accepts a nurse, the patient will invite the nurse to see, share, and touch his or her vulnerability and suffering. One's human presence never leaves one unaffected (Watson, 2010). The nurse enters the patient's world, and the patient is able to identify feelings and solutions, see new directions, and make choices.

When a nurse establishes presence, eye contact, body language, voice tone, listening, and a positive and encouraging attitude act together to create openness and understanding. Establishing presence enhances a nurse's ability to learn from patients, including their hopes, dreams, need for support, and expectations of care. Learning from a patient strengthens a nurse's ability to provide adequate and appropriate nursing care.

It is especially important to establish presence and caring when patients are experiencing stressful events or situations. Awaiting a physician's report of test results, preparing for an unfamiliar procedure, and planning for a return home after serious illness are just a few examples of events in the course of a person's illness that can create unpredictability and dependency on care providers. A nurse's presence and caring help to calm anxiety and fear related to stressful situations. Giving reassurance and thorough explanations about a procedure, remaining at the patient's side, and coaching the patient through the experience all convey a presence that is invaluable to a patient's well-being.

Touch

Patients face situations that are embarrassing, frightening, and painful. Whatever the feeling or symptom, they look to nurses to provide comfort. The use of touch is one comforting approach that reaches out to patients to communicate concern and support (Hanley et al., 2017).

Touch is relational and leads to a connection between nurse and patient. It involves contact and noncontact touch. Contact touch involves obvious skin-to-skin contact and is task-oriented, caring, or protective (Hanley et al., 2017). Before implementing any contact touch, be aware of your patient's cultural practices and past experiences. For some people, a simple touch on the arm may be perceived as invasive, and for victims of abuse a simple touch may be perceived as a threat.

Nurses use task-oriented touch when performing a task or procedure. The skillful and gentle performance of a nursing procedure conveys security and a sense of competence. An expert nurse learns that any procedure is more effective when it is explained and administered carefully and in consideration of any patient concern. For example, if a patient is anxious about having a procedure such as the insertion of a nasogastric tube, offer comfort through a full explanation of the procedure and what the patient will feel. Then perform the procedure safely, skillfully, and successfully. This is done as you prepare the supplies, position the patient, and gently manipulate and insert the nasogastric tube. Throughout a procedure talk quietly with the patient to provide reassurance and support.

Caring touch is a form of nonverbal communication, which successfully influences a patient's comfort and security, enhances self-esteem, increases confidence of caregivers, and improves mental well-being. You express this in the way you hold a patient's hand, give a back massage, or gently position a patient. When using a caring touch, you connect with the patient physically and emotionally.

Protective touch is a form of touch that protects a nurse and/or patient. A patient views it either positively or negatively. The most obvious form of protective touch is in preventing an accident (e.g., holding and bracing a patient to avoid a fall). Protective touch can also protect a nurse emotionally. A nurse withdraws or distances herself or himself from a patient who is unable to tolerate suffering or needs to escape from a situation that is causing tension. When used in this way, protective touch elicits negative feelings in a patient.

Therapeutic touch (TT) is a holistic, evidence-based therapy and is an approved complementary and alternative medicine method (Bagci and Yucel, 2020). It was developed and refined by Dr. Dolores Krieger, PhD, RN, and incorporates the intentional and compassionate use of touch to help patients find their inner balance (Therapeutic Touch International Association, 2019). TT practitioners focus on healing by directing the practitioners' hands on patients' bodies. This complementary therapy is effective in managing anxiety, pain, dementia, and other physical and mental health conditions (Bagci and Yucel, 2020) (see Chapter 32).

Because touch conveys many messages, use it with discretion. Touch itself is a concern when crossing cultural boundaries of either the patient or the nurse (Benner et al., 2010). Ethnographic studies suggest that cultures differ in the extent to which they value physical touch and in its acceptability in different kinds of social relationships (Burleson et al., 2018). Patients generally permit task-oriented touch because most individuals give nurses and physicians a license to enter their personal space to provide care (see Box 7.1). However it is important to inform patients when touch occurs. Know and understand whether patients accept touch and how they interpret your intentions.

Listening

Listening is necessary for meaningful interactions with patients. It is a planned and deliberate act in which the listener is present and engages the patient in a nonjudgmental and accepting manner. You "take in" what a patient says, interpreting and understanding what the patient is saying, and then give back that understanding to the patient. Listening to the meaning of what a patient says helps create a mutual relationship.

True listening leads to knowing and responding to what really matters to a patient and family. Listening, especially when providing end-of-life-care, helps a patient and family caregiver address their concerns and preferences with dignity (Harstade et al., 2018).

Any critical or chronic illness affects all of a patient's life choices and decisions, and sometimes the individual's identity. Being able to tell the story about the illness and its meaning helps a patient break the distress of illness (Borasio and Tamches, 2018; Harstade et al., 2018). The personal concerns that are part of a patient's illness story determine what is at stake for the patient. Caring through listening enables you to become a participant in the patient's life.

To listen effectively you need to silence yourself and listen with an open mind. Remain intentionally silent and concentrate on what the patient has to say. Give patients your full, focused attention as they tell their stories. When a person chooses to tell his or her story, it involves reaching out to another human being (Borasio and Tamches, 2018). Telling the story implies a relationship that develops only if the clinician exchanges his or her story as well. Some professionals do not recognize their own need to be known as part of a clinical relationship (Frank, 1998). Unless a professional acknowledges this need, there is no reciprocal relationship, only an interaction.

Through active listening you begin to truly know your patients and what is important to them. Learning to listen to a patient is sometimes difficult. It is easy to become distracted by tasks at hand, colleagues shouting instructions, or other patients waiting to have their needs met. However, the time you take to listen effectively is worthwhile, in both the information gained and the strengthening of the nurse-patient relationship (Engle, 2010). Listening involves paying attention to an individual's words and tone of voice and entering the individual's frame of reference (see Chapter 24). By observing the expressions and body language of a patient, you find cues to help the patient explore ways to achieve greater peace.

Knowing the Patient

Knowing the patient is an important part of nursing practice. It is a complex process that occurs over time as a nurse cares for multiple patients and it develops within the context of the nurse-patient relationship. Knowing the patient is linked to patient satisfaction and successful outcomes of care (Johansson and Martensson, 2019; Ray and Stargardt., 2020). Knowing the patient is an in-depth knowledge of a patient's pattern of responses within a clinical situation and knowledge of the patient as a person (Tanner et al., 1993). Knowing a patient relates to a nurse's experience with caring for patients, experience in a specific clinical area, and sense of closeness with patients (see Chapter 15). Knowing prepares nurses to recognize patient problems and make appropriate clinical judgments.

One of the five caring processes described by Swanson (1991) is knowing the patient. Knowing emerges from repeated caring relationships between a nurse and patients, in which the nurse engages in a continuous assessment, striving to understand and interpret each patient's needs across all dimensions (Johansson and Martensson, 2019).

Knowing a patient is at the core of clinical decision making and patient-centered care. Through caring, you develop an understanding that helps you to better know the patient as a unique individual, which helps you better analyze cues, identify your patient's main health-related problems, and provide individualized, evidence-based nursing care. Knowing the patient requires you to listen about how a patient's illness, treatment, or rehabilitation affect the patient and family caregiver (Johansson and Martensson, 2019).

Two elements that facilitate knowing a patient are continuity of care and clinical expertise. Knowing is best demonstrated when a nurse works with a patient over time to understand the meaning of an event, such as an illness or loss of function or loss of a loved one (Burgos, 2019). When patient care is fragmented, nurses have limited encounters with patients. This makes it difficult to recognize and know patient patterns and understand how patients are responding to illness and treatment. It also affects knowing a patient's care preferences, compromising patient-centered care (Ray and Stargardt, 2010). Knowing develops over time as a nurse learns the clinical conditions within a specialty and the behaviors and physiological responses of patients. Intimate knowing helps the nurse respond to what really matters to the patient. To know a patient provides the health care team with information to provide patient-focused, team-based interventions that improve patient satisfaction and outcomes (Shippe et al., 2018). Thus, the nurse engages in a caring relationship with the patient that reveals information and cues that facilitate critical thinking and clinical judgments (see Chapter 15).

Factors that contribute to knowing patients include time, continuity of care, teamwork of the nursing staff, trust, and experience. Barriers to knowing a patient are often related to the organizational structure of an agency and economic constraints. Organizational changes that decrease the amount of time that nurses are able to spend with their patients affect nurse-patient relationships. Decreased length of stay also reduces the interactions between nurses and their patients (Zolnierek, 2014).

Many poor outcomes result from not knowing a patient. For example, in the acute care setting, not knowing patients contributes to risk for falls and actual falls. A nurse is less able to recognize common fall risks and identify which risks apply to a specific patient. When nurses do not know patients, they and their families do not understand the complexities of treatment and their participation in care (Johansson and Martensson, 2019; Zolnierek, 2014). Furthermore, patients do not adequately understand their discharge instructions and may administer their home medications or treatments incorrectly. A caring nurse-patient relationship helps you to better know each patient as a unique individual and choose the most appropriate and effective nursing therapies (WCSI, 2021).

Combining a caring relationship with your growing knowledge and experience provides a rich source of meaning when a patient's clinical status changes. Expert nurses develop the ability to detect changes in patients' conditions almost effortlessly; this is a part of knowing patients (Ragan and Kanter, 2017; Benner et al., 2010). Clinical decision making and clinical judgment, perhaps the most important responsibilities of a professional nurse, involve various aspects of knowing a patient: responses to therapies, routines and habits, coping resources, physical capacities and endurance, and body typology and characteristics. Experienced nurses know additional facts about their patients, such as their experiences, behaviors, feelings, and perceptions (Benner et al., 2010). Your patients will experience improved satisfaction and health outcomes when you make clinical decisions within the context of knowing patients well (Chen et al., 2018). When you base care on knowing a patient, the patient perceives care as personalized, comforting, supportive, and healing.

It is important for a beginning nurse to recognize that knowing a patient is more than simply gathering data about one patient's clinical signs and condition. Success in knowing a patient develops over time with patients who present similar health problems. But it begins with caring, enabling you to enter into a social process that includes interaction with members of the health care team; it results in a deep nurse-patient relationship where a patient comes to feel known by you (Ragan and Kanter, 2017; Zolnierek, 2014).

QSEN **Building Competency in Patient-Centered Care** Mrs. Martinez is 72 years of age, has three married sons, and lives in a mother-in-law suite in the home of one son. There are two adult grandchildren who are on their own. Mrs. Martinez's son and daughter-in-law have full-time jobs and are out of the house from 8:00 AM to 6:00 PM each day.

Each summer the other sons and their families visit Mrs. Martinez while the son with whom she lives and his wife go on vacation. Mrs. Martinez's sons and their families spend the holidays together.

Presently Mrs. Martinez is independent. She takes medication for high blood pressure and an irregular heartbeat. At times, these medications make her "light-headed." She also has occasional dizziness from a middle ear problem when she changes position too fast. She is afraid that if she shares this information with her doctor, he would think that she would fall and say she must give up her activities. She equates this with losing her independence.

Given the information about her living situation, current level of independence, and symptoms of light-headedness and dizziness, how do you plan and implement patient-centered care?

Answers to QSEN Activities can be found on the Evolve website.

Spiritual Caring

An individual achieves spiritual health after finding a balance between life values, goals, and belief systems and those of others (see Chapter 35). An individual's beliefs and expectations affect physical well-being.

Research shows that nurses who develop spiritual caring practices early in their career development are able to identify methods to incorporate these practices into routine care and do not perceive variables such as a lack of sufficient time or size of patient assignments as barriers. Establishing a caring relationship with a patient involves interconnectedness between the nurse and the patient. This interconnectedness is why Watson (2008, 2010) describes the caring relationship in a spiritual sense. Spirituality offers a sense of connectedness: intrapersonally (connected with oneself), interpersonally (connected with others and the environment), and transpersonally (connected with the unseen, God, or a higher power). In a caring relationship the patient and the nurse come to know each other so that both move toward a healing relationship by (Brewer and Watson, 2015; WCSI, 2020):

- Mobilizing hope for the patient and the nurse
- Finding an interpretation or understanding of illness, symptoms, or emotions that is acceptable to the patient
- Assisting the patient in using social, emotional, or spiritual resources
- Recognizing that caring relationships connect us human to human, spirit to spirit

Relieving Symptoms and Suffering

Relieving symptoms such as pain, nausea, and suffering is more than giving pain medications, repositioning a patient, cleaning a wound, or providing end-of-life care (see Chapter 36). Reducing symptoms and suffering requires patient-centered caring actions that give a patient comfort, dignity, respect, and peace and that provide comfort and support measures to the family and friends (Baillie et al., 2018).

Through skillful and accurate assessment of a patient's symptoms, your delivery of patient-centered care will improve a patient's level of comfort. You will use multiple interventions to relieve pain (see Chapter 44), nausea, and fatigue. However, knowing about a patient and the meaning of the patient's symptoms guides your care (Baillie et al., 2018). Conveying a quiet, caring presence, touching a patient, or listening helps you to assess and understand the meaning of your patient's discomfort. The caring presence helps you and your patient set desired outcomes for symptom relief.

Human suffering is multifaceted, affecting a patient physically, emotionally, socially, and spiritually. It also affects a patient's family caregivers and other family members (Given and Reinhard, 2017). You may find yourself working with a young family whose newborn baby has multiple developmental challenges. Likewise, you may find yourself working with a family that provides home care for a parent with dementia. In both of these examples, these families' emotional suffering encompasses anger, guilt, fear, or grief. You cannot fix it, but you can provide comfort through a listening, nonjudgmental caring presence. Patients and their families are comforted by a caring listener.

Family Care

Each person experiences life through relationships with others (see Chapter 10). Thus, caring for an individual includes a person's family. As a nurse it is important to know the family and family caregivers as thoroughly as you know the patient (Given and Reinhard, 2017). The family who provides support and care for a patient is an important resource (Fig. 7.2). Success with nursing interventions often depends on the family's willingness to share information about the patient, their acceptance and understanding of therapies, whether the interventions fit with their daily practices, and whether they support and deliver the therapies recommended.

Families of patients with cancer perceive many nurse caring behaviors to be helpful (Box 7.4). It is critical for nurses to ensure a patient's well-being and safety and to help family caregivers be active participants. Although specific to families of patients with cancer, these behaviors offer useful guidelines for developing a caring relationship with all families. Begin a relationship by learning who makes up the patient's family and their roles in the patient's life (Chapter 10). Showing a family that you care for and are concerned about the patient creates an openness that then enables a relationship to form. Caring for the family takes into consideration the context of the patient's illness and the stress it imposes on all members.

REFLECT NOW

Think about a clinical or personal situation in which you needed to provide caring support. Identify the caring behaviors you used. Reflect on your interaction. What was helpful and effective? What could you have done better?

FIG. 7.2 Nurse discusses patient's health care needs with the family.

BOX 7.4 Nurse Caring Behaviors as Perceived by Families of Patients With Cancer

- Providing honest, clear, and accurate information
- Listening to patient and family concerns, complaints, and fears
- Assisting family with implementing advance directives
- Advocating for patient's care preferences and end-of-life decisions
- Involving family in care and teaching the family how to keep the relative physically comfortable
- Informing the patient and family about the types of nursing services and the people who may enter the personal care area
- Providing comfort (e.g., offering warm blanket, rubbing a patient's back)
- Reading patient passages from religious texts, favorite book, cards, or mail
- Assuring the patient that nursing services will be available
- Helping patients do as much for themselves as possible

Data from Maroon AM: Ethical palliative family nursing care: a new concept of caring for patients and families, *JONA's Healthc Law Ethics Regul* 14(4):115, 2012; Lusk JM, Fater K: A concept analysis of patient-centered care, *Nurs Forum* 48(2):89, 2013.

THE CHALLENGE OF CARING

The concept of caring motivates people to become nurses. When nurses commit to being caring individuals, they achieve a meaning and purpose in their lives (Benner et al., 2010). Nurses gain a sense of satisfaction when they know they have made a difference in patients' lives.

Today's health care system presents many challenges for nurses to provide a caring, patient-centered plan of care (Percy and Richardson, 2018; Adams, 2016). Nurses have less time to spend with patients, making it much harder to know who they are. The reliance on technology and cost-effective health care strategies and efforts to standardize and refine work processes all undermine the nature of caring. Nurses often experience compassion fatigue when they are torn between the human caring model and the task-oriented biomedical model, institutional demands, and time constraints (Letourneau et al., 2017). Compassion fatigue negatively affects the health and effectiveness of health care providers and consequently patient care (Cavanagh et al., 2020).

The American Nurses Association (ANA), National League for Nursing (NLN), American Organization of Nurse Executives (AONE), and American Association of Colleges of Nursing (AACN) recommend strategies to reverse the current nursing shortage (see Chapter 1). A number of these strategies have potential for improving the workforce and creating work environments that enable nurses to demonstrate more caring behaviors. In addition, the Robert Wood Johnson Foundation's "Future of Nursing: Campaign for Action" identifies methods to improve both patient care and satisfaction and nurse job satisfaction. This campaign focuses on increasing the amount of time nurses spend with their patients and families. Strategies include greater emphasis on improving the work environment to facilitate more nurse-patient interaction, improving nurse staffing, providing nurses with autonomy over their practice, and promoting increased educational requirements and opportunities (RWJF, 2014).

Health care must become more compassionate to make a positive difference. Nurses play an important role in making care an integral part of health care delivery. This begins when institutions make caring a part of the philosophy and environment of the workplace and incorporate care concepts into standards of nursing care and guidelines for professional conduct.

Finally, nurses need to be committed to caring and willing to establish the relationships necessary with patients and families to provide personal, competent, compassionate, and meaningful nursing care. "Consistent with the wisdom and vision of Nightingale, nursing is a lifetime journey of caring and healing, seeking to understand and preserve the wholeness of human existence and to offer compassionate, informed knowledgeable human caring . . ." (Watson, 2009).

KEY POINTS

- Caring involves a mutual give-and-take and is specific and relational for each nurse-patient encounter.
- Nurses use a variety of caring theories to provide care in a respectful and therapeutic way for patients and family caregivers.
- Current evidence emphasizes what patients perceive from their caregivers and thus provides useful guidelines for practice.
- An ethic of care places the nurse as the patient's advocate, influences the nurse's clinical judgment, and helps guide clinical decision-making regarding ethical dilemmas by attending to relationships and giving priority to each patient's unique personhood.
- Caring is integral to a nurse's ability to establish therapeutic relationships with patients in a respectful and therapeutic manner.
- Presence is a person-to-person interaction, conveying closeness and a sense of caring that involves "being there" and "being with" patients or family caregivers.
- Touch expresses caring through task-oriented, caring, and protective touch.
- Listening is a therapeutic skill that includes interpreting, understanding, and respecting what a patient or family caregiver is saying and expressing that understanding and respect.
- Knowing a patient is at the core of the process the nurse uses to make clinical decisions about patient-centered care.
- Maintaining compassion in all aspects of nursing care contributes to the health and well-being of patients and improves patient and nurse satisfaction.

REFLECTIVE LEARNING

Linda Miller is a new graduate nurse who is assigned to care for Mary Kline, a 48-year-old married woman who has colon cancer. She is one-day post colon cancer surgery and placement of a temporary colostomy. During the preoperative visit, Mary's surgeon indicated that he did not think a colostomy was needed, but he did tell Mary that in some situations a decision is made during surgery to create a temporary colostomy. Mary was surprised and upset to learn after her surgery that she needed to have a temporary colostomy.

- Linda needs to do a history and physical assessment on Mrs. Kline. What caring behaviors should Linda use during the interview?
- During the interview, Mrs. Kline breaks down in tears. Linda starts to leave the room to give her some privacy, but Mrs. Kline asks Linda to "stay and just sit with me." She is asking for Linda's presence. Reflect on and describe the importance of providing presence to Mrs. Kline.
- Mrs. Kline wants to talk about her cancer. She expresses that she is worried that her daughters might inherit a risk for colon cancer. What listening skills should Linda use? Reflect on and describe the importance of each of these listening skills in caring for Mrs. Kline.

REVIEW QUESTIONS

1. A nurse encounters the patient's wife, who is tearful and worried. Her husband was just transferred from his room to the operating room for a complex cardiovascular surgery. The nurse brings the wife a glass of water and encourages her to talk about her fears.

The nurse remains in the room quietly listening. What caring behaviors is the nurse demonstrating? (Select all that apply.)
   1. Touching
   2. Listening
   3. Knowing
   4. Presence
   5. Spiritual care
2. A nurse needs to use clinical judgment before planning and implementing any touch interventions. What does the nurse need to understand about the use of touch? (Select all that apply.)
   1. Some cultures may have specific restrictions about non–skill-based touch.
   2. Touch is a form of nonverbal communication.
   3. Touch reduces only physical pain.
   4. Touch can successfully influence a patient's level of comfort.
   5. There is never a problem with using touch at any time.
3. A young woman comes to a clinic for the first time for a gynecological examination. She asks about the procedure, who will be in the room with her, and does she have to remove all her clothes. Which nursing behavior applies Swanson's caring process of "knowing" the patient?
   1. Sharing feelings about the importance of having regular gynecological examinations
   2. Explaining risk factors for cervical cancer
   3. Recognizing that the patient is modest and maintaining her privacy during the examination
   4. Asking the patient what it means to have a vaginal examination
4. A patient is fearful of upcoming surgery and a possible cancer diagnosis. He discusses his love for the Bible with his nurse, who recommends a favorite Bible verse. Another nurse tells the patient's nurse that there is no place in nursing for spiritual caring. What is the best response by the patient's nurse?
   1. "You're correct; spiritual care should be left to a pastoral care professional."
   2. "You're correct; religion is a personal decision."
   3. "Nurses should explain their own religious beliefs to patients."
   4. "Spiritual, mind, and body connections can affect health."
5. Which of the following are strategies for creating work environments that support nurse caring interventions? (Select all that apply.)
   1. Increasing technological support
   2. Improving flexibility for scheduling
   3. Providing opportunities to discuss care practices
   4. Promoting autonomy of practice
   5. Encouraging increased input concerning nursing functions from health care providers
6. A nurse is caring for a patient newly diagnosed with testicular cancer. He asked the nurse to help him find the meaning of cancer by supporting beliefs about life. This is an example of:
   1. Instilling hope and faith.
   2. Forming a human-altruistic value system.
   3. Cultural caring.
   4. Being with.
7. An example of a nurse caring behavior that families of patients who are acutely ill perceive as important to patients' well-being is:
   1. Making health care decisions for patients.
   2. Having family members provide a patient's total personal hygiene.
   3. Injecting the nurse's perceptions about the level of care provided.
   4. Asking permission before performing a procedure on a patient.
8. A nurse is caring for a patient who has just transferred from an intensive care unit and still has a long hospitalization ahead. Because of the complexity of care and the number of caregivers for this patient, the family members feel disconnected from their loved one

and not part of the care team. Which interventions would demonstrate care by helping family members? (Select all that apply.)
1. Helping family become active participants in care
2. Removing family members from assisting with the patient's personal care
3. Allowing the family to offer opinions on health care decisions for the patient
4. Providing the family opportunities to discuss their concerns with the health care team
5. Planning uninterrupted time for the family and patient to be together

9. A hospice nurse sits at the bedside of a male patient in the final stages of cancer. He and his parents made the decision that he would move home and they would help him in the final stages of his disease. The family participates in his care, but lately the nurse has increased the amount of time spent with the family. Whenever the nurse enters the room or approaches the patient to give care, the nurse touches his shoulder and states, "I am your nurse, and I am here for you." This is an example of what type of touch.
1. Caring touch
2. Protective touch
3. Task-oriented touch
4. Interpersonal touch

10. Match the following caring behaviors with a nursing action.
1. Knowing
2. Being with
3. Doing for
4. Maintaining belief

a. Encouraging a patient or family to use resources and trust previous decisions that have helped to resolve issues.
b. Asking a patient to talk about what the loss of a loved one means for the patient and the family.
c. Telling a family that you understand their anger about the side effects of chemotherapy.
d. Providing an opportunity for a patient's specific religious practice as the patient would do it.

Answers: 1. 2, 4; **2.** 1, 2, 4; **3.** 3, 4; **5.** 2, 3, 4; **6.** 1; **7.** 4; **8.** 1, 4, 5; **9.** 1; **10.** 1b, 2c, 3d, 4a.

Rationales for Review Questions can be found on the Evolve website.

REFERENCES

Adams LY: The conundrum of caring in nursing, *Int J Caring Sci* 9(1):1, 2016.

American Organization of Nurse Executives (AONE): Guiding principles for the role of the nurse in future health care delivery, 2004, 2010, https://www.aonl.org/sites/default/files/aone/role-nurse-future-patient-care.pdf. Accessed May 2021.

Benner P, Wrubel J: *The primacy of caring: stress and coping in health and illness*, Menlo Park, CA, 1989, Addison Wesley.

Benner P, et al.: *Educating nurses: a call for radical transformation*, Stanford, CA, 2010, Carnegie Foundation for the Advancement of Teaching.

Borasio GD, Tamches E: Guest editorial: assessment measures in palliative care: the risk of inflation and the importance of listening to the patient's story, *Palliat Support Care* 12(1), 1, 2018.

Brewer BB, Watson J: Evaluation of authentic human caring professional practices, *JONA* 45(12):622, 2015.

Burgos G: Congruence between nurses' caring behaviors and patient's perceptions of being cared for during disaster responses, *Int J Human Caring* 23(1): 80, 2019.

Colman DE: Evidence based nursing practice, the challenges of health care and diversity, *J Hosp Libr* 19(4): 330, 2019.

Engle M: *I'm here: compassionate communication in patient care*, Orlando, FL, 2010, Phillips Press.

Frank AW: Just listening narrative and deep illness, *Fam Syst Health* 16(3):197, 1998.

Given BA, Reinhard SC: Caregiving at the end of life: the challenges for family caregivers, *Generations J Am Soc Aging* 41(1):50, 2017.

Grant SM et al: Advancing the practice of patient and family-centered care: the central role of nursing leadership, *Nurse Leader*, 17(4): 325, 2019.

Hanley MA, et al.: A practice-based theory of healing through therapeutic touch, *J Hol Nurs* 35(4):369, 2017.

Leininger MM: *Culture care diversity and universality: a theory of nursing*, Pub No 15-2402, New York, 1991, National League for Nursing Press.

Letourneau D, et al.: Humanizing nursing care: an analysis of caring theories through the lens of humanism, *International J Human Caring* 21(1):33, 2017.

Marion L, et al.: Implementing the new ANA standard 8: culturally congruent practice, *Online J Issues Nurs* 22(1):1, 2017.

Markey K, et al.: Understanding nurses' concerns when caring for patients from diverse cultural and ethnic backgrounds, *J Clin Nurs* 27(1/2):e259, 2018.

Moffa C: Caring for novice nurses applying Swanson's Theory of Caring, *Int J Human Caring* 19(1):63, 2015.

Merritt LS et al: International service-learning for nurse practitioner students Enhancing clinical practice skills and cultural competence, *J Nurs Educ* 58(9): 548, 2019

Ortiz MR: Patient-centered care: nursing, knowledge and policy, *Nurse Sci Q* 31(3):291, 2018.

Percy M, Richardson C: Introducing nursing practice to student nurses: how can we promote care compassion and empathy, *Nurse Educ Pract* 29:200, 2018.

Plessis E: Caring presence in practice: facilitating an appreciative discourse in nursing, *Int Nurs Rev* 63(3):377, 2016.

Ragan SL, Kanter E: Learning the patient's story, *Semin Oncol Nurs* 33(5):467, 2017.

Ray J, Stargardt D: Linking hospital consumer assessment of healthcare providers and systems to Swanson Caring Theory: a diagnostic model for improvement, *JONA* 50(4): 216, 2020.

Robert Wood Johnson Foundation (RWJF): *Future of nursing: campaign for action is chalking up successes that will improve patient care*, http://www.rwjf.org/en/about-rwjf/newsroom/newsroom-content/2014/06/campaign-for-action-is-chalking-up-successes-that-will-improve-p.html, 2014. Accessed May 2021.

Therapeutic Touch Internal (TTI) Association : How did therapeutic touch begin?, 2019, https://therapeutic-touch.org/about-us/how-did-therapeutic-touch-being/. Accessed May 2021.

Watson Caring Science Institute (WCSI): *Caring science & human caring theory*, 2021, https://www.watsoncaring-science.org/jean-bio/caring-science-theory/. Accessed May 2021.

Watson J: *The philosophy and science of caring*, Boulder, 2008, University Press of Colorado.

Watson J: Caring science and human caring theory: transforming personal and professional practices of nursing and health care, *J Health Human Serv Adm* 31(4):466, 2009.

Watson J: Caring science and the next decade of holistic healing: transforming self and system from the inside out, *Am Holist Nurses Assoc* 30(2):14, 2010.

RESEARCH REFERENCES

Ackerman L: Caring Science Education: Measuring nurse's caring behaviors, *Intl J Caring Sci.* 12(1): 572, 2019.

Atar NY, Asti T: Attitudes and behaviors of nursing students towards nurse-patient interaction, *Intl J Caring Sci* 13(1): 411, 2020.

Bagci H, Yucel SC: A systematic review of the studies about therapeutic touch after the year 2000, *Intl J Caring Sci*, 132(1): 231, 2020.

Baillie J et al.: Symptom management, nutrition and hydration at end-of-life: a qualitative exploration of patients', carers' and health professionals' experiences and further research questions, *BMC Palliat Care* 17(1):1, 2018.

Burleson MH et al: Perceived cultural acceptability and comfort with affectionate touch: Differences between Mexican Americans and European Americans, *J Soc Pers Relation* 36(3): 1000, 2018.

Cavanagh N et al: Compassion fatigue in healthcare providers: a systematic review and meta-analysis, *Nursing Ethics*, 27(3): 640, 2020.

Chen SY et al: Caring behaviours directly and indirectly affecting nursing student's critical thinking, *Scand J Caring Sci* 32: 197, 2018.

Compton EK et al.: Nurses' caring behaviors, *Clin J Oncol Nurs* 22(2):169, 2018.

da Rocha Rodrigues MG, Sechaud L: Caring models in geriatric rehabilitation: an integrative review, *Holistic Nursing Practice* 33(4): 237, 2019

Dey MM: Relationship of hospitalized elders' perceptions of nurse caring behaviors, type of care unit, satisfaction with nursing care, and health outcome of functional status, *Int J Hum Caring* 20(3):134, 2016.

Duffy JR, et al.: Dimensions of caring: psychometric evaluation of the caring assessment tool, *Adv Nurs Sci* 30(3):235, 2007.

Frankenfield R et al: Caring for staff, *Clin J Onc Nurs* 22(5): 570, 2018.

Hansbrough WB, Georges JM: Validation of the presence of nursing scale using data triangulation, *Nurs Res* 68(6): 439, 2019.

Harstade CW, et al.: Dignity-conserving care actions in palliative care: an integrative review of Swedish research, *Scand J Caring Sci* 32(1):8, 2018.

Hines MW, Gaughan J: Advanced holistic nursing practice narratives, *J Holist Nurs* 35(4):328, 2017.

Johansson B, Martensson KB: Ways of strategies to knowing the patient described by nursing students, *Burs Educ in Prac* 38: 120, 2019.

Komatsu H et al: Effects of a nurse-led medication self-management programme in cancer patients: protocol for a mixed-method randomized controlled trial, *BMC Nursing*, 15(9): 1, 2016.

Labraque LJ, et al.: Nursing students' perception of their own caring behaviors: a multicountry study, *Int J Nurs Knowl* 28(4):225, 2017.

Mohammadipour F, et al.: An exploratory study on the concept of nursing presence from the perspective of

patients admitted to hospitals, *J Clin Nurs* 26(23/24):4313, 2017.

Monsen K, et al.: We can be more caring: a theory for enhancing the experience of being caring as an integral component of prelicensure nursing education, *Int J Hum Caring* 21(1):9, 2017.

Murali KP: End of life Decision-Making: Watson's theory of human caring, Nurs Sci Q 33(1): 73, 2020.

Nightingale S, et al.: The impact of emotional intelligence in health care professionals on caring behaviour towards patients in clinical and long-term care settings: findings from an integrative review, *Int J Nurs Stud* 80:106, 2018.

Ortega Barco MA, de Rodriguez LM: Evaluation of the nursing care offered during the parturition process. Controlled clinical trial of an intervention based on Swanson's theory of caring versus conventional care, *Nurs Res Educ* 36(1):e05, 2018.

Romero-Martin M et al: Systematic review of the nature of nursing care described by using the Caring Behaviours Inventory, *J Clin Nurs* 28: 3734, 2019.

Shippe ND, et al.: Effect of a whole-person model of care on patient experience in patients with complex chronic illness in late life, *Am J Hosp Palliat Care* 35(1):104, 2018.

Sitzman K: Evolution of Watson's human caring science in the digital age, *Int J Human Caring* 21(1):46, 2017.

Su JJ et al: Defining compassionate nursing care, *Nursing Ethics* 27(2): 480, 2020.

Suliman WA et al.: Applying Watson's nursing theory to assess patient perceptions of being cared for in a multicultural environment, *J Nurs Res* 17(4):293, 2009.

Swanson KM: Empirical development of a middle-range theory of caring, *Nurs Res* 40(3):161, 1991.

Swanson KM: Effects of caring, measurement, and time on miscarriage impact and women's well-being, *Nurs Res* 48(6):288, 1999.

Tanner CA, et al. The phenomenology of knowing the patient. *J Nurs Scholarsh* 25:273, 1993.

Wei H et al: The current intervention studies based on Watson's theory of human caring: a systematic review, *Int J of Human Caring*, 23(1): 4, 2019

Wyant RA et al.: Show your stuff and watch your tone: nurses' caring behaviors, *Am J Crit Care* 26(2):111, 2017.

Yagasaki K, Komatsu H: The need for a nursing presence in oral chemotherapy, *Clin J Oncol Nurs* 17(5):512, 2013.

Young K et al: Nurses' experiences of learning to care in practice environments: a qualitative study, *Nurs Educ in Practice* 38: 132, 2019.

Zolnierek CD: An integrative review of knowing the patient. *J Nurs Scholarsh* 46(1):3, 2014.

Caring for Patients With Chronic Illness

Because of advancements in technology and medical treatment, many people are living longer with one or more chronic diseases that affect their daily lives. The increased prevalence of people living longer with multiple complex chronic diseases has greatly affected patients, families, communities, and the health care delivery system. Chronic diseases affect the physical, psychosocial, and economic aspects of a patient and family's life. Changes may occur in a person's interactions and relationships with others as well. Sometimes a disease becomes a person's identity. For example, a patient may be referred to as "the diabetic" or "the cancer patient" instead of a patient living with diabetes mellitus or a person diagnosed with cancer.

To care for patients experiencing chronic diseases, you need to understand not only the physical and psychological implications but also the economic impact. In your role in disease prevention, know the risk factors that contribute to the incidence of chronic disease. The Chronic Care Model provides a framework to guide clinical judgment and decision making in patient care. The roles nurses play in caring for people with chronic diseases include prevention, early detection, and help in identifying effective patient-centered strategies for patients to manage their chronic illnesses.

THE PREVALENCE AND COSTS OF CHRONIC DISEASE

Although they are separate concepts, the terms chronic disease and chronic illness are often used interchangeably. A chronic disease is a pathophysiologic condition that lasts more than 1 year, requires ongoing medical care, and often limits a person's usual activities of daily living due to symptoms of the disease or self-care activities required to manage the disease (CDC, 2021a). Chronic illness refers to a patient's and family's subjective experiences of and responses to a chronic disease (Meiner and Yeager, 2019).

It is estimated that 6 out of every 10 adults in the United States have at least one chronic disease. In addition, 4 out of every 10 adults have two or more chronic conditions (CDC, 2021a). With each additional diagnosed chronic disease, the burden of disease for the individual increases; this translates into additional expenses, such as multiple medications and additional visits to health care providers. Living with two or more chronic diseases often creates the need for patients to make even greater changes to daily activities. Table 8.1 illustrates common chronic diseases listed by body system. Although this is not an

TABLE 8.1   Examples of Chronic Diseases by Body System

Body System	Disease Examples
Cardiac	Hypertension Heart failure Coronary artery disease
Digestive	Cirrhosis of the liver Ulcerative colitis Obesity
Endocrine	Diabetes mellitus
Pulmonary	Chronic bronchitis Emphysema Asthma Allergies
Musculoskeletal	Arthritis Osteoporosis
Neurologic/psychiatric	Alzheimer disease Stroke Parkinson disease Spinal cord injury Systemic lupus Epilepsy Depression Bipolar disorder Multiple sclerosis
Renal	Renal failure
Cancer	Colorectal, breast, cervical, skin, gynecologic
Metabolic	Obesity, metabolic syndrome

TABLE 8.2   Yearly Costs of Chronic Illness Care

Chronic Disease	Yearly Cost of Medical Care in the United States
Cancer care (NCI, n.d.)	$174 billion
Diabetes mellitus (ADA, 2021)	$327 billion
Dementia (AIM, 2020)	$305 billion
Heart disease and stroke (CDC, 2021b)	$214 billion
Obesity (CDC, 2021b)	$147 billion
Arthritis (CDC, 2020a)	$140 billion

exhaustive list, it represents the most common chronic diseases seen in the United States (CDC, 2021a).

The financial burden created by caring for chronic diseases is staggering (Table 8.2). The Centers for Disease Control and Prevention (CDC) (2021b) estimates that 90% of the $3.8 trillion spent on health care in the United States is used to care for people with chronic and mental health diseases. Disease prevention and better symptom management can greatly reduce these costs and potentially save billions of dollars spent yearly on health care (CDC, 2021b). For example, people who have diabetes mellitus spend an average of $16,750 per year to manage their disease, which is 2.3 times higher than what people without Type 2 diabetes mellitus spend on their health care (CDC, 2018a). Type 2 diabetes mellitus is often preventable or can be managed effectively with lifestyle modifications (e.g., dietary changes, regular exercise).

REFLECT NOW

What chronic diseases are most prevalent in your community? Which are preventable? What effect would chronic disease prevention have on the health care dollars spent in your community?

MULTIFACTORIAL NATURE OF CHRONIC DISEASE

Numerous factors come into play when describing how individuals develop chronic disease and the resulting symptoms and impairments. Each patient presents a unique case for how genetic, environmental, and lifestyle factors collide to create disease. The physical and psychological portraits of patients with the same chronic disease will have commonalities but also important differences that will affect your nursing care. Understanding the interrelationship of the factors contributing to chronic disease better enables you to support patients when they suffer chronic diseases. This knowledge prepares you to critically anticipate what to assess and what potential interventions might apply when you make clinical judgments about patient care.

Genetic Factors

Autosomal genetic disorders occur when there is a **genetic mutation** or abnormality in inherited genetic material. Some genetic mutations cause inherited chronic diseases. These disorders fall into two categories: autosomal dominant disorders and autosomal recessive disorders. Autosomal dominant disorders such as Huntington's chorea, familial hypercholesterolemia, and neurofibromatosis occur when a person has one parent with the dominant genetic disorder or a new mutation in a gene occurs (NIH, 2020a). Each child born to a parent who has the dominant disorder has a 50% risk of having the disorder.

Autosomal recessive disorders such as cystic fibrosis and sickle cell anemia occur most commonly when both parents are carriers of the recessive genetic disorder. Although these parents are carriers of the genetic disease, they do not have the disease. Each child born from two parents who carry a recessive disorder has a 25% risk of having the disease. Both autosomal and recessive genetic disorders account for a small percentage of people with chronic diseases.

Influence of Genetics. Although almost all diseases have a genetic component, most are not the result of a single genetic cause (NIH, 2021). Multifactorial inheritance, which includes a combination of genetic factors, environmental elements, and lifestyle choices, increases the risk for the development of most chronic illnesses (NIH, 2021; Rappaport, 2016) (Fig. 8.1). Genetic factors are not modifiable. People are born with genetic material from their parents. Simply inheriting a gene mutation for a disease such as diabetes mellitus, cancer, or hypertension does not guarantee that a person will develop the disease. **Multifactorial inheritance** explains why a person who carries genetic material for developing a chronic illness may or may not eventually be diagnosed with the disease (NIH, 2021).

Family History. Identification of a chronic disease occurrence in a family over several generations is the starting point for determining a person's disease risk. In examining a family disease history, important factors to consider include a multigenerational examination for patterns of the same disease, the age of onset of the disease, and generational frequency of the disorder. If a strong disease pattern is identified in a family history, **genetic counseling** may be indicated. Genetic counselors clarify the risk of disease development based on family history, answer questions about the process, recommend screening tests for the disorder

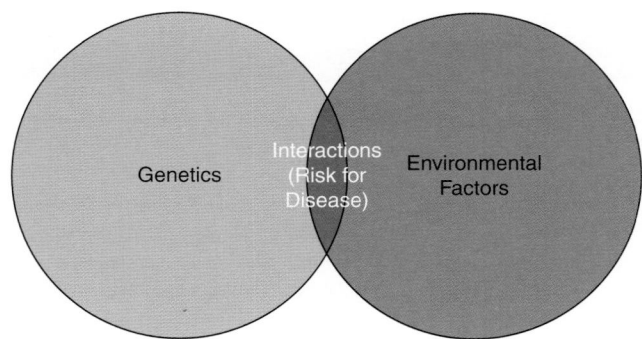

FIG. 8.1 Multifactorial inheritance: interaction of factors promoting chronic disease. (Modified from https://www.genetics.edu.au/publications-and-resources/facts-sheets/fact-sheet-11-environmental-and-genetic-interactions/view. Accessed February 25, 2021.)

if necessary, discuss available genetic testing, and recommend lifestyle changes that may decrease the risk of developing the disease (NIH, 2020b).

Genetic Screening. The science of genetic screening is developing and evolving for chronic diseases. Genetic testing is available for more than 2000 rare and common conditions (NIH, 2020c). There are different types of genetic tests, including (1) diagnostic testing (identifies a genetic condition or disease that is making or in the future will make a person ill), (2) predictive and presymptomatic genetic testing (finds genetic variations that increase a person's chance of developing specific diseases), (3) carrier testing (tells people if they "carry" a genetic change that can cause a disease), and (4) prenatal testing (offered during pregnancy to help identify fetuses that have certain diseases) (NIH, 2020c). These are just a few examples. Diagnostic testing is available for individuals at high risk for developing certain breast and colon cancers (Office of Disease Prevention and Health Promotion [ODPHP], n.d.). Women with a strong family history of breast, ovarian, tubal, or peritoneal cancer may benefit from genetic testing for a *BRCA1* or *BRCA2* mutation (U.S. Preventive Services Task Force, 2019). A positive screen for the *BRCA1* or *BRCA2* genetic mutation indicates the genetic mutation exists in a woman's DNA, placing her at an increased risk for developing one of these cancers. It does not mean that the woman will develop one of these cancers. However, the test results help the woman make informed decisions about her health care and treatment based on scientific data. Knowledge of the presence of a *BRCA1* or *BRCA2* mutation can guide decisions about lifestyle changes, frequency of screening for these cancers, or early preventive therapy such as surgery before cancer develops.

People diagnosed with colon cancer may have an inheritable form of colon cancer called Lynch syndrome (ASCO, 2020). Researchers estimate that 1 in every 300 people carry the gene associated with Lynch syndrome (ASCO, 2020). Because Lynch syndrome is one of the more common hereditary cancer syndromes and because early detection improves survival, genetic screening for this type of colon cancer should be offered to first-degree family members to inform them of the potential risk of developing this cancer. If family members screen positive, more frequent screening for this disease increases the chance of early detection and early treatment to decrease death from this form of colon cancer (ASCO, 2020). Other cancers linked to Lynch syndrome include endometrial, ovarian, small bowel, pancreatic, prostate, urinary tract, liver, kidney, and bile duct cancers. Nurses should provide patient education about recommended cancer screenings related to patients diagnosed with Lynch syndrome (Novinson et al., 2019).

REFLECT NOW

If you had a close relative diagnosed with Lynch syndrome, would you want to have genetic testing? What are the reasons you would want to be tested, and what would prevent you from going for the testing?

Genetic information is also being used to guide care for various chronic diseases, including several types of cancer. Health care providers use testing information to select medications to treat cancer based on how well the medications treated groups of patients with the same cancer type. For some cancers (e.g., lung, colon, melanoma, breast, ovarian), medication choice is often based on the genetic features of a patient's cancer cells (Cleveland Clinic, 2017). Application of knowledge of how genetics impacts people with diseases such as cancer, diabetes mellitus, hypertension, and cardiac disease will continue to be the future focus of research and disease treatment.

Environmental Factors

Unhealthy environments are the cause of more than 12 million deaths worldwide (ODPHP, n.d.). Ongoing exposure to toxic elements within the environment increases the risk for chronic disease such as respiratory diseases, heart disease, and some kinds of cancer (ODPHP, n.d.). Environmental exposure causes long-term health effects, which are associated with significant costs. For example, in the United States, the cost of childhood exposure to lead is estimated at $84 billion per year based on reduced productivity, increased needs for health care and social assistance, and premature mortality associated with lead poisoning (Altarum, 2019). Recognize that cost estimates of any environmental disease in children are probably low because it is difficult to determine the long-term societal losses for children who have cognitive impairment such as IQ loss (Grandjean and Bellanger, 2017).

Researchers are finding that environmental factors ranging from everyday stress to exposure to various chemical agents may alter an individual's DNA. The interaction of environmental toxins and genetic predisposition is probably stronger than genetic risk alone. Public health initiatives focus on recognizing individuals' risks, chemical assessment of toxins, exposure reduction and remediation, monitoring, and avoidance. As a nurse, your role in reducing environmental exposure to toxins involves risk assessment and patient education. Patients are exposed to environmental toxins, such as contaminated water, pesticides, asbestos, mold, heavy metals, and food contamination at home and in the workplace. By identifying exposures and informing individual patients regarding where and how they are being contaminated, you can empower patients to avoid further chemical contamination or to participate in appropriate health promotion activities (Yelton et al., 2020).

Lifestyle and Risk Factors

Many risk factors increase the chance that individuals, families, or communities will develop a chronic illness. Some risk factors are modifiable while others are nonmodifiable (see Chapter 6). The most common modifiable risk factors are lifestyle choices or **risk behaviors** that contribute to the development of chronic illness (e.g., smoking cigarettes, exposure to secondhand smoke, poor nutrition, and excessive alcohol consumption) (CDC, 2021a). Lack of physical activity and obesity are associated with heart disease, obesity, diabetes mellitus, and some cancers (CDC, 2020b). It is estimated that $117 billion in health care costs are spent yearly due to people who choose a sedentary lifestyle (USDHHS, 2015). Chapter 38 discusses current recommendations for daily physical activity for adults.

Tobacco Use. Cigarette smoking or extended exposure to secondhand smoke is the leading cause of preventable death in the United States (USDHHS, 2020). Sixteen different types of cancer have been linked to tobacco use, including lung, mouth and throat, bladder, stomach, and liver (Cancer Council, 2020). Smoking is also linked to pulmonary and cardiovascular disease. Although teens are less likely to smoke cigarettes, the use of electronic cigarettes, or e-cigarettes, is on the rise in both middle and high school teens (CDC, 2020c; see Chapter 12). E-cigarettes contain nicotine and other chemicals that negatively affect a person's health (CDC 2020c). If young people did not start smoking and every smoker stopped smoking, it is estimated that $170 billion could be saved yearly in medical costs (USDHHS, 2020).

Effects of Alcohol. The effects of alcohol on health are directly associated with the pattern, type, and amount of alcohol consumed (WHO, 2021a). Alcohol misuse puts people at increased risk for negative health and social effects. Excessive alcohol use is associated with 1 in 10 deaths in working adults and costs approximately $249 billion yearly in the United States when taking lost productivity, health care expenses, law enforcement, and other costs associated with the criminal justice system into consideration (USDHHS, 2016). Excess consumption of alcohol over a long period of time leads to an increase in chronic disease, including heart disease, liver disease, and several types of cancer.

Nutrition. The rates of chronic diet-related diseases have risen, due in part to changes in lifestyle behaviors. A history of poor eating and physical activity patterns have a cumulative effect and contribute to significant nutrition-related and physical activity–related health challenges that now face the U.S. population (health.gov, 2015). The CDC reports that about half of all adults in the United States have one or more preventable chronic diseases, many of which are related to physical inactivity and eating patterns of poor quality. These diseases include cardiovascular disease, high blood pressure, type 2 diabetes mellitus, certain cancers, and poor bone health (health.gov, 2015). Poor nutritional intake is related to a variety of issues, including limited financial resources, poor access to markets selling high-quality foods, limited transportation, and limited understanding of the components of a healthy diet (see Chapter 45). More than two-thirds of adults and nearly one-third of children and youth are overweight or obese, which highlights the enormous scale of this public health problem (health.gov, 2015). The educational strategies that you can apply to reduce the health risks from poor nutrition are outlined in Table 8.3.

Physical Effects of Chronic Illness

The physical effects and limitations of chronic illness vary greatly, depending on the disease process and treatments required. Determining patients' individual physical needs and providing patient-centered care are essential. For example, a person who is a cancer survivor may have residual side effects from chemotherapy and radiation treatments such as peripheral neuropathy (Knoerl et al., 2018), cardiac or pulmonary toxicity (Kourie and Klastersky, 2017), or cognitive impairment, called chemo brain, which may last for years (American Cancer Society, 2021a). A person who has emphysema may depend on oxygen and have chronic physical changes such as clubbed fingers or a barrel chest. Other common physical symptoms include malnutrition because of difficulty in chewing and digesting food and decreased physical mobility due to poor oxygen reserve (Mete et al., 2018).

One person living with heart failure may need to take two medications every day and eat a no-added-salt diet. Another person with heart failure may be dependent on oxygen and confined to home, take continuous intravenous (IV) medications to increase the heart's ability to

TABLE 8.3	Strategies for Chronic Disease Prevention
Disease	**Strategy**
Obesity	Increasing physical activity, plus reducing intake of foods high in fat and foods and drinks high in sugars, can prevent unhealthy weight gain.
Type 2 diabetes mellitus	Increasing physical activity and maintaining a healthy weight play critical roles in the prevention and treatment of diabetes mellitus.
Cardiovascular disease	Reduced intake of saturated and trans fats; sufficient amounts of (omega-3 and omega-6) polyunsaturated fats, fruits, and vegetables; reduced salt intake; physical activity; and controlling weight can reduce the risk of cardiovascular disease.
Cancer	Maintaining a healthy weight will reduce the risk for cancers of the esophagus, colorectum, breast, endometrium, and kidney. Limiting alcohol intake will reduce the risk for cancers of the mouth, throat, esophagus, liver, and breast. Ensuring an adequate intake of fruits and vegetables should further reduce the risk for oral cavity, esophagus, stomach, and colorectal cancers.
Osteoporosis and bone fractures	An adequate intake of calcium (500 mg/day or more) and vitamin D in populations with high osteoporosis rates helps to reduce fracture risk. Sun exposure and physical activity to strengthen bones and muscles also help to reduce the risk.
Dental disease	Limiting the frequency and amount of sugar consumption and increasing the use of fluoride can prevent tooth decay.

Adapted from World Health Organization: *Diet, nutrition and the prevention of chronic diseases: report of the joint WHO/FAO expert consultation.* WHO Technical Report Series, No. 916 (TRS 916), https://www.who.int/dietphysicalactivity/publications/trs916/summary/en/, 2021. Accessed February 24, 2021.

pump, take eight oral medications per day, and eat a 1-gram sodium diet due to the severity of heart disease. Although these two persons have the same diagnosis, great variations exist regarding their self-care needs.

Psychosocial Needs of Patients with Chronic Illness

A patient's experience with chronic illness encompasses more than the physical symptoms that result from the effects of the illness on different body systems. The emotional response to living with chronic illness varies even more than a patient's physical response. Emotional responses affect how a person perceives and copes with an illness, as well as the person's perceived degree of wellness.

Chronic illness has economic, functional, occupational, psychological, sexual, social, and spiritual effects on patients and families (Chang and Johnson, 2018). Each person with a chronic disease has a unique illness representation (Heid et al., 2018). For example, a woman who feels a lump in her breast might immediately think she has breast cancer. This thought might then stimulate further thoughts of suffering, long-term treatment, and an uncertain outcome, which ultimately results in anxiety and fear. Illness representations are the responses to bodily and functional changes that occur due to an illness that affect a patient's ability to self-manage an illness (Leventhal et al., 2016). To make the clinical decisions needed for patient-centered care, you must learn how to critically assess each patient's unique experience with a chronic illness. This information will then allow you to apply critical thinking and clinical judgment in the way you plan and deliver patient-centered care.

Psychosocial nursing care for patients with chronic illnesses is very complex and involves many aspects of a patient's life. Patients often have physical and mental illnesses at the same time. Medications used to treat physical illnesses can affect a patient's mental health. Likewise, medications used to treat mental illnesses affect a patient's physical health (Parrish, 2018).

Your role in helping patients manage and cope with the psychosocial effects of a chronic illness depends in part on your patients' feelings, relationships with others, and ability to access resources. It is essential to develop a therapeutic relationship with patients to help them manage and discuss their feelings about their chronic illnesses.

Depression. Patients who live with chronic illness often experience depression related to frustration, fear about the future, and loss of control over one's life (Lorig et al., 2020). Patients living with chronic illnesses are at a higher risk of experiencing depression when compared with people who are healthy (Parrish, 2018). Patients who experience depression with chronic illness also often express higher levels of pain, fatigue, and social isolation and withdraw from daily activities, which can impact the entire family (Corvin et al., 2017; Parrish, 2018). Depression associated with a chronic illness can be difficult to manage, and it can negatively affect a patient's ability to adhere to a treatment plan (Corvin et al., 2017).

Social Isolation. Social isolation often occurs as an illness or disability becomes more advanced or severe. A study found that people who lack social connection experience health risks that are similar to people who have an alcohol abuse disorder or who smoke 15 cigarettes a day. In addition, the study found that loneliness and social isolation are twice as harmful to physical and mental health as obesity (Holt-Lunstad, et al., 2015). Some people begin to withdraw as their illnesses become more difficult to manage, have a greater impact on their ability to function, or include symptoms a patient considers to be embarrassing. Managing the symptoms of a chronic illness sometimes becomes so overwhelming that the individual chooses to reduce social interactions with others. For some, it is easier to stay at home, where the environment is more controllable (Meiner and Yeager, 2019). The COVID-19 pandemic offered an example to the world's population of what it is like to become socially isolated over an extended period.

For others, friends and family may withdraw from the individual experiencing chronic illness. Friends sometimes become tired of hearing about a patient's chronic illness experience. Physical and psychosocial limitations created by an illness can make friends and family uncomfortable. Some illnesses (e.g., HIV/AIDS, hepatitis) carry a stigma with them, which often leads to social isolation. Regardless of the cause for social isolation, it is essential to carefully assess patients for social isolation and loneliness and to ensure that their needs for intimacy are met (Meiner and Yeager, 2019; Garcia-Sanjuan et al., 2018).

Loneliness. Although it is natural to feel lonely from time to time, people who regularly feel lonely face significant health risks. Recent U.S. census data show that more than a quarter of the population lives alone—the highest rate ever recorded (Novotny, 2019). In addition, more than half of the population is unmarried, and marriage rates and the number of children per household have declined since the previous census (Novotny, 2019). Couple loneliness with chronic disease and the effects can be disastrous.

In the case of patients with chronic diseases, their beliefs about the benefits of treatment often are related to the degree of loneliness they are experiencing. People who believe in the treatment and its benefits report less loneliness than those who question the benefits of the treatment (Tuncay et al., 2018).

For example, consider you are caring for two different 75-year-old women living with heart failure. One lives alone in a rural area and has limited interaction with her family and friends; the other is married, has a dog, and lives in a neighborhood where she brought up her family and is closely connected with her friends. The woman who lives alone frequently feels lonely. She reports difficulty managing her low-sodium diet and does not believe that the medications for her heart failure are effectively managing her illness. She states she cannot walk or exercise because it is not safe for her to be outside by herself. She copes with her loneliness by eating foods that are high in salt and fat, and she blames herself for her health problems. The woman who is married expresses that she is close to her family and has many good friends. She meets up with other women in the neighborhood to walk her dog at least three to four times a week. She has no difficulty in adhering to her treatment plan, and she has a positive outlook on her future.

People with chronic illness use a variety of personal strengths and strategies to cope with the psychosocial effects of chronic illness (Kristjansdottir, 2018). Internal strengths include being persistent; having a positive outlook; being kind and caring; experiencing positive emotions; being kind toward oneself; reconciling oneself with the situation; and having courage, knowledge, and insight. External strengths include support from family, friends, peers, and health care providers. Self-management strategies include being active, planning and prioritizing, reducing stress, goal setting, and seeking knowledge and help. Encourage patients dealing with chronic illnesses by guiding them to consider personal strengths that can be used to help them cope with the effects of the illness and its related treatment. Help them to find regular activities to participate in that they enjoy (e.g., going to estate sales, volunteering at a local soup kitchen). If your patients live in remote areas, help them to identify other ways to stay connected with others, such as using webcams or other online technology to regularly communicate with others, or scheduling regular times for family and friends to visit them.

QSEN **Building Competency in Patient-Centered Care** Mrs. Jones is a 63-year-old woman who was recently diagnosed with type 2 diabetes mellitus. You are making a home visit to check her progress with the disease. The health record shows that Mrs. Jones is to take an oral hypoglycemic tablet twice a day; eat a low carbohydrate, calorie-controlled diet; exercise daily; and check her blood glucose twice a day using a home glucose monitor. You ask Mrs. Jones, "How are you doing?" She responds, "I am so scared and angry. I hate to even say the word 'diabetes'! I can't go out for lunch with my friends anymore. My neighbor has diabetes and just lost both of her legs. I just can't do all of this! What is going to happen to me?" What is the priority issue with Mrs. Jones? What do you plan to discuss with her first?

Answers to QSEN Activities can be found on the Evolve website.

Growth and Development Considerations

Patients who become chronically ill as children often experience depression and anxiety in adulthood (Secinti et al., 2017). Because the risk for mental health problems in children with chronic illnesses may persist into adulthood, your initial assessment for these issues is critical. Your findings will then guide you in making the clinical judgments needed to address mental health needs as part of a child's chronic illness treatment plan.

Serious chronic illnesses in children often have a negative effect on school attendance as well as their social engagement with other children, thus putting children with chronic illnesses at greater risk for failing to reach their potential at school (Lum et al., 2017). Some children with chronic illnesses experience poorer relationships with their teachers and are at a higher risk of having to repeat grades and achieving lower levels of educational success (Lum et al., 2017). The siblings of these children often have similar experiences, missing more days of school and experiencing changes in their interactions with their peers and teachers (Gan et al., 2017). Chronic illness also greatly affects children's parents, creating intense psychosocial responses, including chronic sorrow, fatigue, and depression (Coughlin and Sethares, 2017). Ensure that you take a family-centered approach when caring for children and their families affected by chronic illness (see Chapter 10). Be empathetic and compassionate while providing family-centered care. Help children and their families understand that the emotions they are experiencing because of the chronic illness are normal (Coughlin and Sethares, 2017). Involving interprofessional teams helps to ensure that the holistic needs of children and their families affected by chronic illnesses are met (Apple, 2017).

When caring for older adults with chronic illness, the focus of care is often on controlling symptoms, maintaining comfort, and preventing crisis (Meiner and Yeager, 2019). Every older adult patient is unique, and the presence of one or more chronic illnesses creates the need for an individualized assessment and critical clinical judgment to plan and implement patient-centered care. Older adults who have chronic illnesses often experience powerlessness and depression because of changes in their body image, changes in their ability to provide self-care, or feelings of loss associated with their illness (Meiner and Yeager, 2019). Having more chronic illnesses is often associated with having more functional limitations and more depressive symptoms (Han, 2018). Older adults who have a negative self-perception of aging often experience more depressive symptoms related to chronic illnesses than those with a positive view of aging (Han, 2018).

Thus, you need to assess an older adult patient with chronic illness for depressive symptoms in addition to the patient's perception of aging to provide a foundation for discussing possible coping strategies (Han, 2018). Using your clinical judgment to develop and implement interventions that maximize your patient's functional ability may also improve coping. Consult as needed with members of the interprofessional health care team, such as physical and occupational therapists, to increase a patient's abilities and decrease functional limitations.

FAMILY CAREGIVERS

Advances in disease management have led to more people living longer with chronic illness. As a result, more than 1 in 6 Americans who work either full-time or part-time are providing care for family members or friends with chronic illnesses or disabilities (Family Caregiver Alliance, 2016a). Family caregivers must learn how to perform new tasks and assume new responsibilities that are often time consuming as well as emotionally, psychosocially, economically, and physically draining.

Individuals who assume the role of family caregiver are at risk for caregiver burden. Family caregivers provide a significant amount of direct and indirect patient care for their family members; as a result, they often fail to address their own personal and health-related concerns (Family Caregiver Alliance, 2016b). They also often receive little help from others, which can lead to anxiety and increased caregiver burden (Moss et al., 2019). Family caregivers report that their personal health worsens over time. Spouses report the largest impact on their health (Family Caregiver Alliance, 2016b). Despite these findings there

have also been population-based studies showing that many caregivers do not report high levels of strain, cope successfully with caregiving, report many psychological benefits from caregiving, and may even experience improved health and reduced mortality because of their caregiving experience (APA, 2015).

Factors that put family caregivers at greatest risk for poor health outcomes include providing care for more than a year, being 65 years of age or older, providing care for a family member who has significant needs, having insufficient resources (knowledge, skills, social support, respite, and community services), caring for someone with Alzheimer disease or other form of dementia, and living with the care recipient (Family Caregiver Alliance, 2016b; APA, 2015).

Because chronic illnesses last a long time and their course is often unknown, the uncertainty related to the illness contributes to the stress of the family caregiver. The experience of the family caregiver is related to the characteristics of the chronic illness (Meiner and Yeager, 2019). For example, a family caregiver may report stress when a patient with cognitive changes no longer recognizes family members. Another family caregiver may experience more difficulty coping and managing caregiving when a patient with cancer experiences a relapse and requires more intense care. Ongoing care of a family member with a chronic illness is physically and emotionally draining. When a family caregiver is the spouse of the patient, the marital relationship may be greatly affected.

Caring for the family caregiver is essential (see Chapters 7 and 10). You must assess the level of a family caregiver's health and caregiving responsibilities. Developing a therapeutic relationship with your patients' family caregivers will enable you to learn more details about their caregiving experiences. Assess the physical, psychosocial, and financial effects of the chronic illness on the patient and family caregiver, and ensure that both members of the caregiving dyad have access to appropriate community resources and services, including respite care, social work, and counseling. Provide patient education when needed (see Chapter 25) and include the patient and family caregiver as a part of the interprofessional health care team (Ates et al., 2018).

THE CHRONIC CARE MODEL

The **Chronic Care Model** provides a framework to guide health care delivery for patients living with chronic illnesses. This model considers the complex nature of factors that affect the care delivery needs of persons with a chronic illness. The Chronic Care Model (Fig. 8.2) illustrates how the community and health care systems interact to influence patient outcomes. The community component focuses on the availability of resources and policies that have the potential to impact health. An effective method to improve preventive health practices includes public policy changes. Examples of these measures include smoke-free legislation, alcohol taxation, or regulations eliminating trans fats in prepared food (Capewell and Capewell, 2018). These policy changes have great potential to enhance preventive health measures and decrease high-risk behaviors associated with the **incidence** (or new cases) of chronic disease. You need to be aware of this type of legislation, which focuses on decreasing exposure to health barriers through public policies and legislative changes.

The health care systems component focuses on how providers can best utilize the resources within their system and provide evidence-based care to improve patient outcomes. Using the chronic care model can improve coordination of planned interprofessional care, improve patient follow-up, and educate patients and families on how to manage patient illnesses. The six essential elements of the Chronic Care Model include (2006-2021 Improving Chronic Illness Care, n.d.):

1. *Community:* Help develop partnerships to enhance the effectiveness of chronic disease management programs. Community partnerships

The Chronic Care Model

Improved Outcomes

FIG. 8.2 The Chronic Care Model. (© 1996-2018 The MacColl Center. The Improving Chronic Illness Care program is supported by The Robert Wood Johnson Foundation, with direction and technical assistance provided by Group Health's MacColl Center for Health Care Innovation. http://www.improvingchroniccare.org/index.php?p=The_Chronic_Care_Model&s=2. Accessed February 25, 2021.)

between health systems and local, state, and national agencies help fill in the gaps that exist in different services and improve patient care.

2. *Self-management support:* Places the patient in the center of disease management. Self-management support requires providers to collaborate with patients, which ultimately empowers patients to take responsibility for and manage their chronic diseases.
3. *Health system:* Needs to constantly attempt to improve the management of chronic illnesses and focus on safety and quality of care.
4. *Delivery system design:* Uses evidence-based care that is patient-centered, preventive in nature, and occurs in a variety of acute, outpatient, and community settings.
5. *Decision support:* Used by health care providers to implement evidence-based guidelines, guide patient education, and encourage patients to participate in their care.
6. *Clinical information systems:* Maintain and share patient health information among providers and patients to ensure effective communication and quality patient care.

Research supports the use of the Chronic Care Model in primary care settings. Llewellyn (2019) reported that barriers and facilitators in implementing this model to manage the primary care of patients with chronic kidney disease focused on readiness and climate of the organization. The focus was on the need for system redesign; the use of volunteers; the health care team's knowledge about evidence-based guidelines in the screening and disease management of patients; attitudes of the health care providers, including confidence in the treatments provided; and economic restrictions. When organizations were able to redesign their systems, the programs employed regular staff and did not rely on volunteers to provide regular care, health care team members were knowledgeable and supportive, and the programs were appropriately funded, implementation of the Chronic Care Model in primary care was successful. Reynolds et al. (2018) identified the primary care chronic disease management interventions most successful in creating positive patient outcomes and disease control. In their systematic review, almost half of the studies demonstrated that *self-management support* was the most effective element from the

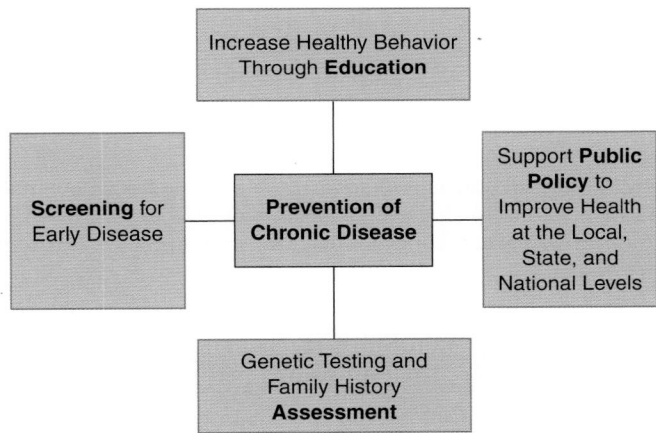

FIG. 8.3 The nurse's role in chronic disease prevention.

model for improving patient outcomes, such as better control of type 2 diabetes mellitus or improved quality of life in patients with arthritis or chronic obstructive pulmonary disease (COPD).

IMPLICATIONS FOR NURSING

The excess illness burden of chronic disease and billions of health care dollars could be saved each year if chronic diseases were prevented (CDC, 2020a). Nursing care of patients experiencing chronic illnesses is complex. It is important to promote healthy lifestyles and detect risks for chronic illness early (Fig. 8.3). You first need to thoroughly assess patients, analyze your findings, and form the clinical judgments needed to identify relevant problems and plan appropriate care. This applies to all patients who are at risk for chronic disease or who are diagnosed with a chronic disease. Helping patients and their family caregivers develop a plan to manage their illness, as well as providing patient education, is essential.

Assessing Patients With Chronic Illnesses

It is important to assess the effect a chronic disease has on your patients. When you collect a nursing history (see Chapters 16 and 30), encourage patients to tell you their stories about their chronic disease and how it affects various aspects of their lives (Tamura-Lis, 2017). The stories your patients tell will provide contextual detail and allow you to better know your patients. As you explore a patient's medical history and treatment, ask open-ended questions such as, "How did that come about?" as opposed to closed-ended questions that require a simple yes or no response (Table 8.4). Let the patient take you on a journey explaining their condition. You might ask, "Tell me how your disease most affects you right now" or "What are the biggest problems you are having now?" Your knowledge of the physical effects of chronic disease coupled with your assessment of a patient's own experience provides data needed for concise problem and nursing diagnosis identification (see Chapter 16). Encourage your patient to tell you stories that also help you better understand the psychosocial aspects of their illness. Be respectful and caring in your approach to encourage open patient communication (Tamura-Lis, 2017).

Adherence. When patients are unable to adhere to a treatment plan, they often experience increased hospital admissions, poor health outcomes, and increased morbidity and mortality. Nonadherence also greatly increases health care expenses. Current estimates of the annual direct health care costs associated with nonadherence to medications range from $100 billion to $300 billion in the United States (Neiman et al., 2017). Improving adherence is a nursing priority and requires an interprofessional approach (Giddens, 2022; Neiman et al., 2017) (Box 8.1).

Wide variation exists from patient to patient regarding adherence to chronic disease management and the effects of treatment on their lives. Adherence depends on the number and type of chronic illnesses, the severity and duration of the chronic illness, and the complexity of a treatment plan. Patients will have different physical symptoms and different pharmacological and nonpharmacological treatments, all of which affect a patient's ability to adhere to a treatment plan. How well a patient with a chronic illness and/or family manages a treatment plan is complex.

Assess adherence by asking patients about how they take medications regularly, follow diet plans, or perform routine exercise. Ask patients to keep diaries and then later check their entries to validate adherence. Having patients create examples of menu plans is another way to determine whether a patient knows how to plan a healthy meal. Family caregivers can also be very helpful in reporting adherence.

Motivational interviewing is a counseling and educational technique that focuses on patient goals and helps people resolve insecurities and ambivalent feelings (e.g., nonadherence) to find the internal motivation

---

TABLE 8.4 Examples of Assessment Questions for Patients Experiencing Chronic Illness

Category	Examples of Questions
Symptoms	Tell me about the symptoms you are experiencing from your illness and its treatment.
	Describe any pain or discomfort you are experiencing.
	Sometimes people with chronic illnesses experience changes in their sleep, appetite, or ability to cope. Describe any changes like these that you are experiencing.
	Tell me about any problems you are having following your treatment plan at home.
Psychosocial problems	How do your family members respond to you now that you have a chronic illness?
	What family members' responses to your chronic illness concern you?
	How has your illness affected the way you see yourself?
	If you have experienced sexual changes because of your illness, which strategies have you tried to make things better? Have these strategies worked?
	Describe any problems you have affording the care your health care provider has prescribed for you.

BOX 8.1 EVIDENCE-BASED PRACTICE

Strategies to Enhance Adherence

PICOT Question: Do interprofessional interventions promote adherence to treatment plans in patients experiencing chronic illness?

Evidence Summary

Chronic diseases require patients and families to make multiple important decisions about their health daily. However, the American health care system does a poor job in supporting self-management of diseases. Patients and providers often express frustration with the approach to chronic disease management, especially due to the many barriers that people who are from underserved populations experience (Lin et al., 2020).

Current evidence supports the use of interprofessional interventions to enhance adherence to chronic disease management. For example, health care coaches with advanced training in behavioral science who maintain ongoing positive patient relationships have been effective in improving adherence in patients with asthma and COPD (George, 2018). The Patient-Care Medical Home (PCMH) is a patient-care delivery model in which a primary care provider facilitates and coordinates interprofessional patient care to assure that patients receive culturally appropriate care when and where they need it. Although patients living with chronic illnesses who use a PCMH recognized by the National Committee for Quality Assurance (NCQA) frequently experience better treatment of their chronic diseases, limited access to care results in reduced patient outcomes in patients from racial minorities (Swietek et al., 2020). In addition to interprofessional care, a patient's social support from family, friends, and peers is an essential component to patient adherence (Arney et al., 2020).

Application to Nursing Practice

- Carefully assess patients who have difficulty adhering to their treatment plan to determine the factors that are preventing them from being successful. For example, ask: "What financial barriers, if any, are interfering with your ability to manage your disease?" "How many medications do you take on a daily basis and when do you take them?" "Describe the role your family plays in helping you manage your illness" (George, 2018; Arney et al., 2020).
- Assess patients' understanding of their chronic diseases and their motivation and ability to change behavior, and provide targeted patient education to help them better manage their chronic illnesses and adhere to their medications (Yazdanpanah et al., 2019).
- Work with the interprofessional health care team across the continuum of care to enhance adherence to chronic disease treatment. For example, providing outpatient clinic visits that include health education; empowering patients to address their medical, physical, emotional, and social challenges; and using face-to-face small group sessions led by peers may be helpful in helping patients adhere to their treatment plans. Exploring incentives to encourage participation, such as free transportation and raffle prizes, may provide motivation for patients experiencing issues surrounding the social determinants of health (Lin et al., 2020).

needed to change their behavior (Psychology Today, 2021) (Chapter 25). Use this approach as a guide, clarifying the patient's strengths and goals, listening to their concerns, boosting their confidence in their ability to change, and eventually collaborating with them on a plan for behavioral change (Souders, 2021).

Some assessment tools measure adherence. A standardized self-reported questionnaire called the Adherence in Chronic Diseases Scale (ACDS) assesses the level of adherence to treatment recommendations in chronically ill adults (Kosobucka et al., 2018). The tool was originally developed and validated in patients with coronary artery disease (CAD) (Kubica et al., 2017). The ACDS includes seven questions that focus primarily on how well a patient manages the medication regimen.

Symptom Management. Symptom management is an ongoing problem for many patients with chronic diseases. Reflect on your knowledge of a chronic disease and previous clinical experiences to explore a patient's presenting symptoms as you conduct a physical examination (see Chapter 30). Ask patients to describe the symptoms that are affecting them the most. For example, if a patient is experiencing pain from peripheral neuropathy from cancer treatment, ask whether the pain is affecting the patient's ability to sleep, and assess the patient's gait and sensation. Explore each symptom that patients identify to gain a complete picture of their health status. Some patients are reluctant to describe or report their symptoms. Be patient, and when you identify a symptom, explore the extent to which it is currently affecting the patient.

Your review of the patient's medical record reveals the type and nature of chronic illness affecting a patient. Focus your physical assessment on the body systems most likely affected to supplement what you learn about symptoms. For example, if a patient states having difficulty breathing, which affects the ability to perform self-care, examine the thorax, assessing lung sounds and degree of excursion.

Tobacco Use. Assess patients to determine their use of tobacco products, including e-cigarettes. Determine the number of times a patient smokes daily and how long the patient has been smoking. Also assess whether the patient lives in an environment where there is secondhand smoke. Your assessment includes the patient's knowledge level about the risks of smoking and the benefits of quitting, and whether the patient has a willingness to stop smoking.

REFLECT NOW

Go to the World Health Organization website and review global policy suggestions to decrease the use of tobacco (https://www.who.int/health-topics/tobacco). How could you use these guidelines when educating a patient about smoking cessation?

Alcohol Consumption. Assess the amount of alcohol patients drink on a typical day and in a typical week. Suspect alcohol misuse if a patient reports excess daily alcohol consumption (more than four drinks for men or more than three drinks a day for women) or excess total alcohol consumption (more than 14 drinks a week for men and more than seven drinks a week for women) (CDC, 2020d). Often patients are reluctant to report the amount of alcohol they drink. The Alcohol Use Disorders Identification Test (AUDIT) is a 10-item screening tool developed by the World Health Organization (WHO) to assess alcohol consumption, drinking behaviors, and alcohol-related problems (Babor et al., 2019). The tool has been tested for its success in identifying patients with drinking problems. Both a clinician-administered version and a self-report version of the AUDIT are available.

Lifestyle. Chronic diseases affect all aspects of a patient's life. Be sure to explore patients' psychological, social, spiritual (see Chapter 35), and sexual (see Chapter 34) needs. If you are unable to identify all your patient's needs on initial assessment, incorporate more detailed assessment questions as you establish rapport and continue to provide care to your patient. Learning how a patient manages care at home is one of the most useful ways to know how an illness affects lifestyle routines. Talk about your patient's daily life and determine the extent to which the chronic illness has affected the patient's ability to perform self-care activities, attend social activities, participate in meals, and obtain adequate sleep. Observe the patient's interactions with family members and friends.

HEALTH PROMOTION AND DISEASE PREVENTION

As a nurse, you need to be actively engaged in health promotion and disease prevention (see Chapter 6). Your approach to patient education will be influenced by a patient's motivation, readiness, and ability to learn, and by the environment where learning will take place (see Chapter 25). Patient education provides information patients require to understand the effects of their lifestyle behaviors on their health, make positive behavioral changes, and lead a healthy lifestyle. Even when patients are diagnosed with a chronic illness, health promotion is important. Understand the nature of a patient's illness as well as the short- and long-term effects of the treatment to guide the topics you choose to teach and the screening interventions you use.

Apply critical thinking in your approach to education. Reflect on standards such as specific evidence-based recommendations that focus on topics such as daily recommended physical activity (see Chapter 38), diet and food choices (see Chapter 45), smoking, and alcohol intake to help patients understand how to prevent the development of chronic disease. Use resources such as the World Health Organization's Global Action Plan for the Prevention and Control of Chronic Noncommunicable Diseases 2013-2030 (WHO, 2020) to help you better understand how people can have healthier lives and to guide your interventions (Fig. 8.4).

Use physical activity guidelines for adults, children, and older adults to provide clear activity goals for all age-groups (ODPHP, 2018; USDHHS, 2018; see Chapter 38). Discuss the importance of both the intensity and frequency of exercise. Encourage patients of all age-groups to engage in at least 150 minutes (2 hours and 30 minutes) to 300 minutes (5 hours) a week of moderate-intensity, or 75 minutes (1 hour and 15 minutes) to 150 minutes (2 hours and 30 minutes) a week of vigorous-intensity aerobic physical activity, or an equivalent combination of moderate- and vigorous-intensity aerobic activity. For patients with chronic disease these goals may be difficult to attain. The USDHHS (2018) recommends that older adults with chronic conditions should consult with their health care providers to understand whether and how their conditions affect their ability to do regular physical activity safely. When older adults cannot do 150 minutes of moderate-intensity aerobic activity a week because of chronic conditions, they should be as physically active as their abilities and conditions allow. People with chronic diseases need to participate in the same amount of activity and muscle-strengthening as healthy people whenever possible (ODPHP, 2018).

Along with routine exercise, help patients make dietary choices that include an intake of appropriate nutrients to promote health and prevent obesity (see Chapter 45). Healthy food choices, which include a variety of fruits and vegetables, grains, fat-free or low-fat dairy, protein,

FIG. 8.4 World Health Organization recommendations to prevent chronic noncommunicable illnesses. (Data from https://www.who.int/ncds/prevention/en/.) Accessed February 25, 2021.)

and oils in an appropriate calorie level, provide balanced nutritional intake (ODPHP, 2020). Controlling sugar, sodium, fat, and alcohol intake assists in weight control. Refer to evidence-based nutritional guidelines, such as the *Dietary Guidelines for Americans*, available at https://health.gov/our-work/food-nutrition, to help guide patient education.

Educate patients about the risks related to using any type of tobacco or smoking product that contains nicotine because of the potential to cause disease (WHO, 2021b). Provide education about the benefits of smoking cessation and ways to stop smoking to promote health. Refer patients to resources such as the American Lung Association (www.lung.org), which has an online resource for smoking cessation called "Freedom from Smoking." This website provides encouragement and ideas about how to stop smoking, as well as information about why and how to stop.

Refer patients to resources and provide information and support about alcohol use when appropriate. For example, the CDC (2020d) and National Institute on Alcohol Abuse and Alcoholism (NIAAA, n.d.) provide online information on how to calculate alcohol intake and how to stop drinking, as well as available resources if patients have excessive alcohol intake.

Screening for Diseases

There are a variety of methods to detect disease in its earliest form. When diseases are detected early, treatment can begin, and the consequences of the disease can often be modified. Implement simple screening measures in children, such as blood pressure screening and height and weight screening to gather basic health information. Encourage all patients to have their blood pressure taken regularly. A person with hypertension usually has no symptoms (American Heart Association, 2021). Without routine blood pressure screening, a patient could have undiagnosed hypertension and without treatment could end up with heart, renal, or cardiovascular disease. The earlier

high blood pressure is recognized through screening, the earlier treatment can begin, and disease can be prevented.

Use health risk assessment data to encourage your patients to have appropriate screenings for diseases such as breast, colon, cervical, and prostate cancer (see Chapter 30). Routine screening at recommended intervals leads to early detection so that if these cancers exist, early treatment with a good prognosis is possible (American Cancer Society, 2021b). Reinforce the need for your patients to routinely participate in these screening processes.

You can also serve as a resource to provide basic information about genetic screening and its benefits based on family history of chronic disease. Genetic counseling is a specialized area of practice. Refer your patients to reliable sources of information, such as the Genetics Home Reference website, available at https://ghr.nlm.nih.gov/ (NIH, 2020d), and to genetic specialists for expert advice when indicated to ensure that patients receive accurate detailed information about the effect of their genetics on their health.

Patient Education and Chronic Disease Self-Management

Patient education and disease self-management focus on the life changes that a person with a chronic illness must make to live well with an illness (Lorig et al., 2003). Living with chronic illnesses requires patients to implement demanding self-care tasks as they learn about their illnesses, how to manage symptoms and emotions, and how to make lifestyle changes to manage their illnesses. Patients are at increased risk of hospitalization or readmission when they are unable to manage their chronic disease at home. Nurses play an instrumental role in patient education to improve home care. When patients are given the tools to manage their illnesses and incorporate healthy behaviors into their daily lives, they usually experience fewer complications and have improved quality of life (CDC, 2018b).

Use your clinical judgment to identify and provide appropriate and tailored patient education to help patients understand their illnesses and related treatment. Follow patient education principles (see Chapter 25) to help patients understand their treatment, medications, diet, activity, and what symptoms to report to their health care provider. Emphasize the consequences when treatment plans are not followed. Prepare patients to implement required self-care activities and assist them in making appropriate changes in their behavior. Ensure that patients receive essential information, starting from the time you first meet them. Include family caregivers as appropriate. The AHRQ Health Literacy Universal Precautions Toolkit (2020) provides a variety of evidence-based tools you can implement to help simplify patient communication to reduce miscommunication, make the health care system easier to navigate, and support patients in improving their health.

Ensure that your patients and their caregivers understand the information provided to them. Only 12% of adults in the United States have the health literacy skills required to manage the complex needs related to their health (AHRQ, 2020). Use teach-back to ensure that patients understand this information before discharge from an acute care setting, before leaving an outpatient clinic setting, or at the conclusion of home care visits (AHRQ, 2020).

Include the interprofessional health care team when providing patient education. Members of the interprofessional team include nurses, pharmacists, dietitians, and health care providers (Fig. 8.5). Together, the team explains and reinforces the necessary health behavior changes needed to manage a chronic illness.

Promoting Adherence

Although frequently researched, interventions designed to promote adherence are not well understood and often do not create changes that are maintained over time (Neiman et al., 2017; Meiner and Yeager, 2019). Many factors affect adherence, including the severity and duration of the illness, the treatment plan, socioeconomic status, patient characteristics (e.g., motivation; personal beliefs about health, illness, and the treatment plan; health literacy; mental health), and characteristics of the health care delivery system (e.g., relationship with health care providers, accessibility) (George, 2018; Yazdanpanah et al., 2019).

Your initial assessment provides information about how a patient feels about his or her health, the desire and ability to change behavior (when change is needed), and personal goals for improving health. Motivational interviewing is very useful in assessing what motivates patients to change. You can advise and assist patients through patient education (see Chapter 25), coaching, providing reminders about treatments (e.g., text messages for taking medications), helping patients establish routines, simplifying treatment plans, being patient advocates, and shared decision making between patients and health care providers (George, 2018; SMRC, 2021). Ongoing follow-up is especially important when your patients' outcomes center on long-lasting behavior change.

Self-Management Education

Self-management education (SME) programs provide evidence-based interventions to help patients with chronic diseases manage their illness and its related symptoms. The Chronic Disease Self-Management Resource Program (CDSMRP) developed by Kate Lorig is one program that has consistently demonstrated improved patient outcomes for patients and their family caregivers by offering small, highly interactive group workshops that are facilitated by highly trained leaders who have health challenges of their own (SMRC, 2021). Small group participants meet for 2.5 hours once a week for 6 weeks in a variety of community settings, such as churches, libraries, clinics, and hospitals. Workshops provide disease-specific information and include the elements of action planning, decision making, and problem solving. Participants identify personal goals and behavioral changes based on their needs and preferences (SMRC, 2021). Current evidence shows that these programs help patients experience improved overall health and use fewer health care resources (Lorig et al., 2016; Cutler et al., 2018).

Refer patients, especially those who are living with multiple chronic diseases, and their caregivers to CDSMRPs whenever possible. Spend time with patients to motivate and promote positive behavioral changes in addition to providing education about disease management. Place your patients at the center of chronic disease management care to enhance patient decision making and motivate change (Cutler et al., 2018). Providing strategies—such as how to deal with fatigue, pain, isolation, gait training, medication management, and effective communication with family, friends, and health care professionals—helps engage patients in making lifestyle changes for their health (Soderlung, 2018).

Many chronic disease management classes and tools that complement patient information and support provided by CDSMRPs are available (SMRC, 2021). Refer patients to disease-specific websites that offer reliable patient education materials and chronic disease guides to encourage maintaining health through consistent self-management (Table 8.5). Some of the free tools provided on these websites help you and other health care professionals better understand current evidence-based care and treatment, while other tools are specifically for patients. Patient tools include information on each disease and disease-management principles (e.g., when to seek medical attention,

FIG. 8.5 Patients may interact with several members of the health care team. (iStock.com/monkeybusinessimages.)

TABLE 8.5	Selected Websites Related to Chronic Illness Management
Chronic Illness(es)	**Organization and Website**
Heart failure Stroke Hypertension	American Heart Association: www.heart.org National Heart, Lung and Blood Institute: https://www.nhlbi.nih.gov/
Cancer	American Cancer Society: www.cancer.org
Emphysema Asthma Lung cancer	American Lung Association: www.lung.org
Diabetes mellitus	American Diabetes Association: www.diabetes.org

how to monitor blood pressure, and diet information). The American Heart Association's website provides a digital tracking mechanism with reminders for patients on when to monitor their blood pressure and a self-assessment of heart failure symptoms, including warning signs that are indicative of deterioration in health and when to seek medical attention.

Public Policy

Nurses are responsible to protect the public. Thus, as a nurse, you need to be aware and supportive of legislation that focuses on controlling external environmental factors that contribute to chronic disease development. Your professional nursing responsibility is awareness and support of public policy that decreases disease burden. Review publications and websites from reputable organizations, such as the American Cancer Society (2021c), about current policies that promote health. For example, your support of a no-smoking law that prohibits smoking in public spaces, such as restaurants and bars, protects everyone who works and visits these spaces by limiting their exposure to secondhand smoke.

You will encounter many patients living with chronic illnesses. Apply critical thinking and sound clinical judgment to promote health by educating patients about the major risk factors that increase the chance they will develop a chronic illness. Promote health and encourage patients to engage in screenings to detect diseases early to identify potential problems and intervene before permanent damage to health occurs. Helping patients understand how their lifestyle choices affect their health has the potential to decrease the occurrence of chronic illness through exercise, healthy food choices, smoking cessation, controlled alcohol intake, and maintaining a healthy weight. Understanding how chronic illnesses affect your patients and their families will help you develop an appropriate patient-centered plan of care to promote optimal patient outcomes.

KEY POINTS

- A chronic disease is a pathophysiologic condition that lasts more than 1 year, requires ongoing medical care, and often limits a person's usual activities of daily living.
- Preventing diseases through screening and education and managing symptoms of chronic illnesses potentially saves billions of dollars spent annually on health care.
- Each patient has a unique interaction among genetic, environmental, and lifestyle factors that influence the development of chronic illness. This explains why a person who carries genetic material for developing a chronic illness may or may not eventually be diagnosed with the disease.
- Poor nutrition and the use of tobacco or alcohol are factors that increase the risk that an individual, family, or community will develop chronic illnesses.
- Patients with the same chronic illness often have different symptoms that affect the patient's ability to function. For example, patients who survive cancer may experience peripheral neuropathy, cardiac or pulmonary toxicity, and/or cognitive impairment.
- Depression, loneliness, and social isolation may negatively influence a patient's ability to cope with chronic illness.
- Regardless of the age of the patient, chronic illnesses affect the entire family. Chronic illnesses often interfere with school attendance and limit educational success, while older adults often experience depression related to impaired functional limitations.
- Family caregivers provide a significant amount of direct and indirect patient care for their family members; as a result, they often fail to address their own personal and health-related concerns. Thus, family caregivers often experience physical, psychosocial, and financial effects of the chronic illness.

- The Chronic Care Model has six elements that emphasize the importance of self-management and provide a framework to help members of the health care team understand how community resources and health care systems impact patient outcomes.
- Nurses use assessment data, including asking patients to tell their stories about their chronic diseases, to help patients make lifestyle changes and learn how to control their illnesses through disease self-management.
- The detection of risk factors and early screening for chronic illness before a disease begins provide opportunities for early intervention to prevent or delay disease onset.
- Teaching healthy lifestyle behaviors provides an opportunity for the nurse to help people identify needed life changes to prevent disease.
- Effective programs that help patients self-manage their chronic diseases provide disease-specific information and help patients make decisions about their care.
- Helping patients understand how to deal with different symptoms related to a chronic disease and its treatment and how to communicate with family, friends, and health care workers assists patients in making lifestyle changes required by their chronic disease.
- Nurses need to be aware of and support public policy that promotes health.

REFLECTIVE LEARNING

- Consider a patient that you cared for recently in clinical practice. What lifestyle choices did this patient make that affected risk factors for developing a chronic disease? What patient education regarding these lifestyle choices did you or could you provide to improve the patient's health?
- Identify someone you know either through your clinical or personal experience who is a family caregiver. What skills did the family caregiver need to learn? What physical, psychosocial, or financial effects is the family caregiver experiencing related to the caregiving experience?
- Evaluate a recent patient's ability to adhere to the treatment plan to manage a chronic disease. What factors affected the patient's ability to follow the treatment plan? What interventions may have enhanced the patient's adherence?

REVIEW QUESTIONS

1. A health system upgraded its electronic health record across all its practice settings to enhance patient care and communication among health care providers. This is an example of which component of the Chronic Care Model?
   1. Health systems
   2. Decision support
   3. Clinical information systems
   4. Community
2. A nurse is providing education to a patient with type 2 diabetes mellitus. Which characteristics does the nurse include in her teaching to explain why type 2 diabetes mellitus is considered a chronic disease? (Select all that apply.)
   1. Type 2 diabetes mellitus lasts throughout a person's life.
   2. Genetic mutations drive the treatment for type 2 diabetes mellitus.
   3. People with type 2 diabetes mellitus have to modify some of their daily activities.
   4. Type 2 diabetes mellitus occurs in elderly people.
   5. People with type 2 diabetes mellitus require ongoing medical care.

3. Which of the family caregivers listed below will the nurse expect to be most at risk for experiencing poor health outcomes?
   1. A 20-year-old daughter caring for a mother who needs help setting up her medications weekly
   2. The 68-year-old spouse of a patient who is experiencing worsening dementia
   3. A 32-year-old parent of a child who has an ear infection
   4. A married couple who is sharing the caregiving responsibilities for a parent who was recently diagnosed with hypertension and coronary artery disease

4. A school nurse is planning a health fair for children in first, second, and third grades to promote healthy behaviors. The most appropriate health screening for this age-group would be: (Select all that apply.)
   1. Providing information about eating fruits and vegetables
   2. Taking the children's blood pressure
   3. Recording the children's height and weight on a growth chart
   4. Asking the students about their family history of cancer
   5. Teaching the students about the risks of secondhand smoke

5. A nurse is providing health promotion information at a health fair for female patients who are diagnosed with cancer. What information should the nurse include? (Select all that apply.)
   1. Recommending that they avoid drinking alcohol to prevent alcohol misuse
   2. Information from the local health department about smoking-cessation classes
   3. The need to avoid physical activity while receiving cancer treatment to lessen fatigue
   4. Strategies to talk with family and friends about the cancer diagnosis and the side effects from their treatment
   5. How nutritional needs may change based on the diagnosis of cancer and its treatment

6. The nurse is caring for a family where there is a strong family history of breast cancer. One of the family members says, "I am afraid of having genetic testing. If it is positive, I know I have cancer." What is the nurse's best response?
   1. "It will help diagnose the cancer early if you have it."
   2. "If the results are positive, it means you have a higher risk for breast cancer, not that you have cancer."
   3. "If it is going to cause you to worry, don't have the screening done."
   4. "I am sure you will be fine. You are a healthy woman."

7. A patient tells the nurse, "My doctor told me to lose weight, exercise, stop smoking, and eat better. I am not sick at all. Why would he tell me that?" The nurse's best response would be:
   1. "Since I was not there to hear the conversation, I am not exactly sure."
   2. "All of these things are behaviors that are good for you and your family. Why not just give it a try?"

   3. "I believe he is trying to get you to think about ways that you can be healthier. All these things help to prevent future health problems."
   4. "Eating a balanced, healthy diet and exercising regularly will help you lose weight. I know stopping smoking is really hard to do."

8. Two nurses are revising a self-management education program to help patients better manage their asthma. What strategies are most important for them to include in the program? (Select all that apply.)
   1. Have patients list the medications they are prescribed to take and describe any problems they are having with their medications.
   2. Create a common set of patient goals that the patients will work toward as a group.
   3. Look for group leaders who are health care providers who are respected by the community.
   4. Provide information on how to balance activities during the day.
   5. Ask patients to discuss how other people in their family react to them now that they have asthma.

9. During a home visit, a patient states, "I am really upset about my heart failure. I can't go out to eat anymore with my friends, I have no energy, and I don't even want to talk on the phone. All I do is focus on how this disease has changed my life and how much time I have left to live." How should the nurse respond? (Select all that apply.)
   1. "Let's talk about going out to lunch. What is making you hesitant about eating with your friends?"
   2. "Tell me about what types of activities you were doing before you knew you had heart failure."
   3. "Eventually you will get used to all of the changes. You are doing OK."
   4. "My mother has heart failure, and she has adjusted to diet, activity, and medication changes."
   5. "How has your heart failure affected your energy level?"

10. Which nursing activities would help a patient self-manage rheumatoid arthritis? (Select all that apply).
    1. Assess the patient's beliefs about rheumatoid arthritis and its effects on activity levels.
    2. Provide a general overview of the different types of arthritis.
    3. Set long-term goals for the patient.
    4. Refer the patient to a support group that helps people with rheumatoid arthritis manage their disease.
    5. Encourage the patient to wait for 2 months before calling the office to set up a follow-up visit.

Answers: 1. 3; **2.** 1, 3, 5; **3.** 2; **4.** 2, 3; **5.** 2, 4, 5; **6.** 2; **7.** 3; **8.** 1, 4, 5; **9.** 1, 2, 5; **10.** 1, 4.

Rationales for Review Questions can be found on the Evolve website.

REFERENCES

Agency for Healthcare Research and Quality (AHRQ): AHRQ health literacy universal precautions toolkit, ed 2. https://www.ahrq.gov/professionals/quality-patient-safety/quality-resources/tools/literacy-toolkit/index.html, 2020. Accessed February 23, 2021.

Altarum: New online tool calculates the cost and economic benefits of preventing childhood lead exposure in the United States, 2019, https://altarum.org/news/new-online-tool-calculates-cost-and-economic-benefits-preventing-childhood-lead-exposure-united. Accessed February 24, 2021.

Alzheimer's impact movement (AIM): Fact sheet, http://act.alz.org/site/DocServer/2012_Costs_Fact_Sheet_version_2.pdf?docID=7161, 2020. Accessed February 23, 2021.

American Cancer Society: Changes in mood or thinking, https://www.cancer.org/treatment/treatments-and-side-effects/physical-side-effects/changes-in-mood-or-thinking.html, 2021a. Accessed February 23, 2021.

American Cancer Society: Stay healthy, https://www.cancer.org/healthy.html, 2021b. Accessed February 23, 2021.

American Cancer Society: Help pass laws to defeat cancer, https://www.cancer.org/involved/volunteer/advocate.html, 2021c. Accessed February 23, 2021.

American Diabetes Association (ADA): The cost of diabetes, https://www.diabetes.org/resources/statistics/cost-diabetes, 2021. Accessed February 23, 2021.

American Heart Association: Why high blood pressure is a "silent killer," 2021, American Heart Association. https://www.heart.org/en/health-topics/high-blood-pressure/why-high-blood-pressure-is-a-silent-killer. Accessed February 23, 2021.

American Psychological Association (APA): Mental and physical health effects of family caregiving, 2015 https://www.apa.org/pi/about/publications/caregivers/faq/health-effects. Accessed February 23, 2021.

American Society of Clinical Oncology (ASCO): Lynch syndrome, https://www.cancer.net/cancer-types/lynch-syndrome, 2020. Accessed June 30, 2020.

Cancer Council: 16 cancers caused by smoking, https://www.cancercouncil.com.au/blog/there-are-16-cancers-that-can-be-caused-by-smoking/, 2020. Accessed February 23, 2021.

Capewell S, Capewell A: An effectiveness hierarchy of preventive interventions: neglected paradigm or self-evident truth? *J Public Health* 40(2):350, 2018. https://doi.org/10.1093/pubmed/fdx055.

Centers for Disease Control and Prevention (CDC): How type 2 diabetes affects your workforce, https://www.cdc.gov/diabetes/prevention/how-type2-affects-workforce.htm?CDC_AA_refVal=https%3A%2F%2F, 2018a. Accessed February 23, 2021.

Centers for Disease Control and Prevention (CDC): Self-management education: learn more. Feel better, https://www.cdc.gov/learnmorefeelbetter/index.htm, 2018b. Accessed February 23, 2021.

Centers for Disease Control and Prevention (CDC): The cost of arthritis in US adults, https://www.cdc.gov/arthritis/data_statistics/cost.htm, 2020a. Accessed February 23, 2021.

Centers for Disease Control and Prevention (CDC): Overweight and obesity, https://www.cdc.gov/obesity/index.html, 2020b. Accessed February 23, 2021.

Centers for Disease Control and Prevention (CDC): Quick facts on the risks of e-cigarettes for kids, teens, and young adults, https://www.cdc.gov/tobacco/basic_information/e-cigarettes/Quick-Facts-on-the-Risks-of-E-cigarettes-for-Kids-Teens-and-Young-Adults.html, 2020c. Accessed February 23, 2021.

Centers for Disease Control and Prevention (CDC): Alcohol and public health, https://www.cdc.gov/alcohol/index.htm, 2020d. Accessed February 23, 2021.

Centers for Disease Control and Prevention (CDC): National center for chronic disease prevention and health promotion: about chronic diseases, http://www.cdc.gov/chronicdisease/about/index.htm, 2021a. Accessed February 23, 2021.

Centers for Disease Control and Prevention (CDC): Health and economic costs of chronic diseases, https://www.cdc.gov/chronicdisease/about/costs/index.htm, 2021b. Accessed February 23, 2021.

Chang E, Johnson A: *Living with chronic illness and disability: principles for nursing practice*, ed 3, Chatswood, NSW, 2018, Elsevier Australia.

Cleveland Clinic: How genetic testing can make your cancer treatment more effective, https://health.clevelandclinic.org/how-genetic-testing-can-make-your-cancer-treatment-more-effective/, 2017. Accessed February 23, 2021.

Family Caregiver Alliance: Caregiver statistics: health, technology, and caregiving resources, https://www.caregiver.org/caregiver-statistics-health-technology-and-caregiving-resources, 2016a. Accessed February 23, 2021.

Family Caregiver Alliance: Caregiver statistics: work and caregiving, https://www.caregiver.org/caregiver-statistics-work-and-caregiving, 2016b. Accessed February 23, 2021.

Giddens J: *Concepts for nursing practice*, ed 3, St Louis, 2022, Elsevier.

Grandjean P, Bellanger M: Calculation of the disease burden associated with environmental chemical exposures: application of toxicological information in health economic estimation, *Environ Health* 6(1):123, 2017.

health.gov: 2015-2020 Dietary Guidelines, 2015, https://health.gov/dietaryguidelines/2015/guidelines/introduction/nutrition-and-health-are-closely-related/. Accessed February 23, 2021.

2006-2021 Improving Chronic Illness Care: *The chronic care model*, n.d., http://www.improvingchroniccare.org/index.php?p=The_Chronic_Care_Model&s=2. Accessed May 9, 2021.

Leventhal H et al.: Modelling management of chronic illness in everyday life: a common-sense approach. *Psychol Topics* 25(1):18, 2016.

Lorig K et al: Self-management education: history, definition, outcomes, and mechanisms, Ann Behav Med 26(1):1, 2003.

Lorig K et al.: *Living a healthy life with chronic conditions*, ed 5, Boulder, CO, 2020, Bull Publishing.

Meiner SE, Yeager JJ: *Gerontologic nursing*, ed 6, St Louis, 2019, Elsevier.

Moss K et al.: Identifying and addressing family caregiver anxiety, *J Hosp Palliat Nurs* 21(1):14, 2019.

National Cancer Institute (NCI): Cancer prevalence and cost of care projections, n.d., https://costprojections.cancer.gov/. Accessed February 23, 2021.

National Institute on Alcohol Abuse and Alcoholism (NIAAA): Rethinking drinking: alcohol and your health, n.d., https://www.rethinkingdrinking.niaaa.nih.gov/. Accessed February 23, 2021.

National Institutes of Health (NIH): What are the different ways in which a genetic condition can be inherited? https://ghr.nlm.nih.gov/primer/inheritance/inheritancepatterns, 2020a. Accessed February 23, 2021.

National Institutes of Health (NIH): What is a genetic consultation? https://ghr.nlm.nih.gov/primer/consult/consultation, 2020b. Accessed February 24, 2021.

National Institutes of Health (NIH): What is genetic testing? https://ghr.nlm.nih.gov/primer/testing/genetictesting, 2020c. Accessed February 23, 2021.

National Institutes of Health (NIH): Genetics home reference, https://ghr.nlm.nih.gov/, 2020d. Accessed February 23, 2021.

National Institutes of Health (NIH): What are complex or multifactorial disorders? https://ghr.nlm.nih.gov/primer/mutationsanddisorders/complexdisorders, 2021. Accessed February 23, 2021.

Novotny A: The risks of social isolation, *Am Psychological Assoc*, 50(5): 2019. https://www.apa.org/monitor/2019/05/ce-corner-isolation. Accessed February 23, 2021.

Office of Disease Prevention and Health Promotion [ODPHP]: *Healthy People 2030*, n.d., US Department of Health and Human Services. https://health.gov/healthypeople. Accessed February 23, 2021.

Office of Disease Prevention and Health Promotion (ODPHP): Physical activity: current guidelines, https://health.gov/paguidelines/second-edition/, 2018. Accessed February 23, 2021.

Office of Disease Prevention and Health Promotion (ODPHP): Food & Nutrition, https://health.gov/our-work/food-nutrition, 2020. Accessed February 23, 2021.

Parrish E: Comorbidity of mental illness and chronic physical illness: a diagnostic and treatment conundrum, *Perspect Psychiatr Care* 54(3):339, 2018.

Psychology Today: Motivational Interviewing, 2021 https://www.psychologytoday.com/us/therapy-types/motivational-interviewing. Accessed February 23, 2021.

Self-Management Resource Center (SMRC): Help your community take charge of its health, https://www.selfmanagementresource.com/, 2021. Accessed February 23, 2021.

Souders B: 17 Motivational Interviewing Questions and Skills, Positive Psychology.com, 2021, https://positivepsychology.com/motivational-interviewing/. Accessed February 23, 2021.

Tamura-Lis W: Reminiscing — a tool for excellent elder care and improved quality of life. *Urol Nurs* 37(3):151, 2017.

US Department of Health and Human Services (USDHHS): Step it up! the surgeon general's call to action to promote walking and walkable communities, https://www.hhs.gov/surgeongeneral/reports-and-publications/physical-activity-nutrition/index.html, 2015. Accessed February 23, 2021.

US Department of Health and Human Services (USDHHS): Facing addiction in America: the surgeon general's report on alcohol, drugs, and health, https://www.hhs.gov/surgeongeneral/reports-and-publications/addiction/index.html, 2016. Accessed February 23, 2021.

US Department of Health and Human Services (USDHHS): Physical activity guidelines for Americans, ed 2, 2018. https://health.gov/paguidelines/second-edition/pdf/Physical_Activity_Guidelines_2nd_edition.pdf. Accessed February 23, 2021.

US Preventive Services Task Force: BRCA-related cancer: risk assessment, genetic counseling, and genetic testing, 2019, https://www.uspreventiveservicestaskforce.org/Page/Document/UpdateSummaryFinal/brca-related-cancer-risk-assessment-genetic-counseling-and-genetic-testing?ds=1&s=cancer, Accessed February 23, 2021.

US Department of Health and Human Services (USDHHS): Smoking cessation: a report of the surgeon general, https://www.hhs.gov/surgeongeneral/reports-and-publications/tobacco/index.html, 2020. Accessed February 23, 2021.

World Health Organization (WHO): Global action plan for the prevention and control of chronic noncommunicable diseases 2013-2030, 2020. https://www.iapb.org/news/consultation-on-ncd-action-plan-and-global-co-ordination-mechanism/. Accessed July 5 2021.

World Health Organization (WHO): Alcohol, https://www.who.int/health-topics/alcohol#tab=overview, 2021a. Accessed February 23, 2021.

World Health Organization (WHO): Tobacco, https://www.who.int/health-topics/tobacco, 2021b. Accessed February 23, 2021.

RESEARCH REFERENCES

Apple RW: Children and adolescents coping with chronic illness and disability, *Int J Child Adolesc Health* 10(4):495, 2017.

Arney JB et al.: The value of peer support for self-management of diabetes among veterans in the Empowering patients in chronic care intervention, *Diabetic Med* 37(5):805, 2020.

Ates M, et al.: Educational needs of caregivers of patients hospitalized in a neurology clinic: results of questionnaire, *Int J Caring Sci* 11(2):968, 2018.

Babor TF, et al.: AUDIT: the alcohol use disorders identification test guidelines for use in primary care, ed 2, Geneva, 2019, World Health Organization.

Coughlin MB, Sethares KA: Chronic sorrow in parents of children with a chronic illness or disability: an integrative literature review, *J Pediatr Nurs* 37:108, 2017.

Corvin J, et al.: Translating research into practice: employing community-based mixed methods approaches to address chronic disease and depression among Latinos, *J Behav Health Serv Res* 44(4):574, 2017.

Cutler S, et al.: Effectiveness of group self-management interventions for persons with chronic conditions: a systematic review, *Medsurg Nurs* 27(6):359, 2018.

Gan LL, et al.: School experiences of siblings of children with chronic illness: a systematic literature review, *J Pediatr Nurs* 33:23, 2017.

Garcia-Sanjuan S, et al.: Understanding life experiences of people affected by Crohn's disease in Spain. A phenomenological approach, *Scand J Caring Sci* 32(1):354, 2018.

George M: Adherence in asthma and COPD: new strategies for an old problem, *Respir Care* 63(6):818, 2018.

Han J: Chronic illnesses and depressive symptoms among older people: functional limitations as a mediator and self-perceptions of aging as a moderator. *J Aging Health* 30(8):1188, 2018, http://dx.doi.org/10.1177/08982643 17711609. Accessed February 23, 2021.

Heid A, et al.: Illness representations of multiple chronic conditions and self-management behaviors in older adults: a pilot study, *Int J Aging Hum Dev* 87(1):90, 2018, http://dx.doi.org/10.1177/0091415018771327. Accessed February 23, 2021.

Holt-Lunstad J et al: Loneliness and Social isolation as risk factors for mortality: a meta-analytic review, *Perspectives on Psychological Science*, 10(2), 2015. https://journals.sagepub.com/doi/10.1177/17456916 14568352. Accessed February 23, 2021.

Knoerl R et al.: Estimating the frequency, severity, and clustering of SPADE symptoms in chronic painful chemotherapy-induced peripheral neuropathy, *Pain Manag Nurs* 19(4):354, 2018.

Kosobucka A, et al.: Adherence to treatment assessed with the Adherence in Chronic Diseases Scale in patients after myocardial infarction, *Patient Prefer Adherence* 12:333–340, 2018.

Kourie HR, Klastersky JA: Physical long-term side-effects in young adult cancer survivors: germ cell tumors model, Curr Opin Oncol 29(4):229, 2017.

Kristjansdottir O, et al.: Personal strengths reported by people with chronic illness: a qualitative study, *Health Expect* 21(4):787, 2018.

Kubica A et al.: The Adherence in Chronic Diseases Scale: a new tool to monitor implementation of a treatment plan, *Folia Cardiol* 12:19, 2017.

Lin AM et al.: Factors associated with participation in the Chronic Disease Self-Management Program: findings from the SUCCEED Trial, Stroke 51(10):2910, 2020. Available at https://www.ahajournals.org/doi/10.1161/STROKEAHA.119.028022. Accessed May 16, 2021.

Llewellyn S: The Chronic Care Model, kidney disease, and primary care: a scoping review, *Nephrol Nurs J* 46(3):301-328, 2019.

Lorig K, et al.: Benefits of diabetes self-management for health plan members: a 6-month translation study, *J Med Internet Res* 18(6):1, 2016.

Lum A, et al.: Understanding the school experiences of children and adolescents with serious chronic illness: a systematic meta-review, *Child Care Health Dev* 43(5):645, 2017.

Mete B et al.: Prevalence of malnutrition in COPD and its relationship with the parameters related to disease severity, *Int J Chron Obstruct Pulmon Dis* 13: 3307–3312, 2018.

Neiman AB et al.: CDC grand rounds: improving medication adherence for chronic disease management — innovations and opportunities, *MMWR* 66(45):1248, 2017.

Novinson D et al.: Increasing awareness of uterine cancer risks and symptoms by using campaign materials from Inside Knowledge: Get the Facts About Gynecologic Cancer, *J Cancer Educ* 34:1190-1197, 2019.

Rappaport S: Genetic factors are not the major causes of chronic diseases, *PLoS One* 11(4):e0154387, 2016.

https://www.ncbi.nlm.nih.gov/pmc/articles/PMC4841510/. Accessed February 23, 2021.

Reynolds R, et al.: A systematic review of chronic disease management interventions in primary care, *BMC Fam Pract* 19(1):11, 2018.

Secinti E et al.: Research review: childhood chronic physical illness and adult emotional health: a systematic review and meta-analysis, *J Child Psychol Psychiatry* 58(7):753, 2017, http://dx.doi.org/10.1111/jcpp.12727. Accessed February 23, 2021.

Soderlung PD: Effectiveness of motivational interviewing for improving physical activity self-management for adults with type 2 diabetes: a review, *Chronic Illn* 14(1):54, 2018.

Swietek KE et al.: Effect of the patient-centered medical home on racial disparities in quality of care, *J Gen Intern Med* 35(8):2304-2313, 2020. Available at: https://link.springer.com/content/pdf/10.1007/s11606-020-05729-x.pdf Accessed May 16, 2021.

Tuncay F et al.: Effects of loneliness on illness perception in persons with a chronic disease, *J Clin Nurs* 27(7–8):e1494, 2018, http://dx.doi.org/10.1111/jocn.14273. Accessed February 23, 2021.

Yazdanpanah Y et al.: Effect of an educational program based on Health Belief Model on medication adherence in elderly patients with hypertension, *Evid Based Care J* 9(1):52, 2019.

Yelton B et al.: How do African-American community members' perceptions about environmental risks of breast cancer compare with the current state of the science? *J Cancer Educ* 2020, https://doi.org/10.1007/s13187-020-01748-8.

9

Cultural Competence

OBJECTIVES

- Explain the relationship between cultural awareness and cultural encounter in the cultural competence model.
- Identify the key concept in the cultural competence model that drives cultural competence.
- Explain the role cultural skill plays in nursing assessment.
- Compare social and cultural influences in health and illness.
- Discuss health disparity and the social determinants that affect it.
- Explain how health care systems can contribute to health disparities.
- Summarize the roles played by communication and self-examination in developing cultural competence.
- Explain the approaches to use in conducting a cultural nursing history and physical assessment.
- Elaborate on how teach-back helps a patient with limited health literacy.
- Explain the principles to apply when using an interpreter.

KEY TERMS

Acculturation
Assimilation
Core measures
Cultural assessment
Cultural awareness
Cultural competence
Cultural desire
Cultural encounter
Cultural knowledge

Cultural respect
Cultural skill
Culturally congruent care
Culture
Emic worldview
Ethnic identity
Etic worldview
Health disparity
Health literacy

Intersectionality
Linguistic competence
Marginalized groups
Oppression
Racial identity
Social determinants of health
Stereotype
Unconscious/implicit bias

MEDIA RESOURCES

http://evolve.elsevier.com/Potter/fundamentals/
- Review Questions
- Case Study with Questions

- Audio Glossary
- Content Updates
- Answers to QSEN Activity and Review Questions

The term **culture** refers to the learned and shared beliefs, values, norms, and traditions of a particular group, which guide our thinking, decisions, and actions (Giger and Haddad, 2021). Culture also refers to ways of relating to one another, language and manner of speaking, work and lifestyle practice, social relationships, values, religious beliefs and rituals, and expression of thoughts and emotions (Ball et al., 2019; Giddens, 2021). Culture is a learned behavior, yet it is constantly changing in response to environmental, biological, political, and social influences.

Every one of us has some type of bias that is culturally driven. Such biases can be referred to as an **unconscious bias** or an **implicit bias**. Unconscious bias refers to a bias we are unaware of and that happens outside our control, which is influenced by our personal background, cultural environment, and personal experiences. Unconscious bias typically directs one to make quick judgments and assessments of people and situations. An implicit bias is similar; however, we are aware of the bias that is present. We are responsible for implicit bias and must recognize and acknowledge our actions as they impact our

behavior, decisions, and patient-centered care provided. One might have a bias toward or against an individual based on culture, such as a bias toward an ethnic group, race, gender, ethnicity, nation, religion, social class, or political party. When you hold a bias toward an individual patient or group of patients, it is very difficult to provide patient-centered transcultural care.

Culturally congruent care or transcultural care emphasizes the need to provide care based on an individual's cultural beliefs, practices, and values; therefore, effective communication is a critical skill in culturally competent care and helps you engage a patient and family in respectful, patient-centered dialogue (Betancourt et al., 2020). A patient-centered approach to providing transcultural care requires you to address your own implicit bias; be respectful of and responsive to individual patient preferences, needs, and values; and ensure that patient values guide all clinical care decisions (Institute for Health Improvement [IHI], 2020a).

This chapter explains the importance of cultural competence and its relationship to patient-centered care. **Cultural competence** means

116

that professional health care must be culturally sensitive, culturally appropriate, and culturally competent to meet the multifaceted health care needs of each person, family, and community (Spector, 2017). Cultural beliefs, values, and practices are learned from birth, first in the home, then in the church or other places where people congregate, and then in educational and other social settings. This cultural learning applies to both you and your patients. The process of cultural competence in delivering health care services is "a culturally conscious model of care in which a healthcare professional continually strives to achieve the ability and availability to effectively work within the cultural context of a client" (family, individual, or community) (Transcultural C.A.R.E. Associates, 2020). It is a process of becoming culturally competent, not being culturally competent (Transcultural C.A.R.E. Associates, 2020). The goal of delivering cultural care is to utilize research findings to provide culturally specific care that is safe and beneficial to the well-being of the diverse population (Betancourt et al., 2020).

The changing demographics of the U.S. population create challenges for the health care system and health care providers. By the year 2060, the U.S. Census Bureau (2020) predicts the following will occur:

- The percentage of racial and ethnic minority groups in the United States is expected to climb to 32% of the population.
- The fastest-growing racial ethnic group in the United States is people whose ancestry is from two or more races, and this group is projected to grow by 200% by 2060.
- The next fastest–growing is the Asian population, which is projected to double, followed by the Hispanic population.
- The population age 65 years and over will increase from 49 million in 2016 to 95 million by the year 2060.

The wealth gap between Blacks and Whites is demonstrated in the fact that Blacks lag behind Whites in homeownership, household wealth, and median income. Additionally, the Centers for Disease Control and Prevention (CDC) (2021) reports that studies show adults who self-report the worst health also have the most limited literacy, numeracy, and health literacy skills. A growing body of evidence shows that individuals with the skills and confidence to become actively engaged in their health care have better health outcomes. Although death rates have declined overall in the United States over the past 50 years, people who are poorly educated and people living in poverty still die at a higher rate from the same conditions than people who are better educated and economically advantaged (Ball et al., 2019). These statistics reveal examples of social determinants of health and cultural factors that influence the health care system and why issues such as health care resource accessibility, patient adherence to medical therapies, patient satisfaction, and health care outcomes are so difficult to manage.

The Joint Commission (TJC), the National Quality Forum (NQF), and the National Commission on Quality Assurance (NCQA) are a few of the influential organizations that have responded to these complexities in health care by implementing new standards focused on cultural competence, health literacy, and patient-centered and family-centered care. These standards recognize that valuing each patient's unique needs improves the overall safety and quality of a patient's care.

WORLDVIEW

Historical and social realities shape an individual's or group's worldview, which determines how people perceive others, how they interact and relate to reality, and how they process information (Betancourt et al., 2020). Worldview is a set of assumptions that begins to develop during childhood and guides how one sees, thinks about, experiences, and interprets the world (Betancourt et al., 2020). It creates a lens through which we view all of life's experiences through our own uniquely tinted view. Our worldview evolves during a lifetime process

How We Develop Our Worldview

CULTURE: Shared experiences and commonalities that have developed and continue to evolve in relation to changing social and political contexts based on multiple social group memberships (Warrier, 2005).

SOCIALIZATION through family, friends, community, peers, schooling, media, work, religious institutions, government, legal system, health care system, etc.

WORLDVIEW

FIG. 9.1 How we develop our worldview. (Copyright © 2011 Barnes-Jewish Hospital Center for Diversity and Cultural Competence.)

of interacting with family, peers, communities, organizations, media, and institutions (Fig. 9.1). It is important for you to advocate for patients based on their worldviews. This requires a thorough ongoing assessment, flexibility, and planning in partnership with each patient to ensure that your care is safe, effective, and culturally sensitive.

In any intercultural encounter there is an insider perspective (emic worldview) and an outsider perspective (etic worldview). For example, a Korean woman requests seaweed soup for her first meal after giving birth. This request puzzles her nurse. The nurse has an emic worldview of professional postpartum care but is an outsider to the Korean culture. As such, the nurse is not aware of the meal's significance to the patient. Conversely, the Korean patient has an etic worldview of American professional postpartum care and assumes that the seaweed soup is available in the hospital. Seaweed can be very expensive and not readily available in health care agencies, so the nurse might offer a substitute of other greens such as kale (Giger and Haddad, 2021). Conflict arises when health care providers interpret the behaviors of patients through their own worldview lens instead of trying to uncover the worldview that guides the behavior of their patients.

A stereotype is an assumed belief regarding a particular group (Giger and Haddad, 2021). It is easy to stereotype various cultural groups after reading general information about their ethnic values, practices, and beliefs. Avoid stereotypes or unwarranted generalizations about any particular group. Avoiding stereotypes prevents an inaccurate patient assessment (Narayan, 2019). Instead, approach each person individually, and ask questions to gain a better understanding of a patient's perspective and needs.

HEALTH DISPARITIES

In 2001 a report by the Institute of Medicine defined quality health care as health care that is safe, effective, patient centered, timely, efficient, and equitable or fair (IOM, 2001). Although the U.S. health care system has improved in most of those areas, the system still does not emphasize equality of care (IHI, 2020a; 2020b). As a result, many health care disparities remain. *Healthy People 2030* defines a health disparity as "a particular type of health difference that is closely linked with social, economic, and/or environmental disadvantage" (Office of Disease Prevention and Health Promotion [ODPHP], 2021) (Box 9.1). Poor health status, disease risk factors, poor health outcomes, and limited access to health care are types of disparities

BOX 9.1   Examples of Health Disparities

- One in six American Indian/Alaska Native (AI/AN) adults aged 45 years and older has experienced a cognitive decline including frequent confusion or memory loss.
- The prevalence of Alzheimer disease and dementia is highest among minorities.
- There are only 33 affordable and adequate public housing units available for every 100 renters identified with very low incomes.
- Adults with low food security have an increased risk for cardiovascular disease.
- Younger African Americans are living with or dying from conditions more common at older ages.
- African Americans 18 to 49 years of age are twice as likely to die from heart disease as Whites, and African Americans aged 35 to 64 years of age are 50% more likely to have high blood pressure than Whites.
- About 1 out of 7 children 2 to 8 years of age has a mental, behavioral, or developmental disorder, such as anxiety, learning problems, or attention-deficit/hyperactivity disorder.
- Children diagnosed with mental, behavioral, or developmental disorders live in rural areas and are faced with greater personal and financial issues than those who live in urbanized areas.
- About 1 in 3 U.S. adults are diagnosed with high blood pressure. African Americans have higher rates than do Whites or Hispanics, and they tend to develop high blood pressure at an earlier age.
- Heart disease ranks as the leading cause of death among American Indians/Alaska Natives (AI/AN).
- Americans living in rural areas have an increased risk of death from heart disease, cancer, unintentional injuries, chronic lower respiratory disease, and stroke than Americans in urban areas.
- Rural residents are more likely than urban residents to smoke, be overweight, and fall short of physical activity recommendations.
- American Indians and Alaska Natives have double the risk of having diabetes.
- Cigarette smoking is the leading risk factor for lung cancer, and African-American men have the highest rates of lung cancer in the United States.

Adapted from Centers for Disease Control and Prevention (CDC): CDC health disparities. https://www.cdc.gov/publichealthgateway/didyouknow/topic/healthdisparities.html, 2019.

that are often interrelated and influenced by the conditions and social context in which people live (CDC, 2019).

Social determinants of health are the conditions in which people are born, grow, live, work, and age that affect health functioning and quality of life outcomes (WHO, 2020; ODPHP, n.d.). The *Healthy People 2030* initiative identifies five categories of social determinants: Economic Stability, Education Access and Quality, Health Care Access and Quality, Neighborhood and Built Environment, and Social and Community Context (ODPHP, n.d.). According to the World Health Organization (WHO) (2020), social determinants of health are mostly responsible for health disparities seen with and between countries. Examples of specific social determinants of health include factors such as age, race, ethnicity, socioeconomic status, access to nutritious food, transportation resources, religion, sexual orientation, level of education. literacy level, disability (physical and cognitive), and geographic location (e.g., access to health care) (CDC, 2019). It is important that you understand how patients' cultural factors and their social determinants of health influence their health disparities. You also need to understand the implications this has on how you provide patient-centered care. According to the U.S. Department of Health and Human Services (USDHHS, n.d.), health care disparities are a public health concern because of the adverse effects on communities.

The 2018 National Healthcare Quality and Disparities Report by the Agency for Healthcare Research and Quality (AHRQ) (2020a) offers some promise regarding health care access and quality. The report noted that

access to health care did not demonstrate significant improvement (2000–2017); however, uninsured rates for Americans decreased over the period of 2010 to 2017. Quality of health care improved overall from 2000 through 2014 to 2017, but the pace of improvement varied. Overall, some disparities were getting smaller, but disparities continue to persist, especially for poor and uninsured populations. People in poor households receive worse care than people in high-income households for almost all quality access measures. Black and Hispanic populations experience worse access to care compared with Whites; however, improvements are noted in the number of Americans with a usual source of consistent medical care. The quality of health care improved generally through 2017 based on quality of measures such as patient safety, healthy living, effective treatment, and trends in care coordination (AHRQ, 2020a).

In addition to disparity among cultural groups, people who are in **marginalized groups** are more likely to have poor health outcomes and die earlier because of a complex interaction among their individual behaviors, environment of the communities in which they live, the policies and practices of health care and governmental systems, and the clinical care they receive (United Health Foundation, 2019). Examples of marginalized groups include people who are LGBTQ+, people of color, people who are physically or mentally challenged, and people who are not college educated. Marginalization places or keeps someone in a powerless or an unimportant position within a society or group. Limited access to health care is one social determinant of health that contributes to health disparities. Access to primary care is an important indicator of broader access to health care services. A patient who regularly visits a primary care provider is more likely to receive adequate preventive care than a patient who lacks such access. Nursing intersects with a variety of people from different cultures; therefore, the awareness of marginalization is critical.

Health care systems and health care providers sometimes contribute significantly to the problem of health care disparities. Disparities have been linked to inadequate resources, poor patient-provider communication, a lack of culturally competent care, and inadequate access to language services (National Quality Forum [NQF], 2021). Populations with a culture that differs from the culture of the health care provider tend to encounter decreased access to care, which leads to poor patient health outcomes (Betancourt et al., 2020). To promote equal treatment for all patients who enter the health care system, we must be deliberate about addressing the impact of health care disparities (NQF, 2021).

Consider this example. *Ms. Millman is a 27-year-old African American. She is overweight and was diagnosed with type 2 diabetes 2 years ago and now requires insulin to control her blood sugar. She became homeless after losing her job and health insurance. She currently lives in housing provided through a neighborhood shelter. Ms. Millman was admitted to the hospital with a blood sugar of 322 mg/dL (her normal targeted range is 80 to 130 mg/dL) and a hemoglobin A_{1c} of 11% (target for Ms. Millman is 7% or less). Hannah, a nursing student, is assigned to care for Ms. Millman. After reading her medical record, Hannah notices that Ms. Millman has come to the emergency department three times during the past 6 months for the same reason. Ms. Millman's previous health care providers documented that she verbalized an understanding of how to manage her diabetes but has difficulty following her treatment plan. Hannah teaches Ms. Millman that it is important to take her insulin as prescribed. She also explains how to make healthy food choices. As Hannah provides patient education, Ms. Millman nods. Hannah gives Ms. Millman a chance to ask questions, but Ms. Millman says she has none.*

In the case study, Ms. Millman has a number of social determinants that affect her health status and ability to manage her diabetes: socioeconomic status (no employment or health insurance, no home, limited financial resources if any), no access to primary care (uses the emergency department), being female, and a questionable literacy problem indicated by her neutral reaction to Hannah's instruction. Hannah needs to consider all these factors to provide Ms. Millman a more culturally competent health care plan.

Intersectionality

Intersectionality is a research and policy model for studying the complexities of people's lives and experiences (Allana et al., 2020). The model looks at how being marginalized affects people's health and access to care. It serves to describe the forces, factors, and power structures that shape and influence life. Intersectionality is a way of understanding and analyzing our complex world by looking at the human experience (Allana et al., 2020). Each of us is at the intersection of two categories: privilege and oppression. Oppression is a formal and informal system of advantages and disadvantages tied to membership in social groups, reinforced by societal norms, biases, interactions, and beliefs (The MSW@USC, 2020). Oppression occurs as individual and group experiences. For example, a patient experiencing oppression has limited access to resources, such as health care, housing, education, employment, and legal services. In contrast, a patient experiencing privilege has no difficulty accessing these resources. Individuals who support the theory of intersectionality believe that we must each determine how privileged and how oppressed we are to understand ourselves, the people around us, and the choices we make. Learning about a culture includes becoming familiar with the heritage of the people and understanding how discrimination, prejudice, and oppression can influence beliefs upheld in everyday life. Then as health care providers, we are better able to identify the nature or source of a patient's health care problems and how best to find solutions. Social groups affect our daily lives, shape our worldview, control our access to resources, and ultimately determine our health outcomes. Whether we live in a disadvantaged community or in a community with access to social power and resources, we all are affected by the system of oppression. Understanding the different levels of oppression and where you stand helps you develop cultural competence (Fig. 9.2).

To apply the intersectionality model to daily nursing practice, think about the following patients who have been diagnosed with type 2 diabetes: a 25-year-old Hispanic woman who is homeless, an 85-year-old African-American retired nurse from rural Alabama, a 32-year-old Latina lesbian executive in San Francisco who is Catholic, and a woman who is an undocumented immigrant from Eastern Europe and has a 3-year-old child with a developmental disability. How may the experiences of each of these patients compare with the experiences of other Americans? How do their experiences with the health care system differ? How does age affect their perspective? How would these answers change if you looked at their lives 15 years ago or 35 years ago? What type of clinical judgment might be needed to individualize care for these patients? These scenarios are likely to draw a wide range of responses. The idea of intersectionality supports a broad view of culture by allowing consideration of a multitude of experiences within the context of power, privilege, and oppression.

RACIAL, ETHNIC, AND CULTURAL IDENTITY

Cultural competence is "a dynamic, fluid, continuous process whereby an individual, system, or health care agency finds meaningful and useful care strategies based on knowledge of the cultural heritage, beliefs, attitudes, and behaviors of those to whom they render care" (Giger and Haddad, 2021, p. 7). Cultural competence is challenging to achieve, but it begins with one's ongoing development, while gaining an awareness of individual racial, ethnic, and cultural identity. That awareness prepares you to better understand patients within the context of their own racial, ethnic, and cultural identity.

As a nurse, you will counsel and comfort patients to help them better understand their health issues (e.g., medication adherence, ability to follow diet restrictions, knowledge of risk factors) and improve their willingness to partner with you in making important behavioral changes when necessary. Reflect on your own sense of how you identify with race and ethnicity within the context of your family, community, and cultural history (Substance Abuse and Mental Health Services Administration [SAMHSA], 2020). Here are two classic definitions. Racial identity is based on one's self-identification with one or more social groups in which a common heritage with a particular racial group is shared (U.S. Census Bureau, 2020). Racial identity and ethnic identity are both components of self-concept that place the focus on being part of a cultural group. Although racial identity and ethnic identity demonstrate the differences between race and ethnicity, they have a shared history, values, and bonds. Research frequently treats racial and ethnic identities as interchangeable (Woo et al., 2019).

These definitions help us to understand how individuals negotiate their own and other cultures in life (SAMHSA, 2020). It is important for you to examine your own racial, ethnic, and cultural identity to better recognize and understand normal and abnormal behavior. If you fail

FIG. 9.2 Ladders of oppression and cultural competence. Each level of the ladder of cultural competence offers a response to the ladder of oppression. Because of the extensiveness and complexity of the systems of oppression, individuals and organizations move up and down both ladders simultaneously. (©2011 Barnes-Jewish Hospital Center for Diversity and Cultural Competence.)

to do this self-examination, you will be more likely to prejudge patients and inaccurately assess their health care problems. A self-examination allows you to understand the cultural factors that shape a patient's life experiences, a patient's health care problems, a patient's behavior, and how a patient might perceive those problems, thus supporting the belief that cultural awareness is essential to healing and building trust in the nurse-patient relationship (Conway-Klassen and Maness, 2017; SAMHSA, 2020).

In addition to one's self-examination regarding racial, ethnic, and cultural identities, one must also understand the process of adaptation when transition occurs. The process of acculturation occurs when an individual or group transitions from one culture and develops traits of another culture (Betancourt et al., 2020; Spector, 2017). In this transition, there will be adaptation to the new cultures, traditions, customs, and language. This can lead to stress when the values of the transitioning culture differ from the accepted traits of another. Assimilation is the process in which the individual adapts to the host's cultural values and no longer prefers the components of the origin culture (Frazer, et al., 2017; Spector, 2017).

The National Institutes of Health (2018) has recently coined the term cultural respect, as opposed to cultural competence. Similar to cultural competence, cultural respect is critical to reducing health disparities and improving access to high-quality health care that is respectful and responsive to the needs of the diverse patient. With the growing number of diverse patient populations, the implementation of culturally respectful care is essential and benefits consumers, stakeholders, and communities, leading to safe and positive health outcomes.

DISEASE AND ILLNESS

People react differently to disease based on their unique cultural perspective. Culture influences our thoughts regarding the way people uniquely define disease and illness. An understanding of the difference between disease and illness allows you to pursue ongoing cultural competence in providing patient care. Illness is the way in which individuals and families react to disease, whereas disease is a malfunctioning of biological or psychological processes. Most health care providers in the United States are primarily educated to treat disease, whereas most individuals seek health care because of their experience with illness. As an example, a patient may have a combination of symptoms that, based on previous experiences with family members and beliefs about illness, the patient believes are untreatable, whereas the patient's physician believes aggressive therapy might offer a cure. Such different perspectives between patients and their health care providers often frustrate patients and providers, fostering a lack of trust, lack of patient adherence to treatment plans, and poor health outcomes. Providing safe, quality care to all patients means taking into consideration both disease and illness (Office of Minority Health [OMH], n.d.).

Culture affects how an individual defines the meaning of illness (see Chapter 6). Some illnesses (e.g., human immunodeficiency virus [HIV], bipolar disorder, cancer, or dementia) are embedded with meaning that is not always based on the physical nature of the condition. Cultural stigma can negatively affect those diagnosed; this can lead to lack of early detection, screening, or diagnosis based on the influence of cultural interpretation and decreased awareness. All illness is socially constructed through the experiences of people—specifically, how individuals come to understand and live with their illnesses (Shiri et al., 2018). This is particularly true with chronic disease. Patients learn the effects of their diseases and how to adapt to live as normally as possible.

Culture also provides the context in which a person interacts with family members, peers, community members, and institutions (e.g., educational, religious, media, health care, legal). Therefore, culture and life experiences shape a person's worldview about health, illness, and health care.

Core Measures

The Centers for Medicare & Medicaid Services (CMS), commercial insurance plans, TJC, Medicare and Medicaid managed-care plans, physician and other care provider organizations, and consumers worked together through the Core Quality Measures Collaborative to identify a set of core measures, which aim to hold health care providers accountable for considering patients' unique cultural perspectives to provide safe quality care (CMS, 2020). The core measures are a set of evidence-based, scientifically researched standards of care (CMS, 2020; TJC, 2020). The core measures are key quality indicators that help health care institutions improve performance, increase accountability, and reduce costs. The measures apply to all patients. The core measures need to be meaningful to patients, consumers, and physicians while reducing variability in outcome measure selection, financial collection burden, and cost (CMS, 2020). There are now two core measure sets: one for adults and one for children (CMS, 2020).

In addition to improving the standard of care, the core measures are intended to reduce health disparities. When hospitals are held accountable to meet the core quality measures, all patients regardless of cultural and socioeconomic status are to be treated equally because the standard of care applies to all. For example, one obstetrics and gynecology core measure is that women are to receive breast cancer screening (CMS, 2020). In another example, patients who present with heart failure are to receive beta blocker therapy for left ventricular systolic dysfunction (CMS, 2020).

A MODEL OF CULTURAL COMPETENCE

Ongoing development of cultural competence will present as your ability to interact effectively with people from different cultures, identifying the need to be respectful and responsive to the health belief practices or linguistic needs of our diverse population (SAMHSA, 2020). Cultural competence is a self-motivated developmental process that evolves over a lifetime as individuals engage with others and learn from their experiences (SAMHSA, 2020). One must look at cultural competence as a journey, not a destination. Campinha-Bacote's model of cultural competence has five interrelated constructs (Transcultural C.A.R.E. Associates, 2020): cultural awareness, cultural knowledge, cultural skill, cultural encounters, and cultural desire. The five constructs provide a framework for you to practice in a culturally competent manner.

- **Cultural awareness** is the process of conducting a self-examination of one's own biases toward other cultures and the in-depth exploration of one's cultural and professional background. It also involves being aware of the existence of documented racism and other "isms" in health care delivery.
- **Cultural knowledge** is the process in which a health care professional seeks and obtains a sound educational base about culturally diverse groups. In acquiring this knowledge, health care professionals must focus on the integration of three specific issues: health-related beliefs and cultural values, care practices, and disease incidence and prevalence.
- **Cultural skill** is the ability to conduct a cultural assessment of a patient to collect relevant cultural data about a patient's presenting problem, as well as accurately conducting a culturally based physical assessment.
- **Cultural encounter** is a process that encourages health care professionals to directly engage in face-to-face cultural interactions and other types of encounters with patients from culturally diverse

backgrounds. A cultural encounter aims to modify a health care provider's existing belief about a cultural group and to prevent possible stereotyping.

- **Cultural desire** is the motivation of a health care professional to "want to" (and not "have to") engage in the process of becoming culturally aware, culturally knowledgeable, and culturally skillful in seeking cultural encounters.

When you provide culturally competent care, you bridge cultural gaps to provide meaningful and supportive care for all patients. Transcultural care is culturally congruent when it fits a person's life patterns, values, and system of meaning. These patterns and meaning are generated by people themselves and not from biased, predetermined criteria. For example, during nursing school you are assigned to care for a female patient who observes Muslim beliefs. You notice the woman's discomfort with several of the male health care providers and you wonder whether this discomfort is related to your patient's religious beliefs. While preparing for clinical, you learn that Muslims differ in their adherence to tradition, but that modesty is an important Islamic ethic that pertains to interaction between the sexes. Thus, you say to the patient, "I know that for many of our Muslim patients, modesty is very important. I want to respect your beliefs; is there some way I can make you more comfortable?" You do not assume that the information will automatically apply to this patient. Instead you combine your knowledge about a cultural group with an attitude of helpfulness and flexibility to provide quality, patient-centered, culturally congruent care. There is great diversity within cultural and racial groups themselves, and knowledge provides a general baseline, which is a great starting point in generating a positive patient outcome based on individual health care needs (Giger and Haddad, 2021).

CULTURAL AWARENESS AND KNOWLEDGE

Cultural awareness requires a self-examination of one's biases toward other cultures and an in-depth exploration of one's own cultural and professional background (Campinha-Bacote, 2002; Younas, 2020). Self-examination helps you to understand your own worldview of how you perceive and engage patients. Before you begin to assess the cultures, races, and ethnicities of your patients and use this information to improve their care, first examine and understand your own cultural history, racial and ethnic heritage, and cultural values and beliefs (Younas, 2020). Every individual is constructed from a unique cultural background, which can influence an individual's opinions, perceptions, beliefs, biases, or thoughts, thus forming a unique individual identity (Giger and Haddad, 2021). When you care for a patient in a health care setting, your cultural beliefs and values meet those of the patient, where each may have a different perspective on health, illness, treatment, and care expectations (Degrie et al., 2017). Nurses who understand themselves and their own cultural groups and perceptions are better equipped to respect patients with diverse belief systems. Being open to understanding a patient's beliefs and forming a partnership is more important than knowing everything about a patient's specific culture (Ball et al., 2019). For example, you are giving discharge instructions to your patient. You notice the patient is avoiding eye contact, and you perceive this as disrespectful or showing disinterest when, in fact, the patient's lack of eye contact is a sign of respect, as some cultures believe the lack of eye contact when in presence of an authority is expected. Becoming culturally aware is a first step in one's ability to provide positive patient-centered care.

There is a recommendation that you begin to gain cultural awareness by not only asking yourself if you hold any biases but also questioning whether there are any "isms" where you work (Transcultural C.A.R.E. Associates, 2020). For example, are there ageism practices in how older adults have their pain treated (e.g., undertreatment)?

Be mindful of such practices so that you can adopt care approaches that minimize biases.

Health care providers gain cultural knowledge by taking time to better understand the populations they serve and obtaining specific cultural knowledge as it relates to help-seeking, treatment, and recovery (SAMHSA, 2020). Cultural knowledge is learning or becoming educated about the beliefs and values of other cultures and diverse ethnic groups (Transcultural C.A.R.E. Associates, 2020). The health care provider must focus on these specific issues: (1) health-related beliefs and cultural values, (2) disease incidence and prevalence, and (3) treatment efficacy (Transcultural C.A.R.E. Associates, 2020). Disease incidence and prevalence differ among ethnic groups. Epidemiological data are needed to guide treatment (Campinha-Bacote, 2002). Treatment efficacy is a critical step for providing care to culturally diverse populations.

One's health-related beliefs and cultural values explain how an illness is interpreted by a patient and will guide health care practices delivered throughout patient care. For example, certain cultures believe in the importance of balance and harmony to stay healthy. Aspects of this concept are evident among the beliefs of many Hispanic, Native American, Asian, and Middle Eastern groups (Ball et al., 2019). Box 9.2 summarizes the naturalistic or holistic balance that many people believe they can achieve by using "hot" and "cold" foods and medicines. However, people from different cultures define "hot" and "cold" differently. For example, people who are of Chinese heritage often uphold the philosophical concept of yin (cold) and yang (hot). To restore (treat) a disturbed balance requires the use of opposites (e.g., a "hot" remedy for a "cold" problem and vice versa). If you know about a specific culture's risks for disease, you can focus your nursing history more appropriately during your assessment. If you learn that an individual believes in a "hot" and "cold" balance when choosing certain foods to eat, support your patient's practices, and adapt this information into the patient's dietary plan.

BOX 9.2	Balance of "HOT" and "COLD"		
Cold Conditions	Hot Treatments	Hot Conditions	Cold Treatments
Cancer	**Foods**	Constipation	**Foods**
Cold, flu	Beef	Diarrhea	Barley water
Earaches	Cereals	Fever	Chicken
Headaches	Chili peppers	Infection	Dairy products
Joint pain	Chocolate	Kidney problems	(bottled milk)
Menses	Eggs	Rash	Fresh vegetables
Pneumonia	Liquor	Sore throat	Tropical fruits
Stomach cramps	Onions	Ulcers	Honey
	Medicines and Herbs		**Medicines and Herbs**
	Anise		Bicarbonate of
	Aspirin		soda
	Castor oil		Milk of Magnesia
	Cinnamon		Orange flower
	Garlic		water
	Ginger root		Sage
	Iron		
	Penicillin		
	Tobacco		

Adapted from Ball JW et al.: *Seidel's guide to physical examination,* ed 9, St Louis, 2019, Elsevier; Giger JN, Haddad LG: *Transcultural nursing: assessment and intervention,* ed 8, St Louis, 2021, Elsevier.

Do not form inappropriate biases or stereotypes when you assess a patient's culture. It is easy to stereotype various cultural groups after reading general information about their ethnic values, practices, and beliefs. Avoid stereotypes or unwarranted generalizations about any particular group that prevents an accurate assessment of an individual's unique characteristics and worldview. Instead approach each person individually, and ask questions to gain a better understanding of a patient's perspective and needs. Stereotyping occurs in two cognitive phases. In the first phase there is an activation of a stereotype when an individual is categorized into a social group. When this occurs, beliefs and prejudices come to mind about what members of that particular group are like (Ball et al., 2019). Stereotypical views eventually occur without awareness automatically. In the second phase, people use these activated beliefs and feelings when they interact with individuals (Ball et al., 2019). Research shows that health care providers activate these stereotypes or unconscious biases routinely when communicating with and providing care to minority individuals (Betancourt et al., 2020). As a result, diagnoses and treatments of patients may be biased even in the absence of the practitioner's intent or awareness.

REFLECT NOW

Consider a patient that you cared for recently. How did the patient's health-related beliefs and cultural values impact the decisions made regarding personal health concerns?

Storytelling

One way to begin to understand a patient's cultural perspective is storytelling. Storytelling conveys culture, combining personal experience with the commonalities of all human experiences (Yan et al., 2020). When you encourage a patient to tell a story or when you tell your own story, you frame important messages in ways that make them memorable for you and your patient. Telling stories engages a nurse and patient in a way that broadens their relational understanding. Use storytelling to explore pertinent health care issues; for example, have patients describe previous surgical experiences, problems with childrearing, or approaches used with self-administration of medications. A story helps identify the real problems affecting a patient's health status and find culturally appropriate ways to intervene (Box 9.3).

Worldview of Providers and Patients

Health care has its own culture of hierarchies, power, values, beliefs, and practices. Most health care providers educated in Western traditions are immersed in the culture of science and biomedicine through their coursework and professional experience. Consequently, they often have a worldview that differs from that of their patients. As a nurse, you need to assume that every patient encounter will be a cross-cultural one.

Patients and all their health care providers bring all their worldviews into the care process. The iceberg analogy is a tool that helps you visualize the visible and invisible aspects of your own worldview (Fig. 9.3). Just as most of an iceberg lies beneath the surface of the water, most aspects of a person's worldview lie outside the person's awareness and are invisible to those around the person. For example, a patient who has willingly agreed to be admitted to the hospital for a serious medical condition requiring surgery may refuse the surgery for religious reasons. In the patient's view, she came to the hospital for help to eliminate the pain and infection from her illness. At the same time, she believes that she needs to seek God for a decision that entails removing a body

BOX 9.3   EVIDENCE-BASED PRACTICE

Use of Storytelling and Patient Involvement in Health Care

PICOT Question: Does the use of storytelling compared with standard assessment approaches among adult and pediatric patients affect patient involvement in selecting health care interventions?

Evidence Summary

A patient's ability to understand the complexities of many health issues and to be able to become engaged in decision making requires the ability to discuss and clarify confusing issues. Storytelling allows patients to reflect on their illness experience and create meaning from it (Hardy and Sumner, 2018; Yan et al., 2020). Storytelling enhances self-management of chronic disease (e.g., cancer, diabetes). A recent study involved patients telling stories about their breast cancer diagnosis (Yan et al., 2020). The shared information allowed clinicians to initiate interventions based on patient experiences of health problems. When patients are able to express their experiences, there is a negotiation with health care providers that leads to a mutual plan of care.

Digital storytelling is also widely used, especially in pediatric patients. Storytelling gives children and adolescents with cancer a platform for making sense of and sharing their cancer experience (Hauer, 2020). Technology can have a significant impact on providing respect, trust, and justice in patient care (Hardy and Sumner, 2018). The act of telling a story is valuable, allowing a patient to initiate the process of reflection to gain understanding of the self and the disease process (Hardy and Sumner, 2018; Hauer, 2020; Yan et al., 2020).

Application to Nursing Practice

- Create a safe, caring, and nonjudgmental environment when using storytelling (Hardy and Sumner, 2018; Hauer, 2020; Yan et al., 2020).
- Storytelling should be participant-centered; give patients substantial control over when and how to tell a story (Yan et al., 2020).
- Use storytelling to clarify issues when performing a cultural assessment.
- When asking a patient to describe major concerns about a health problem, encourage the patient to use storytelling to frame the context of those concerns.
- Tell your own stories about patient experiences (respecting confidentiality and staying professional) to help explain procedures or treatment plans.
- Cognitive behavioral measures such as storytelling can be therapeutic for children (Yan et al., 2020).
- Storytelling allows for expression of emotion and teaching by health care professionals (Hauer, 2020).
- Storytelling empowers patients to use their own voice and confront health concerns (Yan et al., 2020).

part. The patient's health care provider assumes the patient is in the hospital to receive care for a serious illness and is willing to accept any and all treatments to cure the illness. The patient's deeply held religious beliefs about removing a body part are not obvious by assessing for a religious preference. Thus, the nurse needs to conduct a comprehensive cultural assessment to understand how the patient's religious values will affect her willingness to receive care (Box 9.4). These deeply held values reside "underneath the iceberg." The observed behavior (in this case, coming to the hospital) is a visible sign of a person's worldview, but the beliefs, attitudes, knowledge, and experiences that guide the behavior are not visible to others. Conflict arises when health care providers interpret the behaviors of patients through their own worldview lens instead of trying to uncover the worldview that guides the behavior of their patients.

FIG. 9.3 Both nurse and patient act in accordance with their own worldviews. This model was adapted from Campinha-Bacote et al. (2005) Iceberg Analogy. It incorporates the Kleinman (1980) explanatory model. (Copyright © 2011 Barnes-Jewish Hospital Center for Diversity and Cultural Competence.)

CULTURAL SKILL

Collecting a culturally based nursing history, performing a culturally based physical assessment, and using teach-back with plain language are cultural skills that take practice and require you to apply your cultural awareness and knowledge (Box 9.5). It takes time to gather a comprehensive, culturally based nursing history. If you work in a setting such as home health, school nursing, or a health clinic, you will be able to gather more information with each patient visit. When you are in an acute setting, you must focus your assessment on the domains most relevant to a patient's condition and the impending treatment plan. For example, if you know a patient will require extensive postoperative education, it will be important to assess the patient's and family's language, family roles, and health care practices.

Collecting a Patient History

Begin a patient assessment by being mindful that cultural differences will exist. It is important to grasp exactly what the patient means and know exactly what the patient thinks you mean in words and actions (Ball et al., 2019). Do not make assumptions. Listen carefully, let patients tell their stories, rephrase statements for clarity, and validate any assumptions you make about the patient's condition or health care needs with the patient. Make sure you understand the patient's needs and expectations (Degrie et al., 2017). As you perform an assessment, the patient may hesitate to offer beliefs and fears, a hesitancy that can be overcome through respectful, nonjudgmental questioning (see Box 9.4). Have the patient help set the agenda for the visit to help you better understand the patient's needs.

A cultural assessment is intrusive and time consuming and requires a trusting relationship between participants. Each patient encounter is a dynamic process that helps form the meaningful care relationship with the patient (Degrie et al., 2017). Misunderstandings due to inappropriate communication between a health care provider and the patient are a barrier to accessing health care (Betancourt et al., 2020). Misunderstandings occur because of language communication differences between and among participants and differences in interpreting one another's behaviors. Linguistic competence is the ability to communicate effectively and

---

BOX 9.4 Cultural Assessment Guide: Aspects of Understanding

Health Beliefs and Practices
- How does the patient define health and illness? How are feelings concerning pain, fatigue, and illness in general expressed?
- Are particular methods used for the treatment of illness?
- What is the attitude toward preventive health measures such as immunizations?
- Are there restrictions imposed by modesty that must be respected (e.g., constraints related to exposure of parts of the body, discussion of sexual health)?
- What are attitudes toward mental illness, pain, chronic disease, being handicapped, and death and dying?
- Is there a person in the family responsible for health-related decisions?
- Does the patient prefer a health professional of the same gender, age, and ethnic and racial background?

Faith-Based Influences and Special Rituals
- Is there a religion or faith to which the patient adheres?
- Is there a significant person to whom the patient looks for guidance?
- What events, rituals, and ceremonies are important within the life cycle of birth, puberty, marriage, and death?

Language and Communication
- What language is spoken in the home?
- How well does the patient understand spoken and written English?
- Are there special signs of demonstrating respect or disrespect?
- Is touch an acceptable form of communication?

Parenting Styles and Family Roles
- Who makes the decisions in the family?
- What is the composition of the family? How many generations are considered to be a single family?
- What is the role of and attitude toward children in the family?
- When do children need to be disciplined or punished, and how is this done?
- Do family members show physical affection toward each other and their children?
- What major events are important to the family, and how do they celebrate?

Sources of Support Beyond the Family
- Are there ethnic organizations that may influence the patient's approach to health care?
- Are there individuals in the patient's social network that influence perception of health and illness?
- Is there a particular cultural group with which the patient identifies?

Dietary Practices
- What does the family like to eat? Does everyone in the family have similar tastes in food?
- Who is responsible for food preparation?
- Are any foods forbidden by the culture, or are some foods a cultural requirement in observance of a rite or ceremony?
- How is food prepared and eaten?
- Are there periods of required fasting?

Adapted from Ball JW et al.: *Seidel's guide to physical examination*, ed 9, St Louis, 2019, Elsevier.

---

convey information in a manner that is easily understood by diverse audiences. You use transcultural communication skills to interpret a patient's behavior and to behave in a culturally congruent way.

The National Culturally and Linguistically Appropriate Services (CLAS) Standards are intended to advance health equity, improve

BOX 9.5 Transcultural Assessment Model

- Culturally unique individual
- Communication
  - Voice quality
  - Pronunciation and enunciation
  - Use of silence
  - Use of nonverbal communication
  - Touch
- Space
  - Degree of comfort
  - Distance in conversations
  - Definition of space
- Social organization
  - Normal state of health
  - Marital status
  - Number of children
  - Parents alive or deceased
- Time
  - Orientation to time
  - View of time
  - Physiochemical reaction to time
- Environmental control
  - Locus of control
  - Value orientation
- Biological variations
  - Physical assessment
- Nursing assessment
  - Note cultural assimilation
  - Incorporate data into plan of nursing care

Adapted from Giger JN, Haddad LG: *Transcultural nursing: assessment and intervention*, ed 8, St Louis, 2021, Elsevier.

quality, and help eliminate health care disparities by establishing a blueprint to help individuals and health care organizations implement culturally and linguistically appropriate services (Office of Minority Health [OMH], n.d.). The CLAS standards include standards for communication and language assistance. The standards apply when you care for patients who have limited English proficiency and/or other communication needs. Misunderstandings and difficulties in communication often lead to problems with the care relationship and can impact patient outcomes (Betancourt et al., 2020; Degrie et al., 2017). All U.S. health care organizations must meet the following requirements:

- Provide language assistance resources (e.g., trained medical interpreters, qualified translators, telecommunication devices for the deaf) for individuals who have limited English proficiency and/or other communication needs, at no cost to them, to facilitate timely access to all health care and services.
- Inform all individuals of the availability of language assistance services clearly and in their preferred language verbally and in writing.
- Ensure the competence of individuals providing language assistance. Do not use untrained individuals and/or minors as interpreters.
- Provide easy-to-understand print and multimedia materials and signage in the languages commonly used by the populations in the service area.

When you begin a cultural assessment there are some basic questions that can help you explore a patient's culture (Ball et al., 2019):

- What do you call your problem?
- What do you think caused it?
- Why do you think it started when it did?
- What does your sickness do to you?

- How long do you think it will last?
- How different is this problem from the one you had a month ago?
- What is the difference between what we are doing and what you think we should be doing for you?
- Why did you come to us for treatment?
- What benefit do you expect from the treatment?
- How do you typically deal with a problem with your health?

Each question requires an open-ended response, enabling you to gain important details about a patient's perceptions, values, and attitudes. A question might also lead to a useful story. A patient's answer to a question may allow you to explore the patient's cultural background more thoroughly.

After realizing that Ms. Millman needs help to better understand the types of foods that are appropriate for a diabetic diet, Hannah refocuses her assessment on some basic questions. How do you think the foods that you eat affect your diabetes? What does diabetes do to you if your blood sugar becomes too high? What benefit will you get from eating healthy foods? Tell me what you eat during a typical day.

Culture influences how feelings are expressed verbally and nonverbally (Degrie et al., 2017). Verbal and nonverbal communication is an important core of all health care encounters (Betancourt et al., 2020). Touch, facial expressions, eye contact, movement, and body posture all have varying significance. The questions in Box 9.4 can help provide further insight into particular situations and help avoid misunderstanding and miscommunication (Ball et al., 2019).

Assessing Health Literacy

Health literacy is the degree to which individuals have the capacity to obtain, process, and understand basic health information and the services needed to make appropriate health decisions (AHRQ, 2020b). According to the IOM, 90 million adult Americans have limited health literacy, and 20 million Americans speak poor English and 10 million speak none (NIH, n.d.). Limited health literacy can be a problem for anyone. It is important to understand that even people with good literacy skills find that understanding health care information is a challenge. Patients and family members often do not understand medical vocabulary and the basic concepts in health and medicine, such as how the body works or how to navigate the health care system. During your assessment, be alert for patient behaviors that might reflect a literacy deficit, such as having difficulty completing registration forms or health histories, failing to make follow-up appointments, asking few questions during a physical examination, and responding simply "yes" when asked whether explanations are understood. Use health literacy assessment tools to determine the level of a patient's health literacy (AHRQ, 2020b). Examples of these tools include:

- The Short Assessment of Health Literacy—Spanish and English (SAHL-S&E) is an instrument consisting of comparable tests in English and Spanish, with good reliability and validity in both languages (Lee et al., 2010).
- The Rapid Estimate of Adult Literacy in Medicine—Short Form (REALM-SF) is a seven-item word recognition test to provide clinicians with a valid quick assessment of patient health literacy (Arozullah et al., 2007). The REALM-SF has been validated and field-tested in diverse research settings.

Assessing a patient's health literacy level is especially important in planning appropriate patient education approaches (AHRQ, 2020b) (see Chapter 25).

Culturally Based Physical Assessment

When performing a physical assessment, knowledge about a patient directs your physical assessment (see Chapter 30). For example, if you know a patient has had diabetes for many years, you focus on the peripheral vascular and neurologic examination because of the common incidence of circulatory problems and peripheral neuropathy in patients with diabetes. If a patient uses an inhaler for asthma, you perform a more detailed assessment of the lungs compared with what you might do for a healthy patient you see during a routine checkup. Use clinical judgment in performing a culturally based physical assessment, methodically applying critical thinking as you anticipate possible areas of concern.

Similarly, you learn to anticipate physical findings based on a patient's cultural health practices and distinguish physical characteristics of an ethnic or racial group. There are several ways individuals from one cultural group can differ biologically from members of other cultural groups (Giger and Haddad, 2021). For example, Mongolian blue spots are a dark pigmented birthmark that may appear shortly after birth on the buttocks, lower back, arms, or legs of dark skin and should not be mistaken for bruising and a sign of abuse. Another example includes the practices of "coining" and "cupping," which are commonly used by some Asian subcultures to release excess force from the body and restore balance (Ball et al., 2019). The practices leave imprints and markings on the skin that can be wrongly interpreted as signs of abuse or disease. Thus, it is always important to ask patients about their home remedies and practices. Another example of anticipating findings is to consider sickle cell anemia when blood tests reveal laboratory values that show anemia in a patient of African descent. As you become more knowledgeable of different ethnic groups in your practice, you will more readily recognize physical characteristics of conditions unique to those groups.

Teach-Back and Plain Language

Linguistic competence requires the application of health literacy principles in providing readily available, culturally appropriate oral and written language services to patients and families with limited English proficiency (AHRQ, 2019). The dual challenges of caring for patients with limited health literacy and cultural differences are likely to increase with an expanding, increasingly diverse, and older population. Evidence suggests that health care providers who attend to both issues help reduce medical errors and improve adherence, communication between provider and patient and family, and outcomes of care at both individual and population levels (Betancourt et al., 2020). Clear communication is essential for effective delivery of quality and safe health care, but most patients experience significant challenges when communicating with their health care providers.

The use of plain language in communicating with patients makes any information you provide easy to read, understand, and use. Plain language is grammatically correct language that includes complete sentence structure and accurate word usage (National Institutes of Health [NIH], n.d.). The Federal Plain Language Guidelines (PlainLanguage.gov, 2011) provide guidance on improving communication through writing. Clear communication is a priority in providing patient care. Written education must be based on specific patient needs. You can find the tips for writing in plain language from the PlainLanguage.gov website: https://www.plainlanguage.gov/guidelines/. Offering patients clear instructions and educational material written in plain language conveys to a learner exactly what to know without using unnecessary words or expressions.

Use the teach-back method following any patient instruction to confirm that you have explained what a patient needs to know in a manner that the patient understands (Fig. 9.4). The teach-back technique is an ongoing process of asking patients for feedback through explanation or demonstration and of presenting information in a new way until you feel confident that you communicated clearly and that your patient fully understands the information presented (Box 9.6).

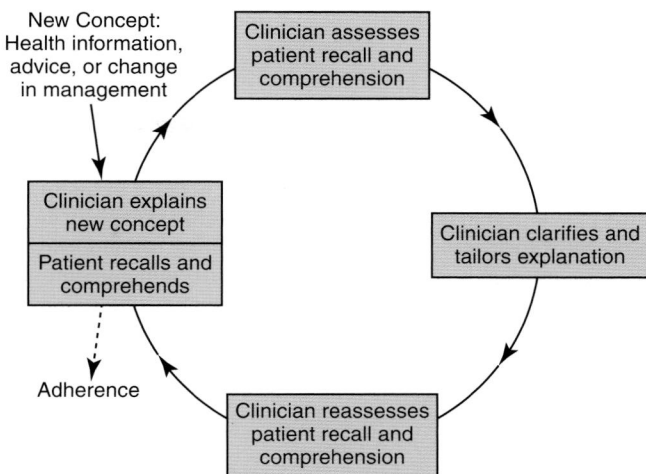

FIG. 9.4 Using the teach-back technique to close the loop. (From the U.S. Health Resources and Services Administration.)

BOX 9.6 PATIENT TEACHING
Medication and Nutritional Adherence

Hannah knows it is important for Ms. Millman to understand her health problems and prescribed treatments. Thus, Hannah plans to use teach-back to ensure that Ms. Millman understands how to effectively manage her diabetes.

Objective
At the end of the teaching session, Ms. Millman will be able to:
- Describe how she plans to make healthy food choices at the shelter and neighborhood store.

Teaching Strategies
- Create a shame-free environment by demonstrating a general attitude of helpfulness.
- Use nonmedical language and define in plain language all medical terms.
- Sit instead of stand and speak slowly.
- Use pictures, models, and written handouts to help Ms. Millman better remember relevant information.
- Have Ms. Millman prepare a meal plan.

Evaluation
Use the principles of teach-back to evaluate patient/family caregiver learning:
- Tell me two strategies that you will use to make healthy food choices when shopping at your neighborhood grocery store.
- We have gone over a lot of information today about changes you plan to make to your diet. In your own words, please review what we talked about. Tell me how you will follow your diet.

When a family caregiver is the recipient of your instruction, use teach-back to confirm learning. You also use teach-back to identify explanations and communication strategies your patients most commonly understand (AHRQ, 2020b).

When using the teach-back technique, do not ask a patient "Do you understand?" or "Do you have any questions?" Instead ask open-ended questions to verify a patient's understanding. Some examples include:
- "I've given you a lot of information (e.g., about your insulin) to remember. Please explain it (e.g., how it affects your blood sugar) to me so that I can be sure that I gave you the information you want and need to take good care of yourself."

- "What will you tell your wife (or husband/partner/child) about the changes we made to your medications today?"
- "We have gone over a lot of information today about how you might change your diet, and I want to make sure I explained everything clearly. In your own words, please review what we talked about. How will you follow this diet at home?"

Teach-back is not intended to test a patient but rather to confirm the clarity of your communication (AHRQ, 2020b). Many patients are embarrassed by their inability to sort out health information or instructions. By regarding teach-back as a test of your communication skills, you take responsibility for the success or failure of the interaction and create a shame-free environment for your patients. Following are helpful hints to consider when trying the teach-back method (AHRQ, 2020b).

- Plan your approach. Think about how you will ask your patient to teach back in a shame-free way. Keep in mind that some situations are inappropriate for teach-back.
- Use handouts, pictures, and models to reinforce your teaching.
- "Chunk and check." Do not wait until the end of the visit to initiate teach-back. Chunk out information into small segments, and have the patient or family caregiver teach it back. Repeat several times during a visit.
- Clarify and check again. If teach-back uncovers a misunderstanding, explain things again using a different approach. Ask patients to teach-back again until they are able to correctly describe the information in their own words. If they parrot your words back to you, they may not have understood.
- Start slowly and use teach-back consistently. Practice. It will take a little time, but once it is part of your routine, teach-back can be done without awkwardness.
- Use the show-me method. When prescribing new medicines or changing a dose, research shows that even when patients correctly say when and how much medicine they will take, many will make mistakes when asked to demonstrate the dose.
- Clarify. If a patient cannot remember or accurately repeat your instructions, clarify your information, and allow the patient to teach it back again (see Box 9.6).

Although it takes time to get used to teach-back, studies show that it does not take longer to perform once it becomes a part of your routine (AHRQ, 2020b). *Box 9.6 provides an example of how Hannah used some of these strategies to educate Ms. Millman on how to manage her diet.*

Working With Interpreters

The National CLAS Standards (OMH, n.d.) ensure that qualified translators (written words) and interpreters (verbal words) are provided to patients with limited English proficiency. The CLAS standards require you to notify patients both verbally and in writing of their rights to receive language assistance. If a health care setting does not have timely access to an interpreter, a more feasible option is the use of a telephone service that provides an on-call trained interpreter connected by phone (Betancourt et al., 2020). Ensure that interpreters are competent in medical terminology and understand issues of confidentiality and impartiality. Do not use a patient's family members to interpret for you or other health care providers. Family members may include their own perceptions or opinions in translation, which can greatly reduce the accuracy of the translated information (Betancourt et al., 2020). When you begin a patient interview with an interpreter present, you should speak in the first person ("I" statements), not the third person (e.g., "tell her," "he said"), and speak directly to the patient, as the interpreter functions as an inconspicuous participant for the conversation. Have the interpreter sit next to or slightly behind the patient. Look at the patient instead of looking at the interpreter and speak in short sentences; then wait for the interpreter to convey them (Betancourt et al., 2020). Avoid using jargon, acronyms, and jokes; attempts at humor are often lost in interpretation. Ask the patient for feedback and clarification at regular intervals. Be observant of the patient's nonverbal and verbal behaviors. At the end of a conversation thank both the patient and the interpreter.

CULTURAL ENCOUNTER

Whenever you directly interact with patients from culturally diverse backgrounds, this interaction is a cultural encounter and has two goals (Campinha-Bacote, 2007; Betancourt et al., 2020). One goal is to communicate in a way that generates a wide variety of responses and to send and receive both verbal and nonverbal communication accurately and appropriately in each culturally different context. The second goal is to continuously interact with patients from culturally diverse backgrounds to validate, refine, or modify existing values, beliefs, and practices about a cultural group.

CULTURAL DESIRE

Engaging with people we perceive as "different" from us can be threatening and difficult. It generally takes more effort and patience than engaging with patients who are more similar to us. Cultural desire refers to having the motivation to engage patients so that you understand them from a cultural perspective. It is the pivotal and key construct of cultural competence, for it is a nurse's desire that evokes the entire process of cultural competence (Transcultural C.A.R.E. Associates, 2020). Cultural desire involves the concept of caring (see Chapter 7). Establishing a caring relationship with a patient requires you to enter into the patient's worldview. Cultural desire includes a genuine passion to be open and flexible with others, to accept differences and build on similarities, and to be willing to learn from others as cultural informants (Transcultural C.A.R.E. Associates, 2020).

You will care for patients who display behaviors that may be in direct moral conflict with your own values (e.g., abortion, substance abuse, spouse abuse). For example, you are asked to care for a young male gang member whose beliefs about violence and respect for life are in direct contrast to yours. Yet you care for this patient nonjudgmentally and with respect. Acquiring the willingness to practice cultural desire requires a respect and acceptance of all human beings. The LEARN Model (Campinha-Bacote, 2003; Ladha et al., 2018) can assist with this process. The mnemonic *LEARN* represents the process of listening, explaining, acknowledging, recommending, and negotiating:

- *Listen* to the patient's perception of the problem. Be nonjudgmental and use encouraging comments, such as "Tell me more" or "I understand what you are saying."
- *Explain* your perception of the problem.
- *Acknowledge* not only the differences between the two perceptions of the problem but also the similarities. Recognize the differences but build on the similarities.
- *Recommendations* must involve the patient.
- *Negotiate* a treatment plan, considering that it is beneficial to incorporate selected aspects of the patient's culture into the plan.

Applying the LEARN mnemonic will help you to reflect at each patient encounter. You recognize that each patient is unique, but you are responsible for understanding what "unique" truly means so that you can engage patients in a patient-centered approach to care.

QSEN **Building Competency in Patient-Centered Care** Mrs. Addelman is 28 years old and 39 weeks pregnant. She has been under medical care since the pregnancy was discovered. At this time, Mrs. Addelman is in labor, and an emergency C-section is needed. She refuses to allow the health care team to prepare her for the C-section until her husband arrives. Her family practices the Muslim faith. What are your concerns related to Mrs. Addelman? What are some steps you, as the nurse, can take to assist?

Answers to QSEN Activities can be found on the Evolve website.

KEY POINTS

- Cultural awareness self-examines the dynamics of personal biases, stereotypes, values, and beliefs related to others different from one's own heritage, while cultural encounter involves directly interacting with patients of a diverse population other than one's own.
- Cultural desire is the pivotal and key construct of cultural competence. It is your desire to engage with patients who have cultural differences that evokes the entire process of cultural competence.
- Cultural skill is the ability to conduct a cultural assessment of a patient to collect relevant cultural data about a patient's presenting problem, as well as accurately conducting a culturally based physical assessment.
- A person's culture and life experiences shape the person's worldview about health, illness, and health care.
- Culture is constantly changing in response to social influences such as lifestyle practices, social relationships, and biases.
- Poor health, disease risk factors, poor health outcomes, and limited access to health care are types of preventable health care disparities often interrelated and influenced by the conditions and social context in which people live.
- Disparities in access to quality health care, preventive health care, and health education contribute to poor population health.
- Social determinants of health are defined by conditions in which people are born, grow, live, work, and age. Social determinants include economic stability, education access and quality, health care access and quality, neighborhood and built environment, and social and community context.
- Health care systems and providers contribute to the problem of health disparities as a result of inadequate resources, poor patient-provider communication, a lack of culturally competent care, system fragmentation, and inadequate access to language services.
- Gaining cultural knowledge and conducting a self-examination allow health care providers to understand the cultural factors that shape patients' life experiences, their health care problems and behavior, and how they might perceive those problems while building a positive nurse-patient relationship.
- Cultural respect is critical to reducing health disparities and improving access to high-quality health care that is respectful and responsive to the needs of a diverse patient.
- Avoid forming inappropriate biases or stereotypes when assessing a patient's needs. Approach each person individually, and ask questions to gain a better understanding of a patient's perspective and needs.
- Ongoing cultural competence and cultural skill are necessary for a nurse to complete a cultural assessment and provide culturally appropriate nursing care for each patient, regardless of the patient's cultural background.

- Knowledge about your patient directs your physical assessment, and the health care provider must learn to anticipate physical findings based on the patient's cultural health practices and the physical characteristics of an ethnic or racial group.
- Teach-back is an ongoing process of asking patients open-ended questions to gather feedback through explanation or demonstration until the health care provider feels confident in the patient's ability to understand and safely apply the new educational content.
- Linguistic competence is the ability to communicate effectively and convey information in a manner that is easily understood by diverse audiences.
- Effective communication is a critical skill in culturally competent care and helps you engage a patient and family in a respectful, patient-centered dialogue. Qualified translators (written words), interpreters (verbal words), and/or the use of a cultural broker (mediator) are options to be utilized to assist with linguistic needs related to effective communication.

REFLECTIVE LEARNING

- Consider a patient that you cared for recently on the clinical unit. How did knowledge of your patient's culture impact your nursing care?
- Discuss some of the social determinants of health that you identified while conducting your assessment of the patient. How have these impacted the health of the patient?
- Review your personal approach to patient education when working with a patient who has a different cultural background from your own. Remember, the teach-back method is a valuable tool for all health care providers to use with each patient. As the health care provider, did you do the following?
  - Use a caring tone of voice and attitude?
  - Display comfortable body language, make eye contact, and sit down at the patient's level?
  - Ask open-ended questions?
  - Take responsibility for making sure the instructions were clear and understood?
  - Use print materials that were reader friendly to support learning?
  - Observe the patient's response to teach-back?

REVIEW QUESTIONS

1. A nurse is seeing all of these patients in the community health clinic. The nurse identifies which patient(s) as having a health disparity? (Select all that apply.)
   1. A patient who has a homosexual sexual preference
   2. A patient unable to access primary care services
   3. A patient living with chronic schizophrenia
   4. A family who relies on public transportation
   5. A patient who has a history of hypertension
2. A 35-year-old woman has Medicaid coverage for herself and two young children. She missed an appointment at the local health clinic to get an annual mammogram because she has no transportation. She gets the annual screening because her mother had breast cancer. Which of the following are social determinants of this woman's health? (Select all that apply.)
   1. Medicaid insurance
   2. Annual screening
   3. Mother's history of breast cancer
   4. Lack of transportation
   5. Woman's age

3. During a nursing assessment a patient displayed several behaviors. Which behavior suggests the patient may have a health literacy problem?
   1. Patient has difficulty completing a registration form at a medical office
   2. Patient asks for written information about a health topic
   3. Patient speaks Spanish as primary language
   4. Patient states unfamiliarity with a newly ordered medicine

4. A nurse desires to communicate with a young woman who is Serbian and who has limited experience with being in a hospital. The nurse has 10 years of experience caring for Serbian women. The patient was admitted for a serious pregnancy complication. Apply the LEARN model and match the nurse's behaviors with each step of the model.

_____ 1. L	a.	The nurse notes that she has learned that fathers can visit mothers at any time in both Serbia and the United States.
_____ 2. E	b.	The nurse shares her perception of the woman's experiences as a patient.
_____ 3. A	c.	The nurse asks the patient how she can maintain bed rest when she returns home.
_____ 4. R	d.	The nurse attends to the patient and listens to her story about hospitals in Serbia.
_____ 5. N	e.	The nurse involves the patient in a discussion of the treatment options for her condition.

5. Health care agencies must provide which of the following based on federal civil rights laws? (Select all that apply.)
   1. Provide language assistance services at all points of contact free of charge.
   2. Provide auxiliary aids and services, such as interpreters, note takers, and computer-aided transcription services.
   3. Use patients' family members to interpret difficult topics.
   4. Ensure that interpreters are competent in medical terminology.
   5. Provide language assistance to all patients who speak limited English or are deaf.

6. A nurse working in a large occupational health clinic knows that many of the workers at her company are marginalized and at risk for poor health outcomes. Which of the following individuals are most likely to be marginalized?
   1. Wives of the employees
   2. The head supervisors of the company
   3. Workers who have a high school education
   4. Workers employed for less than a year at the company

7. A mother is concerned about her child's flulike symptoms. You learn from the health assessment that the mother practices the use of "hot" and "cold" foods to treat ailments. Which of the following foods do you expect the mother to use to treat her child?
   1. Chicken
   2. Yogurt
   3. Fresh fruits
   4. Eggs

8. Which explanation provided by the nurse is the most accurate meaning for "providing culturally congruent care"?
   1. It fits the patient's valued life patterns and set of meanings.
   2. It is the same set of values as those of the health care team member providing daily care.
   3. It holds one's own way of life as superior to those of others.
   4. It redirects the patient to a more socially expected set of values.

9. Which statements made by a nursing student about the teach-back technique show understanding of the technique? (Select all that apply.)
   1. "After teaching a patient how to use an inhaler, I need to use the teach-back technique to test my patient's ability to use the inhaler correctly."
   2. "The teach-back technique is an ongoing process of asking patients for feedback."
   3. "Using teach-back will help me identify explanations and communication strategies that my patients will most commonly understand."
   4. "Using pictures, drawings, and models can enhance the effectiveness of the teach-back technique."
   5. "When doing my patient teaching, I will use plain language to make the material easier to understand for the patient."

10. Match the cultural concepts on the left with the correct definitions on the right.

_____ 1. Etic worldview	a.	Factor that shapes how people perceive others and how they relate to reality
_____ 2. Worldview	b.	Insider's perspective in an intercultural encounter
_____ 3. Cultural desire	c.	A policy model that describes factors and power structures that shape and influence life
_____ 4. Intersectionality	d.	An outsider's perspective in an intercultural encounter
_____ 5. Emic worldview	e.	The motivation of a health care professional to "want to" engage in cultural competence

Answers: 1. 1, 2, 3; **2.** 1, 4, 5; **3.** 1; **4.** 1d, 2b, 3a, 4e, 5c; **5.** 1, 2, 4, 5; **6.** 3; **7.** 4; **8.** 1; **9.** 1, 2, 3, 4, 5; **10.** 1d, 2a, 3e, 4c, 5b.

Rationales for Review Questions can be found on the Evolve website.

REFERENCES

Agency for Healthcare Research and Quality (AHRQ): *What is cultural and linguistic competence*, http://www.ahrq.gov/professionals/systems/primary-care/cultural-competence-mco/cultcompdef.html, 2019. Accessed June 1, 2020.

Agency for Healthcare Research and Quality (AHRQ): *2018 National healthcare quality and disparities report*, https://www.ahrq.gov/research/findings/nhqrdr/nhqdr18/index.html, 2020a. Accessed July 1, 2020.

Agency for Healthcare Research and Quality (AHRQ): *Health Literacy Universal Precautions Toolkit 2nd edition*, September 2020b. Agency for Healthcare Research and Quality, Rockville, MD. https://www.ahrq.gov/health-literacy/quality-resources/tools/

literacy-toolkit/healthlittoolkit2-tool5.html. Accessed April 15, 2021.

Ball JW et al.: *Seidel's guide to physical examination*, ed 9, St Louis, 2019, Elsevier.

Campinha-Bacote J: *The process of cultural competence in the delivery of healthcare services: the journey continues*, ed 5, Cincinnati, OH, 2007, Transcultural C.A.R.E. Associates.

Centers for Disease Control and Prevention (CDC): *Health literacy: Evidence Reviews and Research Summaries*, https://www.cdc.gov/healthliteracy/researchevaluate/evidence-research.html, 2021. Accessed April 13, 2021.

Centers for Disease Control and Prevention (CDC): *Reaching for health equity*, https://www.cdc.gov/healthequity/features/reach-health-equity/index.html, 2019. Accessed July 1, 2020.

Centers for Medicare & Medicaid (CMS): *Core measures*, https://www.cms.gov/Medicare/Quality-Initiatives-Patient-Assessment-Instruments/QualityMeasures/Core-Measures.html, 2020. Accessed July 2, 2020.

Giddens JF: *Concepts for nursing practice*, ed 3, St Louis, 2021, Elsevier..

Giger JN, Haddad LG: *Transcultural nursing: assessment and intervention*, ed 8, St Louis, 2021, Elsevier.

Institute for Health Improvement (IHI): *Across the Chasm: Six Aims for Changing the Health Care System*, http://www.ihi.org/resources/Pages/ImprovementStories/AcrosstheChasmSixAimsforChangingtheHealthCare-System.aspx, 2020a.

Institute for Health Improvement (IHI): *Across the Chasm Aim 6: Health Care Must Be Equitable*, http://www.ihi.org/resources/Pages/ImprovementStories/HealthCareMustBeEquitable.aspx, 2020b.

Institute of Medicine (IOM): *Crossing the quality chasm: a new health system for the 21st century*, Washington DC, 2001, National Academy of Sciences, National Academies Press.

Narayan M: Addressing Implicit Bias in Nursing: A Review, *AJN* 119(7): 37, 2019.

National Institutes of Health (NIH): (n.d.): Clear communication. https://www.nih.gov/institutes-nih/nih-office-director/office-communications-public-liaison/clear-communication, Accessed July 2, 2020.

National Quality Forum (NQF): *Disparities*, http://www.qualityforum.org/Topics/Disparities.aspx, 2021. Accessed April 13, 2021.

Office of Disease Prevention and Health Promotion (ODPHP): *Healthy People 2030 questions and answers*. 2021, U.S. Department of Health and Human Services. https://health.gov/our-work/healthy-people/healthy-people-2030/questions-answers#q9. Accessed April 17, 2021.

Office of Disease Prevention and Health Promotion (ODPHP): Social determinants of health. *Healthy People 2030*. n.d., U.S. Department of Health and Human Services. https://health.gov/healthypeople/objectives-and-data/social-determinants-health. Accessed April 2021.

Office of Minority Health (OMH), U.S. Department of Health and Human Services (USDHHH): (n.d.): National standards for culturally and linguistically appropriate services (CLAS) in health and health care. https://www.thinkculturalhealth.hhs.gov/assets/pdfs/EnhancedNationalCLASStandards.pdf. Accessed July 2, 2020.

Office of Disease Prevention and Health Promotion (ODPHP): Disparities. https://www.healthypeople.gov/2020/about/foundation-health-measures/Disparities, 2020. Accessed July 1, 2020.

PlainLanguage.gov: *Federal plain language guidelines*, https://www.plainlanguage.gov/media/FederalPLGuidelines.pdf, 2011. Accessed July 2, 2020.

Spector R: *Cultural diversity in health and illness*, ed 9, Stamford, CT, 2017, Appleton Lange.

Substance Abuse and Mental Health Services Administration (SAMHSA): *Cultural competence*, https://www.samhsa.gov/section-223/cultural-competency, 2020. Accessed July 2, 2020.

The Joint Commission (TJC): *Measures*, http://www.jointcommission.org/core_measure_sets.aspx, 2020. Accessed July 2, 2020.

The MSW@USC: Diversity toolkit: a guide to discussing identity, power, and privilege, University of Southern California, 2020. https://msw.usc.edu/mswusc-blog/diversity-workshop-guide-to-discussing-identity-power-and-privilege/. Accessed April 14, 2021.

Transcultural C.A.R.E. Associates: The process of cultural competemility in delivery of healthcare services, http://transculturalcare.net/the-process-of-cultural-competence-in-the-delivery-of-healthcare-services/, 2020. Accessed July 1, 2020.

United Health Foundation: *America's health rankings: 2019 annual report*, 2019. https://www.americashealthrankings.org/learn/reports/2019-annual-report. Accessed April 13, 2021.

U.S. Census Bureau: *Demographic turning points for the United States population projection for 2020-2060*, https://www.census.gov/content/dam/Census/library/publications/2015/demo/p25-1143.pdf, 2020. Accessed July 1, 2020.

U.S. Department of Health and Human Services (USDHHS), Office of Minority Health (OMH): (n.d.).: Think cultural health: national standards for culturally and linguistically appropriate services (CLAS) in health and health care. https://www.thinkculturalhealth.hhs.gov/assets/pdfs/EnhancedNationalCLASStandards.pdf Accessed January 2019.

World Health Organization: *Social determinants of health*, http://www.who.int/social_determinants/sdh_definition/en/, 2020. Accessed July 1, 2020.

Younas A: Self-awareness: A tool for providing culturally competent care, *Nursing* 50(2):61, 2020.

RESEARCH REFERENCES

Arozullah AM et al.: Development and validation of a short-form, rapid estimate of adult literacy in medicine, *Med Care* 45:1026, 2007.

Allana S et al.: Intersectionality in Heart failure self-care ignorance is not an option. *Journal of Cardiovascular Nursing* 35(3): 231, 2020.

Betancourt J et al.: Cross-cultural care and communication, *UpToDate*, 2020, https://www.uptodate.com/contents/cross-cultural-care-and-communication. Accessed July 1, 2020.

Campinha-Bacote J: The process of cultural competence in the delivery of health care services: a model of care, *J Transcult Nurs* 13:181, 2002.

Campinha-Bacote J: Many faces: addressing diversity in health care, *Online J Issues Nurs* 8(1), 2003. http://ojin.nursingworld.org/MainMenuCategories/ANAMarketplace/ANAPeriodicals/OJIN/TableofContents/Volume82003/No1Jan2003/

AddressingDiversityinHealthCare.html. Accessed August 9, 2020.

Conway-Klassen J, Maness L: Critical conversations: cultural awareness, sensitivity, and competency, *Clin Lab Sci* 38(1):34, 2017.

Degrie L et al.: How do ethnic minority patients experience the intercultural care encounter in hospitals? A systematic review of qualitative research, *BMC Medical Ethics* 18(2):1, 2017.

Frazer AL et al.: Acculturation dissonance, acculturation strategy, depressive symptoms, and delinquency in Latina/o adolescents, *Child Youth Care Forum* 46:19, 2017.

Hardy P, Sumner T: *Cultivating compassion: how digital storytelling is transforming health care*, ed 2, Cham, Switzerland, 2018, Palgrave MacMillan/Springer.

Hauer J: Pediatric palliative care, *UpToDate*, 2020, https://www.uptodate.com/contents/pediatric-palliative-care. Accessed July 2, 2020.

Ladha T et al.: Cross-cultural communication: Tools for working with families and children. *Paediatr Child Health* 23(1): 66, 2018.

Lee SD et al.: Short assessment of health literacy – Spanish and English: a comparable test of health literacy for Spanish and English speakers, *Health Serv Res* 45(4):1105, 2010.

Shiri FH et al.: Explaining the meaning of cancer stigma from the point of view of Iranian stakeholders: a qualitative study, *Int J Cancer Manag* 11(7):e1, 2018.

Woo B et al.: The role of racial/ethnic identity in the association between racial discrimination and psychiatric disorders: A buffer or exacerbator? *Population Health* 7:100378, 2019.

Yan A et al., Engaging young African American women breast cancer survivors: A novel storytelling approach to identify patient-centred research priorities, *Health Expectations* 23(2):473, 2020.

Family Dynamics

THE FAMILY

Families are important. They are made up of groups of people who have emotional connections with one another and function as a unit. However, the concept, structure, and function of a family unit continue to change over time. Families face many challenges, including the effects of health and illness, childbearing and childrearing, changes in family structure and dynamics, and caring for older family members. Family characteristics or attributes such as durability, resiliency, and diversity help families adapt to these challenges.

Family durability is a system of support and structure within a family that extends beyond the walls of the household. For example, marriages may end in divorce or death, and remarriage may occur, or children may leave home as adults, but in the end the "family" transcends long periods and inevitable lifestyle changes.

Family resiliency is the ability of a family to cope with expected and unexpected stressors. The family's ability to adapt to role and structural changes, family members' developmental milestones, and crises shows resiliency. For example, a family is resilient when the wage earner loses a job and another member of the family takes on that role. A family survives and thrives because of the challenges encountered from stressors.

Family diversity is the uniqueness of each family unit. For example, while one family experiences marriage and has children later in life, another family includes parents with young children and grandparents living in the home. Every person within a family unit has specific needs, strengths, and important developmental considerations (see Chapter 11).

As you care for patients and their families, you are responsible for understanding **family dynamics**, the interactions between and among family members that are affected by a family's makeup (configuration), structure, function, problem solving, and coping capacity. Use this knowledge to build on a patient's and family's strengths and resources (Duhamel, 2017; Umbersome and Thomeer, 2020). The rapidly changing health care delivery system promotes early discharge of patients from acute care settings and referral for home health visits. Living as a family amid an illness is challenging; family functions, communications, and roles are altered (Gross, 2020; Kokonya and Fitzsimons, 2018).

The goal of family-centered nursing care is to address the comprehensive health care needs of the family as a unit and to advocate, promote, support, and provide for the well-being and health of the patient and individual family members (Coats et al., 2018; Orchard et al., 2017). To plan and implement family-centered nursing care, you need to use

FIG. 10.1 Family celebrations and traditions strengthen the role of the family.

critical thinking and clinical judgment to ensure that you provide individualized, family-centered care to meet a family's needs.

Concept of Family

The term *family* suggests a visual image of adults and children living together in a satisfying, harmonious manner (Fig. 10.1). For some this term creates a different image, for example a single parent and children living with a grandparent. Families represent more than a set of individuals, and a family is more than a sum of its individual members (Kaakinen et al., 2018). Families are as diverse as the individuals who compose them. Patients have deeply ingrained values about their families that deserve respect (Gross, 2020).

The specific relationships among patients, families, and health care providers are at the center of patient and family care (Delbanco and Gerteis, 2020). Unfortunately, these relationships are often defined and shaped by the beliefs of health care providers and not the needs of patients and family caregivers. As a nurse, you need to assess for and understand how your patients define their families and how they perceive the general state of member relationships. Think of a **family** as a set of relationships that a patient identifies as family or as a network of individuals who influence one another's lives, whether there are actual biological or legal ties.

Definition: What Is a Family?

Defining *family* initially appears to be a simple undertaking. However, different definitions result in heated debates among social scientists who study the dynamics of families and legislators who set public policies affecting families. The definition of family is significant and affects who is included on health insurance policies, who has access to children's school records, who files joint tax returns, and who is eligible for sick-leave benefits or public assistance programs.

A family is what an individual believes the family to be. It includes a set of interacting individuals who are related through biology or enduring commitments who usually socialize with one another (Kaakinen et al., 2018). For some patients, family includes only people related by marriage, birth, or adoption. To others, aunts, uncles, close friends, and pets are family. Understand that families take many forms and have diverse cultural and ethnic orientations. No two families are alike; each has its own strengths, weaknesses, resources, and challenges. You must care for both the family and the patient. Effective nursing administrators have a clear vision that caring for families is crucial to the mission of their health care agencies and the health of the nation (Orchard et al., 2017).

BOX 10.1   Family Forms

Nuclear Family
A nuclear family consists of two adults (and sometimes one or more children).

Extended Family
An extended family includes relatives (aunts, uncles, grandparents, and cousins) in addition to the nuclear family.

Single-Parent Family
A single-parent family is formed when one parent leaves the nuclear family because of death, divorce, or desertion or when a single person decides to have or adopt a child.

Blended Family
A blended family is formed when parents bring children from previous marriages or other parenting relationships into a new joint-living situation.

Alternative Family
Relationships include multiadult households, grand families (grandparents caring for grandchildren), communal groups with children, "nonfamilies" (adults living alone), and cohabiting partners.

FAMILY FORMS AND CURRENT TRENDS

Family forms are patterns of people considered by family members to be included in a family (Box 10.1). Although all families have some things in common, each family form has unique challenges and strengths. Remain open about who makes up a family to establish a therapeutic relationship with families and to ensure you are aware of a family's resources and concerns.

Families are constantly changing. In some situations, people marry later or delay childbirth. Some choose to have children while others do not have any children. Approximately 49% of people 15 years of age and older are married (U.S. Census Bureau, 2019). However, the number of people living alone is greatly increasing, with approximately 28% of households containing only one person (U.S. Census Bureau, 2019). Calculating divorce rates in the United States is complicated and inaccurate. However, most scholars agree that approximately 50% of marriages will end in divorce (American Psychological Association [APA], 2020). Divorce is becoming less common in younger adults but has doubled since the 1990s in adults age 50 and older (Farris and Bourque, 2020). Remarriage often results in a blended family with a complex set of relationships among all members.

Marital roles are also more complex as families increasingly have two wage earners. About 70% of mothers with children under 18 years of age are in the workforce, and mothers are the primary or sole earner for about 40% of households (Catalyst, 2020; U.S. Bureau of Labor Statistics, 2018). Balancing employment and family life creates a variety of challenges in terms of childcare and household work for parents.

The number of single-parent families appears to be stabilizing. About 27% of children under the age of 18 live with one parent. Although mothers head most single-parent families, father-only families and the number of children living with other relatives are on the rise (U.S. Census Bureau, 2019).

Although there has been a 7% decrease in births in the United States in women under 20 years of age, adolescent pregnancy still remains a concern (Martin et al., 2019). Most adolescent mothers continue to live with their families. An adolescent pregnancy has long-term consequences for the mother. Adolescent mothers may experience problems related to birth, psychological well-being, lack of knowledge about caring for an infant, lack of social support, personal education, and economic strain (Erfina et al., 2019). The overwhelming task of being a parent while still being an adolescent often severely stresses family relationships and resources. Stressors are also placed on adolescent fathers when their partners become pregnant (Chacko, 2020). Adolescent fathers usually have poorer support systems and fewer resources to teach them how to parent. Adolescent fatherhood is associated with lower socioeconomic status, lower educational attainment, and fewer job opportunities (Chacko, 2020). Children of adolescent parents are more likely to have health and cognitive disorders, to have poor academic performance, and to be abused or neglected. In addition, females are more likely to experience an adolescent pregnancy and males are more likely to be incarcerated (Chacko, 2020). Both adolescent parents often struggle with the normal tasks of development and identity but must accept a parenting role that they are not ready for physically, emotionally, socially, and/or financially.

In 2015 the U.S. Supreme Court issued a groundbreaking ruling that found same-sex marriages constitutional. Since this ruling, the number of same-sex marriages continues to increase, and most same-sex couples who live together (61%) are married (Masci et al., 2019). Individuals in same-sex relationships have become more vocal about their legal rights. Public support for same-sex marriage has grown rapidly over the past 10 years (61%) (Masci et al., 2019).

The fastest-growing age-group in America is 65 years of age and older (Mather et al., 2019). In 2016, 49.2 million Americans were 65 years of age or older. This number increased by 33% since 2006 and is expected to almost double to 98 million people in 2060 (Administration for Community Living [ACL] and Administration on Aging [AoA], 2018). This phenomenon, often referred to as the "graying of America," continues to affect the family life cycle, particularly the "sandwich generation"—composed of the children of older adults. These individuals, who are usually in their middle years, must meet their own needs along with those of their children and their aging family members. This balance of needs often occurs at the expense of their own well-being and resources.

More grandparents are raising their grandchildren (U.S. Census Bureau, 2019). This new parenting responsibility is the result of several societal factors, such as military deployment, unemployment, adolescent pregnancy, substance abuse, and divorce resulting in single parenthood.

There are some positive trends emerging in the older-adult population including a rise in educational levels, increased life expectancy, narrowed gender gap in life expectancy, and a drop in poverty levels (Mather et al., 2019).

Factors Influencing Family Forms

Families face many challenges today, including changing structures and roles related to the changing economic status of society. Some families experience challenges related to chronic illness and aging family members. Family caregiving, poverty, homelessness, and domestic violence create challenges for families.

Family Caregivers. The increases in people living with chronic illnesses or disabilities and in the older-adult population have created a greater need for family caregiving (Family Caregiver Alliance [FCA], 2019). Family caregivers are a crucial part of the health care team because they provide most of the physical and emotional care to patients who wish to remain in their homes (FCA, 2019). In 2015 approximately 43.5 million caregivers provided unpaid caregiving to an adult or child. About 34.2 million caregivers cared for a family member who was 50 years of age or older (FCA, 2019). More than one

BOX 10.2 FOCUS ON OLDER ADULTS

Family Caregiver Concerns

- Families often need help to determine their caregiving roles for the various members of the family (e.g., providing additional financial support, designating someone to obtain groceries and medications, providing hands-on physical care).
- Caregivers report loss of income and family savings when one member leaves work to provide care (Meyer, 2020).
- A caregiver's mental health is often at risk, with caregivers reporting an increase in depression, isolation, and stress-related symptoms (Meyer, 2020).
- Caregivers' personal health is at risk, as there is an increase in missed routine screening and management of chronic illness (Meyer, 2020).
- Older adults who have spiritual strength make use of it to make end-of-life decisions and cope with life changes (Moss et al., 2018; Puchalski et al., 2020).
- Social networks and support from family and friends can help mediate the stress experienced by caregivers (Marcum et al., 2020).
- Individualized caregiver education and support are essential. Interprofessional collaboration allows for caregiver education, improved communication, and coping (Off et al., 2019).

in six Americans who work full- or part-time are family caregivers (FCA, 2016). Most working family caregivers rearrange their work schedule, decrease their hours, or take an unpaid leave to meet the caregiving needs of their family member (FCA, 2016). Spouses in their 60s and 70s often are the major caregivers for each other. Older-adult caregivers have special needs (Box 10.2).

Caring for a relative who is frail or chronically ill is an ongoing process in which families must continue to redefine their relationships and roles (DePasquale et al., 2018). Family caregiving occurs within the context of a family and requires more than a simple series of tasks. It encompasses multiple cognitive, behavioral, and interpersonal processes. Caregiving activities include finding resources, providing personal care (bathing, feeding, or grooming), monitoring for complications or side effects of an illness or treatment, and providing instrumental activities of daily living (shopping or housekeeping). Family caregivers also provide ongoing emotional support for their loved ones, making decisions about care options, being a patient advocate, monitoring finances, and maintaining the integrity of the family unit. Whether a husband is caring for his wife or a child is caring for a parent, caregiving is an interactional process. The interpersonal dynamic between family members influences the ultimate quality of caregiving.

Family caregiving can be positive and rewarding, but it can also create caregiver burden and strain. The physical and emotional demands are high. A patient's disease creates changes in the family structure and roles. Family caregivers often do not feel prepared to take on the demands of care for their loved ones. Caregivers have mixed experiences and feelings. Family caregivers often lose some of their social, economic, and physical freedom, which can affect both their mental and their emotional health (Mathias, 2019). In addition, sometimes caregivers do not consider their personal health needs as a high priority and miss routine primary care visits, screenings, and dental care (Meyer, 2020).

Poverty. Although the poverty rate in the United States has been falling since 2014, the impact of poverty on families is profound (Semega et al., 2020). Female single-parent families and families with unrelated individuals are especially vulnerable (Semega et al., 2020). Children continue to be the poorest age-group in America, with the youngest children and children of color being the poorest (Cree et al., 2018). Individuals and families who live in poverty are more likely to be uninsured (Cree et al., 2018).

Although the Affordable Care Act (ACA) improved access to affordable health insurance, the challenge to access appropriate health care continues, especially for individuals and families who are at or near the poverty level (Centers for Disease Control and Prevention [CDC], 2019). When caring for families who live in poverty, be sensitive to their need for independence and help them obtain appropriate financial and health care resources. For example, help a family by providing information about resources within the community to obtain assistance with food, energy bills, dental and health care, and school supplies.

Homelessness. Homelessness is a major public health issue that affects the functioning, health, and well-being of the family and its members (Children's Defense Fund [CDF], 2020). Chronic homelessness is experienced by people who need to use homeless shelters for their long-term housing needs. In contrast, people who experience transitional episodic homelessness need shelter for one stay and for a short period of time (National Coalition for the Homeless, 2019). People who are homeless tend to be younger, with a catastrophic event requiring them to seek shelter.

Adults who are homeless face many health risks. They are more likely to have mental and chronic health problems (U.S. Interagency Council on Homelessness, 2018). Exposure to the elements, poor nutritional status, and poor access to health care affect the health of people who are homeless. They are also vulnerable to physical and emotional violence, injury, and trauma.

Poverty, domestic violence, reduced government support for families with dependent children, and lack of affordable housing contribute to homelessness in families (National Coalition for the Homeless, 2019). Children of families who are homeless are often in fair or poor health and have higher rates of asthma, ear infections, stomach problems, mental illness, poor dental health, and poor immunization documentation. The emergency department often becomes their only access to health care.

Children who are homeless face barriers such as meeting residency requirements for public schools and inability to obtain previous enrollment records when enrolling into and attending a new school. They often lack adult supervision to help them with homework and school-related issues. As a result, they are more likely to drop out of school, develop risky behaviors, and become unemployable (Barnes et al., 2018; National Alliance to End Homelessness, 2020). Homelessness increases the risk for developing long-term health, psychological, and socioeconomic problems, posing a major challenge for our entire society (Barnes et al., 2018; National Alliance to End Homelessness, 2020) (see Chapter 3).

Domestic Violence. Domestic violence includes not only intimate-partner relationships of spousal, live-in partners, and dating relationships but also familial, elder, and child abuse. Emotional, physical, and sexual abuse occurs across all social classes (Futures Without Violence, 2021; Weil, 2020).

Factors associated with family violence are complex and include stress, poverty, social isolation, psychopathology, and learned family behavior. Other factors such as alcohol and drug abuse, pregnancy, sexual orientation, and mental illness increase the incidence of abuse within a family (Futures Without Violence, 2021; Weil, 2020). Although abuse sometimes ends when a person leaves a family environment, negative long-term physical and emotional consequences often linger. One of the consequences includes moving from one abusive situation to another. For example, a child sees marriage as a solution to leave a parents' abusive home and in turn marries a person who continues the abuse in the marriage (Futures Without Violence, 2021; Weil, 2020).

Structure

Structure is based on the ongoing membership of the family and the pattern of relationships, which are often numerous and complex (Kaakinen et al., 2018). Each family has a unique structure and way of functioning. For example, a family member may have relationships with a spouse, child, employer, and work colleagues. Each of these relationships has different demands, roles, and expectations. The multiple relationships and their expectations are often sources of personal and family stress (see Chapter 37).

Structure either enhances or detracts from a family's ability to respond to the expected and unexpected stressors of daily life. Structures that are too rigid or flexible sometimes threaten family functioning. Rigid structures specify who accomplishes different tasks and limit the number of people outside the immediate family allowed to assume these tasks. For example, in one family with a rigid structure, the mother is the only acceptable person to provide emotional support for the children and/or to perform all the household chores. The father is the only acceptable person to provide financial support, maintain the vehicles, do the yard work, and make all the home repairs. A change in the health status of the person responsible for a task places a burden on a rigid family because no other person is available, willing, experienced, or considered acceptable to assume that task. An extremely flexible family structure also presents problems for the family. The absence of stability sometimes prevents other family members from acting during a crisis or rapid change.

Function

Family function is what a family does, such as how a family interacts to socialize younger family members, cooperates to meet economic needs, and relates to the larger society. Family function involves the processes used by a family to achieve its goals (Fig. 10.2). Some processes include communication among family members, goal setting, conflict resolution, caregiving, nurturing, and the use of internal and external resources. Although family members pursue family goals at various times during their development, they need emotional and psychosocial support throughout their life span to be successful.

FAMILY NURSING

Family nursing assumes that all people, regardless of age, are members of some type of family form. The goal of family nursing is to help a family and its individual members reach and maintain maximum health throughout and beyond the illness experience. Family nursing is the focus across all practice settings and is important in all health care environments.

FIG. 10.2 Family recreational activities strengthen family functioning. (Courtesy Bill Branson, National Cancer Institute.)

There are different approaches for family nursing practice. For the purposes of this chapter, family nursing practice has three levels of approaches: (1) *family as context*, (2) *family as patient*, and (3) *family as a system*. Family as a system includes both relational and transactional concepts. All approaches recognize that patient-centered care for one member influences all members and affects family functioning. Families are continually changing. As a result, the need for family support changes over time, and it is important for you to understand that the family is more complex than simply a combination of individual members.

Family as Context

When you view a family as context, the primary focus is on the health and development of an individual member existing within a specific family environment. Although you focus on the health of an individual family member, also assess how much the family provides the individual's basic needs. Needs vary, depending on an individual's developmental level and situation. Consider the family's ability to help your patient meet physical as well as psychological needs when viewing a family as context.

Family as Patient

When you view a family as patient, the family's needs, processes, and relationships (e.g., parenting or family caregiving) are the primary focus of nursing care. Your nursing assessment focuses on family patterns versus characteristics of individual members. Use critical thinking and clinical judgment to concentrate on patterns and processes that are consistent with reaching and maintaining family and individual health. For example, in the case of family caregiving, determine who the family caregivers are, their different roles, and how they interact to meet a patient's needs. Plan care to meet the patient's and family's changing needs. Dealing with overly complex family problems often requires an interprofessional approach. Know the limits of nursing practice and make referrals when appropriate.

Family as a System

Although you make theoretical and practical distinctions between the family as context and the family as patient, they are not necessarily mutually exclusive. When you care for a family as a system, you are caring for each family member (family as context) and the family unit (family as patient), using all available environmental, social, psychological, and community resources.

The following clinical scenario illustrates three levels of approaches to family care.

You are assisting with end-of-life care for David Daniels, who is 35 years old and is a computer programmer. David and his wife, Lisa, have three school-age children. David expressed a wish to die at home. Lisa is on family leave from her job to help David through this period. Both Lisa and David are only children. David's parents are no longer living, but Lisa's mother is committed to staying with the family to help Lisa and David.

When you view this *family as context,* you focus first on the patient (David) as an individual. You assess and meet David's needs at end-of-life, such as comfort, hygiene, and nutrition, as well as his social and emotional needs. You determine how David is coping with knowing his life is coming to an end and how he perceives it will affect his family. When viewing *the family as patient,* you assess and meet the needs of David's wife and children. Determine to what extent the family's basic needs for normal activity, comfort, and nutrition are being met and whether they have resources for emotional and social support. You determine the family's need for rest (especially Lisa's) and their stage of coping (the oldest child shows much anger and fear). You determine the demands placed on David and the family, such as economic survival

and well-being of the children. In addition, you continually assess the family's available resources such as time, coping skills, and energy level to support David through the end-of-life.

When viewing a *family as a system,* you use elements from both the context and patient perspectives and assess the resources available to the family system. Using the knowledge of the family as context, patient, and system, individualize care decisions based on your family assessment and clinical judgment. For example, based on assessment data, you determine that the family is not eating adequately. You also determine that Lisa is experiencing more stress, not sleeping well, and trying to "do it all" regarding her children's school and after-school activities. In addition, Lisa does not want to leave David's bedside when members of their church come to help. You recognize that this family is under enormous stress and that their basic needs such as nutrition, rest, and school activities are not adequately met. As a result, you determine that (1) the family needs help with meals, (2) Lisa needs time to rest, and (3) the family's church is eager to help with David's day-to-day care. Based on these insights, you have a family conference and set up a schedule among Lisa, her mother, and two close church members to provide Lisa with some time away from David's bedside. During the conference, David and Lisa determine when this time will be. Because of the church involvement, members of the church begin to purchase groceries and make all the meals for the family. In addition, other members of the church help with the children's school and after-school activities.

Family and Health

Although American families exist within the same United States culture, there are cultural disparities, and individual family members vary greatly in their experiences, beliefs, and values. When a family is victim to low educational preparation, poverty, and decreased social support, these factors compound one another, magnifying their effect on the health and well-being of the family. Economic stability increases a family's access to adequate health care, creates more opportunity for education, increases good nutrition, and decreases stress (National Coalition for the Homeless, 2019).

The family is the primary social context in which health promotion and disease prevention take place. A family's beliefs, values, and practices strongly influence the family's structure and function. They also affect family communication patterns, roles, and health-promoting practices. Providing culturally appropriate family-centered interventions and teaching can improve family functioning and self-care (Giger and Haddad, 2021).

Some families do not place a high value on good health. In fact, harmful practices are accepted by some families. For example, some families use high-caloric food intake as an acceptable way to cope with stress. Sometimes a family member gives mixed messages about health. For example, a parent chooses to smoke while telling children that smoking is bad for them. Family environment is crucial because health behavior reinforced in early life has a strong influence on later health practices. In addition, the family environment is a crucial factor in an individual's adjustment to a crisis.

Attributes of Healthy Families. The family is a dynamic unit; it is exposed to threats, strengths, changes, and challenges. Some families are crisis proof, whereas others are crisis prone. A crisis-proof, or effective, family combines the need for stability with the need for growth and change. This type of family has a flexible structure that allows different family members to complete tasks and accepts help from outside the family system. The structure is flexible enough to allow adaptability but not so flexible that the family lacks cohesiveness and a sense of stability. An effective family controls the environment and influences the immediate environment of home, neighborhood, and school. An ineffective, or crisis-prone, family lacks or believes it lacks control over its environment.

Hardiness and resiliency moderate a family's stress, thus affecting a family's health. **Family hardiness** includes the internal strengths and durability of the family unit. Psychological hardiness has a direct relationship with the quality of life including characteristics that provide a source of strength against stressful events. Hardiness is demonstrated with a commitment to find meaning and knowledge that life events are controllable and predictable. Challenging situations are seen as an opportunity for growth (Kandi and Zeinali, 2017) Family resilience is demonstrated when there is a high level of spirituality, life satisfaction, low levels of depression, and the ability to withstand life difficulties and stressors (Wakhid et al., 2020). Resources (e.g., adequate income, education) and techniques (e.g., coping resources) that a family or individuals within the family use to maintain a balance or level of health aid in understanding a family's level of resiliency.

Genetic Factors. Genetic factors reflect a family's heredity or genetic susceptibility to diseases that may or may not result in actual development of a disease. The scope of genomics in nursing care is broad and encompasses risk assessment, risk management, counseling and treatment options, and treatment decisions. Clinical applications of genetic and genomic knowledge for nurses have implications for care of people, families, communities, and populations across the life span (National Institutes of Health [NIH], 2020; Raby et al., 2020).

Sometimes identification of genetic factors and genetic counseling help family members decide whether to test for the presence of a disease and/or to have children. Some families choose not to have children; others choose not to know genetic risks and have children; other families choose to know the risk and then determine whether to have children. Some of these diseases (e.g., heart or kidney disease) are manageable. With genetic risks for certain cancers such as some breast cancers, a woman may choose prophylactic bilateral mastectomy to reduce the risk for developing the disease. Families with genetic neurological diseases such as Huntington disease may choose not to have children. When families know of these risks, they can make informed decisions about their lifestyle and health behaviors, are more vigilant about recognizing changes in their health, and in some cases seek medical intervention earlier.

Living With Acute or Chronic Illnesses, Diseases, or Trauma. Any acute or chronic disease influences an entire family economically, emotionally, socially, and functionally. Diseases and illness also affect a family's decision-making and coping resources (see Chapter 6). Hospitalization of a family member is stressful for the whole family. Heath care environments are foreign, physicians and nurses are strangers, the medical language is difficult to understand or interpret, and family members are often separated from one another.

During an acute health crisis that requires hospitalization, family members are sometimes left in waiting rooms to receive information about their loved one. Communication among family members may be misunderstood from fear and worry. Previous family conflicts can rise to the surface, whereas others are suppressed. Interprofessional teams often are helpful in meeting the needs of families experiencing acute health problems.

Chronic illnesses and diseases present continuous challenges for families. Frequently family patterns and interactions, roles, social activities, work and household schedules, economic resources, and other family needs and functions must be reorganized around the chronic illness or disability (see Chapter 8).

Trauma is sudden, unplanned, and sometimes life threatening. Family members often struggle to cope with the challenges of a severe life-threatening event. For example, they often deal with stressors associated with a family member hospitalized in an intensive care environment, anxiety, depression, economic burden, and the impact of the trauma on family functioning and decision making (Newcomb and Hymes, 2017). The powerlessness that family members experience makes them very vulnerable and less able to make important decisions about the health of the family.

When implementing a family-centered care model for patients experiencing acute or chronic illnesses, diseases, or trauma, patients' family members and surrogate decision makers become active partners in decision making and care. Involving family during a hand-off report from one care provider to another, for example, provides an opportunity to involve a patient and family in discussing the present and long-term plan of care (Bigani and Correia, 2018). When possible, patients and family caregivers want to participate in shared decision making about treatment options and ongoing symptom management (Sebern, 2018). Incorporating a patient's and family's cultural beliefs, values, and communication patterns is essential to provide individualized patient/family-centered care (Giger and Haddad, 2020).

In caring for family members, advocate for the patient and family and answer their questions honestly (Gross, 2020; Newcomb and Hymes, 2017). When you do not know the answer, find someone who does. Ensure that the family knows all the members of the health care team. Provide realistic assurance; giving false hope breaks the nurse-patient trust and affects how the family can adjust to "bad news" (Schultz et al., 2017). When a patient is hospitalized, take time to make sure that the family is comfortable. You can bring them something to eat or drink, give them a blanket, or encourage them to get a meal. Sometimes telling a family that you will stay with their loved one while they are gone is all they need to feel comfortable in leaving.

End-of-Life Care. You will encounter families with a member who is terminally ill. Although people equate terminal illness with cancer, many diseases have terminal aspects (e.g., heart failure, pulmonary and renal diseases, and neuromuscular diseases). Although some family members may be prepared for their loved one's death, their need for information, support, assurance, and presence is great (see Chapter 36). Use presence to develop a therapeutic relationship with a patient and family (see Chapter 7). Also use therapeutic communication to enhance family members' relationships with one another and to promote shared decision making (Brooks et al., 2017; Gross, 2020). The more you know about your patient's family, how they interact with one another, their strengths, and their weaknesses, the better. Each family approaches and copes with end-of-life decisions differently. Encourage a patient and family to make decisions about care (e.g., pain control or preferred nonpharmacological comfort measures) and specific therapies. Help a family set up home care if they desire, and make referrals for hospice and other appropriate resources, including grief support. Provide information about the dying process and make sure family members know what to do at the time of death. If you are present at the time of death, be sensitive to a family's needs (e.g., provide for privacy and allow sufficient time for saying goodbyes).

FAMILY-CENTERED CARE AND THE NURSING PROCESS

Nurses interact with families in a variety of community-based and clinical settings. Apply the nursing process and use critical thinking and clinical judgment to develop and implement family-centered nursing care. The approach to the nursing process is the same whether your focus is family as context, patient, or system. When caring for families, use the same process you use with individual patients, but also incorporate the needs and preferences of the family. You use the nursing process to care for an individual within a family (e.g., the family as context) or the entire family (e.g., the family as patient). When initiating the care of families, use these approaches to organize a family-centered approach to the nursing process:

1. Assess all individuals within their family context.
2. Assess the family as patient.
3. Assess the family as a system.

Family Assessment

Using a family-centered approach to assessment allows you to establish a working relationship with the patient and family. A complete assessment provides you a full picture of patient needs as a member of a family and of the family needs as well. If your assessment is complete, it ensures that the patient and family needs are correctly identified and that mutual outcomes and interventions for health care can be established.

Often you will participate in conflict resolution between family members, so each member is able to confront and resolve problems in a healthy way. Ask assessment questions to help the family identify external and internal resources, as necessary. For example, who in the family can run errands to get groceries while the patient is unable to drive? Are there members from the church who can come and provide respite care? Ultimately your aim is to help the family reach a point of optimal function, given the family's resources, capacities, and desire to become healthier.

You play an essential role in helping families adjust to acute, chronic, and terminal illness; however, first you need to understand the family unit and what a patient's illness means to the family members and family functioning. You also need to understand how the illness affects the family structure and the support the family requires (Kaakinen et al., 2018). Although the family as a whole differs from individual members, the measure of family health is more than a summary of the health of all members. The form, structure, function, and health of the family are areas unique to family assessment. Several culturally sensitive tools and models assess or measure family dynamics (Giddens, 2021). Box 10.3 provides examples of family assessment questions based on the Calgary Family Assessment Model (Baldwin, 2020; Shajani and Snell, 2019).

While completing your assessment, consider knowledge of a patient's illness and its potential impact on the family. Because time is limited in many practice settings, it is critical for you to understand how significant a role the family will play in a patient's treatment decisions and recovery. This factor will affect how comprehensive an assessment you conduct. Begin the family assessment by determining a patient's definition of and attitude toward the family. A person's concept of family is highly individualized. The patient's definition will influence how much you are able to incorporate the family into nursing care. When it becomes obvious that family is important for a patient, determine family form and membership by asking whom the patient considers family or with whom the patient shares strong feelings. If the patient is unable to express a concept of family, ask with whom they live, spend time, and share confidences and then ask whether they consider them to be family or like family. To further assess the family structure, ask questions that determine the power structure and patterning of roles and tasks (e.g., "Who decides where to go on vacation?" "How are tasks divided in your family?" "Who mows the lawn?" "Who usually prepares the meals?").

Assess family functions such as the ability to provide emotional support for members, the ability to cope with current health problems or situations, and the appropriateness of its goal setting. Also determine whether the family has sufficient economic resources and whether its social network is extensive enough to provide support.

BOX 10.3 Family Assessment Questions

Family Structure

Determines members of the family, relationships among family members, and the context of the family

- Who are the members of your family? How are they related to you?
- Who lives with you?
- Has anyone recently moved out of your home?
- Is there anyone who does not live with you whom you consider to be family?

Developmental Assessment

Determines how families adapt during predictable and unpredictable changes and difficult times

- What transitions/changes (e.g., recent death, divorce, children leaving/returning home, new births) has your family experienced most recently?
- Are there any members of your family who are having problems (e.g., difficulty in school, acute or chronic illnesses) that are currently affecting your family?
- What aspects of your family do you enjoy the most?
- What plans have you or your family made to care for family members who are in poor health?

Family Functioning

Addresses how individuals behave in relation to one another; includes instrumental aspects, which are routine activities (e.g., making meals, doing laundry), and expressive aspects (e.g., communication, problem solving, roles, influence and power, beliefs)

- Describe a recent problem and how your family resolved it.
- Who is the caregiver for children or older adults?
- What coping strategies does your family use (e.g., exercise, avoidance, overeating, arguing)?
- What are your family beliefs about health/illness, end-of-life care, and advance directives?
- What does your family mean to you?
- How does your family celebrate holidays, birthdays, weddings?
- How do the members of your family manage their health? How do they manage care of a sick family member?
- When someone is ill, who is the caregiver? Is it always the same person?

Cultural Aspects. Always recognize and respect a family's cultural background during your assessment (see Chapter 9). Culture is an important variable when assessing a family because race, ethnicity, language, and norms affect structure, function, health beliefs, values, and the way a family perceives events (Box 10.4). A comprehensive, culturally sensitive family assessment is critical to analyzing cues and forming an understanding of family life, family preferences, current changes in family life, and overall goals and expectations, and to planning family-centered care.

Forming conclusions about families' needs based on cultural backgrounds requires critical thinking and clinical judgment. Developing clinical judgment through the use of critical thinking is important to deliver safe, high-quality, family-centered care (see Chapter 15). It is imperative to remember that categorical generalizations are often misleading. Overgeneralizations in terms of racial and ethnic group characteristics do not lead to greater understanding of a culturally diverse family. Culturally different families vary in meaningful and significant ways; however, neglecting to examine similarities leads to inaccurate assumptions and stereotyping (Giger and Haddad, 2021).

Knowing about a family's culture and the meaning of that culture to a family's structure and functioning, health practices, and family celebrations helps to design family-centered care (see Chapter 9). To determine the influence of culture on a family, ask patients about their

BOX 10.4 CULTURAL ASPECTS OF CARE

Family Nursing

Families have unique perspectives and characteristics, and they have differences in values, beliefs, and philosophies. The cultural heritage of a family or member of the family affects religious, childrearing, and health care practices; recreational activities; and nutritional preferences. Be culturally sensitive and respectful when caring for patients of all cultures. Incorporate individualized cultural preferences into your plan of care so that it is culturally congruent. Design your care to integrate the family preferences, personal values, life patterns, and beliefs of the patient and family into prescribed therapies.

Implications for Patient-Centered Care

- Focus on the needs of the family, and understand the family's beliefs, values, customs, preferences, and roles when designing care. Perception of events and their impact on the family varies across cultural groups. For example, the care of the grandmother may have a great significance to the extended family.
- Family caregiving values, practices, and roles and perceptions of the burden associated with family caregiving vary across cultures (Konerding et al., 2018).
- The family structure sometimes includes multiple generations living together. Intergenerational support and patterns of living arrangements are often related to cultural background (Cohen and Passel, 2018).
- In some cultures, it is a sign of disrespect to place older adults in nursing homes, even when an older-adult family member has severe dementia (Giger and Haddad, 2021).
- Modesty is a strong value among many cultures. Some women bring female family members to health care visits, and a female health care provider must examine the woman.
- In the presence of a critical or terminal illness, some cultures come in groups to pray together with the family at the patient's bedside (Giger and Haddad, 2021).
- Health beliefs differ among various cultures; these differences affect the decisions of a family and its members about when and where to seek help.

REFLECT NOW

Reflect on a family you know that is currently experiencing a life transition. What questions could you ask to assess this family's current needs?

Nursing Diagnoses for Families

After assessing a patient's and family's needs and situation, you identify nursing diagnoses. Several positive and negative diagnoses can be used when caring for families. Examples of nursing diagnoses applicable to family care are:

- *Conflicting Caregiver Attitude*
- *Impaired Family Coping*
- *Risk for Caregiver Stress*
- *Impaired Family Process*
- *Risk for Impaired Parent Child Attachment*
- *Family Able to Participate in Care Planning*
- *Family Knowledge of Disease*

Nursing diagnoses that relate to a family often focus on a family's ability to cope with its current situation. Appropriate use of resources helps a family cope with unexpected events that threaten health and stability. Nursing diagnoses often focus on changes in family processes or roles. For example, a man who is married and has four children is in a motor vehicle accident. He sustained multiple fractures to his lower extremities and pelvis and will be non–weight-bearing for 6 to 8 weeks after discharge. Therefore he cannot go to work and perform many of the activities (e.g., mowing the lawn, taking the children to school) that he normally performs. His spouse is feeling overwhelmed as she develops a plan to meet all the family's needs, which include her husband's needs for rehabilitation. Based on these data, you determine that *Impaired Family Process related to immobility and temporary changes in family roles* is an appropriate nursing diagnosis for this family. Often your assessment will identify multiple interrelated nursing diagnoses for the family.

Planning Family-Centered Care

Once you identify relevant nursing diagnoses, work together with patients and their families to develop plans of care that all members clearly understand and mutually agree to follow. The outcomes you establish need to be concrete and realistic, compatible with the family members' developmental stages (see Chapter 11), and acceptable to family members and their lifestyle.

By offering alternatives for care activities and asking family members for their own ideas and suggestions, you help to include them in the decision making and better meet the patient's needs (Stockwell-Smith et al., 2018). For example, offering options for how to prepare a low-fat diet or how to rearrange the furnishings of a room to accommodate a family member's disability gives a family an opportunity to express their preferences, make choices, and ultimately feel as though they have contributed. Collaborating with other disciplines such as physical therapy and social services increases the likelihood of a comprehensive approach to a family's health care needs, and it ensures better continuity of care. Using other disciplines is particularly important when discharge planning from a health care agency to home or an extended care facility is necessary.

Implementing Family-Centered Care

You will provide family-centered nursing care in a variety of health care settings, whether you are providing health promotion, acute care,

cultural background. Then ask questions concerning cultural practices. For example, "What type of foods do you eat?" "Who cares for sick family members?" "Have you or anyone in your family been hospitalized?" "Did family members remain at the hospital?" "Do you use any health practices of your culture such as acupuncture or meditation?" "What role do grandparents play in raising your children?"

A comprehensive, culturally sensitive family assessment is critical for you to understand family life, family preferences, the current changes within it, and a family's overall goals and expectations. These data provide the foundation for family-centered nursing care (Sousza et al., 2017).

Discharge Planning. Discharge planning begins with the initiation of care and includes the family. You are responsible for an accurate assessment of who will provide caregiving and what will be needed for care in the home at the time of discharge. Consider how the patient's physical and/or cognitive limitations will affect daily living activities and the impact this will have on the family. For example, if a patient who is an older adult is discharged to home after surgery and the patient's spouse cannot perform required dressing changes, you need to find out if anyone else in the family or within their support system is willing and able to do this. If not, you will need to arrange for a home care referral. If the patient also needs exercise and strength training, you consult with the primary health care provider to recommend referral for physical therapy.

or restorative and continuing care. It is important to develop individualized nursing interventions to meet the needs of your patients and their families.

Health Promotion. Although many people learn health behaviors from their families, the primary focus on health promotion has traditionally been on individuals. When implementing family nursing, health promotion interventions are designed to improve or maintain the physical, social, emotional, and spiritual well-being of the family unit and its members (Duhamel, 2017). Health promotion behaviors sometimes need to be tied to the developmental stages of the family members (e.g., adequate prenatal care for the childbearing family or adherence to immunization schedules for the childrearing family). Your interventions need to enable individual members and the total family to reach their optimal levels of wellness.

Whether you provide care for the family as context, patient, or system, evidence-based nursing interventions increase family members' ability to provide care, remove barriers to health care, and perform tasks the family is not currently able to do (Box 10.5). Assist a family in problem solving and express a sense of acceptance and caring by listening carefully to family members' concerns and suggestions.

One of the roles you need to adopt is that of educator (Fig. 10.3). Health education is a process by which a nurse and patient share information (see Chapter 25). Sometimes you recognize family/patient needs for information through direct questioning, but the methods for recognizing these needs are generally subtle. For example, you recognize that a new father is fearful of cleaning his newborn's umbilical cord or that an older-adult woman is not using her cane or walker safely. Respectful communication is necessary. Often you find the subtle needs for information by saying, "I notice you are trying to not touch the umbilical cord. I see that a lot." Or "You use the cane the way I did before I was shown a way to keep from falling or tripping over it; do you mind if I show you?" When you are confident and skillful instead of coming across as an authority on the subject, your patient's defenses are down, making the patient more willing to listen without feeling embarrassed. You will also recognize patient and family learning needs based on a patient's health condition and physical and mental limitations. Your focus as an educator may be on the family caregiver to prepare that person to manage the skills and processes needed to manage a patient's needs within the home.

REFLECT NOW

Think about a time you provided education to a family to help them manage an illness. How did or could you use the teach-back method to evaluate the effectiveness of your teaching?

One approach for achieving outcomes and promoting health is the use of family strengths. Families do not always see their strengths. Help

---

BOX 10.5   EVIDENCE-BASED PRACTICE

Caregiving Education for the Family Caregiver

PICOT Question: Do tailored nursing interventions designed for family caregivers reduce caregiver burden and enhance caregiver well-being?

Evidence Summary

When a family member has an acute or chronic illness or experiences a trauma that changes physical or cognitive function, it is often a major life-changing event that affects all family members. The family faces many changes in family dynamics, social interactions, financial commitments, and emotional support systems (Newcomb and Hymes, 2017; Twaddle and McCormick, 2020). A patient's physical disabilities and altered mental status affect the family caregiver and other members of the family (Weisman de Mamani et al., 2018). As a result, family members report stress and burnout related to the continual demands of the caregiving role (Moriarty et al., 2018). Lower levels of caregiver burden are associated with better mental health in caregivers (Weisman de Mamani et al., 2018). Caregiver coping, especially during hospitalizations, is often influenced by communication with providers, access to the patient, and the presence of staff helping to explain the patient's problems and treatment plan (Newcomb and Hymes, 2017). Providing interventions tailored to the needs of the caregiver reduces caregiver burden and improves caregiver coping and quality of life (Bekdemir and Ilhan, 2019; Weisman de Mamani et al., 2018).

Application to Nursing Practice

- Teach family caregivers to focus on the present moment using mindfulness-based interventions (e.g., meditation, breathing exercises, guided imagery) to reduce caregiver burden and improve mental health. Current evidence shows that mindfulness is often helpful, especially in caregivers for patients with long-term conditions (Hicken et al., 2017; Parkinson et al., 2019; Weisman de Mamani et al., 2018).
- Carefully assess the mental health of the caregiver. Encourage caregivers to discuss their feelings about caregiving responsibilities and help shape their perceptions in a way to improve their mental health (Weisman de Mamani

et al., 2018). For example, if a caregiver states, "I feel trapped by having to bathe my mother," encourage the caregiver to frame this in a more adaptive way, such as "I now have the opportunity to provide care for someone who used to take care of me."
- Encourage family caregivers to remain engaged in a patient's care during hospitalizations (e.g., encourage mobilization, assist with meals, discuss patient education) (Newcomb and Hymes, 2017).
- Teach caregivers for patients living with dementia different ways to cope with and redirect behavioral disturbances associated with dementia to help reduce caregiver burden and distress (Press and Alexander, 2020). In addition, helping caregivers "find a balance" between competing caregiving needs reduces stress and role strain (Hsin-Yun et al, 2021).
- Be aware of and assess for cultural implications of different physical and mental illnesses and their effect on the caregiver. For example, having a mental illness such as schizophrenia is sometimes accompanied by social stigma and isolation in some cultures. Refer caregivers to support groups to encourage them to share their feelings and experiences with others who are in similar situations, and help family members communicate effectively with one another to avoid conflict (Allen, 2020).
- Assess the effect (e.g., physical, mental, financial) of a patient's disability on the family. Provide support and patient education targeted to a patient's and family caregiver's needs. For example, some family caregivers of veterans who have posttraumatic stress disorder (PTSD) and/or traumatic brain injury (TBI) experience greater financial issues and depressive symptoms. Providing emotional support and helping families identify financial resources may reduce caregiver burden and improve coping with PTSD and TBI (Moriarty et al., 2018).
- Use telephone- or Internet-assisted technologies based on family caregiver preferences to provide support and patient education when it is difficult for the caregiver to receive effective support because of geographical constraints (e.g., in rural settings) (Allen, 2020; Hicken et al., 2017).

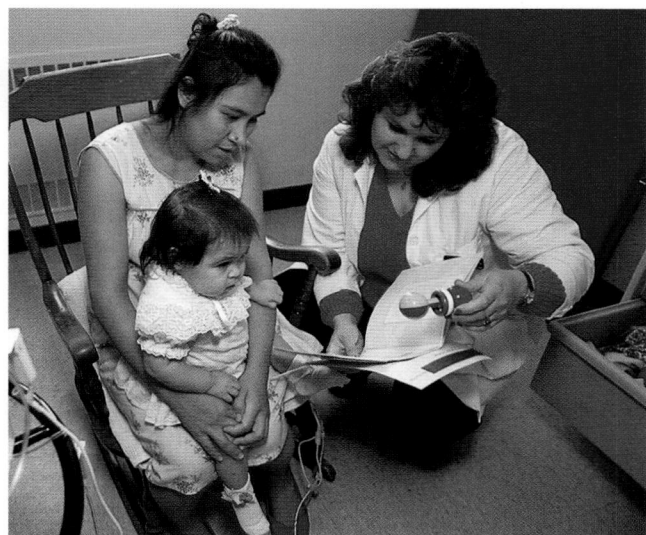

FIG. 10.3 Nurse providing family education. (From Hockenberry MJ, Wilson D, Rodgers CC: *Wong's nursing care of infants and children*, ed 11, St Louis, 2019, Mosby.)

families use their strengths to improve their health and achieve their outcomes. Family strengths may include clear communication, adaptability, healthy childrearing practices, and support and nurturing among family members. Other strengths exist in the form of the use of crisis for growth, a commitment to one another and the family unit, a sense of well-being and cohesiveness, and spirituality. Help the family focus on their strengths instead of on problems and weaknesses. For example, point out that a couple's 30-year marriage has endured many crises and transitions. Therefore they are likely to be able to adapt to this latest challenge. Refer families to health promotion programs aimed at enhancing these strengths as needed. For example, some communities have low-cost fitness activities for children and their families that are designed to reduce the risk for obesity.

Acute Care. The family must be a central focus of nursing care in the acute care setting. It is crucial to emphasize family needs within the context of today's acute health care delivery environment. The complex health care system requires you to be astute, use time wisely, and anticipate the type of interventions needed to support family and patient needs up to and including discharge. The Synergy Model recognizes the importance of the relationship between the nurse and the patient and family to create a healing environment (Byrum et al., 2020; Fournier, 2017). According to this model, when caring for acutely ill patients and their families, integrate your professional knowledge, skills, experiences, and attitudes to meet the needs of patients and their families. Consider the environmental factors that affect the family when planning care. The needs and characteristics of a patient and family drive nursing interventions. When there is synergy between a patient and family and a nurse, optimal patient outcomes result.

Include family caregivers in a patient's care during admission to better prepare them for their role and reduce stress following discharge (Alper et al., 2020). Because hospital stays are shortened, it is important to provide education and encourage families to take an active role in caregiving on admission. For example, if you are caring for a patient who will need to go home with multiple medications, including a subcutaneous injection, provide information to the patient and family about the medications and administration of injections throughout the patient's hospital stay.

One growing area in acute care for family caregivers is end-of-life care. You help family members in their caregiving role by allowing them to participate in decision making, ensuring clear communication between the family and the health care team, and supporting a family's resilience (Harman et al., 2020; Stajduhar et al., 2017). Help family caregivers find home care equipment and community resources and allow them to provide specific aspects of physical care they will need to perform at home. Preparing family members for discharge helps caregiving become a meaningful experience for both caregiver and patient across health care settings.

> **QSEN** **Building Competency in Teamwork and Collaboration** You are caring for the Carlson family. The father, Gary, is a 47-year-old chemical engineer who was diagnosed with amyotrophic lateral sclerosis (Lou Gehrig disease). He is experiencing a progressive degenerative disease affecting his muscles and is now hospitalized with aspiration pneumonia. He continues to weaken and is preparing to be discharged to home with a hospice consultation. His wife, Kathy, is 48 years old and is an information technology specialist. They have two children. Karen is a junior at a local university and lives in the residence hall. Kristen is a high school senior. The family is committed to helping Gary remain at home. Gary has been receiving care from physical therapy, respiratory therapy, the palliative care team, and pastoral care during this hospital stay. What can you do at this time to promote the teamwork and collaboration needed to make Gary's transition to home successful?
>
> Answers to QSEN Activities can be found on the Evolve website.

Discharge Planning. Discharge planning with a family is important during the acute care phase of an illness. An open relationship between you and a patient and family leads to a family-centered plan of care at discharge, including coordination of resources in the community and the patient's home (Gaskin, 2018). For example, when a patient who needs home intravenous (IV) antibiotic therapy is discharged, the family caregiver needs to know how to take care of the peripherally inserted central catheter (PICC) line, how to administer the IV antibiotic, how to recognize complications, and when to contact the home health nurse. Be sure the family caregiver is prepared for discharge and knows where to obtain necessary supplies.

Communication. An acute care setting involves multiple health care providers, and therefore clear communication is essential. It is important for the health care team to use communication techniques that are supportive, clear to understand, and consistent and that advocate for a family's expectations (Stajduhar et al., 2017). In addition, clear communication from the health care team helps to clarify medical terminology and enables the family to understand the health care issues, the types of decisions, and potential health care outcomes (see Chapter 24). Use clear plain language when you communicate, and provide professional interpreters if a patient or family does not speak English.

Help the family identify methods to maintain open lines of communication with you and the interprofessional health care team to anticipate your patient's and family members' needs. For example, when caring for a patient with ovarian cancer, how will you use caring practices to help her spouse inform family members about the patient's progress and plan of care? Identify who makes decisions for the family and consistently go to the decision maker. In some situations the decision maker also needs assistance in developing a method to clearly communicate any decisions. In this electronic age, some families use blogs or social media as a way of providing consistent information. Help the family determine whether this is the best approach for their family needs and structure.

Restorative and Continuing Care. In restorative and continuing care settings, the challenge in family nursing is to maintain patients' functional abilities within the context of the family. This includes having home care nurses help patients remain in their homes following acute injuries, diseases, or illnesses, surgery, or exacerbation of a chronic disease or illness. It also requires finding ways to improve the lives of individuals who are chronically ill or disabled and their families. Work closely with a patient and family to provide well-timed and targeted information, practical guidance, and instructions to help a family caregiver understand the specific care a patient will require in the home (Alper et al., 2020; Macleod et al., 2017).

When a patient's functional status changes, make sure that the home environment will accommodate the patient's strengths and limitations. Make a referral to home care. The patient may require other interprofessional care, such as occupational or physical therapy, as well. Clear, concise, and accurate communication with a home care nurse helps to provide continuity of care and facilitates transition from hospital to home. Educate family members about how they can participate in ongoing care and make changes in the home environment to help the patient be as self-sufficient as possible.

Family Caregiving. You help family caregivers by showing them how to perform specific aspects of physical care (e.g., dressing changes), by helping them find home care equipment (e.g., oxygen therapy), and by identifying other community resources (e.g., respite care facilities, rehab centers). Preparing members of the family for care activities and responsibilities helps caregiving become a meaningful experience for both the caregiver and the patient.

When family members become caregivers, their relationship with the care recipient often changes. Whenever one individual becomes dependent on another family member for care, significant stress affects both the caregiver and the care recipient (Kaakinen et al., 2018). Thus, you have a key role in helping the family caregiver and patient develop communication and problem-solving skills to support the relationships needed for successful caregiving (Zhang, 2018).

Without adequate preparation and support from health care providers, caregiving puts the family at risk. The resilience of caregivers during times of stress can be dependent on their commitment to each other, communication skills, and the capacity to solve problems and make decisions together (Meyer, 2020). If your assessment reveals that the relationship between potential caregivers and care recipients is not supportive, connect the patient and family with community services to provide the patient's caregiving needs.

You support a family caregiver in many ways. For example, listen to a caregiver's stories and help the caregiver continue to meet the demands of the usual lifestyle (e.g., working, raising children). Establish a caregiving schedule that enables all family members to participate, help patients to identify family members who can share the burdens posed by caregiving, and encourage distant relatives to communicate their support. Teach family caregivers to provide physical care for their family member. Recognize that family caregivers also have their own physical and emotional needs. Teach them how to meet their needs (Box 10.6) and set up respite times as appropriate to allow them time to care for themselves (Schaffer et al., 2017; Twaddle and McCormick, 2020).

Connect family caregivers with community resources. National outreach programs such as the Family Caregiver Alliance (https://www.caregiver.org/), Alzheimer's Association (https://www.alz.org/), and Caregiver Action Network (https://caregiveraction.org/) provide information and services that can help improve the lives of family caregivers and the care they provide to their loved ones.

Community resources are organizations that can provide needed services or respite care to give the family caregiver time away from the

---

BOX 10.6   PATIENT TEACHING
Family Caregiving: Caregiver Stress

Objective
- Patient/family will apply two interventions to reduce caregiver role strain.

Teaching Strategies
- Explain to all family caregivers the signs and symptoms of caregiver role strain such as:
  - Change in caregiver's appetite/weight, sleeping, or leisure activities
  - Social withdrawal, irritability, anger, or changes in the caregiver's overall level of health
  - Loss of interest in personal appearance
- Discuss situations in which caregiver role strain may intensify (e.g., if the patient's health status changes or the patient needs to be hospitalized).
- Describe the importance of having family members set up alternating schedules to give the primary caregiver some rest.
- Provide information about community resources for transportation, respite care, and support groups.
- Offer an opportunity to ask questions and, when possible, provide a phone number for questions and assistance.
- Provide family members with the contact information of the patient's health care provider and instruct them to call if the caregiver has health problems, the caregiver seems overly exhausted, or they observe changes in the caregiver's interactions and attention to normal activities.

Evaluation
Use the principles of teach-back to evaluate patient/family caregiver learning:
- "I want to be sure I explained the effects of being a caregiver so you can recognize when you are under stress. Describe two or three effects that caregiving can have on you."
- "Some families I have cared for have trouble coping with all the responsibilities they have with caring for a family member. Can you explain to me what you are planning to do to help you feel less burdened or overwhelmed?"
- "There may be a time when you are going to need to call your mother's health care provider. Where do you plan on keeping the health care provider's contact information? What situations do you imagine might happen that would require you to call the health care provider?"

---

care recipient. Examples of services that are beneficial to families include caregiver support groups, housing and transportation services, food and nutrition services, housecleaning, legal and financial services, home care, hospice, and mental health resources. It is critical that you understand the family's dynamics and their desire for support before referring a family to a community resource. Family caregivers sometimes resist help, feeling obligated to be the sole source of support to the care recipient. Be sensitive to family relationships and help caregivers understand the normalcy of caregiving demands. Given the appropriate resources, family caregivers are able to acquire the skills and knowledge necessary to effectively care for their loved ones within the context of the home while maintaining rich and rewarding personal relationships.

Evaluating the Outcomes of Family Care

Through the Patient's and Family's Eyes. It is important to obtain a family's perspective of the nursing care you provided and compare whether it met the family's expectations and outcomes. If your care did not meet the family's expectations, determine what they believe is missing. Consider short-term and long-term outcomes. Does the family perceive the patient received adequate pain control? Does the family perceive knowing what to do if problems develop at home? Does the family perceive adequate education and support from the health care team? Evaluation is continuous and helps you decide when you need to modify your interventions or make referrals to other members of the health care team.

Patient and Family Outcomes. Evaluation is patient and family centered. When you care for a family as the context, focus on whether patient and family needs were met. Compare the response of a patient and family with the outcomes you set in the patient's plan of care.

When a family is the patient, your measure of family health becomes more than an evaluation of the health of all family members. You continue to focus on the outcomes you set based on the family-centered nursing diagnoses. For example, you evaluate a family's change in functioning and its satisfaction with the new level of functioning to determine whether a family is achieving its outcomes.

When you are caring for a family as a system, your evaluation focuses on the effects that the interventions had on the entire family, including extended family members. For example, if you are caring for an older adult who is receiving chemotherapy for a new cancer diagnosis, you evaluate how frequent trips to the oncology clinic and the cancer diagnosis affect the patient, the spouse, the children, and the grandchildren.

Evaluation is an ongoing process. Use critical thinking, clinical judgment, and clinical decision making to evaluate a family's response to interventions. Often a patient and/or family does not know how to best deliver care. For example, a family does not think that making dietary changes for a patient who is experiencing anorexia and nausea from chemotherapy is being effective. Evaluate the patient's nutritional status (e.g., laboratory values, weight, skin turgor), and explain to the family which evaluation data show that the dietary changes have been effective. Adjust the patient's diet if indicated.

KEY POINTS

- Families are as diverse as the individuals who compose them. Some family members have different beliefs and traditions, even within the same generation.
- Families face many challenges, including changing structures and roles, especially as the laws, economic status, and demographics of society change.
- Family caregiving is an interactive process that occurs within the context of the relationships among its members. Family caregivers are often spouses who are older adults or adult children trying to work full-time and care for aging family members.
- Many factors, including the increased need for family caregivers, poverty, homelessness, and domestic violence, affect family forms and a family's health.
- A family's structure and functioning significantly influence the family's health, health needs, and ability to respond to health problems.
- Your decision to view a family as an important context for an individual family member or to view a family unit as the patient or as a system depends on the situation and the family's needs.
- The family is the primary social context in which health promotion and disease prevention take place. Family members influence one another's health beliefs, practices, and status.
- The concept of family is highly individual; focus the nursing process and nursing care on a patient's attitude and beliefs about family rather than on a traditional definition of family.
- As you provide family-centered care, you use clinical judgment and continually assess, analyze, and reflect on the changing needs and health care goals of patients and their families.

- The outcome of family nursing is to help a family and its individual members reach and maintain maximum health throughout and beyond the illness experience.
- Whether you are caring for a patient with the family as context, patient, or a system, you direct your nursing interventions to increase abilities of family members to function and perform, remove barriers to health care, and do things that the family cannot do for itself.
- Evaluation of nursing care of families is centered on the patient and family. Compare actual responses to care with the outcomes you set in the plan of care and revise the care plan as needed.

REFLECTIVE LEARNING

- Think about a patient you were assigned to care for recently. Describe the patient's family and its structure. What effect did that structure have on your patient's health?
- Interview a peer about his or her family. How do the beliefs and values of your peer's family affect the family's structure, functioning, health practices, and family celebrations?
- Reflect on a patient you cared for who had a family caregiver. What responsibilities did the family caregiver assume for the patient? Describe how the family caregiver coped with the caregiving role. What stressors related to caregiving did the family caregiver experience?

REVIEW QUESTIONS

1. A family includes a mother, a stepfather, two teenage biological daughters of the mother, and a biological daughter of the father. The father's daughter just moved home following the loss of her job in another city. The family is converting a study into a bedroom and is in the process of distributing household chores. Nursing assessment reveals that all members of the family think that their family can adjust to lifestyle changes. This is an example of family:
   1. Diversity
   2. Durability
   3. Resiliency
   4. Configuration
2. A mother and her two children are homeless and enter a free health care clinic. Which statements most likely describe the effects of homelessness on this family? (Select all that apply.)
   1. The children have stability in their education.
   2. The family members may have symptoms of malnutrition, such as anemia.
   3. The family is at a low risk for experiencing violence.
   4. The children are at higher risk for developing ear infections.
   5. All family members may have mental health issues.
3. A nurse is caring for a 66-year-old patient who lives alone and is receiving chemotherapy and radiation for a new cancer diagnosis. He is unable to care for himself because of severe pain and fatigue. He moves into his 68-year-old brother's home so his brother can help care for him. Which assessment findings indicate that this family caregiving situation will be successful? (Select all that apply.)
   1. Both the patient and his brother attend church together regularly.
   2. The brothers are living together and enjoy eating the same foods.
   3. Other siblings live in the same city and are willing to help.
   4. The patient and his brother have a close network of friends.
   5. The patient has obsessive-compulsive disorder and has difficulty throwing away possessions.
4. A family is facing job loss of the father, who is the major wage earner, and relocation to a new city where there is a new job. The children will have to switch schools, and his wife will have to resign

from the job she enjoys. Which of the following contribute to this family's hardiness? (Select all that apply.)
1. Family meetings
2. Established family roles
3. New neighborhood
4. Willingness to change in time of stress
5. Passive orientation to life

5. A patient who is newly divorced states, "Although I'm really scared about what happens next to my children and myself, I know that divorce is not uncommon today." What term does the nurse use in the patient's medical record to describe the characteristic displayed in this statement?
1. Durability
2. End-of-life care
3. Family functioning
4. Family's culture

6. A hospice nurse is caring for a family that is providing end-of-life care for their grandmother, who has terminal breast cancer. The nurse focuses on symptom management for the grandmother and on helping the family with developing coping skills. This approach is an example of which of the following?
1. Family as context
2. Family as patient
3. Family as a system
4. Family as structure

7. A 7-year-old child was recently diagnosed with asthma. A nurse is providing education to the child and her parents about the treatment and management of asthma and changes they need to make in their home environment to promote her health. Which statement made by the parents requires follow-up by the nurse?
1. "We've made an appointment to talk with the school nurse about the change in our child's health."
2. "We forgot to give our daughter her medications before bedtime, so we made a list of her medications to help us remember."
3. "We worked out a schedule to check on her before and after school."
4. "We haven't been spending time with our parents because we're so busy taking care of our daughter."

8. A family consisting of a grandparent, two adults, and three school-age children just immigrated to the United States. They come to a community wellness center to establish health care. Which of the following questions does the nurse ask to assess the family's function? (Select all that apply.)
1. "What does your family do to keep members healthy?"
2. "How does your family usually make decisions?"
3. "What health services are available in your neighborhood?"
4. "Which rituals or celebrations are important for your family?"
5. "Is there a lot of crime in your neighborhood?"
6. "How many parks are there in your community?"

9. A married couple has three children. The youngest child just graduated from college and is moving to a different city to take a job. The other two children left home several years ago. The parents of both spouses are older and are beginning to need help to maintain their home. What assessment questions will help the nurse determine the family's functioning? (Select all that apply.)
1. "Which transitions or changes in your family are you currently experiencing?"
2. "Are your children having any problems that are affecting your family right now?"
3. "Describe a recent family conflict and how your family resolved it."
4. "What coping strategies do you typically use as a family?"
5. "Who is involved in helping care for your parents?"

10. During a visit to a family clinic, a nurse teaches a mother about immunizations, the use of car seats, and home safety for an infant and toddler. Which type of nursing interventions are these?
1. Restorative
2. Health promotion
3. Acute care
4. Growth and development

Answers: 1. 3; 2. 4, 5; 3. 1, 4; 4. 1, 2, 4; 5. 1; 6. 2; 7. 4; 8. 1, 2, 4; 9. 3, 4, 5; 10. 2.

Rationales for Review Questions can be found on the Evolve website.

REFERENCES

Administration for Community Living (ACL) and Administration on Aging (AoA): *2017 profile of older Americans*, https://www.acl.gov/sites/default/files/Aging%20and%20Disability%20in%20America/2017OlderAmericansProfile.pdf, 2018. Accessed August 13, 2020.

Allen L: Palliative care for patients with advanced heart failure: Decision support, symptom management, and psychosocial assistance, *UpToDate*, https://www.uptodate.com/contents/palliative-care-for-patients-with-advanced-heart-failure-indications-and-strategies, 2020. Accessed August 13, 2020.

Alper E et al: Hospital discharge and readmission, *UpToDate*, https://www.uptodate.com/contents/hospital-discharge-and-readmission, 2020. Accessed August 13, 2020.

American Psychological Association (APA): *Marriage & divorce*. https://www.apa.org/topics/divorce/. 2020. Accessed August 2020.

Baldwin L: *Nursing skills for children and young people's mental health*, ed 1, Cham, Switzerland, 2020, Springer.

Catalyst: *Woman in the workforce – Global*. https://www.catalyst.org/research/women-in-the-workforce-global/, 2020. Accessed August 13, 2020.

Centers for Disease Control (CDC): 2019 health, United States, 2018 – Data finder. https://www.cdc.gov/nchs/hus/contents2018.htm?search=Access_to_health_care, 2019. Accessed August 2020.

Chacko M: Pregnancy in adolescents, *UpToDate*, https://www.uptodate.com/contents/pregnancy-in-adolescents, 2020. Accessed August 13, 2020.

Children's Defense Fund (CDF): *The state of America's children® 2020*, https://www.childrensdefense.org/the-state-of-americas-children-2020/ 2020. Accessed August 2020.

Cohen D, Passel JS: *A record 64 million Americans live in multi-generational households*, Pew Research Center, 2018. http://www.pewresearch.org/fact-tank/2018/04/05/a-record-64-million-americans-live-in-multigenerational-households/. Accessed August 13, 2020.

Cree R et al: Health care, family, and community factors associated with mental, behavioral, and developmental disorders and poverty among children aged 2-8 years—United States, 2016. *MMWR Morb Mortal Wkly Rep*, 67: 1377, 2018.

Delbanco T, Gerteis M: A patient-centered view of the clinician-patient relationship, *UpToDate*, https://www.

uptodate.com/contents/a-patient-centered-view-of-the-clinician-patient-relationship. 2020. Accessed August 13, 2020.

Duhamel F: Translating knowledge from a family systems approach to clinical practice: insights from knowledge translation research experiences, *J Fam Nurs* 23(4): 461, 2017.

Family Caregiver Alliance (FCA): *Caregiver statistics: demographics*, https://www.caregiver.org/caregiver-statistics-demographics, 2019. Accessed August 2020.

Family Caregiver Alliance (FCA): *Caregiver statistics: work and caregiving*, https://www.caregiver.org/caregiver-statistics-work-and-caregiving, 2016. Accessed August 2020.

Farris D; Bourque A: *International handbook on the demography of marriage and the family*. (ed 1). Cham, Switzerland, 2020, Springer.

Fournier AL: Creating a sacred space in the intensive care unit at the end of life, *DCCN* 36(2):110, 2017.

Futures Without Violence: *Futures without violence*, http://www.futureswithoutviolence.org/, 2021. Accessed April 19, 2021.

Giddens JF: *Concepts for nursing practice*, ed 3, St Louis, 2021, Elsevier.

Giger J, Haddad L: *Transcultural nursing: Assessment and intervention*, ed 8, St Louis, 2021, Elsevier.

Gross S: Managing family dynamics when caring for older adults. *Nursing2020* 50(4): 57, 2020.

Harman S et al: Palliative care: The last hours and days of life, *UpToDate*, https://www.uptodate.com/contents/palliative-care-the-last-hours-and-days-of-life, 2020. Accessed August 13, 2020.

Kaakinen JR et al.: *Family health care nursing: theory, practice, and research*, ed 6, Philadelphia, 2018, FA Davis.

Martin JA et al.: Births in the United States, *NCHS Data Brief* 346, 2019. https://www.cdc.gov/nchs/products/databriefs/db346.htm. Accessed August 2020.

Mathias D: Improving patient safety by easing caregiver burden, *Nursing2019* 49(1): 63, 2019.

Masci D et al.: *5 facts about same-sex marriage*, https://www.pewresearch.org/fact-tank/2019/06/24/same-sex-marriage/, 2019. Accessed August 2020.

Mather M et al.: *Fact sheet: Aging in the United States*. Washington: DC, Population Reference Bureau, 2019. https://www.prb.org/aging-unitedstates-fact-sheet/ Accessed April 19, 2021.

Meyer F: Psychosocial issues in advanced illness, *UpToDate*, https://www.uptodate.com/contents/psychosocial-issues-in-advanced-illness, 2020. Accessed August 13, 2020.

National Alliance to End Homelessness: *Children and families*, https://endhomelessness.org/homelessness-in-america/who-experiences-homelessness/children-and-families/, 2020. Accessed August 2020.

National Coalition for the Homeless: family homelessness, 2019, https://nationalhomeless.org/issues/families/. Accessed August 2020.

National Institutes of Health (NIH): *What does it mean to have a genetic predisposition to a disease?*, https://ghr.nlm.nih.gov/primer/mutationsanddisorders/predisposition, 2020. Accessed April 2020.

Orchard CA et al.: Collaborative leadership, part 2: the role of the nurse leader in interprofessional team-based practice – shifting from task- to collaborative patient-/family-focused care, *Nurs Leadersh* 30(2): 26, 2017.

Puchalski C et al.: Overview of spirituality in palliative care, *UpToDate*, https://www.uptodate.com/contents/overview-of-spirituality-in-palliative-care, 2020. Accessed August 13, 2020.

Raby B et al: Genetic counseling: Family history interpretation and risk assessment, *UpToDate*, https://www.uptodate.com/contents/genetic-counseling-family-history-interpretation-and-risk-assessment, 2020. Accessed August 13, 2020.

Shajani Z, Snell D: *Wright & Leahy's Nurses and families: a guide to family assessment and intervention*, ed 7, Philadelphia, 2019, FA Davis.

Semega J et al: *Income and Poverty in the United States: 2018 Current Population Reports*, 2020, https://www.census.gov/content/dam/Census/library/publications/2019/demo/p60-266.pdf. Accessed August 14, 2020.

Twaddle M. McCormick E: Palliative care delivery in the home, *UpToDate*, https://www.uptodate.com/contents/palliative-care-delivery-in-the-home, 2020. Accessed August 13, 2020.

U.S. Bureau of Labor Statistics: *Woman in the labor force: a data book*. 2018. Accessed April 19, 2021.

U.S. Census Bureau.: *America's families & living arrangements*, https://www.census.gov/data/tables/2019/demo/families/cps-2019.html. 2019. Accessed April 19, 2021.

U.S. Interagency Council on Homelessness.: *Ending family homelessness*, https://www.usich.gov/goals/families, 2018. Accessed April 19, 2021.

Weil A: Intimate partner violence: Epidemiology and health consequences, *UpToDate*, https://www.uptodate.com/contents/intimate-partner-violence-epidemiology-and-health-consequences, 2020. Accessed August 13, 2020.

RESEARCH REFERENCES

Barnes AJ et al.: Emotional health among youth experiencing family homelessness, *Pediatrics* 141(4):e20171767, 2018.

Bekdemir, A, Ilhan, N.: Predictors of caregiver burden in caregivers of bedridden patients. *The Journal of Nursing Research,* 27(3): e24, 2019.

Bigani DK, Correia AM: On the same page: nurse, patient, and family perceptions of change-of-shift bedside report, *J Pediatr Nurs* 41:84, 2018.

Brooks LA et al.: Communication and decision-making about end-of-life care in the intensive care unit, *Am J Crit Care* 26(4):336, 2017.

Byrum D et al: Developing a synergy model patient acuity tool for admission, discharge and transfer. *American Journal of Critical Care* 29(1): 61, 2020.

Coats H et al.: Nurses' reflections on benefits and challenges of implementing family-centered care in pediatric intensive care units. *Am J Crit Care* 27(1):52, 2018.

DePasquale N.et al.: The family time squeeze: perceived family time adequacy buffers work strain in certified nursing assistants with multiple caregiving roles, *Gerontol* 58(3):546, 2018.

Erfina E et al: Adolescent mothers' experience of transition to motherhood: An integrative review, *International Journal of Nursing Science* 6(2019): 221, 2019.

Gaskin KL: Patterns of transition experience for parents going home from hospital with their infant after first stage surgery for complex congenital heart disease, *J Pediatr Nurs* 41:e23, 2018.

Hicken B et al.: Supporting caregivers of rural veterans electronically (SCORE), *J Rural Health* 33:305, 2017.

Hsin-Yun L et al: Finding a balance in family caregiving for people with dementia: a correlational longitudinal study, *J Adv Nurs* 77(5): 2278, 2021.

Kandi N, Zeinali A: Relationship between personality characteristics, internal locus of control, psychological hardiness and nurses' quality of life, *J Res Dev Nurs Midwifery* 4(1):8, 2017.

Kokonya A, Fitzsimons F: Transition to long-term care: preparing older adults and their families. *Medsurg Nurs* 27(3):143, 2018.

Konerding U et al.: Investigating burden of informal caregivers in England, Finland and Greece: an analysis with the short form of the Burden Scale for Family Caregivers (BSFC-s), *Aging Ment Health* 22(2):280, 2018.

Macleod A et al.: "There isn't an easy way of finding the help that's available." Barriers and facilitators of service use among dementia family caregivers: a qualitative study, *Int Psychogeriatr* 29(5):765, 2017.

Marcum C et al Primary caregivers in a network context, *J Gerontol B Psychol Sci Soc Sci* 75(1): 125, 2020.

Moriarty J et al.: Exploration of factors related to depressive symptomatology in family members of military veterans with traumatic brain injury, *J Fam Nurs* 24(2):184, 2018.

Moss KO et al.: Understanding end-of-life decision-making terminology among African American older adults, *J Gerontol Nurs* 44(2):33, 2018.

Newcomb AB, Hymes RA: Life interrupted: the trauma caregiver experience, *J Trauma Nurs* 24(2):125, 2017.

Off, C et al: Interprofessional caregiver education, training, and wellness in the context of a cohort model for aphasia rehabilitation, *Topics in Language Disorders* 39(1): 5, 2019.

Parkinson, B et al.: Mindfulness for people with long-term conditions and their family caregivers: A systematic review. *Complementary Therapies in Clinical Practice* 34: 76, 2019.

Press D, Alexander M: Safety and societal issues related to dementia. *UpToDate*, https://www.uptodate.com/contents/safety-and-societal-issues-related-to-dementia, 2020. Accessed August 13, 2020.

Schaffer K et al.: Mental and physical health correlates among family caregivers of patients with newly-diagnosed incurable cancer: a hierarchical linear regression analysis. *Support Care Cancer* 25(3):965, 2017.

Schultz RE et al.: Is there hope? Is she there? How families and clinicians experience acute brain injury. *J Palliat Med* 20(2):170, 2017.

Sebern MD: Does an intervention designed to improve self-management, social support and awareness of palliative-care address needs of persons with heart failure, family caregivers and clinicians? *J Clin Nurs* 27(3/4):e643, 2018.

Sousza F et al.: Calgary family assessment model applied in riverside context. *J Nurs UFPE* 11(12):4798, 2017.

Stajduhar K et al.: Bereaved family members' perceptions of the quality of end-of-life care across four types of inpatient care settings. *BMC Palliat Care* 16(1): 59, 2017.

Stockwell-Smith Get al.: Hospital discharge processes involving older adults living with dementia: an integrated literature review. *J Clin Nurs* 27(5/6):e712, 2018.

Umbersome D; Thomeer M: Family matters: Research on family ties and health, 2010 to 2020. *Journal of Marriage and Family* 82: 404, 2020.

Wakhid A et al: Family resilience in the field of nursing: A concept analysis, *Advances in Health Sciences Research* 20: 242, 2020.

Weisman de Mamani A et al.: The interplay among mindfulness, caregiver burden, and mental health in family members of individuals with dementia. *Prof Psychol Res Pract* 49(2):116, 2018.

Zhang Y: Family functioning in the context of an adult family member with illness: a concept analysis. *J Clin Nurs* 27(15/16):3205, 2018.

11

Developmental Theories

OBJECTIVES

- Discuss theoretical underpinnings of growth and development.
- Compare developmental theories.
- Apply developmental theories when assessing patients and identifying nursing diagnoses in the care of patients throughout the life span.

- Explain how nurses use developmental theories to identify patients' needs and guide patient care.

KEY TERMS

Conventional reasoning
Erikson's theory of psychosocial development

Freud's psychoanalytical model of personality development
Kohlberg's theory of moral development

Piaget's theory of cognitive development
Postconventional reasoning
Temperament

MEDIA RESOURCES

http://evolve.elsevier.com/Potter/fundamentals/
- Review Questions
- Case Study with Questions

- Audio Glossary
- Content Updates
- Answers to QSEN Activity and Review Questions

Understanding normal growth and development helps nurses predict, detect, and prevent deviations from patients' expected patterns that may affect their health. Growth encompasses the physical changes that occur from the prenatal period through older adulthood and demonstrates both advancement and deterioration. Development refers to the biological, cognitive, and socioemotional changes that begin at conception and continue throughout a lifetime. Development is dynamic and includes progression. However, in some disease processes development is delayed or regresses.

Individuals have unique patterns of growth and development. The ability to progress through each developmental phase influences the overall health of the individual. The success or failure experienced within a phase affects the ability to complete subsequent phases. If individuals have repeated developmental failures, inadequacies sometimes result. However, when an individual experiences repeated success, health is promoted. For example, a child who does not walk by 20 months demonstrates delayed gross-motor ability that slows exploration and manipulation of the environment. In contrast, a child who walks by 10 months is able to explore and find stimulation in the environment.

When caring for patients, it is important to adopt a life span perspective of human development that considers all developmental stages. Traditionally development focused on childhood; however, an understanding of growth and development throughout the life span gives you a knowledge base that helps in planning questions for health screenings and health history, health promotion and maintenance, and health education for patients.

DEVELOPMENTAL THEORIES

Developmental theories provide a framework for you to identify a patient's normal developmental needs and whether problems exist. For

example, knowledge of Erikson's (1963) psychosocial theory of development allows you to recognize the importance of developing basic trust in the infancy stage. Trust establishes the foundation for all future relationships and is thus a concept to support in any nursing interventions. Developmental theories help nurses use clinical judgment to accurately assess a person's response to an illness and develop an individualized treatment plan. Understanding the specific task or need of each developmental stage guides caregivers in selecting appropriate interventions.

Human development is a dynamic and complex process that cannot be explained by only one theory. This chapter presents biophysical, psychoanalytical/psychosocial, cognitive, and moral developmental theories. Chapters 25 and 35 cover the areas of learning theory for patient teaching and spiritual development.

Biophysical Developmental Theories

Biophysical development is how our physical bodies grow and change. Health care providers compare the changes that occur as a newborn infant grows against established norms. How does the physical body age? What are the triggers that move the body from the physical characteristics of childhood, through adolescence, to the physical changes of adulthood?

Gesell's Theory of Development. Fundamental to Gesell's theory of development is that each child's pattern of growth is unique and the pattern is directed by gene activity (Gesell, 1948). Gesell noted that the pattern of maturation follows a fixed developmental sequence. Sequential development is evident in fetuses, in which there is a specified order of organ system development. Today we know that growth in humans is both cephalocaudal and proximodistal. The cephalocaudal pattern describes the sequence in which growth is fastest at the top (e.g., head and brain develop faster than arm and leg coordination). The proximodistal growth pattern starts at the center of the body and moves toward the extremities (e.g., organ systems in the trunk of the body develop before the arms and legs). Genes direct the sequence of development, but environmental factors also influence development, resulting in developmental changes. For example, genes direct the growth rate in height for an individual, but that growth is only maximized if environmental conditions are adequate. Poor nutrition or chronic disease often affects the growth rate and results in smaller stature, regardless of a person's genetic blueprint. However, adequate nutrition and the absence of disease cannot result in height beyond that determined by heredity.

Psychoanalytical/Psychosocial Theory

Theories of psychoanalytical/psychosocial development describe human development from the perspectives of personality, thinking, and behavior (Table 11.1). Psychoanalytical theory explains development as primarily unconscious and influenced by emotion. Psychoanalytical theorists maintain that these unconscious conflicts influence development through universal stages experienced by all individuals (Berger, 2020).

Sigmund Freud. Freud's psychoanalytical model of personality development states that individuals go through five stages of psychosexual development and that each stage is characterized by sexual pleasure in parts of the body: the mouth, the anus, and the genitals. Freud believed that adult personality is the result of how an individual resolves conflicts between these sources of pleasure and the mandates of reality (Santrock, 2018).

Stage 1: Oral (Birth to 12 to 18 Months). Initially, sucking and oral satisfaction are not only vital to life but also extremely pleasurable in their own rights. Late in this stage the infant begins to realize that the mother/parent is something separate from self. Disruption in the physical or emotional availability of the parent (e.g., inadequate bonding or chronic illness) could affect an infant's development.

Stage 2: Anal (12 to 18 Months to 3 Years). The focus of pleasure changes to the anal zone. Children become increasingly aware of the

pleasurable sensations of this body region with interest in the products of their effort. Through the toilet-training process the child delays gratification to meet parental and societal expectations.

Stage 3: Phallic or Oedipal (3 to 6 Years). The genital organs are the focus of pleasure during this stage. The boy becomes interested in the penis; the girl becomes aware of the absence of the penis, known as *penis envy*. This is a time of exploration and imagination as a child fantasizes about the parent of the opposite sex as the first love interest, known as the *Oedipus* or *Electra complex*. By the end of this stage the child attempts to reduce this conflict by identifying with the parent of the same sex to win recognition and acceptance.

Stage 4: Latency (6 to 12 Years). In this stage Freud believed that children repress and channel sexual urges from the earlier Oedipal stage into productive activities that are socially acceptable. Within the educational and social worlds of the child, there is much to learn and accomplish.

Stage 5: Genital (Puberty Through Adulthood). In this final stage sexual urges reawaken and are directed to an individual outside the family circle. Unresolved prior conflicts surface during adolescence. Once the individual resolves conflicts, that individual is then capable of having a mature adult sexual relationship.

Freud believed that the components of the human personality develop in stages and regulate behavior. These components are the id, the ego, and the superego. The id (i.e., basic instinctual impulses driven to achieve pleasure) is the most primitive part of the personality and originates in the infant. The infant cannot tolerate delay and must have needs met immediately. The ego represents the reality component, mediating conflicts between the environment and the forces of the id. It helps people judge reality accurately, regulate impulses, and make good decisions. Ego is often referred to as one's sense of self. The third component, the superego, performs regulating, restraining, and prohibiting actions. Often referred to as the conscience, the superego is influenced by the standards of outside social forces (e.g., parent or teacher).

Some of Freud's critics contend that he based his analysis of personality development on biological determinants and ignored the influence of culture and experience. Others think that Freud's basic assumptions

TABLE 11.1 Comparison of Major Developmental Theories				
Developmental Stage/Age	**Freud (Psychosexual Development)**	**Erikson (Psychosocial Development)**	**Piaget (Cognitive/ Moral Development)**	**Kohlberg (Development of Moral Reasoning)**
Infancy (birth to 18 months)	Oral stage	Trust vs. mistrust Ability to trust others	Sensorimotor period Progress from reflex activity to simple repetitive actions	
Early childhood/toddler (18 months to 3 years)	Anal stage	Autonomy vs. shame and doubt Self-control and independence	Preoperational period— thinking using symbols Egocentric	Preconventional level Punishment-obedience orientation
Preschool (3-5 years)	Phallic stage	Initiative vs. guilt Highly imaginative	Use of symbols Egocentric	Preconventional level Premoral Instrumental orientation
Middle childhood (6-12 years)	Latent stage	Industry vs. inferiority Engaged in tasks and activities	Concrete operations period Logical thinking	Conventional level Good boy–nice girl orientation
Adolescence (12-19 years)	Genital stage	Identity vs. role confusion Sexual maturity, "Who am I?"	Formal operations period Abstract thinking	Postconventional level Social contract orientation
Young adult		Intimacy vs. isolation Affiliation vs. love		
Adult		Generativity vs. self-absorption and stagnation		
Old age		Integrity vs. despair		

such as the Oedipus complex are not applicable across different cultures. Psychoanalysts today believe that the role of conscious thought is much greater than Freud imagined (Santrock, 2019).

Erik Erikson. Freud had a strong influence on his psychoanalytical followers, including Erik Erikson (1902–1994), who constructed a theory of development that differed from Freud's in one main aspect: Erikson's stages emphasize a person's relationship to family and culture rather than sexual urges (Berger, 2020).

According to **Erikson's theory of psychosocial development**, individuals need to accomplish a particular task before successfully mastering the stage and progressing to the next one. Each task is framed with opposing conflicts, and tasks once mastered are challenged and tested again during new situations or at times of conflict (Hockenberry et al., 2019).

Trust vs. Mistrust (Birth to 12 to 18 months). Establishing a basic sense of trust is essential for the development of a healthy personality. Infants' successful resolution of this stage requires a consistent caregiver who is available to meet their needs. From this basic trust in parents, an infant is able to trust in herself or himself, in others, and in the world (Hockenberry et al., 2019). The formation of trust results in faith and optimism. A nurse's use of anticipatory guidance helps parents cope with the hospitalization of an infant and the infant's behaviors when discharged to home.

Autonomy vs. Sense of Shame and Doubt (18 Months to 3 Years). By this stage, a growing child is more accomplished in some basic self-care activities, including walking, feeding, and toileting. This newfound independence is the result of maturation and imitation. A toddler develops autonomy by making choices. Choices typical for the toddler age-group include activities related to relationships, desires, and playthings. There is also opportunity to learn that parents and society have expectations about these choices. Limiting choices and/or enacting harsh punishment leads to feelings of shame and doubt. A toddler who successfully masters this stage achieves self-control and willpower. A nurse models empathetic guidance that offers support for and understanding of the challenges of this stage. Available choices for the child must be simple in nature and safe.

Initiative vs. Guilt (3 to 6 Years). Children like to pretend and try out new roles. Fantasy and imagination allow them to further explore their environment. Also, at this time they are developing their superego, or conscience. Conflicts often occur between a child's desire to explore and the limits placed on behavior. These conflicts sometimes lead to feelings of frustration and guilt. Guilt also occurs if a caregiver's responses are too harsh. Preschoolers learn to maintain a sense of initiative without imposing on the freedoms of others. Successful resolution of this stage results in direction and purpose. Teaching a child impulse control and cooperative behaviors helps a family avoid the risks of altered growth and development. Preschoolers frequently engage in animism, a developmental characteristic that makes them treat dolls or stuffed animals as if they have thoughts and feelings. Play therapy is also instrumental in helping a child successfully deal with the inherent threats related to hospitalization or chronic illness.

REFLECT NOW

You are observing a group of 4- to 5-year-old children in a hospital play group. You notice that some of the children are applying bandages to their stuffed animals. Think about how you could plan a play activity that may help these children cope with hospitalization.

Industry vs. Inferiority (6 to 12 Years). School-age children are eager to apply themselves to learning socially productive skills and tools. They learn to work and play with their peers. They thrive on their accomplishments and praise. Without proper support for learning new skills or if skills are too difficult, they develop a sense of inadequacy and inferiority. Children at this age need to be able to experience real achievement to develop a sense of competency (see Chapter 12). Erikson believed that an adult's attitudes toward work are traced to successful achievement of this task (Erikson, 1963). During hospitalization it is important for a school-age child to understand the routines and participate, when possible, in treatment (Hockenberry et al., 2019). For example, some children enjoy keeping a record of their intake and output.

Identity vs. Role Confusion (Puberty). Dramatic physiological changes associated with sexual maturation mark this stage. There is a marked preoccupation with appearance and body image. This stage, in which identity development begins with the goal of achieving some perspective or direction, answers the question "Who am I?" Acquiring a sense of identity is essential for adult decision making, such as choice of a vocation or marriage partner. Each adolescent moves in a unique way into society as an interdependent member. Our environment continues to change at a rapid pace, which comes with new social demands and challenges, opportunities, and conflicts that impact the adolescent's emerging identity and separation from family. Erikson held that adolescents' successful mastery of this stage resulted in devotion and fidelity to others and to their own ideals (Hockenberry et al., 2019).

The adolescent does not consistently perceive vulnerability associated with risk-taking behaviors (Fortenberry, 2020). This perceived invulnerability contributes to risk-taking behaviors (Warner, 2018). Nurses have the opportunity to provide education and anticipatory guidance for parents about the changes and challenges and risks to adolescents. When adolescents are hospitalized, help them deal with their illnesses by giving them enough information to help make some decisions about their treatment plan (see Chapter 12).

Intimacy vs. Isolation (Young Adult). Young adults, having developed a sense of identity, deepen their capacity to love others and care for them. They search for meaningful friendships and an intimate relationship with another person. Erikson portrayed intimacy as finding the self and then losing it in another (Santrock, 2019). If the young adult is unable to establish companionship and intimacy, isolation results because of a fear of rejection and disappointment (Berger, 2020). Nurses must understand that during hospitalization a young adult's need for intimacy remains present; thus, young adults benefit from the support of their partner or significant other during this time.

Generativity vs. Self-Absorption and Stagnation (Middle Age). Following the development of an intimate relationship, an adult focuses on supporting future generations. The ability to expand one's personal and social involvement is critical to this stage of development. Middle-age adults achieve success in this stage by contributing to future generations through parenthood, teaching, mentoring, and community involvement. Achieving generativity results in caring for others as a basic strength. Inability to play a role in the development of the next generation results in stagnation (Santrock, 2019). Nurses help adults who are physically ill choose creative ways to foster social development. Middle-age people may find a sense of fulfillment by volunteering in a local school, hospital, or church.

Integrity vs. Despair (Old Age). Many older adults review their lives with a sense of satisfaction, even with their inevitable mistakes. Others see themselves as failures, with their lives marked by despair and regret. Older adults often engage in a retrospective appraisal of their lives. They interpret their lives as a meaningful whole or experience regret because of goals not achieved (Berger, 2020). Because the aging process

FIG. 11.1 Quilting keeps this older adult active.

creates physical and social losses, some adults also suffer loss of status and function (e.g., through retirement or illness). You can enhance feelings of integrity by encouraging older adults to reflect on their meaningful relationships, such as relationships with a higher power, family members, or the community (Shropshire, 2020; Touhy & Jett, 2020). These external struggles are met with internal struggles, such as the search for meaning in life. Meeting these challenges creates the potential for growth and the basic strength of wisdom (Fig. 11.1).

Nurses are in positions of influence within their communities to help people feel valued, appreciated, and needed. Erikson stated, "Healthy children will not fear life, if their parents have integrity enough not to fear death" (Erikson, 1963). Although Erikson believed that problems in adult life resulted from unsuccessful resolution of earlier stages, his emphasis on family relationships and culture offers a broad, life span view of development. As a nurse you will use this knowledge of development as you deliver care in any health care setting.

Theories Related to Temperament. Temperament is a behavioral style that affects an individual's emotional interactions with others. Temperamental traits identified in infancy may continue to influence a child's behavior through middle school (Hockenberry et al., 2019). Personality and temperament are often closely linked, and individuals possess some enduring characteristics into adulthood. The individual differences that children display in responding to their environment significantly influence the ways in which others respond to them and their needs. Knowledge of temperament helps parents better understand their child and can help the child understand and modify their response (Hockenberry et al., 2019).

Most children have one of these three broad temperamental traits—easy, slow to warm up, and difficult (Hockenberry et al., 2019):

- *The easy child*—Easygoing and even-tempered. This child has regular and predictable habits. An easy child is open and adaptable to change and displays a mild to moderately intense mood that is typically positive.
- *The slow-to–warm up child*—Typically displays discomfort when introduced to new situations and needs time to adjust to new environment, authority figures, and expectations. These children respond with tears, somatic complaints, or other maneuvers to avoid the situation (e.g., complaining of a stomachache to avoid going to school).

- *The difficult child*—Highly distracted, active, irritable, and irregular in habits. This child may benefit from "practice," or role playing, to be successful with new skills, situations, or environments.

Knowledge of temperament and how it impacts the parent-child relationship is critical when providing anticipatory guidance for parents. With the birth of a second child, most parents find that the strategies that worked well with the first child no longer work at all. The nurse individualizes counseling to greatly improve the quality of interactions between parents and children (Hockenberry et al., 2019).

Perspectives on Adult Development

Early studies of development focused only on childhood; however, we now know that although the changes come more slowly, people continue to develop new abilities and adapt to shifting environments.

A life span approach accounts for the multiple life events occurring in adulthood. The contemporary life events approach takes into consideration the variations that occur for each individual. This view considers an individual's personal circumstances (health and family support), how a person views and adjusts to changes, and the current social and historical context in which an individual is living. The increase in life expectancy has made popular the life span approach to development (Santrock, 2018). Life span development is lifelong, multidimensional, multidirectional, and contextual. Development is an interaction of biological, sociocultural, and individual factors (Touhy and Jett, 2020).

Cognitive Developmental Theory

Psychoanalytical/psychosocial theories focus on an individual's unconscious thought and emotions; cognitive theories stress how people learn to think and make sense of their world. As with personality development, cognitive theorists have explored both childhood and adulthood. Some of the theories highlight qualitative changes in thinking; others expand to include social, cultural, and behavioral dimensions.

Jean Piaget. Jean Piaget was most interested in the development of children's intellectual organization: how they think, reason, and perceive the world (Piaget, 1952). Piaget's theory of cognitive development includes four periods that are related to age and demonstrate specific categories of knowing and understanding (see also Chapter 12). He built his theory on years of observing children as they explored, manipulated, and tried to make sense out of the world in which they lived. Piaget believed that individuals move from one stage to another seeking cognitive equilibrium or a state of mental balance and that they build mental structures to help adapt to the world (Santrock, 2019). Within each of these primary periods of cognitive development are specific stages (see Table 11.1).

Period I: Sensorimotor (Birth to 2 Years). Infants develop a schema or action pattern for dealing with the environment (Box 11.1). These schemas include hitting, looking, grasping, or kicking. Schemas become self-initiated activities (e.g., the infant learning that sucking achieves a pleasing result generalizes the action to suck fingers, blanket, or clothing). Successful achievement leads to greater exploration. During this stage, children learn about themselves and their environment through motor and reflex actions. They learn that they are separate from the environment and that aspects of the environment (e.g., parents or favorite toy) continue to exist even though those items cannot always be seen. Piaget termed this understanding that objects continue to exist even when they cannot be seen, heard, or touched *object permanence* and considered it one of the child's most important accomplishments.

Period II: Preoperational (2 to 7 Years). During this time children learn to think with the use of symbols and mental images. They exhibit "egocentrism" in that they see objects and people from only one point of view, their own. They believe that everyone experiences the world

Applying Developmental Theory to the Care of Infants

PICOT Question: In infants who are hospitalized, does a change in health care provider attitudes result in improved quality and length of infant sleep?

Evidence Summary

There is a culture within health care agencies that gives sleep a very low priority (Shimko, 2019). Evidence shows that all patients, including infants and children who are hospitalized, lack essential minimal quality sleep (Crawford et al., 2019; Owens, 2020). Routine nursing care, procedures, light, noise, and the environment frequently interrupt a patient's sleep in the health care setting. Crawford et al. (2019) found that nursing staff at a pediatric hospital often interrupted sleep for routine assessments, including vital signs and weights, during the evening hours, while children were sleeping. Using clinical judgment to apply principles of developmental theory and recognizing the importance of parental engagement and health care provider attitudes about the quality of infant sleep may lead to an increased awareness and accelerate changes in the environment to improve the quality of patients' sleep (Crawford et al., 2019; Owens, 2020).

Application to Nursing Practice

- Teach parents the value of sleep and how infant sleep patterns evolve over time (Shimko, 2019).
- Explain to parents how they can assist their infant to develop self-soothing techniques, which will allow the infant to sleep better during the night (Shimko, 2019).
- Limit sleep disruption as much as possible as infants need 16 to 18 hours of sleep per 24 hours (Shimko, 2019; Wise and Glaze, 2020).
- Be flexible in all care provision, including interprofessional rounds (Shimko, 2019).
- As health care providers, be open to the need to change personal perceptions and beliefs about sleep (Shimko, 2019).

FIG. 11.2 Play is important to a child's development.

Period IV: Formal Operations (11 Years to Adulthood). The transition from concrete to formal operational thinking occurs in stages during which there is a prevalence of egocentric thought. This egocentricity leads adolescents to demonstrate feelings and behaviors characterized by self-consciousness: a belief that their actions and appearance are constantly being scrutinized (an "imaginary audience"), that their thoughts and feelings are unique (the "personal fable"), and that they are invulnerable (Santrock, 2018). These feelings of invulnerability frequently lead to risk-taking behaviors, especially in early adolescence. As adolescents share experiences with peers, they learn that many of their thoughts and feelings are shared by almost everyone, helping them to know that they are not so different. As they mature, their thinking moves to abstract and theoretical subjects. They have the capacity to reason with respect to possibilities.

REFLECT NOW

What nursing actions based on developmental theory could you use to promote an adolescent's emotional well-being?

Piaget noted that some aspects of objective performance emerge earlier, and other cognitive abilities can surface later in life. Many adults may not become formal operational thinkers and remain at the concrete stage, and others have cognitive development that goes beyond the stages that Piaget proposed (Santrock, 2018). Assessment of cognitive ability becomes critical as you provide health care teaching to patients and families.

Research in Adult Cognitive Development. Research into cognitive development in adulthood began in the 1970s and continues today. It supports that adults do not always arrive at one answer to a problem but frequently accept several possible solutions. Adults also incorporate emotions, logic, practicality, and flexibility when making decisions. On the basis of these observations, developmentalists proposed a fifth stage of cognitive development termed *postformal thought.* Within this stage adults demonstrate the ability to recognize that answers vary from situation to situation and that solutions need to be sensible. Also, within this stage is a struggle with identity and "finding oneself" (Sinnott, 2017; Sinnott et al., 2020).

One of the earliest to develop a theory of adult cognition was William Perry (1913–1998), who studied college students and found that continued cognitive development involved increasing cognitive

exactly as they do. Early in this stage children demonstrate "animism," in which they personify objects. They believe that inanimate objects have lifelike thought, wishes, and feelings. Their thinking is influenced greatly by fantasy and magical thinking. Children at this stage have difficulty conceptualizing time. Play becomes a primary means by which they foster their cognitive development and learn about the world (Fig. 11.2). Recognize that play helps the child understand the events taking place. Play therapy is a nursing intervention that helps the child work through invasive and intrusive procedures that may occur during hospitalization. In addition, play therapy helps the child who is ill progress developmentally.

Period III: Concrete Operations (7 to 11 Years). Children in this stage are able to perform mental operations. For example, the child thinks about an action that previously was performed physically and is able to describe a process without actually doing it. At this time, children are able to coordinate two concrete perspectives in social and scientific thinking, so they are able to appreciate the difference between their perspective and that of a friend. Reversibility is one of the primary characteristics of concrete operational thought. Children can now mentally picture a series of steps and reverse the steps to get back to the starting point. The ability to mentally classify objects according to their quantitative dimensions, known as *seriation,* is achieved. They are able to correctly order or sort objects by length, weight, or other characteristics. Another major accomplishment of this stage is *conservation,* or the ability to see objects or quantities as remaining the same despite a change in their physical appearance (Santrock, 2018).

flexibility. As adolescents were able to move from a position of accepting only one answer to realizing that alternative explanations could be right, depending on one's perspective, there was a significant cognitive change. Adults change how they use knowledge, and the emphasis shifts from attaining knowledge or skills to using knowledge for goal achievement.

Moral Developmental Theory

Moral development refers to the changes in a person's thoughts, emotions, and behaviors that influence beliefs about what is right or wrong. It encompasses both *interpersonal* and *intrapersonal* dimensions as it governs how we interact with others (Santrock, 2018). Although various psychosocial and cognitive theorists address moral development within their respective theories, the theories of Piaget and Kohlberg are more widely known (see Table 11.1).

Kohlberg's Theory of Moral Development. Kohlberg's theory of moral development expands on Piaget's cognitive theory. Kohlberg interviewed children, adolescents, and adults and found that moral reasoning develops in stages. From an examination of responses to a series of moral dilemmas, he identified six stages of moral development under three levels (Kohlberg, 1981). It is important to note that Kohlberg's theory is applicable from age 4 until adulthood. Children younger than 4 do not understand morality.

Level I: Preconventional Reasoning. Preconventional reasoning is the premoral level, in which there is limited cognitive thinking and an individual's thinking is primarily egocentric. At this stage thinking is mostly based on likes and pleasures. This stage progresses toward having punishment guide behavior. A person's moral reason for acting, the "why," eventually relates to the consequences that the person believes will occur. These consequences come in the form of punishment or reward. It is at this level that children view illness as a punishment for fighting with their siblings or disobeying their parents. Nurses need to be aware of this egocentric thinking and reinforce that the child does not become ill because of wrongdoing.

Stage 1: Punishment and Obedience Orientation. In this first stage a child's response to a moral dilemma is in terms of absolute obedience to authority and rules. A child in this stage reasons, "I must follow the rules; otherwise I will be punished." Avoiding punishment or the unquestioning deference to authority provides motivation to behave. Physical consequences guide right and wrong choices. If the child is caught, it must be wrong; if the child escapes, it must be right.

Stage 2: Instrumental Relativist Orientation. In this stage the child recognizes that there is more than one right view; a teacher has one view that is different from that of the child's parent. The decision to do something morally right is based on satisfying one's own needs and occasionally the needs of others. The child perceives punishment not as proof of being wrong (as in stage 1) but as something that one wants to avoid. Children at this stage follow their parent's rule about being home in time for supper because they do not want to be confined to their room for the rest of the evening if they are late.

Level II: Conventional Reasoning. At level II, conventional reasoning, the person sees moral reasoning based on the personal internalization of societal and others' expectations. A person wants to fulfill the expectations of the family, group, or nation and also develops a loyalty to and actively maintains, supports, and justifies the order. Moral decision making at this level moves from "What's in it for me?" to "How will it affect my relationships with others?" Emphasis is on social rules and a community-centered approach (Berger, 2020). Nurses observe this when family members make end-of-life decisions for their loved ones. Individual members often struggle with this type of moral dilemma. Grief support involves an understanding of the level of moral decision making of each family member (see Chapter 36).

Stage 3: Good Boy–Nice Girl Orientation. The individual wants to win approval and maintain the expectations of one's immediate group. "Being good" is important and defined as having positive motives, showing concern for others, and keeping mutual relationships through trust, loyalty, respect, and gratitude. One earns approval by "being nice." For example, a person in this stage stays after school and does odd jobs to win the teacher's approval.

Stage 4: Society-Maintaining Orientation. During stage 4 individuals expand their focus from a relationship with others to societal concerns. Moral decisions consider societal perspectives. Right behavior is doing one's duty, showing respect for authority, and maintaining the social order. Adolescents who have strong morals choose not to attend a party where they know beer will be served, not because they are afraid of getting caught but because they know that it is not right.

Level III: Postconventional Reasoning. The person finds a balance between basic human rights and obligations and societal rules and regulations in the level of postconventional reasoning. Individuals move away from moral decisions based on authority or conformity to groups to define their own moral values and principles. Individuals at this stage start to look at what an ideal society would be like. Moral principles and ideals come into prominence at this level (Berger, 2020).

Stage 5: Social Contract Orientation. Having reached stage 5, an individual follows the societal law but recognizes the possibility of changing the law to improve society. The individual also recognizes that different social groups have different values but believes that all rational people would agree on basic rights such as liberty and life. Individuals at this stage make more of an independent effort to determine what society *should* value rather than what the society as a group would value.

Stage 6: Universal Ethical Principle Orientation. Stage 6 defines "right" by the decision of conscience in accord with self-chosen ethical principles. These principles are abstract, like the Golden Rule, and appeal to logical comprehensiveness, universality, and consistency (Kohlberg, 1981). For example, the principle of justice requires the individual to treat everyone in an impartial manner, respecting the basic dignity of all people, and guides the individual to base decisions on an equal respect for all. Civil disobedience is one way to distinguish stage 5 from stage 6. Stage 5 emphasizes the basic rights, the democratic process, and following laws without question, whereas stage 6 defines the principles by which agreements will be most just. For example, a person in stage 5 follows a law, even if it is not fair to a certain racial group. An individual in stage 6 may not follow a law if it does not seem just to the racial group.

Kohlberg's Critics. Kohlberg constructed a systemized way of looking at moral development and is recognized as a leader in moral developmental theory. However, critics of his work raise questions about his choice of research subjects. For example, most of Kohlberg's subjects were males raised in Western philosophical traditions. Research attempting to support Kohlberg's theory that moral development and social evolution progressed simultaneously used the stages of moral reasoning as the framework. Results indicated that through stage 1 and 2, investment was with self and not others; stage 3 correlated to investment in family and friends; stage 4 correlated to outside investment other than the self; stage 5 returned to investment with family; and stage 6 returned to investment with all others except self (Mathes, 2019).

Kohlberg has also been criticized for age and gender bias (Gilligan, 2016). Carol Gilligan criticizes Kohlberg for his gender biases. She believes that he developed his theory based on a justice perspective that focused on the rights of individuals. In contrast, Gilligan's research looked at moral development from a care perspective that viewed people in their interpersonal communications, relationships, and concern for others (Gilligan, 2016; Santrock, 2018). Other researchers have examined Gilligan's theory in studies with children and have not found evidence to support gender differences (Santrock, 2018).

Moral Reasoning and Nursing Practice. Nurses need to recognize their own moral reasoning and assess how this impacts their nursing care. Recognizing your own moral developmental level is essential in separating your beliefs from others when helping patients with their moral decision-making process. It is also important to recognize the level of moral and ethical reasoning used by other members of the health care team and its influence on a patient's care plan.

REFLECT NOW

A nurse who believes that all patients deserve the same level of care is caring for a person who is homeless. The case manager, who is responsible for resource allocation, complains about the amount of resources being expended. What types of moral frustration is the nurse encountering, and how might this impact the nursing practice?

Ideally all members of the health care team are on the same level, creating a unified outcome. Research indicates that nurses experience frustration when faced with barriers to doing the right thing rather than confusion over what is the right thing (Rainer et al., 2018).

Knowledge of developmental theories and critical thinking are essential when assessing how and why people respond as they do. From the diverse set of theories included in this chapter, the complexity of human development is evident. No one theory successfully describes all the intricacies of human growth and development. Today's nurse needs to be knowledgeable about several theoretical perspectives when working with patients.

Your assessment of a patient requires a thorough and complete collection of data and an analysis and interpretation of data to form accurate conclusions about a patient's developmental needs. Accurate identification of nursing diagnoses relies on your ability to consider developmental theory and apply clinical judgment during data analysis. You compare normal developmental behaviors with those projected by developmental theory. Examples of nursing diagnoses applicable to patients with developmental problems include *impaired development (infant, child, adolescent, adult), risk for delayed growth,* and *risk for disproportionate growth.*

QSEN Building Competency in Safety Sam is an 84-year-old patient hospitalized for acute abdominal pain. He does not have any local family and lives in an assisted-living community. He is confused and disoriented. How would your knowledge of developmental theories guide your nursing care for Sam in ensuring his safety?

Answers to QSEN Activities can be found on the Evolve website.

Growth and development, as supported by a life span perspective, are multidimensional. The theories included are the basis for a meaningful observation of an individual's pattern of growth and development. They are guidelines for understanding important human processes, and they allow nurses to begin to predict human responses and to recognize deviations from the norm.

KEY POINTS

- Development is dynamic and complex. It is not limited to childhood and adolescence; people grow and develop throughout the life span.
- Developmental theories explain and predict human behavior but approach human growth and development from different perspectives (e.g., cognitive, social, physical). For example, Gesell's theory is based on genetic and physical changes that occur while a person ages, whereas Erikson's theory considers the psychosocial tasks a person needs to accomplish before progressing to the next stage of development.
- You compare expected developmental behaviors with those projected by developmental theory to help you assess and understand your patients' cognitive responses and physical capabilities
- Developmental theories provide important insight for understanding human processes, assist nurses in predicting human responses and deviations from the norm, and guide the selection of appropriate nursing interventions.

REFLECTIVE LEARNING

- Consider a patient experience you encountered recently and describe how you practiced moral reasoning in providing care.
- How did a patient's developmental stage impact the care you provided during a clinical experience?
- Consider two of your patients and compare their cognitive developmental stages. Describe how you adapted your nursing care.

REVIEW QUESTIONS

1. A nurse is aware that preschoolers often display a developmental characteristic that makes them treat dolls or stuffed animals as if they have thoughts and feelings. This is an example of:
   1. Logical reasoning.
   2. Egocentrism.
   3. Concrete thinking.
   4. Animism.
2. A 9-year-old child has a difficult time making friends at school and being chosen to play on teams. He also has trouble completing his homework and, as a result, receives little positive feedback from his parents or teacher. According to Erikson's theory, failure at this stage of development results in: (Select all that apply.)
   1. Feelings of inadequacy.
   2. A sense of guilt.
   3. A poor sense of self.
   4. Feelings of inferiority.
   5. Mistrust.
3. A nurse teaches parents how to have their children learn impulse control and cooperative behaviors. This would be during which of Erikson's stages of development?
   1. Trust versus mistrust
   2. Initiative versus guilt
   3. Industry versus inferiority
   4. Autonomy versus sense of shame and doubt
4. When Ryan was 3 months old, he had a toy train; when his view of the train was blocked, he did not search for it. Now that he is 9 months old, he looks for it, reflecting the presence of:
   1. Object permanence.
   2. Sensorimotor play.
   3. Schemata.
   4. Magical thinking.

5. When preparing a 4-year-old child for a procedure, which method is developmentally most appropriate for the nurse to use?
   1. Allowing the child to watch another child undergoing the same procedure
   2. Showing the child pictures of what will be experienced
   3. Talking to the child in simple terms about what will happen
   4. Preparing the child through play with a doll and toy medical equipment

6. A nurse is caring for a man who is recently retired and who appears withdrawn. He says he is "bored with life." The nurse helps this individual find meaning in life by:
   1. Encouraging him to reflect on his relationships with others.
   2. Encouraging relocation to a new city.
   3. Explaining the need to simplify life.
   4. Encouraging him to adopt a new pet.

7. According to Piaget's cognitive theory, a 12-year-old child is most likely to engage in which of the following activities? (Select all that apply.)
   1. Using building blocks to determine how houses are constructed
   2. Writing a story about a clown who wants to leave the circus
   3. Drawing pictures of a family using stick figures
   4. Writing an essay about patriotism
   5. Hanging out with a best friend

8. Elizabeth, who is having unprotected sex with her boyfriend, comments to her friends, "Did you hear about Kathy? You know, she fools around so much; I heard she was pregnant. That would never happen to me!" This is an example of adolescent:
   1. Imaginary audience.
   2. False-belief syndrome.
   3. Personal fable.
   4. Sense of invulnerability.

9. Which of the following are examples of the conventional reasoning form of cognitive development? (Select all that apply.)
   1. A 35-year-old woman is speaking with you about her recent diagnosis of a chronic illness. She is concerned about her treatment options in relation to her ability to continue to care for her family. As she considers the options and alternatives, she incorporates information, her values, and emotions to decide which plan will be the best fit for her.
   2. A young father is considering whether or not to return to school for a graduate degree. He considers the impact the time commitment may have on the needs of his wife and infant son.
   3. A teenage girl is encouraged by her peers to engage in shoplifting. She decides not to join her peers in this activity because she is afraid of getting caught in the act.
   4. A single mother of two children is unhappy with her employer. She has been unable to secure alternate employment but decides to quit her current job.
   5. A young man drives over the speed limit regularly because he thinks he is an excellent driver and will not get into a car accident.

10. Dave reports being happy and satisfied with his life. What do we know about him?
    1. He is in one of the later developmental periods, concerned with reviewing his life.
    2. He is atypical, since most people in any of the developmental stages report significant dissatisfaction with their lives.
    3. He is in one of the earlier developmental periods, concerned with establishing a career and satisfying long-term relationships.
    4. It is difficult to determine Dave's developmental stage since most people report overall satisfaction with their lives in all stages.

Answers: 1. 4; **2.** 1, 4; **3.** 2; **4.** 1; **5.** 4; **6.** 1; **7.** 2, 5; **8.** 4; **9.** 1, 2, 3; **10.** 4.

Rationales for Review Questions can be found on the Evolve website.

REFERENCES

Berger KS: *The developing person: through the life span,* ed 11, New York, 2020, Worth.

Erikson E: *Childhood and society,* New York, 1963, Norton.

Gesell A: *Studies in child development,* New York, 1948, Harper.

Gilligan C: *In a different voice: Psychological theory and women's development.* Cambridge, Mass: Harvard University Press, 2016.

Hockenberry MJ, Wilson D: *Wong's nursing care of infants and children,* ed 11, St Louis, 2019, Mosby.

Kohlberg L: *The philosophy of moral development: moral stages and the idea of justice,* San Francisco, 1981, Harper & Row.

Piaget J: *The origins of intelligence in children,* New York, 1952, International Universities Press.

Santrock JW: *A topical approach to life span development,* ed 7, New York, 2018, McGraw-Hill.

Santrock JW: *Life span development,* ed 17, New York, 2019, McGraw-Hill.

Touhy TA, Jett K: *Ebersole and Hess' toward healthy aging: human needs and nursing response,* ed 10, St. Louis, 2020, Elsevier.

RESEARCH REFERENCES

Crawford S et al.: Quality of sleep in a pediatric hospital: a descriptive study based on an assessment of interruptions, perceptions, and the environment. *Journal of Nursing Administration,* 49(5): 273-279, 2019.

Fortenberry J: Sexually transmitted infections: Issues specific to adolescents, *UpToDate,* 2020, https://www.uptodate.com/contents/sexually-transmitted-infections-issues-specific-to-adolescents. Accessed April 27, 2021.

Mathes EW: An evolutionary perspective on Kohlberg's theory of moral development. *Curr Psychol,* 2019.

Owens J: Behavioral sleep problems in children, *UpToDate,* https://www.uptodate.com/contents/behavioral-sleep-problems-in-children, 2020. Accessed April 27, 2021.

Rainer J et al.: Ethical dilemmas in nursing: an integrative review, *J Clin Nurs* 27(19/20):3446, 2018.

Shimko A: Sleep in infancy: A concept analysis, *Journal of Pediatric Nursing,* 47:100, 2019.

Shropshire M: Reminiscence intervention for community-dwelling older adults without dementia: a literature review. *Br. J Nurs,* 25(1): 40, 2020.

Sinnott J et al.: Relating flow, mindfulness, cognitive flexibility, and postformal thought: two studies. *J Adult Dev* 27, 1–11, 2020.

Sinnott J: *Identity flexibility in adulthood: perspectives in adult development,* New York, 2017, Springer International Publishing.

Warner TD: Adolescent sexual risk taking: the distribution of youth behaviors and perceived peer attitudes across neighborhood contexts, *J Adolesc Health* 62:226, 2018.

Wise M. Glaze D: Sleep physiology in children, *UpToDate,* https://www.uptodate.com/contents/sleep-physiology-in-children, 2020. Accessed April 27, 2021.

Conception Through Adolescence

OBJECTIVES

- List ways to promote health during pregnancy.
- Discuss common physical and psychosocial changes during the transition of a child from intrauterine to extrauterine life.
- Compare physical changes and growth from conception to adolescence.

- Describe cognitive and psychosocial development from birth through adolescence.
- Explain the role of play in the development of a child.
- Develop ways in which a nurse is able to help parents meet their children's developmental needs.

KEY TERMS

Adolescence	Fetus	Puberty
Apgar score	Infancy	School-age period
Attachment	Neonatal period	Toddlerhood
Embryonic stage	Preembryonic stage	
Fetal stage	Preschool period	

MEDIA RESOURCES

http://evolve.elsevier.com/Potter/fundamentals/
- Review Questions
- Audio Glossary

- Case Study with Questions
- Content Updates
- Answers to QSEN Activity and Review Questions

STAGES OF GROWTH AND DEVELOPMENT

Human growth and development are continuous and complex processes that are typically divided into stages organized by age-groups. Although this chronological division is somewhat arbitrary, it is based on the timing and sequence of developmental tasks that children accomplish in each stage. This chapter focuses on the physical, psychosocial, and cognitive changes, as well as the health risks and health promotion concerns relevant to each stage of growth and development.

SELECTING A DEVELOPMENTAL FRAMEWORK FOR NURSING

Using a family-centered approach that incorporates knowledge of developmental stages and theories (see Chapter 11) provides a framework to appropriately assess and plan care that meets the needs of the child and family. This approach encourages organized care for the child's current level of functioning to motivate self-direction and health promotion. For example, nurses encourage toddlers to make simple choices and to feed themselves to advance their developing autonomy. Nurses recognize that adolescents are developing independence and therefore should feel empowered to participate in decisions regarding their plan of care.

INTRAUTERINE LIFE

From the moment of conception until birth, human development proceeds at a predictable and rapid rate. During gestation, or the prenatal period, the embryo grows from a single cell to a complex, physiological being. All major organ systems develop in utero, with some functioning before birth.

Pregnancy that reaches full term is calculated to last an average of 38 to 40 weeks and is commonly divided into equal phases of 3 months, called *trimesters*. Beginning on the day of fertilization, the first 14 days are referred to as the preembryonic stage, followed by the embryonic stage, which lasts from day 15 until the eighth week. These two stages are then followed by the fetal stage, which lasts from the end of the eighth week until birth (Murray et al., 2019).

The placenta begins development at the third week of the embryonic stage and produces essential hormones that help maintain the pregnancy. The placenta functions as the fetal lungs, kidneys, gastrointestinal tract, and endocrine organ. Because the placenta is extremely porous, noxious materials such as viruses, chemicals, and drugs also pass from mother to child. These agents are called *teratogens* and can cause abnormal development of structures in the embryo. The effect of teratogens on the fetus depends on the developmental stage in which exposure takes place, individual genetic susceptibility, and the extent of the exposure. The embryonic stage is the most vulnerable because all body organs are formed by the eighth week of gestation. Some maternal infections can cross the placental barrier and negatively influence the health of the mother, fetus, or both. It is important to educate women about avoidable sources of teratogens and to help them make healthy lifestyle choices before and during pregnancy.

Health Promotion During Pregnancy

Women who are poorly nourished before pregnancy and continue to consume inadequate nutrients and calories during pregnancy may not be able to meet the nutritional requirements of the fetus. An increase in weight does not always indicate an increase in nutrients. In addition, the pattern of weight gain is important for tissue growth in a mother and fetus. For women who are at normal weight for height, the recommended weight gain during pregnancy is 11 to 15 kg (25–35 lb) over three trimesters (Murray et al., 2019). As a nurse, you are in a key position to provide women with important nutritional education before conception and throughout pregnancy.

Pregnancy presents a developmental challenge that includes physiological, cognitive, and emotional states that are accompanied by stress and anxiety (see Chapter 13). The expectant woman will soon adopt a parenting role, and relationships within the family will change, whether or not there is a partner involved. Pregnancy can be a period of conflict or support; family dynamics have an impact on fetal development. Parental reactions to pregnancy change throughout the gestational period. Listen carefully to concerns expressed by a mother and her partner, and offer support through each trimester.

The age of a woman sometimes plays a role in fertility, the health of the fetus, and maternal health. As women age, the risk of chromosomal defects and infertility challenges increases. Pregnant adolescents often seek prenatal care late in the pregnancy or fail to seek prenatal care for a variety of reasons (Murray et al., 2019). Infants of teenage mothers have an increased risk of prematurity and low birth weight (less than 2500 g or 5.5 lb) (Chacko, 2021; Murray et al., 2019).

Fetal growth and hormonal changes during pregnancy often result in discomfort for the expectant mother. Common concerns expressed include problems such as nausea and vomiting, breast tenderness, urinary frequency, heartburn, constipation, ankle edema, and backache. Always anticipate these discomforts and provide self-care education throughout the pregnancy. Discussing the physiological causes of these discomforts and offering suggestions for safe treatment can be very helpful for expectant mothers and contribute to overall health during pregnancy (Murray et al., 2019).

When assessing a pregnant woman, include questions about the use of complementary and alternative therapies. Some therapies such as herbal supplements can be harmful during pregnancy (Murray et al., 2019). You can promote maternal and fetal health by providing accurate and complete information about health behaviors that support positive outcomes for pregnancy and childbirth.

TRANSITION FROM INTRAUTERINE TO EXTRAUTERINE LIFE

The transition from intrauterine to extrauterine life requires profound physiological changes in the newborn and occurs during the first 24 hours of life. Assessment of the newborn during this period is essential to ensure that the transition is proceeding as expected. Gestational age and development and exposure to depressant drugs before or during labor may influence the newborn's adjustment to the external environment.

Physical Changes

An immediate assessment of the newborn's condition to determine the physiological functioning of the major organ systems occurs at birth.

The most widely used assessment tool is the Apgar score. Heart rate, respiratory effort, muscle tone, reflex irritability, and color are rated to determine the overall status of the newborn. The Apgar assessment generally is conducted at 1 and 5 minutes after birth and is sometimes repeated until the newborn's condition stabilizes. The most extreme physiological change occurs when the newborn leaves the utero circulation and develops independent circulatory and respiratory functioning.

Nursing interventions at birth include maintaining an open airway, stabilizing and maintaining body temperature, and protecting the newborn from infection. The removal of nasopharyngeal and oropharyngeal secretions with suction or a bulb syringe ensures airway patency. Newborns are susceptible to heat loss and cold stress. Because hypothermia increases oxygen needs, it is essential to stabilize and maintain a newborn's body temperature. A healthy newborn may be placed in a radiant warmer, placed directly on the mother's abdomen, or covered in warm blankets with a cap. Preventing infection is a major concern in the care of a newborn, whose immune system is immature. Good handwashing technique is the most important factor in protecting a newborn from infection. You can help prevent infection by instructing parents and visitors to wash their hands before touching the infant.

Psychosocial Changes

After immediate physical evaluation and application of identification bracelets, the nurse promotes early parent-child contact to encourage parent-child attachment. Most healthy newborns are awake and alert for the first hour after birth. This is a good time for parent-child interaction to begin. Skin-to-skin contact and breastfeeding are both early techniques to promote bonding (McKee-Garrett, 2021). If immediate contact is not possible, incorporate it into the care plan as early as possible, which means bringing the newborn to a parent who is ill or bringing the parents to a child who is ill or premature. Attachment begins during pregnancy and continues for many months after birth (Hockenberry et al., 2019).

NEWBORN

The neonatal period is the first 28 days of life. During this stage the newborn's physical functioning is mostly reflexive, and stabilization of major organ systems is the primary task of the body. Behavior is greatly influenced by interaction among the newborn, the environment, and parents/caregivers. For example, a 2-week-old may smile spontaneously and look at the parent's face, eliciting a positive response from the parent. Alternately, the newborn may cry, which is generally a reflexive response to an unmet need such as hunger, fatigue, or discomfort (Hockenberry et al., 2019). If the newborn is crying when hungry, the nurse may counsel the parents to feed the infant on demand rather than on a rigid schedule. Nurses must use knowledge of growth and development to plan care for the parent and newborn.

Physical Changes

Perform a comprehensive nursing assessment as soon as a newborn's physiological functioning is stable, generally within a few hours after birth. At this time, measure height, weight, head and chest circumference, temperature, pulse, and respirations and observe general appearance, body functions, sensory capabilities, reflexes, and responsiveness (McKee-Garrett, 2020). Following a comprehensive physical assessment, assess gestational age and interactions between newborn and parent that indicate successful attachment (Hockenberry et al., 2019).

The average newborn is 2700 to 4000 g (6–9 lb), is 48 to 53 cm (19–21 inches) in length, and has a head circumference of 33 to 35 cm (13–14 inches). Neonates lose up to 10% of birth weight in the first few days of life, primarily through fluid losses by respiration, urination, defecation, and low fluid intake (McKee-Garrett, 2021). They usually

FIG. 12.1 Fontanels and suture lines. (From Hockenberry MJ, et al.: *Wong's nursing care of infants and children,* ed 11, St Louis, 2019, Elsevier.)

regain birth weight by the second week of life, and a gradual pattern of increase in weight, height, and head circumference is evident. Accurate measurement as soon as possible after birth provides a baseline for future comparison (Murray et al., 2019).

Normal physical characteristics of the newborn include the continued presence of lanugo (fine downy hair) on the skin of the back; cyanosis of the hands and feet for the first 24 hours; and a soft, protuberant abdomen. Skin color varies according to racial and genetic heritage and gradually changes during infancy. Molding, or overlapping of the soft skull bones, allows the fetal head to adjust to various diameters of the maternal pelvis and is a common occurrence with vaginal births. The bones readjust within a few days, producing a rounded appearance to the head. The sutures and fontanels are usually palpable at birth. Fig. 12.1 shows the diamond shape of the anterior fontanel and the triangular shape of the posterior fontanel between the unfused bones of the skull. The anterior fontanel usually closes by 12 to 18 months, whereas the posterior fontanel closes by the end of the second or third month.

Assess neurological function by observing the newborn's level of activity, alertness, irritability, and responsiveness to stimuli and the presence and strength of reflexes. Normal reflexes include blinking in response to bright lights, startling in response to sudden loud noises or movement, sucking, rooting, grasping, yawning, coughing, sneezing, swallowing, palmar grasp, plantar grasp, and Babinski. Assessment of these reflexes is vital because the newborn depends largely on reflexes for survival and in response to its environment. Fig. 12.2 shows the tonic neck reflex in the newborn.

Normal behavioral characteristics of the newborn include periods of sucking, crying, sleeping, and activity. Movements are generally sporadic, but they are symmetrical and involve all four extremities. The relatively flexed fetal position of intrauterine life continues as the newborn attempts to maintain an enclosed, secure feeling. Newborns normally watch the caregiver's face, have a nonsocial reflexive smile, and respond to sensory stimuli, particularly the primary caregiver's face, voice, and touch.

Cognitive Changes

Early cognitive development begins with innate behavior, reflexes, and sensory functions (Kotagal, 2020). Newborns initiate reflex activities,

FIG. 12.2 Tonic neck reflex. Newborns assume this position while supine. (From Hockenberry MJ, et al.: *Wong's nursing care of infants and children,* ed 11, St Louis, 2019, Elsevier.)

learn behaviors, and learn their desires. At birth, newborns are able to focus on objects about 20 to 30 cm (8–12 inches) from their faces and perceive forms. Newborns respond to human faces, black-and-white contrasting patterns, and bright colors (Murray et al., 2019). Teach parents about the importance of providing sensory stimulation such as talking to their infant and holding the infant to see the parent's face. This allows newborns to seek or take in stimuli, thereby enhancing learning and promoting cognitive development.

Crying is a means by which newborns communicate to provide cues to parents. Some infants cry because their diapers are wet or they are hungry or want to be held. Others cry just to make noise or because they need a change in position or activity. The crying may frustrate the parents if they cannot see an apparent cause. With the nurse's help, parents learn to recognize the newborn's cry patterns and take appropriate action when necessary.

Psychosocial Changes

During the first month of life most parents and newborns normally develop a strong bond that grows into a deep attachment. Feeding, hygiene, and comfort measures consume much of newborns' waking time. These interactions provide a foundation for the formation of deep attachments. Early on, parents can allow siblings to participate in age-appropriate aspects of the newborn's care (Murray et al., 2019). Family involvement, including siblings, helps support growth and development and promotes nurturing (Fig. 12.3).

If parents or children experience health complications after birth, this may compromise the attachment process. These newborns' behavioral cues are sometimes weak or absent, and caregiving may be less mutually satisfying. When parents are tired or ill, they sometimes have difficulty interpreting and responding to their newborns. Preterm infants and those born with congenital anomalies are often too weak to be responsive to parental cues and require special supportive nursing care. For example, infants born with heart defects tire easily during feedings. Nurses can support parental attachment by pointing out positive qualities and responses of the newborn and acknowledging how difficult the separation can be for parents and newborn.

Health Promotion

Screening. Newborn screening tests are administered before infants leave the health care agency to identify serious or life-threatening conditions before symptoms begin. Results of the screening tests are sent directly to the pediatrician. If a screening test suggests a problem, the infant's health care provider usually follows up with further testing and may refer the infant to a specialist for treatment if needed. Blood tests help detect inborn errors of metabolism (IEMs). These are genetic disorders caused by the absence or deficiency of a substance, usually an enzyme, essential to cellular metabolism that results in abnormal protein, carbohydrate, or fat metabolism. Although IEMs are rare, neonatal screening is done to detect phenylketonuria (PKU), hypothyroidism, galactosemia, and other diseases to allow appropriate treatment that prevents permanent mental retardation and other health problems (McKee-Garrett, 2021).

FIG. 12.3 Siblings should be involved in newborn care. (Copyright © romrodinka/iStock/Thinkstock.)

Studies have indicated that hearing loss is the most common congenital abnormality in newborns. The American Academy of Pediatrics (AAP) recommends universal screening of newborn hearing before discharge or within the first month of life. Early detection of hearing difficulties leads to early treatment and can prevent or decrease developmental delays, especially those related to communication (McKee-Garrett, 2021; Murray et al., 2019).

Car Seats. An essential component of discharge teaching is the use of a federally approved car seat for transporting the newborn from the health care agency or birthing center to home. Automobile injuries are a leading cause of death in children in the United States. Many of these deaths occur when the child is not properly restrained (Hockenberry et al., 2019). Parents need to learn how to fit the child in the restraint and install the car seat properly. All infants and toddlers should ride in a rear-facing car safety seat until they are 2 years of age or until they reach the highest weight or height allowed by the manufacturer or their car safety seat (AAP, 2021a). Placing an infant in a rear-facing restraint in the front seat of a vehicle is extremely dangerous in any vehicle with a passenger-side air bag. Nurses are responsible for providing education on the use of a car seat before discharge from the health care agency.

Sleep and Cribs. In accordance with the recommendations of the AAP (2020a), position infants for sleep on their backs on a firm sleep surface to decrease the risk of sudden infant death syndrome (SIDS) (McKee-Garrett, 2021). Newborns establish their individual sleep-activity cycle, and parents develop sensitivity to their infant's cues. Co-sleeping or bed sharing (see Chapter 43) is associated with an increased risk for SIDS (McKee-Garrett, 2021). Safeguards to reduce the risk for SIDS include proper positioning; removing stuffed animals, soft bedding, crib bumper pads, and pillows; and avoiding overheating the infant. Individuals should avoid smoking during pregnancy and around the infant because it places the infant at greater risk for SIDS (Moon, 2020). Nurses play an important role in educating parents about safe sleeping for infants.

Federal safety standards now prohibit the manufacture or sale of cribs with drop-side rails and require more durable mattress supports and crib slats (AAP, 2020a). New cribs sold in the United States must meet these governmental standards for safety. Unsafe cribs that do not meet the safety standards should be disassembled and thrown away (AAP, 2020a). Parents also need to inspect an older crib to make sure the slats are no more than 6 cm (2.4 inches) apart. The crib mattress should fit snugly, and crib toys or mobiles should be attached firmly with no hanging strings or straps. Instruct parents to remove mobiles as soon as the infant is able to reach them (Hockenberry et al., 2019). Parents need to educate grandparents and other caregivers about the need for safe cribs and bedding.

INFANT

During **infancy**, the period from 1 month to 1 year of age, rapid physical growth and change occur. This is the only period distinguished by such dramatic physical changes and marked development. Psychosocial developmental advances are aided by the progression from reflexive to more purposeful behavior. Interaction between infants and the environment becomes greater and more meaningful for an infant. During this first year of life, you can easily observe the adaptive potential of infants because changes in growth and development occur so rapidly.

Physical Changes

Steady and proportional growth of an infant is more important than absolute growth values. Charts of normal age- and gender-related growth measurements enable you to compare growth with norms for a child's age. For infants born prematurely, norms will be adjusted based on gestational age. Measurements recorded over time are the best way to monitor growth and identify problems. Size increases rapidly during the first year of life; birth weight doubles in approximately 5 months and triples by 12 months. Height increases an average of 2.5 cm (1 inch) during each of the first 6 months and about 1.2 cm (½ inch) each month until 12 months (Hockenberry et al., 2019).

Throughout the first year, an infant's vision and hearing continue to develop. Patterns of body function also stabilize, as evidenced by predictable sleep, elimination, and feeding routines. Some reflexes that are present in the newborn, such as blinking, yawning, and coughing, remain throughout life, whereas others, such as grasping, rooting, sucking, and the Moro or startle reflex, disappear after several months.

Motor development proceeds in a cephalocaudal (head-to-toe) and proximodistal (central-to-peripheral) pattern, as does myelination of nerves (Hockenberry et al., 2019). Gross-motor skills involve large muscle activities and are usually closely monitored by parents, who easily report recently achieved milestones. Newborns can only momentarily hold their heads up, but by 4 months most infants have no head lag. The same rapid development is evident as infants learn to sit, stand, and walk. Fine-motor skills involve small body movements and are more difficult to achieve than gross-motor skills. Maturation of eye-and-hand coordination occurs over the first 2 years of life as infants move from being able to grasp a rattle briefly at 2 months to drawing an arc with a pencil by 24 months. Development proceeds at a variable pace for each individual but usually follows the same pattern and occurs within the same time frame (Table 12.1).

Cognitive Changes

The complex brain development during the first year is demonstrated by an infant's changing behaviors. As stimulation is received through the developing senses of vision, hearing, and touch, the developing brain interprets the stimuli. Thus an infant learns by experiencing and manipulating the environment. Developing motor skills and increasing mobility expand an infant's environment and, with developing visual and auditory skills, enhance cognitive development. For these reasons Piaget (1952) named this first stage of cognitive development, which extends until around the third birthday, the sensorimotor period (see Chapter 11). In this stage of cognitive development, infants explore their world through senses. They learn by experimentation and trial and error. They shake and throw things and put things in their mouths. By the age of 7 to 9 months, they begin to realize that things that can no longer be seen still exist. This is known as *object permanence* and is an important developmental milestone because it demonstrates that their memory is beginning to develop.

Infants need opportunities to develop and use their senses. Assess the appropriateness and adequacy of these opportunities, especially when a child is sick or injured. You must provide alternatives for a child. For example, ill or hospitalized infants sometimes lack the energy to interact with their environment, thereby slowing their cognitive development. Infants need to be stimulated according to their temperament, energy, and age. A nurse may stimulate an infant on tube feeding by offering a pacifier and talking to the child, thereby maximizing development while conserving energy.

Language. Speech is an important aspect of cognition that develops during the first year. Infants proceed from crying, cooing, and laughing to imitating sounds, comprehending the meaning of simple commands, and repeating words with knowledge of their meaning. According to Piaget this demonstrates that an infant is demonstrating some symbolic abilities. By 1 year, infants not only recognize their own names but are also able to say three to five words and understand almost 100 words (Hockenberry et al., 2019). As a nurse, you promote language development by encouraging parents to name objects on which their infant's attention is focused. You also assess the infant's language development to identify developmental delays or potential abnormalities.

Psychosocial Changes
Separation and Individuation. During their first year, infants begin to differentiate themselves from others as separate beings capable of

Age	Gross-Motor Skill	Fine-Motor Skill
Birth to 1 month	Complete head lag persists Cannot sit upright Primitive reflexes present	Reflexive grasp
2–4 months	When prone, lifts head and chest and bears weight on forearms With support, able to sit erect with good head control Can turn from back to side	Holds rattle for short periods but cannot pick it up if dropped Looks at and plays with hands Able to bring objects to mouth
4–6 months	Turns from abdomen to back at 5 months and then back to abdomen at 6 months Can support much of own weight when pulled to stand No head lag when pulled to sit	Grasps objects at will and can drop them to pick up another object Pulls feet to mouth to explore Can hold a bottle
6–8 months	Sits alone without support Bears full weight on feet and can hold on to furniture while standing	Bangs objects together Transfers objects from hand to hand
8–10 months	Scoots or crawls on hands and knees Pulls self to standing position	Picks up small objects Begins to use pincer grasp Shows hand preference
10–12 months	Walks holding onto furniture Stands alone for short periods May attempt first step alone	Can place objects into containers Can turn book pages (more than one page at a time)

TABLE 12.1 Gross-Motor and Fine-Motor Development in Infancy

Adapted from Hockenberry MJ, et al.: *Wong's nursing care of infants and children*, ed 11, St Louis, 2019, Elsevier.

FIG. 12.4 Smiling at and talking to an infant encourage bonding. (From Murray SS, McKinney ES: *Foundations of maternal-newborn and women's health nursing*, ed 6, St Louis, 2014, Saunders.)

acting on their own. Initially infants are unaware of the boundaries of self, but through repeated experiences with the environment they learn where the self ends and the external world begins. As they determine their physical boundaries, they begin to respond to others (Fig. 12.4).

Two- and 3-month-old infants begin to smile responsively rather than reflexively. Similarly, they recognize differences in people when their sensory and cognitive capabilities improve. By 8 months most infants are able to differentiate a stranger from a familiar person and respond differently to the two. Close attachment to their primary caregivers, most often parents, usually occurs by this age. Infants seek out these people for support and comfort during times of stress. The ability to distinguish self from others allows infants to interact and socialize more within their environments. For example, by 9 months infants play simple social games such as patty-cake and peek-a-boo. More complex interactive games such as hide-and-seek involving objects are possible by age 1.

Erikson (1963) described the psychosocial developmental crisis for an infant as trust versus mistrust. During this phase the quality of parent-infant interactions determines development of trust or mistrust. The infant learns to trust self, others, and the world through the relationship between the parent and child and the care the child receives (Hockenberry et al., 2019). During infancy a child's temperament or behavioral style becomes apparent and influences the interactions between parent and child. You can help parents understand their child's temperament and determine appropriate childrearing practices.

Assess the availability and appropriateness of experiences contributing to psychosocial development. Infants who are in a hospital often have difficulty establishing physical boundaries because of repeated bodily intrusions and painful sensations. Limiting these negative experiences and providing pleasurable sensations are interventions that support early psychosocial development. Extended separations from parents complicate the attachment process and increase the number of caregivers with whom the infant must interact. Parents cannot always be present to provide care during hospitalization. When parents are not present, make an attempt to limit the number of different caregivers who have contact with the infant and to follow the parents' directions for care. These interventions foster the infant's continuing development of trust.

Play. Play is important for development of cognitive, social, and motor skills. Much of infant play is solitary and exploratory as infants use their senses to observe and examine their own bodies and objects of interest in their surroundings. Adults facilitate infant learning by planning activities that promote the development of milestones and providing toys that are safe for infants to explore with their mouth and manipulate with their hands such as rattles, wooden blocks, plastic stacking rings, squeezable stuffed animals, and busy boxes.

Health Risks

Injury Prevention. Unintentional injury from all accidents, such as motor vehicle accidents, suffocation, falls, or poisoning, is a major cause of death in children 6 to 12 months old (Kochanek et al., 2019). An understanding of the major developmental accomplishments during this time period allows for injury-prevention planning. As a child achieves gains in motor development and becomes increasingly curious about the environment, constant watchfulness and supervision are critical for injury prevention.

Child Maltreatment. Child maltreatment includes intentional physical abuse or neglect, emotional abuse or neglect, and sexual abuse of children, usually by adults (Boos, 2020; Hockenberry et al., 2019). More children suffer from neglect than any other type of maltreatment. Children of any age can be maltreated, but the youngest are the most vulnerable. In addition, many children experience more than one type of maltreatment. No one profile fits a victim of maltreatment, and the signs and symptoms vary (Box 12.1).

A combination of signs and symptoms or a pattern of injury should arouse suspicion. By law, nurses are mandated reporters and must report suspected child maltreatment to authorities. Children who are hospitalized for maltreatment have the same developmental needs as other children their age (Boos, 2020; Hockenberry et al., 2019).

Health Promotion

Nutrition. The quality and quantity of nutrition profoundly influence an infant's growth and development. Many women have already selected a feeding method well before an infant's birth; others will have questions later in the pregnancy. Nurses are in a unique position to help parents select and provide a nutritionally adequate diet for their infant. Understand that factors such as support, culture, role demands, and previous experiences influence feeding methods (Hockenberry et al., 2019).

BOX 12.1   Warning Signs of Abuse

- Physical evidence of abuse or neglect over time; this includes previous injuries, emergency department visits
- Conflicting or changing stories about the accident or trauma
- Delay in seeking treatment
- Injury blamed on child, sibling, or another party
- History is not compatible with the pattern or degree of injury
- History inconsistent with the child's developmental age (e.g., a 6-month-old burned by turning on the hot water)
- An initial complaint not associated with the signs and symptoms present (e.g., bringing the child to the clinic for a cold when there is evidence of physical trauma)
- Inappropriate response of the child, especially an older child (e.g., not wanting to be touched, looking at caregiver before answering any questions)
- Previous reports of abuse in the family
- Frequent emergency department or clinic visits at multiple facilities

Adapted from Boos S: *Physical child abuse: recognition, UpToDate,* 2020. https://www.uptodate.com/contents/physical-child-abuse-recognition; and Hockenberry MJ, et al.: *Wong's nursing care of infants and children,* ed 11, St Louis, 2019, Elsevier.

Breastfeeding is recommended for infant nutrition because breast milk contains the essential nutrients of protein, fats, carbohydrates, and immunoglobulins that bolster the ability to resist infection. Both the AAP and the U.S. Department of Health and Human Services (USDHHS) recommend human milk for the first year of life (Hockenberry et al., 2019). However, if breastfeeding is not possible or if the parent does not desire it, an acceptable alternative is iron-fortified commercially prepared formula. Recent advances in the preparation of infant formula include the addition of nucleotides and long-chain fatty acids, which augment immune function and increase brain development. The use of whole cow's milk, 2% cow's milk, or alternate milk products before the age of 12 months is not recommended (Duryea, 2020). Also, infants under 4 months of age should not receive supplemental fluids in addition to breast milk or formula, especially water or juice (Hockenberry et al., 2019).

The average 1-month-old infant consumes approximately 18 to 21 ounces of breast milk or formula per day. This amount increases slightly during the first 6 months and decreases after solid foods are introduced. The amount of formula per feeding and the number of feedings vary among infants. The addition of solid foods is not recommended before the age of 6 months because developmentally, infants are not ready for solid food before 6 months. The gastrointestinal tract is not sufficiently mature to handle these complex nutrients, and infants are exposed to food antigens that produce food protein allergies. To identify food sensitivities, one food should be introduced and consumed for approximately 1 week before introducing the next food. This allows for easier identification of which food causes the reaction. The use of fruit juices and nonnutritive drinks such as fruit-flavored drinks or soda should be avoided because these do not provide sufficient and appropriate calories during this period (Duryea, 2020; Hockenberry et al., 2019).

Supplementation. The need for dietary vitamin and mineral supplements depends on an infant's diet. Full-term infants are born with some iron stores. The breastfed infant absorbs adequate iron from breast milk during the first 4 to 6 months of life. After 6 months iron-fortified cereal is generally an adequate supplemental source. Because iron in formula is less readily absorbed than that in breast milk, formula-fed infants need to receive iron-fortified formula throughout the first year.

Fluoride is an essential mineral required for development of healthy teeth. To ensure adequate fluoride ingestion, fluoride is often added to drinking water, toothpaste, and infant formula. Adequate concentrations of fluoride are not available in human milk; however, supplementation in breastfed infants under 6 months of age is generally not needed. In areas where fluoridation of water is inadequate, fluoride supplementation may be indicated. A recent concern is the use of complementary and alternative medical therapies that may or may not be safe for children. Inquire about the use of such products to help the parent determine whether the product is truly safe for the child (Hockenberry et al., 2019).

Immunizations. The widespread use of immunizations has resulted in the dramatic decline of infectious diseases over the past 50 years and therefore is an important factor in health promotion during childhood. Although most immunizations can be given to people of any age, it is recommended that the administration of the primary series begin soon after birth and be completed during early childhood. Vaccines are among the safest and most reliable drugs used. Minor side effects sometimes occur; however, serious reactions are rare. Parents need education regarding the importance of immunizations and common side effects such as low-grade fever and local injection site tenderness. The recommended schedule for immunizations changes as new vaccines are developed and advances are made in the field of immunology. Stay informed of the current policies and direct parents to the primary caregiver for their child's schedule. The AAP maintains the most current schedule on its website (AAP, 2021b). Research documents that infants experience pain with invasive procedures. It is important to be aware of measures such as nonnutritive sucking or swaddling to reduce or eliminate pain with procedures such as an immunization (Azarmnejad et al., 2017; Drutz, 2020).

Sleep. Sleep patterns vary among infants, with many having their days and nights reversed until 3 to 4 months of age. Although young infants may sleep during the day, by 6 months most infants demonstrate nocturnal sleep patterns, sleeping between 9 and 11 hours at night. Most infants take one or two naps a day by the end of the first year. Many parents have concerns regarding their infant's sleep patterns, especially if there is difficulty such as sleep refusal or frequent waking during the night. Carefully assess the individual problem before suggesting interventions to address parents' concern.

QSEN **Building Competency in Patient-Centered Care** Children rely extensively on their parents and caregivers for their daily needs and health care. Describe how a nurse can best engage in family-centered care that respects the values, preferences, and needs of both the child and the family.

Answers to QSEN Activities can be found on the Evolve website.

TODDLER

Toddlerhood is the period from 12 to 36 months of age during which children enjoy increasing independence bolstered by greater physical mobility and cognitive abilities. Toddlers are increasingly aware of their abilities to control and are pleased with successful efforts with this new skill. This success leads them to repeated attempts to control their environments. Unsuccessful attempts at control result in negative behavior and temper tantrums. These behaviors are most common when parents stop the initial independent action. Parents cite these as the most problematic behaviors during the toddler years and at times express frustration with trying to set consistent and firm limits while simultaneously encouraging independence. Nurses and parents should limit the opportunities for a "no" answer, known as *negativism*. For example, do not ask the toddler, "Do you want to take your medicine now?" Instead, tell the child that it is time to take medicine, and offer a choice of water or juice to drink with it.

Physical Changes

The average toddler grows 7.5 cm (3 inches) in height, mostly through elongation of the legs, and gains approximately 1.8 to 2.7 kg (4–6 lb) each year (Hockenberry et al., 2019). The rapid development of motor skills allows the child to participate in self-care activities such as feeding, dressing, and toileting. In the beginning the toddler walks in an upright position with a broad stance and gait, protuberant abdomen, and arms out to the sides for balance. Soon the child begins to navigate stairs, using a rail or the wall to maintain balance while progressing upward, placing both feet on the same step before continuing. Success provides courage to attempt the upright mode for descending the stairs in the same manner. Locomotion skills soon include running, jumping, standing on one foot for several seconds, and kicking a ball. Most toddlers ride tricycles and run well by their third birthday.

Fine-motor capabilities progress from spontaneous scribbling to accurately drawing circles and crosses. By 3 years, the child is usually able to stack a small tower of blocks. Toddlers learn to hold crayons with their fingers rather than with their fists and can imitate vertical and horizontal strokes. They are able to manage feeding themselves with a spoon without rotating it and can drink well from a cup without spilling. Toddlers can turn pages of a book one at a time and can easily turn doorknobs (Hockenberry et al., 2019).

Cognitive Changes

Toddlers increase their ability to remember events and begin to put thoughts into words at about 2 years of age. They recognize that they are separate beings from their mothers, but they are unable to assume the view of another. Toddlers' reasoning is based on their own experience of an event. They use symbols to represent objects, places, and people. Children demonstrate this function as they imitate the behavior of another that they viewed earlier (e.g., pretend to shave like daddy), pretend that one object is another (e.g., use a finger as a gun), and use language to stand for absent objects (e.g., request bottle).

Language. The 18-month-old child uses approximately 10 words. The 24-month-old child has a vocabulary of up to 300 words and is generally able to speak in two-word sentences, although the ability to understand speech is much greater than the number of words acquired (Hockenberry et al., 2019). According to Piaget, the preoperational stage of development begins in toddlerhood. Children begin to think about things more symbolically as their vocabulary develops (Piaget, 1952). "Who's that?" and "What's that?" are typical questions children ask during this period. Verbal expressions such as "me do it" and "that's mine" demonstrate the 2-year-old child's use of pronouns and desire for independence and control. By 36 months, the child can use simple sentences, follow some grammatical rules, and learn to use five or six new words each day. Parents facilitate language development best by talking and reading to their children. Reading to children helps expand their vocabulary, knowledge, and imagination. Screen activities such as television (TV), surface pads, or smartphones should not be used to replace parent-child interaction, as these have been shown to delay language development (Hockenberry et al., 2019; Sices and Augustyn, 2020).

Psychosocial Changes

According to Erikson (1963) a sense of autonomy emerges during toddlerhood. Children strive for independence by using their developing muscles to do everything for themselves and become the master of their bodily functions. Their strong wills are frequently exhibited in negative behavior when caregivers attempt to direct their actions. Temper tantrums result when parental restrictions frustrate toddlers. Parents need to provide toddlers with graded independence, allowing them to do things that do not result in harm to themselves or others. For example, young toddlers who want to learn to hold their own cups often benefit from two-handled cups with spouts and plastic bibs with pockets to collect the milk that spills during the learning process.

Play. During the preoperational stage of development the child's imagination develops, and children begin to discern the difference between past and future, although they still do not grasp more complex concepts such as cause and effect (Piaget, 1952). Socially, toddlers remain strongly attached to their parents and fear separation from them. In their presence they feel safe, and their curiosity is evident in their exploration of the environment. The child continues to engage in solitary play during toddlerhood but also begins to participate in parallel play, which is playing *beside* rather than *with* another child. Play expands the child's cognitive and psychosocial development. It is always important to consider the safety of a toy and whether the toy supports development of the child.

Health Risks

The newly developed locomotion abilities and insatiable curiosity of toddlers make them at risk for injury. Toddlers need close supervision at all times and particularly when in environments that are not childproofed.

Poisonings occur frequently because children near 2 years of age are interested in placing any object or substance in their mouths to learn about it. The prudent parent removes or locks up all possible poisons, including plants, cleaning materials, and medications. These parental actions create a safer environment for exploratory behavior. Lead poisoning continues to be a serious health hazard in the United States. Children may ingest or inhale lead, often from chipping of lead-based paint particles in older homes (Hockenberry et al., 2019).

Toddlers' lack of awareness regarding the danger of water and their newly developed walking skills make drowning a major cause of accidental death in this age-group. Limit setting is extremely important for toddlers' safety. Motor vehicle accidents are a significant cause of death in toddlers (Kochanek et al., 2019). Some of these deaths occurred because children were unrestrained or caregivers failed to use car seat safety guidelines when restraining children (AAP, 2021a; Hockenberry et al., 2019).

Toddlers who become ill and require hospitalization experience stress by the separation from their parents. Nurses encourage parents to stay with their child as much as possible and actively participate in providing care. Creating an environment that supports parents helps greatly in gaining the trust and cooperation of the toddler. Establishing a trusting relationship with the parents often results in toddler acceptance of treatment.

Health Promotion

Nutrition. Childhood obesity and the associated chronic diseases that result are sources of concern for all health care providers. Children establish lifetime eating habits in early childhood, and there is increased emphasis on food choices. They increasingly meet nutritional needs by eating solid foods. The healthy toddler requires a balanced daily intake of bread and grains, vegetables, fruit, dairy products, and proteins. Because the consumption of more than a quart of milk per day usually decreases a child's appetite for these essential solid foods and results in inadequate iron intake, advise parents to limit milk intake to 2 to 3 cups per day. Children should not be offered low-fat or skim milk until age 2 because they need the fat for satisfactory physical and intellectual growth (Duryea, 2020; Hockenberry et al., 2019).

Mealtime has psychosocial and physical significance. If the parents struggle to control toddlers' dietary intake, problem behavior and conflicts can result. Toddlers often develop "food jags," or the desire to eat one food repeatedly. Rather than becoming disturbed by this behavior, encourage parents to offer a variety of nutritious foods at meals and to provide only nutritious snacks between meals. Serving finger foods to toddlers allows them to eat by themselves and to satisfy their need for independence and control. Small, reasonable servings allow toddlers to eat all of their meals.

Toilet Training. Increased locomotion skills, the ability to undress, and development of sphincter control allow toilet training if a toddler has developed the necessary language and cognitive abilities. Assisting parents in the recognition of the child's patterns and urge to urinate and defecate is crucial in determining a child's readiness. The toddler must also be motivated to hold on to please the parent rather than letting go to please the self to successfully accomplish toilet training (Hockenberry et al., 2019). Remind parents that patience, consistency, and a calm attitude, in addition to the child's readiness, are essential to successful toilet training.

PRESCHOOLER

The **preschool period** refers to the years between ages 3 and 5. Children refine the mastery of their bodies and eagerly await the beginning of formal education. Many people consider these the most intriguing years of parenting because children are less negative, more accurately share their thoughts, and more effectively interact and communicate. Physical development occurs at a slower pace than cognitive and psychosocial development.

Physical Changes

Several aspects of physical development continue to stabilize in the preschool years. Children have an average annual weight gain of about 4.5 to 6.5 lb (2–3 kg) and grow 6.5 to 9 cm (2.5–3.5 inches) per year and stand an average of 110 cm (43.5 inches) tall by their fifth birthday. The elongation of the legs results in more slender-appearing children, and little difference exists between the sexes (Hockenberry et al., 2019).

Gross- and fine-motor coordination improves in the preschool years as evidenced by running well, walking up and down steps with ease, and learning to hop. By 5 years they usually skip on alternate feet, jump rope, and begin to skate and swim. Improving fine-motor skills allows intricate manipulations. They learn to copy crosses and squares. Triangles and diamonds are usually mastered between ages 5 and 6 (Hockenberry et al., 2019). Scribbling and drawing help to develop fine-motor skills and the hand-eye coordination needed for the printing of letters and numbers.

Children need opportunities to learn and practice new physical skills. Nursing care of healthy and ill children includes an assessment of the availability of these opportunities. Although children with acute illnesses benefit from rest and exclusion from usual daily activities, children who have chronic conditions or who have been hospitalized for long periods need ongoing exposure to developmental opportunities. The parents and nurses weave these opportunities into the children's daily experiences, depending on their abilities, needs, and energy level.

Cognitive Changes

Preschoolers' cognitive development continues as they accomplish developmental tasks that prepare them for scholastic learning. Much of their development is through imaginative play and interactions with others. Though they begin to recognize others' viewpoints, they remain egocentric in their communication and believe others think as they do. Children have increased social interaction, as is illustrated by the 5-year-old child who offers a bandage to a child with a cut finger.

Preschoolers begin to become aware of cause-and-effect relationships, as illustrated by the statement, "The sun sets because people want to go to bed." Early causal thinking is also evident in preschoolers. For example, if two events are related in time or space, children link them in a causal fashion. For example, the hospitalized child reasons, "I cried last night, and that's why the nurse gave me the shot." As children near age 5, they begin to use or learn to use rules to understand causation. They then begin to reason from the general to the particular. This forms the basis for more formal logical thought. The child now reasons, "I get a shot twice a day, and that's why I got one last night." Children in this stage also believe that inanimate objects have lifelike qualities and are capable of action, as seen through comments such as, "Trees cry when their branches get broken."

Preschoolers' knowledge of the world remains closely linked to concrete (perceived by the senses) experiences. Even their rich fantasy life is grounded in their perception of reality. Preschoolers believe that if a rule is broken, punishment results immediately. During these years they believe that a punishment is automatically connected to an act and do not yet realize that it is socially mediated (Hockenberry et al., 2019).

The greatest fear of this age-group appears to be that of bodily harm. This is evident in children's fear of the dark, animals, thunderstorms, and medical personnel. This fear often interferes with their willingness to allow nursing interventions such as measurement of vital signs. Preschoolers cooperate if they are allowed to help the nurse measure the blood pressure of a parent or to manipulate the nurse's equipment.

Language. Preschoolers' vocabularies continue to increase rapidly; by the age of 5, children have an average of 2100 words that they use to define familiar objects, identify colors, and express their desires and frustrations. They combine four to five words into sentences and use pronouns, prepositions, adjectives, and verbs. Language is more social, and preschoolers often question "Why?" and ask the same question repeatedly until answered. Phonetically similar words such as *die* and *dye* or *wood* and *would* cause confusion in preschool children. Avoid such words when preparing them for procedures, and assess comprehension of explanations.

Psychosocial Changes

The world of preschoolers expands beyond the family into the neighborhood where children meet other children and adults. Their curiosity and developing initiative lead to actively exploring the environment, developing new skills, and making new friends. Preschoolers have a surplus of energy that permits them to plan and attempt many activities that are beyond their capabilities, such as pouring milk from a gallon container into their cereal bowls. Guilt arises within children when they overstep the limits of their abilities and think that they have not behaved correctly. Preschoolers also exhibit magical thinking and believe that if they simply think something, it will happen. Children who in anger wished that their sibling were dead experience guilt if that sibling becomes ill. Children need to learn that "wishing" for something to happen does not make it occur. Erikson (1963) recommends that parents help their children strike a healthy balance between initiative and guilt by allowing them to do things on their own while setting firm limits and providing guidance.

Sources of stress for preschoolers can include changes in caregiving arrangements, starting school, the birth of a sibling, parental marital distress, relocation to a new home, or an illness. During these times of stress, preschoolers sometimes revert to bed-wetting or thumb-sucking and want the parents to feed, dress, and hold them. Reassure parents that these are some of the child's normal coping behaviors. Provide experiences that these children are able to master. Such successes help them return to their prior level of independent functioning. As language skills develop, encourage children to talk about their feelings. Play is also an excellent way for preschoolers to vent frustration or anger and is a socially acceptable way to deal with stress.

Play. The play of preschool children becomes more social after the third birthday as it shifts from parallel to associative play. Children playing together engage in similar if not identical activity; however, there is no division of labor or rigid organization or rules. Most 3-year-old children are able to play with one other child in a cooperative manner in which they make something or play designated roles such as mother and infant. By age 4, children play in groups of two or three, and by 5 years the group has a temporary leader for each activity.

During the preoperational stage of growth and development the child begins to engage in make-believe play (Piaget, 1952). Pretend play allows children to learn to understand others' points of view, develop skills in solving social problems, and become more creative. Some children have imaginary playmates. These playmates serve many purposes, are a sign of health, and allow the child to distinguish between reality and fantasy (Hockenberry et al., 2019).

TV, videos, electronic games, and computer programs also help support development and the learning of basic skills. However, these should be only one part of the child's total play activities. The AAP (2020b) advises no more than 1 hour per day of educational, nonviolent TV programs, which should be viewed by parents or other responsible adults in the home. Limiting TV viewing will provide more time for children to read, engage in physical activity, and socialize with others (Hockenberry et al., 2019).

Health Risks

As fine- and gross-motor skills develop and a child becomes more coordinated with better balance, falls become much less of a problem. Many of the guidelines for injury prevention in the toddler also apply to the preschooler. Children need to learn about safety, and parents need to continue close supervision of activities. Children at this age are great imitators, so parental example is important. For instance, parental use of a helmet while bicycling sets an appropriate example for the preschooler.

Health Promotion

Little research has explored preschoolers' perceptions of their own health. Parental beliefs about health, children's bodily sensations, and their ability to perform usual daily activities help children develop attitudes about their health. Preschoolers are usually quite independent in washing, dressing, and feeding. Alterations in this independence influence their feelings about their own health.

Nutrition. Nutritional requirements for the preschooler vary little from those of the toddler. The average daily intake is 1800 calories. Parents often worry about the amount of food their child is consuming, and this is a relevant concern because of the problem of childhood obesity. However, the quality of the food is more important than quantity in most situations. Preschoolers consume about half of average adult portion sizes. Finicky eating habits are characteristic of the 4-year-old; however, preschoolers engaged in meal preparation are more likely to try new things (Hockenberry et al., 2019).

Sleep. Preschoolers average 12 hours of sleep a night and take infrequent naps. Sleep disturbances are common during these years (Hockenberry et al., 2019). Disturbances range from trouble getting to sleep to nightmares to prolonging bedtime with extensive rituals. Frequently children in this playful age-group have had an overabundance of activity and stimulation. Helping them slow down before bedtime usually results in better sleeping habits.

Vision. Vision screening usually begins in the preschool years and needs to occur at regular intervals. One of the most important tests is to determine the presence of nonbinocular vision or strabismus. Early detection and treatment of strabismus must occur by age 6 to prevent amblyopia (Hockenberry et al., 2019).

REFLECT NOW

Nurses must be careful to recognize their own biases and assumptions when caring for children and families. How can you avoid imposing your beliefs and value system on the families with children that you care for?

SCHOOL-AGE CHILD AND ADOLESCENT

The developmental changes between ages 6 and 18 are diverse and span all areas of growth and development. Children develop, expand, refine, and synchronize physical, psychosocial, cognitive, and moral skills so that the individual is able to become an accepted and productive member of society. The environment in which the individual develops skills also expands and diversifies. Instead of the boundaries of family and close friends, the environment now includes the school, community, and church. With age-specific assessment, you need to review the appropriate developmental expectations for each age-group. You can promote health by helping children and adolescents achieve a necessary developmental balance.

SCHOOL-AGE CHILD

During these "middle years" of childhood from age 6 to about age 12, the foundation for adult roles in work, recreation, and social interaction is laid. Puberty marks the end of these middle years and the beginning of adolescence. Children make great developmental strides during these years as they develop competencies in physical, cognitive, and psychosocial skills.

The school or educational experience expands the child's world and is a transition from a life of relatively free play to one of structured play, learning, and work. The school and home influence growth and development, requiring adjustment by the parents and child. The child learns to cope with rules and expectations presented by the school and peers. Parents have to learn to allow their child to make decisions, accept responsibility, and learn from the experiences of life.

Physical Changes

The rate of growth during these early school years is slow and consistent, a relative calm before the growth spurt of adolescence. The school-age child appears slimmer than the preschooler as a result of changes in fat distribution and thickness. Many children double their weight during these middle-childhood years, and most girls exceed boys in both height and weight by the end of the school years (Hockenberry et al., 2019).

School-age children become more graceful during the school years because their large-muscle coordination improves and their strength doubles. Most children practice the basic gross-motor skills of running, jumping, balancing, throwing, and catching during play, resulting in refinement of neuromuscular function and skills. Individual differences in the rate of mastering skills and ultimate skill achievement become apparent during their participation in many activities and games.

Fine-motor skills improve, which allows proficiency in a wide range of activities, including handwriting, drawing, and playing. Most 6-year-old children are able to hold a pencil and print letters and words; by age 12 a child is able to make detailed drawings and write sentences in script. Painting, drawing, playing computer games, and modeling allow children to practice and improve newly refined skills. The improved fine-motor capabilities of children in middle childhood allow them to become very independent in bathing, dressing, and taking care of other personal needs. They develop strong personal preferences in the way these needs are met. Illness and hospitalization threaten children's control in these areas. Therefore, whenever possible, it is important to allow them to participate in care and maintain as much independence as possible. For example, children can help decide the type of fluids and help keep a record of their intake.

As skeletal growth progresses, a child's body appearance and posture change. Earlier the child's posture was stoop shouldered, with slight lordosis and a prominent abdomen. The posture of a school-age child is more erect. Although the U.S. Preventive Services Task Force (2018) does not recommend screening for scoliosis, the lateral curvature of the spine, other professional groups, including the American Academy of Pediatrics and the American Academy of Orthopaedic Surgeons, recommend screening twice for girls (ages 10 and 12) and once for boys (age 13 or 14). Early treatment of scoliosis can limit progression of the curve and the resulting effects.

Eye shape alters because of skeletal growth. This improves visual acuity, and normal adult 20/20 vision is achievable. Screening for vision and hearing problems is easier, and results are more reliable because school-age children more fully understand and cooperate with the test directions. The school nurse typically assesses the growth, visual, and auditory status of school-age children and refers those with possible deviations to a health care provider such as their family practitioner or pediatrician.

Cognitive Changes

According to Piaget, children begin to transition into the concrete operational stage of growth and development around the age of 7, when they begin to demonstrate logical, more concrete thinking. They become less egocentric and begin to understand that their thoughts and feelings may not be shared by others (Piaget, 1952). Cognitive changes provide the school-age child with the ability to think in a logical manner about the here and now and to understand how one thing relates to another. They are now able to use their developed thinking abilities to experience events without having to act them out (Hockenberry et al., 2019). Their thoughts are no longer dominated by their perceptions; thus their ability to understand the world greatly expands.

School-age children have the ability to concentrate on more than one aspect of a situation. They begin to understand that others do not always see things as they do and even begin to understand another viewpoint. They now have the ability to recognize that the amount or quantity of a substance remains the same even when its shape or appearance changes. For instance, two balls of clay of equal size remain the same amount of clay even when one is flattened and the other remains in the shape of a ball.

The young child is able to separate objects into groups according to shape or color, whereas the school-age child understands that the same element can exist in two classes at the same time. School-age children frequently have collections such as baseball cards or stuffed animals that demonstrate this new cognitive skill. Part of the joy of collecting is the ordering and reordering of items in the collection (Hockenberry et al., 2019).

Language Development. Language growth is rapid during middle childhood. Children improve their use of language and expand their structural knowledge. They become more aware of the rules of syntax, the rules for linking words into phrases and sentences. They also identify generalizations and exceptions to rules. They accept language as a means for representing the world in a subjective manner and realize that words have arbitrary rather than absolute meanings. Children begin to think about language, which enables them to appreciate jokes and riddles. They are not as likely to use a literal interpretation of a word, but rather they reason about its meaning within a context (Hockenberry et al., 2019).

Psychosocial Changes

Erikson (1963) identifies the developmental task for school-age children as industry versus inferiority. During this time children strive to acquire competence and skills necessary for them to function as adults. School-age children who are positively recognized for success feel a sense of worth. Those faced with failure often feel a sense of mediocrity or unworthiness, which sometimes results in withdrawal from school and peers.

School-age children begin to define themselves on the basis of internal more than external characteristics. They begin to define their self-concept and develop self-esteem through ongoing self-evaluation. Interaction with peers allows them to define their own accomplishments in relation to others as they work to develop a positive self-image (Hockenberry et al., 2019).

According to Piaget, school-age children around the age of 11 may begin to enter the fourth and final stage of intellectual development, formal operations. In this stage they begin to ponder abstract relationships. They can formulate hypotheses and consider different possibilities. Piaget believed that this was the final stage of cognitive development and that the continued intellectual development in teenagers and adults depended on the accumulation of knowledge (Piaget, 1952).

Peer Relationships. Group and personal achievements become important to the school-age child. Success is important in physical and cognitive activities. Play involves peers and the pursuit of group goals. Although solitary activities are not eliminated, group play overshadows them. Learning to contribute, collaborate, be a member of a team, and work cooperatively toward a common goal becomes a measure of success (Fig. 12.5).

The school-age child prefers same-sex peers. Peer influence becomes quite diverse during this stage of development, and clubs and peer groups become prominent. School-age children often develop "best friends" with whom they share secrets and with whom they look forward to interacting on a daily basis. Group identity increases as the school-age child approaches adolescence.

Sexual Identity. Freud described middle childhood as the latency period because he believed that children of this period had little interest in their sexuality. In fact, however, children are curious about their sexuality. Children's curiosity about adult magazines or meanings of sexually explicit words is an example of their sexual interest. This is the time for them to have exposure to sex education, including topics about sexual maturation, reproduction, and relationships (Hockenberry et al., 2019).

Stress. Today's children experience more stress than children in earlier generations. Stress comes from parental expectations, peer expectations, the school environment, and violence in the family, school, or community. Some school-age children care for themselves before or after school without adult supervision. Latchkey children sometimes feel increased stress and are at greater risk for injury and unsafe behaviors (Hockenberry et al., 2019). A nurse helps the child cope with stress by helping the parents and child identify potential stressors and designing interventions to minimize stress and the child's stress

FIG. 12.5 School-age children gain a sense of achievement from working and playing with peers. (From Hockenberry MJ, et al.: *Wong's nursing care of infants and children,* ed 11, St Louis, 2019, Elsevier.)

response. Deep-breathing techniques, positive imagery, and progressive relaxation of muscle groups are interventions that most children can learn (see Chapter 37). Include the parent, child, and teacher in the intervention for maximal success.

Virtual Learning

Virtual or online learning is becoming an option for children who for many reasons cannot attend a traditional face-to-face educational environment. Distance learning has been adapted in new ways including new formats for educational lessons. Students will be required to work more independently and should be involved in the development of these activities (Paracha et al., 2020).

Carefully planning the engagement of learners to provide integrated learning should become standard for virtual environment development. This new platform offers learning opportunity with real benefits for learners (Basilaia and Kvavadze, 2020).

To bridge the social distance an online learning platform creates, education should create and implement innovative services to meet the needs of children as social distancing becomes a reality. These digital formats and technologies need to be developed and used to support children's growth and development (Ve, 2020).

Health Risks

Accidents and injuries are a major health problem affecting school-age children (Hockenberry et al., 2019). They are exposed to various environments and less supervision, but their developed cognitive and motor skills make them less likely to sustain unintentional injury. Some school-age children are risk takers and attempt activities that are beyond their abilities. Motor vehicle injuries as a passenger or pedestrian are among the most common in this age-group (Centers for Disease Control and Prevention [CDC], 2020a).

Infections account for the majority of all childhood illnesses. Poverty and the prevalence of illness are highly correlated. Access to primary care is often very limited, and health promotion and preventive health measures are minimal. School nurses play a major role in providing access to meet children's health needs by providing health education and direct care services to children in the school setting.

Health Promotion

Perceptions. During the school-age years, identity and self-concept become stronger and more individualized. Perception of wellness is based on readily observable facts such as presence or absence of illness and adequacy of eating or sleeping. Functional ability is the standard by which personal health and the health of others are judged. Children are aware of their body and are modest and sensitive about being exposed. Always provide for privacy when offering explanations of common procedures.

Health Education. Health education during the school-age years is critical to establish behaviors for a healthy adult life. Promotion of good health practices is a nursing responsibility, and effective health education must be developmentally appropriate. Programs directed at health education are frequently organized and conducted in the school. Effective health education teaches children about their bodies and how choices, such as nutrition and routine exercise, affect their health (Hockenberry et al., 2019).

Health Maintenance. Parents need to recognize the importance of annual health maintenance visits for immunizations, screenings, and dental care. When their school-age child reaches 10 years of age, parents need to begin discussions in preparation for upcoming pubertal changes. Topics include introductory information regarding menstruation, sexual intercourse, reproduction, and sexually transmitted infections (STIs).

Human papillomavirus (HPV) is a widespread virus that will infect nearly 79 million Americans, most in their teens or early 20s (CDC, 2021a). In many individuals, HPV clears spontaneously, but in others it can cause significant consequences. Females can develop cervical, vaginal, and vulvar cancers and genital warts, and males can develop genital warts. Because it is not possible to determine who will or will not develop disease from the virus, the CDC (2021a) recommends routine HPV vaccination for girls and boys, with the first dose given at age 11 to 12. For those who miss this recommended age window, vaccination is still recommended through age 26.

Safety. Because accidents are the leading cause of death and injury in the school-age period, safety is a priority health teaching consideration (Hockenberry et al., 2019). At this age, encourage children to take responsibility for their own safety, such as wearing helmets during bike riding and wearing seat belts when in motor vehicles.

Nutrition. Growth often slows during the school-age period as compared with infancy and adolescence. School-age children are developing eating patterns that are independent of parental supervision. The availability of snacks and fast-food restaurants makes it increasingly difficult for children to make healthy choices. The prevalence of obesity is 18.4% in children ages 6 to 11 years and 20.6% among 12- to 19-year-olds (CDC, 2021b). Childhood obesity has become a prominent health problem, resulting in increased risk for hypertension, diabetes, coronary heart disease, fatty liver disease, pulmonary complications such as sleep apnea, musculoskeletal problems, dyslipidemia, and potential for psychological problems (Hockenberry et al., 2019). Nurses promote healthy lifestyle habits, including nutrition and exercise. School-age children need to participate in educational programs that enable them to plan, select, and prepare healthy meals and snacks. Children need adequate caloric intake in their meals and snacks for growth throughout childhood accompanied by activity for continued gross-motor development.

ADOLESCENT

Adolescence is the period during which the individual makes the transition from childhood to adulthood, usually between ages 13 and 20 years. The term *adolescent* usually refers to psychological maturation of the individual, whereas puberty refers to the point at which reproduction becomes possible. The hormonal changes of puberty result in changes in the appearance of the young person, and cognitive development results in the ability to hypothesize and deal with abstractions. Adjustments and adaptations are necessary to cope with these simultaneous changes and the attempt to establish a mature sense of identity.

Understanding development helps teenagers and parents anticipate and cope with the stresses of adolescence. Nursing activities, particularly education, promote healthy development. These activities occur in a variety of settings and can be developed for the adolescent, parents, or both. For example, a nurse conducts seminars in a high school to provide practical suggestions to a large group of students for solving problems of concern, such as treating acne or making responsible decisions about drug or alcohol use. Similarly, a group education program for parents about how to cope with teenagers would promote parental understanding of adolescent development.

Physical Changes

Physical changes occur rapidly in adolescence. Sexual maturation occurs with the development of primary and secondary sexual characteristics. The four main physical changes are:
1. Increased growth rate of skeleton, muscle, and viscera
2. Sex-specific changes, such as changes in shoulder and hip width

3. Alteration in distribution of muscle and fat
4. Development of the reproductive system and secondary sex characteristics

Wide variation exists between sexes and within the same sex in the timing of physical changes associated with puberty. Girls generally have prepubescent changes 1 to 2 years before boys do (Hockenberry et al., 2019). The rates of height and weight gain are usually proportional, and the sequence of pubertal growth changes is the same in most individuals.

Hormonal changes within the body create change when the body produces gonadotropin-releasing hormones that stimulate ovarian cells to produce estrogen and testicular cells to produce testosterone. These hormones contribute to the development of secondary sex characteristics, such as hair growth and voice changes, and play an essential role in reproduction. The changing concentrations of these hormones are also linked to acne and body odor. Understanding these hormonal changes enables you to reassure adolescents and educate them about body care needs.

Being like peers is extremely important for adolescents (Fig. 12.6). Any deviation in the timing of their physical changes is extremely difficult for them to accept. It is important to provide emotional support for those undergoing early or delayed puberty. Even adolescents whose physical changes are occurring at the normal times seek confirmation of and reassurance about their normalcy.

Height and weight increase during adolescence, with peak height velocity occurring at about 12 years in girls and at about 14 years in boys. Girls' height increases 5 to 20 cm (2–8 inches), and weight increases by 7 to 25 kg (15.5–55 lb). Girls grow less than 2 inches following menarche (the onset of menstruation), reaching their full height by 16 to 17 years of age. Boys' height increases approximately 10 to 30 cm (4–12 inches), and weight increases by 7 to 30 kg (15.5–66 lb). Boys continue to grow taller until 18 to 20 years of age (Hockenberry et al., 2019).

Although individual and sex-related differences exist, growth follows a similar pattern for both sexes. Personal growth curves help nurses assess physical development. However, an individual's sustained progression along the curve is more important than a comparison with the norm.

Cognitive Changes

The adolescent develops the ability to determine and rank possibilities, solve problems, and make decisions through logical operations. The teenager thinks abstractly and deals effectively with hypothetical problems. When confronted with a problem, the adolescent considers an infinite variety of causes and solutions. For the first time the young person moves beyond the physical or concrete properties of a situation and uses reasoning powers to understand the abstract. School-age individuals think about what is, whereas adolescents are able to imagine what might be.

Adolescents are able to think in terms of the future rather than just current events. These newly developed abilities allow an individual to have more insight and skill in playing video, computer, and board games that require abstract thinking and deductive reasoning about many possible strategies. A teenager solves problems requiring simultaneous manipulation of several abstract concepts. Development of this ability is important in the pursuit of an identity. For example, newly acquired cognitive skills allow the teenager to define appropriate, effective, and comfortable sex-role behaviors and to consider their impact on peers, family, and society. A higher level of cognitive functioning makes the adolescent receptive to more detailed and diverse information about sexuality and sexual behaviors. For example, sex education includes an explanation of physiological sexual changes and birth-control measures.

Adolescents also develop the ability to understand how an individual's ideas or actions influence others. Although adolescents have the capability to think as well as adults, they do not have experiences on which to build. It is common for teenagers to consider their parents too narrow-minded or materialistic. At this time adolescents believe that they are unique and the exception, giving rise to their risk-taking behaviors. In other words, they think that they are invincible. For example, adolescents might believe that they are able to drive fast and not have an accident or may argue that e-cigarettes will not affect their health.

Language Skills. Language development is fairly complete by adolescence, although vocabulary continues to expand. The primary focus becomes communication skills that an adolescent uses effectively in various situations. Adolescents need to communicate thoughts, feelings, and facts to peers, parents, teachers, and other people of authority. The skills used in these diverse communication situations vary. Adolescents select the people with whom to communicate, decide on the exact message, and choose the way to transmit it. For example, how teenagers tell parents about failing grades is not the same as how they tell friends. Good communication skills are critical for adolescents in overcoming peer pressure and unhealthy behaviors. The following are some strategies for communicating with adolescents (Hockenberry et al., 2019):

- Provide privacy and a nonthreatening environment. As adolescents become more autonomous, interviews should be conducted without parents present.
- Ensure confidentiality and explain the limitations of confidentiality, such as disclosure of abuse or suicidal ideations.
- Be nonjudgmental and display genuine interest in the adolescent's perspective.
- Ask open-ended questions (see Chapter 24).
- Start with less sensitive topics and then move to more sensitive issues. Asking questions about sex, drugs, and school opens the channels for further discussion.

Psychosocial Changes

The search for personal identity is the major task of adolescent psychosocial development. Teenagers establish close peer relationships or remain socially isolated. Erikson (1963) sees identity (or role) confusion as the prime danger of this stage and suggests that the cliquish behavior and intolerance of differences seen in adolescent behavior are defenses against identity confusion (Erikson, 1968). Adolescents become more emotionally independent from their parents (Hockenberry et al., 2019). In addition, they develop their own ethical systems based on personal values. They begin to make choices about vocation, future education,

FIG. 12.6 Peer interactions help increase self-esteem during puberty. (Copyright © MachineHeadz/iStock/Thinkstock.)

and lifestyle. The various components of total identity evolve from these tasks and compose an adult personal identity that is unique to the individual.

Sexual Identity. Physical changes of puberty enhance achievement of sexual identity (see Chapter 34). The physical evidence of maturity encourages the development of masculine and feminine behaviors. Adolescents depend on these physical clues because they want assurance of maleness or femaleness and they do not wish to be different from peers. Also, development of sexual identity involves identification of sexual orientation. By late adolescence, most individuals identify themselves as heterosexual, and a small number identify as bisexual, gay, or lesbian.

Peer Group Identity. Adolescents seek a group identity because they need self-esteem and acceptance. Similarity in dress or speech is common in teenage groups. Peer groups provide the adolescent with a sense of belonging, approval, and the opportunity to learn acceptable behavior. Popularity with opposite-sex and same-sex peers is important. Supportive peer groups can have a positive influence on health choices; poor peer group selection can lead to poor decision making and negative health outcomes. Nurses should encourage parents to communicate with their adolescents and provide supervision to promote selection of positive peer groups.

Family Identity. Adolescents begin to place more value on peer relationships than on parents. Although financial independence for adolescents is not the norm in American society, many work part-time, using their income to bolster independence. When they cannot have a part-time job because of studies, school-related activities, and other factors, parents can provide allowances for clothing and incidentals, which encourage adolescents to develop decision making and budgeting skills.

Some adolescents and families have more difficulty during these years than others. Adolescents need to make choices, act independently, and experience the consequences of their actions. Nurses help families consider appropriate ways for them to foster the independence of their adolescent while maintaining family structure.

Health Identity. Another component of personal identity is perception of health. This component is of specific interest to health care providers. Healthy adolescents evaluate their own health according to feelings of well-being, ability to function normally, and absence of symptoms (Hockenberry et al., 2019). They also often include health maintenance and health promotion behaviors as important concerns.

Adolescents try new roles, begin to stabilize their identity, and acquire values and behaviors from which their adult lifestyle will evolve. The rapid changes during this period make health promotion programs especially crucial. Adolescents are able to identify behaviors such as smoking and substance abuse as threatening to health in general terms but frequently tend to underestimate the effect of the potentially negative consequences of their own actions. Health promotion strategies should focus not only on reducing risk behaviors but also on maximizing protective factors such as coping and adapting (Hockenberry et al., 2019).

Health Risks

Accidents. In the United States, unintentional injury is the leading cause of death in adolescents. Motor vehicle accidents are the most common cause of death (USDHHS, 2018). Adolescents are at particular risk because of lack of driving experience and risk-taking behaviors such as driving too fast, drinking and driving, or riding with someone under the influence (CDC, 2020b; Hockenberry et al., 2019). The majority of deaths from injury occur in boys. Other frequent causes of

accidental death in teenagers are drowning and the use of firearms. Adolescents think that they are invincible, which leads to risk-taking behaviors. The use of alcohol precedes many injuries, and adolescents continue to be both the victims and perpetrators of violence. An objective for *Healthy People 2030* focuses on preventing violence (e.g., reducing the proportion of public schools that have violent incidents) (Office of Disease Prevention and Health Promotion [ODPHP], n.d.).

Violence and Homicide. Homicide is the second leading cause of death in adolescents in the United States and is the leading cause of death in African-American teenagers (Hockenberry et al., 2019). The Youth Risk Behavior Surveillance System reported that in 2019 more than 7% of students were threatened or injured with a weapon (e.g., gun, club, or knife) on school property (CDC, 2020c). Teenagers are most likely to be killed by an acquaintance or gang member and most often with a firearm. Because having a gun in the home raises the risk of homicide and suicide for adolescents, include assessment of gun presence in the home and discuss gun safety when counseling families (Hockenberry et al., 2019).

Violence among adolescents has become a national concern. School shootings are increasingly common and contribute to stress in childhood and adolescence. Violence includes physical assaults and fighting, threats and intimidation, sexual harassment or violence, human trafficking (Box 12.2), bullying, or theft. Nurses working with adolescents need to be aware of the potential for school violence and include screening questions when providing health care, regardless of the setting.

REFLECT NOW

School violence and school shootings are on the rise in the United States. Reflect on what you now know about an adolescent's development. How can nurses intervene with this age-group to decrease the prevalence of this phenomenon?

Suicide. Suicide is a major leading cause of death in adolescence. In the past 30 years, suicide rates have tripled in children 11 to 14 years of age and have doubled in children 15 to 19 years of age (Kennebeck and Bonin, 2019). Depression and social isolation commonly precede a suicide attempt, but suicide probably results from a combination of several factors. Nurses must be able to identify the factors associated with adolescent depression and suicide risk and precipitating events. Screen for the following changes in behavior:
- Decrease in school performance
- Withdrawal
- Loss of initiative
- Loneliness, sadness, and crying
- Appetite and sleep disturbances
- Verbalization of suicidal thought

If your assessment indicates depression or suicide risk, make immediate referrals to mental health professionals. Guidance helps adolescents focus on the positive aspects of life and strengthen coping abilities.

Substance Abuse. Substance abuse is a concern for all who work with adolescents. Adolescents often believe that mood-altering substances create a sense of well-being or improve level of performance. All adolescents are at risk for experimental or recreational substance use (Hockenberry et al., 2019). The misuse of opioids in high school students has decreased considerably over the past 10 years, and the daily use of marijuana among 12th graders is 6.4% (National Institute on Drug Abuse [NIDA], 2019).

Education Programs to Address Sex Trafficking of Children

PICOT Question: For child and adolescent victims of sex trafficking, will education programs for health care providers and mandatory reporters on the signs and risk factors of sex trafficking victimization improve early identification and intervention?

Evidence Summary

Educational programs on sex trafficking for health care providers are essential to identifying victims and intervening appropriately (Bauer et al., 2019). Sex trafficking of minors is a type of human trafficking involving crimes of a sexual nature committed against children and adolescents. This exploitation occurs when someone uses power, fraud, or coercion to force someone else to commit a commercial sex act, such as prostitution; performing in sexual venues such as strip clubs; survival sex by which a minor performs sex acts for money, food, shelter, or other necessities; pornography; and sex tourism, such as mail-order bride trade or early marriage (Tracy and Macias-Konstantopoulos, 2021; Ulibarri et al., 2017). Because children who are trafficked do not often disclose that they are victims and there is no uniform data collection system in place to track sex trafficking of minors, the prevalence is largely unknown (Bauer et al., 2019; Hartinger-Saunders et al., 2017; Tracy and Macias-Konstantopoulos, 2021).

Traffickers find their victims through social networks, clubs, bars, schools, and on the Internet (sharedhope International, 2021). Victims of sex trafficking come from every demographic, but they typically share risk factors that make them vulnerable to exploitation. Common risk factors include history of abuse or neglect, family violence or dysfunction, poverty, substance misuse, mental health issues, runaway/homelessness, and those who identify as lesbian, gay, bisexual, transgender, queer, or questioning (Greenbaum, 2017; Tracy and Macias-Konstantopoulos, 2021).

Many sex trafficking victims are "trapped and controlled through assault, threats, false promises, perceived sense of protection, isolation, shaming, and debt" (CDC, 2021c), yet many do not recognize they are being trafficked, do not identify themselves as victims (Perkins and Ruiz, 2017), and may even protect their abuser (Hartinger-Saunders et al., 2017). Common health issues of sex trafficking victims include sexually transmitted infections (STIs), HIV/AIDS, pregnancy, physical injury, posttraumatic stress disorder, and depression (Bauer et al., 2019; Greenbaum, 2017; Tracy and Macias-Konstantopoulos, 2021).

Application to Nursing Practice

- Develop educational programs that assist health care providers to identify victims of sex trafficking, including how to safely separate the potential victim from the trafficker and knowledge of immediate resources to protect the victim (Bauer et al., 2019).
- Ensure that mandatory reporters, which include nurses, can recognize the signs of victimization and know how to intervene (Powell et al., 2017).
- Design a "Sex Trafficking Indicator" checklist and educate health care providers on its use (Bauer et al., 2019).
- Use a standardized, evidence-based education program on human trafficking with patient-outcome metrics to educate other health care providers and mandatory reporters to recognize the risk factors and signs of sex traffic victimization (Hartinger-Saunders et al., 2017; Powell et al., 2017).
- Use a framework to help health care providers identify victims, assess their safety, and connect them with resources (Tracy and Macias-Konstantopoulos, 2021).
- Coordinate care and tailor interventions for sex trafficking survivors (Twigg, 2017).
- Lead or participate in research on the best way to educate health care professionals about sex trafficking (Powell et al., 2017).

Tobacco use continues to be a health problem among adolescents. The use of cigarettes by high school students decreased from 15.8% in 2011 to 5.8% in 2019, while the use of electronic cigarettes increased from 1.5% in 2011 to 27.5% in 2019 (CDC, 2020d). This huge increase led to new U.S. Food and Drug Administration (FDA) regulations to reduce the sale of electronic cigarettes to youth (FDA, 2020). Although electronic cigarettes may be less harmful than cigarettes, they should not be considered safe, as they can harm adolescent brain development and increase the presence of cancer-causing chemicals in the body (CDC, 2020e). In addition, vaping has been associated with serious lung problems likely related to irritation or allergic reactions to contaminants (Shmerling, 2019). The increased use of e-cigarettes and vaping does not reduce the addictive or health effects of nicotine use (CDC, 2020d). Nurses must educate teenagers about smoking cessation and the safety risks associated with smoking and substance and alcohol use.

Eating Disorders. Eating disorders include anorexia nervosa, bulimia nervosa, and binge eating disorder. The highest incidence of eating disorders occurs in 15- to 19-year-olds, so routine nutritional screening should be a part of the health care provided to all adolescents. Areas to include in the assessment are past and present diet history, food records, eating habits, attitudes, health beliefs, and socioeconomic and psychosocial factors (Hockenberry et al., 2019). An important psychosocial factor is assessment of an adolescent's perception of body image and self-esteem or any sources of depression (Laporta-Herrero et al., 2018).

Anorexia nervosa is more common in girls and is a clinical syndrome with both physical and psychosocial components of anxiety and depression. People with anorexia nervosa have an intense fear of gaining weight and refuse to maintain body weight at the minimal normal weight for their age and height. Over time this condition affects both physiological and psychosocial function and quality of life (Klein and Attia, 2019).

Bulimia nervosa is most identified with binge eating and behaviors to prevent weight gain. Unlike anorexia, bulimia occurs within a normal weight range; therefore it is much more difficult to detect. Behaviors of individuals with eating disorders include self-induced vomiting, misuse of laxatives and other medications, and excessive exercise. It is important to take a thorough dietary history because, if left undetected and untreated, these disorders lead to significant morbidity and mortality (Hockenberry et al., 2019).

Sexually Transmitted Infections. STIs annually affect millions of sexually active adolescents. This high degree of incidence makes it imperative that sexually active adolescents be screened for STIs even when they have no symptoms. The annual physical examination of a sexually active adolescent includes a thorough sexual history and a careful examination of the genitalia so that STIs are not missed. Be proactive by using the interview process to identify risk factors in the adolescent, and provide education to prevent STIs, including human immunodeficiency virus (HIV) and HPV, and unwanted pregnancies (Hockenberry et al., 2019). As discussed earlier for school-age children, immunization for HPV infection should be considered at this time if not already administered.

Pregnancy. The United States has the highest rate of teenage pregnancy and childbearing annually compared with other industrialized nations (Hockenberry et al., 2019). Adolescent birth rates continue to decline owing to improvements in contraceptive use, the use of long-acting reversible contraception, and safe sex practices (Lindberg et al., 2018). However, adolescent pregnancy continues to be a major social challenge. Adolescent pregnancy occurs across socioeconomic classes, in public and private schools, among all ethnic and religious backgrounds, and in all parts of the country. Pregnant teens need special attention with regard to nutrition, health supervision, and psychological support.

Adolescent mothers also need help in planning for the future and obtaining competent day care for their infants.

Health Promotion

Health Education. Community and school-based health programs for adolescents focus on health promotion and illness prevention. Nurses need to be sensitive to the emotional cues from adolescents before initiating health teaching to know when the teen is ready to discuss concerns. In addition, discussions with adolescents need to be private and confidential. Adolescents define health in much the same way as adults and look for opportunities to reach their physical, mental, and emotional potential. Large numbers of school-based clinics have been developed and implemented to respond to adolescents' needs. Adolescents are much more likely to use these health care services if they encounter providers who are caring and respectful (Hockenberry et al., 2019).

Nurses play an important role in preventing injuries and accidental deaths. For example, discussing alternatives to substance-impaired driving or riding with someone under the influence of drugs or alcohol prepares them to consider alternatives when such an occasion arises. As a nurse, identify adolescents at risk for abuse, provide education to prevent accidents related to substance abuse, and provide resources to those in need of mental health care.

Minority Adolescents. African-American, Hispanic, Latino, Asian, Native American, and Alaskan Native adolescents are the fastest-growing segment in the U.S. population. Minority adolescents experience a greater percentage of health problems and barriers to health care (Hockenberry et al., 2019). Issues of concern for these adolescents living in a high-risk environment include childhood trauma, cyberbullying, death related to violence, unintentional injuries, learning or emotional difficulties, and increased rates of adolescent pregnancy and STIs (Larson et al., 2017). Poverty is a major factor that negatively affects the lives of many minority adolescents. Limited access to health services is common (Duarte et al., 2018). Nurses are able to make a significant contribution to improving access to appropriate health care for adolescents. With knowledge about various cultures and the challenges facing adolescents from minority and at-risk groups, nurses act as advocates to ensure accessibility of appropriate services.

Gay, Lesbian, and Bisexual Adolescents. Sexual orientation refers to patterns of sexual and emotional attraction to persons of the same gender, opposite gender, or both males and females. Although most adolescents identify themselves as heterosexual, many identify themselves as homosexual or bisexual. It is widely known that although some adolescents participate in same-gender sexual activity, they do not necessarily become homosexual as adults (Hockenberry et al., 2019). Adolescents who believe that they have a homosexual or bisexual orientation often try to keep it hidden to avoid any associated stigma, victimization, or bullying. This increases their vulnerability to depression and suicide. If a teen chooses to disclose sexual orientation to you, help the adolescent consider how to discuss with family or friends and to construct a safety plan before telling family or friends in case their response is not supportive (Hockenberry et al., 2019).

KEY POINTS

- Nurses promote the health of pregnant women by addressing nutritional requirements, physical changes, and psychosocial needs.
- At birth, newborns develop independent circulatory and respiratory functioning.
- Promotion of parent-child attachment should begin immediately after birth.

- Physical changes include maturation of organ systems, fine- and gross-motor development, and physical growth. These changes occur in a regular pattern and are monitored to identify developmental concerns.
- Cognitive and psychosocial development throughout childhood is rapid, and a multitude of factors can foster or hinder a child's development.
- Play provides opportunities for development of cognitive, social, and motor skills. Play evolves from solitary to interactive play throughout childhood.
- Through anticipatory guidance, nurses can prepare parents to reduce their children's health risks and to promote achievement of developmental tasks.

REFLECTIVE LEARNING

- Considering what you know about childhood development, how would your approach to assessment of cognitive function be different if a child were of school age versus an adolescent?
- What anticipatory guidance could you provide for a family you cared for to minimize health risks for their preschool child?
- Family support, including financial and child care assistance, for the adolescent mother significantly increases the likelihood that she will complete her education and gain skills for the job market. How can you support these goals for an adolescent mother who does not have sufficient family support?

REVIEW QUESTIONS

1. Which of the following should be included in health teaching for a pregnant patient? (Select all that apply.)
   1. Exposure of the fetus to alcohol, drugs, or tobacco can cause abnormal development.
   2. Nutritional needs increase during pregnancy, and eating healthy foods is important.
   3. Complementary and alternative therapies should always be avoided during pregnancy.
   4. Provide education on self-care to reduce common discomforts of pregnancy, such as nausea.
   5. Recommend birthing classes to prepare the mother for the birthing process.
2. A mother has brought her 6-month-old infant in for a well-child check. Which of her statements indicates a need for further teaching?
   1. "I can start giving her whole milk at about 12 months."
   2. "I can continue to breastfeed for another 6 months."
   3. "I can give her plenty of fruit juice to increase her vitamin intake."
   4. "I can start giving her solid food now, introducing one food at a time."
3. A nurse is teaching the mother of a young infant about prevention of SIDS. Which of the following statements indicates that the teaching has been effective? (Select all that apply.)
   1. "I'll let the baby sleep in bed with me so I can watch her."
   2. "I'll remove stuffed animals and pillows from the crib."
   3. "I'll place my baby on her back for sleep."
   4. "I'll be sure to keep my baby's room cool."
   5. "I'll keep a crib bumper in the bed to prevent drafts."
4. Place the skills in the expected order of gross-motor development in an infant, beginning with the earliest skill.
   1. Can lift head 45 degrees off table, when prone
   2. Pulls self to standing position
   3. Sits upright without support
   4. Rolls from back to abdomen
   5. Rolls from abdomen to back

5. Parents are concerned about their toddler's negativism. To avoid a negative response, which of the following is the best way for a nurse to demonstrate asking the toddler to eat lunch?
   1. "Would you like to eat your lunch now?"
   2. "Would you like to sit at the big table to eat?"
   3. "When would you like to eat your lunch with your friends?"
   4. "Would you like apple slices or applesauce with your sandwich?"

6. As education is moved from the traditional face-to-face to a distance learning environment, what would be the most significant impact on school-age children?
   1. These formats have no significant impact on children.
   2. School-age children do not need to be involved in developing this type of learning.
   3. These formats are easy for children to use and parents to support.
   4. The need for independence increases when working in this format.

7. You are caring for a 4-year-old child who is hospitalized for an infection. He tells you that he is sick because he was "bad." Which is the most correct interpretation of his comment?
   1. Indicative of maladaptive stress response
   2. Representative of his cognitive development
   3. Suggestive of excessive discipline at home
   4. Indicative of his developing sense of inferiority

8. At a well-child examination, the mother comments that her toddler eats little at mealtime, will sit only briefly at the table, and wants snacks all the time. Which of the following should the nurse recommend? (Select all the apply.)
   1. Provide nutritious snacks for a healthy diet.
   2. Offer rewards for eating at mealtimes.
   3. Avoid snacks so she is hungry at mealtime.
   4. Offer finger foods so she can eat as she walks.
   5. Explain to her why eating at mealtime is important.

9. A 15-year-old patient tells the nurse that she is sexually active. What is the best action by the nurse?
   1. Contact her parents to alert them of her need for birth control.
   2. Explain that having sex is not appropriate for her age-group.
   3. Counsel her on safe sex practices and on minimizing health risks.
   4. Ask her to have her partner come to the clinic for STI testing.

10. A 4-month-old infant has not been feeling well for 2 days. Which number on the image identifies the area of the infant's head where the nurse can assess for dehydration?
    1. 1
    2. 2
    3. 3
    4. 4
    5. 5

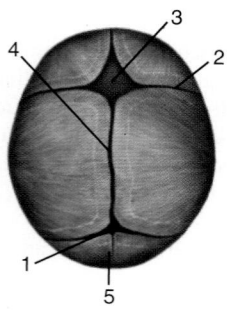

Answers: 1. 1, 2, 4, 5; **2.** 3; **3.** 3, 4, 1, 5, 4, 3; **5.** 4; **6.** 4; **7.** 2; **8.** 1, 4; **9.** 3; **10.** 3

Rationales to Review Questions can be found on the Evolve website.

REFERENCES

American Academy of Pediatrics (AAP): *Make baby's room safe: Parent checklist*, https://www.healthychildren.org/English/safety-prevention/at-home/Pages/Make-Babys-Room-Safe.aspx, 2020a. Accessed April 30, 2021.

American Academy of Pediatrics (AAP): *How to make a family media use plan*, https://www.healthychildren.org/English/family-life/Media/Pages/How-to-Make-a-Family-Media-Use-Plan.aspx, 2020b. Accessed April 30, 2021.

American Academy of Pediatrics (AAP): *Car seats: information for families*, https://www.healthychildren.org/English/safety-prevention/on-the-go/Pages/Car-Safety-Seats-Information-for-Families.aspx, 2021a. Accessed April 30, 2021.

American Academy of Pediatrics (AAP): *Immunization schedules*, https://www.aap.org/en-us/advocacy-and-policy/aap-health-initiatives/immunizations/Pages/Immunization-Schedule.aspx, 2021b. Accessed April 30, 2021.

Bauer R et al.: What health providers should know about human sex trafficking. *Medsurg Nursing* 28(6):347, 2019.

Centers for Disease Control and Prevention (CDC): *Road traffic injuries and deaths – a global problem*. https://www.cdc.gov/injury/features/global-road-safety/index.html, 2020a, Accessed April 29, 2021.

Centers for Disease Control and Prevention (CDC): *Keep teen drivers safe*. https://www.cdc.gov/injury/features/teen-drivers/index. html, 2020b. Accessed April 30, 2021.

Centers for Disease Control and Prevention (CDC): *Preventing school violence*. https://www.cdc.gov/violenceprevention/youthviolence/schoolviolence/fastfact.html, 2020c. Accessed April 30, 2021.

Centers for Disease Control and Prevention (CDC): *Youth and tobacco use*, https://www.cdc.gov/tobacco/data_statistics/fact_sheets/youth_data/tobacco_use/index.htm, 2020d. Accessed April 30, 2021.

Centers for Disease Control and Prevention (CDC): *Electronic cigarettes*, https://www.cdc.gov/tobacco/basic_information/e-cigarettes/index.htm , 2020e. Accessed April 30, 2021.

Centers for Disease Control and Prevention (CDC): *Genital HPV infection: Fact sheet*. https://www.cdc.gov/std/hpv/stdfact-hpv.htm, 2021a. Accessed April 30, 2021.

Centers for Disease Control and Prevention (CDC): *Childhood obesity facts*. https://www.cdc.gov/obesity/data/childhood.html, 2021b. Accessed April 30, 2021.

Center for Disease Control and Prevention (CDC): *Sex trafficking*, https://www.cdc.gov/violenceprevention/sexualviolence/trafficking.html, 2021c. Accessed April 30, 2021.

Erikson EH: *Childhood and society*, ed 2, New York, 1963, Norton.

Erikson EH: *Identity: youth and crises*, New York, 1968, Norton.

Hockenberry M et al.: *Wong's nursing care of infants and children*, ed 11, St Louis, 2019, Elsevier.

Kotagal S: Neurologic examination of the newborn, *UpToDate*, https://www.uptodate.com/contents/neurologic-examination-of-the-newborn, 2020.

McKee-Garrett T: Assessment of the newborn infant, *UpToDate*, https://www.uptodate.com/contents/assessment-of-the-newborn-infant, 2020.

McKee-Garrett T: Overview of the routine management of the healthy newborn infant, *UpToDate*, https://www.uptodate.com/contents/overview-of-the-routine-management-of-the-healthy-newborn-infant?search=Overview%20of%20the%20routine%20management%20of%20the%20healthy%20newborn%20infant&source=search_result&selectedTitle=1~150&usage_type=default&display_rank=1, 2021. Accessed April 30, 2021.

Moon R: *How to keep your sleeping baby safe: AAP policy explained*, American Academy of Pediatrics (AAP). https://www.healthychildren.org/English/ages-stages/baby/sleep/Pages/A-Parents-Guide-to-Safe-Sleep.aspx, 2020. Accessed April 30, 2021.

Murray SS et al.: *Foundations of maternal-newborn and women's health nursing*, ed 7, Philadelphia, 2019, Saunders.

National Institute on Drug Abuse: *Monitoring the future 2019 survey results: Overall findings*. https://www.drugabuse.gov/drug-topics/trends-statistics/infographics/monitoring-future-2019-survey-results-overall-findings, 2019. Accessed April 20, 2021.

Office of Disease Prevention and Health Promotion (ODPHP): Adolescents. *Healthy People 2030*, n.d., U.S. Department of Health and Human Services. https://health.gov/healthypeople/objectives-and-data/browse-objectives/adolescents. Accessed April 30, 2021.

Piaget J: *The origins of intelligence in children*, New York, 1952, International Universities Press.

sharedhope International: *What is sex trafficking?*, https://sharedhope.org/the-problem/what-is-sex-trafficking/, 2021. Accessed April 30, 2021.

Shmerling RH: *Can vaping damage your lungs? What we do (and don't) know*, Harvard Health Publishing. http://

www.health.harvard.edu/blog/can-vaping-damage-your-lungs-what-we-do-and-dont-know-2019090417734, 2019. Accessed April 30, 2021.

U.S. Department of Health and Human Services (USDHHS): *National vital statistics reports* 67(No. 5), 26. https://www.cdc.gov/nchs/data/nvsr/nvsr67/nvsr67_05.pdf, 2018.

U.S. Food and Drug Administration (FDA). *Vaporizers, E-cigarettes, and other electronic nicotine delivery systems (ENDS).* https://www.fda.gov/tobacco-products/products-ingredients-components/vaporizers-e-cigarettes-and-other-electronic-nicotine-delivery-systems-ends, 2020. Accessed April 30, 2021.

U.S. Preventive Services Task Force Recommendation Statement (USPS): Screening for adolescent idiopathic scoliosis. *JAMA* 319(2):165-172, 2018. Available at: https://jamanetwork.com/journals/jama/fullarticle/2668355. Accessed April 29, 2021.

RESEARCH REFERENCES

Azarmnejad E et al.: The effectiveness of familiar auditory stimulus on hospitalized neonates' physiologic responses to procedural pain. *Int J Nurs Practr* 23:e12527, 2017.

Basilaia G, Kvavadze D: Transition to *online education in schools during* a SARS-CoV-2 Coronavirus (COVID-19) pandemic in Georgia, *Pedagogical Research* 5(4), em0060, 2020.

Boos S: Physical child abuse: Recognition, *UpToDate*, https://www.uptodate.com/contents/physical-child-abuse-recognition, 2020.

Chacko M: Pregnancy in adolescents, *UpToDate*, https://www.uptodate.com/contents/pregnancy-in-adolescents , 2021. Accessed April 30, 2021.

Drutz J: Standard immunizations for children and adolescents: Overview, *UpToDate*, https://www.uptodate.com/contents/standard-immunizations-for-children-and-adolescents-overview, 2020. Accessed April 30, 2021.

Duryea T: Dietary recommendations for toddlers, preschool, and school-age children, *UpToDate*, https://www.uptodate.com/contents/dietary-recommendations-for-toddlers-preschool-and-school-age-children, 2020. Accessed April 30, 2021.

Duarte C et al.: Correlation of minority status, cyberbullying, and mental health: a cross-sectional study of 1031 adolescents. *J Child Adolesc Trauma* 11(1):39, 2018.

Greenbaum VJ: Child sex trafficking in the United States: challenges for the healthcare provider. *PLoS Med* 14(11): e1002439, 2017.

Hartinger-Saunders RM et al.: Mandated reporters' perceptions of and encounters with domestic minor sex trafficking of adolescent females in the United States. *Am J Orthopsychiatry* 87(3):195, 2017.

Kennebeck S, Bonin L: Suicidal behavior in children and adolescents: Epidemiology and risk factors, *UpToDate*, https://www.uptodate.com/contents/suicidal-behavior-in-children-and-adolescents-epidemiology-and-risk-factors/print, 2019. Accessed April 30, 2021.

Klein D, Attia E: Anorexia nervosa in adults: Clinical features, course of illness, assessment, and diagnosis, *UpToDate*, https://www.uptodate.com/contents/anorexia-nervosa-in-adults-clinical-features-course-of-illness-assessment-and-diagnosis, 2019. Accessed April 30, 2021.

Kochanek KD et al.: *Deaths-final data for 2017*, National Vital Statistics Report 68(9). https://www.cdc.gov/nchs/data/nvsr/nvsr68/nvsr68_09-508.pdf , 2019. Accessed April 30, 2021.

Laporta-Herrero I et al.: Body dissatisfaction in adolescents with eating disorders. *Eat Weight Disord* 23(3):339, 2018.

Larson S et al.: Chronic childhood trauma, mental health, academic achievement, and school-based health center mental health services. *J School Health* 87(9):675, 2017.

Lindberg LD et al.: Changing patterns of contraceptive use and the decline in rates of pregnancy and birth among U.S. adolescents 2007-2014. *J Adolescent Health* 63(2):253, 2018.

Paracha, S et al: Design, development and evaluation of a virtual environment with children for moral, social & emotional learning. *International Journal of Virtual and Personal Learning Environments*, 10(2), 2020.

Perkins EB, Ruiz C: Domestic minor sex trafficking in a rural state: interviews with adjudicated female juveniles. *Child Adolesc Soc Work J* 34(2):171, 2017.

Powell C et al.: Training U.S. health care professionals on human trafficking: where do we go from here? *Med Educ Online* 22(1): 1267980, 2017.

Sices L, Augustyn: Expressive language delay ("late talking") in young children, *UpToDate*, https://www.uptodate.com/contents/expressive-language-delay-late-talking-in-young-children/print 2020. Accessed April 30, 2021.

Tracy E, Macias-Konstantopoulos W: Human trafficking: Identification and evaluation in the health care setting, *UpToDate*, https://www.uptodate.com/contents/human-trafficking-identification-and-evaluation-in-the-health-care-setting, 2021. Accessed April 30, 2021.

Twigg NM: Comprehensive care model for sex trafficking survivors. *J Nurs Scholarsh* 49(3):259, 2017.

Ulibarri MD et al.: Introduction to special section: research, treatment, and policy regarding trafficking and sexual exploitation of children and adolescents. *J Child Adol Trauma* 10(2):147, 2017.

Ve J: Pediatric mental and behavioral health in the period of quarantine and social distancing with COVID-19. *JMIR Pediatr Parent* 3(2):e19867, 2020.

13

Young and Middle Adults

OBJECTIVES

- Compare young adulthood with emerging adulthood.
- Identify major life events of young and middle adults and the childbearing family.
- Describe developmental tasks of the young adult, the childbearing family, and the middle adult.
- Discuss the significance of marriage and family in the life of the young and middle adult.
- Identify normal physical changes in young and middle adulthood.
- Explore the effects poverty has on the development of young and middle adults.
- Discuss cognitive and psychosocial changes occurring during the young-adult and middle-adult years.
- Explain health concerns of the young adult, the childbearing family, and the middle adult.
- Discuss intimate partner violence (IPV).

KEY TERMS

Braxton Hicks contractions
Climacteric
Doula
Emerging adulthood

Infertility
Lactation
Menopause
Prenatal care

Puerperium
Sandwich generation

MEDIA RESOURCES

http://evolve.elsevier.com/Potter/fundamentals/
- Review Questions
- Audio Glossary

- Case Study with Questions
- Content Updates
- Answers to QSEN Activity and Review Questions

Young and middle adulthood are developmental periods that pose challenges, rewards, and crises. Challenges often include the demands of working and raising families and other crises, such as caring for aging parents or the possibility of job loss in a changing economic environment. Erikson's (1963, 1982) classic works describe the phases of young and middle adulthood and related developmental tasks (see Chapter 11). More recent work has identified emerging adulthood as an additional phase of development in the young adult.

Faced with a societal structure that differs greatly from traditional norms from many years ago, both men and women are assuming different roles in today's society. Men were traditionally the primary supporters of the family. Today many women pursue careers and contribute significantly to their families' incomes. Women comprise half of the workforce. They are the sole or co-breadwinner in half of American families with children. However, women on average earn less than men in almost every occupation. Women from minority groups and those in lower socioeconomic levels have an even greater wage gap (Institute for Women's Policy Research [IWPR], n.d.).

Developmental theories help explain the life events and developmental tasks of the young and middle adult (see Chapter 11). Patients present challenges to nurses who themselves are often young or middle adults coping with the demands of their respective developmental period.

Nurses need to recognize the needs of their patients even if they are not experiencing the same challenges and events.

YOUNG ADULTS

Young adulthood is the period between the late teens and the mid-to-late 30s (Edelman and Kudzma, 2021). In the past several decades researchers identified the developmental phase, emerging adulthood, which occurs from the late teens to mid-20s (Fioretti et al., 2017). This stage of development is unique from young adulthood and extended adolescence. It is a period when individuals face major life transition and decisions with the focus on becoming independent (Butterbaugh et al., 2020). It differs from young adulthood because most young people in their 20s have not made those transitions historically associated with adult status, especially marriage and parenthood. In this stage young adults are faced with the tasks of identity development, who they want to be, and how to attain their goals (Layland et al., 2018).

It is estimated that in 2018 young adults 20 to 34 years of age made up approximately 20% of the population (U.S. Census Bureau, 2021). They tend to adapt well to new experiences and are more ethnically and racially diverse than previous generations. Young adults increasingly move away from their families of origin, establish career goals, and decide whether to marry or remain single and whether to begin families. The exception is for young adults who live in poverty. The number of young people (18–24 years of age) living in poverty has increased over the last several decades, with young adults among the most poverty-prone age-groups since the onset of the Great Recession (Berkeley Public Policy, 2019). This age-group needs additional support as they consider starting college and taking their first jobs,

According to the Pew Research Center (2020), today's emerging adults are history's first "always-connected" generation, with digital technology and social media as major aspects of their lives. However, there is a risk/benefit aspect to "always connected." Individuals acquire information quickly. However, social media are sometimes used to overcome boredom, which may increase a person's risk for feeling socially isolated and disconnected (Stockdale and Coyne, 2020).

Physical Changes

The young adult usually completes physical growth by the age of 20. An exception to this is the pregnant or lactating woman. The physical, cognitive, and psychosocial changes and the health concerns of the pregnant woman and the childbearing family are extensive.

Young adults are usually quite active, experience severe illnesses less frequently than people in older age-groups, tend to ignore physical symptoms, and often postpone seeking health care. Physical strength typically peaks, and physical characteristics of young adults begin to change as middle age approaches. Physical changes in weight and muscle mass often occur as a result of diet, exercise, and lifestyle patterns. Assessment findings are generally within normal limits unless an illness is present.

Cognitive Changes

Critical thinking habits increase steadily through the young-adult years. Formal and informal educational experiences, general life experiences, and occupational opportunities dramatically increase the individual's conceptual, problem-solving, and motor skills. If a young adult was raised in poverty, cognitive functions will differ. Childhood poverty over time is linked to deficits in adult memory and greater psychological distress, including a sense of helplessness and elevated levels of chronic physiological stress (Evans, 2016). Children who are disadvantaged face numerous uncontrollable psychosocial (e.g., family turmoil) and physical (e.g., substandard housing) stressors that may erode a sense of mastery or self-efficacy, rendering children of lower socioeconomic status (SES) vulnerable to helplessness (Evans, 2016).

Identifying an occupational direction is a major task of young adults. When people know their skills, talents, and personality characteristics, educational preparation and occupational choices are easier and more satisfying. Some young adults pursue postsecondary education to attain their occupational goals. Postsecondary education, which includes vocational training (e.g., carpentry, welding) and earned degrees from colleges or universities (e.g., associate, bachelor's, and graduate degrees), is often the entry-level educational requirement for many of the fastest-growing occupations in the United States (U.S. Bureau of Labor Statistics, 2020).

An understanding of how adults learn helps nurses develop patient education plans (see Chapter 25). Adults enter the teaching-learning situation with a background of unique life experiences, including illness and injuries. Their adherence to regimens such as medications, treatments, or lifestyle changes such as smoking cessation involves decision-making processes. When determining the amount of information that an individual needs to make decisions about the prescribed course of therapy, consider factors that possibly affect adherence to the regimen, including educational level, lifestyle habits, socioeconomic factors, and motivation and desire to learn.

Because young adults are continually evolving and adjusting to changes in their homes, workplaces, and social lives, their decision-making processes need to be flexible. The more secure young adults are in their roles, the more flexible and open they are to change. People who are insecure tend to be more rigid in making decisions (Edelman and Kudzma, 2021).

Psychosocial Changes

The emotional health of a young adult is related to the ability to address and resolve personal and social tasks. The young adult is often caught between wanting to prolong some of the freedom of adolescence and assume adult commitments. However, certain trends are relatively predictable. Between the ages of 23 and 28, the person refines self-perception and ability for intimacy. From 29 to 34 the person directs enormous energy toward achievement and mastery of the surrounding world. The years from 35 to 40 are a time of vigorous examination of life goals and relationships. Sometimes as a result of this reexamination people make changes in personal, social, and occupational areas.

Cultural factors such as ethnicity, poverty, language, and social relationships have a sociological and psychological influence in a young adult's life, and these factors pose challenges for nursing care (see Chapter 9). Each person holds individualized definitions of health and illness and the behaviors necessary to stay healthy. Nurses and other health professionals bring with them distinct practices for the prevention and treatment of illness. Knowing too little about a patient's self-perception or beliefs regarding health and illness may create conflict between a nurse and patient.

Changes in the traditional role expectations of both men and women in young adulthood lead to challenges for nursing care. For example, young adults often struggle with balancing job demands, personal relationships, the needs of the family, and socialization (Szkody and McKinney, 2019; Brough et al., 2018). Thus the struggle to balance these factors is a potential source of stress for the young adult, which may affect coping resources, health promotion behaviors, and level of health (Amnie, 2018).

Health is not merely the absence of disease; it also involves wellness in all human dimensions (see Chapter 6). Through patient education the nurse provides a young adult with access to health promotion resources and appropriate referrals to improve coping and health behaviors. The young adult needs to make decisions concerning career, marriage, and parenthood. Although each person makes these decisions based on individual factors, a nurse needs to understand the general principles involved in these aspects of psychosocial development while assessing the young adult's psychosocial status.

Lifestyle. Family history of cardiovascular, renal, endocrine, or neoplastic disease increases a young adult's risk of illness. In addition, young adults, especially young men, are more likely to participate in certain lifestyles that expose them to health risk behaviors, such as dangerous driving practices, smoking, substance abuse, overexposure to sun, binge drinking, and increased unprotected sexual activity (Masiero et al., 2018). Your role in health promotion is to identify unique modifiable factors and provide practical gender-specific and culturally specific patient education and support to reduce unhealthy lifestyle behaviors (Siren and Casier, 2019). These lifestyle changes can include a healthy diet, limited alcohol intake, exercise modifications, use of seat belts, and reduction in risky sex practices.

A personal lifestyle assessment (see Chapter 6) helps nurses and patients identify habits that increase the risk for cardiac, malignant, pulmonary, renal, or other chronic diseases. The assessment includes general life satisfaction, hobbies, and interests; habits such as diet, sleeping, exercise, sexual habits, and use of caffeine, tobacco, alcohol, and illicit drugs; home conditions and pets; economics, including type of health insurance; occupational environment, including type of work and exposure to hazardous substances; and physical or mental stress. Military records, including dates and geographical area of assignments, may also be useful in assessing the young adult for risk factors. Prolonged stress from lifestyle choices increases wear and tear on the adaptive capacities of the body, and stress-related illnesses, such as ulcers, emotional disorders, and infections, sometimes occur (see Chapter 37).

Career. Successful employment is important in the lives of most young adults. In general, young adults with higher education have higher-paying jobs. A good career helps to ensure economic security but also leads to fulfillment, friendships, social activities, support, and respect from co-workers. Individuals who are jobless or are making incomes below the poverty level face serious threats to their well-being.

The average adult under age 35 has an average debt of $67,400. The greatest percentage of that debt is educational. The average millennial household owes $14,800 in student loans (Renzulli, 2020). Therefore many young adults choose a two-career family, which has benefits and liabilities. In addition to increasing the family's financial base, the person who works outside the home is able to expand friendships, activities, and interests. However, stress exists in a two-career family as well. These stressors result from a job transfer of one partner to a new city; increased expenditures of physical, mental, or emotional energy; childcare demands; or household needs. When partners share decision making and responsibilities, the stressors related to a two-career family decrease. For example, some families may decide to limit recreational expenses and instead hire someone to do routine housework.

Sexuality. The development of secondary sex characteristics occurs during the adolescent years (see Chapter 12). Physical development is accompanied by sexual maturation. The young adult usually has emotional maturity to complement the physical ability and therefore is able to develop mature sexual relationships and establish intimacy. Young adults who have failed to achieve the developmental task of personal integration sometimes develop relationships that are superficial and stereotyped (Varcarolis and Dixon, 2020).

The psychodynamic aspect of sexual activity is as important as the type or frequency of sexual intercourse to young adults (see Chapter 34). To maintain total wellness, encourage young adults to assess their sexual activity and practice safe sex. Assist them to realize that their sexual needs and concerns are normal and may change over time (Shaw and Rogge, 2017). When necessary, help to identify risky sexual behaviors, such as unprotected sex or multiple sexual partners. Ensure that these young adults have access to accurate information regarding birth control and the prevention of sexually transmitted infections (STIs).

Childbearing Cycle. Conception, pregnancy, birth, and the **puerperium** are major phases of the childbearing cycle. The changes during these phases are complex. Childbirth education classes can prepare pregnant women, their partners, and other support people to participate in the birthing process (Fig. 13.1). Some health care agencies provide either professional labor support or a lay **doula**, a support person to be present during labor to assist women who have no other source of support. The stress that many women experience after childbirth may have a significant impact on postpartum women's health.

Types of Families. During young adulthood, most individuals experience singlehood and the opportunity to be on their own. Those who eventually marry or establish long-term partnerships encounter several changes as they take on new responsibilities. For example, many couples choose to become parents (Fig. 13.2). Some young adults choose alternative lifestyles, and different family forms emerge (see Chapter 10).

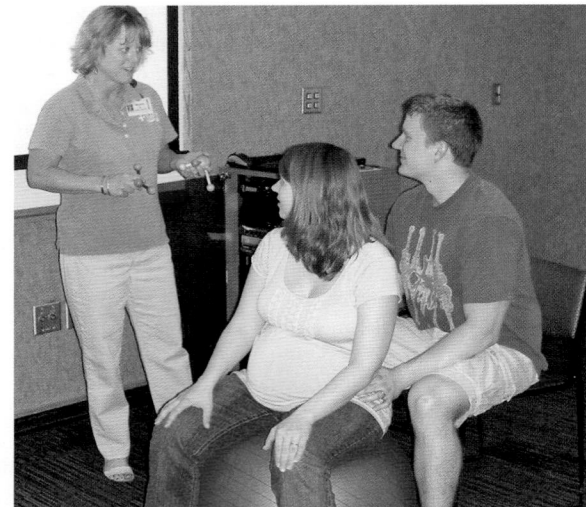

FIG. 13.1 Nurse providing Lamaze class for expectant young adults.

FIG. 13.2 Parent-child nurturing is important in adapting to a newborn. (From Hockenberry MJ et al.: *Wong's nursing care of infants and children,* ed 11, St Louis, 2019, Mosby.)

Singlehood. The social pressure to get married has changed, and some young adults may choose not to marry until their late 20s or early 30s or not at all. For young adults who remain single, parents and siblings become the nucleus for a family. Some view close friends and associates as "family." One cause for the increased single population is the expanding career opportunities for women. Women enter the job market with greater career potential and have greater opportunities for financial independence. More single individuals are choosing to live together outside marriage and become parents either biologically or through adoption. Similarly, many married couples choose to separate or divorce if they find their marital situation unsatisfactory.

Parenthood. Knowledge about sexuality and the availability of contraception help people decide when and if to start a family. Sometimes social pressures encourage young adults to have children. Economic considerations frequently enter into the decision-making process because of the expense of childrearing. Women living in poverty often cannot afford contraceptives and do not know how to prevent pregnancies. General health status and age are also considerations in decisions about parenthood.

Alternative Family Structures and Parenting. Changing norms and values about family life in the United States reveal basic shifts in attitudes about family structure (see Chapter 10). The trend toward greater acceptance of cohabitation without marriage is a factor in the greater numbers of infants being born to single women. In addition, approximately 6 million American children and adults have parents who are lesbian, gay, bisexual, transgender, or queer (LGBTQ+). Approximately 131,000 same-sex households include children under the age of 18 (Rossi, 2018; Bos et al., 2018). The American Academy of Pediatrics (AAP), in recognizing the needs of gay and lesbian parents and their children, published a policy statement supporting adoption of children and the parenting role by same-sex parents (AAP, 2013). When parents demonstrate caring, support, and a positive response to the gender orientation of their child, health outcomes appear to be improved (Forcier and Olson-Kennedy, 2020).

Emotional Health. Young adults need physical and emotional resources and support systems to meet the many challenges, tasks, and responsibilities they face. During psychosocial assessment of young adults, assess for signs of emotional health that support successful maturation in this developmental stage (e.g., satisfaction with personal growth and development, satisfaction with relationships, and attainment of long-term goals related to education, employment, housing, and relationships).

Health Risks

Health risk factors for a young adult originate in the community, lifestyle patterns, and family history. The lifestyle habits that activate the stress response (see Chapter 37) increase the risk of illness. Drug and tobacco use and risky sexual practices place young adults at risk for illnesses or disabilities during their middle- or older-adult years. Young adults may have optimistic bias related to specific behaviors, such as smoking and alcohol consumption. When optimistic bias is present, young adults do not perceive that associated health risks for cancer and chronic cardiac and pulmonary diseases will affect their level of health (Masiero et al., 2018).

In this age-group, smoking is a well-documented risk factor for subsequent pulmonary, cardiac, and vascular diseases in smokers and individuals who are exposed to secondhand smoke. Electronic cigarette (e-cigarette) use or vaping of substances such as tobacco or cannabis has the potential for health risks developing over time because of the inhaled pollutants (Sommerfeld et al., 2018). The nicotine in tobacco is a vasoconstrictor that acts on the coronary arteries, increasing the risk of angina, myocardial infarction, and coronary artery disease. Nicotine also causes peripheral vasoconstriction and leads to vascular problems.

Family History. A family history of a disease sometimes puts a young adult at risk for developing it in the middle- or older-adult years. For example, a young man whose father and paternal grandfather had myocardial infarctions (heart attacks) in their 50s has a risk for a future myocardial infarction. The presence of chronic illnesses such as diabetes mellitus or certain cancers in the family increases the family member's risk of developing the diseases (see Chapter 8). Regular physical examinations and screenings are important because certain conditions such as high blood pressure, high blood glucose, and high cholesterol levels may not have any symptoms in the early stages. In addition, the American Cancer Society (2021) now recommends adults who are at average risk have routine screening for colorectal cancer by age 45 and even earlier screening for individuals with a family history of colorectal cancers. Genomic science and resultant technologies identify people at risk for disease through the use of genetic screening. Understanding the role genomics plays in the health of individuals and families enables clinicians to better advise young adults about current and future health care.

Violent Death and Injury. Violence is a common cause of mortality and morbidity in the young-adult population (Ertl et al., 2019). Factors that predispose individuals to violence, injury, or death include poverty, family breakdown, child abuse and neglect, opioid and other drug use (dealing or illegal use), repeated exposure to violence, and ready access to guns. It is important to perform a thorough psychosocial assessment, including factors such as behavioral patterns, history of physical abuse, education, work history, substance use, and social support systems, to detect personal and environmental risk factors for violence. Death and injury primarily occur from physical assaults, motor vehicle or other accidents, and suicide attempts in young adults (Ertl et al., 2019).

Intimate Partner Violence. Intimate partner violence (IPV), formerly referred to as domestic violence, is a global public health problem. IPV includes physical and sexual violence, stalking, and psychological aggression. It exists along a continuum from a single episode that could have lasting impact on a victim, to ongoing chronic battering (Centers for Disease Control and Prevention [CDC], 2019a). Annually in the United States, approximately 4.8 million women experience intimate partner–related physical assaults and rapes, and men are the victims of approximately 2.9 million intimate partner–related physical assaults (Roberts et al., 2018). Physical injuries from IPV range from minor cuts and bruises to broken bones, internal bleeding, head trauma, and death. IPV is linked to such harmful health behaviors as smoking, alcohol abuse, drug use, and risky sexual activity. Risk factors to look for in an assessment that suggest perpetration of IPV include using drugs or alcohol, especially heavy drinking; unemployment; low self-esteem; gambling; antisocial or borderline personality traits; desire for power and control in relationships; and being a previous victim of physical or psychological abuse (Roberts et al., 2018; CDC, 2019a). An increased risk of violence occurs during the reproductive years, and a pregnant woman has a greater risk of being a victim of IPV than a nonpregnant woman. Women experiencing IPV may be more likely to delay prenatal care and are at increased risk for multiple poor maternal and infant health outcomes, such as low maternal weight gain, infections, high blood pressure, vaginal bleeding, and delivery of a preterm or low-birth-weight infant (Ferdos et al., 2018).

QSEN Building Competency in Patient-Centered Care You are caring for Joan, a 25-year-old patient who has come alone to the clinic because she is experiencing insomnia. Throughout the assessment interview Joan is slightly withdrawn, speaks quietly, and does not make eye contact. She does not work outside the home, and she acknowledges that her relationship with her husband, an engineer who lost his job as a result of downsizing 6 months ago, is "not going well." Physical examination reveals scratches and bruises on Joan's breasts, abdomen, and back. Refer to the Centers for Disease Control and Prevention (CDC) Intimate Partner Violence resource page (https://www.cdc.gov/violenceprevention/intimatepartnerviolence/index.html) to determine which assessment questions, approaches, and tools you can use to determine whether Joan is a victim of IPV. If Joan is experiencing IPV, what resources may help her?

Answers to QSEN Activities can be found on the Evolve website.

Substance Abuse. Substance abuse is a social problem that directly or indirectly contributes to mortality and morbidity in young adults. Substance abuse includes alcohol, drugs, and marijuana. Young adults who are under the influence of substances sometimes are involved in motor vehicle accidents, often resulting in severe injuries, permanent disability, or death to everyone involved in the accident.

Dependence on stimulant or depressant drugs sometimes results in death. Overdose of a stimulant drug ("upper") stresses the cardiovascular and nervous systems to the extent that death occurs. The use of depressants ("downers") can lead to an accidental or intentional overdose and death.

There is an ongoing opioid abuse crisis affecting young adults, which often occurs from overuse of opioid prescriptions. This abuse is the result of the need to take regular and increasing doses of a drug in order to feel good or to avoid feeling bad. The abuse can cause several acute and toxic consequences (Becker and Starrels, 2021; Beneitz and Gil-Alegre, 2017). Addiction is an illness that affects the individual, family, and friends; thus it is important to recommend that family and friends participate in the treatment process (Becker and Starrels, 2021; Kelly et al., 2017).

Substance abuse is difficult to diagnose, particularly in its early stages. Nonjudgmental questions about the use of legal drugs (prescribed drugs, tobacco, and alcohol), soft drugs (marijuana and diazepam), and more problematic drugs (cocaine or heroin) are a routine part of any health assessment. The National Institute on Drug Abuse (NIDA, n.d.) recommends starting a conversation about substance abuse using these questions:

In the past year, how many times have you used the following:
- Alcohol (for men, five or more drinks in a day; for women, four or more drinks in a day)?
- Tobacco products?
- Prescription drugs for nonmedical reasons?
- Illegal drugs?

If the screening test suggests a patient is at risk, there are online tests available for further assessment, including the NIDA-Modified Alcohol, Smoking, and Substance Involvement Screening Test (NM-ASSIST) (NIDA, n.d.). Explain that it is your role as a nurse to convey health recommendations. Recommend quitting before problems (or more problems) develop. Urge patients to talk with their health care providers about the specific medical reasons for quitting (NIDA, n.d.).

Marijuana is one of the most commonly used addictive drugs in the United States, with over 37 million users estimated in 2017. Marijuana use may have a wide range of health effects on the body and brain (CDC, 2018). It affects the parts of the brain responsible for memory, learning, attention, decision making, coordination, emotions, and reaction time (CDC, 2018). People who smoke marijuana as adolescents can have developmental delays that affect the brain. Marijuana also affects women who are pregnant, increasing the risk that their infants will have developmental problems. Educate patients about the risks of marijuana use, and provide patients who are addicted to marijuana information about treatment options.

Caffeine is a naturally occurring legal stimulant that is readily available in a variety of foods and beverages and in over-the-counter medications such as cold tablets or allergy and analgesic preparations. Caffeine stimulates catecholamine release, which in turn stimulates the central nervous system; it also increases gastric acid secretion, heart rate, and basal metabolic rate. This alters blood pressure, increases diuresis, and relaxes smooth muscle. Consumption of large amounts of caffeine results in restlessness, anxiety, irritability, agitation, muscle tremor, sensory disturbances, heart palpitations, nausea or vomiting, and diarrhea in some individuals.

Human Trafficking. A significant social problem is the number of youth and young adults who run away or are homeless. Many risk becoming involved in illegal and dangerous activities to survive, including human trafficking (Ashe-Goins, 2018). The United Nations Office on Drugs and Crime (n.d.) defines human trafficking as the recruitment, transport, transfer, harboring, or receipt of a person by threat or use of force for the purpose of exploitation. Nurses in a variety of settings, such as emergency departments, clinics, and public health agencies, are one of the first lines of health professionals who can identify victims of human trafficking and identify safe living and health care and social resources (Ashe-Goins, 2018; Tracy and Macias-Konstantopoulos, 2021). Although human trafficking is often a hidden crime and accurate statistics are difficult to obtain, estimates indicate that over 80% of trafficking victims are female and 50% are children.

Unplanned Pregnancies. Unplanned pregnancies create stress that may result in adverse health outcomes for the mother, infant, and family. Often young adults have educational and career goals that take precedence over family development. Interference with these goals often affects future relationships and parent-child relationships.

The determination of situational factors that affect the progress and outcome of an unplanned pregnancy is important. Exploration of problems such as financial, career, and living accommodations; family support systems; potential parenting disorders; depression; and coping mechanisms is important in assessing the woman with an unplanned pregnancy.

Sexually Transmitted Infections. STIs are a major health problem in young adults. Examples of STIs include syphilis, chlamydia, gonorrhea, genital herpes, human papillomavirus (HPV), and acquired immunodeficiency syndrome (AIDS). STIs have immediate physical effects such as genital discharge, discomfort, and infection. They also lead to chronic disorders, cancer, infertility, or even death. They remain a major public health problem for sexually active people, with almost half of all new infections occurring in men and women younger than 24 years of age (U.S. Department of Health and Human Services [USDHHS], 2019). Some young adults with STIs also experience IPV. The U.S. Preventive Services Task Force has relevant recommendations for people with STIs and IPV. Safe and effective vaccines are available for some STIs. For example, HPV, which can cause several types of cancer, can be prevented through vaccination with Gardasil or Cervarix, both U.S. Food and Drug Administration (FDA)–approved vaccines for the prevention of HPV. As young people enter sexual relationships, it is important that health care providers acknowledge the normalcy of these relationships and assess which types of sexual activity young-adult patients engage in to determine appropriate screening tests and preventive measures (Hockenberry et al., 2019). Also routinely screen for IPV and refer patients to appropriate community resources.

Environmental or Occupational Factors. A common environmental or occupational risk factor is exposure to work-related hazards or agents that cause diseases and cancer (Table 13.1). Examples include lung diseases, such as silicosis from inhalation of talcum and silicon dust and emphysema from inhalation of smoke. Cancers resulting from occupational exposures may involve the lung, liver, brain, blood, or skin. As a routine part of your assessment, include questions regarding occupational exposure to hazardous material and the safety precautions patients follow.

Health Concerns

Health Promotion. The key to health promotion in young adults is education. Lifestyle choices early on can lead to serious illness or disabilities in the middle- or older-adult years if left uncorrected.

TABLE 13.1 Occupational Hazards/Exposures Associated with Diseases and Cancers

Job Category	Occupational Hazard/Exposure	Work-Related Condition/Cancer
Agricultural workers	Pesticides, infectious agents, gases, sunlight	Pesticide poisoning, "farmer's lung," skin cancer
Anesthetists	Anesthetic gases	Reproductive effects, cancer
Automobile workers	Asbestos, plastics, lead, solvents	Asbestosis[a], dermatitis[b]
Carpenters	Wood dust, wood preservatives, adhesives	Nasopharyngeal cancer, dermatitis[b]
Cement workers	Cement dust, metals	Dermatitis, bronchitis[c]
Dry cleaners	Solvents	Liver disease[c], dermatitis[b]
Dye workers	Dyestuffs, metals, solvents	Bladder cancer, dermatitis[b]
Glass workers	Heat, solvents, metal powders	Cataracts
Hospital workers	Infectious agents, cleansers, latex gloves, radiation	Infections, latex allergies, unintentional injuries
Insulators	Asbestos, fibrous glass	Asbestosis, lung cancer, mesothelioma[a]
Jackhammer operators	Vibration	Raynaud's phenomenon
Lathe operators	Metal dusts, cutting oils	Lung disease, cancer[c]
Office computer workers	Repetitive wrist motion on computers, eyestrain	Tendinitis, carpal tunnel syndrome, tenosynovitis[d]

[a]Singh R, et al.: Assessment of the future mesothelioma disease burden from past exposure to asbestos in ship recycling yards in India, *Int J Hyg Environmental Health*, 225:113478, 2020.
[b]Gaskin, S et al.: What do occupational hygienists really know about skin exposure? *Ann Work Expo Health* 65(2): 219, 2021.
[c]Lytras T, et al.: Cumulative occupational exposures and lung-function decline in two large general population cohorts, *Ann Am Thorac Soc 18*(2): 238, 2021.
[d]Dabbagh A, et al.: Diagnosing carpal tunnel syndrome: Diagnostic test accuracy of scales, questionnaires, and hand symptom diagrams—a systematic review, *J Orthop Sports Phys Ther* 50(11):622, 2020.

For example, young adults are genetically susceptible to certain chronic diseases such as diabetes mellitus and familial hypercholesterolemia (Huether et al., 2020). Knowing the risks associated with family history members is important in motivating an individual to take precautions. Various forms of cancer are becoming more common in young and middle adults. Cancer trends in young adults reflect recent changes in carcinogenic exposures as well as the obesity epidemic in the United States (Sung et al., 2019). From 1995 to 2014 the incidence significantly increased for 6 of 12 obesity-related cancers (multiple myeloma, colorectal, uterine corpus, gallbladder, kidney, and pancreatic cancer) in young adults (25–49 years), with steeper rises in successively younger generations (Sung et al., 2019). Encourage young adults to perform monthly skin, breast, or male genital self-examination (see Chapter 30). Breast cancer is the most common major cancer among women 15 to 39 years of age, with a steadily increasing incidence (Young Survival Coalition, 2021). When breast cancer develops in young-adult women, they face unique challenges (Young Survival Coalition, 2021):

- The possibility of early menopause and body image concerns and sexual dysfunction
- Potential fertility issues (e.g., the risks associated with pregnancy after diagnosis and treatment)
- Needing to sometimes balance raising small children while enduring treatment and subsequent side effects
- Coping with psychosocial issues (e.g., anxiety, depression)

Your role as patient educator is extremely important in teaching all patients about their risks for cancer, the self-examinations available, and current screening recommendations (see Chapter 30). Prolonged exposure to ultraviolet rays of the sun in adolescents and young adults increases the risk for development of skin cancer later in life. Crohn disease, a chronic inflammatory disease of the small intestine, most commonly occurs between 15 and 35 years of age. Many young adults have misconceptions regarding transmission and treatment of STIs. Encourage partners to know one another's sexual history and practices. Be alert for STIs when patients come to clinics with complaints of urological or gynecological

problems (see Chapter 34). Assess young adults for knowledge and use of safe-sex practices and genital self-examinations.

Psychosocial Health. The psychosocial health concerns of the young adult are often related to job (money and job stability) and family stressors. Stress is valuable because it motivates a patient to change. However, if the stress is prolonged and the patient is unable to adapt to the stressor, health problems develop (see Chapter 37). Some mental health disorders such as depression also begin in this age-group. These conditions may manifest during young adulthood, but symptoms and treatment often continue into middle adulthood and beyond (Varcarolis and Dixon, 2020).

Job Stress. Job stress is prevalent in work settings due to relational issues, lack of resources to do the job, and time constraints. Most young adults are able to handle day-to-day crises (Fig. 13.3). Situational job stress can occur when a new boss enters the workplace or a deadline is approaching. Job stress affects health behaviors, and there is often greater use of tobacco and alcohol, poor eating habits, impaired sleeping, and lack of exercise (Wang et al., 2018). Because individuals perceive jobs differently, the types of job stressors, coping strategies, and changes in health behaviors vary from patient to patient (Box 13.1). Your assessment of a young adult includes a description of the usual work performed, changes in job demands, changes in sleep or eating habits, and evidence of an increase in irritability or nervousness.

REFLECT NOW

One of your classmates had a difficult time in yesterday's clinical and is having difficulty participating in the skills lab exercise. During the break she confides that the nurses on the clinical unit don't help her find any equipment, and all she could do last night was think about how "stressful" the clinical site appears to be. What questions could you ask your classmate to better understand the stress she is experiencing? What resources are available that might help her better manage her stress?

FIG. 13.3 The ability to handle day-to-day challenges at work minimizes stress.

BOX 13.1 EVIDENCE-BASED PRACTICE

Assessing for Workplace Job Stress

PICOT Question: Do health promotion behaviors affect workplace job stress in young adults?

Evidence Summary
Job stress is a response to either emotional or physical challenges when workers' capabilities do not match the demands of their jobs (Park and Jang, 2019). It is an important factor affecting the health of the working population. In addition, workplace job stressors affect personal relationships, including those in the home and family. Likewise, relationship, home, and family stressors can affect workplace stressors and subsequently job performance and satisfaction (Padkapayeva et al., 2018). Poor health promotion behaviors have the potential to decrease a person's ability to cope with these stressors. However, research shows that incorporating consistent positive health promotion behaviors, such as workplace exercise and meditation programs, can improve perception of stressors and job performance (Wang et al., 2018; Padkapayeva et al., 2018). In the health care professions, especially the nursing profession, workplace stressors are associated with high nurse turnover and psychosomatic complaints (Williams et al., 2018).

Application to Nursing Practice
- Ask patients about potential job-related stressors and whether these stressors have any impact on work-life balance (Conroy and Tabbenhoff, 2018; Padkapayeva et al., 2018).
- Assess patients' usual and most recent health promotion behaviors (e.g., diet, sleep, exercise habits) (Williams et al., 2018).
- Assist patients in identifying and using personal coping strategies (Brough et al., 2018).
- Help patients identify sources of social and employer support (Brough et al., 2018; Conroy and Tabbenhoff, 2018).
- Partner with patients to identify realistic positive changes in health promotion behaviors (Park and Jang, 2019; Williams et al., 2018).
- Interventions to reduce stress should be geared toward education, wellness promotion, and general health promotion (Kellogg, 2021).

Family Stress. Because of the multiplicity of changing relationships and structures in the emerging young-adult family, stress is frequently high (see Chapter 10). Situational family stressors occur during events such as births, deaths, illnesses, marriages or divorce, and job losses. In the United States, about 23% of families with children under 18 years of age are single-parent families (Pew Research Center, 2019). Stress is related to a number of variables, including the career paths and job stressors for both partners or the single parent, and can lead to dysfunction in the young-adult family (Padkapayeva et al., 2018). When a patient seeks health care and presents stress-related symptoms, you need to assess the family dynamics and for the occurrence of any life-change events.

Each family member has certain predictable roles or jobs. These roles enable a family to function and be an effective part of society. When they change as a result of illness, a situational crisis often occurs. Assess environmental and familial factors, including support systems and coping mechanisms commonly used by family members.

Infertility. According to the American Society for Reproductive Medicine (2021), infertility is the result of a disease (an interruption, cessation, or disorder of body functions, systems, or organs) of the male or female reproductive tract that prevents the conception of a child or the ability to carry a pregnancy to delivery. Infertility evaluation begins after a couple has unprotected intercourse for about 12 months with the failure to conceive. An estimated 10% to 15% of reproductive couples are infertile, and many are young adults. However, approximately half of the couples evaluated and treated in infertility clinics become pregnant. For some infertile couples, a nurse is the first resource they identify. Nursing assessment of the couple experiencing infertility includes comprehensive histories of both the male and female partners to determine factors that have affected fertility and pertinent physical findings (see Chapter 30). Advanced practice nurses often conduct these assessments.

Obesity. Obesity is a major health problem. Approximately 16% of emerging adults are at risk for significant weight gain, which places them at risk for health problems in later life, including cardiovascular diseases, type 2 diabetes, obstructive sleep apnea, certain types of cancer, and osteoarthritis (Johnson and Annesi, 2018). Young adults are half as likely to have obesity as middle-age adults (CDC, 2021a). The CDC (2021a) has also found that, when combining data from 2017 through 2019, non-Hispanic Black adults had the highest prevalence of self-reported obesity (39.8%), followed by Hispanic adults (33.8%) and non-Hispanic White adults (29.9%). In some cases obesity is linked to genetic tendencies. However, it is significantly connected to behaviors such as physical inactivity, poor dietary patterns, medication use, education and skills, and food marketing and promotion (CDC, 2021b). For example, obesity is influenced in young adults by consuming fast food and excessive sugar intake from soft drinks, increases in portion size, and a steady decline in physical activity (Hockenberry et al., 2019). These factors are further complicated by family characteristics, such as parenting style, parents' lifestyles, and environmental factors such as school policies and demographics. Nursing assessment of diet (e.g., types of food, number and size of meals, history of weight gain) and physical activity of young adults is an important part of data collection.

Exercise. People of all ages, both male and female, benefit from regular physical activity (see Chapter 38); however, many young adults spend more time with technology and less time engaged in physical activity. Current guidelines from the American Heart Association (2018) indicate that adults should have a minimum of 2.5 hours of moderate intensity exercise each week. However, a recent study suggests boosting exercise to as much as 5 hours a week may protect against hypertension in midlife, particularly if it is sustained in one's 30s, 40s, and 50s (University of California San Francisco, 2021). Exercise in young adults is important to prevent or decrease obesity and the related chronic health conditions (Berger, 2018). Conduct a thorough musculoskeletal assessment and exercise history (see Chapter 38) to develop a realistic exercise plan. Help patients explore ways to exercise regularly within their daily schedules.

Pregnant Woman and the Childbearing Family. A developmental task for many young-adult couples is the decision to begin a family. Although the physiological changes of pregnancy and childbirth occur only in the woman, cognitive and psychosocial changes and health concerns affect the entire childbearing family, including the baby's father, siblings, and grandparents. Young single-parent families tend to be particularly vulnerable, both economically and socially.

Prenatal Care. Women who are anticipating pregnancy benefit from good health practices before conception, including a balanced diet, folic acid, exercise, dental checkups, prenatal care, avoidance of alcohol, and cessation of smoking once conception occurs. However, women living in poverty or in rural areas often do not have access to prenatal care. The Centers for Medicare and Medicaid Services (CMS, n.d.) describe the lack of access to high-quality maternal health services in rural communities as the result of hospital and obstetric department closures, workforce shortages, and access to care challenges arising from the social determinants of health that have contributed to disparities in maternal health care for rural women and their infants. These access to care challenges can result in a number of negative maternal health outcomes, including premature birth, low birth weight, maternal mortality, severe maternal morbidity, and increased risk of postpartum depression (CMS, n.d.). All pregnant women deserve quality prenatal care.

Prenatal care is the routine examination of the pregnant woman by an obstetrician or advanced practice nurse such as a nurse practitioner or certified nurse-midwife. Prenatal care includes a thorough physical assessment of a pregnant woman during regularly scheduled intervals; provision of information regarding STIs, other vaginal infections, and urinary infections that adversely affect the fetus; and counseling about exercise patterns, diet, and childcare. Regular prenatal care addresses health concerns that may arise during the pregnancy.

Physiological Changes. The physiological changes and needs of the pregnant woman vary with each trimester. Be familiar with them, their causes, and implications for nursing so that you can better inform your patients. All women experience some physiological changes in the first trimester. For example, they commonly have morning sickness, breast enlargement and tenderness, and fatigue. During the second trimester, growth of the uterus and fetus results in some of the physical signs of pregnancy. During the third trimester, increases in Braxton Hicks contractions (irregular, short contractions), fatigue, and urinary frequency occur.

Postpartum. The postpartum period is the time from delivery to approximately 6 weeks afterward. During this time, a woman's body reverts to its prepregnant physical status. Determine the woman's knowledge of and ability to care for both herself and her newborn baby. Assessment of parenting skills and maternal-infant interactions is particularly important. The process of lactation, or breastfeeding, offers many advantages to both the new mother and baby. For the inexperienced mother, breastfeeding can be a source of anxiety and frustration. Be alert for signs that the mother needs information and assistance (e.g., the breastfed baby fails to "latch" onto the mother's breast or infant weight gain is low).

Needs for Education. The entire childbearing family needs education about pregnancy, labor, delivery, breastfeeding, and integration of the newborn into the family structure. Prenatal education promotes

the maintenance of healthy lifestyles during pregnancy, helping expectant mothers manage stress, support a healthy diet, avoid harmful chemicals and situations, recognize warning signs and symptoms that mean something may be wrong with their pregnancy, and prepare for the labor and delivery experience (March of Dimes, 2021).

Psychosocial Changes. Like the physiological changes of pregnancy, psychosocial changes occur at various times during the 9 months of pregnancy and in the puerperium. Table 13.2 summarizes the major categories of psychosocial changes and implications for nursing intervention.

Health Concerns. The pregnant woman and her partner have many health questions. For example, they wonder whether the pregnancy and baby will be normal and whether they have the resources to properly care for the infant. Proper prenatal care has the potential to identify risks and pregnancy problems and meet most of the expectant mother's emotional and physical health needs. For some women, postpartum depression may occur. It is important to educate the mother and family members about common signs, such as overwhelming sadness, mood swings, impaired sleeping, withdrawal, and difficulty bonding with the infant (National Institute of Mental Health [NIMH], n.d.).

TABLE 13.2 Major Psychosocial Changes During Pregnancy

Category	Implications for Nursing
Body image	Morning sickness and fatigue contribute to poor body image.
	Increase in breast size sometimes makes the woman feel more feminine and sexually appealing.
	Encourage her to take extra time with hygiene and grooming, trying new hairstyles and makeup.
	Woman begins to "show" during the second trimester and starts to plan maternity wardrobe.
	Woman has general feeling of well-being when she feels the baby move and hears the heartbeat.
	Woman feels big, awkward, and unattractive during third trimester when fetus is growing more rapidly.
Role changes	Both partners think about and have feelings of uncertainty about impending role changes.
	Both partners have feelings of ambivalence about becoming parents and concern about ability to be parents.
Sexuality	Woman needs reassurance that sexual activity will not harm fetus.
	Woman's desire for sexual activity is influenced by body image.
	Woman sometimes desires cuddling and holding rather than sexual intercourse.
Coping mechanisms	Woman needs reassurance that childbirth and childrearing are natural and positive experiences but are also stressful.
	When indicated, help her to cope with particular stressors such as finding new housing, preparing the nursery, or participating in childbirth classes.
Stresses during puerperium	Woman returns home from hospital fatigued and unfamiliar with infant care.
	Woman experiences physical discomfort or feelings of anxiety or depression.
	Woman may experience subsequent feelings of guilt, anxiety, or possibly a sense of freedom or relief if she must return to work soon after delivery.

Acute Care

Young adults typically require acute care for accidents, substance abuse, exposure to environmental and occupational hazards, stress-related illnesses, respiratory infections, gastroenteritis, influenza, urinary tract infections, and minor surgery. An acute minor illness causes a disruption in life activities of young adults and can increase stress in an already hectic lifestyle. Lack of insurance or underinsurance, dependency, and limitations posed by treatment regimens also increase frustration. To give them a sense of maintaining control of their health care choices, it is important to keep young adults informed about their health status and involve them in health care decisions.

Restorative and Continuing Care

The young adult's need for restorative and continuing care often results from motor vehicle accidents, trauma from violence, or chronic diseases affecting the young-adult population, such as multiple sclerosis, rheumatoid arthritis, AIDS, and cancer. In general, other chronic illnesses such as hypertension, coronary artery disease, and diabetes may not be recognized until later in life. When present, chronic illness or disability threatens a young adult's independence and results in the need to change personal, family, and career goals. Nursing interventions for the young adult faced with chronic illness or disability may need to focus on problems related to sense of identity, establishing independence, reorganizing intimate relationships, and family structure (see Chapter 8).

MIDDLE ADULTS

The U.S. Census Bureau (2021) reports that approximately 37% of the population are middle-age adults (ages 35–64). In middle adulthood an individual can make lasting contributions through involvement with others. During this period personal and career achievements have often already been experienced (see Chapter 11). Many middle adults find joy in helping their children, and other young people become productive and responsible adults (Fig. 13.4). They also begin to help aging parents while being responsible for their own children, placing them in the sandwich generation. Using leisure time in satisfying and creative ways is a challenge that, if met satisfactorily, enables middle adults to prepare for retirement. However, this is a picture of a middle adult with a good income and education. The National Center for Children in Poverty found that children who grow up in poor families are much more likely to be poor in early adulthood, and African-Americans are more likely than Whites to be poor in early and middle adulthood (Saporta Report, 2021). In addition, single female heads of household with children are more likely to live in generational poverty.

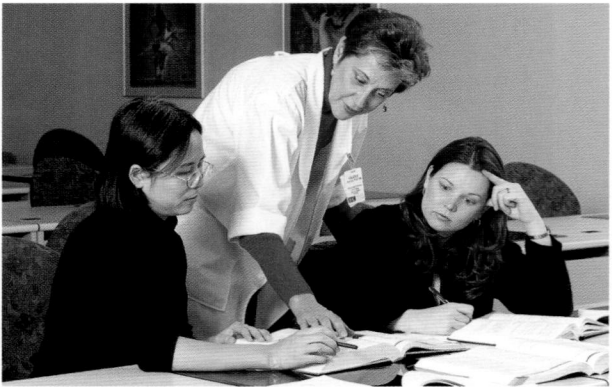

FIG. 13.4 Middle adults enjoy helping young people become productive and responsible adults.

Thus not all middle adults have productive and enriching lives. It is estimated that some 40% of middle-class Americans are at risk of poverty in retirement due to depressed earnings, assets, and increased health care costs (CNBC, 2021). As a result, many middle adults plan to work past the traditional retirement age.

During middle adulthood, men and women adjust to inevitable biological changes. As in adolescence, middle adults use considerable energy to adapt self-concept and body image to physiological realities and changes in physical appearance. High self-esteem, a favorable body image, and a positive attitude toward physiological changes occur when middle adults engage in physical exercise, eat balanced diets, obtain adequate sleep, and follow good hygiene practices that promote vigorous, healthy bodies.

Physical Changes

Major physiological changes occur between 40 and 65 years of age. Because of this it is important to assess the middle adult's general health status. A comprehensive assessment offers direction for health promotion recommendations and planning and implementing any acutely needed interventions. The most visible changes during middle adulthood are graying of the hair, wrinkling of the skin, and thickening of the waist. Decreases in hearing and visual acuity are often evident during this period. Often these physiological changes during middle adulthood have an impact on self-concept and body image. Table 13.3 summarizes abnormal findings to consider when conducting a physical examination (see Chapter 30). The most significant physiological changes during middle age are menopause in women and the climacteric in men.

Perimenopause and Menopause. Menstruation and ovulation occur in a cyclical rhythm in women from adolescence into middle adulthood. Perimenopause is the period during which ovarian function declines, resulting in a diminishing number of ova and irregular menstrual cycles; it generally lasts 1 to 3 years. Menopause is the disruption of this cycle, primarily because of the inability of the neurohormonal system to maintain its periodic stimulation of the endocrine system. The ovaries no longer produce estrogen and progesterone, and the blood levels of these hormones drop markedly. Menopause typically occurs between 45 and 60 years of age (see Chapter 34). Approximately 10% of women have no symptoms of menopause other than cessation of menstruation, 70% to 80% are aware of other changes but have no problems, and approximately 10% experience changes severe enough to interfere with activities of daily living.

Climacteric. The climacteric occurs in men in their late 40s or early 50s (see Chapter 34). Decreased levels of androgens cause the climacteric. Throughout this period and thereafter a man is still capable of producing fertile sperm and fathering a child. However, penile erection is less firm, ejaculation is less frequent, and the refractory period is longer.

Cognitive Changes

Changes in the cognitive function of middle adults are rare except with illness or trauma. Some middle adults enter educational or vocational programs to prepare themselves with new skills and information for entering the job market or changing jobs. The exception again is those who live in poverty. Adults with low income suffer from resource scarcity, environmental instability, and low subjective social status. These factors have been found to trigger a regulatory shift toward the present and the tuning of cognitive skills (Sheehy-Skeffington, 2020). The middle adult in poverty may focus more on immediate needs and short-term decisions, thus hindering the person's achievement of more long-term life goals.

TABLE 13.3 Abnormal Physical Assessment Findings in the Middle Adult

Body System	Assessment Findings
Integument	Very thin skin Rough, flaky, dry skin Lesions
Scalp and hair	Excessive generalized hair loss or patchy hair loss Excessive scales
Head and neck	Large, thick skull and facial bones Asymmetry in movement of head and/or neck Drooping of one side of the face
Eyes	Reduced peripheral vision Asymmetrical position of the light reflex Drooping of the upper lid (ptosis) Redness or crusting around the eyelids
Ears	Discharge of any kind Reddened, swollen ear canals
Nose, sinuses, and throat	Nasal tenderness Occlusion of nostril Swollen and pale pink or bluish-gray nasal mucosa Sinuses tender to palpation or on percussion Asymmetrical movement or loss of movement of uvula Tonsils red or enlarged
Thorax and lungs	Unequal chest expansion Unequal fremitus, hyperresonance, diminished or absent breath sounds Adventitious lung sounds such as crackles and wheezes
Heart and vascular system	Pulse inequality, weak pulses, bounding pulses, or variations in strength of pulse from beat to beat Bradycardia or tachycardia Hypertension Hypotension
Breasts—female	Recent increase in size of one breast Pigskin-like or orange-peel appearance Redness or painful breasts
Breasts—male	Soft, fatty enlargement of breast tissue
Abdomen	Bruises, areas of local discoloration; purple discoloration; pale, taut skin Generalized abdominal distention Hypoactive, hyperactive, decreased, or absent bowel sounds
Female genitalia	Asymmetrical labia Swelling, pain, or discharge from Bartholin glands Decreased tone of vaginal musculature Cervical enlargement or projection into the vagina Reddened areas or lesions in the vagina
Male genitalia	Rashes, lesions, or lumps on skin of shaft of penis Discharge from penis Enlarged scrotal sac Bulges that appear at the external inguinal ring or femoral canal when the patient bears down
Musculoskeletal system	Uneven weight bearing Decreased range of joint motion; swollen, red, or enlarged joint; painful joints Decreased strength against resistance
Neurological system	Lethargy Inadequate motor responses Abnormal sensory system responses: inability to smell certain aromas, loss of visual fields, inability to feel and correctly identify facial stimuli, absent gag reflex

Psychosocial Changes

The psychosocial changes in the middle adult often involve expected events, such as children moving away from home or ongoing changes in employment or career, and unexpected events, such as separation from a partner or the death of a partner or close friend. You need to assess for major life changes and the impact that the changes have on the middle adult's state of physical and emotional health. Include individual psychosocial factors such as coping mechanisms, status of employment, and sources of social support in your assessment.

In the middle-adult years, as children depart from the household, the family enters the postparental family stage. Time and financial demands on the parents typically decrease, and the couple faces the task of redefining their own relationship. It is during this period that many middle adults may take on healthier lifestyles. Assessment of health promotion needs for the middle adult includes regular screening examinations, amount of rest, leisure activities, nutritional intake, and regular exercise. Also assess for the use of tobacco, alcohol, or illicit drugs. Assess the middle adult's social environment, including relationship concerns; communication and relationships with children, grandchildren, and aging parents; and caregiver concerns with parents or an ill spouse.

Career Transition. Career changes occur by choice or as a result of changes in the workplace or society. A most recent example is the effect of the COVID-19 pandemic, which resulted in an estimated 20.5 million Americans being temporarily or permanently out of work (Cunningham, 2021). In recent decades middle adults change occupations more often for a variety of reasons, including limited upward mobility, decreasing availability of jobs, and seeking an occupation that is more challenging. In some cases downsizing, technological advances, or other changes force middle adults to seek new jobs. Such changes, particularly when unanticipated, result in stress that affects health, family relationships, self-concept, and other dimensions (see Chapter 37).

Sexuality. After the departure of their last child from the home, many married couples redefine their relationships and find increased marital and sexual satisfaction. The onset of menopause and the climacteric affect the sexual health of the middle adult. Some women may desire increased sexual activity because pregnancy is no longer possible. Middle-age men and women are able to engage in satisfying sexual relationships (see Chapter 34 for physical changes).

Other factors influencing sexuality during this period include job stress, diminished health of one or both partners, and effects of some prescription medications. For example, antihypertensive agents have side effects that influence sexual desire or functioning. Antihypertensive medications, diuretics, and beta blockers can cause erectile dysfunction (ED) in men (Burcham and Rosenthal, 2019). Sometimes both partners experience sexual dysfunction caused by stresses related to sexual changes or a conflict between their sexual needs and self-perceptions and social attitudes or expectations.

Family Psychosocial Factors. Psychosocial factors involving the family include the stresses of singlehood, marital and relationship changes, transition of the family as children or adult partners leave home, and the care of aging parents.

Singlehood. Many adults over 35 years of age in the United States have never been married (U.S. Census Bureau, 2021). Many are college-educated people who embrace the philosophy of choice and freedom, delayed marriage, and delayed parenthood. Some middle adults choose to remain single but also opt to become parents either biologically or through adoption. Many single middle adults have no relatives but share a family type of relationship with close friends or work associates. Consequently some single middle adults may feel isolated during traditional "family" holidays such as Thanksgiving or Christmas. In times of illness middle adults who choose to remain single and childless rely on other relatives or friends, increasing caregiving demands of family members who also have other responsibilities. Nursing assessment of single middle adults needs to include a thorough assessment of psychosocial factors, including an individual's definition of family and available support systems.

Marital Changes. Marital changes occurring during middle age include death of a spouse or partner, separation, divorce, and the choice of remarrying or remaining single. A widowed, separated, or divorced patient goes through a period of grief and loss in which it is necessary to adapt to the change in marital status. Normal grieving progresses back and forth through a series of phases, and resolution of grief often takes a year or more. Assess the level of coping of the middle adult to the grief and loss associated with life changes (see Chapter 36).

Family Transitions. The departure of the last child from the home is also a stressor. Many parents welcome freedom from childrearing responsibilities, whereas others feel lonely or without direction. *Empty nest syndrome* is the term used to describe the sadness and loneliness that occur when children leave home. Eventually parents need to reassess their marriage and try to resolve conflicts and plan for the future. Occasionally this readjustment phase leads to marital conflicts, separation, and divorce (see Chapter 10).

Care of Aging Parents. Increasing life spans in the United States and Canada have led to increased numbers of older adults in the population. Many middle adults find themselves caught between the responsibilities of caring for dependent children and those of caring for aging and ailing parents. They are part of the sandwich generation.

Most often this responsibility for care of parents and/or in-laws is undertaken by the woman in the family (Evans et al., 2019). The challenges of caregiving are stressful, sometimes forcing the caregiver to choose between the needs of the nuclear family and the needs of the parents and and/or in-laws.

Middle-adult and older-adult parents often have conflicting relationship priorities when older adults strive to remain independent, such as maintaining their own living space or finances. Negotiation and compromise help to define and resolve problems. When meeting family caregivers, take the time to identify the health needs of both groups, and assist the multigenerational family in determining the health and community resources available to them as they make decisions and plans (Liu and Huang, 2018).

Evaluate family relationships to determine family members' perceptions of responsibility, willingness, and perceived loyalty in relation to caring for older-adult members (Ellington et al., 2018). Determine the caregiver's physical and emotional health care needs and incorporate these needs into the plan of care for the patient (Evans et al., 2019).

REFLECT NOW

You are caring for a middle-age couple who have decided to bring the wife's widowed mother, who has stage 4 metastatic breast cancer, to their home for end-of-life care. In order to help the family unit during the early phase of caregiving, think about information you might need, such as expectations the family may have about caregiving, what resources are available to the family, what other resources they might need, and how the family/couple solves problems.

Health Concerns

Health Promotion and Stress Reduction. Because middle adults experience physiological changes and face certain health realities, their perceptions of health and health behaviors are often important factors in maintaining health. It is important that middle adults maintain regular fitness as they grow older. Routine exercise, 20 to 30 minutes 5 or 6 times a week, promotes health (see Chapter 38). For example, there is an association among activity, cardiopulmonary fitness, and long-term health outcomes, especially pertaining to cardiovascular disease (Benck et al., 2018). For women and men with risks for osteoporosis, regular moderate-level physical activity weekly helps to maintain bone health (Huether et al., 2020).

Stress across the life span is a health concern. Today's complex world makes individuals more prone to stress-related illnesses such as heart attacks and hypertension (see Chapter 37). When adults seek health care, nurses in outpatient and home health settings design targeted, culturally appropriate stress management programs focusing on wellness and guide patients to evaluate health behaviors, lifestyle, and environment (Amnie, 2018; Madva, 2018).

Work with the patient to identify approaches to preventing stressful situations, such as habituation, change avoidance, time blocking, time management, and environmental modification (e.g., adding ramps, removing obstacles). Then help the patient to increase stress resistance (e.g., increase self-esteem, improve assertiveness, redirect goal alternatives, and reorient cognitive appraisal). Finally, help patients learn how to avoid the physiological response to stress. Encourage use of relaxation techniques, imagery, yoga, meditation, and biofeedback to recondition the patient's response to stress (see Chapter 37).

Obesity. Obesity is a growing, expensive health concern for middle adults. It is a complicated, multifactorial disease, with genetic, behavioral, socioeconomic, and environmental origins; obesity reduces quality of life and increases the risk for many serious chronic diseases and premature death. The health consequences of obesity include high blood pressure, high blood cholesterol, type 2 diabetes, coronary heart disease, osteoarthritis, and obstructive sleep apnea. *Healthy People 2030* (Office of Disease Prevention and Health Promotion, n.d.) focuses on helping people get enough physical activity and eat the recommended amounts of healthy foods such as fruits, vegetables, and whole grains to reduce obesity, reduce their risk for chronic diseases, and improve their health.

Forming Positive Health Habits. Positive health habits help maintain optimal function and reduce risk for chronic illnesses. Some habits support health (e.g., exercise and brushing and flossing the teeth each day) or prevent disease. It is no longer routine for middle-age women to take calcium and vitamin D supplements. New data note that these supplements are recommended when a vitamin D deficiency is present. The routine use of these supplements does not reduce the risk of fractures (American Bone Health, 2020).

During assessment obtain data on your patient's health behaviors. Learn what is important to a patient with regard to maintaining health. Then determine which behaviors are positive and negative. Examples of positive health behaviors include regular exercise (see Chapter 38), adherence to healthy dietary habits, avoidance of excess consumption of alcohol, participation in routine screening and diagnostic tests for disease prevention and health promotion (e.g., laboratory screening for serum cholesterol or mammography), and lifestyle changes to reduce stress. Other habits involve risk factors to health (e.g., smoking or eating foods with little or no nutritional value).

To help patients form positive health habits, you act as an educator and facilitator. By providing information about how the body functions and how patients can form and change habits relative to their own goals, you raise patients' levels of knowledge regarding the potential impact of behavior on health (Amnie, 2018). Offer positive reinforcement (such as

BOX 13.2 Barriers to Change

External Barriers
- Lack of facilities
- Lack of resources and materials
- Limited social support
- Lack of motivation
- Poor access to care

Internal Barriers
- Lack of knowledge
- Insufficient skills or motivation to change health habits
- Undefined short- and long-term goals

praise and rewards) for health-directed behaviors and decisions. Such reinforcement increases the likelihood that the behavior will be repeated

Help middle adults consider factors such as avoidance of STIs, prevention of opioid and substance abuse, and accident prevention in relation to decreasing health risks. For example, provide patients with information on STI causes, symptoms, and transmission. Discuss methods of protection during sexual activity with a patient in an open and nonjudgmental manner and reinforce the importance of practicing safe sex (see Chapter 34).

Changing poor health habits is hard; recognize that barriers to change exist (Box 13.2). Help patients recognize and modify unsafe and potential health hazards. You must partner with patients and families to minimize or eliminate these barriers.

Health Literacy. Health literacy is defined as the cognitive and social skills that determine the motivation and ability of individuals to gain access to, understand, and use information in ways that promote and maintain good health (see Chapter 25). Health literacy is essential for taking responsibility for one's own health. Lower health literacy may affect the ability to understand basic written health information or to read a prescription bottle correctly (CDC, 2019b). There is a relationship between health literacy and adherence to health-promoting behaviors (e.g., taking medications correctly, exercising), especially in patients with chronic illnesses such as diabetes. Therefore it is important to improve patients' health literacy while providing patient education to enhance health outcomes (Chahardah-Cherik et al., 2018).

People for whom English is a second language are at risk for low health literacy and may be unable to self-manage their health with lifestyle risk-factor modification to prevent the development of chronic diseases (Nierengarten, 2018; Fernandez-Gutierrez et al., 2018). A professional interpreter may be necessary to ensure understanding of health information.

Psychosocial Health

Anxiety. Anxiety is a critical maturational phenomenon related to change, conflict, and perceived control of the environment. Adults often experience anxiety in response to the physiological and psychosocial changes of middle age. Such anxiety motivates an adult to rethink life goals and thus can stimulate productivity. However, for some adults anxiety precipitates psychosomatic illness and preoccupation with death. In this case a middle adult views life as being half or more over and thinks in terms of the time left to live (Varcarolis and Dixon, 2020).

Clearly, a life-threatening illness, marital transition, loss of a spouse or partner, or job stressor increases the anxiety of a patient and family. Use crisis intervention or stress-management techniques to help a patient adapt to the changes of the middle-adult years (see Chapter 37).

Depression. Depression is a mood disorder that manifests in many ways. Although the most frequent age at onset is between ages 14 and

44, it is common among adults in the middle years and has many causes. The risk factors for depression include a family history of depression, being female, being a member of the LGBTQ+ community, a lack of social support, chronic illness, and negative stressful life events (Varcarolis and Dixon, 2020). People with chronic illness or caregivers of family members with chronic and long-term illnesses have a greater level of depression (Madva, 2018). Symptoms vary with the individual and may include depressed mood, loss of interest in activities, impaired concentration, or feelings of worthlessness or guilt. Symptoms can also be nonspecific, such as back pain, weight gain or loss, constipation, headaches, or fatigue. The abuse of alcohol or other substances makes depression worse.

Nursing assessment of a middle adult diagnosed with depression will depend on the setting in which you work. A focused data collection regarding individual and family history of depression, mood changes, cognitive changes, behavioral and social changes, and physical changes is ideal. There are a variety of useful and valid screening tools for depression. Hospitals and other health care agencies often have a preferred depression screening tool. Whichever tool is used, be sure to collect assessment data from both the patient and the patient's family. Family data are often particularly important, depending on the level of depression the middle adult is experiencing (Varcarolis and Dixon, 2020).

Early-Onset Dementia. Early-onset dementia (EOD), or "presenile dementia," defines all dementia-related conditions before age 65 (Elhusein et al., 2020). Depression and anxiety are prominent. As EOD progresses, agitation, apathy, and irritability worsen. EOD has major devastating psychological consequences, affecting people during their productive and leisure years, and also affects family responsibilities. Patients and families need assistance to maintain independence in decision making and activities (Brosch and Farlow, 2020; Sakamoto et al., 2017).

Community Health Programs. Community health programs in clinics, self-help groups, and primary care practices offer services to prevent illness, promote health, and detect disease in the early stages. Nurses make valuable contributions to the health of the community by taking an active part in planning screening and teaching programs and support groups for middle adults (see Chapter 3).

Health education programs promote changes in behavior and lifestyle. As a health teacher, offer information that enables patients to make informed decisions about health practices within the context of health promotion. Make sure that educational programs are culturally appropriate and use simple language (Williams et al., 2018). Changes to more positive health practices during young and middle adulthood lead to fewer or less complicated health problems as an older adult. During health counseling, collaborate with your patients to design a plan of action that addresses their health and well-being. Through objective problem solving you can help your patient grow and change (Edelman and Kudzma, 2021).

Acute Care. Acute illnesses and conditions experienced in middle adulthood are similar to those of young adulthood. However, injuries and acute illnesses in middle adulthood require a longer recovery period because of the slowing of healing processes. In addition, they are more likely to become chronic conditions. For middle adults in the sandwich generation, stress levels also increase as they balance responsibilities related to employment, family life, care of children, and care of aging parents while recovering from an injury or acute illness.

Restorative and Continuing Care. Chronic illnesses affect the roles and responsibilities of middle adults. Some results of chronic illness are strained family relationships, modifications in family activities, increased health care tasks, increased financial stress, the need for housing adaptation, social isolation, medical concerns, and grieving. The degree of disability and a patient's perception of both the illness and the disability determine the extent to which lifestyle changes occur. A few examples of the problems experienced by patients who develop debilitating chronic illness during adulthood include role reversal, changes in sexual behavior, and alterations in self-image. Along with the current health status of a middle adult living with a chronic illness, you need to assess the knowledge base of both the patient and family. This assessment includes the medical course of the illness and the prognosis for the patient. You need to determine the coping mechanisms of the patient and family. In addition, you need to assess adherence to treatment and rehabilitation regimens, evaluate the need for community and social services, and make appropriate referrals.

KEY POINTS

- Emerging adulthood is a stage of development unique from young adulthood and extended adolescence in which individuals face major life transitions and decisions with the focus on becoming independent.
- Emerging adulthood differs from young adulthood because most young people have not made the transitions historically associated with adult status, especially marriage and parenthood. In this stage young adults are faced with the tasks of identity development, who they want to be, and how to attain their goals.
- The young adult who achieves the developmental task of personal integration usually has the emotional maturity to complement the physical ability and therefore is able to develop mature sexual relationships and establish intimacy.
- Adults who have been living in poverty since childhood often are at risk for psychological distress and impaired cognitive skills, which affects their ability to make long-term decisions and adds to their decreased access to health care resources.
- Young female adults are in a stable period of normal physical development, which includes changes related to pregnancy.
- Cognitive development continues throughout the young- and middle-adult years.
- Cognitive changes in middle age are often related to acute illnesses or physical trauma.
- Critical thinking habits such as conceptual skills and problem solving normally increase steadily through the young-adult years.
- The emotional health of young and middle adults is correlated with the ability to address and resolve personal and social problems.
- A family history of a disease sometimes puts a young adult at risk for developing that disease in the middle- or older-adult years.
- Psychosocial changes and health concerns during pregnancy and the postpartum period affect the parents, the siblings, and often the extended family.
- Psychosocial changes for middle adults often include career transition, sexuality, marital changes, family transition, and care of aging parents.
- Health concerns of the young adult usually focus on health promotion habits and fertility and pregnancy issues.
- Health concerns of middle adults commonly involve stress-related illnesses, adoption of positive health habits, and issues with health literacy.
- Intimate partner violence (IPV), formerly referred to as domestic violence, is a global public health problem. It exists along a continuum from a single episode of violence to ongoing battering.

REFLECTIVE LEARNING

- Think about your own health habits.
  - How would you improve them? Select one that you would like to improve.
  - What information would you need in order to be successful in changing this one habit?
- Your friend mentions that her paternal grandmother and uncle are breast cancer survivors. Her father doesn't think he is at risk and hasn't informed his primary care provider about this family history. What do you need to do to prepare for a conversation with your friend to help her gain more information and to critically think about strategies to help her father realize the need to inform his health care provider and do any screenings?
- You are having a coffee break with one of your friends, and you notice bruises on her neck and both wrists. She has shared with you that her boyfriend has a bad temper and tells her she is always wrong. What are the risk factors to look for in an assessment that suggests perpetration of intimate partner violence? How would you proceed to get more information and help your friend?

REVIEW QUESTIONS

1. A nurse is completing an assessment on a 27-year-old female patient. Which questions best assess the psychosocial aspects of this young woman's health? (Select all that apply.)
   1. Do you feel safe in your home and at work?
   2. How many fruits and vegetables do you typically eat every day?
   3. Describe your relationship with your family.
   4. Have you had the vaccine to prevent HPV?
   5. What are your long-term career goals?
2. A 36-year-old patient newly diagnosed with type 1 diabetes shares with you that he is frustrated with the time it takes to prepare meals and monitor his blood sugar. He also is having trouble understanding his insulin schedule. Which of the following suggestions would be most appropriate? (Select all that apply.)
   1. Provide patient education materials that are easy to read.
   2. Refer this patient to a diabetes support group.
   3. Refer the patient to his endocrinologist.
   4. Suggest that the patient make an appointment with a registered dietitian.
   5. Suggest ways to modify his schedule.
3. When assessing the health-related knowledge base of both the middle-age patient with an illness and the family, the assessment should include which of the following? (Select all that apply.)
   1. Medical course of the illness
   2. Prognosis for the patient
   3. Coping mechanisms of the patient and family
   4. Socioeconomic status
   5. Need for community and social services
4. A 50-year-old woman has elevated serum cholesterol levels that increase her risk for cardiovascular disease. The nurse helps this patient control this risk factor by assessing the patient's current diet trends and describing dietary changes to reduce the patient's risk for developing cardiovascular disease. This nursing activity is a form of:
   1. Referral
   2. Counseling
   3. Health education
   4. Stress-management techniques

5. You are caring for a young female patient who is currently homeless. You believe she is experiencing IPV. Your assessment of the patient reveals several socioeconomic factors. Which ones are linked to IPV? (Select all that apply.)
   1. History of smoking marijuana
   2. Income below poverty level
   3. Recent divorce
   4. High school education
   5. Unemployment
6. A home health nurse is caring for a 48-year-old woman with newly diagnosed diabetes mellitus type 2. She is prescribed to take Metformin IR three times a day. The woman lives alone but has a sister who lives just 5 miles away. The doctor orders the patient to measure her blood glucose daily for the next month. Which of the following show the nurse's ability to minimize common barriers to change as she helps this patient manage her diabetes? (Select all that apply.)
   1. Encourages the patient to have an eye examination
   2. Provides a simple-language brochure that explains the long-term implications of diabetes type 2
   3. Tells the patient to always take metformin the same times each day
   4. Informs the patient about availability of a support group in her community
   5. Recommends that the patient's sister be involved in the discussion about medication and glucose monitoring
7. A 48-year-old patient visiting the primary health clinic presents with fatigue and recent weight loss. It is the patient's first visit to the clinic in 2 years. The patient has a family history of cancer and heart disease. During assessment, the nurse finds that the patient has two jobs and works about 12 to 14 hours every weekday. The patient drinks three or four alcoholic drinks a day, relies on fast foods or prepared foods at work, sleeps only 4 to 6 hours a day, and exercises infrequently. The patient takes a nonsteroidal antiinflammatory drug (NSAID) daily for knee pain. Which of the following places this patient at risk for development of a chronic illness later in life? (Select all that apply.)
   1. Working 10 to 12 hours a day
   2. Eating high-calorie and fatty foods
   3. Exercising infrequently
   4. Taking a daily analgesic
   5. Excessive alcohol consumption

8. A 45-year-old woman who is obese tells a nurse that she wants to lose weight. Which assessment findings may be contributing factors to the woman's obesity? (Select all that apply.)
   1. The woman works in an executive position that is very demanding.
   2. The woman says that she has little time to prepare meals at home and eats out at least four nights a week.
   3. The woman works out at the corporate gym at 5 a.m. three mornings per week.
   4. The woman says that she tries to eat "low-cholesterol" foods to help lose weight.
   5. The woman says that she vacations annually.
9. A 34-year-old female executive has a job with frequent deadlines. She notes that when the deadlines appear, she tends to eat high-fat, high-carbohydrate foods. She also explains that she gets frequent headaches and stomach pain during these deadlines. After receiving health education from the nurse, the executive decides to try yoga. In this scenario yoga is best described as which one of the following?
   1. Outpatient referral
   2. Counseling technique
   3. Health promotion activity
   4. Stress-management technique
10. A nurse is completing an assessment on a male patient, age 24. Following the assessment, the nurse notes that his family history is not significant for chronic illnesses, and his physical and laboratory findings are within normal limits. Because of these findings, nursing interventions are directed toward activities related to which of the following? (Select all that apply.)
   1. Instructing him to return in 2 years
   2. Instructing him in secondary prevention
   3. Instructing him in health promotion activities
   4. Instructing him about routine screenings
   5. Instructing him about proper vaccinations

Answers: 1. 1, 3, 5; **2.** 1, 2, 4, 5; **3.** 1, 2, 3, 5; **4.** 3; **5.** 1, 3, 4, 5; **6.** 2, 4, 5; **7.** 2, 3, 5; **8.** 1, 2; **9.** 4; **10.** 3, 4, 5.

Rationales for Review Questions can be found on the Evolve website.

REFERENCES

American Academy of Pediatrics (AAP): Policy statement: promoting the well-being of children whose parents are gay or lesbian, *Pediatrics* 141(4):827, 2013.

American Bone Health: *Guidelines on calcium and vitamin d supplements,* 2020, https://americanbonehealth.org/nutrition/guidelines-calcium-vitamin-d-supplementation/. Accessed August 2020.

American Cancer Society: *Guideline for colorectal cancer screening,* 2021, https://www.cancer.org/cancer/colon-rectal-cancer/detection-diagnosis-staging/acs-recommendations.html. Accessed April 22, 2021.

American Heart Association (AHA): American Heart Association recommendations for physical activity in adults, 2018, http://www.heart.org/HEARTORG/GettingHealthy/PhysicalActivity/FitnessBasics/American-Heart-Association-Recommendations-for-Physical-Activity-in-Adults_UCM_307976_Article.jsp#.VkjC8aSFOpo" http://www.heart.org/HEARTORG/GettingHealthy/PhysicalActivity/FitnessBasics/American-Heart-Association-Recommendations-for-Physical-Activity-in-Adults_UCM_307976_Article.jsp#.VkjC8aSFOpo. Accessed April 2021.

American Society for Reproductive Medicine: *Infertility,* 2021 https://www.asrm.org/topics/topics-index/infertility/. Accessed April 2021.

Ashe-Goins FE: Human trafficking: implications for nurses, *S C Nurse* 25(2):15, 2018.

Berger N: Young adult cancer: influence of the obesity pandemic, *Obesity* 26(4):641, 2018.

Berkeley Public Policy: Poverty among young adults is on the rise, June 2019, https://gspp.berkeley.edu/faculty-and-impact/news/recent-news/poverty-among-young-adults-is-on-the-rise#:~:text=The%20number%20of%20young%20people%20%28ages%2018-24%29%20living, Institute%20for%20the%20Future%20of%20Young%20Americans%20%28BIFYA%29. Accessed April 2021.

Brosch J, Farlow M: Early-onset dementia in adults, *UpToDate,* 2020, https://www.uptodate.com/contents/early-onset-dementia-in-adults.

Burcham JR, Rosenthal LD: *Lehne's pharmacology for nursing care,* ed 10, St Louis, 2019, Elsevier.

Butterbaugh SM et al.: My money and me: attaining financial independence in emerging adulthood through a conceptual model of identity capital

theory, *Contemporary Family Therapy* 42:33, 2020.

Centers for Disease Control and Prevention (CDC): Marijuana and public health: *Health effects,* 2018, https://www.cdc.gov/marijuana/health-effects.html. Accessed April 2021.

Centers for Disease Control and Prevention (CDC): *Preventing intimate partner violence,* 2019a, https://www.cdc.gov/violenceprevention/intimatepartnerviolence/fastfact.html. Accessed August 2020.

Centers for Disease Control and Prevention (CDC): *What is health literacy,* 2019b, https://www.cdc.gov/healthliteracy/learn/index.html. Accessed August 2020.

Centers for Disease Control and Prevention (CDC): *Overweight and obesity: adult obesity prevalence maps,* 2021a, https://www.cdc.gov/obesity/data/prevalence-maps.html. Accessed April, 2021.

Centers for Disease Control and Prevention (CDC): *Overweight and obesity: adult obesity causes & consequences,* 2021b, https://www.cdc.gov/obesity/adult/causes.html. Accessed April 2021.

Centers for Medicare and Medicaid (CMS) *Services: Improving access to maternal health care in rural communities: issue brief,* n.d., https://www.cms.gov/About-CMS/Agency-Information/OMH/equity-initiatives/rural-health/09032019-Maternal-Health-Care-in-Rural-Communities.pdf. Accessed April, 2021.

CNBC: *40% of the American middle class face poverty in retirement, study concludes,* 2021, https://www.cnbc.com/2018/10/12/40percent-of-american-middle-class-face-poverty-in-retirement-study-says.html. Accessed April 2021.

Conroy J, Tabbenhoff B: Workplace stress: name it, reframe it, tame it, *Virginia Nurses Today* 26(1):6, 2018.

Cunningham J: *The pandemic's effect on the economy and workers, national conference of state legislatures,* 2021, https://www.ncsl.org/research/labor-and-employment/the-pandemic-s-effect-on-the-economy-and-workers637463008.aspx. Accessed April 2021.

Edelman C, Kudzma EC: *Health promotion throughout the life span,* ed 10, St Louis, 2021, Elsevier.

Ellington L et al.: Supporting home hospice family caregivers: insights from different perspectives. *Palliat Support Care* 16(2):209, 2018.

Erikson E: *Childhood society,* ed 2, New York, 1963, WW Norton.

Erikson E: *The lifecycle completed: a review,* New York, 1982, WW Norton.

Fioretti C et al.: The role of this listener on the emotional valence of personal memories in emerging adulthood, *J Adult Dev* 24:252, 2017.

Hockenberry MJ et al: *Wong's nursing care of infants and children,* ed 11, St Louis, 2019, Mosby.

Huether S, et al: *Understanding pathophysiology,* ed 7, St Louis, 2020, Mosby.

Institute for Women's Policy Research (IWPR): *Pay equity and discrimination,* n.d., https://iwpr.org/equal-pay-about/. Accessed April 2021.

March of Dimes: *Prenatal education and outreach,* 2021, https://www.marchofdimes.org/mission/prenatal-education-and-outreach.aspx. Accessed April 2021.

National Institute on Drug Abuse: *Talking to patients about their drug use,* n.d., https://www.drugabuse.gov/nidamed-medical-health-professionals/about-addiction-performance-project/addiction-performance-project/talking-to-patients-about-their-drug-use. Accessed August 2020.

National Institute of Mental Health (NIMH): *Postpartum depression,* n.d., https://www.nimh.nih.gov/health/publications/postpartum-depression-facts/index.shtml. Accessed August 2020.

Nierengarten MB: Health literacy: a challenge in diverse populations, 2018, *Contemp Pediatr* 35(1):19, 2018.

Office of Disease Prevention and Health Promotion: Nutrition and healthy eating. *Healthy People 2030,* n.d., U.S. Department of Health and Human Services. https://health.gov/healthypeople/objectives-and-data/browse-objectives/nutrition-and-healthy-eating. Accessed April, 2021.

Pew Research Center: *U.S. has highest rate of children living in single-parent households,* 2019, https://www.pewresearch.org/fact-tank/2019/12/12/u-s-children-more-likely-than-children-in-other-countries-to-live-with-just-one-parent/ Accessed April 2021.

Pew Research Center.: *Social media fact sheet,* https://www.pewresearch.org/internet/fact-sheet/social-media /2020. Accessed August 2020.

Renzulli KA: This is how much debt the average American has now—at every age, *Money* , 2020. http://time.com/money/5233033/average-debt-every-age/. Accessed August 2020.

Rossi N: Commentary on same-sex and different-sex parent households and child health outcomes: additional sources of same-sex parenting stress to consider, *J Dev Behav Pediatrics* 39(2):180, 2018.

Saporta Report: *The effects of generational poverty, sheltering arms,* February 10, 2021, https://saportareport.com/the-effects-of-generational-poverty/thought-leadership/sheltering-arms/ Accessed April 2021.

Sheehy-Skeffington J: The effects of low socioeconomic status on decision-making processes, *Curr Opin Psychol,* 33:183-188, 2020.

Tracy E, Macias-Konstantopoulos W: Human trafficking: Identification and evaluation in the health care setting, *UpToDate,* 2021, https://www.uptodate.com/contents/human-trafficking-identification-and-evaluation-in-the-health-care-setting. Accessed April 2021.

United Nations Office on Drugs and Crime: *Human trafficking FAQs,* n.d. www.unodc.org/unodc/en/human-trafficking/faqs.html. Accessed August 2020.

U.S. Bureau of Labor Statistics: *Bureau of Labor Statistics: occupational outlook handbook,* 2020. www.bls.gov/ooh. Accessed April 2021.

U.S. Census Bureau.: *U.S. Census Bureau Releases 2014-2018 ACS 5-Year Estimates,* Revised 2021. https://www.census.gov/programs-surveys/acs/news/updates/2019.html. Accessed April 2021.

U.S. Department of Health and Human Services (USDHHS): *Centers for disease control and prevention (CDC): sexually transmitted disease surveillance 2018,* 2019, https://www.cdc.gov/std/stats18/STDSurveillance2018-FUll-report.pdf. Accessed August 2020.

University of California San Francisco (UCSF): *Want to be robust at 40-plus? meeting minimum exercise guidelines won't cut it,* 2021, https://www.ucsf.edu/news/2021/04/420281/want-be-robust-40-plus-meeting-minimum-exercise-guidelines-wont-cut-it Accessed April 2021.

Varcarolis EM, Dixon C: *Essentials of psychiatric mental health nursing,* 4 ed, St Louis, 2020, Elsevier.

Young Survival Coalition: *Breast cancer statistics in young adults,* 2021, https://www.youngsurvival.org/learn/about-breast-cancer/statistics. Accessed April 2021.

RESEARCH REFERENCES

Amnie A: An investigation of predictors of self-efficacy to cope with stress and implications for health education practice, *Am J Health Educ* 49(3):155, 2018.

Becker W, Starrels J: Prescription drug misuse: Epidemiology, prevention, identification, and management, *UpToDate,* 2021, https://www.uptodate.com/contents/prescription-drug-misuse-epidemiology-prevention-identification-and-management. Accessed April 2021.

Beneitz MC, Gil-Alegre ME: Opioid addiction: social problems associated and implications of both current and possible future treatments, including polymeric therapeutics for giving up the habit of opioid consumption, *BioMed Res Int* 1, 2017.

Benck L et al.: Association between cardiorespiratory fitness and lung health from young adulthood to middle age, *Am J of Resp and Crit Care Med* 195(9):1236, 2018.

Bos HM et al.: A population-based comparison of female and male same-sex parent and different-sex parent households, *Family Process* 57(1): 148, 2018.

Brough P et al.: Job support, coping, and control: assessment of simultaneous impacts within the occupational stress process, *J Occup Health Psych* 23(2):188, 2018.

Chahardah-Cherik S et al.: The relationship between health literacy and health promoting behaviors in patient with type 2 diabetes, *Int J Community Based Nurs Midwifery* 6(1):65, 2018.

Elhusein B et al.: Early-onset dementia: diagnostic challenges, *BMJ Case Reports,* 13(1): 2020.

Ertl A et al.: Surveillance for violent deaths-national violent death reporting system, 32 states, 2016, *Morbidity and Mortality Weekly Report (MMWR),* 68 (9): 1, 2019, https://www.cdc.gov/mmwr/volumes/68/ss/ss6809a1.htm. Accessed August 2020.

Evans GW: Childhood poverty and adult psychological well-being, *Proc Natl Acad Sci U S A* 113 (52):14949-14952, 2016.

Evans K et al.: The impact of within and between role experiences on role balance outcomes for working sandwich generation women, *Scand J Occup Ther,* 26(3): 184, 2019.

Ferdos J et al.: Association between intimate partner violence during pregnancy and maternal pregnancy complications among recently delivered women in Bangladesh, *Aggress Behav* 44(3):294, 2018.

Forcier M, Olson-Kennedy J: Lesbian, gay, bisexual, and other sexual minoritized youth: Epidemiology and health concerns, *UpToDate,* 2020, https://www.uptodate.com/contents/lesbian-gay-bisexual-and-other-sexual-minoritized-youth-epidemiology-and-health-concerns.

Fernandez-Gutierrez M et al.: Health literacy interventions for immigrant populations: a systematic review, *Int Nurs Rev* 65(1):54, 2018.

Johnson PH, Annesi JJ: Factors related to weight gain/loss among emerging adults with obesity, *Am J Health Behav* 42(3):3, 2018.

Kellogg, MB: Secondary traumatic stress in nursing, *Adv Nurs Sci* 44(2), 157, 2021.

Kelly JF et al.: Coping with the enduring unpredictability of opioid addiction: an investigation of a novel family-focused peer-support organization, *J Subst Abus Treat* 77:193, 2017.

Layland EK et al.: Freedom to explore the self: how emerging adults use leisure to develop identity, *J Positive Psychol* 13(1):78, 2018.

Liu HY, Huang KH: The relationship between family functioning and caregiving appraisal of dementia family caregivers: caregiving self-efficacy as a mediator, *Aging Ment Health* 22(4):558, 2018.

Madva EN: Magnitude and sources of distress in mid-life adults with chronic medical illness: an exploratory mixed-methods analysis, *Psychol Health Med* 23(5):555, 2018.

Masiero M et al.: Optimistic bias in young adults for cancer, cardiovascular and respiratory diseases: a pilot study on smokers and drinkers, *J Health Psych* 23(5):645, 2018.

Padkapayeva K et al.: Gender/sex differences in the relationship between psychosocial work exposures and work and life stress, *Ann Work Expo Health* 62(4):416, 2018.

Park S, Jang MK: Associations between workplace exercise interventions and job stress reduction, *Workplace & Safety,* 67(12); 592, 2019.

Roberts A et al.: Gambling and physical intimate partner violence: results from the national epidemiologic survey on alcohol and related conditions (NESARC), *Am J Addict* 27(1):7, 2018.

Sakamoto et al.: "I'm still here": Personhood and the early-onset dementia experience, *J Geron Nurs* 43(5):12, 2017.

Shaw A, Rogge RD: Symbolic meanings of sex in relationships: developing the meanings of sexual behavior inventory, *Psychol Assess* 29(10):1221, 2017.

Siren A; Casier F: Socio-economic and lifestyle determinants of giving practical support to adult children in the era of changing late life. *Aging and Society* 39(9): 1933, 2019.

Sommerfeld D et al.: Hypersensitivity pneumonitis and acute respiratory distress syndrome from e-cigarette use, *Pediatrics* 164(6):1, 2018.

Stockdale LA, Coyne SM: Bored and online: reasons for using social media, problematic social networking site use, and behavioral outcomes across the transition from adolescence to emerging adulthood, *J Adolesc* 79: 173, 2020.

Sung H et al: Emerging cancer trends among young adults in the USA: analysis of a population-based cancer registry, *Lancet Public Health,* 4(3):e137-e147, 2019.

Szkody E, McKinney C: Indirect effects of social support on psychological health through self-esteem in emerging adulthood, *J Fam Issue* 40(17): 2439, 2019.

Wang S et al.: Job stress in young adults is associated with a range of poorer health behaviors in the childhood determinants of adult health (CDAH) study, *J Occup Environ Med* 60(3):e117, 2018.

Williams HL et al.: Do health promotion, behaviors affect levels of job satisfaction and job stress for nurses in an acute care hospital? *J Nurs Adm* 48(6):342, 2018.

Older Adults

OBJECTIVES

- Identify how common myths and stereotypes about older adults might affect nursing care.
- Discuss how a nurse applies clinical judgment when interpreting signs and symptoms in older adults.
- Explore the common developmental tasks of older adults and the associated nursing implications.
- Identify the impact of common physiological changes of aging.

- Distinguish among delirium, dementia, and depression.
- Discuss issues related to psychosocial changes of aging.
- Explain the multifaceted aspects of elder mistreatment.
- Examine select health concerns of older adults.
- Plan nursing interventions related to the physiological, cognitive, and psychosocial changes of aging.

KEY TERMS

Ageism
Delirium
Dementia
Depression

Elder mistreatment
Gerontological nursing
Gerontology
Reality orientation

Reminiscence
Validation therapy

MEDIA RESOURCES

http://evolve.elsevier.com/Potter/fundamentals/
- Review Questions
- Case Study with Questions

- Audio Glossary
- Content Updates
- Answers to QSEN Activity and Review Questions

People who are 65 years of age are in the lower boundary that society perceives as "old age" in demographics and social policy. However, many older adults consider themselves to be "middle age" well into their seventh decade. Chronological age often has little relation to the reality of aging for an older adult. Each person ages in his or her own way. Every older adult is unique. As a nurse you need to approach each person as an individual.

The number of older adults in the United States is growing quickly. In 2017, there were 50.9 million adults over age 65 in the United States, representing 15.6% of the population or one in seven Americans (Administration on Aging [AOA], 2018). Part of this increase is caused by the increase of the average life span. The number of Americans 65 years of age and older is projected to nearly double to 95 million by 2060 (Population Reference Bureau, 2021). The racial and ethnic diversity of the population over age 65 is also increasing. Between 2014 and 2060, the non-Hispanic white segment of the population is expected to decrease from 77% to 55% (Population Reference Bureau, 2021). As a nurse, you need to consider cultural diversity as an important principle to apply in your care of older adults. The aging of the baby-boom generation and the growth of the population segment over age 85 contribute to the projected increase in the number of older adults. The baby boomers were born between 1946 and 1964. The first baby boomers reached age 65 in 2011. Social and health care programs continue to try to adapt to meet the needs of this growing segment of the population. The challenge is to gain new knowledge and skills to provide culturally sensitive and linguistically appropriate care (see Chapter 9).

VARIABILITY AMONG OLDER ADULTS

Nursing care of older adults poses special challenges because of variations in their physiological, cognitive, and psychosocial health. Older adults also have a wide range of functional ability. Most older adults are active and involved in their communities. A smaller number have lost the ability to care for themselves, are confused or withdrawn, or are unable to make decisions concerning their needs. Most older adults do not live in institutional settings. In 2018, 59% of older adults in noninstitutional settings lived with a spouse/partner (42% of older women, 72% of older men); 28% lived alone (9.3 million women, 4.5 million men); and only 3.1% of all older adults resided in institutions, primarily nursing homes. As would be expected, the percentage of those living in a nursing home increases with age. Only 1% of the 65 to 74 age-group live in a nursing home, while 9% of those 85 and older do (AOA, 2018).

The physical and psychosocial aspects of aging are closely related. A reduced ability to respond to stress, the experience of multiple losses, and the physical changes associated with normal aging combine to place people at high risk for illness and functional deterioration. Most older adults remain functionally independent despite the increasing prevalence of chronic disease. Nursing assessment provides valuable clues to the effects of a disease or illness on a patient's functional status.

Chronic conditions add to the complexity of assessment and care of older adults. Most older people have at least one chronic condition, and many have multiple conditions. Although the interaction of these physical and psychosocial factors may be serious, do not assume that all older adults have signs, symptoms, or behaviors representing disease and decline or that these are the only factors you need to assess. You also need to identify an older adult's strengths and abilities during an assessment and encourage independence as an integral part of your plan of care (Touhy and Jett, 2020).

MYTHS AND STEREOTYPES

Despite ongoing research in the field of gerontology, myths and stereotypes about older adults persist among lay people and health care providers. These include false perceptions about the physical and psychosocial characteristics and lifestyles of older adults. When health care providers hold negative stereotypes about aging, their actions often negatively affect the quality of patient care. Some people stereotype older adults as ill, disabled, and physically unattractive. Others believe that older adults are forgetful, confused, rigid, bored, and unfriendly and that they are unable to understand and learn new information. Yet specialists in the field of gerontology view centenarians, the oldest of the old, as having an optimistic outlook on life, good memories, broad social contacts and interests, and tolerance for others. Although changes in vision or hearing and reduced energy and endurance sometimes affect the process of learning, older adults are lifelong learners.

Stereotypes about lifestyles often include mistaken ideas about living arrangements and finances. Misconceptions about financial status range from beliefs that many are affluent to beliefs that many are poor. According to the U.S. Census Bureau, only 8.1% of people over age 65 had incomes below the poverty level. Older women report a significantly lower income than men. Social Security benefits serve as the primary source of income for most older adults (U.S. Census Bureau, 2020).

In a society that values attractiveness, energy, and youth, these myths and stereotypes lead to the undervaluing of older adults. Some people equate worth with productivity; therefore they think that older adults become worthless after they leave the workforce. Others consider their knowledge and experience too outdated to have any current value. These ideas demonstrate ageism, which is discrimination against people because of increasing age, just as people who are racist and sexist discriminate because of skin color and gender. According to experts in the field of gerontology, ageism typically undermines the self-confidence of older adults, limits their access to care, and distorts caregivers' understanding of the uniqueness of each older adult. Nurses should promote a positive perception regarding the aging process when establishing therapeutic relationships and value the experiences of older adults.

Current laws ban age discrimination. The economic and political power of older adults challenges ageist views. Older adults are a significant proportion of the consumer economy. As voters and activists in various issues, they have a major influence on the formation of public policy. Participation of older adults in voting issues adds a unique perspective on social, economic, and technological issues because they have experienced almost a century of developments. Some older adults lived through or were born during the Great Depression of 1929. They also experienced a world war and wars in Korea, Vietnam, and Iraq and are now experiencing the war on terrorism. They have seen tremendous changes in technology. Changes in health care also impact older adults as the era of the family physician has given way to the age of specialization and managed care. After witnessing the governmental initiatives that established the Social Security system, Medicare, and Medicaid, older adults are currently living with the changes imposed by health care reform.

The implication for nurses is to avoid stereotypes when conducting assessments of patients. It is important to use clinical judgment in a way that objectively assesses a patient's functional, physiological, psychosocial, and emotional status, compare those findings with the patient's normal status, and then decide if health problems exist. The avoidance of stereotypes will also influence the interventions you select for promoting healthy patient outcomes.

NURSES' ATTITUDES TOWARD OLDER ADULTS

It is important to assess your own attitudes toward older adults, your own aging, and the aging of your family, friends, and patients. Nurses' attitudes come from personal experiences with older adults, education, employment experiences, and attitudes of co-workers and employing institutions. Given the increasing number of older adults in health care settings, forming positive attitudes toward them and gaining specialized knowledge about aging and the health care needs of older adults are priorities for all nurses. Positive attitudes are based in part on a realistic portrayal of the characteristics and health care needs of older adults. It is critical for you to respect older adults and actively involve them in care decisions and activities. In the past institutional settings such as hospitals and nursing centers often treated older adults as objects rather than as independent, dignified people. The time has come for nurses to recognize and address ageism by questioning prevailing negative attitudes and stereotypes and reinforcing the realities of aging as they care for older adults in all settings.

> **REFLECT NOW**
>
> Think about how you feel about caring for older adults. Reflect on positive and negative experiences you have had with older adults and how this may affect your nursing care of older adults.

DEVELOPMENTAL TASKS FOR OLDER ADULTS

Theories of aging are closely linked to the concept of developmental tasks appropriate for distinct stages of life (see Chapter 11). Although no two individuals age in the same way, either biologically or psychosocially, there are common developmental tasks for older adults that are associated with varying degrees of change and loss (Box 14.1). More common changes include alterations in health status, loss of significant others, a decreased sense of usefulness, and decreases in socialization, income, and independent living. How older adults adjust to these changes is individualized. For some, adaptation and adjustment are relatively easy. For others, coping with the changes brought on by aging requires the assistance of family, friends, and health care professionals. Be sensitive to the effect of losses on older adults and their families and be prepared to offer support.

> **BOX 14.1 Developmental Tasks for Older Adults**
>
> - Adjusting to changes related to health and physical strength
> - Adjusting to retirement and reduced or fixed income
> - Adjusting to death of a spouse, children, siblings, friends
> - Accepting self as aging person
> - Maintaining satisfactory living arrangements
> - Redefining relationships with adult children and siblings
> - Maintaining quality of life

Older adults learn to adjust to the physical changes that accompany aging. The extent and timing of these changes vary by individual, but as body systems age, changes in appearance and functioning occur. These changes are not associated with a disease; they are normal. However, the presence of disease sometimes alters the timing of the changes or their impact on daily life. The section on physiological changes describes structural and functional changes of aging.

Some older adults, both men and women, find it difficult to accept aging. This is apparent when they understate their ages when asked, adopt younger styles of clothing, or attempt to hide physical evidence of aging with cosmetics. Others deny their aging in ways that are potentially problematic. For example, some older adults deny functional declines and refuse to ask for help with tasks, placing their safety at great risk. Others avoid places and activities designed for their benefit, such as senior citizens' centers and senior health promotion activities, and as a result do not receive the benefits these programs offer. Acceptance of personal aging does not mean retreat into inactivity, but it does require a realistic review of strengths and limitations.

Retirement poses challenges, such as adjusting to the loss of the work role and daily interaction with professional colleagues. Some are able to welcome retirement as a time to pursue new interests and hobbies, volunteer in their communities, continue their education, or start new careers. Retirement plans for others include changing residence by moving to a different city or state or to a different type of housing within the same area. Reasons other than retirement also lead to changes of residence. For example, physical impairments sometimes require relocation to a smaller, single-level home or a nursing center. A change in living arrangements for the older adult usually requires an extended period of adjustment, during which assistance and support from health care professionals, friends, and family members are necessary.

Not all older adults can enjoy retirement. For people age 65 and older, the 2018 poverty rate was 9.7%, representing 5.1 million individuals in poverty (U.S. Census Bureau, 2020). These older adults may continue working well beyond age 65 or place more burden on families who provide care and support.

Many older adults face coping with the death of a spouse, close friend, or partner. In 2018, 32% of all older women were widows, and 11% of older men were widowers (AOA, 2018). They also may need to cope with the deaths of adult children, grandchildren, and lifelong friends. These deaths represent losses and reminders of personal mortality. Coming to terms with them is often difficult. By helping older adults through the grieving process (see Chapter 36), you can help them resolve some of these issues.

Redefining relationships with children continues as older adults experience the challenges of aging. A variety of issues sometimes occur, including control of decision making, dependence, conflict, guilt, and loss. How these issues surface in situations and how they are resolved depend in part on the past relationship between older adults and their adult children. When adult children become their parents' caregivers, they must try to balance the demands of their own children and careers with the many challenges of family caregiving. As adult children and aging parents negotiate the aspects of changing roles, nurses are in the position to act as counselors for the entire family. Helping older adults maintain their quality of life is often a priority. What defines quality of life is unique for each person.

COMMUNITY-BASED AND INSTITUTIONAL HEALTH CARE SERVICES

You will encounter older-adult patients in a wide variety of community and institutional health care settings. Outside of an acute care hospital, nurses care for older adults in clinics, private homes and apartments, retirement communities, adult day care centers, assisted-living residences,

BOX 14.2   FOCUS ON OLDER ADULTS
Selection of a Nursing Center or Home

An important step in the process of selecting a nursing center is to have the patient and any family caregivers visit it. A quality nursing home has the following features:

- Is a home, a place where people live. Residents are encouraged to personalize their rooms. Privacy is respected.
- Is Medicare and Medicaid certified.
- Has adequate, qualified staff members who have passed criminal background checks.
- Does not feel like a hospital. However, the nursing center provides quality care. In addition to assistance with basic activities of daily living such as bathing, dressing, eating, oral hygiene, and toileting, staff regularly help residents with social and recreational activities.
- Offers quality food and mealtime choices.
- Welcomes families when they visit the center. Staff always encourage family involvement, whether families wish to provide information, ask questions, participate in care planning, or help with social activities or physical care.
- Is clean. There are no pervasive odors. The environment feels "homelike."
- Provides active communication from staff to patient and family.
- Attends quickly to resident requests. Staff are actively involved with assisting the residents. They focus on the person, not on the task.

Modified from the Centers for Medicare & Medicaid Services (CMS): *Your guide to choosing a nursing home or other long-term care,* Baltimore, MD, 2019, CMS, https://www.medicare.gov/Pubs/pdf/02174-Nursing-Home-Other-Long-Term-Services.pdf. Accessed July 2020.

and senior living communities (extended care, intermediate care, and skilled nursing facilities). Chapter 2 describes these settings and the services provided in detail.

Sorting through the options for care of older adults can be overwhelming. Nurses and social workers can help older adults and their families by providing information and answering questions as they review care options. Your assistance is especially valuable when patients and families need to make decisions about moving to a nursing center. Some family caregivers consider nursing center placement when in-home care becomes increasingly difficult or when convalescence (recovery) from hospitalization requires more assistance than the family is able to provide. Although the decision to enter a nursing center is never final and a nursing center resident is sometimes discharged to home or another less acute setting, many older adults view the nursing center as their final residence. Results of state and federal inspections of nursing centers are available to the public at the nursing center, online, and at the inspectors' offices. The best way to evaluate the quality of a nursing center is for the patient and family to visit the center and inspect it personally. The Centers for Medicare and Medicaid (CMS, 2019, website http://www.Medicare.gov/NHcompare) provides an excellent resource for you to learn about the quality rating of a nursing center on the basis of health inspections, staffing, and quality measures (Box 14.2). It also offers a nursing center checklist (https://www.medicare.gov/NursingHomeCompare/checklist.pdf).

ASSESSING THE NEEDS OF OLDER ADULTS

Gerontological nursing involves the provision of care that addresses mutually established goals for an older adult, the family, and health care team members. A comprehensive assessment involving clinical judgment that analyzes patients' strengths, limitations, and resources provides a baseline of an older adult's health and functional status. Sound clinical judgment then leads to clinical decisions for selecting appropriate nursing diagnoses and interventions designed to either maintain or enhance physical abilities and activity (see Chapter 38) and to create environments for psychosocial and spiritual well-being (see Chapter 35). To complete a thorough assessment, actively engage older adults and provide adequate time, allowing them to share important information about their past and current health. Caring for older adults often requires creative strategies that will maximize the potential of older adults.

Nursing assessment takes into account three key points to ensure an age-specific approach: (1) the interrelation between physical and psychosocial aspects of aging, (2) the effects of disease and disability on a patient's current functional status, and (3) tailoring the nursing assessment to an older person (Yeager, 2019c). A comprehensive assessment of an older adult takes more time than the assessment of a younger adult because of the longer life and medical history and potential complexity of the history. During the physical examination allow rest periods as needed or conduct the assessment in several sessions if a patient has reduced energy or limited endurance. Review both prescription and over-the-counter medications carefully with each patient.

Sensory changes associated with aging may affect your approach to data gathering. For example, your choice of communication techniques depends on whether an older adult has a visual or hearing impairment. If an older adult is unable to understand your visual or auditory cues when you ask questions or examine the patient, your assessment data will likely be inaccurate or misleading, leading you to incorrectly conclude that the older adult is confused.

Memory deficits, if present, can affect the accuracy and completeness of your assessment. Information contributed by a family member or other caregiver is sometimes necessary to supplement an older adult's recollection of past medical events and information about current self-care habits, medication adherence, allergies, and immunizations. Use tact when involving another person in the assessment interview. The additional person provides supplemental information with the consent of the older adult, but the older adult should remain the primary source of information whenever possible.

During all aspects of an assessment, you are responsible for making careful clinical judgments in how you recognize and interpret signs and symptoms of diseases and patients' laboratory values. Historically, researchers have used younger populations to establish standard signs and norms for disease conditions. However, the classic signs and symptoms of diseases are sometimes absent, blunted, or atypical in older adults (Touhy and Jett, 2020). This is especially true in the cases of bacterial infection, pain, acute myocardial infarction, and heart failure. The masquerading of disease is possibly caused by age-related changes in organ systems and homeostatic mechanisms, progressive loss of physiological and functional reserves, or coexisting acute or chronic conditions. As a result an older adult with a urinary tract infection (UTI) sometimes presents with incontinence, falls, and only a slight elevation of body temperature (within normal limits) instead of having fever, dysuria, frequency, or urgency. Some older adults with pneumonia have tachycardia, tachypnea, and confusion with decreased appetite and functioning, without the more common symptoms of fever and productive cough. Instead of crushing substernal chest pain and diaphoresis, some older adults experience a sudden onset of dyspnea often accompanied by anxiety and confusion when having a myocardial infarction. Variations from the usual norms for laboratory values are sometimes caused by age-related changes in cardiac, pulmonary, renal, and metabolic function. Your ability to make sound clinical judgments requires application of knowledge about what is common in older adults, your assessment findings for a specific patient, and principles for making decisions without bias about aging.

It is important to recognize early indicators of acute illness in older adults. The Fulmer (2019) SPICES framework (Box 14.3) can be used to guide assessment of an older adult. Box 14.4 provides health care

---

BOX 14.3 SPICES Tool for Overall Assessment of Older Adults

S: Sleep disorders
P: Problems with eating or feeding
I: Incontinence
C: Confusion
E: Evidence of falls
S: Skin breakdown

Use clinical judgment to conduct a more in-depth assessment when an older adult demonstrates changes in any of these areas (Fulmer, 2019).

BOX 14.4 Examples of Altered Presentation of Illnesses in Older Adults Occurring in Various Health Care Settings

Hospital
- Confusion is not inevitable. Look for an acute illness, presence of fever, neurological events, new medication, or the presence of risk factors for delirium.
- Many hospitalized older adults have chronic dehydration exacerbated by acute illness (Touhy and Jett, 2020).
- Not all older adults have fevers with infection. Symptoms instead include increased respiratory rate, falls, incontinence, or confusion (Yeager, 2019c).

Nursing Center
- Health care providers often undertreat pain in older adults, especially those with dementia. Look for nonverbal cues of pain presence, such as grimacing or resistance to care (Alderman, 2019).
- Decline in functional ability (even a minor one such as the inability to sit upright in a chair) is a signal of new illness.
- Residents with less muscle mass—both the frail and the obese—are at a much higher risk for toxicity from protein-binding drugs such as phenytoin and warfarin (Yeager, 2019b).
- New urinary and/or fecal incontinence is often a sign of the onset of a new illness.

Ambulatory Care
- Fatigue or a decreased ability to do usual activities is often a sign of anemia, thyroid problems, depression, or neurological or cardiac problems (Yeager, 2019c).
- Severe gastrointestinal problems in older adults do not always present with the same acute symptoms seen in younger patients. Ask about constipation, cramping sensations, and changes in bowel habits.
- Older adults reporting increased dyspnea and confusion, especially those with a cardiac history, need to go to the emergency department because these are the most common manifestations of myocardial infarction in this population (Yeager, 2019c).
- Depression is common among older adults with chronic illnesses. Watch for lack of interest in former activities, significant personal losses, or changes in role or home life.

Home Care
- Investigate all falls, focusing on balance, lower extremity strength, gait, and neurological issues (e.g., loss of sensation).
- Monitor older adults with late-stage heart disease for loss of appetite as an early symptom of impending heart failure (Yeager, 2019c).
- Drug-drug and drug-food interactions in older patients who are seeing more than one provider and taking multiple medications are common. Watch for signs of interactions (Yeager, 2019b).

setting–specific examples of altered presentations of illness. A key principle of providing age-appropriate nursing care is timely detection of these cardinal signs of illness so that early treatment can begin. Mental status changes commonly occur as a result of disease and psychological issues. Some mental changes are often drug related, caused by drug toxicity or adverse drug events.

Falls are complex and often cause life-changing injury (see Chapter 27). They are sometimes costly, affecting functional status or level of independence, and they can be a common event for an older adult. You need to investigate every fall carefully to find out the precipitating event and whether it was related to environmental causes (e.g., surface of a walkway, condition of assist device) or the symptom of a new-onset or existing illness (e.g., dizziness, weak gait). A fall may be the only symptom in new problems with the cardiac, respiratory, musculoskeletal, neurological, urological, and sensory body systems.

Dehydration is common in older adults because of decreased oral intake related to a reduced thirst response and less free water as a consequence of a decrease in muscle mass. Additionally, older adults may decrease their intake to avoid additional trips to the bathroom. This is especially true in those with impaired mobility. When vomiting and diarrhea accompany the onset of an acute illness, an older adult is at risk for further dehydration. Decrease in appetite is a common symptom with the onset of pneumonia, heart failure, and UTI.

Loss of functional ability may be subtle and occur over time, or it may occur suddenly, depending on the underlying cause. Thyroid disease, infection, cardiac or pulmonary conditions, metabolic disturbances, and anemia are common causes of functional decline. The nurse is in a position to recognize even subtle changes in the condition of an older adult. You play an essential role in early identification, referral, and treatment of health problems.

Physiological Changes

Perception of well-being defines quality of life. Understanding an older adult's perceptions about health status is essential for accurate assessment and development of clinically relevant interventions. Older adults' concepts of health generally depend on personal perceptions of functional ability. Therefore older adults engaged in activities of daily living (ADLs) usually consider themselves healthy, whereas those who have physical, emotional, or social impairments that limit their activities perceive themselves as ill.

There are common physiological changes associated with normal aging (Table 14.1). These changes are not pathological in themselves, but they can make older adults more vulnerable to common clinical conditions and diseases (Touhy and Jett, 2020). Some older adults experience all of these changes, and others experience only a few. The body changes continuously with age, and specific effects on particular older adults depend on health, lifestyle, stressors, and environmental conditions. You need to understand these normal, more common changes to provide appropriate care for older adults and help with adaptation to associated changes.

General Survey. Your general survey begins during the initial nurse-patient encounter and includes a quick but careful head-to-toe scan of the older adult that you document in a brief description (see Chapter 30). Initial inspection may reveal some universal aging changes (e.g., facial wrinkles, gray hair, loss of body mass in the extremities, an increase of body mass in the trunk). It is also important at this time to observe general range of joint motion as the patient enters the examination area, status of grooming, and communication skills.

Integumentary System. With aging, the skin loses resilience and moisture. The epithelial layer thins, and elastic collagen fibers shrink and become rigid. Wrinkles of the face and neck reflect lifelong patterns of muscle activity and facial expressions, the pull of gravity on tissue, and diminished elasticity. Spots and lesions are often present on the skin. You need to rule out any premalignant or malignant lesions when examining skin lesions: melanoma, basal cell carcinoma, and squamous cell carcinoma (see Chapter 30). When assessing the skin, ask patients about their hygiene practices. An older adult does not need to take a daily bath, thus the skin may also be dry from excess bathing. Recommend the use of moisturizers to keep the skin more hydrated.

Head and Neck. The facial features of an older adult sometimes become more pronounced from loss of subcutaneous fat and skin elasticity. Facial features may appear asymmetrical because of missing teeth or improperly fitting dentures. In addition, common vocal changes include a rise in pitch and a loss of power and range.

Visual acuity declines with age. This is often the result of retinal damage, reduced pupil size, development of opacities in the lens, or loss of lens elasticity. Presbyopia, a progressive decline in the ability of the eyes to accommodate from near to far vision, is common. More ambient light is necessary for tasks such as reading and other ADLs. When assessing older adults, consider that they have increased sensitivity to the effects of glare. Pupils are smaller and react more slowly. Objects do not appear bright, and older adults may report having difficulty when moving from bright to dark environments. Changes in color vision and discoloration of the lens make it difficult to distinguish between blues and greens and among pastel shades. Dark colors such as blue and black appear the same. Chapter 49 reviews diseases of the older eye, the associated symptoms to look for, and nursing interventions for helping patients adapt to their visual changes.

Auditory changes are often subtle with aging. Most of the time older adults ignore the early signs of hearing loss until friends and family members comment on compensatory attempts, such as either turning up the volume on televisions, asking people to repeat statements, or avoiding social conversations. A common age-related change in auditory acuity is presbycusis. Presbycusis affects the bones of the middle ear and thus the ability to hear high-pitched sounds and conversational speech and is typically bilateral, affecting more men than women. During an examination, you assess whether the patient can respond to your questions or asks you to repeat them frequently. Before you assume a patient has presbycusis, inspect the external auditory canal for the presence of cerumen. Impacted cerumen, a common cause of diminished hearing acuity, is easy to treat.

When a person has a hearing impairment, move to a quiet area to reduce background noise, face the patient, and speak directly in clear, low-pitched tones. When caring for people with visual impairments, sit or stand at eye level and face them. Have them use their assistive devices such as glasses and hearing aids during the assessment. Chapter 49 details techniques to use when communicating with older adults who have sensory deficits.

Salivary secretion is reduced, and taste buds atrophy and lose sensitivity. An older adult is less able to differentiate among salty, sweet, sour, and bitter tastes. The sense of smell also decreases, further reducing taste. Health conditions, treatments, and/or medications often alter taste. It is often a challenge to promote optimal nutrition in an older patient because of the loss of smell and changes in taste.

Thorax and Lungs. Because of changes in the musculoskeletal system, the configuration of the thorax sometimes changes. Respiratory muscle strength begins to decrease, and the anteroposterior diameter of the thorax increases. Vertebral changes caused by osteoporosis lead to dorsal kyphosis, the curvature of the thoracic spine. Calcification of the costal cartilage causes decreased mobility of the ribs. The chest wall

TABLE 14.1	Common Physiological Changes with Aging at a Glance
System	**Common Changes**
Integumentary	Loss of skin elasticity with fat loss in extremities; pigmentation changes; glandular atrophy (oil, moisture, sweat glands); thinning hair, with hair turning gray-white (facial hair: decreased in men, increased in women); slower nail growth; atrophy of epidermal arterioles
Respiratory	Decreased cough reflex and ciliary activity; increased anterior-posterior chest diameter; increased chest wall rigidity; fewer alveoli, increased airway resistance
Cardiovascular	Thickening of blood vessel walls, narrowing of vessel lumen, loss of vessel elasticity, lower cardiac output, decreased number of heart muscle fibers, decreased elasticity and calcification of heart valves, decreased baroreceptor sensitivity, decreased efficiency of venous valves, increased pulmonary vascular tension, increased systolic blood pressure, decreased peripheral circulation
Gastrointestinal	Periodontal disease; decrease in saliva, gastric secretions, and pancreatic enzymes; smooth-muscle changes with decreased peristalsis and small intestinal motility; gastric atrophy; decreased production of intrinsic factor; increased stomach pH; loss of smooth muscle in the stomach; hemorrhoids; rectal prolapse; impaired rectal sensation
Musculoskeletal	Decreased muscle mass and strength, decalcification of bones, degenerative joint changes, dehydration of intervertebral disks, fat tissue increases
Neurological	Degeneration of nerve cells, decrease in neurotransmitters, decrease in rate of conduction of impulses
Sensory	
Eyes	Decreased accommodation to near/far vision (presbyopia), difficulty adjusting to changes from light to dark, yellowing of the lens, altered color perception, increased sensitivity to glare, smaller pupils
Ears	Loss of acuity for high-frequency tones (presbycusis), thickening of tympanic membrane, sclerosis of inner ear, buildup of earwax (cerumen)
Taste	Often diminished, often fewer taste buds
Smell	Often diminished
Touch	Decreased skin receptors
Proprioception	Decreased awareness of body positioning in space
Genitourinary	Fewer nephrons, 50% decrease in renal blood flow by age 80, decreased bladder capacity Male—enlargement of prostate Female—reduced sphincter tone
Reproductive	Male—sperm count diminished, smaller testes, erections less firm and slow to develop Female—decreased estrogen production; degeneration of ovaries; atrophy of vagina, uterus, and breasts; dryness of vaginal mucosa
Endocrine	General—alterations in hormone production with decreased ability to respond to stress Thyroid—diminished secretions Cortisol, glucocorticoids—increased anti-inflammatory hormone Pancreas—increased fibrosis, decreased secretion of enzymes and hormones, decreased sensitivity to insulin
Immune	Thymus decreases in size and volume T-cell function decreases Core temperature elevation is lowered

Modified from Touhy T, Jett K: *Toward Healthy Aging*, ed 10, St Louis, 2020, Elsevier.

gradually becomes stiffer. When you auscultate the lungs you might notice that lung expansion is decreased and that the patient is less able to cough deeply. If kyphosis or chronic obstructive lung disease is present, breath sounds become distant. As a result, an older adult is more susceptible to pneumonia and other bacterial or viral infections.

Heart and Vascular System. Decreased contractile strength of the myocardium results in decreased cardiac output. The decrease is significant when an older adult experiences anxiety, excitement, illness, or strenuous activity. The body compensates for decreased cardiac output by increasing the heart rate during exercise. However, after exercising it may take longer for an older adult's heart rate to return to baseline if the person does not regularly exercise or has underlying cardiac disease. Systolic and/or diastolic blood pressures are sometimes abnormally high. Although a common chronic condition, hypertension is not a normal aging change and predisposes older adults to heart failure, stroke, renal failure, coronary heart disease, and peripheral vascular disease.

Peripheral pulses frequently are still palpable but weaker in lower extremities. Older adults sometimes state that their lower extremities are cold, particularly at night. Changes in the peripheral pulses in the upper extremities are less common.

Breasts. As estrogen production diminishes, the milk ducts of the breasts are replaced by fat, making breast tissue less firm. Decreased muscle mass, tone, and elasticity result in smaller breasts in older women. Atrophy of glandular tissue coupled with more fat deposits results in a slightly smaller, less dense, and less nodular breast. Gynecomastia, enlarged breasts in men, is often the result of medication side effects, hormonal changes, or obesity.

Gastrointestinal System and Abdomen. Aging leads to an increase in the amount of fatty tissue in the trunk and abdomen. Because muscle tone and elasticity decrease, the abdomen becomes more protuberant. Gastrointestinal function changes include a slowing of peristalsis, noted by auscultating reduced bowel sounds, and alterations in secretions. An older adult experiences these changes by becoming less tolerant of certain foods and having discomfort from delayed gastric emptying. Alterations in the lower gastrointestinal tract may be reflected by constipation, flatulence, or diarrhea.

Reproductive System. Changes in the structure and function of the reproductive system occur as the result of hormonal alterations. Women experience a reduced responsiveness of the ovaries to pituitary hormones and a resultant decrease in estrogen and progesterone levels. This may result in the woman having a decreased libido. Hormonal changes can also cause dryness of the vaginal mucosa, causing irritation and pain with intercourse and vaginal examination. During a vaginal examination, the woman may have difficulty assuming the dorsal recumbent position because of musculoskeletal stiffness. Take time with positioning and use a small, well-lubricated vaginal speculum for the exam.

Testosterone lessens with age and sometimes leads to a loss of libido. Aging men also typically experience an erection that is less firm and has a less forceful ejaculation (Touhy and Jett, 2020). Spermatogenesis begins to decline during the fourth decade and continues into the ninth.

Less frequent sexual activity often results from illness, death of a sexual partner, or decreased socialization. However, men and women continue to have sexual desires, thoughts, and actions throughout all decades of life. In a recent University of Michigan/American Association of Retired Persons (AARP) poll involving over 1000 subjects, half of the 65- to 80-year-old men who were surveyed said they were extremely or very interested in sex, compared with 12% of women in that age-group. In addition, only 31% of the women were sexually active compared with 51% of the men (AARP, 2018). Risk factors for sexually transmitted infections (STIs) in older populations include (1) normal sexual changes associated with aging (e.g., increased time to attain an erection, decreased vaginal lubrication, decreases in sexual hormones), (2) psychosocial changes (e.g., loss of partner or spouse and re-entering the dating scene), and (3) risky sexual behaviors, including no or infrequent use of condoms (Johnson, 2013). Screening of older adults for STIs should occur regardless of age based on guidelines such as those from the Centers for Disease Control and Prevention (Johnson, 2013).

Urinary System. Hypertrophy of the prostate gland is frequently seen in older men. This hypertrophy enlarges the gland and places pressure on the neck of the bladder. As a result, urinary retention, frequency, incontinence, and UTIs occur. In addition, prostatic hypertrophy results in difficulty in initiating voiding and maintaining a urinary stream and does not always indicate a malignancy. However, when men develop symptoms of prostatic hypertrophy, it is important that this condition is evaluated by a health care provider to differentiate benign prostatic hypertrophy (BPH) from cancer of the prostate. Cancer of the prostate is the second leading cause of cancer death in American men, behind lung cancer. The American Cancer Society estimates that one in eight men will be diagnosed with prostate cancer and one in 41 will die (ACS, 2021).

Urinary incontinence is an abnormal and typically embarrassing condition. Older women, particularly those who have had children, experience stress incontinence, an involuntary release of urine that occurs when they cough, laugh, sneeze, or lift an object. This is a result of a weakening of the perineal and bladder muscles. Other types of urinary incontinence are urgency, overflow, functional, and mixed incontinence (see Chapter 46). The risk factors for urinary incontinence include age, menopause, diabetes, hysterectomy, stroke, and obesity. It is important that male incontinence also be assessed because men can experience incontinence but are sometimes reluctant to discuss it with their health care providers because they think it is a "woman's disease." Incontinence is not uncommon for men who have had removal of enlarged prostates.

Musculoskeletal System. With aging, muscle fibers become smaller. Muscle strength diminishes in proportion to the decline in muscle mass. Muscle mass begins to decline when individuals reach their 50s; by the time they reach their 80s, muscle mass is typically 30% to 40% of what it was at the age of 30 (Touhy and Jett, 2020). Beginning in the 30s, bone density and bone mass decline in men and women. Older adults who exercise regularly do not lose as much bone and muscle mass or muscle tone as those who are inactive. Osteoporosis, a common condition, is a major public health threat when individuals suffer fractures from falls or other injuries (National Osteoporosis Foundation, 2021). Postmenopausal women experience a greater rate of bone demineralization than older men and lose up to 20% or more of their bone density (National Osteoporosis Foundation, 2021). Women who maintain calcium and vitamin D intake throughout life and into menopause have less bone demineralization than women with low calcium intake. Older men with poor nutrition and decreased mobility are also at risk for bone demineralization.

Neurological System. A decrease in the number and size of neurons in the nervous system begins in the middle of the second decade. Neurotransmitters, chemical substances that enhance or inhibit nerve impulse transmission, change with aging as a result of the decrease in neurons. All voluntary reflexes are slower, and individuals often have less of an ability to respond to multiple stimuli. In addition, older adults frequently report alterations in the quality and the quantity of sleep (see Chapter 43), including difficulty falling asleep, difficulty staying asleep, difficulty falling asleep again after waking during the night, waking too early in the morning, and excessive daytime napping. These problems are believed to be caused by age-related changes in the sleep-wake cycle.

Functional Changes

Physical function is a dynamic process. It changes as individuals interact with their environments. Functional status in older adults includes the day-to-day ADLs involving activities within physical, psychological, cognitive, and social domains. A decline in function is often linked to illness or disease and the degree of chronicity. However, ultimately it is the complex relationship among all of these factors that influences an older adult's functional abilities and overall well-being.

Keep in mind that it may be difficult for older adults to accept the changes that occur in all areas of their lives, which in turn have a profound effect on functional status. Some deny the changes and continue to expect the same personal performance, regardless of age. Conversely some overemphasize them and prematurely limit their activities and involvement in life. The fear of becoming dependent is overwhelming for an older adult who is experiencing functional decline as a result of aging. Educate older adults to promote understanding of age-related changes, appropriate lifestyle adjustments, and effective coping. Factors that promote the highest level of function include a healthy, well-balanced diet; paced and appropriate regular physical activity; regularly scheduled visits with a health care provider; regular participation in meaningful activities; use of stress-management techniques; and avoidance of alcohol, tobacco, or illicit drugs.

Functional status in older adults refers to the capacity for and the safe performance of ADLs and instrumental ADLs (IADLs). It is a sensitive indicator of health or illness in the older adult. ADLs (such as bathing, dressing, and toileting) and IADLs (such as the ability to write a check, shop, prepare meals, or make phone calls) are essential to independent living; therefore carefully assess whether an older adult performs these tasks and how the illness either has changed or threatens to change the way these tasks are completed. Occupational and physical therapists are your best resources for a comprehensive assessment of functional impairment. A sudden change in function, as evidenced by a decline or change in an older adult's ability to perform any one or a combination of ADLs, is often a sign of either an acute illness (e.g., pneumonia, UTI, or electrolyte imbalance) or worsening of a chronic problem (e.g., diabetes or cardiovascular disease) (Touhy and Jett, 2020). An online collection of functional assessment tools used most commonly with older adults is available at the website of the Hartford Institute for Geriatric Nursing, https://consultgeri.org/. When you identify a decline in a patient's functional status, focus your nursing interventions on maintaining, restoring, and maximizing an older adult's functional status to maintain independence while preserving safety and dignity.

Cognitive Changes

A common misconception about aging is that cognitive impairments are widespread among older adults. Because of this misconception, older adults often fear that they are, or soon will be, cognitively impaired. Forgetfulness as an expected consequence of aging is a myth. Some structural and physiological changes within the brain are associated with cognitive impairment. Reduction in the number of brain cells, deposition of lipofuscin and amyloid in cells, and changes in neurotransmitter levels occur in older adults both with and without cognitive impairment. Symptoms of cognitive impairment such as disorientation, loss of language skills, loss of the ability to calculate, and poor judgment *are not* normal aging changes and require you to further assess patients for underlying causes. There are standard assessment forms for determining a patient's mental status, including the Mini-Mental State Exam-2 (MMSE-2), the Mini-Cog, and the clock drawing test (Touhy and Jett, 2020).

The three common conditions affecting cognition are delirium, dementia, and depression (Table 14.2). Distinguishing among these three conditions is challenging. A careful and thorough assessment of older adults with cognitive changes to distinguish among them should

be completed. Select appropriate nursing interventions that are specific to the cause of the cognitive impairment.

Delirium. Delirium, or acute confusional state, is an acute change in attention and awareness that develops over a relatively short time interval and is associated with additional cognitive deficits such as memory deficit, disorientation, or perceptual disturbances (Ali and Cascella, 2021). It is a potentially reversible cognitive impairment (Touhy and Jett, 2020). Delirium is a common phenomenon, occurring in 20% to 70% of hospitalized patients (Ali and Cascella, 2021). Delirium has physiological causes, including electrolyte imbalances, untreated pain, infection, cerebral anoxia, being on mechanical ventilation, hypoglycemia, medication effects, tumors, subdural hematomas, and cerebrovascular infarction or hemorrhage. The condition can be associated with multiple causes. The most common form of delirium, hyperactive delirium, is characterized by agitation, restlessness, emotional lability, and psychotic features such as hallucinations and illusions that often interfere with the delivery of care (Ali and Cascella, 2021). A new onset of delirium should trigger a nurse to assess for signs and symptoms of infections such as pneumonia and UTI. Delirium may also be caused by environmental factors such as sensory deprivation or overstimulation, unfamiliar surroundings, or sleep deprivation, or by psychosocial factors such as emotional distress. Although delirium occurs in any setting, an older adult in the acute care setting is especially at risk because of predisposing factors (physiological, psychosocial, and environmental) in combination with underlying medical conditions. Dementia is an additional risk factor that greatly increases the risk for delirium; it is possible for delirium and dementia to occur at the same time. The presence of delirium is a medical emergency and requires prompt assessment and intervention. Nurses are at the bedside 24/7 and in a position to recognize delirium development and report it. The cognitive impairment usually reverses once health care providers identify and treat the cause of delirium.

TABLE 14.2	Comparison of Clinical Features of Delirium, Dementia, and Depression		
Clinical Feature	**Delirium**	**Dementia**	**Depression**
Onset	Sudden/abrupt; depends on cause	Insidious/slow and often unrecognized	Happens with major life changes; often abrupt but can be gradual
Course	Short, daily fluctuations in symptoms; worse at night, in darkness, and on awakening	Long, no diurnal effects; slow progression over time; some deficits with increased stress	Diurnal effects, typically worse in the morning; situational fluctuations but less than with delirium
Progression	Abrupt	Slow over months and years	Variable; rapid or slow but even
Duration	Hours to less than 1 month; longer if unrecognized and untreated	Months to years	Variable; may be chronic
Consciousness	Reduced/disturbed	Awake	Awake
Alertness	Fluctuates; lethargic or hypervigilant	Generally normal	Normal
Attention	Impaired; fluctuates; inattention	Generally normal	Minimal impairment
Orientation	Generally impaired; severity varies	Generally normal to person but not to place or time	Usually normal
Psychomotor behavior	Variable; hypoactive, hyperactive, or mixed	Normal; some have apraxia	Variable; psychomotor retardation or agitation
Speech	Often incoherent; may call out repeatedly or with the same phrase	Difficulty finding words; perseveration	May be slow
Affect	Variable, but may appear disturbed, frightened	Slowed response; may be labile	Flat

Modified from Touhy T, Jett K: *Toward Healthy Aging*, ed 10, St Louis, 2020, Elsevier.

Dementia. Dementia is a generalized impairment of intellectual functioning that interferes with social and occupational functioning. It is an umbrella term that includes Alzheimer disease (most common type), Lewy body disease, frontal-temporal dementia, and vascular dementia (Alzheimer's Association, 2021). Cognitive function deterioration leads to a decline in the ability to perform basic ADLs and IADLs. Unlike delirium, dementia is characterized by a gradual, progressive, and irreversible decline in cerebral function (Touhy and Jett, 2020). Because of the similarity of some behaviors between delirium and dementia, you need to assess carefully to rule out the presence of delirium whenever you suspect dementia.

Nursing management of older adults with any form of dementia always considers the safety and physical and psychosocial needs of the older adult and the family. These needs change as the progressive nature of dementia leads to increased cognitive deterioration (Fazio et al., 2018). To meet the needs of older adults, individualize nursing care to enhance quality of life and maximize functional performance by improving cognition, mood, and behavior. Persons with dementia may exhibit behaviors, such as wandering, that may be unsafe and puts them at risk for falls and other injuries (see Chapter 27). These behaviors are an expression of an unmet need, such as hunger, pain, anxiety, or the need to void or defecate. Therefore, the nurse should consider the meaning behind a person's actions. Nonpharmacological measures should be used first, before administering medications that may be sedating or have other undesirable effects. Box 14.5 lists general nursing principles for the care of older adults with dementia. Support and education about Alzheimer disease for patients, families, and professionals can be found at the Alzheimer's Association website (www.alz.org).

Depression. Older adults sometimes experience late-life depression, but it is not a normal part of aging. Depression is the most common, yet most undetected and untreated, impairment in older adulthood. It sometimes exists and is exacerbated in patients with other health problems such as stroke, diabetes, dementia, Parkinson disease, heart disease, cancer, and pain-provoking diseases such as arthritis. Loss of a significant loved one or admission to a nursing center sometimes causes depression. Mendoza (2020) explains the nature of depression in the older adult:

> One of the primary factors is loneliness. At this point in life, the person is likely to have experienced multiple losses: family, spouse, friends, pets as well as outliving their own doctors. At some point, there is no one left who knew them from the past. Many of the friends they used to talk to or get together with, if still alive, may have their own problems with transportation, health, functional status, or memory. Giving up a driver's license can have a profound impact on the elderly. They become more dependent and have to rely on others to take them places they want to go.

The Geriatric Depression Scale is an easy-to-use screening tool that can be used in conjunction with an interview with the older adult (Touhy and Jett, 2020). Clinical depression is treatable with medication, psychotherapy, or a combination of both. Electroconvulsive therapy (ECT) is sometimes used for treatment of resistant depression when medications and psychotherapy do not help. Of special note, suicide attempts in older adults are often successful. Suicide rates in all age-groups are on the rise over the past several years; but statistics from the National Council on Aging state that those 85 years of age and older have the highest suicide rate of any age-group (Mendoza, 2020).

Psychosocial Changes

As previously discussed, psychosocial changes occurring during aging involve life transitions. One of those transitions is loss, including retirement and the associated financial changes, changes in roles and relationships, alterations in health and functional ability, changes in one's social network, and relocation. The burden of loss is significant when one becomes older. A study by Massey University (2019) found that in the case of older adults living in poverty, loss is a gradual contributor to poor health. The study identified childhood disadvantage—measured in terms of parents' occupation, quality of housing, access to resources such as clothes and books, and overcrowding in the home—as a factor that is directly related to levels of physical, mental, and social health in older age. If childhood disadvantage leads to limited income and wealth over time, the economic disadvantages in adult life affect the health of older adults (Massey University, 2019).

It is important to assess both the nature of the psychosocial changes that occur in older adults as a result of life transitions and associated losses and the economic well-being of individuals. During your assessment ask how an older adult feels about self, self in relation to others, and self as one who is aging, and ask which coping methods and skills have been beneficial. Areas to address during the assessment include family, intimate relationships, past and present role changes, finances, housing, social networks, activities, access to transportation and health care, wellness habits, and spirituality. Specific topics related to these areas include retirement, social isolation, sexuality, housing and environment, and death.

Retirement. Many often mistakenly associate retirement with passivity and seclusion. In actuality it is a stage of life characterized by transitions and role changes and may occupy 30 or more years of one's life. This transition requires letting go of certain habits and structure and developing new ones (Touhy and Jett, 2020). The psychosocial stresses of retirement are usually related to role changes with a spouse or within the family, loss of the work role, and social isolation. The threat to economic well-being is also a major stressor, with many older adults having inadequate finances. Many older adults delay retirement because of changes in recent years regarding pension plans and the age of eligibility for Social Security benefits (Yoe, 2019). The age of retirement varies, but whether it occurs at age 55, 65, or 75, it is one of the major turning points in life.

Meaningful retirement planning is critical as the population continues to age. Retirement affects more than just the retired. It also affects the spouse, adult children, and even grandchildren. When the spouse is still working, the retired person faces time alone. There may be new expectations of the retired person. For example, a working spouse has new ideas about the amount of housework expected of the retired person. Problems develop when the plans of the retired person conflict with the work responsibilities of the working spouse. The roles of the retiree and the working spouse need clarification. Some adult children expect the retired person to always care for the grandchildren, forgetting that this is a time for the retired person to pursue other personal interests.

Loss of the work role has a major effect on some retired people. When so much of life has revolved around work and the personal relationships at work, the loss of the work role is sometimes devastating. Personal identity is often rooted in the work role, and with retirement individuals need to construct a new identity. They also lose the structure imposed on daily life when they no longer have a work schedule. The social exchanges and interpersonal support that occur in the workplace are lost. In the adjustment to retirement an older adult has to develop a personally meaningful schedule and a supportive social network.

Factors that influence a retired person's satisfaction with life are health status and sufficient income. Positive preretirement expectations also contribute to satisfaction in retirement. You can help the

BOX 14.5 Dementia Care Practice Recommendations

Person-Centered Care
- Know the person as an individual. Assessment should include past social and work history, education, values, interests, and preferences.
- Recognize and accept the person's reality. Do not attempt to reorient the person. Instead, recognize that the person's behavior is a form of communication.
- Support opportunities for meaningful interactions. By knowing the person's preferences, interactions are more likely to be effective and meet the needs of the individual. Promote social interaction when possible.
- Nurture authentic, caring relationships. Focus more on the interaction than the task needing to be accomplished.
- Maintain a supportive community for the person with dementia, the person's family, and staff.

Detection and Diagnosis of Dementia
- Provide information about brain health and related disorders, along with referral to specialists in dementia care.
- Attend to concerns about cognitive changes from family members and other care providers.
- Following a diagnosis of dementia, support and educate the person and family members, including referral to appropriate agencies and support groups.

Person-Centered Assessment and Care Planning
- Ensure that regular ongoing assessments of persons with dementia are conducted. This is an opportunity to support and educate the person, family, and caregivers.
- Involve multiple disciplines when developing a plan of care.
- Regularly evaluate the plan of care for relevance and accuracy.
- Encourage advanced care planning to optimize physical, psychosocial, and fiscal well-being.

Medical Management
- Utilize a holistic approach and manage co-morbidities.
- Encourage nonpharmacological interventions for common behavioral and psychological symptoms.
- Pharmacological measures should be used cautiously and only after attempting nonpharmacological measures. Minimize polypharmacy by decreasing the risk for drug interactions and adverse reactions.

Education and Support of Those Diagnosed With Dementia and Their Families
- Provide education and support early in the disease to better prepare for future events.
- Encourage families and caregivers to work together.
- Educational programming should be culturally sensitive.
- Use technology to reach out to families. Two-way video technology, such as Zoom, Skype, or FaceTime, can be used to enhance family involvement.

Managing Behavioral and Psychological Symptoms of Dementia
- Identify social and environmental triggers of negative behavioral symptoms. Symptoms are individualized responses to the dementia disease process and can vary widely.

- Implement nonpharmacological practices that are tailored to the individual's needs. These include:
  - Sensory practices: aromatherapy, massage, multisensory stimulation, and bright light therapy
  - Psychosocial practices: validation therapy, reminiscence therapy, music therapy, pet therapy, and meaningful activities
  - Structured care protocols (bathing and mouth care)
- Hand in Hand is a training course for direct care providers on safe, effective strategies for caring with persons with dementia.

Supporting Activities of Daily Living
- Allow individuals to be involved in their care to the extent of their cognitive abilities, with a focus on preserving self-dignity.
- Provide limited choices with simple instructions.
- Provide dignity and respect in the toileting process by being attuned to cues indicating a need to void/defecate. Toilet continent individuals on a regular basis.
- Support eating nutritious meals, and consider food preferences. A quiet homelike atmosphere is conducive to adequate nutritional intake. For some, finger foods may be easier to manipulate than feeding oneself with utensils.
- Monitor and support fluid intake.
- Encourage physical activity. Make sure that the environment is safe for mobility, and promote way-finding with pictures or cues.
- Ensure that assistive devices (hearing aids, glasses, dentures) are functioning and used appropriately.

Recommendations for Staffing
- Provide a thorough orientation that focuses on the care of individuals diagnosed with dementia.
- Provide consistent staffing so that the staff members can learn more about the person and so the person and surrounding family can develop relationships with staff members.
- Encourage patients, families, and staff to develop and sustain professional, caring relationships.

Providing a Supportive and Therapeutic Environment
- Promote safety, comfort, and dignity.
- Allow for choice for those with dementia to promote safe independence.

Transitions of Care
- Prepare persons living with dementia and their families for common transitions of care by discussing the risks and benefits of a transfer to a new environment (e.g., care facility, hospital).
- Promote timely and effective communication across care settings. Utilizing transfer reports available in the electronic medical record can enhance the quality and timeliness of information sharing.

Modified from Fazio S, et al: Alzheimer's Association dementia care practice recommendations, *Gerontologist* 58(S1):S1–S9, 2018; Press D, Alexander M: Treatment of dementia, *UpToDate*, 2020, https://www.uptodate.com/contents/treatment-of-dementia.

older adult and family prepare for retirement by discussing with them several key areas, including relations with spouse and children; meaningful activities and interests; building social networks; issues related to income; health promotion and maintenance; and long-range planning, including wills and advance directives. This information should be considered part of your psychosocial assessment and provides context for other concerns expressed by the older adult.

Social Isolation. Many older adults experience social isolation. Isolation is sometimes a choice, the result of a desire not to interact with others, or it is a function of loss of social support. Older adults who experience social isolation become vulnerable to its consequences because of the absence of the support of other adults. Impaired sensory function, functional impairment, chronic illness, reduced mobility, and cognitive changes all contribute to reduced interaction with others and often place an older adult at risk for isolation.

Assess patients' potential for social isolation by identifying their social network, access to transportation, and willingness and desire to interact with others. Consider if depression is linked to social isolation. Use your findings to help a lonely older adult rebuild social networks and reverse patterns of isolation. Many communities have outreach programs designed to make contact with isolated older adults. Outreach programs such as daily telephone calls by volunteers or planned social outings also meet socialization needs. A wide range of organizations welcomes older adults as volunteers and provides the opportunity for them to serve while meeting their socialization or other needs. Churches, colleges, community centers, and libraries offer a variety of programs for older adults that increase the opportunity to meet people with similar interests and needs.

Sexuality. All older adults, whether healthy or frail, need to express their need for intimacy and sexual feelings. Sexuality involves love, warmth, sharing, and touching, not just the act of intercourse. It plays an important role in helping the older adult maintain self-esteem. To help an older adult achieve or maintain sexual health, you need to understand the physical changes in a person's sexual response (see Chapter 34). You need to provide privacy for any discussion of sexuality and maintain a nonjudgmental attitude. Use open-ended questions to elicit information and concerns related to sex and sexuality. Include information about the prevention of sexually transmitted infections. Sexuality and the need to express sexual feelings remain throughout the human life span.

When considering an older adult's need for sexual expression, do not ignore the important need to touch and be touched. Touch is an overt expression with many meanings and is an important part of intimacy (Yeager, 2019a). Touch complements traditional sexual methods or serves as an alternative sexual expression when physical intercourse is not desired or possible. Knowing an older adult's sexual needs allows you to incorporate this information into the nursing care plan. The sexual preferences of older adults are as diverse as those of the younger population. Clearly not all older adults are heterosexual; research is emerging on older adult lesbian, gay, bisexual, and transgender individuals and their health care needs. Nurses often find that they are called on to help other health care professionals understand the sexual needs of older adults. Not all nurses feel comfortable counseling older adults about sexual health and intimacy-related needs. Be prepared to refer older adults to an appropriate professional counselor.

Housing and Environment. Older adults' ability to live independently influences housing choices. In other cases, older adults living in poverty have limited choices for housing. It is difficult to anticipate what services will be needed by an older adult over the course of several years,

especially before significant health problems develop. For example, a housing unit with only one floor and without exterior steps is a prudent choice for an older adult with severe arthritis who has already had lower-extremity joint replacement surgery and anticipates the need for future operations. A broad range of housing options, with numerous variations, exists. The options may be overwhelming to the older adults and their families.

Aging in place, growing older at home, is a concept that is gaining popularity. It is intended to promote successful aging by allowing an older adult to stay in one place while providing the needed supplemental services (National Institutes of Health, 2017). Some aging-in-place initiatives are formal organizations, while others are more loosely organized. Aging in place requires the older adult to anticipate the health and personal services that will be needed and how to access those services, as well as creating a safe physical environment that is accessible in the event of impaired mobility. Some older adults choose to live with family members. Others prefer their own homes or other housing options near their families. Leisure or retirement communities, although expensive, provide older people with living and social opportunities in a one-generation setting. Federally subsidized housing, where available, offers apartments with communal, social, and in some cases food-service arrangements.

During your assessment of a patient's housing and environment, use sound clinical judgment to assess current resources to promote patient safety, independence, and functional ability. Learn what is important to the individual to feel safe. This is important as a recent study has shown that a perception of feeling less safe in one's neighborhood was significantly associated with elevated levels of depressive symptoms; however, perceiving a greater sense of community belonging buffered the relationship with depression (Gonyea et al., 2018). Assessment of physical safety within an older adult's environment includes risks within the environment and the older adult's ability to recognize and respond to the risks (see Chapter 27). Bathroom safety is central in an acceptable environment. The bathroom should have:
- Grab bars that can assist with moving and can be reached in case of a potential or actual fall
- Nonslip surfaces on the floor and tub/shower
- Needed supplies in easy reach
- Minimal obstacles (rugs, furniture, equipment)
- Adequate lighting, especially at night

Other considerations include the removal of clutter and throw rugs to decrease the risk of falls. Lighting should be adequate, particularly in walkways and stairs. Water heaters should not be set higher than 120°F. Smoke and carbon monoxide detectors should be installed and their batteries changed regularly (Health in Aging, 2020).

Housing and environment can either support or hinder physical and social functioning, enhance or impede a person's energy, and complement or tax existing physical changes such as vision and hearing. For example, furnishings with red, orange, and yellow colors are easiest for older adults to see. Shiny waxed floors may appear to be wet. Ensure that door frames and baseboards are an appropriate color that contrasts with the color of the wall to improve perception of the boundaries of halls and rooms, keeping in mind that older adults often have difficulty distinguishing among pastel shades and between green and blue. Walkways leading to the house need to be flat, even, and in good repair, and stairs need to have a color contrast at the edge of the step so that an older person knows where the stair ends. Glare from highly polished floors, metallic fixtures, or windows is difficult for an older adult to tolerate.

Furniture needs to be comfortable and safe. Older adults need to examine furniture carefully for size, comfort, and function before purchasing it. Furniture should have adequate back support and allow a person to get into and out of the chair or sofa easily and safely. Test dining room or kitchen chairs for comfort during meals and for height in relation to the table. Many older adults find that armrests on chairs make sitting down and getting up easier. Older adults often prefer to transfer out of a wheelchair to another chair for meals because some styles of wheelchairs do not allow a person to sit close enough to the table to eat comfortably. Raising the table to clear the wheelchair arms brings the table closer to the older adult but makes it too high to eat comfortably. To make getting out of bed easier and safer, ensure that the height of the bed allows an older adult's feet to be flat on the floor when sitting on the side of the bed.

> **QSEN** **Building Competency in Safety** Mr. Sousa is an energetic 76-year-old man who is ready for discharge from the hospital. He does not "look" 76, as he appears very fit and states that he is active in social activities and volunteering. He was admitted to the hospital 3 days ago for a right total knee replacement and is doing well after surgery; he now walks with the assistance of one person and is using a walker. He is able to walk to the bathroom and has walked 125 feet in the hallway 3 times today. He will get home health care and physical therapy rather than going to the hospital rehabilitation unit. He insists on going home because of his dog, Benji, a black Labrador retriever. Mr. Sousa's daughter is going to pick up Benji from the boarding kennel and take him home. Mr. Sousa's wife of 50 years died recently, leaving him alone at home, but he has been getting along well. His daughter lives within 25 miles of his home and will visit him daily. When considering safety for this patient in the home setting, which assessment questions and teaching approaches and resources can you use to enhance his safety in the home environment?
>
> Answers to QSEN Activities can be found on the Evolve website.

Death. Part of one's life history is the experience of loss through the death of relatives and friends (see Chapter 36). This includes the loss of older generations of families and sometimes, sadly, the loss of a child. However, the death of a spouse or significant other is the loss that most affects the lives of older people. Do not assume that an older adult is comfortable with death. You play a key role in helping older adults understand and cope with loss.

Current evidence supports that older people have a wide variety of attitudes and beliefs about death but fear of their own death is uncommon. Rather they are concerned with the fear of being a burden, experiencing suffering, being alone, or the use of life-prolonging measures (Bub, 2019). The stereotype that the death of an older adult is a blessing does not apply to every older adult. Even as death approaches, many older adults still have unfinished business and are unprepared for it. Families and friends are not always ready to let go of their older significant others. Older adults and family members or friends will often turn to you for assistance. Thus you need knowledge of the grieving process (see Chapter 36), excellent communication skills (see Chapter 24), understanding of legal issues and advance care planning (see Chapter 23), familiarity with community resources, and awareness of one's own feelings, limitations, and strengths as they relate to care of those confronting death.

> **REFLECT NOW**
>
> Reflect on how you would start a conversation with an older adult about end-of-life care, with the intent of determining this person's wishes/goals for care.

ADDRESSING THE HEALTH CONCERNS OF OLDER ADULTS

As the population ages and life expectancy increases, emphasis on health promotion, health maintenance, and disease prevention increases (see Chapter 6). Older adults are becoming more enthusiastic and motivated about healthy lifestyles (AOA, 2018). A number of national programs and projects address preventive practices in the older-adult population. The national initiative *Healthy People 2030* (Office of Disease Prevention and Health Promotion, n.d.) has an overarching goal to improve the health and well-being of older adults. More specifically, *Healthy People 2030* cites the following objectives for older adults:
- General health (improve physical activity for older adults with physical or cognitive health problems, reduce rate of pressure injuries during hospitalization, reduce hospital admissions among older adults with diabetes)
- Dementias (improved awareness and prevention of hospitalizations)
- Foodborne illness (reduce infections caused by *Listeria*, reduce rate of hospital admissions for urinary tract infections)
- Injury prevention (reduce fall-related deaths, reduce the proportion of older adults who use inappropriate medications, reduce emergency department visits due to falls)
- Oral conditions (reduce the proportion of older adults with untreated root surface decay, loss of all teeth, and moderate and severe periodontitis
- Osteoporosis (reduce hip fractures among older adults, increase screening for osteoporosis, increase the proportion of older adults who get treated for osteoporosis after fractures)
- Respiratory disease (reduce the rate of hospital admissions for pneumonia and asthma)
- Sensory or communication disorders (reduce vision loss from age-related macular degeneration)

The challenges of engaging older adults in health promotion and disease prevention are complex and also affect health care providers. Previous health care experiences, personal motivation, health beliefs, culture, health literacy, and non–health-related factors such as transportation and finances often create barriers for older adults. The interests and desires of older adults should be considered when planning health promotion activities as well as when delivering interventions in acute and restorative care (Campbell et al., 2018). Barriers for health care providers include beliefs and attitudes about which services and programs to provide, their effectiveness and the lack of consistent guidelines, and absence of a coordinated approach. Your role is to focus interventions on maintaining and promoting patients' function and quality of life. You can empower older adults to make their own health care decisions and realize their optimum level of health, function, and quality of life (Davis, 2019). Always be open to recognizing an older adult's concerns so that you can adjust a plan of care accordingly.

Learning Needs

Managing the complexities of chronic disease and the cognitive and sensory changes that may be associated with aging add to the challenges of teaching older adults. As you assess the various physical, cognitive, functional, and psychosocial problems of older adults, it is important to also assess their associated learning needs. For example, during a cognitive and psychosocial assessment, you will gain information that indicates a patient's ability to follow a recommended treatment plan. When assessing a patient's medication history, have the patient describe when the medication is taken at home and the dosage. If a patient has slow responses or reaction time when performing physical activities, it is necessary to consider these limitations when teaching new psychomotor skills. During your assessment, carefully consider a patient's learning needs and capability to learn.

Educating Older Adults

Inadequate health literacy disproportionately affects older adults in the United States, causing misunderstanding of health information and subsequent nonadherence, which results in negative outcomes (Cutilli et al., 2018). The World Health Organization (2021) defines health literacy as the ability of individuals to "gain access to, understand and use information in ways which promote and maintain good health" for themselves, their families, and their communities. Older adults expect that the patient education delivered is relevant to their own situation (Touhy and Jett, 2020). It is important to know how to adapt routine patient education strategies based on your assessment to effectively meet the specific learning needs of older adults (Box 14.6). When patients do not receive correct and necessary information from an educational session, they may turn to other sources, such as unreliable Internet sites, or relatives and friends. The information from these sources may be incomplete or inaccurate. You are responsible for providing current and relevant information in a manner that meets the needs of the older adult.

Health Promotion and Maintenance: Physiological Concerns

Patients will have different levels of interest, motivation, and ability to participate in health promotion activities. This is partly the result of the onset of disease as well as the ongoing presence of risks to their health. Your primary role in health promotion and maintenance is health education to ensure quality self-care in the presence of disease and the acquisition of behaviors to minimize health risks.

Use an individualized approach in your care of patients, taking into account a person's beliefs about the importance of staying healthy and remaining independent. The Federal Interagency Forum on Aging-Related Statistics (2020) noted that 24% of women and 20%

of men 65 years and older reported a functional limitation (i.e., difficulty in hearing, vision, cognition, ambulation, self-care, or communication). Difficulties with mobility were the most commonly reported limitation. Some of these disabilities are relatively minor, but others cause people to require assistance to meet important personal needs. The incidence of disability increases with age. Limitations in ADLs limit the ability to live independently. The ADL limitations most often reported include walking, showering and bathing, getting in and out of bed and chair, dressing, toileting, and eating. Healthy Aging in Action is a resource to promote healthy aging and improve health and well-being in later life developed by the National Prevention, Health Promotion, and Public Health Council (2018). Evidence-based health promotion programs are highlighted, including community safety, services and engagement, preventive health services, and fall prevention. General preventive health measures to recommend to older adults include:

- Regular primary care and dental, vision, and hearing visits (if patient has a hearing aid)
- Participation in recommended screening activities as indicated by age (e.g., blood pressure, mammography, depression, vision and hearing, bone density, colonoscopy)
- Immunization for seasonal influenza, tetanus, diphtheria and pertussis, shingles, and pneumococcal disease
- Regular exercise, smoking cessation, and stress management
- Attaining and maintaining target weight
- Eating a low-fat, well-balanced diet or adhering to a specific diet (e.g. diabetic diet, low-sodium diet)
- Moderate alcohol use
- Socialization
- Good handwashing

Those who die from influenzas are predominantly older adults. Providers strongly recommend annual immunization of all older adults for influenza, with special emphasis on residents of assisted living residencies, nursing homes, or long-term care facilities. Other vaccinations, such as those for pneumonia or shingles, are often recommended. In addition, not all older adults are current with their booster injections, and some never received the primary series of injections. Ask patients about their current status of all immunizations, provide information about recommended immunizations, and make arrangements for them to receive immunizations as needed.

Many older adults are interested in their health and are able to take charge of their lives. They want to maintain or improve their health, remain independent, and prevent disability (Fig. 14.1). Initial screenings establish baseline data to determine wellness, identify health needs,

---

BOX 14.6   PATIENT TEACHING

Adapting Instruction for Older Adults With Health Literacy Limitations

Objective
- Patient will implement behaviors to meet specific health care needs (e.g., home safety, wound care, or self-management of chronic conditions).

Teaching Strategies
- Ensure that the patient is ready to learn. Be alert for cues of pain and fatigue.
- Create a comfortable environment (e.g., seating, temperature).
- Adapt teaching materials for culture, language, and health literacy.
- Focus on concrete information about the topic and relate to past experiences as appropriate.
- Use printed materials with large black font on either cream or white paper.
- Use clear, concise language; avoid medical terminology.
- Use pictures, demonstrations, videos, and other methods to augment spoken language.
- Allow the patient time to process information and ask questions.

Evaluation
Use the principles of teach-back to evaluate patient/family caregiver learning:
- Explain three ways that you can improve the safety of your home.
- Show me how to change the dressing on your wound.
- Show me all of your morning medication.

FIG. 14.1 This older adult works part time at a sporting goods store.

and design health maintenance programs. Following initial screening sessions, share with older adults information on nutrition, exercise, medications, stress management, and safety. You can also provide information on specific conditions such as hypertension, arthritis, and diabetes and self-care procedures such as foot and skin care. By providing information about health promotion and self-care, you can significantly improve the health and well-being of older adults.

Heart Disease. Heart disease and cancer are the leading causes of death in older adults (Kochanek et al., 2019). Common cardiovascular disorders are hypertension and coronary artery disease. Hypertension is a silent killer because older adults, especially African Americans, are often unaware that their blood pressure is elevated (see Chapter 29). The fact that hypertension is common does not make it normal or harmless. Only about half of those diagnosed with hypertension have the condition under control. Treatment is linked to reduced incidence of myocardial infarction, chronic kidney disease, stroke, and heart failure. In coronary artery disease, partial or complete blockage of one or more coronary arteries leads to myocardial ischemia and myocardial infarction. The risk factors for both hypertension and coronary artery disease include smoking, obesity, lack of exercise, and stress. Additional risk factors for coronary artery disease include hypertension, hyperlipidemia, and diabetes mellitus (American Heart Association, 2016).

Nursing interventions for the prevention of hypertension and coronary artery disease include patient teaching on weight reduction, exercise, dietary changes, limiting salt and fat intake, stress management, and smoking cessation. Additional patient teaching includes information about medication management, blood-pressure monitoring, and the symptoms indicating the need for emergency care.

Cancer. Nurses educate older adults about patients' risks for cancer and the importance of screening for early detection (e.g., breast and testicular self-exams) and following healthy lifestyle choices (e.g., low-fat diet and avoidance of smoking). It is also important to educate older adults about the signs of cancer and to encourage prompt reporting of nonhealing skin lesions, unexpected bleeding, change in bowel habits, nagging cough, lump in breast or another part of body, change in a mole, difficulty swallowing, and unexplained weight loss.

Chronic Lung Disease. Chronic lung disease, specifically chronic obstructive pulmonary disease (COPD), is the third leading cause of death in those 65 and older (USA Facts, 2020). More women than men die from COPD (American Lung Association, 2021a). Lung injury from inhalants such as tobacco smoke, exposure to secondhand smoke, and fumes from hair dyes, artificial nail products, and paints can lead to COPD, causing airflow blockage and breathing-related difficulty (American Lung Association, 2021a). Because tobacco smoke and exposure to secondhand smoke are key factors in the development and progression of COPD, it is important to provide patients with information about smoking-cessation programs. In addition, depending on the severity of a patient's existing disease, you will teach about proper breathing exercises, how to use inhalers, and techniques for the removal of mucus from the airways (see Chapter 41). Supervised exercise training is a major component of pulmonary rehabilitation programs and is an established safe and effective intervention for improving patients' physical capacity and quality of life (American Lung Association, 2021b).

Stroke (Cerebrovascular Accident). Cerebrovascular accidents (CVAs) are the fourth leading cause of death in the United States and occur as either brain ischemia (inadequate blood supply to areas of brain caused by arterial blockage) or brain hemorrhage (subarachnoid

or intercerebral bleeds). Risk factors include hypertension, hyperlipidemia, diabetes mellitus, history of transient ischemic attacks, and family history of cardiovascular disease (American Stroke Association, 2021). CVAs often impair a person's functional abilities because of paralysis and speech impairment, causing loss of independence. This often leads to the need for family caregivers to assist regularly, or patients are placed in assisted living or nursing centers. The scope of nursing interventions ranges from teaching older adults about risk-reduction strategies to teaching family caregivers the early warning signs of a stroke and ways to support a patient during recovery and rehabilitation.

Smoking. Cigarette smoking is a risk factor for the four most common causes of death in older adults: heart disease, cancer, lung disease, and stroke (American Heart Association, 2016; American Stroke Association, 2021). Smoking is the most preventable cause of disease and death in the United States. Smoking cessation is a health promotion strategy for older adults just as it is for younger adults. In addition to reducing risk, it sometimes stabilizes existing conditions such as COPD and coronary artery disease. Smoking cessation after age 50 reduces the risk of dying prematurely by 50% compared with those who continue to smoke (NCI, 2017). Smoking-cessation programs include individual, group, and telephone counseling and the use of nicotine (gum and patch) or nonnicotine medications. If a patient rejects smoking cessation, suggest at least a reduction in smoking. A recent study among Korean males found that willpower and several disease co-morbidities were related to successful cessation in the middle-age and older adult groups (Kim et al., 2021). If a patient is open to quitting, set a quit or reduction date and a follow-up visit with the older adult to discuss the quit attempt. At follow-up visits, offer encouragement and assistance in modifying the plan, as necessary. Include family members in the plan if possible.

Alcohol Abuse. Studies of alcohol abuse in older adults report two patterns: a lifelong pattern of continuous heavy drinking and a pattern of heavy drinking that begins late in life (Lewis et al., 2018). Alcohol use, high-risk drinking, and alcohol use disorders have increased in the U.S. population and across almost all sociodemographic groups, especially women and older adults (Science Daily, 2017). The National Council on Alcohol and Drug Dependence reports that up to 11% of older adult hospital admissions are because of drug- and alcohol-related issues. (Aging.Com, 2021). About 10% to 15% of people do not start to drink heavily until their later years (Aging.Com, 2021). Frequently cited causes of excessive alcohol use include chronic illness, depression, loneliness, poverty, member of a minority group, and lack of social support.

Alcohol use and late-onset alcohol use disorder (AUD) are often underidentified in older adults (Rosen et al., 2019). The clues of alcohol abuse in the older adult include stress, role/identity loss, loss of a loved one, encouragement/approval by friends, multiple chronic health problems, and coexisting dementia or depression (Emiliussen et al., 2017; Tetrault and O'Connor, 2020). Your suspicion of alcohol abuse increases when there is a history of repeated falls and accidents, social isolation, recurring episodes of memory loss and confusion, failure to meet home and work obligations, a history of skipping meals or medications, and difficulty in managing household tasks and finances. Effectively assessing and intervening for alcohol abuse in an older adult requires sound clinical judgment as to the best time to assess for this issue, the right assessment tool, and coordination of interventions involving the patient, the family, and health care resources (Rosen et al., 2019). Screening tools and resources available for alcohol abuse in older adults include the NIDA Drug Use Screening Tool: Quick Screen and the Helping Patients Who Drink Too Much: A Clinician's Guide (NIAAA). Access to these tools and resources can be found at the

National Institute on Drug Abuse website (https://www.drugabuse.gov/nidamed-medical-health-professionals/screening-tools-resources/chart-screening-tools [NIDA, 2021]). When you suspect that an older adult is abusing alcohol, realize that a variety of treatment options are available. Treatment includes age-specific approaches that acknowledge the stresses experienced by an older adult and encourage involvement in activities that match interests and increase feelings of self-worth. Identifying and treating coexisting depression is also important. The continuum of interventions ranges from simple education about risks to formalized treatment programs that include pharmacotherapy, psychotherapy, and rehabilitation (Rosen et al., 2019).

Nutrition. Lifelong eating habits and situational factors influence how older adults achieve good nutrition. These habits are based in tradition, cultural habits, and preferences. Religious beliefs influence food choices and preparation. Situational factors affecting nutrition include access to grocery stores, finances, physical and cognitive capability for food preparation, and a place to store food and prepare meals. Older adults' levels of activity and clinical conditions affect their nutritional needs. In addition, conditions such as dementia, poor dentition or ill-fitting dentures, dysphagia, and cardiopulmonary, gastrointestinal, renal, or liver diseases impact nutrition. Healthy nutrition for older adults includes appropriate caloric intake and limited intake of fat, salt, refined sugars, and alcohol. When caring for older adults with dementia and other chronic conditions, routinely monitor weight and food intake; provide small, frequent meals and serve food that is easy to eat, such as finger foods (e.g., chicken strips, sandwiches, cut-up vegetables, and fruit); provide assistance with eating; and offer food supplements that the patient likes and are easy to swallow (Brook, 2018). Consult with a registered dietitian when planning nutritional interventions for your patients.

Protein intake is sometimes lower than recommended if older adults have reduced financial resources or limited access to grocery stores. Fat and sodium intake is sometimes higher than usual because older adults can access only quick and convenient frozen meals or they substitute fast-food restaurant meals for meals prepared at home. Home-prepared meals that are fried or made with canned goods also are high in fat and sodium. Some older adults use extra salt and sugar while cooking or at the table to compensate for a diminished sense of taste. Home-delivered meals, such as Meals on Wheels, are an excellent source of nutrition for older adults. Newer online ordering and home delivery services can improve access to quality food sources but may require assistance from family members to order appropriately. These services can be costly.

Dental Problems. Dental problems with natural teeth and dentures are common in older adults. Dental caries, gingivitis, broken or missing teeth, and ill-fitting or missing dentures affect nutritional adequacy, cause pain, and lead to infection. Weight loss may contribute to ill-fitting dentures. Dentures are a frequent problem because the cost is not covered by Medicare, and dentures are quite expensive. Help prevent dental and gum disease through education about routine dental care (see Chapter 40).

Exercise. Older adults need to maintain physical exercise and activity. The primary benefits of exercise include improving and maintaining physical function and muscle strength, as well as promoting a sense of enhanced well-being and quality of life (Qi et al., 2020; Kaushal et al., 2018). Regular daily exercise such as walking builds endurance, increases muscle tone, improves joint flexibility, strengthens bones, reduces stress, and contributes to weight loss. There is some evidence that exercise has some protective effects on cognition and brain health (Tyndall et al., 2018). The United States Department of Health and Human Services (2020) issued *Physical Activity Guidelines for Americans* and includes the following guidelines for older adults:

- Participating in multicomponent physical activity that includes balance training and aerobic and muscle-strengthening activities as part of weekly physical activity
- Determining level of effort for physical activity relative to level of fitness (e.g., knowing target heart rate)
- When chronic conditions exist, understanding whether and how these conditions affect the ability to do regular physical activity safely
- When 150 minutes of moderate-intensity aerobic activity a week is not possible because of chronic conditions, being as physically active as abilities and conditions allow

Many factors influence an individual's willingness to participate in an exercise program. Chapter 38 describes in detail common barriers to activity and exercise. Collaborate with a patient's health care provider before initiating an exercise program to be sure there are no medical contraindications. Exercise programs for sedentary older adults who have not been exercising regularly need to begin conservatively and progress slowly. An exercise program should be appropriate to the older adult's physical ability while being enjoyable, increasing the likelihood of maintaining the program. Developing a habit of routine exercise is beneficial for the physiological effects but also improves mood and quality of life and helps to incorporate activity into a person's lifestyle (Kendrick et al., 2018). Walking is one type of exercise many older adults enjoy (Fig. 14.2). Walking and other low-impact exercises such as riding a stationary exercise bicycle or water exercises in a swimming pool protect the musculoskeletal system and joints. Include exercises in the older adult's daily routine. For example, have an older adult perform arm and leg circles while watching television.

Safety considerations for exercise include wearing supportive shoes and appropriate clothing, drinking water before and after exercising, avoiding outdoor exercise in extreme temperatures, and exercising with a partner. Instruct older adults to stop exercising and seek help if they experience chest pain or tightness, shortness of breath, dizziness or light-headedness, joint pain, or palpitations during exercise.

Falls. There are multiple risks for falls in the older-adult population. Chapter 27 describes in detail the factors contributing to falls and the

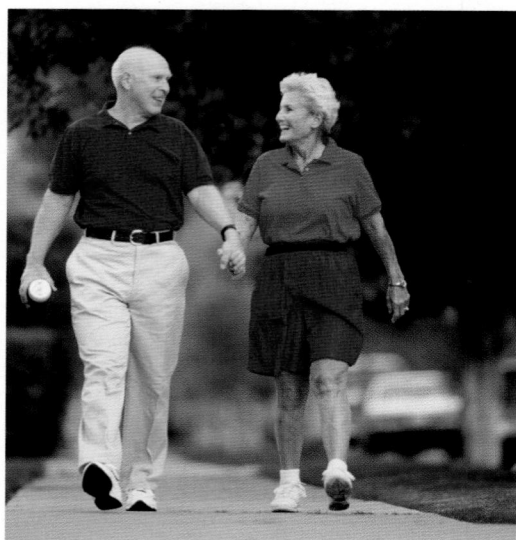

FIG. 14.2 This couple enjoys walking together.

safety concerns of many older adults. Falls are the leading cause of fatal injury and are the most common nonfatal trauma-related reason for hospital admission (National Council on Aging, n.d.). When a fall occurs in an older adult, it may lead to other life-changing events such as hip fracture, spine fracture, or head injury and admission to a nursing center. Fall-related injuries are often associated with a person's preexisting medical conditions such as osteoporosis and bleeding tendencies. Hospitalized older adults require extra attention to decrease the risk of falls (see Chapter 27). Older adults who have fallen will often develop a fear of falling, which in turn often causes them to walk less naturally or to limit their activities, leading to reduced mobility, physical fitness, and independence (Pirrie et al., 2020). Routine exercise and activity can help reduce the risk for falls (Roller et al., 2018; Kaushal et al., 2018).

Sensory Impairments. Because of common sensory impairments experienced by older adults, the promotion of existing sensory function helps ensure that patients live in safe environments. Whenever you provide care activities, make sure that patients wear assistive devices such as a hearing aid or glasses so that they can fully participate in care. Chapter 49 describes in detail the nursing interventions used to maintain and improve sensory function.

Pain. Pain is a symptom and a sensation of distress, alerting a person that something is wrong. It is prevalent in the older-adult population and may be acute or chronic. The consequences of persistent pain include depression, loss of appetite, sleep difficulties, changes in gait and mobility, and decreased socialization. Many factors influence the management of pain, including cultural influences on the meaning and expression of pain for older adults, fears related to the use of analgesic medications, and the problem of pain assessment with older adults who are cognitively impaired. Nurses caring for older adults have to advocate for appropriate and effective pain management (see Chapter 44). Again, the goal of nursing management of pain in older adults is to maximize and maintain function and improve quality of life.

Medication Use. One of the greatest challenges for older adults is safe medication use. Medication categories such as analgesics, anticoagulants, antidepressants, antihistamines, antihypertensives, sedative-hypnotics, and muscle relaxants create a high likelihood of adverse effects in older adults. They are at risk for adverse medication effects because of age-related changes in the absorption, distribution, metabolism, and excretion of drugs, collectively referred to as the process of pharmacokinetics (see Chapter 31). Medications sometimes interact with one another, adding to or negating the effect of another drug. Examples of adverse effects include confusion, impaired balance, dizziness, nausea, and vomiting. Because of these effects, some older adults are unwilling to take medications; others do not adhere to the prescribed dosing schedule, or they try to medicate themselves with herbal and over-the-counter medications.

Polypharmacy, the concurrent use of many medications, increases the risk for adverse drug effects (Box 14.7). Although polypharmacy often reflects inappropriate prescribing, the concurrent use of multiple medications is often necessary when an older adult has multiple acute

---

BOX 14.7 EVIDENCE-BASED PRACTICE

Polypharmacy in Older Adults

PICOT Question: Does the use of a structured medication management program compared with traditional individual provider management affect the incidence of polypharmacy among older adults?

Evidence Summary

Polypharmacy is common among older adults with multiple co-morbidities. It is associated with adverse outcomes, such as adverse drug reactions, falls, increased length of hospital stays, readmission to a hospital soon after discharge, and death (Mizokami et al., 2019; Rochon, 2021). A common risk factor associated with polypharmacy includes patients with cancer and other forms of chronic pain who use opioids to control the pain (Yokota et al., 2019). A large number of community-dwelling older adults have questions about their drug regimens, primarily medication side effects and timing (Mizokami et al., 2019; Rochon, 2021). However, these questions often go unanswered. Many patients also report practical problems primarily related to dosing and remembering instructions that were not written down.

Research has found that formal medication management programs involving a pharmacist and health care provider were beneficial. In one study, patients who were receiving home care services and had medication-related problems (including high-risk drugs affecting the nervous, cardiac, and metabolic systems) received formal consultation. This group had significant reductions in the prescription of potentially inappropriate medications and antipsychotics (Lenander et al., 2018). A nursing home study compared the number and appropriateness of medications before and after implementing *Care by Design*, which used an interprofessional team approach and a physician dedicated to each nursing unit (Andrew et al., 2018). While polypharmacy remained high, a statistically significant reduction in polypharmacy was achieved. Additionally, the number of medications identified by the American Geriatric Society's Beers criteria was reduced; however, the reduction was not statistically significant

(Andrew et al., 2018). One hospital study used an interprofessional team to evaluate appropriateness of medications (Van der Linden et al., 2018). The results demonstrated that the older adults were discharged on fewer medications than they were taking upon admission.

Application to Nursing Practice

- Two tools are useful in guiding the prescription of medications for older adults:
  - The Beers Criteria for Potentially Inappropriate Medication Use in Older Adults (American Geriatrics Society, 2020) helps health care providers recognize potentially inappropriate medications.
  - The Screening Tool of Older Person's Prescriptions and Screening Tool to Alert Doctors to Right Treatment (STOPP-START) screens for drug interactions and potentially inappropriate prescribing in older adults (O'Mahony, 2020; Rochon, 2021). The STOPP-START improves clinical outcomes in older adults with multiple co-morbidities.
- Older adults must maintain an accurate listing of all medications being used. Herbal supplements, vitamins, and over-the-counter medications should be included along with prescription medications (Rochon, 2021).
- If an older adult sees several providers (specialists), there should be one provider who keeps track of the patient's overall medication regimen.
- Older adults can benefit from ongoing education regarding appropriate use of medications and potential adverse effects (Rochon, 2021).
- The use of a systematic approach to medication reviews has been shown to reduce the number of medications prescribed, including potentially inappropriate medications (Andrew et al., 2018; Lenander et al., 2018).
- A number of computer programs and applications can assist with identifying inappropriate medications. These programs are ineffective unless the listing of medications is accurate.

and chronic conditions (Andrew et al., 2018; Rochon, 2021). For example, your patient may be taking one or more medications for hypertension, diabetes, and arthritis. Your role as a nurse is to ensure the greatest therapeutic benefit with the least amount of harm by collaborating with pharmacists and health care providers and educating patients about safe medication use. You need to question the efficacy and safety of combinations of prescribed medications. Advocate for the older adult to prevent adverse reactions. Older adults often use over-the-counter or herbal medications. The mix of over-the-counter and herbal medications with prescription medications can create serious adverse reactions.

For some older adults, safely managing medications is complex and often becomes overwhelming, especially when limited health literacy is an issue. Some take their medications incorrectly because they do not understand the administration instructions, thereby complicating your assessment of medication effects and side effects. Medications that need to be taken more than once or twice a day are a concern because a patient may not remember to take them as scheduled. As a nurse you are in a position to help older-adult patients as they carry out this important self-care activity (see Chapter 31).

The cost of prescriptions is often prohibitive. The Medicare Prescription Drug Benefit, Medicare Part D, is not one plan but a designation of many plans that are approved by the Centers for Medicare and Medicaid Services (CMS, n.d.). Although accompanied by a deductible dependent on the number and expense of the medications prescribed, this benefit is of great help to aging adults. Advocate for patients who need certain medications by working with pharmacies or drug companies to provide the needed medication at less cost. Often a less expensive generic medication will provide the desired effect.

Work collaboratively with older adults and review their medications to ensure safe and appropriate use of all their medications. Teach older adults the names of all medications that they are taking, when and how to take them, and desirable and undesirable effects (Lenander et al., 2018; Rochon, 2021). Pill organizers, bubble packs, and medication calendars help older adults track their doses. Explain how to avoid adverse effects and/or interactions of medications and how to establish and follow an appropriate self-administration pattern. Strategies for reducing the risk for adverse medication effects include reviewing the medications with older adults at each clinic or home visit, examining for potential interactions with food or other medications, simplifying and individualizing medication regimens, taking every opportunity to inform older adults and their family caregivers about all aspects of medication use, and encouraging older adults to question their health care providers about all prescribed and over-the-counter medications (Van der Linden et al., 2018).

The use of medications to manage confusion should be weighed carefully. Sedatives and tranquilizers sometimes prescribed for older adults who are acutely confused often cause or exacerbate confusion and increase risks for falls or other injuries. Carefully monitor patients who receive these medications, taking into account age-related changes in body systems that affect pharmacokinetic activity. When confusion has a physiological cause (such as an infection), health care providers need to treat the cause rather than the confused behavior. When confusion varies by time of day or is related to environmental factors, use creative, nonpharmacological measures such as making the environment more meaningful, providing adequate light, encouraging the use of assistive devices, or even calling friends or family members to let older adults hear reassuring voices.

Health Promotion and Maintenance: Psychosocial Health Concerns

Interventions supporting the psychosocial health of older adults resemble those for middle-adult age-groups. However, older adults face unique concerns, and there are some interventions more crucial for older adults experiencing social isolation, cognitive impairment, or stresses related to retirement, relocation, or approaching death.

Elder Mistreatment. Elder mistreatment is complex, multifaceted, and encompasses a broad range of abuses. It is found across all areas of nursing practice and socioeconomic settings. Elder abuse is defined as an intentional act or failure to act that causes or creates a risk for harm to an older adult (Halphen, 2021). Your ability to screen and assess for it is essential to the safety, health, and well-being of older adults. Types of elder mistreatment include physical abuse, emotional abuse, financial exploitation, sexual abuse, and neglect (intentional and unintentional) (Table 14.3). The U.S. Department of Justice (DOJ) reports at least 10% of adults 65 years of age and older experience some form of elder abuse in a given year, with some older adults simultaneously experiencing more than one type of abuse (U.S. Department of Justice, n.d.). In addition, older adults in rural environments are more likely to exhibit some of the risk factors associated with elder abuse, most commonly dementia (DOJ, n.d.).

Most perpetrators of elder abuse are family caregivers, making abuse cases more complex to identify because of denial, fear of reporting, and the refusal of community services (Rosen et al., 2018). Higher rates of elder mistreatment occur when there is a greater reliance on

TABLE 14.3   Elder Mistreatment: Types, Descriptions, and Examples

Type	Description	Examples
Physical abuse	Occurs when older adults experience illness, pain, or injury as the result of physical force or the threat of physical injury.	Hitting, pushing, slapping, kicking, burning
Psychosocial or emotional abuse	Verbal and nonverbal behaviors that inflict mental pain, anguish, fear, and distress	Humiliation or disrespect, verbal or nonverbal threats, harassment, and geographic or interpersonal isolation
Financial abuse	Illegal taking, misuse, or concealment of money, benefits, property, or assets belonging to an elderly person	Using the elder's money, benefits, belongings, property, or assets for the benefit of someone other than the older adult
Sexual abuse	Nonconsensual sexual contact or activity of any kind; coercing an elder to witness sexual behaviors	Unwanted sexual contact or penetration or noncontact acts, such as sexual harassment
Neglect	Refusal or failure by those responsible to meet basic needs	Refusal or failure to provide basic necessities such as food, water, shelter, clothing, hygiene, and medical care

Modified from Centers for Disease Control and Prevention (CDC), *Preventing elder abuse*, 2020, https://www.cdc.gov/violenceprevention/elderabuse/fastfact.html. Accessed May 2021.

the caregiver because of functional and cognitive impairment. Vulnerable older adults may not reach out for help for fear of further retribution, fear of nursing home placement, or because they have become completely isolated from others.

Elder mistreatment has become the focus of national and international organizations, public and social policy, and research. Established by the U.S. Administration on Aging, the National Center for Elder Abuse (https://ncea.acl.gov/) is a resource center dedicated to the prevention of elder mistreatment. The Elder Justice Act of 2009 is widely regarded as the most comprehensive bill ever passed to address and battle elder mistreatment, providing federal funding to state Adult Protective Services (APS). In most states APS caseworkers are the first responders to reports of abuse, neglect, and exploitation of vulnerable adults. Services include receiving reports of adult abuse, exploitation, or neglect; investigating these reports; case management; monitoring; and evaluation. In addition to casework services, APS arranges medical, social, economic, legal, and housing services, plus law enforcement or other protective emergency or supportive resources (National Center on Elder Abuse, n.d.).

You are in a unique position to screen for elder mistreatment and assess for physical and emotional signs of abuse. A necessary part of your assessment is to complete the interview and assessment privately away from the caregiver. It is definitely a "red flag" if the caregiver refuses to leave the room or area so that you can ask questions confidentially. State laws differ on reporting and investigation of elder mistreatment. However, if you suspect that an older adult is being mistreated, notify your supervisor, who will refer you to the appropriate reporting channels. It is your responsibility to know the reporting provisions of your jurisdiction (Touhy and Jett, 2020). Social workers are excellent resources to assist you.

Therapeutic Communication. Patients accept and respect nurses who meet their expectations of sound knowledge and competence and who communicate effectively about concern for an older adult's welfare. However, you cannot simply enter an older adult's environment and immediately establish a therapeutic relationship. First, you have to be knowledgeable and skilled in communication techniques (see Chapter 24). Sitting down and engaging an older adult eye to eye goes a long way in establishing a therapeutic relationship. Let older adults tell their stories; the result will be access to valuable information enabling you to create a more patient-centered approach to care.

Touch. Touch is a therapeutic tool that can be used to help comfort older adults. It provides sensory stimulation, induces relaxation, provides physical and emotional comfort, conveys warmth, and communicates interest. It is a powerful physical expression of a relationship. In addition, gentle touch is a technique to use when administering any type of procedure that requires physical contact or when repositioning and moving a patient.

Older adults are often deprived of touch when separated from family or friends. An older adult who is isolated, dependent, or ill; who fears death; or who lacks self-esteem has a greater need for touch. You recognize touch deprivation by behaviors as simple as an older adult reaching for the nurse's hand or standing close to the nurse. Unfortunately, older men are sometimes wrongly accused of sexual advances when they reach out to touch others. When you use touch, be aware of cultural variations and individual preferences (see Chapters 7 and 9). Use touch to convey respect and sensitivity. Do not use it in a condescending way such as patting an older adult on the head. When you reach out to an older adult, do not be surprised if the older adult reciprocates.

Reality Orientation. Reality orientation is a communication technique that makes an older adult more aware of person, place, and time. The purposes of reality orientation include restoring a sense of reality; improving the level of awareness; promoting socialization; elevating independent functioning; and minimizing confusion, disorientation, and physical regression. Although you use reality orientation techniques in any health care setting, they are especially useful in the acute care setting. The older adult experiencing a change in environment, surgery, illness, or emotional stress is at risk for becoming disoriented (Chiu et al., 2018). Environmental changes such as bright lights, unfamiliar noises, and lack of windows in specialized units of a hospital often lead to disorientation and confusion. Absence of familiar caregivers is also disorienting. The use of anesthesia, sedatives, tranquilizers, analgesics, and physical restraints in older patients increases disorientation. Anticipate and monitor for disorientation and confusion as possible consequences of hospitalization, relocation, surgery, loss, or illness, and incorporate interventions on the basis of reality orientation into the plan of care.

The principles of reality orientation offer useful guidelines for communicating with individuals who are acutely confused. The key elements of reality orientation include frequent reminders of person, place, and time; the use of familiar environmental aids such as clocks, calendars, and personal belongings; and stability of the environment, routine, and staff (Chiu et al., 2018).

Validation Therapy. Validation therapy is an alternative approach to communication with an older adult who is confused. Whereas reality orientation insists that the confused older adult agree with statements of time, place, and person, validation therapy accepts the description of time and place as stated by the older adult. Do not challenge or argue with statements and behaviors of the older adult. Instead the focus is the emotional aspect of the conversation, which represents an inner need or feeling (Scales, 2018). For example, a patient insists that the day is actually a different day because of high anxiety. Caregivers should acknowledge the distress the individual is experiencing. Validation does not involve reinforcing the older adult's misperceptions; it reflects sensitivity to hidden meanings in statements and behaviors. By listening with sensitivity and validating what the patient is expressing, you convey respect, reassurance, and understanding. Validating or respecting older adults' feelings in the time and place that is real to them is more important than insisting on the literally correct time and place.

Reminiscence. Reminiscence is a method or technique to recall past memories (Shropshire, 2020). Many older adults enjoy sharing past experiences through storytelling. As a therapy, reminiscence uses the recollection of the past to bring meaning and understanding to the present and resolve current conflicts. Looking back to positive resolutions of problems reminds an older adult of coping strategies used successfully in the past. Reminiscing is also a way to express personal identity. Reflection on past achievements supports self-esteem (Scales, 2018). For some older adults the process of looking back on past events uncovers new meanings for those events.

During the assessment process use reminiscence to assess self-esteem, cognitive function, mood, unresolved conflicts, coping ability, and expectations for the future. For example, have a patient talk about a previous loss to assess coping. You can also reminisce during direct care activities. Taking time to ask questions about past experiences and listening attentively conveys to an older adult your attitudes of respect and concern.

Besides its use in one-on-one situations, reminiscence is also effective as a group therapy for older adults to reduce depressive symptoms (Shropshire, 2020; Siverova and Buzgova, 2018). You begin by organizing the group and selecting strategies to start a conversation.

For example, you ask the group to discuss family activities or childhood memories, adapting questions to the group's size, structure, process, goals, and activities to meet its members' needs.

Body Image Interventions. The way older adults present themselves influences body image and feelings of isolation (see Chapter 33). Some physical characteristics of older adulthood such as distinguished-looking gray hair are socially desirable. Other features, such as a lined face that displays character or wrinkled hands that show a lifetime of hard work, are also impressive.

Consequences of illness and aging that threaten an older adult's body image include invasive diagnostic procedures, pain, surgery, loss of sensation in a body part, skin changes, and incontinence. The use of devices such as dentures, hearing aids, artificial limbs, indwelling catheters, ostomy devices, and enteral feeding tubes also affects body image.

Consider the importance an older adult perceives about presenting a socially acceptable image. Also determine how the patient thinks the health condition affects the ability to maintain grooming and hygiene. When older adults have acute or chronic illnesses, the related physical dependence makes it difficult for them to maintain body image. It takes little effort to help older adults adjust their bathing routines and to help them comb their hair, clean their dentures, shave, or change clothing. They usually do not choose to have an objectionable appearance. Be sensitive to odors in the environment. Odors created by urine and some illnesses are often present. By controlling odors you may prevent visitors from shortening their stay or not coming at all.

OLDER ADULTS AND THE ACUTE CARE SETTING

Older adults in the acute care setting need special attention to help them adjust to the acute care environment and meet their basic needs. The acute care setting poses increased risk for adverse events such as delirium, dehydration, malnutrition, health care–associated infections (HAIs), urinary incontinence, and falls. The risk for delirium increases when hospitalized older adults experience immobilization, sleep deprivation, infection, dehydration, pain, sensory impairment, drug interactions, anesthesia, and hypoxia. Nonmedical causes of delirium include unfamiliar surroundings, unfamiliar staff, bed rest, separation from support systems, and stress. Refer to the discussion of delirium, dementia, and depression earlier in the chapter for help in distinguishing among these three conditions. Impaired vision or hearing contributes to confusion and interferes with attempts to reorient an older adult.

When the prevention of delirium fails, nursing management begins with identifying and treating its cause. Supportive interventions include encouraging family visits, providing memory cues (clocks, calendars, and name tags), and compensating for sensory deficits. Reality orientation techniques are often useful.

Older adults are at greater risk for dehydration and malnutrition during hospitalization because of standard procedures such as limiting food and fluids in preparation for diagnostic tests and medications that decrease appetite. The risk for dehydration and malnutrition increases when older adults are unable to reach beverages or feed themselves while in bed or connected to medical equipment. Interventions include getting the patient out of bed, providing beverages and snacks frequently, and including favorite foods and beverages in the diet plan.

The increased risk for HAIs in older adults is associated with the decreased immune system response related to advancing age in addition to other chronic conditions that make older adults more susceptible, along with invasive procedures and devices. The most common HAI are central line–associated bloodstream infections (CLABSIs),

catheter-associated UTIs (CAUTIs), surgical site infection, and ventilator-associated pneumonia (VAP) (CDC, 2021). The leading preventive measure is hand hygiene combined with proper isolation policy and procedures to prevent and control the transmission of infection (see Chapter 28).

Older hospitalized adults are at risk for becoming incontinent of urine (transient incontinence). Causes of incontinence include delirium, untreated UTIs, medications, restricted mobility, or need for assistance to get to the bathroom. Individualized interventions to decrease incontinence include planning voiding opportunities and modification of the environment to improve access to the toilet. It is important to avoid indwelling urinary catheterization (see Chapter 46).

The increased risk for skin breakdown and the development of pressure injuries is related to changes in aging skin and to situations that occur in the acute care setting such as immobility, incontinence, and malnutrition. The key points in the prevention of skin breakdown are using a mattress appropriate for the risk of skin breakdown with proper positioning, reducing shear and friction, providing meticulous skin care and moisture management, and providing nutritional support (see Chapter 48).

Older adults in the acute care setting are also at greater risk for falling and sustaining injuries. The cause of a fall is typically multifactorial and composed of intrinsic or extrinsic factors (see Chapter 27). Sedative and hypnotic medications increase unsteadiness. Lower extremity weakness and general fatigue and deconditioning can make it difficult for a patient to get out of bed. Once the patient does get out of bed, often the patient is unsteady, dizzy, and prone to falling. Medications causing orthostatic hypotension also increase the risk for falls because the blood pressure drops when an older adult gets out of a bed or chair. The increase in urine output from diuretics increases the risk for falling by increasing the number of attempts to get out of bed to void. Pieces of equipment, such as wires from monitors, intravenous tubing, urinary catheters, and other medical devices, become obstacles to safe ambulation. Impaired vision prevents an older adult from seeing tripping hazards such as trash cans.

A safe environment for older adults is a restraint-free environment. Every effort must be made to avoid the use of physical restraints. See Chapter 27 for a detailed discussion of interventions for reducing falls in the health care setting.

OLDER ADULTS AND RESTORATIVE CARE

Restorative care refers to two types of ongoing care: the continuation of recovery from acute illness or surgery that began in the acute care setting and the support of chronic conditions that affect day-to-day functioning. Both types of restorative care take place in private homes and long-term care settings.

Interventions during convalescence from acute illness or surgery aim at regaining or improving patients' prior level of independence in ADLs. Continue interventions that began in the acute care setting and later modify them as convalescence progresses. To achieve this continuation, ensure that discharge information provided by the acute care setting includes information on required ongoing interventions (e.g., exercise routines, wound care routines, medication schedules, and blood glucose monitoring). Interventions also need to address the restoration of interpersonal relationships and activities at either their previous level or the level desired by the older adult. When restorative care addresses chronic conditions, the goals of care include stabilizing the chronic condition and maximizing independence in ADLs.

Interventions to promote independence in ADLs address a person's physical and cognitive ability and safety. The physical ability to perform ADLs requires strength, flexibility, and balance. Make accommodations for impairments of vision, hearing, and touch (see Chapter 49). The cognitive ability to perform ADLs requires the ability to recognize, judge, and remember. Cognitive impairments such as dementia interfere with safe performance of ADLs, although an older adult is still physically capable of the activities. Adapt interventions to promote independence in ADLs to meet the needs and lifestyle of the older adult. Although safety is paramount, an older adult needs to be able to perform ADLs with a level of risk that is acceptable. Collaborate with an occupational therapist, who is trained in selecting the correct type of assistive devices for patients.

Support an older adult's ability to perform IADLs, such as using a telephone, doing laundry, shopping, cleaning the home or apartment, handling money, paying bills, and driving an automobile. To live independently at home or in an apartment, older adults need to be able to perform IADLs, purchase services by outside workers, or have a supportive network of family and friends who routinely help with these tasks. Occupational therapists are an important resource for helping people adapt when IADLs are difficult to perform. Also, it might be appropriate to have a family caregiver assume more responsibility by completing IADLs for patients.

Restorative care measures focus on activities that allow older adults to remain functional and safe within their living environments. Collaborate with an older adult and with family caregivers as necessary to establish priorities of care, determine expected outcomes, and select appropriate interventions. Patient collaboration promotes a patient's understanding about care and minimizes conflicts. Consideration of an older adult's lifetime experiences, values, and sociocultural patterns serves as the basis for planning individual care. When an older adult's cognitive status prevents participation in health care decisions, include the family caregivers. Family and friends are rich sources of data because they knew the older adult before the impairment. Frequently they provide explanations for the older adult's behaviors and suggest methods of management. Thoughtful assessment and planning lead to care interventions that incorporate techniques for addressing normal aging changes, an optimal level of comfort and coping, and promotion of independence in self-care activities.

KEY POINTS

- Nurses must learn to ignore false stereotypes about the physical and psychosocial characteristics of older adults, such as physical disability, poor memory, and inability to learn new information, and instead methodically assess each patient's functional, physiological, psychosocial, and emotional status.
- Because the classic signs and symptoms of diseases are sometimes absent, blunted, or atypical in older adults, sound clinical judgment requires a nurse to anticipate the physiological age-related changes in older adults when interpreting actual assessment findings. There are common developmental tasks for older adults that are associated with varying degrees of change and loss (e.g., maintaining satisfactory living arrangements, the loss of significant others) that nurses must take into consideration when assessing the impact an illness has on the patient.
- Nurses collaborate with older adults in assisting them to achieve their developmental tasks in a healthy manner.
- Common physiological changes associated with normal aging (e.g., loss of skin elasticity, decreased cough reflex, lower cardiac output) are not pathological in themselves but can make older adults more vulnerable to common clinical conditions and diseases.
- It is important to differentiate normal changes in aging with disease manifestations.

- Delirium, dementia, and depression share some common symptoms, but an accurate diagnosis is essential for appropriate management.
- Because of psychosocial changes that occur during older adults' life transitions, nurses learn to assess family dynamics, quality of relationships, past and present role changes, finances, housing, social networks, activities, health and wellness, and spirituality.
- Elder abuse encompasses a broad range of abuses that are most commonly performed by family caregivers, making abuse cases complex to identify because of denial, fear of reporting, and the refusal of community services.
- Because there are different types of elder mistreatment, nurses must be alert to cues of mistreatment and report appropriately.
- Older adults have many health concerns, but they are becoming more enthusiastic and motivated about healthy lifestyles. A nurse is responsible for educating patients on how to better prevent or manage chronic disease and reduce health risks.
- An aim of nursing interventions for older adults is the focus on maintaining maximal functioning and independence.

REFLECTIVE LEARNING

Consider an older patient or an older personal family member or friend and ask yourself these questions:

- Describe how this individual has adapted to the aging process. What are the functional or physical changes? What are the strengths and limitations? Are there any concerns you have about how they are adapting to the aging process?
- What safety concerns might you have for this person? Is the current living arrangement safe? What are the existing environmental and health safety concerns?
- How have you adapted your communication strategies for this person? Was it effective? How could you improve your communication strategies?

REVIEW QUESTIONS

1. A patient's family member is considering having her mother placed in a nursing center. The nurse has talked with the family before and knows that this is a difficult decision. Which of the following criteria does the nurse recommend in choosing a nursing center? (Select all that apply.)
   1. The center needs to be clean, and rooms should look like a hospital room.
   2. Adequate staffing is available on all shifts.
   3. Social activities are available for all residents.
   4. The center provides three meals daily with a set menu and serving schedule.
   5. Staff encourage family involvement in care planning and assisting with physical care.
2. A nurse conducted an assessment of a new patient who came to the medical clinic. The patient is 82 years old and has had osteoarthritis for 10 years and diabetes mellitus for 20 years. He is alert but becomes easily distracted during the assessment. He recently moved to a new apartment, and his pet beagle died just 2 months ago. He is most likely experiencing:
   1. Dementia.
   2. Depression.
   3. Delirium.
   4. Anxiety.

3. A nurse is completing a health history with the daughter of a newly admitted patient who is confused and agitated. The daughter reports that her mother was diagnosed with Alzheimer disease 1 year ago but became extremely confused last evening and was hallucinating. She was unable to calm her, and her mother thought she was a stranger. On the basis of this history, the nurse suspects that the patient is experiencing:
1. Normal aging.
2. Delirium.
3. Depression.
4. Worsening dementia.

4. A 78-year-old male is going through preoperative screening and preparation for his surgery in 1 week. His wife is with him, and initially they both appear anxious. He will be undergoing a colon resection for colon cancer and will have a permanent colostomy. The nurse knows the patient's age and developmental status will affect how the assessment is conducted. The nurse wants to provide a database that will be useful to the nurses in the hospital and therefore applies clinical judgment appropriately through which of the following: (Select all that apply.)
1. While examining the patient, the nurse notes the physical changes of decreased bowel sounds, dry mouth, and reduced skin elasticity are physical changes likely related to the cancer.
2. When the patient has difficult remembering current medications, the nurse asks the wife to supplement information.
3. The nurse anticipates the effect of the colostomy on functioning and asks the patient how he perceives life with a colostomy.
4. While gathering the history of the patient's illness, the nurse anticipates him having the classic signs of fatigue and unexplained weight loss.
5. Knowing that elderly patients have less interest in sexual intimacy, the nurse does not ask about the impact the patient thinks his surgery will have on sexual function.

5. A nurse sees a 76-year-old woman in the outpatient clinic. The patient states that she recently started to notice a glare in the lights at home. Her vision is blurred, and she is unable to play cards with her friends, read, or do her needlework. Which of the following nursing interventions are appropriate? (Select all that apply.)
1. Refer her to an ophthalmologist.
2. Suggest large-print books and playing cards.
3. Reassure her that the visual changes are part of normal aging.
4. Suggest lower-wattage light bulbs to decrease glare.
5. Assess her home environment for safety.

6. A 63-year-old patient is retiring from his job at an accounting firm where he was in a management role for the past 20 years. He has been with the same company for 42 years and was a dedicated employee. His wife is a homemaker. She raised their five children, babysits for their grandchildren as needed, and belongs to numerous church committees. What are the major psychosocial concerns for this patient? (Select all that apply.)
1. The loss of his work role
2. The risk of social isolation
3. A determination on whether the wife will need to start working
4. How the wife may now expect assistance with household tasks and with babysitting the grandchildren
5. The age the patient chose to retire

7. A nurse is assessing an older adult brought to the emergency department following a fall and wrist fracture. The patient lives with her son, is very thin and unkempt, has a Stage 3 pressure injury on her coccyx,

and has old bruising to the extremities in addition to her new bruises from the fall. She defers all of the questions to her caregiver son, who accompanied her to the hospital. What is the nurse's next step?
1. Call social services to begin nursing home placement.
2. Ask the son to step out of the room so that she can complete her assessment.
3. Call adult protective services because you suspect elder mistreatment.
4. Assess the patient's cognitive status.

8. A nurse is participating in a health and wellness event at the local community center. A woman approaches with her father and relates that she is worried that her widowed father is becoming more functionally impaired and may need to move in with her. The nurse asks about his ability to complete activities of daily living (ADLs) by asking which of the following questions? (Select all that apply.)
1. Tell me if you are still driving.
2. Describe any problems you have in sitting or getting up from your toilet.
3. Tell me how often you take a bath during the week and how you bathe.
4. Estimate for me the amount of time you spend exercising each day.
5. Tell me how you do your grocery shopping.

9. A daughter is beginning to assume caregiver responsibility for her 90-year-old widowed father. Her father has hypertension, coronary artery disease, and type 2 diabetes mellitus. Home health services are set for once a week. During the first visit, the daughter expresses concern about all the medications that her father has been prescribed by different doctors and that he has obtained from different pharmacies. The daughter states that her father cannot really tell her what each medication is for or when he should take them. From this initial information the nurse suspects polypharmacy. What medication assessment data are needed? (Select all that apply.)
1. Review all medication prescriptions
2. Match medication prescriptions with the patient's medication bottles or unit-dose blister packs
3. Identify involvement of the caregiver in helping with medication administration
4. Identify and delete duplicate medications
5. Obtain a listing of any over-the-counter medications

10. A nurse is caring for a 76-year-old female patient in the home setting. She just lost her husband from COVID-19 and has four children who live nearby. The patient was an educator and retired only 2 years ago. The nurse applies knowledge of developmental changes and the nature of loss in older adults when assessing which of the following situations? (Select all that apply.)
1. The nature of her relationships with her adult children
2. The total number of medications the patient is taking, including over-the-counter medications
3. The patient's perception of the need for caregiving assistance from the family with activities her husband performed
4. The impact of her husband's death on her monthly income
5. The patient's current physical functional status

Answers: 1. 2, 3, 5; **2.** 2, 3; **4.** 2, 3; **5.** 1, 2, 5; **6.** 1, 4; **7.** 2; **8.** 2, 3; **9.** 1, 2, 3, 5; **10.** 1, 3, 4, 5.

Rationales for Review Questions can be found on the Evolve website.

REFERENCES

Administration on Aging (AOA): *2017 profile of older Americans*, https://www.acl.gov/sites/default/files/Aging%20and%20Disability%20in%20America/2017OlderAmericansProfile.pdf, 2018. Accessed April 2021.

Aging.com: *Alcohol abuse amongst the elderly: a complete guide*, 2021, https://aging.com/alcohol-abuse-amongst-the-elderly-a-complete-guide/. Accessed May 2021.

American Association of Retired Persons (AARP): *Healthy living: two-thirds of older adults are interested in sex, poll says*, 2018, https://www.aarp.org/health/healthy-living/info-2018/older-sex-sexual-health-survey.html. Accessed April 2021.

Alderman J: Pain. In Meiner S, Yeager JJ, editors: *Gerontologic nursing*, ed 6, St. Louis, 2019, Elsevier.

Ali M, Cascella M: *ICU delirium*, StatPearls, 2021 Jan 16, PubMed.Gov, https://pubmed.ncbi.nlm.nih.gov/32644706/ Accessed May 2021.

Alzheimer's Association: *Types of dementia*, 2021, https://www.alz.org/alzheimers-dementia/what-is-dementia/types-of-dementia. Accessed May 2021.

American Cancer Society (ACS): *Key Statistics for prostate cancer*, 2021, https://www.cancer.org/cancer/prostate-cancer/about/key-statistics.html. Accessed April 2021.

American Heart Association: *Understand YOUR risks to prevent a heart attack*, 2016, https://www.heart.org/en/health-topics/heart-attack/understand-your-risks-to-prevent-a-heart-attack. Accessed June 2020.

American Lung Association: *Learn about COPD*, 2021a, https://www.lung.org/lung-health-diseases/lung-disease-lookup/copd/learn-about-copd. Accessed May 2021.

American Lung Association: *Physical activity and COPD*, 2021b, http://www.lung.org/lung-health-and-diseases/lung-disease-lookup/copd/living-with-copd/physical-activity.html. Accessed June 2020.

American Stroke Association: *Stroke risk factors*, 2021, https://www.stroke.org/en/about-stroke/stroke-risk-factors. Accessed May 2021.

Brook S: Nutritional consideration in older adults, *Br J Community Nursing* 23(9):449, 2018.

Bub L: Loss and end-of-life issues. In Meiner S, Yeager JJ, editors: *Gerontologic nursing*, ed 6, St. Louis, 2019, Elsevier.

Centers for Disease Control and Prevention (CDC): *Healthcare infection control practices advisory committee (HICPAC)*, 2021. https://www.cdc.gov/hicpac/index.html. Accessed May 2021.

Centers for Medicare and Medicaid Services (CMS): *Drug coverage—Part D*, (n.d.). http://www.medicare.gov/part-d/index.html. Accessed June 2020.

Centers for Medicare & Medicaid Services (CMS): *Your guide to choosing a nursing home or other long-term care*, Baltimore, MD, 2019, CMS. https://www.medicare.gov/Pubs/pdf/02174-Nursing-Home-Other-Long-Term-Services.pdf. Accessed June 2020.

Davis A: Health promotion and illness/disability prevention. In Meiner S, Yeager JJ, editors: *Gerontologic nursing*, ed 6, St. Louis, 2019, Elsevier.

Fazio S, et al: Alzheimer's Association dementia care practice recommendations, *Gerontologist* 58(S1):S1, 2018.

Federal Interagency Forum on Aging-Related Statistics: *Older Americans 2020: key indicators of well-being*, 2020, https://agingstats.gov/docs/LatestReport/OA20_508_10142020.pdf. Accessed July 2021.

Fulmer T: *Fulmer SPICES: an overall assessment tool for older adults*, https://hign.org/sites/default/files/2020-06/Try_This_General_Assessment_1.pdf, 2019. Accessed July 2020.

Health in Aging: *home safety tips for older adults*, 2020, http://www.healthinaging.org/resources/resource:home-safety-tips-for-older-adults/. Accessed July 2020.

Johnson BK: Sexually transmitted infections and older adults, *J Gerontol Nurs* Nov;39(11):53, 2013.

Kochanek KD: Deaths: Final data for 2017. *National Vital Statistics Reports*: 68(9): 1, 2019, https://www.cdc.gov/nchs/data/nvsr/nvsr68/nvsr68_09-508.pdf. Accessed June 2020.

Massey University: Lifetime effects of poverty take toll in older age, *Medical Press*, August 15, 2019, https://medicalxpress.com/news/2019-08-lifetime-effects-poverty-toll-older.html. Accessed May 2021.

Mendoza MA: Why do the elderly commit suicide? *Psychology Today*, 2020, https://www.psychologytoday.com/us/blog/understanding-grief/202001/why-do-the-elderly-commit-suicide. Accessed May 2021.

National Cancer Institute (NCI): *US National Cancer Institute fact sheet: harms of smoking and health benefits of quitting*. 2017, http://www.cancer.gov/cancertopics/factsheet/Tobacco/cessation. Accessed June 2020.

National Center on Elder Abuse: *Adult protective services*, n.d. https://ncea.acl.gov/What-We-Do/Practice/Intervention-Partners/APS.aspx. Accessed June 2020.

National Council on Aging: *Falls free initiative*, n.d. https://www.ncoa.org/healthy-aging/falls-prevention/falls-free-initiative/. Accessed June 2020.

National Institutes of Health (NIH), National Institute on Aging: *Aging in place: growing old at home*, https://www.nia.nih.gov/health/aging-place-growing-old-home, 2017.

National Institute on Drug Abuse (NIDA): Screening and Assessment Tools Chart, 2021, https://www.drugabuse.gov/nidamed-medical-health-professionals/screening-tools-resources/chart-screening-tools. Accessed July 2021.

National Osteoporosis Foundation: *Bone health basics: get the facts*, https://www.nof.org/preventing-fractures/general-facts/, 2021. Accessed May, 2021.

National Prevention, Health Promotion, and Public Health Council (National Prevention Council): *Healthy aging in action: Advancing the national prevention strategy*, https://www.cdc.gov/aging/pdf/healthy-aging-in-action508.pdf, 2018. Accessed August 2021.

Office of Disease Prevention and Health Promotion: Older adults. *Healthy People 2030*. n.d, U.S. Department of Health and Human Services. https://health.gov/healthypeople/objectives-and-data/browse-objectives/older-adults. Accessed May 2021.

Population Reference Bureau: Fact sheet: *Aging in the United States*, https://www.prb.org/aging-unitedstates-fact-sheet/, 2021. Accessed April 2021.

Science Daily: Increases in alcohol use, especially among women, other groups, *The JAMA Network Journals*, August 2017 https://www.sciencedaily.com/releases/2017/08/170809140254.htm.

Touhy T, Jett K, editors: *Toward healthy aging*, ed 10, St Louis, 2020, Elsevier.

USA Facts: Accidents, cancer and deaths of despair: see how age and location influence US death rates. 2020. https://usafacts.org/articles/americans-causes-of-death-by-age-cdc-data/, Accessed May 2021.

US Census Bureau: *Income and poverty in the United States: 2018*, 2020, https://www.census.gov/content/dam/Census/library/publications/2019/demo/p60-266.pdf. Accessed July 2020.

US Department of Health and Human Services (USDHHS): *Physical activity guidelines for Americans*, 2nd ed, 2020, Office of Disease Prevention and Health Promotion. https://health.gov/paguidelines/second-edition/. Accessed July 12, 2020.

US Department of Justice (DOJ): *Elder abuse statistics*, n.d., https://www.justice.gov/file/1098056/download Accessed May 2021.

World Health Organization: *Health promotion: health literacy: the Mandate for health literacy*, 2021, http://www.who.int/healthpromotion/conferences/9gchp/health-literacy/en/. Accessed May, 2021.

Yeager JJ: Sexuality and aging. In Meiner S, Yeager JJ, editors: *Gerontologic nursing*, ed 6, St. Louis, 2019a, Elsevier.

Yeager JJ: Drugs and aging. In Meiner S, Yeager JJ, editors: *Gerontologic nursing*, ed 6, St. Louis, 2019b, Elsevier.

Yeager JJ: Assessment of the older adult. In Meiner S, Yeager JJ, editors: *Gerontologic nursing*, ed 6, St. Louis, 2019c, Elsevier.

Yoe J: *Why are older people working longer?* U.S. Bureau of Labor Statistics, Monthly Labor Review, July 2019, https://www.bls.gov/opub/mlr/2019/beyond-bls/why-are-older-people-working-longer.htm. Accessed May 2021.

RESEARCH REFERENCES

American Geriatrics Society.: American geriatrics society 2019 updated AGS Beers criteria for potentially inappropriate medication use in older adults, *Am Fam Physician* 101(1): 56, 2020.

Andrew MK et al.: Polypharmacy and use of potentially inappropriate medications in long-term care facilities: does coordinated primary care make a difference, *Int J Pharm Pract* 26:318, 2018.

Campbell J et al.: Assessing statewide need for older adult health promotion services: the Oklahoma experience. *J Soc Serv Res* 44(2):119, 2018.

Chiu HY et al.: Reality orientation therapy benefits cognition in older people with dementia: a meta-analysis, *Int J Nurs Stud* 86:20, 2018.

Cutilli C et al.: Health literacy, health disparities, and sources of health information in U.S. older adults, *Orthop Nurs* 37(1):54, 2018.

Emiliussen J et al.: Identifying risk factors for late-onset (50+) alcohol use disorder and heavy drinking: a systematic review, *Subst Use Misuse* 52(12):1575, 2017.

Gonyea JG et al: Perceptions of neighborhood safety and depressive symptoms among older minority urban subsidized housing residents: the mediating effect of sense of community belonging, *Aging Ment Health*, 22(12):1564, 2018.

Halphen J: Elder abuse, self-neglect, and related phenomena, neglect, and financial exploitation, *UpToDate*, 2021, https://www.uptodate.com/contents/elder-mistreatment-abuse-neglect-and-financial-exploitation.

Kaushal N et al.: The effects of multi-component exercise training on cognitive functioning and health-related quality of life in older adults, *Int J Behav Med* 25(6):617, 2018.

Kendrick D et al.: Keeping active: maintenance of physical activity after exercise programmes for older adults, *Publish Health* 164:118, 2018.

Kim Y et al: Factors associated with successful smoking cessation according to age group: findings of an 11-year Korea national survey *Int J Environ Res Public Health*, 7:18(4):1576, 2021.

Lenander C et al.: Effects of medication reviews on use of potentially inappropriate medications in elderly patients; a cross-sectional study in Swedish primary care, *BMC Health Serv Res* 18:616, 2018.

Lewis B et al.: Drinking patterns and adherence to "low-risk" guidelines among community-residing older adults, *Drug Alcohol Depend* 187(1):285, 2018.

Mizokami F et al: Clinical medication review type III of polypharmacy reduced unplanned hospitalizations in older adults: A meta-analysis of randomized clinical trials, *Geriatr Gerontol Int,* 19: 1275, 2019.

O'Mahony D: STOPP/START criteria for potentially inappropriate medications/potential prescribing omissions in older people: origin and progress, *Expert Review of Clinical Pharmacology,* 13(1): 15, 2020.

Pirrie M et al: Risk of fall and fear of falling in older adults residing in public housing in Ontario, Canada: findings from a multisite observational study, *BMC Geriatrics,* 20(11): 1, 2020.

Qi M et al: Tai Chi combined with resistance training for adults aged 50 years and older: a systemic review: *J Geriatr Phys Ther,* 43(1): 32, 2020.

Rochon P: Drug prescribing for older adults, *UpToDate,* 2021, https://www.uptodate.com/contents/drug-prescribing-for-older-adults. Accessed May 2021.

Roller M et al.: Pilates reformer exercises for fall risk reduction in older adults: a randomized controlled trial, *J Bodyw Mov Ther* 22:983, 2018.

Rosen D et al: Baby boomer's substance abuse and researcher indifference, *J Gerontological Social Work,* 62(1): 16, 2019.

Rosen T et al.: Improving quality of care in hospitals for victims of elder mistreatment: development of the vulnerable elder protection team, *Joint Comm J Qual Patient Saf* 44(3):164, 2018.

Scales K et al.: Evidence-based nonpharmacological practices to address behavioral and psychological symptoms of dementia, *Gerontol* 58(S1):S88–S102, 2018.

Shropshire M: Reminiscence intervention for community-dwelling older adults without dementia: a literature review. *Br. J Nurs,* 25(1): 40, 2020.

Siverova J, Buzgova R: The effect of reminiscence therapy on quality of life, attitudes to ageing, and depressive symptoms in institutionalized elderly with cognitive impairment: a quasi-experimental study, *Int J Ment Health Nurs* 27(5):1430, 2018.

Tetrault J, O'Connor P: Risky drinking and alcohol use disorder: Epidemiology, pathogenesis, clinical manifestations, course, assessment, and diagnosis, *UpToDate,* 2020, https://www.uptodate.com/contents/risky-drinking-and-alcohol-use-disorder-epidemiology-pathogenesis-clinical-manifestations-course-assessment-and-diagnosis.

Tyndall A et al.: Protective effects of exercise on cognition and brain health in older adults. *Exerc Sport Sci Rev* 46(4):215, 2018.

Van der Linden L, et al.: Medication review versus usual care to improve drug therapies in older inpatients not admitted to geriatric wards: a quasi-experimental study (RASP-IGCT), *BMC Geriatr* 18(155), 2018.

Yokota I et al: Risk for polypharmacy in elderly, *Palliative Medicine* 36(7): 598, 2019.

15

Critical Thinking and Clinical Judgment

OBJECTIVES

- Explain the relationship between critical thinking and clinical judgment in nursing practice.
- Interpret the value of applying a clinical judgment model in nursing practice.
- Examine the components of critical thinking in clinical decision making.
- Contrast the differences between basic problem solving and diagnostic reasoning.

- Explain differences in the levels of critical thinking.
- Analyze benefits of clinical experiences that contribute to critical thinking.
- Apply critical thinking attitudes during assessment of a patient condition.
- Explain when to use intellectual standards.
- Evaluate the ability to make accurate clinical decisions.

KEY TERMS

Clinical decision making
Clinical judgment
Critical thinking
Deductive reasoning
Diagnostic reasoning

Evidence-based knowledge
Inductive reasoning
Inference
Intuition
Knowing the patient

Nursing process
Problem solving
Reflection

MEDIA RESOURCES

http://evolve.elsevier.com/Potter/fundamentals/
- Review Questions
- Audio Glossary

- Case Study with Questions
- Content Updates
- Answers to QSEN Activity and Review Questions

Pause for a moment. What goes through your mind when you confront a problem? What do you think about before making a decision? Depending on the nature of the problem or type of decision, you may think about past experiences, reflect on your knowledge about the problem, or consider the time you have and the desire to be accurate, or you might react to intuition. These factors and more involve the critical thinking needed to make a judgment and decide.

A nurse has the role of recognizing patient health-related needs, forming clinical judgments about those needs by using critical thinking, and making timely decisions about when and how to act. Action may involve gathering more data about the patient's problems, deciding to consult with other health care professionals, or delivering an intervention to manage or relieve the problem. Nurses apply critical thinking routinely when making the decisions and clinical judgments needed for optimal patient outcomes.

Every day you think critically without realizing it. If your computer flashes an error warning or your cell phone does not take you to a desired application, you think about the actions you took before the error,

consider possible causes of the problem, and correct a keystroke or reboot the device. If you decide to walk your dogs, go to the door, and notice that it is raining, you decide to change into your raincoat. These simple examples show how you use critical thinking when you make daily decisions.

For a professional nurse, critical thinking is more complicated. You care for patients with unique, complex health care problems that can change within minutes. Critical thinking becomes embedded in your everyday practice, as it involves knowing as much as possible about each patient and sorting out the information into patterns to identify problems, recognize changes, and make appropriate clinical care decisions under pressure. Critical thinking and clinical judgment are essential processes for safe, efficient, and skillful nursing intervention (Papathanasiou et al., 2014). Sound critical thinking enables you to face each new experience and problem involving a patient's care with open-mindedness, confidence, and continual inquiry. It is a process mastered only through experience, commitment, and an active curiosity toward learning.

CLINICAL JUDGMENT IN NURSING PRACTICE

A patient's health care needs initiate the process of clinical judgment and clinical decision making (Dickison et al., 2019). Registered nurses (RNs) are responsible for making accurate and appropriate clinical decisions that ensure patients receive safe, appropriate, timely, and effective nursing interventions. A clinical judgment is defined by the National Council of State Boards of Nursing (NCSBN) as the observed outcome of critical thinking and decision making (NCSBN, 2019). Another definition for clinical judgment is a conclusion about a patient's needs or health problems that leads to taking or avoiding action, using or modifying standard approaches, or creating new approaches based on the patient's response (Tanner, 2006). It is a process that uses nursing knowledge, experience, and critical thinking to observe and assess presenting situations, identify a prioritized patient concern, and generate the best possible evidence-based solutions to make the decisions needed to deliver safe patient care (NCSBN, 2019). Clinical decision making separates professional nurses from technicians or other assistive personnel (AP). For example, an RN observes for changes in a patient's condition, collects and analyzes data about the changes, recognizes and identifies new and potential problems, plans nursing strategies, and takes immediate action when the patient's clinical condition worsens. Nurses direct AP to perform basic aspects of care based on patient need; AP do not have the knowledge or experience to analyze why or when patients' clinical conditions change and what strategies are required. Good clinical decision making requires you to use your judgment in investigating and analyzing all aspects of a clinical problem and then applying scientific and nursing knowledge to choose the best course of action.

Dr. Christine Tanner (2006) described a research-based model of clinical judgment in nursing. It included the following conclusions:

- Clinical judgments are influenced more by a nurse's experience and knowledge than by the objective data about the situation at hand. Experience (such as previous time caring for patients, practicing a skill) is crucial to knowing how to interpret the data.
- Sound clinical judgment partly relies on "knowing the patient" and the patient's typical pattern of responses, as well as engaging with patients about their concerns.
- Clinical judgments are influenced by the context of clinical situations and the culture of patient care settings.
- Nurses use a variety of reasoning approaches in combination, such as problem solving and reflection to understand patient problems and create an individualized plan of care.
- Most patients have health care problems for which there are no clear textbook solutions. Each patient's health problems are unique, a product of the patient's physical health, lifestyle, culture, relationship with family and friends, living environment, and experiences. Therefore, as a nurse, you do not always have a clear picture of a patient's needs and the appropriate actions to take when first meeting a patient. Instead, you must learn to question, wonder, and explore different perspectives and interpretations to find a solution that benefits the patient. With experience you learn to creatively seek new knowledge, act quickly when events change, and make good decisions for patients' well-being.

A Model for Clinical Judgment

Clinical judgments made by thinking critically and making sound decisions are at the core of professional nursing competence. Fig. 15.1 offers a model for clinical judgment that is integrated throughout this textbook. Models help to explain concepts. Critical thinking in nursing is complex; this model explains the many variables involved as you make decisions and clinical judgments about your patients. The model for

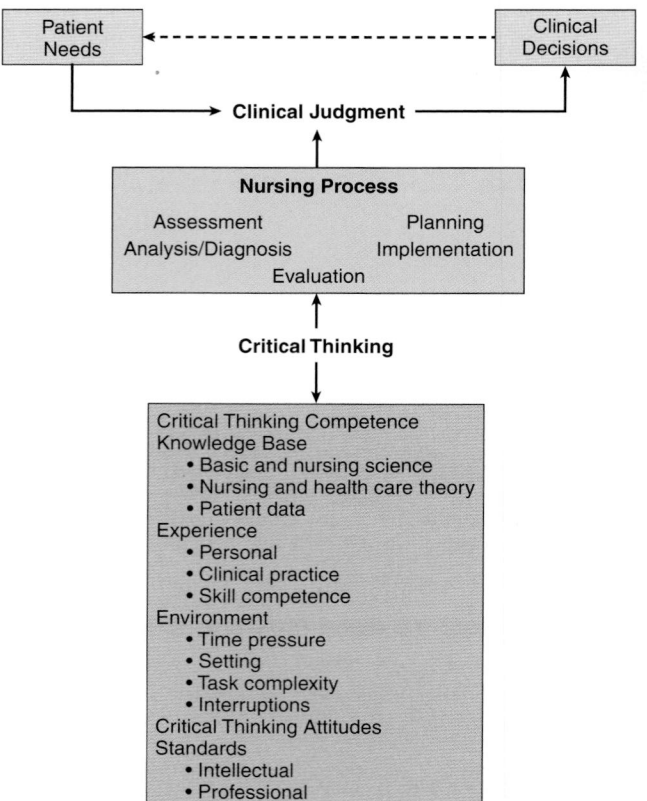

FIG. 15.1 Clinical judgment model for nursing. (Adapted from Kataoka-Yahiro M, Saylor C: A critical thinking model for nursing judgment, *J Nurs Educ* 33:351, 1994; Glaser E: *An experiment in the development of critical thinking*, New York, 1941, Bureau of Publications, Teachers College, Columbia University; Miller M, Malcolm N: Critical thinking in the nursing curriculum, *Nurs Health Care* 11:67, 1990; Paul RW: The art of redesigning instruction. In Willsen J, Blinker AJA, editors: *Critical thinking: how to prepare students for a rapidly changing world*, Santa Rosa, CA, 1993, Foundation for Critical Thinking; Perry W: *Forms of intellectual and ethical development in the college years: a scheme*, New York, 1979, Holt, Rinehart, & Winston; and National Council State Boards of Nursing [NCSBN]: *Next Generation NCLEX News: Clinical Judgment Measurement Model*, Winter 2019. https://www.ncsbn.org/NGN_Winter19.pdf. Accessed March 2, 2020.)

this textbook incorporates research based on previous work by nurse scholars, researchers, and the NCSBN (Kataoka-Yahiro and Saylor, 1994; Miller and Malcolm, 1990; Paul, 1993; NCSBN, 2019).

As you begin your professional nursing education, know that with time, knowledge, and appropriate experiences, you will gain competence in being able to apply the clinical judgment model. The model is not offered for you to try to apply every element or component to each patient situation. But it does contain the elements that allow you to make the right clinical decisions in every type of patient situation. Each patient poses a unique situation for applying the model. For example, when you care for a patient who has respiratory problems because of pneumonia, you will apply knowledge about respiration and oxygenation and the disease pneumonia, physically listen to lung sounds, reflect on criteria as to whether the patient requires airway suctioning, and consider data gathered after interviewing the patient to offer patient-centered care easing anxiety related to shortness of breath. In contrast, when you care for a patient who has respiratory problems because of fractured ribs, you will apply knowledge about ventilation and oxygenation and the pain associated with fractures, examine chest excursion, consider pain relief approaches, and review data gathered after interviewing the patient to offer patient-centered care in promoting pain relief.

The clinical judgment model offers a valuable conceptual approach to understanding the nature of nursing practice. As you enter nursing, consciously consider the model and how you can apply it to each patient for whom you care. Once you become an experienced nurse, your application of elements of the model will be spontaneous, purposeful, and effective in improving patient outcomes.

CRITICAL THINKING

Mr. Lawson is a 68-year-old patient who had abdominal surgery for a colon resection and removal of a tumor yesterday. His nurse, Tonya, finds the patient lying supine in bed with his arms held tightly over his abdomen. His facial expression is tense. Tonya checks the patient's surgical wound, observing the condition of the dressing. She notes that he winces when she gently places her hands to palpate around the surgical incision. She asks Mr. Lawson when he last turned onto his side, and he responds, "Not since last night." Tonya also says, "Show me where you are having pain." The patient points to his incision and says, "It hurts too much to move." Tonya assesses Mr. Lawson with a pain-rating scale. He rates his pain at a 7 on a scale of 0 to 10. Tonya refers to the electronic health record, noting that the patient last received an analgesic 5 hours ago. Tonya considers the information she observed and gathered to determine that the patient's priority problem is pain, in addition to reduced mobility. She decides to take action by administering an analgesic that is ordered to be given as needed every 4 hours and obtaining assistance from the assistive personnel to position the patient more comfortably.

In this case example, Tonya begins by referring to knowledge about abdominal surgery and the effects on the colon when a tumor is removed. She recognizes that a patient problem exists by gathering and assessing information (e.g., clinical data, observation of patient behavior, medical record), analyzing information about the problem (e.g., is it anticipated or unexpected, what cues form patterns?), interpreting the information (reviewing assumptions and evidence, recognizing the patterns), and making conclusions specifically about the problem (diagnosis) so that she can act appropriately. Using critical thinking, Tonya considers what is important in the clinical situation (based on knowledge and experience), imagines and explores alternatives (what to assess further), considers

ethical principles (patient choice about pain control), identifies the patient's problems (pain and mobility), and makes informed decisions about the care of the patient. Tonya forms a clinical judgment by applying **critical thinking**, the ability to think in a systematic and logical manner with openness to question and reflect on the reasoning process. This systematic approach allows her to make appropriate clinical decisions in the patient's care. The aim of critical thinking is the ability to focus on the important issues in any clinical situation and make decisions that produce desired patient outcomes, such as reduced pain and improved mobility for Tonya's patient. *Tonya first learned about the importance of early mobility after surgery when she read the nursing and scientific literature on the concept of mobility and deconditioning. She also learned that pain reduces mobility when she cared for previous patients. When immobility is prolonged, patients become susceptible to complications such as deep vein thrombosis and pneumonia. Applying this knowledge, Tonya decides to implement pain relief measures first so that her patient can become more mobile.*

Critical thinkers question, are honest in facing personal biases, and examine information for answers and deeper meanings in order to understand their patients (Chan, 2013). When core critical thinking competencies are applied, the complex and continuous nature of decision making and clinical judgment becomes clear (Table 15.1). Critical thinking is a way of thinking about clinical situations by asking questions such as:

- Why does the patient have this condition?
- How does the condition normally affect a patient physically and psychologically?
- Are the signs and symptoms shown by the patient what I would expect for the condition or situation?
- Are there signs and symptoms associated with worsening of the condition?
- What do I really know about this patient's situation?
- What other ways can I collect data to help me understand the problem more fully?
- Do I require more information?
- What care options do I have?

When making accurate clinical judgments, nurses rely on a critical thinking process that involves open-mindedness, continual inquiry, and perseverance, combined with a willingness to look at each unique patient situation and determine which identified assumptions are true and relevant. The **nursing process** is described by the American Nurses Association (ANA) as the framework nurses use to apply critical thinking in nursing practice for making clinical decisions (ANA, 2021).

TABLE 15.1	Critical Thinking and Clinical Judgment Skills
Skill	**Nursing Practice Applications**
Interpretation	Be orderly in collecting data about patients. Apply reasoning while looking for patterns to emerge. Categorize the data (e.g., nursing diagnoses [see Chapter 17]). Gather additional data and clarify any data about which you are uncertain.
Analysis	Be open-minded as you analyze information about a patient. Do not make careless assumptions. Do the data reveal a problem or trend that you believe is true, or are there other options?
Inference	Look at the meaning and significance of findings. Are there relationships among findings? Do data about the patient help you see that a problem exists?
Evaluation	Look at all situations objectively. Use objective criteria (e.g., expected outcomes, pain characteristics, learning objectives) to determine results of nursing actions. Reflect on your own behavior.
Explanation	Support your findings and conclusions. Use knowledge and experience to choose strategies to use in the care of patients.
Self-regulation	Reflect on your experiences. Be responsible for connecting your actions with outcomes. Identify the ways you can improve your own performance. What will make you believe that you have been successful?

Adapted from Facione P: Critical thinking: a statement of expert consensus for purposes of educational assessment and instruction. The Delphi report: research findings and recommendations prepared for the American Philosophical Association, ERIC Doc No. ED 315, Washington, DC, 1990, ERIC; and Tanner CA: Thinking like a nurse: a research-based model of clinical judgment in nursing, *J Nurs Educ* 45(6):204, 2006.

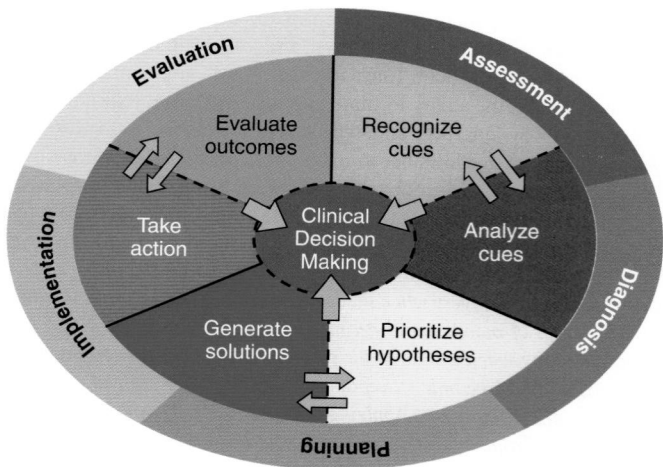

The ANA describes the process as including six steps: assessment, diagnosis, outcome identification, planning, implementation, and evaluation (ANA, 2021). For this text the steps of planning and outcome identification are combined (Fig. 15.2). Six cognitive skills interact, enabling nurses to apply the nursing process in clinical decision making (Dickison et al., 2019). The six cognitive skills are: recognize cues, analyze cues, prioritize problems/diagnoses, generate solutions, take actions, and evaluate outcomes (NCSBN, 2019).

The purpose of the nursing process is to diagnose and treat human responses (e.g., patient symptoms, need for knowledge) to patients' health problems. It encompasses significant actions taken by RNs and forms the foundation of the nurse's clinical decision making (ANA, 2021). Use of the process allows nurses to help patients meet agreed-on outcomes for better health. The format for the nursing process is unique to the discipline of nursing and provides a common language

and process for nurses to "think through" patients' clinical problems (Kataoka-Yahiro and Saylor, 1994). The nursing process requires a nurse to use general and specific critical thinking competencies.

CRITICAL THINKING COMPETENCIES

Critical thinking competencies are the cognitive processes a nurse uses to make judgments about the clinical care of patients (Kataoka-Yahiro and Saylor, 1994). These include general critical thinking, specific critical thinking in clinical situations, and specific critical thinking in nursing. General critical thinking processes are not unique to nursing. They include the scientific method, problem solving, and decision making. Specific critical thinking competencies include diagnostic reasoning and clinical decision making. The specific critical thinking competency in nursing is the nursing process, which incorporates each of the specific critical thinking competencies. Details on performing each step of the nursing process are covered in Chapters 16 through 20.

General Critical Thinking

Scientific Method. The scientific method is a methodical way to solve problems by using reasoning. It is a systematic, ordered approach to gather data and solve problems. Health care researchers, including nurse scientists, use the scientific method when testing research questions (see Chapter 5). The scientific method has five steps:
1. Identify the problem.
2. Collect data.
3. Formulate a question or hypothesis.
4. Test the question or hypothesis.
5. Evaluate results of the test or study.
   Table 15.2 offers an example of a nursing practice issue solved by applying the scientific method in a research study.

Problem Solving. Patients routinely present problems in nursing practice. For example, a home care nurse learns that a patient has difficulty taking her medications regularly. The patient is unable to describe which medications she has taken for the past 3 days. The medication bottles are

TABLE 15.2	Using the Scientific Method to Solve Nursing Practice Questions
Clinical Problem: The incidence of a health care–associated infection (HAI), *Clostridium difficile* infection, has increased on a hospital general medicine unit. The nursing staff on the unit practice committee, an infection control specialist, and a clinical nurse specialist in medicine meet to discuss factors that may be contributing to the problem. They note that visitors are inconsistent in the use of antiseptic hand rubs. A staff member questions whether the use of hand rubs is the best approach for this type of infection.	
Identify the problem.	The incidence of *C. difficile* has increased among patients on a general medicine unit.
Collect data.	Staff members review the literature about the nature of *C. difficile* infection and the hand-hygiene antiseptic techniques recommended to prevent the infection. Staff members search the literature for studies that have investigated hand-hygiene practices of visitors of hospitalized patients. Staff members review performance improvement reports to monitor the occurrence of *C. difficile* on the unit. The infection control specialist is asked to discuss the trends within the hospital in the incidence of *C. difficile*.
Form a research question to study the problem.	Does visitor use of antiseptic hand rub with chlorhexidine versus handwashing with soap and water reduce incidence of *C. difficile* infection in medical patients?
Answer the question.	The nurse specialist and a small team of staff members create a 4-month study approved by the hospital research board. Patients' visitors are asked to use a chlorhexidine rub on their hands before entering and leaving patient rooms. Visitors then switch to handwashing with soap and water the last 2 months of the study. The infection control specialist tracks the incidence of *C. difficile* infection over the 4 months of the study.
Evaluate the results of the study. Does the study answer the research question?	Compare the incidence of *C. difficile* infection for the 2-month period when each hand-hygiene method was used.

labeled and filled. The nurse must solve the problem of why the patient is not following her medication schedule. The nurse knows that when the patient was discharged from the hospital, she had five medications ordered. The patient tells the nurse that she also takes two over-the-counter medications regularly. When the nurse asks her to show the medications that she takes in the morning, the nurse notices that the patient has difficulty seeing the medication labels. The patient can describe the medications that she is to take but is uncertain about the times of administration. The nurse recognizes a problem and recommends having the patient's pharmacy relabel the medications in larger lettering. In addition, the nurse shows the patient examples of pill organizers that will help her sort her medications by time of day for a period of 7 days.

A problem is an unsettled state. Effective **problem solving** requires you to obtain information that clarifies the nature of a problem, suggest possible solutions, and try the solution over time to evaluate that it is effective. In the case of patient care, a solution is an action for a problem. It should be consistently effective so the patient can return to a stable condition or situation. It becomes necessary to try different options if a problem recurs. From the previous example, during a follow-up visit the nurse finds that the patient has organized her medications correctly and is able to read the labels without difficulty. The nurse obtained information that correctly clarified the cause of the patient's problem and tested a solution that proved successful. Having solved a problem in one situation adds to a nurse's experience in practice, which allows the nurse to apply that knowledge in future patient situations (Papathanasiou et al., 2014).

Intuition is one problem-solving approach that relies on one's inner sense. It is the ability to understand something immediately, without the need for conscious reasoning. Intuitive thinking is commonly invoked for well-structured and familiar decision tasks, whereas analytic thinking is triggered for ill-structured and unfamiliar decision tasks (Dickison et al., 2019). For example, we think automatically when we carry out daily routines, but we must consciously think about new tasks or ones that are posing challenges to complete. Intuition is often perceived as being a form of guessing and thus inappropriate when making nursing decisions. However, others view intuition as a legitimate approach to making clinical judgments. Tanner (2006) explained that less experienced nurses, including students, may rely more heavily on analytic reasoning, whereas experienced nurses are more likely to use intuitive reasoning based on their clinical experiences with numerous patients. Experienced nurses sense "red flags" when something goes wrong with a patient, when something just does not look right. Perhaps they have seen the problem before (such as a wound that is separating and forming yellow drainage), or they know to anticipate a problem because of their knowledge base. Responding intuitively enables quick action, but it must then be complemented with thoughtful reasoning and judgment to ensure the proper response has occurred. Intuition is not recommended for beginning nurses because your cognitive level and clinical experience are incomplete and do not allow for valid intuitive decisions (Papathanasiou et al., 2014).

Decision Making. When you face a problem and choose a course of action from several options, you are making a decision. Basic decision making goes hand in hand with problem solving and problem resolution. Following a set of criteria helps you make a thorough and thoughtful decision. The criteria may be personal, based on an organizational policy or standard or, in the case of nursing, based on a professional standard (e.g., ethical standard, standard for confidentiality).

For example, a person makes a decision when choosing a health care provider. The individual must first recognize and define the problem (the need for a health care provider) and assess all options

(e.g., consider a recommended health care provider or choose one whose office is close to home). The person weighs each option against a set of personal criteria (experience, friendliness, reputation, location), tests possible options (talks directly with the different health care providers), considers the consequences of the decision (examines pros and cons of selecting one provider over another), and makes a final decision. Although the set of criteria follows a sequence of steps, decision making involves moving back and forth when considering all criteria. This process leads to informed conclusions that are supported by evidence and reason.

Specific Critical Thinking

Diagnostic Reasoning. Once Tonya gathered information about Mr. Lawson's discomfort and mobility limitation in the case study, **diagnostic reasoning** began. Diagnostic reasoning is a form of decision making that involves being able to understand and think through clinical problems, gather information about the problem, analyze clues or individual cues, understand the meaning of evidence, and know when there is enough information (pattern of data) to make an accurate diagnosis (Resnick, 2016). Once a diagnosis is made, one considers different causes of the problem and then decides on the interventions that best meet the needs of a patient (Resnick, 2016). Accurate problem recognition (e.g., nursing diagnosis, collaborative problem) is necessary before choosing solutions and implementing action. The National Academies of Sciences, Engineering, and Medicine (2015) reports that the right diagnosis is a key aspect of health care because it explains a patient's health problem(s) and informs subsequent health care decisions. It requires you to assign meaning to the behaviors and physical signs and symptoms presented by a patient. *For example, Tonya enters Mr. Lawson's room and finds him to be restless and short of breath, and he tells her, "I have this terrible pain in my chest." What might such a change indicate?* Diagnostic reasoning begins when you interact with a patient or make physical or behavioral observations. An expert nurse sees the context of a patient situation (e.g., Mr. Lawson just had major surgery; has been inactive; and is at risk for blood pooling in the lower extremities, which can cause clots to form in the circulation and then break off and travel to the lung). The nurse observes patterns and themes (e.g., symptoms that include shortness of breath, sharp chest pain, a cough that produces pink mucus, and irregular heart rate), and makes a clinical judgment quickly (e.g., a clot may have dislodged and traveled to the lung's circulation, requiring a quick medical response). The information that a nurse collects and analyzes leads to a diagnosis of a patient's condition (e.g., nursing diagnosis of *Impaired Gas Exchange*). Nurses do not make medical diagnoses, but they do assess and monitor each patient closely and compare a patient's signs and symptoms with those that are common to a medical diagnosis (e.g., in the case of Mr. Lawson, a pulmonary embolus). Nurses think critically to form nursing diagnoses (see Chapter 17). Through diagnostic reasoning, nurses understand the nature of a problem and the patient's response through data assessment and analysis to enable selection of proper therapies.

Often you cannot make a precise diagnosis during your first meeting with a patient. Sometimes you sense that a problem exists but do not have enough data to make a specific diagnosis. Some patients' physical conditions limit their ability to tell you about symptoms. Others choose to not share sensitive and important information during your initial assessment. Some patients' behaviors and physical responses become observable only under conditions not present during your initial assessment. How you interpret this information is part of critical thinking and clinical judgment. When uncertain of a diagnosis, continue to collect data. Critically analyze changing clinical situations until you can determine a patient's unique situation. Any diagnostic conclusions that you make will help health care providers identify the nature of a problem more quickly and select appropriate medical therapies.

Clinical Decision Making. When you face a clinical problem involving a patient and need to choose a course of action from several options, you are making clinical decisions. Clinical decision making focuses on resolving a patient's problem such as a nursing diagnosis (see Chapter 17) (see Fig. 15.1). When you approach a clinical problem, such as a patient who is less mobile and develops an area of redness over the hip, you make a clinical decision that identifies a patient problem (impaired skin integrity in the form of a pressure injury), and through clinical judgment you choose the best nursing interventions (e.g., skin care, special bed surface, and a turning schedule). Nurses make clinical decisions all the time to improve a patient's health or maintain wellness by reducing the severity of the problem or resolving the problem completely.

Effective clinical decision making requires inductive and deductive reasoning and making valid inferences. A nurse faces a problem or situation by critically analyzing data to determine important information and ideas and then discards unnecessary data until a later time (Papathanasiou et al., 2014). Following a set of questions or criteria about the data helps a nurse make thorough and thoughtful decisions (Box 15.1). Socratic questioning is a technique for looking beneath the surface, recognizing and examining assumptions, searching for inconsistencies, examining multiple points of view and biases, and differentiating what one knows from what one merely believes (Papathanasiou et al., 2014). These types of questions are common when a nurse completes an end of shift or reviews a patient's history and progress.

After you answer decision-making questions, you begin to form inferences. A set of assessment facts (e.g., objective clinical findings, diagnostic test results) and observations about a patient leads you to begin making generalizations and to then perform inductive reasoning. When viewed together, the facts and observations suggest a particular interpretation. Inductive reasoning moves from reviewing specific data elements to making an inference by forming a conclusion about the related pieces of evidence. Previous experience with the evidence is also considered. For example, a nurse who observes a patient who has weakness of lower extremities, an unsteady gait, and a previous history of a fall considers previous patients cared for and concludes that this specific patient is at risk for falling. In contrast, deductive reasoning moves from the general to the specific. A nurse will start analysis of the facts and observations from a conceptual viewpoint, such as prioritization of needs according to Nola Pender's health promotion model (see Chapter 6). After collecting data based on the conceptual view, the nurse forms an inference and eventually interprets the patient's condition with respect to that conceptual view (Papathanasiou et al., 2014).

Skilled clinical decision making occurs through knowing the patient (Zolnierek, 2014). Knowing the patient is an in-depth knowledge of a patient's patterns of responses within a clinical situation and knowing the patient as a person (Tanner et al., 1993). It has been found to also apply in health care disciplines other than nursing (McCullough et al., 2016). Although nurses use prior clinical experiences and interactions with patients as key sources of knowledge, these sources are limited for nurses with less experience and in care situations in which the patient's ability to interact may be affected by developmental or cultural factors. Nonetheless, you need to know your patients to develop your clinical expertise. Knowing a patient has two components: a nurse's understanding of a specific patient, and the subsequent selection of interventions. It relates to a nurse's experience with caring for patients, time spent in a specific clinical area, and having a sense of closeness with patients (see Chapter 7). For example, an expert nurse who has worked on a general surgery unit for many years has cared for a patient for the past 2 days. The nurse is familiar with how the patient is progressing physically and mentally. When the patient begins to experience a change (e.g., a slight fall in blood pressure, becoming less responsive), the nurse knows that something is wrong, suspects the patient may be bleeding internally, and takes action. Because of the nurse's clinical experience and knowing the patient, the expert nurse can make a clinical decision and act more quickly than a new nurse can be expected to act.

Knowing the patient offers a nurse "the big picture" and "knowing the whole person" so that suitable patient-centered decisions can be made to protect patients from harm. A critical aspect to knowing patients and thus being able to make timely and appropriate decisions is spending time establishing relationships with them (Zolnierek, 2014). Forming relationships builds your ability to make clinical decisions and enhances your ability to know your patients. Follow these tips:

- Spend enough time during initial and follow-up patient assessments to observe patient behavior and measure physical and psychosocial findings to improve knowledge of your patients. Determine what is important to them and make a positive emotional connection. Patients perceive meaningful time as that involving personal rather than task-oriented conversation.
- Know trends and normative patterns in a patient's clinical condition over time so that you can identify when patients require a change in their treatment plan (Kelley et al., 2013).
- Know a patient's typical behaviors, schedules, and preferences at home to help guide you with their stay in a hospital or extended care setting (Kelley et al., 2013). This allows you to adjust and provide individualized patient-centered care.
- When talking with patients, listen to their accounts of their experiences with illness, watch them, and come to understand how they typically respond (Tanner, 2006).
- Consistently check on patients to assess and monitor problems to help you identify how clinical changes develop over time.
- Ask to have the same patient assigned to you over consecutive days. A nurse-patient relationship develops from getting to know a patient and building a foundation for connecting on the first day

---

BOX 15.1   Clinical Decision-Making Questions

Questions About a Problem
- Is the problem clear and understandable?
- Is the problem important or a priority in the patient's care?
- What does the problem mean to the patient?

Questions About Your Perspective
- Are you looking at the problem from the view of _____? Why?
- How might someone with an opposite view see the problem?
- How does your view compare with that of the patient?

Questions About Assumptions
- You are assuming _____. How does that affect your analysis of the problem? Does it bias you?
- What might you assume instead? Is there another option?

Questions About Evidence
- What evidence (data about patient, scientific evidence about the type of problem) supports your assumption?
- Is there a reason to doubt the evidence? Does it apply to this specific situation?
- What further evidence is needed?

of care, to deepening understanding of the patient and being able to recognize clinical changes on subsequent days.

- Engaging patients in conversations and being able to care for them over time (e.g., days or visits) develops knowing and nurse-patient relationships (Zolnierek, 2014).

Making accurate patient-centered clinical decisions requires you to prioritize your nursing interventions (see Chapter 18). Do not assume that certain health situations produce automatic priorities. For example, a patient who has surgery is anticipated to experience a certain level of postoperative pain, which often becomes a priority for care. However, if the same patient is having severe anxiety that increases pain perception, you need to focus on ways to relieve the anxiety before pain-relief measures will be effective.

Clinical decision making is complicated, especially when nurses work in settings where they are assigned to multiple patients in fast-paced and unpredictable environments. To prioritize patient problems in such situations, use decision criteria that include factors such as the clinical condition of the patient, an examination of the advantages and disadvantages of each option, Maslow's hierarchy of needs (see Chapter 6), the risks involved in treatment delays, environmental factors (time and staff resources available for delegation), and patients' expectations of care to determine which patients have the greatest priorities. For example, a patient who is having a sudden drop in blood pressure along with a change in consciousness requires your immediate attention as opposed to a patient who needs you to collect a urine specimen or one who needs your help to walk down the hallway. Critical thinking in decision making allows you to attend to a patient whose condition is changing quickly and delegate the specimen collection and ambulation to AP. For you to manage the wide variety of problems associated with groups of patients, skillful, prioritized clinical decision making is critical (Box 15.2).

REFLECT NOW

Consider a patient you have been assigned to recently. Based on that individual patient's needs and health problems, what evidence-based information might you seek to provide evidence-based nursing care?

BOX 15.2 Clinical Decision Making for Groups of Patients

- Identify the nursing diagnoses and collaborative problems of each patient (see Chapter 17).
- Analyze the diagnoses/problems and decide which are most urgent based on basic needs, the patients' changing or unstable status, and problem complexity (see Chapter 18).
- Consider the time it will take to care for patients whose problems are of high priority (e.g., do you have the time to restart a critical intravenous [IV] line when medication is due for a different patient?).
- Consider the resources you have to manage each problem, assistive personnel (AP) assigned with you, other health care providers, and patients' family members.
- Involve patients and/or their family as decision makers and participants in care.
- Decide how to combine activities to resolve more than one patient problem at a time.
- Decide which, if any, nursing care procedures to delegate to AP so that you can spend your time on activities requiring professional nursing knowledge.
- Discuss complex cases with other members of the health care team. This ensures a smooth transition in care throughout a patient's health care experience.

LEVELS OF CRITICAL THINKING

Your ability as a nurse to develop and apply critical thinking when making clinical judgments evolves over time. The three levels of critical thinking describe how critical thinking develops (Box 15.3).

Basic Critical Thinking

Beginning nursing students are task oriented. For example, they focus on performing skills and organizing nursing care activities rather than delivering skills within the context of their patients' specific clinical situations. At the basic level of critical thinking a learner trusts that experts have the right answers for every problem. Thinking is concrete and based on a set of rules or principles. For example, as a nursing student you use a hospital procedure manual to confirm how to change an intravenous (IV) dressing. You will follow the procedure step by step without adjusting it to meet a patient's unique needs (e.g., positioning to minimize the patient's pain or mobility restrictions). Your inexperience does not allow you to anticipate how to individualize the procedure when problems arise. A basic critical thinker learns to accept the diverse opinions and values of experts (e.g., instructors and staff nurse preceptors). However, inexperience, weak competencies, and inflexible attitudes restrict a person's ability to move to the next level of critical thinking (Erickson, 2017).

Complex Critical Thinking

Complex critical thinkers begin to rely less on experts and instead trust their own decisions. For example, while teaching a patient how to use an inhaler, you recognize that your patient cannot deliver a dose correctly. Rather than refer to a procedure manual and repeat the same approach, you adapt by offering an inhaler the patient can activate and instruct the patient on how to better coordinate inhaling with delivery of a medication dose. You analyze the clinical situation (e.g., weakness in patient's hands) and examine choices more independently. Critical thinking combined

BOX 15.3 Levels of Critical Thinking

Basic

- Answers to complex problems are perceived as either right or wrong (e.g., when an intravenous [IV] fluid is not infusing correctly, the rate must be regulated correctly).
- A single solution usually resolves each problem (e.g., adjusting the rate instead of trying to position the patient's arm to prevent catheter kinking).
- This is an early step in developing critical thinking.

Complex

- Make clinical decisions more independently.
- Creativity allows nurses to generate many ideas quickly, be able to change viewpoints, and create original solutions to problems.
- Thinking abilities and initiative to look beyond expert opinion begin to change.
- Learn that alternative and perhaps conflicting solutions exist.
- Consider different options from routine procedures.
- Gather additional information and take a variety of different approaches for the same therapy.

Commitment

- Able to consider wider array of clinical alternatives for a patient's situation.
- Recognize that sometimes a proper action is the decision to not act or to delay an action until a later time based on experience and knowledge.
- Able to apply all elements of clinical judgment model almost automatically.

with creativity allows nurses to become more flexible and find original solutions to specific problems when traditional interventions are not effective (Papathanasiou et al., 2014).

When Tonya enters Mr. Lawson's room and finds him to be restless and short of breath, and he tells her, "I have this terrible pain in my chest," she thinks critically. She wonders if something other than the abdominal incision is causing Mr. Lawson's discomfort. She asks Mr. Lawson, "Is the pain you're feeling now different from before I gave you your medication?" The patient tells her that the pain feels sharper, in his chest. Tonya quickly takes a set of vital signs. His heart rate, which was 88 and regular 1 hour ago, is now 102 and irregular. Tonya calls the physician and notifies her of the changes in Mr. Lawson's condition.

Tonya thought outside the box. Rather than assume that Mr. Lawson's continued pain was from his incision, she gathered more data and recognized that the patient possibly was experiencing a life-threatening condition, a pulmonary embolus.

In complex critical thinking each solution has benefits and risks that you weigh before making a final decision. There are options. Thinking becomes more innovative.

Commitment

The third level of critical thinking is commitment (Kataoka-Yahiro and Saylor, 1994). At this level you anticipate when to make choices without assistance from others and accept accountability for decisions made. As a nurse you do more than just consider the complex alternatives that a problem poses. At the commitment level you decide on an action or belief that is based on the available alternatives and support it. Because you take accountability for the decision, you consider the results of the decision and determine whether it was appropriate.

COMPONENTS OF CRITICAL THINKING IN THE CLINICAL JUDGMENT MODEL

The model for clinical judgment presented in this text defines the outcome of critical thinking through the application of the nursing process as clinical judgment. Patient needs initiate the process of clinical judgment, and clinical decisions complete the process (Dickison et al., 2019). The model is relevant to patients' health care problems in a variety of health care settings. The model includes six components of critical thinking in nursing judgment: critical thinking competence (e.g., diagnostic reasoning and clinical decision-making ability), knowledge, experience, environment, attitudes, and standards. The six components combined guide nurses in making sound clinical judgments necessary for relevant and appropriate clinical decisions (Box 15.4). Throughout this text the model helps you to apply critical thinking while using the nursing process. Graphic illustration of the model in the clinical chapters shows you how to apply critical thinking in assessing patients, planning and delivering interventions, and evaluating the results. Applying elements of the model will help you become a more confident and effective professional.

Competence

The critical thinking competencies discussed earlier are essential cognitive processes that guide nurses in applying the nursing process in making accurate clinical judgments. There is an additional competence—the ability to perform nursing skills (e.g., hands-on procedures, physical examination techniques) proficiently (see Chapter 19). When you are still a basic critical thinker you will perform skills carefully and cautiously following policy and procedure. Skills can create a distraction, making it difficult for you as a new nurse to focus on applying the nursing process in an individualized and systematic way. When you become more adept at gathering patient-centered data, identifying patient

BOX 15.4   Components of Critical Thinking in Nursing

I. Critical thinking competence
II. Specific knowledge base
   A. Patient data
   B. Basic and nursing science
   C. Nursing and health care theory
III. Experience
   A. Personal
   B. Clinical practice
   C. Skill competence
IV. Environment
   Time pressure, setting, task, complexity, interruptions
V. Attitudes for critical thinking
   Confidence, independence, fairness, responsibility, risk taking, discipline, perseverance, creativity, curiosity, intellectual integrity, humility
VI. Standards for critical thinking
   A. Intellectual standards
   Clear, precise, specific, accurate, relevant, plausible, consistent, logical, deep, broad, complete, significant, adequate, and fair
   B. Professional standards
      1. Standards of practice
      2. Ethical criteria for nursing judgment
      3. Criteria for evaluation
      4. Professional responsibility

Adapted from Kataoka-Yahiro M, Saylor C: A critical thinking model for nursing judgment, *J Nurs Educ* 33(8):351, 1994; data from Paul RW: The art of redesigning instruction. In Willsen J, Blinker AJA, editors: *Critical thinking: how to prepare students for a rapidly changing world,* Santa Rosa, CA, 1993, Foundation for Critical Thinking; data from National Council of State Boards of Nursing (NCSBN): *Next Generation NCLEX News: Clinical Judgment Measurement Model,* Winter 2019. https://www.ncsbn.org/NGN_Winter19.pdf.

problems, and planning appropriate nursing interventions, you evolve into a complex critical thinker. At that point nursing skills become more like second nature and are adapted to each patient's unique needs. You will develop competence as you continue to practice and perform nursing skills.

Knowledge Base

A nurse's knowledge base varies according to educational experience that includes basic nursing education, continuing education courses, and additional college degrees. A nurse also builds knowledge by reading the nursing literature (especially research-based literature) to maintain current knowledge of nursing science and theory. Evidence-based knowledge, or knowledge based on research or clinical expertise, makes nurses better informed critical thinkers (see Chapter 5). Thinking critically and learning about scientific concepts prepares you to better anticipate and identify patient problems by understanding their origin and nature.

A nurse's knowledge base includes information and theory from the basic sciences, humanities, behavioral sciences, and nursing science. Nurses apply this knowledge in a different way than in other health care disciplines because they think holistically about patient problems. For example, a nurse's broad knowledge base offers a physical, psychological, social, moral, ethical, and cultural view of patients and their health care needs. The depth and extent of scientific knowledge influence a nurse's ability to think critically about nursing problems.

REFLECT NOW

Ask a nurse who works in one of the health care agencies where you have clinicals to spend a moment talking to you about knowing patients. Ask the nurse what they do to know patients. Also discuss the barriers that make knowing patients difficult.

The most critical source of knowledge a nurse applies in critical thinking is patient data. Chapter 16 explores in depth the scope and breadth of patient information needed to fully understand a patient's clinical condition and living situation. Patient data include:

- Observations of patient behavior and clinical signs
- Direct physical examination
- Interviews with patient and family caregivers
- Medical record resources
- Diagnostic data

A complex or committed clinical thinker gathers a thorough but also an appropriate patient-centered database. This means the nurse does not simply gather patient data based on preselected categories found on an assessment recording form. Instead, the nurse applies scientific knowledge to anticipate what assessment data are required for a specific patient. For example, if a patient is known to have diabetes mellitus, a nurse will apply knowledge about the effects of this metabolic disorder and will attend more closely to the patient's actual or expected clinical signs and symptoms. A patient with diabetes mellitus is at risk for circulatory problems, so the nurse assesses peripheral pulses and condition of any existing wound (is it healing?). A patient with diabetes mellitus is also at risk for visual alterations, so a more extensive examination of vision is needed compared with a patient with no known visual risks.

Patient data guide a nurse during assessment. Each piece of data raises questions about the nature of a patient's problem and what additional data are needed. It also creates a picture of an individual and what makes that individual unique. Critical thinking applies knowledge to eventually identify patient problems correctly and promotes a patient-centered approach to care.

Tonya previously earned a bachelor's degree in education and taught high school for 1 year. She is now in her second year as an RN. She is taking additional classes to further her education, including courses in health ethics and population health. Her experience as a staff nurse has allowed her to develop knowledge about a variety of surgical procedures, the effects of different medications, and physical and psychological responses patients typically show to their treatment.

Experience

Nursing is a practice discipline. Clinical learning experiences are necessary to acquire decision-making skills and clinical judgment and to gain competence in performing nursing skills. In clinical situations you learn from observing, sensing, talking with patients and families, providing hands-on care, and reflecting actively on all experiences. Clinical experience is the laboratory for developing and testing approaches that you safely adapt or revise to fit the setting, a patient's unique qualities, and the experiences you have from caring for previous patients. Research has shown that a clinical environment that is safe and encourages free discussion and expression of thought promotes critical thinking (Chan, 2013). With experience you begin to understand clinical situations, anticipate and recognize cues from patients' health data, and interpret the patterns of data as relevant or irrelevant. As experience develops you will identify and build your personal set of cases with identifiable patterns and typical outcomes that can provide valuable background knowledge when dealing with a

current situation (National Health Service [NHS], n.d.). Experience with nursing skills teaches you how to adapt a skill without sacrificing safe principles. Learn to value all patient experiences. Each experience is a stepping stone for building new knowledge, obtaining skills, and inspiring innovative thinking.

When Tonya was finishing her last year in nursing school, she worked as an assistive personnel in a nursing home. She spent considerable time interacting with older-adult patients and giving basic nursing care. Each patient provided her with valuable learning experiences, which she applied in her work with other patients as an RN. Specifically, she developed good interviewing skills, gained an understanding of the importance of the family in an individual's health, and learned to become a patient advocate. She also learned that older adults need more time to perform activities such as eating and bathing; therefore she has adapted these skill techniques.

Environment

Environmental factors (e.g., task complexity, time pressure, work setting, and interruptions) influence clinical decision making (Muntean, 2012). Critical thinking does not occur in a void. Nurses process patient data and knowledge applicable to patients' situations and then critically make judgments, all within the context of patients' conditions and environmental factors. Task complexity is an example. A patient with multiple health problems and/or one who requires numerous nursing procedures performed in a short period of time threatens clinical decision making. Task complexity affects the presentation of cues or patient data, which indirectly affects the decision maker (Muntean, 2012). If a nurse feels time pressure, either because another patient requires attention or because a procedure is due (e.g., medication), attention to making a clear decision is threatened. As a patient's clinical condition changes, expert nurses are able to recognize the change more quickly, consider knowledge pertaining to the situation, judge whether information is adequate, and attend to making a clear decision. An expert nurse will consider the risks and consequences if actions are not taken to improve a patient's clinical course. The more complex a patient and the more frequently clinical changes are displayed, the more challenging it is to be an effective critical thinker.

Timeliness in making decisions affects patient outcomes. A study involving hospitalized patients showed that 60% of cardiac arrests sustained by inpatients could have been prevented, with nearly half of those cases showing clinical signs of deterioration recorded in the preceding 24 hours, but not acted on (as cited in Muntean, 2012). When making a clinical decision you must act in a timely manner when you see a pattern of data suggesting a problem that requires immediate action. A nurse learns the team dynamics of a health care setting, including how and when to communicate, who the leaders of the team are, and expectations the team has for managing problems. Whether a health care setting encourages autonomy is also a factor. Patient harm will occur if you hesitate and do not act on your diagnostic conclusions or judgment.

Tips for critical thinking within the health care environment context include (NHS, n.d.):

- Use the data you have gathered to enlist help, support, and advice from colleagues and the wider interprofessional team.
- Know your own limitations and when you need help.
- Collaborate with colleagues, listen, and be respectful of their ideas.
- Make judgments and prioritize these judgments based on the current patient and do not be distracted by other patients or tasks at the moment.
- Identify a role model who you believe is a competent decision maker. Watch and question how your role model makes decisions: How does your role model find out the information that is needed, make judgments, and decide on a course of action?

Critical Thinking Attitudes

The fifth component of critical thinking is attitudes. Paul (1993) defined 11 attitudes that define the central features of a critical thinker and how a successful critical thinker approaches a problem (see Box 15.4). In a consensus statement on critical thinking in nursing, an international panel of nurse experts defined additional attitudes that included contextual perspective, flexibility, and open-mindedness (Scheffer and Rubenfeld, 2000). Papathanasiou et al. (2014) also describe spiritual courage as a critical thinking attitude.

Mr. Lawson is displaying anxiety. His shortness of breath continues, and Tonya informs him that medical staff are on their way to confirm the nature of his breathing problem. Tonya will display curiosity by seeking further information. Tonya will also use discipline in forming questions and conducting a thorough assessment to find the source of the patient's anxiety.

Attitudes of inquiry involve an ability to recognize that problems exist, to consider the context of those problems, and to recognize that there is a need for evidence to support what you think is true. Critical thinking attitudes are guidelines for how to approach a problem and make the correct decision. Knowing when you need more information, knowing when information is misleading, and recognizing your own knowledge limits are examples of how critical thinking attitudes guide decision making. Table 15.3 summarizes the use of critical thinking attitudes in nursing practice.

Confidence. Confidence is the belief in oneself, one's judgment and psychomotor skills, and one's possession of the knowledge and the ability to think critically. When you are confident, you feel certain about accomplishing a task or goal such as performing a procedure or making a diagnosis. Confidence grows with experience in recognizing your strengths and limitations. You shift your focus from your own needs (e.g., remembering what assessment data mean or how to perform a procedure) to a patient's needs. When you are not confident in knowing whether a patient is clinically changing or in performing a nursing skill, you become anxious about not knowing what to do and may hesitate to make a necessary decision. Always be aware of the extent and limits of your knowledge. If you question the meaning of a clinical situation and you do not know whether the information you have is important, discuss it with your nursing instructor first. Never perform a procedure unless you have the knowledge base and feel confident. Patient safety is a priority. When you are confident, your patients recognize it by how you communicate and the way you perform nursing care. Confidence builds trust between you and your patients.

TABLE 15.3 Critical Thinking Attitudes and Applications in Nursing Practice

Critical Thinking Attitude	Application in Practice
Confidence	The nurse, gaining more experience in reasoning and decision making, does not hesitate to disagree and be troubled, thereby acting as a role model to colleagues (Papathanasiou et al., 2014). Speak with conviction to a patient when you begin an intervention. Do not lead a patient to think that you are unable to perform care safely. Always be well prepared before performing a nursing activity. Encourage a patient to ask questions.
Thinking independently	As you acquire new knowledge and experiences, examine your beliefs under new evidence (Papathanasiou et al., 2014). Be open-minded about different interventions. Read the scientific literature, especially when there are different views on the same subject. Talk with other nurses and share ideas about nursing interventions.
Fairness	Listen to both sides of a discussion. If a patient or family member complains about a co-worker, listen to the story, and speak with the co-worker as well. If a staff member labels a patient uncooperative, assume the care of that patient with openness and a desire to meet the patient's needs.
Responsibility and authority	Ask for help if you are uncertain about how to perform a nursing skill. Refer to a policy and procedure manual to review steps of a skill. Report any problems immediately. Follow standards of practice in your care.
Risk taking	If your knowledge causes you to question a health care provider's order, do so. Be willing to recommend alternative approaches to nursing care when colleagues are having little success with patients, especially if your ideas are supported by scientific evidence.
Discipline	Be thorough in whatever you do. Use known scientific and practice-based criteria for activities such as assessment and evaluation. Take time to be thorough and manage your time effectively.
Perseverance	Be cautious of an easy answer that avoids uncomfortable situations. If co-workers give you information about a patient and some fact seems to be missing, clarify the information or talk to the patient directly. If problems of the same type continue to occur on a nursing division, bring co-workers together, look for a pattern, and find a solution.
Creativity	Look for different approaches if interventions are not working for a patient. For example, a patient in pain may need a different positioning or distraction technique. When appropriate, involve the patient's family in adapting your approaches to care methods used at home.
Curiosity	Always ask why. Be willing to challenge tradition. A clinical sign or symptom often indicates a variety of problems. Explore and learn more about a patient so as to make appropriate clinical judgments.
Integrity	Recognize when your opinions conflict with those of a patient; review your position and decide how best to proceed to reach outcomes that will satisfy everyone. Do not compromise nursing standards or honesty in delivering nursing care.
Humility	Recognize when you need more information to make a decision. When you are new to a clinical division, ask for an orientation to the area. Ask registered nurses (RNs) regularly assigned to the area for assistance with approaches to care.

Thinking Independently. As you gain new knowledge, you learn to consider a wide range of ideas and concepts before making a judgment. You are not limited by what you learn in school but become open-minded to new concepts and interventions (Papathanasiou et al., 2014). This does not mean that you ignore other people's ideas. Instead, you learn to consider all sides of a situation. A critical thinker does not accept another person's ideas without question. When thinking independently, you challenge the ways that others think, and you look for rational and logical answers to problems. You raise important questions about your practice. For example, why is one type of surgical dressing ordered over another, or why do patients on your nursing unit fall? When nurses ask questions and look for the evidence behind clinical problems, they are thinking independently; this is an important aspect of evidence-based practice (see Chapter 5).

Fairness. A critical thinker deals with situations justly. This means that you do not let bias or prejudice affect your decisions. For example, regardless of how you feel about obesity, you do not allow personal attitudes to influence the way you care for a patient who is overweight. Look at a situation objectively and consider all viewpoints to understand the situation completely before making a decision. Having a sense of imagination helps you develop an attitude of fairness. Imagining what it is like to be in your patient's situation helps you see it with new eyes and appreciate its complexity.

Responsibility and Accountability. Responsibility is the knowledge that you are accountable for your decisions, actions, and critical thinking. When caring for patients, you are responsible for correctly performing nursing care activities based on standards of practice. Standards of practice are the minimum level of performance accepted to ensure high-quality care. For example, you do not take shortcuts (work-arounds) when you give a patient a medication (e.g., skipping a step—failing to identify a patient, preparing medication doses for multiple patients at the same time). Professional nurses are responsible for competently performing nursing therapies and making clinical decisions about patients. As a nurse you are answerable or accountable for your decisions, the outcomes of your actions, and knowing the limits and scope of your practice.

Risk Taking. People often associate taking risks with danger. Driving 30 miles an hour over the speed limit is a risk that can result in injury to a driver and an unlucky pedestrian. But risk taking does not always have negative outcomes. Risk taking is desirable, particularly when the result is a positive outcome. A critical thinker will take risks when trying different ways to solve problems. The willingness to take risks, without causing harm to a patient, comes from experiences with similar clinical problems. Trying different approaches to motivating a patient to eat, involving dependent patients more in self-hygiene, or using nonpharmacological approaches to pain relief may pose risk but can be highly beneficial. When taking a risk, follow safety guidelines, analyze any potential dangers to a patient, involve the patient in any decisions, and act in a well-reasoned, logical, and thoughtful manner.

Discipline. A disciplined thinker misses few details when assessing a patient, considering care options and resources, or making decisions about nursing interventions. *For example, Mr. Lawson is experiencing incision and chest pain. Instead of asking the patient only, "How severe is your pain on a scale of 0 to 10?" Tonya knows the need to ask more specific questions about the character of the pain (e.g., "What makes the pain worse?" "Show me exactly where it hurts." "How would you describe the*

pain?"). Being disciplined helps you identify problems more accurately and select the most appropriate interventions.

Perseverance. A critical thinker is determined to find effective solutions to patient care problems. This is especially important when problems remain unresolved or recur. Learn as much as possible about a problem before deciding on various approaches to care. Persevering means to keep looking for more resources until you find a successful approach. It often requires creativity. For example, a patient who is unable to speak following throat surgery poses challenges for a nurse to communicate effectively. Perseverance leads the nurse to try different communication approaches (e.g., message boards or alarm bells) until finding an effective method. A critical thinker who perseveres is not satisfied with minimal effort but works to achieve the highest quality level of care.

Creativity. Creativity involves original thinking. This means that you find solutions outside the standard routines of care while still following standards of practice. Creativity motivates you to think of options and unique approaches. A patient's clinical problems, social support systems, culture, and living environment are examples of factors that can make the simplest nursing procedure more complicated. For example, a home care nurse must find a way to help an older adult patient with arthritis have greater mobility in the home. The patient has difficulty lowering and raising herself in a chair because of pain and limited range of motion in her knees. The nurse uses wooden blocks to elevate the chair legs so that the patient can sit and stand with little discomfort while making sure that the chair is safe to use.

Curiosity. A critical thinker's favorite question is "Why?" As you gather and analyze patient information, data patterns appear that are not always clear. Having a sense of curiosity (asking yourself, "What if?") motivates you to inquire further (e.g., question family or health care provider, review the scientific literature) and investigate a clinical situation so that you get all the information you need to make a decision.

Integrity. Critical thinkers question and test their own knowledge and beliefs. Your personal integrity as a nurse builds trust from your co-workers. Nurses face many dilemmas or problems in everyday clinical practice, and everyone makes mistakes at times. A person of integrity is honest and willing to admit to mistakes or inconsistencies in one's own behavior, ideas, and beliefs. A professional nurse always tries to follow the highest standards of practice.

Humility and Self-awareness. It is important for you to admit to any limitations in your knowledge and skill. Critical thinkers admit what they do not know and try to find the knowledge needed to make proper decisions. It is common for a nurse to be an expert in one area of clinical practice but a novice in another because the knowledge in all areas of nursing is unlimited. A patient's safety and welfare are at risk if you do not admit your inability to deal with a practice problem. Always remain self-aware by clarifying internally your biases, inclinations, strengths, and limitations. Recognize when thinking is being affected by your emotions or self-interest. You must rethink a situation; learn more; and use the new information to form opinions, draw conclusions, and take action.

Mr. Lawson continues to have chest pain and shortness of breath. As Tonya waits for the medical team to arrive, she knows that she is responsible for his welfare until treatment can be initiated. Tonya acts independently by keeping Mr. Lawson comfortable in the chair (to avoid movement that could worsen his condition), explaining steps being taken by the health care team, and gathering additional assessment data. She displays discipline in further assessing Mr. Lawson's condition: rechecking vital signs, observing his abdominal wound and incision, and talking with him to allay anxiety and note if there is a change in consciousness. Tonya knows that she cannot diagnose medically. When the physician arrives, she objectively reports what happened with Mr. Lawson once he sat up in the chair, the symptoms he displayed, and how those symptoms have changed.

Standards for Critical Thinking

The sixth component of critical thinking includes intellectual and professional standards (Kataoka-Yahiro and Saylor, 1994).

Intellectual Standards. Paul (1993) identified intellectual standards (Box 15.5) universal for critical thinking. An intellectual standard is a guideline or principle for rational thought. You apply these standards during all steps of the nursing process. For example, when you consider a patient problem, apply the intellectual standards of preciseness, accuracy, and consistency in measurement to make sure that you have all the data you need to make sound clinical decisions. During planning, apply standards such as logic and significance so that the plan of care is meaningful and relevant to a patient's needs. Routine use of intellectual standards in clinical practice prevents you from performing critical thinking haphazardly.

The physician orders a lung scan and chest x-ray and places Mr. Lawson on bed rest. Blood tests are also ordered in anticipation of placing the patient on anticoagulation (to prevent further clot formation). Tonya asks the physician whether there are risks to be considered regarding Mr. Lawson's wound should the patient receive an anticoagulant (relevant question). She also asks if she can give additional pain medication at this time to manage the patient's surgical incision pain during the x-ray procedures (logical decision). By applying intellectual standards, Tonya is a competent partner in managing the patient's care, showing her ability to anticipate possible clinical problems.

Professional Standards. Professional standards for critical thinking refer to ethical criteria for nursing judgments, evidence-based criteria used for evaluation, and criteria for professional responsibility (Paul, 1993). Professional practice standards improve patient outcomes and maintain a high quality level of nursing care. Using available scientific evidence and best practice guidelines found in professional standards is part of the decision-making process (NHS, n.d.).

Excellent nursing practice reflects ethical standards (see Chapter 22). Being able to focus on a patient's values and beliefs helps you make clinical decisions that are just, respectful of a patient's choices, and beneficial to a patient's well-being. Critical thinkers maintain a sense of self-awareness through conscious awareness of their own beliefs, values, and feelings and the multiple perspectives that patients, family members, and peers present in clinical situations. Critical thinking also requires the use of evidence-based criteria for making clinical judgments. These criteria are sometimes scientifically based on research findings (see Chapter 5) or practice based on standards developed by clinical experts and performance improvement initiatives of an institution. Examples are the clinical practice guidelines developed by individual clinical agencies and national organizations such as the American Association of Critical-Care Nurses (AACN) or the Oncology Nursing Society (ONS). A clinical practice guideline includes standards for the treatment of select clinical conditions such as stroke, deep vein thrombosis, and pressure injuries. Another example is clinical criteria used to categorize clinical conditions, such as the criteria for staging pressure injuries (see Chapter 48) and rating phlebitis (see Chapter 42). Evidence-based evaluation criteria set the minimum requirements necessary to ensure appropriate and high-quality care.

The standards of professional responsibility that a nurse tries to achieve are the standards cited in nurse practice acts, institutional practice guidelines, and professional organizations' standards of practice (e.g., the ANA Standards of Professional Performance [see Chapter 1]). These standards "raise the bar" for the responsibilities and accountabilities that a nurse assumes in guaranteeing high-quality health care to the public.

EVALUATION OF CLINICAL JUDGMENTS

When making clinical decisions about patients, nurses consciously consider if their judgments were accurate and whether the correct and appropriate decisions were made. This is a form of self-evaluation. Evaluation is also a step in the nursing process (see Chapter 20) that methodically determines if nursing care approaches successfully led to desired or expected patient outcomes. Both evaluation processes go hand in hand in developing strong clinical judgment skills.

Reflection

Reflection is like instant replay. It is not intuitive. It involves purposefully visualizing a situation and taking the time to honestly review everything you remember about it. It assists an individual in learning about life situations and experiences that provide a significant means for the person to learn (Galutira, 2018). This reflection allows you to gain new knowledge and raise questions about your practice. Reflection can have an impact on positive outcomes such as personal and professional development, improved quality of care, and improved patient outcomes (Galutira, 2018). When you are engaged in caring for patients, reflective reasoning improves the accuracy of making diagnostic conclusions (see Chapter 17). Reflection goes hand in hand with clinical judgment because to be effective it involves description, critical analysis, synthesis, and evaluation (Galutira, 2018). Gathering information about a patient, reflecting on the meaning of your findings, and exploring the possible meaning of those findings improves

---

BOX 15.5 Intellectual Standards

- Clear—Plain and understandable (e.g., clarity in how one communicates)
- Precise—Exact and specific (e.g., focusing on one problem and possible solution)
- Specific—To mention, describe, or define in detail
- Accurate—True and free from error; getting to the facts (objective and subjective)
- Relevant—Essential and crucial to a situation (e.g., a patient's changing clinical status)
- Plausible—Reasonable or probable
- Consistent—Expressing consistent beliefs or values
- Logical—Engaging in correct reasoning from what one believes in a given instance to the conclusions that follow
- Deep—Containing complexities and multiple relationships
- Broad—Covering multiple viewpoints (e.g., patient and family)
- Complete—Thoroughly thinking and evaluating
- Significant—Focusing on what is important and not trivial
- Adequate (for purpose)—Satisfactory in quality or amount

BOX 15.6   Model for Reflection

REFLECT: This model can be used individually or as a process shared with others.

R—*R*ecall the events. Review the facts about a situation and describe what happened.

E—*E*xamine your responses. Think about or discuss your thoughts and actions at the time of the situation.

F—Acknowledge *f*eelings: Identify any feelings you had during the situation.

L—*L*earn from the experience: Review and highlight what you learned from the situation—for example, your patient's responses and your actions.

E—*E*xplore options: Think about or discuss your options for similar situations in the future.

C—*C*reate a plan of action: Create a plan for how to act in future similar situations.

T—Set a *t*ime: Set a time by which your plan of action will be completed.

Adapted from Barksby J, et al: A new model of reflection for clinical practice, *Nurs Times* 111(34/35):21–23, 2015.

your ability to problem solve. Reflection lessens the guesswork in decision making. Always be cautious in using reflection. Reliance on it can block thinking and not allow you to look at newer evidence or subtle aspects of situations that you have not encountered. Box 15.6 lists steps of a model for using reflection in your practice.

Reflective journaling is a tool for developing self-evaluation skills by consciously clarifying concepts used in nursing practice (Raterink, 2016). It can involve taking time to consciously think through an activity or experience, or it can involve keeping a written record of your clinical experiences in a personal journal. Remember to keep your journal entries confidential so that if someone else reads your journal, patient identity is protected. Returning to the journal after each clinical experience gives you the chance to record the perceptions you had during patient care and better develop the ability to apply theory in practice. Often reflections are on things that go wrong; however, reflecting on things that went well can be just as rewarding and useful to build confidence in your practice (Kiron et al., 2017). Journaling also improves your observational and descriptive skills. Writing skills improve as you learn to clearly describe concepts applied in practice (e.g., suffering, hope, powerlessness). Here are examples of questions to pose in a journal:

- What did I learn from the experience?
- Did I respond appropriately in this situation? If not, how should I have responded?
- What were the consequences of my actions? Whom did they affect and in what way?
- How might I act differently in the future?
- Was I working from tradition or evidence-based practices?

QSEN **Building Competency in Patient-Centered Care** Think about a patient you recently cared for. Describe how you would use each of the elements of the REFLECT model to incorporate principles of patient-centered care.

Answers to QSEN Activities can be found on the Evolve website.

Meeting With Colleagues

A way to develop and evaluate your critical thinking is to regularly meet with colleagues such as fellow students or nurses, faculty members, or preceptors to discuss and examine work experiences and validate decisions. Connecting with others helps you learn that you do not need to know everything because support is available from other colleagues. Willingness to learn from practice and honesty to account for a clinical situation or experience are important. In addition, the persons with whom you share reflection must be trustworthy and approachable (Galutira, 2018). When nurses have a formal means to discuss their experiences, the dialogue allows for questions, differing viewpoints, and sharing of experiences. When they can discuss their practices, the process validates good practice and also offers challenges and constructive criticism.

A discussion of critical incidents—actual or alleged events or situations that create a significant risk of substantial or serious harm to a patient in a clinical setting—is invaluable for developing critical thinking (LaMartina and Ward-Smith, 2014). Many health care agencies conduct safety huddles following a critical incident (e.g., patient fall) in order to learn from the incident and to identify and monitor underlying trends and patterns to allow early detection and prevention in the future.

Concept Mapping

As a nurse you will care for patients who have multiple nursing diagnoses and/or collaborative problems. A concept map is a visual representation of patient problems and interventions that shows their relationships to one another. It is a nonlinear picture of a patient to be used for comprehensive care planning. Research shows that when compared with traditional educational methods, concept mapping can improve students' critical thinking ability as measured with various critical thinking tests and scales (Yue et al., 2017). However, more high-quality studies are needed to support these findings.

Concept maps help you synthesize relevant data about a patient, including assessment data, nursing diagnoses, health needs, nursing interventions, and evaluation measures. Through drawing a concept map, you learn to organize or connect information in a unique way, so the diverse information that you have about a patient begins to form meaningful patterns and concepts. You begin to see a more holistic view of a patient. When you see the relationship between the various patient diagnoses and the data that support them, you better understand a patient's clinical situation. Sample concept maps can be found in the clinical chapters of this text (see Units 5 and 6).

Critical Thinking Synthesis

Critical thinking is a reasoning process by which you cognitively apply and analyze your thoughts, actions, and knowledge to make sound clinical judgments. As a beginning nurse, you will learn the steps of the nursing process and begin to incorporate the elements of critical thinking into your clinical experiences (Fig. 15.3). The two processes are interdependent in making the clinical judgments necessary for appropriate clinical decision making. As a student, you will use a variety of approaches designed to improve your critical thinking competencies (Box 15.7). As an added resource, this text provides a model applied throughout the clinical chapters to show how important critical thinking is in the practice of nursing.

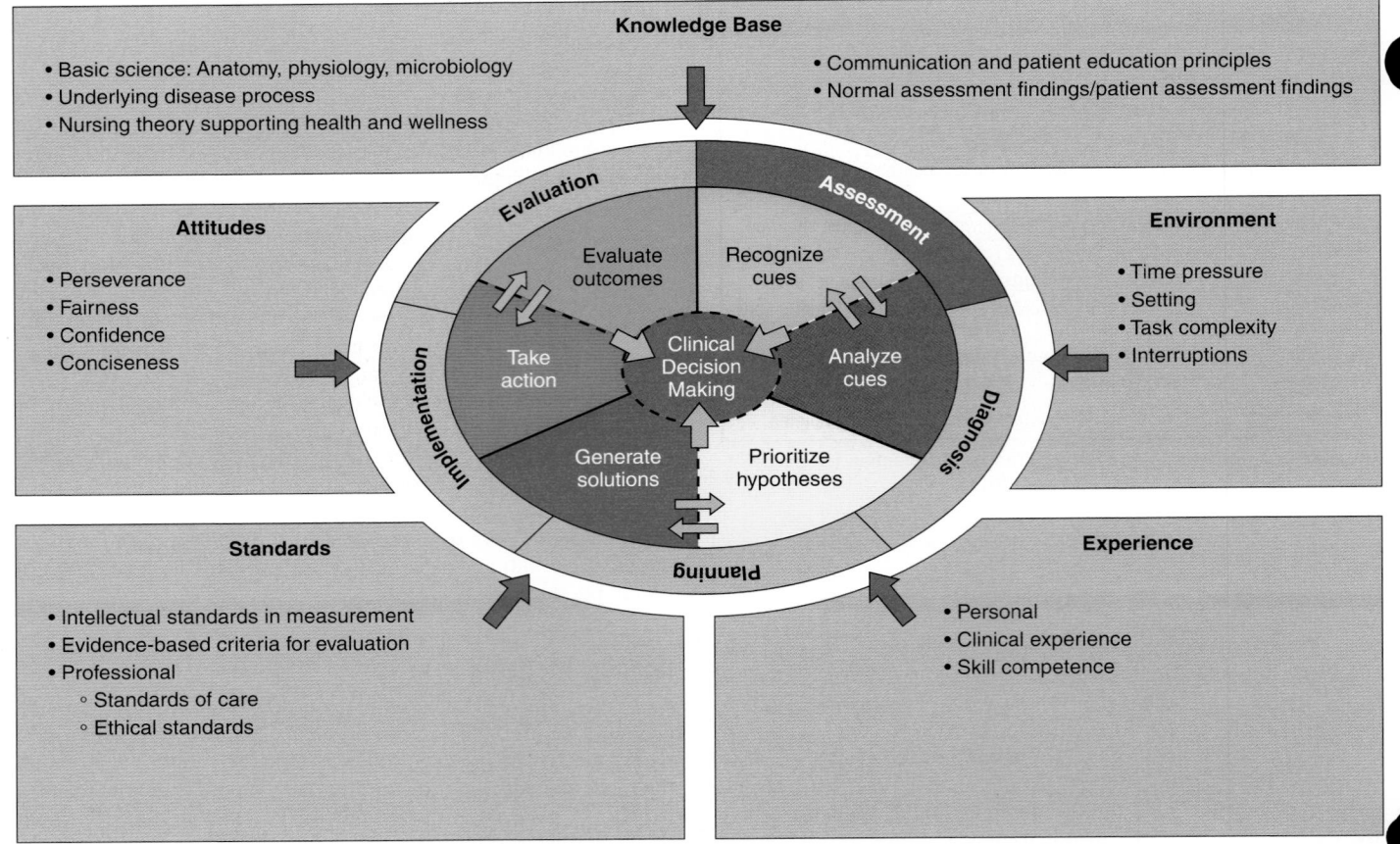

FIG. 15.3 Synthesis of critical thinking with the nursing process. (Clinical Judgment Measurement Model copyright © NCSBN. All rights reserved.)

BOX 15.7   EVIDENCE-BASED PRACTICE

Problem-Based Learning

PICOT Question: Does problem-based learning (PBL) compared with didactic lecture improve critical thinking in undergraduate nursing students?

Evidence Summary

Nursing educational programs must ensure that their students develop critical thinking in order to provide high-quality patient care. The ability of newly graduated health care professionals to think critically and intervene effectively is essential for preventing risks to patient safety (Carvalho et al., 2017). Research investigating teaching approaches for improving critical thinking in undergraduate nurses has used critical thinking tools and conceptual models for measurement. A systematic review of studies examining these teaching approaches found that PBL, including use of case studies, case studies with information integrated from actual patients, concept maps, repeated simulation (not singular), and reflective writing, can improve critical thinking behaviors (Carvalho et al., 2017). However, the studies showed a weak association between PBL and critical thinking measurement

because of how the studies were designed. Studies examining ways to improve students' critical thinking have not been rigorous because they have not studied students over time. One recent clinical trial recommended that PBL combined with a new approach, the Active Learning Model for Critical Thinking (ALMCT), be conducted over an extended time frame (Carbojim et al., 2018). The ALMCT is a set of questions that explores and deepens the meanings, correlations, and search for results through inquiries within the clinical practice or in a clinical case.

Application to Nursing Practice

- Develop concept maps for use with clinical patients and discuss the interrelationships of the nursing process steps with colleagues.
- Use reflective journaling after clinical experiences and before caring for similar types of patients.
- Share clinical case studies with colleagues and examine how critical thinking was applied.

█ KEY POINTS

- A clinical judgment model contains the elements that allow you to make the right clinical decisions in every type of patient situation.
- Clinical judgment is an observed outcome that uses nursing knowledge and experience to observe and assess presenting situations,

identify a prioritized patient concern, and generate the best possible evidence-based solutions to make the decisions needed to deliver safe patient care.
- When striving to make sound clinical judgments, nurses rely on a critical thinking process (the nursing process) that involves open-mindedness, continual inquiry, and perseverance.

- Effective problem solving requires you to obtain information that clarifies the nature of a problem, suggest possible solutions, and try the solution over time compared with diagnostic reasoning, a form of decision making that involves being able to understand and think through clinical problems, analyze individual cues, understand the evidence, and know when there is enough information to make an accurate diagnosis.
- To prioritize patient problems in clinical situations, use decision criteria that include the clinical condition of the patient, a review of the advantages and disadvantages of each option, Maslow's hierarchy of needs, the risks involved in treatment delays, environmental factors, and patients' expectations of care.
- A basic critical thinker is task oriented, whereas a complex critical thinker uses experience to anticipate how to individualize a nursing procedure when problems arise.
- Knowledge is a critical thinking component that prepares you to better anticipate and identify patient problems by understanding their origin and nature.
- With experience, you begin to understand clinical situations, anticipate and recognize cues from patients' health data, and interpret the patterns of data as relevant or irrelevant.
- During the clinical care of patients, apply critical thinking attitudes for how to approach a problem, knowing when you need more information, knowing when information is misleading, and recognizing your own knowledge limits.
- Intellectual standards are guidelines or principles for rational thought to apply during all steps of the nursing process.
- After making a clinical decision, use reflection to consider the meaning of your findings and to explore the possible meaning of those findings in solving a patient problem.

REFLECTIVE LEARNING

A nurse responds to a call light in an assigned patient's room and finds a patient on the floor. The patient is known to have stage III lung cancer and is receiving chemotherapy. The nurse knows from information gathered in electronic health records at the beginning of the shift that the patient has a low platelet count and a history of osteoporosis. The patient has been alert and oriented with stable vital signs. The nurse stands by the patient and makes the following assessments:

- IV fluid still infusing in left forearm
- Patient is lying on right side with hip flexed
- Patient is able to identify day, time, and current location
- Respirations are 26 breaths/min
- Patient reports right hip pain as 8 on a scale of 0 to 10
- A 2.5-cm (1-inch) cut on patient's right hand is bleeding
- Patient states, "I did not hit my head when I slipped and fell down."
- Heart rate is 92 beats/min
- Blood pressure is 142/88 mm Hg
- Patient reports feeling short of breath

1. What assessment information in this patient situation is the most important and of immediate concern for the nurse?
2. Identify three types of critical thinking questions the nurse should raise in this clinical situation.
3. Knowing the patient's diagnosis of lung cancer, what approaches might the nurse use in forming a relationship with this patient that will ultimately lead to appropriate clinical decision making?

REVIEW QUESTIONS

1. A nurse enters a patient's room at the beginning of a shift to assess his condition following a blood transfusion. The nurse cared for the patient on the previous day as well. The patient has several issues he wishes to share with the nurse, who takes time to explore each issue. The nurse also assesses the patient and finds no signs or symptoms of a reaction to the blood product. The nurse observed the patient the prior day and sees a change in his behavior—a reluctance to get out of bed and ambulate. Which of the following actions improve the nurse's ability to make clinical decisions about this patient? (Select all that apply.)
   1. Working the same shift each day
   2. Spending time during the patient assessment
   3. Knowing the early mobility protocol guidelines
   4. Caring for the patient on consecutive days
   5. Knowing the pattern of patient behavior about ambulation
2. Match the concepts for a critical thinker on the left with the application of the term on the right,

Concepts for Critical Thinkers

____ 1. Truth seeking
____ 2. Open-mindedness
____ 3. Analyticity
____ 4. Systematicity

Term Application

a. Anticipate how a patient might respond to a treatment.
b. Organize assessment on the basis of patient priorities.
c. Be objective in asking patient questions.
d. Be tolerant of the patient's views and beliefs.

3. A nurse has seen many cancer patients struggle with pain management because they are afraid of becoming addicted to the medicine. Pain control is a priority for cancer care. By helping patients focus on their values and beliefs about pain control, a nurse can best make clinical decisions. This is an example of:
   1. Creativity
   2. Fairness
   3. Clinical reasoning
   4. Applying ethical criteria
4. The REFLECT model can improve learning after providing patient care. Place the steps of this model in the correct order:
   1. Think about your thoughts and actions at the time of a situation.
   2. Review the knowledge you gained from the experience.
   3. Review the facts of the situation.
   4. Set a schedule for completing your plan of action.
   5. Consider options for handling a similar situation in the future.
   6. Recall any feelings you had at the time of the situation.
   7. Create a plan for future situations.
5. One element of clinical decision making is knowing the patient. Which of the following activities affect a nurse's ability to know patients better? (Select all that apply.)
   1. Caring for similar groups of patients over time
   2. Reading the evidence-based practices appropriate to patients
   3. Learning how patients typically respond to their clinical situations
   4. Observing patients
   5. Engaging with patients experiencing illness
6. A nurse is preparing medications for a patient. The nurse checks the name of the medication on the label with the name of the medication on the health care provider's order. At the bedside, the nurse checks the patient's name against the medication order as well. The nurse is following which critical thinking attitude?
   1. Responsibility
   2. Humility
   3. Accuracy
   4. Fairness

7. A nurse has been caring for a patient with a chronic wound that has not been healing. The nurse talks with a nurse specialist in wound care to find alternative approaches from what the health care provider ordered for dressing the wound. The two decide that because of the patient's allergy to tape, a nonallergenic dressing will be used. The nurse obtains an order from the health care provider for the new dressing. After 2 days there is improvement in the wound. This is an example of which critical thinking standards? (Select all that apply.)
   1. Clarity
   2. Broadness
   3. Relevance
   4. Risk taking
   5. Creativity

8. A nurse is assigned to care for a woman who is expecting her first child. The nurse organizes herself and plans to gather data about the patient by applying Pender's health promotion model, including the patient's characteristics and experiences and situational influences. She plans to observe patient behavior and consider the patient's psychosocial issues. Such data will offer a clear understanding to help the nurse identify the patient's needs. This is an example of which of the following concepts? (Select all that apply.)
   1. Diagnostic reasoning
   2. Deductive reasoning
   3. Inductive reasoning
   4. Assessment
   5. Problem solving

9. A nurse is caring for a patient who has poor pain control. The patient has a history of opioid abuse. During the day, the patient made frequent requests for a pain medication. To make an effective clinical decision about this patient, the nurse needs to ask questions about the data available on the patient to make a thorough and thoughtful decision. The nurse asks herself, "How does my view about the patient's pain tolerance compare with the patient's, and does that pose a problem?" This is an example of:
   1. A question about assumptions
   2. A question about evidence
   3. A question about procedure
   4. A question about perspective

10. A nurse is giving a patient a medication and notices the dosage. From the nurse's experience, the dosage is higher than what is normally given. Which of the following steps should the nurse take to ensure a safe outcome for the patient? (Select all that apply.)
   1. Wait until end of shift when there is time to check dosage with pharmacy reference.
   2. Recognize how the nursing team communicates problems, and consult with charge nurse.
   3. Hold the dose and confer with the ordering health care provider now.
   4. Assess patient knowledge of what has been the routine dose for this medication.
   5. Administer the medication and closely monitor patient response.

Answers: 1. 2, 4, 5; **2.** 1c, 2d, 3a, 4b; **3.** 4; **4.** 3, 1, 6, 2, 5, 7, 4; **5.** 1, 3, 4, 5; **6.** 1; **7.** 3, 4, 5; **8.** 2, 4, 5; **9.** 4; **10.** 2, 3, 4

Rationales for Review Questions can be found on the Evolve website.

REFERENCES

American Nurses Association (ANA): Nursing Scope and Standards of Practice, American Nurses Association. *Nursing: Scope and Standards of Practice* (4th ed.) Silver Spring, MD, 2021, ANA.

Dickison P et al.: Integrating the National Council of State Boards of Nursing Clinical Judgment Model into nursing educational frameworks, *J Nurs Educ* 58(2):72, 2019.

Erickson K: *The importance of critical thinking skills in nursing*, 2017, https://www.rasmussen.edu/degrees/nursing/blog/understanding-why-nurses-need-critical-thinking-skills/, Accessed August 20, 2020.

Galutira GD: Theory of reflective practice in nursing, *Int J Nurs Sci* , 8 (3): 51-56, 2018.

National Academies of Sciences, Engineering, and Medicine: *Improving Diagnosis in Health Care*. Washington, DC, 2015, The National Academies Press.

Kataoka-Yahiro M, Saylor C: A critical thinking model for nursing judgment, *J Nurs Educ* 33(8):351, 1994.

Kiron K, et al.: Reflective practice in health care and how to reflect effectively, *Int J Surg Oncol* 2(6):e20, 2017.

Miller M, Malcolm N: Critical thinking in the nursing curriculum, *Nurs Health Care* 11:67, 1990.

Muntean WJ: Nursing Clinical Decision-Making: A Literature Review, 2012, https://pdfs.semanticscholar.org/ba14/b0d8ef4006ebdd03b73bd62355001f436ee2.pdf?_ga=2.168855393.1787090792.1583439127-756289411.1583439127. Accessed August 20, 2020.

National Health Service (NHS): *Effective practitioner: Clinical decision making*, nd, http://www.effectivepractitioner.nes.scot.nhs.uk/media/254840/clinical%20decision%20making.pdf. Accessed August 20, 2020.

National Council of State Boards of Nursing (NCSBN): *Next Generation NCLEX News: Clinical Judgment Measurement Model*, Winter 2019, https://www.ncsbn.org/NGN_Winter19.pdf. Accessed August 20, 2020.

Paul RW: The art of redesigning instruction. In Willsen J, Blinker AJA, editors: *Critical thinking: how to prepare students for a rapidly changing world*, Santa Rosa, CA, 1993, Foundation for Critical Thinking.

Papathanasiou IV, et al.: Critical thinking: the development of an essential skill for nursing students, *Acta Informatica Med* 22(4):283, 2014.

Raterink G: Reflective journaling for critical thinking development in advanced practice registered nurse students, *J Nurs Educ* 55(2):101, 2016.

Resnick B: Improving care through diagnostic reasoning, *Geriatric Nurs* 37(2):91, 2016.

RESEARCH REFERENCES

Carbojim FDC, et al: Educational intervention to improve critical thinking for undergraduate nursing students: A randomized clinical trial, *Nurse Educ Pract.* 33:121, 2018.

Carvalho DPSRP et al: Strategies used for the promotion of critical thinking in nursing undergraduate education: A systematic review, *Nurse Education Today,* 57(2017): 103, 2017.

Chan ZC: A systematic review of critical thinking in nursing education, *Nurse Educ Today* 33(2013):236, 2013.

Kelley T, et al.: Information needed to support knowing the patient, *ANS Adv Nurs Sci* 36(4):351, 2013.

LaMartina K, Ward-Smith P: Developing critical thinking skills in undergraduate nursing students: the potential for strategic management simulations, *J Nurs Educ Pract* 4(9):155, 2014.

McCullough MB et al: Knowing the patient: A qualitative study on care-taking and the clinical pharmacist-patient relationship, *Research in Social and Administrative Pharmacy*, 12(1): 78, 2016.

Scheffer B, Rubenfeld M: A consensus statement on critical thinking in nursing, *J Nurs Educ* 39:352, 2000.

Tanner CA: Thinking like a nurse: a research-based model of clinical judgment in nursing, *J Nurs Educ* 45(6):204, 2006.

Tanner CA, et al.: The phenomenology of knowing the patient, *J Nurs Scholarsh* 25:273, 1993.

Yue M, et al.: The effectiveness of concept mapping on development of critical thinking in nursing education: a systematic review and meta-analysis, *Nurs Edu Today* 52:87, 2017.

Zolnierek CD: An integrative review of knowing the patient, *J Nurs Scholarsh* 46(1):3, 2014.

Nursing Assessment

OBJECTIVES

- Explain the relationships among assessment, clinical decision making, and clinical judgment.
- Discuss how the two steps involved in nursing assessment are used in practice.
- Differentiate the types of nursing assessments used in practice.
- Examine the components of critical thinking in nursing assessment.
- Analyze practice situations to determine the type of nursing assessment to use.
- Explain how experience in performing nursing skills influences patient assessment.

- Examine how the use of critical thinking attitudes and professional standards yields a comprehensive assessment database.
- Explain the importance of building a nurse-patient relationship when gathering a patient assessment.
- Apply communication techniques when conducting a patient interview.
- Display professionalism during history taking.
- Explain the assessment process.

KEY TERMS

Assessment

Back channeling

Closed-ended questions

Cue

Inference

Nursing health history

Nursing process

Objective data

Open-ended questions

Review of systems (ROS)

Subjective data

Validation

MEDIA RESOURCES

http://evolve.elsevier.com/Potter/fundamentals/
- Review Questions
- Audio Glossary
- Case Study with Questions

- Concept Map Creator
- Content Updates
- Answers to QSEN Activity and Review Questions

Clinical judgment is necessary for you to make informed and timely clinical decisions in nursing practice and patient care (see Chapter 15). Developed by the American Nurses Association (ANA), the steps of the nursing process (assessment, analysis and diagnosis, outcome identification, planning, implementation, and evaluation) (Fig. 16.1) are the essential core of nursing practice that all registered nurses, regardless of role and the population of patients they serve, are expected to competently perform (ANA, n.d.). The process is not linear; instead, it is an ongoing process that evolves as you care for a patient.

Nurses make clinical judgments that combine context-sensitive knowledge with their decision-making experience as part of their work (Dickison, 2019). It is the context-sensitive or patient situational knowledge that a nurse gathers during assessment. The first step of the nursing process, assessment (see Fig. 16.1), involves the collection of as much information as possible about a patient, family, or community. A thorough and comprehensive assessment allows you to sort the data (cues), recognize patterns, and make judgments that allow you to identify the type of health problems your patient is experiencing. Your initial assessment of a patient is critical to identify or confirm as quickly as possible a patient's health problems, but nursing assessment

is ongoing. You will update your assessment of the patient as you continue to provide patient care.

The nursing process enables nurses to deliver holistic, patient-centered care (ANA, n.d.). The Quality and Safety Education for Nurses (QSEN) Institute defines patient-centered care as recognizing a patient or a person selected by the patient as a full partner in providing compassionate and coordinated care based on respect for a patient's preferences, values, and needs (QSEN, 2020). You will learn to use the essential first step of the nursing process, assessment, to learn as much as you can about each patient's health condition and health problems by partnering with patients and their family caregivers in a therapeutic relationship.

Consider the case study introduced in Chapter 15. *Mr. Lawson is displaying anxiety symptoms after having been placed on bedrest while awaiting results of diagnostic testing. Tonya, his nurse, continues monitoring the patient's breathing status and applies oxygen per the health care provider's orders. While monitoring Mr. Lawson's physical status and measuring vital signs, Tonya knows that signs of anxiety include glancing about, poor eye contact, restlessness, and the patient's expression of feeling nervous. She also knows from her knowledge of pathophysiology that pain (chest pain and surgical site pain) can be worsened by anxiety. In addition,*

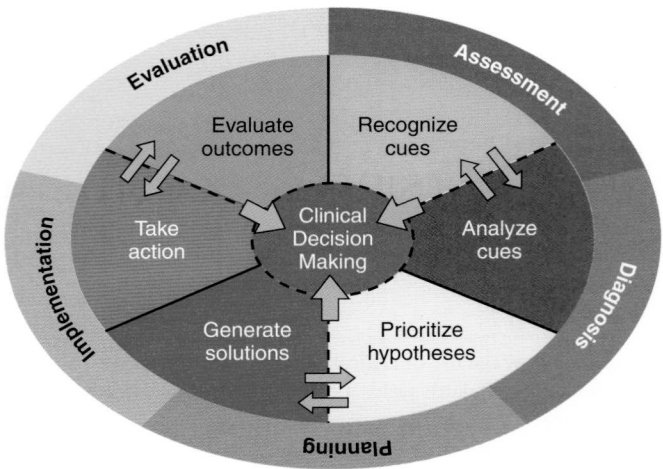

FIG. 16.1 Model for clinical judgment. (Copyright © NCSBN. All rights reserved.)

anxiety is an early sign of a pulmonary embolus. Tonya recognizes that she needs more information about the patient's restlessness. She will display curiosity and discipline by seeking further information, asking Mr. Lawson several questions to learn more about him and the specific nature of his concerns. One area of questioning will be whether Mr. Lawson has a support system.

The nursing process involves scientific reasoning and is essential to clinical judgment. Practicing the five steps of the nursing process ensures a rigorous, systematic, and dynamic way to approach your practice. In the case study involving Tonya and Mr. Lawson, Tonya will gather information to fully understand Mr. Lawson's condition, using behavioral observation, physical examination, and interview techniques. Having an accurate and complete database about a patient allows you to make a clinical judgment in the form of a nursing diagnosis (see Chapter 17) and to make the decisions necessary to plan (see Chapter 18) and implement relevant and appropriate nursing interventions (see Chapter 19). Your assessment also provides the standards for later evaluating the outcomes of care (see Chapter 20). Each time you interact with a patient you apply the nursing process, using critical thinking.

CRITICAL THINKING IN ASSESSMENT

Think about what you do when you study or consider a problem. For example, why is my child or spouse acting this way? You collect data about the problem. In the case of family members behaving differently, you consider their previous behavior, specifically how they are behaving now (voice tone, mannerisms, what they say to you) and perhaps how the behavior is affecting others in the family. You assess the situation. You gather as much information as possible in an effort to understand the true nature of the problem (e.g., my family member does not feel well, is angry, or just received bad news at work). The collection, review, and recognition of data patterns make up the process of assessment.

For you to become competent in applying the nursing process, your assessment must apply all components of critical thinking (Fig. 16.2). Application of critical thinking enables you to be deliberate and systematic in collecting data about your patients. Assessment potentially includes a broad database. The extent of any assessment is based on

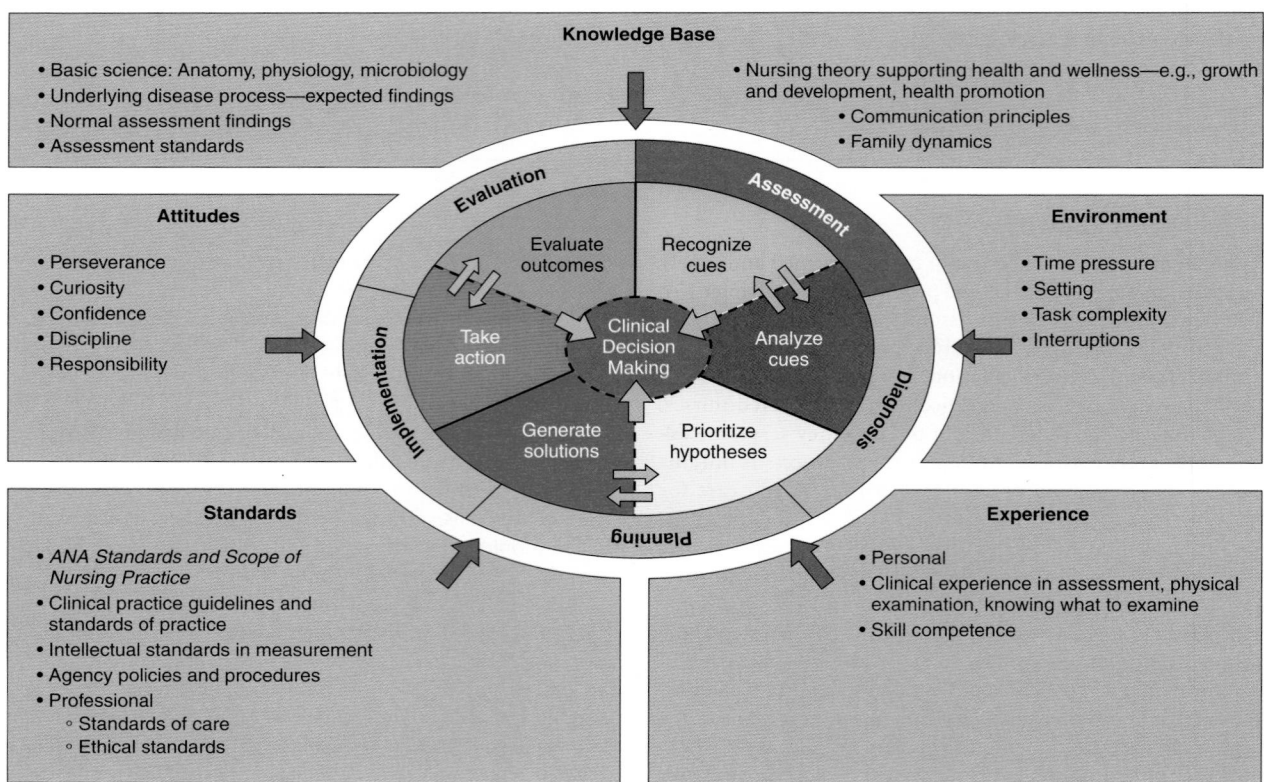

FIG. 16.2 Critical thinking in the assessment of patients. (Clinical Judgment Measurement Model copyright © NCSBN. All rights reserved.)

your judgment, triggered by how a patient is responding (presenting signs and symptoms), whether the patient's condition is urgent, and the time you have to gather data. Assessment is situational. For example, Tonya first assessed Mr. Lawson's surgical postoperative status when she initially met him, knowing that the status of his postoperative recovery including postoperative pain was a priority. But as Mr. Lawson's condition changed, Tonya recognized developing signs and symptoms and assessed for clinical indicators of a possible pulmonary embolus, recognizing that oxygenation was the new priority.

The data you gather during an assessment reveal your patient's current and past health status, functional status, and present and past coping patterns (Carpenito, 2017). Nursing assessment involves two steps:

- Collection of information from a primary source (a patient) and secondary sources (e.g., family caregiver, family members or friends, health professionals, medical record)
- The interpretation and validation of data to determine whether more data are needed or the database is complete

In the case study Tonya collects information from her primary source of data, Mr. Lawson, through observation and asking questions. The diagnostic tests show a small pulmonary embolism, and the physician orders oxygen and an anticoagulant. Once Tonya ensures Mr. Lawson's breathing is stable, she asks the patient to tell her the reason for his restlessness, which continues. He responds by saying, "I didn't know what was happening to me. I was frightened when I couldn't catch my breath." Tonya observes Mr. Lawson's glancing back and forth, closing his eyes to avoid eye contact. She explains the purpose for his oxygen and anticoagulant, then asks, "Is there anything else making you restless?" Mr. Lawson responds, "I feel alone, just not certain what is happening to me." Tonya wants to also learn how Mr. Lawson regularly copes with stress, and asks if he has family support. He responds, "My wife is my support. She's at work but will be here this afternoon, I hope." Tonya plans to try to meet the wife and gather additional relevant data later near the end of her shift. Her assessment will focus on gathering as much information as possible about Mr. Lawson's restlessness, which could ultimately lead her to identify the patient's problem clearly and accurately.

If you practice in a hospital setting, you will usually care for more than one patient, and any of your patients' conditions can change quickly. In the home and community setting, your patients' conditions will also change. Sometimes their changes will be acute, but most often the changes they experience are subtle and develop over time. An assessment database changes whenever a patient's condition changes.

In Mr. Lawson's case, his surgical condition is still a priority. Tonya implemented pain-control strategies shortly after beginning her care, to help him become more mobile so that recovery could proceed. At that time his recovery plan involved early ambulation. Up until the episode of shortness of breath and new chest pain, he had a pain rating at a level of 4 on a scale of 0 to 10 for surgical incision pain. The patient describes the pain as sharp when he most notices it. Tonya observes Mr. Lawson continuing to guard his incision by placing his hand over the wound when he turns in bed. With the patient being restless, she asks him now to rate his incision pain. He replies, "Oh, I guess a 5 or 6. I just hurt all over." Tonya inspects the incision, noting its appearance and whether there is any drainage, and palpates the area to note the degree of tenderness sensed by the patient. Her priorities are assessing the patient's surgical progress, breathing status, pain, and restlessness.

While gathering data about a patient, you synthesize relevant knowledge, recall prior clinical experiences, consider environmental factors influencing your assessment, apply critical thinking standards and attitudes, and use professional standards of practice to direct your assessment in a meaningful and purposeful way (see Fig. 16.2). You apply knowledge from the physical, biological, and social sciences to ask relevant questions and collect a complete history and perform a physical examination. The ability to make clinical decisions requires a broad knowledge base and access to reliable sources of information, as well as working in a supportive environment (Bjørk and Hamilton, 2011). Your ultimate goal in assessment is to gather all of the information necessary to reveal a patient's health care needs.

Tonya knows that Mr. Lawson had a colectomy to remove the part of his colon that had a cancerous tumor. She recalls information from her scientific knowledge about how a colectomy alters gastrointestinal function. This knowledge leads her to assess Mr. Lawson's gastrointestinal status, including bowel sounds, and she asks him if he is passing flatus. Because the colectomy also involves major abdominal surgery, there is the risk for blood clots to form in the legs (venous thrombosis) after surgery. Those blood clots can lead to pulmonary embolus, an urgent clinical condition. Tonya also assesses the circulation in his legs by palpating pulses and noting temperature of the skin.

Types of Assessments

Assessment requires accurate and thorough data collection. There are two types of assessments:

- Patient-centered interview (conducted during a nursing history)
- Periodic assessments (conducted during ongoing contact with patients)

Each type is typically supplemented using physical examination (conducted during an initial nursing history and at any time a patient presents a symptom).

Each type of assessment is either comprehensive or problem focused. Use a patient-centered interview when you conduct a comprehensive nursing history (i.e., a detailed assessment of a patient's physical, psychosocial, cultural, spiritual, and lifestyle needs). Usually you include categories of information in the patient's history that follow a structured database format based on an accepted framework or practice standard. Marjory Gordon's functional health patterns (Gordon, 1994), Nola Pender's health promotion model (Pender, 2015), and the Long Term Care Minimum Data Set (Centers for Medicare and Medicaid Services [CMS], 2012) for residents in certified Medicare long-term care agencies are a few examples. A theory or practice standard provides the categories of information for you to assess. Pender's model is outlined in Chapter 6. Gordon's 11 functional health patterns include health perception and management, nutritional-metabolic, elimination, activity-exercise, sleep-rest, cognitive-perceptual, self-concept, role-relationship, sexuality-reproduction, coping-stress tolerance, and value-beliefs. A health care agency often relies on the nursing history model included in the electronic health record (EHR) as the organizing framework for an assessment. However, EHR frameworks are often medically driven. Frameworks developed from nursing theories are more holistic and patient-centered, providing a more comprehensive patient review. To make a nursing history more patient-centered, focus on what is important to the patient. *Tonya plans to further assess Mr. Lawson's coping-stress tolerance pattern by using the questions included in her agency's EHR assessment form (e.g., coping behaviors and their effectiveness). A nurse who cared for Mr. Lawson on the previous shift validated that the patient continued to be worried about his recovery. Tonya wants to learn more about what the patient knows about recovery from surgery and how Mr. Lawson feels this is affecting him. How does he normally cope? To make the assessment patient-centered, Tonya knows that his response will guide her in deciding how to assess coping resources and determine the type of information to offer to promote coping.*

Periodic problem-focused assessments collected during rounding or while you administer patient care include quick screenings to rule out or follow up on patient problems. For example, an emergency department nurse uses the Airway, Breathing, Circulation, Disability,

TABLE 16.1	Example of Problem-Focused Patient Assessment: Pain	
Problem and Associated Factors	**Questions for Assessment**	**Physical Examination**
Nature of pain	Describe your pain. Tell me how the pain is affecting your daily life.	Observe for nonverbal cues (e.g., facial grimacing, crying).
Precipitating factors causing pain	What causes your pain to get worse during the day? Is your pain associated with movement? Anything else?	Observe if patient demonstrates nonverbal signs of pain during movement (e.g., positioning, swallowing, walking).
Severity of pain	Rate your pain on a scale of 0 to 10.	Inspect area of discomfort. Palpate area for tenderness.

Exposure (ABCDE) approach in all clinical emergencies for immediate assessment and treatment of patients who are injured or critically ill (AusMed, 2020). It is a rapid bedside assessment of a deteriorating/critically ill patient. This quick screening approach allows nurses to assess critical physiological functions and make quick treatment decisions. Another example is a medical-surgical nurse who performs a quick screening of a patient who is demonstrating incisional pain. The quick screening focuses on the patient's incisional pain, which is a priority problem.

Another type of problem-focused approach begins with a patient's presenting situation and specific problematic areas (expected as well as unexpected), such as incisional pain or limited understanding of postoperative recovery. You ask the patient follow-up questions to clarify and expand your assessment so that you better understand the full nature of the problem. Then you perform a physical examination focusing on the same problem areas to confirm your observations. *For example, Tonya focuses on Mr. Lawson's symptoms the first 48 hours after surgery, the expected healing response, and signs of potential complications. She inspects the condition of the patient's surgical wound, looking at the incision for signs of healing. Her assessment focuses also on the patient's cardiothoracic status including lung sounds, vital signs, and the patient's description of breathing, because a pulmonary embolus poses major risks. She also examines the circulation to his lower extremities. Tonya later expands her assessment to determine how Mr. Lawson is adjusting emotionally to surgery, the current complication of possible pulmonary embolus, and his cancer diagnosis.* Table 16.1 offers an example of a problem-focused assessment.

A physical examination can be a problem-specific or comprehensive review of major body systems (see Chapter 30), providing objective data about a patient's clinical status. Portions of a physical examination are typically included in a nursing history (e.g., height and weight, inspection of the skin, lung sounds). You also use physical examination techniques to validate your ongoing observations and gather more data. In Tonya's case, she inspects the suture line and sees normal inflammation but then palpates the incision line for presence of tenderness. Patient symptoms such as pain or shortness of breath will direct you to examine various bodily functions (shortness of breath: lung sounds and chest excursion; nausea: bowel sounds, abdominal distention).

CRITICAL THINKING IN ASSESSMENT

Critical thinking in assessment of a patient's condition involves application of all critical thinking components (Fig. 16.3). All of these sources provide data that interact in a way that presents a story, a patient's health story. As a nurse your role is to interpret the story. *For example, Tonya's scientific knowledge of colectomy and general surgery guides her with respect to what to anticipate (signs of normal healing) and sources of data to use (patient observation and examination, medical record progress notes) in assessing the patient's postoperative condition. Tonya uses the*

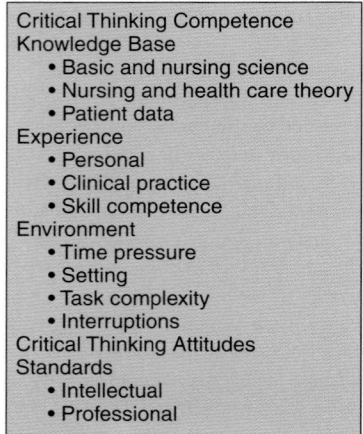

Critical Thinking Competence
Knowledge Base
• Basic and nursing science
• Nursing and health care theory
• Patient data
Experience
• Personal
• Clinical practice
• Skill competence
Environment
• Time pressure
• Setting
• Task complexity
• Interruptions
Critical Thinking Attitudes
Standards
• Intellectual
• Professional

FIG. 16.3 Critical thinking assessment components.

data to begin to interpret whether Mr. Lawson's story is one of normal healing or unexpected complication.

Scientific Data and Theory

Reviewing your textbook and recent nursing, medical, and pharmacological literature about a patient's illness or treatments provides up-to-date information that helps you to identify and anticipate patient needs and to implement evidence-based interventions (see Chapter 19). Knowledge drives your assessment. When you know the scientific nature (e.g., physiology, pathophysiology) of a disease condition, you become aware of the patient behaviors and body systems to assess. The use of scientific and theoretical knowledge increases your awareness of expected signs and symptoms, treatment options, and established standards of therapeutic practice. Always be sure to review the most current evidence-based literature available (see Chapter 5).

Patient Data

A patient is a nurse's primary and best source of information. Patients who are conscious, alert, and able to answer questions appropriately provide the most accurate information. Those with cognitive changes, such as patients who are inattentive or easily distracted, those who are diagnosed with dementia, or who have psychological symptoms such as anxiety or fear, can be less reliable sources. When a patient is not a reliable source, you may refer to the family. The individual identified as a family caregiver is preferred. A patient with limited health literacy has difficulty obtaining, processing, and understanding basic health information, including the questions asked during an assessment (Agency for Healthcare Research and Quality [AHRQ], 2020). A patient with limited health literacy will not always understand some of the questions you use during assessment, especially if you use more clinically focused words or terms or do not speak their language.

BOX 16.1 EVIDENCE-BASED PRACTICE

Assessment of Health Literacy

PICOT Question: In hospitalized adults, does the use of formal literacy screening tools versus asking basic screening questions identify patients with limited health literacy (HL)?

Evidence Summary

HL is essential for patients to manage their own health. HL "universal precautions" involves assuming that all patients have difficulty comprehending health information and accessing health services, thus requiring the presentation of health information to everyone in a clear, easily understood manner (AHRQ, 2020). However, for those with limited HL it is crucial for health care providers to identify patients at risk so that communication-enhancing strategies (e.g., reviewing medications, using diagrams or video-based programs) can be used (Louis et al., 2017).

Numerous instruments are available to assess HL. Although they capture HL comprehensively and measure many factors associated with HL, they are not always useful in clinical practice, especially when time is limited (Altin et al., 2014). Two commonly used instruments include the Rapid Estimate of Adult Literacy in Medicine, Revised (REALM-R) and the Short Test of Functional Health Literacy in Adults (S-TOFHLA) (Louis et al., 2017). The REALM-R includes eight medical terms and the S-TOFHLA includes 36 items. The instruments have been validated for use in hospitals but are cumbersome and/or less likely to be used widely in clinical settings because of their lengthy administration time (S-TOFHLA), the need for a trained administrator because both tools are graded and timed (both), and their "testlike" nature (both) (Louis et al., 2017). An alternative is the Brief Health Literacy Screen (BHLS) (Chew et al., 2008). It is potentially an ideal HL screening tool, especially for hospitalized patients, that is verbally administered to avoid problems with seeing or processing written materials (Louis et al., 2017). A study involving 260 hospitalized

adults involved HL screening using each of the three HL screening tools (Louis et al., 2017). The study showed that if patients are identified as being at risk for low HL with any of the tools, it is appropriate for clinicians to direct appropriate education and counseling resources. Each tool measures different aspects of HL; the S-TOFHLA measures HL-related reading comprehension, whereas the REALM-R measures medical vocabulary fluency (Louis et al., 2017). The BHLS is a self-reported assessment that measures patients' self-perceived HL and ability to navigate the health system, which may not correlate as well with actual HL. Nonetheless, researchers recommend the BHLS to be clinically feasible, and it has high specificity to detect HL (Louis et al., 2017).

Application to Nursing Practice

- Use the literacy screening tools made available at your health care institution with all patients.
  - BHLS questions include: (1) "How often do you have problems learning about your medical condition because of difficulty understanding written information?" (2) "How confident are you in filling out medical forms by yourself?" and (3) "How often do you have someone help you read hospital materials?"
- Follow universal HL precautions (AHRQ, 2020).
- Avoid use of medical jargon.
- Break down information or instructions into small concrete steps.
- Limit the focus of a visit (such as a patient assessment) to three key points that are relevant to the patient and the patient's specific problem.
- Assess a patient's understanding of any instruction by using teach-back.
- Ensure that printed educational information is written at or below a fifth- to sixth-grade reading level.

You will not gather accurate information if a patient does not understand assessment questions. AHRQ (2020) offers tools for assessment of health literacy, including Short Assessment of Health Literacy (Spanish and English), Rapid Estimate of Adult Literacy in Medicine (short form), and Short Assessment of Health Literacy for Spanish Adults (Box 16.1).

Older adults often require more time for assessment than younger patients if their hearing or cognitive function is impaired. However, physiological age and chronological age may not match. It is important to recognize that not all older adults experience the same changes and that changes occur at different rates (Ball et al., 2019). Some older adults have sensory alterations (visual and hearing) that make it more difficult to communicate. Use short (but not leading) questions, keep your language uncomplicated, and listen to a patient carefully (Ball et al., 2019) (Box 16.2). Consult family members, when appropriate, to fill in any gaps in information. Always be attentive, be engaged, and show a caring presence with patients (see Chapter 7). Patients are more likely to fully reveal the nature of health care problems when you show interest, avoid distractions by activities around them, and focus on their concerns.

Types of Patient Data. There are two primary types of patient data: subjective and objective. Subjective data are your patients' verbal descriptions of their health problems gathered during interviews (informal and formal). Subjective data include patient feelings, perceptions, and self-reported symptoms. For example, Mr. Lawson's self-report of pain at the area where his incision slightly separated is an example of subjective data. Only patients provide subjective data relevant to their health condition. The data often reflect physiological, social, or psychological changes. You explore physiological changes through objective physical examination of body systems.

BOX 16.2 FOCUS ON OLDER ADULTS

Approaches for Assessing Older Adults

- Listen patiently; older adults are a rich source of wisdom and experience.
- Allow for pauses and give patients time to tell their story.
- Recognize normal changes associated with aging (see Chapter 14). Older adults' symptoms are often muted or less obvious, vague, or nonspecific compared with younger adults.
- Some patients may not report symptoms because they attribute them to aging or they think nothing can be done for them (Ball et al., 2019).
- If a patient has limited hearing or visual deficits, use nonverbal communication when conducting your interview (see Chapter 49):
  - **Patient-directed eye gaze:** Maintain eye contact with the patient. This allows you or a patient who is speaking to check whether information is understood. It is a signal for readiness to initiate interaction with a patient. Eye contact shows interest in what the other person is saying.
  - **Affirmative head nodding:** This has an important social function. It regulates an interaction (especially when alternate people speak), supports spoken language, and allows for comments on the interaction.
  - **Smiling:** A positive sign that indicates good humor, warmth, and immediacy. Smiles help when first establishing the nurse-patient relationship.
  - **Forward leaning:** This shows awareness, attention, and immediacy. During an interaction it also suggests interest in the person.

Objective data are the findings resulting from observation of patient behavior and clinical signs as well as direct measurement, including what you see, hear, and touch (Ball et al., 2019). Inspecting the condition of a wound, observing a patient walk down the floor, measuring blood pressure (BP), and describing specifically an observed behavior (patient seizure) are examples of objective data.

Objective data are measured on the basis of an accepted standard such as the Fahrenheit or Celsius measure on a thermometer, inches or centimeters on a measuring tape, or a pain rating scale. When you collect objective data, apply critical thinking intellectual standards (e.g., clear, precise, and consistent) so that you can correctly interpret your findings.

Family Caregivers and Significant Others. Family caregivers, other family members, and significant others are primary sources of information for infants or children, critically ill adults, and patients who have intellectual disabilities or cognitive impairments. In cases of severe illness or emergency situations, family members are often your only source of information. The family and significant others are also important secondary sources of information for alert and responsive patients. They confirm findings or identify important health patterns (e.g., whether a patient takes medications regularly or is able to sleep well, and how a patient normally copes with difficulties). Include the family in an assessment when appropriate. Patients do not always want you to question or involve their families. In some cultures, including the family is inappropriate. Some health care agencies require a patient's oral or written permission to collect data from family members. A spouse or close friend who sits in during an assessment can provide another view of a patient's health problems or needs and, more important, tell you when changes in the patient's condition have occurred. Family members are often well informed because of their experiences living with a patient and observing how the patient's health affects daily living activities. They can make important observations about patients' needs that will influence the way you deliver care (e.g., how a patient eats a meal, makes choices, or performs hygiene).

Before her work shift ends, Tonya gets the opportunity to meet Mrs. Lawson. She asks Mr. Lawson if she can update his wife on his current condition. Mr. Lawson agrees. Tonya says, "To begin, Mrs. Lawson, tell me what you know about your husband's current condition." Mrs. Lawson replies, "Well, I know the doctor told us the tumor was cancerous but he thinks he removed it all. We were hoping he would return home in 2 or 3 days." Tonya explains, "Your husband had some chest pain this morning and we have run some tests. You need to speak with his physician, but we are giving him oxygen and a medication to prevent him from having further breathing problems. He is stable right now. Your husband shared with me he feels alone, and he has been restless." Mr. Lawson says, "Yeah, I missed you." Tonya adds, "Tell me how your husband usually deals with stress or uncertainty. Anything you tell us can help us with his care."

Health Care Team. You will often communicate with other health care team members when gathering information about patients. In acute care settings the hand-off report is a method for nurses to communicate the most recent information about patients to nurses or other health care providers on oncoming shifts (see Chapter 26). A hand-off report is defined by The Joint Commission (TJC) as a transfer and acceptance of patient care responsibility achieved through effective communication. It is a real-time process of passing patient-specific information from one caregiver to another or from one team of health care providers to another for the purpose of ensuring the continuity and safety of the patient's care (TJC, 2017a; TJC, 2017b). Hand-offs also occur when patients are transferred from one unit or area of care to another. Effective communication through hand-offs can improve health care providers' perceptions of accuracy and completeness of patient assessment data and the types of interventions provided to patients during a previous shift or level of care. Typically when nurses and other health care providers consult on a patient's condition, each contributes assessment information about the patient. Accurate hand-off information is vital for

you to be able to assess and understand a patient's most current health care needs.

Medical Records. The medical record is a valuable resource for your patient assessment. It contains a patient's medical history, summaries of ongoing assessments and care activities, laboratory and diagnostic test results, current physical findings, and a health care provider's treatment plan. In some cases medical records also contain consultation notes. There are health care agencies that hold electronic health records for all of a patient's visits within an agency system, including inpatient and outpatient. Data in EHRs offer baseline and ongoing objective and subjective information about a patient's response to illness and progress to date. See Chapters 23 and 26 regarding the Health Insurance Portability and Accountability Act (HIPAA) of 1996 Privacy Rule for the protection of patients' health information. Information in a patient's medical record is confidential. The record is a valuable tool to check the consistency and similarities of your own observations and measurements.

Diagnostic Data. An additional source of patient data are the results of diagnostic testing. Serum blood testing, radiological examinations, endoscopic procedures, and specimen analysis are some examples. These data are valuable in confirming observational findings (e.g., if a sample of urine is cloudy in appearance, a specimen of urine examined by a culture test can indicate if infection is present). The data can also direct nurses to explore a patient's condition more fully (e.g., if an x-ray of the chest suggests lung congestion, the nurse will auscultate lung sounds to further determine extent of congestion).

Some patients collect and monitor laboratory data in the home. For example, patients with diabetes mellitus often measure blood glucose daily, and those with asthma measure forced expiratory volumes. Ask patients about their routine results to determine their response to illness and information about the effects of treatment measures. Compare laboratory data with the established norms for a particular test, age-group, and gender.

REFLECT NOW

The next time you assess a patient, consider the data you collect and identify what information is subjective versus objective.
Is the information you collect complete, and if not, how might you gather additional information?

THE NURSE-PATIENT RELATIONSHIP IN ASSESSMENT

Effective communication is the foundation for creating patient-centered relationships that enable patients to tell their stories and nurses to understand patients and the experiences they express (Kourkouta and Papathanasiou, 2014). It requires therapeutic communication skills and the sincere intention of a nurse to understand what concerns a patient (see Chapter 24). Just understanding a patient is insufficient; the nurse must also convey the message that the patient is understandable and that the patient's story is acceptable (Kourkouta and Papathanasiou, 2014). Trust is central to achieving effective patient-centered relationships and necessary to ensure that you are able to learn the information needed to care for a patient.

Typically there is much information to learn about a patient. Regardless of the urgency of a situation or setting, begin by taking quality time to be present with a patient, even if it is for a few minutes. This can be difficult when you are faced with interruptions, the care of other patients, other home visits, or the restricted time given to you in a health care provider's office. Having quality time should occur during admission of a patient to a hospital unit, during rounds when you begin a shift of care, during a follow-up home or clinic visit, or in any encounter with a patient. Connecting with patients by showing interest in their problems and concerns helps you collect a relevant database. Research shows that hearing accounts of patients' health and illness experiences, watching them, and coming to understand how they typically respond develops a type of knowing that fosters sound clinical judgments (Tanner, 2006). Chapter 24 reviews how to establish a nurse-patient relationship and the skills of effective communication.

THE PATIENT-CENTERED INTERVIEW

When conducting an assessment of a patient you will use a combination of interview and observational skills. A patient-centered interview is relationship based and is an organized conversation focused on learning about a patient's concerns and needs. Patient needs are what triggers the process of clinical judgment through the nursing process (see Chapter 15). The interview is designed to encourage patients to discuss their needs from their perspective and focus on priority problem areas. An interview may last less than a minute or several minutes. To gather accurate information from your patient's perspective, you must make every effort to sense the world of an individual patient as the patient senses it (Ball et al., 2019). An empathic, patient-centered interview strengthens a patient's sense of self-esteem and lessens the feelings of helplessness during an episode of illness. Research shows that health care providers' use of good interview skills improves problem detection, diagnostic accuracy, patient satisfaction, patient adjustment to stress and illness, patient recall of information, patient

adherence to therapy, and patient health outcomes (Keifenheim et al., 2015). The most extensive patient-centered interview is the one used during collection of a nursing history. Primary objectives while taking an initial nursing history are to discover details about a patient's concerns, explore expectations for the health care visit, and display genuine interest and partnership.

Interview Preparation

Before you begin an extensive interview (e.g., for a nursing history), be prepared. Review a patient's medical record when information is available. If your interview is performed at patient admission, there may be little information in the record except for an admitting diagnosis and the patient's chief complaint. In other cases, review the previous medical entries or nurses' notes. Were problems identified that remain a part of the patient's treatment plan? Do any of those problems require clarification or follow-up? Does a patient's admitting diagnosis or do other diagnoses suggest lines of questioning? For example, when caring for a patient with a history of chronic lung disease, you include questions about the patient's respiratory status, effects of disease symptoms on lifestyle, and the patient's acceptance and understanding of a chronic disease.

For shorter, ongoing interviews, focus on patient priorities. For example, the information you obtain during a hand-off report at the beginning of a shift will help you frame the clinical questions needed to address the patient's most urgent problems.

Communication Skills. Chapter 24 explores in depth the range of communication skills available to use during interactions with patients. Box 16.3 summarizes effective interview skills to use with patients during assessment interviews.

BOX 16.3 Interview Skills During Patient Assessment

Courtesy
- Greet patients by the name by which they prefer to be addressed. Ask, "Would you prefer I call you by Mrs. Silver or by your first name?" It is all right to shake hands.
- Introduce yourself and explain your role the first time you meet. For example, "My name is Julia, and I will be your nursing student today. I would like to ask you questions about how you are feeling right now. Is that okay with you?"
- Ensure patient that information shared will remain confidential among the health care team.
- Meet and acknowledge visitors in the patient's room and learn their names and roles.
- Sit down next to the patient and do not make an effort to exit the room too soon.
- Ask the patient's permission to conduct an interview in a visitor's presence.
- Try to reduce computer time entering notes; remember key words and record later.

Comfort
- Provide necessary comfort measures before beginning an interview. When patients have symptoms, keep questions short and focused.
- Maintain privacy. Close room curtains or doors and provide a comfortable room temperature.
- Select a location for the interview that is quiet and free of interruptions. Do not answer your mobile phone or pager during an interview unless there is an emergency. If possible, set aside a 10- to 15-minute period when no other activities are planned.
- Avoid making the patient tired. You do not need to complete the interview in one session.

Connection
- Make a good first impression. Do not stare at a computer screen while filling in required data fields or talking on a mobile phone; patients will perceive you to be uncaring or uninterested.
- Stiff formality may inhibit a patient, but being too casual may not instill confidence. Do not be careless with your choice of words; what you think is harmless may seem very important to a patient who is anxious to understand you.
- Begin with open-ended questions that encourage patients to tell their stories (e.g., "How have you been feeling?" "What questions would you like to discuss?")
- Allow patients to fully describe their symptoms without interruption.
- Do not dominate a discussion or assume that you know the nature of a patient's problems. Listen and be attentive.
- Be observant. Note a patient's tone of voice, posture, and level of energy when talking.
- Respect silence and be flexible and open-minded. Let the patient's needs, concerns, or questions guide your follow-up questions. Health problems can have multiple causes; do not leap to conclusions too quickly.

Confirmation
- At the end of an interview, ask the patient to summarize the discussion so that there are no uncertainties. Be open to further clarification or discussion. End by asking if there is anything else the patient wishes to discuss.
- If there are questions you cannot answer, say so and let the patient know that you will return with follow-up if possible.

Adapted from: Ball JW, et al: *Seidel's guide to physical examination: an interprofessional approach*, ed 9, St Louis, 2019, Elsevier.

Phases of the Assessment Interview

When you begin a formal patient-centered interview for the purpose of collecting a nursing history, you will go through the traditional three interview phases: (1) orientation or setting an agenda; (2) working phase—collecting assessment data; and (3) termination of the interview (see Chapter 24). Your ability to complete any one phase will depend on the time you have available and whether the patient's condition changes or declines during the interview.

Orientation and Setting an Agenda. Begin by introducing yourself. Explain why you are collecting data and that you will keep all information confidential. It is important to set an agenda for the interview and explain how you will gather information about a patient's chief concerns or problems (e.g., asking questions and performing a physical examination). Focus on a patient's goals, preferences, and concerns, not your personal agenda. This is a time to ensure your patient feels comfortable speaking with you and becoming an active partner in decisions about care. The professionalism and competence that you show when interviewing strengthens the nurse-patient relationship.

Tonya is doing a follow-up interview the next morning, day 3 postoperatively. Mr. Lawson has been stable since the previous afternoon. He is going to be allowed to sit in a chair today. He is still receiving oxygen and an intravenous (IV) medication to reduce risk of further pulmonary emboli from developing. However, his respirations are stable and he has a normal oxygen saturation. As he continues to recover surgically, Tonya decides to learn more about Mr. Lawson's home situation. She explains, "Mr. Lawson, it looks as if your physician wants you to stay in the hospital a couple of days until we get you stable, but then you will be going home. It's important for us to know more about how you care for yourself at home. Are you comfortable, and can I take a few minutes to talk about your discharge now?" Mr. Lawson replies, "I feel a bit better, and, yes, I've been thinking about some questions I want to ask." Tonya replies, "Good. We'll start there."

Working Phase—Collecting Assessment Data. Whether you are conducting a complete nursing history or gathering ongoing assessment information, the working phase involves gathering accurate, relevant, and complete information about a patient's condition. Beginning an interview with open-ended questions allows patients to describe their concerns and problems clearly. For example, begin by having patients explain the reasons for seeking health care or describe their symptoms or psychological concerns. Ask them to describe what they know about their health problems or to describe their health care expectations. Use attentive listening and summarize key issues to validate your understanding with the patient, and encourage the patient to tell a full story (see Chapter 24). Do not rush to an opinion about what the patient tells you. When a patient describes a symptom, such as dizziness or weakness, clarify what the patient means. For example, say, "Describe how you feel when you are dizzy." Be willing to wait for the patient to respond no matter how long it takes (Muhrer, 2014). If you instead ask direct questions (e.g., "Does the room spin?" or "Do you feel faint?" in the case of dizziness), most patients will say "yes"; however, this may not reveal the true problem. This is important because symptoms often reflect multiple disorders. Dizziness can indicate that the patient has an ear disorder, cardiovascular disease, an anxiety disorder, or a neurological problem. Unless you listen and get a full description of the patient's symptoms and their effect on the patient, you will not identify the true problem.

The verbal cues that a patient expresses will help you stay focused so that you can direct an assessment appropriately. Do not rush a patient. An initial interview is more extensive. Gather information about a patient's concerns and then complete all relevant sections of the nursing history. Ongoing interviews, which occur each time you interact with your patient, do not need to be as

extensive. Organize your time with a patient and focus on priority areas to assess. An ongoing interview also allows you to update a patient's status and concerns, focus on changes previously identified, and review new problems.

Tonya: "Mr. Lawson, you said you had some questions. Can you tell me what they are?"

Mr. Lawson: "Well, I just want to know what's going on. My doctor told me that I wouldn't be able to lift anything heavy for a while, and I'm not sure if I understand. The fact that I'm getting this new medicine, will I need to do something different?"

Tonya notices that Mr. Lawson is having some difficulty with eye contact and remains restless. She focuses on his question. "Let's start with your question about lifting. Tell me what you think that means."

Mr. Lawson: "Well, I suppose it means anything big, but I don't plan to move furniture or do any work around the house until I feel better."

Tonya: "Tell me the types of things you lift regularly at home and approximately how much they weigh."

Mr. Lawson: "Well, when our grandchildren visit, they like to be picked up. We have a pet schnauzer, but he just jumps up on the chair with me. My wife does grocery shopping, but I come out to unload the car."

Tonya: "Anything else?"

Mr. Lawson: "Hmmm, occasionally I lift the laundry basket and take it downstairs."

Tonya: "Okay, and about your medication, yes, you need to know what type of problems to look for when you get home. And you will need to care for your incision. Can you tell me the signs of infection?"

Mr. Lawson: "Not sure I can, but I guess it would hurt more. Is infection common?"

Tonya: "No, but you and your wife need to know the signs, so if something happens once you return home, you can know to call your physician quickly. Has your physician or the nurse practitioner talked to you about incision care?"

Mr. Lawson: "No, they haven't mentioned anything about that yet."

Tonya: "Okay, I'll explain everything you need to know and take the time to be sure you understand. Do you think you learn best by reading information or listening to explanations?"

Mr. Lawson: "I think I do okay with both."

Tonya: "Okay. Is there anything else you wish to discuss?"

Mr. Lawson: "No. It's a lot to take in. I just have trouble not worrying."

Tonya's assessment focuses on the patient's questions and behaviors and how the questions pertain to the information he will need to learn to go home and assume self-care.

> **QSEN** Building Competency in Patient-Centered Care
> Describe how you would conduct a patient-centered interview with Mr. Lawson about his expectations for going home after surgery during the working phase of the interview.
>
> Answers to QSEN Activities can be found on the Evolve website.

Termination Phase. You summarize your discussion with a patient and check for accuracy of the information you collected during the termination phase of an interview. Let your patient know when the interview is coming to an end. For example, say, "I have just two more questions. We'll be finished in a few more minutes." This helps a patient maintain direct attention without being distracted by wondering when the interview will end. This approach also gives the patient an opportunity to ask additional questions. End the interview in a friendly manner, telling the patient when you will return to provide care.

Tonya: "You've given me a good idea of which topics we need to cover and the plans we need to make to get you ready to go home. And we'll include your wife in these decisions if that is okay?"

Mr. Lawson: "Yes, for sure. She always helps me when I need it."

Tonya: "I'll come back after I check on two other patients, okay?"

Mr. Lawson: "Yes, you've already been very helpful."

Interview Techniques. You will use therapeutic communication throughout a nursing history interview. These interview tips are special communication techniques that help you better explore the patient's story. During an interview you want to direct the flow of the discussion so that patients have the opportunity to freely describe their health problems to enable you to get a detailed picture of their needs. Because a patient's report will contain subjective information, validate subjective data later with objective information. For example, if a patient reports difficulty breathing, you will also assess the patient's respiratory rate and lungs sounds during the physical examination.

Observation. Observation is powerful. Observe a patient's verbal and nonverbal behaviors, such as the use of eye contact, body language and positioning, or tone of voice. While observing nonverbal behavior, appearance, and the patient's interaction with the environment, determine whether the data you obtained are consistent with what the patient states verbally. Your observations will lead you to pursue further objective information to form thorough and accurate conclusions. Patients are also observant during interviews. If you establish trust, the patient feels comfortable asking you questions about the health care environment, planned treatments, and diagnostic testing in order to partner with you in making decisions and planning the goals of care.

An important aspect of observation includes a patient's level of function: the physical, developmental, psychological, and social aspects of everyday living. When you observe a patient's level of function, you watch what a patient does when eating, performing hygiene, or making a decision about preparing a medication. Observing a patient perform a function is a more accurate assessment than simply posing a question about whether one can or cannot perform the function.

Open-Ended Questions. During a patient-centered interview try to learn in the patient's own words any concerns or problems, perceived causes for those problems, and any health care goals. Open-ended questions elicit a patient's unique story. An open-ended question gives a patient the ability to decide how much information to disclose (Ball et al., 2019)—for example, "So, tell me more about…." or "What are your concerns about this?" This approach does not lead to a specific answer. You are exploring with the patient. The use of open-ended questions prompts patients to describe a situation in more than just one or two words, allowing patients to actively describe their health status. The open-ended question shows that you want to hear a patient's thoughts and feelings. Listen carefully and do not interrupt the patient. When you interrupt, you will not gather complete information and you also may end up disagreeing with the patient, which is not therapeutic.

Direct Closed-Ended Questions. As you obtain information from a patient about a topic, you will then ask direct closed-ended questions to seek specific information about a problem. Direct questions are not ideal when you wish a patient to be thorough in describing a health problem. However, this problem-seeking technique reveals details needed to identify a patient's specific problems accurately and more fully. For example, a patient reports having indigestion over the course of several days and acknowledges having some diarrhea and loss of appetite. The patient's explanation for the cause relates to a recent series of trips that changed his eating habits. The nurse focuses on the symptoms the patient identifies and the general indigestion problem by asking closed-ended questions that limit answers to one or two

words such as "yes" or "no" or a number or frequency of a symptom. For example, the nurse asks, "How often does the diarrhea occur?" and "Do you have pain or cramping?" This technique requires short answers and clarifies previous information to provide a more comprehensive database. The questions do not encourage patients to volunteer more information than you request.

Leading Questions. These types of interview questions are risky because they can limit the information a patient will provide to what a patient thinks you want to know (Ball et al., 2019). Two examples of leading questions are (1) "It seems to me this is bothering you quite a bit. Is that true?" and (2) "That wasn't very hard to do, do you agree?" When asking how often a symptom or problem occurs, allow a patient to define "often." Do not ask, "It didn't happen too often, did it?" A patient may not understand what you are asking and may say so (Ball et al., 2019).

Back Channeling. Reinforce your interest in what a patient has to say by using good eye contact and listening. Also use back channeling, which includes active listening prompts such as "all right," "go on," or "uh-huh." This technique shows that you have heard what a patient says, are interested in hearing the full story, and are encouraging the patient to give more details.

Probing. As patients tell their stories, encourage a full description without trying to control a story's direction. This requires you to probe with more open-ended questions, such as "Is there anything else you can tell me?" or "What else is bothering you?" Each time a patient offers more detail, probe again until the patient has nothing else to say and has told the full description. Always be observant. If a patient becomes fatigued or uncomfortable, know that it is time to postpone the interview until later.

NURSE'S EXPERIENCE

Experience provides a background for each clinical encounter with a patient. Just as a painter creates a background for the details of a painting, a nurse uses background experiences to put into perspective each patient's clinical situation. Personal experience plays a role. During assessment, consider your own experience with patient situations such as loss, fatigue, loss of a loved one or job, or anxiety over the unknown. Your personal experiences and perceptions can help you understand a patient's situation, as long as you do not allow that experience to bias your findings. Reflect on personal experience to help you explore a patient's situation.

Your experience in caring for patients is one of the most important sources of data. Through clinical experience you observe other patients' behaviors and physical signs and symptoms; track trends, recognize clinical changes, and identify cues; and learn the types of questions to ask, choosing the questions that will give the most useful information. This experience builds your ability to know patients, knowing the pattern of responses shown by similar patients and making appropriate clinical judgments (see Chapter 7).

As a new nurse, use a systematic and analytical method for assessment. Novice nurses usually apply the nursing process in a more linear way. They tend to focus only on data and do not consider the whole context of a patient's situation. New nurses have not had the experiences yet to place each patient situation into context. (For example, after Tonya cares for more patients who have had a colectomy, she can use that experience as context for future patients.) As you gain more clinical practice, you will become more skilled at pulling together all your patient's data. You will make mental connections from previous similar clinical experiences. This will allow you to appropriately use your intuition to form judgments and make effective, patient-centered decisions. That intuition is a feeling of knowing something without conscious use of reason, but is a critical part of clinical decision making (Muntean, 2012). Practical experience and the opportunity to make clinical decisions strengthen your critical thinking.

Experience with nursing skills is also important for accurate assessment. This includes competence in performing an assessment and physical examination. When you have had the opportunity to perform a skill repeatedly you learn what is necessary to adapt a skill without sacrificing safety principles. That experiential knowledge is especially useful in allowing you to anticipate the assessments needed and the steps in preparation that will allow you to perform a skill competently. Be thorough in assessing a patient prior to performing any nursing procedure, including risk factors that affect how the skill is to be performed, patient knowledge of the skill, and patient characteristics that might influence skill outcome.

ENVIRONMENT IN ASSESSMENT

Numerous environmental factors affect the adequacy of an assessment. Consider these factors as part of your critical thinking in performing assessment.

Setting

Always consider the setting where you perform an assessment. An emergency department is a care unit that requires quick, organized thinking as you prioritize the physical and psychological needs of a patient. The severity of each patient's condition guides your assessment. A home care setting permits you to assess an array of conditions (social, financial, cultural) that affect a patient's health status in the home. The setting of a hospital nursing unit affects your assessment depending on how patient rooms are designed, the procedures for nursing activities, and staff resources. Consider these factors as you engage a patient in an assessment. For example, you might choose to delegate a task to assistive personnel so that you can perform an admission assessment of a new patient.

Time Pressure

Time always seems limited in a health care setting. Nurses are challenged with multiple responsibilities. However, unless enough time is spent in patient assessment, you will be unable to identify patient needs accurately. If you learn to value assessment, you will find time to collect essential patient data. As a member of a nursing staff you will become oriented to the personnel and functioning of the unit and aware of the nursing activity of a shift to effectively manage the time (Naya, 2018). For example, you will organize your time to assess each patient based on when hand-off reports occur, when standard procedures (e.g., medication administration) are scheduled, and when specific patients must leave a unit for a procedure. Use each patient **encounter** as a time to perform assessment and focus on the patient priorities. Some tips to use time management for assessment include (Naya, 2018):

- List the care activities that need to be done, including assessment.
- Prioritize these activities.
- Estimate the time needed for each activity.
- Spend the time consciously.
- Cautiously spend the time for unscheduled activities, and learn to say "no."

Task Complexity

Whether it is a patient's physical condition, the numerous procedures to be performed, or both, task complexity affects your ability to perform high-quality assessments. Again, your ability to prioritize patient needs will enable you to manage task complexity. For example, consider a patient with diabetes mellitus who has a risk for infection and circulatory problems by nature of the disease. The patient enters the hospital for the same procedure as Mr. Lawson. But in contrast, this patient develops a surgical wound infection, has more than one IV line for medications, and has the same postsurgical cardiopulmonary risks if the patient remains immobile. In addition, the patient will experience the pain of a surgical wound. A nurse anticipates which priority to address by keenly observing the patient, recognizing clinical changes quickly, and knowing the types of assessments to perform for each type of actual or potential surgical problem. In this case the nurse knows to check the surgical wound frequently as well as the patient's pain status. Routine vital signs might be performed less often if the patient is stable. Assessment of the patient's response to early mobility will also become important.

Interruptions

Research has shown that interruptions occur frequently during medication preparation and administration at the bedside, and these interruptions have been associated with procedural failures and clinical errors (Freitas et al. 2019; Johnson et al., 2017). Medication errors are just one form of adverse event that occurs in hospital settings. Interruptions affect assessment activities as well. When a nurse enters a patient room to administer a medication, assessment is performed to ensure administration safety and accuracy. You must avoid interruptions in order to think critically in anticipation of and during a patient encounter (e.g., medication administration, early ambulation, education). Take a time out and avoid responding to phone calls or questions from others when you perform a necessary patient assessment. Your full attention enables you to observe more subtle signs of a patient's condition and helps you focus on the priorities you selected for an assessment.

CRITICAL THINKING ATTITUDES FOR ASSESSMENT

A thorough patient assessment relies on nurses to apply all critical thinking attitudes. *In the case study involving Mr. Lawson, for example, Tonya is confident in being able to care for Mr. Lawson because of her experience with surgical patients. She applied independent thinking when she recognized Mr. Lawson's developing signs and symptoms suggestive of a major breathing problem and reported them to the health care provider. Tonya has shown discipline in conducting necessary assessments and showed curiosity as she explored Mr. Lawson's knowledge and concerns about discharge.*

STANDARDS IN ASSESSMENT

Intellectual standards guide the manner in which a nurse pursues an assessment. For example, when a home health nurse cares for a 72-year-old patient and notes an unsteady gait, the nurse should recognize immediately that unsteady gait is a fall risk factor. The nurse tries to be precise and specific by having the patient perform a Timed Up and Go test (an evidence-based clinical test for balance) and observes as the patient walks a short distance down the hallway (see Chapter 38). In addition, the nurse assesses the patient's vision to detect visual problems that might contribute to limitations in ambulation. The nurse applies relevance in the assessment by assessing the patient's past history of falls and the condition of his home environment. As you conduct an assessment, reflect on intellectual standards to guide data collection.

Professional standards of practice or clinical guidelines also influence assessment. For example, the Infusion Nurses Society has evidence-based criteria for the signs of phlebitis (inflammation of a vein). A nurse who is caring for a patient with an IV line uses these standard criteria when assessing the patient, by noting the color of the skin at the IV site, palpating temperature of the skin, and inspecting for drainage at the IV site. Standards are useful for comparing your patient's actual assessment findings with what the standard sets as normal or abnormal.

REFLECT NOW

Before your next clinical assignment, consider how to plan a patient-centered interview. In what ways can you connect early with a patient? What questions might be appropriate based on the patient's health situation?

THE NURSING HEALTH HISTORY FORMAT

You have learned how critical thinking applies to the assessment step of the nursing process for forming clinical judgments needed for clinical decisions. The **nursing health history** is a formal method used to collect data about a patient. The format, required content, and length of a nursing health history will vary by health care setting. However, the history typically contains similar categories of information regardless of the setting and EHR software or format. Most health history forms (electronic and written) are structured. However, on the basis of information you gain as you conduct the patient-centered interview, you learn which components of the history to explore fully and which require less detail. As you gain more experience, you will learn to refine and broaden questions as needed to correctly identify a patient's unique needs. Your patient's priorities and needs and the amount of time you have available determine how complete a history will be. A comprehensive history covers all health dimensions (Fig. 16.4).

Cultural Considerations

Obtaining a nursing health history requires cultural competence (see Chapter 9). This involves self-awareness, reflective practice, and knowledge of a patient's core cultural background. It is critical for you to adapt each assessment to the uniqueness of each patient. Cultural humility requires you to recognize your own knowledge limitations and cultural perspective and thus be open to new perspectives (Ball et al., 2019). Without humility you are at risk for being biased and misinterpreting assessment findings.

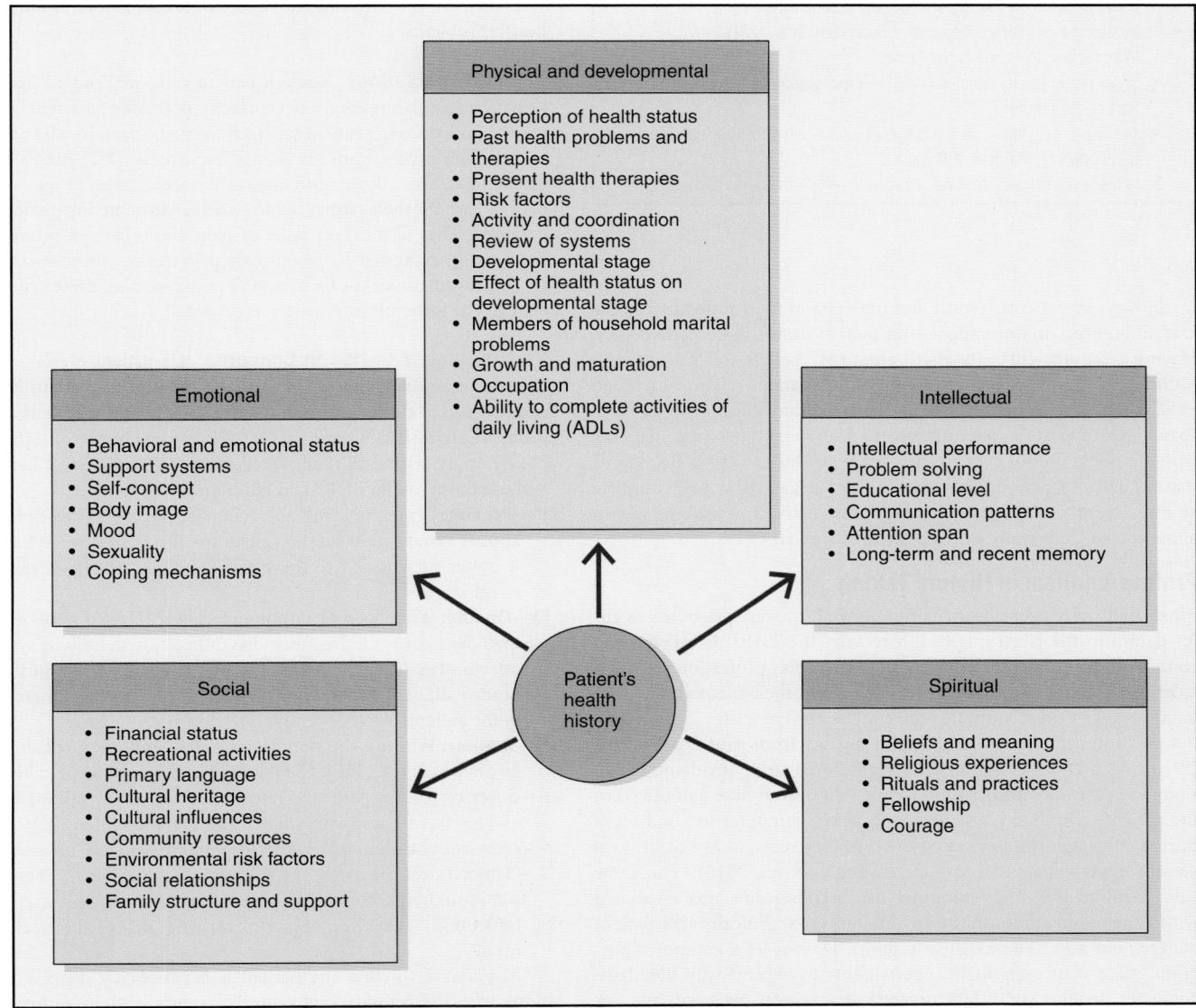

FIG. 16.4 Dimensions for gathering data for a health history.

BOX 16.4   CULTURAL ASPECTS OF CARE

Developing a Patient-Centered Approach

To successfully explore a patient's illness or health care problems, use a patient-centered approach. Elicit patient values, preferences, and expressed needs as part of your clinical interview (QSEN, 2020). Ensure that the interview is inclusive. When patients desire involvement of family members, remove any barriers to having families present (QSEN, 2020). Use a professional interpreter if there is a language difference.

Implications for Patient-Centered Care
- When talking about a patient's illness, try to understand it "through the patient's eyes."
  - What do you think is wrong with you?
  - What worries you most about your illness?
  - How do you define health and illness? How do you feel about pain, your illness, or death?
- When talking about treatments, value a patient's expertise with their own health and symptoms.
  - What should we do to control or eliminate your problem?
  - Which types of treatment do you use at home?
  - What benefits do you expect from the planned treatment?
- Learn about a patient's sources of support (Ball et al., 2019).
  - Who makes decisions in the family?
  - What is the family composition? How many generations are considered part of the family?
  - Are there individuals in the patient's social network that can influence perception of health and illness?
  - Is there a particular cultural group with which the patient identifies?

Show your patients respect and understand their individual needs and differences; do not impose your own attitudes, biases, and beliefs. Having a genuine curiosity about a patient's beliefs and values lays a foundation for a trusting and strong nurse-patient relationship (Ball et al., 2019). For clarity, explain the intent of any questions you have. Avoid stereotypes; the assumptions tied to stereotypes (e.g., patients who are obese do not exercise regularly) can lead to the collection of inaccurate information. Draw on knowledge gained as you complete an assessment and ask questions in a constructive and probing way to allow you to truly know who a patient is (Box 16.4).

Professionalism in History Taking

Most health care agencies use computerized software programs to enter data into the electronic health record (the EHR). In many cases computers are at each patient's bedside. To display professionalism and a caring approach during an interview, look at the patient and not the data categories on a computer screen. Use the computer if you must, but position it in a way that does not distract from your focus on the patient (Ball et al., 2019). In an observational study involving physicians and patients during routine clinic visits, fewer than half (48%) of the patients who had physicians with heavy computer use and focus during clinical encounters rated the care they received as excellent on patient experience surveys (Ratanawongsa et al., 2016). The same study showed that high computer use by physicians was associated with observable communication differences, specifically less patient engagement and more negative rapport. Do not let a computer program guide your assessment. Ask patients to explain why they have come for health care, listen, proceed at a reasonable pace, and ask open-ended questions (Ball et al., 2019).

Components of the Nursing Health History

The nursing history contains several common components. Remember to apply critical thinking to each unique patient situation to ensure the history gathers patient-centered information.

Biographical Information. Biographical information is factual demographic data that include a patient's age, gender, address, insurance information, occupation, working status, marital status, and referral source.

Chief Concern or Reason for Seeking Health Care. The chief concern is a brief statement about why a patient (in the patient's own words) is seeking health care (Ball et al., 2019). This information offers a focus to explore a patient's concerns and issues. Once you learn a patient's chief concerns, you will compare those findings with what you learn during your assessment and physical examination. Often you will learn much more. Ask why a patient is seeking health care (e.g., "Tell me, Ms. Richard, what brought you to the clinic today?"). Once you learn a chief concern, you then gather more comprehensive data and probe for a full description of the patient's health status. Record a patient's response in quotations to indicate a subjective statement. As you explore a patient's reason for seeking health care, you will learn the chronological and sequential history of the patient's health problems.

Patient Expectations. Assess a patient's expectations of health care providers (e.g., being diagnosed correctly, obtaining pain relief, or being treated for a disease). Patient satisfaction can be perceived by patients as poor if their expectations are unmet (see Chapter 2). Patients typically expect to receive information about their treatments, prognosis, and a plan of care for their return home (whether they are inpatients or outpatients). They also expect relief of pain and other symptoms and to have caring expressed by health care providers. After assessing initial patient expectations, use these to later assess whether these expectations changed or were met after care was provided.

Present Illness or Health Concerns. If a patient presents with an illness or symptom, collect essential and relevant data about its nature and course. Go slowly as you try to give context to the present illness or problem, giving it a chronological and sequential framework (Ball et al., 2019). Apply critical thinking intellectual standards (see Chapter 15), and use the acronym PQRST to guide your assessment:

P—**Provokes** (precipitating and relieving factors): How did it come about? What might be the causes for the symptom? What makes it better or worse? Are there activities (e.g., exercise, sleep) that affect it?

Q—**Quality:** What does the symptom feel like? (Have patients explain in their own words.) If the patient has difficulty in describing symptoms, offer probes (e.g., "Is the pain sharp? Dull?" or "Do you feel lightheaded, dizzy, off-balance?"). What does the illness or symptom mean to the patient?

R—**Radiate:** Where is the symptom located? Is it in one place? Does it go anywhere else? Have the patient be as precise as possible.

S—**Severity:** Ask the patient to rate the severity of a symptom on a scale of 0 to 10 (with no symptom at 0 and the worst intensity at 10). This gives you a baseline with which to compare in follow-up assessments.

T—**Time:** Assess the onset and duration of symptoms. When did the symptom first occur? Does it come and go? If so, how often and for how long? What time of day or on what day of the week does it occur?

Also assess whether the patient is experiencing other symptoms along with the primary symptom. For example, does nausea accompany pain? Does the patient have pain along with shortness of breath?

Past Health History. A health history offers a holistic view of a patient's health care experiences and current health habits (see Fig. 16.4). Assess whether a patient has ever been hospitalized or injured or has had surgery. Has any illness or injury limited the patient's ability to function? Include a complete medication history (including past and current prescribed and over-the-counter medications or any herbal supplements) (see Chapter 32). Determine if a patient has a history of allergies, including allergic reactions to food, latex, drugs, or contact agents (e.g., soap). Asking patients whether they have had problems with medications or food clarifies the specific reaction and whether a patient has required treatment. If the patient has an allergy, note the specific reaction and treatment on the assessment form and the special armband provided. Also ask if the patient has ever had a blood product transfusion and whether any reactions occurred.

The history also includes a description of a patient's habits, emotional status, and lifestyle patterns. Assessing for the use of alcohol, tobacco, caffeine, or recreational drugs (e.g., methamphetamine or cocaine) determines a patient's risk for diseases involving the liver, lungs, heart, or nervous system. It is essential to gather information about the type of habit and the frequency and duration of use. Assessing patterns of coping (see Chapter 37), sleep (see Chapter 43), exercise (see Chapter 38), and nutrition (see Chapter 45) are also important when planning nursing care. Your aim is to match a patient's healthy lifestyle patterns with interventions in the plan of care as much as possible.

Family History. The family history includes data about immediate and blood relatives. Your objective is to determine whether a patient is at risk for illnesses of a genetic or familial nature and to identify areas of health promotion and illness prevention (see Chapter 6). A complete and accurate family history guides your risk assessment and recommendations for risk-guided prevention strategies (Orlando et al., 2013). There are clinical screening and treatment guidelines for patients and family members based on risk factors for conditions such as breast and ovarian cancer, colon cancer, venous thrombosis, cardiovascular disease, cerebrovascular disease, and inherited neurological conditions. For example, a patient with a strong family history of breast cancer will be recommended to pursue mammography more often, and female children may be recommended for genetic counseling.

A patient's family history also reveals information about family structure, interaction, support, and function that is useful in planning care, such as when a family caregiver is needed (see Chapter 10). *In the case study, Tonya assesses the level of support that Mrs. Lawson is willing to provide. Mrs. Lawson tells Tonya that the two have been married 32 years and states, "I feel I can do whatever is needed for him. Physically I'm lucky; I'm healthy. I understand he might not like his restrictions, but we'll work together." Tonya's assessment shows a pattern that Mrs. Lawson is supportive and able to help her husband adjust to activity limitations when he returns home. Tonya's assessment allows her to include Mrs. Lawson when she provides patient education.* If a patient's family is not supportive, do not involve the family in care. Stressful family relationships are sometimes a significant barrier when you try to help patients with problems involving loss, self-concept, spiritual health, and personal relationships.

Psychosocial History. A psychosocial history provides information about a patient's support system, which may include a spouse or partner, children, other family members, and friends. The history also includes information about whether a patient has experienced recent loss and ways in which the patient and family typically cope with stress and grief (see Chapters 36 and 37). Behaviors that patients use at home to cope with stress such as walking, reading, or talking with a friend can also be used as nursing interventions if the patient experiences stress while receiving health care.

Spiritual Health. Life experiences and events shape a person's spirituality. The spiritual dimension represents the totality of one's being and is difficult to assess quickly (see Chapter 35). Review with patients their beliefs about life, their source for guidance in acting on beliefs, and the relationship they have with family in exercising their faith. Also assess rituals and religious practices that patients use to express their spirituality. Patients may request availability of these practices while in a health care setting.

Review of Systems. The review of systems (ROS) involves systematic collection of subjective information from patients about the presence or absence of health-related issues in each body system (Ball et al., 2019). During the ROS ask the patient about the normal functioning of each body system and any noted changes. You are more likely to conduct a comprehensive review of all systems during a non-emergent admission to a clinic or an initial home visit. A problem-focused review is common in emergent situations within acute care. When using a structured admission form, you probably will not cover all of the questions for each body system every time you collect a history. When a patient mentions any unexpected signs or symptoms, explore the affected system(s) more in depth. The systems you prioritize for assessment depend on a patient's condition and the urgency in starting care.

Along with the ROS, you conduct a physical examination (see Chapter 30) to further explore and confirm patient information. An accurate history helps focus the physical examination, making it more productive and time efficient. As you gain experience, you will learn to look for more data, challenge any interpretations that you made solely based on the history, and persevere to gather accurate and complete assessment data.

Observation of Patient Behavior. Throughout a nursing history and physical examination closely observe a patient's verbal and nonverbal behaviors and functional status. This information adds depth to your objective database. You determine whether data obtained by observation matches what a patient communicates verbally. For example, a patient expresses no concern about an upcoming diagnostic test but shows poor eye contact, shakiness, and restlessness, all suggesting anxiety and verbal and nonverbal data conflict. Observations direct you to gather additional objective information to make clinical judgments about a patient's condition.

Data Documentation

Record the results of the nursing health history and physical examination in a clear, concise manner using appropriate terminology. This information becomes the baseline for health care providers to identify a patient's nursing diagnoses and health problems, to plan and implement care, and to evaluate a patient's response to interventions. Standardized forms, especially electronic forms, make it easy to enter assessment data as a patient responds to questions. A timely, clear, and concise record is necessary for use by other health care professionals (see Chapter 26). If you do not record an assessment finding or a suspected problem, it is lost and unavailable to anyone else caring for the patient. If information is not specific, the reader is left with only general impressions. Observing and recording patient status are legal and professional responsibilities for all nurses. The nurse practice acts in all states and the ANA Nursing's Social Policy Statement (ANA, 2010) require accurate data collection and recording as independent functions essential to the role of the professional nurse.

Chapter 26 reviews basic rules for accurate and concise documentation of an assessment. When recording data, pay attention to facts and be as descriptive as possible, applying intellectual standards for measurement.

THE ASSESSMENT PROCESS

During the assessment step of the nursing process, you collect data, recognizing and confirming cues that begin to form a picture of a patient's health care problems and needs. *In the case study, Tonya makes rounds near the end of the third postoperative day with Mr. Lawson. Tonya inspects the patient's surgical wound and notices separation of the wound between two sutures at the bottom of the incision. There is a small amount of serous drainage. The area is inflamed, and Tonya asks the patient if the incision is tender when she gently palpates it. Mr. Lawson states, "Ow, that feels sore there. I think I pulled it when I coughed last night." He also rates pain currently as being at a level of 4. Tonya checks the patient's vital signs and notes that his temperature is 37.5°C (99.6°F), slightly above his average temperature of 37.2°C (99.0°F), heart rate is 88 beats/min and regular, and BP is 110/78 mm Hg. Tonya also inspects the IV access site in the patient's left forearm. It is intact, and there are no signs of phlebitis. Tonya reports findings of assessment to the patient's physician.*

Consider Tonya's thought processes as she responds to assessment data cues:
- Separation of wound between two sutures—Data cue.
  - Knowledge—Open wound is potential source of infection.
- Small amount of serous drainage, incision inflamed, tenderness present—Data cues.
  - Knowledge—Signs of surgical site infection (clinical standards) include inflammation, tenderness, and abnormal appearance of drainage.
- Body temperature slightly above patient's normal—Data confirm early indication of infection.
- Inspection of IV site shows no signs of phlebitis—Data are standard criteria for ruling out phlebitis.
  - Knowledge—Any open wound such as an IV site can lead to infection.
- Vital signs normal, pain level is 4 as in previous assessment—Data show stability.

You need to reflect on your knowledge and experience and anticipate sources of data when a patient describes a current problem or concern about a physical sign or symptom. Your thoughtful reflection

will help you gather a relevant and thorough problem-focused or comprehensive assessment. Tonya uses information as she collects it to adapt her approach to assessment. As she gathers data she begins to differentiate important data from all the data collected. She critically interprets assessment data cues to determine whether abnormal findings are present. Her clinical reasoning allows her to make further observations. The cues are the signs and symptoms that a nurse obtains through observation and measurement. You begin to cluster cues that relate together, make inferences, and identify emerging patterns. *In the case of Mr. Lawson, Tonya recognizes the cues that suggest a problem with wound healing and a potential for infection.* Clinical **inference** is part of the clinical decision-making process that occurs before you determine what your patient's problems are. It is the interpretation of the cues and ongoing collection of more data, which involves clinical judgment (Fig. 16.5). As you see patterns in a patient's signs and systems, you may confirm a pattern by adding more data or refute a pattern based on a different assessment finding. Eventually you will interpret the data to identify potential problems and nursing diagnoses from the patient's data (see Chapter 17).

To assess a patient well you critically anticipate, which means that you continuously think about what the data tell you and decide whether more data are needed. Remember to always have supporting signs and symptoms before you make an inference. Your inferences direct you to further questions. Once you ask a patient a question or make an observation, patterns form, and the information branches to an additional series of questions or observations (Fig. 16.6). Knowing how to probe and frame questions using communication and interview techniques is an assessment skill that grows with experience. You learn to decide which questions are relevant to a situation and attend to accurate data interpretation on the basis of inferences and experience.

Validation. Before you complete data interpretation, validate the information you have collected to avoid making incorrect inferences. **Validation** of assessment data is the comparison of data with another source to determine data accuracy. For example, Tonya observed an open inflamed area of the patient's surgical incision and then validated by measuring the patient's body temperature. Making an initial inference is not wrong, but problems result if you do not validate the inference with measurement or by questioning the patient. Compare data in the medical record and consult with other nurses or health care team members to validate

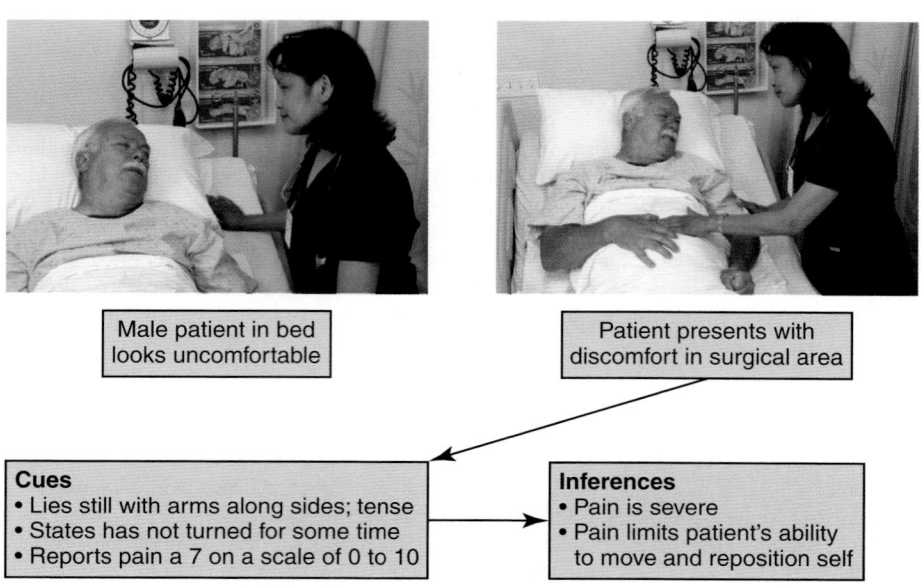

FIG. 16.5 Use of cues to form inferences.

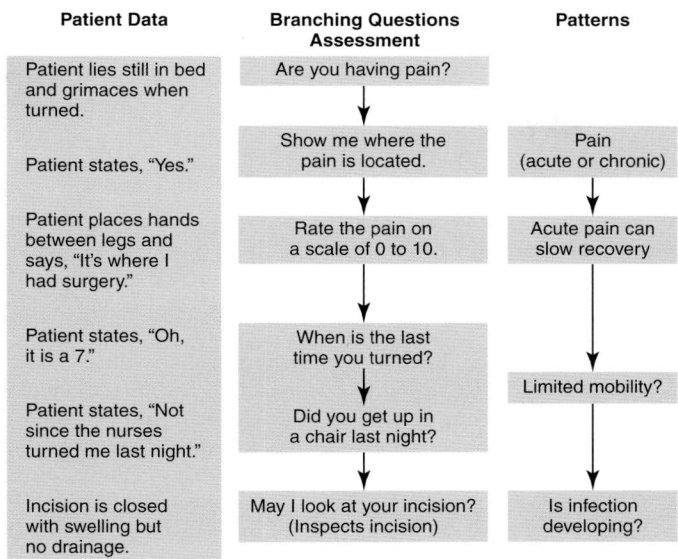

Patient Data	Branching Questions Assessment	Patterns
Patient lies still in bed and grimaces when turned.	Are you having pain?	
Patient states, "Yes."	Show me where the pain is located.	Pain (acute or chronic)
Patient places hands between legs and says, "It's where I had surgery."	Rate the pain on a scale of 0 to 10.	Acute pain can slow recovery
Patient states, "Oh, it is a 7."	When is the last time you turned?	
Patient states, "Not since the nurses turned me last night."	Did you get up in a chair last night?	Limited mobility?
Incision is closed with swelling but no drainage.	May I look at your incision? (Inspects incision)	Is infection developing?

FIG. 16.6 Examples of branching logic for selecting additional assessment questions.

your findings from the physical examination and observation of patient behavior. Often family or friends may also validate your assessment information.

Validation opens the door for gathering more assessment data because it involves clarifying vague or unclear data. Occasionally you need to reassess previously covered areas of the nursing history or gather further physical examination data. Continually analyze to make concise, accurate, and meaningful interpretations. Critical thinking applied to assessment enables you to fully understand a patient's problems, judge the extent of the problems carefully, and discover possible relationships among the problems.

Concept Mapping

Most patients will present with more than one health problem. A concept map is a visual representation that allows you to graphically show the connections among a patient's many health problems. The concept map is a strategy that develops clinical judgement skills, including critical thinking, by helping a learner understand the relationships that exist among patient problems. Educators report that students have expressed that concept mapping activities lead them to develop increased critical thinking skills and to make judgments that lead to better clinical decisions (Khrais, 2017; Yue et al., 2017). Concept maps foster reflection and help students evaluate critical thinking patterns and see the reasons for nursing care. In the case of assessment, it allows a student to readily identify data patterns and see how common data cues may relate to more than one health problem. Your first step in concept mapping is to organize the assessment data you collect. Placing all of the cues together into the clusters that form patterns leads you to the next step of the nursing process, nursing diagnosis (see Chapter 17). Through concept mapping you obtain a holistic perspective of your patient's health care needs, which ultimately leads you to making better clinical decisions. Fig. 16.7 shows the first step in a concept map that Tonya develops for Mr. Lawson as a result of her nursing

CONCEPT MAP

Potential pattern: Comfort problem
- Incision tender on palpation
- Patient reports chest pain and sharp pain over incisional area
- Pain severity ranges from 4 to 6
- Restless
- Guards incision

Potential pattern: Requests information about postoperative care
- Unclear about activity restrictions
- Asks if he will need to "do something to" his incision
- Lifts various objects at home
- Does not know signs of infection

Primary health problem: Colectomy
Priority assessments: Condition of incision, gastrointestinal function, comfort level, knowledge of home care requirements and ability to learn, resources for discharge.

Potential pattern: Altered wound healing
- Has a small separation of wound edges
- Drainage from wound
- Incision tender and inflamed near area of separation

Potential pattern: Worried about condition
- Restless in bed
- Patient states, "I have trouble not worrying"
- Having some difficulty with eye contact

FIG. 16.7 Concept map for Mr. Lawson: Assessment data patterns.

assessment. *Tonya begins to identify cues reflecting patterns of health care problems affecting Mr. Lawson. As a result of the assessment, Tonya sees developing patterns of continued discomfort over the incision, the risk for development of infection, the patient's anxious response to his condition, and the need for instruction about surgical postoperative care.* The next step (see Chapter 17) is to identify specific nursing diagnoses so you can plan appropriate nursing interventions.

KEY POINTS

- Competence in the assessment process involves application of all critical thinking components so that you are deliberate and systematic in collecting data that allow you to make accurate clinical judgments about your patients.
- Nursing assessment involves two steps: (1) the collection of information from as many sources as possible, and (2) the interpretation and validation of data to determine whether more data are needed or if the database is complete to make clinical judgments about patients.
- A nurse will conduct different types of assessments based on a patient's condition and the clinical situation. Patient-centered interviews are conducted during nursing history taking; periodic assessments are conducted during ongoing patient care; and physical examination is a specific skill used to supplement either of the first two types.
- The components of critical thinking guide assessment; with nurses applying knowledge and theory to direct the collection of patient data, consider environmental and time-related factors and then use critical thinking attitudes and standards to make clinical judgments about patient needs.
- The type of an assessment you conduct is based on your judgment, triggered by how a patient is responding (presenting signs and symptoms), whether the patient's condition is urgent, and the time you have to gather data.
- Use the knowledge you gain through your experience to determine when you need to make an adaptation to a skill based on your patient's assessment data.
- Professional standards and clinical guidelines offer a roadmap for what to assess in specific clinical situations.
- Critical thinking attitudes foster the exploration of all data sources in detail to ensure a thorough patient database.
- A patient-centered interview is relationship based and is an organized conversation focused on learning about a patient's concerns and needs.
- Through each phase of an assessment interview, nurses use communication principles and interview techniques that support patient self-expression and encourage full discussion of patient problems and concerns.
- Display professionalism and a caring approach during an interview by looking at the patient and not the data categories on a computer screen.
- The assessment process involves thorough data collection based on critical thinking and the interpretation and validation of the data to ensure that informed and accurate clinical judgments can be made.

REFLECTIVE LEARNING

- A nurse is interviewing a patient to learn more about the patient's arthritis. The nurse inquires, "You have told me you take an antiinflammatory for your arthritis. Tell me how the arthritis affects you."

The patient responds, "I have stiffness in the morning, and I just really ache." The nurse asks, "Which joints are affected?" The patient responds, "My hands, both hands." The nurse says, "Go on." The patient states, "My right hand seems to be the worse; it can get very stiff." The nurse again responds, "Is there anything else you want to share?" Describe the interview techniques used by the nurse in this case example.

- A patient has had diabetes mellitus for 3 years. During a clinic visit the nurse learns the patient is having difficulty describing healthy food choices including appropriate portion sizes. What sources of patient data might the nurse collect to begin understanding the nature of this problem?

- During a home health visit, a patient shares with the nurse, "I have a sore on my foot. Can you take a look at it?" The nurse examines the patient's foot and observes a 2.5-cm (1-inch) gash on the bottom of the left foot; the area is slightly inflamed. The nurse asks, "When did you first notice the sore? Tell me what you think caused it." The patient is uncertain but says, "I sometimes walk around the house in my bare feet. Maybe I picked up something." The nurse further explores, "If you had to rate the pain in your foot on a scale of 0 to 10 with 0 being no pain and 10 being the worst pain, how would you rate it?" Discuss the elements of the PQRST acronym for symptom assessment that the nurse applied in this situation.

REVIEW QUESTIONS

1. A home health nurse is visiting a 62-year-old Hispanic woman diagnosed with type 2 adult-onset diabetes mellitus following a 2-day stay at a local hospital. The physician ordered home health with placement of the patient on a diabetic protocol for education about diabetes mellitus and a new medication and diet counseling. The patient lives with her 73-year-old husband, who has progressive dementia. Their daughter checks on her parents daily, buys groceries, and helps with home maintenance. The nurse conducts an initial history to gather information about the patient's condition. Which of the following data cues combine to reveal a possible health problem? (Select all that apply.)
   1. First time hospitalized
   2. Unable to describe diabetes
   3. Takes antiinflammatory for arthritis
   4. Has limited health literacy
   5. Husband is able to perform self-bathing
   6. Patient unable to identify food sources on prescribed diet
   7. Patient has reduced vision and wears glasses
   8. Patient prescribed an oral hypoglycemic drug

2. Match the assessment activity on the left with the type of assessment on the right.

   ___1. Assessment conducted at beginning of a nurse's shift
   ___2. Review of a patient's chief complaint
   ___3. Completion of admitting history at time of patient admission to a hospital
   ___4. Completion of the Long Term Care Minimum Data Set during an older adult's admission to a nursing home

   A. Problem focused
   B. Comprehensive

3. A nurse initiates a brief interview with a patient who has come to the medical clinic because of self-reported hoarseness, sore throat, and chest congestion. The nurse observes that the patient has a slumped posture and is using intercostal muscles to breathe. The nurse auscultates the patient's lungs and hears crackles in the left lower lobe. The patient's respiratory rate is 22 breaths/min compared with an average of 16 breaths/min during previous clinic visits. The patient tells the nurse, "It's hard for me to get a breath." Which of the following data sets are examples of subjective data? (Select all that apply.)
   1. Heart rate of 22 breaths/min and chest congestion
   2. Lung sounds revealing crackles and use of intercostal muscles to breathe
   3. Patient statement, "It's hard for me to get a breath"
   4. Slumped posture and previous respiratory rate of 16 breaths/min
   5. Patient report of sore throat and hoarseness

4. The nurse asks a patient the following series of questions: "Describe for me how much you exercise each day." "How do you tolerate the exercise?" "Is the amount of exercise you get each day the same, less, or more than what you did a year ago?" This series of questions would likely occur during which phase of a patient-centered interview?
   1. Orientation
   2. Working phase
   3. Data interpretation
   4. Termination

5. A nurse receives a hand-off report for three assigned patients. Using a nursing task list on the EHR, the nurse identifies the care procedures scheduled for the patients. One patient is on the second day after surgery and is stable. Another patient is developing a fever, and diagnostic tests are being conducted to determine the cause. The third patient just returned from surgery and is still on every-30-minutes vital signs. Discuss the ways this nurse can use time management to organize assessment of these patients.

6. A nurse observes a patient walking down the hall with a shuffling gait. When the patient returns to bed, the nurse checks the strength in both of the patient's legs. The nurse applies the information gained to suspect that the patient has a mobility problem. This conclusion is an example of:
   1. Reflection
   2. Clinical inference
   3. Cue
   4. Validation

7. A nurse inspects a patient's sacral pressure injury and notices that the wound is 6 cm (2.4 inches) in diameter with inflammation. The nurse gently applies pressure around the wound, with the patient acknowledging pain. The nurse asks the patient to rate the level of pain on a scale from 0 to 10. A final assessment includes reviewing the electronic health record for how frequently the patient was turned in the last 12 hours.
   Fill in the spaces below to identify the following concepts: assessment activity or cue.
   The nurse inspects (a. _____) a patient's sacral pressure injury and notices that the wound is 6 cm (2.4 inches) in diameter (b. _____) with inflammation (c. _____). The nurse gently applies pressure (d. _____) around the wound, with the patient acknowledging pain (e. _____). The nurse asks the patient to rate the level of pain on a scale (f. _____) from 0 to 10. A final assessment includes reviewing the electronic record (g. _____) for how frequently the patient was turned in the last 12 hours.

8. In preparing to collect a nursing history for a patient admitted for elective surgery, which of the following data are part of the review of present illness in the nursing health history?
   1. Current medications
   2. Patient expectations of planned surgery
   3. Review of patient's family support system
   4. History of allergies
   5. Patient's explanation for what might be the cause of symptoms that require surgery

9. A nurse is conducting a patient-centered interview. Place the statements from the interview in the correct order, beginning with the first statement a nurse would ask.
   1. "You say you've lost weight. Tell me how much weight you've lost in the past month."
   2. "My name is Terry. I'll be the nurse taking care of you today."
   3. "I have no further questions. Is there anything else you wish to ask me?"
   4. "Tell me what brought you to the hospital."
   5. "So, to summarize, you've lost about 6 pounds in the past month, and your appetite has been poor—correct?"

10. Which of the following approaches are recommended when gathering assessment data from an 82-year-old male patient entering a primary care clinic for the first time? (Select all that apply.)
   1. Recognize normal changes associated with aging.
   2. Avoid direct eye contact.
   3. Lean forward and smile as you pose questions.
   4. Allow for pauses as patient tells his story.
   5. Use the list of questions from the clinic assessment form to complete all data.

Answers: 1. 2, 4, 6, 7; **2.** 1A, 2A, 3B, 4B; **3.** 3, 5; **4.** 2; **5.** See Evolve; **6.** 2; **7. a.** assessment activity; **b.** cue; **c.** cue; **d.** assessment activity; **e.** cue; **f.** assessment activity; **g.** assessment activity; **8.** 5; **9.** 2, 4, 1, 5, 3; **10.** 1, 3, 4

Rationales for Review Questions can be found on the Evolve website.

REFERENCES

Agency for Healthcare Research and Quality (AHRQ): *AHRQ Health Literacy Universal Precautions Toolkit*, 2020, https://www.ahrq.gov/health-literacy/quality-resources/tools/literacy-toolkit/index.html. Accessed May 11, 2021.

American Nurses Association (ANA): *Nursing's social policy statement: the essence of the profession*, ed 3, Washington, DC, 2010, The Association.

American Nurses Association (ANA): *The nursing process*, n.d., https://www.nursingworld.org/practice-policy/workforce/what-is-nursing/the-nursing-process. Accessed May 11, 2021.

AusMed: *How to assess a deteriorating/critically ill patient (ABCDE assessment),* 2020, https://www.ausmed.com/cpd/articles/abcde-assessment. Accessed May 11, 2021.

Ball JW et al.: *Seidel's guide to physical examination: an interprofessional approach,* ed 9, St. Louis, 2019, Elsevier.

Bjørk IT, Hamilton GA: *Clinical decision making of nurses working in hospital settings,* 2011, https://www.hindawi.com/journals/nrp/2011/524918/, Article ID 524918. Accessed May 11, 2021.

Carpenito LJ: *Nursing diagnosis: application to clinical practice,* ed 15, Philadelphia, 2017, Lippincott Williams & Wilkins.

Centers for Medicare and Medicaid Services (CMS): *Minimum data set 3.0 Public Reports,* 2012, https://www.cms.gov/Research-Statistics-Data-and-Systems/Computer-Data-and-Systems/Minimum-Data-Set-3-0-Public-Reports. Accessed May 11, 2021.

Dickison P, et al: Integrating the National Council of State Boards of Nursing Clinical Judgment Model into nursing educational frameworks, *J Nurs Educ* 58 (2): 72-78, 2019.

Gordon M: *Nursing diagnosis: process and application,* ed 3, St. Louis, 1994, Mosby.

Kourkouta L, Papathanasiou IV: Communication in nursing practice, *Mater Sociomed* 26(1):65, 2014.

Muhrer JC: History and physical diagnosis. *Nurse Pract* 39(4):30, 2014.

Naya SG: Time management in nursing: hour of need, *International Journal of Caring Sciences,* 11(3):1997, 2018.

Pender NJ et al.: *Health promotion in nursing practice,* ed 7, Upper Saddle River, NJ, 2015, Pearson.

Quality and Safety Education for Nurses Institute (QSEN): *QSEN Competencies,* 2020, https://qsen.org/competencies/pre-licensure-ksas/. Accessed May 11, 2021.

The Joint Commission (TJC): *Sentinel Event Alert: Inadequate hand-off communication,* Issue 58, September 12, 2017a, https://www.jointcommission.org/assets/1/18/SEA_58_Hand_off_Comms_9_6_17_FINAL_(1).pdf. Accessed May 11, 2021.

The Joint Commission: *Eight tips for high quality handoffs,* 2017b, https://www.jointcommission.org/-/media/tjc/documents/resources/patient-safety-topics/sentinel-event/sea_8_steps_hand_off_infographic_2018pdf.pdf?db=web&hash=F4BCE57E34ED03DF76411EB9E302038E. Accessed May 11, 2021.

RESEARCH REFERENCES

Altin SV et al.: The evolution of health literacy assessment tools: a systematic review. *BMC Public Health* 14:1207, 2014.

Chew LD: Validation of screening questions for limited health literacy in a large VA outpatient population. *J Gen Internal Medicine.* 23(5):561, 2008.

Freitas W, et al: Distractions and interruptions in medication preparation and administration in inpatient units, *Rev Eletr Enferm* 21:1207, 2019.

Johnson M et al: The impact of interruptions on medication errors in hospitals: an observational study of nurses, *J Nurs Manag,* 2017, Wiley online library, https://onlinelibrary.wiley.com/doi/abs/10.1111/jonm.12486. Accessed May 29, 2021.

Keifenheim KE et al.: Teaching history taking to medical students: a systematic review. *BMC Med Educ* 15:159, 2015.

Khrais H: The outcomes of integrating concept mapping in nursing education: an integrative review, *Open Journal of Nursing,* 07(11):1335, 2017

Louis A et al.: Screening hospitalized patients for low health literacy—beyond the REALM of possibility?, *Health Educ Behav* 44(3): 360, 2017.

Muntean WJ: Nursing clinical-decision making, a literature review. *National Council of State Boards of Nursing,* 2012. Available at https://www.ncsbn.org/Clinical_Judgment_Lit_Review_Executive_Summary.pdf. Accessed May 11, 2021.

Orlando LA et al.: Development and validation of a primary care-based family health history and decision support program (MeTree). *N C Med J* 74(4):287, 2013.

Ratanawongsa N et al.: Association between clinician computer use and communication with patients in safety-net clinics. *JAMA Internal Med* 176(1):125, 2016.

Tanner CA: Thinking like a nurse: a research-based model of clinical judgment in nursing. *J Nurs Educ* 45(6):204, 2006.

Yue M et al.: The effectiveness of concept mapping on development of critical thinking in nursing education: A systematic review and meta-analysis, *Nurse Education Today,* 52:87, 2017.

Analysis and Nursing Diagnosis

OBJECTIVES

- Explain how the formation of a nursing diagnosis is a factor in clinical judgment.
- Compare a nursing diagnosis with a medical diagnosis and a collaborative problem.
- Discuss the importance of having a standardized language of nursing diagnoses.
- Apply critical thinking in the diagnostic reasoning process.
- Explain the difference between finding data patterns and data interpretation.

- Describe components of a nursing diagnostic statement.
- Critique the different elements of a problem-focused or negative nursing diagnosis versus an at-risk nursing diagnosis.
- Explain how critical thinking applies to prioritization of nursing diagnoses.
- Form a nursing diagnostic statement correctly.
- Identify sources of nursing diagnostic errors.

KEY TERMS

Collaborative problem
Data cluster

International Classification for Nursing Practice (ICNP®)
Medical diagnosis

NANDA International (NANDA-I)
Nursing diagnosis
Risk nursing diagnosis

MEDIA RESOURCES

http://evolve.elsevier.com/Potter/fundamentals/
- Review Questions
- Concept Map Creator
- Case Study with Questions

- Audio Glossary
- Content Updates
- Answers to QSEN Activity and Review Questions

In Chapter 16, you learned that when a patient assessment is performed critically and systematically, the process yields a thorough database. Your knowledge and experience play a role in making clinical judgments about types and sources of data to gather, the depth of information to explore, and the beginning recognition of cues and data patterns. You recognize cues as you analyze significant data from different sources to identify meaningful patterns (Silvestri, 2019). So, why do you need to be able to identify patterns in your patient's assessment data? How does pattern identification benefit a patient? Data patterns lead you to recognize patient problems, in the form of nursing diagnoses, the second step of the nursing process (Fig. 17.1). The American Nurses Association states that "Nursing integrates the art and science of caring and focuses on the protection, promotion, and optimization of health and human functioning; prevention of illness and injury; facilitation of healing; and alleviation of suffering through compassionate presence. Nursing is the diagnosis and treatment of human responses and advocacy in the care of individuals, families, groups, communities, and populations in recognition of the connection of all humanity" (ANA, 2021, p. 1). A key word in this definition is *diagnosis*. A nursing diagnosis is made when a nurse applies all elements of critical thinking in making the clinical judgment that leads to identifying health-related problems or the potential for a patient to develop problems based on patient data. Unless a nurse correctly identifies or diagnoses the nature

of a patient's illness or health condition, a patient's real problems will remain unidentified and untreated. During assessment a nurse constantly sorts data using cognitive reasoning to determine what the data mean. When applying the nursing process, ask yourself, "What are the patterns of data that ultimately point to a clear problem or phenomenon?" This deliberate use of critical thinking will lead you to accurately diagnose a patient's responses to illness.

TYPES OF DIAGNOSES

When making a diagnosis, a clear label or term that is familiar to all health care providers involved in a patient's care is necessary to understand a patient's needs. Consider a patient who is breathing rapidly. This patient could be breathing hard because he is angry, or there could be a physiological reason causing the rapid breathing. The terms *anger* or *impaired breathing* are terms that will prompt nurses to consider similar problem areas: anger is emotional and behavioral versus breathing impairment, which is respiratory or ventilatory in nature. Using standardized terminology provides diagnostic clarity so that all members of the health care team understand a patient's problems and can communicate effectively about them. Using nursing diagnosis in practice is supported by health care technologies. For example, most electronic health records (EHRs) contain standard terminologies that

FIG. 17.1 Nursing Process—Analysis/Diagnosis. (Copyright © NCSBN. All rights reserved.)

nurses and other health care providers use to communicate a patient's condition and the impact of various therapies to the entire interprofessional team. Within nursing practice there are three types of diagnoses or problem statements that nurses must recognize and manage.

Medical Diagnoses

Practitioners started using medical diagnoses to describe the signs and symptoms for many illnesses thousands of years ago. When physicians or certified advanced practice nurses identify and confirm common medical diagnoses such as rheumatoid arthritis or diabetes mellitus today, they know the meanings of the diagnoses, the implications, and the standard approaches for treatment. A medical diagnosis is the identification of a disease condition based on a specific assessment of physical signs and symptoms, a patient's medical history, and the results of diagnostic tests and procedures (Table 17.1). Medical diagnosis is the language health care providers (e.g., physicians, advanced practice nurses) use to communicate a patient's health problems and associated treatments and responses. Physicians and advanced practice nurses, such as nurse practitioners and midwives, are licensed to treat diseases and conditions described in medical diagnostic terms. For example, in the case of diabetes mellitus, health care providers will order various medications and tests such as a hemoglobin A_{1c} (HbA_{1c}) to manage a patient's blood glucose. Nurses will educate the patients about diabetes medication and diet management.

Nursing Diagnosis

A nursing diagnosis is a clinical judgment made by a registered nurse to describe a patient's response or vulnerability to health conditions or life events that the nurse is licensed and competent to treat (NANDA-I, 2018). It is a diagnostic label that classifies an individual's, family's, or community's response to illness so that all nurses, those in regular clinical practice and advanced practice nurses, understand a specific patient's health care needs. Nurses prescribe for and treat patient and group *responses* to situations that include five categories (Carpenito, 2017): pathophysiological (e.g., myocardial infarction, borderline personality), treatment-related (e.g., anticoagulant therapy, dialysis), personal (e.g., dying, divorce), environmental (e.g., overcrowded school, safety barriers in home), and maturational (e.g., peer pressure, parenthood). Just as health care providers make a medical diagnosis, a nurse identifies a nursing diagnosis by analyzing assessment data and recognizing patterns of data associated with a specific problem (see Table 17.1). Nurses cannot treat medical diagnoses; they cannot order an HbA_{1c} or insulin. The exception, of course, is advanced practice nurses. Nurses treat patients' responses to health conditions. A patient with rheumatoid arthritis will have pain and mobility alterations. Nurses provide interventions to minimize and control pain (e.g., application of heat or cold to an injured area) and improve mobility (e.g., implement early mobility protocols). Nursing diagnoses such as *Acute Pain* or *Activity Intolerance* provide clear direction as to the type of nursing interventions (see Chapter 19) nurses are licensed to provide independently.

Collaborative Problems

A collaborative problem is one that requires both medical and nursing interventions to treat (Carpenito, 2017). Nurses practice with other health care professionals to manage certain types of collaborative problems. This involves using physician-prescribed, therapist-recommended, and nursing-prescribed interventions to minimize complications of the events (Carpenito, 2017). For example, in the case of a patient who enters a clinic with an infected leg wound, the patient's health care provider prescribes antibiotics, the nurse monitors for fever and provides wound care, a registered dietitian recommends an appropriate therapeutic diet high in protein, and the patient collaborates by learning good hand hygiene and wound care practices. In the case of a patient who is paralyzed from a spinal cord injury, a nurse uses proper positioning and transfer techniques for patient safety while a physical therapist recommends exercises for the patient's extremities.

All physiological complications are not collaborative problems. If a nurse can prevent the onset of a complication or provide the primary

TABLE 17.1	Comparison of a Medical Diagnosis and a Nursing Diagnosis With Diagnostic and Assessment Findings		
Medical Diagnosis	**Diagnostic Findings**	**Nursing Diagnostic Label**	**Assessment Findings**
Pneumonia	Abnormal lung sounds: crackles, rales	*Impaired Respiratory System Function—Impaired Gas Exchange* (ICN, 2019)	Irregular respirations
	Chest x-ray showing infiltrates		Tachycardia
	Chest pain with productive cough		Orthopnea
	Confusion		Hypercapnia
	Shortness of breath		Diaphoresis
	Positive blood culture for pneumococcus		Productive cough
			Restlessness
			Confusion
			Dyspnea

treatment for it, then the diagnosis is a nursing diagnosis (Carpenito, 2017). For example:

Nurses Can Prevent	Nursing Diagnosis (ICN, 2019)
Pressure injuries	*Risk for Pressure Ulcer*
Aspiration	*Risk for Aspiration*
Nurses Can Treat	**Nursing Diagnosis**
Stage I or II pressure injuries	*Impaired Tissue Integrity*
Swallowing problems	*Impaired Swallowing*
Nurses Cannot Prevent	**Collaborative Problems**
Seizures	Seizures
Bleeding	Bleeding

Interprofessional collaboration in managing patient problems is based on the assumption that when health care providers from various disciplines and patients communicate and consider one another's unique perspectives, they will better manage the multiple factors that influence the health of individuals, families, and communities (Sullivan et al., 2015). It is a process that improves access to health interventions and improves coordination among disciplines, with a focus on more involvement in decision making for individuals and their families (World Health Professions Alliance, 2019). Strong, collaborative interprofessional teams enable members to embrace patient care protocols that are team-based and patient-centered (Moss et al., 2016).

REFLECT NOW

Review the electronic health record of a patient for whom you are assigned to provide care. Look at the list of all health problems identified. Sort those problems out by nursing diagnoses, medical diagnoses, and collaborative problems.

TERMINOLOGIES FOR NURSING DIAGNOSES

Nurses work in a variety of settings, even within a single health care agency such as a hospital. Common terminologies allow you to communicate information about patient problems in a meaningful way that can be understood across all disciplines and care settings. Nursing diagnoses standardize nursing terminology. This allows nurses to specifically identify and discuss patient problems, anticipate the plan of care with associated outcomes, and recognize potential appropriate interventions. Using standard nursing diagnosis terms contributes to effective health care team communication. Health care communicated in unspecific, unclear wording causes inconsistencies due to differences in naming patients' care needs (nursing diagnoses), associated nursing interventions, and expected treatment outcomes among providers, teams, or facilities (Rabelo-Silva et al., 2016).

Standard terminology is a key component of EHRs (see Chapter 26). There are standard interface terminologies recognized by the American Association of Nurses in EHRs (Office of the National Coordinator for Health Information Technology, 2017). These terminologies are concepts used by nurses for describing and documenting the care of patients (Box 17.1). A standard terminology system used across the world is the **International Classification for Nursing Practice (ICNP®)**, which was developed by the International Council of Nurses (ICN, 2019). The ICN is a federation of more than 130 national nurses' associations (NNAs), representing more than 20 million nurses worldwide (ICN, 2020).

BOX 17.1   ANA-Recognized Standard Nursing Terminologies

Interface Terminologies
1. Clinical Care Classification (CCC) System
2. International Classification for Nursing Practice (ICNP)
3. North American Nursing Diagnosis Association International (NANDA-I)
4. Nursing Interventions Classification System (NIC)
5. Nursing Outcomes Classification (NOC)
6. Omaha System
7. Perioperative Nursing Data Set (PNDS)
8. ABC Codes

Adapted from: Office of the National Coordinator for Health Information Technology: Standard Nursing Terminologies: A Landscape Analysis, May 15, 2017, https://www.healthit.gov/sites/default/files/snt_final_05302017.pdf. Accessed May 15, 2021.

It is common for a health care agency to work with vendors of EHRs to create a standard language or set of terminologies unique to the institution. At times these terminologies are based on medical diagnoses only and the opinions or expertise of the agency's health care staff. Nursing diagnosis terminology may or may not be integrated. When it is not integrated, it is up to an individual nurse to specifically identify a patient's relevant nursing diagnoses as they pertain to a patient's health condition.

The nursing diagnosis classification and taxonomy system of **NANDA International (NANDA-I)** was developed in 1982, when nurse educators recognized that assessment data needed to be analyzed and clustered into patterns and interpreted before nurses could make accurate nursing diagnoses (NANDA-I, n.d.). Soon diagnosis became part of the five-step nursing process. The NANDA-I diagnostic classification system has grown to currently include 244 diagnoses (NANDA-I, 2018). You cannot plan and intervene correctly for patients if you do not know your patients' health problems or conditions. The NANDA-I terminology is one system that provides standard, formal diagnostic statements (including definitions, defining characteristics, and related or risk factors). The NANDA-I system aims to achieve the following outcomes (NANDA-I, 2018):

- Provide a precise definition of a patient's human responses to health problems and life processes.
- Develop, refine, and disseminate evidence-based terminology representing clinical judgments by professional nurses.
- Allow nurses to communicate (e.g., verbally and in writing) a plan of care among themselves and with other health care professionals and the public.
- Foster the development of nursing knowledge through research.
- Contribute to the development of informatics and information standards.
- Document care for reimbursement of nursing services.

Many of these same outcomes describe the purposes of the ICNP® system. The ICN developed the International Classification for Nursing Practice (ICNP®) as a unified nursing language system to support standardized nursing documentation at a patient's bedside or point of care (ICN, 2019). It is a wide-ranging, understandable reference terminology that can adapt to multiple purposes (e.g., documentation, research categories, practice guidelines) in different countries and that serves as a primary resource to describe nursing practices (Rabelo-Silva et al., 2016). The World Health Organization (WHO) recognizes ICNP® for classifying patient data and clinical activity in the domain of nursing

---

BOX 17.2 ICNP® Seven Axes With Definitions

- Focus: The area of attention that is relevant to nursing (e.g., pain, homelessness, elimination, life expectancy, knowledge).
- Judgment: Clinical opinion or determination related to the focus of nursing practice (e.g., decreasing level, risk, enhanced, interrupted, abnormal).
- Client: Subject to whom a diagnosis refers and who is the recipient of an intervention (e.g., newborn, caregiver, family, community).
- Action: An intentional process applied to or performed by a client (e.g., educating, changing, administering, monitoring).
- Means: A manner or method of accomplishing an intervention (e.g., bandage, bladder-training technique).
- Location: Anatomical and spatial orientation of a diagnosis or intervention (e.g., posterior, abdomen, school, community health center).
- Time: The point, period, instance, interval, or duration of an occurrence (e.g., admission, childbirth, chronic).

Adapted from Garcia TR, Nobrega MML: The International Classification for Nursing Practice: participation of Brazilian nurses in the project of the International Council of Nurses, *Acta Paul Enferm* 22(Especial - 70 Anos):875, 2009; International Council of Nurses (ICN): Technical Implementation Guide, International Council of Nurses, Geneva, Switzerland, 2018.

---

and for its use in decision making for improving patient health status and health care delivery (WHO, 2017).

The ICNP® classifies nursing phenomena (diagnoses), nursing actions or interventions, and nursing outcomes that describe nursing practice. The ICNP® system currently uses a model that has seven axes (Box 17.2). With multi-axial terminology, terms from different axes are combined to create a concept (Garcia and Nobrega, 2009; ICN, 2018). For example, the term "pain" (from the ICNP® Focus of Nursing Practice Axis) can be combined with "chronic" (from the ICNP® Duration Axis) to create the diagnosis "chronic pain." Nurses and other hospital staff can use the data-based information from ICNP® for planning and managing nursing care, financial forecasting, analysis of patient outcomes, and health policy development (ICN, 2019).

In addition to improving communication among health care providers, using standard nursing terminology creates a scientific knowledge base for nursing. Advances in the discipline of nursing involve the development of interconnections among theory, research, and nursing practice. The use of a clear, well-established terminology system such as nursing diagnoses forms the basis of classification systems in nursing care. Such classification systems help nurses recognize phenomena, make correct decisions, and perform research activities in clinical settings that build new knowledge within the profession of nursing (Mynaříková and Žiaková, 2014).

There are similarities in the language of NANDA-I and the ICNP®. The ICNP® taxonomy or model refers to nursing diagnoses, while NANDA-I officially refers to diagnostic labels. The two classification systems have many of the same labels for certain diagnoses, while there is also much variation in labels describing similar responses to health conditions.

QSEN **Building Competency in Teamwork and Collaboration** A nurse is caring for a 73-year-old patient who fell while in the hospital. The patient has cardiac and respiratory health problems that affect her ability to tolerate exercise. The nurse is attending a discharge planning conference with the physical therapist and social worker. Describe how this nurse can enhance interprofessional collaboration with the other health care providers in the use of nursing diagnoses.

Answers to QSEN Activities can be found on the Evolve website.

CRITICAL THINKING IN ANALYSIS AND NURSING DIAGNOSIS

Having an accurate and complete patient database allows you to make a clinical judgment in the form of a nursing diagnosis and then begin the steps necessary to plan (see Chapter 18) and implement relevant and appropriate nursing interventions (see Chapter 19). Competency in clinical judgment relies on critical thinking. The application of knowledge and experience, the consideration of environmental factors, and the use of critical thinking attitudes and intellectual and professional standards improve analysis and diagnostic accuracy (Fig. 17.2).

When practicing nursing, it is important for you to know the nursing diagnosis classification system used within your nursing program and clinical practice sites. You will also need to become familiar with the definitions, related or causative factors, and the defining characteristics or assessment findings that apply to each diagnosis. It is impossible to memorize the information needed for every type of nursing diagnosis, no matter what system you use. Thus, you need to know how to access this information easily within the agency in which you work. Sources of information about nursing diagnoses include faculty, advanced practice nurses, clinical staff, documentation systems, and practice guidelines.

Diagnostic reasoning analyzes cues connecting data to a patient's clinical presentation (Dickison et al., 2019). Your analysis involves logically explaining a clinical judgment by using patient assessment data to arrive at a nursing diagnosis. You gather a comprehensive set of data, validate your information, analyze the meaning of data looking for patterns, consider whether the data are expected or unexpected, and then add additional data if you find information is lacking. You then interpret the data by identifying clusters or patterns that lead to identification of nursing diagnoses and other problems (Fig. 17.3). The diagnostic process flows from the assessment process and includes decision-making steps. As a nurse, your ability to recognize and analyze cues, prioritize nursing diagnoses, and generate solutions for patients, based in evidence and your personal experiences with patients, will evolve and develop (Dickison et al., 2019).

Data Clustering and Finding Patterns

*In Chapter 16, Tonya is still caring for Mr. Lawson on day 3 postoperatively. He no longer needs supplemental oxygen and he has had no recurrent chest pain. Tonya inspects the patient's surgical wound and notices **separation of the wound between two sutures** at the bottom of the incision. She uses this cue to focus further on the wound, finding a **small amount of serous drainage** and noting that **the area is inflamed**. Tonya considers whether the drainage and inflammation would be expected or unexpected. Her knowledge about normal wound healing tells her serous drainage is normal, as is mild inflammation. But she applies curiosity and considers standard signs of infection to gather more data. Tonya asks the patient whether the incision is tender when she gently palpates it. Mr. Lawson states, "Ow, **that feels sore there**. I think I pulled it when I coughed last night." He also rates **pain at this time as being at a level of 5**. Tonya knows from the previous day that Mr. Lawson's rating of pain at a 5 today is slightly higher than when she cared for him on postoperative day 2. She will continue to use this baseline to determine whether Mr. Lawson's pain increases or not. Tonya's knowledge of the risk for infection (such as a break in skin integrity) leads her to check the patient's vital signs; she notes that his **temperature is 37.5°C (99.6°F), slightly above his average temperature of 37.2°C (99.0°F)**. Tonya is clustering together cues that begin to form a pattern, leading her to monitor the patient more closely for developing signs of infection.*

Your review and analysis of assessment data involve critically organizing all data elements about a patient into meaningful patterns, also

FIG. 17.2 Critical thinking in analysis and diagnosis. (Clinical Judgment Measurement Model copyright © NCSBN. All rights reserved.)

called **data clusters** or sets of assessment findings/defining characteristics. A set of assessment findings is a group of data elements, the signs or symptoms gathered during assessment. Each data element is an objective or subjective sign, symptom, or risk factor that leads you into making a diagnostic conclusion. As you analyze data, you begin to see data elements that offer cues to a type of health problem. For example, a patient with shortness of breath, walking only 100 feet before becoming breathless, and an increased respiratory rate suggest a breathing problem pattern. A patient who reports having no immediate family, who does not initiate conversation, and who just lost his vision shows a coping problem pattern. It is these patterns, or data clusters, that begin to shape a more formal label or description.

While looking for a pattern, compare a patient's data with information that is consistent with normal, healthy patterns (e.g., wound healing). Use accepted norms as the basis for comparison and judgment, norms such as laboratory test values, vital signs, professional standards, and normal physiological limits. Also determine whether the grouped signs and symptoms are expected for a patient (e.g., consider current condition and history) and whether they are within the range of healthy responses. Separate out data that are not within healthy norms to allow you to identify a pattern correctly.

During assessment you collect individual data points either intentionally or unintentionally. An intentional assessment includes the deliberate collection of data through physical examination or interviewing during a health history. Unintentional assessment is noticing data points that are important without planning to collect them (NANDA-I, 2018). *For example, even though Tonya planned on inspecting Mr. Lawson's wound, an unintentional data point is the separation of a surgical wound's edges.* Another example is seeing a patient grimace and hold a body part while you turn and reposition the patient in bed.

Finding a data cluster helps you to think less about individual data points and focus instead on pattern recognition. Your ability to recognize a pattern or cluster comes with knowledge, clinical experience, and intentional practice. At first you will not notice some of the subtleties that exist from observing or examining patients. For example, the first time you look at a patient's surgical wound you will notice the length of an incision and general color of the surrounding skin, but you might not notice an individual suture that has loosened or minor swelling at the end of the incision.

While clustering data, you will find that some data are demographic (e.g., patient's age, gender) and do not necessarily fit a pattern with other data. You also will find data that relate to the cause or nature of a patient's problem (e.g., history of stroke, poor adherence to therapy). A specific assessment finding may apply to one or more patterns of data (e.g., moving a limb slowly can reveal a mobility problem, as well as a problem with comfort). As you recognize data elements, you will cluster or group them together in patterns in a logical way that during interpretation will reveal the nursing diagnoses that describe how a patient is responding to a health condition or life process. Always apply the critical thinking attitude of being curious to ensure you have complete data.

When assessment data reveal risk factors (i.e., the factors that increase a patient's vulnerability to an unhealthy event), you will recognize patterns, compare the patterns with expected data for a risk diagnosis, and then select the correct risk nursing diagnosis.

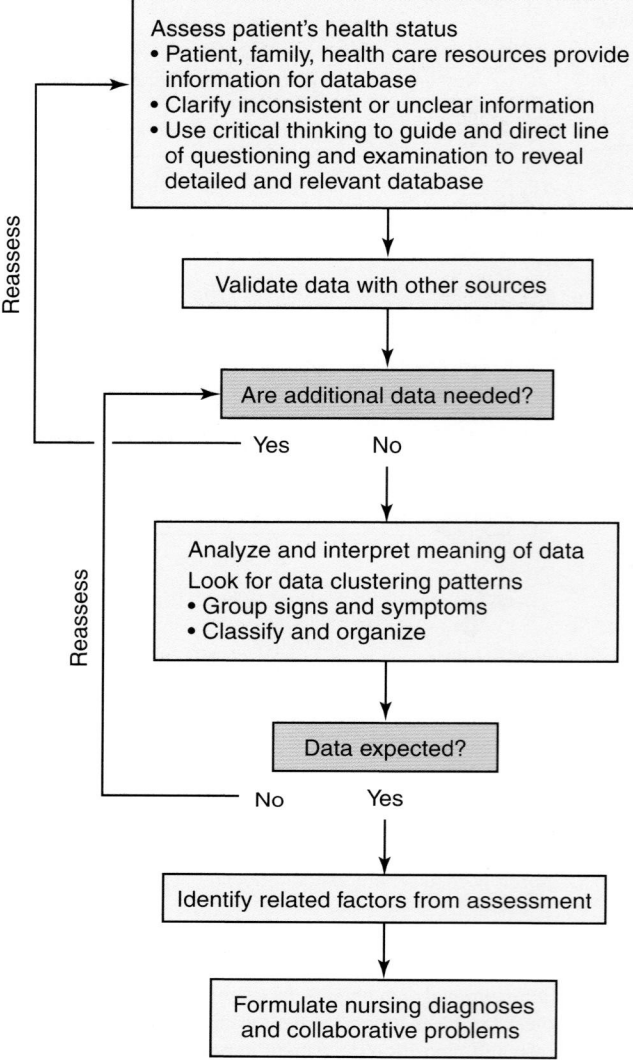

FIG. 17.3 Nursing diagnostic process.

During her assessment Tonya gathered information suggesting that Mr. Lawson possibly has a wound healing problem: open wound edges, drainage (which can foster microorganism growth), tenderness at wound site, and a low-grade fever. The data about Mr. Lawson are cues that form the pattern of possible risk for infection. Selecting a specific diagnosis for this problem area will allow Tonya to develop a relevant and appropriate plan of care.

Data Interpretation

Data interpretation involves placing a label on your data pattern or cluster to clearly identify a patient's response to a health problem. Selecting a diagnosis cannot be casual or simply intuitive. Critical thinking is necessary. Your interpretation of data clusters or patterns leads to the selection of various nursing diagnoses that apply to your patient. It is important to be disciplined in comparing the data in a cluster with the data standards for a diagnosis to come to a reasoned conclusion about a patient's response to a health problem.

In the case of the NANDA-I classification, the data cue standards are the defining characteristics or risk factors (NANDA-I, 2018) used to form a nursing diagnosis. When ICNP® is used as the diagnosis system, the agency where you work will have a set of criteria or standards for the assessment findings and risk factors that form a pattern for a nursing diagnosis (Fig. 17.4). Nurses who use ICNP® in their care settings have contributed to the development of clinically relevant sets of diagnosis, outcome, and intervention statements for a variety of health priorities and delivery settings (Coenen et al., 2012). Users of ICNP® have created catalogs of nursing data subsets for specified health phenomena (nursing diagnoses such as pain), diseases (e.g., HIV/AIDS, depression), care specialties (e.g., palliative care), and care settings (e.g., neonatal nursery). These catalogs are then used to build health information systems (Rabelo-Silva et al., 2016).

Regardless of the diagnostic system you use, you compare your data with the assessment findings standard for select nursing diagnoses to select the specific diagnosis that fits your patient. The recognition of data in a logical cluster or pattern reveals the nursing diagnoses, how a patient is responding to a health condition or life process.

Tonya has a comprehensive set of data about Mr. Lawson. In Chapter 16 she identified that Mr. Lawson has limited knowledge about what his restrictions will be once he returns home. He was unsure of signs of infection, and

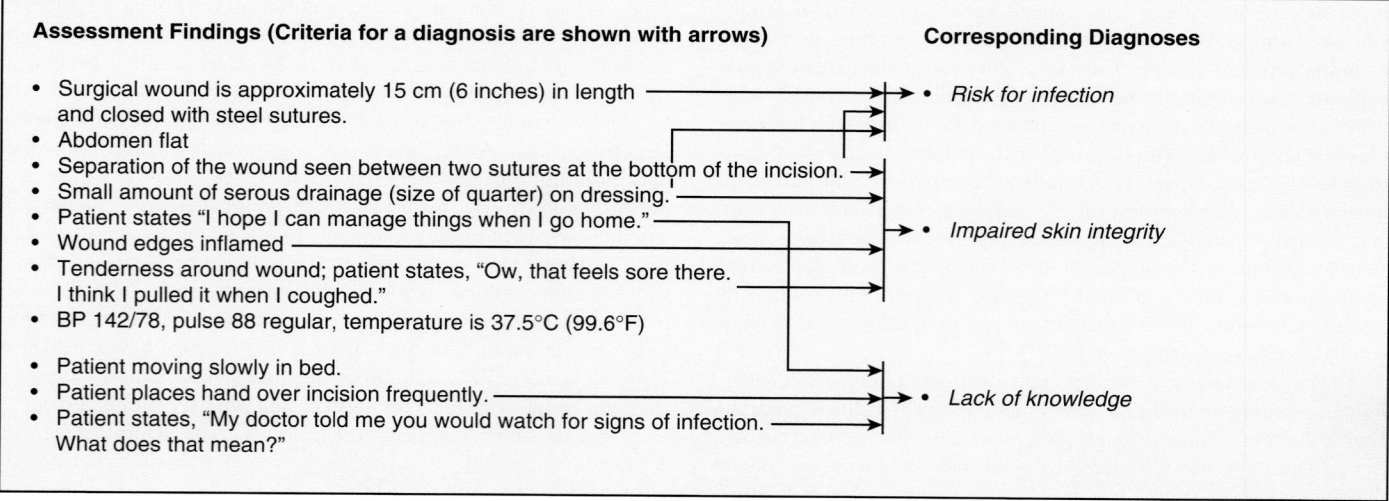

FIG. 17.4 Assessment findings with corresponding diagnoses.

*he asked several questions about his plan of care. Tonya clusters the data she has learned from Mr. Lawson, analyzes the data, and recognizes patterns of a knowledge problem. As Tonya considers Mr. Lawson's request for information, there are different nursing diagnoses for problems related to knowledge, including **Lack of Knowledge, Ready to Learn**, and **Adequate Knowledge**. Knowing the differences among these diagnoses and identifying which one applies comes from thoughtful interpretation of data. **Lack of Knowledge** suggests the patient has insufficient knowledge about a topic or area of interest. **Ready to Learn** implies the patient is motivated and open to learning additional information, while **Adequate Knowledge** implies that the individual has knowledge about a topic but needs further information or reinforcement to strengthen understanding. Mr. Lawson's colectomy is his first experience with major surgery. His earlier questions about lifting and incision care suggest he has limited knowledge of postoperative care.*

Working with similar patients over a period of time helps you recognize patterns of assessment findings, but remember that each patient is unique and requires an individualized diagnostic approach. It can be a challenge to select a diagnosis when assessment findings for two different diagnoses are similar. For example, having insufficient knowledge to set up a medication schedule and being unable to identify the purpose of a medication might be considered assessment findings for the diagnoses of *Lack of Knowledge* (ICN, 2019) or *Impaired Ability To Manage Medication Regime* (ICN, 2019). Further exploration is needed to determine whether a patient's problem is a knowledge issue only or the patient has physical limitations that prevent following a medication schedule. Remember, as you gather data and see clusters or patterns, confirm your data with your source of standards for the diagnostic system you use. It is critical to select the correct diagnosis for each of a patient's health problem responses. *Tonya previously identified Mr. Lawson as having **Acute Pain** from his surgical incision, and he is at **Risk for Infection**. She now makes the clinical judgment that the nursing diagnosis **Lack of Knowledge** also applies to her patient. She will also consider any remaining data to determine whether Mr. Lawson has additional diagnoses. Are there sufficient data to support a continuing problem related to breathing or anxiety?*

Environmental Factors

Just as is the case with assessment (see Chapter 16), environmental factors affect your ability to critically interpret data and correctly identify nursing diagnoses. Communicating accurate and timely medical diagnoses to patients has been shown to be an important component of providing high-quality care; errors in diagnosis threaten high-quality care (Committee on Diagnostic Error in Health Care, 2015). The same holds true for communicating nursing diagnoses to other health care providers and patients; patients must understand their health problems. Various challenges can occur with the tasks and workflow that are required to make a diagnosis. These challenges include problems with the information (amount, accuracy, completeness, appropriateness), communication issues (patients and health care staff), the complexity of the task (multiple patient problem areas), a lack of situational awareness, poor workflow design (admission or transfer process), interruptions, and inefficiencies (Committee on Diagnostic Error in Health Care, 2015). Be mindful of the process of identifying nursing diagnoses by taking the time to make necessary judgments and convey the information to other health care colleagues in a timely manner.

Types of Nursing Diagnostic Statements

NANDA-I categorizes nursing diagnoses into three types: problem-focused, risk diagnosis, and health promotion (NANDA-I, 2018). The ICNP® categorizes diagnoses as positive or negative nursing diagnoses with associated outcomes. The focus of diagnoses from both classifications is similar. Problem-focused nursing diagnoses or

negative diagnoses identify an undesirable human response to existing problems or concerns of a patient. Examples include *Acute Pain* or *Urinary Retention* (NANDA-I, 2018) or *Acute Pain* and *Impaired Urination* (ICN, 2019). Risk nursing diagnoses are diagnoses that apply when there is an increased potential or vulnerability for a patient to develop a problem or complication (NANDA-I, 2018). In the ICN system, an at-risk diagnosis falls under the category of negative nursing diagnoses. Examples include *Risk for Fall* (ICN, 2019) and *Risk for Unstable Blood Pressure* (NANDA-I, 2018). Health promotion nursing diagnoses and positive diagnoses identify the desire or motivation to improve health status through a positive behavioral change. Examples include *Readiness for Enhanced Relationship* and *Readiness for Enhanced Power* (NANDA-I, 2018) and *Positive Family Support* (ICN, 2019). Although many nursing diagnoses are used to identify problems being experienced by individual patients, you will apply some nursing diagnoses to families, groups of individuals, and communities.

Formulating the Diagnostic Statement

The way you phrase or word a nursing diagnostic statement affects how you communicate a patient's problems to other health care staff, which nursing interventions you choose, and how you evaluate patient outcomes. Clarity and precision are essential. When forming a nursing diagnosis, each type of diagnosis has a different format. In the NANDA-I system, a problem-focused nursing diagnostic statement has three parts: a diagnostic label, related factors, and major defining characteristics (NANDA-I, 2018). Risk nursing diagnoses have two segments: a diagnosis and the associated risk factors preceded by the phrase *as evidenced by* (NANDA-I, 2018). Health promotion nursing diagnoses also are written with only two sections: the diagnosis label and defining characteristics or assessment findings. Without the use of the correct format for a nursing diagnosis, the label for the diagnosis is less meaningful and can easily be misunderstood (NANDA-I, 2018).

The same formats can be used for ICNP® diagnoses as well. However, initially selecting a nursing diagnosis in the ICNP system requires that a clinical nurse select at least one term from two axes, namely, the axes "focus" and "judgment" (Rabelo-Silva et al., 2016). The focus is the area of relevance to nursing practice, e.g., physiological status or knowledge, whereas judgment refers to the clinical opinion related to the selected focus, e.g., decreasing level, risk, or enhanced. If you use ICNP® diagnoses, choose among the assessment findings that have formed a pattern for a specific diagnosis; then you can also include a related factor from the data gathered.

Components

- **Diagnostic Label or Diagnosis**—A diagnostic label or diagnosis is the name of a nursing diagnosis approved by NANDA-I, ICNP®, or any other system used by your institution. The NANDA-I system offers definitions for each diagnosis to describe the characteristics of the human response identified.
- **Related Factors**—A patient's response to a health problem is related to a set of conditions that caused or influenced the response. Related factors are etiologies, circumstances, facts, or influences that have a relationship with the nursing diagnosis (NANDA-I, 2018).

    *Tonya uses a critical thinking approach to identify the correct diagnosis that applies to Mr. Lawson's situation. She selects **Lack of Knowledge** as the nursing diagnosis because this is Mr. Lawson's first surgical experience; thus he is unfamiliar with postoperative routines. He has questions about what will occur after surgery. Tonya further clarifies the statement as **Lack of Knowledge regarding postoperative care**. She then selects the related factor as the patient's inexperience. She words the formal diagnosis as*

Lack of Knowledge regarding postoperative care related to inexperience with surgery. This wording will direct other nurses to know the scope of patient education required.

Critically review your assessment data to identify the related factor that applies to your patient. The value of having a related factor in a diagnostic statement is that it directs the type of interventions appropriate for a patient's care. For example, the nursing diagnosis *Body Weight Problem: Overweight* from the ICNP® system could lead a nurse to identify any number of interventions, such as exercise, consulting with a registered dietitian for a low-calorie diet, or counseling a patient about weight management and health. However, a clearer diagnostic statement such as *Body Weight Problem: Underweight related to nausea and inadequate nutrient intake* calls for interventions involving adjustment of the type of diet (e.g., switching from solid foods to liquids), controlling the patient's mealtime environment by eliminating noxious odors, and administering prescribed antiemetics (collaborative intervention).

Related factors for NANDA-I diagnoses have been categorized into four groups: pathophysiological (biological or psychological), treatment-related, situational (environmental or personal), and maturational (Carpenito, 2017). The ICNP® system has not defined sets of possible related factors for nursing diagnoses. A related factor is not intended as a cause-and-effect statement. It instead indicates that the etiology identified in assessment data contributes to or is associated with the patient's diagnosis (Fig. 17.5). Risk diagnoses do not have related factors because you are identifying a vulnerability in a patient for a potential problem; a problem does not yet exist (NANDA-I, 2018).

- **Major Assessment Findings**—Another component of a diagnosis is optional: the listing of major assessment findings. Further clarity can be added to a diagnostic statement if you list major assessment findings or defining characteristics that were used to select a diagnosis.

Highlighting a patient's major assessment findings offers guidelines for how you will evaluate the efficacy of nursing care therapies. For example, in the diagnosis *Body Weight Problem: Underweight related to nausea and inadequate nutrient intake,* adding the phrase "*as evidenced by 4.5-kg (10-lb) weight loss in 1 month and oral pain*" offers more information to plan nursing care. Outcomes for a patient with this problem will include a specific targeted monthly weight gain and the patient's report of reduced or absent oral pain (see Chapter 20).

In the case of Mr. Lawson, Tonya provides clarity to the patient's diagnosis, entering the final diagnostic statement in his plan of care, "*Lack of Knowledge regarding postoperative care related to inexperience with surgery as evidenced by frequent queries about postoperative routines.*"

A complete, accurate diagnostic statement is necessary to deliver appropriate patient-centered care. Table 17.2 shows further examples of the benefits of diagnostic clarity.

Diagnostic Validity

Before finalizing a diagnosis, refer to the official ICNP®, NANDA-I, or classification system used at your agency to ensure accuracy of the diagnostic statement. This is essential for clear communication with all health care team members. Standard diagnostic terminology must be used in any electronic health record using nursing diagnoses. Accurate nursing diagnoses are foundational to the development of an effective, personalized plan of care (Yoost and Crawford, 2020).

FIG. 17.5 Relationship between a diagnosis and related factor or etiology.

TABLE 17.2	Comparison of Interventions for Nursing Diagnoses With Different Related Factors		
Nursing Diagnoses	**Related Factor**	**Assessment Findings**	**Interventions**
Patient A			
Anxiety	Uncertainty over surgery	Patient asks, "What type of pain will I have?" Restless and unable to sleep	Provide detailed instruction about surgery, recovery process, expected postoperative care. Plan formal time for patient to ask questions.
Impaired Mobility	Acute pain	Pain rated a 7 on scale of 0 to 10 Limits movement of right leg	Administer analgesic 30 minutes before planned exercise. Instruct patient on how to splint painful site during activity.
Patient B			
Anxiety	Loss of job	Fired from position 1 month ago Primary source of family income	Consult with social worker to arrange for job counseling. Encourage health promotion activities (e.g., exercise, routine social activities).
Impaired Mobility	Musculoskeletal injury	Weakness in right leg Reduced extension in right leg	Perform active range-of-motion exercises to right leg every 2 hours. Instruct patient on use of 3-point crutch gait.

Prioritization

Nurses' experiences in clinical practice serve to guide their actions and improve their clinical judgment (Dickison et al., 2019). One important form of judgment is prioritization of nursing diagnoses. Silvestri (2019) describes an important aspect of clinical judgment as nurses ranking their hypotheses about patients, prioritizing their concerns and patients' nursing diagnoses. When you begin nursing practice, prioritization of diagnoses is a product of considering a patient's basic needs, making generalizations about what seems more important, and relying on patients and other caregivers to support a priority. However, as you develop clinically, your experience and knowledge about patients' various health problems allow you to be more critical in interpreting which diagnosis is a priority. You are able to see a patient more holistically and recognize how a patient's health problems are interrelated.

*In Mr. Lawson's case, Tonya identified **Lack of Knowledge, Risk for Infection, Anxiety**, and **Acute Pain** as relevant diagnoses. Which is a priority? Tonya knows that unless the patient's pain and anxiety are relieved, he will not be responsive to instructional interventions. But remember that Mr. Lawson also displayed a breathing problem, with diagnostic tests revealing a pulmonary embolus. Over the last 24 hours the patient's breathing status has stabilized, with no additional emboli. Tonya chooses not to select a nursing diagnosis regarding the breathing problem, but will continue monitoring the patient. The patient's pain and anxiety are related, and his anxiety is related to a lack of knowledge and the ability to learn. How Mr. Lawson's diagnoses affect one another will require Tonya to critically prioritize often based on the patient's progressive symptoms with the goal of promoting the patient's surgical recovery.*

The nursing process is dynamic. As a patient's condition changes, there are different priorities and often new or resolved nursing diagnoses. Thus, ongoing critical thinking applied to the process of nursing diagnosis is essential; this involves applying knowledge and experience, recognizing cues reflecting change, exploring the cues further and interpreting new data, and forming sound judgments.

Diagnostic Error

Diagnostic errors by health care professionals may cause harm to patients by preventing or delaying appropriate treatment or by providing unnecessary or harmful treatment (Committee on Diagnostic Error in Health Care, 2015). Errors occur in the nursing diagnostic process during data collection, analysis of data clusters or patterns, and interpretation in choosing a nursing diagnostic statement. Accuracy is a critical thinking element for selection of a nursing diagnosis. Do not skip any of the steps in the nursing diagnostic process, and be sure you complete every step.

Errors in Data Collection. During assessment (see Chapter 16) consistently apply critical thinking in gathering patient data. Apply critical thinking attitudes and intellectual standards while gathering data to avoid inaccurate or missing data. Explore a patient's health problem thoroughly, gathering data on presenting signs and symptoms as well as any findings you might expect for the patient's condition. Be willing to confirm a finding with another nurse. If you think you are missing data or need more data, consider what other questions you might ask the patient or family. Ask yourself whether your physical examination was thorough and relevant to the symptoms a patient reported. Did you explore signs and symptoms based on what you know about the patient's health condition? Be thorough with data collection, and validate that your measurable, objective physical findings support subjective data. For example, when a patient reports "difficulty breathing," you also listen to lung sounds, assess respiratory rate, and measure a patient's chest excursion (see Chapter 30). Current evidence shows that insufficient identification of defining characteristics/assessment findings or related factors is common when making diagnoses (Mynaříková and Žiaková, 2014).

Errors in Data Clustering. Errors occur if you cluster data prematurely, incorrectly, or not at all. Premature clustering occurs when you make a nursing diagnosis before grouping all patient data. For example, a patient reports having occasional incontinence and urinary frequency. You cluster the available data and begin to identify an alteration in urination. Incorrect clustering occurs when you try to make a diagnosis fit a limited set of signs and symptoms that you gather. In this example, further assessment reveals that the patient has urinary incontinence in small volumes with coughing or exercise. The patient does not leak urine at nighttime. The complete data cluster helps you to focus more specifically on a specific type of incontinence problem (e.g., stress versus functional incontinence). Before analyzing your assessment data to identify clusters or patterns, validate the accuracy and completeness of your data one more time. You can do this by reassessing for a particular symptom, confirming data from the health record, or consulting with another nurse. When you are unable to validate data, this is a warning that there may be an inaccurate match between clinical data elements and the nursing diagnosis you want to select.

Errors in Analysis and Interpretation of Data. During analysis and interpretation, be careful to consider any conflicting data elements and determine whether there are sufficient data to form a diagnosis. Remember, a single symptom is insufficient for selecting a nursing diagnosis. For example, a patient who is wincing may be responding to pain, nausea, or even fear, all valid nursing diagnoses.

In the example of the patient displaying symptoms of urinary frequency and occasional incontinence in small volumes following exercise and coughing, a review of assessment findings for associated urinary alteration diagnoses is necessary. The assessment findings identified for this patient best fit criteria for *Stress Incontinence of Urine*. The patient does not leak urine during nighttime or report a constant urge to void, so a nursing diagnosis of *Urge Incontinence of Urine* is probably inappropriate. You learn to sort out the data you have collected and match them with assessment findings standard to a diagnosis to select an appropriate nursing diagnosis. Interpretation is accurate after carefully reviewing nursing diagnoses with similar assessment findings to choose the one that best fits your patient's condition.

Errors in a Diagnostic Statement. Sound clinical reasoning enables you to make the judgment needed to identify an accurate nursing diagnosis. The process then leads to the selection of individualized, specific, and effective nursing interventions (Chapter 19). Successful selection of nursing interventions also depends on having the correct related or etiologic factors or risk factors for a nursing diagnosis. An accurate diagnostic statement with relevant assessment findings guides you and the patient in the selection of appropriate patient outcomes (see Chapter 18). Unfortunately, research shows that nurses are not always methodical in the way they form nursing diagnoses (Box 17.3). You can reduce errors in diagnostic statements by selecting appropriate, concise, and precise language. Be sure that the etiology or related factor is within the scope of nursing practice to diagnose and treat. The following guidelines will assist you in reducing diagnostic errors:

- Identify a patient's response to a health problem, not a medical diagnosis (Carpenito, 2017). A medical diagnosis requires medical interventions; thus, it is inappropriate to include your patient's medical diagnosis in a nursing diagnostic statement. For example, instead of the diagnosis of hypertension, select the nursing diagnosis *Altered Blood Pressure* (ICN, 2019).

BOX 17.3   EVIDENCE-BASED PRACTICE

Sources of Error and Frequency of Nursing Diagnoses Used in Clinical Practice

PICOT Question: Among practicing nurses, what is the level of accuracy in the making of nursing diagnostic statements?

Evidence Summary

Two separate studies conducted internationally examined the most frequently occurring mistakes in nursing diagnostics and the frequency of nursing diagnoses used in clinical practice (Mynaříková and Žiaková, 2014; Johnson et al., 2018). The literature reviews included formal research studies (Johnson et al., 2018) as well as expert reviews and educational texts (Mynaříková and Žiaková, 2014). The use of standard nursing language and nursing diagnosis classification systems has consistently been demonstrated as an essential element that structures nursing documentation and nursing care plans (Johnson et al., 2018). One review found deficiencies in the formation of nursing diagnostic conclusions. This included identification of diagnostic elements (e.g., assessment findings or related factors). In this same study, researchers found that nursing diagnoses are very often determined based on irrelevant or invalid data (Mynaříková and Žiaková, 2014). Studies that examined documentation of nursing diagnoses in a wide variety of settings found that diagnoses pertaining to dysfunctional body functions were more commonly identified, whereas diagnoses from the psychosocial area were identified much less often (Mynaříková and Žiaková, 2014). Because nurses commonly use the same nursing diagnoses for individual medical diagnoses or conditions, they may be less comfortable identifying mental, social, and spiritual diagnoses. For example, any time a patient has a hip replacement, nurses will identify acute pain and impaired mobility regardless of what other data may indicate.

Application to Nursing Practice

- Use critical thinking to improve the accuracy of nursing diagnoses (Johnson et al., 2018).
- Because accuracy in selecting nursing diagnoses involves critical thinking, take the time to analyze data carefully before forming a statement (Mynaříková and Žiaková, 2014).
- Avoid identifying irreversible related factors, which cannot be changed with nursing interventions.
- Do not assume a patient has a nursing diagnosis based on a medical diagnosis. Base your diagnosis selection on complete patient-specific data.
- Focus on the accuracy of nursing data entries. In particular, examine the accuracy, content, and the degree to which nursing notes and diagnoses were based on nursing assessment (Johnson et al., 2018).

- Identify a diagnostic statement rather than a symptom. Identify nursing diagnoses from a cluster of assessment findings and not just a single sign or symptom. One assessment finding is insufficient for diagnosis identification. For example, dyspnea alone does not lead you to a diagnosis. A pattern of dyspnea, reduced chest excursion, and tachypnea are assessment findings for the diagnosis of *Impaired Breathing*.
- Identify a related factor or risk factor treatable through nursing intervention. A diagnostic test or a chronic condition is not an etiology that a nursing intervention is able to treat. A patient with fractured ribs probably has pain when inhaling, impaired chest excursion, and slower, shallow respirations. A chest x-ray may show collapse of alveoli in the affected area. The nursing diagnosis of "*Impaired Breathing related to shallow respirations*" is incorrect. There are no interventions that directly make respirations less shallow. The diagnosis of "*Impaired Breathing related to chest pain from rib fracture evidenced by reduced excursion and dyspnea*" is correct.

Nursing interventions directed toward pain relief will lead to improved breathing.
- Identify a problem caused by the response to a treatment or diagnostic study rather than the treatment or study itself. Patients experience many responses to diagnostic tests and medical treatments. These responses are the focus of nursing care. The patient who has chest pain and is scheduled for a cardiac catheterization possibly has a nursing diagnosis of "*Anxiety related to lack of knowledge about cardiac testing, evidenced by inability to describe cardiac catheterization after repeated questioning.*" An incorrect diagnosis is "*Anxiety related to cardiac catheterization.*"
- Identify a patient response to the equipment rather than the equipment itself. Patients are often unfamiliar with medical technology and its use. The diagnosis of "*Lack of Knowledge regarding the need for cardiac monitoring related to inexperience*" is accurate compared with the statement "*Lack of Knowledge related to cardiac monitoring.*"
- Identify a patient's problems rather than your problems with nursing care. Nursing diagnoses are patient-centered and form the basis for goal-directed care. Consider a patient with a peripheral intravenous (IV) infusion. "*Potential Intravenous Complications related to poor vascular access*" indicates a nursing problem in maintaining the infusion. The diagnosis "*Risk for Infection evidenced by swollen IV site, pain at site, and slowed infusion*" properly centers attention on the patient's potential needs.
- Identify a patient problem rather than a nursing intervention. You plan nursing interventions after identifying a nursing diagnosis. The intervention "Offer bedpan frequently because of incontinence" is not a diagnostic statement. Instead, with the proper assessment data, the correct diagnostic statement would be "*Diarrhea related to food intolerance evidenced by 3 stools daily and soft formed stools.*" A correct diagnosis will more likely result in the selection of appropriate interventions to solve the patient's problem.
- Identify a patient need rather than the goal of care. You establish goals during the planning step of the nursing process (Chapter 18). Goals based on accurate identification of a patient's problems serve as a basis to determine problem resolution. Change the goal-phrased statement of "Patient needs high-protein diet related to potential alteration in nutrition" to "*Impaired Nutritional Intake related to difficulty swallowing evidenced by inability to eat solid foods and painful mouth.*"
- Make professional rather than prejudgmental statements. Base nursing diagnoses on subjective and objective patient data and do not include your personal beliefs and values. Remove your judgment from "*Impaired Skin Integrity related to poor hygiene habits*" by changing the diagnostic statement to read "*Impaired Skin Integrity related to inadequate knowledge about perineal care evidenced by inability to cleanse perineum and inability to explain cleansing techniques.*"
- Avoid legally inadvisable statements in a diagnostic statement (Carpenito, 2017). Statements that imply blame, negligence, or malpractice (see Chapter 23) have the potential to result in a lawsuit. The statement "*Acute Pain related to insufficient medication*" implies an inadequate prescription by a health care provider. Correct problem identification is "*Acute Pain related to insufficient knowledge of analgesic schedule evidenced by self-report of pain intensity and inability to describe dosage plan.*"
- Identify the problem and etiology to avoid a circular statement. Circular statements are vague and give no direction to nursing care. Change the statement "*Impaired Breathing related to shallow breathing*" to identify the real patient problem and cause, "*Impaired Breathing related to incisional pain evidenced by splinting and increased respiratory rate.*"

- Identify only one patient problem in the diagnostic statement. Every problem has different expected outcomes (see Chapter 18). Confusion during the planning of care occurs when you include multiple problems in a nursing diagnosis. It also can result in choosing an insufficient number of nursing interventions or inappropriate interventions. For example, *"Pain and Anxiety related to difficulty in ambulating"* are two diagnoses combined in one nursing diagnosis statement. Two separate diagnoses for *"Pain"* and *"Anxiety"* are more accurate. It is permissible to include multiple etiologies contributing to one patient problem, as in *"Dysfunctional Grief related to diagnosis of a terminal illness and change in family role."*

> **REFLECT NOW**
>
> Share a case summary of assessment findings from a patient you cared for with a student colleague. Compare the nursing diagnoses you made with those your colleague makes. Discuss the similarities and differences.

USE OF NURSING DIAGNOSIS IN PRACTICE

Patients usually present with a variety of health problems, and these problems can cause numerous types of human responses. For example, a medical diagnosis of cerebrovascular accident or stroke often results in altered human responses, including changes in mobility, speech, thought processes, behavioral coping, and family support. Therefore, a single nursing diagnosis such as altered mobility is insufficient to truly design a comprehensive patient-centered approach to care. The assessment findings you obtain will often apply to one or more nursing diagnoses. *We have seen that in the case of Tonya and Mr. Lawson. The patient has nursing diagnoses of **Lack of Knowledge, Anxiety, Acute Pain,** and **Risk for Infection.** Thoroughly interpreting assessment findings leads to a broader picture of a patient's various health responses and how they are related.* One way to communicate the relationships among a patient's multiple nursing diagnoses is through concept mapping. It is a tool that can be helpful to you in your early practice situations.

Concept Mapping

In Chapters 15 and 16 you learned how concept mapping offers a graphic look at the connections among patients' multiple health responses to problems. It is challenging to prioritize and focus on all of a patient's nursing diagnoses. The challenge is compounded when you care for multiple patients in clinical practice. A concept map helps you critically think about a patient's diagnoses and how they relate to one another. Many educators use concept mapping to help students develop critical thinking during clinical practice (Khrais, 2017; Aein and Aliakbari, 2017). Concept mapping organizes and links data about a patient's multiple diagnoses in a logical way. It graphically represents the connections among concepts (e.g., nursing diagnoses, assessment findings, and interventions) that relate to a central subject (the patient's primary health problems). In Fig. 17.6 the dotted lines between nursing diagnoses show that one diagnosis is directly related to another. Concept mapping develops skills that provide nurses with expertise in flexible, individualized, situation-specific problem solving for each patient (Aein and Aliakbari, 2017).

An advantage of a concept map is its central focus on a patient rather than on a disease or health alteration, even though the patient's health problems are central. This holistic focus encourages nurses to concentrate on patients' specific health problems and nursing diagnoses rather than using one approach for all patients with similar problems.

Cultural Relevance in Diagnosis

When you select nursing diagnoses, consider your patients' cultural diversity, including ethnicity, values, beliefs, language, and health practices (see Chapter 9). This includes knowing the cultural differences that affect how your patients define health and illness and their preferences or choices for treatment. For example, Lai et al. (2013) explored how nursing diagnoses affected the quality of professional nursing from the perspective of Taiwanese nurses. Their work found that certain diagnoses were difficult for nurses to apply, considering the cultural beliefs of the traditional Chinese health care setting, which emphasizes holistic harmony and balance. It is important to know yourself, consider your patient's culture, and practice cultural competence to accurately identify a patient's health care problems and to provide patient-centered nursing care. This requires validation of how to identify a patient's diagnosis with the patient.

Consider the example of the ICNP® nursing diagnosis *Conflicting Caregiver Attitude,* where differences of opinion are found to exist between family caregivers of a patient near the end of life. It would be easy to apply your own cultural bias in selecting this diagnosis, depending on your beliefs, past experiences, and comfort in counseling caregivers about death. It would also be easy to apply the diagnosis inappropriately without considering the patient's and family members' values and beliefs. Attitudes and behaviors of families and care providers toward patients and their relationships with patients can affect patients' dignity significantly (Guo and Jacelon, 2014). The inappropriate selection of a nursing diagnosis based on your values or beliefs potentially results in the implementation of interventions that a patient or family caregiver is unlikely to accept. Consider asking these questions to make culturally competent nursing diagnoses:

- How has this health problem affected you and your family?
- What do you believe will help or fix the problem?
- What worries you the most about this problem?
- Which cultural practices do you observe to keep yourself and your family well?
- Let me share how I identify your health problem. Do you agree?

When you ask questions such as these, you use a patient-centered approach that allows you to see a patient's health situation through the patient's eyes. This is necessary to identify relevant assessment data pertaining to a patient's health problems.

CARE PLANNING

Nursing diagnosis provides a universal and standardized way for professional nurses to communicate among themselves and across other health care disciplines. It enhances interprofessional collaboration (see Chapter 18). Diagnoses direct the planning process and the selection of nursing interventions to achieve desired outcomes for patients. Just as a medical diagnosis of diabetes mellitus leads a health care provider to prescribe a low-carbohydrate diet and medication for blood glucose control, the nursing diagnosis of *Impaired Health Maintenance* will lead a nurse to design appropriate educational and social support interventions. In Chapter 18 you will learn how combining nursing diagnostic statements with the Nursing Interventions Classification (NIC) and Nursing Outcomes Classification (NOC) systems facilitates the process of patient-centered care planning. The care plan (see Chapter 18) is a road map for delivering nursing care and demonstrates your accountability for patient care. By making accurate nursing diagnoses, your subsequent care plan communicates a patient's health care responses to problems to all health care professionals and ensures high-quality care.

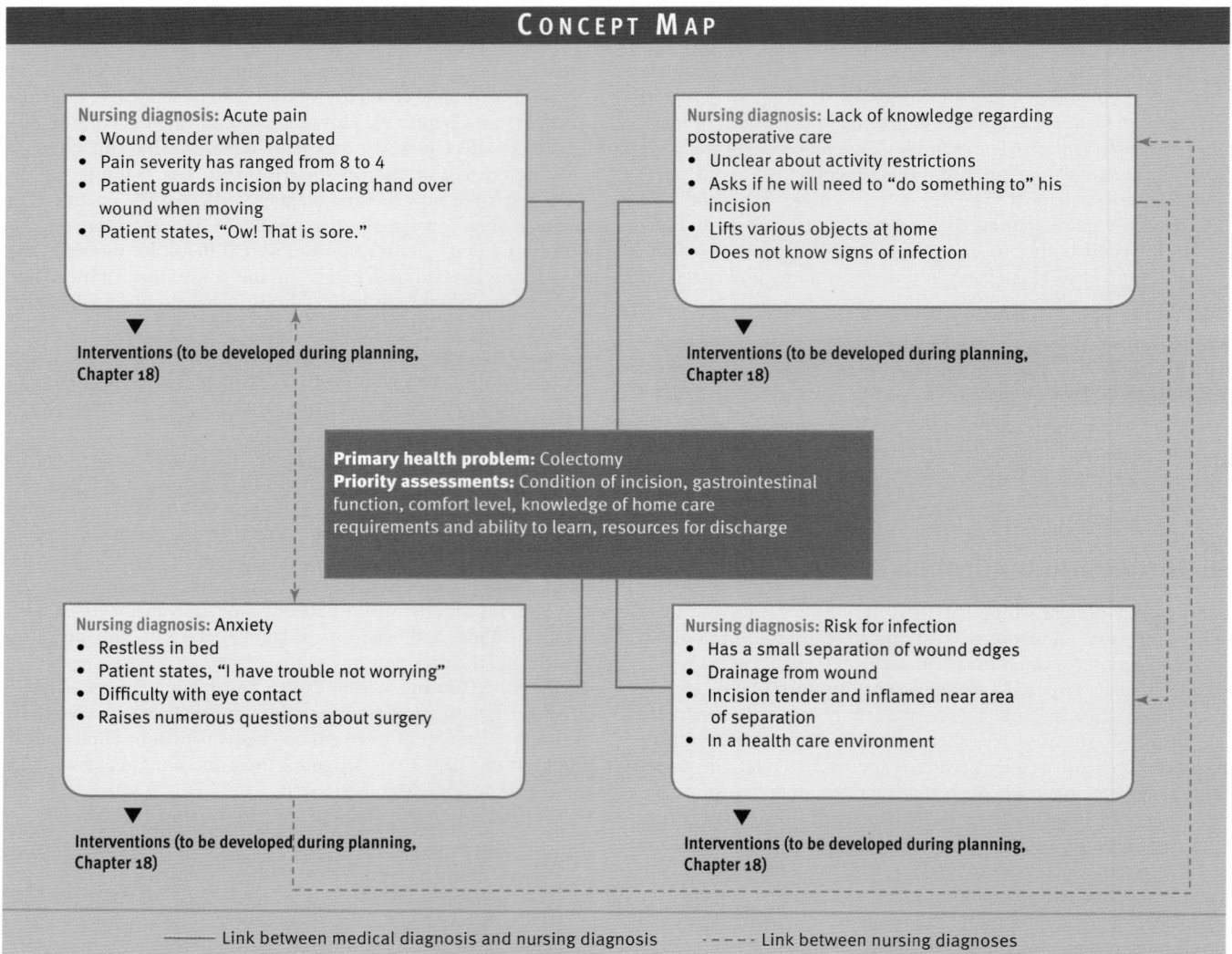

FIG. 17.6 Concept map for Mr. Lawson: Nursing diagnoses identified.

DOCUMENTATION AND INFORMATICS

Accuracy and consistency in the way information is shared among health care providers are essential. Appropriate tools such as the electronic health record (EHR) are needed to ensure continuity, safety, and quality of patient care by enhancing interprofessional communication (Elliot et al., 2018; Keenan et al., 2013) Standardized formats used in EHRs enable nurses and other care providers to share information about the care they provide to sustain life, enable recovery, and promote health. The use of standard, familiar nursing terminology in an EHR helps nurses select nursing diagnoses and interventions in planning patient care and communicating to health care colleagues.

Once you identify a patient's nursing diagnoses, enter them in the EHR of the agency. The agency information system will dictate how the diagnosis is disseminated throughout the record, such as in a formal care plan, a daily task sheet, or nurses' notes. In advanced systems a nurse enters assessment data into the EHR, and the computer software program organizes the data into patterns that enhance the ability to select accurate nursing diagnoses. Once diagnoses are selected, the computer system directs the nurse to outcome and intervention options

to select for the specific patient, allowing for individualized care. Many state-of-the-art EHRs contain nursing diagnoses with NANDA-I diagnoses, related factors, defining characteristics, and Nursing Intervention Classifications (NIC) and Nursing Outcome Classifications (NOC) (NANDA-I, 2018). The ICNP develops catalogs (nursing data subsets) for specified health situations that are used in building health information systems for a variety of settings (Rabelo-Silva, 2016).

Despite the ease and convenience of EHR systems, it is essential to enter the right data so that all health care providers have an accurate database. In a qualitative study examining weaknesses in the flow of patient care information, three themes were identified: (1) variation in nurse documentation and communication; (2) the absence of a centralized care overview in the patient's electronic health record, i.e., easily accessible by the entire care team; and (3) rarity of interdisciplinary communication (Keenan et al., 2013). To manage these weaknesses, follow these tips:

1. Communicate a patient's diagnoses accurately and in a timely manner in the EHR, and document the assessment data confirming the diagnosis.

2. When receiving information from another nurse during a hand-off report, confirm a patient's diagnoses; later, at the end of your shift, communicate the patient's progress.

3. Collaborate with all health care professionals involved in a patient's care, and use nursing diagnoses to convey patient problems.

4. Document priority information, such as the current plan of care (see Chapter 18), and make this easily accessible to all health care team members (Keenan et al., 2013).

KEY POINTS

- A nursing diagnosis is a clinical judgment based on critical analysis and interpretation of data cues that classifies the response to illness by an individual, family, or community.
- Nursing diagnoses provide clear direction as to the types of nursing interventions nurses are licensed to provide independently.
- Nurses cannot treat medical diagnoses; instead, they treat patients' responses to the medical health conditions. The exception to this is advanced practice nurses. Nurses treat patients' responses to health conditions.
- Nurses intervene in collaboration with personnel from other health care professions to manage collaborative problems.
- Using standardized terminology for nursing diagnoses provides diagnostic clarity and effective interprofessional communication and enables nurses to formulate nursing diagnoses and the associated interventions, and to assess the outcomes of nursing care.
- The application of knowledge and clinical experience, the consideration of environmental factors, and the use of critical thinking attitudes and intellectual and professional standards improve diagnostic accuracy.
- The nursing diagnostic reasoning process involves analyzing data gathered about a patient for pattern recognition and validation of available cues. Logically interpreting the data requires making a clinical judgment in selecting an accurate nursing diagnosis.
- The components of a nursing diagnostic statement include a diagnostic label or diagnosis, related factors or etiologies (for problem focused and negative diagnoses), and, as an option, major assessment findings.
- Data analysis involves critically organizing all data elements about a patient into meaningful patterns, also called data clusters or sets of assessment findings/defining characteristics.
- A problem-focused nursing diagnosis or negative diagnosis identifies actual undesirable human response to existing health problems, while a risk nursing diagnosis identifies when there is an increased potential or vulnerability for a patient to develop a problem or complication.
- An important form of clinical judgment is prioritization of nursing diagnoses, demonstrated when nurses apply their experience and knowledge about patients' various health problems to critically interpret which diagnosis is a priority.
- As you recognize data elements from an assessment, you will cluster or group them together in meaningful patterns in a logical way that during interpretation will clearly identify the nursing diagnoses.
- Identify nursing diagnoses from a cluster of assessment findings and not just a single symptom.
- Errors occur in the nursing diagnostic process during data collection; analysis of data, clustering, or pattern formation; and interpretation in choosing a nursing diagnostic statement.

REFLECTIVE LEARNING

After you complete an assessment of a patient in a clinical area or in a simulation laboratory, review your data and apply critical thinking.

- What patterns of data cues appear logically together as you analyze all of the patient information?
- How did your knowledge of the patient's condition influence your assessment activities? What could you have done differently to gather more information?
- As you look at the cues forming each pattern, are there cases in which an individual cue falls into more than one pattern? What does that suggest?

REVIEW QUESTIONS

1. A nurse conducts an assessment of a 42-year-old woman at a health clinic. The woman is married and lives in an apartment with her husband. She reports having frequent voiding and pain when she passes urine. The nurse asks whether she has to go to the bathroom at night, and the patient responds, "Yes." The patient had an episode of diarrhea 1 week ago. She weighs 136 kg (300 lb). The nurse documents the assessment findings listed below. Which of the assessment findings require priority follow-up by the nurse? (Select all that apply.)
   1. The patient has no history of chronic disease.
   2. Patient urinates at night.
   3. Patient reports having difficulty cleansing herself after voiding or passing stool.
   4. Body temperature 38°C (100.4°F)
   5. Recent history of weight gain
   6. Knowledge of perineal care
   7. Last normal bowel movement 2 days ago
   8. Frequency of diarrhea

2. A nurse's assessment reveals a patient having frequent voiding and pain when she urinates. Her body temperature is 38°C (100.4°F). The nurse asks whether she has to go to the bathroom at night, and the patient responds, "Yes." When asked how often, the patient replies, "About three times a night." The nurse asks if having to urinate at night is recent or normal for the patient. The patient explains, "I usually go once a night but that is all." The nurse then asks, "When you feel the need to go, can you reach the toilet in time?" The patient says, "Oh, yes, I can." The nurse asks, "And have you had any leaking of urine?" The patient denies leaking. When asked if she is having any back or abdominal pain, the patient denies discomfort. The nurse then gathers a urine specimen from the patient and inspects its character, noting it is cloudy and foul smelling. Which of the following nursing diagnoses are indicated by cues in this patient's assessment?
   1. *Impaired Kidney Function*
   2. *Impaired Urination*
   3. *Urge Incontinence of Urine*
   4. *Total Urinary Incontinence*

3. A nursing student is working with a faculty member to identify a nursing diagnosis for an assigned patient. The student has assessed that the patient is undergoing radiation treatment to the abdomen, has liquid stool, and the skin is clean and intact. The student selects the nursing diagnosis *Impaired Skin Integrity*. The faculty member explains that the student has made a diagnostic error for which of the following reasons?
   1. Incorrect clustering of data
   2. Wrong diagnosis
   3. Condition is a collaborative problem
   4. Premature ending assessment

4. A nurse assesses a 42-year-old woman at a health clinic. The woman is married and lives in a condo with her husband. She reports having frequent voiding and pain when she urinates. The nurse asks whether she has to go to the bathroom at night, and the patient responds, "Yes, usually twice or more." The patient had an episode of diarrhea 1 week ago. She weighs 136 kg (300 lb) and reports having difficulty cleansing herself after voiding or passing stool. Which of the following demonstrate assessment findings that cluster to indicate the nursing diagnosis *Impaired Urination*. (Select all that apply.)
   1. Age 42
   2. Dysuria
   3. Difficulty performing perineal hygiene
   4. Nocturia
   5. Episode of diarrhea
   6. Weighs 136 kg (300 lb)
   7. Frequent voiding
5. Review the following nursing diagnoses and identify the diagnoses that are stated correctly. (Select all that apply.)
   1. Offer frequent skin care because of *Impaired Skin Integrity*
   2. *Risk for Infection*
   3. *Chronic Pain related to osteoarthritis evidenced by reduced hip range of motion*
   4. *Activity Intolerance related to physical deconditioning evidenced by exertional dyspnea*
   5. *Lack of Knowledge related to laser surgery*
6. A home health nurse completes a home safety assessment. The data reveal that the patient is 71 years old with bilateral cataracts that are causing blurred vision and sensitivity to bright lights. The patient is recovering from a stroke that has caused left-sided weakness of the leg, with an unsteady gait. When talking with the patient, the nurse learns the patient lives alone and fell in the bathroom 4 months ago. Rooms in the home are in disrepair. The nurse identifies nursing diagnoses of *Impaired Vision, Impaired Mobility,* and *Risk for Fall.* Which diagnosis is the nurse's priority? Give a rationale.
7. A nurse is assigned to a new patient admitted to the medical unit. The nurse collects a nursing history and interviews the patient. Place the following steps for making a nursing diagnosis in the correct order.
   1. Consider the context of patient's health problem and select a related factor.
   2. Review assessment findings, noting objective and subjective clinical cues.
   3. Cluster cues that form a pattern.
   4. Gather thorough patient data about the patient's health problem.
   5. Identify the nursing diagnosis.
   6. Consider whether data are expected or unexpected based on the patient's problem.

8. A nurse interviews and conducts a physical examination of a patient that includes the following findings: reduced range of motion of lower hip, reduced strength in left leg, and difficulty turning in bed without assistance. This data set is an example of:
   1. Collaborative data set.
   2. Diagnostic label.
   3. Related factors.
   4. Data cluster.
   5. Validated data set
9. A nurse reviews data gathered regarding a patient's response to a diagnosis of cancer. The nurse notes that the patient is restless, avoids eye contact, has increased blood pressure, and expresses a sense of helplessness. The nurse compares the pattern of assessment findings for *Anxiety* with those of *Fear* and selects *Anxiety* as the correct diagnosis. This is an example of the nurse avoiding an error in which of the following? (Select all that apply.)
   1. Data collection
   2. Data clustering
   3. Data interpretation
   4. Making a diagnostic statement
   5. Outcome setting
10. A nursing assessment reveals a patient in the home setting who has reduced mobility following recovery from a stroke. The patient has weakness in the left leg and arm. The patient has a walker, which he has never used before, and his wife tells the nurse that he is unsteady in using the walker. The patient fell while in the hospital. The physical therapist came to the home, but the wife tells the nurse, "We are not sure how to get my husband upstairs. The therapist explained how to use the walker, but we have questions." The nurse developed the following concept map. Place the links between the nursing diagnoses in the correct direction.

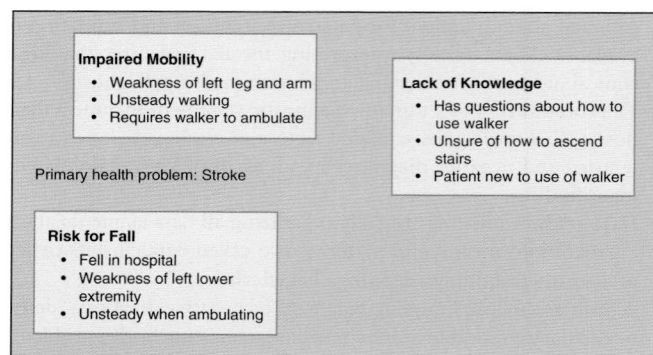

Rationales for Review Questions can be found on the Evolve website.

REFERENCES

American Nursing Association (ANA): *Nursing scope and standards of practice,* ed 4, Washington DC, 2021, American Nurses Association.

Carpenito LJ: *Nursing diagnosis: application to clinical practice,* ed 15, Philadelphia, 2017, Wolters Kluwer.

Committee on Diagnostic Error in Health Care; Board on Health Care Services; Institute of Medicine; The National Academies of Sciences, Engineering, and Medicine; Balogh EP, Miller BT, Ball JR, editors.

Washington, DC, 2015, National Academies Press (US). 2015 Dec 29.

Dickison P et al.: Integrating the National Council of State Boards of Nursing Clinical Judgment Model into nursing educational frameworks, *J Nurs Educ.* 58(2):72, 2019.

Elliot L et al: Standardizing documentation: a place for everything, *MEDSURG Nursing.* 27(1):32, 2018.

Garcia TR, Nobrega MML: The International Classification for Nursing Practice: participation of Brazilian nurses

in the project of the International Council of Nurses, *Acta Paul Enferm* 22(Especial - 70 Anos):875, 2009.

International Council of Nurses (ICN): *Technical Implementation Guide,* International Council of Nurses, Geneva, Switzerland, 2018.

International Council of Nurses (ICN): *Nursing diagnosis and outcome statements – international classification for nursing practice catalogue,* ICN – International Council of Nurses, Geneva, Switzerland, 2019.

International Council of Nurses (ICN): *Who we are*, 2020, https://www.icn.ch/. Accessed May 15, 2021.

Mynaříková E, Žiaková K: The use of nursing diagnoses in clinical practice, *Cent Eur J Nurs Midw* 5(3):117, 2014.

North American Nursing Diagnosis International (NANDA-I): *NANDA international history, momentum and connections*, nd, http://nanda.host4kb.com/article/AA-00240/0/1980-1989.html. Accessed May 15, 2021.

North American Nursing Diagnosis International (NANDA-I): In Herdman TH, Kamitsuru S, editors: *Nursing diagnoses: definitions and classification 2018-2020*, ed 11, 2018. New York, Thieme.

Office of the National Coordinator for Health Information Technology: *Standard nursing terminologies: a landscape analysis*, May 15, 2017, https://www.healthit.gov/sites/default/files/snt_final_05302017.pdf. Accessed May 15, 2021.

Silvestri LA: *White Paper: higher-cognitive-level test questions: a starting point for creating Next-Generation NCLEX® (NGN) test items*, Elsevier, 2019. https://evolve.elsevier.com/education/expertise/next-generation-nclex/higher-cognitive-level-test-questions-a-starting-point-for-creating-next-generation-nclex-ngn-test-items/. Accessed May 15, 2021.

World Health Organization (WHO): *International Classification for Nursing Practice (ICNP)*, 2017, https://www.who.int/standards/classifications/other-classifications/international-classification-for-nursing-practice. Accessed May 15, 2021.

World Health Professions Alliance: *Interprofessional collaborative practice*, 2019, https://www.whpa.org/activities/interprofessional-collaborative-practice. Accessed May 15, 2021.

Yoost B, Crawford L: *Fundamentals of nursing: active learning for collaborative practice*, ed 2, St Louis, 2020, Elsevier.

RESEARCH REFERENCES

Aein F, Aliakbari F: Effectiveness of concept mapping and traditional linear nursing care plans on critical thinking skills in clinical pediatric nursing course, *J Educ Health Promot* 6:13, 2017.

Coenen A et al.: ICNP catalogues for supporting nursing content in electronic health records, *Stud Health Technol Inform* 180:1075, 2012.

Guo Q, Jacelon CS: An integrative review of dignity in end-of-life care, *Palliat Med* 28(7):931, 2014.

Johnson L et al: A systematic literature review of accuracy in nursing care plans and using standardised nursing language, *Collegian*, 25:355, 2018.

Keenan Gl et al: Challenges to nurses' efforts of retrieving, documenting, and communicating patient care information, *J Am Med Inform Assoc* 20(2):245, 2013.

Khrais H: The outcomes of integrating concept mapping in nursing education: an integrative review, *Open J Nurs* 7(11):1335, 2017.

Lai W, et al.: Does one size fit all? Exploring the cultural applicability of NANDA-I nursing diagnoses to Chinese nursing practice. *J Transcult Nurs* 24(1):43, 2013.

Moss E et al.: Registered nurses as interprofessional collaborative partners: creating value-based outcomes, *OJIN*, 21(3), 2016. https://ojin.nursingworld.org/MainMenuCategories/ANAMarketplace/ANAPeriodicals/OJIN/TableofContents/Vol-21-2016/No3-Sept-2016/Registered-Nurses-as-Interprofessional-Collaborative-Partners.html. Accessed May 15, 2021.

Rabelo-Silva ER et al.: Advanced nursing process quality: comparing the international classification for nursing practice (ICNP) with the NANDA international (NANDA-I) and nursing interventions classification (NIC), *J Clin Nurs* 26(3–4):379, 2016.

Sullivan M, et al.: Interprofessional collaboration and education, *AJN* 115(3):47, 2015.

Planning and Outcomes Identification in Nursing Care

OBJECTIVES

- Explain how clinical judgment is integral to the planning process.
- Explain the relationship of planning to nursing diagnosis.
- Examine how critical thinking influences the planning of nursing care.
- Identify factors that influence the prioritization of nursing diagnoses for select patients.
- Examine the relevance of outcomes selected for nursing diagnoses.
- Discuss criteria used in priority setting.

- Use the SMART model for writing outcome statements.
- Explain the factors to consider when selecting interventions for a particular patient diagnosis or problem.
- Discuss the differences between independent and dependent nursing interventions.
- Explain how consultation is conducted in a clinical setting.
- Explain the process of interprofessional collaboration.

KEY TERMS

Consultation
Dependent nursing interventions
Independent nursing interventions
Interprofessional care plans
Interprofessional collaboration

Nurse-sensitive patient outcome
Nursing care plan
Nursing Interventions Classification
Nursing Outcomes Classification
Other provider interventions

Outcome
Planning
Priority setting
Scientific rationale

MEDIA RESOURCES

http://evolve.elsevier.com/Potter/fundamentals/
- Review Questions
- Concept Map Creator

- Case Study with Questions
- Audio Glossary
- Content Updates

How well do you plan? After reviewing the food products in your kitchen pantry, do you make a list and plan meals over the course of a week? As a parent, do you collaborate with a partner after considering your child's activities and plan for what to do over a weekend? How do you plan your expenses for a month? Planning is the process of identifying a problem (e.g., missing food products in the pantry) and making or carrying out a plan of action that is outcome oriented. You select foods you need for the kitchen pantry, plan a trip to the grocery store, and then select and prepare the food products bought to create a desirable and healthy meal.

Planning nursing care is more complicated than preparing for a trip to the grocery because it involves using critical thinking and decision making to form clinical judgments: reviewing a patient's nursing diagnoses and other collaborative problems, prioritizing nursing diagnoses and problems, setting outcomes to guide the plan of care, and choosing relevant interventions for patient care (Ignatavicius, 2019). Judgment lies in making accurate (or appropriate) clinical decisions when prioritizing diagnoses and outcomes and then selecting interventions.

In Chapter 17 you learned the process for identifying relevant and appropriate nursing diagnoses. After analyzing and interpreting a patient's assessment data to identify relevant nursing diagnoses, outcomes identification and planning become the next steps of the nursing process

(Fig. 18.1). Once you identify a diagnosis or problem, you plan a course of action to resolve the problem. You use clinical judgment in performing planning to generate solutions for a patient's care.

*Tonya has been conducting ongoing assessments of Mr. Lawson's health status over the past 3 days and has identified four nursing diagnoses: **Acute Pain** related to trauma of surgical incision, **Lack of Knowledge** regarding postoperative care related to inexperience with surgery, **Anxiety,** and **Risk for Infection.** Tonya is responsible for planning Mr. Lawson's nursing care after identifying relevant nursing diagnoses. The care that she plans will be continually implemented and updated during Mr. Lawson's hospital stay by the other nurses involved in Mr. Lawson's care. If Tonya plans well, the individualized interventions that she selects collaboratively with Mr. and Mrs. Lawson will prepare the patient for recovery and a smooth transition home. Collaboration with the patient and his wife will be critical for a plan of care to be successful.*

CRITICAL THINKING IN PLANNING

Clinical judgment during planning involves use of the six components of critical thinking to guide nurses in making relevant and appropriate clinical decisions (Fig. 18.2). For experienced nurses, planning, including outcomes identification, is a conscious process that occurs rather quickly when nurses are familiar with patients' diagnoses and have

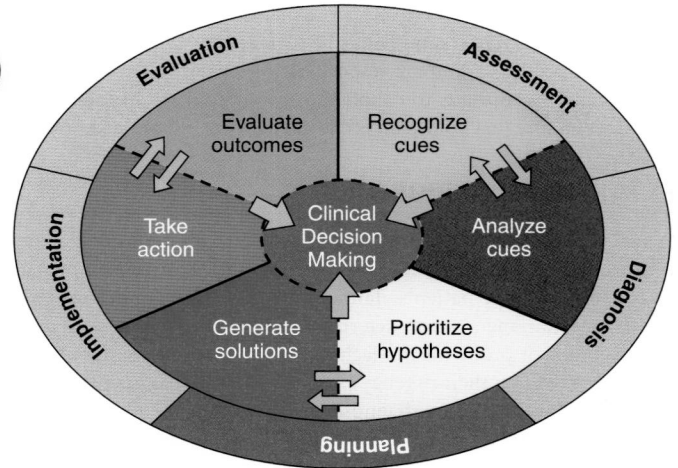

FIG. 18.1 Nursing process—Planning. (Copyright © NCSBN. All rights reserved.)

experience in observing how patients respond to interventions. Anticipation of what occurs in planning is almost automatic. But planning must be patient-centered for each unique patient. Critical thinking offers a methodical way to avoid forming routine plans of care, instead creating an individualized patient-centered plan, developed with the patient's involvement and focused on improving the patient's well-being. You will develop planning skills as your experiences in patient care expand and as you gain competence using the nursing process.

Knowledge

To plan care for a patient, you must apply scientific knowledge of a patient's clinical condition, what you know about the patient from assessment, and nursing knowledge to improve your ability to recognize care priorities (see Fig. 18.2). Use your understanding of the roles of other health care disciplines and available community and family resources to form a plan that is comprehensive and suited to all of a patient's health care problems. A fundamental component of any patient care plan is education of patient or family caregivers, thus requiring knowledge of the teaching and learning process (Chapter 25) and family dynamics (Chapter 10).

In the case study involving Mr. Lawson, Tonya will incorporate what she knows about a colectomy, the anticipated postoperative course following major abdominal surgery, and the pathology of pulmonary embolus when selecting nursing interventions. Recognizing the common postoperative responses, such as pain, wound healing, and return to mobility, will further inform her as she prioritizes her care. Tonya will apply patient education principles as she selects the best approaches for involving the patient and Mrs. Lawson in postoperative instruction.

Environment

Environmental factors within the health care setting will impact the timing and efficiency of any plan of care (see Fig. 18.2). For example, in a hospital setting the model for delivering care (see Chapter 21), the

Knowledge Base
- Patient's data and selected nursing diagnoses
- Anatomy and physiology; pathophysiology of patient's condition
- Normal growth and development
- Evidence-based nursing interventions
- Role of other health care disciplines
- Communication and patient education principles
- Community resources
- Family dynamics
- Delegation principles
- Priority-setting principles

Attitudes
- Perseverance
- Responsibility
- Discipline
- Creativity

Environment
- Time pressure
- Setting
- Health care resources (equipment, personnel)
- Task complexity
- Interruptions

(center diagram) Evaluation — Evaluate outcomes; Assessment — Recognize cues; Analyze cues; Diagnosis; Prioritize hypotheses; Planning; Generate solutions; Take action; Implementation; Clinical Decision Making

Standards
- *ANA Standards and Scope of Nursing Practice*
- Clinical Practice Guidelines and Standards of Practice
- Agency policies and procedures
- Patient-centered outcomes
- Intellectual standards in measurement
- Professional
  - ° Standards of care
  - ° Ethical standards

Experience
- Personal
- Clinical experience
- Skill competence

FIG. 18.2 Critical thinking in planning. (Clinical Judgment Measurement Model copyright © NCSBN. All rights reserved.)

workflow routine of a nursing unit, staffing levels, availability of material resources, and interruptions from other care providers affect the minute-by-minute determination of patient care priorities. In the home health setting, the number of visits scheduled for a day and the availability of family caregivers and resources within a patient's home affect a patient's priorities. Consider all these factors in a plan of care. For example, if a patient's priority is early mobility following hip replacement surgery, does a nursing unit have a physical therapist or trained physical therapy technicians to assist with regular ambulation of patients?

Experience

Your clinical experience will affect your ability to anticipate and recognize when patient problems and priorities change. Judgment grows from witnessing how patients respond to plans of care (see Fig. 18.2). Interventions chosen for a plan of care often include nursing skills or procedures. Your competence in performing these skills will affect patient outcomes. When your experience is limited with respect to the type of patient problem/nursing diagnosis or the interventions that have been recommended by health care providers and nursing colleagues, be willing to ask for assistance.

Standards

Evidence-based knowledge regarding a specific nursing diagnosis or collaborative problem area translates into standards of care applied in patient care. For example, the Infusion Nurses Society has standards of practice that you will use when planning interventions for patients receiving intravenous therapy (Gorski et al., 2021). You use these specific standards while cleansing an intravenous site and managing an infusion to avoid physiologic complications (Chapter 42). Clinical guidelines are commonly developed by a health care agency—guidelines such as early mobility (Chapter 38), prevention of central-line–associated bloodstream infections (Chapter 42), and aspiration precautions (Chapter 45). You incorporate these guidelines as interventions in your plan of care.

Ethical standards are critical, especially when you make decisions involving the patient and family caregiver in planning. Do patients have autonomy in making decisions about their care? Are the interventions chosen in the best interests of a patient? Ethical care is essential in any care plan.

Attitudes

The most effective plans of care are usually creative with respect to incorporating what is known about a patient and individualizing interventions. Creative plans of care enhance efficacy by being more patient-centered. When you establish a plan of care, it is shared with all health care providers. You are responsible for ensuring that the plan is relevant and appropriate. You apply the critical thinking attitude of discipline to be sure that your plan is comprehensive and evidence based.

ESTABLISHING PRIORITIES

When you enter nursing practice, you will care for multiple patients who are influenced by multiple factors (Fig. 18.3). Thus, it is important to collaborate with patients, family caregivers (as applicable), and health care team members to determine the urgency of identified nursing diagnoses or problems for each patient. You prioritize the nursing diagnoses based on their urgency (Ackley et al., 2020). **Priority setting** is the ordering of nursing diagnoses or patient problems to establish the preferred order in which you will implement nursing interventions. As your patients' conditions, diagnoses, and problems change, the order in which you need to implement your interventions also changes. Patients' priorities change sometimes within a matter of minutes. Each time you begin to care for a patient, such as at the beginning of a hospital shift or during a clinic visit, review which diagnoses are priorities. Ongoing patient assessment is critical to determine the status of a patient's nursing diagnoses.

*For example, Tonya provides care to Mr. Lawson on an ongoing basis. **Risk for Infection** becomes a priority when signs or symptoms begin to show a worsening of the condition of the patient's wound. **Pain** is a priority when it interferes with the patient's ability to learn about surgery and when it raises the patient's anxiety. If the patient's wound condition worsens and pain is also on the increase, Tonya must reassess the situation and determine which diagnosis becomes the priority.*

Generally, problem-focused or negative diagnoses take priority over wellness diagnoses, at-risk diagnoses, and health promotion diagnoses. Short-term acute patient care needs and problems typically take priority over longer-term chronic needs (NCLEX, n.d.). Priority setting is not the ordering of a list of care tasks. For example, when you begin a day on a clinical setting, your patient priorities are not based on a list of care activities recorded in the patient's medical record, but instead should be based on the patient's current condition and desired outcomes. Use your nursing and scientific knowledge base to recognize patterns of data from your patient assessment. Then allow certain knowledge triggers to guide you to which diagnoses require intervention and when you need to take action (Ackley et al., 2020). This requires you to identify symptoms that

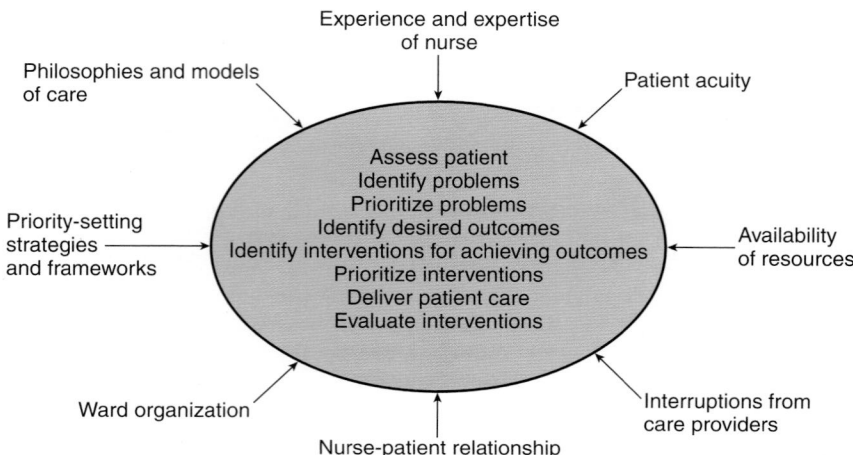

FIG. 18.3 A model for priority setting. (Modified from Hendry C, Walker A: Priority setting in clinical nursing practice, *J Adv Nurs* 47[4]:427, 2004.)

patients have related to their illness, understand which symptom patterns require action, and identify the associated time frame for effective intervention. Some knowledge triggers include pathophysiology or pharmacological information, past experiences with other patients who have had similar problems, and what you know about the patient you are caring for now.

In Mr. Lawson's case, Tonya was initially focused on his postoperative recovery, but when Mr. Lawson developed chest pain and difficulty breathing, the trigger (warning signs caused by possible pulmonary embolus, a complication of surgery) required that she take immediate action.

As you care for a patient or multiple patients, you must deal with certain aspects of care before others. By ranking a patient's nursing diagnoses in order of importance and always monitoring changing signs and symptoms of patient problems, you attend to each patient's most important needs and better organize ongoing care activities. Priorities help you anticipate and sequence nursing interventions.

For example, if there is a time when Mr. Lawson experiences increased pain and signs of heightened anxiety at the same time, Tonya will note the severity of pain and its characteristics and the nature and focus of the patient's anxiety. Considering the influence each problem has on the other, Tonya will decide whether offering a pharmacological intervention is a higher priority than intervening with stress-reducing measures to reduce the patient's anxiety.

You set priorities in collaboration with health care providers, your patients, and family caregivers (when appropriate). Often a health care provider will identify a medical problem, for example, that you did not anticipate and that requires immediate action. You also will select mutually agreed-on priorities with a patient based on the urgency of the problems, the patient's safety, the nature of the treatment indicated, and the relationships among the diagnoses. You establish priorities in relation to the ongoing clinical importance of the patient's diagnoses and problems.

Methods for Prioritizing

As you begin your practice, another helpful way to think of your patient's nursing diagnoses and problems is to categorize them as high, intermediate, or low in importance. Nursing diagnoses that when left untreated result in harm to a patient (e.g., those physiologic needs related to airway status, circulation, safety, and pain) have the highest priorities. Prioritize nursing diagnoses first by considering patients' immediate needs based on ABC (airway, breathing, and circulation) (Ackley et al., 2020). The highest priority can also be determined by using Maslow's hierarchy of needs (see Chapter 6). For example, *Risk for Violence, Impaired Gas Exchange,* and *Impaired Cardiac Function* are examples of high-priority nursing diagnoses that drive the priorities of safety, adequate oxygenation, and adequate circulation. However, it is always important to consider each patient's unique situation. Avoid classifying only physiological nursing diagnoses as high priority.

Consider Mr. Lawson's case. Among his nursing diagnoses, **Acute Pain** *was an initial priority. Tonya knew that she needed to relieve Mr. Lawson's acute pain to promote postoperative recovery. Pain management was also a factor since pain can interfere with a patient's ability to attend to instruction. Now that Mr. Lawson's pain is controlled reasonably well,* **Lack of Knowledge** *becomes a greater priority because of the patient's expressed desire to learn and the urgent need to prepare him adequately for his upcoming discharge.*

Intermediate-priority nursing diagnoses are nonemergent and not life-threatening. *In Mr. Lawson's case,* **Risk for Infection** *is an intermediate diagnosis, unless the time arises when the condition of his wound worsens. The nursing staff will continue to monitor his wound healing, and it is important for Mr. and Mrs. Lawson to learn the signs of infection and understand what to observe once the patient returns home.* In this

case, focused and individualized instruction from all members of the health care team about infection prevention is necessary throughout the patient's hospitalization.

Low-priority nursing diagnoses are not always directly related to a specific illness or prognosis but still affect a patient's future well-being. Many low-priority diagnoses focus on a patient's long-term health care needs.

Mr. Lawson shares a concern with Tonya, "I'm worried about being able to return to work on time." When instructing the patient, Tonya noticed that he was able to attend to what she had to say. However, Tonya knows she has not yet identified fully Mr. Lawson's concerns about returning to work. She will need to assess him more fully, so a nursing diagnosis such as **Anxiety** *may be of low priority at this time. However, if the patient's anxiety is left unaddressed, it could become a higher priority if it interferes with his ability to learn and understand discharge information.*

Ethical care is a part of priority setting (see Chapter 22). When ethical issues cloud priorities, you must maintain an open dialogue with the patient, family members, and other health care providers. For example, when caring for patients with cancer, discuss the situation with them and understand their expectations, understand your professional responsibility in protecting the patients from harm, and know their health care providers' therapeutic or palliative plans of care. These ethical considerations will aid you in selecting which diagnoses are more important. For example, a dying patient's priority of *Fear About Death* may take precedence over *Acute Pain,* even though pain relief might relax the patient. The patient may desire the nurse to withhold medication until the patient can express any fears openly and clearly.

Priorities in Practice

Many factors within the health care environment affect your ability to set priorities (see Fig. 18.3). Nurses should have a plan of action to effectively manage their time, avoid unnecessary interruptions, and avoid helping others when this could potentially jeopardize their patients' priorities of care (NCLEX, n.d.). Remember, colleagues will ask for assistance when their patients have priorities needing immediate attention. That is part of teamwork. But if you are starting to attend to your own patient's priority need when a colleague approaches you, you will need to decide whether you are able to help your colleague or if someone else, such as another nurse, a technician, or an assistive personnel, needs to be found to help.

When you work with assistive personnel (AP), discuss the purpose of each patient's hospitalization, how you expect the patient will look at the end of the shift, the plan for achieving desired outcomes, and how you and the AP will work together to care for the patient. Although you agree on priorities at the beginning of a shift, your patients' priorities will likely change several times before the next shift. The shifts in priorities often happen because your patients' needs will change, as will your patient assignments due to patient discharges, transfers, and admissions.

The same factors that influence your ability to prioritize nursing diagnoses and plan care for groups of patients minute-by-minute also affect your ability to prioritize nursing actions. The nature of nursing work challenges you to attend to a given patient's priorities when you care for more than one patient. The nursing care process is nonlinear. Often you complete an assessment and identify nursing diagnoses for one patient, leave the room to perform an intervention for a second patient, and move on to evaluate the care of a third patient. Nurses exercise "cognitive shifts" (i.e., shifts in attention from one patient to another during the conduct of the nursing process). This shifting of attention occurs in response to changing patient needs, new procedures being ordered, or environmental processes interacting (e.g., call lights, alarms). Because of these cognitive shifts, it becomes important to stay organized and know your patients' priorities. Work from your plan of care, and use patients' priorities to organize the order for delivering interventions and documenting care.

CLINICAL JUDGMENT IN OUTCOMES IDENTIFICATION

A single patient often has multiple nursing diagnoses and collaborative problems. In addition, patients will have medical diagnoses that dictate a variety of interventions you must administer to patients. It thus can be challenging to consistently focus on the outcomes or results you hope to achieve for a patient. An outcome is the effect a health care service or intervention(s) has on the health status of a patient. Outcome measurement is a major factor in how health care agencies measure their level of quality care.

Once you have prioritized a patient's nursing diagnoses, ask the following questions to assist in identifying relevant outcomes:
- Does the patient agree with the outcomes you plan to achieve?
- What is the best approach to address and resolve the nursing diagnosis or problem?
- What does my patient need to achieve (physically, psychologically, socially, and spiritually)?
- How will I know when my patient has achieved an outcome? (How do I measure outcome achievement?)

Raising these questions leads you to select relevant outcomes. Expected outcomes are specific statements of patient behavior or physiological responses that you intend to achieve as a result of your interventions. Outcomes serve two purposes: to set a clear direction for the selection and use of nursing interventions and to set specific measures for evaluating the effectiveness of meeting outcomes.

*In the case of Mr. Lawson, for the nursing diagnosis of **Risk for Infection**, Tonya aims to have the patient remain infection free, preventing a wound infection during his hospitalization. Tonya asks herself, "What does my patient need to achieve?" To make sure Mr. Lawson is infection free, Tonya selects the expected outcomes of the patient being afebrile, without wound drainage, and with wound edges healing by discharge. The measures used to evaluate Mr. Lawson's outcomes will include ongoing measurement of body temperature and inspection of the wound. Tonya also considers, "What is the best approach to address and resolve the **Risk for Infection**?" Based on the diagnosis and outcomes, Tonya selects practices for cleansing and protecting the wound and supporting the patient's nutritional needs.*

Expected outcomes are time limited, measurable ways of determining whether a patient is progressing toward resolution of a nursing diagnosis or problem (Table 18.1). The selection of expected outcomes

and their associated interventions requires consideration of your previous experience with patients who had similar problems and any established standards for clinical problem management. An outcome should meet established intellectual standards by being relevant to patient needs, specific, singular, observable, measurable, and time-limited. You also use critical thinking attitudes in selecting interventions with the greatest likelihood of success.

*Tonya knows that with a nursing diagnosis of **Lack of Knowledge**, Mr. and Mrs. Lawson will require appropriate instruction. She also knows that based on her knowledge of the risks associated with Mr. Lawson's type of surgery, he and his wife will require information about wound care, activity restrictions, and any medications the patient receives. The type of instruction needed to resolve the diagnosis of **Lack of Knowledge** involves informing the patient of his risks and how to avoid them. For Tonya and her health care colleagues to know whether Mr. Lawson understands how to reduce his postoperative risks, the patient must meet expected outcomes. Expected outcomes for resolving Mr. Lawson's lack of knowledge will include:*
- *Mr. Lawson describes activity restrictions to follow by discharge in 48 hours.*
- *Mr. Lawson demonstrates how to cleanse the surgical wound by discharge day.*
- *Mr. Lawson describes three risks for infection in 24 hours.*

Tonya plans to perform teach-back after instruction to determine whether the outcome is met (see Chapter 20). In this case she wishes to have Mr. Lawson learn three different signs of wound infection—wound drainage, fever, and increased tenderness around the wound.

Sometimes achieving an outcome leads to resolution of more than one nursing diagnosis. For example, consider a patient who has experienced traumatic fractures to both arms following a motor vehicle accident. The patient has limited flexion of the elbows bilaterally and difficulty rotating the lower arms. The patient is unable to lift a utensil for eating. The patient has the nursing diagnoses of *Impaired Mobility* and *Impaired Self Feeding*. The outcome of "Patient will achieve improved flexion in elbow (45°)," once achieved, will assist in resolution of both diagnoses.

A patient-centered outcome reflects a patient's highest possible level of wellness and independence in function. It is realistic and individually based on patient needs, abilities, and resources. A patient-centered outcome reflects a patient's specific behavior, not your own goals or the delivery of nursing interventions. For example, a patient who has a pressure injury with the diagnosis *Impaired Skin Integrity* has an outcome of "Pressure injury reduces in diameter by discharge." The outcome is not "Hydrogel dressing applied to pressure injury."

TABLE 18.1	Examples of Expected Outcomes for Mr. Lawson	
Nursing Diagnoses	**Expected Outcomes**
Acute Pain related to trauma of surgical incision	Mr. Lawson reports pain at a level of 3 or below by discharge.
	Mr. Lawson walks to chair with no increase in pain in 24 hours.
Lack of Knowledge regarding postoperative care related to inexperience with surgery	Mr. Lawson describes activity restrictions to follow by discharge in 48 hours.
	Mr. Lawson demonstrates how to cleanse surgical wound by discharge day.
	Mr. Lawson describes three risks for infection in 24 hours.
Risk for Infection	Mr. Lawson is afebrile at discharge.
	Mr. Lawson's wound shows no purulent drainage by discharge.
	Mr. Lawson's wound closes at site of incision separation by discharge.
Anxiety related to uncertainty about recovery	Mr. Lawson verbalizes feeling less anxious about returning home following surgery by discharge.
	Mr. Lawson demonstrates reduced restlessness.

Nurse-Sensitive Outcomes

All health care providers contribute to achievement of patient outcomes. However, nurses monitor and manage patient conditions and diagnose problems that can be treated with nursing interventions. The clinical reasoning and decision making of nurses are key parts of quality health care (Moorhead et al., 2018). Thus, it is essential to measure the patient outcomes that are influenced by nursing care. A **nurse-sensitive patient outcome** is a measurable patient, family, or community behavior or perception that is measured in response to nursing interventions (Moorhead et al., 2018). Nurse-sensitive outcomes are a valid and reliable means to support nursing care quality and performance measurement in health care settings. This includes the evaluation of nursing clinical practice improvement (Heslop and Lu, 2014; Graystone, 2018). The literature identifies nurse-sensitive outcomes within three subcategories: safety, patient-related perception, and patient-related use of health care (Heslop and Lu, 2014). In a similar study, Liu et al. (2014) identified the characteristics of nursing-related patient outcomes. These included: (1) patient functional status (maintained or improved), (2) patient safety (protected or unharmed), and (3) patient satisfaction (patient reporting of comfort and contentment). Examples of nurse-sensitive outcomes are summarized in Box 18.1. In comparison, medical outcomes are primarily influenced by medical interventions. Examples include patient mortality, surgical wound infection, and hospital readmissions. For the nursing profession to become a full participant in clinical research, policy development, and interprofessional collaboration, nurses need to identify and measure patient outcomes influenced by nursing interventions.

Nursing Outcomes Classification

A valuable resource in selecting patient outcomes is the **Nursing Outcomes Classification** (NOC), which links outcomes to NANDA International (NANDA-I) nursing diagnoses (Moorhead et al., 2018). This resource is an option that you can use when selecting outcomes for your patients. For each nursing diagnosis there are multiple evidence-based outcomes. The outcomes have labels for describing the focus of nursing care and include indicators to use to evaluate the success of nursing interventions. The indicators for each NOC outcome allow for measurement at any point on a five-point Likert scale from most negative to most positive (Moorhead et al., 2018). The rating system adds objectivity when evaluating a patient's progress. Using NOC provides consistency in evaluating the effects of nursing interventions over time and across a variety of health care settings. Using a common language for outcomes allows nurses to plan effective patient care and

TABLE 18.2 Examples of Nursing Diagnoses and Suggested NOC Linkages

Nursing Diagnosis	Examples of NOC Outcomes (Consider as Overall Goals)	Outcome Indicators (Expected Outcomes)
Impaired Oral Mucous Membrane	Oral Health	Knowledge of infection management Self-care oral hygiene
	Tissue Integrity	Hydration Infection severity
Activity Intolerance	Activity Tolerance	Oxygen saturation with activity Pulse rate with activity Respiratory rate with activity
	Self-Care Status	Bathes self Dresses self Prepares food and fluid for eating

NOC, Nursing Outcomes Classification.
Adapted from Moorhead S, et al: *Nursing Outcomes Classification (NOC): measurement of health outcomes,* ed 6, St Louis, 2018, Elsevier.

provides a standardized way to measure whether nursing interventions are successful.

What NOC describes as an outcome, such as anxiety level, appetite, or physical comfort, is a very abstract term, which in real clinical practice comes closer to a goal statement. For example, in NOC terminology the outcome for the nursing diagnosis of *Acute Pain* is described as "pain control" or "pain relief," the goal set for Mr. Lawson. The NOC outcome indicators are stated in a manner similar to what most clinicians identify as expected outcomes. In the example of pain control, an expected outcome includes pain severity measured on a pain scale. Table 18.2 offers more examples of how to use NOC terminology for identifying outcome indicators as they relate to nursing diagnoses.

Writing Expected Outcomes

The expected outcomes selected for a nursing diagnosis guide your nursing care. A properly written outcome statement sets the desired physiological, psychological, social, developmental, or spiritual responses that indicate resolution of a patient's health problems. Use the *SMART* acronym (*S*pecific, *M*easurable, *A*ttainable, *R*ealistic, *T*imed) to write outcome statements (Ackley et al., 2020).

1. **Specific**—Outcomes reflect a specific patient behavior or response. For a patient with impaired mobility an outcome statement is: "Patient ambulates in the hall 3 times a day by 4/22." A common error is to write an intervention such as "Ambulate patient in the hall."

   A specific outcome addresses only one behavior or response. For example, an incorrect outcome reads, "Patient's lungs are clear to auscultation, and respiratory rate is 24 breaths/minute by 8/22." How would you evaluate the outcome when you determine that the lungs are clear but the respiratory rate is 28 breaths/min? You would be unable to do so. It is preferable that each outcome be separate. A focus on a single outcome enables you to decide whether you need to modify a plan of care.

2. **Measurable**—You must be able to measure or observe whether a change takes place in a patient's status. Changes occur in physiological findings and in a patient's knowledge, perceptions, and behavior. Examples such as "Body temperature will remain below 37°C (98.6°F)" and "Apical pulse will remain between 60 and 100 beats/min" allow

BOX 18.1 Examples of Nurse-Sensitive Outcomes

- Pressure injury prevalence
- Fall prevalence
- Falls with injury
- Restraint prevalence (vest and limb only)
- Catheter-associated urinary tract infection for patients in the intensive care unit (ICU)
- Central line–associated bloodstream infection rate for patients in the ICU and high-risk nursery (HRN)
- Ventilator-associated pneumonia for patients in the ICU and HRN
- Patient satisfaction
- Patient's perceived level of pain control
- Patient adherence

you to objectively measure physical changes in a patient's status. The outcome statement "Patient's pain is less than 4 on a scale of 0 to 10 in 48 hours" allows you to objectively measure patient perception of pain severity using a pain-rating scale. Do not use vague qualifiers such as "normal," "acceptable," or "stable" in an expected outcome statement. Vague terms result in guesswork in determining a patient's response to care. Terms describing quality, quantity, frequency, length, or weight allow you to evaluate outcomes precisely.

3. **Attainable**—Outcomes are more achievable when you mutually set them with a patient. This ensures that you and your patient agree on the direction and time limits of care. As a patient advocate, apply standards of practice, evidence-based knowledge, safety principles, and basic human needs when helping patients set outcomes. Also use your knowledge about and experience with patients' typical responses to clinical interventions. Always consider patients' desires to recover and their physical and psychological condition to set outcomes.

   For example, Mr. Lawson expressed an interest in knowing what to expect after surgery. Thus Tonya set a mutual outcome for Mr. Lawson to "Describe three risks for infection in 24 hours." Meeting this outcome will prepare Mr. Lawson to monitor his wound healing once discharged. The additional outcome of Mr. Lawson demonstrating how to cleanse his surgical wound by discharge prepares the patient for self-care and prevention of infection. Plus, self-cleansing of the wound is something the patient can perform.

4. **Realistic**—Set expected outcomes that are realistic and relevant for patients. Consider a patient's preferences and needs and the resources of the health care agency, family, and patient. Be aware of a patient's physiological, emotional, cognitive, and sociocultural potential and the economic cost and resources available to reach expected outcomes in a timely manner. For example, are the patient's cultural beliefs reflected in outcomes you set? Does the patient have a family caregiver to assist with an intervention to be performed in the home? You set realistic outcomes within a patient's limitations and abilities. For example, an initial outcome for a patient with a diagnosis of *Self-Care Deficit: Impaired Ability to Perform Hygiene* is "Patient will wash hands and face in 72 hours." Your assessment and collaboration with occupational therapy will determine whether the outcome is realistic for the level of the patient's weakness. Setting realistic outcomes often requires you to communicate them to caregivers in other settings who will assume responsibility for patient care (e.g., home health, rehabilitation).

5. **Timed**—Set a time for each outcome to be met. This helps the health care team collaborate to resolve patient problems. Timed outcomes are road maps toward recovery.

   *For example, the outcome of "Mr. Lawson walks to chair with no increase in pain in 24 hours" and the second outcome, "Mr. Lawson reports pain at a level of 3 or below by discharge," give the health care team time frames for managing and reducing the patient's pain while he is hospitalized. At the time of discharge, evaluation of expected outcomes (e.g., pain-rating score, signs of grimacing, level of movement) shows whether the nursing diagnosis of **Acute Pain** is resolved.*

   Always collaborate with patients to set realistic and reasonable time frames. Time frames also help you and a patient determine whether the patient is making progress at a reasonable rate. If not, you must revise the plan of care. Time frames also promote accountability in delivering and managing nursing care.

Prioritizing Outcomes

The critical thinking processes you use to prioritize outcomes are the same processes you use when prioritizing a patient's nursing diagnoses. Although prioritizing outcomes may seem straightforward when you have progressive time frames for achieving a set of outcomes, it becomes more difficult when an outcome does not have a time frame.

Priority setting includes determining which nursing interventions you plan to use with a patient for meeting outcomes and the order in which you need to implement interventions.

*For example, as Tonya considers the diagnosis of **Acute Pain** for Mr. Lawson, she includes in her plan of care these options: timely administration of an analgesic, repositioning every two hours, and teaching of relaxation exercises. With each clinical encounter, Tonya applies critical thinking to prioritize which intervention to use first. Tonya knows that a certain degree of pain relief is necessary before a patient can participate in relaxation exercises. When she is in the patient's room, she might decide to turn and reposition Mr. Lawson first and then prepare the analgesic. However, if Mr. Lawson expresses that pain is at a high level and he is too uncomfortable to turn, Tonya chooses obtaining and administering the analgesic as her first priority. Later, with Mr. Lawson's pain more under control, she considers whether teaching relaxation exercises is appropriate.*

Involve patients in priority setting whenever possible (Fig. 18.4). Include family caregivers when it is appropriate. Patient-centered care requires you to know a patient's preferences, values, and expressed needs. Sometimes a patient's priorities are different from yours. Resolve those differences through open communication. Consulting with and knowing a patient's concerns do not relieve you of the responsibility to act in a patient's best interests. Always assign priorities based on good nursing judgment.

Role of Health Care Team in Setting Outcomes

Interprofessional collaboration is a complex process involving two or more people from various professional fields to achieve common outcomes for a patient (Mahdizadeh et al., 2015). Many factors are creating an increased need for interprofessional teams. For example, the aging population has resulted in an increased number of people living with multiple complex chronic diseases. Members of the health care team need advanced skills and specialized knowledge to provide comprehensive care to these patients (Nancarrow et al., 2013). The 2003 Institute of Medicine report titled *Health Professions Education: A Bridge to Quality* identified five competencies health care professionals need to reduce errors, three of which are cooperation, communication, and coordination (Jakubowski and Perron, 2018). Interprofessional collaboration is more than a group of health care providers meeting together to discuss a patient. The process involves all health care providers working together while respecting the expertise of those in other disciplines and being aware of the professional roles and responsibilities of other team members (Jakubowski and Perron, 2018).

The elements that must be in place before interprofessional collaboration can be successful are interprofessional education, role

FIG. 18.4 Collaborative outcome setting with patient and family member.

awareness as a member of the team, interpersonal relationship skills, deliberate intervention, and interprofessional teamwork (Jakubowski and Perron, 2018). Nancarrow et al. (2013) add that positive leadership and management attributes, communication structures, personal rewards, appropriate resources and procedures, appropriate skill mix, and clarity of vision are also necessary. Interprofessional team-based care involves care delivered by intentionally created and usually small work groups in health care who are recognized by others as well as by themselves as having a collective identity and shared responsibility for a group of patients (e.g., Rapid Response Team, palliative care team) (Interprofessional Education Collaborative, 2016). Clinical areas that commonly have interprofessional teams are critical care and rehabilitation units.

Nurses play a key role in interprofessional collaboration, especially in communicating patient needs to all members of the health care team, clarifying priorities, and ensuring continuity of care. When interprofessional collaboration functions well, the outcomes are improvements in patient care, patient safety, health care providers' and nurses' satisfaction, cost control, and the reduction in clinical errors (Mahdizadeh et al., 2015).

PLANNING NURSING INTERVENTIONS

Nursing interventions are any treatments or actions based on clinical judgment and knowledge that nurses perform to achieve patient outcomes (Butcher et al., 2018) (see Chapter 19). Each of the clinical chapters in this textbook describes the nursing interventions available for a variety of health problems (see Units 5 and 7). Patient education (see Chapter 25) is a form of nursing intervention suitable for all patients.

Clinical judgment is essential when choosing the appropriate nursing interventions for a patient's plan of care. When you use critical thinking during planning, you can make clinical decisions needed for choosing the nursing interventions most appropriate for a patient's nursing diagnoses and collaborative problems. Choosing suitable nursing interventions requires applying your nursing knowledge and the best scientific evidence for a patient's health problems. Evidence-based practices are supported through research and have demonstrated effectiveness for select clinical problems. Use evidence that is available in the form of clinical guidelines or protocols or evidence you find in the literature to determine the most appropriate interventions for your patients.

In addition to the best available evidence, you also apply your knowledge of what you have learned about your patients and their preferences to select interventions. Patient assessment reveals data about a patient that identifies the related factors or risk factors associated with nursing diagnoses. These same related factors or risk factors are the indicators for choosing interventions. For example, a nursing diagnosis of *Impaired Socialisation related to hearing impairment* will require quite different nursing interventions than *Impaired Socialisation related to impaired mobility* even though the core diagnosis is the same. Application of your knowledge about a patient enhances your ability to choose relevant interventions. You then use critical thinking attitudes for considering how you will deliver interventions, such as the timing of an intervention or creatively involving other resources.

One other critical thinking factor in the selection of nursing interventions is experience. When a nurse gains experience in caring for patients with similar nursing diagnoses or problems and has witnessed those interventions to be successful, the interventions will be used again when the appropriate situation arises. A nurse gains expertise in developing plans of care by learning how certain interventions achieve outcomes through modifying or removing related factors and risk factors. An experienced nurse also knows how to adapt time-tested interventions when a patient poses unique characteristics or problems.

Tonya uses evidence-based practice by identifying a PICOT question to help her select instructional interventions for enhancing Mr. and Mrs. Lawson's knowledge about infection control. She chooses a program available on hospital TV about infection control that the couple can watch in his hospital room. Tonya applies knowledge learned from her PICOT question literature search and chooses the evidence-based visual aid strategy. She plans for the couple to view the TV program when Mrs. Lawson visits. Tonya also chooses interventions based on what she has learned about the related factors behind Mr. Lawson's learning needs. Mr. Lawson has not experienced postoperative care, he is facing restrictions with which he is unfamiliar, and the condition of his incision probably requires wound care at home. Tonya will plan to teach topics that address postoperative risks in a way that will be relevant to Mr. Lawson and his usual routines. She learned that the patient enjoys walking his dog, household maintenance, and gardening. Some of these activities will be limited or not allowed until the patient recovers, and she must address them during instruction.

Types of Interventions

During planning you select interventions designed to help patients move from their present level of health to the level described in the expected outcomes for each nursing diagnosis. Nursing interventions include direct and indirect care measures you provide to individual patients, families, or the community (Butcher et al., 2018). Direct care measures are those treatments or procedures performed through interaction with patients involving the laying-on of hands. Examples include bathing, wound care, and inserting an intravenous catheter. Indirect care measures are those treatments or procedures performed away from patients but on behalf of patients (Butcher et al., 2018). Examples include managing the patient care environment and consultation. In addition, nursing interventions are classified as: nurse-initiated, health care provider–initiated, and other provider–initiated (e.g., pharmacist, respiratory therapist) (Butcher et al., 2018). Some patients require a combination of the three classifications.

Nurse-initiated interventions are the **independent nursing interventions** that a nurse initiates in response to a nursing diagnosis without supervision, direction, or orders from others. Examples include direct care such as positioning patients to prevent pressure injury formation, initiating early mobility protocols, counseling patients for coping with stress, or instructing patients in side effects of medications. Nurse-initiated interventions are autonomous actions based on **scientific rationale**. Such interventions benefit a patient in a predicted way related to nursing diagnoses and patient outcomes (Butcher et al., 2018). Each state within the United States has a nurse practice act that defines the legal scope of nursing practice (see Chapter 23). According to the nurse practice acts in a majority of states, independent nursing interventions pertain to activities of daily living, health education and promotion, and counseling. *Tonya selects the following independent nursing interventions for Mr. Lawson to resolve his acute pain: positioning, relaxation therapy, and exercise promotion.*

Health care provider–initiated interventions are **dependent nursing interventions** that require an order from a health care provider. The interventions are based on a physician's or advanced practice nurse's choices for treating or managing a medical diagnosis. Advanced practice nurses who practice within collaborative agreements with physicians or who are licensed independently by state practice acts are able to write orders for dependent interventions. As a nurse you intervene by carrying out the health care provider's written and/or verbal orders. Administering a medication, implementing an invasive procedure (e.g., inserting a Foley catheter, starting an intravenous [IV] infusion), and preparing a patient for diagnostic tests are examples of health care provider–initiated interventions.

Other provider interventions, or interdependent interventions, are therapies that require the combined knowledge, skill, and expertise of multiple health care providers. Typically, when you plan care for a patient, you review the necessary interventions and determine whether collaboration with other health care disciplines (e.g., social work, rehabilitation, pharmacy) is necessary. A patient care conference with an interprofessional health care team results in the selection of interdependent interventions. Chapter 19 explores in-depth nursing responsibilities for the different types of interventions.

In the case study involving Mr. Lawson, Tonya plans independent interventions to continue to manage Mr. Lawson's pain and to begin teaching him about postoperative care activities. Among the dependent interventions Tonya plans to implement are the administration of an ordered analgesic and wound care. Tonya's other-initiated intervention involves collaborating with the unit discharge coordinator, who will help Mr. and Mrs. Lawson plan for their return home, and the home health department to ensure that the Lawsons have home health visits.

When preparing for health care provider–initiated or other provider–initiated interventions, do not automatically implement the therapies. First, determine whether they are appropriate for each patient. You do this by referring to agency policy and procedure manuals or by asking an RN colleague with more experience. Every nurse faces an inappropriate or incorrect order at some time. The nurse with a strong knowledge base and clinical experience recognizes an error and seeks to correct it. The ability to recognize incorrect therapies is particularly important when administering medications (see Chapter 31) or procedures. Errors occur in writing orders or transcribing them to a documentation form or computer screen. Clarifying an order is competent nursing practice, and it protects a patient and members of the health care team. When you have doubt, clarify any order. When you carry out an incorrect or inappropriate intervention, the error falls as much to you as it does to the person who wrote or transcribed the original order. You are legally responsible for any complications resulting from an error (see Chapter 23).

> **REFLECT NOW**
>
> Consider that Tonya has independent, dependent, and other provider-initiated interventions to perform for Mr. Lawson. How does this affect her prioritization of nursing care for the patient?

Selection of Interventions

During planning do not select interventions randomly based on a diagnostic label. For example, you do not use the same interventions with all patients who have a diagnosis of *Anxiety*. You treat *Anxiety related to the uncertainty of surgical recovery* very differently from *Anxiety related to a threat of loss of job*. When choosing interventions, consider six important factors: (1) desired patient outcomes, (2) characteristics of the nursing diagnosis, (3) research base knowledge for the intervention, (4) feasibility for doing the intervention, (5) acceptability to the patient, and (6) your own competency (Butcher et al., 2018) (Box 18.2).

When developing a plan of care, review resources such as the scientific literature, standard protocols or guidelines, the Nursing Outcomes

---

BOX 18.2 Choosing Nursing Interventions

Desired Patient Outcomes
- Outcomes serve as the criteria against which to judge efficacy of interventions.
- Nursing Outcomes Classification (NOC) outcomes are linked to NANDA Nursing Diagnoses and ICNP® diagnoses with the same label.
- NOC outcomes are also linked to Nursing Interventions Classification (NIC) interventions (Moorhead et al., 2018). Use these resources to develop care plans.

Characteristics of the Nursing Diagnosis
- Choose interventions to alter the etiological (related to) factor or causes of the diagnosis. **Example:** *Acute Pain* related to trauma of surgical incision—choose interventions for Mr. Lawson that relieve swelling and strain on incision site (positioning and turning measures) and that lower pain reception (analgesic).
- When an etiological factor cannot change, direct the interventions toward treating the signs and symptoms (e.g., defining characteristics for a diagnosis). **Example:** *Lack of Knowledge* regarding postoperative care related to inexperience with surgery and impending discharge with self-care needs—choose interventions that provide information that answers Mr. and Mrs. Lawson's questions (e.g., recovery procedures, wound care) and prepares them to monitor Mr. Lawson's progress at home.
- For risk diagnoses, direct interventions at altering or eliminating the risk factors for the diagnosis. **Example:** *Risk for Infection* requires interventions for keeping Mr. Lawson's incisional area clean and free from further trauma, and for maintaining good nutrition.

Research Base
- Be familiar with the research evidence for an intervention and use it for the appropriate patient group and/or setting (see Chapter 5).
- Research evidence in support of a nursing intervention will indicate the effectiveness of using the intervention with certain types of patients.

- When research is unavailable, use scientific principles (e.g., infection control, learning) or consult a clinical expert about your patient.

Feasibility
- A specific intervention has the potential to interact with other interventions provided by the nurse and other health professionals; clarify whether the specific intervention is appropriate.
- Know and be involved in a patient's total plan of care to be aware of interventions that can be performed given the patient's limitations.
- Consider the cost of an intervention and the amount of time required for implementation (in consideration of the patient's condition). **Example:** If you plan to get a patient up into a chair three times a day, will there be staff to assist with the transfer? Is the patient becoming weaker?

Acceptability to the Patient
- When possible, offer a patient a choice of interventions to assist in reaching outcomes.
- Promote informed choice; give patients information about each intervention and how they are expected to participate.
- Consider a patient's values, beliefs, and culture for a patient-centered approach to selecting interventions.

Capability of the Nurse
- Does the nurse understand the scientific rationale for the intervention?
- Does the nurse have the necessary psychosocial and psychomotor skills to complete the intervention?
- Can the nurse function within the specific setting to effectively use health care resources?

Modified from Butcher GM, et al: *Nursing interventions classification (NIC)*, ed 7, St Louis, 2018, Elsevier.

Classification (NOC) and Nursing Interventions Classification (NIC), policy or procedure manuals, other health professionals, or textbooks. As you select interventions, review your patient's needs, priorities, and previous experiences to select the interventions that have the best potential for achieving the expected outcomes.

Nursing Interventions Classification. Just as with the standardized NOC, the Iowa Intervention Project developed a set of nursing interventions that provides a level of standardization to enhance communication of nursing care across all health care settings and to compare outcomes (Butcher et al., 2018). The NIC model includes three levels for ease of use: domains, classes, and the interventions. The seven domains are the highest level (Level 1) of the model, using broad terms (e.g., safety and basic physiological) to organize the more specific classes and interventions (Table 18.3). The second level of the model includes 30 classes or groups of related interventions, which offer useful clinical categories to reference when selecting interventions. An example of a class is *Physical Comfort Promotion.* The third level of the model includes the 565 interventions, defined as any treatment based on clinical judgment and knowledge that a nurse performs to enhance patient outcomes (Butcher et al., 2018) (Box 18.3). The interventions can be used with various diagnostic classifications, including NANDA, ICNP®, and others (Butcher et al., 2018). Each intervention includes a variety of nursing activities from which to choose (Box 18.4) and which a nurse commonly uses in a plan of care. For example, if a patient has a nursing diagnosis of *Acute Pain,* the class of interventions that would apply to the patient is *Physical Comfort Promotion.* That class includes 18 interventions, such as aromatherapy and cutaneous stimulation. Each class has a variety of activities. The intervention for *Pain Management: Acute* has 20 recommended nursing activities, such as ensuring that the patient receives prompt analgesic care and the use of combination analgesics. NIC is a valuable resource for selecting appropriate interventions and activities for your patient. It is evolving and practice-oriented. The classification is comprehensive, including independent and collaborative interventions. It remains your decision to determine which interventions and activities best suit your patient's individualized needs and situation.

SYSTEMS FOR PLANNING NURSING CARE

Systems exist for developing and communicating a nurse's plan of care to other nurses and collaborating health care providers. Using technology and information management systems is related to the quality and safety of patient care (QSEN, 2020). Each of the systems that exist within health care agencies promotes continuity and the use of best practices in patient care.

TABLE 18.3   Examples of Nursing Interventions Classification (NIC) Taxonomy—Domains 1-4 and Accompanying Classes of Interventions

Domain 1	Domain 2	Domain 3	Domain 4
Level 1 Domains			
1. **Physiological: Basic** Care that supports physical functioning	2. **Physiological: Complex** Care that supports homeostatic regulation	3. **Behavioral** Care that supports psychosocial functioning and facilitates lifestyle changes	4. **Safety** Care that supports protection against harm
Level 2 Classes			
A *Activity and Exercise Management:* Interventions to organize or assist with physical activity and energy conservation and expenditure	G *Electrolyte and Acid-Base Management:* Interventions to regulate electrolyte/acid-base balance and prevent complications	O *Behavior Therapy:* Interventions to reinforce or promote desirable behaviors or alter undesirable behaviors	U *Crisis Management:* Interventions to provide immediate short-term help in both psychological and physiological crises
B *Elimination Management:* Interventions to establish and maintain regular bowel and urinary elimination patterns and manage complications caused by altered patterns	H *Drug Management:* Interventions to facilitate desired effects of pharmacological agents	P *Cognitive Therapy:* Interventions to reinforce or promote desirable cognitive functioning or alter undesirable cognitive functioning	V *Risk Management:* Interventions to initiate risk-reduction activities and continue monitoring risks over time
C *Immobility Management:* Interventions to manage restricted body movement and the sequelae	I *Neurologic Management:* Interventions to optimize neurologic function	Q *Communication Enhancement:* Interventions to facilitate delivering and receiving verbal and nonverbal messages	
D *Nutrition Support:* Interventions to modify or maintain nutritional status	J *Perioperative Care:* Interventions to provide care before, during, and immediately after surgery	R *Coping Assistance:* Interventions to assist another to build on own strengths, adapt to a change in function, or achieve a higher level of function	
E *Physical Comfort Promotion:* Interventions to promote comfort using physical techniques	K *Respiratory Management:* Interventions to promote airway patency and gas exchange	S *Patient Education:* Interventions to facilitate learning	
F *Self-Care Facilitation:* Interventions to provide or assist with routine activities of daily living	L *Skin/Wound Management:* Interventions to maintain or restore tissue integrity	T *Psychological Comfort Promotion:* Interventions to promote comfort using psychological techniques	
	M *Thermoregulation:* Interventions to maintain body temperature within a normal range		
	N *Tissue Perfusion Management:* Interventions to optimize circulation of blood and fluids to the tissue		

From Butcher GM, et al: *Nursing interventions classification (NIC),* ed 7, St Louis, 2018, Elsevier.

BOX 18.3 Example of Interventions for Physical Comfort Promotion

Class: Physical Comfort Promotion (Level 2)
- Interventions to promote comfort using physical techniques

Interventions (Examples)
- Aromatherapy
- Cutaneous Stimulation
- Environmental Management
- Heat/Cold Application
- Nausea Management
- Pain Management
- Progressive Muscle Relaxation

Examples of Linked Nursing Diagnoses
- *Acute Pain*
- *Chronic Pain*

From Butcher GM, et al: *Nursing interventions classification (NIC)*, ed 7, St Louis, 2018, Elsevier.

BOX 18.4 Example of an Intervention and Associated Nursing Activities

Intervention—Environmental Management: Comfort
Examples of Activities
- Create a calm and supportive environment.
- Provide a single room if it is the patient's preference to offer quiet and rest.
- Adjust room temperature to that most comfortable for the individual.
- Provide a safe and clean environment.
- Determine sources of discomfort: damp dressing, positioning on tubing, wrinkled linen.
- Position patient to facilitate comfort.
- Provide prompt attention to call lights, which should always be within reach.

From Butcher GM, et al: *Nursing interventions classification (NIC)*, ed 7, St Louis, 2018, Elsevier.

Use of Care Plans in Health Care Agencies

In any health care setting nurses are responsible for providing a nursing plan of care for each patient. The plan of care can take several forms (e.g., individual electronic care plans and standardized care plans). With the growth of EHRs within health care agencies, documentation systems typically include software programs for creating individualized and standard nursing care plans. These programs use standardized nursing language, including nursing diagnostic language (e.g., NANDA or ICNP) and NOC and NIC taxonomies, enabling nurses to clearly identify a plan of care using appropriate nursing diagnoses, outcomes, and interventions. Standardized care plans have typically been developed by a health care agency's clinical experts based on clinical experience and scientific evidence. The standardized plans usually incorporate clinical protocols or guidelines based on common medical or surgical conditions (e.g., prevention of deep vein thrombosis). They outline the nursing care to be provided for patients with such conditions. A standardized language or system enables nurses and other health care providers to quickly identify a patient's needs and situation. Standardization helps prevent errors and omissions in care delivery, reduces duplications in care delivery efforts, and promotes consistency and continuity of care delivery. However, any effort to standardize care should begin with best practices and the option for nurses to customize each plan to the unique needs of each patient.

BOX 18.5 EVIDENCE-BASED PRACTICE
Interprofessional Collaboration and Quality of Care

PICOT Question: How does interprofessional collaboration among health care workers influence quality of patient care?

Evidence Summary
Nurses play critical roles in working alongside other health care professionals and in promoting interprofessional collaboration by their communication skills and positive leadership (Karam et al., 2018). Effective interprofessional collaboration improves access to health interventions and coordination among health care disciplines. It also increases involvement in decision making for individuals and their families (World Health Professions Alliance, 2019). Communication plays a key role, being the central process through which collaboration takes place. Because nurses work with a variety of health care professionals, the ability to build interprofessional collaboration requires the building of trust, mutual respect for professions and individuals, and professional role clarification (Karam et al., 2018). Interprofessional collaboration has been shown to improve workplace environments and quality of care provided to patients (Karam et al., 2018).

Application to Nursing Practice
- When entering into interprofessional collaboration, role negotiation is critical. Clarify your role in the outcomes established by the interprofessional team.
- Establish clear lines of communication and continuity across disciplines. Communication makes possible role negotiation and development in cooperation with others and fosters relationships among the individuals in the team.
- When developing a plan of care for a patient, support a consensus, an implicit understanding of how team members should work together to achieve patient outcomes.
- One adverse effect of using information technology is the encouragement of parallel work practices with less face-to-face collaboration (Reeves et al., 2014). Use hand-off reporting, timely ISBAR communication, and entry of relevant and concise health care record information with members of the interprofessional team.

A **nursing care plan** includes nursing diagnoses, expected outcomes, individualized nursing interventions, and a section for evaluation findings (see Chapter 20). The plan promotes continuity of care and better communication because it informs all health care providers about a patient's needs and interventions and reduces the risk for incomplete, incorrect, or inappropriate care measures. Nurses revise a plan when a patient's status changes. Preprinted standardized care plans and EHR care plans follow a standardized format, but you can individualize each plan to a patient's unique needs. The plan gives all nurses a central document that outlines a patient's diagnoses/problems, the plan of care for each diagnosis/problem, and the outcomes for monitoring and evaluating patient progress. The plan of care communicates nursing care priorities to nurses and other health care providers. It also identifies and coordinates resources for delivering nursing care. For example, in a care plan you list specific supplies necessary to use in a dressing change or names of clinical nurse specialists who are caring for a patient.

In hospitals and community-based settings, patients receive care from more than one nurse, health care provider, or allied health professional. Thus more agencies are developing **interprofessional care plans**, which include contributions from all disciplines involved in patient care (Box 18.5). The interprofessional plan focuses on patient priorities and improves the coordination of all patient therapies and communication among all disciplines.

The Nursing Care Plan provided on the next page is an example of a care plan for Mr. Lawson, using the standard format found throughout this text.

◎ NURSING CARE PLAN

Anxiety

ASSESSMENT

Assessment Activities	*Assessment Findings[a]*
Ask patient to clarify concerns he has about his recovery from surgery.	Patient **reports concern** about his wound not healing and keeping him from being able to return to work in 6 weeks. Has difficulty explaining what to expect during recovery.
Assess patient's cognitive function.	Patient **does not attend** to explanation of risk factors for infection and shows **poor eye contact** when discussing condition.
Observe patient's behaviors during discussion.	Patient is observed to be **irritable** and **displays facial tension** when discussing surgical recovery process.

[a]**Assessment Findings** are shown in **bold** type.

NURSING DIAGNOSIS: Anxiety related to uncertainty over recovery and ability to return to work

PLANNING

Expected Outcomes (NOC)[b]

Anxiety Level

Patient shows less facial tension during discussions about recovery from surgery in 24 hours.

Patient maintains attention during instruction about wound care within 24 hours.

[b]Outcomes classification labels from Moorhead S, et al: *Nursing outcomes classification (NOC)*, ed 6, St Louis, 2018, Elsevier.

INTERVENTIONS (NIC)[c]	**RATIONALE**
Anxiety Reduction	
Use a calm, reassuring approach while explaining expectations for recovery; listen attentively to patient's questions.	For patients to be able to express concerns and ask questions, they must see nurses as being nonthreatening, reliable, and willing to have a human connection (Varcarolis and Fosbre, 2021).
Encourage patient to express concerns.	
Collaborate with health care provider to provide information about wound care, normal progress of wound healing, and signs of poor wound healing as these factors affect expectations for patient's ability to return to work.	Providing information about the processes of surgical recovery helps patients handle symptoms of anxiety (Johnson, 2019).
Teach the patient relaxation exercises (jaw relaxation and total body).	A review of studies involving patients undergoing major abdominal surgery found that patients who used relaxation therapy (jaw relaxation and total body relaxation) may have significantly greater pain relief compared with those who did not use relaxation (Ju et al., 2019).

[c]Intervention classification labels from Bulechek GM, et al., editors: *Nursing interventions classification (NIC)*, ed 7, St. Louis, 2018, Elsevier.

EVALUATION

Evaluation Activity	*Patient Response*
Observe Mr. Lawson's verbal and nonverbal behavior during instructional session.	Mr. Lawson can attend to discussion about his recovery and shows good eye contact. Asks relevant questions and is able to perform relaxation.
Ask Mr. Lawson to describe how his wound is expected to heal during the next two weeks.	Patient is able to describe normal inflammation, how wound should look and feel as it heals, and signs of infection.

Because a care plan includes a patient's outcomes, it is an important part of discharge planning. Thus, you need to involve the family in planning care if the patient is agreeable. The family is often a resource to help a patient meet health care outcomes. In addition, meeting some of the family's needs can improve a patient's level of wellness. Discharge planning is especially important for a patient with a disability or injury that was not present before hospitalization. As a result, the patient must undergo long-term rehabilitation in the community and often will require home health care. Same-day surgeries and earlier discharges from hospitals require you to begin the planning for discharge from the moment the patient enters the health care agency. The complete care plan is the blueprint for nursing action.

Student Care Plans

Student care plans help you learn problem solving using the nursing process, the skills of written communication, and organizational skills for nursing care. Most importantly, a student care plan helps you apply knowledge gained from the scientific literature and the classroom to a practice situation. Students typically write a care plan for each nursing diagnosis, using a table format with columns for assessment findings, expected outcomes, nursing interventions with supporting rationales, and criteria to evaluate outcomes. As with health care agency care plans, the student care plan focuses on supporting interventions with rationales so that students can learn the scientific basis for their practice. Each school uses a different format for student care plans. Often the format used is similar to the one used by the health care agency that provides clinical experiences for the students. The following questions will help you complete a student care plan:

- *What* is the intervention. Is it evidence-based and connected to an outcome?
- *When* should each intervention be implemented?
- *How* should the intervention be performed for the specific patient?

- *Who* should be involved in each aspect of intervention? Is interprofessional collaboration necessary?

Each scientific rationale that you use to support a nursing intervention needs to include a reference, whenever possible, to document the source from the scientific literature. This reinforces the importance of evidence-based nursing practice. It is also important that each intervention be specific and unique to a patient's situation. The planning of nonspecific nursing interventions results in incomplete or inaccurate nursing care, lack of continuity among caregivers, and poor use of resources. Common omissions that nurses make in writing nursing interventions include action, frequency, quantity, method, or person to perform them (see Chapter 19). These errors occur when nurses are unfamiliar with the planning process. In the column of the care plan listing outcomes, evaluate whether each outcome was fully or only partially met. Use the evaluation column to document whether the plan requires revision or when outcomes are met, thus indicating when a nursing diagnosis is no longer relevant to a patient's plan of care (see Chapter 20).

Care Plans for Community-Based Settings

Planning care for patients who are in community-based settings (e.g., clinics or patients' homes) applies the same principles of nursing practice as care plans for patients who are hospitalized. However, in community-based settings you complete a more comprehensive community, home, and family assessment. Ultimately a patient/family unit must be able to provide the majority of health care independently. You design a plan to (1) educate the patient and designated family caregiver about the necessary care techniques and precautions, (2) teach a patient and family caregiver how to integrate care within family activities, and (3) guide the patient and family caregiver on how to assume a greater percentage of care over time. Finally, the plan includes nurses' and the patient's/family caregiver's evaluation of expected outcomes.

Hand-off Reporting

Part of planning is the transferring of essential information (along with responsibility and authority) from one nurse to the next during transitions in care (e.g., end of shift, during a patient transfer to a new care unit, discharge to another setting). Hand-off reporting is a real-time process that offers a health care provider who is accepting the care of a patient the opportunity to ask questions to clarify and confirm important details about a patient's plan of care, patient progress, and continuing needs during the transfer of information. Quality hand-off information enables nurses to quickly recognize changes in patient status and to anticipate risks. Conducting hand-off reports at a patient's bedside, allowing the patient to give input, has a positive impact on patient safety, patient satisfaction, and nurse satisfaction (McAllen et al., 2018). A correctly formulated nursing care plan facilitates a hand-off report as one nurse communicates to another. You learn to focus a report on the patient's nursing care, including patient assessments that need follow-up, current status of treatments, and the patient's expected outcomes. During a hand-off report always provide accurate, up-to-date, and pertinent information to the next nurse assuming patient care. Chapter 26 offers more information on hand-off reporting.

Concept Maps

Because nurses care for patients who have multiple health problems and related nursing diagnoses, it is often unrealistic to have a student written care plan developed for each nursing diagnosis. In addition, care plans usually do not allow you to show the associations among different nursing diagnoses and different nursing interventions. A concept map is a visual representation of all of a patient's nursing diagnoses (including supportive assessment findings) that allows you to diagram interventions for each. A concept map is a working document that makes a patient's diagnoses more meaningful because it shows the cognitive connections you make among assessment findings, diagnoses, and interventions. Using a concept map has been shown to improve self-reflection and critical thinking (Daley et al., 2016). A map shows you the relationships within the nursing process (i.e., how nursing interventions often apply to more than one nursing diagnosis). Concept maps group and categorize nursing concepts to give you a holistic view of your patient's health care needs.

In Chapter 17 you learned how to add nursing diagnostic labels to a concept map. When planning care for each nursing diagnosis, analyze the relationships among the diagnoses. Draw dotted lines between nursing diagnoses to indicate their relationship to one another. It is important for you to make meaningful associations between one concept and another. The links need to be accurate, meaningful, and complete so that you can explain why nursing diagnoses are related.

Fig. 18.5 *shows the progression of Mr. Lawson's concept map, with Tonya incorporating planned interventions for all four nursing diagnoses.*

List nursing interventions to attain the measurable outcomes for each nursing diagnosis either directly on the map or in a separate document. This step corresponds to the planning phase of the nursing process. While caring for a patient, use the map to write the patient's responses to each nursing activity. Also write your clinical impressions regarding the patient's progress toward expected outcomes and the effectiveness of interventions. Keep the concept map with you throughout a clinical day. As you revise the plan, take notes, and add or delete nursing interventions. Use the information recorded on the map to document patient care. Critical thinkers learn by organizing and relating cognitive concepts. Concept maps help you learn the interrelationships among nursing diagnoses to create a unique meaning and organization of information collected.

Critical Pathways

Many hospitals use critical pathways and enhanced recovery after surgery (ERAS) protocols to reduce variations in clinical practice, standardize evidence-based care, reduce patient length of stay, and improve patient outcomes. An ERAS protocol incorporates evidence-based practices and includes a comprehensive projected plan for a patient's journey through the surgical process from preoperative screening to postoperative care (Woolfrey et al., 2018). For example, an ERAS protocol will set time frames for when patients are to progress with mobility, advance diets, receive specific types of medications, and have therapies (such as intravenous infusion, Foley catheterization) discontinued. A pathway is another clinical management tool that provides a road map for best practices based on clinicians' expertise and clinical guidelines shaped by interprofessional teams (Hipp et al., 2016). Traditionally, critical pathways and ERAS protocols have been developed for medical and surgical conditions that are high volume and shown to be consistent and relatively predictable (e.g., total hip replacement, low back pain, palliative care, diabetes mellitus). Although pathways and recovery protocols offer an approach to a consistent workflow, it is still imperative to individualize patient care. There is a risk that clinical pathways can contribute to fragmentation of care if clinicians focus on the disease rather than on the person as a whole (Beaulieu, 2013). Also, it is important to remember that not every patient will fit into a care path; clinical judgment outranks the use of a care path (Lawrence, 2016). Clinical pathways or ERAS protocols need to be updated routinely as new evidence emerges.

REFLECT NOW

Consider three ways that the use of a critical pathway might enhance the quality of a hand-off report.

FIG. 18.5 Concept map for Mr. Lawson: Planning.

CONSULTING WITH HEALTH CARE PROFESSIONALS

You consult with members of the health care team when you face problems in providing nursing or collaborative care or in delivering dependent interventions. A consultation is vital if you need to seek procedural assistance or clinical expertise for a specific problem to ensure a patient receives needed clinical interventions or insights (Stevens et al., 2015). Consultation is a common tool among physicians when patients who are hospitalized require specialty care (e.g. neurology or infectious disease specialist) (Stevens et al., 2020). Consultation can occur at any time, but you usually consult most often during planning and implementation. During these times you are more likely to identify a problem requiring additional knowledge, skills, or resources. One way to initially consult is to use the ISBAR approach, a mechanism for framing conversations, especially critical ones, requiring a clinician's immediate attention and

action (see Chapter 26). ISBAR is an acronym for Identify, Situation, Background, Assessment, and Recommendation (IHI, 2020).

Consultation requires you to be aware of your strengths and limitations as a team member. During a consultation you seek the expertise of a specialist, such as your nursing instructor, a health care provider, or a clinical nurse specialist, to identify ways to handle specific problems in patient management or the planning and implementation of therapies. A nurse in practice will frequently consult with registered dietitians, therapists, and pharmacists. The consultation process offers new insight and specific recommendations for a patient's plan of care. It differs from interprofessional collaboration because it is often a onetime event. However, health care professionals who are consulted in a patient's care often become a collaborating member of the interprofessional team.

An experienced nurse is a valuable consultant when you face an unfamiliar patient care situation such as a new procedure or a patient presenting a set of symptoms that you cannot identify. In clinical nursing, consultation helps to solve problems in the delivery of nursing care. For example, a nursing student consults a clinical specialist for wound care techniques, a home care nurse on how to help a patient adapt to restrictions in the home, or an educator for useful teaching resources. Nurses are consulted for their clinical expertise, patient education skills, or staff education skills. Be prepared before you make a consultation. Consultation is based on the problem-solving approach, and the consultant is the stimulus for change.

QSEN **Building Competency in Teamwork and Collabora-tion** Tonya consults with the unit discharge coordinator, who will help Mr. and Mrs. Lawson plan for their return home. What does Tonya know about Mr. Lawson's situation that should be communicated to the coordinator? Identify three ways the coordinator might be most helpful to the Lawson family.

Answers to QSEN Activities can be found on the Evolve website.

When to Consult

Consultation occurs when you identify a problem that you or the interprofessional team is unable to solve. This process increases your knowledge about a patient's problems and helps you learn skills and use additional resources. A good time to consult with another health care provider is when the exact problem remains unclear. An objective consultant enters a clinical situation and more clearly assesses and identifies the nature of a problem, whether it is patient-, personnel-, or equipment-oriented. Most often you consult with health care providers who are working in your clinical area. However, sometimes you consult over the telephone (Box 18.6).

How to Consult

Begin with your own understanding of a patient's clinical problems. The following list contains important steps to follow in the consultation process.
* Identify the general problem area.
* Choose the appropriate professional, such as another nurse or social worker, to help resolve the problem.

BOX 18.6 **Tips for Making Phone Consultations**

* Have the information you need (e.g., medical record notes, medication sheets, recent nurse summary) available BEFORE you make a call.
* Assess the patient yourself before making the call. For example, when you consult with health care providers, they rely heavily on your assessment so that they can give appropriate advice.
* Address both the clinical history and the patient's perspective, including social and cultural context.
* Give a diagnosis or interpretation of the patient's problem with an explanation or a summary. Use of the ISBAR approach in reporting is helpful (see Chapter 26).
* Understand why you are calling for consultation, and think through some possible solutions. Your experience in caring for the patient allows you to make useful suggestions.

Data from Maison D: Effective communications are more important than ever: a health care provider's perspective, *J Home Care Hospice Professional* 24(3):178, 2006; Males T: In the dark: risks of telephone consultations, *Sessional GP* 4(2):2012, http://www.medicalprotection.org/docs/default-source/pdfs/uk-sessional-gp/oct-2012.pdf. Accessed May 23, 2021.

* Provide a consultant with relevant information and resources about the problem area. Provide a summary of the problem, methods used to resolve the problem so far, and outcomes of these methods. Share information from the patient's medical record, conversations with other nurses, and the patient's family.
* Do not prejudice or influence consultants. Biasing or showing prejudice blocks problem resolution. Avoid bias by not overloading consultants with subjective and emotional conclusions about the patient and the problem.
* Be available to discuss a consultant's findings and recommendations. Provide a private, comfortable atmosphere for the consultant and patient to meet. However, this does not mean that you leave the environment. A common mistake is to turn the whole problem over to the consultant. The consultant is not there to take over the problem but to help you resolve it. Request the consultation for a time when both you and the consultant are able to discuss the patient's situation with minimal interruptions or distractions.
* Incorporate the consultant's recommendations into the care plan. Always give the consultant feedback regarding the outcome of the recommendations.

▌ KEY POINTS

* Clinical judgment during planning involves use of the six components of critical thinking to guide nurses in making relevant and appropriate clinical decisions needed for patient-centered care.
* After identifying a patient's nursing diagnoses and collaborative problems, you begin planning, which involves setting priorities based on patient diagnoses and problems, and then identifying expected outcomes and selecting nursing interventions for each diagnosis.
* Critical thinking offers a methodical approach to individualize a plan of care; it includes the application of knowledge about a patient and the patient's clinical condition, experience with other patients, and knowledge of attitudes and standards. Care plans should be developed with the patient's involvement and focused on improving the patient's well-being.
* Environmental factors within the health care setting impact the timing and efficiency of any plan of care.
* Collaboration with patients and family caregivers, as well as health care team members, aids in determining the priority or urgency of identified nursing diagnoses or problems.
* Determining whether an outcome is relevant to a nursing diagnosis involves asking what is the best approach to address and resolve the nursing diagnosis and what does the patient need to achieve (physically, psychologically, socially, and spiritually).
* Prioritization of nursing diagnoses occurs when you use nursing and scientific knowledge to recognize patterns of data from a patient assessment and allow certain knowledge triggers to guide you to understand which diagnoses require more immediate intervention and when you need to take action.
* One helpful way to prioritize is to think of your patient's nursing diagnoses and problems as high, intermediate, or low in importance.
* By ranking a patient's nursing diagnoses in order of importance and always monitoring changing signs and symptoms of patient problems, you attend to each patient's most important needs and better organize ongoing care activities.
* Outcomes must be measurable so that you can measure or observe whether a change takes place in a patient's physiological status or in a patient's knowledge, perceptions, and behavior.
* A properly written outcome statement sets the desired response that indicates resolution of the patient's health problems. Using the

SMART acronym, each outcome should be *S*pecific, *M*easurable, *A*ttainable, *R*ealistic, and *T*imed.

- Choosing suitable nursing interventions requires applying nursing knowledge and scientific evidence about a patient's health problems, assessment findings about the patient, and experience in caring for patients with similar nursing diagnoses.
- Independent nurse-initiated interventions are autonomous actions based on scientific rationale.
- Dependent nursing interventions require an order from a health care provider to perform.
- You initiate a consult when your patient is experiencing a problem you cannot solve independently as a professional nurse or when you need the advice of another health care professional to provide quality patient care.
- Interprofessional collaboration involves all health care providers working together to achieve common outcomes for a patient, with collaborators respecting the expertise of those in other disciplines and being aware of the professional roles and responsibilities of other team members.

REFLECTIVE LEARNING

Talk with an RN who is assigned to care for one of your patients this week. If possible, ask the RN to give a brief summary of the patient's needs and nursing care provided. After your conversation, consider these questions.
- What was the priority nursing diagnosis or health care problem for the patient the RN cared for?
- Did any one of those priorities change as the RN provided patient care? If so, why?
- What independent and dependent activities did the RN deliver?

REVIEW QUESTIONS

1. Setting priorities for a patient's nursing diagnoses or health problems is an important step in planning patient care. Which of the following statements describe elements to consider in planning care? (Select all that apply.)
   1. Priority setting establishes a preferential order for nursing interventions.
   2. In most cases wellness problems take priority over problem-focused problems.
   3. Recognition of symptom patterns helps in understanding when to plan interventions.
   4. Longer-term chronic needs require priority over short-term problems.
   5. Priority setting involves creating a list of care tasks.
2. Match the elements for correct identification of outcome statements with the SMART acronym terms below.
   ___ 1. Specific
   ___ 2. Measurable
   ___ 3. Attainable
   ___ 4. Realistic
   ___ 5. Timed

   a. Mutually set an outcome a patient agrees to meet.
   b. Set an outcome that a patient can meet based upon physiological, emotional, economic, and sociocultural resources.
   c. Be sure an outcome addresses only one patient behavior or response.
   d. Include when an outcome is to be met.
   e. Use a term in an outcome statement that allows for observation as to whether a change takes place in a patient's status.

3. A nursing student is providing a hand-off report to the RN assuming the patient's care. The nursing student explains, "I ambulated him twice during the shift; he tolerated walking to end of hall and back each time with no shortness of breath. Heart rate was 88 and regular after exercise. The patient said he slept better last night after I closed his door and gave him a chance to have some uninterrupted sleep. I changed the dressing over his intravenous (IV) site and started a new bag of D$_5$½NS." Which intervention is a dependent intervention?
   1. Providing hand-off report at change of shift
   2. Enhancing the patient's sleep hygiene
   3. Administering IV fluids
   4. Taking vital signs
4. A nurse is assigned to care for six patients at the beginning of the night shift. The nurse learns that the floor will be short by one registered nurse (RN) because one of the nurses called in sick. Assistive personnel (AP) from another area is coming to the nursing unit to assist. Because the unit requires hourly rounds on all patients, the nurse begins to make rounds on a patient who recently asked for a pain medication. The nurse is interrupted by another registered nurse who asks about another patient. Which factors in this nurse's unit environment will affect the ability to set priorities? (Select all that apply.)
   1. Policy for conducting hourly rounds
   2. Staffing level
   3. Interruption by staff nurse colleague
   4. Type of hospital unit
   5. Competency of assistive personnel (AP)
5. A nursing student is providing a hand-off report to a registered nurse (RN) who is assuming the patient's care at the end of the clinical day. The student states, "The patient had a good day. His intravenous (IV) fluid is infusing at 124 mL/hr with D$_5$½NS infusing in left forearm. The IV site is intact, and no complaints of tenderness. I ambulated him twice during the shift; he walked to the visitors lounge and back with no shortness of breath, respirations 14, heart rate 88 after returning to chair. He uses his walker without difficulty, gait normal. The patient ate ¾ of his dinner with no gastrointestinal complaints." Which expected outcomes aimed at improving the patient's activity tolerance were discussed in the hand-off? (Select all that apply.)
   1. IV site not tender
   2. Ambulated twice during shift
   3. Uses walker to walk
   4. Walked to visitors lounge
   5. No shortness of breath
   6. Tolerated dinner meal
   7. Patient had a good day
   8. Vital signs after ambulation
6. A nurse on a hospital unit is preparing to hand off care of a patient being discharged to a home health nurse. Match the activities on the left with the hand-off report categories on the right

   Activities
   ___ 1. Use a standard checklist for the report.
   ___ 2. Encourage questions and clarification.
   ___ 3. Offer specific information on how to reduce patient's risks.
   ___ 4. Give report at time when shift has ended and other nurses are requesting information.
   ___ 5. Explain how patient's discharge was delayed by insufficient numbers of staff.
   ___ 6. Organize time by preparing in advance what to report.

   Categories
   a. Strategy for Effective Hand-off
   b. Strategy for Ineffective Hand-off

7. A patient diagnosed with colon cancer has been receiving chemotherapy for six weeks. The patient visits the outpatient infusion center twice a week for infusions. The nurse assigned to the patient is having difficulty accessing the patient's intravenous port used to administer the chemotherapy. Despite attempts to flush the port, it is obstructed. This occurred two weeks earlier as well. What steps should the nurse follow to make a consultation with a member of the IV infusion team? (Select all that apply.)
   1. Ask the IV nurse to come to the infusion center at a time when the nurse starts care for a second patient.
   2. Specifically identify the problem of port obstruction and attempt to flush the port to resolve the problem.
   3. Explain to the IV nurse the frequency in which this port has obstructed in the past.
   4. Tell the IV nurse the problem is probably related to the physician who inserted the port.
   5. Describe to the IV nurse the type and condition of the port currently in use.

8. A nurse assesses a 78-year-old patient who weighs 108.9 kg (240 lb) and is partially immobilized because of a stroke. The nurse turns the patient and finds that the skin over the sacrum is very red and the patient does not feel sensation in the area. The patient has had fecal incontinence on and off for the last two days. The nurse identifies the nursing diagnosis of *Risk for Impaired Skin Integrity*. Which of the following outcomes is appropriate for the patient?
   1. Patient will be turned every two hours within 24 hours.
   2. Patient will have normal formed stool within 48 hours.
   3. Patient's ability to turn self in bed improves.
   4. Erythema of skin will be mild to none within 48 hours.

9. An 82-year-old patient who resides in a nursing home has the following three nursing diagnoses: *Risk for Fall, Impaired Physical Mobility related to pain,* and *Impaired Nutritional Intake related to reduced ability to feed self.* The nursing staff identified several outcomes of care. Match the diagnoses on the left with the appropriate outcome statements on the right.

Diagnoses
___1. *Risk for Fall*
___2. *Impaired Physical Mobility related to pain*
___3. *Impaired Nutritional Intake related to reduced ability to feed self*

Outcomes
a. Patient expresses fewer nonverbal signs of discomfort when walking within 24 hours.
b. Patient increases calorie intake to 2500 calories daily.
c. Patient walks 20 feet using a walker in 24 hours.
d. Patient identifies barriers to remove in the home within 1 week.

10. A student is participating in a postclinical conference with the other students in the clinical group and an instructor. The student states, "My patient has two nursing diagnoses I chose to focus on, *Risk for Impaired Skin Integrity* and *Lack of Knowledge regarding diabetic diet restrictions.* I observed no pressure areas this morning. Because of her weight (100 kg; 220 lb), I turned her every two hours, and we put her on a pressure-relieving surface. We discussed how diabetes mellitus affects her circulation. During the day she had a glucose tolerance test that was normal. We discussed her diet during lunchtime. She completed a menu for a day with food choices that fit her diet. Before the shift was over, I talked with her physician about the patient's medication plan; her blood glucose levels have been higher than desired." Which of the following taken from the student's summary is a nurse-sensitive outcome?
    1. Normal glucose tolerance test
    2. Discussion of diet restrictions
    3. Use of turning and pressure relief
    4. Menu completion with food choices fitting diet
    5. Blood glucose level elevated
    6. Discussion of influence diabetes has on circulation

Answers: 1. 1, 3; **2.** 1c, 2e, 3a, 4b, 5d; **3.** 4, 2, 3, 5; **4.** 2, 3, 5, 4, 5; **5.** 1A, 2A, 3A, 4B, 5B, 6A; **7.** 2, 3, 5; **8.** 4; **9.** 1d, 2 a and c, 3b; **10.** 4.

Rationales for Review Questions can be found on the Evolve website.

REFERENCES

Ackley BJ et al: *Nursing diagnosis handbook,* ed 12, St Louis, 2020, Elsevier.

Beaulieu M: Clinical pathways: Unique contribution of family medicine, *Can Fam Physician* 59(6): 705, 2013.

Butcher GM, et al: *Nursing Interventions Classification* (NIC), ed 7, St Louis, 2018, Elsevier.

Daley BJ et al.: Concept maps in nursing education: a historical literature review and research directions, *J Nurs Educ* 55(11):631, 2016.

Gorski LA et al.: Infusion therapy standards of practice, 8e, *J Infusion Nurs* 44(1S):SI, 2021.

Graystone R: The importance of nurse sensitive outcome measurement, *JONA* 48(11): 533, 2018.

Hipp R. et al. A primer on clinical pathways, *Hosp Pharm* 51(5): 416, 2016.

Ignatavicius D: White Paper: *Using case studies to develop clinical judgment and ensure Next Generation NCLEX® (NGN) success,* St. Louis, 2019, Elsevier.

Institute for Healthcare Improvement (IHI): ISBAR trip tick, 2020 http://www.ihi.org/resources/Pages/Tools/ISBARTripTick.aspx. Accessed May 23, 2021.

Interprofessional Education Collaborative: *Core competencies for interprofessional collaborative practice:*

2016 update, Washington, DC, 2016, https://nebula.wsimg.com/2f68a39520b03336b41038c370497473?AccessKeyId=DC06780E69ED19E2B3A5&disposition=0&alloworigin=1. Accessed May 23, 2021.

Jakubowski TL, Perron TJ: *Reflections on nursing leadership: Interprofessional collaboration improves healthcare,* Sigma, 2018, https://www.reflectionsonnursingleadership.org/features/more-features/interprofessional-collaboration-improves-healthcare. Accessed May 23, 2021.

Johnson, J: Depression after surgery: What you need to know, *Medical News Today* 2019, https://www.medicalnewstoday.com/articles/317616. Accessed May 23, 2021.

Lawrence, L: Finding the care path of least resistance: weighing the risks and rewards of standardizing care, *ASH Clinical News,* 2016, https://www.ashclinicalnews.org/spotlight/finding-the-care-path-of-least-resistance-weighing-the-risks-and-rewards-of-standardizing-care/. Accessed May 23, 2021.

Moorhead S, et al.: *Nursing outcomes classification,* ed 6, St Louis, 2018, Elsevier.

Nancarrow SA, et al.: Ten principles of good interprofessional team work, *Hum Resour Health* 11:19, 2013.

NCLEX: *Establishing Priorities: NCLEX RN,* Registered Nursing.org, n.d., https://www.registerednursing.org/nclex/establishing-priorities/. Accessed May 23, 2021.

QSEN Institute: *QSEN Competencies-patient-centered care,* 2020, https://qsen.org/competencies/pre-licensure-ksas. Accessed May 23, 2021.

Stevens JP et al: Variation in inpatient consultation among older adults in the United States, *J Gen Intern Med* 30(7): 992, 2015.

Stevens JP et al: Association of variation in consultant use among hospitalist physicians with outcomes among medicare beneficiaries, *JAMA Netw* Open, 3(2):e1921750, 2020. https://jamanetwork.com/journals/jamanetworkopen/fullarticle/2761552. Accessed May 23, 2021.

Varcarolis EM, Fosbre CD: *Essentials of psychiatric mental health nursing: a communication approach to evidence-based care,* ed 4, St Louis, 2021, Elsevier.

World Health Professions Alliance: *Interprofessional collaborative practice,* 2019, https://www.whpa.org/activities/interprofessional-collaborative-practice. Accessed May 23, 2021.

RESEARCH REFERENCES

Heslop L, Lu S: Nursing-sensitive indicators: a concept analysis, *J Adv Nurs* 70(11): 2469, 2014.

Ju W et al: Efficacy of relaxation therapy as an effective nursing intervention for post-operative pain relief in patients undergoing abdominal surgery: A systematic review and meta-analysis, *Exp Ther Med* 18(4): 2909, 2019.

Karam M et al: Comparing interprofessional and interorganizational collaboration in healthcare: A systematic review of the qualitative research, *Int J Nurs Stud* 79: 70, 2018.

Liu Y et al.: Patient outcomes in the field of nursing: A concept analysis, *Int J Nurs Sci* 1(1):69, 2014.

Mahdizadeh M. et al: Clinical interprofessional collaboration models and frameworks from similarities to differences: a systematic review, *Global J Health Sci* 7(6): 170, 2015.

McAllen ER et al: Moving shift report to the bedside: an evidence-based quality improvement project, *OJIN*, 23(2), May 2018, https://ojin.nursingworld.org/MainMenuCategories/ANAMarketplace/ANAPeriodicals/OJIN/TableofContents/Vol-23-2018/No2-May-2018/Articles-Previous-Topics/Moving-Shift-Report-to-the-Bedside.html. Accessed May 23, 2021.

Reeves S et al: Interprofessional collaboration and family member involvement in intensive care units: emerging themes from a multi-sited ethnography, *J Interprof Care* 29 (3): 230, 2014.

Woolfrey MR et al.: Optimisation of enhanced rapid recovery after surgery (ERAS) for total joint arthroplasty: A Canadian community hospital perspective, *Orthop Proceed* Vol 98B, No. Supp 20, published online Feb 2018, https://online.boneandjoint.org.uk/doi/abs/10.1302/1358-992X.98BSUPP_20.COA2016-060. Accessed May 23, 2021.

Implementing Nursing Care

- Explain how nursing interventions are related to nursing's scope of practice.
- Explain the factors to consider in determining whether nursing interventions are patient-centered.
- Explain the benefits and limitations of standard nursing interventions.
- Explore the implications for use of standard care bundles.
- Explain how critical thinking influences a nurse's role in the implementation process.
- Discuss the ways in which a nurse anticipates and prevents complications.
- Explain how to balance organizational and patient priorities in time management.
- Explore the three implementation skills as they relate to direct and indirect nursing interventions.
- Critique the factors influencing effective teaching interventions.
- Discuss how to effectively communicate nursing interventions.

KEY TERMS

Activities of daily living (ADLs)
Adverse reaction
Care bundle
Clinical practice guidelines
Counseling
Direct care

Implementation
Indirect care
Instrumental activities of daily living (IADLs)
Interprofessional care plans
Lifesaving measure

Nursing intervention
Patient adherence
Scope of nursing practice
Standing order

MEDIA RESOURCES

http://evolve.elsevier.com/Potter/fundamentals/
- Review Questions
- Concept Map Creator
- Case Study with Questions

- Audio Glossary
- Content Updates
- Answers to QSEN Activity and Review Questions

You first met Tonya and Mr. Lawson in the beginning of this unit (Chapter 15). *Mr. Lawson is a 68-year-old patient who had abdominal surgery for a colectomy and is anticipating discharge in the next two days. His nurse, Tonya, has been developing a plan of care over the time she has cared for Mr. Lawson. The plan has evolved to four different nursing diagnoses:* **Acute Pain, Anxiety, Lack of Knowledge,** *and* **Risk for Infection.** *Mr. Lawson had a pulmonary embolus, an acute health problem, the day following surgery. Since then, his health has stabilized, and now on day 4 he is able to begin walking again. He is taking medication (anticoagulant) to prevent additional emboli. The patient expressed interest in learning about his postoperative activity restrictions and in being able to care for his incision, which has a small separation. Mr. Lawson tells Tonya he is worried about his wound healing and being able to return to work after surgery. Tonya and the other nursing staff have consistently applied the nursing process. After analyzing assessment data, Tonya identified the diagnosis of* **Anxiety** *while planning for Mr. and Mrs. Lawson's discharge education. During implementation Tonya, along with her health care colleagues, will provide planned interventions to achieve the expected outcomes identified in Mr. Lawson's plan of care.* Critical thinking, combined with clinical decision making,

is a part of the clinical judgment process, which is important for the successful implementation of nursing interventions.

The nursing process is not linear. As a nurse your care will often shift quickly between stages of the nursing process (e.g., from implementation to assessment to analysis and diagnosis and back to implementation), based upon the patient's status and presenting needs. For example, a hospital nurse who has been with a patient for several hours will gather assessment data during all patient contacts, reprioritize nursing diagnoses as the patient progresses, reassess the patient as needed, implement a planned intervention, evaluate the patient's response (Chapter 20), consider other planned interventions, and then continue implementation. This example shows how a nurse applies clinical judgment on an ongoing basis and shifts to the step of the nursing process most appropriate at the time. Nurses engage in this cognitive process whenever they provide patient care. The process is even more complex when caring for multiple patients.

Nurses apply critical thinking to carry out nursing interventions using good clinical judgment during **implementation**, the next step of the nursing process (Fig. 19.1). The step of implementation begins after you develop a patient's plan of care. A **nursing intervention** is

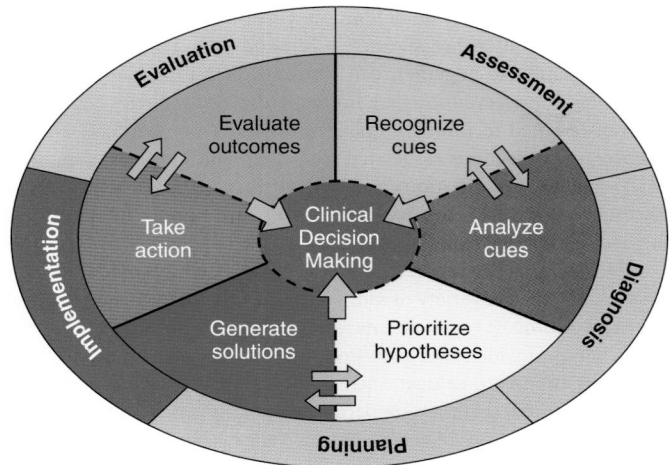

FIG. 19.1 Nursing process—Implementation. (Copyright © NCSBN. All rights reserved.)

any treatment based on clinical judgment and knowledge that a nurse performs to enhance patient outcomes (Butcher et al., 2018). Nursing interventions include direct and indirect care measures, which are either nurse-initiated, health care provider–initiated, or other provider–initiated (see Chapter 18). Ideally a nurse chooses nursing interventions that are evidence based (see Chapter 5), providing the most current, scientifically supported, up-to-date approaches for delivering patient-centered care.

Direct care interventions are treatments nurses provide through interactions with patients or a group of patients (Butcher et al., 2018). For example, a patient receives direct intervention in the form of medication administration, insertion of a urinary catheter, discharge instruction, or counseling during a time of grief. **Indirect care** interventions are treatments performed away from a patient but on behalf of the patient or group of patients (e.g., managing a patient's environment [e.g., safety and infection control]), documentation, and interprofessional collaboration (Butcher et al., 2018) (Fig. 19.2).

Within the **scope of nursing practice**, the American Nurses Association (ANA, n.d.) describes what a nurse is licensed to perform: "Nursing is the protection, promotion, and optimization of health and abilities; prevention of illness and injury; facilitation of healing; alleviation of suffering through the diagnosis and treatment of human response; and advocacy in the care of individuals, families, groups, communities, and populations." The professional scope of practice identifies the nature and intent of nursing interventions for patients, described by Benner (1984) as the domains of practice (Box 19.1). How do the scope of practice, nursing domains, and nursing interventions relate? Here is an example: *For Tonya to promote Mr. Lawson's health status (scope of practice), she provides a teaching-coaching function (domain of practice) by delivering one-to-one patient education sessions using a video program on TV (direct care).*

The challenges and complexities within health care agencies make it difficult for nurses to fully carry out the scope and domains of practice (see Chapter 2). Nurses are required to have effective organizational skills and to maintain competencies in advanced nursing care. In addition, nurses must manage conflict and effectively advocate for patients in challenging interprofessional relationships. Thus it is important for implementation to be patient-centered. Nursing is an art and a science. It is not simply a task-based profession. You must learn to intervene for patients within the context of their unique situations. Consider these factors during implementation:

- Who is the patient?
- How do a patient's attitudes, values, preferences, and cultural background affect how you provide care?

BOX 19.1 Domains of Nursing Practice

- The Helping Role
- The Teaching-Coaching Function
- The Diagnostic and Patient-Monitoring Function
- Effective Management of Rapidly Changing Situations
- Administering and Monitoring Therapeutic Interventions and Regimens
- Monitoring and Ensuring the Quality of Health Care Practices
- Organizational and Work-Role Competencies

From Benner P: *From novice to expert*, Menlo Park, CA, 1984, Addison Wesley.

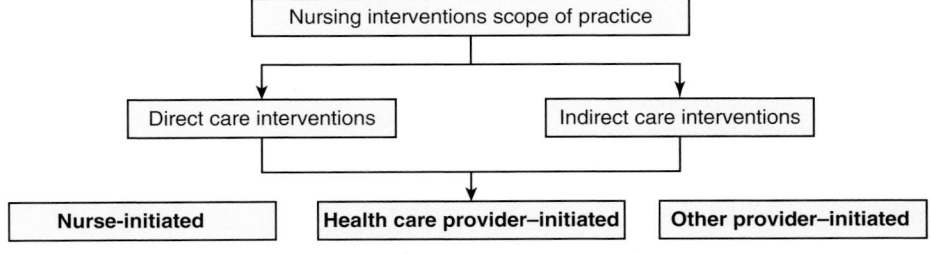

Nursing interventions scope of practice

Direct care interventions | Indirect care interventions

Nurse-initiated | **Health care provider–initiated** | **Other provider–initiated**

Examples of Interventions by Initiation

DOMAINS			
Helping	Conducting family care plan conference		Discharge planning conference
Teaching-Coaching	1:1 instruction, interpersonal skills	1:1 instruction	Exercise, ADL training
Diagnostic/Patient Monitoring	Vital sign monitoring during clinical change	Blood glucose testing	Diet calorie count
Managing Rapidly Changing Situations	Measuring oxygen saturation	Oxygen therapy	Coaching and counseling patient and family during stressful events
Administering/Monitoring Treatments	Pressure injury prevention measures	Wound irrigation	Review of wound culture reports
Monitoring/Ensuring Quality Health Care Practices	Following fall prevention protocol	Monitoring surgical infection rates	Gathering data on fall occurrence
Organizational/Work-Role Competence	Hand-off reporting/delegation	Physician credentialing	Interprofessional rounding

FIG. 19.2 Nursing interventions scope of practice.

- What does an illness mean to a patient and family?
- Which clinical situation requires you to intervene first (what priorities exist)?
- How does a patient perceive the interventions that you will deliver?
- In what way do you best support or show caring as you intervene?

The answers to these questions enable you to deliver care compassionately and effectively with the best outcomes for your patients.

STANDARD NURSING INTERVENTIONS

Although it is critical to implement unique patient-centered interventions for each patient, many health care systems develop sets of standard interventions for more common health care problems. Expert clinical teams typically collaborate to review scientific evidence and current clinical practices to form standard interventions such as clinical protocols, clinical practice guidelines, critical pathways (see Chapter 18), and ERAS (early recovery after surgery) protocols. Standard interventions allow nurses to deliver the most clinically effective care to improve patient outcomes. Many health care agencies incorporate these types of standards into health information documentation systems. Using standard interventions captures patient care information that can be shared across disciplines and care settings, making it easier to measure the quality of care delivered and support ongoing research and analysis (MBL Technologies, 2017).

As a nurse, you are accountable for individualizing standardized interventions based on your patients' needs and preferences. The ANA defines standards of professional nursing practice, while the Quality and Safety Education for Nurses (QSEN) defines skills competencies (QSEN, 2020). These standards are authoritative statements of the duties that all registered nurses (RNs) are expected to perform competently, regardless of role, patient population they serve, or specialty (ANA, 2021) (see Chapter 1).

Clinical Practice Guidelines and Protocols

The Institute of Medicine (IOM, 2011) defines clinical practice guidelines as "statements that include recommendations, intended to optimize patient care, that are informed by a systematic review of evidence and an assessment of the benefits and harms of alternative care options." Guidelines are developed for frequently recurring patient health problems or conditions (e.g., pressure injury prevention, deep vein thrombosis [DVT] prevention, central line–associated bloodstream infection, and management of postoperative surgeries). Clinical guidelines have two parts (Shekelle, 2020):

- The foundation is a systematic review of current research evidence bearing on a clinical question, focused on the strength of the evidence on which clinical decision making for that condition is based.
- A set of recommendations, involving both the evidence and value judgments regarding benefits and harms of alternative care options. Guidelines address how patients with that condition should be managed, everything else being equal.

Expert clinicians within a health care agency formally review the scientific literature and their own standard of practice to develop guidelines and protocols to improve the standard of care at their agency. For example, a hospital develops a rapid-assessment medical protocol to improve the identification and early treatment of patients suspected of having a stroke or sepsis. Some clinical guidelines are developed on a national scale by professional health care organizations. In the case of nursing clinical guidelines, the Association of Critical Care Nurses, the Oncology Nursing Society, and the University of Iowa Hartford Center develop evidence-based practice (EBP) guidelines for their specialties. Well-established clinical guidelines such as those developed by the Infusion Nurses Society (Gorski et al., 2021) are routinely revised and updated.

One form of clinical guideline is a care bundle, a group of interventions related to a disease process or condition. The interventions, when implemented together, can result in better patient outcomes than when the interventions are implemented individually. Care bundles are designed to improve quality of care by preventing the most common complications associated with their conditions or diagnoses. However, there are questions as to the efficacy of bundles on patient outcomes (Box 19.2). You will implement care bundle interventions during your clinical experiences.

Advanced practice registered nurses (APRNs), who provide primary care for patients in a variety of settings, frequently follow diagnostic and treatment protocols for their interventions. A collaborative agreement with a physician identifies protocols for the medical conditions that APRNs are permitted to treat, such as controlled hypertension, and the types of treatment that they are permitted to administer, such as antihypertensive medications. These protocols vary by physician and APRN. APRNs are also able to act independently, developing and applying clinical protocols that outline independent nursing interventions.

BOX 19.2   EVIDENCE-BASED PRACTICE
Use of Care Bundles

PICOT Question: Does the use of care bundles compared with standard practice improve hospitalized patients' recovery outcomes?

Evidence Summary

Care bundles are a set of evidence-based interventions performed collectively with the goal of improving the quality of patient care (Lavallée et al., 2017). Common care bundles include those for deep vein thrombosis, ventilator-associated pneumonia, and surgical site infection (SSI) prevention. A review of studies designed to reduce SSI involved use of core interventions such as antibiotic administration, appropriate hair removal, glycemic (blood glucose) control, and temperature management. The SSI rate in the bundle groups was 7.0% compared with 15.1% in a standard care group. The research showed that surgical care bundles helped reduce the risk of SSI compared with standard care (Tanner et al., 2015). In a review of studies designed to better manage chronic obstructive pulmonary disease, it was found that the use of discharge bundles reduced hospital readmissions, but there was insufficient evidence that care bundles influenced long-term mortality or quality of life (Ospina et al., 2017). Care bundles are becoming more common in acute care hospitals and show promising benefits. However, clinical staff do not always perform all interventions within a bundle (Juknevicius et al., 2012; Kallet, 2019). General benefits of care bundles include simplification of clinical decisions, reduced omissions of interventions, and reduced errors in medical decision making. Lavallée et al. (2017) reviewed 37 studies involving the use of care bundles and reported that the effect of bundles on patient outcomes is uncertain, requiring more research.

Application to Nursing Practice

The following are recommendations when implementing care bundles (Camporota and Brett, 2011).

- Perform the full set of interventions in a care bundle.
- Use clinical judgment when practicing within guidelines of a care bundle.
- If the interventions in a bundle are scientifically sound, perform the interventions, but if the evidence is conflicting, use a critical common-sense approach.
- Consistent use of care bundles for routine and common practices is probably beneficial and unlikely to cause significant harm to patients.
- The optimal balance between care bundle interventions versus individualized care will vary among institutions, depending on staffing and the availability of new research.

Standing Orders

A **standing order** is a preprinted document containing medical orders for routine therapies, monitoring guidelines, and/or diagnostic procedures for specific patients with identified clinical problems. A standing order directs patient care in a specific clinical setting. Licensed prescribing health care providers in charge of care at the time of implementation approve and sign standing orders. These orders reflect health care provider treatment preferences and are common in critical care settings and other specialized acute care settings where patients' needs change rapidly and require immediate attention. An example of such a standing order is one specifying certain medications such as diltiazem and amiodarone for an irregular heart rhythm. After assessing a patient and identifying the irregular rhythm, a critical care nurse gives the specified medication without first notifying the health care provider because the standing order covers the nurse's action. After completing a standing order, the nurse notifies the health care provider. Standing orders are also common in community health settings, where nurses face situations that do not permit immediate contact with a health care provider. Standing orders give nurses legal protection to intervene appropriately in the best interests of patients with rapidly changing needs.

REFLECT NOW

What do you see as a limitation of standard orders when compared with clinical practice guidelines?

Nursing Interventions Classification (NIC)

The NIC system developed by the University of Iowa differentiates nursing practice from that of other health care disciplines (Box 19.3) by offering a language that nurses can use to identify treatments they perform, organize this information into an understandable structure, and provide a language to communicate with patients, families, communities, and all health care providers (Butcher et al., 2018). The NIC interventions offer a level of standardization to enhance communication of nursing care across settings and to compare outcomes. Many health care information systems incorporate the NIC system. By using NIC, you will learn the common interventions recommended for various nursing diagnoses. Chapter 18 describes the NIC system in more detail.

Standards of Practice

When nurses apply the ANA Standards of Professional Nursing Practice (ANA, 2021) in their own practices, it is evidence of the high standard of care provided to patients (see Chapter 1). The standards

BOX 19.3 Purposes of Nursing Interventions Classification (NIC)

1. Standardize the language nurses use to describe sets of actions in delivering patient care.
2. Expand nursing knowledge about connections among nursing diagnoses, treatments, and outcomes.
3. Develop a nursing language for software of health care information systems.
4. Provide a standard set of interventions for effectiveness research, productivity measurement, and competency evaluation.
5. Link with the classification systems of other health care providers.

From Butcher HK, et al: *Nursing interventions classification (NIC)*, ed 7, St Louis, 2018, Elsevier.

are formally reviewed on a regular basis. The newest standards include competencies for establishing professional and caring relationships, using evidence-based interventions and technologies, providing ethical holistic care across the life span to diverse groups, and using community resources and systems. The standards emphasize implementing a timely plan following patient safety goals (ANA, 2021).

Quality and Safety Education for Nurses (QSEN)

The QSEN Institute established standard competencies in knowledge, skills, and attitudes (KSAs) for the preparation of future nurses (QSEN, 2020). The goal of QSEN is to prepare nurses so that they can continuously improve the quality and safety of the health care systems within which they work. Examples of QSEN skills include providing patient-centered care with sensitivity and respect for the diversity of the human experience, initiating effective treatments to relieve pain and suffering, and participating in building consensus or resolving conflict in the context of patient care (QSEN, 2020).

CRITICAL THINKING IN IMPLEMENTATION

Delivering nursing interventions for a patient involves critical thinking, clinical judgment and clinical decision making. Strong clinical reasoning skills lead to the decision making necessary for delivering nursing interventions appropriately for a patient's specific nursing diagnoses. You learn how to implement nursing care by applying appropriate knowledge, experience, environmental factors, attitudes, and standards of care (Fig. 19.3). Delivering nursing interventions is complex. Base your interventions on your scientific knowledge and what you know about a patient, in addition to the social context of the health care setting where you work. Information communicated through interprofessional relationships between nurses and health care providers contributes to nursing judgments for understanding a patient's problems and intervening effectively. Consider the context in which you deliver care to each patient and the many interventions available to make the clinical decisions needed to deliver appropriate care in each clinical situation. Critical thinking allows you to consider the complexity of interventions, changing priorities, alternative approaches, and the amount of time available to act (Table 19.1). Always prepare well before providing any intervention.

*Tonya's use and application of the nursing process continued as she provided care for Mr. Lawson. She initially identified **Acute Pain** and **Risk for Infection** as primary nursing diagnoses. While delivering care to Mr. Lawson, Tonya noticed behavior suggesting **Anxiety** and confirmed her assessment with additional data. Mr. Lawson had an acute pulmonary embolus, requiring Tonya to assess and take immediate action. However, as the condition has stabilized, Tonya has chosen not to identify a nursing diagnosis related to that condition. She continues to monitor the patient's vital signs and administers the anticoagulant (dependent function). Tonya knows the patient's discharge is imminent. The diagnosis of **Lack of Knowledge** regarding postoperative care related to inexperience with surgery has become a priority. The diagnoses are interrelated, and sometimes a planned intervention (e.g., promoting relaxation exercises) treats or modifies more than one of the patient's health problems (anxiety and acute pain). Tonya applies critical thinking and uses her time with Mr. Lawson wisely by anticipating his priorities, applying the knowledge she has about his health problems and the interventions planned, and implementing care strategies skillfully.*

Apply what you have learned during previous clinical experiences to select and implement interventions. Consider which interventions have worked and which have been less successful. What did you do when an intervention was less successful? With experience you become more proficient in anticipating what to expect in each clinical situation

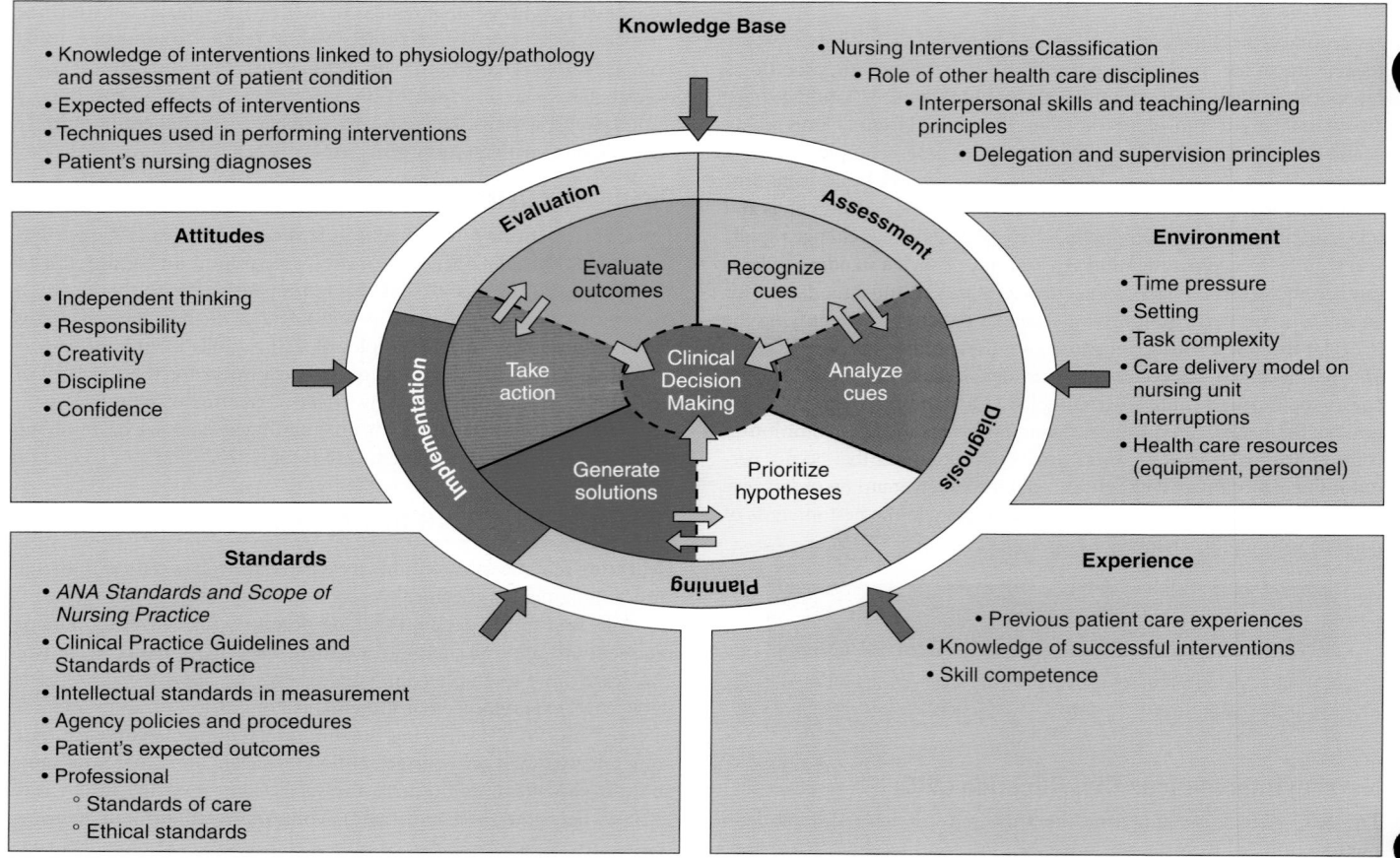

FIG. 19.3 Critical thinking in implementation. (Clinical Judgment Measurement Model copyright © NCSBN. All rights reserved.)

and how to modify your approach. For example, sometimes you need to adapt interventions when you care for older adults. Your knowledge about the changes older adults experience because of physical aging will affect how you deliver interventions. The need for adaptations is also true when patients have common characteristic problems such as mobility restrictions, symptoms (e.g., pain, nausea), and health literacy limitations.

Be aware of professional and agency standards of practice, which offer guidelines for selection of interventions, their frequency and timing, and whether interventions can be delegated. Also be aware of a patient's changing condition and how this impacts selection of interventions. What assessments should you conduct, and what findings do you expect after caring for patients with similar conditions? Once you adjust an intervention, determine a patient's response based on ongoing evaluation (see Chapter 20). Maintain organization and time-management skills to provide safe and effective patient care (see Chapter 21).

Exercise clinical judgment, using critical thinking and decision making, while delivering each intervention: **think before you act.** Consider the resources you have and the scheduling of activities in a health care setting, which often influence when and how to complete an intervention. You are responsible for having the necessary knowledge and clinical competency to perform interventions safely and effectively for your patients. Follow these tips for making decisions during implementation:

- Review the set of all possible nursing interventions for a patient's problem (*e.g., for Mr. Lawson's pain, Tonya considered analgesic administration, positioning and splinting, progressive relaxation, and other nonpharmacological approaches*).

- Review all possible consequences associated with each possible nursing action (*e.g., Tonya considers that the analgesic will relieve pain; have little or insufficient effect; or cause an adverse reaction, including sedating the patient and increasing the risk of falling*).
- Determine the probability of all possible consequences (*e.g., if Mr. Lawson's pain continues to decrease with analgesia and positioning and there have been no side effects, the interventions will likely continue to be successful; however, if the patient continues to remain highly anxious, his pain may not stay relieved, and Tonya needs to consider an alternative*).
- Judge the value of the consequence to the patient (*e.g., if the administration of an analgesic is effective, Mr. Lawson will probably become less anxious and more responsive to postoperative instruction and counseling about his anxiety*).

> **QSEN** Building Competency in Evidence-Based Practice
> Explore the scientific literature for current evidence-based strategies that can reduce anxiety and improve learning in patients following surgery. Which strategies could Tonya provide to best manage Mr. Lawson's anxiety?
>
> Answers to QSEN Activities can be found on the Evolve website.

As you perform a nursing intervention, apply intellectual standards, which are the guidelines for rational thought and responsible action (see Chapter 15). *For example, before Tonya begins to teach Mr. Lawson, she considers how to make her instructions relevant, clear, logical, and complete to promote patient learning.* A critical thinker applies critical thinking attitudes when intervening (see Table 19.1). Confidence in performing

TABLE 19.1 Critical Thinking Elements in Implementation of Nursing Care

Critical Thinking Element	Interventional Activity	Clinical Example
Knowledge		
Anatomy	Perform invasive procedure (e.g., IV catheter insertion).	Apply knowledge of anatomy (e.g., vein distribution in arm) in identifying a vein used for insertion.
Pathophysiology	Perform invasive procedure (e.g., tracheal suctioning).	Apply knowledge of pathology of lung disease (e.g., pneumonia) in determining frequency of suction.
Clinical guideline	Select array of interventions defined by guideline.	Apply elements of clinical bundle for preventing central line–associated bloodstream infection, cleansing IV site, and preventing break in sterile intravenous system.
Communication principles	Provide coaching during a procedure.	Explain to patient in a calming manner each step of nasogastric tube insertion.
Teaching principles	Provide explanations describing purpose and self-care implications of an intervention.	Administer a newly prescribed medication with an explanation of its purpose and implications for safe self-administration, including monitoring effects.
Delegation principles	Organize multiple interventions for a patient (e.g., vital signs, sterile dressing change, early ambulation for postoperative patient).	Select the right task and consider whether patient is stable (Chapter 21); have assistive personnel assist RN with ambulating patient first time.
Experience		
Experience in administering the same intervention for a variety of patients with the same characteristics (e.g., patients with obesity, older adults, patients in pain)	Adapt intervention to a patient's limitation(s) caused by characteristic.	When placing and removing a bedpan, use extra caution in supporting older adult patient's buttocks so that pan does not cause shear or friction against fragile skin.
Skill competence	Perform a new procedure practiced only in simulation lab.	Reflect on your competency and knowledge of procedure; obtain resources (e.g., experienced nurse).
Environment		
Task complexity and interruptions	Administer intervention at a time when no other patient priorities exist and attention is needed for accuracy.	Prepare medication in a no-interruption zone around medication preparation area; temporarily turn off pager (see Chapter 31).
Health care setting	Adapt intervention to conditions existing within setting.	Use surgical asepsis for dressing change of hospitalized patient; teach family caregiver clean technique for dressing change in the home.
Attitudes		
Creativity	Adapt intervention to patient's physical limitation.	Patient with reduced mobility of hands: consult with occupational therapist and use assistive devices for self-feeding.
Confidence	Prepare patient for interventions.	Reflect first on what you know about the reason patient is receiving intervention. Then use clear, calm, confident instructions for how patient can participate and reasons for key steps.
Standards		
Intellectual standard in measurement	Adapt intervention to patient's changing status (relevance).	While a patient is ambulating, anticipate signs of hypotension or unsteady gait; adjust and sit patient in chair when symptoms develop.
	Deliver intervention to target an expected outcome.	Patient has lack of knowledge regarding risk for infection. Provide explanation for specific reasons patient is at risk; do not generalize.

interventions builds trust with patients. Creativity and self-discipline are attitudes that guide you in reviewing, modifying, and implementing interventions. As a beginning nursing student, seek out supervision from faculty or experienced nurses or review agency policy and procedures to guide you in the decision-making process for implementation.

IMPLEMENTATION PROCESS

Many actions that we take occur automatically, with little thinking, such as starting your car and setting the gear to drive, preparing your kids for bedtime, or feeding the pets their dinner. As tasks become

more complicated, more conscious effort is needed to be effective. Implementing nursing interventions is complex. Proper preparation for implementation ensures more efficient, safe, and effective nursing care. Patients often experience adverse events (see Chapter 27) when nurses do not adequately prepare for implementation. The Agency for Healthcare Research and Quality (AHRQ) identifies three categories of adverse events (AHRQ, 2019):

- Preventable adverse events: those that occurred due to error or failure to apply an accepted strategy for prevention
- Ameliorable adverse events: those that, while not preventable, could have been less harmful if care had been different

- Adverse events due to negligence: those that occurred due to care that falls below the standards expected of clinicians

Adverse events can be avoided or minimized with proper preparation and implementation of any intervention. Perform these five preparatory activities: (1) reassess the patient before a procedure, (2) review the nursing care plan and consider whether revision to interventions is necessary based on patient's current condition, (3) organize necessary resources and your delivery of care (especially with multiple patients), (4) anticipate and prevent complications based on what you know about the patient, and (5) implement the intervention(s) correctly.

Tonya visits Mr. Lawson to begin discharge instruction. His wife is present, and Mr. Lawson reports that his incisional pain is currently a level of 3. He makes good eye contact. Tonya checks the patient's blood pressure (in normal range) and helps him sit up in a chair. She sets up the teaching program on the hospital educational TV system and prepares the evidence-based instruction booklets she wants to use to present information on infection control, wound care, and activity restrictions in the home. Because Mr. Lawson still has concerns about returning to work, Tonya wants to incorporate discussion about wound care with expected postoperative recovery. Tonya sees the opportunity of using Mr. Lawson's desire to return to work to increase the likelihood of his adherence to postoperative restrictions. If Mrs. Lawson understands how she can help Mr. Lawson in recovery, positive outcomes should be achieved.

Reassessing a Patient

Assessment is a continuous process that occurs each time you interact with a patient. It involves the collection of **new data**. Reassessment is not the same as repeating a previous assessment to evaluate care or determine a patient's response to an intervention (see Chapter 20). Instead, it is the gathering of additional information to ensure that the plan of care is still complete, current, and appropriate. When you collect new data about a patient, you sometimes identify a new nursing diagnosis or determine that additional interventions might be necessary for not only the new diagnosis but also existing diagnoses. Creating a concept map helps you better understand the relationship among different nursing diagnoses and interventions appropriate to a patient's care (Fig. 19.4). During the initial phase of implementation reassess the patient to confirm that you have selected appropriate interventions. The reassessment helps you decide whether the proposed nursing actions are still appropriate for a patient's level of wellness. *For example, Tonya begins to talk with Mr. and Mrs. Lawson about wound care and the patient's activity restrictions. Mrs. Lawson shares that Mr. Lawson's employer called to ask how he was doing. Tonya notices that Mr. Lawson begins to show more anxiety; as Tonya explains restrictions on lifting, the patient is unable to teach back (repeat information) about what he can and cannot do. Tonya decides to redirect the discussion. She says to Mr. Lawson, "Let's talk about going back to work. Tell me more about when they expect you to return and what your work actually involves." Tonya realizes that to be effective with instruction she needs an attentive learner. Gaining more detail about the patient's work will help him express his concerns while at the same time allow Tonya to explain how activity restrictions fit into daily routines.*

Reviewing and Revising the Existing Nursing Care Plan

After you reassess a patient and determine there is a need to add to or modify the plan of care, you revise the care plan. An out-of-date, incomplete, or incorrect care plan compromises the quality of nursing care. When you gather evaluation data (see Chapter 20) to determine whether previously selected interventions were successful and whether outcomes were met, similar types of revisions can be made. Review and revision of a plan enable you to provide more appropriate and

timely nursing interventions to best meet a patient's needs. Modification of an existing written care plan includes four steps:

1. Revise data in the assessment column to reflect the patient's current status. Date any new data to inform other members of the health care team of the time that the change occurred.
2. Revise the nursing diagnoses and outcomes. Add any new nursing diagnoses that have been identified and select appropriate outcomes. For existing nursing diagnoses, revise related factors or risk factors, the patient's outcomes, and priority interventions as necessary. Date any revisions.
3. Select or revise specific interventions that correspond to the new nursing diagnoses or that are necessary for existing diagnoses. Be sure that revisions reflect the patient's present status.
4. Choose the methods of evaluation that will be used to determine whether the patient achieves expected outcomes.

As Tonya continues to prepare Mr. Lawson for discharge, she evaluates his pain status. His pain has been controlled well on around-the-clock analgesics and use of relaxation. Tonya reassesses whether Mr. Lawson has ever taken analgesics at home and what works best. In consultation with the physician and in preparation for discharge, the physician decides to discontinue the around-the-clock analgesic and orders an analgesic as needed (prn) instead. Tonya plans to explain to Mr. and Mrs. Lawson how best to take a prn medication (see Chapter 25). Tonya also decides to include Mrs. Lawson as a coach to facilitate relaxation exercises for Mr. Lawson.

Preparing for Implementation

Environmental factors play a major role in implementation. Critically consider these factors to implement nursing care activities safely and appropriately. One way to do this is by organizing time and resources. Always be sure that a patient is physically and psychologically ready for any interventions or procedures.

Time Management. Providing patient-centered care is the focus of your nursing practice. You will practice within work environments that are part of the sociocultural context of a health care organization (see Chapter 21). These are busy environments, and you will assume dual roles: a patient care provider and an agency employee. In this dual role you need to be aware of the agency's goals of efficiency and cost control. However, you need to competently provide timely, thoughtful, safe, and efficient care. The ability to manage care in a timely way conveys caring and concern to your patients. Poor patient care results when you are hurried, experience interruptions, or are disorganized. Time devoted to nursing care has three components: physical (the physical amount of time consumed in the completion of nursing activities), psychological (what nursing care patients experience and how they experience it), and sociological (the sequential ordering of events within the daily routines of a practice setting) (Jones, 2010). All components of time occur within the context of an organization and the resources available. As a new nurse, understand that the decisions you make about how your time is allocated, prioritized, and sequenced are always interpreted by the patients you serve (Jones, 2010). Be aware of factors affecting time with patients and apply time-management principles (see Chapter 21).

Tonya decides it is time to examine Mr. Lawson's surgical wound. She wants to maximize her time available with Mr. Lawson. She first checks his comfort level; he is not restless in bed, and he reports his pain level at 4. Tonya encourages Mr. Lawson to begin his relaxation exercise as she inspects the wound. Wanting to use her time efficiently, Tonya describes the appearance of the wound (wound shows no signs of worsening) and discusses activity restrictions needed at home to prevent further wound separation. She also mentions the common signs of infection as it pertains

CONCEPT MAP

Nursing diagnosis: Acute pain
- Wound tender when palpated
- Pain severity has ranged from 4 to 8
- Patient guards incision by placing hand over wound when moving

Interventions
- Administer analgesic prn as ordered
- Educate patient about managing prn medication
- Teach relaxation exercises to be used when pain is in control; include wife as coach

Nursing diagnosis: Lack of knowledge regarding postoperative care
- Unclear about activity restrictions
- Asks if he will need to "do something" to his incision
- Lifts various objects at home
- Does not know signs of infection

Interventions
- Show hospital TV education program on infection control
- Provide a pamphlet outlining postoperative risks
- Demonstrate method for cleansing incision
- Discuss activities not to perform at home because of activity restrictions

Primary health problem: Colectomy
Priority assessments: Condition of incision, gastrointestinal function, comfort level, knowledge of home care requirements and ability to learn, resources for discharge

Nursing diagnosis: Risk for infection
- Has small separation of wound edges
- Drainage from wound
- Incision tender and inflamed near area of separation
- In a health care environment

Interventions
- Have patient and wife view hospital TV education program on signs/symptoms of infection
- Instruct patient and wife on hand hygiene in the home
- Discuss signs and symptoms to report

Nursing diagnosis: Anxiety
- Worried about returning to work on time
- Has not consistently attended to nurse during instruction
- Poor eye contact

Interventions
- Use a calm, reassuring approach during discussions and instruction
- Include Mrs. Lawson in instruction
- Confirm with patient that following postoperative care guidelines will improve likelihood of recovery and ability to return to work

——— Link between medical diagnosis and nursing diagnosis   - - - - Link between nursing diagnoses

FIG. 19.4 Concept map for Mr. Lawson: Implementation.

to Mr. Lawson's wound: increased drainage, yellow or green color of drainage, and increased tenderness or discomfort. She incorporates elements of instruction while examining wound status.

Equipment. Most nursing procedures require some equipment or supplies. Before performing an intervention, decide which supplies you need and determine their availability. Is the equipment in working order to ensure safe use, and do you know how to use it? Place supplies in a convenient location to provide easy access during a procedure. Keep extra supplies available in case of errors or mishaps, but do not open them unless you need them. This controls health care costs, allowing you to be a fiscally responsible member of the health care team. After a procedure return any unopened supplies to storage areas.

REFLECT NOW

Think about a procedure you recently performed in the lab or with an assigned patient. Did you manage your time well in preparing for the skill? What might you have done differently?

Personnel. Nursing care practice models determine how nursing personnel are organized to deliver patient care, including staff RNs, auxiliary staff such as assistive personnel (APs), and RNs in special roles (e.g., nurse specialists). A practice model usually reflects how professional nursing exemplifies the culture of that organization, such as primary nursing, shared governance, or patient-centered care. Common values shared among the various models include nursing autonomy; empowerment; collaboration; evidence-based practice; and cost-effective, quality care. A practice model designates a nurse's role and accountability to patients and other members of the nursing team. For example, a practice model will influence whether APs are assigned to patients or to RNs, two models with very different challenges. When APs are assigned to RNs, each AP knows the RN to whom they are accountable. When APs are assigned to patients, an AP will have to be responsible to more than one RN, often making communication and priority setting difficult. Chapter 21 offers details on the various models of care.

Regardless of the practice model, as a nurse you are responsible for deciding whether to perform an intervention, delegate it to an unlicensed member of the nursing team, or have an RN colleague assist you. Do not make decisions about delegation based only on the intervention your patients need. Your ongoing assessment of each patient, the priorities of care (see Chapter 18), the complexity of an intervention, and the activities occurring in the workplace direct your decision about delegation. You have a legal duty to follow delegation guidelines and to only delegate interventions within the delegate's training and ability according to the state Nurse Practice Act.

Patient care staff should work together as patients' needs demand it. If a patient makes a request such as the use of a bedpan or assistance in feeding, help the patient if you have time rather than trying to find an AP who is in a different room. Nursing staff respect colleagues who show initiative, collaborate, and communicate with one another on an ongoing reciprocal basis as patients' needs change. When interventions are complex or physically difficult, you will need assistance from colleagues. For example, a nurse will be more effective in changing a dressing for a large gaping wound when an AP can assist with patient positioning and handing off supplies.

Environment. A patient's care environment, especially in hospitals, rehabilitation units, and skilled care facilities, needs to be safe and conducive to implementing therapies. Patient safety is your first concern. You can make the environment safer by removing clutter and unnecessary furniture or equipment, creating clear paths for patients to ambulate, and making sure patients' personal items are easily accessible when they lie in bed. If a patient has sensory deficits, physical disabilities, or an alteration in level of consciousness, it is especially important to arrange the environment to prevent injury. For example, provide a patient's assistive devices (e.g., walker or eyeglasses), rearrange furniture and equipment when ambulating a patient, or make sure that the water temperature is not too warm before a bath. Patients benefit most from nursing interventions when surroundings are compatible with care activities. For example, when you need to expose a patient's body parts, do so privately by closing room doors or curtains because the patient will then be more relaxed. Ask visitors to leave as you complete care. Reduce distractions during teaching to enhance a patient's learning opportunities.

The environment influences the ability of nurses to deliver interventions and the ability of patients to heal and recover. Hospitals and other health care settings are using evidence-based design to create healing environments. Evidence-based design (EBD) uses the best available research to construct patient rooms, improve lighting and air quality, reduce noise, provide wayfinding and walking distance guidance, promote hand hygiene, incorporate nature, and accommodate families' needs (Huisman et al., 2012; O'Callaghan and Philip, 2019). The concept is being applied with the building and renovation of hospitals and other care settings. How a nursing unit is designed impacts both patients and care providers. For example, a well-designed hospital

---

BOX 19.4   Physical Environmental Factors That Promote Patient Healing

- Standardization of patient rooms and equipment for making routine tasks simpler, thus decreasing errors.
- Improvement in light illumination in areas where medications are dispensed.
- Effective air quality with improved air-filtration systems.
- Features of a patient room and bath that reduce falls: no slippery floors, appropriate door openings, correct placement of rails and accessories, correct toilet and furniture height, single-bed rooms, easy-to-clean surfaces, automated sinks, and smooth edges in rooms (for easier cleaning).
- Self-supporting systems, such as control over the position of the bed, control over the temperature, control over the lights (including dimmers), control over the sound (music and television), and control over the natural light.
- The use of acuity-adaptable rooms, which limit the need to transfer patients within the hospital when their conditions worsen.
- Privacy and single-patient rooms.
- Decentralization of nurses' stations and supply rooms to allow nurses to spend less time walking and more time treating patients.

Adapted from Henriksen K, et al: The role of the physical environment in crossing the quality chasm, *Jt Comm J Qual Patient Saf* 33(11 Suppl): 68–80, 2007; Agency for Healthcare Research and Quality: *Transforming Hospitals*, 2017, https://www.ahrq.gov/patient-safety/settings/hospital/resource/transform.html. Accessed June 16, 2021.

---

unit can contribute to patient outcomes through reducing errors, improving infection control and safety, offering more privacy, and providing better sleep and comfort (O'Callaghan and Philip, 2019) (Box 19.4).

Patient. Make sure that your patients are physically and psychologically comfortable before you implement care. Physical symptoms such as nausea, dizziness, fatigue, or pain interfere with a patient's full concentration and ability to cooperate. Offer comfort measures before initiating interventions to help patients participate more fully. If you need a patient to be alert, administer a dose of pain medication strong enough to relieve discomfort but not to impair mental faculties (e.g., ability to follow instruction and communicate). If a patient is fatigued, delay ambulation or transfer to a chair until after there has been a chance to rest. Also consider a patient's level of endurance, and plan only the amount of activity that the patient is able to tolerate comfortably.

Awareness of a patient's psychosocial needs helps you create a favorable emotional climate. *Do not rush your care.* Some patients feel reassured by having a significant other present to lend encouragement and moral support. Other strategies include planning sufficient time or multiple opportunities for a patient to work through and ventilate feelings and anxieties. Adequate preparation allows a patient to obtain maximal benefit from each intervention.

Anticipating and Preventing Complications

Risks to patients come from both illness and treatment. Your experience and knowledge of a patient's condition and risk factors enable you to observe for and recognize these risks, adapt your choice of interventions to each situation, assess the relative benefit of the intervention versus the risk, and then take risk-prevention measures. Critical thinking is key to prevent complications. For example, a patient with preexisting left-sided paralysis following a stroke is at risk for developing a pressure injury following orthopedic surgery that requires traction and bed rest. A patient with obesity and diabetes mellitus who has major abdominal surgery is at risk for poor wound healing. Nurses are often the first ones to detect and document changes in patients' conditions. Expert nurses learn to anticipate changes in patient conditions even before confirming that diagnostic signs of complications have developed.

Your knowledge of pathophysiology and experience with previous patients help you identify complications that can occur. A thorough assessment reveals the level of a patient's current risk. The evidence or scientific rationale for how interventions (e.g., pressure-relief devices, repositioning, or wound care) prevent or minimize complications helps you select the most appropriate preventive measures. For example, if a patient who is obese has uncontrolled postoperative pain, the risk for pressure injury development increases because the patient is unwilling or unable to change position frequently. The nurse anticipates when a patient's pain will increase, administers ordered analgesics, and consults with a wound care specialist on the best pressure-relief device to use for removing pressure on the skin and underlying tissue.

Some nursing procedures pose risks. Be aware of potential complications, and take precautions based on your patients' conditions. For example, a patient with an indwelling urinary catheter is at risk for infection. In this case implementing catheter-associated urinary tract infection (CAUTI) care guidelines for UTI prevention reduces infection risk (Chapter 46). Administering oral medications to patients with dysphagia increases their risk for aspiration. Administering medications using a different route may be a better option (Chapter 31).

Identifying Areas of Assistance. Certain patient care situations require you to seek additional personnel, knowledge, or nursing skills. Before beginning care, review the plan to determine whether you need assistance and what kind of help you need. Sometimes you need assistance to perform a procedure, provide comfort measures, or prepare a patient for a diagnostic test. Do not take shortcuts if assistance is not immediately available so as to avoid injury to you and the patient. For example, when you care for a patient who is overweight and immobile, you require additional personnel and transfer equipment to turn and position the patient safely. Be sure to determine in advance the number of additional personnel needed. Discuss your need for assistance with other nurses or the APs.

You will require additional knowledge and skills in situations in which you are less familiar or experienced. For example, seek additional knowledge by accessing a policy and procedure manual before performing a new procedure. Because of the continual growth in health care technology, you may lack the motor skills to use new equipment for a procedure. When you are faced with administering an unfamiliar therapy or operating a new piece of equipment, follow these steps:
1. Seek the information you need to be informed about a procedure. Check the scientific literature for evidence-based information, review resource manuals (e.g., hospital formulary or procedure manuals), or consult with experts (e.g., pharmacists, clinical nurse specialists).
2. Collect all equipment necessary for the procedure to be organized.
3. Consider the consequences of performing the procedure on each specific patient.
4. Have another nurse (e.g., staff nurse, faculty member, clinical nurse specialist) who has completed the procedure correctly and safely provide assistance and guidance.

Requesting assistance occurs frequently in all types of nursing practice. It is a learning process that continues throughout educational experiences and into professional development. One tip is to verbalize with faculty or staff nurse the steps you will take before performing a procedure to improve your confidence and ensure accuracy.

Implementation Skills

Nursing practice requires cognitive, interpersonal, and psychomotor skills as you implement direct and indirect nursing interventions. You apply the appropriate skills to the procedure you perform. Sometimes this requires a mix of skills and good judgment. For example, a nurse is caring for a patient who is prescribed a new medication regimen. The nurse must apply what she knows about adherence and the interpersonal skills that best support the patient in being willing to adhere. The outcome you plan on achieving for a patient influences the skills you use.

Cognitive Skills. Clinical judgment using critical thinking involves cognitive skills. During implementation you apply these skills to ensure that no nursing action is automatic but instead is thoughtful and patient-centered. Carefully consider each clinical situation at hand, interpret the information you observe, decide whether more information is needed, and anticipate a patient's response so that you individualize interventions appropriately. A cognitive skill involves knowing the rationale for therapeutic interventions and understanding normal and abnormal physiological and psychological responses, enabling you to adapt skills when necessary and to properly monitor patients as interventions are performed. Also know the evidence in nursing science to ensure that you deliver current and relevant nursing interventions.

Interpersonal Communication Skills. Interpersonal communication is essential for any nursing intervention (Chapter 24). Apply interpersonal communication skills by developing a trusting relationship, expressing caring, and communicating clearly with patients and their families. Listening is particularly important. Patients want you to hear their stories. Often, they share information that is not only useful for assessment, but also helpful in knowing how best to deliver an intervention. Good interpersonal communication keeps patients informed and engaged in decision making, provides individualized instruction, and supports patients who have challenging emotional needs.

Proper use of interpersonal skills enables you to be perceptive of your patients' verbal and nonverbal communication, understand their needs and desires, and improve your ability to correctly select relevant interventions. As a member of the health care team, communicate patient problems and needs clearly, intelligently, and in a timely way.

Psychomotor Skills. Psychomotor skills require the integration of cognitive and motor activities. For example, when giving an injection, you need to understand anatomy and pharmacology (cognitive) and use good coordination and precision to administer the injection correctly (motor). With time and practice you learn to perform skills correctly, smoothly, and confidently. This is critical in establishing patient trust. You are responsible for acquiring necessary psychomotor skills through your experience in the nursing laboratory, the use of interactive instructional technology, or actual hands-on care of patients. When performing a new skill, assess your level of competency, and obtain the necessary resources to ensure that your patients receive safe treatment.

DIRECT CARE

Nurses provide a wide variety of direct care measures, treatments, or procedures performed through direct interaction with patients. How a nurse applies implementation skills affects the success of any direct care activity. Always be mindful of a patient's clinical condition, your previous experiences, and patient expectations and cultural views as you deliver interventions. All direct care measures require competent safe practice. Show a caring approach when providing direct care.

Activities of Daily Living

Activities of daily living (ADLs) are direct care measures usually performed during a normal day; they include ambulation, toileting, eating,

BOX 19.5   Assisting Patients With Dementia in Performing Activities of Daily Living

- Patients with early dementia may need to be reminded to have a bath or complete other grooming.
- Be present in case patients have problems. For example, be sure the person is soaping and rinsing adequately or eating a complete meal; if not, you may prompt them to do so.
- As dementia progresses, a patient may need to be reminded of specific tasks in a bath (such as soap yourself, rinse yourself) in the right sequence. The objects needed for the bath may need to be prepared for them (basin with water at the right temperature, shaving mug is accessible, towel and clean gown/clothes are on the towel bar).
- Patients may need help for some actions, such as applying soap on the back, washing the toes, or shampooing the hair. Help may be given by guiding the person's wrist or holding the elbow to guide the arm. Patients often are able to do the task if you help them start the task.
- After dementia continues to progress, patients will need help with more difficult tasks, such as tying shoelaces or putting in hearing aids.
- After some days, you may find the person looking at the bath basin in a puzzled way. The amount of assistance needed increases.
- The person may also lose interest in doing anything.
- As dementia progresses, the patient will become more dependent, requiring a bed bath.

Adapted from *Dementia care notes: helping with activities of daily living*, 2020, https://dementiacarenotes.in/caregivers/toolkit/adl/. Accessed June 16, 2021.

dressing, bathing, personal device care, functional mobility (getting into/out of a bed or bathtub), and grooming (Lyon, 2020). A patient's need for assistance with ADLs is temporary, permanent, or rehabilitative. For example, a patient with impaired physical mobility because of bilateral arm casts temporarily needs assistance with eating and bathing. A patient with dementia may initially require coaching to complete tasks, but later requires direct assistance (Box 19.5). A patient with an irreversible cervical spinal cord injury is paralyzed and has a permanent need for full assistance. When patients have difficulty performing ADLs or need to learn new ways to perform self-care activities, occupational and physical therapists play key roles in rehabilitation to restore ADL function.

When patients are experiencing fatigue, a limitation in mobility, confusion, or pain, assistance with ADLs is probably needed. For example, a patient who experiences shortness of breath avoids eating because of associated fatigue. Help the patient by setting up meals, offering to cut up food, and planning for smaller, more frequent meals to maintain nutrition. Assistance with ADLs ranges from partial assistance to complete care. Remember to always respect patients' wishes and determine their preferences. Patients from some cultures prefer to receive assistance with ADLs from family members. If a patient is stable and alert, it is appropriate to allow family to help with care. Most patients want to remain independent in meeting their basic needs. Allow a patient to participate to the level possible. Involving patients in planning the timing and types of interventions boosts their self-esteem and willingness to become more independent.

Instrumental Activities of Daily Living

Illness or disability sometimes alters a patient's ability to be independent in society. Instrumental activities of daily living (IADLs) refer to activities that support daily life and are oriented toward interacting with the environment (e.g., shopping, caring for pets, home maintenance, preparing meals, housecleaning, writing checks, and taking medications) (Lyon, 2020). IADLs are typically more complex than ADLs and generally are managed by occupational therapists. However, nurses within home care and community health settings frequently help patients adapt ways to perform IADLs (such as providing appropriate assistive devices or creating medication organization systems). Often family and friends are excellent resources for helping patients and have found creative ways to assist. In acute care it is important to anticipate how patients' illnesses will affect their ability to perform IADLs so that you can make appropriate referrals to be sure they have the resources they need at home.

Physical Care Techniques

Physical care techniques involve the safe and competent administration of nursing procedures (e.g., turning and positioning, inserting a feeding tube, administering medications, inserting an intravenous catheter, and providing comfort measures) involving hands-on care. The specific knowledge and skills needed to perform these procedures are in subsequent clinical chapters of this text. All physical care techniques require you to protect yourself and patients from injury, use safe patient-handling techniques, use proper infection control practices, stay organized, and follow applicable practice guidelines.

You are responsible to be knowledgeable about the procedure itself, the standard frequency, the associated risks, and the necessary assessments/evaluations before, during, and after performing a skill. Your clinical judgment applies what you know about a procedure with what you know about each patient. Always remain thoughtful of a patient's condition and consider how the patient has responded to the procedure in the past. Know how the procedure is going to affect the patient and which expected outcomes you and the patient desire. For example, if you are going to ambulate a patient, discuss how far you wish the patient to walk and whether there will be opportunity to sit or stop to rest. Ask the patient to tell you if shortness of breath occurs.

In a hospital you perform many procedures each day, often for the first time. Before performing a new procedure, assess the situation and your personal competencies to determine whether you need assistance, new knowledge, or new skills. Performing any procedure correctly requires critical thinking and thoughtful decision making.

Lifesaving Measures

A lifesaving measure is a physical care technique that you use when a patient's physiological or psychological state is threatened (see Chapter 41). The purpose of lifesaving measures is to restore physiological or psychological homeostasis. Such measures include administering emergency medications, instituting cardiopulmonary resuscitation, intervening to protect a patient who is confused or violent, and obtaining immediate counseling from a crisis center for a patient who is severely anxious or suicidal. If a nurse faces a situation requiring emergency measures, the proper nursing actions are to stay with the patient, maintain support, and have another staff member obtain an experienced professional.

Counseling

Counseling is a direct care method that helps patients use problem-solving processes to recognize and manage stress and facilitate interpersonal relationships. As a nurse, you counsel patients to accept actual or impending changes resulting from stress (see Chapter 37). For example, when patients share a problem with you, your role is to talk through their concerns, then direct them to appropriate resources (e.g., social worker, psychologist, pastoral care) to help them sort out the problem. Counseling techniques are an especially helpful resource when caring for patients who are facing terminal or chronic illness. Counseling can involve providing emotional, intellectual, spiritual, and psychological support. Nurses can provide counseling to patients and families who have normal adjustment difficulties and are upset or frustrated, but they are not necessarily psychologically disabled. An example is the stress that a young woman faces when caring for her aging mother. Family caregivers need assistance in adjusting to the physical and emotional demands of caregiving. Sometimes they need to know that respite care (i.e., a break from providing care) is available. Recipients of care also need assistance in adjusting to their disability. Patients with psychiatric diagnoses require therapy from nurses specializing in mental health or from social workers, psychiatrists, or psychologists.

Many counseling techniques foster cognitive, behavioral, developmental, experiential, and emotional growth in patients. Counseling encourages individuals to examine available alternatives and decide which choices are useful and appropriate. When patients are able to examine alternatives, they develop a sense of control and are able to better manage stress.

Teaching

Patient education is key to patient-centered care (Chapter 25). A teaching plan is essential for every patient, especially when patients need to manage health problems they are facing for the first time. Counseling and teaching closely align. Both involve using good interpersonal skills to create a change in a patient's knowledge and behavior. Counseling results in the development of new attitudes, behaviors, and feelings, whereas teaching focuses on growth of knowledge or the acquisition of psychomotor skills.

When you educate patients, respect their expertise with their own health and symptoms, their daily routines, the diversity of their human experiences, their values and preferences as to how they learn, and the importance of shared decision making. As an educator you present health care principles, procedures, and techniques to inform patients about their health status in such a way that patients can adapt what they learn to their daily routines at home to achieve self-care. Emphasis has been placed on patient education in acute care since 2006, when the Hospital Consumer Assessment of Healthcare Providers and Systems (HCAHPS) standardized survey began to be used across the country by hospitals to measure patients' perspectives on hospital care (HCAHPS, 2020). The survey results currently are a standard for measuring and comparing quality of hospitals. Hospitals stress the importance of nurses addressing the topics covered by the survey, including patient education for discharge preparation.

The HCAHPS initiative stresses the importance of patient education. But remember, teaching is an ongoing process of keeping patients informed. Patients want to know why you do what you do. When performing a procedure, engage your patient and explain the procedure, why it is being done, the expected outcomes, and any problems to look for afterward. Encourage patients to ask questions. Here is an example of incorporating teaching in your daily work:

When starting an intravenous (IV) infusion, explain what the IV fluid bag contains, how long the bag should last, sensations the patient will feel if the IV site becomes inflamed, the fact that a small flexible catheter is in the arm, and any potential side effects of medications in the bag. Then explain how the medication will affect the patient's health status and progress.

Teaching takes place in all health care settings (Fig. 19.5). As a nurse you are accountable for the quality of education you deliver. Chapter 25 provides a thorough overview of patient education principles and practices. Follow these basic patient education tips (Nurse Journal, 2020):

- Delegate more responsibilities to support staff so that you can focus on patient education.

FIG. 19.5 Nurse providing discharge instructions.

- Begin to educate patients with every encounter from admission.
- Correct any misinformation based on what a patient already knows.
- Provide information in layman's terms. Use visual activities as often as possible. People remember what they see far more than what they hear or read.
- Question a patient's understanding of the care, and plan for the next lesson. It is all part of the nursing process.
- Use return demonstration when administering care. Involve the patient from the first treatment.
- Ask patients to tell you how they would explain (step by step) their disease or treatment to their spouse, partner, or friend.
- Repeat as needed and build upon the teaching with every opportunity throughout a hospitalization or stay.
- Provide patients with information about signs and symptoms to report to their health care providers, and ensure that they know to do this promptly, without waiting for another crisis to act.

Know your patient; be aware of the cultural and social factors that influence a patient's willingness and ability to learn. It is also important to know your patient's health literacy level (see Chapter 25). Do not assume that patients understand their illness or disease. If they seem uneasy or refuse a treatment, simply ask what concerns them. This gives you the chance to provide further teaching and correct knowledge deficiencies.

Controlling for Adverse Reactions

An **adverse reaction** is a harmful or unintended effect of a medication, diagnostic test, or therapeutic intervention (Chapter 31). Adverse reactions can result from any nursing intervention; thus, learn to anticipate and know which adverse reactions to expect. Nursing actions that control for adverse reactions reduce or counteract a reaction. For example, when applying a moist heat compress, you know that burning the patient's skin is a possible adverse reaction unless you protect the skin. First, assess the condition of the area where you plan to place the compress. Following application of the compress, inspect the area every 5 minutes for any adverse reaction such as excessive reddening of the skin from the heat or skin maceration from the moisture (see Chapter 48). Taking the right precautions can prevent adverse reactions.

When completing a health care provider–directed intervention such as medication administration, always know the potential side effects of the drug. After you administer a medication, evaluate the patient for adverse effects. Also be aware of drugs that counteract the side effects. For example, a patient has an unknown hypersensitivity to penicillin and develops hives after three doses. You record the reaction, stop further administration of the drug, and consult with the health care provider.

You then administer an ordered dose of diphenhydramine, an antihistamine and antipruritic medication, to reduce the allergic response and relieve the itching.

When caring for patients who undergo diagnostic tests, you need to understand the test and any potential adverse effects. Although adverse effects are not common, they do occur. It is important that you recognize the signs and symptoms of an adverse reaction and intervene in a timely manner.

Preventive Interventions

Preventive nursing interventions promote health and prevent illness to avoid the need for acute or rehabilitative health care (see Chapter 2). Changes in the health care system are leading to greater emphasis on health promotion and illness prevention. Primary prevention aimed at health promotion includes wellness education programs, immunizations, and physical and nutritional fitness activities. Secondary prevention focuses on people who are experiencing health problems or illnesses and who are at risk for developing complications or worsening conditions. It includes health screenings and treating early stages of disease. Tertiary prevention involves minimizing the effects of long-term illness or disability, including rehabilitation measures.

INDIRECT CARE

Indirect care measures are nursing treatments or procedures performed away from patients but on behalf of patients (Butcher et al., 2018). Examples include interventions that manage the patient care environment and interprofessional collaborative actions that support the effectiveness of direct care interventions (Butcher et al., 2018) (Box 19.6). Nurses spend much time in indirect unit management activities. Communicating information about patients (e.g., hand-off report, hourly rounding, and consultation) is critical, ensuring that direct care activities are planned, coordinated, and performed with the proper resources. Delegation of care to APs is another indirect care activity (see Chapter 21). When performed correctly, delegation ensures that the right care provider performs the right tasks so that the nurse and APs work together most efficiently for a patient's benefit.

Communicating Nursing Interventions

Any intervention that you provide for a patient is communicated in an electronic, written, or oral format (see Chapter 26). Electronic health records (EHRs) or written charts have sections for individualized interventions that are part of the nursing care plan (see Chapter 18) and a patient's permanent medical record. The record entry usually includes

BOX 19.6   Examples of Indirect Care Activities

- Documentation (electronic or written)
- The act of delegation of care activities to assistive personnel
- Medical order transcription
- Infection control (e.g., proper handling and storage of supplies, use of protective isolation)
- Environmental safety management (e.g., making patient rooms safe)
- Telephone consultations with health care providers
- Hand-off reports to other health care team members
- Collecting, labeling, and transporting specimens
- Transporting patients to procedural areas and other nursing units

From Butcher HK, et al: *Nursing interventions classification (NIC)*, ed 7, St Louis, 2018, Elsevier.

a brief description of pertinent assessment findings, the specific intervention(s), and the patient's response. An EHR or written record validates that you performed a procedure and provides valuable information to subsequent caregivers about the approaches needed to provide successful care. Some agencies have interprofessional care plans (i.e., plans representing the contributions of all disciplines caring for a patient). You enter nursing interventions into the plan, documenting the treatment and patient's response.

Effective communication and good teamwork reduce medical errors and prevent adverse patient outcomes (ECRI Institute, 2019). Miscommunication is often the root cause for most reported adverse or sentinel events that occur in health care organizations. Communication with other health care professionals needs to be timely, accurate, and relevant to a patient's clinical situation. Ineffective or incomplete communication often results in uninformed caregivers, needlessly duplicated interventions, delayed procedures, or tasks that are left undone. Chapter 26 explains the approach for effective hand-off communication. Always be clear, concise, and to the point when you communicate nursing interventions.

Delegating, Supervising, and Evaluating the Work of Other Staff Members

A nurse who develops a patient's care plan frequently does not personally perform all the nursing interventions. Some activities you coordinate and delegate to other members of the health care team, including other RNs, LPNs, or assistive personnel. Delegation is the process for a nurse to direct another person to perform nursing tasks and activities (ANA and National Council of State Boards of Nursing [NCSBN], n.d.). Remember that RNs delegate care tasks but not the nursing process. RNs retain responsibility and accountability for the provision of nursing practice (ANA and National Council of State Boards of Nursing [NCBSN], n.d.). You can assign noninvasive and repetitive interventions to certified nurse assistants and other APs. Such activities include skin care, transfer and mobility skills, hygiene, and vital signs for patients who are stable. Evidence shows that the better the communication and collaborative relationship between a nurse and the delegatee, the better the outcome of the delegation process (National Council of State Boards of Nursing, 2016). Delegation requires clinical judgment and accountability for patient care. The frequency and way nursing care activities are delegated often depend on a nursing unit delivery of care model.

Delegation allows you to use your time more wisely and to have other care providers assist. When you delegate tasks to an AP, you are responsible for ensuring that you assign each task appropriately and that the AP completes each task according to the standard of care. This requires ongoing supervision to be sure the AP has performed the task on time without difficulty. You must be sure that any delegated action was completed correctly, documented, and evaluated. You delegate direct care interventions only to personnel who are competent. Chapter 21 describes the principles to follow in delegation.

ACHIEVING PATIENT OUTCOMES

You implement interventions in a manner to achieve patient outcomes (see Chapter 18). In most clinical situations multiple interventions are needed to achieve select outcomes. In addition, patients' conditions often change minute by minute. Therefore it is important to critically apply principles of care coordination such as good time management, organizational skills, and appropriate use of resources to ensure that you deliver interventions effectively and meet desired outcomes (see Chapter 21). Priority setting is critical in successful implementation. Prioritizing nursing diagnoses and outcomes (Chapters 17 and 18) helps you anticipate and sequence nursing interventions when a patient has multiple nursing diagnoses and collaborative problems.

Another way to help patients achieve their outcomes is to provide interventions that help them adhere to their treatment plan. **Patient adherence** means that patients and families invest time in carrying out required health care treatments. Kardas et al. (2013) explain that adherence is complicated because, in the case of medication adherence, it includes willingness of a patient to implement a regimen (daily drug-taking) and persistence (continuity of treatment) in taking the medication. Research has shown that therapy-related factors (e.g., frequency, strength of treatment) and disease-related factors (e.g., duration) mostly showed no impact on adherence, while analysis of age revealed adherence is lowest in very young and very old people (Gast and Mathes, 2019).

Whether a patient chooses to adhere to a treatment relates in part to the patient's health beliefs and the values and perceptions placed on the treatment. When a treatment is seen as beneficial and making a difference in a patient's quality of life, adherence is more likely. Similarly, when there is a risk of negative consequences if a treatment is not followed, adherence is more likely. Most of the research on patient adherence has focused on medication management and chronic disease management. Studies on medication management suggest that presence of family and social support, as well as the use of simple treatment regimens, favorably impacts adherence. In contrast, socioeconomic factors such as unemployment, poverty, and a lack of or inadequate medical/prescription coverage, as well as a high out-of-pocket cost of drugs, contribute to nonadherence (Kardas et al., 2013; Gast and Mathes, 2019). Interestingly, in several studies education alone has not shown to affect adherence positively, but when education is patient-centered and targeted to a patient's unique situation, there is an impact (Heiney et al., 2019). Interventions that improve adherence have been shown to be technical (e.g., simplification of drug regimen and packaging, pill organizers) and behavioral (e.g., memory aids and reminders). Motivational interviewing techniques and multicomponent approaches (e.g., combining education with specific communication strategies) have also been found to be effective in improving adherence (Kardas et al., 2013; Heiney et al., 2019).

When Tonya presents information to Mr. Lawson about why postoperative restrictions are necessary for wound healing, she does more than give the patient a simple list of "what not to do." Instead, she explains the relationship between the postoperative restrictions and Mr. Lawson's personal pattern of daily activities. She ties education to what she has learned about the patient during assessment (Chapter 16). She explains that if he tries to unload groceries or lift a grandchild, the stress of lifting could cause his wound to open farther. In this way the restrictions are more meaningful and relevant for Mr. Lawson.

To ensure that patients have a smooth transition across different health care settings (e.g., hospital to home and clinic, hospital to rehabilitation agency, or hospital to assisted living), it is important to introduce interventions that patients are willing and able to follow. Adequate and timely discharge planning with collaborative patient and family education are the first steps in promoting a smooth transition from one health care setting to another or to the home. Individualize your care and take into consideration the various factors that influence a patient's health beliefs (see Chapter 6). You are responsible for delivering interventions in a way that reflects your understanding of a patient's health beliefs, culture, lifestyle pattern, and patterns of wellness. In addition, reinforcing successes with the treatment plan encourages a patient to follow the care plan.

KEY POINTS

- The professional scope of nursing practice identifies the nature and intent of the ways nurses intervene, which includes the domains of practice, with each domain including direct and indirect nursing interventions.
- When making decisions as to whether an intervention is patient centered, consider who is the patient; how might the patient's attitudes, values, preferences, and cultural background affect how you provide care; which clinical situation is a priority; and how could you best support or show caring as you intervene.
- Standard nursing interventions such as those in practice guidelines and protocols enable nurses to deliver evidence-based interventions to improve patient outcomes; however, standard interventions must be individualized to a patient's unique needs and clinical status.
- A care bundle is a group of interventions related to a disease condition that when implemented together result in better patient outcomes by preventing the most common complications associated with their condition; however, clinical staff must be consistent in performing all interventions within a bundle.
- Consider the context in which you deliver care to each patient and the many interventions available to make the clinical decisions needed to deliver appropriate care in each clinical situation.
- Critical thinking allows you to consider the complexity of interventions, changing priorities, alternative approaches, and the amount of time available to act.
- Your knowledge of pathophysiology and experience with previous patients helps you identify potential complications that can occur. The evidence or scientific rationale for how interventions prevent or minimize complications helps you select the most appropriate preventive measures.
- Your experience and knowledge of a patient's condition and risk factors enables you to observe for and recognize the risks, adapt your choice of interventions to each situation, assess the relative benefit of the intervention versus the risk, and then take risk-prevention measures.
- When implementing patient care, you must consider an organization's goals of efficiency and cost control while still focusing on competently providing timely, thoughtful, safe, patient-centered care.
- The ability to manage care in a timely way conveys caring and concern to your patients.
- A cognitive skill involves knowing the rationale for therapeutic interventions and understanding normal and abnormal physiological and psychological responses, enabling you to adapt skills when necessary and to properly monitor patients as interventions are performed.
- A psychomotor skill such as suctioning an airway or inserting an intravenous catheter is an integration of cognitive and motor activities that must be delivered competently.
- All three implementation skills are employed together to provide direct and indirect care measures successfully.
- Effective patient education requires you to present health care principles, procedures, and techniques in such a way that patients can adapt what they learn to their personal daily routines at home to achieve self-care.
- When you educate patients, respect their expertise with their own health and symptoms, their daily routines, the diversity of their human experiences, their values and preferences as to how they learn, and the importance of shared decision making.
- Timely, relevant, and accurate communication with other health care professionals prevents misinformation, duplication of interventions, delays in procedures, and uncompleted tasks.

REFLECTIVE LEARNING

After your next clinical experience review the interventions you provided for your patient(s). Focus on those that were the most difficult for you.

- Describe how you applied scientific knowledge and what you knew about the patient in delivering those interventions.
- In what manner did you adapt your interventions to the patient care environment and time management?
- What nursing skills did you apply in your implementation of patient care?

REVIEW QUESTIONS

1. An 80-year-old female patient is admitted to the hospital through the emergency room with acute chest pain. Initial testing shows that the patient had a myocardial infarction. Her current vital signs are BP 156/90; HR 88; respirations 20; she is afebrile. The patient has osteoarthritis, causing chronic pain in both knees. She also has glaucoma. The patient is Bosnian and has been in the United States for 3 years. She requires a professional interpreter at bedside when explanations of treatment are provided. Which of the following factors might require you to adapt the way you assist this patient with ambulation? (Select all that apply.)
   1. Patient is Bosnian
   2. Had a recent myocardial infarction
   3. Respirations 20
   4. Osteoarthritis of both knees
   5. Needs an interpreter
   6. Patient is afebrile

2. A nurse is assigned to five patients, including one who was recently admitted and one returning from a diagnostic procedure. It is currently mealtime. The other three patients are stable, but one has just requested a pain medication. The nurse is working with an assistive personnel. Which of the following are appropriate delegation actions on the part of the nurse? (Select all that apply.)
   1. The nurse directs the assistive personnel to obtain a set of vital signs on the patient returning from the diagnostic procedure.
   2. The nurse directs the assistive personnel to go to the patient in pain and to reposition and offer comfort measures until the nurse can bring an ordered analgesic to the patient.
   3. The nurse directs the assistive personnel to set up meal trays for patients.
   4. The nurse directs the assistive personnel to gather a history from the newly admitted patient about his medications.
   5. The nurse directs the assistive personnel to assist one of the stable patients to sit up in a chair for his meal.

3. A nurse is caring for a patient who is expressing pain. The patient has two analgesics ordered prn for pain and has been using cold applications on his surgical site for pain relief. The last time an analgesic was given was 4 hours ago. The patient is scheduled for a physical therapy visit in 2 hours. Which of the following demonstrate good clinical decision making during intervention? (Select all that apply.)
   1. The nurse reviews the options for pain relief for the patient.
   2. The nurse assesses whether the prn medication, ordered every 4 to 6 hours and last given 4 hours ago, is effective and whether a new type of medication is needed.
   3. The nurse reviews the policy and procedure for the cold application.
   4. The nurse considers how the patient might react if the pain medication is held until an hour before physical therapy.
   5. The nurse delegates the assistive personnel to prepare the patient's medication.

4. A nurse working the evening shift has five patients and is teamed up with an assistive personnel. One of the assigned patients has just returned from surgery, one is newly admitted, and one has requested a pain medication. The patient who has returned from surgery just minutes ago has a large abdominal dressing, is still on oxygen by nasal cannula, and has an intravenous line. One of the other patients has just called out for assistance in setting up a meal tray. Another patient is stable and resting comfortably. Which patient is the nurse's current greatest priority?
   1. Patient in pain
   2. Patient newly admitted
   3. Patient who returned from surgery
   4. Patient requesting assistance with meal tray

5. The nurse is caring for a patient with an abdominal obstruction. The nurse irrigates the patient's nasogastric tube and reports the amount of fluid aspirated from the patient's stomach to the health care provider. The patient has an IV infusing; the nurse changes the transparent dressing over the IV site and instructs the patient to report any tenderness at the site. Which of these interventions is an indirect care measure?
   1. Irrigation of nasogastric tube
   2. Changing of transparent dressing
   3. Instructing patient to report tenderness at IV site
   4. Report of the amount of fluid aspirated

6. Which principle is most important for a nurse to follow when using a clinical practice guideline for an assigned patient?
   1. Knowing the source of the guideline
   2. Reviewing the evidence used to develop the guideline
   3. Individualizing how to apply the clinical guideline for a patient
   4. Explaining to a patient the purpose of the guideline

7. The nurse is visiting a patient who lives alone at home. While talking with the patient's family caregiver, the nurse learns that the patient has been missing doses of medications. The patient currently self-medicates. The nurse wants to perform interventions to improve the patient's adherence. Which of the following will affect how this nurse will make clinical decisions about how to help the patient improve adherence? (Select all that apply.)
   1. Reviewing the family caregiver's understanding of purpose of medications
   2. Determining the value the patient places on taking medications
   3. Reviewing the number of medications and time each is to be taken
   4. Determining patient's perceptions of consequences associated with missing specific medicines
   5. Reviewing the therapeutic actions of the medications

8. The nurse enters a patient's room and finds that the patient was incontinent of liquid stool. Because the patient has recurrent redness in the perineal area, the nurse worries about the risk of the patient developing a pressure injury. The nurse cleanses the patient, inspects the skin, and applies a skin barrier ointment to the perineal area. The nurse consults the wound and ostomy care nurse specialist for recommended skin care measures. Which of the following correctly describe the nurse's actions? (Select all that apply.)
   1. The application of the skin barrier is a dependent care measure.
   2. The call to the wound and ostomy care nurse specialist is an indirect care measure.
   3. The cleansing of the skin is a direct care measure.
   4. The application of the skin barrier is an instrumental activity of daily living.
   5. Inspecting the skin is a direct care activity.

9. Which measures does a nurse follow when being asked to perform an unfamiliar procedure? (Select all that apply.)
   1. Checks scientific literature or policy and procedure
   2. Determines whether additional assistance is needed

3. Collects all necessary equipment
4. Delegates the procedure to a more experienced nurse
5. Considers all possible consequences of the procedure
10. A nurse is conferring with another nurse about the care of a patient with a Stage 2 pressure injury. The two decide to review the clinical practice guideline of the hospital for pressure injury care. The use of a clinical practice guideline achieves which of the following? (Select all that apply.)
   1. Allows nurses to act more quickly and appropriately
   2. Sets a level of clinical excellence for practice

3. Eliminates the need to create an individualized care plan for the patient
4. Incorporates evidence-based interventions for stage II pressure injury
5. Provides for access to patient care information within the electronic health record

9. 1, 2, 3, 5; **10.** 1, 2, 4.

Answers: 1. 2, 4, 5; **2.** 3; **3.** 1, 2, 4; **4.** 3; **5.** 4; **6.** 3; **7.** 2, 4; **8.** 2, 3;

Rationales for Review Questions can be found on the Evolve website.

REFERENCES

Agency for Healthcare Research and Quality (AHRQ): *Patient safety network—adverse events, near misses, and errors,* 2019, https://psnet.ahrq.gov/primer/adverse-events-near-misses-and-errors. Accessed May 28, 2021.

American Nurses Association (ANA): *Scope and standards of practice: nursing,* ed 4, Silver Spring, MD, 2021, American Nurses Association.

American Nurses Association (ANA): *Scope of practice,* n.d., https://www.nursingworld.org/practice-policy/scope-of-practice/. Accessed May 28, 2021.

American Nurses Association (ANA) and National Council of state Boards of nursing (NCSBN): *Joint statement on delegation,* n.d., https://www.ncsbn.org/Delegation_joint_statement_NCSBN-ANA.pdf. Accessed May 28, 2021.

Butcher HK et al., et al.: *Nursing interventions classification (NIC),* ed 7, St Louis, 2018, Elsevier.

ECRI Institute: *Top 10 patient safety concerns for 2019, MiraMed's Healthcare Spotlight,* 2019, https://www.miramedgs.com/blog/top-10-patient-safety-concerns-for-2019-ecri-institute.html#:~:text=%20Top%2010%20Patient%20Safety%20Concerns%20for%202019%3A,concerns%20about%20mobile%20health..%20Although%20mobile...%20More%20. Accessed May 28, 2021.

Hospital Consumer Assessment of Healthcare Providers and Systems (HCAHPS): *HCAHPS,* 2020, https://www.surveyvitals.com/start/hcahps?gclid=EAIaIQobChMI5deBqMCw3AIVBrbACh34_w6VEAAYASAAEgIh7vD_BwE. Accessed May 28, 2021.

Jones TL: A holistic framework for nursing time: implications for theory, practice and research, *Nurs Forum* 45(3):185, 2010.

Lyon S: *Occupational therapy: what to know about ADLs and IADLS,* VeryWell Health, 2020, https://www.verywellhealth.com/what-are-adls-and-iadls-2510011. Accessed May 28, 2021.

MBL Technologies.: *Standard nursing terminologies: a landscape analysis,* 2017, https://www.healthit.gov/sites/default/files/snt_final_05302017.pdf. Accessed May 28, 2021.

National Council of State Boards of Nursing: National Guidelines for Nursing Delegation, *J Nurs Regulation* 7(1):5, 2016.

Nurse Journal: *Tips to improve patient education,* 2020. https://nursejournal.org/community/tips-to-improve-patient-education/, accessed May 28, 2021.

Quality Safety Education for Nurses (QSEN): *QSEN competencies,* 2020, http://qsen.org/competencies/pre-licensure-ksas/. Accessed May 28, 2021.

Shekelle P: Overview of clinical practice guidelines, *Up to Date,* 2020. https://www.uptodate.com/contents/overview-of-clinical-practice-guidelines. Accessed May 28, 2021.

RESEARCH REFERENCES

Benner P: *From novice to expert,* Menlo Park, CA, 1984, Addison-Wesley.

Camporota L, Brett S: Care bundles: implementing evidence or common sense? *Crit Care* 15(3):159, 2011.

Gast A, Mathes T: Medication adherence influencing factors—an (updated) overview of systematic reviews, Systematic Reviews volume 8, Article number: 112, 2019, https://systematicreviewsjournal.biomedcentral.com/articles/10.1186/s13643-019-1014-8. Accessed May 29, 2021.

Gorski LA et al.: Infusion therapy standards of practice, 8th ed, *J Infusion Nurs* 44(1S):S1, 2021.

Heiney SP et al.: A systematic review of interventions to improve adherence to endocrine therapy, *Breast Cancer Res Treat* 173(3):499, 2019.

Huisman ERCM et al.: Healing environment: a review of the impact of physical environmental factors on users, *Build Environ* 58:70, 2012.

Institute of Medicine: *Consensus report—Clinical practice guidelines we can trust,* March 23, 2011, https://pubmed.ncbi.nlm.nih.gov/24983061/ Accessed May 28, 2021.

Juknevicius G et al.: Implementation of evidence-based care bundles in the ICU, *Crit Care* 16(Suppl 1):524, 2012.

Kallet RH: Ventilator bundles in transition: from prevention of ventilator-associated pneumonia to prevention of ventilator-associated events, *Respiratory Care* 64 (8) 994, 2019.

Kardas P al., et al.: Determinants of patient adherence: a review of systematic reviews, *Front Pharmacol,* 2013, https://doi.org/10.3389/fphar.2013.00091.

Lavallée JF: The effects of care bundles on patient outcomes: a systematic review and meta-analysis, *Implement Sci* 12:142, 2017.

O'Callaghan N, et al.: Evidence-based design for neonatal units: a systematic review, *Maternal Health, Neonatology and Perinatology,* 5(6) (2019), https://mhnpjournal.biomedcentral.com/articles/10.1186/s40748-019-0101-0. Accessed May 28, 2021.

Ospina M et al.: A systematic review of the effectiveness of discharge care bundles for patients with COPD, *Thorax* 72:31, 2017.

Tanner J et al.: Do surgical care bundles reduce the risk of surgical site infections in patients undergoing colorectal surgery? A systematic review and cohort meta-analysis of 8,515 patients, *Surgery* 158(1):66, 2015.

Evaluation

OBJECTIVES

- Examine the relationships among critical thinking, clinical judgment, and the evaluation of nursing care.
- Critique how each critical thinking standard influences the evaluation process.
- Explain the difference between evaluative measures and assessment measures.
- Explain the importance of using the correct evaluative measures.
- Analyze the relationship between expected outcomes and evaluation measures when evaluating nursing care.
- Explain how evaluation reveals errors or omissions in care.
- Discuss the process of determining the need to revise a patient's plan of care.

KEY TERMS

Evaluation

Evaluative measures

MEDIA RESOURCES

http://evolve.elsevier.com/Potter/fundamentals/
- Review Questions
- Case Study with Questions
- Audio Glossary
- Content Updates
- Answers to QSEN Activity and Review Questions

Evaluation is the crucial final step of the nursing process that determines whether a patient's condition or well-being improved after nursing interventions were delivered (Fig. 20.1). In the previous chapters of this unit, we discussed how you apply the nursing process to make clinical judgments that allow you to deliver appropriate, evidence-based care to individual patients. Evaluation is part of the process, with nurses utilizing physical examination skills, observation, and communication to determine how a patient responds to the interventions delivered in the plan of care.

Think about some of the ways you perform evaluation in your daily activities. Consider caring for your pet dog or cat. Your pet develops a dislike for its food, which you "assess" by noticing food remaining in the bowl. You "plan" an approach by reviewing new pet food options and determining which food to try next. You then buy a new pet food, which you give to your pet (intervention) for its next meal. You "evaluate" the result of your "intervention" by observing whether your pet eats all its food without problems. The evaluation of nursing care, although more complex, is basically the same process. You perform assessment activities within the context of making measurements after an intervention has been performed to evaluate its efficacy.

It is imperative for nurses to monitor their patients' clinical progress on an ongoing basis. Critical thinking in nursing practice strengthens your clinical performance and reflects your ability to resolve patients' health-related problems (Shu-Yuan et al., 2013). Evaluation monitors the progress of each of your patients. The outcomes identified during planning are the conditions that you measure to determine whether the interventions delivered affected the status of a patient, family, or community. The expected outcomes are the criteria for judging through evaluation the success in delivering nursing care. Nurses are responsible

for evaluating the effect of nursing practice on patient outcomes in the areas of health promotion, injury and illness prevention, and alleviation of suffering (Jones, 2016). Outcome evaluation is a part of every health care agency's quality assessment to determine what clinical practices and nursing care standards are effective.

CLINICAL JUDGMENT AND CRITICAL THINKING IN EVALUATION

Clinical judgment is the cognitive process woven throughout each step of the nursing process. There is little benefit in simply delivering nursing interventions to patients unless you know whether the interventions were sufficient or beneficial. Evaluation is the means for knowing a patient's ongoing health status. A literature review of studies examining critical thinking indicators identified four actions that reflect when a nurse shows competence in performing evaluation (Shu-Yuan et al., 2013):

- Examine the results of care according to clinical data collected.
- Compare achieved effects or outcomes with expected outcomes.
- Recognize errors or omissions.
- Understand a patient situation, reflect on the situation, and correct errors.

The continual comparison of your original assessment data with repeated assessment measures (evaluation data) obtained after an intervention informs you of a patient's status. Consider this example: A patient who presents to a health care provider with a productive cough, fever, and a chest x-ray showing lung consolidation is diagnosed with pneumonia. After the patient completes a course of antibiotics, the health care provider repeats the chest x-ray and looks for an improvement in cough and

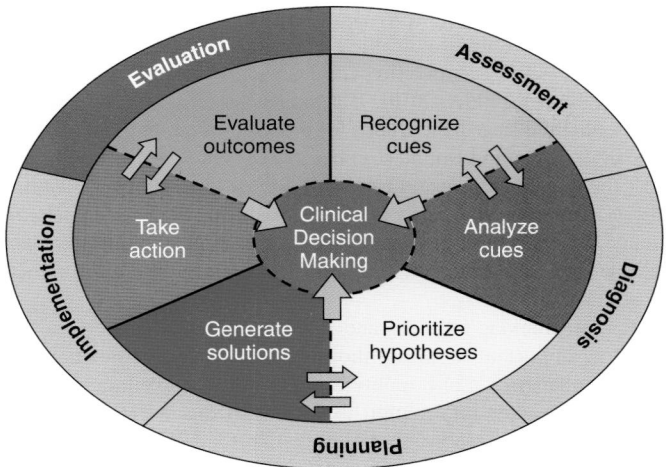

FIG. 20.1 Nursing Process—Evaluation. (Copyright © NCSBN. All rights reserved.)

lowering of body temperature (two original assessments) to evaluate whether the pneumonia has resolved. The nurse follows a similar process. When a nurse cares for a patient with a diagnosis of impaired skin integrity and provides wound care, including application of a warm compress, several steps are involved. The nurse first assesses the appearance of the wound, determines its severity, applies the appropriate form of compress, and returns later to inspect the wound to determine whether the condition has improved. These scenarios depict what ultimately occurs during the process of evaluation: *The nurse performs evaluative measures (e.g., reinspection of the wound) to determine whether a patient met expected outcomes (e.g., decrease in wound drainage within 3 days), not whether nursing interventions were completed.* The expected outcomes established during planning (see Chapter 18) are the standards against which a nurse judges whether wound healing has occurred.

Reflect on the case study with Mr. Lawson and Tonya from the previous chapters in this unit. Mr. Lawson continues to improve following his colectomy. He is going home in a couple of hours. Tonya organizes her care so that she can take the time needed to evaluate the outcomes of her plan of care. Mr. Lawson took two doses of the prn oral analgesic ordered for his pain over the past 8 hours. Thirty minutes after the last dose he rated his pain a 3 on a scale of 0 to 10. He states, "I only really have pain now when I move too quickly." This pain rating has been consistent over the last 24 hours. Mrs. Lawson is in the room, so Tonya takes time to inspect and evaluate Mr. Lawson's wound, describes what she sees, and asks the Lawsons to explain the signs of infection and how to care for the wound at home. Tonya gives the Lawsons the discharge instruction sheet that is part of the standard of care of her nursing unit. She asks Mr. Lawson to explain the types of activity he needs to avoid for the first 2 weeks that he is home.

KNOWLEDGE

Knowledge is a critical thinking element central to evaluation (Fig. 20.2). When a nurse cares for a patient, the nurse's mind acts as a data bank.

Knowledge Base
- Pathophysiology of health condition
- Normal assessment findings
- Characteristics of improved physiological, psychological, socioeconomic, and spiritual status
- Patient's assessment findings, nursing diagnoses, and expected outcomes
- Potential complications associated with health condition and interventions.
  - Characteristics of improved family and group dynamics
  - Community resources

Attitudes
- Perseverance
- Creativity
- Humility
- Responsibility

Environment
- Time pressure
- Setting
- Task complexity
- Interruptions
- Health care resources

Standards
- *ANA Standards and Scope of Nursing Practice*
- Clinical Practice Guidelines and Standards of Practice
- Intellectual standards in measurement
- Agency policies and procedures
- Patient's expected outcomes
- Evidence-based criteria for evaluation
- Professional
  - Standards of care
  - Ethical standards

Experience
- Personal
- Clinical experience with similar interventions
- Clinical experience in seeing change
- Skill competence

FIG. 20.2 Critical thinking in evaluation. (Clinical Judgment Measurement Model copyright © NCSBN. All rights reserved.)

The nurse constantly sorts out knowledge related to the patient's disease or psychological status, the associated signs and symptoms, the nursing diagnoses and collaborative problems associated with the patient's condition, and the interventions delivered in the plan of care. After implementation, the patient's original assessment findings, the outcomes expected, and what measures to use to evaluate care are considered. Clinical judgment is ongoing as a nurse applies knowledge to be able to recognize when patients are progressing, when problems worsen, and when to rethink how to revise the approach to care.

EXPERIENCE

A nurse becomes more expert in evaluation after witnessing the effects of interventions in the past and after witnessing clinical changes. For example, with experience a nurse recognizes the physical appearance of the skin as a pressure injury develops, observes the many nonverbal responses of pain, and observes over time how a patient's ability to ambulate improves. A patient whose physical condition worsens or deteriorates moves from one clinical state to a worse clinical state, which increases the patient's risk for numerous problems (Massey et al., 2017). Because nurses spend more time at a patient's bedside than other health care providers, change recognition is critical. *In the case study, Tonya recognized the physical signs and symptoms of a pulmonary embolus displayed by Mr. Lawson 24 hours after surgery. Her ability to recognize symptoms was a result of her knowledge and experience.*

In an analysis of research studies, Massey et al. (2017) identified three key themes for recognizing patient deterioration: assessing the patient, knowing the patient, and education. Knowing a patient, derived from experience in caring for similar patients or the same patient over time, gives a nurse familiarity with the patient and a heightened awareness of subtle changes in the patient's status (Massey et al., 2017). Nurses recognize patient deterioration based on fully understanding their patients' medical history and current condition, and their previous clinical experience. In addition, nurses who have had more ongoing clinical education and skills training seem to be more perceptive in recognizing clinical change (Massey et al., 2017).

STANDARDS AND ATTITUDES FOR EVALUATION

The American Nurses Association (ANA, 2021) defines standards of professional nursing practice (see Chapter 1), which include standards for the evaluation step of the nursing process. The competencies for evaluation include being systematic and using criterion-based evaluation, collaborating with patients and health care providers, using ongoing assessment data to revise a plan, and communicating results to patients and families. The standards also focus on nurses delivering interventions responsibly and appropriately to minimize unwarranted or unwanted treatment (ANA, 2021).

The criterion-based standards used in evaluation include the expected outcomes identified during planning (see Chapter 18). These outcomes are based on a patient's specific nursing diagnosis and the assessment findings used to form the diagnosis. *For example, in the case of Mr. Lawson, an initial self-reported pain level of 7, his splinting of the incision, and his unwillingness to move around in bed were assessment cues leading to the diagnosis of **Acute Pain**. The outcomes for the diagnosis were focused on removing or relieving assessment cues (e.g., the patient rates pain at a 4 or less on a pain scale of 0-10, has no splinting of incision, and moves freely in bed). Thus the outcomes were standards for the evaluative measures to use in determining Mr. Lawson's progress. Tonya uses the following measures to determine whether Mr. Lawson's pain is relieved: She asks the patient to rate his pain, and she observes his physical movements and breathing.*

Standards for evaluation are also often the outcomes developed from well-established clinical guidelines and protocols. An example is The International Clinical Practice Guideline for pressure injury stages (EPUAP/NPIAP/PPPIA, 2019). If a patient has an identified pressure injury, once it is staged, the criteria for the staging (e.g., appearance, presence of drainage, and wound size) become the outcomes a nurse uses to treat the pressure injury and evaluate response to treatment. The nurse directs interventions toward outcomes of reducing drainage and closing wound edges, criteria in the staging system. Evaluative measures will include inspection of the pressure injury for drainage and measurement of wound diameter.

Critical thinking attitudes and intellectual standards for measurement are important to ensure thorough and accurate evaluation. For example, the attitude of humility is important when you are unsure if you have adequate information to decide whether a patient met the outcome. You are responsible for evaluating the efficacy of your care, which is especially important when you administer critical interventions such as medications, blood products, and intravenous fluids. Clarity, precision, accuracy, and significance are just some of the intellectual standards that make evaluative measures comprehensive.

ENVIRONMENT

As is the case with all steps of the nursing process, environmental factors can promote or disrupt a nurse's ability to evaluate care. You need to spend time in attending to the evaluation process. Delivering interventions in an automatic fashion, without returning to evaluate your patient's results, is irresponsible practice. Use the same principles of environmental control discussed in earlier chapters. Minimize distractions, anticipate the need to evaluate and how it fits in with other care activities, and be thorough when evaluation is complex. Finally, use available resources. You may need help from a more experienced nurse to evaluate patient responses, particularly if you are sensing any kind of worsening condition you have not seen previously.

THE EVALUATION PROCESS

The evaluation process is comprehensive and complex. It requires more than quickly checking whether a patient is stable or not experiencing further problems. Instead, use a methodical approach to determine whether nursing implementation effectively influenced a patient's progress or condition.

Examine Results

Evaluation occurs whenever you have contact with a patient. It is an ongoing process that includes a comparison of before and after an intervention or a comparison after an intervention with an established standard. For example, after assessing a patient's behaviors reflecting anxiety, you offer counseling and instructional support, then compare the behaviors on your initial assessment with those shown after interventions are completed. After a patient undergoes tracheal suctioning, compare the patient's oxygen saturation after suctioning with the presuctioning level and the saturation level you anticipate (e.g., O_2 saturation of at least 95%) to inform you about the efficacy of suctioning and the patient's response to your intervention.

Once you deliver an intervention, you continuously examine results by gathering subjective and objective data from a patient, family, and health care team members (as appropriate). At the same time you reflect on your knowledge regarding a patient's current condition, the treatment, and the resources available for recovery. By also reflecting on previous experiences in caring for similar patients, you are in a better position to know how to evaluate your patient. You can anticipate what to evaluate. You need to have an open mind, keen observation skills, and a neutral perspective to effectively evaluate patient outcomes (Shu-Yuan et al., 2013).

Evaluative Measures. Although you may measure or observe patient data in the same way during the steps of assessment and evaluation, an assessment identifies what, if any, problems exist while an evaluation determines whether the problems you identified during assessment have remained the same, improved, or otherwise changed. **Evaluative measures** are similar to and often the same assessment skills and techniques (e.g., observations, physiological measurements, use of measurement scales, patient interview) you perform during a patient assessment (Fig. 20.3). However, evaluative and assessment measures differ based on when you perform them. Evaluative measures are made after nursing interventions, when you make decisions about a patient's status and progress (Table 20.1).

In many clinical situations it is important to collect evaluative measures over time. You look for trends to determine whether a pattern of improvement or change exists. A onetime observation of a pressure injury is insufficient to determine that the injury is healing. It is important to note a consistency in change. For example, over a period of 3 days has a patient's pressure injury gradually decreased in size, has the amount of drainage declined, and has the redness or inflammation resolved? Recognizing a pattern of improvement or deterioration allows you to reason and decide whether a patient's problems (expressed as nursing diagnoses or collaborative problems) are resolved. This is especially important in the home care or nursing home setting. It may take weeks or even months to determine whether interventions led to

a pattern of improvement. For example, when evaluating a patient's risk for falls over time, has the patient, family, or health care team successfully reduced fall risks in the home, such as eliminating barriers in the home, removing factors impairing the person's vision, or providing direction for the proper use of assistive devices?

It is important to use the right evaluative measure. For example, pain scales are valid and reliable for assessing pain severity (see Chapter 44) and change over time. The pressure injury staging system has specific criteria to accurately stage pressure injuries (see Chapter 48) that allow you to identify whether a treated pressure injury has changed (EPUAP/NPIAP/PPPIA, 2019). The Infusion Nurses Society (INS) (Gorski et al., 2021) has criteria for evaluating IV site phlebitis and infiltration. By using the right measure you are more likely to accurately identify a change, if any, in a patient's condition.

Being able to evaluate behavioral change is more difficult. The information about behavior (e.g., taking medications correctly, following a diet, perceiving less grief) often relies on a patient's self-report. An example of a behavioral measure is any survey or interview that evaluates a patient's ability to perform self-care and achieve self-management. Self-report is a measure of a patient's own perceptions or beliefs and may not truly reflect whether change has occurred. Your willingness to use self-report as an outcome measure of behavior or patient perception reflects trust in the patient. When using self-report, it is important that the patient understands the questions posed and why a verbal response is important to gauge behavioral change.

Patients and their family caregivers need to learn to self-manage their illnesses to improve the quality of their lives. Self-management minimizes the impact of chronic disease or sudden acute illness on a patient's physical health status and functioning. Self-management also enables patients to cope with the psychological effects of an illness. *In Mr. Lawson's case, Tonya planned and implemented educational interventions designed to improve his ability to adopt the behaviors needed for self-care, specifically to follow activity restrictions and perform correct wound care. Tonya evaluates what Mr. Lawson is able to either explain or demonstrate to determine if he has met the expected outcome.* There are relevant, objective, and appropriate evaluative indicators of self-management, including knowledge (information relevant to a patient's situation), independence (independence over areas of health and well-being and other areas that patients feel confident to manage, *and* being independent from others), skills (i.e., ability to manage stress and make decisions), bio-psychosocial markers of health (i.e., quality of life), and positive social networks (Boger et al., 2015) (Table 20.2).

Nursing Outcomes Classification. In Chapter 18 the use of the Nursing Outcomes Classification (NOC) for identifying outcomes was discussed. The classification is a standard nursing language (SNL)

FIG. 20.3 Evaluative measures. Nurse evaluates patient's vital signs.

TABLE 20.1	Evaluative Measures to Determine the Success of Expected Outcomes	
Patient Condition	**Evaluative Measures**	**Expected Outcomes**
Patient has a Stage 2 pressure injury over coccyx, 4 cm diameter, serous drainage.	Inspect color, condition, and location of pressure injury. Measure diameter of pressure injury daily. Note odor and color of drainage from pressure injury.	Erythema is reduced in 2 days. Diameter of injury decreases to 3 cm in 1 week. Injury has no drainage in 2 days.
Following surgery, patient has orders to begin early ambulation protocol. Baseline heart rate 88/min, respirations 18, BP 136/82.	Measure patient's radial pulse after patient ambulates and compare with baseline and the safe maximal heart rate (age-predicted HR max equation equals $208 - [0.7 \times Age]$). Assess respiratory rate during exercise. Observe patient for dyspnea or breathlessness during exercise.	Pulse remains below age-predicted HR during exercise. Pulse rate returns to resting baseline within 10 minutes after exercise. Respiratory rate remains within two breaths of patient's baseline rate. Patient denies feeling of breathlessness.

TABLE 20.2 Self-Management Evaluation

Evaluation Indicator	Examples of Measures
Self-Efficacy	General self-efficacy (GSE) scale; disease-specific self-efficacy scales (e.g., arthritis, diabetes mellitus, cardiac); medication-adherence self-efficacy scale
Health Behavior	Adherence to medication administration (e.g., pill count; number of injections); demonstrated psychomotor skill (e.g., dressing change, self-injection); adherence to medical follow-up visits
Physical Health Status	Clinical indicators (e.g., exercise tolerance, blood pressure control, blood glucose control [HbA$_{1c}$])
Health Service Utilization	Readmission to hospital in 30 days; admission to emergency department
Quality of Life	Quality-of-life scales (e.g., for chronic illness, cancer, chronic pain)
Psychological Indicators	Perceived-stress scale, self-control, or other validated surveys or scales (e.g., Impulsivity Teen Conflict survey)

for the outcomes used in the evaluation step of the nursing process (Box 20.1). The benefits of NOC include (Moorhead et al., 2018):

- Providing a means for nurses and other health care providers to evaluate the status of patients, family, or community.
- Providing an outcome measurement system using standard nursing language (SNL) for all health care settings, specialties, and patients across the life span.

BOX 20.1 EVIDENCE-BASED PRACTICE

Improved Care Plans Using Standard Nursing Language

PICOT Question: Does the use of standard nursing language (SNL) compared with no SNL improve the accuracy of nursing care plans for adult patients?

Evidence Summary

One of the essential characteristics of a quality nursing care plan is accuracy. Nursing care plan content must be comprehensive, which is defined as "documentation according to the different phases of the nursing process," and accurate, which pertains to how precisely the data describe a patient's situation (Thoroddsen et al., 2013). For example, describing a patient's pain as moderate is less accurate than noting the patient's pain severity rating. A nursing care plan must contain accurate nursing diagnoses based on the assessment data gathered from a patient.

An international study involving a systematic review of research examined the impact SNL has on nursing documentation and care plans (Johnson et al., 2018). Nurses use SNL in electronic health care records (EHRs) to label the clinical judgments they make during a nursing assessment. The review of articles concluded that critical thinking improved the accurateness of nursing diagnoses when the nurses used SNL (Johnson et al., 2018). In a separate study involving the use of an SNL continuing education program, it was found that the nurses who completed the program showed improvement in documenting actual nursing diagnoses with the signs and symptoms and etiologies. The nurses also identified risk diagnoses with the risk factors more successfully (Iyanuoluwa et al., 2018).

Application to Nursing Practice

- The consistent use of SNL improves the quality of data collection that enables care providers and health care organizations to evaluate nursing care practices.
- Accuracy of nursing care plans depends on accuracy, content, and degree to which plans are based on data (Johnson et al., 2018).
- In certain EHRs it is increasingly difficult to describe the nursing care that is taking place without SNL (Johnson et al., 2018).
- Using SNL makes documenting nursing care more efficient and facilitates communication of nursing care across health care disciplines and health care environments (Johnson et al., 2018).

- Offering a means to quantify the change in patient status after nursing interventions and to monitor patient progress.

The NOC system includes 540 outcomes, with each outcome having a set of evaluation indicators that describe specific states, perceptions, or behaviors related to the outcome. Each indicator is measured using Likert-type measurement scales (Moorhead et al., 2018) (Table 20.3). The outcome categories are broadly defined, while the indicators (the same as expected outcomes) are more specific and measurable. For example, the outcome category "Comfort Status: Physical" includes indicators such as "symptom control," "physical well-being," and "fluid intake." Five-point Likert-type scales are used with all indicators to demonstrate variability in the state, behavior, or perception patients describe when measuring outcomes. For example, the outcome *Gait* is measured on a scale of "severely compromised to not compromised," while the outcome *Knowledge: Fall Prevention* is measured on a scale of "no knowledge to extensive knowledge." The NOC system was designed to be used with the NANDA-I nursing diagnoses (see Chapter 17) and the Nursing Interventions Classification (NIC) (see Chapter 19). However, the outcome indicators are totally appropriate for use with the International Classification for Nursing Practice (ICNP) diagnoses as well.

QSEN **Building Competency in Informatics** Explain how use of the NOC classification in an electronic health record could improve patient safety. How would such a system help you monitor patient outcomes over time?

Answers to QSEN Activities can be found on the Evolve website.

TABLE 20.3 Examples of Nursing Outcome Classification Outcomes and Indicators

NOC Outcomes	Indicators (Examples)
Anxiety level	Level of restlessness Decreased productivity Level of verbalized anxiety
Knowledge: treatment procedures	Description of treatment procedures Follows restrictions related to procedure Correct use of equipment
Risk control: aspiration	Cleans dentures daily Selects foods based on swallowing ability
Sleep	Hours of sleep Sleep pattern

Adapted from Moorhead S, et al: *Nursing outcomes classification (NOC)*, ed 6, St Louis, 2018, Elsevier.

Compare Achieved Effects with Outcomes. A nursing plan of care includes mutually established nurse-sensitive outcomes relevant to a patient's health status. In Chapter 18 you learned that a nurse-sensitive outcome is a state, behavior, or perception that is measured along a continuum in response to a nursing intervention (Moorhead et al., 2018). During evaluation you use evaluative measures, comparing clinical assessment data, patient behavioral measures, and patient self-report measures collected before implementation with measures gathered after administering nursing care. Next you decide whether the results of care match the expected outcomes for a patient. Critical thinking directs you to analyze the findings from evaluation (Fig. 20.4). Has the patient's condition improved or worsened? Is the patient able to progress, or are there physical factors preventing recovery? Does this patient's motivation or willingness to pursue healthier behaviors influence responses to therapies?

In Mr. Lawson's case the nursing diagnosis of **Anxiety related to uncertainty over ability to return to work** has three established outcomes (Chapter 18):

- Patient shows less facial tension during discussions about recovery from surgery in 24 hours.
- Patient maintains attention during instruction about wound care within 24 hours.
- Patient is able to describe how activity restrictions promote wound healing by discharge.

Tonya has planned and implemented nursing care to prepare Mr. Lawson for a smooth postoperative recovery. She intervenes to minimize his anxiety and provides instruction about his activity restrictions so that he will adhere to his treatment plan. The aim is to achieve adherence so that return to work is realistic. Tonya uses evaluative measures, including observation of the patient's behavior during instruction and then patient self-report of what he understands about normal wound healing. If Tonya's plan of care is successful, the related factor of "uncertainty over ability to return to work" was managed. Tonya will know that because Mr. Lawson was able to attend during instruction and explain how adherence to activity restrictions to promote wound healing will hasten his recovery, one source of anxiety has lessened.

> **REFLECT NOW**
>
> What evaluative measures and outcomes might you anticipate for a patient who has the nursing diagnosis *Risk for Fall*?

Interpreting and Summarizing Findings. A patient's clinical condition often changes during an acute illness. In contrast, chronic illness results in slow, subtle changes, although acute exacerbations can occur. When you compare achieved effects of interventions with outcomes, you interpret or learn to recognize relevant evidence about a patient's condition, even evidence that sometimes does not match clinical expectations. By applying your clinical knowledge and experience, you learn to recognize complications or adverse responses to illness and treatment in addition to expected outcomes.

Careful monitoring and early detection of problems are a nurse's first line of defense. Always make clinical judgments based on your observations of what is occurring with a specific patient and not merely on what happens to patients in general. Because a patient's change in status is not always obvious, you need to gather detailed, patient-specific evaluation measures. Make your evaluation based on your understanding of each patient's behavior, physical status, and reaction to caregivers. Perceptive clinical judgment involves interpreting and summarizing evaluation measures to determine whether a patient's status is improving. Comparing expected and actual findings allows you to interpret and judge a patient's condition and whether predicted changes occurred (Table 20.4). Perform the following steps to objectively evaluate the level of your patient's success in achieving outcomes of care:

1. Examine the outcome criteria to identify the exact desired patient behavior or response.
2. Evaluate a patient's actual behavior or response.
3. Compare the established outcome criteria with the actual behavior or response.

FIG. 20.4 Critical thinking and the evaluation process.

TABLE 20.4   Examples of Objective Evaluation of Outcome Achievement

Outcomes	Patient Response	Evaluation Findings
Patient demonstrates correct hand hygiene by 12/16. Patient describes material to use in dressing change by 12/17. Patient demonstrates dressing change by 12/18.	Patient used antiseptic hand rub correctly to wash hands on 12/16. Patient applied clean gauze correctly and taped securely in place over incision on 12/18.	Patient shows progression toward outcomes and achieved desired behavior.
Coughing is nonproductive by 11/29. Lungs are clear to auscultation by 11/30. Respirations are 20/min by 11/30.	Patient coughed frequently and coughed mucous productively on 11/29 following nebulization. Lungs were clear to auscultation on 11/30. Respirations were 18/min on 11/29.	Patient will require continued nebulizer therapy. Condition is improving.

4. Judge the degree of agreement between outcome criteria and the actual behavior or response.

5. If there is no agreement (or only partial agreement) between the outcome criteria and the actual behavior or response, what is the reason? Why did they not agree? What is your next action?

Evaluation is easier to perform after you care for a patient over a long period or have cared for more than one patient with a similar problem. You are then able to make subtle comparisons of patient responses and behaviors. When you have not cared for a patient over an extended time, evaluation improves by referring to previous experiences or asking colleagues who are familiar with the patient to confirm evaluation findings.

Recognize Errors or Unmet Outcomes

During evaluation the recognition of errors or unmet outcomes requires you to have an open mind, to be patient and confident, and to engage in self-reflection (Shu-Yuan et al., 2013). You cannot assume that your treatment approaches will be successful. You must apply observational skills, critical thinking intellectual standards (see Chapter 15), knowledge, and reflection to recognize the actual results of your care. Reflection is a conscious effort to think about your interventions and outcomes, consider what was positive or challenging, and consider how the plan of care might be revised or done differently in the future. It usually occurs in the presence of a trigger event, which involves a breakdown or perceived breakdown in practice. For example, a nurse observes how a patient reacts to a treatment (e.g., exercise, positioning, or teaching) and realizes that the approach is ineffective. When a nurse reviews a patient's progress and identifies that planned interventions were not done or not completed, this is an example of "missed care" (Ball and Griffiths, 2018). Reflection allows a nurse to recognize how a patient is responding and then adjust interventions accordingly. A nurse will change the frequency of an intervention, change how the intervention is delivered, or select a new intervention based on a patient's response.

Often evaluation reveals patients who have unmet needs. Patients with the same health care problem are not treated the same way. If you mistakenly treat patients the same, you sometimes will make errors in judgment. The systematic use of evaluation provides a way for you to catch these errors. By consistently incorporating evaluation into practice, you minimize errors and ensure that a patient's plan of care is appropriate and relevant and changes according to the patient's specific met and unmet needs.

Correction of Errors

Reflection and subsequent clinical learning are also parts of evaluation. What a nurse gains from caring for patients and carefully evaluating the outcomes of care later contributes to ongoing clinical knowledge development and capacity for making clinical judgments about future

patients (Tanner, 2006). This process helps correct and prevent errors. Reflective reasoning improves the accuracy of clinical decisions and making diagnostic conclusions. This means that, when you gather evaluative measures about a patient, reflection on the findings and exploration about what the findings mean improve your ability to problem solve. Reflection lessens the likelihood that reasoning is based on assumptions or guesswork and increases the likelihood that it is based on objective critical thinking.

REFLECT NOW

Think about an experience in a simulation lab or a recent encounter with a patient. What was your approach and how successful were you? Were there errors made? What might you have done differently to achieve a desired outcome?

Revising the Care Plan

The results of an evaluation help you decide whether to continue, discontinue, or revise the plan of care. The patient and sometimes family members can tell you how interventions helped or did not help (Ackley et al., 2020). This information adds to the evaluative measures you collect. If your patient meets an outcome successfully, either maintain treatment as planned or discontinue that part of the care plan if intervention is no longer required. For example, in the case of a patient achieving a desired level of exercise, you will still continue an exercise regimen. In the case of a patient who is able to demonstrate knowledge of a topic after instruction, further instruction is not needed.

Usually, a change in a patient's condition, needs, or abilities makes alteration of the care plan necessary. This will require you to continue interventions either as planned or less/more often, or you will choose to add interventions focused on the factors affecting outcome achievement. For example, when teaching self-administration of insulin, a nurse discovers that a patient has developed a new problem, a tremor associated with a side effect of a medication. The patient is unable to draw medication from a syringe or inject the needle safely. As a result, the original outcomes of "Patient correctly prepares insulin in a syringe" and "Patient administers insulin injection independently" are no longer appropriate because they cannot be met. The nurse introduces new interventions (instructing a family member in insulin preparation and administration) and revises outcomes—"Family caregiver correctly prepares insulin in syringe" and "Family caregiver administers insulin injection correctly".

When there are unmet or partially met outcomes, or if you determine that perhaps a new problem has developed, reassessment is necessary. A complete reassessment of patient factors relating to an existing nursing diagnosis and etiology is necessary when modifying a plan. If outcomes have not been met, it is helpful to consider the

SMART acronym discussed in Chapter 18 (Ackley et al., 2020). For example, were the outcomes **S**pecific? Were the outcomes **M**easurable? You will often modify or add nursing diagnoses or collaborative problems with appropriate goals and expected outcomes. You then select interventions and redefine priorities of care. Reassessment ensures that the database is accurate and current. It also reveals any missing links (i.e., a critical piece of new information that was overlooked and thus interfered with goal achievement). You sort, validate, and cluster all new data to analyze and interpret differences from the original database (see Chapter 16). An important step in critical thinking in evaluation is to know how a patient is progressing and how problems resolve or worsen.

Tonya evaluates Mr. Lawson's understanding of how activity restrictions aid recovery by using teach-back (see Chapter 25). Tonya states, "I want to know how well you understand your activity restrictions. Describe for me in your own words the restrictions your physician explained." The patient states, "My doctor doesn't want me to do any heavy lifting. It could affect how my wound heals and whether I can get back to work." As Tonya listens to Mr. and Mrs. Lawson further discuss going home, Mrs. Lawson comments, "It will be great for my husband to see the grandkids soon. He's really close to them. He loves playing with the 3-year-old." Tonya uses the evaluative measure of patient self-report during teach-back to determine what Mr. and Mrs. Lawson understand about his activity restrictions. She assessed earlier that the patient enjoys playing with grandkids and picking them up. She revises her instruction to emphasize how lifting children is not an activity Mr. Lawson can perform for several weeks. She adapts her interventions, making her approach more comprehensive.

Discontinuing a Care Plan. After you determine that your patient met the expected outcomes, confirm your evaluation with the patient when possible. If you and the patient agree, you discontinue that part of the care plan. Documentation of a discontinued plan ensures that other nurses will not unnecessarily continue interventions for that part of the plan. Continuity of care assumes that care provided to patients is relevant and timely. You waste time and energy when you do not communicate achieved outcomes with other nurses.

Redefining Diagnoses. After reassessment determine which nursing diagnoses are still accurate for a patient's situation. Critically consider any new assessment cues or changes in previous cues and ask yourself whether you selected the correct diagnosis and if the related factor or risk factor is accurate and current. Then revise the problem list to reflect the patient's changed status. Sometimes you form a new diagnosis or change the prioritization of diagnoses. You base your nursing care on an accurate list of nursing diagnoses. Accuracy is more important than the number of diagnoses selected. As a patient's condition changes, the diagnoses also change.

Revising Expected Outcomes. When revising a care plan, review the expected outcomes for necessary changes. For example, does the time frame for outcomes need to be revised? Does your reassessment reveal an outcome that is unrealistic? Is a more specific measure needed to determine outcome achievement? Examine the appropriateness of outcomes for any unchanged nursing diagnoses, and remember that a change in one health care problem sometimes affects the outcomes for others. *In Mr. Lawson's case, if his anxiety were to worsen again, Tonya would have to revise the plan for managing Mr. Lawson's anxiety and also consider whether her selection of teaching strategies needs to change.* Determining that each expected outcome is realistic for the problem, etiology, and time frame is important.

Revising Interventions. The evaluation of interventions examines two factors: the appropriateness of the intervention selected and the correct application of the intervention. Appropriateness is based on the nursing standards of care for a patient's health problem

(see Chapter 19). Standards of care (i.e., standard interventions, clinical guidelines, care bundles) are the minimum level of care accepted to ensure high-quality patient care. Standards of care define the types of therapies typically administered to patients with defined problems or needs. For example, if a patient who is receiving chemotherapy for leukemia has the nursing diagnosis *Acute Pain related to oral mucosa inflammation from mucositis,* the standard of care established by the nursing department for this problem includes pain-control measures, mouth care guidelines, and diet therapy. Professional organizations such as the Oncology Nursing Society and Association of Critical Care Nurses often have clinical guidelines as standards of care for select health problems. The nurse reviews the standard of care and decides which interventions have been chosen and whether additional ones are required to achieve expected outcomes.

Increasing or decreasing the frequency of an intervention is another approach to ensure better patient outcomes. You adjust frequency of interventions based on a patient's actual response to therapy and your previous experience with similar patients. For example, if a patient continues to have congested lung sounds, you increase the frequency of coughing and deep-breathing exercises to remove secretions and add positioning to ensure airway clearance (see Chapter 41).

During evaluation you find that some planned interventions are designed for an inappropriate level of nursing care. If you need to change the level of care, substitute a different action verb, such as *assist* in place of *provide* or *demonstrate* in place of *instruct.* For example, helping a patient walk requires you to assist the patient during ambulation, whereas providing an assistive device (e.g., a cane or walker) suggests that the patient is more independent. In addition, demonstration requires you to show a patient how a skill is performed rather than simply explaining to the patient how to perform it. Sometimes the level of care is appropriate, but the interventions are unsuitable because of a change in the expected outcome. In this example discontinue the interventions and plan new ones.

Make changes in the plan of care when a patient's response is unfavorable. Consider the nature of the patient's response and consult with other health care team members to make appropriate changes in interventions. Experienced nurses are often excellent resources and can provide valuable insight. Simply changing a care plan is not enough. Implement the new plan and reevaluate the patient's response to the nursing actions. *Evaluation is continuous, occurring through each step of the nursing process.*

DOCUMENT OUTCOMES

Documentation and reporting are important parts of evaluation because it is crucial to share information about a patient's progress and current status with the health care team. Accurate information needs to be present in a patient's medical record and shared during hand-off and ongoing communication so that nurses and other health care team members know whether a patient is progressing and can make ongoing clinical decisions. For example, clearly documented outcomes for new or revised nursing diagnoses are necessary so that all team members are aware of a revised care plan. In settings in which the same nurse will not be providing care throughout a patient's stay, it becomes very important to have consistent, thorough documentation of a patient's progress toward expected outcomes. The use of nursing diagnostic language and the NIC and NOC is becoming more common in electronic medical records, improving the quality, consistency, and accuracy of what is documented. In addition, electronic systems provide linkages to make it easier to interpret cues regarding whether interventions led to expected patient outcomes. When documenting a patient's response to your interventions, describe the interventions, the evaluative measures used, the outcomes achieved, and the continued plan of care. *Here is an example of Tonya's documentation of evaluation of care:*

1430: Instructed patient on importance of handwashing and need to observe surgical wound daily for signs of redness or drainage from incision. Discussed ways to reduce strain on suture line by avoiding lifting any object over 9 kg (20 lb), including his grandchildren. Asked patient to describe when it is necessary to call physician about wound. Patient and wife were able to identify signs of infection and occurrence of pain as reasons to notify physician. Wife was able to demonstrate proper handwashing technique. Patient was able to verbalize several examples of objects not to lift (grandchild, groceries, trash). Provided patient additional instruction in form of pamphlet with outline of wound care steps. Will recommend to home health nurse the need to observe patient and wife perform wound care at home.

Your documentation should present a clear argument from the evaluative data as to whether a patient is progressing. One of the ANA standards for evaluation is to share results of care with patients and their families according to federal and state regulations (ANA, 2021). Keep patients and families informed about the patients' progress. Be aware of guidelines of your agency for the type of clinical information (e.g., diagnostic findings, results of treatment) that you can communicate.

COLLABORATE AND EVALUATE EFFECTIVENESS OF INTERVENTIONS

An important aspect of evaluation is collaboration. Patient-centered care is achieved only when a patient and family are actively involved in the evaluation process. This requires you to consider what is important to your patients, including their values, preferences, and expressed needs. When you identify outcomes in partnership with patients, they become an important resource for being able to tell you whether outcomes are being met. Patients can share their perspective of whether an intervention is successful. For example, a patient knows best whether pain has lessened or whether breathing is easier. The same holds true for the family, who often can recognize changes in patient behavior (such as a change in sleep pattern) sooner than you can because of their familiarity with the patient.

It is essential for nurses to collaborate closely with all members of the health care team during evaluation. Successful collaboration involves interactions in which professionals work together with shared responsibility and interdependence toward achieving patient outcomes. Members of the health care team who contribute to the patient's care also gather evaluative findings. Communicating openly and on a regular basis with the health care team improves the likelihood of staying informed about a patient's responses to care.

Proper evaluation determines the effectiveness of nursing interventions. This includes evaluating whether each patient reaches a level of wellness or recovery that the health care team and patient established in the outcomes of the care plan. In addition, it is important to evaluate whether you have met a patient's expectations of care. Begin by asking patients about their perceptions of care with questions such as "Are you receiving the type of pain relief you expect?" "Do you have enough information to change your dressing when you return home?" "What is your most important need before going home?" Evaluating patient expectations determines a patient's satisfaction with care and strengthens partnering between you and the patient.

BOX 20.2 NDNQI Nurse-Sensitive Outcomes

- Catheter-associated urinary tract infections
- Central line–associated bloodstream infections
- Patient falls (inpatient and ambulatory)
- Patient falls with injury
- Pressure injury rate
- Pain assessment/intervention/reassessment cycles completed
- Peripheral IV infiltration rate
- Physical restraint prevalence
- Ventilator-associated pneumonia rates
- Psychiatric patient assault rates

Adapted from Lockhart L: *Measuring nursing's impact,* Nursing Made Incredibly Easy!: 16(2):55, 2018. https://journals.lww.com/nursingmadeincrediblyeasy/fulltext/2018/03000/measuring_nursing_s_impact.12.aspx; accessed May 30, 2021; National Database of Nursing Quality Indicators (NDNQI): *NDNQI Nursing-Sensitive Indicators,* 2010. https://nursingandndnqi.weebly.com/ndnqi-indicators.html; accessed May 30, 2021.

EVALUATION OF HEALTH CARE

The Centers for Medicaid and Medicare (CMS) do not reimburse health care agencies for the costs associated with treating preventable adverse outcomes such as air embolism, blood incompatibility, or Stages 3 and 4 pressure injuries. The occurrence of such outcomes can be potentially fatal to patients. There are 11 preventable adverse outcomes identified by CMS; four of those (severe pressure injuries, falls and trauma, catheter-associated urinary tract infections [CAUTI], and central line–associated bloodstream infections [CLABSIs]) are nursing-sensitive quality outcomes that can potentially be decreased with greater and better nursing care (Burston et al., 2014; Sung-Heui, 2016). These nursing-sensitive quality outcomes are significant health care problems because they increase patient pain and suffering, prolong hospital stays, and increase health care costs (Burston et al., 2014). The National Database of Nursing Quality Indicators (NDNQI) is the only voluntary nursing quality measurement program. It provides hospitals with unit-level quality performance reports, allowing for comparison of state, national, and regional performance percentiles in the United States. The NDNQI gathers data on several nurse-sensitive outcomes (Box 20.2). Hospitals that achieve Magnet Status are required to gather and report NDNQI data.

As a practicing nurse you will implement clinical guidelines, care bundles, and other evidence-based interventions to prevent these outcomes. Health care organizations gather monthly data on the rates of nursing-sensitive preventable outcomes. All patient care units regularly evaluate their progress in reducing these preventable outcomes and implement ongoing quality improvement efforts (see Chapter 5). A nurse can be most effective in impacting these organization-wide preventable outcomes by delivering patient-centered care and conducting ongoing evaluation of the efficacy of interventions. Learning what is effective for individual patients builds your knowledge of both evidence-based and practical approaches for improving quality of care.

KEY POINTS

- Critical thinking and clinical judgment are integral to evaluation as evidenced by (1) examining the results of care according to clinical data collected; (2) comparing achieved effects with expected outcomes; (3) recognizing errors or omissions; and (4) understanding a patient situation, participating in self-reflection, and correcting errors.

- A nurse applies knowledge about a patient's clinical status, signs and symptoms of health conditions, and anticipated effects of interventions to make the judgment needed to determine whether patients are progressing or problems are worsening.
- Expertise in evaluation relies on experience, requiring a nurse to have witnessed the effects of interventions in the past, to have witnessed clinical change, and then to make evaluative decisions.
- The criterion-based standards used in evaluation are the expected outcomes established during planning.
- Critical thinking attitudes and intellectual standards for measurement are important for ensuring thorough and accurate evaluation.
- Although you may measure or observe patient data in the same way during assessment and evaluation, an assessment identifies what, if any, problems exist, while evaluative measures determine whether the problems you identified during assessment have remained the same, improved, or otherwise changed.
- By using the right evaluative measure, the expected outcome identified during planning, you are more likely to accurately identify whether there has been a change in a patient's condition.
- Standards for evaluation are often outcomes developed from well-established clinical guidelines and protocols.
- During the evaluation phase of the nursing process you perform evaluative measures to compare clinical assessment data, patient behavior, and patient self-reported data collected before implementation with data gathered after administering nursing care to determine whether the results of care match the expected outcomes for a patient.
- The evaluation process involves the use of observational skills, critical thinking, intellectual standards, knowledge, and reflection to recognize errors or omissions so that adjustments to interventions can be made in care plan revision.
- Conducting evaluation involves reviewing evaluative measures to determine whether outcomes are met successfully so that decisions can be made to continue, discontinue, or revise a plan of care.
- When patients do not meet outcomes, you perform a reassessment and identify the factors that interfere with their achievement, which usually involves a change in a patient's condition, needs, or abilities.

REFLECTIVE LEARNING

Tonya organizes herself so that she can take the time needed to evaluate the outcomes of her plan of care. Mr. Lawson has the nursing diagnosis of *Acute Pain related to trauma of surgical incision*. The patient has taken two doses of the prn oral analgesic ordered for his pain over the past 8 hours. Thirty minutes after the last dose Mr. Lawson rated his pain a 3 on a scale of 0 to 10; he states, "I only really notice the pain now when I move too quickly." The pain has been rated 3 over the last 24 hours. An outcome for the patient's goal of achieving pain relief is for pain scores to be at 4 or less. Mrs. Lawson is in the room, so Tonya takes time to give the Lawsons the discharge instruction sheet that is part of the standard of care of her nursing unit. She asks Mr. Lawson to explain the types of activity he must avoid for the first 2 weeks he is at home.

- Describe the type of evaluation measure Tonya uses when asking Mr. Lawson to explain the types of activities he should avoid. What limitations are there in using this type of evaluation measure?
- Explain how Tonya can determine whether the patient's nursing diagnosis of *Acute Pain* has been resolved. Describe how this affects her other priorities.
- Explain how Tonya's evaluation of the patient's ability to learn about activity restrictions can be patient-centered.

REVIEW QUESTIONS

1. A nurse is caring for a 58-year-old patient who had a stroke, causing loss of function of the left leg and reduced movement in the left hand and arm. The patient is alert and able to follow instructions. The patient's dominant side is left. While observing the patient attempt to eat, the nurse notes the patient is unable to use utensils easily in the right hand. The patient is able to lift a glass with the right hand but has trouble opening food containers. Because of weakness on the left side, the patient has limitations in chewing. The nurse identifies a nursing diagnosis of *Self Care Deficit: Impaired Self Feeding*. Which of the following are appropriate nurse-sensitive outcomes for this patient?
   1. Patient provided left-handed assist device
   2. The range of movement in left arm is 20 degrees flexion
   3. Patient opens food container
   4. Patient provided soft diet
   5. Patient gets food onto utensil
   6. Patient able to chew food

2. A nurse who has worked on a cardiac step-down unit for 4 years receives a new patient from the intensive care unit following a 3-day stay for postmyocardial infarction (MI). The nurse knows that the patient is at risk for a recurrent MI, heart failure, arrhythmias, or a stroke. The patient has stable vital signs when arriving at the new unit: pulse 82 and regular, blood pressure (BP) between 120 and 130 over 80 to 90, and denial of chest pain. The nurse checks the patient's IV for proper function, positions the patient comfortably, and explains that the patient will be checked frequently. Sixty minutes after the initial assessment, the nurse responds to the patient's call light. The patient states, "I am not feeling well." Which of the following are evaluative measures the nurse should perform in this situation?
   1. Measurement of BP
   2. Asking patient to self-report location and severity of pain
   3. Asking patient to move both arms and legs
   4. Measurement of heart rate rhythm
   5. Questioning patient about risks following an MI
   6. Asking patient, "Tell me what you mean by not feeling well"

3. A nurse admits a 32-year-old patient for treatment of acute asthma. The patient has labored breathing, a respiratory rate of 28 per minute, and lung sounds with bilateral wheezing. The nurse makes the patient comfortable and starts an ordered intravenous infusion to administer medication that will relax the patient's airways. The patient tells the nurse after the first medication infusion, "I feel as if I can breathe better." The nurse auscultates the patient's lungs and notes decreased wheezing with a respiratory rate of 22 per minute. Which of the following is an evaluative measure? (Select all that apply.)
   1. Asking patient to breathe deeply during auscultation
   2. Counting respirations per minute
   3. Asking the patient to describe how his breathing feels
   4. Starting the intravenous infusion
   5. Auscultating lung sounds

4. A patient has labored breathing, a respiratory rate of 28 per minute, and lung sounds that reveal wheezing bilaterally. The nurse starts an ordered intravenous infusion to administer medication that will relax the patient's airways. When the nurse asks how the patient feels, he responds by saying, "I feel as if I can breathe better." The nurse auscultates the patient's lungs and notes decreased wheezing with a respiratory rate of 22 per minute. Which of the following is a subjective evaluative measure?
   1. Counting respirations per minute
   2. Asking the patient to describe how his breathing feels

3. Observing breathing pattern
4. Auscultating lung sounds
5. Having the patient explain purpose of the IV infusion

5. Which of the following statements correctly describes the evaluation process? (Select all that apply.)
    1. Evaluation involves reflection on the approach to care.
    2. Evaluation involves determination of the completion of a nursing intervention.
    3. Evaluation involves making clinical decisions.
    4. Evaluation requires the use of assessment skills.
    5. Evaluation is performed only when a patient's condition changes.

6. A nurse in a community health clinic has been caring for a young female teenager with Type 1 diabetes mellitus for several months. The expected outcome for this patient is to achieve self-management of insulin administration by discharge. Identify appropriate evaluative measures for self-management for this patient. (Select all that apply.)
    1. Quality of life
    2. Patient satisfaction
    3. Clinic follow-up visits
    4. Adherence to self-administration of insulin
    5. Description of side effects of medications
    6. Patient report of blood glucose level

7. A nurse has been caring for a patient over 2 consecutive days. During that time the patient had an intravenous (IV) catheter in the right forearm. At the end of shift on the second day the nurse inspects the catheter site, observes for redness, and asks whether the patient feels tenderness when the site is palpated. The nurse reviews the medical record from 24 hours ago and finds the catheter site was without redness or tenderness. Which of the activities below reflect the nurse's ability to perform patient evaluation? (Select all that apply.)
    1. Comparing patient response with previous response
    2. Examining results of clinical data
    3. Recognizing error
    4. Self-reflection
    5. Checking medical record for when IV was inserted

8. While receiving a hand-off report, a nurse asks how a patient's condition from a serious infection changed since yesterday. The nurse leaving the shift reports that the patient has two priority nursing diagnoses—fluid imbalance and fever. The receiving nurse begins to provide care by measuring the patient's body temperature, inspecting the condition of the skin, reviewing the intake and output record, and checking the summary notes describing the patient's progress since the day before. The nurse asks an assistive personnel to measure intake and output during the shift. What critical thinking indicators reflect the nurse's ability to perform evaluation? (Select all that apply.)
    1. Checking the summary notes
    2. Asking the leaving RN about the patient's condition
    3. Assigning assistive personnel to measure intake and output
    4. Comparing current outcomes with those set for the patient's goals
    5. Reflecting on patient's progress

9. A nurse in the recovery room is monitoring a patient who had a left knee replacement. The patient arrived in recovery 1 hour ago. The nurse observes the patient to be restless, turning frequently, and groaning; the patient's heart rate is 92 compared with 76 immediately postoperatively. Blood pressure is stable since admission to the recovery room. The nurse reviews the medical orders for analgesic therapy. The nurse notes that the postoperative dose of an ordered analgesic has not yet been given. Which of the following factors is most likely to cause the nurse to reflect on the patient's situation?
    1. The patient is recovering normally.
    2. The nurse observes symptoms of restlessness
    3. The patient's blood pressure trend
    4. The delay in administration of the analgesic

10. A nurse enters a patient's room and begins a conversation. During this time the nurse evaluates how a patient is tolerating a new diet plan. The nurse decides to also evaluate the patient's expectations of care. Which of the following is appropriate for evaluating a patient's expectations of care?
    1. On a scale of 0 to 10 rate your level of nausea.
    2. The nurse weighs the patient.
    3. The nurse asks, "Do you believe that you received the information you needed to follow your diet?"
    4. The nurse states, "Tell me four different foods included in your diet."

Answers: 1. 3, 5, 6; **2.** 1, 2, 4, 6; **3.** 2, 3, 5; **4.** 2, 5; **5.** 1, 3, 4; **6.** 1, 3, 4, 5; **7.** 1, 2; **8.** 1, 2, 4, 5; **9.** 4; **10.** 3.

Rationales for Review Questions can be found on the Evolve website.

REFERENCES

Ackley BJ et al.: *Nursing diagnosis handbook,* ed 12, St Louis, 2020, Elsevier.

American Nurses Association (ANA): *Scope and standards of practice: nursing,* ed 4, Silver Spring, MD, 2021, American Nurses Association.

Ball J, Griffiths P: *Missed nursing care: a key measure for patient safety,* Agency for Healthcare Research and

Quality Patient Safety Network, 2018, https://psnet. ahrq.gov/perspective/missed-nursing-care-key-measure-patient-safety. Accessed May 30, 2021.

Burston S et al.: Nurse-sensitive indicators suitable to reflect nursing care quality: a review and discussion of issues, *J Clin Nurs* 23(13/14):1785, 2014.

Jones T: Outcome measurement in nursing: imperatives, ideals, history, and challenges, *Online J Issues Nurs* 21(2):1, 2016.

Moorhead S et al.: *Nursing outcomes classification (NOC),* ed 6, St Louis, 2018, Elsevier.

RESEARCH REFERENCES

Boger E et al.: Self-management and self-management support outcomes: a systematic review and mixed research synthesis of stakeholder views, *PLoS One* 10(7):e0130990, 2015.

European Pressure Ulcer Advisory Panel (EPUAP) and National Pressure Injury Advisory Panel (NPIAP) and Pan Pacific Pressure Injury Alliance (PPPIA): *Treatment of pressure ulcers/injuries: quick reference guide,* Emily Haesler (ED). EPUAP/NPIAP/PPPIA, 2019.

Gorski LA et al.: Infusion therapy standards of practice, 8e, *J Infusion Nurs* 44(1S):S1, 2021.

Iyanuoluwa O A et al: Effect of standardized nursing language continuing education programme on nurses'

documentation of care at University College Hospital, Ibadan, *Nurs Open* 5(1):37, 2018.

Johnson L et al.: A systematic literature review of accuracy in nursing care plans and using standardised nursing language, *Collegian* 25(3):355, 2018.

Massey D et al: What factors influence ward nurses' recognition of and response to patient deterioration? An integrative review of the literature, *Nurs Open* 4(1):6, 2017.

National Pressure Injury Advisory Panel (NPIAP): *NPIAP position statement on staging—2017 clarifications,* 2017, https://cdn.ymaws.com/npiap.com/resource/resmgr/npuap-position-statement-on-.pdf. Accessed October 31, 2020.

Shu-Yuan C, et al.: Identifying critical thinking indicators and critical thinker attributes in nursing practice, *J Nurs Res* 21(3):204, 2013.

Sung-Heui B: The Centers for Medicare & Medicaid services reimbursement policy and nursing-sensitive adverse patient outcomes, *Nurs Econ* 34(4):161, 2016.

Tanner CA: Thinking like a nurse: a research-based model of clinical judgment in nursing, *J Nurs Educ* 45(6):204, 2006.

Thoroddsen A et al.: Accuracy, completeness and comprehensiveness of information on pressure ulcers recorded in the patient record, *Scand J Caring Sci* 27:84, 2013.

Managing Patient Care

OBJECTIVES

- Explain the characteristics and traits of a transformational leader.
- Compare the types of nursing care delivery models.
- Identify the elements of patient- and family-centered care.
- Discuss the ways in which a nurse manager supports staff involvement in a decentralized decision-making model.
- Distinguish the different elements of the decision-making process.
- Create a plan to develop your own leadership skills.
- Discuss skills needed to coordinate patient care effectively.
- Identify evidence-based methods that ensure accurate communication for building teams.
- Discuss principles to follow in the appropriate delegation of patient care activities.
- Develop a plan to maintain your competence and expand your knowledge throughout your professional nursing career.

KEY TERMS

Accountability
Authority
Autonomy

Case management
Delegation
Patient- and family-centered care

Responsibility
Shared governance
Transformational leadership

MEDIA RESOURCES

http://evolve.elsevier.com/Potter/fundamentals/
- Review Questions
- Case Study with Questions

- Audio Glossary
- Content Updates
- Answers to QSEN Activity and Review Questions

It is important for you to acquire the necessary knowledge and competencies that ultimately allow you to practice as a nurse. The National Council of State Boards of Nursing (NCSBN, 2021) develops licensure examinations for registered nurses (RNs) and licensed practical nurses (LPNs) to ensure entry-level nurses can safely practice nursing. Although nurse practice acts and professional nursing standards vary, you will be expected to possess certain knowledge, skills, and abilities when you enter the nursing profession (Table 21.1). Wherever you practice nursing, you use critical thinking and sound clinical judgment to implement professional standards of care, use health care resources appropriately, use time productively, set priorities, collaborate with the health care team, and apply leadership skills. Delivering nursing care within a health care system is challenging because of the changes that influence health professionals, patients, and health care agencies (see Chapter 2). However, change offers opportunities. As you develop the knowledge and skills to become a nurse, you learn what it takes to effectively manage the patients for whom you care and to take the initiative in becoming a leader among your professional colleagues.

BUILDING A NURSING TEAM

Nurses who work in health care agencies and on units that have cultures that promote autonomy, quality, and collaboration are more satisfied and experience lower levels of moral distress (Hiler et al., 2018; Shimp, 2017). Professional nurses are self-directed and, with proper leadership and motivation, work together to solve complex problems. Your education and commitment to practice nursing within established standards and guidelines help you become part of a cohesive and strong nursing team that values mentoring, integrity, and teamwork. A strong nursing team works together to achieve the best outcomes for patients. Effective team development requires team building and training, trust, communication, and a workplace that facilitates collaboration (Huber, 2018). Patient care units where teamwork is stronger are associated with improved patient safety and nurse well-being (Rosen et al., 2018). Stronger levels of teamwork often contribute to higher levels of job satisfaction among nurses (Kaiser and Westers, 2018).

An empowering work environment brings out the best in nurses. It concentrates on effective patient care systems, supports risk taking and innovation, focuses on results and rewards, and offers professional opportunities for growth and advancement. Building an empowered nursing team begins with the nurse executive, who is often a chief nursing officer. The executive's position within an agency is critical in uniting the strategic direction of an agency with the philosophical values and goals of nursing. The nurse executive is a clinical and business leader who is concerned with maximizing quality of care and cost-effectiveness while maintaining relationships and professional satisfaction of the staff. Perhaps the most important responsibility of the nurse executive is to establish a philosophy for nursing that enables managers and staff to provide quality nursing care.

Effective nurse managers play a critical role in developing successful teams that work together (Huber, 2018; James, 2018; Kivland, 2018)

TABLE 21.1   Entry-Level Nurse Knowledge, Skills, and Abilities

Knowledge	Skills	Abilities
Nursing Process • Steps	Critical Thinking • Consider different health care solutions, conclusions, or approaches to problems	Oral Comprehension • Listen to and understand information and ideas that are spoken
Professional Responsibilities • Ethical principles • Scope of practice • Error reporting and follow-up	Therapeutic Communication • Adapt one's communication style and demonstrate sensitivity to build rapport with others	Dependability • Be reliable, responsible, and accountable • Be punctual and on time
Documentation • Medical terminology and abbreviations • Information to document	Documenting • Document clearly, concisely • Follow documentation standards and policies	Written Expression • Use appropriate words in writing so that others can understand
Focused Assessment • Types of assessments • Evaluation of effectiveness	Focused Assessment • Select appropriate assessment type based on patient problems, symptoms, or diagnosis	Oral Expression • Use appropriate words in speaking • Speak in a way that others can understand
Plan of Care • Methods • Changes in patient conditions	Clinical Judgment • Recognize cues • Take action • Evaluate outcomes	Task and Information Ordering • Implement actions in an order that follows policies and procedures • Set priorities appropriately
Patient Needs Assessment • Methods • Topics	Active Listening • Give full attention and repeat back to clarify information • Ask appropriate questions	Self-sufficiency • Work independently with little assistance from others • Seek assistance appropriately
Patient, Family, and Caregiver Education • Teaching techniques • Evaluation of effectiveness	Patient Education • Help patients interpret health information • Provide information at a level that patients can understand	Speech Clarity • Communicate clearly • Ensure that others can understand what you say
Vital Signs Collection • Techniques and types • Normal and abnormal values • Interventions based on patient values	Patient Monitoring • Recognize changes in patient condition • Anticipate complications or adverse outcomes	Social Confidence • Display self-confidence when working with others
Patient-Centered Care • Holistic principles • Integrating care including patients, families, and caregivers	Problem Solving • Develop and evaluate interventions • Resolve complex problems	Written Comprehension • Read and understand written information and ideas
	Professional Communication • Communicate clearly and concisely • Use appropriate communication styles based on situation	

Modified from National Council of State Boards of Nursing (NCSBN): *Next-Generation NCLEX Project,* 2021, https://www.ncsbn.org/next-generation-nclex.htm; and National Council of State Boards of Nursing (NCSBN): *Strategic Practice Analysis: Executive Summary,* 2018, https://www.ncsbn.org/18-Strategic-Practice-Analysis.pdf; accessed April 5, 2021.

(Box 21.1). The nurse manager who uses **transformational leadership** is focused on change and innovation through team development, serves as a mentor for staff, and develops and supports the moral agency of nurses (Grace, 2018; Huber, 2018). Transformational leaders spend time on the unit with the staff sharing ideas, empowering the staff, supporting opportunities to enhance the team, showing appreciation, recognizing team members for a job well done, and holding team members accountable.

Together a manager and the nursing staff share a philosophy of care for their work unit. A philosophy of care includes the professional nursing staff's values and concerns for the way they view and care for patients. For example, a philosophy addresses the purpose of the nursing unit, how staff members work with patients and families, and the standards of care for the work unit. The selection of a nursing care delivery model and a management structure that both support professional nursing practice is essential to the philosophy of care.

A nurse manager's leadership style affects the work environment and patient outcomes. Contemporary nurse leaders have a shared vision that leads the team to a common goal. Because nurses have specialized knowledge, they need leaders who value and foster the attainment of new knowledge (Huber, 2018). Nurse managers who use interactional and relationship-based leadership styles create a positive work environment by fostering interaction and generating stability to create the energy a team needs to adapt to and grow with a constantly changing health care environment (Huber, 2018).

One contemporary relationship-based leadership style is servant leadership. Servant leaders choose to serve others before they decide to become leaders. Their priority is to put the needs of others first and to promote personal growth and autonomy by ensuring their individual employees' highest priority needs are met (Huber, 2018; Tatsumi, 2019). Servant nurse leaders work closely with their team to understand individual members' strengths and weaknesses. A servant

BOX 21.1 Characteristics of Effective Leaders

- Develop interpersonal trust and ensure effective communication with individuals and teams.
- Have awareness of personal strengths and weaknesses, allowing vulnerabilities to show.
- Take initiative and sustain motivation, especially during times of uncertainty.
- Seek multiple perspectives and opinions to generate options and solutions when problem solving.
- Rebound from setbacks with positivity.
- Understand what they can and cannot change.
- Schedule time and space to regularly reflect, recharge, and reframe.
- Take responsibility for decisions.
- Display caring, understanding, and empathy for others.
- Motivate and empower others.
- Identify need to change and support change effectively.
- Use different leadership styles (e.g., transformational, authentic, value-based) appropriately.

Modified from James AH: Action learning can support leadership development for undergraduate and postgraduate nurses, *Br J Nurs* 27(15):876, 2018; Kivland C: Successfully managing emotions and behavior: emotional intelligence matters more than ever to your leadership career, *Healthc Exec* 33(1):68, 2018; Huber DL: *Leadership & nursing care management*, ed 6, St Louis, 2018, Elsevier.

leader creates teams based on this understanding and ensures that the nurses on a unit are working in the positions that best use their strengths (Tatsumi, 2019). Servant nurse leaders also practice humility. They understand that although they possess a great deal of knowledge, they do not know all the answers. They remain modest and calm, and they give credit to their staff members for successes (Tatsumi, 2019). Effective nurse leaders use a variety of evidence-based strategies to create healthy work environments and lead their teams through change (Box 21.2).

Magnet Recognition Program®

One way of creating an empowering work environment is through the Magnet Recognition Program® (see Chapter 2). The Magnet Recognition Program's Pathway to Excellence Framework® is based on six standards that are crucial to creating a positive practice environment for nurses (American Nurses Credentialing Center [ANCC], n.d.):
- Shared decision making
- Leadership
- Safety
- Quality
- Well-being
- Professional development

A hospital that is Magnet® certified has a transformed culture with a practice environment that is dynamic, autonomous, collaborative, and positive for nurses. The culture focuses on concern for patients. Typically, a Magnet hospital has clinical promotion systems and research- and evidence-based practice programs. The nurses have professional autonomy over their practice and control over the practice environment (Hume and Hall, 2020). A Magnet hospital empowers a nursing team to make changes and be innovative (Nelson-Brantley et al., 2018). Professional nurse councils at the organizational and unit level help to create an empowerment model. This culture and empowerment combine to produce a strong collaborative relationship among team members and improve patient quality outcomes (ANCC, n.d.; Hume and Hall, 2020).

BOX 21.2 EVIDENCE-BASED PRACTICE

Nurses' Work Engagement

PICOT Question: Do nurse leaders who use transformational or relationship-based leadership strategies create healthier work environments and improve patient outcomes?

Evidence Summary
Creating healthy work environments and improving patient outcomes require effective nursing leadership at all levels in an agency, from the nurse executive to the nurse manager to the staff nurses. Effective nurse leaders often use transformational or relationship-based leadership to create workplaces that promote better outcomes for patients and nurses (Alilyyani et al., 2018; Boamah et al., 2018).

Nurses who attend professional leadership development programs have improved collaboration and communication skills, which ultimately lead to a healthy work environment and better patient outcomes (Lacey et al., 2017). Focusing on transformational or relationship-based leadership is supported by current evidence. For example, authentic leadership, a type of relationship-based leadership, has been shown to improve the work environment (e.g., job satisfaction, employee health and well-being) and patient outcomes (Alilyyani et al., 2018). Authentic leaders choose a leadership style consistent with their personalities. They are dedicated to their own growth and build strong relationships with others. Regardless of the leadership strategy used, strong clinical leaders who encourage collaboration and regular interaction among nurse experts within the same health care agency or across different agencies create environments that have a positive impact on patient outcomes, quality of care, and the culture of the workplace (Haines et al., 2018; Wei et al., 2020).

Application to Nursing Practice
- Build positive relationships with colleagues on your nursing unit (Nelson-Brantley, 2018; Wei et al., 2020) as well as with colleagues who work in other health care agencies (Haines et al., 2018).
- Attend professional conferences to stimulate your personal and professional growth and develop your leadership and communication skills (Lacey et al., 2017; Boamah et al., 2018).
- Be engaged with initiatives in your agency that focus on reducing hospital-acquired conditions (e.g., falls, pressure injuries, catheter-associated urinary tract infections) (Lacey et al., 2017).
- Respect the contributions of all members of the health care team and make a conscious commitment to make a positive impact in your workplace every day (Alilyyani et al., 2018; Boamah et al., 2018).

Nursing Care Delivery Models

A nursing care delivery model is designed to help your patients achieve desirable outcomes. Nursing care delivery models contain the common components of nurse-patient relationship, clinical decision making, methods for patient assignments and work allocation, interprofessional communication, and management of the environment of care (Huber, 2018).

Two classic nursing models used to provide patient care in health care agencies are team nursing and primary nursing. In team nursing, care is provided by a group of people led by an RN. The team often includes other RNs, licensed practical nurses, and assistive personnel (APs). To be successful, this model requires effective team leadership, collaboration, and communication (Huber, 2018).

In primary nursing, one RN assumes the responsibility for a caseload of patients from admission to discharge. The same nurse provides care for the same patients throughout their hospitalization. When the nurse is not scheduled to work on the unit, directions are left (e.g., in the plan of care) for other RNs to follow. The model became more popular in the 1970s and early 1980s as hospitals began to employ more RNs. It is typically not practiced today because of the high cost of an all-RN staffing model (Huber, 2018). Total patient care is similar to primary nursing. In this model an RN is responsible for all aspects of care for one or more patients during a shift of care, working directly with patients, families, and health team members.

More common models used today are patient- and family-centered care and case management. Patient- and family-centered care promotes mutual partnerships among the patient, family, and health care team to plan, implement, and evaluate nursing and health. At the center of patient-centered care is the patient or family member as the source of control and full partner in providing care (QSEN Institute, 2020). An RN is the health care leader who assesses patient needs, identifies mutual outcomes, monitors patients for clinical changes, and directs care. The Institute for Patient- and Family-Centered Care identified four core concepts for patient-centered care (IPFCC, n.d.):

1. *Dignity and respect,* ensuring that the care provided is given based on a patient's and family's knowledge, values, beliefs, and cultural backgrounds
2. *Information sharing,* meaning that health care providers communicate and share information so that patients and families receive timely, complete, and accurate information to effectively participate in care and decision making
3. *Participation,* whereby patients and families are encouraged and supported in participating in care and decision making
4. *Collaboration,* demonstrated by the health care leaders collaborating with patients and families in policy and program development, implementation, and evaluation, as well as by patients who are fully engaged in their health care

Nurses support and promote patient engagement and empowerment when using patient- and family-centered communication, bedside shift report, and patient- and family-centered interprofessional rounds (IPFCC, n.d.; Bigani and Correia, 2018).

Case management coordinates and links health care services across all levels of care for patients and their families while streamlining costs and maintaining quality (see Chapter 2). The case-management system is focused on achieving patient outcomes within effective time frames and with available resources (Huber, 2018). Case managers work with patients and families to identify issues and overcome barriers to help patients become healthier (ACMA, n.d.). Current evidence shows case managers link and coordinate health care services with patients and their families while achieving quality cost-effective outcomes (Brown et al., 2017). Case managers, either individually or as part of a team, oversee the management of patients with complex nursing and medical problems (e.g., patients with diabetes mellitus or traumatic brain injury) across all levels of care. Case managers are often advanced practice nurses who, through specific interventions, help to improve patient outcomes, optimize patient safety by facilitating care transitions, decrease length of stay, and lower health care costs. They are accountable for cost management and quality.

For example, a case manager coordinates a patient's acute care in the hospital and follows up with the patient after discharge, either to home, rehabilitation, or a long-term care setting. Case managers do not provide direct care. Instead, they collaborate with direct-care providers and actively coordinate patient discharge planning, ensuring necessary services and resources are available (e.g., home aides, physical therapy) and making cost-efficient choices (e.g., selection of medical equipment or long-term care facilities). Ongoing communication with team members facilitates a patient's transition to home or another health care setting.

Decision Making

Decision making is a critical skill for an effective leader and manager (Huber, 2018). A nurse executive supports nurse managers by advocating

---

BOX 21.3   Responsibilities of a Nurse Manager

- Collaborate with staff to establish annual goals for the unit and the systems needed to accomplish goals (e.g., assignment methods, quality improvement activities, patient education methods).
- Monitor professional nursing standards of practice on the unit.
- Develop an ongoing staff development plan, including one for new employees.
- Recruit new employees (interview and hire).
- Conduct routine staff evaluations.
- Serve as a role model for positive customer service (customers include patients, families, and other health care team members).
- Submit staffing schedules for the unit.
- Advocate for the nursing staff to the administration of the agency.
- Conduct regular patient rounds and problem solve patient or family complaints.
- Establish, monitor, and implement a quality improvement (QI) plan for the unit.
- Review and recommend new equipment for the unit.
- Conduct regular staff meetings.
- Make rounds with health care providers.
- Establish and support staff and interprofessional committees.

---

a nursing governance structure that incorporates staff involvement in forming policies and procedures for decision making needed to achieve agency goals. A skilled nurse manager directs and supports a group of staff in applying an agency's nursing philosophy. Thus, it takes a committed nurse executive, excellent nurse managers, and an empowered nursing staff to create an enriching work environment. Box 21.3 highlights the diverse responsibilities of nursing managers.

Decentralization is a component of the hierarchical level of decision making found in health care agencies. This management approach allows decisions to be made at the staff level. Shared governance is the typical decentralized structure used within health care agencies today (Huber, 2018). This structure creates an environment in which managers and staff become more actively involved in making decisions to shape the identity and determine the success of a health care agency. Working in a decentralized structure has the potential for greater collaborative effort, increased competency of staff, increased staff motivation, and ultimately a greater sense of professional accomplishment and satisfaction (Huber, 2018; Olender et al., 2020).

Progressive agencies achieve more when employees at all levels are empowered and actively involved in decision making. As a result, the role of a nurse manager is critical in the management of effective nursing units or groups. To make shared governance work, managers move decision making down to the lowest level possible. On a nursing unit it is important for all nursing staff members (RNs, LPNs, and LVNs), assistive personnel (AP), and unit secretaries to become engaged and provide input on practice issues and unit operations. They need to be kept well informed of unit and agency initiatives. Giving staff the opportunity to participate in problem-solving activities related to direct patient care and unit activities promotes a high level of employee engagement—a key factor in promoting teamwork and collaboration and a healthy work environment (Olender et al., 2020). Important elements of the decision-making process are responsibility, autonomy, authority, and accountability.

Responsibility refers to the duties and activities that you are employed to perform. A position description outlines your responsibilities as a professional nurse and your expected level of participation as a member of a nursing unit.

Responsibility reflects ownership and obligation. An individual who manages employees distributes responsibility, and the employees accept it. Managers need to ensure that staff clearly understand their responsibilities, particularly in the face of change. For example, when health care agencies participate in work redesign, patient care delivery models change significantly. A manager is responsible for clearly defining an RN's role within a new care delivery model. If decentralized decision making is in place, the professional nursing staff needs to be engaged to define the new RN role. Each RN on the team is responsible for knowing how to communicate with all team members and the process for making decisions on the busy nursing unit. For example, nurses are responsible for completing a nursing assessment of all assigned patients and developing a plan of care that is accessible to all team members (see Chapters 16 to 20). As the staff implements the plan of care, the nurse evaluates whether the plan is successful. This responsibility becomes a work ethic for the nurse in delivering excellent patient care.

Autonomy is freedom of choice and responsibility for the choices. Autonomy consistent with the scope of professional nursing practice maximizes a nurse's effectiveness (Huber, 2018). With clinical autonomy you make independent decisions about patient care, plan patient care within the scope of professional nursing practice, and implement independent nursing interventions (see Chapter 19). Another type of autonomy for nurses is work autonomy. In work autonomy a nurse makes independent decisions about the work of the unit, such as scheduling or unit governance. Autonomy is not an absolute; it occurs in degrees. For example, you have the autonomy to develop and implement a discharge teaching plan based on specific patient needs for your patients and their family caregivers. However, if your unit does not use self-scheduling, you do not have the autonomy to create your own schedule.

Authority refers to the legal ability to perform a task (Huber, 2018). It provides the power for a nurse to make final decisions and give instructions related to the decisions. You use authority to determine whether collaboration was successful. For example, while managing the care of a patient, you discover that one of the members of the health care team, the registered dietitian, did not follow through on a discharge teaching plan. You have the authority to consult with the registered dietitian to understand why the recommendations on the plan of care were not implemented and to review the established plan to ensure that recommended patient teaching is completed.

Accountability refers to individuals being answerable for their actions. It involves follow-up and a reflective analysis of decisions and an evaluation of their effectiveness. It means that as a nurse you take responsibility to provide excellent patient care by following standards of practice and agency policies and procedures. You assume responsibility for the outcomes of the actions, clinical judgments, and omissions in providing patient care. You are not accountable for the overall outcomes of patient care, but you are accountable for what you do (i.e., performing the nursing process, performing nursing procedures correctly, communicating effectively with health care team colleagues, and staying current on nursing practice issues). You will sometimes delegate responsibility, but you remain accountable for the care you delegated. For example, you delegate taking your patient's vital signs to an AP. You are responsible for knowing what your patient's vital signs are normally, for recognizing when the vital signs are in the expected range, and for providing appropriate care (e.g., verifying the temperature and giving acetaminophen as ordered when your patient's temperature is elevated).

Members of a successful nursing unit support the four elements of decision making: responsibility, autonomy, authority, and accountability. An effective nurse manager sets expectations for the staff in how decisions are made. Staff members need to feel comfortable in expressing differences of opinion and challenging ways in which the team functions. Ultimately shared governance helps the staff on a nursing unit to implement its philosophy and vision of professional nursing care.

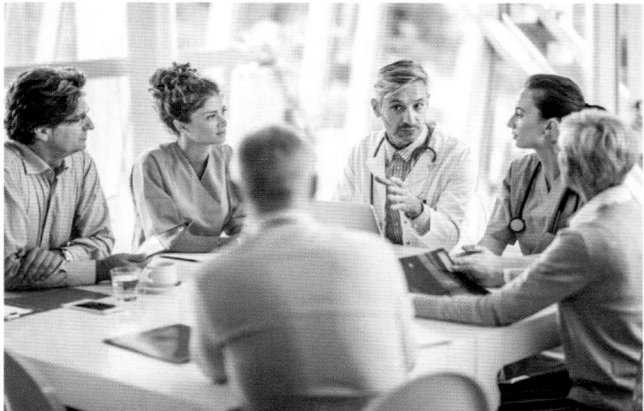

FIG. 21.1 Staff collaborating on practice issues. (Copyright © iStock/skynesher.)

Staff Involvement. When transformational or relationship-based leadership and decentralized decision making exist on a nursing unit, all staff members actively participate in unit activities (Fig. 21.1). Because the work environment promotes participation, all staff members benefit from the knowledge, experience, and skills of the entire work group. If the staff learns to value the pursuit of knowledge and the contributions of colleagues, better patient care results. Recognizing nurses' exceptional work with patients helps reinforce these behaviors, creates a healthy work environment, and reduces nurse burnout (Kelly and Lefton, 2017; Wei et al., 2020). Healthy work environments have nurses who are skilled in communication, promote true collaboration among health care team members, encourage effective decision making, have appropriate levels of staffing to meet patient needs, recognize nurses in a meaningful way, and have an authentic nurse leader (AACN, n.d.). Authentic leadership results in greater nurse empowerment, improved culture and climate, increased implementation of evidence-based practice, better teamwork between nurses and physicians, greater role clarity, and reduced conflict and ambiguity (Baek et al., 2019; Shirey et al., 2019). The nursing manager supports staff involvement through a variety of approaches:

1. **Establishing nursing practice through problem-solving committees or professional shared governance councils.** Staff committees establish and maintain care standards for nursing practice on their unit. Shared governance is a dynamic process that promotes decision making, accountability, and empowerment in staff nurses and enables them to make meaningful and sustainable changes in patient care (Huber, 2018; Porter-O'Grady, 2019). The committees review ongoing clinical care issues, identify problems, apply evidence-based practice in establishing standards of care, develop policy and procedures, implement new practice approaches, resolve patient satisfaction issues, or develop new documentation tools. It is important for the committees to balance their focus between patient outcomes and work issues to ensure quality care on the unit. Quality of care is improved when nurses control their own practice. The committee establishes methods to ensure that all staff have input on practice issues. Managers do not always sit on a committee, but they receive regular reports of committee progress. The nature of work on the nursing unit determines committee membership. At times members of other disciplines (e.g., pharmacy, respiratory therapy, or clinical nutrition) participate in practice committees or shared governance councils.

2. **Interprofessional collaboration among nurses and health care providers.** Interprofessional collaboration among nurses and

health care providers (e.g., medical doctors, physical therapists, respiratory therapists) is critical to the delivery of quality, safe patient care and the creation of a positive work culture for practitioners (McBeth et al., 2017; Interprofessional Education Collaborative [IPEC], 2016). Interprofessional collaboration involves bringing various disciplines together to work with patients and families to deliver quality care (IPEC, 2016). Interprofessional collaboration involves all professions bringing different points of view to the table to identify, clarify, and solve complex patient problems together, providing integrated and cohesive patient care (Goldsberry, 2018). The nurse plays a unique role within the team and is often viewed as the team leader because it is the nurse who takes on the responsibilities of coordination of communication and patient care (QSEN Institute, 2020). Open communication, cooperation, trust, mutual respect, and understanding of team member roles and responsibilities are critical for successful interprofessional collaboration (QSEN Institute, 2020; IPEC, 2016). The IPEC (2016) identified four competencies needed by health care practitioners to be effective team members in interprofessional collaboration. The development of these competencies comes through interprofessional education (Homeyer et al., 2018). Competencies needed for effective interpersonal collaboration include:

- *Values/ethics for interprofessional practice:* Work with individuals of other professions to maintain a climate of mutual respect and shared values.
- *Roles/responsibilities:* Use the knowledge of one's own role and those of other professions to appropriately assess and address the health care needs of patients and to promote and advance the health of populations.
- *Interprofessional communication:* Communicate with patients, families, communities, and professionals in health and other fields in a responsive and responsible manner that supports a team approach to promote and maintain health and prevent and treat disease.
- *Teams and teamwork:* Apply relationship-building values and the principles of team dynamics to perform effectively in different team roles to plan, deliver, and evaluate patient- or population-centered care and population health programs and policies that are safe, timely, efficient, effective, and equitable.

3. **Interprofessional rounding.** Many agencies that focus on patient- and family-centered care conduct interprofessional rounding to encourage patient and family involvement in planning care, to improve patient care coordination, and to enhance communication among the health care team (Bigani and Correia, 2018). During rounding, members of the team meet and share patient information, answer questions asked by other team members, discuss a patient's clinical progress and plans for discharge, and focus all team members on the same patient outcomes and goals (Prystajecky et al., 2017; McBeth, 2017). Interprofessional rounding improves decision making, nurses' job satisfaction, and quality of care (Ashcraft et al., 2017). For interprofessional rounding to be successful, health care team members need to be flexible and open to ideas, questions, and suggestions offered by others.

4. **Staff communication.** A manager's greatest challenge, especially if a work group is large, is communication with staff. It is difficult to make sure that all staff members receive consistent, clear, accurate, and timely information. Lack of communication about planned changes often leads to mistrust among staff members. However, a manager cannot assume total responsibility for all communication. An effective manager uses a variety of approaches to communicate quickly and accurately to all staff. For example, many managers distribute biweekly or monthly newsletters of ongoing unit or agency activities. Minutes of committee meetings are usually in an accessible location for all staff to read or are sent to individuals via e-mail. When the team needs to discuss important issues regarding the operations of the unit, the manager conducts staff meetings. When the unit has practice- or quality-improvement committees, each committee member has the responsibility to communicate directly to a select number of staff members. Thus, all staff members are contacted and given the opportunity to provide input.

5. **Staff education.** A professional nursing staff needs to always grow in knowledge. It is impossible to remain knowledgeable about current medical and nursing practice trends without ongoing education. A nurse manager is responsible for making learning opportunities available, so staff members remain competent in their practice and empowered in their clinical decision making. This involves planning in-service programs, sending staff to continuing education classes and professional conferences, and having staff present case studies or evidence-based practice issues during staff meetings. Staff members are responsible for pursuing educational opportunities for relicensure/recertification and changing information regarding their patient population.

LEADERSHIP SKILLS FOR NURSING STUDENTS

It is important to prepare yourself for leadership roles from the time you decide to become a nurse. Begin by being a dependable, respectful, and competent team member. As a nursing student you are responsible and accountable for the care you give to your patients. This translates into being prepared with the knowledge you need for making sound clinical judgments. Learn to consult with faculty and nursing staff to obtain guidance and feedback. Use your critical thinking to learn from mistakes, work closely with professional nurses, and try to improve your performance during each patient interaction. Clinical judgment applied through use of the nursing process allows you to make appropriate clinical decisions (see Chapter 15). These clinical decisions focus on meeting the needs of your patients while considering their preferences, considering alternatives to problems, understanding the rationale for performing nursing interventions, and evaluating the effectiveness of care. Clinical experiences develop your clinical judgment and critical thinking (Benner et al., 2010). Important leadership skills to learn include clinical care coordination, team communication, delegation, and knowledge building.

> **REFLECT NOW**
>
> Think about what you have learned about leadership development so far. Create a personal plan you can use to help you develop your own leadership skills.

Clinical Care Coordination

You acquire necessary knowledge and skills so that you can deliver patient care competently and safely. Most nursing students begin by caring for one patient. However, as your skills in clinical judgment and reasoning and clinical decision making improve, you will care for groups of patients and for patients with more complex needs. To coordinate the clinical care of patients safely and effectively, you need to learn how to recognize and analyze your patient's assessment cues, generate solutions to patient problems, make clinical decisions, set priorities, delegate safely, gain organizational skills, use resources, manage time, and evaluate your patient's outcomes (Dickison et al., 2019). Clinical care coordination requires you to use critical reflection and reasoning and clinical judgment (Benner et al., 2010). These are important first steps in developing a caring relationship with a patient.

Use a critical thinking approach, applying previous knowledge and experience to the decision-making process (see Chapter 15).

Clinical Judgment. You will use clinical judgment and make clinical decisions through application of the nursing process (see Chapters 16 to 20). You begin caring for a patient by conducting a focused but complete assessment so that you know your patient and can make accurate clinical judgments (see Chapter 16). Knowing the patient involves more than gathering formal assessment data. Knowing develops over time after caring for patients with similar patterns of responses to illness and being able to anticipate health problems. Your initial contact with a patient is an important first step in developing a caring relationship. Encouraging patients to share their stories about their health problems is very useful (e.g., say, "Tell me how you are dealing with . . ." or "Can you share what has been your biggest problem since becoming ill?"). After obtaining a thorough assessment and analyzing assessment data for cues to identify a patient's nursing diagnoses and problems, you develop a plan of care, implement nursing interventions, and evaluate patient outcomes. The process requires clinical decision making using a critical thinking approach (Dickison et al., 2019) (see Chapter 15).

Sound clinical judgment ensures therapeutic nursing care, especially when a patient's condition changes. It is important to be thorough. Learn to attend and listen to the patient, look for any cues (obvious or subtle) that point to a pattern of findings, and direct your assessment to explore the pattern further. Never hesitate to ask for assistance when a patient's condition changes.

Priority Setting. After forming a picture of a patient's total needs, you set priorities by deciding which patient needs or problems need attention first (see Chapter 18). Priority setting is not the ordering of a list of care tasks but rather a way to organize your care. Recognizing cues from your assessment database and your knowledge helps you understand which diagnoses require intervention and the associated time frame to intervene effectively (Ackley and Ladwig, 2020). It is important to set priorities whenever you provide patient care because it allows you to see the most important issues, as well as the relationships among patient problems, and to avoid delays in taking action, which could lead to serious complications for a patient. When a patient is experiencing a serious physiological or psychological problem, the priority becomes clear. You need to act immediately to stabilize the patient's condition.

Nurses prioritize care in different ways. If you use Maslow's hierarchy of needs, you meet a patient's physiological needs such as oxygen, food, water, sleep, and elimination first. Once physiological needs are met, you help patients meet their higher-level needs, such as safety, security, belonging, esteem, and self-actualization. To prioritize your care, evaluate and weigh each competing task by reflecting on the following three questions:
- Is this a life-threatening situation? Will this patient or another patient be endangered if this task is not done immediately or is left for later?
- Is this task essential to patient or staff safety?
- Is this task essential to the patient's plan of care?

When prioritizing care, you need to understand the "big picture" of your patient's problems and expected outcomes. Once you know all your patient's problems, determine the relationships among the problems. Remember that setting priorities is a dynamic process; it changes frequently (Alfaro-Lefevre, 2020). Always give high priority to patient and family caregiver safety (e.g., fall prevention, safe medication administration, and patient education needs). Use the following steps to classify problems into one of three priority levels, and use this information to help you set priorities (Alfaro-Lefevre, 2020):
1. Assign high priority to first-level problems using *ABC*+VL (**a**irway, **b**reathing, **c**ardiac and circulation problems, **v**ital signs concerns, and **l**ife-threatening laboratory values), and attend to these immediately.

2. Next address second-level problems, which immediately follow the first level and include concerns such as changes in mental status, untreated medical issues, acute pain, acute elimination problems, abnormal laboratory results, and risks.
3. Then tend to third-level problems, which are health problems other than those at the first two levels, such as long-term issues in health management, rest, and family coping.

Many patients have all three levels of problems, requiring you to make careful clinical judgments in choosing a course of action. High priority needs demand immediate attention. When a patient has diverse priority needs, it helps to focus on the basic needs. For example, a patient who returns to his room after ambulating down the hall is short of breath. The dietary assistant arrives in the room to deliver a meal tray. Instead of immediately helping with the meal, you position the patient comfortably in bed, offer basic hygiene measures, and then evaluate breathlessness. The patient is likely to become more interested in eating after becoming more comfortable. The patient also is more receptive to any instruction you need to provide.

Eventually you will be required to meet the priority needs of a group of patients. This means that you need to know the priorities of each patient within the group, assessing each patient's needs as soon as possible while addressing high priorities first. Use information from the change-of-shift or hand-off report, the patient acuity classification system, and information from the medical record to determine which patient to assess first. Over time you learn to spontaneously rank patients' needs by priority or urgency. Priorities do not remain stable but change as a patient's condition changes. It is important to think about the resources available, to be flexible in recognizing that priority needs often change, and to consider how to use time wisely.

You also set priorities based on your patient's expectations. Sometimes you establish an excellent plan of care; however, if a patient resists certain therapies or disagrees with your approach, your care will not be effective or safe. Be caring and work closely with a patient and family caregiver when setting priorities to establish trust and cooperation.

> **REFLECT NOW**
>
> Think about a patient you cared for recently. How did you prioritize the care you provided your patient? Did you provide care that was effective and efficient? What could you have done differently to improve your prioritization?

Organizational Skills. Implementing a plan of care requires you to be effective and efficient. Effective use of time means doing the right things, whereas efficient use of time means doing things right. Learn to become efficient by combining various nursing activities (i.e., doing more than one thing at a time). For example, during medication administration or while obtaining a specimen, combine therapeutic communication, teaching interventions, assessment, and evaluation. Always establish and strengthen relationships with patients and use any patient contact as an opportunity to convey important information. Patient interaction gives you the chance to show caring and interest. Always attend to a patient's behaviors and responses to therapies to assess whether new problems are developing and to evaluate responses to interventions.

It is easier to provide patient care if you are organized. A well-organized nurse approaches any procedure by having all the necessary equipment available and making sure that the patient is prepared. If the patient is comfortable and well informed, the procedure will probably go smoothly. Sometimes you need help from colleagues to perform or complete a procedure. Keep the work area organized and complete preliminary steps before asking colleagues for assistance.

Although you plan and deliver care based on established priorities, events sometimes occur that interfere with your plans. For example, just as you begin to bathe a patient, an x-ray technician enters to take a chest x-ray film. Once the technician takes the x-ray, a phlebotomist arrives to draw a blood sample. In this case your priorities conflict with the priorities of other health care personnel. It is important to always keep a patient's needs at the center of attention. If the patient experienced symptoms earlier that required a chest x-ray film and laboratory work, it is important to be sure that the diagnostic tests are completed. In another example a patient is waiting to visit family, and a chest x-ray film is a routine order. The patient's condition is stable, and the x-ray technician is willing to return later to shoot the film. In this case attending to the patient's hygiene and comfort so that family members can visit is the higher priority.

Use of Resources. Appropriate use of resources is an important aspect of clinical care coordination. Resources include members of the health care team. In any setting providing patient care occurs more smoothly when staff members work together. Never hesitate to have staff help you, especially when there is an opportunity to make a procedure or activity more comfortable and safer for patients. For example, you often need assistance in turning, positioning, and ambulating patients when patients have mobility limitations. Having a staff member such as an AP assist with handling equipment and supplies during complicated procedures such as catheter insertion or dressing changes makes procedures more efficient. In addition, you need to recognize personal limitations and use professional resources for assistance. For example, you assess a patient and find relevant clinical signs and symptoms but are unfamiliar with the physical condition. Consulting with an experienced RN confirms findings and ensures that you take the proper course of action for the patient. Leaders know their limitations and seek professional colleagues for guidance and support.

Time Management. Shorter hospital stays, early discharges, same-day surgeries, and increasing complexity in patients' needs create stress for nurses as they work to meet patient needs in hospital settings (Huber, 2018). One way to manage this stress is to use time-management skills. These skills involve learning how, where, and when to use your time. Because you have a limited amount of time with patients, it is essential to remain goal oriented and use time wisely. Managing yourself better leads to better time management and reduces the risk of developing burnout (de Oliveira et al., 2019). Effective time management includes being prepared, being organized, and managing priorities.

Make efficient and effective use of your time by remaining focused on your patient's outcomes. However, you also need to learn how to establish personal goals and realistic time frames. For example, you are caring for two patients on a busy surgical nursing unit. One had surgery the day before, and the other will be discharged the next day. The first patient's outcomes center on restoring physiological function that is impaired because of surgery. The second patient's outcomes focus on adequate preparation to assume self-care at home. In reviewing the therapies required for both patients, you learn how to organize your time so that you complete your nursing care, and your patients achieve their outcomes. Anticipate when care will be interrupted for medication administration and diagnostic testing and determine the best time for planned therapies such as dressing changes, patient education, and patient ambulation. Delegating tasks is another way to help improve time management.

One useful time-management skill involves making a to-do list. When you begin to work with patients, it helps to make a list that

sequences the nursing activities you need to perform. The hand-off report at the change of shift helps you prioritize activities based on what you learn about a patient's condition and the care provided before you arrived on the unit.

Consider activities that have specific time limits in terms of addressing patient needs such as administering a pain medication before a scheduled procedure or instructing patients before their discharge home. You also analyze the items on the list that are scheduled by agency policies or routines (e.g., medications or intravenous [IV] tubing changes). Note which activities need to be done on time and which activities you can do at your discretion. Administer medication within a specific schedule, but you can also perform other activities while in the patient's room. Finally, estimate the amount of time needed to complete the various activities. Activities requiring the assistance of other staff members usually take longer because you need to plan around their schedules.

Good time management also involves setting goals to help you complete one task before starting another. You will always deliver care to a group of patients, moving back and forth between patients as needs and priorities change. If possible, complete an activity started with one patient before moving on to the next. Care is less fragmented, and you are better able to focus on what you are doing for each patient. As a result, you will be less likely to make errors. Time management requires you to anticipate the activities of the day and combine activities when possible. When you practice good time management, you focus on organization and setting priorities. Other strategies include keeping your work area clean and clutter free and trying to decrease interruptions as you are completing tasks. Box 21.4 summarizes principles of time management.

Evaluation. Evaluation is one of the most important aspects of clinical care coordination (see Chapter 20). You constantly evaluate a patient's condition and progress toward an expected patient outcome. Evaluation is an ongoing process. It does not occur only at the end of an activity. Once you assess a patient's needs and implement interventions for a patient's problem, immediately evaluate whether the interventions

---

BOX 21.4   Principles of Time Management

Goal setting: Review a patient's outcomes and care that needs to be accomplished for the day as well as any goals you have for activities, such as completing documentation, attending a patient care conference, giving a hand-off report, or preparing medications for administration.

Time analysis: Reflect on how you use your time. While taking care of patients, keep track of how you use your time in different activities. This helps you become more aware of how well organized you really are and areas you may need to improve upon.

Priority setting: Set the priorities that you have established for patients within set time frames. For example, determine when the best time is to have teaching sessions, plan ambulation, and provide rest periods based on what you know about a patient's condition. For instance, if a patient is nauseated or in pain, it is not a good time for a teaching session.

Interruption control: Everyone needs time to socialize or discuss issues with colleagues. However, do not let this interrupt important patient care activities such as medication administration (see Chapter 31), ordered treatments, or teaching sessions. Use time during report, mealtime, or team meetings to your advantage. In addition, plan time to help fellow colleagues so that it complements your patient care schedule.

Evaluation: At the end of each day take time to think and reflect about how effectively you used your time. If you are having difficulties, discuss them with an instructor or a more experienced staff member.

BOX 21.5 Key TeamSTEPPS® Principles

Team Structure: Identify the complex parts of the health care system that work together effectively to promote patient safety.

Communication: Use structured processes to exchange information clearly and accurately among members of the health care team.

Leadership: Ensure that all members of the health care team understand the team's actions, receive information about changes, and have the resources needed to perform their jobs.

Situation Monitoring: Actively assess any situation to gather information, improve your understanding, or maintain awareness to support the functioning of the team.

Mutual Support: Understand the responsibilities and workload of all team members so that you can anticipate and support their needs.

Modified from Pocket Guide: TeamSTEPPS. Content last reviewed January 2020. Agency for Healthcare Research and Quality, Rockville, MD. https://www.ahrq.gov/teamstepps/instructor/essentials/pocketguide.html. Accessed April 5, 2021.

BOX 21.6 SBAR As a Communication Tool

Case Study: You administered 1 tablet of oxycodone HCl 5 mg/ibuprofen 400 mg PO to a patient 30 minutes ago for postsurgical pain. You return to the patient's room to evaluate the effectiveness of the medication 30 minutes later. The patient rates his pain as an 8 on a scale of 0–10. You use SBAR to contact the patient's health care provider.

Situation: The patient is rating his pain as an 8 on a scale of 0–10. He had his pain medication 30 minutes ago.

Background: The patient had a knee replacement and returned from the postanesthesia care unit 6 hours ago. He has 1 tablet of oxycodone HCl 5 mg/ibuprofen 400 mg PO ordered every 6 hours. This is the first pain medication he has taken since being admitted to the unit.

Assessment: His current medication order is not sufficiently managing the patient's pain. He does not want to sit up or move because of the pain he is experiencing.

Recommendation: It might be helpful to change the pain medication order for the patient.

were effective and the patient's response. The process of evaluation compares actual patient outcomes with expected outcomes. For example, you assess a foot ulcer of a patient who has diabetes mellitus to determine whether healing has progressed since the last clinic visit. When expected outcomes are not met, evaluation reveals the need to continue current therapies for a longer period, revise approaches to care, or introduce new therapies. As you care for a patient throughout the day, anticipate when to return to the bedside to evaluate care (e.g., 30 minutes after an oral medication was administered, 15 minutes after an IV fluid has begun infusing, or 60 minutes after discussing discharge instructions with the patient and family caregiver).

Focusing on evaluation of a patient's progress lessens the chance of becoming distracted by the tasks of care. It is common to assume that staying focused on planned activities ensures that you will perform care appropriately. However, task orientation does not ensure positive patient outcomes. Learn that at the heart of good organizational skills is the constant inquiry into a patient's condition and progress toward an improved level of health.

Team Communication

Effective communication is critical to all teams (QSEN Institute, 2020). As part of a health care team, you are responsible for using open, professional communication. Regardless of the setting, an enriching professional environment is one in which staff members respect one another's ideas, share information, and keep one another informed (Kaiser and Westers, 2018).

Some health care agencies use evidence-based teamwork principles to improve communication, teamwork, and patient safety. The Team-STEPPS® system provides training for all health care staff to guide communication, increase team awareness, and eliminate barriers to patient safety (AHRQ, 2019). Use TeamSTEPPS® principles to promote professional communication and teamwork in your practice setting (Box 21.5).

Strategies to improve your communication with health care providers include addressing the colleague by name, having the patient and medical record available when discussing patient issues, focusing on the patient problem, and being professional and assertive but not aggressive or confrontational. One way of fostering good team communication is to understand the roles and responsibilities of everyone on the health care team (AHRQ, 2019). A professional nurse treats colleagues with respect, listens to the ideas of other staff members without interruption,

explores the way other staff members think, and is honest and direct while communicating. Part of good communication is clarifying what others are saying and building on the merits of your colleagues' ideas. An effective team knows that it can count on all members when needs arise.

Sharing expectations of what, when, and how to communicate is a step toward establishing a strong work team (AHRQ, 2019). Examples of effective team communication strategies include briefings or short discussions among team members, group rounds on patients, callouts to share critical information such as vital signs with all team members at the same time, and check-backs to restate what a person has said to verify understanding of information. The two-challenge rule allows concerns about safety to be voiced twice. Some patient care settings use different tools to communicate a change in a patient's condition. For example, some use the CUS Tool, which means I am **C**oncerned, I am **U**ncomfortable, and this is a **S**afety issue (AHRQ, 2019). Another tool often used by health care agencies to share information is Situation-Background-Assessment-Recommendation (SBAR) (Box 21.6; see Chapter 27) (AHRQ, 2019). When using electronic communication, it is important to communicate the appropriate information to the correct person, always maintaining patient privacy and confidentiality.

QSEN **Building Competency in Teamwork and Collaboration**

You are caring for Mrs. Saucer, who had a stroke 3 days ago. Upon your initial assessment, she was oriented, smiling, and joking with her visitors. You enter her room 2 hours later and find that Mrs. Saucer remains oriented, but she is tearful, and her emotional status has changed. She states, "I'm not sure what is wrong with me. I feel so much different than I did earlier today." Your intuition tells you that although Mrs. Saucer's physical status and orientation have not changed, there is something that is not quite right. You know that even the slightest neurological change in a patient who has had a stroke could be a sign of worsening neurological status. Using the CUS tool, how would you communicate this change in status to Mrs. Saucer's health care provider?

Answers to QSEN Activities can be found on the Evolve website.

Delegation

The art of effective delegation is a skill to observe and practice to improve your own management skills. **Delegation** is the process of assigning part of your responsibility to another qualified person in a specific situation (NCSBN and ANA, 2019). Your state's Nurse Practice

Act, along with principles of authority, accountability, and responsibility, provides the basis for effective delegation. Effective delegation results in the achievement of quality, safe patient care; improved efficiency; increased productivity; empowered staff; and skill development (Yoder-Wise, 2019). For example, asking a staff member to obtain an ordered specimen while you administer a patient's pain medication effectively prevents a delay in the patient gaining pain relief. Delegation also provides job enrichment. You show trust in colleagues by delegating tasks to them and showing staff members that they are important players in the delivery of care (Riisgaard et al., 2017). Successful delegation is important to the quality of the relationship you have with all team members, including LPNs and APs (Lyman et al., 2017). Delegating a task that you dislike doing or would not do yourself creates negative feelings and poor working relationships. For example, if a patient asks to be placed on a bedpan and there are no urgent care issues, you assist the patient rather than leave the room to find the LPN or AP. Remember that even though the delegation of a task transfers the responsibility and authority to another person, you are accountable for the delegated task.

As a nurse you are responsible and accountable for providing care to patients and delegating care activities to others (Huber, 2018). Use the five rights of delegation to ensure you stay within an RN's legal scope of practice (Box 21.7). Never delegate clinical reasoning, nursing judgment (e.g., the steps of the nursing process of assessment, diagnosis, planning, intervention, and evaluation or patient teaching), and critical decision making to APs (NCSBN and ANA, 2019). Remember that when you delegate to another member of the health care team,

you delegate tasks, not patients. Although LPNs can manage most patient care on their own, do not give APs sole responsibility for the care of patients. One way to accomplish safe delegation is to conduct rounds with LPNs and APs who are assigned to work with you. APs attend to basic patient needs (e.g., hygiene, meal assistance, ambulation), while LPNs can provide basic direct nursing care (e.g., observe and report clinical changes, perform wound care, and ADLs). You delegate care based on assessment findings and priority setting.

As a leader of the health care team, you give clear instructions, effectively prioritize patient needs and therapies, and give staff timely and meaningful feedback. Do not automatically delegate a task because it is a task. Rather, delegate it because it is appropriate for LPNs or APs to perform it. For example, as a nurse, you are always responsible for the assessment of a patient's ongoing status; however, if a patient is stable, you delegate administration of medications (exception: IV medications in most states) to the LPN and the taking of vital signs to the AP.

Effective delegation begins with knowing which skills you can delegate. Thus, you need to be familiar with the Nurse Practice Act of your state, agency policies and procedures, and agency job descriptions for LPNs and APs. These standards define the necessary level of education and competency of all staff and contain specific guidelines regarding which tasks or activities you can delegate. A job description identifies required education, as well as the types of tasks LPNs and APs can perform either independently or with direct supervision. Agency policies define the training required for APs. Procedures detail who is qualified to perform a given nursing procedure, whether supervision is necessary, and the type of reporting required.

As a professional nurse you cannot delegate without considering the implications. Assess the patient and determine a plan of care before identifying which tasks someone else can perform. Determine how much supervision is necessary. For example, you are working with an AP who was recently hired. When deciding which tasks to delegate to the AP, determine whether the patient has a complicating factor that makes your assistance necessary. Ask the AP, "Is this the first time you have performed this task?" "Have you cared for patients with similar needs?" "Have you had the chance to do this skill during orientation?" If you decide delegation of the skill is possible, you need to evaluate whether the AP performed the task properly and whether the desired outcomes were met after the AP completes the task.

Efficient delegation requires ongoing communication (i.e., sending clear messages and listening so that all participants understand expectations regarding patient care) (Huber, 2018). Provide clear instructions and desired outcomes when delegating tasks. Focus your instructions on the procedure itself, what will be accomplished, when it should be completed, and the unique needs of the patient. You also communicate when and which information to report such as expected observations and specific patient concerns (NCSBN and ANA, 2019). Communication is a two-way process in delegation; thus, create a trusting relationship so that the staff you work with (e.g., LPNs, APs) feel comfortable and are able to ask questions and clarify your expectations (NCSBN and ANA, 2019). Effective communication, shared decision making, and sharing of knowledge promote safe patient care (Okoli et al., 2020). As you become more familiar with a staff member's competency, trust builds, and the staff member needs fewer instructions. Always clarify patients' specific needs.

When delegating patient care, you evaluate a staff member's performance, achievement of the patient's outcomes, the communication process used, and any problems or concerns that occurred (NCSBN and ANA, 2019). For example, when a newly hired AP performs a task correctly and does a good job, it is essential to provide praise and recognition. If a staff member's performance is unsatisfactory, give constructive

---

BOX 21.7 The Five Rights of Delegation

Right Task

The right tasks to delegate are ones that are included in the delegatee's job description or are included in the health care agency's policies and procedures. Policies and procedures need to describe expectations, limits, and required competency training for the activity.

Right Circumstance

Consider the patient's status. The patient needs to be stable for you to delegate tasks. The delegatee must report changes in patient condition to the licensed nurse. The licensed nurse must reassess and evaluate the situation and appropriateness of delegation when a patient's condition changes.

Right Person

The licensed nurse, employer, and delegatee are all responsible for ensuring the delegatee has the knowledge and skills required to perform the activity.

Right Directions and Communication

Give a clear, concise description of a task, including its objective, limits, and expectations. Communication needs to be ongoing between the licensed nurse and delegatee. The delegatee is responsible for asking questions to clarify information.

Right Supervision and Evaluation

Provide appropriate monitoring, evaluation, intervention as needed, and feedback. The licensed nurse must follow up with the delegatee at the end of the activity to evaluate patient outcomes, be available and ready to intervene when appropriate, and ensure appropriate documentation.

Modified from National Council of States Boards of Nursing and American Nurses Association (NCSBN & ANA): *National guidelines for nursing delegation,* 2019, https://www.ncsbn.org/NGND-PosPaper_06.pdf. Accessed April 5, 2021.

and appropriate feedback. Always give specific feedback regarding any mistakes that staff members make, explaining how to avoid the mistake or a better way to handle the situation. Giving feedback in private is professional and preserves the staff member's dignity. When giving feedback, focus on what can be changed, choose only one issue at a time, and give specific details. Frequently when a staff member's performance does not meet expectations, it is the result of inadequate training or assignment of too many tasks. In this case, review the procedure and offer demonstration or even recommend additional training with the education department. If too many tasks are being delegated, this might be a nursing practice issue. All staff need to discuss the appropriateness of delegation on their unit. Sometimes staff need help to learn how to prioritize. In some cases, you discover that you are overdelegating. It is your responsibility to complete documentation of the delegated task. Here are a few tips on appropriate delegation to assistive personnel (AP) (Yoder-Wise, 2019; NCSBN and ANA, 2019):

- *Assess the knowledge and skills of the person to whom you are delegating:* Assess the person's knowledge and skills by asking open-ended questions that elicit conversation and details about what the person knows (e.g., "How do you usually apply the cuff when you measure a blood pressure?" or "Tell me how you prepare the tubing before you give an enema").
- *Match tasks to the person's skills:* Know which tasks and skills the training program includes for APs in your agency. Determine whether APs have learned critical thinking, such as recognizing when a patient is in harm or understanding the difference between normal clinical findings and changes to report.
- *Communicate clearly:* Always provide clear directions by describing a task, the desired outcome, and the time within which the AP needs to complete the task. Never give instructions through another staff member. Make APs feel as though they are part of the team. Begin requests for help with *please* and end with *thank you*. For example, "I'd like you to please help me by getting Mr. Floyd up to ambulate before lunch. Be sure to check his blood pressure before he stands and record it in his chart. Thank you for your help." Ask the AP to report back to you after completing the task.
- *Listen attentively:* Listen to an AP's response after you provide directions. Does the AP feel comfortable in asking questions or requesting clarification? Does the AP understand your request? Ask the AP for suggestions in patient care and listen to the response. Be especially attentive if the AP is helping another nurse. Help sort out priorities.
- *Provide feedback:* Always give the AP feedback regarding performance, regardless of outcome. Let the AP know of a job well done. A "thank you" increases the likelihood of the AP helping in the future. If an outcome is undesirable, find a private place to discuss what occurred, any miscommunication, and how to achieve a better outcome in the future.

Knowledge Building

As a professional and accountable nurse, you are responsible for lifelong learning and maintaining your competency (Kaulback, 2020). Lifelong learning allows you to continuously provide safe, effective, quality care. A leader recognizes that there is always something new to learn. Opportunities for learning occur with each patient interaction, each encounter with a professional colleague, and each meeting or class session in which health care professionals meet to discuss clinical care issues. People always have different experiences and knowledge to share. Listen to the contributions of others, and value the information they share. In-service programs, workshops, professional conferences, professional reading, and taking classes to further your education offer innovative and current information on the rapidly changing world of health care. To be a safe and competent nurse you need to actively pursue learning opportunities, both formal and informal, and to respectfully interact with the professional colleagues you encounter.

KEY POINTS

- A transformational leader develops effective teams on the nursing unit, empowers staff members, communicates effectively with the nursing team, and guides and supports the nursing team in shared decision making.
- Nursing care delivery models vary according to the responsibility and autonomy of the nurse in coordinating care delivery and the roles other staff members play in assisting with care.
- Patient- and family-centered care is composed of the core concepts of respect and dignity, information sharing, participation of family members, and collaboration.
- Shared governance, a type of decentralized decision-making model, empowers nursing staff to make decisions about how they practice and deliver patient care.
- Important elements of professional nursing and the decision-making process include responsibility (activities you perform), autonomy (freedom of choice), authority (your legal ability to perform a task), and accountability (being answerable for your actions).
- Nursing students and nurses develop their own leadership skills by being responsible and accountable, thinking critically, reflecting upon and learning from mistakes, and being an engaged member of the health care team.
- You will use a variety of skills to coordinate patient care. For example, to prioritize patient care, evaluate and weigh each competing task by reflecting on whether the patient is in a life-threatening situation, whether the task is essential to patient or staff safety, and whether the task is essential to the patient's plan of care.
- Use evidence-based communication strategies such as SBAR and CUS to accurately communicate patient problems to other members of the health care team.
- Effective delegation requires effective communication skills and improves productivity and job enrichment. Using the five rights of delegation helps you delegate care appropriately.
- You need to maintain your competence and expand your knowledge throughout your career in a variety of ways, including learning from others, attending workshops and professional conferences, and pursuing formal as well as informal educational opportunities.

REFLECTIVE LEARNING

- Reflect on a recent clinical experience. Which nursing care delivery model was used in this setting? Based on the goals of this care delivery model, was it effective? What challenges do you think the team may experience with this model?
- Describe how you used clinical judgment to prioritize care for a recent patient or group of patients during a recent clinical or simulation experience. What factors influenced your decisions? How effective was your care and the decisions you made? Reflecting on this experience, is there anything you would have done differently? Explain your answer.
- Reflect on a clinical experience. What are some examples of teamwork and collaboration you witnessed? Did you observe any situations in which the health care team did not work well together? If so, what do you think caused this situation and what could be done to improve the work environment to reduce conflict and improve patient care? What effect did the lack of teamwork have on your patient?

REVIEW QUESTIONS

1. At 1300 the registered nurse (RN) says to the assistive personnel (AP), "You did a good job transferring Mr. Harvey into his chair this morning at 0830. I saw that you recorded how long he stayed in his chair. I saw that Mr. Harvey did not have any shoes or nonslip slippers on, though. For safety, the next time you transfer a patient into a chair, you need to make sure that the patient wears slippers or shoes. Please get Mr. Harvey up in his chair again by 1500." Which characteristics of positive feedback did the RN use when talking to the AP? (Select all that apply.)
   1. Feedback is given immediately.
   2. Feedback focuses on one issue.
   3. Feedback offers concrete details.
   4. Feedback identifies ways to improve.
   5. Feedback focuses on changeable things.
   6. Feedback is specific about what is done incorrectly only.

2. A nurse received change-of-shift reports on these four patients and starts rounding. Which patient does the nurse need to focus on as a priority?
   1. A patient who had abdominal surgery 2 days ago and is requesting pain medication
   2. A patient admitted yesterday with atrial fibrillation who now has a decreased level of consciousness
   3. A patient with a wound drain who needs teaching before discharge in the early afternoon
   4. A patient going to surgery for a mastectomy in 3 hours who has a question about the surgery

3. A nurse asks an AP to help the patient in Room 418 walk to the bathroom right now. The nurse tells the AP that the patient needs the assistance of one person and the use of a walker. The nurse also tells the AP that the patient's oxygen can be removed while he goes to the bathroom but to make sure that when it is put back on, the flowmeter is still at 2 L. The nurse also instructs the AP to make sure the side rails are up and the bed alarm is reset after the patient gets back in bed. Which of the following components of the "Five Rights of Delegation" were used by the nurse? (Select all that apply.)
   1. Right task
   2. Right circumstance
   3. Right person
   4. Right directions and communication
   5. Right supervision and evaluation

4. While administering medications, a nurse realizes that a prescribed dose of a medication was not given. The nurse acts by completing an incident report and notifying the patient's health care provider. Which of the following is the nurse exercising?
   1. Authority
   2. Responsibility
   3. Accountability
   4. Decision making

5. Which task is appropriate for a registered nurse (RN) to delegate to an AP?
   1. Determining whether the patient understands the preoperative preparation required before the surgery in the morning
   2. Administering the ordered antibiotic to the patient before surgery
   3. Obtaining the patient's signature on the surgical informed consent
   4. Helping the patient to the bathroom before leaving for the operating room

6. A nurse performs the following four steps in delegating a task to an AP. Place the steps in the correct order of appropriate delegation.
   1. Do you have any questions about walking with Mr. Malone?
   2. Before you take him for his walk to the end of the hallway and back, please take and record his pulse rate.
   3. In the next 30 minutes please assist Mr. Malone in Room 418 with his afternoon walk.
   4. I will make sure that I check with you in about 40 minutes to see how the patient did.

7. Which example demonstrates a nurse performing the skill of evaluation?
   1. The nurse explains the side effects of the new blood pressure medication ordered for the patient.
   2. The nurse asks a patient to rate pain on a scale of 0 to 10 before administering a pain medication.
   3. After completing a teaching session, the nurse observes a patient drawing up and administering an insulin injection.
   4. The nurse changes a patient's leg ulcer dressing using aseptic technique.

8. The nurse manager from the surgical unit was awarded the nursing leadership award for practice of transformational leadership. Which of the following are characteristics or traits of transformational leadership displayed by the award winner? (Select all that apply.)
   1. The nurse manager regularly rounds on staff to gather input on unit decisions.
   2. The nurse manager sends thank-you notes to staff in recognition of a job well done.
   3. The nurse manager sends memos to staff about decisions that the manager has made regarding unit policies.
   4. The nurse manager has an "innovation idea box" to which staff are encouraged to submit ideas for unit improvements.
   5. The nurse manager develops a philosophy of care for the staff.

9. A new nurse graduate is in orientation on a surgical unit and is being mentored by an experienced nurse. Which action completed by the new nurse graduate requires intervention by the experienced nurse? (Select all that apply.)
   1. The new nurse stops documenting about a dressing change to take a patient some water.
   2. The new nurse gathered the medications for two different patients at the same time.
   3. The new nurse asked an AP to help transfer a patient from the bed to a wheelchair before discharge.
   4. The new nurse educates a patient about pain management when administering a pain medication to a patient.
   5. The new nurse gathers all equipment necessary to start a new IV site before entering a patient's room.

10. JoAnn, a nurse, is calling a patient's health care provider about a problem that her patient, Ms. Ducote, is having during a blood transfusion. The health care agency uses the SBAR system in reporting patient problems. Put the statements in the correct order according to the SBAR system.
    1. I think she might need a diuretic ordered. Is it possible for you to come see her soon? Is there anything else you would like for me to do right now?
    2. This is JoAnn. I am caring for Ms. Ducote. She is having labored breathing and her heart rate is higher now than it was an hour ago. She is receiving the second unit of her blood transfusion. She says she is having trouble catching her breath.

3. Ms. Ducote had surgery earlier yesterday to remove a tumor in the colon. Her hemoglobin was 9.6 grams/dL, and her hematocrit was 33.6% this morning. Her first ordered unit of packed red blood cells infused over 90 minutes, and she is 30 minutes into receiving her second unit of blood now. She states she takes furosemide 20 mg every morning at home. She does not currently have an order for furosemide.

4. The patient denies pain, and her vital signs are as follows: B/P 150/98 mm Hg; pulse 118; respiratory rate 28; temperature 98.8° F (37.1° C). I think she is showing signs of fluid volume overload.

Answers: 1. 2, 3, 4, 5; **2.** 2; **3.** 1, 2, 3, 4; **4.** 3; **5.** 4; **6.** 3, 2, 4, 1; **7.** 3; **8.** 1, 2, 4; **9.** 1, 2; **10.** 2, 3, 4, 1.

Rationales to Review Questions can be found on the Evolve website.

REFERENCES

Ackley BJ, Ladwig G: *Nursing diagnosis handbook*, ed 12, St Louis, 2020, Elsevier.

Agency for Healthcare Research and Quality (AHRQ): *About TeamSTEPPS®*, https://www.ahrq.gov/teamstepps/about-teamstepps/index.html, 2019. Accessed April 5, 2021.

Alfaro-Lefevre R: *Critical thinking, clinical reasoning, and clinical judgment: a practical approach*, ed 7, St Louis, 2020, Saunders.

American Association of Critical Care Nurses (AACN): *Healthy work environments*, n.d., https://www.aacn.org/nursing-excellence/healthy-work-environments. Accessed April 5, 2021.

American Case Management Association (ACMA): What is case management? n.d., https://www.acmaweb.org/section.aspx?sID=136. Accessed April 5, 2021.

American Nurses Credentialing Center (ANCC): Magnet Recognition Program ®, n.d., https://www.nursingworld.org/organizational-programs/magnet/. Accessed April 5, 2021.

Ashcraft S et al: Interprofessional clinical rounding: effects on processes and outcomes of care, *Journal for Healthcare Quality* 39(2):85-94, doi: 10.1097/JHQ.0000000000000039, 2017.

Benner P et al.: *Educating nurses: a call for radical transformation*, San Francisco, CA, 2010, Josey-Bass.

Dickison P et al: Integrating the National Council of State Boards of Nursing Clinical Judgment Model into nursing educational frameworks, *J Nurs Educ* 58(2):72-78, 2019.

Goldsberry JW: Advanced practice nurses leading the way: interprofessional collaboration, *Nurse Educ Today* 65(1), 2018.

Grace P: Enhancing nurse moral agency: the leadership promise of doctor of nursing practice preparation, *Online J Issues Nurs* 23(1):1, 2018.

Huber DL: *Leadership and nursing care management*, ed 6, St Louis, 2018, Saunders.

Hume L, Hall M: Sustaining a positive practice environment after Pathway to Excellence® designation, *Nursing Management* 51(2):6-9, 2020, doi: 10.1097/01.NUMA.0000651208.47176.91 Available at https://journals.lww.com/nursingmanagement/Fulltext/2020/02000/Sustaining_a_positive_practice_environment_after.2.aspx. Accessed April 5, 2021.

Institute for Patient and Family Centered Care (IPFCC): Patient- and family-centered care, n.d., http://www.ipfcc.org/about/pfcc.html. Accessed April 5, 2021.

Interprofessional Education Collaborative (IPEC): *Core competencies for interprofessional collaborative practice: 2016 update*, Washington, DC: Interprofessional Education Collaborative, 2016, https://www.ipecollaborative.org/ipec-core-competencies. Accessed April 5, 2021.

James AH: Action learning can support leadership development for undergraduate and postgraduate nurses, *Br J Nurs* 27(15):876, 2018.

Kivland C: Successfully managing emotions and behavior: emotional intelligence matters more than ever to your leadership career, *Healthc Exec* 33(1):68, 2018.

National Council of State Boards of Nursing (NCSBN): *NCSBN: leading regulatory excellence*, https://www.ncsbn.org/index.htm, 2021. Accessed April 5, 2021.

National Council of States Boards of Nursing and American Nurses Association (NCSBN & ANA): *National guidelines for nursing delegation*, 2019, https://www.ncsbn.org/NGND-PosPaper_06.pdf. Accessed April 5, 2021.

Porter-O'Grady T: Principles for sustaining shared/professional governance in nursing, *Nursing Management* 50(1):36, 2019. Available at: https://journals.lww.com/nursingmanagement/FullText/2019/01000/Principles_for_sustaining_shared_professional.8.aspx. Accessed April 5, 2021.

QSEN Institute: *QSEN competencies*, http://qsen.org/competencies/pre-licensure-ksas/, 2020. Accessed April 5, 2021.

Tatsumi CL: The nurse as servant leaders: guiding others in caring advocacy, *Beginnings* 39(4):6-14, 2019.

Yoder-Wise PS: *Leading and managing in nursing*, ed 7, St Louis, 2019, Elsevier.

RESEARCH REFERENCES

Alilyyani B et al.: Antecedents, mediators, and outcomes of authentic leadership in healthcare: a systematic review, *Int J Nurs Stud* 83:34, 2018.

Baek H et al: Authentic leadership, job satisfaction and organizational commitment: the moderating effect of nurse tenure, *J Nurs Manage* 27(8): 1655, 2019.

Bigani DK, Correia AM: On the same page: nurse, patient, and family perceptions of change-of-shift bedside report, *J Pediatr Nurs* 41:84, 2018.

Boamah SA et al.: Effect of transformational leadership on job satisfaction and patient safety outcomes, *Nurs Outlook* 66(2):180, 2018.

Brown K et al.: Grandparents raising grandchildren with disabilities: assessing health status, home environment and impact of a family support case management model, *Int Public Health* 9(2):181, 2017.

de Oliveira SM et al: Prevention actions of burnout syndrome in nurses: an integrating literature review, *Clin Pract Epidemiol Ment Health*, 15:64, 2019.

Haines MM et al.: Improving the quality of healthcare: a cross-sectional study of the features of successful clinical networks. *Public Health Research & Practice*, 2018, https://doi.org/10.17061/phrp28011803. Available at: https://www.phrp.com.au/issues/december-2018-volume-28-issue-4/improving-the-quality-of-healthcare-a-cross-sectional-study-of-the-features-of-successful-clinical-networks/. Accessed April 5, 2021.

Hiler CA et al.: Predictors of moral distress in a US sample of critical care nurses, *Am J Crit Care* 27(1): 59, 2018.

Homeyer S et al.: Effects of interprofessional education for medical and nursing students: enablers, barriers and expectations for optimizing future interprofessional collaboration—a qualitative study, *BMC Nurs* 17(13), doi: 10.1186/s12912-018-0279-x. eCollection, 2018.

Kaiser JA, Westers JB: Nursing teamwork in a health system: a multisite study. *J Nurs Manage* 26(5):555, 2018.

Kaulback MK: Correlating self-directed learning abilities to lifelong learning orientation in baccalaureate nursing students, *Nurse Educator* 45(6):347-351, 2020 –doi: 10.1097/NNE.0000000000000803, available at: https://journals.lww.com/nurseeducatoronline/Citation/2020/11000/Correlating_Self_directed_Learning_Abilities_to.25.aspx. Accessed April 5, 2021.

Kelly LA, Lefton C: Effect of meaningful recognition on critical care nurses' compassion fatigue, *Am J Crit Care* 26(6):438, 2017.

Lacey SR et al: Driving organizational change from the bedside: the AACN Clinical Scene Investigator Academy, *Crit Care Nurse* 37(4):e12, 2017.

Lyman B et al.: Organizational learning in a cardiac intensive care unit, *DCCN* 36(2):78, 2017.

McBeth CL et al: Interprofessional huddle: one children's hospital's approach to improving patient flow, *Pediatr Nurs* 43(2):71, 2017.

Nelson-Brantley HV et al.: Nurse executives leading change to improve critical access hospital outcomes: a literature review with research-informed recommendations, *Online J Rural Nurs Health Care* 18(1):148, 2018.

Okoli C et al.: Shared decision making between patients and healthcare providers and its association with favorable health outcomes among people living with HIV, *AIDS Behav*, 2020, https://doi.org/10.1007/s10461-020-02973-4. Accessed April 5, 2021.

Olender, L et al.: The impact of interprofessional shared governance and a caring professional practice model on staff's self-report of caring, workplace engagement, and workplace empowerment over time, *JONA: The Journal of Nursing Administration* 50(1):52-58, 2020, doi: 10.1097/NNA.0000000000000839. Available at: https://journals.lww.com/jonajournal/Abstract/2020/01000/The_Impact_of_Interprofessional_Shared_Governance.12.aspx. Accessed April 5, 2021.

Prystajecky M et al: A case study of healthcare providers' goals during interprofessional rounds, *J Interprof Care* 31(4):463, 2017.

Riisgaard H et al: Associations between degrees of task delegation and job satisfaction of general practitioners and their staff: a cross-sectional study, *BMC Health Serv Res* 17:44, 2017.

Rosen MA et al.: Teamwork in healthcare: key discoveries enabling safer, high-quality care, *Am Psychol* 73(4): 433-450, 2018.

Shimp KM: Systematic review of turnover/retention and staff perception of staffing and resource adequacy related to staffing, *Nurs Econ* 35(5):239, 2017.

Shirey M et al.: Integration of authentic leadership lens for building high performing interprofessional collaborative practice teams, *Nurs Admin Q* 43(2): 101-112, 2019.

Wei H et al.: The impact of nurse leadership styles on nurse burnout: a systematic literature review, *Nurse Leader* 18(5):439-450, 2020.

22

Ethics and Values

OBJECTIVES

- Discuss the role of ethics in professional nursing.
- Utilize values clarification when you apply ethics in practice.
- Explain the principles and approaches commonly used in health care ethics discussions.
- Compare and contrast the difference between an ethical dilemma and moral distress.
- Apply a stepwise approach to ethical problems.
- Discuss contemporary ethical issues that nurses face.

KEY TERMS

Accountability
Advocacy
Autonomy
Beneficence
Bioethics
Casuistry

Code of ethics
Confidentiality
Deontology
Ethics
Ethics of care
Feminist ethics

Fidelity
Justice
Morals
Nonmaleficence
Utilitarianism
Value

MEDIA RESOURCES

http://evolve.elsevier.com/Potter/fundamentals/
- Review Questions
- Case Study with Questions

- Audio Glossary
- Content Updates
- Answers to QSEN Activity and Review Questions

Ethics is the study of what is right and wrong with our conduct. It concerns our obligations to individuals, groups, and society. Acts that are ethical reflect a commitment to standards that individuals, professions, and societies strive to meet. When decisions must be made about health care, understandable disagreement can occur among health care professionals, families, patients, friends, and people in the community. The right thing to do can be difficult to determine, particularly when individual values, beliefs, and perceptions conflict. This chapter describes concepts that will help you embrace the role of ethics in your professional life and promote resolution when ethical problems develop. Use your critical thinking and clinical judgment skills with ethical decision making when working through ethical problems with patients and families.

BASIC TERMS IN HEALTH ETHICS

Ethical issues differ from legal issues. Legal issues are resolved by reference to laws that are usually concrete and publicly determined. Breaking a law results in a public consequence, such as a ticket for speeding or jail time for stealing. However, ethics has a broader base of interest than the law, referring more to issues of behavior and character. The terms *ethics* and *morals* are sometimes used interchangeably. Morals usually refer to judgment about behavior, based on specific beliefs, and ethics refers to the study of the ideals of right and wrong behavior.

Values play an important role in understanding ethics. A value is a deeply held personal belief about the worth a person holds for an idea, a custom, or an object. The values that a person holds reflect cultural and social influences. For example, a person who makes a living in a rural place may value the environment differently than someone who visits rural areas for recreation. Ethical codes grow from shared values, negotiated and discussed over time through religious groups, ethnic groups, or work groups. As you enter the nursing profession, you undergo a similar process of learning shared values. Clarity about your values and your own point of view will guide you in making effective ethical decisions.

The study of bioethics represents a branch of ethics within the field of health care. The study of bioethics has grown over the last 50 years, beginning with the emergence of technologies related to organ transplant. When researchers perfected kidney transplant procedures in the early 1970s, only a limited number of kidneys were available for transplant compared with the number of patients in need. This lack of resources became an immediate ethical concern. The health care community in the

United States began to address this issue by means of ethical discussion in local and national groups.

Changing medical technologies continue to require societies to face difficult ethical questions. Why should we do genetic testing for diseases we cannot cure? How shall we define quality of life? Who should decide? How are scarce medical resources allocated and by whom? In the study of bioethics, health care professionals agree to negotiate these difficult and important questions by referring to a common set of ethical principles.

An understanding of the concepts common in ethical discourse will help you participate thoughtfully in discussions with others and may help you shape your own thoughts about ethical issues. The application of the concepts is fundamental to developing skills in ethical decision making. During the ethical decision-making process, you will apply the concepts of autonomy, beneficence, nonmaleficence, justice, and fidelity.

Autonomy

Autonomy refers to freedom from external control. In health care the concept applies to respect for the autonomy of patients. It can also apply to agency respect for the autonomy of health care professionals. A commitment to respect the autonomy of others is a fundamental principle of ethical practice.

Respect for patient autonomy refers to the commitment to include patients in decisions about all aspects of care (Burkhardt and Alvita, 2021). It is a key feature of patient-centered care. In respecting patient autonomy, you acknowledge and protect a patient's independence. Respect for autonomy reflects a movement away from paternalistic patient care in which health care providers made all decisions. Involving patients in decisions about their care is now standard practice. We often demonstrate respect for patient autonomy through the informed consent process. Rather than the health care team making choices about patients' care, the team's role is to inform patients about risks and benefits of treatment options and then, with the patients, determine a plan of care that matches their goals and values. In many cases (e.g., surgery and diagnostic procedures), the consent of a patient is documented by the patient's signature.

Another way nurses show respect for patient autonomy is by explaining nursing procedures such as obtaining a blood pressure or administering medications. Nurses also demonstrate respect for patient autonomy by supporting patients who raise questions about procedures and by ensuring that they get the information they request. In addition, your conversations with patients and families can help them to articulate their preferences, values, and goals. Clarifying what is important to them is a key step in making autonomous health care decisions.

Respect for professional autonomy refers to the relationship between members of the health care team and the agencies in which they work. What happens when a health care professional is asked to perform duties that conflict with a religious or personal belief? Health care agencies have developed policies that accommodate respect for health care professionals by finding a way to reassign duties when this conflict occurs. However, the reassignment is conducted so that the patient is protected from abandonment and patient care is not compromised. What happens when an individual employee takes issue with policies or practices of an agency and is concerned that a practice is unsafe? Employees may be concerned about reporting information because of potential retaliation. Some health care agencies have an anonymous reporting system for this reason. Agency whistleblower protections prohibit retaliation against an employee who makes a legitimate report about clinical safety issues. These protections represent expressions of respect for professional autonomy.

Beneficence

Beneficence refers to taking positive actions to help others (Burkhardt and Alvita, 2021). The concept of beneficence is fundamental to the practice of nursing and medicine. The agreement to act with beneficence implies that the best interests of the patient remain more important than self-interest. It implies that nurses practice primarily as a service to others, even in the details of daily work.

Nonmaleficence

Maleficence refers to harm or hurt. Nonmaleficence refers to the avoidance of harm or hurt. In health care, ethical practice involves not only the will to do good but the equal commitment to do no harm (Burkhardt and Alvita, 2021). A health care professional tries to balance the risks and benefits of care while striving at the same time to do the least harm possible. A bone marrow transplant procedure may offer a chance at cure, but the process involves periods of suffering, and it may not be possible to guarantee a positive outcome. Decisions about the best course of action can be difficult and uncertain precisely because nurses agree to avoid harm at the same time as they commit to promoting benefit.

Justice

Justice refers to fairness and the distribution of resources (Burkhardt and Alvita, 2021). The term is most often used in discussions about access to health care, including the just distribution of scarce services and resources. Discussions about health insurance, hospital locations and services, and organ transplants generally are among the issues that cite the concept of justice. The term itself is open to interpretation, as people interpret fairness differently. Does the concept of justice mean that health care resources should be available to those who have earned them? Or should they be distributed equally? Should those with a greater need for resources receive more than others? Especially as health care costs continue to rise, the issue of justice remains a critical part of the discussion about health care reform and access to care.

The term *just culture* refers to the promotion of open discussion without fear of recrimination whenever mistakes, especially those involving adverse events, occur or nearly occur. Blame is withheld at least at first so that system issues and other elements can be investigated for their contributions to the error. By fostering open discussion about errors, members of the health care team become more richly informed participants, able to design new systems that prevent harm.

Fidelity

Fidelity refers to faithfulness or the agreement to keep promises (Doherty, 2020). As a nurse you have a duty to be faithful to the patients you care for, to the health care agency you work for, and to yourself. If you assess a patient for pain and offer a plan to manage the pain, the standard of fidelity encourages you to initiate the interventions in the plan as soon as possible and to monitor the patient's response to the nursing interventions. Fidelity is honored when we strive to provide excellent care to all patients, including those whose values are different from our own. We recognize a professional duty to apply the same skills and knowledge to the care of patients and families, regardless of their background, lifestyle, or past or present choices. When our need to exercise our own autonomy leads us to remove ourselves from a particular treatment or situation, fidelity demands that we not abandon the patient but instead find an equally qualified professional to provide the care we are unable to provide.

Our duty to be faithful to the health care agency employing us means that we follow the policies and procedures set forth or, in the event that the policy or procedure is not appropriate, seek to correct it and improve the standard of care provided by the health care agency. Finally, fidelity to oneself is honored when we attend to our own needs for emotional support, mentoring, or continuing education. Honoring our commitment to ourselves is essential to the delivery of safe and effective care to patients.

PROFESSIONAL NURSING CODE OF ETHICS

A code of ethics is a set of guiding principles that all members of a profession accept. It is a collective statement about the group's expectations and standards of behavior. The American Nurses Association (ANA) established its first Code of Ethics for Nursing in 1950, and the organization has continued to review and revise it periodically. The provisions of the Code of Ethics describe the nurse's obligation to the patient, the role of the nurse as a member of the health care team, and the duties of the nurse to the profession and to society (ANA, 2015). A few of the key principles in the code include advocacy, responsibility, accountability, and confidentiality.

Advocacy

Advocacy refers to the application of one's skills and knowledge for the benefit of another person. Lawyers are sometimes called "advocates" because they use their expertise to advance their clients' best interests. As a nurse you advocate for the health, safety, and rights of patients, including their right to privacy and their right to refuse treatment (Harding et al., 2020). Your special relationship with patients provides you with knowledge that is specific to your role as a registered nurse and as such with the opportunity to make a unique contribution to understanding a patient's point of view.

Responsibility

The word *responsibility* refers to a willingness to respect one's professional obligations and to follow through. As a nurse you are responsible for your actions, the care you provide, and the tasks that you delegate to others. This responsibility also means maintaining your competence to provide care and seeking guidance when you are uncertain of your skills and knowledge. You also demonstrate responsibility by applying your workplace's policies and procedures to the care you provide.

Accountability

Accountability refers to answering for your own actions. You ensure that your professional actions are explainable to your patients and your employer. Health care agencies also exercise accountability by monitoring individual and agency compliance with national standards established by agencies such as The Joint Commission (TJC). TJC establishes national patient safety guidelines to ensure patient and workplace safety through consistent, effective nursing practices (TJC, 2021). The ANA promotes ethical decision making by setting standards for collaborative interprofessional communication (ANA, 2015).

Confidentiality

Patients have the right to keep their personal health information private. Confidentiality refers to the health care team's obligation to respect patient privacy. Confidentiality is a fundamental part of the trusting

relationship between a nurse and a patient (Doherty, 2020). Federal legislation known as the Health Insurance Portability and Accountability Act of 1996 (HIPAA) mandates confidentiality and protection of patients' personal health information. The legislation defines the rights and privileges of patients for protection of privacy. It establishes fines for violations (USDHHS, 2021). In practice, you cannot share information about a patient's medical condition or personal information with anyone who is not involved in the care of the patient. HIPAA calls this the "right to know." HIPAA also regulates communication of patient information contained in medical records (see Chapter 26).

VALUES

Nursing is a work of intimacy. Nursing practice requires you to be in contact with patients physically, emotionally, psychologically, and spiritually. In most other intimate relationships, you choose to enter the relationship, anticipating that at least some of your values will align with those of the other person. But as a nurse you agree to provide care to your patients solely on the basis of their need for your services. The ethical concepts of beneficence and fidelity shape the practice of health care and distinguish it from other common human relationships such as friendship, marriage, and employer-employee. By its very nature, relationships in health care sometimes occur in the presence of conflicting values.

A value is a deeply held belief about the worth of an idea, attitude, custom, or object that affects choices and behaviors. While values reflect cultural and social influences, they can change over time as individuals become part of different groups. For example, you have personal values from your family, education, and other experiences, and then, as a nurse, you develop professional values as a member of the nursing profession and the health care team. Recognizing your own values is like seeing the bubble you live in; most of the time, we look at the world through the lens of our values without acknowledging them. Values are intrinsic to our view of the world. Learning to appreciate your values as your own individual perspective is the first step to working effectively with other health care professionals, patients, and families whose values are different.

Values Clarification

Ethical dilemmas almost always occur in the presence of conflicting values. To resolve ethical conflicts, one needs to distinguish among value, fact, and opinion. Facts are supported by objective data, and opinions are views or ideas that are not necessarily based on facts. Sometimes people have such strong values that they consider them to be facts. However, when people express a strong emotional reaction, this is often a sign that their values are threatened. Sometimes people are so passionate about their values that they become judgmental in a way that intensifies conflict. Clarifying values—your own, your patients', your co-workers'—is an important and effective part of ethical discourse.

Examine the cultural values exercise in Box 22.1. The values in the exercise are in neutral terms so that you can appreciate how differing values need not indicate "right" or "wrong." For example, for some people it is important to remain silent and stoic in the presence of great pain, and for others it is important to talk about it to understand and control it. Identifying values as something separate from facts can help you understand others even when there are differences that set you apart.

APPROACHES TO ETHICS

Historically, health care ethics constituted a search for fixed standards that would determine correct actions. Over time ethics has grown into a field of study that is more flexible and is filled with differences of

The column on the right contains statements describing an opinion; the column on the left contains statements describing the opposite opinion. Neither statement is right, nor is it wrong. These statements reflect opinion, not necessarily fact. If people from a variety of cultures were given this questionnaire, some would strongly agree with the beliefs on the right and others with the opinions on the left. Read each statement and reflect on your own values and opinions. Circle 1 if you strongly agree with the statement on the left and 2 if you moderately agree. Circle 4 if you strongly agree with the statement on the right and 3 if you moderately agree.

Statement	Rank	Statement
Preparing for the future is an important activity and reflects maturity.	1 2 3 4	Life has a predestined course. The individual should follow that course.
Vague answers are dishonest and confusing.	1 2 3 4	Vague answers are sometimes preferred because they avoid embarrassment and confrontation.
Punctuality and efficiency are characteristics of a person who is both intelligent and concerned.	1 2 3 4	Punctuality is not as important as maintaining a relaxed atmosphere, enjoying the moment, and being with family and friends.
When in severe pain, it is important to remain strong and not to complain too much.	1 2 3 4	When in severe pain, it is better to talk about the discomfort and express frustration.
It is self-centered and unwise to accept a gift from someone you do not know well.	1 2 3 4	It is an insult to refuse a gift when it is offered.
Addressing people by their first name shows friendliness.	1 2 3 4	Addressing people by their first name is disrespectful.
Direct questions are usually the best way to gain information.	1 2 3 4	Direct questioning is rude and could cause embarrassment.
Direct eye contact shows interest.	1 2 3 4	Direct eye contact is intrusive.
Ultimately the independence of the individual must come before the needs of the family.	1 2 3 4	The needs of the individual are always less important than the needs of the family.

Modified from Renwick GW, Rhinesmith SH: *An exercise in cultural analysis for managers,* Chicago, 1995, Intercultural Press.

opinion and deeply meaningful efforts to understand human interaction. The following review introduces you to some of the philosophical approaches to ethics that you may encounter during ethical discussions in health care settings. These approaches can be intentionally adopted to help you interpret and address ethical problems in practice. *To illustrate how these approaches work, consider a situation in which a nurse is caring for an older adult, Stella, who has dementia and whose son, David, does not adhere to the unit's visitation policy, namely, that he leave her bedside for half an hour during change of shift.*

Deontology

Deontology proposes a system of ethics that is perhaps most familiar to health care practitioners. Deontology defines actions as right or wrong based on their adherence to rules and principles such as fidelity to promises, truthfulness, and justice (Burkhardt and Alvita, 2021). Instead of looking at consequences of actions to determine whether

they are right or wrong, deontology examines a situation for the existence of essential right or wrong. *In the situation of Stella and David, the nurse applying a deontology approach may see the right action as seeking help in enforcing the visitation policy. Her fidelity to the health care agency supports a duty to enforce its regulations. Making an exception for David when other family members are following the rules is an injustice.*

Deontology requires a mutual understanding of justice, autonomy, and goodness. But it still leaves room for confusion to surface. The principle of respect for autonomy can be complicated when dealing with children and patients, like Stella, who may be unable to voice their preferences. *If Stella stated clearly that she desired David's presence at all times, a respect for her autonomy could be the guiding principle. In this case, the nurse should advocate for an exception to the visitation policy.* A commitment to respect the "rightness" of autonomy is a guiding principle in deontology, but adherence to the principle alone does not always provide clear answers for complicated situations.

Utilitarianism

A utilitarian system of ethics proposes that the value of something is determined by its usefulness. This philosophy is sometimes called *consequentialism* because its main emphasis is on the outcome or consequence of action. The greatest good for the greatest number of people is the guiding principle for determining right action in a utilitarian system (Burkhardt and Alvita, 2021). As with deontology, utilitarianism relies on the application of a certain principle (i.e., measures of "good" and "greatest"). The difference between utilitarianism and deontology is the focus on outcomes. Utilitarianism measures the effect that an act will have; deontology looks at the act itself and judges its "rightness" by the rules or principles it upholds.

In the case of Stella and David, a nurse applying a utilitarian approach may determine that resolving the issue about David's visit should be done in a manner that creates the least risk of disturbing the rest of the patients and the other staff members on the unit. The nurse interprets the greatest good for the greatest number as the absence of conflict and thus negotiates an exception to the visitation policy. While violating the policy is unacceptable in a deontological approach because that action itself is not good, in utilitarianism, if the outcome—a peaceful interaction with the son—is good, then the action itself is correct.

As with deontology, the utilitarian approach has some flaws, mainly that it can be taken too far. Do the ends always justify the means? A classic example in health care is the idea of removing organs from a perfectly healthy person to save the lives of seven other people who are awaiting transplantation. Seven people are more than one, so the outcome is good, but does that make the action, killing that one person, right? In addition, people have conflicting definitions of "greatest good." As with deontology, utilitarianism provides guidance, but it does not guarantee agreement.

Casuistry

Casuistry, or case-based reasoning, turns away from conventional principles of ethics as a way to determine best actions and focuses instead on the details of a situation. People who take this approach to ethics find similar precedent cases and determine a course of action on the basis of what was done to manage that prior situation (Bleyer, 2020). *A nurse applying this approach to the case of Stella and David would consider past instances in which families were permitted to stay at the bedside, even during change of shift, or other instances in which families made a similar request but were asked to follow the policy as it stands. A key step in applying this approach is comparing the details of Stella and David's situation, such as her prognosis and his ability to contribute to her care, to determine which prior situation is the closest match.*

A weakness of the casuistry approach is that finding a similar precedent case may be challenging, particularly in complex situations with unique features.

Feminist Ethics

Noting the limitations of deontology and utilitarianism, scholars who focused on differences between men and women, especially women's points of view, developed a critique of conventional ethical philosophies. Called feminist ethics, this view holds that the natural caring for others is the basis for moral behavior; it places an emphasis on caring relationships and a strong sense of responsibility (Fromme, 2020). Those with a feminist perspective tend to concentrate more on practical solutions than on theory and to ask questions about the people involved and their relationships rather than looking to underlying principles.

For Stella and David, a nurse taking the feminist approach might look for a power imbalance and seek to take action that addresses it. Is David's presence at the bedside intimidating for Stella? Are staff members seeking to enforce the policy assuming a position of unjustified power over David? These questions, which may not surface in a traditional approach, will help determine the action that is right from a feminist ethics perspective.

Critics of feminist ethics worry about the lack of appeal to traditional ethical principles. Without guidance from concepts such as autonomy and beneficence, they argue, solutions to ethical questions will depend too much on subjective judgment.

Ethics of Care

The ethics of care offers an alternative view to utilitarianism and deontology. Similar to feminist ethics, care-based ethics focuses on understanding relationships, personal narratives, and the context in which ethical problems arise. Unlike feminist ethics, ethics of care emphasizes the role of the decision maker in the situation. With deontology and utilitarianism, the decision maker is detached and objective, gathering facts, identifying principles, or predicting outcomes. In the ethics of care, nurses participate in clinical ethics consultation, with patient advocacy being a top priority (Atkinson et al., 2020). This philosophy often resonates with nurses who, in their intimate experiences with patients, are often making ethical decisions while engaged in caring relationships.

A nurse taking the ethics of care approach with Stella and David first learns more about the relationships involved in the current situation and then identifies the course of action that best supports them. Stella and David have a relationship with each other, and the nurses caring for Stella also have a relationship with each of them. What action, allowing David to stay or asking that he leave, will have the best impact on those relationships? Are there additional actions, such as listening to David's reasons for wanting to stay, that might have a positive impact on these relationships?

NURSING POINT OF VIEW

All patients in health care systems interact with nurses at some point, and they interact in ways that are unique to nursing. Nurses generally engage with patients over longer periods of time than do health care providers from other disciplines. They are involved in intimate physical acts such as bathing, feeding, and special procedures. As a result, patients and families may feel more comfortable in revealing information or in asking questions they have not shared with other health care providers. Details about family life, information about coping styles, personal preferences, and details about fears and insecurities are likely to come out during the course of nursing interventions. Your ability to shape your care based on this special knowledge provides an indispensable contribution to the overall care of your patient.

FIG. 22.1 Nurses collaborate with other professionals in making ethical decisions.

Today patient care involves collaboration with other disciplines. Therapists, health care providers, surgeons, social workers, and pharmacists are some of the interprofessional team members who will provide care to patients with you and bring their own points of view. In addition, managers and administrators from many different professional backgrounds contribute to ethical discourse with their knowledge of systems, distribution of resources, financial possibilities, and limitations (Fig. 22.1).

> ### REFLECT NOW
>
> Consider a time in which you disagreed with a family member or a friend about the correct action to take in a situation. What factors helped you or prevented you from honestly expressing your own point of view? What did it feel like to listen to the other person's perspective?

Types of Ethical Problems

Two common ethical problems that nurses encounter are ethical dilemmas and moral distress (Burkhardt and Alvita, 2021). As an example, take a situation in which a nursing student working with an older adult finds that the patient refuses to take her morning pills. "I won't take a single one until you give me my hormone medicine." The patient has several medical problems, but none of her morning pills fit the description of "hormone medicine." In relating the issue to another member of the health care team, she is advised, "Why don't you go in there with one of the pills she needs and tell her it is her hormone pill? Then she'll cooperate with you."

Ethical Dilemma. The nursing student immediately feels conflicted by this advice. If the student follows the suggestion, the student can accomplish the task of administering the medications, a task that is in the patient's best interest and so could be justified by the principle of beneficence. At the same time, the student feels uncomfortable lying to the patient. Lying to her is a violation of the patient's autonomy, a betrayal of her trust. This interpretation of the situation is a classic example of an ethical dilemma. The student cannot do both options—take the advice to lie so that the patient gets the benefit of the medications *and* be truthful in identifying the pills to the patient. An ethical problem is called a dilemma when two opposing courses of action can both be justified by ethical principles (Burkhardt and Alvita, 2021).

Moral Distress. Now imagine the same situation with a change in details. The person the nursing student consults for help is the patient's health care provider, and the advice to lie about the pills feels to the student like a specific direction—not so much a suggestion but more of an order. At the same time, envision that at this moment during the clinical day, there is no one else the student can turn to for help. The student was told by her clinical instructor about the need to be more efficient in completing tasks and the medications were due to be given 30 minutes ago. Given the pressure of time and the source of the advice, the student might feel compelled to lie to the patient. But what if, based on her values, the student feels that action is morally wrong? Now the student is at risk for moral distress, a different ethical problem. In moral distress, instead of competing options for action, the nurse feels the need to take a specific action while believing that action to be wrong (Burkhardt and Alvita, 2021).

Distinguishing between ethical dilemmas and moral distress is important to achieving resolution. When the problem is a dilemma, with two opposing but justifiable options, often the application of the nursing process will include identifying more options. For example, the student might be able to succeed in giving the patient her medications without lying if the student builds trust with the patient by spending time with her. With moral distress, as this example shows, the environment often contributes to the problem. Discuss situations that generate moral distress with another person when they are identified. Additional resources, such as nursing colleagues, managers, and other health care professionals, can work together to address the factors that contribute to moral distress (Box 22.2).

Processing an Ethical Problem

Resolving an ethical problem is similar to the nursing process in its methodical approach to a clinical issue. However, it differs from the nursing process in that it requires negotiation of differences of opinion and clarity about situations where there may not be a single right answer. Finding clarity and consensus can occur when the following elements remain essential to the process: the presumption of goodwill on the part of all participants, strict adherence to confidentiality, patient-centered decision making, and the welcome participation of families and primary caregivers.

Because they involve values and obligations, ethical problems can raise troubling emotions. Processing an ethical problem begins with recognizing that an ethical problem exists (Doherty, 2020). Sometimes communication problems look like ethical problems, and taking the time to speak openly and listen to others achieves resolution. You then gather pertinent information about the case, including recent clinical evaluations, the views of colleagues, and the values and perspectives of the patient and family involved. Examining your personal values at this point can help to differentiate between fact and opinion, an important part of the process. Once information is gathered and ethical elements identified, developing a statement of the problem will facilitate discussion. The next step, listing all possible courses of action, requires some creativity and is best done in a conversation with others. Deciding on an action and implementing it sometimes requires courage. The final step is an evaluation of the outcome (Doherty, 2020) (Box 22.3).

BOX 22.2 EVIDENCE-BASED PRACTICE

Moral Distress

PICOT Question: Do strategies that build moral resilience reduce moral distress among acute care nurses?

Evidence Summary

Moral distress describes the anguish experienced when a person feels unable to act according to closely held core values. Evidence indicates that causes of moral distress among critical care nurses include quality of life concerns for patients, lacking a voice in documentation, difficulty with their advocacy role, ambiguity between the guidelines of care and limitation of licensure, trying to implement personal values to provide care, communication issues when full disclosure has not been implemented with the patient and family, and role conflict between goals of care and barriers to care delivery (Burton et al., 2020). Nurses need to be aware of moral distress, which is foundational to developing strategies for moral resilience (Burton et al., 2020). While multiple studies document the existence of moral distress and its association with aspects of the work environment, interventions to address moral distress are an area of evolving research (Burton et al., 2020). Strategies to address moral distress consider not only the individual experiencing the problem but also the work environment. Health care agencies often offer services such as an ethics resource or a moral distress service to specifically address the needs of nurses. Sonya et al. (2020) described a Moral Distress Consult Service that is accessible in the hospital and helps address pervasive or persistent issues that are causing moral distress. The American Association of Critical-Care Nurses (AACN) created the Standards for Establishing and Sustaining Healthy Work Environments and an Assessment Tool that health care teams can use to identify and address gaps (AACN, 2016). Moral resilience is the ability to grow and even gain confidence from adverse and complex ethical problems. While further study is needed, deliberate attention to building moral resilience among nurses may reduce their susceptibility to moral distress.

Application to Nursing Practice

- Develop and practice skilled communication. Learning to talk with colleagues, patients, and families in a professional manner that conveys a desire to share your own views and an openness to theirs can help prevent conflicts and reduce moral distress.
- Identify resources available to help you reduce moral distress. Find out whether your hospital has an ethics committee or other resource for support and how that resource is consulted.
- Find a mentor or leader on your unit with a particular skill in examining ethical problems to help you process ethical situations.
- Create a culture of moral resiliency with targeted formal and informal support and education for staff (Burton et al., 2020).
- Collaborate with health care administrators regarding ways to better understand, recognize, and manage patient and nurse factors related to moral distress (Burton et al., 2020).
- Design education programs to assist nurses to recognize and respond to stressful situations (Burton et al., 2020).
- Educate staff members on how to use their voices to communicate constructively and confidently about morally challenging situations (Burton et al., 2020).
- Evaluate existing programs, including just-in-time support, a health care ethics residency, and moral resiliency training (Burton et al., 2020).

If the process involves a family conference or changes in the treatment plan, you document all relevant information in the medical record. Some agencies use a special ethics consultation form to structure documentation. However, if the ethical concern does not directly affect patient care, you may document the discussion in meeting minutes or in an e-mail to those involved in the discussion.

BOX 22.3 Key Steps in the Resolution of an Ethical Dilemma

Step 1: Ask: Is this an ethical problem?

Step 2: Gather information relevant to the case. Patient, family, health care agency, and social perspectives are important sources of relevant information.

Step 3: Identify the ethical elements in the situation by clarifying values and recognizing the principals involved. Distinguish among fact, opinion, and values.

Step 4: Name the problem. A clear, simple statement of the problem is not always easy, but it helps to ensure effectiveness in the final plan and facilitates discussion.

Step 5: Identify possible courses of action. Access others for their input and be creative in identifying different options.

Step 6: Create and implement an action plan. Gather support from others and identify an alternative action if the chosen one does not achieve resolution.

Step 7: Evaluate the action plan to determine whether further action is needed or if lessons learned in this experience can be applied forward.

To review the process of ethical decision making, consider the following situation:

You are caring for Miguel, an 18-year-old with type 1 diabetes mellitus. Another nurse tells you that his parents are supportive, involved, and knowledgeable about his condition, but Miguel is mostly angry and is not interested in diabetes education. You walk into the room and find that a friend from Miguel's high school is visiting and has brought in candy and other snacks that contradict Miguel's prescribed diet. What is the best action to take?

- **Step 1.** Ask: Is this an ethical problem?

While feeling uncertain about how to respond can be an indication of an ethical problem, not all uncertainty involves values and obligations. Some uncertainty can resolve with asking for advice or gathering more information. When strong emotions are triggered and when you are in a situation in which the action you take will demonstrate your personal or professional values, then you may have an ethical problem. If the problem is an ethical dilemma, you will likely feel conflicted between opposing courses of action, each of which seems right in some ways and wrong in others. Moral distress often manifests as anger or frustration (Burton et al., 2020).

In this case, more clinical information alone will not resolve the problem; you know that Miguel's health could be harmed if he ate all the candy and snacks his friends brought him. You may feel angry that Miguel is threatening his own health, which, as a member of the health care team, you feel obligated to protect. At the same time, you may also value Miguel's autonomy; he is technically an adult and has a right to select his diet, as long as he is informed of the risks and benefits. If you feel compelled to allow him to enjoy the snacks his friend brought while also feeling that it is wrong to do so, the situation may become morally distressing. There could be an ethical dilemma because two opposing actions—to try to stop Miguel from eating the snacks or to leave him alone—can both be justified. The situation is an ethical problem.

- **Step 2.** Gather information that is relevant to the case.

Resolution of ethical problems can come from unlikely sources. Helpful information may include clinical information about the patient's current state of health, literature about his disease process, and information about his religious, cultural, and family background. A key strategy in gathering information is to ask open-ended questions and take time to listen. Because our interpretation of a situation is based on our own values, we need focused interaction to hear the perspectives of others.

A review of Miguel's chart shows that his diabetes is poorly controlled. There is a note from the hospital's diabetes education program indicating that Miguel and his parents were given information about a diabetic diet and appeared to understand the information. There is also a note by the social worker concerned that Miguel is having trouble accepting this diagnosis.

- **Step 3.** Identify the ethical elements in the problem and examine your values.

Part of the goal is to accurately identify your own perspective, and an equally critical goal is to form respect for the perspectives of others. Consider whether the principles discussed earlier support a particular course of action. Take a moment to examine whether there are relationships involved that need to be supported or that could be adversely affected by actions to resolve the problem.

Reflect on your values. You want to ensure that Miguel manages his diabetes because you value his health. At the same time, you recognize that as a teenager, he wants the freedom to make his own choices, unrestrained by his disease process. You value him as a person and recognize that in addition to his physical health problems, he has developmental needs. Beneficence, the obligation to do good, supports you in seeking the action that is best for Miguel. The concept of autonomy supports actions that respect his right to make his own choices, while fidelity to the health care team supports actions that adhere to the current treatment plan.

- **Step 4.** Name the problem.

This step is harder than it sounds and often goes better if you involve others—either a friend, another nurse, or the health care team. While it is possible to develop a statement that specifically describes the problem on your own, speaking aloud encourages you to use the right language and allows you to get feedback from others. As you will find in Step 5, you may need to collaborate in later steps too, so identifying someone to talk to at this step may facilitate a faster resolution.

After reviewing Miguel's medical record, you find a colleague who has a few minutes to hear your story. As you talk to her, you say, "On the one hand, I want to go in there and take away that food because he really shouldn't have it, and I know he knows that. On the other hand, I can see where he may be trying to show his independence from his parents and do things that other teenagers do." You arrive at the conclusion that you have an ethical dilemma between acting with beneficence to protect Miguel's health and respecting his autonomy.

- **Step 5.** Identify possible courses of action.

In a dilemma, there are two courses of action that can be justified, but they are opposing, so it is often helpful to think of other options. At this stage, it is important to know your resources. Ask yourself what the options are, and also ask who is available to help. Like most aspects of health care, ethics is best managed as a team and not in isolation. Knowing the resources available to help you with ethical problems is similar to knowing the resources for clinical issues. Box 22.4 lists some of the resources to consider.

As you talk to your colleague, you identify the option of taking a tough stance with Miguel and removing the food and the option of avoiding his room and pretending to be unaware of his behavior. Your colleague points out that another option is to ask him about his behavior but in a kind way, not punitive or threatening. You also consider calling in Miguel's health care provider to talk to him, calling his parents and asking that they intervene, or pulling Miguel's friend out of the room and explaining to him that he needs to leave and take the food with him because he is disrupting Miguel's care.

BOX 22.4   Resources to Address Ethical Problems

Nursing colleagues—to listen to the problem, offer alternative actions, and help you articulate the issue. Giving and receiving support from other nurses promotes a positive work environment.

Nurse leaders—may include a preceptor, charge nurse, manager, educator, or advanced practice registered nurse. They may have faced and managed similar situations and so have guidance to offer. They can also access other resources within the hospital.

Members of the interprofessional team—includes physicians, social workers, registered dietitians, therapists, pharmacists, and chaplains. All may be interacting with the patient or are aware of the situation that you are facing. Hearing their perspectives can help you to identify the problem and consider solutions.

Consultation services—may include ethics committees and palliative care specialists. Ethics committees often gather members of the team with divergent views and facilitate productive conversation. Palliative care consult services are a resource in some health care agencies for the management of seriously ill patients.

Professional organizations—often set standards for nursing practice and have web-based resources to help you develop knowledge and skills in ethical analysis.

Boards of Nursing—can help address questions about scope of practice and competency.

• **Step 6.** Create and implement an action plan and carry it out.

Often through the process of articulating the problem and listing the options, the course of action that is the best fit becomes clear. Rather than determining a single action to take, it may be helpful to select what to do first and then what to do later if that first step is ineffective in achieving resolution. For instance, if in identifying options for action you decide to call on a particular resource, such as a manager, for help, you may also decide that if the manager validates the issue, you will go on to consult the hospital ethics committee.

This step requires courage. Because ethics deals with values and obligations, unpleasant emotions such as fear and anger can occur. As much as possible, focus on your desired outcome, which is resolution of the ethical issue, to help you enact the plan.

You decide to take your colleague's advice and go to the room to speak to Miguel. If that is ineffective, then you will call on other members of the health care team. Your colleague helps you to plan the words you will use. Despite your nervousness, you enter the room and tell Miguel, "I don't want to stop you from enjoying your friend's visit, but I'm concerned about the snacks he brought. I know you've had education about your diet. Can we talk about that?"

Miguel shrugs and says, "I don't really care." You then ask, "Well, what do you care about?" Miguel looks surprised. His friend smiles and says the name of a computer game Miguel likes. "That's what Miguel cares about," the friend says. A conversation ensues among you, Miguel, and his friend, and for the first time Miguel seems content rather than sullen and angry. After the conversation, you ask Miguel if his friend can take the snacks with him when he leaves, telling him, "It sounds as if you have things to do that are better than being in the hospital, and these snacks won't help you get out of here." Miguel nods and helps you pack the food back into the friend's grocery bag.

• **Step 7.** Evaluate the action plan.

This is the step where you decide whether further action is needed or resolution has been achieved. If the evaluation shows that the issue has

resolved, be sure to consider what aspects of your actions and the actions of others made that happen. These are lessons to apply in the future. If the situation is not resolved, then further action is required.

In evaluating the outcome with Miguel, you realize that spending a few minutes to learn more about him made it easier to negotiate the removal of the snacks. He came to trust you because of the interest you showed in him as a person; this is often more effective than education that tells patients what they can and cannot do. This is a strategy you can apply in the future.

Ethics Committees

Most hospitals have an ethics committee devoted to the teaching and processing of ethical issues and dilemmas. An ethics committee involves individuals from different disciplines and backgrounds who support health care agencies with three major functions: providing clinical ethics consultation, developing and/or revising policies pertaining to clinical ethics and hospital policy (e.g., advance directives, withholding and withdrawing life-sustaining treatments, informed consent, organ procurement), and facilitating education about topical issues in clinical ethics. In most agencies, any person seeking ethical advice, including nurses, physicians, health care providers, patients, and family members, can request access to an ethics committee.

Ethics committees often conduct their work by calling a meeting with the members of the team and the patient and family involved in the situation. When you attend an ethics meeting, be sure to articulate a personal point of view and at the same time show respect for the points of view of others. A successful meeting is one in which every perspective is heard. Sometimes these meetings result in consensus around a specific course of action; other times the meeting ends without a clear plan but with an improved understanding of one another's perspectives.

You may also process ethical issues in settings other than a committee. Nurses provide insight about ethical problems at family conferences, staff meetings, or even in one-on-one meetings. As a member of a health care community, regardless of your work setting, you can reduce the risk for moral distress by promoting discourse even when disagreements or confusion are profound. You will find it helpful when engaged in these conversations to assume that all the participants want to do good, even if they may have different ideas about what that means.

QSEN **Building Competency in Patient-Centered Care** You are assigned to care for a 75-year-old patient who is readmitted to the hospital after having knee surgery a week ago. He was brought to the hospital by ambulance because his family could not wake him up. In the emergency department, he responds well to treatment for opioid overdose, becoming more awake and alert. When you enter the room to do an initial assessment, the daughter expresses anger at her father's situation, namely that he was discharged after surgery with "too much medication." She states her belief that the care on the last hospital stay was "really inappropriate, especially since the news tells us we are in an opioid crisis." How will a focus on patient-centered care help you address this patient's needs and the daughter's concern?

Answers to QSEN Activities can be found on the Evolve website.

ISSUES IN HEALTH CARE ETHICS

Ethical issues change as society and technologies change, but common denominators remain: the basic process used to address the issues and your responsibility to deal with them. The following section describes a few of the many current sources of ethical concerns.

Social Media

The access to Internet-based social networks, such as Facebook, Twitter, Snapchat, YouTube, and Instagram, may present ethical challenges for nurses. On the one hand, social media can be a supportive source of information about patient care or professional nursing activities and can provide you with emotional support when you encounter hardships at work. Social media can also be a source of support to your patients, to connect with friends and loved ones who cannot be physically present. On the other hand, the risk to patient privacy with social media is great (NCSBN, 2018). Posting information or pictures about patients, even without specific identifiers, is a violation of confidentiality.

Interaction between health care professionals and patients on social media is also problematic. Online "friendship" with a patient risks clouding your ability to remain objective in your clinical perceptions. This crosses the professional boundary between the patient and professional, and the relationship becomes more personal. The public nature of online interactions poses the additional risk that other users will recognize the nature of your relationship with the patient and learn more than they should about that person's health (NCSBN, 2018). Workplace policies may help to answer questions you have about when and where it is appropriate to engage in social media. In addition, the ANA (n.d.) has created a webpage with principles to guide nurses' use of social media (see https://www.nursingworld.org/social/).

Quality of Life

Quality of life is deeply personal. Health care researchers use quality-of-life measures to scientifically define the value and benefits of medical interventions. Any intervention creates a burden for the patient and family, and this must be offset by the benefit that they will receive from that care. Injections of flu vaccine, for instance, cause pain, but the short-term nature of this burden is offset by the large benefit of potentially avoiding infection with the flu or spreading of the flu, which are low-quality experiences. A more complex intervention, such as a 6-month course of chemotherapy, creates a greater burden and so impacts the quality of the patient's life to a greater degree. That impact is acceptable if the treatment outcome is a return to quality of life, based on the patient's definition. In the event that the treatment is unlikely to result in a quality of life that the patient finds acceptable, a different plan of care is considered.

Objective measures of quality of life can include the age of a patient, the patient's ability to live independently, or the ability to contribute to society in a gainful way. Subjective measures involve asking patients to identify their priorities, what they enjoy, and what matters most to them. Increasingly, scientists incorporate not just observed measurement but also patient self-reports about quality of life and other outcomes, referred to as Patient-Reported Outcomes. As a nurse, you can facilitate conversations about treatment choices by encouraging patients to articulate their definition of quality of life.

REFLECT NOW

What matters most to you and so should be included in your own personal definition of quality of life? What roles, relationships, or activities are you engaged in that are most meaningful to you?

Care at the End of Life

Providing care to patients at the end of life and to those with serious illness who may be nearing end of life is a frequent source of ethical problems. While everyone can agree that a "good death" is desirable, there are a variety of opinions about what a "good death" looks like. In addition, patients and families may have goals for end of life, such as adequate pain control or being with family, but expect that this will happen much later and not now. Predictions about health outcomes are not always accurate; thus health care providers may have difficulty conveying to patients with serious illness that end of life is at hand. Because views about death and dying are part of deeply held spiritual and cultural beliefs, conflicts about end-of-life care are common in health care. These conflicts can occur between members of the health care team and among patients, families, and team members (Fromme, 2020).

The term *futile* refers to something that is hopeless or serves no useful purpose. In health care discussions, the term *futile* refers to interventions unlikely to produce benefit for a patient (Fromme, 2020). For example, if a patient is dying of a condition with little or no hope of recovery, almost any intervention beyond symptom management and comfort measures is seen as futile. In this situation an agreement to label an intervention as futile can help the health care team members, families, and patients turn to palliative care measures as a more constructive approach to the situation (see Chapter 36).

Access to Health Care

Access to health care is an ethical issue of justice (Burkhardt and Alvita, 2021). The questions of "Is health care a right that everyone can claim?" and "How can we best divide the health care resources we have?" involve fairness and justice. In the United States, the cost of care is such that few can afford services unless they are enrolled in an insurance plan. In some cases, health insurance is provided as a benefit of employment. Those who do not have employer-based health insurance may qualify for state-based Medicaid programs on the basis of need or for Medicare, a federal insurance program available to all individuals age 65 and older. Because of conflicting views about what is fair and because of its effect on everyone, access to health care is a controversial issue.

While the nature of insurance coverage varies, most plans allow an individual to access some basic preventive care and more expensive urgent services when unexpected changes in health occur. In the latter part of the 20th century, as health care costs increased at a dramatic rate, the number of people with insurance declined. In 2010, the Affordable Care Act (ACA) was passed to create regulations that control costs and improve the availability of insurance. This legislation has facilitated access to care for millions of formerly uninsured individuals in the United States. According to a 2019 report by the National Health Center for Health Statistics, part of the U.S. Department of Health and Human Services, the number of uninsured people in the United States declined by 18 million between 2010 and 2018 (Cohen et al., 2019). The ACA also offered changes in payment for services to reward practices that reduce harm and promote quality outcomes. The aim of this part of the legislation was to expand access to less expensive preventive health services and so to reduce the incidence of expensive, burdensome chronic illness. How people access health care in the United States will continue to evolve. Staying knowledgeable about affordable care in your community as a way to ensure healthy outcomes is an important part of your role as advocate for your patients and will reflect your ethical commitment to justice (Box 22.5).

The courage and intelligence to act as both an advocate for patients and a professional member of the health care community come from a committed effort to learn and understand ethical principles. As a professional nurse, you provide a unique point of view regarding patients, the systems that support patients, and the agencies that make up the health care system. You have an obligation and a privilege to articulate that point of view. Learning how to identify and discuss ethical issues is necessary to exercise this privilege. Review and consideration of various ethical principles help you form personal points of view, a necessary skill in the negotiation of difficult ethical situations.

BOX 22.5 CULTURAL ASPECTS OF CARE

Access to Affordable Health Care

Since the implementation of the Affordable Care Act, more residents in the United States have access to care than ever before. But according to the 2018 National Healthcare Quality and Disparities Report (QDR), people of color, ethnic minorities, and low-income residents are "disproportionately represented among those with access problems." Reports from the QDR reveal that lack of health insurance is the most significant contributing factor to poor quality of care (AHRQ, 2020).

Implications for Patient-Centered Care
- Issues of justice and the just distribution of resources help to inform the discussion about access to care and its effect on health care outcomes.
- Health outcomes often correlate directly to health care access.
- Know and respect patients' cultural practices regarding health promotion and health care needs (see Chapter 9).
- Identify culturally appropriate resources for patients and families in their communities.

KEY POINTS

- Learning and applying the language of ethics is an essential element of nursing practice.
- Understanding our own values and encouraging patients, families, and colleagues to clarify their values promote productive discussion of ethical problems.
- You apply fundamental concepts such as autonomy, justice, fidelity, and beneficence to ethical decision making.
- Approaches to ethics include deontology, utilitarianism, and a relationship-based perspective.
- In an ethical dilemma, a nurse faces two equally justifiable courses of action, whereas in moral distress the nurse feels unable to take the action that is correct.
- Using a systematic approach similar to the nursing process promotes resolution of ethical issues. While the specific ethical issues nurses face evolve and change over time, the values and obligations remain constant.
- Although ethical issues often change with changes in technology and society, common ethical issues surrounding nursing practice include the use of social media as a nursing professional, determining the burdens and benefits of treatment on a patient's quality of life, providing care at the end of life, and challenges regarding patients' access to health care.

REFLECTIVE LEARNING

- Do you think there are situations in which maintaining confidentiality and withholding private information are not the right actions? Discuss why.
- Think about your first impression of a patient early in the day, when you first met. How did this impression change over the course of spending a shift involved in that patient's care? How do you think this change in your perspective relates to your ethical obligations as a nurse?
- What questions might you ask a patient if you wanted to better understand the patient's view of quality of life?

REVIEW QUESTIONS

1. The nurse is caring for a patient who needs a liver transplant to survive. This patient has been out of work for several months, does not have health insurance, and cannot afford the procedure. Which of the following statements speaks to the ethical elements of this case?
   1. The health care team should select a plan that considers the principle of justice as it pertains to the distribution of health care resources.
   2. The patient should enroll in a clinical trial of a new technology that can do the work of the liver, similar to the way dialysis treats kidney disease.
   3. The social worker should look into enrolling the patient in Medicaid, since many states offer expanded coverage.
   4. A family meeting should take place in which the details of the patient's poor prognosis are made clear to his family so that they can adopt a palliative approach.
2. When designing a plan for pain management for a patient following surgery, the nurse assesses that the patient's priority is to be as free of pain as possible. The nurse and patient work together to identify a plan to manage the pain. The nurse continually reviews the plan with the patient to ensure that the patient's priority is met. If the nurse's actions are driven by respect for autonomy, what aspect of this scenario best demonstrates this action?
   1. Assessing the patient's pain on a numeric scale every 2 hours
   2. Asking the patient to establish the goal for pain control
   3. Using alternative measures such as distraction or repositioning to relieve the pain
   4. Monitoring the patient for oversedation as a side effect of his pain medication
3. The application of deontology does not always resolve an ethical problem. Which of the following statements best explains one of the limitations of deontology?
   1. The emphasis on relationships feels uncomfortable to decision makers who want more structure in deciding the best action.
   2. The single focus on power imbalances does not apply to all situations in which ethical problems occur.
   3. In a diverse community it can be difficult to find agreement on which principles or rules are most important.
   4. The focus on consequences rather than on the "goodness" of an action makes decision makers uncomfortable.
4. The *ethics of care* suggests that ethical dilemmas can best be solved by attention to relationships. How does this differ from other approaches to ethical problems? (Select all that apply.) Ethics of care:
   1. pays attention to the context in which caring occurs.
   2. is used only by nurses because it is part of the Nursing Code of Ethics.
   3. requires understanding the relationships between involved parties.
   4. considers the decision maker's relationships with other involved parties.
   5. is an approach that suggests a greater commitment to patient care.
   6. considers the decision maker to be in a detached position outside the ethical problem.
5. The following are steps in the process to help resolve an ethical problem. What is the best order of these steps to achieve resolution?
   1. List all the possible actions that could be taken to resolve the problem.
   2. Articulate a statement of the problem or dilemma that you are trying to resolve.
   3. Develop and implement a plan to address the problem.
   4. Gather all relevant information regarding the clinical, social, and spiritual aspects of the problem.
   5. Take time to clarify values and identify the ethical elements, such as principles and key relationships involved.
   6. Recognize that the problem requires ethics.

6. Which social media uses can be implemented with patients and families without violating confidentiality? (Select all that apply.)
    1. Social media can be used to provide supportive information.
    2. Results such as x-ray results can easily be sent via social media.
    3. Family and friends who cannot be present can connect with the patient.
    4. All health information can be shared on social media.
    5. Social media should never be used with patients and families.
7. Resolution of an ethical problem involves discussion with the patient, the patient's family, and participants from appropriate health care disciplines. Which statement best describes the role of the nurse in the resolution of ethical problems?
    1. To articulate the nurse's unique point of view, including knowledge based on clinical and psychosocial observations
    2. To study the literature on current research about the possible clinical interventions available for the patient in question
    3. To hold a point of view but realize that respect for the authority of administrators and health care providers takes precedence over personal views
    4. To allow the patient and the health care provider private time to resolve the dilemma on the basis of ethical principles
8. Which statements reflect the difficulty that can occur for agreement on a common definition of the word *quality* when it comes to quality of life? (Select all that apply.)
    1. Community values influence definitions of quality, and they are subject to change over time.
    2. Individual experiences influence perceptions of quality in different ways, making consensus difficult.
    3. The value of elements such as cognitive skills, ability to perform meaningful work, and relationship to family is difficult to quantify using objective measures.
    4. Statistical analysis is difficult to apply when the outcome cannot be quantified.
    5. Whether a person has a job is an objective measure, but it does not play a role in understanding quality of life.

9. Which statements properly apply an ethical principle to justify access to health care? (Select all that apply.)
    1. Access to health care reflects the commitment of society to principles of beneficence and justice.
    2. If low income compromises access to care, respect for autonomy is compromised.
    3. Access to health care is a privilege in the United States, not a right.
    4. Poor access to affordable health care causes harm that is ethically troubling because nonmaleficence is a basic principle of health care ethics.
    5. If a new drug is discovered that cures a disease but at great cost per patient, the principle of justice suggests that the drug should be made available to those who can afford it.
10. Match the following actions (1 through 4) with the terms (a through d) listed below:

    ____1. You see an open medical record on the computer and close it so that no one else can read the record without proper access.
    ____2. You administer a once-a-day cardiac medication at the wrong time, but nobody sees it. However, you contact the provider and your nurse manager and follow agency procedure.
    ____3. A patient at the end of life wants to go home to die, but the family wants every care possible. The nurse contacts the primary care provider about the patient's request.
    ____4. You tell your patient that you will return in 30 minutes to give him his next pain medication.

    a. Advocacy
    b. Responsibility
    c. Accountability
    d. Confidentiality

Answers: 1. 1; **2.** 2; **3.** 3; **4.** 1, 3; **4.** 1, 3; **5.** 6, 4, 5, 2, 1, 3; **6.** 1, 3; **7.** 1; **8.** 1, 2, 4; **9.** 1, 2, 4; **10.** 1d, 2c, 3a, 4b.

Rationales for Review Questions can be found on the Evolve website.

REFERENCES

Agency for Healthcare Research and Quality (AHRQ): *2018 National Healthcare Quality and Disparities Report*, 2020. https://www.ahrq.gov/research/findings/nhqrdr/nhqdr18/index.html. Accessed April 24, 2021.

American Nurses Association (ANA*): Responsibility for nursing judgments, decisions, and actions. guide to the code of ethics for nurses with interpretive statements: development, interpretation, and application*, 2015. https://www.nursingworld.org/nurses-books/guide-to-the-code-of-ethics-for-nurses-with-interpretive-statements-develo/. Accessed April 25, 2021.

Burkhardt M, Alvita N: *Ethical competence in nursing practice: competencies, skills and decision making*, New York, 2021, Springer Publishing Company.

Cohen RA, et al: *Health insurance coverage: early release of estimates from the National Health Interview Survey*, 2019. https://www.cdc.gov/nchs/data/nhis/earlyrelease/insur201905.pdf. Accessed August 16, 2020.

Doherty RF: *Ethical dimensions in the health professions*, ed 7, St Louis, 2020, Elsevier.

Harding M, et al: *Lewis's medical-surgical nursing: Assessment and management of clinical problems*, ed 11, Philadelphia, 2020, Elsevier.

Fromme E: *Ethical issues in palliative care*, UpToDate, 2020. https://www.uptodate.com/contents/ethical-issues-in-palliative-care/print. Accessed August 16, 2020.

National Council of State Boards of Nursing (NCSBN): *A nurse's guide to the use of social media*, 2018. https://

www.ncsbn.org/NCSBN_SocialMedia.pdf. Accessed August 16, 2020.

The Joint Commission (TJC): *2021 National Patient Safety Goals*, Oakbrook Terrace, IL, 2021, The Commission. https://www.jointcommission.org/standards/national-patient-safety-goals/. Accessed April 22, 2021.

US Department of Health and Human Services (USDHHS): *HIPAA for professionals*, 2021. https://www.hhs.gov/hipaa/for-professionals/index.html. Accessed August 25, 2021.

RESEARCH REFERENCES

American Association of Critical-Care Nurses: *AACN standards for establishing and sustaining healthy work environments*, ed 2, Aliso Viejo, CA, 2016, The Association.

Atkinson S, et al: Patient rights at the end of life: the ethics of aid-in-dying, *Prof Case Manag* 25(2):77, 2020.

Bleyer B: Casuistry: on a method of ethical judgement in patient care, *HEC Forum* 32:211, 2020.

Burton M, et al: Moral distress: defined and described by neonatal and pediatric critical care nurses in a quaternary care free-standing pediatric hospital. *Dimens Crit Care Nurs* 39(2):101, 2020.

Sonya D, et al: Addressing moral distress in critical care nurses: a systemized literature review of intervention studies, *Connect: The World of Critical Care Nursing* 13(2), 2020.

Legal Implications in Nursing Practice

OBJECTIVES

- Compare the effects of constitutional, statutory, civil, and criminal law on nursing practice.
- Describe how standards of nursing care shape your nursing practice.
- Discuss how federal statutes promote patient safety and affect nursing practice.
- Explain how state laws and regulations affect nursing practice.
- Summarize guidelines that affect nurses in the workplace.
- Determine nursing actions most often associated with nursing malpractice.
- Define the standard of proof required to establish a nurse's negligence.
- Discuss how risk management, performance improvement (PI), and quality improvement (QI) reduce a nurse's legal risk for negligence and malpractice.
- Identify proactive measures nurses can take to help reduce their legal risks in the workplace.

KEY TERMS

Administrative law
Battery
Case law
Civil law
Common law
Constitutional law
Criminal law
Defamation of character
Durable power of attorney for health care (DPAHC)

Informed consent
Intentional tort
Libel
Malpractice
Neglect
Negligence
Nurse delegation
Nurse practice acts
Occurrence report
Professional licensure defense

Quasi-intentional torts
Risk management
Scope of nursing practice
Slander
Standard of proof
Standards of nursing care
Statutory law
Torts
Unintentional torts

MEDIA RESOURCES

http://evolve.elsevier.com/Potter/fundamentals/
- Review Questions
- Audio Glossary

- Case Study with Questions
- Content Updates
- Answers to QSEN Activity and Review Questions

Safe evidence-based and competent nursing practice requires nurses to know laws, regulations, and policies that help to frame the health care system and nursing practice. They include state nurse practice acts, the scope and standards of nursing care, and the code of ethics for nursing practice. Understanding where you fit in the health care system demands clinical judgment skills. Society expects safe health care delivery, especially from nurses, who typically are perceived as being part of the most ethical and trusted profession (Gaines, 2021). As patient care becomes more complex and practice innovations and new health care technologies emerge, the principles of negligence and malpractice liability are being applied to challenging new situations. Therefore you need to know laws governing nursing practice to provide evidence-based care that keeps the patient at the center of decision making.

LEGAL LIMITS OF NURSING

Sources of Law

Many types of law govern nursing practice, including constitutional law, statutory law, common law, administrative law, and case law. Knowing these sources of law informs your practice and identifies why it is important to provide current evidence-based care when working with your patients.

Constitutional law is derived from federal and state constitutions. For example, in the United States a constitutional right afforded to every citizen is the right to refuse treatment (Furrow et al., 2018). As a nurse, you must understand the rights of your patients to refuse treatment even when you may not agree with their decisions.

Statutory law is derived from statutes passed by the U.S. Congress and state legislatures. These laws are either civil or criminal. **Civil laws** protect the rights of individuals and provide for fair and equitable treatment when civil wrongs or violations occur (Furrow et al., 2018; Pozgar, 2020). Nurse practice acts are civil state laws that define nursing and the standards nurses must meet within individual states. Your state's nurse practice act defines a nurse's scope of practice, the educational requirements you must have to be a nurse, and how to obtain licensure as a nurse in your state (Oyeleye, 2019; Pozgar, 2020). Nurse practice acts also distinguish nursing from other health professions (e.g., medicine, therapists, and alternative medicine providers).

Criminal laws protect society and provide punishment for crimes, which are defined by municipal, state, and federal legislation (Furrow et al., 2018). Typically, actions that violate criminal laws are defined as either misdemeanors or felonies. Criminal mistreatment of adults who are vulnerable is an example of criminal statutory law. Criminal mistreatment is classified as either a misdemeanor or a felony offense depending on the severity of harm done to a patient who is vulnerable.

Administrative law, or regulatory law, more clearly defines expectations of civil and criminal laws. For example, a nurse practice act, as a civil statutory law, states that you have a duty to care for your patients. Regulations typically state that duty means you will observe, assess, diagnose, plan, intervene, and evaluate patient care. Providing current, evidence-based care is essential to meeting nursing statutory duty and regulations. Regulatory law also describes the process to report incompetent or unethical nursing conduct to the State Board of Nursing or Nursing Commission. A nurse who does not report unethical or incompetent conduct violates regulatory law. Nurses can appeal violations to the State Board of Nursing or the Nursing Commission. In comparison, criminal mistreatment statutes have regulations to determine the intent of the person who commits the crime. The degree of offense often distinguishes whether the person intentionally committed the mistreatment, knew or should have known harm would result, or did not consider that harm would result. Nurses who are accused of violating a regulatory law typically knew or should have known that their actions could result in patient harm.

Common law originates from decisions that were made in the absence of law. For example, the right to privacy is implied in the U.S. Constitution. Thus patient confidentiality originated as common law. Prior to the passage of multiple related laws, a patient's right to confidentiality, which prevents nurses and health care providers from sharing patient information with others who are not caring for the patient, was implied through common law (Furrow et al., 2018; Busch, 2019; McGuire et al., 2019).

Case law describes decisions made in legal cases that were resolved in courts. After a case is presented to a judge or jury, there is a report of the issue, facts, findings, and subsequent decision that was made to resolve the issue. For example, in *Jefferson v Mercy Hospital and Medical Center* (2018), the guardian of the estate of Ms. Turner alleged that her health care providers did not meet the standard of practice when caring for a tracheostomy required to assist her to breathe. Subsequently she died. At trial the jury concurred and awarded the estate $22 million. After an appeal and a lengthy analysis, the court awarded in favor of the estate for $7 million in light of past damages, but it denied the request for future damages in the amount of $15 million.

Scope and Standards of Nursing

The scope of nursing practice defines nursing and reflects the values of the nursing profession. Standards of nursing care reflect the knowledge and skill ordinarily possessed and used by nurses to perform within the scope of practice (Furrow et al., 2018; American Nurses Association [ANA], 2021) (see Chapter 1). Standards of nursing care are derived from health care laws, best practice guidelines, white papers written by professional organizations, evidence-based nursing knowledge, and citizen advocacy groups.

The ANA and specialty nursing organizations develop standards for nursing practice, the code of ethics for nurses, and policy statements. For example, the scope of nursing and 17 standards of practice that describe what nurses do are published by the ANA (2021). Nursing is defined, and the responsibilities and expectations of a registered nurse (RN) are clearly explained. They define the scope, function, and role of nurses in practice and guide your practice. Sometimes they are used as standards when legal actions are taken against nurses.

Nursing policies and procedures within health care agencies are based on the scope and standards of nursing practice (ANA, 2021). They must reflect current best practices and the evidence that supports the processes for the procedures and policies that they describe. The Joint Commission (TJC) (2021a) requires written nursing policies and procedures that are accessible on all nursing units. Agency policies and procedures must conform to state and federal laws and community standards (TJC, 2021a; Furrow et al., 2018).

For example, bedside report is a best practice for health care settings because it places patients at the center of decision making and emphasizes the importance of clear communication with patients and their families and the health care team. When a hospital establishes a policy and procedure to implement bedside hand-off reporting, the nurse who is transferring care of a patient to another nurse, the nurse accepting the care of the patient, and the patient should be involved in the reporting process. If the nurses decide not to follow the policy and procedure and conduct the report without including the patient, the nurses are not following the policy and procedure. Thus the nurses may be at risk for litigation, especially if harm occurs to the patient because of not following the hospital's policy. Thus it is important to know the scope and standards of nursing practice as well as the health care agency's policies and procedures intended to implement them.

FEDERAL STATUTES AFFECTING NURSING PRACTICE

Use your knowledge of federal statutes and regulations to help guide your clinical judgment in nursing practice. Typically these statutes and regulations are linked to Medicare and Medicaid reimbursement, and they are often expanded when states pass laws that increase application of the federal statute to other situations. Therefore you need to consider federal statutes in the context of how they are implemented in each state. Ultimately statutes and regulations influence the context of the health care settings in which you practice, affecting the decisions you make about patient care (Dickison et al., 2019). For example, the Omnibus Reconciliation Act of 1986 mandated that skilled nursing facility residents be given rights, including but not limited to being able to vote, receiving visitors privately, receiving a 30-day notice of discharge before moving from the facility, and being able to participate in meetings to develop their plan of care. Many states subsequently passed laws by which these same rights were given to patients in retirement homes, assisted-living facilities, and adult family homes. Thus if you are caring for patients in an assisted-living facility in a state that provides for these patients' rights, you need to include your patients and their preferences when planning their care (Fig. 23.1) and ensure they are given the opportunity to vote.

Patient Protection and Affordable Care Act

The Patient Protection and Affordable Care Act (PPACA) was passed in 2010. Its name was later changed to the Affordable Care Act (ACA). The ACA is characterized by four themes embedded in nursing practice: (1) consumer rights and protections, (2) affordable health care

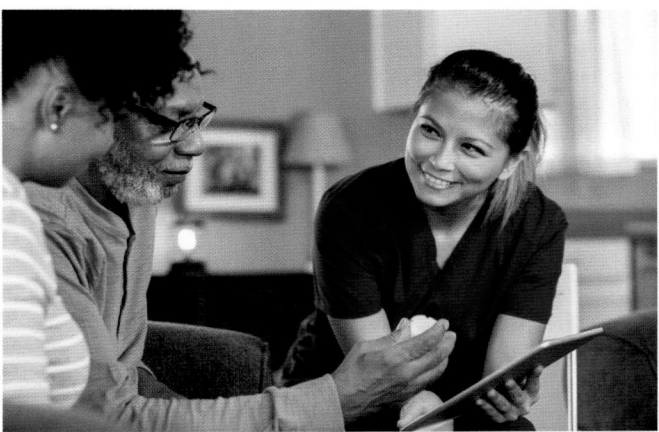

FIG. 23.1 Nurses ensure patients' rights by including patients and family caregivers in planning care. (Copyright © iStock.)

coverage, (3) increased access to care, and (4) quality of care that meets the needs of patients. The ACA has been challenged in court many times since its enactment. Examples of issues discussed in court around the ACA include mandatory enrollment in health care insurance and eligibility for insurance for patients with a preexisting condition.

A new Patient's Bill of Rights, created by the ACA, prohibits patients from being denied health care coverage because of prior existing conditions, limits on the amount of care for those conditions, and/or an accidental mistake in paperwork when a patient got sick (PPACA, 2010). The ACA intended to reduce overall medical costs by (1) providing tax credits, (2) increasing insurance company accountability for premiums and rate increases, and (3) increasing the number of choices available to patients to select insurers that best meet their needs. In addition, the ACA increased access to health care. Patients now receive recommended preventive services such as screenings for cancer, blood pressure, and diabetes without having to pay copays or deductibles. The ACA improved Medicare coverage for vulnerable populations by improving access to care and prescriptions, decreasing costs of medications, extending the life of the Medicare Trust Fund until 2024, and addressing fraud and abuse in billing practices (U.S. Department of Health and Human Services [USDHHS], 2021).

The ACA reduced the number of uninsured Americans from over 44 million people in 2013, right before the act's health care coverage provisions began, to just below 27 million people in 2016. However, starting in 2017 the number of uninsured people started to increase again, with 28.9 million nonelderly individuals being uninsured in 2019 (KFF, 2020). The number of uninsured people remains substantially lower compared with 2010 (KFF, 2020). The high cost of medical insurance and not having access to medical coverage through an employer are the main reasons people remain uninsured. Other adults are ineligible for financial assistance for health care coverage, especially those who live in states that did not expand Medicaid coverage. Those who remain uninsured typically are in families that have at least one family member who works, are in families that have a low income (especially below 200% of the federal poverty level), and are adults under 65 years of age. People of color have a higher risk of being uninsured when compared with non-Hispanic White people (KFF, 2020).

The ACA is politically charged and frequently debated. Thus, like all statutes, the ACA has the potential to change. For example, the Centers for Medicare and Medicaid Services (CMS, 2019) proposed changes to the ACA to increase the affordability of coverage, to allow people the choice to join Qualified Health Plans (QHPs) that do not cover termination of pregnancy services, and to provide greater flexibility in how

people shop for QHPs. In 2019, the 5th Circuit of the U.S. Court of Appeals ruled that requiring all Americans to have health care coverage was unconstitutional (Caffrey, 2019). The U.S. Supreme Court upheld the constitutionality of the ACA in spring 2021 (*California et al. v. Texas et al.*, 2021).

It is especially important that nurses have current factual knowledge, voice their opinions to appropriate legislators about issues that affect health care, and provide accurate information to patients when they seek guidance about their health care. Nurses are often at the center of those decisions with their patients. It is critical that when helping patients make decisions about their care, the decisions are clinically sound and based on the patient's preferences, values, and beliefs.

Emergency Medical Treatment and Active Labor Act

The Emergency Medical Treatment and Active Labor Act (EMTALA, 1986) prohibits the transfer of patients from private to public hospitals without appropriate screening and stabilization. It is intended to prevent patient dumping. This act ensures that patients are medically screened when they come to the emergency department or the hospital. Staff must assess all patients who enter the hospital and cannot discharge or transfer them until their conditions stabilize. Exceptions to this provision include if a patient requests transfer or discharge in writing after receiving information about the benefits and risks of the transfer or if a health care provider certifies that the benefits of transfer outweigh the risks.

Health Insurance Portability and Accountability Act

The Health Insurance Portability and Accountability Act (HIPAA, 1996) provides rights to patients and protects employees. It includes standards regarding accountability in the health care setting. Notably, it establishes patient rights regarding privacy of their health care information and records.

HIPAA established a patient's right to consent to the use and disclosure of protected health information (PHI), to inspect and copy one's medical record, and to amend mistaken or incomplete information (Privacy Rights Clearinghouse, 2014). It limits who can access a patient's record. It establishes the basis for privacy and confidentiality concerns, viewed as two basic rights within the U.S. health care system. Privacy is the right of patients to keep personal information from being disclosed. Confidentiality protects private patient information once it is disclosed in health care settings. Nurses help health care agencies protect patients' rights to privacy and confidentiality. Although HIPAA does not require extreme measures such as soundproof rooms in hospitals, it does mean that nurses and health care providers need to avoid discussing patients in public areas (e.g., hallways, elevators, cafeteria) and provide reasonable levels of privacy when communicating with and about patients in any manner. Thus nurses must be especially vigilant to ensure that patients are afforded the privacy they are entitled to and that is mandated in law. For example, message boards used to post daily patient care information in patient rooms or patient care units cannot contain information revealing a patient's medical condition.

Health care information privacy is also protected by standards set by the CMS for hospitals and health care providers who participate in Medicare and Medicaid (CMS, 2020; Furrow et al., 2018). These standards require that hospitals and health care providers give notice to patients of their rights regarding decisions about their care, grievances regarding their care management, personal freedom and safety, confidentiality, access to their own medical records, and freedom from physical or chemical restraints that are not clinically necessary. In addition, many state laws allow patients to access their medical records. Exceptions apply to psychotherapy notes or when a health care provider has determined that access would result in harm to the patient or another party (Privacy Rights Clearinghouse, 2014).

Health Information Technology Act

The Health Information Technology for Economic and Clinical Health Act (HITECH Act, 2009) was passed with HIPAA in response to new technology and social media. HITECH expands the principles extended under HIPAA, especially when a security breach of PHI occurs. Under the HITECH Act, nurses must ensure that patient PHI is not inadvertently conveyed on social media and that protected data are not disclosed other than as permitted by patients (Box 23.1). *Best practice, regardless of patient consent, is to never post patient information on social media.* Electronic data are accessible, regardless of assurances to the contrary. Civil and criminal sanctions may be brought against both a nurse and an organization if either or both violate HIPAA or the HITECH Act. Report violations of patient confidentiality to your supervisor.

Americans With Disabilities Act

The Americans With Disabilities Act (ADA) of 1990 and amended in 2008 is a civil rights statute that protects the rights of people with physical or mental disabilities (American Disabilities Act National Network [ADANN], 2021). The ADA prohibits discrimination and ensures equal opportunities for people with disabilities in employment, state and local government services, public accommodations, commercial facilities, and transportation. It is enforced by the Office of Equal Employment Opportunity.

As defined by the statute and the U.S. Supreme Court, a disability is a mental or physical condition that substantially limits a major life activity, including seeing, hearing, speaking, walking, breathing, performing manual tasks, learning, caring for oneself, and/or working. Employers must provide reasonable accommodations to employees or applicants who are qualified to hold a job. Reasonable accommodations enable a person to perform the essential functions of a job (ADANN, 2021). Consider the case of Bryan, a nurse who has a hearing disability and who may require accommodations to work safely. Under the ADA, Bryan is not required to report his hearing disability. Rather, he is able to make the choice whether to tell others of his disability. Under the ADA requirements, Bryan's employer must consider his needs and must provide reasonable accommodations, such as a special stethoscope that allows for amplification of sounds, to allow him to practice nursing safely.

Although the ADA protects health care workers who have disabilities in the workplace, several cases have held that health care providers must disclose if they are human immunodeficiency virus (HIV)–positive. However, health care workers cannot discriminate against patients who are HIV-positive (Furrow et al., 2018).

Mental Health Parity and Addiction Equity Act

The Mental Health Parity and Addiction Equity Act (MHPAEA, 1996) was originally passed in 1996. Amendments were passed in 2008, then it was amended by the Health Care and Education Reconciliation Act of 2010 and it eventually became a part of the ACA (CMS, n.d.). The MHPAEA requires health insurance companies to provide coverage for mental health and substance use disorder (SUD) treatment, just as they do for medical coverage. The ACA extended these requirements to small group and individual health insurance plans (U.S. Department of the Treasury, 2013). The ACA requires parity (the state or condition of being equal) in the provision of 10 specific services, including mental health, behavioral health, and SUD services. Insurers may not discriminate or deny coverage to patients with mental illness or SUD because of preexisting conditions.

The Mental Health and Substance Use Disorder Parity Task Force facilitates coordination of services among federal agencies and ensures that consumers receive the care and treatment they require. The Task Force improved awareness of the benefits that parity for mental health and SUD provide. For example, to increase transparency, the Task Force has helped stakeholders (e.g., insurers, regulators, and consumers) understand what equality means in relation to treatment of mental health illnesses and SUDs. The Task Force also provides resources to ensure that coverage is consistent with the intent of the MHPAEA (https://www.hhs.gov/programs/topic-sites/mental-health-parity/index.html).

Patients are admitted either voluntarily or involuntarily to a mental health or SUD unit. Involuntary admission to a mental health center usually occurs when patients are a danger to themselves (e.g., patients who are suicidal) or others. Typically a mental health professional (MHP) makes this decision in the emergency room. In some states, patients with an SUD can also be placed in a treatment center by an SUD professional if they are a danger to themselves or others. In either case, the professional who assessed the patient, a court-appointed guardian ad litem, a family member, or another interested party can ask the court to determine whether a longer stay is required to protect the patient from continuing to harm self or others. A judge may order the patient to be hospitalized for 21 more days for treatment. From a legal perspective this is viewed as taking away a patient's constitutional rights. Nurses must clearly and accurately document the patient's behaviors. The court will review this evidence when making its decisions (Furrow et al., 2018; Barr et al., 2019). Under constitutional law, having the right to move from place to place is at the very basis of being a U.S. citizen. When removing that constitutionally protected right, the case must be made that not doing so would result in significant or deadly harm.

When patients attempt suicide within health care settings, it is typically alleged that nurses failed to provide appropriate individualized care, supervise the patient adequately, and adhere to existing policies and procedures to keep the patient safe. When providing care to patients with mental illnesses and SUDs, consider the scope and standards of nursing care as well as the specific statutes and regulations associated with their care. You also need to know your agency's policies and procedures when caring for patients at risk of harm. Integrate this

---

BOX 23.1   EVIDENCE-BASED PRACTICE

Social Media and Legal Liability

PICOT Question: Do nurses who use social media put themselves at greater risk for legal liability compared with nurses who do not use social media?

Evidence Summary

Social media are used today to reach millions of patients, colleagues, and peers. They are a useful tool for interprofessional communication, promoting collaboration, disseminating information, and providing education. Nurses are ultimately responsible and accountable for understanding the use, implications, policies, and guidelines associated with the use of social media (NCSBN, 2018; Reinbeck and Antonacci, 2019). The National Council of State Boards of Nursing (NCSBN, 2018) and the International Nurse Regulator Collaborative (INRC) identified nurses' behaviors for appropriate use of social media. Nurses who follow current professional guidelines and laws can use social media to enhance their practice and do not place themselves at greater risk for liability (NCSBN, 2018; Reinbeck and Antonacci, 2019).

Application to Nursing Practice
- Understand the risks and benefits of using social media (NCSBN, 2018).
- Maintain professional boundaries (NCSBN, 2018).
- Present a professional image in all social media interactions (Reinbeck and Antonacci, 2019).
- Maintain privacy and confidentiality of patient information (NCSBN, 2018).
- Understand the implications of identifying yourself as a nurse (NCSBN, 2018).
- Know state laws and agency policies governing use of social media (NCSBN, 2018).

knowledge to provide evidence-based nursing and to ensure that your documentation reflects the care you provided.

Patient Self-Determination Act

The Patient Self-Determination Act (PSDA, 1991) requires health care institutions to provide written information to patients concerning their rights to make decisions about their care, including the right to refuse treatment and to formulate an advance directive. A patient's record must indicate whether a patient has signed an advance directive and include a copy of the directive if it is available. Patients must also be offered information about advance directives.

An advance directive is a document developed by patients that instructs others to do tasks before, during, and after their death. At a minimum, an advance directive includes a statement of a patient's wishes if a respiratory or cardiac arrest occurs and a copy of the patient's **durable power of attorney for health care (DPAHC)**. Instructions regarding care before or during cardiac or respiratory arrest should be signed by either a physician or a nurse practitioner. Unless otherwise specified by state law, the document should be treated as an order; it may direct whether to provide lifesaving measures such as cardiopulmonary resuscitation (CPR) or to provide comfort care only.

Most DPAHCs begin with a statement that says the designated person can make decisions when the patient becomes incapacitated. This means that patients cannot be bypassed—they retain the ability and the right to make their own decisions whenever they can. This is true whether they are at home, in the emergency room, or in an inpatient setting. Decisional capacity is the patient's ability to make choices about care. The health care provider, working in conjunction with information from nurses and family members, can make the determination of decisional capacity. The power of attorney for health care may not be asked and cannot make health care decisions until a provider makes an assessment that the patient no longer has the capacity to make decisions. The assessment that triggers the beginning of the DPAHC should be reflected in the medical record.

When the physician or nurse practitioner is unable to determine capacity or there is disagreement regarding the patient's capacity, a competency hearing is conducted in court on the patient's behalf. As in involuntary commitment hearings, the court is asked to deny a U.S. citizen the constitutional right to make decisions, which essentially takes away all rights and privileges provided as a U.S. citizen. When a patient is determined to be incompetent, a guardian is appointed to make decisions regarding care the patient will or will not receive. No other person, including family members or providers, has the power to override the guardian's decisions. To do so, that person must return to court and explain why the guardian's decision should not be honored. Thus, under the PSDA and state-specific statutes, advance directives that include a DPAHC and orders whether or not to provide resuscitation must be clear and in compliance with law. Nursing care is individualized based on the patient's instructions and on the state in which the patient resides at the time a directive is implemented. The DPAHC's ability to make decisions for the patient ends at the time of death. Therefore it is important that patients and their families arrange their after-life care in advance when possible.

Living wills also include information about a patient's preferences regarding end-of-life care (Furrow et al., 2018; Touhy and Jett, 2022). Some include physician orders about sustaining life, such as use of enteral feedings. Others contain information on whether to initiate CPR on cessation of breathing. It is important to thoroughly read documents titled "living will." They are based on values of informed consent, patient autonomy over end-of-life decisions, truth telling, and control over the dying process. A patient must be capable to make decisions regarding health care treatment when creating a living will. Many resources are

available to help create a living will. For example, Five Wishes is an organization that helps patients write their directives when responding to five questions (https://fivewishes.org/). The questions help patients identify a DPAHC, the kind of medical treatment wanted or not wanted, comfort measures they wish to receive, how they want to be treated by those around them, and what they want those who love them to know. Providing this information and assisting patients in recording their wishes is rewarding for the patient, empowering to their loved ones, and humbling to the nurses who help them.

Patients make difficult decisions when writing a living will. Sometimes family and friends have difficulty in understanding and adhering to those decisions. The ethical doctrine of autonomy, which has been upheld in court, ensures a patient the right to refuse medical treatment. For example, courts upheld a patient's right to refuse medical treatment in *Bouvia v Superior Court* (1986). Courts have also upheld the right of a legally competent patient to refuse medical treatment for religious reasons. The U.S. Supreme Court stated in the *Cruzan v Director of Missouri Department of Health* case (1990) that "we assume that the U.S. Constitution would grant a constitutionally protected competent person the right to refuse lifesaving hydration and nutrition." In the Terri Schiavo case (*Schindler & Schindler v Schiavo*, 2003), Schiavo's husband, who was her legal guardian, argued that his wife would not want to have her life artificially prolonged. Her parents disagreed and wanted her to continue to receive artificial nutrition and hydration. The court noted that it understood "why a parent who had raised and nurtured a child from conception would hold out hope that some level of cognitive function remained." However, after more than 10 years, the court upheld the guardianship court's initial decision to allow Ms. Schiavo's husband, as her guardian, to make medical decisions on her behalf in the absence of her wishes being known before her death.

In cases involving a patient's right to refuse or withdraw medical treatment, the courts balance the patient's interest with the interest of the state in protecting life, preserving medical ethics, preventing suicide, and protecting innocent third parties. Children are generally innocent third parties. Although the courts will not force adults to undergo treatment refused for religious reasons, they will grant an order allowing hospitals and health care providers to treat children of parents or groups who have denied consent for treatment of their minor children for religious reasons. This is based on the legal doctrine of *parens patriae* in which the state or government makes decisions on behalf of those who are unable to make decisions for themselves.

In addition to patient refusals of treatment, nurses frequently encounter "do not resuscitate" (DNR) or "no code" DNR orders. The state of New York was the first to develop legislation based on the recommendations of the New York State Task Force on Life and the Law in 1986. These recommendations, which went into effect in 1988, allow competent adults to authorize a DNR order (Golden, 1988). Documentation that the health care provider has consulted with the patient and/or family is required before writing a DNR order in the patient's medical record (Furrow et al., 2018; Touhy and Jett, 2022). Patient conditions change, and patients have the right to change their minds. The health care provider needs to review DNR orders with the patient periodically to assure that the order reflects current wishes.

When patients have living wills or advance directives, remember that the "do not resuscitate" designation does not mean "do not care." Although the patient has made the choice to refuse CPR and other acts (stated on DNR order) in the event of a cardiopulmonary arrest, you must provide patient care and meet the patient's needs. Health care providers are required to make every effort to revive patients who arrest and do not have a DNR order. Some states offer DNR Comfort Care and DNR Comfort Care Arrest protocols. Protocols in these instances list specific actions that health care providers will take when providing CPR.

CPR is an emergency treatment provided without patient consent (see Chapter 41). Health care providers perform CPR when needed unless there is a DNR order in the patient's chart. The statutes assume that all patients want to be resuscitated unless there is a written DNR order in the medical record. Legally, capable adult patients consent to a DNR order verbally or in writing after receiving the appropriate information from the health care provider. Be familiar with the DNR protocols of your state.

REFLECT NOW

You are caring for a patient who is terminally ill and has a "do not resuscitate" order, but the medical record does not have an entry regarding the physician's discussion with the patient prior to writing the order. How would you respond if the patient has a cardiac arrest? How would your response differ if the patient were 8 versus 80 years old?

Uniform Anatomical Gift Act

The Uniform Anatomical Gift Act (UAGA) (2006) was first passed in 1968 and was revised in 1987 and 2006. The UAGA provides the foundation for the national organ donation system. Patient autonomy, individual autonomy, and public trust remain the ethical principles on which organ donation occurs. An individual who is at least 18 years of age can make an organ donation (defined as a "donation of all or part of a human body to take effect upon or after death"). Donors make the gift in writing. In many states, adults sign the back of their driver's license, indicating consent to organ donation.

In most states Required Request laws mandate that at the time of admission to a hospital a qualified health care provider must ask all patients over age 18 whether they are an organ or tissue donor. If the answer is affirmative, the health care provider obtains a copy of the document. If the answer is negative, the health care provider discusses the option to make or refuse an organ donation and places such documentation in the patient's medical record. In most states there is a law requiring that at the time of death a qualified health care provider ask a patient's family members to consider organ or tissue donation (National Organ Transplant Act, 1984). Individuals are approached in the following order: (1) spouse, (2) adult son or daughter, (3) parent, (4) adult brother or sister, (5) grandparent, and (6) guardian. The health care provider who certifies death is not involved in the removal or transplantation of organs (see Chapter 36).

The National Organ Transplant Act (1984) prohibits the purchase or sale of organs (Korobkin, 2017). The act provides civil and criminal immunity to the hospital and health care provider who perform in accordance with the act. It also protects the donor's estate from liability for injury or damage that results from the use of the gift. Organ transplantation is extremely expensive. Patients in end-stage renal disease are eligible for Medicare coverage for a kidney transplant. Sometimes private insurance pays for other transplants. The United Network for Organ Sharing (UNOS) has a contract with the federal government and sets policies and guidelines for the procurement of organs. Recently UNOS changed policy regarding transplant eligibility. The patient with the most urgent need for a transplant will have first claim on any organ from a compatible donor within a 150-mile radius, then a 250-mile radius, and on up to a 500-mile radius (Luthi, 2018). This process will continue with the priority given to the sickest people. Older laws based on geographical proximity arguably reduced access to many critically ill people. Geography is still a factor, but patient need is now the priority

(Luthi, 2018). Be familiar with your role as a nurse defined by the policies and procedures of your agency regarding organ donation.

The Omnibus Budget Reconciliation Act (1986)

The Omnibus Reconciliation Act (OBRA) of 1986 significantly altered the way in which health care is provided to older adults. It focused on patient rights, quality of life, quality of care, and the physical environment in which patients live. One change focused on the use of restraints intended to change older-adult behavior.

OBRA 1986 addressed the use of both physical and chemical restraint use (see Chapter 14). The legal definition of a restraint is any manual method, physical or mechanical device, or material or equipment that immobilizes or reduces the ability of a patient to move freely, with a chemical restraint including the use of medication (e.g. antipsychotics) to alter the behavior of a patient (CMS, 2020). The use of restraints has been associated with serious complications and even death. The CMS (2008), ANA (2012), and TJC (2021b) set standards to reduce the use of all types of restraints in health care settings. All patients have a U.S. constitutional right to be free from seclusion and physical or chemical restraints, except on rare occasions, to ensure the safety of patients, staff, and others in emergency situations.

Application of a physical restraint or administration of a chemical restraint must be the intervention of last resort and not the first intervention of choice when a patient is nonadherent, aggressive, or combative. Chapter 27 describes interventions for a restraint-free environment and the conditions that ultimately allow restraints to be ordered. You must know current evidence-based and legal procedures related to both the use of restraints and discontinuation. It is critical to know who can legally order the use of restraints, the assessments required, and the length of time for which restraints can be used. You are required to continuously monitor patients who are restrained or secluded to ensure they are safe. A physician, nurse practitioner, physician assistant, or RN who has been trained in CMS restraint and seclusion requirements is required to assess the patient face to face within 1 hour or less of applying the restraints (CMS, 2020).

Restraints can be used (1) only to ensure the physical safety of the patient or other patients, (2) when less restrictive interventions are unsuccessful, and (3) only on the written order of a health care provider (CMS, 2020). The regulations also describe documentation of restraint use and follow-up assessments. Litigation from improper restraint use may include allegations of unlawful imprisonment and/or harm associated with injury due to restraint use (Pozgar, 2020). Knowing when and how to use restraints correctly is key (see Chapter 27).

STATE STATUTES AFFECTING NURSING PRACTICE

State law directs how health care will be delivered and regulates and licenses health care agencies and health care professionals providing care to citizens within the state. Therefore when harm occurs to patients, malpractice suits are filed primarily under state law, actions are taken against facilities to no longer operate, and charges are made against a nurse's license when it is determined that the nurse contributed to the harm. Sometimes federal statutes affect state laws. In *Gibbons v Ogden* (1824) the U.S. Supreme Court established that regulation and licensure of local matters belong to the states under powers afforded to them under the U.S. Constitution. Nursing licenses are issued and enforced by states.

Nurse Practice Acts

Nurse practice acts are state laws intended to protect citizens, make nurses accountable, and ensure that care is consistent with best practices within the scope and standards of nursing. Creation of a state board of nursing, sometimes called the nursing commission, is part of a state nurse practice act. Members of the boards and the boards' responsibilities are written in the statutes and in the regulations that more clearly delineate their duties. State boards of nursing educate the public and nurses as the profession changes. For example, white papers to clarify administration of conscious sedation by a nurse have been shared with stakeholders when practice acts are revised or challenged. State boards regulate and disseminate information related to nursing practice.

The State Board of Nursing or Nursing Commission licenses all RNs in the state in which they practice. The requirements for licensure vary among states. States use the National Council Licensure Examinations (NCLEX®) for nursing examinations. Legally, a license to practice nursing is considered a privilege and not a right. Licensure permits people to offer special skills to the public, and it also provides legal guidelines for protection of the public.

The Nurse Licensure Compact (NLC) enables a nurse to practice in multiple states under one license; an individual license from each participating state is not required (National Council of State Boards of Nursing [NCSBN], 2021). Having an NLC license allows nurses to provide telehealth care when the nurse works in one state and the patient is in another state. It also facilitates care when nurses cross state lines to provide care during emergencies. As practice acts change, more states are participating in the NLC process (NCSBN, 2021).

The State Board of Nursing investigates, suspends, and/or revokes a license if a nurse's conduct violates the state's Nurse Practice Act. For example, nurses who wrongfully administer a medication that results in permanent harm to a patient may have a restriction placed on their license. If this occurs and the nurse has an NLC license, other states may also investigate and take action in their jurisdictions, even though the act occurred in another state. Actions taken in other states may be less severe, worse, or the same as that taken in the originating state where the violation occurred. In part, this demonstrates the importance of having professional liability insurance.

While a license may be considered a privilege, it is also a means by which a person is employed. As such, when penalties are taken against a nurse's license, statutes regarding right to employment may be triggered to protect the person's ability to work. Thus actions taken to restrict, suspend, and/or revoke a nursing license may become daunting to the nurse who wishes to remain in practice.

The State Board of Nursing must provide notice and follow due process before revoking or suspending a license. Notice means that affirmative actions are taken to inform the nurse that a charge has been made and will be investigated by the Board. It also means that reasonable efforts will be made to inform the nurse of the date, time, and place where an action may be taken to restrict, suspend, or revoke the nurse's license. Due process means that the state is required to inform the nurse of the allegations and the investigation process, including who is being asked to provide information about the allegations. The name of the complainant is disclosed only under court order when anonymity is requested. Nurses should attend and respond to allegations during hearings regarding any allegations. They may and should request an attorney to represent and defend them in a hearing. Hearings for suspension or revocation of a license do not occur in court. Usually a panel of professionals conducts the hearing. Most states provide administrative and judicial review of these cases after nurses have exhausted all other forms of appeal. Actions and decisions by state boards of nursing are published and accessible by health care agencies and the public. When administrative appeals have been exhausted, nurses can bring their cases forward to the court for review of the actions taken by the Board in their respective states.

Professional licensure defense is expensive when nurses do not have insurance that covers the costs of keeping their licenses to practice

nursing. Nurses often presume that either their personal or their employer's malpractice insurance will include costs of defending and retaining their nursing license. In most instances this is not true. Professional licensure defense insurance is a contract between a nurse and an insurance company. When a complaint is made to a state board of nursing, an action is initiated that could result in a restriction, suspension, or revocation of the nurse's license to practice. When a nurse specifically has professional licensure defense insurance, the nurse notifies the company. In response, the company will refer the nurse to an attorney, usually a nurse attorney, who will then represent the nurse when interacting with the state board. The insurance company will cover costs of representing the nurse when responding to allegations the state board is investigating.

Health Care Acts and Informed Consent

Health care acts within each state describe and define the minimum standards of care that will be provided within their geographical region. These acts and the regulations associated with them are interrelated with other laws governing the practice of nursing, such as expectations regarding informed consent.

A patient's signed consent form is necessary for admission to a health care agency, performance of invasive procedures such as intravenous central line insertion, surgery, some treatment programs such as chemotherapy, and participation in research studies (Furrow et al., 2018). State laws designate individuals who are legally able to give consent to medical treatment (Medical Patient Rights Act, 1994). Nurses need to know the law in their states and be familiar with the policies and procedures of their employing agency regarding consent (Box 23.2). Special consideration is used when a patient is deaf, is illiterate, or speaks a foreign language. A professional interpreter must be present in person or remotely to explain the terms of consent. A family member or acquaintance who speaks a patient's language should not interpret health information. Make every effort to help a patient make an informed choice.

In addition, health care acts have been amended to include more specific direction to ensure that patients receive information that the typical person would reasonably want to know when providing consent to medical care. Informed consent is a patient's agreement to have a medical procedure after receiving full disclosure of risks, benefits, alternatives, and consequences of refusal (Furrow et al., 2018; Pozgar, 2020). Informed consent requires a health care provider to disclose information in terms a patient can understand to make an informed choice (Cruzan, 1990; Furrow et al., 2018). Failure to obtain consent in situations other than emergencies can result in a claim of battery.

Informed consent is part of the health care provider–patient relationship. It must be obtained and witnessed when the patient is not under the influence of medication such as opioids. In most situations, obtaining patients' informed consent does not fall within the nurse's responsibility. The person responsible for performing the procedure is responsible for obtaining the informed consent.

Key elements of informed consent include the following (Furrow et al., 2018):

1. The patient receives an explanation of the procedure or treatment.
2. The patient receives the names and qualifications of people performing and assisting in the procedure.
3. The patient receives a description of the serious harm, including death, that may occur as a result of the procedure and anticipated pain and/or discomfort.
4. The patient receives an explanation of alternative therapies to the proposed procedure or treatment and the risks of doing nothing.
5. The patient knows of the right to refuse the procedure or treatment without discontinuing other supportive care.

BOX 23.2 Statutory Guidelines for Legal Consent for Medical Treatment

Those who may consent to treatment are governed by state law but generally include the following:

I. Adults
A. Any competent individual 18 years of age or older for himself or herself
B. Any parent for an unemancipated minor
C. Any guardian for a ward
D. Any adult for the treatment of a minor brother or sister (if an emergency and parents are not present)
E. Any grandparent for a minor grandchild (in an emergency and if parents are not present)

II. Minors
A. Ordinarily minors may not consent to medical treatment without a parent. However, emancipated minors may consent to medical treatment without a parent. Emancipated minors include:
 1. Minors who are designated emancipated by a court order
 2. Minors who are married, divorced, or widowed
 3. Minors who are in active military service
B. Unemancipated minors may consent to medical treatment if they have specific medical conditions.
 1. Pregnancy and pregnancy-related conditions. (Various states differ in characterizing a pregnant minor as either emancipated or unemancipated. Know your state's rules in this matter.)
 2. A minor parent for a custodial child
 3. Sexually transmitted infection (STI) information and treatment
 4. Substance abuse treatment
 5. Outpatient and/or temporary sheltered mental health treatment
C. The issue of emancipated or unemancipated minors does not relieve the health care provider's duty to attempt to obtain meaningful informed consent.

---

6. The patient knows of the right to refuse the procedure or treatment even after the procedure has begun.

Nurses witness consent; they do not obtain consent for procedures performed by others (Furrow et al., 2018). A nurse's signature as a witness to the consent means that the patient appeared to voluntarily give consent, that the patient appeared capable to give consent, and that the patient signed the consent form in the nurse's presence. If you suspect that a patient does not understand or did not voluntarily and/or knowingly give consent, notify the health care provider and nursing supervisor. To ensure valid consent, contact the medical director when necessary. If a patient refuses the treatment, ensure that documentation of the rejection is written, signed, and witnessed. Nursing students cannot and should not under any circumstances be responsible for or be asked to witness the signing of consent forms because of the legal nature of the document.

Parents are usually the legal guardians of pediatric patients and the ones who typically sign consent forms for treatment. Occasionally a parent or guardian refuses treatment for a child. For example, you are caring for a child whose parents do not want their child to receive the measles, mumps, rubella (MMR) vaccine. The court may intervene on the child's behalf. Courts generally consider the child's ultimate safety and well-being as the most important factors. Under these circumstances, the court may also order the child to be vaccinated under the doctrine of *parens patriae,* in the best interests of the child and those who may be exposed to the disease if the unvaccinated child is exposed to and develops measles.

In some instances, obtaining informed consent is difficult. For example, if a patient is unconscious, you must obtain consent from a person legally authorized to give it on the patient's behalf. Sometimes a patient has legally designated surrogate decision makers through special power of attorney documents or court guardianship procedures. In emergencies, if it is impossible to obtain consent from the patient or an authorized person, a health care provider may perform a procedure required to benefit the patient or save a life without liability for failure to obtain consent. In such cases the law assumes that the patient would wish to be treated.

Patients with mental illnesses or SUDs must also give consent. They have the right to refuse treatment until a court has determined legally that they are incompetent to decide for themselves. Informed consent is one aspect of health care statutes. Implications related to informed consent are influenced by many related statutes.

Good Samaritan Laws

Good Samaritan laws encourage health care professionals to assist in emergencies (Furrow et al., 2018). These laws limit liability and offer legal immunity if a nurse helps at the scene of an accident. For example, if you stop at the scene of an automobile accident and give appropriate emergency care such as applying pressure to stop hemorrhage, you are acting within accepted standards, even though proper equipment is unavailable. If the patient subsequently develops complications due to your actions, you are immune from liability if you acted without gross negligence (Furrow et al., 2018; Good Samaritan Act, 1997). Although Good Samaritan laws provide immunity to a nurse who does what is reasonable to save a person's life, if you perform a procedure exceeding your scope of practice and for which you have no training, you are liable for injury that may result from that act. You should only provide care that is consistent with your level of knowledge and experience. In addition, once you have committed to providing emergency care to a patient, you must stay with that patient until you can safely transfer the patient's care to someone who can provide needed care, such as emergency medical technicians (EMTs) or emergency department staff. If you leave a patient without properly transferring or handing off that patient to a capable person, you may be liable for patient abandonment and responsible for any injury sustained after you leave (Furrow et al., 2018; Pozgar, 2020).

Public Health Laws

Public health laws affect individuals, populations, and communities. They may be either federal or state statutes that are intended to improve the health of people. State legislatures enact statutes under health codes, which describe the requirements for reporting communicable diseases, school immunizations, and other conditions intended to promote health and reduce health risks in communities. The Centers for Disease Control and Prevention (CDC) (http://www.CDC.gov) and the Occupational Safety and Health Administration (OSHA) (http://www.osha.gov) provide guidelines on a national level for safe and healthy communities and work environments. Public health laws protect populations, advocate for the rights of people, regulate health care and health care financing, and ensure professional accountability for care provided.

Nurses have the legal duty to provide care to protect public health (see Chapter 3). These laws include reporting suspected abuse and neglect of a child, older adult, or victim of domestic violence; reporting communicable diseases; ensuring that patients in the community have received recommended immunizations; and reporting other health-related issues to protect public health. In most states all nurses are mandatory reporters of abuse or neglect of patients when they have reasonable suspicion to believe an individual is at risk of harm. In most states, **neglect** means a pattern of conduct by a person with a duty of care to provide services that maintain the physical and/or mental health of a child or vulnerable adult (Adigun et al., 2020). It may also be a one-time act that is a clear and present danger to another's health, welfare, or safety. Neglect does not usually require that a nurse intentionally acts to harm a patient; rather, the nurse knew or should have known that neglect would occur under the circumstances. Abuse means the willful act or inaction that inflicts injury, confinement, intimidation, or punishment on a child or an adult. Of note in situations of neglect or abuse, the standard of proof to report is that a nurse has a reasonable suspicion that the person may be at risk of harm. Nurses must place the health and safety of the patient above that of the caregiver when making the decision to report. Health care professionals who do not report instances when they have suspicion of abuse or neglect may be liable for civil or criminal legal action. Some state boards of nursing now require mandatory continuing education on abuse and neglect for license renewal or before obtaining a new nursing license.

Termination of Pregnancy

In the case of *Roe v Wade* (1973) the U.S. Supreme Court ruled that there is a fundamental right to privacy, which includes a woman's decision to terminate a pregnancy. The court ruled that during the first trimester a woman could end her pregnancy without state regulation because the risk of natural mortality from abortion is less than with normal childbirth. During the second trimester the state has an interest in protecting maternal health, and it enforces regulations regarding the person terminating the pregnancy and the agency where it is done. By the third trimester, when the fetus becomes viable, the interest of the state is to protect the fetus; therefore it prohibits termination except when necessary to save the mother.

In *Webster v Reproductive Health Services* (1989), the court substantially narrowed *Roe v Wade*. Some states require viability tests before conducting abortions. Other states require a minor's parental consent or a judicial decision that the minor is mature and can self-consent, whereas other states do not require parental consent. Recently some states have passed "heartbeat" laws, which state that a pregnancy may not be terminated after a heartbeat is heard. Thus it is critical to know the law in your state related to termination of pregnancy before working in this area of practice.

Physician-Assisted Suicide

Providing end-of-life care in today's world is challenging for health care professionals because people are living longer (see Chapter 36). The Oregon Death With Dignity Act (1994) was the first statute that legislatively defined "death with dignity," sometimes called *physician-assisted suicide*. The statute stated that competent individuals with a terminal disease could make an oral and written request for medication to end their life in a humane and dignified manner. A terminal disease is defined as an "incurable and irreversible disease that has been medically confirmed and will, within reasonable medical judgment, produce death within 6 months."

The ANA (2019) believes that nurses' participation in assisted suicide violates the code of ethics for nurses. The American Association of Colleges of Nursing (AACN) has historically supported the International Council of Nurses' mandate to ensure an individual's peaceful end of life. The positions of these two national organizations are not considered contradictory and require nurses to approach a patient's end of life with openness to listening to a patient's expressions of fear and to attempt to control a patient's pain during the last months of life. You need to know your state's laws and ensure that your practice falls within the laws' requirements.

The Uniform Determination of Death Act

Many legal issues surround the event of death, including a basic definition of the actual point at which a person is legally dead. The definitions vary by state law. There are two standards for the determination of death. The cardiopulmonary standard requires irreversible cessation of circulatory and respiratory functions. The whole-brain standard requires irreversible cessation of all functions of the entire brain, including the brainstem. Most states have statutes like the proposed language in the Uniform Determination of Death Act (National Conference of Commissioners on Uniform State Laws, 1980). It states that health care providers can use either the cardiopulmonary or the whole-brain definition to determine death. Be aware of legal definitions of death in your state because you need to document relevant information when the patient is in your care. Nurses have a specific legal obligation to treat the deceased person's remains with dignity (see Chapter 36). Wrongful handling of a deceased person's remains causes emotional harm to the surviving family.

NURSING WORKFORCE GUIDELINES

Statutes and agency policies and procedures help to protect health care providers and patients. They promote safety in the workplace and influence your nursing practice, patient assignments, and how you delegate nursing care. These laws and policies also provide guidelines for nursing students. You need to be aware of the laws, policies, and procedures that affect your practice, and follow them as you plan to care for patients.

Staffing and Nurse-to-Patient Ratios

Adequate staffing is required to ensure patient safety and satisfaction with care. Nurse-to-patient ratios are determined in different ways. Legal issues occur when there are not enough nurses to provide competent care or when nurses work excessive overtime. In the case of *Spires v Hospital Corporation of America* (2006), poor patient care due to insufficient RN staffing resulting in the death of a patient was alleged. This suit emphasized the potential seriousness of short staffing and the importance of nurses' asserting employee rights.

Some states require that nursing committees in acute care settings determine safe staffing based on the needs of patients admitted to their facilities. While staffing committees have worked to determine appropriate staffing needs, employers have inappropriately asked some committees to make budgetary recommendations to pay for the staffing. In California, fixed nurse-patient ratios in acute care settings are mandated by law. The safe staffing ratio debate is occurring throughout the country and demands close attention by all nurses (ANA, n.d.b).

Nursing Assignments

Nurses are sometimes required to work on a unit where they do not typically care for patients. In this practice, often called "floating," nurses temporarily work in another area because there are not enough nurses to care for the number of patients and the acuity of the patients' needs on that unit at that time. If you are asked to float, you must inform the supervisor if you do not have the required education or experience to care for the patients assigned to you. You should request and receive an orientation to the unit. Supervisors are responsible to give staff nurses assignments that they can handle safely. Before accepting employment, learn the policies of the agency regarding floating and understand what is expected (ANA, n.d.a).

Patient Abandonment

Patient abandonment occurs when a nurse refuses to provide care for a patient after having established a patient-nurse relationship. Before having established that relationship, a nurse may refuse an assignment when (1) the nurse lacks the knowledge or skill to provide competent care; (2) care exceeding the nurse practice act is expected; (3) health of the nurse or the nurse's unborn child is directly threatened by the type of assignment; (4) orientation to the unit has not been completed and safety is at risk; (5) the nurse clearly states and documents a conscientious objection on the basis of moral, ethical, or religious grounds; or (6) the nurse's clinical judgment is impaired as a result of fatigue, resulting in a safety risk for the patient (ANA, 2021; ANA, 2015; Nurses Service Organization [NSO], 2017).

When refusing an assignment, it is important to give your immediate supervisor specific reasons for the refusal and to determine whether other alternatives, such as reassignment, are available. Document in your personal notes the specifics of the incident, the date and time it occurred, to whom you reported it, and actions you took to ensure that patients were safe and that you did not abandon your patients.

Nurse Delegation

Some state boards of nursing or nursing commissions specifically define responsibilities of the licensed practical nurse (LPN), RN, and advanced practice RNs and develop position statements and guidelines to help RNs and LPNs delegate safely (NCSBN, 2016; NCSBN and ANA, 2019). The process of nurse delegation is defined in nurse practice acts; regulations vary from state to state. In general, nurse delegation means that an RN educates, observes, and verifies that a nonregistered nurse (e.g., LPN, nurse assistant, or assistive personnel) can do a specific task that is usually completed by an RN (see Chapter 21). Several requirements ensure patient safety when delegating care. The RN retains responsibility to communicate clearly and supervise care received by a patient and to periodically reassess whether nurse delegation continues to be appropriate (Fig. 23.2). Delegated tasks may include hygiene care, ambulation assistance, vital signs, or blood glucose monitoring. RNs can usually delegate administration of medications to LPNs. It is important to know delegation requirements, including caregiver education and experience requirements, and the role and responsibilities of the RN. Just as RNs can delegate to non-RNs, LPNs can usually delegate tasks to other members of the health care team, such as certified nursing assistants (CNAs) or assistive personnel. Tasks delegated by LPNs often involve basic patient care (e.g., helping with ambulation, meeting patients' hygiene needs, and taking vital signs).

Nursing Students

Nursing students are liable if their actions exceed their scope of practice and cause harm to patients. Regardless of intent, students are expected to know what they can and cannot do when providing care to patients. If a student harms a patient as a direct result of a lack of action, the student, instructor, hospital or health care agency, and university or educational institution generally share the liability for the incorrect action. Nursing students should never be assigned to perform tasks for which they are unprepared, and instructors should supervise them carefully as they learn new skills. Although nursing students are not employees of a hospital, the agency has a responsibility to monitor their acts. They are expected to perform as professional nurses would in providing safe patient care. Faculty members are usually responsible for instructing and observing students, but in some situations staff nurses serving as preceptors share these responsibilities. Every nursing school should provide clear definitions of preceptor and faculty responsibility. It is equally important that nursing preceptors be aware of state laws applicable to nursing students, faculty, and the educational institution when supervising students.

Nursing students should perform only tasks that have been delegated to them and that are included in their titled job description when they are employed in health care settings (e.g., as nursing assistants, medication technicians). For example, if a student who also works as a medication technician has learned to administer intramuscular (IM) medications in a nursing class, the student cannot administer IM injections when working as a medication technician unless this is allowed under the state's Nurse Practice Act and the student's job description. If a staff nurse assigns a nursing student work without regard for the student's ability to safely conduct the task defined in the job description, the staff nurse is also liable. Nursing students employed in an agency as nurse's aides must refuse to perform tasks that are not included in their job description or agency's policies. Nursing students also should refuse to perform tasks that they are not prepared to complete safely. The student employee must tell the supervisor so that the task can be assigned to an appropriate health care professional. Patient safety is essential. Nursing students must ensure that their actions meet the scope of nursing required of them. Their actions must meet the standards of practice required for safe care of a patient whether they are at school, in the community, or employed at a health care agency. Although nursing students may have learned how to do a nursing task, it does not mean that they can safely perform the task on a patient independently. Err on the side of caution. Do not exceed your scope of practice whether you are a nurse's aide, nursing assistant, medication assistant, nursing student medication technician, or an employee with any other title.

FIG. 23.2 Nurses must communicate clearly and supervise care delegated to nonregistered nurses. (Copyright © iStock.)

> ### REFLECT NOW
>
> Consider your role as a nursing student as it is defined in your state's Nurse Practice Act. What are you required to do when working in a hospital? In your state, is it different if you are working in a skilled nursing facility or nursing home? What about if you are in a retirement center? What can you do in one place that you cannot do in another?

LEGAL IMPLICATIONS AND REDUCING YOUR LEGAL RISKS

Some patients or their families, especially those who experience poor health outcomes, believe that care provided by nurses failed to fall within the scope of nursing practice or failed to meet the standards of nursing practice. Sometimes in these cases, patients or their families file torts or lawsuits in the courts, alleging that the nurses knew, or should have known, that their behavior was less than what a reasonably prudent nurse would do under similar circumstances.

Torts

Torts are civil wrongful acts or omissions of care made against a person or property. They are classified as intentional, quasi-intentional, or unintentional.

Intentional torts are deliberate acts against a person or property that may result in both civil and criminal actions. Assault is an intentional threat toward another person that places the person in reasonable fear of harmful, imminent, or unwelcome contact (Furrow et al., 2018). No actual contact is required for an assault to occur. For example, if a nurse threatens to give a patient an injection or to restrain a patient while having an x-ray taken when the patient has refused consent, the nurse's action is considered an assault. Likewise, assault occurs when a patient threatens a nurse. Battery is any intentional offensive touching without consent or lawful justification (Furrow et al., 2018). The contact can be harmful to the patient and cause an injury, or it merely can be offensive to the patient's personal dignity. In the example of a nurse threatening to give a patient an injection without the patient's consent, if the nurse gives the injection, it is battery. Battery also results if a health care provider performs a procedure that goes beyond the scope of a patient's consent. For example, if a patient gives consent for an appendectomy and the surgeon performs a tonsillectomy, battery has occurred. The key component is the patient's consent. False imprisonment occurs when a patient is restrained without a legal reason. False imprisonment happens when nurses restrain a patient in a confined area, preventing the ability to move freely in a bed, chair, room, or other area in which the patient wishes to be (Furrow et al., 2018; Yeung et al., 2019).

Quasi-Intentional Torts. Quasi-intentional torts are acts in which a person may not intend to cause harm to another but does. Typically, the person invades another's privacy or in some way defames another's character. Quasi-intentional torts are alleged when a person should have known that harm to another person could occur.

Invasion of privacy is usually the release of a patient's health care information to an unauthorized person, such as a member of the press, the patient's employer, the patient's family, or online. HIPAA and the HITECH Act privacy standards have raised awareness of the need for health care professionals to provide confidentiality and privacy. The information that is in a patient's medical record is a confidential communication that may be shared only with health care providers to provide treatment. This includes electronic communication by e-mail, text, or other devices. All communications become part of the health care record and must be considered confidential. They may not be released without permission of the patient. Individuals who insist on receiving information without patient consent must immediately be referred to a supervisor. It is not within the nurse's scope of practice to determine when information should or should not be disclosed.

Defamation of character is the publication of false statements that result in damage to a person's reputation. Slander occurs when one speaks falsely about another. For example, if a nurse tells people erroneously that a patient has gonorrhea and the disclosure affects the patient's business, the nurse is liable for slander. Libel is the written defamation of character (e.g., charting false defamatory entries in a medical record) (Furrow et al., 2018; Philo et al., 2019-2020).

Unintentional Torts. Unintentional torts arise when a person is harmed and the person inflicting the harm knew, or should have known, that these actions were less than the accepted scope and standard of practice.

Negligence is conduct that falls below the generally accepted standard of care of a reasonably prudent person (Furrow et al., 2018). Anyone, including people not in the medical field, can be liable for negligence. Nurses are negligent when they had a duty of care that is breached and their patient is physically harmed. A reasonably prudent nurse under similar circumstances would have provided care differently. The law establishes the standard of care to protect others against an unreasonably great risk of harm (Furrow et al., 2018). Negligent acts, such as hanging the wrong intravenous solution for a patient or applying a warm compress that causes a burn, often result in disciplinary action by the State Board of Nursing and a lawsuit for negligence against the nurse and the employer. Most lawsuits allege negligence.

Malpractice is a type of negligence. A person being held liable for malpractice must be a professional. Certain criteria are necessary to establish nursing malpractice: (1) the nurse (defendant) owed a duty of care to the patient (plaintiff), (2) the nurse did not carry out or breached that duty, (3) the patient was injured as a result of the breach in duty, and (4) damages or remedies are allowed under state law to "make the person whole" in the eyes of the court. Even though nurses do not intend to injure patients, some patients file claims of malpractice if nurses give care that does not meet the appropriate standards. Most malpractice and professional licensure claims occur in hospital settings. Common causes of malpractice against nurses include failure to follow the standard of care (e.g., not implementing a pressure injury or fall prevention protocol), failure to communicate important information to another health care provider, failure to document appropriately, failure to assess and monitor a patient, and inappropriate delegation of nursing tasks.

More health care agencies are using medication administration technology, such as bar coding, to try to reduce medication administration errors (see Chapter 31). However, the capacity to override or work around intended safeguards has contributed to significant harm to patients. It is essential that you always follow the policies and procedures of your agency and never override safeguards intended to promote safe patient care.

Malpractice is a type of negligence. Malpractice sometimes involves failing to check a patient's identification correctly before administering blood and then giving the blood to the wrong patient. It also involves administering a medication to a patient even though the medical record contains documentation that the patient has an allergy to that medication. In general, courts define nursing malpractice as the failure to use a degree of skill or learning ordinarily used under the same or similar circumstances by members of the nursing profession (Furrow et al., 2018).

Another area of potential risk is associated with the use of electronic monitoring devices. No monitor is reliable all the time. Therefore do not depend on them completely. Continually assess a patient to determine the accuracy of electronic monitoring. There are also electrical hazards to nurses and patients. Biomedical engineers check equipment to ensure that it is in proper working order and that a patient will not receive an electrical shock.

The best way for nurses to avoid malpractice is to follow evidence-based standards of care, deliver care competently, and communicate in a timely manner with other health care providers. You also avoid malpractice by developing a caring rapport with patients and thoroughly documenting assessments, interventions, and evaluation of care. Generate and act on your spirit of inquiry to provide the best care in conjunction with your patients' preferences and values. Know and follow the policies and procedures of the agency where you work. Be sensitive to your patients' risks and the common sources of patient injury such as pressure injuries, falls, and medication errors. Finally, communicate with your patients; explain all tests, medications, and treatments in language they understand; document understanding of patient education; and listen to your patients' concerns about treatments. You are accountable to report any significant changes in your patient's condition in a timely manner to the health care provider and to document these changes in the patient's electronic health record (EHR) (see Chapter 26). Timely and truthful documentation is important to provide communication necessary among health care team members. Documentation must be accurate (Furrow et al., 2018). In the EHR, ensure that assessments are complete and consistent with those completed previously. Ensure that you conduct your own assessment rather than copying the previous assessment in the patient's medical record to ensure accuracy of information. Investigate and do not override safeguards built into each program to alert you to concerns such as black box warnings when administering medications. Notify other team members in a timely manner when changes in condition are triggered within the record. If you are named in a malpractice suit, you need to know your rights and understand the legal process (Box 23.3). Work with your health care agency's legal team and be sure to advocate for yourself.

BOX 23.3   Anatomy of a Lawsuit

The lawsuit process varies because of differences in state laws and civil procedure rules. However, lawsuits typically follow a similar process.

- A civil action begins with a **complaint** that is accompanied by a summons. The complaint is developed by an attorney and outlines what the defendant nurse did wrong and, because of that alleged negligence, how the plaintiff was injured and what the plaintiff believes should occur because of the negligence (e.g., pay damages).
- The defendant (the nurse) has to **answer** within a specified amount of time (e.g., 3 weeks). In the answer, the nurse admits or denies each allegation in the petition and if the defendant has any claims against the plaintiff.
- The parties involved in the lawsuit exchange documents and information during **discovery.** The discovery period can last for months to years depending on the state. In this phase, discovery occurs in three different ways:
  - **Interrogatories:** Written questions requiring answers under oath. Typically opposing counsel requests a list of possible witnesses, insurance experts, and which health care providers the plaintiff saw before and after the event.
  - **Requests for document productions:** Opposing parties request relevant documents, pictures, or related materials such as medical records for treatment before and after the event; agency policies and procedures; and all e-mails, texts, and other social media communications about the incident.
  - **Depositions:** Questions are posed to opposing parties, witnesses, and expert witnesses under oath to obtain all relevant, nonprivileged information about the case. Experts establish the elements of the case and the applicable standard of care.
- The opposing parties will meet after the discovery phase to discuss the possibility of resolving the case before it goes to trial. An arbitrator, who is an impartial third party, may be used during this process. The court typically is not involved in this type of settlement. If the parties cannot come to a resolution or a settlement, then the case goes to trial.
- During the **trial** the attorneys for both sides present evidence and arguments for their side. The plaintiff and defendant make opening statements and then the plaintiff presents evidence to support the case. The defense can question or cross-examine each witness. After the plaintiff rests the case, the defense can present evidence and witnesses to counter the plaintiff's case. A settlement may be agreed on at any point during the case. If no settlement is made by the end of the trial, either the judge or the jury determines the resolution.
- Either or both parties can **appeal** the decision to a higher court.

Adapted from Bookman K and Zane, RD: Surviving a medical malpractice lawsuit, *Emerg Med Clin North Am* 38(2):539–548, 2020; FindLaw: *What to expect—a lawsuit chronology*, 2016. https://www.findlaw.com/litigation/filing-a-lawsuit/what-to-expect-a-lawsuit-chronology.html. Accessed April 17, 2021.

An agency must maintain its medical records according to specific statutes and accreditation regulations. Nurses' notes are an important part of the medical record because they contain substantial evidence needed to understand the care received by a patient. If records are lost, incomplete, or altered, there is a presumption that negligent care caused a patient's injuries. In addition, incomplete or illegible records make a health care provider less credible or believable. Determine changes in patient conditions documented by prior nursing staff, and document timely responses to those changes. In addition, it is essential to provide and document patient decision making; the patient is the primary decision maker, regardless of setting, when care is provided. EHRs record every time a person accesses them. Thus there is an electronic record whenever you view, document, or alter them. In addition, EHRs can be retrieved and compared as they existed in real time from one moment to another. When making a late entry into an electronic record, it is essential that the amended note be entered as such; never delete and then reenter different language representative of the same date and time as had been previously erased. Regardless of intent, the record subsequently may be considered altered to protect the agency and hide information from the court regarding care received or not received by the patient.

Standard of Proof

The standard of proof is typically what a reasonably prudent nurse would do under similar circumstances in the geographical area in which the alleged breach occurred. Malpractice is the result of nursing care falling below a standard of care. In a malpractice lawsuit, it is typically required that the nurse had a duty of care (i.e., nurse practice act), that the duty was breached (i.e., nursing regulations), that physical harm occurred (i.e., testimony and records), and that in that state the awarding of damages or monetary compensation is allowed. The standard of proof in this case is the degree to which the evidence must show that a duty of care was violated, resulting in harm to the patient (Bookman and Zane, 2020; Frank and Danks, 2019).

During a malpractice suit, a nurse's actual conduct is compared with nursing standards of care (i.e., scope and standards of nursing care [ANA, 2021; ANA, 2015]) to determine whether the nurse acted as any reasonably prudent nurse would act under the same or similar circumstances (Furrow et al., 2018; Philo et al., 2019-2020). For example, if a patient is burned from a warm compress application, negligence is determined by reviewing whether the nurse followed the correct procedure for applying the compress. If a procedure was not followed, the policy is reviewed. It there is no policy, this could reflect a systemic problem because the nurses are not provided information regarding current evidence-based knowledge to guide them on how to appropriately apply warm compresses. There is a greater possibility that other patients are at risk for, or have already had, burns due to erroneous application of warm compresses. The scope and standards of nursing practice are also being violated; subsequently, litigation would encompass more than failure to simply follow a procedure. The policies and procedures that guide your practice need to be updated regularly by the nursing department and reflect current best practice evidence. When you follow your agency's policies and procedures, you ensure that your care is similar to what other reasonable, prudent nursing colleagues would provide under the same or similar circumstances.

Malpractice Insurance

Malpractice insurance is a contract between an insurance company and a nurse or employer. It is intended to cover costs incurred when a patient sues the employer and/or the nurse. Malpractice insurance provides for a defense of the nurse and the employer in a lawsuit. The insurance company pays for costs, attorney's fees, settlement, and other related fees generated in the representation of the nurse. It covers the costs to the patient; it does not cover the costs when a complaint is filed with the state licensing board. These are two different actions, and different laws apply. Therefore it is suggested that nurses carry both professional licensure defense and malpractice insurance or one policy that specifically includes both actions. It is also often recommended that nurses have their own personal liability insurance policy. Relying on your employer's malpractice insurance is often inadequate.

Health care agencies have insurance intended to provide financial assistance when it is alleged that a patient was permanently harmed in one of their facilities. As an employee or agent of the agency, the actions of the nurse when caring for the patient are examined. It is important to remember in these cases that the lawyer is representing the employer and not the nurse. The insurance provided by the employing agency covers nurses only while they are working within the scope of their employment.

Nurse Experts

When a case that involves nursing care is filed, a nursing expert will often testify about the standards of nursing care as applied to the facts of a case (Box 23.4). An expert has education and experience related to the alleged complaint of the patient and accurately and concisely describes the pertinent scope and standards of practice required of a nurse under similar circumstances (Grant and Ballard, 2018). For example, when a patient sustains an injury from a fall, a nurse with experience in risk management and fall prevention will be asked to consult as an expert on the case. The expert nurse must determine that no conflict of interest exists before accepting a case. For example, the expert nurse could not work for either party's employer. The expert will review all evidence before giving an opinion, including relevant

laws and regulations, policies and procedures, patient records, other expert reports, and depositions. Depositions are interviews in which lawyers can ask questions of others who are under oath to provide honest and complete answers. These interviews are transcribed by a court reporter who is present during the sessions. For example, opposing counsel will depose the expert nurse. During the deposition, the nurse will respond to the questions that are asked. The court reporter will record the session in writing, on audio recording, and sometimes on video recording. Within a couple of weeks, the deposition document will be given to all parties to make corrections. Once completed, the document is finalized and will be entered into the case record (Furrow et al., 2018). Nurse experts base their opinions on existing standards of practice established by nurse practice acts, federal and state licensing laws, TJC standards, professional organizations, institutional policies and procedures, job descriptions, and current evidence-based literature. When reviewing a case a nurse expert determines if the nurse in question met the same standards as other nurses practicing in similar settings and under similar circumstances; they do not make legal decisions. Specialized nurses such as critical care nurses, wound care specialists, or surgical nurses have specially defined standards of care and skills. Ignorance of the law or of standards of care is not a defense against malpractice (Furrow et al., 2018). All nurses are required to know valid, reliable, and credible evidence that is applicable to their practice and the settings in which they work, including current standards of care and the policies and procedures of their employing agency (ANA, 2021; TJC, 2021c).

One of the first and most important cases to discuss a nurse's liability was *Darling v Charleston Community Memorial Hospital* (1965). It involved an 18-year-old man with a fractured leg. The emergency department physician applied a cast with insufficient padding. The man's toes became swollen and discolored, and he developed decreased sensation. He reported the decreased sensation to nursing staff many times. Although the nurses recognized the symptoms as signs of impaired circulation, they failed to tell their supervisor that the physician did not respond to their calls or the patient's needs. Gangrene developed, and the man's leg was amputated. Although the physician was held liable for incorrectly applying the cast, the nursing staff were also held liable for failing to adhere to the standards of care for monitoring and reporting the patient's symptoms. Even though the nurses attempted to contact the physician, the jury and subsequent judges held that when the physician failed to respond, the nurses should have acted on behalf of the patient's safety, followed the chain of command, and obtained assistance from the charge nurse, nursing supervisor, and the chief medical officer to make sure that the patient received appropriate care. Almost every state uses this 1965 Illinois Supreme Court case as a legal precedent.

Reducing Legal Risks

Health care agencies, nurses, health care providers, and other health care employees need to take appropriate actions to reduce their legal risks. In addition to being aware of the actions taken at the organizational level by your employer, it is important that you remain involved in the nursing profession to reduce your personal legal risk.

Risk Management and Performance/Quality Improvement

Risk-management, performance improvement (PI), and quality improvement (QI) programs help to reduce a nurse's legal risk for malpractice and negligence because they help to identify potential hazards and eliminate them before harm occurs. Risk management involves several components, including identifying possible risks, analyzing them, acting to reduce the risks, and evaluating the steps

---

BOX 23.4   Proof of Negligence

- The nurse owed a duty of care to the patient.
- The nurse did not carry out the duty or breached it (failed to use that degree of skill and learning ordinarily used under the same or similar circumstances by members of the profession).
- The patient was physically injured or harmed because the nurse breached the duty.
- The patient's injury resulted in compensable damages that can be qualified as medical bills, lost wages, and pain and suffering.

Common Sources of Negligence

Be aware of the following common negligent acts that have resulted in lawsuits against hospitals and nurses (Frank and Danks, 2019; Grant and Ballard, 2018):

- Failure to follow the standard of care
- Failure to communicate (e.g., failure to notify the health care provider of abnormal assessment data or significant changes in a patient's status)
- Failure to document care and evaluation of care provided to the patient
- Failure to assess and/or monitor, including making a nursing diagnosis
- Failure to act as a patient advocate
- Failure to properly delegate and supervise care
- Failure to initiate the chain of command (e.g., failure to address a concern about a team member's conduct that negatively affects a patient's safety or well-being)
- Failure to manage and maintain an adequate hospital information system
- Failure to administer medications correctly (e.g., not following the seven rights of medication administration; failure to administer an intramuscular injection correctly)
- Failure to follow policies and procedures (e.g., failure to implement fall prevention protocol)

taken to reduce them (TJC, 2021c). PI and QI place emphasis on human performance, work processes, and organizational structure (Auton, 2018; Health Catalyst Editors, 2019). These programs promote a "just culture" environment that encourages honest disclosure and system-wide resolution to prevent occurrence or recurrence of circumstances surrounding a concern. QI, PI, and risk-management procedures are essential; they require documentation of information to facilitate resolution of questions regarding care.

Nurses often assume the role of risk manager. For example, surgeons rely on operating room nurses to compare the consent form with the indicated and prepped surgical site for accuracy. TJC's Universal Protocol helps prevent errors due to patients undergoing the wrong operation or having surgery performed on the wrong site (TJC, 2021c). The protocol requires mandatory time-outs before beginning any surgery. Nurses are responsible to implement this protocol whenever an invasive surgical procedure is performed, regardless of setting (see Chapter 50).

Patient safety and improved care are the goals of QI, PI, and risk management (TJC, 2021c). Professional groups such as the Institute of Medicine focus on patient safety as major goals. *Never events* are preventable errors, which include falls, urinary tract infections from improper use of catheters, and pressure injuries (Agency for Healthcare Research and Quality [AHRQ], 2019). The federal government and health care insurance companies have developed policies to withhold reimbursement for never events (AHRQ, 2019) (see Chapter 27). All inpatient health care settings conduct routine monthly monitoring of the incidence of never events, and health care staff are expected to maintain standards for prevention of these events. When trending shows an increase in never events, QI and PI activities are quickly implemented. Know your agency's policies and procedures to help develop a system and culture of patient safety.

One tool used in risk management is the occurrence report or incident report. Occurrence reporting provides a database to determine deviations from standards of care, to identify corrective measures needed to prevent recurrence, and to alert risk management to a potential claim. Examples of an occurrence include patient or visitor falls or injury; failure to follow health care provider orders; a significant complaint by patient, family, health care provider, or other hospital department; an error in technique or procedure; and a malfunctioning device or product. The health care worker involved most directly in the occurrence completes the report. Agencies generally have specific guidelines to direct health care providers in how to complete occurrence reports. A report is confidential and separate from the health care record. However, it is discoverable by court order during a legal proceeding. Risk managers work with nurses to provide safe care and to determine how to prevent recurrence of circumstances when a patient is potentially or actually harmed.

QSEN Building Competency in Quality Improvement You are a member of your unit's task force focusing on quality improvement and reduction in never events. The chairperson explains to the task force that quality improvement relates to data collection, evaluation, and improvement in patient outcomes. One of the nurses asks, "How can we reduce the number of occurrence reports being filed on the unit related to patient falls?" How would you respond?

Answers to QSEN Activities can be found on the Evolve website.

Professional Involvement

As a professional nurse, it is important to implement actions in your own practice that will help reduce your legal risk. Develop and use your clinical judgment to identify patient needs and make sound clinical decisions. Remain present for your patients. Assess them carefully, use critical thinking to analyze cues, and identify patterns and needs. Respond to patient needs in a timely manner. Provide accurate patient education and verify that your patients understand your instructions. Ensure that your patients understand their treatment plans and have been provided the opportunity to give informed consent when required. Document clearly and in a timely manner and alert your patient's health care provider when your patient's health status changes. Avoid posting information about your patients or your workplace on social media. Clarify unclear medical orders, implement and follow your agency's policies, and speak up if you have concerns about patient safety. Many environmental (e.g., resources, patient observations, task complexity, cultural considerations) and individual (e.g., knowledge, skills, level of experience) factors come into play when caring for patients with complex health needs. Use your understanding of these factors along with analytical and nonanalytical reasoning to develop accurate conclusions that are evidence based and will most likely result in positive patient outcomes (Dickison et al., 2019).

It is also essential to remain aware of current issues in health care. Become involved in professional organizations and committees that define the standards of care for nursing practice. If current laws, rules and regulations, or policies under which nurses practice are not evidence based, advocate to ensure that the scope of nursing practice is defined accurately. Be willing to represent nursing and the patient's perspective in the community as well. The voice of nursing is powerful and effective when the organizing focus is the protection and welfare of the public entrusted to nurses' care.

KEY POINTS

- Constitutional law gives patients the right to refuse treatment, and your state's Nurse Practice Act, a statutory law, defines the scope of nursing practice and the standards you must meet within that state to ensure safe, evidence-based, and competent nursing practice.
- The scope and standards of nursing practice, created by various professional organizations and health care agencies, define nursing and reflect the responsibilities, knowledge, and skills ordinarily expected from nurses.
- Federal statutes are typically linked to Medicare and Medicaid reimbursement, are intended to enhance patient safety, and greatly influence nursing practice. For example, the Patient Self-Determination Act (PSDA) requires health care institutions to provide information to patients regarding their rights to make informed decisions about their care, including the right to create an advance directive.
- State health care acts outline which individuals may provide informed consent for a patient to have invasive procedures or to participate in a research study.
- Different states have different laws that affect care at the beginning and end of life that do not always align with nursing standards. For example, although some states have laws that allow assisted suicide, the American Nurses Association (ANA) believes that helping patients end their lives is against the nursing code of ethics.
- A variety of guidelines affect nursing practice in the workplace and address issues such as patient-to-nurse ratios, nursing assignments, delegation, and the supervision of nursing students in clinical agencies.
- Worsening pressure injuries, failure to contact the health care provider as conditions change, and medication errors often trigger complaints of negligence or malpractice against nurses.
- When a nurse's performance is questioned, the standard of proof in nursing is typically what a reasonably prudent nurse would do

under similar circumstances in the geographical area in which the alleged breach occurred.

- Risk-management, performance improvement (PI), and quality improvement (QI) activities enhance patient safety and reduce a nurse's legal risk by identifying potential safety issues, implementing actions to prevent patient harm, and evaluating the effects of these actions on patient outcomes.
- It is important to know your Nurse Practice Act, to implement and follow agency policies and procedures, to delegate care appropriately, and to follow staffing and delegation guidelines to reduce your legal risk when practicing nursing.

REFLECTIVE LEARNING

You are working in an outpatient clinic where you meet a 34-year-old married mother of two small children who is seeing the doctor for numbness and tingling in her right leg. Over the next 6 months, she has critically high glucose levels, she does not take her medication, and the provider is significantly concerned. She continues to have numbness and tingling that migrate from her left hip, leg, and foot. The physician orders scans of her leg and lower spine. Each scan is negative. She continues to have pain and numbness and tingling in her neck, back, and legs. During her most recent visit, the provider ordered a scan of her thoracic spine and right knee. One week later, the patient e-mails the provider that although the knee scan was completed, no one has contacted her about the other scan. The nurse checks the record and responds, "My bad. I missed it. I'll order it now." The next day the patient unexpectedly appears at the clinic, where you observe her staggering at the desk and slurring her speech, asking to see you. You and the receptionist place her immediately into a wheelchair. After being assessed, she is admitted to the hospital, where she is diagnosed with slow bleeding into the spinal column. The patient has irreparable damage to the spine and will be quadriplegic for the remainder of her life.

- What standards of practice apply in this scenario? Does this situation establish negligence? Specifically, what are the duty, the breach in duty, the permanent harm, and damages in this case?
- What is the standard of proof that would be applied to this situation to determine whether the nurse is liable for the harm incurred by this patient? Make a case for either side.
- Using your clinical judgment to guide you (see Chapter 15), identify which environmental and individual factors led to the poor patient outcome. Which assessment findings were missed or not reported? What actions could have been taken by the nurse or other health care providers that may have prevented this situation from happening?

REVIEW QUESTIONS

1. A nurse is planning care for a patient going to surgery. Who is responsible for informing the patient about the surgery along with possible risks, complications, and benefits?
   1. Family member
   2. Surgeon
   3. Nurse
   4. Nurse manager
2. A woman has severe life-threatening injuries, is unresponsive, and is hemorrhaging following a car accident. The health care provider ordered 2 units of packed red blood cells to treat the woman's anemia. The woman's husband refuses to allow the nurse to give his wife the blood for religious reasons. What is the nurse's responsibility?
   1. Obtain a court order to give the blood.
   2. Convince the husband to allow the nurse to give the blood.

3. Call security and have the husband removed from the hospital.
4. Gather more information about the wife's preferences and determine whether the husband has her power of attorney for health care.

3. A nurse sends a text message to the oncoming nurse that states, "Mr. Kodro in room 3348-1 refused to take his sertraline hydrochloride as ordered this morning because he said he was feeling better." What should the oncoming nurse do? (Select all that apply.)
   1. Add this information to the board hanging at the patient's bedside.
   2. Tell the nurse who sent the text that the text is a HIPAA violation.
   3. Inform the nursing supervisor.
   4. Forward the text to the charge nurse.
   5. Thank the nurse for sending the information.
4. Which of the following actions, if performed by an RN, could result in both criminal and administrative law sanctions against the nurse? (Select all that apply.)
   1. Reviewing the EHR of a family member who is a patient in the same hospital on a different unit
   2. Refusing to provide health care information to an older adult's child
   3. Reporting suspected abuse and neglect of children
   4. Applying physical restraints without a written order
   5. Completing an occurrence report on the unit
5. A nurse received a bedside report at the change of shift with the night-shift nurse and the patient. The nursing student assigned to the patient asks to review the patient's medical record. The nurse lists patients' medical diagnoses on the message boards in the patients' rooms. Later in the day the nurse discusses the plan of care for a patient who is dying with the patient's family. Which of these actions describes a violation of HIPAA?
   1. Discussing patient conditions at the bedside at the change of shift
   2. Allowing the nursing student to review the assigned patient's chart before providing care during the clinical experience
   3. Posting medical information about the patient on a message board in the patient's room
   4. Releasing patient information regarding terminal illness to family when the patient has given permission for information to be shared
6. A patient is in skeletal traction and has a plaster cast due to a fractured femur. The patient experiences decreased sensation and a cold feeling in the toes of the affected leg. The nurse observes that the patient's toes have become pale and cold but forgets to document and report this to the health care provider because one of the nurse's other patients experienced cardiac arrest at the same time. Two days later the patient in skeletal traction has an elevated temperature, and he is prepared for surgery to amputate the leg below the knee. Which of the following statements regarding a breach of duty apply to this situation? (Select all that apply.)
   1. Failure to document a change in assessment data
   2. Failure to provide discharge instructions
   3. Failure to provide patient education about cast care
   4. Failure to use proper medical equipment ordered for patient monitoring
   5. Failure to notify a health care provider about a change in the patient's condition
7. A man who is homeless enters the emergency department seeking health care. The health care provider indicates that the patient needs to be transferred to the city hospital for care before assessing the patient. This action is most likely a violation of which of the following laws?
   1. Health Insurance Portability and Accountability Act (HIPAA)
   2. Americans With Disabilities Act (ADA)

3. Patient Self-Determination Act (PSDA)
4. Emergency Medical Treatment and Active Labor Act (EMTALA)

8. A home health nurse notices significant bruising on a 2-year-old patient's head, arms, abdomen, and legs. The patient's mother describes the patient's frequent falls. What is the best nursing action for the home health nurse to take?
   1. Document her findings and treat the patient.
   2. Instruct the mother on safe handling of a 2-year-old child.
   3. Contact a child abuse hotline.
   4. Discuss this story with a colleague.

9. Which of the following statements indicate that the new nursing graduate understands ways to remain involved professionally? (Select all that apply.)
   1. "I am thinking about joining the health committee at my church."
   2. "I need to read newspapers, watch news broadcasts, and search the Internet for information related to health."
   3. "I will join nursing committees at the hospital after I have completed orientation and better understand the issues affecting nursing."

4. "Nurses do not have very much voice in legislation in Washington, DC, because of the nursing shortage."
5. "I will go back to school as soon as I finish orientation."

10. You are working on a patient care unit and observe several other nurses who are not following the agency's policy when preparing and administering medications. When you ask them to explain why they are doing this, they state the new medication administration technology installed on the unit takes too much time to use, so they are using workarounds to get their patient medications administered on time. Which is the best action to take first?
    1. Discuss the situation with the nursing manager.
    2. Call a colleague who works at another institution to talk about the problem.
    3. Look for a position on a different nursing unit.
    4. Say nothing and begin your work.

Answers: 1. 2; 4; 3; 2. 4; 1; 4; 5; 3; 6. 1; 5; 7. 4; 8. 3; 9. 1, 2, 3; **10.** 1.

Rationales for Review Questions can be found on the Evolve website.

REFERENCES

Adigun OO, et al: *Abuse and neglect,* 2020. https://www.ncbi.nlm.nih.gov/books/NBK436015/. Accessed April 17, 2021.

Agency for Healthcare Research and Quality (AHRQ): *Never events,* U.S. Department of Health and Human Services, 2019. https://psnet.ahrq.gov/primers/primer/3/Never-Events. Accessed April 18, 2021.

American Disabilities Act National Network (ADANN): *What is the American with Disabilities Act (ADA)?* 2021. https://adata.org/learn-about-ada. Accessed April 17, 2021.

American Nurses Association (ANA): *Position statement: reduction of patient restraint and seclusion in health care settings,* Silver Spring, MD, 2012, Author. https://www.nursingworld.org/practice-policy/nursing-excellence/official-position-statements/id/reduction-of-patient-restraint-and-seclusion-in-health-care-settings/. Accessed April 18, 2021.

American Nurses Association (ANA): *Nursing: scope and standards of practice,* ed 4, Silver Spring, MD, 2021, The Association.

American Nurses Association (ANA): *Position Statement: risk and responsibility in providing nursing care,* Silver Spring, MD, 2015, The Association. https://www.nursingworld.org/~4af23e/globalassets/docs/ana/ethics/riskandresponsibilitypositionstatement2015.pdf. Accessed April 16, 2021.

American Nurses Association Ethics Advisory Board: ANA Position Statement: The nurse's role when a patient requests medical aid in dying, *OJIN Online J Issue Nurs* 24(3), 2019. https://ojin.nursingworld.org/MainMenuCategories/ANAMarketplace/ANAPeriodicals/OJIN/Columns/ANA-Position-Statements/Nurses-Role-Medical-Aid-in-Dying.html. Accessed November 2021.

American Nurses Association (ANA): *Nurse staffing.* n.d.a. https://www.nursingworld.org/practice-policy/advocacy/state/nurse-staffing/. Accessed April 17, 2021.

American Nurses Association (ANA): *Position statement: questions to ask about safe staffing before accepting employment,* Silver Spring, MD, n.d.b. https://www.nursingworld.org/practice-policy/workforce/questions-to-ask-about-safe-staffing-before-accepting-employment/. Accessed April 17, 2021.

Auton G: *A new framework for healthcare performance improvement,* 2018, https://www.hfma.org/topics/article/61619.html. Accessed April 18, 2021.

Barr L, et al: Promoting positive and safe care in forensic mental health inpatient settings: evaluating critical

factors that assist nurses to reduce the use of restrictive practices, *Int J Ment Health Nurs* 28(4):888, 2019.

Bookman K, Zane, RD: Surviving a medical malpractice lawsuit, *Emerg Med Clin North Am* 38(2):539–548, 2020.

Busch C: Implementing personalized law: personalized disclosures in consumer law and data privacy law, *Univ Chic Law Rev* 86(2):309, 2019. https://www.jstor.org/stable/26590557. Accessed April 16, 2021.

Caffrey M: *Federal appeals court strikes down ACA individual mandate,* AJMC, December 18, 2019. https://www.ajmc.com/newsroom/federal-appeals-court-strikes-down-aca-individual-mandate. Accessed April 17, 2021.

California et al., v. Texas et al. No. 19-840, June 17, 2021. https://www.supremecourt.gov/opinions/20pdf/19-840_6jfm.pdf. Accessed September 7, 2021.

Centers for Medicare and Medicaid Services (CMS): *Revisions to Medicare conditions of participation,* 482. Bethesda, MD, 2008, U.S. Department of Health and Human Services, p 13.

Centers for Medicare and Medicaid Services (CMS): *Patient Protection and Affordable Care Act; HHS notice of benefit and Payment parameters for 2020,* 2019. https://www.federalregister.gov/documents/2019/01/24/2019-00077/patient-protection-and-affordable-care-act-hhs-notice-of-benefit-and-payment-parameters-for-2020. Accessed April 17, 2021

Centers for Medicare and Medicaid Services (CMS): *State operations manual appendix a—survey protocol, regulations and interpretive guidelines for hospitals,* 2020. https://www.cms.gov/Regulations-and-Guidance/Guidance/Manuals/downloads/som107ap_a_hospitals.pdf. Accessed April 17, 2021.

Centers for Medicare and Medicaid Services (CMS): *The Mental Health Parity and Addiction Equity Act (MHPAEA),* n.d. https://www.cms.gov/CCIIO/Programs-and-Initiatives/Other-Insurance-Protections/mhpaea_factsheet. Accessed April 18, 2021.

Dickison P, et al: Integrating the National Council of State Boards of Nursing clinical judgment model into nursing educational frameworks, *J Nurs Educ* 58(2):72, 2019.

Furrow BR, et al: *Health law: cases, materials and problems,* ed 8, St. Paul, MN, 2018, West Academic Publishing.

Frank L, Danks J: Perianesthesia nursing malpractice: reducing the risk of litigation, *J Perianesth Nurs* 34(3):463, 2019.

Gaines K: *Nurses ranked most trusted profession 19 years in a row,* 2021. https://nurse.org/articles/nursing-ranked-most-honest-profession/. Accessed May 15, 2021.

Grant PD, Ballard DC: *Law for nurse leaders,* ed 2, Springer Publishing Company, 2018, New York, NY, https://books.google.com/books?hl=en&lr=&id=RXQkDwAAQBAJ&oi=fnd&pg=PA51&dq=nursing+malpractice+and+negligence&ots=y2nBWdu0yy&sig=YiIL022FE8A8v6TQ7ZwhGtcEk7w#v=onepage&q=nursing%20malpractice%20and%20negligence&f=false. Accessed April 18, 2021.

Golden S: Do not resuscitate orders: a matter of life and death in New York, *J Contemp Health Law Policy* 4(1):449, 1988.

Health Catalyst Editors: *The top six examples of quality improvement in healthcare,* 2019. https://www.healthcatalyst.com/insights/top-examples-quality-improvement-healthcare. Accessed April 18, 2021.

Henry J, Kaiser Family Foundation (KFF): *Key facts about the uninsured population,* 2020. https://www.kff.org/uninsured/fact-sheet/key-facts-about-the-uninsured-population/. Accessed April 17, 2021.

Korobkin R: Property rights and the control of human biospecimens. In Lynch HF, et al., editors: *Specimen science: ethics and policy implications,* Cambridge, MA, 2017, The MIT Press.

Luthi S: *U. S. Organ transplant rules get an overhaul,* Modern Healthcare, December 7, 2018. https://www.modernhealthcare.com/article/20181207/NEWS/181209931/u-s-organ-transplant-rules-get-an-overhaul. Accessed April 17, 2021.

McGuire AL, et al: Who owns the data in a medical information commons? *J Law Med Ethics* 47(1):62, 2019.

National Council of State Boards of Nursing (NCSBN): *White paper: national guidelines for nursing delegation,* 2016. https://www.ncsbn.org/NCSBN_Delegation_Guidelines.pdf. Accessed April 18, 2021.

National Council of State Boards of Nursing (NCSBN): *White paper: a nurse's guide to the use of social media,* 2018. https://www.ncsbn.org/NCSBN_SocialMedia.pdf. Accessed April 17, 2021.

National Council of State Boards of Nursing (NCSBN) and American Nurses Association (ANA): *National guidelines for nursing delegation,* 2019. https://www.ncsbn.org/NGND-PosPaper_06.pdf. Accessed April 18, 2021.

National Council of State Boards of Nursing (NCSBN): *Nurse Licensure Compact (NLC),* 2021. https://www.ncsbn.org/nurse-licensure-compact.htm. Accessed April 17, 2021.

Nurses Service Organization (NSO): *When to refuse an assignment,* 2017. Affinity Insurance Services. https://www.nso.com/Learning/Artifacts/Articles/when-to-refuse-an-assignment. Accessed April 17, 2021.

Oyeleye OA: The nursing licensure compact and its disciplinary provisions: what nurses should know, *Online J Issues Nurs* 24(2), 2019. http://dx.doi.org/10.3912/OJIN.Vol24No02PPT09.

Philo H, et al: *Lawyers desk reference,* ed 10, Eagan, MN, 2019-2020, Thomson Reuters.

Pozgar GD: *Legal and ethical issues for health professionals,* ed 5, Burlington, MA, 2020, Jones & Bartlett Publishing.

Privacy Rights Clearinghouse: *The HIPAA privacy rule: patients' rights,* 2014, https://www.privacyrights.org/consumer-guides/hipaa-privacy-rule-patients-rights. Accessed April 17, 2021.

Reinbeck D, Antonacci J: Tech notes. How nurses can use social media to their advantage, *Nursing* 49(5):61, 2019.

The Joint Commission (TJC): *Comprehensive accreditation manual for hospitals: the official handbook*, Oak Brook Terrace, IL, 2021a, The Joint Commission.

The Joint Commission (TJC): *Restraint and seclusion—enclosure beds, side rails and mitts. Is an enclosure bed, side rails or hand mitts a restraint?* 2021b. https://www.jointcommission.org/en/standards/standard-faqs/critical-access-hospital/provision-of-care-treatment-and-services-pc/000001668/. Accessed April 17, 2021.

The Joint Commission (TJC): *2021 National patient safety goals,* Oakbrook Terrace, IL, 2021c, The Commission. https://www.jointcommission.org/en/standards/national-patient-safety-goals/. Accessed April 16, 2021.

Touhy TA, Jett F: *Ebersole and Hess' gerontological nursing and healthy aging,* ed 6, St Louis, 2022, Elsevier.

U.S. Department of Health and Human Services (USDHHS): *About the Affordable Care Act,* 2021, https://www.hhs.gov/healthcare/about-the-aca/index.html. Accessed April 17, 2021.

U.S. Department of the Treasury: Final rules under the Paul Wellstone and Pete Domenici Mental Health Parity and Addiction Equity Act (MHPAEA) of 2008; technical amendment to external review for multi-state plan program; final rule, *Federal Register* Document number 2013-27086, 2013. https://www.federalregister.gov/documents/2013/11/13/2013-27086/final-rules-under-the-paul-wellstone-and-pete-domenici-mental-health-parity-and-addiction-equity-act. Accessed April 17, 2021.

Yeung AS, et al: *Capacity assessment and involuntary commitment in psychiatric and medical settings: clinical, legal and cultural considerations,* 2019. https://www.ncbi.nlm.nih.gov/pubmed/31265769. Accessed April 17, 2021.

STATUTES

Americans with Disabilities Act (ADA), 42 USC §§121.010-12213 (1990)

Emergency Medical Treatment and Active Labor Act (EMTALA), 42 USC §1395 (dd) (1986)

Good Samaritan Act, IL Compiled Statutes, 745 ILCS 49/ (1997)

Health Insurance Portability and Accountability Act of 1996 (HIPAA), Public Law No. 104 (1996)

Health Information Technology for Economic and Clinical Health Act (HITECH Act) 45 C.F.R. § 164.304.n8

Health Information Technology for Economic and Clinical Health Act (HITECH Act), Pub. L. No. 111-5, 123 Stat. 115 (Feb. 17, 2009), § 13401(a) (codified at 42 U.S.C. § 17931(a); 45 C.F.R. § 160.103)

Medical Patient Rights Act, IL Compiled Statutes, 410 ILCS 50 (1994)

Mental Health Parity Act of 1996, 29 USC §1885 (1996)

National Conference of Commissioners on Uniform State Laws. (1980). *Amendments to Uniform Brain Death Act, Uniform Determination of Death Act.* Chicago, 1980, Author.

National Organ Transplant Act.: *Public Law* 98, 1984

Omnibus Budget Reconciliation Act of 1986 (Federal Nursing Home Reform Act). Retrieved from https://www.govtrack.us/congress/bills/99/hr5300. Accessed July 30, 2020

Oregon Death With Dignity Act, Ore Rev Stat §§127.800-127.897 (1994)

Patient Protection and Affordable Care Act (PPACA), 42 USC 18001 (2010)

Patient Self-Determination Act, 42 CFR 417 (1991)

Uniform Anatomical Gift Act (2006)

CASES

Bouvia v Superior Court, 225 Cal Rptr 297 (1986)

Cruzan v Director of Missouri Department of Health, 497 U.S. 261 (1990)

Darling v Charleston Community Memorial Hospital, 33 Ill 2d 326 (Ill 1965)

Gibbons v Ogden, 22 U.S. 1, 6 L. Ed. 23, 1824 U.S. LEXUS 370 – Supreme Court, 1824

Jefferson v Mercy Hospital and Medical Center, 2018 IL App (1st) https://cases.justia.com/illinois/court-of-appeals-first-appellate-district/2018-1-16-2219.pdf?ts=1517965779. Accessed April 16, 2021

Roe v Wade, 410 U.S. 113 (1973)

Schindler R, Schindler M, Appellants v: Michael Schiavo, as guardian of the person of Theresa Marie Schiavo, appellee, https://scholar.google.com/scholar_case?case=14050841824849133847&q=Terri+Schiavo&hl=en&as_sdt=4,10,60&as_ylo=2000&as_yhi=2019. Accessed April 17, 2021

Spires v Hospital Corporation of America, 28 U.S.C. §1391(b) Kansas (2006), W. L. 1642701 (2006)

Webster v Reproductive Health Services, 492 U.S. 490 (1989)

Communication

OBJECTIVES

- Identify ways to apply critical thinking and clinical judgment to the communication process.
- Summarize approaches in communication that reflect caring.
- Explain the five levels of communication with patients.
- Summarize features of the circular transactional model of communication.
- Explain features of the verbal communication process.
- Identify key aspects of the nonverbal communication process.
- Identify a nurse's communication approaches within the four phases of a nurse-patient helping relationship.
- Identify desired outcomes of nurse–health care team member relationships.

- Describe patient-centered assessment approaches to use when caring for patients with a variety of needs.
- Engage in effective communication techniques to enhance assessment of older adults.
- Demonstrate therapeutic communication while interacting with patients.
- Identify opportunities to improve communication with patients while giving care.
- Implement nursing care measures for patients with special communication needs.
- Evaluate the effectiveness of your communication with others.

KEY TERMS

Active listening
Assertiveness
Autonomy
Channel
Circular transactional model
Closed-ended question
Communication
Complementary

Empathy
Environment
Feedback
Interpersonal variables
Lateral violence
Message
Motivational interviewing
Open-ended question

Perceptual biases
Receiver
Referent
Sender
Stereotypes
Symmetrical
Therapeutic communication

MEDIA RESOURCES

http://evolve.elsevier.com/Potter/fundamentals/
- Review Questions
- Audio Glossary

- Case Study with Questions
- Content Updates
- Answers to QSEN Activity and Review Questions

COMMUNICATION AND NURSING PRACTICE

Communication is a lifelong learning process. Nurses are often included in their patients' and families' intimate journeys from the miracle of birth to the mystery of death. As a nurse your aim is to communicate with patients and families by developing meaningful and helping relationships. Within those relationships you apply critical thinking and clinical judgment to collect relevant assessment data, analyze the nature of patient's health problems, provide education and counseling, and interact purposefully during nursing interventions. The use of therapeutic communication promotes personal growth and helps patients reach their health-related outcomes. Despite the complexity of technology and the multiple demands on nurses' time, it is the intimate moment of connection between a nurse and a patient that makes all the difference in the quality of care provided. Communication is essential to establish nurse-patient relationships and deliver high-quality patient-centered care.

Patient safety also requires effective communication among all members of the health care team as patients move from one caregiver to another or from one care setting to another. Effective team communication skills promote working relationships that improve patient outcomes, increase patient satisfaction, and reduce the risk of errors (Sethi and Rani, 2017). These same skills are essential to ensure patient safety and optimum patient care (Koosey et al., 2020). Competent communication maintains effective relationships within the entire sphere of professional practice and meets legal, ethical, and clinical standards of care. The qualities and behaviors of therapeutic communication described in this chapter characterize professionalism in caring relationships.

Communication and Interpersonal Relationships

Caring relationships formed by a nurse and those affected by the nurse's practice are at the core of nursing (see Chapter 7). All behavior communicates, and all communication influences behavior. Nurses demonstrate caring by being with, doing for, and promoting patient well-being (Lillykutty and Samson, 2018). The following nursing actions are examples that reflect caring:

- Becoming sensitive and supportive to self and others
- Being present and encouraging the expression of positive and negative feelings
- Developing healing relationships
- Instilling faith and hope
- Promoting interpersonal teaching and learning
- Promoting patient advocacy
- Providing for nursing care needs in a supportive way
- Respecting and allowing for spiritual expression

Being able to relate to others is important for interpersonal communication. This includes the ability to take initiative in establishing and maintaining communication, to be authentic (oneself), and to respond appropriately to others. Effective interpersonal communication also requires a sense of mutuality (i.e., a belief that the nurse-patient relationship is a partnership and that both are equal participants). Nurses recognize and accept that people are very complex and ambiguous. Often more is communicated than first meets the eye, and patient responses are not always what you expect. Each patient is a unique individual, with specific communication needs. Nurses learn to embrace a nonjudgmental, holistic view of people and understand the need for effective, supportive communication and human interaction. When patients and nurses work together, much can be accomplished. Patient- and family-centered communication, such as involving patients in conversations about care, contributes to a culture of safety (Sandström et al., 2019). When these conversations occur at the bedside, providing for privacy is essential.

Therapeutic communication occurs within a healing relationship between a nurse and patient (Arnold and Boggs, 2020). Like any powerful therapeutic agent, a nurse's communication can result in both harm and good. Every nuance of posture, every small expression and gesture, every word chosen, every attitude held—all have the potential to hurt or heal, affecting others through the transmission of human energy. Knowing that intention and behavior directly influence health gives nurses the ethical responsibility to do no harm to those entrusted to their care. Respect the potential power of communication and do not misuse communication carelessly to hurt, manipulate, or coerce others. Skilled communication empowers others to express what they believe and make their own choices; these are essential aspects of the individualized healing process. Nurses have wonderful opportunities to bring about good things for themselves, their patients, and their colleagues through therapeutic communication.

Developing Communication Skills

Gaining expertise in communication requires both an understanding of the communication process and reflection about one's communication experiences as a nurse. Nurses who develop their critical thinking and clinical judgment make the best communicators. They form therapeutic relationships, using their understanding of culture and previous experiences to gather relevant and comprehensive information about their patients. These nurses then draw on theoretical knowledge about communication and integrate this knowledge with knowledge previously learned through personal clinical experience. Nurses interpret messages received from others to obtain new information, correct misinformation, analyze findings to make clinical judgments, and plan patient-centered care that promotes patient understanding (Arnold and Boggs, 2020; Dickison et al., 2019).

Critical thinking attitudes and ethical standards of care, when applied correctly, lead to clinical decisions that promote effective communication. When you consider a patient's problems, it is important to apply critical thinking through the nursing process and make clinical judgments to improve communication in all aspects of patient care (Arnold and Boggs, 2020; Dickison et al., 2019). For example, curiosity motivates a nurse to communicate and learn more about a person. Patients are more likely to communicate with nurses who express an interest in them. The critical thinking attitudes of perseverance and creativity motivate a nurse to assess patients more thoroughly, identify health care needs, and communicate and identify innovative solutions. A self-confident attitude is important because a nurse who conveys confidence and comfort while communicating more readily establishes an interpersonal caring relationship. In addition, an independent attitude and understanding of the environment encourage a nurse to communicate with colleagues and share ideas about nursing interventions. Integrity allows nurses to recognize when their opinions conflict with others (e.g., patients, co-workers), review positions of those involved, and decide how to communicate to reach mutually beneficial decisions. It is also very important for a nurse to communicate responsibly and ask for help if uncertain or uncomfortable about an aspect of patient care. An attitude of humility is necessary to recognize when you need to better communicate and intervene with patients, especially related to their cultural needs (Borden, 2018).

It is challenging to understand human communication within interpersonal relationships. Each individual bases perceptions about information received through the five senses of sight, hearing, taste, touch, and smell (Arnold and Boggs, 2020). An individual's culture, experiences, and education also influence perception. Critical thinking applied during any patient interaction helps to overcome perceptual biases or stereotypes that interfere with accurately perceiving and interpreting messages from others. It is the accurate interpretation of messages that leads to relevant questions to pose, appropriate clarification, and ultimately the right clinical decisions for patients. People often incorrectly assume that they understand an individual's culture. They tend to distort or ignore information that goes against their expectations, preconceptions, or stereotypes (Borden, 2018). Being aware of and thinking critically about personal communication habits will help you learn to control these tendencies and become more effective in developing interpersonal relationships, which will help you make sound clinical judgments.

You become more competent in the nursing process as your communication skills develop. You learn to integrate communication skills throughout the nursing process as you collaborate with patients, family caregivers, and health care team members to achieve outcomes of care (Box 24.1). Use communication skills to gather, analyze, and interpret information and accomplish the work of each step of the process. Although the nursing process is a reliable framework for patient care, it requires effective interpersonal communication and sound clinical judgment (see Chapter 15).

Patients often experience high levels of anxiety when they are ill or receiving treatment. Nurses use self-awareness, motivation, empathy, and social skills to build helping therapeutic relationships with patients (Arnold and Boggs, 2020). Patients' emotions can negatively influence their self-care behaviors. When you understand a patient's perceptions and motivations, you can help the patient make healthy behavior changes.

The nature of the communication process requires you to constantly decide what, when, where, why, and how to convey a message. A nurse's clinical decision making is always contextual (i.e., the unique

---

BOX 24.1   Communication Throughout the Nursing Process

Assessment
- Verbal interviewing and history taking
- Visual and intuitive observation of nonverbal behavior
- Visual, tactile, and auditory data gathering during physical examination
- Written medical records, diagnostic tests, and literature review

Analysis and Nursing Diagnosis
- Analysis and interpretation of assessment findings
- Identification and validation of health care needs and priorities via verbal discussion with patient
- Documentation of nursing diagnosis

Planning and Outcomes Identification
- Interpersonal or small-group health care team planning sessions
- Interpersonal collaboration with patient and family to determine expected outcomes and implementation methods
- Written documentation of expected outcomes
- Written or verbal referral to health care team members

Implementation
- Delegation, discussion, and collaboration with interprofessional health care team
- Verbal, visual, auditory, and tactile health teaching activities
- Provision of support via therapeutic communication techniques
- Written documentation of patient's response to nursing interventions in medical record

Evaluation
- Acquisition of verbal and nonverbal feedback
- Comparison of actual and expected outcomes
- Identification of factors affecting outcomes
- Modification and update of care plan
- Verbal and/or written explanation of care plan revisions to patient

---

BOX 24.2   Challenging Communication Situations

- People who speak and/or understand little English
- People who are silent or withdrawn and have difficulty expressing feelings or needs
- People who are sad and depressed
- People who require assistance with visual or speech disabilities (special needs)
- People who are angry or confrontational and cannot listen to explanations
- People who are uncooperative and resent being asked to help others
- People who are talkative or lonely and want someone to be with them all the time
- People who are demanding and expect others to meet their requests
- People who are frightened, anxious, and having difficulty coping
- People who have cognitive disorders such as dementia or are confused and disoriented
- People who are flirtatious or sexually inappropriate

Levels of Communication

Nurses use different levels of communication in their professional role. A competent nurse uses a variety of techniques in each level.

Intrapersonal communication is a powerful form of communication that you use as a professional nurse. This level of communication is also called *self-talk*. People's thoughts and inner communications strongly influence perceptions, feelings, behavior, and self-esteem. Always be aware of the nature and content of your own thinking. Positive self-talk provides a mental rehearsal for difficult tasks or situations so that you can deal with them more effectively and with increased confidence (Arnold and Boggs, 2020). You use intrapersonal communication to develop self-awareness and a positive self-esteem to enhance appropriate self-expression. Positive self-talk can diminish cognitive distortions that lead to a decrease in self-esteem and affect your ability to work with patients. Transforming statements from "I'm scared to work with this type of patient" into "This is my opportunity to learn about this patient, and I can ask for help when it's needed" is an example of positive self-talk.

Interpersonal communication is one-on-one interaction between a nurse and another person that occurs face to face or via text or other electronic format. It is the level most frequently used in nursing situations and lies at the heart of nursing practice. It takes place within a social context and includes all the symbols and cues used to give and receive meaning. Because meaning resides in people and not in words, messages received are sometimes different from intended messages. Nurses work with people who have different opinions, experiences, values, and belief systems than their own. Therefore it is important to validate meaning or mutually negotiate it between participants. For example, when you use the teach-back method, you interact with a patient by asking questions to assess your patient's understanding and clarify misinterpretations when providing information about a health concern (see Chapter 25). This method verifies how well you explained the information to your patient; it does not test your patient's knowledge (Agency for Healthcare Research and Quality [AHRQ], 2020). Meaningful interpersonal communication results in an exchange and clarification of ideas, problem solving, expression of feelings, decision making, achieving outcomes, team building, and personal growth.

Small-group communication is the interaction that occurs when a small number of people meet. This type of communication is usually outcome oriented and requires an understanding of group dynamics. When nurses work on committees with nurses or participants from

---

features of any situation influence the nature of the decisions made). For example, the explanation of the importance of following a prescribed diet to a patient with a newly diagnosed medical condition differs from the explanation to a patient who has repeatedly chosen not to follow diet restrictions. Effective communication techniques are easy to learn, but their application is difficult. Deciding which techniques best fit each unique nursing situation is challenging because it requires critical thinking in deciding among techniques that are appropriate versus inappropriate. Communicating with patients and families about illness such as cancer or advance care planning can be stressful. Nurses may experience grief and fatigue related to emotional exhaustion when discussing these topics, especially when they have developed a bond with patients or families (Sullivan et al., 2019). However, discussing these important and sensitive topics can increase the quality of life for patients and family members.

Throughout this chapter, brief clinical examples will guide you in learning how to use effective communication techniques. Situations that challenge your clinical decision-making skills (Box 24.2) and call for careful use of therapeutic techniques involve a variety of human behaviors. Because the best way to acquire and develop effective communication skills is through practice, it is useful for you to discuss and role-play these scenarios before experiencing them in the clinical setting. Effective communication and collaboration are imperative for success.

other disciplines and participate in patient care conferences, they use a small-group communication process. Communication in these situations should be organized, concise, and complete. All participating disciplines are encouraged to contribute and provide feedback. Good communication skills help each participant better meet a patient's needs and promote a safer care environment.

Public communication is interaction with an audience. Nurses often provide information to groups about health-related topics, present scholarly work to colleagues at conferences, or lead classroom discussions with peers or students. Public communication requires special adaptations in eye contact, gestures, voice inflection, and the use of media materials to communicate messages effectively. Effective public communication increases audience knowledge about health-related topics, health issues, and other issues important to the nursing profession.

Electronic communication is the use of technology to create ongoing relationships with patients and their health care team. Secure messaging provides an opportunity for frequent and timely communication with a patient's physician or nurse via a patient portal. An electronic portal enables patients to stay engaged and informed, though the empathetic nature of the therapeutic relationship with the health care team may be more challenging (Brandt et al., 2018). It is important to follow professional communication guidelines when communicating electronically with patients. For example, avoid using text written in all capital letters, use language your patient will understand, and be sure to sign your messages with your professional credentials (Crossley et al., 2020; Manfrida et al., 2017).

ELEMENTS OF THE COMMUNICATION PROCESS

Communication is an ongoing and continuously changing process as you interact with someone. You are changing, the people with whom you are communicating are changing, and your environment is also continually changing. Nursing situations have many unique aspects that influence the nature of communication and interpersonal relationships such as the urgency of a patient's condition, the time available for interaction, and the patient's own unique perception of that situation. As a professional you will use critical thinking to focus on each aspect of communication so that your interactions are purposeful and effective.

Circular Transactional Model

The circular transactional model includes several elements: the referent, sender and receiver, message, channels, context or environment in which the communication process occurs, feedback, and interpersonal variables (Fig. 24.1). In this model each person in the communication interaction is both a speaker and a listener and can be simultaneously sending and receiving messages. Both parties view the perceptions, attitudes, and potential reactions to a sent message. Communication is continuous and interactive. Feedback from the receiver or environment enables the communicators to correct or validate the communication. This model also describes the role relationship of the communicators as complementary and symmetrical. Complementary role relationships function with one person holding an elevated position over the other person. Symmetrical relationships are more equal. A complementary role occurs when a nurse provides education to a patient about a new medication or therapy. A group of patients discussing their plans after discharge is an example of a symmetrical role relationship (Arnold and Boggs, 2020).

Referent.
The referent motivates one person to communicate with another. In a health care setting, sights, sounds, sensations, perceptions, and ideas are examples of cues that initiate the communication process. Knowing a stimulus or referent that initiates communication

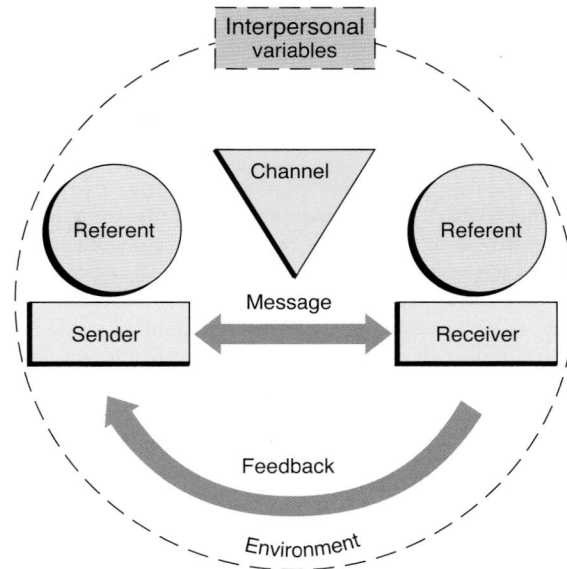

FIG. 24.1 Circular transactional model of communication.

allows you to develop and organize messages more efficiently. For example, a patient's request for help prompted by difficulty in breathing causes a different response than does a patient's request for pain medication.

Sender and Receiver. The sender is the person who encodes and delivers a message, and the receiver is the person who receives and decodes the message. The sender puts the message into verbal and nonverbal symbols that the receiver can understand (Arnold and Boggs, 2020). The sender's message acts as a referent for the receiver. Transactional communication involves the role of sender and receiver switching back and forth between nurse and patient. A decoding process includes the receiver interpreting the meaning of the word symbols. Active listening is important to accurately decode and understand a message. The more the sender and receiver have in common and the closer the relationship, the more likely it is that they will accurately perceive one another's meaning and respond accordingly (Arnold and Boggs, 2020). Establishing rapport with a patient ensures more effective communication, which ultimately improves your clinical judgment and decision making.

Message. The message is the content of the communication. It contains verbal and nonverbal expressions of thoughts and feelings. Effective messages are clear, direct, timely, and in understandable language. Individuals with cognitive disorders (e.g., confusion, dementia) or communication barriers may need assistance (e.g., hearing aids, interpreters, or pictures) to clarify information to understand messages sent and received. Personal perceptions may also distort the receiver's interpretation of a message. As a nurse you send effective messages by expressing clearly, directly, calmly, and in a manner familiar to a patient. You determine the need for clarification by watching a listening patient for nonverbal cues that suggest confusion or misunderstanding. Communication is difficult when participants have different levels of education and health care literacy and experience. For example, statements such as "Your incision is healing well without purulent drainage" means the same as "Your wound edges are close together, and because I see no drainage there is no sign of infection," but the latter is easier to understand. You can also send messages in writing. Regardless of how you communicate, make sure your patients are able to understand the meaning of your communication.

Channels. Individuals use communication channels to send and receive messages through visual, auditory, and tactile senses. Facial expressions send visual messages; spoken words travel through auditory channels. Touch uses tactile channels. Individuals usually understand a message more clearly when the sender uses more channels to send it.

Feedback. Feedback is the message a sender receives from the receiver. It indicates the extent to which the receiver understood the meaning of the sender's message. Feedback occurs continuously between a sender and receiver. A sender seeks verbal and nonverbal feedback to evaluate the receiver's response and effectiveness of a communicated message. The type of feedback a sender or receiver gives depends on factors such as background, prior experiences, education, attitudes, cultural beliefs, and self-esteem. A sender and receiver need to be sensitive and open to each other's messages, to clarify the messages, and to modify behavior accordingly for successful communication.

Interpersonal Variables. Interpersonal variables are factors within both the sender and receiver that influence communication. Perception provides a uniquely personal view of reality formed by an individual's culture, expectations, and experiences. Each person senses, interprets, and understands a communicated message differently. A nurse says, "You haven't been talking very much since your family left. Is there something on your mind?" One patient may perceive the nurse's question as caring and concerned; another perceives the nurse as invading privacy and is less willing to talk. Cultural humility enables you to recognize that you do not completely understand your patient's culture and allows you to explore the interpersonal variables such as educational and developmental level, sociocultural background, values and beliefs, emotions, gender, physical health status, and roles and relationships that affect how a patient communicates. Interpersonal variables associated with a patient's illness, such as pain, anxiety, and medication effects, also affect nurse-patient communication.

Environment. The environment is the setting for sender-receiver interaction. An effective communication setting provides participants with physical and emotional comfort and safety. Noise, temperature extremes, distractions, and lack of privacy or space create confusion, tension, and discomfort. Environmental distractions are common in health care settings and interfere with messages sent between people. You control the environment as much as possible to create favorable conditions for effective communication.

FORMS OF COMMUNICATION

Messages are conveyed verbally and nonverbally, concretely and symbolically. As people communicate, they express themselves through words, movements, voice inflection, facial expressions, and use of space. These elements work in harmony to enhance a message, or conflict with one another to contradict and confuse it.

Verbal Communication

Verbal communication uses spoken or written words. Verbal language is a code that conveys specific meaning through a combination of words. The most important aspects of verbal communication are presented in the following paragraphs.

Vocabulary. Communication is unsuccessful if senders and receivers cannot translate one another's words and phrases. When you care for a patient who speaks another language, a professional interpreter is necessary. Even those who speak the same language use subcultural variations of certain words (e.g., *dinner* means a noon meal to one person and the last meal of the day to another). Medical jargon (technical terminology used by health care providers) sounds like a foreign language to patients unfamiliar with the health care setting. Limiting use of medical jargon to conversations with other health care team members improves communication. Children have a more limited vocabulary than adults and often use special words to describe bodily functions or a favorite blanket or toy. Teenagers often use words in unique ways that are unfamiliar to adults.

Denotative and Connotative Meaning. Some words have several meanings. Individuals who use a common language share the denotative meaning: *baseball* has the same meaning for everyone who speaks English, but *code* denotes cardiac arrest primarily to health care providers. The connotative meaning is the shade or interpretation of the meaning of a word influenced by the thoughts, feelings, or ideas that people have about the word. For example, health care providers tell a family that a loved one is in serious condition, and the family believes that death is near; but to nurses *serious* simply describes the nature of the illness. You need to select words carefully, avoiding easily misinterpreted words, especially when explaining a patient's medical condition or therapy, and obtain feedback as to what the patient or family understood. Even a much-used phrase such as "I'm going to take your vital signs" may be unfamiliar to an adult or frightening to a child. "I'm going to check your blood pressure, heart rate, and temperature" may be more appropriate.

Pacing. Conversation is more successful at an appropriate speed or pace. Speak moderately slowly and enunciate clearly. Talking rapidly, using awkward pauses, or speaking excessively slowly and deliberately conveys an unintended message. Long pauses and rapid shifts to another subject give the impression that you are hiding the truth. Think before speaking, and develop an awareness of the rhythm of your speech to improve pacing.

Intonation. Tone of voice dramatically affects the meaning of a message. Depending on intonation, even a simple question or statement expresses enthusiasm, anger, concern, or indifference. Be aware of voice tone to avoid sending unintended messages. For example, communication is inhibited if a patient interprets your patronizing tone of voice as condescending. Similarly, a working colleague may sense your mistrust from a patronizing response. A patient's tone of voice provides information about emotional state or energy level.

Clarity and Brevity. Effective communication is simple, brief, and direct. For certain populations such as the elderly, fewer words result in less confusion. Speak slowly, enunciate clearly, and use brief examples to make explanations easier to understand. Repeating important parts of a message also clarifies communication. Phrases such as "right" or "Okay?" at the end of every sentence does not achieve clarity. Use sentences and words that express an idea simply and directly. For example, "Where is your pain?" is much better than "I would like you to describe for me the location of your discomfort."

Timing and Relevance. Timing is critical in communication. Even though a message is clear, poor timing prevents it from being effective. For example, you do not begin routine teaching when a patient is in severe pain or emotional distress. Often the best time for interaction is when a patient expresses an interest in communicating. If messages are relevant or important to the situation at hand, they are more effective. When a patient is facing emergency surgery, discussing the risks of smoking is less relevant than explaining presurgical procedures or clarifying the patient's fears. Face-to-face time while performing assessments, administering medications, or performing procedures offers an excellent opportunity to talk with patients and provide support or education. Patients report improved satisfaction, understanding, and perception of safety when nurses and the interprofessional health care team participate in bedside rounding and communicate information about the plan of care (Real et al., 2020).

Nonverbal Communication

Nonverbal communication includes the five senses and everything that does not involve the spoken or written word. Nonverbal aspects of communication such as voice tone, eye contact, and body positioning are often as important as verbal messages (Lorié, 2017). Nonverbal communication is unconsciously motivated and more accurately indicates a person's intended meaning than spoken words (Varcarolis and Fosbre, 2021). When there is incongruity between verbal and nonverbal communication, the receiver usually "hears" the nonverbal message more so than the true message.

All nonverbal communication is important, but interpreting it is often problematic. Sociocultural background is a major influence on the meaning of nonverbal behavior. In the United States, with its diverse cultural communities, nonverbal messages between people of different cultures are easily misinterpreted. Assessing and responding to nonverbal messages appropriately are important for accurate assessment and evaluation of nursing care.

Personal Appearance. Personal appearance includes physical characteristics, facial expression, and manner of dress and grooming. These factors are a powerful means of nonverbal communication. In the health care setting, research shows that patients prefer that nurses employed in an agency all wear a single uniform and that the "RN" or "LPN" tag be displayed prominently (Pawlowski et al., 2019). Many health care agencies restrict how much jewelry you can wear and whether certain types of tattoos need to be covered. For hygienic reasons nurses should have long hair pulled back and off the shoulders and short clean fingernails. Remember, first impressions are largely based on appearance. Nurses learn to develop a general impression of patient health and emotional status through appearance, and patients develop a general impression of the nurse's professionalism and caring in the same way.

Posture and Gait. Posture and gait (manner or pattern of walking) can be forms of self-expression. The way people sit, stand, and move reflects attitudes, emotions, self-concept, and health status. For example, an erect posture and a quick, purposeful gait communicate a sense of well-being and confidence. Leaning forward conveys attention. A slumped posture and slow, shuffling gait indicate depression, illness, or fatigue.

Facial Expression. The face is the most expressive part of the body. Facial expressions convey emotions such as surprise, fear, anger, happiness, and sadness. Some people have an expressionless face, or flat affect, which reveals little about what they are thinking or feeling. An inappropriate affect is a facial expression that does not match the content of a verbal message (e.g., smiling when describing a sad situation). People are sometimes unaware of the messages their expressions convey. For example, a nurse frowns in concentration while doing a procedure, and the patient interprets this as anger or disapproval. Patients closely observe nurses. Consider the impact your facial expression could have on a person who asks, "Am I going to die?" The slightest change in the eyes, lips, or facial muscles reveals your feelings. Although it is hard to control all facial expressions, try to avoid showing shock, disgust, dismay, or other distressing reactions in a patient's presence.

Eye Contact. Eye contact is a fundamental aspect of nonverbal communication and social interaction (Jongerius et al., 2020). People signal readiness to communicate through eye contact. Maintaining eye contact during conversation shows respect, engagement, and willingness to listen. Eye contact also allows people to closely observe one another. People's experience of eye contact can be influenced by many factors, such as the presence of a third person, the distance from the other person's face, or the perceiver's visual acuity (Jongerius et al., 2020). Lack of eye contact sometimes indicates anxiety, defensiveness, discomfort, or lack of confidence in communicating. However, people from some cultures consider eye contact intrusive, threatening, or harmful and minimize or avoid its use (see Chapter 9). Always consider a person's culture and personal preferences when interpreting the meaning of eye contact. Eye movements communicate feelings and emotions. Looking down on a person establishes authority, whereas interacting at the same eye level indicates equality in the relationship. Maintaining the same eye level as an angry person helps establish autonomy over the situation or concern.

Gestures. Gestures emphasize, punctuate, and clarify the spoken word. Gestures alone carry specific meanings, or they create messages with other communication cues. A finger pointed toward a person communicates several meanings, but when accompanied by a frown and stern voice, the gesture becomes an accusation or a threat. Pointing to an area of pain is sometimes more accurate than describing its location.

Sounds. Sounds such as sighs, moans, groans, or sobs also communicate feelings and thoughts. Combined with other nonverbal communication, sounds help clarify messages. They have several interpretations. For example, moaning can convey pleasure or suffering, and crying can communicate happiness, sadness, or anger. Validate nonverbal messages with patients to interpret them accurately. For example, "I notice you frowning as you move. Are you having pain?"

Territoriality and Personal Space. Territoriality is the need to gain, maintain, and defend one's right to space. Territory is important because it provides people with a sense of privacy, identity, security, and control. It is sometimes separated and made visible to others, as with a fence around a yard or a curtain around a bed in a hospital room. Personal space is invisible and individual and travels with a person. During interpersonal interaction people maintain varying distances between one another, depending on their culture, the nature of their relationship, and the situation. When personal space becomes threatened, people respond defensively and communicate less effectively. Situations dictate whether the interpersonal distance between nurse and patient is appropriate. Box 24.3 provides examples of nursing actions within communication zones (Varcarolis and Fosbre, 2021). Nurses frequently move into patients' territory and personal space because of the nature of caregiving. You need to convey confidence, gentleness, and respect for privacy, especially when your actions require intimate contact or involve a patient's vulnerable zone.

Metacommunication. *Metacommunication* is a broad term that refers to all factors that influence communication. Awareness of influencing factors helps people better understand what is communicated (Arnold and Boggs, 2020). For example, a nurse observes a young patient holding his body rigidly, and his voice is sharp as he says, "Going to surgery is no big deal." The nurse replies, "You say having surgery doesn't bother you, but you look and sound tense. I'd like to hear more about how you're feeling." Awareness of the tone of the verbal response and the nonverbal behavior results in further exploration of the patient's feelings and concerns.

BOX 24.3 Zones of Personal Space

Zones of Personal Space
Intimate Distance (0–18 Inches)
- Holding a crying infant
- Performing physical assessment
- Bathing, grooming, dressing, feeding, and toileting a patient
- Changing a patient's surgical dressing

Personal Distance (18–40 Inches)
- Sitting at a patient's bedside
- Taking a patient's nursing history
- Teaching an individual patient

Social Distance (4–12 Feet)
- Giving directions to visitors in the hallway
- Asking whether families need assistance from the patient doorway
- Giving verbal report to a group of nurses

Public Distance (12 Feet and More)
- Speaking at a community forum
- Lecturing to a class of students
- Testifying at a legislative hearing

Special Zones of Touch
Social Zone (Permission Not Needed)
- Hands, arms, shoulders, back

Consent Zone (Permission Needed)
- Mouth, wrists, feet

Vulnerable Zone (Special Care Needed)
- Face, neck, front of body

Intimate Zone (Permission and Great Sensitivity Needed)
- Genitalia, rectum

BOX 24.4 Phases of the Helping Relationship

Preinteraction Phase
Before meeting a patient:
- Review available data, including the medical and nursing history (e.g., ability of patient to communicate, pathology of any speech mechanisms, medications affecting mood, reports of previous behavior problems).
- Talk to other caregivers who have information about the patient.
- Anticipate health concerns or issues that arise.
- Identify a location and setting that fosters comfortable, private interaction.
- Plan enough time for the initial interaction.

Orientation Phase
When you and a patient meet and get to know each other:
- Set the tone for the relationship by adopting a warm, empathetic, caring manner. Sit down next to the patient if possible.
- Recognize that the initial relationship is often superficial, uncertain, and tentative.
- Expect the patient to test your competence and commitment.
- Let the patient know when to expect the relationship to be terminated.
- Closely observe the patient and expect to be closely observed by the patient.
- Begin to make inferences and form judgments about patient messages and behaviors.
- Assess the patient's health status.
- Prioritize the patient's problems and identify expected outcomes.
- Clarify the patient's and your roles.
- Form contracts with the patient that specify who will do what.

Working Phase
When you and a patient work together to solve problems and accomplish outcomes:
- Encourage and help the patient express feelings about health.
- Encourage and help the patient with self-exploration.
- Provide information needed to understand and change behavior.
- Collaborate with the patient to set individualized outcomes.
- Take action to meet the outcomes set with the patient.
- Use therapeutic communication skills to facilitate successful interactions.
- Use appropriate self-disclosure and confrontation.

Termination Phase
During the ending of the relationship:
- Remind the patient that termination is near.
- Evaluate achievement of expected outcomes with the patient.
- Reminisce about the relationship with the patient.
- Separate from the patient by relinquishing responsibility for care.
- Achieve a smooth transition for the patient to other caregivers as needed.

PROFESSIONAL NURSING RELATIONSHIPS

Your application of knowledge, understanding of human behavior and communication, and commitment to ethical behavior create professional relationships. Having a philosophy based on caring and respect for others helps you be more successful in establishing relationships of this nature.

Nurse-Patient Caring Relationships

Caring therapeutic relationships are the foundation of clinical nursing practice. In such relationships you assume the role of a professional who cares about each patient and the patient's unique health needs, human responses, and patterns of living. Therapeutic relationships promote a psychological climate for positive change and growth, such as your patients' ability to attain health-related outcomes (Arnold and Boggs, 2020). The outcomes of a therapeutic relationship focus on a patient achieving optimal personal growth related to personal identity, ability to form relationships, and ability to satisfy needs and achieve personal goals (Varcarolis and Fosbre, 2021). There is an explicit time frame, a goal-directed approach, and a high expectation that what you discuss together is kept confidential among only members of the health care team involved in a patient's care. You establish, direct, and take responsibility for the interaction, and a patient's needs take priority over your needs. Your nonjudgmental acceptance of a patient is an important characteristic of the relationship. Acceptance conveys a willingness to hear a message or acknowledge feelings. It does not mean that you always agree with the other person or approve of the patient's decisions or actions. A caring relationship between you and a patient does not just happen; you create it with skill and trust.

There is a natural progression of four goal-directed phases that characterize the nurse-patient relationship (Box 24.4). The relationship often begins before you meet a patient and continues until the caregiving relationship ends. Even a brief interaction uses an abbreviated version of preinteraction, orientation, working, and termination (Varcarolis and Fosbre, 2021). For example, a nursing student gathers patient information to prepare in advance for caregiving, meets the patient and establishes trust, accomplishes health-related outcomes through use of the nursing process, and says goodbye at the end of the day.

Socializing is an important initial component of interpersonal communication. It helps people get to know one another and relax. It is easy, superficial, and not deeply personal, whereas therapeutic interactions are often more intense, difficult, and uncomfortable. A nurse often uses social conversation to lay a foundation for a closer relationship: "Hi, Mr. Simpson, I hear it's your birthday today. May I ask how old you are?" A friendly, informal, and warm communication style establishes trust, but you need to move beyond social conversation to talk about issues or concerns affecting the patient's health. During social conversation, some patients ask personal questions such as those about your family or place of residence. Students often wonder whether it is appropriate to reveal such information. The skillful nurse uses judgment about what to share and provides minimal information or deflects such questions with gentle humor and refocuses conversation back to the patient.

In a therapeutic relationship, it may be helpful to encourage patients to share personal stories. Sharing stories is called *narrative interaction*. Through listening to stories, you begin to understand the context of others' lives and learn what is meaningful for them from their perspective. For example, a nurse listens to a patient's perception of what it means to refuse medication treatment for breast cancer and is then better able to articulate the patient's wishes. Taking adequate time to listen to patients' stories positively affects the patient care experience (Sethi and Rani, 2017). This information is not usually revealed with a standard history form that elicits short answers.

As a nurse, you can also tell stories to enhance communication. Telling good stories frames important messages you wish to send and makes messages memorable for your patients. Purposeful storytelling brings across factual information along with a human-interest perspective that draws on an individual's emotions, such as a patient's desire to get well or feel a sense of hope. Be mindful not to divulge confidential information while using a story to illustrate a point. Emotions play a significant role in helping adults learn the ability to grasp new ideas.

Motivational Interviewing

Motivational interviewing (MI) is a technique that encourages patients to share their thoughts, goals, beliefs, fears, and concerns with the aim of changing their behavior. MI provides a way of working with patients who may not seem ready to make behavioral changes that are considered necessary by their health practitioners. You can use it to evoke change talk, which links to improved patient outcomes (Brown et al., 2018; Magil et al., 2019). For example, an interviewer uses information about a patient's personal goals with respect to maintaining health to promote the patient's adherence to a new medication or an exercise plan, or adopt an alcohol moderation program. It is important to incorporate what the patient wants or perceives is important to be successful in achieving change. The interviewing is delivered in a nonjudgmental, guided communication approach. When using MI, a nurse tries to understand a patient's motivations and values using an empathic and active listening approach. The nurse identifies differences between a patient's current health goals and behaviors and current health status. The patient is supported even though a phase of resistance and ambivalence often occurs. Communication then focuses on recognizing the patient's strengths and supporting those strengths to make positive changes. This can result in dramatic improvements in health outcomes and patient satisfaction (Newman-Casey et al., 2020).

Nurse-Family Relationships

Many nursing situations, especially those in community and home care settings, require you to form caring relationships with entire families. The same principles that guide one-on-one helping relationships also apply when the patient is a family unit, although communication within families requires additional understanding of the complexities of family dynamics, needs, and relationships (see Chapter 10).

Nurse–Health Care Team Relationships

Effective communication with other members of the health care team affects patient outcomes, patient safety, and the work environment (Hannawa, 2018). Problems occur when communication is inconsistent, inaccurate, not timely, and incomplete. Patients moving from one nursing unit to another or from one provider to another are situations in which miscommunication can easily occur. To address this risk, health care providers provide detailed hand-off reports at the end of shifts or when patients transfer from one unit to another or from acute care to long-term care settings to ensure a safe and smooth transition in care (Gettis et al., 2019; Streelman and Staffileno, 2021). Standardized discharge or transfer procedures and forms help reduce the risk of errors during patient transitions. Timely follow-up after discharge or transfer is also appropriate.

The acronym *SACCIA* is one way to assist nurses in communicating effectively with other team members. The acronym stands for *Sufficiency, Accuracy, Clarity, Contextualization, and Interpersonal Adaptation.* For example, consider a situation in which a charge nurse is preparing for a change of shift on an inpatient rehabilitation unit. She is preparing to report to a nurse who is a new graduate but has been working on the unit for 4 weeks. The charge nurse is reporting about the condition and care plan for a 72-year-old man who experienced a stroke 1 week ago that left him with right-sided weakness and a slight aphasia. The charge nurse's report must have the following:

- Sufficiency—enough detail to explain the patient's current condition, what occurred during the past shift, and plans for the next shift.
- Accuracy—a review of the patient's physical progress and ability to communicate with the presence of aphasia. Any behaviors pertinent to the patient's motivation for rehabilitation should be objectively described, as well as any factors related to the patient's age that impact care.
- Clarity—the report should be concise with the essential information needed to continue the patient's care without risk of errors or duplicating care activities.
- Contextualization and Interpersonal Adaptation—The charge nurse uses the typical bedside shift approach to communicate to the new nurse, adjusts explanations to the experience level of the nurse, and encourages the nurse to ask any questions for clarification.

Use of a common language such as the SBAR technique for communicating critical information is another method for improving the perception of communication and information about patients among health care providers (Institute for Healthcare Improvement [IHI], 2021; Stewart, 2017). This technique is a popular communication tool that standardizes communication between health care providers. SBAR is the acronym for *Situation, Background, Assessment, and Recommendation* (IHI, 2021). Some organizations have added an *Identify* step (ISBAR) into the SBAR process. The Identify step is used when health care providers do not actively know one another. They start with an introduction, a description of their location, and their role in caring for the patient (IHI, 2021). The use of these easy-to-remember, orderly techniques relays relevant information in a structured and timely manner. Evidence identifies nursing actions that increase the effectiveness of nurse-to-nurse interaction and interprofessional communication (Box 24.5).

BOX 24.5   EVIDENCE-BASED PRACTICE

Standardized Bedside Nursing Hand-Off Reporting

PICOT Question: In the hospital setting, what are the outcomes of the practice of standardized bedside hand-off reporting during transitions in patient care compared with unstandardized hand-off reporting?

Evidence Summary

Many of the adverse events that occur during hospitalization may have been prevented with a complete and effective hand-off report conducted by nurses and other health care professionals with effective training (Simonovic et al., 2019; Sun et al., 2020; Tortosa-Alted et al., 2021). Nurse-to-nurse bedside hand off reporting is used as a tool to improve patient safety and continuity of care to promote positive patient outcomes (Kim et al., 2021). A recent integrative review of studies evaluating the effectiveness of bedside hand-off reporting showed that bedside nursing hand-off reporting reduced the incidence of patient falls, pressure injuries, and medication errors in addition to improving communication (Hada and Coyer, 2021). Bedside reporting is most effective when guidelines, standards, and expectations of the hand-off report are established and followed by all hospital staff (Kim et al., 2021; Tortosa-Alted et al., 2021). The quality of bedside hand-off reporting is often influenced by the nurse's level of education, duration of hospital employment, and acceptance of the hand-off reporting procedure, as well as the setting in which the reporting occurs (Kim et al., 2021; Tortosa-Alted et al., 2021).

Application to Nursing Practice

- Nurses who do not completely and accurately communicate during nurse-to-nurse handovers create miscommunication that can lead to patient care errors (Kim et al., 2021).
- Using bedside nurse-to-nurse shift reporting helps provide continuity of care (Kim et al., 2021).
- To use bedside hand-off reporting effectively, nurses and other hospital staff need to receive education and training on a standardized approach to this intervention (Kim et al., 2021; Tortosa-Alted et al., 2021).
- Ensure that hand-off reporting occurs at the patient's bedside and that the environment is conducive to the process. For example, ensure that the environment is calm, quiet, respectful, ensures patient privacy, and provides an opportunity for patients and family caregivers to participate during the report (Tortosa-Alted et al., 2021; Simonovic et al., 2019).

QSEN   Building Competency in Patient-Centered Care You are assigned to work with Mr. Rodriguez, a patient with a recent fracture of the femur, who is having surgery later today. Mr. Rodriguez fractured his femur on the job as a landscaper. He is a legal immigrant whose family is from Mexico. Mr. Rodriguez speaks English but has limited literacy. The registered nurse (RN) providing a hand-off report to you gives the relevant objective data about the patient. As an aside, the RN complains about how demanding and difficult the patient has been and how she does not believe people like him belong here, and she berates his insistence on the inclusion of a family member in all conversations. You recognize that providing patient-centered care, including integration of many dimensions of care, as well as respect for diverse cultural, ethnic, and social backgrounds, may contribute to positive patient care outcomes. What possible values, preferences, and needs may the patient be experiencing? Describe communication strategies and approaches that you would use with this patient to facilitate effective patient-centered care. How should every nurse recognize and address personally held beliefs and attitudes about patients from diverse backgrounds?

Answers to QSEN Activities can be found on the Evolve website.

Lateral Violence. Professional nursing care requires nurses to interact with members of the nursing team and interprofessional health care providers. Communication focuses on team building, facilitating group processes, collaborating, consulting, delegating, supervising, leading, and managing (see Chapter 21). Social, informational, and therapeutic interactions help team members build morale, accomplish goals, and strengthen working relationships. Lateral violence or workplace bullying between colleagues sometimes occurs and includes behaviors such as withholding information, being hypercritical, raising blame or making put-downs, criticizing without solutions, excluding, and using nonverbal expressions of disapproval such as raising eyebrows or making faces. Lateral violence adversely affects the work environment, leading to job dissatisfaction, a decreased sense of value, poor teamwork, poor retention of qualified nurses, and nurses leaving the profession (Bambi et al., 2019). Lateral violence can be a precursor to compassion fatigue when health care workers perceive a threat during interactions with colleagues and react emotionally rather than communicating intentionally in a professional manner.

Lateral violence interferes with effective health care team communication, jeopardizes patient safety, and interferes with attainment of desired patient outcomes (Bambi et al., 2019). Intimidation decreases the likelihood that a nurse will report a near-miss event, question an order, or act to improve the quality of patient care. There must be zero tolerance of lateral violence. Develop skills in conflict management and assertive communication to stop the spread of lateral violence in the workplace. Mentors can help new nurses learn skills to address the perpetrators of bullying. Mentors can also be a personal support for nurses and serve as a role model for the department. The nurse experiencing lateral violence can also use additional techniques such as the following:

- When the behavior occurs, address it in a calm manner.
- Describe how the behavior affects your functioning.
- Ask for the abuse to stop.
- Notify the manager to get support for the situation.
- Avoid gossiping about the situation or the person with other staff.
- Plan for taking action in the future.
- Document the incidents in detail in your personal notes, not patient records.

Nurse-Community Relationships

Many nurses form relationships with community groups by participating in local organizations, volunteering for community service, or becoming politically active. As a nurse, learn to establish relationships with your community to be an effective change agent. Providing clear and accurate information to members of the public is the best way to prevent errors, reduce resistance, and promote change. Communication within the community occurs through channels such as neighborhood newsletters, health fairs, public bulletin boards, newspapers, radio, television, and electronic information sites. Use these forms of communication to share information and discuss issues important to community health (see Chapter 3).

ELEMENTS OF PROFESSIONAL COMMUNICATION

Professional appearance, demeanor, and behavior are important in establishing trustworthiness and competence. A professional is expected to be clean, neat, well groomed, conservatively dressed, and odor free. Visible tattoos and piercings may not be considered acceptable in some professional settings. Professional behavior reflects warmth, friendliness, confidence, and competence. Professionals speak in a clear, well-modulated voice; use good grammar; listen to others; help and support colleagues; and communicate effectively. Being on time, organized, well prepared, and equipped for the responsibilities of the nursing role also communicate professionalism.

AIDET® is a technique developed by the Studer Group (2021) to enable health care workers to provide accurate and timely professional communication to patients and families while focusing on excellent patient service. It is a technique commonly used in hospitals today. The acronym stands for *A*cknowledge, *I*ntroduce, *D*uration, *E*xplain, and *T*hank you. When using AIDET, you first acknowledge the person standing in front of you with a positive attitude and make the person feel comfortable. Introduce yourself and let the person know what your role is in the department and in the person's care. It is important to always wear a name badge when working in a health care setting. When possible, give a patient or family an idea of how long a procedure may take. This keeps the patient informed of any delays that may occur. It is also helpful to let a patient know how long it will take to get results if they are related to testing. When explaining procedures, describe what the patient will experience with the treatment, procedure, or test. Inform the patient of any safety precautions. When using AIDET, thank patients for coming to your organization for care and let them know how much you enjoyed working with them (Studer Group, 2021).

Courtesy

Common courtesy is part of professional communication. Often a nurse is the first health care professional a patient or family meets, and it is important to present a courteous, competent, and professional impression. To practice courtesy, knock on the door before entering a patient's hospital or examination room and say hello and goodbye to patients. State your purpose, address people by name, and say "please" and "thank you" to team members as well as patients and families. Introduce yourself and state your title. When a nurse is discourteous or unprofessional, others perceive that nurse as rude or insensitive. It sets up barriers to forming helping relationships between nurse and patient and causes friction among team members.

Use of Names

Always introduce yourself. Failure to give your name and status (e.g., nursing student, RN, or licensed practical nurse) or to acknowledge a patient creates uncertainty about an interaction and conveys an impersonal lack of commitment or caring. Making eye contact and smiling are ways to recognize others. Addressing people by name conveys respect for human dignity and uniqueness. Because using last names is respectful in most cultures, nurses usually use a patient's last name in an initial interaction and then use the first name if the patient requests it. Ask how your patients and co-workers prefer to be addressed, and honor their personal preferences. Using first names is appropriate for infants, young children, patients who are confused or unconscious, and close team members. Avoid terms of endearment such as "honey," "dear," "grandma," or "sweetheart." Even the closest nurse-patient relationships rarely progress to identities beyond first names. Avoid referring to patients by diagnosis, room number, or another attribute when interacting with colleagues or family members at the bedside, which is demeaning and sends the message that you do not care enough to know the person as an individual.

Trustworthiness

Trust is relying on someone without doubt or question. Being trustworthy means helping others without hesitation. To foster trust, communicate warmth and demonstrate consistency, reliability, honesty, competence, and respect. Sometimes it is not easy for a patient to ask for help. Trusting another person involves risk and vulnerability, but it also fosters open, therapeutic communication and enhances the expression of feelings,

thoughts, and needs. When trust exists, patients are more likely to share their stories with you. Without trust a nurse-patient relationship rarely progresses beyond social interaction and superficial care. Avoid dishonesty at all costs. Withholding key information, lying, or distorting the truth violates both legal and ethical standards of practice. Sharing personal information or gossiping about others sends the message that you cannot be trusted and damages interpersonal relationships.

Autonomy and Responsibility

Autonomy is being self-directed and independent in accomplishing outcomes and advocating for others. Professional nurses make choices and accept responsibility for the outcomes of their actions (Varcarolis and Fosbre, 2021). They take initiative in problem solving and communicate in a way that reflects the importance and purpose of a therapeutic conversation (Arnold and Boggs, 2020). It important for professional nurses to recognize and advocate for their patients' autonomy.

Assertiveness

Assertiveness allows you to express feelings and ideas without judging or hurting others. Assertive behavior includes appropriate eye contact; nonverbal communication that reflects interest, honesty, and active listening; spontaneous verbal responses with a confident voice; and culturally sensitive use of touch and space. An assertive nurse communicates self-assurance; communicates feelings; takes responsibility for choices; and is respectful of others' feelings, ideas, and choices (Gultekin et al., 2018). Assertive behavior increases self-esteem and self-confidence, increases the ability to develop satisfying interpersonal relationships, and increases outcome attainment. Assertive individuals make decisions and control their lives more effectively than nonassertive individuals. They deal with criticism and manipulation by others and learn to say no, set limits, and resist intentionally imposed guilt. Assertive responses contain "I" messages such as "I want," "I need," "I think," or "I feel" (Arnold and Boggs, 2020). Nurses often experience ethical issues that may make it difficult to use their assertiveness skills for fear of retaliation (e.g., identifying an error made by another health care provider). In such a situation the individual needs to take steps to resolve this ethical dilemma (see Chapter 22).

❖ NURSING PROCESS

Apply critical thinking during the nursing process in your care of patients. The nursing process provides a clinical decision-making approach for you to form clinical judgments and develop and implement a patient-centered, individualized plan of care. You will use the nursing process for all patients. However, with respect to communication, the nursing process guides care for patients who need special assistance with communication.

◆ Assessment

During the assessment process, use critical thinking to make the clinical judgments necessary to thoroughly assess each patient and critically analyze findings to ensure that you make patient-centered clinical decisions required for safe nursing care.

Through the Patient's Eyes. Many internal and external factors affect a patient's ability to communicate (Box 24.6). Assessing these factors relevant to your patient achieves a patient-centered approach that helps you make clinical judgments and appropriate decisions during the communication process. Patient-centered care requires careful assessment of a patient's values; preferences; and cultural, ethnic, and social backgrounds. During assessment, a nurse also explores any personal biases and experiences that might affect the

---

BOX 24.6 Assessment: Factors Influencing Communication

Psychophysiological Context (Internal Factors Affecting Communication)
- Physiological status (e.g., pain, hunger, nausea, weakness, dyspnea)
- Emotional status (e.g., anxiety, anger, hopelessness, euphoria)
- Growth and development status (e.g., age, developmental tasks)
- Unmet needs (e.g., safety/security, love/belonging)
- Attitudes, values, and beliefs (e.g., meaning of illness experience)
- Perceptions and personality (e.g., optimist/pessimist, introvert/extrovert)
- Self-concept and self-esteem (e.g., positive or negative)

Relational Context (Nature of the Relationship Among Participants)
- Social, helping, or working relationship
- Level of trust among participants
- Level of caring expressed
- Level of self-disclosure among participants
- Shared history of participants
- Balance of power and control

Situational Context (Reason for Communication)
- Information exchange
- Goal achievement
- Problem resolution
- Expression of feelings (e.g., grief, anger, fear)

Environmental Context (Physical Surroundings in Which Communication Occurs)
- Privacy level
- Noise level
- Comfort and safety level
- Distraction level

Cultural Context (Sociocultural Elements That Affect an Interaction)
- Educational level of participants
- Language and self-expression patterns
- Customs and expectations

---

ability to form a therapeutic relationship. If the nurse cannot resolve any bias related to a patient, care should be transferred to another individual. Seek to understand the patient's viewpoint as you provide patient-centered care.

Environmental Factors. The environment has a significant impact on communication between nurses and other health care providers and patients. While completing a patient assessment, environmental factors such as noise and distractions (e.g., phones ringing, text messages, electronic pumps and monitors beeping, people talking) greatly affect your ability to establish a therapeutic relationship with patients. Ensuring privacy and confidentiality, reducing distractions, and making the environment as comfortable as possible positively affect your communication with patients.

Physical and Emotional Factors. It is especially important to assess the psychophysiological factors that influence communication. Changes in health status and human responses limit communication. People with hearing or visual impairments often have difficulty receiving messages (see Chapter 49). Facial trauma, laryngeal cancer,

or endotracheal intubation often prevents movement of air past vocal cords or mobility of the tongue, resulting in inability to articulate words. An extremely breathless person needs to use oxygen to breathe rather than speak. People with aphasia after a stroke or in late-stage Alzheimer disease cannot understand or form words. Some mental illnesses such as psychoses or depression cause patients to jump from one topic to another, constantly verbalizing the same words or phrases or exhibiting a slowed speech pattern. People with high anxiety are sometimes unable to perceive environmental stimuli or hear explanations. Patients who are unresponsive or heavily sedated cannot send or respond to verbal messages.

Review of a patient's medical record provides relevant information about the patient's ability to communicate. The medical history and physical examination document physical barriers to speech, neurological deficits, and pathophysiology affecting hearing or vision. Reviewing a patient's medication record is also important. For example, opiates, antidepressants, neuroleptics, hypnotics, or sedatives may cause a patient to slur words or use incomplete sentences. The nursing progress notes in the electronic health record (EHR) sometimes reveal other factors that contribute to communication difficulties, such as the absence of family members to provide more information about a patient who is confused.

Remaining attentive and establishing eye contact allows you to communicate effectively to determine patients' ability to attend to, interpret, and respond to stimuli. If patients have difficulty communicating, determine the cause of the difficulty and assess the effect of the problem. Patients who are unable to speak are at risk for injury unless you identify an alternate communication method. If barriers exist that make it difficult to communicate directly with patients, family or friends become important sources concerning the patients' communication patterns and abilities.

Gender. Gender influences how we think, act, feel, and communicate. Men tend to use less verbal communication but are more likely to initiate communication and address issues more directly. They are also more likely to talk about issues. Women tend to disclose more personal information and use more active listening, answering with responses that encourage the other person to continue the conversation. It is important for you to recognize a patient's gender communication pattern.

Developmental Factors. Aspects of a patient's growth and development also influence nurse-patient interaction. For example, an infant's self-expression is limited to crying, body movement, and facial expression, whereas older children express their needs more directly. Adapt assessment and communication techniques to the special needs of infants, children, and their parents. Depending on a child's age, include the parents, child, or both as sources of information about the child's health. Giving a young child toys or other distractions allows parents to give you their full attention. Children are especially responsive to nonverbal messages. Sudden movements, loud noises, or threatening gestures are frightening. Children often prefer to make the first move in interpersonal contacts and do not like adults who stare or look down at them. A child who has received little environmental stimulation possibly is behind in language development, thus making communication more challenging.

Age alone does not determine an adult's capacity for communication. Communicate with older adults on an adult level and avoid patronizing or speaking in a condescending manner. Avoid sudden shifts from subject to subject. Hearing loss and visual impairments are changes that may occur during aging that contribute to communication barriers (Mormer et al., 2020). Modify your assessment approach with older adults who have motor, cognitive, or sensory impairments (Box 24.7).

BOX 24.7 FOCUS ON OLDER ADULTS

Tips for Improved Communication With Older Adults Who Have Hearing Loss

- Determine if the patient uses hearing aids, glasses, or other adaptive equipment.
- Make sure the patient knows that you are talking.
- Face the patient at eye level, be sure that your face/mouth is visible, and do not chew gum.
- Speak clearly but do not exaggerate lip movement or shout.
- Speak a little more slowly but not excessively slowly.
- Choose a quiet, well-lit environment with minimal distractions.
- Allow time for the patient to respond. Do not assume that a patient who does not reply or takes a long time to reply is being uncooperative.
- Give the patient a chance to ask questions.
- Keep communication short and to the point. Ask one question at a time.

Data from Arnold E, Boggs KU: *Interpersonal relationships: professional communication skills for nurses,* ed 8, St Louis, 2020, Saunders; and Blevins S: Nurses as educators: teaching patients with hearing loss, *Medsurg Nurs* 24(2):128, 2015.

Encouraging older adults to share life stories and reminisce about the past has a therapeutic effect and increases their sense of well-being, which can enhance the details of your assessment. It is sometimes also helpful to include a patient's family and friends and to become familiar with a patient's favorite topics for conversation.

REFLECT NOW

As you think back on a recent experience interacting with a patient or family member, describe the unique personal factors that you observed. How should you tailor your own communication to create an effective interaction?

◆ Analysis and Nursing Diagnosis

Most individuals experience difficulty with some aspect of communication. Using clinical judgment, analyze your assessment findings, and look for patterns or cues to help you identify nursing diagnoses or collaborative problems surrounding patient communication.

For example, some patients lack skills in attending, listening, responding, and self-expression because of illness, treatment effects, or cultural or language barriers. The primary nursing diagnostic label used to describe a patient with limited or no ability to communicate verbally is *Impaired Verbal Communication.* This occurs when your analysis reveals your patient is experiencing difficulty receiving, processing, transmitting, or using symbols for a variety of reasons. Use this diagnosis if your patient is unable to articulate words or experiences inappropriate verbalization, difficulty in forming words, and difficulty in comprehending (International Council of Nurses, 2019). This diagnosis is useful for a wide variety of patients with special problems and needs related to communication, such as impaired perception, reception, and articulation. Although a patient's primary problem is *Impaired Verbal Communication,* the associated difficulty in self-expression or altered communication patterns may also contribute to other nursing diagnoses such as:

- Communication Barrier
- Difficulty Coping
- Powerlessness
- Impaired Socialisation

Assessment findings in a patient with *Impaired Verbal Communication* typically reveal factors associated with a communication disorder, which often include physiological, mechanical, anatomical, psychological, cultural, or developmental factors. Accuracy in identifying and analyzing assessment findings is necessary so that you select interventions that effectively resolve the source of the diagnostic problem. For example, you manage the diagnosis of *Impaired Verbal Communication related to cultural difference (Hispanic heritage)* very differently from the diagnosis of *Impaired Verbal Communication related to hearing loss.*

◆ Planning and Outcomes Identification

Once you have identified the nature of a patient's communication issues, consider several factors when designing the care plan. Use critical thinking to reflect on your experiences in communicating with others. Your experiences and analysis of situations, whether communication was effective or not, will help you plan care for patients who are experiencing an alteration in communication.

Consider the environment while planning care. When the focus is on practicing communication approaches, arrange for a quiet, private place that is free of distractions such as television or visitors. When the nature of a patient's problem is psychosocial, role-playing, for example, may be a care option. Meet basic comfort and safety needs before introducing new communication methods and techniques. Allow adequate time for practice. Participants need to be patient with themselves and one another to achieve effective communication. Motivation is a factor in improving communication, and patients often require encouragement to try different approaches that involve significant change. It is especially important to involve the patient and family in decisions about the plan of care to determine whether suggested methods are acceptable.

Outcomes. Once you identify a diagnosis, select an outcome that is relevant, measurable, and achievable for the patient, such as being able to express needs or achieving understanding of physical condition. Ensure that the expected outcomes are specific and measurable. For example, outcomes for a patient possibly include the following:

- Patient initiates conversation about diagnosis or health care problem.
- Patient is able to attend to appropriate stimuli.
- Patient conveys clear and understandable messages with health care team.
- Patient expresses increased satisfaction with the communication process.

At times you care for patients whose difficulty in sending, receiving, and interpreting messages interferes with healthy interpersonal relationships. In this case impaired communication is a contributing factor to other nursing diagnoses such as *Impaired Socialisation* or *Difficulty Coping.* Plan interventions to help these patients improve their communication skills. Expected outcomes for a patient in this situation possibly include demonstrating the ability to appropriately express needs, feelings, and concerns; communicating thoughts and feelings more clearly; engaging in appropriate social conversation with peers and staff; and increasing perceived feelings of autonomy and assertiveness.

Setting Priorities. Establish nursing care priorities for communication based on assessment data, your knowledge of similar problems, the nursing diagnoses identified, and the outcomes of care. Physiologic needs often seem to take priority, but if a patient has a communication problem, the two may go hand in hand. For example, if it is urgent to manage a patient's problem with impaired airway clearance, it may be necessary to simultaneously plan the need to allay the patient's fear or anxiety as you initiate airway interventions.

It is essential to always maintain an open line of communication so that a patient can express emergent needs or problems. This sometimes involves an intervention as simple as keeping the nurse call system in reach for a patient restricted to bed or providing communication augmentative devices (e.g., message board or Braille computer). When you plan to have lengthy interactions with a patient, it is important to address physical care priorities first so that the discussion is not interrupted. Make the patient comfortable by ensuring that any symptoms are under control and elimination needs have been met.

Teamwork and Collaboration. To ensure an effective plan of care, you will sometimes collaborate with other health care team members who have expertise in communication strategies. Speech-language pathologists help patients with aphasia and dysphagia, professional interpreters are necessary for patients who speak a foreign language, and mental health nurse specialists help angry or highly anxious patients to communicate more effectively.

◆ Implementation

In carrying out any plan of care, apply clinical judgment in selecting communication techniques that are appropriate for a patient's individual needs. Before learning how to adapt communication methods to help patients with serious communication impairments, it is necessary to learn the communication techniques that serve as the foundation for professional communication. It is also important to understand communication techniques that create barriers to effective interaction and how to adapt your communication in different patient situations.

Therapeutic Communication Techniques. Therapeutic communication techniques are specific responses that encourage the expression of feelings and ideas and convey acceptance and respect. These techniques apply in a variety of different situations. Although some of the techniques seem artificial at first, skill and comfort increase with practice. Tremendous satisfaction results from developing therapeutic relationships that achieve desired patient outcomes.

Active Listening. Active listening means being attentive to what a patient is saying both verbally and nonverbally. It facilitates patient communication. Inexperienced nurses sometimes feel the need to talk to prove that they know what they are doing or to decrease anxiety (Varcarolis and Fosbre, 2021). It is often difficult at first to be quiet and really listen. Also, many health care settings use computers for data entry, and thus it is too easy to be distracted if you try to talk and work at a computer at the same time. Active listening enhances trust because you communicate acceptance and respect for a patient. The SURETY Model is one model you can use to facilitate attentive listening and therapeutic communication with your patients (Stickley, 2011).

- **S**—*S*it at an angle facing the patient. Sitting at a slight angle to the patient creates a nonconfrontational seating arrangement that is conducive to communication. This posture conveys the message that you are there to listen and are interested in what the patient is saying.
- **U**—*U*ncross legs and arms. This position suggests that you are "open" to what the patient says. A "closed" position such as crossing arms conveys a defensive attitude, possibly provoking a similar response in the patient.
- **R**—*R*elax. It is important to communicate a sense of being relaxed and comfortable with the patient. Restlessness communicates a lack of interest and a feeling of discomfort to the patient.
- **E**—*E*ye contact. Establish and maintain intermittent eye contact to convey your involvement in and willingness to listen to what the patient is saying (Fig. 24.2). Absence of eye contact or shifting the eyes gives the message that you are not interested in what the patient is saying.

FIG. 24.2 Maintain eye contact when communicating with patients. (Copyright © iStock.)

- **T**—*T*ouch. Use touch that is respectful to communicate empathy and understanding to the patient. Ensure that your use of touch is therapeutic and acceptable to the patient.
- **Y**—*Y*our intuition. Trust your intuition as you grow in confidence to individualize, adapt, and apply communication techniques in your interpersonal encounters with your patients.

Sharing Observations. Nurses make observations by commenting on how the other person looks, sounds, or acts. Stating observations often helps a patient communicate without the need for extensive questioning, focusing, or clarification. This technique can help start a conversation with a patient who is quiet or withdrawn. Do not state observations that will embarrass or anger a patient, such as telling someone, "You look a mess!" Even if you make such an observation with humor, the patient can become resentful.

Sharing observations differs from making assumptions, which means drawing unnecessary conclusions about the other person without validating them. Making assumptions puts a patient in the position of having to contradict you. Examples include interpreting a patient's fatigue as depression or assuming that untouched food indicates lack of interest in meeting nutritional intake goals. Making observations is a gentler and safer technique: "You look tired . . .," "You seem different today . . .," or "I see you haven't eaten anything."

Sharing Empathy. Empathy is the ability to understand and accept another person's reality, accurately perceive feelings, and communicate this understanding to the other. This is a therapeutic communication technique that enables you to understand a patient's situation, feelings, and concerns (Lorié, 2017). To express empathy, you reflect that you understand and feel the importance of the other person's communication. Empathetic understanding requires you to be sensitive and imaginative, especially if you have not had similar experiences. Strive to be empathetic in every situation because it is a key to unlocking concern and communicating support for others. Statements reflecting empathy are highly effective because they tell a person that you heard both the emotional and the factual content of the communication. Empathetic statements are neutral and nonjudgmental and help establish trust in difficult situations. For example, a nurse says to an angry patient who has low mobility after a stroke, "It must be very frustrating to not be able to do what you want."

Sharing Hope. Nurses recognize that hope is essential for healing and learn to communicate a "sense of possibility" to others. Appropriate encouragement and positive feedback are important in fostering hope and self-confidence and for helping people achieve their potential and reach their goals. Foster hope by commenting on the positive aspects of the other person's behavior, performance, or response. Sharing a vision of the future and reminding others of their resources and strengths also strengthen hope. Reassure patients that there are many kinds of hope and that meaning and personal growth can come from illness experiences. For example, a nurse says to a patient discouraged about a poor prognosis, "I believe that you'll find a way to face your situation because I've seen your courage and creativity."

Sharing Humor. Humor is an important but often underused resource in nursing interactions. It is a coping strategy that can reduce anxiety and promote positive feelings (Mota Sousa et al., 2019). It is a perception and attitude in which a person can experience joy even when facing difficult times. It provides emotional support to patients and professional colleagues and humanizes the illness experience. It enhances teamwork and relieves tension. Bonds develop between people who laugh together (Mills et al., 2019). Patients use humor to release tension, cope with fear related to pain and suffering, communicate a fear or need, or cope with an uncomfortable or embarrassing situation. The aim of using humor as a health care provider is to bring hope and joy to a situation and enhance a patient's well-being and the therapeutic relationship (Mota Sousa et al., 2019). It makes you seem warmer and more approachable. Use humor during the orientation phase to establish a therapeutic relationship and during the working phase as you help a patient cope with a situation.

You will care for patients from different cultural backgrounds. Humor often has a cultural context. When you interact with patients, be sensitive and realize that they may misunderstand or misinterpret jokes and statements meant to be humorous, and you may decide that humor is inappropriate for a particular patient (Giger and Haddad, 2021). It is never appropriate, with any patient, to joke about sexual orientation, race, economic status, disability, or any cultural attribute.

Health care professionals sometimes use a kind of dark, negative humor after difficult or traumatic situations to deal with unbearable tension and stress. This coping humor has a high potential for misinterpretation as uncaring by people not involved in the situation. For example, nursing students are sometimes offended and wonder how staff are able to laugh and joke after unsuccessful resuscitation efforts. When nurses use coping humor within earshot of patients or their loved ones, great emotional distress results.

Sharing Feelings. Emotions are subjective feelings that result from one's thoughts and perceptions. Feelings are not right, wrong, good, or bad, although they are pleasant or unpleasant. If individuals do not express feelings, stress and illness may worsen. Help patients express emotions by making observations, acknowledging feelings, encouraging communication, giving permission to express "negative" feelings, and modeling healthy emotional self-expression. At times patients will direct their anger or frustration prompted by their illness toward you. Do not take such expressions personally. Acknowledging patients' feelings communicates that you listened to and understood the emotional aspects of their illness situation.

When you care for patients, be aware of your own emotions because feelings are difficult to hide. Students sometimes wonder whether it is helpful to share feelings with patients. Sharing emotions makes nurses seem more human and brings people closer. It is appropriate to share feelings of caring or even to cry with others if you are in control of the expression of these feelings and express them in a way that does not burden the patient or break confidentiality. Patients are perceptive and sense your emotions. It is usually inappropriate to discuss personal emotions such as anger or sadness with patients. A social support system of colleagues is helpful. Employee assistance programs, peer group meetings, and the use of interprofessional teams, such as social work and pastoral care, provide other means for nurses to safely express feelings away from patients.

FIG. 24.3 The nurse uses touch to communicate.

Using Touch. Because of modern fast-paced technical environments in health care, nurses face major challenges in bringing the sense of caring and human connection to their patients (see Chapters 7 and 32). Touch is one of the most potent and personal forms of communication. It expresses concern or caring to establish a feeling of connection and promote healing (Varcarolis and Fosbre, 2021). Touch conveys many messages, such as affection, emotional support, encouragement, tenderness, and personal attention. When performing nursing procedures, a gentle approach to touch conveys competence. Comfort touch such as holding a hand is especially important for patients who are vulnerable or experiencing severe illness with its accompanying physical and emotional losses (Fig. 24.3).

Some students initially find giving intimate care to be stressful, especially when caring for patients of the opposite gender. They learn to cope with intimate contact by changing their perception of the situation. Because much of what nurses do involves touching, you need to learn to be sensitive to others' reactions to touch and use it wisely. When performing a nursing procedure that involves touching sensitive areas of the body, let the patient know what you are going to do before touching. For example, as you prepare to provide perineal hygiene or cleanse a site for a urinary catheter insertion say, "I am going to gently pull the skin around the area where you urinate so I can get a better view and cleanse correctly. This will not be painful." Touch should always be as gentle or as firm as needed and delivered in a comforting, nonthreatening manner. Sometimes you withhold touch for highly suspicious or angry persons who respond negatively or even violently to you.

Nurses need to be aware of patients' nonverbal cues and ask permission before touching them to ensure that touch is an acceptable way to provide comfort. Some individuals may be sensitive to physical closeness and uncomfortable with touch. When this occurs, share the information with other nurses who will care for the patient. Nurses should be aware of a patient's concern and act accordingly. A nod, gesture, body position, or eye contact can also convey interest and acceptance of touch, which promotes a bonding moment with a patient (Varcarolis and Fosbre, 2021).

Using Silence. It takes time and experience to become comfortable with silence. Most people have a natural tendency to fill empty spaces with words, but sometimes these spaces really allow time for a nurse and patient to observe one another, sort out feelings, think about how to say things, and consider what has been communicated. Silence prompts some people to talk. It allows a patient to think and gain insight (Varcarolis and Fosbre, 2021). In general, allow a patient to break the silence, particularly when the patient has initiated it.

Silence is particularly useful when people are confronted with decisions that require much thought. For example, it helps a patient gain the necessary confidence to share the decision to refuse medical treatment. It also allows the nurse to pay attention to nonverbal messages, such as worried expressions or loss of eye contact. Remaining silent demonstrates patience and a willingness to wait for a response when the other person is unable to reply quickly. Silence is especially therapeutic during times of profound sadness or grief.

Providing Information. Providing relevant information tells other people what they need or want to know so that they are able to make decisions, experience less anxiety, and feel safe and secure. It is also an integral aspect of health teaching (see Chapter 25). It usually is not helpful to hide information from patients, particularly when they seek it. If a health care provider chooses to withhold information, it becomes your role to explain and clarify a situation with the patient so as to not conflict with the health care provider's choice. However, patients have a right to know about their health status and what is happening in their environment. Information of a distressing nature needs to be communicated with sensitivity, at a pace appropriate to a patient's ability to absorb it, and in general terms at first: "John, your heart sounds have changed from earlier today, and so has your blood pressure. I'll let your doctor know." A nurse provides information that enables others to understand what is happening and what to expect: "Mrs. Evans, John is getting an echocardiogram right now. This test uses painless sound waves to create a moving picture of his heart structures and valves and should tell us the effect, if any, of his murmur on his heart."

Clarifying. To check whether you understand a message accurately, restate an unclear or ambiguous message to clarify the sender's meaning. In addition, ask the other person to rephrase it, explain further, or give an example of what the person means. Without clarification you may make invalid assumptions and miss valuable information. Despite efforts at paraphrasing, you still may not understand a patient's message. Let the patient know if this is the case: "I'm not sure I understand what you mean by 'sicker than usual.' What is different now?"

Focusing. Focusing involves centering a conversation on key elements or concepts of a message. If conversation is vague or rambling or patients begin to repeat themselves, focusing is a useful technique. Do not use focusing if it interrupts patients while they are discussing important issues. Rather, use it to guide the direction of conversation to important areas: "We've talked a lot about your medications; now let's look more closely at the trouble you're having in taking them on time."

Paraphrasing. Paraphrasing is restating another's message more briefly using one's own words. Through paraphrasing you send feedback that lets patients know that they are actively involved in the search for understanding and clarity. Accurate paraphrasing requires practice. If the meaning of a message is changed or distorted through paraphrasing, communication becomes ineffective. For example, a patient says, "I've been overweight all my life and never had any problems. I can't understand why I need to be on a diet." Paraphrasing this statement by saying "You don't care if you're overweight" is incorrect. It is more accurate to say, "You're not convinced that you need to make different food choices because you've stayed healthy."

Validation. Validation is a technique that nurses use to recognize and acknowledge a patient's thoughts, feelings, and needs. Patients and families know they are being heard and taken seriously when the caregiver addresses their issues. For example, a nurse validates a patient's comments by saying, "Tell me if I understand your concerns regarding your surgery. You're worried that you will not be able to do some of the things you could do before your surgery." This type of statement enables a nurse to convey empathy and interest in the patient's thoughts, feelings, and perceptions.

Asking Relevant Questions. Ask relevant questions to seek information needed for decision making. Ask only one question at a time, and fully explore one topic before moving to another area. During patient assessment you ask questions that follow a logical sequence and usually proceed from general to more specific. **Open-ended questions** allow patients to take the conversational lead and introduce pertinent information about a topic. For example, "Tell me what is your biggest problem at the moment?" Use focused questions when more specific information is needed in an area: "How has your pain affected your life at home?" Allow patients to respond fully to open-ended questions before asking more focused questions. **Closed-ended questions** elicit a yes, no, or one-word response: "How many times a day are you taking pain medication?" Although they are helpful during assessment, they are generally less useful during therapeutic exchanges.

Sometimes asking too many questions is dehumanizing. Seeking factual information does not allow a nurse or patient to establish a meaningful relationship or deal with important emotional issues. It is a way for a nurse to ignore uncomfortable areas in favor of more comfortable, neutral topics. A useful exercise is to try to converse without asking the other person a single question. By using techniques such as giving general leads ("Tell me about . . ."), making observations, paraphrasing, focusing, and providing information, you discover important information that would have remained hidden if you had limited the communication process to questions alone.

Summarizing. Summarizing is a concise review of key aspects of an interaction. It brings a sense of satisfaction and closure to an individual conversation and is especially helpful during the termination phase of a nurse-patient relationship. By reviewing a conversation, participants focus on key issues and add relevant information as needed. Beginning a new interaction by summarizing a previous one helps patients recall topics discussed and shows that you analyzed their communication. Summarizing also clarifies expectations, as in this example of a nurse manager who has been working with an unsatisfied employee: "You've told me a lot of things about why you don't like this job and how unhappy you've been. We have also come up with some possible ways to make things better. You have agreed to try some of them and let me know if any help."

Self-Disclosure. Self-disclosures are subjectively true personal experiences about the self that are intentionally revealed to another person. This is not therapeutic for a nurse; rather it shows a patient that the nurse understands his experiences and that they are not unique. You choose to share experiences or feelings that are like those of the patient and emphasize both the similarities and differences. This kind of self-disclosure is indicative of the closeness of the nurse-patient relationship and indicates respect for the patient. You offer self-disclosure as an expression of sincerity and honesty; it is an aspect of empathy (Lorié, 2017). Self-disclosures need to be relevant and appropriate and made to benefit the patient rather than yourself. Use them sparingly so that the patient is the focus of the interaction.

Confrontation. When you confront someone in a therapeutic way, you help the other person become more aware of inconsistencies in feelings, attitudes, beliefs, and behaviors (Varcarolis and Fosbre, 2021). This technique improves patient self-awareness and helps the patient recognize growth and deal with important issues. Use confrontation only after you have established trust and do it gently with sensitivity: "You say you've already decided what to do, yet you're still talking a lot about your options."

Nontherapeutic Communication Techniques. Certain communication techniques hinder or damage professional relationships. These specific techniques are referred to as *nontherapeutic* or *blocking* and often cause others to activate defenses to avoid being hurt or negatively affected. Nontherapeutic techniques discourage further expression of feelings and ideas and engender negative responses or behaviors in others.

Asking Personal Questions. "Why don't you and John get married?" "Is it true your wife does not agree with your decision?" Asking personal questions that are not relevant to a situation simply to satisfy your curiosity is inappropriate professional communication. Such questions are nosy, invasive, and unnecessary. If patients wish to share private information, they will. To learn more about a patient's interpersonal roles and relationships, ask questions such as "How would you describe your relationship with John?"

Giving Personal Opinions. "If I were you, I would put your mother in a nursing home." When a nurse gives a personal opinion, it takes decision making away from the other person. It inhibits spontaneity, stalls problem solving, and creates doubt. Personal opinions differ from professional advice. At times people need suggestions and help to make choices. Suggestions that you present are options; the other person makes the final decision. Remember that the problem and its solution belong to the other person and not to you. A much better response is "Let's talk about the options available for your mother's care." The nurse also should not make promises to a patient about situations that require collaboration. For example, "I cannot recommend that you stop taking the medications because of your side effects, but I would be happy to inform your primary care provider and ask whether a change in medication is appropriate."

Changing the Subject. "Let's not talk about your problems with the insurance company. It's time for your walk." Changing the subject when another person is trying to communicate a story is rude and shows a lack of empathy. It blocks further communication, and the sender then withholds important messages or fails to openly express feelings. In some instances, changing the subject serves as a face-saving maneuver. If this happens, reassure the patient that you will return to the concerns: "After your walk let's talk some more about what's going on with your insurance company."

Automatic Responses. "Older adults are always confused." "Administration doesn't care about the staff." Automatic responses are often triggered by stereotypes that are generalized beliefs held about people. Making stereotyped remarks about others reflects poor nursing judgment and threatens nurse-patient or team relationships. A cliché is a stereotyped comment such as "You can't win them all" that tends to belittle the other person's feelings and minimize the importance of the person's message. These automatic phrases communicate that you are not taking concerns seriously or responding thoughtfully. Another kind of automatic response is parroting (i.e., repeating what the other person has said word for word). Parroting is easily overused and is not as effective as paraphrasing. A simple "Oh?" gives you time to think if the other person says something that takes you by surprise.

A nurse who is task oriented automatically makes the task or procedure the entire focus of interaction with patients, missing opportunities to communicate with them as individuals and meet their needs. Task-oriented nurses are often perceived as cold, uncaring, and unapproachable. When students first perform technical skills, it is difficult to integrate therapeutic communication because of the need to focus on the procedure. In time you learn to integrate communication with high-visibility tasks and accomplish a procedure or action more effectively.

False Reassurance. "Don't worry; everything will be all right." When a patient is seriously ill or distressed, you may be tempted to offer hope with statements such as "You'll be fine" or "There's nothing to worry about." When a patient is reaching for understanding, false reassurance discourages open communication. Offering reassurance not supported by facts does more harm than good. Although you are trying to be kind, it has the secondary effect of helping you avoid the other person's distress, and it tends to block conversation and discourage further expression of feelings. To use a more facilitative response you can say "It must be difficult not to know what the surgeon will find. What can I do to help?"

Sympathy. "I'm so sorry about your mastectomy; you probably feel devastated." Sympathy is concern, sorrow, or pity felt for another person. A nurse often takes on a patient's problems as if they were his or her own. Sympathy is a subjective look at another person's world that prevents a clear perspective of the issues confronting that person. If a nurse overidentifies with a patient, objectivity is lost, and the nurse is unable to help the patient work through the situation (Varcarolis and Fosbre, 2021). Although sympathy is a compassionate response to another's situation, it is not as therapeutic as empathy. A nurse's own emotional issues sometimes prevent effective problem solving and impair good judgment. A more empathetic approach is "The loss of a breast is a major change. Do you feel comfortable talking about how it will affect your life?"

Asking for Explanations. "Why are you so anxious?" Some nurses are tempted to ask patients why they believe, feel, or act in a certain way. Patients frequently interpret "why" questions as accusations or think nurses know the reasons and are simply testing them. Regardless of a patient's perception of your motivation, asking "why" questions causes resentment, insecurity, and mistrust. If you need additional information, it is best to phrase a question to avoid using the word "why." For example, "You seem upset. What's on your mind?" is more likely to help an anxious patient communicate.

Approval or Disapproval. "You should not even think about stopping your cancer treatments." Do not impose your own opinions, attitudes, values, beliefs, and moral standards on others while in the professional helping role. Other people have the right to be themselves and make their own decisions. Judgmental responses often contain terms such as *should, ought, good, bad, right,* or *wrong.* Agreeing or disagreeing sends the subtle message that you have the right to make value judgments about patient decisions. Approving implies that the behavior being praised is the only acceptable one. Often a patient shares a decision with you not to seek approval but to provide a means to discuss feelings. Disapproval implies that the patient needs to meet your expectations or standards. Instead, help patients explore their own beliefs and decisions. For example, the response "Have you had the opportunity to talk to your doctors about stopping cancer treatments? Tell me more about your thoughts" gives the patient a chance to express ideas or feelings without fear of being judged.

Defensive Responses. "No one here would intentionally lie to you." Becoming defensive in the face of criticism implies that the other person has no right to an opinion. The sender's concerns are ignored when the nurse focuses on the need for self-defense, defense of the health care team, or defense of others. When patients express criticism, listen to what they have to say. Listening does not imply agreement. Listen nonjudgmentally to discover reasons for a patient's anger or dissatisfaction. By avoiding a defensive attitude, you are able to defuse anger and uncover deeper concerns. A better response would be "You believe that people are dishonest with you. It must be hard to trust anyone."

Passive or Aggressive Responses. "Things are bad, and there is nothing I can do about it." "Things are falling apart, and it is all your fault." Passive responses serve to avoid conflict or sidestep issues. They reflect feelings of sadness, depression, anxiety, powerlessness, and hopelessness. Aggressive responses provoke confrontation at the other person's expense. They reflect feelings of anger, frustration, resentment, and stress. Nurses who lack assertive skills also use triangulation (i.e., complaining to a third party rather than confronting the problem or expressing concerns directly to the source). This lowers team morale and draws others into the conflict situation. Assertive communication is a far more professional approach for a nurse to take.

Arguing. "How can you say you didn't sleep a wink when I heard you snoring all night long?" Challenging or arguing against perceptions denies that they are real and valid. A skillful nurse gives information or presents reality in a way that avoids argument, with a statement such as "You feel as if you did not get any rest at all last night, even though I thought you slept well since I heard you snoring."

REFLECT NOW

Learning to avoid nontherapeutic communication techniques is difficult, as they are often a part of everyday conversation. As you reflect on a recent conversation with a patient, which nontherapeutic communication techniques did you catch yourself using? What therapeutic response could you have used?

Special Communication Considerations

Sociocultural Considerations. Culture influences thinking, feeling, behaving, and communicating. Be aware of the typical patterns of interaction that characterize various ethnic groups, but do not allow this information to bias your response. Take time to talk with, listen to, and know each patient individually (e.g., does the patient feel comfortable with eye contact or in sharing information with others?). Respect the individuality of each patient and adapt your communication techniques based on patient preferences. For example, you will approach a patient who is open and willing to discuss private family matters very differently from a patient who is reluctant to reveal personal or family information to strangers.

People from other countries do not always speak or understand English. Those who speak English as a second language often have trouble with self-expression or language comprehension. To practice cultural sensitivity in communication, understand that people of different ethnic origins use different degrees of eye contact, personal space, gestures, loud voice, pace of speech, touch, silence, and meaning of language. Make a conscious effort not to interpret messages through your cultural perspective, but to consider the communication within the context of the other individual's background. Avoid stereotyping, patronizing, and making fun of other cultures. Language and cultural barriers are not only frustrating but also dangerous, causing delay in care (Box 24.8).

Speech and Language Considerations. Throughout your nursing career, you will care for many patients who have difficulty communicating for various reasons. Interacting with people who have speech or language impairments requires special thought and sensitivity. Use appropriate interventions based on patient needs to adapt your communication techniques. Box 24.9 lists methods available to encourage, enhance, restore, or substitute for verbal communication. Be sure that a patient is physically able to use the chosen method and that it does not cause frustration by being too complicated or difficult.

Patients who speak little or no English present challenges for nurse-patient communication. Federal and state laws require that hospitals that receive federal funding, including Medicare, Medicaid, and the State Children's Health Insurance Plan (SCHIP), are required to provide interpretation services to facilitate communication, which improves patient safety and patient outcomes. If you are unable to provide on-site interpreters, use telephone interpretation services. Use of family members, friends, or bilingual staff members to interpret for patients is strongly discouraged. Language is not the only barrier. Cultural differences also lead to misunderstanding and have been identified as an important factor affecting patient satisfaction (Sethi and Rani, 2017).

Changes in sensory function also affect communication. Hearing loss, which affects approximately 16% of the U.S. population, can make communicating with patients challenging (Centers for Disease Control and Prevention [CDC], 2018). The incidence of hearing loss increases with age. Some patients with impaired hearing use hearing aids or sign language to communicate. Vision loss also affects communication and presents a challenge for many individuals, particularly

---

🌐 BOX 24.8   CULTURAL ASPECTS OF CARE

Cultural Diversity and Communication

- Differences in language comprehension may impede understanding and negatively affect the quality and safety of nursing care.
- Even among native speakers, variability in word usage, vocabulary, and literacy may skew patient and nurse understanding.
- Differences in nonverbal communication styles may create misunderstanding or discomfort, including practices regarding personal space, privacy, eye contact, and touch.
- Among people of different cultures, decision-making authority for patient care decisions may vary.
- Variability in religious and spiritual beliefs affects how individuals perceive the health care experience.
- Incorporating the patient's beliefs and practices into the health care situation contributes to a patient-centered care experience.

Implications for Patient-Centered Care
- Understand your own cultural values and biases.
- Assess the patient's primary language and level of fluency in English.
- Speak directly to the patient even if an interpreter is present.
- Nodding or statements such as "Okay" do not necessarily mean that the patient understands.
- Provide written information in English and primary language.
- Learn about other cultures, especially those commonly encountered in your work area.
- Incorporate the patient's communication methods or needs into plan of care.

---

over the age of 65. Vision loss is among the top 10 disabilities in the United States. It affects activities of daily living, sometimes leading to depression and isolation (CDC, 2020).

Patients who have had a stroke or laryngectomy may require communication aids such as a writing or picture board or a special call system. Such patients benefit greatly when you adapt communication techniques to their unique circumstances, developmental level, or cognitive and sensory deficits.

When communicating with a patient who is experiencing cognitive impairment, determine what strategies the family finds effective. Use other techniques such as pictures or demonstration to help you communicate as needed. Use the following ABC mnemonic (Schlögl and Jones, 2020) when interacting with patients and family caregivers to facilitate as much clarity of understanding as possible without causing undue frustration related to conveying a message that is too complex:

1. **A**ttend mindfully: Reflect on how you typically communicate and align your nonverbal communication with your spoken message.
2. **B**ehave calmly: Ensure you convey respect when communicating with your patients by approaching them from the front, respecting your patient's personal space, putting yourself at the patient's eye level, avoiding making sudden movements, and projecting a calm and positive attitude. Ensure that your body language does not convey frustration, anger, or impatience.
3. **C**ommunicate clearly: Use short and simple questions and gestures to help underline your words. Allow your patient time to respond to your questions.

◆ Evaluation

Evaluate the effectiveness of your own communication by videotaping practice sessions with peers or by making process recordings—written records of your verbal and nonverbal interactions with patients. Process recording analysis reveals how to improve personal communication techniques to make them more effective. Box 24.10 contains a sample

BOX 24.9 Special Communication Approaches

Patients Who Do Not Speak English
- Speak to patient in normal tone of voice.
- Establish method for patient to ask for assistance (nurse call system).
- Provide a professional interpreter as needed.
- Avoid using family members, especially children, as interpreters.
- Use communication board, pictures, or cards.
- Translate words from native language into English list for patient to make basic requests.
- Have dictionary (e.g., English/Spanish) available if patient can read.

Patients Who Have a Hearing Impairment
- Check for hearing aids and glasses.
- Reduce environmental noise.
- Get patient's attention before speaking.
- Face patient with mouth visible.
- Do not chew gum.
- Speak at normal volume—do not shout.
- Rephrase rather than repeat if misunderstood.
- Provide a sign-language interpreter if indicated.

Patients Who Are Visually Impaired
- Check for use of glasses or contact lenses.
- Identify yourself when you enter the room and notify the patient when you leave the room.
- Speak in a normal tone of voice.
- Do not rely on gestures or nonverbal communication.
- Use indirect lighting, avoiding glare.
- Use at least 14-point print.

Patients Who Cannot Speak Clearly (Aphasia, Dysarthria, Muteness)
- Listen attentively, be patient, and do not interrupt.
- Ask simple questions that require "yes" or "no" answers.
- Allow time for understanding and response.
- Use visual cues (e.g., words, pictures, and objects) when possible.
- Allow only one person to speak at a time.
- Encourage patient to converse.
- Let patient know if you have not understood.
- Collaborate with speech therapist as needed.
- Use communication aids: letter boards, flash cards, computer-generated speech program.

Patients Who Have a Cognitive Impairment
- Use simple sentences and avoid long explanations.
- Ask one question at a time.
- Allow time for patient to respond.
- Be an attentive listener.
- Include family and friends in conversations, especially in subjects known to patient.
- Use picture or gestures that mimic the action desired.

Patients Who Are Unresponsive
- Call patient by name during interactions.
- Communicate both verbally and by touch.
- Speak to patient as though he or she can hear.
- Explain all procedures and sensations.
- Provide orientation to person, place, and time.
- Avoid talking about patient to others in his or her presence.

BOX 24.10 Sample Communication Analysis

Nurse: Good morning, Mr. Simpson."
(Smiles, approaches bed holding clipboard)
Acknowledged by name, social greeting to begin conversation
Patient: "What's good about it?"
(Arms crossed over chest, frowning, direct stare)
Nonverbal signs of anger
Nurse: "You sound unhappy."
(Pulls up chair and sits at bedside)
Sharing observation, nonverbal communication of availability
Patient: "You'd be unhappy, too, if nobody would answer your questions. That girl wouldn't tell me my blood sugar."
(Angry voice tone, challenging expression)
Further expression of feelings facilitated by nurse making accurate observation
Nurse: "This hospital has a fine staff, Mr. Simpson. I'm sure no one would intentionally keep information from you."
Feeling threatened and being defensive, a nontherapeutic technique
Nurse: "I'm going to test your glucose in a minute, and I'll tell you the results."
(Does test) "Your blood sugar was 350."

Providing information, demonstrating trustworthiness
Patient: "I'm so afraid complications will set in since my blood sugar is high."
(Stares out window)
Feels free to express deeper concerns, but they are hard to face
Nurse: "What kinds of things are you worried about?"
Open-ended question to seek information
Patient: "I could lose a leg, like my mother did, or go blind or have to live hooked up to a kidney machine for the rest of my life."
Nurse: "You've been thinking about all kinds of things that could go wrong, and it adds to your worry not to be told what your blood sugar is."
Summarizing to let patient "hear" what he has communicated
Patient: "I always think the worst."
(Shakes head in exasperation)
Expressing insight into his "inner dialogue"
Nurse: "I'll pass along to the technician that it's okay to tell you your glucose levels. And later this afternoon I'd like us to talk more about some things you can do to help avoid these complications and set some goals for controlling your glucose."
Providing information, encouraging collaboration, and goal setting

communication analysis of such a record. Analysis of a process recording enables you to evaluate the following:
- Determine whether you encouraged openness and allowed the patient to "tell his or her story," expressing both thoughts and feelings.
- Identify any missed verbal or nonverbal cues or conversational themes.
- Examine whether your responses facilitated or blocked the patient's efforts to communicate.
- Determine whether your responses were positive and supportive or superficial and judgmental.

- Examine the type and number of questions asked.
- Determine the type and number of therapeutic communication techniques used.
- Discover any missed opportunities to use humor, silence, or touch.

Through the Patient's Eyes. One form of evaluation is to determine a patient's perception of the success of the plan of care in facilitating communication. You determine together which strategies or interventions were effective and which patient changes (behaviors or perceptions) resulted because of the interventions. Ask the patient whether you and other members of the interprofessional health care team met expectations. For example, does the patient believe that nurses responded in a timely way when the nurse call system was activated? Does the patient feel able to express needs clearly with the new communication techniques that were introduced? Is the patient satisfied with the information that has been provided about his condition or hospitalization? Successful nursing care related to patients' communication needs results in clear and effective communication between patients and all members of the health care team and can favorably impact patient satisfaction and the delivery of safe care.

Patient Outcomes. If expected outcomes for the patient's plan of care are not met or if progress is unsatisfactory, you determine which factors influenced the outcomes and modify the plan of care. If your evaluation data indicate that a patient perceives difficulty in communicating, you explore contributing factors so that they can be addressed. For example, if using a pen and paper is frustrating for a patient who is nonverbal and whose handwriting is shaky, you revise the care plan to include the use of a picture board instead. Possible questions you ask when a patient does not meet expected outcomes include:

- You seem to be having difficulty communicating right now. What do you think is contributing to this?
- You are telling me that you do not feel anxious right now, but your face appears tense. Help me better understand how you are feeling right now.
- You seem frustrated with the use of pencil and paper to communicate. Would you like to try a letter board or a picture board to see whether either of these is easier for you to use?

Evaluation of the communication process helps nurses gain confidence and competence in interpersonal skills. Becoming an effective communicator greatly increases your professional satisfaction and success. There is no skill more basic, and no tool more powerful.

KEY POINTS

- Nurses use critical thinking in communication by considering past experiences and knowledge and by interpreting messages received from others to obtain new information, correct misinformation, and make clinical judgments for patient-centered care.
- Nursing actions that reflect caring in communication include being present and encouraging the expression of positive and negative feelings, instilling faith and hope, and promoting patient advocacy.
- Nurses use the five levels of communication in their interactions: intrapersonal, interpersonal, small group, public, and electronic.
- The circular transactional model of communication demonstrates the ever-changing nature of communication, and includes the referent, sender and receiver, message, channels, feedback, interpersonal variables, and environment.
- Verbal communication involves spoken or written words, and the vocabulary, meaning, pacing, tone, clarity, brevity, timing, and relevance of a message.
- Nonverbal communication, which occurs through the five senses and includes everything except the written or spoken word, is unconsciously motivated and more accurately indicates a person's intended meaning than spoken words,
- There is a natural progression of four goal-directed phases—preinteraction, orientation, working, and termination—that characterize the nurse-patient relationship, even during a brief interaction.
- Effective health care team communication using an approach modeled by the acronym *SACCIA*—Sufficiency, Accuracy, Clarity,

Contextualization, and Interpersonal Adaptation—promotes working relationships that promote safe and effective care.

- Taking a patient-centered approach by seeking a patient's viewpoints and being aware of your own personal biases will help you assess and identify your patients' communication needs.
- Adapting your communication approach with older adults, such as encouraging them to share life stories and reminisce about the past, can enhance your assessment and promote an effective nurse-patient relationship.
- Use of both professional and therapeutic communication techniques contributes to achievement of patient outcomes. Practicing these techniques is essential in your development as a nurse.
- Nontherapeutic communication techniques damage professional and caring relationships; therefore pay attention to your own communication to remove these blocking techniques from your responses.
- Patients with special communication needs require you to use specific techniques to facilitate mutual understanding, such as listening intently without interruption and ensuring patients use special devices to hear and see messages clearly.
- Being aware of and analyzing the outcomes of your conversations with patients and the health care team and adapting your communication approach as needed helps ensure that patients meet their outcomes effectively.

REFLECTIVE LEARNING

- Compare and contrast the similarities and differences in factors that affect communication among two patients that you have cared for recently, and describe how you altered your own communication style to create an effective nurse-patient communication.
- Describe a recent interaction you witnessed between a nurse and other health care providers or a nurse and a patient. What verbal and nonverbal communication did you see during this exchange? What could have improved the effectiveness of the conversation?
- Describe a recent patient care or personal experience in which there was *Impaired Verbal Communication*. What were the impairments that you observed? How did or could you adjust communication to provide for mutual understanding and respect?

REVIEW QUESTIONS

1. When working with an older adult who is hearing-impaired, the use of which techniques would improve communication? (Select all that apply.)
   1. Check for needed adaptive equipment.
   2. Exaggerate lip movements to help the patient lip-read.
   3. Give the patient time to respond to questions.
   4. Keep communication short and to the point.
   5. Communicate only through written information.
2. A patient has gone through a number of treatment changes during a shift of care. During the hand-off report, the nurse plans to communicate effectively with the nurse who will be caring next for the patient for which of the following reasons? (Select all that apply.)
   1. To improve the nurse's status with the health team members
   2. To reduce the risk of errors to the patient
   3. To provide an optimum level of patient care
   4. To improve patient outcomes
   5. To prevent issues that need to be reported to outside agencies
3. A nurse is using motivational interviewing with a patient. What outcomes does the nurse expect? (Select all that apply.)
   1. Gain an understanding of the patient's health goals.

2. Direct the patient to avoid poor health choices.
3. Recognize the patient's strengths and support the patient's efforts.
4. Provide assessment data that can be shared with families to promote change.
5. Identify differences in patient's health outcomes and current behaviors.

4. Which techniques demonstrate a therapeutic response to an adult patient who is anxious? (Select all that apply.)
   1. Matching the rate of speech to be the same as that of the patient
   2. Providing good eye contact
   3. Demonstrating a calm presence
   4. Spending time attentively with the patient
   5. Assuring the patient that all will be well

5. A nurse prepares to contact a patient's health care provider about a change in the patient's condition. Put the following statements in the correct order using SBAR (Situation, Background, Assessment, and Recommendation) communication.
   1. "She is a 53-year-old woman who was admitted 2 days ago with pneumonia and was started on levofloxacin at 5 p.m. yesterday. She states she has a poor appetite; her weight has remained stable over the past 2 days."
   2. "The patient reported feeling very nauseated after her dose of levofloxacin an hour ago."
   3. "Is it possible to make a change in antibiotics, or could we give her a nutritional supplement before her medication?"
   4. "The patient started to complain of nausea yesterday evening and vomited several times during the night."

6. A patient states, "I don't have confidence in my doctor. She looks so young." What is the nurse's therapeutic response?
   1. Tell me more about your concern.
   2. You have nothing to worry about. Your doctor is perfectly competent.
   3. You can go online and see how others have rated your doctor. I do that.
   4. You should ask your doctor to tell you her background.

7. The nurse applying effective communication skills throughout the nursing process should: (Place the following interventions in the correct order.)
   1. Validate health care needs through verbal discussion with the patient.

2. Compare actual and expected patient care outcomes with the patient.
3. Provide support through therapeutic communication techniques.
4. Complete a nursing history using verbal communication techniques.

8. A nurse works with a patient using therapeutic communication during all phases of the therapeutic relationship. Place the nurse's statements in order according to these phases.
   1. The nurse states, "Let's work on learning injection techniques."
   2. The nurse is mindful of biases and knowledge in working with the patient with B$_{12}$ deficiency.
   3. The nurse summarizes progress made during the nursing relationship.
   4. After providing introductions, the nurse defines the scope and purpose of the nurse-patient relationship.

9. Which strategies should a nurse use to facilitate a safe transition of care during a patient's transfer from the hospital to a skilled nursing facility? (Select all that apply.)
   1. Collaboration between staff members from sending and receiving departments
   2. Requiring that the patient visit the facility before a transfer is arranged
   3. Using a standardized transfer policy and transfer tool
   4. Arranging all patient transfers during the same time each day
   5. Relying on family members to share information with the new facility

10. What outcome demonstrates the effective use of silence as a therapeutic communication technique?
    1. The nurse feels like there was enough time to be therapeutic when communicating with the patient.
    2. The patient states a preference to talk with another staff member.
    3. The patient perceives having gained insight into the issue after the conversation.
    4. The patient was able to drift off to sleep more easily.

Answers: 1. 1, 3, 4; **2.** 2, 3, 4; **3.** 1, 3, 5; 4, 2, 3, 4; **5.** 4, 5; 1B, 2A, 3R; **6.** 1; **7.** 4, 1, 3, 2; **8.** 2, 4, 1, 3; **9.** 1, 3; **10.** 3.

Rationales to Review Questions can be found on the Evolve website.

REFERENCES

Agency for Healthcare Research and Quality (AHRQ): *Health literacy universal precautions toolkit*, ed 2, 2020. https://www.ahrq.gov/health-literacy/improve/precautions/tool5.html. Accessed April 24, 2021.

Arnold E, Boggs KU: *Interpersonal relationships: professional communication skills for nurses*, ed 8, St Louis, 2020, Saunders.

Borden E: Looking within: using cultural humility in communications, *Oncol Nurse Advis* 9(1):28, 2018.

Brandt C, et al: Determinants of successful eHealth coaching for consumer lifestyle changes: qualitative interview study among health care professionals, *JMIR* 20(7):76, 2018.

Centers for Disease Control and Prevention (CDC): CDC estimates U.S. hearing loss prevalence at 16 percent. *ASHA Leader* 23(2):14, 2018.

Centers for Disease Control and Prevention (CDC): *Vision loss: a public health problem*, 2020. https://www.cdc.gov/visionhealth/basic_information/vision_loss.htm. Accessed April 24, 2021.

Dickison P, et al: Integrating the national council of state boards of nursing clinical judgment model into nursing educational frameworks, *J Nurs Educ* 58(2):72, 2019.

Giger JN, Haddad LC: *Transcultural nursing: assessment and intervention*, ed 8, St. Louis, 2021, Elsevier.

Gultekin A, et al: The effect of assertiveness education on communication skills given to nursing students, *Int J Caring Sci* 11(1):395, 2018.

Hannawa AF: "SACCIA Safe Communication": five core competencies for safe and high-quality care, *J Patient Saf Risk Manag* 23(3):99, 2018.

Institute for Healthcare Improvement (IHI): *ISBAR trip tick*, 2021. http://www.ihi.org/resources/Pages/Tools/ISBARTripTick.aspx. Accessed April 24, 2021.

International Council of Nurses: International Classification for Nursing Practice (ICNP®). *Nursing diagnosis and outcome statements*, 2019. https://www.icn.ch/sites/default/files/inline-files/ICNP2019-DC.pdf. Accessed April 24, 2021.

Koosey S, et al: National patient safety consortium: learning from large-scale collaboration, *Healthc Q* 22:10, 2020.

Lillykutty MJ, Samson R: Insights from Kristen M Swanson's Theory of Caring, *AJNER* 8(1):173, 2018.

Manfrida G, et al: Connected: recommendations and techniques in order to employ internet tools for the

enhancement of online therapeutic relationships. Experiences from Italy, *Contemp Fam Ther* 39(4):314, 2017.

Mills CB, et al: No laughing matter: workplace bullying, humor orientation, and leadership styles, *Workplace Health Saf* 67(4):159, 2019.

Pawlowski P, et al: Nursing dress code and perception of a nurse by patients, *Nurs 21st Cent* 18(1):60, 2019.

Schlögl M, Jones CA: Maintaining our humanity through the mask: mindful communication during COVID-19, *J Am Geriatr Soc* 68(5):E12, 2020. https://www.ncbi.nlm.nih.gov/pmc/articles/PMC7262056/. Accessed April 24, 2021.

Sethi D, Rani MK: Communication barrier in health care setting as perceived by nurses and patient, *Int J Nurs Educ* 9(4):30, 2017.

Stewart KR: SBAR, communication, and patient safety: an integrated literature review, *Medsurg Nurs* 26(5): 297, 2017.

Stickley T: From SOLER to SURETY for effective nonverbal communication, *Nurse Educ Pract* 11:395, 2011.

Streelman M, Staffileno BA: Reducing readmissions one handoff at a time: standardizing report from acute care to the post-acute care setting, *Medsurg Nurs* 30(2):83, 2021.

Studer Group: *AIDET patient communication,* 2021. https://www.studergroup.com/aidet. Accessed April 24, 2021.

Varcarolis E, Fosbre CD: *Essentials of psychiatric mental health nursing,* ed 4, St Louis, 2021, Elsevier.

RESEARCH REFERENCES

Bambi S, et al: Negative interactions among nurses: an explorative study on lateral violence and bullying in nursing work settings, *J Nurs Manag* 27(4):749, 2019.

Brown M, et al: Therapist-client interactions in motivational interviewing: the effect of therapists' utterances on client change talk, *Alcohol* 53(4):408, 2018.

Crossley SA, et al: Predicting the readability of physicians' secure messages to improve health communication using novel linguistic features: findings from the ECLIPPSE study, *J Commun Healthc* 13(4):344, 2020.

Gettis MA, et al: Bedside report: nursing handoffs impact outcomes for caregivers, healthcare providers, and organizations, *Worldviews Evid Based Nurs* 16(6):495, 2019.

Hada A, Coyer F: Shift-to-shift nursing handover interventions associated with improved inpatient outcomes—falls, pressure injuries and medication administration errors: an integrative review. *Nurs Health Sci* 23(2):337, 2021.

Jongerius C, et al: The measurement of eye contact in human interactions: a scoping review, *J Nonverbal Behav* 44:363, 2020.

Kim JH, et al: Patient safety culture and handoff evaluation of nurses in small and medium-sized hospitals. *Int J Nurs Sci* 8(2021):58, 2021.

Lorié A: Culture and nonverbal expressions of empathy in clinical settings: a systematic review, *Patient Educ Couns* 100(3):411, 2017.

Magil M, et al: Motivational interviewing technical process and moderated relational process with underage young adult heavy drinkers, *Psychol Addict Behav* 33(2):128, 2019.

Mormer E, et al: Hearing loss and communication among hospitalized older adults: prevalence and recognition, *J Gerontol Nurs* 46(6):34, 2020.

Mota Sousa LM, et al: Humor intervention in the nurse-patient interaction, *Rev Bras Enferm* 72(4):1136, 2019.

Newman-Casey PA, et al: A glaucoma-specific brief motivational interviewing training program for ophthalmology para-professionals: assessment of feasibility and initial patient impact, *Health Commun* 35(2):233, 2020.

Real K, et al: Patient perceptions and real-time observations of bedside rounding team communication: the interprofessional teamwork innovation model (ITIM), *Jt Comm J Qual Patient Saf* 46(7):400, 2020.

Sandström P, et al: 'I want to know why and need to be involved in my own care …': a qualitative interview study with liver, bile duct or pancreatic cancer patients about their experiences with involvement in care, *Support Care Cancer* 27(7):2561, 2019.

Simonovic S, et al: Bedside shift report enhances patient satisfaction for Hispanic and public insurance patients and improves visibility of leadership in obstetric and postpartum settings. *J Nurs Pract Appl Rev Res* 9(2):4, 2019.

Sullivan CE, et al: Reducing compassion fatigue in inpatient pediatric oncology nurses, *Oncol Nurs Forum* 46(3):338, 2019.

Sun C, et al: Exploring practices of bedside shift report and hourly rounding: is there an impact on patient falls? *J Nurs Adm* 50(6):355, 2020.

Tortosa-Alted R, et al: Emergency handover of critical patients: a systematic review. *Int Emerg Nurs* 56(2021):100997, 2021.

Patient Education

OBJECTIVES

- Identify the three purposes of patient education.
- Explain how the Speak Up Initiatives from The Joint Commission (TJC) promote patient participation in learning.
- Compare the communication process with the steps of the teaching process.
- Critique when nurses use the different domains of learning during patient instruction.
- Explore how basic learning principles influence a patient's learning.
- Identify factors that influence an adult's readiness to learn.
- Critique factors within a patient care environment that promote learning.
- Explain the relationship between self-efficacy and health promotion.

- Explain how clinical judgment influences delivery of patient education.
- Summarize how a nurse integrates assessment data regarding a patient's learning needs, motivation, readiness, and ability to learn to develop individualized teaching strategies.
- Compare the nursing and teaching processes.
- Explain the relevance of assessing a patient's health literacy.
- Explain how to prioritize outcomes for patient education.
- Create a teaching plan that progresses logically and promotes learning.
- Design an environment conducive for learning for patients who have low health literacy.
- Apply the teach-back method during evaluation of a teaching plan.

KEY TERMS

Affective learning
Analogies
Attentional set
Cognitive learning
Health literacy

Learning
Learning objective
Motivation
Psychomotor learning
Reinforcement

Return demonstration
Self-efficacy
Teach-back
Teaching

MEDIA RESOURCES

http://evolve.elsevier.com/Potter/fundamentals/
- Review Questions
- Audio Glossary

- Case Study with Questions
- Content Updates
- Answers to QSEN Activity and Review Questions

Patient education is one of the most important nursing interventions in any health care setting. Shorter hospital stays, increased demands on nurses' time, an increased number of patients living with chronic illnesses, and the need to give acutely ill patients meaningful information quickly emphasize the importance of high-quality patient education. As nurses try to find the best way to educate patients, the public has become more assertive in seeking knowledge about health concerns, understanding health, and finding resources available within the health care system. Through education, nurses empower their patients to prevent acute and chronic disease, decrease disability, and improve wellness (Miller and Stoeckel, 2019). Patient education is a component of the Teaching-Learning domain of nursing practice (see Chapter 19), aimed at enhancing a patient's quality of life, improving self-care, reducing hospital admissions, and improving treatment adherence (Flanders, 2018).

Patients have the right to know and be informed about their health risks, diagnoses, prognoses, and available treatments to help them make intelligent, informed decisions about their health and lifestyle. Part of patient-centered care is to make the appropriate clinical judgments

needed to identify patients' educational needs and then integrate educational approaches that acknowledge patients' understanding of their own health. A well-designed, comprehensive teaching plan provides a good fit with each patient's unique learning needs and ultimately changes behaviors to improve patient outcomes. In due course the information gained helps patients make informed decisions about their care and become healthier and more independent (Flanders, 2018).

PURPOSES OF PATIENT EDUCATION

The primary goal of patient education is to help individuals, families, or communities achieve optimal levels of health (Miller and Stoeckel, 2019). Patient education through active patient participation and decision making is essential for providing safe, patient-centered care (Quality and Safety Education for Nurses [QSEN], 2020). In addition, providing education about preventive health care helps reduce health care costs for individuals. Patients learn ways to change their lifestyles (e.g., diet, exercise, stop smoking) to prevent chronic disease and reduce the effects of chronic illnesses and associated medical care. Because most patients now know more about their health, they want to be actively involved in their health maintenance. Comprehensive patient education includes three important purposes, each involving a separate phase of health care: health promotion and illness prevention, health restoration, and coping.

Maintenance and Promotion of Health and Illness Prevention

As a nurse you are a visible, competent resource for patients who want to improve their physical and psychological well-being. In the school, home, clinic, or workplace you provide information and skills to help patients adopt healthier behaviors. For example, in childbearing classes you teach expectant parents about physical and psychological changes in a woman. After learning about normal childbearing, the mother who applies new knowledge is more likely to eat healthy foods, engage in physical exercise, and avoid substances that can harm the fetus. An adult with obesity and a family history of diabetes can learn about the effects diabetes has on health and adopt improved diet and exercise habits to avoid development of the disease. Success in patient education is not the ability of a patient to simply recall information that is provided, but also the ability of the patient to incorporate knowledge into everyday life activities in a way that promotes health.

Restoration of Health

Patients recovering from and adapting to changes resulting from illness or injury often seek information about their conditions and need information and skills to help them regain or maintain their levels of health. Nurses who work in home health and rehabilitation settings have the opportunity to educate patients using strategies that promote self-care. However, some patients find it difficult to adapt to illness and become disinterested in learning. As a nurse you learn to identify patients' willingness to learn and motivate your patients' interest in learning (Bastable, 2019). The family often is a vital part of a patient's return to health if a patient chooses to involve them. Family caregivers usually require as much education as patients, including information on how to perform skills within the home. If you exclude a family from a teaching plan, conflicts can occur. However, do not assume that a family caregiver should be involved; assess the patient-family relationship before providing education for family caregivers.

Coping With Impaired Functions

Not all patients fully recover from illness or injury. In addition, patients with preexisting mental illness or those who have lower literacy skills have difficulty understanding patient education (Bastable, 2019). Many patients with impaired function need to learn to cope with permanent health alterations. New knowledge and skills are often necessary for patients to continue activities of daily living. For example, a patient loses the ability to speak after larynx surgery and needs to learn new ways of communicating. Changes in function are physical and/or psychosocial of the patient. In the case of serious disability such as following a stroke or a spinal cord injury, the patient's family (as defined by the patient) needs to understand and accept many changes in the physical capabilities of the patient. The family's ability to provide support results in part from education, which begins as soon as you identify the patient's needs and the family displays a willingness to help. Teach family members to help the patient with health care management (e.g., giving medications through gastric tubes and doing passive range-of-motion exercises). Families of patients with alterations such as alcohol use disorder, intellectual disability, or substance abuse disorder learn to adapt to the emotional effects of these chronic conditions and provide psychosocial support to facilitate the patient's health. Comparing a realistic desired level of health with the actual state of health enables you to identify deficits and needs and then plan effective teaching programs.

TEACHING AND LEARNING

It is impossible to separate teaching from learning. Teaching is the concept of imparting knowledge through a series of directed activities. It consists of a conscious, deliberate set of actions that help individuals gain new knowledge, change attitudes, adopt new behaviors, or perform new skills (Billings and Halstead, 2020). An effective educator is knowledgeable about the subject matter and patient teaching principles in order to provide individuals with guidance, appropriately set the learning pace, and creatively introduce concepts to successfully achieve the objectives of new knowledge, behaviors, or changed attitudes.

Learning is defined as a "conscious or unconscious permanent change in behavior as a result of a lifelong, dynamic process by which individuals acquire new knowledge, skills, and/or attitudes that can be measured and can occur at any time or in any place through exposure to environmental stimuli" (Bastable, 2019). It is a process of both understanding and applying newly acquired concepts. For example, an adult exhibits learning when he demonstrates how to set up his weekly pillbox correctly. He shows transfer of learning when he demonstrates how to set up his wife's pillbox. Teaching and learning begin when a person identifies a need for knowing or acquiring an ability to do something. Teaching is most effective when it responds to a learner's needs. An educator assesses these needs by asking questions and determining a learner's interests. Interpersonal communication is essential for successful teaching (see Chapter 24).

Role of the Nurse in Teaching and Learning

Nurses are legally responsible for providing education to all patients, regardless of gender, culture, age, literacy level, religion, or any other defining characteristics (Bastable, 2019). The American Hospital Associated published the document *The Patient Care Partnership* in 2003 to help patients understand what their expectations should be with regards to being patients within hospitals (AHA, 2003). The document indicates that patients have the right to participate in making informed decisions about their care. The information required to make informed decisions must be accurate, complete, and relevant to patients' needs, language, and health literacy. Medicare (Medicare.gov, n.d.) also has standards for residents' rights in nursing homes, including the right to be informed about one's medical condition and medications and the right to see one's own doctor.

The Joint Commission's (TJC's) Speak Up campaign helps patients understand their rights when receiving medical care and supports them to become more active participants in their care by asking questions (TJC, 2021a). The process makes them more aware of their rights and increases the chance that they will get the care they need when they need it. The program offers the following Speak Up tips to help patients become more involved in their treatment (TJC, 2019):

- **S**peak up if you have questions or concerns. If you still do not understand, ask again. It is your body, and you have a right to know.
- **P**ay attention to the care you get. Always make sure that you are getting the right treatments and medicines from the right health care professionals. Do not assume anything.
- **E**ducate yourself about your illness. Learn about the medical tests that are prescribed and your treatment plan so you can make informed decisions.
- **A**sk a trusted family member or friend to be your advocate (adviser or supporter).
- **K**now about your new medicine(s) and why you take them. Medication errors are the most common health care mistakes.

BOX 25.1 EVIDENCE-BASED PRACTICE

Effectiveness of the Teach-Back Method to Reduce Hospital Readmissions

PICOT Question: In adult patients who are discharged from the hospital, does use of the teach-back method compared with standard review of teaching content result in fewer hospital readmissions?

Evidence Summary

There is a nationwide focus on how to improve care transitions from the hospital to home or treatment center, such as a nursing home or rehabilitation center. The Centers for Medicare and Medicaid Services (CMS) has sponsored more than 100 projects to explore the best practice in terms of care transitions. Specifically, researchers have examined the frequency of hospital readmissions, reflecting concern over how well patients are prepared for discharge. There has been some improvement on this issue. The frequency of Medicare patients being readmitted within 30 days of discharge dropped from 16.7% in 2010 to 15.7% in 2017 (Rau, 2019). Effective education that includes ensuring the patient understands the discharge plan may decrease the likelihood of readmission by 30% (Almkuist, 2017). One approach to ensuring patient understanding is the teach-back method. A recent systematic review and meta-analysis of discharge education with the teach-back method for hospitalized patients yielded only three studies. However, the combined results showed a 45% reduction in 30-day readmission rates (Oh et al., 2021). Research has also involved patients with ambulatory care conditions, showing that patient teach-back is associated with a reduced risk of hospitalization, especially among patients with cardiovascular diseases and type 2 diabetes mellitus (Hong et al, 2019).

A systematic review of patients with chronic disease identified improved outcomes in disease-specific knowledge, adherence, and self-efficacy, with a positive but inconsistent trend in improved self-care and reduction of hospital readmission rates when patients understood discharge information (Ha et al., 2016). Some studies focused on specific patient diagnoses, such as heart failure, while other studies have looked at generalized patient populations. For example, heart failure affects approximately 6.2 million people (CDC, 2020). A study of the National Readmission Database showed that 18.2% of patients hospitalized for heart failure had a readmission within 30 days, and 31.2% of patients with heart failure had a readmission within 90 days (Khan et al., 2021). Almkuist et al. (2017) conducted a systematic review of patients with heart failure and found that using the teach-back method during discharge reduced readmission rates and improved self-care abilities and increased the patient's and family's knowledge about a specific disease. Use of teach-back is a standard approach for evaluating patient understanding of instructions. Its use reduces the complexity of health care by increasing patient understanding of health information and enhancing support for patients at all degrees of health literacy (AHRQ, 2020).

Application to Nursing Practice

- To implement teach-back, you ask patients or family members to explain in their own words what they need to know or do (AHRQ, 2020).
- Implement the teach-back method when teaching about complex chronic illnesses, such as diabetes, asthma, and heart failure (Oh et al, 2021; Almkuist, 2017).
- Examples of teach-back questions include (AHRQ, 2017):
  - "Just to be safe, I want to make sure we are on the same page. Can you tell me . . .?"
  - "I want to make sure that I explained things clearly. Can you explain to me . . .?"
  - "Can you show me how you would use your . . . (e.g., inhaler, blood pressure manometer) at home?"
- Not using the teach-back method can lead to gaps in understanding between health care providers, patients, and family caregivers.

- *U*se a hospital, clinic, surgery center, or other type of health care organization that you have researched or checked carefully.
- *P*articipate in all decisions about your care. You are the center of the health care team.

The Speak Up program also offers materials and messages that patients have found to be well organized and succinct, and that have a visual component (TJC, 2021a). Patients are advised that they have a right to be informed about the care they will receive, obtain information about care in their preferred language, know the names of their caregivers, receive treatment for pain, receive an up-to-date list of current medications, and expect that they will be heard and treated with respect.

Your role as a nurse is to teach information that patients and their families need and understand. You will learn in the nursing process section of this chapter how to identify patients' learning needs, identify the primary problems associated with those needs, and select the appropriate teaching interventions. When you value and provide education, patients are better prepared to assume health care responsibilities. Nursing research about patient education strategies supports the positive impact of patient education on patient outcomes (Box 25.1).

Teaching as Communication

The teaching process closely parallels the communication process (see Chapter 24) (Fig. 25.1). Effective teaching depends in part on effective interpersonal communication. An educator applies each element of the communication process while providing information to learners. Thus the educator and learner become involved together in a teaching process that increases the learner's knowledge and skills.

The Communication Process

FIG. 25.1 The communication process.

The steps of the teaching process are similar to those of the communication process. You use patient requests for information or identify a need for information because of a patient's health restrictions, recent diagnosis of an illness, or a recent injury. Then you identify specific learning objectives to describe the behaviors the learner will exhibit as a result of successful instruction (Bastable, 2019). Those objectives serve the same role as outcomes when delivering physical and psychological care (see Chapter 18).

The nurse begins as the sender who conveys a message to the patient (see Fig. 25.1). Many intrapersonal variables influence your style and approach. Attitudes, values, emotions, cultural perspective, and knowledge influence the way information is delivered. Past experiences with teaching are also helpful for choosing the best way to present necessary content.

The receiver in the teaching-learning process is the learner. A number of intrapersonal variables affect a patient's motivation and ability to learn. Patients are ready to learn when they express a desire to do so and are more likely to receive your message when they understand the content. Attitudes, anxiety, physical symptoms, health literacy, and values influence the ability to understand a message. The ability to learn depends on factors such as emotional and physical health, education, cultural perspective, patients' values about their health, the stage of development, and previous knowledge.

Effective communication involves feedback from the sender and receiver. An effective educator delivers instruction and then provides a mechanism (e.g., teach-back) for evaluating the success of a teaching plan by gaining feedback from the receiver (Bastable, 2019). If the feedback demonstrates learning, the educator returns feedback in the form of reinforcement. This type of response reinforces health behavior and promotes continued self-management. You provide feedback both during and at the completion of each instructional encounter. Feedback needs to affirm the level of success of the learner in achieving objectives (i.e., the learner successfully verbalizes information or provides a return demonstration of skills learned). Feedback you receive from the learner indicates the effectiveness of instruction and whether you need to modify your approach.

DOMAINS OF LEARNING

Learning occurs in three domains: cognitive (understanding), affective (attitudes), and psychomotor (motor skills) (Bastable, 2019). The most effective learning takes place when all three of these domains are used (Miller and Stoeckel, 2019). Your use of all domains will depend on the instructional topic required. You often work with patients who need to learn in each domain. For example, a patient who has undergone surgery for colon cancer and who has to manage an ostomy needs to learn how the ostomy is affected by diet, medications, and activity (cognitive domain). In addition, this same patient begins to learn coping skills to accept the change in body image created by the ostomy (affective domain). The patient with an ostomy also needs to learn how to change an ostomy pouch and provide skin care (psychomotor domain). An effective educator will find ways to incorporate instructional methods that merge domains. For example, while changing an ostomy pouch the nurse explains the steps but also explores the patient's feelings about the ostomy. The characteristics of learning within each domain influence your teaching and evaluation methods. Understanding each learning domain prepares you to select proper teaching techniques and apply the basic principles of learning (Box 25.2).

Cognitive Learning

Cognitive learning occurs when an individual gains information to further develop intellectual abilities, mental capacities, understanding, and thinking processes (Bastable, 2019). Bloom's revised taxonomy of six cognitive behaviors is a hierarchy that increases in complexity (Anderson and Krathwohl, 2001; Krathwohl, 2002) (Fig. 25.2). The taxonomy is used to assess learning at a variety of cognitive levels and to then use strategies to promote higher-order thought in students by building on lower-level cognitive skills. Each simpler skill is a prerequisite to mastery of the next more complex one. For example, knowledge or remembering has to be mastered before someone can master the higher level of understanding or comprehension. Each of the cognitive behaviors is divided into subcategories. For example, remembering (formerly *Knowledge*) includes factual, conceptual, procedural, and metacognitive knowledge (Krathwohl, 2002). The revised taxonomy for cognitive learning includes:

- Remember (formerly *Knowledge*): Recognizing or recalling knowledge from memory

---

BOX 25.2 Appropriate Teaching Methods Based on Domains of Learning

Cognitive
- Discussion (one-on-one or group)
  - Involves nurse and one patient or a nurse with several patients
  - Promotes active participation and focuses on topics of interest to patient
  - Allows peer support
  - Enhances application and analysis of new information
- Lecture
  - Is more formal method of instruction because it is educator controlled
  - Helps learner acquire new knowledge and gain comprehension
- Question-and-answer session
  - Addresses patient's specific concerns
  - Helps patient apply knowledge
- Role-play, discovery
  - Allows patient to actively apply knowledge in controlled situation
  - Promotes synthesis of information and problem solving
- Independent project (computer-assisted instruction), field experience
  - Allows patient to assume responsibility for completing learning activities at own pace
  - Promotes analysis, synthesis, and evaluation of new information and skills

Affective
- Role-play
  - Allows expression of values, feelings, and attitudes
- Discussion (group)
  - Allows patient to receive support from others in group
  - Helps patient learn from others' experiences
  - Promotes responding, valuing, and organization
- Discussion (one-on-one)
  - Allows discussion of personal, sensitive topics of interest or concern

Psychomotor
- Demonstration
  - Provides presentation of procedures or skills by nurse
  - Permits patient to incorporate modeling of nurse's behavior
  - Allows nurse to control questioning during demonstration
- Practice
  - Gives patient opportunity to perform skills using equipment in a controlled setting
  - Provides repetition
- Return demonstration
  - Permits patient to perform skill as nurse observes
  - Provides excellent source of feedback and reinforcement
  - Assists in determining patient's ability to correctly perform a skill or technique
- Independent projects, games
  - Requires teaching method that promotes adaptation and origination of psychomotor learning
  - Permits learner to use new skills

- Understand (formerly *Comprehension*): Constructing meaning from different types of messages or activities, such as interpreting, exemplifying, classifying, summarizing, inferring, comparing, or explaining
- Apply: Carrying out or using a procedure through executing or implementing
- Analyze: Breaking materials or concepts into parts, then determining how the parts relate to one another or how they interrelate, or how the parts relate to an overall structure or purpose
- Evaluate: Making judgments based on criteria and standards through checking and critiquing

FIG. 25.2 Bloom's taxonomy: Bloom versus Anderson/Krathwohl. (From Wilson LO: *Bloom's taxonomy revised,* 2020. https://thesecondprinciple.com/essential-teaching-skills/blooms-taxonomy-revised/ Accessed June 6, 2021).

- Create (formerly *Synthesis*): Putting elements together to form a coherent or functional whole; reorganizing elements into a new pattern or structure through generating, planning, or producing

Affective Learning

Affective learning deals with learning how to express feelings and emotions and to develop values, attitudes, and beliefs needed toward improving health (Billings and Halstead, 2020). Values clarification (see Chapter 22) is an example of affective learning. The affective domains of learning were developed by Krathwohl, Bloom, and Masia (Krathwohl et al., 1956) The simplest behavior in affective learning is receiving, and the most complex is characterizing. Affective learning includes the following (Wilson, 2021):

- Receiving: Learner is passive (not engaged) but is alert and willing to receive information.
- Responding: Requires active participation. This refers to a learner's active attention to stimuli, verbal and nonverbal responses, and motivation to learn.
- Valuing: Attaching worth and value to the acquired knowledge (e.g., new coping skills) as demonstrated by the learner's behavior through acceptance, preference, or commitment.
- Organizing: Developing a value system. Learner internalizes values and beliefs involving (1) the conceptualization of values and (2) the organization of a value system.
- Characterizing: Highest level of internalization. Acting and responding with a consistent value system; requires introspection and self-examination of one's own values in relation to an ethical issue or particular experience.

Psychomotor Learning

Psychomotor learning involves the development of manual or physical skills, such as learning how to walk or how to type on a computer (Billings and Halstead, 2020; Wilson, 2021). The simplest behavior in the hierarchy is fundamental (depending on the hierarchical model), whereas the most complex is origination. Psychomotor learning includes the following:

- Fundamental: Skills, movements, or behaviors related to walking, running, jumping, pushing, pulling, and manipulating. They are often components for more complex actions.
- Perception: Skills related to kinesthetic (bodily movements), visual, auditory, tactile (touch), or coordination abilities as they are related to the ability to take in information from the environment and react.

- Guided response: Early stages of learning a particular skill under the guidance of an instructor that involves imitation and practice of a demonstrated act.
- Mechanism: Higher level of behavior in which a person gains confidence and proficiency in performing a skill that is more complex or involves several more steps than a guided response.
- Complex overt response: Smoothly and accurately performing a motor skill that requires complex movement patterns.
- Adaptation: Motor skills are well developed and movements can be modified when unexpected problems occur.
- Origination: Using existing psychomotor skills to create new movement patterns and perform them as needed in response to a particular situation or problem.

When assessing a patient's knowledge, clinical situation, and learning needs, consider the patient's current level within the domain(s) you choose to focus on instructionally. Select teaching approaches that will aid the patient in achieving a higher level of performance in that domain. For example, before teaching a patient how to use a walker, assess the fundamental skills: Can the patient walk independently or bear weight? Then use strategies to progress the patient to guided response, the behavior in which the patient uses the walker with assistance. As the patient gains confidence in using the walker, the patient will progress to mechanism, which is the behavior that shows patient proficiency in using the walker.

BASIC LEARNING PRINCIPLES

To teach effectively and efficiently you must know the principles that influence how a person learns (Bastable, 2019). Achievement of the desired learning outcomes (objectives) depends on a number of principles, including an individual's motivation, readiness and ability to learn, and the environment where learning will take place. The ability to learn depends on physical and cognitive attributes, developmental level, physical wellness, and intellectual thought processes. All of these principles influence your teaching approach.

A person's learning style often affects preferences for learning. People process information in a number of ways: through seeing, touch, and hearing; reflecting and acting; reasoning logically and intuitively; and analyzing and visualizing. Effective teaching plans incorporate a combination of activities that target a variety of learning styles (Savage et al., 2017; Miller and Stoeckel, 2019). When you tailor your teaching approach to meet your patient's needs and learning style, you optimize your patient's learning experience.

Motivation to Learn

Motivation is an internal state (e.g., an idea, emotion, or a physical need) that helps arouse, direct, and sustain human behavior (Miller and Stoeckel, 2019). A patient's motivation to learn is influenced by a belief in the need to know something. Patients who need knowledge for survival have a stronger motivation to learn than patients who need it for promoting health (Bastable, 2019). Unfortunately, not all people are interested in maintaining health. Many do not adopt new health behaviors or change unhealthy behaviors unless they perceive a disease as a threat, overcome barriers to changing health practices, and see the benefits of adopting a healthy behavior. For example, some patients with lung disease continue to smoke. A person's therapy is more effective when the person believes that health is important and that the therapy will improve health.

Motivational interviewing (MI) is a counseling and educational technique that focuses on a patient's perceived goals and helps people resolve insecurities and ambivalent feelings (e.g., nonadherence) to find the internal motivation needed to change their behavior (SAMHSA, 2018; *Psychology Today*, n.d.). It is patient centered, based on the principle that the motivation for change must come from the patient rather than the health care provider. As health care providers we may think we know what a patient "needs to learn." However, if the information we choose to deliver does not meet a patient's own personal goals or values, teaching efforts are often ineffective. Studies have shown that this intervention works well with individuals who start off unmotivated or unprepared for change (*Psychology Today*, n.d.; Faghihian et al., 2020).

Current evidence shows MI is effective in addressing lifestyle behaviors such as diet, exercise, and smoking cessation, as well as the psychosocial needs of patients living with cancer (Spencer and Wheeler, 2016). The technique also helps patients manage type 2 diabetes and arterial hypertension (Steffen et al., 2021). MI is also effective in outpatient care settings with improvement in patient adherence to oral chemotherapy and self-efficacy for adherence to drug therapy as well as screening for breast and cervical cancer (Cakmak and Kapucu, 2021; Chan and So, 2021). The objective of MI is not to solve a patient's problem or even to develop a plan. MI aims to encourage a patient's autonomy in decision making, with the clinician acting as a guide—clarifying patients' strengths and aspirations, listening to their concerns, boosting their confidence in their ability to change, and eventually collaborating with them on a plan for behavioral change (Souders, 2021). MI interview questions are also useful in the assessment process for determining patients' learning needs. The role of the interviewer is primarily to evoke a conversation about change and commitment (*Psychology Today*, n.d.).

Use of Theory to Enhance Motivation and Learning.
Health education often involves changing attitudes and values that are not easy to change simply through transfer of information. Using theory-based interventions when developing patient education plans can be very useful. Learning theories focus on how individuals learn. Such theories are typically based on learning research. The use of theory facilitates the teaching-learning process by creating the desired climate for learning and guiding the selection of appropriate instructional strategies. Because patient education is complex, there are different theories and models available to guide it (Table 25.1). Using a theory that matches a patient's problems and personal learning preferences helps you select interventions that have the best chance of helping the patient become an active participant.

Among the various theories, social learning theory is one of the most useful approaches to patient education. It considers the personal characteristics of the learner, behavioral patterns, and the environment and guides the educator in developing effective teaching interventions that motivate and enhance learning (Bastable, 2019). According to social learning theory, a person's state of mind and intrinsic motivational factors (i.e., sense of accomplishment, pride, or confidence) reinforce behaviors and influence learning (Miller and Stoeckel, 2019). This type of internal reward system allows a person to attain desired outcomes and avoid undesired outcomes, resulting in improved motivation. Self-efficacy, a concept included in social learning theory, refers to a person's perceived ability to successfully complete a task. When people believe that they can achieve a particular behavior, they are more likely to perform the behavior consistently and correctly. Motivational interviewing techniques incorporate self-efficacy principles.

Self-efficacy beliefs come from four sources: verbal persuasion, vicarious experience, enactive mastery experience, and psychological and affective states (Bandura, 1997; Miller and Stoeckel, 2019). For example, a nurse who is teaching a child recently diagnosed with asthma how to correctly use an inhaler expresses personal belief in the child's ability to use the inhaler (verbal persuasion). Then the nurse demonstrates how to use the inhaler (vicarious experience). Once the demonstration is complete, the child uses the inhaler (enactive mastery experience). As the child's wheezing and anxiety decrease after the correct use of the inhaler, the child experiences positive feedback, further enhancing confidence to use it (physiological and affective states). Interventions such as these enhance perceived self-efficacy, which in turn improves the achievement of desired outcomes.

Self-efficacy is a concept included in many health promotion theories because it often is a strong predictor of healthy behaviors and because many interventions improve self-efficacy, resulting in improved lifestyle choices (Bandura, 1997). For example, Kate Lorig (2015), as the previous director of the Stanford Patient Education Research Center (now the Self-Management Resource Center), developed a Chronic Disease Self-Management Program based on self-efficacy theory. The program uses skill mastery, modeling, reinterpretation, and social persuasion to enhance a person's self-efficacy. Dr. Lorig's programs have been especially effective for patients with diabetes or chronic lung problems and those in cardiac rehabilitation (see Chapter 8). When nurses implement interventions to enhance self-efficacy, their patients frequently experience positive outcomes. For example, researchers associated increased self-efficacy scores and increased achievement of health goals when patients had follow-up education through telephone encounters over a period of 6 months (Zhou et al., 2018). In another study, researchers found that a self-care education program was effective at reducing all unplanned readmissions in patients with heart failure (Boyde et al., 2018).

Cultural Factors.
Knowing your patients' cultural preferences (see Chapter 9) and health beliefs (see Chapter 6) helps you develop patient-centered interventions that will motivate your patients to learn. Carefully assess a patient's cultural needs and preferences for instructional methods to enhance learning and adherence. Using a model such as ACCESS helps you to focus on cultural factors that influence patient education outcomes. The six ACCESS model components are (Purnell and Fenkl, 2019):

1. **Assessment** of a patient's lifestyle, health beliefs, cultural traditions, and health practices
2. **Communication** with an awareness of the many variations in verbal and nonverbal responses
3. **Cultural** negotiation and compromise that encourages awareness of characteristics of a patient's culture and one's own biases
4. **Establishment** of respect for a patient's cultural beliefs and values; creating a caring rapport
5. **Sensitivity** to how patients from diverse backgrounds perceive their care needs and the patterns of communication they use
6. **Safety** that enables patients to feel culturally secure and avoids disempowerment of their cultural identity

TABLE 25.1   Learning Theories

Learning Theory	Definition	Application
Cognitive Dissonance	Individuals desire consistency and will make necessary changes and adaptations to gain that consistency (Festinger, 1957). Cognitive dissonance refers to a situation involving conflicting attitudes, beliefs, or behaviors that produces mental discomfort leading to an alteration in one of the attitudes, beliefs, or behaviors to reduce the discomfort and restore life balance (McCleod, 2018).	A patient with a recent myocardial infarction (MI) faces stressors associated with potential and actual health risks and changes needed as result of diagnosis. There are lifelong implications. The patient needs to change beliefs, attitudes, and values to regain consistency in life during recovery.
Health Belief Model	Patients will perceive a certain susceptibility and severity of their disease. Modifying factors include knowledge, as well as demographics and social and psychological variables. Likelihood of action is based on the perceived barriers and benefits of the situation (Hochbaum, 1958). The Health Belief Model is a framework for motivating people to take positive health actions that uses the desire to avoid a negative health consequence as the prime motivation.	How a patient who has an MI copes with illness will depend on all modifying factors. If the patient does not feel threatened, believes there will not be a benefit from interventions, or is not confident that the interventions will be effective in the management of the condition, the patient may not be as receptive to teaching.
Transtheoretical Model of Change	Model is used to define how individuals initiate change in their lives, progress through those changes, and process and maintain behaviors. There are five stages in the model: precontemplation, contemplation, preparation, action, and maintenance (Prochaska, et al., 1998).	If a patient has experienced serious damage to the heart and requires cardiac rehabilitation, there are lifestyle changes to consider, such as diet, exercise, and medication management. With each stage of the model the patient makes decisions weighing the pros and cons and probable outcomes. Positive outcomes must outweigh negative aspects of change.
Self-Efficacy	Model focuses on the patient's belief in the ability to make and maintain changes and positive outcomes in the patient's life (Bandura, 1977). Self-efficacy is based on self-confidence and is a good indicator for motivation to make behavioral changes.	A patient who is discharged home with an MI must provide some level of self-care. Break down any skill into manageable steps with encouragement and support from others. The patient moves from self-doubt and anxiety to comfort and confidence in own abilities.
Health Promotion	Model is based on the premise that characteristics and experiences of an individual affect actions specific to behaviors and in turn affect outcomes specific to behavior (Pender, 1975). The model applies general information from social learning theory to build on the nursing perspective of the holistic patient.	The behaviors of a patient who has an MI are driven by prior health promotion behaviors, as well as personal factors (biological, psychological, and sociocultural). Patients must be active participants in initiating and maintaining health promotion.

Adapted from Syx RL: The practice of patient education: the theoretical perspective, *Orthop Nurs* 27(1):50, 2008.

Active Participation. Learning occurs when a patient is motivated to be actively involved in an educational session (Edelman and Kudzma, 2018). A patient's involvement in learning implies an eagerness to acquire knowledge or skills. It also improves the opportunity for the patient to make decisions during teaching sessions. For example, when teaching car seat safety during a parenting class, hold a teaching session in the parking lot where the participants park their cars. Encourage active participation by providing the learners with several different car seats for them to place in their cars. At the completion of this session, the parents are able to determine which type of car seat fits best in their cars and which is the easiest to use. This provides participants with the information needed to purchase the appropriate car seat.

Readiness to Learn

Readiness to learn is based on a patient's willingness to engage in learning (Miller and Stoeckel, 2019). Many factors affect readiness to learn. A loss of health is usually very difficult for patients to accept. Grief is a complex process that patients experience during illness and loss (see Chapter 36). The process of grieving gives individuals time to adapt psychologically to the emotional and physical implications of their illnesses or loss. Readiness to learn is affected by each stage of grieving (Table 25.2). Patients cannot learn when they are unwilling or unable to accept a loss or their illness. Appropriately timed teaching using the right approaches during the grieving process facilitates adjustment to illness, loss, or disability.

A patient's physical health status also affects readiness to learn. Patients move along a continuum of health. As a patient moves along this continuum, the readiness to learn changes as well (Miller and Stoeckel, 2019). For example, a patient who is acutely ill is concerned with survival and will likely be most interested in a treatment plan before learning about long-term implications of illness. After a stroke, a patient will be most ready to learn about self-care skills when the patient is receiving rehabilitation care.

An **attentional set** is the mental state that allows a learner to focus on and comprehend a learning activity. Before learning anything, patients must be able to pay attention to or concentrate on the information to be learned. Physical discomfort, anxiety, confusion, and environmental distractions influence the ability to concentrate. Therefore determine a patient's level of comfort before beginning a teaching plan, and ensure that the patient is able to focus on the information. As anxiety increases, a patient's ability to pay attention often decreases. A mild level of anxiety can be conducive to learning. However, a high level of anxiety prevents learning from occurring. At times when a patient is unable to attend, a family caregiver often becomes the recipient of education. Simple facts, rather than detailed teaching strategies, are most important during these times. For example, a patient in pain is receptive

TABLE 25.2 Psychosocial Adaptation to Illness, Grief, and Learning

Stage	Patient's Behavior	Learning Implications for Nurse and Family Caregiver	Rationale
Denial or disbelief	Patient avoids discussion of illness ("I'm fine; nothing is wrong with me"), withdraws from others, and disregards physical restrictions. Patient suppresses and distorts information that has not been presented clearly.	Provide support, empathy, and careful explanations of all procedures while they are being done. Remain available and accessible for discussion. Explain situation to family or significant other if appropriate. Teach in present tense (e.g., explain current therapy).	Patient is not prepared to deal with problem. Any attempt to convince or tell patient about illness or loss results in further anger or withdrawal. Provide only information patient pursues or absolutely requires.
Anger	Patient blames and directs anger toward nurse or others.	Do not argue with patient. Listen to concerns. Use good eye contact. Teach in present tense. Reassure family and significant others that patient's anger is normal.	Patient needs opportunity to express feelings and anger; patient is still not prepared to face future.
Bargaining	Patient offers to live better life in exchange for promise of better health. ("If God lets me live, I promise to quit smoking.")	Continue to introduce only reality. Teach only in present tense.	Patient is still unwilling to accept limitations.
Resolution	Patient begins to express emotions openly, realizes that illness has created changes, and begins to ask questions.	Encourage expression of feelings. Find out what patient wants to learn. Begin to share information needed for future and set aside formal times for discussion.	Patient begins to perceive need for assistance and is ready to be responsible for learning.
Acceptance	Patient recognizes reality of condition, actively pursues information, and strives for independence.	Focus teaching on future skills and knowledge required. Continue to teach about present occurrences. Involve family/significant other in teaching information for discharge.	Patient is more easily motivated to learn. Acceptance of illness reflects willingness to deal with its implications.

to learning about how to use a patient-controlled analgesia pump but not how to use crutches.

Ability to Learn

A patient's developmental level and cognitive and physical capabilities influence the ability to learn. In addition, the learning environment is a significant factor affecting learning ability.

Developmental Capability. Cognitive development influences a patient's ability to learn. You can be a competent educator, but if you do not consider a patient's intellectual abilities, your teaching is unsuccessful. Learning, like developmental growth, is an evolving process. Assess a patient's level of knowledge and intellectual skills (e.g., simple problem solving, decision making, applying a concept such as infection control in the home) before beginning a teaching plan. Learning occurs more readily when new information complements existing knowledge. For example, measuring liquid or solid food portions requires the ability to perform mathematical calculations. When caring for a patient in the home setting, first determine whether the patient understands what a portion consists of and then observe the patient prepare the liquid or solid food. Reading a medication label or discharge instructions requires reading and comprehension skills. Assessing a patient's health literacy will help determine the patient's existing ability.

Learning in Children. The capability for learning and the type of behaviors that children are able to learn depend on the child's maturation (see Chapter 12). Without proper physiological, motor, language, and social development, many types of learning cannot take place. In addition, every child learns in different ways. However, learning occurs in children of all ages. Intellectual growth moves from the concrete to

the abstract as the child matures. Therefore information presented to children needs to be understandable, and the expected outcomes must be realistic based on the child's developmental stage (Box 25.3). Remember that a child's developmental stage may not correspond to the child's chronological age. Use teaching methods that are evidence-based. Some evidence-based teaching strategies include using visuals in explanations, providing examples for multi-step problems, giving students time to practice doing new things, and giving feedback (Killian, 2019). Use teaching aids that are developmentally appropriate (Fig. 25.3). Learning occurs when behavior changes as a result of experience or growth (Miller and Stoeckel, 2019).

Adult Learning. Teaching adults differs from teaching children. Adults are able to critically reflect on their current situation but sometimes need help to see their problems and change their perspectives. Because adults become independent and self-directed as they mature, they are often able to identify their own learning needs (Billings and Halstead, 2020). Learning needs come from problems or tasks that result from real-life situations. Although adults tend to be self-directed learners, they often become dependent in new learning situations, such as receiving a new diagnosis or being prescribed a new medication. The amount of information you provide and the amount of time you spend with an adult patient varies depending on the patient's personal situation and readiness to learn. An adult's readiness to learn is often associated with developmental stage and other events that are occurring in life. Help patients resolve any needs they perceive as important so that learning can occur.

Adults have a wide variety of personal life experiences. Adult learners do best when asked to both use their previous experiences and apply new knowledge to solve real-life problems (Billings and Halstead, 2020). Adult learners are more successful when they view the information as

BOX 25.3 Teaching Methods Based on Patient's Developmental Capacity

Infant
- Keep routines (e.g., feeding, bathing) consistent.
- Hold infant firmly while smiling and speaking softly to convey sense of trust.
- Have infant touch different textures (e.g., soft fabric, hard plastic).

Toddler
- Use play to teach procedure or activity (e.g., handling examination equipment, applying bandage to doll).
- Offer picture books that describe story of children in hospital or clinic.
- Use simple words such as "cut" instead of "laceration" to promote understanding.

Preschooler
- Use role-play, imitation, and play to make learning fun.
- Encourage questions and offer explanations. Use simple explanations and demonstrations.
- Encourage children to learn together through pictures and short stories about how to perform hygiene.

School-Age Child
- Teach psychomotor skills needed to maintain health. (Complicated skills such as learning to use a syringe take considerable practice.)
- Offer opportunities to discuss health problems and answer questions.

Adolescent
- Help adolescent learn about feelings and need for self-expression.
- Use teaching as collaborative activity.
- Allow adolescents to make decisions about health and health promotion (safety, sex education, substance abuse).
- Use problem solving to help adolescents make choices.

Young or Middle Adult
- Encourage participation in teaching plan by setting mutual goals.
- Encourage independent learning.
- Offer information so adult understands effects of health problem.

Older Adult
- Teach when patient is alert and rested.
- Involve adult in discussion or activity.
- Focus on wellness and person's strength.
- Use approaches that enhance patient's reception of stimuli when there is a sensory impairment (see Chapter 49).
- Keep teaching sessions short.

FIG. 25.3 The nurse uses developmentally appropriate food models to teach healthy eating behaviors to the school-age child. (Copyright © iStock.com/alkir.)

personally relevant and important to their daily lives (Billings and Halstead, 2020). For example, if you instruct a patient to limit certain activities after surgery, learn what activities a person normally performs that may conflict with the restrictions. Find ways that will help the patient adhere to the restrictions. Assessing what an adult patient currently knows or does and what the patient wants to know and setting mutual learning objectives improve the outcomes of patient education (Bastable, 2019).

Health Literacy and Learning Disabilities. Research shows that not only is health literacy a strong predictor of a person's health status, but it is also a stronger predictor compared with several other factors, including age, income, employment status, educational level, and race (Parnell, 2015; National Library of Medicine [NLM], n.d.). The World Health Organization (WHO, 2021) defines **health literacy** as the cognitive and social skills that determine the ability of individuals to gain access to, understand, and use information in ways that promote and maintain good health. The Centers for Disease Control and Prevention (CDC) define personal health literacy as the degree to which individuals have the ability to find, understand, and use information and services to inform health-related decisions and actions for themselves and others (CDC, 2021a). Health literacy pertains not only to a patient's ability to read and comprehend health-related information but also to having the skills to problem solve, articulate, and make appropriate health care decisions (Parnell, 2015; CDC, 2021a). People most likely to be at risk for low health literacy include older adults, minority populations, immigrant populations, people of low income, people without a high school education, and people with chronic mental and/or physical health conditions (NLM, n.d.). According to the National Assessment of Adult Literacy, 9 out of 10 adults struggle to understand and use health information if it is unfamiliar, is complex, or uses jargon (CDC, 2021b). This means 90% of the population is at risk for lacking the skills needed to manage their health and prevent disease. To compound the problem, research has shown that health materials are often written at complex levels that are not understandable and exceed not only the general public's reading level but also the reading level of average high school graduates (Parnell, 2015; CDC, 2021c). This discrepancy results in unsafe health care. Health literacy is one of the most important predictors of health outcomes. Low health literacy can lead to more emergency department visits, along with more hospital admissions and readmissions (Miller and Stoeckel, 2019). To ensure patient safety, all health care providers need to ensure that information is presented clearly and in a culturally sensitive manner (TJC, 2019). Many people need printed health information at a fifth-grade level or lower, and people often read at a level or two lower than their highest level of education (Miller and Stoeckel, 2019).

Physical Capability. Readiness to learn often depends on a patient's level of physical development and overall physical health. Many factors impair the ability to learn, including preexisting physical or mental illness, fatigue, body temperature, electrolyte imbalance, oxygenation status, and blood glucose level. To learn psychomotor skills a patient must possess a certain level of strength, coordination, and sensory acuity. For example, it is useless to teach a patient to transfer from a bed to a wheelchair if the patient has insufficient upper body strength. An older patient with poor eyesight or the inability to grasp objects tightly cannot learn to apply an elastic bandage. Therefore do not overestimate the patient's physical development or status. The following physical characteristics are necessary to learn psychomotor skills:

- Size (patient's height and weight should match the task to be performed or the equipment being used)
- Strength (ability of the patient to follow a strenuous exercise program)
- Coordination (dexterity needed for complicated motor skills such as using utensils or changing a bandage)
- Sensory acuity (visual, auditory, tactile, gustatory, and olfactory; sensory resources needed to receive and respond to messages taught)

Determining a patient's ability to perform psychomotor skills is best assessed by a physical therapist or occupational therapist. Also, consider how a patient adapts any physical limitations to performing skills at home.

Any condition or symptom (e.g., pain, nausea, or fatigue) that depletes a patient's energy also impairs the ability to learn. For example, a patient who spends a morning having rigorous diagnostic studies is unlikely to be able to learn later in the day because of fatigue. Postpone teaching when an illness becomes aggravated by complications such as a high fever or respiratory difficulty. As you work with a patient, assess energy level by noting the patient's willingness to communicate, the amount of activity initiated, and responses to questions. Temporarily stop teaching if the patient needs rest. You achieve better outcomes when patients are physically able to actively participate in learning.

Learning Environment

Factors in the physical environment where teaching takes place make learning either a pleasant or a difficult experience (Bastable, 2019). The ideal setting helps a patient focus on the learning task. The number of people included in the teaching session; the need for privacy; the room temperature; and the lighting, noise, ventilation, and furniture in the room are important factors when choosing a setting. The ideal environment for learning is well lit and has good ventilation, appropriate furniture, and a comfortable temperature. A darkened room interferes with a patient's ability to watch your actions, especially when demonstrating a skill or using visual aids such as posters or pamphlets. A room that is cold, hot, or stuffy makes a patient too uncomfortable to focus on the information being presented.

It is also important to choose a quiet setting. A quiet setting offers privacy; infrequent interruptions are best. Provide privacy even in a busy hospital by closing cubicle curtains or taking the patient to a quiet spot. Family caregivers often need to share in discussions in the home setting. However, patients who are reluctant to discuss the nature of the illness when others are in the room benefit from receiving education in a room separate from household activities, such as a bedroom.

Teaching a group of patients requires a room that allows everyone to be seated comfortably and within hearing distance of the educator. Make sure that the size of the room does not overwhelm the group. Arranging the group to allow participants to observe one another further enhances learning. More effective communication occurs as learners observe others' verbal and nonverbal interactions.

CLINICAL JUDGMENT IN PATIENT EDUCATION

Because patient education is very complicated given the patient and the information you plan to teach, critical thinking paired with good clinical judgment is necessary. Your knowledge of a patient's health condition and the patient information you gain from assessment will allow you to predict the topic and level of instruction required. In addition your clinical judgment will allow you to determine the best time for teaching, the resources to use, and how to engage the patient. To be an effective educator, you need to do more than just pass on facts. Carefully determine what patients already know, what they need to know, and their learning preferences, and then find the time to educate them when they are ready to learn. Your experience in patient education will be invaluable in matching patient educational needs with the right instructional approaches and knowing when to deliver them.

Critical thinking in patient education involves standards. Patient education has long been a standard for professional nursing practice. All state nurse practice acts recognize that patient teaching falls within the scope of nursing practice (Bastable, 2019). In addition, various accrediting agencies set guidelines for providing patient education in health care institutions. For example, TJC (2021b) sets standards for patient and family education. These standards require nurses and all health care providers to assess patients' learning needs and provide education on a variety of topics, including medications, nutrition, use of medical equipment, pain management, and the patient's plan of care. Other standards include professional organizations' clinical guidelines and protocols, which often include educational topics that are standards of care for select patient conditions. Implementing patient education standards successfully requires collaboration among health care professionals and enhances patient safety.

The environment as a learning principle was discussed earlier. However, the health care setting itself is a significant factor in a nurse's success in being able to provide patient education. In acute care settings, patients' lengths of stay have been on the decline for many years. Patients are sicker when hospitalized. Thus the quality time available for teaching in acute care is very limited. Managing this requires you to identify patients' potential learning needs as early as possible following hospital admission. This is easier when a patient has a condition that is seen routinely on a patient care unit. For example, patients who undergo major joint replacement have very specific guidelines to follow after discharge, and nurses can begin education early. In contrast, patients whose conditions are more complicated or unclear may not have obvious learning needs until a day before discharge. In clinic, home care, and rehabilitation settings, nurses have more time to identify patients' learning needs and to provide comprehensive ongoing education. In an acute care setting, learn the resources a patient has (e.g., family caregivers) as early as possible, engage those individuals early in instruction, and confirm with patients and family caregivers what is most important for them to learn and be prepared to return home.

❖ NURSING PROCESS

Apply critical thinking when performing the nursing process so you can provide a patient-centered teaching plan. There are distinct similarities between the nursing process and the teaching process. During the assessment phase of the nursing process, you determine a patient's health care needs (see Unit 3). Like the nursing process, the teaching process requires assessment—in this case identifying a patient's learning needs, motivation, and ability to learn. Your findings regarding the knowledge, skill, or behavioral change that a patient needs to learn will lead to a nursing diagnostic statement. An example is *Lack of*

Knowledge regarding a newly diagnosed condition or status related to insufficient information (e.g., *Lack of Knowledge related to insufficient information about postoperative recovery*). A diagnosis such as *Anxiety* will often identify factors interfering with learning. Instead of outcomes, you develop specific learning objectives for a teaching plan. The nursing and teaching processes differ in that the nursing process requires assessment of all sources of data to determine a patient's total health care needs. The teaching plan focuses on a patient's learning needs as they relate to the patient's health and functional status, and on a patient's motivation, ability, and readiness to learn.

Implementation involves the use of appropriate patient-centered and evidence-based teaching strategies. Incorporate learning principles as they specifically apply to each patient, to ensure that your patient acquires the necessary knowledge and skills. Finally, the teaching process requires an evaluation of learning, including patient feedback based on learning objectives. Table 25.3 compares the teaching and nursing processes.

◆ Assessment

Through the Patient's Eyes. When providing patient education, it is important to partner with the patient to ensure safe, compassionate, and coordinated care (QSEN, 2020). This means that during the assessment you determine a patient's expectations for learning and expectations for any teaching encounter. What type of information does the patient (or family caregiver) perceive will be needed to maintain self-care at home or in a transitional care setting? What type of information is needed to enable the patient to monitor recovery correctly? Assess the patient's preferences, values, and expressed needs in order to see the health care situation through the patient's eyes (QSEN, 2020). In this way you gain a better appreciation of your patient's knowledge, expectations, and preferences for learning. Teaching will be more effective.

Learning Needs. Learning needs are defined as "gaps in knowledge that exist between a desired level of performance and the actual level of performance" (Miller and Stoeckel, 2019). Box 25.4 provides examples of specific assessment questions to use in determining a patient's unique learning needs.

Sometimes nurses use formal educational assessment tools to determine their patients' perceived learning needs. At other times they identify their patients' expectations during routine assessments. Patients often identify their own learning needs on the basis of the

implications of living with their illness. For example, a patient diagnosed with Parkinson disease learns that it is progressive and needs to know how to adapt to the physical changes that develop.

To identify patients' learning needs, assess what patients view as important information to know. A patient who has a need to know something is likely to be receptive to information presented. For example, new parents need to know how to care for their baby. Therefore they are often very receptive to information about infant care (e.g., how to feed the infant and make sure that the infant gets enough sleep).

Determine information that is critical for patients to learn. Reflect on your knowledge of the physiological and pathological effects of various diseases and the impact those effects have on health management. Learning needs change, depending on a patient's current health status. Because health status is dynamic, assessment is an ongoing activity. Assess the following:
- Information or skills needed by a patient to perform self-care and to understand the implications of a specific health problem. For example, you teach a young man who has just entered high school how to prevent sexually transmitted infections (STIs).
- Patient experiences (e.g., new or recurring problem, past hospitalization) that influence the motivation and need to learn.
- Information that family caregivers require to support the patient's needs. The amount of information needed depends on the patient's health status and extent of a family member's role in helping the patient.

Motivation to Learn. Ask questions to identify and define a patient's motivation. These questions determine whether a patient is prepared and willing to learn. Assess the following factors:
- Behavior (e.g., attention span, tendency to ask questions, memory, and ability to concentrate during the teaching session).
- Health beliefs and sociocultural background: Norms, values, experiences, and traditions all influence a patient's beliefs and values about health and various therapies, communication patterns, and perceptions of time (see Chapter 9).
- Perception of the severity and susceptibility of a health problem and the benefits and barriers to treatment.
- Identification of patient outcomes for learning, which must originate from the patient and not be imposed from outside by health care providers.

TABLE 25.3 Comparison of the Nursing and Teaching Processes

Basic Steps	Nursing Process	Teaching Process
Assessment	Collect data about patient's physical, psychological, social, cultural, developmental, and spiritual needs from patient, family, diagnostic tests, medical record, nursing history, and literature.	Gather data about patient's physical and psychological health condition (problems requiring patient management), learning needs, motivation, ability to learn, health literacy, and teaching resources from patient, family, learning environment, medical record, nursing history, and literature.
Nursing diagnosis	Identify appropriate nursing diagnoses on basis of assessment findings.	Identify patient's learning needs on basis of three domains of learning. Nursing diagnoses may identify learning needs or conditions that interfere with learning.
Planning and outcomes identification	Develop an individualized care plan. Set diagnosis priorities on basis of patient's expected outcomes. Collaborate with patient on care plan.	Establish learning objectives stated in behavioral terms. Identify priorities regarding learning needs. Collaborate with patient about teaching plan. Identify type of teaching method(s) to use.
Implementation	Perform nursing care therapies. Include patient as active participant in care. Involve family/significant other in care as appropriate.	Implement teaching methods. Actively involve patient in learning activities. Include family caregiver as appropriate.
Evaluation	Identify success in meeting expected outcomes of nursing care. Alter interventions as indicated when outcomes are not met.	Determine outcomes of teaching-learning process. Measure patient's achievement of learning objectives. Reinforce information as needed.

BOX 25.4　Nursing Assessment Questions

Motivation to Learn

- Tell me what is most important for you to learn about _____?
- If you had one habit that you wanted to change to improve your health, what would that be?
- What goal for your health would you like to set that you are willing to achieve?
- Listen reflectively—let patients express their thoughts and then, instead of telling them what they need to learn, capture the essence of what they have said, with the purpose of eliciting conversation and helping them arrive at an idea for change.

Readiness to Learn

- Describe for me any physical discomfort or anxiety you may be feeling.
- Assess patient's ability to attend to questions raised during assessment.

Ability to Learn

- Assess patient's developmental status in relationship to being able to intellectually understand instruction.
- Assess if patient uses visual or auditory aids.
- Assess if the patient has physical characteristics that make learning psychomotor skills difficult.

Previous Learning and Identification of Learning Needs and Preferences

- What do you know about your illness and your treatment plan?
- Which experiences have you had in the past that are similar to those you are experiencing now?
- Together we can choose the best way for you to learn about your disease. How can I best help you?
- When you learn new information, do you prefer to have it given to you in pictures or written down in words?
- When you give someone directions to your house, do you tell the person how to get there, write out the instructions, or draw a map?

Self-Management

- Tell me how you believe your illness will affect your current lifestyle?
- Which barriers currently exist that prevent you from managing your illness the way you would like to manage it?
- What role do you believe your health care providers should take in helping you manage your illness or maintain health?
- How involved do you want a family member to be in the management of your illness? Who is that family member?

Cultural and Spiritual Influences

- Which cultural or spiritual beliefs do you have about your illness and its treatment?

For Family Caregivers

- When are you available to help, and how do you plan to help your loved one?
- Your spouse needs some help. How do you feel about learning how to assist?
- Tell me how you feel about performing the care activities that your family member requires.
- Do you think you will need some assistance to provide the right type of support for your family member? If so, what information about home care would be helpful?

- Perceived ability to perform needed health behaviors.
- Desire to learn.
- Attitudes about health care providers (e.g., role of patient and nurse in making decisions).
- Learning style preference: As the nurse, any educational effort will be more effective if the chosen method of instruction aligns with your patient's preferred learning style (Billings and Halstead, 2020). Education may require more than one instructor, as each instructor may excel at different types of teaching (verbal versus role-playing). Patients who are visual-spatial learners enjoy learning through pictures, visual charts, or any exercise that allows them to visualize concepts. The verbal/linguistic learner demonstrates strength in the language arts and therefore prefers learning by listening to or reading information. Kinesthetic learners process knowledge by moving and participating in hands-on activities. Role-play and return demonstrations are popular activities for the kinesthetic learner. Patients who learn through logical-mathematical reasoning think in terms of cause and effect and respond best when required to predict logical outcomes. If a patient is unable to identify a preferred learning style, delivering a combination of strategies will be more effective than just focusing on one type of learning style.

Readiness and Ability to Learn. Determine a patient's physical and cognitive ability to learn. Health care providers often underestimate patients' cognitive and physical deficits. Assess the following factors:

- Cognitive function, including memory, knowledge, association, and judgment.
- The cognitive domain of learning currently mastered by a patient. If you know your instruction will involve a cognitive skill, for example, first assess what a patient knows about the topic. Based on Bloom's taxonomy, knowledge or remembering has to be mastered before someone can master the higher level of understanding or comprehension. For example, a patient who has type 1 diabetes mellitus must learn knowledge about insulin and its effects before you can educate the patient to understand implications for adherence. Assess a patient's current level within the domain(s) you choose to focus on instructionally. Consider what approaches to use to aid the patient in achieving a higher level of performance in that domain.
- The psychomotor domain of learning currently mastered by a patient. Assess physical strength, endurance, movement, dexterity, and coordination (see Chapter 30) if you anticipate educating patients about psychomotor skills. For example, determine the extent to which a patient can perform skills by having the patient practice with equipment that will be used in self-care at home.
- Sensory deficits, such as visual or hearing loss, that can affect a patient's ability to understand or follow instruction (see Chapter 49).
- Patient's reading level: This is often difficult to assess because patients who are functionally illiterate are often able to conceal it by using distractors such as not having the time to read or not being able to see the print. Two ways to assess a patient's reading level and level of understanding are to ask the patient to read instructions from an educational handout and then explain their meaning or to complete a health literacy screening tool (see the discussion of health literacy later).
- Patient's developmental level, which influences the selection of teaching approaches (see Box 25.6). Consider age-appropriate abilities.
- Pain, fatigue, depression, anxiety, or other physical or psychological symptoms that interfere with the ability to maintain attention and participate: In acute care and rehab settings a patient's physical condition can easily prevent a patient from learning.

You are creating a teaching plan for your local community regarding road safety. The plan will be presented at a weekly community safety class for older adults and for a group of sixth graders at a local school. How do you differentiate your teaching plan for adults versus children?

Environmental Factors. Assess the environment for any barriers to learning. Assess the following environmental factors:

- Distractions or persistent noise: A quiet area is essential for focusing on the topic and effective learning.
- Comfort of the room, including ventilation, temperature, lighting, furniture, and size.
- Room facilities and available equipment.

Resources for Learning. A patient often requires the support of family members or significant others. Determine who is the patient's primary family caregiver. If this support is necessary, assess the readiness and ability of family caregivers to learn the information necessary and to physically be able to provide for the care of the patient. Also review resources within the home environment and community. Assess the following:

- Patient's willingness to have family caregivers involved in the teaching plan and provide health care: Information about a patient's health care is confidential unless the patient chooses to share it. Sometimes it is difficult for a patient to accept the help of family caregivers, especially when bodily functions are involved.
- Family caregiver's perceptions and understanding of a patient's illness and its implications: Conflict occurs in a teaching plan if the family caregiver's perceptions do not match those of the patient.
- Family caregiver's willingness and ability to participate in care: If a patient chooses to share health status information with family members, they need to be responsible, willing, and physically and cognitively able to assist in care activities such as bathing or administering medications. Not all family members meet these requirements.
- Resources, including financial or material, such as having the ability to obtain health care equipment.
- Knowledge of community resources, such as cardiac rehabilitation support groups.
- Teaching tools, including brochures, audiovisual materials, or posters: Materials should be current, be written clearly and logically, and match the patient's reading level.

Health Literacy. Because health literacy influences how you deliver teaching strategies, it is critical for you to assess a patient's health literacy before providing instruction. Assessing health literacy is challenging, especially in busy clinical settings where often there is little time to conduct a thorough assessment. TJC has a standard for the interprofessional team to identify a patient's health literacy needs and provide appropriate education to those people who have special health literacy needs (Jordan, 2016).

To assess health literacy, ask patients to perform simple literacy skills. For example, can a patient read a medication label back to you correctly? After you give a simple 1-minute explanation of a diet or exercise program, can the patient explain it back to you? Can a patient correctly describe the information provided in a written handout? A variety of screening tools are available to test literacy. The Agency for Healthcare Research and Quality (AHRQ, 2020) offers tools for assessment of health literacy, including Short Assessment of Health Literacy

(Spanish and English), Rapid Estimate of Adult Literacy in Medicine (REALM) (short form), and Short Assessment of Health Literacy for Spanish Adults. However, because these tools are self-reports for health literacy and thus subjective, researchers suggest other assessment methods be combined with literacy tools, such as interviews and observations, to increase the authenticity and objectivity of the data (Liu et al., 2018). The Brief Health Literacy Screen (BHLS) is an effective health literacy screening tool that is verbally administered to avoid problems with patients seeing or processing written materials on an assessment tool (Louis et al., 2017).

In addition to health literacy, assess patients for learning disabilities. For example, many self-care behaviors require an understanding of mathematics, including computation and fractions. If a learning disability impairs a patient's ability to effectively use mathematical skills, teaching is challenging, especially when trying to teach about complex medication dosages and frequencies. Although not considered a learning disability, attention-deficit/hyperactivity disorder (ADHD) also affects a patient's ability to learn. Patients with ADHD frequently experience inattention, hyperactivity, and impulsivity, which makes it difficult for them to stay focused during educational sessions, making learning challenging (CDC, 2021d).

Patients who have low health literacy or learning disabilities may be ashamed of not being able to understand you and often try to mask their inability to comprehend information. Therefore make sure that you are sensitive and maintain a therapeutic relationship with your patients while assessing their ability to learn. Appreciating the unique qualities of your patients helps to ensure safe and effective patient care (QSEN, 2020).

◆ Analysis and Nursing Diagnosis

After assessing information related to a patient's motivation, readiness, and ability to learn, interpret data and cluster assessment findings to form diagnoses that reflect specific learning needs or factors affecting the ability to learn (Box 25.5). Accurate diagnosis ensures that teaching will be directed at the appropriate health problem and any risks or related factors. If a patient has several learning needs, the nursing diagnoses guide priority setting. When the nursing diagnosis is *Lack of Knowledge,* the diagnostic statement describes the specific type of learning need and its cause (e.g., *Lack of Knowledge* regarding a surgical procedure). Providing a related factor (e.g., related to lack of recall and exposure to information) for a problem-oriented or negative diagnosis offers further specificity in how to design teaching strategies. Patients often require education to support resolution of their various health problems. Examples of nursing diagnoses that indicate a need for education include the following:

- Decisional Conflict
- Lack of Knowledge (Affective, Cognitive, Psychomotor)

BOX 25.5 Nursing Diagnostic Process

Lack of Knowledge (Psychomotor) Regarding Use of Crutches Related to Lack of Experience

Assessment Activities	Assessment Findings
Have patient describe what he knows about how to walk with crutches.	Patient states that he has not received information about use of crutches.
Have patient demonstrate ability to stand and bear weight.	Determines if patient has fundamental psychomotor skill needed to learn crutch walking.
Assess patient's level of attentiveness; observe behavior during discussion.	Patient remains attentive and asks questions about how to use crutches.

- Impaired Health Maintenance
- Impaired Ability to Manage Dietary/Exercise Regimen
- Self-Care Deficit

When you can manage or eliminate health care problems through education, the related factor of a diagnostic statement is *Lack of Knowledge.* For example, an older-adult woman is having difficulty managing a medication regimen that involves a number of newly prescribed medications that she has to take at different times of the day. The nursing diagnosis is *Impaired Health Maintenance regarding scheduling of medications related to lack of knowledge.* In this case educating the patient about her medications and the correct dosage schedules improves her ability to schedule and take them as directed. When you identify conditions that cause barriers to effective learning (e.g., nursing diagnosis of *Acute Pain* or *Activity Intolerance),* teaching is inappropriate. In these cases delay teaching until the nursing diagnosis is resolved or the health problem is controlled.

◆ Planning and Outcomes Identification

After determining the nursing diagnoses that identify a patient's learning needs, develop a teaching plan, determine expected outcomes, and involve the patient in selecting learning experiences. Expected outcomes of an education plan are learning objectives. They guide the choice of teaching strategies and approaches with a patient. Patient participation ensures a more relevant, meaningful plan.

Outcomes. Outcomes or learning objectives identify what a patient needs to achieve to gain a better understanding of a health care topic and to better manage illness (e.g., "achieves ostomy self-care"). Outcomes describe the specific behaviors that a patient must achieve, such as "empties colostomy bag correctly" and "describes diet options to reduce diarrhea." When developing outcomes, conditions or time frames need to be realistic and meet the patient's needs (e.g., "will identify the side effects of aspirin by discharge"). Consider conditions under which the patient or family will typically perform the behavior (e.g., "will walk from bedroom to bathroom using crutches"). Include the patient when establishing learning outcomes, and serve as a resource in setting the minimum criteria for success.

In some health care settings nurses develop teaching plans in the electronic health record. The teaching plan includes standard topics for instruction, resources (e.g., equipment, teaching booklets, and referrals to special educational programs), recommendations for involving family, and objectives of the teaching plan. Some plans are very detailed, whereas others are in outline form. Use the plan to provide continuity of instruction. The more specific the plan, the easier it is to follow.

The setting influences the complexity of any teaching plan. In an acute care setting, plans are concise and focused on the primary learning needs of the patient because there is limited time for teaching. Home care and outpatient clinic teaching plans are usually more comprehensive in scope because you often have more time to instruct patients and patients are often less anxious in outpatient settings.

Setting Priorities. Include a patient when determining priorities for patient education. Base priorities on a patient's nursing diagnoses or collaborative problems and the outcomes established. Priorities also depend on what a patient perceives to be most important, anxiety or physical comfort level, and the amount of time available to teach. You set a patient's learning needs in order of priority. For example, a patient recently diagnosed with coronary artery disease needs to be prepared to respond quickly when problems develop. The diagnosis *Lack of Knowledge regarding newly diagnosed illness* has an outcome of "patient will identify correct way to take nitroglycerin for chest pain." The same diagnosis also has an outcome of "patient will develop diet plan low

in saturated fat." The patient benefits most by first learning about the correct way to take nitroglycerin and how long to wait before calling for help when chest pain occurs. Once you assist in meeting patient priority needs related to basic survival, you can discuss other topics such as exercise and nutritional changes.

Timing. When is the right time to teach? Before a patient enters a hospital? When a patient first enters a clinic? At discharge? At home? Each is appropriate because patients continue to have learning needs before they enter a hospital or outpatient treatment center and for as long as they stay in the health care system. Plan teaching activities for a time when a patient is most attentive, receptive, and alert, and organize the patient's activities to provide time for rest and teaching-learning interactions.

In acute care settings, timing instruction is sometimes difficult because the emphasis is on a patient's timely discharge from a hospital. For example, it takes several hours after surgery for a patient to be alert and comfortable enough to learn. By the time a patient feels ready to learn, discharge is already scheduled. Limited time is available for short teaching sessions and opportunity for patient feedback. Therefore, to improve patient outcomes, when you work in an outpatient testing setting (for example), anticipate a patient's educational needs upon entry to the hospital to have surgery, and involve family caregivers if possible. Often when a patient has elective surgery, education occurs preoperatively (see Chapter 50).

Although prolonged teaching sessions reduce concentration and learner attentiveness, make sure that teaching sessions are not too brief. A patient needs time to comprehend the information and give feedback. It is easier for patients to tolerate and retain interest in the material during frequent sessions lasting 10 to 15 minutes. However, factors such as shorter hospital stays and lack of insurance reimbursement for outpatient education sessions often necessitate longer teaching sessions. Follow-up care in the form of referrals to home health or rehab can help provide continuity of instruction after a patient goes home.

The frequency of teaching sessions depends on a learner's abilities and the complexity of the material. For example, a child newly diagnosed with diabetes requires more visits to an outpatient center than the older adult who has had diabetes for 15 years and lives at home. Make sure that intervals between teaching sessions are not so long that the patient forgets information. Home care nurses frequently reinforce learning during home visits after patients are discharged from the hospital.

Organizing Teaching Material. An effective educator carefully considers the order of information to present. When a nurse has an ongoing relationship with a patient, as in the case of home health or case management, an outline of content helps organize information into a logical sequence. Material needs to progress from simple to complex because a person must learn the simple facts and concepts before learning how to make associations or complex interpretations of ideas. Staff nurses in acute care settings often focus on the simpler, more essential concepts, whereas home health nurses can better address complex issues. For example, a nurse plans to teach a wife how to feed her husband, who has a gastric tube. The nurse will first teach the wife how to measure the tube feeding and manipulate the equipment. Once the wife has accomplished this, instruction on how to administer the feeding will occur.

Begin instruction with essential content because patients are more likely to remember information that you teach early in a teaching session. For example, immediately after surgical removal of a malignant breast tumor, a patient has many learning needs. To ensure that all essential material is covered, start with content considered to be high priority, such as how to monitor an incision site for signs of infection. Deal with the emotional aspects of a cancer diagnosis, and complete the teaching session with informative but less critical content, such as how often follow-up appointments will occur. Repetition reinforces learning. A concise summary of key content helps the learner remember the most important information (Bastable, 2019). Using instructional materials that contain the same summaries is very helpful.

Teamwork and Collaboration. During planning choose appropriate teaching methods that match the topics to be presented. Encourage the patient to offer suggestions about timing and methods, and make referrals to other health care professionals (e.g., registered dietitians and physical, speech, or occupational therapists) when appropriate. As a nurse you are the member of the health care team primarily responsible for ensuring that all patient educational needs are met. However, sometimes patient needs are highly complex. In these cases identify appropriate health system educational resources available in the patient's community during planning. Examples of resources for patient education include diabetes education clinics, cardiac rehabilitation programs, prenatal classes, and support groups. When patients receive education and support from these types of resources, the nurse obtains a referral order (if necessary), encourages patients to attend educational sessions, and reinforces information taught. Resources that specialize in a particular health need (e.g., wound care or ostomy specialists) are integral to successful patient education.

REFLECT NOW

Your patient is a 44-year-old single man who was recently hospitalized due to an embolic stroke with residual left-sided weakness. He is left-handed and does not currently have any fine motor skills on the left side. He was found to have untreated hypertension and high cholesterol, so he was started on clopidogrel for secondary stroke prevention along with lisinopril for hypertension and atorvastatin for high cholesterol. What disciplines would you include when providing his discharge education?

◆ Implementation

The implementation methods for patient education depend on the accuracy of the nursing diagnoses identified for a patient's learning needs and your ability to critically think and judge if alterations need to be made in teaching strategies. Just as a patient's condition can change clinically, a patient's ability to learn can change. When you provide instruction you must continually assess how a patient is responding and judge if it is appropriate to continue instruction, adapt a strategy, or delay.

You create a teaching plan based on a patient's nursing diagnoses. Carefully evaluate the learning objectives, and determine which teaching and learning principles most effectively and efficiently help the patient meet expected outcomes. Each interaction with a patient is an opportunity to teach, whether you are taking vital signs, administering a medication, or providing comfort measures. Use evidence-based interventions to create an effective learning environment.

Maintaining Learning Attention and Participation. Active participation is key to learning. People learn better when more than one of the senses is stimulated. Audiovisual aids, group discussion, and role-playing are good teaching strategies. By actively experiencing a learning event, a person is more likely to retain knowledge. An educator's actions also increase learner attention and interest. When conducting a discussion with a learner, an educator stays active by changing the tone and intensity of the voice, making eye contact, and using gestures that accentuate key points of discussion. An effective educator engages learners, includes active learning strategies, and talks and moves among a group rather than remaining stationary

behind a lectern or table. A learner remains interested in an educator who is actively enthusiastic about the subject under discussion.

When a patient is anxious or inattentive, implement strategies such as relaxation and deep breathing to decrease the patient's anxiety (see Chapter 37). Have the patient practice these skills before instruction to improve comprehension and understanding once you begin instruction (Bastable, 2019). Also remember to manage any symptoms, such as pain or nausea, before beginning a teaching session so that a patient can better relax during instruction.

Building on Existing Knowledge and Ability. A patient learns best on the basis of preexisting cognitive, psychomotor, and affective intellectual and physical abilities. An assessment of the patient's learning needs will reveal the cognitive, psychomotor, or affective levels of learning that must take place. An educator is more effective when presenting information that builds on a learner's existing level. For example, a patient who has lived with multiple sclerosis for several years is able to remember, understand, and apply considerable information about the disease, its physical effects, and how to adapt self-care. The patient's wife provides valuable backup when needed. However, the patient is beginning a new medication that is given subcutaneously. Neither the patient nor his wife have experience giving an injection. Therefore new cognitive information about the medication is needed and psychomotor skills are required to self-administer an injection. Multiple sclerosis typically causes weakness and tremors in the hands. The nurse caring for the patient has already assessed that the patient has limited dexterity in the hands and difficulty picking up the syringe. The proper approach to implementation will require the nurse to teach the patient and his wife together how to prepare the medication and give an injection. Having a one-on-one discussion and reinforcing the information with a teaching pamphlet builds the patient's ability to understand and apply information about the new medication if problems develop. The nurse thus individualizes the teaching plan by building on the patient's previous knowledge and physical ability and incorporates the wife into the teaching plan.

Teaching Approaches. A nurse's teaching approach is different from teaching methods. Some situations require an educator to be directive. Others require a nondirective approach. An effective educator concentrates on the task and uses teaching approaches appropriate to the learner's needs. A learner's needs and motives frequently change over time. An effective educator is always aware of the need to modify teaching approaches.

Telling. Use the telling approach when there is limited time for teaching information (e.g., preparing a patient for an emergent diagnostic procedure). If a patient is highly anxious but it is vital for information to be given, telling is effective. When using telling, the nurse outlines the task that a patient will perform and gives simple, explicit instructions. There is no opportunity for feedback with this method.

Participating. In the participating approach a nurse and patient set objectives and become involved in the learning process together. The patient helps decide content, and the nurse guides and counsels the patient with pertinent information. In this method there is opportunity for discussion, feedback, mutual outcome setting, and revision of the teaching plan. For example, a parent caring for a child with leukemia must learn how to care for the child at home and recognize problems that need to be reported immediately. The parent and nurse collaborate on developing an appropriate teaching plan for how to recognize, understand and manage complications, maintain a healthy diet for the child, and maximize the child's ability to remain active. After each teaching session is completed, the parent and nurse review the objectives together, determine whether the objectives were met, and plan what will be covered in the next session.

Entrusting. The entrusting approach provides a patient the opportunity to manage self-care. The aim of the instructional approach is to provide the knowledge and skills that enable a patient to accept responsibilities and perform tasks correctly and consistently. The nurse observes the patient's progress and remains available to assist without introducing more new information. For example, a patient has been managing type 2 diabetes well for 10 years with oral medications, diet, and exercise. However, 1 year ago his diabetes changed, and it was difficult to control his hemoglobin A_{1c} level (which reflects glucose control). As a result, the oral medications were discontinued and insulin was added to his self-management plan. After initial instruction on dose management and injections, the nurse now monitors the patient's A_{1c} level monthly, offers reinforcement, and asks the patient if any new learning needs have developed. The nurse trusts that the patient has become self-sufficient with managing insulin doses and injections.

Reinforcing. Reinforcement requires the use of a stimulus to increase the probability of a desired response. A learner who receives reinforcement before or after a desired learning behavior is more likely to repeat that behavior. Reinforcers are positive or negative. Positive reinforcement such as a smile or verbal praise promotes desired behaviors. Although negative reinforcement such as frowning or criticizing can decrease an undesired response, it may also discourage participation and cause the learner to withdraw (Bastable, 2019). The effects of negative reinforcement are less predictable and often undesirable.

Reinforcers can come in the form of social acknowledgments (e.g., nods, smiles, words of encouragement), pleasurable activities (e.g., walks or play time), and tangible rewards (e.g., toys or food). Choosing an appropriate reinforcer to alter behavior requires careful observation of an individual's response to specific stimuli. When a nurse works with a patient, most reinforcers are social; however, material reinforcers may work well with young children. In adults, reinforcement is more effective when the nurse has established a therapeutic relationship with the patient. Whatever the form, it is important that reinforcement closely follow the desired behavior. Timing is essential so that a clear correlation between the desired behavior and reward is established (Bastable, 2019).

Incorporating Teaching With Nursing Care. Many nurses find that they are able to teach more effectively while delivering nursing care. This becomes easier as you gain confidence in your clinical skills. In addition, by recognizing environmental factors that might create barriers to any teaching session, teaching while delivering care is more efficient and time sensitive. For example, while hanging blood, you explain to the patient why the blood is necessary and the symptoms of a transfusion reaction that need to be reported immediately. Another example is to explain the side effects of a medication while administering it. An informal, unstructured style relies on the positive therapeutic relationship between nurse and patient, which fosters spontaneity in the teaching-learning process. Teaching during routine care is efficient and cost-effective (Fig. 25.4).

Instructional Methods. Choose instructional methods that match a patient's learning needs, the time available for teaching, the setting, the resources available, and your comfort level with teaching. Skilled educators are flexible in altering teaching methods according to a learner's responses. An experienced educator uses a variety of techniques and teaching aids. Specific teaching strategies should include open-ended questioning and problem-solving exercises (see Box 25.2). For example, when teaching patients about new medications:

- Have the patient consider the action of the medication and its effects. Is there a better time of day to take the medication, matching time with the patient's daily schedule?
- Have the patient interpret what to do if a dose of medication is missed for a day.

FIG. 25.4 Teaching postoperative care while walking with the patient uses time efficiently. (Copyright © iStock.com/kali9.)

- Have the patient develop a method to organize medications for a day, when multiple medications are prescribed.

Do not expect to be an expert educator when first entering nursing practice. Learning to become an effective educator takes time and practice and an active willingness to involve your patients. When first starting to teach patients, it helps to remember that patients perceive you as an expert. However, this does not mean that they expect you to have all of the answers. It simply means that they expect that you will keep them appropriately informed. Effective nurses keep the teaching plan simple and focused on patients' needs.

Verbal One-on-One Discussion. The most common method of instruction is a one-on-one verbal discussion. This approach involves sharing information directly with a patient. Verbal education of patients and family members requires an interprofessional approach that takes into account patients' learning styles, literacy, and culture to apply clear communication and instructional methods. This approach typically is done in an informal manner, allowing a patient to ask questions and share concerns. Speaking with a health care provider one on one is a preferred educational modality for many patients. However, education is ineffective if any verbal instruction is not done well. Apply critical thinking to be sure any instructional information is accurate, timely, complete, and relevant to patient needs. Be sure information is clear. Research has shown that verbal communication is often partly understood, misunderstood, or misinterpreted (Marcus, 2014). Performing teach-back is an effective way to determine a patient's level of understanding your instructions. Nurses today often do not have the time to fully listen to patients and engage in good-quality verbal instruction. The Brigham and Women's Faulkner Hospital (BWFH) Patient/Family Education Committee reviewed research on verbal instruction and developed the EDUCATE Model, which includes the following elements (Marcus, 2014):

- **E**nhance comprehension and retention—Collaborate with a patient to create a question list so that the patient can ask questions and you can answer them. Follow the teaching strategies in Box 25.6.
- **D**eliver patient-centered education—Talk *with*, and not *at*, a patient. Learn patients' values and preferences for education about their health. Practice empathetic skills, especially when the view of the patient is different from that of the provider.

BOX 25.6 PATIENT TEACHING

Teaching a Patient With Literacy or Learning Disability Problems

Objective
- Patient will perform desired behaviors accurately.

Teaching Strategies
- Establish trust with patient before beginning the teaching-learning session.
- Face patient when speaking. Sit at the patient's level to maintain eye contact.
- Speak slowly and invite patient participation. Encourage patient to ask questions and be involved in the conversation during visits and to be proactive in own health care.
- Use simple terminology. If necessary, explain medical terms using basic one- or two-syllable words. Use common words that you would use to explain medical information to your friends or family, such as stomach or belly instead of abdomen.
- Keep teaching sessions short and to the point and minimize distractions. Include the most important information at the beginning of the session and emphasize one to three key points.
- Teach in increments and organize information into sections.
- Provide teaching materials written in plain language that reflect the reading level of the patient, with attention given to short words and sentences, large type, and simple format (generally, information written on a fifth-grade reading level is recommended for adult learners).
- Show graphics: Draw pictures, use illustrations, or demonstrate with three-dimensional models. All pictures and models should be simple, designed to demonstrate only the important concepts, without detailed anatomy.
- Relate practical information to personal experiences or real-life situations.
- Use simple analogies or stories to personalize messages.
- Model appropriate behavior and use role-playing to help patient learn how to ask questions and ask for help effectively.
- Frequently ask patient for feedback to determine whether information is comprehended.
- Ask for return demonstrations, use the teach-back method, and clarify instructions when needed.
- Keep motivation high and recognize progress with positive reinforcement.
- Reinforce the most important information at the end of the session.
- Schedule teaching sessions at frequent intervals.

Evaluation
Use the principles of teach back to evaluate patient/family caregiver learning:
- I want to make sure I explained this information clearly. Please tell me why it is important for you to manage your illness.
- We discussed how it will be important for you to prepare a diet at home with the right type of foods. Let me see you prepare a sample menu for a breakfast, lunch, and dinner.

Data from Bastable S: *Nurse as educator: principles of teaching and learning for nursing practice*, ed 5, Burlington, 2017, Jones & Bartlett; and Agency for Healthcare Research and Quality (AHRQ): *AHRQ Health Literacy Universal Precautions Toolkit*, 2020, https://www.ahrq.gov/health-literacy/quality-resources/tools/literacy-toolkit/index.html. Accessed June 2021.

- **U**nderstand the learner—Build instruction based on what the patient already knows and wants to learn. Attend to nonverbal messages as you instruct the patient and gather feedback.
- **C**ommunicate clearly and effectively—Follow the teaching strategies in Box 25.6.
- **A**ddress health literacy.
- Measure outcomes of **T**eaching and **E**ducation—Know what is effective, adapt the approach based on the patient's ability to learn. Use teach-back.

Group Instruction. You may choose to teach patients in groups because of the advantages associated with group teaching. Groups are an economical way to teach a number of patients at one time. Patients are able to interact with one another and learn from the experiences of others. Learning in a group of six or fewer is most effective and avoids distracting behaviors (Bastable, 2019; Van Zant and Volpe, 2018). Group-based instruction benefits include deeper understanding, longer retention, increased social support, and more active participation (Bastable, 2019). Small-group instruction can provide a comfortable environment and boost the confidence of students who might not otherwise participate in a lesson or activity (Van Zant and Volpe, 2018). Group instruction often involves both lecture and discussion. Lectures are highly structured and efficient in helping groups of patients learn standard content about a subject. A lecture does not ensure that learners are actively thinking about the material presented; thus discussion and practice sessions are essential. After a lecture, learners need the opportunity to share ideas and seek clarification. Group discussions allow patients and families to learn from one another as they review common experiences. A productive group discussion helps participants solve problems and arrive at solutions toward improving each member's health. To be an effective group leader, you guide participation. Acknowledging a look of interest, asking questions, and summarizing key points foster group involvement. However, not all patients benefit from group discussions; sometimes the physical or emotional level of wellness makes participation difficult or impossible.

Preparatory Instruction. Patients frequently face unfamiliar tests or procedures that create significant anxiety about the procedure and outcome. Providing information about procedures often decreases anxiety because this gives patients a better idea of what to expect during their procedures, enhancing their sense of control. The known is less threatening than the unknown. Follow these guidelines for giving preparatory explanations:
- Describe physical sensations during a procedure. For example, when drawing a blood specimen, explain that the patient will feel a sticking sensation as the needle punctures the skin.
- Describe the cause of the sensation, preventing misinterpretation of the experience. For example, explain that a needlestick burns because the alcohol used to clean the skin enters the puncture site.
- Prepare patients only for aspects of the experience that others have commonly noticed. For example, explain that it is normal for a tight tourniquet to cause a person's hand to tingle and feel numb.
- Be sure the patients know when the results will be available and who will give them the results of their tests and/or procedures.

A cognitive regulation technique called "reappraisal" can be effective in reducing anticipatory anxiety. This cognitive change strategy involves changing the meaning of a stimulus in a way that alters its emotional impact (Yoshimura et al., 2014). It allows people to change an underlying appraisal that contributes to negative emotions (Troy et al., 2018). For example, rather than saying to a patient during the insertion of an intravenous catheter, "You are going to feel a stick," say instead, "The catheter I am about to place in your arm will be our way of giving you the fluids and medications you need." Reappraisal typically includes reconsideration or reframing of an emotional event in less emotional terms (Yoshimura et al., 2014). It has important short-term effects on the experience of both negative and positive emotions (Troy et al., 2018).

Demonstrations. Use demonstrations when teaching psychomotor skills such as preparing a syringe, bathing an infant, crutch walking, or taking a pulse. Demonstrations are most effective when learners first observe the educator and during a **return demonstration** have the chance to practice the skill. Combine a demonstration with discussion to clarify concepts and feelings. An effective demonstration requires advanced planning:
1. Position the learner to provide a clear view of the skill being performed so the learner can see each step of the demonstration easily.

2. Assemble and organize the equipment. Make sure that all equipment works.
3. Perform each step slowly and accurately in sequence while analyzing the knowledge and skills involved, and allow the patient to handle the equipment.
4. Review the rationale and steps of the procedure.
5. Encourage the patient to ask questions to ensure understanding of each step.
6. Judge proper speed and timing of the demonstration on the basis of the patient's cognitive abilities and anxiety level.
7. Demonstrate mastery of the skill by having the patient perform a return demonstration under the same conditions that will be experienced at home or in the place where the skill is to be performed. For example, when a patient needs to learn to walk with crutches, simulate the home environment. If the patient's home has stairs, the patient would practice going up and down a staircase in the hospital.

Analogies. Learning occurs when an educator translates complex language or ideas into words or concepts that a patient understands. Analogies supplement verbal instruction with familiar images that make complex information more real and understandable. For example, when explaining arterial blood pressure, use an analogy of the flow of water through a hose. Follow these general principles when using analogies:

- Be familiar with the concept.
- Know the patient's background, experience, and culture so that you can make an analogy relevant.
- Keep the analogy simple and clear.

Role-playing. During role-playing people are asked to play themselves or someone else. Patients learn required skills and feel more confident in being able to perform them independently. The technique involves rehearsing a desired behavior. For example, a nurse who is teaching a parent how to respond to a child's behavior pretends to be a child who is having a temper tantrum. The parent responds to the nurse who is pretending to be the child. Afterward the nurse evaluates the parent's response and determines whether an alternative approach would have been more appropriate. The nurse gathers feedback from the parent about the response and perception of the role-playing.

Simulation. Simulation is a useful technique for teaching problem solving, application, and independent thinking. During individual or group discussion you pose a pertinent problem or situation for patients to solve. For example, patients with heart disease plan a meal that is low in cholesterol and fat. The patients in the group decide which foods are appropriate. You ask the group members to present their diet, providing an opportunity to identify mistakes and reinforce correct information.

Illiteracy and Other Disabilities.
Patients with low health literacy, illiteracy, and learning disabilities have an impaired ability to analyze instructions or synthesize information. Many of these patients have not acquired or are unable to acquire the problem-solving skills of drawing conclusions and inferences from experience, and they do not ask questions to obtain or clarify information that has been presented. Using strategies to enhance health literacy creates a more patient-centered approach to health education and can have a significant impact on patient outcomes (Edelman and Kudzma, 2018) (see Box 25.6). You help patients with limited health literacy learn effectively by creating a safe, shame-free environment, using clear and purposeful communication techniques, using visual aids to reinforce spoken material, and taking special care to evaluate patient understanding of the content.

Sometimes patients have sensory deficits that affect how you present information (see Chapter 49). For example, patients who are deaf may require a sign language interpreter. Not all people who are deaf read lips. Therefore it is very important to provide clear written materials that match the patients' reading level. Visual impairments also affect the

teaching strategy you use. Many people who are blind have acute listening skills. Avoid shouting, and announce your presence to patients with visual impairments before approaching them. If the patient has partial vision, use colors and a print font size (14-point font or larger) that the patient is able to see. Be sure to use proper lighting. Other helpful interventions include audio recording teaching sessions and providing structured, well-organized instructions (Bastable, 2019).

QSEN Building Competency in Patient-Centered Care You are assessing a 62-year-old patient named Betty at an outpatient neurology clinic; Betty was recently discharged from the hospital following an ischemic stroke. Betty was recently started on several new medications for secondary stroke prevention, including medications for high cholesterol, high blood pressure, and thrombolytic therapy. While reviewing her medications, you find that she has difficulty understanding printed teaching sheets. Betty discloses to you, "I had to drop out of school when I was 13 years old to take care of my younger siblings. I really haven't been to the doctor since my old doctor retired and I didn't like his replacement, and that was over 10 years ago." When asked where she keeps her medication, Betty shows you a grocery bag that has prescription bottles inside, and it includes both current and expired prescriptions. Which assessment questions and teaching strategies, approaches, and tools do you need to enhance Betty's learning and ability to take her medications as prescribed?

Answers to QSEN Activities can be found on the Evolve website.

Cultural Diversity. Accept a patient's cultural background and belief system and be prepared to offer culturally sensitive approaches in a patient's native language (see Chapter 9 and Box 25.7). Be careful not to generalize or stereotype patients solely on the basis of their culture. Collaborate with other nurses and educators to develop appropriate teaching approaches, and ask people from their cultural group to help

---

🌐 BOX 25.7 CULTURAL ASPECTS OF CARE
Patient Education

Sociocultural norms, values, and traditions often determine the importance of different health education topics and the preference for one learning approach over another. Educational efforts are especially challenging when patients and educators do not speak the same language or when written materials are not culturally sensitive and are written above patients' reading abilities.

Implications for Patient-Centered Care
- Develop cultural awareness to establish and maintain respectful relationships with culturally diverse patients to encourage trust and communication (Bastable, 2019) (see Chapter 9).
- Implement the National CLAS Standards (https://thinkculturalhealth.hhs.gov/clas), a set of 15 action steps intended to advance health equity, improve quality, and help eliminate health care disparities (U.S. Department of Health and Human Services [USDHHS], n.d.).
- When you and the patient do not speak the same language, use trained and certified health care interpreters to provide health care information.
- Recognize that sociocultural factors influence a patient's perception of health and illness and how patients seek health care information (Bastable, 2019).
- Nurses need to have access to a variety of culturally diverse health care resources and should select teaching strategies that are relevant to the individual patient.

by sharing their values and beliefs. Ethnic nurses are excellent resources who are able to provide input through their experiences to improve the care provided to members of their own community.

In addition, be aware of intergenerational conflicts of values. This occurs when immigrant parents uphold their traditional values and their children, who are exposed to American values in social encounters, develop beliefs similar to those of their American peers. Consider this conflict in values when providing information to families or groups who have members from different generations. To enhance patient education in culturally diverse populations, know when and how to provide education while respecting cultural values. Modify teaching to accommodate for cultural differences. Research has shown that health outcomes are improved when education is given in the context of each person's specific cultural beliefs and practices (Bastable, 2019).

Using Teaching Tools. Many teaching tools are available for patient education. Selection of the right tool depends on the instructional method, a patient's learning needs, and the ability to learn (Table 25.4).

For example, a printed pamphlet is not the best tool to use for a patient with poor reading comprehension, but an audio recording is a better choice. A printed pamphlet is not the preferred tool if the patient actively uses the Internet to find information. Health care agencies often provide clinicians with access to a variety of teaching resources. Be knowledgeable about what is available in your agency to better serve your patients. Also, if patients show interest in seeking information about their health from the Internet, inform them of the most reliable sources. For example, the American Cancer Society, American Lung Association, American Heart Association, and CDC offer excellent information for laypeople.

Special Needs of Children and Older Adults. Children, adults, and older adults learn differently. Adapt your teaching strategies to each learner. Children pass through several developmental stages (see Unit 2). In each developmental stage children acquire new cognitive and psychomotor abilities that respond to different types of teaching methods. Incorporate parental input in planning health education for children.

TABLE 25.4 Teaching Tools for Instruction

Description	Learning Implications
Written Materials	
Printed and Online Materials	
Written teaching tools available as pamphlets, booklets, brochures (font size of 14 recommended for older adults) (Office of Disease Prevention and Health Promotion [ODPHP], 2016)	Material needs to be easy to read. Information needs to be accurate and current. Method is ideal for understanding complex concepts and relationships.
Programmed Instruction	
Written sequential presentation of learning steps requiring that learners answer questions and educators tell them whether they are right or wrong	Instruction is primarily verbal, but the educator sometimes uses pictures or diagrams. Method requires active learning, giving immediate feedback, correcting wrong answers, and reinforcing right answers. Learner works at own pace.
Computer Instruction	
Use of programmed instruction format in which computers store response patterns for learners and select further lessons on basis of these patterns (programs can be individualized)	Method requires reading comprehension, psychomotor skills, and familiarity with computer.
Nonprint Materials	
Diagrams	
Illustrations show interrelationships by means of lines and symbols	Method demonstrates key ideas, summarizes, and clarifies key concept.
Graphs (Bar, Circle, or Line)	
Visual presentations of numerical data	Graphs help learner grasp information about single concept quickly.
Charts	
Highly condensed visual summary of ideas and facts that highlights series of ideas, steps, or events	Charts demonstrate relationship of several ideas or concepts. Method helps learners know what to do.
Pictures	
Photographs or drawings used to teach concepts in which the third dimension of shape and space is not important	Photographs are more desirable than diagrams because they more accurately portray the details of the real item.
Physical Objects	
Use of actual equipment, objects, or models to teach concepts or skills	Models are useful when real objects are too small, large, or complicated or are unavailable. Allows learners to manipulate objects that they will use later in skill.
Other Audiovisual Materials	
Slides, audiotapes, television, and videotapes used with printed material or discussion	Materials are useful for patients with reading comprehension problems and visual deficits.

Older adults experience numerous physical and psychological changes as they age (see Chapter 14). These changes not only increase their educational needs but also create barriers to learning unless adjustments are made in instructional interventions. Sensory changes such as visual and hearing changes require adaptation of teaching methods to enhance functioning (Touhy and Jett, 2020). Older adults learn and remember effectively if you pace the learning properly and if the material is relevant to the learner's needs and abilities. Although many older adults have slower cognitive function and reduced short-term memory, you facilitate learning in several ways to support behaviors that maximize the individual's capacity for self-care (Box 25.8). Include family members who assume care for the patient. However, be sensitive to a patient's desire for assistance because offering unwanted support often results in negative outcomes and perceptions of nagging and interference. Not all relationships between older adults and other family members are therapeutic.

BOX 25.8 FOCUS ON OLDER ADULTS

Providing Patient Education

Facilitate learning by using the following teaching strategies when providing patient education to older adults:

- Promote concentration and learner readiness by scheduling teaching sessions when the patient is comfortable and well rested. Provide medication for pain relief when necessary. Ensure that the patient is not drowsy from medication during the education session.
- Create a casual and relaxed learning environment.
- Establish personalized, realistic short-term learning objectives/outcomes.
- Provide sufficient lighting with low glare.
- If using visual aids or written materials to supplement instruction, assess the patient's reading ability and make sure that information is printed in a large-size font and in a color that contrasts with the background (e.g., black 14-point print on matte white paper). Avoid blues and greens because these colors can become more difficult to distinguish with age.
- To accommodate for hearing loss, present information slowly and in a clear, low tone of voice. Eliminate any extraneous noises and directly face the learner when speaking. Do not place your hand near your mouth while a hearing-impaired patient is trying to hear (or lip-read) instructions. Mustaches can make lip reading difficult for a hearing-impaired patient.
- Encourage the use of prosthesis (i.e., glasses, hearing aid), and ensure proper fit and working condition.
- Allow sufficient time to process and comprehend new information.
- Build on existing knowledge and present content in a way that relates to relevant past life experiences.
- Make information meaningful by using concrete examples that apply to current situations.
- Present only the most significant information to avoid overwhelming the learner. Use repetition to reinforce content.
- When giving instructions or teaching a new skill, give concise, step-by-step directions. Assess understanding of each step before moving ahead.
- Provide regular positive reinforcement.
- Keep teaching sessions short and allow for frequent breaks. Schedule follow-up sessions as needed to ensure learning.
- Conclude with a brief summary and allow sufficient time for questions and feedback.

Data from Touhy TA, Jett KF: *Ebersole and Hess' toward healthy aging*, ed 10, St Louis, 2020, Elsevier; and Edelman C, Kudzma EC: *Health promotion throughout the life span*, ed 9, St Louis, 2019, Elsevier.

◆ Evaluation

Through the Patient's Eyes. An important part of evaluation is to determine whether the patient's expectations, identified during assessment, were met. You engage patients to determine if they perceive having learned what they expected. For example, "Tell me if you are happy with the information you now have to check your blood pressure at home." "We want to be sure you feel you can follow your activity restrictions at home; tell me if you feel that way." Or "Is there anything further you would like to learn about your medicines?"

Be sure their expectations have been fully met. Does the patient have the sense that self-care can be maintained based on the information received? It is important to evaluate through the patient's eyes, considering the type of situations and environments that patients return to after receiving care. Evaluation helps the educator determine adequacy of teaching. If expectations have not been met, you revise the plan of care and offer additional instruction or reinforcement.

Patient Outcomes. Evaluation of any instructional approach involves measuring whether learning objectives were met. You gather data to measure whether the patient has the new knowledge, behaviors, or skills that education aimed to provide. You observe a patient's performance of any expected behavior or skill. You also ask evaluative questions, phrased carefully, then guide the patient to identity or describe information so that you can determine whether the established outcomes and learning objectives were met. For example, you might say, "Tell me specifically the times of day you are to take this new medication" or "We discussed the safety risks in your home; tell me how you plan to remove them." Consider these questions as you evaluate a patient's education plan.

- Were the patient's outcomes realistic and observable?
- Is the patient able to perform the behavior or skill in the natural setting (e.g., home)?
- How well is the patient able to answer questions about the topic?
- Does the patient continue to have problems understanding the information or performing a skill? If so, how can you change the interventions to enhance knowledge or skill performance?

Evaluate a patient's learning in a timely manner so that you can make adjustments or changes as needed. A nurse is legally responsible for providing accurate, timely patient information that promotes continuity of care; therefore it is essential to document the outcomes of teaching. Documentation of patient teaching also supports quality improvement efforts, meets TJC standards, and promotes third-party reimbursement. Teaching flow sheets and written plans of care are excellent records that document the plan, implementation, and evaluation of learning.

Teach-back. It is imperative to assess whether a patient understands the information delivered during an educational session. One way to evaluate patient understanding is with the teach-back method. Teach-back is an evidence-based health literacy intervention that promotes patient engagement, patient safety, adherence, and quality. The goal of teach-back is to ensure that you have explained medical information clearly so that patients and their families understand what you communicated to them (AHRQ, 2020).

Teach-back is a closed-loop communication technique that assesses patient retention of the information given during a teaching session. To perform teach-back, ask the patient to explain material that was discussed, such as the role of diet and exercise in managing blood glucose levels, or to demonstrate a skill, such as self-monitoring blood glucose. The response allows you to determine the degree to which the patient remembers and understands what was taught or demonstrated. Use nonjudgmental language so that patients do not feel tested (Flanders, 2018). For example, say, "I want to be certain that I taught this well.

Can you please describe some symptoms of a stroke?" Examples of teach-back prompts and questions include:

1. "Tell me in your own words how you will take this medication at home."
2. "Tell me some of the side effects that you should watch for."
3. "When will you call the office regarding your blood pressure?"
4. "Please show me how to request a refill of this medication online."

If the patient has difficulty recalling the material or demonstrating a skill, modify and repeat the content and reassess retention. Also, take ownership of the teaching experience by responding, "I must not have explained stroke symptoms very well. Let me try again." Patient understanding is confirmed when the patient can accurately restate the information in own words (Bastable, 2019).

KEY POINTS

- The three purposes of patient education are health promotion and illness prevention, health restoration, and coping with impaired function.
- The Joint Commission's (TJC's) Speak Up initiatives help patients understand their rights when receiving medical care and support them to become more active participants in their care by asking questions of health care providers.
- Steps of the teaching process are similar to those of the communication process.
- Just as effective communication involves feedback from the sender and receiver, an effective educator delivers instruction and then provides a mechanism (e.g., teach-back) for evaluating the success of a teaching plan by gaining feedback from the receiver.
- The most effective teaching plan often includes all three domains of learning: cognitive (understanding), affective (attitudes), and psychomotor (motor skills). Nurses consider the patient's needs and learning preferences and the content of what the patient needs to know to select the appropriate domain.
- Motivation to learn is influenced by an individual's belief in the need to know something; the more important people believe information to be, the stronger their motivation is to learn.
- An adult's readiness to learn is affected by health status, attentional set, and acceptance of the illness experience.
- The ability to learn depends on physical and cognitive attributes, developmental level, physical wellness, and intellectual thought processes. A person's learning style affects preferences for learning.
- The ideal environment for learning is well lit and has good ventilation, appropriate furniture, and a comfortable temperature.
- Self-efficacy is a concept included in many health promotion theories because it often is a strong predictor of motivation to learn healthy behaviors. People who have self-efficacy for health-promoting behaviors believe they can accurately complete a particular health behavior and are more likely to perform the behavior consistently and correctly.
- Knowledge of a patient's health condition and the patient information you gain from assessment during the nursing process allows you to critically select the topic and level of instruction required and allows you to determine the best time for teaching and how to engage the patient.
- A nurse assesses a patient's current level within a learning domain and then selects approaches to use to aid the patient in achieving a higher level of performance in that domain.
- The characteristics of learning within each domain influence your teaching and evaluation methods. Understanding each learning domain prepares you to select proper teaching techniques and apply the basic principles of learning.
- The nursing and teaching processes differ in that the nursing process requires assessment of all sources of data to determine a patient's total health care needs. The teaching plan focuses on a patient's learning needs as they relate to the patient's health status, as well as on a patient's motivation, ability, and readiness to learn.
- Health literacy is one of the most important predictors of health outcomes because it influences whether an individual has the skills needed to manage health and prevent disease.
- A nurse bases educational priorities on a patient's nursing diagnoses, outcomes established for the patient and the patient's perception of what information is most important, anxiety or physical comfort level, and the amount of time available to teach.
- When planning a teaching session, remember that patients need to learn essential content first. Learning progresses from simple to complex; thus learners need to acquire simpler knowledge and skills within a learning domain before they can master more complex knowledge and skills.
- Nurses promote learning in patients with limited health literacy by creating a safe, shame-free environment, communicating clearly, using visual aids to reinforce spoken information, and carefully evaluating the patient and family caregivers' understanding of the content.
- At the end of a teaching session, a nurse uses the teach-back technique to evaluate learning by asking the patient to explain the material that was discussed or demonstrate a skill.

REFLECTIVE LEARNING

- Consider a member of your family or a friend who has some type of health issue. Review what you would assess about the individual to determine learning needs, and then summarize your conclusion about the person's ability and motivation to learn.
- After you complete a clinical assignment with a recent patient, reflect on how you determined if the patient understood the care you provided and any information you shared.
- Select a student colleague, and together develop a case study of a patient requiring health instruction. Using the case study, describe the learning domains relevant to what the patient's educational needs are. Then identify three approaches for instructing the patient.

REVIEW QUESTIONS

1. A nurse who works in an outpatient chemotherapy infusion center is assigned to the care of a 56-year-old male patient who is receiving chemotherapy for colon cancer. This is the patient's first clinic visit. The nurse reviews the patient's medical record and sees a note about the patient receiving instruction on how chemotherapy treats cancer, but the note does not summarize the patient's response. The doctor makes a quick visit and tells the patient, "We will get your treatment started today and we will be checking your blood each week for any problems." The doctor leaves and the patient asks the nurse, "What are the blood tests for?" To determine this patient's learning needs, what should the nurse assess? (Select all that apply.)
   1. Medical record summary of the stage of the cancer
   2. The patient's behavior as the nurse interacts with him
   3. The patient's level of knowledge about chemotherapy effects
   4. The number of treatments the patient will be receiving
   5. The patient's health literacy
   6. The patient's self-description of severity of his cancer
   7. The date of the medical record note describing patient instruction

2. A nurse who works in an outpatient chemotherapy infusion center is assigned to the care of a 56-year-old male patient who is receiving chemotherapy for colon cancer. This is the patient's first clinic visit. The nurse reviews the patient's medical record and sees a note about the patient receiving instruction on how chemotherapy treats cancer; the note does not summarize the patient's response. The nurse's assessment reveals that the patient is motivated to learn more about his chemotherapy and is alert and currently feeling well. The nurse has prepared the first infusion, regulated it, and now takes time to begin instruction. Which teaching approaches are best suited for this situation?
   1. Use an entrusting approach in explaining how to monitor for side effects of chemotherapy.
   2. Bring the patient together with two other patients in the clinic and conduct a group discussion.
   3. Provide verbal one-on-one instruction, with the patient participating in selection of content.
   4. Present the patient with a problem situation involving a serious side effect and have the patient decide what to do.

3. A 26-year-old patient visits a medical clinic and asks a nurse to provide instruction on how to perform a breast self-examination. "My mom had cancer so I want to learn how." Which domains are required to learn this skill? (Select all that apply.)
   1. Affective domain
   2. Sensory domain
   3. Cognitive domain
   4. Attentional domain
   5. Psychomotor domain

4. A patient suddenly experienced a severe headache with numbness and decreased movement in the left arm. An emergency brain scan confirmed a cerebral vessel clot. With a stroke confirmed, the emergency room physician consults with a neurosurgeon to schedule an emergent angiogram to remove the clot. Which teaching approach is most appropriate for explaining to the patient what to expect from the procedure?
   1. Selling approach
   2. Telling approach
   3. Entrusting approach
   4. Participating approach

5. A nurse is teaching an older-adult patient about ways to detect a melanoma. Which of the following are age-appropriate teaching techniques for this patient? (Select all that apply.)
   1. Speak in a low tone.
   2. Begin and end the session with the most important information regarding melanoma.
   3. Provide a pamphlet about melanoma with large font in blues and greens.
   4. Use basic one- or two-syllable medical terms.
   5. Provide specific information in frequent, small amounts.
   6. Speak quickly so that you do not take up much of the patient's time.

6. A 55-year-old man has been in the hospital for over a week following surgical complications. The patient has had limited activity but is now ordered to begin a mobility program. The patient just returned from several diagnostic tests and tells the nurse he is feeling fatigued. The nurse prepares to instruct the patient on the mobility program protocol. Which of the following learning principles will likely be affected by this patient's condition?
   1. Motivation to learn

2. Developmental stage
3. Stage of grief
4. Readiness to learn

7. A patient recovering from open heart surgery is taught how to cough and deep breathe using a pillow to support or splint the chest incision. Following the teaching session, which of the following is the best way for the nurse to evaluate whether learning has taken place?
   1. Verbalization of steps to use in splinting
   2. Selecting from a series of flash cards the images showing the correct technique
   3. Return demonstration
   4. REALM test

8. A patient's cultural background affects the motivation for learning. Using the ACCESS model, match the nursing approach with the correct model component.

ACCESS Model

Component	Nursing Approach
___1. Assessment	A. Help patients feel culturally secure and able to maintain their cultural identity.
___2. Communication	
___3. Cultural	B. Remain aware of verbal and nonverbal responses.
___4. Establishment	
___5. Sensitivity	C. Be aware of how patients from diverse backgrounds perceive their care needs.
___6. Safety	
	D. Become aware of your patient's culture and your own cultural biases.
	E. Learn about the patient's health beliefs and practices.
	F. Show respect by creating a caring rapport.

9. A nurse is preparing to teach a patient who has sleep apnea how to use a continuous positive airway pressure (CPAP) machine at night. Which action is most appropriate for the nurse to perform first?
   1. Allow patient to manipulate machine and look at parts.
   2. Provide a teach-back session.
   3. Set mutual goals for the education session.
   4. Discuss the purpose of the machine and how it works.

10. Which of the following scenarios demonstrate that patient learning has taken place? (Select all that apply.)
    1. A patient listens to a nurse's review of the warning signs of a stroke.
    2. A patient describes how to set up a pill organizer for newly ordered medicines.
    3. A patient attends a spinal cord injury support group.
    4. A patient demonstrates how to take his blood pressure at home.
    5. A patient reviews written information about resources for cancer survivors.

Answers: 1. 2, 3, 5, 6; **2.** 3; **3.** 3, 5; **4.** 2, 5; **5.** 1, 2, 5; **6.** 4; **7.** 3; **8.** 1E, 2B, 3D, 4F, 5C, 6A; **9.** 3; **10.** 2, 4.

Rationales for Review Questions can be found on the Evolve website.

REFERENCES

Agency for Healthcare Research and Quality (AHRQ): *Teach-back intervention: quick start guide*, 2017. https://www.ahrq.gov/patient-safety/reports/engage/interventions/teachback.html. Accessed June 4, 2021.

Agency for Healthcare Research and Quality (AHRQ): AHRQ *Health literacy universal precautions toolkit*, 2020. https://www.ahrq.gov/health-literacy/quality-resources/tools/literacy-toolkit/index.html. Accessed June 4, 2021.

American Hospital Association: *The patient care partnership*, 2003. https://www.aha.org/system/files/2018-01/aha-patient-care-partnership.pdf. Accessed June 4, 2021.

Bandura A: Self-efficacy: toward a unifying theory of behavioral change, *Psychol Rev* 84(2):191, 1977. https://doi.org/10.1037/0033-295X.84.2.191.

Bandura A: *Self-efficacy: the exercise of control*, New York, 1997, WH Freeman.

Bastable SB: *Nurse as educator: principles of teaching and learning for nursing practice*, ed 5, Burlington, 2019, Jones & Bartlett.

Billings DM, Halstead JA: *Teaching in nursing: a guide for faculty*, ed 6, St Louis, 2020, Elsevier.

Centers for Disease Control and Prevention (CDC): *Heart failure*, 2020. https://www.cdc.gov/heartdisease/heart_failure.htm. Accessed June 7, 2021.

Centers for Disease Control and Prevention (CDC): *What is health literacy?* 2021a. https://www.cdc.gov/healthliteracy/learn/index.html. Accessed June 6, 2021.

Centers for Disease Control and Prevention: *Talking points about health literacy*, 2021b. https://www.cdc.gov/healthliteracy/shareinteract/TellOthers.html. Accessed June 6, 2021.

Centers for Disease Control and Prevention: *Health literacy: develop and test materials*, 2021c. https://www.cdc.gov/healthliteracy/developmaterials/index.html. Accessed June 7, 2021.

Centers for Disease Control and Prevention (CDC): *Attention-deficit hyperactivity disorder*, 2021d. https://www.cdc.gov/ncbddd/adhd/index.html. Accessed June 7, 2021.

Edelman C, Kudzma EC: *Health promotion throughout the life span*, ed 9, St Louis, 2018, Elsevier.

Festinger L: *A theory of cognitive dissonance*, Palo Alto, CA, 1957, Stanford University Press.

Flanders SA: Effective patient education: evidence and common sense, *Medsurg Nurs* 27(1):55, 2018.

Jordan LM: *Health literacy made simple*, The Joint Commission: accreditation ambulatory care, 2016. https://www.jointcommission.org/-/media/deprecated-unorganized/imported-assets/tjc/system-folders/topics-library/health-literacy-pcmhpdf.pdf?db=web&hash=E0384547146B5345A7258D94DF545D13#:~:text=2%20%C2%A9%20Copyright%2C%20The%20Joint%20Commission.%20What%20is,and%20services%20needed%20to%20make%20appropriate%20health%20decisions. Accessed June 6, 2021.

Killian S: *6 High impact teaching strategies*, 2019. https://www.evidencebasedteaching.org.au/high-impact-teaching-strategies/. Accessed June 7, 2021.

Krathwohl DR, et al: *Taxonomy of educational objectives: the classification of educational goals. Handbook II: affective domain*, New York, 1956, David McKay Co., Inc.

Krathwohl DR: A revision of Bloom's taxonomy: an overview, *Theory Pract* 41(4), Autumn 2002, College of Education, The Ohio State University. https://www.depauw.edu/files/resources/krathwohl.pdf. Accessed July 2020.

Lorig K: Chronic disease self-management program: insights from the eye of the storm, *Front Public Health* 2:253, 2015.

McCleod S: *Cognitive dissonance*, 2018. https://www.simplypsychology.org/cognitive-dissonance.html. Accessed June 6, 2021.

Medicare.gov: *Your rights and protections as a nursing home resident*, n.d. https://downloads.cms.gov/medicare/Your_Resident_Rights_and_Protections_section.pdf. Accessed June 4, 2021.

Miller M, Stoeckel P: *Client education: theory and practice*, ed 3, Sudbury, MA, 2019, Jones & Bartlett.

National Library of Medicine (NLM): *Health literacy*, n.d. https://nnlm.gov/initiatives/topics/health-literacy#toc-5. Accessed June 6, 2021.

Office of Disease Prevention and Health Promotion ODPHP): *Health literacy on line-display content clearly on the page*, 2016. https://health.gov/healthliteracyonline/display/full/. Accessed June 6, 2021.

Parnell TA: *Health literacy in nursing: providing person-centered care*, New York, 2015, Springer Publishing.

Pender NJ: A conceptual model for preventive health behavior, *Nurs Outlook* 23(6):385, 1975.

Prochaska JO, et al: The transtheoretical model of behavior change. In Shumaker SS, Schron EB, editors: *The handbook of health behavior change*, ed 2, New York, 1998, Springer Publishing, pp 59.

Psychology Today: Motivational Interviewing, n.d. https://www.psychologytoday.com/us/therapy-types/motivational-interviewing. Accessed June 6, 2021.

Purnell LD, Fenkl E: *Guide to culturally competent health care*, ed 4, Philadelphia, 2019, F.A. Davis.

Quality and Safety Education for Nurses (QSEN): Competency KSAs (pre-licensure), 2020. http://qsen.org/competencies/pre-licensure-ksas/#patient-centered_care. Accessed June 4, 2021.

Rau J: *New round of medicare readmission penalties hits 2,583 hospitals, Kaiser Health News*, October 1, 2019. https://khn.org/news/hospital-readmission-penalties-medicare-2583-hospitals/. Accessed June 4, 2021.

Souders B: *17 Motivational interviewing questions and skills*, Positive Psychology.com, 2021. https://positivepsychology.com/motivational-interviewing/. Accessed June 6, 2021.

Substance Abuse and Mental Health Services Administration (SAMHSA): *Empowering change: motivational interviewing*, 2018. https://www.samhsa.gov/homelessness-programs-resources/hpr-resources/empowering-change. Accessed June 6, 2021.

The Joint Commission (TJC): *Speak up about your care*, 2019. https://www.jointcommission.org/-/media/tjc/documents/resources/speak-up/speak-ups/about-your-care/speak-up-about-your-care-infographic-2019-85x11.pdf. Accessed June 4, 2021.

The Joint Commission (TJC): *Speak up campaigns*, 2021a. https://www.jointcommission.org/resources/for-consumers/speak-up-campaigns/. Accessed June 4, 2021.

The Joint Commission (TJC): *Joint Commission comprehensive accreditation manual for hospitals*, 2021b, The Commission.

Touhy TA, Jett KF: *Ebersole and Hess' toward healthy aging*, ed 10, St. Louis, 2020, Elsevier.

U.S. Department of Health and Human Services – Office of Minority Health (USDHHS): *National CLAS standards*, n.d. https://www.thinkculturalhealth.hhs.gov/clas. Accessed June 6, 2021.

Van Zant S, Volpe N: *Small group instruction: how to make it effective*, 2018, Consortium on Reaching Excellence in Education. https://www.corelearn.com/small-group-instruction-blog/. Accessed June 6, 2021.

Wilson LO: *Three domains of learning – cognitive, affective, psychomotor, the second principle*, 2021. https://thesecondprinciple.com/instructional-design/threedomainsoflearning/. Accessed June 4, 2021.

World Health Organization (WHO): *Health promotion. Track 2: health literacy and health behavior*, 2021. http://www.who.int/healthpromotion/conferences/7gchp/track2/en/. Accessed June 6, 2021.

RESEARCH REFERENCES

Almkuist KD: Using teach-back method to prevent 30-day readmissions in patients with heart failure: a systematic review, *MedSurg Nurs* 26(5):309, 2017.

Anderson LW, Krathwohl DR, editors: *A taxonomy for learning, teaching, and assessing: a revision of Bloom's taxonomy of educational objectives*, Boston, 2001, Allyn & Bacon.

Boyde M, et al: Self-care educational intervention to reduce hospitalizations in heart failure: a randomized controlled trial, *Eur J Cardiovasc Nurs* 17(2):178, 2018.

Cakmak HSG, Kapucu S: The effect of educational follow-up with the motivational interview technique on self-efficacy and drug adherence in cancer patients using oral chemotherapy treatment: a randomized controlled trial, *Semin Oncol Nurs* 37(2):151140, 2021. https://doi.org/10.1016/j.soncn.2021.151140.

Chan DN, So WKW: Effectiveness of motivational interviewing in enhancing cancer screening uptake amongst average-risk individuals: a systematic review, *Int J Nurs Stud* 113(2021):103786, 2021. https://doi.org/10.1016/j.ijnurstu.2020.103786.

Faghihian R, et al: Impact of motivational interviewing on early childhood caries: a systematic review and meta-analysis, *J Am Dent Assoc* 151(9):650, 2020.

Ha Dinh TT, et al: The effectiveness of the teach-back method on adherence and self-management in health education for people with chronic disease: a systematic review, *JBI Database System Rev Implement Rep* 14(1):210, 2016.

Hochbaum GM: Public participation in medical screening programs: a sociopsychological study, *PHS Publication No. 572*, Washington, DC, 1958, US Government Printing Office.

Hong YR, et al: Teach-back experience and hospitalization risk among patients with ambulatory care sensitive conditions: a matched cohort study, *J Gen Intern Med* 34(10):2176, 2019.

Khan MS, et al: Trends in 30- and 90-day readmission rates for heart failure, *Circ Heart Fail* 14(4):e008335, 2021, https://www.ahajournals.org/doi/10.1161/CIRCHEARTFAILURE.121.008335.

Liu H, et al: Assessment tools for health literacy among the general population: a systematic review, *Int J Environ Res Public Health* 15(8):1711, 2018.

Louis A, et al: Screening hospitalized patients for low health literacy—Beyond the REALM of possibility? *Health Educ Behav* 44(3):360, 2017.

Marcus C: Strategies for improving the quality of verbal patient and family education: a review of the literature and creation of the EDUCATE model, *Health Psychol Behav Med* 2(1):482, 2014.

Oh EG, et al: Effectiveness of discharge education with the teach-back method on 30-day readmission: a systematic review, *J Patient Saf* 17(4):305, 2021, https://pubmed.ncbi.nlm.nih.gov/30882616/. Accessed June 6, 2021.

Savage K, et al: Preferences in learning styles and modes of information delivery in patients receiving first-day education for radiation therapy, *J Med Imaging Radiat Sci* 48(2):193, 2017.

Spencer JC, Wheeler SB: A systematic review of motivational interviewing interventions in cancer patients and survivors, *Patient Educ Couns* 99(7):1099, 2016.

Steffen PS, et al: Motivational interviewing in the management of type 2 diabetes mellitus and arterial hypertension in primary health care: an RCT, *Am J Prev Med* 60(5):e203, 2021.

Troy AS, et al: Cognitive reappraisal and acceptance: effects on emotion, physiology, and perceived cognitive costs, *Emotion* 18(1):58, 2018.

Yoshimura S, et al: Neural basis of anticipatory anxiety reappraisals, *PLoS ONE* 9(7):e102836, 2014.

Zhou Y, et al: Effects of a nurse-led phone follow-up education program based on the self-efficacy among patients with cardiovascular disease, *J Cardiovasc Nurs* 33(1):E15, 2018.

Informatics and Documentation

OBJECTIVES

- Identify the purposes of a health care record.
- Explain the relationship between documentation and financial reimbursement for health care.
- Discuss legal guidelines for documentation.
- Identify ways to maintain confidentiality of health care record data.
- Explain the guidelines for quality documentation.
- Predict what will happen with the inappropriate use of abbreviation(s) in health care documentation.
- Explain the different types of forms nurses use in documentation.
- Summarize the elements to include when documenting a patient's discharge plan.
- Explain the elements to include in documentation of telephone conversations with providers.
- Discuss the relationship between informatics and high-quality health care.
- Discuss the specific competencies in informatics for new graduate nurses entering the workforce.

KEY TERMS

Accreditation
Acuity rating system
Case management
Charting by exception (CBE)
Clinical decision support system (CDSS)
Clinical information system (CIS)
Clinical practice guidelines (CPG)
Computerized provider order entry (CPOE)
Critical pathways
Diagnosis-related group (DRG)

Documentation
Electronic health record (EHR)
Electronic health record system (EHRS)
Electronic medical record (EMR)
Firewall
Flow sheets
Health care informatics
Health care information system (HIS)
Health information technology (HIT)
Health record

Incident report (occurrence report)
Meaningful use
Narrative documentation
Nursing clinical information system (NCIS)
Nursing informatics
Password
Protected health information (PHI)
Standardized care plans
Variances

MEDIA RESOURCES

http://evolve.elsevier.com/Potter/fundamentals/
- Review Questions
- Audio Glossary
- Case Study with Questions
- Content Updates
- Answers to QSEN Activity and Review Questions

Documentation is a key communication strategy that produces a written account of pertinent patient data, clinical decisions and interventions, and patient responses in a health record. Documentation in a patient's health record is a vital aspect of nursing practice. Health care documentation consists of all information entered into a health record, which may be electronic, paper, or a combination of both formats. Nursing documentation systems should reflect current standards of nursing practice and minimize the risk of errors. Documentation systems need to be flexible enough to allow members of the health care team to efficiently document and retrieve clinical data, track patient outcomes, and facilitate continuity of care. Information in a patient's record provides a detailed account of the level of quality of care delivered. The quality of care, the standards of regulatory agencies and nursing practice, the reimbursement structure in the health care system, and legal guidelines make documentation and reporting an extremely important nursing responsibility.

The information you enter into a patient's individual medical record communicates within the patient's integrated health record the type and frequency of patient care delivered and provides accountability for the care you implemented. This information is then available for all members of the health care team in all settings to review.

It is necessary to document all the nursing care you provide for each patient, including assessment data, nursing problems or diagnoses, interventions, and evaluation of patient responses, in the health record. Your data enable providers and outside reviewers of the medical record to track a patient's clinical course. In 2008 the Centers for Medicare and Medicaid Services (CMS) implemented a policy under which hospitals are no longer reimbursed for the treatment of 11 specific hospital-acquired conditions (HACs) or preventable adverse events, commonly known as "never events" (CMS, 2020). Four of these preventable adverse events are considered "nurse-sensitive": Stage 3 and 4 pressure injuries, falls with injury, catheter-associated urinary tract infections (CAUTIs), and central line–associated blood-stream infections (CLABSIs) (Daniels et al., 2020; Hommel et al., 2020). Identifying the progress of a patient and how events develop is crucial to clinical care and ultimately hospital reimbursement. It is also crucial that your documentation accurately reflects the status of the patient and responses to interventions, especially on admission, transfer, or discharge. You use critical thinking and clinical judgment to ensure that you complete your documentation accurately and completely.

PURPOSES OF THE HEALTH CARE RECORD

The health care record is a valuable source of data for all members of the health care team. Data entered into the health care record serve many purposes, including facilitating interprofessional communication among health care providers and providing a legal record of care provided and justification for financial billing and reimbursement of care. Data are also used to audit, monitor, and evaluate care provided to support the process needed for quality and performance improvement (Wager et al., 2017; Wu et al., 2019). In addition, the health care record is a resource for education and research. There are privacy and ethical considerations to address when accessing health care information and when health records serve as resources for nursing and health care education and for research data (Misto et al., 2020).

INTERPROFESSIONAL COMMUNICATION WITHIN THE HEALTH RECORD

The health care record provides a way for members of the interprofessional health care team to communicate about multiple aspects of patient care, including patient needs and response to care and therapies; clinical decision making; and the content and outcomes of consultations, patient education, and discharge planning. Information communicated in the health care record allows health care providers to know a patient thoroughly, facilitating safe, effective, timely, and patient-centered clinical decision making. The health care record is the most current and accurate, continuous source of information about a patient's health care status, allowing the plan of care to be clear to anyone who accesses the record. To enhance communication and promote safe patient care, you document assessment findings and patient information as soon as possible after you provide care (e.g., immediately after providing a nursing intervention or completing a patient assessment). The quality of patient care depends on your ability to communicate with other members of the health care team (see Chapter 24). When a plan is not communicated to all members of the health care team, care becomes fragmented, tasks are repeated, and delays or omissions in care often occur. The health record is an important means of communication because it is a confidential, permanent, legal documentation of information relevant to a patient's health care. The record is an ongoing current and accurate account of a patient's health care status and is available to all members of the health care team.

The record is one resource that prepares the health care provider to know a patient thoroughly so that timely and appropriate care decisions can be made. All health records contain the following information:
- Patient identification and demographic data
- Existence of "living will" or "durable power of attorney for health care" documents
- Informed consent for treatment and procedures
- Admission data
- Nursing diagnoses or problems and the nursing or interprofessional care plan
- Record of nursing care treatment and evaluation
- Medical history
- Medical diagnoses

- Therapeutic orders, including code status (i.e., provider order for "do not resuscitate")
- Medical and interprofessional progress notes (including treatments administered)
- Physical assessment findings
- Diagnostic study results
- Patient education
- Summary of operative procedures
- Discharge summary and plan

Legal Documentation

Accurate documentation is one of the best defenses for legal claims associated with nursing care. Documentation is an important professional responsibility. To limit liability, your documentation needs to follow agency standards, which include a clear description of individualized and outcome-directed nursing care you provide based on your nursing assessment. Always document patient care in a timely manner, following agency standards. Documenting all aspects of the nursing process is a critical nursing responsibility that limits nursing liability by providing evidence that you maintained or exceeded practice standards while taking care of patients (Harding et al., 2020; Office of the National Coordinator for Health Information Technology [ONC], 2020).

Mistakes in documentation can result in malpractice, including the following: (1) failing to record pertinent health or medication information, (2) failing to record nursing actions, (3) failing to record medication administration, (4) failing to record medication reactions or changes in patients' conditions, (5) incomplete or illegible records, and (6) failing to document discontinued medications. Table 26.1 provides guidelines for avoiding these mistakes and gives some examples of basic criteria for legally sound documentation in a health record.

Reimbursement

Documentation of patient care by all members of the health care team allows one to determine the severity of a patient's illness, the intensity of services received, and the quality of care provided during an episode of care. Insurance companies use this information to determine payment or reimbursement for health care services. Diagnosis-related groups (DRGs) are classifications based on a patient's primary and secondary medical diagnoses that are used as the basis for establishing Medicare reimbursement for patient care provided by a health care agency. Health care agencies are reimbursed a predetermined dollar amount by Medicare for each DRG. Private insurance carriers and auditors from federal agencies review records to determine the reimbursement that a patient or a health care agency receives (Bauder et al., 2017; Heflin, 2021). Accurate documentation of nursing services provided, as well as the supplies and equipment used in a patient's care, clarifies the type of treatment a patient received and supports accurate and timely reimbursement to a health care agency and/or patient.

Auditing and Monitoring

The quality of patient care depends on the ability of all members of the interprofessional team to communicate effectively and in a timely manner. As a member of that team, you are held accountable for the accuracy of the documentation you enter into the patient's record. Regulations from agencies such as The Joint Commission (TJC) and CMS require health care agencies to monitor and evaluate the quality and appropriateness of patient care (TJC, 2021; CMS, 2021). Audits of health records offer information on recurrent health care problems, specific patient incidents, and whether health care providers follow standards of care. Health care record audits help to identify areas for improvement and staff development. For example, a quality improvement (QI) nurse may monitor a unit's records to determine whether

TABLE 26.1 Legal Guidelines for Documentation

Guidelines for Electronic and Written Documentation	Rationale	Correct Action
Do not document retaliatory or critical comments about a patient or care provided by another health care professional. Do not enter personal opinions.	Statements can be used as evidence for nonprofessional behavior or poor quality of care.	Enter only objective and factual observations of a patient's behavior or the actions of another health care professional. Quote all patient statements.
Correct all errors promptly.	Errors in recording can lead to errors in treatment or may imply an attempt to mislead or hide evidence.	Avoid rushing to complete documentation; be sure that information is accurate and complete.
Record all facts.	Record must be accurate, factual, and objective.	Be certain that each entry is thorough. A person reading your documentation needs to be able to determine that a patient received adequate care.
Document discussions with providers that you initiate to seek clarification regarding an order that is questioned.	If you carry out an order that is written incorrectly, you are just as liable for prosecution as the health care provider.	Do not record "physician made error." Instead document that "Dr. Smith was called to clarify order for analgesic." Include the date and time of the phone call, with whom you spoke, and the outcome.
Document only for yourself.	You are accountable for information that you enter into a patient's record.	Never enter documentation for someone else (exception: if caregiver has left unit for the day and calls with information that needs to be documented; include date and time of entry and reference specific date and time to which you are referring and name of source of information in entry; include that the information was provided via telephone).
Avoid using generalized, empty phrases such as "status unchanged" or "had good day."	This type of documentation is subjective and does not reflect patient assessment.	Use complete, concise descriptions of assessments and care provided so that documentation is objective and factual.
Begin each entry with date and time and end with your signature and credentials.	Ensures that the correct sequence of events is recorded; signature documents who is accountable for care delivered.	Do not wait until the end of shift to record important changes that occurred several hours earlier; sign each entry according to agency policy (e.g., M. Marcus, RN).
Protect the security of your password for computer documentation.	Maintains security and confidentiality of patient health records.	Once logged into a computer, do not leave computer screen unattended. Log out when you leave the computer. Make sure that a computer screen is not accessible for public viewing.
Do not erase or scratch out errors made while recording.	Charting becomes illegible: it appears as if you were attempting to hide information or deface a written record.	Draw single line through error, write word "error" above it, and sign your name or initials and date it. Then record note correctly.
Do not leave blank spaces or lines in a written nurse's progress note.	Allows another person to add incorrect information in open space.	Chart consecutively, line by line; if space is left, draw a line horizontally through it and place your signature and credentials at the end.
Record all written entries legibly using black ink. Do not use pencils, felt-tip pens, or erasable ink.	Illegible entries are easily misinterpreted, causing errors and lawsuits; ink from felt-tip pen can smudge or run when wet and may destroy documentation; erasures are not permitted in clinical documentation; black ink is more legible when records are photocopied or scanned.	Write clearly and include appropriate abbreviations using black ink.

nurses consistently and accurately document implementation of fall precautions or evaluation of pain management interventions. Any deficiencies identified are shared with all members of the nursing staff so that changes in policy or practice can occur.

Education

Health care records are a rich source of information about a patient's health care. Reading the record of a patient for whom you are assigned to care is an effective way to learn the nature of a patient's condition and response to treatment. Over time, as you care for patients with similar diagnoses or problems, the information gained from those

patients' records allows you to identify patterns and trends and to build your clinical knowledge (Fig 26.1). As you identify patterns associated with specific diseases and conditions, you are able to anticipate the type of care your patients require and how patients respond to treatment.

Research

De-identification is a process used to prevent a person's identity from being connected with information. For example, when a data form is used to collect information from a health record, a patient's name or Social Security number is not entered; instead, a random number is

FIG. 26.1 Nursing students and nursing faculty at computer screens reviewing records.

used for labeling and categorizing the form. De-identified data obtained from health records can be used for statistical analysis (e.g., frequency of clinical disorders, complications, use of specific medical and nursing therapies, clinical outcomes achieved during care for specific illnesses, and patient mortality). Analysis of the data contributes to evidence-based nursing practice and high-quality health care (LoBiondo-Wood and Haber, 2021). After obtaining appropriate approval from an institutional review board (IRB) of a health care agency or hospital, a nurse researcher reviews patients' records in a research study to collect information on a particular health problem. For example, if a nurse researcher suspects that early ambulation decreases the complication rate in postoperative patients, the researcher could review the records of select surgical patients to compare the rates of postoperative complications following early versus late ambulation.

The Shift to Electronic Documentation

Historically, health care professionals documented on paper health care records. Paper records were episode oriented, with a separate record created for each patient visit to a health care agency. Because a health care provider could not easily review a previous record, key information such as patient allergies, current medications, and complications from treatment were lost from one episode of care (e.g., hospitalization or clinic visit) to the next, jeopardizing a patient's safety (Hebda et al., 2019).

To facilitate communication among health care providers and improve patient safety, the American Recovery and Reinvestment Act (ARRA) of 2009 set a goal that all health care records would be kept electronically as of 2014 (Hebda et al., 2019). Since 2011 the Health Information Technology for Economic and Clinical Health Act (HITECH), enacted under Title XIII of ARRA, has been a major driver in the adoption and use of electronic health records (EHRs) across the United States. HITECH established provisions to promote the meaningful use of health information technology (HIT) to improve the quality and value of health care (U.S. Department of Health & Human Services [USDHHS], 2017). Meaningful use requires that use of an electronic health record system (EHRS) results in improved quality, safety, and efficiency of health care; increases health care consumers' active involvement in their care; increases coordination of health care delivery; advances public health; and safeguards the privacy and security of personal health records (Rathert et al., 2019; Stimson & Bodruff, 2017). By 2014 the goal of the ARRA was to have all health care records maintained electronically. Although the goal has not been fully met, the ONC (2018) reported the following:

- Ninety-six percent of all nonfederal acute care hospitals possessed certified HIT.
- Small rural and critical access hospitals had the lowest rates at 93%.
- Ninety-nine percent of large hospitals (more than 300 beds) had certified HIT, and 97% of medium-sized hospitals (more than 100 beds) had certified HIT.

Although the terms *EHR* and *EMR* have been used interchangeably in practice, there are differences between them. The term electronic health record (EHR) has become the favored term for an individual's lifetime computerized record; it means both the displayed or printed record. The addition of an "S" at the end of the acronym *(EHRS)* indicates the supporting software system. The term electronic medical record (EMR) refers to a patient's record within an integrated health care information system for an individual visit to a health care provider's office or for an individual admission to an acute care setting that allows for seamless documentation of the progression of care. To meet agreed-on standards, EHRs are expected to have the following attributes or components (Hebda et al., 2019):

- Provide a longitudinal or lifetime patient record by linking all patient data from previous health care encounters.
- Contain a problem list that indicates current clinical problems for each health care encounter, the number of occurrences associated with all past and current problems, and the current status of each problem.
- Use accepted standardized measures to evaluate and record health status and functional levels.
- Provide a method for documenting the clinical reasoning or rationale for diagnoses and conclusions that allows clinical decision making to be tracked by all providers who access the record.
- Support confidentiality, privacy, and audit trails.
- Provide continuous access to authorized users at any time and allow multiple health care providers access to customized views of patient data at the same time.
- Support links to local or remote information resources such as databases using the Internet or intranet resources based within an agency.
- Support the use of decision analysis tools.
- Support direct entry of patient data by providers.
- Include mechanisms for measuring the cost and quality of care.
- Support existing and evolving clinical needs by being flexible and expandable.

A unique feature of an EHR is its ability to integrate all patient information into one record, regardless of the number of times a patient enters a health care system. An EHR also includes results of diagnostic studies that may include diagnostic images (e.g., x-ray or ultrasound images) and decision support software programs. Because an unlimited number of patient records potentially can be stored within an EHR system, health care providers can access clinical data to identify quality issues, link interventions with positive outcomes, and make evidence-based decisions (Atasoy et al., 2019). The key advantages of an EHR for nursing include a means for nurses to compare current clinical data about a patient with data from previous health care encounters, maintain ongoing symptom management, and provide an ongoing record of health education provided to a patient and the patient's response to that information (Karp et al., 2019; Ozkaynak, et al., 2017).

Maintaining Privacy, Confidentiality, and Security of the Health Care Record

Nurses are legally and ethically obligated to keep information about patients confidential. Only members of the health care team who are directly involved in a patient's care have legitimate access to a patient's health record. You discuss a patient's diagnosis, treatment, assessment, and any personal conversations only with members of the health care team who are specifically involved in the patient's care. Do not share information with other patients or with health care team members who are not caring for the patient. Patients have the right to request copies of their medical record and read the information. Each agency has policies that describe how medical records are shared with patients or other people who request them. In most situations, patients are required to give written permission for release of their medical information.

The Health Insurance Portability and Accountability Act (HIPAA) of 1996 was the first federal legislation to provide protection for patient records; it governs all areas of patient information and management of that information. To eliminate barriers that potentially delay access to care, HIPAA requires providers to notify patients of privacy policies and to obtain written acknowledgment from patients indicating they received this information. Under HIPAA, the Privacy Rule requires that disclosure or requests regarding health information be limited to the specific information required for a particular purpose (Hebda et al., 2019). For example, if you need a patient's home telephone number to reschedule an appointment, access to the health record is limited solely to telephone information. Of equal importance under HIPAA is the Security Rule, which specifies administrative, physical, and technical safeguards for 18 specific elements of **protected health information (PHI)** in electronic form (USDHHS, 2020).

Nurses are permitted to use health records for data gathering, research, or continuing education as long as records are used as specified and permission is granted from an institutional review board (for research) or appropriate administrative department. When you are a student learning in a clinical setting, maintaining patient confidentiality and adhering to HIPAA are required as part of professional practice. You can review patient health records only for information needed to provide safe and effective patient care. For example, when you are assigned to care for a patient, you need to review the patient's health record and the interprofessional plan of care. You *do not* share this information with classmates (except for clinical conferences) and *do not* access the health records of other patients on the unit. Access to an EHR is traceable through user log-in information. It is unethical to view health records of other patients, and breaches of confidentiality will lead to disciplinary action by employers and potentially dismissal from work or nursing school. To protect patient confidentiality, you must ensure that any electronic or written materials you use in your student clinical practice *do not* include patient identifiers (e.g., name, room number, date of birth, demographic information). *Never* print material from an EHR for personal use; any information printed must be for professional use only and should not include identifiable information.

Privacy, Confidentiality, and Security Mechanisms

There are legal implications associated with the use of electronic documentation. It is possible for anyone to access a computer within a health care agency and gain information about almost any patient. Under HIPAA, ensuring appropriate access to and confidentiality of personal health information is the responsibility of all persons working in health care. Personal health information is individually identifiable information relating to an individual's past, present, or future health status that is created, collected, transmitted, or maintained by a HIPAA-covered entity in relation to the provision of health care, payment for health care services, or use in health care operations (USDHHS, 2020). Protection of information and computer systems is one of your top priorities.

Most computer information system security mechanisms use a combination of logical and physical restrictions to protect information.

For example, an automatic sign-off is a safety mechanism that logs a user off a computer system after a specified period of inactivity (Hebda et al., 2019). Other security measures include firewalls and the installation of antivirus and spyware-detection software. A **firewall** is a combination of hardware and software that protects private network resources (e.g., the information system of the agency) from outside hackers, network damage, and theft or misuse of information.

Physical security measures include placing computers or file servers in restricted areas or using privacy filters for computer screens that are visible to visitors or other people who should not have access to the information displayed. This form of security has limited benefit, especially if an agency uses mobile wireless devices such as notebooks, tablets, personal computers (PCs), and smartphones. These devices are easily misplaced or lost, and at risk for falling into the wrong hands.

Access or log-in codes along with passwords are frequently used for authenticating authorized access to electronic records. A **password** is a collection of alphanumeric characters and symbols that a user types into a computer sign-on screen before accessing a program after the entry and acceptance of an access code or username. Strong passwords use combinations of letters, numbers, and symbols that are difficult to guess. When using a health care agency computer system, it is essential that you do not share your computer password with anyone under any circumstances. A good system requires frequent changes in personal passwords to prevent unauthorized persons from tampering with records. A password does not appear on the computer screen when it is typed, and it should not be known to anyone but the user and information system administrators (Hebda et al., 2019). Most health care personnel are given access only to patients in their work area. Some staff (e.g., administrators or risk managers) have authority to access all patient records. To protect patient privacy, health care agencies track who accesses patient records and when they access them. Failure to adhere to HIPAA can result in civil and criminal penalties for health care agencies and providers. Depending on the nature of a violation, civil penalties can result in minimal fines of $100 per violation and maximum fines of $50,000 per violation with an annual maximum of $1.5 million (American Medical Association, 2021). Thus employers have policies for disciplinary action.

Handling and Disposing of Information

Maintaining the confidentiality of health records is a fundamental responsibility of all members of the health care team. It is essential to safeguard any information that is printed from the record or extracted for report purposes. For example, you print a copy of a nursing activities work list to use in planning your shift while providing patient care. You refer to information on the list and write notes to record into the computer and share later during the hand-off report. Information on the list is protected health information (PHI); you must not leave it in view of unauthorized persons. Destroy (e.g., shred or place in a locked receptacle designated for collection of material that is to be shredded) anything that is printed when the information is no longer needed. Nursing students should not print information from the health record to take away from the clinical agency to complete written assignments for clinical course assignments. Instead, transcribe patient information needed for clinical assignments to academic forms or notebooks directly while viewing the health record on the computer screen or the physical chart. You must de-identify all patient data that is transcribed onto forms or used for academic papers for clinical courses in nursing school. Any information that is transcribed and must be removed from the clinical setting and any documents that must be printed out must be kept secure and destroyed through shredding or disposal in a locked receptacle as soon as possible.

Historically, information printed from a patient record and/or faxed to other health care providers has been the primary source for accidental, unauthorized disclosure of PHI. All papers containing PHI must be destroyed after use or after being faxed. Sometimes nurses are responsible for erasing from a computer hard drive files that contain calendars, schedules for surgery or diagnostic procedures, or other daily records that contain PHI (Hebda et al., 2019). You are responsible to know and follow disposal policies for these types of records in the agency where you work.

Health care agencies and departments should have policies for the use of fax machines that specify the kinds of information that can be faxed, who can receive faxed information, where information can be sent, and the process used to verify that information was sent to and received by the appropriate person or persons. Information sent by fax should not exceed what was requested or required for immediate clinical needs. Following are steps to enhance fax security (Neppe and Gerck, 2019):

- Always use a cover page.
- For any new recipient, verify the number with a test fax before sending PHI.
- Follow agency policies for storing, copying, and disposing of faxes containing PHI.
- Use a fax machine designated exclusively for PHI, and keep it separate from other fax machines.
- Fax machines must be located in secure, nonpublic areas.
- There must be a robust process in place for password creation and password changes.
- Providers must be able to prove that their agency has implemented policies and procedures to protect PHI.
- After faxing something, ensure that the document receipt printed.
- Consider using secure email technologies such as Zsentry.com, which automatically date and time stamp faxes.

STANDARDS AND GUIDELINES FOR QUALITY NURSING DOCUMENTATION

Whether the transfer of patient information occurs through verbal reports or electronic or written documents, you need to follow basic guidelines and standards for nursing documentation. Every health care agency has standards that govern the type of information nurses document and for which they are held accountable. Agency standards or policies often dictate the frequency of documentation, such as how often you record a nursing assessment or a patient's level of pain. You are responsible for knowing the standards of care for every nursing procedure and the standards for providing complete and accurate documentation. Information in patient health records can be used as evidence in a court of law to demonstrate whether nursing standards of practice were, or were not, met.

In addition, your documentation needs to conform to the standards of the National Committee for Quality Assurance (NCQA) and accrediting bodies such as TJC to maintain agency accreditation and to minimize liability. Health care agencies usually incorporate accreditation standards into policies and revise documentation

systems and forms to suit these standards. Current documentation standards require that all patients admitted to a health care agency be assessed for physical, psychosocial, environmental, self-care, spiritual, cultural, knowledge level, and discharge planning needs. Your documentation needs to demonstrate application of the nursing process, describe clinical decision making, and include evidence of patient and family teaching and discharge planning (TJC, 2021). In addition to HIPAA standards, health care documentation is affected by standards from state and federal regulatory agencies, the Department of Justice, and CMS.

Guidelines for Quality Documentation

Quality nursing documentation enhances efficient, individualized patient care and has five important characteristics: factual, accurate, current, organized, and complete. It is easier to maintain these characteristics in your documentation if you continually seek to express ideas clearly and succinctly by doing the following:
- Stick to the facts.
- Write in short sentences.
- Use simple, short words.
- Avoid the use of jargon or abbreviations.

Factual. A factual record contains clear descriptive, objective information about what a nurse observes, hears, palpates, and smells. Avoid vague terms such as *appears, seems,* or *apparently.* These words suggest you are stating an opinion; they do not accurately communicate facts and do not inform other caregivers about the details regarding the behaviors exhibited by a patient. Objective data are obtained through direct observation and measurement and include description of a patient's behaviors—for example, "*BP 90/50, heart rate 115 and regular, patient diaphoretic and holding both hands over abdominal dressing.*" The only subjective data included in the record are statements made by a patient. When recording subjective data, document a patient's exact words within quotation marks whenever possible. Include objective data to support subjective data so that your documentation is as descriptive as possible. For example, instead of documenting "*the patient seems anxious,*" provide objective signs of anxiety and document the patient's statement about the feelings experienced: "*Patient's heart rate 110 beats/min, respiratory rate is slightly labored at 22 breaths/min, and patient states, 'I feel very nervous.'*"

Accurate. Using exact measurements establishes accuracy and helps you determine whether a patient's condition has changed in a positive or negative way. For example, a description such as "*Intake, 360 mL of water*" is more accurate than "*Patient drank an adequate amount of fluid.*" Documenting that an abdominal incision is "*Approximated, 5 cm in length without redness, drainage, or edema*" is more descriptive than "*Large abdominal incision healing well.*" Documentation of concise data is clear and easy to understand. Avoid using unnecessary words and irrelevant detail. For example, the fact that the patient is watching television is necessary only when this activity is significant to the patient's status and plan of care. Examples of criteria for documentation or reporting specific situations can be found in Table 26.2.

Appropriate Use of Abbreviations in Health Care Documentation. Use abbreviations carefully to avoid misinterpretation and promote patient safety. TJC (2020) maintains a list of "do not use" abbreviations to promote patient safety (Table 26.3). In addition, TJC requires that health care agencies develop a list of standard abbreviations, symbols, and acronyms to be used by all members of the health care team when documenting or communicating patient care and treatment. To minimize errors, spell out abbreviations in their entirety when they become confusing.

TABLE 26.2   Examples of Criteria for Documentation and Reporting

Topic	Criteria to Report or Record
Subjective assessment data	Patient's description of episode in quotation marks (e.g., "*I feel like an elephant is sitting on my chest, and I can't catch my breath.*") Describe in patient's own words the onset, location, description of condition (severity, duration, frequency, precipitating, aggravating, and relieving factors) (e.g., "*The pain in my left knee started last week after I knelt on the ground. Every time I bend my knee, I have a shooting pain on the inside of the knee.*").
Objective assessment data (e.g., rash, tenderness, breath sounds, or descriptions of patient behavior [e.g., anxiety, confusion, hostility])	Onset, location, description of condition (e.g., 11:00: 2-cm raised pale, red area noted on back of left hand). Precipitating factors, behaviors exhibited (e.g., Physician informed patient of diagnosis, patient pacing in room, avoiding eye contact with nurse), patient statements (e.g., repeatedly stating, "*I have to go home now*").
Nursing interventions, treatments, and evaluation (e.g., enema, bath, dressing change)	Time administered, equipment used, patient's response (subjective and objective responses) compared with previous treatment (e.g., denied incisional pain during abdominal dressing change, ambulated 300 feet in hallway without assistance).
Medication administration	At time of administration when using a computerized bar-code medication administration program (or immediately after administration), document time medication given; medication name, dose, route; preliminary assessment (e.g., pain level, vital signs); patient response, or effect of medication (e.g., 1500: Reports "*throbbing headache all over my head.*" Rates pain at 6 (scale 0–10). Tylenol 650 mg given PO. 1530: Patient reports pain level 2 (scale 0–10) and states, "*the throbbing has stopped.*"
Patient and/or family teaching	Information presented; method of instruction (e.g., discussion, demonstration, videotape, booklet); and patient response, including questions and evidence of understanding such as teach-back, return demonstration, or change in behavior.
Discharge planning	Measurable expected outcomes, progress toward goals, need for referrals.

TABLE 26.3   The Joint Commission's Official "Do Not Use" List[a] of Abbreviations

Do Not Use	Potential Problem	Use Instead
U, u (unit)	Mistaken for "0" (zero), the number "4" (four), or "cc"	Write "unit."
IU (International Unit)	Mistaken for "IV" (intravenous) or the number "10" (ten)	Write "International Unit."
Q.D., QD, q.d., qd (daily) Q.O.D., QOD, q.o.d., qod (every other day)	Mistaken for each other Period after the Q mistaken for "I" and the "O" mistaken for "I"	Write "daily." Write "every other day."
Trailing zero (X.0 mg)[b] Lack of leading zero (.X mg)	Decimal point is missed	Write X mg. Write 0.X mg.
MS MSO$_4$ and MgSO$_4$	Can mean morphine sulfate or magnesium sulfate Confused for one another	Write "morphine sulfate." Write "magnesium sulfate."

From https://www.jointcommission.org/facts_about_do_not_use_list/, 2020. Accessed May 26, 2021.
[a]Applies to all orders and all medication-related documentation that is handwritten (including free-text computer entry) or on pre-printed forms.
[b]Exception: A "trailing zero" may be used only where required to demonstrate the level of precision of the value being reported, such as for laboratory results, imaging studies that report size of lesions, or catheter/tube sizes. It may not be used in medication orders or other medication-related documentation.

Correct spelling demonstrates a level of competency and attention to detail. Many terms are easily misinterpreted (e.g., *dysphagia* or *dysphasia*). Some spelling errors can result in serious treatment errors (e.g., the names of medications such as lamotrigine and lamivudine or hydromorphone and hydrocodone are similar). Transcribe medication information carefully to ensure a patient receives the correct medication.

All health care record entries should be dated and timed, and the author of each entry must be clearly identified (TJC, 2021). Each entry in a patient's record must end with the caregiver's full name or initials and credentials/title/role, such as "Jane Cook, RN." If initials are used in a signature, the full name and credentials/title/role of the individual needs to be documented at least once in the health care record to allow others to readily identify that individual. As a nursing student, enter your full name and nursing student abbreviation, such as "David Jones, NS" or "David Jones, SN." The abbreviation for *nursing student* varies between *NS* for *nursing student* or *SN* for *student*

nurse. Include information about your educational institution at the end of your signature when required by agency policy.

Current. Timely entries are essential in a patient's ongoing care, as delays in documentation can lead to unsafe patient care. Many health care agencies keep records or computers near a patient's bedside to facilitate immediate documentation of information. Document the following activities or findings at the time of occurrence:
- Vital signs
- Pain assessment
- Administration of medications and treatments
- Preparation for diagnostic tests or surgery, including preoperative checklist
- Change in patient's status, treatment provided, and who was notified (e.g., health care provider, manager, patient's family)
- Admission, transfer, discharge, or death of a patient
- Patient's response to treatment or intervention

FIG. 26.2 Comparison of 24 hours of military time with the hourly positions for civilian time on the clockface.

Most health care agencies use military time, a 24-hour system that avoids misinterpretation of a.m. and p.m. times (Fig. 26.2). Instead of two 12-hour cycles in standard time, the military clock is one 24-hour time cycle. The military clock ends with midnight at 2400 and begins at 1 minute after midnight as 0001. For example, 10:22 a.m. is 1022 military time, and 10:22 p.m. is 2222 military time.

Organized. Documentation is more effective when notes are concise, clear and to the point, and presented in a logical order. To document notes about complex situations in an organized fashion, first think about the situation, and then make decisions about what information and words you need to include before beginning to enter data in the health care record. Application of your critical thinking and clinical judgment skills to the nursing process will help you document clearly and comprehensively in a logical order. For example, an organized entry would describe a patient's pain, your assessment and interventions, and the patient's response to treatment.

Complete. Be sure the information within a recorded entry or a report is complete, containing appropriate and essential information. Follow established criteria and standards for thorough communication within the health care record or when reporting certain health problems or nursing activities.

METHODS OF DOCUMENTATION

There are several documentation methods for recording patient assessment data and progress notes. Regardless of whether documentation is entered electronically or on paper, each health care agency selects a documentation system that reflects the philosophy of nursing at that agency. The same system is used throughout a specific agency and sometimes is used throughout a health care system as well.

Documentation of Patient Assessment Data

Within the EHR, nurses routinely document patient physiological data and routine care using **flow sheets** (graphic records) that are organized by body system and navigated through use of the computer mouse with a series of tabs or rows (Fig. 26.3). These forms allow you to quickly and easily enter assessment data about a patient, such as vital signs, admission and/or daily weights, and percentage of meals eaten.

They also facilitate the documentation of routine, repetitive care, such as hygiene measures, ambulation, and safety and restraint checks. These documents provide current patient information accessible to all members of the health care team and help team members quickly see patient trends over time.

Describe any routine data in greater detail when a change in a patient's functional ability or status occurs. For example, if your patient's blood pressure, pulse, and respirations are elevated above expected values after a walk down the hall, you would first complete and record a focused assessment in the flow sheet, and then document additional, detailed information about the patient's status and response to the walk in the appropriate place in the health care record using narrative free text within the flow sheet, or in a narrative progress note.

Progress Notes. Health care team members monitor and record the progress made toward resolving a patient's problems in progress notes. Health care providers write narrative progress notes in one of several formats or structured notes within the EHR. Notes either take the form of traditional narrative documentation or make use of precise formats such as (1) focus charting, incorporating data, action, and response (DAR); (2) SOAP notes, identifying interprofessional problems; or (3) notes with a specific nursing focus, identifying nursing problems or diagnoses (PIE). See Box 26.1 for examples of nursing documentation using these formats. Narrative documentation is the format traditionally used by nurses and health care providers to record patient assessment, clinical decisions, and care provided; it consists of a storylike format to document information. In an electronic nursing information system, this is accomplished through the use of free text entry or menu selections (Hebda et al., 2019). An example of a comprehensive narrative note written by a nurse looks like this:

> 1915: Adhering to bed rest as ordered. Left lower extremity is swollen; calf circumference is 76 cm (30 inches). Areas of redness that are warm and tender to touch are noted over anterior 3 cm by 4 cm (1.2–1.6 inches) and medial areas 3 cm by 3 cm (1.2 by 1.2 inches) of left leg. Left lower leg elevated on one pillow. Heparin infusing at 1400 units/hr via 20-gauge peripheral IV in left lower forearm. Site without redness, swelling, or drainage. Verbalizes sharp throbbing leg pain rated at 8 on a 0-to-10 scale. Pedal pulses 3+ bilaterally. Capillary refill in toes of both feet is less than 3 seconds. Oxycodone/acetaminophen 2 tablets (PO) given for pain as ordered. Chris Banks, RN.
>
> 2000: States, "The pain medication really helped." Rates pain in left lower leg at 4 on a 0-to-10 scale. Comfort level goal is 4/10. Chris Banks, RN.

Although the nursing patient assessment flow sheet section of the EHR allows users to enter descriptive details through the use of short, narrative comments, these sections of the EHR are primarily designed to allow the use of multiple checkboxes or drop-down lists. When entering a narrative progress note in the EHR, be clear and accurate when describing subjective and objective patient assessment findings, as well as any interventions performed to resolve patient problems and maintain patient safety. Health care providers review nursing documentation for details about changes in a patient's condition, and use of narrative documentation within the EHR may provide more detail than charting by exception when trying to document complex situations. EHRs that enable all health care providers to easily retrieve important patient information from narrative notes, as well as flow sheet data, may augment clinician communication and interprofessional understanding for patient care (Bardach et al., 2017; Wu et al., 2019).

Respiratory Assessment

☐ No assessment required at this time

Respiratory Pattern
Mark All That Apply:

- ☑ Even
- ☑ Effortless
- ☐ Uneven
- ☐ Labored
- ☐ Deep

Respiratory Effort
Mark All That Apply:

- ☐ Dyspnea/shortness of breath
- ☐ Shortness of breath on exertion
- ☐ Increased chest expansion
- ☐ Orthopnea
- ☐ Use of accessory muscles

Lung Auscultation

Left Lateral

Mark the breath sounds heard at this location

Left Lateral:
- ○ Clear
- ○ Fine crackles
- ◉ Coarse crackles
- ○ Rhonchi
- ○ Rales
- ○ Wheeze
- ○ Diminished
- ○ Absent

Wheeze Description:
- ○ Inspiratory
- ○ Expiratory
- ○ Throughout

Respiratory Pattern and Breath Sounds Notes:

Oxygenation

- ☑ Oxygen in use
- ◉ Amount of oxygen in L/min: 2
  - Or
- ○ Amount of oxygen in %

Oxygen delivery system:
- ○ Room Air
- ○ Aerosol
- ◉ Nasal Cannula
- ○ Non-rebreather Mask
- ○ Partial Rebreather Mask

Oxygenation Notes:

Oxygenation evaluation:
- ○ Continuous pulse oximetry
- ◉ Intermittent pulse oximetry

Respiratory/breathing support:
Mark All That Apply:
- ☐ Nebulizer treatment
- ☑ Incentive spirometer

Incentive spirometer best effort (mL): 700

Suctioning
- ☐ Periodic
- ☐ Frequent suctioning with bulb syringe

Amount: -SELECT-
Color: -SELECT-
Consistency: -SELECT-
Odor: -SELECT-

FIG. 26.3 Example of documentation of nursing assessment of respiratory system within the electronic health record (EHR). (Copyright © Elsevier 2019. SimChart® www.evolve.elsevier.com.)

BOX 26.1 **Examples of Nursing Documentation in Different Formats**

Narrative Note
- **Patient states,** "My leg is so swollen. I'm worried about this blood clot." Is asking questions about medications and how DVT will be treated. Alert and oriented; responds appropriately to instruction. Discussed importance of bed rest and the reason for treatment with heparin infusion. Explained need for daily blood tests to check anticoagulation levels. Provided brochure on anticoagulation therapy for DVT. Used teach-back method to validate patient understanding; he is able to describe that the heparin infusion will be stopped when his PT/INR is therapeutic on warfarin and he can expect to take warfarin for about 6 months after discharge until clot is resolved.

PIE
- A PIE note has a specific nursing focus.
- **P: Nursing problem or diagnosis**—*Lack of Knowledge* related to inexperience with disease condition
- **I: Interventions that will be used to address the problem**—Provided brochure on anticoagulation therapy for DVT. Explained rationale for bed rest and daily blood tests to check anticoagulation levels. Explained that heparin infusion will be stopped when PT/INR is at therapeutic level and that he can expect to take warfarin for about 6 months until clot resolves.
- **E: Nursing evaluation**: Patient states, "I'm worried about the blood clot, but I understand how it is being treated." Able to teach back and verbalize that the heparin infusion will be stopped when PT/INR tests are "normal." Also states that he expects to take warfarin for about 6 months until clot in leg dissolves.

Focus Charting
- Uses a DAR format to report problems. DAR notes address patient concerns such as a sign or symptom, condition, nursing diagnosis, behavior, significant event, or change in condition.
- **D: Data** (subjective and objective)—Patient states, "My leg is so swollen. I'm worried about this blood clot. Do you know how they are going to treat it?"
- **A: Action or nursing intervention**—Provided brochure on anticoagulation therapy for DVT. Explained rationale for bed rest and daily blood tests to check anticoagulation levels. Explained that heparin infusion will be stopped when PT/INR is at therapeutic level.
- **R: Response of the patient**—Able to teach back and verbalized that heparin infusion will be stopped when PT/INR reaches "normal level" and that he can expect to take warfarin for 6 months after discharge until clot is fully resolved.

SOAP Note—Used By All Health Care Disciplines
- **S: Subjective**—Patient states, "My leg is so swollen. I'm worried about this blood clot. Do you know how they are going to treat it?"
- **O: Objective**—Patient asking question about medications and how DVT will be treated. Alert and oriented; responds appropriately to instruction.
- **A: Assessment**—Patient lacks knowledge regarding anticoagulation therapy, seeking information about therapy.
- **P: Plan**: Discussed importance of bed rest and the reason for treatment with heparin infusion. Provided brochure on anticoagulation therapy for DVT. Explained rationale for bed rest and daily blood tests to check anticoagulation levels. Explained that heparin infusion will be stopped when PT/INR is at therapeutic level and that he can expect to take warfarin for about 6 months until clot resolves.

REFLECT NOW

What patient situations have you observed in the clinical setting that might be more appropriately documented through use of a narrative note versus use of flow sheet documentation within the EHR? Think of a recent patient situation you observed that you believe should be documented in narrative fashion. Practice writing a narrative note about that situation, and ask your clinical faculty to review and comment on your work.

Charting by Exception

The philosophy behind charting by exception (CBE) is that all standards for normal assessment findings or for routine care activities are met unless otherwise documented. Exception-based documentation systems incorporate standards of care and use clearly, predefined statements for the nursing documentation of "normal" body system findings. These normal findings, called "within defined limits" (WDL) or "within normal limits" (WNL), consist of written criteria for a "normal" assessment for each body system. Documentation within a computerized system allows nurses to select a WDL statement or to choose other statements from a drop-down menu that allow description of any unexpected assessment findings or assessment findings that deviate from the WDL definition (Elliott et al., 2018). Well-designed flow sheets are a key part of a good exception-based documentation system within the EHR. However, this form of documentation also calls for use of narrative notes concerning any significant indicator of the patient's condition or change in status, any subsequent interventions, and the patient's response (Nurses Service Organization, 2018). When an exception occurs, if a nurse's note offers few explanations, little description of key findings, or no mention of periodic patient checks, a patient's lawyer could claim negligence on the part of the nurse (Nurses Service Organization, 2018).

The SBAR or ISBAR format is a commonly used framework for a narrative note when exceptions occur. Both are also popular formats for verbal reporting (see Chapter 24). When changes in a patient's condition develop, you must include a narrative progress note that provides a thorough and precise description of the effects of the changes on the patient and the actions taken to address those changes.

COMMON RECORD-KEEPING FORMS WITHIN THE ELECTRONIC HEALTH RECORD

Nurses use a variety of electronic or paper forms for the type of information routinely documented within the EHR. The categories or data fields within a form are usually derived from agency standards of practice or guidelines established by accrediting agencies.

Admission Nursing History Form

A nurse completes a nursing history form when a patient is admitted to a nursing unit. The fields in the form guide you through a comprehensive assessment to identify relevant nursing diagnoses or problems (see Chapters 16 and 30). Completion of this form provides baseline data that you use for comparison when a patient's condition changes.

Patient Care Summary

Many computerized documentation systems generate a patient care summary document that you review (and sometimes print) for each patient at the beginning and/or end of each shift to use as a worksheet for organizing care and in giving the hand-off report (Fig. 26.4). The document automatically updates and provides the most current information that was entered into the EHR and usually includes the following information:
- Basic demographic data (e.g., age, religion)
- Health care provider's name
- Primary medical diagnosis

ELECTRONIC HEALTH RECORD

SimChart®

Rae, Lisa   MRN: 7761384   Room: 322   Health Care Provider: L Moore, MD

Sex: Female   Weight: 110 lb   Code Status: Full   BMI: 17.8   Hospital Floor: Medical-Surgical

Age: 78 years   Height: 5' 6"   Allergies: NKA   Diet: 3 g sodium restriction

Patient Summary

- Authority for Admission
- Admission History
- History and Physical
- Orders
- MAR
- Vital Signs
- Assessments
- Basic Nursing Care
- Provider Notes
- Nursing Notes
- Laboratory-Diagnostics
- Patient Teaching

Summary

Risk Alerts

Fall Risk:
No Data Entered

Pressure Sore Risk:
No Data Entered

Obstructive Sleep Apnea Risk:
No Data Entered

Basic Information

Code Status:
Full code

Isolation Status:
No Data Entered

Allergies:
NKA

Alerts:
No Data Entered

Problem List

Medical Diagnosis:
Primary Diagnosis: Hypotension
Secondary Diagnosis: Mechanical fall
Tertiary Diagnosis:
No Data Entered

Nursing Diagnosis:
No Data Entered

Patient Monitoring

Chart Time	Temperature (F)	Pulse (Beats/min)	Respiration (Resp/min)	Blood Pressure (mmHg)	Oxygen Saturation (%)
Mon 10:40	98.6	84	18	94/70	93

Pain: Mon | 11:40 Numeric pain level: 5   Intake: 200 mL

Blood Glucose: No Data Entered   Output: 250 mL

Active Invasive Items

IV Lines:
Mon | 10:40 **Right Median Cubital (Antecubital)**
Peripheral

Active Wounds

Lesions   Mon | 10:40   **Right Hip**
Bruising (contusion)

FIG. 26.4 Example of sections/information available in an electronic health record (EHR). Copyright © Elsevier 2019. SimChart® www.evolve.elsevier.com.)

- Medical and surgical history
- Current orders from the health care provider (e.g., dressing changes, ambulation, glucose monitoring)
- Nursing care plan
- Nursing orders (e.g., education needed, symptom relief measures, counseling)
- Scheduled tests and procedures
- Safety precautions used in a patient's care
- Factors that affect patient independence with activities of daily living
- Nearest relative/guardian or person designated as a patient's health care power of attorney to contact in an emergency
- Emergency code status (e.g., indication of do-not-resuscitate order)
- Allergies

Care Plans

Many computerized documentation systems include standardized care plans or clinical practice guidelines (CPGs) to facilitate the creation and documentation of a nursing and/or interprofessional plan of care (see Chapter 18). Each standardized plan facilitates safe and consistent care for an identified problem by describing or listing agency standards and evidence-based guidelines that are easily accessed and included within a patient's EHR (Khokhar et al., 2017; Macieira et al., 2019). After completing a nursing assessment, you identify and select the standardized plans that are appropriate for the patient and are to be included in the individualized plan of care. Most computer documentation systems allow these care plans to be modified by creating individualized interventions and outcomes for each patient.

Standardized care plans are useful when conducting QI audits. They also improve continuity of care among professional nurses. When they are used, the nurse still remains responsible for providing individualized care to each patient. Standardized care plans cannot replace a nurse's clinical judgment and decision making. You update care plans on a regular basis to ensure that the documents are appropriate and evidence-based.

Discharge Summary Forms

Nurses help ensure cost-effective care and appropriate reimbursement by preparing patients for a safe, effective, and timely discharge from a health care agency. Developing a comprehensive plan for a safe discharge relies on interprofessional discharge planning. This process includes identification of key clinical outcomes and appropriate timelines for reaching them, the appropriate level of care for discharge, and all necessary resources.

Ideally discharge planning begins at admission, which requires partnering with the patient and family caregiver to identify outcomes for recovery and potential discharge needs. Nursing and other health care professionals then begin to plan with the patient for discharge to the appropriate level of care. Consideration is given to the support services (i.e., home care, physical therapy) required and whether any health care equipment is needed in the home setting. Involvement of the patient and family in the discharge planning process ensures that they have the necessary information and resources to return home or move to the next level of care. Discharge documentation includes medications, diet, community resources, follow-up care, and the name

---

BOX 26.2   Discharge Summary Information

- Use clear, concise descriptions in patient's own language.
- Provide step-by-step description of how to perform a procedure (e.g., home medication administration). Reinforce explanation with printed instructions for the patient to take home.
- Provide a detailed list of all prescribed medications.
- Identify precautions to follow when performing self-care or procedures (e.g., dressing change) or taking medications.
- Review any restrictions that may relate to activities of daily living (e.g., bathing, ambulating, and driving).
- Review signs and symptoms of complications to report to health care provider.
- List names and phone numbers of health care providers and community resources for the patient to contact.
- Identify any unresolved problem(s), including plans for follow-up and continuous treatment.
- List actual time of discharge, mode of transportation, and who accompanied patient.

BOX 26.3   Guidelines for Telephone and Verbal Orders

- Only authorized staff (who are identified in a written policy by each agency) receive and record telephone and verbal orders.
- Clearly identify the patient's name, room number, and diagnoses.
- Use clarification questions to avoid misunderstandings. Ask health care provider to repeat a word or phrase if needed.
- Document "TO" (telephone order) or "VO" (verbal order), including date and time, name of patient, the complete order; the name and credentials of the health care provider giving the order(s); and your name and credentials as the nurse taking the order.
- Read back all orders prescribed to the health care provider who gave them and document "TORB" (telephone order read back) when signing your name and credentials.
- Follow agency policies; some agencies require TOs and VOs to be reviewed and signed by two nurses.
- The health care provider cosigns each TO and VO within the time frame required by each agency (usually 24 hours).

---

of a person to contact for questions or in case of an emergency. All of this information is included in a discharge summary document that is printed out and given to the patient on discharge. The information remains in the EHR as a record of the discharge teaching that was provided (Box 26.2).

DOCUMENTING COMMUNICATION WITH PROVIDERS AND UNIQUE EVENTS

Telephone Calls

Document every phone call you make to a health care provider. Your documentation needs to include when the call was made, the number called, who made the call, who was called, to whom information was given, what information was given, and what information was received. For example: *"08/25/2021 (2130): Called Dr. Banks' office at 123-456-7890. Spoke with L. Matthews, RN, who will inform Dr. Banks that Mr. Andrews' potassium level drawn at 2000 was 5.9 mEq/dL. Informed that Dr. Banks will call back after he is finished seeing his current patient. R. Jenner, RN."*

Telephone and Verbal Orders

Telephone orders (TOs) occur when a health care provider gives therapeutic orders over the phone to a registered nurse (RN). Verbal orders (VOs) occur when a health care provider gives therapeutic orders to an RN face-to-face while they are standing in proximity to each other. The potential for verbal orders to be misunderstood, misheard, or transcribed incorrectly makes them error prone, particularly given different care provider accents, dialects, and drug name pronunciations (Institute for Safe Medication Practices [ISMP], 2017). Use of VOs is discouraged except in urgent or emergent situations. TOs and VOs should be used only when absolutely necessary and not for the sake of convenience for the health care provider. In some situations, it is wise to have a second person listen on the telephone line as a TO is given by a health care provider; some agency policies require this. Check your agency's policy. Box 26.3 provides guidelines that promote accurate documentation of TOs or VOs.

A nurse receiving a TO or VO enters the complete order into the computer by using the computerized provider order entry (CPOE) software or writes it out on a physician's order sheet for entry into the computer as soon as possible. TJC requires that the receiver of a VO or TO record it and read (not repeat) it back to the prescriber. This helps ensure that one has not only heard an order correctly but also transcribed it accurately (ISMP, 2017). For example, document a TO as follows: *"09/30/2021 (1015), Change IV fluid to Lactated Ringers with potassium 20 mEq/L to run at 125 mL/h. TO: Dr. Knight/K. Day, RN, telephone order read back (TORB)."* The health care provider later verifies the TO or VO legally by cosigning it within a time frame (e.g., 24 hours) set by agency policy.

Incident or Occurrence Reports

An incident or occurrence is any event that is not consistent with the routine, expected care of a patient or the standard procedures in place on a health care unit or within an agency (Chapter 23). Examples include patient falls, needlestick injuries, medication administration errors, accidental omission of ordered therapies, a visitor losing consciousness, and any circumstances that lead to injury or pose a risk for patient injury such as a "near miss." There are several definitions for "near miss"; however, there is consensus that this term should be used to indicate incidents in which a patient is exposed to a hazardous situation with the potential to cause harm but in which, for a variety of reasons (luck or early detection), no harm did occur (Agency for Healthcare Research and Quality [AHRQ], 2019).

An incident report or occurrence report is completed whenever an incident occurs. Analysis of incident reports helps to identify system and/or individual human issues in which educational or in-service programs or changes in policies and procedures are needed to reduce the risk of future occurrences. Incident reports are an important part of the QI program of a unit or agency; however, they are not part of the health care record. Incident reports contain confidential information; distribution of the report is limited to the individuals responsible for reviewing the forms.

Follow agency policy when completing an incident report and file the report with your agency's risk-management department. When an incident occurs, document an objective description of what happened, what you observed, and the follow-up actions taken, including notification of the patient's health care provider in the patient's health care record. Remember to evaluate and document the patient's response to the incident in the health care record as well. Do not label this as an "incident," "near miss," or "sentinel event" in the health care record, and do not make any reference to these types of documents. A notation about an incident, near miss, or sentinel event report in a patient's health care record makes it easier for a lawyer to argue that the reference makes the incident report part of the health care record and therefore admissible for attorney review.

ACUITY RATING SYSTEMS

Nurses use acuity rating systems to determine the hours of care and number of staff required for a given group of patients every shift or every 24 hours. A patient's acuity level, usually determined by the assessment data an RN enters into a computer program, is based on the type and number of nursing interventions (e.g., intravenous [IV] therapy, wound care, or ambulation assistance) required by that patient over a 24-hour period. Although acuity ratings are not part of a patient's health care record, nursing documentation within the health care record provides evidence that supports the assessment of an acuity rating for an individual patient.

The acuity level is a classification that compares one or more patients with another group of patients. An acuity system classifies patients from 1 (independent in all but one or two aspects of care; almost ready for discharge) to 5 (totally dependent in all aspects of care; requiring intensive care). Using this system, a patient returning from surgery requiring frequent monitoring and extensive care has an acuity level of 3, compared with another patient awaiting discharge after a successful recovery from surgery who has an acuity level of 1. Accurate acuity ratings justify the number and qualifications of staff needed to safely care for patients. The patient-to-staff ratios established for a unit depend on a composite gathering of 24-hour acuity data for all patients receiving care.

DOCUMENTATION IN THE LONG-TERM HEALTH CARE SETTING

Long-term health care settings include skilled nursing facilities (SNFs), in which patients receive 24-hour-a-day care, including housing, meals, specialized (skilled) nursing care, and treatment services; and long-term care facilities, in which patients with chronic conditions receive 24-hour-a-day care, including housing, meals, personal care, and basic nursing care. Requirements for documentation in these facilities are governed by individual state regulations, TJC, and CMS. CMS mandates use of the Resident Assessment Instrument (RAI), which includes the Minimum Data Set (MDS) and the Care Area Assessment (CAA), to document data in long-term care facilities. MDS assessment forms are completed on admission and then periodically within specific guidelines and time frames for all residents in certified nursing homes (Yurkofsky and Ouslander, 2020). MDS data also determine the reimbursement level under the Prospective Payment System for Medicare Part A residents in an SNF (see Chapter 2).

Communication among nurses; social workers; dietitians; and recreational, speech, physical, and occupational therapists is essential. Documentation in the long-term care setting supports an interprofessional approach to the assessment and planning process for all patients. Adherence to state and federal requirements as well as reimbursement for care provided in a long-term care facility is dependent on accurate completion of the required documentation to justify the care provided (Hebda et al., 2019).

DOCUMENTATION IN THE HOME HEALTH CARE SETTING

Documentation in the home care setting is different from other areas of nursing. The use of laptop and tablet computers makes it possible for home health care records to be available in multiple locations (i.e., the patient's home and the home care agency). This system improves accessibility to information and facilitates interprofessional collaboration. Medicare has specific guidelines to establish eligibility for home care reimbursement. Information used for reimbursement is gathered from documentation of care provided in the home care setting. Documentation is the quality control and the justification for reimbursement from Medicare, Medicaid, or private insurance companies. Information in the home care health care record includes patient assessment, referral and intake forms, the interprofessional plan of care, a list of medications, and reports to third-party payers. Nurses document all their services for payment (e.g., direct skilled care, patient teaching, skilled observation, and evaluation visits) (TJC, 2021).

Nurses use two different data sets to document clinical assessments and care provided in the home care setting. Assessment using the Outcome and Assessment Information Set (OASIS) is required for all patients 18 years of age and older (with the exception of patients receiving prenatal or postnatal care) who are receiving skilled care through a home health agency that is reimbursed by Medicare or Medicaid. OASIS includes a comprehensive admission assessment and allows for the calculation of clinical, functional, and service scores that provide justification for reimbursement of services. The Omaha System is a research-based, comprehensive, standardized taxonomy or classification designed to enhance practice, documentation, and information management. It consists of three components (Problem Classification Scheme, Intervention Scheme, and Problem Rating Scale for Outcomes) and provides a useful model for comprehensive evaluation of the quality of nursing care provided in the home care setting (Eardley et al., 2018; Hebda et al., 2019).

CASE MANAGEMENT AND USE OF CRITICAL PATHWAYS

The case management model incorporates an interprofessional approach to delivery and documentation of patient care (see Chapter 2). Critical pathways (also known as clinical pathways, practice guidelines, or CareMap tools) are interprofessional care plans that identify patient problems, key interventions, and expected outcomes within an established time frame (Busse et al., 2019). Critical pathway documents facilitate integration of care because all members of the health care team use the same document to monitor a patient's progress during each shift or, in the case of home care, every visit. Evidence-based critical pathways can improve patient outcomes. For example, use of critical pathways has been shown to improve adherence to evidence-based guidelines for administration of antibiotics for community-acquired pneumonia (Eekholm et al., 2020).

Unexpected outcomes and interventions not specified within a critical pathway are called variances. A variance occurs when the activities on the critical pathway are not completed as predicted or a patient does not meet the expected outcomes. Variances sometimes result from a change in a patient's health or because of other health complications not associated with the primary reason for which a patient requires care. Once you identify a variance, you modify the patient's care to meet the needs associated with the variance. A positive variance occurs when a patient makes progress faster than expected (e.g., an indwelling urethral catheter is discontinued a day earlier than anticipated according to the critical pathway). An example of a negative variance is when a patient develops pulmonary complications after surgery, requiring oxygen therapy and monitoring with pulse oximetry. Variances to expected outcomes are documented with a progress note (Box 26.4). Documentation allows trends to be identified and analyzed, which can provide data to develop an effective action plan for responding to identified patient problems. Over time, health care teams sometimes revise critical pathways if similar variances recur.

BOX 26.4   Example of Variance Documentation

An RN working in the case management role is using a critical pathway for "Routine Postoperative Care" for a 56-year-old man who had abdominal surgery yesterday. One of the expected outcomes for postoperative day 1 on the critical pathway document is "Afebrile with lungs clear bilaterally." This patient has an elevated temperature, his breath sounds are decreased bilaterally in the bases of both lobes of the lungs, and he is slightly confused.

The following is an example of how the RN case manager documents this variance on the pathway:

"Breath sounds diminished bilaterally at the bases. T-100.4; P-92; R-28/min; pulse oximetry 84% on room air. Daughter states he is "confused" and did not recognize her when she arrived a few minutes ago. Oxygen 2 L via nasal cannula started per standing orders. Oxygen saturation improved to 92% after 5 minutes. Dr. Lopez notified of change in status. Daughter remains at bedside."

INFORMATICS AND INFORMATION MANAGEMENT IN HEALTH CARE

Health information technology (HIT) is the use of information systems and other information technology to record, monitor, and deliver patient care, and to perform managerial and organizational functions in health care (Hebda et al., 2019). The focus of HIT is the patient and the process of care, and the goal of using HIT is to enhance the quality and efficiency of care provided.

Health Care Information System

A health care information system (HIS) consists of "computer hardware and software dedicated to the collection, storage, processing, retrieval, and communication of patient care information in a healthcare agency" (Hebda et al., 2019). An HIS consists of two major types of information systems: a clinical information system and an administrative information system. Together the two systems operate to make the entry and communication of data and information more efficient. Individual health care agencies sometimes use one or several clinical information systems and administrative information systems. Administrative information systems include databases such as payroll, financial, and QI systems (Hebda et al., 2019).

Clinical Information System

A clinical information system (CIS) (also known as a patient care information system) is a large, computerized database management system that is used to access patient data needed to plan, implement, and evaluate care (Hebda et al., 2019). A CIS can include monitoring systems; order entry systems; and laboratory, radiology, and pharmacy systems. A monitoring system often includes devices that automatically monitor and record biometric measurements (e.g., vital signs and oxygen saturation) in acute care, critical care, and specialty care areas. Some of these devices can be programmed to electronically send measurements directly to a nursing documentation system, decreasing nursing workload.

One example of an order entry system is a computer program that allows nurses to order supplies and services from another department, such as sterile supplies from the central supply department. This eliminates the use of written order forms and expedites the delivery of needed supplies to a nursing unit. Another example is a computerized provider order entry (CPOE) system that allows health care providers to directly enter standardized, legible, and complete orders for patient care into a medical record from any computer in the HIS. Advanced CPOE systems have built-in clinical decision support tools and alerts to help a health care provider select the most appropriate medication or

diagnostic test and automatically check for drug interactions, medication allergies, and other potential problems (HealthIT.gov, 2018; Zhu and Weingart, 2020). The direct entry of orders by providers eliminates safety issues related to illegible handwriting and transcription errors. In addition, a CPOE system potentially speeds the implementation of ordered diagnostic tests and treatments, which contributes to high-quality care and better patient outcomes. A CPOE system improves reimbursements because some orders require preapprovals from insurance plans. CPOE, when integrated with an electronic practice management system, can flag orders that require preapproval, helping a health care agency reduce denied insurance claims (HealthIT.gov, 2018). Use of a CPOE system has been shown to improve productivity and cost-effectiveness in the communication and implementation of health care provider orders. More important, most CPOE systems have significant potential to reduce medication errors associated with inappropriate drug use and dosing (Hebda et al., 2019).

Nursing Clinical Information Systems

A well-designed nursing clinical information system (NCIS) incorporates the principles of nursing informatics to support the work that nurses do by facilitating documentation of nursing process activities and offering resources for managing nursing care delivery. It is important for nurses to be able to access computer programs easily, review patients' medical histories and health care provider orders, and then go to the patients' bedsides to conduct comprehensive assessments. Once you complete an assessment, you enter data into the computer terminal at the patient's bedside and develop a plan of care from the information gathered. This allows you to quickly share the plan of care with your patient and other health care providers. You will periodically return to the computer to check on laboratory test results, administer medications (Box 26.5), and document the care you deliver. The computer screens and optional pop-up windows make it easy to locate information, enter and compare data, and make changes.

NCISs have two designs. The nursing process design is the most traditional. It organizes documentation within well-established formats such as admission and postoperative assessment problem lists, care plans, intervention lists or notes, and discharge planning instructions. The nursing process design facilitates the following:

- Generation of a nursing work list that outlines routine scheduled care activities for a patient
- Documentation of routine aspects of patient care such as hygiene, positioning, fluid intake and output, wound care measures, and blood glucose measurements
- Progress note entries: narrative notes, charting by exception, and/or flow sheets
- Documentation of medication administration (see Chapter 31)

More advanced systems incorporate standardized nursing languages such as the International Classification for Nursing Practice (ICNP), the North American Nursing Diagnosis Association International (NANDA-I) nursing diagnoses, the Nursing Interventions Classification (NIC), and the Nursing Outcomes Classification (NOC) into the software (Hebda et al., 2019).

The other model for an NCIS is the protocol or critical pathway design (Hebda et al., 2019). This design facilitates interprofessional management of information because all health care providers use evidenced-based protocols or critical pathways to document the care they provide. The information system allows a user to select one or more appropriate protocols for a patient. An advanced system merges multiple protocols, using a master protocol or path to direct patient care activities. Standard health care provider order sets are included in the protocols and automatically processed. The system also integrates appropriate information into the medication delivery process to enhance patient safety. In addition, the system identifies variances of

Effect of Electronic Health Record (EHR) Documentation on Nursing Practice

PICOT Question: For nurses working in acute care settings, what is the effect of using the electronic health record (EHR) on reducing medication errors and improving patient outcomes?

Evidence Summary

Medication administration is a complex process that requires many steps (e.g., medication prescription, transcription, dispensing, nursing preparation, and administration). Members of the health care team make multiple decisions and take a variety of actions throughout the process. Errors can occur at any step (Mieiro et al., 2019).

Medication errors greatly affect patient outcomes. For example, experts estimate that in the United States, 7000 to 9000 people die every year because of medication errors, and hundreds of thousands of other patients experience adverse reactions to their medications that often go unreported (Mieiro et al., 2019; Tariq et al., 2021). Furthermore, adverse drug events cause about 19% of inpatient injuries in the United States (Zhu and Weingart, 2020). Caring for patients who experience medication errors costs more than $40 billion every year (Tariq et al., 2021). Additionally, medication errors decrease patient satisfaction, create a lack of trust in the health care team, and can cause physical and psychosocial pain (Tariq et al., 2021).

Because medication administration is complex and involves many different members of the health care team, evidence shows that implementing an EHR and a multisystem approach that includes health care providers, nurses, and the health care system can help prevent medication errors (Holmgren et al., 2020; Zhu and Weingart, 2020). Using computerized provider order entry (CPOE) helps to standardize practice, improves the legibility of orders and alerts, enhances communication, and updates health care providers on side effects, drug-drug interactions, and new orders (Holmgren et al., 2020; Zhu and Weingart, 2020). Technology that integrates CPOE with bar coding medications, often results in reduced medication errors, which improves patient outcomes (Burkoski et al., 2019). Other strategies that have been shown to reduce medication errors include medication reconciliation, limiting nurse interruptions during medication preparation and administration, and providing tailored medication education that begins during hospitalization and continues after discharge (Alper et al., 2020; Huckels-Baumgart et al., 2021; Crannage et al., 2020).

Application to Nursing Practice

- Be vigilant and follow agency policies surrounding medication administration. Avoid taking short cuts when using bar coding and other technologies and limit interruptions to enhance medication administration safety (Burkoski et al., 2019; Huckels-Baumgart et al., 2021).
- Document medication administration accurately in the patient's electronic health record to improve communication among the health care team and reduce medication errors (Holmgren et al., 2020; Zhu and Weingart, 2020).
- Provide frequent individualized patient education and use teach-back to ensure that patients and family caregivers understand their medications (Alper et al., 2020; Crannage et al., 2020; Zhu and Weingart, 2020).

the anticipated outcomes on the protocols as documentation is entered. This provides all caregivers the ability to analyze variances and offer an accurate clinical picture of a patient's progress.

Advantages of a Nursing Clinical Information System. Anecdotal reports and descriptive studies suggest that NCISs offer important advantages to nurses in practice. According to Hebda et al. (2019), some specific advantages include:

- Better access to information

- Enhanced quality of documentation through prompts
- Reduced errors of omission
- Reduced hospital costs
- Increased nurse job satisfaction
- Adherence to requirements of accrediting agencies (e.g., TJC)
- Development of a common clinical database
- Enhanced ability to track records

Many NCISs include content-importing technologies that allow the use of templates, macros, automated data points, and the ability to copy forward either parts of or entire nursing shift assessments that enable nurses to quickly document their assessment or the care they provided. These features have benefits and risks associated with their use. When allergy and current medication lists are automatically imported into nursing admission documentation from a previous health care agency encounter, you need to meticulously review this information for accuracy and update it as needed to avoid documentation errors and patient safety concerns. When nursing shift assessment data are copied forward from a previous shift or day, you must update the documentation so that it accurately reflects a patient's current clinical status (Lowry et al., 2017).

Clinical Decision Support Systems

A **clinical decision support system (CDSS)** is a computer program that aids and supports clinical decision making. The knowledge base within a CDSS contains rules and logic statements that link information required for clinical decisions to generate tailored recommendations for individual patients; the recommendations are presented to health care providers as alerts, warnings, or other information for consideration (Hebda et al., 2019: Sutton et al., 2020). For example, an effective CDSS notifies health care providers of patient allergies before a medication order is entered using CPOE to increase patient safety during the medication-ordering process.

CDSSs also improve nursing care. When patient assessment data are combined with patient care guidelines, nurses are better able to implement evidence-based nursing care. These programs are called a *nursing clinical decision support system (NCDSS)* when used to support nursing decisions.

An example of an NCDSS is a program that requires entry of data regarding a patient's risk factors for falls and provides evidence-based alternatives for fall prevention interventions. The interventions are displayed through the decision support system and are selected for the plan of care, thus supporting clinical decision making (Sutton et al., 2020). Use of nursing-specific CDSSs has not been implemented as often as CDSSs in other disciplines. However, CDSSs are in development for acute care nursing settings.

Nursing Informatics

You need to be knowledgeable in the science and application of nursing informatics. **Nursing informatics** is the specialty that integrates nursing science, computer science, and information science to manage and communicate data, information, knowledge, and wisdom in nursing and informatics practice (American Nursing Informatics Association, 2021). Nursing informatics is recognized as a specialty area of nursing practice at the graduate level. Nurses who specialize in informatics have advanced knowledge in information management and demonstrate proficiency with informatics to support all areas of nursing practice, including QI, research, project management, and system design (American Nursing Informatics Association, 2021). Through the application of nursing informatics, technology is put to practical use to enhance bedside care and education. It offers an efficient and effective nursing information system that facilitates the integration of data, information, and knowledge to support patients, nurses, and other providers in patient care decision making.

Informatics Competencies for Nursing Graduates Entering the Workforce

Nursing competence in health care informatics is a priority because of the wide usage of electronic documentation among health care providers and agencies across the United States. You need informatics competencies to deliver safe and efficient care and to facilitate the implementation of evidence-based practice. Professional organizations such as the American Association of Colleges of Nursing (AACN) (2021), the National League for Nursing (2021), and the Quality and Safety Education for Nurses (QSEN) Institute (2020) recommend that all nurses at all educational levels acquire competence in informatics and the use of information technology.

QSEN defines the scope of RN competencies for informatics as "the use of information and technology to communicate, manage knowledge, mitigate error, and support decision making" and outlines specific knowledge, skills, and attitudes that nursing students need to learn to use informatics technology to provide patient care in an effective and safe manner (QSEN Institute, 2020). Competence in informatics is not the same as computer competency. To become competent in informatics, you must use evolving methods of discovering, retrieving, and using information in practice (Hebda et al., 2019). Patients' records contain multiple types of data, and you need to know how to record, interpret, and report data and use critical thinking and clinical judgment to apply your knowledge when providing patient care. You must also recognize when information is needed and have the skills to find, evaluate, and use that information effectively. QSEN competencies in informatics for prelicensure nursing students are outlined in Box 26.6.

As a nurse you need to know how to use clinical databases within your agency and apply the information so that you can deliver safe, high-quality, appropriate patient care. You will collect data, including numbers, characters, or facts, according to a perceived need for analysis and possible action. You gain knowledge from gathering and using information from several sources. For example, you review several consecutive assessments of a wound documented within the EHR. Reviewing changes in the descriptions of the wound's edges, color of drainage, and measurements over several days allows you to evaluate and identify a pattern that indicates that the wound is not healing. Based on evidence available in the scientific literature, you apply knowledge of wound care principles and intervene to develop new nursing interventions to manage the patient's wound and promote healing.

> **QSEN** **Building Competency in Informatics** A patient diagnosed with a deep vein thrombosis (DVT) in the left lower leg was admitted 3 days ago and has been receiving a continuous heparin infusion of 1300 units/hr via a peripheral IV catheter located in the left lower forearm. You are the RN caring for this patient from 1500 to 2300 today, and you learn during the hand-off report that the patient's most recent partial thromboplastin time (PTT) is 70 seconds, indicating that the current dose of heparin infusing at 1300 units/h is therapeutic (Pagana et al., 2019). The outcome for this patient is to establish therapeutic anticoagulation levels by using warfarin (an oral anticoagulant) so that the heparin infusion can be discontinued. The patient will be discharged with a prescription for warfarin, which will be taken daily for 6 months until the DVT has resolved. The patient received the first dose of warfarin 10 mg orally (PO) yesterday evening.
>
> The patient's next dose of warfarin 10 mg PO is due at 1800. You log on to the computer located in the patient's room at that time and open the medication administration record in the patient's EHR. As you scan the package of warfarin using the bar-code medication administration function, a warning statement pops up on the computer screen: "Review most recent PT/INR results before administration." You switch screens in the EHR to review the patient's laboratory results and note that the patient's most recent prothrombin time (PT) was 21 seconds, and the international normalized ratio (INR) was 2.3, indicating that the dose of warfarin that the patient received yesterday was too high and that the patient has a critically increased risk for bleeding (Pagana et al., 2019). The abnormal results are displayed in a red font in the EHR, and a notation reading "Critical Value" is displayed next to each of the results displayed in red. What does the warning statement that popped up on the computer screen represent? What is the most appropriate action for you to take in this situation?
>
> Answers to QSEN Activities can be found on the Evolve website.

BOX 26.6 QSEN Competencies for Informatics

QSEN Competency in Informatics: Use information and technology to communicate, manage knowledge, mitigate error, and support decision making.

Knowledge:
Explain why information and technology skills are essential for safe patient care.

Skills:
Seek education about how information is managed in care settings before providing care.
Apply technology and information management tools to support safe processes of care.

Attitudes:
Appreciate the necessity for all health professionals to seek lifelong, continuous learning of information technology skills.

Knowledge:
Identify essential information that must be available in a common database to support patient care.
Contrast benefits and limitations of different communication technologies and their impact on safety and quality.

Skills:
Navigate the electronic health record.
Document and plan patient care in an electronic health record.
Employ communication technologies to coordinate care for patients.

Attitudes:
Value technologies that support clinical decision making, error prevention, and care coordination.
Protect confidentiality of protected health information in electronic health records.

Knowledge:
Describe examples of how technology and information management are related to the quality and safety of patient care.
Recognize the time, effort, and skill required for computers, databases, and other technologies to become reliable and effective tools for patient care.

Skills:
Respond appropriately to clinical decision-making supports and alerts.
Use information management tools to monitor outcomes of care processes.
Use high-quality electronic sources of health care information.

Attitudes:
Value nurses' involvement in design, selection, implementation, and evaluation of information technologies to support patient care.

From QSEN Institute: *QSEN competencies,* 2020. http://qsen.org/competencies/pre-licensure-ksas/#informatics. Accessed June 3, 2021.

KEY POINTS

- The health care record facilitates interprofessional communication, provides a legal and financial record of care, aids in clinical education and research, and guides professional and agency performance improvement.
- Nursing documentation supports reimbursement to health care agencies through accurate accounting of the use of services and equipment and medications administered.
- Effective nursing documentation limits liability through objective description of what happened to a patient and clearly indicates that individualized, outcome-directed nursing care was provided based on nursing assessment.
- A variety of methods, such as limiting who can access electronic health records, firewalls, spyware detection software, automatic sign-offs, and the use of strong passwords are used to secure the confidentiality of PHI in the EHR.
- Only members of the health care team who are directly involved in a patient's care have legitimate access to a patient's health record; follow agency policies that describe the sharing of medical records.
- Quality documentation is factual, accurate, detailed, and timely, and incorporates precise measurements, correct spelling, and proper use of abbreviations.
- Patient safety is enhanced when health care professionals eliminate the use of dangerous abbreviations, acronyms, symbols, and dose designations from their documentation.
- Nurses use a variety of forms when admitting patients, providing nursing care, and discharging patients to document patient care. Documentation requires nurses to be skilled in the use of checklists, flow sheets, and narrative notes regardless of whether they document electronically or on paper.
- Documentation of a safe plan for discharge includes information given on medications, diet, community resources, follow-up care, and contact information for whom to call with questions or in case of an emergency.
- When information relevant to care is communicated by telephone, documentation includes when the call was made, the number called, who made the call, who was called, to whom information was given, what information was given, what information was received, and verification of information through use of a read-back process.
- Health care informatics facilitates the integration of data, information, knowledge, and wisdom to support patients, nurses, and other providers in decision making in all roles and settings.
- Nursing students must develop the knowledge, skills, and attitudes that will enable them to use information and technology to communicate, manage knowledge, mitigate error, and support decision making. For example, nursing students need to know how to document in an EHR, value technologies that support clinical decision making, and respond appropriately to clinical decision-making alerts.

REFLECTIVE LEARNING

- Describe the actions you will take to protect the privacy of patient information if you need to print information from an EHR during clinical to complete your clinical paperwork after returning to campus.

- Using a recent clinical experience, describe how a CDSS could support evidence-based practice, allowing you to make decisions that would result in safe and effective nursing actions.
- Imagine there is an increased incidence of pressure injuries among the patients on the unit where you have clinical. Describe what data you could collect from the agency's nursing information system to determine why these patients are at greater risk for skin breakdown and what factors related to the nursing care provided on the unit are influencing the prevalence of hospital-acquired pressure injuries. Discuss why this information is important to collect.

REVIEW QUESTIONS

1. A nurse contacts the health care provider about a change in a patient's condition and receives several new orders for the patient over the phone. When documenting telephone orders in the EHR, what should the nurse do?
   1. Print out a copy of all telephone orders entered into the EHR in order to keep them in personal records for legal purposes.
   2. "Read back" all telephone orders to the health care provider over the phone to verify all orders were heard, understood, and transcribed correctly before entering the orders in the EHR.
   3. Record telephone orders in the EHR but wait to implement the order(s) until they are electronically signed by the health care provider who gave them.
   4. Implement telephone order(s) immediately but insist that the health care provider come to the patient care unit to personally enter the order(s) into the EHR within the next 24 hours.
2. You are a nurse who is working in an agency that has recently implemented an EHR. Which of the following are acceptable practices for maintaining the security and confidentiality of EHR information? (Select all that apply.)
   1. Using a strong password and changing your password frequently according to agency policy
   2. Allowing a temporary staff member to use your computer username and password to access the electronic record
   3. Ensuring that work lists (and any other data that must be printed from the EHR) are protected throughout the shift and disposed of in a locked receptacle designated for documents that are to be shredded when no longer needed
   4. Ensuring that the patient information that is displayed on the computer monitor that you are using is not visible to visitors and other health care providers who are not involved in that patient's care
   5. Remaining logged into a computer to save time if you only need to step away to administer a medication
3. When documenting an assessment of a patient's cardiac system in an EHR, the nurse uses the computer mouse to select the "WNL" statement to document the following findings: *"Heart sounds S1 & S2 auscultated. Heart rate between 80 and 100 beats/min, and regular. Denies chest pain."* This is an example of using which of the following documentation formats?
   1. Focus charting incorporating data, action, and response (DAR)
   2. Problem-intervention-evaluation (PIE)
   3. Charting by exception (CBE)
   4. Narrative documentation

4. The nurse works at an agency where military time is used for documentation and needs to document that a patient was medicated for pain after midnight. Identify the correct military time to document medication administered at 12:05 a.m.

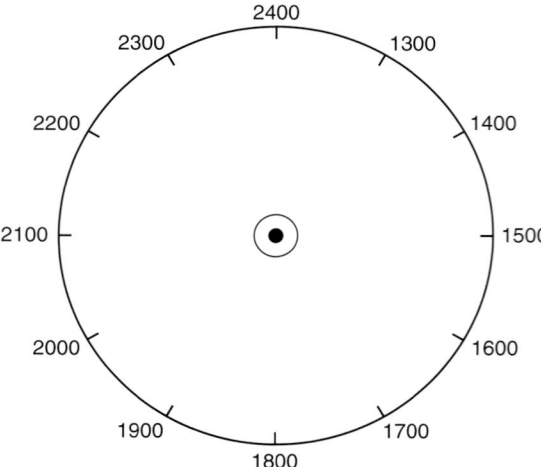

1. 2405
2. 0005
3. 2205
4. 1205

5. The nurse who works at the local health care agency is transferring a patient to an acute rehabilitation center in another town. To complete the transfer, information from the patient's EHR must be printed and faxed to the acute rehabilitation center. Which of the following actions are appropriate for the nurse to take to maintain privacy and confidentiality of the patient's information when faxing this information? (Select all that apply.)
   1. Confirm that the fax number for the acute rehabilitation center is correct before sending the fax.
   2. Use the encryption feature on the fax machine to encode the information and make it impossible for staff at the acute rehabilitation center to read the information unless they have the encryption key.
   3. Fax the patient's information without a cover sheet so that the person receiving the information at the acute rehabilitation center can identify it more quickly.
   4. After sending the fax, place the information that was printed out in a standard trash can after ripping it into several pieces.
   5. After sending the fax, place the information that was printed out in a secure canister marked for shredding.

6. The nurse is administering a dose of metoprolol to a patient and is completing the steps of bar-code medication administration within the EHR. As the bar-code information on the medication is scanned, an alert that states, "Do not administer dose if apical heart rate (HR) is <60 beats/min or systolic blood pressure (SBP) is <90 mm Hg" appears on the computer screen. The alert that appeared on the computer screen is an example of what type of system?
   1. Electronic health record (EHR)
   2. Charting by exception
   3. Clinical decision support system (CDSS)
   4. Computerized provider order entry (CPOE)

7. The nurse is writing a narrative progress note. Identify each of the following statements as subjective data (S) or objective data (O):
   1. April 24, 2021 (0900)
   2. Repositioned patient on left side.
   3. Medicated with hydrocodone-acetaminophen 5/325 mg, 2 tablets PO.
   4. "The pain in my incision increases every time I try to turn on my right side."
   5. S. Eastman, RN
   6. Surgical incision right lower quadrant, 3 inches in length, well approximated, sutures intact, no drainage.
   7. Rates pain 7/10 at location of surgical incision.

8. The nurse is discussing the advantages of using CPOE with a nursing colleague. Which statement best describes the major advantage of a CPOE system within an EHR?
   1. CPOE reduces the time necessary for health care providers to write orders.
   2. CPOE reduces the time needed for nurses to communicate with health care providers.
   3. Nurses do not need to acknowledge orders entered by CPOE in an EHR.
   4. CPOE improves patient safety by reducing transcription errors.

9. The nurse is reviewing health care provider orders that were handwritten on paper when all computers were down during a system upgrade. Which of the following orders contains an inappropriate abbreviation included on TJC's "do not use" list and should be clarified with the health care provider?
   1. Change open midline abdominal incision daily using wet-to-moist normal saline and gauze.
   2. Lorazepam 0.5 mg PO every 4 hours prn anxiety
   3. Morphine sulfate 1 mg IVP every 2 hours prn severe pain
   4. Insulin aspart 8u SQ every morning before breakfast

10. The nurse is changing the dressing over the midline incision of a patient who had surgery. Assessment of the incision reveals changes from what was documented by the previous nurse. After documenting the current wound assessment, the nurse contacts the surgeon by telephone to discuss changes in the incision that are of concern. Which of the following illustrates the most appropriate way for the nurse to document this conversation?
    1. Health care provider notified about change in assessment of abdominal incision. T. Wright, RN
    2. 09-3-21: Notified the surgeon by phone that there is a new area of redness around the patient's incision. T. Wright, RN
    3. 1015: Contacted the surgeon and notified about changes in abdominal incision. T. Wright, RN
    4. 09-3-21 (1015): Surgeon contacted by phone. Notified about new area of bright red erythema extending approximately 1 inch around circumference of midline abdominal incision and oral temperature of 101.5 F. No orders received. T. Wright, RN

Rationales for Review Questions can be found on the Evolve website.

REFERENCES

Agency for Healthcare Research and Quality: *Patient Safety Network: Adverse events, near misses, and errors,* 2019. https://psnet.ahrq.gov/primers/primer/34/Adverse-Events-Near-Misses-and-Errors. Accessed May 31, 2021.

Alper E, et al: *Hospital discharge and readmission.* UpToDate, 2020. https://www.uptodate.com/contents/hospital-discharge-and-readmission. Accessed May 31, 2021.

American Association of Colleges of Nursing (AACN): *AACN essentials,* 2021. https://www.aacnnursing.org/Education-Resources/AACN-Essentials. Accessed June 3, 2021.

American Medical Association: *HIPAA violations & enforcement,* 2021. https://www.ama-assn.org/practice-management/hipaa/hipaa-violations-enforcement. Accessed May 31, 2021.

American Nursing Informatics Association: *Mission statement of the American Nursing Informatics Association,* 2021. https://www.ania.org/sites/default/files/assets/documents/factSheet.pdf. Accessed June 3, 2021.

Busse R, et al: *Improving healthcare quality in Europe: Characteristics, effectiveness, and implementation of different strategies,* WHO Regional Office for Europe, Copenhagen, Denmark, 2019, WHO.

Centers for Medicare and Medicaid Services (CMS): *Hospital-acquired conditions,* 2020. https://www.cms.gov/Medicare/Medicare-Fee-for-Service-Payment/HospitalAcqCond/Hospital-Acquired_Conditions. Accessed May 31, 2021.

Centers for Medicare and Medicaid Services (CMS): *Clinical quality measures basics,* 2021. https://www.cms.gov/regulations-and-Guidance/Legislation/EHRIncentivePrograms/ClinicalQualityMeasures.html. Accessed May 31, 2021.

Eardley D, et al: The Omaha System as a structured instrument for bridging nursing informatics with public health nursing education: a feasibility study, *Comput Inform Nurs* 36(6):275, 2018.

Elliott L, et al: Standardizing documentation: a place for everything. *Medsurg Nurs* 27(1):32, 2018.

Harding M, et al: *Lewis's medical-surgical nursing: assessment and management of clinical problems,* ed 11, St Louis, 2020, Elsevier.

HealthIT.gov: *What is computerized provider order entry?* 2018. https://www.healthit.gov/faq/what-computerized-provider-order-entry. Accessed May 31, 2021.

Hebda T, et al: *Handbook of informatics for nurses and health care professionals,* ed 6, New York, 2019, Pearson.

Institute for Safe Medication Practices (ISMP): *Despite technology, verbal orders persist, read back is not widespread, and errors continue,* 2017. https://www.ismp.org/resources/despite-technology-verbal-orders-persist-read-back-not-widespread-and-errors-continue. Accessed May 31, 2021.

Khokhar A, et al: Framework for mining and analysis of standardized nursing care plan data, *West J Nurs Res* 39(1):20, 2017.

LoBiondo-Wood G, Haber J: *Nursing research: methods and critical appraisal for evidence-based practice,* ed 10, St. Louis, 2021, Elsevier.

Lowry S, et al: An overview of clinical decision support systems: benefits, risks, and strategies for success, *NPJ Digit Med* 3:17, 2020.

National League for Nursing (NLN): *Informatics,* 2021. http://www.nln.org/professional-development-programs/teaching-resources/toolkits/informatics-teaching/informatics. Accessed June 3, 2021.

Nurses Service Organization: *Charting by exception: the legal risks,* 2018. https://www.nso.com/Learning/Artifacts/Articles/Charting-by-exception-the-legal-risks. Accessed May 31, 2021.

Office of the National Coordinator for Health Information Technology (ONC): *Strategy on reducing burden relating to the use of health IT and EHRs,* 2020. https://www.healthit.gov/topic/usability-and-provider-burden/strategy-reducing-burden-relating-use-health-it-and-ehrs. Accessed May 31, 2021.

Office of the National Coordinator for Health Information Technology (ONC): *Health IT dashboard: percent of*

hospitals, by type, that possess certified health IT, 2018. dashboard.healthit.gov/quickstats/pages/certified-electronic-health-record-technology-in-hospitals.php. Accessed May 31, 2021.

Pagana K, et al: *Mosby's diagnostic and laboratory test reference,* ed 13, St Louis, 2019, Elsevier.

QSEN Institute: *QSEN competencies: informatics,* 2020. http://qsen.org/competencies/pre-licensure-ksas/#informatics. Accessed May 31, 2021.

Sutton RT, et al: An overview of clinical decision support systems: benefits, risks, and strategies for success, *Digit Med* 3:17, 2020. https://www.nature.com/articles/s41746-020-0221-y. Accessed June 3, 2021.

Stimson CE, Bodruff AL: Daily electronic health record reports meet meaningful use requirements, improve care efficiency, and provide a layer of safety for trauma patients, *J Trauma Nurs* 24(1):53, 2017.

Tariq RA, et al: Medication dispensing errors and prevention, *Stat Pearls,* 2021. https://www.ncbi.nlm.nih.gov/books/NBK519065/. Accessed June 3, 2021.

The Joint Commission (TJC): *2021 comprehensive accreditation manual for hospitals,* Oakbrook, Illinois, 2021, The Joint Commission.

The Joint Commission (TJC): *The Joint Commission's official "do not use" list of abbreviations,* 2020. https://www.jointcommission.org/-/media/tjc/documents/resources/patient-safety-topics/patient-safety/do_not_use_list_9_14_18.pdf. Accessed November 5, 2021.

US Department of Health & Human Services (USDHHS): *HITECH Act enforcement final rule,* 2017. https://www.hhs.gov/hipaa/for-professionals/special-topics/hitech-act-enforcement-interim-final-rule/index.html. Accessed June 3, 2021.

US Department of Health & Human Services (USDHHS): *The security rule,* 2020. https://www.hhs.gov/hipaa/for-professionals/security/index.html. Accessed June 3, 2021.

Wager KA, et al: *Health care information systems: a practical approach for health care management,* ed 4, San Francisco, CA, 2017, Jossey-Bass.

RESEARCH REFERENCES

Atasoy H, et al: The digitization of patient care: a review of the effects of electronic health records on health care quality and utilization, *Annu Rev Public Health* 40(1), 487, 2019.

Bardach SH, et al: Perspectives of health care practitioners: an exploration of interprofessional communication using electronic medical records, *J Interprof Care* 31(3):300, 2017.

Bauder R, et al: A survey on the state of health care upcoding fraud analysis and detection, *Health Serv Outcomes Res Methodol* 17(1):31, 2017.

Burkoski V, et al: Closed-loop medication system: leveraging technology to elevate safety, *Nurs Leadersh* 32:17, 2019.

Crannage AJ, et al: Implementation of a discharge education program to improve transitions of care for patients at high risk of medication errors, *Ann Pharmacother* 54(6):561, 2020.

Daniels M, et al: What nursing sensitive outcomes have been studied to-date among patients cared for in intensive care units? Findings from a scoping review, *Int J Nurs Stud* 102:103491, 2020.

Eekholm S, et al: Gaps between current clinical practice and evidence-based guidelines for treatment and care of older patients with community-acquired pneumonia: a descriptive cross-sectional study. *BMC Infect Dis* 20:73, 2020.

Heflin M: *Geriatric health maintenance,* UpToDate, 2021. https://www.uptodate.com/contents/geriatric-health-maintenance. Accessed May 26, 2021.

Holmgren AJ, et al: Assessing the safety of electronic health records: a national longitudinal study of medication-related decision support, *BMJ Qual Saf* 29:52, 2020.

Hommel A, et al: Exploring the incidence and nature of nursing-sensitive orthopaedic adverse events: a multicenter cohort study using Global Trigger Tool, *Int J Nurs Stud* 102, 2020.

Huckels-Baumgart, et al: Separate medication preparation rooms reduce interruptions and medication errors in the hospital setting: a prospective observational study, *J Patient Saf* 17(3):e161, 2021.

Karp E, et al: Changes in efficiency and quality of nursing electronic health record documentation after implementation of an admission patient history essential data set, *Comput Inform Nurs* 37(5):260, 2019.

Macieira T, et al: Secondary use of standardized nursing care data for advancing nursing science and practice: a systematic review, *J Am Med Inform Assoc* 26(11):1401, 2019.

Mieiro DB, et al: Strategies to minimize medication errors in emergency units: an integrative review, *Rev Bras Enferm* 72(Suppl 1):307, 2019. https://www.scielo.br/j/reben/a/gMgPrcLkFvyq3VvCz6KJhKH/?lang=en. Accessed June 3, 2021.

Misto K, et al: Interprofessional evidence-based strategies to enhance provider and patient interactions during electronic health record use, *J Nurs Prof Develop* 36(3):134, 2020.

Neppe V, Gerck E: Privacy of communications: faxes are not usually HIPAA compliant. An editorial perspective, *J Psychol Clin Psych* 10(6):249, 2019.

Ozkaynak M, et al: Use of electronic health records by nurses for symptom management in inpatient settings: a systematic review, *Comput Inform Nurs* 35(9):465, 2017.

Rathert C, et al: Seven years after meaningful use: physicians' and nurses' experiences with electronic health records, *Health Care Manage Rev* 44(1):30, 2019.

Riva S, et al: Evaluation of medication errors in electronic medical prescriptions and proposal for correction, *Res Biomed Eng* 36:59, 2020.

Wu MW, et al: Evaluation of electronic health records on the nursing process and patient outcomes regarding fall and pressure injuries, *Comput Inform Nurs* 37(11):573, 2019.

Yurkofsky M, Ouslander J: *Medical care in skilled nursing facilities (SNFs) in the United States,* UpToDate, 2020. https://www.uptodate.com/contents/medical-care-in-skilled-nursing-facilities-snfs-in-the-united-states. Accessed May 31, 2021.

Zhu J, Weingart S: *Prevention of adverse drug events in hospitals,* UpToDate, 2020. https://www.uptodate.com/contents/prevention-of-adverse-drug-events-in-hospitals. Accessed August 18, 2020.

27

Patient Safety and Quality

OBJECTIVES

- Describe the complex nature of clinical judgment for nurses delivering patient-centered care for patients' improved safety.
- Explain the rationale for vulnerable populations being at risk for threats to safety.
- Discuss common environmental hazards and methods for preventing them.
- Describe how a nurse assists patients in managing safety risks in the home.
- Discuss how an individual's developmental stage creates safety risks.
- Conduct an assessment of mobility alterations that pose risks for falling.

- Conduct a fall risk assessment in a health care agency setting.
- Describe ways to prevent procedure-related accidents.
- Describe assessment activities that identify the psychosocial status of patients as it pertains to their safety.
- Explain the role critical thinking and clinical judgment play in planning care for a patient's safety needs.
- Discuss how to select environmental interventions for fall prevention for the hospital and home environment.
- Identify evidence-based alternatives to restraints for patients who are alert, oriented, and low risk.
- Identify factors to assess before and during placement of patients in physical restraints.

KEY TERMS

Aura	Restraint	Seizure precautions
Immunization	Root cause analysis	Status epilepticus
Poison	Seizure	Workplace violence

MEDIA RESOURCES

http://evolve.elsevier.com/Potter/fundamentals/
- Review Questions
- Audio Glossary
- Case Study with Questions
- Concept Map Creator

- Video Clips
- Skills Performance Checklists
- Content Updates
- Answers to QSEN Activity and Review Questions

Mrs. Cohen is 78 years old and lives at home. The patient is recovering from a stroke (10 days ago) affecting her left arm and leg. She also has some slurring of speech. Mrs. Cohen lives alone but receives regular help from her daughter and son, who both live within 5 miles of the patient. She is scheduled for home physical therapy starting this week. Kylie is Mrs. Cohen's assigned home health nurse and will be making her first visit today.

Safety is the freedom from psychological and physical injury, and is a basic human need. Individuals seeking health care, regardless of setting, present numerous conditions that place them at risk for being unsafe. An individual's home or workplace environment, comorbid health conditions, attitudes and beliefs about safety, and economic resources all affect safety within the home. In the health care environment, presence of individuals with infectious disease, the patient's own comorbid conditions, layout and barriers within health care settings,

and infection control practices of staff all affect an individual's vulnerability to some form of injury.

Reducing the risk of harm associated with the delivery of health care is a national health care policy priority. Patient safety is one of the primary drivers behind health care staff education, clinical practice guidelines formation, and policy and procedure development. The World Health Organization (WHO, 2021) offers a simple definition of patient safety: the prevention of errors and adverse effects to patients associated with health care. As part of the health care team, professional nurses engage in all activities that support a patient-centered safety culture. Health care agencies use a variety of processes and approaches to improve the quality of care delivered to patients. Much of the force behind the focus on safety comes from regulatory and accrediting agencies such as the Centers for Medicare and Medicaid Services (CMS) and

The Joint Commission (TJC). The Joint Commission's 2021 National Patient Safety Goals include standards such as identifying patients correctly, using medicines correctly, and preventing infection (TJC, 2021a). The annual standards are for all health care institutions and are specifically directed at reducing the risk of medical errors. A culture of safety within a health care agency is important for minimizing adverse events even as nurses perform complex and hazardous work. The Agency for Healthcare Research and Quality (AHRQ, 2019) describes key features of a "culture of safety":

- Acknowledgment of the high-risk nature of an organization's activities and the determination to achieve consistently safe operations
- A blame-free environment where individuals are able to report errors or near misses without fear of reprimand or punishment
- Encouragement of collaboration across levels of employees and disciplines to seek solutions to patient safety problems
- Organizational commitment of resources to address safety concerns

As members of the health care team, nurses are professionally responsible for engaging in activities that support a patient-centered safety culture.

A TJC safety alert emphasizes the importance of identifying and reporting unsafe conditions before they cause harm, trusting that other health care staff and leadership will act on the report, and taking personal responsibility for one's actions to create a safety culture within a health care organization (TJC, 2018). Organizations that support a culture of safety continually focus on performance improvement based on risk management monitoring, empowerment of employees to actively participate in safety activities of the organization, and empowerment of employees to complete safety reports to design safer work environments (see Chapter 23).

With the myriad of factors influencing patients' safety risks and the emphasis of health care agencies to enforce a patient-centered safety culture, critical thinking applied to sound clinical judgment is essential. You must reflect and analyze your knowledge about safety, patients' safety risks, and conditions presented in each clinical situation, in order to provide safe and competent nursing care. Partnership with patients is an important factor. Patient-centered care promotes safety and requires you to recognize your patients or their designees as the source of control and full partners in providing compassionate and coordinated care based on respect for patient preferences, values, and needs (QSEN, 2020). The National Academy of Medicine's scientific panel defined patient and family engaged care (PFEC) as care planned, delivered, managed, and continuously improved in active partnership with patients and their families to ensure integration of their health and health care goals, preferences, and values (Frampton et al., 2017). It is difficult to achieve positive patient outcomes without nurses actively involving patients and families in safety promotion.

SCIENTIFIC KNOWLEDGE BASE

Environmental Safety

A patient's environment includes physical and psychosocial factors that influence or affect the life and survival of that patient. This broad definition of environment crosses the continuum of care for settings in which a nurse and patient interact, such as a hospital, long-term care agency, clinic, community center, school, and home. A safe environment protects the staff as well, allowing them to function optimally. Vulnerable populations are especially at risk for alterations in safety because of reduced access to health care, fewer resources, and increased morbidity. Those vulnerable groups most affected include infants, children, older adults, individuals with a chronic disease or a physical or mental disability, individuals who

have difficulty communicating, and individuals who have a low income or are homeless (Joszt, 2018). A safe environment meets basic needs, reduces physical hazards as well as the transmission of pathogens, and controls pollution.

Basic Human Needs. Physiological needs, including the need for oxygen, nutrition, and optimum temperature, influence a person's safety. According to Maslow's hierarchy of needs, these basic needs must be met before physical and psychological safety and security can be addressed (see Chapter 6).

Oxygen. Supplemental oxygen is sometimes needed to meet a person's oxygenation needs. Patients who require supplemental oxygen in health care settings are at risk because oxygen is highly flammable. Fire can occur when a patient on oxygen therapy chooses to smoke or is exposed to a heat source. Strict codes regulate the use and storage of medical oxygen in health care agencies. This is not the case in home environments. Chapter 41 describes how to administer oxygen safely in the home and provides information you can offer patients and family caregivers who manage oxygen therapies. Oxygen can build up in a home and on a patient's clothing and hair. If a person smokes in an environment that has supplemental oxygen, such as a house, even a small spark can cause a fire that will spread very quickly, resulting in extensive burns and even death. It is essential that no one smokes in a home, apartment, or room equipped with supplemental oxygen.

Know factors in a patient's environment that decrease the amount of available oxygen. An improperly functioning heating system is a hazard in the home. A furnace, fireplace, or stove that is not properly vented introduces carbon monoxide (CO) into the environment. CO affects oxygenation by binding strongly with hemoglobin, preventing the formation of oxyhemoglobin and reducing the supply of oxygen delivered to tissues. Low concentrations of oxygen cause nausea, dizziness, headache, and fatigue. Unintentional, non–fire-related (UNFR) CO poisoning is one of the most common causes of poisoning in the United States. The Centers for Disease Control and Prevention (CDC, 2020a) reports that every year approximately 50,000 people in the United States visit the emergency department because of accidental CO poisoning.

Nutrition. Meeting nutritional needs of patients requires knowledge about healthy food and food safety. Chapter 45 details the principles of balanced nutrition. Health care agencies are required to meet State Board of Health regulations for the storage, preparation, and provision of food to patients. In the home some patients do not know how to properly refrigerate, store, and prepare food. The CDC (2020b) estimates that 48 million people get sick from a foodborne illness, 128,000 are hospitalized, and 3000 die each year. When you care for patients returning home or if you work in home health, educate them about food safety principles. Also, patients require an adequate, clean water supply for drinking and to wash fresh produce and dishes. If a patient does not prepare or store foods properly, this increases the risk for infections and food poisoning from norovirus or bacteria such as *Escherichia coli*, *Salmonella*, or *Listeria*.

Temperature. Temperature extremes that frequently occur during the winter and summer pose safety risks for vulnerable populations. Exposure to severe cold for prolonged periods causes frostbite and accidental hypothermia. Older adults, the young, patients with cardiovascular conditions, patients who have ingested drugs or alcohol in excess, and people who are homeless are at high risk for hypothermia. In contrast, exposure to extreme heat changes the electrolyte balance of the body and raises the core body temperature, potentially resulting in heatstroke or heat exhaustion. Chronically ill patients, older adults, infants, and marathon runners are at great risk for injury from extreme heat.

Common Environmental Hazards. Environmental hazards in the home and at work threaten a person's safety and often result in physical or psychological injury or death. In 2016, unintentional injuries became the third leading cause of death in the United States (Kochanek et al., 2017). Motor vehicle accidents, poisonings, and falls were the leading causes of unintentional injuries. Additional environmental hazards include fire and disasters. In the work setting, repetitive motion injuries, vehicle accidents, falling objects, and falls are common causes of injuries. A nurse's role is to educate patients about the common safety hazards in the home and at work, teaching them how to prevent injury and emphasizing the hazards to which patients are the most vulnerable.

Motor Vehicle Accidents. Vehicle design and equipment such as seat belts, airbags, laminated windshields, and accident prevention systems have improved vehicular safety. State laws relating to licensing of young drivers, safety belt use, child restraint use, and motorcycle helmets exist for driver protection. It is important that children ride in child safety seats and booster seats appropriate for their age and weight and type of car. The American Academy of Pediatrics (AAP) (Durbin and Hoffman, 2018) recommends the following:

- Infants and toddlers should ride in a rear-facing car safety seat as long as possible, until they reach the highest weight or height allowed by their seat (see manufacturer's directions). Most convertible seats have limits that will allow children to ride rear-facing for 2 years or more.
- Once they are facing forward, children should use a forward-facing car safety seat with a harness for as long as possible, until they reach the height and weight limits for their seats. Many seats can accommodate children up to 29.5 kg (65 lb) or more.
- When children exceed these limits, they should use a belt-positioning booster seat until the vehicle's lap and shoulder seat belt fits properly. This is often when they have reached at least 144.8 cm (4 feet, 9 inches) in height and are 9 to 12 years of age.
- When children are old enough and large enough to use the vehicle seat belt alone, they should always use lap and shoulder seat belts for optimal protection.
- All children 12 years of age and younger should be restrained in the rear seats of vehicles for optimal protection.

According to the CDC (2020c), the risk of motor vehicle accidents is higher among 16- to 19-year-old drivers than any other age-group, with motor vehicle crashes being the leading cause of death for this age-group. Adolescents often underestimate dangerous situations or are unable to recognize hazardous situations (e.g., texting or talking on a phone while driving). In addition, they tend to speed and allow shorter headways, ride with intoxicated drivers, drive at night, and drive after using alcohol or drugs. Adolescents also have the lowest rate of seat belt use.

Older-adult drivers are keeping their licenses longer and driving more miles than in the past. Driving is an important way in which older adults remain independent. But there are often risks, the longer an older adult drives. Age-related decline in vision and cognitive functioning (ability to reason and remember) and physical changes affect driving abilities of some older adults (CDC, 2020d). Ways to promote safety among older-adult drivers include:

- Exercise regularly to increase strength and flexibility.
- Ask the physician or pharmacist to review medications—both prescription and over-the-counter—to reduce side effects and interactions.
- Have eyes checked by an eye doctor at least once a year and wear glasses and corrective lenses as required.
- Drive during daylight and in good weather.
- Plan the route before driving. Find the safest route, with well-lit streets, intersections with left-turn arrows, and easy parking.
- Leave a large following distance between the car and the car in front.
- Avoid distractions in the car, such as listening to a loud radio, talking or texting on the phone, and while eating.
- Consider potential alternatives to driving, such as riding with a friend, or ride-share.

Poison. A poison is any substance that impairs health or results in death when ingested, inhaled, injected, or absorbed into the body. Poisons often impair the function of every major organ system. Almost any substance is poisonous if too much is taken. Sources of poison in a person's home often include medicines, solid or liquid cleaning substances, gases, and vapors. Toddlers, preschoolers, and young school-age children are at greatest risk because of their curiosity; they often ingest household cleaning solutions, medications, or personal hygiene products in the home. Medications are commonly packaged in containers that hold multiple doses. As a result a child who is able to open a medicine container has access to multiple tablets or capsules. Emergency treatment is necessary when a person ingests a poisonous substance or comes into contact with a chemical that is absorbed through the skin. Every day, over 300 children in the United States ages 0 to 19 are treated in an emergency department as a result of being poisoned (CDC, 2019a). A poison control center is the best resource for patients and parents needing information about the treatment of an accidental poisoning. The nationwide poison control hotline center phone number is 1-800-222-1222.

Although lead has not been used in house paint or plumbing materials since the U.S. Consumer Product Safety Commission banned it in 1978, some older homes still contain high lead levels. Soil and water systems are sometimes contaminated. Lead is emitted into the environment from industrial sources and contaminated sites, such as former lead smelters (Environmental Protection Agency [EPA], 2020). Poisoning occurs from swallowing or inhaling lead. Fetuses, infants, and children are more vulnerable to lead poisoning than adults because their bodies absorb lead more easily, and small children are more sensitive to the damaging effects of lead. Exposure to excessive levels of lead affects a child's growth or causes learning and behavioral problems and brain and kidney damage.

Falls. A fall is an event that results in a person coming to rest inadvertently on the ground or floor or other lower level (WHO, 2018). Falls have been a major health problem, ranking as the second leading cause of accidental or unintentional injury deaths worldwide (WHO, 2018). Falls contribute to disability, lost work time and, in the case of many older adults, long-term care and institutionalization. Fall prevention has been a major quality health care initiative for community-dwelling older adults, as well as those in health care settings.

Falls are multifactorial; numerous factors increase the risk of falls. Older adults have the highest risk of death or serious injury following a fall (WHO, 2018). Other risk factors include (WHO, 2018; National Institute on Aging, 2017):

- Occupations at elevated heights or other hazardous working conditions
- Alcohol or substance use
- Socioeconomic factors, including poverty, overcrowded housing, sole parenthood, or young maternal age
- Underlying medical conditions, such as neurological, cardiac (orthostatic hypotension), or other disabling conditions
- Polypharmacy and side effects of medications
- Physical inactivity and loss of balance, particularly among older adults
- Poor mobility (impaired balance, gait, coordination), cognition, and vision, particularly among those living in an institution, such as a nursing home or chronic care facility

- Unsafe environments (e.g., broken stairs, icy sidewalks, inadequate lighting, throw rugs, exposed electrical cords, barriers along walking paths, and improper devices for ambulation)
- Foot problems that cause pain, and unsafe footwear such as backless shoes or high heels

Health care agencies throughout the country carefully monitor the incidence of falls and fall-related injuries as part of their ongoing performance improvement work. Some of the agencies that provide education, monitoring guidelines, and fall prevention resources include:

- TJC—https://www.jointcommission.org
- Institute for Healthcare Improvement (IHI)—www.ihi.org
- U.S. Department of Veterans Affairs Center for Patient Safety—https://www.patientsafety.va.gov/index.asp?_ga=2.255699786. 35041262.1543845065-460341664.1543845065
- U.S. Department of Health and Human Services—www.hhs.gov

Falls often lead to serious injuries such as fractures or internal bleeding. Patients most at risk for injury are those with osteoporosis or with bleeding tendencies resulting from disease or medical treatments. Fear of falling is a concern of community-dwelling older adults, and many avoid activities because of their fear.

Fire. The U.S. Fire Administration (USFA) reported a total of 379,600 residential fires in 2018, with the top two causes being cooking (50.7%) and heating (9.4%) (USFA, 2021). The improper use of cooking equipment and appliances, particularly stoves and space heaters, is a major cause of in-home fires and fire injuries. Unintentional, careless fires are the third most common type of fires, often involving improper disposal of cigarettes or use of candles. Nurses play a role in educating the public about fire prevention measures.

Fires occur in health care agencies each year, with most occurring in nursing homes, followed by mental health agencies, hospitals, and hospices. Because patients in health care agencies are sick, disabled, or elderly, health care staff must know how to protect patients and respond to fires appropriately. Health care agencies have routine fire drills to measure staff responsiveness and understanding of fire safety protocols (National Fire Protection Association [NFPA], 2017).

Disasters. Natural disasters such as floods, tsunamis, hurricanes, tornadoes, and wildfires are a major cause of death and injury. These types of disasters may result in death and can leave many people homeless. Every year millions of Americans are affected by natural disasters and their terrifying consequences. Bioterrorism is another cause of disaster and refers to biological agents (microbes or toxins) used as weapons to further personal or political agendas. A bioterrorist attack could be caused by virtually any pathogenic microorganism. The agents of greatest concern are anthrax (a bacterium) and smallpox (a virus). Both can be lethal. Anthrax is not communicable from direct contact but is transmitted in spores that become aerosolized. Smallpox is readily transmitted from person-to-person contact. Symptoms caused by these pathogens vary depending on how the person was exposed but generally occur within 7 days of the exposure. Health care agencies that are accredited by TJC must demonstrate that they have proper plans and response mechanisms in place if a disaster occurs. The hospitals conduct annual disaster-preparedness exercises and must monitor the following six critical factors

- Communication
- Resources (supplies) and assets
- Safety and security
- Staff responsibilities
- Utilities management
- Patient clinical and support activities

Health care agencies have routine disaster drills to ensure staff are educated and trained in the appropriate responses.

Transmission of Pathogens. Pathogens and parasites pose an ongoing threat to an individual's safety (see Chapter 28). Both patients and health care providers are at risk for exposure to pathogens. A pathogen is any microorganism capable of producing an illness. The most common means of transmission of pathogens is by the hands. For example, if an individual infected with hepatitis A does not wash their hands thoroughly after having a bowel movement, the risk for transmitting the disease to others during food preparation is increased. Nurses must educate patients about their unique risks for developing infection, such as immunosuppression from medications, chronic disease, or older age.

When a patient acquires an infection in a health care setting, it is called a nosocomial infection or health care–acquired infection (HAI). An HAI is one not present in a patient at the time of admission to a health care agency but that develops during the course of the stay. Health care agencies have standards for infection prevention in a variety of clinical situations, such as prevention of surgical site infections or catheter-associated urinary tract infections. The most effective method for limiting the transmission of pathogens in health care is the medically aseptic practice of hand hygiene (see Chapter 28). It is important that you adhere to the practice of hand hygiene, follow standard and transmission-based isolation precautions, and educate patients, visitors and family caregivers about the importance of using hand hygiene in all aspects of their lives.

Immunizations. Childhood vaccination is one of the most effective public health strategies to control and prevent disease (Ventola, 2016). Immunization reduces, and in some cases prevents, the transmission of disease from person to person. Recently, however, some parents have shown concerns about immunizing their children. For example, some parents have had concerns that autism might be linked to the vaccines children receive, but studies have shown that there is no link between receiving vaccines and developing autism (CDC, 2020f). Another parental concern has been whether the timing of the 2-month and 4-month vaccinations is associated with sudden infant death syndrome (SIDS), which commonly occurs in that same time frame. Studies have found that vaccines do not cause and are not linked to SIDS (CDC, 2020f). As of 2017, early childhood vaccination rates in the United States for the recommended seven-vaccine series (diphtheria, tetanus, pertussis, polio, measles, mumps, rubella) (CDC, 2020g) was at 70.4%. Rates were the highest for polio (92.7%) and the measles, mumps, rubella combination (91.5%). Adherence to childhood vaccinations is a problem for vulnerable populations. Historically, African-American children are less likely to be fully vaccinated than White or Hispanic children, and children in families with incomes below the poverty level were less likely than those in families with incomes at or above the poverty level to receive the combined-series vaccination. Vaccination rates also vary regionally in states, with several allowing for personal belief/philosophical exemptions (Frew and Lutz, 2017). Missed well-child visits are a primary driver of undervaccinated children (Blue Cross Blue Shield, 2021). Nurses play a role in informing parents about the importance of adhering to vaccination schedules for their children.

Access the AAP current immunization schedule at https://www.aap.org/en-us/advocacy-and-policy/aap-health-initiatives/immunizations/Pages/Immunization-Schedule.aspx

Adults require regular vaccinations depending on their age, job, lifestyle, travel, or health conditions (CDC, 2019b). For example, older adults are at risk for infectious disease if not regularly immunized for the flu and pneumonia. People in this age-group should also consult with their health care providers about receiving the vaccine for shingles, as it is recommended for healthy adults age 50 years and older (CDC, 2019b). Health care workers who are at risk for being exposed to blood or other body fluids should receive the three-dose series of vaccinations for hepatitis B.

REFLECT NOW

Think about the members of your family and identify any physical hazards that each member is likely to encounter.

NURSING KNOWLEDGE BASE

Factors Influencing Patient Safety

Nursing science informs us about numerous factors influencing patient safety, including developmental factors, common individual risk factors, and the risks existing in the home and health care environments. This source of knowledge equips nurses to be well informed to take an aggressive preventive approach to promoting patient safety.

Developmental Stages and Risks. A patient's developmental stage can create threats to safety because of lifestyle, cognitive and mobility status, sensory impairments, and safety awareness. With this information safety-prevention programs are tailored to address the needs, preferences, and life circumstances of particular age-groups. Unfortunately, all age-groups are subject to physical and mental abuse. Child abuse, domestic violence, and elder abuse are serious threats to safety (see Chapters 11 to 14).

Infant, Toddler, and Preschooler. Injuries are the leading cause of death in children over 1 year of age. The nature of the injury sustained is closely related to normal growth and development. For example, because of improved motor skills, coordination, and balance, preschoolers are less prone to falls than toddlers (Hockenberry et al., 2019). Infants and toddlers explore the environment and, because of their increased level of oral activity, put objects in their mouths. This increases their risk for poisoning or aspiration and choking on foreign material such as small toys. Parents do not always recognize the danger in seemingly harmless items, such as remote control devices and keyless remote door openers for vehicles. Button batteries if swallowed can cause serious injury or death (National Safety Council, 2021).

A safe sleep environment for an infant involves placing the infant on the back on a firm mattress in a safety-approved crib that is free of pillows, toys, and blankets, as these are suffocation hazards. Instruct patents about the hazards of sleeping with an infant in bed, on the sofa, or on the floor (AAP, 2021a).

Fortunately, preschoolers are generally less reckless and are aware of potential dangers such as hot objects or sharp instruments (Hockenberry et al., 2019). Limited physical coordination in preschoolers contributes to falls from riding bicycles and using playground equipment. Other injuries include burns and drowning. Most drowning or near-drowning incidents happen when a child falls into a pool or is left alone in the bathtub (National Safety Council, 2021). Accidents involving children are largely preventable. But accident prevention requires health education for parents and the removal of dangers in the home and outside play areas whenever possible.

School-Age Child. School-age children enter a period of less intense emotions, secure in their dependency on parents and family and with self-confidence tempered by a more realistic perspective. They have energy to explore the environment beyond the home and to gradually increase the scope of interpersonal interaction (Hockenberry et al.,

2019). When a child enters school, the environment expands to include the school, transportation to and from school, school friends, and after-school activities. School-age children are learning how to perform more complicated motor activities and often are uncoordinated. They are also expanding their cognitive and psychosocial skills. A child at this age needs to learn to cope with the rules and expectations of schools and peers. School-age children involved in team and contact sports may not consistently follow the rules for playing safely and may fail to use protective safety equipment, such as helmets and other protective gear. School-age children are exposed to more environments in which they need protection, they have less supervision, and they take more responsibility as they participate in a more adult world (Hockenberry et al., 2019).

The incidence of school violence, including fighting; bullying, cyberbullying, weapon use, and physical, sexual, and psychological abuse; and violence against oneself (intentional nonsuicidal self-injury) has increased. Nearly 9% of high school students reported being in a physical fight on school property one or more times during the 12 months before the 2017 CDC's Youth Risk Behavior Survey (CDC, 2020h). Violence in any form disrupts a child's ability to learn and may have a negative effect on health throughout life (National Association of School Nurses, 2018). School nurses are able to recognize the multiple factors that may increase or decrease a youth's risk of becoming a perpetrator or victim of school violence and may be able to identify students at risk (Box 27.1).

Adolescent. As children enter adolescence, they develop greater independence and a sense of identity. Adolescents begin to separate

BOX 27.1 Risk Factors for Violence

Individual Risk Factors
- History of violent victimization
- Disabilities: attention deficits, hyperactivity, learning disorders
- History of early aggressive behavior
- Substance abuse
- Low IQ
- Poor behavioral control
- High emotional distress
- History of treatment for emotional problems
- Antisocial beliefs and attitudes
- Exposure to violence and conflict in the family

Family Risk Factors
- Authoritarian childrearing attitudes
- Harsh, lax, or inconsistent disciplinary practices
- Low parental involvement
- Low emotional attachment to parents or caregivers
- Low parental education and income
- Parental substance abuse or criminality
- Dysfunctional family
- Poor monitoring and supervision of children

Peer and Social Risk Factors
- Association with delinquent peers
- Gang participation
- Social rejection by peers
- Lack of involvement in conventional activities
- Poor academic performance
- Low commitment to school and school failure

Adapted from National Association of School Nurses: *School violence—the role of the school nurse,* https://www.cdc.gov/ViolencePrevention/youthviolence/riskprotectivefactors.html. Accessed January 21, 2021.

emotionally from their families, and peer groups begin to have a stronger influence. Adolescents typically have wide variations that swing from childlike to mature behavior. They test their boundaries by trying risky behaviors. Experimentation with the use of tobacco, alcohol, and other substances is common. Trends such as the current opioid epidemic have alerted school communities to the dangers of prescription painkillers. Without appropriate health literacy skills, misinformed parents and students can overlook or downplay the risks of substance use. Environmental clues of substance abuse include the presence of drug-oriented magazines, beer and liquor bottles, or drug paraphernalia and the wearing of long-sleeved shirts in hot weather. Psychosocial clues include failing grades, change in dress, absenteeism from school, isolation, and changes in interpersonal relationships. Substance abuse increases the risks for accidents such as drowning and motor vehicle accidents.

Adolescents are at risk for suicide because of feelings of decreased self-worth and hopelessness. Risk factors include (Kaslow, 2021):

- A recent or serious loss, such as the death of a family member, a friend, or a pet.
- A psychiatric disorder, particularly a mood disorder, such as depression, or a trauma- and stress-related disorder.
- Prior suicide attempts.
- Alcohol and other substance abuse disorders, as well as getting into a lot of trouble, having disciplinary problems, or engaging in high-risk behaviors
- Struggling with sexual orientation in an environment that is not respectful of or accepting of that orientation.
- A family history of suicide, as well as a history of domestic violence, child abuse, or neglect.
- Lack of social support. A child who doesn't feel support from significant adults in her life, as well as her friends, can become isolated.
- Bullying. It is known that being a victim of bullying is a risk factor, but there is also some evidence that children who are bullies may be at increased risk for suicidal behavior.
- Access to lethal means, such as firearms and pills.

Adult. The threats to an adult's safety are often related to lifestyle habits. For example, a person who uses alcohol excessively is at greater risk for motor vehicle accidents or sustaining an injury at home. People who smoke long-term have a greater risk of cardiovascular or pulmonary disease because of the inhalation of smoke and the effect of nicotine on the circulatory system. Likewise, the adult experiencing a high level of stress is more likely to have an accident or illness such as headaches, gastrointestinal (GI) disorders, and infections.

Older Adult. The physiological changes associated with aging, the effects of multiple medications, psychological and cognitive changes, and the effects of acute or chronic disease increase an older adult's risk for falls and other types of accidents (e.g., burn injuries, vehicular crashes). More than one out of four adults 65 years of age and older fall each year, but fewer than half tell their health care providers (CDC, 2017a). Falls are the major cause of injury leading to disability and death among adults 65 years of age and older. Once a patient falls, the risk of falling a second time is increased (CDC, 2017a).

There are multiple reasons for cognitive changes in older adults. Some cognitive changes are a natural part of aging. For example, an older adult may walk into a room and forget the purpose of going to the room or begin to leave the home and find the car keys are misplaced. However, there are also reasons for abnormal cognitive changes that need to be assessed in the older adult. For example, the changes may be associated with treatment for a disease process (such as chemotherapy for cancer). Lange et al. (2018) studied patients who were 65 years of age or older with newly diagnosed early-stage breast cancer (EBC).

The researchers noted five significant patterns of cognitive decline and impairment after the patients had completed their treatments.

Dementia is a clinical syndrome caused by neurodegeneration and characterized by progressive deterioration in cognitive ability and capacity for independent living. There are approximately 5.7 million people living with dementia in the United States (Alzheimer's Association, 2018). The number of dementia cases (e.g., Alzheimer disease, vascular dementia) are expected to rise as life expectancy increases.

Dementia limits the cognitive ability to process information that normally allows people to perform tasks and prevent injury. Older adults who develop dementia often develop wandering. Wandering is the meandering, aimless, or repetitive locomotion that exposes a person to harm and is often in conflict with boundaries (such as doors), limits, or obstacles (Herdman and Kamitsuru, 2018). Wandering is dangerous. Individuals can walk away from home or off care units or enter restricted or closed areas without the knowledge of caregivers. Interrupting a wandering patient can increase their distress. Family caregivers, as well as professional caregivers, must apply safety principles to reduce patients' tendencies to wander and to provide safe living environments.

Mind wandering is very common for all adults. It is a condition in which thoughts do not remain focused on a task at hand (e.g., listening to a sermon, driving, walking a familiar route in neighborhood). Instead, thoughts range widely and spontaneously across other topics. It tends to occur during tasks that do not require sustained attention (American Psychological Association [APA], 2020). When mind wandering occurs in older adults it can have negative functional consequences, such as falls, and impaired task performance because it is distracting. In a study by Nagamatsu et al. (2013), falls were associated with an increased frequency of mind wandering, involving an inability to actively control attention to align with current behavioral goals while simultaneously inhibiting task-unrelated thoughts. The tendency to mind wander poses an obstacle for individuals to safely navigate their environments.

Individual Risk Factors. An individual's safety is threatened by numerous factors including comorbidities; workplace culture; lifestyle; impaired mobility; sensory, cognitive, or communication impairment; limited economic resources; and the lack of safety awareness. The impact of these common risk factors offers a knowledge base to help nurses anticipate patient risks.

Workplace Culture. There are numerous factors within a workplace that affect an individual's adherence to safety practices. Whether an organization has a safety culture, the attitudes and beliefs of workers, and the availability of equipment to keep workers safe influence adherence. An example for health care workers is adherence to the use of personal protective equipment (PPE). The 2008 report by the Institute of Medicine (IOM) still has relevance today with regard to the range of factors that impact PPE-related behaviors and adherence (IOM, 2008). These factors are organized into three categories:

1. *Individual factors,* such as knowledge, beliefs, attitudes, perception of risk, history, and sociodemographics
2. *Environmental factors,* including availability of equipment and negative-pressure rooms
3. *Organizational factors,* such as management's expectations and performance feedback, workplace policies, and training and education programs

These same factors can apply to a variety of work settings. Nurses who work in occupational health and safety can apply these factors when developing training and education programs for their work colleagues.

Lifestyle. Some lifestyle choices increase safety risks. People who drive or operate machinery while under the influence of chemical substances (drugs or alcohol), who work at dangerous jobs (construction, utility repair, law enforcement), who text while driving, or who are general risk takers are at greater risk of injury. Also, people experiencing stress, anxiety, fatigue, or alcohol or drug withdrawal, or those taking prescribed medications are sometimes more accident prone because of physical effects of these conditions. For example, an individual who is overly fatigued or very dizzy from a medication becomes preoccupied about symptoms and fails to notice the source of potential accidents, such as cluttered stairs or a stop sign.

Impaired Mobility. A patient with impaired mobility has many kinds of safety risks. Muscle weakness, paralysis, abnormal gait, and poor coordination or balance are major factors in placing patients at risk for falls. Immobilization predisposes patients to physical deconditioning and emotional hazards, which in turn further restrict mobility and independence (see Chapter 39). People who are physically challenged are at greater risk for injury when entering motor vehicles and buildings that are not handicap accessible.

Sensory, Cognitive, or Communication Impairment. Cognitive impairments associated with delirium, dementia, and depression alter concentration and attention span and cause impaired memory and orientation changes. Patients with these alterations become easily confused about their surroundings and are more likely to have falls and burns. This is a common problem when such patients temporarily or permanently move to a health care setting. Patients with visual, hearing, tactile, or communication impairment, such as aphasia or a language barrier, are not always able to perceive potential dangers or express their need for assistance (see Chapter 49). Patients with reduced health literacy are unable to understand the information needed to make the decisions required for providing safe home environments.

Economic Resources. People with lower incomes (including the homeless) are more likely to have behavioral health issues, such as depression or substance use problems, that place them at risk for injury. They also do not have access to the health care resources (such as medications and treatments) that those with higher incomes have (see Chapter 9). Those who are homeless are less likely to have a regular source of health care and are more likely to forgo needed care. Homeless individuals also likely do not have a safe place to stay. When a patient who has a lower income enters a health care agency, ensure that you assess all of the patient's resources and safety risks.

Lack of Safety Awareness. Some patients are unaware of or inexperienced in following safety precautions in the home or workplace. Examples of behaviors reflecting lack of awareness include not keeping medicine or poisons away from children, not reading the expiration dates on food products, and not using safety equipment at work. You cannot assume a patient's knowledge about a safety topic. There are also patients who believe safety information is not relevant to their situation or who simply choose to ignore it. As a nurse, one of the first areas to assess is a patient's understanding of any safety risks and the approaches needed to minimize the effects of those risks. Sound clinical judgment requires understanding a patient's perspective of safety as well as the risks posed by any physical condition.

Risks in Health Care Agencies. The prevention of medical errors continues to be one of the most pressing health care challenges in the nation. Medical errors occur when planned actions are not completed as intended or wrong plans of care are used. They occur in all health care settings. Be aware of the organizational and regulatory patient safety measures that have been established in the health care setting where you work. The AHRQ lists 20 tips for patients to become partners and help prevent medical errors (AHRQ, 2020a). The patient fact sheet can be viewed at the AHRQ website, https://www.ahrq.gov/patients-consumers/care-planning/errors/20tips/index.html.

TJC and CMS emphasize error prevention and patient safety. Their Speak Up campaign encourages patients to take a role in preventing health care errors by becoming active, involved, and informed participants on the health care team (TJC, 2021b). For example, patients are encouraged to ask health care workers whether they have washed their hands before providing care. The National Patient Safety Goals of TJC (TJC, 2021a) highlight specific improvements in patient safety and ongoing problematic areas in health care. These evidence-based recommendations require health care agencies to focus their attention on a series of specific actions.

Another national organization, the National Quality Forum (NQF), leads the national collaboration among health care agencies and the public to improve health and health care quality through measurement (NQF, 2021a).The NQF brings key public- and private-sector leaders together to establish national priorities and goals to achieve health care that is safe, effective, patient centered, timely, efficient, and equitable. In addition, the organization creates NQF-endorsed standards used to measure and report on the quality and efficiency of health care in the United States. Many of the NQF measurement standards for patient safety (e.g., patient falls with injury, incidence of pressure injuries, and central line–associated bloodstream infection [CLABSI]) are standards for judging the quality of care of health care organizations. Among the safety measures, the NQF endorsed a select list of serious reportable events (SREs) that include a range of clinical settings where patients receive care, including office-based practices, ambulatory surgery centers, and skilled nursing facilities (NQF, 2021b) (Box 27.2). The 29 events are a major focus of health care providers for patient safety initiatives.

CMS selects some SREs as their *Never Events* (CMS, 2019) (Box 27.3). Many of the hospital-acquired conditions (e.g., fall or Stage 3 pressure injury) are nurse-sensitive indicators, meaning that a nurse directly affects their development. These indicators are the focus of performance improvement efforts by nursing departments across the country. The NQF released 34 Safe Practices for Better Healthcare (last updated in 2010) that are effective in reducing the occurrence of adverse health care events across a variety of environments (NQF, 2021c). Scientific evidence supports the effectiveness of these practices in reducing the occurrence of adverse health care events.

Health care agencies often conduct a failure mode and effect analysis (FMEA) to identify problems with health care processes and products before they occur. When an actual or potential adverse event occurs, the nurse or health care provider involved completes an incident or occurrence report. An incident report is a confidential document that completely describes any patient accident occurring on the premises of a health care agency (see Chapter 23). Reporting allows an organization to identify trends or patterns throughout the agency and areas to improve. Focusing on the root cause of an event instead of the individual involved promotes a culture of safety that helps in specifically identifying what contributed to an error. The evidence shows that the use of evidence-based practices can have a favorable impact on patient safety. The strongest evidence exists for interventions that are effective in preventing delirium, adverse drug events, infections, and falls (Zegers et al., 2016).

Procedure-Related Accidents. Procedure-related accidents are caused by health care providers and include medication administration errors, improper application of external devices, and accidents related to improper performance of procedures such as urinary catheter insertion or transferring patients without use of safe patient-handling techniques. Strictly following policies and procedures or

BOX 27.2   National Quality Forum Serious Reportable Events in Health Care

1 Surgical or Invasive Procedure Events
A. Surgery or other invasive procedure performed on the wrong site (updated)
B. Surgery or other invasive procedure performed on the wrong patient
C. Wrong surgical or other invasive procedure performed on a patient (updated)
D. Unintended retention of a foreign object in a patient after surgery or other invasive procedure (updated)
E. Intraoperative or immediately postoperative/postprocedure death in an ASA Class 1 patient (updated)

2 Product or Device Events
A. Patient death or serious injury associated with the use of contaminated drugs, devices, or biologics provided by the health care setting (updated)
B. Patient death or serious injury associated with the use or function of a device in patient care, in which the device is used or functions other than as intended (updated)
C. Patient death or serious injury associated with intravascular air embolism that occurs while being cared for in a health care setting (updated)

3 Patient Protection Events
A. Discharge or release of a patient/resident of any age who is unable to make decisions to other than an authorized person (updated)
B. Patient death or serious injury associated with patient elopement (disappearance) (updated)
C. Patient suicide, attempted suicide, or self-harm that results in serious injury, while being cared for in a health care setting (updated)

4 Care Management Events
A. Patient death or serious injury associated with a medication error (e.g., errors involving the wrong drug, wrong dose, wrong patient, wrong time, wrong rate, wrong preparation, or wrong route of administration) (updated)
B. Patient death or serious injury associated with unsafe administration of blood products (updated)
C. Maternal death or serious injury associated with labor or delivery in a low-risk pregnancy while being cared for in a health care setting (updated)
D. Death or serious injury of a neonate associated with labor or delivery in a low-risk pregnancy (new)

E. Patient death or serious injury associated with a fall while being cared for in a health care setting (updated)
F. Any Stage 3, Stage 4, and unstageable pressure injuries acquired after admission/presentation to a health care setting (updated)
G. Artificial insemination with the wrong donor sperm or wrong egg (updated)
H. Patient death or serious injury resulting from the irretrievable loss of an irreplaceable biological specimen (new)
I. Patient death or serious injury resulting from failure to follow up or communicate laboratory, pathology, or radiology test results (new)

5 Environmental Events
A. Patient or staff death or serious injury associated with an electric shock in the course of a patient care process in a health care setting (updated)
B. Any incident in which systems designated for oxygen or other gas to be delivered to a patient contain no gas or the wrong gas, or are contaminated by toxic substances (updated)
C. Patient or staff death or serious injury associated with a burn incurred from any source in the course of a patient care process in a health care setting (updated)
D. Patient death or serious injury associated with the use of physical restraints or bedrails while being cared for in a health care setting (updated)

6 Radiological Events
A. Death or serious injury of a patient or staff associated with the introduction of a metallic object into the magnetic resonance imaging (MRI) area (new)

7 Potential Criminal Events
A. Any instance of care ordered by or provided by someone impersonating a physician, nurse, pharmacist, or other licensed health care provider (updated)
B. Abduction of a patient/resident of any age (updated)
C. Sexual abuse/assault on a patient or staff member within or on the grounds of a health care setting (updated)
D. Death or serious injury of a patient or staff member resulting from a physical assault (i.e., battery) that occurs within or on the grounds of a health care setting (updated)

Copyright © 2021 National Quality Forum.
ASA, American Society of Anesthesiologists.

BOX 27.3   The Centers for Medicare and Medicaid Services Hospital-Acquired Conditions (Present-on-Admission Indicator)

For discharges occurring on or after October 1, 2008, hospitals will not receive additional payment for cases in which one of the selected conditions was not present on admission:
• Foreign object retained after surgery
• Air embolism
• Blood incompatibility
• Pressure injury Stage 3 or 4
• Falls and trauma (fracture, dislocation, intracranial injury, crushing injury, burn, electric shock)
• Catheter-associated urinary tract infections
• Vascular catheter-associated infections

• Manifestations of poor glycemic control (diabetic ketoacidosis, nonketotic hyperosmolar coma, hypoglycemic coma, secondary diabetes with ketoacidosis, secondary diabetes with hyperosmolarity)
• Surgical site infections following:
  • Mediastinitis following coronary artery bypass graft
  • Certain orthopedic procedures (spine, neck, shoulder, elbow)
  • Bariatric surgery for obesity (laparoscopic gastric bypass, gastroenterostomy, laparoscopic gastric restrictive surgery)
  • Cardiac implantable medical device
  • Deep-vein thrombosis (DVT)/pulmonary embolism (PE) following certain orthopedic procedures (total knee replacement, hip replacement)
  • Iatrogenic pneumothorax with venous catheterization

From Centers for Medicare and Medicaid Services (CMS): *Hospital-acquired conditions (present on admission indicator),* 2019, http://www.cms.gov/HospitalAcqCond/06_Hospital-Acquired_Conditions.asp. Accessed January 21, 2021.

standards of nursing practice prevent these accidents. All staff need to be aware that distractions and interruptions contribute to procedure-related accidents and need to be limited, especially during high-risk procedures such as intravenous (IV) medication administration. One valuable approach is to take a time-out, similar to what occurs in operating room settings. When performing high-risk procedures or those with which you are less experienced performing, take a short time-out, reflect on what is to be done, review your knowledge, and refer to a policy and procedure manual if needed.

Equipment-Related Accidents. Equipment-related accidents result from an electrical hazard or malfunction, disrepair, or misuse of equipment. To avoid rapid infusion of IV fluids, for example, nurses use programmed infusion pumps with free-flow protection. To avoid accidents, do not operate medical equipment without adequate instruction. If you find a faulty piece of equipment, replace it with properly working equipment, place a tag on the faulty one, take it out of service, and then promptly report malfunction to the appropriate department. Assess potential electrical hazards at the bedside to reduce the risk of electrical fires, electrocution, or injury from faulty equipment. Clinical engineering staff in health care settings regularly make safety checks of equipment. Agencies must report all suspected medical device–related deaths to the U.S. Food and Drug Administration (FDA, 2020) and the product manufacturer.

Chemical Exposure. Both patients and health care workers face serious environmental health risks within health care agencies. An example of a risk to health care workers is exposure to various forms of chemicals. Chemicals found in some medications (e.g., chemotherapy), anesthetic gases, cleaning solutions, and disinfectants are potentially toxic if ingested, absorbed into the skin, or inhaled. A health care provider or family caregiver who becomes exposed to a chemotherapeutic agent, especially one in liquid form, has an increased risk for leukemia, other cancers, and adverse reproductive outcomes and chromosomal damage (CDC, 2017b). If you are exposed to a chemical, access Material Safety Data Sheets (MSDSs) that contain detailed information about the chemical, the precautions for safe handling and use, health hazards related to exposure, first aid guidelines, and steps for containment and removal in case of release or spillage. MSDSs are required resources available in any health care agency (OSHA, n.d.a). Always know the location of the MSDSs and how to follow safety guidelines within your agency.

Falls. A report from the Health Research and Educational Trust (HRET, 2016) commissioned by TJC noted that an estimated 700,000 to 1,000,000 people fall in U.S. hospitals each year and that 30% to 35% of those patients sustain an injury as a result of the fall, and approximately 11,000 falls are fatal. A fall may result in fractures, bruises, lacerations, or internal bleeding, leading to increased diagnostic tests and treatments, extended hospital stays, and discharge to rehabilitation or long-term care instead of home. Falls have been identified by the CMS as a preventable event that should never occur. Therefore the CMS in October 2008 stopped reimbursing hospitals for costs related to patient falls (Fehlberg et al., 2017). Fall prevention is a priority of all health care settings. It requires a culture of safety in which all health care providers are mindful of the fall risks existing within health care settings combined with the fall risks created by patients' health conditions and are proactive in providing fall prevention strategies.

Falls are clearly multifactorial. Many different conditions can contribute to a single patient fall (Berry and Kiel, 2021). The risk factors for falls include two categories: patient related (intrinsic) and hospital environment and working process related (extrinsic). The intrinsic factors are predisposing factors, whereas extrinsic factors increase the susceptibility of an individual to fall. In international and national studies examining risk factors for falls, common risks are found for all patients (Berry and Kiel, 2021; HRET, 2016; Severo et al., 2014) (Table 27.1).

To anticipate a patient's fall risk, health care agencies use validated fall risk assessment tools that include risk factors that have been identified from the scientific literature. The number of risks identified for a specific patient is computed into a fall risk score—for example, high, medium, and low. The most common risk assessment tools used in hospitals are the Morse Fall Scale, the STRATIFY scale, and the Hendrich II Fall Risk Model (Berry and Kiel, 2021; Severo et al., 2014). Once a patient's fall risks are identified, your responsibility is to partner with the patient to confirm those risks and to select evidence-based interventions (usually multiple strategies) that appropriately target the patient's risks (Berry and Kiel, 2021).

Universal Fall Precautions are called "universal" because they apply to all patients regardless of fall risk. Universal Fall Precautions revolve around keeping a patient's environment safe and comfortable. Although the choice of which precautions to emphasize may vary by health care agency, a starting list has been recommended by the AHRQ (2018):

- Familiarize the patient with the environment.
- Have the patient demonstrate call light use.
- Maintain call light within reach.
- Keep the patient's personal possessions within patient safe reach.
- Have sturdy handrails in patient bathrooms, rooms, and hallways.
- Place the hospital bed in low position when a patient is resting in bed; raise bed to a comfortable height when the patient is transferring out of bed.
- Keep hospital bed brakes locked.
- Keep wheelchair wheel locks in "locked" position when stationary.
- Keep nonslip, comfortable, well-fitting footwear on the patient.
- Use night lights or supplemental lighting.
- Keep floor surfaces clean and dry. Clean up all spills promptly.
- Keep patient care areas uncluttered.
- Follow safe patient-handling practices.

Fall prevention is not simple. Even after adopting Universal Fall Precautions, it is recommended that additional individualized interventions be used based on patients' fall risks. However, there is still no conclusive evidence for any set of interventions that will consistently prevent falls, even though numerous individual nursing fall prevention interventions have been tested (Fehlberg et al., 2017). The AHRQ (2018) recommends these tips:

- Fall prevention must be balanced with other priorities for the patient. The patient is usually not in the hospital because of falls, so attention is naturally directed elsewhere. Yet a fall in a sick patient can be disastrous and prolong recovery.
- Fall prevention must be balanced with the need to mobilize patients. It may be tempting to leave patients in bed to prevent falls, but patients need to transfer and ambulate to maintain their strength and to avoid complications of bed rest.
- Fall prevention is one of many activities needed to protect patients from harm during their hospital stay. How should fall prevention be reinforced while maintaining enthusiasm for other priorities, such as infection control?
- Fall prevention is interprofessional. All health care providers need to cooperate to prevent falls. How should the right information about a patient's fall risks get to the right member of the team at the right time?
- Fall prevention needs to be individualized.

Each patient has a different set of fall risk factors, so critical thinking must be applied during assessment to identify each patient's unique needs. For example, patients with urinary urgency will benefit from diuretics given in the early morning and from use of bedside toilets.

TJC's Center for Transforming Healthcare aims to prevent inpatient falls with injury (HRET, 2016). Seven hospitals in the United States worked with the center and successfully reduced total number of

TABLE 27.1 Risk Factors for Falls or Injuries to Hospitalized Patient	
Intrinsic Factors	**Extrinsic Factors**
History of Previous Fall	***Communication Issues***
Behavioral	• Frequency of rounding
• Patient does not seek assistance for toileting	• Inconsistent or incomplete communication of patient risk for falls between
• Patient did not know, forgot, or chose not to use call light	caregivers
Altered Cognition	***Education Issues***
• Dementia, sedation, delirium	• Fall prevention education for patient and family is not used or is inconsis-
• Patient awareness and acknowledgment of own risk for falls	tently used
Altered Mobility	• Improper performance of procedures or taking short cuts
• Lower extremity weakness	***Physical Hazards***
• Abnormal gait	• Liquids on floor
• Shuffling and stumbling	• Electrical cords near walking path
• Requires assistance with mobility and/or assistive device	• Uses intravenous (IV) pole to walk
Sensory Deficit	• Improper application of medical devices (e.g., wears compression stocking
• Unable to see walking path clearly	with cords)
• Reduced visual field	***Competency***
Medications	• Increased use of restraints (Miake-Lye et al., 2013)
• Benzodiazepines	• Improper fitting of assistive devices
• Antipsychotics	• Improper supervision of patient
• Antidepressants	• Decreased efforts by hospital staff to mobilize patients (Miake-Lye et al.,
• Opiates	2013)
• Barbiturates	• Inappropriate or no footwear
• Antihistamines	
• Anticonvulsants	
• Sedatives	
• Antihypertensives	
• Diuretics	
Toileting Problems	
• Takes diuretics	
• Has urgency or frequency	
Disease Conditions Causing:	
• Dizziness	
• Peripheral neuropathy	
• Pain (especially in lower extremities)	
• Hypotension	

falls and falls with injury by creating awareness among staff, empowering patients to take an active role in their own safety, using validated fall risk assessment tools, engaging patients and their families in fall safety programs, providing hourly rounding that includes proactive toileting, and engaging all hospital staff to ensure that no patient walks unaccompanied (HRET, 2016).

Workplace Safety. Violence is a familiar occurrence in health care settings. The sources of violence include patients, visitors, intruders, and co-workers. The National Institute for Occupational Safety and Health (NIOSH, 2020) defines workplace violence as the act or threat of violence, ranging from verbal abuse to physical assault, directed toward persons at work or on duty. The impact of workplace violence ranges from psychological issues (e.g., posttraumatic stress disorder [PTSD], compassion fatigue) to physical injury or death. When subjected to workplace violence, health care staff experience anger, frustration, fear, stress, and irritability.

In a publication entitled "Workplace Violence Against Health Care Workers in the United States," data from the Bureau of Labor Statistics showed that health care workers are nearly 4 times more likely than others to require time away from work as a result of violence (Campbell, 2019). However, workplace violence occurs on a continuum. Bullying, verbal threats, and name calling are common. In health care settings, patients are most commonly the source of

violence resulting from hitting, kicking, beating, and shoving (OSHA, 2015). Risk factors for workplace violence caused by patients include working with patients who have a history of violence, overcrowded waiting areas, poor lighting in hallways, working in isolation from co-workers, inadequate security staff, work setting located in a high-crime neighborhood, having a mobile workplace, transporting or lifting patients, and presence of firearms (OSHA, 2015). Many incidents of violence are not reported, but violence can be prevented with proper safety policies and environmental adaptations.

> **QSEN** **Building Competency in Safety** A nurse is caring for a patient who is receiving chemotherapy. The patient becomes confused and pulls out her IV line, and the chemotherapy drug leaks into the bed linens and all over the floor. What risks are posed for this patient? What risks are posed for the nurse? How should the nurse manage the situation?
>
> Answers to QSEN Activities can be found on the Evolve website.

While planning for her first home visit with Mrs. Cohen, Kylie reflects on what she knows about cerebrovascular accidents (CVAs) (strokes) and their impact on motor function and speech. Her assessment will include an examination of the patient's neurological and musculoskeletal systems. She also considers the patient's age, knowing that being 78 places the patient at risk for injury due to normal physical and cognitive changes. She plans on assessing the patient's economic resources, family support, and the home environment to ensure a thorough assessment can be conducted.

CRITICAL THINKING

Because patient safety involves the different factors each patient brings to a clinical situation, you must anticipate what to assess and also recognize that such factors as well as environmental factors can differ or change quickly. Successful critical thinking requires a synthesis of knowledge, experience, environmental factors, critical thinking attitudes, and intellectual and professional standards. Sound clinical judgments require you to anticipate the information, analyze the data, and make decisions regarding your patient's care (Fig. 27.1).

For example, in the case of Kylie, she will assess the physical condition of Mrs. Cohen because Kylie knows a stroke potentially causes loss of or reduction in motor function, resulting in impaired gait and balance, which can create a risk for Mrs. Cohen to fall.

Clinical experience is invaluable to a nurse who has cared for patients with conditions that pose safety risks. A nurse benefits from seeing how a condition affects a patient and how any interventions prove successful. Experience also plays a role when nurses search to find ways to engage patients effectively. Patient engagement yields more information about how an individual perceives, accepts, and understands safety issues.

Critical thinking enhances a nurse's ability to make clinical decisions about patient safety through routine application of critical thinking attitudes and intellectual standards. Both attitudes and standards serve to guide nurses in making comprehensive and patient-centered safety assessments so that accurate diagnoses can be made.

Environmental factors affect patient safety. A nurse must critically anticipate what common conditions pose safety risks in the home or health care setting and then determine if such conditions exist in a patient's current environment. It is much like being a radar detector, looking for broken equipment, uneven floor surfaces, or poor lighting—conditions that create safety risks. Patients are often in very dependent situations, relying on nurses to detect such risks. A nurse also considers how to avoid environmental disruptions that can negatively influence attending to patient care needs. For example, a phone call or request from a colleague can delay a nurse from returning to the room of a patient left on a bedside commode. Unless the nurse attends to the patient and ignores the distractions, the patient could fall while returning to bed unassisted.

Sound clinical judgment involves nurses applying evidence-based knowledge and standards of practice for meeting patient safety needs. The American Nurses Association (ANA) standards for nursing practice address the nurse's responsibility in maintaining patient safety. TJC (2021a) also provides numerous standards for safety. Every acute

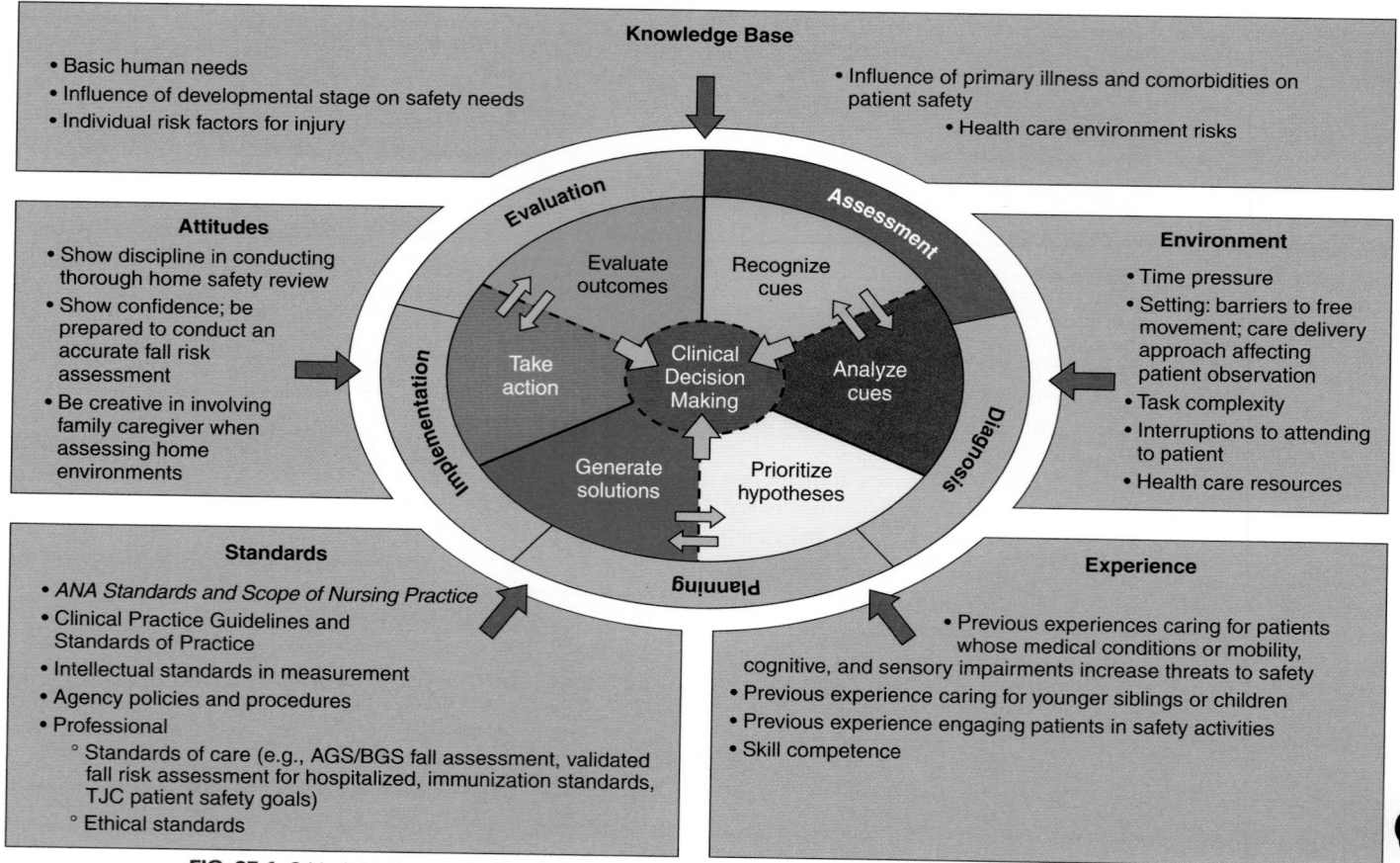

FIG. 27.1 Critical thinking model for assessing safety. *AGS,* American Geriatrics Society; *ANA,* American Nurses Association; *BGS,* British Geriatrics Society; *TJC,* The Joint Commission. (Clinical Judgment Measurement Model copyright © NCSBN. All rights reserved.)

care agency has standards developed in the form of either policies and procedures or clinical guidelines for fall prevention, fire safety, and electric and chemical safety.

REFLECT NOW

Reflect on your last clinical experience. What risks to patient safety did you observe? Describe interventions taken to reduce risks to patient safety.

❖ NURSING PROCESS

When you apply the critical thinking elements to the nursing process, you will make sound clinical judgments for the clinical decisions needed to maintain or promote patient safety.

◆ Assessment

During the assessment process thoroughly assess each patient and the environment and critically analyze findings and compare findings with those expected, to ensure that you have a thorough database needed to make patient-centered clinical decisions for safe patient care.

Through the Patient's Eyes. Patients expect to be safe in health care settings and in their homes. However, sometimes a patient's view of what is safe is different from that of the nurse and the standards associated with safety in the health care environment. For example, when patients from an ethnic minority need to be hospitalized, they have to leave their familiar context behind (e.g., families, usual daily activities) and enter an unknown and frightening environment (Degrie et al., 2017). Individuals have different perceptions of safety. Therefore you cannot make decisions based on your own bias as to what is safe. For this reason your nursing assessment needs to be patient centered; this includes (1) a patient's own perceptions of risk factors, (2) a patient's values and beliefs about safety, (3) a patient's concerns about being in a health care setting, (4) a patient's knowledge of how to adapt to safety risks, and (5) information about a patient's previous experience with accidents. Consult with family caregivers when appropriate.

Patients and their families are your partners; involve them in any safety assessment. Patients often recognize when medical errors occur or when they feel at risk. Data collected from a research study involving over 19,000 patients from 11 countries revealed that patients often report poor coordination of care: 10.9% of the patients reported that test results or medical records were not available, 19.6% perceived they had received conflicting information from care providers, and 10.5% reported that tests were ordered that had been performed before (Schwappach, 2014).

Nursing History and Examination. A nursing history (see Chapter 30) includes data about a patient's medical history, medications, psychosocial and cultural background, and presence of fall risk factors to determine whether any underlying conditions pose threats to safety (Box 27.4). A physical examination focuses on bodily functions that can affect a patient's mobility and ability to interact safely in their environment. For example, an assessment with a safety focus includes a patient's cognitive status, gait, lower-body muscle strength and coordination, balance, and visual and hearing status. A cardiovascular assessment is critical when patients have poor activity tolerance, making them vulnerable to injuries. For example, a patient with severe shortness of breath has an unstable stance. You assess the patient's balance and gait by observing the patient walk in the room; do not rely on the patient's self-report. Review a

BOX 27.4 Nursing Assessment Questions

Perceptions of Safety
- Tell me what it means to feel safe.
- Describe any changes you think should be made to improve your safety at work and at home.

Lifestyle
- Do you use any assistive devices, such as a wheelchair, walker, or cane, to help you move or get around? Did someone show you how to use them safely? (Have patient demonstrate use.)
- Describe for me any difficulties you have with bathing, dressing, or toileting.
- Explain how you prepare meals at home (e.g., use stove and appliances safely).
- Do you do your own laundry? How do you do this, and where are these appliances located?
- Describe the types of social activities you engage in.
- Do you drive a car or motorcycle? When do you normally drive? How far?
- How often do you wear a seat belt when in the car or a helmet when on your bike?

Medication History
- Which medications (prescription, over-the-counter, herbal) do you take?
- Has your doctor or pharmacist reviewed your medicines with you in the last year?
- Describe for me any side effects that you have after taking your medications.

History of Falls
- Have you ever fallen or tripped over anything in your home? Have you had any near misses?
- Tell me what you think caused you to fall. Which activity were you performing before the fall?
- Have you ever sustained an injury from a fall? What was it and how did it happen?
- Did you have any symptoms right before you fell? What were they?

Home Maintenance and Safety
- Who does your simple home maintenance or minor home repairs?
- Who shovels your snow? Mows your lawn?
- Do you feel safe in your home? Describe anything in your environment that makes you feel unsafe.
- If you have an emergency at home, whom can you call for help?
- How do you feel about modifying your home to make it safer?

patient's developmental status as you analyze physical and cognitive assessment information. For example, if a patient is an adolescent, does the patient show risk factors for suicide or drug and alcohol abuse? Review the patient's medication history and any planned procedures that pose risks. For example, the use of diuretics increases frequency of voiding and results in a patient having to go to the toilet more often. Frequent toileting is a risk factor for falls, especially when patients get out of bed quickly without assistance.

Psychosocial and Cultural Background. The intercultural care encounter between patients and health care providers in the agency setting is challenging. It occurs suddenly because of an unplanned illness, and it is necessary and inevitable during the hospitalization because of the various cultures represented by health care workers. This is true for all patients. The possibility of providing good intercultural care in this context is also challenged by language barriers, lower health literacy and higher socioeconomic stressors in ethnic minority groups, scarcity of hospital resources (time, money, and people), differences in cultural traditions, differences in understanding illness and treatment, and negative attitudes among patients and caregivers (Degrie et al., 2017).

Home care or outpatient care is also challenging, but the context may be less threatening if a patient is discharged in relatively stable condition, placing fewer demands on family caregivers and professional caregivers by the nature of the patient's condition being more stable. Whenever a provider enters the patient's environment, cultural competency is critical (see Chapter 9).

Your assessment must include a review of a patient's cultural perspective, health literacy, and perception of health and safety. For example, ask the question, "What does it mean for you to be safe?" The patient may have a focus on his community, the family dynamics of keeping a member safe, or the interior of the home. The patient's feedback will be invaluable, especially when attempting any health promotion strategies along with education interventions. Does a patient consider taking safety precautions beneficial? What do the precautions mean to a patient? Does the patient normally wear a seat belt, drive within speed limits, or wear protective gear for sports or work activities? In the health care agency setting, what is the time frame in which a patient expects a nurse to respond to a call light? To understand patient expectations about safety, you must help patients express treatment preferences and care needs. This is more difficult when patients who speak a foreign language are too shy to speak or when they are inhibited to ask questions on a deeper level owing to language barriers (Degrie et al., 2017). Use of a professional interpreter is critical for learning how these patients perceive safety precautions and whether they understand how to participate in their care.

Health Care Environment. When caring for patients within a health care setting, determine whether any hazards exist in the immediate care environment:

- Does the placement of equipment (e.g., drainage bags, IV pumps) or furniture pose barriers when the patient tries to ambulate?
- Does the positioning of the bed allow the patient to reach items on a bedside table or stand easily? Does the patient need help with ambulation?
- Is there a gait belt or an assistive device available for when the patient ambulates?
- Are health care workers and family visitors following hand hygiene guidelines?
- Are there multiple tubes or IV lines?
- Is the nurse call system within reach?

Contact the clinical engineering staff if there are questions as to whether equipment is functioning properly and in good condition.

Risk for Medical Errors. Be alert to factors within your own work environment that create conditions in which medical errors are more likely to occur. Distractions during medication preparation or nursing procedures increase the risk for error. Common distractions include phone calls, alarms, or staff needing assistance. It is your responsibility to recognize the potential problem any distraction might cause (such as delayed treatment; delay in responding to patient request). Studies show that overwork and fatigue, particularly when working consecutive 12-hour shifts, cause a significant decrease in alertness and concentration, leading to errors (Geiger-Brown et al., 2012). You may have little control over the length of shifts you work. However, be mindful if you sense developing fatigue and be vigilant to maintain attention to your tasks. It is important for you to be aware of risk factors in the workplace and to include checks and balances when working under stress. For example, to reduce the chance for a medical error, you need to verify a patient's identity by using two identifiers (e.g., name and birthday or name and medical record number) according to agency policy before beginning any procedure or administering a medication (see Chapter 31) (TJC, 2021a).

Disasters. Hospitals must be prepared to respond to and care for a sudden influx of patients at the time of a community disaster, such as a pandemic or bioterrorist attack. Be prepared to make accurate and timely assessments in any type of setting. Initially a bioterrorist attack is likely to resemble a natural outbreak. Acutely ill patients representing the earliest cases after a covert attack seek care in emergency departments. Patients less ill at the onset of an illness possibly seek care in primary care settings. Rapid detection of a bioterrorism attack occurs through syndrome surveillance and reporting of suspected cases. The early signs of a bioterrorism-related illness often include nonspecific symptoms (e.g., nausea, vomiting, diarrhea, fever, confusion) that may persist for several days before the onset of more severe disease. Patients who experience these early (prodromal) symptoms often seek outpatient care and are assigned nonspecific diagnoses such as "viral syndrome."

It is important that your nursing assessment and ultimate interventions help individuals focus on avoiding losses and reducing their risk for injury associated with disasters. The Federal Emergency Management Agency (http://www.fema.gov/) and the American Red Cross (http://www.redcross.org/) provide nationwide education to help community members prepare for disasters of all types.

REFLECT NOW

Go to the CDC website (https://www.cdc.gov/homeandrecreationalsafety/pubs/english/booklet_eng_desktop-a.pdf) and conduct a home risk assessment on your own home or the home of someone you know who is 65 years of age or older. Once completed, think about how to minimize safety risks.

Patient's Home Environment. Access to appropriate supportive care technologies and home health care services depends in part on where patient homes are located, the types of spaces available for care in the home, and whether basic services (such as utilities, Internet) are reliable (Albert, 2010). No two homes are alike. Homes differ in their spaces available for care but also in the willingness of family caregivers to make the adaptations needed to work with health care staff to provide care. The home environment is nested in social and cultural layers that may lead to different home care outcomes, even with similar patients and common home environments (Albert, 2010). Your nursing assessment must identify the potential for disruption of family relations when a patient requires home health care services and assisting family members to reconcile the demands of home care with the needs of other family members.

When caring for a patient in the home, complete a home hazard assessment. A thorough hazard assessment includes all the rooms in a home and the outdoor entrance areas. Give special focus to the room where a patient will receive care from a family caregiver (e.g., bedroom or living room). Each room assessment covers topics such as adequacy of lighting (inside and outdoors), condition of flooring and walking surfaces, presence of safety devices (e.g., alarms, side rails on steps, safety bars in bathtubs), and placement of furniture or other items that can create barriers. Know where medications and cleaning supplies are located. Walking through the home with the patient and discussing how daily activities are normally conducted and whether the environment poses problems are important. Additional assessment includes the presence of locks on doors and windows. Getting a sense of a patient's routines helps you recognize less obvious hazards. It is also important to learn the patient's willingness to make changes in the environment. This is also true for a family caregiver. Decisions on changing the environment require the patient's full participation.

Assessment for risk of foodborne illness includes assessing a patient's knowledge of food preparation and storage practices. For example, does a patient know to check expiration dates of prepared food and milk products? Are the foods in the refrigerator fresh and not spoiled? Does the patient clean fresh fruits and vegetables correctly before eating them? Assess for clinical signs of infection by conducting an examination of GI and central nervous system function, observing for a fever, and analyzing the results of cultures of feces and emesis. Further assessment includes inspecting the food and water sources and assessing the patient's and family members' handwashing practices.

Assessment of the environmental comfort of a patient's home includes a review of when the patient normally has heating and cooling systems serviced. Does the patient have a functional furnace or space heater? Does the home have air conditioning or fans? Inform patients who use space heaters of the risk for fires. Are smoke detectors and CO detectors up-to-date and functional, and are fire extinguishers present and placed strategically throughout the home and checked routinely?

When patients live in older homes, encourage them to have inspections for lead in paint, dust, or soil. Because lead also comes from the solder or plumbing fixtures in a home, patients need to have water from each faucet tested. Local health offices will help homeowners locate a trained lead inspector who takes samples from various locations and has them analyzed at a laboratory for lead content.

Risk for Falls. As you assess both a patient's health care and home environments, you simultaneously consider presence of fall risks. The identification of fall risks (e.g., impaired balance, reduced visual acuity) is essential to determine the targeted interventions needed to prevent falls. There are many fall risk–assessment instruments used by health care agencies. Most tools include risk categories based on age, fall history, elimination habits, high-risk medications, mobility, and cognition. Some include assessment for presence of patient care equipment (such as indwelling catheter or IV infusion) that makes mobility awkward. At a minimum the assessment needs to be completed on admission, following a change in a patient's condition, after a fall, and when the patient is transferred (AHRQ, 2018). Patients who are at risk for falling require ongoing assessments. When a patient has a previous history of falling, ask about the nature of the fall and what the patient thinks precipitated it. Focus the assessment on that information to determine whether a condition or risk persists. In many cases family members are important resources in assessing a patient's fall risk. Families often can report on the patient's level of confusion and ability to ambulate or safely toilet. Based on the results of a fall risk assessment, you will implement Universal Fall Precautions and other evidence-based interventions for fall prevention. It is very important that you inform the patient and family members about the fall risks that you identify from the assessment. Often, younger patients are not aware of how medications and treatments cause dizziness, orthostatic hypotension, or changes in balance. When patients are unaware of their risks, they are less likely to ask for assistance. If family members are informed, they will often call for help (when they are visiting patients) to be sure that patients have appropriate assistance.

In the primary care setting the American Geriatrics Society (AGS) and British Geriatrics Society (BGS) have a clinical practice guideline for fall risk assessment and management (AGS/BGS, 2011; Huntzinger, 2010) (Fig. 27.2). The guideline recommends screening all adults aged 65 years of age and older for fall risk annually. This screening consists of asking patients whether they have fallen 2 or more times in the past year or sought medical attention for a fall, or, if they have not fallen, whether they feel unsteady when walking. Patients who answer positively to any of these questions are at increased risk for falls and should receive further assessment (Phelan et al., 2015). People who have fallen once without injury should have their balance and gait evaluated; those with gait or balance abnormalities should receive additional assessment.

Kylie is greeted at the door by Mrs. Cohen's daughter Meg. Kylie enters Mrs. Cohen's home and immediately begins observing the room, looking at the condition of the room and noting any safety hazards. She is taken to the patient's living room where there are multiple throw rugs and two piles of magazines on the floor, near an armchair. Kylie recalls from past experience assessing patient homes that this is an area to focus on. Meg then leads Kylie into the patient's bedroom, where she finds Mrs. Cohen sitting in a chair next to the bed. The bedroom is dimly lit. Kylie introduces herself and states, "I am happy to meet you, Mrs. Cohen. My name is Kylie, and I'm your home health nurse. I want to get to know you a bit better to find out what ways we can help you. Does that seem okay with you?" Mrs. Cohen responds, "Well, Meg helps me a lot, but with this stroke, I know we can use your help." Kylie says, "Good. Let me start by asking you a few questions. Tell me what you most want us to help you with." Mrs. Cohen responds, "The doctor put me on several new medicines. If my kids can't be here, I need to know how to take them right. I want to get my strength back in my arm and leg so I can walk." Kylie states, "Helping with your medicines and getting you to walk again. That is a good plan. Now tell me, have you fallen at home anytime in the last 12 months before your stroke?" Mrs. Cohen says, "Ah, let me think. . . ." Meg answers, "Mom, remember you slipped in the living room and landed on your hip about 4 months ago? Fortunately you weren't hurt." Kylie asks, "Is your living room the place where you spend most of your time?" Mrs. Cohen replies, "Yes, I do." Kylie continues her fall risk assessment and examines Mrs. Cohen's strength and ability to stand (a walker was provided by the hospital physical therapy staff). Kylie knows from past experience that allowing patients to self-report their ability to walk is often misleading. Assessment needs to involve the patient actually walking. Mrs. Cohen is able to stand but has obvious weakness of the left leg, and her left hand grasp is weak. When she takes one step, Kylie notes that she drags her left foot. Mrs. Cohen can use her left arm but has difficulty moving the walker forward. Kylie explains to Mrs. Cohen, "Your safety at home is my concern. Your stroke has caused a weakness that adds to your risk of falling. I want to discuss this more, but first I would like to check your home for safety conditions. Is that okay?" Mrs. Cohen says, "Yes, please do."

Psychosocial Resources. Because numerous factors influence patient safety, a safety assessment is not comprehensive unless it includes a review of a patient's psychosocial and economic resources. If a family caregiver is involved in the care of a patient, learn that individual's knowledge and understanding of a patient's needs, willingness and physical ability to assist, and understanding of how to perform care activities. Determine if a patient has the economic resources to ensure safety; can the patient afford medications, assistive devices, or needed home repairs? If a patient has no primary family caregiver, who within the immediate community is available to assist?

As Kylie observes Mrs. Cohen, she says to Meg, "Tell me how often you are here to help your mom." Meg responds, "Well, right now I've moved into her extra bedroom until she gets more strength. PT is coming tomorrow. My brother comes over after work when he can." Kylie asks, "Do you agree with your mom that managing her medicines and helping her to walk are her main needs?" Meg responds, "Yes, I think so. I worry about her when she'll have to be alone again." Kylie asks, "Do you believe that it is unsafe for her?" Meg answers, "Well, I know she wants to be at home. The doctors wanted her to go to rehab, but she insisted on coming home."

◆ Analysis and Nursing Diagnosis

Apply critical thinking as you gather assessment data, recognize any cues among assessment findings, and begin to identify patterns in the data. Your analysis of any data patterns, including risk factors, will allow you to make the clinical judgment needed for identifying relevant nursing diagnoses (Box 27.5). In addition to the accurate clustering of assessment data, an important part of formulating nursing diagnoses is identifying the relevant related factor (when a diagnosis is *negative* or problem focused) or risk factors (when a diagnosis is a risk diagnosis). You choose interventions that treat or modify the related factor *or* risk for the diagnosis to be resolved. For example, the

FIG. 27.2 American Geriatrics Society/British Geriatrics Society Clinical Practice Guideline Fall Prevention Algorithm, 2011. (From American Geriatrics Society (AGS)/British Geriatrics Society (BGS): Summary of the updated American Geriatrics Society/British Geriatrics Society Clinical Practice Guideline for Prevention of Falls in Older Persons, Panel on Prevention of Falls in Older Persons, American Geriatrics Society and British Geriatrics Society, *J Am Geriatr Soc* 2011. https://geriatricscareonline.org/ProductAbstract/updated-american-geriatrics-societybritish-geriatrics-society-clinical-practice-guideline-for-prevention-of-falls-in-older-persons-and-recommendations/CL014. Accessed June 22, 2021.)

nursing diagnosis of *Risk for Fall* might be associated with altered mobility or a visual alteration as a risk factor. Altered mobility will lead you to select such nursing interventions as range-of-motion (ROM) exercises; more frequent supervised ambulation; or teaching the proper use of safety devices such as side rails, canes, or crutches. If visual impairment is the risk factor, select different interventions, such as keeping the living area well lit; orienting the patient to the surroundings; or keeping eyeglasses clean, close to the patient, and well protected. When you do not identify the correct risk factors for the diagnosis *Risk for Fall*, using inappropriate interventions or omitting proper interventions may increase a patient's risk for falling. Examples of additional nursing diagnoses for patients with safety risk include the following:

- Risk for Injury
- Impaired Cognition: Confusion
- Lack of Knowledge
- Risk for Poisoning

Kylie analyzes her assessment findings so far. She knows that she will continue her assessment during her next home visit. Currently she recognizes a pattern with Mrs. Cohen's age, history of previous fall, reduced strength and impaired balance, and environmental hazards as risks for the diagnosis of **Risk for Fall.** *The patient's weakness of left leg, reduced ability to move her walker forward, weakened hand grip, and dragging her foot are assessment findings for* **Impaired Mobility.** *Kylie plans to assess more fully the ability of Mrs. Cohen to remain in her home alone safely. She will collaborate with the physical therapist on this assessment. For now, she sees the patient's interest in learning and being able to regain strength, and her cognitive clarity in being able to ask questions, as a pattern of findings for* **Health Seeking Behaviour.**

BOX 27.5   Nursing Diagnostic Process

Risk for Fall

Assessment Activities	Assessment Findings
Observe patient's posture, range of motion, gait, strength, balance, and body alignment.	Decrease in left lower extremity strength; drags left foot, left hand grasp weak while holding walker, demonstrates unsteady gait, impaired balance when standing
Assess patient's visual acuity—ability to read, identify distant objects.	Reports difficulty seeing at night Vision blurred, unable to identify near objects without glasses
Complete a home hazard appraisal.	Poorly lighted home Excessive amount of furniture in living room Rugs not secure throughout home No grab bars in bath

◆ Planning and Outcomes Identification

Critical thinking is an important tool in patient safety. Patients with actual or potential risks to safety receive patient-centered interventions that prevent and minimize the specific threats to their safety. Knowledge of a patient's existing health condition and how it poses safety risks, the severity of those risks, and the resources a patient has to minimize risks informs a nurse as to how to critically plan care for each nursing diagnosis. When health promotion is a nurse's focus, knowledge gained during assessment of a patient's beliefs and attitudes about safety will ensure that chosen interventions are patient centered. Professional standards such as Universal Fall Precautions or standards from the AGS are key components to any plan for fall prevention.

Findings from a nurse's environmental assessment are critical for planning safety strategies. The condition of a patient's home and surroundings or the observed presence of hazards within a health care setting must be considered in any plan of care. When you prepare for any procedure, consider safety principles. Ask yourself, can care tasks be safely delegated or do you require the assistance of assistive personnel to perform a procedure correctly? Time plays a role in your approach to care. For example, if a patient is on fall precautions, you must be attentive and certain that the patient's needs are responded to in a timely manner. If you delay returning to a patient in the bathroom, on a bedpan, or sitting in a chair, a patient who is independent or restless might get up alone without assistance and fall.

Design interventions to help patients feel safe to move about and interact freely within their environment. The plan of care addresses all aspects of patient needs and uses resources of the health care team and the community when appropriate. Critically synthesize information from multiple sources (Fig. 27.3). Also reflect on previous experiences in which patients benefited from safety interventions. Such experience helps you adapt approaches with each new patient. Applying critical thinking attitudes such as creativity helps you to collaborate with a patient in planning interventions that are relevant and most useful, particularly when making changes in the home environment.

Outcomes. You collaborate with a patient, family caregiver, and other members of the health care team when setting outcomes during the planning process (see the Nursing Care Plan). The patient who actively participates in reducing threats to safety becomes more alert to potential hazards and is more likely to adhere to the plan. Make sure that

FIG. 27.3 Critical thinking model for planning safety. *ANA,* American Nurses Association; *CMS,* Centers for Medicare and Medicaid Services. (Clinical Judgment Measurement Model copyright © NCSBN. All rights reserved.)

◎ NURSING CARE PLAN

Risk for Fall

ASSESSMENT

Assessment Activities	Assessment Findings[a]
Conduct a home hazard assessment.	Kitchen table is cluttered with unopened mail and papers. **Throw rugs are on floors**; bathroom and bedroom **lighting are poor** (40-watt bulbs); bathtub **lacks grab bars.**
Observe gait and posture.	Patient able to bear weight on right (dominant) leg. **Leans forward when holding walker. Moves left leg slowly, drags left foot, weak left hand grasp.**
Assess medications prescribed.	Patient is taking an **antihypertensive, diuretic**, calcium and vitamin D, and thyroid medication.

[a]Assessment findings are shown in bold type.

NURSING DIAGNOSIS: Risk for Fall

PLANNING

Expected Outcomes (NOC)[b]

Knowledge: Personal Safety

Patient and daughter will identify personal and environmental risks for falls in 1 week.

Patient and daughter will select prevention methods to avoid falls in home at conclusion of teaching session (2 weeks).

Fall Prevention Behavior

Patient will not fall in 1 month.

[b]Outcome classification labels from Moorhead S et al: *Nursing outcomes classification (NOC)*, ed 6, St Louis, 2018, Elsevier.

INTERVENTIONS (NIC)[c]	RATIONALE
Fall Prevention	
Review findings from a home hazard assessment with patient and her daughter, and collaborate with an occupational therapist on proposed changes: removal of throw rugs, placement of grab bars in bathroom; increased lighting intensity in rooms (75 watt).	Home hazard assessment highlights extrinsic factors that lead to falls and that can be changed. Home modifications, when delivered by occupational therapists, can reduce falls among high-risk community-dwelling older adults (Stark et al., 2017).
Discuss with patient and daughter the normal changes of aging, specific effects of recent stroke and associated risks for injury, and how to reduce risks.	Education regarding hazards reduces fear of falling (Olsen and Bergland, 2014).
Collaborate with physical therapist to begin appropriate exercises for strengthening upper and lower extremities. Follow physical therapy guidelines for use of walker.	Safe use of assistive device reduces fall risk. Health care providers must emphasize importance of walker use for injury prevention through patient education to promote personal relevance, proper fitting, and training (Luz et al., 2017).
Consult with physical therapist and occupational therapist to assess need for endurance training and use of assistive devices for kyphosis, left-sided weakness, and gait.	A multicomponent exercise intervention composed of strength, endurance, and balance training has been shown to be the best strategy to improve rate of falls, gait ability, balance, and strength performance in physically frail older adults (Cadore et al., 2013).

[c]Intervention classification labels from Butcher HK, et al: *Nursing interventions classification (NIC)*, ed 7, St Louis, 2018, Elsevier.

EVALUATION

Evaluation Activities	Patient Response
Ask patient and daughter to identify fall risks and the plan for changes in home.	Patient identifies previous fall and left-sided weakness as fall risks. Patient identified the piles of magazines and mail cluttered in family room and throw rugs on floors as safety hazards. Daughter identified bathroom hazards, including bathroom lighting and lack of grab bars.
Ask patient and daughter to identify fall prevention strategies planned for home	Patient and daughter agree to remove throw rugs in rooms. Son states he will help install lighting and grab bars.
Reassess if patient has experienced a fall in the last month.	Patient has not experienced a fall.

outcomes for each nursing diagnosis are measurable and realistic, with consideration of the resources available to the patient. Focus outcomes on removing risks or managing the related factors contributing to a nursing diagnosis. Examples include:

- Patient remains injury free at 1 month.
- Patient adopts safety precautions at work in 1 week.
- Patient removes environmental barriers in the home in 1 month.

Kylie sets the outcome of "Patient will not fall in 1 month" for the diagnosis **Risk for Fall.** *Kylie hopes to extend the time parameter for the outcome, but she knows Mrs. Cohen has a high risk for falls as she recovers from the CVA. Fall prevention will be a priority in the initial weeks. The outcome for* **Impaired Mobility,** *"Patient will ambulate correctly with walker in 2 weeks," is ambitious for Mrs. Cohen. The patient has obvious weakness on her left side, but Kylie plans to collaborate with the physical therapist, the patient, and Mrs. Cohen's children to plan rehab strategies for strengthening Mrs. Cohen's walking ability. As for the diagnosis of* **Health Seeking Behavior,** *Kylie sets the outcome of "Patient will identify personal fall risks in 1 week." Kylie intends to make fall prevention the patient's first priority because during these next few weeks, with the patient's instability following a stroke, safe mobility is key. She plans to*

CONCEPT MAP

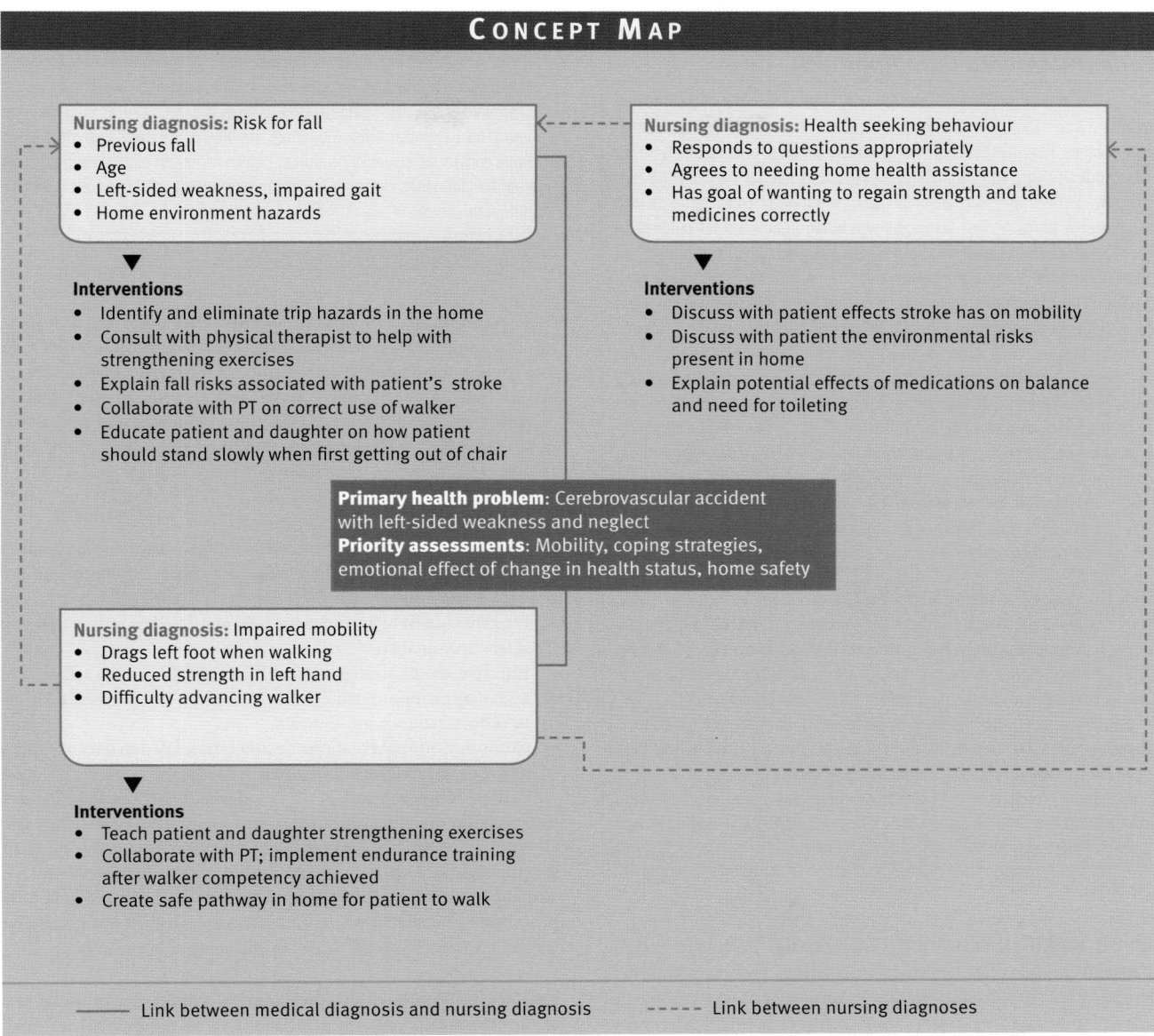

Nursing diagnosis: Risk for fall
- Previous fall
- Age
- Left-sided weakness, impaired gait
- Home environment hazards

Interventions
- Identify and eliminate trip hazards in the home
- Consult with physical therapist to help with strengthening exercises
- Explain fall risks associated with patient's stroke
- Collaborate with PT on correct use of walker
- Educate patient and daughter on how patient should stand slowly when first getting out of chair

Nursing diagnosis: Health seeking behaviour
- Responds to questions appropriately
- Agrees to needing home health assistance
- Has goal of wanting to regain strength and take medicines correctly

Interventions
- Discuss with patient effects stroke has on mobility
- Discuss with patient the environmental risks present in home
- Explain potential effects of medications on balance and need for toileting

Primary health problem: Cerebrovascular accident with left-sided weakness and neglect
Priority assessments: Mobility, coping strategies, emotional effect of change in health status, home safety

Nursing diagnosis: Impaired mobility
- Drags left foot when walking
- Reduced strength in left hand
- Difficulty advancing walker

Interventions
- Teach patient and daughter strengthening exercises
- Collaborate with PT; implement endurance training after walker competency achieved
- Create safe pathway in home for patient to walk

——— Link between medical diagnosis and nursing diagnosis   ----- Link between nursing diagnoses

FIG. 27.4 Concept map for Ms. Cohen. *PT,* Physical therapist.

center patient education on fall prevention initially. Then she will transition and begin to spend time with medication adherence, because the patient is anxious to learn.

Setting Priorities. During assessment a nurse learns a great deal about a patient. Once nursing diagnoses have been established, the nurse uses clinical judgment and applies knowledge about the patient to prioritize diagnoses and the interventions chosen for the plan of care. Fig. 27.4 shows a concept map for Mrs. Cohen. The map demonstrates the interrelationship of all nursing diagnoses. Diagnoses pertaining to patient safety are often the main priority for patients. However, when caring for patients who do not understand safety risks or who are reluctant to engage and participate in their own safety, other priorities may arise. For example, if a patient does not understand why a neurological condition poses risks to safety, targeted education about risks pertaining to gait, balance, or coordination disturbances might be needed.

Select priorities based on the severity or immediacy of risk, the patient's developmental stage, level of health, lifestyle preferences, and cultural needs (Box 27.6). Planning involves an understanding of a patient's need to maintain independence within physical and cognitive capabilities. Build consensus with the patient and family (when appropriate) as to the type of interventions to deliver (QSEN, 2020). Collaborate to establish ways to maintain or encourage the patient's active involvement within the home and health care environment. Patient and family caregiver education is also an important intervention to plan for reducing safety risks over the long term.

REFLECT NOW

Consider a patient you cared for recently. How did you prioritize meeting the patient's safety needs?

BOX 27.6 CULTURAL ASPECTS OF CARE

A Patient-Centered Care Approach

Hospitalization places patients at risk for injury in an unfamiliar and confusing environment. The experience is usually at least minimally frightening. Normal life cues such as a bed without side rails and the direction one usually takes to the bathroom are absent. Thought processes and coping mechanisms are affected by illness and its accompanying emotions. Thus patients are more vulnerable to injury. This vulnerability is often intensified for patients of diverse backgrounds. It is a nurse's responsibility to diligently protect all patients, regardless of their socioeconomic status and cultural background. Most adverse events are related to failures of communication. Be sensitive and aware of patients who have low health literacy as you perform assessments and attempt to implement safe care measures. Screen all patients for health literacy. Ensure that you use an approach that recognizes a patient's cultural background so that you ask appropriate questions to reveal health behaviors and risks. Be aware of cultural beliefs about physical restraints when caring for patients who need them. A physical restraint can be seen as a significant threat by anyone who comes from a culture of violence. Patient safety is enhanced when you consider the whole person and value seeing each care situation through "the patient's eyes" and not just through your own perspective. Some specific patient-centered safety guidelines about the use of restraints follow.

Implications for Patient-Centered Care

- When restraints are needed, assess their meaning to the patient and the family. Some cultures may find restraints to be disrespectful. Similarly, some survivors of war or persecution or those with posttraumatic stress disorder may view restraints as imprisonment or punishment.
- Collaborate with family members in accommodating a patient's cultural perspectives about restraints. Removing the restraints when family members are present shows respect and caring for the patient.
- Know agency protocols when you identify potential areas for negotiation with the patient's/family's preferences for using restraints, including having family members stay with the patient.

Teamwork and Collaboration. Collaboration with the patient, family caregiver, and other health care providers, such as social work and occupational and physical therapy, becomes an important part of a patient's plan of care. For example, a patient in a hospital often needs to go to an inpatient rehabilitation center to gain strength and endurance before being discharged home. Or, nurses will work with physical therapists who make home visits to deliver therapies. An occupational therapist is helpful in the home setting for making recommendations for installation of stairway railings, slip-resistant surfacing in the bathroom, or use of assistive aids for activities of daily living (ADLs) (Stark et al., 2017). Communication with all participants in the plan of care is essential.

You communicate risk factors and the plan of care with the patient, family caregiver, and other health care providers, including other disciplines and nurses on other shifts. Be sure assistive personnel (AP) are familiar with any risk factors that may affect how they provide care. Permanent dry-erase boards in a hospital or long-term care setting are often installed in patient rooms. Use these boards to communicate pertinent patient information such as fall risks, activity level, level of assistance needed with activity, and any fall prevention interventions (when relevant) to all health care providers. A standard approach to communication such as ISBAR or SBAR ([Introduction], Situation, Background, Assessment, Recommendation, Request, or Readback) helps you obtain and organize information about patients when problems develop (see Chapter 24).

Patients need to be able to identify, select, and know how to use resources within their communities (e.g., neighborhood block homes, local police departments, and neighbors willing to check on their well-being) that enhance safety. Make sure that the patient and family caregiver understand the need for these resources and how to contact these resources, and determine whether they are willing to make changes that promote their safety.

◆ Implementation

QSEN (2020) outlines recommended skills to ensure nurse competency in patient safety. Among these skills are those involving safe nursing practice during direct care:

- Effective use of technology and standardized practices that support safety and quality.
- Effective use of strategies to reduce risk of harm to self or others.
- Use of appropriate strategies (e.g., forcing functions and checklists) to reduce reliance on memory.
- Communicate observations or concerns related to hazards and errors to patients, families, and the health care team.

Critical thinking and clinical judgment go hand in hand when directing nursing interventions toward maintaining a patient's safety in all types of health care settings. Reflect on your knowledge of a patient's specific risks and always anticipate and look for environmental hazards and approaches for avoiding those hazards. You will implement health promotion and illness prevention measures in the community setting, whereas prevention is a priority in the acute care setting.

Health Promotion. Health promotion requires a person to be in a safe environment and practice a lifestyle that minimizes risk of injury. A nurse's choice of interventions will depend in part on knowledge gathered about the patient's cultural values about health and a safe environment. There are passive and active strategies aimed at health promotion. Passive strategies include public health measures (e.g., public education about disease outbreaks and neighborhood safety, issuing travel restrictions and screening travelers) and governmental legislative interventions (e.g., sanitation and clean water laws) (see Chapter 3). Active strategies are those in which an individual is actively involved through changes in lifestyle (e.g., engaging in better nutritional health or exercise programs, wearing seat belts) and participation in wellness programs.

Nurses can promote individual and community health by supporting legislation, acting as positive role models, and working in community-based settings. Being culturally competent within a community setting arises from established trust with community members. Environmental conditions and community practices influence whether a person can focus on healthy behaviors. Therefore community and home health nurses must assess and recommend safety measures that fit patients' homes, schools, neighborhood settings, and workplaces.

Developmental Interventions

Infant, Toddler, and Preschooler. Growing, curious children need adults to protect them from injury. Nurses play a key role in educating parents about reducing risks of disease and injuries to children, and teaching ways to promote safety in the home (Table 27.2). Evidence-based interventions that are effective for improving childhood immunization rates include reminder/recall systems (postcard, letter, telephone, or combination) and outreach, case management, home visits, and in-home vaccinations for hard-to-reach populations (Frew and Lutz, 2017). The AAP (2021b) recommends these additional steps for vaccine-hesitant parents:

- Listen to parents' concerns and acknowledge them in a nonconfrontational manner. This increases their willingness to listen to a health care provider's views.

- Partner with parents in decision making. Make sure the parent understands the information about vaccines. Clarify and reaffirm parents' correct beliefs and modify misconceptions.
- Discuss the benefits of vaccines and the possibility of adverse events. Be open about what is known about immunizations and what is not known.
- Stress the number of lives saved by immunization, as a positive approach.

Nurses working in prenatal and postpartum settings routinely incorporate safety into the care plans of childbearing families. Community health nurses assess the home and show parents how to promote safety.

TABLE 27.2 Interventions to Promote Safety for Children and Adolescents

Intervention	Rationale
Infants and Toddlers	
Keep soft objects, toys, crib bumpers, and loose bedding out of an infant's sleep area. Make sure nothing covers the baby's head.	Reduces risk of sudden infant death syndrome. Possibility exists for these items to cause risk of suffocation, strangulation, or entrapment.
Use a firm sleep surface, such as a mattress in a safety-approved crib covered by a fitted sheet.	Reduces suffocation.
Prepare an infant's sleep area next to where parents sleep. An infant should not sleep in an adult bed, on a couch, or on a chair alone or with a parent or anyone else.	Provides a safe sleep area.
Infants should be immunized and have regular health checkups.	Evidence suggests that immunization reduces the risk of SIDS and other preventable diseases.
Do not attach pacifiers to string or ribbon and place around a child's neck.	Items increase risk for choking.
Follow all instructions for preparing and storing formula.	Proper formula preparation and storage prevent contamination. Follow product directions for proper concentration of formula. Undiluted formula causes fluid and electrolyte disturbances; much-diluted formula does not provide sufficient nutrients.
Use large, soft toys without small parts such as buttons.	Small parts become dislodged, and choking and aspiration can occur.
Do not leave the mesh sides of playpens lowered; spaces between crib slats need to be less than 6 cm (2⅜ inches) apart.	Possibility exists for a child's head to become wedged in the lowered mesh side or between crib slats, and asphyxiation may occur.
Never leave crib sides down or infants unattended on changing tables or in infant seats, swings, strollers, or high chairs.	Infants and toddlers roll or move and fall from changing tables or out of accessories such as infant seats or swings.
Do not use infant seats and swings when the child becomes too active or physically too big. In addition, only use seats and swings according to the manufacturer's directions.	When physically active or too big, the child can fall out of or tip over these accessories and sustain an injury.
Never leave a child alone in the bathroom, tub, or near any water source (e.g., pool).	Supervision reduces risk for accidental drowning.
Baby-proof a home; remove small or sharp objects and toxic or poisonous substances, including plants; install safety locks on floor-level cabinets.	Infants explore their world with their hands and mouth. Choking and poisoning can occur.
Remove plastic bags from the cleaners or grocery store from the home.	Removal reduces risk for suffocation from plastic bags.
Cover electrical outlets.	Reduces opportunity for crawling infants to insert objects into outlets and experience an electrical shock.
Install keyless locks (e.g., deadbolts) on doors above a child's reach, even when they are standing on a chair.	Deadbolts prevent a toddler from leaving the house and wandering off. Keyless locks allow for rapid exit in case of fire.
Caregivers need to learn cardiopulmonary resuscitation (CPR) and the Heimlich maneuver.	Ensures preparation for acute emergencies such as choking.
Preschoolers	
Teach children to swim at an early age, but always provide supervision near water.	Swimming is a useful skill that can save a child's life. However, all children need constant supervision.
Teach children how to cross streets and walk in parking lots. Instruct them to never run out after a ball or toy.	Pedestrian accidents involving young children are common.
Teach children not to talk to, go with, or accept any item from a stranger.	Avoiding strangers reduces the risk of injury and stranger abduction.
Teach children basic physical safety rules: proper use of safety scissors, never running with an object in their mouth or hand, and never attempting to use the stove or oven unassisted.	Risk of injury is lower if children know basic safety procedures.

Continued

TABLE 27.2 Interventions to Promote Safety for Children and Adolescents—cont'd

Intervention	Rationale
Preschoolers—cont'd	
Teach children not to eat items found in the street or grass (e.g., mushroom, weeds).	Avoids risk for possible poisoning.
Remove doors from unused refrigerators and freezers. Instruct children not to play or hide in a car trunk or unused appliances.	If a child cannot freely exit from appliances and car trunks, asphyxiation can occur.
School-Age Children	
Teach children proper bicycle and skateboard safety, including use of helmet and rules of the road.	Reduces injuries from falling off a bike or skateboard or being hit by a car.
Teach children proper techniques for specific sports and the need to wear proper safety gear.	Using proper techniques can prevent injuries.
Teach children not to operate electrical equipment while unsupervised.	If an electrical mishap were to occur, no one would be available to help.
Do not allow children access to firearms or other weapons. Keep all firearms in locked cabinets.	Children are often fascinated by firearms and often try to play with them.
Adolescents	
Encourage enrollment in driver education classes.	Many injuries in this age-group are related to motor vehicle accidents.
Provide information about the effects of smoking and using alcohol and drugs.	Adolescents are highly prone to risk-taking behaviors and peer pressure.
Refer adolescents to community- and school-sponsored activities.	The adolescent needs to socialize with peers, yet needs some supervision.
Encourage mentoring relationships between adults and adolescents.	Adolescents are in need of role models after whom they can pattern their behavior.
Teach them safe use of the Internet.	Avoids overuse and possible exposure to inappropriate websites.

Modified from Hockenberry M, Wilson D: *Wong's nursing care of infants and children*, ed 11, St Louis, 2019, Elsevier.

School-Age Child. School-age children increasingly explore their environment (see Chapter 12). They have friends outside their immediate neighborhood, and they become more active in school, church, and community activities. The school-age child needs specific teaching regarding safety in school and at play. See Table 27.2 for nursing interventions to help guide parents in providing for the safety of school-age children.

Adolescent. Risks to the safety of adolescents involve many factors outside the home because much of their time is spent away from home and with their peer group (see Chapter 12). Adults who serve as positive role models for adolescents provide examples of how to behave, set expectations, and provide education to minimize risks to the adolescent's safety. Because of peer pressure this age-group is at risk for alcohol and drug use. In addition, this age-group has a high incidence of suicide. Be aware of the risks posed at this time and be prepared to teach adolescents and their parents the measures needed to prevent accidents and injury. You can also help parents be aware of ways to minimize risk of adolescent suicide, including the promotion of good problem-solving abilities (e.g., conflict with peers); support for strong connections to their families, friends, and people in the community; restricted access to highly lethal means of suicide; and demonstration of cultural and religious beliefs that discourage suicide and that support self-preservation (Kaslow, 2021).

Adult. Risks to young and middle-age adults frequently result from lifestyle factors such as childrearing, high stress levels, inadequate nutrition, use of firearms, excessive alcohol intake, and substance abuse (see Chapter 13). In this fast-paced society there also appears to be more expression of anger, which can quickly precipitate accidents related to "road rage." Help adults understand their safety risks and guide them in making lifestyle modifications by referring them to resources such as classes to help quit smoking or for stress management, including employee-assistance programs. Also encourage adults to exercise regularly, maintain a healthy diet, practice relaxation techniques, and get adequate sleep (see Chapter 43).

Older Adult. Nursing interventions for older adults reduce patients' risk for falls and other accidents and compensate for the physiological changes of aging (Box 27.7). The AGS (2011) developed an algorithm for fall prevention (see Fig. 27.2). Use this resource to reduce risks in the home. Provide information about neighborhood resources to help an older adult maintain an independent lifestyle. Older adults frequently relocate to new neighborhoods and need to become acquainted with new resources, such as modes of transportation, church schedules, and food resources (e.g., Meals on Wheels).

Educate older adults about safe driving tips (e.g., driving shorter distances, using side and rearview mirrors carefully, and looking behind them toward their "blind spot" before changing lanes). If hearing is a problem, encourage the patient to keep a window rolled down while driving or to reduce the volume of the radio. Counseling is often necessary to help older patients decide when to stop driving. At that time help locate resources in the community that provide transportation.

Burns and scalds are also more apt to occur with older people because they sometimes forget and leave hot water running or become confused when turning the dials on a stove or other heating appliance. Nursing measures for preventing burns minimize the risk from impaired vision. Hot-water faucets and dials are color coded to make it easier for an adult to know which is hot and which is cold. Reducing the temperature of the hot water heater is also very beneficial.

Many older adults love to walk. Reduce pedestrian accidents for older adults and all other age-groups by persuading people to wear reflectors on garments when walking at night; to stand on the sidewalk and not in the street when waiting to cross a street; to always cross at corners and not in the middle of the block (particularly if the street is a major one); to cross with the traffic light and not against it; and to look left, right, and left again before entering the street or crosswalk. Also encourage people to assess their walking route for hazards such as unequal or damaged walkways, unrestrained dogs, and excessive toys; all of these increase the risk for falls.

Environmental Interventions. A thorough patient assessment reveals the environmental threats existing in a patient's home and whether a patient has inherent risks to be prone to injury. Applying this information

BOX 27.7 FOCUS ON OLDER ADULTS

Physiological Changes of Aging and Their Effect on Patient Safety

Physiological changes accompany aging. Older adults experience visual and hearing alterations, slowed reaction time, and decreased range of motion, flexibility, and strength. Reflexes are slowed in addition to the ability to respond to multiple stimuli. Memory can become impaired, and nocturia and incontinence are more frequent in older adults. The family plays a significant role in the care of older adults. There are an estimated 53 million family caregivers in the United States, approximately 19% of the U.S. adult population (National Alliance for Caregiving, 2021). In addition, 24% of family caregivers care for more than one person. Educate family members on how to best support the older adult.

The high prevalence of chronic conditions in older adults results in the use of a high number of prescription and over-the-counter medications. Coupled with age-related changes in pharmacokinetics, there is a greater risk of serious adverse effects. Medications typically prescribed for older adults include anticholinergics, diuretics, anxiolytic and hypnotic agents, antidepressants, antihypertensives, vasodilators, analgesics, and laxatives, all of which pose risks or interact to increase the risk for falls.

Implications for Practice

- Encourage family caregivers to allow older adults to remain as independent as possible.
- Offer family caregivers resources from the Centers for Disease Control and Prevention (CDC) on the STEADI (Stopping Elderly Accidents, Deaths, and Injuries) fall prevention program (CDC, 2021a), available at https://www.cdc.gov/steadi/index.html.
- Encourage annual vision and hearing examinations and frequent cleaning of glasses and hearing aids as a means of preventing falls and burns.
- Teach safety tips for avoiding automobile accidents. Sometimes driving needs to be restricted to daylight hours or temporarily or permanently suspended.
- Encourage supervised strengthening and balance exercise classes targeted for older adults.
- Install safety features in the home such as grab bars and smoke alarms.
- Be sure that adults know how to use assistive devices (e.g., walkers and canes) correctly. Consult with a physical therapy staff member.
- Consult with an occupational therapist to help patients make adaptations needed to feed, bathe, and toilet independently.
- Institute a regular toileting schedule for a patient. A recommended frequency is every 2 or 3 hours. Give diuretics in the morning. Provide assistance, along with adequate lighting, to patients who need to go to the bathroom at night.
- Encourage patients to use medication organizers, which can be purchased at any drugstore at a very reasonable cost. Fill these dispensers once a week with the proper medications to be taken at a specific time during the day.
- Review a patient's drug profile to ensure that these drugs are used cautiously, and assess the patient regularly for any adverse effects that increase fall risk.

results in nursing interventions directed at eliminating environmental threats associated with a person's basic needs and general preventive measures.

Basic Needs. When administering oxygen, take appropriate precautions to prevent fire. In home settings, post "No Smoking" and "Oxygen in Use" signs. Do not use oxygen around electrical equipment or flammable products. Store oxygen tanks upright in carts or stands to prevent tipping or falling over. Chapter 41 outlines guidelines for proper oxygen administration. In the home setting a home medical provider and home health nurse educate patients who require oxygen about safe oxygen use.

Fire safety in the home requires education of patients and families about the importance of purchasing modern space heaters that include safety features, placing smoke detectors and CO detectors strategically throughout the home, and keeping multipurpose fire extinguishers in close proximity to the kitchen and workshop areas. Recommend that patients have annual inspections of heating systems, chimneys, and fuel-burning appliances. CO detectors are not expensive but are not a replacement for proper use and maintenance of fuel-burning appliances. Space heaters are a fire risk. Instruct patients on proper use in the home (Electrical Safety Foundation International, 2015):

- Be sure a space heater has a label showing that it is listed by a recognized testing laboratory.
- Before using any space heater, read the manufacturer's instructions carefully.
- Inspect heaters for cracked or broken plugs or loose connections before each use. If frayed, worn, or damaged, do not use the heater.
- Never leave a space heater unattended. Turn it off when you're leaving a room or going to sleep, and do not let pets or children play too close to a space heater.
- *Do not* use space heaters to warm bedding, cook food, dry clothing, or thaw pipes.
- Install smoke alarms on every floor of your home and outside all sleeping areas.
- Place space heaters correctly; keep at least 3 feet away from anything that can burn, including papers, clothing, and rugs.
- Plug space heaters directly into a wall outlet. Do not use an extension cord or power strip, which could overheat and result in a fire.

Food safety requires a patient and family to understand the principles of food preparation and storage. Patients should follow four basic food safety tips (CDC, 2020b):

1. Wash hands and food preparation and cooking surfaces often. This includes washing cooking utensils and cutting boards thoroughly.
2. Do not cross-contaminate food while preparing or while stored in a refrigerator. Keep raw meat, poultry, seafood, and their juices away from other foods. Use separate cutting boards. Rinse fruits and vegetables thoroughly.
3. Cook food to the proper temperature. Refrigerate leftovers promptly.
4. Be sure a patient living at home has a functioning refrigerator with a freezer compartment to keep perishable foods fresh. Keep a refrigerator below 40°F, and know when to throw leftovers or opened containers of food away.

Fall Safety in the Home. Modifications in the home environment easily reduce the risk of falls. Collaborate with patients and family caregivers to make changes based on their home fall risk assessment and the patient's risk factors. For example, remove all obstacles (e.g., furniture, piles of magazines or boxes) from halls and other heavily traveled areas. Be sure that end tables are secure and have stable, straight legs. Place nonessential items in drawers to eliminate clutter. Patients who have problems stumbling or tripping should never have small area rugs in the home. If small area rugs are used, secure them with a nonslip pad or skid-resistant adhesive strips. Make sure that carpeting on the stairs is secured with carpet tacks. If patients have a history of falling and live alone, recommend that they wear an electronic safety alert device. When activated by the wearer, this device alerts a monitoring site to call emergency services for assistance.

Observe patients using assistive devices (e.g., canes, walkers) in the home to ensure the devices are held and used correctly. Inform patients about how to keep these devices in safe working order.

General Preventive Measures. Neighborhood safety is important. Often patients are not aware of basic safety tips. Proper lighting and locks on windows and doors help reduce the risk of injury from crime. The local police department and community organizations often have

BOX 27.8 PATIENT TEACHING
Prevention of Electrical Hazards

Objective
- Patient will recognize and eliminate electrical hazards in the home.

Teaching Strategies
- Discuss how to check for grounding of electrical appliances and other equipment.
- Provide examples of common hazards: frayed cords, damaged equipment, and overloaded outlets.
- Discuss guidelines to prevent electrical shocks:
  - Use extension cords only when necessary and use electrical tape to secure the cord to the floor, preferably against baseboards.
  - Do not run wires under carpeting.
  - Grasp the plug, not the cord, when unplugging items.
  - Keep electrical items away from water.
  - Do not operate unfamiliar equipment.
  - Disconnect items before cleaning.

Evaluation
Use the principles of teach-back to evaluate patient/family caregiver learning:
- I want to be sure I explained the fire hazards that I found in your home clearly. What electrical hazards exist in your home right now, and what steps can you take to eliminate them?
- What can you do in your home to prevent getting an electrical shock?

BOX 27.9 PATIENT TEACHING
Correct Use of a Fire Extinguisher in the Home

Objective
- Patient will use a fire extinguisher in the home correctly.

Teaching Strategies
- Discuss how to choose a correct location for an extinguisher: Place on each level of the home, near an exit, in clear view, away from stoves and heating appliances, and above the reach of small children.
- Keep a fire extinguisher in the kitchen, near the furnace, and in the garage.
- Make sure that patients read instructions after purchasing the extinguisher and that they know how often to review the instructions.
- Describe considerations to make before using a fire extinguisher. Attempt to fight the fire only when all occupants have left the home, the fire department has been called, the fire is confined to a small area, there is an exit route readily available, the extinguisher is the right type for the fire, and the patient knows how to use it.
- Instruct the patient to memorize the mnemonic *PASS*:
  - **P**ull the pin to unlock handle.
  - **A**im low at the base of the fire.
  - **S**queeze the handles.
  - **S**weep the unit from side to side (see Fig. 27.6C).

Evaluation
Use the principles of teach-back to evaluate patient/family caregiver learning:
- When would it be appropriate to use a fire extinguisher at home?
- Explain for me what the mnemonic *PASS* means.

---

safety classes available for residents to learn how to take precautions to minimize the chance of becoming involved in a crime. For example, some useful tips include always parking the car near a bright light or busy public area, carrying a whistle attached to the car keys, keeping car doors locked while driving, and always paying attention while driving to notice if anyone starts to follow the car.

Accidental home fires typically result from smoking in bed, placing cigarettes in trash cans, grease fires, improper use of candles or space heaters, or electrical fires resulting from faulty wiring or appliances. Teach patients and families how to reduce the risk of electrical injury in the home (Box 27.8) and how to use a home fire extinguisher (Box 27.9). To reduce the risk of fires in the home, counsel patients to quit smoking or to smoke outside the home. Have them inspect the condition of cooking equipment and appliances, particularly irons and stoves. Have patients with visual deficits install dials with large numbers or symbols on temperature controls. Make sure that smoke detectors are in strategic positions throughout the home so that the alarm will alert the occupants in a home in case of fire. All patients, even young children, need to know the phrase "stop, drop, and roll," which describes what to do when a person's clothing or skin is burning.

Help parents reduce the risk of accidental poisoning by teaching them to keep hazardous substances such as medications, cleaning fluids, and batteries out of the reach of children. Drug and other substance poisonings in adolescents and adults are commonly related to suicide attempts or drug experimentation. Teach parents that calling a poison control center for information before attempting home remedies will save their child's life. Guidelines for accepted interventions for accidental poisonings are available to teach a parent or guardian (Box 27.10). Older adults are also at risk for poisoning because diminished eyesight may cause an accidental ingestion of a toxic substance. In addition, the impaired memory of some older adults results in an accidental overdose of prescription medications. In health care settings it is important for you to know how to respond when exposure to a poisonous

substance occurs. In addition, adhere to guidelines for intervening in accidental poisoning.

Be sure that a patient's home medications are kept in their original containers and labeled in large print. Recommend the use of medication organizers that are filled once a week by the patient and/or family caregiver. Have patients keep poisonous substances out of the bathroom and discard old or unused medications appropriately.

To prevent the transmission of pathogens, nurses teach aseptic practices. Medical asepsis, which includes hand hygiene and environmental cleanliness, reduces the transfer of organisms (see Chapter 28). Patients and family members need to learn how to perform thorough hand hygiene (handwashing or use of a hand rub) and when to use it (i.e., before and after caring for a family member, before food preparation, before preparing a medication for a family member, after using the bathroom, and after contacting any bodily fluids). Patients also need to know how to dispose of infectious material such as wound dressings and used needles in the home setting. Heavy plastic containers such as hard, colored plastic liquid detergent bottles are excellent for needle disposal. The FDA (2018) recommends a two-step process:
- Place all needles and other sharps (e.g., lancets) in a sharps container immediately after use.
- Dispose of used sharps disposal containers according to community guidelines, including drop box or supervised collection sites, household hazardous waste collection sites, mail-back programs, or residential special waste pickup services.

Acute and Restorative Care. Safety is a priority within hospital and long-term care settings. Nurses implement various measures including fall prevention strategies, prevention of injuries from use of restraints and side rails, and precautions to prevent procedure-related accidents, fires, and exposure to poisoning and electrical hazards. Special precautions are

BOX 27.10 Intervening in Accidental Poisoning

If the individual collapses, has a seizure, has trouble breathing, or cannot be awakened: Call 9-1-1 *immediately* (National Capital Poison Center, n.d.). Initiate CPR if indicated until emergency personnel arrive. If patient has normal breathing, position the victim with head turned to the side to reduce risk for aspiration.

The National Capital Poison Center (n.d.) reports that there are first aid measures that make a difference if accomplished within seconds to minutes of the poison exposure.

- Have the person drink a small amount of water or milk immediately, before getting Poison Control assistance, if:
  - The product swallowed is burning, irritating or caustic, AND
  - The person is conscious, not having convulsions, and able to swallow
- If the person is conscious and alert, go online at https://www.poison.org/ or call the national toll-free poison control center number (1-800-222-1222) before trying any intervention. Post this number in a visible area in the home. A Web-based tool, webPOISONCONTROL® online, is available to get specific recommendations for your case based on age, substance, and amount taken.
- Poison control centers have information needed to treat poisoned patients or offer referral to treat. The administration of ipecac syrup or induction of vomiting is no longer recommended for routine home treatment of poisoning.
- Check for signs or symptoms of ingestion of harmful substance, such as nausea, vomiting, foaming at the mouth, drooling, difficulty breathing, sweating, and lethargy.
- Stop exposure to the poison. Have the person empty the mouth of pills, plant parts, or other material.
- If poisoning is caused by skin or eye contact, irrigate the skin or eye with copious amounts of cool tap water for 15 to 20 minutes continuously.
- For an inhalation exposure, safely remove the victim from the potentially dangerous environment.
- Identify the type and amount of substance ingested to help determine the correct type and amount of antidote needed.
- Never induce vomiting if the victim has ingested the following poisonous substances: lye, household cleaners, hair care products, grease or petroleum products, furniture polish, paint thinner, or kerosene.

Adapted from Hockenberry MJ, Wilson D: *Wong's essentials of pediatric nursing,* ed 11, St Louis, 2019, Elsevier; American Academy of Pediatrics, Committee on Injury, Violence and Poison Prevention: Gastrointestinal decontamination of the poisoned patient, *Pediatr Emerg Care* 24(3):176, 2008.

BOX 27.11 EVIDENCE-BASED PRACTICE

Fall Prevention

PICOT Question: Does a multifactorial fall-intervention program compared with single interventions reduce the incidence of falls among hospitalized adult patients?

Evidence Summary

Falls are the most common adverse events that are reported in hospitalized older adults (Slade et al., 2017). Falls in hospitals are associated with longer length of stay and poorer patient outcomes. An individualized patient assessment and multifactorial interventions that include aerobic exercises, strength training, mobility strategies, medication management, consumer and staff education, provision of effective assistive devices, and environmental modifications have been shown to reduce falls in hospitals (Slade et al., 2017). In the community setting, falls are also a frequent occurrence. Research shows that multifactorial and individual exercise interventions are associated with fall-related benefits. However, evidence was most consistent across multiple fall-related outcomes for exercise; specifically, benefits were shown involving gait, balance, or functional training lasting approximately 12 months, with the most common frequency of three exercise sessions per week (Guirguis-Blake et al., 2018).

Application to Nursing Practice

- Promote early mobility in hospitalized patients (see Chapter 38) and collaborate with physical therapist to ensure that appropriate gait training (if needed) and assistive device are used.
- Implement Universal Fall Precautions for all acute care patients, and then tailor multi-interventions specific to patient's own fall risk factors.
- Adopt hourly "purposeful" rounding with nurses intentionally using a standard checklist of actions (e.g., checking patient need for pain management, elimination needs, current satisfaction) for each patient (HRET, 2016; Daniels, 2016; Touhy and Jett, 2022).
- Benefits have been gained from using checklists that incorporate hospital-approved fall prevention interventions. The checklist has shown promise for improving nursing staff's adherence to each intervention and on the incidence of falls. Checklists can be used during change-of-shift hand-offs to determine whether all prevention interventions are in place before accepting care of a patient (Johnston and Magnan, 2019).
- In the community setting, evidence-based exercise programs have been shown to be effective. Efficacy is clearly associated when exercise is delivered by accredited exercise instructors (Fuzhong et al., 2016). The Centers for Disease Control and Prevention (CDC) makes an evidence-based toolkit available through the Stopping Elderly Accidents, Deaths, and Injuries (STEADI) program (CDC, 2020i; Touhy and Jett, 2022).

also necessary to prevent injury in patients susceptible to having seizures. Radiation exposure injuries are also a specific safety concern in hospitals. Clinical judgment plays a role in how these measures are adopted. For example, a patient who demonstrates dementia and restless behavior receives different interventions from those that a patient who had a stroke receives. How any given intervention is performed depends on a nurse's original and ongoing assessment findings. For example, as a patient who had a stroke becomes better able to bear weight on the affected leg, the nurse will adapt the safe handling technique needed to safely ambulate the patient. In the case of a patient with dementia, basic safe handling is used along with interventions that reduce wandering.

Nurses are responsible for making a patient's bedside safe. Explain and demonstrate to patients how to use the call light or nurse call system device, and always place the device close to the patient. Respond quickly to call lights and bed/chair alarms. Keep the environment free from clutter and barriers (e.g., other furniture) around the bedside.

Fall Prevention. Patient falls continue to be a top adverse event in health care agencies, often resulting in injury and even death. Falls are

also a serious concern in skilled nursing and long-term care settings. Implementing a fall prevention plan for a patient begins with the nurse and patient partnering in recognizing the patient's fall risks. A comprehensive fall prevention approach includes a fall risk assessment of every patient, conducted routinely (see hospital policy) until a patient's discharge. Many health care agencies have implemented hourly/purposeful rounding to reduce falls (Box 27.11). It is a proactive, systematic, nurse-driven, evidence-based intervention that helps nurses anticipate and address patient needs before incidents (e.g., falls) occur. In addition, most agencies apply yellow color-coded wristbands to patients' wrists to communicate to all health care providers that a patient is at a higher risk for falling. The American Hospital Association recommends that all member hospitals standardize colors of their alert wristbands: red for allergy, yellow for fall risk, and purple for do not resuscitate

(Lalande, 2014). This single step is designed to improve communication and drastically reduce medical errors. Most hospitals have adopted this practice. However, wristbands can be difficult to discern at a distance, in low light, or when obscured, and can go unnoticed during a crisis (Wood and Bagian, 2011); therefore additional measures are needed

Patient-centered care applying critical thinking is an important component of any fall reduction plan. While partnering with patients and families, a fall reduction plan incorporates knowledge about the patient, standards of practice, and the patient's environment to individualize nursing interventions (see Skill 27.1). For example, if a patient routinely has postural hypotension, the nurse will place the bed in the low position and have the patient dangle the feet on the side of bed for 3 to 5 minutes before ambulation. A patient with a history of urinary urgency or incontinence should be provided a bedside commode instead of being expected to walk to the bathroom unassisted. Gait belts and additional safety equipment should be used as needed when moving, transferring, and ambulating patients (see Chapter 38).

When patients use assistive aids such as canes, crutches, or walkers, it is important to routinely check the condition of rubber tips and the integrity of the aid. In addition, it is important to ensure that patients use their devices correctly. Remove excess furniture and equipment and instruct patients to wear rubber-soled shoes or slippers for walking or transferring. Safety bars near toilets, locks on beds and wheelchairs (Fig. 27.5), and a nurse call system are additional safety features found in health care settings.

Another area of fall risk includes wheelchair-related falls involving older adults or patients with disabilities. Patients who use wheelchairs can experience falls, pressure injuries, and even choking if seat belts used on wheelchairs are applied too loosely, enabling a patient's torso to slide down and the belt to become a choking hazard. Transporting patients without proper application or engagement of safety features such as anti-tip bars, brakes, or side rails may lead to patient ejection, collisions, or entrapped limbs (Robson Forensic, 2016). An example of a wheelchair characteristic that increases risk for falls is having smaller and harder front wheels that cause a chair to tip when striking uneven terrain (such as an uneven floor surface moving into an elevator). Tripping over the front foot or leg rest and leaning over the back of a wheelchair to engage or disengage the wheel lock are common causes of injury. Wheelchair prescription, posture, training, and maintenance are critical components of safety education for patients who use

FIG. 27.5 Wheelchair with safety locks and anti-tip bars.

wheelchairs routinely. Transferring a patient from a bed to a wheelchair encompasses the same steps and principles used when transferring patients from a standard chair (see Chapter 38).

Kylie begins interventions by partnering with Mrs. Cohen and Meg on how to adapt the home to make it safer for Mrs. Cohen to walk with the walker. She begins by referring to Mrs. Cohen's personal plan and explaining Mrs. Cohen's fall risks. Kylie explains, "You said your plan was to be able to become stronger and walk again. To do that, we need to work together to reduce your risk for falling. Having fallen before, your age, and the effects of your stroke place you at risk. Your medicine for blood pressure can also cause you to become dizzy when you first stand." Mrs. Cohen responds, "I thought my medicine was meant to keep me from having another stroke?" Kylie responds, "It is, but it also has what we call a side effect. It may sometimes cause your blood pressure to drop when you stand up after sitting or lying down, making you dizzy. I am going to show you and Meg how to manage that." Meg states, "I guess we need to be cautious." Kylie responds, "Yes. Plus, the reduced strength in your mom's legs, her slow gait, and the fact she tends to drag her foot are all fall risk factors. But we will work with physical therapy to improve her gait and hopefully minimize or eliminate the foot drag. Now let us also go over together how we can make it safer for you, Mrs. Cohen, to walk in your home. To begin, whenever you stand from the chair or bed to begin walking, I want you to go slow, take time to just stand up straight and notice if you feel dizzy. If not, then it is safe to begin walking. This helps lessen the effects of your blood pressure medicine."

Restraints. Patients who are confused or agitated or who repeatedly try to remove medical devices (e.g., IV lines, urinary catheters, or wound dressings) may temporarily require physical restraints to keep them safe. In the nursing home environment, research has shown that restraints are used when there are increases in the degree of care dependency as well as mobility limitations (Hofmann et al., 2015). A physical restraint is any manual method, physical or mechanical device, material, or equipment that immobilizes or reduces the ability of a patient to move arms, legs, body, or head freely. A restraint does not include devices such as orthopedically prescribed devices, protective helmets, or methods that involve physically holding a patient to conduct an examination or test, protecting a patient from falling out of bed, or permitting a patient to participate in activities without risk of physical harm (TJC, 2020a; TJC, 2020b). Chemical restraints are medications such as anxiolytics and sedatives used to manage a patient's behavior and are not a standard treatment for a patient's condition. Restraints are not a solution to a patient problem, but rather a temporary means to provide safety. You must use all alternatives before placing patients in restraints. Federal and state laws prohibit Medicare- and Medicaid-certified nursing homes from using restraints unless they are medically needed. Only in emergencies can restraints be applied without a resident's or family member's informed consent.

Patients who are confused or disoriented, who repeatedly wander or fall, or who try to remove medical devices may require the temporary use of restraints to keep them safe. *However, the use of alternatives to restraints is preferred, and if a restraint is required, use the least restrictive type (e.g., soft mitt versus a limb restraint).* Individualize your choice of a restraint alternative based on each patient's situation (Box 27.12). An interprofessional approach that includes individualized assessments and development of structured treatment plans reduces restraint use. *The optimal goal for all patients is a restraint-free environment.*

The use of restraints is associated with serious complications resulting from immobilization, such as pressure injuries, pneumonia, constipation, and incontinence. Loss of self-esteem, humiliation, and agitation are also serious problems. In some cases, death has resulted because of restricted breathing and circulation. A study from Australia revealed that neck compression and entrapment by a restraint was the

BOX 27.12 Alternatives to Restraints

- Orient patients and family members to the environment; explain all procedures.
- Provide companionship and supervision; use trained sitters; adjust staffing and involve family.
- Offer diversional activities: music, puzzles, activity aprons, folding towels. Use ideas of the patient and/or family.
- Assign confused or disoriented patients to rooms near nurses' stations, and observe frequently.
- Use de-escalation, time-out, and other verbal intervention techniques when managing aggressive behaviors.
- Provide visual and auditory stimuli (e.g., family pictures, a clock, music).
- Remove cues that promote leaving the room (e.g., close doors to block view of stairs; do not allow inpatient to wear street clothes).
- Promote relaxation techniques and normal sleep patterns.
- Institute exercise and ambulation schedules as allowed by patient's condition.
- Attend frequently to patient's needs for toileting, food and liquid, and pain management.
- Camouflage intravenous lines with clothing, stockinette, or Kling gauze dressing.
- Evaluate all medication effects and ensure timely and effective pain management.
- Discontinue bothersome treatments (e.g., nasogastric tubes or Foley catheters) as soon as possible.
- Use protective devices such as hip pads, helmet, skidproof slippers, and nonskid strips near bed.

mechanism of harm in all reported cases, resulting in patient asphyxia (Bellenger et al., 2017). Because of these risks, legislation and regulatory standards have reduced the use of restraints. TJC and CMS enforce standards for safe use of restraint devices. Many health care agencies have eliminated the use of the once-common jacket (vest) restraint (Ealey and Cameron, 2016). Another standard involves staff training. All direct care staff must receive training in a health care setting's restraint and seclusion policies and procedures, and all staff who may be involved in the use of restraints must be trained in safe use of mechanical restraint devices (CMS, 2020).

For patients who continue to try to ambulate without assistance, use low beds and electronic bed/chair alarms (see Skill 27.1). A low bed places patients in a position to more easily rise to a standing position from the side of the bed and lowers the distance to the floor if a fall does occur. An alarm device warns nursing staff that a patient is attempting to leave a bed or chair unassisted. There are a variety of devices, including one with a knee band that sounds an alarm when the patient reaches a near-vertical position. An infrared type of alarm is affixed to a headboard or bedframe, allowing a patient to move freely in a bed. If a patient tries to leave the bed, the infrared beam detects motion and sends out an alarm. Alarm devices help avoid physical restraints and, when responded to promptly, can prevent patient falls and subsequent injuries.

When restraints are required to protect a patient (or nursing staff from being assaulted), involve the patient and family caregiver in the decision to use them. Help patient and family adapt to this change by explaining the purpose of the restraint, expected care while the patient is in restraints, and that the restraint is temporary and protective. For legal purposes, know agency-specific policy and procedures for appropriate use and monitoring of restraints. The use of a restraint must be clinically justified and part of a patient's prescribed medical treatment and plan of care. A health care provider's order based on a face-to-face assessment of a patient is required (TJC, 2020a). The order must be current (within 24 hours), stating the type and location of the

restraint, and must specify the duration and circumstances (e.g., preventing removal of medical device) under which it will be used. For restraints applied for violent or self-destructive behavior, a health care provider must assess the patient within 60 minutes. The orders need to be renewed within a specific time frame according to agency policy. In hospitals each original restraint order and renewal is limited to 4 hours for adults (18 years of age and older), 2 hours for children 9 through 17 years of age, and 1 hour for children younger than 9 years of age (CMS, 2020; TJC, 2020a). Orders may be renewed to the time limits for a maximum of 24 consecutive hours. Restraints are not to be ordered on an as-needed basis (prn).

Nurses are responsible for making ongoing assessments of patients who are restrained. After a restraint is applied, monitor a patient closely (i.e., every 15 minutes for a violent patient and every 2 hours for a nonviolent patient). Monitoring should include vital signs, skin integrity underneath the restraint, nutrition, hydration, circulation to an extremity, range-of-motion (ROM), hygiene, elimination needs, cognitive functioning, psychological status, and need for restraint. In this case, clinical judgment is again important. For example, an older adult who has loose and fragile skin requires that skin integrity be checked more often. Remove restraints periodically per agency policy. Continuously assess patients who are violent via audio or video monitors when available.

Skill 27.2 includes guidelines for the proper use and application of restraints. Their use must meet one of the following objectives:

- Reduce the risk of patient injury from falls.
- Prevent interruption of therapy such as traction, IV infusions, nasogastric (NG) tube feeding, or Foley catheterization.
- Prevent patients who are confused or combative from removing life-support equipment.
- Reduce the risk of injury to others by the patient.

Collaborate with other members of the health care team to design a restraint-free environment for patients. The goal is to discontinue the use of restraints as soon as possible.

Side Rails. When used correctly, side rails help to increase a patient's mobility and/or stability when repositioning or moving in bed or moving from bed to chair. Although side rails are the most commonly used physical restraint, they increase the risk of falls when patients attempt to get out of bed or crawl over a rail. Side rails also can lead to patients becoming caught, trapped, entangled, or strangled, especially in those who are frail, elderly, or confused (FDA, 2017). Therefore an assessment of a patient's mobility and responsiveness to instructions helps determine whether using a side rail is safe. The same bedrail may have the effect of restraining one individual but not another, depending on the patient's condition. For example, if a patient shows considerable independence and a reluctance to follow instructions, a side rail could be dangerous. Patients have been known to climb out of bed over raised side rails.

When a patient has a route to exit a bed safely and to maneuver freely within the bed, side rails are not considered a restraint. For example, raising only the two side rails at the top of a bed so that the lower part of the bed is open gives a patient room to exit the bed safely. Side rails used to prevent a patient such as one who is sedated from falling out of bed are not considered a restraint. Always know agency policy about the use of side rails. Be sure a bed is in the lowest position possible when side rails are raised. Check the condition of rails; bars between the bedrails need to be closely spaced to prevent entrapment. A potential exists for trapping a person's head and body in gaps and openings between the bedframe and mattress.

The use of side rails alone for a patient who is disoriented usually causes more confusion and further injury. Frequently a patient who is confused or determined to get out of bed because of pain or toileting

FIG. 27.6 Correct use of a fire extinguisher. (A) **P**ull pin. (B) **A**im at base of fire. (C) **S**queeze handles and **S**weep from side to side to coat area evenly.

needs tries to climb over a side rail or out at the foot of the bed. Either attempt often results in a fall. To reduce a patient's confusion, focus your interventions first on the cause, such as a response to a new medication, dehydration, or pain. Frequently nurses mistake a patient's attempt to explore the environment or to self-toilet as confusion. Additional safety measures include the use of a low bed with a nonskid mat placed alongside the bed on the floor. A low bed reduces the distance between the bed and floor, facilitating a roll rather than a fall from the bed.

Fires. Although smoking is not allowed in health care agencies and long-term care settings, smoking-related fires continue to pose a significant risk because of unauthorized smoking in beds or bathrooms. Institutional fires also may result from an electrical or anesthetic-related fire. The best intervention is to prevent fires. Nursing measures include complying with the smoking policies of an agency and keeping combustible material away from heat sources. Box 27.13 highlights fire intervention guidelines in health care agencies. Health care agencies are required to have practice fire drills annually.

If a fire occurs in a health care agency, protect patients from immediate injury, report the exact location of the fire, contain it, and extinguish it if possible. Fig. 27.6 demonstrates the process of using an extinguisher. Agencies have fire doors that are held open by magnets and close automatically when a fire alarm sounds. It is important to keep equipment from blocking these doors. All personnel evacuate patients when appropriate. Patients who are close to a fire, regardless of its size, are at risk of injury and need to be moved to another area. If a patient is on life support, maintain their respiratory status manually with a bag-valve-mask device (e.g., Ambu bag) (see Chapter 41) until they are moved away from the fire. Direct all ambulatory patients to walk by themselves to a safe area. In some cases, they can help move patients in wheelchairs. For patients who cannot get out of bed, move them from the scene of a fire by using a stretcher, their bed, or a wheelchair. Try to avoid carrying patients. If you overextend your physical limits for lifting, injuring yourself results in further injury to the patient. If fire department personnel are on the scene, they help evacuate the patients.

Electrical Hazards. Much of the equipment used in health care settings is electrical and must be well maintained. The clinical engineering departments of hospitals inspect biomedical equipment such as hospital beds, infusion pumps, and ventilators regularly. You know that a piece of equipment is safe to use when you see a safety inspection sticker with an expiration date. Decrease the risk for electrical injury and fire by using properly grounded and functional electrical equipment. The ground prong of an electrical outlet carries stray electrical current back to the ground. Remove and designate for repair equipment that is not in proper working order or that sparks when plugged in, and notify the appropriate hospital staff.

Seizures. Patients who have experienced some form of neurological injury or metabolic disturbance are at risk for a seizure. A seizure is

hyperexcitation and disorderly discharge of neurons in the brain. This leads to a sudden, violent, involuntary series of muscle contractions that is episodic, causing loss of consciousness, falling, tonicity (rigidity of muscles), and clonicity (jerking of muscles). During a seizure, patients are at risk for musculoskeletal or head injury as a result of a fall or striking a body part against a hard object. Patients with a history of seizures are placed on seizure precautions so that if a seizure occurs, the risk of injury can be minimized.

Know the signs and symptoms of seizures. A generalized tonic-clonic, or grand mal, seizure lasts approximately 2 minutes (no longer than 5) and is characterized by a cry and loss of consciousness with falling, tonicity, clonicity, and incontinence. Before a convulsive episode a few patients report an aura, which serves as a warning or sense that a seizure is about to occur. An aura is often a bright light or a smell or taste. During a seizure the patient often experiences shallow breathing, cyanosis, and loss of bladder and bowel control. A postictal phase follows the seizure, during which the patient has amnesia or confusion and falls into a deep sleep. A person in the community needs immediate medical attention. Call 9-1-1 if a person has repeated seizures, if a seizure lasts 5 minutes or longer, if one seizure occurs right after another without the person regaining consciousness between seizures, if seizures occur closer together than usual for that person, if breathing is difficult or the person appears to be choking, if the seizure occurs in water, or if an injury is suspected (Epilepsy Foundation of America, 2020). Instruct family members in the steps to take when a patient experiences a seizure (Epilepsy Foundation of America, 2020):

- **STAY** with the person and start timing the seizure. STAY until the person is awake and alert.
  - Remain calm. Talk calmly and reassuringly to the person during and after the seizure; it will help as they recover from the seizure.
  - Check for medical ID.
  - Look at your watch and time the seizure from the beginning to the end of the active seizure. Timing the seizure will help you determine if emergency help is needed.
  - Although most seizures last only a few minutes, some may start with minor symptoms but lead to loss of consciousness or a fall that could cause injury.
- Keep the person **SAFE**.
  - Move or guide away from harmful or sharp objects.
  - If a person is wandering or confused, help guide them away from dangerous situations such as away from traffic, train or subway platforms, heights, or sharp objects.
  - Encourage other people to step back and give the person some room. Waking up to a crowd can be embarrassing and confusing for a person after a seizure.
  - Ask someone to stay nearby in case further help is needed.
  - Do not give water, pills, or food to swallow until the person is awake.
- Turn the person onto their **SIDE** if they are not awake and aware.
  - Make the person as comfortable as possible; loosen tight clothes around neck.
  - If the person is aware, help them sit down in a safe place.
  - If the person is at risk of falling or having a convulsive seizure or tonic-clonic seizure:
    - Lay them down on the floor.
    - Put something small and soft under the head.
    - Turn the person on the side, with the mouth pointing toward the ground.

Prolonged or repeated seizures indicate status epilepticus, a medical emergency that requires intensive monitoring and treatment. It is important that you observe the patient carefully before, during, and after the seizure so that you can document the episode accurately. Seizure precautions encompass nursing interventions to protect a patient from traumatic injury, to position for adequate ventilation and drainage of oral secretions, and to provide privacy and support following a seizure (Box 27.14).

Disasters. As a nurse, be prepared to respond and care for a sudden influx of patients during a disaster. TJC (2020a) requires hospitals to have emergency-management plans that address the identification of possible emergency situations, their probable impact, maintenance of an adequate amount of supplies, and a formal response plan that includes actions to be taken by staff and steps to restore essential services and resume normal operations following the emergency. Infection control practices are critical in the event of a biological attack.

You manage all patients with suspected or confirmed bioterrorism-related illnesses with Standard Precautions (see Chapter 28). Additional precautions including Airborne Precautions or contact isolation are needed for diseases such as smallpox and pneumonic plague. In the case of coronavirus disease 2019 (COVID-19), the CDC (2020e) recommends:

1. Isolate symptomatic patients as soon as possible.
2. Set up separate, well-ventilated triage areas, place patients with suspected or confirmed COVID-19 in private rooms with the door closed and with private bathrooms (as possible).
3. Reserve airborne infection isolation rooms for patients with COVID-19 undergoing aerosol-generating procedures and for care of patients with pathogens transmitted by the airborne route (e.g., tuberculosis, measles, varicella).

BOX 27.14 Tips for Protecting Patients During a Seizure

1. When a seizure begins, note the time, stay with the patient, and call for help. Track duration of seizure. Notify health care provider immediately.
2. Position patient safely. If standing or sitting, ease the patient safely to the floor and protect head by cradling in your lap or placing a pad under head.
3. Do not lift patient from floor to bed while seizure is in progress. Clear surrounding area of furniture and anything else that is hard or sharp.
4. If patient is in bed, remove pillows and raise side rails.
5. If possible, turn patient onto one side, head tilted slightly forward.
6. Do not restrain patient; hold limbs loosely. Loosen clothing. Remove eyeglasses.
7. Never force apart a patient's clenched teeth. Do not place any objects into patient's mouth such as fingers, medicine, tongue depressor, or airway when teeth are clenched. **Insert a bite-block or oral airway in advance only if you recognize the possibility of a tonic-clonic seizure.**
8. Stay with patient, observing sequence and timing of seizure activity.
9. As patient regains consciousness, reorient and reassure. Assist patient to position of comfort in bed with side rails up (one rail down for easy exit) and bed in lowest position.
10. Conduct a head-to-toe evaluation: inspect the oral cavity for breaks in mucous membranes from bites or broken teeth; look for bruising of skin or injury to bones and joints.

---

4. When entering the room of a patient with known or suspected COVID-19, adhere to Standard Precautions and use a respirator (or face mask if a respirator is not available), gown, gloves, and eye protection.

Preventing Workplace Violence. Being able to work in a safe environment is central to job satisfaction. As a nurse, be aware of your risks of being exposed to violence in the setting where you work. Nurses do not always know what acts constitute violence. A study involving nurses in emergency departments found that nurses often underreport violence, and as a direct result resources are not recognized or provided (Stene et al., 2015). It is important to recognize the patients who are most likely to enact violence. Jackson et al. (2014) reported from an observational study, conducted in an acute care setting, six key behaviors that predict patient violence: (1) increased volume of speech, (2) irritability, (3) prolonged or intense glaring, (4) mumbling, (5) abusive language toward caregivers (e.g., name calling, swearing), and (6) pacing around waiting area or bed. In a study that reviewed hospital incident reports involving patient violence, health care staff reported these causal factors for violence (Arnetz et al., 2015):

- Patient behavior—cognitive impairment and demanding to leave
- Patient care issues—use of needles, pain/discomfort, and physical transfers
- Situational events—restraints (holding or use of physical or chemical restraint), transitions in care, intervening (attempts to stop a patient from acting), and redirecting (helping a patient back into bed or back to hospital room)

Be aware of your own behavior. Research has shown that health care providers contribute to the onset of violence. In one study patients and staff reported similar perceptions and emotions regarding the episodes of violence in which they were involved (Shafran-Tikva et al., 2017). Of the 4047 statements elicited in the study's staff survey regarding the eruption of violence, 39% referred to staff behavior. In addition, 35% of the staff respondents reported that their own behavior contributed to the creation of the most severe violent episode in which they were involved, and 48% stated that staff behavior contributed to violent episodes (Shafran-Tikva et al., 2017). Half of the reasons stated by physicians and nurses for violence eruption were related to patient dissatisfaction with the quality of service, the degree of staff professionalism, or an unacceptable comment of a staff member (Shafran-Tikva et al., 2017).

Assessment tools are available for nurses to predict patients who are likely to act violently (see agency procedure). If you face a violent situation, use the following tips for reducing violence (Crisis Prevention Institute [CPI], 2021):

- Be nonjudgmental and empathic of the patient's feelings. Whatever the patient's problem is, it can be highly important to them.
- Respect personal space.
  - Stand 1½ to 3 feet away from a patient who is escalating. This helps reduce a patient's anxiety and can help you prevent acting-out behavior.
  - If you must enter personal space to provide care, first explain what you are doing and why.
- Use nonthreatening nonverbal communication.
  - While losing control, a patient does not listen to you and instead reacts to your nonverbal communication (see Chapter 24).
  - Keep your voice tone, facial expressions, and movements neutral.
- Do not overreact. Stay calm, rational, and professional. Use positive thoughts, such as "I can manage this."
- Focus on feelings.
  - Some people cannot identify how they really feel in a situation. Watch and listen carefully for the patient's real message.
- Redirect or refocus any challenging questions, such as "Why does it always take so long for the doctor to see me?" or "Who's going to make me go to that test?"
  - Restate your request or directive; do not ignore the patient.
  - Bring the discussion back to how you can work together.
- Set limits.
  - If patients become belligerent, defensive, or disruptive, give them clear, simple, enforceable limits.
  - Speak clearly, and offer a positive choice.
- Choose wisely what you insist on.
  - Be thoughtful in deciding which rules are negotiable and which are not. For example, if a patient is unwilling to walk at a given time, can you let the patient choose a better time?
- Allow silence for reflection.
  - Silence gives a person a chance to think about what is happening and how to proceed.
- Allow time for the patient to make a decision. Give patients a few moments *to think through what you have said.* A person's stress increases when they feel rushed.

If you find that you work in a setting where violence is common, be sure to take care of yourself. Dealing with patients who are potentially violent is stressful and sometimes dangerous. Find positive ways to care for yourself away from work by using stress-management approaches (see Chapter 37).

REFLECT NOW

Consider the following situation. You are caring for a 10-year-old child who has recently been diagnosed with acute lymphocytic leukemia. The child has started receiving treatment and is experiencing many side effects. The child's father is extremely angry about his child's diagnosis and perceives that family and friends are not providing appropriate support. You walk into the patient's room to administer a medication and the father begins to yell at you because he believes you are not providing appropriate care to his child. How would you respond to the father at this time? Role-play your response with a peer.

◆ Evaluation

Through the Patient's Eyes. Patient-centered care involves a thoughtful evaluation of a patient's perspective related to safety and whether expectations were met. Once again, you think critically, considering what you know about a patient's conditions, any physical or cognitive limitations, and the patient's psychosocial perceptions and expectations of care. Ask the patient questions such as "Are you satisfied with the changes you have chosen to make for your home? Do you feel safer because of the changes? Tell me how you feel now; are you still afraid of falling? In what way could we make you feel safer?" Involve the family in your evaluation, especially if they live with the patient and provide assistance in the home.

Patient Outcomes. Evaluation involves monitoring a patient's response to actual care delivered by the health care team based on the expected outcomes (Fig. 27.7). It requires clinical judgment. You reflect on knowledge originally obtained from the patient assessment and compare evaluative findings for each nursing diagnosis to determine whether the outcomes of care have been met. Is there improvement? Is there a decline? Perhaps there is no change. If your patient meets the outcomes, the nursing diagnosis is resolved, and your nursing interventions were effective and appropriate. If not, determine whether new safety risks to the patient have developed or whether previous risks remain. For example, if the patient has another fall, reassess the conditions surrounding that fall and determine whether contributing factors can be removed or managed. The patient and family need to participate to find permanent ways to reduce risks to safety. When patient outcomes are not met, ask the following questions:

- What factors led to your fall/injury?
- Help me understand what makes you feel unsafe in your environment.
- What questions do you have about your safety?
- Do you need help locating community resources to help make your home safer?
- What changes have you recently experienced that you believe contribute to your risk for falling or lack of safety?

Continually reassess a patient's and family's need for additional support services, such as home care, physical therapy, counseling, and further teaching. A safe environment is essential to promoting, maintaining, and restoring health. Overall, your expected outcomes include a safe physical environment and a patient whose expectations have been met, who is knowledgeable about safety factors and precautions, and who is free from injury.

Before ending her first visit, Kylie assesses Mrs. Cohen's knowledge of her medications and their purpose. Mrs. Cohen replies, "I know both of the medicines help lower my blood pressure. One of them makes me go to the bathroom more often. I take each medicine once a day." Taking these two medicines along with her vitamin supplements should make for an easy routine. Kylie has Mrs. Cohen and Meg review the best times to take the medicine (morning) and tells them she will check their success in managing the medicines at her next visit. Kylie finishes her visit with an explanation of Mrs. Cohen's fall risks and how she and her children can help to make the home safer. Mrs. Cohen agrees to the changes, and Meg states, "This is definitely doable. We'll start immediately." To ensure the patient understands the instructions, Kylie asks, "Tell me one final time, Mrs. Cohen, why are you at risk for falling?" Mrs. Cohen responds, "Well, the weakness from my stroke, and the fact I fell before." Kylie probes: "Anything else?" Mrs. Cohen answers, "Ah, you said I need to use the walker correctly or it can cause a fall." Kylie says, "That is correct. Also, remember that your age and your medicine for blood pressure place you at risk." Mrs. Cohen responds, "Oh yes, now I remember." Kylie then says, "When I visit you next week, I will review how well you stayed on schedule with your medicines and I will be sure to reinforce the exercises physical therapy will be showing you." Mrs. Cohen replies, "That sounds good."

FIG. 27.7 Critical thinking model for evaluation of safety. *ANA,* American Nurses Association; *CMS,* Centers for Medicare and Medicaid Services. (Clinical Judgment Measurement Model copyright © NCSBN. All rights reserved.)

SAFETY GUIDELINES FOR NURSING SKILLS

Ensuring patient safety is an essential role of the professional nurse. Use sound clinical judgment by communicating clearly with members of the health care team, assessing and analyzing patient's clinical findings and incorporating the patient's priorities of care and preferences. Use the best evidence, applying professional standards, when selecting interventions to use in patient care delivery. When performing the skills in this chapter, remember the following points to ensure safe, individualized patient care:

- Anticipate a patient's fall risks based on your assessment and knowledge of physiological and behavioral factors when choosing fall prevention strategies.

- Involve patients and families in the selection of fall prevention strategies to improve adherence.
- Always try restraint alternatives first before using a restraint. Involve family in your approach.
- Implement fall prevention protocols and provide patient and family education about fall prevention.

SKILL 27.1   FALL PREVENTION IN HEALTH CARE SETTINGS

Delegation and Collaboration

The skill of assessing and communicating a patient's risks for falling cannot be delegated to assistive personnel (AP). Skills used to prevent falls can be delegated. Direct the AP by:

- Explaining a patient's specific fall risks and associated prevention measures needed to minimize risks.
- Explaining environmental safety precautions to use.
- Explaining specific patient behaviors (e.g., disorientation, wandering) that are precursors to falls and that should be reported immediately.

Equipment

- Standardized and valid fall risk assessment tool (HRET, 2016; TJC, 2020a)
- Hospital bed with side rails; *Option:* low bed
- Wedge cushion
- Nurse call system
- Gait belt for assisting with ambulation
- Wheelchair and seat belt (as needed)
- Optional safety devices: bed alarm pad, no slip floor mat, head protective gear, hip protector

Continued

SKILL 27.1   FALL PREVENTION IN HEALTH CARE SETTINGS—cont'd

STEPS	RATIONALE

ASSESSMENT

1. Identify patient using at least two identifiers (e.g., name and birthday or name and medical record number) according to agency policy.

Ensures correct patient. Complies with The Joint Commission standards and improves patient safety (TJC, 2021a).

2. Review medical record and determine if patient has a recent history of a fall and risks for injury (ABCs) (IHI, 2021):
   - **A**ge over 85
   - **B**one disorders (e.g., metastasis, osteoporosis)
   - **C**oagulation disorders (e.g., leukemia, thrombocytopenia, anticoagulant use)
   - **S**urgery (specifically thoracic or abdominal surgery or lower limb amputation)

Conditions increase likelihood of serious injury from a fall such as fracture or internal hemorrhage.

3. Assess patient and family caregiver health literacy.

Ensures patient has the capacity to obtain, communicate, process, and understand basic health information (CDC, 2021b).

4. Perform hand hygiene. Assess for fall risks using a validated fall risk assessment tool. Compute fall risk score. Perform fall risk assessment in general acute care settings on admission, on transfer from one unit to another, with a significant change in a patient's condition, or after a fall (AHRQ, 2018).

Reduces transmission of microorganisms. A variety of intrinsic physiological factors predispose patients to falls. Fall risk tools based on the risk factors of a population (e.g., older adult, oncology, or neurological patient) are more likely sensitive to predicting falls.

CLINICAL JUDGMENT: *Implement a standardized cognitive assessment tool and integrate into fall risk assessment tool if cognitive assessment is not included in the fall risk assessment (HRET, 2016).*

5. Continue with a comprehensive individualized patient assessment and consider patient's unique intrinsic fall risks (TJC, 2020a) (see Table 27.1)

Reveals all factors placing patient at a fall risk.

6. Use the Banner Mobility Assessment Tool (BMAT) (Boynton et al., 2014; Matz, 2019) or perform the Timed Up and Go (TUG) test (CDC, 2017c; Berry and Kiel, 2021) if patient is able to ambulate. At a minimum, observe an ambulatory patient walk in room (with or without help).

The BMAT assesses four functional tasks to identify the level of mobility a patient can achieve, revealing if assistance is needed (Boynton et al., 2014; Matz, 2019). The TUG test measures the progress of balance, sit to stand, and walking.

CLINICAL JUDGMENT: *Do not ask patient to provide a self-report of balance, gait, or ability to ambulate. Your direct observation will be more accurate.*

7. Assess patient's pain severity (use rating scale ranging 0 to 10).

Pain, especially when it is associated with lower extremities (e.g., arthritis, injury) is a fall risk factor.

8. Ask patient or family caregiver if patient has a history of recent falls or other injuries within the home. Assess previous falls using the acronym SPLATT (Touhy and Jett, 2022).
   - **S**ymptoms at time of fall
   - **P**revious fall
   - **L**ocation of fall
   - **A**ctivity at time of fall
   - **T**ime of fall
   - **T**rauma after fall

Symptoms are helpful in identifying cause for fall. Onset, location, and activity offer details on how to prevent future falls.

9. Review patient's medications (including over-the-counter [OTC] medications and herbal products) for drugs that create risk for falls (see Table 27.1). Compare those drugs with ones on the Beers Criteria® lists (AGS, 2019).

Drugs commonly cause drowsiness. The AGS Beers Criteria® lists include certain medications worth discussing with patients because the medications may not be the safest or most appropriate options for older adults (AGS, 2019). The five lists included in the AGS Beers Criteria® describe particular medications with scientific evidence suggesting that they should be:
   1. Avoided by most older people (outside of hospice and palliative care settings)
   2. Avoided by older people with specific health conditions
   3. Avoided in combination with other treatments because of the risk for harmful drug-drug interactions
   4. Used with caution because of the potential for harmful side effects
   5. Dosed differently or avoided among people with reduced kidney function, which affects how the body processes medicine

10. Assess for polypharmacy (unnecessary use of multiple [five or more] and/or redundant medications in management of the same condition and drugs inappropriate for condition).

Over a 2-year period, polypharmacy was significantly associated with 21% increased rate of falls in a study involving adults older than 60 years (Dhalwani et al., 2017).

STEPS	RATIONALE
11. Assess patient's fear of falling: consider if patient is female; is older; or has a lower level of education, chronic illness (more than three chronic illnesses), poor subjective health, functional impairment, a history of falling, or depression.	These are factors found to be associated with a severe fear of falling (Park et al., 2017).
12. Assess condition of any assistive devices or equipment used by patient (e.g., legs on bedside commode, end tips on a walker).	Equipment in poor repair increases risk for fall.
13. Use patient-centered approach to determine what patient already knows about risks for falling. Show patient and family caregiver results of fall risk assessment and explain significance of risk factors. Explain how a plan for fall prevention will be developed.	Allows you to determine content to include in fall prevention education.
14. Assess patient's goals or preferences for how to implement fall prevention strategies.	Matching your approach with patient goals will likely improve patient's participation. Initial commitment from a learner is critical. The learner processes information just collected from the assessment and articulates the plan (Chinai et al., 2018).
15. If patient has a fall risk, apply color-coded wristband (see illustration). Some agencies institute fall risk signs on doors; others may use color-coded socks or gowns.	Color-coded yellow bands, socks, and gowns are easily recognizable.
16. If patient is in a wheelchair, assess the level of comfort, fatigue, boredom, mental status, or level of engagement with others.	These factors can cause patient to make an attempt to exit wheelchair without help.

PLANNING

1. Provide privacy. Be sure patient is comfortable.	Maintains patient dignity and respect.
2. Perform hand hygiene. Prepare equipment, making sure all is functional.	Reduces transmission of microorganisms. A well-equipped room with functioning equipment promotes safety.
3. Explain safety measure to be taken as they pertain to patient's specific fall risks. Also plan for time to discuss fall prevention in the home. *Option:* Some agencies use a patient acknowledgment form for a patient to personally acknowledge the fall risks (HRET, 2016).	Clear, concise information with explanations of purpose, benefits, and expectations results in increased patient participation.
4. Educate patients and family caregivers on medication side effects that increase risk for falls (HRET, 2016).	Patients on multiple medications are often unaware of risk factors.

IMPLEMENTATION

1. Conduct hourly purposeful rounds on all patients to determine status of pain, be proactive in offering assist to toilet, assess comfort of position, and assess need to relocate personal items for easy reach; provide pain relief intervention.	Use of purposeful and timely patient rounding has been shown to reduce falls and encourage team communication (Daniels, 2016). Patients who fall have been shown to not seek help while toileting (HRET, 2016).
2. Implement early mobility protocols within health care agency. Follow protocols to ensure patient increases level of mobility progressively. Consider use of accelerometers, small devices that can be worn by a patient and quantify biomechanical body movement and number of steps per shift (Growdon et al., 2017).	A patient's functional decline (loss of the ability to perform self-care activities or ADLs) may result from deconditioning, which is associated with inactivity (Gorman et al., 2014; Grass et al., 2018). Deconditioning is a risk for hospitalized patients who spend most of their time in bed, even when they are able to walk.
3. Implement Universal Fall Precautions.	
a. Adjust bed to low position with wheels locked (AHRQ, 2018). Place nonslip padded floor mat at exit side of bed.	Height of bed allows ambulatory patient to get in and out of bed easily and safely. Mats provide nonslippery surface for preventing falls and injuries.
b. Encourage use of properly fitted skid-proof footwear (AHRQ, 2018).	Prevents falls from patient slipping on floor.

STEP 15 A color coded "fall risk" armband alerts health care staff to patient's risk of falling.

Continued

SKILL 27.1 FALL PREVENTION IN HEALTH CARE SETTINGS—cont'd

STEPS	RATIONALE
c. Orient patient to surroundings. Explain nurse call system and routines to expect in plan of care (AHRQ, 2018; HRET, 2016).	Orientation to room and plan of care provides familiarity with environment and activities to anticipate.

CLINICAL JUDGMENT: *Agencies with successful fall prevention programs have implemented a patient agreement form to use call light for all ambulation (HRET, 2016). Be sure agreement has been signed.*

(1) Provide patient's hearing aid and glasses. Be sure that each is functioning and clean (AHRQ, 2018). If patient complains of visual or hearing problems, refer to appropriate health care provider.	Enables patient to remain alert to conditions in environment.
(2) Place nurse call system in an accessible location within patient's reach (see illustration). Explain and demonstrate how to use system at bedside and in bathroom. Have patient perform return demonstration.	Knowledge of location and use of call system is essential for patient to be able to call for help quickly. Reaching for an object when in bed can lead to an accidental fall.
(3) Explain to patient/family caregiver when and why to use nurse call system (e.g., report pain, assistance needed to get out of bed or go to bathroom) (HRET, 2016). Provide clear instructions regarding mobility restrictions.	Increases likelihood that patient/family caregiver will call for help and of nurse being able to respond to patient's needs in a timely way.
d. Safe use of side rails:	
(1) Explain to patient and family caregiver reason for patient to use side rails: moving and turning in bed, comfort and security, easy access to call system (FDA, 2017).	Promotes a feeling of comfort and security. Aids in turning and repositioning and provides easy access to bed controls (FDA, 2017).
(2) Check agency policy regarding side rail use.	
i. Patients who are dependent and less mobile: In two–side rail bed, keep both rails up. (**NOTE:** Rails on newer hospital beds allow for room at foot of bed for patient to safely exit bed.) In four–side rail bed, leave only two upper rails up.	Side rails are restraint devices if they restrict a patient's freedom of movement and therefore do not promote the individual's independent functioning (TJC, 2020b).
ii. Patient able to get out of bed independently: In four–side rail bed, leave two upper side rails up. In two–side rail bed, keep only one rail up.	Allows for safe exit from bed.
e. Make patient's environment safe:	
(1) Remove excess equipment, supplies, and furniture from rooms and halls.	Reduces likelihood of falling or tripping over objects.
(2) Keep floors free of clutter and obstacles (e.g., IV pole, electrical cords), particularly path to bathroom (AHRQ, 2018).	Reduces likelihood of falling or tripping over objects.
(3) Coil and secure excess electrical, telephone, and any other cords or tubing.	Reduces risk of entanglement.
(4) Clean all spills on floors promptly (AHRQ, 2018). Post sign indicating wet floor. Remove sign when floor is dry (usually done by housekeeping).	Reduces risk of falling on slippery, wet surfaces.
(5) Ensure adequate glare-free lighting; use a night-light at night.	Glare may be problem for older adults because of vision changes.
(6) Have assistive devices (e.g., cane, walker, bedside commode) on exit side of bed. Have chair back of a bedside commode placed against wall of room if possible.	Provides added support when transferring out of bed. Stabilizes commode.

STEP 3c(2) Nurse call system within bed.

STEPS	RATIONALE
(7) Arrange personal items (e.g., water pitcher, telephone, reading materials, dentures) within patient's easy reach and in logical way (AHRQ, 2018).	Facilitates independence and self-care; prevents falls related to reaching for hard-to-reach items.
(8) Secure locks on beds, stretchers, and wheelchairs (AHRQ, 2018).	Prevents accidental movement of devices during patient transfer.
4. Use a proper size mattress or mattress with raised foam edges (FDA, 2017).	Prevents patients from being trapped between the mattress and rail.
a. Reduce the gaps between the mattress and side rails (FDA, 2017)	Prevent patient entrapment.
5. Provide comfort measures, offer ordered analgesics for patients experiencing pain, preferably around the clock.	Pain can cause patients to exit bed and has been associated with an increase in falls (Patel et al., 2014). Be cautious, as opioids further increase fall risk.
6. Interventions for patients at **moderate-to-high risk for falling** (based on fall risk assessment):	
a. Prioritize call-light responses to patients at high risk; use a team approach, with all staff knowing responsibility to respond.	Ensures rapid response by care provider when patient calls for help; decreases chance of patient trying to get out of bed on own.
b. Establish elimination schedule; use bedside commode when appropriate.	Proactive toileting keeps patients from being unattended with sudden urge to use toilet.

CLINICAL JUDGMENT: *Toileting is a common event leading to a patient's fall (Berry and Kiel, 2021). Caution: Bedside commode reduces distances patient must walk to toilet, but patient still requires caregiver assistance to commode.*

STEPS	RATIONALE
c. Stay with patient during toileting (standing outside bathroom door; next to bedside commode). Increase availability and use of raised toilet seats, toilet safety frames/grab bars (VA Healthcare, 2015).	Patients often try to get up to stand and walk back to their beds from the bathroom without help. Raised seats make it easier to sit on or sit up from toilet. Toilet frames and grab bars can be grasped to provide support when standing and sitting.
d. Place patient in a geri chair or wheelchair with wedge cushion. Use wheelchair only for transport, not for sitting an extended time.	Maintains alignment and comfort and makes it difficult to exit chair.
e. Provide hip protectors, which are padded shorts or underwear that are worn over or in place of underwear (used more often in long-term care settings).	Prevents fractures by distributing the force of a fall on the hip to the softer tissue around the buttocks and thigh (U.S. Department of Veterans Affairs, 2019).
f. Consider use of a low bed that has lower height than standard hospital bed. Apply nonskid floor mats (U.S. Department of Veterans Affairs, 2019).	Low beds may reduce fall-related injuries by making it difficult for patients with lower extremity weakness or pain in lower joints to exert effort needed to stand. Mats prevent slipping when walking and standing.
g. Activate a bed alarm or surveillance system, such as a camera monitoring system for patient (VA Healthcare, 2015).	Alarm activates when patient rises off sensor. Alarm sounds alert to staff. Camera can detect falls.

CLINICAL JUDGMENT: *Use judgment in choosing use of a bed alarm. Bed alarms alert nursing staff so that if a patient exits a bed, a quick response may prevent a fall (Potter et al., 2017). If a patient exits a bed quickly and falls, the alarm alerts staff to respond so that further injury does not occur while patient lies on floor. However, bed and chair alarms can restrict patient activity. Reports have shown that patients perceive that an alarm makes them feel restrained (Growdon et al., 2017). Determine if use of bed or chair alarm is limiting frequency of patient getting up and remaining active. The use of many alarm devices (IV alarm, bed alarm, electrocardiographic monitor) can result in sound dispersion and alarm fatigue among health care providers; the health care providers may ignore the alarm, resulting in a fall event (Ward-Smith, 2015).*

STEPS	RATIONALE
h. Confer with physical therapist about gait training, strength and balance training, and regular weight-bearing activities.	Exercise can reduce falls, fall-related fractures, and several risk factors for falls in individuals with low bone density and older adults. Strength and balance training reduces the rate of injurious falls in older adults (Uusi-Rasi et al., 2015).
i. Use sitters or restraints only when alternatives are exhausted.	A sitter is a nonprofessional staff member or volunteer who stays in a patient room to closely observe patients who are at risk for falling. Restraints should be used only as a final option (see Skill 27.2).
j. Consider having patient wear head protective gear (e.g., oncology patient or patients at risk for bleeding).	Contains impact-resistant material within the hat that surrounds the head and protects against head injury.
7. When ambulating a patient, have patient wear a gait belt or use a walking sling and walk along the patient's side (see Chapter 38).	Safe patient-handling techniques allow for safe patient ambulation and prevention of injury to you and patient.
8. Safe use of wheelchair:	
a. Be sure that wheelchair is correct fit for patient: Patient thighs are level while sitting, feet flat on floor; back of chair comes up to mid-shoulder, elbows rest on armrests without leaning over or tucking arms in, and 2 finger widths of space between patient and side of chair.	Correctly fitted chair promotes comfort, making it less likely for patient to try to exit it.

Continued

SKILL 27.1   FALL PREVENTION IN HEALTH CARE SETTINGS—cont'd

STEPS	RATIONALE
b. Transfer patient to wheelchair using safe handling techniques. Use a wedge cushion in chair (see illustration).	Cushion prevents patient from slipping out of chair.
c. Back wheelchair into and out of elevator or door, leading with large rear wheels first (see illustration).	Prevents smaller front wheels from catching in crack between elevator and floor, causing chair to tip.
d. Manage patient's pain and do not allow them to sit in wheelchair for an extended amount of time; provide alternative sitting option.	Reduces restlessness and discomfort that can lead to wheelchair exit.
9. Schedule oral medication administration for at least 2 hours prior to bedtime (HRET, 2016).	Reduces risk created by medications that can cause patients to have to use bathroom during night.
10. After implementing safety strategies, help patient to comfortable position.	Reduces restlessness and desire to exit bed.
11. Raise side rails (as appropriate) and lower bed to lowest position.	Promotes safety and prevents falls.
12. Place nurse call system in an accessible location within patient's reach.	Ensures patient can call for assistance if needed and promotes safety and prevents falls.
13. Dispose of all contaminated supplies in appropriate receptacle, remove and dispose of gloves, and perform hand hygiene.	Reduces transmission of microorganisms. Use appropriate disposal receptacle if patient is on hazardous drugs.
14. Continue hourly purposeful rounding.	Reduces patient anxiety, lessens need for patient to exit bed independently

EVALUATION

1. Ask patient/family caregiver to identify patient's fall risks.	Demonstrates learning.
2. Ask patient/family caregiver to describe fall prevention interventions to implement in the home.	Demonstrates learning. **NOTE:** Visit by health care provider in home is necessary to confirm that interventions were implemented.
3. Evaluate patient's ability to use assistive devices such as walker or bedside commode at different times during the day	Adjustments in devices may become necessary. Evaluating at different times can help identify strengths and weaknesses.
4. Evaluate for changes in motor, sensory, and cognitive status and review if any falls or injuries have occurred.	May require different interventions to be added. Fall outcomes determine success of plan.
5. Evaluate patient's level of pain using a pain rating scale.	Determines if patient's pain is under adequate control.
6. **Use Teach-Back:** "I want to be sure I explained clearly to you why you are at risk to fall. Tell me some of those reasons." Revise your instruction now or develop a plan for revised patient/family caregiver teaching if patient/family caregiver is not able to teach back correctly.	Teach-back is an evidence-based health literacy intervention that promotes patient engagement, patient safety, adherence, and quality. The goal of teach-back is to ensure that you have explained medical information clearly so that patients and their families understand what you have communicated to them (AHRQ, 2020b).

STEP 8b Wheelchair with footplates raised and wedge cushion in place.

STEP 8c Nurse backing wheelchair into elevator.

UNEXPECTED OUTCOMES AND RELATED INTERVENTIONS

1. Patient/family caregiver unable to identify fall risks or fall prevention strategies.
   - Reinforce identified risks and review safety measures with patient and family caregiver.
   - Consider using other instructional options.
2. Patient found on floor after falling.
   - Call for assistance.
   - Assess patient for injury and stay with the patient until help arrives.
   - Notify primary health care provider and family caregiver.
   - Complete an agency occurrence or sentinel event report (see agency policy)
   - Conduct a postfall huddle/debrief as soon as possible after the fall. Involve staff at all levels and the patient if possible. Discuss whether appropriate interventions were in place, considerations as to why fall occurred, staffing at time of fall, which environment of care factors were in place, and how care plan will change (VA Healthcare, 2015; HRET, 2016).

RECORDING AND REPORTING

- Record patient's specific fall risks and fall prevention interventions in electronic health record (EHR) or chart. Use whiteboards in patient rooms to communicate patient fall risks to all staff (HRET, 2016).
- Document in nurses' notes what patient is able to explain or not explain about fall risks and interventions taken.
- If fall occurs, complete an agency safety event or incident report, noting objective details of a fall (time, location, patient's condition, treatment, treatment response). Do not place the report in patient's medical record.
- Use a hand-off communication tool that includes specific patient risks for falls and falls with injury between caregivers (include AP). Discuss patient-specific interventions taken (HRET, 2016).
- Report immediately to the health care provider if patient sustains a fall or an injury.

SKILL 27.2 APPLYING PHYSICAL RESTRAINTS

Delegation and Collaboration
The skill of assessing a patient's behavior, orientation to the environment, need for restraints, and appropriate use of restraints cannot be delegated. The application and routine checking of a restraint can be delegated to assistive personnel (AP). CMS (2020) requires training of all direct care staff who apply restraints. Instruct the AP about:
- Appropriate restraint to use and correct placement of restraint.
- When and how to change patient's position and provide ROM exercises, hydration, toileting, skin care, and time for socialization.
- When to report signs and symptoms of patient not tolerating restraint and what to do.

Equipment
- Proper-sized restraint
- Padding (if needed)

STEPS	RATIONALE
ASSESSMENT	
1. Identify patient using at least two identifiers (e.g., name and birthday or name and medical record number) according to agency policy.	Ensures correct patient. Complies with The Joint Commission standards and improves patient safety (TJC, 2021a).
2. Review medical record to assess for underlying cause(s) of agitation and cognitive impairment that may lead to patient-initiated medical device removal (Boltz et al., 2020).	Physiological alterations might lead to accidental patient-initiated medical device removal (Boltz et al., 2020). Identification of conditions might lead to more appropriate medical or pharmacological treatment, eliminating need for restraints.
a. If there is abrupt change in perception, attention, or level of consciousness, perform hand hygiene. Assess for respiratory and neurological alterations, fever and sepsis, hypoglycemia and hyperglycemia, alcohol or substance withdrawal, and fluid and electrolyte imbalance.	Reduces transmission of microorganisms. Factors can develop quickly that affect patient cognition.
b. Notify health care provider of change in mental status and compromised physiological status.	Health care provider must determine if change in status results in behavior that necessitates temporary use of restraint.
3. Obtain baseline or premorbid cognitive function from family caregivers.	Excellent sources of information for patient's behavior patterns and past history.
4. Establish whether patient has history of dementia or depression (Boltz et al., 2020).	Cognitively impaired are at risk for exiting bed without asking for assistance.
5. Review medications that can cause risk for falling (Boltz et al., 2020; AGS, 2019) and changes in mental status.	Medications can alter cognition, cause drowsiness, result in postural hypotension, and create other risks.
6. Review current laboratory values (e.g., electrolytes, blood glucose, blood culture, urinalysis).	May reveal a fluid and electrolyte imbalance or other problems such as a blood glucose imbalance or an infection, all of which can cause sudden confusion in the elderly (Wang et al., 2016; Meiner and Yeager, 2019).

Continued

SKILL 27.2   APPLYING PHYSICAL RESTRAINTS—cont'd

STEPS	RATIONALE
7. Assess patient's current behavior (e.g., confusion, disorientation, agitation, restlessness, combativeness, inability to follow directions, or repeated removal of therapeutic devices). Does patient create a risk to other patients?	If patient's behavior continues despite treatment or restraint alternatives, use of least restrictive restraint might be indicated.

CLINICAL JUDGMENT: *In the case of alcohol withdrawal, resistance against restraints can increase temperature, produce rhabdomyolysis, and cause physical injury (Hoffman and Weinhouse, 2020).*

8. If restraint alternatives failed earlier, confer with health care provider. Review agency policies and state laws regarding restraints. **Obtain current health care provider's order for restraint,** including purpose, type, location, and time or duration of restraint. Determine if signed consent for use of restraint is necessary (long-term care). For nonviolent/non–self-destructive patients, orders are renewed per agency policy.	A restraint order that is being used for violent or self-destructive behavior has a definite time limit (e.g., every 4 hours for adults, every 2 hours for children and adolescents ages 9–17); these orders may be renewed according to the prescribed time limits for a maximum of 24 consecutive hours (CMS, 2020). A health care provider's order for least restrictive type of restraint is required (CMS, 2020).

CLINICAL JUDGMENT: *A licensed independent health care provider responsible for the care of the patient evaluates the patient in person within 1 hour of the initiation of restraint used for the management of **violent or self-destructive behavior** that jeopardizes the physical safety of the patient, staff, or others. A registered nurse, advanced practice nurse, or physician assistant may conduct the in-person evaluation if they are trained in accordance with requirements and consults with the aforementioned health care provider after the evaluation as determined by hospital policy (CMS, 2020).*

9. Review manufacturer instructions for restraint application. Determine most appropriate size restraint. Be familiar with all devices	Incorrect sizing and application of restraint device can result in patient injury or death.
10. Assess patient's or family caregiver's health literacy and then determine knowledge about use of restraints and experience.	Ensures patient has the capacity to obtain, communicate, process, and understand basic health information (CDC, 2021b).
11. Assess patient's goals or preferences for how skill is to be performed or what patient expects.	Allows care to be individualized to patient.

PLANNING

1. Perform hand hygiene. Prepare restraint; make sure it is intact.	Reduces transmission of microorganisms. Ensures restraint is in condition for correct use.
2. Provide patient privacy, and drape as appropriate for comfort.	Promotes patient comfort.
3. Explain to patient and family caregiver the choice of restraint, how it will be applied, length of time it is to be used, and procedure for ongoing assessment.	Promotes patient/family cooperation and helps to minimize any anxiety.

IMPLEMENTATION

1. Adjust bed to proper height and lower side rail on side of patient contact. Be sure that patient is comfortable and in proper body alignment.	Allows you to reposition patient during restraint application without injuring self or patient. Proper alignment prevents contracture formation when restraints are in place.
2. Inspect area where restraint is to be placed. Note if there is any nearby tubing or device. Assess condition of skin, sensation, adequacy of circulation, and range of joint motion.	Restraints sometimes compress and interfere with functioning of devices or tubes. Assessment provides baseline to monitor patient's response to restraint.
3. Pad skin and bony prominences (as necessary) that will be under restraint.	Reduces friction and pressure from restraint to skin and underlying tissue.
4. Apply proper-size restraint. **Note:** Refer to manufacturer directions. a. *Mitten restraint:* Thumbless mitten device restrains patient's hands. Place hand in mitten, being sure that Velcro strap is around wrist and not forearm (see illustration).	Prevents patient from dislodging or removing medical device, removing dressings, or scratching. Hand mitts are considered a restraint if (TJC, 2020b): 1. The mitts are pinned or otherwise attached to the bed/bedding, or wrist restraints are also used, and/or 2. The mitts are applied so tightly that the patient's hands or finger are immobilized, and/or 3. The mitts are so bulky that the patient's ability to use the hands is significantly reduced, and/or 4. The mitts cannot be easily removed intentionally by the patient in the same manner they were applied by staff, considering the patient's physical condition and ability to accomplish the objective.

CLINICAL JUDGMENT: *Mittens are considered a restraint alternative if untethered and patient is physically and cognitively able to remove the mitt.*

STEPS	RATIONALE
b. *Elbow restraint (freedom splint):* Restraint consists of rigidly padded fabric that wraps around arm and is closed with Velcro. The upper end has a clamp that hooks to sleeve of patient's gown or shirt (see illustration). Insert arm so elbow joint rests against padded area, keeping joint extended. Secure restraint to bedframe.	The restraint makes it difficult to remove or disrupt a medical device near the face or neck. It does not impede removal of abdominal or urinary medical devices. With freedom sleeves, patients have difficulty bending their arms. The sleeves may not prevent a patient from removing IV lines (Rose, 2015).
c. *Belt or body restraint:* Have patient in sitting position in bed. Apply belt over clothes, gown, or pajamas. Be sure to place restraint at waist, not chest or abdomen. Slot in belt may be positioned in front for limited movement or rear for increased movement. Remove wrinkles or creases in clothing. Bring ties through slots in belt. Help patient lie down in bed. Have patient roll to side and avoid applying belt too tightly. Ensure that straps secured to bedframe are snug so belt does not slide to sides of bed (see illustration).	Restrains center of gravity and prevents patient from rolling off stretcher or bed, or sitting up while on stretcher or bed. Tight application interferes with ventilation if belt moves up over abdomen or chest. Belt restraint is good option for confused or impulsive patients who are continually trying to get out of bed after repeated redirection, when it is unsafe for them to get up unaided (Rose, 2015).
d. *Soft extremity (ankle or wrist) restraint:* Restraint made of soft quilted material or sheepskin with foam padding. Wrap limb restraint around wrist or ankle with soft part toward skin and secure snugly (not tightly) in place with Velcro strap. Insert two fingers under secured restraint (see illustration).	Appropriate for patients who are becoming increasingly agitated, cannot be redirected with distraction, and keep trying to remove needed medical devices (Rose, 2015). Restraint designed to immobilize one or all extremities. Tight application interferes with circulation and potentially causes neurovascular injury.

CLINICAL JUDGMENT: *Patient with wrist and/or ankle restraints is at risk for aspiration if positioned supine. Place patient in lateral position or with head of bed elevated rather than supine.*

STEP 4a Mitten restraint. (From Sorrentino SA, Remmert LN: *Mosby's workbook for nursing assistants,* ed 10, St Louis, 2021, Elsevier.)

STEP 4b Freedom elbow restraint. (Copyright © Mosby's Clinical Skills: Essentials collection.)

STEP 4c Properly applied belt restraint allows patient to turn in bed. (From Sorrentino SA, Remmert LN: *Mosby's textbook for nursing assistants,* ed 10, St Louis, 2021, Elsevier.)

Continued

SKILL 27.2	APPLYING PHYSICAL RESTRAINTS—cont'd

STEPS	RATIONALE
5. Attach restraint straps to part of bedframe that moves when raising or lowering head of bed. Be sure that straps are secure. *Do not attach to side rails.* Attach restraint to chair frame for patient in chair or wheelchair, being sure that buckle is out of patient's reach.	Properly positioned strap does not tighten and restrict circulation when bed is raised or lowered.
6. Secure restraints on bedframe with quick-release buckle (see illustration). *Do not tie strap in a knot.* Be sure that buckle is out of patient reach.	Allows for quick release in emergency.
7. Double-check and insert two fingers under secured restraint one more time. Assess proper placement of restraint, including skin integrity, pulses, skin temperature and color, and sensation of restrained body part. Place bed in lowest position after restraint(s) applied.	Provides baseline to later evaluate if injury develops from restraint. Provides safest environment in which to leave a patient who is restrained.
8. Perform hand hygiene. Remove restraint at least every 2 hours (TJC, 2020b) or more frequently as determined by agency policy. Reposition patient, provide comfort and toileting measures, and evaluate patient condition each time. If patient is agitated, violent, or noncompliant, remove one restraint at a time and/or have staff assistance while removing restraints.	Provides opportunity to attend to patient's basic needs and determine need for continuation of restraints. A temporary, directly supervised release of a restraint that occurs for the purpose of caring for a patient's needs (e.g., toileting, feeding, or ROM exercises) is **not** considered a discontinuation of the restraint (CMS, 2020).

CLINICAL JUDGMENT: *Restraints cannot be ordered prn. If a patient was recently released from restraint, and exhibits behavior that can be handled only through the reapplication of restraint or seclusion, a new order is required (CMS, 2020).*

CLINICAL JUDGMENT: *Do not leave a patient who is violent or aggressive unattended while restraints are off. Monitoring of violent/self-destructive patients placed in restraints is continuous (by way of video or audio) versus every 2 hours for nonviolent/non–self-destructive patients.*

STEPS	RATIONALE
9. Place nurse call system in an accessible location within patient's reach.	Ensures patient can call for assistance if needed and promotes safety and prevents falls.
10. Leave bed or chair with wheels locked. Raise side rails (as appropriate) and lower bed to lowest position.	Prevents bed or chair from moving if patient tries to get out. If patient falls with bed in lowest position, this reduces chance of injury. Promotes safety and prevents falls.
11. Dispose of all contaminated supplies in appropriate receptacle, remove and dispose of gloves, and perform hand hygiene.	Reduces transmission of microorganisms. Use appropriate disposal receptacle if patient is on hazardous drugs.

EVALUATION

STEPS	RATIONALE
1. After restraint application, evaluate patient's response to restraints: a. *Patients who are not violent:* Conduct evaluation for signs of injury (e.g., circulation, ROM, vital signs, skin condition), behavior and psychological status, and readiness for discontinuation (frequency based on agency policy) (TJC, 2020b). b. *Patients who are violent/self-destructive:* Conduct same evaluation every 15 minutes. Perform visual checks if patient is too agitated to approach (TJC, 2020b).	Frequent evaluation prevents injury to patient and ensures removal of restraint at earliest possible time. Frequency of monitoring guides staff in determining appropriate intervals for evaluation based on patient's needs and condition, type of restraint used, risk associated with use of chosen intervention, and other relevant factors.

STEP 4d Soft extremity restraint. Check restraint for constriction by inserting two fingers under restraint.

STEP 6 Quick release buckle.

STEPS	RATIONALE
2. Evaluate patient's need for toileting, nutrition and fluids, and hygiene, and release restraint at least every 2 hours.	Prevents injury to patient and attends to basic needs.
3. Evaluate patient for any complications of immobility.	Early detection of skin irritation, restricted breathing, or reduction in mobility prevents serious adverse events.

4. Renewal of restraints (CPI, 2021; CMS, 2020):
   a. Patients who are not violent may have renewal of restraints based on hospital policy. However, the restraint must be discontinued at the earliest possible time, regardless of the scheduled expiration of the order.
   b. Patients who are violent/self-destructive may have restraints renewed within the following limits:
    • 4 hours for adults 18 years of age or older
    • 2 hours for children and adolescents 9 to 17 years of age
    • 1 hour for children under 9 years of age
   Orders may be renewed according to the time limits for a maximum of 24 consecutive hours.
	Ensures that restraint application continues to be medically appropriate.

5. Examine IV catheters, urinary catheters, and drainage tubes to determine that they are positioned correctly and that therapy remains uninterrupted.	Reinsertion is uncomfortable and increases risk for infection or interrupts therapy.
6. **Use Teach-Back:** "We've talked about the reason we're using restraints on your father. Tell me that reason. I want to be sure you understand." Revise your instruction now or develop a plan for revised family caregiver teaching if family caregiver is not able to teach back correctly.	Teach-back is an evidence-based health literacy intervention that promotes patient engagement, patient safety, adherence, and quality. The goal of teach-back is to ensure that you have explained medical information clearly so that patients and their families understand what you have communicated to them (AHRQ, 2020b).

UNEXPECTED OUTCOMES AND RELATED INTERVENTIONS

1. Patient experiences impaired skin integrity.
   - Evaluate need for continued use of restraint and if alternatives can be used.
   - If restraint is still needed, be sure that it is applied correctly and provide adequate padding.
   - Check skin under restraint for abrasions, and remove restraints more often. Provide appropriate skin care and change wet or soiled restraints.
2. Patient becomes more confused or agitated.
   - Determine cause of behavior and eliminate if possible; consult with health care provider.
   - Determine need for more or less sensory stimulation and make any stimulation meaningful.
   - Reorient as needed and try restraint-free options.
3. Patient has neurovascular injury (e.g., cyanosis, pallor, and coldness of skin or complains of tingling, pain, or numbness).
   - Remove restraint immediately, stay with patient, and have health care provider notified.
   - Protect extremity from further injury.

RECORDING AND REPORTING

- Record restraint alternatives used and patient's response, patient's current behavior and medical condition, level of orientation, and patient or family caregiver's statement of understanding of the purpose of restraint and consent for application (if required by facility).
- Record in nurses' notes and restraint flow sheet the placement and purpose of restraint, type and location of restraint, condition of skin under restraint, time applied, ongoing assessment findings, and time restraint ended.
- Record patient's behavior after restraint application. Record times patient was assessed, attempts to use alternatives to restraint and patient's response, times restraint was released (temporarily and permanently), and patient's response when restraint was removed.
- Document evaluation of patient learning.
- Report any injury resulting from a restraint to registered nurse in charge and health care provider immediately
- During hand-off report, note the location and type of restraint, last time assessment was conducted, and findings.

▮ KEY POINTS

- Clinical judgment is complex when promoting safety because it requires understanding a patient's perspective of safety as well as the risks posed by any physical conditions.
- Vulnerable populations (e.g., infants, children, older adults, persons with chronic disease) are especially at risk for alterations in safety because of reduced access to health care, fewer resources, and increased morbidity.
- Common environmental hazards to safety include vehicle accidents, poisonings, conditions causing falls, and fire hazards.
- A nurse's role in managing environmental hazards is to educate patients about the common hazards in the home and at work, teaching them how to prevent injury and emphasizing the hazards to which patients are the most vulnerable.
- A patient's developmental stage can create threats to safety because of lifestyle choices, cognitive and mobility status, sensory impairments, and safety awareness.

- Use the Banner Mobility Assessment Tool (BMAT) or Timed Up and Go (TUG) test to determine a patient's ability to walk, need for assistance, and progress of balance, sit to stand, and walking.
- Conduct a fall risk assessment in a hospital by using a validated tool containing major risk categories such as age, fall history, elimination habits, high-risk medications, mobility, and cognition. At a minimum, conduct the assessment on admission, following a change in a patient's condition, after a fall, and when the patient is transferred to a new health care setting.
- A procedure-related accident is less likely to occur when you strictly follow policies and procedures or standards of nursing practice, and when you minimize distractions and interruptions.
- An assessment of psychosocial factors that influence patient safety must include a review of a patient's health literacy, cultural background, and perception of health and safety.
- Patients with actual or potential risks to safety require you to make clinical judgments necessary in selecting the patient-centered interventions that prevent and minimize the specific threats to safety.
- It is important to learn a patient's routines and willingness to make changes in the environment, because decisions on ways to change the environment require the patient's full participation.
- Evidence-based alternatives to physical restraints include offering diversional activities, using de-escalation techniques, providing visual and auditory stimuli, and promoting relaxation techniques.
- Before applying restraints, review the medical record for underlying cause(s) of agitation and cognitive impairment, assess whether the patient has a history of dementia or depression, and review medications and current laboratory values.
- When a patient is in a physical restraint, assess the placement of the restraint, and note skin integrity, pulses, skin temperature and color, and sensation of the restrained body part.

REFLECTIVE LEARNING

On her second visit to Mrs. Cohen's home, Kylie decides to take time to speak specifically with Meg. Kylie says, "You told me last week that you have moved into your mom's extra bedroom until she gets more strength. You said you were worried about her being alone. And I believe physical therapy visited last week as well?" Meg responds, "Yes. I've been here now about 10 days. PT came Thursday and began some exercises to make Mom's legs stronger for walking. My husband asked how long I might remain here."

- What further assessment information in this situation is the most important and of immediate concern for Kylie? [Recognize Cues]
- Meg says, "After watching PT I worry whether I can help my mom like I'm supposed to when she walks. What if she falls? Also, I haven't been getting much sleep since I've been here." Kylie responds, "Tell me what you think affects your sleep." Meg says, "I don't know, I just feel like I may not be doing enough." What family member conditions are consistent with this assessment information? [Analyze Cues]
- Which nursing diagnoses are most likely applicable in this caregiver situation? Which diagnoses are the most serious or the highest priority? [Prioritize Diagnoses]
- What actions might Kylie take to achieve desired outcomes for Meg and would likely benefit Mrs. Cohen as well? [Generate Solutions]
- Discuss three actions Kylie might implement to assist Mrs. Cohen. In what priority order should they be implemented? Explain. [Take Action]
- What evaluative measures would indicate that Kylie's actions were effective? [Evaluate Outcomes]

REVIEW QUESTIONS

1. You are caring for a patient in an intensive care unit (ICU) who has pulled out his own IV line. You have tried restraint alternatives. Which of the following would you assess to determine appropriateness or reason to physically restrain the patient? (Select all that apply.)
   1. Health care provider's order
   2. Patient's current behavior
   3. Current medications
   4. Health literacy
   5. Presence of fever
   6. Serum electrolytes
   7. Age
2. You complete a fall risk assessment on your assigned patient, who is 45 years old and has a history of cocaine use and liver failure. His laboratory results show an elevated prothrombin time. You determine that the patient is at high risk for falling. Which of the following measures are targeted to his fall risk status? (Select all that apply.)
   1. Using skid-proof footwear
   2. Scheduling any oral medications at least 2 hours before bedtime
   3. Placing a low bed in room
   4. Placing the nurse call system within patient's reach
   5. Using a bed exit alarm
   6. Providing patient with a protective head helmet when in chair or walking
3. During a home health visit a nurse observes a patient preparing lunch. Which of the following are safe practices to follow in the safe preparation and storage of food? (Select all that apply.)
   1. Always use a single cutting board to prepare foods for cooking.
   2. Refrigerate leftovers as soon as possible.
   3. Always buy vegetables in packages marked "prewashed."
   4. Cook meats to the proper temperature.
   5. Wash hands thoroughly before food preparation.
4. A nurse enters the hospital room of a patient who had a total knee replacement the day before and is sitting in a chair. The nurse is preparing to return the patient to bed. Which of the following pose potential safety risks? (Select all that apply.)
   1. A current safety inspection sticker is on the IV fluid pump.
   2. A walker is positioned near the patient's bedside.
   3. The hospital bed is in the high position.
   4. There is no gait belt at the bedside.
   5. The overbed table with the patient's glasses is positioned against the wall opposite the end of the bed.
5. Match the patient fall risks on the left with the correct risk factor category on the right.
   ___1. A 42-year-old patient who is recovering from anesthesia refuses assistance with walking to the bathroom.
   ___2. A 60-year-old patient with a history of falling in the last 6 months.
   ___3. A patient's walking path has spilled fruit juice on the floor.
   ___4. A 68-year-old patient recovering from a colon resection uses an IV pole to walk.
   ___5. Patient is unable to identify own fall risks.
   ___6. The physical therapist has not yet fitted a 62-year-old patient for a prescribed walker.

   A. Intrinsic risk
   B. Extrinsic risk

6. A nurse working on a surgery floor is assigned four patients. The nurse assesses each patient, noting behaviors and physical signs and symptoms. Which of the following patients is more likely to be violent toward the nurse?
   1. The first patient maintains eye contact with the nurse, is calm during the nurse's assessment, and asks questions frequently.
   2. The second patient is very drowsy, loses attention when the nurse asks questions, and mumbles when speaking.
   3. The third patient moves nervously in bed, swears and grimaces when trying to cough, and speaks in a low volume.
   4. The fourth patient speaks in a loud voice and becomes irritable when the nurse arrives to help walk the patient.

7. Match the intervention for promoting child safety on the left with the correct developmental stage on the right.
   1. Teach children proper bicycle and skateboard safety.
   2. Teach children how to cross streets and walk in parking lots.
   3. Teach children proper techniques for specific sports.
   4. Teach children not to operate electric toothbrushes while unsupervised.
   5. Teach children not to talk to or go with a stranger.
   6. Teach children not to eat items found in the grass.

   A. School-age child
   B. Preschooler

8. The nurse finds a 68-year-old woman wandering in the hallway and exhibiting confusion. The patient says she is looking for the bathroom. Which interventions are appropriate for this patient? (Select all that apply.)
   1. Ask the health care provider to order a restraint.
   2. Recommend insertion of a urinary catheter.
   3. Provide scheduled toileting rounds every 2 to 3 hours.
   4. Institute a routine exercise program for the patient.

5. Keep the bed in high position with side rails down.
6. Keep the pathway from the bed to the bathroom clear.

9. Place the following steps for applying a wrist restraint in the correct order:
   1. Pad the skin overlying the wrist.
   2. Insert two fingers under the secured restraint to be sure that it is not too tight.
   3. Be sure that the patient is comfortable and in correct anatomical alignment.
   4. Secure restraint straps to bedframe with quick-release buckle.
   5. Wrap limb restraint around wrist or ankle with soft part toward skin and secure snugly.

10. Match the fall prevention intervention on the left with the scientific rationale on the right.
    ___1. Prioritize nurse call system responses to patients at high risk.
    ___2. Place patient in a wheelchair with wedge cushion.
    ___3. Establish elimination schedule with bedside commode.
    ___4. Use a low bed for patient.
    ___5. Provide a hip protector.
    ___6. Place nonskid floor mat on floor next to bed.

    A. Maintains comfort and makes exit difficult
    B. Makes it difficult for patients with lower extremity weakness to stand
    C. Reduces slipping when walking
    D. Reduces fall impact
    E. Ensures rapid response for help
    F. Reduces chance of patient trying to get out of bed on own

Answers: 1. 1, 2, 3, 5, 6; **2.** 2, 3, 5, 6; **3.** 2, 4, 5; **4.** 3, 4, 5; **5.** 1A, 2A, 3B, 4B, 5A, 6B; **6.** 4; **7.** A: 1, 2, 3; B: 4, 5, 6; **8.** 3, 4, 6; **9.** 3, 1, 5, 2, 4; **10.** 1E, 2A, 3F, 4B, 5D, 6C.

Rationales for Review Questions can be found on the Evolve website.

REFERENCES

Agency for Healthcare Research and Quality (AHRQ): *20 tips to help prevent medical errors: a patient fact sheet,* 2020a. https://www.ahrq.gov/patients-consumers/care-planning/errors/20tips/index.html. Accessed January 21, 2021.

Agency for Healthcare Research and Quality (AHRQ): *Health literacy universal precautions toolkit 2nd edition,* 2020b. https://www.ahrq.gov/professionals/quality-patient-safety/quality-resources/tools/literacy-toolkit/healthlittoolkit2-tool5.html. Accessed January 25, 2021.

Agency for Healthcare Research and Quality (AHRQ): *Preventing falls in hospitals,* 2018. https://www.ahrq.gov/professionals/systems/hospital/fallpxtoolkit/index.html. Accessed on January 21, 2021.

Agency for Healthcare Research and Quality (AHRQ): *Culture of safety,* 2019. https://psnet.ahrq.gov/primers/primer/5/Culture-of-Safety. Accessed June 2, 2020.

Agency for Healthcare Research and Quality (AHRQ): *Health literacy universal precautions toolkit 2nd edition,* 2020b. https://www.ahrq.gov/professionals/quality-patient-safety/quality-resources/tools/literacy-toolkit/healthlittoolkit2-tool5.html. Accessed January 25, 2021.

Albert SM: *The role of human factors in healthcare. Chapter 11 impact of cultural, social, and community environments on home care,* Washington, DC, 2010, The National Academies Press.

Alzheimer's Association: 2018 Alzheimer's disease facts and figures, *Alzheimers Dement* 14:367–429, 2018.

American Academy of Pediatrics: *Safe sleep: recommendations,* 2021a. https://www.aap.org/en-us/advocacy-and-policy/aap-health-initiatives/safe-sleep/Pages/Safe-Sleep-Recommendations.aspx. Accessed January 21, 2021.

American Academy of Pediatrics (AAP): *Immunizations: vaccine hesitant parents,* 2021b. https://www.aap.org/en-us/advocacy-and-policy/aap-health-initiatives/immunizations/Pages/vaccine-hesitant-parents.aspx.

American Geriatrics Society (AGS): *For older people, medications are common; updated ags beers criteria® aims to make sure they're appropriate, too,* 2019. https://www.americangeriatrics.org/media-center/news/older-people-medications-are-common-updated-ags-beers-criteriar-aims-make-sure. Accessed January 23, 2021.

American Geriatrics Society (AGS) British Geriatrics Society (BGS), Panel on Prevention of Falls in Older Persons, American Geriatrics Society and British Geriatrics Society: Summary of the Updated American Geriatrics Society/British Geriatrics Society clinical practice guideline for prevention of falls in older persons, *J Am Geriatr Soc* 59:148–157, 2011. https://geriatricscareonline.org/ProductAbstract/updated-american-geriatrics-societybritish-geriatrics-society-clinical-practice-guideline-for-prevention-of-falls-in-older-persons-and-recommendations/CL014. Accessed June 22, 2021.

American Psychological association (APA): *APA dictionary of psychology,* 2020. https://dictionary.apa.org/mind-wandering. Accessed January 21, 2021.

Blue Cross Blue Shield: *Early childhood vaccination trends in America,* 2021. https://www.bcbs.com/the-health-of-america/reports/early-childhood-vaccination-trends-america. Accessed January 21, 2021.

Boltz M, et al: *Evidence-based geriatric nursing protocols for best practice,* ed 6, New York, 2020, Springer Publishing Company.

Campbell R: Environmental Health and Safety solutions, 2019, https://ei1.com/2019/06/27/increased-risk-workplace-violence-in-the-healthcare-industry/. Accessed January 21, 2021.

Centers for Disease Control and Prevention (CDC): *Important facts about falls,* 2017a. https://www.cdc.gov/homeandrecreationalsafety/falls/adultfalls.html. Accessed June 3, 2020.

Centers for Disease Control and Prevention (CDC): *Antineoplastic drug administration – effects of organizational safety practices and perceived safety climate on Use of exposure controls and adverse events,* 2017b. https://www.cdc.gov/niosh/topics/healthcarehsps/antidrugeffects.html. Accessed June 4, 2020.

Centers for Disease Control and Prevention (CDC): *Assessment: timed up and go,* 2017c. https://www.cdc.gov/steadi/pdf/TUG_test-print.pdf. Accessed January 25, 2021.

Centers for Disease Control and Prevention (CDC): *Poisoning prevention,* 2019a. https://www.cdc.gov/

safechild/poisoning/index.html. Accessed January 22, 2021.

Centers for Disease Control and Prevention (CDC): *What vaccines are recommended for you*, 2019b. https://www.cdc.gov/vaccines/adults/rec-vac/index.html. Accessed January 22, 2021.

Centers for Disease Control and Prevention (CDC): *Carbon monoxide, (CO) poisoning prevention*, 2020a. https://www.cdc.gov/nceh/features/copoisoning/index.html. Accessed January 21, 2020.

Centers for Disease Control and Prevention (CDC): *Foodborne germs and illnesses*, 2020b. https://www.cdc.gov/foodsafety/foodborne-germs.html. Accessed January 21, 2021.

Centers for Disease Control and Prevention (CDC): *Teen drivers: get the facts*, 2020c. https://www.cdc.gov/motorvehiclesafety/teen_drivers/teendrivers_factsheet.html. Accessed June 2, 2020.

Centers for Disease Control and Prevention (CDC): *Older adult drivers*, 2020d. https://www.cdc.gov/motorvehiclesafety/older_adult_drivers/index.html.

Centers for Disease Control and Prevention (CDC): *Corona virus disease 2019 (COVID 19): interim infection prevention and control recommendations for patients with suspected or confirmed coronavirus disease 2019 (COVID-19) in healthcare settings*, 2020e. https://www.cdc.gov/coronavirus/2019-ncov/hcp/infection-control-recommendations.html. Accessed January 22, 2021.

Centers for Disease Control and Prevention (CDC): *Common vaccine questions and safety concerns*, 2020f. https://www.cdc.gov/vaccinesafety/concerns/index.html. Accessed January 21, 2021.

Centers for Disease control and Prevention (CDC): *Immunization*, 2018; reviewed 2020g. https://www.cdc.gov/nchs/fastats/immunize.htm. Accessed January 21, 2021.

Centers for Disease Control and Prevention (CDC): *About school violence*, 2020h. https://www.cdc.gov/violenceprevention/youthviolence/schoolviolence/index.html. Accessed January 21, 2021.

Centers for Disease Control and Prevention (CDC): *STEADI-Older adult fall prevention*, 2021a, https://www.cdc.gov/steadi/index.html. Accessed July 28, 2021.

Centers for Disease Control and Prevention (CDC): *What is health literacy*, 2021b, https://www.cdc.gov/healthliteracy/learn/index.html. Accessed January 23, 2021.

Centers for Medicare and Medicaid Services (CMS): *State operations manual appendix a - survey protocol, regulations and interpretive guidelines for hospitals*, 2020. https://www.cms.gov/Regulations-and-Guidance/Guidance/Manuals/downloads/som107ap_a_hospitals.pdf. Accessed January 25, 2021.

Centers for Medicare and Medicaid Services (CMS): *Hospital-acquired conditions (present on admission indicator)*, 2019. http://www.cms.gov/HospitalAcqCond/06_Hospital-Acquired_Conditions.asp. Accessed January 21, 2021.

Chinai SA, et al: Taking advantage of the teachable moment: a review of learner-centered clinical teaching models, *West J Emerg Med* 19(1):28, 2018.

Crisis Prevention Institute (CPI): *CPI's top 10 de-escalation tips*, 2021. https://www.crisisprevention.com/Blog/October-2017/CPI-s-Top-10-De-Escalation-Tips-Revisited. Accessed January 22, 2021.

Durbin DR, Hoffman BD, Council on Injury, Violence, and Poison Prevention: Child passenger safety, *Pediatrics* 142(5):e20182460, 2018. https://pediatrics.aappublications.org/content/142/5/e20182460. Accessed January 21, 2021.

Ealey R, Cameron E: *Restraints: patient safety and regulatory compliance – extended version*, 2016, SSRN. http://dx.doi.org/10.2139/ssrn.2712831. Accessed June 10, 2020.

Environmental Protection Agency (EPA): *Learn about lead*, 2020. https://www.epa.gov/lead/learn-about-lead. Accessed January 21, 2021.

Epilepsy Foundation of America: *Seizure first aid*, 2020. https://www.epilepsy.com/sites/core/files/atoms/files/SFA%20Flier_HQ_8.5x11_PDF.pdf. Accessed January 21, 2021.

Electrical Safety Foundation International: *Space heater safety tips*, 2015. https://www.esfi.org/resource/space-heater-safety-tips-146. Accessed January 22, 2021.

Fehlberg EA, et al: Impact of the CMS no-pay policy on hospital-acquired fall prevention related practice patterns, *Innov Aging* 1(3):igx036, 2017.

Frampton SB, et al: *Harnessing evidence and experience to change culture: a guiding framework for patient and family engaged care*, Washington, DC, 2017, Discussion Paper, National Academy of Medicine. https://nam.edu/wp-content/uploads/2017/01/Harnessing-Evidence-and-Experience-to-Change-Culture-A-Guiding-Framework-for-Patient-and-Family-Engaged-Care.pdf. Accessed January 21, 2021.

Gorman G, et al: Physical activity, exercise and aging, *Wellbeing* 4(7):1–19, 2014.

Growdon ME, et al: Viewpoint: the tension between promoting mobility and preventing falls in the hospital, *JAMA Intern Med* 177(6):759, 2017.

Health Research & Educational Trust (HRET): *Preventing patient falls: a systematic approach from the joint commission center for transforming healthcare project*, Chicago, IL, 2016, Health Research & Educational Trust. http://www.hpoe.org/Reports-HPOE/2016/preventing-patient-falls.pdf. Accessed January 21, 2021.

Herdman TH, Kamitsuru S, editors: *NANDA International nursing diagnoses: definitions and classification*, ed 11, New York, 2018, Thieme, pp 2018–2020.

Hockenberry MJ, et al: *Wong's nursing care of infants and children*, ed 11, St Louis, 2019, Elsevier.

Hoffman RS, Weinhouse GL: *Management of moderate and severe alcohol withdrawal syndromes*, Up-to-date, 2020. https://www.uptodate.com/contents/management-of-moderate-and-severe-alcohol-withdrawal-syndromes. Accessed January 25, 2021.

Huntzinger A: AGS releases guideline for prevention of falls in older persons, *Am Fam Physician* 82(1):81–82, 2010. https://www.aafp.org/afp/2010/0701/p81.html. Accessed January 22, 2021.

Institute for Healthcare Improvement (IHI): *The ABCs of reducing harm from falls*, 2021. http://www.ihi.org/resources/Pages/ImprovementStories/ABCsofReducingHarmfromFalls.aspx. Accessed January 22, 2021.

Insurance Institute for Highway Safety (IIHS): *Fatality facts 2018 – Yearly Snapshot*, vol A, Arlington, 2019. https://www.iihs.org/iihs/topics/t/general-statistics/fatalityfacts/overview-of-fatality-facts.

Joszt L: *5 vulnerable populations in healthcare*, 2018, AJMC. https://www.ajmc.com/newsroom/5-vulnerable-populations-in-healthcare. Accessed January 21, 2020.

Kaslow N: *Teen suicides: what are the risk factors*? 2021. https://childmind.org/article/teen-suicides-risk-factors/. Accessed January 21, 2021.

Kochanek KD, et al: *Mortality in the United States, 2016*, Centers for Disease Control and Prevention: National Center for Health Statistics, 2017. https://www.cdc.gov/nchs/products/databriefs/db293.htm. Accessed January 21, 2021.

Lalande F: *Standardization of color-coded alerts: time for a national effort*, 2014, Patient Safety and Quality Healthcare. https://www.psqh.com/news/standardization-of-color-coded-alerts-time-for-a-national-effort/#:,:text5The%20American%20Hospital%20Association's%20recommended,John%20Companies%2C%202011). Accessed January 22, 2021.

Matz M: *Patient handling and mobility assessments*, ed 2, the facility guidelines institut, 2019. https://www.fgiguidelines.org/wp-content/uploads/2019/10/FGI-Patient-Handling-and-Mobility-Assessments_191008.pdf.

Meiner SE, Yeager JJ: *Gerontologic nursing*, ed 6, St. Louis, 2019, Elsevier.

National Alliance for Caregiving: *2020 report: caregiving in the US 2020*, 2021. https://www.caregiving.org/caregiving-in-the-us-2020/. 2021. Accessed January 22, 2021.

National Association of School Nurses: *School violence - the role of the school nurse: position statement*, 2018. https://www.nasn.org/advocacy/professional-practice-documents/position-statements/ps-violence.

National Capital Poison Center: *Poison control: first aid instructions for poisonings*, n.d. https://www.poison.org/articles/first-aid. Accessed January 22 2021.

National Fire Protection Association [NFPA]: *Fires in healthcare facilities*, 2017. https://www.nfpa.org/News-and-Research/Data-research-and-tools/Building-and-Life-Safety/Fires-in-Health-Care-Facilities. Accessed January 21, 2021.

National Institute on Aging: *Prevent falls and fractures*, 2017. https://www.nia.nih.gov/health/prevent-falls-and-fractures. Accessed January 21, 2021

National Institute for Occupational Safety and Health (NIOSH): *Workplace violence prevention for nurses*, 2020. https://www.cdc.gov/niosh/topics/violence/training_nurses.html. Accessed January 20, 2021.

National Safety Council: *Child safety*, 2021. https://www.nsc.org/home-safety/safety-topics/child-safety. Accessed January 21, 2021.

National Quality Forum (NQF): *NQF's mission and vision*, Washington, DC, 2021a. https://www.qualityforum.org/about_nqf/mission_and_vision/.

National Quality Forum (NQF): *List of SRE's*, Washington, DC, 2021b. https://www.qualityforum.org/Topics/SREs/List_of_SREs.aspx.

National Quality Forum (NQF): *Patient safety: safe practices - 2010*, Washington DC, 2021c. http://www.qualityforum.org/Projects/Safe_Practices_2010.aspx. Accessed January 21, 2021.

Occupational Safety and Health Administration (OSHA): *Hazard communication*, n.d. a, United States Department of Labor. https://www.osha.gov/dsg/hazcom/. Accessed January 21, 2021.

Occupational Safety and Health Administration (OSHA): *Workplace violence in healthcare - understanding the challenge*, 2015. https://www.osha.gov/Publications/OSHA3826.pdf. Accessed January 21, 2021.

Quality and Safety Education for Nurses (QSEN): *QSEN competencies: patient-centered care*, NC, 2020, University of North Carolina at Chapel Hill, Chapel Hill. http://qsen.org/competencies/pre-licensure-ksas/#patient-centered_care. Accessed January 21, 2020.

Robson Forensic: *Patient transport – expert article on injuries in healthcare facilities*, 2016. http://www.robsonforensic.com/articles/patient-transport-expert-witness. Accessed January 22, 2021.

Rose C: Choosing the right restraint, *Am Nurse Today* 10(1):28, 2015, https://www.americannursetoday.com/choosing-restraints/. Accessed January 25, 2021.

Stene J, et al: Workplace violence in the emergency department: giving staff the tools and support to report, *Perm J* 19(2):e113, 2015.

The Joint Commission: *Sentinel event alert - developing a reporting culture: learning from close calls and hazardous conditions*, (60), 2018. https://www.jointcommission.org/assets/1/18/SEA_60_Reporting_culture_FINAL.pdf. Accessed January 21, 2021.

The Joint Commission (TJC): *Comprehensive accreditation manual for hospitals*, Oakbrook Terrace, IL, 2020a, The Commission.

The Joint Commission (TJC): *Restraint and seclusion - enclosure beds, side rails and mitts*, 2020b. https://www.jointcommission.org/en/standards/standard-faqs/critical-access-hospital/provision-of-care-treatment-and-services-pc/000001668/. Accessed January 25, 2021.

The Joint Commission (TJC): *2021 National patient safety goals*, Oakbrook Terrace, IL, 2021a, The Commission. https://www.jointcommission.org/en/standards/national-patient-safety-goals/. Accessed January 21, 2021.

The Joint Commission (TJC): *Speak up campaigns*, 2021b. https://www.jointcommission.org/speakup.aspx. Accessed January 21, 2021.

Touhy T, Jett K: *Ebersole and Hess' gerontological nursing & healthy aging*, ed 6, St Louis, 2022, Elsevier.

U.S. Department of Veterans Affairs: *VA national center for patient safety – falls toolkit*, 2019. https://www.patientsafety.va.gov/professionals/onthejob/falls.asp. Accessed January 25, 2021.

U.S. Fire Administration (USFA): *U.S. fire statistics*, 2021. https://www.usfa.fema.gov/data/statistics/#causesR. Accessed January 21, 2021.

U.S. Food and Drug Administration (FDA): *A guide to bed safety bed rails in hospitals, nursing homes and home health care: the facts*, 2017. https://www.fda.gov/medicaldevices/productsandmedicalprocedures/generalhospitaldevicesandsupplies/hospitalbeds/ucm123676.htm. Accessed January 22, 2021.

U.S. Food and Drug Administration (FDA): *Best way to get rid of used needles and other sharps*, 2018. https://www.fda.gov/medicaldevices/productsandmedicalprocedures/homehealthandconsumer/consumerproducts/sharps/ucm263240.htm. Accessed January 22, 2021.

U.S. Food and Drug Administration (FDA): *Report a problem to the FDA*, 2020. https://www.fda.gov/safety/report-problem-fda?utm_campaign5 OCPharmacy&utm_medium5FDA-facebook-rxwiki&utm_source5OCPharmacy. Accessed January 21, 2021.

VA Healthcare: *Implementation guide for fall injury reduction, va national center for patient safety reducing preventable falls and fall-related injuries*, 2015. https://www.patientsafety.va.gov/docs/fallstoolkit14/falls_implementation_%20guide%20_02_2015.pdf. Accessed January 25, 2021.

Ventola CL: Immunization in the United States: recommendations, barriers, and measures to improve compliance, part 1: childhood vaccinations, *P T* 41(7):426, 2016.

Veterans Administration (VA): *Healthcare: implementation guide for fall injury reduction*, 2015. https://www.patientsafety.va.gov/docs/fallstoolkit14/falls_implementation_%20guide%20_02_2015.pdf. Accessed January 25, 2021.

Ward-Smith P, et al: Effectiveness of a bed alarm system to predict falls in an acute care setting, *Clin Nurs Stud* 3(1):1–4, 2015.

World Health Organization (WHO): *Falls*, 2018. http://www.who.int/news-room/fact-sheets/detail/falls. Accessed January 21, 2021.

World Health Organization: *Patient Safety*, 2021. http://www.euro.who.int/en/health-topics/Health-systems/patient-safety. Accessed June 2, 2020.

RESEARCH REFERENCES

Arnetz JE, et al: Understanding patient-to-worker violence in hospitals: a qualitative analysis of documented incident reports, *J Adv Nurs* 71(2):338, 2015.

Bellenger E, et al: Physical restraint deaths in a 13-year national cohort of nursing home residents, *Age Ageing* 46(4):688, 2017.

Berry S, Kiel D: *Falls: prevention in nursing care facilities and the hospital setting*, UpToDate, 2021. http://www.uptodate.com/contents/falls-prevention-in-nursing-care-facilities-and-the-hospital-setting. Accessed June 22, 2021.

Boynton T, et al: Implementing a mobility assessment tool for nurses: a nurse-driven assessment tool reveals the patient's mobility level and guides SPHM technology choices, *Am Nurse Today* 13, 2014. https://americannursetoday.com/wp-content/uploads/2014/09/ant9-Patient-Handling-Supplement-821a_Implementing.pdf. Accessed January 23, 2021.

Cadore EL, et al: Effects of different exercise interventions on risk of falls, gait ability, and balance in physically frail older adults: a systematic review, *Rejuvenation Res* 16(2):105, 2013.

Daniels J: Purposeful and timely nursing rounds: a best practice implementation project, *JBI Database System Rev Implement Rep* 14(1): 248, 2016.

Degrie L, et al: How do ethnic minority patients experience the intercultural care encounter in hospitals? A systematic review of qualitative research, *BMC Medical Ethics*, 18(1):2, 2017.

Dhalwani NN, et al: Association between polypharmacy and falls in older adults: a longitudinal study from England, *BMJ Open* 7:e016358, 2017. https://bmjopen.bmj.com/content/7/10/e016358. Accessed January 22, 2021.

Frew PM, Lutz CS: Interventions to increase pediatric vaccine uptake: an overview of recent findings, *Hum vaccin immunother* 13(11):2503, 2017.

Fuzhong L, et al: Exercise and fall prevention: narrowing the research-to-practice gap and enhancing integration of clinical and community practice, *J Am Geriatr Soc* 64(2):425, 2016.

Geiger-Brown J, et al: Sleep, sleepiness, fatigue, and performance of 12-hour shift nurses, *Chronobiol Int* 29(2):211, 2012.

Grass G, et al: Feasibility of early postoperative mobilization after colorectal surgery: a retrospective cohort study, *Int J Surg* 56:161, 2018.

Guirguis-Blake JM, et al: Interventions to prevent falls in older adults: updated evidence report and systematic review for the US Preventive Services Task Force, US Preventive Services Task Force Evidence Report, *JAMA*, 319(16):1705, 2018.

Hofmann H, et al: Use of physical restraints in nursing homes: a multicentre cross-sectional study, *BMC Geriatr* 15:129, 2015.

Institute of Medicine (IOM): *2000 To err is human: building a safer health system*, Washington, DC, 2008 National Academy Press. Preparing for an influenza pandemic: Personal protective equipment for healthcare workers. Washington, DC: The National Academies Press.

Jackson D, et al: Cues that predict violence in the hospital setting: findings from an observational study, *Collegian* 21:65, 2014.

Johnston M, Magnan MS: Using a fall prevention checklist to reduce hospital falls results of a quality improvement project, *AJN* 119(3):43, 2019.

Lange M, et al: Cognitive changes after adjuvant treatment in older adults with early-stage breast cancer, *Oncologist* 24(9), 62, 2019.

Luz C, et al: Do canes or walkers make any difference? Nonuse and fall injuries, *Gerontologist* 57(2):211, 2017.

Miake-Lye IM, et al: Inpatient fall prevention programs as a patient safety strategy: a systematic review, *Ann Intern Med* 158(5 Pt 2):390, 2013.

Nagamatsu LS, et al: Mind-wandering and falls risk in older adults, *Psychol Aging* 28(3):685, 2013.

Olsen CF, Bergland A: The effect of exercise and education on fear of falling in elderly women with osteoporosis and a history of vertebral fracture: results of a randomized controlled trial, *Osteoporos Int* 25(8):2017, 2014.

Park JI, et al: Risk factors associated with the fear of falling in community-living elderly people in Korea: role of psychological factors, *Psychiatry Investig* 14(6):894, 2017.

Patel KV, et al: High prevalence of falls, fear of falling, and impaired balance among older adults with pain in the United States: findings from the 2011 National Health and Aging Trends Study, *J Am Geriatr Soc* 62(10):1844, 2014.

Phelan EA, et al: Assessment and management of fall risk in primary care settings, *Med Clin North Am* 99(2):281, 2015.

Potter P, et al: Evaluation of sensor technology to detect fall risk and prevent falls in acute care, *Jt Comm J Qual Patient Saf* 43(8):414, 2017.

Schwappach DLB: Risk factors for patient-reported medical errors in eleven countries, *Health Expect* 17(3):321, 2014.

Severo IM, et al: Risk factors for falls in hospitalized adult patients: an integrative review, *Rev Esc Enferm USP* 48(3):537, 2014.

Shafran-Tikva S, et al: Violence against physicians and nurses in a hospital: how does it happen? A mixed-methods study, *Isr J Health Policy Res* 6:59, 2017.

Slade SC, et al: Effects of falls prevention interventions on falls outcomes for hospitalized adults: protocol for a systematic review with meta-analysis, *BMJ Open* 7(11):e017864, 2017, https://www.ncbi.nlm.nih.gov/pmc/articles/PMC5695509/. Accessed January 21, 2021.

Stark S, et al: Protocol for the home hazards removal program (HARP) study: a pragmatic, randomized clinical trial and implementation study, *BMC Geriatr*, 17:90, 2017. https://bmcgeriatr.biomedcentral.com/articles/10.1186/s12877-017-0478-4. Accessed January 21, 2021.

Uusi-Rasi K, et al: Exercise and vitamin D in fall prevention among older women: a randomized clinical trial, *JAMA Intern Med* 175(5):703, 2015.

Wang L, et al: Electrolyte disorders and aging: risk factors for delirium in patients undergoing orthopedic surgeries, *BMC Psychiatry* 16:418, 2016.

Wood SD, Bagian JP: A cognitive analysis of color-coded wristband use in health care, *Proc Hum Factors Ergon Soc Annu Meet* 55(1):281, 2011.

Zegers M, et al: Evidence-based interventions to reduce adverse events in hospitals: a systematic review of systematic reviews, *BMJ Open* 6(9):e012555, 2016.

Infection Prevention and Control

OBJECTIVES

- Explain the relationship between the infection chain and transmission of infection.
- Identify the normal defenses of the body against infection.
- Outline the events in the inflammatory response.
- Summarize the outcomes that result from the transmission of health care–associated infections.
- Analyze data to identify cues for patients most at risk for infection.
- Compare the signs/symptoms of a localized infection with those of a systemic infection.
- Explain the difference between medical and surgical asepsis.

- Select an intervention to prevent infection for each element of the infection chain.
- Explain the rationale for Standard Precautions.
- Demonstrate proper procedures for hand hygiene.
- Explain procedures for each isolation category.
- Apply personal protective equipment properly in the correct order.
- Explain how infection control measures differ in the home versus the hospital.
- Explain the postexposure process for health care workers after exposure to hepatis.

KEY TERMS

Aerobic
Anaerobic
Asepsis
Bactericidal
Bacteriostasis
Broad-spectrum antibiotics
Colonization
Communicable disease
Cough etiquette
Disinfection
Endogenous infection
Exogenous infection

Hand hygiene
Handwashing
Health care–associated infections (HAIs)
Iatrogenic infections
Immunocompromised
Infection
Infectious
Invasive
Localized
Medical asepsis
Multidrug-resistant organism
Pathogens

Reservoir
Standard Precautions
Sterile field
Sterilization
Suprainfection
Surgical asepsis
Susceptibility
Systemic
Vector
Virulence

MEDIA RESOURCES

http://evolve.elsevier.com/Potter/fundamentals/
- Review Questions
- Video Clips
- Concept Map Creator
- Concept Care Map

- Case Study with Questions
- Skills Performance Checklists
- Audio Glossary
- Content Updates
- Answers to QSEN Activity and Review Questions

Mrs. Andrews is a 76-year-old woman who lives alone and enjoys meeting regularly, when able, with women from her church for lunch and Bible study. Mrs. Andrews has type 2 diabetes mellitus that is controlled with oral hypoglycemic medications and diet. She also has urinary incontinence and degenerative disk disease. Mrs. Andrews was admitted to the hospital to have surgery on her lower spine. Kathy Jackson is a nursing student assigned to care for Mrs. Andrews postoperatively. Kathy knows that on the first postoperative day, care for Mrs. Andrews will be focused on pain control, improving Mrs. Andrews' mobility, and prevention of infection. Kathy also listens to Mrs. Andrews' concerns related to her urinary incontinence, her recovery from surgery, and her ability to care for herself at home. When Kathy assesses Mrs. Andrews, Kathy finds that

Mrs. Andrews is experiencing pain along her incision and difficulty log-rolling over to her side in bed. Mrs. Andrews also rates her pain as 6 out of 10. Mrs. Andrews needs to wear a brace when she is out of bed and needs an incisional dressing change because of contamination from urinary incontinence. The health care provider removes the dressing, leaving the incision open to air. The physical therapist plans to help Mrs. Andrews learn how to transfer to a chair after breakfast.

The incidence of infectious diseases such as AIDS, influenza, pneumonia, COVID-19, measles, and sexually transmitted infections are a significant public health problem in the United States and around the world (Centers for Disease Control and Prevention [CDC], 2021h). In 2016 there were 15.5 million visits to physician offices, with infectious and parasitic diseases as the primary diagnosis (CDC, 2021h). Multiple factors affect the spread of infectious diseases, such as humans' susceptibility, drug resistance, human tendency to avoid vaccination, and drug immunosuppression. The effects of infectious disease are constantly evolving; an infection that is considered a national or global threat one year could be eliminated the next (Contagion Live, 2019). For example, the opioid crisis has increased the number of people diagnosed with infective endocarditis because of IV injections, subsequently requiring cardiac valve replacements (CDC, 2021h). As a nurse it is critical to understand how infections develop, your patients' risk(s) for infection, and how to institute preventive measures.

The incidence of patients who develop infections as the direct result of contact with health care personnel is an increasing health problem. Based on a large sample of U.S. acute care hospitals, a CDC survey found that, on any given day, about 1 in 25 patients who are hospitalized have at least one health care–associated infection (HAI) (CDC, 2018b). Current trends, public awareness, and rising costs of health care have increased the importance of infection prevention and control. The Joint Commission (TJC) (2021) views HAIs as a patient safety issue. Nurses are essential to infection prevention and control by creating safe health care environments for patients, families, and health care staff. Patients in all health care settings are at risk for acquiring infections because of lower resistance to **pathogens**; increased exposure to pathogens, some of which may be resistant to most antibiotics; and **invasive** procedures. Health care workers are at risk for exposure to pathogens because of contact with patient blood, body fluids, and contaminated equipment and surfaces. By practicing basic infection prevention and control techniques, you avoid spreading pathogens to patients and sustaining an exposure when providing direct care.

Patients and their families need to be able to recognize sources of infection and understand measures used to protect themselves. Patient teaching must include basic information about infection, the various modes of transmission, and appropriate methods of prevention, such as hand hygiene and covering the mouth during a cough.

Health care workers protect themselves from contact with infectious material, sharps injury, and/or exposure to communicable diseases by applying knowledge of the infectious process and using appropriate personal protective equipment (PPE). Increases in multidrug-resistant organisms (MDROs), HAIs, and concern about diseases such as COVID-19 (SARS-CoV-2), hepatitis B virus (HBV) and hepatitis C virus (HCV), human immunodeficiency virus (HIV) infection, and tuberculosis (TB) require a greater emphasis on infection prevention and control techniques (CDC, 2019a, 2020e, 2021a).

SCIENTIFIC KNOWLEDGE BASE

Nature of Infection

It is important to know the difference between an infection and a colonization. An **infection** results when a pathogen invades tissues and begins growing within a host. **Colonization** is the presence and growth of microorganisms within a host but without tissue invasion or damage (Tweeten, 2018). Disease or infection results only if the pathogens multiply and alter normal tissue function. Some **infectious** diseases such as viral meningitis and pneumonia have a low risk or no risk for transmission. Although these illnesses can be serious for patients, they do not pose a risk to others, including caregivers.

If an infectious disease can be transmitted directly from one person to another, it is termed a **communicable disease** (Tweeten, 2018). If the pathogens multiply and cause clinical signs and symptoms, the infection is symptomatic. If clinical signs and symptoms are not present, the illness is termed asymptomatic. HCV is an example of a communicable

disease that can be asymptomatic. It is most efficiently transmitted through the direct passage of blood into the skin from a percutaneous exposure, even if the source patient is asymptomatic (CDC, 2018a, 2020b).

Chain of Infection

The presence of a pathogen does not mean that an infection will occur. Infection occurs in a cycle that depends on the presence of all of the following elements:
- An infectious agent or pathogen
- A reservoir or source for pathogen growth
- A port of exit from the reservoir
- A mode of transmission
- A port of entry to a host
- A susceptible host

Infection can develop if this chain remains uninterrupted (Fig. 28.1). Preventing infections involves patients' self-care activities or nurses' actions that will break the chain of infection.

Infectious Agent. Microorganisms include bacteria, viruses, fungi, and protozoa (Table 28.1). Microorganisms on the skin are either resident flora or transient flora. Resident organisms (normal flora) are permanent residents of the skin and within the body, where they survive and multiply without causing illness (CDC, 2019a; World Health Organization [WHO], 2009). The potential for microorganisms or parasites to cause disease depends on the number of microorganisms present; their **virulence**, or ability to produce disease; their ability to enter and survive in a host; and the susceptibility of the host. Resident skin microorganisms are not virulent. However, they can cause serious infection when surgery or other invasive procedures allow them to enter deep tissues or when a patient is severely **immunocompromised** (has an impaired immune system).

Transient microorganisms attach to the skin when a person has contact with another person or object during normal activities. For example, when you touch a contaminated gauze dressing or cleanse a patient following a diarrheal episode, transient bacteria adhere to your skin. These organisms may be readily transmitted unless removed using hand hygiene. If hands are visibly soiled with proteinaceous material or care is being provided to a patient with a spore-borne

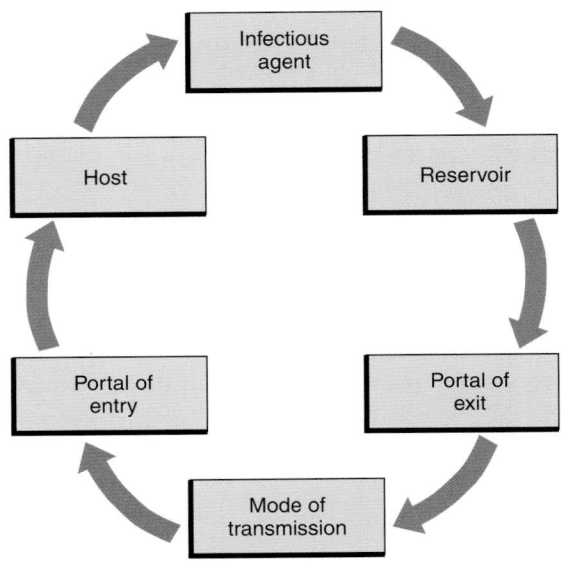

FIG. 28.1 Chain of infection.

TABLE 28.1 Infections and Common Causative Organisms

Infection Site	Common Organisms
Bronchitis	*S. pneumoniae, H. influenzae,* respiratory viruses
Device-related	Coagulase-negative staphylococci, *Corynebacterium* sp.
Empyema	*S. aureus,* streptococci, anaerobes
Endocarditis	*S. viridans, S. aureus,* enterococci
Gastroenteritis	*Salmonella* sp., *Shigella* sp., *Campylobacter* sp.
Meningitis	*E. coli* O157:H7, viruses
Pelvic inflammatory disease	*H. influenzae, N. meningitides, S. pneumoniae*
Peritonitis	*C. trachomatis, N. gonorrhoeae, Bacteroides* sp., Enterobacteriaceae
Pneumonia (community)	*S. pyogenes,* respiratory viruses
Pneumonia (health care–associated)	*S. pneumoniae, H. influenzae, M. pneumoniae, C. pneumoniae,* M. tuberculosis
Osteomyelitis	*Pseudomonas* sp., *S. aureus,* Enterobacteriaceae
Septic arthritis	*S. aureus*
Septicemia	*S. aureus, N. gonorrhoeae*
Skin	*S. pneumoniae, H. influenzae, S. pyogenes, S. aureus*
Urinary tract	*S. aureus, S. pyogenes, Candida* sp., dermatophytes

Modified from Brown M: Microbiology basics. In Grota P, editor: *APIC text of infection control and epidemiology,* Washington, DC, 2018, Association for Professionals in Infection Control and Epidemiology.

infection such as anthrax (*Bacillus anthracis*) or *Clostridium difficile* (*C. difficile*), washing with soap and water is the preferred practice (CDC, 2021c). If hands are not visibly soiled, use of an alcohol-based hand product or handwashing with soap and water is acceptable for disinfecting hands of health care workers. Hand hygiene is the most effective way to break the chain of infection (CDC, 2019a; WHO, 2009).

Reservoir. A reservoir is a place where microorganisms survive, multiply, and await transfer to a susceptible host. Common reservoirs are humans and animals (hosts), insects, food, water, and organic matter on inanimate surfaces (fomites). Frequent reservoirs for HAIs include health care workers, especially their hands; patients; equipment; and the environment. Human reservoirs are divided into two types: those with acute or symptomatic disease and those who show no signs of disease but are carriers of it. Humans can transmit microorganisms in either case. Animals, food, water, insects, and inanimate objects can also be reservoirs for infectious organisms. To thrive, organisms require a proper environment, including appropriate food, oxygen, water, temperature, pH, and light. A common way food becomes a reservoir is when it is not properly stored or refrigerated.

Food. Microorganisms require nourishment. Some such as *Clostridium perfringens,* the microbe that causes gas gangrene, thrive on organic matter. Others such as *Escherichia coli* consume undigested foodstuff in the bowel. Carbon dioxide and inorganic material such as soil provide nourishment for other organisms.

Oxygen. Aerobic bacteria require oxygen for survival and for multiplication sufficient to cause disease. Aerobic organisms cause more infections in humans than anaerobic organisms. An example of an aerobic organism is *Staphylococcus aureus.* Anaerobic bacteria thrive where little or no free oxygen is available. Anaerobes typically cause infections deep within the pleural cavity, in a joint, or in a deep sinus tract. An example of an anaerobic organism is *Bacteroides fragilis,* an organism that is part of the normal flora of the human colon but that can cause infection if displaced into the bloodstream or surrounding tissue following surgery or injury.

Water. Most organisms require water or moisture for survival. For example, a frequent place for microorganisms is the moist drainage from a surgical wound. Some bacteria assume a form, called a *spore,* that is resistant to drying and can live on inanimate surfaces for long periods. A common spore-forming bacterium is *C. difficile,* an organism that causes antibiotic-induced diarrhea.

Temperature. Microorganisms can live only in certain temperature ranges. Each species of bacteria has a specific temperature at which it grows best. The ideal temperature for most human pathogens is 20° to 43°C (68° to 109°F). For example, *Legionella pneumophila* grows best in water at 25° to 42°C (77° to 108°F). Cold temperatures tend to prevent growth and reproduction of bacteria (bacteriostasis). A temperature or chemical that destroys bacteria is bactericidal.

pH. The acidity of an environment determines the viability of microorganisms. Most microorganisms prefer an environment within a pH range of 5.0 to 7.0. Bacteria thrive in urine with an alkaline pH.

Light. Microorganisms thrive in dark environments such as those under dressings and within body cavities.

Portal of Exit. After microorganisms find a site to grow and multiply, they need to find a portal of exit if they are to enter another host and cause disease. Portals of exit include sites such as blood, skin and mucous membranes, respiratory tract, genitourinary (GU) tract, gastrointestinal (GI) tract, and transplacental (mother to fetus). Ebola virus, for example, is transmitted through direct contact with the blood or body fluids of a person who is sick with Ebola. However, droplets (e.g., splashes or sprays) of respiratory or other secretions from a person who is sick with Ebola can also be infectious. Therefore, certain precautions (called Standard, Contact, and Droplet Precautions) are recommended to prevent the transmission of the virus from patients who are sick with Ebola (CDC, 2021b). In the case of COVID-19, the virus is spread in three main ways (CDC, 2021f):

- Breathing in air when close to an infected person who is exhaling small droplets and particles that contain the virus.
- Having these small droplets and particles that contain virus land on the eyes, nose, or mouth, especially through splashes and sprays such as a cough or sneeze.
- Touching the eyes, nose, or mouth with hands that have the virus on them.

Skin and Mucous Membranes. The skin is considered a portal of exit because any break in the integrity of the skin and mucous membranes allows pathogens to exit the body. This may be exhibited by the presence of purulent drainage.

Respiratory Tract. Pathogens that infect the respiratory tract, such as the influenza virus, are released from the body when an infected person sneezes or coughs.

Urinary Tract. Normally urine is sterile. However, when a patient has a urinary tract infection (UTI), microorganisms exit during urination.

Gastrointestinal Tract. The mouth is one of the most bacterially contaminated sites of the human body, but most of the organisms are normal floras. A common flora in the stomach is *Helicobacter pylori,* the organism that can cause peptic ulcers. *Lactobacillus* and *Enterococcus* are bacteria found in the duodenum. Organisms that are normal floras in one person can be pathogens in another. For example, organisms exit when a person expectorates saliva. In addition, gastrointestinal portals of exit include emesis, bowel elimination, drainage of bile via surgical wounds, or drainage tubes.

Reproductive Tract. The female reproductive tract contains normal microbial flora that are developmentally and age related. *Lactobacilli* are typically the dominant organism in adult females, but other organisms present in the vagina include staphylococci, *Coryneform* bacteria, *Candida*, and *Streptococcus*. Organisms such as *Neisseria gonorrhoeae* and HIV exit through a man's urethral meatus or a woman's vaginal canal during sexual contact.

Blood. The blood is normally a sterile body fluid; however, in the case of communicable diseases such as HBV, HCV, or HIV, it becomes a reservoir for pathogens. Organisms exit from wounds, venipuncture sites, hematemesis, and bloody stool.

Modes of Transmission. Each disease has a specific mode of transmission. Often, you are able to do little about the infectious agent or the susceptible host, but by practicing infection prevention and control techniques such as hand hygiene and use of PPE, you interrupt the mode of transmission (Box 28.1). The same microorganism is sometimes transmitted by more than one route. For example, varicella zoster (chickenpox) is spread by the airborne route in droplet nuclei or by direct contact.

The major route of transmission for pathogens identified in the health care setting is the unwashed hands of the health care worker (CDC 2020a; WHO, 2009). Equipment used within the environment (e.g., a stethoscope, blood pressure cuff, or bedside commode) often becomes a source for the transmission of pathogens.

Portal of Entry. Organisms enter the body through the same routes they use for exiting. For example, during venipuncture when a needle pierces a patient's skin, organisms enter the body if proper skin preparation is not performed first. Factors such as a depressed immune system that reduce body defenses enhance the chances of pathogens entering the body.

Susceptible Host. Susceptibility to an infectious agent depends on an individual's degree of resistance to pathogens. Although everyone is constantly in contact with large numbers of microorganisms, an infection does not develop until an individual becomes susceptible to the strength and numbers of the microorganisms. A person's natural defenses against infection and certain risk factors (e.g., age, nutritional status, presence of chronic disease, trauma, and smoking) affect susceptibility (resistance) (Tweeten, 2018). Organisms such as *S. aureus* with resistance to key antibiotics are becoming more common in all health care settings but especially in acute care. The increased resistance of antibiotics in all health care settings is due to inappropriate prescribing of antibiotics and lack of infection control actions (CDC, 2021e).

The Infectious Process

By understanding the chain of infection, you have knowledge that is vital in preventing infections. When a patient is at risk for an infection, take precautions to break the infection chain. If a patient acquires an infection, observe for the signs and symptoms and take appropriate action to prevent its spread. Infections follow a progressive course (Box 28.2).

If an infection is localized (e.g., a wound infection), a patient usually experiences localized symptoms such as pain, tenderness, warmth, and redness at the wound site. An infection that affects the entire body instead of just a single organ or part is systemic and can become fatal if undetected and untreated.

The course of an infection influences the level of nursing care provided. The nurse is responsible for implementing infection control

practices, properly administering antibiotics, monitoring the response to drug therapy (see Chapter 31), using proper hand hygiene, following Standard Precautions, and using Isolation Precautions when necessary. Supportive therapy includes providing adequate nutrition and rest to bolster defenses of the body against the infectious process. The course of care for the patient often has additional effects on body systems affected by the infection.

Defenses Against Infection. The body has natural defenses that protect against infection. Normal floras, body system defenses, and inflammation are all nonspecific defenses that protect against microorganisms

---

BOX 28.1 Modes of Transmission

Contact
Direct
- Person-to-person (fecal, oral) physical contact between source and susceptible host.
- A health care provider's hands become contaminated by touching germs present on a patient, medical equipment, or high-touch surfaces, and the health care worker then carries the germs on the hands and spreads to a susceptible person.

Indirect
- Personal contact of susceptible host with contaminated inanimate object (e.g., needles or sharp objects, soiled linen, dressings, environment).

Droplet
- An infected person coughs or sneezes, creating droplets that carry germs short distances (within approximately 6 feet). These germs can land on a susceptible person's eyes, nose, or mouth and can cause infection (e.g., pertussis or meningitis).

Airborne
- Organisms are carried in droplet nuclei or residue or evaporated droplets suspended in air during coughing or sneezing. Germs are aerosolized by medical equipment or by dust from a construction zone (e.g., nontuberculous mycobacteria or *Aspergillus*).

Vehicles
- Contaminated items. For example, sharps injuries can lead to infections (e.g., HIV, HBV, HCV) when bloodborne pathogens enter a person through a skin puncture by a used needle or sharp instrument.
- Water
- Drugs, solutions
- Blood
- Food (improperly handled, stored, or cooked; fresh or thawed meats)

Vector
- External mechanical transfer (flies)
- Internal transmission such as parasitic conditions between **vector** and host such as:
  - Mosquito
  - Louse
  - Flea
  - Tick

Modified from Tweeten S: General principles of epidemiology. In Grota P, editor: *APIC text of infection control and epidemiology,* Washington, DC, 2018, Association for Professionals in Infection Control and Epidemiology; Centers for Disease Control and Prevention (CDC): How infections spread, 2016, https://www.cdc.gov/infectioncontrol/spread/index.html. Accessed June 29, 2020.

BOX 28.2 Course of Infection by Stage

Incubation Period

Interval between entrance of pathogen into body and appearance of first symptoms (e.g., chickenpox, 14 to 16 days after exposure; common cold, 1 to 2 days; influenza, 1 to 4 days; measles, 10 to 12 days; mumps, 16 to 18 days; Ebola 2 to 21 days (CDC, 2021b).

Prodromal Stage

Interval from onset of nonspecific signs and symptoms (malaise, low-grade fever, fatigue) to more specific symptoms. (During this time microorganisms grow and multiply, and patient may be capable of spreading disease to others.) For example, herpes simplex begins with itching and tingling at the site before the lesion appears.

Illness Stage

Interval when patient manifests signs and symptoms specific to type of infection. For example, strep throat is manifested by sore throat, pain, and swelling; mumps is manifested by high fever and parotid gland swelling.

Convalescence

Interval when acute symptoms of infection disappear. (Length of recovery depends on severity of infection and patient's host resistance; recovery may take several days to months.)

---

regardless of prior exposure. If any of these body defenses fail, an infection usually occurs and leads to a serious health problem.

Normal Flora. The body normally contains microorganisms that reside on the surface and deep layers of skin, in the saliva and oral mucosa, and in the GI and GU tracts. A person normally excretes trillions of microbes daily through the intestines. Normal floras do not usually cause disease when residing in their usual area of the body but instead participate in maintaining health.

Normal floras of the large intestine exist in large numbers without causing illness. They also secrete antibacterial substances within the walls of the intestine. The normal floras of the skin exert a protective, bactericidal action that kills organisms landing on the skin. The mouth and pharynx are also protected by floras that impair growth of invading microbes. Normal floras maintain a sensitive balance with other microorganisms to prevent infection. Any factor that disrupts this balance places a person at increased risk for acquiring a disease. For example, the use of **broad-spectrum antibiotics** for the treatment of infection can lead to **suprainfection**. A suprainfection develops when broad-spectrum antibiotics eliminate a wide range of normal flora organisms, not just those causing infection. When normal bacterial floras are eliminated, body defenses are reduced, which allows disease-producing microorganisms to multiply, causing illness (Arnold, 2018).

Body System Defenses. A number of body organ systems have unique defenses against infection (Table 28.2). The skin, respiratory tract, and GI tract are easily accessible to microorganisms. Pathogenic organisms can adhere to the surface skin, be inhaled into the lungs, or be ingested with food. Each organ system has defense mechanisms physiologically suited to its specific structure and function. For example, the lungs cannot completely control the entrance of microorganisms. However, the airways are lined with moist mucous membranes and cilia, hairlike projections that rhythmically beat to move mucus or cellular debris up to the pharynx to be expelled through swallowing.

Inflammation. The cellular response of the body to injury, infection, or irritation is termed *inflammation*. Inflammation is a protective vascular reaction that delivers fluid, blood products, and nutrients to an area of injury. The process neutralizes and eliminates pathogens or dead (necrotic) tissues and establishes a means of repairing body cells and tissues. Signs of localized inflammation include swelling, redness, heat, pain or tenderness, and loss of function in the affected body part. When inflammation becomes systemic, other signs and symptoms develop, including fever, increased white blood cells (WBCs), malaise, anorexia, nausea, vomiting, lymph node enlargement, or organ failure.

Physical agents, chemical agents, or microorganisms trigger the inflammatory response. Mechanical trauma, temperature extremes, and radiation are examples of physical agents. Chemical agents include external and internal irritants such as harsh poisons or gastric acid. Sometimes microorganisms also trigger this response.

After tissues are injured, a series of well-coordinated events occurs. The inflammatory response includes vascular and cellular responses, formation of inflammatory exudates (fluid and cells that are discharged from cells or blood vessels [e.g., pus or serum]), and tissue repair.

Vascular and Cellular Responses. Acute inflammation is an immediate response to cellular injury. Rapid vasodilation occurs, allowing more blood to be delivered near the location of the injury. The increase in local blood flow causes the redness and localized warmth at the site of inflammation.

Injury causes tissue damage and possibly necrosis. As a result, the body releases chemical mediators that increase the permeability of small blood vessels, and fluid, protein, and cells enter interstitial spaces. The accumulation of fluid appears as localized swelling (edema). Another sign of inflammation is pain; it is caused by the swelling of inflamed tissues, which increases pressure on nerve endings. As a result of the physiological inflammatory response, the involved body part may have a temporary loss of function. For example, a localized infection of the hand causes the fingers to become swollen, painful, and discolored. Joints become stiff because of swelling, but function of the fingers returns when inflammation subsides.

During the cellular response of inflammation, WBCs arrive at the site. WBCs pass through blood vessels and into the tissues. Phagocytosis is a process that involves the destruction and absorption of bacteria. Through the process of phagocytosis, specialized WBCs, called neutrophils and monocytes, ingest and destroy microorganisms or other small particles. If inflammation becomes systemic, other signs and symptoms develop. Leukocytosis, or an increase in the number of circulating WBCs, is the response of the body to WBCs leaving blood vessels. In the adult a serum WBC count is normally 5,000 to 10,000/mm^3 but typically rises to 15,000 to 20,000/mm^3 and higher during inflammation. Fever is caused by phagocytic release of pyrogens from bacterial cells, which causes a rise in the hypothalamic set point (see Chapter 29).

Inflammatory Exudate. Accumulation of fluid, dead tissue cells, and WBCs forms an exudate at the site of inflammation. Exudate may be serous (clear, like plasma), sanguineous (containing red blood cells), or purulent (containing WBCs and bacteria). Usually the exudate is cleared away through lymphatic drainage. Platelets and plasma proteins such as fibrinogen form a meshlike matrix at the site of inflammation to prevent its spread.

Tissue Repair. When there is injury to tissue cells, healing involves the defensive, reconstructive, and maturative stages (see Chapter 48). Damaged cells eventually are replaced with healthy new cells. The new cells undergo a gradual maturation until they take on the same structural characteristics and appearance as the previous cells. If inflammation is chronic, tissue defects sometimes fill with fragile granulation tissue that eventually takes the form of a scar at the completion of the healing process. The scar and surrounding tissues are not as strong as normal tissue and may be more susceptible to injury from pressure, shear, or friction; this increases the risk for pressure injury development (see Chapter 48).

TABLE 28.2 Natural Defense Mechanisms Against Infection

Defense Mechanisms	Action	Factors That May Alter Defense Mechanisms
Skin		
Intact multilayered surface (first line of defense against infection)	Provides barrier to microorganisms and antibacterial activity	Cuts, abrasions, puncture wounds, areas of maceration
Shedding of outer layer of skin cells	Removes organisms that adhere to outer layers of skin	Failure to bathe regularly, improper handwashing technique
Sebum	Contains fatty acid that kills some bacteria	Excessive bathing
Mouth		
Intact multilayered mucosa	Provides mechanical barrier to microorganisms	Lacerations, trauma, extracted teeth
Saliva	Washes away particles containing microorganisms Contains microbial inhibitors (e.g., lysozyme)	Poor oral hygiene, dehydration
Eye		
Tearing and blinking	Provides mechanisms to reduce entry (blinking) or help wash away (tearing) particles containing pathogens, thus reducing dose of organisms	Injury, exposure—splash/splatter of blood or other potentially infectious material into eye
Respiratory Tract		
Cilia lining upper airway, coated by mucus	Traps inhaled microbes and sweeps them outward in mucus to be expectorated or swallowed	Smoking, high concentration of oxygen and carbon dioxide, decreased humidity, cold air
Macrophages	Engulf and destroy microorganisms that reach alveoli of lung	Smoking
Urinary Tract		
Flushing action of urine flow	Washes away microorganisms on lining of bladder and urethra	Obstruction to normal flow by urinary catheter placement, obstruction from growth or tumor, delayed micturition
Intact multilayered epithelium	Provides barrier to microorganisms	Introduction of urinary catheter, continual movement of catheter in urethra can facilitate migration of organisms to bladder
Gastrointestinal Tract		
Acidity of gastric secretions	A gastric fluid pH of 1 to 2 is deleterious to many microbial pathogens	Administration of antacids Inhibition of acid secretion by various drugs
Rapid peristalsis in small intestine	Prevents retention of bacterial contents	Delayed motility resulting from impaction of fecal contents in large bowel or mechanical obstruction by masses
Vagina		
At puberty normal flora causing vaginal secretions to achieve low pH	Inhibits growth of many microorganisms	Antibiotics and oral contraceptives disrupting normal flora

Health Care–Associated Infections

Patients in health care settings, especially hospitals and long-term care facilities, have an increased risk of acquiring infections. **Health care–associated infections (HAIs)** result from the delivery of health services in a health care agency. They occur as the result of invasive procedures, antibiotic administration, the presence of **multidrug-resistant organisms** (MDROs), and breaks in infection prevention and control activities. The number of health care employees having direct contact with a patient, the type and number of invasive procedures, the therapy received, and the length of hospitalization further influence the risk of infection. Major sites for HAIs include surgical or traumatic wounds, urinary and respiratory tracts, and the bloodstream (Box 28.3).

HAIs significantly increase the cost of health care. This is especially true in older adults, who have increased susceptibility to these infections because of their affinity to chronic disease and the aging process (Box 28.4). Extended stays in health care institutions, increased disability, increased costs of antibiotics, and prolonged recovery times add to the expenses both of the patient and the health care institution and funding bodies (e.g., Medicare). Costs for HAIs are often not reimbursed; as a result, prevention has a beneficial financial impact and is an important part of patient care. TJC lists several national safety goals focusing on the care of older adults (e.g., preventing infection after surgery and ensuring that older adults receive influenza and pneumonia vaccines) (TJC, 2021).

Patients who develop HAIs often have multiple illnesses, are older adults, or are poorly nourished and may have a compromised immune system; thus, they are more susceptible to infections. In addition, many patients have a lowered resistance to infection because of underlying medical conditions (e.g., diabetes mellitus or cancer) that impair or damage the immune response of the body. Invasive treatment devices such as IV catheters or indwelling urinary catheters impair or bypass the natural defenses of the body against microorganisms. Critical illness increases patients' susceptibility to infections, especially multidrug-resistant bacteria. Meticulous hand hygiene practices, the use of chlorhexidine washes for bathing and personal hygiene care, advances in intensive care unit (ICU) infection prevention, and the creation of evidence-based bundles help to prevent these infections (Deprez et al., 2019; Donskey and Deshpande, 2016).

BOX 28.3   Examples of Sites for and Causes of Health Care–Associated Infections

Improperly performing hand hygiene increases patient risk for all types of health care–associated infections.

Urinary Tract
- Unsterile insertion of urinary catheter
- Improper positioning of the drainage tubing
- Open drainage system
- Catheter and tube becoming disconnected
- Drainage bag port touching contaminated surface
- Improper specimen collection technique
- Obstructing or interfering with urinary drainage
- Urine in catheter or drainage tube being allowed to reenter bladder (reflux)
- Repeated catheter irrigations
- Improper perineal hygiene

Surgical or Traumatic Wounds
- Improper skin preparation before surgery (e.g., shaving versus clipping hair; not performing a preoperative bath or shower)
- Failure to clean skin surface properly
- Failure to use aseptic technique during operative procedures and dressing changes
- Use of contaminated antiseptic solutions

Respiratory Tract
- Contaminated respiratory therapy equipment
- Failure to use aseptic technique while suctioning airway
- Improper disposal of secretions

Bloodstream
- Contamination of intravenous (IV) fluids by tubing
- Insertion of drug additives to IV fluid
- Addition of connecting tube or stopcocks to IV system
- Improper care of needle insertion site
- Contaminated needles or catheters
- Failure to change IV access at first sign of infection or at recommended intervals
- Improper technique during administration of multiple blood products
- Improper care of peritoneal or hemodialysis shunts
- Improperly accessing an IV port

BOX 28.4   FOCUS ON OLDER ADULTS

Risks for Infection

- An age-related functional deterioration in immune system function, termed immune senescence, increases the susceptibility of the body to infection and slows overall immune response (Meiner and Yeager, 2019; Pawelec, 2018).
- Older adults are less capable of producing lymphocytes to combat challenges to the immune system. When antibodies are produced, the duration of their response is shorter, and fewer cells are produced (Roach, 2018).
- Risks associated with the development of infections or health care–associated infections in older patients include poor nutrition and unintentional weight loss, lack of exercise, poor social support, and low serum albumin levels (Meiner and Yeager, 2019).
- Flu and pneumonia vaccinations are recommended for older adults to reduce their risk for infectious diseases.
- Teach older adults and their families how to reduce the risk for infections by using proper hand hygiene practices.

HAIs are either exogenous or endogenous. An **exogenous infection** comes from microorganisms found outside the individual, such as *Salmonella*, *Clostridium tetani*, and *Aspergillus*. These microorganisms do not exist as normal floras. An **endogenous infection** occurs when part of the patient's flora becomes altered and an overgrowth occurs (e.g., staphylococci, enterococci, yeasts, and streptococci). This often happens when a patient receives broad-spectrum antibiotics that alter the normal floras. When sufficient numbers of microorganisms normally found in one body site move to another site, an endogenous infection develops. The number of microorganisms needed to cause an HAI depends on the virulence of the organism, the susceptibility of the host, and the body site affected.

Iatrogenic infections are a type of HAI caused by an invasive diagnostic or therapeutic procedure. For example, procedures such as a bronchoscopy and treatment with broad-spectrum antibiotics increase the risk for certain infections. Use clinical judgment when practicing aseptic techniques during the performance of procedures. Consider a patient's condition and the risks for infection, and follow basic infection prevention and control policies and procedures as well as interventions unique to the patient's needs to reduce the risk of HAIs. Always anticipate how the approach to care increases or decreases the patient's risk for infection.

REFLECT NOW

What are the nursing strategies you can use to break the chain of infection when you care for a patient at risk for a urinary tract infection?

NURSING KNOWLEDGE BASE

Body substances such as feces, urine, and wound drainage contain potentially infectious microorganisms. Thus health care workers are at risk for exposure to microorganisms during routine care activities in the hospital and/or home setting (Fiutem, 2018). The meticulous use of specific infection prevention practices reduces the risk of cross-contamination and transmission of infection to noninfected patients when caring for a patient with a known or suspected infection.

Serious infections are ongoing challenges to clinicians, and they create physical and emotional responses, including feelings of anxiety, frustration, loneliness, and anger in patients and/or their families (Currie et al., 2018). These feelings worsen when patients are isolated to prevent transmission of a microorganism to other patients or health care staff. Isolation disrupts normal social relationships with visitors and caregivers. Patient safety is usually an additional risk for a patient on isolation precautions (Monsees, 2018). For example, an older patient with a chronic illness is more at risk for an HAI. When family members fear the possibility of developing the infection, they may avoid contact with the patient. Some patients perceive the simple procedures of proper hand hygiene and gown and glove use as evidence of rejection. Help patients and families reduce some of these feelings by discussing the disease process, explaining isolation procedures, and maintaining a friendly, understanding manner.

When establishing a plan of care, it is important to know how a patient reacts to an infection or infectious disease. The challenge is to identify and support behaviors that maintain human health or prevent infection.

Factors Influencing Infection Prevention and Control

Multiple factors influence a patient's susceptibility to infection. It is important to understand how each of these factors alone or in combination increases this risk. When more than one factor is present, a patient's susceptibility often increases, which affects length of stay, recovery time, and/or overall level of health following an illness. Understanding these factors helps you to analyze assessment data and cues, identify priority problems, decide on patient outcomes, and deliver patient-centered care for a patient who has an infection or is at risk for one.

Age. Throughout life a person's susceptibility to infection changes. For example, an infant has immature defenses against infection. Born with only the antibodies provided by the mother, an infant's immune system is incapable of producing the necessary immunoglobulins and WBCs to adequately fight some infections. However, breastfed infants often have greater immunity than bottle-fed infants because they receive their mother's antibodies through the breast milk. As the child grows, the immune system matures, but the child is still susceptible to organisms that cause the common cold, intestinal infections, and infectious diseases such as mumps, measles, and chickenpox (if not vaccinated). Since 2000, there has been a major effort to vaccinate all children against all infectious diseases for which vaccines are available. As a result, vaccine-preventable disease levels are at or near record lows (CDC, 2018e).

The young or middle-age adult has refined defenses against infection. Viruses are the most common cause of communicable illness in young or middle-age adults. Young women are most likely to develop urinary tract infections (UTIs), vaginal yeast infections, and human papillomavirus (HPV). Although UTIs are relatively uncommon in men, prostatitis (infection of the prostate gland) affects men of all ages but tends to be more common in men 50 or younger (Mayo Clinic, 2021).

Defenses against infection change with aging (Roach, 2018). The immune response, particularly cell-mediated immunity, declines. Older adults also undergo alterations in the structure and function of the skin, urinary tract, and lungs. For example, the skin loses its turgor, and the epithelium thins. As a result, it is easier to tear or abrade the skin, which increases the potential for invasion by pathogens. In addition, older adults who are hospitalized or reside in an assisted-living or residential care facility are at risk for airborne infections. Ensuring that health care workers are vaccinated against influenza reduces the transmission of this illness in older adults (CDC, 2021g).

Sex. Women and men differ in their immune responses to infections (Ingersol, 2017). Only recently have the biological pathways responsible for these sex-based differences in the manifestations of infectious diseases been researched. Besides genetic factors, these differences can be explained through the greatly divergent and changing levels of sex steroid hormones and their interplay with the immune system. Estrogens promote (but androgens suppress) immune responses during infections and after vaccination. They also increase the risk for autoimmune diseases (Gubbels Bupp et al., 2018). In vaccinated adults, sex-related differences have been observed in immunogenicity (ability of an antigen to provoke an immune response in the body of a human) and clinical effectiveness of influenza, pneumococcal, tetanus, diphtheria, and herpes zoster vaccines (Gubbels Bupp et al., 2018).

Nutritional Status. A patient's nutritional health directly influences susceptibility to infection. A reduction in the intake of protein and other nutrients such as carbohydrates and fats reduces body defenses against infection and impairs wound healing (see Chapter 48). Patients with illnesses or problems that increase protein requirements, such as extensive burns and febrile conditions, are at further risk. For example, patients who have undergone surgery require increased protein. A thorough diet history is necessary. Determine a patient's normal daily nutrient intake and whether preexisting problems such as nausea, impaired swallowing, or oral pain alter food intake. Confer with a registered dietitian to assist in calculating the calorie count of foods ingested.

Stress. The body responds to emotional or physical stress by the general adaptation syndrome (see Chapter 37). During the alarm stage the basal metabolic rate increases as the body uses energy stores. Adrenocorticotropic hormone increases serum glucose levels and decreases unnecessary antiinflammatory responses through the release of cortisone. If stress continues or becomes intense, elevated cortisone levels result in decreased resistance to infection. Continued stress leads to exhaustion, which causes depletion in energy stores, and the body has no resistance to invading organisms. The same conditions that increase nutritional requirements, such as surgery or trauma, also increase physiological stress.

Disease Process. Patients with diseases of the immune system are at particular risk for infection. Leukemia, AIDS, lymphoma, and aplastic anemia are conditions that compromise a host by weakening defenses against infectious organisms. For example, patients with leukemia are unable to produce enough WBCs to fight off infection. Patients with HIV are often unable to ward off simple infections and are prone to opportunistic infections.

Patients with chronic diseases such as diabetes mellitus and multiple sclerosis are also more susceptible to infection because of general debilitation and nutritional impairment. Diseases that impair body system defenses such as emphysema and bronchitis (which impair ciliary action and thicken mucus), cancer (which alters the immune response), and peripheral vascular disease (which reduces blood flow to injured tissues) increase susceptibility to infection. Patients with burns have a high susceptibility to infection because of the damage to skin surfaces. The greater the depth and extent of the burns, the higher is the risk for infection.

Kathy plans her care for Mrs. Andrews for the next day. She spends time reading to increase her knowledge of degenerative disk disease and spinal surgery and how patients progress with mobility after surgery. Because Mrs. Andrews just had surgery, Kathy reviews information on risk factors for complications after surgery, paying attention to ways to prevent infection in patients after surgery and how best to manage pain following back surgery. Kathy also reads about wound healing after surgery so that she can develop an appropriate plan of care for Mrs. Andrews. She also knows that Mrs. Andrews has type 2 diabetes mellitus, so Kathy wants to know more about how diabetes affects wound healing. Kathy reads up on the importance of nutrition in diabetes and wound healing so that she can help Mrs. Andrews select foods that are needed for healing.

REFLECT NOW

Consider the care of an older adult patient who is receiving chemotherapy for a recent cancer diagnosis. What risk factors for infection would you need to address when planning care for this patient?

❖ NURSING PROCESS

Your clinical judgment in the care of patients with infection will involve applying the nursing process and critical thinking so that you can make appropriate clinical decisions for a patient-centered approach to care.

◆ Assessment

Perform a thorough assessment of each patient, including a patient's current condition, any history of previous health problems involving

TABLE 28.3 Host Characteristics Influencing Susceptibility to and Severity of Disease

Characteristic	Examples
Age	"Childhood diseases" (e.g., measles, chickenpox) are seen more frequently in children, whereas chronic diseases, such as heart disease or chronic obstructive pulmonary disease, occur more frequently in older patients.
Sex	Reproductive diseases are sex-specific. Sex influences immune response and susceptibility to certain infections.
Ethnicity	Tay-Sachs disease occurs in Jews of European descent.
Socioeconomic status	Socioeconomic status influences the ability to purchase food, pay for immunizations, and obtain health care services.
Marital status	Some studies of stress-related diseases have shown marital status to be a factor influencing susceptibility.
Lifestyle	Homelessness increases susceptibility due to poor nutrition and exposure to pathogens.
Heredity	Sickle cell anemia influences susceptibility.
Nutritional status	Inadequate nutrition reduces immune function.
Occupation	Coal miners are at risk for black lung. Prison guards or social workers involved with immigrants or asylum seekers originating from areas with a high tuberculosis (TB) prevalence are at risk for contacting TB.
Immunization status	Those who have not been vaccinated for measles are at risk for the disease.
Diagnostic/therapeutic procedures	Patients who have had an organ transplant have an increased risk of infection.
Medications	Steroid use increases the risk of infection.
Pregnancy	Women who are pregnant and are positive for tuberculosis are more likely to reactivate.
Trauma	Injury may provide a portal of entry for organisms and triggers an inflammatory response that may increase the risk of infection.

Modified from Tweeten SM: General principles of epidemiology. In Grota P, editor: *APIC text of infection control and epidemiology,* Washington, DC, 2018, Association for Professionals in Infection Control and Epidemiology.

infection, and potential risks posed in the patient's current environment. As you conduct your assessment, apply knowledge of the infectious process, the patient's diagnosed medical problem(s), and your previous experience with patients with infection to focus on your physical examination.

Through the Patient's Eyes. Determine how patients feel about their illness or risk for infection. Has a patient had experiences in the past that will affect expectations for care? For example, a patient undergoing a second surgical procedure might have different expectations than a patient who is having surgery for the first time regarding the prevention of wound infection. Perhaps there were problems the first time with intravenous management or care of the patient's dressing that will cause the patient who is having the second surgical procedure to be anxious and set greater expectations. Also assess a patient's knowledge of risk factors that increase the susceptibility for developing an infection (Table 28.3) to help you plan appropriate patient education.

Some patients with infection have a variety of problems, including physical, psychological, social, or economic needs. Patients with chronic or serious infection, especially communicable infections such as TB or AIDS, experience psychological and social problems from self-imposed isolation or rejection by friends and family. Ask the patient how an infection affects the ability to maintain relationships and perform activities of daily living. Determine whether chronic infection has drained the patient's financial resources. Ask about the patient's expectations of care and preferences (e.g., how a procedure should be performed), and determine how much the patient wants to be involved in planning care. Some patients and their families wish to know more about the disease process, whereas others want to know only the interventions necessary to treat the infection. Encourage patients to verbalize their expectations so that you are able to establish interventions to meet patients' priorities.

Risk Factors. A review of a patient's clinical condition can begin with the identification of risk factors. Ask specific questions to determine the patient's and family's awareness of any risks for infection (Box 28.5). Assess the patient's age, nutritional status, presence of chronic illnesses or stress, and presence of disease processes to identify factors that influence

BOX 28.5 Nursing Assessment Questions

Risk Factors
- Tell me what vaccinations you have received in the last 5 years.
- Describe for me any illnesses or diseases that you have and those for which you receive treatment.
- Tell me about any recent diagnostic testing you have undergone, such as colonoscopy or cystoscopy.
- Describe what you normally eat during a day.

Possible Existing Infections
- Do you have or feel as if you have a fever?
- Do you have any cuts or wounds with drainage?
- Do you have any pain/burning during urination?
- Do you have a cough? Is there any sputum?

Recent Travel History
- Have you traveled outside the United States in the past 6 months?
- Are you a resident of or have you traveled within the past 21 days to a country where an Ebola outbreak is occurring (CDC, 2021b)?
- Were any of the people you visited or traveled with ill?

Medication History
- List for me the medications you are currently taking.
- Describe for me the doses of each medication you are supposed to take daily.
- Describe any over-the-counter medications or herbals that you are currently taking.

Stressors
- Tell me about any major lifestyle change occurring, such as the loss of employment or place of residence, divorce, or disability.

susceptibility to infection. Gather information about each factor through your interview and the patient's medical history.

Clinical Appearance. Perform a physical assessment (see Chapter 30) of a patient, examining areas involved in an infection as well as areas where risk of infection exists. The signs and symptoms of infection may

TABLE 28.4 Laboratory Tests to Screen for Infection

Laboratory Value	Normal (Adult) Values	Indication of Infection
White blood cell (WBC) count	5000-10,000/mm³	Increased in acute infection, decreased in certain viral or overwhelming infections
Erythrocyte sedimentation rate	Up to 15 mm/hr for men and 20 mm/hr for women	Elevated in presence of inflammatory process
Iron level	80-180 mcg/mL for men 60-160 mcg/mL for women	Decreased in chronic infection
Cultures of urine and blood	Normally sterile, without microorganism growth	Presence of infectious microorganism growth
Cultures and Gram stain of wound, sputum, and throat	No WBCs on Gram stain, possible normal flora	Presence of infectious microorganism growth and WBCs on Gram stain
Differential Count (Percentage of Each Type of White Blood Cell)		
Neutrophils	55%-70%	Increased in acute suppurative (pus-forming) infection, decreased in overwhelming bacterial infection (older adult)
Lymphocytes	20%-40%	Increased in chronic bacterial and viral infection, decreased in sepsis
Monocytes	2%-8%	Increased in protozoan, rickettsial, and tuberculosis infections
Eosinophils	1%-4%	Increased in parasitic infection
Basophils	0.5%-1.5%	Normal during infection

Adapted from Pagana KD, et al: *Mosby's diagnostic and laboratory test reference*, ed 14, St Louis, 2019, Elsevier.

be local or systemic. Localized infections are most common in areas of skin or mucous membrane breakdown, such as surgical and traumatic wounds, pressure injuries, oral lesions, and abscesses.

To assess an area for localized infection, first inspect it for redness, warmth, and swelling caused by inflammation. Because there may be drainage from open lesions or wounds, wear clean gloves. Infected drainage may be yellow, green, or brown, depending on the pathogen. For example, green nasal secretions often indicate a sinus infection. Ask the patient about pain or tenderness around the site. Some patients experience tightness and pain caused by edema. If the infected area is large enough, movement is restricted. Gentle palpation of an infected area usually results in some degree of tenderness. Wear personal protective equipment (PPE), especially protective eyewear and a surgical mask, when there is a risk for splash or spray with blood or body fluids.

Systemic infections cause more generalized symptoms than local infection. These symptoms often include fever, fatigue, nausea/vomiting, and malaise. Lymph nodes that drain the area of infection often become enlarged, swollen, and tender during palpation. For example, an abscess in the peritoneal cavity causes enlargement of lymph nodes in the groin. An infection of the upper respiratory tract causes cervical lymph node enlargement. If an infection is serious and widespread, all major lymph nodes may enlarge.

Systemic infections sometimes develop after treatment for localized infection has failed. Be alert for changes in a patient's level of activity and responsiveness. As systemic infections develop, an elevation in body temperature can lead to episodes of increased heart and respiratory rates and low blood pressure. Involvement of major body systems produces specific symptoms. For example, a pulmonary infection results in a productive cough with purulent sputum. A UTI results in cloudy, foul-smelling urine.

An infection does not always present with typical signs and symptoms in all patients. For example, in some older adults an infection may be advanced before it is identified. Because of the aging process, there is a reduced inflammatory and immune response. Older adults have increased fatigue and diminished pain sensitivity. A reduced or absent fever response often occurs from chronic use of aspirin or nonsteroidal antiinflammatory drugs. Atypical symptoms such as confusion, incontinence, or agitation may be the only symptoms of an infectious illness (Roach, 2018). For example, as many as 20% of older adults with pneumonia do not have the typical signs and symptoms of fever, shaking,

chills, and colored productive sputum. Often the only symptoms are an unexplained increase in heart rate, confusion, or generalized fatigue. A pneumonia vaccine is available and recommended for all people with chronic respiratory problems and those over 65 years of age.

Status of Defense Mechanisms. As you conduct your physical assessment, determine the status of normal defense mechanisms against infection. For example, any break in the skin such as an ulcer on the foot of a patient who has diabetes is a potential site for infection. Any reduction in the primary or secondary defenses of the body against infection, such as a weakened ability to cough, places a patient at increased risk.

Medical Therapy. Some drugs and medical therapies compromise immunity, increasing the risk for infection. Assess your patient's medication history to determine whether the patient takes any medications that increase infection susceptibility (see Box 28.5). This includes any over-the-counter medications and herbal supplements. A review of therapies received within the health care setting further reveals risks. For example, adrenal corticosteroids, prescribed for several conditions, are antiinflammatory drugs that cause protein breakdown and impair the inflammatory response against bacteria and other pathogens. Corticosteroids and TNF (tumor necrosis factor) inhibitors are two medications that increase the chance of getting a fungal infection (CDC, 2020c). Cytotoxic and antineoplastic drugs attack cancer cells but also cause the side effects of bone marrow depression and normal cell toxicity, which affects the response of the body against pathogens.

Travel History. Review a patient's recent travel history to determine possible exposure to communicable diseases. Also assess whether any immediate family members have traveled and presented risks to the patient (see Box 28.5). A person's exposure depends on the presence of infectious agents in the area visited. The risk of becoming infected will vary according to the purpose of the trip and the itinerary within the area; the standards of accommodation, hygiene, and sanitation; and the behavior of the traveler (WHO, 2020).

Laboratory Data. Review laboratory data as soon as the results are available. Laboratory values such as increased WBCs and/or a positive blood culture often indicate infection (Table 28.4). However, laboratory values are not enough to detect infection. It is possible that a contaminated specimen was collected because of poor technique (e.g., a blood sample is mixed with IV fluid because it has been improperly collected from an indwelling line; a urine specimen is contaminated because of poor perineal cleansing). You need to assess other clinical signs of infection. A culture result may show growth of an organism in the absence of infection. For example, in the older adult bacterial growth in urine without clinical symptoms does not always indicate the presence of a UTI (Roach, 2018). Also know that laboratory values often vary from laboratory to laboratory. Be sure to know the standard range of laboratory values for the laboratory in your facility.

Kathy's previous experience with caring for patients after surgery helps her assess Mrs. Andrews' pain levels, knowing that it is important to treat the patient's pain after surgery. Mrs. Andrews rated her pain an 8 out of 10 but said that the pain medication helped to make the pain tolerable at a rating of 2 out of 10. When the pain is more acute, Mrs. Andrews is less willing to move or get up to the chair. Kathy also auscultates Mrs. Andrews' lungs to make sure that she is not developing postoperative atelectasis. Mrs. Andrews' vital signs are BP 126/76, P 78, R 14, and T 37.1° C (98.8°F). After the health care provider removes Mrs. Andrews' incisional dressing, Kathy notes that the edges of the incision are approximated and that there is no redness or drainage from the wound. Kathy is present when the physical therapist helps Mrs. Andrews into the chair. The patient's gait is slow, and Kathy notes that Mrs. Andrews grimaces and moans when getting into her back brace and moving into the chair. Kathy also notes that she was unsteady on her feet and that it took two people to transfer Mrs. Andrews the first time. Kathy consults with the physical and occupational therapist on how she can assist Mrs. Andrews with her mobility. Once the patient is settled in the chair, Kathy focuses her attention on the environment in Mrs. Andrews' room, rearranging furniture and items so that they are within Mrs. Andrews' reach in the chair. Mrs. Andrews states, "It was really hard to get up. I am not sure how I will be able to take care of myself at home if I cannot walk very well. It was also awfully hard for me to turn over in bed last night because of the pain. I hope that I do not hurt that much when I get home." Mrs. Andrews also states, "I am worried about my incision getting wet and then infected because I have these continued problems of not being able to hold my urine." Kathy notes in the medical record that Mrs. Andrews' perineal area was slightly red.

REFLECT NOW

What questions would you ask a patient who just returned from a mission trip from another country when assessing for a possible infection?

◆ Analysis and Nursing Diagnosis

During assessment gather objective data, such as inspection of an open incision or a record of reduced caloric intake, and subjective data, such as a patient's complaint of tenderness over a surgical wound site. Data interpretation involves analyzing the assessment data carefully, looking for cues and clusters of assessment findings or risk factors that create a pattern. This pattern suggests a specific nursing diagnosis (Box 28.6). Once you have identified the nursing diagnosis, you can identify expected patient outcomes and select appropriate nursing interventions for the plan of care for the patient. While there are other possible nursing diagnoses for patients with problems related to infection prevention and control, the nursing diagnoses in the following paragraphs and the following list represent examples of diagnoses commonly associated with infection prevention and control:

- Risk for Infection
- Impaired Nutritional Status: Deficient Food Intake

BOX 28.6   Nursing Diagnostic Process

Risk for Infection

Assessment Activities	Assessment Findings
Check results of laboratory tests.	WBC count 5000/mm^3
Review current medications.	Patient receiving antibiotics and oral antidiabetic medications
Identify potential sites of infection.	IV catheter in right forearm, in place for 3 days
	Foley catheter draining cloudy amber-colored urine

IV, Intravenous; *WBC*, white blood cell.

- Impaired Oral Mucous Membrane
- Social Isolation
- Impaired Tissue Integrity

It is necessary to validate data, such as inspecting the integrity of a wound more carefully, and to review laboratory findings to confirm a diagnosis. Success in planning appropriate nursing interventions depends on the accuracy of the diagnostic statement and the ability to meet the patient's needs. A patient will have assessment findings for a problem-focused or a negative diagnosis and/or risk factors for a risk diagnosis. You individualize the diagnosis with the addition of an accurate *related* factor in the diagnostic statement. Accuracy ensures appropriate interventions are chosen. For example, minimizing the risk for infection in a patient with a diagnosis of *Impaired Oral Mucous Membrane related to mouth breathing* requires frequent and proper oral hygiene measures. Minimizing the risk for infection in a patient with a nursing diagnosis of *Impaired Nutritional Status: Deficient Food Intake related to inability to absorb nutrients* requires good nutritional support and fluid balance. At-risk diagnoses such as *Risk for Infection* require careful identification of relevant risk factors.

Kathy analyzes the data that she has gathered from her morning assessment on Mrs. Andrews. She recognizes that her findings—an incision dressing wet from urine, wound edges approximated with no redness or drainage, Mrs. Andrews' age, and her use of glucocorticoids and diabetes mellitus— form a cluster of cues that lead Kathy to the nursing diagnosis of **Risk for Infection** *as the priority problem. The cues also lead Kathy to make an interrelated nursing diagnosis of* **Impaired Skin Integrity** *related to the surgical incision. The patient's pain and limitations from the effects of spinal surgery make* **Impaired Mobility** *a relevant diagnosis. Kathy knows from her reading that Mrs. Andrews has multiple risk factors that contribute to poor wound healing and could lead to a wound infection. Kathy also recognizes that Mrs. Andrews' previous statements about her incision, pain, and discharge to home show that Mrs. Andrews is experiencing a problem with* **Anxiety***.*

◆ Planning and Outcomes Identification

During the planning step of the nursing process, develop a plan of care for each of the patient's nursing diagnoses. Clinical judgment at this step is important because you reflect on previous experiences and environmental factors and apply knowledge and critical thinking attitudes and standards in selecting the most appropriate nursing interventions. Integrate assessment data with knowledge about a patient's condition and the resources and therapies available for infection prevention and control to develop an individualized plan of care. Match the patient's needs with evidence-based interventions that are supported and recommended in the clinical and research literature. Patients often have multiple nursing diagnoses that are interrelated, and one diagnosis often impacts the other diagnoses. A concept map (Fig. 28.2) is a useful

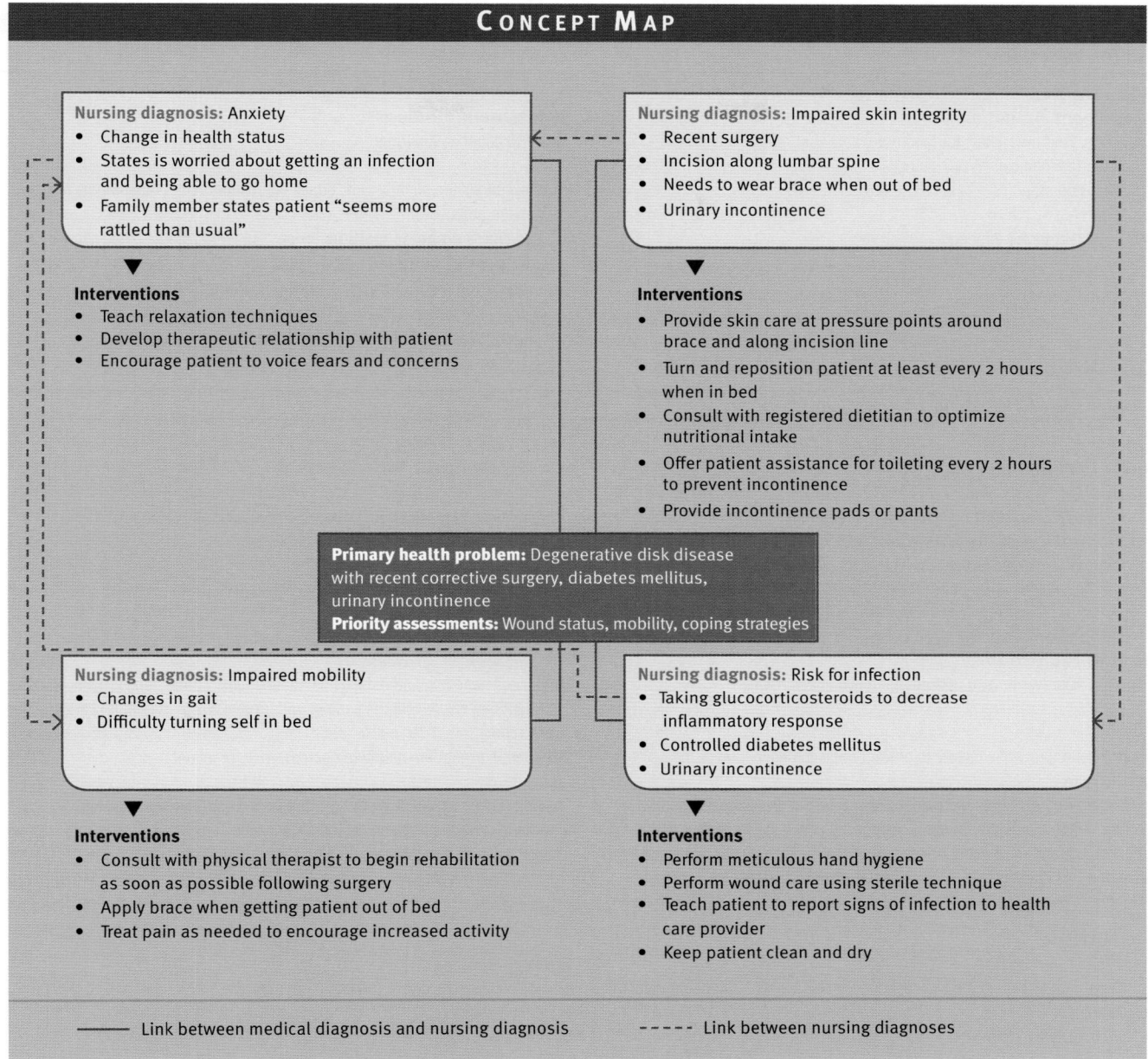

FIG. 28.2 Concept map for Mrs. Andrews.

tool to organize patient care and show how the patient's medical diagnosis, assessment data, and nursing diagnoses are interrelated.

Prior experience with other patients and your own personal experience are valuable when selecting interventions for infection prevention and control. For example, you may have cared for a patient who developed a wound infection after surgery and you used medical and surgical asepsis during dressing changes and procedures to care for the wound. Your previous patient experiences can also help you recognize best practices for infection prevention. Your experiences in the health care agency reinforce your knowledge of the importance of proper hand hygiene and agency policies on infection prevention and control.

It is also important to recognize environmental factors that impact infection prevention and control. For example, when you are working with a patient, you are checking the patient's room, making sure it is clean and organized and that the patient's belongings are within reach.

You want to make sure you are uninterrupted when performing sterile procedures so that the risk for contamination of the sterile field is minimized. Also, you can work with other members of the health care team to develop a plan to help reduce the incidence of a specific infection, such as CAUTI, on the unit that you are assigned to for your clinical experience. Consider the patient's culture and preferences when planning patient-centered interventions.

Outcomes. Partner with the patient and family to identify expected outcomes and develop a mutually agreed-on plan of care based on the patient's nursing diagnoses (see the Nursing Care Plan). Use clinical judgment to establish realistic outcomes that align with the patient's expectations and preferences. Develop a plan that sets realistic outcomes, so interventions are purposeful, direct, and measurable. For example, when you care for a patient with broken skin and obesity, the nursing

◎ NURSING CARE PLAN

Risk for Infection

ASSESSMENT

Assessment Activities

Review Mrs. Andrews' chart for laboratory data that reflect infection (e.g., white blood cell [WBC] count).

Inspect incision area.

Review risk factors for infection.

Assessment Findings[a]

The WBC count is 9500/mm³.

Incision edges are slightly pink; edges approximated but edematous; no drainage noted.

Has had type 2 **diabetes mellitus** for past 16 years; states blood sugars have been **"poorly controlled"** for the past year. Dietary assessment reflects **malnutrition** before surgery. Is **taking a glucocorticosteroid,** which reduces inflammation and suppresses the immune system.

Had had problems with **urinary incontinence** for the past year.

[a]**Assessment Findings** are shown in bold type.

NURSING DIAGNOSIS: Risk for infection

PLANNING

Expected Outcomes (NOC)[b]

Immune Status

Mrs. Andrews has no signs or symptoms of infection (e.g., remains afebrile; incision intact; edges approximated; no redness, swelling, or drainage).

Knowledge: Infection Management

Mrs. Andrews demonstrates appropriate hand hygiene before discharge.

[b]Outcome classification labels from Moorhead S, et al.: *Nursing outcomes classification (NOC),* ed 6, St Louis, 2018, Elsevier.

INTERVENTIONS (NIC)[c]

Infection Protection

Teach Mrs. Andrews how to perform hand hygiene correctly.

Monitor Mrs. Andrews frequently to prevent urine contamination of the incision site.

Provide Mrs. Andrews with incontinence panties that she wears at home.

Help Mrs. Andrews identify a family member to check the incision until it is healed, and teach Mrs. Andrews and the family member signs and symptoms of infection.

RATIONALE

Meticulous hand hygiene reduces bacterial counts on the hands (Hass, 2018). Patient can easily come in contact with organisms in the health care environment that can cause infection.

Offer bedpan/restroom hourly to decrease risk for incontinence.

Absorbent padding will wick away urine from Mrs. Andrews' incision.

Mrs. Andrews will be unable to visualize incision since it is on her back; she will need a family member to help monitor healing of the surgical site.

[c]Intervention classification labels from Butcher HK, et al.: *Nursing interventions classification (NIC),* ed 7, St Louis, 2018, Elsevier.

EVALUATION

Evaluation Activities

Observe incision site for signs of infection (e.g., redness, warmth, and wound discharge).

Ask Mrs. Andrews to demonstrate how she will wash her hands at home.

Patient Response

Incision shows no signs of infection: redness, warmth, or drainage.

Mrs. Andrews demonstrates correct hand hygiene procedure.

---

diagnosis of *Risk for Infection* requires you to implement skin and wound care measures to promote healing. The expected outcome of "absence of drainage" sets an expected outcome for measuring the patient's improvement. Examples of additional outcomes of care applicable to patients with infection or to prevent infection include the following:

- The patient demonstrates proper hand hygiene prior to discharge.
- The patient identifies the signs and symptoms of wound infection.
- The patient is afebrile upon discharge.
- The patient's wound edges are approximated at time of discharge.

REFLECT NOW

How would you begin to identify expected outcomes with a patient in the hospital who is experiencing an infection?

Setting Priorities. Establish priorities for each diagnosis and related outcomes of care. For example, you are caring for a patient with cancer who develops an open wound and is unable to tolerate solid foods. The priority of administering therapies to promote wound healing such as improved nutritional intake overrides the goal of educating the patient to assume self-care therapies at home. When this patient's condition improves, the priorities change, and patient education will then become an essential intervention. Patient priorities change quickly, especially in the acute care environment. In the home setting, priorities may remain appropriate for weeks at a time.

After identifying **Risk for Infection** as the priority for Mrs. Andrews, Kathy starts to plan patient-centered personal care based on Mrs. Andrews' preferences when possible. Together, Kathy and Mrs. Andrews identify two outcomes— that Mrs. Andrews can demonstrate proper hand hygiene and that she has no signs or symptoms of infection at discharge. Kathy develops a care plan to decrease the risk of infection. Another priority for Mrs. Andrews

BOX 28.7 CULTURAL ASPECTS OF CARE

Implications for Infection Control and Isolation Procedures

Various cultural practices and beliefs present challenges to health care providers when infection control and isolation procedures are needed. Patients' health care practices and beliefs influence their decisions to seek treatment for an infection or to use methods to prevent infections. In the United States cities and rural areas have immigrant populations that sometimes hold on to the health care practices of their countries of origin. Some members of the immigrant population may come from war-torn countries where health care was limited and infections were rampant. In addition, some of these patients may fear isolation equipment, which for some may indicate that they have a deadly disease or that harm will come to them or their families. It is important to meet the cultural needs of the patients but also to integrate best practices related to infection control and, when needed, isolation procedures. Although gender-congruent caregivers are important for many cultures, the cultural aspects of care for infection control must expand beyond that premise (Giger and Haddad, 2021; San Patten and Associates, 2016).

Implications for Patient-Centered Care

- Assess a patient's literacy and identify the best method for communication and patient teaching for the patient and family. This may include a community elder, an interpreter, or a family member.
- Determine initially whether the patient has any signs of fear, anxiety, or confusion about the condition and treatment plan.
- Reinforce that infection control and isolation procedures are designed for patient safety. Use simple language to explain.
- Explain each item used for infection control and isolation procedures, and obtain feedback from the patient to determine the level of understanding.
- Be aware that in some cultures touch from a person who is not a family member is not appropriate. Prepare the patient by explaining why you need to touch; when possible, ask permission. For example, say, "I need to check your arm that has an IV line. May I do that now?"
- If the patient seems fearful of the isolation equipment, continually reinforce why you are wearing the equipment.
- Using culturally sensitive care, identify unique approaches to help patients who are on isolation precautions understand why the precautions are necessary. Answer any questions, and allay the fear of patients and families.

is her diagnosis of **Anxiety**. Kathy also plans interventions that will help Mrs. Andrews decrease her anxiety and feel more ready to go home. By reducing anxiety, these interventions may also reduce her discomfort.

Teamwork and Collaboration. The development of a care plan includes prevention and infection control practices provided by multiple disciplines. Select interventions in collaboration with the patient, the family caregiver, and health care providers such as the registered dietitian or respiratory therapist. Know the patient's sociocultural preferences to help you identify how to provide the most appropriate types of interventions (Box 28.7). In addition, consult with an expert in infection control in planning the patient's care. Before discharge, consult with case management to complete a home assessment and identify home health needs. Case managers work with the patient, family, and home care services to ensure that the transition from the hospital goes smoothly and that a safe discharge plan is in place. If the patient is being discharged with an open wound from an infection, consultation with a wound care specialist (see Chapter 48) can help the patient with wound management at home.

When care continues into the patient's home, the home health nurse plans to ensure that the home environment supports good infection prevention and control practices. For example, if a patient does not have running water yet requires wound care, even simple hand hygiene with soap and water is difficult to achieve. Home health nurses instruct patients to perform hand hygiene with either bottled water and soap or alcohol-based hand products. In addition, in the home it is common to use clean instead of sterile asepsis. Consult with the patient's health care provider if you have questions about proper aseptic technique.

Four days after surgery Mrs. Andrews has done well and is scheduled for discharge home. Kathy provides education to Mrs. Andrews on signs and symptoms of infection, wound care, urinary incontinence prevention, and diet for wound healing. Kathy makes a referral to home health services to arrange for nursing visits and in-home assistance for Mrs. Andrews' bathing. Kathy collaborates with physical therapy and occupational therapy to improve Mrs. Andrews' mobility. Mrs. Andrews' married daughter lives in town and plans on helping her mother after surgery and taking her to physical therapy and health care provider appointments. Kathy plans on involving Mrs. Andrews' daughter in the discharge teaching and discharge planning.

◆ Implementation

By identifying relevant nursing diagnoses and expected outcomes and implementing a patient-centered plan of care with appropriate evidence-based measures, you can effectively reduce the risk of infection and aggressively manage an existing infection.

Health Promotion. Use clinical judgment and critical thinking to prevent an infection from developing or spreading. In the home and community settings, review with and teach patients and their family caregivers about ways to strengthen a potential host's defenses against infection. Nutritional support, rest, personal hygiene, maintenance of physiological protective mechanisms, and recommended immunizations protect patients. Explain how to perform infection prevention and control principles such as hand hygiene and methods for proper disposal of medical waste. Based on your assessment of a patient's cultural practices, integrate infection prevention and control measures into the patient's daily lifestyle practices.

Nutrition. Nutritional requirements for your patients vary depending on their age and condition. A proper diet helps the immune system function and consists of a variety of foods from all food groups (see Chapter 45). Collaborate with registered dietitians, the patient, and the family to select the correct foods. Recommend ways to prepare foods that the patient will enjoy. Teach patients the importance of a proper diet in maintaining immunity and preventing infection.

Hygiene. Personal hygiene measures (see Chapter 40) reduce microorganisms on the skin and maintain the integrity of mucous membranes such as the mouth and vagina. Patients and family caregivers need to understand techniques for cleansing the skin and how to avoid the spread of microorganisms in body secretions or excretions. For example, teach female patients how to wash their perineum from clean to dirty, from the urethra down toward the rectum, using a clean washcloth with each wipe. Another example is to teach patients the proper technique to cleanse around a wound (see Chapter 48).

Immunization. The CDC's Advisory Committee on Immunization Practices recommends routine vaccination by age 24 months against 14 potentially serious illnesses (CDC, 2018d). Immunization programs for infants and children have historically decreased the occurrence of childhood diphtheria, whooping cough, and measles. In 2017, coverage with most recommended vaccines among children 19 to 35 months of age remained stable and high, but coverage was lower in more rural areas and among children who were uninsured or on Medicaid (CDC, 2018d). A small but increasing proportion of children received no vaccines by age 24 months (CDC, 2018d).

More recently developed vaccines for meningococcal pneumonia and rotavirus provide immunity to adults and children. Another important vaccine for adults is the shingles vaccine. Recombinant zoster vaccine (RZV, Shingrix) has been in use since 2017 and is recommended by the CDC's Advisory Committee on Immunization Practices (ACIP) as the preferred shingles vaccine (CDC, 2018f). Inform patients that their risk of shingles increases as they get older and that just because they may have had shingles does not mean they cannot acquire the virus a second time. Advise parents about the advantages of immunizations but also make them aware of the contraindications for certain vaccines, especially in pregnant and lactating women. You can access the most current immunization schedules at http://www.cdc.gov/vaccines/schedules/hcp/index.html.

Adequate Rest and Regular Exercise. Adequate rest and regular exercise help prevent infection. Physical exercise increases lung capacity, circulation, energy, and endurance. It also decreases stress and improves appetite, sleeping, and elimination. Help patients with a schedule that balances regular exercise with the need for rest and sleep.

Acute Care. Treatment of an infectious process includes eliminating infectious organisms and supporting a patient's defenses. To identify the causative organisms, you will collect specimens of body fluids such as sputum or drainage from infected body sites for lab cultures. When the disease process or causative organism is identified, the health care provider prescribes the most effective treatment (e.g., antimicrobials). As a nurse you will implement supportive infection control measures.

Systemic infections require measures to prevent complications of fever (see Chapter 29). Maintaining intake of fluids prevents dehydration resulting from diaphoresis. The patient's increased metabolic rate requires an adequate nutritional intake, which may be provided through IV parenteral nutrition. Rest preserves energy for the healing process.

Localized infections often require measures to assist removal of debris to promote healing. You perform skills of wound care to remove infected drainage (e.g., irrigation, wound dressing debridement) from wound sites and support the integrity of healing wounds (see Chapter 48). When changing a dressing, wear a mask and goggles or a mask with a face shield if splashing or spraying with blood or body fluids is anticipated. Apply gloves to reduce the transmission of microorganisms into the wound. Apply special dressings to facilitate removal of drainage and promote healing of wound margins. Sometimes a surgeon will insert drainage tubes to remove infected drainage from body cavities (see Chapter 48). Use medical and surgical aseptic techniques appropriately to manage wounds and ensure correct handling of all drainage or body fluids.

During the course of infection, support the patient's body defense mechanisms. For example, if a patient has diarrhea, maintain skin integrity by frequent cleansing of the skin, application of a skin-barrier cream, and frequent repositioning to prevent breakdown and the entrance of additional microorganisms. Other routine hygiene measures such as cleaning the oral cavity and bathing protect the skin and mucous membranes from invasion and overgrowth of organisms.

Medical Asepsis. Asepsis is the absence of pathogenic (disease-producing) microorganisms. Aseptic technique refers to the practices/procedures that help reduce the risk for infection. The two types of aseptic technique are medical and surgical asepsis. Basic medical aseptic techniques break the chain of infection. Use these techniques for all patients, even when no infection is diagnosed. Aggressive preventive measures are highly effective in reducing HAIs. Hand hygiene, use of personal protective equipment, and routine environmental cleaning are examples of medical asepsis. Principles of medical asepsis are also commonly followed in the home; for example, hand hygiene is performed with soap and water before preparing food, after using the bathroom, or after touching what are interpreted as dirty objects. It is important to include cultural or social beliefs of the patient and family.

Control or Elimination of Infectious Agents. With the increased use of disposable equipment, nurses are often less aware of disinfection and sterilization procedures. The proper cleaning, disinfection, and sterilization of contaminated objects significantly reduce and/or eliminate microorganisms (Chetan, 2018). In health care agencies a sterile processing department is responsible for the disinfection and sterilization of reusable supplies and equipment. However, nurses sometimes need to perform these functions in the home care setting. Many principles of cleaning and disinfection also apply to the home, so it is important to educate patients and family caregivers on these techniques.

Cleaning. Cleaning is the removal of organic material (e.g., blood) or inorganic material (e.g., soil) from objects and surfaces (Chetan, 2018). In general, cleaning involves the use of water, a detergent/disinfectant, and proper mechanical scrubbing. Cleaning occurs before disinfection and sterilization procedures.

When an object comes in contact with an infectious or potentially infectious material, it is contaminated. If the object is disposable, it is discarded. Reusable objects need to be cleaned thoroughly before reuse and then either disinfected or sterilized according to manufacturer recommendations. Failure to follow manufacturer recommendations transfers liability from the manufacturer to the health care agency if an infection results from improper processing.

Apply protective eyewear (or a face shield) and utility (dishwashing style) gloves when cleaning equipment that is soiled by organic material such as blood, fecal matter, mucus, or pus. Protective barriers provide protection from potentially infectious organisms. A brush and detergent or soap are necessary for cleaning. The following steps ensure that an object is clean:

1. Rinse the contaminated object or article with cold running water to remove organic material. Hot water causes the protein in organic material to coagulate and stick to objects, making removal difficult.
2. After rinsing, wash the object with soap and warm water. Soap or detergent reduces the surface tension of water and emulsifies dirt or remaining material. Rinse the object thoroughly.
3. Use a brush to remove dirt or material in grooves or seams. Friction dislodges contaminated material for easy removal. Open hinged items for cleaning.
4. Rinse the object in warm water.
5. Dry the object and prepare it for disinfection or sterilization if indicated by classification of the item (i.e., critical, semicritical, or noncritical).
6. The brush, gloves, and sink used to clean the equipment are considered contaminated and are cleaned and dried according to policy.

Disinfection and Sterilization. Disinfection and sterilization use both physical and chemical processes that disrupt the internal functioning of microorganisms by destroying cell proteins. Disinfection describes a process that eliminates many or all microorganisms, with the exception of bacterial spores, from inanimate objects (Chetan, 2018). There are two types of disinfection: (1) the disinfection of surfaces, and (2) high-level disinfection, which is required for some patient care items such as endoscopes and bronchoscopes. Sterilization eliminates or destroys all forms of microbial life, including spores (Chetan, 2018). Sterilization methods include processing items using steam, dry heat, hydrogen peroxide plasma, or ethylene oxide (ETO). The decision to clean, clean and disinfect, or sterilize depends on the intended use of a contaminated item (Box 28.8). Be familiar with the policies and procedures of your health care agency for cleaning, handling, and delivering care items for eventual disinfection and sterilization. Workers in the central processing area who are specially trained in disinfection and sterilization perform most of the procedures. The following factors influence the efficacy of the disinfecting or sterilizing method:

- *Concentration of solution and duration of contact.* A weakened concentration or shortened exposure time lessens its effectiveness.
- *Type and number of pathogens.* The greater the number of pathogens on an object, the longer the required disinfecting time.
- *Surface areas to treat.* All dirty surfaces and areas need to be fully exposed to disinfecting and sterilizing agents. The type of surface is an important factor. Is the surface porous or nonporous?
- *Temperature of the environment.* Disinfectants tend to work best at room temperature.
- *Presence of soap.* Soap causes certain disinfectants to be ineffective. Thorough rinsing of an object is necessary before disinfecting.
- *Presence of organic material.* Disinfectants become inactivated unless blood, saliva, pus, or body excretions are washed off.

Table 28.5 lists processes for disinfection and sterilization and their characteristics. Some delicate instruments requiring sterilization cannot tolerate steam and must be processed with gas or plasma.

Protection of the Susceptible Host. A patient's resistance to infection improves as you protect normal body defenses against infection. Intervene to maintain the normal reparative processes of the body (Box 28.9). Nurses also protect themselves and others through the use of isolation precautions.

Control or Elimination of Reservoirs of Infection. To control or eliminate the numbers and types of organisms in reservoir sites, eliminate sources of body fluids, drainage, or solutions that possibly harbor microorganisms. Eliminating reservoirs of infection (e.g., emptying urinary drainage bags, keeping food refrigerated and stored), controlling portals of exit and entry (e.g., using antiseptic wipes on IV tubing ports), and avoiding actions that transmit microorganisms prevent bacteria from finding a new site in which to grow (Box 28.10). Be aware of the state regulations for the handling and disposal of

BOX 28.8 Categories for Sterilization, Disinfection, and Cleaning

Critical Items

Items that enter sterile tissue or the vascular system present a high risk of infection if they are contaminated with microorganisms, especially bacterial spores. *Critical items* must be *sterile.* These items include:
- Surgical instruments
- Cardiac or intravascular catheters
- Urinary catheters
- Implants

Semicritical Items

Items that come in contact with mucous membranes or nonintact skin also present a risk. These objects must be free of all microorganisms (except bacterial spores). *Semicritical items* must be *high-level disinfected (HLD)* or *sterilized.* These items include:
- Respiratory and anesthesia equipment
- Endoscopes
- Endotracheal tubes
- GI endoscopes
- Diaphragm fitting rings

After rinsing, dry items and store in a manner to protect from damage and contamination.

Noncritical Items

Items that come in contact with intact skin but not mucous membranes must be clean. *Noncritical items* must be *disinfected.* These items include:
- Bedpans
- Blood pressure cuffs
- Bedrails
- Linens
- Stethoscopes
- Bedside trays and patient furniture
- Food utensils

TABLE 28.5 Examples of Disinfection and Sterilization Processes

Characteristics	Examples of Use
Moist Heat Steam is moist heat under pressure. When exposed to high pressure, water vapor reaches a temperature above boiling point to kill pathogens and spores.	Autoclave sterilizes heat-tolerant surgical instruments and semicritical patient care items.
Chemical Sterilants—High-Level Disinfection (HLD) A number of chemical disinfectants are used in health care. These include alcohols, chlorines, formaldehyde, glutaraldehyde, hydrogen peroxide, iodophors, phenolics, and quaternary ammonium compounds. Each product performs in a unique manner and is used for a specific purpose.	Chemicals disinfect heat-sensitive instruments and equipment such as endoscopes and respiratory therapy equipment.
Ethylene Oxide (ETO) Gas This gas destroys spores and microorganisms by altering the metabolic processes of cells. Fumes are released within an autoclave-like chamber. ETO gas is toxic to humans, and aeration time varies with products.	This gas sterilizes most medical materials.
Boiling Water Boiling is least expensive for use in the home. Bacterial spores and some viruses resist boiling. It is not used in health care agencies.	Boiling is commonly used in the home for items such as urinary catheters, suction tubes, and drainage collection devices.

BOX 28.9   Infection Prevention and Control: Protecting the Susceptible Host

Protecting Natural Defense Mechanisms

- Regular bathing removes transient microorganisms from the surface of the skin. Lubrication helps keep the skin hydrated and intact. In many intensive care settings, a chlorhexidine (CHG) bath is recommended if there is a risk for *methicillin-resistant Staphylococcus aureus* (MRSA) or other resistant bacteria (CDC, 2019c; Popovich, 2017).
- Perform regular oral hygiene. Saliva contains enzymes that promote digestion and has a bactericidal action to maintain control of bacteria. Flossing removes tartar and plaque that cause germ infection.
- Maintain an adequate fluid intake to promote normal urine formation and a resultant outflow of urine to flush the bladder and urethral lining of microorganisms.
- For patients who are physically dependent or immobilized, encourage routine coughing and deep breathing to keep lower airways clear of mucus.
- Encourage proper immunization of children or adult patients who are exposed to certain infectious microorganisms. Children are vaccinated for measles, mumps, rubella, chickenpox, diphtheria, and other vaccine-preventable diseases. Adults need a seasonal flu (influenza) vaccine every year. Every adult should get the Tdap (tetanus, diphtheria, pertussis) vaccine once if they did not receive it as an adolescent to protect against pertussis (whooping cough), and then a Td (tetanus, diphtheria) booster shot every 10 years (CDC, 2019e).
- Adults 50 years of age or older should consult with their physicians about recommended additional vaccines in the context of any preexisting conditions. In general, however, older adults should receive the shingles vaccine, pneumococcal polysaccharide vaccine (PPSV23) (recommended for all adults 65 years of age or older, and for adults younger than 65 years who have certain health conditions), and pneumococcal conjugate vaccine (PCV13), which protects against serious pneumococcal disease and pneumonia (recommended for all adults with a condition that weakens the immune system, cerebrospinal fluid leak, or cochlear implant).

Maintaining Healing Processes

- Promote intake of adequate fluids and a well-balanced diet containing essential proteins, vitamins, carbohydrates, and fats. Use measures to increase the patient's appetite.
- Promote a patient's comfort and sleep so that energy stores are replaced daily.
- Help the patient learn techniques to reduce stress.

BOX 28.10   Infection Prevention and Control to Reduce Reservoirs of Infection

Bathing

- Use soap and water to remove drainage, dried secretions, or excess perspiration.

Dressing Changes

- Change dressings that become wet and/or soiled (see Chapter 48).

Contaminated Articles

- Place tissues, soiled dressings, or soiled linen in fluid-resistant bags for proper disposal.

Contaminated Sharps

- Place all needles, safety needles, and needleless systems into puncture-proof containers, which should be located at the site of use. Federal law requires the use of needle-safe technology. Blood tube holders are single use only (OSHA, 2012a).

Bedside Unit

- Keep table surfaces clean and dry.

Bottled Solutions

- Do not leave bottled solutions open.
- Keep solutions tightly capped.
- Date bottles when opened and discard in 24 hours.

Surgical Wounds

- Keep drainage tubes and collection bags patent to prevent accumulation of serous fluid under the skin surface.

Drainage Bottles and Bags

- Wear gloves and protective eyewear if splashing or spraying with contaminated blood or body fluids is anticipated.
- Empty and dispose of drainage suction bottles according to agency policy.
- Empty all drainage systems on each shift unless otherwise ordered by a health care provider.
- Never raise a drainage system (e.g., urinary drainage bag) above the level of the site being drained unless it is clamped off.

---

medical (infectious) waste. Occupational Safety and Health Administration (OSHA) regulations address the handling and disposal of blood and body fluids that potentially pose a risk for the transmission of bloodborne pathogens. These regulations defer to state laws and regulations (OSHA, 2012a).

Control of Portals of Exit/Entry. To control organisms exiting via the respiratory tract, cover your mouth or nose when coughing or sneezing. Teach patients, health care staff, patients' families, and visitors about respiratory hygiene or cough etiquette. The use of posters and written material explaining cough etiquette to learners is beneficial. Cough etiquette has become more important because of concern for transmission of respiratory infections such as Coronavirus-19 (COVID-19), *Mycobacterium tuberculosis*, severe acute respiratory syndrome (SARS), and H1N1 influenza (CDC, 2019a). The elements of respiratory hygiene and cough etiquette are summarized in Table 28.6 (CDC, 2019a).

Another way of controlling the exit of microorganisms is by using Standard Precautions (see Table 28.6) when handling body fluids such as urine, feces, and wound drainage. Wear clean gloves if there is any chance of contact with any blood or body fluids and perform hand

hygiene after providing care. Be sure to bag contaminated items (e.g., linen placed in fluid-resistant linen bags) appropriately.

Many measures that control the exit of microorganisms also control their entrance. Maintaining the integrity of skin and mucous membranes reduces the chances of microorganisms reaching a host. Keep a patient's skin well lubricated by using lotion as appropriate. Patients who are immobilized and debilitated are particularly susceptible to skin breakdown. Do not position patients on tubes or objects that cause breaks in the skin. It is important to turn and position patients before their skin becomes reddened. Frequent oral hygiene prevents the drying of mucous membranes. A water-soluble ointment keeps a patient's lips well lubricated.

After elimination instruct women to clean the rectum and perineum by wiping from the urinary meatus toward the rectum. Cleaning in a direction from the least to the most contaminated area helps reduce GU infections. Meticulous and frequent perineal care is especially important in older-adult women who wear disposable incontinence pads.

Another cause for entrance of microorganisms into a host is improper handling and management of urinary catheters and drainage sets (see Chapter 46) (Box 28.11). Keep the point of connection between a catheter and drainage tube closed and intact. If such systems are closed, their contents are considered sterile. Outflow spigots on drainage bags

TABLE 28.6 Centers for Disease Control and Prevention Isolation Guidelines

STANDARD PRECAUTIONS (TIER ONE) FOR USE WITH ALL PATIENTS

- Standard Precautions apply to blood, blood products, all body fluids, secretions, excretions (except sweat), nonintact skin, and mucous membranes.
- Perform hand hygiene before direct contact with patients; between patient contacts; after contact with blood, body fluids, secretions, and excretions and with equipment or articles contaminated by them; and immediately after gloves are removed.
- When hands are visibly soiled or contaminated with blood or body fluids, wash them with either a nonantimicrobial soap or antimicrobial soap and water.
- When hands are not visibly soiled or contaminated with blood or body fluids, use an alcohol-based hand rub to perform hand hygiene.
- Wash hands with nonantimicrobial or antimicrobial soap and water if contact with spores (e.g., *Clostridium difficile*) is likely to have occurred.
- Do not wear artificial fingernails or extenders if duties include direct contact with patients at high risk for infection and associated adverse outcomes.
- Wear gloves when touching blood, body fluids, secretions, excretions, nonintact skin, mucous membranes, or contaminated items or surfaces. Remove and dispose of gloves and perform hand hygiene between patient care encounters and when going from a contaminated to a clean body site.
- Wear PPE when your anticipated patient interaction is likely to involve contact with blood or body fluids.
- A private room is unnecessary. Check with the infection prevention and control professional of your agency.
- Discard all contaminated sharp instruments and needles in a puncture-resistant container. Health care agencies must make needleless devices available. Activate the mechanical safety device, if present. If needle recapping is necessary, use the one-handed scoop method and dispose of the capped needle as soon as possible.
- Respiratory hygiene and cough etiquette: Have patients cover the nose or mouth when sneezing or coughing; use tissues to contain respiratory secretions and dispose in nearest waste container; perform hand hygiene after contact with respiratory secretions and contaminated objects or materials; contain respiratory secretions with procedure or surgical mask; sit at least 3 feet away from others if coughing.

TRANSMISSION-BASED PRECAUTIONS (TIER TWO) FOR USE WITH SPECIFIC TYPES OF PATIENTS

Category	Disease	Barrier Protection
Airborne Precautions (Droplets <5 μm)	Measles, chickenpox (varicella), disseminated herpes zoster, *Mycobacterium tuberculosis*, rubeola	Private room; negative-pressure airflow of at least 6-12 exchanges per hour via HEPA filtration; mask or respiratory protection device, N95 respirator
Droplet Precautions (Droplets >5 μm; being within 3 feet of the patient)	Influenza, adenovirus, group A streptococcus, *Neisseria meningitides*, pertussis, rhinovirus, mycoplasma pneumoniae, pertussis, diphtheria, pneumonic plague, rubella, mumps, respiratory syncytial virus	Private room or cohort patients; mask or respirator (refer to agency policy)
Contact Precautions (Direct patient or environmental contact)	Colonization or infection with multidrug-resistant organisms, such as VRE and MRSA, *Clostridium difficile*, shigella and other enteric pathogens, major wound infections, herpes simplex, scabies, varicella zoster (disseminated), respiratory syncytial virus	Private room or cohort patients (see agency policy); gloves, gowns
Protective environment	Allogeneic hematopoietic stem cell transplants	Private room; positive airflow with ≥12 air exchanges per hour; HEPA filtration for incoming air; mask, gloves, gowns

HEPA, High-efficiency particulate air; *MRSA,* methicillin-resistant *Staphylococcus aureus*; *PPE,* personal protective equipment; *VRE,* vancomycin-resistant enterococcus.
Modified from Centers for Disease Control and Prevention (CDC): *2007 Guideline for Isolation Precautions: Preventing Transmission of Infectious Agents in Healthcare Settings,* Washington, DC, 2019, https://www.cdc.gov/infectioncontrol/guidelines/isolation/index.html, accessed August 10, 2020; Association of periOperative Registered Nurses (AORN): *AORN guidelines for perioperative practice,* Denver, 2020; U.S. Food and Drug Administration (FDA): *Safely using sharps (needles and syringes) at home, at work and on travel,* 2018, https://www.fda.gov/medicaldevices/productsandmedicalprocedures/homehealthandconsumer/consumerproducts/sharps/default.htm, accessed June 29, 2020.

should also remain closed to prevent entrance of bacteria. Minimize movement of the catheter at the urethra by stabilizing it with tape or a securing device to reduce the chance of microorganisms ascending the urethra into the bladder. Do not share urine-measuring containers among patients. Sometimes you care for patients with closed drainage systems that collect wound drainage, bile, or other body fluids. Make sure that the site from which a drainage tube exits remains clear of excess moisture or accumulated drainage. Keep all tubing connected throughout use and open drainage receptacles only when it is necessary to discard or measure the volume of drainage (see Chapter 46).

Control of Transmission. Effective prevention and control of infection requires you to remain aware of the modes of transmission of microorganisms and ways to control them. The use of Standard Precautions (see Table 28.6) for all patients is a step toward preventing transmission of

infection. In any health care setting a patient usually has a personal set of care items. Sharing bedpans, urinals, bath basins, and eating utensils among patients easily leads to cross-infection by indirect contact. When using a stethoscope, always wipe off the bell, diaphragm, and ear tips with a disinfectant such as an alcohol wipe before proceeding to the next patient. Diaphragms and ear tips are a common location for staphylococcal organisms (Adesanya et al., 2017). In facilities where HAI diarrhea occurs, electronic thermometers are not recommended for rectal temperatures. You usually use oral or tympanic thermometers to assess temperature. When patients are on contact isolation, you use equipment to measure vital signs, such as thermometers and blood pressure cuffs, that are disposable or dedicated only to be used for that patient.

Always be careful when handling exudate such as urine, feces, emesis, and blood. Contaminated fluids easily splash while being

BOX 28.11   EVIDENCE-BASED PRACTICE

Daily Unit Rounds to Reduce CAUTI

PICOT Question: Does the implementation of routine root cause analysis compared with routine daily rounds affect the incidence of catheter-associated urinary tract infections?

Evidence Summary

Among urinary tract infections (UTI) acquired in the hospital, approximately 75% are associated with a urinary catheter. Between 10% and 25% of patients receive urinary catheters during their hospital stay (CDC, 2018b; Fekete, 2020). The most important risk factor for developing a catheter-associated urinary tract infection (CAUTI) is prolonged use of the urinary catheter (Perrin et al., 2021). CAUTIs are common in hospitals across the United States. Hospitals have demonstrated a high use of urinary catheters as well as high CAUTI rates for several years. Because CAUTIs are usually preventable, numerous studies have examined strategies for decreasing CAUTI rates. Strategies have included the development of CDC guidelines for the prevention of CAUTIs (CDC, 2019b), the use of a CAUTI guide with questions regarding proper indwelling catheter use (Fletcher et al., 2016), and the development of a safety program for reducing CAUTI incidence in hospitals (AHRQ, 2015). Evidence-based strategies to reduce the incidence of CAUTIs include daily huddles to justify urinary catheter placement and education of nursing staff to generate awareness of why and how CAUTIs occur and strategies to prevent them (Graziano-Husser et al., 2018). Root cause analyses (RCAs) to review CAUTI cases, including identifying patients' key CAUTI risk factors, reviewing the necessity of the catheter, determining if appropriate culturing was completed, and identifying challenges and concerns the staff experienced related to the appropriate care and maintenance of the urinary catheter have also led to a decrease in the incidence of CAUTIs (Graziano-Husser et al., 2018; Letica-Kriege et al., 2019).

Application to Nursing Practice

- Insert catheters only when indicated, such as acute urinary retention or strict output monitoring (Graziano-Husser et al., 2018).
- Leave catheters in place only if needed and remove within 24 hours unless there are appropriate indications for continued use (AHRQ, 2015).
- Ensure that only properly trained persons insert and maintain urinary catheters (AHRQ, 2015).
- Insert urinary catheters using aseptic technique and sterile equipment (CDC, 2019b).
- Following aseptic insertion, maintain a closed drainage system (CDC, 2019b).
- Use hand hygiene and Standard (or appropriate isolation) Precautions.

discarded in toilets or hoppers. Empty urinals and bedpans at water level to reduce the risk of splash or splatter, and wear gloves and protective eyewear. Appropriately dispose of disposable soiled items in trash bags. Dispose of items contaminated with large amounts of blood in biohazard bags. Know the location of biohazard bags; it will differ among facilities. Handle laboratory specimens from all patients as if they were infectious, and place them in designated biohazard containers or bags for transport or disposal. Because certain microorganisms travel easily through the air, do not shake linens or bedclothes. Dust with a treated or dampened cloth to prevent dust particles from entering the air.

To prevent transmission of microorganisms through indirect contact, do not allow soiled items and equipment to touch your clothing. A common error is to carry dirty linen in the arms against your uniform. Use fluid-resistant linen bags or carry soiled linen with hands held out

from the body. Cover laundry hampers and empty them before they become overloaded. **Never put clean or soiled linens on the floor.**

Hand Hygiene. The most effective basic technique in preventing and controlling the transmission of infection is hand hygiene (see Skill 28.1) (Hass, 2018; WHO, 2021). Hand hygiene is a general term that applies to four techniques: handwashing, antiseptic hand wash, antiseptic hand rub, or surgical hand antisepsis. Handwashing is defined by the CDC (2019a) as the vigorous, brief rubbing together of all surfaces of lathered hands followed by rinsing under a stream of warm water for 15 seconds. The fundamental principle behind handwashing is to remove microorganisms mechanically from the hands and rinse with water. Handwashing does not kill microorganisms.

An antiseptic hand wash means washing hands with warm water and soap or other detergents containing an antiseptic agent; some antiseptics kill bacteria and some viruses. An antiseptic hand rub means applying an antiseptic hand-rub product to all surfaces of the hands to reduce the number of microorganisms present. Ethanol-based hand antiseptics containing 60% to 90% alcohol appear to be the most effective against common pathogens found on the hands (CDC, 2015b). Alcohol-based products are more effective for standard handwashing or hand antisepsis (nonsoiled hands) by health care workers than regular soap or antimicrobial soaps (CDC, 2019a). Surgical hand antisepsis is an antiseptic hand-wash or hand-rub technique that surgical personnel perform before surgery to eliminate transient flora and reduce resident hand flora. Antiseptic detergent preparations have persistent antimicrobial activity (CDC, 2019a; WHO, 2009).

According to WHO (2009), hand cleansing practices are likely to be established in the first 10 years of a person's life. This imprinting affects an individual's attitudes about hand cleansing throughout life. This is called inherent hand hygiene (WHO, 2009). Attitudes toward handwashing in situations such as the delivery of health care are called elective handwashing practices (WHO, 2009). In many patient populations, inherent and elective handwashing is influenced by cultural factors. Thus, hand hygiene is often performed for hygienic reasons, rituals, and symbolic reasons. It is important to learn the significance hand hygiene holds for an individual.

The use of alcohol-based hand rubs is recommended by the CDC (2019a) to improve hand-hygiene practices, protect health care workers' hands, and reduce the transmission of pathogens to patients and personnel in health care settings. Alcohols have excellent germicidal activity and are as effective as soap and water. However, alcohol-based hand antiseptics are ineffective on hands that are visibly dirty or contaminated with organic material (CDC, 2020e). WHO (2017) recommends the following hand-hygiene guidelines:

1. When hands are visibly dirty, when hands are soiled with blood or other body fluids, before eating, and after using the toilet, wash hands with water and either a nonantimicrobial or antimicrobial soap.
2. Wash hands if exposed to spore-forming organisms such as *C. difficile*, *Bacillus anthracis*, or *Norovirus* (CDC, 2020d).
3. If hands are not visibly soiled (WHO, 2021), use an alcohol-based, waterless antiseptic agent for routinely decontaminating hands in the following clinical situations:
   - Before, after, and between direct patient contact (e.g., taking a pulse, lifting a patient)
   - Before putting on sterile gloves and before inserting invasive devices such as a peripheral vascular catheter or urinary catheter
   - After contact with body fluids or excretions, mucous membranes, nonintact skin, and wound dressings (even if gloves are worn)
   - When moving from a contaminated to a clean body site during care
   - After contact with surfaces or objects in the patient's room (e.g., overbed table, IV pump)
   - After removing gloves (CDC, 2019a)

Remember, contaminated hands of health care workers are a primary source of infection transmission in health care settings. It is recommended that health care workers have well-manicured nails and refrain from wearing artificial nails to reduce microorganism transmission.

Infection can easily be transmitted by visitors of patients in health care settings. A study by Birnbach et al. (2015) included hand-hygiene observations of visitors and collection of cultures as visitors entered patient rooms. Thirty-five of 55 visitors did not perform hand hygiene before entering the patient room, and all 55 visitors agreed to providing hand cultures. All the cultures from visitors not doing hand hygiene grew a significantly higher number of bacteria than the cultures from visitors doing hand hygiene. The study demonstrates the need for education of visitors on the importance of hand hygiene and evaluation of corresponding changes in hand hygiene behavior. Instruct patients and visitors about proper hand-hygiene technique, the reason for it, and the times for performing it. If health care is to continue at home, teach patients and family caregivers to wash their hands before eating or handling food; after handling contaminated equipment, linen, or organic material; and after elimination. In health care settings, encourage visitors to wash their hands before eating or handling food; after coming in contact with infected patients; and after handling contaminated equipment, patient furniture, or organic material (CDC, 2020a).

You are responsible for providing the patient and family with a safe environment. The CDC (2020a) launched a Clean Hands Save Lives Campaign that highlights for consumers the five simple and effective steps (Wet, Lather, Scrub, Rinse, Dry) to take to reduce the spread of diarrheal and respiratory illnesses and thus to stay healthy. Many hospitals encourage patients to follow the recommendations of TJC's "Speak Up" campaign. TJC and the Centers for Medicare and Medicaid Services urge patients to take a role in preventing health care errors by becoming active, involved, and informed participants on the health care team. The program features brochures, posters, and buttons on a variety of patient safety topics. One recommendation is to have patients speak up to be sure health care providers have cleaned their hands or put on gloves when providing care.

The effectiveness of infection prevention practices such as hand hygiene depends on the conscientiousness and consistency in using proper technique by all health care providers. It is human nature to forget key procedural steps or, when hurried, to take shortcuts that break aseptic procedures. However, failure to adhere to basic procedures places patients at risk for infections that can seriously impair recovery or lead to death.

Isolation and Isolation Precautions. In 2007 the Hospital Infection Control Practices Advisory Committee (HICPAC) of the CDC published revised guidelines for isolation precautions. HICPAC recommended that facilities modify the guidelines according to need and as dictated by federal, state, or local regulations. The guidelines contain recommendations for respiratory hygiene/cough etiquette as part of Standard Precautions. The CDC recommendations contain two tiers of precautions (see Table 28.6). The first and most important tier is called Standard Precautions, which are designed to be used for the care of all patients, in all settings, regardless of risk or presumed infection status. Standard Precautions are the primary strategies (including barrier precautions) for prevention of infection transmission and apply to contact with blood, body fluids, nonintact skin, mucous membranes, and equipment or surfaces contaminated with potentially infectious materials. In the acute care setting, nurses follow Standard Precautions in all aspects of care. This includes barrier precautions and the appropriate use of PPE such as gowns, gloves, masks, eyewear, and other protective devices or clothing. The choice of barriers depends on the task being performed and the patient's disease. Standard Precautions apply to all patients because every patient has the potential to transmit infection via blood and body fluids, and the risk for infection transmission is unknown. Respiratory hygiene/cough etiquette applies to any person with signs of respiratory infection, including cough, congestion, rhinorrhea, or increased production of respiratory secretions, when entering a health care site. Educating health care staff, patients, and visitors to follow respiratory hygiene/cough etiquette protects both patients and health care workers.

The second tier of precautions (see Table 28.6) includes precautions designed for the care of patients who are known or suspected to be infected or colonized with microorganisms transmitted by droplet, airborne, or contact routes (Berends and Walesa, 2018; CDC, 2019a). There are four types of transmission-based precautions, which are based on the mode of transmission of a disease: *Airborne, Droplet, Contact,* and *Protective Environment Precautions.* These precautions are for patients with highly transmissible pathogens. The protective environment category is designed for patients who have undergone transplants and gene therapy, making them highly vulnerable to infection (CDC, 2019a).

- *Contact Precautions:* Used for direct and indirect contact with patients and their environment. Direct contact refers to the care and handling of contaminated body fluids. Contact Precautions require a gown and gloves. An example includes blood or other body fluids from an infected patient that enter the health care worker's body through direct contact with compromised skin or mucous membranes. Indirect contact involves the transfer of an infectious agent through a contaminated intermediate object such as contaminated instruments or hands of health care workers. The health care worker may transmit microorganisms from one patient site to another if hand hygiene is not performed between patients (CDC, 2019a).

- *Droplet Precautions:* Focus on diseases that are transmitted by large droplets (greater than 5 microns) expelled into the air and by being within 3 feet of a patient. Droplet Precautions require the wearing of a surgical mask when within 3 feet of the patient, proper hand hygiene, and some dedicated-care equipment. An example is a patient with influenza.

- *Airborne Precautions:* Focus on diseases that are transmitted by smaller droplets, which remain in the air for longer periods of time. Airborne Precautions require a specially equipped room with a negative airflow referred to as an *airborne infection isolation room.* Air is not returned to the inside ventilation system but is filtered through a high-efficiency particulate air (HEPA) filter and exhausted directly to the outside. For example, all health care personnel wear an N95 respirator every time they enter the room of a patient with TB.

- *Protective environment:* Focuses on a very limited patient population, all of whom are highly susceptible to infection because of an underlying condition or treatment. This form of isolation requires a specialized room with positive airflow. The airflow rate is set at greater than 12 air exchanges per hour, and all air is filtered through a HEPA filter. One example of a patient requiring a protective environment is a patient who received a kidney transplant. The patient wears a mask when leaving the hospital room during transportation to x-ray.

In the example of COVID-19, OSHA recommends that health care workers use a combination of Standard Precautions, Contact Precautions, Airborne Precautions, and eye protection (e.g., goggles, face shields) to protect against exposure to the virus (United States Department of Labor, n.d.). Patients are placed in airborne infection isolation rooms, when available.

Health care agencies are required to have the capability of isolating patients. However, not all communicable diseases require placing a patient in a special private room. You can conduct many isolation practices in standard rooms using barrier precautions.

Because of the resurgence of TB, the CDC (2019a) developed guidelines to prevent its transmission to health care workers and stresses the importance of isolation for the patient with known or suspected TB in a special negative-pressure room. Close the doors to the patient's room to control the direction of airflow. You must wear a special high-filtration particulate respirator on entering a respiratory isolation room. A respirator must be fitted to your facial size and characteristics. When worn correctly, particulate respirators and masks have a tighter face seal and filter at a higher level than routine surgical masks.

MDROs such as methicillin-resistant *Staphylococcus aureus* (MRSA), vancomycin-resistant enterococcus (VRE), and *C. difficile* are more common as a cause of colonization and HAIs. MDROs have developed a resistance to one or more broad-spectrum antibiotics, making the organisms hard to treat effectively. Major efforts have been in place for a number of years to reduce the incidence of HAIs caused by these dangerous organisms. For example, evidence shows that there has been a significant decrease in central line–associated bloodstream infections, catheter-associated urinary tract infections, and hospital-acquired *C. difficile* (CDC, 2021d). Unlike MRSA and VRE, *C. difficile* (which is transmitted by the fecal-oral route) is harder to eliminate from the environment. It is a spore-forming microorganism, meaning it can remain on surfaces (e.g., bedside table, stethoscope) in a dormant state for long periods. To reduce the risk of cross-contamination among patients, use Contact Precautions in addition to Standard Precautions when caring for patients with MDROs.

Regardless of the type of isolation or barrier protection you use, follow these basic principles when caring for patients:
- Understand how certain diseases are transmitted and which protective barriers to use.
- Use thorough hand hygiene before entering and leaving the room of a patient in isolation.
- Dispose of contaminated supplies and equipment in a manner that prevents spread of microorganisms to other people as indicated by the mode of transmission of the organism.
- Protect all people who might be exposed during transport of a patient outside the isolation room.

Psychological Implications of Isolation. Consider the psychological effects of being in an isolation room. Many patients find positive aspects of being in a single room; however, the overall experience of isolation is commonly viewed negatively (Purssell et al., 2020). Isolation imposes barriers to the expression of a patient's identity and normal interpersonal relationships and affects the delivery of quality care. When a patient requires isolation in a private room, a sense of loneliness sometimes develops because normal social relationships become disrupted. This situation can be psychologically harmful, especially for children. A study noted that patients in isolation experienced more depression and anxiety and were less satisfied with their care (Sprague et al., 2016). Patients' body images become altered as a result of the infectious process. Some feel unclean, rejected, lonely, or guilty. Infection prevention and control practices further intensify these beliefs of difference or undesirability. Isolation disrupts normal social relationships with visitors and caregivers. Take the opportunity to listen to a patient's concerns or interests. If you rush care or show a lack of interest in a patient's needs, the patient feels rejected and even more isolated.

Before you institute isolation measures, the patient and family need to understand the nature of the disease or condition, the purposes of isolation, and steps for following specific precautions. If they are able to participate in maintaining infection prevention and control practices, the chances of spreading the infection decrease. Teach the patient and family to perform hand hygiene and use barrier protection if appropriate. Demonstrate each procedure; be sure to give the patient and family

an opportunity for practice. It is also important to explain how infectious organisms are transmitted so that the patient and family understand the difference between contaminated and clean objects. Explaining and demonstrating these procedures, especially hand hygiene, help the family to consistently practice correct hand hygiene and prescribed isolation measures (Singh et al., 2017).

Take measures to improve a patient's sensory stimulation during isolation. Make sure that the room environment is clean and pleasant. Open drapes or shades and remove excess supplies and equipment. Listen to the patient's concerns or interests. Mealtime is a particularly good opportunity for conversation. Providing comfort measures such as repositioning, a back massage, or a warm sponge bath increases physical stimulation. Depending on the patient's condition, encourage the patient to walk around the room or sit up in a chair. Recreational activities such as board games, reading, and playing cards are options for keeping a patient mentally stimulated.

Explain to the family the patient's risk for depression or loneliness. Encourage visiting family members to avoid expressions or actions that convey revulsion or disgust related to infection prevention and control practices. Discuss ways to provide meaningful stimulation.

The Isolation Environment. Private rooms used for isolation sometimes provide negative-pressure airflow to prevent infectious particles from flowing out of a room to other rooms and the air handling system. Special rooms with positive-pressure airflow are also used for patients who are immunocompromised, such as recipients of transplanted organs. On the door or wall outside the room a nurse posts a card listing precautions for the isolation category in use according to health care agency policy. The card is a handy reference for health care personnel and visitors and alerts anyone who enters the room that special precautions must be followed.

An area immediately outside an isolation room or an adjoining anteroom needs to contain hand hygiene and PPE supplies. Soap and antiseptic (antimicrobial) solutions also should be available. Personnel and visitors perform hand hygiene before entering a patient's room and again before leaving the room. If toilet facilities are unavailable, there are special procedures for handling portable commodes, bedpans, or urinals.

All patient care rooms, including those used for isolation, should contain an impervious bag for soiled or contaminated linen and a trash container with plastic liners. Impervious receptacles prevent transmission of microorganisms by preventing leaking and soiling of the outside surface. A disposable rigid container needs to be available in the room to discard used sharps such as safety needles and syringes.

Remain aware of infection prevention and control techniques while working with patients in protected environments. You need to feel comfortable performing all procedures and yet remain conscious of infection prevention and control principles. Depending on the microorganism and mode of transmission, assess which articles or equipment to take into an isolation room. For example, the CDC (2016b) recommends the dedicated use of articles such as stethoscopes, sphygmomanometers, and thermometers in the isolation room of a patient infected or colonized with VRE. Do not use these devices on other patients unless the devices are first adequately cleaned and disinfected.

Personal Protective Equipment. The PPE, specialized clothing or equipment (e.g., gowns, masks or respirators, protective eyewear, and gloves) that you wear for protection against exposure to infectious materials, should be readily available in a patient care area (CDC, 2016b). You choose the equipment to use depending on the task to be performed.

Gowns. The primary reason for gowning is to prevent soiling clothes during contact with a patient. Gowns or cover-ups protect health care personnel and visitors from coming in contact with infected material and blood or body fluids. Gowns are often required, depending on the expected amount of exposure to infectious material. Gowns used for barrier protection are made of a fluid-resistant material. Change gowns immediately if damaged or heavily contaminated.

Isolation gowns usually open at the back and have ties or snaps at the neck and waist to keep the gown closed and secure. Gowns need to be long enough to cover all outer garments. Long sleeves with tight-fitting cuffs provide added protection. No special technique is required for applying clean gowns if they are fastened securely. However, carefully remove gowns to minimize contamination of the hands and uniform, and discard them after removal.

Masks. Masks provide respiratory protection. Wear full-face protection (with eyes, nose, and mouth covered) when you anticipate splashing or spraying of blood or body fluid into the face. Also wear masks when working with a patient placed on Airborne or Droplet Precautions. If a patient is on Airborne Precautions for TB, apply an OSHA-approved respirator-style mask. The mask protects you from inhaling microorganisms and small-particle droplet nuclei that remain suspended in the air from a patient's respiratory tract. The surgical mask protects a wearer from inhaling large-particle aerosols that travel short distances (3 feet). When caring for patients on Droplet or Airborne Precautions, apply a mask (surgical or respirator) when entering the isolation room.

At times, a patient who is susceptible to infection wears a mask to prevent inhalation of pathogens. Patients on Droplet or Airborne Precautions who are transported outside their rooms need to wear a surgical mask to protect other patients and personnel. Masks prevent transmission of infection by direct contact with mucous membranes (CDC, 2019a). A mask discourages the wearer from touching the eyes, nose, or mouth (Box 28.12).

If a person wears glasses, the top edge of the mask fits below the glasses so that they do not cloud over as the person exhales. Keep talking to a minimum while wearing a mask to reduce respiratory airflow. A mask that becomes moist does not provide a barrier to microorganisms and is ineffective. You need to discard it. Never reuse a disposable mask. Warn patients and family members that a mask can cause a sensation of smothering. If family members become uncomfortable, they should leave the room and discard the mask.

Specially fitted respiratory protective devices (N95 respirator masks) are required when caring for patients on Airborne Precautions such as patients with known or suspected TB (Fig. 28.3) (CDC, 2005; 2019a). The mask must have a higher filtration rating than regular surgical masks and be fitted snugly to prevent leakage around the sides. Be aware of health care agency policy regarding the type of respiratory protective device required. Special fit testing is required to establish the size and ability of the nurse to wear this type of mask (CDC, 2005).

BOX 28.12   PROCEDURAL GUIDELINES

Applying a Disposable Mask

Delegation and Collaboration

The skill of applying a disposable mask can be delegated to assistive personnel (AP). The nurse informs AP to:
- Put on the mask following the appropriate steps.
- Change the mask if it becomes moist or contaminated.
- Remove the mask when leaving the patient's room.

Equipment

Disposable mask

Procedural Steps

1. Find top edge of mask (some have a thin metal strip along edge). Pliable metal fits snugly against bridge of nose. Others offer an occlusive fit that does not require an adjustment.
2. Hold mask by top two strings or loops. Secure two top ties at top of back of head (see illustration), with ties above ears. (*Alternative:* Slip loops over each ear.)

3. Tie two lower ties snugly around neck with mask well under chin (see illustration).
4. Gently pinch upper metal band around bridge of nose.
   NOTE: Change mask when it becomes wet, moist, or contaminated.
5. Remove mask by untying *bottom* mask strings and then top strings; pull mask away from face and drop into trash receptacle. (Do not touch outer surface of mask.)

STEP 3 Securing lower ties of a tie-on mask.

STEP 2 Securing top two ties of a tie-on mask.

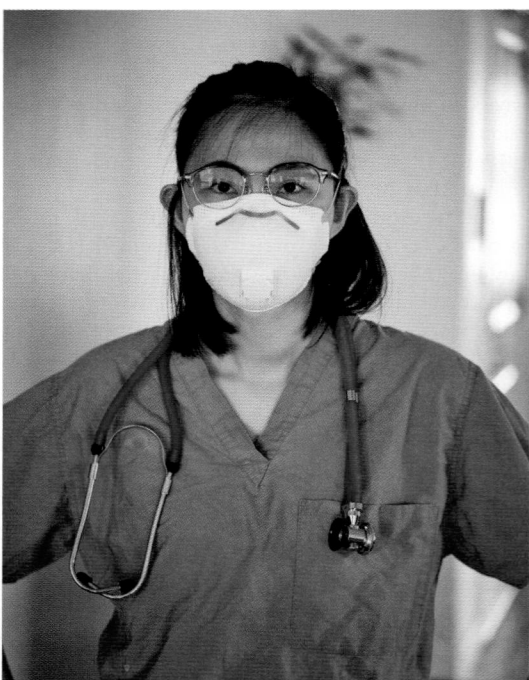

FIG. 28.3 N95 respirator mask with filter. (Copyright © iStock/RichLegg.)

Eye Protection. Use either special glasses or goggles when performing procedures that generate splash or splatter. Examples of such procedures include irrigation of a large abdominal wound or insertion of an arterial catheter when the nurse assists a health care provider. A nurse who wears prescription glasses uses removable, reusable, or disposable side shields over them (OSHA, 2011). Eyewear is available in the form of plastic glasses or goggles. The eyewear needs to fit snugly around the face so that fluids cannot enter between the face and the glasses.

Gloves. Gloves help to prevent the transmission of pathogens by direct and indirect contact. The CDC (2019a) notes that you need to wear clean gloves when touching blood, body fluid, secretions, excretions (except sweat), moist mucous membranes, nonintact skin, and contaminated items or surfaces. Follow these guidelines:

- Change and dispose of gloves and perform hand hygiene between tasks and procedures on the same patient after contact with material that contains a high concentration of microorganisms.
- Remove and dispose of gloves promptly after use, before touching noncontaminated items and environmental surfaces, and before going to another patient.
- Perform hand hygiene immediately after removing gloves to avoid transfer of microorganisms to other patients or environments.

To reduce the incidence of health care providers developing a sensitivity or allergy to the latex in gloves, health care agencies provide nonlatex gloves to employees. Most health care agencies are working to become latex free to protect health care providers and patients.

Box 28.13 describes the steps to follow for applying full PPE. During a procedure, be sure PPE remains in place. If you notice a break or tear in a glove while providing care, change gloves. If you do not plan to have additional contact with a patient after a care activity, reapplying gloves is unnecessary. Perform hand hygiene when gloves are removed.

Instruct family members visiting patients on isolation precautions on how to apply gloves properly. Demonstrate the application of gloves to family members and explain the reason for the use of gloves. Emphasize the importance of performing hand hygiene after removing gloves.

Specimen Collection. Many laboratory studies are often necessary when a patient is suspected of having an infectious or communicable disease (Box 28.14). You collect body fluids and secretions suspected of containing infectious organisms for culture and sensitivity tests. After a specimen is sent to a laboratory, the laboratory technologist identifies the microorganisms growing in the culture. Additional test results indicate the antibiotics to which the organisms are resistant or sensitive. Sensitivity reports determine which antibiotics used in treatment are effective and need to be ordered for treatment.

Obtain all culture specimens using clean gloves and sterile equipment. Blood cultures are taken from two separate venipuncture sites and before initiation of antimicrobials. Collecting fresh material such as wound drainage from the site of infection ensures that neighboring microbes do not contaminate a specimen. Seal all specimen containers tightly to prevent spillage and contamination of the outside of the container.

Bagging Trash or Linen. Bagging contaminated items prevents accidental exposure of personnel and contamination of the surrounding environment. Double bagging is not recommended (CDC, 2019a). A single intact, standard-size linen bag that is not overfilled and that is tied securely is adequate to prevent infection transmission. Check the color code of bag that your agency uses for bagging these items.

Transporting Patients. Before transferring patients to wheelchairs or stretchers, give them clean gowns to serve as robes. Patients infected with organisms transmitted by the airborne route normally leave their rooms only for essential purposes such as diagnostic procedures or surgery. A patient with an airborne infection must wear a mask when leaving the room. Notify personnel in diagnostic or procedural areas or the operating room of the type of isolation precautions the patient requires. Some patients being transported drain body fluids onto a stretcher or wheelchair. Use an extra layer of sheets to cover the stretcher or seat of the wheelchair. Be sure to clean the equipment with an approved germicide after patient use and before another patient uses the shared equipment.

QSEN Building Competency in Evidence-Based Practice
You are asked to participate on a unit-based team to help your fellow health care workers be more adherent to hand hygiene before and after patient care. Your unit's current rate of adherence to hand hygiene is 74%, and the unit manager has been directed by administration to improve the rate by the next quarter. Your team meets, and many team members offer opinions on how best to improve the unit hand-hygiene adherence rates, but no one is sure where to start. You know that implementing an evidence-based plan will be more successful than a trial and error approach. How can you guide the team in a way that will provide an evidence-based approach to the problem?

Answers to the QSEN Activities can be found on the Evolve website.

Role of the Infection Control Professional. An infection control professional is a valuable resource for helping nurses control HAIs. These professionals are specially trained in infection prevention and control. They are responsible for advising health care personnel regarding infection prevention and control practices and monitoring infections within the hospital. An infection control professional's responsibility often includes (Friedman, 2018):

- Collection and analysis of infection data
- Evaluation of products and procedures
- Development and review of policies and procedures
- Consultation on infection risk assessment, prevention, and control strategies (includes activities related to occupational health, construction, and emergency management)

BOX 28.13 PROCEDURAL GUIDELINES

Caring for a Patient on Isolation Precautions

Delegation and Collaboration

The skill of caring for a patient on isolation precautions can be delegated to assistive personnel (AP). However, it is the nurse who assesses the patient's status and isolation indications. Instruct AP about:

- Reason patient is on isolation precautions
- Use of the correct personal protective equipment (PPE) for the specific isolation type
- Precautions about bringing equipment into the patient's room
- Reporting abnormal findings and any high-risk behaviors (e.g., patient does not adhere to secretion control when coughing)
- Special precautions regarding individual patient needs such as transportation to diagnostic tests

Equipment

PPE—gloves, gowns, masks, protective eyewear, or face shield—is determined by the type of isolation that is needed. Other patient care equipment depends on procedures performed in room (e.g., hygiene items; disposable blood pressure [BP] cuff, thermometer, and stethoscope; sharps container; soiled linen bag; and trash receptacle).

Procedural Steps

1. Assess patient's health history for isolation indications (e.g., tuberculosis [TB], diarrhea, major draining wound or purulent cough).
2. Review laboratory test results (e.g., wound culture; acid-fast bacillus [AFB] smears) to identify the type of microorganism for which the patient is isolated and whether the patient is immunocompromised.
3. Review agency policies and precautions necessary for the specific isolation system and consider care measures you will perform and necessary equipment to use while in the patient's room.
4. Review nurses' notes or speak with colleagues regarding patient's emotional state and adjustment to isolation.
5. Determine whether patient has latex allergy to avoid sensitivity or allergic reaction. If allergy exists, refer to agency policy to provide full latex-free care.
6. Perform hand hygiene and prepare all equipment that you need to take into patient's room. In some cases, equipment remains in the room (stethoscope or BP cuff).
7. Prepare for entrance into isolation room. Ideally, before applying PPE, step into patient's room and stay by door. Introduce yourself and explain the care that you are providing. If this is not possible, apply PPE outside of room.
   a. Apply cover gown, being sure that it covers all outer garments. Pull sleeves down to wrist. Tie securely at neck and waist (see illustration).

STEP 7a Tie gown at waist.

   b. Apply either surgical mask or fitted respirator around mouth and nose. (Type depends on type of precautions and agency policy.) You must have a medical evaluation and be fit tested before using a respirator (OSHA, 2011).
   c. If needed, apply eyewear, goggles, or face shield securely around face and eyes. If prescription glasses are worn, side shield may be used.
   d. Apply clean gloves. (**NOTE:** Wear unpowdered latex-free gloves if you, patient, or another health care worker has a history of latex allergy.) Secure glove cuffs over edge of gown sleeves (see illustration).

STEP 7d Apply gloves over gown sleeves.

8. Enter patient's room. Arrange supplies and equipment. (If equipment will be removed from room for reuse, place on clean paper towel.)
9. Identify patient using at least two identifiers (e.g., name and birthday or name and medical record number) according to agency policy (TJC, 2021).
10. Assess patient's or family caregiver's knowledge, experience, and health literacy.
11. Explain purpose of isolation and necessary precautions for patient and family to take. Offer opportunity to ask questions. Discuss types of activities patient may wish to do to try to stay occupied. Assess for evidence of emotional problems that can occur from isolation. If TB precautions are in use, instruct patient to cover mouth with tissue when coughing and to wear disposable surgical mask when leaving room.
12. Assess vital signs (see Chapter 29).
    a. If patient is infected or colonized with a resistant organism (e.g., vancomycin-resistant enterococci, methicillin-resistant *Staphylococcus aureus* or *Clostridium difficile*), use disposable equipment that remains in room. This includes thermometer, stethoscope, and BP cuff.
    b. If stethoscope is to be reused, clean diaphragm or bell with alcohol. Set aside on clean surface.
    c. Use individual electronic or disposable thermometer.

CLINICAL JUDGMENT: If disposable thermometer indicates a fever, assess for other signs/symptoms. Confirm fever using an alternative thermometer. Do not use electronic thermometer if patient is suspected or confirmed to have *C. difficile* (Amitra et al., 2018).

13. Administer medications (see Chapter 31).
    a. Give oral medication in wrapper or cup.
    b. Dispose of wrapper or cup in plastic-lined receptacle.
    c. Wear gloves when administering an injection.
    d. Discard safety needle and syringe or uncapped needle into sharps container.
    e. Place reusable syringe (e.g., Carpujet) on a clean towel for eventual removal and disinfection.
    f. If you are not wearing gloves and hands come into contact with contaminated article or body fluids, perform hand hygiene as soon as possible.
14. Administer hygiene, encouraging patient to discuss questions or concerns about isolation. Provide informal teaching at this time.

Continued

BOX 28.13   PROCEDURAL GUIDELINES—cont'd

Caring for a Patient on Isolation Precautions

a. Avoid allowing isolation gown to become wet. Carry wash basin out away from gown; avoid leaning against any wet surface.

b. Help patient remove own gown; discard in leakproof linen bag.

c. Remove linen from bed; avoid contact with isolation gown. Place in linen bag according to agency policy.

d. Provide clean bed linen and a set of towels.

e. Remove and dispose of gloves, perform hand hygiene, and reglove if further care is necessary.

15. Collect specimens.

a. Place specimen containers on clean paper towel in patient's bathroom. Follow procedure for collecting specimen of body fluids.

b. Transfer specimen to container without soiling outside of container. Label specimen in front of patient. All specimen containers must be placed in a double-sided, self-sealing polythene bag with one compartment containing the laboratory request form and the other the specimen (Nukifora, 2015).

c. Perform hand hygiene and reglove if additional procedures are needed.

d. Check label on specimen with patient at bedside for accuracy. Send to laboratory. Be sure containers are labeled with a biohazard label (see illustration).

STEP 15d Specimen container placed in biohazard bag.

16. Assist patient to comfortable position. Place nurse call system in an accessible location within patient's reach. Instruct patient in its use.

17. Raise side rails (as appropriate) and lower bed to lowest position.

18. Dispose of linen, trash, and disposable items.

a. Empty trash bag as it becomes full.

b. Use sturdy, moisture-resistant single bags to contain soiled articles. Use double bag if outside of bag is contaminated.

c. Tie bags securely at top in knot (see illustration).

STEP 18c Tie trash bag securely.

19. Retrieve and clean nondedicated reusable equipment. Clean any contaminated surfaces (see health care agency policy).

20. Resupply room as needed. Have a staff member outside the isolation room hand you new supplies.

21. Explain to patient when you plan to return to room. Ask whether patient requires any personal care items, books, or magazines.

22. Leave isolation room. The order for removing PPE depends on what was needed for the type of isolation. The sequence listed is based on full PPE being required.

a. Remove and dispose of gloves. Remove one glove by grasping cuff and pulling glove inside out over hand. With ungloved hand tuck finger inside cuff of remaining glove and pull it off, inside out (see illustration).

STEP 22a Remove glove.

b. Remove eyewear/face shield or goggles. Dispose in receptable.

c. Untie waist and neck strings of gown. Allow gown to fall from shoulders. Remove hands from sleeves without touching outside of gown. Hold gown inside at shoulder seams and fold inside out. Discard in laundry bag if fabric, or in trash receptacle if gown is disposable.

d. Remove mask: If mask loops over your ears remove from ears and pull away from face. For a tie-on mask, untie *bottom* mask strings; hold strings; untie *top* strings, pull mask away from face, and drop it into trash receptacle. Do not touch outer surface of mask (see illustration).

STEP 22d Remove mask.

e. Perform hand hygiene.

f. Leave room and close door if necessary. (Make sure that door is closed if patient is on airborne precautions).

g. Dispose of all contaminated supplies and equipment in a manner that prevents spread of microorganisms to other people (see health care agency policy).

BOX 28.14   Specimen Collection Techniques[a]

Ensure that all specimen containers used have the biohazard symbol on the outside (Pagana et al., 2019). Also follow agency policy in confirming proper labeling of all specimen containers (i.e., labeling in front of patient [TJC, 2021]).

Wound Specimen

Perform hand hygiene and apply clean gloves. Clean site with sterile water or saline before wound specimen collection with a clean swab. Wipe from edges outward to remove old exudate (see Chapter 48). Remove and dispose of gloves, perform hand hygiene, and apply new pair of gloves. Use a sterile cotton-tipped swab or syringe to collect as much drainage as possible. Have clean test tube or culture tube on clean paper towel. After swabbing center of wound site, grasp collection tube with a paper towel. Carefully insert swab without touching outside of tube. After securing top of tube, label specimen container with patient name and identifying information with patient present. Then transfer tube into labeled biohazard bag for transport and perform hand hygiene.

Blood Specimen

(This procedure is often performed by a laboratory technician.)

Wearing gloves, clean venipuncture site with antiseptic swab; move the first swab back and forth on horizontal plane, another swab on the vertical plane, and the last swab in a circular motion from site outward for 5 cm (2 inches), lasting a total of 30 seconds. Allow area to dry. Clean tops of culture bottles for 15 seconds with agency-approved cleansing solution. Use a 20-mL needle-safe syringe and collect up to 10 to 15 mL of blood per culture bottle (check health care agency policy). Perform venipuncture at two different sites to decrease likelihood of both specimens being contaminated with skin flora. Place blood culture bottles on a clean paper towel on bedside table or other surface; swab off bottle tops with alcohol. Inject an appropriate amount of blood into each bottle. If collecting aerobic and anaerobic specimens, inject blood into the aerobic bottle first and the anaerobic bottle second. Transfer labeled specimen into clean, labeled biohazard bag for transport. Remove and dispose of gloves and perform hand hygiene.

Stool Specimen

Wearing gloves, use clean cup with seal top (need not be sterile) and a tongue blade to collect a small amount, approximately 2 to 3 cm (1 inch) of stool. Place cup on clean paper towel in patient's bathroom. Using tongue blade, collect needed amount of feces from patient's bedpan. Transfer feces to cup without touching outside surface of cup. Dispose of tongue blade and place seal on cup. Transfer labeled specimen into clean labeled biohazard bag for transport. Remove and dispose of gloves and perform hand hygiene.

Urine Specimen

Apply gloves. Cleanse needleless port on urinary catheter and, using a needle-less safety syringe, collect 1 to 5 mL of urine. Fill sterile specimen tube and place on clean paper towel in patient's bathroom. If the patient is not catheterized, instruct the patient to follow the procedure to obtain a clean voided specimen (see Chapter 46). Secure top of transfer container, label container in front of patient, and place in a biohazard bag with label attached. Remove and dispose of gloves and perform hand hygiene.

[a]Health care agency policy may differ on types of containers and amounts of specimen material required.

- Educational efforts directed at interventions to reduce infection risks
- Education of patients and families
- Implementation of changes mandated by regulatory, accrediting, and licensing agencies (includes reporting communicable diseases to health departments)
- Application of epidemiological principles, including activities directed at improving patient outcomes using implementation science

FIG. 28.4 Five Moments for Hand Hygiene. (From World Health Organization: *About SAVE Lives: Clean Your Hands: 5 moments for hand hygiene,* 2021, https://www.who.int/campaigns/world-hand-hygiene-day. Accessed November 2021.)

- Antimicrobial management
- Participation in research projects
- Monitoring antibiotic-resistant organisms in the institution

Infection Prevention and Control for Hospital Personnel. Health care workers are continually at risk for exposure to infectious microorganisms. Numerous efforts have been made by health care agencies to improve health care provider adherence to hand hygiene, including increased access to automatic alcohol-based hand sanitizers, posted reminders, and sensor monitoring of sanitizer use. The WHO recently released a new initiative for improving adherence of health care workers to hand hygiene. The WHO's Five Moments for Hand Hygiene has emerged from the WHO Guidelines on Hand Hygiene in Health Care to add value to any hand hygiene improvement strategy (WHO, 2021). The Five Moments defines the key moments for hand hygiene, overcoming misleading language and complicated descriptions (Fig. 28.4).

Patient Education. Often patients need to learn to use infection prevention and control practices at home (Box 28.15). Preventive technique becomes almost second nature to the nurse who practices it daily. However, patients are less aware of factors that promote the spread of infection or ways to prevent its transmission. The home environment may not always lend itself to infection prevention and control. Often you help a patient adapt according to the resources available to maintain hygienic techniques. Generally, patients in a home care setting have a decreased risk of infection because of decreased exposure to resistant organisms such as those found in a health care setting and fewer invasive procedures. However, it is important to educate patients and their family caregivers about infection prevention and control techniques.

Surgical Asepsis. Surgical asepsis or sterile technique prevents contamination of an open wound, serves to isolate an operative or procedural area from an unsterile environment, and maintains a sterile field for surgery or procedural intervention. Surgical asepsis includes procedures used to eliminate all microorganisms, including pathogens and spores, from an object or area (Chetan, 2018). In surgical asepsis an area or object is considered contaminated if touched by any object that is not sterile. It demands the highest level of aseptic technique and requires that all areas be kept free of infectious microorganisms.

BOX 28.15   PATIENT TEACHING

Infection Prevention and Control

Objective
- Patient and/or family caregiver will use proper infection prevention and control practices when performing a clean dressing change.

Teaching Strategies
- Demonstrate proper hand hygiene, explaining that the patient and/or caregiver needs to perform hand hygiene before and after all treatments and whenever contact is made with infected body fluids.
- Instruct patient and/or caregiver about the signs and symptoms of wound infection and when to notify the health care provider.
- Instruct patient and/or caregiver to place contaminated dressings and other disposable items containing infectious body fluids in impervious plastic or brown paper bags. Place needles in metal or hard plastic containers, such as coffee cans or laundry detergent bottles, and tape the openings shut. *Some states have specific requirements for sharps disposal. Check local regulations.*
- Instruct patient and/or caregiver to separate linen soiled with wound drainage from other laundry. Wash in warm water with detergent. There are no special recommendations for setting a dryer temperature (CDC, 2019a).

Evaluation
Use the principles of teach-back to evaluate patient/family caregiver learning:
- Tell me what you will do to decrease the spread of infection at home. Show me how you do hand hygiene before the dressing change.
- Show me how you would change your dressing.
- Tell me three signs or symptoms of wound infection that you will watch for. Tell me the signs and symptoms that you might develop that would require you to call your health care provider.

Use surgical asepsis in the following situations:
- During procedures that require intentional perforation of the patient's skin, such as insertion of peripheral IV catheters or a central IV line
- When the integrity of the skin is broken as a result of trauma, surgical incision, or burns
- During invasive procedures, such as the insertion of a urinary catheter or the insertion of surgical instruments into sterile body cavities (e.g., placement of a wound drain)

Although surgical asepsis is common in the operating room, labor and delivery area, and major diagnostic/procedural areas, you also use surgical aseptic techniques at a patient's bedside (e.g., when inserting IV or urinary catheters, suctioning the tracheobronchial airway, and sterile dressing changes). A nurse in an operating room follows a series of steps to maintain sterile technique, including applying a mask, protective eyewear, and a cap; performing a surgical hand scrub; and applying a sterile gown and gloves. In contrast, a nurse performing a dressing change at a patient's bedside only performs hand hygiene and applies sterile gloves. For certain procedures (e.g., changing a central line dressing) the nurse also uses a mask and gown (see agency policy). Regardless of the procedures followed or the setting, the nurse always recognizes the importance of strict adherence to aseptic principles (Iwamoto and Post, 2018).

Patient Preparation for a Sterile Procedure. Because surgical asepsis requires exact techniques, you need to have the patient's full cooperation. Therefore, assess a patient's understanding of the sterile procedure, and explain the reasons for not moving or interfering with the procedure. Certain patients fear moving or touching objects during a sterile procedure, whereas others try to help. Explain how you will perform a procedure and what the patient can do to avoid contaminating sterile items, including the following:
- Avoid sudden movements of body parts covered by sterile drapes.
- Refrain from touching sterile supplies, drapes, or the nurse's gloves and gown.
- Avoid coughing, sneezing, or talking over a sterile area.

Certain sterile procedures last an extended time. Assess a patient's needs and anticipate factors that may disrupt a procedure. If a patient is in pain, administer ordered analgesics about a half-hour before a sterile procedure begins. Ask whether the patient needs to use the bathroom or a bedpan. Often patients must assume relatively uncomfortable positions during sterile procedures. Help a patient assume the most comfortable position possible. Finally, a patient's condition sometimes results in actions or events that contaminate a sterile field. For example, a patient with a respiratory infection transmits organisms by coughing or talking. Anticipate such a problem and place a surgical mask on the patient before the procedure begins.

Principles of Surgical Asepsis. Performing sterile aseptic procedures requires a work area in which objects can be handled with minimal risk of contamination. A sterile field provides a sterile surface for placement of sterile equipment. It is an area considered free of microorganisms and consists of a sterile kit or tray, a work surface draped with a sterile towel or wrapper, or a table covered with a large sterile drape (Murphy, 2018). When beginning a surgically aseptic procedure, nurses follow certain principles to ensure maintenance of asepsis. Failure to follow these principles places patients at risk for infection. The following principles are important:
1. *A sterile object remains sterile only when touched by another sterile object.* This principle guides you in placement of sterile objects and how to handle them.
   a. Sterile touching sterile remains sterile (e.g., use sterile gloves or sterile forceps to handle objects on a sterile field).
   b. Sterile touching clean becomes contaminated (e.g., if the tip of a syringe or other sterile object touches the surface of a clean disposable glove, the object is contaminated).
   c. Sterile touching contaminated becomes contaminated (e.g., when you touch a sterile object with an ungloved hand, the object is contaminated).
   d. Sterile state is questionable (e.g., when you find a tear or break in the covering of a sterile object). Discard it regardless of whether the object itself appears untouched.
2. *Only sterile objects may be placed on a sterile field.* All items are properly sterilized before use. Sterile objects are kept in clean, dry storage areas. The package or container holding a sterile object must be intact and dry. A package that is torn, punctured, wet, or open is considered unsterile.
3. *A sterile object or field out of the range of vision or an object held below a person's waist is contaminated.* Never turn your back on a sterile field or tray or leave it unattended. Contamination can occur accidentally by a dangling piece of clothing or an unknowing patient touching a sterile object. Any object held below waist level is considered contaminated because it cannot always be viewed. Keep sterile objects in front with the hands as close together as possible.
4. *A sterile object or field becomes contaminated by prolonged exposure to air.* Avoid activities that create air currents such as excessive movements or rearranging linen after a sterile object or field becomes exposed. When you open sterile packages, it is important to minimize the number of people walking into an area. Microorganisms also travel by droplet through the air. Do not talk, laugh, sneeze, or cough over a sterile field or when gathering and using sterile equipment. When opening sterile packages, hold the item or

piece of equipment as close as possible to the sterile field without touching the sterile surface.

5. When a sterile surface comes in contact with a wet, contaminated surface, the sterile object or field becomes contaminated by capillary action. If moisture leaks through the protective covering of a sterile package, microorganisms travel to the sterile object. When stored sterile packages become wet, discard the objects immediately or send the equipment for resterilization. When working with a sterile field or tray, you may have to pour sterile solutions. Any spill is a source of contamination unless on a sterile surface that moisture cannot penetrate. Urinary catheterization trays contain sterile supplies that rest in a sterile plastic container. In contrast, if you place a piece of sterile gauze in its wrapper on a patient's bedside table and the table surface is wet, the gauze is considered contaminated.

6. *Fluid flows in the direction of gravity.* A sterile object becomes contaminated if gravity causes a contaminated liquid to flow over the surface of the object. To avoid contamination during a surgical hand scrub, hold your hands above your elbows. This allows water to flow downward without contaminating your hands and fingers. The principle of water flow by gravity is also the reason for drying from fingers to elbows, with hands held up, after the scrub.

7. *The edges of a sterile field or container are considered contaminated.* Frequently you place sterile objects on a sterile towel, drape, or tray (Fig. 28.5). Because the edge of the drape touches an unsterile surface such as a table or bed linen, a 2.5-cm (1-inch) border around the drape is considered contaminated. Objects placed on the sterile field need to be *inside* this border. The edges of sterile containers become exposed to air after they are open and thus are contaminated. After you remove a sterile needle from its protective cap or forceps from a container, the objects must not touch the edge of the container.

Performing Sterile Procedures. Assemble all the equipment that will be needed before a procedure. Have a few extra supplies available in case objects accidentally become contaminated. Do not leave a sterile area, because you will not know if the area was contaminated during your absence. Before a sterile procedure, explain each step so that the patient can cooperate fully. If an object becomes contaminated during the procedure, do not hesitate to discard it immediately.

Donning and Removing Caps, Masks, and Eyewear. Wear a surgical mask and eyewear without a cap for any sterile procedures on a general nursing unit. Eyewear is worn as a part of Standard Precautions if there is a risk of fluid or blood splashing into your eyes. For sterile surgical procedures, you first apply a clean cap that covers all your hair and then the surgical mask and eyewear. A mask must fit snugly around the face and nose. After wearing a mask for several hours, the area over the

mouth and nose often becomes moist. Because moisture promotes the growth of microorganisms, change the mask if it becomes moist.

Protective glasses or goggles fit snugly around the forehead and face to fully protect the eyes. Wear eyewear only for procedures that create the risk of body fluids splashing into the eyes. Remove PPE in the following order: gloves, face shield or goggles, gown, and mask or respirator (CDC, 2015a). After removing all PPE, perform hand hygiene.

Opening Sterile Packages. Sterile items such as syringes, gauze dressings, or catheters are packaged in paper or plastic containers and are impervious to microorganisms if they are dry and intact. These items have expiration labels on the packages. Do not use an item after the expiration date. Some institutions wrap reusable supplies (e.g., operating room instruments) in a double thickness of paper, linen, or muslin. These packages are permeable to steam and thus allow for steam autoclaving. Sterile items are kept in clean, enclosed storage cabinets and separated from dirty equipment.

Sterile supplies that have been autoclaved have chemical tapes indicating that a sterilization process has taken place. The tapes change color during the process. Failure of the tapes to change color means that the item is not sterile. Health care agencies follow the principles of event-related sterility, a concept that items are considered sterile if the packaging is uncompromised (Jefferson and Young, 2018). Never use a sterile item if the packaging is open or soiled, shows evidence that the package has been wet, or has dropped to the floor. Before opening a sterile item, perform hand hygiene. Inspect the supplies for package integrity and sterility, and assemble the supplies in the work area, such as the bedside table or treatment room, before opening packages. A bedside table or countertop provides a large, clean working area for opening items. Keep the work area above waist level. Do not open sterile supplies in a confined space where contamination might occur.

Opening a Sterile Item on a Flat Surface. You must open sterile packages without contaminating the contents. Commercially packaged items are usually designed so that you must tear away or separate only the paper or plastic cover. Hold the item in one hand while pulling the wrapper away with the other (Fig. 28.6). Take care to keep the inner contents sterile before use. You may use a sterile wrapper from a commercial kit or a sterile paper or linen wrapper from an institutional pack to create a sterile field on which to work. Use the inner surface of the package (except for the 2.5-cm [1-inch] border around the edges) as a sterile field to add sterile items. You can grasp the 2.5-cm (1-inch) border to maneuver the field on a table surface (see Skill 28.2).

Opening a Sterile Item While Holding It. To open a small sterile item, hold the package in your nondominant hand while opening the top flap and pulling it away from you. Using the dominant hand, carefully open the sides and innermost flap away from the enclosed sterile item in the same order as opening a sterile item on

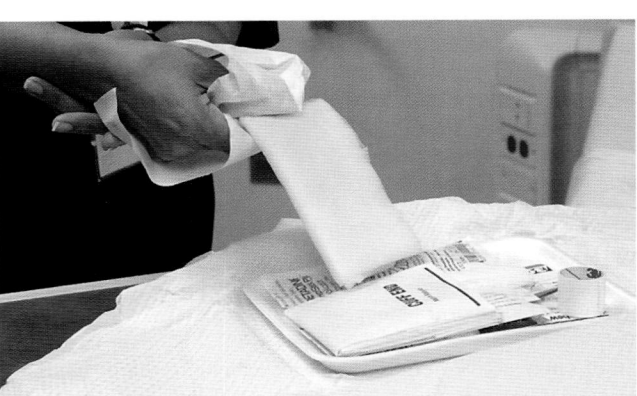

FIG. 28.5 Placing sterile item on sterile field.

FIG. 28.6 Nurse opens sterile package on work area above waist level.

a flat surface (see Skill 28.2). You open the item in a hand so that you can pass it to a person wearing sterile gloves or transfer it to a sterile field.

Preparing a Sterile Field. When performing sterile procedures, you need a sterile work area that provides room for handling and placing sterile items. A **sterile field** is an area free of microorganisms that is prepared to receive sterile items. You prepare the field by using the inner surface of a sterile wrapper as the work surface or by using a sterile drape or dressing tray. After creating the surface for the sterile field, add sterile items by placing them directly on the field or transferring them with sterile forceps (see Skill 28.2). Discard an object that comes in contact with the 2.5-cm (1-inch) border.

Sometimes you will wear sterile gloves while preparing items on a sterile field. If you do this, you can touch the entire drape, but sterile items must be handed over by an assistant. The gloves cannot touch the wrappers of sterile items.

Pouring Sterile Solutions. Often you need to pour sterile solutions into sterile containers. A bottle containing a sterile solution is sterile on the inside and contaminated on the outside; the neck of the bottle is also contaminated, but the inside of the bottle cap is considered sterile. After you remove the cap or lid, hold it in your hand or place its sterile side (inside) up on a *clean* surface. This means that you can see the inside of the lid as it rests on the table surface. Never rest a bottle cap or lid on a sterile surface. The outer edge of the cap is unsterile and contaminates the surface. Placing a sterile cap down on an unsterile surface increases the chances of the inside of the cap becoming contaminated.

Hold the bottle with its label in the palm of the hand to prevent the possibility of the solution wetting and fading the label. Keep the edge of the bottle away from the edge or inside of the receiving container. Pour the solution slowly to avoid splashing the underlying drape or field. Never hold the bottle so high above the container that even slow pouring causes splashing. Hold the bottle outside the edge of the sterile field. Any remaining fluids should be discarded. The edge of a container is considered contaminated after the contents have been poured. Reuse of open containers may contaminate solutions due to drops contacting unsterile areas and then running back over container openings (AORN, 2020).

Surgical Scrub. Patients undergoing operative procedures are at an increased risk for infection. Nurses working in operating rooms perform surgical hand antisepsis (see Skill 28.3) to decrease and suppress the growth of skin microorganisms under gloved hands in case of glove tears. A surgical hand scrub must eliminate the transient flora and reduce the resident flora on the hands. For maximum elimination of bacteria, remove all jewelry and keep the nails clean and short. Do not wear chipped nail polish, artificial nails, or extenders because they often hold a greater number of bacteria (AORN, 2020; WHO, 2009). Nurses who have active skin infections, open lesions or cuts, or respiratory infections should be excluded from the surgical or procedure team.

During surgical hand antisepsis the nurse scrubs from fingertips to elbows with an antiseptic soap before each surgical procedure. Research studies vary on the optimum duration of a surgical hand scrub (WHO, 2009). Chlorhexidine gluconate has been found to be more effective than povidone-iodine as a cleansing agent, although both can be found in health care agencies. Thus, the type of product used for cleansing will influence the time required for hand antisepsis (CDC, 2019a). The traditional scrub time in the United States for both the initial and the subsequent scrub is 5 minutes, but research has shown effectiveness can be gained when scrubs are performed for 2, 3, and 6 minutes (WHO, 2009). Follow the operating room policy or the manufacturer recommendation for scrub solutions. For many years preoperative handwashing protocols required nurses to scrub with a brush. However, this practice damages the skin. Scrubbing

FIG. 28.7 Sterile glove cuffs pulled over surgical gown cuffs.

with a disposable sponge or combination sponge-brush reduces bacterial counts on the hands as effectively as scrubbing with a brush. However, several studies suggest that neither a brush nor a sponge is necessary to reduce bacterial counts on the hands, especially when using an alcohol-based product (CDC, 2008).

Applying Sterile Gloves. Sterile gloves are an additional barrier to bacterial transfer. There are two gloving methods: open and closed. Nurses who work on general nursing units use open gloving before procedures such as dressing changes or urinary catheter insertions. In the open-glove technique, your hands slide all the way through the sleeves out beyond the cuffs of the gown (if worn). The closed-gloving method, performed after applying a sterile gown, is practiced in operating rooms and special procedure areas. In the closed-glove technique, your hands remain inside the sleeves and do not touch the cuffs. The cuffs of the gloves are pulled over the the cuffs of the surgical gown (Fig. 28.7). Make sure to select the proper glove size; the glove should not stretch so tightly that it can tear easily, yet it must be tight enough that you can pick up objects easily.

Donning a Sterile Gown. Nurses wear sterile gowns when assisting at the sterile field in the operating room, delivery room, and special procedure areas. It allows a nurse to handle sterile objects and also be comfortable with less risk of contamination. The sterile gown acts as a barrier to decrease shedding of microorganisms from skin surfaces into the air and thus prevents wound contamination. Nurses caring for patients with large open wounds or assisting health care providers during major invasive procedures (e.g., inserting an arterial catheter) also wear sterile gowns. The circulating nurse generally does not wear one.

Do not apply a sterile gown until after applying a mask and surgical cap and completing surgical handwashing. Pick up the gown from a sterile pack, or have an assistant hand the gown to you. Only a certain portion of the gown (i.e., the area from the anterior waist to, but not including, the collar and the anterior surface of the sleeves) is considered sterile. The back of the gown, the area under the arms, the collar, the area below the waist, and the underside of the sleeves are not sterile because you cannot keep these areas in constant view and ensure their sterility.

Exposure Issues. Patients and health care personnel, including housekeepers and maintenance personnel, are at risk for acquiring infections from accidental needlesticks. In the past, a stray needle lying in bed linen or carelessly thrown into a wastebasket served as a prime source for exposure to bloodborne pathogens. With the passage of the Needlestick Safety and Prevention Act in 2000 (OSHA, 2012b) and the implementation of safety needle devices, the incidence rate of sharps injuries has decreased. All sharps must now be either needle safe or needleless. After administering an injection or inserting an IV catheter, place the used

BOX 28.16 Hepatitis B Vaccination and Postexposure Follow-Up After Hepatitis C and Human Immunodeficiency Virus Exposure

Hepatitis B Vaccination

- Health care employers shall make available the hepatitis B vaccine and vaccination series to all employees who may have occupational exposures. Employees who decline the vaccine must sign a declination form. Evaluation and follow-up care are available to all employees who have been exposed.
- Hepatitis B vaccinations are made available to employees within 10 working days of assignment—this means before starting to provide patient care and after receiving education and training on the vaccine.
- A blood test (titer) is offered in some facilities 1 to 2 months after completing the three-dose vaccine series (check the health care agency policy).
- Vaccine is offered at no cost to employees. At present the vaccine does not require any boosters.
- After exposure, no treatment is needed if there is a positive blood titer on file. If no positive titer is on file, follow CDC guidelines.

Exposure to Hepatitis C Virus

- If the source patient is positive for hepatitis C virus (HCV), the employee receives a baseline test.
- At 4 weeks after exposure the employee should be offered an HCV-RNA test to determine whether the employee contracted HCV.
- If positive, the employee starts treatment.
- There is no prophylactic treatment for HCV after exposure.
- Early treatment for infection can prevent chronic infection.

Exposure to Human Immunodeficiency Virus

- If the patient is positive for human immunodeficiency virus (HIV) infection, a viral load study should be performed to determine the amount of virus present in the blood.
- If the exposure meets the CDC criteria for HIV PEP, it should be started as soon as possible, preferably within 24 hours after the exposure (CDC, 2015c).

All medical evaluations and procedures, including the vaccine and vaccination series and evaluation after exposure (prophylaxis), are made available at no cost to at-risk employees.

A confidential written medical evaluation will be available to employees with exposure incidents.

CDC, Centers for Disease Control and Prevention; *PEP*, postexposure prophylaxis; *RNA*, ribonucleic acid.
From Occupational Safety and Health Administration: Occupational Safety and Health Act of 2001, 2004, 2005, http://www.cdc.gov.

needle safety device in a puncture-resistant box (see Chapter 31). Sharps boxes must be at the site of use; this is an OSHA requirement (OSHA, 2012b).

HBV and HCV are the infections most commonly transmitted by contaminated needles (Box 28.16). Report any contaminated needlestick immediately. Additional criteria for exposure reporting include blood or other potentially infectious materials (OPIMs) that come into direct contact with an open area of the skin, blood or OPIM that is splashed into a health care worker's eye or mouth or up the nose, and cuts with a sharp object that is covered with blood or OPIM.

Follow-up for risk of acquiring infection begins with source patient testing. Access to testing the source patient is stated in the testing law for each state. Some states have deemed consent, which means that the state has granted the patient's consent to be tested. Other states require that the patient consent to testing for the presence of bloodborne pathogens.

Know the testing policies in the agency and state in which you practice. Health care agencies and workers' compensation require exposed employees to complete an injury report and seek appropriate treatment if needed. The need for treatment is linked to the results of a risk assessment and the testing of the patient. Test the patient for HIV, HBV, and HCV. If positive for HIV or HCV, testing for syphilis may be indicated because of the incidence of coinfection (CDC, 2019d). It is required that an employee is given the patient's testing results when an exposure occurs. This is *not* a violation of the Health Insurance Portability and Accountability Act (HIPAA) of 1996. Both the CDC and OSHA state that this information must be given to the exposed health care worker contingent on the health care worker's willingness to be tested.

Testing the employee at the time of the exposure is not needed immediately unless required by the state testing law. If the patient tests positive for a bloodborne pathogen or if the source patient is unknown, prophylactic treatment is recommended for the employee.

Exposures also occur involving nonbloodborne pathogens. Airborne and droplet diseases pose a risk to the nonimmune nurse. The CDC (2018c) has published a list of recommended immunizations and vaccinations for health care workers, including hepatitis B vaccine; TB testing; annual influenza vaccine; measles, mumps, and rubella (MMR); chickenpox vaccine; and tetanus, diphtheria, and pertussis. Employee health should review your health history and offer appropriate prevention. Declination forms are needed if these are declined (OSHA, 2012a),

Working with Mrs. Andrews, Kathy implemented the plan of care the two of them developed based on Mrs. Andrews' expectations. Kathy practiced good hand hygiene to decrease the risk of infection. She regularly cleaned the incision per agency policy and made sure that Mrs. Andrews used the incentive spirometer to help prevent postoperative atelectasis. Kathy made sure to keep Mrs. Andrews clean and dry to prevent urine from contaminating the incision. Kathy provided teaching to Mrs. Andrews and her daughter on the signs and symptoms of infection and when to contact the health care provider. Kathy also taught Mrs. Andrews proper hand hygiene. Kathy spent time with Mrs. Andrews, talking about her concerns regarding discharge and making sure that all of her questions were answered. Using therapeutic communication during their conversations, Kathy was able to decrease Mrs. Andrews' anxiety about discharge. Kathy also helped Mrs. Andrews explore ways to stay connected to her circle of friends once she is home. As part of the plan, Kathy made the referral to home health services, which provided additional assurance to Mrs. Andrews that she would be able to be at home. Kathy also worked with physical and occupational therapy to help Mrs. Andrews become more mobile and able to care for herself at home. Mrs. Andrews stated, "It's important for me to continue to be independent at home." During their sessions together, Kathy administered the patient-ordered analgesic and 30 minutes later helped Mrs. Andrews complete range-of-motion exercises and sit in a chair.

◆ Evaluation

Measure the success of infection prevention and control techniques by determining whether you achieved the outcomes for reducing or preventing infection identified in the patient's plan of care. Document the patient's response to therapies for infection prevention and control. A clear description of any signs and symptoms of systemic or local infection is necessary to give all nurses a baseline for comparative evaluation. Also determine if the patient's expectations for care were met.

Through the Patient's Eyes. Patients generally expect to be safe and protected when receiving health care. Ask patients whether their expectations for care have been met. A patient at risk for infection needs to understand the measures needed to reduce or prevent microorganism growth and spread. Providing patients and/or family caregivers the opportunity to discuss infection prevention and control measures or to demonstrate procedures such as hand hygiene reveals their ability to understand and adhere to therapy. Be sure that you understand the patient's perceptions of how infection spreads, the expectations for self-care, and how it can affect the patient as you evaluate the results of your instruction. Sometimes patients require new information or previously instructed information needs reinforcement, especially if the patient is being discharged with a urinary catheter or open wound. Help the patient identify concerns and determine what is needed to safely transition to care in the home. Attentive listening to your patients and their families determines their level of satisfaction with care and whether the plan of care met their expectations. Maintain open communication, and give your patients an opportunity to express new expectations, their level of satisfaction, and care concerns as they prepare for discharge.

Patient Outcomes. A comparison of a patient's response before and after an infection control measure, such as the absence of fever or wound infection, is an example of an expected outcome for measuring the success of nursing interventions. Compare the patient's response, such as a decrease in fever, with the expected outcomes identified in the nursing care plan. Observe wounds during dressing changes to determine the degree of wound healing. Monitor patients, especially those at risk, for signs and symptoms of infection. For example, a patient who has undergone a surgical procedure is at risk for infection at the surgical site and other invasive sites such as the venipuncture site or central line sites. In addition, the patient is at risk for a respiratory tract infection because of decreased mobility and for a UTI if an indwelling catheter is present. Observe all invasive and surgical sites for swelling, erythema (redness), or purulent drainage. Monitor breath sounds for changes and observe sputum character for change in color or consistency. Review laboratory test results for leukocytes. For example, leukocytosis in the urine often indicates a UTI. The patient and family need to practice proper hand-hygiene techniques when interacting with any care-related equipment or when the family is interacting with the patient. You evaluate their ability to follow medical asepsis through direct observation, while monitoring the patient's outcomes such as absence of fever or wound drainage. The absence of signs or symptoms of infection is the expected outcome of infection prevention and control.

Kathy is working with Mrs. Andrews, her daughter, and the health care team on finalizing plans for Mrs. Andrews' discharge. To evaluate the plan of care, Kathy first asks Mrs. Andrews whether she was satisfied with her care and whether her expectations for her care were met. Mrs. Andrews stated that she was satisfied with her participation in planning her care and that her preferences were considered when planning care. Mrs. Andrews tells Kathy, "My care was good. Everyone was attentive and listened to me when I had questions or concerns. The nurses did a good job keeping my pain at a low score, usually 2 out of 10." Kathy also evaluated Mrs. Andrews' anxiety about going home and caring for herself. When Kathy asked Mrs. Andrews about how she felt about going home, Mrs. Andrews stated, "I think I am ready to go home. I feel so much stronger now after working with physical and occupational therapy. I know my daughter is coming every day to check on me. Also knowing that a home health nurse and aide are coming has helped with my anxiety. I know that I will be getting good care at home." Kathy also was concerned about Mrs. Andrews' continued risk for infection after discharge. As part of the teaching, Mrs. Andrews was able to demonstrate proper hand hygiene and tell Kathy the signs and symptoms of infection. Mrs. Andrews' daughter also explained to Kathy what the indications were for calling the health care provider. Kathy set up Mrs. Andrews' return visits with the surgeon and her primary health care provider prior to discharge.

Kathy also worked with Mrs. Andrews on her urinary incontinence. Kathy taught Mrs. Andrews how to perform Kegel exercises, and Mrs. Andrews tells Kathy that she plans on continuing the exercise after she is home. She wants to try to prevent her incision from getting contaminated with urine. Mrs. Andrews' daughter also purchased the incontinence underwear that Kathy recommended to try to help keep Mrs. Andrews' incision area dry.

SAFETY GUIDELINES FOR NURSING SKILLS

Ensuring patient safety is an essential role of the professional nurse. Use sound clinical judgment by communicating clearly with members of the health care team, assessing and analyzing the patient's clinical findings, and making appropriate clinical decisions about the patient's priorities of care and preferences. Use the best evidence, applying professional standards, when selecting interventions to use in patient care delivery. When performing the skills in this chapter, remember the following points to ensure safe, patient-centered care.

- Apply Standard Precautions when performing all nursing care activities.
- Use clean gloves when you anticipate contact with body fluids and nonintact skin or mucous membranes when there is a risk of drainage.
- Use gown, mask, and eye protection when there is a risk for splash.
- Keep bedside table surfaces clutter-free, clean, and dry when performing aseptic procedures.
- Clean all equipment that is shared between patients.
- Ensure that patients cover mouth and nose when coughing or sneezing, use tissues to contain respiratory secretions, and dispose of tissues in waste receptacle.

SKILL 28.1   HAND HYGIENE

Delegation and Collaboration
The skill of hand hygiene is performed by all caregivers. Hand hygiene is not optional.

Equipment
- Antiseptic hand rub
  - Alcohol-based waterless antiseptic
- Handwashing
  - Easy-to-reach sink with warm running water
  - Antimicrobial or regular soap
  - Paper towels
  - Disposable nail cleaner *(optional)*

STEP	RATIONALE

ASSESSMENT

1. Inspect surface of hands for breaks or cuts in skin or cuticles. Cover any skin lesions with a dressing before providing care. If lesions are too large to cover, you may be restricted from direct patient care.
2. Inspect hands for visible soiling.
3. Inspect condition of nails. Natural tips should be no longer than 0.625 cm (¼ inch) long. Be sure that fingernails are short, filed, and smooth.

Open cuts or wounds can harbor high concentrations of microorganisms. Agency policy may prevent nurses from caring for high-risk patients if open lesions are present on hands (WHO, 2021).
Visible soiling requires handwashing with soap and water (CDC, 2021c).
Microorganisms can live under artificial nails after handwashing and using an alcohol-based sanitizer, and artificial nails should not be worn by health care providers having direct contact with patients (CDC, 2021c).

PLANNING

1. Organize supplies. Ensure that a filled hand sanitizer dispenser and/or a sink with running water and soap is available.

Having needed hand-hygiene supplies readily available and visible increases hand-hygiene adherence.

IMPLEMENTATION

1. Push wristwatch and long uniform sleeves above wrists. Avoid wearing rings. If worn, remove during hand hygiene.
2. Antiseptic hand rub
   a. Following manufacturer directions, dispense ample amount of product into palm of one hand (see illustration).
   b. Rub hands together covering all surfaces of hands and fingers with antiseptic (see illustration).
   c. Rub hands together (approximately 20 seconds) until alcohol is dry. Allow hands to dry completely before applying gloves.
3. Handwashing using regular or antimicrobial soap:
   a. Stand in front of sink, keeping hands and uniform away from sink surface. (If hands touch sink during handwashing, repeat sequence.)
   b. Turn on water. Turn on faucet (see illustration). It is best if sinks have knee, foot, or electronic sensor controls.

   c. Avoid splashing water against uniform.
   d. Regulate flow of water so that temperature is warm.
   e. Wet hands and wrists thoroughly under running water. Keep hands and forearms lower than elbows during washing.
   f. Apply the amount of antiseptic soap recommended by the manufacturer and rub hands together (see illustration).

Provides complete access to fingers, hands, and wrists. The skin underneath jewelry may carry a higher bacterial count (AORN, 2020).

Use enough product to cover hands thoroughly.

Ensures even bacteriostatic action.

Provides enough time for product to work (CDC, 2021c).

Inside of sink is a contaminated area. Reaching over sink increases risk of touching edge, which is contaminated.
Knee pads within operating room and treatment areas are preferred to prevent hand contact with faucet. Faucet handles are likely to be contaminated with organic debris and microorganisms (AORN, 2020).
Microorganisms travel and grow in moisture.
Warm water removes less of protective oils on hands than hot water.
Hands are most contaminated parts to wash. Water flows from least to most contaminated area, rinsing microorganisms into sink.
Ensure that all surfaces of hands and fingers are cleaned.

CLINICAL JUDGMENT: *The decision whether to use an antiseptic soap or an alcohol-based hand rub depends on whether the hands are visibly soiled, the type of infectious microorganism, the procedure you will perform, and the patient's immune status.*

g. Perform hand hygiene using plenty of lather and friction for at least 15 seconds (some agencies recommend 20 seconds) (CDC, 2021c). Interlace fingers and rub palms and back of hands with circular motion at least five times each. Keep fingertips down to facilitate removal of microorganisms.

Soap cleans by emulsifying fat and oil and lowering surface tension. Friction and rubbing mechanically loosen and remove dirt and transient bacteria. Interlacing fingers and thumbs ensures that all surfaces are cleaned. Adequate time is needed to expose skin surfaces to antimicrobial agent.

STEP 2a Apply waterless antiseptic to hands.

STEP 2b Rub hands thoroughly.

Continued

SKILL 28.1   HAND HYGIENE—cont'd

STEP	RATIONALE
h. Areas underlying fingernails are often soiled. Clean them with fingernails of other hand and additional soap or with disposable nail cleaner.	Area under nails can be highly contaminated, which increases risk for transmission of infection from nurse to patient.
i. Rinse hands and wrists thoroughly, keeping hands down and elbows up (see illustration).	Rinsing mechanically washes away dirt and microorganisms.
j. Dry hands thoroughly from fingers to wrists with paper towel or single-use cloth.	Drying from cleanest (fingertips) to least clean (wrist) avoids contamination. Drying hands prevents chapping and roughened skin. Do not tear or cut skin under or around nail.
k. If paper towel is used, discard in proper receptacle.	Prevents transfer of microorganisms.
l. To turn off hand faucet, use clean, dry paper towel; avoid touching handles with hands (see illustration). Turn off water with foot or knee pedals (if applicable).	Wet towel and hands allow transfer of pathogens from faucet by capillary action.
m. If hands are dry or chapped, use small amount of lotion or barrier cream.	Helps to minimize skin dryness. Only use lotions or creams approved by your health care agency as they have been selected to not interact with hand sanitizing products (CDC, 2021c).

EVALUATION

1. Inspect surface of hands for obvious signs of dirt or other contaminants.	Determines whether hand hygiene is adequate.
2. Inspect hands for dermatitis or cracked skin.	Breaks in skin integrity increase risk for transmission of microorganisms.

UNEXPECTED OUTCOMES AND RELATED INTERVENTIONS

1. Hands or areas under fingernails remain soiled.
  • Repeat handwashing with soap and water.
2. Repeated use of soaps or antiseptics causes dermatitis or cracked skin.
  • Rinse and dry hands thoroughly after using soap and water; avoid excessive amounts of soap or antiseptic; try various products.
  • Use approved hand lotions or barrier creams that will not interfere with hand sanitizing products (CDC, 2021c).

STEP 3b Turn on water.

STEP 3f Lather hands thoroughly.

STEP 3i Rinse hands.

STEP 3l Turn off faucet.

RECORDING AND REPORTING

- It is unnecessary to document handwashing.
- Report dermatitis, psoriasis, and/or cuts to your agency's employee health or infection control department.

HOME CARE CONSIDERATIONS

- Evaluate the handwashing facilities in a patient's home, including the availability of warm running water and soap, to determine the potential for contamination, how close the facilities are to the patient, and available supplies in the area.
- Anticipate the need for alternative handwashing products such as alcohol-based hand rubs and/or detergent-containing towels.
- Instruct the patient and primary caregiver in proper techniques and situations for handwashing. Use teach-back to confirm learning.

| SKILL 28.2 | PREPARATION OF STERILE FIELD |

Delegation and Collaboration

Nurses prepare sterile fields for some sterile procedures, such as urinary catheter insertion and performing tracheostomy care and suctioning, while other health care providers usually prepare sterile fields in the operating room (see agency's policy). The skill of preparing a sterile field cannot be delegated to assistive personnel (AP). The nurse can direct the AP to:

- Help with patient positioning and obtain any necessary supplies.

Equipment

- Sterile pack (commercial or facility wrapped)
- Sterile drape or kit that will be used as a sterile field
- Sterile gloves (if not included in kit)
- Sterile solution and equipment specific to procedure
- Waist-high table/countertop surface
- Appropriate personal protective equipment (PPE): gown, mask, cap, protective eyewear (see agency policy)

STEP	RATIONALE

ASSESSMENT

1. Identify patient using at least two identifiers (e.g., name and birthday or name and medical record number) according to agency policy.

Ensures correct patient. Complies with The Joint Commission standards and improves patient safety (TJC, 2021).

2. Assess type of aseptic technique needed for procedure.

Some procedures require medical, whereas others require surgical aseptic technique.

3. Assess patient's comfort, positioning, oxygen requirements, and elimination needs before preparing for procedure.

Certain procedures requiring a sterile field may last a long time. Anticipates patient's needs so that patient can relax and avoid any unnecessary movement that might disrupt procedure.

4. Assess patient for latex allergies.

A review of the patient's health history may reveal a latex allergy. Determine the need to use latex-free supplies.

5. Assess patient's or family caregiver's knowledge, experience, and health literacy.

Ensures patient has the capacity to obtain, communicate, process, and understand basic health information (CDC, 2021i).

6. Assess patient's prior experience with the sterile procedure and feelings about procedure.

Reveals need for patient support.

7. Assess patient's goals or preferences for how skill is to be performed or what patient expects.

Allows care to be individualized to patient.

PLANNING

1. Complete all other nursing interventions (e.g., medication administration, hygiene) before beginning procedure.

Prepare sterile field as close as possible to time of use to reduce potential for contamination (AORN, 2020).

2. Suggest that visitors step out of room briefly during procedure. Discourage movement of staff assisting with procedure.

Traffic or movement can increase potential for contamination through spread of microorganisms by air currents.

3. Close room door and bedside curtain.

Provides patient privacy. Surgical preparation often includes full or partial skin exposure before draping.

4. Anticipate supplies needed for procedure

Ensures availability of equipment before procedure and prevents break in sterile technique. Not all sterile kits contain sufficient amounts or types of supplies needed for all procedures. Failure to have the proper supplies may cause you to leave sterile field, increasing risk for contamination and potential need to set up another sterile field. (**Note:** Povidone-iodine and chlorhexidine are not considered sterile solutions and require separate work surfaces for preparation).

5. Arrange equipment/supplies at bedside or in a location convenient to the procedure. Check sterile package integrity for punctures, tears, discoloration, moisture, or any other signs of contamination. Check the expiration date. Check sterile package for sterilization indicator (marker that changes color when exposed to heat or steam).

Ensures more efficient procedure. Inspection of packaging ensures that sterile field is not contaminated (AORN, 2020).

Continued

SKILL 28.2   PREPARATION OF STERILE FIELD—cont'd

STEP	RATIONALE
6. Position patient comfortably for specific procedure to be performed. If a body part is to be examined or treated, position patient so that area is accessible. Have AP help with positioning as needed.	Patient should be able to lie still in one position comfortably during procedure. Movement can disrupt the sterile field.
7. Provide an explanation of procedure.	Preparing patient for procedure improves adherence and decreases patient stress.
8. Instruct patient (and family caregiver, if present) not to touch work surface or equipment during procedure.	Prevents contamination of sterile field. Promotes patient understanding and cooperation.

IMPLEMENTATION

1. Perform hand hygiene (see Skill 28.1.)	Reduces number of microorganisms on hands, thus reducing transmission to patient. Do not allow rinse water to run down arms onto clean hands (i.e., arms are considered dirty).
2. Apply PPE as needed (check agency policy).	PPE controls microorganism transmission.
3. Select a clean, flat, dry work surface above waist level.	A dry surface is needed for a sterile field. A sterile object placed below a person's waist is considered contaminated.
4. Prepare sterile work surface.	
a. Use sterile commercial kit or package containing sterile items.	
(1) Place sterile kit or package on the prepared work surface.	
(2) Open outside cover (see illustration) and remove package from dust cover. Place on work surface.	Outside of kit is not sterile. Inner kit remains sterile.
(3) Grasp outer surface of tip of outermost flap.	Outer surface of package is considered unsterile. There is a 2.5-cm (1-inch) border around any sterile drape or wrap that is considered contaminated and can be touched with clean fingers.
(4) Open outermost flap away from body, keeping arm outstretched and away from sterile field (see illustration).	Reaching over sterile field contaminates it.
(5) Grasp outside surface of edge of first side flap.	Outer border is considered unsterile.
(6) Open side flap, pulling to side, allowing it to lie flat on table surface. Keep arm to side and not over sterile surface (see illustration).	Drape or wrapper should lie flat, so it does not accidentally rise up and contaminate inner surface or sterile contents.
(7) Repeat Step (6) for second side flap (see illustration).	

STEP 4a(2) Open outside cover of sterile kit.

STEP 4a(4) Open outermost flap of sterile kit away from body.

STEP	**RATIONALE**

(8) Grasp outside border of last and innermost flap (see illustration). Stand away from sterile package and pull flap back, allowing it to fall flat on table. Kit is ready to be used.

Outer border is considered unsterile.
Never reach over a sterile field.

b. Open sterile linen-wrapped package.

  (1) Place package on clean, dry, flat work surface above waist level.

Sterile items placed below waist level are considered contaminated.

  (2) Remove sterilization tape seal and unwrap both layers following same steps (see Steps 4a [2] through 4a [8]) as for sterile kit (see illustration).

Linen-wrapped items have two layers. The first is a dust cover. The second layer must be opened to view sterilization indicator.

  (3) Use opened package wrapper as sterile field.

Inside of package wrapper is considered sterile.

c. Prepare sterile drape.

  (1) Place pack containing sterile drape on flat, dry surface and open as described (see Steps 4a [2] through 4a[8]) for sterile package.

Packaged drape remains sterile.

  (2) Apply sterile gloves (*optional,* see agency policy). The outer 2.5-cm (1-inch) border of drape may be touched without wearing gloves.

Sterile object remains sterile only when touched by another sterile object. Gloves are not necessary as long as fingers grasp the 2.5-cm (1-inch) unsterile border of the drape.

  (3) Using fingertips of one hand, pick up folded top edge of drape along 2.5-cm (1-inch) border. Gently lift drape up from its wrapper without touching any object. Discard wrapper with other hand.

If sterile object touches any nonsterile object, it becomes contaminated.

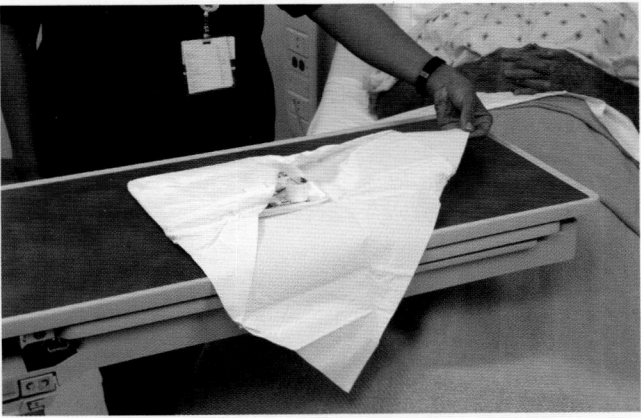

STEP 4a(6) Open first side flap, pulling to side.

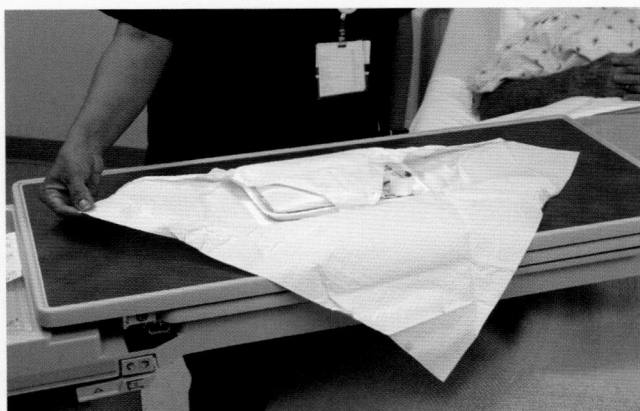

STEP 4a(7) Open second side flap, pulling to side.

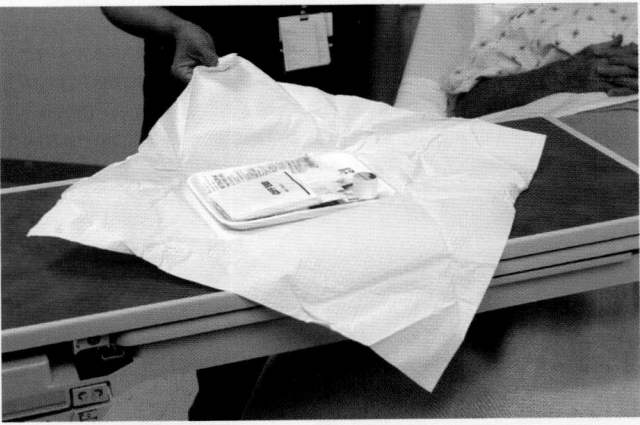

STEP 4a(8) Open last and innermost flap.

STEP 4b(2) Open sterile linen-wrapped package.

Continued

SKILL 28.2	PREPARATION OF STERILE FIELD—cont'd

STEP	RATIONALE
(4) With other hand, grasp an adjacent corner of drape and hold it straight up and away from body. Allow drape to unfold, keeping it above waist and work surface and away from body (see illustration).	An object held below a person's waist or above chest is contaminated. Drape can now be placed properly with two hands.
(5) Holding drape, position bottom half over top half of intended work surface (see illustration).	Proper positioning prevents nurse from reaching over sterile field.
(6) Allow top half of drape to be placed over bottom half of work surface (see illustration). Sterile field is ready to use.	Proper positioning creates flat, sterile work surface for placement of sterile supplies.

CLINICAL JUDGMENT: *Use slow movements when setting up sterile drapes. Fast movements can stir up dust, lint, and infectious microorganisms, which can contaminate the sterile field.*

---

5. Add sterile items to sterile field.	
a. Open sterile item (following package directions) while holding outside wrapper in nondominant hand.	Use of nondominant hand frees dominant hand for unwrapping outer wrapper.
b. Carefully peel wrapper over nondominant hand.	Item remains sterile. Inner surface of wrapper covers hand, making it sterile.
c. Be sure that the wrapper does not fall onto the sterile field. Place the item onto the field at an angle (see illustration). **Do not hold arms over sterile field.**	Secured wrapper edges prevent flipping wrapper and contaminating contents of sterile field (AORN, 2020).
	Skin is a source of bacteria and shedding.
d. Dispose of outer wrapper.	Disposal prevents accidental contamination of sterile field.
6. Pour sterile solutions.	
a. Verify contents and expiration date of solution.	Verification ensures proper solution and sterility of contents.
b. Place receptacle for solution near table/work surface edge. Sterile kits have cups or plastic molded sections into which fluids can be poured.	Proper placement prevents reaching over sterile field during pouring of solution.
c. Remove sterile seal and cap from bottle in upward motion.	Upward movement prevents contamination of bottle lip.

STEP 4c(4) Grasp corners of sterile drape, then hold up and away from body. (From Elsevier: *Clinical Skills: Essentials Collection*, St Louis, 2021, Mosby.)

STEP 4c(5) Position bottom half of sterile drape over top half of work space. (From Elsevier: *Clinical Skills: Essentials Collection*, St Louis, 2021, Mosby.)

STEP 4c(6) Allow top half of drape to be placed over bottom half of work surface. (From Elsevier: *Clinical Skills: Essentials Collection*, St Louis, 2021, Mosby.)

STEP 5c Add items to sterile field.

STEP	RATIONALE
d. With solution bottle held away from field and bottle lip 2.5 to 5 cm (1 to 2 inches) above inside of sterile receiving container, slowly pour needed amount of solution into container. Hold bottle with label facing palm of hand (see illustration).	Edge and outside of bottle are considered contaminated. Slow pouring prevents splashing. Sterility of contents cannot be ensured if cap is replaced. Prevents label from becoming wet and illegible.

CLINICAL JUDGMENT: *When liquids permeate sterile field or barrier, it is called a strikethrough, resulting in contamination of the sterile field.*

STEP	RATIONALE
7. Help patient to comfortable position.	Promotes patient comfort and safety.
8. Place nurse call system in an accessible location within patient's reach.	Ensures patient can call for assistance if needed.
9. Raise side rails (as appropriate) and lower bed to lowest position.	Promotes patient safety.
10. Dispose of all contaminated supplies in appropriate receptacle, remove and dispose of gloves, and perform hand hygiene.	Reduces transmission of infection.

EVALUATION

1. Observe for breaks in sterile technique throughout the procedure.	A break in sterile technique requires you to repeat the procedure.
2. **Use Teach-Back:** "I want to be sure I explained the procedure that I just performed and steps I took to prevent any infection. Please tell me in what way the procedure will help you." Revise your instruction now or develop a plan for revised patient/family caregiver teaching if patient/family caregiver is not able to teach back correctly.	Teach-back is an evidence-based health literacy intervention that promotes patient engagement, patient safety, adherence, and quality. The goal of teach-back is to ensure that you have explained medical information clearly so that patients and their families understand what you have communicated to them (AHRQ, 2020).

UNEXPECTED OUTCOMES AND RELATED INTERVENTIONS

1. Sterile field contacts contaminated object or liquid splatters onto drape, causing strikethrough.
   - Discontinue field preparation and start over with new equipment.
2. Sterile item falls off sterile field.
   - Have a colleague open another package containing new sterile item. With your gloves still on, grasp item and add it to the sterile field. If field becomes contaminated, a new sterile field needs to be established.

RECORDING AND REPORTING

- Record the procedure performed and that sterile technique was used.
- Discuss with nurses and other pertinent health care providers the sterile procedure performed, outcome, patient's response, and any necessary follow-up.

STEP 6d Pour solution into receiving container on sterile field.

SKILL 28.3	SURGICAL HAND ASEPSIS

Delegation and Collaboration

The skill of surgical hand asepsis can be delegated to properly trained surgical technicians (know the state Nurse Practice Act).

Equipment

- Deep sink with foot or knee controls for dispensing water and soap (faucets should be high enough for hands and forearms to fit comfortably)

- Antimicrobial agent approved by the health care agency
- Surgical scrub sponge with plastic nail pick *(optional)*
- Paper face mask, cap or hood, surgical shoe covers
- Sterile towel
- Sterile pack containing sterile gown
- Protective eyewear (glasses or goggles)

Continued

SKILL 28.3	SURGICAL HAND ASEPSIS—cont'd

STEP	RATIONALE

ASSESSMENT

1. Consult manufacturer policy regarding required length of time and antiseptic to use for hand antisepsis. Chlorhexidine has been found to be more effective than povidone iodine (WHO, 2009).
2. Remove bracelets, rings, and watches.

3. Be sure that fingernails are short, clean, and healthy. Artificial nails should be removed. Natural nails should be less than ¼ inch long from fingertip.

Guidelines vary regarding ideal time needed and antiseptic to use for surgical scrub. Most facilities in the United States follow 3 to 5 minutes for hand scrub (AORN, 2016).

Jewelry may harbor or protect microorganisms from removal. Allergic skin reactions may occur as a result of scrub agent or glove powder accumulating under jewelry (Association of Surgical Technologists [AST], 2017).

Long nails and chipped or old polish increase the number of bacteria residing on nails. Long fingernails can puncture gloves, causing contamination. Artificial nails are known to harbor gram-negative microorganisms and fungus (AORN, 2020; CDC, 2021c).

CLINICAL JUDGMENT: *Remove nail polish if chipped or worn longer than 4 days because it is likely to harbor microorganisms* (AORN, 2020).

4. Inspect condition of cuticles, hands, and forearms for abrasions, cuts, or open lesions.

These conditions increase likelihood of more microorganisms residing on skin surfaces. Broken skin permits microorganisms to enter layers of the skin, providing deeper microbial breeding grounds (AORN, 2020).

PLANNING

1. Apply surgical shoe covers, cap or hood, face mask, and protective eyewear (depends on procedure; see agency policy).

Mask prevents escape into air of microorganisms that can contaminate hands. Other protective wear prevents exposure to blood and body fluid splashes during the procedure.

IMPLEMENTATION

1. Turn on water using knee or foot controls and adjust to comfortable temperature.
2. Prescrub wash/rinse: Wet hands and arms under running lukewarm water and lather with detergent to 5 cm (2 inches) above elbows. (Hands need to be above elbows at all times.)

3. Rinse hands and arms thoroughly under running water. Remember to keep hands above elbows.
4. Under running water clean under nails of both hands with nail pick. Discard after use (see illustration).
5. Surgical hand scrub (with sponge)
   a. Wet clean sponge and apply antimicrobial agent. Visualize each finger, hand, and arm as having four sides. Wash all four sides effectively. Scrub the nails of one hand with 15 strokes. Scrub the palm, each side of thumb and fingers, and posterior side of hand with 10 strokes each.
   b. Divide the arm mentally into thirds: scrub each third 10 times (AORN, 2020) (see illustration). Some health care agency policies require scrub by total time (e.g., 3 to 5 minutes) rather than number of strokes (AORN, 2016). Rinse sponge and repeat sequence for the other arm. A two-sponge method may be substituted (check health care agency policy).

Knee or foot controls prevent contamination of hands after scrub.

Water runs by gravity from fingertips to elbows. Hands become cleanest part of upper extremity. Keeping hands elevated allows water to flow from least to most contaminated areas. Washing a wide area reduces risk of contaminating overlying gown that the nurse later applies.

Rinsing removes transient bacteria from fingers, hands, and forearms.

Removes dirt and organic material that harbor large numbers of microorganisms.

Friction loosens resident bacteria that adhere to skin surfaces. Ensures coverage of all surfaces. Scrubbing is performed from cleanest area (hands) to marginal area (upper arms).

Eliminates transient microorganisms and reduces resident hand flora.

STEP 4 Clean under fingernails.

STEP	RATIONALE
c. Discard sponge. Flex arms and rinse from fingertips to elbows in one continuous motion, allowing water to run off at elbow (see illustration).	Hands remain the cleanest part of upper extremities.
d. Turn off water with foot or knee control, with hands elevated in front of and away from body. Enter operating room suite by backing into room.	Keeps hands free of microorganisms.
e. Approach sterile setup; grasp sterile towel, taking care not to drip water onto sterile setup.	Water contaminates sterile setup.
f. Bending slightly at waist, keeping hands and arms above waist and outstretched, grasp one end of sterile towel and dry one hand, moving from fingers to elbow in a rotating motion (see illustrations).	Avoids sterile towel from contacting unsterile scrub attire and transferring contamination to hands. Dry skin from cleanest (hands) to least clean (elbows).
g. Repeat drying method for other hand by carefully reversing towel or using a new sterile towel.	Prevents accidental contamination.
h. Drop towel into linen hamper or circulating nurse's hand.	Prevents accidental contamination.
6. *Optional:* Brushless antiseptic hand rub	
a. After prescrub wash (see Step 2), dry hands and forearms thoroughly with paper towel.	Promotes reduction in microorganisms on all surfaces of hands and arms.
b. Dispense 2 mL of antimicrobial agent hand preparation into palm of one hand. Dip fingertips of opposite hand into hand preparation and work it under nails. Spread remaining hand preparation over hand and up to just above elbow, covering all surfaces (see illustrations).	
c. Using another 2 mL of hand preparation, repeat with other hand.	
d. Dispense another 2 mL of hand preparation into either hand and reapply to all aspects of both hands up to wrist. Allow to dry thoroughly before donning gloves.	Ensures complete antiseptic coverage of all hand surfaces.
7. Proceed with sterile gowning (see agency policy).	

STEP 5b Scrub forearms.

STEP 5c Rinse arms.

STEP 5f A, Grasp sterile towel. **B,** Drying sequence.

Continued

SKILL 28.3	SURGICAL HAND ASEPSIS—cont'd

STEP	RATIONALE

STEP 6b Application of antimicrobial agent for brushless hand scrub. Nurse using 3M Avagard. (Photos courtesy 3M Health Care.)

EVALUATION

1. After procedure is completed, remove gloves and inspect hands for dermatitis or cracked skin.	Breaks in skin integrity increase risk for transmission of microorganisms during future care activities

RECORDING AND REPORTING

- It is not necessary to record or report this procedure.
- Report any skin dermatitis to employee health or infection control per agency policy.

SKILL 28.4	OPEN GLOVING

Delegation and Collaboration

Assisting with skills that include the application and removal of sterile gloves may be delegated to assistive personnel (AP). However, most procedures that require the use of sterile gloves cannot be delegated to AP. The nurse instructs the AP about:
- The reason sterile gloves are being used for a specific procedure.

Equipment

- Package of proper-size sterile gloves, latex or synthetic nonlatex. If patient has a latex allergy, ensure that gloves are latex free and powder free.

STEP	RATIONALE

ASSESSMENT

1. Consider the type of procedure to be performed and consult agency policy on use of sterile gloves. In some facilities, double gloving is recommended for the operating room and if exposure to blood, body fluids, or infectious microorganisms is anticipated (AORN, 2020).	Ensures proper use of sterile gloves. Evidence supports the use of double gloving and double gloving with an indicator glove system to decrease the risk of percutaneous injury and therefore be an effective barrier to bloodborne pathogen exposure (AORN, 2020).
2. Consider patient's risk for infection (e.g., preexisting condition, immunosuppressed, type of procedure).	Knowledge of risk directs you to follow necessary precautions (e.g., use of additional protective barriers) if necessary.
3. Select correct size and type of gloves and examine glove package to determine whether it is dry and intact with no visible stains.	Torn or wet package is considered contaminated. Visible stains on package indicate previous contamination by water or other liquid.
4. Use nonpowdered gloves.	The FDA passed a ruling that powdered gloves may no longer be used due to increased risks of hypersensitivity and allergic reactions (FDA, 2016).
5. Inspect condition of hands for cuts, hangnails, open lesions, or abrasions. In some settings, you can cover any open lesion with a sterile, impervious transparent dressing (check agency policy). In some cases, presence of such lesions may prevent you from participating in a procedure.	Cuts, abrasions, and hangnails tend to ooze serum, which possibly contains pathogens. Breaks in skin integrity permit microorganisms to enter and increase the risk for infection for both patient and nurse (AORN, 2020).

6. Assess patient for the following risk factors before applying latex gloves:
   a. Previous reaction to the following items within hours of exposure: adhesive tape, dental or face mask, golf club grip, ostomy bag, rubber band, balloon, bandage, elastic underwear, intravenous (IV) tubing, rubber gloves, condom.
   b. Personal history of asthma, contact dermatitis, eczema, urticaria, rhinitis.
	Risk factors determine level of patient's risk for latex allergy.
	Items are known to lead to latex allergy.
	
	Patients with a history of these conditions are at higher risk of having a reaction.

STEP	RATIONALE
c. History of food allergies, especially avocado, banana, peach, chestnut, raw potato, kiwi, tomato, papaya.	Patients with a history of food allergies are at higher risk of developing a reaction.
d. Previous history of adverse reactions during surgery or dental procedure.	Previous history suggests allergic response.
e. Previous reaction to latex product.	Previous reaction suggests allergic response.
7. Assess patient's or family caregiver's knowledge, experience, and health literacy.	Ensures patient has the capacity to obtain, communicate, process, and understand basic health information (CDC, 2021i).
8. Assess patient's prior experience with the procedure and feelings about procedure.	Reveals need for patient support.
9. Assess patient's goals or preferences for how skill is to be performed. Assess patient's expectations.	Allows care to be individualized to patient.

PLANNING

1. Explain procedure to patient.	Reduces anxiety and promotes cooperation.
2. Obtain and organize equipment for patient procedure.	Having needed supplies readily available decreases time patient needs to be exposed. Ensures more efficient procedure.
3. Perform hand hygiene (see Skill 28.1).	Reduces number of microorganisms on hands, thus reducing transmission to patient. Do not allow rinse water to run down arms onto clean hands (i.e., arms are considered dirty).
4. Close room door and bedside curtain.	Provides patient privacy.
5. Position patient comfortably for specific procedure to be performed. If a body part is to be examined or treated, position patient so that area is accessible.	Patient should be able to lie still in one position comfortably during procedure. Movement can disrupt the sterile field.

IMPLEMENTATION

1. Apply sterile gloves.	
a. Remove outer glove package wrapper by carefully separating and peeling apart sides (see illustration).	Proper removal prevents inner glove package from accidentally opening and touching contaminated objects.
b. Grasp inner package and place on clean, dry, flat surface at waist level. Open package, keeping gloves on inside surface of wrapper (see illustration).	Sterile object held below waist is contaminated. Inner surface of glove package is sterile.
c. Identify right and left glove. Each glove has a cuff approximately 5 cm (2 inches) wide. Glove dominant hand first.	Proper identification of gloves prevents contamination by improper fit. Gloving of dominant hand first improves dexterity.
d. With thumb and first two fingers of nondominant hand, grasp glove for dominant hand by touching only inside surface of cuff.	Inner edge of cuff will lie against skin and thus is not sterile.
e. Carefully pull glove over dominant hand, leaving a cuff and being sure that cuff does not roll up wrist. Be sure that thumb and fingers are in proper spaces (see illustration).	If outer surface of glove touches hand or wrist, it is contaminated.
f. With gloved dominant hand, slip fingers underneath cuff of second glove (see illustration).	Cuff protects gloved fingers. Sterile touching sterile prevents glove contamination.
g. Carefully pull second glove over fingers of nondominant hand (see illustration).	Contact of gloved hand with exposed hand results in contamination.
h. After second glove is on, interlock hands together and hold away from body above waist level until beginning procedure (see illustration).	Ensures smooth fit over fingers and prevents contamination.

CLINICAL JUDGMENT: *Do not allow fingers and thumb of gloved dominant hand to touch any part of exposed nondominant hand. Keep thumb of dominant hand abducted back.*

STEP 1a Open outer glove package wrapper.

STEP 1b Open inner glove package on work surface.

Continued

SKILL 28.4   OPEN GLOVING—cont'd

STEP	RATIONALE

STEP 1e Pick up glove at cuff of dominant hand and insert fingers. Pull glove completely over dominant hand (example is for left-handed person).

STEP 1f Pick up glove for nondominant hand.

STEP 1g Pull second glove over nondominant hand.

STEP 1h Interlock gloved hands.

2. Perform sterile procedure.
3. Remove and dispose of gloves.
   a. Grasp outside of one cuff with other gloved hand; avoid touching wrist.
   b. Pull glove off, turning it inside out, and place it in gloved hand.
   c. Take fingers of bare hand and tuck inside remaining glove cuff (see illustration). Peel glove off inside out and over previously removed glove. Discard both gloves in trash receptacle.
   d. Perform thorough hand hygiene.

Procedure minimizes contamination of underlying skin.
Outside of glove does not touch skin surface.
Fingers do not touch contaminated glove surface.

Hand hygiene protects health care provider from contamination resulting from any unseen tears or pinholes in gloves.

4. Help patient to comfortable position.
5. Place nurse call system in an accessible location within patient's reach.
6. Raise side rails (as appropriate) and lower bed to lowest position.
7. Dispose of all contaminated supplies in appropriate receptacle; perform hand hygiene.

Promotes patient comfort and safety.
Ensures patient can call for assistance if needed.
Promotes patient safety.
Reduces transmission of microorganisms.
Use appropriate disposal receptacle if patient on hazardous drugs.

EVALUATION

1. Assess patient for signs/symptoms of infection, focusing on area treated.
2. Assess patient for signs/symptoms of latex allergy.
3. **Use Teach-Back:** "I want to be sure I explained why I used sterile gloves for this procedure. Please explain to me why I needed to use sterile gloves." Revise your instruction now or develop a plan for revised patient/family caregiver teaching if patient/family caregiver is not able to teach back correctly.

Improper sterile technique contributes to development of an infection.
Assessment establishes baseline for patient's reaction to latex.
Teach-back is an evidence-based health literacy intervention that promotes patient engagement, patient safety, adherence, and quality. The goal of teach-back is to ensure that you have explained medical information clearly so that patients and their families understand what you have communicated to them (AHRQ, 2020).

STEP 3c Remove second glove by turning it inside out.

UNEXPECTED OUTCOMES AND RELATED INTERVENTIONS

1. Patient develops localized signs of infection (e.g., urine becomes cloudy or odorous; wound becomes painful, edematous, or reddened).
- Contact health care provider and implement appropriate interventions as prescribed.

2. Patient develops systemic signs of infection (e.g., fever, malaise, increased white blood cell count).
- Contact health care provider and implement appropriate interventions as prescribed.

3. Patient develops allergic reaction to latex.
- Immediately remove source of latex, if known.
- Bring emergency equipment to bedside. Have epinephrine injection ready for administration and be prepared to initiate IV fluids and oxygen.
- Alert the health care team following agency protocol.

RECORDING AND REPORTING

- No recording or reporting is required for sterile gloving.
- Record the procedure performed and patient's response.
- Discuss with nurses and other pertinent health care providers the sterile procedure performed, patient's response, outcome, and any necessary follow-up.

▋ KEY POINTS

- Transmission of infection can occur if the six elements of the infection chain are present and uninterrupted.
- Normal body flora and body system defenses help the body resist infection by reducing the number of pathogenic organisms.
- The vascular response to acute inflammation includes rapid vasodilation, allowing more blood to be delivered near the location of the injury. The increase in local blood flow causes the redness and localized warmth at the site of inflammation, and the body releases chemical mediators that increase the permeability of small blood vessels, which leads to edema of interstitial spaces. The cellular response results in an increase in WBCs to the site of inflammation. If the inflammation becomes systemic, cellular responses result in increased WBCs in the bloodstream.
- Health care–associated infections lead to adverse patient events and signifcantly higher health care costs that are often not reimbursed.
- Multiple factors influence a patient's susceptibility to infection; patients may have one or more of these factors. Careful analysis of data and cues allow you to recognize patient risks such as poor nutrition, stress, chronic disease, and treatments that compromise the immune response.
- Signs of localized infection are more targeted and include swelling, redness, pain, and restriction of movement in the affected body part, whereas the signs and symptoms of systemic inflammation are more generalized and include fever, fatigue, nausea/vomiting, malaise, and lymph nodes that are enlarged, swollen, and tender.
- You use basic medical aseptic techniques such as handwashing and use of barrier precautions with all patients to break the chain of infection.
- Surgical asepsis, such as sterile gloving, is a more stringent technique than medical asepsis.
- Proper handling and management of urinary catheters and drainage sets prevents infection by eliminating a potential portal of entry for microorganisms.
- Proper storage and refrigeration of food prevents a reservoir of infection from developing in food.
- Standard Precautions are applied in all patient care activities to prevent patients and health care workers from transmitting infection even in the absence of disease.
- Hand hygiene using antiseptic hand rub or washing with soap and water is the most effective basic technique in preventing and controlling infection transmission. Hands must remain in contact with antimicrobial agent long enough to clean hand surfaces.
- Transmission-based precautions, including airborne, droplet, contact, and protective environment, are used in addition to Standard Precautions for patients with highly transmissible pathogens. For example, Airborne Precautions focus on diseases that are transmitted by large

droplets expelled into the air and by being within 3 feet of a patient, requiring use of a surgical mask when within 3 feet of the patient, proper hand hygiene, and dedicated personal protective equipment.

- Proper application of personal protective equipment protects the patient and health care worker from transmission of pathogens. When entering isolation, apply a cover gown first, followed by a surgical mask or respirator, then eyewear or face shield and, finally, clean gloves.
- In the home setting, educating patients and caregivers on infection prevention is critical, adapting interventions to a patient's unique home environment.
- Health care workers believed to have been exposed to hepatitis B will receive the vaccine and vaccination series. A blood test (titer) is offered in some health care settings.

▌ REFLECTIVE LEARNING

Mrs. Andrews was readmitted to the hospital 2 weeks after her surgery because she started having increased pain in her incision area. Kathy was able to provide care for Mrs. Andrews again during her readmission. Kathy assesses Mrs. Andrew's incision and notes that it is red, swollen, and warm. Mrs. Andrews has a low-grade fever (38° C [100.4° F]). Mrs. Andrews states, "I am not sure what is wrong with me, but my lower back really hurts, and I am not able to walk very well. I am having trouble finding a comfortable position to sleep. I also have not felt much like eating the past three days." Kathy discusses the situation with Mrs. Andrews' nurse and surgeon. After examining Mrs. Andrews, the surgeon determines Mrs. Andrews has an infection of her incision. The surgeon takes the patient to surgery to open and clean the wound of drainage. Upon Mrs. Andrews' return to the nursing unit the surgeon orders wound irrigation with normal saline and dressing changes three times a day. Mrs. Andrews is to remain on bed rest until tomorrow morning.

- What assessment information in Mrs. Andrews' situation is the most important or of immediate concern? (Recognize Cues)
- Considering Mrs. Andrews' situation, what environmental, organizational, or other factors are influencing infection control and prevention for Mrs. Andrews? (Analyze Cues)
- Considering the assessment data and history, what would be the priority nursing problem in caring for Mrs. Andrews at this time? (Prioritize Diagnoses)
- Identify two expected outcomes for Mrs. Andrews. Consider Mrs. Andrews' situation, and describe what nursing and medical interventions could be used to achieve the expected outcomes. (Generate Solutions)
- Which nursing and medical interventions should have priority when implementing the care plan for Mrs. Andrews? (Take Action).
- Considering the implementation of the plan of care for Mrs. Andrews, what assessment data should be gathered to evaluate whether the interventions were effective? (Evaluate Outcomes)

▌ REVIEW QUESTIONS

1. A patient who has been placed on Contact Precautions for *Clostridium difficile* (*C. difficile*) asks you to explain what he should know about this organism. Which statements made by the patient show an understanding of the patient teaching? (Select all that apply.)
   1. "The organism is usually transmitted through the fecal-oral route."
   2. "Hands should always be cleaned with soap and water rather than the alcohol-based hand sanitizer."
   3. "Everyone coming into the room must wear a gown and gloves."
   4. "While I am in Contact Precautions, I cannot leave the room."
   5. "*C. difficile* dies quickly once outside the body."

2. A patient is diagnosed with meningitis. Which type of isolation precaution is *most* appropriate for this patient?
   1. Reverse isolation
   2. Droplet Precautions
   3. Standard Precautions
   4. Contact Precautions

3. A patient is placed on Airborne Precautions for pulmonary tuberculosis. The nurse notes that the patient seems to be angry, but the nurse recognizes that this is a normal response to isolation. Which is the nurse's best intervention?
   1. Provide a dark, quiet room to calm the patient.
   2. Reduce the level of precautions to keep the patient from becoming angry.
   3. Explain the reasons for isolation procedures and provide meaningful stimulation.
   4. Limit family and other caregiver visits to reduce the risk of spreading the infection.

4. Which type of personal protective equipment should the nurse wear when caring for a pediatric patient who is placed on Airborne Precautions for confirmed chickenpox/herpes zoster? (Select all that apply.)
   1. Disposable gown
   2. N95 respirator mask
   3. Face shield or goggles
   4. Disposable mask
   5. Gloves

5. The infection control nurse has asked the staff to work on reducing the number of iatrogenic infections on the unit. Which of the following actions on the nurses' part would contribute to reducing health care–acquired infections? (Select all that apply.)
   1. Teaching correct handwashing to assigned patients
   2. Using correct procedures in starting and caring for an intravenous infusion
   3. Providing perineal care to a patient with an indwelling urinary catheter
   4. Isolating a patient on antibiotics who has been having loose stool for 24 hours
   5. Decreasing a patient's environmental stimuli to decrease nausea

6. Which of the following actions by the nurse demonstrate the practice of core principles of surgical asepsis? (Select all that apply.)
   1. The front and sides of the sterile gown are considered sterile from the waist up.
   2. Keep the sterile field in view at all times.
   3. Consider the outer 2.5 cm (1 inch) of the sterile field as contaminated.
   4. Only health care personnel within the sterile field must wear personal protective equipment.
   5. After cleansing the hands with antiseptic rub, apply clean disposable gloves.

7. Put the following steps for removal of protective barriers after leaving an isolation room in order.
   1. Remove and dispose of gloves.
   2. Perform hand hygiene.
   3. Remove eyewear or goggles.
   4. Untie bottom and then top mask strings and remove from face.
   5. Untie waist and neck strings of gown. Remove gown, rolling it onto itself without touching the contaminated side.

8. A patient is diagnosed with a multidrug-resistant organism (MDRO) in his surgical wound and asks the nurse what this means. What is the nurse's best response? (Select all that apply.)
   1. There is more than one organism in the wound that is causing the infection.
   2. The antibiotics the patient has received are not strong enough to kill the organism.
   3. The patient will need more than one type of antibiotic to kill the organism.
   4. The organism has developed a resistance to one or more broad-spectrum antibiotics, indicating that the organism will be hard to treat effectively.
   5. There are no longer any antibiotic options available to treat the patient's infection.
9. Which of these statements are true regarding disinfection and cleaning? (Select all that apply.)
   1. Proper cleaning requires mechanical removal of all soil from an object or area.
   2. Routine environmental cleaning is an example of medical asepsis.
   3. When cleaning a wound, wipe around the wound edge first and then clean inward toward the center of the wound.
   4. Cleaning in a direction from the least to the most contaminated area helps reduce infections.
   5. Disinfecting and sterilizing medical devices and equipment involve the same procedures.
10. The nurse assesses the following data from a patient with diabetes mellitus who is 4 days postoperative for repair of an abdominal aortic aneurysm. Which assessment finding is of greatest concern for the nurse?
   1. Vesicular breath sounds in the lung bases
   2. Temperature 38.5° C (101.4° F)
   3. Incision pain rating of 6 out of 10
   4. Blood glucose of 164 mg/dL

Answers: 1. 1, 2, 3; 2. 2, 3; 3. 4, 1, 2, 5; 5. 1, 2, 3; 6. 2, 3; 7. 1, 3, 5, 4, 2; 8. 2, 4; 9. 1, 2, 4; 10. 2.

Rationales for Review Questions can be found on the Evolve website.

REFERENCES

Agency for Healthcare Research and Quality (AHRQ): *Toolkit for reducing catheter-associated urinary tract infections in hospital units: implementation guide*, 2015. https://www.ahrq.gov/sites/default/files/publications/files/implementation-guide_0.pdf. Accessed July 25, 2020.

Agency for Healthcare Research and Quality (AHRQ): *Health literacy universal precautions toolkit 2nd edition*, Rockville, MD, 2020, Agency for Healthcare Research and Quality. https://www.ahrq.gov/health-literacy/quality-resources/tools/literacy-toolkit/healthlittoolkit2-tool5.html. Accessed July 25, 2020.

Arnold F: Antimicrobials and resistance. In Grota P, editor: *APIC text of infection control and epidemiology*. Washington, DC, 2018, Association for Professionals in Infection Control and Epidemiology.

Association of Perioperative Nurses: *Guidelines for perioperative practice*, Denver, 2016, AORN.

Association of periOperative Registered Nurses (AORN): *Guidelines for perioperative practice*, Denver, 2020, AORN.

Association of Surgical Technologists (AST): *AST guidelines for best practices for wearing jewelry*, 2017. http://www.ast.org/uploadedFiles/Main_Site/Content/About_Us/Standard%20Wearing%20Jewelry.pdf. Accessed July 2, 2020.

Berends C, Walesa B: Isolation precautions (transmission precautions). In Grota P, editor: *APIC text of infection control and epidemiology*, Washington, DC, 2018, Association for Professionals in Infection Control and Epidemiology.

Centers for Disease Control and Prevention (CDC): *Guideline for preventing the transmission of mycobacterium tuberculosis in health-care facilities*, Washington, DC, 2005, CDC.

Centers for Disease Control and Prevention (CDC): *Hospital infection control practice advisory committee and the HICPAC/SHEA/APIC/IDSA: hand hygiene task force guidelines for hand hygiene in health care settings*, Atlanta, 2008, Centers for Disease Control and Prevention.

Centers for Disease Control (CDC): *Example of safe donning and removal of personal protective equipment (PPE)*, 2015a. https://www.cdc.gov/infectioncontrol/guidelines/isolation/appendix/ppe.html. Accessed September 2021.

Centers for Disease Control and Prevention (CDC): *Norovirus guidelines for healthcare settings*, 2015b.

https://www.cdc.gov/infectioncontrol/guidelines/norovirus/index.html. Accessed August 10, 2020.

Centers for Disease Control and Prevention (CDC): *Updated US Public Health Service guidelines for the management of occupational exposures to HIV and recommendations for postexposure prophylaxis*, Washington, DC, 2015c, CDC.

Centers for Disease Control and Prevention (CDC): *CDC vital signs: making health care safer*, 2016a. https://www.cdc.gov/vitalsigns/pdf/2016-08-vitalsigns.pdf. Accessed August 10, 2020.

Center for Disease Control and Prevention (CDC): *Transmission-based precautions*, 2016b. https://www.cdc.gov/infectioncontrol/basics/transmission-based-precautions.html. Accessed June 29, 2020.

Centers for Disease Control and Prevention (CDC): *HAI data and statistics*, 2018a. https://www.cdc.gov/hai/surveillance/index.html. Accessed June 29, 2020.

Centers for Disease Control and Prevention (CDC): *Healthcare-associated infections, HAI data*, 2018b. https://www.cdc.gov/hai/data/index.html.

Centers for Disease Control and Prevention (CDC): *Recommended vaccines for healthcare workers*, 2018c. https://www.immunize.org/catg.d/p2017.pdf. Accessed August 10, 2020.

Centers for Disease Control and Prevention (CDC): *Vaccination coverage among children aged 19-35 months: United States 2017*, 2018d. https://www.cdc.gov/mmwr/volumes/67/wr/mm6740a4.htm. Accessed August 11, 2020.

Centers for Disease Control and Prevention (CDC): *Vaccination laws*, 2018e, CDC. https://www.cdc.gov/phlp/publications/topic/vaccinationlaws.html. Accessed August 10, 2020.

Centers for Disease Control and Prevention (CDC): *What everyone should know about shingles vaccine*, 2018f. https://www.cdc.gov/vaccines/vpd/shingles/public/index.html. Accessed July 2, 2020.

Centers for Disease Control and Prevention (CDC): *2007 Guideline for isolation precautions: preventing transmission of infectious agents in healthcare settings*, Washington, DC, 2019a, CDC. https://www.cdc.gov/infectioncontrol/guidelines/isolation/index.html. Accessed August 10, 2020.

Centers for Disease Control and Prevention (CDC): *Guidelines for the prevention of catheter-associated*

urinary tract infections, CDC, 2019b. https://www.cdc.gov/infectioncontrol/pdf/guidelines/cauti-guidelines-H.pdf. Accessed June 23, 2021.

Centers for Disease Control and Prevention (CDC): *Precautions to prevent the spread of MRSA in healthcare settings*, 2019c. http://www.cdc.gov/mrsa/index.html. Accessed June 29, 2020.

Centers for Disease Control and Prevention (CDC): *2015 Sexually transmitted disease treatment guidelines*, 2019d. https://www.cdc.gov/mmwr/pdf/rr/rr6403.pdf. Accessed November 2021.

Centers for Disease Control and Prevention (CDC): *Vaccine information for adults: what vaccines are recommended for you*, 2019e. https://www.cdc.gov/vaccines/adults/rec-vac/index.html.

Centers for Disease Control and Prevention (CDC): *Handwashing: clean hands save lives*, 2020a. http://www.cdc.gov/handwashing/. Accessed June 29, 2020.

Centers for Disease Control and Prevention (CDC): *Hepatitis overview and statistics*, 2020b. https://www.cdc.gov/hepatitis/hcv/hcvfaq.htm#section2. Accessed June 29, 2020.

Centers for Disease Control and Prevention (CDC): *Medications that weaken your immune system and fungal infections*, 2020c. https://www.cdc.gov/fungal/infections/immune-system.html. Accessed June 29, 2020.

Centers for Disease Control and Prevention (CDC): *Show me the science—when to use hand sanitizers*, 2020d. http://www.cdc.gov/handwashing/show-me-the-science-hand-sanitizer.html. Accessed June 29, 2020.

Centers for Disease Control and Prevention (CDC): *When and how to wash your hands*, 2020e. http://www.cdc.gov/features/handwashing. Accessed June 29, 2020.

Centers for Disease Control and Prevention (CDC): *Disease or condition of the week: coronavirus disease 2019 (COVID-19)*, 2021a. https://www.cdc.gov/dotw/covid-19/index.html. Accessed June 22, 2021.

Centers for Disease Control and Prevention (CDC): *Ebola virus disease*, 2021b. http://www.cdc.gov/vhf/ebola/index.html. Accessed June 29, 2020.

Centers for Disease Control and Prevention (CDC): *Hand hygiene in healthcare settings: healthcare providers*, 2021c. https://www.cdc.gov/handhygiene/providers/index.html. Accessed June 28, 2021.

Centers for Disease Control and Prevention (CDC): *Healthcare-associated infections: data portal*, 2021d.

https://www.cdc.gov/hai/data/portal/index.html. Accessed September 2021.

Centers for Disease Control and Prevention (CDC): *Healthcare settings: about healthcare settings and antibiotic resistance*, 2021e. https://www.cdc.gov/drugresistance/solutions-initiative/healthcare.html.

Centers for Disease Control and Prevention (CDC): *How COVID-19 spreads*, 2021f. https://www.cdc.gov/coronavirus/2019-ncov/prevent-getting-sick/how-covid-spreads.html. Accessed June 23, 2021.

Centers for Disease Control and Prevention (CDC): *Influenza vaccination information for health care workers*, 2021g. https://www.cdc.gov/flu/professionals/healthcareworkers.htm. Accessed July 2, 2020.

Centers for Disease Control and Prevention (CDC): *National Center for Health Statistics: infectious diseases*, 2021h. https://www.cdc.gov/nchs/fastats/infectious-disease.htm. Accessed June 22, 2021.

Centers for Disease Control and Prevention (CDC): *What is health literacy*, 2021i. https://www.cdc.gov/healthliteracy/learn/index.html. Accessed October 2021.

Chetan J: Cleaning, disinfection and sterilization. In Grota P, editor: *APIC text of infection control and epidemiology*, Washington, DC, 2018, Association for Professionals in Infection Control and Epidemiology.

Contagion Live: *Top 5 infectious disease concerns to watch in 2019*, January 1, 2019. https://www.contagionlive.com/news/top-5-infectious-disease-concerns-to-watch-in-2019. Accessed June 30, 2020.

Fiutem C: Risk factors facilitating transmission of infectious agents. In Grota P, editor: *APIC text of infection control and epidemiology*, Washington, DC, 2018, Association for Professionals in Infection Control and Epidemiology.

Food and Drug Administration (FDA): *Banned devices; ban powdered surgeon's gloves, powdered patient examination gloves, and absorbable powder for lubricating a surgeon's glove*, 2016. Docket No. FDA-2015-N-5017. https://www.fda.gov/downloads/aboutfda/reportsmanuals forms/reports/economicanalyses/ucm532959.pdf. Accessed June 30, 2020.

Friedman C: Infection prevention and control programs. In Grota P, editor: *APIC text of infection control and epidemiology*, Washington, DC, 2018, Association

for Professionals in Infection Control and Epidemiology.

Giger J, Haddad L: *Transcultural nursing: assessment and intervention*, ed 8, St. Louis, 2021, Elsevier.

Gubbels Bupp MR, et al: The confluence of sex hormones and aging on immunity, *Front Immunol* 9(Article 1269):1, 2018. https://www.frontiersin.org/articles/10.3389/fimmu.2018.01269/full. Accessed July 2, 2020.

Hass J: Hand hygiene. In Grota P, editor: *APIC text of infection control and epidemiology*, Washington, DC, 2018, Association for Professionals in Infection Control and Epidemiology.

Ingersoll MA: Sex differences shape the response to infectious diseases, *PLoS Pathog* 13(12):e1006688, 2017. https://www.ncbi.nlm.nih.gov/pmc/articles/PMC5746274/. Accessed July 2, 2020.

Iwamoto P, Post M: Aseptic technique. In Grota P, editor: *APIC text of infection control and epidemiology*, Washington, DC, 2018, Association for Professionals in Infection Control and Epidemiology.

Jefferson J, Young M: Sterile processing. In Grota P, editor: *APIC text of infection control and epidemiology*, Washington, DC, 2018, Association for Professionals in Infection Control and Epidemiology.

The Joint Commission (TJC): *2021 National Patient Safety Goals*, Oakbrook Terrace, IL, 2021, The Commission. https://www.jointcommission.org/en/standards/national-patient-safety-goals/. Accessed July 1, 2021.

Mayo Clinic: *Prostatitis*, 2021. https://www.mayoclinic.org/diseases-conditions/prostatitis/symptoms-causes/syc-20355766. Accessed June 23, 2021.

Meiner S, Yeager JJ: *Gerontologic nursing*, ed 6, St. Louis, 2019, Elsevier.

Monsees E: Patient safety. In Grota P, editor: *APIC text of infection control and epidemiology*, Washington, DC, 2018, Association for Professionals in Infection Control and Epidemiology.

Murphy R: Surgical services. In Grota P, editor: *APIC text of infection control and epidemiology*, Washington, DC, 2018, Association for Professionals in Infection Control and Epidemiology.

Nucifora K: *The importance of proper specimen collection and handling*, 2015. https://www.labtestingmatters.org/from-the-bench/the-importance-of-proper-specimen-collection-and-handling/. Accessed June 30, 2020.

Occupational Safety and Health Administration (OSHA): Respiratory protective devices: final rules and notice, *Fed Regist* 33606, 2011.

Occupational Safety and Health Administration (OSHA): Enforcement procedures for the occupational exposure to bloodborne injury final rule, *Fed Regist* 33606, 2012a.

Occupational Safety and Health Administration (OSHA): Needlestick Safety and Prevention Act, *Fed Regist* 19934, 2012b.

Pagana KD, et al: *Mosby's diagnostic & laboratory test reference*, ed 14, St. Louis, 2019, Elsevier.

Pawelec G: Age and immunity: what is "immunosenescence"? *Exp Gerontol* 105:4–9, 2018.

Popovich KJ: Another look at CHG bathing in a surgical intensive care unit, *Ann Transl Med* 5(1):13, 2017.

Roach R: Geriatrics. In Grota P, editor: *APIC text of infection control and epidemiology*, Washington, DC, 2018, Association for Professionals in Infection Control and Epidemiology.

San Patten and Associates: *International literature review for newcomer, migrant and refugee health*, 2016, The Interagency Coalition on AIDs and Development. http://www.icad-cisd.com/pdf/NMRH/NMRH-International-Lit-Review-FINAL.pdf. Accessed June 29, 2020.

Tweeten SM: General principles of epidemiology. In Grota P, editor: *APIC text of infection control and epidemiology*, Washington, DC, 2018, Association for Professionals in Infection Control and Epidemiology.

US Department of Labor: *COVID-19 control and prevention: healthcare workers and employers*, n.d. https://www.osha.gov/coronavirus/control-prevention/healthcare-workers. Accessed June 25, 2021.

World Health Organization (WHO): *WHO guidelines on hand hygiene in healthcare*, Geneva, Switzerland, 2009, WHO Press.

World Health Organization (WHO): *Health risks when travelling*, 2020. https://www.who.int/ith/other_health_risks/infectious_diseases/en/. Accessed June 29, 2020.

World Health Organization (WHO): *SAVE LIVES- clean your hands: annual global campaign*, 2021, https://www.who.int/campaigns/world-hand-hygiene-day. Accessed November 2021.

RESEARCH REFERENCES

Adesanya OA, et al: Bacterial contamination of stethoscopes at a tertiary care hospital in southwestern Nigeria, *Afr J Clin Exp Microbiol* 8(2):59, 2017.

Amitra J, et al: Evaluation of the potential for electronic thermometers to contribute to spread of healthcare-associated pathogens, *Am J Infect Control* 46(6):708, 2018.

Birnbach DJ, et al: An evaluation of hand hygiene in an intensive care unit: are visitors a potential vector for pathogens? *J Infect Public Health* 8(6):570, 2015.

Currie K, et al: Understanding the patient experience of health care–associated infection: A qualitative systematic review, *Am J Infect Control* 46(8):936, 2018.

DePrez B, et al: Implementation of chlorhexidine gluconate bathing to reduce HAIs: A nurse leader-led evidence-based practice change, *Nurs Manage* 50(11):13–17, 2019.

Donskey E, Deshpande A: Effect of chlorhexidine bathing in preventing infections and reducing skin burden and environmental contamination: a review of the literature, *Am J Infect Control* 44(Suppl 5):17, 2016.

Fekete T: *Catheter-associated urinary tract infection in adults*, 2020, UpToDate. https://www.uptodate.com/contents/catheter-associated-urinary-tract-infection-in-adults.

Fletcher K, et al: Qualitative validation of the CAUTI Guide to patient safety assessment tool, *Am J Infect Control* 44(10):1102, 2016.

Graziano-Husser J, et al: Does including front line staff in root cause analyses reduce the incidence of catheter associated urinary tract infections? *Am J Infect Control* 46(Suppl 6):S77, 2018.

Letica-Kriege AS, et al: Identifying the risk factors for catheter-associated urinary tract infections: a large cross-sectional study of six hospitals, *BMJ Open* 9(1):e022137, 2019.

Perrin K, et al: Catheter-associated urinary tract infection (CAUTI) in the NeuroICU: identification of risk factors and time-to-CAUTI using a case-control design, *Neurocrit Care* 34(1):271, 2021.

Purssell E, et al: Impact of isolation on *hospitalised* patients who are infectious: systematic review with meta-analysis, *BMJ Open* 10:e030371, 2020.

Singh AT, et al: Just a friendly reminder...improving visitor hand hygiene practice with a simple verbal cue, *Pediatrics* 140(1 MeetingAbstract):22, 2017.

Sprague E, et al: Patient isolation precautions: are they worth it? *Can Respir J* 5352625, 2016.

Vital Signs

OBJECTIVES

- Identify when it is appropriate to assess each vital sign.
- Evaluate a patient's disease process, cognition, age, and other factors when selecting sights for temperature, pulse, and blood pressure assessments.
- Select nursing measures that promote heat loss and heat conservation.
- Summarize physiological changes associated with fever.
- Analyze a patient's body temperature.
- Analyze a patient's radial and apical pulses.
- Evaluate the significance of a pulse deficit.
- Analyze a patient's respirations.
- Explain the benefits and precautions involving self-measurement of blood pressure.
- Analyze a patient's blood pressure.
- Explain factors that cause variations in SpO_2 values.
- Analyze a patient's oxygenation status (SpO_2), using pulse oximetry.
- Summarize factors that cause variations in body temperature, pulse, oxygen saturation (SpO_2), capnography, respirations, and blood pressure measurement.
- Discuss how clinical judgment is essential in identifying when to measure vital signs.
- Determine when it is appropriate to delegate vital sign measurements to assistive personnel.
- Evaluate the effectiveness of nursing interventions to promote or maintain normal vital signs.
- Demonstrate accurate recording and reporting of vital sign measurements.

KEY TERMS

Afebrile
Antipyretics
Auscultatory gap
Blood pressure
Bradycardia
Capnography
Conduction
Convection
Core temperature
Diaphoresis
Diastolic pressure
Dysrhythmia
Eupnea
Evaporation
Febrile

Fever
Fever of unknown origin (FUO)
Frostbite
Heat exhaustion
Heatstroke
Hematocrit
Hypertension
Hyperthermia
Hypotension
Hypothermia
Hypoxemia
Malignant hyperthermia
Nonshivering thermogenesis
Orthostatic hypotension
Oxygen saturation

Postural hypotension
Pulse deficit
Pulse pressure
Pyrexia
Pyrogens
Radiation
Shivering
Sphygmomanometer
Systolic pressure
Tachycardia
Thermoregulation
Ventilation
Vital signs

MEDIA RESOURCES

http://evolve.elsevier.com/Potter/fundamentals/

- Review Questions
- Video Clips
- Case Study with Questions

- Skills Performance Checklists
- Audio Glossary
- Content Updates
- Answers to QSEN Activity and Review Questions

The most frequent and routine measurements obtained by health care providers are those of temperature, pulse, blood pressure (BP), respiratory rate, and oxygen saturation. These measurements reflect a patient's health status by indicating the effectiveness of circulatory, respiratory, neural, and endocrine body functions. Because of their importance, they are referred to as vital signs (VS). Pain, a subjective symptom, is often called another vital sign and is frequently measured with the others (see Chapter 44).

Measurement of vital signs provides data to determine a patient's usual state of health (baseline data). Many factors such as the temperature of the environment, the patient's physical exertion, and the effects of illness cause vital signs to change, sometimes outside an acceptable range. Vital signs can reveal both sudden changes in a patient's condition and changes that occur progressively over time. Any difference between a patient's normal baseline measurement and present vital signs may indicate the need for nursing therapies and medical interventions. Vital signs are also important in evaluating a patient's response to therapy—for example, how a patient with a fever responds to antipyretics, how a patient in pain responds to opioids, or how a patient with hypertension responds to medication. An alteration in vital signs signals a change in physiological function. Assessment of vital signs provides data to identify nursing diagnoses, implement planned interventions, and evaluate outcomes of care.

Vital signs are a quick and efficient way of monitoring a patient's condition or identifying problems and evaluating their response to interventions. When you learn the physiological variables influencing vital signs and recognize the relationship of their changes to one another and to other physical assessment findings, you can make precise determinations about a patient's health status and the need for medical or nursing interventions. Vital signs and other physiological measurements are the basis for clinical judgment and decision making. Many agencies adopt Early Warning Scores (EWS) determined by vital signs data entered into the electronic health record (EHR) to alert nurses to potential changes in a patient's condition. An EWS system responds to multiple vital sign parameters at the same time and identifies at-risk patients at the first sign of a subtle change in vital signs (IHI, 2020).

GUIDELINES FOR MEASURING VITAL SIGNS

Vital signs are a part of the assessment database. You include them in a complete physical assessment (see Chapter 30), routinely per a health care provider's order, or obtain them individually to assess a patient's condition. Establishing a database of vital signs during a routine physical examination serves as a baseline for future assessments.

As a nurse, you will apply critical thinking in clinical judgment to monitor a patient's vital signs. A patient's condition determines when, where, how, and by whom vital signs are measured. You need to measure them correctly, and at times you appropriately delegate their measurement. You also need to know expected values (Box 29.1), interpret your patient's values, communicate findings appropriately, and begin interventions as needed. Use the following guidelines to incorporate measurements of vital signs into nursing practice:

- Measuring vital signs is your responsibility. Use critical thinking and clinical judgment to determine when it is safe and appropriate to delegate these measurements in selected situations (e.g., in stable patients). However, it is your responsibility to review the data from the measurement of vital signs, interpret their significance, and critically think through decisions about interventions.
- Devices (e.g., sphygmomanometer) for measuring vital signs are often shared among patients. Cleaning each device carefully between patients decreases patients' risk of infection.
- Assess equipment to ensure that it is working correctly to provide accurate findings.
- Select equipment on the basis of the patient's condition and characteristics (e.g., do not use an adult-size BP cuff for a child).
- Know the patient's usual range of vital signs. These values can differ from the acceptable range based on a patient's age or health status. The patient's usual values serve as a baseline for comparison with later findings. Thus you are able to detect a change in condition over time.
- Know your patient's health history, therapies, and prescribed and over-the-counter medications. Some illnesses or treatments cause predictable changes in vital signs. Some medications affect one or more vital signs.

- Control or minimize environmental factors that affect vital signs. For example, assessing a patient's temperature in a warm, humid room may yield a value that is not a true indicator of the condition.
- Use an organized, systematic approach. Each vital sign procedure requires a step-by-step approach to ensure accuracy.
- On the basis of a patient's condition, collaborate with health care providers to decide the frequency of vital sign assessment. In the hospital health care providers order a minimum frequency of vital sign measurements for each patient. As a patient's physical condition worsens, it is often necessary to monitor more frequently, such as every 5 to 10 minutes. As a nurse, you must use critical thinking to form a clinical judgment as to when more frequent vital sign assessments are necessary (Box 29.2).

BOX 29.1   Vital Signs

Acceptable Ranges for Adults

Temperature Range
Average temperature range: 36° to 38°C (96.8° to 100.4°F)
Average oral/tympanic: 37°C (98.6°F)
Average rectal: 37.5°C (99.5°F)
Axillary: 36.5°C (97.7°F)

Pulse
60 to 100 beats/min, strong and regular

Pulse Oximetry (SpO$_2$)
Normal: SpO$_2$ ≥95%

Respirations
12 to 20 breaths/min, deep and regular

Blood Pressure
Systolic <120 mm Hg
Diastolic <80 mm Hg
Pulse pressure: 30 to 50 mm Hg

Capnography (EtCO$_2$)
Normal: 35-45 mm Hg

BOX 29.2   When to Measure Vital Signs

- On admission to a health care agency
- When assessing a patient during home care visits
- In a clinic setting before a health care provider examines the patient and after any invasive procedures
- In a hospital on a routine schedule according to the health care provider's order or hospital standards of practice
- Before, during, and after a surgical procedure or invasive diagnostic/treatment procedure
- Before, during, and after a transfusion of any type of blood product
- Before, during, and after the administration of medication or therapies that affect cardiovascular, respiratory, or temperature-control functions
- Before, during, and after nursing interventions influencing a vital sign (e.g., before and after a patient previously on bed rest ambulates, before and after the patient performs range-of-motion exercises)
- When a patient reports nonspecific symptoms of physical distress (e.g., feeling "funny" or "different")
- When a patient's general physical condition changes (e.g., loss of consciousness or increased intensity of pain)

- Use vital sign measurements to determine indications for medication administration. For example, give certain cardiac drugs only within a range of pulse or BP values. Administer antipyretics when temperature is elevated outside the acceptable range for the patient. Know the acceptable vital sign ranges for your patients before administering medications.
- Analyze the results of vital sign measurements on the basis of a patient's condition and past health history.
- Verify and communicate significant changes in vital signs. Baseline measurements provide a starting point for identifying and accurately interpreting possible changes. When vital signs appear abnormal, have another nurse or health care provider repeat the measurement to verify readings. Inform the charge nurse or health care provider immediately, document findings in your patient's record, and report changes to nurses during hand-off communication (TJC, 2021).
- Educate the patient or family caregiver in vital sign assessment and the significance of findings.

BODY TEMPERATURE

Physiology

Body temperature is the difference between the amount of heat produced by body processes and the amount lost to the external environment.

Heat Produced − Heat Lost = Body Temperature. Despite extremes in environmental conditions and physical activity, temperature-control mechanisms of humans keep body core temperature (temperature of the deep tissues) relatively constant (Fig. 29.1). However, surface temperature varies, depending on blood flow to the skin and the amount of heat lost to the external environment. Sites reflecting core temperature are more reliable indicators of body temperature than sites reflecting surface temperatures (Kiekkas et al., 2019).

The site of temperature measurement (oral, rectal, tympanic membrane, temporal artery, esophageal, pulmonary artery, axillary, or even urinary bladder) is one factor that determines a patient's temperature. For healthy young adults, the average oral temperature is 37°C (98.6°F). In the older adult population the average core temperature ranges from 35° to 36.1°C (95° to 97°F) as a result of changes in temperature regulation.

The time of day also affects body temperature, with the lowest temperature at 6:00 a.m. and the highest temperature at 4:00 p.m. in healthy people. Invasive measurements obtained with a pulmonary artery or esophageal catheter are considered core temperatures, whereas axillary temperatures are reflective of the surface temperature of the body. It is important to remember that a consistent body temperature measurement from a single site allows you to monitor patterns of your patient's body temperature. As you assess and analyze your patient's body temperature, observe and document temperature trends and collaborate with the health care team to determine whether a specific body temperature measurement site is more appropriate.

Body Temperature Regulation. Physiological and behavioral mechanisms regulate the balance between heat lost and heat produced, or thermoregulation. For the body temperature to stay constant and within an acceptable range, various mechanisms maintain the relationship between heat production and heat loss. Apply knowledge of temperature-control mechanisms to promote temperature regulation.

Neural and Vascular Control. The hypothalamus, located between the cerebral hemispheres, controls body temperature the same way a thermostat works in the home. A comfortable temperature is the "set point" at which a heating system operates. In the home a drop in environmental temperature activates the furnace, whereas a rise in temperature shuts the system down.

The hypothalamus senses minor changes in body temperature. The anterior hypothalamus controls heat loss, and the posterior hypothalamus controls heat production. When nerve cells in the anterior hypothalamus become heated beyond the set point, impulses are sent out to reduce body temperature. Mechanisms of heat loss include sweating, vasodilation (widening) of blood vessels, and inhibition of heat production. The body redistributes blood to surface vessels to promote heat loss.

If the posterior hypothalamus senses that body temperature is lower than the set point, the body initiates heat-conservation mechanisms. Vasoconstriction (narrowing) of blood vessels reduces blood flow to the skin and extremities to reduce heat loss. Compensatory heat production is stimulated through voluntary muscle contraction and muscle shivering. When vasoconstriction is ineffective in preventing additional heat loss, shivering begins. Disease or trauma to the hypothalamus or the spinal cord, which carries hypothalamic messages, causes serious alterations in temperature control.

Heat Production. Temperature regulation depends on normal heat production processes. Heat produced by the body is a by-product of metabolism, which is the chemical reaction in all body cells. Activities requiring additional chemical reactions increase the metabolic rate. As metabolism increases, additional heat is produced. When metabolism decreases, less heat is produced. Heat production occurs during rest, voluntary movements, involuntary shivering, and nonshivering thermogenesis.

- Basal metabolism accounts for the heat produced by the body at absolute rest. The average basal metabolic rate (BMR) depends on the body surface area. Thyroid hormones also affect the BMR. By promoting the breakdown of body glucose and fat, thyroid hormones increase the rate of chemical reactions in almost all cells of the body. When large amounts of thyroid hormones are secreted, the BMR can increase 100% above normal. The absence of thyroid hormones reduces the BMR by half, causing a decrease in heat production. The male sex hormone testosterone increases BMR. Men have a higher BMR than women.
- Voluntary movements such as muscular activity during exercise require additional energy. The metabolic rate increases during activity, sometimes causing heat production to increase up to 50 times normal.
- Shivering is an involuntary body response to temperature differences in the body. The skeletal muscle movement during shivering requires significant energy. Shivering sometimes increases heat production 4 to 5 times greater than normal. The heat that is produced helps equalize the body temperature, and the shivering ceases. In vulnerable patients shivering seriously drains energy sources, resulting in further physiological deterioration.

FIG. 29.1 Ranges of normal temperature values and abnormal body temperature alterations.

- **Nonshivering thermogenesis** occurs primarily in neonates because they cannot shiver (Hockenberry et al., 2019). A limited amount of vascular brown tissue, present at birth, is metabolized for heat production.

Heat Loss. Heat loss and heat production occur simultaneously. The structure of the skin and exposure to the environment result in constant, normal heat loss through radiation, conduction, convection, and evaporation.

Radiation is the transfer of heat from the surface of one object to the surface of another without direct contact between the two. As much as 85% of the surface area of the human body radiates heat to the environment. Peripheral vasodilation increases blood flow from the internal organs to the skin to increase radiant heat loss. Peripheral vasoconstriction minimizes radiant heat loss. Radiation increases as the temperature difference between the objects increases. Radiation heat loss can be considerable during surgery when the patient's skin is exposed to a cool environment. However, if the environment is warmer than the skin, the body absorbs heat through radiation.

The patient's position enhances radiation heat loss (e.g., standing exposes a greater radiating surface area, and lying in a fetal position minimizes heat radiation). Help promote heat loss through radiation by removing clothing or blankets. Covering the body with dark, closely woven clothing decreases the amount of heat lost from radiation.

Conduction is the transfer of heat from one object to another with direct contact. Solids, liquids, and gases conduct heat through contact. When the warm skin touches a cooler object, heat is lost. Conduction normally accounts for a small amount of heat loss. Applying an ice pack or bathing a patient with a cool cloth increases conductive heat loss. Applying several layers of clothing reduces conductive loss. The body loses heat by conduction when it makes contact with materials cooler than skin temperature (e.g., application of an ice pack).

Convection is the transfer of heat away by air movement. A fan promotes heat loss through convection. The rate of heat loss increases when moistened skin comes into contact with slightly moving air.

Evaporation is the transfer of heat energy when a liquid is changed to a gas. The body continuously loses heat by evaporation. Approximately 600 to 900 mL a day evaporates from the skin and lungs, resulting in water and heat loss. By regulating perspiration or sweating, the body promotes additional evaporative heat loss. When body temperature rises, the anterior hypothalamus signals the sweat glands to release sweat through tiny ducts on the surface of the skin. During physical exercise over 80% of the heat produced is lost by sweat evaporation.

Diaphoresis is visible perspiration primarily occurring on the forehead and upper thorax, although it occurs in other places on the body. For each hour of exercise in hot conditions up to 2 L of body fluid can be lost in sweat. Excessive evaporation causes skin scaling and itching and drying of the nares and pharynx. A lowered body temperature inhibits sweat gland secretion. Individuals who have a congenital absence of sweat glands or a serious skin disease that impairs sweating are unable to tolerate warm temperatures because they cannot cool themselves adequately.

Skin in Temperature Regulation. The skin regulates temperature through insulation of the body, vasoconstriction (which affects the amount of blood flow and heat loss to the skin), and temperature sensation. The skin, subcutaneous tissue, and fat keep heat inside the body. Individuals with more body fat have more natural insulation than do slim and muscular individuals.

The way the skin controls body temperature is similar to the way an automobile radiator controls engine temperature. An automobile engine generates a great deal of heat. Water is pumped through the engine to collect the heat and carry it to the radiator, where a fan transfers the heat from the water to the outside air. In the human body the internal organs produce heat; during exercise or increased sympathetic stimulation (such as in the stress response) the amount of heat produced is greater than the usual core temperature. Blood flows from the internal organs, carrying heat to the body surface. The skin has many blood vessels, especially the areas of the hands, feet, and ears. Blood flow through these vascular areas of the skin varies from minimal flow to as much as 30% of the blood ejected from the heart. Heat transfers from the blood, through vessel walls, and to the surface of the skin and is lost to the environment through heat-loss mechanisms. The core temperature of the body remains within safe limits.

The degree of vasoconstriction determines the amount of blood flow and heat loss to the skin. If the core temperature is too high, the hypothalamus inhibits vasoconstriction, thus blood vessels dilate, and more blood reaches the surface of the skin. On a hot, humid day the blood vessels in the hands are dilated and easily visible. In contrast, if the core temperature becomes too low, the hypothalamus initiates vasoconstriction, and blood flow to the skin lessens to conserve heat.

Behavioral Control. Healthy individuals maintain a comfortable body temperature when exposed to temperature extremes. The ability of a person to control body temperature depends on (1) the degree of temperature extreme, (2) the person's ability to sense feeling comfortable or uncomfortable, (3) thought processes or emotions, and (4) the person's mobility or ability to remove or add clothes. Individuals are less able to control body temperature if any of these abilities are lost. For example, infants are able to sense uncomfortable warm conditions but need help to change their environment. Older adults sometimes need help to detect cold environments and minimize heat loss. Illnesses, a decreased level of consciousness, or impaired thought processes result in an inability to recognize the need to change behavior for temperature control. When temperatures become extremely hot or cold, health-promoting behaviors such as removing or adding clothing have a limited effect on controlling temperature.

Factors Affecting Body Temperature

Many factors affect body temperature. Changes in body temperature within an acceptable range occur when physiological or behavioral mechanisms alter the relationship between heat production and heat loss. Be aware of these factors and how they impact body temperature regulation when assessing for and evaluating temperature variations.

Age. At birth, the newborn leaves a warm, relatively constant environment and enters one in which temperatures fluctuate widely. Temperature-control mechanisms are immature. An infant's temperature responds drastically to changes in the environment. Take extra care to protect newborns from environmental temperatures. A newborn loses up to 30% of body heat through the head and therefore needs to wear a cap to prevent heat loss (Hockenberry et al., 2019). When protected from environmental extremes, the newborn's body temperature is usually within 35.5° to 37.5°C (95.9° to 99.5°F).

Temperature regulation is unstable until children reach puberty. The usual temperature range gradually drops as individuals approach older adulthood. The older adult has a narrower range of body temperatures than the younger adult. Oral temperatures of 35°C (95°F) are sometimes found in older adults in cold weather. However, the average body temperature of older adults is approximately 35° to 36.1°C (95° to 97°F). Older adults are particularly sensitive to temperature extremes because of deterioration in control mechanisms, particularly poor vasomotor control (control of vasoconstriction and vasodilation), reduced amounts of subcutaneous tissue, reduced sweat gland activity, and reduced metabolism.

Exercise. Muscle activity requires an increased blood supply and carbohydrate and fat breakdown. Any form of exercise increases metabolism and heat production and thus body temperature. Prolonged strenuous exercise such as long-distance running temporarily raises body temperature.

Hormone Level. Women generally experience greater fluctuations in body temperature than men. Hormonal variations during the menstrual cycle cause body temperature fluctuations. Progesterone levels rise and fall cyclically during the menstrual cycle. When progesterone levels are low, the body temperature is a few tenths of a degree below the baseline level. The lower temperature persists until ovulation occurs. During ovulation greater amounts of progesterone enter the circulatory system and raise the body temperature to previous baseline levels or higher. These temperature variations help to predict a woman's most fertile time to achieve pregnancy.

Body temperature changes also occur in women during menopause (cessation of menstruation). Women who have stopped menstruating often experience periods of intense body heat and sweating lasting from 30 seconds to 5 minutes. During these periods skin temperature can increase as much as 4°C (7.2°F), referred to as hot flashes. This is caused by the instability of the vasomotor controls for vasodilation and vasoconstriction.

Circadian Rhythm. Body temperature normally changes 0.5° to 1°C (0.9° to 1.8°F) during a 24-hour period. However, temperature is one of the most stable rhythms in humans. The temperature is usually lowest between 1:00 a.m. and 4:00 a.m. (Fig. 29.2). During the day body temperature rises steadily to a maximum temperature value at about 4:00 p.m. and then declines to early-morning levels. Temperature patterns are not automatically reversed in individuals who work at night and sleep during the day. It takes 1 to 3 weeks for the cycle to reverse. In general the circadian temperature rhythm does not change with age.

Stress. Physical and emotional stress increase body temperature through hormonal and neural stimulation (see Chapter 37). These physiological changes increase metabolism, which increases heat production. A patient who is anxious about entering a hospital or a health care provider's office often has a higher normal temperature.

Environment. Environment influences body temperature. When placed in a warm room a patient may be unable to regulate body temperature by heat-loss mechanisms, and the body temperature may elevate. If a patient is outside in the cold without warm clothing or in an operating room, body temperature may be low as a result of extensive radiant and conductive heat loss. Environmental temperatures affect infants and older adults more often because their temperature-regulating mechanisms are less efficient.

Temperature Alterations. Changes in body temperature outside the usual range are related to excessive heat production, excessive heat loss, minimal heat production, minimal heat loss, or any combination of these alterations.

Fever. Fever, or pyrexia, occurs because heat-loss mechanisms are unable to keep pace with excessive heat production, resulting in an abnormal rise in body temperature. In general, a fever is a temperature above 100.4°F (38°C) for an adult or child, depending on the type of thermometer used (Ward, 2020; Mayo Clinic, 2019b). The height of a child's fever is not always the best indicator of whether the child needs to be treated. Instead, it is important to note how a child behaves and appears because fever is usually accompanied by other symptoms (Ward, 2020). These are the cutoffs for fever in children using different types of thermometers (Seattle Children's Hospital, 2020):
- Rectal (bottom), ear, or forehead temperature: 38.0°C (100.4°F) or higher
- Oral (mouth) temperature: 37.8°C (100°F) or higher
- Under the arm (armpit) temperature: 37.2°C (99°F) or higher
- *Caution:* Ear temperatures are inaccurate before 6 months of age.

A single temperature reading does not always indicate a fever (Bijur et al., 2016). In addition to physical signs and symptoms of infection, fever determination is based on several temperature readings at different times of the day compared with the usual value for that person at that time.

A true fever results from an alteration in the hypothalamic set point. Pyrogens such as bacteria and viruses elevate body temperature by acting as antigens to trigger the immune system. The hypothalamus reacts to raise the set point, and the body responds by producing and conserving heat. Several hours pass before the body temperature reaches the new set point. During this period, a person experiences the physical signs and symptoms of chills, shivers, and feeling cold, even though the body temperature is rising (Fig. 29.3). The chill phase resolves when the new set point, a higher temperature, is achieved. During the next phase, the plateau, the chills subside, and the person feels warm and dry. If the new set point is "overshot" or the pyrogens are removed (e.g., destruction of bacteria by antibiotics), the third phase of a febrile episode occurs. The hypothalamus set point drops, initiating heat-loss responses. The skin becomes warm and flushed because of vasodilation. Diaphoresis assists in evaporative heat loss. When the fever "breaks," the patient becomes afebrile.

FIG. 29.2 Temperature cycle for 24 hours.

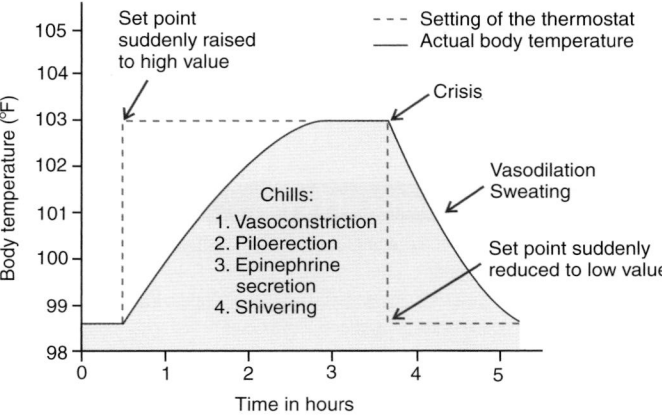

FIG. 29.3 Effect of changing set point of hypothalamic temperature control during a fever. (Modified from Hall JE, Hall ME: *Guyton and Hall textbook of medical physiology*, ed 14, Philadelphia, 2021, Elsevier.)

Fever is an important defense mechanism. Mild temperature elevations as high as 39°C (102.2°F) enhance the immune system of the body. However, during a fever, cellular metabolism increases, and for every 1°C rise in body temperature, the body's chemical reactions increase 10% (Mogensen et al., 2018a, 2018b). During a febrile episode white blood cell production is stimulated. Increased temperature reduces the concentration of iron in the blood plasma, suppressing the growth of bacteria. Fever also fights viral infections by stimulating interferon, the natural virus-fighting substance of the body.

The body responds to the increase in metabolic needs during a fever by increasing heart and respiratory rates. The increased metabolism uses energy to produce additional heat. If a patient has a cardiac or respiratory problem, the stress of a fever is great. A prolonged fever weakens a patient by exhausting energy stores. Increased metabolism requires additional oxygen. If the body cannot meet the additional oxygen demand, cellular hypoxia (inadequate oxygen) occurs. Myocardial hypoxia produces angina (chest pain). Cerebral hypoxia produces confusion. When water loss through increased respiration and diaphoresis is excessive, the patient is at risk for fluid volume deficit. Dehydration is a serious problem for older adults and children with low body weight. Maintaining optimum fluid volume status is an important nursing action (see Chapter 42).

Fevers and fever patterns serve a diagnostic purpose. Fever patterns differ, depending on the causative pyrogen (Box 29.3). The increase or decrease in pyrogen activity results in fever spikes and declines at different times of the day. The duration and degree of fever depend on the strength of the pyrogen and the ability of the individual to respond. The term fever of unknown origin (FUO) refers to a fever with an undetermined cause.

Hyperthermia. An elevated body temperature related to the inability of the body to promote heat loss or reduce heat production is hyperthermia. Whereas fever is an upward shift in the set point, hyperthermia results from an overload of the thermoregulatory mechanisms (Mechem, 2019). Any disease or trauma to the hypothalamus impairs heat-loss mechanisms. Malignant hyperthermia is a hereditary condition of uncontrolled heat production that occurs when susceptible individuals receive certain general anesthesia medications (see Chapter 50).

Heatstroke. Heat depresses hypothalamic function. Prolonged exposure to the sun or a high environmental temperature overwhelms the heat-loss mechanisms of the body. These conditions cause heatstroke, defined as a body temperature of 40°C (104°F) or more accompanied by hot, dry skin and central nervous system abnormalities, such as delirium, convulsions, or coma (Hifumi et al., 2018). Heatstroke is a dangerous heat emergency with a high mortality rate. There are two groups of heatstroke. Exertional heatstroke develops in able-bodied individuals, such as athletes, soldiers, or laborers who are performing rigorous physical activities. In contrast, nonexertional heatstroke can develop during low-level physical activities among

elderly, ambulatory individuals with comorbidities (e.g., diabetes or cardiovascular disease) (Mechem, 2019). Also at risk are those who take medications (e.g., phenothiazines, anticholinergics, diuretics, amphetamines, and beta-adrenergic receptor antagonists) that decrease the ability of the body to lose heat.

Signs and symptoms of heatstroke include giddiness, confusion, delirium, excessive thirst, nausea, muscle cramps, visual disturbances, and even incontinence. Vital signs reveal a body temperature sometimes as high as 45°C (113°F), with an increase in heart rate (HR) and lowering of BP. The most important sign of heatstroke is hot, dry skin. Victims of heatstroke do not sweat because of severe electrolyte loss and hypothalamic malfunction. If the condition progresses, a patient with heatstroke becomes unconscious, with fixed, nonreactive pupils. Permanent neurological damage occurs unless cooling measures are rapidly started.

Heat Exhaustion. Heat exhaustion is caused by environmental heat exposure and presents with profuse diaphoresis that results in excess water and electrolyte loss. A patient exhibits signs and symptoms of deficient fluid volume (see Chapter 42).

Hypothermia. Heat loss during prolonged exposure to cold overwhelms the ability of the body to produce heat, causing hypothermia. Hypothermia is classified by core temperature measurements (Table 29.1). Hypothermia contributes to poor patient outcomes such as increased infection complications, clotting disorders, and prolonged length of hospitalization (Zafren and Mechem, 2020). Preventing hypothermia increases patient comfort and prevents complications.

Hypothermia can be unintentional, such as falling through the ice of a frozen lake, or intentionally induced during surgical or emergency procedures to decrease metabolism and the body's need for oxygen. Accidental hypothermia usually develops gradually and goes unnoticed for several hours. Older adults are more susceptible to accidental hypothermia (Zafren and Mechem 2020). When skin temperature drops below 34°C (93.2°F), the patient suffers uncontrolled shivering, loss of memory, depression, and poor judgment. As the body temperature falls, HR, respiratory rate, and BP also fall. The skin becomes cyanotic. Patients experience cardiac dysrhythmias and loss of consciousness and are unresponsive to painful stimuli if hypothermia progresses. In severe cases a person demonstrates clinical signs similar to those of death (e.g., lack of response to stimuli and extremely slow respirations and pulse). Assessment of core temperature is critical when you suspect hypothermia (Zafren and Mechem, 2020). A special low-reading thermometer is required because standard devices do not register below 35°C (95° F).

Frostbite occurs when the body is exposed to subnormal temperatures. Ice crystals form inside the cells, and permanent circulatory and tissue damage occurs. Areas particularly susceptible to frostbite are the earlobes, tip of the nose, and fingers and toes. The injured area becomes white, waxy, and firm to the touch. The patient loses sensation in the affected area. Interventions include gradual warming measures, analgesia, and protection of the injured tissue.

BOX 29.3   Patterns of Fever

Sustained: A constant body temperature continuously above 38°C (100.4°F) that has little fluctuation

Intermittent: Fever spikes interspersed with usual temperature levels (Temperature returns to acceptable value at least once in 24 hours.)

Remittent: Fever spikes and falls without a return to acceptable temperature levels

Relapsing: Periods of febrile episodes and periods with acceptable temperature values (Febrile episodes and periods of normothermia are often longer than 24 hours.)

TABLE 29.1   Classification of Hypothermia by Core Temperature

	Celsius	Fahrenheit
Mild	32°–35°	90.0°–95°
Moderate	28°–32°	82°–90°
Severe	<28°	<82°

From Zafren K, Mechem CC: *Accidental hypothermia in adults,* UpToDate, 2020, https://www.uptodate.com/contents/accidental-hypothermia-in-adults. Accessed August 2020.

❖ NURSING PROCESS

Apply clinical judgment, using the nursing process and critical thinking to provide appropriate patient care. The nursing process provides a clinical decision-making approach for you to develop and implement an individualized patient-centered plan of care.

Knowledge of the physiology of body temperature regulation is essential to assess and evaluate a patient's response to temperature alterations and to intervene safely. Implement independent nursing measures to increase or minimize heat loss, promote heat conservation, and increase comfort. These measures complement the effects of medically ordered therapies during illness. You also provide education to family members, parents of children, or other caregivers.

◆ Assessment

During the assessment process thoroughly assess each patient and critically analyze findings to ensure that your clinical judgment leads to the patient-centered clinical decisions required for safe nursing care.

Through the Patient's Eyes. Identify your patient's values, beliefs, current treatments, preferences, and expectations regarding fever management. When possible, select the temperature site preferred by the patient. Include the patient's preferences when selecting nonpharmacological interventions for hyperthermia (e.g., cooling blankets, tepid baths, fans).

Temperature Measurement Sites. Core and surface body temperature can be measured at several sites. Intensive care units use the core temperatures of the pulmonary artery, esophagus, and urinary bladder. These measurements require the use of continuous invasive devices placed in body cavities or organs and continually display readings on an electronic monitor.

Use a thermometer for the mouth, rectum, tympanic membrane, or temporal artery to obtain intermittent temperature measurements. Axillary temperature measurements, obtained by placing a thermometer under the axillae, require longer measurement time and are inconsistent in measuring fever in infants. The use of noninvasive skin temperature sensors or chemically prepared thermometer patches is helpful to screen infants for temperature alterations (Hockenberry et al., 2019).

Oral, rectal, and skin temperature sites rely on effective blood circulation at the measurement site. The heat of the blood is conducted to the thermometer probe. Tympanic temperature relies on the radiation of body heat to an infrared sensor. Because the tympanic membrane shares the same arterial blood supply as the hypothalamus, it is a core temperature. Temporal artery measurements detect the temperature of cutaneous blood flow.

To ensure accurate temperature readings, measure each site correctly (see Skill 29.1). The temperature obtained varies, depending on the site used, but it is usually between 36°C (96.8°F) and 38°C (100.4°F). Rectal temperatures are usually 0.5°C (0.9°F) higher than oral temperatures. Each of the common temperature measurement sites has advantages and disadvantages (Table 29.2). Choose the safest and most accurate site for each patient. When possible, use the same site when repeated measurements are necessary.

Thermometers. Two types of thermometers are available for measuring body temperature: electronic and disposable. The mercury-in-glass thermometer, once the standard device, has been eliminated from health care agencies because of the environmental hazards of mercury. However, some patients may still use mercury-in-glass thermometers at home. When you find a mercury-in-glass thermometer in the home, teach the patient about safer temperature devices and encourage the disposal of mercury products at appropriate neighborhood hazardous

disposal locations. Disposable digital thermometers are readily available for use in the home setting. Home disposable thermometers are useful for temperature screening but are less accurate than nondisposable electronic thermometers.

Each device measures temperature using the Celsius or Fahrenheit scale. Electronic thermometers convert the temperature scales by activating a switch. When it is necessary to convert temperature readings, use the following formulas:
1. To convert Fahrenheit to Celsius, subtract 32 from the Fahrenheit reading and multiply the result by 5/9.

$$C = (F - 32) \times \frac{5}{9}$$

$$\text{Example} : 40° \, C = (104° \, F - 32) \times \frac{5}{9}$$

2. To convert Celsius to Fahrenheit, multiply the Celsius reading by 9/5 and add 32 to the product.

$$F = \left(\frac{9}{5} \times °C\right) + 32$$

$$\text{Example} : 104°F = \left(\frac{9}{5} \times 40°C\right) + 32°$$

Electronic Thermometer. The electronic thermometer consists of a rechargeable battery-powered display unit, a thin wire cord, and a temperature-processing probe covered by a disposable probe cover (Fig. 29.4A). Separate unbreakable reusable probes with single-use disposable covers are available for oral and rectal use. Electronic thermometers provide two modes of operation: a 4-second predictive temperature and a 3-minute standard temperature. Nurses use the 4-second predictive mode, which improves measurement accuracy. A sound signals, and a reading appears on the display unit when the peak temperature reading has been measured.

Another form of electronic thermometer is used exclusively for tympanic temperature. An otoscope-like speculum with an infrared sensor tip detects heat radiated from the tympanic membrane (Fig. 29.4B). The tip is covered by a single patient-use cover. Within seconds of placement in the auditory canal, a sound signals, and a reading appears on the display unit when the peak temperature reading has been measured.

There is an electronic thermometer that measures the temperature of the superficial temporal artery. A handheld scanner with an infrared sensor tip detects the temperature of cutaneous blood flow by sweeping the sensor across the forehead and just behind the ear (Fig. 29.4C). After scanning is complete, a reading appears on the display unit. Temporal artery temperature is a reliable noninvasive measure of core temperature.

The greatest advantages of electronic thermometers are that their readings appear within seconds and that they are easy to read. The plastic sheath is unbreakable and ideal for children. Their expense is a major disadvantage. Maintaining cleanliness of the probes is an important consideration. For example, if improperly cleaned between patients, gastrointestinal contamination of a rectal probe causes disease transmission. Wipe the thermometer device daily with alcohol and the thermometer probe with an alcohol swab after each patient, paying particular attention to the ridges where the probe cover is secured to the probe.

Chemical Dot Thermometers. Single-use or reusable chemical dot thermometers (Fig. 29.4D) are thin strips of plastic with a temperature sensor at one end. The sensor consists of a matrix of chemically impregnated dots that change color at different temperatures. In the Celsius version there are 50 dots, each representing a temperature increment of 0.1°C, over a range of 35.5°C to 40.4°C. The Fahrenheit version has 45 dots with increments of 0.2°F and a range of 96°F to 104.8°F.

TABLE 29.2 Advantages and Disadvantages of Select Temperature Measurement Sites

Site Advantages	Site Limitations
Oral	
Easily accessible—requires no position change	Causes delay in measurement if patient recently ingested hot/cold fluids or foods, smoked, or is receiving oxygen by mask/cannula
Comfortable for patient	Not for patients who had oral surgery, trauma, history of epilepsy, or shaking chills
Provides accurate surface temperature reading	Not for infants, small children, or patients who are confused, unconscious, or uncooperative
Reflects rapid change in core temperature	Risk of body fluid exposure
Reliable route to measure temperature in patients who are intubated	
Tympanic Membrane	
Easily accessible site	More variability of measurement than with other core temperature devices
Found to be most accurate method in critically ill patients when compared with oral, axillary, and rectal (Mogensen et al., 2018a).	Requires removal of hearing aids before measurement
Minimal patient repositioning required	Requires disposable sensor cover with only one size available
Obtained without disturbing, waking, or repositioning patients	Otitis media and cerumen impaction distorts readings
Used for patients with tachypnea without affecting breathing	Not used in patients who have had surgery of the ear or tympanic membrane
Sensitive to core temperature changes	Does not accurately measure core temperature changes during and after exercise
Very rapid measurement (2 to 5 seconds)	Does not obtain continuous measurement
Unaffected by oral intake of food or fluids or smoking	Affected by ambient temperature devices such as incubators, radiant warmers, and facial fans
Not influenced by environmental temperatures	Use in infants older than 6 months (Seattle Children's Hospital, 2020) and children under 3 years of age; use care to position device correctly because anatomy of ear canal makes it difficult to position.
	Inaccuracies reported caused by incorrect positioning of handheld unit
Rectal	
Argued to be more reliable when oral temperature is difficult or impossible to obtain	Lags behind core temperature during rapid temperature changes
	Not for patients with diarrhea, rectal disorders, or bleeding tendencies or those who had rectal surgery
	Requires positioning and is often a source of patient embarrassment and anxiety
	Risk of body fluid exposure and injury to rectal lining
	Requires lubrication
	Not for routine vital signs in newborns
	Readings influenced by impacted stool
Skin	
Inexpensive	Measurement lags behind other sites during temperature changes, especially during hyperthermia
Provides continuous reading	Adhesion impaired by diaphoresis or sweat
Safe and noninvasive	Reading affected by environmental temperature
Used for neonates	Cannot be used for patients with allergy to adhesives
Temporal Artery	
Easy to access without position change	Inaccurate with head covering or hair on forehead
Very rapid measurement	Affected by skin moisture such as diaphoresis or sweating
Comfortable with no risk of injury to patient or nurse	
Eliminates need to disrobe or be unbundled	
Comfortable for patient	
Used as a screening tool for infants and young children; it is not predictable for fever (Hockenberry et al., 2019)	
Reflects rapid change in core temperature	
Sensor cover not required	
Axillary	
Safe and inexpensive	Long measurement time
Recommended for infants younger than 1 month old (Hockenberry et al., 2019)	Requires continuous positioning
	Measurement lags behind core temperature during rapid temperature changes
	Not recommended for detecting fever
	Requires exposure of thorax that can result in temperature loss, especially in newborns
	Affected by exposure to environment, including time to place the thermometer
	Underestimates core temperature

FIG. 29.4 (A) Electronic thermometer with disposable probe. (B) Genius 3 Tympanic Thermometer. (C) Temporal artery thermometer. (D) Chemical dot disposable single-use thermometer. (**A** Courtesy Hillrom; **B** Copyright © 2018 Courtesy of Cardinal Health UK Ltd.; **C** Copyright iStock/guvendemir.)

Chemical dots on the thermometer change color to reflect the temperature reading, usually within 60 seconds. Most are for single use. In one reusable brand for a single patient, the chemical dots return to their original color within a few seconds. Chemical dot thermometers are for oral use and are useful for screening temperatures, especially in infants, young children, and patients who are intubated. Chemical dot thermometers often underestimate oral temperature by 0.4°C (0.7°F) or more. Use an electronic thermometer to confirm measurements made with a chemical dot thermometer when treatment decisions are involved. Chemical dot thermometers are useful when caring for patients who have sores in the mouth or who are on protective isolation to avoid the need to take electronic instruments into patient rooms (see Chapter 28).

Another disposable thermometer useful for screening temperature is a temperature-sensitive patch or tape. Applied to the forehead or abdomen, chemical-sensitive areas of the patch change color at different temperatures. This type of thermometer can also be affected by environmental temperature.

REFLECT NOW

You are planning interventions for a patient with hyperthermia who has entered the emergency department. How will the patient's physical characteristics influence your care plan?

◆ Analysis and Nursing Diagnosis

After concluding your assessment, identify patterns or clusters of assessment data to form a nursing diagnosis (Box 29.4). For example, a decrease in body temperature, shivering, skin cool to touch, tachycardia,

---

BOX 29.4 Nursing Diagnostic Process

Impaired Thermoregulation Related to Aging and Inability to Adapt to Environmental Temperature

Assessment Activities	Assessment Findings
Review patient's health history.	85-year-old woman with history of dementia; living in an unventilated apartment during heat wave
Obtain vital signs, including temperature, pulse (see Skill 29.2), respirations (see Skill 29.3), SpO_2 (see Skill 29.4).	Increased body temperature above usual range Tachycardia Tachypnea SpO_2 = 88%
Palpate skin.	Warm, dry skin
Observe patient's appearance and behavior while talking and resting.	Confusion Mild shivering Flushed skin

and lowered SpO_2 indicate the nursing diagnosis of *Hypothermia*. State a nursing diagnosis as either an at-risk or problem-focused (negative) temperature alteration. Implement actions to minimize or eliminate risk factors if the patient has an at-risk diagnosis. Examples of additional nursing diagnoses for patients with body temperature alterations include the following:

- Impaired Thermoregulation
- Risk for Impaired Thermoregulation
- Hyperthermia
- Fever
- Chronic Fever

Once you determine a nursing diagnosis, accurately select the related factor for problem-focused (negative) diagnoses. The related factor allows you to develop/set appropriate expected outcomes and select appropriate nursing interventions. In the example of hyperthermia, a related factor of *vigorous activity* results in interventions that are much different from those used with a related factor of *decreased ability to perspire.*

◆ Planning and Outcomes Identification

During planning, integrate the knowledge gathered from assessment and the patient's clinical condition to develop an individualized plan of care. Match the patient's needs with interventions that are supported and recommended in the clinical research literature.

Outcomes. The plan of care for a patient with alteration in temperature must include relevant and measurable patient outcomes. This requires collaboration with the patient and family caregiver in setting patient-centered outcomes while selecting nursing interventions. Establish expected outcomes to measure progress toward returning or maintaining the body temperature to an acceptable range. In cases in which the temperature alteration requires helping patients modify their home environment, outcomes may include increasing ventilation in the home or obtaining appropriate clothing to wear in cold weather. When the patient has an altered body temperature, the expected outcome may be to regain normal range of body temperature. In the example of a patient who has an elevated fever and excessive diaphoresis, maintaining fluid and electrolyte balance is a priority. In this example, an outcome of care is to achieve a balance between the patient's intake and output over the next 24 hours.

Setting Priorities. Your knowledge of temperature regulation and the patient's nursing diagnoses and disease process will support your clinical judgment in setting priorities of care. The severity of a temperature alteration and its effects, together with the patient's general health status, influence your priorities in the patient's care. Safety is a top priority. Often other medical problems complicate the care plan. For instance, body temperature imbalance affects body requirements for fluids. However, patients with cardiac problems often have difficulty tolerating required fluid replacement therapy.

Teamwork and Collaboration. Patients at risk for imbalanced body temperature require an individualized care plan directed at maintaining normothermia and reducing risk factors. For example, it is important to establish the outcome that a patient who is homeless can explain appropriate actions to take (e.g., fluid intake, type of clothing) and available community resources to use (e.g., cooling stations) during a heat wave. In contrast, an older adult living at home may need encouragement and reminders from family to use fans or window air conditioner units and to drink appropriate amounts of fluids. Teach the patient and caregiver the importance of thermoregulation and actions to take during excessive environmental heat. Education is particularly important for parents, who need to know how to take action at home and whom to call (e.g., health care provider's office, home care nurse) when an infant or child develops a temperature imbalance.

◆ Implementation

Health Promotion. By maintaining balance between heat production and heat loss you promote the health of patients at risk for imbalanced body temperature. Consider patient activity, temperature of the environment, and appropriate clothing. Teach patients to avoid strenuous exercise in hot, humid weather; to drink fluids such as water or clear fruity juices before, during, and after exercise; and to wear lightweight, loose-fitting, light-colored clothes. Also teach patients to avoid exercising in areas with poor ventilation, to wear a protective covering over the head when outdoors, and to expose themselves to hot climates gradually.

Prevention is key for patients at risk for hypothermia. It involves educating patients, family members, and friends. Patients at risk include the very young; the very old; and individuals debilitated by trauma, stroke, diabetes mellitus, drug or alcohol intoxication, and sepsis. Patients who are mentally ill or handicapped sometimes fall victim to hypothermia because they are unaware of the dangers of cold conditions. Individuals with inadequate home heating, shelter, diet, or clothing are also at risk. Fatigue, dark skin color, malnutrition, and hypoxemia contribute to the risk of frostbite.

Prevention is also the focus for individuals at risk for heatstroke, with prevention strategies such as using air conditioners (despite client concerns with utility bills); limiting outdoor activities during the day; drinking ample fluids; wearing loose-fitting and light-colored clothing; knowing medication side effects that may cause fluid losses, decrease sweating, or decrease heart rate; and never leaving impaired adults or children in a car unattended (Peiris et al., 2017).

Acute Care

Fever. When an elevated body temperature develops, initiate interventions to treat fever. The objective of therapy is to increase heat loss, reduce heat production, and prevent complications. The choice of interventions depends on the cause; adverse effects; and the strength, intensity, and duration of the temperature elevation. The health care provider attempts to determine the cause of the elevated temperature by isolating the causative pyrogen. Sometimes it is necessary to obtain culture specimens for laboratory analysis such as urine, blood, sputum, and wound sites to determine the microorganism and select appropriate antibiotics (see Chapter 28). Frequently an antibiotic may be ordered after the cultures have been obtained. Administering antibiotics destroys pyrogenic bacteria and eliminates body stimulus for the elevated temperature. Nurses are essential in assessing and implementing temperature-reducing strategies (Box 29.5).

BOX 29.5   Nursing Interventions for Febrile Patients

Interventions (Unless Contraindicated by Medical Condition)

- Obtain cultures of body fluids such as urine, sputum, or blood (before beginning antibiotics) if ordered.
- Obtain blood culture specimens to coincide with temperature spikes when the antigen-producing organism is most prevalent (check agency policy).
- Minimize heat production: reduce frequency of activities that increase oxygen demand such as excessive turning and ambulation; allow rest periods; limit physical activity.
- Maximize heat loss: reduce external covering on patient's body without causing shivering; keep patient, clothing, and bed linen dry.
- Satisfy requirements for increased metabolic rate: provide supplemental oxygen therapy as ordered to improve oxygen delivery to body cells; provide measures to stimulate appetite and offer well-balanced meals; provide fluids (at least 8 to 10 [8-oz] glasses for patients with normal cardiac and renal function) to replace fluids lost through insensible water loss and sweating.
- Promote patient comfort: encourage oral hygiene because oral mucous membranes dry easily from dehydration; control temperature of the environment without inducing shivering; apply damp cloth to patient's forehead.
- Identify onset and duration of febrile episode phases: examine previous temperature measurements for trends.
- Initiate health teaching as indicated.
- Control environmental temperature to 21° to 27°C (70° to 80°F).

Most fevers in children are of a viral origin, last only briefly, and have limited effects. However, children still have immature temperature-control mechanisms, and temperatures can rise rapidly. Dehydration and febrile seizures occur during rising temperatures of children between 6 months and 3 years of age. Febrile seizures are unusual in children over 5 years old. The extent of the temperature, often exceeding 38.8°C (101.8°F), seems to be a more important factor in regard to seizures than the rapidity of the temperature increase (Hockenberry et al., 2019). Children are at particular risk for fluid volume deficit because they can quickly lose large amounts of fluids in proportion to their body weight. It is important to maintain accurate intake and output records, weigh patients daily, encourage fluids, and provide regular mouth/oral care.

Sometimes a fever is a hypersensitivity response to a drug. Drug fevers are often accompanied by other allergy symptoms such as rash or pruritus (itching). Treatment involves withdrawing the medication, treating any skin integrity impairment, and educating the patient and family about the allergy.

Antipyretics are medications that reduce fever. Acetaminophen and nonsteroidal anti-inflammatory drugs such as ibuprofen, salicylates, and indomethacin reduce fever by increasing heat loss. Medications containing salicylates, such as aspirin, should never be given to children as there is an association between Reye syndrome and aspirin use (Hockenberry et al., 2019). Although not used to treat fever, corticosteroids reduce heat production by interfering with the hypothalamic response. It is important to remember that steroids mask signs and symptoms of infection (Burchum and Rosenthal, 2019; Frenkel et al., 2018). Therefore patients who are prescribed steroids need to be monitored closely, especially if they are at risk for infection.

Nonpharmacological therapies for fever increase heat loss by evaporation, conduction, convection, or radiation. Make sure that nursing measures to enhance body cooling do not stimulate shivering. Shivering is counterproductive and increases energy expenditure up to 400%. Tepid sponge baths, bathing with alcohol-water solutions, applying ice packs to axillae and groin areas, and cooling fans were previously used to reduce fever; however, *avoid these therapies because they lead to shivering*. When patients shiver, the body temperature will increase and there is no advantage of these methods over antipyretic medications.

Blankets cooled by circulating water delivered by motorized units increase conductive heat loss. Follow manufacturer instructions for applying these hypothermia blankets because of the risk for skin breakdown and "freeze burns." Placing a bath blanket between the patient and the hypothermia blanket and wrapping distal body parts (fingers, toes, and genitalia) reduces the risk of injury to the skin and tissue from hypothermia therapy. Wrapping the patient's extremities reduces the incidence and intensity of shivering. Medications such as meperidine or butorphanol reduce shivering.

Heatstroke. Heatstroke first aid treatment includes moving the patient to a cooler environment; removing excess body clothing; placing cool, wet towels over the skin; and using oscillating fans to increase convective heat loss. Emergency medical treatment also includes administering intravenous (IV) fluids, irrigating the stomach and lower bowel with cool solutions, and applying hypothermia blankets.

Hypothermia. The priority treatment for hypothermia is to prevent a further decrease in body temperature. Removing wet clothes, replacing them with dry ones, and wrapping patients in blankets are key nursing interventions. In emergencies away from a health care setting, have the patient lie under blankets next to a warm person. A conscious patient benefits from drinking hot liquids such as soup and by avoiding alcohol and caffeinated fluids. It is also helpful to keep the head covered, to place the patient near a fire or in a warm room, or to place heating pads next to areas of the body (head and neck) that lose heat the quickest.

REFLECT NOW

You implement an order for acetaminophen for an elderly patient with a fever of 100.6°F. What additional measures can you implement to improve comfort care? What vital sign changes do you expect if your interventions are successful?

Restorative and Continuing Care. Educate the patient with a fever about the importance of taking and continuing any antibiotics as directed until the course of treatment is completed. Children and older adults are at risk for deficient fluid volume because they can quickly lose large amounts of fluids in proportion to their body weight. Provide education on signs of dehydration such as dry mouth, sunken eyes, and decreased urine output. Identifying preferred fluids and encouraging oral fluid intake are important ongoing nursing interventions.

◆ Evaluation

Through the Patient's Eyes. Evaluate your patients' perspectives about the care provided. Are they satisfied with the outcomes of care or does the care plan need to be modified? Including patients in the evaluation demonstrates that you value their perspective and contributes to patient safety.

Patient Outcomes. Evaluate all nursing interventions by comparing the patient's actual response to the expected outcomes of the care plan. Use your clinical judgment in determining whether the outcomes were achieved; if they were not achieved, revise the care plan when necessary. After an intervention, measure the patient's temperature to evaluate for change. In addition, use other evaluative measures such as palpating the skin and assessing pulse and respirations. If therapies are effective, body temperature returns to an acceptable range, other vital signs stabilize, and the patient reports a sense of comfort.

PULSE

The pulse is the palpable bounding of blood flow in a peripheral artery. Blood flows through the body in a continuous circuit. The pulse is an indirect indicator of circulatory status.

Physiology and Regulation

Electrical impulses originating from the sinoatrial (SA) node travel through heart muscle to stimulate cardiac contraction. Approximately 60 to 70 mL of blood enters the aorta with each ventricular contraction (stroke volume [SV]). With each SV ejection, the walls of the aorta distend, creating a pulse wave that travels rapidly toward the distal ends of the arteries. The pulse wave moves 15 times faster through the aorta and 100 times faster through the small arteries than the ejected volume of blood. When a pulse wave reaches a peripheral artery, you can feel it by palpating the artery lightly against underlying bone or muscle. The number of pulsing sensations occurring in 1 minute is the pulse rate.

The volume of blood pumped by the heart during 1 minute is the cardiac output, the product of HR and the ventricular SV. In an adult the heart normally pumps 5000 mL of blood per minute. A change in HR or SV does not always change the output of the heart or the amount of blood in the arteries. For example, if a person's HR is 70 beats/min and the SV is 70 mL, the cardiac output is 4900 mL/min (70 beats/min × 70 mL/beat).

If the HR drops to 60 beats/min and the SV rises to 85 mL/beat, the cardiac output increases to 5100 mL or 5.1 L/min (60 beats/min × 85 mL/beat).

Mechanical, neural, and chemical factors regulate the strength of ventricular contraction and the SV. SV depends on the time available to fill the ventricle with blood. When the contraction strength or SV cannot be altered, a change in HR causes a change in cardiac output. As HR increases, there is less time for the ventricular chambers of the heart to fill. When SV cannot change when the HR increases, the BP will decrease. As HR slows, filling time is increased, and BP increases.

An abnormally slow, rapid, or irregular pulse alters cardiac output. Assess the ability of the heart to meet the demands of body tissue for nutrients by palpating a peripheral pulse or using a stethoscope to listen to heart sounds (apical pulse) (see Skill 29.2).

❖ NURSING PROCESS

◆ Assessment of Pulse

Assessing a patient's peripheral pulses determines the integrity of the cardiovascular system. You can assess any artery for pulse rate, but you typically use the radial artery because it is easy to palpate. When a patient's condition suddenly worsens and cardiac output declines significantly, peripheral pulses weaken and are difficult to palpate. In this situation, the carotid artery site is recommended for quickly finding and assessing the pulse. The heart continues to deliver blood through the carotid artery to the brain as long as possible.

The radial and apical locations are the most common sites for pulse rate assessment. Use the radial pulse to teach patients how to monitor their own HRs (e.g., athletes, individuals taking cardiac medications, and patients starting a prescribed exercise regimen). If the radial pulse is abnormal or intermittent resulting from dysrhythmias or if it is inaccessible because of a dressing or cast, assess the apical pulse. When a patient takes medication that affects the HR, the apical pulse provides a more accurate assessment of heart function. The brachial or apical pulse is the best site for assessing an infant's or a young child's pulse because other peripheral pulses are deep and difficult to palpate accurately.

Assessment of other peripheral pulse sites such as the brachial or femoral artery is unnecessary when routinely obtaining vital signs.

You assess other peripheral pulses when conducting a complete physical, when surgery or treatment has impaired blood flow to a body part, or when there are clinical indications of impaired peripheral blood flow (see Chapter 30). Table 29.3 summarizes additional pulse locations.

Use of a Stethoscope. Assessing the apical rate requires a stethoscope. The five major parts of the stethoscope are the earpieces, binaurals, tubing, bell chest piece, and diaphragm chest piece (Fig. 29.5). The plastic or rubber earpieces should fit snugly and comfortably in your ears. The binaurals should be angled and strong enough that the earpieces stay firmly in the ears without causing discomfort. To ensure the best reception of sound, the earpieces follow the contour of the ear canal, pointing toward the face when the stethoscope is in place.

The polyvinyl tubing is flexible and 30 to 45 cm (12 to 18 inches) in length. Longer tubing decreases the transmission of sound waves. Thick-walled and moderately rigid tubing eliminates the transmission of environmental noise and prevents the tubing from kinking, which distorts sound-wave transmission. Stethoscopes have single or dual tubes.

The chest piece consists of a bell and a diaphragm that you rotate into position. The diaphragm or bell needs to be in proper position during use to hear sounds through the stethoscope. With the earpieces in your ears, tap lightly on the diaphragm to determine which side of the chest piece is functioning. The diaphragm is the circular, flat portion of the chest piece covered with a thin plastic disk. It transmits high-pitched sounds created by the high-velocity movement of air and blood. Auscultate bowel, lung, and heart sounds with the diaphragm. Place the stethoscope directly on the skin because clothing obscures the sound. Position the diaphragm to make a tight seal, and press firmly against the patient's skin (Fig. 29.6A). Do not use your thumb to hold the diaphragm in place because you may hear your pulse being transmitted through it.

The bell is the bowl-shaped chest piece usually surrounded by a rubber ring. The ring avoids chilling patients with cold metal when placed on the skin. The bell transmits low-pitched sounds created by the low-velocity movement of blood. Auscultate heart and vascular sounds with the bell. Apply the bell lightly, resting the chest piece on the skin (Fig. 29.6B).

TABLE 29.3   Pulse Sites

Site	Location	Rationale for Selection
Temporal	Over temporal bone of head, above and lateral to eye	Easily accessible site used to assess pulse in children
Carotid	Along medial edge of sternocleidomastoid muscle in neck	Easily accessible site used during physiological shock, cardiac arrest, or when other sites are not palpable
Apical	Fourth to fifth intercostal space at left midclavicular line	Site used to auscultate for apical pulse
Brachial	Groove between biceps and triceps muscles at antecubital fossa	Site used to assess status of circulation to lower arm and to auscultate blood pressure
Radial	Radial or thumb side of forearm at wrist	Common site used to assess character of pulse peripherally and status of circulation to hand
Ulnar	Ulnar or little finger side of forearm at wrist	Site used to assess status of circulation to hand; also used to perform an Allen's test
Femoral	Below inguinal ligament, midway between symphysis pubis and anterior superior iliac spine	Site used to assess character of pulse during physiological shock or cardiac arrest when other pulses are not palpable; used to assess status of circulation to leg
Popliteal	Behind knee in popliteal fossa	Site used to assess status of circulation to lower leg
Posterior tibial	Inner side of ankle, below medial malleolus	Site used to assess status of circulation to foot
Dorsalis pedis	Along top of foot, between extension tendons of great and first toe	Site used to assess status of circulation to foot

Compressing the bell against the skin reduces low-pitched sound amplification and creates a "diaphragm of skin." Some stethoscopes have one chest piece that combines features of the bell and diaphragm. When you use light pressure, the chest piece is a bell; exerting more pressure converts the bell into a diaphragm.

The stethoscope is a delicate instrument and requires proper care for optimal function. Remove the earpieces regularly and clean them of cerumen (earwax). Clean the bell and diaphragm between patients thoroughly with an antiseptic swab to remove microorganisms. Clean the tubing regularly with mild soap and water. A study examined the cross-contamination of physicians' hands with methicillin-resistant *Staphylococcus aureus* (MRSA) microorganisms following a physical examination of patients. The study showed that the contamination level of the stethoscope was substantial after a single physical examination and can result in cross-contamination and hospital-acquired infections (HAIs) (Marcos et al., 2019; Medical Environment Update, 2019).

Character of the Pulse. Assessment of the radial pulse includes measuring the rate, rhythm, strength, and equality. When auscultating an apical pulse, assess rate and rhythm only.

Rate. Before measuring a pulse, review the patient's baseline rate for comparison (Table 29.4). Some health care providers prefer to make baseline measurements of the pulse rate as a patient assumes a sitting, standing, and lying position. Postural changes affect the pulse rate because of alterations in blood volume and sympathetic activity. The HR temporarily increases when a person changes from a lying to a sitting or standing position.

When assessing the pulse, consider the variety of factors influencing the heart rate (Table 29.5). A single factor or a combination of these factors often causes significant changes. If you detect an abnormal rate while palpating a peripheral pulse, the next step is to assess the apical rate. The apical rate requires auscultation of heart sounds, which provides a more accurate assessment of cardiac contraction.

Assess the apical rate by listening to heart sounds (see Chapter 30). Identify the first and second heart sounds (S_1 and S_2). At normal slow rates S_1 is low pitched and dull, sounding like a "lub." S_2 is higher pitched and shorter, creating the sound "dub." Count each set of "lub-dub" as one heartbeat. Using the diaphragm or bell of the stethoscope, count the number of lub-dubs occurring in 1 minute.

Peripheral and apical pulse rate assessment often reveals variations in HR. Two common abnormalities in pulse rate are tachycardia and bradycardia. Tachycardia is an abnormally elevated HR, above 100 beats/min in adults. Bradycardia is a slow rate, below 60 beats/min in adults.

An inefficient contraction of the heart that fails to transmit a pulse wave to the peripheral pulse site creates a pulse deficit. To assess a pulse deficit, you and a colleague assess radial and apical rates simultaneously and then compare rates (see Skill 29.2). The difference between the apical and radial pulse rates is the pulse deficit. For example, an apical rate

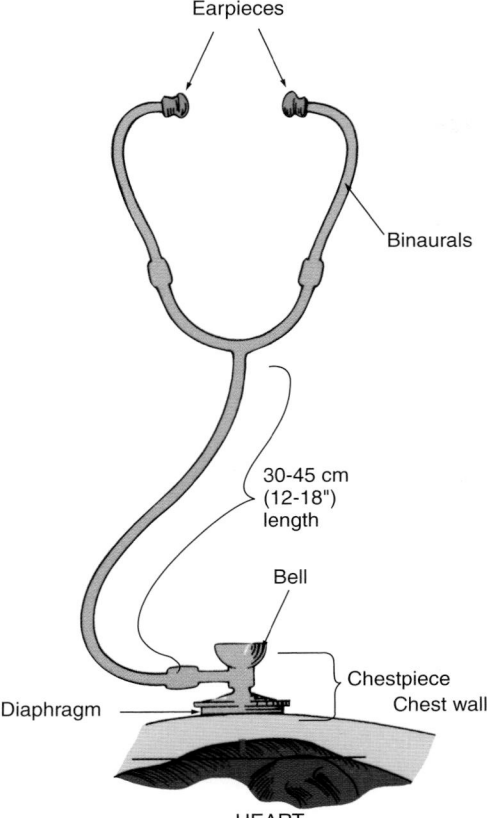

FIG. 29.5 Parts of stethoscope.

FIG. 29.6 (A) Place the diaphragm firmly and securely when auscultating high-pitched lung and bowel sounds. (B) The bell must be placed lightly on the skin to hear low-pitched vascular and heart sounds.

TABLE 29.4	Acceptable Ranges of Heart Rate
Age	**Heart Rate (beats/min)**
Infant	120-160
Toddler	90-140
Preschooler	80-110
School-age child	75-100
Adolescent	60-90
Adult	60-100

TABLE 29.5   Factors Influencing Heart Rate

Factor	Increases Pulse Rate	Decreases Pulse Rate
Exercise	Short-term exercise	Heart conditioned by long-term exercise, resulting in lower resting pulse and quicker return to resting level after exercise (AHA, 2021)
Temperature	Fever and heat	Hypothermia
Acute pain	Increased sympathetic activity increases heart rate, stroke volume, and peripheral resistance, all of which increase myocardial work and oxygen demand.	Effect of chronic pain on heart rate varies; parasympathetic stimulation increased by unrelieved severe pain lowers heart rate
Emotions	Sympathetic stimulation increased by anxiety affects heart rate.	
Medications	Positive chronotropic drugs such as epinephrine	Negative chronotropic drugs such as digitalis; beta-adrenergic and calcium channel blockers
Hemorrhage	Sympathetic stimulation increased by loss of blood	
Postural changes	Standing or sitting	Lying down
Pulmonary conditions	Diseases causing poor oxygenation such as asthma, chronic obstructive pulmonary disease (COPD)	

of 92 with a radial rate of 78 leaves a pulse deficit of 14 beats. Pulse deficits are often associated with abnormal rhythms.

Rhythm. Normally a regular interval occurs between each pulse or heartbeat. An interval interrupted by an early or late beat or a missed beat indicates an abnormal rhythm, or **dysrhythmia**. A dysrhythmia threatens the ability of the heart to provide adequate cardiac output, particularly if it occurs repetitively. You identify a dysrhythmia by palpating an interruption in successive pulse waves or auscultating an interruption between heart sounds. If a dysrhythmia is present, assess the regularity of its occurrence and auscultate the apical rate (see Chapter 30). Dysrhythmias are described as regularly irregular or irregularly irregular.

To document a dysrhythmia, the health care provider often orders an electrocardiogram (ECG), Holter monitor, or telemetry monitor. An ECG records the electrical activity of the heart for a 12-second interval. This test requires placement of electrodes across a patient's chest followed by recording of the heart rhythm. A patient wears a Holter monitor to record and store 24 hours of electrical activity. Access to the information recorded is not available until after the 24 hours have passed and the data are reviewed. Cardiac telemetry provides continuous monitoring of the electrical activity of the heart transmitted to a stationary monitor. Telemetry permits continuous observation of heart rhythm during all of a patient's daily activities and thus allows for immediate treatment if the rhythm becomes erratic or unstable.

Children often have a sinus dysrhythmia, which is an irregular heartbeat that speeds up with inspiration and slows with expiration.

This is a normal finding that you can verify by having the child hold their breath; the HR usually becomes regular.

Strength. The strength or amplitude of a pulse reflects the volume of blood ejected against the arterial wall with each heart contraction and the condition of the arterial vascular system leading to the pulse site. Normally the pulse strength remains the same with each heartbeat. Document the pulse strength as bounding (4); full or strong (3); normal and expected (2); diminished or barely palpable (1); or absent (0). Include assessment of pulse strength in the assessment of the vascular system (see Chapter 30).

Equality. Assess radial pulses on both sides of the peripheral vascular system, comparing the characteristics of each. A pulse in one extremity is sometimes unequal in strength or absent in many disease states (e.g., thrombus [clot] formation). Assess all symmetrical pulses simultaneously except for the carotid pulse. *Never measure the carotid pulses simultaneously because excessive pressure occludes blood supply to the brain.*

◆ Analysis and Nursing Diagnosis

Pulse assessment determines the general state of cardiovascular health and the response of the body to other system imbalances. Tachycardia, bradycardia, and dysrhythmias are important assessment data that support many nursing diagnoses, including the following examples:
- Activity Intolerance
- Dehydration
- Hypervolaemia
- Impaired Cardiac Function
- Impaired Peripheral Tissue Perfusion

◆ Planning, Outcomes Identification, and Implementation

The nursing care plan includes independent, individualized patient-centered nursing interventions based on the nursing diagnoses identified and the risk factors or related factors. For example, the assessment findings of an abnormal HR in response to activity, exertional dyspnea, and a patient's verbal report of fatigue lead to a diagnosis of *Activity Intolerance.* When the related factor is *inactivity following a prolonged illness,* use clinical judgment to select and develop interventions to focus on increasing the patient's daily exercise routine. If the diagnosis has a related factor of *sedentary lifestyle,* interventions include an exercise routine with adaptations during activities of daily living that increase the patient's overall activity level. In ill and hospitalized patients activity and exercise are beneficial in reducing the length of hospital stays, reducing complications, and restoring health. Chapter 38 details standards for promoting early activity and exercise. A patient-centered plan of care is key to developing an exercise plan to which a patient will adhere. Match reccommended activities with a patent's activity preferences (e.g. walking, cycling, swimming) when possible. Educate patients about the benefits of exercise and how to measure heart rate during exercise. Patients who are placed on medications to improve heart function should also learn how to measure their own pulse.

A patient's nursing diagnoses will often develop as a result of medical conditions, such as heart failure, chronic lung diseases, or myocardial infarction. Therefore the plan of care includes dependent interventions that focus on the timely administration of medications (e.g., cardiotonics, beta-adrenergic blocking agents, and oxygen) and careful management of fluid balance.

◆ Evaluation

Patient Outcomes. Once a plan of care is implemented, evaluate the patient's outcomes, which will involve evaluation of the character of the pulse in response to interventions. For example, if a patient is beginning to ambulate after prolonged immobility, measure the pulse as the patient ambulates and when ambulation is completed to identify any change. Basically, the patient's target pulse rate is about 50% to 70% of the maximum heart rate during moderate exercise (American Heart Association [AHA], 2021). Exercise intensity is a subjective measure of how hard physical activity feels to a person while exercising (Mayo Clinic, 2019a). It is important to always ask patients how they feel, especially when exercising the first time after a prolonged illness or surgery. For example, during low to moderate exercise a patient may perceive that breathing quickens but is not out of breath. The patient may develop a light sweat after about 10 minutes of activity (Mayo Clinic, 2019b). A more objective measure of activity tolerance is measuring a patient's actual heart rate compared with the patient's target heart rate. The target heart rate is useful for evaluating a patient's exercise intensity and tolerance (see Chapter 50).

RESPIRATION

Respiration is the exchange of respiratory gases, oxygen (O_2) and carbon dioxide (CO_2), between cells of the body and the atmosphere (see Chapter 41). Three processes of respiration are: ventilation (i.e., mechanical movement of gases into and out of the lungs); diffusion (i.e., movement of oxygen and carbon dioxide between the alveoli and the red blood cells); and perfusion (i.e., distribution of red blood cells to and from the pulmonary capillaries).

Analyzing respiratory efficiency requires integrating assessment data from all three processes. Assess ventilation by determining respiratory rate, depth, rhythm, and end-tidal carbon dioxide ($EtCO_2$) value. Assess diffusion and perfusion by determining oxygen saturation (SpO_2).

Physiological Control

Breathing generally is a passive process. Normally a person thinks little about it. The respiratory center in the brainstem regulates the involuntary control of respirations. Adults normally breathe in a smooth, uninterrupted pattern 12 to 20 times a minute.

The body regulates ventilation using levels of CO_2, O_2, and hydrogen ion concentration (pH) in the arterial blood. The most important factor in the control of ventilation is the level of CO_2 in the arterial blood. An elevation in the CO_2 level causes the respiratory control system in the brain to increase the rate and depth of breathing. The increased ventilatory effort removes excess CO_2 (hypercarbia) by increasing exhalation. However, patients with chronic lung disease have ongoing hypercarbia. For these patients chemoreceptors in the carotid artery and aorta become sensitive to hypoxemia, or low levels of arterial O_2. When arterial oxygen levels fall, these receptors signal the brain to increase the rate and depth of ventilation. Hypoxemia thus helps to control ventilation in patients with chronic lung disease. However, when arterial oxygen levels fall below 88%, supplemental low-dose oxygen may be required. Continuous long-term oxygen administration improves survival of patients with COPD (Koczulla et al., 2018).

Mechanics of Breathing

Although breathing is normally passive, muscular work is involved in moving the lungs and chest wall. Inspiration is an active process. During inspiration, the respiratory center sends impulses along the phrenic nerve, causing the diaphragm to contract. Abdominal organs move downward and forward, increasing the length of the chest cavity to move air into the lungs. The diaphragm moves approximately 1 cm ($4/10$ inch), and the ribs retract upward from the midline of the body approximately 1.2 to 2.5 cm ($\frac{1}{2}$ to 1 inch). During a normal, relaxed breath, a person inhales 500 mL of air. This amount is referred to as the tidal volume. During expiration the diaphragm relaxes, and the abdominal organs return to their original positions. The lung and chest wall return to a relaxed position (Fig. 29.7). Expiration is a

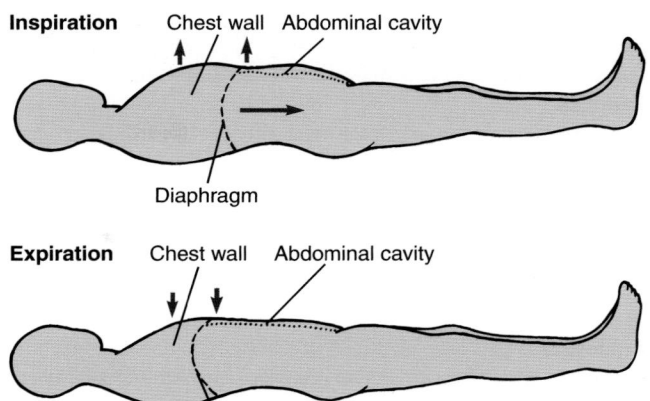

FIG. 29.7 Illustration of diaphragmatic and chest wall movement during inspiration and expiration.

passive process. Sighing interrupts the normal rate and depth of ventilation, eupnea. The sigh, a prolonged deeper breath, is a protective physiological mechanism for expanding small airways and alveoli not ventilated during a normal breath.

The accurate assessment of respirations depends on the recognition of normal thoracic and abdominal movements. During quiet breathing the chest wall gently rises and falls. Contraction of the intercostal muscles between the ribs or contraction of the muscles in the neck and shoulders (the accessory muscles of breathing) is not visible.

❖ NURSING PROCESS

◆ Assessment of Ventilation

Respirations are the easiest of all vital signs to assess, but they are often the most haphazardly measured. Do not estimate respirations. Accurate measurement requires observation and palpation of chest wall movement.

A sudden change in the character of respirations is important. Altered breathing tends to be the first sign of clinical deterioration and is one of the most important indicators for predicting patient outcomes (Takayama et al., 2019). Because respiration is tied to the function of numerous body systems, consider all variables when changes occur (Box 29.6). For example, a decrease in respirations occurring in a patient after head trauma often signifies injury to the brainstem.

Do not let a patient know that you are assessing respirations. When a patient is aware of the assessment, the patient can change the rate and depth of breathing (Hill et al., 2018). Quietly observe the patient's breathing and when appropriate begin to count the rate. Assess respirations immediately after measuring pulse rate, with your hand still on the patient's wrist as it rests over the chest or abdomen. When assessing a patient's respirations, keep in mind the patient's usual ventilatory rate and pattern, the influence any disease or illness has on respiratory function, the relationship between respiratory and cardiovascular function, and the influence of therapies on respirations. The objective measurements of respiratory status include the rate and depth of breathing and the rhythm of ventilatory movements (see Skill 29.3).

Respiratory Rate. Observe a full inspiration and expiration when counting ventilation or respiration rate. The usual respiratory rate varies with age (Table 29.6). The usual range of respiratory rate declines throughout life. A patient's respiratory rate can be used to help predict

BOX 29.6   Factors Influencing Character of Respirations

Exercise
- Exercise increases rate and depth to meet the need of the body for additional oxygen and to rid the body of CO_2.

Acute Pain
- Pain alters rate and rhythm of respirations; breathing becomes shallow.
- Patient inhibits or splints chest wall movement when pain is in area of chest or abdomen.

Anxiety
- Anxiety increases respiration rate and depth as a result of sympathetic stimulation.

Smoking
- Chronic smoking changes pulmonary airways, resulting in increased rate of respirations at rest when not smoking.

Body Position
- A straight, erect posture promotes full chest expansion.
- A stooped or slumped position impairs ventilatory movement.
- Lying flat prevents full chest expansion.

Medications
- Opioid analgesics, general anesthetics, and sedative hypnotics depress rate and depth.
- Amphetamines and cocaine sometimes increase rate and depth.
- Bronchodilators slow rate by causing airway dilation.

Neurological Injury
- Injury to brainstem impairs respiratory center and inhibits respiratory rate and rhythm.

Hemoglobin Function
- Decreased hemoglobin levels (anemia) reduce oxygen-carrying capacity of the blood, which increases respiratory rate.
- Increased altitude lowers amount of saturated hemoglobin, which increases respiratory rate and depth.
- Abnormal blood cell function (e.g., sickle cell disease) reduces ability of hemoglobin to carry oxygen, which increases respiratory rate and depth.

TABLE 29.6   Acceptable Ranges of Respiratory Rate

Age	Rate (breaths/min)
Newborn	30-60
Infant (6 months)	30-50
Toddler (2 years)	25-32
Child	20-30
Adolescent	16-20
Adult	12-20

TABLE 29.7   Alterations in Breathing Pattern

Alteration	Description
Bradypnea	Rate of breathing is regular but abnormally slow (less than 12 breaths/min).
Tachypnea	Rate of breathing is regular but abnormally rapid (greater than 20 breaths/min).
Hyperpnea	Respirations are labored, increased in depth, and increased in rate (greater than 20 breaths/min) (occurs normally during exercise).
Apnea	Respirations cease for several seconds. Persistent cessation results in respiratory arrest.
Hyperventilation	Rate and depth of respirations increase. Hypocarbia sometimes occurs.
Hypoventilation	Respiratory rate is abnormally low, and depth of ventilation is depressed. Hypercarbia sometimes occurs.
Cheyne-Stokes respiration	Respiratory rate and depth are irregular, characterized by alternating periods of apnea and hyperventilation. Respiratory cycle begins with slow, shallow breaths that gradually increase to abnormal rate and depth. The pattern reverses; breathing slows and becomes shallow, concluding as apnea before respiration resumes.
Kussmaul's respiration	Respirations are abnormally deep, regular, and increased in rate.
Biot's respiration	Respirations are abnormally shallow for two to three breaths, followed by irregular period of apnea.

a risk for cardiac arrest. For example, a respiratory rate greater than 27 breaths/min in an adult is a better predictor of cardiac arrest within 72 hours than heart rate or blood pressure (Kelly, 2018).

The apnea monitor is a device that aids respiratory rate assessment. This device uses leads attached to a patient's chest wall; the leads sense movement. The absence of chest wall movement triggers the apnea alarm. Apnea monitoring is used often with infants in the hospital and at home to observe the risk for prolonged apneic events.

Ventilatory Depth. Assess the depth of respirations by observing the degree of excursion or movement of the chest. Describe ventilatory movements as deep or shallow, normal, or labored. A deep respiration involves a full expansion of the lungs with full exhalation. Respirations are shallow and difficult to observe when only a small quantity of air passes through the lungs. Use more objective techniques if you observe that chest excursion is unusually shallow (see Chapter 30). Table 29.7 summarizes types of breathing patterns.

Ventilatory Rhythm. Determine breathing pattern by observing the chest or the abdomen. Diaphragmatic breathing results from the contraction and relaxation of the diaphragm, and you observe it best by watching abdominal movements. Healthy men and children usually demonstrate diaphragmatic breathing. Women tend to use thoracic muscles to breathe, assessed by observing movements in the upper chest. Labored respirations usually involve the accessory muscles of respiration visible in the neck. When something such as a foreign body interferes with the movement of air in and out of the lungs, the intercostal spaces retract during inspiration. A longer expiration phase is evident when the outward flow of air is obstructed (e.g., asthma, chronic obstructive pulmonary disease [COPD]).

With normal breathing a regular time interval occurs after each respiratory cycle. Infants tend to breathe less regularly. A young child often breathes slowly for a few seconds and then suddenly breathes more rapidly. Respiration is regular or irregular in rhythm.

FIG. 29.8 Portable pulse oximeter with digit probe.

◆ Assessment of Diffusion and Perfusion

Assess the respiratory processes of diffusion and perfusion by measuring the oxygen saturation of the blood. Blood flow through the pulmonary capillaries delivers red blood cells for oxygen attachment. After oxygen diffuses from the alveoli into the pulmonary blood, most of the oxygen attaches to hemoglobin molecules in red blood cells. Red blood cells carry the oxygenated hemoglobin molecules through the left side of the heart and out to the peripheral capillaries, where the oxygen detaches, depending on the needs of the tissues.

The percent of hemoglobin that is bound with oxygen in the arteries is the percent of saturation of hemoglobin (or SaO_2). It is usually between 95% and 100% (Pagana et al., 2019). It is affected by factors that interfere with ventilation, perfusion, or diffusion (see Chapter 41). The saturation of venous blood (SvO_2) is lower because the tissues have removed some of the oxygen from the hemoglobin molecules. Factors that interfere with or increase tissue oxygen demand affect SvO_2, which is usually between 65% and 75%.

Measurement of Arterial Oxygen Saturation. A pulse oximeter permits the indirect, noninvasive measurement of oxygen saturation (see Skill 29.4) by measuring the hemoglobin saturation in peripheral blood. The pulse oximeter is a probe with a light-emitting diode (LED) connected by a cable to an oximeter (Fig. 29.8). The LED emits light wavelengths that the oxygenated and deoxygenated hemoglobin molecules absorb differently. A photodetector in the probe detects the amount of oxygen bound to hemoglobin molecules, and the oximeter calculates the peripheral saturation (SpO_2). A saturation greater than 92% is acceptable while a saturation of 75% or less is considered a critical value as the tissues are unable to extract enough oxygen to carry out vital functions. Values obtained with pulse oximetry are less accurate at saturations less than 70% (Pagana et al., 2019).

Selecting the appropriate pulse oximeter probe is important to reduce measurement error. Pulse oximetry measurement of SpO_2 is simple and painless and has few of the risks associated with more invasive measurements of oxygen saturation such as arterial blood gas sampling. A vascular, pulsatile area is needed to detect the change in the transmitted light when making measurements with a finger probe. Conditions that decrease arterial blood flow, such as peripheral vascular disease, hypothermia, pharmacological vasoconstrictors, hypotension, or peripheral edema, affect accurate determination of oxygen saturation in these areas. Factors that affect light transmission or peripheral arterial pulsations affect the ability of the photodetector to measure SpO_2 correctly (Box 29.7).

For patients with decreased peripheral perfusion, apply an earlobe or forehead sensor (Seifi et al., 2018). Earlobe probes have greater accuracy at lower saturations and are least affected by peripheral vasoconstriction. Disposable sensor pads come in a variety of sizes and are used for a variety of sites, including the forehead, the bridge of an adult's nose, or the sole of an infant's foot. These pads are less likely than the spring-loaded probes to cause pressure injuries. Oxygen saturation measurement using a forehead probe is quicker than finger probes and more accurate in conditions that decrease blood flow.

Capnography. Capnography is the measurement of exhaled carbon dioxide throughout exhalation. At the end of exhalation, the $EtCO_2$ measurement approximates the $PaCO_2$ in a healthy patient, normally 35 to 45 mm Hg. In nonintubated patients $EtCO_2$ can be obtained from a special nasal cannula (see Chapter 41) connected to a monitor that detects the percentage of carbon dioxide exhaled at the end of each respiratory cycle. The $EtCO_2$ can be used to assess respiratory and cardiac status, whereas interpretation of a continuous recording, or capnogram, can detect changes in ventilation.

◆ Analysis and Nursing Diagnosis

During assessment of respiration you obtain data on your patient's respiratory rate, pattern, and depth of breathing, lung sounds, SpO_2, and $EtCO_2$. In addition, you collect assessment parameters on the quality of ventilation, diffusion, and perfusion (see Chapters 30 and 41). Use relevant assessment cues to determine the nature of a patient's problem and nursing diagnoses. For example, the assessment findings of tachycardia, dyspnea, restlessness, and an increase in CO_2 level are assessment findings for a nursing diagnosis of *Impaired Gas Exchange*. Related factors could include *alveolar capillary membrane changes from infection* or *a ventilator-perfusion imbalance*. Altered respirations are key assessment findings for other nursing diagnoses, including the following:
- Activity Intolerance
- Hyperventilation

- Impaired Airway Clearance
- Impaired Gas Exchange

◆ Planning, Outcomes Identification, and Implementation

The nursing care plan includes individualized patient-centered outcomes and interventions based on the nursing diagnoses identified and the related factors. A patient's outcomes should be measurable and realistic in regard to the patient's condition. For example, an outcome of improved airway clearance is more likely achievable for a postoperative patient with temporary reduced ventilation from pain compared with a patient who has chronic bronchitis and copious lung secretions. If a patient has *Impaired Gas Exchange*, an expected outcome will likely include improved oxygen saturation within a set time frame.

You select interventions (e.g., coughing, positioning, and fluid management) on the basis of the related factor. As in the case of pulse alterations, medical diagnoses associated with respiratory changes require dependent nursing interventions, including pharmacologic agents such as bronchodilators. Chapter 41 details oxygen therapies.

Teamwork and Collaboration. Patients with or at risk for impaired respiration and ventilation often require interventions from other disciplines. When patients need oxygen support, respiratory therapists are excellent resources to help a patient use supplemental oxygen equipment. For a patient with severe impairment in respiration and ventilation, a mechanical ventilator may be required. In this case, the respiratory therapist is essential to set up the ventilator and to assist in the care of the patient (see Chapter 41).

◆ Evaluation

Patient Outcomes. After providing interventions designed to improve a patient's activity tolerance, breathing pattern, and/or gas exchange, evaluate patient outcomes by reassessing the respiratory rate, ventilatory depth, rhythm, and SpO_2. Consider the physiological changes expected from nursing interventions as you evaluate patient outcomes. For example, after suctioning secretions from a patient's airway, the respiratory rate should decrease and the respiratory depth should increase. The administration of bronchodilators, which relax constricted airways, can reduce respiratory rate and improve respiratory depth.

BLOOD PRESSURE

Blood pressure (BP) is measured on virtually all patients receiving health care. Accurate measurement of BP is essential to guide patient management, determine a patient's response to interventions, and prevent adverse outcomes (AACN, 2016). Blood pressure is the force exerted on the walls of an artery by the pulsing blood under pressure from the heart. Systemic or arterial BP, the BP in the system of arteries in the body, is a good indicator of cardiovascular health. Blood flows throughout the circulatory system because of pressure changes. It moves from an area of high pressure to one of low pressure. The contraction of the heart forces the blood under high pressure into the aorta. The peak pressure, or systolic pressure, occurs when the ventricles of the heart contract and force blood under high pressure into the aorta. When the ventricles relax, the heart fills, and the pressure of blood in the arteries is the diastolic pressure. Diastolic pressure is the minimal pressure exerted against the arterial walls at all times.

The standard unit for measuring BP is millimeters of mercury (mm Hg). The measurement indicates the height to which the BP raises a column of mercury. Record BP with the systolic reading before the diastolic reading (e.g., 120/80). The difference between systolic and diastolic pressure is the pulse pressure. For example, for a BP of 120/80, the pulse pressure is 40.

Recent validation and testing of automated oscillometric devices demonstrate that these devices provide accurate BP measurement and are capable of accurately measuring serial BP to record patient responses to treatment. Both auscultatory methods are considered acceptable for measuring BP in children and adolescents as well (Muntner et al., 2019).

Physiology of Arterial Blood Pressure

Blood pressure reflects the interrelationships of cardiac output, peripheral vascular resistance, blood volume, blood viscosity, and artery elasticity. Your knowledge of these hemodynamic variables helps in the assessment of BP alterations.

Cardiac Output. The BP depends on the cardiac output. When volume increases in an enclosed space such as a blood vessel, the pressure in that space rises. Thus, as cardiac output increases, more blood is pumped against arterial walls, causing the BP to rise. Cardiac output increases as a result of an increase in HR, greater heart muscle contractility, or an increase in blood volume. Changes in HR occur faster than changes in heart muscle contractility or blood volume. A rapid or significant increase in HR decreases the filling time of the heart, which decreases the volume in the left ventricle, and BP decreases.

Peripheral Resistance. The BP depends on peripheral vascular resistance. Blood circulates through a network of arteries, arterioles, capillaries, venules, and veins. Arteries and arterioles are surrounded by smooth muscle that contracts or relaxes to change the size of the lumen. The size of arterial lumens changes to adjust blood flow to the needs of local tissues. For example, when a major organ needs more blood, the peripheral arteries constrict, decreasing their supply of blood. More blood becomes available to the major organ because of the resistance change in the periphery. Normally arteries and arterioles remain partially constricted to maintain a constant flow of blood. Peripheral vascular resistance is the resistance to blood flow determined by the tone of vascular musculature and diameter of blood vessels. The smaller the lumen of a vessel, the greater is the peripheral vascular resistance to blood flow. As resistance rises, arterial BP rises. When vessels dilate and resistance falls, arterial BP falls.

Blood Volume. Blood pressure depends on the volume of circulating blood. Most adults have a circulating blood volume of 5000 mL. Normally the blood volume remains constant. However, an increase in blood volume exerts more pressure against arterial walls. For example, the rapid, uncontrolled infusion of IV fluids elevates BP. When a person's circulating blood volume falls, as in the case of hemorrhage or dehydration, the BP also falls.

Viscosity. The thickness or viscosity of blood affects the ease with which blood flows through small vessels. The hematocrit, or percentage of red blood cells in the blood, determines blood viscosity. When the hematocrit rises and blood flow slows, arterial BP increases. The heart contracts more forcefully to move the viscous blood through the circulatory system.

Elasticity. Normally the walls of an artery are elastic and easily distensible. As pressure within the arteries increases, the diameter of vessel walls increases to accommodate the pressure change. The ability of arteries to dilate prevents wide fluctuations in BP. However, in certain diseases such as arteriosclerosis, the vessel walls lose their elasticity and are replaced by fibrous tissue that cannot stretch well. Reduced elasticity results in greater resistance to blood flow. As a result, when the left ventricle ejects its SV, the vessels no longer yield to pressure. Instead a given volume of blood is forced through the rigid arterial walls, and the systemic pressure rises. Systolic pressure is more significantly elevated than diastolic pressure as a result of reduced arterial elasticity.

Each hemodynamic factor significantly affects the others. For example, as arterial elasticity declines, peripheral vascular resistance increases. The complex control of the cardiovascular system normally prevents any single factor from permanently changing the BP. For example, if the blood volume falls, the body compensates with an increased vascular resistance.

Factors Influencing Blood Pressure

Blood pressure is not constant. With many influencing factors one BP measurement cannot adequately reflect a patient's health status. Even under the best conditions, BP changes from heartbeat to heartbeat. BP trends, not individual measurements, guide nursing interventions. Understanding these factors ensures a more accurate interpretation of BP readings.

Age. Normal BP levels vary throughout life (Table 29.8). BP increases during childhood. You assess the level of a child's or adolescent's BP with respect to their percentile of height and their age (Hockenberry et al., 2019). Larger children (heavier and/or taller) have higher BPs than smaller children of the same age. During adolescence BP continues to vary according to body size. An adult's BP tends to rise with advancing age. The optimal BP for a healthy, middle-age adult is less than 120/80 mm Hg. A systolic value of 120 to 129 and a diastolic value greater than 80 is considered to be an elevated blood pressure (Whelton et al., 2018).

TABLE 29.8 Average Optimal Blood Pressure for Age

Age	Blood Pressure (mm Hg)
Newborn (3000 g [6.6 lb.])	40 (mean)
1 month	85/54
1 year	95/65
6 years[a]	105/65
10-13 years[a]	110/65
14-17 years[a]	119/75
18 years and older	<120/<80

[a]In children and adolescents, hypertension is defined as blood pressure that on repeated measurement is at the 95th percentile or greater adjusted for age, height, and gender.
Data from Whelton et al.: Guideline for the prevention, detection, evaluation, and management of high blood pressure in adults: report of the American College of Cardiology/American Heart Association Task Force on Clinical Practice Guidelines, 2018, *Hypertension* 71(6): e13, 2018.

Stress. Emotional stress (e.g., anxiety and fear) and acute pain result in sympathetic stimulation, which increases HR, cardiac output, and vascular resistance. The effect of sympathetic stimulation increases BP.

Ethnicity and Genetics. Ethnic and genetic characteristics influence blood pressure. The prevalence of hypertension (high blood pressure) in African Americans in the United States is among the highest in the world. In addition, more than 40% of non-Hispanic African American men and women have high blood pressure (AHA, 2017a; AHA, 2016). Heart disease develops earlier in African Americans, and high blood pressure is a factor in more than 50% of all related deaths.

However, other ethnic groups are at risk as well. In a study involving prevalence of hypertension among Asian and Hispanic adults in New York City, two major racial/ethnic minority groups had higher odds of hypertension than non-Hispanic whites: non-Hispanic black and Asian individuals (Fei et al., 2017). There is a need for specifically targeted interventions for hypertension because of ethnic differences (Fei et al., 2017).

Genetic factors also contribute to a patient's blood pressure. Assess the patient's family history for early hypertension and any complications related to hypertension. Individuals with a family history of high blood pressure may share common environments and other potential factors that increase their risk of hypertension (CDC, 2020).

Gender. There is no clinically significant difference in BP levels between males and females. After puberty males tend to have higher BP readings. After menopause women tend to have higher BP levels than men of similar age. There are no specific guidelines for treating hypertension in men and women. However, numerous human studies have shown differences in the mechanisms responsible for blood pressure control between the sexes (Reckelhoff, 2018). Both men and women require education on the risk for hypertension and hypertension-related complications.

Daily Variation. Blood pressure varies throughout the day, with lower BP during sleep between midnight and 3:00 a.m. Between 3:00 a.m. and 6:00 a.m. there is a slow and steady rise in BP. When a patient awakens, there is an early-morning surge. It is highest during the day between 10:00 a.m. and 6 p.m. No two individuals have the same pattern or degree of variation.

Medications. Some medications directly or indirectly affect BP. Before BP assessment ask whether the patient is receiving antihypertensive, diuretic, or other cardiac medications, which lower BP (Table 29.9). Another class of medications that lowers BP is opioid analgesics. Vasoconstrictors and an excess volume of IV fluids increase BP.

TABLE 29.9 Antihypertensive Medications

Medication Type	Example	Action
Diuretics	Furosemide, spironolactone, metolazone, polythiazide, hydrochlorothiazide	Lowers blood pressure by reducing resorption of sodium and water by the kidneys, thus lowering circulating fluid volume
Beta-adrenergic blockers	Atenolol, nadolol, timolol maleate, metoprolol	Combines with beta-adrenergic receptors in the heart, arteries, and arterioles to block response to sympathetic nerve impulses; reduces heart rate and thus cardiac output
Vasodilators	Hydralazine hydrochloride, minoxidil	Acts on arteriolar smooth muscle to cause relaxation and reduce peripheral vascular resistance
Calcium channel blockers	Diltiazem, verapamil hydrochloride, nifedipine, nicardipine	Reduces peripheral vascular resistance by systemic vasodilation
Angiotensin-converting enzyme (ACE) inhibitors	Captopril, enalapril, lisinopril, benazepril	Lowers blood pressure by blocking the conversion of angiotensin I to angiotensin II, preventing vasoconstriction; reduces aldosterone production and fluid retention, lowering circulating fluid volume
Angiotensin-II receptor blockers (ARBs)	Losartan, olmesartan	Lowers blood pressure by blocking the binding of angiotensin II, which prevents vasoconstriction

TABLE 29.10   Categories of BP in Adults[a]

BP Category	SBP		DBP
Normal	<120 mm Hg	and	<80 mm Hg
Elevated	120-129 mm Hg	and	<80 mm Hg
Hypertension			
Stage 1	130-139 mm Hg	or	80-89 mm Hg
Stage 2	≥140 mm Hg	or	≥90 mm Hg

[a]Individuals with SBP and DBP in two categories should be designated to the higher BP category.
BP indicates blood pressure (based on an average of ≥ careful readings obtained on ≥2 occasions, as detailed in diastolic blood pressure (DBP) and systolic blood pressure (SBP).
Data from Whelton et al: Guideline for the prevention, detection, evaluation, and management of high blood pressure in adults, *J Am Coll Cardiol* 71(19):2199-2269, 2018.

TABLE 29.11   Recommendations for Blood Pressure Follow-Up

Initial Blood Pressure	Follow-Up Recommended[a]
Normal	Recheck in 1 year.
Elevated	Recheck in 3-6 months.[b]
Stage 1 hypertension	Evaluate therapy within 3-6 months.[b]
Stage 2 hypertension	Evaluate therapy within 1 month.[b] For those with higher pressure (e.g., >180/110 mm Hg), evaluate and treat immediately or within 1 week, depending on clinical situation and complications.

[a]Modify the scheduling of follow-up according to reliable information about past blood pressure measurements, other cardiovascular risk factors, or target organ damage.
[b]Provide advice about lifestyle modifications.
Data from Whelton PK et al: Guideline for the prevention, detection, evaluation, and management of high blood pressure in adults—executive summary, *J Am Coll Cardiol* 71:(19): 2199, 2018.

Activity and Weight. A period of moderate exercise can reduce BP for several hours afterward. An increase in oxygen demand by the body during activity increases BP. Inadequate exercise frequently contributes to weight gain, and obesity is a factor in the development of hypertension.

Smoking. Smoking results in vasoconstriction, a narrowing of blood vessels. BP rises when a person smokes and returns to baseline about 15 minutes after stopping smoking.

Hypertension

The most common alteration in BP is hypertension. Hypertension is often asymptomatic. Hypertension is a major factor underlying death from heart attack and stroke. Experts have determined criteria for the categories of hypertension (Whelton et al., 2018). Elevated blood pressure, a designation for patients at high risk for developing hypertension, is between 120 and 129 mm Hg systolic BP (SBP) and less than 80 mm Hg diastolic BP (DBP). In these patients early intervention by adoption of healthy lifestyles reduces the risk of or prevents hypertension. Stage 1 hypertension is defined as an SBP from 130 mm Hg to 139 mm Hg or a DBP from 80 to 89 mm Hg. Stage 2 hypertension is defined as an SBP of 140 or greater or a DBP of 90 or greater. The diagnosis of hypertension in adults requires the average of two or more readings taken at each of two or more visits after an initial screening (Table 29.10).

One BP measurement revealing a high systolic or diastolic BP does not qualify as a diagnosis of hypertension. However, if you assess a high reading (e.g., 150/90 mm Hg), encourage the patient to practice a healthy lifestyle, such as exercise and a low-fat, low-sodium diet, with plenty of fresh fruits and vegetables, and to return for another checkup within 3 to 6 months (Table 29.11). Hypertension increases the risk of hypertension-related illness, including stroke, heart attack, and damage to kidneys, retinas, and the peripheral nervous system. The categories of hypertension determine nonpharmacological and pharmacological intervention.

Hypertension is associated with thickening and loss of elasticity in the arterial walls. Peripheral vascular resistance increases within thick and inelastic vessels. The heart continually pumps against greater resistance. As a result, blood flow to vital organs such as the heart, brain, and kidney decreases with untreated or chronic hypertension.

Multiple risk factors are associated with hypertension. Modifiable risk factors include obesity, cigarette smoking, heavy alcohol consumption, and high sodium (salt) intake. A sedentary lifestyle and continued exposure to stress are also linked to hypertension. The incidence of hypertension is greater in patients with diabetes and in older adults. Hypertension contributes to deaths from strokes and myocardial infarctions (heart attacks).

Hypotension

Hypotension is present when the systolic BP falls to 90 mm Hg or below. Although some adults have a low BP normally, for most individuals low BP is an abnormal finding associated with illness.

Hypotension occurs because of the dilation of the arteries in the vascular bed, the loss of a substantial amount of blood volume (e.g., hemorrhage), or the failure of the heart muscle to pump adequately (e.g., myocardial infarction). Hypotension associated with pallor, skin mottling, clamminess, confusion, increased HR, or decreased urine output is life threatening and is reported to a health care provider immediately.

When a healthy individual changes from a lying–to sitting–to standing position, the peripheral blood vessels in the legs constrict. When standing, the lower extremity vessels constrict, preventing the pooling of blood in the legs caused by gravity. Thus an individual normally does not feel any symptoms when standing. Orthostatic hypotension, also referred to as postural hypotension, occurs when a normotensive person develops symptoms (e.g., light-headedness or dizziness) and a drop in systolic pressure by at least 20 mm Hg or a drop in diastolic pressure by at least 10 mm Hg within 2 to 5 minutes of quiet standing or 5 minutes of supine rest (Palma and Kaufmann, 2020). Orthostatic hypotension occurs when patients are unable to constrict their lower extremity blood vessels to maintain their BP. Patients who are dehydrated, anemic, or have recent blood loss are at risk for orthostatic hypotension, particularly in the morning (Palma and Kaufmann, 2020). Orthostatic changes in vital signs are effective indicators of blood volume depletion. Some medications cause orthostatic hypotension, especially in young patients and older adults. Orthostatic hypotension is a risk factor for falls, especially among older adults with hypertension.

❖ NURSING PROCESS

◆ Assessment of Blood Pressure

Arterial BP measurements are obtained either directly (invasively) or indirectly (noninvasively). The direct method requires the insertion of a thin catheter into an artery. Tubing connects the catheter with electronic hemodynamic monitoring equipment. The monitor displays a constant arterial pressure waveform and reading. Because of the risk of

FIG. 29.9 Guidelines for proper blood pressure cuff size. Cuff width 20% more than upper-arm diameter or 40% of circumference and two-thirds of arm length.

TABLE 29.12 Common Errors in Blood Pressure Assessment

Error	Effect
Bladder or cuff too wide	False-low reading
Bladder or cuff too narrow or too short	False-high reading
Cuff wrapped too loosely or unevenly	False-high reading
Deflating cuff too slowly	False-high diastolic reading
Deflating cuff too quickly	False-low systolic and false-high diastolic reading
Arm below heart level	False-high reading
Arm above heart level	False-low reading
Arm not supported	False-high reading
Stethoscope that fits poorly or impairment of examiner's hearing, causing sounds to be muffled	False-low systolic and false-high diastolic reading
Stethoscope applied too firmly against antecubital fossa	False-low diastolic reading
Inflating too slowly	False-high diastolic reading
Repeating assessments too quickly	False-high systolic reading
Inadequate inflation level	False-low systolic reading
Multiple examiners using different sounds for diastolic readings	False-high systolic and false-low diastolic reading

sudden blood loss from an artery, invasive BP monitoring is used only in intensive care settings. The common indirect methods require either a sphygmomanometer and stethoscope with auscultation or an automated oscillometric device without auscultation. The technique for measuring BP by auscultation is described in Skill 29.5.

Blood Pressure Equipment for Auscultation. Before assessing BP, make sure that you are comfortable using the equipment. For more than half a century health care settings relied on a sphygmomanometer and stethoscope to measure BP by auscultation. A **sphygmomanometer** includes a pressure manometer, an occlusive cuff that encloses an inflatable rubber bladder, and a pressure bulb with a release valve that inflates the bladder manually. The aneroid manometer has a glass-enclosed circular gauge containing a needle that registers millimeter calibrations. Before using the aneroid model, make sure that the needle points to zero and that the manometer is correctly calibrated. Aneroid sphygmomanometers require biomedical calibration every 6 months to verify their accuracy.

An occlusive cuff comes in different sizes. The size selected is proportional to the circumference of the limb being assessed (Fig. 29.9). Ideally the width of the cuff is 40% of the circumference (or 20% wider than the diameter) of the midpoint of the limb on which the cuff is used to measure BP. The bladder enclosed within the cuff should encircle at least 80% of the upper arm. Many adults require a large adult cuff. A regular-size cuff holds a bladder in the width of 12 to 13 cm (4.8 to 5.2 inches) and the length of 22 to 23 cm (8.5 to 9 inches). An improperly fitting cuff produces inaccurate BP measurements (Table 29.12). It is important that there is no clothing under the blood pressure cuff, as clothing can impede blood pressure cuff fit and distort auscultatory sounds.

Measure a blood pressure in the arm by placing the lower edge of the cuff above the antecubital fossa, allowing room for positioning the stethoscope bell or diaphragm over the brachial artery. Using the forearm when a larger cuff is not readily available is not recommended and can result in an overestimate of systolic blood pressure up to 20 mm Hg (Brown et al., 2019; Schimanski et al., 2014). The release valve of the sphygmomanometer needs to be clean and freely movable in either direction. A closed valve holds the pressure constant. A sticky valve makes pressure cuff deflation hard to regulate.

Auscultation. The best environment for BP measurement by auscultation is a quiet room at a comfortable temperature. Although the patient may lie or stand, sitting is the preferred position. In most cases BP readings obtained with the patient in the supine, sitting, and standing positions are similar.

The patient's position during routine BP determination needs to be the same during each measurement to permit a meaningful comparison of values. Before obtaining the patient's BP, attempt to control factors responsible for artificially high readings such as pain, anxiety, or exertion. The patient's perception that the physical or interpersonal environment is stressful affects the BP measurement. BP measurements taken at the patient's place of employment or in a health care provider's office are often higher than those taken at the patient's home.

During the initial assessment obtain and record the BP in both arms. Normally there is a difference of 5 to 10 mm Hg between the arms. In subsequent assessments, measure the BP in the arm with the higher pressure. Pressure differences greater than 10 mm Hg indicate vascular problems and are reported to the health care provider or nurse in charge.

Ask the patient to state their usual BP. If the patient does not know, inform them after measuring and recording it. This is a good opportunity to educate a patient about optimal values of BP, risk factors for developing hypertension, and dangers of hypertension.

Indirect measurement of arterial BP works on a basic principle of pressure. Blood flows freely through an artery until an inflated cuff applies pressure to tissues and causes the artery to collapse. After release of the cuff pressure, the point at which blood flow returns and sound appears through auscultation is the systolic pressure.

In 1905 Korotkoff, a Russian surgeon, first described the sounds heard over an artery distal to the BP cuff when the cuff was deflated. The first sound is a clear rhythmic tapping corresponding to the pulse rate that gradually increases in intensity. *Onset of the sound corresponds to the systolic pressure.* A blowing or swishing sound occurs as the cuff continues to deflate, resulting in the second sound. As the artery distends there is turbulence in blood flow. The third sound is a crisper and more intense tapping. The fourth sound becomes muffled and low pitched as the cuff is further deflated. At this point the cuff pressure has fallen below the pressure within the vessel walls; *this sound is the diastolic pressure in infants and children.* The fifth sound marks the disappearance of sound. *In adolescents and adults the fifth sound corresponds with the diastolic pressure* (Fig. 29.10). In some patients the sounds are clear and distinct. In others only the beginning and ending sounds are clear.

The manual auscultatory method for BP measurement requires clinical judgment and clinical skill when selecting and applying the blood pressure cuff and reading the systolic and diastolic values and is prone to observer bias (Brown et al., 2019). Obtaining an accurate measurement is essential because BP assessment results in many medical decisions and nursing interventions. There are several sources for error (see Table 29.12). When you are unsure of a reading, have a colleague reassess the BP.

The American Heart Association recommends recording two numbers for a BP measurement: the point on the manometer when you hear the first sound for systolic and the point on the manometer when you hear the fifth sound for diastolic. Some health care agencies recommend recording the point when you hear the fourth sound as well, especially for patients with hypertension. Divide the numbers by slashed lines (e.g., 120/70 or 120/100/70). Note the arm used to measure the BP (e.g., right arm [RA] 130/70) and the patient's position (e.g., sitting).

Orthostatic Hypotension. Assess for orthostatic hypotension during measurements of vital signs by obtaining BP and pulse in sequence with the patient supine, sitting, and standing. Obtain BP readings

within 3 minutes after the patient changes position. In most cases orthostatic hypotension is detected within a minute of standing. If it occurs, help the patient to a lying position and notify the health care provider or nurse in charge. While obtaining orthostatic measurements, continually monitor for changes in pulse rate and observe for other symptoms of hypotension such as fainting, weakness, blurred vision, or light-headedness. Orthostatic hypotension is a risk factor for falls, especially among elderly patients who take antihypertensive medications (Shields et al., 2020; Shaw et al., 2019). When recording orthostatic BP measurements, record the patient's position in addition to the BP measurement (e.g., 140/80 mm Hg supine, 132/72 mm Hg sitting, 108/60 mm Hg standing). The skill of orthostatic blood pressure measurements cannot be delegated; this skill requires ongoing assessment and clinical judgment when anticipating the patient's physiologic response to changing positions from lying to sitting or sitting to standing when patients are at risk for orthostatic hypotension.

Ultrasonic Stethoscope. When you are unable to auscultate sounds because of a weakened arterial pulse, you can use an ultrasonic stethoscope (see Chapter 30). This stethoscope allows you to hear low-frequency systolic sounds. You frequently use this device when measuring the BP of infants and children or low BP in adults.

Palpation. Indirect measurement of BP by palpation is useful for patients whose arterial pulsations are too weak to create sounds that are audible by auscultation. Severe blood loss and decreased heart contractility are examples of conditions that result in BPs too low to auscultate accurately. In these cases you can assess the systolic BP by palpation (see Skill 29.5, Step 10). The diastolic BP is difficult to determine by palpation. When using the palpation technique, record the systolic value and how you measured it (e.g., RA 90/-, palpated, supine).

In some patients with hypertension the sounds are usually heard over the brachial artery when the cuff pressure is high and disappear as pressure is reduced and then reappear at a lower level. This temporary disappearance of sound is the auscultatory gap. It typically occurs between the first and second sounds. The gap in sound covers a range of 40 mm Hg and thus causes an underestimation of systolic pressure or overestimation of diastolic pressure. The examiner needs to be certain to inflate the cuff high enough to hear the true systolic pressure before the auscultatory gap. Palpation of the radial artery helps to determine how high to inflate the cuff. The examiner inflates the cuff 30 mm Hg above the pressure at which the radial pulse was palpated. Record the range of pressures in which the auscultatory gap occurs (e.g., BP RA 180/94 mm Hg with an auscultatory gap from 180 to 160 mm Hg, sitting).

Equipment for Oscillometric Measurement. More common today is the use of automated electronic oscillometric devices that do not require use of a stethoscope for auscultation. The devices include an electronic monitor with a pressure sensor, a digital display, and an upper arm cuff (Fig. 29.11). An electrically driven pump raises the pressure in the cuff (MHRA, 2019). There are also devices that fit around a patient's wrist. Devices usually have an adjustable set inflation pressure, or they will automatically inflate to the appropriate level, usually about 30 mm Hg above an estimated systolic reading (MHRA, 2019). When started, the device automatically inflates, then deflates the cuff and displays the systolic and diastolic values. These devices rely on oscillometric principle to measure mean blood pressure and apply a manufacturer- and device-specific algorithm to estimate systolic and diastolic blood pressure.

Blood Pressure Measurement Using Oscillometric Device. Many different styles of electronic oscillometric devices are available to determine BP automatically. Place the arm cuff around the upper arm,

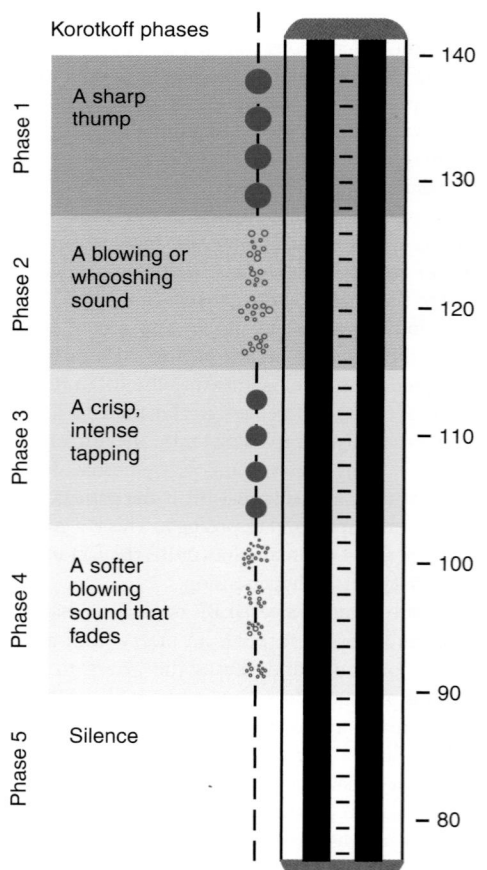

FIG. 29.10 The sounds auscultated during blood pressure measurement can be differentiated into five phases. In this example blood pressure is 140/90 mm Hg.

Korotkoff phases

Phase 1	A sharp thump
Phase 2	A blowing or whooshing sound
Phase 3	A crisp, intense tapping
Phase 4	A softer blowing sound that fades
Phase 5	Silence

FIG. 29.11 Automatic blood pressure monitor.

just above the brachial artery. A push of a button activates the inflation of the cuff. The electronic pressure sensor detects the vibrations caused by the rush of blood through an artery (Box 29.8). Once a BP is sensed, a reading appears on the electronic display. Oscillometric devices are mercury-free, lightweight, compact, portable, easy to use, and offer no observer bias (MHRA, 2019). More of these devices can be found in physician offices and clinics and even on hospital inpatient units. The devices are particularly useful when frequent BP assessment is necessary, such as in patients who are critically ill or unstable, during or after invasive procedures, or when therapies require frequent monitoring (e.g., IV heart and BP medications). Box 29.9 lists conditions that are not appropriate for automatic BP devices. If a BP result is questionable based on a patient's condition, ensure accurate BP measurement by obtaining manual measurements using auscultation with a sphygmomanometer

Blood Pressure Assessment in Children.

Blood pressure measurement in the ambulatory setting begins at 3 years of age during every wellness visit. For otherwise healthy children, BP need only be measured annually rather than during every health care encounter (Hockenberry et al., 2019; Flynn et al., 2017). If a child has obesity, diabetes mellitus, renal disease, or vascular problems, obtain readings during every health encounter (Flynn et al., 2017). BP in children changes with growth and development. The prevalence of BP elevations and hypertension in children, especially among children who are overweight, has increased (Flynn et al., 2017). Help parents understand the importance of routine BP screening to detect children who are at risk for hypertension. The measurement of BP in infants and children is difficult for several reasons:

- Different arm size requires careful and appropriate cuff size selection. Do not choose a cuff on the basis of the name of the cuff. An "infant" cuff can be too small for some infants.
- Readings are difficult to obtain in restless or anxious infants and children. Allow at least 15 minutes for children to recover from recent activities and become less apprehensive. The child's cooperation is

increased when you or the parent have prepared them for the unusual sensation of the BP cuff. Most children understand the analogy of a "tight hug on your arm."
- Placing the stethoscope too firmly on the antecubital fossa causes errors in auscultation. Sounds are difficult to hear in children because of low frequency and amplitude. A pediatric stethoscope bell is often helpful.

Lower Extremity Blood Pressure.

Dressings, casts, IV catheters, or arteriovenous fistulas or shunts can make the upper extremities inaccessible for BP measurement. If this is the case, then you need to obtain the BP in a lower extremity. Comparing upper-extremity BP with that in the legs is also necessary for patients with certain cardiac and BP abnormalities. The popliteal artery, palpable behind the knee in the popliteal space, is the site for auscultation or oscillometric measurement. The cuff needs to be wide and long enough to allow for the larger girth of the thigh. Placing the patient in a prone position is best. If such a position is impossible, ask the patient to lie supine and flex the knee slightly for easier access to the artery (AACN, 2016). Position the cuff 2.5 cm (1 inch) above the popliteal artery, with the bladder over the posterior aspect of the midthigh (Fig. 29.12). The procedure is identical to brachial artery measurement. Systolic pressure in the legs is usually higher by 10 to 40 mm Hg than in the brachial artery, but the diastolic pressure is the same.

Self-Measurement of Blood Pressure.

Electronic monitoring devices allow individuals to measure their own BPs in their home with the push of a button. The devices are mercury-free, lightweight, compact, portable, easy to use, and have no observer bias (MHRA, 2019). The most common portable home devices are electronic digital readout devices that do not require use of a stethoscope. The electronic devices are easy to manipulate but require frequent recalibration, more than once a year.

Stationary automatic BP devices are often found in public places such as grocery stores, fitness clubs, airports, or work sites. Users simply rest their arms within the inflatable cuff of the machine, which contains a pressure sensor. A visual display tells users their BP within 60 to 90 seconds. The reliability of the stationary machines is limited. BP values can vary by 5 to 10 mm Hg or more (for both systolic and diastolic values) compared with pressures taken with a manual sphygmomanometer.

Self-measurement of BP has several benefits. Sometimes elevated BP is detected in individuals previously unaware of a problem. Individuals with prehypertension provide information about the pattern of BP values to their health care provider. Patients with hypertension benefit from participating actively in their treatment through self-monitoring, which helps adherence with treatment (Ringrose et al., 2019). The disadvantages of self-measurement include improper use of the device and risk of inaccurate readings. Some patients are needlessly alarmed with one elevated reading. Some patients with hypertension become overly conscious of their BP and inappropriately self-adjust medications.

◆ Analysis and Nursing Diagnosis

The assessment of BP along with pulse assessment determines the general state of cardiovascular health and responses to other system imbalances. For example, the assessment findings of hypotension, bradycardia or tachycardia, edema, fatigue, or weight gain lead to a diagnosis of *Impaired Cardiac Output*. Related factors might include deconditioning or altered fluid intake. Hypotension, hypertension, orthostatic hypotension, and narrow or wide pulse pressures are assessment findings of certain nursing diagnoses, including the following:

- Activity Intolerance
- Anxiety
- Impaired Cardiac Output
- Fluid Imbalance
- Acute Pain

BOX 29.8 PROCEDURAL GUIDELINES

Noninvasive Electronic Blood Pressure Measurement

Delegation and Collaboration

The skill of blood pressure measurement using an electronic blood pressure machine can be delegated to assistive personnel (AP) unless the patient is considered unstable (i.e., hypotensive). The nurse instructs the AP by:

- Explaining the frequency of measurement and which extremity to use.
- Reviewing how to select appropriate-size blood pressure cuff for designated extremity and appropriate cuff for the machine.
- Reviewing patient's usual blood pressure and directing AP to report significant changes or abnormalities to the nurse.

Equipment

Electronic oscillometric blood pressure machine, blood pressure cuff of appropriate size as recommended by manufacturer, pen and vital sign flow sheet or electronic health record (EHR) per agency policy.

Procedural Steps

1. Identify patient using at least two identifiers (e.g., name and birthday or name and medical record number), according to agency policy (TJC, 2021).
2. Assess need to measure blood pressure (see Skill 29.5 Assessment Steps 2 through 5), and determine patient's baseline blood pressure.
3. Determine appropriateness of using electronic blood pressure measurement. Patients with irregular heart rate, known hypertension, peripheral vascular disease, seizures, tremors, and shivering are not candidates for the device (Wang et al., 2016).
4. Perform hand hygiene. Determine best site for cuff placement; inspect the condition of the extremities.
5. Collect and bring appropriate equipment to patient's bedside. Select appropriate cuff size for patient extremity. Electronic blood pressure cuff and device must be matched by manufacturer and are not interchangeable.
6. Assist patient to comfortable position, either lying or sitting. Plug device into electrical outlet and place it near patient, ensuring that connector hose between cuff and machine reaches.
7. Locate on/off switch and turn on machine to enable device to self-test computer systems.
8. Remove constricting clothing to ensure proper cuff application.
9. Prepare blood pressure cuff by manually squeezing all the air out of the cuff and connecting it to connector hose.
10. Perform hand hygiene. Wrap flattened cuff snugly around extremity, verifying that only one finger can fit between cuff and patient's skin. Make sure that "artery" arrow marked on outside of cuff is placed correctly (see illustration).

STEP 10 Aligning blood pressure cuff arrow with brachial artery.

11. Verify that connector hose between cuff and machine is not kinked. Kinking prevents proper inflation and deflation of cuff.

12. Following manufacturer directions, set frequency control for automatic or manual and press the start button. The first blood pressure measurement pumps cuff to a peak pressure of approximately 180 mm Hg. After this pressure is reached, the machine begins a deflation sequence that determines the blood pressure. The first reading determines peak pressure inflation for additional measurements.
13. When deflation is complete, digital display provides most recent values and flashes time in minutes that have elapsed since the measurement occurred (see illustration).

STEP 13 Digital electronic blood pressure display. (Image courtesy of Hillrom.)

> **CLINICAL JUDGMENT:** If unable to obtain blood pressure with electronic device, verify machine connections (e.g., plugged into working electrical outlet, hose-cuff connections tight, machine on, correct cuff). Repeat electronic blood pressure; if unable to obtain, use auscultatory technique (see Skill 29.5).

14. Set frequency of measurements and upper and lower alarm limits for systolic, diastolic, and mean blood pressure readings. Intervals between measurements can be set from 1 to 90 minutes. A nurse determines frequency and alarm limits on the basis of patient's acceptable range of blood pressure, nursing judgment, and health care provider order.
15. Obtain additional readings at any time by pressing the start button. Pressing the cancel button immediately deflates the cuff.
16. If frequent measurements are required, the cuff may be left in place. Remove it at least every 2 hours to assess the integrity of the underlying skin and, if possible, alternate measurement sites.

> **CLINICAL JUDGMENT:** Frequent measurement by electronic blood pressure machines increases the risk of extremity pressure injuries, especially in vulnerable elders, patients with paralysis, and patients with peripheral vascular diseases. Patients with abnormal bleeding tendencies are at risk for microvascular rupture from repeated inflations. Inspect the skin under the blood pressure cuff at regular intervals, depending on the frequency of use.

17. When patient no longer requires frequent blood pressure monitoring:
    a. Assist patient in return to comfortable position and cover upper arm or leg if previously clothed to restore comfort and provide sense of well-being.
    b. Place nurse call system within reach, and instruct patient in its use to promote safety and prevent falls.
    c. Raise side rails (as appropriate) and lower bed to lowest position to promote safety and prevent falls.
    d. Wipe cuff with agency-approved disinfectant to reduce transmission of infection. Clean and store electronic blood pressure machine.

BOX 29.8 PROCEDURAL GUIDELINES—cont'd
Noninvasive Electronic Blood Pressure Measurement

18. Perform hand hygiene.
19. Compare electronic blood pressure readings with auscultatory measurements to verify accuracy of electronic device. Electronic measurements can underestimate measurements (Drawz, 2017).
20. Inform patient of blood pressure reading.
21. **Use Teach-Back:** "I want to be sure I explained why you need to keep your arm straight while the machine is taking your blood pressure. Tell me

why it is important to remain still." Revise your instruction now or develop a plan for revised patient/family caregiver teaching if patient/family caregiver is not able to teach back correctly.
22. Record blood pressure, site assessed, and use of electronic device; record any signs or symptoms of blood pressure alterations.
23. Notify nurse in charge or health care provider of abnormal findings.

BOX 29.9 Patient Conditions Not Appropriate for Electronic Blood Pressure Measurement

- Irregular heart rate
- Known hypertension
- Peripheral vascular obstruction (e.g., clots, narrowed vessels)
- Shivering
- Seizures
- Excessive tremors
- Inability to cooperate
- Blood pressure less than 90 mm Hg systolic

FIG. 29.12 Lower extremity blood pressure cuff positioned above popliteal artery at midthigh with knee flexed.

BOX 29.10 PATIENT TEACHING
Health Promotion

Objective
- Patient identifies measures to promote cardiovascular health.

Teaching Strategies
- Instruct patient about the importance of diet, exercise, and remaining tobacco free.
- Demonstrate self-assessment of heart rate using the carotid pulse. Patients taking certain prescribed cardiac medications need to learn to assess their own pulse rate to detect side effects of medications. Patients undergoing cardiac rehabilitation need to learn to assess their own pulse rate to determine their response to exercise.
- Instruct patient about normal blood pressure values, risk factors for hypertension, and usual lack of hypertension symptoms.
- Demonstrate how to obtain blood pressure to the patient/patient's family caregiver using an appropriate-size blood pressure cuff for home use:
  - Do not take a measurement over clothing (AHA, 2017b).
  - Sit correctly with your back straight and supported (on a dining chair, rather than a sofa). The feet should be flat on the floor and the legs should not be crossed (AHA, 2017b).
  - Measure at the same time each day, after patient has had a brief rest, and in the same position and arm each time pressure is taken.
  - Take two or three readings 1 minute apart, and record the results at each measurement (AHA, 2017a; AHA, 2017b).

Evaluation
Use the principles of teach-back to evaluate patient/family caregiver learning:
- Tell me three activities you will do to promote cardiovascular health.
- Observe patient obtaining carotid pulse rate.
- Observe patient or family caregiver's measurement of blood pressure.

◆ Planning, Outcomes Identification, and Implementation

The nursing care plan includes individualized patient-centered interventions based on the nursing diagnosis identified and the related factors. The related factor guides the choice of nursing interventions.

Health Promotion. The emphasis on health promotion and maintenance and early discharge from hospital settings has resulted in an increase in the need for patients and their families to monitor vital signs in the home and to know how to take medications correctly for management of cardiovascular problems. Teaching considerations affect all vital sign measurements. Incorporate them within the patient's plan of care (Box 29.10).

When patients are diagnosed with an elevated blood pressure or hypertension, educate them about BP values, long-term follow-up care and therapy, the usual lack of symptoms (the fact that it may not be "felt"), the ability of therapy to control but not cure high BP, and a

consistently followed treatment plan that ensures a relatively normal lifestyle (Whelton et al., 2018; AHA, 2017a).

Consumers can learn to use self-measurement devices if they have the information needed to perform the procedure correctly and if they know when to seek a health care provider (Ringrose et al., 2019). Advise patients of possible inaccuracies in the BP devices, help them understand the meaning and implications of readings, and teach them proper measurement techniques. Encourage them to record the date of their BP readings to assess BP over time and to share findings with their health care provider.

When considering how to teach patients and their families about vital sign measurements and their importance and significance, a patient's age is an important factor. With an increase in the older-adult population there is a greater need for family caregivers to be aware of changes that are unique to older adults. Box 29.11 identifies some of these variations.

BOX 29.11   FOCUS ON OLDER ADULTS

Factors Affecting Vital Signs of Older Adults

Temperature

- The temperature of older adults is at the lower end of the normal temperature range, 36° to 36.8°C (96.8° to 98.3°F) orally and 36.6° to 37.2°C (98° to 99°F) rectally. Therefore temperatures considered within normal range sometimes reflect a fever in an older adult. In an older adult fever is present when a single oral temperature is over 37.8°C (100°F); repeated oral temperatures are over 37.2°C (99°F); rectal temperatures are over 37.5°C (99.5°F); or temperature has increased more than 1°C (2°F) over baseline.
- Older adults are very sensitive to slight changes in environmental temperature because their thermoregulatory systems are not as efficient.
- A decrease in sweat gland reactivity in the older adult results in a higher threshold for sweating at high temperatures, which leads to hyperthermia and heatstroke.
- Be especially attentive to subtle temperature changes and other manifestations of fever in this population such as tachypnea, anorexia, falls, delirium, and overall functional decline.
- Older adults without teeth or with poor muscle control may be unable to close their mouths tightly to obtain accurate oral temperature readings.

Pulse Rate

- If it is difficult to palpate the pulse of an obese older adult, a Doppler device provides a more accurate reading.
- Pedal pulses are often difficult to palpate in older adults.
- The older adult has a decreased heart rate at rest.
- It takes longer for the heart rate to rise in the older adult to meet sudden increased demands that result from stress, illness, or excitement. Once elevated, the pulse rate takes longer to return to normal resting rate.
- Heart sounds are sometimes muffled or difficult to hear in older adults because of an increase in air space in the lungs.

Blood Pressure

- Older adults who have lost upper arm mass, especially the frail elderly, require special attention to selection of a smaller-size blood pressure cuff.
- Older adults sometimes have an increase in systolic pressure related to a decrease in vessel elasticity, whereas the diastolic pressure remains the same, resulting in a wider pulse pressure.
- Instruct older adults to change position slowly and wait after each change to avoid postural hypotension and prevent injuries.
- The skin of older adults is more fragile and susceptible to cuff pressure during frequent measurements. More frequent assessment of skin under the cuff or rotating blood pressure sites is recommended.

Respirations

- Aging causes ossification of costal cartilage and downward slant of ribs, resulting in a more rigid rib cage, which reduces chest wall expansion. Kyphosis and scoliosis that occur in older adults also restrict chest expansion and decrease tidal volume.
- Older adults depend more on accessory abdominal muscles during respiration than on weaker thoracic muscles.
- The respiratory system matures by the time a person reaches 20 years of age and begins to decline in healthy individuals after the age of 25. Despite this decline older adults are able to breathe effortlessly as long as they are healthy. However, sudden events that require an increased demand for oxygen (e.g., exercise, stress, illness) create shortness of breath in the older adult.
- Identifying an acceptable pulse oximeter probe site is difficult with older adults because of the likelihood of peripheral vascular disease, decreased cardiac output, cold-induced vasoconstriction, and anemia.

◆ Evaluation

Patient Outcomes. Know a patient's baseline trend when evaluating blood pressure values in response to therapies. Know the expected effects of an intervention for blood pressure alterations. For example, if a patient is receiving an antihypertensive medication or an increased infusion of IV fluids, has the BP responded appropriately? The antihypertensive medication should lower BP while an increase in fluids can raise the BP. Evaluate outcomes of teaching interventions by having patients or family caregivers explain the importance of BP measurement and BP medications. Request a demonstration of the blood pressure measurement device.

Recording Vital Signs. Special electronic and paper graphic flow sheets exist for recording vital signs (see Chapter 26). Identify institution procedure for documenting on a graphic. In addition to the actual vital sign values, record in the nurses' notes any accompanying or precipitating symptoms, such as chest pain and dizziness with changes in pulse rate, abnormal BP, shortness of breath with abnormal respirations, or flushing and diaphoresis with elevated temperature. Document any interventions initiated as a result of vital sign measurement such as administration of oxygen therapy, cooling blankets, or an antihypertensive medication.

Patients being managed on clinical pathway often have vital sign values listed as outcomes. If a vital sign value is above or below the anticipated outcome, write a variance note to explain the nature of the variance and the nursing course of action. For example, a path for a patient who has undergone lung surgery often has an outcome during the postoperative period of "afebrile." If the patient has a fever, the

nurse's variance note addresses possible sources of fever (e.g., retained pulmonary secretions) and nursing interventions (e.g., increased suctioning, postural drainage, or hydration).

QSEN Building Competency in Informatics The team leader notifies you that your patient has achieved a critical Early Warning Score (EWS), a computer-generated value that reflects a patient's condition on the basis of the vital signs entered by the assistive personnel (AP) within the past 15 minutes. After completing a focused assessment of the patient, you review the vital signs and compare the most recent with baseline readings. Which vital signs that are included in the EWS indicate a potential change in the patient's condition? Which actions should you take next?

Baseline Vital Signs	Vital Signs During the Past 15 Minutes
Heart rate 86 beats/min and regular	Heart rate 92 beats/min and regular
Blood pressure 120/84 mm Hg in right arm via electronic blood pressure machine	Blood pressure 92/76 mm/Hg in right arm via electronic blood pressure machine
Oxygen saturation 95% on 2 L nasal cannula	Oxygen saturation 89% on 2 L nasal cannula
Respiratory rate 16 breaths/min, regular and deep	Respiratory rate 22 breaths/min, regular and deep
Temperature 37.2°C (98.9°F) via temporal artery	Temperature 37.6°C (99.6°F) via temporal artery

Answers to QSEN Activities can be found on the Evolve website.

SAFETY GUIDELINES FOR NURSING SKILLS

Ensuring patient safety is an essential role of the professional nurse. Use sound clinical judgment by communicating clearly with members of the health care team, assessing and analyzing the patient's clinical findings, and incorporating the patient's priorities of care and preferences. Use the best evidence, applying professional standards, when selecting interventions to use in patient care delivery. When performing the skills in this chapter, remember the following points to ensure safe, patient-centered care.

- If a device for measuring vital signs is shared among patients, clean each device carefully between patients to decrease risk of infection.

- Blood pressure cuffs and pulse oximetry sensors can apply excessive pressure on fragile skin. Rotating sites during repeated measurements decreases risk for skin breakdown.
- Analyze trends for measuring vital signs, and report abnormal findings to the health care provider.
- Determine the frequency for measuring vital signs on the basis of the patient's condition.
- Determine a patient's status before delegating a vital sign skill.

SKILL 29.1   MEASURING BODY TEMPERATURE

Delegation and Collaboration

The skill of temperature measurement can be delegated to assistive personnel (AP). The nurse instructs the AP by:

- Communicating the appropriate route, device, and frequency of temperature measurement.
- Explaining any precautions needed in positioning the patient (e.g., for rectal temperature measurement).
- Reviewing the patient's usual temperature values and significant changes to report to the nurse.

Equipment

- Thermometer (selected on the basis of site used, see Table 29.2)
- Soft tissue or wipe
- Alcohol swab
- Water-soluble lubricant (for rectal measurements only)
- Pen and vital sign flow sheet, record form, or electronic health record (EHR)
- Clean gloves *(optional)*, plastic thermometer sleeve, disposable probe or sensor cover
- Towel

STEP	RATIONALE
ASSESSMENT	
1. Identify patient using at least two identifiers (e.g., name and birthday or name and medical record number) according to agency policy.	Ensures correct patient. Complies with The Joint Commission standards and improves patient safety (TJC, 2021).
2. Review patient's electronic health record (EHR) to determine need to measure patient's body temperature:	
a. Note patient's risks for temperature alterations:	Certain conditions place patients at risk for temperature alterations and require more frequent temperature measurement and nursing assessment.
• Expected or diagnosed infection	
• Open wounds or burns	
• White blood cell count below 5000/mm³ or above 12,000/mm³	
• Immunosuppressive drug therapy	
• Injury to hypothalamus	
• Exposure to temperature extremes	
• Blood product infusion	
• Hypothermia or hyperthermia therapy	
b. Determine previous baseline temperature and measurement site (if available) from patient's EHR.	Allows you to assess for change in condition. Provides comparison with future temperature measurements.
3. Assess patient's or family caregiver's knowledge, experience, and health literacy.	Ensures patient has the capacity to obtain, communicate, process, and understand basic health information (CDC, 2021).
4. Perform hand hygiene.	Reduces transmission of microorganisms.
5. Assess for signs and symptoms that indicate a temperature alteration:	Physical signs and symptoms alert you to alterations in body temperature.
• *Hyperthermia:* Decreased skin turgor, dry mucous membranes; tachycardia; hypotension; decreased venous filling; concentrated urine	
• *Heatstroke:* Body temperature of 40°C (104°F) or more (Hifumi et al., 2018); hot, dry skin; tachycardia; hypotension; muscle cramps; visual disturbances; confusion or delirium	
• *Hypothermia:* Pale skin; skin cool or cold to touch; bradycardia and dysrhythmias; uncontrollable shivering; reduced level of consciousness; shallow respirations	
6. Assess for factors that normally influence temperature by reviewing EHR or questioning patient:	Allows you to accurately assess for presence and significance of temperature alteration.
• Age	Older adults have narrower range of temperature than younger adults.

CLINICAL JUDGMENT: *No single temperature is normal for all individuals. A temperature within an acceptable range in an adult may reflect a fever in an older adult. Undeveloped temperature-control mechanisms in infants and children cause temperature to rise and fall rapidly.*

• Exercise	Muscle activity increases metabolism, which increases heat production and raises temperature.

Continued

| SKILL 29.1 | MEASURING BODY TEMPERATURE—cont'd |

STEP	RATIONALE
• Hormones	Women have wider temperature fluctuations than men because of menstrual cycle hormonal changes, because body temperature varies during menopause, and because women have thicker layer of subcutaneous fat.
• Stress	Stress elevates temperature.
• Environmental temperature	Infants and older adults are more sensitive to environmental temperature changes.
• Medications	Some drugs impair or promote sweating, vasoconstriction, or vasodilation or interfere with ability of hypothalamus to regulate temperature. Oxygen administered by nasal cannula greater than 6 L can result in inaccurate temperature measurement using the oral and temporal route (Mason et al., 2017)
• Daily fluctuations	Body temperature normally changes 0.5° to 1°C (0.9° to 1.8°F) during 24-hour period. Temperature is lowest during early morning. Most patients have maximum temperature elevation around 4 p.m.; temperature falls gradually during night.
7. Determine appropriate measurement site and device for patient (see Table 29.2). Use disposable thermometer for patient on isolation precautions.	Determines whether patient's status contraindicates selection of a specific method or site.
8. Assess patient's knowledge, prior experience with temperature measurement, and feelings about procedure.	Reveals need for patient instruction and/or support.
9. Assess patient's preferences (e.g., position) for how skill is to be performed or what patient expects.	Allows care to be individualized to patient.

PLANNING

STEP	RATIONALE
1. Obtain and organize equipment for temperature measurement at bedside.	Ensures an organized approach for body temperature measurement.
2. Provide privacy: draw curtain around bed and/or close room door. Prepare bedside environment for patient safety.	Maintains patient comfort and removes barriers that may interfere with procedure.
3. If measuring oral temperature, verify that patient has not had anything to eat or drink and has not chewed gum or smoked within the past 20 minutes.	Oral food and fluids, smoking, and gum can alter oral temperature measurement (Mason et al., 2017)
4. Explain to patient the way you will measure temperature and the importance of maintaining proper position until reading is complete.	Promotes patient cooperation and increases compliance. Patients are often curious about their temperatures and should be cautioned against prematurely removing thermometer to read results.

IMPLEMENTATION

STEP	RATIONALE
1. Perform hand hygiene. Help patient to a comfortable position that provides easy access to temperature measurement site.	Reduces transmission of infection. Ensures patient's comfort and accuracy of temperature reading.
a. Sitting or lying supine (oral, tympanic, temporal, axillary)	
b. Side lying with upper leg flexed (rectal)	
2. Obtain temperature reading.	
a. Oral temperature (electronic):	
(1) *Optional:* Apply clean gloves when there is risk for exposure to respiratory secretions or facial or mouth wound drainage.	An oral probe cover is removable without physical contact; thus does not require gloves.
(2) Remove thermometer pack from charging unit. Attach oral thermometer probe stem (blue tip) to thermometer unit. Grasp top of probe stem, being careful not to apply pressure on ejection button.	Charging provides battery power. Ejection button releases plastic cover from probe stem.
(3) Slide disposable plastic probe cover over thermometer probe stem until cover locks in place (see illustrations).	Soft plastic cover will not break in patient's mouth and prevents transmission of infection between patients.
(4) Ask patient to open mouth; gently place thermometer probe under tongue in posterior sublingual pocket lateral to center of lower jaw (see illustration).	Heat from superficial blood vessels in sublingual pocket produces temperature reading. Oral inflammatory process can cause false elevations in temperature (Mason et al., 2017). With electronic thermometer, temperatures in right and left posterior sublingual pocket are significantly higher than in area under front of tongue.
(5) Ask patient to hold thermometer probe with lips closed.	Maintains proper position of thermometer during recording.
(6) Leave thermometer probe in place until audible signal indicates completion and patient's temperature appears on digital display; remove thermometer probe from under patient's tongue. Note temperature reading.	Probe must stay in place until signal occurs to ensure accurate reading.
(7) Push ejection button on thermometer probe stem to discard plastic probe cover into appropriate receptacle. Return thermometer probe stem to storage position of thermometer unit.	Reduces transmission of microorganisms. Protects probe stem from damage. Returning thermometer probe stem automatically causes digital reading to disappear.
(8) If wearing gloves, remove, dispose in appropriate receptacle, and perform hand hygiene.	Reduces transmission of infection.

STEP	RATIONALE

STEP 2a(3) Disposable plastic cover is placed over probe.

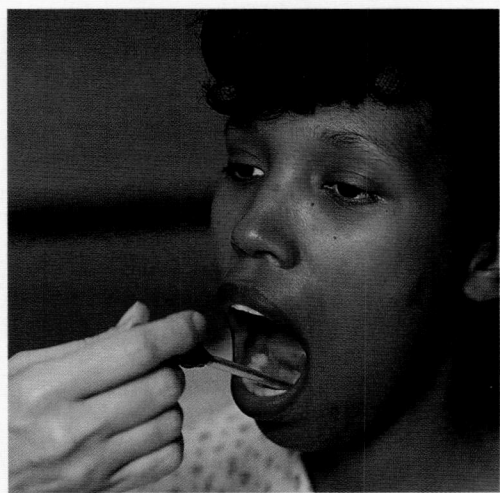

STEP 2a(4) Probe placed under tongue in posterior sublingual pocket.

b. Rectal temperature (electronic):

(1) With patient in side-lying position and upper leg flexed, move aside bed linen to expose only anal area. Keep patient's upper body and lower extremities covered with sheet or blanket.

Maintains patient's privacy, minimizes embarrassment, and promotes comfort.

(2) Apply clean gloves. Cleanse anal region when feces and/or secretions are present. Remove soiled gloves, perform hand hygiene, and reapply clean gloves.

Maintains Standard Precautions when exposed to items soiled with body fluids (e.g., feces).

(3) Remove thermometer pack from charging unit. Attach rectal thermometer probe stem (red tip) to thermometer unit. Grasp top of probe stem, being careful not to apply pressure on ejection button.

Ejection button releases plastic cover from probe stem.

(4) Slide disposable plastic probe cover over thermometer probe stem until cover locks in place.

Soft plastic probe cover prevents transmission of infection between patients.

(5) Using a single-use package, squeeze a liberal amount of lubricant on tissue. Dip probe cover of thermometer, blunt end, into lubricant, covering 2.5 to 3.5 cm (1 to 1½ inches) for adult.

Lubrication minimizes trauma to rectal mucosa during insertion. Using a tissue allows adequate lubrication of probe.

CLINICAL JUDGMENT: *Rectal temperatures are contraindicated in infants younger than 1 month old due to risk of rectal perforation (Hockenberry et al., 2019).*

Continued

SKILL 29.1   MEASURING BODY TEMPERATURE—cont'd

STEP	RATIONALE
(6) With nondominant hand separate patient's buttocks to expose anus. Ask patient to breathe slowly and relax.	Fully exposes anus for thermometer insertion. Relaxes anal sphincter for easier thermometer insertion.
(7) Gently insert thermometer into anus in direction of umbilicus 3.5 cm (1½ inches) for adult (see illustration). Do not force thermometer.	Ensures adequate exposure against blood vessels in rectal wall.

CLINICAL JUDGMENT: *If you cannot adequately insert thermometer into rectum or resistance is felt during insertion, remove thermometer, and consider alternative method for obtaining temperature. Never force a rectal thermometer.*

(8) Once positioned, hold thermometer probe in place until audible signal indicates completion and patient's temperature appears on digital display; remove thermometer probe from anus. Note temperature reading.	Probe must stay in place until signal occurs to ensure accurate reading.
(9) Push ejection button on thermometer stem to discard plastic probe cover into appropriate receptacle. Wipe probe stem with an alcohol swab, paying particular attention to ridges where probe stem connects to probe. Allow probe stem to dry (10 to 20 seconds) and return probe stem to recording unit.	Reduces transmission of microorganisms. Protects probe stem from damage. Returning thermometer probe stem automatically causes digital reading to disappear.
(10) Clean patient's anal area with soft tissue to remove lubricant or feces and discard tissue. Perform perineal hygiene as needed. Replace gown and linen.	Reduces transmission of microorganisms. Provides for comfort and hygiene. Maintains patient's privacy and minimizes embarrassment.
(11) Remove and dispose of gloves in appropriate receptacle. Perform hand hygiene.	Reduces transmission of infection.

c. Axillary temperature (electronic):

(1) With patient in supine or sitting position, move clothing or gown away from shoulder and arm.	Maintains patient's privacy, minimizes embarrassment, and promotes comfort. Exposes axilla for correct thermometer probe placement.
(2) Remove thermometer pack from charging unit. Attach oral thermometer probe stem (blue tip) to thermometer unit. Grasp top of thermometer probe stem, being careful not to apply pressure on ejection button.	Charging provides battery power. Ejection button releases plastic cover from probe stem.
(3) Slide disposable plastic probe cover over thermometer stem until cover locks in place.	Soft plastic probe cover prevents transmission of infection between patients.
(4) Raise patient's arm away from torso. Inspect for skin lesions and excessive perspiration; if needed, dry axilla or select alternative site. Insert thermometer probe into center of axilla (see illustration), lower arm over probe, and place arm across patient's chest.	Maintains proper position of thermometer against blood vessels in axilla. Thermometer probe must be completely surrounded by tissue for accurate measurement (Mason et al., 2017).

CLINICAL JUDGMENT: *Do not use axilla if skin lesions are present because local temperature is sometimes altered, and area may be painful to touch.*

STEP 2b(7) Probe inserted into anus. (Copyright © *Mosby's Clinical Skills: Essentials Collection.*)

STEP	RATIONALE

STEP 2c(4) Insert thermometer probe into center of axilla.

(5) Once thermometer probe is positioned, hold it in place until audible signal indicates completion and patient's temperature appears on digital display; remove thermometer probe from axilla. Note temperature reading.

Thermometer probe must stay in place until signal occurs to ensure accurate reading.

(6) Push ejection button on thermometer stem to discard plastic probe cover into appropriate receptacle. Return thermometer stem to storage position of recording unit and perform hand hygiene.

Returning thermometer stem to storage position automatically causes digital reading to disappear. Protects stem from damage.

(7) Replace linen or gown. Perform hand hygiene.

Restores comfort and sense of well-being. Reduces infection transmission.

d. Tympanic membrane temperature:

(1) Help patient to assume comfortable position with head turned toward side, away from you. If patient has been lying on one side, use upper ear. Note whether there is an obvious presence of cerumen (earwax) in patient's ear canal.

Ensures comfort and facilitates exposure of auditory canal for accurate temperature measurement. Heat trapped in ear facing down causes false-high temperature reading. Cerumen impedes lens cover of speculum. Switch to other ear or select alternative measurement site.

(2) Obtain temperature from patient's right ear if you are right-handed and from patient's left ear if you are left-handed.

The less acute the angle of approach, the better the probe seal.

(3) Remove thermometer handheld unit from charging base, being careful not to apply pressure to ejection button.

Charging base provides battery power. Removal of handheld unit from base prepares it to measure temperature. Ejection button releases plastic probe cover from thermometer tip.

(4) Slide disposable speculum cover over otoscope-like lens tip until it locks in place. Be careful not to touch lens cover.

Soft plastic probe cover prevents transmission of infection between patients. Lens cover should not have dust, fingerprints, or cerumen obstructing optical pathway.

(5) Insert speculum into ear canal following manufacturer instructions for tympanic probe positioning (see illustration):

Correct positioning of probe with respect to ear canal allows maximal exposure of tympanic membrane.

(a) Pull ear pinna backward, up, and out for an adult. For children less than 3 years of age, pull pinna down and back; point covered probe toward midpoint between eyebrow and sideburns. For children older than 3 years, pull pinna up and back (Hockenberry et al., 2019).

Ear tug straightens external auditory canal, allowing maximum exposure of tympanic membrane and therefore correctly positioning speculum (Hockenberry et al., 2019).

(b) Fit speculum tip snug in canal, pointing toward nose.

Gentle pressure seals ear canal from ambient air temperature, which alters readings as much as 2.8°C (5°F).

Optional: Move thermometer in figure-eight pattern.

Some manufacturers recommend movement of speculum tip in figure-eight pattern that allows sensor to detect maximum tympanic membrane heat radiation.

(6) Once positioned, press scan button on handheld unit. Leave speculum in place until audible signal indicates completion and patient's temperature appears on digital display.

Pressing scan button causes detection of infrared energy. Speculum probe tip must stay in place until device has detected infrared energy noted by audible signal.

Continued

SKILL 29.1 **MEASURING BODY TEMPERATURE—cont'd**

STEP	RATIONALE
(7) Carefully remove speculum from auditory meatus. Note temperature. Push ejection button on handheld unit to discard speculum cover into appropriate receptacle.	Reduces transmission of infection. Automatically causes digital reading to disappear.
(8) If temperature is abnormal or second reading is necessary, replace probe cover and wait 2 minutes before repeating in same ear or repeat measurement in other ear. Consider an alternative temperature site or instrument.	Lens cover must be free of cerumen to maintain optical path. Time allows ear canal to regain usual temperature.
(9) Return handheld unit to thermometer base.	Protects sensor tip from damage.
(10) Perform hand hygiene.	Reduces transmission of infection.
e. Temporal artery temperature:	
(1) Ensure that forehead is dry; dry with towel if needed.	Moisture and diaphoresis interfere with thermometer sensor (Mason et al., 2017).
(2) Place sensor firmly on patient's forehead.	Firm contact avoids measurement of ambient temperature.
(3) Press red scan button with your thumb. Slowly slide thermometer straight across forehead while keeping sensor flat and firmly on skin (see illustration). Keeping scan button depressed, lift sensor after sweeping forehead and touch sensor on neck just behind earlobe. Read temperature when clicking sound during scanning stops. Release scan button.	Thermometer continuously scans for highest temperature when scan button is depressed. Area behind earlobe is less affected by diaphoresis and verifies temperature.
(4) Gently clean sensor with alcohol swab and return to charging storage unit.	Maintains battery charge of thermometer unit.
(5) Perform hand hygiene.	Prevents transmission of infection.
3. Inform patient of temperature reading and record per agency policy.	Promotes participation in care and understanding of health status.
4. Determine that patient is in a comfortable position.	Restores comfort and sense of well-being.
5. Place nurse call system in an accessible location within patient's reach.	Ensures patient can call for assistance if needed and promotes safety and prevents falls.
6. Raise side rails (as appropriate) and place bed in lowest position.	Promotes safety and prevents falls.

EVALUATION

1. If you are assessing a patient's temperature for the first time, establish it as baseline if it is within acceptable range.	Used to compare future temperature measurements.
2. Compare temperature reading with patient's previous baseline and acceptable temperature range for patient's age-group.	Body temperature fluctuates within narrow range; comparison reveals presence of abnormality. Improper placement or movement of thermometer can cause inaccuracies. Second measurement confirms initial findings of abnormal body temperature.
3. If patient has fever, take temperature approximately 30 minutes after administering antipyretics and every 4 hours until temperature stabilizes.	Determines whether temperature begins to fall in response to therapy.
4. Use Teach-Back. "I want to be sure I explained how to check your child's temperature at home. Show me how to swipe his forehead using the temporal thermometer." Revise your instruction now or develop a plan for revised patient/family caregiver teaching if patient/family caregiver is unable to teach back correctly.	Teach-back is an evidence-based health literacy intervention that promotes patient engagement, patient safety, adherence, and quality. The goal of teach-back is to ensure that you have explained medical information clearly so that patients and their families understand what you have communicated to them (AHRQ, 2020).

STEP 2d(5) Tympanic thermometer with probe cover inserted into auditory canal.

STEP 2e(3) Scanning the forehead with a temporal artery thermometer.

UNEXPECTED OUTCOMES AND RELATED INTERVENTIONS

1. Patient has temperature 1°C (1.8°F) or more above usual range.
   Initiate measures to lower body temperature:
   - Cool room environment.
   - Reduce external covering on patient's body to promote heat loss, but do not induce shivering.
   - Keep clothing and bed linen dry.
   - Apply hypothermia blanket as ordered.
   - Limit physical activity and sources of emotional stress.
   - Administer antipyretics as ordered.
   - Prevent or control spread of infection.
   - Increase fluid intake to at least 3 L daily (unless contraindicated).
2. Patient has temperature 1°C (1.8°F) or more below usual range.
   Initiate measures to raise body temperature:
   - Remove wet clothing or linen.
   - Apply warm blankets and, unless contraindicated, offer warm liquids.
   - Apply hyperthermia blankets if ordered.
3. Unable to obtain temperature.
   - Reassess correct placement of temperature probe or sensor.
   - Choose alternative temperature measurement site.
   - Obtain alternative temperature measurement device.

RECORDING AND REPORTING

- Record temperature and route and any signs or symptoms of temperature alteration in the EHR.
- Record temperature after administration of specific therapies, such as blood or blood product transfusions.
- Document your evaluation of patient learning.
- Report type of temperature, abnormal findings, and any measures used to reduce or increase temperature to health care provider.

HOME CARE CONSIDERATIONS

- Assess temperature and ventilation of patient's environment to determine existence of any environmental condition that influences patient's temperature.

SKILL 29.2   ASSESSING APICAL AND RADIAL PULSE

Delegation and Collaboration

The skill of apical pulse measurement cannot be delegated to assistive personnel (AP). This measurement is often taken when you suspect an irregularity in the radial pulse or when a patient's condition requires more accurate pulse assessment.

The skill of radial pulse measurement can be delegated to assistive personnel (AP) if a patient's condition is stable. The skill cannot be delegated when a patient's condition is unstable because the patient is at high risk for acute or serious cardiac problems or when the nurse is evaluating a patient's response to a treatment or medication. The nurse instructs the AP by:

- Indicating the appropriate site for measuring pulse rate; the frequency of measurement; and factors related to the patient history such as risk for abnormally slow, rapid, or irregular pulse.
- Reviewing the patient's usual pulse rate and specific changes or abnormalities to report to the nurse.

Equipment

- Stethoscope
- Wristwatch with second hand or digital seconds display
- Pen and vital sign flow sheet in chart or electronic health record (EHR)
- Alcohol swab

STEP	RATIONALE

ASSESSMENT

Apical pulse or radial pulse:

1. Identify patient using at least two identifiers (e.g., name and birthday or name and medical record number) according to agency policy.

   Ensures correct patient. Complies with The Joint Commission standards and improves patient safety (TJC, 2021).

2. Review patient's EHR to determine need to assess pulse: Assess for history of the following: heart or peripheral vascular disease, onset of sudden chest pain or acute pain from any site, invasive cardiovascular diagnostic tests, surgery, sudden infusion of large volume of intravenous (IV) fluid, internal or external hemorrhage, administration of medications that alter heart function.

   Certain conditions are risk factors for pulse alterations. A history of peripheral vascular disease often alters pulse rate and quality.

3. Assess patient's or family caregiver's knowledge, experience, and health literacy.

   Ensures patient has the capacity to obtain, communicate, process, and understand basic health information (CDC, 2021).

Continued

SKILL 29.2	**ASSESSING APICAL AND RADIAL PULSE—cont'd**

STEP	**RATIONALE**
4. Review EHR or question patient about factors that normally influence pulse rate and rhythm:	Allows you to anticipate factors that alter pulse, ensuring an accurate interpretation.
• Age (see also Table 29.4)	Newborn's heart rate (HR) ranges from 120-140 beats/min at rest; by age 2 pulse rate slows to 70 to 120 beats/min; by adolescence rate varies between 60 and 90 beats/min and remains so throughout adulthood (Hockenberry et al., 2019).
• Exercise	Physical activity increases HR; a well-conditioned patient may have a slower-than-usual resting HR that returns more quickly to resting rate after exercise.
• Position changes	HR increases temporarily when changing from lying to sitting or standing position.
• Medications	Antidysrhythmics, sympathomimetics, and cardiotonics affect rate and rhythm of pulse; large doses of opioid analgesics can slow HR; general anesthetics slow HR; central nervous system stimulants such as caffeine can increase HR (Burchum and Rosenthal, 2019).
• Temperature	Fever or exposure to warm environments increases HR; HR declines with hypothermia.
• Sympathetic stimulation	Emotional stress, anxiety, or fear stimulates sympathetic nervous system, which increases HR.
5. Assess patient's baseline heart rate from medical record if available.	Baseline provides measure to determine any change in patient's clinical condition.
6. Perform hand hygiene. Assess for physical signs and symptoms of altered cardiac function such as dyspnea, fatigue, chest pain, orthopnea, syncope, palpitations, edema of dependent body parts.	Reduces transmission of infection. Physical signs and symptoms indicate alteration in conduction of cardiac electrical impulses, cardiac output, or stroke volume, all of which can affect radial pulse and rhythm.
7. If obtaining apical pulse, determine any report of latex allergy. If patient has latex allergy, ensure that stethoscope is latex free.	Reduces risk of allergic reaction to stethoscope.
8. Assess patient's knowledge, prior experience with pulse measurement, and feelings about procedure.	Reveals need for patient instruction and/or support.
9. Assess patient's goals or preferences for how skill is to be performed or what patient expects.	Allows care to be individualized to patient.

PLANNING

1. Provide privacy for patient; if necessary, draw curtain around bed and/or close door. Prepare bedside environment for patient safety.	Maintains privacy and minimizes embarrassment, helping patient relax. Removes barriers that may interfere with patient care.
2. Obtain and organize equipment for pulse measurement at bedside.	Ensures an organized approach for assessing pulse.
3. Explain to patient that you will assess radial pulse rate or apical pulse rate. Encourage patient to relax as much as possible. If patient has been active, wait 5 to 10 minutes before assessing pulse rate. If patient has been smoking or ingesting caffeine, wait 15 minutes before assessing pulse rate.	Anxiety, activity, smoking, and caffeine elevate heart rate.

IMPLEMENTATION
1. Apical pulse

a. Perform hand hygiene.	Reduces transmission of infection.
b. Have patient assume a sitting or supine position. Locate anatomical landmarks to identify point of maximal impulse (PMI), also called *apical impulse* (see Chapter 30). The heart is located behind and to left of sternum with base at top and apex at bottom. Find angle of Louis just below suprasternal notch between sternal body and manubrium; it feels like a bony prominence (see illustration A). Slip fingers down each side of angle to find second intercostal space (ICS) (see illustration B). Carefully move fingers down left side of sternum to fifth ICS and laterally to left midclavicular line (MCL) (see illustration C). A light tap felt within area 1 to 2.5 cm (½ to 1 inch) of PMI is reflected from apex of heart (see illustration D).	Provides easy access to pulse sites. Use of anatomical landmarks allows correct placement of stethoscope over apex of heart. This position enhances ability to hear heart sounds clearly. If unable to palpate PMI, reposition patient on left side. In presence of serious heart disease, you may locate PMI to left of MCL or at sixth ICS. PMI may not be palpated in obese adults or patients with severe pulmonary disease that has changed shape of thorax.
c. Place diaphragm of stethoscope in palm of hand for 5 to 10 seconds.	Warming of metal or plastic diaphragm prevents patient from being startled and promotes comfort.
d. Place diaphragm of stethoscope over PMI at fifth ICS, at left MCL, and auscultate for normal S_1 and S_2 heart sounds (heard as "lub-dub") (see illustrations).	Allow stethoscope tubing to extend straight without kinks that would distort sound transmission. Normal sounds S_1 and S_2 are high pitched and best heard with diaphragm.

STEP	RATIONALE
e. When you hear S₁ and S₂ with regularity, use second hand of watch and begin to count rate; when sweep hand hits number on dial, start counting with zero, then one, two, and so on.	Apical rate is determined accurately only after you can auscultate sounds clearly. Timing begins with zero. Count of one is first sound auscultated after timing begins.
f. If apical rate is regular, count for 30 seconds and multiply by 2.	You can assess regular apical rate within 30 seconds.

CLINICAL JUDGMENT: *When HR is irregular or patient is receiving cardiovascular medication, count for a full 1 minute (60 seconds). An irregular rate is more accurately assessed when measured over longer interval.*

STEP 1b (A) Nurse locates sternal notch. (B) Nurse locates second intercostal space. (C) Nurse locates fifth intercostal space. (D) Nurse locates point of maximal impulse at fifth intercostal space at left midclavicular line.

STEP 1d (A) Location of point of maximal impulse (PMI) in adult. (B) Listening to PMI in adult.

Continued

SKILL 29.2	ASSESSING APICAL AND RADIAL PULSE—cont'd

STEP	RATIONALE
g. Note regularity of any dysrhythmia (S_1 and S_2 occurring early or late after previous sequence of sounds) (e.g., every third or every fourth beat is skipped).	Regular occurrence of dysrhythmia within 1 minute indicates inefficient contraction of heart and potential alteration in cardiac output.

CLINICAL JUDGMENT: *If apical rate is abnormal or irregular, repeat measurement or have another nurse conduct measurement. Original measurement may be incorrect. Second measurement confirms initial findings of an abnormal HR.*

STEP	RATIONALE
h. Replace patient's gown and bed linen.	Restores comfort and promotes sense of well-being.
2. Radial pulse	
a. Perform hand hygiene and help patient to assume a supine or sitting position.	Provides easy access to pulse sites.
b. If patient is supine, place the forearm straight alongside or across lower chest or upper abdomen (see illustration A). If sitting, bend patient's elbow 90 degrees and support lower arm on chair or on your arm. Place tips of first two or middle three fingers of hand over groove along radial or thumb side of patient's inner wrist (see illustration B). Slightly extend or flex wrist with palm down until you note strongest pulse.	Fingertips are most sensitive parts of hand to palpate arterial pulsation. Your thumb has pulsation that interferes with accuracy.
c. Lightly compress pulse against radius, losing pulse initially; relax pressure so that pulse becomes easily palpable.	Pulse assessment is more accurate when using moderate pressure. Too much pressure occludes pulse and impairs blood flow.
d. Determine strength of pulse. Note whether thrust of vessel against fingertips is bounding (4+); full, strong (3+); expected (2+); barely palpable, diminished (1+); or absent, not palpable (0).	Strength reflects volume of blood ejected against arterial wall with each heart contraction. Accurate description of strength improves communication among nurses and other health care providers.
e. After palpating a regular pulse, look at watch second hand and begin to count rate. Count the first beat after the second hand hits the number on the dial; count as one, then two, and so on.	Rate is determined accurately only after pulse has been palpated. Timing begins with zero. Count of one is first beat palpated after timing begins.
f. If pulse is regular, count rate for 30 seconds and multiply total by 2.	A 30-second count is accurate for rapid, slow, or regular pulse rates.

CLINICAL JUDGMENT: *If pulse is irregular, count rate for a full 60 seconds. Assess frequency and pattern of irregularity and compare radial pulses bilaterally. An inefficient contraction of the heart can fail to transmit a pulse wave, resulting in an irregular pulse. A marked difference in pulse rate between radial sites may indicate that arterial flow is compromised to one extremity, and as a nurse you need to take action.*

STEP	RATIONALE
3. Assist patient to comfortable position.	Promotes comfort and sense of well-being.
4. Discuss findings with patient.	Promotes participation in care and understanding of health status.
5. Place nurse call system in an accessible location within patient's reach.	Ensures patient can call for assistance if needed and promotes safety and prevents falls.
6. Raise side rails (as appropriate) and lower bed to lowest position.	Promotes safety and prevents falls.
7. Store reusable equipment. Perform hand hygiene.	Reduces transmission of infection.

EVALUATION

1. If assessing a patient's pulse for first time, establish apical or radial rate as baseline if it is within an acceptable range.	Used to compare future pulse assessments.
2. Compare apical or radial rate and character with patient's previous baseline and acceptable range of HR for patient's age.	Allows you to assess for change in patient's condition and for presence of cardiac alteration.

STEP 2b (A) Pulse check with patient's forearm at side with wrist extended. (B) Hand placement for pulse check.

STEP	RATIONALE
3. Use Teach-Back: "I want to be sure I explained why it is important to check your heart rate at home. Tell me which medication you are taking that would decrease your heart rate." Revise your instruction now or develop a plan for revised patient/family caregiver teaching if patient/family caregiver is not able to teach back correctly.	Teach-back is an evidence-based health literacy intervention that promotes patient engagement, patient safety, adherence, and quality. The goal of teach-back is to ensure that you have explained medical information clearly so that patients and their families understand what you have communicated to them (AHRQ, 2020).

UNEXPECTED OUTCOMES AND RELATED INTERVENTIONS

1. Adult patient's apical or radial pulse is greater than 100 beats/min (tachycardia).
   - Identify related data, including fever, pain, fear or anxiety, recent exercise, low blood pressure, blood loss, or inadequate oxygenation.
   - Observe for signs and symptoms associated with abnormal cardiac function, including dyspnea, fatigue, chest pain, orthopnea, syncope, palpitations, edema of body parts.
2. Patient's apical or radial pulse is less than 60 beats/min (bradycardia).
   - Assess for factors that decrease HR such as beta blockers and antiarrhythmic drugs.
   - Observe for signs and symptoms associated with abnormal cardiac function, including dyspnea, fatigue, chest pain, orthopnea, syncope, palpitations, edema of body parts, or dizziness.
   - Have another nurse assess apical pulse.
   - Report findings to nurse in charge and/or health care provider. It may be necessary to withhold prescribed medications that alter HR until health care provider can evaluate need to adjust dosage.
3. Patient's apical pulse is irregular.
   - Assess for signs and symptoms of decreased cardiac output.
   - Report findings to nurse in charge and/or health care provider, who may order an electrocardiogram to detect cardiac conduction alteration.
4. Patient's radial pulse is irregular.
   Assess for Pulse Deficit.
   - One nurse auscultates apical pulse while a second provider simultaneously palpates radial pulse; one nurse begins 60-second pulse count by calling out loud when both should begin to count pulses. The two pulse rates are compared.
   - If pulse count differs by more than 2, a deficit exists. Assess for other signs and symptoms of decreased cardiac output (see Chapter 30).

RECORDING AND REPORTING

- In the EHR, record pulse rate and character routinely and after administration of specific therapies.
- Record any signs and symptoms of alteration in cardiac function.
- Document your evaluation of patient learning.
- Report bradycardia, tachycardia, or irregular pulse to nurse in charge or health care provider immediately.

HOME CARE CONSIDERATIONS

- Talk with patient and family caregiver to determine educational needs to self monitor pulse.
- Assess home environment to determine room that affords quiet environment for auscultating apical rate.

SKILL 29.3 ASSESSING RESPIRATIONS

Delegation and Collaboration

The skill of counting respirations can be delegated to assistive personnel (AP) unless the patient is considered unstable (i.e., complaints of dyspnea, excessive airway secretions). The nurse instructs the AP by:
- Communicating the frequency of measurement and factors related to patient history or risk for increased or decreased respiratory rate or irregular respirations.
- Reviewing any unusual respiratory values and significant changes to report to the nurse.

Equipment
- Wristwatch with second hand or digital seconds display
- Pen and vital sign flow sheet in chart or electronic health record (EHR)

STEP	RATIONALE
ASSESSMENT	
1. Identify patient using at least two identifiers (e.g., name and birthday or name and medical record number) according to agency policy.	Ensures correct patient. Complies with The Joint Commission standards and improves patient safety (TJC, 2021).
2. Assess patient's or family caregiver's knowledge, experience, and health literacy.	Ensures patient or family caregiver has the capacity to obtain, communicate, process, and understand basic health information (CDC, 2021).
3. Review patient's electronic health record (EHR) or question patient regarding factors that influence the patient's respirations. • Fever	Allows you to anticipate factors that influence respirations, ensuring a more accurate interpretation. Elevated body temperature increases oxygen demand and increases respiration rate and depth.

Continued

SKILL 29.3   ASSESSING RESPIRATIONS—cont'd

STEP	RATIONALE
• Recent exercise	Respirations increase in rate and depth to meet need for additional oxygen and rid body of carbon dioxide.
• Anxiety	Increases oxygen demand and respiratory rate and depth because of sympathetic nervous system stimulation.
• Diseases/trauma of chest wall or muscles	Certain conditions (e.g., fractured ribs, thoracic surgery, asthma, chronic lung disease) affect inspiration and/or expiration.
• Constrictive chest or abdominal dressings	Dressings can restrict ease with which a patient is able to breathe deeply.
• Acute pain	Pain increases oxygen demand and alters rate and rhythm of respirations; breathing becomes shallow. Patient inhibits or splints chest wall movement when pain is in area of chest or abdomen.
• Smoking	Chronic smoking changes pulmonary airways, resulting in increased respiratory rate at rest when not smoking.
• Medications	Opioid analgesics, general anesthetics, and sedative hypnotics depress rate and depth; amphetamines and cocaine increase rate and depth; bronchodilators cause dilation of airways, which ultimately slows respiratory rate.
• Body position	Standing or sitting erect promotes full ventilatory movement and lung expansion; stooped or slumped posture impairs ventilatory movement; lying flat prevents full chest expansion.
• Neurological injury	Damage to brainstem impairs respiratory center and inhibits rate and rhythm.
• Anemia, decreased hemoglobin	Decreased hemoglobin levels lower amount of oxygen carried in blood, which results in increased respiratory rate to increase oxygen delivery.
• Increased altitude	An increase in altitude lowers the amount of saturated hemoglobin, which increases respiratory rate and depth.

4. Review EHR and assess pertinent laboratory/clinical values:

   a. *Arterial blood gases (ABGs):* Normal ranges (values vary slightly among agencies) (Pagana et al., 2019):
      - pH, 7.35–7.45
      - $PaCO_2$, 35–45 mm Hg
      - HCO_3, 22–28 mEq/L
      - PaO_2, 80–100 mm Hg
      - SaO_2, 95%–100%

   Rationale: ABG values measure arterial blood pH, partial pressure of oxygen and carbon dioxide, and arterial oxygen saturation, which reflect patient's ventilation and oxygenation status (see Chapter 41).

   b. *Pulse oximetry (SpO_2):* Normal SpO_2 ≥95%–100%; less than 90% is a clinical emergency (see Skill 29.4).

   Rationale: SpO_2 less than 90% is often accompanied by changes in respiratory rate, depth, and rhythm.

   c. *Complete blood count (CBC):* Normal ranges for adults (values vary among agencies) (Pagana et al., 2019):
      - Hemoglobin: 14–18 g/100 mL, males; 12–16 g/100 mL, females
      - Hematocrit: 42%–52%, males; 37%–47%, females
      - Red blood cell count: 4.7–6.1 million/mm^3, males; 4.2–5.4 million/mm^3, females

   Rationale: CBC measures concentration of hemoglobin. Decreased hemoglobin levels lower amount of oxygen carried in blood, which results in increased respiratory rate to increase oxygen delivery.

5. Determine previous baseline respiratory rate (if available) from patient's record.

   Rationale: Assesses for change in condition. Provides comparison with future respiratory measurements.

6. Perform hand hygiene. Assess for signs and symptoms of respiratory alterations such as:
   - Bluish or cyanotic appearance of nail beds, lips, mucous membranes, and skin
   - Restlessness, irritability, confusion, reduced level of consciousness
   - Pain during inspiration
   - Labored or difficult breathing
   - Orthopnea
   - Use of accessory muscles
   - Adventitious breath sounds (see Chapter 30)
   - Inability to breathe spontaneously
   - Thick, frothy, blood-tinged, or copious sputum production

   Rationale: Reduces transmission of infection. Physical signs and symptoms indicate alterations in respiratory status (see Chapter 30).

STEP	RATIONALE

PLANNING

1. Provide privacy; close curtains or room door. Organize and set up any equipment needed to perform procedure. Prepare bedside environment for patient safety.

Promotes relaxation and provides privacy. Ensures more efficiency when completing an assessment.

2. Position patient in a comfortable position, preferably sitting or lying with the head of the bed elevated 45 to 60 degrees.

Sitting erect promotes full ventilator movement. A position of discomfort causes patient to breath more rapidly.

3. If patient has been active, wait 5 to 10 minutes before assessing respirations.

Exercise increases respiratory rate and depth. Assessing respirations while patient is at rest allows for objective comparison of values.

CLINICAL JUDGMENT: *Assess patients with difficulty breathing (dyspnea) such as those with heart failure or abdominal ascites or in late stages of pregnancy in the position of greatest comfort. Repositioning may increase the work of breathing, which increases respiratory rate.*

---

4. Calm patient, encourage to relax.

Patient should not be aware of your intent to count respirations. Relaxation ensures more normal rate will be measured.

5. Be sure that patient's chest is visible. If necessary, move bed linen or gown. Perform hand hygiene.

Ensures clear view of chest wall and abdominal movements. Reduces transmission of microorganisms.

6. In an adult, assess respirations after pulse rate (see Skill 29.2).

Inconspicuous assessment after pulse assessment prevents patients from consciously or unintentionally altering rate and depth of breathing.

IMPLEMENTATION

1. With patient's arm in relaxed position across abdomen or lower chest, leave fingertips on the wrist, or place your hand directly over patient's upper abdomen.

A similar position used during pulse assessment allows respiratory rate assessment to be inconspicuous. Patient awareness of monitoring reduces respiratory rate by 2 breaths per minute (Hill et al., 2018). Patient's or your hand rises and falls during respiratory cycle.

2. Observe complete respiratory cycle (one inspiration and one expiration).

Rate is accurately determined only after viewing a complete respiratory cycle. An inspiratory breath is half as long as an expiratory breath (Rolfe, 2019).

3. After observing a cycle, look at second hand of watch and begin to count rate: when sweep hand hits number on dial, begin time frame, counting one with first full respiratory cycle.

Timing begins with count of one. Respirations occur more slowly than pulse; thus timing does not begin with zero.

4. If rhythm is regular, count number of respirations in 30 seconds and multiply by 2. If rhythm is irregular, less than 12, or greater than 20, count for **1 full minute** (Box 29.12).

Respiratory rate is equivalent to number of respirations per minute. Suspected irregularities require assessment for at least 1 minute (see Table 29.7). Shorter count durations overestimate respiratory rate by 2 to 4 breaths (Takayama et al., 2019).

5. Note depth of respirations by observing degree of chest wall movement while counting rate. In addition, assess depth by palpating chest wall excursion or auscultating posterior thorax after you have counted rate (see Chapter 30). Describe depth as shallow, normal, or deep.

Character of ventilatory movement reveals specific disease states restricting volume of air from moving into and out of lungs.

BOX 29.12 EVIDENCE-BASED PRACTICE

Reliability in Assessing Respiratory Rate

PICOT Question: Do nurses who count respirations of adult patients for 15 or 30 seconds accurately assess the respiratory rate compared with nurses who count respirations for 60 seconds?

Evidence Summary

Respiratory compromise is a common and potentially dangerous complication in hospitalized patients and is a strong predictor of adverse events and correlated with in-hospital mortality (Lamberti, 2020). Respiratory rate has been labeled the most important vital sign as it is the most sensitive indicator of clinical acute deteriorations; however, it is often neglected in clinical practice (Elliott and Baird, 2019). Many Early Warning Scores (EWS) include respiratory rate measurements. Therefore it is important that respiratory rate be measured accurately and reliably. Brabrand et al. (2018) presented experienced nurses with five 60-second patient videos and asked them to measure respiratory rate. In each case measurements had a wide range of more than 10 breaths per minute. Daw et al. (2017) conducted a similar study using 169 emergency room pediatric patients. Three health care professionals—a nurse, physician, and respiratory therapist—measured respiratory rate. Measurements varied from 11 breaths below to 18 breaths above the known respiratory rate. Higher respiratory rates resulted in less agreement. Nurses who count for 15 seconds and multiply by 4 or count for 30 seconds and multiply by 2 round down or round up, which contributes to the measurement error. Convenient electronic devices exist for pulse, blood pressure, oxygen saturation, and temperature for prompt and accurate measurement. Respiratory rate remains a subjective assessment full of human error.

Application to Nursing Practice

- 15-second assessments of respiratory rates are unreliable.
- High and irregular respiratory rates require a 60-second assessment of respiratory rate.
- Pulse oximetry values are a component of respiratory assessment, but a stand-alone measure, and should not take the place of assessing respiratory rate (Elliott and Baird, 2019).
- Obtaining routine respiratory assessment helps identify early respiratory compromise (Lamberti, 2020).
- Abnormal respiratory rates should be reassessed before initiating therapies.

Continued

SKILL 29.3   ASSESSING RESPIRATIONS—cont'd

STEP	RATIONALE
6. Note rhythm of ventilatory cycle. Normal breathing is regular and uninterrupted. Do not confuse sighing with abnormal rhythm.	Character of ventilations reveals specific types of alterations. Periodically, people unconsciously take single deep breaths or sighs to expand small airways prone to collapse.

CLINICAL JUDGMENT: *Any irregular respiratory pattern or periods of apnea (cessation of respiration over 5 seconds) are symptoms of underlying disease in an adult; report this to the health care provider or nurse in charge. Further assessment and immediate intervention are often necessary.*

STEP	RATIONALE
7. Replace bed linen and patient's gown.	Restores comfort and promotes sense of well-being.
8. Assist patient to comfortable position.	Promotes comfort and sense of well-being.
9. Inform patient of respiratory rate and record per agency policy	Promotes participation in care and understanding of health status.
10. Place nurse call system in an accessible location within patient's reach.	Ensures patient can call for assistance if needed and promotes safety and prevents falls.
11. Raise side rails (as appropriate) and lower bed to lowest position.	Promotes safety and prevents falls.
12. Perform hand hygiene.	Reduces transmission of infection.

EVALUATION

1. If assessing a patient's respirations for the first time, establish rate, rhythm, and depth as baseline if within acceptable range.	Used to compare future respiratory assessments.
2. Compare respirations with patient's previous baseline and usual rate, rhythm, and depth.	Allows you to assess for changes in patient's condition and presence of respiratory alterations.
3. Correlate respiratory rate, depth, and rhythm with data obtained from pulse oximetry and ABG measurements if available.	Evaluation of ventilation, perfusion, and diffusion is interrelated.
4. **Use Teach-Back:** "I want to be sure I explained why you need to take deep breaths after your surgery. Tell me why deep breathing is important." Revise your instruction now or develop a plan for revised patient/family caregiver teaching if patient/family caregiver is not able to teach back correctly.	Teach-back is an evidence-based health literacy intervention that promotes patient engagement, patient safety, adherence, and quality. The goal of teach-back is to ensure that you have explained medical information clearly so that patients and their families understand what you have communicated to them (AHRQ, 2020).

UNEXPECTED OUTCOMES AND RELATED INTERVENTIONS

1. Adult patient's respiratory rate is below 12 breaths/min (bradypnea) or above 20 breaths/min (tachypnea). Breathing pattern is irregular (see Table 29.7). Depth of respirations is increased or decreased. Patient complains of dyspnea.
   - Assess for related factors, including obstructed airway, abnormal breath sounds, productive cough, restlessness, anxiety, and confusion (see Chapter 30).
   - Help patient to supported sitting position (semi- or high-Fowler's) unless contraindicated.
   - Provide oxygen as ordered (see Chapter 41).
   - Assess for environmental factors that influence patient's respiratory rate such as secondhand smoke, poor ventilation, or gas fumes.
   - Notify health care provider or nurse in charge if alteration continues.
2. Patient demonstrates Kussmaul's, Cheyne-Stokes, or Biot's respirations (see Table 29.7).
   - Notify health care provider for additional evaluation and possible medical intervention.

RECORDING AND REPORTING

- Record respiratory rate and character, noting any abnormalities.
- Record respiratory rate after administration of specific therapies.
- Record type and amount of oxygen therapy if used by patient during assessment.
- Document your evaluation of patient learning.
- Report bradypnea, tachypnea, abnormal depth, or rhythm to nurse in charge or health care provider immediately.

HOME CARE CONSIDERATIONS

- Assess for environmental factors in the home that influence respiratory rate such as secondhand smoke, poor ventilation, gas or fireplace fumes, dust, and pets.

SKILL 29.4   MEASURING OXYGEN SATURATION (PULSE OXIMETRY)

Delegation and Collaboration

The skill of SpO$_2$ measurement cannot be delegated when patients are unstable. In stable patients the skill of SpO$_2$ measurement can be delegated to assistive personnel (AP). The nurse instructs the AP by:

- Communicating specific factors related to the patient that can falsely lower SpO$_2$.
- Informing AP about appropriate sensor site and probe and about reporting any skin irritation from probe placement to nurse.
- Notifying about frequency of SpO$_2$ measurements for a specific patient.
- Instructing AP to notify the nurse immediately of any reading lower than SpO$_2$ of 95% or value for specific patient.

- Instructing to refrain from using pulse oximetry to obtain heart rate because oximeter will not detect an irregular pulse.

Equipment

- Oximeter
- Oximeter probe appropriate for patient and recommended by oximeter manufacturer
- Acetone or nail-polish remover if needed
- Pen and vital sign flow sheet in chart or the EHR as per agency policy

STEP	RATIONALE

ASSESSMENT

1. Identify patient using at least two identifiers (e.g., name and birthday or name and medical record number) according to agency policy.

   Ensures correct patient. Complies with The Joint Commission standards and improves patient safety (TJC, 2021).

2. Determine previous baseline SpO$_2$ (if available) from patient's medical record.

   Provides basis for comparison and assists in the assessment of current status and evaluation of interventions.

3. Determine need to assess patient's oxygen saturation:

   Certain conditions place patients at risk for decreased oxygen saturation.

   a. Review the EHR to identify conditions that can cause decreased oxygen saturation, including acute or chronic compromised respiratory function, recovery from general anesthesia or conscious sedation, traumatic injury to chest wall, collapse of lung tissue, ventilator dependence, or a change in oxygen therapy.

4. Assess patient's or family caregiver's knowledge, experience, and health literacy.

   Ensures patient has the capacity to obtain, communicate, process, and understand basic health information (CDC, 2021).

5. Perform hand hygiene. Assess for signs and symptoms of alteration in oxygen saturation such as altered respiratory rate, depth, or rhythm; abnormal breath sounds (see Chapter 30); cyanotic appearance of nail beds, lips, mucous membranes; restlessness, irritability, confusion; reduced level of consciousness; and labored or difficult breathing.

   Reduces transmission of infection. Physical signs and symptoms often indicate low oxygen saturation.

6. Assess for factors that influence measurement of SpO$_2$ (e.g., oxygen therapy, respiratory therapy such as postural drainage and percussion, hemoglobin level, hypotension, temperature, nail polish, and medications such as bronchodilators).

   Allows you to accurately assess oxygen saturation variations.

7. Determine whether patient has a latex allergy.

   Disposable adhesive sensors may contain latex.

8. Determine most appropriate patient-specific probe site (e.g., finger, toe, earlobe, forehead, nose) for sensor placement by evaluating capillary refill (see Chapter 30). If capillary refill is greater than 2 seconds, select alternative site.

   Sensor requires pulsating vascular bed to identify light-absorbing hemoglobin molecules. Patients requiring vasopressors or who are critically ill may have increased peripheral capillary refill; forehead sensors are preferred. Moisture and black or brown nail polish alter readings. Motion artifact is the most common cause of inaccurate measurements. Clip-on probe may be too small for obese patient.

9. Assess patient's knowledge, prior experience with pulse oximetry, and feelings about procedure.

   Reveals need for patient instruction and/or support.

10. Assess patient's goals or preferences for how skill is to be performed or what patient expects.

    Allows care to be individualized to patient.

PLANNING

1. Provide privacy and prepare bedside environment for patient safety.

   Maintains patient comfort and removes barriers that may interfere with procedure.

2. Obtain and organize appropriate supplies at the patient's bedside.

   Ensures an organized approach for oxygen saturation measurement.

3. Explain to patient the way you will measure oxygen saturation and the importance of breathing normally until reading is complete.

   Promotes patient cooperation and increases adherence. Prevents large fluctuations in minute ventilation and possible error in SpO$_2$ readings.

IMPLEMENTATION

1. Perform hand hygiene.

   Prevents transmission of infection.

2. Position patient in a comfortable position, preferably sitting or lying with the head of the bed elevated 45 to 60 degrees.

   Sitting erect promotes full ventilation. A position of discomfort causes patient to breath more rapidly.

3. Attach sensor to monitoring site (see illustrations). If using finger, remove fingernail polish from digit with acetone or polish remover. Instruct patient that clip-on probe will feel like a clothespin on the finger but will not hurt.

   Nail polish falsely alters saturation.

CLINICAL JUDGMENT: *Do not attach probe to finger, ear, or bridge of nose if area is edematous or skin integrity is compromised. Do not use earlobe and bridge of nose sensors for infants and toddlers because of skin fragility. Do not attach sensor to fingers that are hypothermic. Select ear or bridge of nose if adult patient has a history of peripheral vascular disease. Do not use disposable adhesive sensors if patient has a latex allergy. Do not place sensor on same extremity as electronic blood pressure cuff because blood flow to finger will be interrupted temporarily when cuff inflates and cause inaccurate reading that can trigger alarms.*

4. Once sensor is in place, turn on oximeter by activating power. Observe pulse waveform/intensity display and audible beep. Correlate oximeter pulse rate with patient's radial pulse.

   Pulse waveform and audible beep enables detection of valid pulse. Pitch of audible beep is proportional to SpO$_2$ value. Correlating pulse rates ensures oximeter accuracy; difference requires reassessment of sensor placement site.

5. Leave sensor in place 10 to 30 seconds or until oximeter readout reaches constant value and pulse display reaches full strength during each cardiac cycle. Inform patient that oximeter alarm will sound if sensor falls off or patient moves it. Read SpO$_2$ on digital display.

   Sensor alarm may frighten patient or visitors.

Continued

SKILL 29.4	MEASURING OXYGEN SATURATION (PULSE OXIMETRY)—cont'd
STEP	**RATIONALE**

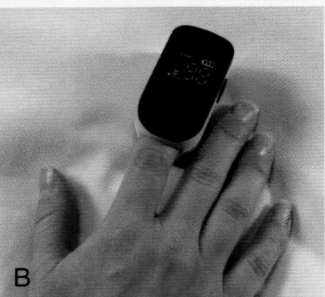

STEP 3 (A) Pulse oximetry machine. (B) Clip-on pulse oximetry sensor.

STEP	RATIONALE
6. For continuous SpO₂ monitoring: • Verify SpO₂ alarm limits preset by manufacturer at a low of 85% and a high of 100%. • Determine limits for SpO₂ and pulse rate as indicated by patient's condition. • Verify that alarms are on. • Assess skin integrity under sensor probe every 2 hours; relocate sensor at least every 4 hours and more frequently if skin integrity is altered or tissue perfusion compromised.	Sensor tension and sensitivity to disposable sensor adhesive cause skin irritation and lead to disruption of skin integrity.
7. If you plan intermittent checking or spot-checking of SpO₂, remove probe and turn oximeter power off. Clean sensor and store sensor in appropriate location.	Prevents transmission of infection. Sensor probes are vulnerable to damage. Cleansing reduces transmission of microorganisms.
8. Assist patient to comfortable position.	Restores comfort and promotes a sense of well-being.
9. Discuss results with patient.	Promotes participation in care and understanding of health.
10. Place nurse call system in an accessible location within patient's reach.	Ensures patient can call for assistance if needed and promotes safety and prevents falls.
11. Raise side rails (as appropriate) and lower bed to lowest position.	Promotes safety and prevents falls.
12. Discard disposable equipment and perform hand hygiene.	Prevents transmission of infection.

EVALUATION

1. If assessing a patient's oxygen saturation for the first time, establish it as baseline if within acceptable range.	Used to compare future SpO₂ measurements.
2. Compare SpO₂ reading with patient's previous baseline and acceptable values. Note use of oxygen therapy, which can affect SpO₂.	Allows you to assess for changes in patient's condition and presence of respiratory alterations.
3. Correlate SpO₂ with SaO₂, obtained from ABG measurements if available.	Documents reliability of noninvasive assessment.
4. Correlate reading with data obtained from respiratory rate, depth, and rhythm assessment (see Skill 29.3).	Measurements assessing ventilation, perfusion, and diffusion are interrelated.
5. **Use Teach-Back:** "I want to be sure I explained the reasons for a falsely low oxygen saturation. Can you tell me two ways you could cause a reading to be false? Revise your instruction now or develop a plan for revised patient/family caregiver teaching if patient/family caregiver is unable to teach back correctly.	Teach-back is an evidence-based health literacy intervention that promotes patient engagement, patient safety, adherence, and quality. The goal of teach-back is to ensure that you have explained medical information clearly so that patients and their families understand what you have communicated to them (AHRQ, 2020).

UNEXPECTED OUTCOMES AND RELATED INTERVENTIONS

1. SpO₂ is less than 90%.
   - Verify that oximeter sensor is intact and properly applied.
   - Observe for signs and symptoms of decreased oxygenation such as anxiety, restlessness, or tachycardia.
   - Verify that supplemental oxygen is delivered as ordered and that system is functioning properly.
   - Assist patient to a position that maximizes ventilator effort (e.g., position an obese patient in a high-Fowler position).
   - Report SpO₂ to nurse in charge or health care provider to initiate appropriate evaluation and treatment.
2. Sensor device results in pressure injury.
   - Change type or location of sensor device. Rotate oximetry probe sites more frequently.
   - Increase frequency of skin assessment under sensor.

RECORDING AND REPORTING

- In EHR, record type and amount of oxygen therapy used by patient during assessment, SpO₂ readings, and any signs or symptoms of alterations in oxygenation.
- Document your evaluation of patient learning.
- Report alterations in SpO₂ to health care provider.

SKILL 29.5   MEASURING BLOOD PRESSURE BY AUSCULTATION

Delegation and Collaboration

The skill of BP measurement can be delegated to assistive personnel (AP) unless the patient is considered unstable (i.e., hypotensive). The nurse instructs the AP by:

- Explaining the appropriate limb for measurement, BP cuff size, and equipment (manual or electronic) to be used.
- Communicating the frequency of measurement and factors to consider during measurement, such as risk for orthostatic hypotension.
- Reviewing the patient's usual BP values and significant changes or abnormalities to report to the nurse.

Equipment

- Aneroid sphygmomanometer
- Cloth or disposable vinyl pressure cuff of appropriate size for patient's extremity (see Planning Step 2)
- Stethoscope
- Alcohol swab
- Pen and vital sign flow sheet in chart or electronic health record (EHR)

STEP	RATIONALE
ASSESSMENT	
1. Identify patient using at least two identifiers (e.g., name and birthday or name and medical record number) according to agency policy.	Ensures correct patient. Complies with The Joint Commission standards and improves patient safety (TJC, 2021).
2. Review patient's electronic health record (EHR) to assess for risk factors for blood pressure alterations:	Certain conditions place patients at risk for BP alteration.
• History of cardiovascular disease	
• Renal disease	
• Diabetes mellitus	
• Circulatory shock (hypovolemic, septic, cardiogenic, or neurogenic)	
• Acute or chronic pain	
• Rapid intravenous (IV) infusion of fluids or blood products	
• Increased intracranial pressure	
• Postoperative status	
• Gestational hypertension	
3. Assess patient's or family caregiver's knowledge, experience, and health literacy.	Assures patient has the capacity to obtain, communicate, process, and understand basic health information (CDC, 2021).
4. Assess for factors that influence BP:	Allows you to anticipate factors that influence BP, ensuring a more accurate interpretation.
• Age	Acceptable values for BP vary throughout life. Older patients experience greater "white coat" effect as BP increases when in the presence of a provider (Kallioinen et al., 2017).
• Gender	During and after menopause women often have higher BPs than men of same age.
• Daily (diurnal) variation	BP varies throughout day; pressure is highest during the day between 10:00 a.m. and 6:00 p.m. and lowest in early morning.
• Position	BP falls as individual moves from lying to sitting or standing position; acceptable postural variations are less than 10 mm Hg (Hale et al., 2017).
• Exercise	Increases in oxygen demand by body during activity increases BP. BP can be increased if patient does not rest at least 15 minutes before measurement (Kallioinen et al., 2017).
• Weight	Obesity is an independent predictor of hypertension.
• Sympathetic stimulation	Pain, anxiety, or fear stimulates sympathetic nervous system, causing BP to rise. A full bladder increases systolic and diastolic BP (Kallioinen et al., 2017).
• Medications	Antihypertensives, diuretics, beta-adrenergic blockers, vasodilators, calcium channel blockers, angiotensin-converting enzyme (ACE) inhibitors, angiotensin receptor blockers (ARBs), and antidysrhythmics lower BP; opioids and general anesthetics also cause a drop in BP (Burchum and Rosenthal, 2019).
• Smoking	Smoking results in vasoconstriction, a narrowing of blood vessels. SBP and DBP rise acutely and return to baseline approximately 20-30 minutes after stopping smoking, 30 minutes after snuff chewing, and 40-60 minutes after a nicotine tablet (AHA, 2015; Muntner et al., 2019).
• Ethnicity	Incidence of hypertension is higher in African Americans and Hispanics than in European Americans. African Americans tend to develop more severe hypertension at an earlier age and have twice the risk for the complications of hypertension (i.e., stroke and heart attack). Hypertension-related deaths are also higher among African Americans (Moughrabi, 2017).
• Temperature	Cold exposure increases systolic BP (Kallioinen et al., 2017).

Continued

SKILL 29.5	MEASURING BLOOD PRESSURE BY AUSCULTATION—cont'd

STEP	RATIONALE
5. Perform hand hygiene. Assess for signs and symptoms of BP alterations (especially patients at high risk for hypertension): headache (usually occipital), flushing of face, nosebleed, and fatigue in older adults. Hypotension is associated with dizziness; mental confusion; restlessness; pale, dusky, or cyanotic skin and mucous membranes; and cool, mottled skin over extremities.	Reduces transmission of infection. Physical signs and symptoms indicate alterations in BP. Hypertension is often asymptomatic until pressure is very high.
6. Determine best site for BP assessment. Remove clothing over blood pressure cuff placement area. Avoid applying cuff to extremity when IV fluids are infusing, an arteriovenous shunt or fistula is present, breast or axillary surgery has been performed on that side, or patient has a peripherally inserted central catheter or midline catheter (AACN, 2016). In addition, avoid applying cuff to traumatized or diseased extremity or one that has a cast or bulky bandage. Use lower extremities when brachial arteries are inaccessible.	Inappropriate site selection may result in poor amplification of sounds, causing inaccurate readings. Clothing underneath the cuff can distort cuff fit and placement and impede auscultation. Application of pressure from inflated cuff bladder temporarily impairs blood flow and can further compromise circulation in extremity that already has impaired blood flow.

CLINICAL JUDGMENT: *For a patient who has had a mastectomy or lumpectomy, do not use the involved arm(s) for BP measurement if lymphedema is present (AACN, 2016).*

7. Determine previous baseline BP and site (if available). Determine any report of latex allergy.	Assesses for change in condition. Provides comparison with future BP measurements. If patient has latex allergy, verify that stethoscope and BP cuff are latex free.
8. Assess patient's knowledge, prior experience with blood pressure measurement, and feelings about procedure.	Reveals need for patient instruction and/or support.
9. Assess patient's goals or preferences for how skill to be performed or what patient expects.	Allows care to be individualized to patient.

PLANNING

1. Provide privacy and prepare bedside environment for patient safety.	Maintains patient comfort and removes barriers that may interfere with procedure.
2. Select appropriate cuff size with a bladder of an adequate size, capable of going around the arm as recommended (see Fig 29.9) (AACN, 2016; Muntner et al., 2019). Ensure that sphygmomanometer or electronic blood pressure machine is in patient's room.	Use of improper cuff can cause measurement errors (Mickley et al., 2018; AACN, 2016) (see Table 29.12).
3. Ensure that patient has not exercised, ingested caffeine, or smoked for 30 minutes before assessing BP.	Exercise causes false elevation in BP. Smoking increases BP immediately and for up to 15 minutes. Caffeine increases BP for up to 3 hours (James et al., 2014).
4. Explain to patient that you will measure BP. Have patient assume sitting or lying position. Allow the patient to rest 3-5 minutes before obtaining a BP (Mickley et al., 2018). Ask patient not to speak while you are measuring BP.	Reduces anxiety that falsely elevates readings. Deep breathing lowers BP. Talking to a patient during assessment increases BP. A higher BP measurement occurs if the patient has not rested or relaxed (Mickley et al., 2018). Systolic and diastolic BPs of hypertensive and normotensive patients increase with talking (AACN, 2016).

IMPLEMENTATION

1. Perform hand hygiene. Clean stethoscope earpieces and diaphragm with alcohol swab.	Reduces transmission of infection. Cleansing of stethoscope pieces before and after patient use has the potential to reduce HAIs (Marcos et al., 2019).
2. Position patient.	
a. *Upper extremity:* With patient sitting or lying, position forearm at heart level with palm turned up (see illustration). Support arm on a table or under your arm. If sitting, support back and instruct patient to keep feet flat on floor without legs crossed. If supine, patient should not have legs crossed.	If arm is extended and not supported, patient will perform isometric exercise that can increase diastolic pressure. Placement of arm above level of heart causes false-low reading; arm below the level of the heart creates a false-high reading (Kallioinen et al., 2017; AACN, 2016). Not supporting the arm can falsely elevate systolic BP (AACN, 2016). BP readings measured with the back unsupported are higher than those with the back supported (Ringrose et al., 2017). Legs crossed at the knees can significantly increase BP (Kallioinen et al., 2017).

CLINICAL JUDGMENT: *There are special circumstances (such as bilateral arm trauma or bilateral arm lymphedema) when the upper extremities cannot be used for blood pressure measurement.*

b. *Lower extremity:* When upper extremities are inaccessible, obtain a lower extremity BP measurement. (1) **Calf BP:** Position the patient supine. (2) **Thigh BP:** If the patient cannot be placed prone, position the patient supine with knee slightly bent (AACN, 2016).	Allows for application of blood pressure cuff and placement of stethoscope over dorsalis pedis (calf measurement) and popliteal artery (thigh measurement).

STEP	RATIONALE

STEP 2a Patient's forearm supported on bed. (*Copyright © Mosby's Clinical Skills: Essentials Collection.*)

CLINICAL JUDGMENT: *If patients with unstable vital signs, spinal surgeries, or orthopedic injuries cannot tolerate the prone position for thigh BP measurement, consult health care provider to determine whether a calf BP measurement is acceptable.*

CLINICAL JUDGMENT: *Patients with spinal cord injuries may be placed on rotational support surfaces. If thigh BP measurements are ordered, time the assessment of the thigh BP measurement for when the support surface rotates the patient to the prone position.*

---

3. Expose extremity (arm or leg) fully by removing constricting clothing. Cuff may be placed over a sleeve as long as stethoscope rests on skin (Kallioinen et al., 2017).

   Ensures proper cuff application. Thin clothing (<5 mm) does not impact cuff inflation or BP measurements (Zhang et al., 2019).

4. Palpate brachial artery (arm, see illustration A) or popliteal artery (thigh) or dorsalis pedis artery or posterior tibial artery (calf).

   Brachial artery measurement: With cuff fully deflated, position bladder of cuff 2-3 cm (1.25 inch) above antecubital fossa, at the level of the right atrium (midpoint of the sternum), above artery by centering arrows marked on cuff over artery (AACN, 2016; Muntner et al., 2019) (see illustration B). If cuff does not have any center arrows, estimate center of bladder and place this center over artery. With cuff fully deflated, wrap it evenly and snugly around upper arm (see illustration C) or lower extremity.

   Brachial artery is along groove between biceps and triceps muscles above elbow at antecubital fossa. Popliteal artery is just below patient's thigh, behind knee.

   Dorsalis pedis artery is on the top of the patient's foot, midpoint between the ankle and toes. The posterior tibial artery is behind the knee and above the Achilles tendon.

   Placing bladder directly over artery ensures that you apply proper pressure during inflation. Loose-fitting cuff causes false-high readings.

CLINICAL JUDGMENT: *When a patient has a thigh BP measurement ordered, position cuff 2-3 cm (0.78 to 1.2 inch) above popliteal fossa (AACN, 2016).*

---

5. Position manometer gauge vertically at eye level. You should be no farther than 1 meter (approximately 1 yard) away.

   Looking up or down at scale can result in distorted readings.

6. Auscultate BP.

   a. Two-step method:

   (1) Relocate brachial or popliteal pulse. Palpate artery distal to cuff with fingertips of nondominant hand while inflating cuff rapidly to pressure 30 mm Hg above point at which pulse disappears. Slowly deflate cuff and note point when pulse reappears. Deflate cuff fully and wait 30 seconds.

   Estimating prevents false-low readings. Determine maximal inflation point for accurate reading by palpation. If unable to palpate artery because of weakened pulse, use ultrasonic stethoscope (see Chapter 30). Deflating the cuff completely prevents venous congestion and false-high readings.

   (2) Place stethoscope earpieces in ears, and be sure that sounds are clear, not muffled.

   Ensure that each earpiece follows angle of ear canal to facilitate hearing.

   (3) Relocate artery and place bell or diaphragm chest piece of stethoscope over it. Do not allow chest piece to touch cuff or clothing.

   Proper stethoscope placement ensures best sound reception. Stethoscope improperly positioned causes muffled sounds that often result in false-low systolic and false-high diastolic readings. The stethoscope bell or diaphragm can be used for auscultatory readings (Muntner et al., 2019). The bell provides better sound reproduction, whereas the diaphragm is easier to secure with fingers and covers a larger area. Placing the stethoscope under the cuff increases the systolic and decreases the diastolic BP measurement (Kallioinen et al., 2017).

   (4) Close valve of pressure bulb clockwise until tight. Quickly inflate cuff to 30 mm Hg above patient's estimated systolic pressure.

   Tightening valve prevents air leak during inflation. Rapid inflation ensures accurate measurement of systolic pressure.

Continued

SKILL 29.5   MEASURING BLOOD PRESSURE BY AUSCULTATION—cont'd

STEP	RATIONALE

STEP 4 (A) Palpating brachial artery. (B) Aligning blood pressure cuff arrow with brachial artery. (C) Blood pressure cuff wrapped around upper arm. (Copyright © *Mosby's Clinical Skills: Essentials Collection*.)

(5) Slowly release pressure bulb valve, and allow manometer needle to fall at rate of 2 to 3 mm Hg/second.

A too-rapid decline decreases systolic BP and increases diastolic BP measurement (Kallioinen et al., 2017).

(6) Note point on manometer when you hear first clear sound. Sound will slowly increase in intensity.

First sound reflects systolic BP.

(7) Continue to deflate cuff gradually, noting point at which sound disappears in adults. Note pressure to nearest 2 mm Hg. Listen for 20 to 30 mm Hg after last sound and allow remaining air to escape quickly.

Beginning of last or fifth sound is indication of diastolic pressure in adults (Thomas and Pohl, 2020). In children distinct muffling of sounds indicates diastolic pressure (Thomas and Pohl, 2020).

b. One-step method:

(1) Place stethoscope earpieces in ears, and be sure that sounds are clear, not muffled.

Earpieces should follow angle of ear canal to facilitate hearing.

(2) Locate brachial or popliteal artery, and place bell or diaphragm chest piece of stethoscope over it. Do not allow chest piece to touch cuff or clothing.

Proper stethoscope placement ensures optimal sound reception. Stethoscope improperly positioned causes muffled sounds that often result in false readings. Bell provides better sound reproduction, whereas diaphragm is easier to secure with fingers and covers a larger area. Placing the stethoscope under the cuff increases the systolic and decreases the diastolic BP measurement (Kallioinen et al., 2017).

(3) Close valve of pressure bulb clockwise until tight. Quickly inflate cuff to 30 mm Hg above patient's usual systolic pressure.

Tightening valve prevents air leak during inflation. Inflation above systolic level ensures accurate measurement of systolic pressure.

(4) Slowly release pressure bulb valve and allow manometer needle to fall at rate of 2 to 3 mm Hg/second. Note point on manometer when you hear first clear sound. Sound will slowly increase in intensity.

A too-rapid decline decreases systolic BP and increases diastolic BP measurement (Kallioinen et al., 2017). First sound reflects systolic pressure.

(5) Continue to deflate cuff gradually, noting point at which sound disappears in adults. Note pressure to nearest 2 mm Hg. Listen for 10 to 20 mm Hg after last sound and allow remaining air to escape quickly.

Beginning of fifth sound is indication of diastolic pressure in adults (Thomas and Pohl, 2020). In children distinct muffling of sounds indicates diastolic pressure (Thomas and Pohl, 2020).

7. The American Heart Association recommends average of two sets of BP measurement, 2 minutes apart. Use second set of BP measurements as baseline. If readings are different by more than 5 mm Hg, additional readings are necessary.

Two sets of BP measurements help to prevent false-positive readings based on patient's sympathetic response (alert reaction). Averaging minimizes effect of anxiety, which often causes first reading to be higher than subsequent measures (Kallioinen et al., 2017). Systolic BP in leg is generally higher than in arm, but diastolic BP is same.

STEP	RATIONALE

8. Remove cuff from patient's arm or leg unless patient condition requires repeated measurements.

Continuous cuff inflation causes arterial occlusion, resulting in numbness and tingling of patient's arm/leg.

9. If this is first assessment of patient, repeat procedure on other arm or leg.

Comparison of BP in both arms and legs detects circulatory problems. (Normal difference of 5 to 10 mm Hg exists between arms.) Use arm with higher pressure for repeated measurements (AACN, 2016).

10. Assess systolic BP by palpation:
 a. Follow Steps 2-5.
 b. Relocate and then continually palpate brachial, radial, or popliteal artery with fingertips of one hand. Inflate cuff to pressure 30 mm Hg above point at which you can no longer palpate pulse.

Ensures accurate detection of true systolic pressure once pressure valve is released.

CLINICAL JUDGMENT: *If unable to palpate artery because of weakened pulse, use a Doppler ultrasonic stethoscope (see Chapter 30).*

 c. Slowly release valve and deflate cuff, allowing manometer needle to fall at rate of 2 mm Hg/second. Note point on manometer when pulse is again palpable, which indicates systolic pressure.

A too-rapid decline falsely decreases systolic BP measurement (Kallioinen et al., 2017). Palpation helps identify systolic pressure only.

 d. Deflate cuff rapidly and completely. Remove cuff from patient's extremity unless patient condition requires repeated measurements.

Continuous cuff inflation causes arterial occlusion, resulting in numbness and tingling of extremity.

11. Assist patient return to comfortable position and cover upper arm or leg if previously clothed.

Restores comfort and provides sense of well-being.

12. Inform patient of blood pressure, and record the reading per agency policy. Discuss findings with patient.

Promotes participation in care and understanding of health status.

13. Place nurse call system in an accessible location within patient's reach.

Ensures patient can call for assistance if needed and promotes safety and prevents falls.

14. Raise side rails (as appropriate) and lower bed to lowest position.

Promotes safety and prevents falls.

15. Clean earpieces and diaphragm of stethoscope with alcohol swab as needed. Wipe cuff with agency-approved disinfectant if used between patients. Perform hand hygiene.

Reduces transmission of microorganisms.
Controls transmission of microorganisms when nurses share stethoscope (Marcos et al., 2019).

EVALUATION

1. If assessing a patient's BP for first time, establish baseline BP if it is within acceptable range.

Used to compare future BP measurements.

2. Compare BP reading with patient's previous baseline and usual BP for patient's age.

Allows you to assess for change in condition. Provides comparison with future BP measurements.

3. Use Teach-Back: "I want to be sure I explained why it is important to stand up slowly since you are taking blood pressure medications. Tell me which of your medications might make you dizzy if you stand up too fast." Revise your instruction now or develop a plan for revised patient/family caregiver teaching if patient/family caregiver is not able to teach back correctly.

Teach-back is an evidence-based health literacy intervention that promotes patient engagement, patient safety, adherence, and quality. The goal of teach-back is to ensure that you have explained medical information clearly so that patients and their families understand what you have communicated to them (AHRQ, 2020).

UNEXPECTED OUTCOMES AND RELATED INTERVENTIONS

1. Patient's BP is above acceptable range.
 - Repeat measurement in other extremity and compare findings. When a clinically significant difference greater than 10 mm Hg exists, use the arm with the higher pressure (AACN, 2016).
 - Verify correct size and placement of BP cuff.
 - Have another nurse repeat measurement in 1 to 2 minutes.
 - Observe for related symptoms that are not apparent unless BP is extremely high, including headache, facial flushing, nosebleed, and fatigue in an older patient.
 - Report BP to nurse in charge or health care provider to initiate appropriate evaluation and treatment.
 - Administer antihypertensive medications as ordered.

2. Patient's BP is below acceptable range.
 - Position patient in supine position to enhance circulation, and restrict activity that decreases BP further.
 - Assess for signs and symptoms associated with hypotension, including tachycardia; weak, thready pulse; weakness; dizziness; confusion; and cool, pale, dusky, or cyanotic skin.
 - Assess for factors that contribute to low BP, including hemorrhage, dilation of blood vessels resulting from hyperthermia, anesthesia, or medication side effects.
 - Report BP to nurse in charge or health care provider to initiate appropriate interventions.
 - Increase rate of IV infusion or administer vasoconstriction drugs if ordered.
 - If patient stabilizes, assess for postural hypotension.

3. Unable to obtain BP reading.
 - Determine that no immediate crisis is present by obtaining pulse and respiratory rate.
 - Assess for signs and symptoms of decreased cardiac output; if present, notify nurse in charge or health care provider immediately.
 - Use alternative sites or procedures to obtain BP: use Doppler ultrasonic instrument (see Chapter 30); palpate systolic BP.

RECORDING AND REPORTING

- In the EHR, record BP, extremity assessed, method of assessment, and any signs and symptoms of BP alterations.
- Record measurement of BP after administration of specific therapies.
- Document assessment of patient learning.
- Report elevated or low blood pressure, a difference of more than 20 mm Hg between extremities or more than 20 mm Hg drop in systolic blood pressure or a 10 mm Hg drop in diastolic blood pressure when rising from a supine to a sitting or standing position.

HOME CARE CONSIDERATIONS

- Assess home noise level to determine room that provides most quiet environment for assessing BP.
- Consider use of an electronic BP cuff for home if patient has hearing difficulties, sufficient financial resources, and adequate dexterity.
- Blood pressure taken in the home may differ from the measurements assessed in a health care agency because the equipment and environment are different.
- Home blood pressure readings predict cardiovascular events and are particularly useful for monitoring the effects of treatment.

KEY POINTS

- For the body temperature to stay constant and within an acceptable range, various mechanisms maintain the relationship between heat production and heat loss.
- Body temperature will decrease using measures that increase radiation, evaporation, convection, and conduction of heat.
- Fever serves as an important mechanism to enhance the immune system's ability to fight infection.
- Fever increases metabolism, which requires additional energy and oxygen.
- Vital sign assessment requires an organized approach.
- Patient age, gender, activity, medications, and health status influence vital signs.
- Measurement location and time of day influence vital signs.
- Acceptable vital signs fall within a normal range, with infant and children values higher for pulse and respirations and lower in blood pressure, compared with adults.
- Changes related to aging influence the vital sign values of older adults.
- Assessment of a child's vital signs requires you to consider that the brachial or apical pulse is the best site for assessing an infant's or a young child's pulse, and when measuring respirations, infants tend to breathe less regularly.
- Self-measurement of blood pressure helps patients adhere to treatment regimens, but findings should not be used for treatment decisions.
- Document route and site when measuring temperature, blood pressure, pulse, and oxygen saturation.
- When vital signs are above or below expected values, enter a note in the patient's record regarding the finding, any intervention, and the patient's response.
- Vital signs can be delegated to assistive personnel when the patient's condition is stable; however, the skill of apical pulse measurement cannot be delegated.

REFLECTIVE LEARNING

- Review a patient you recently cared for and identify if there were assessment findings to support changing the frequency of vital sign measurement. If so, consider the rationale.
- Consider your knowledge and/or experiences with the delegation of vital signs. Identify patient assessment findings that support and do not support the delegation of this skill to the assistive personnel (AP).

- Imagine a clinical experience in which the division to which you are assigned has an increase in hospital-acquired infections (HAIs). Consider the vital sign measurement equipment you should use and how it prevents the spread of infection.

REVIEW QUESTIONS

1. A 52-year-old woman is admitted with pneumonia, dyspnea, and discomfort in her left chest when taking deep breaths. She has smoked for 35 years and recently lost over 4.5 kg (10 lb). She is started on intravenous antibiotics, high-protein shakes, and 2 L O_2 via nasal cannula. Her vital signs at the start of treatment are HR 112, BP 138/82, RR 22, tympanic temperature 37.9°C (100.2°F), and oxygen saturation 94%. Which of the vital signs taken 4 hours later reflect a positive outcome of the treatment interventions? (Select all that apply.)
   1. Temperature: 37°C (98.6°F)
   2. Radial pulse: 98
   3. Respiratory rate: 18
   4. Oxygen saturation: 96%
   5. Blood pressure: 134/78
2. The licensed practical nurse (LPN) provides you with the shift hand-off vital signs on four of your patients. Based on your knowledge of the pathophysiology of each patient's illness, use clinical judgment to prioritize, in order, the follow-up patient assessments to be made.
   1. 84-year-old man recently admitted with pneumonia, RR 28, SpO2 85%
   2. 54-year-old woman admitted after surgery for repair of a fractured arm, BP 160/86 mm Hg, HR 72
   3. 63-year-old man with venous ulcers from diabetes, temperature 37.3°C (99.1°F), HR 84
   4. 77-year-old woman with left mastectomy 36 hours ago, temperature 38.3°C (101°F), pulse 110, RR 22, BP 148/62
3. A patient has been hospitalized for the past 48 hours with a fever of unknown origin. His medical record indicates tympanic temperatures of 38.7°C (101.6°F) at 0400, 36.6°C (97.9°F) at 0800, 36.9°C (98.4°F) at 1200, 37.6°C (99.6°F) at 1600, and 38.3°C (100.9°F) at 2000. How would the nurse describe this pattern of temperature measurements?
   1. Usual range of circadian rhythm measurements
   2. Sustained fever pattern
   3. Intermittent fever pattern
   4. Resolving fever pattern

4. A patient presents in the clinic with dizziness and fatigue. The assistive personnel (AP) reports a slow but regular radial pulse of 44. Place the following care activities in priority order.
   1. Have AP obtain a blood pressure.
   2. Request that the patient lie on the clinical stretcher.
   3. Assess the patient's apical pulse for a full minute.
   4. Prepare to administer cardiac-stimulating medications as ordered.
   5. Obtain oxygen saturation (SpO$_2$).
5. Which of the following patients are at most risk for tachypnea? (Select all that apply.)
   1. Patient just admitted with four rib fractures
   2. Woman who is 9 months pregnant
   3. A patient admitted with hypothermia
   4. Postoperative patient waking from general anesthesia
   5. Three-pack–per-day smoker with pneumonia
6. Which number marks the location where the nurse would auscultate the point of maximal impulse (PMI)?
   1. 1
   2. 2
   3. 3
   4. 4
   5. 5
   6. 6

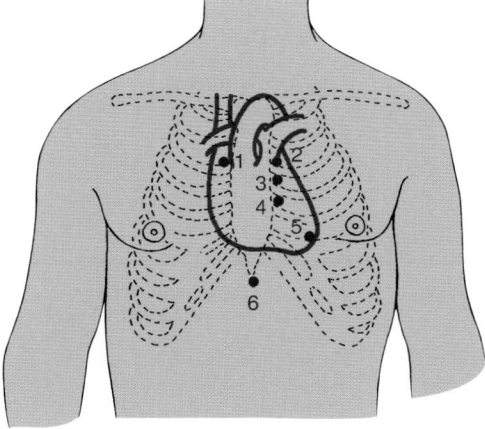

7. During admission of an obese patient with heart failure the assistive personnel (AP) reports to the nurse that the blood pressure (BP) is 140/76 on the left arm and 128/72 on the right arm. What actions do you take on the basis of this information? (Select all that apply.)
   1. Notify the health care provider immediately.
   2. Repeat the measurements on both arms using a stethoscope.

3. Ask the patient whether she has taken her blood pressure medications recently.
   4. Obtain blood pressure measurements on lower extremities.
   5. Review the patient's record for her baseline vital signs.
8. The assistive personnel (AP) informs the nurse that the electronic blood pressure machine on the patient who has recently returned from surgery after removal of her gallbladder is flashing a blood pressure of 65/46 and alarming. Place the care activities in priority order.
   1. Press the start button of the electronic blood pressure machine to obtain a new reading.
   2. Obtain a manual blood pressure with a stethoscope.
   3. Check the patient's pulse distal to the blood pressure cuff.
   4. Assess the patient's mental status.
   5. Remind the patient not to bend her arm with the blood pressure cuff.
9. A healthy adult patient tells the nurse that he obtained his blood pressure in "one of those quick machines in the mall" and was alarmed that it was 152/72. He immediately repeated the measurement, and the value was 158/80. His normal BP value ranges from 114/72 to 118/78. The nurse obtains a blood pressure of 116/76. What would account for the blood pressure of 152/72? (Select all that apply.)
   1. Cuff too small on the device
   2. Arm positioned above heart level
   3. Slow inflation of the cuff by the machine
   4. Patient did not remove his long-sleeved shirt
   5. Insufficient time between measurements
10. A patient with heart failure is one-day postoperative for major abdominal surgery. When the nurse and the assistive personnel raise the head of the bed to sit the patient on the side of the bed before ambulation, the patient immediately complains of dizziness and nausea. What are your immediate actions? (Select all that apply.)
    1. Lower the head of the bed and return the patient to the supine position.
    2. Obtain vital signs.
    3. Encourage the patient to try to sit on the side of the bed and then stand.
    4. Allow the patient to rest for 20 to 30 minutes.
    5. Raise the head of the bed again and obtain blood pressure readings.

Answers: 1. 1, 2, 3, 4; **2.** 1, 4, 2, 3; **3.** 4, 2, 1, 3, 5, 4; **4.** 5, 1, 2, 5; **6.** 5; **7.** 2, 5; **8.** 4, 1, 3, 2, 5; **9.** 1, 4, 5; **10.** 1, 2, 4, 5.

Rationales for Review Questions can be found on the Evolve website.

REFERENCES

AACN Practice Alert: Obtaining accurate noninvasive blood pressure measurements in adults, *Crit Care Nurse* 36(3):e12, 2016. https://www.aacn.org/clinical-resources/practice-alerts/obtaining-accurate-noninvasive-blood-pressure-measurements-in-adults. Accessed June 2020.

Agency for Healthcare Research and Quality (AHRQ): *Teach-Back: intervention. Quick start guide full page*, Rockville, MD, March 2020, Agency for Healthcare Research and Quality. https://www.ahrq.gov/health-literacy/quality-resources/tools/literacy-toolkit/healthlittoolkit2-tool5.html.

American Heart Association (AHA): *More than half of all African-Americans have high blood pressure under new diagnostic guidelines*, 2017a. https://www.heart.org/en/news/2018/05/01/more-than-half-of-all-african-americans-have-high-blood-pressure-under-new-diagnostic-guidelines. Accessed August 2020.

American Heart Association (AHA): *High blood pressure and African Americans*, 2016. https://www.heart.org/en/health-topics/high-blood-pressure/why-high-blood-pressure-is-a-silent-killer/high-blood-pressure-and-african-americans. Accessed August 2020.

American Heart Association (AHA): *Monitoring your blood pressure at home*, 2017b. https://www.heart.org/en/health-topics/high-blood-pressure/understanding-blood-pressure-readings/monitoring-your-blood-pressure-at-home. Accessed August 2020.

American Heart Association (AHA): *Target heart rates chart*, 2021. https://www.heart.org/en/healthy-living/fitness/fitness-basics/target-heart-rates. Accessed July 2021.

Brown JL, et al: Considerations for accurate blood pressure measurement in clinical care and research, *J Vasc Nurs* 37(4):274, 2019.

Burchum JR, Rosenthal LD: *Lehne's pharmacology for nursing care*, ed 10, St. Louis, 2019, Elsevier.

Centers for Disease Control and Prevention (CDC): *Know your risk for high blood pressure*, 2020. https://www.cdc.gov/bloodpressure/risk_factors.htm?CDC_AA_refVal5https%3A%2F%2Fwww.cdc.gov%2Fbloodpressure%2Ffamily_history.htm. Accessed June 2020

Centers for Disease Control and Prevention (CDC): *What is health literacy*, 2021. https://www.cdc.gov/healthliteracy/learn/index.html. Accessed October 2021.

Drawz P: Clinical implications of different blood pressure measurement techniques, *Curr Hypertens Rep* 19:54, 2017.

Hale G, et al: Treatment of primary orthostatic hypotension, *Ann Pharmacother* 51(5):417, 2017.

Hifumi T, et al: Heat stroke, *J Intensive Care* 6:30, 2018. https://www.ncbi.nlm.nih.gov/pmc/articles/PMC5964884/.

Hockenberry MJ, et al: *Wong's nursing care of infants and children*, ed 11, St. Louis, 2019, Elsevier.

Institute for Healthcare Improvement (IHI): *Early Warning Systems: scorecards that save lives*, 2020. http://www.ihi.org/resources/Pages/ImprovementStories/EarlyWarningSystemsScorecardsThatSaveLives.aspx. Accessed June 2020.

James P, et al: Evidence-based guideline for the management of high blood pressure in adults: report from the panel members appointed to the Eighth Joint National Committee (JNC8), *JAMA* 311:507, 2014.

Kelly C: Respiratory rate 1: why accurate measurement and recording are crucial, *Nurs Times* 114(4):23, 2018.

Lamberti J: Respiratory monitoring in general care units, *Respir Care* 65(6):870, 2020.

Mason T, et al: Equivalence study of two temperature-measurement methods in febrile adult patients with cancer, *Oncol Nurs Forum* 44(2):e82, 2017.

Mayo Clinic: *Exercise intensity: how to measure it*, 2019a, Mayo Foundation for Medical Education and Research. https://www.mayoclinic.org/healthy-lifestyle/fitness/in-depth/exercise-intensity/art-20046887. Accessed August 2020.

Mayo Clinic: *Fever: first aid*, 2019b. https://www.mayoclinic.org/first-aid/first-aid-fever/basics/art-20056685. Accessed August 2020.

Mechem A: *Severe nonexertional hyperthermia (classic heat stroke) in adults*, 2019, UpToDate. https://www.uptodate.com/contents/severe-nonexertional-hyperthermia-classic-heat-stroke-in-adults. Accessed August 2020.

Medical Environment Update: Get the alcohol out: your stethoscopes are dirtier than you think they are, *Med Environ Update* 29(2):7, 2019.

Medicines and Healthcare Products Regulatory Agency (MHRA): *Blood pressure measurement devices*, 2019. https://assets.publishing.service.gov.uk/government/uploads/system/uploads/attachment_data/file/841944/BP_monitoring_2019_v2.2.pdf. Accessed June 2020.

Mickley J, et al: Pilot application of varied equipment and procedural techniques to determine clinical blood pressure measurements, *J Diagn Med Sonogr* 34(6):447–447, 2018.

Mogensen C, et al: Forehead or ear temperature measurement cannot replace rectal measurements, except for screening purposes, *BMC Pediatr* 18(1):15, 2018a. doi:10118/s12887-018-0994-1.

Mogensen C, et al: Ear measurement of temperature is only useful for screening for fever in an adult emergency department, *BMC Emerg Med* 18(1):51, 2018b.

Moughrabi S: Nonadherence to hypertensive medications in African American adolescents, *Pediatr Nurs* 43:223, 2017.

Muntner P, et al: American Heart Association Scientific Statement: Measurement of blood pressure in humans, *Hypertension* 73:e35–e66, 2019.

Pagana DK, et al: *Mosby's diagnostic & laboratory test reference*, ed 14, St. Louis, 2019, Elsevier.

Palma J, Kaufmann H: *Mechanisms, causes, and evaluation of orthostatic hypotension*, 2021, UpToDate. https://www.uptodate.com/contents/mechanisms-causes-and-evaluation-of-orthostatic-hypotension. Accessed July 2021.

Peiris AN, et al: Heat stroke, *JAMA* 318(24):2503, 2017.

Reckelhoff JF: Gender differences in hypertension, *Curr Opin Nephrol Hypertens* 27(3):176, 2018.

Rolfe S: The importance of respiratory rate monitoring, *Br J Nurs* 228(8):504–508, 2019. doi:10.12968/bjon.2019.28.8.504.

Seattle Children's Hospital: *Fever-how to take the temperature*, 2020. https://www.seattlechildrens.org/conditions/a-z/fever-how-to-take-the-temperature/. Accessed June 2020.

Seifi S, et al: Accuracy of pulse oximetry in detection of oxygen saturation in patients admitted to the intensive care unit of heart surgery: comparison of finger, toe, forehead and earlobe probes, *BMC Nurs* 17:15, 2018. doi:10.1186/s12912-018-0283-1.

Shields S, et al: Orthostatic vital signs assessment for reducing falls, *MEDSURG Nurs* 29(3):169, 2020.

The Joint Commission (TJC): *2021 National Patient Safety Goals*, Oakbrook Terrace, IL, 2021, The Commission. http://www.jointcommission.org/standards/national-patient-safety-goals/. Accessed July 2021.

Thomas G, Pohl MA: *Blood pressure measurement in the diagnosis and management of hypertension in adults*, 2020, UpToDate. https://www.uptodate.com/contents/blood-pressure-measurement-in-the-diagnosis-and-management-of-hypertension-in-adults. Accessed August 15, 2020.

Wang X, et al: How to evaluate BP measurements using the oscillometric method in atrial fibrillation: the value of pulse rate variation, *Hypertens Res* 39:588, 2016.

Ward MA: *Patient education: fever in children (beyond the basics)*, 2020, UpToDate. https://www.uptodate.com/contents/fever-in-children-beyond-the-basics. Accessed August 15, 2020.

Zafren K, Mechem CC: *Accidental hypothermia in adults*, 2020, UpToDate. https://www.uptodate.com/contents/accidental-hypothermia-in-adults. Accessed August 15, 2020.

RESEARCH REFERENCES

Bijur P, et al: Temperature measurement in the adult emergency department: oral, tympanic membrane and temporal artery temperatures versus rectal temperature, *Emerg Med J* 33:843, 2016.

Brabrand M, et al: Measurement of respiratory rate by multiple raters in a clinical setting is unreliable: a cross-sectional simulation study, *J Crit Care* 44:404, 2018.

Daw W, et al: Poor inter-observer agreement in the measurement of respiratory rate in children: a prospective observational study, *BMJ Paediatr Open* 1:e000173, 2017.

Elliott M, Baird J: Pulse oximetry and the enduring neglect of respiratory rate assessment: a commentary on patient surveillance, *Br J Nurs* 28(19):1256, 2019.

Fei K, et al: Racial and ethnic subgroup disparities in hypertension prevalence, New York City Health and Nutrition Examination Survey, 2013–2014, *Prev Chronic Dis* 14:160478, 2017. https://www.cdc.gov/pcd/issues/2017/16_0478.htm. Accessed August 15, 2020.

Flynn JT, et al: Clinical practice guideline for screening and management of high blood pressure in children and adolescents, *Pediatrics* 140(3):e20171904, 2017. http://pediatrics.aappublications.org/content/140/3/e20171904. Accessed August 15, 2020.

Frenkel A, et al: Estimations of a degree of steroid induced leukocytosis in patients with acute infections, *Am J Emerg Med* 36(5):749, 2018.

Hill A, et al: The effects of awareness and count duration on adult respiratory rate measurements: an experimental study, *J Clin Nurs* 27:546, 2018.

Kallioinen N, et al: Sources of inaccuracy in the measurement of adult patients' resting blood pressure in clinical settings: a systematic review, *J Hypertens* 35:421, 2017.

Kiekkas P, et al: Temporal artery thermometry in pediatric patients: systematic review and meta-analysis, *J Pediatr Nurs* 46:89–99, 2019.

Koczulla A, et al: Long-term oxygen therapy, *Dtsch Arztebl Int* 115(51–52):871, 2018.

Marcos PS, et al: Comparative assessment of the effectiveness of three disinfection protocols for reducing bacterial contamination of stethoscopes, *Infect Control Hosp Epidemiol* 41:120, 2019.

Ringrose J, et al: Patient perceptions of ambulatory blood pressure monitoring testing, tolerability, accessibility, and expense, *J Clin Hypertens* 22(1):16, 2020.

Ringrose J, et al: The effect of back and feet support on oscillometric blood pressure measurements, *Blood Press Monit* 22(4):213, 2017.

Schimanski K, et al: Comparison study of upper arm and forearm non-invasive blood pressures in adult emergency department patients, *Int J Nurs Stud* 51(12):1575, 2014.

Shaw BH, et al: Relationship between orthostatic hypotension, frailty, falling and mortality in elderly care home residents, *BMC Geriatr* 19(1):1, 2019.

Takayama A, et al: A comparison of methods to count breathing frequency, *Respir Care* 64(5):555, 2019.

Whelton PL, et al: Guideline for the prevention, detection, evaluation, and management of high blood pressure in adults, *J Am Coll Cardiol* 71(19):2199, 2018.

Zhang X, et al: Evidence-based nursing practice on the influences of different clothing thicknesses on blood pressure measurement of patients, *Clin Nurs Res* 33(13):2198, 2019.

Health Assessment and Physical Examination

- Explain the rationale for understanding the purpose of a physical assessment.
- Explain how cultural diversity influences a nurse's approach in performing a health assessment.
- List techniques for preparing a patient physically and psychologically before and during an examination.
- Explain interview techniques used to enhance communication during history taking.
- Plan environmental preparations before an examination.
- Identify data to collect from the nursing history before an examination.
- Demonstrate the techniques used with each physical assessment skill.

- Discuss normal physical findings in a young, middle-age, and older adult.
- Propose ways to incorporate health promotion and health teaching into an examination.
- Use physical assessment skills during routine nursing care.
- Summarize physical measurements made in assessing each body system.
- Identify self-screening examinations commonly performed by patients.
- Identify preventive screenings and the appropriate age(s) for each screening to occur.

KEY TERMS

Adventitious sounds
Alopecia
Aphasia
Apical impulse or point of maximal impulse (PMI)
Arcus senilis
Atrophied
Auscultation
Borborygmi
Bruit
Cerumen
Clubbing
Conjunctivitis
Distention
Dysrhythmia
Ectropion
Edema

Entropion
Erythema
Excoriation
Goniometer
Hypertonicity
Hypotonicity
Indurated
Inspection
Jaundice
Kyphosis
Lordosis
Malignancy
Murmurs
Nystagmus
Olfaction
Orthopnea
Osteoporosis

Ototoxicity
Palpation
Percussion
Peristalsis
PERRLA
Petechiae
Polyps
Ptosis
Scoliosis
Stenosis
Striae
Syncope
Thrill
Turgor
Ventricular gallop
Vocal or tactile fremitus

MEDIA RESOURCES

- Review Questions
- Audio Glossary
- Case Study with Questions

- Video Clips
- Content Updates
- Answers to QSEN Activity and Review Questions

Completing a health assessment and physical examination is an important step toward providing safe and competent nursing care. The nurse is in a unique position to determine each patient's current health status, distinguish variations from the norm, and recognize improvements or deterioration in the patient's condition. Nurses apply clinical judgment when they recognize cues and interpret assessment findings related to each patient's behavioral and physical presentation. You perform health assessments and physical examinations to identify health patterns and evaluate each patient's response to treatments and therapies.

You gather assessment data about patients' past and current health conditions in a variety of ways, using a comprehensive or focused approach, depending on the patient situation. Nurses perform assessments at health fairs, at screening clinics, in a health provider's office, in acute care agencies, or in patients' homes. Depending on the outcome of an assessment, a nurse considers evidence-based recommendations for care based on a patient's preferences and values, the health provider's clinical expertise, or personal experience.

A complete health assessment involves a nursing history (see Chapter 16) and behavioral and physical examination. Through the health history interview you gather subjective data about a patient's condition. Objective data are obtained while observing a patient's behavior and overall presentation. The data collected during the history help to focus your physical examination appropriately. Gather additional objective data through a head-to-toe body system review during the physical examination, focusing on problem areas. You make clinical judgments based on all the gathered data to create an individualized plan of care for each situation. With accurate data you create a patient-centered care plan, identifying the nursing diagnoses, desired patient outcomes, and nursing interventions.

PURPOSES OF THE PHYSICAL EXAMINATION

Nurses conduct physical examinations for many reasons, such as an initial evaluation in triage for emergency care; for routine screening to promote wellness behaviors and preventive health care measures; to determine eligibility for health insurance, military service, or a new job; or to admit a patient to a hospital or long-term care facility. After considering a patient's current condition, a nurse selects a focused physical examination on a specific system or area. For example, when a patient is having a severe asthma episode, the nurse first focuses on the pulmonary and cardiovascular systems so that treatments can begin immediately. When the patient is no longer at risk for a poor outcome or injury, the nurse performs a more comprehensive examination of the other body systems.

For patients who are hospitalized, a nurse integrates the collection of physical assessment data during routine patient care, validating findings with what is known about the patient's health history. For example, on entering a patient's room a nurse may notice behavioral patient cues that indicate sadness or may observe swallowing difficulties while administering medications. Use the physical examination to do the following:

- Gather baseline data about a patient's health status.
- Supplement, confirm, or refute subjective data obtained.
- Identify and confirm nursing diagnoses.
- Make clinical decisions about a patient's changing health status and management.
- Evaluate the outcomes of care.

Cultural Sensitivity

Respect the cultural differences among patients from a variety of backgrounds when completing an examination. It is important to remember that cultural differences influence patient behaviors. Consider the patient's health beliefs, use of alternative therapies, nutritional habits, relationships with family, and comfort with physical closeness during the examination and history. These factors will affect both your approach and the type of findings you might expect.

Be culturally aware and avoid stereotyping based on gender, race, education, or other cultural factors. There is a difference between cultural and physical characteristics. Learn to recognize common characteristics and disorders among members of ethnic populations within the community (Giger and Haddad, 2021). It is equally important to recognize variations in physical characteristics, such as in the skin and musculoskeletal system. Recognize the impact of cultural difference in racial and ethnic aspects. Be aware of cultural humility

and recognize your own knowledge deficits related to different cultures. Consider how the illness may affect the patient, adaptations that may be needed for the physical assessment, mode of communication, health beliefs and practices, familial relationships, and nutritional practices (Ball et al., 2019). By addressing cultural diversity, you show respect for each patient's uniqueness, leading to higher-quality care and improved clinical outcomes (see Chapter 9).

PREPARATION FOR EXAMINATION

Physical examination is a routine and integral part of a patient assessment. In many care settings a head-to-toe physical assessment is required daily. You perform a reassessment when a patient's condition changes and as it improves or worsens. In some health care settings, such as during a home health visit, a focused physical examination is preferred. A proper physical examination will take into consideration cultural aspects, infection control, preparation of the environment, patient position, age of the patient, equipment, and explanation of assessment procedures. This will provide a smooth physical examination with few interruptions. A disorganized approach could cause errors and incomplete findings. Safety for patients who are confused should be a priority; never leave a patient who is confused or combative alone during an examination.

Infection Control

Some patients present with open skin lesions, infected wounds, or other communicable diseases. Use Standard Precautions throughout an examination (see Chapter 28). When an open sore or microorganism is present, wear gloves to reduce contact with contaminants. If a patient has excessive drainage or there is a risk of splashing from a wound, use additional personal protective equipment, such as an isolation gown or eye shield. Follow the agency's hand hygiene policies before initiating and after completing a physical assessment.

Although most health care agencies make nonlatex gloves available, it is your responsibility to identify latex allergies in patients and use equipment items that are latex free. By recognizing risk factors for latex allergies, patients remain free of a natural rubber latex (NRL) allergy. Three types of allergic responses appear with NRL. The most immediate is an immunological reaction. This is a type I response, for which the body develops antibodies known as *immunoglobulin E* that can lead to an anaphylactic response. The second is type IV (delayed-type) hypersensitivity, which is T cell mediated and appears 6 to 48 hours after exposure (Harding et al., 2020). Irritant contact dermatitis is a nonallergic reaction and presents with dry, irritated, or fissured skin. The severity of the response varies among individuals. Table 30.1 provides a short list of products that contain latex and suggests available alternatives.

Environment

A respectful, considerate physical examination requires privacy. In the acute setting nurses perform assessments in a patient's room, whereas examination rooms are used in clinics or offices. In the home the examination is performed in a space where privacy can be established, such as the patient's bedroom.

Examination spaces need to be well equipped for any procedures. Adequate lighting is necessary to properly illuminate body parts. The hospital room can be secured for privacy so that patients are comfortable discussing their condition. Eliminate extra noise and take precautions to prevent interruptions from others. The room must be warm enough to maintain comfort.

Depending on the body part being assessed, it may be difficult to perform a selected assessment skill when a patient is in bed or on a stretcher. Special examination tables make positioning easier and body

TABLE 30.1 Products Containing Latex and Nonlatex Substitutes[a]

Products Containing Latex	Nonlatex Substitutes
Medical Equipment	
Disposable gloves	Vinyl, nitrile, or neoprene gloves
Blood pressure cuffs	Covered cuffs
Stethoscope tubing	Covered tubing
Intravenous injection ports	Needleless system, stopcocks, covered latex ports
Tourniquets	Latex-free or cloth-covered tourniquets
Syringes	Glass syringes
Adhesive tape	Nonlatex tapes
Oral and nasal airways	Nonlatex tubes
Endotracheal tubes	Hard plastic tubes
Catheters	Silicone catheters
Eye goggles	Silicone eye goggles
Anesthesia masks	Silicone masks
Respirators	Nonlatex respirators
Rubber aprons	Cloth-covered aprons
Wound drains	Silicone drains
Medication vial stoppers	Stoppers removed
Household Items	
Rubber bands	String; latex-free bands
Erasers	Silicone erasers
Motorcycle and bicycle handgrips	Handgrips removed or covered
Carpeting	Other types of flooring
Swimming goggles	Silicone construction
Shoe soles	Leather shoes
Expandable fabric (e.g., waistbands)	Fabric removed or covered
Dishwashing gloves	Vinyl gloves
Condoms	Nonlatex condoms
Diaphragms	Synthetic rubber diaphragms
Balloons	Mylar balloons
Pacifiers and baby bottle nipples	Silicone, plastic, or nonlatex pacifiers and nipples

[a]This is not a complete list but is intended to provide examples of products and alternatives.
Adapted from Ball JW, et al: *Mosby's guide to physical examination,* ed 9, St Louis, 2019, Elsevier; and U.S. National Library of Medicine Medline Plus: *Latex allergies: for hospital patients,* 2020. https://medlineplus.gov/ency/patientinstructions/000499.htm. Accessed August 27, 2020.

areas more easily accessible. By helping patients on and off examination tables, injury can be avoided. Examination tables can be uncomfortable; elevate the head of the table about 30 degrees. A small pillow helps with head and neck comfort. If the examination is completed in the patient room, raise the height of the patient's bed to be able to reach the patient more comfortably.

Equipment

Perform hand hygiene thoroughly before handling equipment and starting an examination. Arrange any necessary equipment so that it is

BOX 30.1 Equipment and Supplies for Physical Assessment

- Cervical brush or broom devices (if needed)
- Cotton applicators
- Disposable pad/paper towels
- Drapes/cover
- Eye chart (e.g., Snellen chart)
- Flashlight and spotlight
- Forms (e.g., physical, laboratory)
- Gown for patient
- Nonlatex gloves (clean)
- Ophthalmoscope
- Otoscope
- Papanicolaou (Pap) liquid preparation (if needed)
- Percussion (reflex) hammer
- Pulse oximeter
- Ruler
- Scale with height measurement rod
- Specimen containers, slides, wooden or plastic spatula, and cytological fixative (if needed)
- Sphygmomanometer and cuff
- Sterile swabs
- Stethoscope
- Tape measure
- Thermometer
- Tissues
- Tongue depressors
- Tuning fork
- Vaginal speculum (if needed)
- Water-soluble lubricant
- Watch with second hand or digital display

readily available and easy to use. Prepare equipment as appropriate (e.g., warm the diaphragm of the stethoscope between the hands before applying it to the skin). Be sure that equipment functions properly before using it (e.g., ensure that the ophthalmoscope and otoscope have good batteries and light bulbs). Box 30.1 lists typical equipment used during a physical examination.

Physical Preparation of the Patient

Show respect for a patient by ensuring that physical comfort needs, such as using the restroom, are met before starting the examination. An empty bladder and bowel facilitate a more comfortable examination of the abdomen, genitalia, and rectum. Collect urine or fecal specimens at this time if needed.

Physical preparation involves making certain that patient privacy is maintained with proper dress and draping. The patient in the hospital is probably wearing a hospital gown. In the clinic or health care provider's office the patient needs to undress and usually is provided a disposable paper cover or gown. If the examination is limited to certain body systems, it is not always necessary for the patient to undress completely. Provide the patient privacy and plenty of time to undress to lessen the patient's anxiety. After changing, the patient sits or lies down on the examination table with a light drape over the lap or lower trunk. Make sure that drafts are eliminated, temperature is controlled, and blankets are provided. Routinely ask whether the patient is comfortable.

Positioning. During the examination ask the patient to assume proper positions so that body parts are accessible and the patient stays comfortable. Table 30.2 lists the preferred positions for each part of the examination and contains figures illustrating the positions. Patients' abilities to assume positions depend on their physical strength, joint mobility, ease of breathing, age, and degree of wellness. After explaining a position, help the patient to assume it correctly. Take care to maintain respect and show consideration by adjusting the drapes so that only the area examined is accessible. During the examination, a patient may need to assume more than one position. To decrease the number of position changes, organize the examination so that all techniques requiring a sitting position are completed first, followed by those that require a supine position next, and so forth. Use extra care when positioning older adults with disabilities and limitations.

TABLE 30.2 Positions for Examination

Position	Areas Assessed	Rationale	Limitations
Sitting	Head and neck, back, posterior thorax and lungs, anterior thorax and lungs, breasts, axillae, heart, vital signs, and upper extremities	Sitting upright provides full expansion of lungs and better visualization of symmetry of upper body parts.	Physically weakened patient sometimes is unable to sit. Use supine position with head of bed elevated instead.
Supine	Head and neck, anterior thorax and lungs, breasts, axillae, heart, abdomen, extremities, pulses	This is normally a relaxed position. It provides easy access to pulse sites.	If patient becomes short of breath easily, raise head of bed.
Dorsal recumbent	Head and neck, anterior thorax and lungs, breasts, axillae, heart, abdomen	Position is for abdominal assessment because it promotes relaxation of abdominal muscles.	Patients with painful disorders are more comfortable with knees flexed.
Lithotomy[a]	Female genitalia and genital tract	Position with knees abducted provides maximal exposure of female genitalia and facilitates insertion of vaginal speculum.	Lithotomy position is embarrassing and uncomfortable; thus, examiner minimizes time that patient spends in it. Keep patient well draped.
Prone	Musculoskeletal system	Position is only for assessing extension of hip joint, skin, and buttocks.	Patients with respiratory difficulties do not tolerate this position well.
Lateral recumbent	Heart Rectum and Vagina	Side lying position aids in detecting murmurs. Flexion of hip and knee improves exposure of rectal and perineal area.	Patients with respiratory difficulties do not tolerate this position well. Joint deformities hinder patient's ability to bend hip and knee.
Knee-chest[a]	Rectum	Position provides maximal exposure of rectal area.	This position is embarrassing and uncomfortable.

[a]Some patients with arthritis or other joint deformities are unable to assume this position.

Psychological Preparation of a Patient

Many patients find an examination stressful or tiring, or they experience anxiety about possible findings. A thorough explanation of the purpose and steps of each assessment lets a patient know what to expect and how to cooperate. Adapt your explanations to the patient's level of understanding, and encourage questions and comment on any discomfort. Convey an open, professional approach while remaining relaxed. A quiet, formal demeanor inhibits a patient's ability to communicate, but a style that is too casual may cause doubt of an examiner's competence (Ball et al., 2019).

Consider cultural or social norms when performing an examination on a person of the opposite gender. When this situation occurs, another person of the patient's gender or a culturally approved family member needs to be in the room. By taking this step you demonstrate cultural awareness for a patient's individual needs. As a side benefit, the second person acts as a witness to the conduct of the examiner and the patient should any question arise.

During the examination watch the patient's emotional responses by observing whether the patient's facial expressions show fear or concern or whether body movements indicate anxiety. When you remain calm, the patient is more likely to relax. Especially if the patient is weak or elderly, it is necessary to pace the examination, pausing at intervals to ask how the patient is tolerating the assessment. If the patient feels all right, the examination can proceed. However, do not force the patient to cooperate based on your schedule. Postpone the examination when needed; your findings may be more accurate when the patient can cooperate and relax.

Assessment of Age-Groups

Use different interview styles and approaches to physical examination for patients of different age-groups. When assessing children, show sensitivity and anticipate a child's perception of the examination as a strange and unfamiliar experience. Routine pediatric examinations focus on health promotion and illness prevention, particularly for well children who receive competent parenting and have no serious health problems (Hockenberry and Wilson, 2019). This examination focuses on growth and development, sensory screening, dental examination, and behavioral assessment. When examining children, the following tips help in data collection:

- Gather all or part of the history on infants and children from parents or guardians. Use open-ended questions to allow parents to share more information and describe more of the children's situation. This will allow observation of parent-child interactions. Older children can be interviewed and provide details about their health history and severity of symptoms.
- Gain a child's trust before doing any type of an examination. Perform the examination in a nonthreatening area. Talk and play with the child first. Do the visual parts of the examination before touching the child. Start the examination from the periphery and then move to the center (e.g., start with the extremities before moving to the chest).
- Because parents sometimes think the examiner is testing them, offer support during the examination and do not pass judgment.
- Call children by their first names and address the parents as "Mr.," "Mrs.," or "Ms." rather than by their first names unless instructed differently.
- Treat adolescents as adults and individuals because they tend to respond best when treated as such. Remember that adolescents have the right to confidentiality. After talking with parents about historical information, speak alone with adolescents.

A comprehensive health assessment and examination of older adults includes physical data; family relationships; religious and occupational pursuits; and a review of the patient's cognitive, affective, and social level. An important aspect is to assess the patient's ability to perform basic activities of daily living (e.g., bathing, grooming) and complex instrumental activities of daily living (e.g., making a phone call).

Throughout an examination, recognize that older adults often present with subtle or atypical signs and symptoms (Touhy and Jett, 2020). Principles to follow during examination of an older adult include the following:

- Do not stereotype about aging patients' level of cognition. Most older adults are reliable historians and can adapt to change and learn about their health.
- Recognize that some older adults have sensory or physical limitations that affect how quickly they can be interviewed and examinations can be conducted. It might be necessary to plan for more than one examination session. Sometimes it helps to give patients an initial health questionnaire before they come to a clinic or office.
- Perform the examination with adequate space; this is especially important for patients with mobility aids such as a cane or walker.
- During the examination use patience, allow for pauses, and observe for details. Let patients tell their stories and explore any symptoms or problems they reveal. Recognize normal physiological and behavioral changes that are characteristic of later life.
- Giving certain types of health information is stressful for older patients. Some view illness as a threat to independence and a step toward institutionalization.

- Be aware of the location of the closest bathroom in case the patient has an urgent need to eliminate.
- Be alert to signs of increasing fatigue, such as sighing, grimacing, irritability, leaning against objects for support, and drooping head and shoulders.

> ### REFLECT NOW
>
> As the nurse preparing to begin the physical examination, verbalize your opening statement to your older-adult patient. Reflect on your knowledge of culture, aging, and developing a safe environment of trust. What nursing strategies should you use during the physical examination?

ORGANIZATION OF THE EXAMINATION

Assess each body system during a physical examination. Use judgment to ensure that an examination is relevant and includes the correct assessments. Patients with focused symptoms or needs require only parts of an examination—for example, when a patient comes to a clinic with symptoms of a severe chest cold, a neurological assessment is not usually required. When a patient is admitted to the hospital, you perform a complete examination at the time of admission and at least once each day to maintain and monitor the patient's baseline. Agency guidelines may define the components of a complete examination (see agency policy). A patient in the community seeks screening for specific conditions, often dependent on the age or health risks listed in Table 30.3.

Follow a systematic routine when you perform a physical examination to avoid missing important findings. A head-to-toe approach includes all body systems, and the examiner recalls and performs each step in a predetermined order. For an adult, the examination begins with an assessment of the head and neck and progresses methodically down the body to incorporate all body systems. The following tips help keep an examination well organized:

- Compare both sides of the body for symmetry. A degree of asymmetry is occasionally normal (e.g., the biceps muscles in the dominant arm are sometimes more developed than the same muscles in the nondominant arm).
- If the patient is seriously ill, first assess the systems of the body most at risk for being abnormal. For example, complete a cardiovascular assessment first when caring for a patient with chest pain.
- If the patient becomes fatigued, offer rest periods between assessments.
- Perform painful procedures near the end of an examination.
- Record assessments in specific terms in the electronic or paper record. A standard form allows for recording information in the same sequence in which it is gathered.
- Use common and accepted medical terms and abbreviations to keep notes accurate, brief, and concise.
- Record quick notes during the examination to avoid delays. DO NOT conduct the examination from the computer terminal by simply asking patient questions; focus on the correct hands-on examination techniques. Complete any larger documentation notes at the end of the examination.

TECHNIQUES OF PHYSICAL ASSESSMENT

The four techniques used in a physical examination are inspection, palpation, percussion, and auscultation.

Inspection

To inspect, carefully look, listen, and smell to distinguish normal from abnormal findings. To do so, you must be aware of any personal visual,

TABLE 30.3   Recommended Preventive Screenings

Disease or Condition	Age-Group	Screening Measures
Breast cancer[a] (women at average risk)	Ages 40–44	Should have the choice to start annual breast cancer screening with mammograms if they wish to do so. The risks of screening as well as the potential benefits should be considered.
		Monthly breast self-examination (BSE) dependent on health care provider recommendations (not recommended by ACS).
	Ages 45–54	Monthly BSE dependent on health care provider recommendations (not recommended by ACS).
		Should get mammogram every year.
	Ages 55 and older	Should switch to mammograms every 2 years or have the choice to continue yearly screening.
		Women with a personal history of breast cancer, a family history of breast cancer, a genetic mutation known to increase the risk of breast cancer (such as *BRCA*), and women who have had radiation therapy to the chest before the age of 30 are at a higher risk for breast cancer, not average risk. These women require earlier and more extensive screening.
Colon/rectal cancer[b]	Ages 45 and older	Men and women need to have one of the following sensitive tests that look for signs of cancer: fecal occult blood test (FOBT) or flexible sigmoidoscopy (FSIG) or colonoscopy. Earlier screening is necessary if risk factors exist.
Ear disorders	All ages	Periodic hearing checks as needed.
	Over age 65	Regular hearing checks.
Eye disorders	Age 40 and under	Complete eye examination every 3–5 years (more if positive history for eye disease [e.g., diabetes mellitus]).
	Ages 40–64	Complete eye examination every 2 years to screen for conditions that may go unnoticed (e.g., glaucoma). Annual eye examinations if patient has diabetes mellitus.
	Age 65 and older	Complete eye examination every year.
Heart/vascular disorders	Men ages 45–65	Regular measurement of total blood cholesterol levels, lipids, and triglycerides; blood pressure screenings. (If patient has risk factors for coronary artery disease [CAD], blood pressure screening needs to begin at age 20–35 for men, 20–45 for women.)
	Women ages 45–65	
Obesity	All ages	Periodic height and weight measurements.
Oral cavity/pharyngeal disorders/cancer	All ages (children, adults, older adults)	Regular dental examinations every 6 months.
Ovarian cancer[c]	Age 18 and up or on becoming sexually active	Annual pelvic examinations by health care provider. (This screening rarely detects ovarian cancer unless it is in its advanced stage. Those at high risk need to have a thorough pelvic examination, a transvaginal ultrasound, and a blood test [tumor marker CA 125]) (ACS, 2020b).
Prostate cancer[b]	Age 50 and up	Men who have at least a 10-year life expectancy need to have a digital rectal examination (DRE) and prostate-specific antigen (PSA) blood test annually. Men at high risk require earlier screening.
Skin cancer[b]	Ages 20–40	See specialist every 3 years.
	Over 40	Annual skin checkups with biopsy of suspicious lesions.
Testicular cancer[b]	Age 15 and up	Monthly testicular self-examination (TSE).
Uterine cancer[b,d]	Screening begins 3 years after having vaginal intercourse but not later than age 21	Annual pelvic examination by health care provider plus annual Papanicolaou (Pap) test.[d]
Cervical cancer[e]	An annual Pap test is no longer recommended by the American Cancer Society (ACS, 2020b).	
	Ages 21–29	Pelvic examination by health care provider plus Pap test with cytology every 3 years; human papillomavirus (HPV) needed only if Pap test result is abnormal (ACS, 2020b).
	Ages 30–65	Preferred screening is with a Pap test combined with an HPV test every 5 years. This is called co-testing (ACS, 2020b).
	Over 65	No testing needed if previous regular testing was competed and normal. If at high risk for cervical cancer or previous incidence, then screening should be continued (ACS, 2020b).
Endometrial cancer	Same as for cervical cancer	Endometrial biopsy at age 35 for high-risk patients (those with or at risk for hereditary nonpolyposis colon cancer [HNPCC]). (At menopause women at average and high risk need to be informed about signs and symptoms to report.)

ACS, American Cancer Society.
[a]Data from American Cancer Society (ACS): *Breast cancer early detection and diagnosis,* 2021. https://www.cancer.org/cancer/breast-cancer/screening-tests-and-early-detection/american-cancer-society-recommendations-for-the-early-detection-of-breast-cancer.html , 2021. Accessed July 12, 2021.
[b]American Cancer Society (ACS): *Cancer A-Z,* n.d. https://www.cancer.org/cancer.html. Accessed August 27, 2020.
[c]Data from American Cancer Society (ACS): *Can ovarian cancer be found early?* 2020, https://www.cancer.org/cancer/ovarian-cancer/detection-diagnosis-staging/detection.html?_ga=2.29301694.34924562.1540912089-41350218.1539106062. Accessed August 27, 2020.
[d]Data from American Cancer Society (ACS): *Uterine sarcoma early detection, diagnosis, and staging,* 2020. https://www.cancer.org/cancer/uterine-sarcoma/detection-diagnosis-staging/detection.html. Accessed August 27, 2020.
[e]Data from American Cancer Society (ACS): *Screening tests for cervical cancer,* 2020. https://www.cancer.org/cancer/cervical-cancer/detection-diagnosis-staging/screening-tests.html. Accessed August 30, 2020.

TABLE 30.4 Assessment of Characteristic Odors

Odor	Site or Source	Potential Causes
Alcohol	Oral cavity	Ingestion of alcohol, diabetes mellitus
Ammonia	Urine	Urinary tract infection, renal failure
Body odor	Skin, particularly in areas where body parts rub together (e.g., underarms and under breasts)	Poor hygiene, excess perspiration (hyperhidrosis), foul-smelling perspiration (bromhidrosis)
	Wound site	Wound abscess
	Vomitus	Abdominal irritation, contaminated food
Feces	Vomitus/oral cavity (fecal odor)	Bowel obstruction
	Rectal area	Fecal incontinence
Foul-smelling stools in infant	Stool	Malabsorption syndrome
Halitosis	Oral cavity	Poor dental and oral hygiene, gum disease
Sweet, fruity ketones	Oral cavity	Diabetic acidosis
Stale urine	Skin	Uremic acidosis
Sweet, heavy, thick odor	Draining wound	*Pseudomonas* (bacterial) infection
Musty odor	Casted body part	Infection inside cast
Fetid, sweet odor	Tracheostomy or mucous secretions	Infection of bronchial tree (*Pseudomonas* bacteria)

hearing, or olfactory deficits. It is important to deliberately practice this skill and learn to recognize all the possible pieces of data that can be gathered through inspection alone. **Inspection** occurs when interacting with a patient, watching for nonverbal expressions of emotional and mental status, and assessing physical movements and structural components. Most important, be deliberate and pay attention to detail. Follow these guidelines to achieve the best results during inspection:

- Make sure that adequate lighting is available, either direct or indirect.
- Use a direct lighting source (e.g., a penlight or lamp) to inspect body cavities.
- Inspect each area for size, shape, color, symmetry, position, and abnormality.
- Position and expose body parts as needed so that all surfaces can be viewed but privacy can be maintained.
- When possible, check for side-to-side symmetry by comparing each area with its match on the opposite side of the body.
- Validate findings with the patient.

While assessing a patient, recognize the nature and source of body odors (Table 30.4). An unusual odor often indicates an underlying pathology. **Olfaction** helps to detect abnormalities. For example, when a patient's breath has a sweet, fruity odor, assess for signs of diabetes mellitus. Continue to inspect various parts of the body during the entire physical examination. Palpation may be used concurrently with inspection, or it may follow in a more deliberate fashion.

Palpation

Palpation involves using the sense of touch to gather information. Through touch you make judgments about expected and unexpected findings of the skin or underlying tissue, muscle, and bones. For example, you palpate the skin for temperature, moisture, texture, turgor, tenderness, and thickness and the abdomen for tenderness, distention, or masses. Use different parts of the hand to detect different characteristics (Table 30.5). The palmar surface of the hand and finger pads is more sensitive than the fingertips and is used to determine position, texture, size, consistency, masses, fluid, and crepitus (Fig. 30.1A). Assess body temperature by using the dorsal surface or back of the hand (Fig. 30.1B). Vibration is best felt on the palmar surface of the hand and fingers (Fig. 30.1C).

Touching a patient is a personal experience for both you and the patient. Display respect and concern throughout an examination. Before palpating consider the patient's condition and ability to tolerate the assessment techniques, paying close attention to areas that are painful or tender. In addition, always be conscious of the environment and any threats to the patient's safety.

Prepare for palpation by warming hands, keeping fingernails short, and using a gentle approach. Palpation proceeds slowly, gently, and deliberately. Encourage the patient to relax, and help the patient feel comfortable, because tense muscles make assessment more difficult. To promote relaxation, have the patient take slow, deep breaths and place both arms along the sides of the body. Ask the patient to point to more sensitive areas, watching for nonverbal signs of discomfort. *Palpate tender areas last.*

Two types of palpation, light and deep, are used for physical examination. Perform light palpation by placing the hand on the body part being examined; it also involves pressing inward about 1 cm (½ inch). Light, superficial palpation of structures such as the abdomen gives the patient the chance to identify areas of tenderness (Fig. 30.2A). Inquire about areas of tenderness and assess them further for potentially serious pathologies. Use deep palpation to examine the condition of organs such as those in the abdomen (Fig. 30.2B). Depress the area under examination approximately 4 cm (2 inches) (Ball et al., 2019), using one or both hands (bimanually). When using bimanual palpation, relax one hand (sensing hand) and place it lightly over the patient's skin. The other hand (active hand) helps apply pressure to the sensing hand. The lower hand does not exert pressure directly and thus remains sensitive to detect organ characteristics. For safety, deep palpation should be used with caution in a patient with discomfort in the area to be palpated.

Percussion

Percussion involves tapping the skin with the fingertips to vibrate underlying tissues and organs. The vibration travels through body tissues, and the character of the resulting sound reflects the density of the underlying tissue. The denser the tissue, the quieter is the sound. By knowing how various densities influence sound, it is possible to locate organs or masses, map their edges, and determine their size. An abnormal sound from what is expected in that area suggests a mass or substance such as air or fluid

TABLE 30.5   Examples of Characteristics Measured by Palpation

Area Examined	Criteria Measured	Portion of Hand to Use
Skin	Temperature	Dorsum of hand/fingers
	Moisture	Palmar surface
	Texture	Palmar surface
	Turgor and elasticity	Grasping with fingertips
	Tenderness	Finger pads/palmar surface of fingers
	Thickness	Palmar surface
Organs (e.g., liver and intestine)	Size	Entire palmar surface of hand or palmar surface of fingers
	Shape	
	Tenderness	
	Absence of masses	
Glands (e.g., thyroid and lymph)	Swelling	Pads of fingertips
	Symmetry and mobility	
Blood vessels (e.g., carotid, or femoral artery)	Pulse amplitude	Palmar surface/pads of fingertips
	Elasticity	
	Rate	
	Rhythm	
Thorax	Excursion	Palmar surface
	Tenderness	Finger pads/palmar surface of fingers
	Fremitus	Palmar or ulnar surface of entire hand

FIG. 30.1 (A) Radial pulse is detected with pads of fingertips, the most sensitive part of the hand. (B) Dorsum of hand detects temperature variations in skin. (C) Bony part of palm at base of fingers detects vibrations.

within an organ or body cavity. The skill of percussion is used more often by advanced practice nurses than by nurses in daily practice at the bedside.

Auscultation

Auscultation involves listening to sounds the body makes to detect variations from normal. Some sounds such as speech and coughing can be heard without additional equipment, but a stethoscope is necessary to hear internal body sounds.

Internal body sounds are created by blood, air, or gastric contents as they move against the body structures. For example, normal heart sounds are created when the heart valves close, moving blood to the next part of the cardiovascular system. Normal sounds for each body system are discussed later in this chapter. Learn to recognize abnormal sounds after learning normal variations. Becoming more proficient in auscultation occurs by knowing the types of sounds each body structure makes and the location in which the sounds are heard best.

To auscultate internal sounds, you need to hear well, have a good stethoscope, and know how to use it properly (see Chapter 29). Nurses

with hearing disorders can obtain stethoscopes with extra sound amplification. There are two aspects to the stethoscope. The bell is best for hearing low-pitched sounds such as vascular and certain heart sounds, and the diaphragm is best for listening to high-pitched sounds such as bowel and lung sounds.

By practicing with the stethoscope, you become proficient at using it and realize when sounds are clear and when there are extraneous sounds. Extraneous sounds created by rubbing against the tubing or chest piece interfere with auscultation of body organ sounds. By deliberately producing these sounds, you learn to recognize and disregard them during the actual examination. Box 30.2 lists ways to practice using the stethoscope and techniques for caring for the stethoscope. Describe any sound you hear using the following characteristics:

- Frequency indicates the number of sound wave cycles generated per second by a vibrating object. The higher the frequency, the higher the pitch of a sound, and vice versa.
- Loudness refers to the amplitude of a sound wave. Auscultated sounds range from soft to loud.

A

B

FIG. 30.2 (A) During light palpation, gentle pressure against underlying skin and tissues can detect areas of irregularity and tenderness. (B) During deep palpation, depress tissue to assess condition of underlying organs.

- Quality refers to sounds of similar frequency and loudness from different sources. Terms such as *blowing* or *gurgling* describe the quality of sound.
- Duration means the length of time that sound vibrations last. The duration of sound is short, medium, or long. Layers of soft tissue dampen the duration of sounds from deep internal organs.

Auscultation requires concentration and practice. While listening, know which sounds are expected in certain parts of the body and what causes the sounds. Expected sounds are discussed in each body system section of this chapter. After understanding the cause and character of normal auscultated sounds, it becomes easier to recognize abnormal sounds and their origins.

GENERAL SURVEY

When a patient first enters an examination room, observe the patient's walk and general appearance and be attentive to behavior and dress. A general survey of the patient's presentation and behavior provides information about characteristics of an illness, the patient's ability to function independently, body image, emotional state, recent changes in weight, and developmental status. If there are abnormalities or problems, assess the affected body system more closely during the full examination. As you explore any problem areas, allow patients to tell their stories of any symptoms. Open-ended questions encourage a full explanation of the symptom timeline and its effects on the patient's functioning.

General Appearance and Behavior

Assess appearance and behavior while preparing the patient for the examination. For this review include:
- *Gender and race:* A person's gender affects the type of examination performed and the order of the assessments. Different physical features are related to gender and race. Certain illnesses are more likely to affect a specific gender or race (e.g., the incidence of skin cancer is more common in Whites than in Blacks, the rate of prostate cancer is higher in Black men than in White men, and cancer

BOX 30.2 Use and Care of the Stethoscope

- Ensure that the earpiece follows the contour of the ear canals. Learn which fit is best for you by comparing amplification of sounds with the earpieces in both directions.
- Place the earpieces in your ears with the tips turned toward the face. *Lightly* blow into the diaphragm. Again, place the earpieces in your ears, this time with the ends turned toward the back of the head. *Lightly* blow into the diaphragm. You will find that you hear clearer sounds with the earpiece turned toward the face. After you have learned the right fit for the loudest amplification, wear the stethoscope the same way each time.
- Put on the stethoscope and *lightly* blow into the diaphragm. If the sound is barely audible, *lightly* blow into the bell. Sound is carried through only one part of the chest piece at a time. If the sound is greatly amplified through the diaphragm, the diaphragm is in position for use. If the sound is barely audible through the diaphragm, the bell is in position for use. Rotation of the diaphragm and bell places the chest piece in the desired position. Leave the diaphragm in position for the next exercise.
- Place the diaphragm over the anterior part of your chest. Ask a friend to speak in a normal conversational tone. Environmental noise seriously detracts from hearing the noise created by body organs. When using a stethoscope, the patient and the examiner need to remain quiet.
- Put on the stethoscope and gently tap the tubing. It is often difficult to avoid stretching or moving the stethoscope tubing. The examiner is in a position so that the tubing hangs free. Moving or touching the tubing creates extraneous sounds.
- *Care of the stethoscope:* Remove earpieces regularly and clean; remove cerumen (earwax). Keep the bell and diaphragm free of dust, lint, and body oils. Keep the tubing away from body oils. Avoid draping the stethoscope around the neck next to the skin. Clean daily or after soiling by wiping the entire stethoscope (e.g., diaphragm, tubing) with alcohol. Be sure to dry all parts thoroughly. Follow manufacturer recommendations.
- *Infection control:* Harmful bacteria such as gram-positive bacilli, methicillin-resistant *Staphylococcus aureus* (MRSA), non-*aureus Staphylococcus*, *Enterobacter cloacae,* and methicillin-sensitive *S. aureus* can be transferred from patient to patient when using portable equipment such as stethoscopes. Clean the stethoscope (diaphragm/bell) *before* reuse on another patient. Using a disinfectant such as isopropyl alcohol (with or without chlorhexidine), benzalkonium, or sodium hypochlorite is effective in reducing the number of bacterial colonies. Hand foam serves this purpose well. Earpieces of stethoscopes are sources of transferable bacteria. When you inadvertently touch your ears and care for the patient, potential pathogens could contaminate the earpieces. Using hand hygiene before and after patient contact decreases the risk of transmitting microorganisms from your ear to your patient. Follow the institution's infection control guidelines, especially Contact Precautions, to decrease this risk.

of the bladder occurs at a higher rate in men than in women) (American Cancer Society [ACS], 2020a).
- *Age:* Age influences normal physical characteristics and a person's ability to participate in some parts of the examination.
- *Signs of distress:* Sometimes obvious signs or symptoms indicate pain (grimacing, splinting painful area), difficulty breathing (shortness of breath, sternal retractions), or anxiety. Set priorities and examine the related physical areas first.
- *Body type:* Observe whether the patient appears trim and muscular, obese, or excessively thin. Body type reflects the level of health, age, and lifestyle.
- *Posture:* Normal standing posture shows an upright stance with parallel alignment of the hips and shoulders. Normal sitting posture

involves some degree of rounding of the shoulders. Observe whether the patient has a slumped, erect, or bent posture, which reflects mood or pain. Changes in older-adult physiology often result in a stooped, forward-bent posture, with the hips and knees somewhat flexed and the arms bent at the elbows.

- *Gait:* Observe as the patient walks into the room or stands at the bedside (if the patient is ambulatory). Note whether movements are coordinated or uncoordinated. A person normally walks smoothly, with the arms swinging freely at the sides, each leg moving through with a heel to toe placement, and the head and face leading the body. Note if the feet touch the floor correctly or is there any dragging of a foot.
- *Body movements:* Observe whether movements are purposeful, noting any tremors involving the extremities. Determine whether any body parts are immobile.
- *Hygiene and grooming:* Note the patient's level of cleanliness by observing the appearance of the hair, skin, and fingernails. Determine whether the clothes are clean. Grooming depends on the patient's cognitive and emotional function, daily or social activities, financial resources, and occupation. Observe for excessive use of cosmetics or colognes that could indicate a change in self-perception.
- *Dress:* Culture, lifestyle, socioeconomic level, and personal preference affect the selection and wearing of clothing. However, you assess whether the clothing is appropriate for the temperature, weather conditions, or setting. People who are depressed or mentally ill may not be able to select proper clothing, and an older adult might tend to wear extra clothing because of sensitivity to cold.
- *Body odor:* An unpleasant body odor can result from physical exercise, poor hygiene, or certain disease states. Validate any odors that might indicate a health problem.
- *Affect and mood:* Affect is how a person appears to others. Patients express mood or emotional state verbally and nonverbally. Determine whether verbal expressions match nonverbal behavior and whether the mood is appropriate for the situation. By maintaining eye contact you can observe facial expressions while asking questions.
- *Speech:* Normal speech is understandable and moderately paced and shows an association with the person's thoughts. However, emotion or neurological impairment sometimes causes rapid or slowed speech. Observe whether the patient speaks in a normal tone with clear inflection of words.
- *Signs of patient abuse:* During the examination observe whether the patient fears a spouse or partner, a caregiver, a parent, or an adult child. Abuse of children, women, and older adults is a growing health problem. Consider any obvious physical injury or neglect as a sign of possible abuse (e.g., evidence of malnutrition or presence of bruising on the extremities or trunk) (World Health Organization [WHO], 2021). Abuse occurs in many forms: physical, mental, emotional, sexual, social, and financial or economic. Observe the behavior of the individual for any signs of frustration, explanations that do not fit the physical presentation, or signs of injury. Most states mandate a report to a social service center when abuse or neglect is suspected (Box 30.3). It is difficult to detect abuse because victims often do not report that they are in abusive situations. If you suspect abuse, find a way to interview the patient in private; patients are more likely to reveal any problems when the suspected abuser is absent from the room. It is imperative that you, the health care team, and the proper authorities help the patient find safe housing or seek protection from the abuser because the risk for further abuse is high once the victim has reported it or tries to leave the abusive situation.

- *Substance abuse:* Unusual or inconsistent behavior may be an indicator of substance abuse, which can affect all socioeconomic groups. Although a single patient visit to a clinic does not always reveal the problem, investigate unusual behaviors further with a well-focused history and physical examination. Always approach the patient in a caring and nonjudgmental way; substance abuse involves both emotional and lifestyle issues. Box 30.4 lists characteristics of patients who should be further assessed for potential substance abuse. A tool such as the online Tobacco, Alcohol, Prescription Medication, and Other Substance Use (TAPS) tool can be used to assess a patient's risk for substance abuse (National Institute on Drug Abuse [NIDA], 2018). If you suspect that alcohol abuse is a major problem, the CAGE questionnaire provides a useful set of questions to guide assessment. CAGE is an acronym for the following:
  - Have you ever felt the need to **Cut down** on your drinking or drug use?
  - Have people **Annoyed** you by criticizing your drinking or drug use?
  - Have you ever felt bad or **Guilty** about your drinking or drug use?
  - Have you ever used or had a drink first thing in the morning as an **Eye-opener** to steady your nerves or feel normal?

When assessing adolescents, there are brief online tools to screen substance use, such as the Brief Screener for Tobacco, Alcohol, and Other Drugs (BSTAD) and Screening to Brief Intervention (S2BI) (NIDA, 2019). Among older adults, risk factors for development of alcohol-related problems include chronic medical disorders, sleep disorders, social isolation, loneliness, bereavement, and acute or chronic pain.

Vital Signs

After completing the general survey, measure the patient's vital signs. Measurement of vital signs is more accurate if completed before beginning positional changes or movements. If there is a chance that the vital signs are inaccurate when you first take them, recheck them later during the rest of the examination. Assess for pain, the fifth vital sign, whenever you take a patient's vital signs.

Height and Weight

The relationship of height and weight reflects a person's general health status. Assess every patient to identify whether the patient is at a healthy weight, underweight, overweight, or obese. Weight is routinely measured during health screenings, visits to physicians' offices or clinics, and on admission to the hospital. Infants and children are measured for both height and weight at each health care visit to assess for healthy growth and development. If older adults are underweight, difficulty with feeding and other functional activities is a possibility. Measuring height and weight of older adults, along with obtaining a dietary history (Box 30.5), shows risk factors for chronic diseases.

Assess a patient's weight and height and look for trends in weight changes (loss or gain). A patient's weight normally varies daily because of fluid loss or retention. Use the nursing history to identify possible causes for a change in weight (Table 30.6). For example, a downward trend in an older adult who is frail indicates a serious reduction in nutritional reserves. Ask the patient to report current height and weight, along with a history of any substantial weight gain or loss. A weight gain of 0.9 to 1.4 kg (2–3 lb) in 1 day indicates fluid-retention problems. A weight loss is considered significant if the patient has lost more than 5% of body weight in 6 months to a year (Mayo Clinic, 2021).

When a patient is hospitalized, daily weight is measured at the same time of day and on the same scale (Ball et al., 2019). This allows an

BOX 30.3 Clinical Indicators of Abuse

Physical Findings	Behavioral Findings
Child Abuse	
Vaginal or penile discharge	Problem sleeping or eating, anxiety, depression
Blood on underclothing	Fear of certain people or places
Pain, itching, or unusual odor in genital area	Play activities recreate the abuse situation
Genital injuries	Regressed behavior
Difficulty sitting or walking	Sexual acting out
Pain while urinating; recurrent urinary tract infections	Knowledge of explicit sexual matters
Foreign bodies in rectum, urethra, or vagina	Preoccupation with others' or own genitals
Sexually transmitted infections	Profound and rapid personality changes
Pregnancy in young adolescent	Rapidly declining school performance
	Poor relationship with peers
Intimate Partner Violence	
Injuries and trauma inconsistent with reported cause	Overuse of health services
Multiple injuries involving head, face, neck, breasts, abdomen, and genitalia (black eyes, orbital fractures, broken nose, fractured skull, lip lacerations, broken teeth, vaginal tears)	Thoughts of or attempted suicide
	Eating or sleeping disorders
X-ray films showing old and new fractures in different stages of healing	Anxiety and panic attacks
Abrasions, lacerations, bruises/welts	Pattern of substance abuse (follows physical abuse)
Burns from cigarettes or other cause	Low self-esteem
Human bites	Depression, problems with eating or sleeping
Unexplained injuries (e.g., bruises, fractures, and welts)	Sense of helplessness
Strangulation marks on neck from rope burns or bruises; throat pain, voice changes, trouble swallowing; damage to hyoid bone	Guilt
	Smoking
Stress-related disorders such as irritable bowel syndrome, exacerbation of asthma, or chronic pain	Stress-related complaints (headache, anxiety)
	Financial dependence on abuser
	Isolation from others
	Unsafe sexual behaviors
Older-Adult Abuse	
Injuries and trauma inconsistent with reported cause (scratch, bruise, or bite)	Dependent on caregiver
Hematomas, bruises at various stages of resolution	Physically and/or cognitively impaired
Unexplained bruises or welts, pattern bruises	Combative, verbally aggressive
Burns	Wandering
Bruises, chafing, excoriation on wrist or legs (restraints)	Minimal social support
Fractures inconsistent with cause described	Prolonged interval between injury and medical treatment
Dried blood	Life circumstances do not match size of patient's estate
Overmedication or undermedication	Uncommunicative or isolated
Exposure to severe weather, cold or hot	
Torn, bloody underwear or vaginal and anal bruises	
Sunken eyes or loss of weight	
Extreme thirst	
Bed sores	

Data from Halphen J, Dyer C: *Elder mistreatment: abuse, neglect, and financial exploitation, UpToDate,* 2020. https://www.uptodate.com/contents/elder-mistreatment-abuse-neglect-and-financial-exploitation. Accessed August 28, 2020; Hockenberry MJ, Wilson P: *Wong's nursing care of infants and children,* ed 10, St Louis, 2019, Elsevier; and Weil A: *Intimate partner violence: diagnosis and screening, UpToDate,* 2020. https://www.uptodate.com/contents/intimate-partner-violence-diagnosis-and-screening/print. Accessed August 28, 2020.

objective comparison of subsequent weights. Accuracy of weight measurement is important because health care providers base medical and nursing decisions (e.g., drug dosage, medications) on changes.

Several different scales are available for use. Patients capable of bearing their own weight use a standing scale. You calibrate a standard platform scale by moving the large and small weights to zero. Through adjustment of the calibrating knob, the balance beam is leveled and steadied. The patient stands on the scale platform and remains still as you adjust the largest solid weight to the 50-lb or 22.5-kg increment under the patient's weight. Next, the smaller weight is moved to balance the scale at the nearest ¼ pound or 0.1 kg (Ball et al., 2019).

Electronic scales are calibrated automatically each time they are used and automatically display the weight within seconds.

Bed and chair scales are available for patients who are unable to bear weight. Newer electronic hospital beds have built-in electronic scales for weighing patients who are not able to get out of bed.

You can use a basket or platform scale to weigh infants. Keep the room warm to prevent chills. Before weighing the infant, clean the infant scale and place a light cloth or paper cover on the surface to prevent cross-infection from urine or feces. Place a dry diaper on the scale and zero the scale so that the weight of the items on the scale will not be represented in the infant's weight. Once the scale is at zero, the

BOX 30.4   Indicators of Substance Abuse

Among adolescents and adults: Agitation; inappropriate behavior; problems thinking clearly, remembering, and paying attention; poor coordination; seizure; respiratory depression; coma; asphyxiation; aspiration; pulmonary edema; cardiac arrhythmias; immune system impairment; self-inflicted trauma; and suicidal ideation

Red Flags
- The risk of suicide, seizures, and violent behavior is high among substance abusers.
- Intoxicated patients, particularly those with phencyclidine (PCP) or methamphetamine intoxication, are at significant risk for becoming agitated and violent, placing themselves and others at risk for injury.

Observe for Combinations or Repetition of These Behaviors
- Frequently misses appointments
- Frequently requests written excuses for absence from school or work
- Drops out of school
- Chief complaints of insomnia, "bad nerves," or pain that do not fit a particular pattern
- Reports lost prescriptions (e.g., tranquilizers or pain medications) or asks for frequent refills
- Frequent emergency department visits
- History of changing health care providers or brings in medication bottles prescribed by several different providers
- History of gastrointestinal bleeding, peptic ulcers, pancreatitis, cellulitis, or frequent pulmonary infections
- Frequent sexually transmitted infections (STIs), complicated pregnancies, multiple abortions, or sexual dysfunction
- Complaints of chest pains or palpitations or has a history of admissions to rule out heart attacks
- History of activities that place the patient at risk for human immunodeficiency virus (HIV) infection (multiple partners, multiple rapes)
- Family history of addiction; history of childhood sexual, physical, or emotional abuse; or social and financial or marital problems
- Intimate partner violence

Data from Bukstein O: *Substance use disorder in adolescents: epidemiology, pathogenesis, clinical manifestations and consequences, course, assessment, and diagnosis, UpToDate,* 2020. https://www.uptodate.com/contents/substance-use-disorder-in-adolescents-epidemiology-pathogenesis-clinical-manifestations-and-consequences-course-assessment-and-diagnosis. Accessed August 28, 2020; Dugosh K, Cacciola J: *Clinical assessment of substance use disorders, UpToDate,* 2020. https://www.uptodate.com/contents/clinical-assessment-of-substance-use-disorders/print; National Institute on Drug Abuse: *Drugs, brains and behavior: the science of addiction,* 2020. https://www.drugabuse.gov/publications/drugs-brains-behavior-science-addiction/introduction. Accessed August 28, 2020.

BOX 30.5   Dietary History for Older Adults

- Does the older adult need or have help shopping for or preparing meals?
- Is income adequate for food purchasing? Are food stamps or public assistance required?
- Does the older adult ever skip meals?
- Are the five primary food groups from MyPlate (fruits, grains, protein, vegetables, dairy) represented in the daily diet (see Chapter 45) (USDA, n.d.)? Females 60 years of age and older require about 1600 to 2200 calories per day, and males 60 years of age and older require about 2000 to 2600 calories per day (U.S. Department of Agriculture [USDA] and U.S. Department of Health and Human Services [USDHHS], 2020).
- Does the older adult take nutritional supplements such as multivitamins?
- Does the older adult take any medication affecting appetite or absorption of nutrients?
- Does the older adult have any religious or cultural beliefs and practices that influence diet?
- Does the older adult have a special diet, food intolerances, or allergies? Does the older adult's diet contain an unusual amount of alcohol, sweets, or fried food?
- Does the older adult have problems with chewing, swallowing, or salivation?
- Does the older adult have gastrointestinal problems that interfere with food intake?
- Does the older adult eat meals alone or with others? Sharing meals with friends and family can help increase food enjoyment and promote adequacy of dietary intake for older adults (USDA and USDHHS, 2020).

Data from Meiner SE, Yeager JJ: *Gerontologic nursing,* ed 6, St Louis, 2019, Elsevier; and U.S. Department of Agriculture and U.S. Department of Health and Human Services. *Dietary guidelines for Americans, 2020-2025,* 9th Edition. December 2020. Available at DietaryGuidelines.gov. Accessed July 8, 2021.

naked infant can be placed on the scale and the diaper secured. When placing an infant in a basket or on a platform, hold a hand lightly above the infant to detect movements and prevent accidental falls. Measure an infant's weight in both ounces and grams.

In patients who can stand, measure height by having them remove their shoes. The standing surface should be clean. Use a measuring rod attached vertically to a weight scale or use a tape ruler on the wall. As the patient stands erect, place a flat surface on the head that is even with the vertical measure. Then read the number on the scale or ruler that indicates the height in centimeters or inches.

Remove the shoes of a patient who cannot bear weight and position the patient (such as an infant) supine on a firm surface. When measuring an infant, hold the head and make sure that the legs are straight at the knees. After positioning the infant, use a tape measure to measure length from the head to the bottom of the feet (Fig. 30.3). Record the infant's length to the nearest 0.5 cm (¼ inch).

SKIN, HAIR, AND NAILS

The integumentary system refers to the skin, hair, scalp, and nails. To assess, you first gather a health history to guide your examination and use the techniques of inspection and palpation.

Skin

Begin an assessment of the skin by focusing on the health history questions found in Table 30.7. Then inspect all visible skin surfaces; assess less visible surfaces when you examine other body systems. Use the senses of sight, smell, and touch while inspecting and palpating the skin.

Assessment of the skin reveals the patient's health status related to oxygenation, circulation, nutrition, local tissue damage, and hydration. Check the condition of the patient's skin to determine the need for nursing care. If there is an alteration in integumentary status, then adequate nutrition and hydration may become priority goals of therapy (see Chapter 45).

Every patient has a risk for skin impairment in a hospital setting. This risk increases in certain situations, such as excessive pressure against the skin when the patient is immobile, reactions to various medications used in treatment, and moisture if the patient is incontinent or has wound drainage. Patients at high risk are those who have neurological impairments, chronic illnesses, decreased mental status, poor tissue oxygenation, low cardiac output, or inadequate nutrition

TABLE 30.6   Nursing History for Assessment of Weight

Assessment	Rationale
Ask about total weight lost or gained; compare with usual weight; note time period for loss and whether it was planned (e.g., gradual, sudden, desired, or undesired).	Assessment determines severity of problem and reveals whether weight change is related to disease process, change in eating pattern, or pregnancy. The point at which unexplained weight loss becomes a medical concern is not exact. Many health care providers agree that a medical evaluation is called for if a patient loses more than 5% of body weight in 6 months to a year, especially if patient is an older adult (Mayo Clinic, 2021).
If weight loss desired, ask about eating habits, diet plan followed, food preparation, calorie intake, appetite, exercise pattern, support group participation, weight goal.	Assessment helps to determine appropriateness of diet plan followed.
If weight loss undesired, ask about anorexia; vomiting; diarrhea; thirst; frequent urination; and change in lifestyle, activity, and stress levels.	Assessment focuses on problems that cause weight loss (e.g., gastrointestinal problems).
Assess whether patient has noted changes in social aspects of eating: more meals in restaurants, rushing to eat meals, stress at work, or skipping meals.	Lifestyle changes sometimes contribute to weight changes.
Assess whether patient takes chemotherapy, diuretics, insulin, fluoxetine, prescription and nonprescription appetite suppressants, laxatives, oral hypoglycemics, or herbal supplements (weight loss); steroids, oral contraceptives, antidepressants, insulin (weight gain).	Weight gain or loss is a side effect of these medications.
Assess for preoccupation with body weight or body shape, such as fasting, never feeling thin enough, unusually strict caloric intake or restrictions, laxative abuse, induced vomiting, amenorrhea, excessive exercise, alcohol intake.	Excesses indicate an eating disorder.

FIG. 30.3 Measurement of infant length. (From Murray SS, McKinney ES: *Foundations of maternal-newborn and women's health nursing*, ed 7, St Louis, 2019, Elsevier.)

or those who have had orthopedic or vascular injuries. Patients who are homebound, in nursing homes, or in extended-care facilities are often at risk for pressure injuries, depending on their level of mobility and the presence of chronic illness. Routinely assess the skin of all patients, especially those at risk, to look for primary or initial lesions that develop. Without identification and appropriate care, primary lesions can quickly deteriorate to become secondary lesions that require more extensive nursing care. For example, the development of a pressure injury lengthens a hospital stay unless it is prevented or discovered and treated early (see Chapter 48).

Adequate lighting is required when assessing the skin. Daylight is the best choice for identifying variations in skin color, especially for detecting skin changes in patients with dark skin. When sunlight is unavailable, fluorescent lighting is the next best choice. Room temperature also affects skin assessment. A room that is too warm causes superficial vasodilation, resulting in increased redness of the skin. A cool environment causes a sensitive patient to develop cyanosis around the lips and nail beds (Ball et al., 2019).

Although you inspect the skin over each part of the body during an examination, it is helpful to make a brief but careful overall visual sweep of the entire body. This approach provides a good idea of the distribution and extent of any lesions and the overall symmetry of skin color. Inspect all skin surfaces, making a point to do so when examining other body systems. Often overlooked, inspection of the feet is essential for patients with poor circulation or diabetes mellitus. If any abnormalities are found during an examination, palpate the involved areas. Use disposable gloves for palpation if open, moist, or draining lesions are present.

Throughout the examination remain alert for skin odors. Black and White adolescents and adults ordinarily have body odor because they have a greater number of functioning apocrine glands. In contrast, Asians and Native Americans/American Indians often do not (Ball et al., 2019). Fig. 30.4 illustrates a normal cross-section of the skin.

Color. Skin color varies from body part to body part and from person to person. Despite individual variations, it is usually uniform over the body. Table 30.8 lists common variations. Normal skin pigmentation ranges in tone from ivory or light pink to ruddy pink in light skin and from light to deep brown or olive in dark skin. In older adults, pigmentation increases unevenly, causing discolored skin. While inspecting the skin, be aware that cosmetics or tanning agents sometimes mask normal skin color.

The assessment of color first involves areas of the skin not exposed to the sun, such as the palms of the hands. Note whether the skin is unusually pale or dark. Areas exposed to the sun, such as the face and arms, are darker. It is more difficult to note changes such as pallor or cyanosis in patients with dark skin. Usually color hues are most evident in the palms, soles of the feet, lips, tongue, and nail beds. Areas of increased (hyperpigmentation) and decreased (hypopigmentation) color are common. Skin creases and folds are darker than the rest of the body in patients with dark skin.

TABLE 30.7   Nursing History for Skin Assessment

Assessment	Rationale
Ask patient about history of changes in skin: dryness, scaliness, pruritus, sores, rashes, lumps, color, texture, odor, and lesion that does not heal.	Patient is best source to recognize change. Usually skin cancer is first noticed as a localized change in skin color. Scaly lesions are an early indication of precancerous lesions.
Consider whether patient has the following history: fair, freckled, ruddy complexion; light-colored hair or eyes; tendency to burn easily.	Characteristics are risk factors for skin cancer.
Determine whether patient works or spends excessive time outside. If so, ask whether patient wears sunscreen and the level of protection.	Exposed areas such as face and arms are more pigmented than rest of body. The American Cancer Society (2020a) recommends sun safety and use of sunscreen and lip balm with broad-spectrum protection and a sun protection factor (SPF) of 30 or higher and not sunbathing or indoor tanning.
Determine whether patient has noted lesions, rashes, or bruises.	Most skin changes do not develop suddenly. Change in character of lesion can indicate cancer. Bruising indicates trauma or bleeding disorder.
Question patient about frequency of bathing and type of soap used.	Excessive bathing and use of harsh soaps cause dry skin.
Ask whether patient has had recent trauma to skin.	Some injuries cause bruising and changes in skin texture.
Determine whether patient has history of allergies.	Skin rashes commonly occur from allergies.
Ask whether patient uses topical medications or home remedies on skin.	Incorrect use of topical agents causes inflammation or irritation.
Ask whether patient goes to tanning parlors, uses sunlamps, or takes tanning pills.	Overexposure of skin to these irritants can cause skin cancer.
Ask whether patient has family history of serious skin disorders such as skin cancer or psoriasis.	Family history can reveal information about patient's condition.
Determine whether patient works with creosote, coal, tar, petroleum products, arsenic compounds, or radium.	Exposure to these agents creates risk for skin cancer.

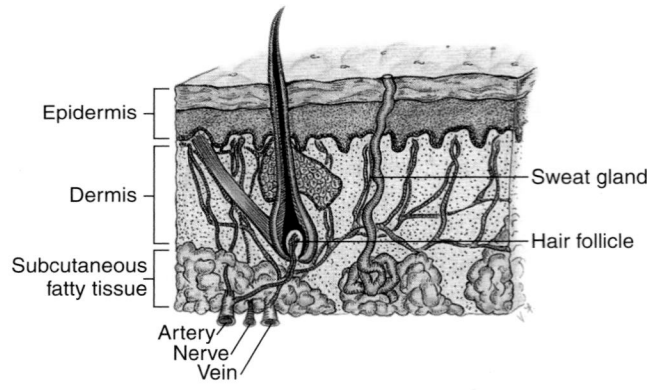

FIG. 30.4 Cross-section of skin reveals three layers: epidermis, dermis, and subcutaneous fatty tissues.

Inspect sites where abnormalities are more easily identified. For example, pallor is more evident in the face, buccal (mouth) mucosa, conjunctiva, and nail beds. Observe for cyanosis (bluish discoloration) in the lips, nail beds, palpebral conjunctivae, and palms. In recognizing pallor in a patient with dark skin, observe that normal brown skin appears to be yellow-brown and normal black skin appears to be ashen gray. Also assess the lips, nail beds, and mucous membranes for generalized pallor; if pallor is present, the mucous membranes are ashen gray. Assess for cyanosis in a patient with dark skin in areas where pigmentation occurs the least (conjunctiva, sclera, buccal mucosa, tongue, lips, nail beds, and palms and soles). In addition, verify these findings with clinical manifestations (Ball et al., 2019).

Discoloration of the skin occurs on different areas of the body for varying reasons. A patient's sclera is the best site to inspect for jaundice (yellow-orange discoloration). Normal reactive hyperemia, or redness, is most often seen in regions exposed to pressure, such as the sacrum, heels, and greater trochanter. Inspect for any patches or areas of skin color variation. Localized skin changes such as pallor or erythema (red discoloration) indicate circulatory changes. It is difficult to observe erythema in a patient with dark skin; therefore palpate the area for heat and warmth to note the presence of skin inflammation. For example, you notice an area of erythema in a patient with dark skin that is caused by localized vasodilation resulting from a sunburn, inflammation, or fever. Compare the area with a different part of the skin to detect a difference in temperature. An area of an extremity that appears unusually pale results from arterial occlusion or edema. Be sure to ask whether the patient has noticed any changes in skin coloring.

There is also a pattern of findings associated with patients who are chemically dependent or abuse intravenous (IV) drugs (Table 30.9). It is sometimes difficult to recognize signs and symptoms through an isolated examination. A patient who takes repeated IV injections has edematous, reddened, and warm areas along the arms and legs. This pattern suggests recent injections. Areas of old injection sites appear as hyperpigmented and shiny or scarred.

Moisture. The hydration of skin and mucous membranes helps to reveal body fluid imbalances, changes in the environment of the skin, and regulation of body temperature. Moisture refers to wetness and oiliness. The skin is normally smooth and dry. Skinfolds such as the axillae are normally moist. Minimal perspiration or oiliness is often present (Ball et al., 2019). Increased perspiration can be associated with activity, exposure to warm environments, obesity, anxiety, or excitement. Use ungloved fingertips to palpate skin surfaces. Observe for dullness, dryness, crusting, and flaking that resembles dandruff when the skin surface is lightly rubbed. Excessively dry skin is common in older adults because their sebaceous and sweat gland activity decreases, reducing perspiration (Ball et al., 2019). Other factors causing dry skin include lack of humidity, exposure to sun, smoking, stress,

TABLE 30.8 Skin Color Variations

Color	Condition	Causes	Assessment Locations
Bluish (cyanosis)	Increased amount of deoxygenated hemoglobin (associated with hypoxia)	Heart or lung disease, cold environment	Nail beds, lips, mouth, skin (severe cases)
Pallor (decrease in color)	Reduced amount of oxyhemoglobin	Anemia	Face, conjunctivae, nail beds, palms of hands
	Reduced visibility of oxyhemoglobin resulting from decreased blood flow	Shock	Skin, nail beds, conjunctivae, lips
Loss of pigmentation	Vitiligo	Congenital or autoimmune condition causing lack of pigment	Patchy areas on skin over face, hands, arms
Yellow-orange (jaundice)	Increased deposit of bilirubin in tissues	Liver disease, destruction of red blood cells	Sclera, mucous membranes, skin
Red (erythema)	Increased visibility of oxyhemoglobin caused by dilation or increased blood flow	Fever, direct trauma, blushing, alcohol intake	Face, area of trauma, sacrum, shoulders, other common sites for pressure injuries
Tan-brown	Increased amount of melanin	Suntan, pregnancy	Areas exposed to sun: face, arms, areolas, nipples

TABLE 30.9 Physical Findings of the Skin Indicative of Substance Abuse

Skin Finding	Commonly Associated Drug
Diaphoresis	Sedative hypnotic (including alcohol)
Spider angiomas	Alcohol, stimulants
Burns (especially fingers)	Alcohol
Needle marks	Opioids
Contusion, abrasions, cuts, scars	Alcohol, other sedative hypnotics, intravenous (IV) opioids
"Homemade" tattoos	Cocaine, IV opioids (prevents detection of injection sites)
Vasculitis	Cocaine
Red, dry skin	Phencyclidine (PCP)

Adapted from Burchum J, Rosenthal L, *Lehne's pharmacology for nursing care,* ed 10, St Louis, 2019, Elsevier; and Dugosh K, Cacciola J: *Clinical assessment of substance use disorders, UpToDate,* 2019. https://www.uptodate.com/contents/clinical-assessment-of-substance-use-disorders/print. Accessed July 8, 2021.

excessive perspiration, and dehydration. Excessive dryness worsens existing skin conditions such as eczema and dermatitis. Patients with large abdominal skinfolds are at high risk for moisture within the skinfolds. Excessive moisture may cause maceration of the skin or softening of the tissues, resulting in an increased risk for breakdown (see Chapter 48).

Temperature. The temperature of the skin depends on the amount of blood circulating through the dermis. Increased or decreased skin temperature indicates an increase or decrease in blood flow. An increase in skin temperature often accompanies localized erythema or redness of the skin. A reduction in skin temperature often accompanies pallor and reflects a decrease in blood flow. Remember that a cold or excessively warm examination room can cause changes in the patient's skin temperature and color.

Accurately assess temperature by palpating the skin with the dorsum or back of the hand and compare symmetrical body parts. Normally the skin temperature is warm. Sometimes it is the same throughout the body, and other times it varies in one area. Always assess skin temperature for patients at risk of having impaired circulation, such as after a cast application or vascular surgery. A Stage 1 pressure injury can be identified early by noting warmth over an area of erythema on the skin (see Chapter 48).

Texture. Texture refers to the appearance of the surface of the skin and how the deeper layers feel. By palpating lightly with the fingertips, you determine whether the patient's skin is smooth or rough, thin or thick, tight or supple, and *indurated* (hardened) or soft. The texture of the skin is normally smooth, soft, even, and flexible in children and adults. However, the texture is usually not uniform throughout, with thicker texture over the palms of the hand and soles of the feet. In older adults the skin becomes wrinkled and leathery because of a decrease in collagen, subcutaneous fat, and sweat glands.

Localized skin changes result from trauma, surgical wounds, or lesions. When there are irregularities in texture such as scars or indurations, ask the patient about recent injury to the skin. Deeper palpation sometimes reveals irregularities such as tenderness or localized areas of induration, which can be caused by an injury or repeated injections.

Turgor. *Turgor* refers to the elasticity of the skin. To assess skin turgor, grasp a fold of skin on the back of the forearm or sternal area with the fingertips and release (Fig. 30.5). Normally the skin loses its elasticity with age, but fluid balance can also affect skin turgor. Edema or dehydration diminishes turgor and makes the skin tauter. Because the skin on the back of the hand is normally loose and thin, turgor is not assessed reliably at that site (Ball et al., 2019). Normally the skin lifts easily and falls immediately back to its resting position. When turgor is poor, it stays pinched and shows tenting. Evaluate the ease with which the skin moves and the speed at which it returns to its resting state. Failure of the skin to reassume its normal contour or shape indicates dehydration. A patient with poor skin turgor does not have resilience to the normal wear and tear on the skin, and a decrease in turgor predisposes the patient to skin breakdown.

FIG. 30.5 Assessment for skin turgor.

freckles or age-related changes such as skin tags, senile keratosis (thickening of skin), cherry angiomas (ruby-red papules), and atrophic warts. Lesions that are primary occur as an initial spontaneous sign of a pathological process, such as with an insect bite. Secondary lesions result from later formation or trauma to a primary lesion, such as a pressure injury. When you find a lesion, collect standard information about its color, location, texture, size, shape, type, grouping (clustered or linear), and distribution (localized or generalized). Next observe for any exudate, odor, amount, and consistency. Measure the size of the lesion in centimeters by using a small, clear, flexible ruler. Measure each lesion for height, width, and depth.

Palpation helps determine the mobility, contour (flat, raised, or depressed), and consistency (soft or indurated) of a lesion. Certain types of lesions present characteristic patterns. For example, a tumor is usually an elevated, solid lesion larger than 2 cm (1 inch). Primary lesions such as macules and nodules come from some stimulus to the skin (Box 30.6). Secondary lesions such as ulcers occur as alterations in primary lesions. After you identify a lesion, thoroughly inspect it in good lighting. Palpate gently, covering the entire area of the lesion. If it is moist or draining fluid, wear gloves during palpation and pay attention to whether the patient identifies any areas of tenderness.

Skin (cutaneous) malignancies are the most common neoplasms. For this reason, you need to complete a thorough skin assessment on all patients. Cancerous lesions have distinct features and over time undergo changes in color and size (Box 30.7). Basal cell carcinoma is most common in areas exposed to the sun and frequently occurs with a history of sun damage; it almost never spreads to other parts of the body. Squamous cell carcinoma is more serious than basal cell and develops on the outer layers of sun-exposed skin; these cells may travel to lymph nodes and throughout the body. Malignant melanoma, a skin cancer that develops from melanocytes, begins as a mole or other area that has changed in appearance and is usually located on normal skin. (**Note:** Melanoma also can originate in noncutaneous primary sites, including mucosal epithelium [gastrointestinal (GI) tract], retinas, and leptomeninges.) In African Americans (more than in other races) it can also appear under fingernails or on the palms of the hands and soles of the feet. Use the *ABCDE* mnemonic to assess the skin for any type of carcinoma (ACS, 2020a):

- *Asymmetry*—Look for an uneven shape. One half of mole does not match the other half.
- *Border irregularity*—Look for edges that are blurred, notched, or ragged.
- *Color*—Look for pigmentation that is not uniform; variegated areas of blue, black, and brown and areas of pink, white, gray, blue, or red are abnormal.
- *Diameter*—Look for areas greater than 6 mm (about the size of a typical pencil eraser).
- *Evolution*—A change in appearance over time.

Vascularity. The circulation of the skin affects color in localized areas and leads to the appearance of superficial blood vessels. Vascularity occurs in localized pressure areas when patients remain in one position. Vascularity appears reddened, pink, or pale (see Chapter 48). With aging, capillaries become fragile and more easily injured. Petechiae are nonblanching, pinpoint-size, red or purple spots on the skin caused by small hemorrhages in the skin layers. Many petechiae have no known cause, but some may indicate serious blood-clotting disorders, drug reactions, or liver disease.

Edema. Edema is present when areas of the skin become swollen or edematous from a buildup of fluid in the tissues. Direct trauma and impairment of venous return are two common causes of edema. Inspect edematous areas for location, color, and shape. The formation of edema separates the surface of the skin from the pigmented and vascular layers, masking skin color. Edematous skin also appears stretched and shiny. Palpate edematous areas to determine mobility, consistency, and tenderness. When pressure from the examiner's fingers leaves an indentation in the edematous area, it is called pitting edema. To assess the degree of pitting edema, press the edematous area firmly with the thumb for several seconds and release. The depth of pitting, recorded in millimeters, determines the degree of edema (Ball et al., 2019). For example, 1+ edema equals a 2-mm depth, 2+ edema equals a 4-mm depth, 3+ equals 6 mm, and 4+ equals 8 mm (Fig. 30.6).

Lesions. The term *lesion* refers broadly to any unusual finding of the skin surface. Normally the skin is free of lesions, except for common

FIG. 30.6 Assessing for pitting edema. (From Ball JW, et al: *Seidel's guide to physical examination*, ed 9, St Louis, 2019, Elsevier.)

BOX 30.6 Types of Primary Skin Lesions

Macule: Flat, nonpalpable change in skin color; smaller than 1 cm (0.4 inch; e.g., freckle, petechiae)

Papule: Palpable, circumscribed, solid elevation in skin; smaller than 1 cm (0.4 inch; e.g., elevated nevus)

Nodule: Elevated solid mass, deeper and firmer than papule; 1–2 cm (0.4–0.7 inch; e.g., wart)

Tumor: Solid mass that extends deep through subcutaneous tissue; larger than 1–2 cm (0.4–0.7 inch; e.g., epithelioma)

Wheal: Irregularly shaped, elevated area or superficial localized edema; varies in size (e.g., hive, mosquito bite)

Vesicle: Circumscribed elevation of skin filled with serous fluid, smaller than 1 cm (0.4 inch; e.g., herpes simplex, chickenpox)

Pustule: Circumscribed elevation of skin similar to vesicle but filled with pus; varies in size (e.g., acne, staphylococcal infection)

Ulcer: Deep loss of skin surface that extends to dermis and frequently bleeds and scars; varies in size (e.g., venous stasis ulcer)

Atrophy: Thinning of skin with loss of normal skin furrow, with skin appearing shiny and translucent; varies in size (e.g., arterial insufficiency)

Report abnormal lesions to the health care provider for further examination. Because ultraviolet light of the sun or tanning beds increases the risk for development of skin cancers, teach patients about the risks that exist. In addition, using individualized teaching materials, teach patients how to perform a skin self-examination (Box 30.8).

Hair and Scalp

Assess a patient's hair during all parts of the examination. Two types of hair cover the body: soft, fine, vellus hair, which covers the body; and coarse, long, thick terminal hair, which is easily visible on the scalp, axillae, and pubic areas and in the facial beard on men. First obtain health history information listed in Table 30.10. Prepare to inspect the condition and distribution of hair and the integrity of the scalp by first obtaining a good light source.

Inspection. During inspection explain that it is necessary to separate parts of the hair to detect abnormalities. Wear a pair of clean gloves if open lesions or lice are noted.

First inspect the color, distribution, quantity, thickness, texture, and lubrication of body hair. Scalp hair is coarse or fine and curly or straight; it should be shiny, smooth, and pliant. While separating sections of scalp hair, observe characteristics of color and coarseness. Color varies from very light blond to black to gray and is sometimes altered by rinses or dyes. In older adults the hair sometimes becomes dull gray, white, or yellow.

Be aware of the normal distribution of hair growth in a man and a woman. At puberty, an increase in the amount and distribution of hair occurs for both genders. During the aging process the hair may thin over the scalp, axillae, and pubic areas. Facial hair of older men decreases. A woman with hirsutism has hair growth on the upper lip, chin, and cheeks, with vellus hair becoming coarser over the body; this may be related to an endocrine disorder. For some a change in hair growth negatively affects body image and emotional well-being. The amount of hair covering the extremities is sometimes reduced because of aging, or it could result from arterial insufficiency that could reduce hair growth over the lower extremities. In the United States and some other cultures,

BOX 30.7 Skin Malignancies

Basal Cell Carcinoma
- 0.5- to 1-cm (0.2–0.4 inch) crusted lesion that is flat or raised and has a rolled, somewhat scaly border
- Frequent appearance of underlying, widely dilated blood vessels within the lesion

Squamous Cell Carcinoma
- Occurs more often on mucosal surfaces and nonexposed areas of skin than basal cell
- 0.5- to 1.5-cm (0.2–0.6 inch) scaly lesion sometimes ulcerated or crusted; appears frequently and grows more rapidly than basal cell

Melanoma
- 0.5- to 1-cm (0.2–0.4 inch) brown, flat lesion; appears on sun-exposed or nonexposed skin; variegated pigmentation, irregular borders, and indistinct margins
- Ulceration, recent growth, and recent changes in long-standing mole are ominous signs

Illustrations from Belcher AE: *Cancer nursing,* St Louis, 1992, Mosby; Habif TP: *Clinical dermatology: a color guide to diagnosis and therapy,* ed 3, St Louis, 1996, Mosby; and Zitelli BJ, et al: *Zitelli and Davis' atlas of pediatric physical diagnosis,* ed 7, St Louis, 2018, Saunders.

women commonly shave their legs and axilla, although shaving remains a matter of personal preference among women from all cultures.

Assess for causes of changes in the thickness, texture, and lubrication of scalp hair. At times these are a result of febrile illnesses or scalp diseases that result in hair loss. Conditions such as thyroid disease alter the condition of the hair, making it fine and brittle. Hair loss (**alopecia**) or thinning of the hair is usually related to genetic tendencies, endocrine disorders such as diabetes mellitus, thyroiditis, and menopause. Poor nutrition causes stringy, dull, dry, and thin hair. The oil of sebaceous

BOX 30.8 PATIENT TEACHING

Skin Assessment

Objective
- Patient will perform a monthly self-examination of the skin.
- Patient will identify factors that increase the risk of skin cancer.
- Patient will follow hygiene practices aimed at maintaining skin integrity.

Teaching Strategies
- Instruct patient to conduct a complete monthly self-examination of the skin, noting moles, blemishes, and birthmarks. Tell patient to inspect all skin surfaces. Cancerous melanomas start as small, molelike growths that increase in size, change color, become ulcerated, and bleed (see Box 30.7).
- Tell patient to report to a health care provider any change in skin lesions or a sore that does not heal.
- Instruct patient to report any lesion that bleeds or fails to heal to a health care provider. Especially instruct older adults, who tend to have delayed wound healing.
- Encourage the use of sunscreen and lip balm with broad-spectrum protection and a sun protection factor (SPF) of 30 or higher (ACS, 2020a).
- To treat excessively dry skin, tell patient to avoid hot water, harsh soaps, and drying agents such as rubbing alcohol.
- Apply moisturizers (mineral oil) to the skin regularly to reduce itching and drying, and wear cotton clothing.

Evaluation
Use the principles of teach-back to evaluate patient/family caregiver learning:
- Observe patient perform skin assessment.
- Have patient describe signs of skin cancer and measures to take to prevent skin cancer.

TABLE 30.10 Nursing History for Hair and Scalp Assessment

Assessment	Rationale
Ask if patient is wearing a wig or hairpiece; if so, ask the patient to remove it.	Wigs or hairpieces interfere with inspection of hair and scalp. (Patient sometimes requests to omit this part of examination.)
Determine whether patient has noted change in growth, loss of hair, change in texture or color, or presence of skin lesion or scaliness (see Skin Assessment).	Change often occurs slowly over time. Lesions may indicate cancerous lesions.
Identify type of hair-care products used for grooming.	Excessive use of chemical agents and burning of hair causes drying and brittleness.
Determine whether patient has had chemotherapy (drugs that cause hair loss) recently or taken a vasodilator (minoxidil) for hair growth.	Chemotherapeutic agents kill cells that rapidly multiply, such as tumor and normal hair cells. Minoxidil causes excessive hair growth.
Has patient noted changes in diet or appetite?	Nutrition influences condition of hair.

FIG. 30.7 Head lice infestation. (From Dinulos JGH: *Habif's clinical dermatology: a color guide to diagnosis and therapy*, ed 7, St Louis, 2021, Elsevier.)

glands lubricates the hair, but excessively oily hair is associated with androgen hormone stimulation. Dry, brittle hair occurs with aging and excessive use of chemical agents.

Normally the scalp is smooth and inelastic with even coloration. Carefully separate strands of hair and thoroughly inspect the scalp for lesions, which are not easy to notice in thick hair. Note the characteristics of any scalp lesion (see Skin Assessment). For lumps or bruises, ask whether the patient has experienced recent head trauma. Moles on the scalp are common, but they can bleed because of vigorous combing or brushing. Dandruff or psoriasis frequently causes scaliness or dryness of the scalp. Teach the patient to perform hair and scalp hygiene practices (Box 30.9).

Careful inspection of hair follicles on the scalp and pubic areas can reveal lice or other parasites. The three types of lice are *Pediculus humanus capitis* (head lice), *Pediculus humanus corporis* (body lice), and *Pediculus pubis* (crab lice). The presence of lice does not mean that a person practices poor hygiene. Lice spread easily, especially among children who play closely together. Head and crab lice attach their eggs to hair. The tiny eggs look like oval particles of dandruff, although the lice themselves are difficult to see (Fig. 30.7). Head and body lice are exceedingly small with grayish-white bodies, whereas crab lice have red legs. To better identify infestations, observe for small, red, pustular eruptions in the hair follicles and areas where skin surfaces meet, such as behind the ears and in the groin. A person often has intense itching of the scalp, especially on the back of the head or neck. Combing with a fine-tooth comb reveals the small oval-shaped lice; if lice are discovered, immediate treatment is required (see Chapter 40).

Nails

The condition of the nails reflects a person's general health, state of nutrition, occupation, and habits of self-care. Before assessing the nails, gather a brief history (Table 30.11). The most visible part of the nail is the nail plate, the transparent layer of epithelial cells covering the nail bed (Fig. 30.8). The vascularity of the nail bed creates the underlying color of the nail. The semilunar whitish area at the base of the nail bed is called the *lunula*, from which the nail plate grows.

Inspection and Palpation. Inspect the nail bed for color, length, symmetry, cleanliness, and configuration. The shape and condition of the nails can give clues to pathophysiological problems. Assess the thickness and shape of the nail, its texture, the angle between the nail and the nail bed, and the condition of the lateral and proximal nail folds around the nail. When inspecting the nails, you gather a sense of a patient's hygiene practices. The nails are normally transparent, smooth, well rounded, and convex, with a nail bed angle of about 160 degrees (Box 30.10). A larger angle and softening of the nail bed indicate chronic oxygenation problems. The surrounding cuticles are normally smooth, intact, and without inflammation. When you assess for basic care of the nails, you recognize that nail biting, stains, and jagged edges either represent poor nail care or are caused by habits or occupational exposure to grease or dirt. Jagged, bitten, or broken nail edges or cuticles predispose a patient to localized infection.

When palpating, expect to find a firm nail base, and check for any abnormalities such as erythema or swelling. For patients with impaired circulation, especially observe for early signs of infection or open lesions. To palpate, gently grasp the patient's finger and observe the color of the nail bed. The nail bed and nails appear pink with white nail tips in White patients. In patients with darker skin, the nail beds are darkly pigmented with a blue or reddish hue. A brown or

TABLE 30.11 Nursing History for Nail Assessment	
Assessment	**Rationale**
Ask whether patient has experienced recent trauma or changes in nails (splitting, breaking, discoloration, thickening).	Trauma changes shape and growth of nail. Systemic conditions cause changes in color, growth, and shape.
Has patient had other symptoms of pain, swelling, presence of systemic disease with fever, or psychological or physical stress?	Alterations sometimes occur slowly over time.
Question patient's nail care practices. Determine whether patient has acrylic nails or silk wraps.	Change in nails can be caused by local or systemic problem. Acrylic nails and silk wraps are areas for fungal growth.
Determine whether patient has risks for nail or foot problems (e.g., diabetes mellitus, peripheral vascular disease, older adulthood, obesity).	Chemical agents cause drying of nails. Improper care damages nails and cuticles. Vascular changes associated with diabetes mellitus and peripheral vascular disease reduce blood flow to peripheral tissues; foot lesions and thickened nails are common. Some older adults have trouble performing foot and nail care because of poor vision, lack of coordination, or inability to bend over. Patients who are obese often have difficulty bending.

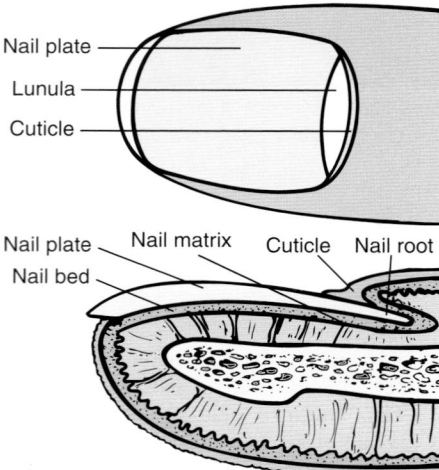

FIG. 30.8 Components of nail unit. (From Lewis SL, et al: *Medical-surgical nursing*, ed 9, St Louis, 2014, Mosby.)

BOX 30.10   Abnormalities of the Nail Bed

Normal nail: Approximately 160-degree angle between nail plate and nail

Clubbing: Change in angle between nail and nail base (eventually larger than 180 degrees); nail bed softening with nail flattening; often enlargement of fingertips
Causes: Chronic lack of oxygen: heart or pulmonary disease

Beau lines: Transverse depressions in nails indicating temporary disturbance of nail growth (nail grows out over several months)
Causes: Systemic illness such as severe infection; nail injury

Koilonychia (spoon nail): Concave curves
Causes: Iron deficiency anemia, syphilis, use of strong detergents

Splinter hemorrhages: Red or brown linear streaks in nail bed
Causes: Minor trauma, subacute bacterial endocarditis, trichinosis

Paronychia: Inflammation of skin at base of nail
Causes: Local infection, trauma

black pigmentation is normal with longitudinal streaks (Fig. 30.9). Trauma, cirrhosis, diabetes mellitus, and hypertension cause splinter hemorrhages; vitamin, protein, and electrolyte changes cause various lines or bands to form on the nail beds.

Nails normally grow at a constant rate, but direct injury or generalized disease changes growth patterns. With aging the nails of the fingers and toes become harder and thicker, longitudinal striations develop, and the rate of nail growth slows. In older adults with insufficient calcium the nails become more brittle and dull and turn opaque yellow, and the cuticle becomes thick and wide.

Calluses and corns commonly are found on the toes or fingers. A callus is flat and painless, resulting from a thickening of the epidermis. Friction and pressure from shoes cause corns, usually over bony prominences. During the examination instruct the patient in proper nail care (Box 30.11).

HEAD AND NECK

An examination of the head and neck includes assessment of the head, eyes, ears, nose, mouth, pharynx, and neck (lymph nodes, carotid arteries, thyroid gland, and trachea). Assessment of the head and neck uses inspection, palpation, and auscultation. Many times, you will inspect and palpate the head and neck at the same time.

Head

Inspection and Palpation. The nursing history screens for intracranial injury and local or congenital deformities (Table 30.12). Inspect the patient's head, noting the position, size, shape, and contour. The head is normally held upright and midline to the trunk. A patient who tilts the head to one side may have unilateral hearing or visual loss or

TABLE 30.12   Nursing History for Head Assessment

Assessment	Rationale
Determine whether patient experienced recent head trauma. If so, assess state of consciousness after injury (when consciousness returns and 5 minutes later), duration of unconsciousness, and predisposing factors (e.g., seizure, poor vision, blackout).	Trauma is major cause of lumps, bumps, cuts, bruises, or deformities of scalp or skull. Loss of consciousness following head injury indicates possible brain injury.
Ask whether patient has history of headache; note onset, duration, character, pattern, and associated symptoms.	Character of headache helps to reveal causative factors such as sinus infection, migraine, or neurological disorders.
Determine length of time patient has experienced neurological symptoms.	Duration of signs or symptoms reveals severity of problem.
Review patient's occupational history for use of safety helmets.	Nature of some occupations creates a risk for head injury.
Ask whether patient participates in contact sports, cycling, rollerblading, or skateboarding.	These activities require use of safety helmets.

FIG. 30.9 Pigmented bands in nail of patient with dark skin. (From Dinulos JGH: *Habif's clinical dermatology: a color guide to diagnosis and therapy*, ed 7, St Louis, 2021, Elsevier.)

muscle weakness in the neck. A horizontal jerking or bobbing may indicate a tremor.

Note the patient's facial features, looking at the eyelids, eyebrows, nasolabial folds, and mouth for shape and symmetry. It is normal for slight asymmetry to exist. If there is facial asymmetry, note whether all features on one side of the face are affected or if only a part of the face is involved. Various neurological disorders (e.g., facial nerve paralysis) affect different nerves that innervate muscles of the face.

Examine the size, shape, and contour of the skull. The skull is generally round with prominences in the frontal area anteriorly and the occipital area posteriorly. Trauma typically causes local skull deformities. In infants a large head results from congenital anomaly or the buildup of cerebrospinal fluid in the ventricles (hydrocephalus). Some adults have enlarged jaws and facial bones resulting from acromegaly, a disorder caused by excessive secretion of growth hormone. Palpate the skull for nodules or masses. Gently rotate the fingertips down the midline of the scalp and along the sides of the head to identify abnormalities. Palpate the temporomandibular joint (TMJ) space bilaterally. Place the fingertips just anterior to the tragus of each ear. The fingertips should slip into the joint space as the patient's mouth opens to gently palpate the joint spaces. Normally the movements should be smooth, although it is not unusual to hear or feel a clicking, grating, or snapping in the TMJ, indicating degenerative joint disease (Ball et al., 2019).

BOX 30.11   PATIENT TEACHING

Nail Assessment

Objective
- Patient will properly care for fingernails, feet, and toenails.

Teaching Strategies
- Instruct patient to cut nails only after soaking them for about 10 minutes in warm water. (**Exception:** Patients with diabetes mellitus or peripheral vascular disease are warned against soaking nails because this can cause maceration of the skin, leading to infection. Long-term soaking also dries out the hands and feet; dry, cracked skin leads to infection.)
- Caution patient against over-the-counter preparations to treat corns, calluses, or ingrown toenails.
- Instruct patient to cut nails straight across and even with tops of fingers or toes. Tell patients with diabetes mellitus to file rather than cut nails (see Chapter 40).
- Instruct patient to shape nails with a file or emery board.
- If patient has diabetes mellitus:
  - Wash feet daily in warm water and carefully dry them, especially between toes. Inspect feet each day in good lighting, looking for dry places and cracks in skin. Soften dry feet by applying a cream or lotion such as Nivea, Eucerin, or Alpha Keri.
  - Do not put lotion between toes; moisture between toes allows microorganisms to grow, leading to infections.
  - Caution patient against using sharp objects to poke or dig under toenail or around the cuticle.
  - Have patient see a podiatrist for treatment of ingrown toenails and nails that are thick or tend to split.

Evaluation
Use the principles of teach-back to evaluate patient/family caregiver learning:
- Show me how you are going to clean and moisturize your hands and feet.
- Explain the measures that you will take to avoid injury to your feet.

Eyes

Examination of the eyes includes assessment of visual acuity, visual fields, extraocular movements, and external and internal eye structures. Fig. 30.10 shows a cross-section of the eye. The eye assessment detects visual alterations and determines the general level of assistance that patients require when ambulating or performing self-care activities. Some patients with visual problems also need special aids for reading educational materials or instructions (e.g., medication labels). Table 30.13 reviews the nursing history for an eye examination. Box 30.12 describes common types of visual problems.

TABLE 30.13   Nursing History for Eye Assessment

Assessment	Rationale
Determine whether patient has history of eye disease (e.g., glaucoma, retinopathy, cataracts), eye trauma, diabetes mellitus, hypertension, or eye surgery.	Some diseases or trauma cause risk for partial or complete visual loss. Patient may have had surgery for a visual disorder.
Determine problems that prompted patient to seek health care. Ask patient about eye pain, photophobia (sensitivity to light), burning or itching, excess tearing or crusting, diplopia (double vision) or blurred vision, awareness of a "film" or "curtain" over field of vision, floaters (small black spots that seem to float across field of vision), flashing lights, or halos around lights.	Common symptoms of eye disease indicate need for health care provider.
Determine whether there is family history of eye disorders or diseases.	Certain eye problems such as glaucoma or retinitis pigmentosa are inherited.
Review patient's occupational history and recreational hobbies. Are safety glasses worn?	Performance of close, intricate work causes eye fatigue. Working with computers causes eye strain. Certain occupational tasks (e.g., working with chemicals) and recreational activities (e.g., fencing, motorcycle riding) place people at risk for eye injury unless they take precautions.
Ask if patient wears glasses or contacts and, if so, how often.	Patients need to wear glasses or contacts during certain parts of examination for accurate assessment.
Determine when patient last visited ophthalmologist or optometrist.	Date of last eye examination reveals level of preventive care patient takes.
Assess medications patient is taking, including eyedrops or ointment.	Determines need to assess patient's knowledge of medications. Certain medications cause visual symptoms.

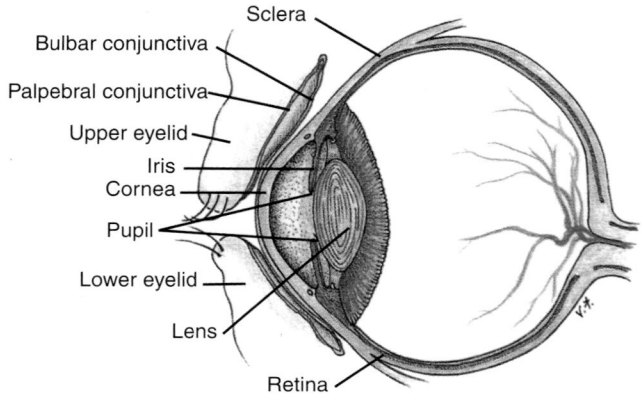

FIG. 30.10   Cross-section of eye.

Labels: Sclera, Bulbar conjunctiva, Palpebral conjunctiva, Upper eyelid, Iris, Cornea, Pupil, Lower eyelid, Lens, Retina

Visual Acuity. Assessing visual acuity (i.e., the ability to see small details) tests central vision. The easiest way to assess near vision is to ask patients to read printed material under adequate lighting. If patients wear glasses, make sure that they wear them during the assessment. Asking patients to read aloud also helps to assess literacy. If the patient has difficulty reading, move to the next step.

Assessment of distant vision requires using a Snellen chart (paper chart or projection screen). The chart should be well lit. Test vision without corrective lenses first. Have the patient sit or stand 6.1 meters (20 feet) away from the chart and try to read all the letters, beginning at any line with both eyes open. Then have the patient read the line with each eye separately (patient covers the opposite eye with an index card or eye cover to avoid applying pressure to the eye). Note the smallest line on which the patient can read all of the letters correctly, and record the visual acuity for that line. Repeat the test with the patient wearing corrective lenses. Complete the test rapidly enough that the patient does not memorize the chart (Ball et al., 2019). If a patient is unable to read, use an E chart or one with pictures of familiar objects. Instead of reading letters, patients tell which direction each E is pointing or the name of the object.

The Snellen chart has standardized numbers at the end of each line of the chart. The numerator is the number 20, or the distance the patient stands from the chart. The denominator is the distance from which the normal eye can read the chart. Normal visual acuity is 20/20. The larger the denominator, the poorer the patient's visual acuity. For example, a value of 20/40 means that the patient, standing 20 feet away, can read a line that a person with normal vision can read from 40 feet away. Record visual acuity for each eye and both eyes and record whether the test was performed with or without correction (including glasses or contact lenses).

If patients cannot read even the largest letters or figures of a Snellen chart, test their ability to count upraised fingers or to distinguish light. Hold a hand 31 cm (1 foot) from the patient's face and have the patient count the upraised fingers. To check light perception, shine a penlight into the eye and turn off the light. If the patient notes when the light is turned on or off, light perception is intact.

Assess near vision by asking the patient to read a handheld card containing a vision screening chart. The patient holds the card a comfortable distance (31.7–35.5 cm [about 12½–14 inches]) from the eyes and reads the smallest line possible. This part of the examination is a good time to discuss the need for routine eye examinations (Box 30.13).

Extraocular Movements. Six small muscles guide the movement of each eye. Both eyes move parallel to one another in each of the six directions of gaze (Fig. 30.11). To assess extraocular movements, a patient sits or stands, and the nurse faces the patient from 60 cm (2 feet) away. The nurse holds a finger at a comfortable distance (15–31 cm [6–12 inches]) from the patient's eyes. While the patient maintains the head in a fixed position facing forward, the nurse directs the patient to follow with the eyes only as the nurse's finger moves to the right, left, and diagonally up and down to the left and right. The nurse moves the finger smoothly and slowly within the normal field of vision.

As the patient gazes in each direction, observe for parallel eye movement, the position of the upper eyelid in relation to the iris, and the presence of abnormal movements. As the eyes move through each direction of gaze, the upper eyelid covers the iris only slightly. Nystagmus, an involuntary, rhythmical oscillation of the eyes, occurs because of local injury to eye muscles and supporting structures or a disorder

BOX 30.12 Common Eye and Vision Problems

Hyperopia

Hyperopia is farsightedness, a refractive error in which rays of light enter the eye and focus behind the retina. People can clearly see distant objects but not close objects.

Myopia

Myopia is nearsightedness, a refractive error in which rays of light enter the eye and focus in front of the retina. People can clearly see close objects but not distant objects.

Presbyopia

Presbyopia is impaired near vision in middle-age and older adults caused by loss of elasticity of the lens and associated with the aging process.

Retinopathy

Retinopathy is a noninflammatory eye disorder resulting from changes in retinal blood vessels. It is a leading cause of blindness.

Strabismus

Strabismus is a (congenital) condition in which both eyes do not focus on an object simultaneously; these eyes appear crossed. Impairment of the extraocular muscles or their nerve supply causes strabismus.

Cataracts

A cataract is an increased opacity of the lens, which blocks light rays from entering the eye. Cataracts sometimes develop slowly and progressively after age 35 or suddenly after trauma. They are one of the most common eye disorders. Most older adults (65 years old and older) have some evidence of visual impairment from cataracts.

Glaucoma

Glaucoma is intraocular structural damage resulting from elevated intraocular pressure. Obstruction of the outflow of aqueous humor causes this. Without treatment the disorder leads to blindness.

Macular Degeneration

Macular degeneration is associated with aging and results in severe loss of a patient's central vision. It is the leading cause of blindness and low vision in the United States in those 65 years of age and older (CDC, 2021a). There is no cure, but there are injections and laser treatments that may slow the progression.

BOX 30.13 PATIENT TEACHING

Eye Assessment

Objective
- Patient will follow recommendations for regular eye examinations and prevention of injury.

Teaching Strategies
- Explain recommended frequency for eye testing with a Snellen chart and examination (see Table 30.3).
- Describe the typical symptoms of eye disease.
- Instruct older adult to take the following precautions because of normal vision changes: avoid or use caution while driving at night, increase lighting in the home to reduce risk of falls, and paint the first and last steps of a staircase and the edge of each of the other steps a bright color to aid depth perception.
- Remind patient that wearing protective eyewear prevents injury from debris and splashes.

Evaluation
Use the principles of teach-back to evaluate patient/family caregiver learning:
- Tell me how often you should schedule an eye examination.
- Describe for me the symptoms you should watch for and when you should call the health care provider.
- Tell me what changes you are making in your home that will improve your safety.

Adapted from Ball JW, et al: *Seidel's guide to physical examination,* ed 9, St Louis, 2019, Elsevier.

of the cranial nerves innervating the muscles. Initiate nystagmus in patients with normal eye movements by having them gaze to the far left or right.

Visual Fields. Normally all objects in the periphery can be seen as a person looks straight ahead. To assess visual fields, direct the patient to stand or sit 60 cm (2 feet) away at eye level. The patient gently closes or covers one eye (e.g., the left) and looks at your eye directly opposite. You close your opposite eye (in this case the right) so that the field of vision is superimposed on that of the patient. Next move a finger equidistant between you and the patient outside the field of vision and slowly bring it back into the visual field. The patient indicates when the examiner's finger is observed. If you see the finger before the patient does, a part of the patient's visual field is reduced. To test temporal field vision, hold an object or your finger slightly behind the patient. Repeat the procedure for each field of vision for the other eye. Patients with visual field problems are at risk for injury because they cannot see all the objects in front of them. Older adults commonly have loss of peripheral vision caused by changes in the lens.

External Eye Structures. To inspect external eye structures, stand directly in front of the patient at eye level and ask the patient to look at your face.

Position and Alignment. Assess the position of the eyes in relation to each other. Normally they are parallel to each other. Bulging eyes (exophthalmos) usually indicate hyperthyroidism. Crossed eyes (strabismus) result from neuromuscular injury or inherited abnormalities. Tumors or inflammation of the orbit often cause abnormal eye protrusion. For the remainder of the eye examination have the patient remove contact lenses.

Eyebrows. Inspect the eyebrows for size, extension, texture of hair, alignment, and movement. Normally the eyebrows are symmetrical. Coarseness of hair and failure to extend beyond the temporal canthus possibly reveals hypothyroidism. Thin brows may be a result of waxing or plucking. Aging causes loss of the lateral third of the eyebrows. To assess movement, ask the patient to raise and lower the eyebrows. The brows normally raise and lower symmetrically. An inability to move them indicates a facial nerve paralysis (cranial nerve VII).

Eyelids. Inspect the eyelids for position; color; condition of the surface; condition and direction of the eyelashes; and the patient's ability to open, close, and blink. When the eyes are open in a normal position, the lids cover the sclera above the iris but not the pupil. The lids are also close to the eyeball. An abnormal drooping of the lid over the pupil is called ptosis (pronounced "toe-sis") and is caused by edema or impairment of the third cranial nerve. In the older adult ptosis results from a loss of elasticity that accompanies aging. An older adult frequently has lid margins that turn out (ectropion) or in (entropion). Entropion sometimes leads to the lashes of the lid irritating the conjunctiva and cornea, increasing the risk of infection. Normally the eyelashes are distributed evenly and curved outward away from the eye. An erythematous or yellow lump (hordeolum or stye) on the follicle of an eyelash indicates an acute suppurative inflammation.

FIG. 30.11 Six directions of gaze. Direct patient to follow finger movement through each gaze. *CN,* Cranial nerve.

FIG. 30.12 The lacrimal apparatus secretes and drains tears, which moisten and lubricate eye structures.

FIG. 30.13 Chart depicting pupillary size in millimeters.

To inspect the surface of the upper lids, ask the patient to close the eyes while observing for lid tremors. Normally the lids are smooth and the same color as the surrounding skin. Redness indicates inflammation or infection. Lid edema is sometimes caused by allergies or heart or kidney failure. Edema of the eyelids prevents them from closing. Inspect any lesions for typical characteristics and discomfort or drainage. Wear clean gloves if drainage is present.

The lids normally close symmetrically. Their failure to close exposes the cornea to drying. This condition is common in unconscious patients or those with facial nerve paralysis. To inspect the lower lids, ask the patient to open the eyes again while you look for the same characteristics noted for the upper lids. Normally a patient blinks involuntarily and bilaterally up to 20 times a minute. The blink reflex lubricates the cornea. Report absent, infrequent, rapid, or monocular (one-eyed) blinking.

Lacrimal Apparatus. The lacrimal gland (Fig. 30.12), located in the upper outer wall of the anterior part of the orbit, is responsible for tear production. Tears flow from the gland across the surface of the eye to the lacrimal duct, which is in the nasal corner or inner canthus of the eye. The lacrimal gland is sometimes the site of tumors or infections and should be inspected for edema and redness. Palpate the gland gently to detect tenderness; normally tenderness cannot be felt.

The nasolacrimal duct sometimes becomes obstructed, blocking the flow of tears. Observe for evidence of edema in the inner canthus. Gentle palpation of the duct at the lower eyelid just inside the lower orbital rim causes a regurgitation of tears.

Conjunctivae and Sclerae. The bulbar conjunctiva covers the exposed surface of the eyeball up to the outer edge of the cornea. Observe the sclera under the bulbar conjunctiva; normally it has the color of white porcelain in patients with light skin and is light yellow in patients with dark skin. Sclerae become pigmented and appear either yellow or green if liver disease is present.

Take care when inspecting the conjunctivae. For adequate exposure of the bulbar conjunctiva, retract the eyelids without placing pressure directly on the eyeball. Gently retract both lids, with the thumb and index finger pressed against the lower and upper bony orbits. Ask the patient to look up, down, and from side to side. Many patients begin to blink, making the examination difficult. Inspect for color, texture, and the presence of edema or lesions. Normally the conjunctivae are free of erythema. The presence of redness indicates an allergic or infectious conjunctivitis. Bright red blood in a localized area surrounded by normal-appearing conjunctiva usually indicates subconjunctival hemorrhage. Conjunctivitis is a highly contagious infection. It is easy to spread the crusty drainage that collects on eyelid margins from one eye to the other. When drainage is present, wear clean gloves during the examination and perform proper hand hygiene before and after the eye examination.

Corneas. The cornea is the transparent, colorless part of the eye covering the pupil and iris. From a side view it looks like the crystal of a wristwatch. While the patient looks straight ahead, inspect the cornea for clarity and texture while shining a penlight obliquely across its entire surface. The cornea is normally shiny, transparent, and smooth. In older adults it loses its luster. Any irregularity in the surface indicates an abrasion or tear that requires further examination by a health care provider. Both conditions are very painful. Note the color and details of the underlying iris. In an older adult the iris becomes faded. A thin white ring along the margin of the iris, called an arcus senilis, is common with aging but is abnormal in anyone under age 40. To test for the corneal blink reflex, see the cranial nerve test section of this chapter.

Pupils and Irises. Observe the pupils for size, shape, equality, accommodation, and reaction to light. They are normally black, round, regular, and equal in size (3–7 mm in diameter) (Fig. 30.13). The iris should be clearly visible.

FIG. 30.14 (A) To check pupillary reflexes the nurse first holds penlight to side of patient's face. (B) Illumination of pupil causes pupillary constriction.

FIG. 30.15 Fundus of White patient (A) and Black patient (B). (Courtesy MEDCOM, Cypress, CA.)

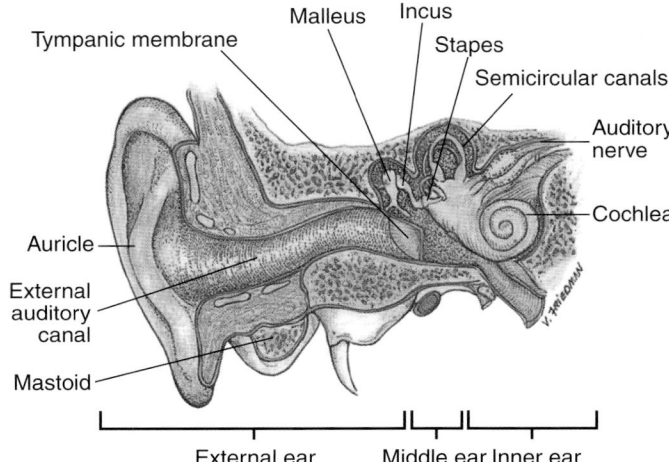

FIG. 30.16 Structures of external, middle, and inner ear.

Cloudy pupils indicate cataracts. Dilated pupils result from glaucoma, trauma, neurological disorders, eye medications (e.g., atropine), or withdrawal from opioids. Inflammation of the iris or use of drugs (e.g., pilocarpine, morphine, or cocaine) causes constricted pupils. Pinpoint pupils are a common sign of opioid intoxication. Shining a beam of light through the pupil and onto the retina stimulates the third cranial nerve, causing the muscles of the iris to constrict. Any abnormality along the nerve pathways from the retina to the iris alters the ability of the pupils to react to light. Changes in intracranial pressure, lesions along the nerve pathways, locally applied ophthalmic medications, and direct trauma to the eye alter pupillary reaction.

Test pupillary reflexes (to light and accommodation) in a dimly lit room. Instruct the patient to avoid looking directly at the light. While the patient looks straight ahead, bring a penlight from the side of the patient's face, directing the light onto the pupil (Fig. 30.14). A directly illuminated pupil constricts, and the opposite pupil constricts consensually. Observe the quickness and equality of the reflex. Repeat the examination for the opposite eye.

To test for accommodation, ask the patient to gaze at a distant object (the far wall) and then at a test object (finger or pencil) held approximately 10 cm (4 inches) from the bridge of the patient's nose. The pupils normally converge and accommodate by constricting when looking at close objects. The pupillary responses are equal. Testing for accommodation is important only if the patient has a defect in the pupillary response to light (Ball et al., 2019). If assessment of pupillary reaction is normal in all tests, record the abbreviation **PERRLA** (pupils equal, round, reactive to light, and accommodation).

Internal Eye Structures. The examination of the internal eye structures using an ophthalmoscope is beyond the scope of new graduate nurses' practice. Advanced nurse practitioners use the ophthalmoscope to inspect the fundus (Fig. 30.15), which includes the retina, choroid, optic nerve disc, macula, fovea centralis, and retinal vessels. Patients in greatest need of an examination are those with diabetes mellitus, hypertension, and intracranial disorders or trauma.

Ears

The ear assessment determines the integrity of ear structures and hearing acuity. The three parts of the ear are the external, middle, and inner ear (Fig. 30.16). Inspect and palpate external ear structures, which consist of the auricle, outer ear canal, and tympanic membrane (eardrum). The ear canal is normally curved and approximately 2.5 cm (1 inch) long in an adult. It is lined with skin containing fine hairs, nerve endings, and glands secreting cerumen. The middle ear is inspected with an otoscope. It is an air-filled cavity containing the three bony ossicles (malleus, incus, and stapes). The eustachian tube connects the middle ear to the nasopharynx. Pressure between the outer atmosphere and the middle ear is stabilized through this tube. Finally, the inner ear is tested

TABLE 30.14 Nursing History for Ear Assessment

Assessment	Rationale
Ask whether patient has experienced ear pain, itching, discharge, vertigo, tinnitus (ringing in ears), or change in hearing.	These signs and symptoms indicate infection, postural vertigo, or hearing loss.
If patient had recent hearing problem, note onset, contributing factors, affected ear, and effect on activities of daily living.	Helps determine nature and severity of hearing problem.
Assess risks for hearing problem. • *Infants/children:* Hypoxia at birth, meningitis, birth weight less than 1500 g, family history of hearing loss, congenital anomalies of skull or face, nonbacterial intrauterine infections (rubella, herpes), maternal drug use, excessively high bilirubin level, head trauma • *Adolescents:* Frequent exposure to loud music from concerts, car radios, and cell phone or iPods while wearing headphone, earbuds, or other devices • *Adults:* Exposure to industrial or recreational noise, genetic disease (Ménière disease), neurodegenerative disorder	Risk factors predispose patient to permanent hearing loss. It is difficult to assess infant's hearing status with examination only.
Determine patient's exposure to loud noises at work and availability of protective devices. Does patient understand benefit of using devices?	Prolonged noise exposure causes temporary or permanent hearing loss.
Note behaviors indicative of hearing loss, such as failure to respond when spoken to, requests to repeat comments, leaning forward to hear, and child's inattentiveness or use of a monotonous voice tone.	People with hearing loss cope with sensory deficit through a variety of behavioral cues.
Assess whether patient takes large doses of aspirin or other ototoxic drugs (e.g., aminoglycosides, furosemide, streptomycin, cisplatin, ethacrynic acid).	Medications have side effects of hearing loss.
Determine whether patient uses hearing aid.	Determination allows you to assess patient's ability to care for device and adjust voice tone to communicate.
Determine whether patient has repeated history of cerumen buildup in ear.	Cerumen impaction is common cause for conduction deafness.

by measuring a patient's hearing acuity. The inner ear contains the cochlea, vestibule, and semicircular canals. Assessing the ears determines the integrity of ear structures and the condition of hearing. Use nursing history data to identify patients' risks for hearing disorders (Table 30.14).

Understanding the mechanisms for sound transmission helps identify the nature of hearing disorders. Sound travels through the ear by air and bone conduction. Nerve impulses from the cochlea travel to the auditory nerve (eighth cranial nerve) and the cerebral cortex. Disorders of the ear result from several types of problems, including mechanical dysfunction (blockage by cerumen or foreign body), trauma (foreign bodies or noise exposure), neurological disorders (auditory nerve damage), acute illnesses (viral infection), and toxic effects of medications.

Auricles. With the patient sitting comfortably, inspect the size, shape, symmetry, landmarks, position, and color of the auricle (Fig. 30.17). The auricles are normally of equal size and level with each other. The upper point of attachment is in a straight line with the lateral canthus, or corner of the eye. The position of the auricle is almost vertical. Ears that are low set or at an unusual angle are a sign of chromosomal abnormality such as Down syndrome. Ear color is usually the same as that of the face, without moles, cysts, deformities, or nodules. Redness is a sign of inflammation or fever. Extreme pallor indicates frostbite.

Palpate the auricles for texture, tenderness, and skin lesions. Auricles are normally smooth and without lesions. If a patient has pain, gently pull the auricle, press on the tragus, and palpate behind the ear over the mastoid process. If palpating the external ear increases the pain, an external ear infection is likely. If palpating the auricle and tragus does not influence the pain, the patient may have a middle ear infection. Tenderness in the mastoid area indicates mastoiditis.

Inspect the opening of the ear canal for size and presence of discharge. If discharge is present, wear clean gloves. A swollen or occluded

FIG. 30.17 Anatomical structures of auricle.

meatus is not normal. A yellow, waxy substance called cerumen is common. Yellow or green, foul-smelling discharge indicates infection or a foreign body.

Ear Canals and Eardrums. Observe the deeper structures of the external and middle ear with the use of an otoscope. A special ear speculum attaches to the handle of the ophthalmoscope. For best visualization select the largest speculum that fits comfortably in the patient's ear. Before inserting the speculum, check for foreign bodies in the opening of the auditory canal.

Make sure that the patient avoids moving the head during the examination to avoid damage to the canal and tympanic membrane. Infants and

FIG. 30.18 Otoscopic examination. (From Wilson S, Giddens J: *Health assessment for nursing practice,* ed 7, St Louis, 2022, Elsevier.)

young children might need to be held securely to prevent movement. Lay infants supine with head turned to one side and arms held securely at the sides. Have young children sit on their parents' laps with their legs held between the parents' knees.

Turn on the otoscope by rotating the dial at the top of the handle. To insert the speculum properly, ask the patient to tip the head slightly toward the opposite shoulder. Hold the handle of the otoscope in the space between the thumb and index finger, supported on the middle finger. This leaves the ulnar side of the hand to rest against the patient's head, stabilizing the otoscope as you insert it into the canal (Ball et al., 2019). There are two ways to grip the otoscope: (1) hold the handle along the patient's face with the fingers against the face or neck, and (2) lightly brace the inverted otoscope against the side of the patient's head or cheek. This latter grip, used with children, prevents accidental movement of the otoscope deeper into the ear canal. Insert the scope while pulling the auricle upward and backward in the adult and older child (Fig. 30.18). This maneuver straightens the ear canal. For infants, the auricle should be pulled down and back.

Insert the speculum slightly down and forward 1 to 1.5 cm (½ inch) into the ear canal. Take care not to scrape the sensitive lining, which is painful. The ear canal normally has little cerumen and is uniformly pink with tiny hairs in the outer third of the canal. Observe for color, discharge, scaling, lesions, foreign bodies, and cerumen. Normally cerumen is dry (light brown to gray and flaky) or moist (dark yellow or brown) and sticky. Dry cerumen is common in Asians and Native Americans (Ball et al., 2019). A reddened canal with discharge is a sign of inflammation or infection. In older adults accumulated cerumen is a common problem; buildup creates a mild hearing loss. During the examination ask the patient about methods used to clean the ear canal (Box 30.14).

The light from the otoscope allows visualization of the tympanic membrane. Know the common anatomical landmarks and their appearances (Fig. 30.19). Gently move the otoscope so that the entire tympanic membrane and its periphery are visible. Because the tympanic membrane is angled away from the ear canal, the light from the otoscope appears as a cone shape rather than a circle. A ring of fibrous cartilage surrounds the oval membrane. The umbo is near the center of the membrane, behind which is the attachment of the malleus. The underlying short process of the malleus creates a knoblike structure at the top of the drum. Check carefully to make sure that there are no tears or breaks in the membrane. The normal tympanic membrane is

BOX 30.14 PATIENT TEACHING
Ear Assessment

Objective
- Patient will follow preventive guidelines for screening of hearing loss and proper cleaning technique for the ears.

Teaching Strategies
- Explain that noise-induced hearing loss can lead to communication difficulties, learning difficulties, pain or ringing in the ears (tinnitus), distorted or muffled hearing, and an inability to hear some environmental sounds and warning signals.
- Encourage patients to adopt behaviors to protect their hearing (CDC, 2021b):
  - Avoid or limit exposure to excessively loud sounds.
  - Turn down the volume of music systems.
  - Move away from the source of loud sounds when possible.
  - Use hearing protection devices when it is not feasible to avoid exposure to loud sounds or to reduce them to a safe level.
- Instruct patient in the proper way to clean the outer ear (see Chapter 40), avoiding use of cotton-tipped applicators and sharp objects such as hairpins, which cause impaction of cerumen deep in the ear canal or trauma.
- Tell patient to avoid inserting pointed objects into the ear canal.
- Encourage patients over age 65 to have regular hearing checks. Explain that a reduction in hearing is a normal part of aging (see Chapter 49).
- Instruct family members of patients with hearing loss to avoid shouting; to speak more slowly and with lower tones; and to be sure that the patient is able to see the speaker's face.

Evaluation
Use the principles of teach-back to evaluate patient/family caregiver learning:
- Describe two ways to protect hearing while you are home.
- Show me how you will safely clean your ears.
- Tell me how often you should have your hearing checked.

FIG. 30.19 Normal right tympanic membrane. (Courtesy Dr. Richard A. Buckingham, Abraham Lincoln School of Medicine, University of Illinois, Chicago.)

translucent, shiny, and pearly gray. It is free from tears or breaks. A pink or red bulging membrane indicates inflammation. A white color reveals pus behind it. The membrane is taut, except for the small triangular pars flaccida near the top. If cerumen is blocking the tympanic membrane, warm water irrigation safely removes the wax.

Hearing Acuity. A patient with a hearing loss often fails to respond to conversation. The three types of hearing loss are conduction, sensorineural,

TABLE 30.15   Tuning Fork Tests

Tests and Steps	Rationale
Weber Test (Lateralization of Sound) Hold fork at its base and tap it lightly against heel of palm. Place base of vibrating fork on midline vertex of patient's head or middle of forehead (see illustration *A*). Ask patient whether sound is heard equally in both ears or better in one ear (lateralization).	Patient with normal hearing hears sound equally in both ears. In conduction deafness, sound is heard best in impaired ear. In sensorineural hearing loss, sound is heard better in normal ear.
Rinne Test (Comparison of Air and Bone Conduction) Place stem of vibrating tuning fork against patient's mastoid process (see illustration *B*). Begin counting the interval with your watch. Ask patient to tell you when sound is no longer heard; note number of seconds. Quickly place still-vibrating tines 1 to 2 cm (½–1 inch) from ear canal and ask patient to tell you when sound is no longer heard (see illustration *C*). Continue counting time the sound is heard by air conduction. Compare number of seconds the sound is heard by bone conduction versus air conduction.	Patient should hear air-conducted sound twice as long as bone-conducted sound (2:1 ratio). For example, if patient hears bone-conducted sound for 10 seconds, air-conducted sound should be heard for an additional 10 seconds. In conduction deafness patient hears bone conduction longer than air conduction in affected ear. In sensorineural loss patient hears air conduction longer than bone conduction in affected ear, but at less than a 2:1 ratio (Ball et al., 2019).

and mixed. A conduction loss interrupts sound waves as they travel from the outer ear to the cochlea of the inner ear because the sound waves are not transmitted through the outer and middle ear structures. Causes of a conduction loss include swelling of the auditory canal and tears in the tympanic membrane. A sensorineural loss involves the inner ear, auditory nerve, or hearing center of the brain. Sound is conducted through the outer and middle ear structures, but the continued transmission of sound becomes interrupted at some point beyond the bony ossicles. A mixed loss involves a combination of conduction and sensorineural loss. Patients working or living around loud noises and those who listen to loud music are at risk for hearing loss.

Older adults experience an inability to hear high-frequency sounds and consonants (e.g., *S*, *Z*, *T*, and *G*). Deterioration of the cochlea and thickening of the tympanic membrane cause older adults to gradually lose hearing acuity. They are especially at risk for hearing loss caused by ototoxicity (injury to auditory nerve) resulting from high maintenance doses of antibiotics (e.g., aminoglycosides).

To conduct a hearing assessment, have the patient remove any hearing aid if worn. Note the responses to questions. Normally the patient responds without excessive requests to have the questions repeated. If a hearing loss is suspected, check the patient's response to the whispered voice. Test one ear at a time while the patient occludes the other ear with a finger. Ask the patient to gently move the finger up and down during the test in response to the whispered sound. While standing 31 to 60 cm (1–2 feet) from the testing ear, speak while covering the mouth so that the patient is unable to read lips. After exhaling fully, whisper softly toward the unoccluded ear, reciting random numbers with equally accented syllables, such as *nine-four-ten*. If necessary, gradually increase voice intensity until the patient correctly repeats the numbers. Then test the other ear for comparison. Ball et al. (2019) report that patients normally hear numbers clearly when whispered, responding correctly at least 50% of the time.

If a hearing loss is present, test the hearing using a tuning fork. A tuning fork of 256 to 512 hertz (Hz) is most commonly used. The tuning fork allows for comparison of hearing by bone conduction with that of air conduction. Hold the base of the tuning fork with one hand without touching the tines. Tap the fork lightly against the palm of the other hand to set it in vibration (Table 30.15).

TABLE 30.16 Nursing History for Nose and Sinus Assessment

Assessment	Rationale
Ask whether patient has had trauma to nose.	Trauma causes septal deviation and asymmetry of external nose.
Ask whether patient has history of allergies, nasal discharge, epistaxis (nosebleeds), or postnasal drip.	History is useful in determining source or nature of nasal and sinus drainage.
If there is history of nasal discharge, assess color, amount, odor, duration, and associated symptoms (e.g., sneezing, nasal congestion, obstruction, or mouth breathing).	Aids in ruling out presence of infection, allergy, or drug use.
Assess for history of nosebleed, including site, frequency, amount of bleeding, treatment, and difficulty stopping bleeding.	Characteristics sometimes reveal trauma, medication use, or excessive dryness as causative factors.
Ask whether patient uses nasal spray or drops, including type, amount, frequency, and duration of use.	Overuse of certain over-the-counter nasal preparations causes physical change in mucosa. Normal saline nasal drops are safe to use.
Ask whether patient snores at night or has difficulty breathing.	Difficulty breathing or snoring indicates septal deviation or obstruction.

Nose and Sinuses

Use inspection and palpation to assess the integrity of the nose and sinuses. The patient sits during the examination. A penlight allows for gross examination of each naris. A more detailed examination requires use of a nasal speculum to inspect the deeper nasal turbinates. Do not use a speculum unless a qualified practitioner such as a nurse educator or an advanced practice nurse is present. Table 30.16 lists components of the nursing history.

Nose. When inspecting the external nose, observe for shape, size, skin color, and the presence of deformity or inflammation. The nose is normally smooth and symmetrical, with the same skin color as the face. Recent trauma sometimes causes edema and discoloration. If swelling or deformities exist, gently palpate the ridge and soft tissue of the nose by placing one finger on each side of the nasal arch and gently moving the fingers from the nasal bridge to the tip. Note any tenderness, masses, or underlying deviations. Nasal structures are usually firm and stable.

Air normally passes freely through the nose when a person breathes. To assess patency of the nares, place a finger on the side of the patient's nose and occlude one naris. Ask the patient to breathe with the mouth closed. Repeat the procedure for the other naris.

While illuminating the anterior nares, inspect the mucosa for color, lesions, discharge, swelling, and evidence of bleeding. If discharge is present, apply gloves. Normal mucosa is pink and moist without lesions. Pale mucosa with clear discharge indicates allergy. A mucoid discharge indicates rhinitis. An infection (viral or bacterial) results in yellowish or greenish discharge. Habitual use of intranasal cocaine and opioids causes puffiness and increased vascularity of the nasal mucosa. For the patient with a nasogastric tube, routinely check for local skin breakdown (excoriation) of the naris, characterized by redness and skin sloughing.

To view the septum and turbinates, have the patient tip the head back slightly to provide a clear view. Illuminate the septum and observe for alignment, perforation, or bleeding. Normally the septum is close to the midline and thicker anteriorly than posteriorly. The turbinates are covered with mucous membranes that warm and moisten inspired air. Normal mucosa is pink and moist, without lesions. A deviated septum obstructs breathing and interferes with passage of a nasogastric tube. Perforation of the septum often occurs after repeated use of intranasal cocaine. Note any polyps (tumorlike growths) or purulent drainage.

Sinuses. Examination of the sinuses involves palpation. In cases of allergies or infection, the interior of the sinuses becomes inflamed and swollen. The most effective way to assess for tenderness is by externally

FIG. 30.20 Palpation of maxillary sinuses.

palpating the frontal and maxillary facial areas (Fig. 30.20). Palpate the frontal sinus by exerting pressure with the thumb up and under the patient's eyebrow. Gentle, upward pressure elicits tenderness easily if sinus irritation is present. Do not apply pressure to the eyes. If sinus tenderness is present, the sinuses may be transilluminated. However, this procedure requires advanced experience. Box 30.15 describes teaching guidelines during nose and sinus assessment.

Mouth and Pharynx

Assess the mouth and pharynx to detect signs of overall health. Determine a patient's oral hygiene needs and therapies needed for dehydration, restricted intake, oral trauma, or oral airway obstruction. To assess the oral cavity, use a penlight and tongue depressor or gauze square. Wear clean gloves during the examination. Have the patient sit or lie down. Assess the oral cavity also while administering oral hygiene (see Chapter 40). Table 30.17 describes the nursing history for assessment of the mouth and pharynx.

Lips. Inspect the lips for color, texture, hydration, contour, and lesions. With the patient's mouth closed, view the lips from end to end. Normally

BOX 30.15 PATIENT TEACHING

Nose and Sinus Assessment

Objective

- Patient will explain self-care measures to maintain sinus integrity and minimize loss of olfaction.

Teaching Strategies

- Caution patient against overuse of over-the-counter nasal sprays, which leads to "rebound" effect, causing excess nasal congestion.
- Instruct parents in care of a child with nosebleeds: have child sit up and lean forward to avoid aspiration of blood, apply pressure to the anterior nose with the thumb and forefinger as the child breathes through the mouth, and apply ice or a cold cloth to the bridge of the nose if pressure fails to stop bleeding.
- Instruct older adults with loss of olfaction to follow safety precautions:
  - Install smoke detectors on each floor of their home.
  - Ask others to advise them when food smells pungent.
- Instruct older adults to always check dated labels on food to ensure against spoilage.

Evaluation

Use the principles of teach-back to evaluate patient/family caregiver learning:
- Show me how you will instill the nasal spray you purchased at the pharmacy.
- Show me the techniques that you will use to stop a nosebleed.
- Show me the smoke detector locations in your home and how you check to make sure they are working properly.

they are pink, moist, symmetrical, and smooth (Fig. 30.21). Lip color in a patient with dark skin varies from pink to plum. Have female patients remove their lipstick before the examination. Anemia causes pallor of the lips, with cyanosis caused by respiratory or cardiovascular problems. Cherry-colored lips indicate carbon monoxide poisoning. When you inspect any lesion, consider the potential of it being an infection, irritation, or skin cancer.

Buccal Mucosa, Gums, and Teeth. Ask the patient to clench the teeth and smile to observe teeth occlusion. The upper molars normally

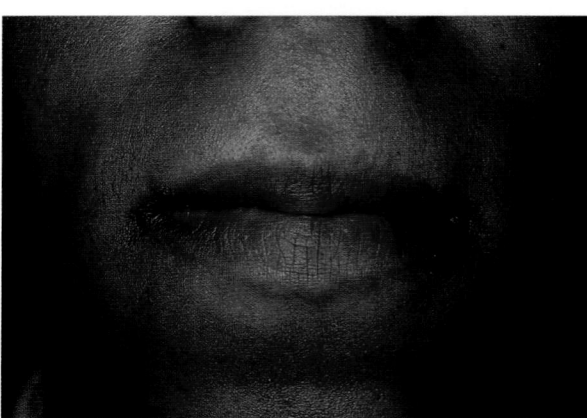

FIG. 30.21 Lips are normally pink, symmetrical, smooth, and moist.

TABLE 30.17 Nursing History for Mouth and Pharyngeal Assessment

Assessment	Rationale
Determine whether patient wears dentures or retainers and whether they are comfortable.	Patient needs to remove dentures to visualize and palpate gums. Ill-fitting dentures chronically irritate mucosa and gums.
Determine whether patient has had recent change in appetite or weight.	Symptoms may result from painful mouth conditions or poor oral hygiene.
Determine if patient has history of human papilloma virus HPV16.	HPV16 contributes more to the incidence rate of oral cancers, particularly in the posterior part of the mouth (oropharynx, tonsils, the base of the tongue) and many times does not produce visible lesions or discolorations that have historically been the early warning signs of the disease process in the anterior (front) of the mouth (Oral Cancer Foundation, 2021).
Determine whether patient uses tobacco products: • Smoking cigarettes, cigars, or pipe; smokeless tobacco; chewing tobacco and snuff • E-cigarettes or vapor cigarettes	Tobacco use in any form (smoked and smokeless) increases the risk for oral-pharyngeal cancer (ACS, 2020a). Long-term smokeless tobacco users have an increased risk for cancer of the gums and cheeks (ACS, 2020a). Electronic nicotine delivery systems (e-cigarettes) are on the rise in adolescents and may contribute to the use of combustible tobacco products because the flavorings desensitize the lungs' negative response to nicotine inhalation (ACS, 2020a; Cancer.Net, 2019).
Review history for alcohol consumption.	Oral and pharyngeal cancers are more common in people who use alcohol. Those who both smoke and drink have a 30 times greater risk of developing oral cancer than others (ACS, 2020a; Oral Cancer Foundation, 2021).
Assess dental hygiene practices, including use of fluoride toothpaste, frequency of brushing and flossing, and frequency of dental visits.	Assessment reveals patient's need for education and/or financial support. Periodontal disease has a higher prevalence in older adults who have history of high plaque buildup, use tobacco, and visit the dentist infrequently.
Ask whether patient has pain from chewing or eating. If so, ask whether mouth lesions are present, including duration and associated symptoms.	Pain is often associated with broken teeth, teeth grinding, or temporomandibular joint problems. Extra care is needed during oral hygiene administration.
Review a patient's medical history for a previous diagnosis of the human papilloma virus (HPV).	HPV, particularly HPV-16, has been definitively implicated as a risk for oral cancers, particularly those that occur in the back of the mouth (oropharynx, base of tongue, tonsillar pillars and crypt, and the tonsils themselves) (ACS, 2020a; Oral Cancer Foundation, 2021).

BOX 30.16 PATIENT TEACHING

Mouth and Pharynx Assessment

Objective
- Patient will practice proper oral hygiene/dental care measures and identify symptoms of oral cancer.

Teaching Strategies
- Discuss proper techniques for oral hygiene, including brushing and flossing (see Chapter 40).
- Explain the early warning signs of oral cavity and pharynx cancer that should be checked by a health care professional, including a mouth sore that bleeds easily and does not heal, a lump or thickening in the cheek, a white or red patch on the mucosa that persists, a sore throat or a feeling that something is caught in the throat, numbness of the tongue or other area of the mouth, or a swelling of the jaw that causes dentures to not fit (Oral Cancer Foundation, 2021).
- Late symptoms of oral cancer are difficulty in chewing, swallowing, or moving the tongue or jaw (ACS, 2020a).
- Encourage regular dental examination every 6 months for children, adults, and older adults.

Evaluation
Use the principles of teach-back to evaluate patient/family caregiver learning:
- Show me the technique you use to brush your teeth.
- Explain to me how often you should have regular dental checkups.
- Tell me the warning signs of mouth cancer and when you should call the health care provider.

FIG. 30.22 Inspection of inner oral mucosa of lower lip.

FIG. 30.23 Retraction of buccal mucosa allows for clear visualization.

rest directly on the lower molars, and the upper incisors slightly override the lower incisors. A symmetrical smile reveals normal facial nerve function.

Inspect the teeth to determine the quality of dental hygiene (Box 30.16). Note the position and alignment of the teeth. To examine the posterior surface of the teeth, have the patient open the mouth with the lips relaxed. Use a tongue depressor to retract the lips and cheeks, especially when viewing the molars. Note the color of teeth and presence of dental caries (cavities), tartar, and extraction sites. Normal, healthy teeth are smooth, white, and shiny. A chalky white discoloration of the enamel is an early indication of caries formation. Brown or black discolorations indicate the formation of caries. A stained yellow color is from tobacco use; coffee, tea, and colas cause a brown stain. In the older adult loose or missing teeth are common because bone resorption increases. An older adult's teeth often feel rough when tooth enamel calcifies. Yellow or darkened teeth are also common in the older adult because of the general wear and tear that exposes the darker underlying dentin.

To view the mucosa and gums, ask the patient to first remove any dental appliance. View the inner oral mucosa by having the patient open and relax the mouth slightly, and then gently retract the lower lip away from the teeth (Fig. 30.22). Repeat this process for the upper lip. Inspect the mucosa for color; hydration; texture; and lesions such as ulcers, abrasions, or cysts. Normally the mucosa is glistening, pink, smooth, and moist. Some common small, yellow-white raised lesions on the buccal mucosa and lips are Fordyce spots, or ectopic sebaceous glands (Ball et al., 2019). If lesions are present, palpate them gently with a gloved hand for tenderness, size, and consistency.

To inspect the buccal mucosa, ask the patient to open the mouth, and then gently retract the cheeks with a tongue depressor (Fig. 30.23). View the surface of the mucosa from right to left and top to bottom.

A penlight illuminates the most posterior part of the mucosa. Normal mucosa is glistening, pink, soft, moist, and smooth. Varying shades of hyperpigmentation are normal in 10% of Whites after age 50 and as many as 90% of Blacks by the same age. For patients with normal pigmentation, the buccal mucosa is a good site to inspect for jaundice and pallor. In older adults the mucosa is normally dry because of reduced salivation. Thick white patches (leukoplakia) are often a precancerous lesion seen in heavy smokers and alcoholics. Palpate for any buccal lesions by placing the index finger within the buccal cavity and the thumb on the outer surface of the cheek. Patients who smoke cigarettes, cigars, or pipes and those who use smokeless tobacco have an increased risk of oral, pharyngeal, laryngeal, and esophageal cancer. These individuals may have leukoplakia or other lesions anywhere in their oral cavity (e.g., lips, gums, or tongue) at an early age. These usually appear as cream-white patches throughout the inner mouth area.

Inspect the gums (gingivae) for color, edema, retraction, bleeding, and lesions while retracting the cheeks. Healthy gums are pink, smooth, and moist and fit tightly around each tooth. Patients with dark skin often have patchy pigmentation. In older adults the gums are usually pale. Using clean gloves, palpate the gums to assess for lesions, thickening, or masses. Normally there is no tenderness. Spongy gums that bleed easily indicate periodontal disease and vitamin C deficiency. If a patient has loose or mobile teeth, swollen gums, or pockets containing debris at the tooth margins, a dental referral is necessary to check for periodontal disease or gingivitis.

FIG. 30.24 Undersurface of tongue is highly vascular.

FIG. 30.25 Hard palate is located anteriorly in roof of mouth.

FIG. 30.26 Penlight and tongue depressor allow visualization of uvula and posterior soft palate.

Tongue and Floor of Mouth. Carefully inspect the tongue on all sides and the floor of the mouth. Have the patient relax the mouth and stick the tongue out halfway. Note any deviation, tremor, or limitation in movement. This tests hypoglossal nerve function. If a patient protrudes the tongue too far, it elicits the gag reflex. When the tongue protrudes, it lies midline. To test for tongue mobility, ask the patient to raise it up and move it from side to side. It should move freely.

Using a penlight for illumination, examine the tongue for color, size, position, texture, and coatings or lesions. A normal tongue is medium or dull red in color, moist, slightly rough on the top surface, and smooth along the lateral margins. The undersurface of the tongue and the floor of the mouth are highly vascular (Fig. 30.24). Take extra care to inspect this area, a common site for oral cancer lesions. The patient lifts the tongue by placing its tip on the palate behind the upper incisors. Inspect for color, swelling, and lesions such as nodules or cysts. The ventral surface of the tongue is pink and smooth, with large veins between the frenulum folds. To palpate the tongue, explain the procedure and ask the patient to protrude it. Grasp the tip with a gauze square and gently pull it to one side. With a gloved hand palpate the full length of the tongue and the base for any areas of hardening or ulceration. Varicosities (swollen, tortuous veins) are common in the older adult and rarely cause problems.

Palate. Have the patient extend the head backward, holding the mouth open, to inspect the hard and soft palates. The hard palate, or roof of the mouth, is located anteriorly. The whitish hard palate is dome shaped. The soft palate extends posteriorly toward the pharynx. It is normally light pink and smooth. Observe the palates for color, shape, texture, and extra bony prominences or defects (Fig. 30.25). A bony growth, or exostosis, between the two palates is common.

Pharynx. Perform an examination of pharyngeal structures to rule out infection, inflammation, or lesions. Have the patient tip the head back slightly, open the mouth wide, and say "ah" while you place the tip of a tongue depressor on the middle third of the tongue. Take care not to press the lower lip against the teeth. By placing the tongue depressor too far anteriorly, the posterior part of the tongue mounds up, obstructing the view. Placing the tongue depressor on the posterior tongue elicits the gag reflex.

With a penlight first inspect the uvula and soft palate (Fig. 30.26). Both structures, which are innervated by the tenth cranial (vagus) nerve, should rise centrally as the patient says "ah." Examine the anterior and posterior pillars, soft palate, and uvula. View the tonsils in the cavities between the anterior and posterior pillars and note the presence

or absence of tissue. The posterior pharynx is behind the pillars. Normally pharyngeal tissues are pink and smooth and well hydrated. Small irregular spots of lymphatic tissue and small blood vessels are normal. Note edema, petechiae (small hemorrhages), lesions, or exudate. Patients with chronic sinus problems frequently exhibit a clear exudate that drains along the wall of the posterior pharynx. Yellow or green exudate indicates infection. A patient with a typical sore throat has a red and edematous uvula and tonsillar pillars, with possible presence of yellow exudate.

Neck

Assessment of the neck includes assessing the neck muscles, lymph nodes of the head and neck, carotid arteries, jugular veins, thyroid gland, and trachea (Fig. 30.27). You may postpone the examination of the jugular veins and carotid arteries until the vascular system assessment. Inspect and palpate the neck to determine the integrity of its structures and examine the lymphatic system. An abnormality of superficial lymph nodes sometimes reveals the presence of an infection or **malignancy**. Examine the lymphatic system region by region during the assessment of other body systems (head and neck, breast, genitalia, and extremities). Examination of the thyroid gland and trachea also aids in ruling out malignancies. Perform this examination with the patient sitting. The sternocleidomastoid and trapezius muscles outline the areas of the neck, dividing each side of the neck into two triangles.

TABLE 30.18   Nursing History for Neck Assessment

Assessment	Rationale
Assess for history of recent cold, infection, or enlarged lymph nodes or exposure to radiation or toxic chemicals.	Colds or infections cause temporary or permanent lymph node enlargement. Lymph nodes are also enlarged in various diseases such as cancer.
If there is an enlarged lymph node, consider reviewing history of intravenous drug use, hemophilia, sexual contact with people infected with human immunodeficiency virus (HIV), history of blood transfusion, multiple and indiscriminate sexual contacts, or male with homosexual or bisexual activities.	These are risk factors for HIV infection.
Ask whether patient has had history of neck pain with restriction in movement.	This indicates muscle strain, head injury, local nerve injury, or enlarged or swollen lymph node.
Ask whether patient has had change in temperature preference (more or less clothing); swelling in neck; change in texture of hair, skin, or nails; or change in emotional stability.	Symptoms indicate thyroid disease.
Ask whether patient has history of hypothyroidism or hyperthyroidism, takes thyroid medication, or has a family history of thyroid disease.	Disease or medications influence tissue growth of gland.
Review medical history of pneumothorax (collapsed lung) or bronchial tumor.	Conditions place patient at risk for tracheal displacement or lateral deviation.

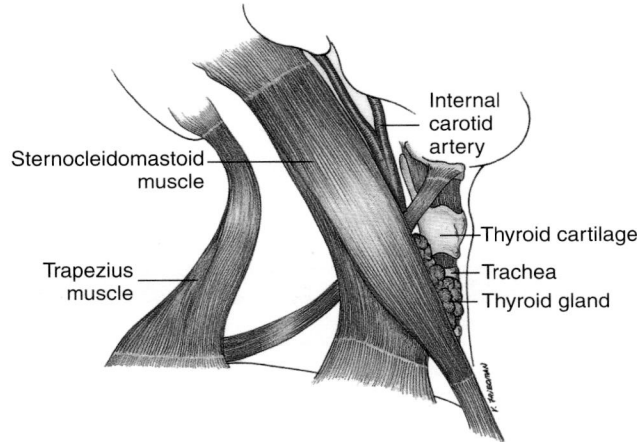

FIG. 30.27 Anatomical position of major neck structures. Note triangles formed by sternocleidomastoid muscle, lower jaw, and anterior neck anteriorly and sternocleidomastoid muscle, trapezius muscle, and lower neck posteriorly.

The anterior triangle contains the trachea, thyroid gland, carotid artery, and anterior cervical lymph nodes. The posterior triangle contains the posterior lymph nodes. Table 30.18 reviews the nursing history for the head and neck examination.

Neck Muscles. First inspect the neck in the usual anatomical position, with slight hyperextension. Observe for symmetry of the neck muscles. Ask the patient to flex the neck with the chin to the chest, hyperextend the neck backward, and move the head laterally to each side and then sideways with the ear moving toward the shoulder. This tests the sternocleidomastoid and trapezius muscles. The neck normally moves without discomfort. Perform other tests for muscle strength and function during assessment of the musculoskeletal system.

Lymph Nodes. An extensive system of lymph nodes collects lymph from the head, ears, nose, cheeks, and lips (Fig. 30.28). The immune system protects the body from foreign antigens, removes damaged cells from the circulation, and provides a partial barrier to growth of malignant cells within the body. Assessing the lymph nodes is critical in detecting a patient's risk for a compromised immune system, which is often linked to allergies, human immunodeficiency virus (HIV) infection, autoimmune disease (e.g., lupus erythematosus), or serious infection.

With the patient's chin raised and head tilted slightly, first inspect the area where lymph nodes are distributed and compare both sides. This position stretches the skin slightly over any possible enlarged nodes. Inspect visible nodes for edema, erythema, or red streaks. Nodes normally are not visible.

Use a methodical approach to palpate the lymph nodes to avoid overlooking any single node or chain. The patient relaxes with the neck flexed slightly forward. Inspect and palpate both sides of the neck for comparison. During palpation either face or stand to the side of the patient for easy access to all nodes. Use the pads of the middle three fingers of each hand to gently palpate in a circular motion over the nodes (Fig. 30.29). Check each node methodically in the following sequence: occipital nodes at the base of the skull, postauricular nodes over the mastoid, preauricular nodes just in front of the ear, retropharyngeal nodes at the angle of the mandible, submandibular nodes, and submental nodes in the midline behind the mandibular tip. Try to detect enlargement and note the location, size, shape, surface characteristics, consistency, mobility, tenderness, and warmth of the nodes. If the skin is mobile, move it over the area of the nodes. It is important to press underlying tissue in each area and not simply move the fingers over the skin. However, if you apply excessive pressure, you miss small nodes and destroy palpable nodes.

To palpate supraclavicular nodes, ask the patient to bend the head forward and relax the shoulders. Palpate these nodes by hooking the index and third fingers over the clavicle lateral to the sternocleidomastoid muscle. Palpate the deep cervical nodes only with the fingers hooked around the sternocleidomastoid muscle.

Normally lymph nodes are not easily palpable. However, small, mobile, nontender nodes are common. Lymph nodes that are large, fixed, inflamed, or tender indicate a problem such as local infection, systemic disease (e.g., autoimmune problem), or neoplasm (Ball et al., 2019) (Box 30.17). When you find enlarged nodes, explore the adjacent areas and regions that they drain. Tenderness almost always indicates inflammation. A problem involving a lymph node of the head and neck means an abnormality in the mouth, throat, abdomen, breasts, thorax, or arms. These are the areas drained by the head and neck nodes.

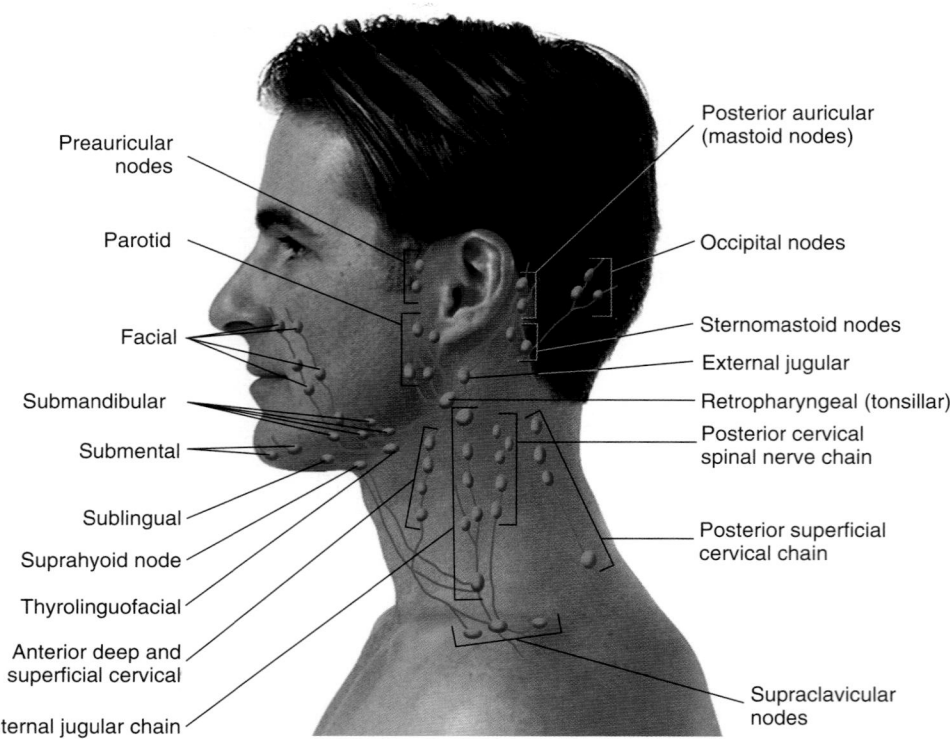

FIG. 30.28 Palpable lymph nodes in head and neck. (From Ball JW, et al: *Seidel's guide to physical examination,* ed 9, St Louis, 2019, Mosby.)

FIG. 30.29 (A) Palpation of preauricular lymph nodes. (B) Palpation of supraclavicular lymph nodes.

BOX 30.17   PATIENT TEACHING

Neck Assessment

Objective
- Patient will take proper preventive action if a mass in the neck is noted.

Teaching Strategies
- Stress the importance of regular adherence with the medication schedule to patients with thyroid disease.
- Instruct patient about the lymph nodes and how infection commonly causes node tenderness and mild enlargement.
- Instruct patient to call a health care provider when he or she notices a fixed, enlarged lump or mass in the neck.
- Teach patient the risk factors for HIV infection and other sexually transmitted diseases.

Evaluation
Use the principles of teach-back to evaluate patient/family caregiver learning:
- Tell me what signs and symptoms in the neck area would require you to contact your health care provider.

HIV, Human immunodeficiency virus.

Thyroid Gland. The thyroid gland lies in the anterior lower neck, in front of and to both sides of the trachea. The gland is fixed to the trachea, with the isthmus overlying the trachea and connecting the two irregular, cone-shaped lobes (Fig. 30.30). Inspect the lower neck overlying the thyroid gland for obvious masses, symmetry, and any subtle fullness at the base of the neck. Ask the patient to hyperextend the neck, which helps tighten the skin for better visualization. Offer the patient a glass of water and, while observing the neck, have the patient

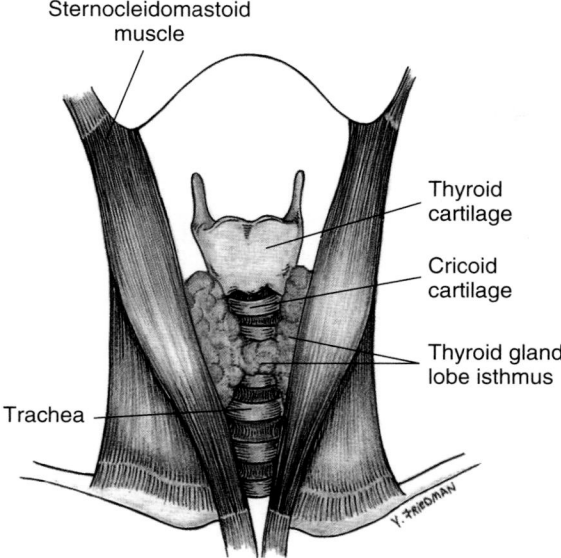

Sternocleidomastoid
muscle

Thyroid
cartilage

Cricoid
cartilage

Thyroid gland
lobe isthmus

Trachea

FIG. 30.30 Anatomical position of thyroid gland.

swallow. This maneuver helps to visualize an abnormally enlarged thyroid. Normally the thyroid cannot be visualized. Advanced practice nurses examine the thyroid by palpating for more subtle masses.

Carotid Artery and Jugular Vein. This part of the examination is described under examination of the vascular system (see later section).

Trachea. The trachea is a part of the upper respiratory system that you directly palpate. It is normally located in the midline above the suprasternal notch. Masses in the neck or mediastinum and pulmonary abnormalities cause displacement laterally. Have the patient sit or lie down during palpation. Determine the position of the trachea by palpating at the suprasternal notch, slipping the thumb and index fingers to each side. Note if the finger and thumb shift laterally. Do not apply forceful pressure because this elicits coughing.

THORAX AND LUNGS

Accurate physical assessment of the thorax and lungs requires review of the ventilatory and respiratory functions of the lungs. Diseases of the lungs affect other body systems. For example, the brain is extremely sensitive to oxygen levels. When a patient has reduced oxygenation, changes in level of consciousness and mental alertness result. Use data from all body systems to determine the nature of pulmonary alterations. You use inspection, palpation, and auscultation to examine the thorax and lungs. Diagnostic equipment such as x-ray films, magnetic resonance imaging (MRI), and computed tomography (CT) scans create little need for the use of percussion as an assessment measure. Risk factors for lung disease are reviewed at the time of respiratory assessment (Box 30.18).

First identify the landmarks of the chest to assess the thorax and lungs correctly (Fig. 30.31). A patient's nipples, angle of Louis, suprasternal notch, costal angle, clavicles, and vertebrae are key landmarks that provide a series of imaginary lines for sign identification. Keep a mental image of the location of the lobes of the lung and the position of each rib (Fig. 30.32). Your understanding of the anatomical structures ensures a thorough assessment of the anterior, lateral, and posterior thorax.

Locate the position of each rib to visualize the lobe of the lung being assessed. To begin, find the angle of Louis at the manubriosternal

BOX 30.18   PATIENT TEACHING
Lung Assessment

Objective
- The patient will practice preventive care measures for lung health.

Teaching Strategies
- Explain risk factors for chronic lung disease and lung cancer, including cigarette smoking; history of smoking for over 20 years; exposure to environmental pollution; and radiation exposure from occupational, medical, and environmental sources. Exposure to radon and asbestos also increases risk. Other risk factors include exposure to certain metals (e.g., arsenic, cadmium, chromium), some organic chemicals, and tuberculosis. Exposure to secondhand cigarette smoke increases risk for nonsmokers (ACS, 2020a).
- Share brochures on lung cancer, asthma, and chronic obstructive pulmonary disease (COPD) from American Cancer Society with patient and family.
- Instruct patient with asthma to identify and tell family members and friends which triggers cause asthma episodes.
- Instruct patient with asthma on proper use of inhaler and how to measure peak expiratory flow rate.
- Discuss warning signs of lung cancer, such as a persistent cough, sputum streaked with blood, chest pains, and recurrent attacks of pneumonia or bronchitis.
- Counsel older adult about benefits of receiving influenza and pneumonia vaccinations because of a greater susceptibility to respiratory infection.
- Instruct patient with COPD how to perform coughing and pursed-lip breathing exercises.
- Refer people at risk for tuberculosis to visit clinics or health care centers for skin testing.

Evaluation
Use the principles of teach-back to evaluate patient/family caregiver learning:
- Tell me three risk factors for lung disease and lung cancer.
- Describe for me the warning signs of lung cancer.
- Show me how to use your inhaler and measure peak expiratory flow rate.
- Explain to me the importance of receiving a pneumonia and annual influenza vaccine.
- Show me how you perform your deep breathing and coughing exercises.

junction. The angle is a visible and palpable angulation of the sternum and is the point at which the second rib articulates with the sternum. Count the ribs and intercostal spaces (between the ribs) from this point. The number of each intercostal space corresponds to that of the rib just above it. The spinous process of the third thoracic vertebra and the fourth, fifth, and sixth ribs help to locate the lobes of the lung laterally. The lower lobes project laterally and anteriorly (see Fig. 30.32B). Posteriorly the tip or inferior margin of the scapula lies approximately at the level of the seventh rib (see Fig. 30.32C). After identifying the seventh rib, count upward to locate the third thoracic vertebra and align it with the inner borders of the scapula to locate the posterior lobes.

Ensure that the patient is undressed to the waist, and that the room has good lighting when performing your assessment. Begin with the patient sitting to assess the posterior and lateral chest if possible. Have the patient sit or lie down for assessment of the anterior chest. Table 30.19 reviews the nursing history for lung examination. Before beginning the thoracic examination, observe for any signs or symptoms in other body systems that indicate pulmonary problems. Reduced mental alertness, nasal flaring, somnolence, and cyanosis are examples of assessed signs that indicate oxygenation problems.

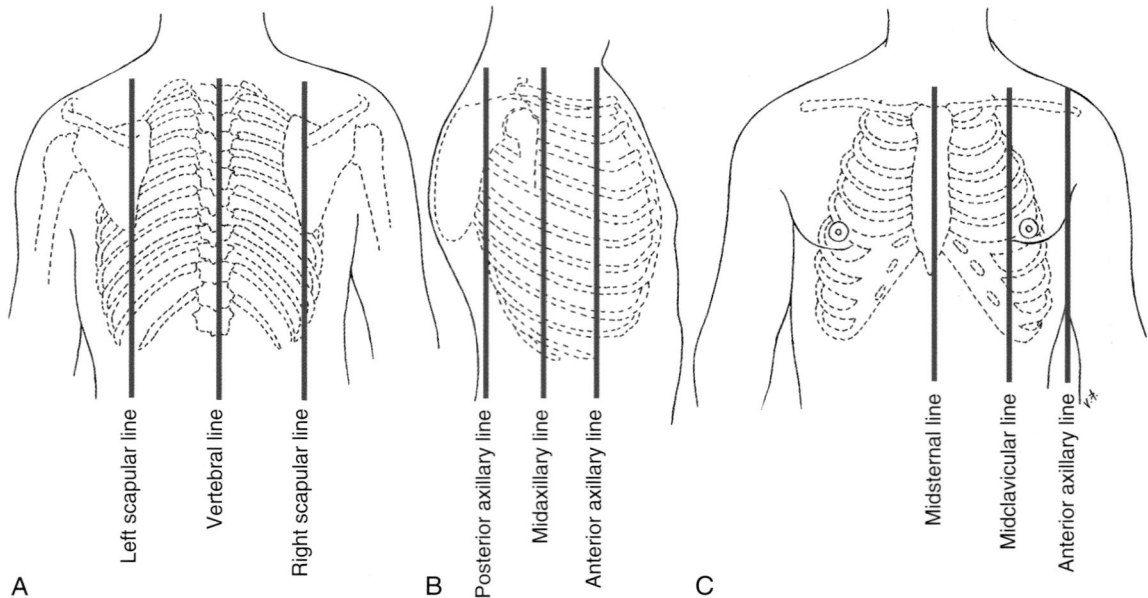

FIG. 30.31 Anatomical chest wall landmarks. (A) Posterior chest landmarks. (B) Lateral chest landmarks. (C) Anterior chest landmarks.

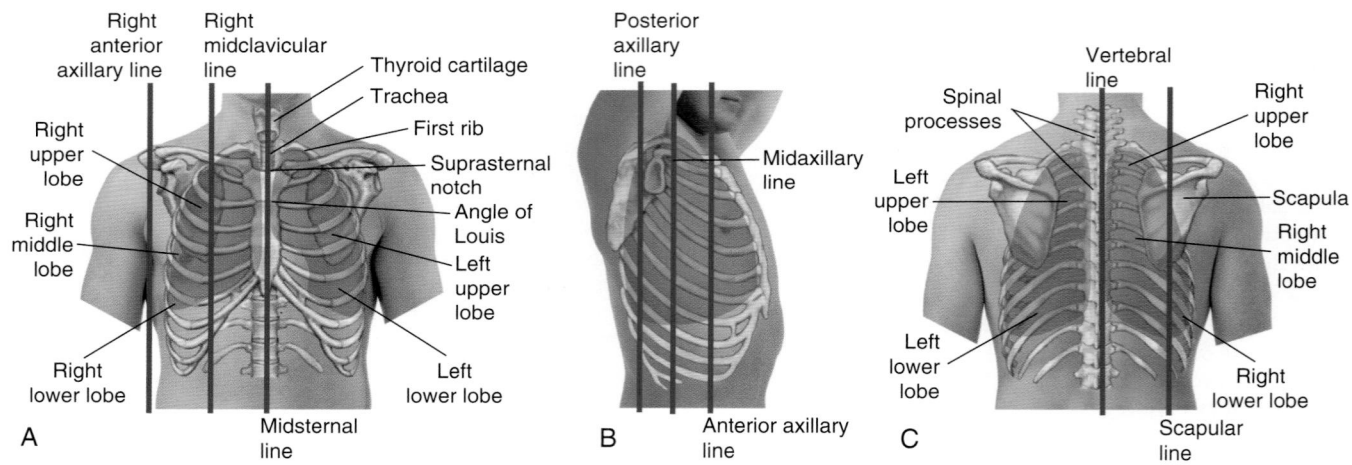

FIG. 30.32 Position of lung lobes in relation to anatomical landmarks. (A) Anterior position. (B) Lateral position. (C) Posterior position. (From Ball JW, et al: *Seidel's guide to physical examination,* ed 9, St Louis, 2019, Elsevier.)

Posterior Thorax

Inspect the posterior thorax by observing the shape and symmetry of the chest from the patient's back and front. Note the anteroposterior diameter. Body shape or posture significantly impairs ventilatory movement. Normally the chest contour is symmetrical, with the anteroposterior diameter one-third to one-half of the transverse, or side-to-side, diameter. A barrel-shaped chest (anteroposterior diameter equals transverse diameter) characterizes aging and chronic lung disease. Infants have an almost round shape. Congenital and postural alterations cause abnormal contours in which a patient may lean over a table or splint the side of the chest because of a breathing problem. Pain sometimes causes a patient to splint or hold the chest wall and bend toward the affected side, resulting in impaired ventilatory movement.

Standing at a midline position behind the patient, look for deformities, position of the spine, slope of the ribs, retraction of the intercostal spaces during inspiration, and bulging of the intercostal spaces during expiration. The scapulae are normally symmetrical and closely attached to the thoracic wall. The normal spine is straight without lateral deviation. Posteriorly the ribs tend to slope across and down. The ribs and intercostal spaces are easier to see in a thin person. Normally no bulging or active movement occurs within the intercostal spaces during breathing. Bulging indicates that a patient is using great effort to breathe.

Also assess the rate and rhythm of breathing. Observe the thorax as a whole. It normally expands and relaxes regularly with equal movement bilaterally. In healthy adults the normal respiratory rates vary from 12 to 20 respirations per minute.

TABLE 30.19 Nursing History for Lung Assessment

Assessment	Rationale
Assess history of tobacco or marijuana use, including type of tobacco, duration, and amount (Pack-years = Number of years smoking × Number of packs per day), age started, efforts to quit, and length of time since smoking stopped.	Smoking is a risk factor for lung cancer, heart disease, cerebrovascular disease, emphysema, or chronic bronchitis. It accounts for a significant percentage of all cancer deaths (ACS, 2020a).
Ask whether patient has had a *persistent cough* (productive or nonproductive), *sputum streaked with blood, voice change, chest pain,* shortness of breath, **orthopnea**, dyspnea during exertion or at rest, poor activity tolerance, or *recurrent attacks of pneumonia or bronchitis.*	Symptoms of cardiopulmonary alterations help localize objective physical findings. (Warning signals for lung cancer are in italic type.) The diaphragm of the lungs expands more easily when the individual is sitting upright, as for patients who must be in an upright position to breathe.
Determine whether patient works in environment containing pollutants (e.g., asbestos, arsenic, coal dust) or requiring exposure to radiation. Does patient have exposure to secondhand smoke?	These risk factors increase chance for various lung diseases.
Review history for known or suspected human immunodeficiency virus (HIV) infection; substance abuse; low income; or being homeless, a resident or employee of a nursing home or shelter, a recent prison inmate, a family member of a tuberculosis (TB) patient, or an immigrant to the United States from a country where TB is prevalent.	These are risk factors for TB.
Ask whether patient has history of persistent cough, hemoptysis, unexplained weight loss, fatigue, night sweats, or fever.	These are risk factors for both TB and HIV infection.
Does patient have history of chronic hoarseness?	Hoarseness indicates laryngeal disorder or abuse of cocaine or opioids (sniffing).
Assess history of allergies to pollens, dust, or other airborne irritants and to foods, drugs, or chemical substances.	Symptoms such as choking feeling, bronchospasm with respiratory stridor, wheezes on auscultation, and dyspnea are often caused by allergic response.
Review family history for cancer, TB, allergies, or chronic obstructive pulmonary disease.	Conditions place patient at risk for lung disease.
Ask whether patient has had a pneumonia or influenza vaccine and a TB test; if not, educate on the need to do so.	The very young, the very old, and those with chronic respiratory problems or immunosuppressive diseases are at increased risk for respiratory disease.

FIG. 30.33 (A) Hand position for palpation of posterior thorax excursion. (B) As patient inhales, movement of chest excursion separates thumbs.

Palpation of the posterior thorax provides further information about a patient's health status. Palpate the thoracic muscles and skeleton for lumps, masses, pulsations, and unusual movement. If the patient voices pain or tenderness, avoid deep palpation. Fractured rib fragments could be displaced against vital organs. Normally the chest wall is not tender. If there is a suspicious mass or swollen area, lightly palpate it for size, shape, and the typical qualities of a lesion.

To measure chest excursion or depth of breathing, stand behind the patient and place the thumbs along the spinal processes at the 10th rib, with the palms lightly contacting the posterolateral surfaces. Place thumbs 5 cm (2 inches) apart, pointing toward the spine with fingers pointing laterally (Fig. 30.33A). Press the hands toward the spine so that a small skinfold appears between the thumbs. Do not slide the hands over the skin. Instruct the patient to exhale and then take a deep breath. Note movement of the thumbs during inhalation (see Fig. 30.33B). Chest excursion is symmetrical, separating the thumbs 3 to 5 cm (1¼–2 inches). Reduced chest excursion may be caused by pain, postural deformity, or fatigue. In older adults, chest movement normally declines because of costal cartilage calcification and respiratory muscle atrophy.

During speech, the sound created by the vocal cords is transmitted through the lungs to the chest wall. The sound waves create vibrations that you palpate externally. These vibrations are called **vocal or tactile fremitus**. The accumulation of mucus, the collapse of lung tissue, or the presence of one or more lung lesions blocks the vibrations from reaching the chest wall.

To palpate for tactile fremitus, use a firm, light touch, and place the palmar surfaces of the fingers or the ulnar part of the hand over symmetrical intercostal spaces, beginning at the lung apex (Fig. 30.34A).

FIG. 30.34 (A–C) Systematic pattern (posterior-lateral-anterior) is followed when palpating and auscultating thorax.

Ask the patient to say "ninety-nine" or "one-one-one." Palpate both sides simultaneously and symmetrically (from top to bottom) for comparison or use one hand, quickly alternating between the two sides (Ball et al., 2019). Normally a faint vibration is present as a patient speaks. If fremitus is faint, ask the patient to speak in a louder or lower tone of voice. Normally fremitus is symmetrical. Vibrations are strongest at the top, near the level of the tracheal bifurcation. Strong vibrations through the chest wall occur in crying infants.

Use auscultation to assess the movement of air through the tracheobronchial tree and detect mucus or obstructed airways. Normally air flows through the airways in an unobstructed pattern. Recognizing the sounds created by normal airflow allows you to detect sounds caused by airway obstruction. Follow the same systematic approach you used for palpation when auscultating the lungs (see Fig. 30.34A).

Place the diaphragm of the stethoscope firmly on the skin, over the posterior chest wall between the ribs (Fig. 30.35). Have the patient fold the arms in front of the chest and keep the head bent forward while taking slow, deep breaths with the mouth slightly open. Listen to an entire inspiration and expiration at each position of the stethoscope. If sounds are faint, as in a patient who is obese, ask the patient to breathe harder and faster temporarily. Breath sounds are much louder in children because of their thin chest walls. The bell works best in children because of a child's small chest. Auscultate for normal breath sounds and abnormal or adventitious sounds (Fig. 30.36). Normal breath sounds differ in character, depending on the area you are auscultating

and the age of the patient. Bronchovesicular and vesicular sounds are normally heard over the posterior thorax (Table 30.20).

Abnormal sounds result from air passing through moisture, mucus, or narrowed airways. They also result from alveoli suddenly reinflating or an inflammation between the pleural linings of the lung. Adventitious sounds often occur superimposed over normal sounds. The four types of adventitious sounds are crackles, rhonchi, wheezes, and pleural friction rub (see Fig. 30.36). Each sound has a specific cause and typical auditory features (Table 30.21). During auscultation note the location and characteristics of the sounds and listen for the absence of breath sounds (found in patients with collapsed or surgically removed lobes).

If there are abnormalities in tactile fremitus or auscultation, perform the vocal resonance tests (spoken and whispered voice sounds). Place the stethoscope over the same locations used to assess breath sounds and have the patient say "ninety-nine" in a normal voice tone. Normally the sound is muffled. If fluid is compressing the lung, the vibrations from the patient's voice are transmitted to the chest wall, and the sound becomes clear (bronchophony). Then ask the patient to whisper "ninety-nine." The whispered voice is usually faint and indistinct. Certain lung abnormalities cause the whispered voice to become clear and distinct (whispered pectoriloquy).

Lateral Thorax

After assessing the posterior thorax, move to the lateral sides of the chest. The patient sits during examination of the lateral chest whenever possible. Have the patient raise the arms to improve access to lateral thoracic structures. Use inspection, palpation, and auscultation skills to examine the lateral thorax (see Fig. 30.34B). Do not assess excursion laterally. Normally the breath sounds you hear are vesicular.

Anterior Thorax

Inspect the anterior thorax for the same features as the posterior thorax. The patient sits or lies down with the head elevated. Observe the accessory muscles of breathing: sternocleidomastoid, trapezius, and abdominal muscles. The accessory muscles move little with normal passive breathing. However, patients who use a great deal of effort to breathe as a result of strenuous exercise or pulmonary disease (e.g., chronic obstructive pulmonary disease) rely on the accessory and abdominal muscles to contract to inhale and exhale. Some patients who require great effort produce a grunting sound.

Observe the width of the costal angle. It is usually larger than 90 degrees between the two costal margins. Observe a patient's breathing pattern. Normal breathing is quiet and barely audible near the open mouth. You most often assess respiratory rate and rhythm anteriorly. The male patient's respirations are usually diaphragmatic,

FIG. 30.35 Use diaphragm of stethoscope to auscultate breath sounds.

FIG. 30.36 Schema of breath sounds in the ill and well patient. (From Ball JW, et al: *Seidel's guide to physical examination,* ed 9, St Louis, 2019, Elsevier.)

ILL

Rhonchi: coarse, low-pitched; may clear with cough

Wheeze: whistling, high-pitched bronchus
Bronchial: coarse, loud; heard with consolidation
Rub: scratchy, high-pitched
Crackles: fine crackling, high-pitched

WELL

Bronchial: coarse, loud

Bronchovesicular: combination bronchial and vesicular, normal in some areas

Vesicular: low-pitched, breezy

TABLE 30.20 Normal Breath Sounds

Description	Location	Origin
Vesicular Vesicular sounds are soft, breezy, and low pitched. Inspiratory phase is 3 times longer than expiratory phase.	Best heard over periphery of lung (except over scapula)	Created by air moving through smaller airways
Bronchovesicular Bronchovesicular sounds are blowing sounds that are medium pitched and of medium intensity. Inspiratory phase is equal to expiratory phase.	Best heard posteriorly between scapulae and anteriorly over bronchioles lateral to sternum at first and second intercostal spaces	Created by air moving through large airways
Bronchial Bronchial sounds are loud and high pitched with hollow quality. Expiration lasts longer than inspiration (3:2 ratio).	Heard only over trachea	Created by air moving through trachea close to chest wall

TABLE 30.21 Adventitious Breath Sounds

Sound	Site Auscultated	Cause	Character
Crackles	Most common in dependent lobes: right and left lung bases	Random, sudden reinflation of groups of alveoli; disruptive passage of air through small airways. Can result from pneumonia, heart failure, chronic lung disease.	Fine crackles are high-pitched fine, short, interrupted crackling sounds heard during end of inspiration; usually not cleared with coughing. Medium crackles are lower, moister sounds heard during middle of inspiration; not cleared with coughing. Coarse crackles are loud, bubbly sounds heard during inspiration; not cleared with coughing.
Rhonchi (sonorous wheeze)	Primarily heard over trachea and bronchi; if loud enough, able to be heard over most lung fields	Muscular spasm, fluid, or mucus in larger airways; new growth (e.g., tumor) or external pressure causing turbulence	Loud, low-pitched, rumbling, coarse sounds are heard either during inspiration or expiration; sometimes cleared by coughing.
Wheezes (sibilant wheeze)	Heard over all lung fields	High-velocity airflow through severely narrowed or obstructed airway. Common in asthma and bronchitis.	High-pitched, continuous musical sounds are like a squeak heard continuously during inspiration or expiration; usually louder on expiration.
Pleural friction rub	Heard over anterior lateral lung field (if patient is sitting upright)	Inflamed pleura; parietal pleura rubbing against visceral pleura. Common in viral infections (e.g., flu).	Dry, rubbing, or grating quality is heard during inspiration or expiration; does not clear with coughing; loudest over lower lateral anterior surface.

Data from Ball JW, et al: *Seidel's guide to physical examination,* ed 9, St Louis, 2019, Elsevier.

TABLE 30.22 Nursing History for Heart Assessment

Assessment	Rationale
Determine history of smoking, alcohol intake, caffeine intake, use of prescription and recreational drugs, exercise habits, and dietary patterns and intake (including fat and sodium intake).	Smoking; alcohol ingestion; cocaine use; lack of regular exercise; intake of foods high in carbohydrates, fats, and cholesterol are risk factors for cardiovascular disease. Caffeine can cause heart dysrhythmias.
Determine whether patient is taking medications for cardiovascular function (e.g., antidysrhythmics, antihypertensives) and knows their purpose, dosage, and side effects.	Knowledge allows nurse to assess adherence with drug therapies. Medications sometimes affect vital sign values.
Assess for chest pain or discomfort, palpitations, excess fatigue, cough, dyspnea, leg pain or cramps, edema of feet, cyanosis, fainting, and orthopnea. Ask whether symptoms occur at rest or during exercise.	These are key symptoms of heart disease. Cardiovascular function is sometimes adequate during rest but not during exercise. Positions affect how well lungs can expand.
If patient reports chest pain, determine whether it is cardiac in nature. Anginal pain is usually a deep pressure or ache that is substernal and diffuse, radiating to one or both arms, neck, or jaw.	Assessment determines nature of pain and need to initiate care immediately.
Determine whether patient has stressful lifestyle. Which physical demands and/or emotional stressors exist?	Repeated exposure to stress increases risk for heart disease.
Assess family history for heart disease, diabetes mellitus, high cholesterol levels, hypertension, stroke, or rheumatic heart disease.	Factors increase risk for heart disease.
Ask patient about history of heart trouble (e.g., heart failure, congenital heart disease, coronary artery disease, dysrhythmias, murmurs).	Knowledge reveals patient's level of understanding of condition. Preexisting condition influences examination techniques used and findings to expect.
Determine whether patient has preexisting diabetes mellitus, lung disease, obesity, or hypertension.	These disorders alter heart function.

whereas in female patients they are more costal. Accurate assessment occurs as the patient breathes passively.

Palpate the anterior thoracic muscles and skeleton for lumps, masses, tenderness, or unusual movement. The sternum and xiphoid are relatively inflexible. Place the thumbs parallel approximately along the costal margin 6 cm (2½ inches) apart with the palms touching the anterolateral chest. Push the thumbs toward the midline to create a skinfold. As the patient inhales deeply, the thumbs normally separate approximately 3 to 5 cm (1¼–2 inches), with each side expanding equally.

Assess tactile fremitus over the anterior chest wall. Anterior findings differ from posterior findings because of the heart and female breast tissue. Fremitus is felt next to the sternum at the second intercostal space, at the level of the bronchial bifurcation. It decreases over the heart, lower thorax, and breast tissue.

Auscultation of the anterior thorax follows a systematic pattern (see Fig. 30.34C) comparing right and left sides. This allows you to compare lung sounds in one region on one side of the body with sounds in the same region on the opposite side of the body.

If possible, have the patient sit to maximize chest expansion. Give special attention to the lower lobes, where mucous secretions commonly gather. Listen for bronchovesicular and vesicular sounds above and below the clavicles and along the lung periphery. In addition, auscultate for bronchial sounds, which are loud, high pitched, and hollow sounding, with expiration lasting longer than inspiration (3:2 ratio). This sound is normally heard over the trachea.

HEART

Compare your assessment of a patient's heart with findings from the vascular assessment (see later section). Alterations in either system sometimes manifest as changes in the other. Some patients with signs or symptoms of heart (cardiac) problems have a life-threatening condition requiring immediate attention. In this case act quickly and conduct only the parts of the examination that are necessary. Conduct

FIG. 30.37 Anatomical position of heart.

a more thorough assessment when the patient is more stable. The nursing history (Table 30.22) provides data to help interpret physical findings.

Assess the cardiac system through the anterior thorax. Form a mental image of the exact location of the heart (Fig. 30.37). In the adult it is in the center of the chest (precordium), behind and to the left of the sternum, with a small section of the right atrium extending to the right of the sternum. The base of the heart is the upper part, and the apex is the bottom tip. The surface of the right ventricle composes most of the anterior surface of the heart. A section of the left ventricle shapes the left anterior side of the apex. The apex touches the anterior chest wall at approximately the fourth to fifth intercostal space just medial to the left midclavicular line. This is the **apical impulse or point of maximal impulse (PMI)**.

An infant's heart is positioned more horizontally. The apex of the heart is at the third or fourth intercostal space, just to the left of the midclavicular line. By the age of 7 a child's PMI is in the same location

FIG. 30.38 Cardiac cycle. *AVC,* Aortic valve closes; *AVO,* aortic valve opens; *ECG,* electrocardiogram; *MVC,* mitral valve closes; *MVO,* mitral valve opens.

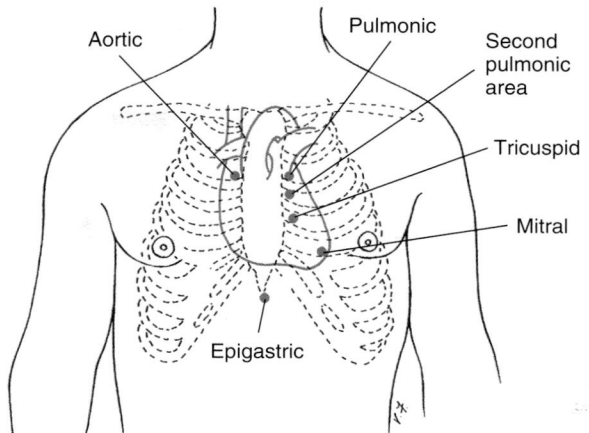

FIG. 30.39 Anatomical sites for assessment of cardiac function.

as the adult's. In tall, slender people the heart lies more vertically and centrally. In shorter or stockier individuals, the heart tends to lie more to the left and horizontally (Ball et al., 2019).

To assess the heart, you need a clear understanding of the cardiac cycle and associated physiological events (Fig. 30.38). The heart normally pumps blood through its four chambers in a methodical, even sequence. Events on the left side occur just before those on the right. As blood flows through each chamber, the valves open and close, the pressures within chambers rise and fall, and the chambers contract. Each event creates a physiological sign. Both sides of the heart function in a coordinated fashion.

There are two phases to the cardiac cycle: systole and diastole. During systole, the ventricles contract and eject blood from the left ventricle into the aorta and from the right ventricle into the pulmonary artery. During diastole, the ventricles relax, and the atria contract to move blood into the ventricles and fill the coronary arteries.

Heart sounds occur in relation to physiological events in the cardiac cycle. As systole begins, ventricular pressure rises and closes the mitral and tricuspid valves. Valve closure causes the first heart sound (S_1), often described as "lub." The ventricles then contract, and blood flows through the aortic and pulmonary valves into circulation. After the ventricles empty, ventricular pressure falls below that in the aorta and pulmonary artery. This allows the aortic and pulmonic valves to close, causing the second heart sound (S_2), described as "dub." As ventricular pressure continues to fall, it drops below that of the atria. The mitral and tricuspid valves reopen to allow ventricular filling. When the heart attempts to fill an already distended ventricle, a third heart sound (S_3) can be heard, as with heart failure. An S_3 is considered abnormal in adults over 31 years of age but can often be heard normally in children and young adults. It can also be present among women in the late stages of pregnancy. A fourth heart sound (S_4) occurs when the atria contract to enhance ventricular filling. An S_4 is often heard in healthy older adults, children, and athletes, but it is not normal in adults. Because S_4 also indicates an abnormal condition, report it to a health care provider.

Inspection and Palpation

Provide a relaxed and comfortable environment for the examination. Explain the assessment procedure to help decrease a patient's anxiety.

An anxious or uncomfortable patient can have mild tachycardia, which leads to inaccurate findings.

Use the skills of inspection and palpation simultaneously. Begin the examination with the patient in the supine position or with the upper body elevated 45 degrees. Patients with heart disease frequently experience shortness of breath while lying flat. Stand at the patient's right side. Do not let the patient talk, especially when auscultating heart sounds. Good lighting in the room is essential.

Direct your attention to the anatomical sites best suited for assessment of the cardiac area. During inspection and palpation look for visible pulsations and exaggerated lifts and palpate for the apical impulse and any source of vibrations (thrills). Follow an orderly sequence, beginning with assessment of the base of the heart (top) and moving toward the apex (bottom). First inspect the angle of Louis, which lies between the sternal body and manubrium, and feel the ridge in the sternum approximately 5 cm (2 inches) below the sternal notch. Slip the fingers along the angle on each side of the sternum to feel adjacent ribs. The intercostal spaces are just below each rib. The second intercostal space allows identification of each of the six anatomical landmarks (Fig. 30.39). The second intercostal space on the right is the *aortic area,* and the left second intercostal space is the *pulmonic area.* You need to use deeper palpation to feel the spaces in obese or heavily muscled patients. After locating the pulmonic area, move the fingers down the patient's left sternal border to the third intercostal space, called the *second pulmonic area.* The *tricuspid area* is located at the fourth or fifth intercostal space along the sternum. To find the *apical* or *mitral area,* locate the fifth intercostal space just to the left of the sternum and move the fingers laterally to the left midclavicular line. Locate the apical area with the palm of the hand or the fingertips. Normally you feel the apical impulse as a light tap in an area 1 to 2 cm (½–1 inch) in diameter at the apex (Fig. 30.40). Another landmark is the epigastric area at the tip of the sternum. Palpate there if you suspect aortic abnormalities.

Locate the six anatomical landmarks of the heart and inspect and palpate each area. Look for the appearance of pulsations, viewing each area over the chest at an angle to the side. Normally you do not see pulsations except perhaps at the PMI in thin patients or at the epigastric area because of abdominal aorta pulsation. Use the proximal halves of the four fingers together and alternate this with the ball of the hand to palpate for pulsations. Touch the areas gently to allow movements to lift the hand. Normally no pulsations or vibrations are felt in the second, third, or fourth intercostal spaces. Loud murmurs cause a vibration.

FIG. 30.40 Palpation of apical pulse.

Just medial to the left midclavicular line, at the fourth or fifth intercostal space, is the PMI. If you cannot locate it with the patient in a supine position, have the patient roll onto the left side, moving the heart closer to the chest wall. Estimate the size of the heart by noting the diameter of the PMI and its position relative to the midclavicular line. In cases of serious heart disease, the cardiac muscle enlarges, with the PMI found more to the left of the midclavicular line. The PMI is sometimes difficult to find in the older adult because the chest deepens in its anteroposterior diameters. It is also difficult to find in muscular or overweight patients. An infant's PMI is located near the third or fourth intercostal space. It is easy to palpate because of the child's thin chest wall.

Auscultation

You may hear normal heart sounds, extra heart sounds, and/or murmurs during auscultation of the heart. Concentrate on detecting the normal low-intensity sounds created by valve closures. Before auscultating the heart, eliminate all sources of room noise and explain the procedure to reduce the patient's anxiety. Follow a systematic pattern, beginning at the aortic area and inching the stethoscope across each of the anatomical sites. Listen for the complete cycle ("lub-dub") of heart sounds clearly at each location. Repeat the sequence with the bell of the stethoscope. Sometimes you will have a patient assume three different positions during the examination to hear sounds clearly (Fig. 30.41): sitting up and leaning forward (good for all areas and to hear high-pitched murmurs), supine (good for all areas), and left lateral recumbent (good for all areas; best position to hear low-pitched sounds in diastole).

Learn to identify the first (S_1) and second (S_2) heart sounds. At normal rates S_1 occurs after the long diastolic pause and before the short systolic pause. S_1 is high pitched, dull in quality, and heard best at the apex. If it is difficult to hear S_1, time it in relation to the carotid pulsation. S_2 follows the short systolic pause and precedes the long diastolic pause; it is best heard at the aortic area.

Auscultate for rate and rhythm after hearing both sounds clearly. Each combination of S_1 and S_2 or "lub-dub" counts as one heartbeat. Count the rate for 1 minute and listen for the interval between S_1 and S_2 and then the time between S_2 and the next S_1. A regular rhythm involves regular intervals of time between each sequence of beats. There is a distinct silent pause between S_1 and S_2. Failure of the heart to beat at regular successive intervals is a **dysrhythmia**. Some dysrhythmias are life threatening.

When assessing an irregular heart rhythm, compare apical and radial pulse rates simultaneously to determine whether a pulse deficit exists. Auscultate the apical pulse first and then immediately palpate the radial pulse (one examiner present). When two examiners are present,

FIG. 30.41 Sequence of patient positions for heart auscultation. (A) Sitting. (B) Supine. (C) Left lateral recumbent.

assess the apical and radial rates at the same time (see Chapter 29). When a patient has a pulse deficit, the radial pulse is slower than the apical pulse because ineffective contractions fail to send pulse waves to the periphery. Report a difference in pulse rates to the health care provider immediately.

Assess for extra heart sounds at each auscultatory site. Use the bell of the stethoscope and listen for low-pitched extra heart sounds such as S_3 and S_4 gallops, clicks, and rubs. Auscultate over all anatomical areas. S_3, or a **ventricular gallop**, occurs after S_2. It is caused by a premature rush of blood into a ventricle that is stiff or dilated as a result of heart failure and hypertension. The combination of S_1, S_2, and S_3 sounds like "Ken-TUCK-y."

S_4, or an atrial gallop, occurs just before S_1 or ventricular systole. The sound of an S_4 is like that of "TEN-nes-see." Physiologically it is caused by an atrial contraction pushing against a ventricle that is not accepting blood because of heart failure or other alterations. You can hear extra heart sounds more easily with the patient lying on the left side and the stethoscope at the apical site.

The final part of the auscultation examination includes assessment for heart murmurs. **Murmurs** are sustained swishing or blowing sounds heard at the beginning, middle, or end of the systolic or diastolic phase. They are caused by increased blood flow through a normal valve, forward flow through a stenotic valve or into a dilated vessel or heart chamber, or backward flow through a valve that fails to close. A murmur is asymptomatic or a sign of heart disease (Box 30.19). It is common in children. Keep the following factors in mind when auscultating to detect murmurs:

- When a murmur is detected, auscultate the mitral, tricuspid, aortic, and pulmonic valve areas for placement in the cardiac cycle (timing); the place it is heard best (location); radiation; loudness; pitch; and quality.
- If a murmur occurs between S_1 and S_2, it is a systolic murmur.
- If it occurs between S_2 and the next S_1, it is a diastolic murmur.
- The location of a murmur is not necessarily directly over the valves. Experience with hearing murmurs helps with better understanding

of where each type of murmur is best heard. For example, mitral murmurs are best heard at the apex of the heart.
- To assess for radiation, listen over other areas in addition to where it is heard best. Murmurs can also be heard over the neck or back.
- Intensity or loudness is related to the rate of blood flow through the heart or the amount of blood regurgitated. Feel for a thrust or intermittent palpable sensation at the auscultation site in serious murmurs. A **thrill** is a continuous palpable sensation that resembles the purring of a cat. Intensity is recorded using the following grades (Ball et al., 2019):
  - *Grade 1:* Barely audible in a quiet room
  - *Grade 2:* Quiet but clearly audible
  - *Grade 3:* Moderately loud
  - *Grade 4:* Loud, with associated thrill
  - *Grade 5:* Very loud; thrill easily palpable
  - *Grade 6:* Very loud; audible with stethoscope not in contact with chest; thrill palpable and visible

A murmur is low, medium, or high in pitch, depending on the velocity of blood flow through the valves. A low-pitched murmur is best heard with the bell of the stethoscope. If the murmur is best heard with the diaphragm, it is high pitched. The quality of a murmur refers to its characteristic pattern and sound. A crescendo murmur starts softly and builds in loudness. A decrescendo murmur starts loudly and becomes less intense.

Vascular System

Examination of the vascular system includes measuring the blood pressure and assessing the integrity of the peripheral vascular system. Table 30.23 reviews the nursing history data collected before the examination. Use the skills of inspection, palpation, and auscultation. Perform parts of the vascular examination during other body system assessments. For example, check the carotid pulse after palpating the cervical lymph nodes. Assess the skin, as part of the vascular system, for signs and symptoms of arterial and venous insufficiency.

BOX 30.19 PATIENT TEACHING

Heart Assessment

Objective
- Patient will describe risk factors for heart disease and take appropriate steps to eliminate risks from lifestyle.

Teaching Strategies
- Explain risk factors for heart disease, including high dietary intake of saturated fat or cholesterol, lack of regular aerobic exercise, smoking, excess weight, stressful lifestyle, hypertension, and family history of heart disease.
- Refer patient (if appropriate) to resources available for controlling or reducing risks (e.g., nutritional counseling, exercise class, stress-reduction programs).
- Teach patient to eat a well-rounded healthy diet. Explain that a healthy pattern emphasizes variety, including fruits and vegetables, whole grains, low-fat dairy products, skinless poultry and fish, nuts, and legumes, and nontropical vegetable oils. Limit saturated and trans fats, sodium, red meats, sweets, and sugar-sweetened beverages (American Heart Association [AHA], 2020).
- Encourage patient who is over 20 years old to have cholesterol checked every 4 to 6 years. A complete cholesterol test, also called a lipid profile, will give the results of High-density lipoprotein (HDL; "good") cholesterol, low-density lipoprotein (LDL; "bad") cholesterol, triglycerides, and total blood cholesterol. The health care provider will look at these numbers in relation to the patient's other risk factors to assess overall cardiovascular risk (AHA, 2020).
- Encourage patient to discuss with health care provider the need for periodic C-reactive protein (CRP) testing. CRP levels assess a patient's risk for cardiovascular disease.
- Advise patient to avoid cigarette smoke because nicotine causes vasoconstriction.
- Advise patient to quit smoking to lower the risk for coronary heart disease and coronary vascular disease.
- Patients who are at risk benefit from taking a daily low dose of aspirin. Consult health care provider before starting therapy.

Evaluation
Use the principles of teach-back to evaluate patient/family caregiver learning:
- List for me the risk factors for heart disease.
- Show me the meal plan you developed that helps you follow a diet low in cholesterol and saturated fat.
- Describe for me how you have reduced risk factors for heart disease in your life.

TABLE 30.23 Nursing History for Vascular Assessment

Assessment	Rationale
Determine whether patient experiences leg cramps; numbness or tingling in extremities; sensation of cold hands or feet; pain in legs; or swelling or cyanosis of feet, ankles, or hand.	These signs and symptoms indicate vascular disease.
If patient experiences leg pain or cramping in lower extremities, ask whether walking or standing for long periods or sleeping aggravates or relieves it.	Relationship of symptoms to exercise clarifies whether problem is vascular or musculoskeletal. Pain caused by vascular condition tends to increase with activity. Musculoskeletal pain usually is not relieved when exercise ends.
Ask patients whether they wear tight-fitting garters, socks, or hosiery and sit or lie in bed with legs crossed.	Tight hosiery around lower extremities and crossing legs can impair venous return.
Reconsider previous heart risk factors (e.g., smoking, exercise, nutritional problems).	These predispose patient to vascular disease.
Assess medical history for heart disease, hypertension, phlebitis, diabetes mellitus, or varicose veins.	Circulatory and vascular disorders influence findings gathered during examination.

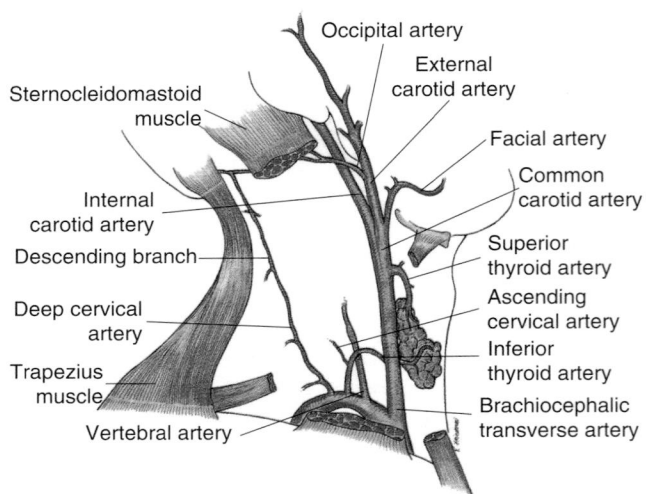

FIG. 30.42 Anatomical position of carotid artery.

FIG. 30.43 Palpation of internal carotid artery along margin of sterno-cleidomastoid muscle.

Blood Pressure

When auscultating blood pressure, know that readings between the arms vary by as much as 10 mm Hg and tend to be higher in the right arm (Ball et al., 2019). Always record the higher reading. Repeated systolic readings that differ by 15 mm Hg or more suggest atherosclerosis or disease of the aorta.

Carotid Arteries

When the left ventricle pumps blood into the aorta, the arterial system transmits pressure waves. The carotid arteries reflect heart function better than peripheral arteries because their pressure correlates with that of the aorta. The carotid artery supplies oxygenated blood to the head and neck (Fig. 30.42). The overlying sternocleidomastoid muscle protects it.

To examine the carotid arteries, have the patient sit or lie supine with the head of the bed elevated 30 degrees. Examine one carotid artery at a time. If both arteries are occluded simultaneously during palpation, the patient loses consciousness because of inadequate circulation to the brain. *Do not palpate or massage the carotid arteries vigorously* because the carotid sinus is located at the bifurcation of the common carotid arteries in the upper third of the neck. This sinus sends impulses along the vagus nerve. Stimulating it causes a reflex drop in heart rate and blood pressure, which causes **syncope** or circulatory arrest. This is a particular problem for older adults.

Begin inspection of the neck for obvious pulsation of the artery. Have the patient turn the head slightly away from the artery being examined. Sometimes the wave of the pulse is visible. The carotid is the only site for assessing the quality of a pulse wave. An absent pulse wave indicates arterial occlusion (blockage) or **stenosis** (narrowing).

To palpate the pulse, ask the patient to look straight ahead or turn the head slightly toward the side you are examining. Turning relaxes the sternocleidomastoid muscle. Slide the tips of the index and middle fingers around the medial edge of the sternocleidomastoid muscle. Gently palpate to avoid occlusion of circulation (Fig. 30.43).

The normal carotid pulse is localized and strong rather than diffuse. It has a thrusting quality. As a patient breathes, no change occurs. Rotating the neck or going from a sitting to a supine position does not change the quality of the carotid impulse. Both carotid arteries are normally equal in pulse rate, rhythm, and strength and are equally elastic. Diminished or unequal carotid pulsations indicate atherosclerosis or other forms of arterial disease.

FIG. 30.44 Occlusion or narrowing of the carotid artery disrupts normal blood flow. The resultant turbulence creates a sound (bruit) that is auscultated.

The carotid is the most commonly auscultated pulse. Auscultation is especially important for middle-age or older adults or patients suspected of having cerebrovascular disease. When the lumen of a blood vessel is narrowed, it disturbs blood flow. As blood passes through the narrowed section, it creates turbulence, causing a blowing or swishing sound. The blowing sound is called a **bruit** (pronounced "brew-ee") (Fig. 30.44).

Place the bell of the stethoscope over the carotid artery at the lateral end of the clavicle and the posterior margin of the sternocleidomastoid muscle. Have the patient turn the head slightly away from the side being examined (Fig. 30.45). Ask the patient to hold the breath for a moment so that breath sounds do not obscure a bruit. Normally you do not hear any sounds during carotid auscultation. Palpate the artery lightly for a thrill (palpable bruit) if you hear a bruit.

FIG. 30.45 Auscultation for carotid artery bruit.

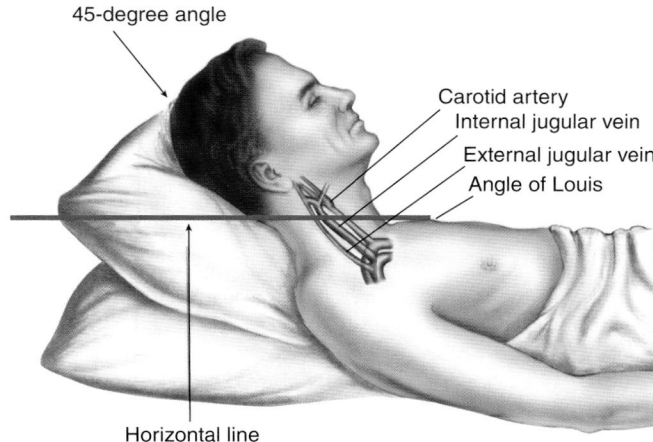

FIG. 30.46 Position of patient to assess jugular vein distention. (From Thompson JM, et al: *Mosby's manual of clinical nursing*, ed 5, St Louis, 2001, Mosby.)

Jugular Veins

The most accessible veins for examination are the internal and external jugular veins in the neck. Both veins drain bilaterally from the head and neck into the superior vena cava. The external jugular vein lies superficially and is just above the clavicle. The internal jugular vein lies deeper, along the carotid artery.

It is best to examine the right internal jugular vein because it follows a more direct anatomical path to the right atrium of the heart. The column of blood inside the internal jugular vein serves as a manometer, reflecting pressure in the right atrium. The higher the column, the greater is the venous pressure. Raised venous pressure reflects right-sided heart failure.

Normally, when a patient lies in the supine position, the external jugular vein distends and becomes easily visible. In contrast, the jugular veins normally flatten when the patient changes to a sitting or standing position. However, for some patients with heart disease the jugular veins remain distended when sitting.

Venous pressure is influenced by blood volume (i.e., the capacity of the right atrium to receive blood and send it to the right ventricle and the ability of the right ventricle to contract and force blood into the pulmonary artery). Any factor resulting in greater blood volume within the venous system results in elevated jugular venous pressure. You can observe for elevation in jugular venous pressure by using the following steps:

1. Have the patient lie flat in the supine position. Expose the neck and upper thorax. Use a pillow to align the head. Avoid neck hyperextension or flexion to ensure that the vein is not stretched or kinked (Fig. 30.46). Observe for engorgement of the jugular veins.
2. Gradually raise the head of the bed until the jugular venous pulsations become evident between the angle of the jaw and the clavicle. **Note:** Palpating a carotid pulse helps to distinguish venous pulsations from carotid palpations. The jugular pulse can only be visualized, not palpated.
3. Inspect the jugular veins. Usually pulsations are not evident with the patient sitting up. As the patient slowly leans back into a supine position, the level of venous pulsations begins to rise above the

TABLE 30.24	Indicators for Assessing Local Blood Flow	
Indicator	**Rationale**
Systemic diseases (e.g., arteriosclerosis, atherosclerosis, diabetes mellitus)	Diseases change integrity of walls of arteries and smaller blood vessels.
Coagulation disorders (e.g., thrombosis, embolus)	Blood clot causes mechanical obstruction to blood flow.
Local trauma or surgery (e.g., contusion, fracture, vascular surgery)	Direct manipulation of vessels or localized edema impairs blood flow.
Application of constricting devices (e.g., casts, dressings, elastic bandages, restraints)	Constriction causes tourniquet effect, impairing blood flow to areas below site of constriction.

level of the manubrium as much as 1 or 2 cm (½–1 inch) as the patient reaches a 45-degree angle.

Peripheral Arteries and Veins

To examine the peripheral vascular system, first assess the adequacy of blood flow to the extremities by measuring arterial pulses and inspecting the condition of the skin and nails. Next assess the integrity of the venous system. Assess the arterial pulses in the extremities to determine sufficiency of the entire arterial circulation.

Factors such as coagulation disorders, local trauma or surgery, constricting casts or bandages, and systemic diseases impair circulation to the extremities (Table 30.24). Discuss risk factors and ways to monitor for circulatory problems with the patient (Box 30.20).

Peripheral Arteries. Examine each peripheral artery using the distal pads of your second and third fingers. The thumb helps anchor the brachial and femoral arteries. Apply firm pressure but avoid occluding a pulse. When a pulse is difficult to find, it helps to vary pressure and feel all around the pulse site. Be sure not to palpate your own pulse.

Routine vital signs usually include assessment of the rate and rhythm of the radial artery because it is easily accessible. Count the pulse for either 30 seconds or a full minute, depending on the character

BOX 30.20 PATIENT TEACHING
Vascular Assessment

Objective
- Patient with vascular insufficiency will avoid activities that worsen circulatory status.

Teaching Strategies
- Instruct patient with risk or evidence of vascular insufficiency in the lower extremities to avoid tight clothing over the lower body or legs, to avoid sitting or standing for long periods, to avoid sitting with legs crossed, to walk regularly, and to elevate feet when sitting.
- Advise patient to avoid or stop the smoking of cigarettes, cigars, or pipes or the use of nicotine products (e.g., chewing tobacco, nicotine patches or gum) because nicotine causes vasoconstriction. Offer a referral to a reliable stop-smoking program.
- Instruct patient with hypertension about the benefits of regular monitoring of blood pressure (daily, weekly, or monthly). Teach patient how to use home monitoring kits.

Evaluation
Use the principles of teach-back to evaluate patient/family caregiver learning:
- Explain to me what precautions you are taking to avoid further decrease in your peripheral circulation.
- Explain to me what your normal limits for blood pressure are. Tell me when you would contact your health care provider.
- Show me how you take your blood pressure at home.

FIG. 30.47 (A) Anatomical positions of brachial, radial, and ulnar arteries. (B) Palpation of radial pulse. (C) Palpation of ulnar pulse. (D) Palpation of brachial pulse.

of the pulse. Always count an irregular pulse for 60 seconds. With palpation, the pulse waves are normally felt at regular intervals. When an interval is interrupted by an early, a late, or a missed beat, the pulse rhythm is irregular. During cardiac emergencies health care providers usually assess the carotid artery because it is accessible and most useful in evaluating heart activity. To check local circulatory status of tissues (e.g., when a leg cast is in place or following vascular surgery), palpate the peripheral arteries long enough to note that a pulse is present.

Assess each peripheral artery for elasticity of the vessel wall, strength, and equality. The arterial wall normally is elastic, making it easily palpable. After depressing the artery, it springs back to shape when the pressure is released. An abnormal artery is hard, inelastic, or calcified.

The strength of a pulse is a measurement of the force at which blood is ejected against the arterial wall. Some examiners use a scale rating from 0 to 4 for the strength of a pulse (Ball et al., 2019):
0: Absent, not palpable
1: Pulse diminished, barely palpable
2: Expected
3: Full, increased
4: Bounding, aneurysmal

Measure all peripheral pulses for equality and symmetry. Compare the left radial pulse with that of the right, and so on. Lack of symmetry indicates impaired circulation, such as a localized obstruction or an abnormally positioned artery.

In the upper extremities the brachial artery channels blood to the radial and ulnar arteries of the forearm and hand. If circulation in this artery becomes blocked, the hands do not receive adequate blood flow. If circulation in the radial or ulnar arteries becomes impaired, the hand still receives adequate perfusion. An interconnection between the radial and ulnar arteries guards against arterial occlusion (Fig. 30.47A).

To locate pulses in the arm, have the patient sit or lie down. Find the radial pulse along the radial side of the forearm at the wrist. Thin individuals have a groove lateral to the flexor tendon of the wrist. Feel

the radial pulse with light palpation in the groove (see Fig. 30.47B). The ulnar pulse is on the opposite side of the wrist and feels less prominent (see Fig. 30.47C). Palpate the ulnar pulse when evaluating arterial insufficiency to the hand.

To palpate the brachial pulse, find the groove between the biceps and triceps muscle above the elbow at the antecubital fossa (see Fig. 30.47D). The artery runs along the medial side of the extended arm. Palpate it with the fingertips of the first three fingers in the muscle groove.

The femoral artery is the primary artery in the leg, delivering blood to the popliteal, posterior tibial, and dorsalis pedis arteries (Fig. 30.48A). An interconnection between the posterior tibial and dorsalis pedis arteries guards against local arterial occlusion.

Find the femoral pulse with the patient lying down with the inguinal area exposed (see Fig. 30.48B). The femoral artery runs below the inguinal ligament, midway between the symphysis pubis and the anterosuperior iliac spine. Sometimes deep palpation is necessary to feel the pulse. Bimanual palpation is effective in patients who are obese. Place the fingertips of both hands on opposite sides of the pulse site. Feel a pulsatile sensation when the arterial pulsation pushes the fingertips apart.

The popliteal pulse runs behind the knee. Have the patient slightly flex the knee with the foot resting on the examination table or assume a prone position with the knee slightly flexed (see Fig. 30.48C) and leg muscles relaxed. Palpate with the fingers of both hands deeply into the popliteal fossa, just lateral to the midline. The popliteal pulse is difficult to locate.

With the patient's foot relaxed, locate the dorsalis pedis pulse. The artery runs along the top of the foot in line with the groove between the extensor tendons of the great toe and first toe (see Fig. 30.48D). To find the pulse, place the fingertips between the first and second toes and slowly move up the dorsum of the foot. This pulse is sometimes congenitally absent.

Find the posterior tibial pulse on the inner side of each ankle (Fig. 30.48E). Place the fingers behind and below the medial malleolus (ankle bone). With the foot relaxed and slightly extended, palpate the artery.

FIG. 30.48 (A) Anatomical position of femoral, popliteal, dorsalis pedis, and anterior and posterior tibial arteries. (B) Palpation of femoral pulse. (C) Palpation of popliteal pulse. (D) Palpation of dorsalis pedis pulse. (E) Palpation of posterior tibial pulse.

Ultrasound Stethoscopes. If a pulse is difficult to palpate, an ultrasound (Doppler) stethoscope is a useful tool that amplifies the sounds of a pulse wave. Factors that weaken a pulse or make palpation difficult include obesity, reduction in the stroke volume of the heart, diminished blood volume, or arterial obstruction. Apply a thin layer of transmission gel to the patient's skin at the pulse site or directly onto the transducer tip of the probe. Turn on the volume control and place the tip of the transducer at a 45- to 90-degree angle on the skin (Fig. 30.49). Move the transducer until you hear a pulsating "whooshing" sound that indicates that arterial blood flow is present.

REFLECT NOW

How would you respond if while completing an assessment you found a severe abnormality in a body system? Think through your body language, facial expression, and the conversation you would have with the patient through this situation. What further assessments might you need to complete?

Tissue Perfusion. The condition of the skin, mucosa, and nail beds offers useful data about the status of circulatory blood flow. Examine the face and extremities, looking at the color of the skin, lips, mucosa, and nail beds. Bluish color of lips or nail beds or a decrease in pallor sometimes indicates cyanosis. When cyanosis is present, obtain a patient's oxygen saturation to determine the severity of the problem (see Chapter 29). Health care providers sometimes order additional blood tests to further evaluate oxygenation status. Examination of the nails involves inspection for **clubbing**, a bulging of the tissues at the nail base, which causes an abnormal curvature of the nail. Clubbing suggests a chronic problem such as emphysema and congenital heart disease.

Inspect the lower extremities for changes in color, temperature, and condition of the skin, indicating either arterial or venous alterations (Table 30.25). Ask if the patient has pain in the legs. If an arterial occlusion is present, the patient will experience pain distal to the occlusion. The five *P*s—pain, pallor, pulselessness, paresthesias, and paralysis—characterize an occlusion. Venous congestion causes tissue changes that indicate an inadequate circulatory flow back to the heart.

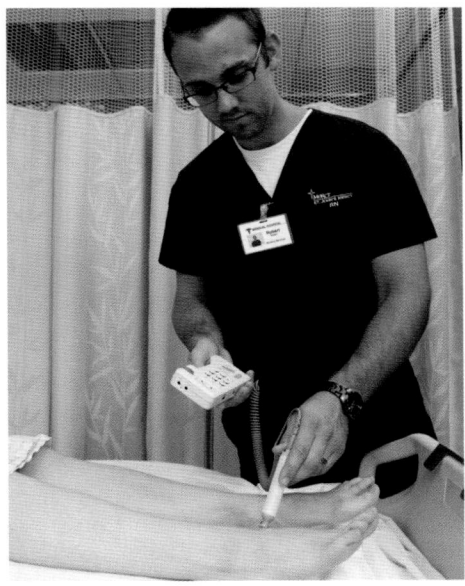

FIG. 30.49 Ultrasound stethoscope in position on the pedal pulse.

TABLE 30.25   Signs of Venous and Arterial Insufficiency

Assessment Criterion	Venous	Arterial
Color	Normal or cyanotic	Pale; worsened by elevation of extremity; dusky red when extremity is lowered
Temperature	Normal	Cool (blood flow blocked to extremity)
Pulse	Normal	Decreased or absent
Edema	Often marked	Absent or mild
Skin changes	Brown pigmentation around ankles	Thin, shiny skin; decreased hair growth; thickened nails

While examining the lower extremities, also inspect skin and nail texture; hair distribution on the lower legs, feet, and toes; the venous pattern; and scars, pigmentation, or ulcers. Absence of hair on the legs may indicate circulatory insufficiency; remember to consider whether the patient has shaved legs or wears tight socks, which can lead to a decrease in hair on the legs. Chronic recurring ulcers of the feet or lower legs are a serious sign of circulatory insufficiency and require a health care provider's intervention. Palpate the skin of the legs and feet for color, temperature, and edema. Capillary refill, the time it takes the capillary bed to fill after it is occluded by pressure, determines adequacy of peripheral blood flow to the digits (Ball et al., 2019). To perform capillary refill time, blanch a fingernail bed by pressing over it with a finger for several seconds, release the pressure, then observe the time elapsed before nail color returns to normal (Ball et al., 2019). Refill time is normally less than 2 seconds. Problems with vascular flow result in a refill time greater than 2 seconds (Ball et al. 2019).

Peripheral Veins. Assess the status of the peripheral veins by asking the patient to assume sitting and standing positions. Assessment includes inspection and palpation for varicosities, peripheral edema, and phlebitis. Varicosities are superficial veins that become dilated, especially when the legs are in a dependent position. They are common in older adults because the veins normally fibrose, dilate, and stretch. They are also common in people who stand for prolonged periods. Varicosities in the anterior or medial part of the thigh and the posterolateral part of the calf are abnormal.

Dependent edema around the area of the feet and ankles is a sign of venous insufficiency or right-sided heart failure. It is common in older adults and people who spend a lot of time standing (e.g., waitresses, security guards, and nurses). To assess for pitting edema, use the index finger to press firmly for several seconds and release over the medial malleolus or the shins. A depression left in the skin indicates edema. Grading 1+ through 4+ characterizes the severity of the edema (see Fig. 30.6).

Phlebitis is an inflammation of a vein that occurs commonly after trauma to the vessel wall, infection, immobilization, and prolonged insertion of IV catheters. To assess for phlebitis in the leg, inspect the calves for localized redness, tenderness, and swelling over vein sites. Gentle palpation of calf muscles reveals warmth, tenderness, and firmness of the muscle. Unilateral edema of the affected leg is one of the most reliable findings of phlebitis. The Homan sign is not a reliable indicator of phlebitis or deep vein thrombosis (DVT) and is present in other conditions (Bauer, 2021). To confirm DVT, other diagnostic tests are used whether or not the Homan sign is positive.

Lymphatic System

Assess the lymphatic drainage of the lower extremities during examination of the vascular system or during the female or male genital examination. Superficial and deep nodes drain the legs, but only two groups of superficial nodes are palpable. With the patient supine, palpate the area of the superficial inguinal nodes in the groin area (Fig. 30.50A). Then move the fingertips toward the inner thigh, feeling for any inferior nodes. Use a firm but gentle pressure when palpating over each lymphatic chain. Multiple nodes normally are not palpable, although a few soft nontender nodes are not unusual. Enlarged, hardened, tender nodes reveal potential sites of infection or metastatic disease.

In the upper extremities, lymph is carried by the collecting ducts from the upper extremities to the subclavian lymphatic trunk. To assess this lymph system, gently palpate the epitrochlear nodes, located on the medial aspect of the arms near the antecubital fossa (see Fig. 30.50B). The proximal part of the upper extremity lymph system is located in the axilla and is usually assessed during examination of the breasts.

FIG. 30.50 (A) Lymphatic drainage for lower extremities. (B) Lymphatic drainage for upper extremities. (From Ball JW, et al: *Seidel's guide to physical examination*, ed 9, St Louis, 2019, Mosby.)

BREASTS

It is important to examine the breasts of both female and male patients. Men have a small amount of glandular tissue in the breast, which is a potential site for the growth of cancer cells. In contrast, the majority of the female breast is glandular tissue.

Female Breasts

It is estimated there will be 281,550 new cases of female breast cancer in 2021 in the United States along with 43,600 deaths (NCI, n.d.). The disease is second to lung cancer as the leading cause of death in women with cancer. Early detection is the key to cure.

Table 30.3 outlines the ACS (2021) guidelines for the early detection of breast cancer in women at average risk. The ACS (2021; 2020a) recommends that women who are at high risk for breast cancer based on certain factors should get an MRI scan and a mammogram every year. This includes women who:
- Have a lifetime risk of breast cancer of about 20% to 25% or greater, according to risk assessment tools that are based mainly on family history
- Have a known *BRCA1* or *BRCA2* gene mutation
- Have a first-degree relative (parent, brother, sister, or child) with a *BRCA1* or *BRCA2* gene mutation and have not had genetic testing themselves
- Had radiation therapy to the chest when they were between 10 and 30 years of age

BOX 30.21   Breast Self-Examination

Procedure
- Help patient identify the appropriate time of the month to perform breast self-examination (BSE).
- Describe normal findings and what findings require notification of health care provider.
- Teach patient the steps to perform BSE:
  1. Examine your right breast. Lie on your back and place your right arm behind your head. The examination is best completed lying down, not standing up, because when you lie down the breast tissue spreads evenly over the chest wall and is as thin as possible, making it much easier to feel all of it.
  2. Use finger pads of the three middle fingers on your left hand to feel for lumps in the right breast. Use overlapping dime-size circular motions of the finger pads to feel the breast tissue. Use three different levels of pressure to feel all the breast tissue. Light pressure is needed to feel the tissue closest to the skin, medium pressure to feel a little deeper, and firm pressure to feel the tissue closest to the chest and ribs. It is normal to feel a firm ridge in the lower curve of each breast, but you should tell your health care provider if you feel anything else out of the ordinary. If you are not sure how hard to press, discuss this with your health care provider. Use each pressure level to feel the breast tissue before moving on to the next spot.
  3. Move around the breast in an up-and-down pattern starting at an imaginary line drawn straight down your side from the underarm and moving across the breast to the middle of the chest bone (sternum or breastbone). Be sure to check the entire breast area, going down until you feel only ribs

and up to the neck or collarbone (clavicle). Evidence shows that the up-and-down pattern is the most effective pattern for covering the entire breast.
  4. Repeat self-examination in the left breast, putting your left arm behind your head and examining the left breast as noted in Steps 1 to 3.
  5. While standing in front of a mirror with your hands pressing firmly down on your hips, look at your breasts, observing for any changes in size, shape, contour, dimpling, redness, or scaliness of the nipple or breast tissue. Pressing down on your hips contracts the chest wall muscles and enhances any breast changes.
  6. Examine each underarm while sitting or standing and with your arm only slightly raised so that you can feel any lumps or changes in this area easily. Raising your arm straight tightens the tissue in this area, making it harder to examine.

  NOTE: If implants are present, help the patient determine the edges of each implant and how to evaluate each breast.
- Instruct patient to call the health care provider if she finds a lump or other abnormality.
- Use Teach-Back to evaluate patient/family caregiver learning: "I want to be sure I explained to you how to conduct a breast self-examination. Can you show me how to conduct an examination on both of your breasts?" Document your evaluation of patient learning. Revise your instruction or develop a plan for revised patient teaching to be implemented at an appropriate time if patient is not able to teach back correctly.

Images from Silvestri LA, Silvestri AE: *Saunders comprehensive review for the NCLEX-PN® Examination,* ed 7, St Louis, 2019, Elsevier.

Monthly breast self-examination (BSE) is no longer recommended by the ACS (2021) for women at any age because there is limited evidence to benefits in locating cancerous tumors, but other health care agencies encourage BSE as an important option for women (National Breast Cancer Foundation, n.d.). Encourage women to ask what their personal physician recommends. If a female patient chooses to perform BSE, assess the method she uses and when she does the examination in relation to her menstrual cycle (Box 30.21). The best time for a BSE is the fourth through seventh days of the menstrual cycle or right after the menstrual cycle ends, when the breasts are no longer swollen or tender from hormone elevations. If the woman does not menstruate (e.g., due to pregnancy or menopause), advise her to check her breasts on the same day each month.

TABLE 30.26 Nursing History for Breast Assessment

Assessment	Rationale
Determine whether woman is over age 40; has a personal or family history of breast cancer, especially with the *BRCA1* or *BRCA2* inherited gene mutations; early-onset menarche (before age 12) or late-age menopause (after age 55); has never had children or gave birth to first child after age 31; or has recently used oral contraceptives.	These are risk factors for breast cancer (ACS, 2020a; ACS, 2021).
Ask whether patient (both sexes) has noticed lump, thickening, pain, or tenderness of breast; discharge, distortion, retraction, or scaling of the nipple; or change in size of breast.	Potential signs and symptoms of breast cancer allow nurse to focus on specific areas of breast during assessment.
Determine patient's use of medications (oral contraceptives, digitalis, diuretics, steroids, or estrogen). Determine patient's caffeine intake.	Some medications cause nipple discharge. Hormones and caffeine cause fibrocystic changes in breast.
Determine patient's level of activity, alcoholic intake, and weight.	Breast cancer incidence rates correlate with being overweight or obese (postmenopausal), physical inactivity, and consumption of alcoholic beverages (ACS, 2021).
Ask whether patient performs monthly breast self-examination (BSE). If so, determine time of month she performs examination in relation to menstrual cycle. Have her describe or demonstrate method used.	Nurse's role is to educate patient about breast cancer and correct techniques for BSE.
If patient reports a breast mass, ask about length of time since she first noticed the lump. Does lump come and go, or is it always present? Have there been changes in the lump (e.g., size, relationship to menses), and are there associated symptoms?	Assessment helps to determine nature of mass (e.g., breast cancer versus fibrocystic disease).

BOX 30.22 Normal Changes in the Breast During a Woman's Life Span

Puberty (8–20 Years)
Breasts mature in five stages. One breast may grow more rapidly than the other. The ages at which changes occur and rate of developmental progression vary.

Stage 1 (Preadolescent)
This stage involves elevation of the nipple only.

Stage 2
The breast and nipple elevate as a small mound, and the areolar diameters enlarge.

Stage 3
There is further enlargement and elevation of the breast and areola, with no separation of contour.

Stage 4
The areola and nipple project into the secondary mound above the level of the breast (does not occur in all girls).

Stage 5 (Mature Breast)
Only the nipple projects, and the areola recedes (varies in some women).

Young Adulthood (20–31 Years)
Breasts reach full (nonpregnant) size. Shape is generally symmetrical. Breasts are sometimes unequal in size.

Pregnancy
Breast size gradually enlarges to 2 to 3 times the previous size. Nipples enlarge and become erect. Areolas darken, and diameters increase. Superficial veins become prominent. The nipples expel a yellowish fluid (colostrum).

Menopause
Breasts shrink. Tissue becomes softer, sometimes flabby.

Older Adulthood
Breasts become elongated, pendulous, and flaccid as a result of glandular tissue atrophy. The skin of the breasts tends to wrinkle, appearing loose and flabby.
Nipples become smaller and flatter and lose erectile ability. They sometimes invert because of shrinkage and fibrotic changes.

Data from Touhy TA, Jett KF: *Ebersole and Hess' toward healthy aging,* ed 10, St Louis, 2020, Elsevier; Hockenberry MJ, Wilson P: *Wong's nursing care of infants and children,* ed 10, St Louis, 2019, Elsevier; and Ball JW, et al: *Seidel's guide to physical examination,* ed 9, St Louis, 2019, Elsevier.

Older women require special attention when reviewing the need for regular BSE. Unfortunately, many older women ignore changes in their breasts, assuming that they are a part of aging. In addition, physiological factors affect the ease with which older women perform a BSE. Musculoskeletal limitations, diminished peripheral sensation, reduced eyesight, and changes in joint range of motion (ROM) limit palpation and inspection abilities.

The patient's history (Table 30.26) reveals normal developmental changes and signs of breast disease. Because of its glandular structure, the breast undergoes changes during a woman's life. Knowing these changes (Box 30.22) allows complete and accurate assessment. Encourage both men and women to observe their breasts for changes and to report any changes to their health care provider.

Inspection. Have the patient remove the top gown or drape to allow simultaneous visualization of both breasts. Have her stand or sit with her arms hanging loosely at her sides. If the patient chooses to perform BSE, place a mirror in front of her if possible during inspection so that she sees what to look for when performing a BSE. Describe observations or findings in relation to imaginary lines that divide the breast into four quadrants and a tail. The lines cross at the center of the nipple. Each tail extends outward from the upper outer quadrant (Fig. 30.51).

Inspect the breasts for size and symmetry. Normally they extend from the third to the sixth ribs, with the nipple at the level of the fourth intercostal space. It is common for one breast to be smaller. However, inflammation or a mass causes a difference in size. As a woman ages,

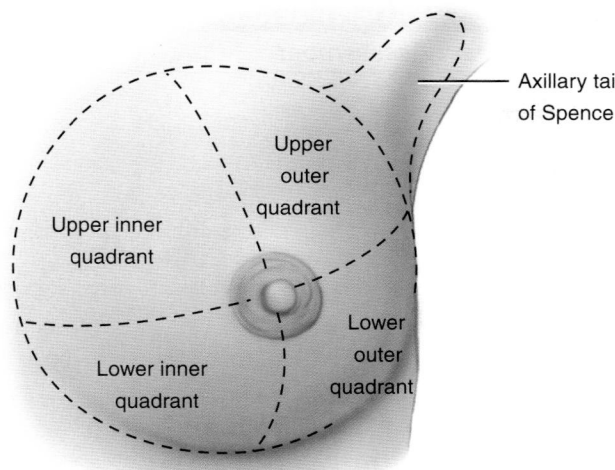

FIG. 30.51 Quadrants of left breast and axillary tail of Spence. (From Shiland BJ: *Medical terminology and anatomy for coding*, ed 3, St Louis, 2017, Mosby.)

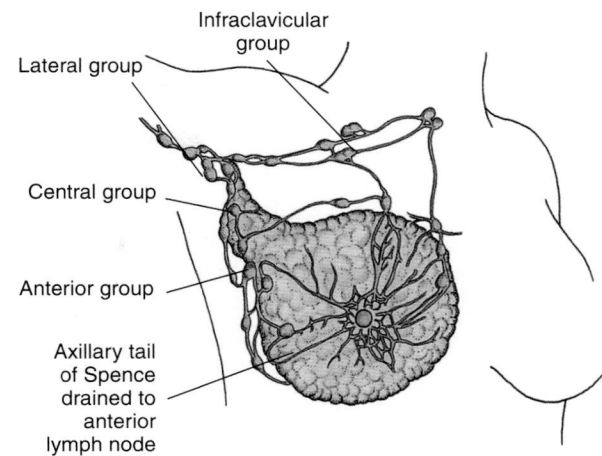

FIG. 30.52 Anatomical position of axillary and clavicular lymph nodes.

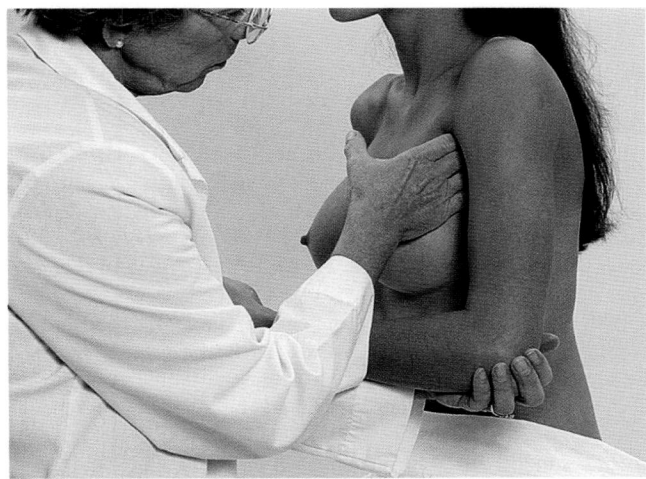

FIG. 30.53 Support patient's arm and palpate axillary lymph nodes. (From Wilson S, Giddens J: *Health assessment for nursing practice*, ed 7, St Louis, 2022, Elsevier.)

the ligaments supporting the breast tissue weaken, causing the breasts to sag and the nipples to lower.

Observe the contour or shape of the breasts and note masses, flattening, retraction, or dimpling. Breasts vary in shape from convex to pendulous or conical. Retraction or dimpling can result from invasion of underlying ligaments by tumors. The ligaments fibrose and pull the overlying skin inward toward the tumor. Edema also changes the contour of the breasts. To bring out retraction or changes in the shape of breasts, ask the patient to assume three positions: raise arms above the head, press hands against the hips, and extend arms straight ahead while sitting and leaning forward. Each maneuver causes a contraction of the pectoral muscles, which accentuates the presence of any retraction.

Carefully inspect the skin for color; venous pattern; and the presence of lesions, edema, or inflammation. Lift each breast when necessary to observe lower and lateral aspects for color and texture changes. The breasts are the color of neighboring skin, and venous patterns are the same bilaterally. Venous patterns are easily visible in thin or pregnant women. Women with large breasts often have redness and excoriation of the undersurfaces caused by rubbing of skin surfaces.

Inspect the nipple and areola for size, color, shape, discharge, and the direction in which the nipples point. The normal areolas are round or oval and nearly equal bilaterally. Color ranges from pink to brown. In light-skinned women the areola turns brown during pregnancy and remains dark. In dark-skinned women the areola is brown before pregnancy (Ball et al., 2019). Normally the nipples point in symmetrical directions, are everted, and have no drainage. If the nipples are inverted, ask whether this has been a lifetime history. A recent inversion or inward turning of the nipple indicates an underlying growth. Rashes or ulcerations are not normal on the breast or nipples. Note any bleeding or discharge from the nipple. Clear yellow discharge 2 days after childbirth is common. While inspecting the breasts, explain the characteristics you see. Teach patients the significance of abnormal signs or symptoms.

Palpation. Use palpation to assess the condition of underlying breast tissue and lymph nodes. Breast tissue consists of glandular tissue, fibrous supportive ligaments, and fat. Glandular tissue is organized into lobes that end in ducts that open onto the surface of the nipple. The largest part of glandular tissue is in the upper outer quadrant and

tail of each breast. Suspensory ligaments connect to skin and fascia underlying the breast to support the breast and maintain its upright position. Fatty tissue is located superficially and to the sides of the breast.

A part of the lymph system, the breasts drain into axillary lymph nodes. If cancerous lesions metastasize (spread), the nodes commonly become involved. Study the location of supraclavicular, infraclavicular, and axillary nodes (Fig. 30.52). The axillary nodes drain lymph from the chest wall, breasts, arms, and hands. A tumor of one breast sometimes involves nodes on the same and opposite sides.

To palpate the lymph nodes, have the patient sit with her arms at her sides and muscles relaxed. While facing the patient and standing on the side you are examining, support her arm in a flexed position and abduct it from the chest wall. Place the free hand against the patient's chest wall and high in the axillary hollow. With the fingertips press gently down over the surface of the ribs and muscles. Palpate the four areas of the axilla and the axillary nodes with the fingertips, gently rolling soft tissue (Fig. 30.53).

Normally lymph nodes are not palpable. Carefully assess each area and note their number, consistency, mobility, and size. One or two small, soft, nontender palpable nodes are normal. An abnormal palpable node

FIG. 30.54 Patient lies flat with arm abducted and hand under head to help flatten breast tissue evenly over chest wall. Each breast is palpated in a systematic fashion. (From Wilson S, Giddens J: *Health assessment for nursing practice,* ed 7, St Louis, 2022, Elsevier.)

feels like a small mass that is hard, tender, and immobile. Continue to palpate along the upper and lower clavicular ridges. Reverse the procedure for the patient's other side.

It is sometimes difficult for a patient to learn to palpate for lymph nodes. Lying down with the arm abducted makes the area more accessible. Instruct the patient to use her left hand for the right axillary and clavicular areas. Take the patient's fingertips and move them in the proper fashion. Then have the patient her right hand to palpate for nodes on the left side.

With the patient lying supine and one arm under the head and neck (alternating with each breast), palpate her breast tissue (Fig. 30.54). The supine position allows the breast tissue to flatten evenly against the chest wall. The position of the arm and hand further stretches and positions breast tissue evenly. Place a small pillow or towel under the patient's shoulder blade to further position breast tissue. Palpate the tail of Spence.

The consistency of normal breast tissue varies widely. The breasts of a young patient are firm and elastic. In an older patient the tissue sometimes feels stringy and nodular. A patient's familiarity with the texture of her own breasts is especially important. Teach patients about strategies to promote breast health (Box 30.23).

If a mass is palpated by you or the patient, examine the opposite breast to ensure an objective comparison of normal and abnormal tissue. Use the pads of the first three fingers to compress breast tissue gently against the chest wall, noting tissue consistency. Perform palpation systematically in one of three ways: (1) using a vertical technique with the fingers moving up and down each quadrant; (2) clockwise or counterclockwise, forming small concentric circles with the fingers along each quadrant and the tail; or (3) palpating from the center of the breast in a radial fashion, returning to the areola to begin each spoke (Fig. 30.55). Whichever approach you use, be sure to cover the entire breast and tail, directing attention to any areas of tenderness. Use a bimanual technique when palpating large, pendulous breasts. Support the inferior part of the breast in one hand while using the other hand to palpate breast tissue against the supporting hand.

During palpation note the consistency of breast tissue. It normally feels dense, firm, and elastic. With menopause breast tissue shrinks and becomes softer. The lobular feel of glandular tissue is normal. The lower edge of each breast sometimes feels firm and hard. This is the normal inframammary ridge and not a tumor. It helps to move the patient's hand so that she can feel normal tissue variations. Palpate abnormal

BOX 30.23 PATIENT TEACHING
Female Breast Assessment

Objective
- Patient will follow prevention and detection practices to ensure breast health.

Teaching Strategies
- Have patient perform return demonstration of breast self-examination (BSE), and offer the opportunity to ask questions (see Box 30.21).
- Explain recommended frequency of mammography and assessment by the patient's health care provider.
- Discuss signs and symptoms of breast cancer.
- Discuss signs and symptoms of benign (fibrocystic) breast disease.
- Inform a woman who is obese or has a family history of breast cancer that she is at higher risk for the disease (ACS, 2020a; ACS, 2021). Encourage dietary changes, including limiting meat consumption to well-trimmed, lean beef, pork, or lamb; removing skin from cooked chicken before eating it; selecting tuna and salmon packed in water and not oil; and using low-fat dairy products.
- Encourage patient to reduce intake of caffeine. Although this approach is controversial, it can reduce symptoms of benign (fibrocystic) breast disease.

Evaluation
Use the principles of teach-back to evaluate patient/family caregiver learning:
- Tell me when was your last mammogram? Explain to me how often you should get a mammogram.
- Describe for me the signs and symptoms of breast cancer and when you should contact your health care provider.

masses to determine location in relation to quadrants, diameter in centimeters, shape (e.g., round, or discoid), consistency (soft, firm, or hard), tenderness, mobility, and discreteness (clear or unclear boundaries).

Cancerous lesions are hard, fixed, nontender, irregular in shape, and usually unilateral. A common benign condition of the breast is benign (fibrocystic) breast disease. Bilateral lumpy, painful breasts and sometimes nipple discharge characterize this condition. Symptoms are more apparent during the menstrual period. When palpated, the cysts (lumps) are soft, well differentiated, and movable. Deep cysts feel hard.

Give special attention to palpating the nipple and areola. Palpate the entire surface gently. Use the thumb and index finger to compress the nipple and note any discharge. During the examination of the nipple and areola, the nipple sometimes becomes erect with wrinkling of the areola. These changes are normal. Continue by positioning the patient and examining the other breast.

Male Breasts

Fewer than 1% of all breast cancers are diagnosed in men. In 2019, about 2670 new cases of invasive breast cancer will be diagnosed in men (BreastCancer.org, 2019). Inspect the nipple and areola for nodules, edema, and ulceration. An enlarged male breast results from obesity or glandular enlargement. Breast enlargement in young males results from steroid use. Fatty tissue feels soft, whereas glandular tissue is firm. Use the same techniques to palpate for masses used in examination of the female breast. Because breast cancer in men is relatively rare, routine self-examinations are unnecessary. Breast tumors are often not found in men until late; thus men have a lower survival rate than women (BreastCancer.org, 2019). However, men who have a first-degree relative (e.g., mother or sister) with breast cancer are at risk for breast cancer and may be scheduled by their health care provider for routine mammograms.

FIG. 30.55 Various methods for palpation of breast. (A) Palpate from top to bottom in vertical strips. (B) Palpate in concentric circles. (C) Palpate out from center in wedge sections.

TABLE 30.27 Nursing History for Abdominal Assessment	
Assessment	**Rationale**
If patient has abdominal or low back pain, assess character of pain in detail (location, onset, frequency, precipitating factors, aggravating factors, type of pain, severity, course).	Pattern of characteristics of pain helps determine its source.
Carefully observe patient's movement and position, including lying still with knees drawn up, moving restlessly to find comfortable position, and lying on one side or sitting with knees drawn to chest.	Positions assumed by patient reveal nature and source of pain, including peritonitis, renal stone, and pancreatitis.
Assess normal bowel habits and stool character; ask whether patient uses laxatives.	Data compared with physical findings help identify cause and nature of elimination problems.
Determine whether patient has had abdominal surgery, trauma, or diagnostic tests of gastrointestinal (GI) tract.	Surgical or traumatic alterations of abdominal organs cause changes in expected findings (e.g., position of underlying organs). Diagnostic tests change character of stool.
Assess whether patient has had recent weight changes or intolerance to diet (e.g., nausea, vomiting, cramping, especially in last 24 hours).	Data can indicate alterations in upper GI tract (stomach or gallbladder) or lower colon.
Assess for difficulty in swallowing, belching, flatulence (gas), bloody emesis (hematemesis), black or tarry stools (melena), heartburn, diarrhea, or constipation.	These characteristic signs and symptoms indicate GI alterations.
Ask whether patient takes antiinflammatory medication (e.g., aspirin, ibuprofen, steroids) or antibiotics.	Pharmacological agents cause GI upset or bleeding.
Ask patient to locate tender areas before examination begins.	Assess painful areas last to minimize discomfort and anxiety.
Inquire about family history of cancer, kidney disease, alcoholism, hypertension, or heart disease.	Data can reveal risk for alterations identifiable during examination.
Determine whether female patient is pregnant; note last menstrual period.	Pregnancy causes changes in abdominal shape and contour.
Assess patient's usual intake of alcohol.	Chronic alcohol ingestion causes GI and liver problems, including liver, colon, and pancreatic cancer (ACS, 2020a).
Review patient's history for the following: health care occupation, hemodialysis, intravenous drug user, household or sexual contact with hepatitis B virus (HBV) carrier, heterosexual person with more than one sex partner in previous 6 months, sexually active homosexual or bisexual male, international traveler in area of high HBV infection rate.	Risk factors for HBV exposure.

ABDOMEN

The abdominal examination is complex because of the number of organs located within and near the abdominal cavity. A thorough nursing history (Table 30.27) helps interpret physical signs. The examination includes an assessment of structures of the lower GI tract in addition to the liver, stomach, uterus, ovaries, kidneys, and bladder. Abdominal pain is one of the most common symptoms that patients report when seeking medical care. An accurate assessment requires matching patient history data with a careful assessment of the location of physical symptoms.

Assess the organs anteriorly and posteriorly. A system of landmarks helps map out the abdominal region. The xiphoid process (tip of the sternum) is the upper boundary of the anterior abdominal region. The symphysis pubis marks the lower boundary. Divide the abdomen into four imaginary quadrants (Fig. 30.56A); refer to assessment findings and record them in relation to each quadrant. Posteriorly the lower ribs and heavy back muscles protect the kidneys, which are located

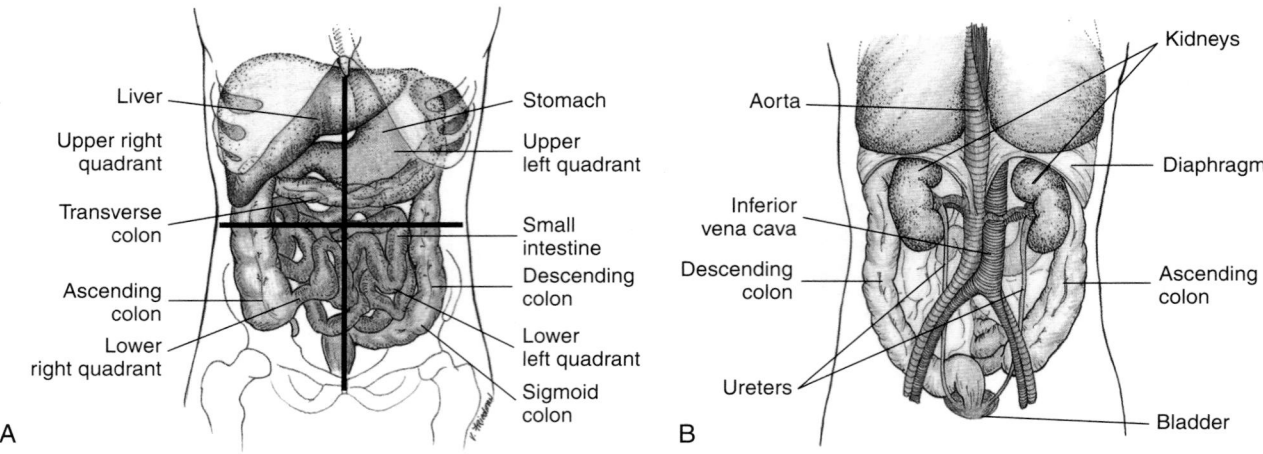

FIG. 30.56 (A) Anterior view of abdomen divided by quadrants. (B) Posterior view of abdominal section.

from the T12 to L3 vertebrae (see Fig. 30.56B). The costovertebral angle formed by the last rib and vertebral column is a landmark used during kidney palpation.

During the abdominal examination, the patient needs to relax. A tightening of abdominal muscles hinders palpation. Ask the patient to void before beginning. Be sure that the room is warm, and drape the upper chest and legs. The patient lies supine or in a dorsal recumbent position with the arms at the sides and knees slightly bent. Place small pillows beneath the knees. If the patient places the arms under the head, the abdominal muscles tighten. Proceed calmly and slowly, being sure that there is adequate lighting. Expose the abdomen from just above the xiphoid process down to the symphysis pubis. Warm hands and stethoscope further promote relaxation. Ask the patient to report pain and point out tender areas. Assess tender areas last.

The order of an abdominal examination differs slightly from previous assessments. Begin with inspection and follow with auscultation. By completing palpation last there is less chance of altering the frequency and character of bowel sounds. Be sure to have a tape measure and marking pen available during the examination.

Inspection

Make it a habit to observe the patient during routine care activities. Note posture and look for evidence of abdominal splinting: lying with the knees drawn up or moving restlessly in bed. A patient free from abdominal pain does not guard or splint the abdomen. To inspect the abdomen for abnormal movement or shadows, stand on the patient's right side and inspect from above the abdomen. After sitting or stooping down to look across the abdomen, assess abdominal contour. Direct the examination light over the abdomen.

Skin. Inspect the skin over the abdomen for color, scars, venous patterns, lesions, and striae (stretch marks). The skin is subject to the same color variations as the rest of the body. Venous patterns are normally faint, except in thin patients. Striae result from stretching of tissue by obesity or pregnancy. Artificial openings indicate drainage sites resulting from surgery (see Chapter 50) or an ostomy (see Chapters 46 and 47). Scars reveal evidence of past trauma or surgery that has created permanent changes in underlying organ anatomy. Bruising indicates accidental injury, physical abuse, or a type of bleeding disorder. If needle marks or bruises are present, ask whether the patient self-administers injections (e.g., low-molecular-weight heparin or insulin). Unexpected findings include generalized color changes such as jaundice

or cyanosis. Shiny abdominal skin with a taut (tight) appearance can indicate ascites.

Umbilicus. Note the position; shape; color; and signs of inflammation, discharge, or protruding masses. A normal umbilicus is flat or concave, with the color the same as that of the surrounding skin. Underlying masses cause displacement of the umbilicus. An everted (pouched-out) umbilicus usually indicates distention. Hernias (protrusion of abdominal organs through the muscle wall) cause upward protrusion of the umbilicus. Normally the umbilical area does not emit discharge.

Contour and Symmetry. Inspect for contour, symmetry, and surface motion of the abdomen, noting any masses, bulging, or distention. A flat abdomen forms a horizontal plane from the xiphoid process to the symphysis pubis. A round abdomen protrudes in a convex sphere from the horizontal plane. A concave abdomen appears to sink into the muscular wall. Each of these findings is normal for the individual patient if the shape of the abdomen is symmetrical. In older adults there is often an overall increased distribution of adipose tissue. The presence of masses on only one side, or asymmetry, can indicate an underlying pathological condition.

Intestinal gas, a tumor, or fluid in the abdominal cavity causes distention (swelling). When distention is generalized, the entire abdomen protrudes. The skin often appears taut, as if it were stretched over the abdomen. When gas causes distention, the flanks (side muscles) do not bulge. However, if fluid is the source of the problem, the flanks bulge. Ask the patient to roll onto one side. A protuberance forms on the dependent side if fluid is the cause of the distention. Ask the patient whether the abdomen feels unusually tight. Be careful not to confuse distention with obesity. In obesity the abdomen is large, rolls of adipose tissue are often present along the flanks, and the patient does not complain of tightness in the abdomen. If distention is expected, measure the abdomen by placing a tape measure around it at the level of the umbilicus (this may require the patient to roll side to side as you position the tape measure). Consecutive measurements show any increase or decrease in distention. Use a marking pen to indicate the location of the tape measure.

Enlarged Organs or Masses. Observe the contour of the abdomen while asking the patient to take a deep breath and hold it. Normally the contour remains smooth and symmetrical. This maneuver forces the diaphragm downward and reduces the size of the abdominal cavity. Any enlarged organs in the upper abdominal cavity (e.g., liver or

BOX 30.24 EVIDENCE-BASED PRACTICE

Detection of Gastrointestinal Complications

PICOT Question: Does a comprehensive gastrointestinal (GI) assessment in adult patients with general medical problems identify and/or prevent complications during hospitalization?

Evidence Summary

A well-performed, complete GI assessment can identify the type of changes that lead to complications and guide care of the patient. The subjective component of the GI assessment requires questions to determine history, daily routine, food consumption, elimination patterns, and discomfort. It is recommended to use multiple objective assessment techniques such as auscultation, inspection, and palpation as well as more detailed tests such as computed tomography (CT), ultrasound, endoscopy, and real-time bowel sound analysis using acoustic sensors (Kendall and Moreira, 2020). Using only one component of the examination, such as auscultation of bowel sounds, is not a good indicator of complications. Bowel sounds can vary greatly depending on the patient situation. An increase in the frequency of bowel sounds can present because the patient is chewing gum (Frazer et al., 2018), or an increase in blood sugar can slow motility and decrease the frequency of bowel sounds (Ladopoulos et al., 2018). Over the years the physical GI examination has been scaled down while imaging techniques

have increased. Scales such as the Sequential Organ Failure Assessment (SOFA) and GI failure (GIF) score can be used in combination with a physical examination to help identify complications (Moonen et al., 2018).

GI complications contribute to a high risk of mortality, increased length of stay, and medical costs (Frazer et al., 2018). Current and preexisting conditions, such as obesity, advancing age, chronic alcohol use, altered fluid and electrolytes, or kidney issues, make the patient more likely to experience GI complications (Bond and Hallmark, 2018).

Application to Nursing Practice

- GI complications are common in patients admitted to the hospital (Kendall and Moreira, 2020).
- Conduct a complete GI assessment, including subjective and objective information, because an assessment finding as minor as hiccups can be an indication of a complication (Bond and Hallmark, 2018).
- Auscultation of bowel sounds should be completed but should not be the sole indicator of a complication (Kendall and Moreira, 2020).
- Movement, such as ambulation and change in position, can help decrease GI complications in patients.

---

spleen) descend below the rib cage to cause a bulge. Perform a closer examination with palpation. To evaluate the abdominal musculature, have the patient raise the head. This position causes superficial abdominal wall masses, hernias, and muscle separations to become more apparent.

Movement or Pulsations. Inspect for movement. Normally men breathe abdominally, and women breathe more costally. A patient with severe pain has diminished respiratory movement and tightens the abdominal muscles to guard against the pain. Closely inspect for peristaltic movement and aortic pulsation by looking across the abdomen from the side. These movements are visible in thin patients; otherwise no movement is present.

Auscultation

Auscultate before palpation during the abdominal assessment because manipulation of the abdomen alters the frequency and intensity of bowel sounds. Ask patients not to talk. Patients with GI tubes connected to suction need them temporarily turned off before beginning an examination.

Bowel Motility. Peristalsis, or the movement of contents through the intestines, is a normal function of the small and large intestine. Bowel sounds are the audible passage of air and fluid that peristalsis creates. Place the warmed diaphragm of the stethoscope lightly over each of the four quadrants. Normally air and fluid move through the intestines, creating soft gurgling or clicking sounds that occur irregularly 5 to 35 times per minute (Ball et al., 2019). It normally takes 5 to 20 seconds to hear a bowel sound. However, it takes 5 minutes of continuous listening before determining that bowel sounds are absent (Ball et al., 2019). Auscultate all four quadrants to be sure that you do not miss any sounds. The best time to auscultate is between meals. Sounds are generally described as normal, audible, absent, hyperactive, or hypoactive. Absent sounds indicate a lack of peristalsis, possibly the result of late-stage bowel obstruction; paralytic ileus; or peritonitis. Absent or hypoactive bowel sounds may be normal after surgery following general anesthesia. Hyperactive sounds are loud, "growling"

BOX 30.25 PATIENT TEACHING

Abdominal Assessment

Objective
- Patient will maintain normal bowel elimination.

Teaching Strategies
- Explain factors that promote normal bowel elimination such as diet (fruits, vegetables, fiber), regular exercise, limited use of over-the-counter drugs causing constipation, establishment of regular elimination schedule, and a good fluid intake (see Chapter 47). Stress importance for older adults.
- Caution patients about the dangers of excessive use of laxatives or enemas.
- Instruct patient to have acute abdominal pain evaluated by a health care provider.

Evaluation
Use the principles of teach-back to evaluate patient/family caregiver learning:
- Describe for me how often you have a bowel movement and what the stool looks like.
- Describe for me the high-fiber foods that you have added to your diet.

---

sounds called borborygmi, which indicate increased GI motility and can be caused by inflammation of the bowel, anxiety, diarrhea, bleeding, excessive ingestion of laxatives, and reaction of the intestines to certain foods. Assessment findings vary based on patient situation and level of care (Box 30.24). Teach patients practices that promote normal elimination patterns (Box 30.25).

Vascular Sounds. Bruits indicate narrowing of the major blood vessels and disruption of blood flow. The presence of bruits in the abdominal area can reveal aneurysms or stenotic vessels. Use the bell of the stethoscope to auscultate in the epigastric region and each of the four quadrants. Normally there are no vascular sounds over the aorta (midline through the abdomen) or femoral arteries (lower quadrants).

FIG. 30.57 Light palpation of abdomen.

FIG. 30.58 Deep palpation of abdomen.

You can hear renal artery bruits by placing the stethoscope over each upper quadrant anteriorly or over the costovertebral angle posteriorly. Report a bruit immediately to a health care provider.

Kidney Tenderness. With the patient sitting or standing erect, use direct or indirect percussion to assess for kidney inflammation. With the ulnar surface of the partially closed fist, percuss posteriorly the costovertebral angle at the scapular line. If the kidneys are inflamed, the patient feels tenderness during percussion.

Palpation

Palpation primarily detects areas of abdominal tenderness, distention, or masses. As your skill base increases, learn to palpate for specific organs by using light and deep palpation.

Use light palpation over each abdominal quadrant to detect areas of tenderness. Initially avoid areas previously identified as problem spots. Lay the palm of the hand with fingers extended and approximated lightly on the abdomen. Explain the maneuver to the patient and, with the palmar surface of the fingers, depress approximately 1.3 cm (½ inch) in a gentle dipping motion (Fig. 30.57). Avoid quick jabs, and use smooth, coordinated movements. If the patient is ticklish, first place the patient's hand on the abdomen with your hand on the patient's; continue this until the patient tolerates palpation.

Use a systematic palpation approach for each quadrant and assess for muscular resistance, distention, tenderness, and superficial organs or masses. Observe the patient's face for signs of discomfort. The abdomen is normally smooth with consistent softness and nontender without masses. In contrast to firm muscles found among young adults, an older adult often lacks abdominal tone. Guarding or muscle tenseness sometimes occurs while palpating a sensitive area. If tightening remains after the patient relaxes, peritonitis, acute cholecystitis, or appendicitis is sometimes the cause. It is easy to detect a distended bladder with light palpation because the bladder lies below the umbilicus and above the symphysis pubis. Routinely check for a distended bladder if the patient has been unable to void (e.g., because of anesthesia or sedation; the patient has been incontinent; or an indwelling urinary catheter is not draining well).

With practice and experience, perform deep palpation to delineate abdominal organs and detect less obvious masses. You need short fingernails. It is important for the patient to be relaxed while the hands depress approximately 2.5 to 7.5 cm (1–3 inches) into the abdomen (Fig. 30.58). Never use deep palpation over a surgical incision, over tender organs, or on abnormal masses. Deep pressure causes tenderness

in a healthy patient over the cecum, sigmoid colon, aorta, and the midline near the xiphoid process (Ball et al., 2019).

Survey each quadrant systematically. Palpate masses for size, location, shape, consistency, tenderness, pulsation, and mobility. Test for rebound tenderness by pressing a hand slowly and deeply into the involved area and letting go quickly; if discomfort is present, then the test is positive. Be careful with this examination technique if pain is present. Rebound tenderness occurs in patients with peritoneal irritation such as occurs in appendicitis; pancreatitis; or any peritoneal injury causing bile, blood, or enzymes to enter the peritoneal cavity.

Aortic Pulsation. Palpate with the thumb and forefinger of one hand deeply into the upper abdomen just left of the midline to assess aortic pulsation. Normally a pulsation is transmitted forward. If the aorta is enlarged because of an aneurysm (localized dilation of a vessel wall), the pulsation expands laterally. Do not palpate a pulsating abdominal mass. When enlargement from an aneurysm is present, palpate this area only lightly, referring the finding to the health care provider. In patients who are obese, it is often necessary to palpate with both hands, one on each side of the aorta.

FEMALE GENITALIA AND REPRODUCTIVE TRACT

Examination of the female genitalia can be embarrassing to a patient unless you use a calm, relaxed approach. The gynecological examination is one of the most difficult experiences for adolescents. A person's cultural background further adds to apprehension. For example, female Mexican Americans have a strong social value that women do not expose their bodies to men or even to other women. Similarly, Chinese Americans believe that the examination of genitalia is offensive. Muslim women value respect for female modesty. Establishing privacy, draping carefully, and using a calm approach is essential for all patients.

Provide a thorough explanation of the reason for the procedures used in an examination. The lithotomy position assumed during the examination is an added source of embarrassment and can increase anxiety. A patient is more comfortable when you use correct positioning and draping. Be sure to explain each part of the examination in advance so that patients anticipate necessary actions. Adolescents sometimes choose to have parents present in the examination room.

Sometimes a patient requires a complete examination of the female reproductive organs, including assessing the external genitalia and performing a vaginal examination. You can examine external genitalia while performing routine hygiene measures or when preparing to insert

TABLE 30.28 Nursing History Assessment for Female Genitalia and Reproductive Tract Assessment

Assessment	Rationale
Determine whether patient has had previous illness (e.g., STIs) or surgery involving reproductive organs.	Illness or surgery influences appearance and position of organs being examined.
Determine whether patient has received HPV vaccine.	HPV increases patient's risk for development of cervical cancer.
Review menstrual history, including age at menarche, frequency and duration of menstrual cycle, character of flow (e.g., amount, presence of clots), presence of dysmenorrhea (painful menstruation), pelvic pain, dates of last two menstrual periods, and premenstrual symptoms.	This information helps to reveal level of reproductive health, including normalcy of menstrual cycle.
Ask patient to describe obstetrical history, including each pregnancy and history of abortions or miscarriages.	Observed physical findings vary, depending on woman's history of pregnancy.
Determine whether patient uses safe sex practices; have patient describe current and past contraceptive practices and problems encountered. Discuss risk of STIs and HIV infection.	Use of certain types of contraceptives influences reproductive health (e.g., sensitivity reaction to spermicidal jelly). Sexual history reveals risk for and understanding of STIs.
Assess whether patient has signs and symptoms of vaginal discharge, painful or swollen perianal tissues, or genital lesions.	These signs and symptoms may indicate STI or other pathological condition.
Determine whether patient has symptoms or history of genitourinary problems, including burning during urination, frequency, urgency, nocturia, hematuria, incontinence, or stress incontinence (see Chapter 46).	Urinary problems are associated with gynecological disorders, including STIs.
Ask whether patient has had signs of bleeding outside of normal menstrual period or after menopause or has had unusual vaginal discharge.	These are warning signs for cervical and endometrial cancer or vaginal infection.
Determine whether patient has history of HPV (condyloma acuminatum, herpes simplex, or cervical dysplasia), has multiple sex partners, smokes cigarettes, has had multiple pregnancies, or was young at first intercourse.	These are risk factors for cervical cancer (ACS, 2020a).
Ask if patient has a strong personal or family history of breast or ovarian cancer; women who have had breast cancer or who have tested positive for inherited mutations in *BRCA1* or *BRCA2* genes are at increased risk. Other medical conditions associated with increased risk include pelvic inflammatory disease and Lynch syndrome. The use of estrogen alone as menopausal hormone therapy has been shown to increase risk. Tobacco smoking increases the risk of mucinous ovarian cancer. Heavier body weight may be associated with increased risk of ovarian cancer.	These are risk factors for ovarian cancer (ACS, 2020a).
Determine whether patient is postmenopausal, is obese, has abdominal fat, or is infertile. Assess whether patient received menopausal estrogen therapy, had late menopause, never had children, or has a history of polycystic ovary syndrome. Tamoxifen, a drug used to reduce breast cancer risk, increases the risk slightly because it has estrogen-like effects on the uterus. Medical conditions that increase the risk include Lynch syndrome and diabetes.	These are risk factors for endometrial cancer (ACS, 2020a).

HIV, Human immunodeficiency virus; *HPV,* human papillomavirus (HPV) vaccine; *STI,* sexually transmitted infection.

a urinary catheter. An internal examination is part of each woman's preventive health care; even though ovarian cancer incidence has declined, it was estimated that 21,750 new cases would occur in 2020 (ACS, 2020b).

Adolescents and young adults are examined because of the growing incidence of sexually transmitted infections (STIs). The average age of menarche among young girls has declined, and the majority of male and female teenagers are sexually active by age 19 (Hockenberry and Wilson, 2019). It is important to assess a patient's level of anxiety when obtaining the nursing history (Table 30.28). Combine rectal and anal assessments with the pelvic examination, as the patient is situated in a lithotomy or dorsal recumbent position.

Preparation of the Patient

As a new nurse you are responsible for assisting a patient's health care provider with a pelvic examination. For a complete examination the following equipment is needed: examination table with stirrups, vaginal speculum of correct size, adjustable light source, sink, clean disposable gloves, sterile cotton swabs, glass slides, plastic or wooden spatula, cervical brush or broom device, cytological fixative, and culture plates or media (Ball et al., 2019).

Make sure that the equipment is ready before the examination begins. Ask the patient to empty her bladder so that the uterus and ovaries are readily palpable. Often it is necessary to collect a urine specimen. Help the patient to the lithotomy position in bed or on an examination table for the external genitalia assessment. Assist her into stirrups for a speculum examination. Have a woman stabilize each foot in a stirrup and slide the buttocks down to the edge of the examining table. Place a hand at the edge of the table and instruct the patient to move until touching the hand. The patient's arms should be at her sides or folded across the chest to prevent tightening of abdominal muscles.

Sometimes women who have pain or a deformity of the joints are unable to assume a lithotomy position. In this situation have the patient abduct only one leg or have another person assist in separating the patient's thighs. In addition, use the side-lying position with the patient on the left side with the right thigh and knee drawn up to her chest.

Give the patient a square drape or sheet. She holds one corner over her sternum, the adjacent corners fall over each knee, and the fourth corner covers the perineum. After the examination begins, lift the drape over the perineum. A male examiner always needs to have a female attendant present during the examination, whereas a female examiner may choose to work alone. An additional woman should be present based on the patient's preferences.

External Genitalia

You can perform this examination independently of a health care provider. Make sure that the perineal area is well illuminated. Follow standard precautions and wear clean gloves to prevent contact with infectious organisms. The perineum is sensitive and tender; do not touch the area suddenly without warning a patient. It is best to touch the inner thigh first before touching the perineum.

While sitting at the end of the examination table or bed, inspect the quantity and distribution of hair growth. Preadolescents have no pubic hair. During adolescence hair grows along the labia, becoming darker, coarser, and curlier. In an adult hair grows in a triangle over the female perineum and along the medial surfaces of the thighs. The underlying skin is free of inflammation, irritation, or lesions.

Inspect surface characteristics of the labia majora. The skin of the perineum is smooth, clean, and slightly darker than other skin. The mucous membranes appear dark pink and moist. The labia majora can be gaping or closed, appear dry or moist, and are usually symmetrical. After childbirth, the labia majora separate, causing the labia minora to become more prominent. When a woman reaches menopause, the labia majora become thinned; they become atrophied in older age. The labia majora are normally without inflammation, edema, lesions, or lacerations.

To inspect the remaining external structures, use your nondominant hand and gently place the thumb and index finger inside the labia minora and retract the tissues outwardly (Fig. 30.59). Be sure to have a firm hold to avoid repeated retraction against the sensitive tissues. Use the other hand to palpate the labia minora between the thumb and second finger. On inspection the labia minora are normally thinner than the labia majora, and one side is sometimes larger. The tissue feels soft on palpation and without tenderness. The size of the clitoris varies, but it normally does not exceed 2 cm (1 inch) in length and 0.5 cm (¼ inch) in width. Look for atrophy, inflammation, or adhesions. If inflamed, the clitoris is a bright cherry red. In young women it is a common site for an abnormal finding such as syphilitic lesions, or chancres, which appear as small open ulcers that drain serous material.

Inspect the urethral orifice carefully for color and position. It is normally intact without inflammation. The urethral meatus is anterior to the vaginal orifice and is pink. It appears as a small slit or pinhole opening just above the vaginal canal. Note any discharge, polyps, or fistulas.

Inspect the vaginal orifice for inflammation, edema, discoloration, discharge, and lesions. Normally the opening is a thin, vertical slit, and the tissue is moist. While inspecting the vaginal orifice, note the condition of the hymen, which is just inside the opening. In the virgin female the hymen restricts the opening of the vagina, but the tissue retracts or disappears after sexual intercourse or with normal growth in adolescence (Ball et al., 2019).

Inspect the anus, looking for lesions and hemorrhoids (see the discussion of the rectal examination). After completion of the external examination, dispose of examination gloves and offer the patient soft disposable cloths for perineal hygiene.

Patients who are at risk for contracting an STI need to learn to perform a genital self-examination (Box 30.26). The purpose of the examination is to detect any signs or symptoms of an STI. Many people do not know that they have an STI (e.g., chlamydia), and some STIs (e.g., syphilis) remain undetected for years.

Speculum Examination of Internal Genitalia

An examination of the internal genitalia requires much skill and practice. Advanced nurse practitioners and primary care providers perform this examination. As a nursing student you observe the procedure or assist the examiner by helping the patient with positioning, handing off specimen supplies, and providing emotional support for the patient.

The examination involves use of a plastic or metal speculum consisting of two blades and an adjustment device. The examiner inserts the speculum into the vagina to assess the internal genitalia for cancerous lesions and other abnormalities. During the examination, the examiner collects a specimen for a Papanicolaou (Pap) test for cervical and vaginal cancer. The cervix is inspected for color, position, size, surface characteristics, and discharge (Ball et al., 2019).

MALE GENITALIA

An examination of the male genitalia assesses the integrity of the external genitalia (Fig. 30.60), inguinal ring, and canal. Because the incidence of STIs in adolescents and young adults is high, an assessment of the genitalia needs to be a routine part of any health maintenance examination for this age-group (Box 30.27). The examination begins by having the patient void. Make sure the examination room is warm. During the examination have the patient stand or lie supine with the chest, abdomen, and lower legs draped. Apply clean gloves.

Use a calm, gentle approach to lessen the patient's anxiety. The position and exposure of the body during the examination is embarrassing for some men. To minimize his anxiety, it often helps to offer explanation of the steps of examination so that he anticipates all actions. Manipulate the genitalia gently to avoid causing erection or discomfort. Obtain a thorough history (Table 30.29) before the examination, ensuring that the assessment is complete.

Sexual Maturity

First note the sexual maturity of the patient by observing the size and shape of the penis and testes; the size, color, and texture of the scrotal skin; and the character and distribution of pubic hair. The testes first increase in size in preadolescence and there is no pubic hair. By the end of puberty, the testes and penis enlarge to adult size and shape, and

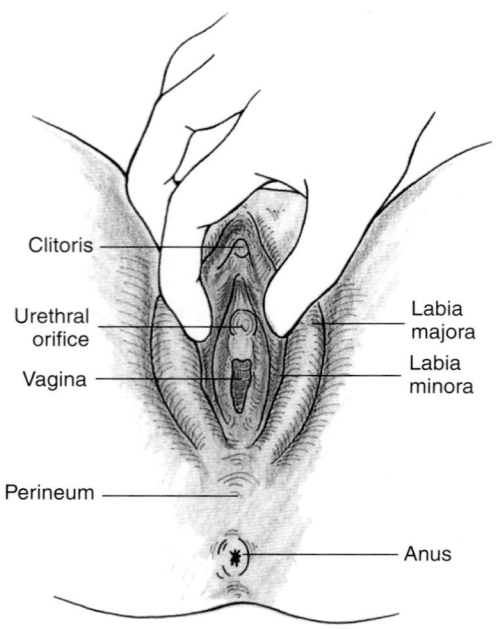

FIG. 30.59 Female external genitalia.

BOX 30.26 PATIENT TEACHING

Female Genitalia and Reproductive Tract Assessment

Objective
- Patient will use measures to maintain sexual health and prevent acquisition and transmission of sexually transmitted infections (STIs).

Teaching Strategies
- Instruct patient about purpose and recommended frequency of Papanicolaou (Pap) smears and gynecological examinations. Explain that a pelvic examination is needed yearly for women who are sexually active or over the age of 21. Patients are screened more often if certain risk factors exist such as a weak immune system, multiple sex partners, smoking, or a history of infections (e.g., human papillomavirus [HPV]).
- Counsel patient with an STI about the implications of diagnosis and treatment.
- Teach measures to prevent STIs: male partner's use of condoms, restricting number of sexual partners, avoiding sex with people who have several other partners, and perineal hygiene measures.
- Counsel young males and females and their parents about genital HPV infection and the need to receive the HPV vaccine before becoming sexually active. The vaccine is recommended for preteen boys and girls at age 11 or 12 (CDC, 2019a; CDC, 2019b). Adolescent boys and girls who did not start or finish the HPV vaccine series when they were younger should get it now. Young women can get an HPV vaccine through age 26, and young men can get vaccinated through age 21 (CDC, 2019a; CDC, 2019b).
- Instruct in genital self-examination (GSE). Using a mirror, position self to examine the area covered by the pubic hair. Spread the hair apart, looking for bumps, sores, or blisters. Also look for any warts, which appear as small, bumpy spots and enlarge to fleshy, cauliflower-like lesions. Next spread the outer vaginal lips apart and look at the clitoris for bumps, blisters, sores, or warts. Look at both sides of the inner vaginal lips. Inspect the area around the urinary and vaginal opening for bumps, blisters, sores, or warts.
- Explain warning signs of STIs: pain or burning on urination, pain during sex, pain in pelvic area, bleeding between menstruation, itchy rash around vagina, and abnormal vaginal discharge.
- Tell patients with an STI to inform sexual partners of the need for an examination.
- Reinforce the importance of performing perineal hygiene (as appropriate).

Evaluation
Use the principles of teach-back to evaluate patient/family caregiver learning:
- Explain to me the reason for getting the HPV vaccination for your child.
- Explain to me why it is important for you to get a routine gynecological examination and Pap test.
- Describe measures you can take to prevent transmission of an STI.
- Since you were diagnosed with an STI, describe for me the safe sexual practices that you are using to prevent further infections.

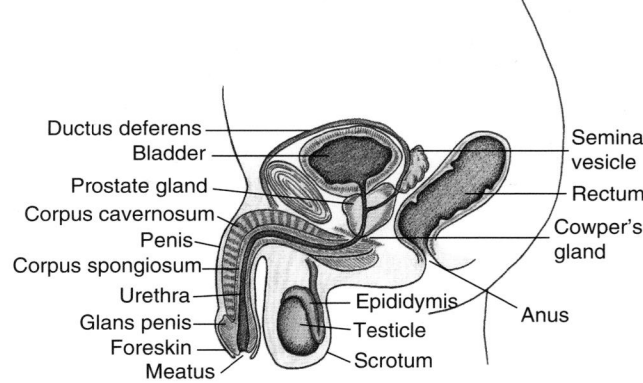

FIG. 30.60 External and internal male sex organs.

BOX 30.27 PATIENT TEACHING

Male Genitalia Assessment

Objective
- Patient will use measures to maintain sexual health and prevent acquisition and transmission of sexually transmitted infections (STIs).

Teaching Strategies
- Teach patient how to perform genital self-examination (see Box 30.28).
- Counsel patient who has an STI about diagnosis implications and treatment.
- Explain warning signs of STIs: pain on urination and during sex, abnormal penile discharge (different from usual), swollen lymph nodes, or rash or ulcer on skin or genitalia.
- Teach measures to prevent STIs: HPV immunization, use of condoms, avoiding sex with infected partner, restricting number of sexual partners, avoiding sex with people who have multiple partners, and using regular perineal hygiene.
- Recommend HPV vaccine for preteen boys age 11 or 12; young men can get vaccinated through age 21 (CDC, 2019a; CDC, 2019b).
- Tell patients with an STI to inform their sexual partners of the need to have an examination.
- Instruct patient to seek treatment as soon as possible if partner becomes infected with an STI.

Evaluation
Use the principles of teach-back to evaluate patient/family caregiver learning:
- Describe measures you can take to prevent the spread of an STI.
- Since you were diagnosed with an STI, describe for me the safe sexual practices that you are using to prevent further infections.

---

scrotal skin darkens and becomes wrinkled. Hair becomes coarser and more abundant in the pubic area. The penis has no hair, and the scrotum has very little hair (Fig. 30.61). Also inspect the skin covering the genitalia for lice, rashes, excoriations, or lesions. Normally it is clear, without lesions.

Penis

To inspect penile surfaces, manipulate the genitalia or have the patient assist. Inspect the shaft, corona, prepuce (foreskin), glans, and urethral meatus. The dorsal vein is apparent on inspection. In uncircumcised males retract the foreskin to reveal the glans and urethral meatus. The foreskin usually retracts easily. A small amount of white, thick smegma

sometimes collects under this foreskin. Obtain a culture if abnormal discharge is present. The urethral meatus is slitlike in appearance and positioned on the ventral surface just millimeters from the tip of the glans. In some congenital conditions the meatus is displaced along the penile shaft. The area between the foreskin and glans is a common site for venereal lesions. Gently compress the glans between the thumb and index finger; this opens the urethral meatus for inspection of lesions, edema, and inflammation. Normally the opening is glistening and pink without discharge. Palpate any lesion gently to note tenderness, size, consistency, and shape. When inspection and palpation of the glans are complete, pull the foreskin down to its original position.

Continue by inspecting the entire shaft of the penis, including the undersurface, looking for lesions, scars, or edema. Palpate the shaft between the thumb and first two fingers to detect localized areas of

TABLE 30.29   Nursing History for Male Genitalia Assessment

Assessment	Rationale
Review normal urinary elimination pattern, including frequency of voiding; history of nocturia; character and volume of urine; daily fluid intake; symptoms of burning, urgency, and frequency; difficulty starting stream; and hematuria (see Chapter 46).	Urinary problems are directly associated with genitourinary problems because of anatomical structure of men's reproductive and urinary systems.
Assess patient's sexual history and use of safe sex habits (multiple partners, infection in partners, failure to use condom).	Sexual history reveals risk for and understanding of sexually transmitted diseases (STIs) and human immunodeficiency virus (HIV).
Determine whether patient has received the human papillomavirus (HPV) vaccine.	HPV is associated with genital warts in males and can lead to cervical cancer in females (CDC, 2019a).
Determine whether patient has had previous surgery or illness involving urinary or reproductive organs, including STI.	Alterations resulting from disease or surgery are sometimes responsible for symptoms or changes in organ structure or function.
Ask whether patient has noted penile pain or swelling, genital lesions, or urethral discharge.	These signs and symptoms may indicate STI.
Determine whether patient has noticed heaviness or painless enlargement of testis or irregular lumps.	These signs and symptoms are early warning signs for testicular cancer.
If patient reports an enlargement in the inguinal area, assess whether it is intermittent or constant, associated with straining or lifting, and painful; and whether pain is affected by coughing, lifting, or straining at stool.	Signs and symptoms reflect potential inguinal hernia.
Ask whether patient has difficulty achieving erection or ejaculation; also review whether patient is taking diuretics, sedatives, antihypertensives, or tranquilizers.	These medications influence sexual performance.

FIG. 30.61 Appearance of male genitalia. (A) Circumcised. (B) Uncircumcised. (From Ball JW et al: *Seidel's guide to physical examination,* ed 9, St Louis, 2019, Mosby.)

surface. The scrotal skin is usually loose, and the surface is coarse. The scrotal skin is more deeply pigmented than body skin. Tightening of the skin or loss of wrinkling reveals edema. The size of the scrotum normally changes with temperature variations because the dartos muscle contracts in cold and relaxes in warm temperatures. Lumps in the scrotal skin are commonly sebaceous cysts.

Testicular cancer is a solid tumor common in young men ages 18 to 34 years. Early detection is critical (ACS, 2018a). Explain testicular self-examination (see Box 30.28) while examining the patient. The testes are normally sensitive but not tender. The underlying testicles are normally ovoid and approximately 2 to 4 cm (1–1½ inches) in size. Gently palpate the testicles and epididymis between the thumb and first two fingers. The testes feel smooth, rubbery, and free of nodules. The epididymis is resilient. Note the size, shape, and consistency of the organs. The most common symptoms of testicular cancer are a painless enlargement of one testis and the appearance of a small, hard palpable lump, about the size of a pea, on the front or side of the testicle. In the older adult the testicles decrease in size and are less firm during palpation. Continue to palpate the vas deferens separately as it forms the spermatic cord toward the inguinal ring, noting nodules or swelling. It normally feels smooth and discrete.

Inguinal Ring and Canal

The external inguinal ring provides the opening for the spermatic cord to pass into the inguinal canal. The canal forms a passage through the abdominal wall, a potential site for hernia formation. A hernia is a protrusion of a part of intestine through the inguinal wall or canal. Sometimes an intestinal loop enters the scrotum. Have the patient stand during this part of the examination.

During inspection ask the patient to strain or bear down. The maneuver helps to make a hernia more visible. Look for obvious bulging in the inguinal area. Complete the examination by palpating for inguinal lymph nodes. Normally small, nontender, mobile horizontal nodes are palpable. Any abnormality indicates local or systemic infection or malignant disease.

hardness or tenderness. A patient who has lain in bed for a prolonged time sometimes develops dependent edema in the penis shaft.

It is important for any male patient to learn to perform a genital self-examination to detect signs or symptoms of STIs, especially men who have had more than one sexual partner or whose partner has had other partners. It is common for men to have an STI but not be aware of it; self-examination is a routine part of self-care (Box 30.28).

Scrotum

Be particularly cautious while inspecting and palpating the scrotum because the structures lying within the scrotal sac are very sensitive. The scrotum is divided internally into two halves. Each half contains a testicle, epididymis, and the vas deferens, which travels upward into the inguinal ring. Normally the left testicle is lower than the right. Inspect the size, shape, and symmetry of the scrotum while observing for lesions or edema. Gently lift the scrotum to view the posterior

BOX 30.28 Male Genital Self-Examination

All men 15 years and older need to perform this examination monthly using the following steps.

Genital Examination

- Perform the examination after a warm bath or shower when the scrotal skin is less thick.
- Stand naked in front of a mirror, hold the penis in your hand, and examine the head. Pull back the foreskin if uncircumcised to expose the glans.
- Inspect and palpate the entire head of the penis in a clockwise motion, looking carefully for any bumps, sores, or blisters (bumps and blisters may be light colored or red, resemble pimples).
- Look also for any genital warts.
- Look at the opening (urethral meatus) at the end of the penis for discharge (see illustration).
- Look along the entire shaft of the penis for the same signs.
- Be sure to separate pubic hair at the base of the penis and carefully examine the skin underneath.

Testicular Self-Examination

- Look for swelling or lumps in the skin of the scrotum while looking in the mirror.
- Use both hands, placing the index and middle fingers under the testicles and the thumb on top (see illustration).
- Gently roll the testicle, feeling for lumps, swelling, soreness, or a harder consistency.
- Find the epididymis (a cordlike structure on the top and back of the testicle; it is not a lump).
- Feel for small, pea-size lumps on the front and side of the testicle. Abnormal lumps are usually painless.
- Call your health care provider for abnormal findings.

Illustrations from Ball JW, et al: *Seidel's guide to physical examination,* ed 9, St Louis, 2019, Elsevier.

TABLE 30.30 Nursing History for Rectal and Anal Assessment

Assessment	Rationale
Determine whether patient has experienced bleeding from rectum, black or tarry stools (melena), rectal pain, or change in bowel habits (constipation or diarrhea).	These are warning signs of colorectal cancer or other gastrointestinal alterations.
Determine whether patient has personal or strong family history of colorectal cancer, polyps, or chronic inflammatory bowel disease. Ask whether patient is over age 40.	These are risk factors for colorectal cancer (ACS, 2020a).
Assess dietary habits, including high fat intake, diet high in processed or red meats, or deficient fiber content (inadequate fruits and vegetables).	Bowel cancer is often linked to dietary intake of fat or insufficient fiber intake (ACS, 2020a).
Determine whether patient is obese, is physically inactive, smokes, or consumes alcohol.	These are risk factors for colorectal cancer (ACS, 2020a).
Determine whether patient has undergone screening for colorectal cancer (digital examination, fecal occult blood test, flexible sigmoidoscopy, and colonoscopy).	Undergoing this screening reflects understanding and adherence with preventive health care measures.
Assess medication history for use of laxatives or cathartic medications.	Repeated use causes diarrhea and eventual loss of intestinal muscle tone.
Assess for use of codeine or iron preparations.	Codeine causes constipation. Iron turns the color of feces black and tarry.
Ask male patient whether he has experienced weak or interrupted urine flow, inability to urinate, difficulty starting or stopping urine flow, polyuria, nocturia, hematuria, or dysuria. Does patient have continuing pain in lower back, pelvis, or upper thighs?	These are warning signs of prostate cancer (ACS, 2020a). Symptoms also suggest infection or prostate enlargement.

RECTUM AND ANUS

A good time to perform the rectal examination is after the genital examination. Usually this examination is not performed for young children or adolescents. It detects colorectal cancer in its early stages. The rectal examination also detects prostatic tumors in men. Collect a health history (Table 30.30) to detect the patient's risk for bowel or rectal disease (men and women) or prostate disease (men). Teach the patient about the purpose of the examination (Box 30.29).

The rectal examination is uncomfortable; explaining all steps helps a patient relax. Use a calm, slow-paced, gentle approach during the examination. Female patients remain in the dorsal recumbent position following genitalia examination or they assume a side-lying position. The best way to examine men is to have the patient stand and bend over forward with hips flexed and upper body resting across an examination table. Examine a patient who cannot stand in the lateral recumbent position. Use nonlatex clean gloves.

BOX 30.29 PATIENT TEACHING
Rectal and Anal Assessment

Objective
- Patient will be able to identify symptoms of colorectal and prostatic cancer.

Teaching Strategies
- Discuss the guidelines of the American Cancer Society (ACS, 2020a) for early detection of colorectal cancer. **Beginning at age 45,** both men and women of average risk should use one of these screening tests (ACS, 2018b):
  - Fecal occult blood test (FOBT) or fecal immunochemical test (FIT) annually
  - Stool DNA test performed every 3 years
  - Flexible sigmoidoscopy (FSIG): Visual inspection of the rectum and lower colon with a hollow, lighted tube performed by a health care provider every 5 years *OR*
  - Double-contrast barium enema every 5 years if recommended by health care provider
  - Colonoscopy every 10 years if recommended
  - Computed tomography (CT) colonoscopy every 5 years if recommended
- Individuals at increased risk should discuss options with their health care provider.

- Discuss warning signs of colorectal cancer (see Table 30.30).
- Discuss with male patient the ACS guidelines (ACS, 2020a) for early detection of prostate cancer:
  - For men age 50 and older, digital rectal examination (DRE) and prostate-specific antigen test (PSA). The ACS recommends that men who have at least a 10-year life expectancy should have an opportunity to make an informed decision with their health care provider about whether to be screened for prostate cancer after receiving information about the potential benefits, risks, and uncertainties of testing.
- Discuss warning signs of prostate cancer.

Evaluation
Use the principles of teach-back to evaluate patient/family caregiver learning:
- Tell me what screening tests for colorectal cancer that you have had done and when they were completed.
- Describe for me the warning signs of colorectal and prostate cancer and when you should contact your health care provider.

Inspection

Using the nondominant hand, gently retract the buttocks to view the perianal and sacrococcygeal areas. Perianal skin is smooth, more pigmented, and coarser than skin over the buttocks. Inspect anal tissue for skin characteristics, lesions, external hemorrhoids (dilated veins that appear as reddened protrusions), ulcers, fissures and fistulas, inflammation, rashes, or excoriation. Anal tissues are moist and hairless, and the voluntary external muscle sphincter holds the anus closed. Next ask a patient to bear down as though having a bowel movement. Any internal hemorrhoids or fissures appear at this time. Use clock referents (e.g., 3 o'clock or 8 o'clock) to describe the location of findings. Normally there is no protrusion of tissue.

Digital Palpation

Examine the anal canal and sphincters with digital palpation, and in male patients palpate the prostate gland to rule out enlargement. Usually, advanced practitioners perform this part of the examination. This technique is not discussed here.

MUSCULOSKELETAL SYSTEM

The musculoskeletal assessment can be performed as a separate examination or integrated with other parts of the total physical examination. In addition, you can assess the patient's movements while performing other nursing care measures such as bathing or positioning. The assessment of musculoskeletal function focuses on determining range of joint motion, muscle strength and tone, and joint and muscle condition. Assessing musculoskeletal integrity is especially important when a patient reports pain or loss of function in a joint or muscle. Because muscular disorders are often the result of neurological disease, you may choose to perform a simultaneous neurological assessment.

While examining a patient's musculoskeletal function, visualize the anatomy of bone and muscle placement and joint structure (see Chapter 38). Joints vary in degree of mobility, depending on the type of joint.

For a complete examination expose the muscles and joints, so they are free to move. Have the patient assume a sitting, supine, prone, or standing position while you assess specific muscle groups. Table 30.31 lists the information gathered in the nursing history.

General Inspection

Observe a patient's gait when he or she enters the examination room. When the patient is unaware of the nature of your observation, gait is more natural. Later have the patient walk in a straight line away from and returning to the point of origin. Note how the patient walks, sits, and rises from a sitting position. Normally patients walk with the arms swinging freely at the sides, the feet placed one at a time (heel to toe), and the head leading the body. Older adults often walk with smaller steps and a wider base of support. Note foot dragging, limping, shuffling, and the position of the trunk in relation to the legs.

Observe the patient from the side and while facing the patient in a standing position. The normal standing posture is upright with parallel alignment of the hips and shoulders (Fig. 30.62). There is an even contour of the shoulders, level scapulae and iliac crests, alignment of the head over the gluteal folds, and symmetry of extremities. While observing from the side of the patient, note the normal cervical, thoracic, and lumbar curves. Holding the head erect is normal. As the patient sits, some degree of rounding of the shoulders is normal. Older adults tend to assume a stooped, forward-bent posture with the hips and knees somewhat flexed and arms bent at the elbows, raising the level of the arms.

Common postural abnormalities include kyphosis, lordosis, and scoliosis (Fig. 30.63). Kyphosis, or hunchback, is an exaggeration of the posterior curvature of the thoracic spine. This postural abnormality is common in older adults. Lordosis, or swayback, is an increased lumbar curvature. A lateral spinal curvature is called scoliosis. Loss of height is frequently the first clinical sign of osteoporosis, in which height loss occurs in the trunk as a result of vertebral fracture and collapse. Osteoporosis is a systemic skeletal condition that is noted to include both decreased bone mass and deterioration of bone tissue, making bones fragile and at risk for fracture (Ball et al., 2019). Osteopenia, characterized by low bone mass of the hip, puts people at risk for osteoporosis, fractures, and potential complications later in life. Approximately 80% of people with osteoporosis are women (CDC, 2020). It can affect any age-group, including children. Teach patients ways to reduce the chance of developing this disease (Box 30.30).

During general inspection look at the extremities for overall size, gross deformity, bony enlargement, alignment, and symmetry. Normally there is bilateral symmetry in length, circumference, alignment,

TABLE 30.31 Nursing History for Musculoskeletal Assessment

Assessment	Rationale
Determine whether patient is involved in competitive sports (particularly involving collision and contact), fails to warm up adequately prior to exercise, is in poor physical condition, or has had a rapid growth spurt (adolescents).	These are risk factors for sports injury.
Assess for risk factors of osteoporosis. Uncontrollable risk factors: • Over age 50 • Female • Nulliparous • Menopause before age 45 • Family history of osteoporosis • Low body weight/being small and thin/constant dieting • Broken bones or height loss Controllable risk factors: • Not getting enough calcium (less than 500 mg) and vitamin D • Not eating enough fruits and vegetables • Getting too much protein, sodium, and caffeine • Having an inactive lifestyle • Smoking • Drinking too much alcohol • Losing weight Long-term use of certain medications: aluminum-containing antacids; antiseizure medicines such as phenytoin or phenobarbital; aromatase inhibitors such as anastrozole, exemestane and letrozole; cancer chemotherapeutic drugs; and heparin	These are risk factors for osteoporosis (U.S. Preventive Services Task Force [USPSTF], 2018).
Ask patient to describe history of problems in bone, muscle, or joint function (e.g., recent fall, trauma, lifting of heavy objects, history of bone or joint disease with sudden or gradual onset, location of alteration).	History helps to assess nature of musculoskeletal problem.
Assess nature and extent of pain, including location, duration, severity, predisposing and aggravating factors, relieving factors, and type.	Pain frequently accompanies alterations in bone, joints, or muscle. This has implications not only for comfort, but also for ability to perform activities of daily living.
Assess patient's normal activity pattern, including type of exercise routinely performed.	Provides baseline in assessment. Sedentary lifestyle and lack of appropriate exercise increase bone loss and risk of fractures.
Determine how alteration influences ability to perform activities of daily living (e.g., bathing, feeding, dressing, toileting, ambulating) and social functions (e.g., household chores, work, recreation, sexual activities).	The extent to which patient can perform self-care determines the level of nursing care. Type and degree of restriction in continuing social activities influence topics for patient education and ability of nurse to identify alternative ways to maintain function.
Assess height loss of woman over age 50 by subtracting current height from recall of maximum adult height. Refer to physician for bone density examination (women 65 years and older).	Measurement is useful screening tool to predict osteoporosis. Bone measurement testing recommended by USPSTF (2018).

and position and in the number of skinfolds (Ball et al., 2019). A general review can identify areas requiring a more specialized assessment.

Palpation

Apply gentle palpation to all bones, joints, and surrounding muscles during a complete examination. For a focused assessment examine only the involved area. Note any heat, tenderness, edema, or resistance to pressure. The patient should not feel any discomfort when you palpate. Muscles should be firm.

Range of Joint Motion

The examination includes comparison of both active and passive ROM. Ask the patient to put the major joint showing limitation in movement through active and passive full ROM (see Chapter 38). Measuring ROM in all joints is not necessary if the patient demonstrates good joint movement and no problems have been identified. Learn the correct terminology, the normal range of each joint, and the

extent to which you can move the patient's joints (Table 30.32). Teach the patient how to move through each ROM by demonstrating the ROM when possible. To assess ROM passively, ask the patient to relax, and then passively assist movement of the extremities through their ROM. Compare the same body parts for equality in movement. Fig. 30.64 shows an example of ROM positions for the hand and wrist. Do not force a joint into a painful position. ROM is equal between contralateral joints. If a patient is scheduled for surgery involving a joint, assess the patient's normal range to determine a baseline for assessing later change.

Joints are typically free from stiffness, instability, swelling, or inflammation. There should be no discomfort when applying pressure to bones and joints. In older adults, joints often become swollen and stiff, with reduced ROM resulting from cartilage erosion and fibrosis of synovial membranes (see Chapter 38). If a joint appears swollen and inflamed, palpate it for warmth. A goniometer is an instrument with two flexible arms and a 180-degree protractor in the center. It is

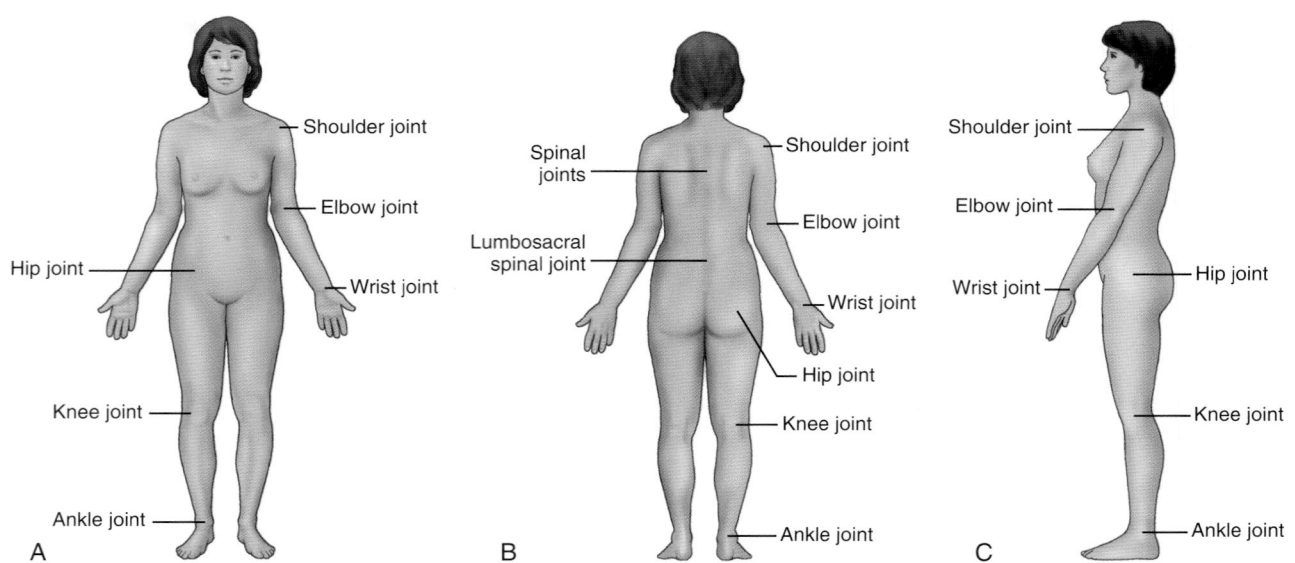

FIG. 30.62 Inspection of overall body posture. (A) Anterior view. (B) Posterior view. (C) Lateral view. (From Muscolino: JE: *Kinesiology: the skeletal system and muscle function,* ed 3, St Louis, 2017, Elsevier.)

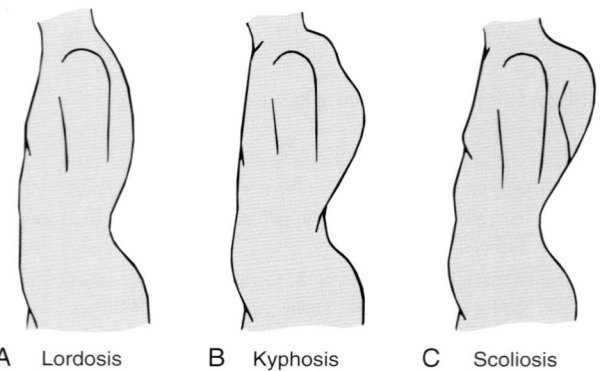

| A   Lordosis | B   Kyphosis | C   Scoliosis |

FIG. 30.63 Common postural abnormalities. (A) Lordosis. (B) Kyphosis. (C) Scoliosis.

frequently used by physical and occupational therapists to measure the precise degree of motion in a joint and is mainly for patients who have a suspected reduction in joint movement.

Muscle Tone and Strength

Assess muscle strength and tone during ROM measurement. Integrate these findings with those from the neurological assessment. Note muscle tone, the slight muscular resistance felt as you move the relaxed extremity passively through its ROM.

Ask the patient to allow an extremity to relax or hang limp. This is often difficult, particularly if the patient feels pain in it. Support the extremity and grasp each limb, moving it through the normal ROM (Fig. 30.65). Normal tone causes a mild, even resistance to movement through the entire range.

If a muscle has increased tone, or **hypertonicity**, there is considerable resistance with any sudden passive movement of a joint. Continued movement eventually causes the muscle to relax. A muscle that has little tone (**hypotonicity**) feels flabby. The involved extremity hangs loosely in a position determined by gravity.

For assessment of muscle strength, have the patient assume a stable position. The patient performs maneuvers demonstrating strength of

BOX 30.30   PATIENT TEACHING

Health Promotion to Prevent Osteoporosis in Women

Objective
- Patient will follow measures to prevent or minimize osteoporosis.

Teaching Strategies
- Recommend women age 65 and older for routine screening for osteoporosis (USPSTF, 2018). Recommend men for screening as well; they are at risk for development of osteoporosis equally as they age.
- To reduce bone demineralization, instruct older adults in a proper exercise program (e.g., weight-bearing, muscle-strengthening, and balance-training exercises) to be followed 3 or more times a week.
- Encourage intake of calcium to meet the recommended daily allowance. Increased vitamin D aids calcium absorption.
- Recommendation for calcium supplements for adults over age 25 is 1000 to 1500 mg/day. Instruct patient to take no more than 500 mg of calcium at one time.
- Instruct older adults and those with osteoporosis in proper body mechanics and range-of-motion and moderate weight-bearing exercises (e.g., swimming and walking) to minimize trauma and subsequent fracture of bones.
- Instruct older patients to pace activities to compensate for loss in muscle strength.

Evaluation
Use the principles of teach-back to evaluate patient/family caregiver learning:
- Show me how you maintain correct posture when you are sitting, standing, and walking.
- Describe for me what therapies you use for preventing osteoporosis.
- Show me how you do your range-of-motion exercises.

major muscle groups (Table 30.33). Use a grading scale of 0 to 5 to compare symmetrical muscle pairs for strength (Table 30.34). The arm on the dominant side normally is stronger than the arm on the nondominant side. In older adults a loss of muscle mass causes bilateral weakness, but muscle strength remains greater in the dominant arm or leg.

FIG. 30.64 Range of motion of hand and wrist. (A) Metacarpophalangeal flexion and hyperextension. (B) Finger flexion: thumb to each fingertip and to base of little finger. (C) Finger flexion, fist formation. (D) Finger abduction. (E) Wrist flexion and hyperextension. (F) Wrist radial and ulnar movement. (From Ball JW et al: *Seidel's guide to physical examination,* ed 9, St Louis, 2019, Mosby.)

TABLE 30.32 Terminology for Normal Range-of-Motion Positions

Term	Range of Motion	Examples of Joints
Flexion	Movement decreasing angle between two adjoining bones; bending of limb	Elbow, fingers, knee
Extension	Movement increasing angle between two adjoining bones	Elbow, knee, fingers
Hyperextension	Movement of body part beyond its normal resting extended position	Head
Pronation	Movement of body part so that front or ventral surface faces downward	Hand, forearm
Supination	Movement of body part so that front or ventral surface faces upward	Hand, forearm
Abduction	Movement of extremity away from midline of body	Leg, arm, fingers
Adduction	Movement of extremity toward midline of body	Leg, arm, fingers
Internal rotation	Rotation of joint inward	Knee, hip
External rotation	Rotation of joint outward	Knee, hip
Eversion	Turning of body part away from midline	Foot
Inversion	Turning of body part toward midline	Foot
Dorsiflexion	Flexion of toes and foot upward	Foot
Plantar flexion	Bending of toes and foot downward	Foot

Examine each muscle group. Ask the patient to first flex the muscle you are examining and then to resist when you apply an opposing force against that flexion. It is important to not allow the patient to move the joint. Gradually increase pressure to a muscle group (e.g., elbow extension). Have the patient resist the pressure you apply by attempting to move against resistance (e.g., elbow flexion) until instructed to stop. Vary the amount of pressure applied and observe the joint move. If you identify a weakness, compare the size of the muscle with its opposite counterpart by measuring the circumference of the muscle body with a tape measure. A muscle that has **atrophied** (reduced in size) feels soft and boggy when palpated.

NEUROLOGICAL SYSTEM

The neurological system is responsible for many functions, including initiation and coordination of movement, reception and perception of sensory stimuli, organization of thought processes, control of speech, and storage of memory. A close integration exists between the neurological system and all other body systems. For example, urine production relies in part on the adequacy of blood flow to the kidneys and on neural control, which affects the size of arterioles supplying the kidneys.

A full assessment of neurological function requires much time and attention to detail. For efficiency, integrate neurological measurements with other parts of the physical examination. For example, test cranial nerve function while assessing the head and neck. Observe mental and emotional status during the initial interview.

Consider many variables when deciding the extent of the neurological examination. A patient's level of consciousness influences the ability to follow directions. General physical status influences tolerance to assessment. A patient's chief complaint or presenting problem also helps determine the

FIG. 30.65 Assessing muscle tone.

TABLE 30.33 Maneuvers to Assess Muscle Strength

Muscle Group	Maneuver
Neck (sternocleidomastoid)	Place hand firmly against patient's upper jaw. Ask patient to turn head laterally against resistance.
Shoulder (trapezius)	Place hand over midline of patient's shoulder, exerting firm pressure. Have patient raise shoulders against resistance.
Elbow	
Biceps	Pull down on forearm as patient attempts to flex arm.
Triceps	As you flex patient's arm, apply pressure against forearm. Ask patient to straighten arm.
Hip	
Quadriceps	When patient is sitting, apply downward pressure to thigh. Ask patient to raise leg up from table.
Gastrocnemius	Patient sits while examiner holds shin of flexed leg. Ask patient to straighten leg against resistance.

TABLE 30.34 Muscle Strength

Muscle Function Level	Grade	% Normal	Lovett Scale
No evidence of contractility	0	0	0 (zero)
Slight contractility, no movement	1	10	T (trace)
Full range of motion, gravity eliminated[a]	2	25	P (poor)
Full range of motion with gravity	3	50	F (fair)
Full range of motion against gravity, some resistance	4	75	G (good)
Full range of motion against gravity, full resistance	5	100	N (normal)

Adapted from Ball JW, et al: *Seidel's guide to physical examination,* ed 9, St Louis, 2019, Elsevier.
[a]Passive movement.

TABLE 30.35 Nursing History for Neurological Assessment

Assessment	Rationale
Determine whether patient uses analgesics, alcohol, sedatives, hypnotics, antipsychotics, antidepressants, nervous system stimulants, or recreational drugs.	These medications alter level of consciousness or cause behavioral changes. Abuse sometimes causes tremors, ataxia, and changes in peripheral nerve function.
Determine whether patient has recent history of seizures/convulsions: clarify sequence of events (aura, fall to ground, motor activity, loss of consciousness); character of any symptoms; and relationship of seizure to time of day, fatigue, or emotional stress.	Seizure activity often originates from central nervous system alteration. Characteristics of seizure help determine its origin.
Screen patient for symptoms of headache, tremors, dizziness, vertigo, numbness or tingling of body part, visual changes, weakness, pain, or changes in speech. Presence of any symptom requires more detailed review (onset, severity, precipitating factors, or sequence of events).	These symptoms frequently originate from alterations in central or peripheral nervous system function. Identification of specific patterns aids in diagnosis of pathological condition.
Discuss with patient's family any recent changes in patient's behavior (e.g., increased irritability, mood swings, memory loss, change in energy level).	Behavioral changes sometimes result from intracranial pathological states.
Assess patient for history of change in vision, hearing, smell, taste, or touch.	Major sensory nerves originate from brainstem. These symptoms help to localize nature of problem.
If an older patient displays sudden acute confusion (delirium), review history for drug toxicity (anticholinergics, diuretics, digoxin, cimetidine, sedatives, antihypertensives, antiarrhythmics), serious infections, metabolic disturbances, heart failure, and severe anemia.	Delirium is one of the most common mental disorders in older people. Condition is always potentially reversible (see Box 30.32).
Review history for head or spinal cord injury, meningitis, congenital anomalies, neurological disease, or psychiatric counseling.	Factors cause neurological symptoms or behavioral changes to develop, focusing assessment on possible cause.

need for a thorough neurological assessment. Patients with a headache or a recent loss of function in an extremity need a complete neurological review. Table 30.35 lists the data collected in the nursing history. You will need the following items for a complete examination:

- Reading material
- Vials containing aromatic substances (e.g., vanilla extract and coffee)
- Opposite tip of cotton swab or tongue blade broken in half
- Snellen eye chart
- Penlight
- Vials containing sugar, salt, lemon with applicators
- Tongue blade

BOX 30.31 Mini-Mental State Examination Sample Questions

- Orientation to time
  "What is the date?"
- Registration
  "Listen carefully. I am going to say three words. Say them back after I stop. Ready? Here they are: HOUSE (pause), CAR (pause), LAKE (pause). Now repeat these words back to me."
  (Repeat up to 5 times but score only the first trial.)
- Naming
  "What is this?" (Point to a pencil or pen.)
- Reading
  "Please read this and do what it says." (Show examinee the words on the stimulus form.)
  Close Your Eyes

Reproduced by special permission of the publisher, Psychological Assessment Resources, Inc., 16204 North Florida Avenue, Lutz, FL 33549, from *Mini-Mental State Examination*, by Marshal Folstein and Susan Folstein, Copyright 1975, 1998, 2001 by Mini Mental, LLC, Inc. Published 2001 by Psychological Assessment Resources, Inc. Further reproduction is prohibited without permission of PAR, Inc. The MMSE can be purchased from PAR, Inc. by calling (800) 331-8378 or (813) 968-3103.

BOX 30.32 Clinical Criteria for Delirium

Definition: An acute disturbance of consciousness that is accompanied by a change in cognition. It is not caused by a preexisting or evolving dementia. Delirium develops over a short period of time, usually hours to days, and tends to fluctuate during the day. It is usually a direct physiological consequence of a general medical condition. It is most common in older adults but occasionally occurs in younger patients.

- There is reduced clarity of awareness of the environment.
- Ability to focus, sustain, or shift attention is impaired (questions must be repeated).
- Irrelevant stimuli easily distract the person.
- There is an accompanying change in cognition (memory impairment, disorientation, or language disturbance).
- Recent memory commonly is affected.
- Disorientation usually occurs, with patient disoriented to time, place, or person.
- Language disturbance involves impaired ability to name objects or ability to write; speech is sometimes rambling.
- Perceptual disturbances include misinterpretations, delusions, or visual and auditory hallucinations. Neurological signs include tremor, unsteady gait, asterixis, or myoclonus.

Reprinted with permission from the *Diagnostic and statistical manual of mental disorders,* ed 5, text revision. Copyright © 2013, American Psychiatric Association.

- Two test tubes, one filled with hot water and the other with cold water
- Cotton balls or cotton-tipped applicators
- Tuning fork
- Reflex hammer

Mental and Emotional Status

You learn a great deal about mental capacities and emotional state simply by interacting with a patient. Ask questions during an examination to gather data and observe the appropriateness of emotions and thoughts. Special assessment tools are designed to assess a patient's mental status. The Mini-Mental State Examination (MMSE) is an instrument that measures orientation and cognitive function (Folstein and Folstein, 1975). The questions in Box 30.31 offer examples of questions found on the MMSE. The maximum score on the MMSE is 31. Patients with scores of 21 or less generally reveal cognitive impairment requiring further evaluation.

To ensure an objective assessment, consider a patient's cultural and educational background, values, beliefs, and previous experiences. Such factors influence response to questions. An alteration in mental or emotional status reflects a disturbance in cerebral functioning. The cerebral cortex controls and integrates intellectual and emotional functioning. Primary brain disorders, medication, and metabolic changes are examples of factors that change cerebral function.

Delirium is an acute mental disorder that occurs among patients who are hospitalized. Obtain a thorough history of a patient's behavior before delirium develops to recognize the condition early. Family members are usually a good resource. It is characterized by confusion, disorientation, and restlessness. It is often a sign of an impending or underlying physical illness in older adults; it may be related to serious injury, impaired senses, poor pain management, medications, or restraint use (Ball et al., 2019). The acute condition differs from dementia, a more progressive, organic mental disorder such as Alzheimer disease. You need to recognize the difference so that you can try to learn the underlying cause of delirium. Fortunately, the condition often reverses when it is correctly assessed and the underlying cause is treated (e.g., central nervous system [CNS], metabolic, or cardiopulmonary disorders; systemic illnesses; or sensory deprivation or overload). To avoid misdiagnosis, you need to adequately assess mental status. Frequently patients who develop delirium are labeled with "sundown syndrome" because the delirium frequently worsens at night. Many practitioners mistake this as being common with old age. Children can also be vulnerable to delirium due to illness, medications, trauma, or surgery (Hockenberry and Wilson, 2019). Box 30.32 summarizes clinical criteria for delirium.

Level of Consciousness. A person's level of consciousness exists along a continuum from full awakening, alertness, and cooperation to unresponsiveness. Talk with the patient, asking questions about events involving concerns about any health problems. A fully conscious patient responds to questions quickly and expresses ideas logically. With a lowering of a patient's consciousness, use the Glasgow Coma Scale (GCS) for an objective measurement of consciousness on a numerical scale (Table 30.36). The patient needs to be as alert as possible before testing. Take care when using the scale if the patient has sensory losses (e.g., vision or hearing). The GCS allows evaluation of a patient's neurological status over time. The higher the score, the better the patient's neurological function. Ask short, simple questions such as "What is your name?" "Where are you?" and "What day is this?" Also ask the patient to follow simple commands such as "Move your toes."

If the patient is not conscious enough to follow commands, try to elicit the pain response. Apply firm pressure with the thumb over the root of the patient's fingernail. The normal response to the painful stimuli is withdrawal of the body part from the stimulus. A patient with serious neurological impairment exhibits abnormal posturing in response to pain. A flaccid response indicates the absence of muscle tone in the extremities and severe injury to brain tissue.

Behavior and Appearance. Behavior, moods, hygiene, grooming, and choice of dress reveal pertinent information about mental status. Remain perceptive of a patient's mannerisms and actions during the entire physical assessment. Note nonverbal and verbal behaviors. Does

TABLE 30.36 Glasgow Coma Scale

(The total score is the sum of the scores in the three categories.)

Action	Response	Score
Eyes open	Spontaneously	4
	To speech	3
	To pain	2
	None	1
Best verbal response	Oriented	5
	Confused	4
	Inappropriate words	3
	Incomprehensible sounds	2
	None	1
Best motor response	Obeys commands	6
	Localized pain	5
	Flexion withdrawal	4
	Abnormal flexion	3
	Abnormal extension	2
	Flaccid	1
	TOTAL SCORE	**3 to 15**

the patient respond appropriately to directions? Does the patient's mood vary with no apparent cause? Does the patient show concern about appearance? Is the hair clean and neatly groomed, and are the nails trimmed and clean? The patient should behave in a manner expressing concern and interest in the examination. The patient should make eye contact with you and express appropriate feelings that correspond to the situation. Normally the patient shows some degree of personal hygiene.

Choice and fit of clothing reflect socioeconomic background or personal taste rather than deficiency in self-concept or self-care. Avoid being judgmental and focus assessment on the appropriateness of clothing for the weather. Older adults sometimes neglect their appearance because of finances, reduced vision, a lack of energy, or depression.

Language. Normal cerebral function allows a person to understand spoken or written words and express the self through written words or gestures. Assess the patient's voice inflection, tone, and manner of speech. Normally a patient's voice has inflections, is clear and strong, and increases in volume appropriately. Speech is fluent. When communication is clearly ineffective (e.g., omission or addition of letters and words, misuse of words, or hesitations), assess for aphasia. Injury to the cerebral cortex results in aphasia.

The two types of aphasia are sensory (or receptive) and motor (or expressive). With receptive aphasia a person cannot understand written or verbal speech. With expressive aphasia a person understands written and verbal speech but cannot write or speak appropriately when attempting to communicate. A patient sometimes has a combination of receptive and expressive aphasia. Assess language capabilities when a patient is communicating ineffectively. Some simple assessment techniques include the following:
- Point to a familiar object and ask the patient to name it.
- Ask the patient to respond to simple verbal and written commands such as "Stand up" or "Sit down."
- Ask the patient to read simple sentences out loud.

Normally a patient names objects correctly, follows commands, and reads sentences correctly.

Intellectual Function

Intellectual function includes memory (recent, immediate, and past), knowledge, abstract thinking, association, and judgment. Testing each aspect of function involves a specific technique. However, because cultural and educational background influences the ability to respond to test questions, do not ask questions related to concepts or ideas with which a patient is unfamiliar.

Memory. Assess immediate recall and recent and remote memory. Patients demonstrate immediate recall by repeating a series of numbers (e.g., *7, 4, 1*) in the order they are presented or in reverse order. Patients normally recall a series of five to eight digits forward and four to six digits backward.

First ask to test the patient's memory. Then state clearly and slowly the names of three unrelated objects. After mentioning all three, ask the patient to repeat each. Later in the assessment ask the patient to repeat the three words again. The patient should be able to identify them. Another test for recent memory involves asking the patient to recall events occurring during the same day (e.g., what was eaten for breakfast). Validate information with a family member.

To assess past memory, ask the patient to recall mother's maiden name, a birthday, or a special date in history. It is best to ask open-ended rather than simple yes-or-no questions. A patient usually has immediate recall of such information. With older adults do not interpret hearing loss as confusion. Good communication techniques are essential throughout the examination to ensure that a patient clearly understands all directions and testing.

Knowledge. Assess knowledge by asking how much the patient knows about the illness or the reason for seeking health care. A knowledge assessment allows you to determine a patient's ability to learn or understand. If there is an opportunity to teach, test a patient's mental status by asking for feedback during a follow-up visit.

Abstract Thinking. Interpreting abstract ideas or concepts reflects the capacity for abstract thinking. For an individual to explain common phrases such as "A stitch in time saves nine" or "Don't count your chickens before they're hatched" requires a higher level of intellectual function. Note whether a patient's explanations are relevant and concrete. A patient with altered mental status probably interprets the phrase literally or merely rephrases the words.

Association. Another higher level of intellectual functioning involves finding similarities or associations between concepts: a dog is to a beagle as a cat is to a Siamese. Name related concepts and ask the patient to identify their associations. Ask questions that are appropriate to the patient's level of intelligence, using simple concepts.

Judgment. Judgment requires a comparison and evaluation of facts and ideas to understand their relationships and form appropriate conclusions. Attempt to measure the patient's ability to make logical decisions with questions such as "Why did you seek health care?" or "What would you do if you became ill at home?" Normally a patient makes logical decisions.

Cranial Nerve Function

To assess cranial nerve function, you may test all 12 cranial nerves, a single nerve, or a related group of nerves. A dysfunction in one nerve reflects an alteration at some point along the distribution of the cranial nerve. Measurements used to assess the integrity of organs within the head and neck also assess cranial nerve function. A complete assessment involves testing the 12 cranial nerves in their numerical order.

TABLE 30.37   Cranial Nerve Function and Assessment

Number	Name	Type	Function	Method
I	Olfactory	Sensory	Sense of smell	Ask patient to identify different nonirritating aromas such as coffee and vanilla.
II	Optic	Sensory	Visual acuity	Use Snellen chart or ask patient to read printed material while wearing glasses.
III	Oculomotor	Motor	Extraocular eye movements: inward, up and inward, up and outward, down and outward	Assess six directions of gaze.
			Pupil constriction and dilation	Measure pupillary reaction to light reflex and accommodation.
			Opening the eye	
IV	Trochlear	Motor	Downward, inward eye movements	Assess six directions of gaze.
V	Trigeminal	Sensory and motor	Sensory nerve to skin of face	Lightly touch cornea with wisp of cotton. Assess corneal reflex. Measure sensation of light pain and touch across skin of face.
			Motor nerve to muscles of jaw	Palpate temples as patient clenches teeth.
VI	Abducens	Motor	Lateral movement of eyeballs	Assess six directions of gaze.
VII	Facial	Sensory and motor	Facial expression	As patient smiles, frowns, puffs out cheeks, and raises and lowers eyebrows, look for asymmetry.
			Taste	Have patient identify salty or sweet taste on front of tongue.
VIII	Auditory	Sensory	Hearing	Assess ability to hear spoken word.
IX	Glossopharyngeal	Sensory and motor	Taste	Ask patient to identify sour or sweet taste on back of tongue.
			Ability to swallow	Use tongue blade to elicit gag reflex.
X	Vagus	Sensory and motor	Sensation of pharynx	Ask patient to say "ah." Observe movement of palate and pharynx.
			Movement of vocal cords	Assess speech for hoarseness.
			Parasympathetic innervation to glands of mucous membranes of the pharynx, larynx, organs in the neck, thorax (heart and lungs), and abdomen	Assess heart rate, presence of peristalsis.
XI	Spinal accessory	Motor	Movement of head and shoulders	Ask patient to shrug shoulders and turn head against passive resistance.
XII	Hypoglossal	Motor	Position of tongue	Ask patient to stick out tongue to midline and move it from side to side.

To remember the order of the nerves, use this simple phrase: "On old Olympus' towering tops, a Finn and German viewed some hops." The first letter of each word in the phrase is the same as the first letter of the names of the cranial nerves listed in order (Table 30.37).

Sensory Function

The sensory pathways of the CNS conduct sensations of pain, temperature, position, vibration, and crude and finely localized touch. Different nerve pathways relay the sensations. Most patients require only a quick screening of sensory function unless there are symptoms of reduced sensation, motor impairment, or paralysis. The risk of skin breakdown is greater in a patient with impaired sensation. When assessing decreased sensation, complete a skin assessment of the area affected by the sensory loss. In addition, teach the patient to avoid pressure, thermal, and/or chemical trauma to the area.

Normally a patient has sensory responses to all stimuli that are tested and feels sensations equally on both sides of the body in all areas. Assess the major sensory nerves by knowing the sensory dermatome zones (Fig. 30.66). Some areas of the skin are innervated by specific dorsal root cutaneous nerves. For example, if assessment reveals reduced sensation when checking for light touch along an area of the skin (e.g., the lower neck), this determines in general where a neurological lesion exists (e.g., fourth cervical spinal cord segment).

Perform all sensory testing with the patient's eyes closed so that the patient is unable to see when or where a stimulus touches the skin (Table 30.38). Then touch the patient's skin in a random, unpredictable order to maintain attention and prevent detection of a predictable pattern. Ask the patient to describe when, what, and where each stimulus is felt. Compare symmetrical areas of the body while applying stimuli to the patient's arms, trunk, and legs.

Motor Function

An examination of motor function includes assessments made during the musculoskeletal examination. In addition, you assess the patient's cerebellar function. The cerebellum coordinates muscular activity, maintains balance and equilibrium, and controls posture.

Coordination. To avoid confusion, demonstrate each maneuver and have the patient repeat it, observing for smoothness and balance in

FIG. 30.66 Dermatomes of body (body surface areas innervated by particular spinal nerves); C1 usually has no cutaneous distribution. (A) Anterior view. (B) Posterior view. It appears that there is a distinct separation of surface area controlled by each dermatome, but there is almost always overlap between spinal nerves. (From Ball JW, et al: *Seidel's guide to physical examination*, ed 9, St Louis, 2019, Mosby.)

movements (Box 30.33). In older adults, normally slow reaction time causes movements to be less rhythmical.

To assess fine-motor function, have the patient extend the arms out to the sides and touch each forefinger alternately to the nose (first with eyes open, then with eyes closed). Normally a patient alternately touches the nose smoothly. Performing rapid, rhythmical, alternating movements demonstrates coordination in the upper extremities. While sitting, the patient begins by patting the knees with both hands. Then the patient alternately turns up the palm and back of the hands while continuously patting the knees. Normally patients perform the maneuver smoothly and regularly with increasing speed.

An additional maneuver for upper extremity coordination involves touching each finger with the thumb of the same hand in rapid sequence. A patient moves from the index finger to the little finger and back, with one hand tested at a time. The dominant hand is slightly less awkward when performing this movement. Movement is smooth and in succession.

Test lower extremity coordination with the patient lying supine, legs extended. Place a hand at the ball of the patient's foot. The patient taps the hand with the foot as quickly as possible. Test each foot for speed and smoothness. The feet do not move as rapidly or evenly as the hands.

Balance. Use one or two of the following tests to assess balance and gross-motor function. When examining an adult for balance and equilibrium, be aware of the risk for falls. Some older adults need help with this part of the examination.

Have the patient perform a Romberg test by standing with feet together, arms at the sides, both with eyes open and eyes closed. Protect the patient's safety by standing at the side; observe for swaying. Expect slight swaying of the body in the Romberg test. A loss of balance (positive Romberg) causes a patient to fall to the side. Normally the patient does not break the stance.

Have the patient close the eyes, with arms held straight at the sides, and stand on one foot and then the other. Normally patients can maintain balance for 5 seconds with slight swaying. Another test involves asking the patient to walk a straight line by placing the heel of one foot directly in front of the toes of the other foot.

Reflexes

Eliciting reflex reactions provides data about the integrity of sensory and motor pathways of the reflex arc and specific spinal cord segments. Assessment of reflexes does not determine higher neural center functioning but helps to assess peripheral spinal nerve function. Fig. 30.67

TABLE 30.38 Assessment of Sensory Nerve Function

Function	Equipment	Method	Precautions
Pain	End of paper clip or wooden end of cotton applicator	Ask patients to voice when they feel dull or sharp sensation. Alternately apply sharp and blunt ends of the paper clip or broken cotton applicator to surface of skin. Note areas of numbness or increased sensitivity.	Remember that areas where skin is thick such as heel or sole of foot are less sensitive to pain.
Temperature	Two test tubes, one filled with hot water and another with cold	Touch skin with tube. Ask patient to identify hot or cold sensation.	Omit test if pain sensation is normal.
Light touch	Cotton ball or cotton-tip applicator	Apply light wisp of cotton to different points along surface of skin. Ask patients to voice when they feel a sensation.	Apply at areas where skin is thin or more sensitive (e.g., face, neck, inner aspect of arms, top of feet and hands).
Vibration	Tuning fork	Apply stem of vibrating fork to distal interphalangeal joint of fingers and interphalangeal joint of great toe, elbow, and wrist. Have patients voice when and where they feel vibration.	Be sure that patient feels vibration and not merely pressure.
Position		Grasp finger or toe, holding it by its sides with thumb and index finger. Alternate moving finger or toe up and down. Ask patient to state when finger is up or down. Repeat with toes.	Avoid rubbing adjacent appendages as you move finger or toe. Do not move joint laterally; return to neutral position before moving again.
Two-point discrimination	Two ends of paper clips	Lightly apply one or both ends of paper clips simultaneously to the surface of the skin. Ask patients whether they feel one or two pricks. Find the distance at which patient can no longer distinguish two points.	Apply blade tips to same anatomical site (e.g., fingertips, palm of hand, or upper arms). Minimum distance at which patient discriminates two points varies (2–8 mm on fingertips).

BOX 30.33 PATIENT TEACHING

Neurological Assessment

Objective
- Patient and family or significant others will understand relationship of patient's behavioral and mental changes to physical status.

Teaching Strategies
- Explain to family caregiver the implications of any behavioral or mental impairment shown by patient.
- If patient has sensory or motor impairments, explain measures to ensure safety (e.g., wearing glasses or hearing aids, use of ambulation aids or safety bars in bathrooms or stairways) (see Chapter 49).
- Teach older adult to plan enough time to complete tasks because reaction time is slow.
- Teach older adult to observe skin surfaces for areas of trauma because pain perception is reduced.

Evaluation
Use the principles of teach-back to evaluate patient/family caregiver learning:
- Describe for me behaviors that can indicate a neurological impairment.
- Describe for me the safety measures you are using to avoid injury because of your sensory and motor limitations.
- Explain to me why it is important as an older adult that you inspect your skin surface regularly.

FIG. 30.67 Pathway of reflex arc.

traces the pathway of the reflex arc. Each muscle contains a small sensory unit called a *muscle spindle*, which controls muscle tone and detects changes in the length of muscle fibers. Tapping a tendon with a reflex hammer stretches the muscle and tendon, lengthening the spindle. The spindle sends nerve impulses along afferent nerve pathways to the dorsal horn of the spinal cord segment. Within milliseconds the

TABLE 30.39   Assessment of Common Reflexes

Type	Procedure	Normal Reflex
Deep Tendon Reflexes		
Biceps	Flex patient's arm up to 45 degrees at elbow with palms down. Place your thumb in antecubital fossa at base of biceps tendon and your fingers over biceps muscle. Strike biceps tendon with reflex hammer.	Flexion of arm at elbow
Triceps	Flex patient's arm at elbow, holding arm across chest, or hold upper arm horizontally and allow lower arm to go limp. Strike triceps tendon just above elbow.	Extension at elbow
Patellar	Have patient sit with legs hanging freely over side of table or chair or have patient lie supine and support knee in a flexed 90-degree position. Briskly tap patellar tendon just below patella.	Extension of lower leg
Achilles	Have patient assume same position as for patellar reflex. Slightly dorsiflex patient's ankle by grasping toes in palm of your hand. Strike Achilles tendon just above heel at ankle malleolus.	Plantar flexion of foot
Cutaneous Reflexes		
Plantar	Have patient lie supine with legs straight and feet relaxed. Take handle end of reflex hammer and stroke lateral aspect of sole from heel to ball of foot, curving across ball of foot toward big toe.	Plantar flexion of all toes
Abdominal	Have patient stand or lie supine. Stroke abdominal skin with base of cotton applicator over lateral borders of rectus abdominis muscle toward midline. Repeat test in each abdominal quadrant.	Contraction of rectus abdominis muscle with pulling of umbilicus toward stimulated side

impulses reach the spinal cord and synapse to travel to the efferent motor neuron in the spinal cord. A motor nerve sends the impulses back to the muscle, causing the reflex response.

The two categories of normal reflexes are deep tendon reflexes, elicited by mildly stretching a muscle and tapping a tendon, and cutaneous reflexes, elicited by stimulating the skin superficially. Grade reflexes as follows (Ball et al., 2019):

0: No response
1+: Sluggish or diminished
2+: Active or expected response
3+: More brisk than expected, slightly hyperactive
4+: Brisk and hyperactive with intermittent or transient clonus

When assessing reflexes, have the patient relax as much as possible to avoid voluntary movement or tensing of muscles. Position the limbs to slightly stretch the muscle being tested. Hold the reflex hammer loosely between the thumb and fingers so it can swing freely, and tap the tendon briskly (Fig. 30.68). Compare the responses on corresponding sides. Normally the older adult presents with diminished reflexes. Reflexes are hyperactive in patients with alcohol, cocaine, or opioid intoxication. Table 30.39 summarizes common deep tendon and cutaneous reflexes.

FIG. 30.68 Position for eliciting patellar tendon reflex. Lower leg normally extends.

AFTER THE EXAMINATION

Record findings from the physical assessment either during the examination or after it has been completed. If you document while performing an examination, do not allow this to distract you. It is important to attend to the patient to observe the patient's response to any examination technique. Special forms are available to record data both electronically and on printed forms. Review all findings before helping patients dress, in case it is necessary to recheck any information or gather additional data. Integrate physical assessment findings into the plan of care.

After completing an assessment, give the patient time to dress. A patient in a hospital sometimes needs help with hygiene and returning to bed. When the patient is comfortable, it helps to share a summary of the assessment findings. If the findings have revealed serious abnormalities such as a mass or highly irregular heart rate, consult the patient's health care provider before revealing them. It is the health care provider's responsibility to make definitive medical diagnoses. Explain the type of abnormality found and the need for the health care provider to conduct an additional examination.

Delegate the cleanup of the examination area to assistive personnel (AP) if needed. Use infection control practices to remove materials or instruments soiled with potentially infectious wastes. If the patient's bedside was the examination site, clear away soiled items from the bedside table and make sure that the bed linen is dry and clean. A patient appreciates a clean gown and the opportunity to wash the face and hands. Place the nurse call system within reach of the patient and raise the side rails as appropriate. Afterward be sure to perform hand hygiene.

Be sure to record a complete assessment. Review the documents for accuracy and thoroughness. Communicate significant findings to appropriate personnel, either verbally or in the patient's written care plan.

QSEN Building Competency in Safety A 38-year-old female patient presents to the examination room via a wheelchair. You notice that she is frail, her feet are curled up into the chair, and both of her arms are across her stomach and pressing into her stomach in a firm manner. The patient is sitting in the fetal position within the wheelchair. When you ask her whether she needs help getting on the table in the examination room, she answers in Spanish and you see tears in her eyes. She is accompanied by a younger woman who explains that the patient said, "My stomach hurts, and I don't think I can get to the table." Which aspects of the QSEN competency of Safety would be used to best care for this patient throughout the entire physical examination related to culture and physical assessment of the abdomen? How does the competency of patient-centered care play a role in the patient's safety?

Answers to QSEN Activities can be found on the Evolve website.

KEY POINTS

- Knowing the purpose of an overall assessment is important so that you can focus and organize the history and physical on the patient's primary problems and concerns.
- Consideration of a patient's cultural background may affect whether you make adaptations in the physical assessment and mode of communication while assessing in the context of a patient's health beliefs and practices and nutritional practices.
- Prepare a patient for a physical examination by having an organized approach for the entire assessment to ensure the mental and physical comfort of the patient.
- You prepare a patient psychologically for an examination by offering a thorough explanation of the purpose and steps of each assessment technique, letting a patient know what to expect and how to cooperate.
- Using open-ended, focused questions helps you gather current information and history to complete a full assessment. Open-ended questions encourage a full explanation of a symptom timeline and its effects on the patient's functioning.
- Before an examination, set up the room, gather all needed equipment, and make sure the room is a comfortable temperature for the patient.
- Through the health history interview, you gather subjective data about a patient's condition and objective data from observations of a patient's behavior and overall presentation. These data allow you to focus a physical examination appropriately.
- Each assessment area has different techniques that must be performed correctly to detect any normal and abnormal findings that you will use to interpret data.
- Recognize that the normal aging process affects physical and assessment findings in older adults.
- Converse with the patient during each part of an examination. Teaching health promotion activities related to the area being assessed is a good way to build a relationship of trust and to promote the patient's knowledge of healthy behaviors.
- Physical assessment can be incorporated into routine care. For example, skin assessment can be completed while helping the patient transfer or prepare for bathing.
- Patients should be encouraged to perform regular self-screening examinations for breast, testicular, and skin cancers.
- A patient in the community may seek screening for specific health conditions that are often dependent on age or health risks, such as breast cancer (mammogram age 55 years and older), colorectal cancer (age 45 years and older), ear disorders (periodic tests at all ages), and obesity (all ages).

REFLECTIVE LEARNING

- Describe the order in which you completed the assessment on a patient that you cared for during your last clinical rotation. Explain the rationale for completing the assessment in this manner.
- Describe any abnormal assessment findings you obtained when assessing your patient during your clinical experience. What might these findings indicate? Describe the steps you took after obtaining the abnormal findings.
- Consider a patient that you cared for on the clinical unit. Describe how this patient's assessment findings varied based on age.

REVIEW QUESTIONS

1. A patient has been admitted from the emergency department (ED) with a primary problem of abdominal pain. Diagnostic tests performed in the ED are pending. The nurse focuses an examination on the abdomen and uses the following techniques. Which technique is correct?
   1. Perform auscultation first.
   2. Have patient place folded arms under the head.
   3. Palpate the patient's painful area first.
   4. Observe the contour of the abdomen while asking the patient to take a deep breath and hold it.
2. Which number corresponds to the area of the chest where you would auscultate for the tricuspid valve?

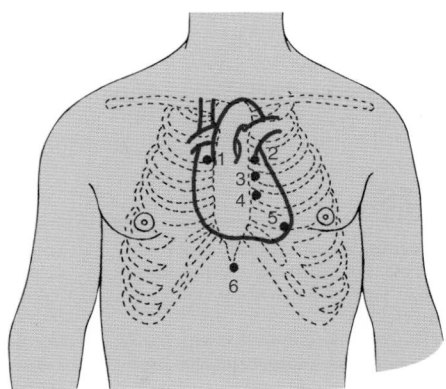

3. The nurse is assessing a patient who returned 1 hour ago from surgery for an abdominal hysterectomy. Which assessment finding would require immediate follow-up?
   1. Auscultation of an apical heart rate of 76
   2. Absence of bowel sounds on abdominal assessment
   3. Respiratory rate of 8 breaths/min
   4. Palpation of dorsalis pedis pulses with strength of +2
4. Which statement made by a patient who is at average risk for colorectal cancer indicates an understanding about teaching related to early detection of colorectal cancer?
   1. "I'll make sure to schedule my colonoscopy annually after the age of 60."
   2. "I'll make sure to have a colonoscopy every 2 years."
   3. "I'll make sure to have a flexible sigmoidoscopy every year once I turn 55."
   4. "I'll make sure to have a fecal occult blood test annually once I turn 45."
5. The nurse is teaching a patient to prevent heart disease. Which information should the nurse include? (Select all that apply.)
   1. Add salt to every meal.
   2. Talk with your health care provider about taking a daily low dose of aspirin.

3. Work with your health care provider to develop a regular exercise program.
4. Limit saturated and trans fats, sodium, red meats, sweets, and sugar-sweetened beverages.
5. Review strategies to encourage the patient to quit smoking.

6. The nurse is assessing the cranial nerves. Match the cranial nerve with its related function.

Cranial Nerves	Cranial Nerve Function
____1. XII Hypoglossal	a. Motor innervation to the muscles of the jaw
____2. V Trigeminal	
____3. VI Adducens	b. Lateral movement of the eyeballs
____4. IV Trochlear	c. Sensation of the pharynx
____5. X Vagus	d. Downward, inward eye movements
	e. Position of the tongue

7. The nurse is teaching a patient how to perform a testicular self-examination. Which statement made by the patient indicates a need for further teaching?
   1. "I'll recognize abnormal lumps because they are very painful."
   2. "I'll start performing testicular self-examination monthly after I turn 15."
   3. "I'll perform the self-examination in front of a mirror."
   4. "I'll gently roll the testicle between my fingers."

8. The nurse is observing the patient for general appearance and behavior. What assessments might indicate that the patient is in pain? (Select all that apply). The patient:
   1. is slumped in the bed.
   2. responds to questions by making eye contact.
   3. is short of breath and breathing rapidly.
   4. protects and splints the left arm.
   5. is alert and oriented.

9. A patient has undergone surgery for a femoral artery bypass. The surgeon's orders include assessment of dorsalis pedis pulses. The nurse will use which of the following techniques to assess the pulses? (Select all that apply.)
   1. Place the fingers behind and below the medial malleolus.
   2. Have the patient slightly flex the knee with the foot resting on the bed.
   3. Have the patient relax the foot while lying supine.
   4. Palpate the groove lateral to the flexor tendon of the wrist.
   5. Palpate along the top of the foot in a line with the groove between the extensor tendons of the great and first toes.

10. Which of the following are normal findings you should find during a physical exam? (Select all that apply.)
    1. Jugular vein flattens when a patient sits up.
    2. A swooshing sound is normally heard when auscultating a carotid artery.
    3. Upon palpation, a lymph node is normally tender.
    4. Normal sitting posture involves some degree of rounding of the shoulders.
    5. Normally there is no bulging within the intercostal spaces during breathing.

Answers: 1. 4; **2.** 4; **3.** 4; **4.** 5; **5.** 2, 3, 4; **6.** 1e, 2a, 3b, 4d, 5c; **7.** 1; **8.** 1, 3, 4; **9.** 3, 5; **10.** 1, 4, 5.

Rationales for Review Questions can be found on the Evolve website.

REFERENCES

American Cancer Society (ACS): *Risk factors for testicular cancer,* 2018a. https://www.cancer.org/cancer/testicular-cancer/causes-risks-prevention/risk-factors.html. Accessed August 28, 2020.

American Cancer Society (ACS): *Colorectal cancer screening guidelines,* 2018b. https://www.cancer.org/health-care-professionals/american-cancer-society-prevention-early-detection-guidelines/colorectal-cancer-screening-guidelines.html. Accessed August 28, 2020.

American Cancer Society (ACS): *Cancer facts and figures,* 2020a. https://www.cancer.org/content/dam/cancer-org/research/cancer-facts-and-statistics/annual-cancer-facts-and-figures/2020/cancer-facts-and-figures-2020.pdf. Accessed August 28, 2020.

American Cancer Society (ACS): *Can ovarian cancer be found early?* 2020b. https://www.cancer.org/cancer/ovarian-cancer/detection-diagnosis-staging/detection.html?_ga=2.29301694.34924562.1540912089-41350218.1539106062. Accessed August 28, 2020.

American Cancer Society (ACS): *American Cancer Society recommendations for the early detection of breast cancer,* 2021. https://www.cancer.org/cancer/breast-cancer/screening-tests-and-early-detection/american-cancer-society-recommendations-for-the-early-detection-of-breast-cancer.html. Accessed July 12, 2021.

American Heart Association (AHA): *What your cholesterol levels mean,* 2020. https://www.heart.org/en/health-topics/cholesterol/about-cholesterol/what-your-cholesterol-levels-mean. Accessed August 28, 2020.

Ball JW, et al: *Seidel's guide to physical examination,* ed 9, St. Louis, 2019, Mosby.

BreastCancer.org: *Men with breast cancer have lower survival rates than women,* 2019. https://www.breastcancer.org/research-news/men-with-bc-have-lower-survival-rates#:~:text=While%20breast%20cancer%20in%20men%20is%20rare%2C%20it,getting%20breast%20cancer%20is%20about%201%20in%20833. Accessed July 12, 2021.

Cancer.Net: *Health risks of e-cigarettes, smokeless tobacco, and waterpipes,* Alexandria, VA, 2019, American Society of Clinical Oncology. https://www.cancer.net/navigating-cancer-care/prevention-and-healthy-living/stopping-tobacco-use-after-cancer-diagnosis/health-risks-e-cigarettes-smokeless-tobacco-and-waterpipes. Accessed August 28, 2020.

Centers for Disease Control and Prevention (CDC): *HPV vaccine,* 2019a. http://www.cdc.gov/hpv/parents/vaccine.html. Accessed August 28, 2020.

Centers for Disease Control and Prevention (CDC): *Vaccines and immunizations: HPV vaccine questions and answers.* 2019b. http://www.cdc.gov/vaccines/vpd-vac/hpv/vac-faqs.htm. Accessed August 28, 2020.

Centers for Disease Control and Prevention: *Genomics and prevention health: Does osteoporosis run in your family?* 2020. https://www.cdc.gov/genomics/disease/osteoporosis.htm#:~:text=Osteoporosis%20is%20more%20common%20in%20women.%20It%20affects,they%20have%20it%20until%20they%20break%20a%20bone. Accessed July 13, 2021.

Centers for Disease Control and Prevention (CDC): *Learn about age-related macular degeneration,* 2021a. https://www.cdc.gov/visionhealth/resources/features/macular-degeneration.html. Accessed July 8, 2021.

Centers for Disease Control and Prevention (CDC): *Loud noise can cause hearing loss,* 2021b. https://www.cdc.gov/nceh/hearing_loss/. Accessed July 10, 2021.

Giger J, Haddad L: *Transcultural nursing: assessment and intervention,* ed 8, St. Louis, 2021, Elsevier.

Harding M, et al: *Lewis's medical-surgical nursing: assessment and management of clinical problems,* ed 11, St. Louis, Missouri, 2020, Elsevier.

Hockenberry MJ, Wilson P: *Wong's nursing care of infants and children,* ed 10, St. Louis, 2019, Elsevier.

Mayo Clinic: *Symptoms: unexplained weight loss,* 2021. https://www.mayoclinic.org/symptoms/unexplained-weight-loss/basics/definition/sym-20050700#:~:text=The%20point%20at%20which%20unexplained%20weight%20loss%20becomes,a%20year%2C%20especially%20if%20you%27re%20an%20older%20adult. Accessed July 8, 2021.

National Breast Cancer Foundation: *Breast self-exam,* n.d. https://www.nationalbreastcancer.org/breast-self-exam. Accessed August 28, 2020.

National Cancer Institute (NCI): *Surveillance, epidemiology and end results program, cancer stat facts: female breast cancer,* n.d. https://seer.cancer.gov/statfacts/html/breast.html. July 12, 2021

National Institute on Drug Abuse (NIDA): *Screening tools for adolescent substance use,* 2019. https://www.drugabuse.gov/nidamed-medical-health-professionals/screening-tools-resources/screening-tools-for-adolescent-substance-use. Accessed August 28, 2020.

National Institute on Drug Abuse (NIDA): *New clinician screening tool available for substance use,* 2018. https://www.drugabuse.gov/news-events/news-releases/2018/06/new-clinician-screening-tool-available-substance-use. Accessed August 28, 2020.

Oral Cancer Foundation: *Oral cancer facts,* 2021. https://oralcancerfoundation.org/facts/. Accessed July 10, 2021.

Touhy T, Jett K: *Ebersole and Hess' towards healthy aging,* ed 10, St. Louis, 2020, Elsevier.

U.S. Department of Agriculture (USDA): *Start simple with MyPlate*, n.d. https://www.choosemyplate.gov/eathealthy/start-simple-myplate. Accessed August 28, 2020.

U.S. Department of Agriculture, U.S. Department of Health and Human Services: *Dietary guidelines for Americans*, 2020-2025, ed 9, December 2020.

U.S. Preventive Services Task Force (USPSTF): Screening for osteoporosis to prevent fractures, US Preventive Services Task Force recommendation statement, *JAMA* 319(24):2521, 2018.

World Health Organization (WHO): *Understanding and addressing violence against women*, 2021. https://www.who.int/reproductivehealth/topics/violence/vaw_series/en/. Accessed July 8, 2021.

RESEARCH REFERENCES

Bauer K: *Clinical presentation and diagnosis of the nonpregnant adult with suspected deep vein thrombosis of the lower extremity*, 2021, *UpToDate*. https://www.uptodate.com/contents/clinical-presentation-and-diagnosis-of-the-nonpregnant-adult-with-suspected-deep-vein-thrombosis-of-the-lower-extremity. Accessed July 12, 2021.

Bond L, Hallmark B: Educating nurses in the intensive care unit about gastrointestinal complications, *Crit Care Nurs Clin North Am* 30(1):75, 2018.

Folstein MF, Folstein S: "Mini-mental state": a practical method for grading the cognitive state of patients for the clinician, *J Psychiatr Res* 12(3):189, 1975.

Frazer C, et al: Gastrointestinal motility problems in critically ill patients, *Crit Care Nurs Clin North Am* 30(1):109, 2018.

Kendall J, Moreira M: *Evaluation of the adult with abdominal pain in the emergency department*, 2020, UpToDate. https://www.uptodate.com/contents/evaluation-of-the-adult-with-abdominal-pain-in-the-emergency-department. Accessed August 28, 2020.

Ladopoulos T, et al: Gastrointestinal dysmotility in critically ill patients, *Ann Gastroenterol* 3(31):273, 2018.

Moonen P, et al: The black box revelation: monitoring gastrointestinal function, *Anaesthesiol Intensive Ther* 50(1):72, 2018.

31

Medication Administration

Patients with health problems use a variety of strategies to restore or maintain their health. One strategy they often use is medication, a substance used in the diagnosis, treatment, cure, relief, or prevention of health problems. No matter where patients receive health care (i.e., hospitals, clinics, or home), nurses play an essential role in preparing, administering, and evaluating the effects of medications. Family caregivers, friends, or home care personnel often administer medications when patients cannot administer them themselves at home. In all settings nurses are responsible for evaluating the effects of medications on the patient's ongoing health status, providing education about medications and side effects, encouraging adherence to the medication regimen, and evaluating the patient's and family caregiver's ability to administer medications.

SCIENTIFIC KNOWLEDGE BASE

Because medication administration and evaluation are a critical part of nursing practice, nurses need to understand the actions and effects of all medications taken by their patients. Administering medications safely requires sound clinical judgment based on an understanding of legal aspects of health care, pharmacology, pharmacokinetics (the movement of drugs in the human body), the life sciences, pathophysiology, human anatomy, and mathematics.

Medication Legislation and Standards

Federal Regulations. The U.S. government protects the health of the people by ensuring that medications are safe and effective. The first American law to regulate medications was the Pure Food and Drug Act. This law requires all medications to be free of impure products. Subsequent legislation created standards related to safety, potency, and efficacy. Currently the U.S. Food and Drug Administration (FDA) enforces medication laws that ensure that all medications on the market undergo vigorous testing before they are sold to the public. Federal medication laws also control medication sales and distribution; testing, naming, and labeling; and the use of controlled substances. Official publications such as the *United States Pharmacopeia* (USP) and the *National Formulary* set standards for medication strength, quality, purity, packaging, safety, labeling, and dose form. In 1993 the FDA instituted the MedWatch program. This voluntary program encourages nurses and other health care professionals, by completing the Medwatch form, to report when a medication, product, or medical event causes serious harm to a patient. The form is available on the MedWatch website (FDA, 2021a).

State and Local Regulation of Medication. State and local medication laws must conform to federal legislation. States often have additional controls, including control of substances not regulated by the federal government. Local governmental bodies regulate the use of alcohol and tobacco.

Health Care Agencies and Medication Laws. Health care agencies establish individual policies to meet federal, state, and local regulations. The size of the agency, the services it provides, and the professional personnel it employs influence these policies. Agency policies are often more restrictive than governmental controls. For example, a common agency policy is the automatic discontinuation of narcotics after a set number of days. Although a health care provider can reorder the narcotic, this policy helps to control unnecessarily prolonged medication therapy because it requires the health care provider to regularly review the need for the medication.

Medication Regulations and Nursing Practice. State nurse practice acts (NPAs) define the scope of nurses' professional functions and responsibilities. Most NPAs are purposefully broad so that nurses' professional responsibilities are not limited. Health care agencies can interpret specific actions allowed under NPAs, but they cannot modify, expand, or restrict the intent of the act. The primary intent of NPAs is to protect the public from unskilled, undereducated, and unlicensed personnel.

A nurse is responsible for following legal provisions when administering controlled substances such as opioids, which are carefully controlled through federal and state guidelines. Violations of the Controlled Substances Act are punishable by fines, imprisonment, and loss of nurse licensure. Hospitals and other health care agencies have policies for the proper storage and distribution of narcotics (Box 31.1).

BOX 31.1   Guidelines for Safe Opioid (Narcotic) Administration and Control

- Store all narcotics in a locked, secure cabinet or container (e.g., computerized, locked cabinets are preferred).
- Maintain a running count of opioids by counting them whenever dispensing them. If you find a discrepancy, correct it and report it immediately.
- Use a special inventory record each time an opioid is dispensed. Records are often kept electronically and provide an accurate ongoing count of narcotics used, wasted, and remaining.
- Use the record to document the patient's name, date, time of medication administration, name of medication, and dosage. If the agency keeps a paper record, the nurse dispensing the medication signs the record. If the agency uses a computerized system, the computer records the nurse's name.
- A second nurse witnesses disposal of the unused part if a nurse gives only part of a dose of a controlled substance. Computerized systems record the nurses' names electronically. If paper records are kept, both nurses sign their names on the form.
- Follow agency policy for appropriate waste of opioids. Do not place wasted parts of medications in sharps containers.

Pharmacological Concepts

Medication Names. Some medications have as many as three different names. The chemical name of a medication provides an exact description of its composition and molecular structure. Nurses rarely use chemical names in clinical practice. An example of a chemical name is *N*-acetyl-*para*-aminophenol, which is commonly known as Tylenol. The manufacturer that first develops the medication gives the generic or nonproprietary name, with United States Adopted Names (USAN) Council approval (American Medical Association [AMA], 2021). Acetaminophen is an example of the generic name for Tylenol. The generic name becomes the official name listed in official publications such as the USP. The trade name, brand name, or proprietary name is the name under which a manufacturer markets a medication. The trade name has the symbol (™) at the upper right of the name, indicating that the manufacturer has trademarked the name of the medication (e.g., Panadol™ and Tempra™).

Manufacturers choose trade names that are easy to pronounce, spell, and remember. Many companies produce the same medication, and similarities in trade names are often confusing. Be careful to obtain the exact name and spelling for each medication you administer to your patients. Because similarities in medication names are a common cause of medical errors, the Institute for Safe Medication Practices (ISMP) (2019a; 2020a) publishes a list of medications that are frequently confused with one another. The ISMP recommends the use of FDA-approved tall-man or mixed-case letters when possible (e.g., aMILoride versus amLODIPine) to help health care providers easily recognize the difference between these commonly confused medications.

Classification. Medication classification indicates the effect of a medication on a body system, the symptoms a medication relieves, or its desired effect. Usually, each class contains more than one medication that is used for the same type of health problem. For example, patients who have asthma often take a variety of medications, such as beta$_2$-adrenergic agonists, to control their illness. The beta$_2$-adrenergic classification contains more than 15 different medications (Burchum and Rosenthal, 2019). Some medications are in more than one class. For example, aspirin is an analgesic, an antipyretic, and an antiinflammatory medication.

Medication Forms. Medications are available in a variety of forms, or preparations. The form of the medication determines its route of administration. The composition of a medication enhances its absorption and metabolism. Many medications come in several forms, such as tablets, capsules, elixirs, and suppositories. When administering a medication, be certain to use the proper form (Table 31.1).

Pharmacokinetics as the Basis of Medication Actions

For a medication to be useful therapeutically, it must be taken into a patient's body; be absorbed and distributed to cells, tissues, or a specific organ; and alter physiological functions. Pharmacokinetics is the study of how medications enter the body, reach their site of action, metabolize, and exit the body. You use knowledge of pharmacokinetics

when timing medication administration, selecting the route of administration, and evaluating a patient's response.

Absorption. Absorption occurs when medication molecules pass into the blood from the site of medication administration. The route of administration, ability of the medication to dissolve, blood flow to the site of administration, body surface area (BSA), and lipid solubility of the medication influence a medication's absorption.

Route of Administration. Each route of medication administration has a different rate of absorption. When applying medications on the skin, absorption is slow because of the physical makeup of the skin. Because orally administered medications pass through the gastrointestinal (GI) tract, the overall rate of absorption is usually slow. Medications placed on

TABLE 31.1   Forms of Medication

Form	Description
Medication Forms Commonly Prepared for Administration by Oral Route	
Solid Forms	
Caplet	Shaped like capsule and coated for ease of swallowing
Capsule	Medication encased in gelatin shell
Tablet	Powdered medication compressed into hard disk or cylinder; in addition to primary medication, contains binders (adhesive to allow powder to stick together), disintegrators (to promote tablet dissolution), lubricants (for ease of manufacturing), and fillers (for convenient tablet size)
Enteric-coated tablet	Coated tablet that does not dissolve in stomach; coatings dissolve in intestine, where medication is absorbed
Liquid Forms	
Elixir	Clear fluid containing water and/or alcohol; often sweetened
Extract	Syrup or dried form of pharmacologically active medication, usually made by evaporating solution
Aqueous solution	Substance dissolved in water and syrups
Aqueous suspension	Finely dissolved medication particles dispersed in liquid medium; when suspension is left standing, particles settle to bottom of container
Syrup	Medication dissolved in a concentrated sugar solution
Tincture	Alcohol extract from plant or vegetable
Other Oral Forms and Terms Associated With Oral Preparations	
Troche (lozenge)	Flat, round tablets that dissolve in mouth to release medication; not meant for ingestion
Aerosol	Aqueous medication sprayed and absorbed in mouth and upper airway; not meant for ingestion
Sustained release	Tablet or capsule that contains small particles of a medication coated with material that requires a varying amount of time to dissolve
Medication Forms Commonly Prepared for Administration by Topical Route	
Ointment (salve or cream)	Semisolid, externally applied preparation, usually containing one or more medications
Liniment	Usually contains alcohol, oil, or soapy emollient applied to skin
Lotion	Semiliquid suspension that usually protects, cools, or cleanses skin
Paste	Medication preparation that is thicker than ointment; absorbed through skin more slowly than ointment; often used for skin protection
Transdermal disk or patch	Medicated disk or patch absorbed through skin slowly over long period of time (e.g., 24 hours)
Medication Forms Commonly Prepared for Administration by Parenteral Route	
Solution	Sterile preparation that contains water with one or more dissolved compounds
Powder	Sterile particles of medication that are dissolved in a sterile liquid (e.g., water, normal saline) before administration
Medication Forms Commonly Prepared for Instillation Into Body Cavities	
Intraocular disk	Small, flexible oval (similar to contact lens) consisting of two soft, outer layers and a middle layer containing medication; slowly releases medication when moistened by ocular fluid
Suppository	Solid dosage form mixed with gelatin and shaped in form of pellet for insertion into body cavity (rectum or vagina); melts when it reaches body temperature, releasing medication for absorption

the mucous membranes and respiratory airways are absorbed quickly because these tissues contain many blood vessels. Intramuscular (IM) and subcutaneous medications are absorbed more quickly than oral medications, with IM injections entering the bloodstream more quickly than medications in subcutaneous injections. Intravenous (IV) injection produces the most rapid absorption because medications are available immediately when they enter the systemic circulation.

Ability of a Medication to Dissolve. The ability of an oral medication to dissolve depends largely on its form or preparation. The body absorbs solutions and suspensions already in a liquid state more readily than tablets or capsules. Acidic medications pass through the gastric mucosa rapidly. Medications that are basic are not absorbed before reaching the small intestine.

Blood Flow to the Site of Administration. The blood supply to the site of administration will determine how quickly the body can absorb a medication. Medications are absorbed as blood comes in contact with the site of administration. The richer the blood supply to the site of administration, the faster a medication is absorbed.

Body Surface Area. When a medication comes in contact with a large surface area, it is absorbed at a faster rate. This helps explain why most of medications are absorbed in the small intestine rather than the stomach (Burchum and Rosenthal, 2019).

Lipid Solubility. Because the cell membrane has a lipid layer, highly lipid-soluble medications cross cell membranes easily and are absorbed quickly. Another factor that often affects medication absorption is whether food is in the stomach. Some oral medications are absorbed more easily when administered between meals because food changes the structure of a medication and sometimes impairs its absorption. When some medications are administered together, they interfere with each other, impairing the absorption of both medications.

Safe medication administration requires knowledge of factors that alter or impair absorption of prescribed medications. You need to understand medication pharmacokinetics, a patient's health history, physical examination data, and knowledge gained through daily patient interactions. Use your knowledge and agency policy to plan medication administration times that will promote optimal absorption. For example, plan medication administration times around meals (e.g., before or after meals) when medications interact with food. When they interact with one another, make sure that you do not give them at the same time. Consult and collaborate with your patient's health care provider or a pharmacist when setting medication times to ensure that the patient achieves the therapeutic effect of all medications. Before administering any medication, check pharmacology books, medication references, or package inserts or consult with pharmacists to identify medication-medication or medication-food interactions.

Distribution. After a medication is absorbed, it is distributed within the body to tissues and organs and ultimately to its specific site of action. The rate and extent of distribution depend on the physical and chemical properties of the medication and the physiology of the person taking it.

Circulation. Once a medication enters the bloodstream, it is carried throughout the tissues and organs. How fast it reaches a site depends on the vascularity of the various tissues and organs. Conditions that limit blood flow or blood perfusion inhibit the distribution of a medication. For example, patients with heart failure have impaired circulation, which slows medication delivery to the intended site of action. Therefore the effectiveness of medications in these patients is often delayed or altered.

Membrane Permeability. Membrane permeability refers to the ability of a medication to pass through tissues and membranes to enter target cells. To be distributed to an organ, a medication must pass

through all of the tissues and biological membranes of the organ. Some membranes serve as barriers to the passage of medications. For example, the blood-brain barrier allows only fat-soluble medications to pass into the brain and cerebrospinal fluid. Because of this, central nervous system infections often require treatment with antibiotics injected directly into the subarachnoid space in the spinal cord. Some older adults experience adverse effects (e.g., confusion) because of the change in the permeability of the blood-brain barrier, with easier passage of fat-soluble medications.

Protein Binding. The degree to which medications bind to serum proteins such as albumin affects their distribution. Most medications partially bind to albumin, reducing the ability of a drug to exert pharmacological activity. The unbound or "free" medication is its active form. Older adults and patients with liver disease or malnutrition have decreased albumin in the bloodstream. Because more medication is unbound in these patients, they are at risk for an increase in medication activity, toxicity, or both.

Metabolism. After a medication reaches its site of action, it becomes metabolized into a less active or an inactive form that is easier to excrete. Biotransformation occurs under the influence of enzymes that detoxify, break down, and remove biologically active chemicals. Most biotransformation occurs within the liver, although the lungs, kidneys, blood, and intestines also metabolize medications. The liver is especially important because its specialized structure oxidizes and transforms many toxic substances. The liver degrades many harmful chemicals before they become distributed to the tissues. If a decrease in liver function occurs, such as with aging or liver disease, a medication is usually eliminated more slowly, resulting in its accumulation. Patients are at risk for medication toxicity if organs that metabolize medications are not functioning correctly. For example, a small sedative dose of a barbiturate sometimes causes a patient with liver disease to lapse into a coma.

Excretion. After medications are metabolized, they exit the body through the kidneys, liver, bowel, lungs, and exocrine glands. The chemical makeup of a medication determines the organ of excretion. Gaseous and volatile compounds such as nitrous oxide and alcohol exit through the lungs. Deep breathing and coughing (see Chapter 41) help patients eliminate anesthetic gases more rapidly after surgery. The exocrine glands excrete lipid-soluble medications. When medications exit through sweat glands, the skin often becomes irritated, requiring you to teach patients good hygiene practices (see Chapter 40). If a medication is excreted through the mammary glands, there is a risk that a nursing infant will ingest the chemicals. Check the safety of any medication used in women who are breastfeeding.

The GI tract is another route for medication excretion. Medications that enter the hepatic circulation are broken down by the liver and excreted into the bile. After chemicals enter the intestines through the biliary tract, the intestines resorb them. Factors that increase peristalsis (e.g., laxatives and enemas) accelerate medication excretion through the feces, whereas factors that slow peristalsis (e.g., inactivity and improper diet) often prolong the effects of a medication.

The kidneys are the main organs for medication excretion. Some medications escape extensive metabolism and exit unchanged in the urine. Others undergo biotransformation in the liver before the kidneys excrete them. Maintenance of an adequate fluid intake (50 mL/kg/h) promotes proper elimination of medications for the average adult. If a patient's renal function declines, the kidneys cannot adequately excrete medications. Thus the risk for medication toxicity increases. Health care providers usually reduce medication doses when this happens.

Types of Medication Action

Medications vary considerably in the way they act and their types of action. Patients do not always respond in the same way to each successive dose of a medication. Sometimes the same medication causes very different responses in different patients. Therefore you need to understand all the effects that medications you administer have on patients.

Therapeutic Effects. The therapeutic effect is the expected or predicted physiological response caused by a medication. For example, nitroglycerin reduces cardiac workload and increases myocardial oxygen supply. Some medications have more than one therapeutic effect. For example, prednisone, a steroid, decreases swelling, inhibits inflammation, reduces allergic responses, and prevents rejection of transplanted organs. Knowing the desired therapeutic effect for each medication allows you to provide patient education and accurately evaluate the desired effect of a medication.

Adverse Effects. Every medication can harm a patient. Undesired, unintended, and often unpredictable responses to medication are referred to as adverse effects. Adverse medication effects range from mild to severe. Some happen immediately, whereas others develop over time. Be alert and assess for unusual individual responses to medications, especially with newly prescribed medications. Patients most at risk for adverse medication reactions include the very young and older adults, pregnant women, patients taking multiple medications, patients who are extremely underweight or overweight, and patients with renal or liver disease. If adverse effects are mild and tolerable, patients often remain on the medications. However, if these effects are not tolerated and are potentially harmful, stop giving the medication immediately. When adverse responses to medications occur, the health care provider discontinues the medication immediately. Health care providers report adverse effects to the FDA using the MedWatch program (FDA, 2021a).

Side Effects. A side effect is a predictable and often unavoidable adverse effect produced at a usual therapeutic dose. For example, some antihypertensive medications cause impotence in men. Side effects range from being harmless to causing serious symptoms or injury. If the side effects are serious enough to negate the beneficial effects of the therapeutic action of the medication, the health care provider discontinues the medication. Patients often stop taking medications because of side effects, the most common of which are anorexia, nausea, vomiting, constipation, drowsiness, and diarrhea.

Toxic Effects. Toxic effects often develop after prolonged intake of a medication or when a medication accumulates in the blood because of impaired metabolism or excretion. Excess amounts of a medication within the body sometimes have lethal effects, depending on its action. For example, toxic levels of morphine, an opioid, cause severe respiratory depression and death. Antidotes are available to treat specific types of medication toxicity. For example, naloxone, an opioid antagonist, reverses the effects of opioid toxicity.

Idiosyncratic Reactions. Medications sometimes cause unpredictable effects such as an idiosyncratic reaction, in which a patient overreacts or underreacts to a medication or has a reaction different from normal. For example, a child who receives diphenhydramine, an antihistamine, becomes extremely agitated or excited instead of drowsy. At present it is not possible to predict whether a patient will have an idiosyncratic response to a medication.

Allergic Reactions. Allergic reactions are unpredictable responses to a medication. Some patients become immunologically sensitized to the initial dose of a medication. With repeated administration the patient develops an allergic response to it, its chemical preservatives, or a metabolite. The medication or chemical acts as an antigen, triggering

TABLE 31.2	Mild Allergic Reactions
Symptom	**Description**
Urticaria (hives)	Raised, irregularly shaped skin eruptions with varying sizes and shapes; eruptions have reddened margins and pale centers
Rash	Small, raised vesicles that are usually reddened; often distributed over entire body
Pruritus	Itching of skin; accompanies most rashes
Rhinitis	Inflammation of mucous membranes lining nose; causes swelling and clear, watery discharge

FIG. 31.1 Allergy identification bracelet (A) and medal (B). (A from istock.com/monkeybusinessimages; B from Scully C: *Medical problems in dentistry*, ed 6, St Louis, 2010, Elsevier.)

the release of the antibodies in the body. A patient's medication allergy symptoms vary, depending on the individual and the medication (Table 31.2). Among the different classes of medications, antibiotics cause a high incidence of allergic reactions. Severe or anaphylactic reactions, which are life threatening, are characterized by sudden constriction of bronchiolar muscles, edema of the pharynx and larynx, and severe wheezing and shortness of breath. Immediate medical attention is required to treat anaphylactic reactions. A patient with a known history of an allergy to a medication needs to avoid taking that medication in the future and wear an identification bracelet or medal (Fig. 31.1), which alerts nurses and other health care providers to the allergy if a patient is unable to communicate when receiving medical care.

Medication Interactions. When one medication modifies the action of another, a medication interaction occurs. Medication interactions are common when individuals take several medications. Some medications increase or diminish the action of others or alter the way another medication is absorbed, metabolized, or eliminated from the body. When two medications have a **synergistic effect**, their combined effect is greater than the effect of the medications when given separately. For example, alcohol is a central nervous system depressant that has a synergistic effect on antihistamines, antidepressants, barbiturates, and narcotic analgesics. Sometimes a medication interaction is desired. Health care providers often combine medications to create an interaction that has a beneficial effect. For example, a patient with high blood pressure takes several medications such as diuretics and vasodilators that act together to control blood pressure when one medication is not effective on its own.

Medication Tolerance and Dependence. Medication tolerance occurs over time. It is usually noted clinically when patients receive more and more medication (higher doses) to achieve the same therapeutic effect. Medications that produce tolerance include opium alkaloids (e.g., morphine), nitrates, and ethyl alcohol. Patients hospitalized for acute illnesses usually do not develop medication tolerance. It may take a month or longer for tolerance to occur.

Medication tolerance is not the same as medication dependence. Two types of medication dependence (addiction) exist: physical and psychological. In psychological dependence a patient desires the medication for benefit other than the intended effect. Physical dependence is a physiological adaptation to a medication that manifests with intense physical disturbance when the medication is withdrawn. If a patient is dependent on alcohol, a higher-than-usual medication dose is necessary to achieve the desired effect of the medication.

Nurses and other health care professionals play an important role in the care of patients with drug addiction. Patients need to be approached with positive attitudes so that the patient may be more open to learning about treatment options. Using the newest evidence-based treatment options can help patients with addictions receive the care and treatment they need.

Timing of Medication Dose Responses

Medications administered intravenously enter the bloodstream and act immediately, whereas those given through other routes take time to enter the bloodstream and have an effect. The quantity and distribution of a medication in different body compartments change constantly. Medications are ordered at various times, depending on when their response begins, becomes most intense, and ceases.

The **minimum effective concentration (MEC)** is the plasma level of a medication below which the effect of the medication does not occur. The toxic concentration is the level at which toxic effects occur. When a medication is prescribed, the goal is to achieve a constant blood level within a safe **therapeutic range**, which falls between the MEC and the toxic concentration (Fig. 31.2). When a medication is administered repeatedly, its serum level fluctuates between doses. The highest level is called the **peak** concentration, and the lowest level is called the **trough** concentration. After reaching its peak, the serum concentration of the medication falls progressively. With IV **infusions** the peak concentration occurs quickly, but the serum level also begins to fall immediately. Doses of some medications (e.g., vancomycin) are based on peak and trough serum levels. The trough level is generally drawn 30 minutes before the medication is administered, and the peak level is drawn whenever the medication is expected to reach its peak concentration. The time it takes for a medication to reach its peak concentration varies, depending on the pharmacokinetics of the medication.

All medications have a **biological half-life**, which is the time it takes for excretion processes to lower the serum medication concentration by half. To maintain a therapeutic plateau, a patient needs to receive regular fixed doses. For example, pain medications are most effective for some cancer

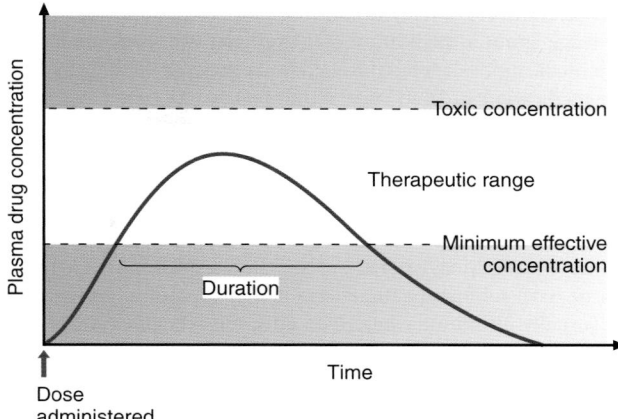

FIG. 31.2 The therapeutic range of a medication occurs between the minimum effective concentration and the toxic concentration. (From Burchum JR, Rosenthal LD: *Pharmacology for nursing care*, ed 10, St Louis, 2019, Elsevier.)

TABLE 31.3   Common Dosage Administration Schedules

Dosage Schedule (Meaning)	Abbreviation
Before meals	AC, ac
As desired	ad lib
Twice each day	BID, bid
After meals	PC, pc
Whenever there is a need	prn
Every morning, every a.m.	q am
Every hour	Qh
Every day	Daily
Every 4 hours	q4h
4 times per day	QID, qid
Give immediately	STAT, stat
3 times per day	TID, tid

patients when they are given around-the-clock (ATC) rather than when a patient intermittently complains of pain because the body maintains an almost constant level of pain medication (Burchum and Rosenthal, 2019). After an initial medication dose, the patient receives each successive dose when the previous dose reaches its half-life. The patient and nurse need to follow regular dosage schedules and administer prescribed doses at correct intervals. Know the following time intervals of medication action to anticipate the effect of a medication:

1. *Onset of medication action:* Time it takes after you administer a medication for it to produce a therapeutic effect
2. *Peak action:* Time it takes for a medication to reach its highest effective peak concentration
3. *Trough:* Minimum blood serum concentration of medication reached just before the next scheduled dose
4. *Duration of action:* Length of time during which a medication is present in a concentration great enough to produce a therapeutic effect
5. *Plateau:* Blood serum concentration reached and maintained after repeated, fixed doses

You and your patient follow prescribed doses and dosage intervals (Table 31.3). Health care agencies usually set schedules for medication administration. However, you can change this schedule based on your knowledge about a medication. For example, you work at an agency where medications ordered once a day are given at 0800. Your patient has a medication ordered once a day that works better when given before bedtime; therefore you adjust the time to give the medication, accordingly, based on agency policy. Acute care agencies also follow guidelines from the ISMP to determine safe, effective, and timely administration of medications (ISMP, 2011; ISMP, 2020a). According to the guidelines, health care agencies determine whether medications are time critical. Medications that are time critical most likely cause harm or have subtherapeutic effects if they are not administered on time (usually 30 minutes before or after the scheduled dose). Non–time-critical medications most likely do not cause harm if they are given within 1 to 2 hours before or after the scheduled time. You need to administer time-critical medications at a precise time, within 30 minutes before or after their scheduled time. You administer non–time-critical medications within 1 to 2 hours of their scheduled time. Ensure that you follow your agency medication policies about the timing of medications to ensure that your patients receive their medications at the right time (Furnish and Wagner, 2020; ISMP, 2011).

When you teach patients about dosage schedules, use familiar language. For example, when teaching a patient about twice-daily medication dosing, instruct the patient to take the medication in the morning and again in the evening. Knowledge of the time intervals of medication action help you anticipate the effect of the medication (Table 31.4). With this knowledge, instruct the patient when to expect a response.

Routes of Administration

The route prescribed for administering a medication depends on the properties and desired effect of the medication and the patient's physical and mental condition (Table 31.5). Work with the health care provider to determine the best route for a patient's medication.

QSEN Building Competency in Evidence-Based Practice A nursing student is caring for a patient being treated for multiple fractures after a recent fall. The health care provider writes a new medication order for morphine sulfate liquid suspension 20 mg orally STAT and then q4h as needed for pain. The patient is having difficulty swallowing pills because of the trauma; therefore the medication is ordered in liquid suspension.

1. What does the student need to know about morphine sulfate before administering it?
2. Four unit-dose containers of liquid morphine sulfate arrive on the patient care unit. The labels on the medication say: "40 mg morphine sulfate/5 mL." The student will need to waste some of the liquid morphine before administering it to the patient. What are the procedures for wasting a narcotic?
3. While being supervised by nursing faculty, the student collects the appropriate equipment to administer the medication, performs hand hygiene, prepares the medication, takes it to the patient at the correct time, and uses two unique patient identifiers to ensure that this is the right patient. Which step does the student need to take next in administering the medication?

Answers to QSEN Activities can be found on the Evolve website.

Oral Routes. The oral route is the easiest and the most commonly used route of medication administration. Medications are given by mouth and swallowed with fluid. Oral medications have a slower onset of action and a more prolonged effect than parenteral medications. Patients generally prefer the oral route.

Sublingual Administration. Some medications (e.g., nitroglycerin) are readily absorbed after being placed under the tongue to dissolve (Fig. 31.3). Instruct patients not to swallow a medication given by the

TABLE 31.4 Terms Associated With Medication Actions

Term	Meaning
Onset	Time it takes after a medication is administered for it to produce a response
Peak	Time it takes for a medication to reach its highest effective concentration
Trough	Minimum blood serum concentration of medication reached just before the next scheduled dose
Duration	Time during which medication is present in concentration great enough to produce a response
Plateau	Blood serum concentration of medication reached and maintained after repeated fixed doses

sublingual route or drink anything until the medication is completely dissolved to ensure that the medication will have the desired effect.

Buccal Administration. Administration of a medication by the buccal route involves placing the solid medication in the mouth against the mucous membranes of the cheek until it dissolves (Fig. 31.4). Teach patients to alternate cheeks with each subsequent dose to avoid mucosal irritation. Warn patients not to chew or swallow the medication or to take any liquids with it. A buccal medication acts locally on the mucosa or systemically as it is swallowed in a person's saliva.

Parenteral Routes. Parenteral administration involves injecting a medication into body tissues. The following are the four major sites of injection:

1. **Intradermal (ID):** Injection into the dermis just under the epidermis
2. **Subcutaneous:** Injection into tissues just below the dermis of the skin
3. **Intramuscular (IM):** Injection into a muscle
4. **Intravenous (IV):** Injection into a vein

Some medications are administered into body cavities through other routes, including epidural, intrathecal, intraosseous, intraperitoneal, intrapleural, and intraarterial. Nurses usually are not responsible for the administration of medications through these advanced techniques. Whether or not you administer a medication, you remain responsible for monitoring the integrity of the medication delivery system, understanding the therapeutic value of the medication, and evaluating a patient's response to the therapy.

Epidural. Epidural medications are administered in the epidural space via a catheter, which is placed by a nurse anesthetist or an anesthesiologist. This route is used for the administration of regional analgesia for surgical procedures (see Chapters 44 and 50). Nurses who have advanced education in the epidural route can administer medications by continuous infusion or a bolus dose.

Intrathecal. Physicians and specially educated nurses administer intrathecal medications through a catheter surgically placed in the subarachnoid space or one of the ventricles of the brain. Intrathecal medication administration often is a long-term treatment.

Intraosseous. The intraosseous method of medication administration involves the infusion of medication directly into the bone marrow. It is used most often in infants and toddlers who have poor access to their intravascular space or when an emergency arises and IV access is impossible.

Intraperitoneal. Medications administered into the peritoneal cavity are absorbed into the circulation. Chemotherapeutic agents, insulin, and antibiotics are administered in this fashion.

TABLE 31.5 Factors Influencing Choice of Administration Routes

Advantages by Route	Disadvantages and Contraindications
Oral, Buccal, Sublingual Routes	
Convenient and comfortable	Oral route is avoided when patient has alterations in gastrointestinal (GI) function (e.g., nausea, vomiting), reduced GI motility (after general anesthesia or bowel inflammation), and surgical resection of the GI tract.
Economical	
Easy to administer	
Often produce local or systemic effects	Oral administration is contraindicated in patients unable to swallow (e.g., patients with neuromuscular disorders, esophageal strictures, mouth lesions).
Rarely cause anxiety for patient	Oral administration is contraindicated in patients who are unconscious, confused, or unable or unwilling to swallow or hold medication under tongue.
	Oral medications cannot be administered when patients have gastric suction; are contraindicated before some tests or surgery.
	Oral medications sometimes irritate lining of GI tract, discolor teeth, or have unpleasant taste.
	Gastric secretions destroy some medications.
Parenteral Routes (Subcutaneous, Intramuscular, Intravenous, Intradermal)	
Can be used when oral medications are contraindicated	There is risk of introducing infection.
More rapid absorption than with topical or oral routes	Some medications are expensive.
Intravenous (IV) infusion provides medication delivery when patient is critically ill or long-term therapy is necessary; if peripheral perfusion is poor, IV route preferred over injections	Some patients experience pain from repeated needlesticks.
	Subcutaneous, intramuscular (IM), and intradermal (ID) routes are avoided in patients with bleeding tendencies.
	There is risk of tissue damage.
	IM and IV routes have higher absorption rates, thus placing patient at higher risk for reactions.
	They often cause considerable anxiety in many patients, especially children.
Topical Routes	
Skin	
Primarily provides local effect	Patients with skin abrasions are at risk for rapid medication absorption and systemic effects.
Painless	Medications are absorbed through skin slowly.
Limited side effects	
Transdermal	
Prolonged systemic effects with limited side effects	Medication leaves oily or pasty substance on skin and sometimes soils clothing.
Mucous Membranes[a]	
Therapeutic effects provided by local application to involved sites	Mucous membranes are highly sensitive to some medication concentrations.
Aqueous solutions readily absorbed and capable of causing systemic effects	Patients with ruptured eardrum cannot receive ear irrigations.
	Insertion of rectal and vaginal medication often causes embarrassment.
Potential route of administration when oral medications are contraindicated	Rectal suppositories contraindicated if patient has had rectal surgery or if active rectal bleeding is present.
Other Routes	
Inhalation	
Provides rapid relief for local respiratory problems	Some local agents cause serious systemic effects.
Used for introduction of general anesthetic gases	
Intraocular Disk	
Route advantageous because it does not require frequent administration as eyedrops do	Local reactions are possible; medication is expensive.
	Patients must be taught to insert and remove disk.
	Contraindicated in eye infections.

[a] Includes eyes, ears, nose, vagina, rectum, and ostomy.

Intrapleural. A syringe and needle or a chest tube are used to administer intrapleural medications directly into the pleural space. Chemotherapeutic agents are the most common medications administered via this method. Physicians also instill medications that help resolve persistent pleural effusion to promote adhesion between the visceral and parietal pleura. This is called *pleurodesis*.

Intraarterial. Intraarterial medications are administered directly into the arteries. Intraarterial infusions are common in patients who have arterial clots and receive clot-dissolving agents. A nurse manages a continuous infusion of the clot-dissolving agent and carefully monitors the integrity of the infusion to prevent inadvertent disconnection of the system and subsequent bleeding.

Other methods of medication administration that are usually limited to physician administration are intracardiac, an injection of a medication directly into cardiac tissue, and intraarticular, an injection of a medication into a joint.

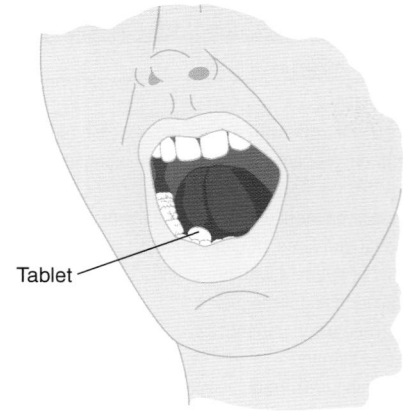

FIG. 31.3 Sublingual administration of a tablet.

FIG. 31.4 Buccal administration of a tablet.

Topical Administration. Medications applied to the skin and mucous membranes generally have local effects. You apply topical medications to the skin by painting or spreading the medication over an area, applying moist dressings, soaking body parts in a solution, or giving medicated baths. Systemic effects often occur if a patient's skin is thin or broken down, the medication concentration is high, or contact with the skin is prolonged. A **transdermal disk** or patch (e.g., nitroglycerin, scopolamine, and estrogens) has systemic effects. The disk secures the medicated ointment to the skin. These topical applications are left in place for as little as 12 hours or up to 7 days.

You apply topical medications to mucous membranes in the following ways:

1. Direct application of a liquid or ointment (e.g., eyedrops, gargling, or swabbing the throat)
2. Insertion of a medication into a body cavity (e.g., placing a suppository in rectum or vagina or inserting medicated packing into vagina)
3. Instillation of fluid into a body cavity (e.g., eardrops, nose drops, or bladder and rectal **instillation** [fluid is retained])
4. Irrigation of a body cavity (e.g., flushing eye, ear, vagina, bladder, or rectum with medicated fluid [fluid is not retained])
5. Spraying a medication into a body cavity (e.g., instillation into nose and throat)

Inhalation Route. The deeper passages of the respiratory tract provide a large surface area for medication absorption. Nurses administer inhaled medications through the nasal and oral passages or endotracheal

or tracheostomy tubes. Endotracheal tubes enter the patient's mouth and end in the trachea, whereas tracheostomy tubes enter the trachea directly through an incision made in the neck. Inhaled medications are readily absorbed and work rapidly because of the rich vascular alveolar capillary network present in the pulmonary tissue. Many inhaled medications have local or systemic effects.

Intraocular Route. **Intraocular** medication delivery involves inserting a medication similar to a contact lens into a patient's eye. The eye medication disk has two soft outer layers that have medication enclosed in them. The nurse inserts the disk into the patient's eye, much like a contact lens. The medication remains in the eye for up to 1 week.

Systems of Medication Measurement

Safely administering medications requires the ability to compute medication doses accurately and measure medications correctly. A careless mistake in placing a decimal point or adding a zero to a dose can lead to a fatal error. Check every dose carefully before giving a medication.

The health care industry in the United States uses primarily the metric system of measurement for medication therapy. Globally most nations use the metric system as their standard of measurement. However, the household system may still be used in medication orders when health care providers write prescriptions, or orders for medications, that are to be administered at home by patients in household measures. Current safety recommendations include that a household measure can be listed in parentheses in an order immediately following the metric measure, such as 5 mL (1 teaspoonful) (Consumer Med Safety, 2021). Health care providers rarely use the apothecary system, a measurement system that includes ounces, pounds, and pints.

Metric System. As a decimal system, the metric system is the most logically organized. You convert and compute metric units using simple multiplication and division. Each basic unit of measurement is organized into units of 10. Multiplying or dividing by 10 forms secondary units. In multiplication the decimal point moves to the right; in division the decimal moves to the left. For example:

$$10 \text{ mg} \times 10 = 100 \text{ mg}$$

$$10 \text{ mg} \div 10 = 1 \text{ mg}$$

The basic units of measurement in the metric system are the meter (length), the liter (volume), and the gram (weight). For medication calculations, use only the volume and weight units. The metric system uses lowercase or capital letters or a combination of lowercase and capital letters to designate basic units:

Gram = g or GM
Liter = l or L
Milligram = mg
Milliliter = mL

A system of Latin prefixes designates subdivision of the basic units: *deci-* (1/10 or 0.1), *centi-* (1/100 or 0.01), and *milli-* (1/1000 or 0.001). Greek prefixes designate multiples of the basic units: *deka-* (10), *hecto-* (100), and *kilo-* (1000). When writing medication doses in metric units, health care providers and nurses use fractions or multiples of a unit. Convert fractions to decimals.

$$500 \text{ mg or } 0.5 \text{ g, not } \frac{1}{2} \text{ g}$$

$$10 \text{ mL or } 0.01 \text{ L, not } \frac{1}{100} \text{ L}$$

Many actual and potential medication errors happen with the use of fractions and decimal points. Follow practice standards when medications are ordered in fractions to prevent these errors. For example, to

TABLE 31.6 Equivalents of Measurement

Metric	Household
1 mL	15 drops (gtt)
5 mL	1 teaspoon (tsp)
15 mL	1 tablespoon (tbsp)
30 mL	2 tablespoons (tbsp)
240 mL	1 cup (c)
480 mL (approximately 500 mL)	1 pint (pt)
960 mL (approximately 1 L)	1 quart (qt)
3785 mL (approximately 4 L)	1 gallon (gal)

make the decimal point more visible, a leading zero is *always* placed in front of a decimal (e.g., use 0.25, *not* .25). *Never* use a trailing zero (i.e., a zero after a decimal point) because if a health care worker does not see the decimal point, the patient may receive 10 times more medication than prescribed (e.g., use 5, *not* 5.0) (ISMP, 2017a).

Household Measurements. Most people are familiar with household measures, which include liquid measures such as drops, teaspoons, tablespoons, cups, pints, and quarts. Even though household measurements are convenient and familiar, they are inaccurate. Dose errors have occurred when household measures are used (ISMP, 2020a; Consumer Med Safety, 2021). As a result, the ISMP recommends a best practice for all oral liquids that are not commercially available as unit-dose products. The liquids should be dispensed by the pharmacy in an oral syringe using metric measurement (ISMP, 2020a). The ISMP also recommends that patients or family caregivers purchase oral liquid dosing devices (oral syringes, cups, or droppers) that display only the metric scale. Encourage patients to never use household measuring devices with liquid medications (Table 31.6). Today's over-the-counter (OTC) liquid medications almost always have their own measuring devices (Consumer Med Safety, 2021).

Solutions. Nurses use solutions of various concentrations for injections, irrigations, and infusions. A solution is a given mass of solid substance dissolved in a known volume of fluid or a given volume of liquid dissolved in a known volume of another fluid. When a solid is dissolved in a fluid, the concentration is in units of mass per units of volume (e.g., g/L, mg/mL). You can also express a concentration of a solution as a percentage. For example, a 10% solution is 10 g of solid dissolved in 100 mL of solution. A proportion also expresses concentrations. A $\frac{1}{1000}$ solution represents a solution containing 1 g of solid in 1000 mL of liquid or 1 mL of liquid mixed with 1000 mL of another liquid.

REFLECT NOW

You are teaching a family caregiver of a 5-year-old about administering an oral antibiotic after discharge. What are some important concepts to teach the family caregiver about administering oral medications to children in the home?

NURSING KNOWLEDGE BASE

In 1999 the Institute of Medicine (IOM) published the book *To Err Is Human: Building a Safer Health System.* This book created national awareness about the effect of medical errors within the health care

BOX 31.2 EVIDENCE-BASED PRACTICE
Preventing Medication Errors

PICOT Question: In health care agencies, does the use of computerized prescription order entry (CPOE), automated medication dispensers (AMDs), and bar-code medication administration (BCMA) during medication administration decrease the incidence of medication errors made by nurses when compared with nurses who do not use these technologies?

Evidence Summary
Medication errors account for 1.5 million adverse medication events annually in the U.S. (Leapfrog Group, 2018). Preventable medication errors in all health care settings cost approximately $21 billion dollars a year (Leapfrog Group, 2018). A systematic review found that optimal implementation of an AMD system provided the benefits of decreased medication errors, decreased medication administration time, and reduction in costs (Batson et al., 2021). One study found that after the implementation of BCMA, medication errors were reduced by 43.5% (Thompson et al., 2018). When there is a problem with the BCMA system design, workflow is interrupted and workarounds and policy deviations occur, which increases the incidence of medication errors (McBee et al., 2019; Mulac et al., 2021). Therefore the use of a well-designed BCMA reduces workarounds and policy deviations, decreases medication errors, and reduces harm from serious medication errors (McBee et al., 2019; Mulac et al., 2021). Research has shown that 90% of medication errors occurred at the ordering and transcribing steps of the medication process (AHRQ, 2019). The use of CPOE is a strategy to reduce medication errors that occur from ordering the wrong medication, medication dose, or frequency, as well as errors from transcription of poorly handwritten medication orders (AHRQ, 2019). A multisystem approach, including the provider, nurse, and health care system, should be used to prevent medication errors (Batson et al., 2021; Zhu and Weingart, 2020).

Application to Nursing Practice
- Everyone administering medications should review the medication list at each patient encounter.
- Be vigilant when handling and administering high-risk medications.
- Consider medications as the cause of any new symptoms.
- When possible, use CPOE to (AHRQ, 2019; Poly et al., 2020; Rochon, 2021):
  - Standardize practice
  - Improve legibility of orders
  - Alert and update health care providers on side effects, drug-drug interactions, and new orders
- Use an electronic medical record when possible and interface this with CPOE if available to improve communication and alert all providers to administration times (AHRQ, 2019; Zhu and Weingart, 2020).
- Bar-coding medications linked to patient identification bracelets improves safety and provides one last opportunity to identify a medication error.
- Work with the health care agency to identify workflow and policy issues with the BCMA that lead to workarounds (McBee et al., 2019; Mulac et al., 2021).
- Avoid all interruptions during bar-coding administration to reduce errors (Bonafide et al., 2020).
- Medication reconciliation identifies medication discrepancies and prevents errors.
- Address nonadherence issues for patients such as fear of addiction (Apter, 2021).
- Patient, family caregiver, and provider education can be used to prevent medication errors (Apter, 2021; Zhu and Weingart, 2020).

system. According to the FDA (2019) there are over 100,000 reported medication errors each year.

Nurses play an important role in patient safety, especially in medication administration. The safe administration of medications is also an important topic for current nursing researchers (Box 31.2). As a nurse you need to know how to calculate medication doses accurately and understand the different roles that members of the health care team play in prescribing and administering medications. Apply your knowledge and clinical judgment to provide safe medication administration.

Clinical Calculations

To administer medications safely, you need to understand basic mathematics skills to calculate medication doses, mix solutions, and perform a variety of other activities. This is important because medications are not always dispensed in the unit of measure in which they are ordered. Medication companies package and bottle medications in standard dosages. For example, a patient's health care provider orders 20 mg of a medication that is available only in 40-mg vials. Nurses frequently convert available units of volume and weight to desired doses. You use equivalents when performing other nursing actions such as when calculating patients' intake and output and IV flow rates. You are responsible for converting available units of volume and weight to the desired doses. Know the approximate equivalents in all major measurement systems. After you calculate a medication dose, use critical thinking to assess that your dose was calculated correctly.

Conversions Within One System.
Converting measurements within one system is relatively easy; simply divide or multiply in the metric system. To change milligrams to grams, divide by 1000, moving the decimal 3 points to the left.

$$1000 \text{ mg} = 1 \text{ g}$$
$$350 \text{ mg} = 0.35 \text{ g}$$

To convert liters to milliliters, multiply by 1000 or move the decimal 3 points to the right.

$$1 \text{ L} = 1000 \text{ mL}$$
$$0.25 \text{ L} = 250 \text{ mL}$$

To convert units of measurement within the household system, consult an equivalence table. For example, when converting fluid ounces to quarts, you first need to know that 32 ounces is the equivalent of 1 quart. To convert 8 ounces to a quart measurement, divide 8 by 32 to get the equivalent, ¼ or 0.25 quart.

Conversion Between Systems.
The conversion between systems is becoming less common because of the ISMP (2020a) recommendations for use of the metric system for liquid medication dosing. Even though health care providers are encouraged to order using the metric system, you may encounter a situation in which you calculate the correct dose of a medication by converting weights or volumes from one system of measurement to another. For example, metric units are sometimes converted to equivalent household measures for medication administration at home. To convert from one measurement system to another, always use equivalent measurements. Tables of equivalent measurements are available in all health care agencies. The pharmacist is also a good resource.

Dose Calculations.
Dosage calculation methods include the ratio and proportion method, the formula method, and dimensional analysis. Use the method that is the most logical and comfortable for you. Use this same method consistently. Before you begin any calculation, make a mental estimate of the approximate and reasonable dosage. If your estimate does not closely match the answer you calculate, you need to recheck your math before preparing and administering the medication. Many nursing students feel uncomfortable or anxious when they need to do medication calculations. To enhance accuracy and decrease your anxiety, think critically about the steps you go through when calculating medications, and practice doing calculations to feel more confident about your math skills.

Most health care agencies require a nurse to double-check calculations with another nurse before giving medications, especially when the risk for giving the wrong medication dose is high (e.g., heparin or insulin). Always have another nurse or health care professional double-check your work if the answer to a medication calculation seems unreasonable or inappropriate.

The Ratio and Proportion Method. A ratio indicates the relationship between two numbers separated by a colon (:). The colon in the ratio indicates the need to use division. Think of a ratio as a fraction; the number to the left is the numerator, and the number to the right is the denominator. For example, the ratio 1:2 is the same as 1/2. A proportion is an equation that has two ratios of equal value. Write a proportion in one of three ways:

Example 1: 1:2 = 4:8
Example 2: 1:2::4:8
Example 3: 1/2 = 4/8

In a proportion the first and last numbers are called the *extremes,* and the second and third numbers are called the *means.* When multiplying the extremes, the answer is the same as when multiplying the means. For example, in the previous proportions, multiplying the extremes ($1 \times 8 = 8$) yields the same result as multiplying the means ($2 \times 4 = 8$). Because of this relationship, if you know three of the numbers in the proportion, calculating the unknown fourth number is easy. The numbers need to all be in the same unit and system of measurement. To solve a calculation using the ratio and proportion method, first estimate the answer in your mind. Then set up the proportion, labeling all the terms. Put the terms of the ratio in the same sequence (e.g., mg:mL = mg:mL). Cross-multiply the means and the extremes and divide both sides by the number before the *x* to obtain the dosage. *Always* label the answer; if the answer is not close to your estimate, recheck the calculation.

Example: The health care provider orders 500 mg of amoxicillin to be administered in a gastric tube every 8 hours. The bottle of amoxicillin is labeled 400 mg/5 mL. Use the following steps to calculate how much amoxicillin to give:

1. **Estimate the answer:** The amount to be given is a little more than the labeled dose per 5 mL (unit dose) that is provided in the solution; therefore the answer is a little more than 5 mL.
2. **Set up the** proportion:

$$\frac{400 \text{mg}}{5 \text{mL}} = \frac{500 \text{mg}}{x \text{mL}}$$

3. **Cross-multiply the means and the extremes:**
$$400x = 500 \times 5$$
$$400x = 2500$$

4. **Divide both sides by the number before *x*:**
$$\frac{400x}{400} = \frac{2500}{400}$$
$$x = \frac{2500}{400}$$
$$x = 6.25 \text{ mL}$$

5. **Compare the estimate in Step 1 with the answer in Step 4:** The answer (6.25 mL) is close to the estimated amount (a little more than 5 mL). Therefore you prepare and administer 6.25 mL in the patient's gastric tube.

The Formula Method. Using the formula method requires you to first memorize the formula. Estimate the answer and then place all the information from the medication order into the formula. Label all the parts of the formula and ensure that all measures in the formula are in the same units and system of measurement before calculating the dosage. If the measures are not in the same measurement system, convert the numbers to the same system before calculating the dose. Calculate and label the answer and compare the answer with the estimated answer. If the estimate is not similar to the answer, recheck the calculation. Use the following basic formula when using the formula method:

$$\frac{\text{Dose ordered}}{\text{Dose on hand}} \times \text{Amount on hand} = \text{Amount to administer}$$

The dose ordered is the amount of medication prescribed. The dose on hand is the dose (e.g., mg, units) of medication supplied by the pharmacy. The amount on hand is the basic unit or quantity of the medication that contains the dose on hand. For solid medications, the amount on hand is often one capsule; the amount of liquid on hand is sometimes 1 mL or 1 L, depending on the container. For example, a liquid medication comes in the strength of 125 mg per 5 mL. In this case 125 mg is the dose on hand, and 5 mL is the amount on hand. The amount to administer is the actual amount of medication the nurse administers. Always express the amount to administer in the same unit as the amount on hand.

Example: The health care provider orders morphine sulfate 2 mg IV. The medication is available in a vial containing 10 mg/mL. The formula is applied as follows:

1. **Estimate the answer:** The medication is a liquid; therefore the answer will be in milliliters (mL). The amount to be given is less than ½ of the available dose on hand; therefore the answer will be less than ½ mL.

2. **Set up the formula:**

$$\frac{\text{Dose ordered}}{\text{Dose on hand}} \times \text{Amount on hand} = \text{Amount to administer}$$

$$\frac{2\,\text{mg}}{10\,\text{mg}} \times \text{mL} = \text{Amount to administer}$$

3. **Calculate the answer:**

$$\frac{2\,\text{mg}}{10\,\text{mg}} \times 1\,\text{mL} = 0.2\,\text{mL}$$

4. **Compare the estimate in Step 1 with the answer in Step 3:** The answer is less than ½ mL; therefore it is close to the estimated answer. Prepare 0.2 mL of the medication in a syringe and administer it to the patient.

Dimensional Analysis. Dimensional analysis is the factor-label or the unit-factor method. There is no need to memorize a formula because only one equation is needed, and the same steps are used in solving every medication calculation. Nursing students who use dimensional analysis to calculate medication dosages often find it easier to calculate medications than when they use the formula method. Use the following steps to calculate medication doses by dimensional analysis:

1. Identify the unit of measure that you need to administer. For example, if you are giving a pill, you usually give a tablet or a capsule; for parenteral or liquid oral medications, the unit is milliliters.
2. Estimate the answer.
3. Place the name or appropriate abbreviation for *x* on the left side of the equation (e.g., *x* tab, *x* mL).
4. Place available information from the problem in a fraction format on the right side of the equation. Place the abbreviation or unit that matches what you are going to administer (determined in Step 1) in the numerator.
5. Look at the medication order and add other factors into the problem. Set up the numerator so it matches the unit in the previous denominator.

6. Cancel out like units of measurement on the right side of the equation. You should end up with only one unit left in the equation, and it should match the unit on the left side of the equation.
7. Reduce to the lowest terms if possible and solve the problem or solve for *x*. Label your answer.
8. Compare your estimate from Step 1 with your answer in Step 2.

Example: The health care provider orders 0.45 g penicillin V potassium through a gastric tube. The vial label reads: penicillin V potassium 125 mg/5 mL.

1. **Identify the unit of measure that you need to administer.** This medication is given in a gastric tube, which is a liquid medication; therefore the answer will be in milliliters (mL).
2. **Estimate the answer.** The medication order is more than 3 times but less than 4 times the unit dose in the vial; therefore the answer is more than 15 mL but less than 20 mL.
3. **Place the name or appropriate abbreviation for *x* on the left side of the equation.**

$$x\,\text{mL} =$$

4. **Place available information from the problem in a fraction format on the right side of the equation.** Because the medication will be administered in milliliters, place mL in the numerator.

$$x\,\text{mL} = \frac{5\,\text{mL}}{125\,\text{mg}}$$

5. **Look at the medication order and add other factors into the problem.** Set up the numerator so it matches the unit in the previous denominator. The order is for 0.45 g, and the medication is available in 125-mg bottles. Knowing that 1 g = 1000 mg, add this conversion to the calculation.

$$x\,\text{mL} = \frac{5\,\text{mL}}{125\,\text{mg}} \times \frac{1000\,\text{mg}}{1\,\text{g}} \times \frac{0.45\,\text{g}}{1}$$

6. **Cancel out like units of measurement on the right side of the equation.**

$$x\,\text{mL} = \frac{5\,\text{mL}}{125\,\cancel{\text{mg}}} \times \frac{1000\,\cancel{\text{mg}}}{1\,\cancel{\text{g}}} \times \frac{0.45\,\cancel{\text{g}}}{1}$$

7. **Reduce to the lowest terms if possible and solve the problem or solve for *x*.** Label your answer.

$$x\,\text{mL} = \frac{5 \times 1000 \times 0.45}{125}$$

$$x = \frac{2250}{125}$$

$$x = 18\,\text{mL}$$

8. **Compare the estimate from Step 2 with the answer in Step 7.** The calculated answer is 18 mL, which is between 15 mL and 20 mL. This matches the estimate made in Step 2. Prepare and administer 18 mL of medication as ordered.

Pediatric Doses. Current evidence shows that children are at a much higher risk for experiencing a medication error than adults, and medication errors in children have a much greater chance of causing serious and even fatal consequences. To prevent medication errors in children (Beal, 2017; Hockenberry et al., 2019; Zhu and Weingart, 2020):

- Use only the metric system on prescriptions, medication labels, and dosing instruments.
- Never administer medications using household spoons.
- Round all dosing instructions to the nearest 0.1, 0.5, or 1 mL.

- Medication needs to be tailored based on age, weight, and body mass index (BMI).
- Provide education using hands-on demonstration and return demonstration.
- Consider using picture-based education if low health literacy is a possibility.

Calculating children's medication doses requires caution (Hockenberry et al., 2019). Even small errors or discrepancies in medication amounts can negatively affect a child's health. A child's age, weight, and maturity of body systems affect the ability to metabolize and excrete medications. Nurses sometimes have difficulty in evaluating a child's response to a medication, especially when the child cannot communicate verbally. For example, a side effect of vancomycin is ototoxicity, which affects hearing acuity. If a child cannot talk yet, it is challenging to assess for ototoxicity. Use the following guidelines when calculating pediatric doses:

1. Most pediatric medications are ordered in milligrams per kilogram (mg/kg). Therefore weigh the patient in kilograms before administering medications. Avoid converting the patient's weight from pounds to kilograms to prevent errors.
2. Pediatric doses are usually a lot smaller than adult doses for the same medication. You frequently use micrograms and small syringes (e.g., tuberculin or 1 mL).
3. IM doses are very small and usually do not exceed 1 mL in small children or 0.5 mL in infants.
4. Subcutaneous dosages are also very small and do not usually exceed 0.5 mL.
5. Most medications are not rounded to the nearest tenth. Instead, they are rounded to the nearest thousandth.
6. Measure dosages that are less than 1 mL in syringes that are marked in tenths of a milliliter if the dosage calculation comes out even and does not need to be rounded. Use a tuberculin syringe for medication preparation when the medication needs to be rounded to the nearest thousandth.
7. Estimate the patient's dose before beginning the calculation; label and compare the answer with the estimate before preparing the medication.
8. To determine if a dose is safe before giving the medication, compare and evaluate the amount of medication ordered over 24 hours with the recommended dosage.

Different formulas and methods are used to calculate medication dosages in children. The two most common methods of calculating pediatric dosages are based on a child's weight or BSA. BSA is used in rare situations (e.g., determining chemotherapy doses). Refer to a pediatric or pharmacology resource and consult with the patient's health care provider or the pharmacist if you must calculate a medication based on BSA.

Most of the time you calculate medications based on a child's weight. You can use the ratio and proportion method, the formula method, or dimensional analysis to calculate a pediatric dose using body weight. Refer to the previous sections on ratio and proportion, formula method, and dimensional analysis to select the method easiest for you to use.

Health Care Provider's Role

A physician, nurse practitioner, or physician's assistant prescribes medications by writing an order on a form in a patient's medical record, in an order book, or on a legal prescription pad. Some health care providers use a desktop, laptop, or handheld electronic device to enter medication orders. Many health care agencies implement computerized physician order entry (CPOE) to handle medication orders to decrease medication errors (Zhu and Weingart, 2020). In these systems the health care provider completes all computerized fields before

---

> ### BOX 31.3   Guidelines for Telephone and Verbal Orders
>
> - Only authorized staff receive and record telephone or verbal orders. The health care agency identifies in writing the staff who are authorized.
> - Clearly identify patient's name, room number, and diagnosis.
> - Read back all orders to health care provider (TJC, 2021).
> - Use clarification questions to avoid misunderstandings.
> - Write "TO" (telephone order) or "VO" (verbal order), including date and time, name of patient, and complete order; sign the name of the health care provider and nurse.
> - Follow agency policies; some agencies require documentation of the "read-back" or require two nurses to review and sign telephone or verbal orders.
> - The health care provider co-signs the order within the time frame required by the agency (usually 24 hours; verify agency policy).

the order for the medication is filled, thus avoiding incomplete or illegible orders.

Sometimes a health care provider orders a medication by telephone or by talking to a nurse in person. An order for a medication or medical treatment made over the telephone is called a *telephone order*. If the order is given verbally to the nurse, it is called a **verbal order**. When a verbal or telephone order is received, the nurse who took the order writes the complete order or enters it into a computer, reads it back, and receives confirmation from the health care provider to confirm accuracy. The nurse indicates the time and the name of the health care provider who gave the order, signs it, and follows agency policy to indicate that it was read back. The health care provider countersigns the order later, usually within 24 hours after giving it. Follow guidelines for taking telephone or verbal orders for medications safely (Box 31.3). Agency policies vary regarding personnel who can take telephone or verbal orders. Nursing students cannot take medication orders of any kind. They give newly ordered medications only after a registered nurse (RN) has written and verified the order.

Common abbreviations are often used when writing orders. Abbreviations indicate dosage frequencies or times, routes of administration, and special information for giving the medication (see Table 31.3). Medication errors frequently involve the use of abbreviations. Table 31.7 lists abbreviations that are associated with a high incidence of medication errors. Do *not* use these abbreviations when documenting medication orders or other information about medications (ISMP, 2017a; The Joint Commission [TJC], 2020). Sometimes abbreviations used by different agencies vary. Check agency policy to determine which abbreviations are acceptable to use and their meaning.

> **QSEN** **Building Competency in Safety** The health care provider has written the following orders for a 4-year-old patient with otitis media of the right ear. Which orders do you need to clarify before administering the medication? Provide a rationale for your answers and rewrite the order so that it follows the ISMP current medication order safety guidelines.
>
> Floxin otic solution AS twice a day
>
> Amoxicillin 25 mg/kg/day in divided doses
>
> Acetaminophen 1 teaspoon for fever greater than 38.3°C (101°F)
>
> Answers to QSEN Activities can be found on the Evolve website.

Types of Orders in Acute Care Agencies

A medication cannot be given to a patient without a health care provider order. The frequency and urgency of medication administration forms the basis for medication orders. Some conditions change the

TABLE 31.7 Prohibited and Error-Prone Abbreviations[a]

The abbreviations, symbols, and dose designations found in this table have been reported to the Institute for Safe Medication Practices (ISMP) through the USP-ISMP Medication Error Reporting Program as being frequently misinterpreted and involved in harmful medication errors. They should NEVER be used when communicating medical information. This includes internal communications, telephone/verbal prescriptions, computer-generated labels, labels for medication storage bins, medication administration records, and pharmacy and prescriber computer order entry screens. The Joint Commission (TJC) has established a National Patient Safety Goal that specifies that certain abbreviations must appear on the "do not use" list of the accredited organization; they are highlighted with a superscript letter b ([b]). However, we hope that you will consider others beyond the minimum TJC requirements. By using and promoting safe practices and educating one another about hazards, we can better protect our patients.

Abbreviations	Intended Meaning	Misinterpretation	Correction
μg	Microgram	Mistaken as "mg"	Use "mcg"
AD, AS, AU	Right ear, left ear, each ear	Mistaken as OD, OS, OU (right eye, left eye, each eye)	Use "right ear," "left ear," or "each ear"
OD, OS, OU	Right eye, left eye, each eye	Mistaken as AD, AS, AU (right ear, left ear, each ear)	Use "right eye," "left eye," or "each eye"
BT	Bedtime	Mistaken as "BID" (twice daily)	Use "bedtime"
HS	Half-strength	Mistaken as bedtime	Use "half-strength" or "bedtime"
hs	At bedtime, hours of sleep	Mistaken as half-strength	Use "bedtime" or "half-strength"
IU[b]	International unit	Mistaken as IV (intravenous) or 10 (ten)	Use "units"
o.d. or OD	Once daily	Mistaken as "right eye" (OD—oculus dexter), leading to oral liquid medications administered in the eye	Use "daily"
Per os	By mouth, orally	The "os" can be mistaken as "left eye" (OS—oculus sinister)	Use "PO," "by mouth," or "orally"
q.d. or QD[b]	Every day	Mistaken as q.i.d., especially if the period after the "q" or the tail of the "q" is misunderstood as an "I"	Use "daily"
qhs	Nightly at bedtime	Mistaken as "qhr" or every hour	Use "nightly"
SC, SQ, sub q	Subcutaneous	SC mistaken as SL (sublingual); SQ mistaken as "5 every"; the "q" in "sub q" has been mistaken as "every" (e.g., a heparin dose ordered "sub q 2 hours before surgery" misunderstood as every 2 hours before surgery)	Use "subcut" or "subcutaneously"
TIW or tiw	3 times a week	Mistaken as "3 times a day" or "twice in a week"	Use "3 times weekly"
U or u[b]	Unit	Mistaken as the number 0 or 4, causing a 10-fold overdose or greater (e.g., 4 U seen as "40" or 4 u seen as "44"); mistaken as "cc" so dose given in volume instead of units (e.g., 4 u seen as 4 cc)	Use "unit"

Dose Designations and Other Information

Trailing zero after decimal point (e.g., 1.0 mg)[c]	1 mg	Mistaken as 10 mg if the decimal point is not seen	Do not use trailing zeros for doses expressed in whole numbers
"Naked" decimal point (e.g., .5 mg)[b]	0.5 mg	Mistaken as 5 mg if the decimal point is not seen	Use zero before a decimal point when the dose is less than a whole unit
Abbreviations such as mg. or mL. with a period following the abbreviation	mg mL	The period is unnecessary and could be mistaken as the number 1 if written poorly	Use mg, mL, etc. without a terminal period

Drug Name Abbreviations

HCl	Hydrochloric acid or hydrochloride	Mistaken as potassium chloride (the "H" is misinterpreted as "K")	Use complete drug name unless expressed as a salt of a drug
HCT	Hydrocortisone	Mistaken as hydrochlorothiazide	Use complete drug name
HCTZ	Hydrochlorothiazide	Mistaken as hydrocortisone (seen as HCT250 mg)	Use complete drug name
MgSO4[b]	Magnesium sulfate	Mistaken as morphine sulphate	Use complete drug name
MS, MSO4[b]	Morphine sulfate	Mistaken as magnesium sulphate	Use complete drug name
PCA	Procainamide	Mistaken as patient-controlled analgesia	Use complete drug name

Stemmed Drug Names

"Nitro" drip	nitroglycerin infusion	Mistaken as sodium nitroprusside infusion	Use complete drug name

Continued

Abbreviations	Intended Meaning	Misinterpretation	Correction
Symbols			
3	Dram	Symbol for dram mistaken as "3"	Use metric system
×3d	For 3 days	Mistaken as "3 doses"	Use "for three days"
> and <	Greater than and less than	Mistaken as opposite of intended; mistakenly use incorrect symbol; "<10" mistaken as "40"	Use "greater than" or "less than"
@	At	Mistaken as "2"	Use "at"
&	And	Mistaken as "2"	Use "and"
+	Plus or and	Mistaken as "4"	Use "and"
°	Hour	Mistaken as a zero (e.g., q2° seen as q20)	Use "hr," "h," or "hour"

TABLE 31.7   Prohibited and Error-Prone Abbreviations—cont'd

aApplies to all orders and medication-related documentation that is handwritten (including free-text computer entry or on preprinted forms).
bThese abbreviations are included on TJC "minimum list" of dangerous abbreviations, acronyms, and symbols that must be included on the "do not use" list of an organization.
cException: A "trailing zero" may be used only where required to show precision of a reported value (e.g., laboratory test results), in studies that report the size of lesions, or for catheter and tube sizes. A trailing zero cannot be used in medication orders or medication-related documentation (ISMP, 2017a).
From The Joint Commission (TJC): *Official "Do not use" list,* 2020. https://www.jointcommission.org/-/media/tjc/documents/fact-sheets/do-not-use-list-8-3-20.pdf?db=web&hash=2489CB1616A30CFFBDAAD1FB3F8021A5&hash=2489CB1616A30CFFBDAAD1FB3F8021A5. Accessed August 17, 2021.

status of a patient's medication orders. For example, in some agencies a patient's preoperative medications are discontinued automatically, and the health care provider writes new medication orders after surgery (see Chapter 50). Agency policies that surround medication orders vary. Nurses need to be aware of and follow these policies.

Standing Orders or Routine Medication Orders. A standing order is carried out until the health care provider cancels it by another order or a prescribed number of days elapse. Some standing orders indicate a final date or number of treatments or doses. Know your agency's policies surrounding the discontinuation of standing orders. The following are examples of standing orders:

Tetracycline 500 mg PO q6h

Decadron 10 mg daily × 5 days

prn Orders. Sometimes the health care provider orders a medication to be given only when a patient requires it. This is a prn order. Use objective and subjective assessment (e.g., severity of pain, body temperature) and clinical judgment in determining whether the patient needs the medication. An example of a prn order is:

Morphine sulfate 2 mg IV q2h prn for incisional pain

This order indicates that the patient needs to wait at least 2 hours between doses and can take the medication if experiencing pain at the incision. When administering prn medications, document assessment findings to show why the patient needs the medication and the time of administration. Frequently evaluate the effectiveness of the medication, and record evaluation data appropriately. Unclear orders for prn medications that include a range (e.g., morphine sulfate IM 5–10 mg every 4–6 hours) are a source of medication errors. If a range order is written, ensure that the order follows agency policy for these types of orders. An example of a safer range order is to increase morphine dosage 50% to 100% if pain is moderate to severe based on use of the agency pain scale.

When multiple prn medications with the same action are ordered, the orders need to identify when to use each medication and how to use the medications in relationship to each other. The order below

provides an example of a safe prn order for two medications used for treatment of constipation:

Docusate 100 mg PO TID prn constipation for two days and if no results then administer magnesium hydroxide 30 mL PO prn constipation

Single (One-Time) Orders. Sometimes a health care provider orders a medication to be given once at a specified time. This is common for preoperative medications or medications given before diagnostic examinations. The following is an example of a single order:

Lorazepam 1 mg IV on call to MRI

STAT Orders. A STAT order signifies that a single dose of a medication is to be given immediately and only once. STAT orders are often written for emergencies when a patient's condition changes suddenly. For example:

Hydralazine 10 mg IV STAT

Now Orders. A now order is more specific than a one-time order and is used when a patient needs a medication quickly but not right away, as in a STAT order. When receiving a now order, the nurse has up to 90 minutes to administer the medication. Only administer now medications one time. For example:

Vancomycin 1 g IV piggyback now

Prescriptions. The health care provider writes prescriptions for patients who are to take medications outside the agency. The prescription includes more detailed information than a medication order because the patient needs to understand how to take the medication and when to refill the prescription if necessary. Some agencies require health care providers to write prescriptions for controlled substances on a special prescription pad that is different (e.g., a different color) than the prescription pad used for other medications.

Pharmacist's Role

The pharmacist prepares and distributes prescribed medications. Pharmacists work with nurses, physicians, and other health care providers to evaluate the effectiveness of patients' medications. They are responsible for filling prescriptions accurately and being sure that prescriptions are valid. Pharmacists in health care agencies rarely mix compounds or solutions, except in the case of IV solutions. Most medication companies deliver medications in a form ready for use. Dispensing the correct medication, in the proper dosage and amount, with an accurate label is the pharmacist's main task. Pharmacists also provide information about medication side effects, toxicity, interactions, and incompatibilities.

Distribution Systems

Systems for storing and distributing medications vary. Health care agencies have a special area for stocking and dispensing medications. Examples of storage areas include special medication rooms, portable locked carts, computerized medication cabinets, and individual storage units next to patients' rooms. Medication storage areas need to be locked when unattended.

Unit Dose. A unit-dose system is a storage system that varies by health care agency. Pharmacists provide the medications in single-unit packages that contain the ordered dose of medication that a patient receives at one time. Nurses distribute the medications to patients. Each tablet or capsule is wrapped separately. Usually no more than a 24-hour supply of medication is available at any given time. Some unit-dose systems use carts containing a drawer with a 24-hour supply of medications for each patient. Each drawer is labeled with the name of the patient in the patient's designated room. At a designated time each day, the pharmacist or a pharmacy technician refills the drawers in the cart with a fresh medication supply. The cart also contains limited amounts of prn and stock medications for special situations. Controlled substances are not kept in an individual patient drawer. Instead, they are kept in a larger locked drawer to keep them secure. The unit-dose system reduces medication errors, decreases the amount of medication that is stocked in patient care areas, and saves time for nurses and pharmacists.

Automated Medication Dispensing Systems. Automated medication dispensing systems (AMDSs) are used throughout the country (Fig. 31.5). The systems within an agency are networked with one another and with other agency computer systems (e.g., computerized medical record). AMDSs control the dispensing of all medications, including narcotics. Each nurse accesses the system by entering a security code. Some systems require bio-identification as well. In these systems you place your finger on a screen to access the computer. You select the patient's name and medication profile before the AMDS dispenses a medication. In these systems you can select the desired medication, dosage, and route from a list displayed on the computer screen. The system causes the drawer containing medication to open, records it, and charges it to the patient. Systems that are connected to the patient's computerized medical record then record information about the medication (e.g., medication name, dose, time) and the nurse's name in the patient's medical record. The bar-code medication administration (BCMA) system is often used with AMDSs. BCMA requires nurses to scan bar codes to identify the patient, the medication, and an identification tag of the nurse administering the medication before recording this information in the patient's computerized medical record. Agencies that implement AMDSs with BCMA often reduce the incidence of medication errors (see Box 31.2).

Special Handling of Controlled Substances

As a nurse, you are responsible for following all legal regulations when administering controlled substances (medications with potential for abuse). Controlled substances must be properly stored to prevent diversion. Violations of the Controlled Substances Act may result in fines, imprisonment, and loss of license. Health care agencies have policies for

FIG. 31.5 Automated medication dispensing system (AMDS). (From Davis K, Guerra T: *Mosby's pharmacy technician: principles and practice,* ed 5, St Louis, 2019, Elsevier.)

the proper storage and distribution of controlled substances, including opioids. Most agencies use computerized systems for medication access and distribution.

Handling Chemotherapy Medications

A common treatment for cancer is chemotherapy, antineoplastic drugs that act by killing cells that divide rapidly, one of the main properties of most cancer cells. Chemotherapy is administered in both IV and oral forms. In 2016 the American Oncology Association in conjunction with the Oncology Nursing Society (ONS) updated the chemotherapy administration standards to improve both patient and nurse safety related to administration of these medications (ONS, 2018; ONS, 2019). Nurses must undergo certification to administer IV chemotherapy. However, oral chemotherapy is becoming more common and can be administered by any RN.

Oral chemotherapy has the same exposure risks to health care providers, patients, and their family caregivers as IV forms (Neuss et al., 2017). Physically touching a chemotherapy tablet is dangerous. Chemotherapy is highly toxic not only to cancer cells but also to normal cells. Chemotherapy drugs cause DNA damage leading to cell death or cell growth arrest. The damage to others may not be known for months or years because the injuries could include cancer, birth defects, or immune dysfunction. It is critical for health care providers, patients, and family caregivers to use proper protective techniques to avoid exposure to oral chemotherapy tablets.

A patient excretes chemotherapy chemicals through urine, stool, vomit, sweat, and saliva. When patients self-administer chemotherapy at home, families should be warned of the dangers of exposure. For example, patients' toilets should be double-flushed after use, during and for 48 hours after discontinuing chemotherapy. Toilets are a hazard for children and pets.

Accidental exposure to oral chemotherapeutic agents can occur during handling (i.e., unpacking, storage, handling, administration, and disposal) (Neuss et al., 2017). Guidelines for health care providers, patients, and family caregivers to handle these drugs safely and appropriately are essential:

- In health care agencies, cytotoxic agents should be stored in a designated area per the manufacturer's instructions and separate from noncytotoxic agents.
- Use gloves that have been tested for chemotherapy or hazardous medication use and double glove when indicated when preparing and handling chemotherapy medications and after handling agent or bodily secretions (Eisenberg, 2018; ONS, 2018).
- Perform thorough hand hygiene before and after glove application.
- Do not crush, cut, or split chemotherapy drugs.
- Use separate equipment to prepare chemotherapy and regular medications. Nurses must now use closed-system transfer devices when administering IV chemotherapy (Eisenberg, 2018).
- The health care agency must have a spill policy in place (Eisenberg, 2018).
- All disposable protective clothing is considered a single-use item (Eisenberg, 2018). Protective clothing, as well as any disposable materials used while handling chemotherapeutic agents, should be disposed of as cytotoxic waste according to the local waste disposal regulatory guidelines.
- Any clothes or sheets that have body fluids on them should be washed in a washing machine—not by hand. Wash them twice in hot water with regular laundry detergent. Do not wash them with other clothes. If they cannot be washed right away, seal them in a plastic bag.

Nurse's Role

Administering medications requires unique nursing knowledge, clinical judgment, and skills. You first determine that the medication ordered is the correct medication. As a nurse you need to assess the patient's ability to self-administer medications, determine whether a patient should receive a medication at a given time, administer medications correctly, and then closely monitor their effects. Do not delegate any part of the medication administration process to assistive personnel (AP) and use the nursing process to integrate medication therapy into care.

Patient and family caregiver education about proper medication administration and monitoring is an integral part of your role. Begin instruction about medications that the patient will be taking home as soon as possible. This often does not occur until the day of discharge, but if you can obtain this information sooner, the patient will benefit.

Medication Errors

The National Coordinating Council for Medication Error Reporting and Prevention (2021) defines a medication error as any preventable event that may cause inappropriate medication use or jeopardize patient safety. Medication errors include inaccurate prescribing, administering the wrong medication, giving the medication using the wrong route or time interval, administering extra doses, and/or failing to administer a medication. Preventing medication errors is essential. The process of administering medications has many steps and involves many members of the health care team. Because nurses play an essential role in preparing and administering medications, they need to be vigilant in preventing errors

---

BOX 31.4 Steps to Take to Prevent Medication Errors

- Follow the seven rights of medication administration.
- Prepare medications for only one patient at a time.
- Be sure to read labels at least 3 times (comparing medication administration record [MAR] with label): (1) when removing medication from storage, (2) before taking to patient's room, and (3) before giving medication.
- Use at least two patient identifiers every time you administer medications (e.g., patient name, birthday, agency number) whenever administering a medication (TJC, 2021).
- Do not allow any other activity to interrupt administration of medication to a patient (e.g., phone call, pager, discussion with other staff).
- Double-check all calculations and other high-risk medication administration processes (e.g., patient-controlled analgesia) and verify with another nurse.
- Question unusually large or small doses.
- Do not interpret illegible handwriting; clarify with the health care provider.
- Document all medications as soon as they are given.
- When you have made or discovered an error, reflect on what went wrong and ask how you could have prevented it. Complete an occurrence report per agency policy.
- Evaluate the context or situation in which a medication error occurred. This helps to determine whether nurses have the necessary resources for safe medication administration.
- When repeated medication errors occur within a work area, identify and analyze the factors that may have caused the errors and take corrective action.
- Attend in-service education programs on the medications you commonly administer.
- Ensure that you are well rested when caring for patients. Nurses make more errors when they are tired.
- Involve and educate patients when administering medications. Address patients' concerns about medications before administering them (e.g., concerns about their appearance or side effects).
- Follow established agency policies and procedures when using technology to administer medications (e.g., automated medication dispensing system [AMDS] and bar-code scanning). Medication errors occur when nurses "work around" the technology (e.g., override alerts without thinking about them) (Zhu and Weingart, 2020).

(Box 31.4). Advances in health care informatics have helped to decrease the occurrence of medication errors (Box 31.5).

Medication errors can be caused by many factors, such as technology work-arounds, the design of medication labels, and medication distribution systems. When an error occurs, the patient's safety and well-being are the top priorities. You first assess and examine the patient's condition and notify the health care provider of the incident as soon as possible. Once the patient is stable, report the incident to the appropriate person in the agency (e.g., manager or supervisor). You are responsible for preparing and filing an occurrence or incident report as soon as possible after the error occurs. The report includes patient identification information; the location and time of the incident; an accurate, factual description of what occurred, and the actions taken; and your signature. The occurrence report is not a permanent part of the medical record and is not referred to anywhere in a patient's medical record to legally protect the nurse and health care agency (see Chapters 23 and 26). Occurrence reports track incident patterns and indicate the need to implement quality improvement actions.

Report all medication errors that reach the patient, including those that do not cause harm. You also need to report near misses. For example,

BOX 31.5 Informatics and Medication Safety

Many medication errors occur when a nurse incorrectly administers medications at the patient's bedside. The following innovations and advances in technology have helped reduce the number of medication errors in nursing practice.

- Networked computers allow all the patient's health care providers to see a current list of ordered and discontinued medications.
- Internet and intranet access allows nurses and other health care providers to access current information about medications (e.g., indications, desired effects, adverse effects) and specific agency policies that address medication administration (e.g., how fast to administer an intravenous [IV] push medication, how to administer medications through a nasogastric tube).
- In some agencies health care providers use computerized physician order entry (CPOE), allowing them to enter medication orders directly into a networked computer system or a personal handheld computer (Zhu and Weingart, 2020).
- Automated medication dispensers (AMDs) and electronic medication administration records (eMARs) help with medication reconciliation, administration, and documentation (Zhu and Weingart, 2020).
- Bar-coding technology requires nurses to scan the medication, the patient's identification bracelet, and the nurse's identification badge before administering the medication, which helps ensure the seven rights of medication administration.

Application to Nursing Practice

- Actively participate in selecting and evaluating advanced technologies and creating nursing policies and protocols used for medication administration.
- Always follow agency policies when administering medications.
- Implement agency policies when the technology cannot be used (e.g., during down time or power outages).
- Follow manufacturer guidelines for care of electronic equipment, and report problems with technology immediately.

BOX 31.6 Process for Medication Reconciliation

1. **Obtain, Verify, Document:** Obtain a comprehensive and current list of a patient's medications whenever the patient experiences a change in health care setting (e.g., during admission, transfer, discharge). Include all current prescriptions, over-the-counter (OTC) medications, and homeopathic products.
2. **Consider and Compare:** Review what the patient was taking at home or preadmission, and make sure that the list of medications, dosages, and frequencies is accurate. Compare this list to the current ordered medications and treatment plan to ensure accuracy. Include family caregiver in this discussion when appropriate.
3. **Reconcile:** Compare new medication orders with the current list; investigate any discrepancies with the patient's health care provider. Document any changes.
4. **Communicate:** Ensure that all the patient's health care providers have the most updated list of medications. Communicate and verify changes in medications as with the patient.

Data from Zhu J, Weingart S: *Prevention of adverse drug events in hospitals, UpToDate,* 2020. https://www.uptodate.com/contents/prevention-of-adverse-drug-events-in-hospitals. Accessed August 17, 2021.

accepting the patient. The nurse on the rehabilitation unit reconciles the patient's medications when the patient is discharged with the home health nurse. Many agencies have computerized or written forms to facilitate the process of medication reconciliation. The process is challenging and takes a lot of time and concentration. Eliminate distractions and go slowly when reconciling patients' medications. Always clarify information when needed and question for accuracy. Accurate medication reconciliation requires consulting with the patient, family caregivers, other clinicians, pharmacists, and other members of the health care team.

CRITICAL THINKING

Knowledge

Successful critical thinking requires a synthesis of knowledge, experience, environmental factors, critical thinking attitudes, and intellectual and professional standards. Sound clinical judgment requires you to anticipate the information, analyze the data, and make decisions regarding your patient's care. You use knowledge from many disciplines when administering medications. Your knowledge helps you understand why a medication is prescribed for a patient and how it will alter the patient's physiology to have a therapeutic effect. For example, in physiology you learn that potassium is a major intracellular ion. When patients do not have enough potassium in their body (hypokalemia), they experience signs and symptoms such as muscle fatigue or weakness. In some cases, severe hypokalemia is fatal because of associated cardiac dysrhythmias. Prescribed medications help to restore the patient's potassium level to normal, which relieves the signs and symptoms of hypokalemia. In another example, knowledge about child development indicates that children often associate medication administration with a negative experience. Use principles from child development to ensure that the child cooperates with the medication experience.

Patients take a variety of medications, and new medications are constantly approved. As a result, you will not always understand all the medications ordered for a patient. Critical thinkers admit what they do not know and acquire the knowledge needed to safely administer unfamiliar medications. This means that when you do not know all the medications you need to administer, you will consult a reliable source (e.g., a more expert nurse, pharmacist, the health care provider, or a reference book) *before* administering the medication.

you are caring for a patient who has a urinary tract infection and is allergic to sulfa medications. The patient's health care provider orders trimethoprim/sulfamethoxazole (TMP/SMZ). You know TMP/SMZ contains sulfa. You contact the health care provider before you administer the medication to obtain an order for a different medication. This type of medication error is a near miss because it did not actually reach the patient. All health care workers, including nurses, need to feel comfortable in reporting an error and not fear repercussions from managers or administrators. Even when a patient suffers no harm from a medication error, the agency can still learn why the mistake occurred and what can be done to avoid similar errors in the future.

Some medication errors happen when patients experience a transition in care, such as when a patient is admitted or discharged from a health care agency, is transferred from an intensive care unit to a general patient care unit, or sees a new health care provider. During these times, the risk of unintended changes in medication orders increases. Therefore reconciling medication information is a key Hospital National Patient Safety Goal (TJC, 2021). During medication reconciliation, nurses, pharmacists, and other health care providers compare the medication that a patient is taking currently with what the patient should be taking and any newly ordered medications (Box 31.6). Throughout this process you identify and resolve orders that are duplicated and omitted. You also evaluate the risk for unintended medication interactions. Creating and maintaining an accurate list of all patient medications helps to ensure safe and effective patient care. For example, when you admit a patient who is having a hip replacement to an orthopedic unit, you compare the medications that the patient took at home with those ordered in the agency. When the patient is discharged to a rehabilitation unit, you communicate the patient's current medications with the nurse who is

Experience

Nursing students have limited experience with medication administration as it applies to professional practice. Clinical experiences give you opportunities to use the nursing process as it applies to medication administration. As you gain experience, your psychomotor skills ("the how-to") become more refined. However, psychomotor skills represent a small part of medication administration. Patient attitudes, knowledge, physical and mental status, and responses make medication administration a complex responsibility.

Attitudes

Use critical thinking to administer medications safely. Be disciplined and take adequate time to prepare and administer medications. Take the time to read your patient's medical record before administering medications, and carefully review the patient's history, physical examination findings, and orders. Look up medications that you do not know in a medication reference and determine why each patient is taking each of the prescribed medications. Every step of safe medication administration requires a disciplined attitude and a comprehensive, systematic approach. Following the same procedure each time medications are administered ensures safe administration.

Responsibility and accountability are other critical thinking attitudes essential to safe medication administration. Accept full accountability and responsibility for all actions surrounding the administration of medications. Do not assume that a medication that is ordered for a patient is the correct medication or the correct dose. Be responsible for knowing that the medications and doses ordered are correct and appropriate. You are accountable if you give an ordered medication that is not appropriate for a patient. It is important for you to be familiar with each medication, including its therapeutic effect, usual dosage, anticipated changes in laboratory data, and side effects. You are also responsible for ensuring that patients or caregivers who administer medications have been properly informed about all aspects of self-administration (TJC, 2021). If you determine that a patient cannot self-administer medications safely, design interventions such as involving family caregivers to ensure safe administration.

Environment

Determine environmental factors that will affect patient care. Prior to assessment, review the patient's medical record for new information (e.g., specific medication practices; new orders for medical equipment or therapies). Avoid time conflicts; for example, determine if additional personnel are needed for certain care activities or if additional therapies, medical equipment, or devices increase the length of time needed to administer medications.

Standards

Standards are actions that ensure safe nursing practice. Standards for medication administration are set by health care agencies and the nursing profession. Agency policy sets limits on a nurse's ability to administer medications in certain units of the acute care setting. Sometimes nurses are limited by certain medication routes or dosages. Most agencies have nursing procedure manuals and formularies that contain policies that define the types of medications nurses can and cannot administer. The types and dosages of some medications that nurses deliver vary from unit to unit within the same agency. For example, phenytoin, a medication for treating seizures, may be administered by mouth or IV push. In large dosages phenytoin affects heart rhythm. Because of this, some agencies place limits on how much nurses can administer to a patient on a nursing unit that does not have the ability to monitor a patient's heart rate and rhythm. Not all health care providers are aware of the limitations and sometimes prescribe medications that nurses cannot give in a particular health care setting. Recognize these limitations and inform the health care provider accordingly. Take appropriate actions to ensure that patients receive medications as prescribed and within the time prescribed in the appropriate environment.

Professional standards such as *Nursing: Scope and Standards of Practice* (American Nurses Association [ANA], 2021) (see Chapters 1 and 23) apply to the activity of medication administration. To prevent medication errors, follow the seven rights of medication administration consistently every time you administer medications. Many medication errors can be linked in some way to an inconsistency in adhering to these seven rights:

1. The right medication
2. The right dose
3. The right patient
4. The right route
5. The right time
6. The right documentation
7. The right indication

Right Medication. A medication order is required for every medication that you administer to a patient. Sometimes health care providers write orders by hand in the patient's medical record. Alternatively, some agencies use CPOE. CPOE allows a health care provider to order medications electronically, eliminating the need for written orders and enhancing medication safety (Zhu and Weingart, 2020). Regardless of how a medication order is received, the nurse compares the health care provider's written orders with the medication administration record (MAR) or electronic MAR (eMAR) when it is ordered initially. Nurses verify medication information whenever new MARs (or eMARs) are created or distributed or when patients transfer from one nursing unit or health care setting to another.

Once you determine that information on a patient's MAR is accurate, use it to prepare and administer medications. When preparing medications from bottles or containers, compare the label of the medication container with the MAR 3 times: (1) before removing the container from the drawer or shelf, (2) as the amount of medication ordered is removed from the container, and (3) at the patient's bedside before administering the medication to the patient. Never prepare medications from unmarked containers or containers with illegible labels (TJC, 2021). With unit-dose prepackaged medications, check the label with the MAR when taking medications out of the medication dispensing system. Finally, verify all medications at the patient's bedside with the patient's MAR and use at least two identifiers before giving the patient any medications (TJC, 2021).

Patients who self-administer medications need to keep them in their original labeled containers, separate from other medications, to avoid confusion. To enhance accuracy and patient safety, many health care agencies require that nurses administer all medications rather than letting patients self-administer. Because the nurse who administers the medication is responsible for any errors related to it, nurses administer only the medications they prepare. You cannot delegate preparation of medication to another person and then administer the medication to the patient. If a patient questions the medication, do not ignore these concerns. A patient or a family caregiver familiar with a patient's medications often knows whether a medication is different from those received before. In most cases a patient's medication order has changed; however, sometimes patient questions reveal an error. When this occurs, withhold the medication, and recheck it against the health care provider's orders. If a patient refuses a medication, discard it rather than returning it to the original container. Unit-dose medications can be saved if they are not opened. If a patient refuses opioid or any controlled substance, follow proper agency procedure by having someone else witness the "wasted" medication.

Right Dose. The unit-dose system is designed to minimize errors. When preparing a medication from a larger volume or strength than needed or when the health care provider orders a system of measurement different from that which the pharmacy supplies, the chance of error increases. You need to have another qualified nurse check the calculated doses when performing medication calculations or conversions. Prepare medications using standard measurement devices such as graduated cups, syringes, and scaled droppers to measure medications accurately. Educate patients to use similar measurement devices at home, such as measuring spoons with metric calibrations rather than household teaspoons and tablespoons, which are inaccurate.

Medication errors occur when pills need to be split. Studies show that the accuracy of split tablets is questionable, even if a tablet is scored (ISMP, 2018a). In addition, in the home setting patients may assume that tablets in containers have already been split when they have not been or may split them again when they have been split already (ISMP, 2018a). The FDA (2020) developed suggestions to help patients split pills. They include ensuring that the tablet is designed to be split, using a tablet splitter, not splitting the entire prescription at one time, and determining whether the patient has the motor dexterity and visual acuity to split tablets. If possible, health care providers need to avoid ordering medications that require splitting.

Tablets are sometimes crushed and mixed with food. Be sure to completely clean a crushing device before crushing the tablet. Remnants of previously crushed medications increase the concentration of a medication or result in the patient receiving part of a medication that was not prescribed. Mix crushed medications with very small amounts of food or liquid (e.g., a single tablespoon). Do not use a patient's favorite foods or liquids because medications alter their taste and decrease the patient's desire for them. This is especially a concern for pediatric patients.

Not all medications are suitable for crushing. Some medications (e.g., extended-release capsules) have special coatings to prevent them from being absorbed too quickly. These medications should not be crushed. Refer to the "Do Not Crush List" (ISMP, 2020b) to ensure that a medication is safe to crush.

Right Patient. Medication errors often occur because a patient gets a medication intended for another patient. An important step in safe medication administration is being sure that you give the right medication to the right patient. It is difficult to remember every patient's name and face. Before administering a medication, use at least two patient identifiers (TJC, 2021). Acceptable patient identifiers include the patient's name, the medical record number assigned by a health care agency, or a telephone number. Do not use the patient's room number or physical complaint as an identifier. To identify a patient correctly, you usually compare the patient identifiers on the MAR with the patient's identification bracelet while at the patient's bedside. If an identification bracelet becomes smudged or illegible or is missing, obtain a new one. All agencies in all health care settings need to use a system that verifies the patient's identification with at least two identifiers before administering medications and other treatments.

Patients do not need to state their names and other identifiers when you administer medications. Collect patient identifiers reliably when the patient is admitted to a health care setting. Once the identifiers are assigned to the patient (e.g., putting identifiers on an armband and placing the armband on the patient), you use the identifiers to match the patient with the MAR, which lists the correct medications. Asking patients to state their full names and identification information provides a third way to verify that the nurse is giving medications to the right patient.

In addition to using two identifiers, some agencies use BCMA to help identify the right patient (Fig. 31.6). This system requires nurses to scan a personal bar code that is commonly placed on their name tag

FIG. 31.6 Nurse using bar-code scanner to identify patient during medication administration.

first. Then the nurse scans a bar code on the single-dose medication package. Finally, the nurse scans the patient's armband. All this information is then stored in a computer for documentation purposes. This system helps eliminate medication errors because it provides another step to ensure that the right patient receives the right medication (Zhu and Weingart, 2020).

Right Route. Always consult the health care provider if an order does not include a route of administration. Likewise alert the health care provider immediately if the specified route is not the recommended route. Recent evidence shows that medication errors involving the wrong route are common. For example, when nurses need to prepare an oral medication in a syringe, the risk to administer the medication via the wrong route (e.g., intravenously) is very high and often results in fatal consequences. Therefore the ISMP (2020a) recommends that pharmacists, *not nurses,* prepare all oral medications that are not prepared commercially as a unit product to enhance patient safety.

The accidental IV injection of a liquid designed for oral use produces local complications, such as sterile skin abscess, or systemic effects, such as a fatality. If you work in a setting that requires you to prepare oral medications, use only enteral syringes (e.g., ENFit) when you prepare oral medications. Enteral syringes often use a color different from the parenteral syringes and are clearly labeled for oral or enteral use. The syringe tips of enteral syringes will not connect with parenteral medication administration systems. Needles do not attach to enteral syringes, and the syringes cannot be inserted into any type of IV line. Label the syringe after preparing the medication and be sure to remove any caps from the tip of an oral syringe before administering the medication.

Right Time. To administer medications safely, you need to know why a medication is ordered for certain times of the day and whether you can alter the time schedule. For example, two medications are ordered, one q8h (every 8 hours) and the other 3 times a day. Both medications are scheduled for 3 times within a 24-hour period. You need to give the q8h medication every 8 hours ATC to maintain therapeutic blood levels of the medication. In contrast, you need to give the 3-times-a-day medication at 3 different times while the patient is awake. Each agency has a recommended time schedule for medications ordered at frequent intervals. You can alter these recommended times if necessary or appropriate.

The health care provider often gives specific instructions about when to administer a medication. A preoperative medication to be given "on call" means that you give the medication when the operating room staff members notify you that they are coming to get a patient for surgery. Give a medication ordered PC (after meals) within half an hour after a meal, when a patient has a full stomach. Give a STAT medication immediately.

Give priority to time-critical medications that must act and therefore be given at certain times. Hospitals designate which medications are time critical and which are non–time critical (ISMP, 2011; ISMP, 2020a). You administer time-critical medications within 30 minutes before or after their scheduled time. For example, give insulin (a time-critical medication) at a precise interval before a meal. Give antibiotics 30 minutes before or after they are scheduled ATC to maintain therapeutic blood levels. Give all routinely ordered non–time-critical medications within 1 to 2 hours before or after the scheduled time or per agency policy (Furnish and Wagner, 2020; ISMP, 2011).

Some medications require a nurse's clinical judgment in deciding the proper time for administration. Administer a prn sleeping medication when a patient is prepared for bed. In addition, use clinical judgment when administering prn analgesics. For example, you may need to obtain a STAT order from the health care provider if a patient requires a medication before the prn interval has elapsed. Always document when you call a patient's health care provider to obtain a change in a medication order.

Before discharge from the agency setting, evaluate a patient's need for home care, especially if the patient was admitted to the agency because of a problem with medication self-administration. Patients often leave the agency with a basic knowledge of their medications but are unable to remember or implement this knowledge once back home. Before patients are discharged from the agency, evaluate whether the medications are adequate or prescribed at therapeutic levels for them.

At home, some patients take several medications throughout the day. Help to plan schedules based on preferred medication intervals, the pharmacokinetics of the medications, and the patient's daily schedule. For patients who have difficulty remembering when to take medications, make a chart that lists the times to take each one, or prepare a special container to hold each timed dose.

Right Documentation. Nurses and other health care providers use documentation to communicate with one another. Many medication errors result from inaccurate documentation. Always document medications accurately at the time of administration and identify any inaccurate documentation before you give medications.

Before you administer a medication, ensure that the MAR clearly shows:
- *The patient's full name*
- *The full name of the ordered medication (without abbreviations of medication names)*
- *The time the medication is to be administered*
- *The dosage, route, and frequency of administration*

Common problems with medication orders include incomplete information; inaccurate dosage form or strength; illegible order or signature; incorrect placement of decimals, leading to the wrong dosage; and nonstandard terminology. If there is any question about a medication order because it is incomplete, illegible, vague, or not understood, contact the health care provider before administering the medication. The health care provider is responsible to provide accurate, complete, and understandable medication orders. If the health care provider is unable to do this, nurses implement agency policy (usually a "chain of command" policy) to determine whom to contact until they resolve issues related to patients' medications. You are responsible to begin this chain of command to ensure that patients receive the correct medication. You are also responsible for documenting any preassessment data required with certain medications such as a blood pressure measurement for antihypertensive medications or laboratory values, as in the case of warfarin, before giving the medication.

After administering a medication, immediately document which medication was given on a patient's MAR per agency policy to verify that it was given as ordered. Inaccurate documentation, such as failing to document giving a medication or documenting an incorrect dose, leads to errors in subsequent decisions about patient care. For example, errors in documentation about insulin often result in negative patient outcomes. Consider the following situation: a patient receives insulin before breakfast, but the nurse who gave the insulin forgot to document it. The nurse caring for the patient goes home, and you are the patient's new nurse for the day. You notice that the insulin is not documented, you assume that the previous nurse did not give the insulin, and you give the patient another dose of insulin. Approximately 2 hours later, the patient experiences a low blood glucose level, which results in seizure activity. Accurate documentation and following up with the nurse from the previous shift to verify that the insulin was given as ordered would have prevented this situation from happening.

Never document that you have given a medication until you have actually given it. Document the name of the medication, the dose, the time of administration, and the route on the MAR. Also document the site of any injections and the patient's responses to medications, either positive or negative. Notify a patient's health care provider of any negative responses to medications, and document the time, date, and name of the health care provider who was notified in the patient's medical record. The efforts you make to ensure proper documentation help provide safe care.

Maintaining Patients' Rights. In accordance with The Joint Commission's *SpeakUp* Campaign (TJC, 2019) and because of the potential risks related to medication administration, a patient has the following rights:
- To be informed about their care.
- To make decisions about their care.
- To refuse care.
- To be listened to by the caregivers.
- To receive information in a way that meets their individual needs.

Know these rights and handle all patient and family caregiver questions courteously and professionally. Do not become defensive if a patient refuses medication therapy, recognizing that every person of consenting age has a right to refusal.

Right Indication. A seventh right of medication administration that would enhance the safety of every medication order, the *right indication,* is being considered for inclusion into the rights of medication administration (Grissinger, 2019). Indication-based prescribing would narrow medication choices, dosage forms, and dosing regimens, which reduces the risk of a wrong medication being chosen (Grissinger, 2019; Rochon, 2021). In addition, indication-based prescribing would empower and educate patients, which can improve medication adherence. Communication would be improved between the interprofessional team and the patients and family caregivers. Medication reconciliation would improve, as indication-based prescribing would aid in preventing represcribing.

❖ NURSING PROCESS

Apply the nursing process and use a critical thinking approach in your care of patients. The nursing process provides a clinical decision-making approach for you to make clinical judgments and develop and implement a patient-centered, individualized plan of care.

◆ Assessment

Thoroughly assess each patient and critically analyze findings to ensure that you make patient-centered clinical decisions required for safe nursing care.

Through the Patient's Eyes. Use professional knowledge, skills, and attitudes to provide compassionate and coordinated care. Consider patients' preferences and values while determining their need for and possible responses to medication therapy. Assess their experiences and encourage them to express their beliefs, feelings, and concerns about their medications. For example, ask them how their religious or family backgrounds influence their beliefs about taking medications. Putting patients in the center of their care helps you to see the situation through their eyes and contributes to safe medication administration. Begin your assessment by asking a variety of questions to help you better understand your patients' current medication management routine, their ability to afford medications, and their beliefs and expectations about medications.

History. Before you administer medications, review a patient's medical history to help you understand the indications or contraindications for medication therapy. Some illnesses place patients at risk for adverse medication effects. For example, if a patient has a gastric ulcer, medications containing aspirin increase the likelihood of bleeding. Long-term health problems (e.g., diabetes or arthritis) require specific medications. This knowledge helps you anticipate the type of medications that a patient requires. A patient's surgical history also sometimes indicates the need for medications. For example, after a thyroidectomy a patient requires thyroid hormone replacement.

Allergies. Inform the other members of the health care team if a patient has a history of allergies to medications and foods. Many medications have ingredients also found in food sources. For example, propofol, which is used for anesthesia and sedation, includes egg lecithin and soybean oil as inactive ingredients. Patients who have an egg or soy allergy should not receive propofol (Skidmore-Roth, 2021). In most health care settings patients wear identification bands listing medication and food allergies. Ensure that all your patient's allergies and their allergic reactions are documented appropriately in the patient's medical record (e.g., history and physical, MAR) to facilitate communication of this essential information to members of the health care team.

Medications. Ask your patients questions to find out about each medication they take (Box 31.7). Possible questions include: How

BOX 31.7 Nursing Assessment Questions

- Which prescription and nonprescription medications do you take? What herbal and nutritional supplements do you take? When do you take them? How do you take them? Do you have a list of medications from your pharmacy or health care provider's office?
- Why do you take these medications?
- Which side effects do you experience? Which of the side effects bother you or affect you negatively?
- What have you been told to do if a side effect develops?
- Have you ever stopped taking your medications? If so, why?
- What do you do to help remember to take your medications?
- Do you have any allergies to medications or foods? If so, which ones? Describe what happens when you take the medication or eat the food.
- Describe your normal eating patterns. Which foods and at what times do you normally eat?
- How do you pay for your medications? Do you sometimes have to stretch your budget to afford them or space them out to save money?
- What questions do you have about your medications?

long have you been taking these medications? What is the current dosage of each medication? Do you experience side effects or adverse effects from your medications? In addition, review the action, purpose, normal dosage, routes, side effects, and nursing implications for administering and monitoring each medication. You often need to consult several resources such as pharmacology textbooks; medication manuals available on a computer, electronic tablet, or AMDS; nursing journals; the *Physicians' Desk Reference* (PDR); medication package inserts; and pharmacists to gather necessary information. As a nurse you are responsible for knowing as much as possible about each medication your patients take.

Diet History. A diet history reveals a patient's normal eating patterns and food preferences. Use your patient's diet history to plan an effective and individualized medication dosage schedule. Teach your patient to avoid foods that interact with medications. In addition, provide education when your patients take medications that need to be taken before, with, or after meals.

Patient's Perceptual or Coordination Problems. Patients with perceptual, fine-motor, or coordination limitations often have difficulty self-administering medications. For example, a patient who takes insulin to manage blood glucose and has arthritis has difficulty manipulating a syringe. Assess the patient's ability to prepare doses and take medications correctly. If a patient is unable to self-administer medications, assess whether a family caregiver or friends are available to help, or make a home care referral.

Patient's Current Condition. The ongoing physical or mental status of a patient affects whether a medication is given and how it is administered. *Assess a patient carefully before giving any medication.* For example, check a patient's blood pressure before giving an antihypertensive. A patient who is vomiting is unable to take medications by mouth. Notify the patient's health care provider when this happens. Assessment findings serve as a baseline in evaluating the effects of medication therapy.

Patient's Attitude About Medication Use. A patient's attitudes about medications (e.g., benefit, risk, likelihood to cure) sometimes reveal a level of medication dependence or medication avoidance.

🌐 BOX 31.8 **CULTURAL ASPECTS OF CARE**

Influences in Medication Administration

Health beliefs vary by culture and often influence how patients manage and respond to medication therapy (Giger and Haddad, 2021). Significant differences in attitudes, regional differences, and socioeconomic status affect a patient's adherence to or preference for medication therapy. Some cultures attach different symbolic meanings to medications and medication therapy. Herbal remedies and alternative therapies are common in various cultures and ethnic groups and sometimes interfere with prescribed medications (Saper, 2021). Some people stop taking medications when their symptoms are resolved, even if the medications are still needed for management of a chronic illness. In addition, health beliefs often differ markedly between health providers and patients, further affecting a patient's adherence to medical therapy (Ball et al., 2019). In addition to the psychosocial aspect of medication therapy, pharmacological research has shown that differences in medication response, metabolism, and side effects may be affected by patients' ethnicity, genetics, gender, and age (Ball et al., 2019).

Implications for Patient-Centered Care

- Assess cultural beliefs, attitudes, and values when administering medications and teaching patients about self-administration.
- Establish trust with patients and resolve conflicts between medications and cultural beliefs to achieve optimal patient outcomes (Ball et al., 2019).
- Investigate whether the patient practices any alternative therapies or is taking any herbal preparations (Saper, 2021).
- Consider cultural influences on medication response, metabolism, and side effects if a patient is not responding to medication therapy as expected. Confer with the patient's health care provider because a change in the patient's medication is sometimes necessary.
- Assess food preferences that may interfere with patients' medication therapy (Betancourt et al., 2021; Saper, 2021).

Some patients do not express their feelings about taking a medication, particularly if dependence is a problem. Listen carefully when patients describe how they use medications to identify evidence of dependence or avoidance. Also, be aware that cultural beliefs about Western medicine sometimes interfere with medication adherence (Box 31.8; see Chapter 9).

Factors Affecting Adherence to Medication Therapy. Many complex factors affect a patient's ability to adhere to prescribed medication therapy. For example, a patient's knowledge and understanding of medication therapy influence the willingness or ability to follow a medication regimen. If a patient has a history of poor adherence (e.g., frequently missed doses or failure to fill prescriptions), investigate whether the patient can afford prescribed medications, and review resources available for the purchase of medications if indicated. Also determine whether the patient understands the purpose of the medication, the importance of regular dosage schedules, proper administration methods, and the possible side effects. Without adequate funding, knowledge, and motivation, adherence to medication schedules is unlikely (Ball et al., 2019).

Patient's Learning Needs. Health-related information is difficult to understand because of the use of technical terminology. Serious errors can occur when patients do not understand information about their medications. Assess patients' health literacy regarding medication administration to determine their need for instruction (Betancourt et al., 2021) (see Chapter 25). Have the patient explain the medication schedule of a typical day. Have the patient read a medication label and

explain what it includes. Health literacy also includes numeracy. Have a patient show how to give a medication dose if it is necessary to split a pill or use more than one in a container. Consider patient responses to your medication assessment questions such as those listed in Box 31.7. When a patient is unable to answer questions about medications appropriately, assess health literacy.

REFLECT NOW

Using Box 31.8, how would you begin to assess the learning needs of a patient who has his or her own unique cultural, spiritual, or religious beliefs about medication administration?

◆ Analysis and Nursing Diagnosis

Assessment provides data about the patient's condition, ability to self-administer medications, and medication adherence. Analyze these data for cues that will help you determine a patient's actual or potential problems with medication therapy. Certain data are assessment findings that, when clustered together, reveal actual nursing diagnoses. For example, *Complex Medication Regimen related to complexity of medication schedule* is indicated when patients have a complex medication schedule and admit to having difficulty integrating their medications into their daily routine. This list of nursing diagnoses may apply during medication administration in a variety of settings:

- Impaired Health Maintenance
- Lack of Knowledge (Medication)
- Nonadherence (Medication Regimen)
- Adverse Medication Interaction
- Complex Medication Regimen (Polypharmacy)

After selecting the diagnosis, identify the related factor (if applicable) that drives the selection of nursing interventions. In the example of *Nonadherence,* the related factors of *financial barriers* versus *lack of knowledge about the regimen* require different interventions. If a patient's nursing diagnosis is related to inadequate finances, you collaborate with family caregivers, social workers, case managers, or community agencies to connect the patient with necessary financial resources and develop a medication regimen the patient can afford. If the related factor is *lack of knowledge,* you implement a teaching plan with appropriate follow-up.

◆ Planning and Outcomes Identification

Always organize your care activities to ensure the safe administration of medications. Take your time when preparing and administering medications to decrease the risk of errors. It is important to minimize distractions or interruptions when preparing and administering medications (Suclupe et al., 2020). If possible, do not answer text messages or phone calls during medication administration (Bonafide et al., 2020). No-Interruption Zones (NIZs) have been recommended to reduce distractions and interruptions during medication administration (Freitas et al., 2019). NIZs are created by placing signs, red tape, or some type of border on the floor around medication carts or areas. Nurses standing in these areas are not to be interrupted.

Outcomes. Establishing expected outcomes contributes to patient safety and allows for effective use of time during medication administration. For example, a nurse establishes the following expected outcomes for a patient with newly diagnosed type 2 diabetes who has the diagnosis of *Lack of Knowledge related to insufficient medication information*:
Outcomes:

> The patient verbalizes understanding of desired and adverse effects of medications.

The patient states signs, symptoms, and treatment of hypoglycemia.
The patient can monitor blood glucose levels to determine whether it is safe to take medication or an alteration in dose is needed.
The patient prepares a dose of ordered medication.
The patient describes a daily routine that will integrate timing of medication with daily activities.

Setting Priorities. Prioritize care when administering medications. Use patient assessment data to determine which medications to give first, whether it is time to evaluate a patient's response to a medication, or whether it is appropriate to administer prn medications. For example, if a patient is in pain, it is important to provide pain medication as soon as possible. If the patient's blood pressure is elevated, administer the blood pressure medication before other medications. Nurses also prioritize when providing patient education about medications. Provide the most important information about the medications first. For example, hypoglycemia is a serious side effect of insulin. A patient taking insulin needs to be able to identify and treat hypoglycemia immediately; therefore first teach how to recognize and treat hypoglycemia before teaching how to administer an injection.

Teamwork and Collaboration. Collaboration during medication administration is essential. You need to collaborate with a patient's family caregivers whenever possible. Family caregivers and significant others often reinforce the importance of medication schedules when a patient is at home. Nurses often collaborate with patients' health care providers, pharmacists, and case managers to ensure that patients can afford their medications. On discharge ensure that patients know where and how to obtain medications. Be sure that patients can read medication labels and medication teaching information. Some patients also need to understand how to calculate dosages and prepare complex medication regimens. Collaborate with community resources (e.g., agency on aging, public health department, medical interpreters) when patients have significant literacy issues or difficulty in understanding medication instructions (see Chapter 25).

◆ **Implementation**

Health Promotion. In promoting or maintaining a patient's health, nurses identify factors that improve or diminish well-being. Health beliefs, personal motivation, socioeconomic factors, and habits influence a patient's adherence with medications. Several nursing interventions promote adherence to the medication regimen and foster independence. Teach a patient and family caregiver about the benefit of a medication and the knowledge needed to take it correctly. Integrate a patient's health beliefs and cultural practices into the treatment plan. Help a patient and family caregiver establish a medication routine that fits into the patient's normal schedule. Make referrals to community resources if a patient is unable to afford or cannot arrange transportation to obtain necessary medications.

Patient and Family Caregiver Teaching. Some patients take medications incorrectly or not at all because they do not understand their medications. When this happens, you need to provide patient education using language your patient understands (see Chapter 25). Include information about the purpose, actions, timing, dosages, and side effects of medications. Many health care agencies offer easy-to-read teaching sheets written at the sixth-grade level about specific types of medications. Patients need to know how to take medications properly and the risks associated when they fail to do so. For example, after receiving a prescription for an antibiotic, a patient needs to understand the importance of taking the full prescription. Failure to do this can lead to a worsening of the condition and the development of bacteria resistant to the medication. Current recommendations suggest the use

---

BOX 31.9 PATIENT TEACHING

Safe Insulin Administration

Objective
- Patient will correctly self-administer subcutaneous insulin.

Teaching Strategies
- Teach patient how to determine whether insulin is expired.
- Instruct patient to keep medication in its original labeled container and refrigerated if needed.
- Demonstrate how to prepare insulin in a syringe; ensure that patient can draw up the correct amount of insulin.
- Coach patient through the steps of administering subcutaneous insulin injection.
- Demonstrate how to rotate insulin injection sites.
- Instruct patient how to determine the amount of insulin required based on the results of home capillary glucose monitoring as ordered by the health care provider.
- Show patient how to keep a daily log for insulin injections, including results of home capillary glucose monitoring, type and amount of insulin given, expiration date on insulin vial, time of insulin injection, and injection site used.

Evaluation
Use the principles of teach-back to evaluate patient/family caregiver learning:
- Describe for me the procedure you use at home for determining the correct dose of insulin you need.
- Please show me how you draw up your insulin based on your capillary glucose monitoring result. Show me how you select your injection site and administer your insulin.
- Review your log with me so I can evaluate it for completeness.

---

of teach-back as a method to confirm patient learning and improve health care provider education (Betancourt et al., 2021). Have the patient explain the topic about which you instructed, so you can confirm understanding.

Nurses teach patients how to administer their medications correctly. For example, teach a patient how to measure a liquid medication accurately. Provide special education to patients who depend on daily injections (Box 31.9). The patient learns to prepare and administer an injection correctly using aseptic technique. Teach family caregivers how to give injections in case the patient becomes ill or physically unable to handle a syringe. Provide specially designed equipment such as syringes with enlarged calibrated scales or medications with labels in braille when patients have visual alterations.

Patients need to know the symptoms of medication side effects or toxicity. For example, patients taking anticoagulants learn to notify their health care providers immediately when signs of bleeding or bruising develop. Inform family caregivers or friends of medication side effects such as changes in behavior because they are often the first to recognize these effects. Patients cope better with problems caused by medications if they understand how and when to act. All patients need to learn the basic guidelines for medication safety, which ensure the proper use and storage of medications in the home.

Acute Care. Patients are often hospitalized to receive expert nursing assessment and documentation of responses to medications. When a nurse receives a medication order, several nursing interventions are essential for safe and effective medication administration.

Receiving, Transcribing, and Communicating Medication Orders. A medication order is required to administer any medication to a patient. In the absence of CPOE, health care providers handwrite orders onto order sheets in a patient's chart. If orders are handwritten, be sure that medication names, dosages, and symbols are legible. Clarify and then rewrite any unclear or illegible transcribed orders.

The process of verifying medical orders varies among health care agencies. Nurses follow agency policy and current national patient safety standards when receiving, transcribing, and communicating medication orders. *Nursing students are prohibited from transcribing or receiving verbal and telephone orders.*

Medication orders need to contain all the elements in Box 31.10. If a medication order is incomplete, inform the health care provider and ensure completeness before carrying it out. Nurses read back verbal or telephone orders to health care providers to ensure that the correct order is obtained. The RN follows agency policy regarding receiving, recording, and transcribing verbal and telephone orders. In general, the health care provider must sign them within 24 hours.

Nurses and pharmacists check all medication orders for accuracy and thoroughness several times during the transcription process. They also take patients' current problems, treatments, laboratory values, and other prescribed medications into consideration. Once the nurse and pharmacist determine that a medication order is safe and appropriate, it is placed on the appropriate medication form, usually called the *MAR*. The MAR is either printed on paper or available electronically. An electronic version of the MAR is called an *eMAR*. Whether it is handwritten, printed from a computer, or in an electronic version, it includes the patient's name, room, and bed number; medical record number; medical and food allergies; other patient identifiers (e.g., birthday); and medication name, dose, frequency, and route and time of administration. Each time a medication dose is prepared, the nurse refers to the MAR.

It is essential to verify the accuracy of every medication you give to your patients with the patients' orders. If the medication order is incomplete, incorrect, or inappropriate or if there is a discrepancy between the original order and the information on the MAR, consult with the health care provider. Do not give a medication until you are

certain that you can follow the seven rights of medication administration. When you give the wrong medication or an incorrect dose, *you* are legally responsible for the error.

Accurate Dose Calculation and Measurement. You calculate each dose when preparing medications. To avoid calculation errors, pay close attention to the process of calculation and avoid interruptions from other people or nursing activities. Ask another nurse to double-check your calculations against the health care provider's order if you are in doubt about the accuracy of your calculation or if you are calculating a new or unusual dose.

Avoidance of Distractions. Current evidence shows that distractions or hurrying during medication preparation administration increases the risk of medication errors (Westbrook et al., 2017). Suggestions to reduce distraction include signage identifying the medication administration area, development of a checklist that includes all the components of medication administration, an educational program for nursing staff, and wearing some identifying clothing (e.g., vest) when preparing medications (Freitas et al., 2019; Palese et al., 2019; Westbrook et al., 2017).

REFLECT NOW

Observe two RNs administering medications on the clinical unit to which you are assigned. What types of distractions occurred while the RNs were setting up medications? What can you take away from this experience to help you safety set up and administer medications in the future?

Correct Administration. For safe administration follow the seven rights of medication administration. Verify the patient's identity by using at least two patient identifiers (TJC, 2021). In the acute care setting identifiers are usually on a patient's armband. Carefully compare patient identifiers with the MAR to ensure that you are giving the medication to the right patient. Use aseptic technique and proper procedures when handling and giving medications, and perform necessary assessments (e.g., heart rate for antidysrhythmic medications) before administering a medication to a patient. Carefully monitor a patient's response to a medication, especially when the first dose of a new medication is administered.

Recording Medication Administration. Follow all agency policies when documenting medication administration. After administering a medication, appropriately document the name of the medication, dose, route, and exact time of administration immediately. Include the site of any injections per agency policy.

If a patient refuses a medication or is undergoing tests or procedures that result in a missed dose, explain the reason that a medication was not given in the nurses' notes. Some agencies require the nurse to circle the prescribed administration time on the medication record or to notify the health care provider when a patient misses a dose. Be aware of the effects that missing doses may have on a patient (e.g., with hypertension or diabetes). Coordinating care with health care providers and other services when testing or diagnostic procedures are being completed helps ensure patient safety and therapeutic control of the disease.

Restorative Care. Because of the numerous types of restorative care settings, medication administration activities vary. Patients with cognitive or functional limitations often require a nurse to fully administer all medications. In the home care setting patients usually administer their own medications or receive assistance from family caregivers. Regardless of the type of medication activity, the nurse is responsible for instructing

---

BOX 31.10 Components of Medication Orders

A medication order needs to have all the following parts:

Patient's full name: A patient's full name distinguishes the patient from other people with the same last name. In the acute care setting patients are sometimes assigned special identification numbers (e.g., medical record number) to help distinguish patients with the same names. This number is often included on the order form.

Date and time that the order is written: The day, month, year, and time need to be included. Designating the time that an order is written clarifies when certain orders are to start and stop. If an incident occurs involving a medication error, it is easier to document what happened when this information is available.

Medication name: A health care provider orders a medication by its generic or trade name. Correct spelling is essential to prevent confusion with medications with similar spelling.

Dosage: The amount or strength of the medication is included.

Route of administration: A health care provider uses only accepted abbreviations for medication routes. Accuracy is important to ensure that patients receive medications by the intended route.

Time and frequency of administration: A nurse needs to know what time and how frequently to administer medications. Orders for multiple doses establish a routine schedule for medication administration.

Signature of health care provider: The signature makes an order a legal request.

patients and family caregivers in medication action, administration, and side effects. The nurse is also responsible for monitoring adherence with medication and determining the effectiveness of medications that have been prescribed.

Special Considerations for Administering Medications to Specific Age-Groups. A patient's developmental level is a factor to consider when administering medications. Knowledge of developmental needs helps you anticipate responses to medication therapy.

Infants and Children. In many pediatric settings the standard of practice is to have another nurse verify all pediatric dose calculations before administration. All children require special psychological preparation before receiving medications. A child's parents are often valuable resources for determining the best way to give a child medication. Sometimes it is less traumatic for a child if a parent gives the medication, and the nurse supervises. Supportive care is necessary if a child is expected to cooperate. Explain the procedure to a child, using words appropriate to the child's level of comprehension. Long explanations increase a child's anxiety, especially for painful procedures such as an injection. Providing a child with choices, when possible, can result in greater success. For example, saying "It's time to take your pill now. Do you want it with water or juice?" allows a child to make a choice. Do not give the child the option of not taking a medication. After the medication has been administered, praise the child and offer a simple reward such as a star or token. Tips for administering medication to children are in Box 31.11.

Older Adults. Adverse medication events occur in 22% or more of older-adult patients presenting to health care agencies (Rochon, 2021).

The most common serious manifestations include falls, orthostatic hypotension, heart failure, and delirium. Older adults require special nursing considerations during medication administration (Box 31.12). Be vigilant when administering medications and know the physiological changes of aging (Fig. 31.7) so that you can anticipate adverse reactions. Nurses can collaborate with health care providers to minimize adverse medication events in older adults by discontinuing medications, prescribing new medications sparingly, reducing the number of prescribers, and frequently reconciling medications (Rochon, 2021).

Polypharmacy. Polypharmacy is the use of multiple medications, the use of potentially inappropriate or unnecessary medications, or the use of a medication that does not match a diagnosis (Touhy and Jett, 2021). For example, polypharmacy exists when a patient takes two medications from the same chemical class to treat the same illness. Suspect polypharmacy if your patient uses two or more medications with the same or similar actions to treat several illnesses simultaneously and mixes nutritional supplements or herbal products with medications. Older adults also often experience polypharmacy when they seek relief from a variety of symptoms (e.g., pain, constipation, insomnia, and indigestion) by using OTC preparations. Sometimes polypharmacy is unavoidable. For example, some patients need to take more than one medication to control their high blood pressure. When a patient experiences polypharmacy, the risk of adverse reactions and medication interactions with other medications and food is increased.

Because many older adults have chronic health problems, polypharmacy is common. However, it is also becoming more common in children and patients with mental illnesses. Taking OTC medications frequently, lack of knowledge about medications, incorrect beliefs about medications, and visiting several health care providers to treat different illnesses increase the risk for polypharmacy. To minimize risks associated with polypharmacy, frequent communication among health care providers is essential to make sure that the patients' medication regimen is as simple as possible (Rochon, 2021).

BOX 31.11 Tips for Administering Medications to Children

Oral Medications
- Liquids are safer to swallow than pills to avoid aspiration.
- Use calibrated droppers for administering liquids to infants; the use of straws often helps older children or patients who have difficulty swallowing pills.
- Offer juice, a soft drink, or frozen juice bar, if allowed, after the child swallows a medication.
- When mixing medications in other foods or liquids, use only a small amount. The child may refuse to take all of a larger mixture.
- Avoid mixing a medication in a child's favorite foods or liquids because the child may later refuse them.
- A plastic disposable oral syringe is the most accurate device for preparing liquid doses, especially those less than 10 mL. (Cups, teaspoons, and droppers are inaccurate.)

Injections
- Use caution when selecting intramuscular (IM) injection sites. Infants and small children have underdeveloped muscles. Follow agency policy.
- Children are sometimes unpredictable and uncooperative. Make sure that someone (preferably another nurse) is available to restrain a child if needed. Have the parent act as a comforter, not restrainer, if restraint is necessary.
- Always awaken a sleeping child before giving an injection.
- Distracting a child with conversation, bubbles, or a toy reduces pain perception.
- If time allows, apply a lidocaine ointment (e.g., eutectic mixture of local anesthetics [EMLA] cream) to an injection site before the injection to reduce pain perception during the injection.

Adapted from Hockenberry MJ, et al: *Wong's nursing care of infants and children,* ed 11, St Louis, 2019, Elsevier.

BOX 31.12 FOCUS ON OLDER ADULTS
Safety in Medication Administration

- Frequently review a patient's medication history, including use of over-the-counter medications, and consult with health care provider to simplify the medication therapy plan whenever possible (Rochon, 2021).
- Keep instructions clear and simple, provide memory aids (e.g., calendar, medication schedule), and ensure that written information about medications is in print large enough for a patient to see (Rochon, 2021; Touhy and Jett, 2021).
- Assess functional status (including vision, hand grasp, fine-motor skills) to determine whether patient will require assistance in taking medications (Touhy and Jett, 2021).
- Some older adults have a greater sensitivity to medications, especially those that act on the central nervous system. Carefully monitor patients' responses to medications and anticipate dosage adjustments as needed (Touhy and Jett, 2021).
- If patient has difficulty swallowing a capsule or tablet, ask the health care provider to substitute a liquid medication or instruct patient to place medication on the front of the tongue and then swallow fluid to help wash it to the back of the throat. If the patient continues to have problems, have the patient try taking medication with a very small amount of semisolid food (e.g., applesauce) (Touhy and Jett, 2021).
- Teach alternatives to medications such as a proper diet instead of vitamins and exercise instead of laxatives (Rochon, 2021; Touhy and Jett, 2021).

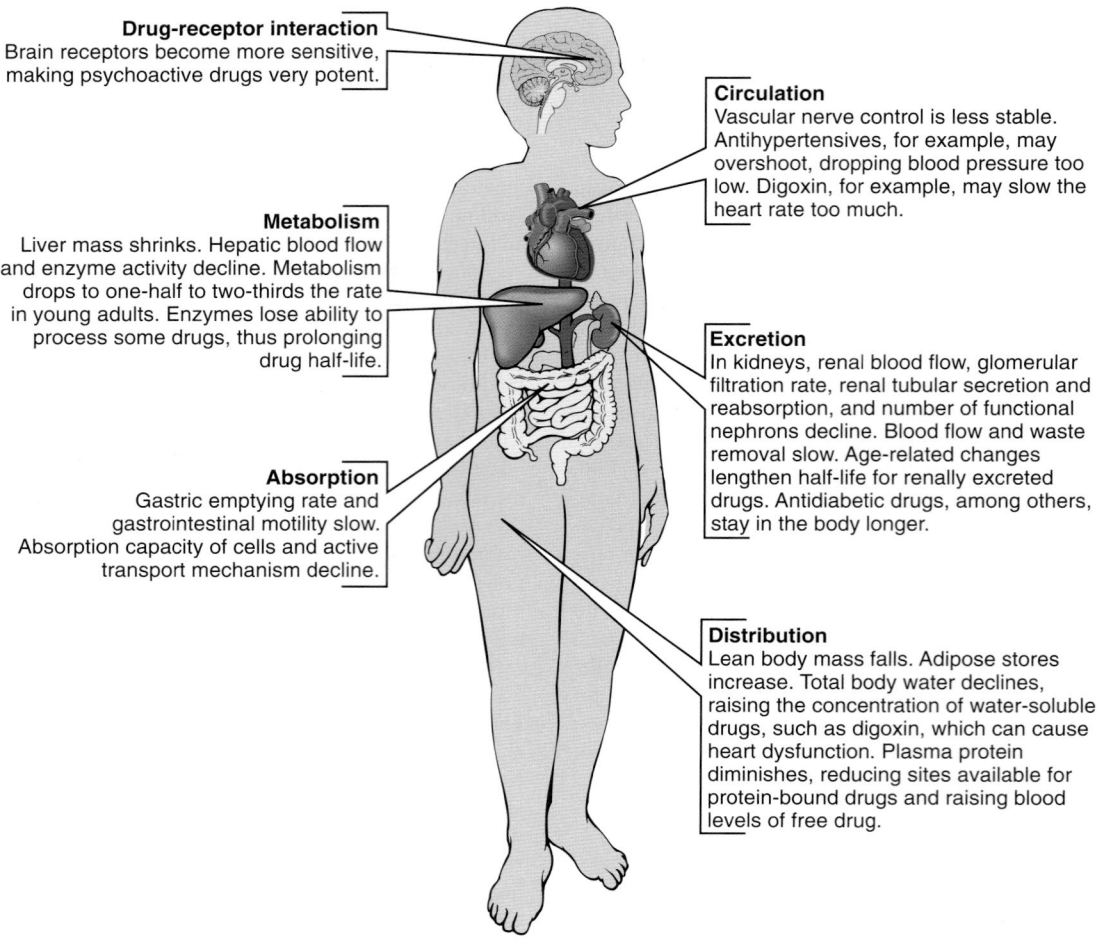

Drug-receptor interaction
Brain receptors become more sensitive, making psychoactive drugs very potent.

Circulation
Vascular nerve control is less stable. Antihypertensives, for example, may overshoot, dropping blood pressure too low. Digoxin, for example, may slow the heart rate too much.

Metabolism
Liver mass shrinks. Hepatic blood flow and enzyme activity decline. Metabolism drops to one-half to two-thirds the rate in young adults. Enzymes lose ability to process some drugs, thus prolonging drug half-life.

Excretion
In kidneys, renal blood flow, glomerular filtration rate, renal tubular secretion and reabsorption, and number of functional nephrons decline. Blood flow and waste removal slow. Age-related changes lengthen half-life for renally excreted drugs. Antidiabetic drugs, among others, stay in the body longer.

Absorption
Gastric emptying rate and gastrointestinal motility slow. Absorption capacity of cells and active transport mechanism decline.

Distribution
Lean body mass falls. Adipose stores increase. Total body water declines, raising the concentration of water-soluble drugs, such as digoxin, which can cause heart dysfunction. Plasma protein diminishes, reducing sites available for protein-bound drugs and raising blood levels of free drug.

FIG. 31.7 Effects of aging on medication metabolism. (From Lewis SM, et al: *Medical-surgical nursing*, ed 9, St Louis, 2014, Mosby.)

◆ Evaluation

Evaluation of medication administration is an essential role of professional nursing that requires assessment skills; clinical judgment; analysis; and knowledge of medications, physiology, and pathophysiology. You need to thoroughly and accurately gather data to complete a holistic evaluation. The goal of safe and effective medication administration is met when a patient responds appropriately to medication therapy and assumes responsibility for self-care. When patients do not achieve expected outcomes of medication therapy, investigate possible reasons, and determine appropriate revisions to the plan of care.

Through the Patient's Eyes. Evaluation is more effective when you value your patients' participation. It is important to partner with your patients and include them in the evaluation process. Ensure that they understand and can safely administer their medications. For example, if you are caring for a child who needs an inhaler, be sure to watch the patient use the inhaler. To determine whether patients understand their medication schedules, ask them to explain when they take their medications and whether they can take them as prescribed. When patients struggle with their medication schedule, determine barriers to adherence (e.g., cost, lack of knowledge) and remove these barriers if possible. Also remember that patients have different values and define health differently. These values and beliefs influence their perception of the effectiveness of their medications. Therefore ask patients to describe this effectiveness. Ask whether they are satisfied with their medications and how they make them feel. Use patients' statements and responses to questions (e.g., "I feel less anxious now") when determining the effectiveness of medications. Including patients in the evaluation process empowers them and helps them become more actively involved in their care.

Patient Outcomes. A patient's clinical condition can change minute by minute. Use knowledge of the desired effect and common side effects of each medication to compare expected outcomes with actual findings. A change in a patient's condition is often physiologically related to changes in health status or results from medications or both. Be alert for reactions in a patient taking several medications. To evaluate patient responses to medications, nurses use a variety of measures such as direct observation of physiological measures (e.g., blood pressure or laboratory values), behavioral responses (e.g., agitation), and rating scales (e.g., rating on a pain or nausea scale). The type of measurement used varies with the medication action being evaluated, the reading skill and knowledge level of the patient, and the patient's cognitive and psychomotor ability. The most common type of measurement is physiological. Examples of physiological measures are blood pressure, heart rate, and visual acuity. Nurses also use patient statements as evaluative measures. Table 31.8 contains examples of expected outcomes, and corresponding evaluative measures.

TABLE 31.8	Example Evaluation for Patient Outcomes	
Expected Outcomes	**Evaluative Measure with Example**
Patient and family caregiver describe information about medication, dosage, schedule, purpose, and adverse effects.	Written measurement: Have patient write out medication schedule for a 24-hour period. Oral questioning: Use teach-back and ask patient to describe purpose, dosage, and adverse effects of each prescribed medication.
Patient and family caregiver identify situations that require medical intervention.	Oral questioning: Use teach-back and have family caregiver describe what to do when a patient has adverse effects from a medication.
Patient and family caregiver demonstrate appropriate administration technique.	Direct observation: Have patient complete return demonstration by filling insulin syringe and administering injection.
Patient follows prescribed treatment regimen.	Anecdotal notes: Have family caregiver keep log of patient's adherence to therapy for 1 week.
Patient performs administration techniques correctly.	Direct observation: Observe patient instilling eyedrops.
Patient identifies available resources for obtaining necessary medication.	Oral questioning: Use teach-back and ask family caregiver to identify how to contact local pharmacy or community clinic for necessary medications.

MEDICATION ADMINISTRATION

A sound knowledge base and clinical judgment are required for medications to be administered safely. Nurses need to be prepared to administer medications through a variety of routes.

Oral Administration

The easiest and most desirable route for administering medications is by mouth (see Skill 31.1). Patients usually can self-administer oral medications. Food sometimes affects a medication's absorption. Thus you give oral medications on an empty stomach if absorption is decreased by food. Likewise, give medications with meals if absorption is enhanced by food (Burchum and Rosenthal, 2019). Most tablets and capsules need to be swallowed and administered with approximately 60 to 240 mL of fluid (as allowed).

Oral medication administration is contraindicated in some situations (see Table 31.5). Many medications interact with nutritional and herbal supplements. You need to be knowledgeable about these interactions to determine the best time to give oral medications.

An important precaution to take when administering any oral preparation is to protect patients from aspiration. Aspiration occurs when food, fluid, or medication intended for GI administration inadvertently enters the respiratory tract. Protect a patient from aspiration by assessing the ability to swallow. Box 31.13 provides techniques that protect patients from aspiration. Proper positioning is essential. Position a patient in a seated position at a 90-degree angle when administering oral medications if not contraindicated by the patient's condition. Usually having the patient slightly flex the head in a chin-down position reduces aspiration. Use a multidisciplinary approach (e.g., speech-language pathologist, registered dietitian, and occupational therapist) to determine the best techniques for patients who have difficulty swallowing.

Special consideration is needed when administering medications to patients with enteral or small-bore feeding tubes (Box 31.14). Failing to follow current evidence-based recommendations from the American Society for Parenteral and Enteral Nutrition (ASPEN) can result in tube obstruction, reduced medication effectiveness, and increased risk of medication toxicity (Boullata et al., 2017). Tubing misconnections continue to cause patient injury because tubes with different functions can be connected with Luer connectors (Malone et al., 2019). In response to this issue the International Organization for Standardization (IOS, 2020) has developed tubing connector standards in which the enteral connector will no longer be Luer compatible (ISMP, 2020a). An enteral-only connector (ENFit) is available, and health care agencies have changed enteral nutrition practices, policies, procedures, and processes per the new guidelines. Before giving a medication by this route, verify

BOX 31.13 Protecting a Patient From Aspiration

- Allow patient to self-administer medications if possible.
- Know the signs of dysphagia (difficulty swallowing): cough, change in voice tone or quality after swallowing, delayed swallowing, incomplete oral clearance or pocketing of food, regurgitation.
- Assess patient's ability to swallow and cough by checking for presence of gag reflex and then offering 50 mL of water in 5-mL allotments. Stop if patient begins to cough.
- Prepare oral medication in form that is easiest to swallow.
- Position the patient in an upright seated position at a 90-degree angle with feet on the floor, hips and knees at 90 degrees, head midline, and back erect if possible and if not contraindicated by the patient's condition.
- Suggest that the patient slightly flex the head in a chin-down position before swallowing.
- Prepare oral medications in the form that is easiest to swallow.
- If patient has unilateral (one-sided) weakness, place medication in stronger side of mouth.
- Administer pills one at a time, ensuring that each medication is properly swallowed before next one is introduced.
- Thicken regular liquids or offer fruit nectars if patient cannot tolerate thin liquids.
- Some medications can be crushed and mixed with pureed foods if necessary. Refer to a medication reference to identify medications that are safe to crush.
- Avoid straws because they decrease the control the patient has over volume intake, which increases risk of aspiration.
- Have patient hold and drink from a cup if possible.
- Time medications, if possible, to coincide with mealtimes or when patient is well rested and awake.
- Administer medications using another route if risk of aspiration is severe (see agency policy).

that the location of the tube (e.g., stomach or jejunum) is compatible with medication absorption. For example, iron dissolves in the stomach and is mostly absorbed in the duodenum. If it is administered through a jejunal tube, it has poor bioavailability.

Use liquid medications when possible. When liquid medications are unavailable, crush simple tablets or open capsules and dilute them in water. Pierce a gel cap with a sterile needle and empty the contents into 30 mL of warm water or other solution as designated by the manufacturer of the medication. You can dissolve gel caps in warm water, but this often takes 15 to 20 minutes. Only use oral syringes when preparing medications for this route to prevent accidental parenteral administration. Flush tubes

BOX 31.14 PROCEDURAL GUIDELINES

Administering Medications Through an Enteral Tube (Nasogastric Tube, G-Tube, J-Tube, or Small-Bore Feeding Tube)

Delegation and Collaboration

The skill of administering medications by enteral feeding tubes cannot be delegated to assistive personnel (AP). The nurse instructs the AP to:

- Keep the head of the bed elevated a minimum of 30 degrees (preferably 45 degrees) for 1 hour after medication administration; follow agency policy.
- Report immediately to the nurse coughing, choking, gagging, or drooling of liquid or dissolved pills.
- Report to the nurse any occurrence of possible medication side effects (specific to medication).

Equipment

Medication administration record (MAR) (electronic or printed), appropriate medication syringe or 60-mL Asepto syringe for large-bore tubes only, enteral-only connector (ENFit) designed to fit the specific enteral tube (see illustration), gastric pH test strip (scale of 0 to 11.0), graduated container, medication to be administered, pill crusher if medication in tablet form, water (or sterile water for patients who are immunocompromised), tongue blade or straw to stir dissolved medication, clean gloves, and pulse oximeter (for evaluation)

Enteral-only connector.

Procedural Steps

1. Check accuracy and completeness of each MAR or computer printout with health care provider's written medication order. Check patient's name, medication name and dosage, route of administration, and time for administration. Clarify incomplete or unclear orders with health care provider before administration.
2. Review pertinent information related to medication, including action, purpose, normal dose and route, side effects, time of onset and peak action, indication, and nursing implications.
3. Assess for any contraindications to receiving enteral medications, including presence of bowel inflammation, reduced peristalsis, recent gastrointestinal (GI) surgery, and gastric suction that cannot be turned off.
4. Avoid complicated medication schedules that often interrupt enteral feedings. Use alternative routes of medication administration if possible (e.g., transdermal, rectal, intravenous [IV]).
   a. Determine where medication is absorbed and ensure that point of absorption is not bypassed by feeding tube. For example, some medications such as antacids are absorbed in stomach, not jejunum.
   b. Determine whether medication interacts with enteral feeding. If so, hold the feeding for at least 30 minutes before giving the medication (see agency policy or consult pharmacist).

5. Assess patient's medical, medication, and diet history and history of allergies. List patient's food and medication allergies on each page of the MAR, and prominently display it on the patient's medical record per agency policy. When patient has allergy, provide allergy bracelet. If you identify contraindications, withhold medication, and inform health care provider.
6. For a patient who has had surgery, review the postoperative orders for type of enteral tube care.
7. Check with pharmacy for availability of liquid preparation for patient's medications. The health care provider may need to change dosage form.
8. Assess patient's or family caregiver's knowledge, experience, and health literacy.
9. Perform hand hygiene. Gather and review physical assessment data (e.g., bowel sounds, abdominal distention) and laboratory data (e.g., renal and liver function) that may influence medication administration.
10. Before administration of enteral medications, verify placement of feeding tube according to agency policy and determine that tube is placed in the stomach or small intestine correctly.
11. Assess patient's knowledge, prior experience with enteral medications, and feelings about procedure.
12. Assess patient's goals or preferences for how skill is to be performed or what patient expects.
13. Perform hand hygiene. Collect equipment and MAR.
14. Prepare medications for instillation into feeding tube. Attend to procedure and avoid distractions. Check medication label against MAR 2 times—when removing medication from unit dose or automated medication dispensing system (AMDS) and before leaving medication preparation area. *These are the first and second checks for accuracy.* Fill graduated container with 50 to 100 mL of tepid water. Use sterile water for patients who are immunocompromised or critically ill (Boullata et al., 2017).

CLINICAL JUDGMENT: Whenever possible, use liquid medications instead of crushed tablets. If you must crush tablets, flush the tubing before and after the medication administration to prevent the medication from adhering to the inside of the tube. In addition, make sure that concentrated medications are thoroughly diluted. Never add crushed medications directly to a tube feeding (Boullata et al., 2017).

   a. *Tablets:* Crush each tablet into a fine powder, using pill-crushing device or two medication cups. Dissolve each tablet in separate cup of 30 mL of warm water.
   b. *Capsules:* Apply clean gloves. Ensure that contents of capsule (granules or gelatin) can be expressed from covering (consult with pharmacist). Open capsule or pierce gel cap with sterile needle and empty contents into 30 mL of warm water (or solution designated by drug company). Gel caps dissolve in warm water, but this may take 15 to 20 minutes. Remove and dispose of gloves.
   c. Prepare liquid medication (prepared by pharmacy in appropriate syringe).
   d. Perform hand hygiene.
15. Take medication(s) to patient at correct time (see agency policy). Consider if medication is time critical. During administration apply seven rights of medication administration.
16. Identify patient using at least two identifiers (e.g., name and birthday or name and medical record number) according to agency policy. Compare identifiers with information on patient's MAR or medical record (TJC, 2021).
17. At patient's bedside again compare MAR or computer printout with names of medications on medication labels and patient name. Ask patient about any allergies. *This is the third check for accuracy.*

BOX 31.14   PROCEDURAL GUIDELINES—cont'd

Administering Medications Through an Enteral Tube (Nasogastric Tube, G-Tube, J-Tube, or Small-Bore Feeding Tube)

18. Explain procedure to patient and discuss purpose of each medication, action, and possible adverse effects. Allow patient to ask any questions about medications.
19. Help patient to sitting position. Elevate head of bed to minimum of 30 degrees and preferably 45 degrees (unless contraindicated) or sit patient up in a chair (Boullata et al., 2017).
20. If continuous enteral tube feeding is infusing, adjust infusion pump setting to hold tube feeding.
21. Perform hand hygiene. Apply clean gloves. Check placement of feeding tube by observing gastric contents and checking pH of aspirate contents. *Gastric pH less than 5.0 is a good indicator that tip of tube is correctly placed in stomach* (Boullata et al., 2017; Judd, 2020).
22. Check for gastric residual volume (GRV). Draw up 10 to 30 mL of air into a 60-mL syringe and connect syringe to feeding tube. Flush tube with air and pull back slowly to aspirate gastric contents. Determine GRV using either scale on syringe or a graduated container. If GRV exceeds 500 mL, hold feeding for 2 hours and recheck (Boullata et al., 2017) (check agency policy). When GRV is excessive, hold medication and contact health care provider. Some health care agencies prohibit measurement of GRV for small-bore feeding tubes (Judd, 2020).
23. Irrigate the tubing.
    a. Pinch or clamp enteral tube and remove syringe. Draw up 30 mL of water into syringe. Reinsert tip of syringe into tube, release clamp, and flush tubing. Clamp tube again and remove syringe.
    b. Using the appropriate enteral connector, attach to enteral tube.
24. Remove bulb or plunger of syringe and reinsert syringe into tip of feeding tube.
25. Administer dose of first liquid or dissolved medication by pouring into syringe. Allow to flow by gravity.

CLINICAL JUDGMENT: Verify that the connector meets the International Organization for Standardization (IOS) tubing connector standards (Boullata et al., 2017; IOS, 2020). Do not attach the enteral tubing to a standardized Luer syringe or needleless device (FDA, 2018; IOS, 2020).

CLINICAL JUDGMENT: Sometimes it is necessary to transfer oral medications into a medication cup for enteral administration. If medication does not flow freely, raise the height of the syringe to increase the rate of flow

or try having the patient change position slightly because the end of the feeding tube may be against the gastric mucosa. If these measures do not improve the flow, a gentle push with bulb of Asepto syringe or plunger of the syringe may facilitate flow of fluid.

   a. If giving only one dose of medication, flush tubing with 30 to 60 mL of water after administration.
   b. To administer more than one medication, give each separately and flush between medications with 15 to 30 mL of water.
   c. Follow last dose of medication with 30 to 60 mL of water.
26. Clamp proximal end of feeding tube if tube feeding is not being administered, and cap end of tube.
27. When continuous tube feeding is being administered by infusion pump, follow medication administration policy for turning off feedings prior to administering medications. If medications are not compatible with feeding solution, hold feeding for additional 30 to 60 minutes (Boullata et al., 2017).
28. Help patient to comfortable position and keep head of bed elevated, if not contraindicated, for 1 hour (see agency policy).
29. Place nurse call system in an accessible location within patient's reach.
30. Raise side rails (as appropriate) and lower bed to lowest position.
31. Dispose of soiled supplies, rinse graduated container and syringe with tap water, remove and dispose of gloves, and perform hand hygiene.
32. Document name of medication, dose, route, and time administered on MAR. Document patient's response in nurses' notes of MAR in the electronic health record (EHR) or chart.
33. Record patient teaching and validation of patient's understanding on flow sheet or nurses' notes in EHR or chart.
34. Observe patient for signs of aspiration such as choking, gurgling, gurgling speech, breath sounds, and difficulty breathing.
35. Return within 30 minutes to evaluate patient's response to medications.
36. **Use Teach-Back:** "I want to be sure I explained clearly why your father must take his medications through his feeding tube. Tell me why he is receiving his medications through his feeding tube." Revise your instruction now or develop a plan for revised patient/family caregiver teaching if patient/family caregiver is not able to teach back correctly. Determines patient's/family caregiver's level of understanding of instructional topic.

---

with at least 30 mL of water before and after giving medications. When administering more than one medication at a time, give each separately and flush between medications with 15 to 30 mL of water. Determine whether medications need to be given on an empty stomach or if they are compatible with the patient's enteral feeding. If a medication needs to be given on an empty stomach or is incompatible with the feeding (e.g., phenytoin, carbamazepine, warfarin, fluoroquinolones, proton pump inhibitors), hold the feeding for at least 30 minutes before or 30 minutes after medication administration. Verify the time with a medication reference or consult with a pharmacist. Monitor the patient closely for adverse reactions. The risk for drug-drug interactions is high when two or more medications are given via this route because they can interact together as soon as they are administered.

Topical Medication Applications

Topical medications are medications that are applied locally, most often to intact skin. They come in many forms (see Table 31.1). They are also applied to mucous membranes.

Skin Applications. Because many locally applied medications such as lotions, pastes, and ointments create systemic and local effects, apply these medications with gloves and applicators. Use sterile technique if a patient has an open wound. Skin encrustation and dead tissues harbor microorganisms and block contact of medications with the tissues to be treated. Before applying medications, clean the skin thoroughly by washing the area gently with soap and water, soaking an involved site, or locally debriding tissue.

Apply each type of medication according to directions to ensure proper penetration and absorption. When applying ointments or pastes, spread the medication evenly over the involved surface and cover the area well without applying an overly thick layer. Health care providers sometimes order a gauze dressing to be applied over the medication to prevent soiling clothes and wiping away the medication. Lightly spread lotions and creams onto the surface of the skin; rubbing often causes irritation. Apply a liniment by rubbing it gently but firmly into the skin. Dust a powder lightly to cover the affected area with a thin layer.

Some topical medications are applied in the form of a transdermal patch that remains in place for an extended amount of time (e.g., 12 hours or 7 days). Before applying a new patch, don disposable gloves and remove the old one. Medication remains on the patch even after its recommended duration of use. Nurses and patients have inadvertently left old transdermal patches in place, resulting in the patient receiving an overdose of the medication. For example, patients who use fentanyl transdermal patches for pain management can experience respiratory depression, coma, and death when the patches are not removed. In addition, some people, especially children, have experienced life-threatening harm from accidental exposure to fentanyl patches that were not disposed of properly. Many patches are clear, which makes them difficult to see. Carefully assess the patient's skin and be sure to remove the existing patch before applying a new one. Follow these guidelines to ensure safe administration of transdermal or topical medications:

- When taking a medication history or reconciling medications, specifically ask patients if they take any medications in the forms of patches, topical creams, or any route other than the oral route.
- When applying a transdermal patch, ask the patient whether there is an existing patch.
- Wear disposable clean gloves when removing and applying transdermal patches.
- If the dressing or patch is difficult to see (e.g., clear), apply a noticeable label to the patch.
- Document on the MAR the location on the patient's body where the medication was placed.
- Document removal of the patch or medication on the MAR. Fold sticky sides of the patch together and dispose of the patch in a childproof container. There are exceptions; a fentanyl patch, an adhesive patch that delivers a potent pain medication through the skin, comes with instructions to flush used or leftover patches (FDA, 2021b). Always read package directions.

Nasal Instillation. Patients with nasal sinus alterations sometimes receive medications by spray, drops, or tampons (Box 31.15). The most common form of nasal instillation is via decongestant spray or drops, used to relieve symptoms of sinus congestion and colds. Caution patients to avoid abuse of medications because overuse leads to a rebound effect in which the nasal congestion worsens. When excess decongestant solution is swallowed, serious systemic effects also develop, especially in children. Saline drops are safer than nasal preparations that contain sympathomimetics (e.g., oxymetazoline or phenylephrine) as a decongestant for children.

It is easier to have patients self-administer sprays because they can control the spray and inhale as the medication enters the nasal passages. For patients who use nasal sprays repeatedly, check the nares for irritation. When used to treat a sinus infection, position patients to permit the nasal medication to reach the affected sinus. A health care provider treats severe nosebleeds with packing or nasal tampons, which are treated with epinephrine, to reduce blood flow.

Eye Instillation. Some patients use OTC eyedrops and ointments such as artificial tears and vasoconstrictors (e.g., Visine and Murine). Other patients, especially older adults, receive prescribed ophthalmic medications for eye conditions such as glaucoma or after cataract extraction. Age-related problems, including poor vision, hand tremors, and difficulty grasping or manipulating containers, affect an older adult's ability to self-administer eye medications. Educate your patients and family caregivers about the proper techniques for administering them (see Skill 31.2). Evaluate a patient's and family caregiver's ability to self-administer through a return demonstration of the procedure. Show patients each step for instilling eyedrops to help them understand the procedure. Follow these principles when administering eye medications:

- Avoid instilling any form of eye medications directly onto the cornea. The cornea of the eye has many pain fibers and thus is very sensitive to anything applied to it.
- Avoid touching the eyelids or other eye structures with eyedroppers or ointment tubes. The risk of transmitting infection from one eye to the other is high.
- Use eye medication only for the patient's affected eye.
- Never allow a patient to use another patient's eye medications.

Intraocular Administration. One less common way to administer eye medications is by the intraocular route (see Skill 31.2). These medications resemble a contact lens. You place the medication into the conjunctival sac, where it remains for up to 1 week. You need to teach patients how to insert and remove the disk and to monitor for adverse medication reactions.

Ear Instillation. Because internal ear structures are very sensitive to temperature extremes, you need to instill eardrops at room temperature to prevent vertigo, dizziness, or nausea. Although the structures of the outer ear are not sterile, sterile solutions are used in case the eardrum is ruptured. The entrance of nonsterile solutions into middle ear structures often results in infection.

If a patient has ear drainage, check with the health care provider to be sure that the patient does not have a ruptured eardrum before instilling the drops. Never occlude or block the ear canal with the dropper or irrigating syringe. Forcing medication into an occluded ear canal creates pressure that injures the eardrum. Box 31.16 provides guidelines for administering eardrops.

Ear irrigations are performed when the external ear canal becomes occluded with cerumen that cannot be removed by more conservative measures such as wax softeners. Typically, an irrigation is performed only when the patient has a hearing deficit or ear discomfort or if it is necessary to visualize the tympanic membrane. You should not perform an ear irrigation if there is a history of middle ear infection in the last 6 weeks, if the patient has undergone *any* form of ear surgery, if the patient has a perforation, or if there is a history of a mucous discharge in the last year.

Vaginal Instillation. Vaginal medications are available as suppositories, foam, jellies, or creams. Solid, oval-shaped suppositories (Fig. 31.8) are packaged individually in foil wrappers and are sometimes stored in the refrigerator to prevent them from melting. After a suppository is inserted into the vaginal cavity, body temperature causes it to melt and be distributed and absorbed. Foam, jellies, and creams are administered with an applicator inserter (Box 31.17).

Insert the suppository with a gloved hand in accordance with Standard Precautions (see Chapter 28). Patients often prefer administering their own vaginal medications and need privacy. Because vaginal medications are often given to treat infection, discharge is usually foul smelling. Follow aseptic technique and offer the patient frequent opportunities to maintain perineal hygiene (see Chapter 40).

Rectal Instillation. Rectal suppositories are thinner and more bullet shaped than vaginal suppositories. The rounded end prevents anal trauma during insertion. Rectal suppositories contain medications that exert local effects such as promoting defecation or systemic effects such as reducing nausea. They are stored in a refrigerator until administered. Sometimes it is necessary to clear the rectum with a small cleansing enema before inserting a suppository (Box 31.18).

BOX 31.15 PROCEDURAL GUIDELINES

Administering Nasal Medications

Delegation and Collaboration

The skill of administering nasal medications cannot be delegated to assistive personnel (AP). The nurse instructs the AP about:

- Potential side effects of medications and to report their occurrence to the nurse.
- Reporting any bloody nasal drainage to the nurse.

Equipment

Medication administration record (MAR) (electronic or printed), prepared medication with clean dropper or spray container, facial tissue, small pillow *(optional)*, washcloth *(optional)*, clean gloves

Procedural Steps

1. Check accuracy and completeness of each MAR with health care provider's medication order. Check patient's name and medication name, dosage, route (which sinus), and time of administration. Clarify incomplete or unclear orders with health care provider before administration.
2. Review pertinent information related to medication, including action, purpose, normal dose and route, side effects, time of onset and peak action, and nursing implications.
3. Assess patient's medical history (e.g., hypertension, heart disease, diabetes, and hyperthyroidism), medication history, and history of allergies. List medication allergies on each page of the MAR and prominently display any allergies on the patient's medical record per agency policy. When patient has allergy, provide allergy bracelet.
4. Assess patient's or family caregiver's knowledge, experience, and health literacy.
5. Perform hand hygiene. Using a penlight, inspect condition of nose and sinuses. Palpate sinuses for pain or tenderness (see Chapter 30). Note type of drainage if present.
6. Assess patient's knowledge, prior experience with the use of nasal instillation and technique for instillation, and feelings about procedure.
7. Assess patient's goals or preferences for how skill is to be performed or what patient expects.
8. Perform hand hygiene. Collect appropriate equipment and MAR.
9. Prepare medications for instillation. Attend to procedure to avoid distractions. Check label of medication against MAR 2 times (see Skill 31.1). Preparation usually involves checking label when removing nasal drops or sprays out of storage and before leaving preparation area. Check expiration date on container. *These are the first and second checks for accuracy.* Perform hand hygiene.

10. Take medication(s) to patient at correct time (see agency policy). Consider whether medication is time critical. During administration, apply seven rights of medication administration.
11. Identify patient using two identifiers (e.g., name and birthday or name and medical record number) according to agency policy (TJC, 2021). Compare identifiers with information on patient's MAR or medical record.
12. At patient's bedside again compare MAR or computer printout with names of medications on medication labels and patient name. Ask patient about any allergies. *This is the third accuracy check.*
13. Explain procedure to patient and sensations to expect. Discuss purpose of each medication, action, and possible adverse effects. Allow patient to ask any questions about medications. Patients who self-instill medications may be allowed to give drops under nurse's supervision (check agency policy). Tell patients receiving nasal instillation that they may experience burning or stinging of mucosa or choking sensation as medication trickles into throat.
14. Arrange supplies and medications at bedside. Perform hand hygiene and apply clean gloves (if nasal drainage is present).
15. Gently roll or shake container. Instruct patient to clear or blow nose gently unless contraindicated (e.g., risk of increased intracranial pressure or nosebleeds).
16. *Administer nasal drops:*
    a. Help patient to supine position and position head properly.
        (1) For access to posterior pharynx, tilt patient's head backward.
        (2) For access to ethmoid or sphenoid sinus, tilt head back over edge of bed or place small pillow under patient's shoulder and tilt head back (see illustration).
        (3) For access to frontal and maxillary sinus, tilt head back over edge of bed or pillow with head turned toward side to be treated (see illustration).
    b. Support patient's head with nondominant hand.
    c. Instruct patient to breathe through mouth.
    d. Hold dropper 1 cm (½ inch) above nares and instill prescribed number of drops toward midline of ethmoid bone.
    e. Have patient remain in supine position 5 minutes.
    f. Offer facial tissue to blot runny nose, but caution patient against blowing nose for several minutes.
17. *Administer nasal spray:*
    a. Help patient into upright position with head tilted slightly forward.

STEP 16a(2) Position for instilling nose drops into ethmoid or sphenoid sinus.

STEP 16a(3) Position for instilling nose drops into frontal and maxillary sinus.

Continued

BOX 31.15 PROCEDURAL GUIDELINES—cont'd

Administering Nasal Medications

b. Instruct or assist patient to insert tip of nasal spray into appropriate nares and occlude other nostril with finger. Point spray tip toward side and away from center of nose.

c. Have patient spray medication into nose while inhaling. Help patient remove nozzle from nose and instruct to breathe out through the mouth.

d. Offer facial tissue to blot runny nose, but caution patient against blowing nose for several minutes.

CLINICAL JUDGMENT: Some medications are designed for one spray per dose. Examples include calcitonin, desmopressin, and sumatriptan. It is essential to ensure that the patient understands the correct number of sprays to use per dose to prevent overdosing.

18. Help patient to a comfortable position after medication is absorbed.
19. Place nurse call system in an accessible location within patient's reach.
20. Raise side rails (as appropriate) and lower bed to lowest position.
21. Dispose of all contaminated supplies in appropriate receptacle, remove and dispose of gloves, and perform hand hygiene.
22. Document name of medication, dose, route, and time of administration on MAR.

23. Observe patient for onset of side effects 15 to 30 minutes after administration.
24. Ask whether patient can breathe through nose after decongestant administration. It may be necessary to have patient occlude one nostril at a time and breathe deeply.
25. Reinspect condition of nasal passages between instillations.
26. Ask patient to describe risks of overuse of decongestants and methods for administration.
27. Feedback ensures that patient can self-administer medications properly.
28. Have patient demonstrate self-administration of nasal medication.
29. Record patient response to medication, patient teaching, and validation of patient understanding and self-administration on flow sheet or nurses' notes in electronic health record (EHR) or chart.
30. **Use Teach-Back:** "I want to be sure I explained your nasal spray correctly. Can you tell me the best time for you to use this spray? What side effects may you get from using the spray?" If patient self-administers medications at home, state, "Show me how you're going to take this medication at home." Revise your instruction now or develop plan for revised teaching if patient/family caregiver is not able to teach back correctly. Determines patient's/family caregiver's level of understanding of instructional topic.

BOX 31.16 PROCEDURAL GUIDELINES

Administering Ear Medications

Delegation and Collaboration

The skill of administering ear medications cannot be delegated to assistive personnel (AP). The nurse instructs the AP about:

- Potential side effects of medications and to report their occurrence.
- The potential for dizziness or irritation after administration of ear medications.

Equipment

Medication administration record (MAR) (electronic or printed)

Drops: Medication bottle with dropper, cotton-tipped applicator, cotton balls, clean gloves if drainage is present

Irrigation: Irrigating solution and syringe, kidney basin, towel

Procedural Steps

1. Check accuracy and completeness of each MAR with health care provider's medication order. Check patient's name, medication name and dosage, route, and time for administration. Clarify incomplete or unclear orders with health care provider before administration.
2. Review pertinent information related to medication, including action, purpose, normal dose, and route (one or both ears), side effects, time of onset and peak action, and nursing implications.
3. Assess patient's medical history, medication history, and history of allergies (including latex). List medication allergies on each page of the MAR and prominently display any allergies on the patient's medical record per agency policy. When patient has allergy, provide allergy bracelet.
4. Perform hand hygiene. Assess condition of external ear structures (see Chapter 30). This may be done just before medication instillation (apply clean gloves if drainage is present).
5. Determine whether patient has any symptoms of ear discomfort or hearing impairment.
6. Assess patient's level of consciousness (LOC) and ability to follow directions.

7. Assess patient's or family caregiver's knowledge, experience, and health literacy.
8. Assess patient's knowledge, prior experience with ear medication, and feelings about procedure.
9. Assess patient's goals or preferences for how skill is to be performed or what patient expects.
10. Assess patient's ability to manipulate and hold ear dropper.
11. Perform hand hygiene. Collect appropriate equipment and MAR.
12. Prepare medications for instillation. Attend to procedure and avoid distractions. Check label of medication against MAR 2 times (see Skill 31.1). Take eardrops out of refrigerator and rewarm to room temperature before administering to patient. Preparation usually involves checking label when removing eardrops out of storage and before leaving preparation area. Check expiration date on container. *These are the first and second checks for accuracy.* Perform hand hygiene.
13. Take medication(s) to patient at correct time (see agency policy). Consider whether medication is time critical. During administration apply seven rights of medication administration.
14. Arrange supplies at bedside.
15. Identify patient using at least two identifiers (e.g., name and birthday or name and medical record number) according to agency policy (TJC, 2021). Compare identifiers with information on patient's MAR or medical record.
16. At patient's bedside again compare MAR or computer printout with names of medications on medication labels and patient name. Ask patient about any allergies. *This is the third check for accuracy.*
17. Explain procedure to patient and sensations to expect. Discuss purpose of each medication, action, and possible adverse effects. Allow patient to ask any questions about the medications. Patients who self-instill medications may be allowed to give drops under nurse's supervision (check agency policy).

BOX 31.16 PROCEDURAL GUIDELINES—cont'd

Administering Ear Medications

18. Perform hand hygiene.
19. *Administer eardrops:*
    a. Perform hand hygiene. Position patient on side (if not contraindicated) with ear to be treated facing up, or patient may sit in chair or at bedside. *Option:* Apply clean gloves if ear drainage is present.
    b. If cerumen or drainage occludes outermost part of ear canal, wipe out gently with cotton-tipped applicator (see illustration) or washcloth. Take care not to force cerumen into canal.

STEP 19b Always clean only outer canal. Do not push cerumen or secretions into ear.

    c. Hold the container in the palm of your hands for a few minutes to warm the contents to body temperature. Then, if the eardrops are in a cloudy suspension, shake bottle for about 10 seconds.
    d. Straighten ear canal by pulling pinna up and back to 10 o'clock position (adult or child older than age 3) or down and back to 6- to 9-o'clock position (child under age 3) (see illustration).

STEP 19d Pull pinna up and back for adults and children older than 3 years.

    e. Instill prescribed drops holding dropper 1 cm (½ inch) above ear canal. Avoid contact of dropper tip against external ear canal.
    f. Ask patient to remain in side-lying position for a few minutes. Apply gentle massage or pressure to tragus of ear with finger (see illustration).
    g. If ordered, gently insert part of cotton ball into outermost part of canal. Do not press cotton into canal.
    h. Remove cotton after 15 minutes. Help patient to comfortable position after drops are absorbed.

STEP 19f Nurse applies gentle pressure to tragus of ear after instilling drops.

20. *Administer ear irrigations:*
    a. Assess the tympanic membrane or review medication record for history of eardrum perforation, which contraindicates ear irrigation.
    b. Help patient into sitting position or lying position with head tilted or turned toward affected ear. Place towel under patient's head and shoulder and have patient hold basin under affected ear.
    c. Fill irrigating syringe with solution (approximately 50 mL) at room temperature.
    d. Gently grasp auricle and straighten ear by pulling pinna down and back for children younger than 3 years or upward and outward for patients 3 years of age and older.
    e. Slowly instill irrigating solution by holding tip of syringe 1 cm (½ inch) above opening of ear canal. Allow fluid to drain out during instillation. Continue until you use all solution.
21. Clean area and put supplies away.
22. Help patient to comfortable position.
23. Place nurse call system in an accessible location within patient's reach.
24. Raise side rails (as appropriate) and lower bed to lowest position.
25. Dispose of all contaminated supplies in appropriate receptacle, remove and dispose of gloves, and perform hand hygiene.
26. Record medication, concentration, dose or strength, number of drops, site of application (left, right, or both ears), and time of administration on MAR immediately after administration.
27. Observe response to medication by assessing hearing changes, asking whether symptoms are relieved, and noting any side effects or discomfort felt.
28. Ask patient to discuss purpose of medication, action, side effects, and technique of administration.
29. Record patient response to medication, patient teaching, and validation of patient understanding and self-administration on flow sheet or nurses' notes in electronic health record (EHR) or chart.
30. **Use Teach-Back:** "I want to be sure I clearly showed you how to administer eardrops. Let's take this time we have for you to show me how to place eardrops in your right ear." Revise your instruction now or develop a plan for revised patient/family caregiver teaching if patient/family caregiver is not able to teach back correctly. Determines patient's/family caregiver's level of understanding of instructional topic.

FIG. 31.8 Vaginal suppositories *(right)* are larger and more oval than rectal suppositories *(left)*. (From Lilley LL, et al: *Pharmacology and the nursing process,* ed 9, St Louis, 2020, Elsevier.)

Administering Medications by Inhalation

Medications administered with handheld inhalers are dispersed through an aerosol spray, mist, or powder that penetrates lung airways. The alveolar-capillary network absorbs medications rapidly.

Pressurized metered-dose inhalers (pMDIs), breath-actuated metered-dose inhalers (BAIs), and dry powder inhalers (DPIs) deliver medications that produce local effects such as bronchodilation. Some medications create serious systemic side effects. pMDIs use a chemical propellant to push the medication out of the inhaler and require the patient to apply approximately 5 to 10 lb of pressure to the top of the canister to administer the medication. Children or older adults with chronic respiratory diseases often use pMDIs. These two populations

---

BOX 31.17   PROCEDURAL GUIDELINES

Administering Vaginal Medications

Delegation and Collaboration

The skill of administering vaginal medications cannot be delegated to assistive personnel (AP). The nurse instructs the AP about:

- Potential side effects of medications and to report their occurrence to the nurse.
- Reporting any change in comfort level or new or increased vaginal discharge or bleeding to the nurse.

Equipment

Medication administration record (MAR) (electronic or printed); vaginal cream, foam, jelly, tablet, suppository, or irrigating solution; applicators (see Fig. 31.8 and Fig. 31.9) (if needed); clean gloves; tissues; towels and/or washcloths; perineal pad; drape or sheet; water-soluble lubricants; bedpan; irrigation or douche container (if needed); gooseneck lamp *(optional)*

Procedural Steps

1. Check accuracy and completeness of each MAR with health care provider's medication order. Check patient's name, medication name and dosage, route, and time for administration. Clarify incomplete or unclear orders with health care provider before administration.
2. Review pertinent information related to medication, including action, indication, purpose, normal dose and route, side effects, time of onset and peak action, and nursing implications.
3. Assess patient's medical and medication history and history of allergies. List medication allergies on each page of the MAR and prominently display any allergies on the patient's medical record per agency policy. When patient has allergy, provide allergy bracelet.
4. Assess patient's or family caregiver's knowledge, experience, and health literacy.

FIG. 31.9 *From top:* Vaginal cream with applicator, applicator, and vaginal suppository. (From Lilley LL, et al: *Pharmacology and the nursing process,* ed 9, St Louis, 2020, Elsevier.)

5. Perform hand hygiene and apply clean gloves. During perineal care inspect condition of vaginal tissues; note if drainage is present. Remove and dispose of gloves and perform hand hygiene.
6. Ask whether patient is experiencing any symptoms of pruritus, burning, or discomfort.
7. Assess patient's knowledge, prior experience with vaginal medications, and feelings about procedure.
8. Assess patient's goals or preferences for how skill is to be performed or what patient expects.
9. Assess patient's ability to manipulate applicator, suppository, or irrigation equipment and to properly position self to insert medication (may be done just before insertion).
10. Perform hand hygiene. Collect appropriate equipment and MAR.
11. Prepare suppository for administration. Attend to the procedure and avoid distraction. Preparation usually involves checking the label when removing suppository from refrigerator and before leaving preparation area. Check expiration date on container. *These are the first and second checks for accuracy.* Perform hand hygiene.
12. Take medication(s) to patient at correct time (see agency policy). Consider whether medication is time critical. During administration apply seven rights of medication administration.
13. Identify patient using at least two identifiers (e.g., name and birthday or name and medical record number) according to agency policy (TJC, 2021). Compare identifiers with information on patient's MAR or medical record.
14. At patient's bedside again compare MAR or computer printout with names of medications on medication labels and patient name. Ask patient about any allergies. *This is the third check for accuracy.*
15. Explain procedure to patient. Be specific if patient plans to self-administer medication. Discuss purpose of each medication, action, and possible adverse effects. Allow patient to ask any questions about medication.
16. Close door or pull curtain. Perform hand hygiene and apply clean gloves. Have patient void (using bathroom agencies or bedpan). Help her lie in dorsal recumbent position. Patients with restricted mobility in knees or hips may lie supine with legs abducted.
17. Keep abdomen and lower extremities draped.
18. Be sure that vaginal orifice is well illuminated by room light. Otherwise position portable gooseneck lamp.
19. *Insert vaginal suppository:*
    a. Remove suppository from wrapper and apply liberal amount of water-soluble lubricant to smooth or rounded end (see illustration). Be sure that suppository is at room temperature. Lubricate gloved index finger of dominant hand.

BOX 31.17 PROCEDURAL GUIDELINES—cont'd

Administering Vaginal Medications

STEP 19a Lubricate tip of suppository.

STEP 19c Angle of vaginal suppository insertion.

b. With nondominant gloved hand gently separate labial folds in front-to-back direction.

c. With dominant gloved hand insert rounded end of suppository along posterior wall of vaginal canal the entire length of finger (7.5–10 cm [3–4 inches]) (see illustration).

d. Withdraw finger and wipe away remaining lubricant from around orifice and labia with tissue or cloth.

e. Remove and dispose of gloves and perform hand hygiene.

20. *Apply cream or foam:*

a. Perform hand hygiene and apply clean gloves. Fill cream or foam applicator following package directions.

b. With nondominant gloved hand gently separate labial folds.

c. With dominant gloved hand gently insert applicator approximately 5 to 7.5 cm (2–3 inches). Push applicator plunger to deposit medication into vagina (see illustration).

d. Withdraw applicator and place on paper towel. Wipe off residual cream from labia or vaginal orifice with tissue or cloth.

e. Remove and dispose of gloves and perform hand hygiene.

21. *Administer irrigation or douche:*

a. Place patient on bedpan with absorbent pad underneath.

b. Be sure that irrigation or douche fluid is at body temperature. Run fluid through container nozzle (priming the tubing).

c. Perform hand hygiene and apply gloves.

STEP 20c Applicator inserted into vaginal canal. Plunger pushed to instill medication.

d. Gently separate labial folds and direct nozzle toward sacrum, following floor of vagina.

e. Raise container approximately 30 to 50 cm (12–20 inches) above level of vagina. Insert nozzle 7 to 10 cm (3–4 inches). Allow solution to flow while rotating nozzle. Administer all irrigating solution.

f. Withdraw nozzle and help patient to comfortable sitting position.

g. Allow patient to remain on bedpan for a few minutes. Clean perineum with soap and water.

h. Help patient off bedpan. Dry perineal area.

i. Remove and dispose of gloves and perform hand hygiene.

22. Instruct patient who received suppository, cream, or tablet to remain on her back for at least 10 minutes.

23. If using an applicator, wash with soap and warm water, rinse, air-dry, and then store for future use.

24. Offer perineal pad when patient resumes ambulation.

25. Help patient to comfortable position.

26. Place nurse call system in an accessible location within patient's reach.

27. Raise side rails (as appropriate) and lower bed to lowest position.

28. Dispose of all contaminated supplies in appropriate receptacle, remove and dispose of gloves, and perform hand hygiene.

29. Record the medication, dosage, route, and actual time and date of administration on MAR immediately after administration, not before. Include initials or signature.

30. Thirty minutes after administration perform hand hygiene and apply clean gloves. Then inspect condition of vaginal canal and external genitalia. Assess vaginal discharge if present. Remove and dispose of gloves and perform hand hygiene.

31. Question patient regarding continued pruritus, burning, discomfort, or discharge.

32. Ask patient to discuss purpose, action, and side effects of medication.

33. Record patient response to medication, patient teaching, and validation of patient understanding and self-administration of suppository on flow sheet or nurses' notes in electronic health record (EHR) or chart.

34. **Use Teach-Back:** "I want to be sure I explained how to use the vaginal cream applicator. Tell me how you will draw the correct amount of cream into the applicator." Revise your instruction now or develop a plan for revised patient/family caregiver teaching if patient/family caregiver is not able to teach back correctly. Determines patient's/family caregiver's level of understanding of instructional topic.

BOX 31.18   PROCEDURAL GUIDELINES

Administering Rectal Suppositories

Delegation and Collaboration

The skill of rectal medication administration cannot be delegated to assistive personnel (AP). The nurse instructs the AP to:

- Report expected fecal discharge or bowel movement to the nurse.
- Report the occurrence of any potential side effects of medications to the nurse.
- Inform the nurse of any rectal pain or bleeding.

Equipment

Medication administration record (MAR) (electronic or printed); rectal suppository; water-soluble lubricating jelly; clean gloves; tissue; drape

Procedural Steps

1. Check accuracy and completeness of each MAR or computer printout with health care provider's written medication order. Check patient's name, medication name and dosage, route of administration, and time of administration. Clarify incomplete or unclear orders with health care provider before administration.
2. Review pertinent information related to medication, including action, purpose, normal dose and route, side effects, time of onset and peak action, indication, and nursing implications.
3. Review patient's medical history (e.g., history of rectal surgery or bleeding, cardiac problems), medication history, and history of allergies. List medication allergies on each page of the MAR and prominently display the list of allergies on the patient's medical record per agency policy. When patient has allergy, provide allergy bracelet.
4. Review any presenting signs and symptoms of gastrointestinal (GI) alterations (e.g., constipation or diarrhea).
5. Assess patient's or family caregiver's knowledge, experience, and health literacy.
6. Assess patient's ability to hold suppository and position self to insert medication.
7. Review patient's knowledge, prior experience with rectal medication, and feelings about procedure.
8. Assess patient's goals or preferences for how skill is to be performed or what patient expects.
9. Perform hand hygiene. Collect appropriate equipment and MAR.
10. Prepare suppository for administration. Attend to procedure and avoid distraction. Check label of medication against MAR 2 times (see Skill 31.1). Preparation usually involves checking label when taking suppository out of refrigerator and before leaving preparation area. Check expiration date on container. *These are the first and second checks for accuracy.*
11. Take medication(s) to patient at correct time (see agency policy). Consider whether medication is time critical. During administration apply seven rights of medication administration.
12. Identify patient using at least two identifiers (e.g., name and birthday or name and medical record number) according to agency policy (TJC, 2021). Compare identifiers with information on patient's MAR or medical record.
13. At patient's bedside again compare MAR or computer printout with names of medications on medication labels and patient name. Ask patient about any allergies. *This is the third check for accuracy.*
14. Explain procedure to patient. Be specific if patient wishes to self-administer medication. Discuss purpose of each medication, action, and possible adverse effects. Allow patient to ask any questions about the medications. Explain procedure if patient plans to self-administer medication.
15. Perform hand hygiene. Arrange supplies at bedside and apply clean gloves. Close door or pull curtain.
16. Help patient assume left side-lying position with upper leg flexed upward.
17. If patient has mobility impairment, help into lateral position. Obtain help to turn patient and use pillows under upper arm and leg.

18. Keep patient draped with only anal area exposed.
19. Examine condition of anus externally. *Option:* Palpate rectal walls as needed (e.g., if impaction is suspected) (see Chapter 30). If you palpate rectal walls, dispose of gloves by turning them inside out and placing them in proper receptacle if they become soiled. Otherwise keep gloves on your hands and proceed to Step 20.
20. Perform hand hygiene and apply new pair of clean gloves (if previous gloves were soiled and discarded).

   CLINICAL JUDGMENT: Do not palpate patient's rectum if there is a recent history of rectal surgery. A suppository is contraindicated in the presence of active bleeding and diarrhea (Burchum and Rosenthal, 2019).

21. Remove suppository from foil wrapper and lubricate rounded end with water-soluble lubricant. Lubricate gloved index finger of dominant hand. If patient has hemorrhoids, use liberal amount of lubricant and touch area gently.
22. Ask patient to take slow, deep breaths through mouth and relax anal sphincter.
23. Retract patient's buttocks with nondominant hand. With gloved index finger of dominant hand, insert suppository gently through anus, past internal sphincter, and against rectal wall, 10 cm (4 inches) in adults (see illustration) or 5 cm (2 inches) in infants and children. You should feel rectal sphincter close around your finger.

STEP 23 Inserting rectal suppository past sphincter and against rectal wall. (From Williams P: *Fundamental concepts and skills for nursing*, ed 6, St. Louis, 2022, Elsevier.)

   CLINICAL JUDGMENT: Do not insert suppository into a mass of fecal material; this will reduce effectiveness of medication.

24. *Option:* A suppository may be given through a colostomy (not ileostomy) if ordered. Patient should lie supine. Use small amount of water-soluble lubricant for insertion.
25. Withdraw finger and wipe patient's anal area.
26. Ask patient to remain flat or on side for 5 minutes.
27. Discard gloves by turning them inside out and dispose of all contaminated supplies in appropriate receptacle, remove and dispose of gloves, and perform hand hygiene.
28. Help patient to comfortable position.

BOX 31.18 PROCEDURAL GUIDELINES—cont'd

Administering Rectal Suppositories

29. Place nurse call system in an accessible location within patient's reach.
30. Raise side rails (as appropriate) and lower bed to lowest position.
31. If suppository contains laxative or fecal softener, place nurse call system within reach so that patient can obtain help to reach bedpan or toilet.
32. If suppository was given for constipation, remind patient *not* to flush commode after bowel movement, so you can observe characteristics of stool.
33. Record the medication, dosage, route, and actual time and date of administration on MAR immediately after administration, not before. Include initials or signature.
34. Return to bedside within 5 minutes to determine whether suppository was expelled.
35. Ask whether patient experienced localized anal or rectal discomfort during insertion.

36. Evaluate patient at time of peak medication effect for relief of symptoms for which medication was prescribed.
37. Record patient response to medication, patient teaching, and validation of patient understanding of self-administration of suppository on flow sheet or nurses' notes in electronic health record (EHR) or chart.
38. **Use Teach-Back:** "I want to be sure I explained clearly to you how to insert a rectal suppository. Describe the steps you will follow to insert the suppository." Revise your instruction now or develop a plan for revised patient/family caregiver teaching if patient/family caregiver is not able to teach back correctly. Determines patient's/family caregiver's level of understanding of instructional topic.

have diminished hand strength; therefore it is essential to assess whether they have enough strength to use the pMDI.

Sometimes patients use a spacer with the pMDI. A spacer is a tube that is 10.16 to 20.32 cm (4–8 inches) in length that attaches to the pMDI and allows the particles of medication to slow down and break into smaller pieces. This helps the medication get deeper into the lungs and enhances absorption. Spacers are helpful when a patient has difficulty coordinating the steps involved in self-administering medications. However, patients who do not use their spacers correctly do not receive the full effect of the medication. BAIs and DPIs do not use spacers.

BAIs release medication when a patient raises a lever and inhales. Release of the medication depends on the strength of the patient's breath on inspiration, and a BAI is a good choice for patients who have difficulty in using pMDIs because it eliminates the need for hand-breath coordination (Hess and Dhand, 2020a).

DPIs hold dry powder medication and create an aerosol when the patient inhales through a reservoir that contains a dose of the medication. The reservoir holds a dose of the medication. Compared with MDIs, DPIs deliver more medication to the lungs (Burchum and Rosenthal, 2019). Some DPIs are unit dosed. These inhalers require patients to load a single dose of medication into the inhaler with each use. Other DPIs hold enough medication for 1 month. DPIs require less manual dexterity. Because the device is activated with the patient's breath, there is no need to coordinate puffs with inhalation. However, the medication inside the DPI can clump if the patient is in a humid climate, and some patients cannot inspire fast enough to administer the entire dose of the medication.

Patients who receive medications by inhalation frequently have chronic respiratory disease such as chronic asthma, emphysema, or bronchitis. Different respiratory problems require different inhaled medication. For example, patients with asthma usually receive antiinflammatory medications because asthma is primarily an inflammatory disease, whereas patients with chronic obstructive pulmonary disease (COPD) receive bronchodilators because they usually have problems with bronchoconstriction. Inhaled medications are also often described as "rescue" or "maintenance" medications. Rescue medications are short acting and taken for immediate relief of acute respiratory distress. Maintenance medications are used on a daily schedule to prevent acute respiratory distress. The effects of maintenance medications start within hours of administration and last for a longer time period than rescue medications. Some inhalers contain combinations of rescue and maintenance medications. Because patients depend on inhaled medications for disease control and because current evidence shows that many patients do not use their inhalers correctly, nurses need to teach and reteach their patients about their safe and effective use (Gerald and Dhand, 2020) (see Skill 31.3).

One important aspect of patient teaching is to help the patient determine when the MDI, BAI, or DPI is empty and needs to be replaced. Floating an MDI in water to determine how much medication is left is not recommended because extra propellant causes the container to float even if no medication remains in the inhaler. Devices that count down the number of remaining doses are available for MDIs. Some DPIs have mechanisms that indicate how many doses are left. However, these mechanisms are not always accurate. To calculate how long medication in an inhaler will last, divide the number of doses in the container by the number of doses the patient takes per day. For example, a patient is to take albuterol 2 puffs 4 times a day. The canister has a total of 200 puffs. Complete the following calculation to determine how long the MDI will last:

$$2 \text{ puffs} \times 4 \text{ times a day} = 8 \text{ puffs per day}$$

$$200 \text{ puffs} \div 8 \text{ puffs per day} = 25 \text{ days}$$

The canister in this example will last 25 days. To ensure that the patient does not run out of medication, teach the patient to refill it at least 7 to 10 days before it runs out.

Administering Medications by Irrigation

Some medications irrigate or wash out a body cavity and are delivered through a stream of solution. Irrigations most commonly use sterile water, saline, or antiseptic solutions on the eye, ear, throat, vagina, or urinary tract. Use aseptic technique if there is a break in the skin or mucosa. Use clean technique when the cavity to be irrigated is not sterile, as in the case of the ear canal or vagina. Irrigations cleanse an area, instill a medication, or apply hot or cold to injured tissue (see Chapter 48).

Parenteral Administration of Medications

Parenteral administration of medications is the administration of medications by injection into body tissues. This is an invasive procedure that is performed using aseptic techniques (Box 31.19). A risk of infection occurs after a needle pierces the skin.

Each type of injection requires certain skills to ensure that the medication reaches the proper location. The effects of a parenteral medication develop rapidly, depending on the rate of medication absorption. You must closely observe a patient's response to parenteral medications.

BOX 31.19   Preventing Infection During an Injection

- To prevent contaminating the solution, draw up medication quickly. Do not allow ampules to stand open.
- To prevent needle contamination, avoid letting a needle touch contaminated surfaces (e.g., outer edges of ampule or vial, outer surface of needle cap, nurse's hands, countertop, table surface).
- To prevent syringe contamination, avoid touching length of plunger or inner part of barrel. Keep tip of syringe covered with cap or needle.
- To prepare skin, wash with soap and water if soiled with dirt, drainage, or feces, and dry. Use friction and a circular motion while cleaning with an antiseptic swab. Swab from center of site and move outward in a 5-cm (2-inch) radius.

FIG. 31.10 Types of syringes: (A) 5-mL syringe; (B) 3-mL syringe; (C) tuberculin syringe marked in 0.01 (hundredths) for doses less than 1 mL; (D) insulin syringe marked in units (50).

FIG. 31.11 Parts of a syringe and needle.

Equipment. You will administer parenteral medications by using a needle and a syringe, available in a variety of sizes. Each is designed to deliver a certain volume of a medication to a specific type of tissue. Determine the appropriate size of syringe, length and gauge of needle, volume of solution, and medication route based on the quantity and type of medication prescribed and the body size of a patient. Most syringes come with needleless systems or safety needles that help prevent needlestick injuries.

Syringes. Syringes consist of a cylindrical barrel with a tip designed to fit the hub of a hypodermic needle and a close-fitting plunger. Syringes are single use, disposable, and classified as being Luer-Lok or non–Luer-Lok. This terminology is based on the design of the tip of the syringe. Luer-Lok syringes have needles that are twisted onto the tip and lock themselves in place (Fig. 31.10A–B). This design prevents the inadvertent removal of the needle. Non–Luer-Lok syringes (Fig. 31.10C–D) have needles that slip onto the tip. Syringes come with or without a sterile needle and with a needleless sharp with engineered sharps injury protection (SESIP) device.

Syringes come in a variety of sizes, from 0.5 to 60 mL. It is unusual to use a syringe larger than 5 mL for an injection. A 1- to 3-mL syringe is usually adequate for a subcutaneous or IM injection (Fig. 31.10B). A larger volume creates discomfort. Use larger syringes to administer certain IV medications and to irrigate wounds or drainage tubes. Syringes often come prepackaged with a needle attached. However, you sometimes change a needle based on the route of administration and size of a patient.

The tuberculin syringe (see Fig. 31.10C) is calibrated in sixteenths of a minim and hundredths of a milliliter and has a capacity of 1 mL. Use a tuberculin syringe to prepare small amounts of medications (e.g., ID or subcutaneous injections). A tuberculin syringe is also useful when preparing small, precise doses for infants or young children.

Insulin syringes (see Fig. 31.10D) hold 0.3 mL to 1 mL, and low-dose insulin syringes (30 units per 0.3 mL or 50 units per 0.5 mL) hold 0.3 mL to 1 mL. Insulin syringes come with preattached needles and are calibrated in units. Most insulin syringes are U-100s, designed for use with U-100–strength insulin. Each milliliter of solution contains 100 units of insulin.

Fill a syringe by pulling the plunger outward while the needle tip remains immersed in the prepared solution. Touch only the outside of the syringe barrel and the handle of the plunger to maintain sterility. Avoid letting any unsterile object touch the tip or inside of the barrel, the hub, the shaft of the plunger, or the needle.

Needles. Some needles come packaged in individual sheaths to allow flexibility in choosing the right needle for a patient, whereas others are preattached to standard-size syringes. Most needles are made of stainless steel, and all are disposable. A needle has three parts: the hub, which fits onto the tip of a syringe; the shaft, which connects to the hub; and the bevel, or slanted tip (Fig. 31.11). The tip of a needle, or the bevel, is always slanted. When the needle is injected into tissue, the bevel creates a narrow slit that quickly closes when the needle is removed to prevent leakage of medication, blood, or serum. Long, beveled tips are sharper and narrower, minimizing discomfort when entering tissue used for subcutaneous or IM injections.

Most needles vary in length from ¼ to 3 inches (Fig. 31.12). Choose the needle length according to a patient's size and weight and the type of tissue into which the medication is to be injected. Current evidence suggests that needle length should be based on a patient's weight (Holliday et al., 2019). There should be a 5-mm depth of muscle penetration for an IM injection (Hibberd et al., 2021). A child or slender adult generally requires a shorter needle. Use longer needles (1–1½ inches) for IM injections and a shorter needle (⅜ – ⅝ inch) for subcutaneous injections. As the needle gauge becomes smaller, the diameter becomes larger. The selection of a gauge depends on the viscosity of fluid to be injected or infused.

Disposable Injection Units. Single-dose, prefilled, disposable syringes are available for some medications. You do not need to prepare medication doses except perhaps to expel unneeded portions of medication or

FIG. 31.12 Hypodermic needles *(top to bottom)*: 18 gauge, 1½-inch length; 21 gauge, 1½-inch length; 22 gauge, 1½-inch length; 23 gauge, 1-inch length; and 25 gauge, ⅝-inch length.

air. However, it is important to check the medication and concentration carefully because prefilled syringes appear very similar. Prefilled unit-dose systems such as Tubex and Carpuject include reusable plastic syringe holders and disposable, prefilled, sterile, glass cartridge units (Fig. 31.13). To assemble a prefilled system, place the cartridge barrel first into the plastic syringe holder. Following manufacturer's instructions, turn the plunger rod to the left (counterclockwise) and the lock to the right (clockwise) until it "clicks." Finally, remove the needle guard and advance the plunger to expel air and excess medication, as with a regular syringe. The cartridge may be used with SESIP needles. After administering a medication, dispose of the glass cartridge safely in a puncture-proof and leak-proof container. This design reduces the risk for needlestick injury.

Preparing an Injection From an Ampule. Ampules contain single doses of medication in a liquid. They are available in several sizes, from 1 mL to 10 mL or more (Fig. 31.14A). An ampule is made of glass with a constricted neck that must be snapped off to allow access to the medication. A colored ring around the neck indicates where the ampule is prescored so that you can break it easily. Carefully aspirate the medication into a syringe (see Skill 31.4) with a filter needle. Filter needles must be used when preparing medication from a glass ampule to prevent glass particles from being drawn into the syringe (Painchart et al., 2018). *Do not* use a filter needle to administer a medication. Place an appropriate-size needle on the syringe after withdrawing the medication.

Preparing an Injection From a Vial. A vial is a single-dose or multidose container with a rubber seal at the top (see Fig. 31.14B). A metal cap protects the seal until it is ready for use. Vials contain liquid or dry forms of medications. Medications that are unstable in solution are packaged dry. The vial label specifies the solvent or diluent used to dissolve the medication and the amount of diluent needed to prepare a desired medication concentration. Normal saline and sterile distilled water are commonly used to dissolve medications.

Unlike the ampule, the vial is a closed system, and air needs to be injected into it to permit easy withdrawal of the solution. Failure to inject air when withdrawing creates a vacuum within the vial that makes withdrawal difficult. If concerned about drawing up parts of the

FIG. 31.13 (A) Carpuject syringe and prefilled sterile cartridge with needle. (B) Assembling the Carpuject. (C) Cartridge slides into syringe barrel. Turn and lock syringe into cartridge. (D) Screw plunger into end of cartridge. Expel excess medication to obtain accurate dose (not pictured).

rubber stopper or other particles into the syringe, use a filter needle when preparing medications from vials (ISMP, 2019b). Some vials contain powder, which is mixed with a diluent during preparation and before injection (see Skill 31.4). After mixing multidose vials, make a label that includes the date and time of mixing and the concentration of medication per milliliter. Some multidose vials require refrigeration after the contents are reconstituted.

FIG. 31.14 (A) Medication in ampules. (B) Medication in vials.

FIG. 31.15 (A) Injecting air into vial A. (B) Injecting air into vial B and withdrawing dose. (C) Withdrawing medication from vial A; medications are now mixed.

Mixing Medications. If two medications are compatible, it is possible to mix them in one injection if the total dose is within accepted limits. This prevents a patient from having to receive more than one injection at a time. Most nursing units have charts that list common compatible medications. If there is any uncertainty about medication compatibilities, consult a pharmacist or a medication reference.

Mixing Medications From a Vial and an Ampule. When mixing medication from both a vial and ampule, prepare medication from the vial first. Using the same syringe and filter needle, next withdraw medication from the ampule. Nurses prepare the combination in this order because it is not necessary to add air to withdraw medication from an ampule.

Mixing Medications From Two Vials. Apply these principles when mixing medications from two vials:
1. Do not contaminate one medication with another.
2. Ensure that the final dose is accurate.
3. Maintain aseptic technique.

Use only one syringe with a needle or needleless access device attached to mix medications from two vials (Fig. 31.15). Aspirate the volume of air equivalent to the dose of the first medication (vial A) (Fig. 31.15A). Inject the air into vial A, making sure that the needle does not touch the solution. Withdraw the needle and aspirate air equivalent to the dose of the second medication (vial B). Inject the volume of air into vial B (Fig. 31.15B). Immediately withdraw the medication from vial B into the syringe and insert the needle back into vial A, being careful not to push the plunger and expel the medication within the syringe into the vial. Withdraw the desired amount of medication from vial A into the syringe (Fig. 31.15C). After withdrawing the necessary amount, withdraw the needle and apply a new safety needle or needleless access device suitable for injection.

Insulin Preparation. Insulin is the hormone used to treat diabetes mellitus. It is administered by injection because the GI tract breaks down and destroys an oral form of insulin. Most patients with diabetes mellitus who take insulin injections learn to administer their own injections. In the United States and Canada, health care providers usually prescribe insulin in concentrations of 100 units per milliliter of solution. This is called *U-100 insulin*. Insulin is also commercially available in concentrations of 500 units per milliliter of solution; it is called *U-500 insulin*. U-500 insulin is 5 times as strong as U-100 insulin and is used only in rare cases when patients are very resistant to insulin. Insulin injection guidelines have been developed and modified over the past several years in response to increasing evidence and research about best practices for patient assessment and site selection (Weinstock, 2021a; Weinstock, 2021b). Based on this evidence:
- Use the same technique for both insulin syringes and insulin pens.
- For most adults, a 4-mm needle is sufficient for the injection.

- If an insulin pen is used, after injection keep the needle in place for 10 seconds to avoid leakage.
- Do not aspirate the injection, which is especially important with insulin pens to prevent leakage of medication.
- Because insulin is absorbed rapidly through the abdominal wall, the abdomen is your first choice for sites when using rapid-acting insulin.

Use the correct syringe when preparing insulin. Use a 100-unit insulin syringe or an insulin pen to prepare U-100 insulin. Until recently there was no syringe designed to prepare U-500 insulin, and many medication errors resulted with this kind of insulin. To prevent errors, ensure that the health care provider order for U-500 specifies units and that the patient is taught the difference between U-500 and U-100 syringes (Consumer Med Safety, 2018; ISMP, 2017b). Verify every injection you prepare with another nurse before administering it. Additional safety measures common with U-500 insulin include listing the insulin as being concentrated in computerized medication dispensing systems, making health care providers and pharmacists verify that a patient is to receive U-500 insulin when it is ordered, and stocking U-500 insulin with U-500 syringes on patient care units only when it is ordered for a specific patient (ISMP, 2017b; Weinstock, 2021a).

Insulin is classified by rate of action, including rapid-acting, short-acting, intermediate-acting, and long-acting types. To provide safe and effective care, you need to know the onset, peak, and duration for each of your patients' ordered insulin doses. Refer to a medication reference or consult with a pharmacist if you are unsure of this information. Regular insulin is the only type of insulin that can be given intravenously.

A patient with diabetes mellitus sometimes requires more than one type of insulin. For example, by receiving a short-acting (regular) and intermediate-acting (NPH) insulin, a patient receives more sustained control of blood glucose levels over 24 hours. The timing of insulin injections attempts to imitate the normal pattern of insulin release from the pancreas. Some insulins come in a stable premixed solution (e.g., 70/30 insulin is 70% NPH [intermediate] and 30% regular), eliminating the need to mix the insulins in a syringe. Other patients use an insulin pen. The insulin pen provides multiple doses and allows a patient to dial in the dose, avoiding the need to use a syringe for insulin preparation. Research shows that different types of a patient's blood cells can enter into the insulin pen after an injection. Several U.S. health care agencies recently reported that the same insulin pen was inadvertently used on multiple patients, exposing the patients to bloodborne illnesses (e.g., human immunodeficiency virus [HIV], hepatitis B, and hepatitis C). Therefore the ISMP (2017b) recommends that insulin pens be used only at home and that inpatient settings provide an insulin pen for a single patient use.

Insulin is ordered by a specific dose at select times. Correction or correctional insulin, also known as sliding-scale insulin, provides a dose of insulin based on the patient's blood glucose level (Box 31.20). The term *correctional insulin* is preferred because it indicates that small doses of rapid- or short-acting insulin are needed to correct a patient's elevated blood sugar.

Before drawing up insulin doses, gently roll all cloudy insulin preparations between the palms of the hands to resuspend the insulin.

Do not shake insulin vials, shaking causes bubbles to form. Bubbles take up space in the syringe and alter the dose.

If more than one type of insulin is required to manage the patient's diabetes, you mix two different types of insulin into one syringe *if* they are compatible (Box 31.21). If regular and intermediate-acting insulins are ordered, prepare the regular insulin first to prevent it from becoming contaminated with the intermediate-acting insulin. Use the following principles when mixing insulins (Association of Diabetes Care & Education Specialists (ADCES), 2020; ISMP, 2017b; Wexler, 2021):

- Patients whose blood glucose levels are well controlled on a mixed-insulin dose need to maintain their individual routine when preparing and administering their insulin.
- Do not mix insulin with any other medications or diluents unless approved by the health care provider.
- Never mix insulin glargine or insulin detemir with other types of insulin.
- Inject rapid-acting insulins mixed with NPH insulin within 15 minutes before a meal.
- Verify insulin doses with another nurse while you are preparing the injection.

Administering Injections

Each injection route differs based on the type of tissues the medication enters. The characteristics of the tissues influence the rate of medication

---

BOX 31.20 Example of Correction Insulin Order

Give regular U-100 insulin subcutaneously:
2 units for glucose 150 to 200 mg/dL
4 units for glucose 201 to 275 mg/dL
Call for glucose greater than 275 mg/dL

Clinical scenario: Before lunch patient's blood glucose level is 201 mg/dL. After referring to patient's correction insulin order, what is the correct amount of insulin the nurse should administer?

BOX 31.21 PROCEDURAL GUIDELINES

Mixing Two Types of Insulin in One Syringe

Delegation and Collaboration

The skill of mixing two types of insulin in one syringe cannot be delegated to assistive personnel (AP). The nurse directs the AP about:

- Potential side effects of medications and the need to immediately report their occurrence to the nurse.

Equipment

Medication administration record (MAR) (printed or electronic); insulin vials, insulin syringe, antiseptic swab

Procedural Steps

1. Check accuracy and completeness of MAR or computer printout with health care provider's written medication order. Check patient's name, medication name and dosage, route of administration, and time of administration. Clarify incomplete or unclear orders with health care provider before administration.
2. Review medication and medical history (e.g., type of diabetes, reason for elevated blood sugar) and allergies to medications, food, and latex.
3. Verify insulin labels carefully against MAR before preparing the dose to ensure that you give the correct type of insulin. *This is the first check for accuracy.*
4. Perform hand hygiene.
5. If patient takes insulin that is cloudy, roll the bottle of insulin between the hands to resuspend the insulin preparation.
6. Wipe off tops of both insulin vials with alcohol swabs and allow to dry.
7. Verify insulin dosages against MAR a second time. *This is the second accuracy check.*
8. If mixing rapid- or short-acting insulin with intermediate-acting insulin, take insulin syringe and aspirate volume of air equivalent to dose to be withdrawn from intermediate-acting insulin first. If two intermediate-acting insulins are mixed, it makes no difference which vial you prepare first.

9. Insert needle and inject air into vial of intermediate-acting insulin. Do not let the tip of the needle touch the insulin.
10. Remove the syringe from the vial of intermediate-acting insulin without aspirating medication.
11. With the same syringe, inject air equal to the dose of rapid- or short-acting insulin into the vial and withdraw the correct dose into the syringe.
12. Remove the syringe from the rapid- or short-acting insulin and get rid of air bubbles to ensure accurate dosing.
13. After verifying insulin dosages with MAR a third time, show insulin prepared in syringe to another nurse to verify that you prepared correct dosage of insulin. *This is the third accuracy check.* Determine which point on syringe scale indicates combined units of insulin measure by adding the number of units of both insulins together (e.g., 5 units regular + 10 units NPH = 15 units total).
14. Place the needle of the syringe back into the vial of intermediate-acting insulin. Be careful not to push plunger and inject insulin in syringe into the vial.
15. Invert the vial and carefully withdraw the desired amount of insulin into syringe.
16. Withdraw needle and check fluid level in syringe. Keep needle of prepared syringe sheathed or capped until ready to administer medication. Show another nurse the syringe to verify that you prepared the correct dose.
17. Dispose of soiled supplies in proper receptacle. Place empty vials in puncture-proof and leak-proof container and perform hand hygiene.
18. Because rapid- or short-acting insulin binds with intermediate-acting insulin, which reduces the action of the faster-acting insulin, administer mixture within 5 minutes of preparing it.

Adapted from Weinstock R: General principles of insulin therapy in diabetes mellitus, *UpToDate*, 2020a. http://www.uptodate.com/contents/general-principles-of-insulin-therapy-in-diabetes-mellitus. Accessed August 17, 2021.

absorption, affecting the onset of medication action. Before injecting a medication, know the volume of the medication to administer, the characteristics and viscosity of the medication, and the location of anatomical structures underlying injection sites (see Skill 31.5).

If you do not administer injections correctly, negative patient outcomes result. Failure to select an injection site in relation to anatomical landmarks results in nerve or bone damage during needle insertion. Inability to maintain stability of the needle and syringe unit can result in pain and tissue damage. If you fail to aspirate the syringe before injecting an IM medication, the medication may be injected accidentally directly into an artery or vein. Injecting too large a volume of medication for the site selected causes extreme pain and results in local tissue damage.

Many patients, particularly children, fear injections. Patients with serious or chronic illness often are given several injections daily. Minimize discomfort in the following ways:

- Use a sharp-beveled needle in the smallest suitable length and gauge.
- Position a patient as comfortably as possible to reduce muscular tension.
- Select the proper injection site, using anatomical landmarks.
- Apply a vapocoolant spray (e.g., Fluori-Methane spray or ethyl chloride) or topical anesthetic (e.g., eutectic mixture of local anesthetics [EMLA] cream) to the injection site before giving the medication when possible (see agency policy).
- Divert the patient's attention from the injection through conversation using open-ended questioning.
- Insert the needle quickly and smoothly to minimize tissue pulling.
- Hold the syringe steady while the needle remains in tissues.
- Inject the medication slowly and steadily.

Subcutaneous Injections. Subcutaneous injections involve placing medications into the loose connective tissue under the dermis (see Skill 31.5). Because subcutaneous tissue is not as richly supplied with blood as the muscles, medication absorption is somewhat slower than with IM injections. Physical exercise or application of hot or cold compresses influences the rate of drug absorption by altering local blood flow to tissues. Any condition that impairs blood flow is a contraindication for subcutaneous injections. Because subcutaneous tissue contains pain receptors, a patient often experiences slight discomfort.

The best subcutaneous injection sites include the outer posterior aspect of the upper arms, the abdomen from below the costal margins to the iliac crests, and the anterior aspects of the thighs (Fig. 31.16). The

site most frequently recommended for heparin injections is the abdomen (Fig. 31.17). Alternative subcutaneous sites for other medications include the scapular areas of the upper back and the upper ventral or dorsal gluteal areas. The injection site you choose needs to be free of skin lesions, bony prominences, and large underlying muscles or nerves.

The administration of low-molecular-weight heparin (LMWH) (e.g., enoxaparin) requires special considerations. When injecting the medication, use the right or left side of the abdomen at least 5 cm (2 inches) from the umbilicus (the patient's "love handles") and pinch the injection site as you insert the needle. Administer LMWH in its prefilled syringe with the attached needle, and do not expel the air bubble in the syringe before giving the medication.

Use U-100 insulin syringes with preattached 31- to 25-gauge needles when giving U-100 insulin and U-500 insulin syringes when giving U-500 insulin. The use of individual patient insulin pens is recommended for all insulin administration (ISMP 2017b; Weinstock 2021a; Weinstock, 2021b). Recommended sites for insulin injections include the upper arm and the anterior and lateral parts of the thigh, buttocks, and abdomen. Rotating injections within the same body part (intrasite rotation) provides more consistency in the absorption of the insulin. For example, if a patient receives morning insulin in the right arm, give the next injection in a different place in the same arm. The injections are to be given at least 2.5 cm (1 inch) away from the previous site. Injection sites should not be used again for at least 1 month. The rate of insulin absorption varies based on the site; the abdomen has the quickest absorption, followed by the arms, thighs, and buttocks (Weinstock, 2021a).

Subcutaneous tissue is sensitive to irritating solutions and large volumes of medications. Therefore you administer only small volumes (0.5–1.5 mL) of water-soluble medications subcutaneously to adults. You give smaller volumes up to 0.5 mL to children (Hockenberry et al., 2019). Hardened, painful lumps called *sterile abscesses* occur under the skin if medication collects within the tissues.

A patient's body weight indicates the depth of the subcutaneous layer. Choose the needle length and angle of insertion based on a patient's weight and an estimation of the amount of subcutaneous tissue (Larkin et al., 2018). Nurses typically use a 25-gauge, ⅝-inch (16-mm) needle inserted at a 45-degree angle (Fig. 31.18) or a ½-inch (12-mm) needle inserted at a 90-degree angle to administer subcutaneous medications to a normal-size adult patient. Some children require only a ½-inch needle. If the patient is obese, pinch the tissue and use a needle long enough to insert through fatty tissue at the base of the skinfold. Patients who are

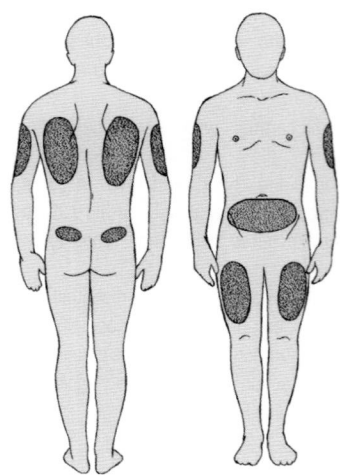

FIG. 31.16 Sites recommended for subcutaneous injections.

FIG. 31.17 Giving subcutaneous heparin in abdomen.

FIG. 31.18 Comparison of angles of insertion for intramuscular (90 degrees), subcutaneous (45–90 degrees), and intradermal (15 degrees) injections.

FIG. 31.19 Insulin injection pen. (From Lewis SM, et al: *Medical-surgical nursing,* ed 10, St Louis, 2017, Elsevier.)

FIG. 31.20 Jet injection system is held perpendicular to skin. (Image courtesy Pharmajet. All rights reserved.)

FIG. 31.21 Subcutaneous device. (Image courtesy IntraPump Infusion Systems. All rights reserved.)

thin often do not have sufficient tissue for subcutaneous injections; the upper abdomen is usually the best site in this case. To ensure that a subcutaneous medication reaches the subcutaneous tissue, follow this rule: If you can grasp 2 inches (5 cm) of tissue, insert the needle at a 90-degree angle; if you can grasp 2.5 cm (1 inch) of tissue, insert the needle at a 45-degree angle.

Research in insulin administration shows that insulin needles that are 5/16 inch (8 mm) or longer often enter the muscles of men and people with a BMI of 25 or less. Shorter (3/16-inch or 4- to 5-mm) needles were associated with less pain, adequate control of blood sugars, and minimal leakage of medication (ISMP, 2017b). Accordingly, when administering insulin, you should use needles of 31 gauge (4–6 mm) administered at a 90-degree angle to reduce pain and achieve adequate control of blood sugars with minimal adverse effects for people of all BMIs, including children (Levitsky and Misra, 2020; Weinstock, 2021a).

Several technologies are available for administration of subcutaneous injections. *Injection pens* are a technology that patients can use to self-administer medications (e.g., epinephrine, insulin, or interferon) subcutaneously (Fig. 31.19). They offer a convenient delivery method using prefilled, disposable cartridges. The patient pinches the skin, inserts the needle, and injects a predetermined medication dose. Teaching is essential to ensure that patients use the correct injection technique and deliver the correct dose of medication. Patients need to be taught the importance of purging the pen before a dose is given. The disadvantages to this technology include increased risk for needlestick injury and users' lack of knowledge and skill in administration technique (ISMP, 2017b). The *needleless jet injection system* administers subcutaneous medications without the use of needles. Needle-free injections use high pressure to penetrate the skin with the medication into the subcutaneous tissue (Fig. 31.20). Another advance in subcutaneous injection is the *subcutaneous injection device* (e.g., insuflon) (Fig. 31.21), which is inserted into the subcutaneous tissue; the needle is then removed, leaving the cannula in the tissue to provide an avenue for administering medications for up to 3 days without having to puncture the skin with each injection.

Intramuscular Injections. The IM injection route deposits medication into deep muscle tissue, which has a rich blood supply, allowing medication to be absorbed faster than by the subcutaneous route. However, there is a risk for injecting medications directly into blood vessels. Any factor that interferes with local tissue blood flow affects the rate and extent of medication absorption. In addition, if a medication is not injected correctly into a muscle, complications can arise such as abscess, hematoma, ecchymosis, pain, and vascular and nerve injury (Vicdan et al., 2019).

The viscosity of the medication, injection site, and patient's weight, gender, and amount of adipose tissue influence needle size selection (Strohfus et al., 2018). Determine needle gauge according to the medication to be administered. Some medications such as hepatitis B and tetanus, diphtheria, and pertussis (Tdap) immunizations are given only intramuscularly.

Use a longer and heavier-gauge needle to pass through subcutaneous tissue and penetrate deep muscle tissue (see Skill 31.5). A patient's BMI and the amount of adipose tissue influence needle size selection. You must choose the needle length and site of injection based on the size of the muscle, the thickness of adipose tissue at the injection site, the volume to be administered, the injection technique, and the depth below the muscle surface to be injected (Centers for Disease Control and Prevention [CDC], 2021a; Davidson and Bertram, 2019). Investigate other medication routes, especially when IM injections are ordered for patients who are obese (Larkin et al., 2018). Note that the most common IM injections are immunizations.

The angle of insertion for an IM injection is 90 degrees (see Fig. 31.18). Muscle is less sensitive to irritating and viscous medications. A normal, well-developed adult patient tolerates 3 mL of medication into a larger muscle without severe muscle discomfort (Lilley et al., 2020). Larger volumes of medication (4–5 mL) are unlikely to be absorbed properly. Children, older adults, and patients who are thin tolerate only 2 mL of an IM injection. Do not give more than 1 mL to small children and older infants, and do not give more than 0.5 mL to smaller infants (Hockenberry et al., 2019).

Assess a muscle before giving an injection. Properly identify the site for the IM injection by palpating bony landmarks and be aware of the potential complications associated with each site. The site needs to be free of tenderness because repeated injections in the same muscle cause severe discomfort. With the patient relaxed, palpate the muscle to rule out any hardened lesions. Minimize discomfort during an injection by helping a patient assume a position that helps to reduce muscle strain. Other interventions such as distraction and applying pressure to an IM site decrease pain during an injection.

Rotate IM injection sites to decrease the risk for tissue hypertrophy. Emaciated or atrophied muscles absorb medication poorly; thus, avoid their use when possible. The Z-track method, a technique for pulling the skin during an injection, is recommended for IM injections (Strohfus et al., 2018). It prevents leakage of medication into subcutaneous tissues, seals medication in the muscle, and minimizes irritation. To use the Z-track method, apply the appropriate-size needle to the syringe and select an IM site, preferably in a large, deep muscle such as the ventrogluteal. Pull the overlying skin and subcutaneous tissues approximately 2.5 to 3.5 cm (1–1½ inches) laterally to the side with the ulnar side of the nondominant hand. Hold the skin in this position until you have administered the injection (Fig. 31.22A). After cleaning a site, inject the needle deeply into the muscle. To reduce injection site discomfort, there is no longer any need to aspirate after the needle is injected when *administering vaccines* (CDC, 2021a). It is the nurse's responsibility to follow agency policy for aspirating vaccines after inserting the needle. Keep the needle inserted for 10 seconds to allow the medication to disperse evenly. Release the skin after withdrawing the needle. This leaves a zigzag path

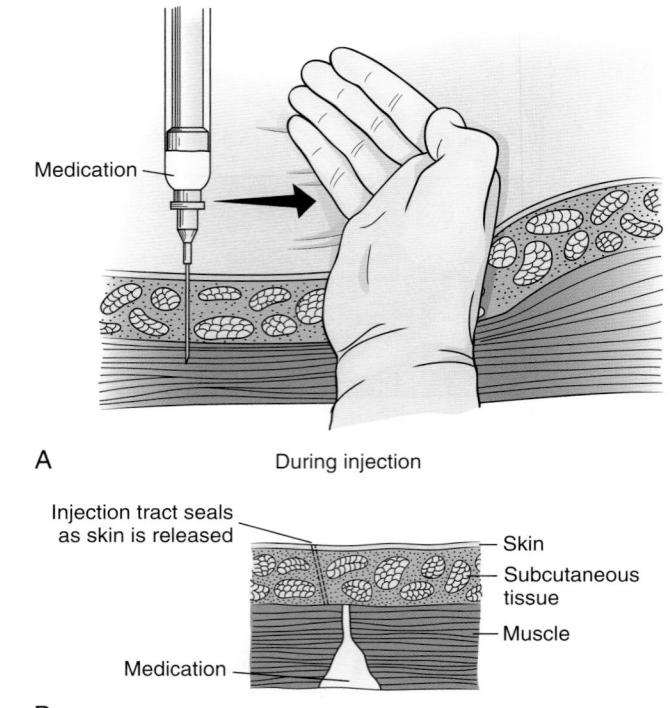

FIG. 31.22 (A) Pulling on overlying skin during intramuscular injection moves tissue to prevent later tracking. (B) Z-track method of injection prevents deposit of medication into sensitive tissue.

that seals the needle track wherever tissue planes slide across one another see (Fig. 31.22B). The medication is sealed in the muscle tissue.

Sites. When selecting an IM site, consider the following: Is the area free of infection or necrosis? Are there local areas of bruising or abrasions? What are the locations of underlying bones, nerves, and major blood vessels? What volume of medication is to be administered? Each site has different advantages and disadvantages.

Ventrogluteal. The ventrogluteal muscle involves the gluteus medius; it is situated deep and away from major nerves and blood vessels. This site is the preferred and safest site for all adults, children, and infants, especially for medications that have larger volumes and are more viscous and irritating (Drutz, 2021; Hockenberry et al., 2019; Strohfus et al., 2018; Vicdan et al., 2019).

Locate the ventrogluteal muscle by positioning the patient in a supine or lateral position. One way to locate the ventrogluteal muscle use is by the "V" method. You position a patient in a supine or lateral position with the knee and hip flexed to relax the muscle. Use your right hand for the left hip and your left hand for the right hip. For example, if you are administering the injection into the patient's left hip, place the palm of your right hand over the greater trochanter of the patient's hip with your wrist perpendicular to the femur. Then move your thumb toward the patient's groin and your index finger toward the anterior superior iliac spine. Extend or open your middle finger back along the iliac crest toward the patient's buttock. The index finger, middle finger, and iliac crest form a V-shaped triangle, with the injection site in the center of the triangle (Fig. 31.23) (Larkin et al., 2018). To relax this muscle, help patients to lie on their side or back, flexing the knee and hip.

There has been some evidence to suggest that the "V" technique is not always reliable because of differences in nurses' hand structure and patients' body structure, especially when a patient is obese (Larkin et al., 2018).

FIG. 31.23 (A) Landmarks for ventrogluteal site. (B) Locating ventrogluteal site in patient. (C) Giving intramuscular injection in ventrogluteal muscle using Z-track method.

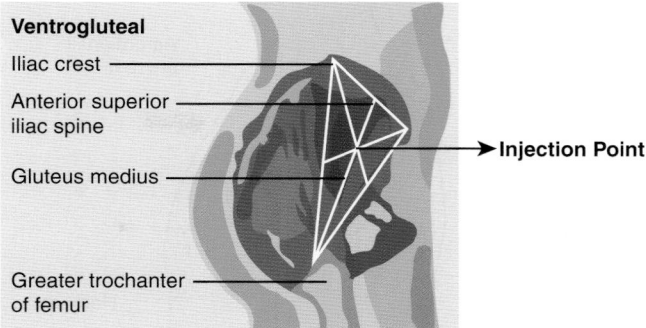

Ventrogluteal

Iliac crest
Anterior superior iliac spine
Gluteus medius
Injection Point
Greater trochanter of femur

FIG. 31.24 Determination of intramuscular injection site using the G method. (From Kaya N, et al: The reliability of site determination methods in ventrogluteal area injection: a cross-sectional study, *Int J Nurs Stud* 52:355, 2015.)

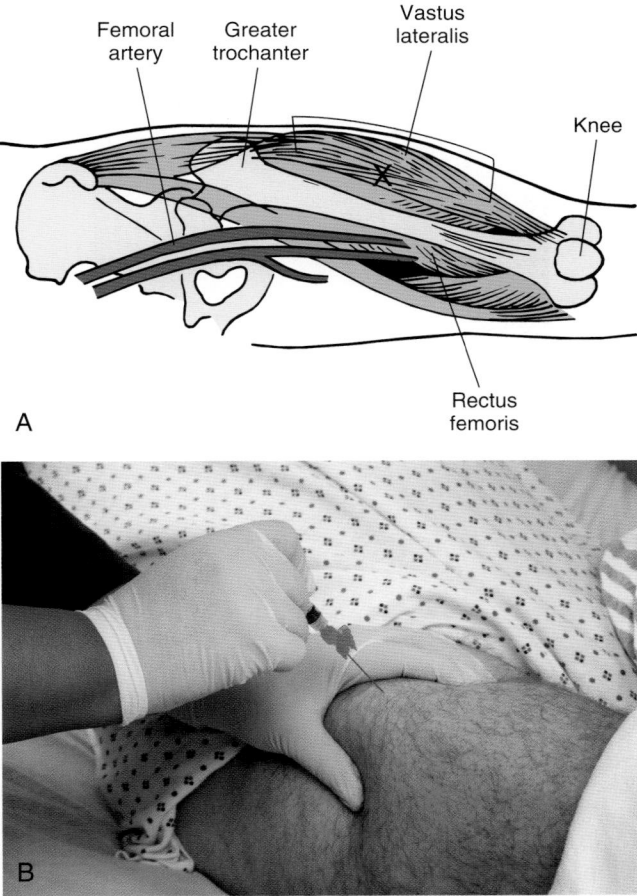

FIG. 31.25 (A) Landmarks for vastus lateralis site. (B) Giving intramuscular injection in vastus lateralis muscle.

The "G" method, or geometric method, is another option for identifying the correct ventrogluteal site (Fig. 31.24). With a patient in the side-lying position, you reference three bone prominences and draw imaginary lines between the ends of the bones (Kara et al., 2015). You imagine lines drawn from the patient's greater trochanter to the iliac crest, and then to the anterior superior iliac spine, and from the greater trochanter to the anterior superior iliac spine. A triangle is created by the imaginary lines. After that, draw median lines from every single corner of triangle to the opposite side.

The convergence point of the three median lines is the center for the triangle, the needle entry point for IM injections (Kaya et al., 2015).

Vastus Lateralis. The vastus lateralis muscle is another injection site used in adults and is the preferred site for administration of biologicals (e.g., immunizations) to infants, toddlers, and children (CDC, 2021a; Hockenberry et al., 2019). The muscle is thick and well developed; it is located on the anterolateral aspect of the thigh. It extends in an adult from a hand breadth above the knee to a hand breadth below the greater trochanter of the femur (Fig. 31.25). Use the middle third

FIG. 31.26 (A) Landmarks for deltoid site. (B) Giving intramuscular injection in deltoid muscle.

of the muscle for injection. The width of the muscle usually extends from the midline of the thigh to the midline of the outer side of the thigh. With young children or patients who are cachectic, it helps to grasp the body of the muscle during injection to ensure that the medication is deposited in muscle tissue. To help relax the muscle, ask the patient to lie flat with the knee slightly flexed and foot externally rotated or to assume a sitting position.

Deltoid. Although the deltoid site is easily accessible, the muscle is not well developed in many adults. There is potential for injury because the axillary, radial, brachial, and ulnar nerves and the brachial artery lie within the upper arm under the triceps and along the humerus (Fig. 31.26A). *Carefully assess the condition of the deltoid muscle, consult medication references for suitability of medication, and carefully locate the injection site using anatomical landmarks.* Use this site for small medication volumes (less than 2 mL); administration of routine immunizations in toddlers, older children, and adults; or when other sites are inaccessible because of dressings or casts (CDC, 2021a).

Locate the deltoid muscle by fully exposing the patient's upper arm and shoulder and asking the patient to relax the arm at the side or by

supporting the patient's arm and flexing the elbow. Do not roll up any tight-fitting sleeve. Allow the patient to sit or lie down. Palpate the lower edge of the acromion process, which forms the base of a triangle in line with the midpoint of the lateral aspect of the upper arm. The injection site is in the center of the triangle, about 3 to 5 cm (1–2 inches) below the acromion process (see Fig. 31.26B). You locate the apex of the triangle by placing four fingers across the deltoid muscle, with the top finger along the acromion process. The injection site is 3 finger widths below the acromion process.

Intradermal Injections. ID injections typically are used for skin testing (e.g., tuberculin screening and allergy tests). Because these medications are potent, they are injected into the dermis, where blood supply is reduced, and medication absorption occurs slowly. Some patients have a severe anaphylactic reaction if medications enter the circulation too rapidly. You need to choose skin-testing sites that allow you to easily assess for changes in color and tissue integrity. ID sites need to be lightly pigmented, free of lesions, and relatively hairless. The inner forearm and upper back are ideal locations.

Use a tuberculin or small hypodermic syringe for skin testing. The angle of insertion for an ID injection is 5 to 15 degrees (see Fig. 31.18), and the bevel of the needle is pointed up. As you inject the medication, a small bleb resembling a mosquito bite appears on the surface of the skin. If a bleb does not appear or if the site bleeds after needle withdrawal, there is a good chance that the medication entered subcutaneous tissues. In this situation, test results will not be valid.

Safety in Administering Medications by Injection

Needleless Devices. Approximately 5.6 million health care workers in the United States are at risk of occupational exposure to bloodborne pathogens such as HIV and the hepatitis B virus (Occupational Safety and Health Administration [OSHA], n.d.). Occupational exposure often occurs through accidental needlesticks and sharps injuries. Needlestick injuries commonly occur when health care workers recap needles, mishandle IV lines and needles, or leave needles at a patient's bedside. Exposure to bloodborne pathogens is one of the deadliest hazards to which nurses are exposed daily. Most needlestick injuries are preventable with the implementation of safe needle devices. The Needlestick Safety and Prevention Act mandates the use of special needle safety devices to reduce the frequency of needlestick injuries.

Safety syringes have a sheath or guard that covers a needle immediately after it is withdrawn from the skin (Fig. 31.27). This eliminates the chance for a needlestick injury. The syringe and sheath are disposed of together in a receptacle. Use needleless devices whenever possible to reduce the risk of needlestick and sharps injuries (OSHA, n.d.). Always dispose of needles and other instruments considered sharps into clearly marked, appropriate containers (Fig. 31.28). Containers need to be puncture proof and leak proof. Never force a needle into a full needle disposal receptacle. Never place used needles and syringes in a wastebasket, in your pocket, on a patient's meal tray, or at the patient's bedside. Box 31.22 summarizes the recommendations for the prevention of needlestick injuries.

Intravenous Administration. Nurses administer medications intravenously by the following methods:
1. Infusion of large volumes of IV fluid containers that contain medications mixed, labeled, and dispensed by pharmacy
2. Injection of a bolus or small volume of medication through an existing IV infusion line or intermittent venous access (heparin or saline lock)
3. Piggyback infusion of a solution containing the prescribed medication and a small volume of IV fluid through an existing IV line

FIG. 31.27 Needle with plastic guard to prevent needlesticks. (A) Position of guard before injection. (B) After injection guard locks in place, covering needle.

FIG. 31.28 Sharps disposal using only one hand.

In all three methods a patient has either an existing IV infusion running continuously or an IV access site for intermittent infusions. Most policies and procedures list who can administer IV medications and in which patient care units they can be given. These policies are based on the medication, capability and availability of staff, and the type of monitoring equipment available.

Chapter 42 describes the technique for performing venipuncture and establishing continuous IV fluid infusions. Medication administration is only one reason for supplying IV fluids. IV fluid therapy is used primarily for fluid replacement in patients unable to take oral fluids and as a means of supplying electrolytes and nutrients.

Data from Occupational Safety and Health Administration (OSHA): Bloodborne pathogens and needlestick prevention, n.d., https://www.osha.gov/bloodborne-pathogens. Accessed August 17, 2021.

When using any method of IV medication administration, observe patients closely for symptoms of adverse reactions. After a medication enters the bloodstream, it begins to act immediately, and there is no way to stop its action. Because of the rapid onset of action, take special care to avoid errors in dose calculation and preparation. Carefully follow the seven rights of safe medication administration, double-check medication calculations with another nurse, and know the desired action and side effects of every medication you give. If the medication has an antidote, make sure that it is available during administration. When administering potent medications, assess vital signs before, during, and after infusion. There are situations in which it is recommended to do an independent double check of a medication dosage, especially high-risk medications given via the IV route. The ISMP (2019c) describes how to do an independent double check:

- A double check must be conducted independently by a second person. A single person preparing and checking a medication is likely to see what is expected to be seen, even if an error has occurred.
- Two people must *separately* check each component of the work process. For example, a pharmacist calculates a dose, prepares a syringe of medication, and compares the product to the order; then a nurse *independently* checks the order, calculates the dose, and compares the results with the dispensed product for verification.
- Two people are unlikely to make the same mistake if they work independently. Holding up a syringe and a vial while saying "This is 5 units of insulin; can you check it?" is ineffective. The person asking for the double check must not influence the individual checking the product in any way.
- Use a double check only for very selective high-risk tasks or high-alert medications (not all) that most warrant their use (see agency policy).
- Fewer double checks performed strategically at the most vulnerable points of the medication use process are more effective than too many.

Administering medications by the IV route has advantages. Nurses often use this route in emergencies when a fast-acting medication needs to be delivered quickly. The IV route is also best when it is necessary to give medications to establish constant therapeutic blood levels.

Some medications are highly alkaline and irritating to muscle and subcutaneous tissue. These medications cause less discomfort when given intravenously. Because IV medications are immediately available to the bloodstream once they are administered, verify the rate of administration with a medication reference or a pharmacist before giving them to ensure that you give them safely over the appropriate amount of time. Patients experience severe adverse reactions if IV medications are administered too quickly.

Large-Volume Infusions. In the past, nurses often mixed medications into large volumes of IV fluids (500–1000 mL). However, today's safety standards and scientific evidence no longer support this practice (Gorski, 2018; Gorski et al., 2021; TJC, 2021). Safety risks such as incorrect calculation, poor aseptic technique, incorrect labeling, pump programming errors, lack of medication knowledge, and mix-up with another medication occur when nurses prepare medications in IV containers on patient care units (Gorski, 2018). Box 31.23 summarizes current best practices for preparation and administration of IV medication.

Pharmacies prepare medications in large volumes (500 or 1000 mL) of compatible IV fluids such as normal saline or lactated Ringer solution. Vitamins and potassium chloride are two types of medications often added to IV fluids. Continuous infusion carries a risk: if the IV fluid is infused too rapidly, the patient is at risk for medication overdose and circulatory fluid overload.

Nurses mix medications into IV fluids only in emergency situations. The nurse *never* prepares high-alert medications (e.g., heparin, dopamine, dobutamine, nitroglycerin, potassium, antibiotics, or magnesium) on a patient care unit. Check with a pharmacist before mixing a medication in an IV container. If a pharmacist confirms that you need to prepare the medication, ask another nurse to verify your medication calculations and

have that nurse watch you during the entire procedure to ensure that you prepare the medication safely. First ensure that the IV fluid and medication are compatible. Then prepare the medication in a syringe (see Skill 31.4) using strict aseptic technique. *Do not* add medications to IV bags that are already hanging because there is no way to tell the exact concentration of the medication. Add medications *only* to new IV bags.

When administering medications in large IV infusions, regulate the IV rate according to the health care provider's order. Monitor patients closely for adverse reactions to the medication and fluid volume overload. Also check the site frequently for infiltration and phlebitis (see Chapter 42).

Intravenous Bolus. An IV bolus, or "push," involves introducing a concentrated dose of a medication directly into the systemic circulation (see Skill 31.6). IV push medications are given through either an existing continuous IV infusion or an intermittent venous access (commonly called a *saline lock*). A saline lock is an IV catheter with a small "well" or chamber covered by a rubber cap. An IV catheter can be converted into a lock by inserting a special rubber-seal injection cap into the end of the catheter. Use of a lock saves time by eliminating constant monitoring of an IV line. It also offers better mobility, safety, and comfort for patients by eliminating the need for a continuous IV line. After you administer an IV bolus through an intermittent venous access, flush with a normal saline solution to keep it patent.

Because a bolus requires only a small amount of fluid to deliver the medication, it is an advantage when the amount of fluid that the patient can take is restricted. The IV bolus, or "push," is the most dangerous method for administering medications because there is no time to correct errors. In addition, a bolus may cause direct irritation to the lining of blood vessels. Before administering a bolus, confirm placement of the IV line. Never give a medication intravenously if the insertion site appears swollen or edematous or the IV fluid cannot flow at the proper rate. Accidental injection of a medication into the tissue around a vein causes pain, sloughing of tissue, and abscesses, depending on the composition of the medication. Medications that carry a risk of adverse effects if administered too quickly should be diluted and administered as a piggyback or via an infusion pump.

Verify the rate of administration of IV push medication by using agency guidelines or a medication reference manual. Follow these strategies to reduce harm from rapid IV push medications (Gorski, 2018; ISMP, 2018b; ISMP, 2019b):

- Use commercially available or pharmacy-prepared IV push medication whenever possible.
- Do not dilute IV push medications unless recommended by the manufacturer, agency policy, or reference literature.
- IV push medications should be administered at the rate recommended by the manufacturer, agency policy, or reference literature.
- Appropriately label clinically prepared syringes.
- Determine the rate needed and amount of time involved to administer the medication.
- Identify all incompatibilities (i.e., drug or solution) with existing infusions.
- Review the amount of medication that a patient will receive each minute, the recommended concentration, and the rate of administration. For example, if a patient is to receive 6 mL of a medication over 3 minutes, give 2 mL of the IV bolus medication every minute.
- Understand the purpose of the medication and any potential adverse reactions related to the rate and route of administration. Some IV medications can only be given IV push safely when a patient is being monitored continuously for dysrhythmias, blood pressure changes, or other adverse effects. Therefore you can push some medications only in specific areas within a health care agency (e.g., critical care unit). Confirm agency guidelines regarding requirements for special monitoring.

BOX 31.23   Best Practices for Administration of Intravenous Solutions and Medications

- Review medication orders for standardized concentrations and dosages of medication.
- Use standardized procedures for ordering, preparing, and administering intravenous (IV) medications.
- Administer solutions and medications prepared and dispensed from the pharmacy or as the commercially prepared form when possible.
- Never prepare high-alert medications (e.g., heparin, dopamine, dobutamine, nitroglycerin, potassium, antibiotics, or magnesium) on a patient care unit.
- Review medication order for use of standardized infusion concentrations of "high-alert" medications.
- Standardize the storage of IV medications.
- Use the mnemonic *CATS PRRR* to help remember safety checks for administering IV medications: *C,* compatibilities; *A,* allergies; *T,* tubing correct; *S,* site checked; *P,* pump safety checked; *R,* right rate; *R,* release clamps; *R,* return and reassess the patient.
- Use standardized label practices. Bold patient name, generic medication name, and patient-specific dose.
- Correctly use technology such as intelligent-infusion devices, bar code–assisted medication administration, and electronic medication administration record.

Adapted from Gorski L: *Phillips*'s manual of I.V. therapeutics: evidence-based practice for infusion therapy, ed 7, Philadelphia, 2018, FA Davis; Gorski LA et al.: Infusion therapy standards of practice, 8th edition, *J Infusion Nurs* 44(1S):S1, 2021; and The Joint Commission (TJC): *2021 National Patient Safety Goals,* Oakbrook Terrace, IL, 2021, The Joint Commission. http://www.jointcommission.org/standards_information/npsgs.aspx. Accessed August 17, 2021.

Volume-Controlled Infusions. Another way of administering IV medications is through small amounts (50–100 mL) of compatible IV fluids. The fluid is within a secondary fluid container separate from the primary fluid bag. The container connects directly to the primary IV line or to separate tubing that inserts into the primary line (see Skill 31.7). Three types of containers are volume-control administration sets (e.g., Volutrol or Pediatrol), piggyback sets, and syringe pumps. Using volume-controlled infusions has several advantages:

- It reduces risk of rapid-dose infusion by IV push. Medications are diluted and infused over longer time intervals (e.g., 30–60 minutes).
- It allows for administration of medications (e.g., antibiotics) that are stable for a limited time in solution.
- It allows for control of IV fluid intake.

Piggyback. A piggyback is a small (25–250 mL) IV bag or bottle connected to a short tubing line that connects to the *upper* Y-port of a primary infusion line or to an intermittent venous access (Fig. 31.29). The label on the medication follows the ISMP IV piggyback medication label format (ISMP, 2019d) (Fig. 31.30). The piggyback tubing is a microdrip or macrodrip system (see Chapter 42). The set is called a *piggyback* because the small bag or bottle is higher than the primary infusion bag or bottle. In the piggyback setup the main line does not infuse when the piggybacked medication is infusing. The port of the primary IV line contains a back-check valve that automatically stops flow of the primary infusion once the piggyback infusion flows. After the piggyback solution infuses and the solution within the tubing falls below the level of the primary infusion drip chamber, the back-check valve opens, and the primary infusion again flows.

Volume-Control Administration. Volume-control administration (e.g., Buretrol) sets are small (150-mL) containers that attach just below the primary infusion bag or bottle. The set is attached and filled in a manner similar to that used with a regular IV infusion. Follow package directions for priming sets (see Chapter 42).

Syringe Pump. The syringe pump is battery operated and allows medications to be given in very small amounts of fluid (5–60 mL) within controlled infusion times using standard syringes.

Intermittent Venous Access. An intermittent venous access (commonly called a *saline lock*) is an IV catheter capped off on the end with a small chamber covered by a rubber diaphragm or a specially designed cap. Special rubber-seal injection caps usually accept needle safety devices (see Chapter 42). Advantages to intermittent venous access include the following:

- Cost savings resulting from the omission of continuous IV therapy
- Effectiveness of nurse's time enhanced by eliminating constant monitoring of flow rates
- Increased mobility, safety, and comfort for the patient

FIG. 31.29 Piggyback setup.

John Jones ❶	❷ Room 2647
MR# 123456 ❸	

Hydrocortisone ❹   **100 mg** ❻
(SOLU-CORTEF) ❺

In D5W ❼   IVPB ❽
Total Volume   50 mL ❾

Exp: 12/31/2020 ❿❷   RPh Initials: *AMH* ⓫

Deaconess Hospital Pharmacy ⓭
Infuse medication over 20-30 minutes ⓮
⓯

1. **Patient name**
2. Location
3. Second identifier
   (Date of birth, financial #,
   encounter #, medical record #)
4. **Generic name**
5. BRAND name
6. **Patient dose**
7. Diluent
8. Route
9. Total volume
10. Bar code
11. Initials as needed
12. Expiration date as needed in a
    MM/DD/YYYY format
13. Pharmacy information if required
14. Comments
15. Other information as required
    by state or federal law

FIG. 31.30 Intravenous piggyback medication with label.

Before administering an IV bolus or piggyback medication, assess the patency and placement of the IV site. After the medication has been administered through an intermittent venous access, the access must be flushed with a solution to keep it patent. In general, normal saline is an effective flush solution for peripheral catheters. Some agencies require the use of heparin. Nurses need to verify and follow agency policies regarding the care and maintenance of the IV site.

Administration of Intravenous Therapy in the Home. Sometimes patients need IV therapy at home. Common infusions that patients receive include antimicrobials, chemotherapy, total parenteral nutrition, biological therapy, and other medications (Gorski, 2018). Most patients typically receive their home IV therapy through a long-term central venous catheter (CVC) (see Chapter 42). Home health nurses assess patients' responses to the medication, monitor the CVC site, and teach patients and their family caregivers how to administer infusions and maintain the CVC.

Carefully assess patients and their family caregivers to determine their ability to manage IV therapy at home. Begin instruction on IV care management as soon as you know that a patient will have IV therapy at home. Your instruction often begins while a patient is hospitalized. Patients and family caregivers need to learn how to check their catheter for signs of complications and to flush, lock, and ensure the patency of the IV catheter (Gorski, 2018). If the patient has a tunneled catheter (see Chapter 42), site care including dressing changes may be taught as well. Patients also need to know when to notify the home care nurse or health care provider. Plan to teach patients and their family caregivers how to maintain IV administration equipment, including the infusion pump.

SAFETY GUIDELINES FOR NURSING SKILLS

Ensuring patient safety is an essential role of the professional nurse. Use sound clinical judgment by communicating clearly with members of the health care team, assessing, and analyzing the patient's clinical findings and incorporating the patient's priorities of care and preferences. Use the best evidence, applying professional standards, when selecting interventions to use in patient care delivery. When performing the skills in this chapter, remember the following points to ensure safe, patient-centered care.

Follow these guidelines to ensure safe medication administration:

- Be vigilant during medication administration. Avoid distractions while preparing all medications. NIZs have been recommended to reduce distractions during medication preparation and administration (Freitas et al., 2019). NIZs are created by placing signs, red tape, or tile borders on the floor around medication carts or areas. Nurses standing in these zones are not to be interrupted.
- Be sure that your patients receive the appropriate medications.
- Know why your patient is receiving each medication; know what you need to do before, during, and after medication administration; and evaluate the effectiveness of medications and any adverse effects.
- Verify that medications have not expired by checking labels.
- Use at least two identifiers before administering medications and check against the MAR. Follow agency policy for patient identification.
- Before medication administration, it is critical to ensure that all information is correct. You should check for accuracy three times:
  1. The first check is when the medications are pulled or retrieved from the automated dispensing machine, the medication drawer, or whatever system is in place at the agency.
  2. The second check is when preparation of the medications for administration takes place.
  3. The final check occurs at the patient's bedside just before medications are given.

- Clarify unclear medication orders and ask for help whenever you are uncertain about an order or calculation. Consult with your peers, pharmacists, and other health care providers, and be sure that you have resolved all concerns related to medication administration before preparing and giving medications.
- Use the technology (e.g., bar scanning, eMARs) available in your agency when preparing and giving medications. Follow all policies related to use of the technology, and do not use work-arounds. A *work-around* bypasses a procedure, policy, or problem in a system. Nurses who use work-arounds fail to follow agency protocols, policies, or procedures during medication administration in an attempt to get medications administered to patients in a timelier fashion.
- Use strict aseptic technique during parenteral medication preparation and administration.
- Educate patients about each medication they take while you are administering medications. It is important for a patient to know each medication with respect to purpose, daily dose and when to take the medications, most common side effects, and the problems to report to the health care provider. Make sure that you answer all their questions before administering medications. Educate family caregivers if appropriate.
- Most of the time you cannot delegate medication administration. Ensure that you follow standards set by the nurse practice act in your state and guidelines established by your health care agency. Licensed practical nurses or licensed vocational nurses usually can administer medications via the oral (po), subcutaneous, IM, and ID routes. Sometimes they can give medications intravenously if they have had special training and if the medications are not high-alert medications. Some states also allow certified medical assistants to administer some types of medications (e.g., oral medications) in long-term care agencies.
- Follow safety guidelines to prevent needlestick injuries. Use engineered devices and dispose of all sharps in safety containers.

SKILL 31.1   ADMINISTERING ORAL MEDICATIONS

Delegation and Collaboration

The skill of administering oral medications cannot be delegated to assistive personnel (AP). The nurse instructs the AP about:

- Potential side effects of medications and to report their occurrence.
- Informing nurse if patient condition changes or worsens (e.g., pain, itching, or rash) after medication administration.

Equipment

- Automated, computer-controlled medication dispensing system or medication cart
- Disposable medication cups (mL only cup)
- Glass of water, juice, or preferred liquid and drinking straw
- Pill-crushing device *(optional)*
- Paper towels
- MAR (electronic or printed)
- Clean gloves (if handling an oral medication)

STEPS	RATIONALE

ASSESSMENT

1. Check accuracy and completeness of each MAR or computer printout with health care provider's written medication order. Check patient's name, medication name and dosage, route of administration, and time of administration. Clarify incomplete or unclear orders with health care provider before administration.

The order sheet is the most reliable source and only legal record of medications that patient is to receive. Ensures that patient receives the correct medications (Palese et al., 2019). Transcription errors are a source of medication errors (Zhu and Weingart, 2020).

2. Review pertinent information related to medication, including action, purpose, normal dose and route, side effects, time of onset and peak action, indications, and nursing implications.

Allows you to anticipate effects of medication and observe patient's response.

3. Assess for any contraindications to patient receiving oral medication, including being on nothing by mouth (NPO) status, inability to swallow, nausea/vomiting, bowel inflammation, reduced peristalsis, recent GI surgery, gastric suction, and decreased level of consciousness (LOC). Notify health care provider if any contraindications are present.

Alterations in GI function can interfere with medication absorption, distribution, and excretion. Patients with GI suction do not receive actions of oral medications because the medications are suctioned from the GI tract before they are absorbed.

4. Assess patient's medical, medication, and diet history, and history of allergies. List any medication allergies on each page of MAR and prominently display on patient's medical record. When allergies are present, patient should wear an allergy bracelet.

These factors influence how certain medications act. Information reveals previous problems with medication administration. Allergy alert helps prevent adverse events.

5. Perform hand hygiene. Gather and review physical assessment findings, including patient's weight (in metric units), vital signs, and laboratory data that influence medication administration, such as results of renal and liver function studies.

Many medication doses are based on patient's weight. Physical examination findings or laboratory data may contraindicate medication administration. Renal and liver function status affects metabolism and excretion of medications (Burchum and Rosenthal, 2019).

6. Assess patient's or family caregiver's knowledge, experience, and health literacy.

Ensures patient or family caregiver has the capacity to obtain, communicate, process, and understand basic health information (CDC, 2021b).

7. Assess risk for aspiration using a dysphagia screening tool if available (see Chapter 45). Protect patient from aspiration by assessing swallowing ability.

Aspiration occurs when food, fluid, or medication intended for GI administration is inadvertently administered into the respiratory tract. Patients with altered ability to swallow are at higher risk for aspiration (Bartlett, 2021; Forough et al., 2018).

8. Assess patient's symptoms before initiating medication therapy.

Provides information to evaluate desired effect of medication.

9. Assess patient's preference for fluids and determine whether medications can be given with these fluids. Maintain fluid restrictions as prescribed.

Some fluids interfere with medication absorption (e.g., dairy products affect tetracycline). Offering fluids during medication administration is an excellent way to increase patient's fluid intake. Fluids ease swallowing and facilitate absorption from the GI tract. However, if fluid restriction exists, skillful planning of fluid intake must coordinate with medication times and types of medications.

10. Assess patient's knowledge, prior experience regarding health and medication use, medication schedule, ability to prepare medications, and feelings about procedure.

Determines patient's and family caregiver's need for medication education and guidance to achieve medication adherence.

Reveals need for patient instruction and/or support.

11. Assess patient's goals or preferences for how skill is to be performed or what patient expects.

Allows care to be individualized to patient.

PLANNING

1. Perform hand hygiene. Collect appropriate equipment and MAR.

Promotes time management and efficiency when preparing medications for all patients.

2. Plan preparation to avoid interruptions. Create a quiet environment. Do not take phone calls or talk with others. Follow agency No-Interruption Zone (NIZ) policy.

Interruptions contribute to medication errors (Freitas et al., 2019; Palese et al., 2019) (see Box 31.4).

IMPLEMENTATION

1. Prepare medications.

   a. Perform hand hygiene. Arrange medication tray and cups in medication preparation area or move medication cart to position outside patient's room.

   Reduces transfer of microorganisms. Organization of equipment saves time and reduces error.

   b. Log on to AMDS or unlock medicine drawer or cart.

   Medications are safeguarded when locked in cabinet, cart, or AMDS.

   c. Perform hand hygiene and prepare medications for *one patient at a time* using aseptic technique. Follow the seven rights of medication administration. Keep all pages of MAR or computer printouts for one patient together or look at only one patient's eMAR screen.

   Ensures that medications remain sterile. Prevents preparation errors.

   d. Select correct medication from AMDS, unit-dose drawer, or stock supply. Compare name of medication on label with MAR or computer printout (see illustration). Exit AMDS after removing medication.

   Reading label and comparing it against transcribed order reduces errors. Exiting AMDS ensures no one else can remove medications using your identify. *This is the first check for accuracy.*

   e. Check or calculate medication dose as necessary. Double-check any calculation. Check expiration date on all medications and return outdated medication to pharmacy.

   Double-checking pharmacy calculations reduces risk for error. Agency policy may require you to check calculations of certain medications such as insulin with another nurse. Expired medications may be inactive or harmful to patient.

Continued

SKILL 31.1   **ADMINISTERING ORAL MEDICATIONS—cont'd**

STEPS	**RATIONALE**
f. If preparing a controlled substance, check record for previous medication count and compare current count with available supply. Controlled medications may be stored in computerized locked cart.	Controlled substance laws require nurses to carefully monitor and count dispensed controlled medications (e.g., opioids).
g. Prepare solid forms of oral medications.	
(1) To prepare unit-dose tablets or capsules, place packaged tablet or capsule directly into medication cup without removing wrapper. Administer medications only from containers with labels that are clearly marked.	Wrappers maintain cleanliness and identify medication name and dose, which can facilitate teaching.
(2) When using a blister pack, "pop" medications through foil or paper backing into a medication cup (see illustration).	Packs provide a 1-month supply, with each "blister" usually containing a single dose.
(3) If it is necessary to give half the dose of medication, pharmacy should split, label, package, and send medication to unit. If you must split medication, use clean, gloved hand to cut with clean pill-cutting device. Only cut tablets that are prescored by the manufacturer (line traverses the center of the tablet).	Reduces contamination of the tablet. In health care agencies, only pharmacy should split tablets to ensure patient safety (ISMP, 2018a). If a tablet is FDA approved to be split, this information will be printed in the "HOW SUPPLIED" section of the manufacturer's package insert.
(4) Place all tablets or capsules that patient will receive in one medicine cup, except for those requiring preadministration assessments (e.g., pulse rate or blood pressure). Place those medications in separate additional cup with wrapper intact.	Keeping medications that require preadministration assessments separate from others serves as a reminder and makes it easier to withhold medications, as necessary.
(5) If patient has difficulty swallowing and liquid medications are not an option, use a pill-crushing device. Clean device before using. If device is unavailable, place medication between two cups, and grind and crush (see illustration). Mix ground tablet in small amount (teaspoon) of soft food (custard or applesauce).	Large tablets are often difficult to swallow. A ground tablet mixed with palatable soft food is usually easier to swallow.

CLINICAL JUDGMENT: *Not all medications can be crushed safely. Consult with a pharmacist or the ISMP Do Not Crush List (ISMP, 2020b).*

STEP 1d Nurse compares label of medication with transcribed medication order on computerized medication administration record (MAR).

STEP 1g(2) Place tablet from blister pack into medicine cup without removing wrapper.

STEP 1g(5) Crushing tablet with pill-crushing device.

STEPS	RATIONALE

h. Prepare liquids.

   (1) Use unit-dose container with correct amount of medication. Gently shake container. Administer medication packaged in a single-dose cup directly from the single-dose cup. Do not pour medicine into another cup.

Using unit-dose container with correct dosage of medication provides most accurate dose of medication (ISMP, 2020a). Shaking container ensures that medication is mixed before administration.

   (2) Unit-dose oral syringe (see illustration): Be sure to use only oral syringes marked "Oral Use Only" dispensed by pharmacy.

Ensures that all oral medications that are not commercially available as unit-dose products are dispensed by the pharmacy in an oral syringe (ISMP, 2020a).

CLINICAL JUDGMENT: *Based on current best practice (ISMP, 2020a), liquid medications that are not available or are not in correct dose in a unit-dose container should be dispensed by the pharmacy in special oral syringes marked "Oral Use Only." These syringes do not connect to any type of parenteral (e.g., IV) tubing. In addition, current evidence shows that liquid measuring devices on patient care units result in inaccurate dosing. Having oral medications prepared in the pharmacy ensures that you give the most accurate dose of a medication possible and prevents parenteral administration of oral medications.*

---

i. Return stock containers or unused unit-dose medications to shelf or drawer. Label medication cups and poured medications with patient's name before leaving medication preparation area. Do not leave medications unattended.

Ensures that correct medications are prepared for correct patient.

j. Before going to patient's room, compare patient's name and name of medication on label of prepared medications with MAR.

Comparing labels a second time reduces errors. *This is the second check for accuracy.*

2. Administer medications.

  a. Take medication to patient at correct time (see agency policy). Medications that require exact timing include STAT doses, first-time or loading doses, and one-time doses. Give time-critical scheduled medications (e.g., antibiotics, anticoagulants, insulin, anticonvulsants, or immunosuppressive agents) at exact time ordered (no more than 30 minutes before or after scheduled dose). Give non–time-critical scheduled medications within a range of 1 or 2 hours of scheduled dose (ISMP, 2011). During administration apply seven rights of medication administration.

Hospitals must adopt medication administration policy and procedure for timing of medication administration that considers nature of the prescribed medication, specific clinical application, and patient needs (USDHHS, 2011; ISMP, 2011). Time-critical scheduled medications are those for which early or delayed administration of maintenance doses of greater than 30 minutes before or after the scheduled dose may cause harm or result in substantial suboptimal therapy or pharmacological effect. Non–time-critical medications are those for which early or delayed administration within a specified range of either 1 or 2 hours should not cause harm or result in substantial suboptimal therapy or pharmacological effect (USDHHS, 2011; ISMP, 2011).

  b. Identify patient using at least two identifiers (e.g., name and birthday or name and medical record number) according to agency policy. Compare identifiers with information on patient's MAR or medical record.

Ensures correct patient. Complies with The Joint Commission standards and improves patient safety (TJC, 2021).

  c. At patient's bedside, again compare MAR or computer printout with name of medication on medication labels and patient name. Ask patient about any allergies.

This is the third check for accuracy and ensures that patient receives correct medication.

Confirms patient's allergy history.

  d. Explain the purpose of each medication, action, and most common adverse effects. Allow sufficient time for patient to ask questions. Include family caregiver if appropriate.

Patient has the right to be informed, and patient and family caregiver understanding of each medication improves adherence with medication therapy.

STEP 1h(2) Use special oral medication syringes to prepare small amounts of liquid medications.

Continued

SKILL 31.1   ADMINISTERING ORAL MEDICATIONS—cont'd

STEPS	RATIONALE
e. Perform hand hygiene. Perform necessary preadministration assessment (e.g., blood pressure, pulse) for specific medications. Ask patient again about any allergies.	Reduces transmission of microorganisms. Determines whether specific medications should be withheld at that time. Confirms patient's allergy history.

CLINICAL JUDGMENT: *If patient expresses concern regarding accuracy of a medication, do not give the medication. Explore patient's concern and verify health care provider's order before administering. Listening to patient's concerns may prevent a medication error.*

f. Help patient to sitting or Fowler position. Use side-lying position if patient is unable to sit. Have patient stay in this position for 30 minutes after administration.	Decreases risk for aspiration during swallowing.
g. *For tablets:* Patient may wish to hold solid medications in hand or cup before placing in mouth. Offer water or preferred liquid to help patient swallow medications.	Patient can become familiar with medications by seeing each medication. Choice of fluid can improve fluid intake.
h. *For orally disintegrating formulations (tablets or strips):* Remove medication from packet just before use. Do not push tablet through foil. Place medication on top of patient's tongue. Caution against chewing it.	Orally disintegrating formulations begin to dissolve when placed on tongue. Water is not needed. Careful removal from packaging is necessary because tablets and strips are thin and fragile.
i. *For sublingually administered medications:* Have patient place medication under tongue and allow it to dissolve completely (see Fig. 31.3). Caution patient against swallowing tablet.	Medication is absorbed through blood vessels of undersurface of tongue. If swallowed, it is destroyed by gastric juices or rapidly detoxified by liver, preventing therapeutic blood level.
j. *For buccally administered medications:* Have patient place medication in mouth against mucous membranes of cheek and gums until it dissolves (see Fig. 31.4).	Buccal medications act locally or systemically as they are swallowed in saliva.

CLINICAL JUDGMENT: *Avoid administering anything by mouth, including other oral medications, until orally disintegrating buccal or sublingual medication is completely dissolved.*

k. *For powdered medications:* Mix with liquids at bedside and give to patient to drink.	When prepared in advance, powdered medications thicken; some even harden, making swallowing difficult.
l. *For crushed medications mixed with food:* Give each medication separately in teaspoon of food.	Ensures that patient swallows all of medicine. *Never mix medication in a meal serving of food.*
m. *For lozenge:* Caution patient against chewing or swallowing lozenges.	Lozenges act through slow absorption through oral mucosa, not gastric mucosa.
n. *For effervescent medication:* Add tablet or powder to glass of water. Administer immediately after dissolving.	Effervescence improves unpleasant taste and often relieves GI problems.
o. If patient is unable to hold medications, place medication cup or oral syringe to lips and gently introduce each medication into mouth one at a time. Administer each tablet or capsule one at a time. Inject liquid from oral syringe slowly. A spoon can also be used to place pill in patient's mouth. Do not rush or force medications.	Administering a single-dose tablet, capsule, or oral syringe dose eases swallowing and decreases risk for aspiration.
p. Stay until patient swallows each medication completely or takes it by the prescribed route. Ask patient to open mouth if uncertain whether medication has been swallowed.	Ensures that patient receives ordered dose. If left unattended, patient may not take dose or may save medications, causing health risks.
q. For highly acidic medications (e.g., aspirin), offer patient a nonfat snack (e.g., crackers) if not contraindicated by the patient's condition.	Reduces gastric irritation. Fat content of foods may delay medication absorption.
r. Help patient to a comfortable position.	Restores comfort and sense of well-being.
s. Stay with patient for several minutes and observe for any allergic reactions.	Dyspnea, wheezing, and circulatory collapse are signs of severe anaphylactic reaction.
3. Place nurse call system in an accessible location within patient's reach.	Ensures patient can call for assistance if needed and promotes safety and prevents falls.
4. Raise side rails (as appropriate) and lower bed to lowest position.	Promotes safety and prevents falls.
5. Dispose of all contaminated supplies in appropriate receptacle, remove and dispose of gloves, and perform hand hygiene.	Reduces transmission of microorganisms. Use appropriate disposal receptacle if patient is on hazardous drugs.

EVALUATION

1. Return within an appropriate time to evaluate patient's response to medications, including therapeutic effects, side effects or allergic reactions, and adverse effects.	Evaluates therapeutic benefit of medication and helps to detect onset of side effects or allergic reactions. Sublingual medications act in 15 minutes; most oral medications act in 30 to 60 minutes.
2. Ask patient or family caregiver to identify medication name and explain purpose, indication, action, dose schedule, and potential side effects.	Determines level of knowledge gained by patient and family caregiver.
3. **Use Teach-Back:** "I want to be sure I showed you how to use your sublingual nitroglycerin. Show me where you will place the tablet in your mouth." Revise your instruction now or develop a plan for revised patient/family caregiver teaching if patient/family caregiver is not able to teach back correctly.	Teach-back is an evidence-based health literacy intervention that promotes patient engagement, patient safety, adherence, and quality. The goal of teach-back is to ensure that you have explained medical information clearly so that patients and their families understand what you communicated to them (Agency for Healthcare Research and Quality [AHRQ], 2020).

UNEXPECTED OUTCOMES AND RELATED INTERVENTIONS

1. Patient exhibits adverse effects (e.g., side effect, toxic effect, allergic reaction).
   - Notify health care provider and pharmacy.
   - Withhold further doses.
   - Assess vital signs.
   - Symptoms such as urticaria, rash, pruritus, rhinitis, and wheezing may indicate an allergic reaction and need for emergency medications.
   - Add allergy information to patient's medical record.
2. Patient refuses medication.
   - Assess reason for patient refusing medication.
   - Provide further instruction
   - Do not force patient to take medications.
   - Document and notify health care provider.
3. Patient or family caregiver is unable to explain medication information.
   - Further assess patient's or family caregiver's knowledge of medications and guidelines for medication safety.
   - Further instruction or different approach to instruction is necessary.

RECORDING AND REPORTING

- Record medication, dose, route, and time administered on patient's MAR immediately *after* administration, not before. Include initials or signature.
- If you do not administer the medication, record reason on flow sheet or nurses' notes in electronic health record (EHR) or chart and follow agency policy for noting withheld medication.
- Record patient response to medication, instructions (including teach-back), and validation of understanding on flow sheet or nurses' notes in EHR or chart.
- Report adverse effects and patient response and/or withheld medications to nurse in charge or health care provider.

| SKILL 31.2 | ADMINISTERING OPHTHALMIC MEDICATIONS | ▶ |

Delegation and Collaboration

The skill of administering eye medications cannot be delegated to assistive personnel (AP). The nurse instructs the AP about:

- The specific potential side effects of medications and to report their occurrence.
- The potential for temporary burning or blurring of vision after administration of eye medications.

Equipment

- Appropriate medication (eyedrops with sterile dropper, ointment tube, or medicated intraocular disk)

- Clean gloves (for eyedrops)
- MAR (electronic or printed)

Eyedrops/Ointment

- Eyedrops or ointment
- Cotton balls or facial tissue
- Warm water and washcloth
- Eye patch and tape *(optional)*

| STEPS | RATIONALE |

ASSESSMENT

STEPS	RATIONALE
1. Check accuracy and completeness of each MAR or computer printout with health care provider's written medication order. Check patient's name, medication name and dosage, route of administration, and time of administration. Clarify incomplete or unclear orders with health care provider before administration.	The order sheet is the most reliable source and only legal record of medications that patient is to receive. Ensures that patient receives the correct medications (Palese et al., 2019). Transcription errors are a source of medication errors (Palese et al., 2019).
2. Review pertinent information related to medication, including action, purpose, normal dose and route, side effects, time of onset and peak action, indication, and nursing implications.	Allows you to anticipate effects of medication and observe patient's response.
3. Assess patient's medical and medication history and history of allergies. List any medication allergies on each page of the MAR and prominently display it on the patient's medical record per agency policy. When allergies are present, patient should wear allergy bracelet.	Factors influence how certain medications act. Reveals patient's need for medication. Allergy alert prevents adverse effects.
4. Assess patient's or family caregiver's knowledge, experience, and health literacy.	Ensures that patient and family caregiver have the capacity to obtain, communicate, process, and understand basic health information (CDC, 2021b).
5. Perform hand hygiene. Assess condition of external eye and structures (see Chapter 30). This may be done just before medication instillation (if drainage is present, apply clean gloves).	Provides baseline to determine whether local response to medications occurs. Also indicates need to clean eye before medication application.
6. Determine whether patient has any symptoms of eye discomfort or visual impairment.	Certain eye medications act to either lessen or increase these symptoms.
7. Assess patient's LOC and ability to follow directions.	If patient becomes restless or combative during procedure, greater risk for accidental eye injury exists.

Continued

SKILL 31.2	**ADMINISTERING OPHTHALMIC MEDICATIONS—cont'd**

STEPS	**RATIONALE**
8. Assess patient's and family caregiver's knowledge regarding medication therapy and patient's desire to self-administer medication.	Indicates need for health teaching. Motivation influences teaching approach.
9. Assess patient's goals or preferences for how skill is to be performed or what patient expects	Allows care to be individualized to patient.
10. Assess patient's ability to manipulate and hold dropper or ocular disk.	Reflects patient's ability to learn to self-administer medication.

PLANNING

1. Perform hand hygiene. Collect appropriate equipment and MAR	Promotes time management and efficiency when preparing medications for all patients.
2. Plan preparation to avoid interruptions. Create a quiet environment. Do not take phone calls or talk with others. Follow agency No-Interruption Zone (NIZ) policy.	Interruptions contribute to medication errors (Freitas et al., 2019; Palese et al., 2019) (see Box 31.4).

IMPLEMENTATION

1. Prepare medications for *one patient at a time*. Attend to procedure and avoid distraction. Check label of medication against MAR 2 times, when removing medication from unit dose or AMDS and before leaving preparation area (see Skill 31.1). Prepare eyedrops by taking container out of refrigerator and rewarming to room temperature before administering to patient. Check expiration date on container. Perform hand hygiene.	Warming eyedrops reduces eye irritation. *These are the first and second checks for accuracy.* Process ensures that right patient receives right medication.
2. Take medication(s) to patient at correct time (see agency policy). Medications that require exact timing include STAT doses, first-time or loading doses, and one-time doses. Give time-critical scheduled medications (e.g., antibiotics, anticoagulants, insulin, anticonvulsants, or immunosuppressive agents) at exact time ordered (no more than 30 minutes before or after scheduled dose). Give non–time-critical scheduled medications within a range of 1 or 2 hours of scheduled dose (ISMP, 2011). During administration apply seven rights of medication administration.	Hospitals must adopt medication administration policy and procedure for timing of medication administration that considers nature of the prescribed medication, specific clinical application, and patient needs (USDHHS, 2011; ISMP, 2011). Time-critical scheduled medications are those for which early or delayed administration of maintenance doses of greater than 30 minutes before or after the scheduled dose may cause harm or result in substantial suboptimal therapy or pharmacological effect. Non–time-critical medications are those for which early or delayed administration within a specified range of either 1 or 2 hours should not cause harm or result in substantial suboptimal therapy or pharmacological effect (USDHHS, 2011; ISMP, 2011).
3. Identify patient using at least two identifiers (e.g., name and birthday or name and medical record number) according to agency policy. Compare identifiers with information on patient's MAR or medical record.	Ensures correct patient. Complies with The Joint Commission standards and improves patient safety (TJC, 2021).
4. At patient's bedside again compare MAR or computer printout with names of medications on medication labels and patient name. Ask patient about any allergies.	*This is the third check for accuracy* and ensures that patient receives correct medication. Confirms patient's allergy history.
5. Discuss purpose of each medication, action, and possible adverse effects. Allow patient to ask any questions about the medications. Patients who self-instill medications may be allowed to give drops under nurse's supervision (check agency policy).	Patient has right to be informed, and patient's understanding of each medication improves adherence to medication therapy.
6. Tell patients receiving eyedrops (e.g., mydriatics) that vision will be blurred temporarily and that sensitivity to light may occur.	May relieve patient's anxiety.

CLINICAL JUDGMENT: *Instruct and reinforce that patient should not drive or operate machinery or perform any activity that requires clear vision until vision and sensitivity to light return to normal.*

7. Instill eye medications.	
a. Perform hand hygiene and apply clean gloves. Ask patient to lie supine or sit back in chair with head slightly hyperextended, looking up.	Position provides easy access to eye for medication instillation and minimizes drainage of medication into tear duct.

CLINICAL JUDGMENT: *Do not hyperextend the neck of a patient with cervical spine injury.*

b. If drainage or crusting is present along eyelid margins or inner canthus, gently wash away. Soak any dried crusts with warm, damp washcloth or cotton ball over eye for several minutes. Always wipe clean from inner to outer canthus (see illustration). Remove gloves and perform hand hygiene.	Soaking allows easy removal of crusts without applying pressure to eye. Cleaning from inner to outer canthus avoids entrance of microorganisms into lacrimal duct (Burchum and Rosenthal, 2019).
c. Explain that there might be temporary burning sensation from drops.	Corneas are highly sensitive.
d. Instill eyedrops.	
(1) Hold clean cotton ball or tissue in nondominant hand on patient's cheekbone just below lower eyelid.	Cotton or tissue absorbs medication that escapes eye.

STEPS	RATIONALE

(2) With tissue or cotton ball resting below lower lid, gently press downward with thumb or forefinger against bony orbit, exposing conjunctival sac. Never press directly against patient's eyeball.

Prevents pressure and trauma to eyeball and prevents fingers from touching eye.

(3) Ask patient to look at ceiling. Rest dominant hand on patient's forehead; hold filled medication eyedropper approximately 1 to 2 cm (½–1 inch) above conjunctival sac.

Action moves cornea up and away from conjunctival sac and reduces blink reflex. Prevents accidental contact of eyedropper with eye and reduces risk of injury and transfer of microorganisms to dropper (ophthalmic medications are sterile).

(4) Drop prescribed number of drops into conjunctival sac (see illustration).

Conjunctival sac normally holds 1 or 2 drops. Provides even distribution of medication across eye.

(5) If patient blinks or closes eye, causing drops to land on outer lid margins, repeat procedure.

Drops must enter conjunctival sac to achieve therapeutic effect.

(6) When administering drops that have systemic effects, apply gentle pressure to patient's nasolacrimal duct with clean tissue for 30 to 60 seconds over each eye, one at a time (see illustration). Avoid pressure directly against patient's eyeball.

Prevents overflow of medication into nasal and pharyngeal passages. Prevents absorption into systemic circulation (Lilley et al., 2020).

(7) After instilling drops, ask patient to close eyes gently.

Helps distribute medication. Squinting or squeezing eyelids forces medication from conjunctival sac (Lilley et al., 2020).

e. Instill ophthalmic ointment.

(1) Holding applicator above lower lid margin, apply thin ribbon of ointment evenly along inner edge of lower eyelid on conjunctiva (see illustration) from inner to outer canthus.

Reduces transmission of infection. Distributes medication evenly across eye and lid margin.

(2) Have patient close eye and rub lid lightly in circular motion with cotton ball if not contraindicated. Avoid placing pressure directly against patient's eyeball.

Further distributes medication without traumatizing eye.

(3) If excess medication is on eyelid, gently wipe it from inner to outer canthus.

Promotes comfort and prevents trauma to eye.

STEP 7b Clean eye, washing from inner to outer canthus before administering drops or ointment.

STEP 7d(4) Hold eyedropper over lower conjunctival sac.

STEP 7d(6) Apply gentle pressure against nasolacrimal duct after giving eye medications.

STEP 7e(1) Nurse applies ointment along inner edge of lower eyelid from inner to outer canthus.

Continued

SKILL 31.2   ADMINISTERING OPHTHALMIC MEDICATIONS—cont'd

STEPS	RATIONALE
(4) If patient needs an eye patch, apply clean one by placing it over affected eye so that entire eye is covered. Tape securely without applying pressure to eye.	Clean eye patch reduces risk of infection.
f. Insert intraocular disk.	
(1) Open package containing disk. Gently press your fingertip against disk so that it adheres to your finger. It may be necessary to moisten gloved finger with sterile saline. Position convex side of disk on your fingertip.	Allows you to inspect disk for damage or deformity.
(2) With your other hand gently pull patient's lower eyelid away from eye. Ask patient to look up.	Prepares conjunctival sac for receiving medicated disk and moves sensitive cornea away.
(3) Place disk in conjunctival sac so that it floats on sclera between iris and lower eyelid (see illustration).	Ensures delivery of medication.
(4) Pull patient's lower eyelid out and over disk (see illustration). You should not be able to see disk at this time. Repeat if you can see disk.	Ensures accurate medication delivery.
8. Remove intraocular disk.	
a. Perform hand hygiene and apply clean gloves. Gently pull downward on lower eyelid using your nondominant hand.	Exposes disk.
b. Using forefinger and thumb of your dominant hand, pinch disk and lift it out of patient's eye (see illustration).	
9. Help patient to comfortable position.	Restores comfort and sense of well-being.
10. Place nurse call system in an accessible location within patient's reach.	Ensures patient can call for assistance if needed and promotes safety and prevents falls.
11. Raise side rails (as appropriate) and lower bed to lowest position.	Promotes safety and prevents falls.
12. Dispose of all contaminated supplies in appropriate receptacle, remove and dispose of gloves, and perform hand hygiene.	Reduces transmission of microorganisms. Use appropriate disposal receptacle if patient is on hazardous drugs.

EVALUATION

1. Observe response to medication by assessing visual changes, asking whether symptoms are relieved, and noting any side effects or discomfort felt.	Evaluates effects of medication.
2. Ask patient to discuss purpose of medication, indication, action, side effects, and technique of administration.	Determines patient's level of understanding.
3. Use Teach-Back: "I want to be sure I showed you how to insert the intraocular disk. Show me how to insert it into your left eye." Revise your instruction now or develop a plan for revised patient/family caregiver teaching if patient/family caregiver is not able to teach back correctly.	Teach-back is an evidence-based health literacy intervention that promotes patient engagement, patient safety, adherence, and quality. The goal of teach-back is to ensure that you have explained medical information clearly so that patients and their families understand what you communicated to them (AHRQ, 2020).

UNEXPECTED OUTCOMES AND RELATED INTERVENTIONS

1. Patient complains of burning or pain or experiences local side effects (e.g., headache, bloodshot eyes, local eye irritation). Medication concentration and patient's sensitivity both influence chances of side effects developing.
   - Eyedrops may have been instilled onto cornea, or dropper touched surface of eye.
   - Notify health care provider for possible adjustment in medication type and dosage.
2. Patient experiences systemic effects from drops (e.g., increased heart rate and blood pressure from epinephrine, decreased heart rate and blood pressure from timolol).
   - Notify health care provider immediately.
   - Remain with patient. Assess vital signs.
   - Withhold further doses.
3. Patient or family caregiver is unable to explain medication information or steps for administering eyedrops or has trouble manipulating dropper.
   - Repeat instructions as appropriate. Include return demonstration.

STEP 7f(3) Place intraocular disk in conjunctival sac between iris and lower eyelid.

STEP 7f(4) Gently pull patient's lower eyelid over disk.

STEP 8b Carefully pinch disk to remove it from patient's eye.

RECORDING AND REPORTING

- Record medication, concentration, dose or strength, number of drops, site of application (e.g., right eye, left eye, or both eyes), and time administered on MAR immediately after administration, not before. Include initials or signature.
- Record patient teaching (including teach-back) and validation of understanding on flow sheet or nurses' notes in EHR or chart.
- Record objective data related to tissues involved (e.g., redness, drainage, irritation), any subjective data (e.g., pain, itching, altered vision), and patient's response to medications. Note evidence of any side effects experienced on flow sheet or nurses' notes in EHR or chart.
- Report adverse effects and patient response and/or withheld medications to nurse in charge or health care provider.

SKILL 31.3 — USING METERED-DOSE INHALERS (MDIs) OR DRY POWDER INHALERS (DPIs)

Delegation and Collaboration

The skill of administering inhaled medications cannot be delegated to assistive personnel (AP). The nurse instructs the AP about:

- Potential side effects of medications and to report their occurrence to the nurse.
- Reporting breathing difficulty (e.g., paroxysmal, or sustained coughing, audible wheezing) to the nurse.

Equipment

- Inhaler device with medication canister (MDI, breath-actuated inhaler [BAI], or DPI)) (Fig. 31.31)
- Spacer device such as AeroChamber or InspirEase *(optional for MDI)*
- Facial tissues *(optional)*
- MAR (electronic or printed)
- Stethoscope
- Pulse oximeter *(optional)*

STEPS	RATIONALE

ASSESSMENT

1. Check accuracy and completeness of each MAR or computer printout with health care provider's written medication order. Check patient's name, medication name and dosage, route of administration, and time of administration. Clarify incomplete or unclear orders with health care provider before administration.

The order sheet is the most reliable source and only legal record of medications that patient is to receive. Ensures that patient receives the correct medications (Palese et al., 2019). Transcription errors are a source of medication errors (Palese et al., 2019).

2. Review pertinent information related to medication, including action, purpose, normal dose and route, side effects, time of onset and peak action, indication, and nursing implications.

Allows you to anticipate effects of medication while observing patient's response.

3. Assess patient's medical and medication history and history of allergies. List medication allergies on each page of the MAR and prominently display it on the patient's medical record. When allergies are present, patient should wear an allergy bracelet.

Factors influence how certain medications act. Reveals patient's need for medication.

Allergy alert helps prevent adverse effects.

4. Assess patient's or family caregiver's knowledge, experience, and health literacy.

Ensures patient or family caregiver has the capacity to obtain, communicate, process, and understand basic health information (CDC, 2021b).

5. Perform hand hygiene. Assess respiratory status and auscultate breath sounds (see Chapter 30). Also assess exercise tolerance; does patient develop shortness of breath easily?

Reduces transmission of microorganisms. Establishes baseline of airway status for comparison during and after treatment.

6. Measure the patient's peak expiratory flow rate using a peak flow meter. Have patient measure if doing so at home. Use patient's peak flow meter if available (see Chapter 41).

A peak flow meter is used to measure air flow or peak expiratory flow rate and aids in monitoring airway status of patients with chronic asthma (American Academy of Allergy, Asthma, and Immunology [AAAAI], 2020; Hess and Dhand, 2020b).

7. Assess patient's symptoms before initiating medication therapy.

Provides information to evaluate desired effect of medication.

8. Assess patient's ability to hold, manipulate, and depress canister and inhaler.

Any impairment of grasp or presence of hand tremors interferes with patient's ability to depress canister within inhaler. Spacer device is often necessary with an MDI.

FIG. 31.31 Types of inhalers. (A) Metered-dose inhaler (MDI). (B) Breath-actuated inhaler (BAI). (C) Dry powder inhaler (DPI).

Continued

SKILL 31.3	USING METERED-DOSE INHALERS (MDIs) OR DRY POWDER INHALERS (DPIs)—cont'd

STEPS	RATIONALE
9. If patient was previously instructed in self-administration, have patient demonstrate how to use the device.	Patients who have adequate understanding of how to use an inhaler may forget the procedure. Ongoing assessment of inhaler technique identifies areas for further education and reinforcement (AAAAI, 2020).
10. Assess patient's readiness and ability to learn and use inhaler. Determine type of device patient may prefer, considering portability, access to obtain, and cost. Ask questions about medication and its availability. Determine whether patient is alert, able to participate in own care, and is not fatigued, in pain, or in respiratory distress.	When selecting an aerosol delivery device, consider several factors, such as medication availability and administration time, patient age and ability to use the device correctly, portability of device, convenience in both outpatient and inpatient settings, and costs, as well as health care provider and patient preference (AAAAI, 2020; Hess and Dhand, 2020b). In some situations, mental or physical limitations affect patient's ability to learn and methods used for instruction.
11. Assess patient's knowledge and understanding of disease and purpose and action of prescribed medications.	Knowledge of disease is essential for patient to realistically understand when to use inhaler.
12. Assess patient's goals or preferences for how skill is to be performed or what patient expects.	Allows care to be individualized to patient.

PLANNING

1. Perform hand hygiene. Collect appropriate equipment and MAR.	Promotes time management and efficiency when preparing medications for all patients.
2. Plan preparation to avoid interruptions. Create a quiet environment. Do not take phone calls or talk with others. Follow agency No-Interruption Zone (NIZ) policy.	Interruptions contribute to medication errors (Freitas et al., 2019; Palese et al., 2019) (see Box 31.4).

IMPLEMENTATION

1. Prepare medications for inhalation. Attend to procedure and avoid distraction. Check label of medication against MAR 2 times, when removing inhaler from unit dose or AMDS and before leaving medication preparation area (see Skill 31.1). Preparation usually involves taking inhaler device out of storage and into patient room. Check expiration date on container. Perform hand hygiene.	*These are the first and second checks for accuracy.* Process ensures that right patient receives right medication.
2. Take medication to patient at correct time (see agency policy). Medications that require exact timing include STAT dose, first-time or loading doses, and one-time doses. Give time-critical scheduled medications (e.g., antibiotics, anticoagulants, insulin, anticonvulsants, or immunosuppressive agents) at exact time ordered (no more than 30 minutes before or after scheduled dose). Give non–time-critical scheduled medications within a range of 1 or 2 hours of scheduled dose (ISMP, 2011). During administration apply seven rights of medication administration.	Hospitals must adopt medication administration policy and procedure for timing of medication administration that considers nature of the prescribed medication, specific clinical application, and patient needs (USDHHS, 2011; ISMP, 2011). Time-critical scheduled medications are those for which early or delayed administration of maintenance doses of greater than 30 minutes before or after the scheduled dose may cause harm or result in substantial suboptimal therapy or pharmacological effect. Non–time-critical medications are those for which early or delayed administration within a specified range of either 1 or 2 hours should not cause harm or result in substantial suboptimal therapy or pharmacological effect (USDHHS, 2011; ISMP, 2011).
3. Identify patient using at least two identifiers (e.g., name and birthday or name and medical record number) according to agency policy. Compare identifiers with information on patient's MAR or medical record.	Ensures correct patient. Complies with The Joint Commission standards and improves patient safety (TJC, 2021).
4. At patient's bedside again compare MAR or computer printout with names of medications on medication labels and patient name. Ask patient about any allergies.	*This is the third check for accuracy* and ensures that patient receives correct medication. Confirms patient's allergy history.
5. Help patient to sit up into high-Fowler position or up in chair.	This position makes it easier to use inhaler.
6. Discuss purpose of each medication, action, and possible adverse effects. Allow patient to ask any questions about the medications. Warn about overuse of inhaler and side effects.	Patient has right to be informed, and patient's understanding of each medication improves adherence to medication therapy.
7. Explain procedure to patient. Be specific if patient wishes to self-administer medication. Allow adequate time for patient to manipulate inhaler, canister, and/or spacer device (if provided). Explain where and how to set up at home.	Patient must be familiar with how to use equipment.
8. Explain and demonstrate steps for administering MDI without spacer.	Simple one-on-one instruction and demonstration of step-by-step administration allow patient to ask questions at any point during procedure and increase patient adherence to inhaler use (Apter, 2021; Schmitz et al., 2019).
a. Insert MDI canister into holder. Then remove mouthpiece cover from inhaler.	

CLINICAL JUDGMENT: *If using an MDI that is new or has not been used for several days, push a "test spray" into the air to prime the device before using. This ensures that the MDI is patent and that the metal canister is positioned properly.*

STEPS	**RATIONALE**
b. Shake inhaler well for 2 to 5 seconds (five or six shakes).	Aerosolizes fine particles of medication.
c. Have patient hold inhaler in dominant hand.	Easier position to activate device.
d. Instruct patient to position inhaler in one of two ways:	
(1) Have patient close mouth around mouthpiece with opening toward back of throat, closing lips tightly around it (see illustration). Do not block the mouthpiece with the teeth or tongue.	Proper positioning of inhaler is essential to administering medication correctly.
(2) Position inhaler mouthpiece 2 to 4 cm (1–2 inches) in front of widely opened mouth (see illustration), with opening of inhaler toward back of throat. Lips should not touch inhaler.	Directs aerosol spray toward airway. This is best way to deliver medication without a spacer.
e. While holding the mouthpiece away from the mouth, have patient take deep breath and exhale completely.	Empties lung volume and prepares airway to receive medication.
f. With inhaler positioned correctly, be sure patient holds inhaler with thumb at mouthpiece and index and middle fingers at top. This is a three-point or lateral hand position.	MDIs are easier to activate when patients use a three-point or lateral hand position to activate canister (Burchum and Rosenthal, 2019).
g. Instruct patient to tilt head back slightly and inhale slowly and deeply through mouth for 3 to 5 seconds while depressing canister fully.	Medication is distributed to airways during inhalation.
h. Have patient hold breath for as long as comfortable, up to 10 seconds.	Allows aerosol spray droplets to reach deeper branches of airways.
i. Have patient remove MDI from mouth before exhaling and exhale slowly through nose or pursed lips.	Keeps small airways open during exhalation.
9. Explain and demonstrate steps to administer MDI using spacer device.	Simple one-on-one instruction and demonstration of step-by-step administration allows patient to ask questions at any point during procedure and increases patient adherence to inhaler use (Apter, 2021; Schmitz et al., 2019).
a. Remove mouthpiece cover from MDI and mouthpiece of spacer device.	Inhaler fits into end of spacer device.
b. Shake inhaler well for 2 to 5 seconds (five or six shakes).	Aerosolizes fine particles of medication.
c. Insert MDI into end of spacer device.	Spacer device traps medication released from MDI; patient then inhales medication from device. These devices resolve hand-breath coordination difficulty to improve delivery of correct dose of inhaled medication (Burchum and Rosenthal, 2019).
d. Instruct patient to place spacer device mouthpiece in mouth and close lips. Do not insert beyond raised lip on mouthpiece. Avoid covering small exhalation slots with lips.	Medication should not escape through mouth.
e. Have patient take a deep breath, exhale, and then breathe normally through spacer device mouthpiece (see illustration).	Allows patient to empty lungs and relax before delivering medication.
f. Instruct patient to depress medication canister 1 time, spraying 1 puff into spacer device.	Spacer contains fine spray and allows patient to inhale more medication. The spacer increases medication delivery and deposition of the medication on the oropharyngeal mucosa (Burchum and Rosenthal, 2019).
g. Have patient breathe slowly and fully through mouth for 5 seconds.	Ensures that particles of medication are distributed to deeper airways.
h. Instruct patient to hold full breath for 10 seconds.	Ensures full medication distribution through airways.
i. Have patient remove MDI and spacer and then exhale.	

STEP 8d(1) Patient opens lips and places inhaler mouthpiece in mouth with opening toward back of throat.

STEP 8d(2) Patient positions inhaler mouthpiece 2 to 4 cm (1–2 inches) from widely open mouth. This is considered the best way to deliver medication without a spacer.

Continued

SKILL 31.3	USING METERED-DOSE INHALERS (MDIs) OR DRY POWDER INHALERS (DPIs)—cont'd

STEPS	RATIONALE

10. Explain steps to administer a DPI or BAI.
   a. If DPI has an external counter, note number indicated.
         Determines doses remaining.
   b. Remove mouthpiece cover. *Do not shake* inhaler.
   c. Prepare medication. Some DPIs require loading medication before administration; some require rotation of a lever to load medication or insertion of a capsule; and some require insertion of a disk into inhaler device. Follow manufacturer's specific instructions.
         Primes inhaler, ensuring that medication is delivered to patient effectively.
   d. Have patient take a breath and exhale away from the inhaler.
         Prevents loss of powder.
   e. Have patient position mouthpiece of DPI between lips and inhale quickly and deeply through mouth (see illustration).
         Keeps medication from escaping through mouth. Forceful inhalation creates an aerosol.
   f. Have patient hold breath for 5 to 10 seconds.
         Distributes medication.

11. Instruct patient to wait 20 to 30 seconds between inhalations (if same medication) or 2 to 5 minutes between inhalations (if different medications). Be sure patient inhales correct number of prescribed puffs.
         Medications must be inhaled sequentially. Always administer bronchodilators before steroids so that dilators can open airway passages (Burchum and Rosenthal, 2019).

12. Instruct patient to not repeat inhalations before next scheduled dose.
         Medications are prescribed at intervals during day to provide constant medication levels and minimize side effects. Beta-adrenergic MDIs are used either on an "as-needed" basis or regularly every 4 to 6 hours.

13. Warn patients that they may feel gagging sensation in throat caused by droplets of medication on pharynx or tongue.
         This occurs when medication is sprayed and inhaled incorrectly.

14. About 2 minutes after last dose, instruct patient to rinse mouth with warm water and spit water out.
         Steroids may alter normal flora of oral mucosa and lead to development of fungal infection. Rinsing out patient's mouth reduces risk of fungal infection (Hess and Dhand, 2020b).

15. Instruct patient how to clean the inhaler.
         Removes residual medication and reduces transmission of microorganisms.
   a. Once a day remove MDI canister and cap from the mouthpiece. Do not wash the canister or immerse it in water. Run warm tap water through the top and bottom of the plastic mouthpiece for 30 to 60 seconds. Make sure that inhaler is completely dry before reusing. Do not get valve mechanism of canister wet.
         Water damages valve mechanism of canister. Accumulation of medication around mouthpiece interferes with proper medication distribution during use.
   b. Instruct patient to clean mouthpiece of MDI and spacer twice a week with a mild dishwashing soap, rinse thoroughly, and dry completely before storage.
         Provides better antimicrobial removal. Pressurized metered-dose inhalers (pMDIs) are potential reservoirs for bacteria.

16. Help patient to comfortable position.
         Restores comfort and sense of well-being.

17. Place nurse call system in an accessible location within patient's reach.
         Ensures patient can call for assistance if needed and promotes safety and prevents falls.

18. Raise side rails (as appropriate) and lower bed to lowest position.
         Promotes safety and prevents falls.

19. Dispose of all contaminated supplies in appropriate receptacle, remove and dispose of gloves, and perform hand hygiene.
         Reduces transmission of microorganisms. Use appropriate disposal receptacle if patient is on hazardous drugs.

EVALUATION

1. Auscultate patient lungs, listen for abnormal breath sounds, and obtain peak flow measures if ordered.
         Determines patient response to medication.

2. Have patient explain and demonstrate steps in use and cleaning of inhaler.
         Return demonstration provides feedback for measuring patient's learning.

3. Ask patient to explain medication schedule and dose of medication.
         Improves likelihood of adherence to therapy.

STEP 9e Using spacer device with a metered-dose inhaler (MDI).

STEP 10e Have patient place mouthpiece of dry powder inhaler (DPI) between lips.

STEPS	RATIONALE
4. Ask patient to describe side effects of medication and criteria for calling health care provider.	Allows patient to recognize signs of overuse and need to seek medical support when medications are ineffective.
5. **Use Teach-Back:** "I want to be sure I clearly showed you how to use your inhaler. Let's take this time; show me how you will use the inhaler to take your medicine." Revise your instruction now or develop a plan for revised patient/family caregiver teaching if patient/family caregiver is not able to teach back correctly.	Teach-back is an evidence-based health literacy intervention that promotes patient engagement, patient safety, adherence, and quality. The goal of teach-back is to ensure that you have explained medical information clearly so that patients and their families understand what you communicated to them (AHRQ, 2020).

UNEXPECTED OUTCOMES AND RELATED INTERVENTIONS

1. Patient's respirations are rapid and shallow; breath sounds indicate wheezing.
- Evaluate vital signs and respiratory status.
- Notify health care provider.
- Reassess type of medication and/or delivery method.

2. Patient needs bronchodilator more than every 4 hours (may indicate respiratory problem).
- Reassess type of medication and delivery methods needed.
- Notify health care provider.

3. Patient experiences cardiac dysrhythmias (e.g., light-headedness, syncope), especially if receiving beta-adrenergic medications.
- Withhold all further doses of medication.
- Evaluate cardiac and pulmonary status (see Chapter 30).
- Notify health care provider for reassessment of type of medication and delivery method.

RECORDING AND REPORTING

- Record medication administered, dose or strength, number of inhalations, and actual time administered immediately after administration, not before. Include initials or signature.
- Record patient and family caregiver teaching (use of teach-back) and validation of understanding on flow sheet or nurses' notes in EHR or chart.
- Record on flow sheet or nurses' notes in EHR or chart the patient's response to inhaled medication (e.g., respiratory rate and pattern, breath sounds), evidence of side effects (e.g., arrhythmia, patient's feelings of anxiety), and patient's ability to use inhaler.
- Report adverse effects and patient response and/or withheld medications to nurse in charge or health care provider.

SKILL 31.4   PREPARING INJECTIONS: AMPULES AND VIALS

Delegation and Collaboration
The skill of preparing injections from ampules and vials cannot be delegated to assistive personnel (AP).

Equipment
Medication in an Ampule
- Syringe, needle, and filter needle
- Small sterile gauze pad or alcohol swab

Medication in a Vial
- Syringe and two needles
- Needles:
  - Needleless blunt-tip vial-access cannula or needle (with safety sheath) for drawing up medication (if needed)
  - Filter needle if indicated

- Small sterile gauze pad or alcohol swab
- Diluent (e.g., 0.9% sodium chloride or sterile water if indicated)

Both
- SESIP safety needle for injection
- MAR or computer printout
- Medication in vial or ampule
- Puncture-proof container for disposal of syringes, needles, and glass

STEPS	RATIONALE
ASSESSMENT	
1. Check accuracy and completeness of each MAR or computer printout with health care provider's written medication order. Check patient's name, medication name and dosage, route of administration, and time of administration. Clarify incomplete or unclear orders with health care provider before administration.	The order sheet is the most reliable source and only legal record of medications that patient is to receive. Ensures that patient receives the correct medications (Palese et al., 2019). Transcription errors are a source of medication errors (Palese et al., 2019).
2. Review pertinent information related to medication, including action, purpose, normal dose and route, side effects, time of onset and peak action, indication, and nursing implications.	Allows you to anticipate effects of medication while observing patient's response.
3. Assess patient's medical and medication history and history of allergies. List medication allergies on each page of the MAR and prominently display it on the patient's medical record. When allergies are present, patient should wear an allergy bracelet.	Factors influence how certain medications act. Reveals patient's need for medication. Allergy alert helps prevent adverse effects.

Continued

| **SKILL 31.4** | **PREPARING INJECTIONS: AMPULES AND VIALS—cont'd** |

STEPS	**RATIONALE**
4. Review medication reference information for action, purpose, side effects, and nursing implications.	Allows you to administer medication properly and monitor patient's response.
5. Assess patient's body build, muscle size, weight, and viscosity of medication if giving subcutaneous or IM medication.	Determines type and size of syringe and needle for injection.

PLANNING

1. Perform hand hygiene. Collect appropriate equipment and MAR.	Promotes time management and efficiency when preparing medications for all patients.
2. Plan preparation to avoid interruptions. Create a quiet environment. Do not take phone calls or talk with others. Follow agency No-Interruption Zone (NIZ) policy. Keep all pages of MAR or computer printouts for one patient together or look at only one patient's eMAR at a time.	Interruptions contribute to medication errors (Freitas et al., 2019; Palese et al., 2019) (see Box 31.4).

IMPLEMENTATION

1. Perform hand hygiene and prepare medications.	
a. If using a medication cart, move it outside patient's room.	Organization of equipment saves time and reduces error.
b. Unlock medication drawer or cart or log onto AMDS.	Medications are safeguarded when locked in cabinet, cart, or AMDS.
c. Select correct medication from stock supply or unit-dose drawer. Compare label of medication with MAR computer printout or computer screen.	Reading label and comparing it with transcribed order reduce errors. *This is the first check for accuracy.*
d. Check expiration date on each medication, one at a time.	Medications used past their expiration date are sometimes inactive, less effective, or harmful to patients.
e. Calculate medication dose, as necessary. Double-check your calculation. In the case of high-risk medications ask another nurse to perform an independent double check of dosage (see agency policy).	Double-checking may help reduce error. Independent double checks should be used only for very selective high-alert medications (not all) that most warrant their use (ISMP, 2019c).
f. If preparing a controlled substance, check record for previous medication count and compare with supply available.	Controlled substance laws require careful monitoring of dispensed narcotics.
g. Do not leave medications unattended.	Nurse is responsible for safekeeping of medications.
2. Prepare ampule.	
a. Tap top of ampule lightly and quickly with finger until fluid moves from its neck (see illustration).	Dislodges any fluid that collects above neck of ampule. All solution moves into lower chamber.
b. Place small gauze pad around neck of ampule (see illustration).	Protects fingers from trauma as glass tip is broken off. Do not use opened alcohol swab to wrap around top of ampule because alcohol may leak into ampule.
c. Snap neck of ampule quickly and firmly away from hands (see illustration).	Protects your fingers and face from shattering glass.
d. Draw up medication quickly, using filter needle long enough to reach bottom of ampule to access medication.	System is open to airborne contaminants. Filter needles filter out any fragments of glass (Painchart et al., 2018).

STEP 2a Tapping ampule moves fluid down neck. **STEP 2b** Gauze pad placed around neck of ampule. **STEP 2c** Neck snapped away from hands.

STEPS	RATIONALE
e. Hold ampule upside down or set it on flat surface. Insert filter needle into center of ampule opening. Do not allow needle tip or shaft to touch rim of ampule.	Broken rim of ampule is considered contaminated. When ampule is inverted, solution dribbles out if needle tip or shaft touches rim of ampule.
f. Aspirate medication into syringe by gently pulling back on plunger (see illustration).	Withdrawal of plunger creates negative pressure within syringe barrel, which pulls fluid into syringe.
g. Keep needle tip under surface of liquid. Tip ampule to bring all fluid within reach of needle.	Prevents aspiration of air bubbles.
h. If you aspirate air bubbles, do not expel air into ampule.	Air pressure forces fluid out of ampule, and medication will be lost.
i. To expel excess air bubbles, remove needle from ampule. Hold syringe vertically with needle pointing up. Tap side of syringe to cause bubbles to rise toward needle. Draw back slightly on plunger and push plunger upward to eject air. Do not eject fluid.	Withdrawing plunger too far removes it from barrel. Holding syringe vertically allows fluid to settle in bottom of barrel. Pulling back on plunger allows fluid within needle to enter barrel so that fluid is not expelled. Then expel air at top of barrel and within needle.
j. If syringe contains excess fluid, use sink for disposal. Hold syringe vertically with needle tip up and slanted slightly toward sink. Slowly eject excess fluid into sink. Recheck fluid level in syringe by holding it vertically.	Safely disperses excess medication into sink. Position of needle allows you to expel medication without having it flow down needle shaft. Rechecking fluid level ensures proper dose.
k. Cover needle with its safety sheath or cap. Replace filter needle with regular SESIP needle.	Minimizes needlesticks. Filter needles cannot be used for injection.
3. Prepare vial containing a solution.	
a. Remove cap covering top of unused vial to expose sterile rubber seal. If a multidose vial has been used before, cap is already removed. Firmly and briskly wipe surface of rubber seal with alcohol swab and allow it to dry.	Vial comes packaged with cap that cannot be replaced after seal removal. Not all medication manufacturers guarantee that rubber seals of unused vials are sterile. Swabbing with alcohol reduces transmission of microorganisms. Allowing alcohol to dry prevents alcohol from coating needle and mixing with medication.
b. Pick up syringe and remove needle cap or cap covering needleless access device (see illustration). Pull back on plunger to draw amount of air into syringe equivalent to volume of medication to be aspirated from vial.	Injecting air into vial prevents buildup of negative pressure in vial when aspirating medication.

STEP 2f (A) Medication aspirated with ampule inverted. (B) Medication aspirated with ampule on flat surface.

Bevel

Protective cap

Needle shaft

Activator-assist lever

STEP 3b (A) Needleless system. (B) Safety needle system. (C) Detail of safety needle system. (A and B courtesy and © Becton, Dickinson and Company.)

Continued

SKILL 31.4	PREPARING INJECTIONS: AMPULES AND VIALS—cont'd

STEPS	RATIONALE

CLINICAL JUDGMENT: *Some medications and agencies require use of a filter needle when preparing medications from vials. Check agency policy or medication reference. If you use a filter needle to aspirate medication, you need to change it to a regular SESIP needle of the appropriate size to administer medication (Antoszyk, 2018).*

c. With vial on flat surface, insert tip of needle or needleless device through center of rubber seal (see illustration). Apply pressure to tip of needle during insertion. Label the syringe with the name of the medication and dose.	Center of seal is thinner and easier to penetrate. Using firm pressure prevents dislodging rubber particles that could enter vial or needle. Syringe needs to be labeled before medication is placed in the syringe to prevent any possible mix up with syringe filled with something other than the medication (TJC, 2021).
d. Inject air into air space of vial, holding on to plunger. Hold plunger firmly; plunger is sometimes forced backward by air pressure within vial.	Injection of air creates vacuum needed to get medication to flow into syringe. Injecting into air space of vial prevents formation of bubbles and an inaccurate dose.
e. Invert vial while keeping firm hold on syringe and plunger. Hold vial between thumb and middle fingers of nondominant hand. Grasp end of syringe barrel and plunger with thumb and forefinger of dominant hand to counteract pressure in vial.	Inverting vial allows fluid to settle in lower half of container. Position of hands prevents forceful movement of plunger and permits easy manipulation of syringe.
f. Keep tip of needle or needleless device below fluid level.	Prevents aspiration of air.
g. Allow air pressure from vial to fill syringe gradually with medication. If necessary, pull back slightly on plunger to obtain correct amount of medication.	Positive pressure within vial forces fluid into syringe.
h. When you obtain desired volume, position needle or needleless device into air space of vial; tap side of syringe barrel gently to dislodge any air bubbles (see illustration). Eject any air remaining at top of syringe into vial.	Forcefully striking barrel while needle is inserted in vial may bend needle. Accumulation of air displaces medication and causes dose errors.
i. Remove needle or needleless access device from vial by pulling back on barrel of syringe.	Pulling plunger rather than barrel causes plunger to separate from barrel, resulting in loss of medication.
j. Hold syringe at eye level at 90-degree angle to ensure correct volume and absence of air bubbles. Remove any remaining air by tapping barrel to dislodge any air bubbles. Draw back slightly on plunger; then push it upward to eject air. Do not eject fluid. Recheck volume of medication.	Holding syringe vertically allows fluid to settle in bottom of barrel. Tapping dislodges air to top of barrel. Pulling back on plunger allows fluid within needle to enter barrel so that you do not expel fluid. You then expel air at top of barrel and within needle.

CLINICAL JUDGMENT: *When preparing medication from single-dose vial, do not assume that volume listed on label is total volume in vial. Some manufacturers provide small amount of extra liquid, expecting loss during preparation. Be sure to draw up only desired volume.*

k. Before you inject medication into patient's tissue, change needle with regular SESIP to appropriate gauge and length according to route of medication administration.	Inserting needle through rubber stopper dulls beveled tip. New needle is sharper and, because no fluid is along shaft, does not track medication through tissues. Filter needles cannot be used for injection.
l. Cover needle with its safety sheath or cap.	Minimizes needlesticks.
m. For multidose vial, make label that includes date of opening, concentration of medication per milliliter, and your initials.	Ensures that nurses will prepare future doses correctly. You discard some medications within a certain time frame after mixing.

STEP 3c Insert safety needle through center of vial diaphragm (with vial flat on table).

STEP 3h Hold syringe upright; tap barrel to dislodge air bubbles.

STEPS	RATIONALE

4. Prepare vial containing powder (reconstituting medications).

a. Remove cap covering vial of powdered medication and cap covering vial of proper diluent. Firmly swab both rubber seals with alcohol swab and allow alcohol to dry.

Allowing alcohol to dry prevents it from coating needle and mixing with medication.

b. Draw up manufacturer suggestion for volume and type of diluent into syringe following Steps 3b through 3j.

Prepares diluent for injection into vial containing powdered medication.

c. Insert tip of needle or needleless device through center of rubber seal of vial of powdered medication. Inject diluent into vial. Remove needle.

Diluent begins to dissolve and reconstitute medication.

d. Mix medication thoroughly. Roll in palms. Do not shake.

Ensures proper dispersal of medication throughout solution and prevents formation of air bubbles.

e. Reconstituted medication in vial is ready to be drawn into new syringe. Read label carefully to determine dose after reconstitution.

Once you add diluent, concentration of medication (mg/mL) determines dose you give. Reading medication label carefully decreases medication errors.

f. Draw up reconstituted medication into syringe. Insert needleless device/needle into vial. Do not add air. Then follow Steps 3e through 3l.

Prepares medication for administration.

CLINICAL JUDGMENT: *Some agencies require that doses of certain medications (e.g., insulin and heparin) be checked using an independent double check by another nurse (ISMP, 2019c). Check policies and procedures before administering medication.*

5. Compare label of medication with MAR, computer screen, or computer printout.

This is the second check for accuracy.

6. Dispose of soiled supplies. Place broken ampule and/or used vials and used needle or needleless device in puncture- and leak-proof container. Clean work area and perform hand hygiene.

Proper disposal of glass and needle prevents accidental injury to staff. Controls transmission of infection.

EVALUATION

1. Just before administering medication to patient, compare MAR with label of prepared medication and compare dose in syringe with desired dose.

Ensures that dose is accurate. This is the third check for accuracy.

UNEXPECTED OUTCOMES AND RELATED INTERVENTIONS

1. Air bubbles remain in syringe.
- Expel air from syringe and add medication to it until you prepare correct dose.

2. Incorrect dose of medication is prepared.
- Discard prepared dose.
- Prepare correct new dose.

SKILL 31.5   ADMINISTERING INJECTIONS

Delegation and Collaboration

The skill of administering injections cannot be delegated to assistive personnel (AP). The nurse instructs the AP about:
- Potential medication side effects and allergic responses and the need to report their occurrence along with any changes in patient's vital signs or LOC (e.g., sedation).

Equipment
All Injections
- Small gauze pad
- Alcohol swab
- Vial or ampule of medication or skin test solution
- Clean gloves
- MAR (electronic or printed)
- Puncture-proof container for sharps

- Proper size syringe and sharps with SESIP needle:
  - *Subcutaneous*: syringe (1- to 3-mL) and needle (25- to 27-gauge, ⅛- to ⅝-inch)
  - *Immunizations*: 23- to 25-gauge, ⅝-to 1 ½-inch needle (CDC, 2021a)
  - *Subcutaneous U-100 insulin*: insulin syringe (1 mL) with preattached needle (28- to 31-gauge, ¼- to ⅝-inch)
  - *Subcutaneous U-500 insulin*: 1 mL tuberculin (TB) syringe with needle (25- to 27-gauge, ½- to ⅝-inch)
  - *Intramuscular (IM):* Syringe 2 to 3 mL for adult, 0.5 to 1 mL for infants and small children
  - *Intradermal (ID):* 1-mL tuberculin syringe with needle (25- to 27-gauge, ½- to ⅝-inch)
  - Needle gauge often depends on length of needle; administer biological and medication in aqueous solution with a 22- to 25-gauge needle.
  - Needle length typically corresponds to site of injection, age, gender, and size of patient. Refer to the following guidelines for vaccine administration; length needed may vary outside of these guidelines for patients who are smaller or larger than average.

Continued

SKILL 31.5   ADMINISTERING INJECTIONS—cont'd

NEEDLE LENGTH FOR IMMUNIZATIONS (BASED ON CDC 2021a GUIDELINES)

Site	Child	Adult
Ventrogluteal	Not recommended	1½ inches
Vastus lateralis	⅝–1¼ inch	⅝–1 inch
Deltoid	⅝–1 inch	1–1½ inches

Gender—Male	Gender—Female	Needle Length
Less than 130 lb	Less than 130 lb	⅝–1 inch
130–152 lb	130–152 lb	1 inch
153–260 lb	153–200 lb	1–1½ inches
260+ lb	200+ lb	1½ inches

Age-Group	Needle Length	Site
Neonates[a]	⅝ inch (16 mm)[b]	Vastus lateralis
Infants, 1–12 months	1 inch (25 mm)	Vastus lateralis
Toddlers, 1–2 years	1–1¼ inches (25–32 mm)	Vastus lateralis[c]
	⅝[b]–1 inch (16–25 mm)	Deltoid muscle of arm
Children, 3–10 years	⅝[b]–1 inch (16–25 mm)	Deltoid muscle of arm[c]
	1–1¼ inches (25–32 mm)	Vastus lateralis
Children, 11–18 years	⅝[b]–1 inch (16–25 mm)	Deltoid muscle of arm[c]
	1–1½ inches (25–38 mm)	Vastus lateralis
Men and women, less than 60 kg (130 lb)	1 inch (25 mm)	Deltoid muscle of arm
Men and women, 60–70 kg (130–152 lb)	1 inch (25 mm)	Deltoid muscle of arm
Men, 70–118 kg (152–260 lb)	1–1½ inches (25–38 mm)	Deltoid muscle of arm
Women, 70–90 kg (152–200 lb)	1–1½ inches (25–38 mm)	Deltoid muscle of arm
Men, greater than 118 kg (260 lb)	1½ inches (38 mm)	Deltoid muscle of arm
Women, greater than 90 kg (200 lb)	1½ inches (38 mm)	Deltoid muscle of arm

[a]First 28 days of life.
[b]If skin is stretched tightly and subcutaneous tissues are not bunched.
[c]Preferred site.

STEPS	RATIONALE

ASSESSMENT

1. Check accuracy and completeness of each MAR with health care provider's medication order. Check patient's name, medication name and dosage, and route and time of administration. Clarify incomplete or unclear orders with health care provider before administration.

The order sheet is the most reliable source and only legal record of medications that patient is to receive. Ensures that patient receives the correct medications (Palese et al., 2019). Transcription errors are a source of medication errors (Palese et al., 2019).

2. Assess patient's medical and medication history and history of allergies. List medication allergies on each page of the MAR and prominently display any allergies on the patient's medical record. When allergies are present, patient should wear an allergy bracelet.

Factors influence how certain medications act. Reveals patient's need for medication.

Allergy alert helps prevent adverse effects.

3. Review medication reference information for medication action, purpose, normal dose, side effects, time and peak of onset, and nursing implications. In the case of an intradermal injection, review expected reaction and/or anticipated effects when testing skin with specific allergen and appropriate time to read site.

Allows you to administer medication safely and monitor patient's response to therapy. Type of reaction to an immunization depends on patient's ability to mount a cell-mediated immune response. Knowledge of expected and adverse reactions to skin testing helps you determine for which symptoms to monitor, how frequently, and when to reassess patient.

4. Assess patient's symptoms before initiating medication therapy.

Provides information to evaluate desired effect of medication.

5. Assess for contraindications to injections.
   a. For ID injections
      (1) Reduced local tissue perfusion. Assess for history of severe adverse reactions that occurred after previous ID injection.

Decreased tissue perfusion reduces absorption of ID medications. Prior history of severe reactions increases the risk for future severe reactions.

   b. For subcutaneous injections
      (1) Assess for factors such as circulatory shock or reduced local tissue perfusion. Assess adequacy of patient's adipose tissue.

Reduced tissue perfusion interferes with medication absorption and distribution. Physiological changes of aging or patient illness often influence amount of subcutaneous tissue that patient possesses.

STEPS	RATIONALE

c. For IM injections

(1) Assess for factors such as muscle atrophy, reduced blood flow, or circulatory shock.

Atrophied muscle absorbs medication poorly. Factors interfering with blood flow to muscles impair medication absorption.

6. Assess patient's or family caregiver's knowledge, experience, and health literacy.

Ensures patient or family caregiver has the capacity to obtain, communicate, process, and understand basic health information (CDC, 2021b).

7. Assess patient's knowledge of purpose and expected response to medication or skin testing.

Patients need to know when to return for follow-up reading of skin test and when and how to report any reaction. Poses implications for patient education.

8. Assess patient's knowledge about medication.

Determines whether there is a need for patient education.

9. Assess patient's goals or preferences for how skill is to be performed or what patient expects.

Allows care to be individualized to patient.

10. For subcutaneous insulin or heparin, assess relevant laboratory results (e.g., blood glucose, partial thromboplastin).

Provides baseline for measuring medication response.

11. Observe patient's previous verbal and nonverbal responses toward injection.

Anticipating patient's anxiety allows you to use distraction to reduce pain awareness.

12. Check expiration date on medication.

Dose potency increases or decreases when expired.

PLANNING

1. Perform hand hygiene. Collect appropriate equipment and MAR

Promotes time management and efficiency when preparing medications for all patients.

2. Plan preparation to avoid interruptions. Create a quiet environment. Do not take phone calls or talk with others. Follow agency No-Interruption Zone (NIZ) policy. Keep all pages of MAR or computer printouts for one patient together or look at only one patient's eMAR at a time.

Interruptions contribute to medication errors (Freitas et al., 2019; Palese et al., 2019) (see Box 31.4).

IMPLEMENTATION

1. Prepare medications for injection. Attend to procedure and avoid distraction. Check label of medication against MAR 2 times, when removing medication from unit dose or AMDS and before leaving medication preparation area (see Skill 31.1). Perform hand hygiene.

Ensures that medication is sterile. Preventing distractions reduces medication preparation errors. *These are the first and second checks for accuracy* and ensure that correct medication is administered. Reduces transmission of microorganisms. Hand hygiene decreases transfer of microorganisms.

2. Take medications to patient at correct time (see agency policy). Medications that require exact timing include STAT doses, first-time, loading, and one-time doses. Give time-critical scheduled medications (e.g., antibiotics, anticoagulants, insulin, anticonvulsants, or immunosuppressive agents) at exact time ordered (within 30 minutes before or after scheduled dose). Give non–time-critical scheduled medications within a range of either 1 or 2 hours of scheduled doses (ISMP, 2011). Apply the seven rights of medication administration throughout medication administration.

Ensures intended therapeutic effect and adheres to professional standards. Hospitals need to adopt a medication administration policy and procedure for the timing of medication administration that considers patient needs, prescribed medication, and specific clinical indications (USDHHS, 2011; ISMP, 2011). Time-critical scheduled medications are medications in which early or delayed administration of maintenance doses of more than 30 minutes before or after the scheduled dose may cause harm or result in suboptimal therapy or pharmacological effect. Non–time-critical medications are medications in which early or delayed administration of 1 to 2 hours should not cause harm or result in suboptimal therapy or pharmacological effects (USDHHS, 2011; ISMP, 2011).

3. Close room curtain or door.

Provides privacy.

4. Identify patient using at least two identifiers (e.g., name and birthday or name and medical record number) according to agency policy. Compare identifiers with information on patient's MAR or medical record.

Ensures correct patient. Complies with The Joint Commission standards and improves patient safety (TJC, 2021).

5. At patient's bedside, compare MAR or computer printout with names of medications on medication labels and patient name. Ask patient about any allergies.

This is the third accuracy check and ensures that patient receives correct medication. Confirms patient's allergy history.

6. Discuss purpose of each medication and/or skin test, action, and possible adverse effects. Allow patient to ask any questions. Tell patient that injection will cause slight burning or sting. An intradermal injection will create a small bleb on the skin.

Patient has right to be informed, and patient's understanding of each medication improves adherence to medication therapy. Helps minimize patient's anxiety.

7. Perform hand hygiene and apply clean gloves. Keep sheet or gown draped over body parts not requiring exposure.

Reduces transmission of microorganisms. Draping the patient provides privacy.

8. Select appropriate injection site. Inspect skin surface over sites for bruises, inflammation, or edema.

Injection sites need to be free of abnormalities that interfere with medication absorption. Sites used repeatedly become hardened from lipohypertrophy (increased growth in fatty tissue). Do not use an area that is bruised or has signs associated with infection.

a. Intradermal (ID):

(1) Note lesions or discolorations of skin. If possible, select site 3 to 4 finger widths below antecubital space and a hand width above wrist. If you cannot use forearm, inspect upper back. If necessary, use sites for subcutaneous injections.

An ID site needs to be clear, so you can see results of skin test and interpret them correctly (Kowal and DuBuske, 2020).

Continued

SKILL 31.5 ADMINISTERING INJECTIONS—cont'd

STEPS	RATIONALE

b. Subcutaneous:

   (1) Do not use an area that is bruised or has signs associated with infection. Palpate sites and avoid those with masses or tenderness. Be sure that needle is correct size by grasping skinfold at site with thumb and forefinger. Measure fold from top to bottom. Make sure that needle is one-half length of fold.

   You can mistakenly give subcutaneous injections in muscle, especially in abdomen and thigh sites. Appropriate size of needle ensures that you inject medication into subcutaneous tissue (Drutz, 2021).

   (2) When administering insulin or heparin, use abdominal injection sites first, followed by thigh injection site. Choose site on right or left side of abdomen at least 5 cm (2 inches) away from umbilicus.

   Risk for bruising is not affected by site.

c. IM:

   (1) Note integrity and size of muscle and palpate for tenderness or hardness. Avoid these areas. If injections are given frequently, rotate sites. Use ventrogluteal site if possible.

   Ventrogluteal is preferred injection site for adults. It is also preferred site for children of all ages (Drutz, 2021; Hockenberry et al., 2019; Strohfus et al., 2018). The anterolateral thigh can be used for children of all ages.

9. Help patient to comfortable position:

  a. ID: Have patient extend elbow and support it and forearm on flat surface.

  Stabilizes injection site for easiest accessibility.

  b. Subcutaneous: Have patient relax arm, leg, or abdomen, depending on site selection.

  Relaxation of site minimizes discomfort.

  c. IM: Position patient depending on site chosen (e.g., sit or lie flat, on side, or prone).

  Reduces strain on muscle and minimizes discomfort of injections.

CLINICAL JUDGMENT: *Ensure that medical condition (e.g., circulatory shock, orthopedic surgery) does not contraindicate patient's position for injection.*

---

10. Relocate site using anatomical landmarks. For subcutaneous insulin, rotate site within anatomical area (e.g., abdomen) and systematically rotate sites within area.

Injection into correct anatomical site prevents injury to nerves, bones, and blood vessels.

11. Clean site with an antiseptic swab. Apply swab at center of site and rotate outward in circular direction for approximately 5 cm (2 inches) (see illustration). *Option for IM injection*: Apply EMLA cream on injection site at least 1 hour before IM injection or use vapocoolant spray (e.g., ethyl chloride) just before injection (see agency policy).

Mechanical action of swab removes secretions containing microorganisms.

Decreases pain at injection site.

12. Hold swab or gauze between third and fourth fingers of nondominant hand.

Gauze or swab remains readily accessible when withdrawing needle after injection.

13. Remove needle cap or sheath from needle by pulling it straight off.

Preventing needle from touching sides of cap prevents contamination.

14. Hold syringe between thumb and forefinger of dominant hand:

  a. ID: Hold syringe with bevel of needle pointing up.

  With bevel up, medication is less likely to be deposited into tissues below dermis.

  b. Subcutaneous and IM: Hold as dart, palm up (see illustration).

  Quick, smooth injection requires proper manipulation of syringe parts.

STEP 11 Clean site with circular motion.

STEP 14b Hold syringe as if grasping a dart.

STEPS	RATIONALE

15. Administer injection:

  a. ID

    (1) With nondominant hand stretch skin over site with forefinger or thumb.

        Needle pierces tight skin more easily.

    (2) With needle almost against patient's skin, insert it slowly with bevel up at 5- to 15-degree angle until resistance is felt. Advance needle through epidermis to approximately 3 mm (⅛ inch) below skin surface. You will see needle tip through skin.

        Ensures that needle tip is in dermis. You obtain inaccurate results if you do not inject needle at correct angle and depth.

    (3) Inject medication slowly. Normally you feel resistance. If not, needle is too deep; remove and begin again.

        Slow injection minimizes discomfort at site. Dermal layer is tight and does not expand easily when solution is injected.

    (4) While injecting medication, note that small bleb approximately 6 mm (¼ inch) in diameter (resembling mosquito bite) appears on surface of skin (see illustration). Instruct patient that this is normal finding.

        Bleb indicates that medication is deposited in dermis.

  b. Subcutaneous

    (1) For average-size patient, pinch skin with nondominant hand.

        Needle penetrates taut skin more easily than loose skin. Pinching skin elevates subcutaneous tissue and desensitizes area.

    (2) Inject needle quickly and firmly at 45- to 90-degree angle (see Fig. 31.18). Release skin. *Option:* If using injection pen or administering heparin, continue to pinch skin while injecting medication.

        Quick, firm insertion minimizes discomfort. (Injecting medication into compressed tissue irritates nerve fibers.) Correct angle prevents accidental injection into muscle.

    (3) For patient who is obese, pinch skin at site and inject needle at 90-degree angle below tissue fold.

        Patients who are obese have fatty layer of tissue above subcutaneous layer.

    (4) After needle enters site, grasp lower end of syringe barrel with nondominant hand to stabilize it. Move dominant hand to end of plunger and slowly inject medication over several seconds (see illustration). When giving heparin, inject over 30 seconds (Hull et al., 2019). Avoid moving syringe.

        Movement of syringe may displace needle and cause discomfort. Slow injection of medication minimizes discomfort.

CLINICAL JUDGMENT: *Aspiration after injecting a subcutaneous medication is not necessary. Piercing a blood vessel in a subcutaneous injection is very rare. Aspiration after injecting heparin and insulin is not recommended (CDC, 2021a; Lilley et al., 2020).*

---

  c. IM

    (1) Position ulnar aspect of your nondominant hand just below site and pull skin approximately 2.5 to 3.5 cm (1–1½ inches) down or laterally to administer in a Z-track. Hold position until medication is injected (see Fig. 31.22). With dominant hand inject needle quickly at 90-degree angle into muscle (see Fig. 31.18).

        Z-track creates zigzag path through tissues that seals needle track to avoid tracking of medication. Use Z-track for all IM injections (Strohfus et al., 2018). A quick, dartlike injection reduces discomfort.

    (2) *Option:* If patient's muscle mass is small, grasp body of muscle between thumb and fingers.

        Ensures that medication reaches muscle mass (CDC, 2021a; Hockenberry et al., 2019; Strohfus et al., 2018).

STEP 15a(4) Injection creates small bleb.

STEP 15b(4) Inject medication slowly.

Continued

SKILL 31.5	ADMINISTERING INJECTIONS—cont'd

STEPS	RATIONALE
(3) After needle pierces skin, still pulling on skin with nondominant hand, grasp lower end of syringe barrel with fingers of nondominant hand to stabilize it. Move dominant hand to end of plunger. Avoid moving syringe.	Smooth manipulation of syringe reduces discomfort from needle movement. Skin remains pulled until after medication is injected to ensure Z-track administration.
(4) Pull back on plunger 5 to 10 seconds. If no blood appears, inject medicine slowly, at rate of 1 mL/10 seconds. **NOTE:** Do not aspirate if administering immunizations (CDC, 2021a).	Aspiration of blood into syringe indicates possible placement of needle into a vein. Slow injection rate reduces pain and tissue trauma and reduces chance of leakage of medication back through needle track (Hockenberry et al., 2019). The CDC (2021a) no longer recommends aspiration when administering an immunization.

CLINICAL JUDGMENT: *If blood appears in syringe, remove needle, and dispose of medication and syringe properly. Prepare another dose of medication for injection.*

STEPS	RATIONALE
(5) Once medication is injected, wait 10 seconds; then smoothly and steadily withdraw needle, release skin, and apply gauze gently over site.	Allows time for medication to absorb into muscle before removing syringe. Dry gauze minimizes discomfort associated with alcohol on nonintact skin.
16. Apply gentle pressure to site. Do not massage site. Apply bandage if needed.	Massage causes underlying tissue damage. Massaging ID site disperses medication into underlying tissue layers and alters test results.
17. Help patient to comfortable position.	Restores comfort and sense of well-being.
18. Place nurse call system in an accessible location within patient's reach.	Ensures patient can call for assistance if needed and promotes safety and prevents falls.
19. Raise side rails (as appropriate) and lower bed to lowest position.	Promotes safety and prevents falls.
20. Dispose of all contaminated supplies in appropriate receptacle, remove and dispose of gloves, and perform hand hygiene.	Reduces transmission of microorganisms. Use appropriate disposal receptacle if patient is on hazardous drugs.
21. Stay with patient and observe for any allergic reactions.	Dyspnea, wheezing, and circulatory collapse are signs of severe anaphylactic reaction, which is life-threatening emergency.

EVALUATION

1. Return to room in 15 to 30 minutes and ask whether patient feels any acute pain, burning, numbness, or tingling at injection site.	After an ID injection, continued discomfort could indicate injury to underlying tissue. After a subcutaneous or IM injection, continued discomfort may indicate injury to underlying bones or nerves.
2. After an ID injection ask patient to discuss implications of skin testing and signs of hypersensitivity.	Patient's ability to recognize signs of skin testing helps to ensure timely reporting of results.
3. Inspect ID bleb. *Option:* Use skin pencil and draw circle around perimeter of injection site. Read TB test site at 48 to 72 hours; look for induration (hard, dense, raised area) of skin around injection site of (CDC, n.d.):	Determines whether reaction to antigen occurs, indication positive for tuberculosis or tested allergens. Site must be read at various intervals to determine test results. Pencil marks make site easy to find. You determine results of skin testing at various times, based on type of medication used or type of skin testing completed. Manufacturer directions determine when to read test results. Degree of reaction varies based on patient condition.

- 15 mm or more in patients with no known risk factors for tuberculosis
- 10 mm or more in patients who are recent immigrants; intravenous (IV) drug users; residents and employees of high-risk settings; patients with certain chronic illnesses; children younger than 4 years of age; and infants, children, and adolescents exposed to high-risk adults
- 5 mm or more in patients who are HIV positive, have fibrotic changes on chest x-ray film consistent with previous tuberculosis infection, have had organ transplants, or are immunosuppressed

CLINICAL JUDGMENT: *When a patient does not return for reading of the TB test within 72 hours, the patient needs to have the test repeated.*

4. Inspect subcutaneous or IM site, noting any bruising or induration. Document bruising or induration if present. Notify health care provider and provide warm compress to site.	Bruising or induration indicates complication associated with injection. Document findings and notify health care provider.
5. Observe patient's response to medication at times that correlate with onset, peak, and duration of medication. Review laboratory results as appropriate (e.g., blood glucose, partial thromboplastin).	Adverse effects of parenteral medications develop rapidly. Evaluate effect of medication on basis of onset, peak, and duration of action.
6. **Use Teach-Back**: "I want to be sure I explained about your injection. Can you explain why you need this injection and the side effects to watch for and report to me if they occur?" Revise your instruction now or develop plan for revised patient/family caregiver teaching if patient/family caregiver is not able to teach back correctly.	Teach-back is an evidence-based health literacy intervention that promotes patient engagement, patient safety, adherence, and quality. The goal of teach-back is to ensure that you have explained medical information clearly so that patients and their families understand what you communicated to them (AHRQ, 2020).

UNEXPECTED OUTCOMES AND RELATED INTERVENTIONS

1. Raised, reddened, or hard zone (induration) forms around an ID test site.
   - Notify patient's health care provider.
   - Document sensitivity to injected allergen or positive test if tuberculin skin testing was completed.
2. Patient has adverse reaction with signs of urticaria, pruritus, wheezing, and dyspnea.
   - Notify patient's health care provider immediately.
   - Follow agency policy for appropriate response to medication reactions (e.g., administration of antihistamine such as diphenhydramine or epinephrine).
   - Add allergy information to patient's record.
3. Patient complains of localized pain, numbness, tingling, or burning at injection site, indicating possible injury to nerve or tissues.
   - Assess injection site.
   - Document findings.
   - Notify patient's health care provider.

RECORDING AND REPORTING

- Record medication, dose, route, site, time, and date on MAR in the EHR or chart immediately after administration, not before. Correctly sign MAR according to agency policy.
- Record patient teaching, validation of understanding, and patient's response to medication in the EHR or chart.
- Record area of ID injection and appearance of skin in the EHR or chart.
- Report any undesirable effects from injection to patient's health care provider and document adverse effects in record.
- Document immunizations in patient's permanent record, including date of administration, vaccine manufacturer and lot number, expiration date, name and title of the person who administered the vaccine and the address of the agency where the permanent record will reside, vaccine information statement (VIS) and date printed on the VIS, and date VIS given to patient or parent/guardian (CDC, 2021a).

SKILL 31.6   ADMINISTERING MEDICATIONS BY INTRAVENOUS BOLUS

Delegation and Collaboration

The skill of administering medications by IV bolus cannot be delegated to assistive personnel (AP). The nurse directs the AP about:
- Potential medication actions and side effects and to immediately report their occurrence to the nurse.
- Reporting any patient complaints of moisture or discomfort around IV insertion site.
- Obtaining required vital signs and reporting them to the nurse.

Equipment
- Watch with second hand
- Clean gloves
- Antiseptic gloves
- Medication in vial or ampule
- Proper-size syringes for medication and saline flush with needleless device or SESIP needle (21- to 25- gauge)
- IV lock: Vial of normal saline flush solution (saline recommended [Gorski, 2018]); if agency continues to use heparin flush, the most common concentration is 10 units/mL; check agency policy.
- MAR or computer printout
- Puncture-proof container

STEPS	RATIONALE

ASSESSMENT

1. Check accuracy and completeness of each MAR or computer printout with health care provider's written medication order. Check patient's name, medication name and dosage, route of administration, and time of administration. Clarify incomplete or unclear orders with health care provider before administration.

The order sheet is the most reliable source and only legal record of medications that patient is to receive. Ensures that patient receives the correct medications (Palese et al., 2019). Transcription errors are a source of medication errors (Palese et al., 2019).

CLINICAL JUDGMENT: *Some IV medications can be pushed safely only when a patient is monitored continuously for dysrhythmias, blood pressure changes, or other adverse effects. Therefore some medications can be pushed only in specific patient care units. Confirm agency guidelines.*

---

2. Assess patient's medical and medication history and history of allergies. List medication allergies on each page of the MAR and prominently display any allergies on the patient's medical record. When allergies are present, patient should wear an allergy bracelet.

Determines need for medication or possible contraindications for medication administration. IV bolus delivers medication rapidly. Allergic response is immediate.

3. Review medication reference information for medication action, purpose, side effects, normal dose, time of peak onset, how slowly to give medication, and nursing implications such as need to dilute medication or administer it through a filter.

Knowledge of medication allows you to give it safely and monitor patient's response to therapy.

4. If you give medication through an existing IV line, determine compatibility of medication with IV fluids and any additives within IV solution.

IV medication is not always compatible with IV solution and/or additives, and a new site may need to be initiated.

5. Assess patient's symptoms before initiating medication therapy.

Provides information to evaluate desired effects of medication.

Continued

SKILL 31.6	ADMINISTERING MEDICATIONS BY INTRAVENOUS BOLUS—cont'd

STEPS	RATIONALE
6. Assess patient's or family caregiver's knowledge, experience, and health literacy.	Ensures patient or family caregiver has the capacity to obtain, communicate, process, and understand basic health information (CDC, 2021b).
7. Perform hand hygiene. (Apply clean gloves if risk of contact with body fluids.) Assess condition of IV needle insertion site for signs of infiltration or phlebitis.	Reduces transmission of microorganisms. Do not administer medication if site is edematous or inflamed.
8. Assess patency of patient's existing IV infusion line or saline lock (see Chapter 42).	For medication to reach venous circulation effectively, IV line must be patent, and fluids must infuse easily.
9. Assess patient's knowledge, prior experience with IV medications, and feelings about procedure.	Reveals need for patient instruction and/or support.
10. Assess patient's goals or preferences for how skill is to be performed or what patient expects.	Allows care to be individualized to patient.

PLANNING

1. Perform hand hygiene. Collect appropriate equipment and MAR.	Reduces transmission of microorganisms. Ensures organized procedure.
2. Follow agency No-Interruption Zone (NIZ) policy. Prepare medications for one patient at a time. Keep all pages of MAR or computer printouts for one patient together or look at only one patient's eMAR at a time.	Interruptions contribute to medication errors (Freitas et al., 2019; Palese et al., 2019) (see Box 31.4).

IMPLEMENTATION

1. Prepare medications for IV bolus administration. Attend to procedure and avoid distraction. Check label of medication against MAR 2 times, when removing medication from unit dose or AMDS and before leaving medication preparation area. Perform hand hygiene.	Ensures that medication is sterile. *These are the first and second checks for accuracy* and ensure that correct medication is administered. Reduces transmission of microorganisms.

CLINICAL JUDGMENT: *Some IV medications require dilution before administration. Verify with agency policy or pharmacy if dilution is permitted. If a small amount of medication is given (e.g., less than 1 mL), dilute medication in small amount (e.g., 5 mL) of normal saline or sterile water so that it does not collect in the "dead spaces" (e.g., Y-site injection port, IV cap) of the IV delivery system.*

2. Take medication(s) to patient at correct time (see agency policy). Medications that require exact timing include STAT doses, first-time or loading doses, and one-time doses. Give time-critical scheduled medications (e.g., antibiotics, anticoagulants, insulin, anticonvulsants, or immunosuppressive agents) at exact time ordered (no more than 30 minutes before or after scheduled dose). Give non–time-critical scheduled medications within a range of 1 or 2 hours of scheduled dose (ISMP, 2011). During administration apply seven rights of medication administration.	Hospitals must adopt medication administration policy and procedure for timing of medication administration that considers nature of the prescribed medication, specific clinical application, and patient needs (USDHHS, 2011; ISMP, 2011). Time-critical scheduled medications are those for which early or delayed administration of maintenance doses of greater than 30 minutes before or after the scheduled dose may cause harm or result in substantial suboptimal therapy or pharmacological effect. Non–time-critical medications are those for which early or delayed administration within a specified range of either 1 or 2 hours should not cause harm or result in substantial suboptimal therapy or pharmacological effect (USDHHS, 2011; ISMP, 2011).
3. Close room curtain or door.	Provides privacy.
4. Identify patient using at least two identifiers (e.g., name and birthday or name and medical record number) according to agency policy. Compare identifiers with information on patient's MAR or medical record.	Ensures correct patient. Complies with The Joint Commission standards and improves patient safety (TJC, 2021).
5. At patient's bedside again compare MAR or computer printout with names of medications on medication labels and patient name. Ask patient about any allergies.	*This is the third check for accuracy* and ensures that patient receives correct medication. Confirms patient's allergy history.
6. Discuss purpose of each medication, action, and possible adverse effects. Allow patient to ask questions. Explain that you will give medication through existing IV line. Encourage patient to report symptoms of discomfort at IV site.	Keep patient informed of planned therapies, minimizing anxiety. Patients who verbalize pain at IV site help detect IV infiltrations early, lessening damage to surrounding tissue.
7. Perform hand hygiene and apply clean gloves.	Reduces transmission of microorganisms.
8. IV push (existing IV line):	
a. Select injection port of IV tubing closest to patient. Use needleless injection port.	Follows provisions of Needle Safety and Prevention Act of 2001 (OSHA, n.d.).

CLINICAL JUDGMENT: *Never administer IV medications through tubing that is infusing blood, blood products, or parenteral nutrition solutions.*

b. Clean injection port with antiseptic swab. Allow to dry.	Prevents transfer of microorganisms during blunt cannula insertion.
c. Connect syringe to IV line: Insert needleless tip of syringe containing medication through center of port (see illustration).	Prevents introduction of microorganisms. Prevents damage to port diaphragm and possible leakage from site.
d. Occlude IV line by pinching tubing just above injection port (see illustration). Pull back gently on plunger of syringe to aspirate for blood return.	Final check ensures that medication is being delivered into bloodstream.

STEPS	RATIONALE

CLINICAL JUDGMENT: *In the case of smaller-gauge IV needles, blood return sometimes is not aspirated even if IV line is patent. If IV site does not show signs of infiltration and IV fluid is infusing without difficulty, give IV push.*

e. Release tubing and inject medication within amount of time recommended by agency policy, pharmacist, or medication reference manual. Use watch to time administrations (see illustration). You can pinch IV line while pushing medication and release it when not pushing medication. Allow IV fluids to infuse when not pushing medication.

Ensures safe medication infusion. Rapid injection of IV medication can be fatal. Allowing IV fluids to infuse while pushing IV medication enables medication to be delivered to patient at prescribed rate.

f. After injecting medication, withdraw syringe and recheck IV fluid infusion rate.

Injection of bolus may alter rate of fluid infusion. Rapid fluid infusion can cause circulatory fluid overload.

g. If IV medication is incompatible with IV fluids, stop IV fluids, clamp IV line, and flush with 10 mL of normal saline or sterile water (see agency policy). Then give IV bolus over appropriate amount of time and flush with another 10 mL of normal saline or sterile water at *same rate* as medication was administered.

Allows IV bolus to be administered without risks associated with IV incompatibilities. Ensure that agency guidelines permit flushing lines with incompatible medications. A new site may need to be initiated.

STEP 8c Connect syringe to intravenous line with needleless blunt cannula tip.

STEP 8d Occlude intravenous tubing above injection port.

STEP 8e Use watch to time intravenous push medication.

Continued

SKILL 31.6	ADMINISTERING MEDICATIONS BY INTRAVENOUS BOLUS—cont'd

STEPS	RATIONALE
h. If IV line that currently is hanging is a medication, disconnect it and administer IV push medication as outlined in Step 9. Verify agency policy for stopping IV fluids or continuous IV medications. If unable to stop IV infusion, start new IV site (see Chapter 42) and administer medication using IV push (IV lock) method.	Avoids giving patient sudden bolus of medication in existing IV line.
9. IV push (IV lock):	
a. Prepare flush solutions according to agency policy.	
(1) *Saline flush method (preferred method):* Prepare two syringes filled with 2 to 3 mL of normal saline (0.9%). Many agencies do not provide prefilled normal saline syringes for flushing IV lines.	Normal saline is effective in keeping IV locks patent and is compatible with wide range of medications (Gorski, 2018).
(2) Heparin flush method (prepare heparin flush and saline syringe according to agency policy).	
b. Administer medication:	
(1) Clean injection port with antiseptic swab.	Prevents transfer of microorganisms during needle insertion.
(2) Insert needleless tip of syringe with normal saline 0.9% through center of injection port of IV lock.	
(3) Pull back gently on syringe plunger and check for blood return.	Indicates if needle or catheter is in vein.
(4) Flush IV site with normal saline by pushing slowly on plunger.	Clears needle and reservoir of blood. Flushing without difficulty indicates patent IV line.

CLINICAL JUDGMENT: *Carefully observe the area of skin above the IV catheter. Note any puffiness or swelling as the IV site is flushed, which could indicate infiltration into the vein, requiring removal of catheter.*

STEPS	RATIONALE
(5) Remove saline-filled syringe.	
(6) Clean injection port with antiseptic swab.	Prevents transmission of microorganisms.
(7) Insert needleless tip of syringe containing prepared medication through injection port of IV lock.	Allows administration of medication.
(8) Inject medication within amount of time recommended by agency policy, pharmacist, or medication reference manual. Use watch to time administration.	Many medication errors are associated with IV pushes being administered too quickly. Following guidelines for IV push rates promotes patient safety.
(9) After administering bolus, withdraw syringe.	
(10) Clean injection port with antiseptic swab.	Prevents transmission of microorganisms.
(11) Flush injection port.	
(a) Attach syringe with normal saline and inject flush at same rate that medication was delivered.	Flushing IV line with saline prevents occlusion of IV access device and ensures that all medication is delivered. Flushing IV site at same rate as medication ensures that any medication remaining within IV needle is delivered at the correct rate.
10. Help patient to comfortable position.	Restores comfort and sense of well-being.
11. Discard uncapped needle or needle enclosed in safety shield and attached syringe into puncture- and leak-proof receptacle.	Prevents injury to patients and health care personnel. Recapping needles increases risk for needlestick injury (OSHA, n.d.).
12. Place nurse call system in an accessible location within patient's reach.	Ensures patient can call for assistance if needed and promotes safety and prevents falls.
13. Raise side rails (as appropriate) and lower bed to lowest position.	Promotes safety and prevents falls.
14. Dispose of all contaminated supplies in appropriate receptacle, remove and dispose of gloves, and perform hand hygiene.	Reduces transmission of microorganisms. Use appropriate disposal receptacle if patient is on hazardous drugs.

EVALUATION

1. Observe patient closely for adverse reactions during administration and for several minutes thereafter.	IV medications act rapidly.
2. Observe IV site during injection for sudden swelling and for 48 hours after IV push.	Swelling indicates infiltration into tissue surrounding vein. Signs of infiltration may not occur for 48 hours.
3. Assess patient's status after giving medication to evaluate effectiveness of the medication.	Some IV bolus medications can cause rapid changes in patient's physiological status, thus requiring careful monitoring and assessment and possibly future laboratory testing (e.g., vasopressors and antiarrhythmics require blood pressure and heart rate monitoring, and heparin requires laboratory studies after administration to determine therapeutic levels).
4. Use Teach-Back: "I want to be sure I explained to you why you are receiving this IV medication. Can you explain to me what the medication is for and when to call the nurse?" Revise your instruction now or develop a plan for revised patient/family caregiver teaching if patient/family caregiver is not able to teach back correctly.	Teach-back is an evidence-based health literacy intervention that promotes patient engagement, patient safety, adherence, and quality. The goal of teach-back is to ensure that you have explained medical information clearly so that patients and their families understand what you communicated to them (AHRQ, 2020).

UNEXPECTED OUTCOMES AND RELATED INTERVENTIONS

1. Patient develops adverse reaction to medication.
   - Stop delivering medication immediately and follow agency policy or guidelines for appropriate response to allergic reaction (e.g., administration of antihistamine such as diphenhydramine or epinephrine) and reporting of adverse medication reactions.
   - Notify patient's health care provider of adverse effects immediately.
   - Add allergy information to patient's record.
2. IV site shows symptoms of infiltration or phlebitis (see Chapter 42).
   - Stop IV infusion immediately or discontinue access device and restart in another site.
   - Determine how much damage IV medication can produce in subcutaneous tissue.
   - Provide IV extravasation care as indicated by agency policy; use a medication reference and consult pharmacist to determine appropriate follow-up care.

RECORDING AND REPORTING

- Immediately record medication administration, including medication, dose, route, time instilled, and date and time administered on MAR in the EHR or chart. Include initials or signature.
- Record patient's medication response in nurses' notes.
- Record patient teaching and validation of understanding on the flow sheet or nurses' notes in the EHR or chart.
- Report any adverse reactions to patient's health care provider. Patient's response sometimes indicates need for additional medical therapy.

| SKILL 31.7 | ADMINISTERING INTRAVENOUS MEDICATIONS BY PIGGYBACK, VOLUME-CONTROL ADMINISTRATION SETS, AND MINI-INFUSION (SYRINGE) PUMPS |

Delegation and Collaboration
The skill of administering IV medications by piggyback, intermittent infusion sets, and mini-infusion (syringe) pumps cannot be delegated to assistive personnel (AP). The nurse directs the AP about:
- Potential medication actions and side effects and to immediately report their occurrence to the nurse.
- Reporting any patient complaints of moisture or discomfort around IV insertion site.
- Reporting any change in patient's condition or vital signs to the nurse.

Equipment
- Adhesive tape *(optional)*
- Antiseptic swab
- Clean gloves
- IV pole
- MAR or computer printout

- Puncture-proof container
- Labels—all tubing, IV bags, medications

Piggyback or Mini-Infusion (Syringe) Pump
- Medication prepared in 5- to 250-mL labeled infusion bag or syringe
- Prefilled syringe containing normal saline flush solution (for saline lock only)
- Short microdrip, macrodrip, or syringe IV tubing set, with blunt-end needleless cannula attachment
- Needleless device
- Syringe pump if indicated

Volume-Control Administration Set
- Volutrol or Buretrol
- Infusion tubing with needleless system attachment
- Syringe (1–20 mL)
- Vial or ampule of ordered medication

STEPS	RATIONALE

ASSESSMENT

1. Check accuracy and completeness of each MAR or computer printout with health care provider's written medication order. Check patient's name, medication name and dosage, route of administration, and time of administration. Clarify incomplete or unclear orders with health care provider before administration.

The order sheet is the most reliable source and only legal record of medications that patient is to receive. Ensures that patient receives the correct medications (Palese et al., 2019). Transcription errors are a source of medication errors (Palese et al., 2019).

2. Assess patient's medical and medication history and history of allergies. List medication allergies on each page of the MAR and prominently display any allergies on the patient's medical record. When allergies are present, patient should wear an allergy bracelet.

Determines need for medication or possible contraindications for medication administration. IV bolus delivers medication rapidly. Allergic response is immediate.

3. Review medication reference information for medication action, purpose, side effects, normal dose, time of peak onset, how slowly to give medication, and nursing implications such as need to dilute medication or administer it through a filter.

Allows you to administer medication safely and monitor patient's response to therapy.

4. If you give medication through existing IV line, determine compatibility of medication with IV fluids and any additional additives within IV solution.

IV medication is sometimes not compatible with IV solution and/or additives.

CLINICAL JUDGMENT: *Never administer IV medications through tubing that is infusing blood, blood products, or parenteral nutrition solutions.*

Continued

SKILL 31.7	ADMINISTERING INTRAVENOUS MEDICATIONS BY PIGGYBACK, VOLUME-CONTROL ADMINISTRATION SETS, AND MINI-INFUSION (SYRINGE) PUMPS—cont'd

STEPS	RATIONALE
5. Perform hand hygiene. Assess patency and placement of patient's existing IV infusion line or saline lock (see Chapter 42).	Do not administer medication if site is edematous or inflamed. For medication to reach circulation effectively, IV line must be patent, and fluids must infuse easily.

CLINICAL JUDGMENT: *If patient's IV site is saline locked, clean the port with alcohol and assess the patency of the IV line by flushing it with 2 to 3 mL of sterile sodium chloride.*

6. Assess patient's symptoms before initiating medication therapy.	Provides information to evaluate desired effects of medication.
7. Assess patient's or family caregiver's knowledge, experience, and health literacy.	Ensures patient or family caregiver has the capacity to obtain, communicate, process, and understand basic health information (CDC, 2021b).
8. Assess patient's knowledge, prior experience with IV medications, and feelings about procedure.	Reveals need for patient instruction and/or support.
9. Assess patient's goals or preferences for how skill is to be performed or what patient expects.	Allows care to be individualized to patient.

PLANNING

1. Perform hand hygiene. Collect appropriate equipment and MAR.	Reduces transmission of microorganisms. Ensures organized procedure.
2. Follow agency No-Interruption Zone (NIZ) policy. Prepare medications for one patient at a time. Keep all pages of MAR or computer printouts for one patient together or look at only one patient's eMAR at a time.	Interruptions contribute to medication errors (Freitas et al., 2019; Palese et al., 2019) (see Box 31.4).

IMPLEMENTATION

1. Prepare medications for IV administration. Attend to procedure and avoid distraction. Check label of medication against MAR 2 times, when removing medication from unit dose or AMDS and before leaving medication preparation area. Pharmacy prepares piggyback and prefilled syringes. You will prepare medication for a volume administration set. Perform hand hygiene.	Ensures that medication is sterile. *These are the first and second checks for accuracy* and ensure that correct medication is administered. Reduces transmission of microorganisms.
2. Take medication(s) to patient at correct time (see agency policy). Medications that require exact timing include STAT doses, first-time or loading doses, and one-time doses. Give time-critical scheduled medications (e.g., antibiotics, anticoagulants, insulin, anticonvulsants, or immunosuppressive agents) at exact time ordered (no more than 30 minutes before or after scheduled dose). Give non–time-critical scheduled medications within a range of 1 or 2 hours of scheduled dose (ISMP, 2011). During administration apply seven rights of medication administration.	Hospitals must adopt medication administration policy and procedure for timing of medication administration that considers nature of the prescribed medication, specific clinical application, and patient needs (USDHHS, 2011; ISMP, 2011). Time-critical scheduled medications are those for which early or delayed administration of maintenance doses of greater than 30 minutes before or after the scheduled dose may cause harm or result in substantial suboptimal therapy or pharmacological effect. Non–time-critical medications are those for which early or delayed administration within a specified range of either 1 or 2 hours should not cause harm or result in substantial suboptimal therapy or pharmacological effect (USDHHS, 2011; ISMP, 2011).
3. Close room curtain or door.	Provides privacy.
4. Identify patient using at least two identifiers (e.g., name and birthday or name and medical record number) according to agency policy. Compare identifiers with information on patient's MAR or medical record.	Ensures correct patient. Complies with The Joint Commission standards and improves patient safety (TJC, 2021).
5. At patient's bedside again compare MAR or computer printout with names of medications on medication labels and patient name. Ask patient about any allergies.	*This is the third check for accuracy* and ensures that patient receives correct medication. Confirms patient's allergy history.
6. Discuss purpose of each medication, action, and possible adverse effects. Allow patient to ask any questions. Explain that you will give medication through existing IV line. Encourage patient to report symptoms of discomfort at site.	Keep patient informed of planned therapies, minimizing anxiety. Patients who verbalize pain at IV site help detect IV infiltrations early, lessening damage to surrounding tissues.
7. Perform hand hygiene and apply clean gloves. Administer infusion:	Reduces transmission of microorganisms.
a. Piggyback infusion:	
(1) Connect infusion tubing to medication bag (see Chapter 42). Fill tubing by opening regulator flow clamp. Once tubing is full, close clamp and cap end of tubing.	Filling infusion tubing with solution and freeing air bubbles prevent air embolus. Capping reduces transmission of microorganisms.
(2) Hang piggyback (see illustration) medication bag above level of primary fluid bag. (Use hook to lower main bag.) Primary line continues to infuse.	Height of fluid bag affects rate of flow to patient.
(3) Connect tubing of piggyback infusion to appropriate connector on upper Y-port of primary infusion line:	Connection allows IV medication to enter main IV line.
(a) *Needleless system:* Wipe off needleless port of main IV line with alcohol swab, allow to dry, and insert cannula tip of piggyback infusion tubing.	Use needleless connections to prevent accidental needlestick injuries (Gorski et al., 2021; OSHA, n.d.).

STEPS	RATIONALE
(b) *Normal saline lock:* Follow steps to flush and prepare lock (see Skill 31.6). Wipe off port with alcohol swab, let dry, and insert tip of piggyback infusion tubing via needleless access (see illustrations).	Flushing of lock ensures patency.
(4) Regulate flow rate of medication solution by adjusting regulator clamp or IV pump infusion rate. Infusion times vary. Refer to medication reference or agency policy for safe flow rate.	Provides slow, safe, intermittent infusion of medication and maintains therapeutic blood levels.
(5) Once medication has infused:	
(a) *Continuous infusion:* Check flow rate of primary infusion. Primary infusion automatically begins after piggyback solution is empty.	Back-check valve on piggyback prevents flow of primary infusion until medication infuses. Checking flow rate ensures proper administration of IV fluids.
(b) *Normal saline lock:* Disconnect tubing, clean port with alcohol, and flush IV line with 2 to 3 mL of sterile 0.9% sodium chloride. Maintain sterility of IV tubing between intermittent infusions.	
(6) Regulate continuous main infusion line to ordered rate.	Infusion of piggyback sometimes interferes with main line infusion rate.
(7) Leave IV piggyback and tubing in place for future medication administration (see agency policy) or discard it and the uncapped needle/needle enclosed safety shield of flushing syringe in puncture- and leak-proof container.	Establishing secondary line produces route for microorganisms to enter main line. Repeated changes in tubing increase risk for infection transmission.
b. Volume-control administration set (e.g., Volutrol):	
(1) Fill Volutrol with desired amount of IV fluid (50–100 mL) by opening clamp between Volutrol and main IV bag (see illustration).	Small volume of fluid dilutes IV medication and reduces risk of fluid infusing too rapidly.
(2) Close clamp and check to be sure that clamp on air vent Volutrol chamber is open.	Prevents additional leakage of fluid into Volutrol. Air vent allows fluid in Volutrol to exit at regulated rate.
(3) Clean injection port on top of Volutrol with antiseptic swab.	Prevents introduction of microorganisms during needle insertion.

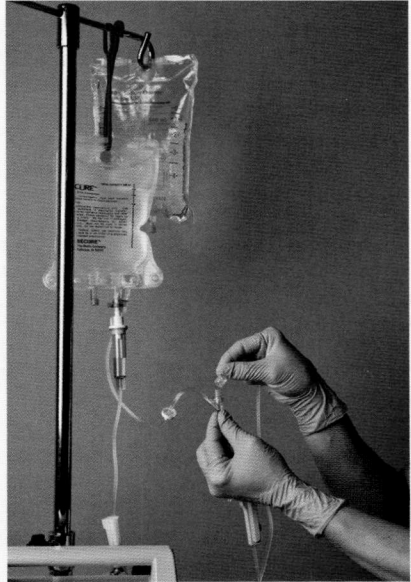

STEP 7a(2) Small-volume minibag for piggyback infusion.

STEP 7a(3)(b) (A) Needleless lock cannula system. (B) Blunt-ended cannula inserts into port and locks.

Continued

SKILL 31.7	ADMINISTERING INTRAVENOUS MEDICATIONS BY PIGGYBACK, VOLUME-CONTROL ADMINISTRATION SETS, AND MINI-INFUSION (SYRINGE) PUMPS—cont'd

STEPS	RATIONALE
(4) Remove needle cap or sheath and insert needleless syringe or syringe needle through port and inject medication (see illustration). Gently rotate Volutrol between hands.	Rotating mixes medication with solution to ensure equal distribution in Volutrol.
(5) Regulate IV infusion rate to allow medication to infuse in time recommended by agency policy, pharmacist, or medication reference manual.	For optimal therapeutic effect, medication should infuse in prescribed time interval.
(6) Label Volutrol with name of medication; dosage; total volume, including diluent; and time of administration following ISMP (2019d) safe-medication label format.	Alerts nurses to medication being infused. Prevents other medications from being added to Volutrol.
(7) If patient is receiving continuous IV infusion, check infusion rate after Volutrol infusion is complete.	Ensures appropriate rate of administration.
(8) Dispose of uncapped needle or needle enclosed in safety shield and syringe in puncture- and leak-proof container. Discard supplies in appropriate container. Perform hand hygiene.	Prevents accidental needlesticks (OSHA, n.d.). Reduces transmission of microorganisms.

c. Mini-infusion (syringe) pump administration:

(1) Connect prefilled syringe to mini-infusion tubing; remove end cap of tubing.	Special tubing designed to fit syringe delivers medication to main IV line.
(2) Carefully apply pressure to syringe plunger, allowing tubing to fill with medication.	Ensures that tubing is free of air bubbles to prevent air embolus.
(3) Place syringe into mini-infusion pump (follow product directions) and hang on IV pole. Be sure that syringe is secured.	Secure placement is needed for proper infusion.
(4) Connect end of mini-infusion tubing to main IV line or saline lock:	Establishes route for IV medication to enter main IV line.
(a) *Existing IV line:* Wipe off needleless port on main IV line with alcohol swab, allow to dry, and insert tip of mini-infusion tubing through center of port.	Needleless connections reduce risk for accidental needlestick injuries (OSHA, n.d.).
(b) *Normal saline lock:* Follow steps to flush and prepare lock (see Skill 31.6). Wipe off port with alcohol swab, allow to dry, and insert tip of mini-infusion tubing.	Flushing of lock ensures patency.
(5) Set pump to deliver medication within time recommended by agency policy, pharmacist, or medication reference manual. Press button on pump to begin infusion.	Pump automatically delivers medication at safe, constant rate based on volume in syringe.
(6) Once medication has infused:	
(a) *Main IV infusion:* Check flow rate. Infusion automatically begins to flow once pump stops. Regulate infusion to desired rate as needed.	Maintains patent primary IV fluids.
(b) *Normal saline lock:* Disconnect tubing, clean port with alcohol, and flush IV line with 2 to 3 mL of sterile 0.9% sodium chloride. Maintain sterility of IV tubing between intermittent infusions.	
(c) Dispose of uncapped needle or needle enclosed in safety shield of flushing syringe in puncture- and leak-proof container. Discard supplies in appropriate container. Perform hand hygiene.	

STEP 7b(1) Fill volume-control administration device.

STEP 7b(4) Medication injected into device.

STEPS	RATIONALE
8. Help patient to comfortable position.	Restores comfort and sense of well-being
9. Place nurse call system in an accessible location within patient's reach.	Ensures patient can call for assistance if needed and promotes safety and prevents falls.
10. Raise side rails (as appropriate) and lower bed to lowest position.	Promotes safety and prevents falls.
11. Dispose of all contaminated supplies in appropriate receptacle, remove and dispose of gloves, and perform hand hygiene.	Reduces transmission of microorganisms. Use appropriate disposal receptacle if patient is on hazardous drugs.
12. Stay with patient for several minutes and observe for any allergic reactions.	Dyspnea, wheezing, and circulatory collapse are signs of severe anaphylactic reaction.

EVALUATION

1. Observe patient for signs or symptoms of adverse reaction.	IV medications act rapidly.
2. During infusion periodically check infusion rate and condition of IV site.	IV must remain patent for proper medication administration. Infiltration of IV site requires discontinuing infusion.
3. Ask patient to explain purpose and side effects of medication.	Evaluates patient's understanding of instruction.
4. Use Teach-Back: "I want to be sure I explained to you the reason for this IV medication. Can you explain to me why you are receiving the medication and what to report to the nurse?" Revise your instruction now or develop a plan for revised patient/family caregiver teaching if patient/family caregiver is not able to teach back correctly.	Teach-back is an evidence-based health literacy intervention that promotes patient engagement, patient safety, adherence, and quality. The goal of teach-back is to ensure that you have explained medical information clearly so that patients and their families understand what you communicated to them (AHRQ, 2020).

UNEXPECTED OUTCOMES AND RELATED INTERVENTIONS

1. Patient develops adverse or allergic reaction to medication.
- Stop medication infusion immediately.
- Follow agency policy or guidelines for appropriate response to allergic reaction (e.g., administration of antihistamine such as diphenhydramine or epinephrine) and reporting of adverse medication reactions.
- Notify patient's health care provider of adverse effects immediately.
- Add allergy information to patient record per agency policy.

2. Medication does not infuse over established time frame.
- Determine reason (e.g., improper calculation of flow rate, poor positioning of IV needle at insertion site, infiltration).
- Take corrective action as indicated by agency policy or health care provider.

3. IV site shows signs of infiltration or phlebitis (see Chapter 42).
- Stop IV infusion and discontinue access device.
- Treat IV site as indicated by agency policy.
- Insert new IV catheter if therapy continues.
- For infiltration determine how harmful IV medication is to subcutaneous tissue. Provide IV extravasation care (e.g., injecting phentolamine around IV infiltration site) as indicated by agency policy or consult pharmacist to determine appropriate follow-up care.

RECORDING AND REPORTING

- Immediately record medication administration, including medication, dose, route, time instilled, and date and time administered on MAR in the EHR or chart. Include initials or signature.
- Record volume of fluid in medication bag or syringe pump as fluid intake.
- Record patient teaching and validation of understanding on the flow sheet or nurses' notes in the EHR or chart.
- Report any adverse reactions to patient's health care provider. Patient's response sometimes indicates need for additional medical therapy.

■ KEY POINTS

- Administering medications safely requires an understanding of the legal aspects of health care.
- Apply knowledge of the four major pharmacokinetic processes—medication absorption, distribution, metabolism, and excretion—to time medication administration, select the route of administration, and evaluate a patient's response.
- When a medication is prescribed, the goal is a constant blood level within a safe therapeutic range.
- Prompt recognition and reporting of adverse medication events prevents serious patient injury.
- In health care agencies, patients with known medication allergies have their allergy information recorded in a clearly identifiable place.
- The route prescribed for administering a medication depends on the medication's properties and desired effect and on a patient's physical and mental condition.
- Metric units are easy to convert and calculate using simple multiplication and division, with each basic unit of measurement organized into units of 10.
- A health care provider prescribes a patient's medications, and the pharmacist prepares and distributes the prescribed medications. Nurses, physicians, and other health care providers work together to evaluate the effectiveness of medication therapy.
- Distractions may cause a medication error. Distractions include a page, phone call, or request from a colleague or patient that draws away, disturbs, or diverts attention from a current desired task or that forces attention on a new task, at least temporarily.

- The seven rights of medication administration include the right medication, right dose, right patient, right route, right time, right documentation, and right indication.
- Medications that are time critical most likely cause harm or have subtherapeutic effects if they are not administered on time (usually 30 minutes before or after the scheduled dose).
- Before administering medications, perform a physical assessment, which will reveal physical findings for any indications or contraindications for medication therapy.
- Responsibilities of medication administration include knowing medication therapeutics, assessing a patient before administration, calculating doses, administering medications using the seven rights, monitoring and evaluating medication effects, and assessing a patient's ability to self-administer medications.
- For patient safety, it is essential that you refer to the MAR each time you prepare a medication and have it available at the patient's bedside when administering medications.
- Collaboration with patients and their family caregivers is essential, particularly if patients will require assistance with self-administration and if medication regimens are complicated.
- Evaluation of medication administration is an essential role of professional nursing that requires assessment skills, clinical judgment, analysis, and knowledge of medications, physiology, and pathophysiology.

■ REFLECTIVE LEARNING

- You are a new nurse and have started a staff nurse position on a busy medical-surgical unit. You must administer many medications to four different patients throughout the shift and feel overwhelmed. How would you organize safe medication administration for these patients?
- Consider all the nonparenteral routes of medication your patients may be receiving during their admission to a health care agency. Consider the need for different approaches to administering these medications. When might it be acceptable to allow a patient to administer medications via some of these routes themselves?
- Consider a time when you were caring for patients who required a variety of routes for administering IV medication. How might you ensure you are correctly assessing for medication compatibility, rate of infusion, and route of administration?

■ REVIEW QUESTIONS

1. A nurse is administering an oral tablet to a patient. Which of the following steps is the second check for accuracy in determining the patient is receiving the right medication?
   1. Logging on to AMDS or unlocking medicine drawer or cart.
   2. Before going to patient's room, comparing patient's name and name of medication on label of prepared drugs with MAR.
   3. Selecting correct medication from ADMS, unit-dose drawer, or stock supply and comparing name of medication on label with MAR or computer printout.
   4. Comparing MAR or computer printout with names of medications on medication labels and patient name at patient's bedside.
2. The health care provider has written the following orders. Which order(s) does the nurse need to clarify before administering the medication? (Select all that apply.)
   Provide a rationale for your answers and rewrite the incorrect order(s) to follow the ISMP current medication order safety guidelines.

1. Timoptic .25% solution 1 drop OD BID
2. Metoprolol 12.50 mg QD
3. Insulin Glargine 6 u SC twice a day
4. Enalapril 2.5 mg. PO 3 times a day, hold for systolic blood pressure <100

3. An older adult states that she cannot see her medication bottles clearly to determine when to take her prescription. What actions should the nurse take to help the older adult patient? (Select all that apply.)
   1. Provide a dispensing system for each day of the week.
   2. Provide larger, easier-to-read labels.
   3. Tell the patient what is in each container.
   4. Have a family caregiver administer the medication.
   5. Use teach-back to ensure that the patient knows what medication to take and when.
4. Which of the following guidelines must a nurse use for taking verbal or telephone orders? (Select all that apply).
   1. Follow the health care agency guidelines regarding authorized staff who may receive and record verbal or telephone orders.
   2. Clearly identify patient's name, room number, and diagnosis.
   3. Read back all orders to health care provider.
   4. Use clarification questions to avoid misunderstandings.
   5. Write "VO" (verbal order) or "TO" (telephone order), including date and time, name of patient, and complete order; sign the name of the health care provider and nurse.
5. Which aspects of the patient's care related to the administration of heparin can the nurse delegate to the nursing AP? (Select all that apply):
   1. Notify the nurse if there are any signs of bleeding.
   2. Assess the vital signs for possible symptoms of bleeding.
   3. Assess bleeding sites and apply appropriate pressure to the sites.
   4. Notify the nurse if there is blood noted in the patient's urine.
   5. Notify the nurse if there is oozing from any puncture sites.
6. The nurse is administering an IV push medication to a patient who has a compatible IV fluid running through IV tubing. Place the following steps in the appropriate order.
   1. Release tubing and inject medication within amount of time recommended by agency policy, pharmacist, or medication reference manual. Use watch to time administration.
   2. Select injection port of IV tubing closest to patient. Whenever possible, injection port should accept a needleless syringe. Use IV filter if required by medication reference or agency policy.
   3. After injecting medication, release tubing, withdraw syringe, and recheck fluid infusion rate.
   4. Connect syringe to port of IV line. Insert needleless tip or small-gauge needle of syringe containing prepared drug through center of injection port.
   5. Clean injection port with antiseptic swab. Allow to dry.
   6. Occlude IV line by pinching tubing just above injection port. Pull back gently on syringe plunger to aspirate blood return.
7. A nurse is administering an MDI with a spacer to a patient with COPD. Place the steps of the procedure in the correct order.
   1. Insert MDI into end of spacer.
   2. Perform a respiratory assessment.
   3. Remove mouthpiece from MDI and spacer device.
   4. Place the spacer mouthpiece into patient's mouth and instruct patient to close lips around the mouthpiece.
   5. Depress medication canister, spraying 1 puff into spacer device.
   6. Shake inhaler for 2 to 5 seconds.
   7. Instruct patient to hold breath for 10 seconds.
   8. Instruct patient to breathe in slowly through mouth for 3 to 5 seconds.

8. A patient is to receive medications through a small-bore nasogastric feeding. Which nursing actions are appropriate? (Select all that apply.)
1. Verifying tube placement after medications are given
2. Mixing all medications together to give all at once
3. Using an enteral tube syringe to administer medications
4. Flushing tube with 30 to 60 mL of water after the last dose of medication
5. Checking for gastric residual before giving the medications
6. Keeping the head of the bed elevated for 30 to 60 minutes after the medications are given

9. Place the steps of administering an intradermal injection in the correct order.
1. Inject medication slowly.
2. Note the presence of a bleb.
3. Advance needle through epidermis to 3 mm.
4. Using nondominant hand, stretch skin over site with forefinger.
5. Insert needle at a 5- to 15-degree angle into the skin until resistance is felt.
6. Cleanse site with antiseptic swab.

10. After receiving an IM injection in the deltoid, a patient states, "My arm really hurts. It's burning and tingling where I got my injection." What should the nurse do next? (Select all that apply.)
1. Assess the injection site.
2. Administer an oral medication for pain.
3. Notify the patient's health care provider of assessment findings.
4. Document assessment findings and related interventions in the patient's medical record.
5. This is a normal finding, so nothing needs to be done.
6. Apply ice to the site for relief of burning pain.

Answers: 1. 2; **2.** 1, 2, 3, 4; **3.** 1, 2, 5; **4.** 1, 2, 3, 4, 5; **5.** 1, 4, 5; **6.** 2, 5, 4, 6, 1, 3; **7.** 2, 1, 3; **8.** 3, 4, 5, 6; **9.** 6, 4, 5, 3, 1, 2; **10.** 1, 3, 4

Rationales for Review Questions can be found on the Evolve website.

REFERENCES

Agency for Healthcare Research and Quality (AHRQ): *Computerized provider order entry*, 2019. https://psnet.ahrq.gov/primer/computerized-provider-order-entry. Accessed August 17, 2021.

Agency for Healthcare Research and Quality (AHRQ): *Health Literacy Universal Precautions Toolkit 2nd edition*, Rockville, MD, March 2020, Agency for Healthcare Research and Quality. https://www.ahrq.gov/health-literacy/quality-resources/tools/literacy-toolkit/healthlittoolkit2-tool5.html. Accessed August 17, 2021.

American Academy of Allergy, Asthma & Immunology (AAAI): *Peak flow meter*, 2020. https://www.aaaai.org/conditions-and-treatments/library/asthma-library/peak-flow-meter. Accessed August 17, 2021.

American Medical Association (AMA): *Procedure for USAN name selection*, 2021. https://www.ama-assn.org/procedure-usan-name-selection. Accessed August 17, 2021.

American Nurses Association (ANA): *Nursing: scope and standards of practice*, ed 4, Silver Spring, MD, 2021, The Association.

Association of Diabetes Care & Education Specialists (ADCES): *Learning how to inject insulin*, 2020. https://www.diabeteseducator.org/docs/default-source/legacy-docs/_resources/pdf/general/Insulin_Injection_How_To_AADE.pdf. Accessed August 17, 2021.

Ball J, et al: *Seidel's guide to physical examination: an interprofessional approach*, ed 9, St. Louis, 2019, Elsevier.

Beal J: Pediatric medication errors, *Am J Matern Child Nurs* 42(2):116, 2017.

Burchum J, Rosenthal L: *Lehne's pharmacology for nursing care*, ed 10, St. Louis, 2019, Elsevier.

Centers for Disease Control and Prevention (CDC): *Mantoux tuberculin skin testing*, n.d. https://www.cdc.gov/tb/education/mantoux/pdf/Mantoux_TB_Skin_Test.pdf. Accessed August 17, 2021.

Center for Disease Control and Prevention (CDC): *Vaccine administration: general best practice guidelines for immunization: best practices guidance of the Advisory Committee on Immunization Practices (ACIP)*, 2021a. https://www.cdc.gov/vaccines/hcp/acip-recs/general-recs/administration.html#. Accessed August 17, 2021.

Centers for Disease Control and Prevention (CDC): *What is health literacy?* 2021b. https://www.cdc.gov/healthliteracy/learn/index.html. Accessed August 17, 2021.

Consumer Med Safety: *Humulin R-500 insulin errors*, 2018, Institute for Safe Medicine Practices. https://www.ismp.org/sites/default/files/attachments/2018-11/u-500-insulinfinal.pdf. Accessed August 17, 2021.

Consumer Med Safety: *Tips for measuring liquid medicines safely*, 2021, Institute for Safe Medicine Practices. http://www.consumermedsafety.org/tools-and-resources/medication-safety-tools-and-resources/taking-your-medicine-safely/measure-liquid-medications. Accessed August 17, 2021.

Eisenberg S: USP <800> and strategies to promote hazardous drug safety, *J Infus Nurs* 41(1):12, 2018.

Giger J, Haddad L: *Transcultural nursing: assessment and intervention*, ed 8, St. Louis, 2021, Elsevier.

Gorski L: *Phillips's manual of I.V. therapeutics: evidence-based practice for infusion therapy*, ed 7, Philadelphia, PA, 2018, FA Davis.

Hockenberry MJ, et al: *Wong's nursing care of infants and children*, ed 11, St. Louis, 2019, Elsevier.

Institute for Safe Medication Practices (ISMP): *ISMP acute care guidelines for timely administration of scheduled medications*, 2011. http://www.ismp.org/Tools/guidelines/acutecare/tasm.pdf. Accessed August 17, 2021.

Institute for Safe Medication Practices (ISMP): *ISMP's list of error-prone abbreviations, symbols, and dose designations*, 2017a. https://www.ismp.org/recommendations/error-prone-abbreviations-list. Accessed August 17, 2021.

Institute for Safe Medication Practices (ISMP): *ISMP guidelines for optimizing safe subcutaneous insulin use in adults*, Horsham, PA, 2017b, The Institute for Safe Medication Practices.

Institute for Safe Medication Practices (ISMP): *The breakup: errors when altering oral solid dosage forms*, 2018a. https://www.ismp.org/alerts/breakup-errors-when-altering-oral-solid-dosage-forms. Accessed August 17, 2021.

Institute for Safe Medication Practices (ISMP): *Part II: survey results suggest action is needed to improve safety with adult IV push medications*, 2018b. https://www.ismp.org/resources/part-ii-survey-results-suggest-action-needed-improve-safety-adult-iv-push-medications. Accessed August 17, 2021.

Institute for Safe Medication Practices (ISMP): *List of confused drug names*, 2019a. https://www.ismp.org/recommendations/confused-drug-names-list. Accessed August 17, 2021.

Institute for Safe Medication Practices (ISMP): *IV push gap analysis tool (GAT) helps uncover national priorities for safe injection practices*, 2019b. https://www.ismp.org/resources/iv-push-gap-analysis-tool-gat-helps-uncover-national-priorities-safe-injection-practices. Accessed August 17, 2021.

Institute for Safe Medication Practices (ISMP): *Independent double checks: worth the effort if used judiciously and properly*, 2019c. https://www.ismp.org/resources/independent-double-checks-worth-effort-if-used-judiciously-and-properly. Accessed August 17, 2021.

Institute for Safe Medication Practices (ISMP): *Guidelines for safe electronic communication of medication information*, 2019d. https://www.ismp.org/resources/guidelines-safe-electronic-communication-medication-information. Accessed August 17, 2021.

Institute for Safe Medication Practices (ISMP): *2020-2021 targeted medication safety best practices for hospitals*, 2020a. https://www.ismp.org/sites/default/files/attachments/2020-02/2020-2021%20TMSBP-%20FINAL_1.pdf. Accessed August 17, 2021.

Institute for Safe Medication Practices (ISMP): *Oral dosage forms that should not be crushed*, 2020b. https://www.ismp.org/recommendations/do-not-crush. Accessed August 17, 2021.

International Organization for Standardization (IOS): *Enteral feeding systems: design and testing*, 2020. https://www.iso.org/obp/ui/#iso:std:iso:20695:ed-1:v1:en. Accessed August 17, 2021.

Leapfrog Group: *Bar code medication administration*, 2018. https://www.leapfroggroup.org/sites/default/files/Files/Leapfrog-Castlight_BCMA_Final.pdf. Accessed August 17, 2021.

Lilley LL, et al: *Pharmacology and the nursing process*, ed 9, St. Louis, 2020, Elsevier.

Malone A, et al: *ASPEN enteral nutrition handbook*, ed 2, Silver Spring, MD, 2019, ASPEN.

National Coordinating Council for Medication Error Reporting and Prevention (NCCMERP): *What is a medication error?* 2021. http://www.nccmerp.org/about-medication-errors. Accessed August 17, 2021.

Occupational Safety and Health Administration (OSHA): *Bloodborne pathogens and needlestick prevention*, n.d. https://www.osha.gov/SLTC/bloodbornepathogens/index.html. Accessed August 17, 2021.

Oncology Nurses Society (ONS): *Toolkit for safe handling of hazardous drugs for nurses in oncology*, 2018. https://www.ons.org/sites/default/files/2018-06/ONS_Safe_Handling_Toolkit_0.pdf. Accessed August 17, 2021.

Oncology Nurses Society (ONS): *Ensuring healthcare worker safety when handling hazardous drugs*, 2019. https://www.ons.org/make-difference/ons-center-advocacy-and-health-policy/position-statements/ensuring-healthcare. Accessed August 17, 2021.

Skidmore-Roth L: *Mosby's 2021 nursing drug reference*, ed 34, St. Louis, 2021, Elsevier.

The Joint Commission (TJC). *Speak up for your rights,* 2019. https://www.jointcommission.org/-/media/tjc/ documents/resources/speak-up/speak-ups/for-your-rights/speak-up-for-your-rights-85-x-11_.pdf. Accessed October 11, 2021.

The Joint Commission (TJC): *Do not use list,* 2020. https:// www.jointcommission.org/-/media/tjc/documents/fact-sheets/do-not-use-list-8-3-20.pdf?db=web&hash= 2489CB1616A30CFFBDAAD1FB3F8021A5&hash= 2489CB1616A30CFFBDAAD1FB3F8021A5. Accessed August 17, 2021.

The Joint Commission (TJC): *2021 National Patient Safety Goals,* Oakbrook Terrace, IL, 2021, The Commission. https://www.jointcommission.org/en/standards/national-patient-safety-goals/. Accessed August 17, 2021.

Touhy TA, Jett KF: *Ebersole and Hess' gerontological nursing & healthy aging,* ed 6, St. Louis, 2021, Elsevier.

U.S. Department of Health and Human Services, Centers for Medicare & Medicaid (USDHHS): *Updated guidance on medication administration, Hospital Appendix A of State Operations Manual,* Baltimore, 2011, Department of Health and Human Services.

U.S. Food and Drug Administration (FDA): *Reducing risks through standards developments for medical device connectors,* 2018. https://www.fda.gov/medical-devices/ medical-device-connectors/reducing-risks-through-standards-development-medical-device-connectors. Accessed August 17, 2021.

U.S. Food and Drug Administration (FDA): *Working to reduce medication errors,* 2019. https://www.fda.gov/ drugs/drug-information-consumers/working-reduce-medication-errors. Accessed August 17, 2021.

U.S. Food and Drug Administration (USFDA): *Tablet scoring: nomenclature, labeling, and data for evaluation,* 2020. https://www.fda.gov/regulatory-information/search-fda-guidance-documents/tablet-scoringnomenclature-labeling-and-data-evaluation. Accessed August 17, 2021.

U.S. Food and Drug Administration (USFDA): *MedWatch: the FDA safety information and adverse event reporting program,* 2021a. https://www.fda.gov/safety/medwatch/ default.htm. Accessed August 17, 2021.

U.S. Food and Drug Administration (USFDA): *Where and how to dispose of unused medicines,* 2021b. https://www. fda.gov/consumers/consumer-updates/where-and-how-dispose-unused-medicines. Accessed August 17, 2021.

RESEARCH REFERENCES

Apter A: *Asthma education and self-management,* 2021, UpToDate. https://www.uptodate.com/contents/ asthma-education-and-self-management. Accessed August 17, 2021.

Antoszyk A, et al: Usability of the ranibizumab 0.5 mg prefilled syringe: Human factors studies to evaluate critical task completion by healthcare professionals, *PDA J Pharm Sci Technol* 72:411, 2018.

Bartlett J: *Aspiration pneumonia in adults,* 2021, UpToDate. https://www.uptodate.com/contents/aspiration-pneumonia-in-adults. Accessed August 17, 2021.

Batson S, et al: Automation of in-hospital pharmacy dispensing: a systematic review, *Eur J Hosp Pharm* 28(2):58, 2021.

Betancourt J: *Cross-cultural care and communication,* 2021, UpToDate. https://www.uptodate.com/contents/ cross-cultural-care-and-communication#!. Accessed August 17, 2021.

Bonafide C, et al: Association between mobile telephone interruptions and medication administration errors in a pediatric intensive care unit, *JAMA Pediatr* 174(2):162, 2020.

Boullata J, et al: ASPEN safe practices for enteral nutrition therapy, *J Parenter Enteral Nutr* 41(1):15, 2017.

Davidson K, Bertram J: Best practice for deltoid intramuscular injections in older adults: study in cadavers, *J Nurs Educ Pract* 9(9):92, 2019.

Drutz J: *Standard immunizations for children and adolescents: overview,* 2021, UpToDate. https://www.uptodate.com/ contents/standard-immunizations-for-children-and-adolescents-overview. Accessed August 17, 2021.

Forough A, et al: Nurses' experiences of medication administration to people with swallowing difficulties in aged care agencies: a systematic review protocol, *JBI Database System Rev Implement Rep* 15(4):932, 2018.

Freitas W, et al. Distractions and interruptions in medication preparation and administration in inpatient units, *Rev Eletr Enferm* 21:1, 2019.

Furnish C, Wagner S: Evaluation of medication administration timing-Are we meeting our goals? *J Pharm Pract* 19:897, 2020.

Gerald L, Dhand R: *Patient education: inhaler techniques in adults (Beyond the Basics),* 2020, UpToDate. https:// www.uptodate.com/contents/inhaler-techniques-in-adults-beyond-the-basics. Accessed August 17, 2021.

Gorski LA, et al: Infusion therapy standards of practice, 8th edition, *J Infus Nurs* 44(1S):S1, 2021.

Grissinger M. Is an indication-based prescribing system in our future? *P T* 44(5):232, 2019.

Hull R, et al: *Heparin and LMW heparin: dosing and adverse effects,* 2019, UpToDate. https://www.uptodate. com/contents/heparin-and-lmw-heparin-dosing-and-adverse-effects/print.

Hess D, Dhand R: *Delivery of inhaled medication in adults,* 2020a, UpToDate. https://www.uptodate.com/contents/ delivery-of-inhaled-medication-in-adults. Accessed August 17, 2021.

Hess D, Dhand R: *The use of inhaler devices in adults,* 2020b, UpToDate. https://www.uptodate.com/contents/the-use-of-inhaler-devices-in-adults. Accessed August 17, 2021.

Hibberd P, et al: *Standard immunizations for nonpregnant adults,* 2021, UpToDate. https://www.uptodate.com/ contents/standard-immunizations-for-nonpregnant-adults. Accessed August 17, 2021.

Holliday R, et al: Body mass index: a reliable predictor of subcutaneous fat thickness and needle length for ventral gluteal intramuscular injections, *Am J Ther* 26(1):e72, 2019.

Judd M: Confirming nasogastric tube placement in adults, *Nursing* 50(4):43, 2020.

Kara D, et al: Using ventrogluteal site in intramuscular injections is a priority or an alternative? *Int J Caring Sciences* 8(2):507, 2015.

Kaya N, et al: The reliability of site determination methods in ventrogluteal area injection: a cross-sectional study, *Int J Nurs Stud* 52:355, 2015.

Kowal K, DuBuske L: *Overview of skin testing for allergic disease,* 2020, UpToDate. https://www.uptodate.com/ contents/overview-of-skin-testing-for-allergic-disease/ print. Accessed August 17, 2021.

Larkin T, et al: Influence of gender, BMI, and body shape on theoretical injection outcome at the ventrogluteal and dorsogluteal sites, *J Clin Nurs* 27(1/2):e242, 2018.

Levitsky, L, Misra M: *Overview of the management of type 1 diabetes mellitus in children and adolescents,* 2020, UpToDate. https://www.uptodate.com/contents/ management-of-type-1-diabetes-mellitus-in-children-and-adolescents. Accessed August 17, 2021.

McBee ME, et al: What you need to know about bar-code medication administration, *J Nurs Interprof Leadersh Qual Saf* 2(2):1, 2019.

Mulac A, et al: Barcode medication administration technology use in hospital practice: a mixed-methods observational study of policy deviations, *BMJ Qual Saf.* Epub ahead of print: July 20, 2021. doi:10.1136/ bmjqs-2021-013223.

Neuss M, et al: 2016 updated American Society of Clinical Oncology/Oncology Nursing Society chemotherapy administration safety standards, including standards for pediatric oncology, *ONF* 44(1):3, 2017.

Painchart L, et al: Particulate contamination associated with the manipulation of drugs in glass ampules: a literature review, *Ann Pharm Fr* 76(1):3, 2018.

Palese A, et al: "I am administering medication-please do not interrupt me": Red tabards preventing interruptions as perceived by surgical patients, *J Patient Saf* 15(1):30, 2019.

Poly TN, et al: Appropriateness of overridden alerts in computerized physician order entry: systematic review. *JMIR Med Inform* 8(7):e15653, 2020.

Rochon P: *Drug prescribing for older adults,* 2021, UpToDate. https://www.uptodate.com/contents/ drug-prescribing-for-older-adults. Accessed August 17, 2021.

Saper R: *Overview of herbal medicine and dietary supplements,* 2021, UpToDate. https://www.uptodate. com/contents/overview-of-herbal-medicine-and-dietary-supplements. Accessed August 17, 2021.

Schmitz D, et al: Imperative instruction for pressurized metered-dose inhalers: provider perspectives, *Resp Care* 64(3):292, 2019.

Suclupe S, et al: Medication errors in prescription and administration in critically ill patients, *J Adv Nurs* 76(5):1192, 2020.

Strohfus P, et al: Evidence calls for practice change in intramuscular injection techniques, *J Nurs Educ Pract* 8(2):83, 2018.

Thompson KM, et al: Implementation of bar-code medication administration to reduce patient harm, *Mayo Clin Proc Innov Qual Outcomes* 2(4):342, 2018.

Vicdan A, et al: Evaluation of the training given to the nurses on the injection application to the ventrogluteal site: a quasi-experimental study. *Int J Caring Sci* 12(3):1467, 2019.

Weinstock R: *General principles of insulin therapy in diabetes mellitus,* 2021a, UpToDate. http://www. uptodate.com/contents/general-principles-of-insulin-therapy-in-diabetes-mellitus. Accessed August 17, 2021.

Weinstock R: *Management of blood glucose in adults with type 1 diabetes mellitus,* 2021b, UpToDate. https://www. uptodate.com/contents/management-of-blood-glucose-in-adults-with-type-1-diabetes-mellitus/print. Accessed August 17, 2021.

Westbrook J, et al: Effectiveness of a 'Do not interrupt' bundled intervention to reduce interruptions during medication administration: a cluster randomized controlled feasibility study, *BMJ Qual Saf* 26(9):734, 2017.

Wexler D: *Patient education: type 2 diabetes: insulin treatment (beyond the basics),* 2021, UpToDate. https:// www.uptodate.com/contents/type-2-diabetes-insulin-treatment-beyond-the-basics. Accessed August 17, 2021.

Zhu J, Weingart S: *Prevention of adverse drug events in hospitals,* 2020, UpToDate. https://www.uptodate.com/ contents/prevention-of-adverse-drug-events-in-hospitals. Accessed August 17, 2021.

Complementary, Alternative, and Integrative Therapies

OBJECTIVES

- Explain the difference between complementary and alternative therapies.
- Discuss integrative health care as applied to nursing practice.
- Summarize the need for additional research to support the use of complementary therapies.
- Identify the clinical applications of relaxation therapies.
- Identify complementary therapies that nurses can independently implement in their nursing practice.
- Explain the relaxation response and its effect on somatic ailments.
- Summarize the principles and effectiveness of imagery, meditation, and breathwork.

- Explain the purpose and principles of biofeedback.
- Discuss the methods of and the psychophysiological responses to therapeutic touch.
- Explain the principles and applications of acupuncture.
- Compare safe and unsafe herbal therapies.
- Discuss the relationship between patient involvement and the effectiveness of complementary therapies.
- Explain why you need to appropriately evaluate a patient's response to complementary therapies.

KEY TERMS

Acupoints
Acupuncture
Allopathic or biomedicine
Alternative therapies
Biofeedback
Chiropractic therapy
Complementary therapies
Creative visualization
Cupping

Imagery
Integrative health care
Integrative nursing
Integrative therapies
Meditation
Moxibustion
Passive relaxation
Pilates
Progressive relaxation

Qi gong
Relaxation response
Stress response
Tai chi
Therapeutic touch (TT)
Traditional Chinese medicine (TCM)
Vital energy (*qi*)
Whole medical systems
Yin and yang

MEDIA RESOURCES

http://evolve.elsevier.com/Potter/fundamentals/
- Review Questions
- Case Study with Questions

- Audio Glossary
- Content Updates
- Answers to QSEN Activity and Review Questions

With few exceptions, the general health of North American people has steadily improved over the course of the past century, as evidenced by lower mortality rates and increased life expectancies. Changes in knowledge, technology, science, and health care have altered the course of many illnesses. Although allopathic or biomedicine (conventional Western medicine) is quite effective in treating numerous physical ailments (e.g., bacterial infections, structural abnormalities, and acute emergencies), it is generally less effective in decreasing stress-induced illnesses, managing symptoms of chronic disease, caring for the emotional and spiritual needs of individuals, and improving quality of life and general well-being. As a result, patients continue to seek complementary (nonbiomedical) treatments in increasing numbers, integrating these therapies with biomedicine.

The most recent comprehensive national survey estimates that between 33.2% and 50.6% of the U.S. population integrate complementary and biomedical treatments to reduce symptom burden and improve overall well-being (Clarke et al., 2015). In part, this use corresponds to (1) a desire for less invasive, less toxic, "more natural" treatments; (2) lack of satisfaction with biomedical treatments; (3) an increasing desire by patients to take a more active role in their treatment process; (4) beliefs that a combination of treatments (biomedical and complementary) results in better overall results; (5) the increased number of research articles in journals such as *Journal of Alternative and Complementary Medicine* and *Journal of Holistic Nursing;* and (6) beliefs and values that are consistent with an approach to health that incorporates the mind, body, and spirit or a holistic approach (Koithan, 2018). Fortunately, primary care physicians are recommending complementary health approaches (CHAs). An analysis of a survey administered to office-based physicians found that massage therapy was the most commonly recommended CHA (30.4%), followed by chiropractic/osteopathic manipulation (27.1%), herbs/nonvitamin supplements (26.5%), yoga (25.6%), and acupuncture (22.4%) (Stussman et al., 2020).

COMPLEMENTARY AND INTEGRATIVE THERAPIES

The National Institutes of Health/National Center for Complementary and Integrative Health (NIH/NCCIH, 2021) identifies complementary and integrative approaches as an array of health care approaches with a history of use or origins outside of mainstream or conventional medicine. Complementary therapies are therapies used together with conventional treatment recommended by a person's health care provider. As the name implies, complementary therapies complement conventional treatments. Many of them, such as therapeutic touch, hypnotherapy, and chiropractic therapy, contain diagnostic and therapeutic methods that require special training. Others, such as guided imagery and breathwork, are easily learned and applied. Complementary therapies also include relaxation; exercise; massage; reflexology; prayer; biofeedback; creative therapies, including art, music, or dance therapy; meditation; and herbs/supplements (Lindquist et al., 2018). Another term to describe interventions used in this fashion, particularly by licensed health care providers, is integrative therapies (Kreitzer and Koithan, 2018).

When nonpharmacological therapies such as exercise, chiropractic, and herbal supplements are used in place of conventional pharmacological or other medical procedures, they are considered alternative therapies (NIH/NCCIH, 2021). These therapies then become primary treatments, replacing biomedical care. For example, consider a person with chronic pain who uses yoga to encourage flexibility and relaxation at the same time in which analgesics or nonsteroidal antiinflammatory drugs are prescribed. Both sets of interventions are based on conventional pathophysiology and anatomy while acknowledging the mind-body connection that contributes to the physiological pain response. In this case, yoga is used as a complementary intervention. However, when that same patient decides to use a meditative practice that includes yoga and other lifestyle changes rather than medication, yoga now becomes an alternative therapy and is perceived as more helpful than an allopathic approach for chronic pain. Some patients, particularly those from different cultural backgrounds, may choose to use whole medical systems, such as traditional Chinese medicine (TCM), Ayurveda, or naturopathy, as alternative systems of care to biomedicine. When used in this fashion, these approaches are always considered alternative because they are based on completely different philosophies and life systems than those used by allopathic medicine. Table 32.1 presents types of complementary therapies.

Because of the increased interest in complementary therapies, many educational institutions, including medical and nursing schools, have integrated conventional "biomedical" education with programs that incorporate complementary therapy content. These integrative health care programs graduate practitioners who recommend a full spectrum of possible treatments, both biomedical and complementary. In an integrative health care system consumers are treated by a team of providers consisting of both biomedical and complementary practitioners. More fully defined, integrative health care emphasizes the importance of the relationship between practitioner and patient; focuses on the whole person; is informed by evidence; and makes use of appropriate therapeutic approaches, health care professionals, and disciplines to achieve optimal health (Rakel, 2018).

Nurses have historically practiced in an integrative fashion; a review of nursing theory (see Chapter 4) reveals the values of holism, relational care, and evidence-informed practice. Until recently, nursing identified its practice as holistic rather than integrated. Holistic nursing treats the mind-body-spirit of a patient, using interventions such as relaxation therapy, music therapy, touch therapies, and guided imagery (Helming et al., 2020). The American Holistic Nurses Association maintains Standards of Holistic Nursing Practice, which defines and establishes the scope of holistic practice and describes the level of care expected from a holistic nurse (AHNA/ANA 2019).

Kreitzer and Koithan (2018) challenge the profession to embrace its long-standing roots of integrative care, standing alongside colleagues to help transform the current health care system and operationalize our collective wisdom to offer whole person care that is patient-centered, relationship-based, and supported by evidence that incorporates the best of all possible interventions. Grounded in six principles, integrative nursing is defined as "a way of being-knowing-doing that advances the health and well-being of persons, families, and communities through caring-healing relationships. Integrative nurses use evidence to inform traditional and emerging interventions that support whole person/whole systems healing" (Kreitzer and Koithan, 2018).

Increasing interest in integrative health care is evident in the increased number of publications in respected health care journals and the continued support of research. The mission of the National Institutes of Health/National Center for Complementary and Integrative Health (NIH/NCCIH, 2021) supports the investigation of the benefits and safety of complementary interventions. Although the body of evidence about complementary therapies is growing, limited data make it difficult to establish the benefits of specific therapies. Reasons are varied but reflect the growing and developing nature of the science. More rigorous research is needed, especially randomized trials. Therefore nurses need to weigh the risk and benefits of each intervention and consider the following when recommending complementary therapies: (1) the history of each therapy (many have been used by cultures for thousands of years to support health and ameliorate suffering); (2) nursing's history and experience with a particular therapy; (3) other forms of evidence reporting outcomes and safety data, including case study and qualitative research; and (4) the cultural influences and context for certain patient populations.

This chapter discusses several types of complementary therapies, including a description, the clinical applications, and the limitations of each therapy. The therapies are organized into two categories. The first are nursing-accessible therapies that you can begin to learn and apply in patient care. The second category includes training-specific therapies such as chiropractic therapy or acupressure that a nurse cannot perform without additional training and/or certification.

REFLECT NOW

Reflect on your own life experiences. Do you personally use a variety of therapeutic strategies (e.g., massage for a sore back or neck), and do your own practices influence your acceptance of this approach to care?

NURSING-ACCESSIBLE THERAPIES

Some complementary therapies and techniques are general in nature and use natural processes (e.g., breathing, thinking and concentration, presence, movement) to help people feel better and cope with both acute and chronic conditions (Box 32.1). You can learn about these techniques and integrate them into your independent nursing practice with patients (Climaco et al., 2019). Nursing accessible therapies challenge you to reflect on your nursing knowledge, knowledge about the patient's disease process, expected therapies, and expected response to treatment. It is important that you understand your patient's condition to determine the most appropriate complementary therapy. Use clinical judgment to analyze ongoing patient assessment data and to evaluate your patient's response to therapies. This analysis is essential in determining the appropriateness and usefulness of any complementary

TABLE 32.1   Complementary Therapies

Types	Definitions
Biologically Based Therapies *(Natural products)*	
Dietary supplements	Defined by the Dietary Supplement Health and Education Act of 1994 and used to supplement dietary/nutritional intake by mouth; contain one or more dietary ingredients, including vitamins, minerals, herbs, or other botanical products
Herbal medicines	Plant-based therapies used in whole systems of medicine or as individual preparations by allopathic providers and consumers for specific symptoms or issues
Macrobiotic diet	Predominantly a vegan diet (no animal products except fish); initially used in the management of a variety of cancers; emphasis placed on whole cereal grains, vegetables, and unprocessed foods
Mycotherapies	Fungi-based (mushroom) products
Orthomolecular medicine (megavitamin)	Increased intake of nutrients such as vitamin C and beta-carotene; treats cancer, schizophrenia, autism, and certain chronic diseases such as hypercholesterolemia and coronary artery disease
Probiotics	Live microorganisms (in most cases, bacteria) that are similar to beneficial microorganisms found in the human gastrointestinal system; also called *good bacteria*
The "Zone"	Dietary program that requires eating protein, carbohydrate, and fat in a 30:40:30 ratio—30% of calories from protein, 40% from carbohydrate, and 30% from fat; used to balance insulin and other hormones for optimal health
Energy Therapies *(Use or manipulation of energy fields)*	
Acupuncture	Traditional Chinese method of producing analgesia or altering the function of a body system by inserting thin needles along a series of lines or channels, called meridians; direct needle manipulation of energetic meridians influences deeper internal organs by redirecting *qi*
Healing touch	Biofield therapy; uses gentle touch directly on or close to body to influence and support the human energy system and bring balance to the whole body (physical, spiritual, emotional, and mental); a formal educational and certification system provides credentials for practitioners
Reiki therapy	Biofield therapy derived from ancient Buddhist rituals; practitioner places hands on or above a body area and transfers "universal life energy," providing strength, harmony, and balance to treat a patient's health disturbances
Therapeutic touch	Biofield therapy involving direction of a practitioner's balanced energies in an intentional manner toward those of a patient; practitioner's hands lay on or close to a patient's body
Magnet therapy	Bioelectromagnetic therapy; devices (magnets) applied to the body surface, producing a measurable magnetic field; used primarily to alleviate pain associated with musculoskeletal injuries or disorders
Manipulative and Body-Based Methods *(Involve movement of body with focus on body structures and systems)*	
Acupressure	Applying digital pressure in a specified way on designated points on the body to relieve pain, produce analgesia, or regulate a body function
Chiropractic medicine	Manipulating the spinal column; includes physiotherapy and diet therapy
Massage therapy	Manipulating soft tissue through stroking, rubbing, or kneading to increase circulation, improve muscle tone, and provide relaxation
Simple touch	Touching the patient in appropriate and gentle ways to make connection, display acceptance, and give appreciation
Mind-Body Interventions *(Honor connections between thoughts and physiological functioning using emotion to influence health and well-being)*	
Art therapy	Using art to reconcile emotional conflicts, foster self-awareness, and express patients' unspoken and frequently unconscious concerns about their disease
Biofeedback	Process providing a person with visual or auditory information about autonomic physiological functions of the body such as muscle tension, skin temperature, and brain wave activity through the use of instruments
Breathwork	Using a variety of breathing patterns to relax, invigorate, or open emotional channels
Guided imagery	Concentrating on an image or series of images to treat pathological conditions
Meditation	Self-directed practice for relaxing the body and calming the mind using focused rhythmic breathing
Music therapy	Using music to address physical, psychological, cognitive, and social needs of individuals with disabilities and illnesses; improves physical movement and/or communication, develops emotional expression, evokes memories, and distracts people who are in pain
Tai chi	Incorporating breath, movement, and meditation to cleanse, strengthen, and circulate vital life energy and blood; stimulate the immune system; and maintain external and internal balance

Continued

TABLE 32.1   Complementary Therapies—cont'd

Types	Definitions
Yoga	Focuses on body musculature, posture, breathing mechanisms, and consciousness; goal is attainment of physical and mental well-being through mastery of body achieved through exercise, holding of postures, proper breathing, and meditation
Movement Therapies *(Eastern or Western approaches to promote well-being)*	
Dance therapy	Intimate and powerful medium because it is a direct expression of the mind and body; treats persons with social, emotional, cognitive, or physical problems
Feldenkrais method	A complementary therapy based on establishment of good self-image through awareness and correction of body movements; integrates the understanding of the physics of body movement patterns with an awareness of the way people learn to move, behave, and interact
Pilates	A system of exercises (e.g., mat and special apparatus) and body movement used to strengthen, lengthen, and improve the voluntary control of muscles and muscle groups, especially those used for posture and core strengthening; awareness of breathing and precise movements are integral components
Whole Medical Systems *(Complete systems of theory and practice that have evolved independently from or parallel to conventional biomedicine)*	
Ayurvedic medicine	One of the oldest systems of medicine, practiced in India since the first century AD. There are eight branches of Ayurvedic medicine, including internal medicine; surgery; treatment of head and neck disease; gynecology, obstetrics, and pediatrics; toxicology; psychiatry; elder care and rejuvenation; and sexual vitality. Treatments balance the doshas using a combination of dietary and lifestyle changes, herbal remedies and purgatives, massage, meditation, and exercise.
Homeopathic medicine	Developed in Germany and practiced in the United States since the mid-1800s. It is a system of medical treatments based on the theory that certain diseases can be cured by giving small, highly diluted doses of substances that in a healthy person would produce symptoms like those of the disease. Prescribed substances called *remedies* are made from naturally occurring plant, animal, or mineral substances and are used to stimulate the vital force of the body so that it can heal itself.
Latin American traditional healing	*Curanderismo* is a Latin American traditional healing system that includes a humoral model for classifying food, activity, drugs, and illnesses and a series of folk illnesses. The goal is to create a balance between the patient and the environment, thereby sustaining health.
Native American traditional healing	Tribal traditions are individualistic, but similarities across traditions include the use of sweating and purging, herbal remedies, and ceremonies in which a shaman (a spiritual healer) makes contact with spirits to ask their direction in bringing healing to people to promote wholeness and healing.
Naturopathic medicine	A system of therapeutics focused on treating the whole person and promoting health and well-being rather than an individual disease. Therapeutics include herbal medicine, nutritional supplementation, physical medicine, homeopathy, lifestyle counseling, and mind-body therapies with an orientation toward assisting the person's internal capacity for self-healing (vitalism).
Traditional Chinese medicine (TCM)	An ancient healing tradition identified in the first century AD focused on balancing yin/yang energies. It is a set of systematic techniques and methods, including acupuncture, herbal medicines, massage, acupressure, moxibustion (use of heat from burning herbs), *qi gong* (balancing energy flow through body movement), cupping, and massage. Fundamental concepts are from Taoism, Confucianism, and Buddhism.

therapies. Sometimes changes to health care provider–prescribed therapies, such as medication doses, are needed when complementary therapies alter physiological responses and lead to therapeutic responses (Sandvik et al., 2020; Ringdahl et al., 2018).

Complementary therapies teach individuals ways to change their behavior to help alter physical responses to stress and improve symptoms such as muscle tension, gastrointestinal discomfort, pain, or sleep disturbances. Active patient involvement is a primary principle for these therapies; individuals achieve better responses if they commit to practice the techniques or exercises daily. Therefore to achieve effective outcomes, match the therapeutic strategies with an individual's acceptance of the therapy, health condition, lifestyle, their personal beliefs and values, and the context within which the care is to be delivered (acute or community-based).

Relaxation Therapy

People face situations in everyday life that evoke the **stress response** (see Chapter 37). The mind modifies the biochemical functions of the major organ systems in response to feedback. Thoughts and feelings influence the production of chemicals (i.e., neurotransmitters, neurohormones, and peptides) that circulate throughout the body and convey messages via cells to various systems within the body. The stress response is a good example of the way in which systems cooperate to protect an individual from harm. Physiologically, the cascade of changes associated with the stress response causes increased heart and respiratory rates; tightened muscles; increased metabolic rate; and a general sense of foreboding, fear, nervousness, irritability, and negative mood. Other physiological responses include elevated blood pressure; dilated pupils; stronger cardiac contractions; and increased levels of blood glucose, serum cholesterol, circulating free fatty acids, and triglycerides. Although these responses prepare a person for short-term stress, the effects on the body from long-term stress may include structural damage and chronic illness such as angina, tension headaches, cardiac arrhythmias, pain, ulcers, and atrophy of the immune system organs (Voss and Kreitzer, 2018).

The **relaxation response** reduces generalized cognitive, physiological, and/or behavioral arousal. The process of relaxation elongates the muscle fibers, reduces the neural impulses sent to the brain, and thus

BOX 32.1 EVIDENCE-BASED PRACTICE

Use of Complementary Therapies in Treating Chronic Back Pain

PICOT Question: Do complementary therapies safely and effectively reduce pain and discomfort in patients with chronic back pain?

Evidence Summary
Pain is a complex phenomenon for a patient with chronic back pain. It involves psychological, biological, and sociological factors in a patient's and family's life. Frequently these patients are prescribed analgesics to control the pain. As the pain continues or worsens, the dosage and types of medications increase, which increases patients' risks for adverse drug effects (Whedon et al., 2018; Globe et al., 2016). Several systematic reviews analyzing the use of complementary therapies to control pain show that many of these therapies, such as relaxation, focused breathing, and therapeutic touch, are effective in pain control (Bagci and Yucel, 2020; dos Santos Felix et al., 2019). Nurses' knowledge and use of complementary therapies such as mindfulness, relaxation, and breathing techniques aid in reducing pain and improving comfort (Koithan, 2018; Hilton et al., 2017).

Application to Nursing Practice
- Use evidence-based complementary therapy clinical practice guidelines to develop individualized patient-centered interventions for pain control (Globe et al., 2016; Qaseem et al., 2017).
- Integrate complementary therapies, such as meditation and relaxation exercises, into a patient's plan of care and patient education needs (Koithan, 2018; Hilton et al., 2017).
- When appropriate, help patients with chronic back pain learn tai chi to improve balance, control pain, and reduce the fear or risk of falling (Huang et al., 2019).
- Instruct patients and family caregivers on the use of specific complementary therapies as comfort measures (e.g., relaxation or prescribed physical therapy). Provide time for the patients and family caregivers to practice these techniques (Qaseem et al., 2017; dos Santos Felix, 2019).

decreases the activity of the brain and other body systems. Decreased heart and respiratory rates, blood pressure, and oxygen consumption and increased alpha brain activity and peripheral skin temperature characterize the relaxation response. The relaxation response occurs through a variety of techniques that incorporate a repetitive mental focus and the adoption of a calm, peaceful attitude (Bee et al., 2018).

Relaxation helps individuals develop cognitive skills to reduce the negative ways in which they respond to situations within their environment. Cognitive skills include the following:
- Focusing (the ability to identify, differentiate, maintain attention on, and return attention to simple stimuli for an extended period)
- Passivity (the ability to stop unnecessary goal-directed and analytic activity) ·
- Receptivity (the ability to tolerate and accept experiences that are uncertain, unfamiliar, or paradoxical)

The long-term goal of relaxation therapy is for people to continually monitor themselves for indicators of tension and consciously let go and release the tension contained in various body parts.

Progressive relaxation training teaches the individual how to effectively rest and reduces tension in the body. The person learns to detect subtle localized muscle tension sequentially, one muscle group at a time (e.g., the upper arm muscles, the forearm muscles). In doing so the individual learns to differentiate among high-intensity tension (strong fist clenching), very subtle tension, and relaxation (Bee et al., 2018). A person practices this activity using different muscle groups. One active progressive relaxation technique involves the use of slow,

deep abdominal breathing while tightening and relaxing an ordered succession of muscle groups, focusing on the associated bodily sensations while letting go of extraneous thoughts. When guiding a patient, you may decide to begin with the muscles in the face, followed by those in the arms, hands, abdomen, legs, and feet. Conversely you may also guide a patient to tense and relax muscles, beginning with the feet and working up the body.

The goal of passive relaxation is to still the mind and body intentionally without the need to tighten and relax any particular body part. One effective passive relaxation technique incorporates slow abdominal breathing exercises while imagining warmth and relaxation flowing through specific body parts such as the lungs or hands. Passive relaxation is useful for persons for whom the effort and energy expenditure of active muscle contracting leads to discomfort or exhaustion.

Clinical Applications of Relaxation Therapy. Research shows relaxation techniques effectively lower blood pressure and heart rate, decrease muscle tension, improve well-being, and reduce symptom distress in persons experiencing a variety of situations (e.g., complications from medical treatments, pain, cancer and other chronic illnesses, or loss of a significant other) (dos Santos Felix et al., 2019; Nayeri et al., 2020). Research also indicates that relaxation, alone or in combination with imagery, yoga (Fig. 32.1), and music, reduces pain, opioid use, and anxiety in intensive care patients (Sandvik et al., 2020; Montero-Marin et al., 2019). Other benefits of relaxation include the reduction of depression (Pospos et al., 2018) and breathlessness in persons with chronic respiratory illnesses (Brighton et al., 2019). Nurses apply clinical judgment in deciding which relaxation techniques are most appropriate for a patient (vigorous versus passive) and the times to best utilize the therapies (e.g., before a painful procedure or diagnostic test).

Relaxation enables individuals to exert control over their lives. Some experience a decreased feeling of helplessness and a more positive psychological state overall. For example, relaxation also reduces workplace stress experienced by nurses working on nursing units. Deep-breathing exercises, centering, and focusing attention often lead to improved staff satisfaction, staff relationships and communication, and workload perceptions (Montero-Marin et al., 2019; Clarke et al., 2009). Nursing units that incorporate relaxation activities into daily routines experience reduced turnover and improved patient satisfaction scores (Kreitzer and Zbrowsky, 2018).

Limitations of Relaxation Therapy. During relaxation training individuals learn to differentiate between low and high levels of muscle tension. During the first months of training sessions, when a person is

FIG. 32.1 Yoga is a discipline that focuses on muscles, posture, breathing, and consciousness.

learning how to focus on body sensations and tensions, there are reports of increased sensitivity in detecting muscle tension. Usually, these feelings are minor and resolve as the person continues with the training. However, be aware that on occasion some relaxation techniques may result in continued intensification of symptoms or the development of new symptoms. New symptoms may indicate progression of an existing condition or a new illness. When these occur, completely assess the new symptoms, and notify the health care provider of the symptoms and your assessment findings.

An important consideration when choosing any type of relaxation technique is the physiological and psychological status of the individual. Some patients with advanced disease such as cancer or acquired immunodeficiency syndrome (AIDS) seek relaxation training to reduce their stress response. However, techniques such as active progressive relaxation training require a moderate expenditure of energy, which often increases fatigue and limits an individual's ability to complete relaxation sessions and practice. Therefore, active progressive relaxation is inappropriate for patients with advanced disease or those who have decreased energy reserves. Passive relaxation or guided imagery is more appropriate for these individuals.

> ### REFLECT NOW
>
> Reflect on a time when you were experiencing a substantial stress response. What physical and mental/cognitive sensations did you feel? What strategies (passive or progressive) did you use to relax or reduce this stress response?

Meditation and Breathing

Meditation is any activity that limits stimulus input by directing attention to a single unchanging or repetitive stimulus so that the person is able to become more aware of self (Nayeri et al., 2020; Gross et al., 2018). It is a general term for a wide range of practices that involve relaxing the body and stilling the mind. Although meditation has its roots in Eastern religious practices (Hinduism, Buddhism, and Taoism), conventional health care providers began to recognize its healing potential in the early 1970s (Gross et al., 2018). According to Benson (1975), the four components of meditation are (1) a quiet space, (2) a comfortable position, (3) a receptive attitude, and (4) a focus of attention. Meditation is described as a process that anyone can use to calm down, cope with stress, and, for those with spiritual inclinations, feel as one with God or the universe.

Meditation is different from relaxation; the purpose of meditation is to become "mindful," increasing our ability to live freely and escape destructive patterns of negativity. Meditation is self-directed; it does not necessarily require a teacher and can be learned from books or audiotapes (Kabat-Zinn, 2018). Guided meditation techniques involve slow, relaxed, deep abdominal breathing that evokes a restful state, lowers oxygen consumption, reduces respiratory and heart rates, improves feelings of well-being, and reduces anxiety (Nayeri et al., 2020).

Clinical Applications of Meditation. Research supports the clinical benefits of meditation. For example, meditation reduces overall systolic and diastolic blood pressures and significantly reduces hypertensive risk (Park and Han, 2017). It also successfully reduces relapses in alcohol treatment programs (Wilson et al., 2017). Patients with cancer who use mindfulness-based cognitive therapies often experience less depression, anxiety, and distress and report an improved quality of life (Carlson, 2017). Patients who have posttraumatic stress disorders and chronic pain also benefit from mindfulness meditation (Cushing and Braun, 2018).

In addition, meditation increases productivity, improves mood, increases a sense of identity, and lowers irritability (Bee et al., 2018).

Considerations for the appropriateness of meditation include the person's degree of self-discipline; it requires ongoing practice to achieve lasting results. Most meditation activities are easy to learn and do not require memorization or particular procedures. Patients typically find mindfulness and meditation self-reinforcing. The peaceful, positive mental state is usually pleasurable and provides an incentive for individuals to continue to meditate.

Limitations of Meditation. Although meditation contributes to improvement in a variety of physiological and psychological ailments, it is contraindicated for some people. For example, a person who has a strong fear of losing control will possibly perceive it as a form of mind control and thus will be resistant to learning the technique. Some individuals also become hypertensive during meditation and require a much shorter session than the average session of 15 to 20 minutes.

Meditation may also increase the effects of certain drugs. Therefore monitor individuals learning meditation closely for physiological changes related to their medications. Prolonged practice of meditation techniques sometimes reduces the need for antihypertensive, thyroid-regulating, and psychotropic medications (e.g., antidepressants and antianxiety agents). In these cases, adjustment of the medication is necessary (Gross et al., 2018).

Imagery

Imagery, or visualization, is a mind-body therapy that uses the conscious mind to create mental images to stimulate physical changes in the body, improve perceived well-being, and/or enhance self-awareness. Frequently imagery, combined with some form of relaxation training, facilitates the effect of the relaxation technique. Imagery can be self-directed, in which individuals create their own mental images, or guided, during which a practitioner leads an individual through a particular scenario (Schaub and White, 2022). When guiding an imagery exercise, direct the patient to begin slow abdominal breathing while focusing on the rhythm of breathing (see Chapter 44). Then direct the patient to visualize a specific image such as ocean waves coming to shore with each inspiration and receding with each exhalation. Next instruct the patient to take notice of the smells, sounds, and temperatures being experienced. As the imagery session progresses, instruct the patient to visualize warmth entering the body during inspiration and tension leaving the body during exhalation. Individualize imagery scenarios for each patient to ensure that the image does not evoke negative memories or feelings.

Imagery often evokes psychophysiological responses such as alterations in gastric secretions, body chemistry, internal and superficial blood flow, wound healing, and heart rate/heart rate variability (dos Santos Felix et al., 2019). Although most imagery techniques involve visual images, they also include the auditory, proprioceptive, gustatory, and olfactory senses. An example of this involves visualizing a lemon being sliced in half and squeezing the lemon juice on the tongue. This visualization produces increased salivation as effectively as the actual event. People typically respond to their environment according to the way they perceive it and by their own visualizations and expectancies. Therefore you need to help patients individualize imagery based on their preferences and expectations (Schaub and White, 2022).

Creative visualization is one form of self-directed imagery that is based on the principle of mind-body connectivity (i.e., every mental image leads to physical or emotional changes) (Gawain, 2016). Box 32.2 lists patient teaching strategies for creative visualization.

Clinical Applications of Imagery. Imagery has applications in a number of pediatric and adult patient populations. For example, it helps

BOX 32.2 PATIENT TEACHING

Creative Visualization

Objective
- The patient will demonstrate skills in creative visualization.

Teaching Strategies
- Ask patient to create a clear image that is personally pleasing, such as a beach, favorite garden, or a frequently visited vacation destination. Although it is sometimes difficult to develop a visual image, if the patient views the goals of the imagery with clear thoughts and in the present tense, the patient will be more successful in creating an effective image.
- Have the patient frequently visualize the image.
- Instruct patient to use this visualization during relaxing states and throughout the day but particularly before bedtime or on wakening, when the mind usually is more relaxed.
- Have the patient repeat encouraging statements while focusing on the image. This helps the patient to alleviate any doubts about the ability to achieve established goals.

Evaluation
Use the principles of teach-back to evaluate patient/family caregiver learning:
- Describe how you will select your visual image.
- Describe for me when you plan to use visualization.
- I want to be sure I described this therapy well. Please explain to me the steps you are going to take to practice visualization.

to control or relieve pain, reduces symptoms associated with stress, and improves sleep (Nayeri et al., 2020; Sandvik et al., 2020). It also aids in the relief and management of symptoms associated with chronic conditions such as asthma, cancer, sickle cell anemia, migraines, autoimmune disorders, atrial fibrillation, functional urinary disorders, menstrual and premenstrual syndromes, gastrointestinal disorders such as irritable bowel syndrome and ulcerative colitis, and rheumatoid arthritis (Fitzgerald and Langevin, 2018).

Limitations of Imagery. Imagery is a behavioral intervention that has relatively few side effects (Schaub and White, 2022). Guided imagery along with relaxation techniques is effective in managing postoperative pain (dos Santos Felix et al., 2019). Some patients with chronic obstructive pulmonary disease (COPD) and asthma experience increased airway constriction when using guided imagery (Volpato et al., 2015). Thus you need to closely monitor patients when using this therapy.

TRAINING-SPECIFIC THERAPIES

Training-specific therapies are complementary treatments that nurses administer only after completing a specific course of study and training. These therapies require postgraduate certificates or degrees indicating completion of additional education and training, national certification, or additional licensure beyond the registered nurse (RN) to practice and administer them. Several training-specific therapies (e.g., biofeedback, Pilates, and acupuncture) are very effective and often recommended by conventional health care providers (NIH/NCCIH, 2021; Qaseem et al., 2017). However, other therapies (e.g., homeopathy and naturopathy) have not been adequately studied, and their effectiveness in many conditions has been questioned (NIH/NCCIH, 2021). Although many of these complementary therapies elicit positive effects, all therapies carry some risk, particularly when used in conjunction with conventional medical therapies. Therefore, you need advanced knowledge to effectively talk about them with patients and provide education about their safe use.

Biofeedback

Biofeedback is a mind-body technique that uses instruments to teach self-regulation and voluntary self-control over specific physiological responses. Electronic or electromechanical instruments measure, process, and provide information to patients about their muscle tension, cardiac activity, respiratory rates, brain-wave patterns, and autonomic nervous system activity. This information, or feedback, is given in physical, physiological, auditory, and/or visual feedback signals that increase a person's awareness of internal processes that are linked to illness and distress. Biofeedback therapies are used to change thinking, emotions, and behaviors, which in turn support beneficial physiological changes, resulting in improved health and well-being. For example, patients connected to a biofeedback device sometimes hear a sound if their pulse rate or blood pressure increases out of their therapeutic zone. Practitioners then help patients interpret these sounds and use a variety of breathing, relaxation, and imaging exercises to gain voluntary control over their racing heart or their increasing systolic blood pressure.

Biofeedback is an effective addition to more traditional relaxation programs because it immediately demonstrates to patients their ability to control some physiological responses and the relationship among thoughts, feelings, and physiological responses (Fig. 32.2). It helps individuals focus on and monitor specific body parts. Biofeedback helps patients control the physiological functions that are most difficult to control by providing immediate feedback about which stress relaxation behaviors work most effectively. Eventually patients notice positive physiological changes without the need for instrument feedback.

Clinical Applications of Biofeedback. Biofeedback in a variety of forms has application in numerous situations, with evidence supporting its effectiveness dating back to the 1980s. A study of systematic reviews revealed that in a large number of trials biofeedback can reduce headache pain and can provide benefit as an adjunctive therapy to men experiencing urinary incontinence after a prostatectomy (Kondo et al., 2019). The same researchers found consistent evidence although across fewer trials suggesting that biofeedback may improve fecal incontinence and stroke recovery. There is insufficient evidence to draw conclusions about effects for many conditions, including bruxism, labor pain, and Raynaud's disease (Kondo et al., 2019).

One of the most critical components of any behavioral program is adherence to the treatment regimen. Patients who adhere to the treatment regimen have more positive results.

FIG. 32.2 A patient using biofeedback can visually see how relaxation affects physiological functions. (From Okeson JP: *Management of temporomandibular disorders and occlusion*, ed 8, St Louis, 2020, Elsevier.)

Limitations of Biofeedback. Although biofeedback produces effective outcomes in select patients, there are several precautions, particularly in those with psychological or neurological conditions. During biofeedback sessions the repressed emotions or feelings for which coping is difficult sometimes surface. For this reason, practitioners who offer biofeedback need to be trained in more traditional psychological methods or have qualified professionals available for referral. In addition, long-term use of biofeedback sometimes lowers blood pressure, heart rates, and other physiological parameters. As with other biobehavioral interventions, monitor patients closely to determine the need for medication adjustments.

Traditional Chinese Medicine

Traditional Chinese medicine (TCM) is a whole system of medicine that began as an ethnic healing system approximately 3600 years ago. Chinese medicine views health as "life in balance," which manifests as lustrous hair, a radiant complexion, engaged interactions, a body that functions without limitations, and emotional balance. Health promotion encourages a healthy diet, moderate regular exercise, regular meditation/introspection, healthy family and social relationships, and avoidance of environmental toxins such as cigarette smoke.

Several concepts and principles guide the TCM system of assessment, diagnosis, and intervention. The most important of these is the concept of yin and yang, which represent opposing yet complementary phenomena that exist in a state of dynamic equilibrium. Examples are night/day, hot/cold, and shady/sunny. Yin represents cold, shade, and inhibition, whereas yang represents fire, light, and excitement. Yin also represents the inner part of the body, specifically the viscera, liver, heart, spleen, lung, and kidney, whereas yang represents the outer part, specifically the bowels, stomach, and bladder. Harmony and balance in every aspect of life are the keys to health, including yin/yang balance. Practitioners believe that disease occurs when there is an imbalance in these two paired opposites. Imbalance occurs as excess or deficiencies in three areas: external (six "evils" linked to weather and climate, including wind, cold, fire, damp, summer heat, and dryness), internal (originate in emotions and affect different organs, such as anger [liver], joy [heart], or fear [kidney]), or neither internal nor external (congenital weak constitutions, such as birth defects, trauma, overexertion, excessive sexual activity, poor-quality diet, and poisons). Imbalance ultimately leads to disruption of vital energy, qi, which then compromises the body-mind-spirit of the person, causing "disease." Disruptions in qi along the meridians can be systematically evaluated and treated by TCM practitioners.

TCM is an individualized treatment system based on a very specific assessment process. Practitioners use four methods to evaluate a patient's condition: observing, hearing/smelling, asking/interviewing, and touching/palpating. In TCM, outward manifestations reflect the internal environment. For example, the color, shape, and coating of the tongue reflect the general condition of the internal organs. The pulses provide information about the condition and balance of qi, blood, yin and yang, and internal organs. Therapeutic modalities include acupuncture, Chinese herbs, tui na massage, moxibustion (burning moxa, a cone or stick of dried herbs that have healing properties on or near the skin), cupping (placing a heated cup on the skin to create a slight suction), tai chi (originally a martial art that is now viewed as a moving meditation in which patients move their bodies slowly, gently, and with awareness while breathing deeply), qi gong (originally a martial art, now viewed as a series of carefully choreographed movements or gestures that are designed to promote and manipulate the flow of qi within the body), lifestyle modifications, and dietary changes.

Clinical Applications of Traditional Chinese Medicine. In spite of widespread use of TCM in Asia, evidence about its effectiveness as a whole system of care is limited. Most research in this field focuses on the study of individual treatment components of TCM such as acupuncture and herbal therapies.

Tai chi is effective in patients with balance disorders and in older adults. Patients with vestibular (inner ear) and other balance disorders benefit from an improvement in balance and a reduction in falls (Huang et al., 2019). In addition, group tai chi exercises are effective in residential care settings to reduce both the fear of falling and actual falls (Purdie, 2019). Some evidence shows that TCM is helpful in treating fibromyalgia (Nayeri et al., 2020).

Limitations of Traditional Chinese Medicine. TCM is not currently regulated in most states, although acupuncture is regulated. The federal government recognizes the Accreditation Commission for Acupuncture and Oriental Medicine (ACAOM) as responsible for accrediting schools that teach acupuncture and TCM, and approximately one-third of the states that license acupuncture require graduation from an ACAOM-accredited school. The National Certification Commission for Acupuncture and Oriental Medicine (NCC/AOM, n.d.) offers a certification examination for acupuncture and Chinese herbal and manipulative therapies. Refer patients requesting TCM to a qualified practitioner found at http://www.nccaom.org/find-a-practitioner-directory/.

There is some concern about the safety of Chinese herbal treatments that are used in teas, remedies, and supplements. The U.S. Food and Drug Administration (FDA) does not regulate, inspect, or ensure that the ingredients of these herbs are safe and without toxins. Recent reports about these products suggest that many Chinese herbs interact with other traditional medications, such as those associated with aspirin, clopidogrel, and other cardiovascular medications (Xiao et al., 2019; Aykan and Aykan, 2019). Further, these herbs can be very powerful, interacting with drugs and causing serious complications (Burchum and Rosenthal, 2019). When assessing a person using TCM, you always need to ask about the full complement of therapies, including the types of herbs that the patient is using. Some patients consider these as teas or dietary additives, powders, or supplements and not as over-the-counter medications.

Acupuncture

As a key component of TCM, acupuncture is an ancient practice shared by other Asian systems of care. When applied outside the system practice of TCM, acupuncture is viewed as a mind-body therapy and is referred to as medical acupuncture. In the United States, medical acupuncture is often provided as an individual treatment by conventionally trained physicians, nurses, chiropractors, dentists, and acupuncturists for many chronic conditions. Many states now have regulations and licensure requirements to practice as an acupuncturist.

Acupuncture regulates or realigns the vital energy (qi), which flows like a river through the body in channels that form a system of pathways called meridians. Twelve primary and eight secondary meridians are used by medical acupuncturists. An obstruction in these channels blocks energy flow in other parts of the body. Acupuncturists insert needles in specific areas along the channels called acupoints, through which the qi can be influenced and flow reestablished. Application of heat or weak electrical currents enhances the effects of the needles.

Clinical Applications of Acupuncture. Current evidence shows that acupuncture modifies the body's response to pain and how pain is processed by central neural pathways and cerebral function (NIH/NCCIH, 2021). Acupuncture is effective for low back pain, myofascial pain (e.g., temporomandibular joint disorder and trigeminal neuralgia), chemotherapy-induced nausea and vomiting (along with oral antiemetics), tension headaches, migraine prevention, and postoperative pain (Koppelman, n.d.; Nayeri et al., 2020;

Reinstein et al., 2017). It is also used to treat gastrointestinal disorders, menopausal hot flashes, clinical depression (with antidepressants), and posttraumatic stress disorder with varying effectiveness (Koppelman, n.d.; NIH/NCCIH, 2021).

Limitations of Acupuncture. Acupuncture is a safe therapy when the practitioner has the appropriate training and uses sterilized needles. Although needle complications occur, they are rare if the practitioner takes appropriate steps to ensure the safety of the equipment and the patient. Reported complications include infections resulting from inadequately sterilized needles or those that are left in place for an extended length of time, broken needles, puncture of an internal organ, bleeding, fainting, seizures, and posttreatment drowsiness.

Caution is necessary when using acupuncture with pregnant patients and those who have a history of seizures, are carriers of hepatitis, or are infected with human immunodeficiency virus (HIV). Treatment is contraindicated in persons who have bleeding disorders and skin infections. Further, semipermanent needles should not be used with patients who have valvular heart disease because of the increased risk of infection. Electroacupuncture is not recommended for persons with a pacemaker or for those who have cardiac arrhythmias or epilepsy or who are pregnant (Fontaine, 2018).

Therapeutic Touch

Therapeutic touch (TT), developed in the 1970s by Delores Krieger and Dora Kunz, is one of the "touch therapies" identified by NIH/NCCIH. It affects the energy fields that surround and penetrate the human body with the conscious intent to help or heal (Bagci and Yucel, 2020; Helming et al., 2022). Nurses include this therapy in all aspects of care. Other touch therapies include acupressure, healing touch (HT), and reiki. Blending ancient Eastern traditions with modern nursing theory, TT uses the energy of the provider to positively influence the patient's energy field (see Chapter 7).

TT consists of placing the practitioner's open palms either on or close to the body of a person (Fig. 32.3). It occurs in five phases: centering, assessing, unruffling, treating, and evaluating. To begin, the practitioner centers physically and psychologically, becoming fully present in the moment and quieting outside distractions. Then the practitioner scans the body of the patient with the palms (roughly 5 to 15 cm [2 to 6 inches] from the body) from head to toe. While assessing the energetic biofield of the patient, the practitioner focuses on the quality of the *qi*, identifying areas of accumulated energetic tensions, uneasiness, sluggishness, or congestion that manifest as sensations of congestion, pressure, warmth, coolness, blockage, pulling or drawing, or static or tingling. The practitioner then redirects these energetic patterns to harmonize distressed areas or to stimulate movement of *qi* in areas that are stuck and congested. Using long, downward strokes over the energy fields of the body, the practitioner touches the body or maintains the hands in a position a few inches away from the body. The final phase consists of evaluating the patient, reassessing the energy field to ensure that energy is flowing freely, and determining additional outcomes and responses to the treatment (Nayeri et al., 2020: Krieger, 1975, 1979).

Clinical Applications of Touch Therapies. The evidence supporting the effectiveness of touch therapies, including therapeutic and healing touch, is inconclusive, although it may be effective in treating pain in adults and children, dementia, trauma, and anxiety during acute and chronic illnesses (Baldwin and Trent, 2017). Box 32.3 summarizes the importance of touch in older adults.

Limitations of Touch Therapies. Although touch therapies cause very few complications or side effects, they may be contraindicated in certain patient populations. For example, people who are sensitive to

FIG. 32.3 During a therapeutic touch session, the practitioner intentionally directs energy to facilitate the patient's healing process.

BOX 32.3　FOCUS ON OLDER ADULTS
The Importance of Touch

- Touch is a primal need, as necessary as food, growth, or shelter. Touch is like a nutrient transmitted through the skin, and "skin hunger" is like a form of malnutrition that has reached epidemic proportions in the United States, especially among older adults (Bagci and Yucel, 2020; Hanley et al., 2017).
- Older adults need touch as much as or more than any other age-group. However, older adults often experience "skin hunger." Older adults often have fewer family members or friends to touch them at a time when simple touch may enhance communication, especially when other senses are reduced (Helming et al., 2022).
- Simple touch helps older adults feel more connected to and accepted by those around them and more in tune with their environment. Touch enhances self-esteem and sense of worth (Umbreit and Johnson, 2018).
- Nurses who react adversely to skin changes caused by aging often find it difficult to touch older adults. This reluctance communicates a negative message to the older adult (Fontaine, 2018). Therefore, be aware of your own reactions to touch when caring for older adults to ensure a therapeutic approach to patient-centered care.
- Be mindful of a patient's own acceptance of touch. Ask permission to hold a hand or give a hug. Once you form a relationship with a patient, touch can usually be more spontaneous.

human interaction and touch (e.g., those who have been physically abused or have psychiatric disorders) often misinterpret the intent of the treatment and feel threatened and anxious by it. Determining whether your patient has experienced trauma is important before using touch therapies (see https://www.samhsa.gov/trauma-violence for additional information). Other patients, including women who are pregnant, neonates, patients with cardiovascular and neurological instabilities, or patients who are dying, sometimes are sensitive to energy repatterning. Sessions with these populations need to be time limited and particularly gentle (Umbreit and Johnson, 2018).

Pilates

Pilates involves a system of exercises based on six basic principles: centering, concentration, control, precision, flow of movement, and breathing. These exercises are appropriate for patients across the life span and are designed to improve muscle strength, coordination, balance, and in some situations functional status. A study of children and adolescents who had musculoskeletal pain or limited muscle function noted that Pilates improved their flexibility, muscle strength, postural control, and balance (Hornsby and Johnston, 2020). Adults and older adults with chronic back and/or neck pain benefited from Pilates. When compared with using aerobic exercises, this age-group reported better pain control and improved muscle strength and coordination with the Pilates exercises (de Oliveira et al., 2019).

A lack of balance increases a person's risk of falling; this is especially true for older adults. A systematic review of Pilates in older adults documented that Pilates exercises improved personal balance and functional status. What was interesting about this systematic review is that these improvements occurred when Pilates exercises were completed only once a week (Casonatto and Yamacita, 2020). The benefits of Pilates may encourage exercise in patients who are reluctant to start an exercise program, especially those with underlying conditions and changes in functional status.

Chiropractic Therapy

Chiropractic therapy, a manipulative or body-based therapy, was developed in 1895 in Iowa. The central belief of the chiropractic profession is that body structure (primarily that of the spine and spinal cord) and the ability of the body to function normally are closely related. Thus when the spine is misaligned, energy flow is impeded, and the innate healing abilities of the body are impaired. Chiropractic therapy aims to normalize the relationship between structure and function by a series of joint manipulations (Laoudikou and McCarthy, 2020). Practitioners use their hands or a device to provide manipulation, which is the application of a controlled, sudden forceful movement to a joint, moving it beyond its passive range of motion. Often manipulations are combined with additional therapeutic modalities, including ice and heat, electrical stimulation, deep tissue massage, joint immobilization, lifestyle counseling, and medications.

Chiropractic care is a popular form of complementary therapy in the United States; 8.4% of the adult population and 3.3% of the pediatric population visit chiropractors each year, representing almost 20 million health care visits (Clarke et al., 2015). Chiropractic care is often covered by insurance plans, including Medicare and Medicaid.

Clinical Applications of Chiropractic Therapy. The basic goals of chiropractic therapy focus on restoring structural and functional imbalances. Chiropractors believe that structure and function coexist with one another and that alterations or distortions in structure ultimately lead to abnormalities in function. A major structural problem that chiropractors treat is vertebral (neck/back) subluxation with its accompanying symptom of pain.

Chiropractic therapy improves acute pain and disability in some patients. This therapy is sometimes effective over longer periods to reduce acute and subacute low back pain and joint pain caused by osteoarthritis. Chiropractic treatments for low back pain are effective in reducing pain, restoring function, and reducing pharmacological intervention (Whedon et al., 2018). Chiropractic care is also effective in treating asthma in children and adolescents (Driehuis et al., 2019).

Patients with cancer have pain management challenges; a patient-centered plan of care that incorporates chiropractic treatments along with standard cancer treatment and pain control interventions can help reduce musculoskeletal and muscle pain (Laoudikou and McCarthy, 2020).

Limitations of Chiropractic Therapy. Although chiropractic therapies are safe for a variety of conditions, chiropractors do not treat several diseases or conditions with manipulation. Bone and joint infections require pharmacological or surgical intervention because the structural integrity of the bone is compromised if excessive force is used. Other contraindications include acute myelopathy, fractures, dislocations, rheumatoid arthritis, and osteoporosis.

Some risks are associated with chiropractic therapy. A variety of injuries, ranging in severity from mild adverse responses (e.g., mild transient headache, increased pain and stiffness) to more serious injuries (e.g., vertebral artery dissection), have been reported (Shekelle et al., 2017). Degree and risk of injury depend on the type of manipulation performed, location of the manipulation (cervical spine is more susceptible to serious injury), overall health of the patient, and expertise of the provider. When educating patients about chiropractic care, advise patients to check the educational and licensure credentials of chiropractors, and review with them typical treatments and possible complications.

Natural Products and Herbal Therapies

It is estimated that approximately 25,000 plant species are used medicinally throughout the world. It is the oldest known form of medicine, and archeological evidence suggests that herbal remedies have been used for over 60,000 years. Herbal medicines are a prominent part of health care among indigenous populations worldwide. Interest in natural products also continues to increase in countries where biomedicine is dominant (Clarke et al., 2015).

Nonvitamin, nonmineral natural products are used by 18% of the U.S. population to prevent disease and illness and to promote health and well-being. A natural product is a chemical compound or substance produced by a living organism and includes herbal medicines (also known as botanicals), dietary supplements, vitamins, minerals, mycotherapies (fungi-based products), essential oils (aromatherapy), and probiotics. Many are sold over the counter as dietary supplements. The most frequently used products are fish oil/omega-3 fatty acids, glucosamine, probiotics/prebiotics, melatonin, coenzyme Q10, echinacea, cranberry, garlic, ginseng, and ginkgo biloba (Clarke et al., 2015).

Herbal medicines are not approved for use as drugs and are not regulated by the FDA. For this reason, many are sold as foods or food supplements. The Dietary Supplement Health and Education Act (1994) allows companies to sell herbs as dietary supplements as long as there are no health claims written on their labels. Natural products in the United States are prepared primarily from plant materials. They are provided as tinctures or extracts, elixirs, syrups, capsules, pills, tablets, lozenges, powders, ointments or creams, drops, and suppositories.

Clinical Applications of Herbal Therapy. A number of herbs are safe and effective for a variety of conditions (Table 32.2). For some women menopausal depression significantly impedes daily and social activities. Pharmacological support does offer some relief. However, the use of oral Chinese herbal medicine (OCHM) in combination reduced patient's self-report of depressive symptoms and improved the quality of life (Wang et al., 2018). Another study investigated curcumin—a yellow plant substance associated with turmeric as well as ginger. Curcumin appears to have a potent antiinflammatory effect, with suggested use in cancer prevention and progression, as well as in other chronic conditions. Clinical trials have recently found that

TABLE 32.2 Safe or Effective Herbs Determined By Non–United States Regulatory Authorities

Common Name and Uses	Effects	Potential Drug Interactions
Aloe vera		
Skin disorders, including burns, inflammation, and acute injuries (used topically)	Acceleration of wound healing	Furosemide and loop diuretics
GI ulcerations, including Crohn's disease and ulcerative colitis (taken orally)	Unknown mechanism, although there is a known laxative effect	May enhance the effects of laxatives when taken orally
Chamomile		
Inflammatory diseases of GI and upper respiratory tracts	Antiinflammatory	Drugs that cause drowsiness (alcohol, barbiturates, benzodiazepines, narcotics, antidepressants)
Generalized anxiety disorder	Calming agent	
Echinacea		
Upper respiratory tract infections	Stimulant of immune system	Antirejection drugs and other drugs that weaken immune system
		May interact with antiretrovirals and other drugs used in the treatment of HIV/AIDS
Feverfew		
Wound healing	Antiinflammatory	Warfarin and other anticoagulants
Arthritis	Inhibition of serotonin and prostaglandins	Aspirin and ibuprofen
Garlic		
Elevated cholesterol levels	Inhibition of platelet aggregation	Warfarin and blood thinners
Hypertension		Saquinavir and other anti-HIV drugs
Ginger		
Nausea and vomiting	Antiemetic	Warfarin and anticoagulants
		Aspirin and NSAIDs
Ginkgo		
Alzheimer disease and dementia	Memory improvement, although these effects are now in question given results in two recent clinical trials	Warfarin and anticoagulants
		Aspirin and NSAIDs
Licorice Root		
GI disorders, including gastric ulcers and hepatitis C	Unknown	Corticosteroids and other immunosuppressive drugs
		Digoxin
		Antihypertensive drugs
Saw Palmetto		
Benign prostatic hyperplasia	Prevention of conversion of testosterone to dihydrotestosterone (needed for prostate cell multiplication)	Finasteride and antiandrogen drugs
Chronic pelvic pain	Unknown mechanism	None known
Valerian		
Sleep disorders, mild anxiety, and restlessness	Central nervous system depression	Barbiturates and other sleep medications
		Alcohol
		Antihistamines

AIDS, Acquired immunodeficiency disease; *GI,* gastrointestinal; *HIV,* human immunodeficiency virus; *NSAIDs,* nonsteroidal antiinflammatory drugs.
Data from National Institutes of Health/National Center for Complementary and Integrative Health: *Herbs at a glance,* n.d. https://nccih.nih.gov/health/herbsataglance. Accessed September 12, 2021.

TABLE 32.3 Unsafe Herbs

Common Name	Effects	Comments
Calamus (Indian type most toxic)	Fever Digestive aid	Contains varying amounts of carcinogenic *cis*-isoasarone Documented cases of kidney damage and seizures with oral preparations
Chaparral	Anticancer Used for bronchitis in traditional healing systems (Native American and Hispanic folk medicine) Found in "natural" weight-loss products	No proven efficacy Induces severe liver toxicity in some cases Severe uterine contractions
Coltsfoot	Antitussive	Contains carcinogenic pyrrolizidine alkaloids Hepatotoxic
Comfrey	Wound healing and acute injuries Used for antiinflammatory effects in osteoarthritis and rheumatoid arthritis	Contains carcinogenic pyrrolizidine alkaloids May induce venoocclusive disease Hepatotoxic
Ephedra (ma huang)	Central nervous system stimulant Bronchodilator Cardiac stimulation Weight loss	Unsafe for people with hypertension, diabetes, or thyroid disease Avoid consumption with caffeine
Life root	Menstrual flow stimulant	Hepatotoxic
Pokeweed	Antirheumatic Anticancer	Do not use with children, but many websites state that it is safe with observation and monitoring as well as proper dosing; often used with folk remedies and in Native American healing

Data from National Institutes of Health/National Center for Complementary and Integrative Health: *Herbs at a glance,* n.d., http://nccam.nih.gov/health/herbsataglance.htm. Accessed June 2020; Therapeutic Research Center: *Foods, herbs, and supplements,* 2021, https://naturalmedicines.therapeuticresearch.com/databases/food,-herbs-supplements.aspx. Accessed June 4, 2021; and U.S. Pharmacopeia, 2020, from http://www.usp.org/. Accessed October 4, 2020.

curcuminoids are effective in lowering fasting blood sugars in persons with dysglycemia, including prediabetes and other metabolic syndromes (Melo et al., 2018).

Limitations of Herbal Therapy. Simply because a product is "natural" does not make it "safe." Although herbal medicines provide beneficial effects for a variety of conditions, a number of problems exist. Because they are not regulated, concentrations of the active ingredients vary considerably. Contamination with other herbs or chemicals, including pesticides and heavy metals, is also problematic. Not all companies follow strict quality control and manufacturing guidelines that set standards for acceptable levels of pesticides, residual solvents, bacterial levels, and heavy metals. For this reason, teach patients to purchase herbal medicines only from reputable manufacturers. This means that labels on herbal products need to contain the scientific name of the botanical, the name and address of the actual manufacturer, a batch or lot number, the date of manufacture, and the expiration date. Using natural products that have been verified by the United States Pharmacopeia (USP) is another way to ensure product safety, quality, and purity. Look for the USP Verified Dietary Supplement mark on product labels when buying or recommending natural products.

Some herbs also contain toxic products that have been linked to cancer. Table 32.3 lists several unsafe herbs. Some herbal substances contain powerful chemicals. As with any other medication, examine herbs for interaction and compatibility with other prescribed or over-the-counter substances that are being used simultaneously.

THE INTEGRATIVE NURSING ROLE

The interest in complementary therapies and an integrative approach to care continues to increase, fueled in part by the explosion in opioid addictions, the increase in chronic disease, and the need to consider nonpharmacological treatment options (National Academies of Sciences, Engineering, and Medicine, 2017). In North America and Europe, professional groups increasingly support the use of complementary therapies and monitor research in this area. The American College of Physicians issued new clinical practice guidelines for the management of acute, subacute, and chronic low back pain in 2017, recommending the use of nonpharmacological interventions that include tai chi, yoga, and other mind/body techniques (Qaseem et al., 2017). The Joint Commission's pain assessment and management standards require accredited agencies to offer nonpharmacological (complementary) therapy to effectively manage patients' pain (TJC, 2021). All providers, including nurses, need to encourage open, honest dialogue with patients about the use of complementary therapies. Providers also need to actively engage patients to accept integrative care to prevent disease, manage illness, and improve whole person well-being by employing the full spectrum of possible therapeutics rather than relying solely on surgery or drugs.

The integrative approach to health care is consistent with nursing's patient-centered, relationship-based legacy, which is focused on whole person well-being and health. Nurses have the potential for becoming essential participants in this type of health care delivery system. Many nurses already practice the use of touch, relaxation techniques, imagery, and breathwork and practice using the principles of integrative nursing (Kreitzer and Koithan, 2018). Familiarize yourself with the evidence in each modality that you incorporate into your practice. Know which patients are most likely to benefit from each therapy, when to use the various therapies, which complications might occur, and which precautions are needed when using these therapies.

In addition, you need enough knowledge to discuss the full range of biomedical and complementary therapeutic options so that you can help patients make informed health care decisions. Always ask patients directly about their use of complementary therapies, including self-care activities such as yoga, meditation, or dietary supplements. Be knowledgeable about the evidence for different complementary therapies so that you can make appropriate recommendations about which therapies are possibly useful for patients. Know about the different credentialing processes and how to refer patients to competent providers. Understand thoroughly the potential benefits and risks so that information is clearly and fully disclosed. Be knowledgeable, so you can give advice to patients about when to seek conventional care and when it is safe to consider complementary care services. For example, if a patient has right lower abdominal pain, nausea, and vomiting, be suspicious of conditions such as appendicitis or colitis and recommend consultation with a health care provider. However, if the patient has a chronic gastrointestinal disorder and has a diagnosis of irritable bowel syndrome, the patient may benefit from relaxation and herbal therapy. Be aware of the safety precautions for each complementary therapy and incorporate these in your teaching plans. Finally, understand your state Nurse Practice Act with regard to complementary therapies, and practice only within the scope of these laws.

Nurses work very closely with their patients and are in the unique position of becoming familiar with a patient's spiritual and cultural viewpoints. They are often able to determine which complementary therapies are more appropriately aligned with these beliefs and offer recommendations accordingly. Being knowledgeable about complementary therapies will help you provide accurate information to patients and other health care professionals.

QSEN **Building Competency in Patient-Centered Care** You are caring for Carmen, a 48-year-old woman with stage III breast cancer. She was discharged from the hospital 2 days ago and is readmitted for treatment of an infection in her suture line and around her drain site. Just before changing her dressings, you notice that she is more withdrawn and unwilling to speak more than one or two words and only to answer direct questions. When you question her further, she states that she cannot stop thinking about her future and fears that "this will be how it's going to be ... one hospital visit after another." She also says that she is concerned about the amount of pain medication that she's taking and that she's "tired of feeling drowsy and out of it" when her family comes to visit but doesn't know how else to manage her fear and pain. Which complementary and integrative approaches would you offer Carmen to improve her level of comfort? Are there strategies that would help address her fears of the future and begin to view it in a more positive light?

Answers to QSEN Activities can be found on the Evolve website.

▌ KEY POINTS

- Complimentary or integrative health care programs use the full complement of treatment approaches (biomedical and complementary) to provide patient-centered care to patients.
- Alternative therapy uses complementary therapies *in place of* conventional medical and pharmacological treatment; alternative therapies are the primary treatment that replaces biomedical care.
- The stress response is an adaptive response that allows individuals to respond to stressful situations.
- A chronic stress response is often maladaptive, leading to chronic muscle tension, mood changes, and immune changes.
- Some complementary therapies require commitment and regular involvement by the patient to be most effective and have prolonged beneficial outcomes.
- Continuously evaluate a patient's response to complementary therapies, as medication doses may need to change based on physiological responses.

- Complementary therapies accessible to nursing include relaxation, meditation and mindfulness techniques, and imagery. Evidence supports their use to decrease the effects of stress and improve overall patient well-being.
- Relaxation is an effective treatment for many patients. For example, relaxation can lower blood pressure, reduce cancer-related symptoms, manage depression and breathlessness, and reduce pain, opioid use, and anxiety. Nurses use clinical judgment to determine which relaxation techniques to use and when to use them with patients.
- Biofeedback is a mind-body technique that uses instruments to teach self-regulation and voluntary self-control over specific physiological responses. Biofeedback therapies are used to change thinking, emotions, and behaviors, which in turn support beneficial physiological changes, resulting in improved health and well-being.
- Therapeutic touch is a "touch therapy" that nurses include in many aspects of care. Other touch therapies include acupressure, healing touch (HT), and reiki, which blend ancient Eastern traditions with modern nursing theory.
- Acupuncture regulates *qi*, which flows through the body in medians. Acupuncturists insert needles in specific areas to influence and reestablish the flow of *qi*. Acupuncture is used to treat a variety of symptoms such as pain, chemotherapy-induced nausea and vomiting, and migraine and tension headaches.
- Many complementary therapies require additional education and certification, including biofeedback, touch therapies (therapeutic touch, reiki, and healing touch), and acupuncture.
- Herbal medicines are not approved for use as drugs and are not regulated by the FDA. A number of herbs are safe and effective for a variety of conditions. Some herbal medicines can be contaminated with prescribed medications, and it is important to understand the actions of herbal medicines and any potential interactions with patients' prescribed medications.
- Although there is increasing evidence to support the use of complementary therapies, additional research of sufficient quality and rigor is needed.

▌ REFLECTIVE LEARNING

- You are completing a preoperative admission assessment for a patient. What assessment information do you need to determine whether your patient uses any natural products or complementary therapies?
- Reflect on a recent clinical experience. Were there any situations in which a complementary or integrative approach to care would be helpful or perhaps inappropriate? For example, think about whether a complementary therapy would be useful in the emergency department and in end-of-life care.
- Reflect on several relaxation techniques discussed in this chapter. How would these techniques help you prepare for your current courses and clinical experiences?

▌ REVIEW QUESTIONS

1. When planning patient education, it is important to remember that patients with which of the following illnesses may find relief in complementary therapies?
   1. Lupus and diabetes mellitus
   2. Ulcers and hepatitis
   3. Heart disease and pancreatitis
   4. Chronic back pain and arthritis
2. Which complementary therapies are most easily learned and applied by a nurse? (Select all that apply.)
   1. Therapeutic massage therapy
   2. Traditional Chinese medicine

3. Progressive relaxation
4. Breathwork and guided imagery
5. Therapeutic touch

3. While planning care for a patient, a nurse understands that providing integrative care includes treating which of the following?
   1. Disease, spirit, and family interactions
   2. Desires and emotions of the patient
   3. Mind-body-spirit of patients and their families
   4. Muscles, nerves, and spine disorders

4. Which cognitive skills can a patient develop while practicing relaxation? (Select all that apply.)
   1. Increasing an ability to focus attention for an extended period of time
   2. Limiting stimuli that come into one's field of vision
   3. Stopping a focus on unnecessary goal-directed activity
   4. Being able to tolerate experiences that are uncertain
   5. Building relationships with significant others

5. A nurse is caring for a patient with chronic arthritis pain. The patient wants to add some complementary therapies to help with pain management. Which therapies might be most effective for controlling pain? (Select all that apply.)
   1. Biofeedback
   2. Acupuncture
   3. Therapeutic touch
   4. Chiropractic therapy
   5. Herbal medicines

6. A nurse is caring for a patient experiencing a stress response. The nurse plans care with the knowledge that systems respond to stress in what manner? (Select all that apply.)
   1. Always fail and cause illness and disease
   2. Protect an individual from harm in the short term
   3. React the same way for all individuals
   4. Cause negative responses over time
   5. Tolerate the stress response indefinitely

7. Meditation may intensify the effects of which of these medications? (Select all that apply.)
   1. Steroid medications
   2. Insulin
   3. Thyroid-regulating medications
   4. Cough syrups
   5. Antihypertensive medications

8. Which of the following statements best explains therapeutic touch (TT)?
   1. Intentionally mobilizes energy to balance, harmonize, and repattern the recipient's biofield
   2. Intentionally heals tissue damage or corrects certain disease symptoms
   3. Is overwhelmingly effective in many conditions
   4. Is completely safe and does not warrant any special precautions

9. Which statement most accurately describes intervention(s) offered by TCM providers?
   1. Uses acupuncture as its primary intervention modality
   2. Uses many modalities based on the individual's needs
   3. Uses primarily herbal remedies and exercise
   4. Is the equivalent of medical acupuncture

10. The nurse manager of a community clinic arranges for staff in-services about various complementary therapies available in the community. What is the purpose of this training? (Select all that apply.)
    1. Nurses play an essential role in the safe use of complementary therapies.
    2. Nurses are often asked for recommendations and strategies that promote well-being and quality of life.
    3. Nurses learn how to provide all of the complementary modalities during their basic education.
    4. Nurses play an essential role in patient education to provide information about the safe use of these healing strategies.
    5. Nurses appreciate the cultural aspects of care and recognize that many of these complementary strategies are part of a patient's life.

Answers: 1. 4; 2. 3, 4; 3. 3; 4. 1, 3, 4; 5. 1, 2, 3, 4; 6. 2, 4; 7. 3, 5; 8. 1; 9. 2; 10. 1, 2, 4, 5.

Rationales for Review Questions can be found on the Evolve website.

REFERENCES

American Holistic Nursing Association/American Nurses Association: *Holistic nursing: scope and standards of practice*, ed 3, Silver Spring, MD, 2019, American Nurses Publishing.

Benson H: *The relaxation response*, New York, 1975, Avon.

Burchum JR, Rosenthal LD: *Lehne's pharmacology for nursing care*, ed 10, St. Louis, 2019, Elsevier.

Climaco LC, et al: Getting to know the integrative and complementary practices in health: educational workshop, *J Nurs UFPE* 13(4):1167, 2019.

Fontaine K: *Complementary and integrative therapies for nursing practice*, ed 5, Upper Saddle River, NJ, 2018, Prentice Hall.

Gawain S: *Creative visualization: use the power of your imagination to create what you want in your life*, Novato, CA, 2016, New World Library.

Gross C, et al: Meditation. In Lindquist R, et al., editors: *Complementary and alternative therapies in nursing*, ed 8, New York, 2018, Springer.

Hanley MA, et al: A practice-based theory of healing through therapeutic touch, *J Holist Nurs* 35(4):369, 2017.

Helming M, et al: *Dossey and Keegan's holistic nursing: a handbook for practice*, ed 8, Boston, MA, 2022, Jones & Bartlett.

Kabat-Zinn J: *Falling awake: how to practice mindfulness in everyday life*, New York, 2018, Hachette Books.

Koithan M: Concepts and principles of integrative nursing. In Kreitzer MJ, Koithan M, editors: *Integrative nursing*, ed 2, New York, 2018, Oxford Press.

Krieger D: Therapeutic touch: the imprimatur of nursing, *Am J Nurs* 25:784, 1975.

Krieger D: Searching for evidence of physiological change, *Am J Nurs* 79:660, 1979.

Kreitzer MJ, Koithan M: *Integrative nursing*, ed 2, New York, 2018, Oxford Press.

Lindquist R, et al: *Complementary and alternative therapies in nursing*, ed 8, New York, 2018, Springer.

National Academies of Sciences: *Engineering, and medicine: pain management and the opioid epidemic: balancing societal and individual benefits and risks of prescription opioid use*, Washington, DC, 2017, The National Academies Press.

National Certification Commission for Acupuncture and Oriental Medicine (NCC/AOM): n.d. https://www.nccaom.org/. Accessed September 12, 2021.

National Institutes of Health/National Center for Complementary and Integrative Health (NIH/NCCIH): 2021. https://nccih.nih.gov/. Accessed September 12, 2021.

Purdie N: Tai Chi to prevent falls in older adults, *Br J Community Nurs* 24(11):L 550, 2019.

Rakel D: *Integrative medicine*, ed 4, Philadelphia, 2018, Elsevier Saunders.

Ringdahl D, et al: Integrative nursing practice. In Kreitzer MJ, Koithan M, editors: *Integrative nursing*, ed 2, New York, 2018, Oxford Press.

Schaub B, White M. Imagery. In Helming M, et al., editors: *Dossey and Keegan's holistic nursing: a handbook for practice*, ed 8, Boston, MA, 2022, Jones & Bartlett.

Voss M, Kreitzer MJ: Stress, resilience, and wellbeing. In Kreitzer MJ, Koithan M, editors: *Integrative nursing*, ed 2, New York, 2018, Oxford Press.

RESEARCH REFERENCES

Aykan DA, Aykan AC: Factors associated with the concomitant use of cardiovascular drugs and dietary herbal products: a cross-sectional study, *J Cardiovasc Pharmacol Ther* 24(2):146, 2019.

Bagci H, Yucel SC: A systematic review of the studies about therapeutic touch after the year 2000, *Int J Caring Sci* 13(1):2312, 2020.

Baldwin AL, Trent NL: An integrative review of scientific evidence for reconnective healing, *J Altern Complement Med* 23(8):590, 2017.

Bee SM, et al: Relaxation therapies. In Lindquist R, et al., editor: *Complementary and alternative therapies in nursing*, ed 8, New York, 2018, Springer.

Brighton LJ, et al: Holistic services for people with advanced disease and chronic breathlessness: a systematic review and meta-analysis, *Thorax* 74(3):270, 2019. https://www.ncbi.nlm.nih.gov/pmc/articles/PMC6467249/. Accessed September 12, 2021.

Carlson LE: Distress management through mind-body therapies in oncology, *J Natl Cancer Inst Monogr* 2017(52):37, 2017.

Casonatto J, Yamacita CM: Complementary therapies in medicine, *Complement Ther Med* 48:102232, 2020.

Clarke T, et al: Trends in the use of complementary health approaches among adults: United States, 2002–2012, *Natl Health Stat Report* 79:1, 2015. https://www.ncbi.nlm.nih.gov/pmc/articles/PMC4573565/. Accessed September 12, 2021.

Cushing RM, Braun KL: Mind-body therapy for military veterans with post-traumatic stress disorder: a systematic review, *J Altern Complement Med* 24(2):106, 2018.

de Oliveira NTB, et al: Effectiveness of the Pilates method versus aerobic exercises in the treatment of older adults with chronic low back pain: a randomized controlled trial protocol, *BMC Musculoskelet Disord* 20(1):1, 2019.

dos Santos Felix MM, et al: Relaxation therapy with guided imagery for postoperative pain management: an integrative review, *Pain Manag Nurs* 20:3, 2019.

Driehuis F, et al: Spinal manual therapy in infants, children and adolescents: a systematic review and meta-analysis on treatment indication, technique and outcomes, *J Clin Chiropr Pediatr* 18(2):1603, 2019.

Globe G, et al: Clinical practice guidelines: chiropractic care for low back pain, *J Manipulative Physiol Ther* 39(1):1, 2016.

Huang HW, et al: Impact of Tai Chi exercise on balance disorders: a systematic review, *Am J Audiol* 28:391, 2019.

Hilton L, et al: Mindfulness meditation for chronic pain: systematic review and meta-analysis, *Ann Behav Med* 51(2):199, 2017.

Hornsby E, Johnston LN: Effect of Pilates intervention on physical function of children and youth: a systematic review, *Arch Phys Med Rehabil* 101(2):317, 2020.

Kondo K, et al: Efficacy of biofeedback for medical conditions: an evidence map, *J Gen Intern Med* 34(12):2883, 2019. https://www.ncbi.nlm.nih.gov/pmc/articles/PMC6854143/. Accessed September 12, 2021.

Koppelman MH: Acupuncture: an overview of scientific evidence, n.d. https://www.evidencebasedacupuncture.org/acupuncture-scientific-evidence/. Accessed September 12, 2021.

Kreitzer MJ, Zbrowsky T: Creating optimal healing environments. In Lindquist R, et al., editors: *Complementary and alternative therapies in nursing*, ed 8, New York, 2018, Springer.

Laoudikou MT, McCarthy PW: Patients with cancer. Is there a role for chiropractic? *J Can Chiropr Assoc* 64(1):32, 2020.

Melo I, et al: Curcumin or combined curcuminoids are effective in lowering the fasting blood glucose concentrations of individuals with dysglycemia: systematic review and meta-analysis of randomized controlled trials, *Pharmacol Res* 128:137, 2018.

Montero-Marin J, et al: Meditation techniques v. relaxation therapies when treating anxiety: a meta-analytic review, *Psychol Med* 49:2118, 2019.

Nayeri ND, et al: The effect of complementary and alternative medicines on quality of life in patients with breast cancer: a systematic review, *Indian J Palliat Care* 26L:95, 2020.

Park SH, Han KS: Blood pressure response to meditation and yoga: a systematic review and meta-analysis, *J Altern Complement Med* 23(9):685, 2017.

Pospos S, et al: Web-based tools and mobile applications to mitigate burnout, depression, and suicidality among healthcare students and professionals: a systematic review, *Acad Psychiatry* 42(1):109, 2018.

Qaseem A, et al: Noninvasive treatments for acute, subacute, and chronic low back pain: a clinical practice guideline from the American College of Physicians, *Ann Intern Med* 166(7):514, 2017.

Reinstein AS, et al: Acceptability, adaptation, and clinical outcomes of acupuncture provided in the emergency

department: a retrospective pilot study, *Pain Med* 18(1):169, 2017.

Sandvik RK, et al: Pain relief from nonpharmacological interventions in the intensive care unit: a scoping review, *J Clin Nurs* 29:1488, 2020.

Shekelle PG, et al: The effectiveness and harms of chiropractic care for the treatment of acute neck and lower back pain: a systematic review, *VA ESP Project #05-226*, 2017.

Stussman BJ, et al: U.S. physician recommendations to their patients about the use of complementary health approaches, *J Altern Complement Med* 26(1):25–33, 2020. https://www.ncbi.nlm.nih.gov/pmc/articles/PMC6998052/. Accessed September 12, 2021.

The Joint Commission (TJC): *Pain assessment and management standards*, 2021. https://www.jointcommission.org/resources/patient-safety-topics/pain-management-standards-for-accredited-organizations/. Accessed September 12, 2021.

Umbreit A, Johnson L: Healing touch. In Lindquist R, et al., editor: *Complementary and alternative therapies in nursing*, ed 8, New York, 2018, Springer.

Volpato E, et al: Relaxation techniques for people with chronic obstructive pulmonary disease: a systematic review and a meta-analysis, *Evid Based Complement Alternat Med* 628365, 2015. https://www.ncbi.nlm.nih.gov/pmc/articles/PMC4539049/. Accessed September 12, 2021.

Wang J, et al: Adjuvant therapy of oral Chinese herbal medicine for menopausal depression: a systematic review and meta-analysis, *Evid Based Complement Alternat Med* 2018:7420394, 2018.

Whedon JM, et al: Association between utilization of chiropractic services for treatment of low back pain and risk of adverse drug effects, *J Manipulative Physiol Ther* 41(5):383, 2018.

Wilson AD, et al: Mindfulness-based interventions for addictive behaviors: implementation issues on the road ahead, *Psychol Addict Behav* 31(8):888, 2017.

Xiao M, et al: Impact of the Chinese herbal medicines on dual antiplatelet therapy with clopidogrel and aspirin: pharmacokinetic and pharmacodynamics outcomes and related mechanisms in rats, *J Ethnopharmacol* 235:100, 2019.

33

Self-Concept

OBJECTIVES

- Discuss factors that influence the components of self-concept and self-esteem.
- Identify stressors that affect self-concept and self-esteem.
- List the components of self-concept as related to psychosocial and cognitive developmental stages.
- Analyze ways in which a nurse's self-concept and nursing actions affect a patient's self-concept and self-esteem.
- Use sound clinical judgment to design evidence-based care for patients with disturbed body image, altered self-concept, low self-esteem, and role conflict.
- Examine cultural considerations that affect self-concept and self-esteem.

KEY TERMS

Body image
Identity
Identity confusion
Role ambiguity

Role conflict
Role overload
Role performance
Role strain

Self-concept
Self-esteem
Sick role

MEDIA RESOURCES

http://evolve.elsevier.com/Potter/fundamentals/
- Review Questions
- Audio Glossary
- Case Study with Questions

- Concept Map Creator
- Content Updates
- Answers to QSEN Activity and Review Questions

Mrs. Johnson is 52 years old and is recovering from a left radical mastectomy. She is in her room requesting that the curtains remain drawn at the window and lights off. She does not initiate any interaction with hospital staff when they enter her room. Kathryn Kline is a senior nursing student assigned to care for Mrs. Johnson throughout her hospital stay.

Self-concept is an individual's view of self. It is subjective and involves a complex mixture of unconscious and conscious thoughts, adaptive development, cultural identify, coping style, attitudes, and perceptions (Cicero, 2020). Self-concept, or how one *thinks* about oneself, directly affects self-esteem, or how one *feels* about oneself. Although the terms *self-concept* and *self-esteem* often are used interchangeably, nurses need to differentiate the two so that they correctly and completely assess a patient and develop an individualized plan of care based on a patient's needs.

Patients face a variety of health problems that threaten their self-concept and self-esteem. A loss of bodily function, decline in activity tolerance, and difficulty in managing a chronic illness are examples of situations that change a patient's self-concept. Your sound clinical judgment is essential to selecting the correct nursing interventions to help your patient adapt and adjust to alterations in self-concept. As the components of self-concept strengthen, patients gain successful coping strategies and improved health-related quality of life and health outcomes (Zhou et al., 2020).

SCIENTIFIC KNOWLEDGE BASE

A positive self-concept, especially a positive physical self-concept, is a key component to one's mental health and psychological well-being (Garn et al., 2020). The development and maintenance of self-concept and self-esteem begin at a young age and continue across the life span. Not only do parents and other primary caregivers influence the development of a child's self-concept and self-esteem, but research suggests that self-concept clarity is transmitted from parents to children (Esnaola and Sesé, 2020; Garn et al., 2020). In addition, individuals learn and internalize cultural influences on self-concept and self-esteem in childhood and adolescence. There is a significant emphasis on fostering a school-age child's self-concept. In general, young children tend to rate themselves more highly than they rate other children, suggesting that their view of themselves is positively inflated (Thomaes et al., 2017). Adolescence is a

FIG. 33.1 Adolescents' participation in group activities can foster self-esteem. (iStock.com/hraun.)

particularly critical developmental period when many variables, including school, family, and friends, affect self-concept and self-esteem (Rosenberg, 1965). The adolescent experience can adversely affect self-esteem, often more strongly for girls than for boys. Boys often have a better overall self-concept than girls, particularly in physical and social domains (Agrahari and Kinra, 2017; Esnaola and Sesé, 2020). During puberty adolescent girls are more sensitive about their appearance and how others view them (Garn et al., 2020; Vartanian et al., 2018). It is during adolescence that the search for an enduring sense of self turns into a core developmental task influenced by biological changes (e.g., puberty) and psychosocial changes (e.g., new interactions with peers and modifications in parent-adolescent relationships) (Erikson, 1963). During adolescence, individuals may rethink their previous sense of self and experiment with new roles and life plans. Therefore it is important to assess changes in identity formation and self-esteem among early, middle, and late adolescence because changes in self-concept occur over time (Fig. 33.1).

Most individuals cope with the transition from childhood through adolescence to adulthood successfully and become healthy and productive adults (Centers for Disease Control and Prevention [CDC], 2020). Job satisfaction and overall performance in adulthood are also linked to self-esteem. Self-enhancing opportunities such as exploring new ideas, solving problems in creative ways, and learning new skills predict job satisfaction and commitment and promote self-concept clarity and self-esteem (Touhy and Jett, 2020). Sometimes when individuals lose a job, their sense of self diminishes, they lose motivation to be socially active, and they even become depressed. They lose their job identity, altering their self-perceptions and self-care practices. Establishing a stable sense of self that transcends relationships and situations is a developmental goal of adulthood.

Cultural variations in self-concept and self-esteem across the life span affect health behaviors. In adolescent girls, culture, class, and self-esteem serve as protective factors against risk-taking behaviors, including unhealthy sexual behaviors (Cicero, 2020; Wilkins and Miller, 2017). Similarly, cultural identity of older adults is one of the major elements of self-concept and self-esteem (Touhy and Jett, 2020). Be aware of the cultural perspectives of aging when providing patient care. Sensitivity to factors that affect self-concept and self-esteem in diverse cultures is essential to ensure an individualized approach to health care.

There is a close relationship between how individuals view themselves and their perception of their health. Lower self-esteem is a risk factor that leaves one vulnerable to health problems, whereas higher self-esteem and strong social relationships support good health (Varcarolis and Fosbre, 2021). A patient's belief in personal health often enhances self-concept. Statements such as "I can get through anything" or "I've never been sick a day in my life" indicate that a person's thoughts about personal health are positive. Illness, hospitalization, and surgery affect self-concept. Chronic illness often affects the ability to provide financial support and maintain relationships, which then affects an individual's self-esteem and perceived identity and roles. Negative perceptions regarding health status are reflected in such statements as "It's not worth it anymore" or "I'm a burden to my family." Chronic illness affects identity and body image as reflected by verbalizations such as "I'll never get any better" or "I can't stand to look at myself anymore."

What individuals think and how they feel about themselves affect the way in which they approach self-care physically and emotionally and how they care for others. A person's behaviors are generally consistent with both self-concept and self-esteem. Individuals who have a poor self-concept often do not feel in control of situations and worthy of care, which influences decisions regarding health care. Patients often have difficulty making even simple decisions, such as what to eat. Knowledge of variables that affect self-concept and self-esteem is critical to provide effective treatment.

> **REFLECT NOW**
>
> Reflect on a statement a patient made recently about identity, body image, role performance, or self-esteem to which you felt unprepared to respond.

NURSING KNOWLEDGE BASE

Nursing research and research from the social sciences have contributed significantly to knowledge about how to care for the social and emotional needs of patients. This broad knowledge base provides nurses with a holistic view of patients, thus promoting high-quality patient care that best meets the self-concept needs of each patient and family. Understanding a patient's self-concept is a necessary part of all nursing care (Varcarolis and Fosbre, 2021).

Factors Influencing the Development of Self-Concept

The development of self-concept is a complex lifelong process that involves many factors. Erikson's psychosocial theory of development (Erikson, 1963) remains beneficial in understanding key tasks that individuals face at various stages of development. Each stage builds on the tasks of the previous stage. Successful mastery of each stage leads to a solid sense of self (Box 33.1).

Learn to recognize an individual's challenges when trying to achieve an age-appropriate developmental stage or the individual's regression to an earlier stage in a period of crisis. This understanding allows you to individualize care and determine appropriate nursing interventions. Self-concept is always changing and can be based on some of the following factors:

- Sense of competency
- Perceived reactions of others to one's body
- Ongoing perceptions and interpretations of the thoughts and feelings of others
- Personal and professional relationships
- Academic and employment-related identity
- Personality characteristics that affect self-expectations
- Perceptions of events that have an impact on self

BOX 33.1 Self-Concept: Developmental Tasks

Trust Versus Mistrust (Birth to 18 Months)
- Ability to trust others
- Develops trust following consistency in caregiving and nurturing interactions
- Distinguishes self from environment

Autonomy Versus Shame and Doubt (18 Months to 3 Years)
- Begins to communicate likes and dislikes
- Self-control and independence in thoughts and actions
- Appreciates body appearance and function (e.g., dressing, feeding, talking, and walking)

Initiative Versus Guilt (3–5 Years)
- Highly imaginative
- Identifies with a gender
- Enhances self-awareness
- Increases language skills, including identification of feelings

Industry Versus Inferiority (6–12 Years)
- Engages in tasks and activities
- Incorporates feedback from peers and teachers
- Increases self-esteem with new skill mastery (e.g., reading, mathematics, sports, music)
- Aware of strengths and limitations

Identity Versus Role Confusion (12–19 Years)
- Accepts body changes/maturation
- Sexual maturity
- Examines attitudes, values, and beliefs; establishes goals for the future
- Feels positive about expanded sense of self

Intimacy Versus Isolation (Young Adult to Mid-40s)
- Has stable, positive feelings about self
- Affiliation versus love
- Experiences successful role transitions and increased responsibilities

Generativity Versus Self-Absorption (Adult: Mid-40s to Mid-60s)
- Able to accept changes in appearance and physical endurance
- Reassesses life goals
- Shows contentment with aging

Integrity Versus Despair (Mid-Late 60s to Death)
- Feels positive about life and its meaning
- Interested in providing a legacy for the next generation

- Socioeconomic status
- Mastery of prior and new experiences
- Cultural identity

Self-esteem usually increases in early and middle childhood, fluctuates or remains constant in adolescence, increases strongly in young adulthood, continues to increase in middle adulthood, and peaks between ages 60 and 70 years. Depending on self-concept clarity, self-esteem diminishes or stays constant in old age with a sharp drop in very old age. In some situations this drop in self-esteem is closely related to loss of friends and loved ones, functional status, and independence (Orth et al., 2018). Although this pattern varies, in general it holds true across gender, socioeconomic status, and culture.

Children often report high self-esteem because their sense of self is inflated by a variety of extremely positive sources, and periodic declines may be associated with shifts to more realistic information about the self. Adolescence is a time of marked maturational changes and shifting levels of self-esteem that set the stage for rises in self-concept from adolescence to young adulthood (Esnaola and Sesé, 2020; Garn et al., 2020).

Erikson's (1963) emphasis on the generativity stage explains the rise in self-esteem and self-concept in adulthood (see Chapter 11). The individual focuses on being increasingly productive and creative at work while at the same time promoting and guiding the next generation. On the basis of Erikson's stages of development, a decline in self-concept in later adulthood reflects a diminished need for self-promotion and a shift in self-concept to a more modest and balanced view of self. Many report a decline in self-esteem in later adulthood caused in part by physical and emotional changes associated with aging, but older adults with self-concept clarity demonstrate psychological well-being. When aging is associated with deterioration of health, nursing interventions must focus on health behavior changes to promote self-care and self-concept (Touhy and Jett, 2020). Identifying specific nursing interventions to address the unique needs of patients at various life stages is essential.

Components and Interrelated Terms of Self-Concept

A positive self-concept gives a sense of meaning, wholeness, and consistency to a person. A healthy self-concept provides a high degree of stability, which generates positive feelings toward self. The components of self-concept are identity, body image, and role performance.

Identity. Identity involves the internal sense of individuality, wholeness, and consistency of a person over time and in different situations. It implies being distinct and separate from others. Being "oneself" or living an authentic life is the basis of true identity. Children learn culturally accepted values, behaviors, and roles through identification and modeling. They often gain an identity from self-observations and from what individuals tell them. An individual first identifies with parenting figures and later with other role models such as teachers or peers (Hockenberry et al., 2019). Relationships with parents, teachers, and peers have unique and combined effects on young children's general, academic, and social self-concept. To form an identity, a child must be able to bring together learned behaviors and expectations into a coherent, consistent, and unique whole (Erikson, 1963).

The achievement of identity is necessary to develop intimate relationships because individuals express identity in relationships with others (Varcarolis and Fosbre, 2021). Sexuality is a part of identity, and its focus differs across the life span. For example, as an adult ages, the focus shifts from procreation to companionship, physical and emotional intimacy, and pleasure seeking (Touhy and Jett, 2020). Gender identity is a person's private view of maleness or femaleness; gender role is the masculine or feminine behavior exhibited. This image and its meaning depend on culturally determined values (see Chapters 9 and 34).

Cultural differences in identity exist (Box 33.2). Cultural identity develops from identification and socialization within an established group and through the experience of integrating the response of individuals outside the group into one's self-concept. Differences in cultural identity exist through identification with traditions, customs, and rituals within one's cultural group. When cultural identity is central to self-concept and is positive, cultural pride and self-esteem tend to be strong. In contrast, internalization of prejudice and devaluation of one's ethnic and racial minority group can result in social isolation, which can negatively influence self-concept (Cicero, 2020; Benninger and Savahl, 2017). An individual who experiences discrimination, prejudice, or environmental stressors such as low-income or high-crime neighborhoods can conceptualize himself or herself differently than an individual who experiences privilege. One's perception of social class also affects self-esteem (Wilkins and Miller, 2017).

⊕ BOX 33.2 CULTURAL ASPECTS OF CARE

Promoting Self-Concept and Self-Esteem in Culturally Diverse Patients

Early in growth and development an individual develops cultural identity within the context of family (Betancourt et al., 2020). As an individual matures, the cultural aspects of self-concept are reinforced through social, family, or cultural experiences. In addition, a person's self-concept is strengthened or questioned through political, social, or cultural influences experienced in the home, school, and workplace environments. Positive or negative cultural role modeling, identity, and past experiences influence self-care, self-concept, and self-esteem. Socioeconomic status is a strong predictor of a positive self-image (Easterbrook et al., 2020). As social media evolved, researchers noted that public social media comments (e.g., Facebook, Twitter) had a significant impact on self-concept (Cicero, 2020; Eleuteri et al., 2017). Bullying, including cyberbullying, is one type of youth violence that threatens young people's self-concept and well-being. Nationwide, electronic bullying is rising, particularly among youth of color, including through e-mail, chat rooms, instant messaging, websites, and texting (CDC, 2020).

Implications for Patient-Centered Care

- Develop an open, nonrestrictive attitude for assessing and encouraging cultural practices to improve patients' self-concept.
- Understand that the relationship among self-esteem, stress, and social support can facilitate the development of nursing strategies to promote effective coping in culturally diverse adolescents (Bleidorn et al., 2016).
- Ask patients what they think is important to help them feel better or gain a stronger sense of self.
- Encourage cultural identity and pride by collaborating with patients and family about self-care practices and offering treatment choices (Cicero, 2020).
- Facilitate culturally sensitive health promotion activities that address at-risk behaviors (e.g., smoking, vaping, drinking, eating disorder risks, premature sexual experiences, excessive and violent video gaming) identified through evidence-based practice (Eleuteri et al., 2017).
- When completing a social history, a priority nursing action is the assessment of child and adolescent coping strategies, conflict resolution, and stress management as they relate to the use of social media and texting (CDC, 2020).

FIG. 33.2 An individual's appearance influences self-concept. (iStock.com/katleho Seisa.)

Body Image. Body image involves attitudes related to the body, including physical appearance, structure, or function. Feelings about body image include those related to sexuality, femininity and masculinity, youthfulness, health, and strength. These mental images are not always consistent with a person's actual physical structure or appearance (Fig. 33.2). Some body image distortions have deep psychological origins, such as the eating disorder anorexia nervosa. Other alterations occur as a result of situational events, such as the loss or change in a body part. Be aware that most men and women experience some degree of dissatisfaction with their bodies, which affects body image and overall self-concept. Individuals often exaggerate disturbances in body image when a change in health status occurs. The way others view a person's body and the feedback offered are also influential.

Normal developmental changes such as puberty and aging have a more apparent effect on body image than on other aspects of self-concept. Hormonal changes during adolescence influence body image. The development of secondary sex characteristics and the changes in body fat distribution have a tremendous impact on an adolescent's self-concept. For both male and female adolescents, appearance comparisons can result in a negative body image that affects health behaviors, including disordered eating and exercise

(Vartanian et al., 2018). For example, an adolescent girl may have a distorted body image and view herself as fat, which signals an eating disorder. Your assessment may reveal that an adolescent engages in self-harmful behaviors such as cutting; self-mutilation can indicate self-concept and self-esteem issues that warrant nursing intervention (Varcarolis and Fosbre, 2021). A threat to body image and overall self-concept can affect adherence to recommended health regimens, including diet, exercise, health screening practices, and taking medications as prescribed. Changes associated with aging (e.g., menopause; wrinkles; graying hair; and decrease in visual acuity, hearing, and mobility) also affect body image in middle-aged and older women (Watt and Konnert, 2020).

Cultural and societal attitudes and values influence body image. Culture and society dictate the accepted norms of body image and influence one's attitudes. Cultural background and social class play an integral role in self-esteem in adolescent girls and are reflected in differences in satisfaction with body image and appearance (Wilkins and Miller, 2017). Body image is more favorable in cultures in which girls describe more reasonable views about physical appearance, report less social pressure for thinness, and have less tendency to base self-esteem on body image. Low self-concept clarity increases vulnerability to body image issues as a result of the internalization of the thin ideal and appearance-related social comparisons (Vartanian et al., 2018). Values such as ideal body weight and shape and attitudes toward piercing and tattoos are culturally based. American society emphasizes youth, beauty, and wholeness. Western cultures have been socialized to dread the normal aging process, whereas Eastern cultures view aging positively and respect older adults. Body image issues are often associated with impaired self-concept and self-esteem.

Role Performance. Role performance is the way in which individuals perceive their ability to carry out significant roles (e.g., parent, supervisor, partner, or close friend). Normal changes associated with maturation result in changes in role performance. For example, when a man has a child, he becomes a father. The new role of father requires many changes in behavior if the man is going to be successful. Roles that individuals follow in given situations involve socialization, expectations, or standards of behavior. The patterns are stable and change only minimally during adulthood.

Ideal societal role behaviors are often hard to achieve in real life. Individuals have multiple roles and personal needs that sometimes conflict. Successful adults learn to distinguish between ideal role expectations and realistic possibilities. To function effectively in multiple roles, a person must know the expected behavior and values, desire to conform to them, and be able to meet the role requirements. Fulfillment of role expectations leads to an enhanced sense of self. Difficulty or failure to meet role expectations leads to deficits and often contributes to decreased self-esteem or altered self-concept.

Self-Esteem. Because how one thinks about oneself (self-concept) affects how one feels about oneself (self-esteem), you need to understand both concepts. Self-esteem is an individual's overall feeling of self-worth or how individuals value, like, and accept themselves and is considered to be one of the critical elements that affect future behavioral choice and action (Lee et al., 2018). When self-esteem is positive, one feels capable, worthwhile, and competent. A person's self-esteem is related to the person's evaluation of effectiveness at school, within the family, and in social settings. A person with a low or negative self-esteem is more likely to engage in risky behaviors such as substance abuse. During preteen years through the early young adult years, the evaluation of others also influences a person's self-esteem (Lee et al., 2018; Sukamti et al., 2019).

Considering the relationship between a person's actual self-concept and the person's ideal self enhances understanding of that person's self-esteem. The ideal self consists of the aspirations, goals, values, and standards of behavior that a person considers ideal and strives to attain. In general, a person whose self-concept comes close to matching the ideal self has high self-esteem, whereas a person whose self-concept varies widely from the ideal self suffers from low self-esteem (Varcarolis and Fosbre, 2021). Once established, basic feelings about the self tend to be constant, even though a situational crisis can temporarily affect self-esteem.

Factors Influencing Self-Concept

A self-concept stressor is any real or perceived change that threatens identity, body image, or role performance (Fig. 33.3). An individual's perception of the stressor is the most important factor in determining the individual's response. The ability to reestablish balance following a stressor is related to numerous factors, including the number of stressors, duration of the stressor, and health status (see Chapter 37). Stressors challenge a person's adaptive capacities. Changes that occur in physical, spiritual, emotional, sexual, familial, and sociocultural health affect self-concept. Being able to successfully adapt to stressors is likely to lead to a positive sense of self, whereas failure to adapt often leads to a negative self-concept.

Any change in health is a stressor that potentially affects self-concept. A physical change in the body sometimes leads to an altered body image, affecting identity and self-esteem (Tonsing and Ow, 2018; Varcarolis and Fosbre, 2021). Chronic illness often alters role performance, which changes an individual's identity and self-esteem. An essential process in the adjustment to loss is the development of a new self-concept. A loss of a partner can lead to a loss of identity and lower self-esteem. Unlike the loss in self-esteem shown in vulnerable older adults, the resiliency demonstrated in some older adults may reflect more sophisticated cognitive strategies to manage losses (Touhy and Jett, 2020).

The stressors created as a result of a crisis also affect a person's health (see Chapter 37). If the resulting identity confusion, disturbed body image, low self-esteem, or role conflict is not relieved, illness can result. For example, the diagnosis of cancer places additional demands on a person's established living pattern. It changes a person's self-appraisal and self-satisfaction with body image, overall quality of life, and physical, emotional, and social functioning (Tonsing and Ow, 2018; Zhou et al., 2020). It is important to assess self-esteem, effectiveness of coping strategies, and social support in all patients. During self-concept crises, supportive and educational resources are valuable in helping a person learn new ways of coping with and responding to the stressful event or situation to maintain or enhance self-concept.

Identity Stressors. Identity stressors affect an individual throughout life, but adolescents are particularly vulnerable. Adolescents need to adjust to the physical, emotional, and mental changes of increasing maturity, which may result in insecurity and anxiety. Adolescents also develop academic and psychosocial competence at this time. The use of social media also affects identity development as adolescents attempt to navigate relationships and express themselves in a way others will accept and like (Eleuteri et al., 2017).

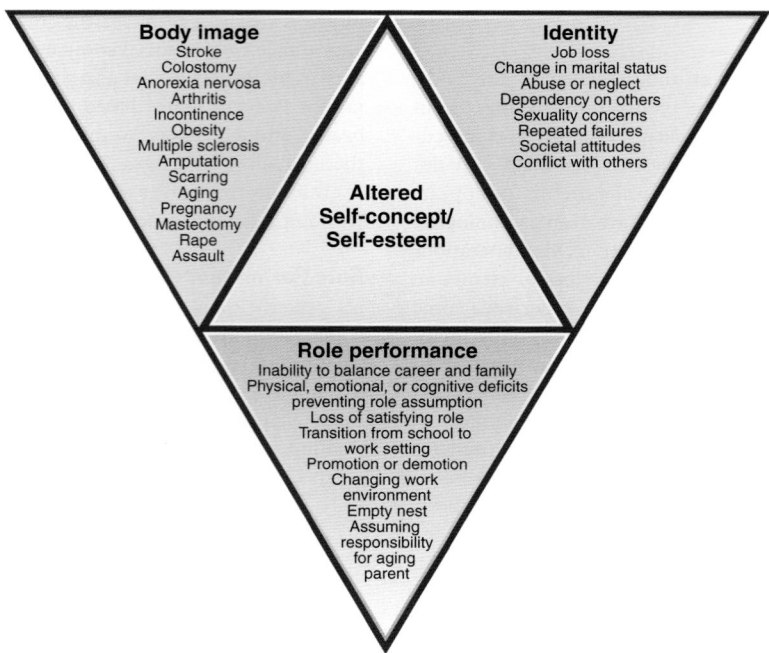

FIG. 33.3 Common stressors that influence self-concept.

Compared with an adolescent, an adult generally has a more stable identity and thus a more firmly developed self-concept (Orth et al., 2018). Cultural and social stressors rather than personal stressors have more impact on an adult's identity. For example, an adult has to balance career and family or make choices regarding honoring religious traditions from one's family of origin. Identity confusion results when people do not maintain a clear, consistent, and continuous consciousness of personal identity. Inability to adapt to identity stressors can result in identity confusion regardless of stage of life.

Body Image Stressors. A change in the appearance, structure, or function of a body part are stressors that require a body image adjustment. An individual's perception of the change and the relative importance placed on body image affect the significance of a loss of function or change in appearance (Zhou et al., 2020). For example, a woman's perception of body image may incorporate sexual characteristics (e.g., reproductive organs, breasts). Therefore the diagnosis and treatment for breast or uterine cancer is significant because it often results in loss of a breast, uterus, or ovary. These losses can result in a woman's perceived loss of femininity or wholeness (Jabłoński et al., 2019). Changes in the appearance of the body such as an amputation, facial disfigurement, or scars from burns are obvious stressors affecting body image. Mastectomy and colostomy are surgical procedures that alter the appearance and function of the body, yet the changes typically are not apparent to others when the individual is dressed. Although potentially undetected by others, these changes significantly affect the individual. Even some elective changes such as breast augmentation or reduction affect body image. Chronic illnesses such as heart and renal disease affect body image because the body no longer functions at an optimal level. The patient has to adjust to a decrease in activity tolerance that affects the ability to perform normal activities of daily living. In addition, pregnancy, significant weight gain or loss, pharmacological management of illness, or radiation therapy changes body image. Negative body image often leads to adverse health outcomes.

The response of society to physical changes in an individual often depends on the conditions surrounding the alteration. Some social changes have allowed the public to respond more favorably to illness and altered body image. For example, the media frequently present positive stories about people adjusting in a healthy manner to serious injuries, debilitating illness, or chronic disease (e.g., surfer Bethany Hamilton with her loss of a limb, actor Michael J. Fox with Parkinson disease, and singer and actress Selena Gomez with lupus). These stories change public awareness and the perception of what constitutes a disability, and provide positive role models for individuals undergoing self-concept stressors and their families, friends, and society as a whole. In light of the growing epidemic of obesity in Western cultures, parents and health care providers need to address weight-management issues without causing further injury to body image. Providing a social environment that focuses on health and fitness rather than a drive for thinness for girls or muscularity for boys can potentially increase adolescents' and young adults' satisfaction with their bodies.

Role Performance Stressors. Throughout life a person undergoes numerous role changes. Situational transitions occur when parents, spouses, children, or close friends die or people move, marry, divorce, or change jobs. It is important to recognize that a shift along the continuum from illness to wellness is as stressful as a shift from wellness to illness. Any of these transitions may lead to role conflict, role ambiguity, role strain, or role overload.

Role conflict results when a person has to simultaneously assume two or more roles that are inconsistent, contradictory, or mutually exclusive. For example, when a middle-age woman with teenage children assumes responsibility for the care of her older parents, conflicts occur in relation to being both a parent to her children and the child of her parents. Negotiating a balance of time and energy between her children and parents creates role conflicts (see Chapter 13). The perceived importance of each conflicting role influences the degree of conflict experienced. The sick role involves the expectations of others and society regarding how an individual behaves when sick. Role conflict occurs when general societal expectations (take care of yourself and you will get better) and the expectations of co-workers (need to get the job done regardless of illness) collide. The conflict of taking care of oneself while getting everything done is often a major challenge.

Role ambiguity involves unclear role expectations, which makes people unsure about what to do or how to do it, creating stress and confusion. Role ambiguity is common in the adolescent years. Parents, peers, and the media pressure adolescents to assume adultlike roles; yet many lack the resources to move beyond the role of a dependent child. Role ambiguity is also common in employment situations. In complex, rapidly changing, or highly specialized organizations, employees often become unsure about job expectations.

Role strain combines role conflict and role ambiguity. Some express role strain as a feeling of frustration when a person feels inadequate or unsuited to a role such as providing care for a disabled child or a family member with dementia or terminal cancer (see Chapter 14).

Role overload involves having more roles or responsibilities within a role than are manageable. This is common in an individual who unsuccessfully attempts to meet the demands of work and family while carving out some personal time. Often during periods of illness or change, those involved either as the one who is ill or as a significant other find themselves in role overload. Role overload may occur with the "Sandwich Generation" who are trying to take care of older family members while caring for their own family and maintain a career (see Chapter 13).

Self-Esteem Stressors. Individuals with high self-esteem generally are more resilient and better able to cope with demands and stressors than those with low self-esteem (Lee et al., 2018). Low self-worth contributes to feeling unfulfilled and disconnected from others. Decreased self-worth potentially can result in depression and unremitting uneasiness or anxiety. Young adults, ages 18 to 29, have the highest rates of depression, which negatively affects self-esteem as well as self-efficacy (Reed-Fitzke, 2020).

Illness, surgery, or accidents that change life patterns also influence feelings of self-worth. Chronic illnesses such as arthritis, cancer, and cardiac disease require changes in accepted and long-assumed behavioral patterns. Female children and adolescents with chronic illness are particularly vulnerable to low self-esteem. The more the chronic illness interferes with the person's ability to engage in activities contributing to feelings of worth or success, the more it affects self-esteem.

Self-esteem stressors vary with developmental stages. Perceived inability to meet parental expectations, harsh criticism, inconsistent discipline, and unresolved sibling rivalry reduce the level of self-worth of children. A developmental milestone such as pregnancy introduces unique self-esteem stressors and has significant health care implications. Self-esteem and health behaviors are intertwined, as self-esteem helps guide health behaviors and organize health-related actions (Tonsing and Ow, 2018). Stressors affecting the self-esteem of an adult include failure in work and unsuccessful relationships. Self-esteem stressors in older adults include health problems, declining socioeconomic status, decreasing physical functioning and independence, loss of spouse and friends, and declining social support (Box 33.3).

The Effect of Family on Self-Concept Development

The family plays a key role in creating and maintaining the self-concepts of its members. Children develop a basic sense of who they are from their family caregivers. A child also gains accepted norms for thinking, feeling, and behaving from family members (Hockenberry et al., 2019).

BOX 33.3 FOCUS ON OLDER ADULTS

Enhancing Self-Esteem in Older Adults

In some older adults, self-esteem can be negatively affected by a number of life changes. However, in other individuals aging promotes improved coping strategies that protect against the declining feelings of low self-esteem, despite the physical, emotional, social, and financial changes often associated with aging (Orth et al., 2018). High levels of self-esteem and sexual quality of life are associated with successful aging in postmenopausal women (Touhy and Jett, 2020). Nursing interventions aimed at enhancing self-concept and self-esteem in older adults are essential, particularly during illness, injury, or disability. Encouraging physical exercise can enhance the global well-being needed for successful aging and health-related quality of life (Hsu and Lu, 2018). Changing negative attitudes toward the elderly on the part of health care providers is essential to ensure positive patient outcomes (Touhy and Jett, 2020).

Implications for Practice

- Thoroughly assess a patient's physical complaints, and if no physical explanation exists, encourage the patient to verbalize concerns (e.g., anxiety, fear, insecurity, loneliness).
- Clarify what the life changes mean and the effect on self-esteem. Allow opportunity for patient and family to discuss perceptions of health problems, declining socioeconomic status, spousal loss or bereavement, and loss of social support following retirement (Heflin, 2020).

- Conduct supportive conversations to understand challenges to the patient's perceptions of body image adjustments as part of aging and changes associated with illness, injury, or disability (Hsu and Lu, 2018).
- Help patient identify positive coping mechanisms and describe why they are effective. Encourage family to support effective strategies (Varcarolis and Fosbre, 2021).
- Help patient identify negative coping mechanisms and describe why they are ineffective.
- Identify and provide patient-centered resources to help patient learn new positive coping mechanisms, including lifestyle self-care practices (Leão et al., 2017).
- Encourage the use of storytelling and review of old photographs.
- Modify nursing interventions with patients experiencing dementia to support self-concept; recognize that self-concept in early dementia is largely intact (Touhy and Jett, 2020).
- Take time to actively listen to and accept a patient's feelings, being respectful and praising healthy behaviors.
- Allow additional time to complete tasks. Reinforce the older adult's efforts at independence.

BOX 33.4 EVIDENCE-BASED PRACTICE

Self-Concept and the Impact on Adolescent Drinking Behaviors and Drug Use

PICOT Question: How does self-concept influence substance abuse in at-risk adolescents?

Evidence Summary

For some individuals, the stages of adolescence and young adulthood increase the risk for substance abuse (Bukstein, 2020; Lee et al., 2018). Adolescents experience changes in their physical appearance, social interactions, confidence, and independence. At times, these changes are perceived as overwhelming, and they all have the potential to influence self-concept. In addition, adolescents are very influenced by peer group acceptance (Agrahari and Kinra, 2017; Bukstein, 2020). A low self-concept may precede or perhaps increase risky behavior, such as adolescent drinking (Eleuteri et al., 2017; Bartsch et al., 2017). Because many teens engage in risky behaviors, such as teen drinking and drug use, helping youth develop a healthy self-concept and healthy behaviors can prevent these risks and future impact on health (CDC, 2020). In 2019 the CDC reported that 5% to 13% of middle school students drank alcohol for the first time before the age of 11, 13% of high school students reported drinking one drink of alcohol a day, 14% reported binge drinking, and 15% reported current marijuana or synthetic marijuana use. In addition, 14.5% of students had taken prescription pain medicine without a health care provider's prescription or differently than how the prescriber told them to use it. Nationwide, 8% of high school students had smoked cigarettes and 14% had used an electronic vapor product on at least 1 day during the 30 days before the survey (CDC, 2020). Identifying risk and protective factors is important when creating drinking, cigarette and electronic vapor products, and drug prevention programs (Eleuteri et al., 2017). Enhancing

opportunities to learn skills to increase self-compassion, self-awareness, resiliency, and self-worth, as well as to improve relationships with peers and families, may reduce the risk behaviors in adolescents (Bartsch et al., 2017).

Application to Nursing Practice

- Identifying risk factors for early drug and alcohol use, including genetic predisposition, family environment, and cultural identity, must be a priority for health care providers.
- Substance abuse prevention efforts should include stress management and improvement in self-esteem (Cao and Liang, 2020; CDC, 2020; Bukstein, 2020).
- A priority nursing action is the assessment of child and adolescent coping strategies. Appropriate techniques include effective communication, conflict resolution, and stress management (Leão et al., 2017).
- Implement individualized coping skills training and family health education to assist in improving adolescent self-esteem (Sukamti et al., 2019).
- Participation in physical exercise and youth sports programs helps adolescents gain peer support and improve coping strategies and self-concept (Garn et al., 2020).
- Help families, peers, and teachers learn how to provide social support to instill personal pride and life satisfaction, which promotes self-concept and the use of protective factors against risk behaviors such as drinking and drug abuse (Cao and Liang, 2020; Benninger and Savahl, 2017).
- Family, social, and behavioral factors are important issues to address during preadolescence and adolescence (Benninger and Savahl, 2017; Varcarolis and Fosbre, 2021).

Sometimes well-meaning statements or advice can cultivate negative self-concepts in children. Parents are important influences on a child's development, yet variations in parenting approach depend on the culture. Specifically, a child's positive self-esteem and school achievement are fostered by parents who respond in a firm, consistent, and warm manner. High levels of parental support and parental monitoring are related to greater self-esteem and reduced risk behaviors. Positive

communication and social support foster self-esteem and well-being in adolescence. Parents who are harsh, are inconsistent, or have low self-esteem themselves often behave in ways that foster negative self-concepts in their children, which can influence negative health practices, such as substance abuse (Box 33.4). Change in self-concept demands an evidence-based practice approach supported by the entire health care team.

Nurse's Effect on Patient's Self-Concept

Your acceptance of a patient with an altered self-concept can promote positive change. Often this simply involves sitting and listening to a patient and forming a therapeutic relationship. When a patient's physical appearance has changed, it is likely that both the patient and the family look to nurses and observe their verbal and nonverbal responses and reactions to the changed appearance. You need to remain aware of your own feelings, ideas, values, expectations, and judgments. Self-awareness is critical in understanding and accepting others. Your self-concept and professional identity are enhanced from a public perception of nurses' image; work environment; education; and professional, social, and cultural values (Leão et al., 2017). Positive self-esteem, interprofessional collaboration, and counseling support services can help to protect nurses from burnout and emotional exhaustion, which in turn assists nurses to deliver high-quality patient care (Barnett et al., 2019; Manomenidis et al., 2017). Before you care for patients, assess and clarify the following self-concept issues about yourself:

- Thoughts and feelings about lifestyle, health, and illness
- Awareness of how your nonverbal communication affects patients and families
- Personal values and expectations and how these affect patients
- Ability to accept differences in health beliefs and values
- Ability to convey a nonjudgmental attitude toward patients and families
- Preconceived attitudes toward differences in self-concept and self-esteem

Some patients with a change in body appearance or function are extremely sensitive to the verbal and nonverbal responses of the health care team. A positive, matter-of-fact approach to care provides a model for the patient and family to follow. For example, when you observe a positive change in a patient's behavior, such as a change to more healthy eating, acknowledge the change and tell the patient the positive change you observed, such as a decrease in weight.

Nurses have a significant effect on patients by conveying genuine interest and acceptance. Building a trusting nurse-patient relationship that incorporates both the patient and family in the decision-making process enhances self-concept and self-esteem. It is important that health care providers understand the degree to which self-esteem affects patient outcomes, and including self-concept and self-esteem issues in the planning and delivery of care influences positive patient outcomes. You can individualize your approach by highlighting a patient's unique needs and incorporating alternative health care practices or methods of spiritual expression into the plan of care.

Your nursing care significantly affects a patient's body image. For example, the body image of a woman following a mastectomy is positively influenced by showing acceptance of the mastectomy scar. On the other hand, a nurse who has a shocked or disgusted facial expression contributes to the woman developing a negative body image. Patients closely watch the reactions of others to their wounds and scars, and it is very important to be aware of your responses toward the patient. Statements such as "This wound is healing nicely" or "This tissue looks healthy" are affirmations for the body image of the patient. Nonverbal behaviors convey the level of caring that exists for a patient and affect self-esteem. Anticipate personal reactions, acknowledge them, and focus on the patient instead of the unpleasant task or situation. Nurses who put themselves in the patient's situation incorporate measures to ease embarrassment, frustration, anger, and denial.

Kathryn knew she needed to review her knowledge about breast cancer and care of the postmastectomy patient. However, Kathryn also recognized that this type of surgery has many psychosocial as well as physiological implications. She reviewed the literature on psychological adjustment following a cancer diagnosis and radical mastectomy. To add to her knowledge base she contacted the local chapter of the American Cancer Society for literature on recovery and support for breast cancer survivors. After Kathryn reviewed the information about the physical and emotional needs of a patient with newly diagnosed breast cancer, she outlined a few assessment strategies and questions.

CRITICAL THINKING

Any patient with actual changes in or threats to body image is at risk for experiencing stress, which can result in anxiety, depression, and other physical and psychosocial problems. Sound clinical judgment in applying critical thinking during the nursing process ensures safe and appropriate care. During assessment (Fig. 33.4) consider all critical thinking elements that will enable you to make the clinical judgments necessary to identify appropriate nursing diagnoses.

In the case of self-concept, it is essential to integrate knowledge from nursing and other disciplines, including self-concept theory, communication principles, the impact of illness on self-concept, and a consideration of developmental and cultural and factors. Previous experience in caring for patients with self-concept alterations helps to individualize care. Self-concept profoundly influences a person's response to illness. A critical thinking approach to care is essential.

REFLECT NOW

Describe a situation you encountered recently in which your own self-concept or self-esteem negatively influenced the care you provided.

❖ NURSING PROCESS

Apply the nursing process and use critical thinking in your care of patients. The nursing process provides a clinical decision-making approach for you to develop and implement an individualized plan of care.

◆ Assessment

During assessment, your skills of interviewing, listening to what your patient is saying, and observing your patient's nonverbal behaviors are critical to collecting complete and appropriate data about your patient's perception of self-concept and its components. Use sound clinical judgment to thoroughly assess your patient and critically analyze findings to ensure that you make patient-centered, clinical decisions required for safe nursing care.

When assessing self-concept and self-esteem, first focus on each component of self-concept (identity, body image, and role performance). Then determine the patient's perceptions of these factors to reveal the level of self-esteem. Assessment also includes identifying the patient's self-concept stressors (see Fig. 33.3), the number and intensity of stressors, and observing the range of behaviors suggesting an altered self-concept (Box 33.5), and identifying coping resources and patterns. Gathering comprehensive assessment data requires the critical synthesis of information from multiple sources (see Fig. 33.4). In addition to direct questioning (Box 33.6), gather much of the data regarding self-concept through

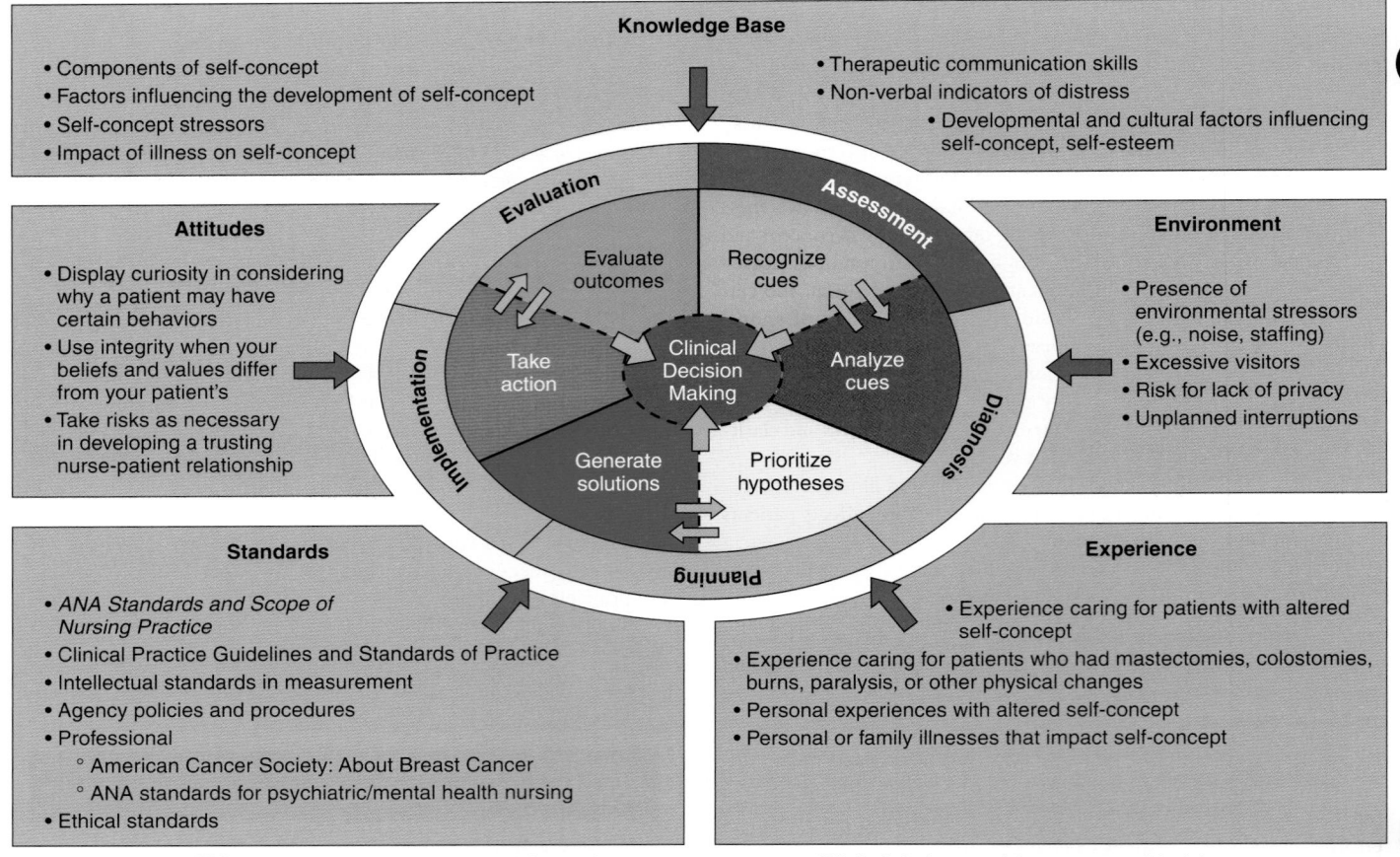

FIG. 33.4 Critical thinking model for self-concept assessment. (Clinical Judgment Measurement Model copyright © NCSBN. All rights reserved.)

BOX 33.5 Behaviors Suggestive of Altered Self-Concept

- Avoidance of eye contact
- Slumped posture
- Unkempt appearance
- Overly apologetic
- Hesitant speech
- Overly critical or angry
- Frequent or inappropriate crying
- Negative self-evaluation
- Excessively dependent
- Hesitant to express views or opinions
- Lack of interest in what is happening
- Passive attitude
- Difficulty in making decisions
- Self-harm behaviors

BOX 33.6 Nursing Assessment Questions

Nature of the Problem
- How would you describe yourself?
- Which aspects of your appearance do you like?
- Tell me about the things you do that make you feel good about yourself.
- Tell me about your primary roles. How effective are you at carrying out each of these roles? Do you feel good about these roles?

Onset and Duration
- When did you start to think or feel differently about yourself?
- How long have you struggled with _____ (specify identity, body image, role performance, or self-esteem)?
- Can you remember a time when you felt good about yourself?
- When did your primary roles change? What are the changes?

Effect on Patient
- Tell me how your _____ (e.g., loss of a breast, loss of hand function, fatigue) affects your roles and independence.
- What impact does your self-esteem have on your relationships?
- How does your self-esteem affect other areas of your life, such as decision making, socializing with friends?
- Have you considered hurting yourself (specify self-mutilation, suicidal gestures)?

observation of the patient's nonverbal behavior and by paying attention to the content of the patient's conversations. Take note of the manner in which patients talk about the people in their lives because this provides clues to both stressful and supportive relationships and key roles the patient assumes. Use knowledge of developmental stages to determine which areas are likely to be important to the patient, and inquire about these aspects of the person's life. For example, ask a 70-year-old patient about his life and what has been important to him. The individual's conversation likely provides data relating to role performance, identity, stressors, and coping patterns, all of which affect self-concept.

Through the Patient's Eyes. An important factor in assessing self-concept is the person's view of his or her health condition and its influence on self-concept. Give patients the opportunity to tell their stories of how they perceive their illness or condition affecting their self-concept, including their identity, their image of themselves, and their ability to lead a normal lifestyle. Assess their expectations of health care by asking them how interventions will make a difference and the differences they expect. For example, a nurse teaching relaxation exercises to a patient who is experiencing anxiety related to an upcoming diagnostic study asks the patient about his expectations of the relaxation exercise that they have been practicing together. The patient's response gives the nurse valuable information about his perception regarding the efficacy of the interventions and the potential need to modify the nursing approach.

Environment. Take time to assess the impact of environmental factors on a patient's self-concept. Are there excessive factors, such as noise, interruptions in care, or unplanned or overzealous visitors? In any health care setting a patient's privacy is essential, and maintaining a patient's privacy must be a priority of care, especially following trauma or major surgery. Ask your patients about how these factors affect their physical and emotional comfort. In addition, determine from your patients their individualized goals for controlling environmental issues to improve care.

Coping Behaviors. Assessment of a patient's coping behaviors includes a review of internal and external resources. Knowledge of how a patient has dealt with stressors in the past provides insight into the patient's style of coping. Patients do not address all issues in the same way, but they often use a familiar coping pattern for newly encountered stressors. Identify previous coping strategies to determine whether these patterns have contributed to healthy functioning or created more problems. For example, the use of drugs or alcohol during times of stress often creates additional stressors (see Chapter 37).

QSEN **Building Competency in Patient-Centered Care** You are caring for a patient who is recovering from a stroke. As you prepare to assess his self-esteem and self-concept, which questions might you ask him and his family to identify the factors that currently are influencing his self-esteem and self-concept?

Answers to QSEN Activities can be found on the Evolve website.

Significant Others. Exploring resources and strengths such as availability of significant others or prior use of community resources is important in formulating a realistic and effective plan of care. Valuable information comes from conversations with family and significant others. Significant others sometimes have insights into the person's way of dealing with stressors. They also have knowledge about what is important to the person's self-concept. The way in which a significant other talks about the patient and the significant other's nonverbal behaviors provide information about which kind of support is available for the patient.

This is Mrs. Johnson's first postoperative day. Prior to starting care, Kathryn reviewed the medical record, organized her assessment plan, and reviewed the patient's progress so far. Kathryn enters Mrs. Johnson's room and notices the environment, a darkened room with the window curtains pulled shut and lights off. The breakfast tray appeared untouched.

Kathryn notes that Mrs. Johnson had one dose of pain medication postoperatively more than 12 hours ago, as "patient did not request any pain medication" was noted in the medical record. When Kathryn enters Mrs. Johnson's darkened room, she notices that the patient is curled up on her right side, crying with her eyes closed, and she does not acknowledge Kathryn. Kathryn sits at eye level with Mrs. Johnson and asks about her pain level and its location. Mrs. Johnson explains she has incisional pain and rates it 9 out of 10. Kathryn suggests to Mrs. Johnson that she might be more comfortable if she receives something for pain, and Mrs. Johnson agrees. Kathryn administers the analgesic and tells Mrs. Johnson she will leave her alone for 30 minutes to allow the medication to reach its peak effect.

When Kathryn returns, Mrs. Johnson is not crying and has raised the head of her bed. Mr. Johnson is present, and the patient comments that the pain medication helped her discomfort and pain, which is now 3 out of 10. Kathryn explains to Mrs. Johnson that she is going to be providing care for her during her hospitalization, and she wants to complete an assessment to identify Mrs. Johnson's care needs. However, she explains to Mrs. and Mr. Johnson that before doing the physical assessment and physical care, she wants to hear what Mrs. Johnson is feeling and asks if Mrs. Johnson is willing to talk. Mrs. Johnson asks to have her husband remain in the room.

Mrs. Johnson shares her breast cancer story with Kathryn. It started with a routine mammogram 1 month ago in which an abnormality was noted. Following diagnostic screening, scans, and testing it was determined that surgery was needed. During surgery, two lymph nodes were positive for cancer, which resulted in a radical mastectomy. She thought she was just going to have a lumpectomy, so the radical mastectomy was a surprise. Mr. and Mrs. Johnson acknowledge that this all happened so fast, they did not have time to really think about it or process it.

Kathryn sits quietly and listens to Mrs. Johnson' story and asks her to describe how she thinks this diagnosis and surgery affect her life. Mrs. Johnson starts crying and says she has a strong 30-year marriage, but really can't talk to her husband because he cries when he thinks of her having cancer. Mr. Johnson is also crying at her bedside. Her friends know and want to help by talking about the cancer and people who have had treatment and reconstruction. Right now she just worries that cancer treatment and reconstruction will not work and "all this talking just makes me more anxious."

Through her tears she tells Kathryn that she cannot even look at her chest, at its bandages and drains, because to her they are symbols of her disfigurement. She states," I don't think I feel good as a person, let alone a woman. Heaven knows what my chest will look like after the bandages are removed. I don't want to see it." She knows that people are giving her information about her care, treatment, and reconstruction, but she feels that she is getting too much information to make decisions. Mr. Johnson acknowledges that he really understands her feelings and wants to partner with her in this journey, but he too admits that it was a lot for their family to process in a short period of time.

Following this discussion with the couple, Mrs. Johnson says that she is more comfortable physically and Kathryn can proceed with the postoperative physical assessment. Mr. Johnson leaves to go home and check on their family dog.

REFLECT NOW

Reflect on how you could improve your self-concept assessment skills.

BOX 33.7 Nursing Diagnostic Process

Situational Low Self-Esteem

Assessment Activities	Assessment Findings
Ask patient to explain thoughts and feelings about self.	Patient is tearful and reports negative thoughts about self. She states she does not want any visitors, except her husband.
Observe patient's behavior. Ask family whether the patient is experiencing emotional or behavioral changes.	Patient is crying and wants a darkened room. Spouse describes withdrawal and avoidance of discussing surgery or looking at the dressing. He describes wife as unable to make decisions.
Determine whether patient has had issues with self-esteem in the past and her plans to improve her self-esteem.	Patient and husband deny any lack of confidence, self-concept, or self-esteem issues during their marriage. She and her husband are willing to think about counseling.

◆ Analysis and Nursing Diagnosis

Clinical judgment involves use of critical thinking to analyze assessment findings. Consider the knowledge you have about a patient's condition and assessment findings to differentiate normal versus abnormal findings. Making nursing diagnoses about self-concept is complex. Rely on your knowledge and previous experience and apply appropriate nursing and professional standards. Use sound clinical judgment to completely organize, review, and analyze assessment cues to formulate a nursing diagnosis (Box 33.7).

Some assessment findings are relevant for more than one nursing diagnosis For example, a patient expresses feelings of fear, uncertainty, indecision, lack of confidence, and inadequacy. These assessment cues support *Anxiety* and *Situational Low Self-Esteem*. Realizing that the patient's assessment findings can be for more than one nursing diagnosis guides you in validating and differentiating the underlying problems. To further support *Anxiety* as a nursing diagnosis, consider whether the person has any of the following assessment findings: increased muscle tension, shakiness, a sense of feeling unsure, or restlessness. These clusters of assessment findings suggest *Anxiety* as an appropriate diagnosis. On the other hand, if the patient expresses negative self-appraisal, including inability to cope with situations or events and difficulty in making decisions, these findings suggest that *Situational Low Self-Esteem* is more appropriate. To further aid in differentiating between the two provisional diagnoses, information regarding recent events in the person's life and how the person has viewed himself or herself in the past provide insight into the most appropriate nursing diagnosis. As you analyze all assessment findings, priority nursing diagnoses become evident and help to direct relevant nursing interventions to improve a patient's self-concept.

Validate the nursing diagnosis by sharing observations with the patient and allowing the patient to verify perceptions. This approach often results in the patient providing additional data, which further clarifies the situation. For example, "I noticed that you jumped when I touched your arm. Are you feeling uneasy today?" allows the patient to verify anxiety and to describe any concerns.

Recurring data from the assessment relate to Mrs. Johnson's perception of her body following surgery. Mrs. Johnson does not want to see her surgical site, feels disfigured, and says she does not feel good as a person, let alone as a woman. Analysis of these assessment findings support the nursing diagnosis **Disturbed Body Image related to negative view of self after mastectomy.** *She says that she is not sleeping well, is restless,*

and does not have relief from the patient-controlled analgesia (PCA) pump; she does acknowledge that following the analgesia administered by Kathryn, her pain was much better. **Acute Pain related to mastectomy incision** *is also a priority diagnosis. Mrs. Johnson is getting a lot of information about treatment and reconstruction and probably advice from well-meaning friends, and this increases her worries and anxiety. These assessment findings support the nursing diagnosis* **Anxiety related to success of future treatment.** *All the information she is getting increases her feeling of not being able to cope. All this information about treatment compounded with the unexpected diagnosis affects her decision making, and she stated that she feels "useless." These assessment findings support the nursing diagnosis* **Situational Low Self-Esteem related to breast cancer diagnosis.**

The following list provides examples of other self-concept–related nursing diagnoses:
- Disturbed Personal Identity
- Impaired Role Performance
- Situational Low Self-Esteem
- Chronic Low Self-Esteem

◆ Planning and Outcomes Identification

During planning, use critical thinking to synthesize knowledge, environment, experience, critical thinking attitudes, and standards (Fig. 33.5). Use sound clinical judgment to make the clinical decisions needed for a patient's plan of care (see the Nursing Care Plan). The information gained regarding the factors affecting the patient's perceived self-concept enables you to select appropriate interventions. Alterations in self-concept are often very personal and private, and privacy in a health care environment is hard to protect. There are threats to protected health information and unexpected interruptions during care. Be proactive in identifying environmental factors that impact privacy, and resolve risks in a timely manner. Think about how your past experiences will help to improve your competency in planning care for patients with self-concept issues. Use professional nursing scope and standards of practice (e.g., American Nurses Association [ANA], 2021) and established ethical and evidence-based practice guidelines from professional and community-based organizations to select effective nursing interventions.

Another method to help plan care is a concept map. The concept map (Fig. 33.6) shows the relationship of a primary health problem (postoperative bilateral radical mastectomy) and four nursing diagnoses and several interventions. The concept map shows the interrelationships between the nursing diagnoses and nursing interventions. In certain patients a single nursing intervention can be effective for more than one diagnosis.

Outcomes. Develop an individualized plan of care for each nursing diagnosis. Work collaboratively with the patient to identify outcomes of care, making sure that outcomes are individualized, realistic, and measurable. Consult with the patient about whether they are achievable, and help the patient identify ways in which they can be achieved. Consultation with significant others, mental health clinicians, and community resources results in a more comprehensive and workable plan. When you collaborate with the patient to identify outcomes, consider the data necessary to demonstrate how the patient's problem would change if the nursing diagnosis were managed. For example, a patient is diagnosed with *Situational Low Self-Esteem related to a recent job layoff.* Examples of outcomes to support the patient's self esteem may include:
- Patient describes three areas of her life in which she is functioning well.
- Patient states that that losing her job is not reflective of her worth as a person.
- Patient attends a support group for recently unemployed executives.

FIG. 33.5 Critical thinking model for self-concept planning. (Clinical Judgment Measurement Model copyright © NCSBN. All rights reserved.)

Setting Priorities. Establishing priorities includes using therapeutic communication to address self-concept issues, which ensures that the patient's ability to address physical needs is maximized. Collaborate with the patient and family to identify strengths and limitations, and provide resources and education to turn limitations into strengths. Patient teaching creates understanding of the normalcy of certain situations (e.g., nature of a chronic disease; change in relationships; effect of a loss). Often, once patients understand their situations, their sense of hopelessness and helplessness is lessened.

Sound clinical judgment is needed to develop a care plan for a patient with an alteration in self-concept. Supportive and individualized interventions help a patient adapt to some of the stressors that led to the self-concept disturbance and support and reinforce the development of coping methods. Often a patient perceives a situation as overwhelming and feels hopeless about returning to the level of previous functioning. The patient often needs time to adapt to physical and emotional changes but can work toward progressive improvement in self-concept and self-esteem.

REFLECT NOW

Reflect about some self-concept priorities for an adolescent with facial trauma following a motor vehicle accident.

Teamwork and Collaboration. Collaborate with the health care team and the patient's family and significant others. A patient's perceptions of family and significant others are important to incorporate into the plan of care. Individuals who have experienced prior issues with self-concept before the current episode of treatment have often established a system of support that includes mental health clinicians, clergy, and other community resources. However, before including any family member or significant others, consider the patient's desires for their involvement and cultural norms regarding who most frequently makes decisions in the family (Cicero, 2020).

Patients who are experiencing threats to or alterations in self-concept often benefit from collaboration with mental health and community resources to promote increased awareness. Additional resources include physical therapy, occupational therapy, behavioral health, social services, and pastoral care (Easterbrook et al., 2020). Knowledge of available resources allows appropriate referrals.

Kathryn discusses the plan of care with Mrs. Johnson. She and Mrs. Johnson agree to plan patient-centered personal hygiene care. The first priority is managing her current pain level, and the second priority is to respect Mrs. Johnson's unwillingness to look at her incisional area at this time. Her pain remains less than 3/10, and Kathryn reinforces the pain-control outcome below 5/10 with Mrs. Johnson and tells her to let Kathryn or another nurse know when the pain is 5/10. Another outcome is to increase Mrs. Johnson's ability to perform self-care hygiene so as to reduce anxiety and begin to adapt to her disturbed body image.

◎ **NURSING CARE PLAN**

Disturbed Body Image

ASSESSMENT

Assessment Activities	*Assessment Findings*[a]
Identify body image concerns (e.g., sexual role, femininity). Ask how the loss of her breast has affected her sense of self.	Mrs. Johnson **looks away, shakes her head**, and states, "**I feel like less of a woman**. My husband says I'll always be attractive in his eyes, but I don't believe him. I really **find it hard to talk** with him."
Observe Mrs. Johnson's mood and affect and her nonverbal communication and interactions with others.	Mrs. Johnson demonstrates intermittent eye contact, frequent **crying when alone,** pulling hospital gown tightly across chest, and superficial conversations with family members.
Assess Mrs. Johnson's involvement in self-care activities.	Mrs. Johnson is unable to decide when to bathe, comb her hair, or apply her usual makeup. **She avoids looking in a mirror.**
Ask Mrs. Johnson if she would like opportunities to participate in treatment activities.	**Mrs. Johnson avoids** looking at or touching her chest and **does not ask questions** about her condition. "I don't know if I want to do anything right now."

[a]Assessment findings are shown in bold type.

NURSING DIAGNOSIS: Disturbed body image related to negative view of self after mastectomy

PLANNING

Expected Outcomes (NOC)[b]

Self-Esteem

Mrs. Johnson meets basic grooming and hygiene needs within 2 days.

Mrs. Johnson verbalizes improved feelings of self-acceptance and self-worth by discharge.

Body Image

Mrs. Johnson demonstrates positive adjustments to changes in body appearance, such as grooming and applying some makeup, by discharge.

[b]Outcome classification labels from Moorhead S, et al: *Nursing Outcomes Classification (NOC): measurement of health outcomes*, ed 6, St Louis, 2018, Elsevier.

INTERVENTIONS (NIC)[c]	**RATIONALE**
Self-Esteem Enhancement	
Use communication techniques to facilitate a safe and comfortable environment for the patient to discuss her self-esteem issues.	A therapeutic nurse-patient relationship promotes positive patient outcome, including the patient assuming responsibility for her own care (Varcarolis and Fosbre, 2021).
Engage patient in discussion about her feelings about her self-image and how community support programs are beneficial.	Mastectomy affects psychosocial functioning especially in self-esteem and body image. Changes in self-esteem and body image are strong predictors of depression. Community programs and in some cases mindfulness exercises give the patient skills to cope with these changes (Franco et al., 2020).
Provide opportunities for patient to use previous self-care practices to cope with the stress of cancer and a mastectomy.	Promoting self-care practices, apparel, makeup, usual sleep practice, exercise, and nutrition enhances coping and self-esteem (Jabłoński et al., 2019).
Body Image Enhancement	
Provide patient-centered care to support acceptance of alterations in physical appearance.	Postmastectomy threat to body image affects an overall perception of patient's quality of life (Zhou et al., 2020). Self-concept often influences self-care practices and acceptance of changes in physical appearance (Varcarolis and Fosbre, 2021).

[c]Intervention classification labels from Butcher HK, et al: *Nursing Interventions Classification (NIC)*, ed 7, St Louis, 2018, Elsevier.

EVALUATION

Evaluation Activities	*Patient Response*
Ask Mrs. Johnson how effective she feels in her ability to identify and express feelings verbally and nonverbally.	Mrs. Johnson reports, "I've been able to talk with my husband, even about my concerns that he won't find me attractive anymore."
Monitor changes in Mrs. Johnson's statements about herself.	Mrs. Johnson is making fewer negative comments and evaluating body image more realistically but remains dissatisfied with appearance.
Observe Mrs. Johnson's participation in self-care related to mastectomy.	Mrs. Johnson is more assertive in completing basic hygiene; applying makeup, styling her hair, and looking at her mastectomy scar.

CONCEPT MAP

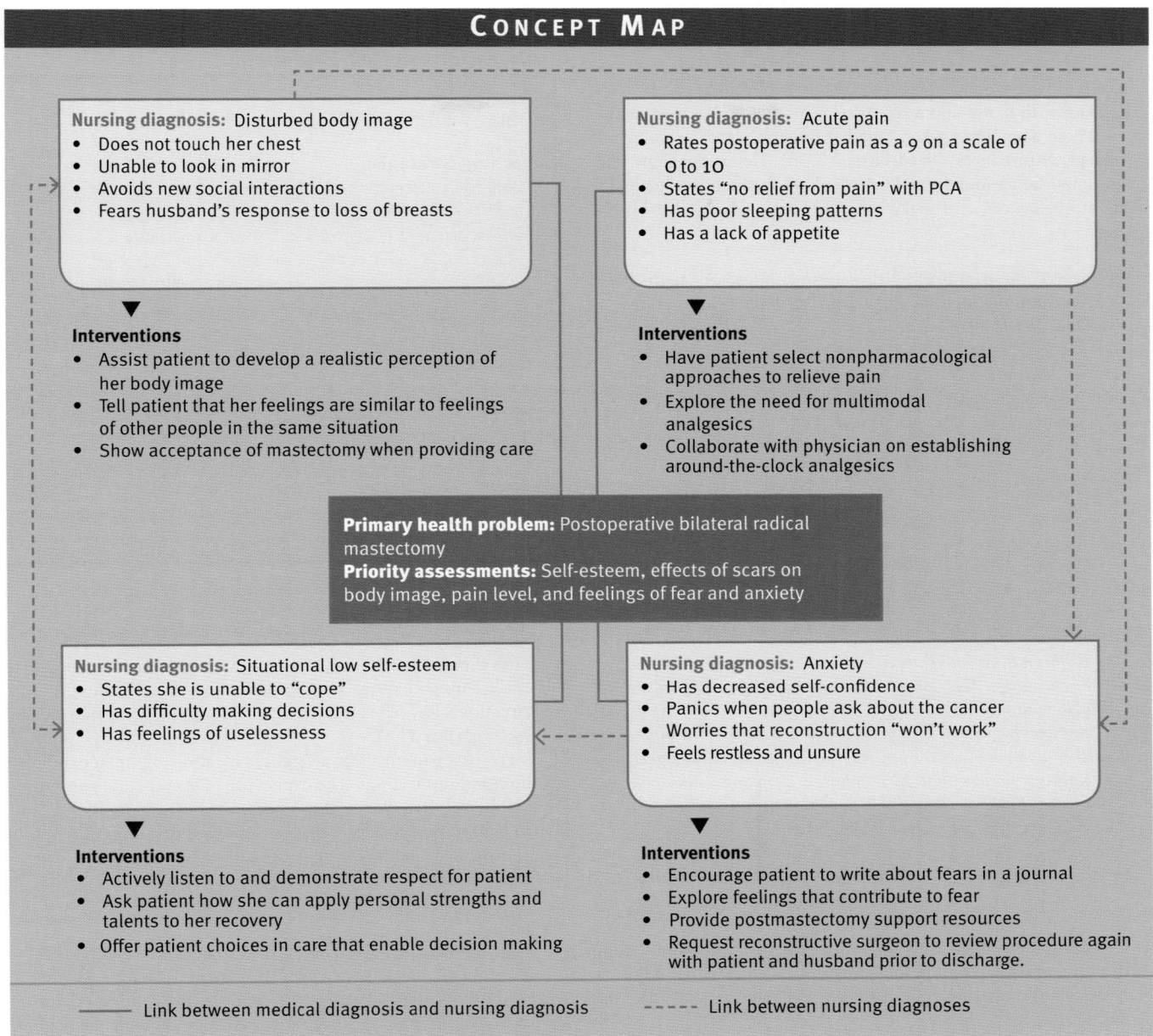

Nursing diagnosis: Disturbed body image
- Does not touch her chest
- Unable to look in mirror
- Avoids new social interactions
- Fears husband's response to loss of breasts

Interventions
- Assist patient to develop a realistic perception of her body image
- Tell patient that her feelings are similar to feelings of other people in the same situation
- Show acceptance of mastectomy when providing care

Nursing diagnosis: Acute pain
- Rates postoperative pain as a 9 on a scale of 0 to 10
- States "no relief from pain" with PCA
- Has poor sleeping patterns
- Has a lack of appetite

Interventions
- Have patient select nonpharmacological approaches to relieve pain
- Explore the need for multimodal analgesics
- Collaborate with physician on establishing around-the-clock analgesics

Primary health problem: Postoperative bilateral radical mastectomy
Priority assessments: Self-esteem, effects of scars on body image, pain level, and feelings of fear and anxiety

Nursing diagnosis: Situational low self-esteem
- States she is unable to "cope"
- Has difficulty making decisions
- Has feelings of uselessness

Interventions
- Actively listen to and demonstrate respect for patient
- Ask patient how she can apply personal strengths and talents to her recovery
- Offer patient choices in care that enable decision making

Nursing diagnosis: Anxiety
- Has decreased self-confidence
- Panics when people ask about the cancer
- Worries that reconstruction "won't work"
- Feels restless and unsure

Interventions
- Encourage patient to write about fears in a journal
- Explore feelings that contribute to fear
- Provide postmastectomy support resources
- Request reconstructive surgeon to review procedure again with patient and husband prior to discharge.

——— Link between medical diagnosis and nursing diagnosis   ----- Link between nursing diagnoses

FIG. 33.6 Concept map for Mrs. Johnson. *PCA,* Patient-controlled analgesia.

To begin to achieve this outcome, Kathryn collaborates with Mrs. Johnson and an oncology nurse specialist to identify postmastectomy hygiene needs. Mr. Johnson is also included in the plan of care to assist his wife with physical (e.g., hygiene, dressing changes) and emotional needs following discharge. Mr. Johnson is also provided resources for the spouse of a patient who has breast cancer.

◆ **Implementation**

When caring for a patient with alterations in self-concept, strong communication skills and a therapeutic nurse-patient relationship are central to implementing patient-centered care. To identify effective nursing interventions, consider each nursing diagnosis and use sound clinical judgment to individualize interventions that treat the diagnosis. Collaborating with members of the health care team maximizes the comprehensiveness of the approach to self-concept issues. Regardless of the health care setting, it is important to work with patients and their families or significant others to promote a healthy self-concept. For example, select nursing interventions that help patients regain or restore the elements that contribute to a strong and secure sense of self. The approaches chosen vary according to the level of care required.

Health Promotion. Work with patients to help them develop healthy lifestyle behaviors that contribute to a positive self-concept. For example, develop interventions to support adaptation to stress, such as proper nutrition, regular exercise within the patient's capabilities, and adequate sleep and rest. In addition, teach the patient stress-reducing practices to contribute to a healthy self-concept (Varcarolis and Fosbre, 2021). Nurses are in a unique position to identify lifestyle practices that put a person's self-concept at risk. For example, a young teacher visits a clinic because she is unable to sleep and is experiencing anxiety. In gathering the nursing history, the nurse identifies lifestyle practices such as too little rest; many life changes occurring simultaneously, such as a breakup with fiancé and a recent relocation; and excessive use of alcohol. These data, when taken together, suggest actual or potential self-concept disturbances (Reed-Fitzke, 2020). Determine how the patient views the various lifestyle elements to facilitate the patient's insight into behaviors, and make referrals or provide needed health teaching.

Acute Care. *Kathryn prioritized two nursing diagnoses:* **Acute Pain related to mastectomy incision** *and* **Disturbed Body Image related to negative view of self after mastectomy.** *From previous clinical experiences and postclinical conferences, Kathryn has learned that postoperative care is more than just pain control; often patients must also deal with changes in their body appearance. Even when patients are prepared for physical postoperative changes, dealing with the actual changes is complex. In the case of Mrs. Johnson, her self-esteem and body image are affected by the surgery.*

Kathryn plans pain control for Mrs. Johnson. Kathryn tells Mrs. Johnson that managing acute pain often provides patients with physical energy and emotional energy for care. She explains the pain-control plan from her surgeon and gives Mrs. Johnson a written schedule for when she can have pain medication. Kathyryn also helps Mrs. Johnson use relaxation, which she often practices at home, to help ease her discomfort.

Kathryn knows that Mrs. Johnson is not ready to view her incisional area, and Kathryn must make appropriate adjustments when providing hygiene. She encourages Mrs. Johnson to do as much of the hygiene as she is comfortable with and then Kathryn will complete the other areas. As Kathryn completes hygiene in the left chest and arm region, she also takes time to further assess the surgical site, surgical drains, and drainage. During care, Kathryn notices that Mrs. Johnson is taking some looks at the surgical area. Kathryn chooses not to comment but continues to let Mrs. Johnson look at the area as she is comfortable.

In the acute care setting the nature of an illness or trauma and the treatment and/or diagnostic procedures are potential threats to a patient's self-concept. These threats often result in anxiety and/or fear. In the acute care setting there is often more than one stressor, thus increasing the overall stress level for the patient and family. You need to address a patient's numerous stressors, assisting with modification of lifestyle and offering interventions for adaptation to changes in functioning (e.g., assist devices).

Nurses in the acute care setting encounter patients who face the need to adapt to an altered body image because of surgery or other physical change. With shortened lengths of stay, addressing these needs is difficult to do while in acute care; therefore appropriate follow-up and referrals, including home care, are essential. Remain sensitive to the patient's level of acceptance of any changes. Forcing confrontation with a change before the patient is ready likely will delay acceptance. Signs that a person is receptive to accepting a change include asking questions related to how to manage a particular aspect of what has happened or looking at the changed body area. As the patient expresses readiness to integrate the body change into the self-concept, let the patient know about support groups that are available, and offer to make the initial contact.

Restorative and Continuing Care. Often in a home care environment a nurse has the opportunity to work with a patient to attain a more positive self-concept. Interventions are based on the premise that the patient first develops insight and self-awareness concerning problems and stressors and then acts to solve the problems and cope with

---

BOX 33.8 PATIENT TEACHING
Alterations in Self-Esteem

Objective
- Patient will discuss ways to improve situational low self-esteem.

Teaching Strategies
- Have patient identify strengths and weaknesses and reinforce strengths and successes.
- Discuss situations in which patient's stress may intensify.
- Explore coping resources patient can apply to current problem.
- Provide information needed to allow patient to better care for self.
- Incorporate any psychiatric comorbidities (e.g., depression, anxiety) and alterations to self-esteem and body image when planning patient education sessions.
- Collaborate with patient to identify alternative solutions and new strategies (e.g., communication skills, decision-making skills, healthy coping strategies).

Evaluation
Use the principles of teach-back to evaluate patient/family caregiver learning.
- Describe the new communication skills you have tried since we last met.
- Tell me about the decisions about your care that you have made this week.
- Which coping strategies are you using now?

---

the stressors. One way to achieve this is by helping to reframe the patient's thoughts and feelings in a more positive way. Incorporate this approach into patient teaching for alterations in self-concept, including situational low self-esteem, that sometimes are present in the home care setting (Box 33.8).

Increase a patient's self-awareness by allowing open exploration of thoughts and feelings. The expert use of therapeutic communication skills helps to clarify the expectations of a patient and family. Open exploration makes the situation less threatening for a patient and encourages behaviors that expand self-awareness. Use a nonjudgmental approach when accepting a patient's thoughts and feelings, help the patient clarify interactions with others, and be empathic.

Help the patient apply coping mechanisms most suitable for the health problem. Work closely with the patient to analyze adaptive and maladaptive responses, contrast alternatives, and continue to use coping strategies that are most effective. Collaborate with the patient to identify alternative solutions and expected outcomes to facilitate real change. Design opportunities that result in success, reinforce the patient's skills and strengths, and help to find needed assistance. Encourage the patient to commit to decisions and actions to achieve expected outcomes by teaching the patient to move away from ineffective coping mechanisms and develop successful coping strategies. Supporting attempts that are helpful is essential because with each success a patient is motivated to make another attempt.

◆ Evaluation

Sound clinical judgment is important when evaluating a patient's response to care. Frequent and complete evaluation will assist in determining the effectiveness of the nursing interventions for improving self-concept. Apply critical thinking during evaluation to document patient response to nursing interventions and determine if the outcomes were achieved (Fig. 33.7).

Through the Patient's Eyes. Collaborate with the patient and family caregiver, if appropriate, during the evaluation process. Review whether

Knowledge Base
- Patient's assessment findings, nursing diagnoses, and expected outcomes
- Components of positive self-concept
- Behaviors reflecting self-concept

- Impact of illness stressors on self-concept
- Available community resources
- Expected effects of interventions

Attitudes
- Use confidence when evaluating patient outcomes for improved self-concept
- Exhibit perseverance to find successful therapies if the patient has a permanent alteration affecting body image

Environment
- Presence of environmental stressors (e.g., noise, visitors)
- Risk for lack of privacy
- Unplanned interruptions

Standards
- *ANA Standards and Scope of Nursing Practice*
- Clinical Practice Guidelines and Standards of Practice
- Intellectual standards in measurement
- Agency policies and procedures
- Professional
  - American Cancer Society: About Breast Cancer
  - ANA standards for psychiatric/mental health nursing
  - Community resource standards of practice
- Ethical standards

Experience
- Experience caring for patients with altered self-concept
- Experience caring for patients who had mastectomies, colostomies, burns, paralysis, or other physical changes
- Personal experiences with altered-self concept
- Personal or family illnesses that impact self-concept

(Center wheel) Evaluation / Assessment / Diagnosis / Planning / Implementation; Evaluate outcomes, Recognize cues, Take action, Clinical Decision Making, Analyze cues, Generate solutions, Prioritize hypotheses

FIG. 33.7 Critical thinking model for self-concept evaluation. (Clinical Judgment Measurement Model copyright © NCSBN. All rights reserved.)

their expectations were met. If expectations were not met, ask what the patient would like to have changed. Determine if the patient perceives satisfaction with relationships with health care providers and the planned interventions. Does the patient and/or family caregiver feel that the patient education was sufficient? Do they have enough information to continue some of the interventions at home? A patient's perception of a supportive relationship with caregivers often results in satisfaction with the care provided and a willingness to continue prescribed interventions in the home setting.

Patient Outcomes. Expected outcomes for a patient with a self-concept disturbance include displaying behaviors indicating a positive self-concept, verbalizing statements of self-acceptance, and validating acceptance of a change in appearance or function. Key observational indicators of a patient's self-concept are nonverbal behaviors (Varcarolis and Fosbre, 2021). For example, a patient who initially had difficulty in making eye contact now demonstrates a more positive self-concept by making more frequent eye contact during conversation. Social interaction, adequate self-care, acceptance of changes resulting from illnesses or operations, and statements indicating understanding of patient education indicate progress. Investing in satisfying hobbies, getting physical exercise, exerting choices in daily life, understanding their own needs during transitions, and adapting to life circumstances are evidence of self-esteem and self-efficacy in older adults (Orth et al., 2018; Touhy and Jett, 2020). A positive attitude toward rehabilitation and increased movement toward independence facilitate a return to preexisting roles at work or at home. Patterns of interacting also reflect changes in self-concept.

For example, a patient who has been hesitant to express personal views more readily offers opinions and ideas as self-esteem increases.

Kathryn includes Mr. and Mrs. Johnson in evaluating the outcomes of her nursing care. Mr. and Mrs. Johnson both admit this is a hard adjustment. On the second postoperative day they are able to discuss with the oncology nurse specialist the concerns they both have with each other. Also, Mr. Johnson is able to connect with the community breast cancer support group for patients, spouses, and families.

Pain control improves by the third postoperative, discharge day. Mrs. Johnson's pain has been below 3/10 for the last 24 hours and she is prescribed oral analgesics. She works with the oncology nurse specialist and views her incision, and she understands what normal healing should look like and postoperative dressing and drain care. She performs a return demonstration of dressing and drain care, as she will need to do this for 3 days until she returns to the surgeon. She is also able to state any complications that require a phone call to the surgeon. The oncology nurse specialist answers questions about the reconstruction process. Mrs. Johnson comments that she feels less anxious and she has more knowledge about decisions ahead.

If the patient status changes and the outcomes of care sometimes become unrealistic or inappropriate, revise the plan as needed. Reflect on past successful experiences with other patients. Often adjustment to major changes in self-concept or its components can take a year or longer. Educate the patient and family that because this period is long, it does not suggest that the patient is having a problem adjusting to the change. Changes in self-concept take time. Although change is often slow, care of a patient with a self-concept disturbance is rewarding.

Look for signs that the patient has reduced some stressors and that some behaviors have become more adaptive. If initial outcomes regarding self-concept are not met, individualize care using the following questions:

- Tell me what you will do if you are not able to return to work (may substitute "school" or "home") as planned.
- What will you do if you are not feeling any better about yourself in 2 weeks? Do you have an individual to contact and talk to about these feelings?
- What strategies are you using to improve how you view yourself and your perception of how others view you? Are you happy with these strategies?
- How will you know that your sense of worth is improving?

KEY POINTS

- Components of self-concept including identity, body image, and role performance can be affected by developmental milestones and life events.
- Self-concept and self-esteem stressors include developmental and relationship changes, illness (particularly chronic illness involving changes in what were normal activities), surgery, accidents, and the responses of other individuals to changes resulting from these events.
- Self-concept and self-esteem change with developmental milestones and the person's response to those events.
- Health care providers can influence a patient's self-concept.
- A health care provider's self-concept is influenced by the practice environment and is positively affected by effective teamwork.
- Be aware of how cultural variations affect a patient's self-concept and self-esteem and incorporate culturally sensitive interventions.
- Assessing a patient's self-concept includes obtaining information about the patient's perception of self, family's and significant other's perceptions, and coping strategies.
- Planning care for self-concept alterations must include collaboration with the patient in identifying measurable outcomes and methods to help patients achieve these outcomes of care.
- Implementing nursing interventions for self-concept disturbance involves using evidence-based care to expand the patient's self-awareness, encourage self-exploration, aid in self-evaluation, and help patients achieve outcomes of care.
- Evaluation for self-concept alterations must include the patient's response to nursing interventions and perceptions of changes in self-concept in addition to the health care evaluation of change.

REFLECTIVE LEARNING

From the ongoing case study in this chapter, you know that Mrs. Johnson is 52 years old and is recovering from a left radical mastectomy. She is in her room requesting that the curtains remain drawn at the window and lights off. She doesn't initiate any interaction with hospital staff when they enter her room. She cries frequently and tells her nurse that she cannot even look at her chest, at its bandages and drains, because to her they are symbols of her disfigurement. She states, "I don't think I feel good as a person, let alone as a woman. Heaven knows what my chest will look like after the bandages are removed. I don't want to see it." She does not request medication, and often her pain increases to 9/10 prior to administration of pain medication; following administration her pain level drops to 3/10.

Mrs. Johnson had a routine mammogram 1 month ago and an abnormality was noted. Following diagnostic screening, scans, and testing, it was determined that surgery was needed. During surgery, two lymph nodes were positive for cancer, which resulted in a radical mastectomy. She thought she was just going to have a lumpectomy, so the radical mastectomy was unexpected.

*An initial self-concept nursing diagnosis was **Disturbed Body Image** related to negative view of self after mastectomy. However, Mrs. Johnson also said that she is not sleeping well and is restless. She still has some **Acute Pain** related to mastectomy incision, and this is a priority diagnosis.*

Mrs. Johnson is ready for discharge and will recover at home. Her husband will be home with her and they are planning to go to the community breast cancer support group together.

- Think about the type of additional assessment data that would indicate Mrs. Johnson is at increased risk for ongoing low self-esteem during discharge and recovery at home. (Recognize Cues)
- Considering the fact that Mrs. Johnson is discharged to home and is in the recovery phase of an unexpected radical mastectomy, identify additional assessment data and cues that support additional nursing diagnoses. (Analyze Cues)
- Consider all the information in the case study, care plan, and concept map and the additional postdischarge nursing diagnoses you just identified. What are the priority home care needs for Mrs. Johnson? (Prioritize Diagnoses)
- Review the case study information, Mrs. Johnson's nursing care plan, and the concept map. Describe additional nursing interventions to help resolve any ongoing situational low self-esteem during recovery at home. (Generate Solutions)
- Continue to review the case study, care plan, concept map, and discharge needs, and from the list below identify the appropriate nursing intervention to help reduce Mrs. Johnson's anxiety during recovery at home. List in order of priority, with number 1 being the most important. (Take Action)
  1. Teach and, if needed, demonstrate comfort measures for postoperative incisional pain.
  2. Provide community health resources.
  3. Provide time for Mrs. Johnson to discuss her fears and concerns.
  4. Encourage Mr. and Mrs. Johnson to identify and discuss strategies they learned through the community breast cancer support group to comfort one another.
  5. Teach Mrs. Johnson techniques regarding basic hygiene care, methods for dressing changes, pain management, and other needs.
- Evaluate the discharge plan. What criteria support achievement of discharge expected outcomes or support revision? (Evaluate Outcomes)

REVIEW QUESTIONS

1. A 50-year-old woman is recovering from a bilateral mastectomy. She refuses to eat, discourages visitors, and pays little attention to her appearance. One morning the nurse enters the room to see the patient with her hair combed and makeup applied. Which of the following is the best response from the nurse?
   1. "What's the special occasion?"
   2. "You must be feeling better today."
   3. "This is the first time I've seen you look this good."
   4. "I see that you've combed your hair and put on makeup."
2. A 30-year-old patient diagnosed with major depressive disorder has a nursing diagnosis of *Situational Low Self-Esteem related to negative view of self*. Which of the following are appropriate interventions by the nurse? (Select all that apply.)
   1. Encourage reconnecting with high school friends.
   2. Role-play to increase assertiveness skills.
   3. Focus on identifying strengths and accomplishments.
   4. Provide time for journaling to explore underlying thoughts and feelings.
   5. Explore new job opportunities.

3. A patient who is depressed is crying and verbalizes feelings of low self-esteem and self-worth, such as "I'm such a failure. I can't do anything right." What is the nurse's best response?
   1. Remain with the patient until the patient validates feeling more stable.
   2. Tell the patient that this is not true and that every person has a purpose in life.
   3. Review recent behaviors or accomplishments that demonstrate skill ability.
   4. Reassure the patient that you know how he or she is feeling and that things will get better.

4. A 20-year-old patient diagnosed with an eating disorder has a nursing diagnosis of *Situational Low Self-Esteem*. Which of the following nursing interventions are appropriate to address self-esteem? (Select all that apply.)
   1. Offer independent decision-making opportunities.
   2. Review previously successful coping strategies.
   3. Provide a quiet environment with minimal stimuli.
   4. Support a dependent role throughout treatment.
   5. Increase calorie intake to promote weight stabilization.

5. The nurse can increase a patient's self-awareness and self-concept through which of the following actions? (Select all that apply.)
   1. Helping the patient define personal problems clearly
   2. Allowing the patient to openly explore thoughts and feelings
   3. Reframing the patient's thoughts and feelings in a more positive way
   4. Having family members assume more responsibility during times of stress
   5. Recommending self-help reading materials

6. Which of the following assessment findings support the nursing diagnosis of an altered self-concept? (Select all that apply.)
   1. Uneven gait
   2. Slumped posture
   3. Avoidance of eye contact
   4. Frequent use of the call light
   5. Poor personal hygiene

7. A nurse in an outpatient setting is performing an admission assessment on a 77-year-old woman who was suddenly widowed 3 weeks ago. During the health history the patient tells the nurse that at times she "feels lost and isolated" and says she "does not feel like participating in previous social or hobby activities." She says she "just doesn't feel like her usual self." The nurse needs to understand that which of the following most directly influences the patient's current self-concept?

1. Attitude and behaviors of relatives providing care
2. Caring behaviors of the nurse and health care team
3. Level of education, economic status, and living conditions
4. Adjustment to role change, loss of loved ones, and physical energy

8. A nurse is working with an older adult who recently moved to an assisted-living center because of declining physical capabilities and socialization. Which nursing interventions are directed at promoting self-esteem in this patient? (Select all that apply.)
   1. Commending the patient's efforts at completing self-care tasks
   2. Assuming that the patient's physical complaints are attention-seeking measures
   3. Encouraging the patient to add personal items to the residence
   4. Minimizing time discussing memories and past achievements with the patient
   5. Providing decision-making opportunities to join the center's daily activities program

9. A nurse is caring for a 40-year-old man who was diagnosed with Crohn's disease several years ago, resulting in numerous hospitalizations each year for the past 3 years. Which of the following behaviors interfere with the developmental tasks of middle adulthood? (Select all that apply.)
   1. Sends birthday cards to friends and family
   2. Refuses visitors while hospitalized
   3. Self-absorbed in physical and psychological issues
   4. Performs self-care activities
   5. Communicates feelings of inadequacy

10. When assessing a patient's adjustment to the role changes brought about by a medical condition such as a stroke, which of the following are critical assessment questions? (Select all that apply.)
    1. What are your thoughts about returning to work?
    2. What questions do you have about your medications?
    3. How has your health affected your relationship with your partner?
    4. What level of physical activity are you able to perform?
    5. What concerns do you have about another stroke?

Answers: 1. 4; 2. 3, 4; 3. 1; 4. 1, 2; 5. 1, 2, 3; 6. 2, 3; 7. 4; 8. 1, 3, 5; 9. 2, 3, 5; 10. 1, 3.

Rationales for Review Questions can be found on the Evolve website.

REFERENCES

American Nurses Association: *Nursing: scope and standards of practice*, ed 4, Silver Spring, MD, 2021, American Nurses Association.

Centers for Disease Control and Prevention: *Youth risk behavior surveillance system (YRBSS)*, 2020. https://www.cdc.gov/healthyyouth/data/yrbs/index.htm. Accessed June 25, 2021.

Erikson E: *Childhood and society*, ed 2, New York, 1963, WW Norton.

Hockenberry M, et al: *Wong's nursing care of infants and children*, ed 11, St Louis, 2019, Elsevier.

Rosenberg M: *Society and the adolescent self-image*, Princeton, NJ, 1965, Princeton University Press.

Touhy TA, Jett KF: *Ebersole and Hess' toward healthy aging: human needs and nursing response*, ed 10, St Louis, 2020, Elsevier.

Varcarolis EM, Fosbre CD: *Essentials of psychiatric mental health nursing*, ed 4, St Louis, 2021, Elsevier.

RESEARCH REFERENCES

Agrahari SK, Kinra A: A comparative study on self-concept of adolescent boys and girls, *Indian J Posit Psychol* 8(4):519, 2017.

Barnett MD, et al: Meaning in life and self-esteem help hospice nurses withstand prolonged exposure to death, *J Nurs Manag* 27:775, 2019.

Bartsch LA, et al: Self-esteem and alcohol use among youths, *J Child Adolesc Subst Abuse* 26(5):414, 2017.

Benninger E, Savahl S: The children's Delphi: considerations for developing a programme for promoting children's self-concept and well-being, *Child Fam Soc Work* 22(2):1094, 2017.

Betancourt J, et al: Cross-cultural care and communication, *UpToDate*, 2020. https://www.uptodate.com/contents/cross-cultural-care-and-communication. Accessed June 25, 2021.

Bleidorn W, et al: Age and gender differences in self-esteem—a cross-cultural window, *J Pers Soc Psychol* 111:396, 2016.

Bukstein O: *Approach to treating substance use disorder in adolescents*, 2020, *UpToDate*. https://www.uptodate.com/contents/approach-to-treating-substance-use-disorder-in-adolescents. Accessed June 25, 2021.

Cao Q, Liang Y: Perceived social support and life satisfaction in drug addicts: self-esteem and loneliness as mediators, *J Health Psychol* 25(7):976, 2020.

Cicero D: Measurement invariance of the self-concept clarity scale across race and sex, *J Psychopathol Behav Assess* 42:296, 2020.

Easterbrook M, et al: Socioeconomic status and the structure of the self-concept, *Br J Soc Psychol* 59(1):66, 2020.

Eleuteri S, et al: Identity, relationships, sexuality, and risky behaviors of adolescents in the context of social media, *Sex Relat Ther* 32(3–4):354, 2017.

Esnaola I, Sesé A: The development of multiple self-concept dimensions during adolescence, *J Res Adolesc* 30(Suppl 1):100, 2020.

Franco C, et al: Improving psychosocial functioning in mastectomized women through a mindfulness-based program: *flow meditation*, *Int J Stress Manag* 27(1):74, 2020.

Garn AC, et al: Moderate-to-vigorous physical activity as a predictor of changes in physical self-concept in adolescents, *Health Psychol* 39(3):190, 2020.

Heflin M: *Geriatric health maintenance*, *UpToDate*, 2020. https://www.uptodate.com/contents/geriatric-health-maintenance. Accessed June 25, 2021.

Hsu Y, Lu FJH: Older adults' physical exercise and health-related quality of life: the mediating role of physical self-concept, *Educ Gerontol* 44(4):247, 2018.

Jabłoński MC, et al: Exploring the relationship between the body self and the sense of coherence in women after surgical treatment for breast cancer, *Psychooncology* 28(1):54, 2019.

Leão ER, et al: Stress, self-esteem, and well-being among female health professionals: a randomized clinical trial on the impact of a self-care intervention mediated by the senses, *PLoS ONE* 12(2):e0172455, 2017.

Lee CH, et al: Longitudinal trajectory of the relationship between self-esteem and substance abuse from adolescence to young adulthood, *J Sch Health* 88(1):9, 2018.

Manomenidis G, et al: Is self-esteem actually the protective factor in nursing burnout? *Int J Caring Sci* 10(3):1348, 2017.

Orth U, et al: Development of self-esteem from age 4 to 94 years: a meta-analysis of longitudinal studies, *Psychol Bull* 144(10):1045, 2018.

Reed-Fitzke K: The role of self-concepts in emerging adult depression: a systematic research synthesis, *J Adult Dev*, 27:36, 2020.

Sukamti N, et al: The influence of coping skills training and family health education on self-esteem among adolescents in substance abuse prevention, *Enferm Clin*, 29(Suppl 2):532, 2019.

Thomaes S, et al: Why most children think well of themselves, *Child Dev* 88(6):1873, 2017.

Tonsing KN: Ow R: Quality of life, self-esteem, and future expectation of adolescent and young adult cancer survivors, *Health Soc Work* 43(1):15, 2018.

Vartanian LR, et al: Risk and resiliency factors related to body dissatisfaction and disordered eating: the identity disruption model, *Int J Eat Disord* 51:322, 2018.

Watt AD, Konnert CA: Body satisfaction and self-esteem among middle-aged and older women: the mediating roles of social and temporal comparisons and self-objectification, *Aging Ment Health* 24(5):797, 2020.

Wilkins AC, Miller SA: Secure girls: class, sexuality, and self-esteem, *Sexualities* 20(7):815, 2017.

Zhou K, et al: Body image mediated the relationship between post-surgery needs and health-related quality of life among women with breast cancer: a cross-sectional study, *Health Qual Life Outcomes* 18(1):1, 2020.

Sexuality

OBJECTIVES

- Explain key concepts of sexual development across the life span.
- Identify patient risk factors in the area of sexual health.
- Discuss a nurse's role in maintaining or enhancing a patient's sexual health.
- Identify personal attitudes, beliefs, and biases related to sexuality.
- Assess a patient's sexuality and sexual health within the context of a patient's lifestyle.
- Compare causes of sexual dysfunction.
- Formulate appropriate nursing diagnoses for patients with alterations in sexuality.

- Create a patient-centered plan of care to help patients meet achievable and measurable outcomes of care to enhance their sexual health.
- Use your critical thinking and clinical judgment when helping patients meet their sexual needs.
- Select appropriate patient-centered nursing interventions using clinical judgment to promote sexual health.
- Evaluate patient outcomes related to sexual health needs.

KEY TERMS

Bisexual

Contraception

Gay

Gender identity

Infertility

Lesbian

Sexual dysfunction

Sexual health

Sexual identity

Sexual orientation

Sexuality

Sexually transmitted infections (STIs)

Transgender

MEDIA RESOURCES

http://evolve.elsevier.com/Potter/fundamentals/

- Review Questions
- Case Study with Questions
- Concept Map Creator

- Audio Glossary
- Content Updates
- Answers to QSEN Activity and Review Questions

Mr. Clements is 65 years old and had a myocardial infarction (MI) 3 days ago. He has hypertension, which is treated with propranolol. Mr. Clements is married and lives with his wife. Mrs. Clements is visiting her husband. She has expressed concern with her sister about Mr. Clement's health and the couple's ability to continue having a sexual relationship. She has not shared this with health care staff.

Joshua, a 30-year-old nursing student, is caring for Mr. Clements. Joshua knows from reading his textbook that changes in health status often result in stressors that can affect a person's sexuality. Joshua also is aware that some antihypertensive medications cause side effects such as decreased sex drive or impotence. He plans to begin caring for Mr. Clements by using his clinical judgment to assess the patient's sexual health and identify if there are any stressors that are affecting Mr. and Mrs. Clements. He will individualize nursing interventions that support their adaptation to this change in health status.

Sexuality is a broad term that refers to all aspects of being sexual, including how you identity yourself sexually and with whom you choose to be intimate. It is a part of who you are as a person and is important for overall health. Sexuality includes a person's thoughts and feelings about the body, gender identity, romantic and erotic attachments toward

others, and attitudes toward sexual functioning. Our sexual health is based on our ability to form healthy relationships with others. Sex is considered a basic physiological need, and sexual intimacy throughout the life span is equally important for sexual health. Healthy sexuality enables people to develop and maintain their fullest potential.

Sexuality is important for overall health. Even though discussion of sexual topics is more prominent in the media, individuals generally do not understand sexual health and the impact of disease and associated treatments. Although patients may be hesitant to bring up their concerns, they often share their feelings when a nurse addresses sexuality in a relaxed, matter-of-fact manner.

Expression of an individual's sexuality is influenced by interactions among biological, social, psychological, spiritual, religious, economic, political, historical, and cultural factors (World Health Organization [WHO], 2018). Within this complex context, values, attitudes, and beliefs as well as behaviors and relationships with others influence sexuality.

Sexuality differs from *sexual health*. According to WHO (WHO, 2018; WHO, 2021), **sexual health** is a state of physical, emotional, mental, and social well-being in relation to sexuality and is not merely the absence of disease or dysfunction. Sexual health requires a positive and respectful approach to sexuality and sexual relationships, as well as the possibility of having pleasurable and safe sexual experiences that are free of coercion, discrimination, and violence. People who are sexually healthy have a positive and respectful approach to sexuality and sexual relationships.

It is important to apply clinical judgment in care for a patient's sexuality and sexual health. To feel comfortable addressing sexuality, you use therapeutic communication skills (see Chapter 24) and your knowledge about all aspects of sexuality, including values and issues surrounding sexuality. Religious teachings, cultural influences on male or female roles, beliefs about sexual orientation, and social and environmental climates influence the values systems for both patients and health care providers.

SCIENTIFIC KNOWLEDGE BASE

A broad knowledge base allows you to have a holistic view of patients, thus promoting high-quality patient care that best meets the sexuality and sexual health needs of each patient and family. A sound scientific knowledge base regarding sexuality provides you with the necessary information to accurately interpret your patients' needs and to help them achieve sexual health. A basic understanding of sexual development, sexual identity and sexual orientation, contraception, and sexually transmitted infections (STIs) is necessary.

Sexual Development

Sexuality changes as a person grows and develops. Each stage of development brings changes in sexual functioning and the role of sexuality in relationships. Sexuality is a complex process that involves many factors. It begins at birth and continues throughout life. Erikson's (1963) psychosocial theory of development helps you understand key tasks that individuals face at various stages of development. Early researchers focused on sexuality from adolescence to middle age, but we now understand that sexuality is already in progress at birth and continues throughout life, including into old age (LeVay et al., 2019).

Infancy and Early Childhood. The first several years of life are crucial in the development of sexuality and gender identity. Young children are curious about physical differences, and they learn through the senses (e.g., touch) (National Center on the Sexual Behavior of Youth [NCSBY], n.d.). Children imitate the behavior of other children and adults, and whether a child repeats a sexual behavior is often related to how caregivers respond to that behavior (NCSBY, n.d.). Children become aware of differences between the sexes, begin to perceive that they identify a gender, and interpret the behaviors of others as socially consistent with genders (LeVay et al., 2019).

School-Age Years. Puberty is a time in the lives of school-age children in which their bodies begin to change in many ways, allowing them to be capable of reproducing (NCSBY, n.d.). Puberty is a time that brings many changes in children's bodies, minds, emotions, and relationships with others. It is an important time of life and in many cultures is honored through coming-of-age rituals during adolescence (NCSBY, n.d.). This can be a difficult time for caregivers such as parents, educators, and peer groups who serve as role models and influence how to relate to other people. Preadolescent children often segregate by sex, which minimizes heterosexual activities and facilitates same-sex sexual behaviors. This early sexual behavior is not indicative of sexual orientation (LeVay et al., 2019). Because school-age children continue to be curious, typical childhood sexual play is normal. But caregivers need to know which behaviors are not normal. School-age children do not obsess about sexual activity or practice more advanced sexual behaviors such as intercourse or oral

sex. Intrusive, planned, forced, or aggressive sexual acts are not part of typical or normal sex play of children but are instead problem behaviors (NCSBY, n.d.). School-age children have questions about the physical and emotional aspects of sex. They need accurate information from home and school about changes in their bodies and emotions and what to expect as they move into adolescence. Parents often find it uncomfortable to communicate with their children about bodily changes and sexuality; thus children often turn to other sources of information that may be inaccurate, such as sexual information and troublesome values from other youth and from movies, magazines, song lyrics, the Internet, and television (NCSBY, n.d.).

Puberty/Adolescence. Adolescence is often marked by increased sexual interest (LeVay et al., 2019). Adolescents function within a powerful peer group, with the almost constant anxiety of "Am I normal?" and "Will I be accepted?" (Fig. 34.1). They face many decisions and need accurate information on topics such as body changes, sexual activity and identity, emotional responses within sexual relationships, STIs, contraception, and pregnancy. Both developmental disabilities and medical conditions can affect children's sexual development. Health care professionals and family members often are unsure how to understand, accept, and respond to sexual development in individuals with disabilities. Many adolescents with developmental disabilities may wish to date or otherwise be in intimate relationships with other youths. Unfortunately, the youth are less likely to have been provided developmentally appropriate sexual education (NCSBY, n.d.).

The status of sexual health education varies throughout the United States and is insufficient in many areas. In most states, fewer than half of high schools teach all 20 sexual health topics recommended by the Centers for Disease Control and Prevention (CDC, 2019). In addition, sex education is not starting early enough; in no state did more than half of middle schools teach all 20 sexual health topics recommended by the CDC. Finally, sex education has been declining over time. The percentage of U.S. schools in which students are required to receive instruction on prevention of human immunodeficiency virus (HIV) also significantly decreased (CDC, 2019).

Adolescence is often a time when individuals explore their sexual identity and primary sexual orientation (LeVay et al., 2019). Adolescents often face significant stress related to sexual identity. They benefit from education about sexuality and sexual health issues, including STIs such as HIV and chlamydia (CDC, 2019).

In the United States almost 40% of high school students reported that they had sexual intercourse at least one time, and 10% of high

FIG. 34.1 Adolescents function within a powerful network of peers as they explore their sexual identity. (© bikeriderlondon.)

school students had four or more sexual partners (Kann et al., 2018). The use of social media influences adolescent sexuality because it may be the first opportunity for adolescents to explore their sexuality freely. Adolescents who engage in risky sexual behaviors may experience negative health outcomes such as STIs and unintended pregnancy (LeVay et al., 2019). Research shows higher rates of STIs among some racial or ethnic minority groups compared with Whites. However, it is important to understand that these higher rates are not caused by ethnicity or heritage but by social conditions such as poverty, large gaps between the rich and the poor, fewer jobs, and low education levels (CDC, 2020e). These factors make it more difficult for people to stay sexually healthy.

If an adolescent practices a pattern of risk-taking behavior, it tends to be established and to continue throughout life. Parents need to be educated and understand the importance of providing factual information, sharing their values, and promoting sound decision-making skills. Adolescents and parents often disagree about whether they talked about sexual issues, which reinforces the need for clear communication (Grossman et al., 2017). Parents and guardians need to know that, even with the best guidance and information, adolescents make their own decisions and need to be held accountable for them. Support from peers, family, school counselors, clergy, nurses, and other health professionals is important during this time.

Young Adulthood. Although young adults have matured physically, they continue to explore and mature emotionally in relationships. Intimacy and sexuality are issues for all young adults, whether they are in a sexual relationship, choose to abstain from sex, remain single by choice, or are not in a committed relationship. Sexual activity is often defined as a basic need, and healthy sexual desire is channeled into forms of intimacy throughout a lifetime. At times, young adults require support and education or psychotherapy to achieve satisfying sexual relationships.

Middle Adulthood. Changes in physical appearance in middle adulthood sometimes lead to concerns about sexual attractiveness. In addition, actual physical changes related to aging affect sexual functioning. Decreasing levels of estrogen in perimenopausal women lead to diminished vaginal lubrication and decreased vaginal elasticity. Both of these changes often lead to dyspareunia, or the occurrence of pain during intercourse. Decreasing levels of estrogen may also result in a decreased desire for sexual activity. As men age, they are likely to experience changes such as an increase in the postejaculatory refractory period and delayed ejaculation. Anticipatory guidance regarding these normal changes, using vaginal lubrication, and creating time for caressing and tenderness ease concerns regarding sexual functioning. Some aging adults also need to adjust to the impact of chronic illness, medications, aches, pains, and other health concerns about sexuality. Older adults who report being highly satisfied with their sex lives also tend to be satisfied with their lives (Skałacka and Gerymski, 2019).

Later in the adult years some individuals need to adjust to the social and emotional changes associated with children moving away from home. This results in either a time of renewed intimacy between partners or a time when formerly intimate partners realize that they no longer care for one another or have common interests. In either case, when children leave home, intimate relationships usually change.

Older Adulthood. Sexuality in older adults is an important aspect of health that often is overlooked by health care providers. Studies show a positive correlation between sexual activity and physical health in older adults (Touhy and Jett, 2021). Research indicates that many older adults are more sexually active than previously thought and engage in high-risk sexual encounters, resulting in a steady increase of HIV and STI rates (Box 34.1).

BOX 34.1   FOCUS ON OLDER ADULTS

Sexuality in Older Adults

- Sexuality and continued interest in sex throughout middle and late life are usually associated with good physical health.
- Physiological changes with aging that influence sexual response are multifactorial and related to various factors, including circulation and hormones.
- Issues with the aging sexual response are often related to illnesses and side effects from medications.
- Older adults are often reluctant to discuss sexual problems with health care providers.
- Older adults who live in extended-care facilities often lose their privacy and experience a decline in physical and cognitive abilities that affects their sexual expression. People who live in assisted-living facilities have more privacy and are often able to live as couples.
- As the population ages and remains healthy, increasing numbers of older lesbian, gay, bisexual, transgender, queer, questioning, asexual, and others (LGBTQ+) people remain sexually active.
- Increased availability of treatments for male and female sexual dysfunction contributes to continued sexual activity throughout the life span.
- Older sexually active adults are at risk for contracting sexually transmitted infections. Because the risk of pregnancy is not an issue, older adults often do not recognize the need for protected sex when becoming active with new and/or multiple partners.

From Touhy TA, Jett K: Ebersole and Hess' gerontological nursing and healthy aging, ed 6, St Louis, 2021, Elsevier.

Factors that determine sexual activity in older adults include present health status, medications, past and present life satisfaction, and the status of marital or intimate relationships. Nurses working with older adults need to assess the sexual identity, sexual interest and functioning, and general perception of sexual health of their patients and plan accordingly (Touhy and Jett, 2021). It is essential to maintain a nonjudgmental attitude and convey that sexual activity is normal in later years. It is important to have adequate knowledge about sexuality across the life span and to be aware of your own attitudes and beliefs while promoting sexual health in older adults (Komlenac et al., 2019). Patients achieve positive outcomes when their health care team promotes an environment that encourages a culture of acceptance, enhances sexual health knowledge, and adopts positive attitudes toward the sexuality of the older adult (Bauer et al., 2019).

To be effective in promoting sexual health, you need to understand the normal sexual changes that occur as people age. The excitement phase prolongs in both men and women, and it usually takes longer for them to reach orgasm. The refractory time following orgasm is also longer. Both males and females experience a reduced availability of sex hormones. Men often have erections that are less firm and shorter acting. Women usually do not have difficulty maintaining sexual function unless they have a medical condition that impairs their sexual activity. Typically the infrequency of sex in older women is related to the age, health, and sexual function of their partner. Women continue to experience changes related to menopause, and those with problems related to urinary incontinence often experience embarrassment during intercourse. Individuals who have physically disabling conditions often need information about which positions are more comfortable when having sexual intercourse (LeVay et al., 2019).

Sexual Identity and Sexual Orientation

Sexual identity is how a person thinks about himself or herself sexually. It includes gender identity, gender role, and sexual orientation.

Gender identity is a person's private view of maleness and femaleness, and gender role is the male and female behavior a person exhibits. Assessing one's sexual orientation, defined as a person's gender identity in relation to the gender to which they are attracted, and gender identity requires you to acknowledge and accept the LGBTQ+ (lesbian, gay, bisexual, transgender, queer, questioning, asexual, and others) continuum (Landry and Kensler, 2019).

As a person grows and develops, so does his or her sexuality. Knowledge of sexual development and changes throughout the life span is essential for you as a nurse. An adult has achieved physical maturation but is continuing to explore and define emotional maturation in relationships. Even into adulthood people continue to struggle with questions about who they are, how they want to present themselves, and what type of partners they find most attractive. As a nurse, it helps to have a clear sense of your own sexual identity because it influences your ability to form open relationships, which is needed to support patients' sexual health. You will provide care to individuals whose sexual orientation and sexual identity are heterosexual (attracted to different-sex partners), lesbian or gay (same-sex partners; women-women and men-men, respectively), bisexual (having both same and other-gendered partners), transgender (people whose gender identity or expression is different from their sex at birth), queer (an umbrella term representing all individuals who fall out of the gender and sexuality binary), questioning (exploring one's sexual orientation or identity), asexual or aromantic (does not experience sexual or romantic attraction), fluid (fluctuating mix of options), pansexual (sexual attraction to members of all gender identities/expressions), and cisgender (gender identity, gender expression, and biological sex all align), as well as qualities uniquely defined by your patient (American Psychological Association [APA], 2020). You will also care for patients who are involved in intimate relationships with several partners and for patients whose sexual relationships occur outside of marriage or a committed relationship. You may not learn a great deal about a patient's sexual preferences, even if you ask direct questions. As a caregiver you must learn to accept a person's sexual orientation and sexual identity and help individuals understand the implications that their health condition has on maintaining healthy sexual relationships and on achieving positive health outcomes.

Sexuality Stressors. As a nurse you work with patients who are making decisions or dealing with issues related to sexuality on a regular basis. For example, people of all ages face reproductive health issues, including contraception, infertility, sexual performance and dysfunction, and sexual satisfaction. Understanding some of the decisions and issues that patients face increases your effectiveness in helping them reach their maximum level of sexual health.

LGBTQ+ individuals have unique stressors related to their sexual identity and sexual orientation, which is the emotional, romantic, or sexual attraction to others. Peer, family, and social support is often lacking. Nurses need to be culturally competent and knowledgeable in how to eliminate health disparities and improve interventions and outcomes for patients who are in vulnerable populations, including the LGBTQ+ community. Nurses are in a unique position to support patients and provide education and resources based on their individual needs. Patients who are LGBTQ+ experience barriers to health care that include fear of discrimination, insensitivity, and lack of knowledge about LGBTQ+-specific health needs. This may create negative feelings around getting tested and treated for STIs (CDC, 2020e). Individuals in this population are at high risk for STIs, depression, suicide, and victimization (Landry and Kensler, 2019; Johns et al., 2019; Pachankis et al., 2020). Research has also shown that young gay and bisexual men who have sex with older partners are at a greater risk for HIV infection because an older partner is more likely to have had more sexual partners or other risks and is more likely to be infected with HIV (CDC, 2020b).

Health care providers should specifically explain during assessment of patients that it is important to disclose sexual preferences and behaviors because many patients do not make the connection between sexuality and physical health (Komlenac et al., 2019). Alterations in sexual health occur from a variety of situations such as illness, infertility, trauma, and abuse. Sexual dysfunction involves problems with desire, arousal, or orgasm. Erectile dysfunction (ED) is a common problem among older men. It is generally related to chronic diseases such as diabetes, kidney disease, alcohol dependence, depression, neurological disorders, vascular insufficiency, and diseases of the prostate (Touhy and Jett, 2021). In addition, side effects of medications or medical conditions also contribute to sexual dysfunction. Examples of common medications that can cause sexual dysfunction include statins, antihypertensives, antidepressants, antipsychotics, and benzodiazepines.

Older-adult women can also experience sexual dysfunction. For example, in a study of older women who experienced a stroke, sexuality was affected by negatively impacting self-concept and by limiting the ways in which sexuality could be expressed (Lever and Pryor, 2017). The causes of sexual dysfunction are both physiological and psychological. Sometimes the cause of a dysfunction cannot be identified or is a result of a combination of several factors.

Because sexual dysfunction sometimes results from the use of medications, it is important to include a discussion of sexual side effects in patient teaching. Your patient is more likely to adhere to a treatment plan if you discuss side effects of medications that alter sexual function with both partners and if the patient is able to make an informed decision. It is also important to ask if patients are continuing to take those medications that are causing any sexual side effects. A patient's health greatly influences sexual response (from desire to arousal to orgasm). The availability of sexual performance–enhancing medications such as sildenafil and tadalafil has changed the lives of many couples. These medications treat ED but are contraindicated in men with coronary artery disease or those taking common cardiac drugs.

Changing physical appearance and concerns about physical attractiveness affect sexual functioning. Many older adults remain sexually active. Some older adults face health concerns and societal attitudes that make it difficult for them to continue sexual activity. Although declining physical abilities may sometimes make sex as they knew it painful or impossible, with intervention older adults are able to experiment with and learn alternative ways of sexual expression.

Hormonally stimulated changes brought on by developmental maturation are also stressors that affect sexuality across the life span. Menarche, the onset of menstrual cycle in girls, is occurring at an earlier age in the United States, and some adolescent girls are unaware that it is normal to grow pubic, underarm, and body hair and deposit more fat on their hips and breasts, all of which also affect body image.

As boys approach puberty, physical changes include nocturnal emissions and ejaculation, increasing sexual desire, and increased hygiene needs. Mutually monogamous relationships, delayed sexual debut, and the consistent use of latex condoms reduce the risk of STIs as well as unplanned pregnancies (CDC, 2020b). Therefore patient teaching needs to include instruction on sexual health and decision making, breast and testicular self-examinations, and prevention of sexually transmitted infections (STIs), which are spread through oral, anal, or vaginal sexual contact.

Older women experiencing menopause, including the cessation of menstrual periods, experience changes in vaginal lubrication and sexual interest. Most menopausal women recognize the importance of maintaining an active sex life and are able to maintain a satisfying sex life.

TABLE 34.1 Signs and Symptoms That Indicate Possible Current Sexual Abuse or a History of Sexual Abuse

Types of Findings	Symptoms Often Found in Children	Symptoms Often Found in Adults
Injuries and/or physical signs	Bruises, bleeding, soreness, infection, or irritation of external genitalia, anus, mouth, or throat Sexually transmitted infections Recurrent urinary tract infections Unintended pregnancy Chronic pain Difficulty walking or sitting Unusual odor in genital area Penile discharge Torn, stained, or bloody underclothing	Welts, bruising, swelling, scars, burns, or lacerations on arms, legs, breasts, or abdomen Wounds that do not match the patient's "story" Multiple bruises in various stages of healing Vaginal or rectal bleeding Fractures of face, nose, ribs, or arms Trauma to labia, vagina, cervix, or anus Vomiting or abdominal tenderness
Behavior, nonverbal and/or vague somatic complaints	Physical aggression Sexual acting out Excessive masturbation Expressions of low self-esteem Poor school performance Poor peer relationships Sleep disturbances Social withdrawal and excessive daydreaming Running away from home Substance abuse or suicide attempts	Facial grimacing Absence of facial response or flat affect Anxiety Depression Panic attacks Difficulty sleeping Slow, unsteady gait

Data from Hockenberry MJ, Wilson D: *Wong's nursing care of infants and children,* ed 11, St Louis, 2019, Elsevier; Touhy TA, Jett K: *Ebersole and Hess' gerontological nursing and healthy aging,* ed 6, St Louis, 2021, Elsevier.

However, many report a reduced sex drive, decreased sexual interest, and mood changes that can benefit from intervention by a health care provider. (Touhy and Jett, 2021). Postmenopausal women who report good health and have an intimate partner tend to be satisfied with their sexual health (Harder et al., 2019).

Sexual abuse, assault, and rape also affect self-concept and sexuality. Certain findings or clues, such as the interaction between the patient and partner, suggest abuse (Table 34.1). Controlling behaviors such as speaking for the person or refusing to leave him or her alone with a caregiver are suggestive of emotional and perhaps physical or sexual abuse. Patients need to be interviewed privately when abuse is suspected. A patient will probably not admit to problems of abuse with the abuser present. Asking questions that are direct yet compassionate when sexual abuse is suspected is helpful: "Are you in a relationship in which someone is hurting you?" or "Have you ever been forced to have sex when you didn't want to?" When you recognize or report abuse, mobilize treatment immediately for the survivor of sexual violence and the family. The most important factor to consider is the safety of the survivor.

> **REFLECT NOW**
>
> Reflect on a statement a patient made recently about sexuality and how you could have improved your response.

NURSING KNOWLEDGE BASE

Use clinical judgment, applying basic nursing knowledge when addressing patients' sexual health needs. Draw from the following areas of nursing knowledge: sociocultural dimensions of sexuality, decisional issues, and alterations in sexual health.

Factors Influencing Sexuality

Sociocultural Dimensions of Sexuality. People assign different meanings to sexuality based on their culture, gender expression, education, socioeconomic status, and religion. Society plays a powerful role in shaping sexual values and attitudes and in supporting specific expression of sexuality in its members.

Each cultural and social group has its own set of rules and norms that guide sexual behavior, sexual health, and the willingness to discuss this private part of life. For example, cultural norms influence how people find partners, whom they choose as partners, how they relate to one another, how often they have sex, and what they do when they have sex. Personal beliefs enable certain practices and prohibit others (Box 34.2).

Impact of Pregnancy and Menstruation on Sexuality. Sexual interest and activity of women and their partners vary during pregnancy and menstruation. Some cultures encourage sexual intercourse or male-female contact during menstruation and pregnancy, but others strictly forbid it. Research has not found any physiological contraindication to intercourse during menstruation or during most pregnancies. Female sexual interest tends to fluctuate during pregnancy, with increased interest during the second trimester and often decreased interest during the first and third trimesters. There is often a decrease in libido during the first trimester because of nausea, fatigue, and breast tenderness. During the second trimester, blood flow to the pelvic area increases to supply the placenta, resulting in increased sexual enjoyment and libido. During the third trimester the increased abdominal size often makes finding a comfortable position difficult (LeVay et al., 2019).

Discussing Sexual Issues

Sexuality is a significant part of each person's being, yet sexual assessment and interventions are not always included in health care. The area

BOX 34.2   CULTURAL ASPECTS OF CARE

Cultural Factors and Human Immunodeficiency Virus (HIV)

All sexually active individuals are at risk for HIV; however, some races and cultures have higher infection rates. Black/African-American gay and bisexual men account for the largest number of HIV diagnoses, followed by Hispanic/Latino gay and bisexual men, and then White gay and bisexual men. Over time, diagnoses in White gay and bisexual men have decreased, while diagnoses in Latino and Black gay and bisexual men have risen (HIV.gov, 2021). African Americans continue to experience the greatest burden of HIV compared with other races and ethnicities, accounting for 45% of HIV diagnoses. Similarly, Hispanics/Latinos are also disproportionately affected by HIV, as they have been found to represent about 22% of HIV diagnoses (CDC, 2018; HIV.gov, 2021).

The Youth Risk Behavior Surveillance System (YRBSS) monitors health risk behaviors that contribute to the leading causes of death and disability among youth. The most recent YRBSS data reveal that low rates of HIV testing, higher use of substances paired with sexual activity, low rates of condom use, and multiple sexual partners lead to a youth's increased risk of becoming HIV positive. Only 9% of high school students have been tested for HIV. Only 15% of male students who had sexual contact with other males had ever been tested for HIV. About 20% of male students who had sexual contact with other males drank alcohol or used drugs before their most recent sexual intercourse, compared with 19% of all students who were currently sexually active. Nationally, 46% of all sexually active high school students and 48% of male students who had sexual contact with other males did not use a condom the last time they had sexual intercourse. Nearly one-quarter (24%) of male students who had sexual contact with other males reported that they had had sexual intercourse with four or more persons during their lives, compared with 10% of all students who had never had sexual contact (CDC, 2020b).

Older adults also are a high-risk population. Almost half of the people with HIV who live in the United States were 50 years of age and older in 2016. People over 50 accounted for 17% of the 38,739 new HIV diagnoses in the United States. Among people aged 50 and older, Blacks/African Americans accounted for 41% of all new HIV diagnoses. Whites accounted for 35%, Hispanics/Latinos accounted for 19%, and other races/ethnicities accounted for the other 5%. Among people aged 50 and older, nearly half of new HIV diagnoses were among gay and bisexual men, 15% were among heterosexual men, 25% were among heterosexual women, and 9% were among people who inject drugs. Of those people 55 years of age and older who have HIV, 50% have been living with HIV for 4.5 years before being diagnosed, which is the longest delay in diagnosis of any age-group (CDC, 2020c). This delay in diagnosis increases the risk of older adults transmitting HIV to others and often results in greater health implications at diagnosis.

Health care providers need to consider cultural values and their influence on sexual practices when working with diverse populations. It is important for nurses to develop and implement HIV prevention programs in the communities most affected by HIV. The Centers for Disease Control and Prevention (CDC) has committed to funding from 2017 to 2022 for community-based organizations to provide HIV testing to young gay and bisexual men and transgender youth of color, with the goals of identifying previously undiagnosed HIV infections and linking those who have HIV to care and prevention services. CDC grants have also been targeted to deliver effective prevention and evidence-based interventions for antiretroviral therapy adherence for older Americans (Kann et al., 2018).

Implications for Patient-Centered Care
- Establish a therapeutic relationship with a patient/family before discussing sexual health (Varcarolis and Fosbre, 2021).
- Provide both males and females written and verbal information in their primary language regarding contraception, sexually transmitted infections (STIs), and HIV testing and management options (CDC, 2018).
- Target adolescents by expanding education on STIs, HIV, and contraception in middle- and high-school curricula (CDC, 2019).
- Increase HIV testing at community clinics and offer combined laboratory work for STIs and HIV to promote acceptance (CDC, 2021a).
- Promote cultural-specific and bilingual multimedia and community education about HIV risk-reduction strategies (CDC, 2018).

of sexuality is often emotionally charged for nurses and patients. Sometimes nurses avoid discussing sexual issues with patients because they lack information or have different values than their patients. Nurses need to explore their personal level of discomfort and develop a plan to address it. If you are uncomfortable discussing topics related to sexuality, the patient is unlikely to share sexual concerns with you. You need to be aware of your personal beliefs before discussing sexuality with your patients.

Decisional Issues

Nurses are advocates and can assist individuals in making decisions about health concerns affecting their sexuality.

Promoting or Preserving Sexual Health

Contraception. Decisions patients make regarding contraception or preventing pregnancy have far-reaching effects on their lives. Pregnancy, whether planned or unplanned, significantly affects the life of the parent or parents and their support network. Effects are physical, interpersonal, social, financial, and societal. The choice to use contraception is multifaceted and not completely understood. Factors that affect the effectiveness of contraception include the type of method used, the couple's understanding of the method, the consistency of use, and adherence to the requirements of the chosen method. Choice of contraception method varies in relation to the age, ethnicity, marital status, income, education, sexual orientation, and previous pregnancies of the woman. Mobile apps are available to help patients and health professionals monitor reproductive health (e.g., to remind you when to take oral contraceptives, when to replace your transdermal patch or vaginal ring, or when your most fertile time is occurring).

Numerous contraceptive options are available to sexually active couples today. They provide varying levels of protection against unwanted pregnancies. Some methods do not require a prescription, whereas others require a prescription or some other type of intervention from a health care provider. Methods that are effective for contraception do not always reduce the risk of STIs. For example, the pill and intrauterine contraceptive device (IUD) are effective as birth control but not for protection from STIs. A latex condom should be used during each act of intercourse to reduce the risk of STIs. Effectiveness varies with each contraceptive method and the consistency of use. Unplanned pregnancies occur because contraceptives are not used, are used inconsistently, or are used improperly. As a nurse, you serve an important role in discussing contraceptive options with patients. Although reasons for recent declines in teen pregnancy are not totally clear, evidence suggests that these declines are due to more teens abstaining from sexual activity and more teens who are sexually active using birth control than in previous years. However, the U.S. teen pregnancy rate is substantially higher than in other Western industrialized nations, and racial/ethnic differences persist (Kann et al., 2018).

Nonprescription Contraceptive Methods. Nonprescription methods for contraception include abstinence, barrier methods, and timing of intercourse with regard to a woman's ovulation cycle. Although abstinence from sexual intercourse is 100% effective in preventing pregnancy, it is often difficult for both men and women to use consistently. Any act of unprotected intercourse potentially results in pregnancy and exposure to STIs.

Barrier methods include over-the-counter spermicidal products and condoms. Spermicidal products (e.g., creams, jellies, foams, and sponges) are put into the vagina before intercourse to create a spermicidal barrier between the uterus and ejaculated sperm. A latex condom is a thin rubber sheath that fits over the penis to prevent entrance of sperm into the vagina. A diaphragm is a barrier method to prevent pregnancy, which must be used with a spermicide with each sexual encounter. Vaginal spermicides and condoms are most effective when instructions are followed carefully; their combined use is more effective in preventing pregnancy than the use of either one alone.

Nonprescription methods of contraception based on the physiological changes of the menstrual cycle include the rhythm, basal body temperature, cervical mucus, and fertility-awareness methods. Couples who use these methods need to understand the female partner's reproductive cycle and the subtle signs and signals that her body gives during the cycle. To prevent pregnancy, couples abstain from sexual intercourse during designated fertile periods.

Contraceptive Methods That Require a Health Care Provider's Intervention. Contraceptive methods that require the intervention of a health care provider include hormonal contraception, IUDs, the diaphragm, the cervical cap, and sterilization. Hormonal contraception is available in several forms: oral contraceptive pills, vaginal contraceptive rings, hormonal injections, subdermal implant, transdermal skin patches, and IUDs. Hormonal contraception alters the hormonal environment to prevent ovulation, thicken cervical mucus, and thin the lining of the uterus.

An IUD is a plastic device inserted by a health care provider into the uterus through the cervical opening. IUDs contain either copper or progesterone, and some contain a progestin hormone called levonorgestrel that is often used in birth-control pills. The primary mechanism by which both types of IUDs prevent pregnancy is to stop the sperm from fertilizing an egg. The release of progesterone may also increase cervical mucus thickness and alter the lining of the uterus.

The diaphragm is a round, rubber dome that has a flexible spring around the edge. It is used with a contraceptive cream or jelly and is inserted in the vagina so that it provides a contraceptive barrier over the cervical opening. A woman needs to be refitted after a significant change in weight (4.5-kg [10-lb] gain or loss) or pregnancy. The cervical cap functions like the diaphragm; however, it covers only the cervix. It may be left in place longer, and some perceive it as more comfortable than the diaphragm.

Sterilization is the most effective contraception method other than abstinence. Female sterilization, or tubal ligation, involves cutting, tying, or otherwise ligating the fallopian tubes. In male sterilization, or vasectomy, the vas deferens, which carries the sperm away from the testicles, is cut and tied. Both a tubal ligation and a vasectomy usually are considered permanent surgical procedures, although reversal is possible and unintended pregnancies have been reported.

Abortion. Nineteen percent of all established pregnancies in the United States end in abortion; it is estimated that 1 in 3 American women will have an abortion by the age of 45. Young single women, low-income women, and people of color are disproportionately represented (LeVay et al., 2019). Recently abortion rates are declining, with women in their twenties having the most abortions (Kann et al., 2018). The safety and

availability of abortions in the United States improved after the 1973 Supreme Court decision *Roe v Wade,* which established the right of every woman to have an abortion. Abortions are safer and less costly when performed in the early weeks of pregnancy.

Abortion is a hotly debated issue. Women and their partners who face an unwanted pregnancy may consider it as an option. If caring for a patient contemplating abortion, provide an environment in which the patient is able to discuss the issue openly, allowing exploration of various options with an unwanted pregnancy. Discuss religious, social, and personal issues in a nonjudgmental manner with patients. Reasons for choosing an abortion vary and include terminating an unwanted pregnancy or aborting a fetus known to have birth defects. When a woman chooses abortion as a way of dealing with an unwanted pregnancy, the woman and often her partner experience a sense of loss, grief, and/or guilt.

Be aware of personal values related to abortion. As a nurse you are entitled to your personal views. You should not be forced to participate in counseling or procedures contrary to your beliefs and values. It is essential to choose specialties or places of employment where personal values are not compromised and the care of a patient in need of health care is not jeopardized.

Prevention of Sexually Transmitted Infections. Responsible sexual behavior includes knowing one's sexual partner and the partner's sexual history, being able to openly discuss drug-use history with the partner, not allowing drugs or alcohol to influence decision making and sexual practices, and using STI and contraceptive protective devices.

The incidence of STIs continues to increase. Approximately 20 million people in the United States are diagnosed with an STI each year, with the highest incidence occurring in men who have sex with men, bisexual men, and youths between the ages of 15 and 24 (CDC, 2021a). However, according to the CDC (2020e), in the United States STIs are a major public health challenge among women, who disproportionately bear the long-term consequences of STIs. For example, each year untreated STIs cause infertility, and untreated syphilis in pregnant women results in infant death in up to 40% of cases. The prevalence of STIs is a major health concern. Poverty, access to health care, and sexual practices contribute to disparities in the STI rates. Commonly diagnosed STIs include syphilis, gonorrhea, chlamydia, trichomoniasis, and infection with the human papillomavirus (HPV) and herpes simplex virus (HSV) type 2 (genital warts and genital herpes, respectively).

As the name implies, STIs are transmitted from infected individuals to partners during intimate sexual contact. The site of transmission is usually genital, but sometimes it is oral-genital or anal-genital. People most likely to be infected share one key characteristic: unprotected sex with multiple partners. Gonorrhea, chlamydia, syphilis, and pelvic inflammatory disease (PID) are caused by bacteria and are usually curable with antibiotics. Patients need to take antibiotics for the full course of treatment. However, an emerging concern is that some of these bacterial infections (e.g., gonorrhea and syphilis) are now developing antibiotic-resistant strains. Infections such as HSV types 1 and 2, HPV, and HIV are caused by viruses and cannot be cured.

A major problem in dealing with STIs is finding and treating the people who have them. Some people do not know that they are infected because symptoms are sometimes absent or go unnoticed. This is especially common in women. If symptoms do occur, they can go away even though the infection may remain (CDC, 2020e). Common symptoms of an STI include discharge from the vagina, penis, anus, or throat; pain during sex or when urinating; and unexplained rash or lesions. Because sexual behavior often includes the whole body rather than just the genitalia, many parts of the body are potential sites for an STI, including the perineum, anus, and rectum.

Furthermore, any contact with another person's body fluids around the head or an open lesion on the skin, anus, or genitalia can transmit an STI (LeVay et al., 2019).

Sometimes people do not seek treatment because they are embarrassed to discuss sexual symptoms or concerns. Often they are hesitant to talk about their sexual behavior if they believe that it is not "normal." Any sexual behavior that embarrasses a patient often hinders the detection of an STI. Develop communication skills and an accepting, nonjudgmental attitude to provide effective care for those diagnosed with one. Detect valuable clues about an STI by establishing trust, talking with patients in a matter-of-fact manner, and asking questions in a caring manner. Assess attitudes toward sexuality and adjust the intervention to make it acceptable to the patient's sexual value system.

Human Immunodeficiency Virus Infection. HIV is a bloodborne pathogen present in most body fluids of infected individuals. Transmission occurs when there is an exchange of body fluid. Primary routes of transmission include contaminated intravenous (IV) needles, anal intercourse, vaginal intercourse, oral-genital sex, and transfusion of blood and blood products.

The natural history of HIV progresses in three stages. The primary infection stage lasts for about a month after the virus is contracted. During this time the person often experiences flulike symptoms. Then he or she enters the clinical latency phase, which has no symptoms of infection. HIV antibodies appear in the blood about 6 weeks to 3 months after infection. With treatment, individuals with HIV may never have their disease progress to AIDS and can live a long, full life. If left untreated, people who are infected with HIV live about 10 years. The last stage, acquired immunodeficiency syndrome (AIDS), happens when a person begins to·show symptoms of the disease. AIDS is a serious, debilitating, and eventually fatal disease. Antiretroviral therapy (ART) or highly active antiretroviral therapy (HAART) and having an experienced HIV clinician greatly increase the survival time of people who live with HIV/AIDS (CDC, 2021a,e).

Human Papillomavirus Infection. HPV is the most common STI in the United States. An estimated 50% to 75% of sexually active men and women acquire HPV at some point in their lives, with 14 million new infections occurring annually. Most HPV infections are asymptomatic and self-limiting; most infected people eventually clear the virus from their bodies and become noninfectious to others in a couple of years (LeVay et al., 2019). However, certain types can cause cervical cancer in women and anogenital cancers and genital warts in both men and women. HPV is spread through direct contact with warts, semen, and other body fluids from others who have the disease. The textured warts often have a cauliflower appearance and are most common on the penis and scrotum in men and the vagina and cervix in women. Although there is screening available for cervical cancer for women, there is no screening for the other cancers caused by HPV infection, such as cancers of the mouth and throat, anus and rectum, penis, vagina, or vulva (CDC, 2020d).

The HPV vaccination provides safe, effective, and lasting protection against the HPV infections that most commonly cause cancer (CDC, 2020d). The Gardasil 9 vaccine is recommended for males and females in early adolescence (ages 11 or 12 years old) to decrease the risk for cancers associated with HPV, including genital warts and cancers of the cervix, vagina, vulva, penis, anus, and throat (CDC, 2020d). The greatest benefit occurs when individuals receive the vaccines before sexual activity or exposure to the virus. Two doses of the 9-valent HPV vaccine are recommended for preteens, and three doses are advised for older adolescents and young adults. Misinformation remains prevalent and affects rates of vaccination (Box 34.3).

Chlamydia. The bacterium *Chlamydia trachomatis* causes chlamydia. It is the most reported infectious disease in the United States, affecting about

---

BOX 34.3 EVIDENCE-BASED PRACTICE

Barriers Associated With Consenting to the Human Papillomavirus Vaccine

PICOT Question: Does providing education about the human papillomavirus (HPV) vaccine to parents, preteens, and adolescents influence their decision to receive the HPV vaccine?

Evidence Summary

The Gardasil-9 vaccine targets nine types of HPV, including the specific HPVs linked to cancer and warts. It is recommended for all youths ages 11 to 26 years, but vaccination rates in the United States are low. Parental acceptance of the vaccine influences vaccination status, and parents have voiced concern that the vaccine is unsafe or that it will encourage risky sexual behavior despite evidence indicating otherwise (LeVay et al., 2019; Niu et al., 2020). Less research has been conducted on male vaccination adherence, but barriers such as lack of knowledge concerning health risks, confusion about the need for vaccination of boys as well as girls, and provider recommendation to parents have all been shown to affect vaccination rates in males. A study found that individuals who used social media for health purposes and who received patient-centered communication and education about the HPV vaccine had improved perceptions about the efficacy of the vaccine (Niu et al., 2020). Another study by Potts and Southard (2020) involved a one-group, pretest/posttest design, with participants viewing an HPV education video. The study assessed participants' attitudes, knowledge, and intent to vaccinate before and after viewing the video. The result was that participants' attitudes toward HPV/HPV vaccine improved while knowledge increased. Intent to receive the vaccine increased by 31% after viewing the HPV educational video (Potts and Southard, 2020).

Application to Nursing Practice

- Share evidence-based patient-centered information in person and on social media about the effectiveness of the HPV vaccine to encourage vaccine acceptance among parents and youth (Niu et al., 2020).
- Recommend HPV vaccination in the same way and on the same day that you recommend other routinely recommended vaccines for preteen patients at age 11 or 12 years (CDC, 2020d).
- Look for innovative ways to educate parents about HPV (Potts and Southard, 2020).
- Discuss the benefits of the vaccine with parents and youths ages 11 to 26 years and offer catch-up vaccines as needed.
- Reduce parental concerns by sharing evidence supporting that vaccine administration does not increase sexual activity or risk behaviors (Niu et al., 2020).
- Teach safe sex practices to youth and their parents (Niu et al., 2020).

---

3 million Americans each year (CDC, 2021b). Chlamydia is spread by contact with fluids from the infected site. The infection can be transmitted during the birthing process and cause conjunctivitis and pneumonia in newborns. It frequently infects the cervix and, if left untreated, can cause PID, ectopic pregnancy, and infertility from damage to the female reproductive organs. Most people do not realize that they are infected with chlamydia because it causes few symptoms (CDC, 2020a). Therefore the CDC recommends annual screening for all sexually active women up to age 25. High-risk populations are people who have multiple sex partners or are infected with other STIs and men who have sex with men.

Syphilis. Syphilis is caused by the bacterium *Treponema pallidum.* It is commonly spread through contact with an infected person's sores during vaginal, anal, or oral sexual activity and enters the body through minor cuts or abrasions in the skin or mucus membranes. Syphilis is divided into four stages. During the primary stage, an individual typically has firm, round, and painless sores at the site of the original infection, usually around or in the genitals, anus, rectum, or mouth. The symptoms of secondary syphilis include a skin rash, swollen lymph nodes, and fever. Because the symptoms of primary and secondary syphilis are mild, people who are infected may not realize they have syphilis. When a person enters the latent phase, there are no signs or symptoms of the disease. Significant medical problems affecting the heart, brain, nervous system, eye, and other organs are associated with tertiary syphilis, the fourth stage (CDC, 2021c).

Currently syphilis is a significant public health concern. The incidence of primary and secondary syphilis has increased 71% since 2014 (CDC, 2021b). Mothers who are infected with syphilis can transmit the disease to their unborn children, resulting in congenital syphilis (CS). The number of CS cases has quadrupled in recent years (CDC, 2021d). CS can cause significant health risks to a newborn (e.g., bone deformities, severe anemia, hepatomegaly, splenomegaly, blindness, deafness), and up to 40% of babies born to mothers who have not been treated for syphilis may be stillborn or die after birth (CDC, 2021d). Prevention is key. Patient education about reducing the risk of getting syphilis before and during pregnancy and testing women for syphilis at their first prenatal visit are essential. Babies born with CS need immediate treatment to help prevent the development of serious health problems (CDC, 2021d).

Alterations in Sexual Health

Infertility. Infertility is the inability to conceive after 1 year of unprotected intercourse. People experiencing infertility have special needs. Some experience a sense of failure and think that their bodies are defective. Sometimes the desire to become pregnant grows until it permeates most waking moments. Some individuals become preoccupied with creating just the right circumstances for conception. With advances in reproductive technology, people experiencing infertility face many choices that involve religious and ethical values and financial limitations.

Choices include adoption, medical assistance with fertilization, or deciding to remain childless. Organizations such as RESOLVE: The National Organization of Infertility, a national support group for people with infertility, provide support and offer referral sources.

Sexual Abuse. Sexual abuse is a widespread health problem. Abuse occurs in all socioeconomic, age, and ethnic groups, and in men and women. Most often it is at the hands of an intimate partner or family member. Sexual abuse has far-ranging effects on physical and psychological functioning. Sometimes it begins, continues, or even intensifies during pregnancy. Cues that raise a question of possible sexual abuse in women include extreme jealousy and refusal to leave a woman's presence. The overall appearance is sometimes that of a very concerned and caring partner when the underlying reason for this behavior is very different.

Nurses are in an ideal position to assess occurrences of sexual violence, help patients confront these stressors, and educate individuals regarding community services. Nurses are mandated reporters who must report suspected child and elder abuse to the proper authorities per state laws. When you suspect or recognize abuse, mobilize support for the victim and the family. When there is abuse, all family members usually require therapy to promote healthy interactions and relationships.

Patients who have been raped need to work through the crisis before feeling comfortable with intimate expressions of affection. The partner needs to know how to help and support the patient. Children who have been molested sexually need to be identified and be able to share their story and know they are not at fault. The parents need to understand that their response is critical to how the child reacts and adapts.

Personal and Emotional Conflicts. Ideally sex is a natural, spontaneous act that passes easily through several recognizable physiological stages and ends in one or more orgasms. In reality this sequence of events is more the exception than the rule. You will care for patients who have problems with one or more of the stages of sexual activity, including the feeling of wanting sex, the physiological processes and emotions of having sex, and the feelings experienced after sex. For example, some women and men who are taking antidepressants report that their ability to reach orgasm is negatively affected.

Sexual Dysfunction. The incidence of sexual dysfunction in the general population is estimated to be as high as 40% in men and 60% to 80% in women (Touhy and Jett, 2021). It is more prevalent in men and women with poor emotional and physical health (Box 34.4). Sometimes the exact cause cannot be determined.

The incidence of ED increases with age but can occur in men under 40 (LeVay et al., 2019). Risk factors are similar to those for heart disease (e.g., diabetes mellitus, hyperlipidemia, hypertension, hypothyroidism, chronic renal failure, smoking, obesity, alcohol abuse, and lack of exercise). The etiology of ED is often multifactorial. Neurogenic problems, medications, or endocrine or psychogenic factors can cause it. An age-related decrease in testosterone often results in decreased tone of the erectile tissues.

One of the most common problems affecting women of all ages is hypoactive sexual desire disorder (HSDD). Biological, organic, or psychosocial factors can contribute to the incidence of HSDD. Chronic medical conditions such as breast or gynecological cancers and hormonal fluctuations, pain, or depression and anxiety can contribute to a decreased interest in sexual intimacy (LeVay et al., 2019).

The Nurse's Influence on the Patient's Sexuality

Your professional behavior will influence how willing a patient is to express sexual concerns and partner with you and other health care providers in finding successful therapeutic interventions. When you consider the sexuality of patients, think about your own knowledge and values regarding sexual development, sexual orientation, sexual response, STIs, contraception, and alterations in sexual health. Also consider your knowledge base about communication (see Chapter 24). Your own sexuality, sexual experiences, and communication style are valuable when trying to understand your patient's experiences. Do not convey negative feelings to patients verbally or nonverbally.

BOX 34.4 Illnesses and Medications That Affect the Sexual Health of Men and Women

Illnesses	Medications
• Diabetes mellitus	• Antibiotics and antivirals
• Cancer (e.g., prostate, breast, colon, ovarian, testicular, rectal)	• Antihyperlipidemics
• Neuropathy	• Antihypertensives
• Spina bifida	• Antiglycemics
• Spinal cord injury	• Antiarthritics
• Heart disease (e.g., unstable angina, uncontrolled hypertension)	• Antiparkinson agents
• Chronic obstructive pulmonary disease	• Analgesics
• Human immunodeficiency virus infection	• Antidepressives
• Substance abuse	• Anxiolytics
• Depression	• Antipsychotics
• Anxiety	• Diuretics

Data from Touhy TA, Jett K: Ebersole and Hess' gerontological nursing and healthy aging, ed 6, St Louis, 2021, Elsevier.

Attempts at self-exploration teach us about our bodies and the potential for providing pleasure. Your attitude about masturbation may have stemmed from personal experience or from values or beliefs communicated by other people. Games such as "doctor" and "nurse" may have provided early sex play and exploration. In addition, your own sexual experiences add to understanding the complexities of a first sexual encounter or the challenges of sexual interactions when you are or an intimate partner is ill. In addition to personal experiences related to sexuality, nurses use what they have learned through working with other patients to develop trust with current patients.

After identifying that Mr. Clements and his wife have concerns related to their sexual relationship, Joshua reflects on his knowledge of sexual development and stressors commonly experienced by older adults. He understands that older adults are sometimes hesitant or embarrassed to discuss sexual concerns with others. He plans to develop a therapeutic relationship with Mr. and Mrs. Clements and use his nursing knowledge to direct his assessment. In addition to completing a physical assessment, Joshua plans to use a caring and compassionate approach with a combination of direct and open-ended questions to allow Mr. and Mrs. Clements the opportunity to express their concerns to help identify factors affecting their sexual functioning.

CRITICAL THINKING

Successful clinical judgment requires the application of critical thinking, synthesizing knowledge, experience, information gathered from patients, critical thinking attitudes, and intellectual and professional standards. Sound clinical judgments require you to anticipate information, analyze assessment data, and make appropriate clinical decisions regarding

patient care. Fig. 34.2 shows the clinical judgment model for assessing patients' sexuality to form nursing diagnoses.

In the case of sexuality, integrate knowledge from nursing and other disciplines. Have a thorough understanding of safe sex practices and the risks and behaviors associated with sexual problems to anticipate how to assess a patient and interpret findings. Use previous experiences to provide care for patients with sexual issues in a more reflective and helpful way.

Patients have customs and values that are different from your own. Professional standards require respect for each patient as an individual. Critical thinking attitudes such as integrity require you to recognize when personal opinions and values conflict with those of the patient and to consider how to proceed in a way that is mutually beneficial. Be aware of your own biases, opinions, and competency in discussing concerns related to a patient's sexuality. If you are not comfortable or do not have the knowledge or ability to discuss a patient's concerns, be prepared to make consultations to other health care professionals who specialize in this area. The health care environment often affects how comfortable a patient will be to discuss sexual concerns with you. For example, a patient will likely feel more comfortable discussing sexual concerns in a quiet, private environment rather than a busy emergency room setting.

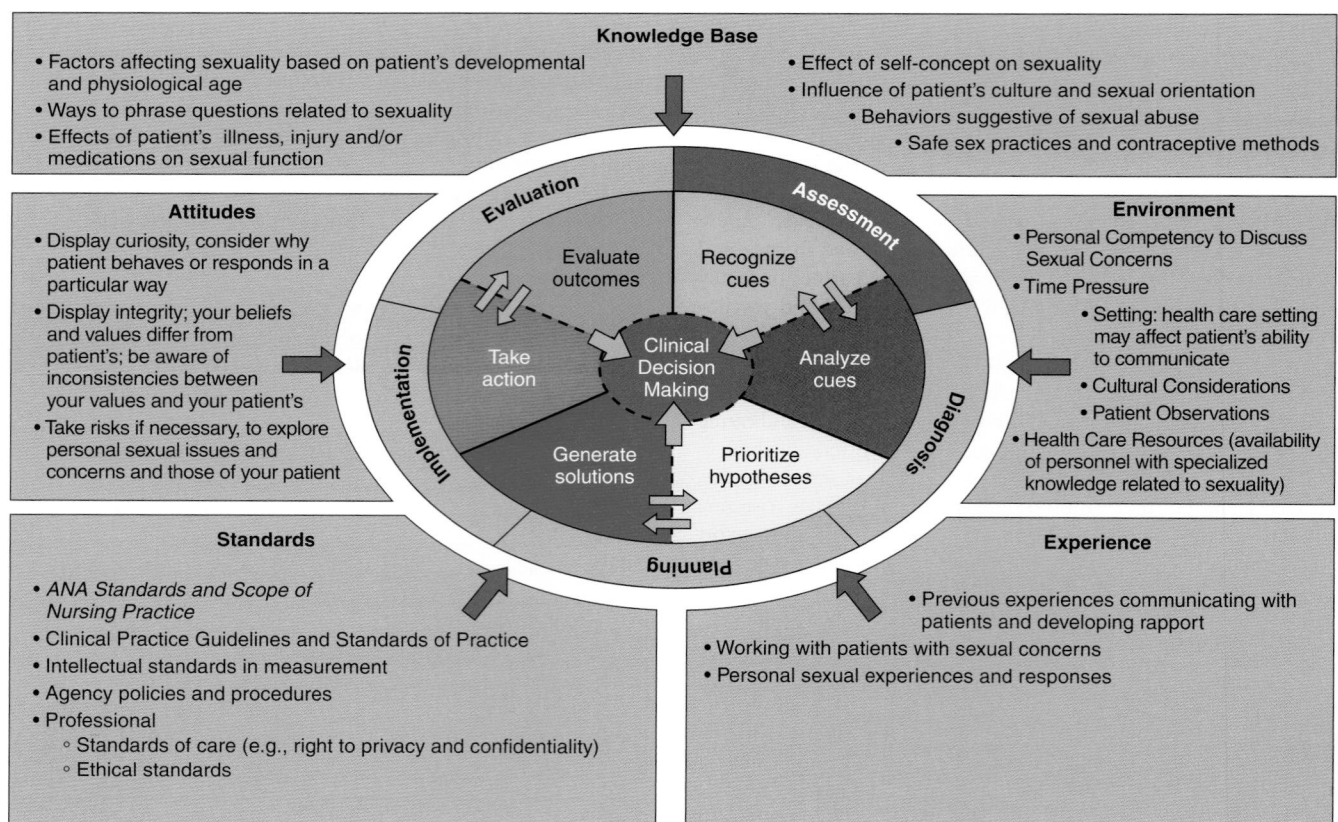

FIG. 34.2 Critical thinking model for sexuality assessment. (Clinical Judgment Measurement Model copyright © NCSBN. All rights reserved.)

❖ NURSING PROCESS

Apply critical thinking in the nursing process as you form the clinical judgments needed to provide care to your patients. The nursing process provides a clinical decision-making approach to help you develop and implement an individualized plan of care. Assess all relevant factors, including physical, environmental, psychological, social, and cultural factors, to determine a patient's needs or health problems that affect sexual well-being. The nursing role in addressing sexual concerns ranges from ongoing assessment to providing information, counseling, and referral. Keep in mind that you are not expected to have answers to all identified sexual issues and concerns.

◆ Assessment

During the assessment process thoroughly assess each patient and critically analyze findings to ensure that you make patient-centered clinical decisions required for safe nursing care.

Through the Patient's Eyes.
As in any patient assessment, it is important to understand a patient's expectations regarding care. Questions such as "What would you like to know about how your health problem might affect your sexual needs?" "What would you like to have happen regarding your sexual health problems?" and "What initial steps do you want to take?" help a patient identify desired outcomes. It is important to set aside personal views and consider a patient's needs and preferences for care.

Environmental Factors.
Discussions surrounding sexuality are very personal and private. Therefore it is essential to conduct your assessment in an appropriate setting that ensures a patient's privacy and is free from interruptions. Ensure that the room temperature is comfortable and lighting is appropriate. Observe a patient's emotional responses throughout the assessment.

Maintain an environment that conveys respect. Be alert for signs of anxiety and be prepared to pause your assessment based on your patient's response. Some agencies require that you have another staff member (e.g., another nurse) present when completing physical assessments of the breasts, genitalia, and reproductive tract. In addition, some states have parental involvement laws that require you to include a child or adolescent's parent while providing care such as contraceptive services and sexual health education. Follow agency policies and maintain a calm and nonjudgmental environment during your assessment. If you suspect your patient is being abused, do *not* ask the patient about any abusive behaviors in the presence of the suspected abuser. Provide privacy and obtain information in a protective environment.

Factors Affecting Sexuality.
In gathering a sexual history consider physical, functional, relationship, lifestyle, developmental, and self-esteem factors that influence sexual functioning. Sexual desire varies among individuals; some people want and enjoy sex every day, whereas others want sex only once a month, and still others have no sexual desire and are quite comfortable with that fact. Sexual desire becomes an issue if the person wants to satisfy it more often, if he or she believes that it is necessary to measure up to some cultural norm, or if there is a discrepancy between the sexual desires of the partners in a relationship.

Ask patients to describe factors that typically influence their sexual desire. Knowing a patient's medical history and probing for information are helpful. For example, minor illness, medications, and fatigue often decrease sexual desire. Lifestyle factors such as the use or abuse of alcohol, lack of sleep, lack of time, or the demands of caring for a new baby are other influencing factors. For example, working parents sometimes feel so overburdened that they perceive sexual advances from a partner as an additional demand on them. Confirm factors that

potentially affect sexual desire and determine with the patient the extent to which sexual function is impaired.

Consider how self-concept issues (see Chapter 33), including gender identity, body image, role performance, and self-esteem, affect a patient's sexuality and how these factors relate to a patient's condition. For example, poor body image associated with chronic disease magnifies feelings of rejection. This often results in diminished or absent sexual desire.

Issues in a relationship often affect sexual desire. After the initial glow of a new relationship has faded, some couples find that they have major differences in their values or lifestyles. Ask couples to describe how close they feel to each other and how often they interact on an intimate level. Assess communication patterns between sexual partners to determine sexual satisfaction within a relationship.

Sexual Health History.
Most patients want to know how medications, treatments, and surgical procedures influence their sexual relationship even though they often do not ask questions. With experience nurses recognize that most patients welcome the opportunity to talk about their sexuality, especially when they are experiencing difficulties. The classic PLISSIT model (Annon, 1976), which was later expanded to the Ex-PLISSIT model (Davis and Taylor, 2006), provides an approach that nurses can use to assess sexuality in patients (Fig 34.3). The acronym *PLISSIT* indicates four levels of intervention:
- **P**ermission to discuss sexuality issues
- **L**imited **I**nformation related to sexual health problems being experienced
- **S**pecific **S**uggestions—only when the nurse is clear about the problem
- **I**ntensive **T**herapy—referral to professional with advanced training if necessary

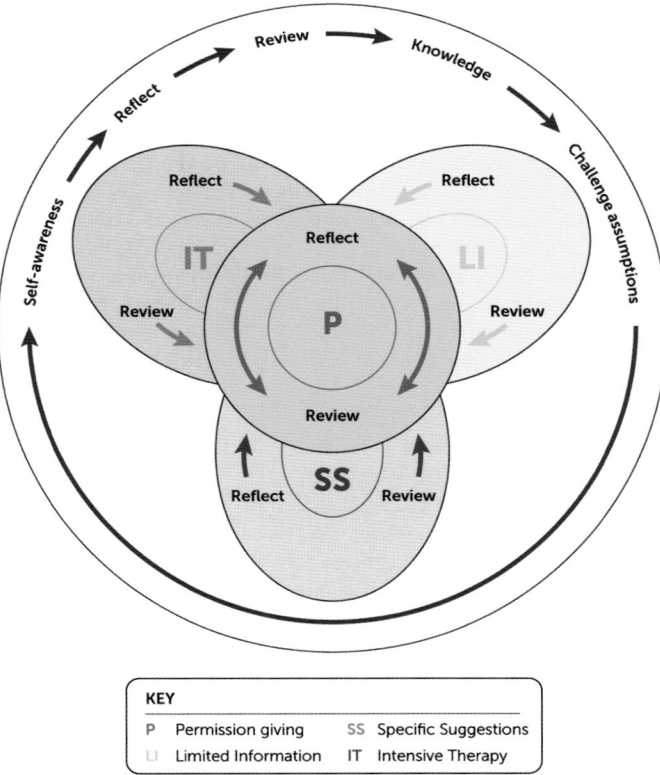

KEY		
P Permission giving	SS	Specific Suggestions
LI Limited Information	IT	Intensive Therapy

FIG. 34.3 The Ex-PLISSIT model is an extension of Annon's original PLISSIT model. (Reproduced from Davis S, Taylor B: From PLISSIT to Ex-PLISSIT. In David S, editor: *Rehabilitation: the use of theories and models in practice.* Edinburgh, 2006, Churchill Livingstone.)

BOX 34.5   Nursing Assessment Questions

- Describe your level of sexual activity for me.
- With whom do you have sex: men, women, or both?
- How many sexual partners do you have (or have you ever had)?
- Tell me how you feel about the sexual aspects of your life.
- Tell me about any changes you have noticed in the way you feel about yourself.
- How has your illness, medication, or surgery affected your sex life?
- It is not unusual for people with your condition to be experiencing some sexual changes. Do you have any concerns?
- Are you in a relationship in which someone is hurting you?
- Has anyone ever forced you to have sex against your will?
- Tell me what you know about safe sex practices, use of contraceptives, or prevention of sexually transmitted infections.
- Tell me the safe sex practices that you follow.

The revised Ex-PLISSIT model emphasizes the importance of permission giving at all stages. Thus the new level includes permission giving at its core, which normalizes sexuality and gives patients the opportunity to ask questions and voice concerns to nurses and other health care providers who use this model (Taylor and Davis, 2007). Using permission giving ensures that the assessment data you gather address the needs and concerns of your patient.

Incorporate assessment questions related to sexuality in the nursing history (Box 34.5). Using an opening statement puts a patient at ease when introducing these questions (e.g., "Sex is an important part of life, and a person's health status often affects sexuality. Many people have questions and concerns about their sexual health. What questions or concerns do you have?"). Use knowledge of developmental stages to determine which areas are likely to be important for your patient. For example, when gathering a sexual history from an older adult, it is important to keep in mind that some have difficulty in discussing intimate details with health care providers.

Nurses who conduct sexual assessments of children and adolescents face special challenges. Use age-appropriate language that is accurate and understandable. Also promote normal development, avoid minimizing problems, and screen for sexual concerns while making the child or adolescent feel at ease. The sexual counseling of minors raises ethical and legal issues regarding a patient's rights to health care and education on the one hand and a parent's or guardian's right to supervise information on the other. Children and adolescents frequently respond when they know that having questions related to sexuality is normal. Being open, positive, and interested when introducing sexual questions is helpful.

Considering the prevalence of intimate partner violence, it is important to ask questions exploring potential abusive relationships. Address these questions in private. Recognizing both subjective and objective signs and symptoms of abuse in children and adults helps to identify this too-common problem (see Table 34.1).

Some individuals are too embarrassed or do not know how to ask sexual questions directly. Look for clues that a person has questions. For example, a patient expresses concern about how his or her partner will respond now or makes a sexual comment or joke. Observing for and listening to concerns about sexuality takes practice. With experience you develop skill in clarifying and paraphrasing to help individuals express sexual concerns. By including sexuality in the nursing history, you acknowledge that it is an important component of health and create an opportunity for a person to discuss sexual concerns.

Sexual Dysfunction. Many illnesses, injuries, medications, and aging changes have a negative effect on sexual health, which results in either temporary or permanent sexual dysfunction. Apply knowledge about

conditions and medications that frequently cause sexual dysfunction while assessing a patient's own condition (see Box 34.4). Be aware of the possible risks for physical problems. You will explore any problems the patient begins to identify. Some patients bring up the topic of sexual dysfunction. Other times you will discover issues as the patient answers other nursing history questions.

REFLECT NOW

Reflect on a statement one of your patients made about sexuality and how you could have improved your response.

Physical Assessment. A physical examination helps assess the cause of sexual concerns or problems and usually provides the best opportunity to teach an individual about sexual health issues. In examining a woman's breasts and the external and internal genitalia, you have the opportunity to assess the woman's reaction, answer questions, provide information about the examination of anatomical and physiological structures, and teach a woman how to perform breast self-examination. During physical assessment of a male patient's genitalia, you can teach the patient how to perform testicular self-examination (see Chapter 30). Knowledge of normal scrotal anatomical structures helps men detect signs of testicular cancer. Instruct both men and women on signs and symptoms of STIs during the examination when patients' histories suggest risks for them.

As Joshua prepares to assess Mr. Clements, Joshua closes the door to the room to ensure privacy. Joshua recently completed a clinical rotation at the STI Clinic at the local public health department. That experience emphasized the importance of using a caring, open, and compassionate approach when caring for patients who have sexual concerns. Joshua uses his experiences there as well as his understanding of the Ex-PLISSIT model to develop assessment questions that will help Mr. Clements feel at ease and to identify factors affecting Mr. Clements' sexual concerns. Joshua begins his assessment by stating, "I know that some people have concerns about their sexuality after having a heart attack. Mr. Clements, do you have any concerns you would like to discuss right now?" Mr. Clements states, "Yes. I'm worried about having sex with my wife now that I've had a heart attack. I haven't been able to have sex with her since I started on my high blood pressure medicine, and now this.... My wife is worried, and I just don't think I can enjoy having sex anymore. I know she wants to have sex; I just can't do it right now. I hope she doesn't leave me. What if I never am able to have sex with my wife again?"

◆ Analysis and Nursing Diagnosis

After completing an assessment, you apply critical thinking to begin analyzing assessment data. Your analysis of assessment cues and application of clinical judgment lead you to identify a patient's nursing diagnoses and collaborative problems. Assessment findings related to sexuality often include the patient's concerns about sexual health, history of surgery of reproductive organs, changes in appearance or body image, a history of or current physical or sexual abuse, chronic illness, or developmental milestones. To make a nursing diagnosis related to sexual dysfunction, consider anatomical, physiological, sociocultural, ethical, and situational issues thoroughly. Possible nursing diagnoses related to sexual functioning include:

- Problematic Sexual Behavior
- Difficulty Coping
- Lack of Knowledge of Contraception
- Impaired Sexual Functioning
- Risk for Impaired Reproductive Function

Clarify assessment findings and ensure that the patient perceives a problem or difficulty with sexuality (Box 34.6). Determining the contributing factors or risk factors helps you plan effectively and select the appropriate nursing interventions. For example, nursing interventions appropriate for the nursing diagnosis of *Impaired Sexual Functioning* will differ for different contributing factors. *Impaired Sexual Functioning related to misinformation about the risk of sexually transmitted infections* requires counseling and education on how to maintain safe sexual practices. In contrast, patients who experience *Impaired Sexual Functioning related to physical abuse* need counseling and referral to community resources (e.g., crisis services and physical abuse support group).

*After completing his assessment, Joshua uses critical thinking to begin to analyze the assessment data. Joshua looks for common findings that cluster together to indicate the priority nursing diagnoses that most accurately describe the problems Mr. Clements is currently experiencing. Joshua first makes the nursing diagnosis of **Impaired Sexual Functioning** after considering the statements Mr. Clements made about his inability to have sexual intercourse with his wife since he started taking his antihypertensive medication. Joshua analyzes Mr. Clements' statements regarding concerns that he is not going to be able to have sex with his wife combined with the possibility that his wife may leave him, and determines that the nursing diagnosis* Fear *is also appropriate at this time.*

◆ Planning and Outcomes Identification

Critical thinking ensures that a patient's plan of care integrates all that a nurse knows about an individual's sexuality. In planning care, remember that patients must feel safe in the environment for your care to be effective. Maintain a patient's dignity and identity at all times. For example, to convey respect for the patient's gender identity preferences, ask the patient about preferred pronouns and use the patient's preferred pronouns in all interactions.

Recognize your own knowledge, biases, and competency in addressing a patient's sexual concerns. Include professional standards when developing a plan of care. Plan to include nurses, social workers and other health care providers who have competence in providing care to patients with complicated needs related to their sexual health as needed.

Outcomes. Use critical thinking to synthesize information from multiple resources and make the decisions needed for an individualized plan of care (Fig. 34.4) for each nursing diagnosis (see the Nursing Care Plan).

BOX 34.6 Nursing Diagnostic Process

Impaired Sexual Functioning

Assessment Activities	Assessment Findings
Review medical and medication history	History of hypertension History of uncomplicated myocardial infarction (MI) Takes propranolol
Have patient describe sexual problems	Less interested in having intercourse with wife since taking propranolol Rarely has sexual intercourse with wife Sometimes has trouble having an erection
Patient's fears and concerns	Fearful will have chest pain or another MI while having intercourse

---

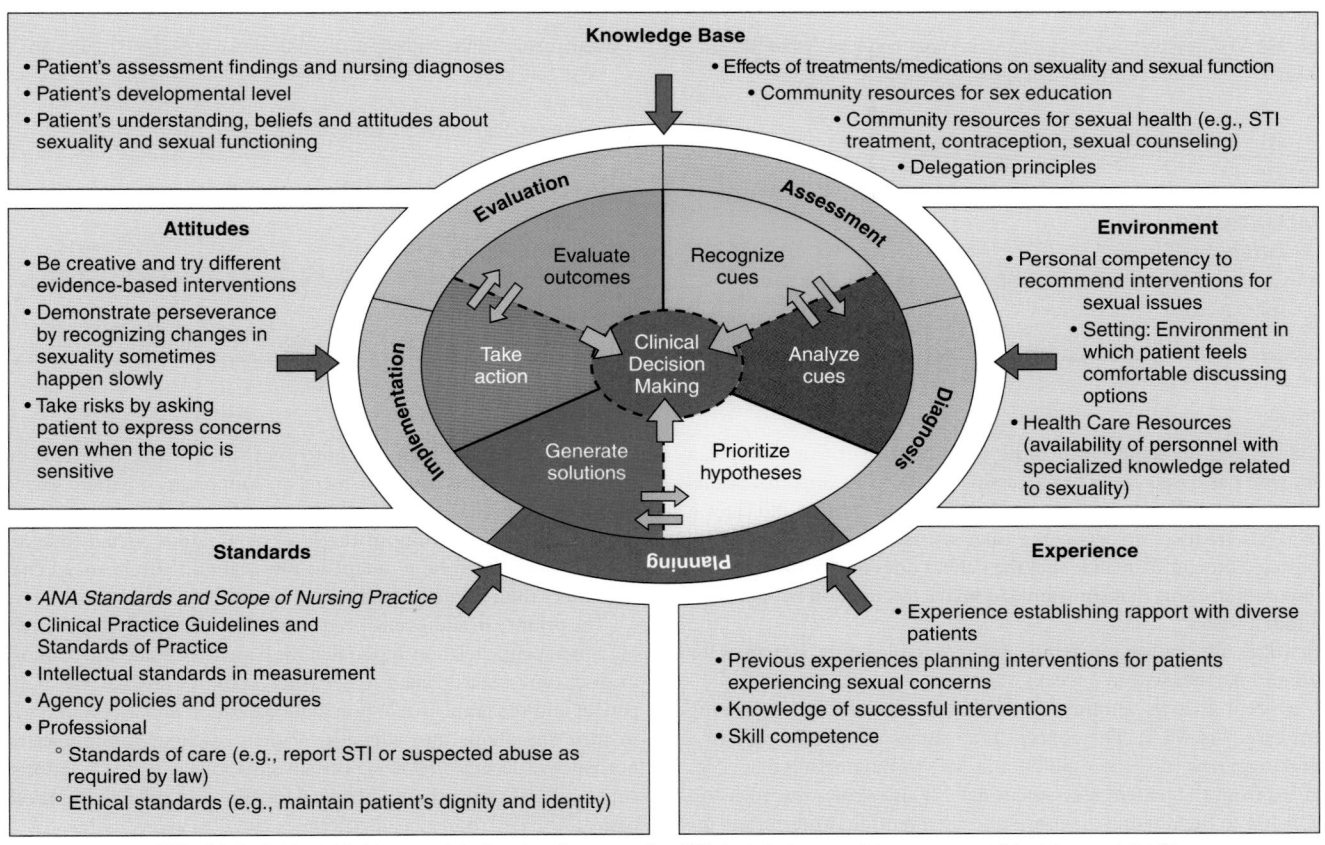

Knowledge Base

- Patient's assessment findings and nursing diagnoses
- Patient's developmental level
- Patient's understanding, beliefs and attitudes about sexuality and sexual functioning

- Effects of treatments/medications on sexuality and sexual function
- Community resources for sex education
- Community resources for sexual health (e.g., STI treatment, contraception, sexual counseling)
- Delegation principles

Attitudes

- Be creative and try different evidence-based interventions
- Demonstrate perseverance by recognizing changes in sexuality sometimes happen slowly
- Take risks by asking patient to express concerns even when the topic is sensitive

Environment

- Personal competency to recommend interventions for sexual issues
- Setting: Environment in which patient feels comfortable discussing options
- Health Care Resources (availability of personnel with specialized knowledge related to sexuality)

Standards

- *ANA Standards and Scope of Nursing Practice*
- Clinical Practice Guidelines and Standards of Practice
- Intellectual standards in measurement
- Agency policies and procedures
- Professional
  - ° Standards of care (e.g., report STI or suspected abuse as required by law)
  - ° Ethical standards (e.g., maintain patient's dignity and identity)

Experience

- Experience establishing rapport with diverse patients
- Previous experiences planning interventions for patients experiencing sexual concerns
- Knowledge of successful interventions
- Skill competence

Evaluation — Evaluate outcomes
Assessment — Recognize cues
Implementation — Take action
Clinical Decision Making
Analyze cues — Diagnosis
Generate solutions
Prioritize hypotheses
Planning

FIG. 34.4 Critical thinking model planning for sexuality. (Clinical Judgment Measurement Model copyright © NCSBN. All rights reserved.)

◎ NURSING CARE PLAN

Impaired Sexual Functioning

ASSESSMENT

Assessment Activities

Ask Mr. Clements whether his interest in sex has changed since he started taking propranolol.

Ask Mr. Clements whether he has had difficulties with an erection.

Ask Mr. Clements what concerns or fears he has about resuming his sexual relationship with his wife now that he has had a myocardial infarction (MI).

Assessment Findings[a]

He responds that he has been **less interested in having sexual intercourse with his wife** since he started to take propranolol.

He states that since he started to take propranolol, he **sometimes has trouble having an erection.**

He states that he is afraid that after discharge he will have chest pain or another heart attack if he has sexual intercourse with his wife.

[a]Assessment findings are shown in bold type.

NURSING DIAGNOSIS: Impaired sexual functioning related to altered body function (side effects of propranolol) and lack of knowledge

PLANNING

Expected Outcomes (NOC)[b]

Sexual Functioning

Patient expresses renewed sexual interest within 2 weeks.

Patient will express mutually satisfying sexual relationship with wife within 1 month.

[b]Outcome classification labels from Moorhead S, et al: Nursing Outcomes Classification (NOC): measurement of health outcomes, ed 6, St Louis, 2018, Elsevier.

INTERVENTIONS (NIC)[c]

Sexual Counseling

Establish trust and respect with Mr. Clements. Offer privacy during conversations.

Discuss possible effects of MI and propranolol on sexual functioning and safe resumption of sexual activity.

Include Mrs. Clements in discussions about sexual issues as frequently as possible and when appropriate.

Anxiety Reduction

Encourage Mr. Clements to express fears about resuming sexual activity and assure him that others who have had MIs experience similar fears.

RATIONALE

Establishing trust and offering privacy express sense of caring, increasing likelihood of patient's ability to express concerns (Varcarolis and Fosbre, 2021).

Discussion enhances understanding about reasons for sexual difficulties and provides safe guidelines for resumption of sexual intercourse following MI.

Including partner in the plan of care can enhance personal and intimate relationships and improve health outcomes (Boothby et al., 2018).

Sexual dysfunction sometimes occurs after an MI because of anxiety and/or from side effects of medications. Knowing that feelings and fears are normal helps decrease anxiety and encourages return of sexual activity outcomes (Boothby et al., 2018).

[c]Intervention classification labels from Butcher HK, et al: Nursing Interventions Classification (NIC), ed 7, St Louis, 2018, Elsevier.

EVALUATION

Evaluation Activities

Ask Mr. Clements whether he and his wife are satisfied with their sexual relationship during return office visit.

Patient Response

Mr. Clements reports that his interest in sex is back to normal and that he is able to have an erection.

Mr. Clements reports he and his wife are satisfied with their relationship.

Set realistic and measurable outcomes with the patient. For example, a patient who has dyspareunia has a nursing diagnosis of *Impaired Sexual Functioning related to decreased sexual desire.* Your patient indicates a desire to have reduced anxiety and greater satisfaction with sexual activity. Expected outcomes include that the patient does the following:

- Discusses stressors that contribute to sexual dysfunction with partner within 2 weeks
- Identifies alternative, satisfying, and acceptable sexual practices for self and partner within 4 weeks

A concept map is another method that is useful in organizing patient care (Fig. 34.5). The concept map shows the relationship of a medical diagnosis (decreased libido and MI) to the nursing diagnoses identified from the patient assessment data. It also shows the links and relationship to the nursing diagnosis and interventions appropriate for each diagnosis. For example, *Difficulty Coping* affects and contributes to *Withdrawn Behavior,* and as long as the patient has difficulty coping, the withdrawn behavior continues or perhaps worsens.

Setting Priorities. Expected outcomes and nursing interventions for patients with sexual concerns focus on supporting a patient's need for intimacy and sexual activity. Patients often feel overwhelmed and hopeless about returning to the level of previous sexual functioning and usually need time to adapt to physical and psychosocial changes that affect their sexuality and sexual health.

The priority in addressing needs related to sexuality includes establishing a therapeutic relationship so that the patient feels safe and comfortable in discussing issues related to sexuality. Look for strengths in both the patient and the family while providing education and access to resources to turn limitations into strengths. Patient teaching communicates the normalcy of feelings following certain situations (e.g., the diagnosis of a chronic illness or the change in sexual function). In collaboration with the patient, you determine a patient's needs and plan accordingly.

A patient's current problems and needs help you determine the priorities related to his or her sexual health. Priorities for sexual health often include resuming sexual activities. For example, if a woman is

CONCEPT MAP

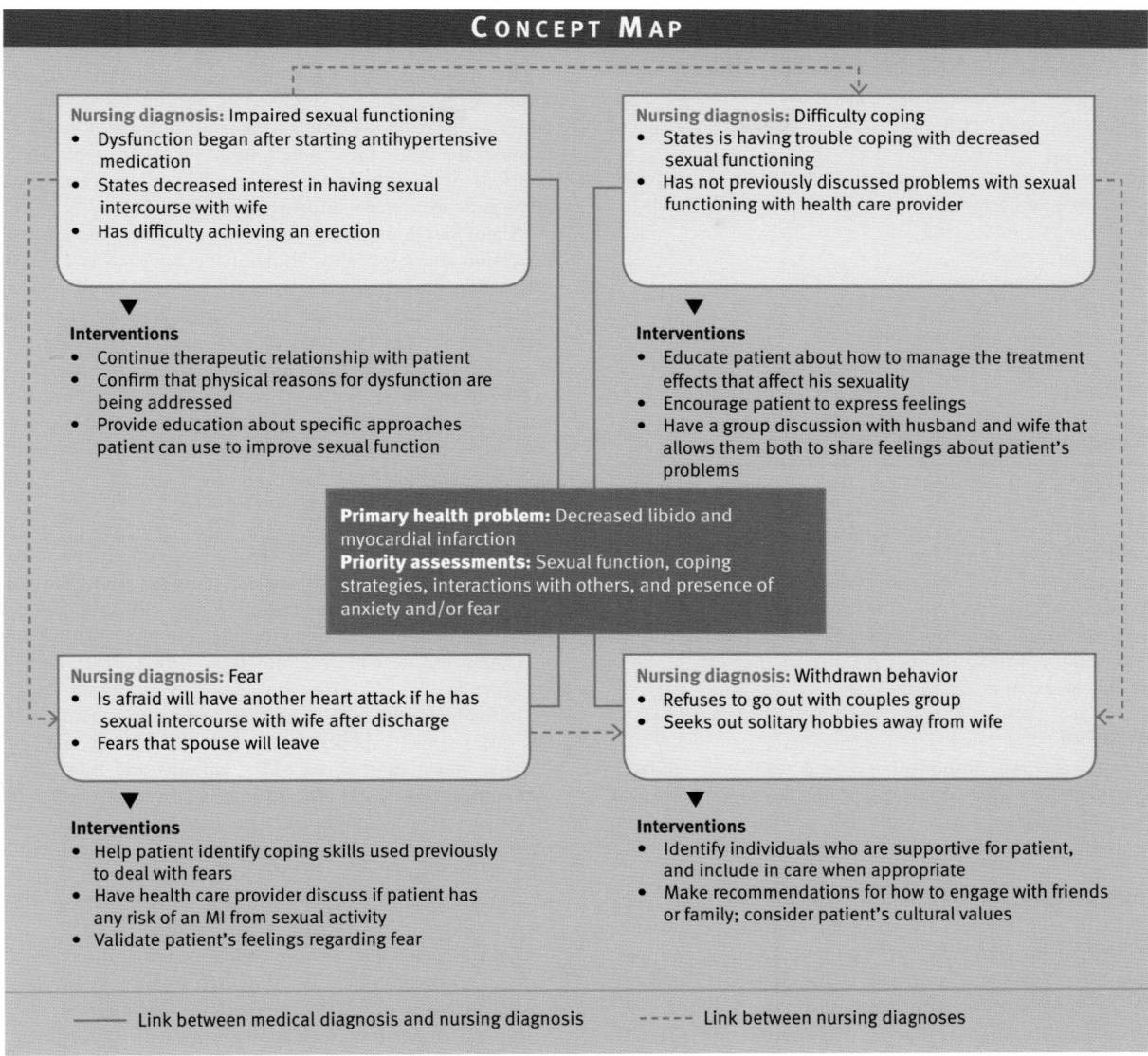

Nursing diagnosis: Impaired sexual functioning
- Dysfunction began after starting antihypertensive medication
- States decreased interest in having sexual intercourse with wife
- Has difficulty achieving an erection

Interventions
- Continue therapeutic relationship with patient
- Confirm that physical reasons for dysfunction are being addressed
- Provide education about specific approaches patient can use to improve sexual function

Nursing diagnosis: Difficulty coping
- States is having trouble coping with decreased sexual functioning
- Has not previously discussed problems with sexual functioning with health care provider

Interventions
- Educate patient about how to manage the treatment effects that affect his sexuality
- Encourage patient to express feelings
- Have a group discussion with husband and wife that allows them both to share feelings about patient's problems

Primary health problem: Decreased libido and myocardial infarction
Priority assessments: Sexual function, coping strategies, interactions with others, and presence of anxiety and/or fear

Nursing diagnosis: Fear
- Is afraid will have another heart attack if he has sexual intercourse with wife after discharge
- Fears that spouse will leave

Interventions
- Help patient identify coping skills used previously to deal with fears
- Have health care provider discuss if patient has any risk of an MI from sexual activity
- Validate patient's feelings regarding fear

Nursing diagnosis: Withdrawn behavior
- Refuses to go out with couples group
- Seeks out solitary hobbies away from wife

Interventions
- Identify individuals who are supportive for patient, and include in care when appropriate
- Make recommendations for how to engage with friends or family; consider patient's cultural values

——— Link between medical diagnosis and nursing diagnosis   - - - - - Link between nursing diagnoses

FIG. 34.5 Concept map for Mr. Clements.

recovering from a mastectomy and is having problems resuming an intimate relationship with her spouse because of problems related to body image, you help her adapt to and cope with the changes in her body image associated with the mastectomy. Once the patient's issues related to body image are resolved, she is better able to restore intimacy with her spouse and address her sexual health needs.

QSEN Building Competency in Teamwork and Collaboration
Mr. Clements asks what lifestyle changes he will need to make after discharge from the hospital. You know that patients with cardiovascular problems often require an interprofessional approach to achieve optimal recovery, and you arrange for consultation with different health professionals. You inform Mr. Clements that he will work with a team of experts, including cardiologists, physical therapists, dietitians, and counselors. Assure him that you will share your assessment data and plan of care with the team and will recommend nurses who can remain involved in his outpatient care. Discuss how each of these professionals will contribute to Mr. Clements' care during and after hospitalization.

Answers to QSEN Activities can be found on the Evolve website.

Teamwork and Collaboration. You often collaborate with other health care providers and make referrals to community resources when planning care for a patient's sexual health needs (Box 34.7). Raise awareness of sexual issues, clarify patient concerns, and/or provide information. Nurses who have specialized education in sexual functioning and counseling provide more intensive sex therapy. Know the limits of your knowledge base and include other health care providers, such as sex therapists, clinical psychologists, and social workers as appropriate, to meet patients' needs for sexual health. For example, conflicts in marriage usually require intensive treatment with a mental health professional or certified sex therapist. When caring for a woman who is currently in an abusive relationship, collaborate with special women's shelters that provide counseling and serve as a safe place for her while further plans are made.

*After analyzing assessment cues, Joshua works with Mr. Clements to identify that **Impaired Sexual Functioning** is the priority nursing diagnosis. After discussing the plan of care with Mr. Clements, Joshua determines that Mr. Clements is hoping to experience a renewed sexual interest in his wife and to reestablish a mutually satisfying sexual relationship with his wife following discharge from the hospital. Joshua*

BOX 34.7   Examples of Community Resources Relating to Sexuality

- Community and free clinics offering contraceptive information and resources
- Health department (often for both family planning and sexually transmitted infections)
- Groups that provide education and services for those with specific health conditions include the following:
  - American Diabetes Association
  - American Heart Association
  - Muscular Dystrophy Association
  - Muscular Sclerosis Society
  - Sexual abuse support groups and hotlines
  - Women's shelters (for those who are at risk of continued physical and/or sexual abuse)
  - Resolve: The National Infertility Association
  - North American Menopause Society

focuses his interventions on providing education to Mr. Clements and his wife about the effects of Mr. Clements' medical diagnoses and medications on his sexual functioning. Joshua also determines that it is essential to help Mr. Clements feel more comfortable in having a sexual relationship with his wife by helping manage his anxiety and fear of having another MI during sexual intercourse.

◆ Implementation

Promote sexual health as a component of overall health and wellness by identifying patients at increased risk, providing appropriate information, helping individuals gain insight into their problems, and exploring methods to deal with them effectively.

Health Promotion. How you respond to patients who have experienced changes in sexuality sets the stage for how they come to see themselves. The patient with a change in body functioning or appearance is often extremely sensitive to verbal and nonverbal responses. Building a trusting nurse-patient relationship and appropriately including a patient in decision making will support most patients' healthy sexuality. Sometimes individualized approaches, including supporting the use of alternative healing techniques or methods of spiritual expression, help a patient adapt to changes in sexual health.

Helping patients maintain or gain sexual health involves considering factors that influence sexual satisfaction. Educate patients about measures for contraception, safe sex practices, and prevention of STIs. Regular breast self-examinations, mammograms, and Papanicolaou (Pap) smears are important sexual health measures for women; testicular self-examinations are important for men. Offer the 9-valent HPV vaccine to males and females who are between 11 and 26 years of age (CDC, 2020d). The vaccine is safe for girls as young as 9 years old and is recommended for females ages 11 to 26 if they have not already completed the three required injections. Booster doses currently are not recommended. The vaccine is most effective if administered before sexual activity or exposure.

Exploring an individual's values, discussing levels of satisfaction, and providing sex education require therapeutic communication skills. Structure the environment and timing to provide privacy, comfort, and uninterrupted time. For example, when discussing methods of contraception with a woman, provide education in a private area with the patient fully dressed rather than in the examination room when the patient is only partially clothed.

Topics of education vary and often are related to a patient's developmental level. For example, a nurse talks to school-age children regarding the appearance of breast buds or pubic hair. When discussing sexual health with patients of childbearing age, always consider a patient's cultural and religious beliefs regarding contraception. The discussion includes the desire for children, usual sexual practices, and acceptable methods of contraception. Review all methods of contraception to allow patients to make informed decisions.

Major developmental events (e.g., puberty, menopause) prompt education about sexuality. Situational crises such as a life change with pregnancy, illness, divorce, extreme financial stress, placement of a spouse in a nursing home, or loss and grief affect sexuality. Some effects last for days, months, or years and are often minimized when the individual is prepared for possible changes in sexual functioning.

Demonstrate recognition, acceptance, and respect for an older adult's sexuality by displaying a willingness to openly discuss sex and sexuality-related concerns. Strategies that enhance sexual functioning include the following (LeVay et al., 2019).

- Avoid alcohol (in excess) and tobacco.
- Eat well-balanced meals.
- Plan sexual activity for times when the couple feels rested.
- Take pain medication if needed before sexual intercourse.
- Use pillows and alternate positioning to enhance comfort.
- Encourage touch, kissing, hugging, and other tactile stimulation.
- Communicate concerns and fears with partner and health care provider.

Individuals who have more than one sex partner or whose partner has other sexual experiences need to learn about safe sex practices. Provide information about STI symptoms and transmission, use of condoms, and risky sexual activities (e.g., trauma from penile-anal sex). To prevent HIV infection, teach patients to avoid having multiple sex partners and to use condoms correctly to reduce the risk of HIV/AIDS (Box 34.8). Role-playing is useful in helping a person learn to say no or in negotiating with a partner to use a condom. When discussing safe sex, consider patients' physical and emotional health.

Encourage patients to have regular health and screening examinations to maintain sexual health. Often asymptomatic STIs are diagnosed during a physical examination with appropriate laboratory work. Annual health examinations provide an opportunity to discuss contraception and safe sex practices. However, some people do not seek annual health examinations routinely. For example, some women frequently do not have breast examinations, mammograms, and cervical cancer screening because of religious and cultural beliefs about modesty. Develop a therapeutic relationship with patients and provide culturally sensitive educational materials that are written at an appropriate reading level (see Chapter 25). Barriers to reproductive health services include cultural beliefs, access to health care, and low health literacy.

Acute Care. Illness and surgery create situational stressors that often affect a person's sexuality. During periods of illness individuals experience major physical changes, the effects of drugs or treatments, the emotional stress of a prognosis, concern about future functioning, and separation from significant others. Never assume that sexual functioning is not a concern merely because of the presence of other major physical problems, an individual's age, or the severity of prognosis. After identifying concerns, address them in the context of the patient's value system and a realistic view of how health problems will affect the patient.

When a patient identifies sexual concerns, initiate discussion and education appropriately. Refer to appropriate outpatient resources if

BOX 34.8 PATIENT TEACHING

Using a Condom Correctly

Objective
- Patient will verbalize correct use of a condom.

Teaching Strategies
- Develop a trusting relationship with patient.
- Explain to patient to always use a latex or rubber condom when having vaginal, oral, or anal sex and to store condoms in a cool, dry place away from sunlight.
- Encourage patient to read the label on the condom package to check the expiration date and ensure that the condom protects against sexually transmitted infections.
- Instruct patient to never reuse a condom or use a damaged condom.
- Explain how to apply the condom correctly (e.g., put it on as soon as the penis is hard and before vaginal, anal, or oral contact; gently squeeze any air out from the tip of the condom, leaving space for semen; unroll the condom to the base of the penis).
- Teach patient to pull out right after ejaculating and hold onto the condom when pulling out.
- Instruct patient to use only water-based lubricants (e.g., K-Y Jelly) to prevent the condom from breaking; do not use petroleum jelly, massage oils, body lotions, or cooking oil.

Evaluation
Use the principles of teach-back to evaluate patient/family caregiver learning:
- Tell me where you store your condoms.
- What would you do if you noticed that a condom you just opened had a slit in it?

needed. Help patients anticipate how their illness or disease will change over time and the adjustments that will be necessary to achieve sexual fulfillment.

After identifying the priority nursing diagnosis and working with Mr. Clements to identify appropriate outcomes, Joshua uses his personal experience as well as the current evidence to select interventions to help Mr. Clements achieve his outcomes. Based on what Joshua has learned, he knows that the priority intervention is to establish a trusting relationship and provide a private setting for their conversations before providing patient education and helping Mr. Clements manage his anxiety. While Joshua is discussing the side effects of antihypertensive medications on sexual functioning, an assistive personnel (AP) enters the room to deliver Mr. Clements' lunch tray. Joshua pauses instruction until the AP leaves and asks Mr. Clements, "I see your lunch is here. Would you like to continue our discussion while you eat, or would you prefer for me to come back after you finish your lunch?" Mr. Clements responds, "Please let's continue our discussion while I eat and before my wife returns this afternoon to visit me."

Restorative and Continuing Care. You need to establish relationships with couples to encourage honest and open discussions about sexual health during restorative or continuing care. Address needs that have been identified in the sexual health history using the basic model such as Ex-PLISSIT (see Fig. 34.3). Management of sexual concerns is important when promoting sexual intimacy and providing closeness and closure between partners at the end of life.

In the home environment it is important to provide information on how an illness limits sexual activity and give ideas for adapting or facilitating sexual activity. Interventions range from giving permission for a partner to lie in bed and hold a patient to coordinating nursing

care and medications to provide opportunity for privacy and intimacy. Often nurses help individuals create an environment that is comfortable for sexual activity in the home. This sometimes involves making recommendations for ways to arrange the bedroom to accommodate physical limitations. For example, some individuals who are in a wheelchair prefer being able to move the chair close to the side of the bed at an angle that allows for more ease in touching and caressing. Suggestions regarding how to accommodate barriers such as Foley catheters or drainage tubes contribute to sexual activity.

Long-term care facilities need to make proper arrangements for privacy during residents' sexual experiences (LeVay et al., 2019). The ideal situation is to set up a pleasant room that is used for a variety of activities that the resident is able to reserve for private visits with a spouse or partner. If this is not possible, arrange for the roommate of a patient to be somewhere else to allow a couple time alone. Never leave patients alone in a situation in which injury is possible.

◆ Evaluation

Through the Patient's Eyes. Evaluate patients' perceptions of nursing interventions to determine whether their expectations have been met. Clinical judgment ensures that you apply what is known about sexuality and a patient's unique situation. Focus on patients' identified sexual concerns and ask if their concerns have been addressed.

When possible, arrange for follow-up discussions with the patient and/or partner to determine whether they were satisfied with your approaches. Sexuality is felt more than observed, and sexual expression requires an intimacy that you cannot observe.

Patient Outcomes. Evaluate whether your patient achieved the expected outcomes established in the plan of care (Fig. 34.6). Ask patients questions about risk factors, sexual concerns, and their level of satisfaction. Observe behavioral cues such as eye contact, posture, and extraneous hand movements that indicate comfort or suggest continued anxiety or concern as topics are addressed. Anticipate the need to modify expectations with an individual and partner when evaluating outcomes. Sometimes you need to establish more appropriate time frames in which to achieve target outcomes. Ask patients to define what is acceptable and satisfying while considering the partner's level of sexual satisfaction. When outcomes are not met, begin to ask questions to determine appropriate changes in interventions. Examples of questions include the following:
- What other questions do you have about your sexual health?
- Did you experience less pain during sexual intercourse after taking your pain medication?
- Which positions did you find most comfortable when you had sexual intercourse? Which positions were most awkward?
- What barriers are preventing you from discussing your feelings and fears with your partner?

Joshua follows up with Mr. Clements by phone approximately 2 weeks after discharge to evaluate the outcomes of Mr. Clements' care. Joshua uses clinical judgment along with his therapeutic communication skills while applying the Ex-PLISSIT model when asking Mr. Clements about his perceptions of his care. Joshua says, "Sometimes when patients who have had a heart attack go home, they are anxious about resuming sexual activity with their spouses. How are you and Mrs. Clements doing? Have you had a chance to talk with her about your concerns?" Mr. Clements states, "I really appreciate what you did for me while I was in the hospital. I understand now that my feelings are normal. I have had a chance to discuss my fears with my wife and explain to her the sexual side effects of my medications. She understands and we are so much happier with our relationship. Thank you so much."

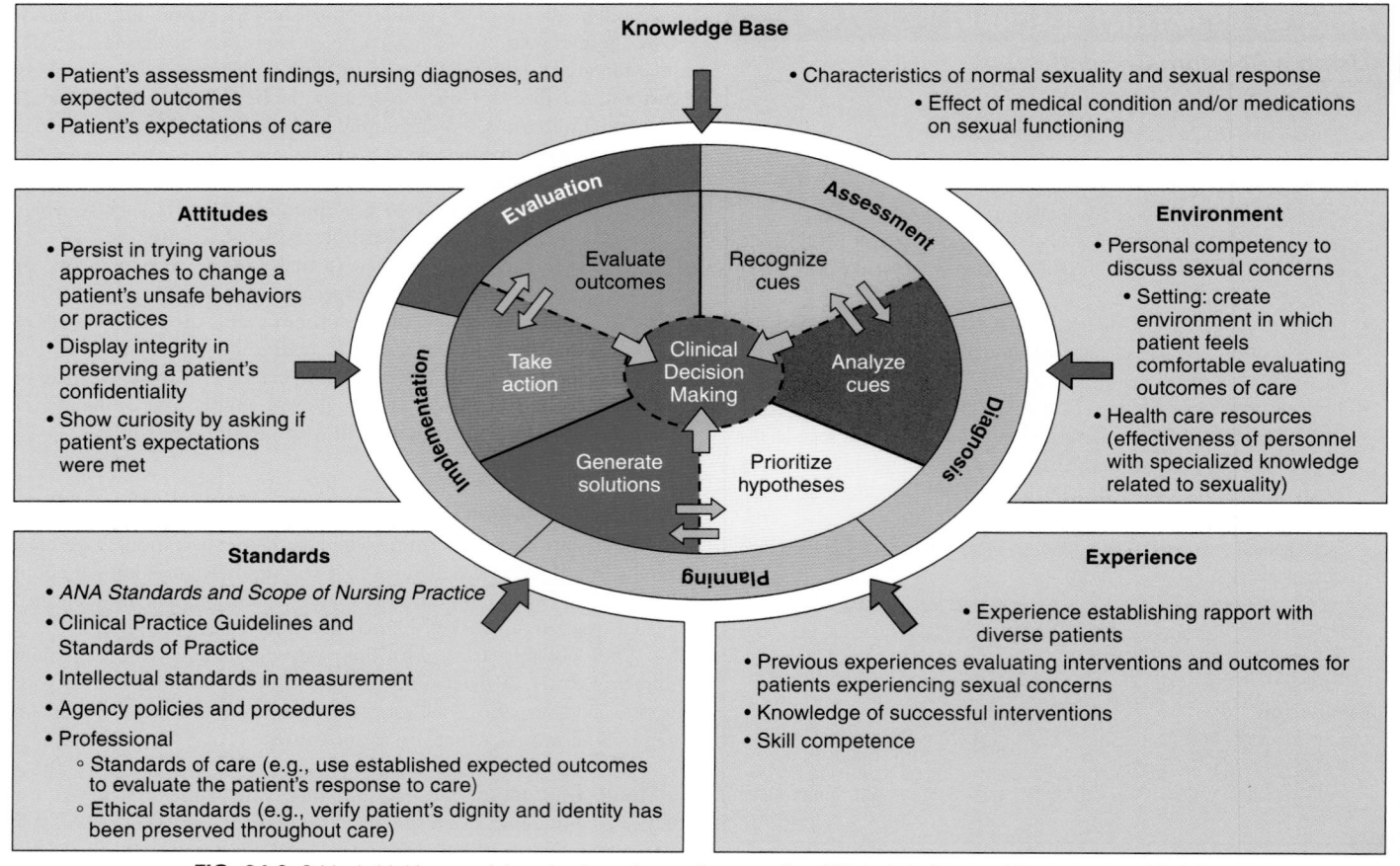

FIG. 34.6 Critical thinking model evaluation of care for sexuality. (Clinical Judgment Measurement Model copyright © NCSBN. All rights reserved.)

KEY POINTS

- Sexual health involves physical and psychosocial aspects and contributes to an individual's sense of self-worth and positive interpersonal relationships.
- Patient risk factors for STIs include risky behaviors, including substance use, low rates of condom use, and multiple partners.
- Building a trusting nurse-patient relationship and appropriately including a patient in decision making supports patients' ability to manage sexual health problems.
- Nurses must be knowledgeable about all aspects of sexuality, including how their own values and issues surrounding sexuality affect patient-centered care.
- Because sexuality is related to all dimensions of health, address sexual concerns or problems as a routine part of nursing care.
- Thoroughly assessing for potential causes of sexual dysfunction, such as the effects of physical problems and medications or altered self-concept, promotes effective treatment.
- Nursing diagnoses related to alterations in sexuality demonstrate the interface between physical and psychological issues.
- To develop an individualized plan of care, collaborate with patients to identify realistic and measurable outcomes of care.
- Expert communication and understanding a patient's nonverbal communication will result in compassionate care surrounding sexuality and sexual health.

- Consider your patient's development stage, personal situation, ethical issues, emotional conflicts, and health status to help you identify appropriate patient-centered nursing interventions to enhance a patient's sexual health.
- Patients who experience improved communication with their partner and establishment or return to a mutually satisfying sex life often perceive that they achieved their outcomes of care following alterations in sexual health.

REFLECTIVE LEARNING

Joshua is now completing a clinical rotation at the health clinic on his university's campus where he meets Cai, a 20-year-old college student of Asian American descent studying mechanical engineering. Cai comes to the campus health clinic after having experienced flulike symptoms with progressive fatigue for several weeks. He tells Joshua that he is gay and has had multiple sexual partners over the past 4 years. Cai has told his sister that he is gay, but he has not yet disclosed his sexual orientation to his parents.

- What assessment data are the most important for Joshua to collect at this time? What strategies would help Joshua establish a therapeutic relationship to put Cai at ease discussing the intimate aspects of his life? State examples of nonjudgmental questions Joshua could ask Cai to determine this information. (Recognize Cues)
- What sexual health conditions and concerns are consistent with Cai's assessment data? (Analyze Cues)

- What is Cai's priority sexual health concern? (Prioritize Diagnoses)
- What might be appropriate outcomes of Cai's care? Which nursing actions and interventions would help Cai achieve these outcomes? Which actions should Joshua plan to avoid because they are irrelevant or potentially harmful? (Generate Solutions)
- Which nursing actions are most appropriate to address Cai's sexual concerns? Describe how Joshua should implement them and place them in order of the highest priority to the lowest priority. (Take Action)
- What evaluative statements made by Cai would indicate that the actions to help Cai achieve enhanced sexual health were effective? Describe alternative actions that could be taken if Cai did not indicate that he met his outcomes of care. (Evaluate Outcomes)

REVIEW QUESTIONS

1. A 16-year-old female tells the school nurse that she does not need the HPV vaccine since her partner always uses condoms. The best response by the nurse to this statement is:
   1. "Latex condoms are the most effective way to eliminate the risk of HPV transmission."
   2. "Your parents may not want you to receive the HPV vaccine since it has been shown to increase sexual risk taking and sexual activity."
   3. "The HPV 9-valent vaccine is recommended for males and females even if they use condoms because it targets the specific viruses that cause cancer and genital warts."
   4. "You are past the recommended age to receive the vaccine."
2. An adolescent who is pregnant for the first time is at her initial prenatal visit. The women's health nurse practitioner (WHNP) informs the patient that she will be screening her for STIs. The patient replies, "I know I don't have an STI because I don't have any symptoms." Which responses by the WHNP would be appropriate? (Select all that apply.)
   1. "Untreated STIs can cause serious complications in pregnancy, so we routinely screen pregnant women."
   2. "Bacterial STIs do not usually cause symptoms, or you could have an asymptomatic viral STI."
   3. "Chlamydia screening is recommended for all sexually active women up to age 25 even if asymptomatic."
   4. "People between the ages of 15 and 24 are often asymptomatic and have the highest incidence of STIs."
   5. "There is no need then to screen for infection since you aren't having any problems or symptoms."
3. A nurse who recently graduated from nursing school is providing discharge instructions to a patient who had an MI. The nurse knows that sexual issues are common after an MI but feels uncomfortable bringing up this topic. What is the best way for the nurse to handle this situation? (Select all that apply.)
   1. Instruct the patient to avoid discussing sexual concerns with his or her partner after discharge.
   2. Avoid discussing the topic unless the patient brings it up.
   3. Ask a more experienced nurse to cover this with the patient and learn from the example.
   4. Plan to attend conferences or training soon on how to discuss such issues.
   5. Provide a patient teaching sheet about how to prevent contacting STIs.

4. A nurse is caring for an older adult patient who is moving into a nursing home. The nurse plans care for this patient with the understanding that:
   1. The patient cannot be sexually active since he is moving into a nursing home.
   2. The patient may want opportunities for privacy to maintain an intimate relationship with his partner.
   3. There is no need to take a sexual history since most older adults are uncomfortable discussing intimate details of their lives.
   4. Older adults in nursing homes usually do not participate in sexual activity.
5. The nurse is providing education on STIs to a group of older adults. The nurse knows that further teaching is needed when the participants make which statements? (Select all that apply.)
   1. "I don't need to use condoms since there is no risk for pregnancy."
   2. "I should be screened for an STI each time I'm with a new partner."
   3. "I know I'm not infected because I don't have discharge or sores."
   4. "I was tested for STIs last year, so I know I'm not infected."
   5. "The infection rate in older adults is low because most are not sexually active."
6. The nurse is providing community education about how the sexual response changes with age. Which statement made by one of the adults indicates the need for further information?
   1. "Health problems such as diabetes, chronic obstructive pulmonary disease, and hypertension have little effect on sexual functioning and desire."
   2. "It usually takes longer for both sexes to reach an orgasm."
   3. "Most of the normal changes in function are related to alteration in circulation and hormone levels."
   4. "Many medications can interfere with sexual function."
7. The nurse is assessing a 28-year-old female patient being admitted to the hospital for orthopedic surgery to stabilize a broken ankle. Which assessment findings indicate potential sexual abuse? (Select all that apply.)
   1. Bruises are present on legs, arms, and back that are in various stages of healing.
   2. The patient's boyfriend will not leave her bedside and answers assessment questions directed to the patient.
   3. The patient states she has no difficulties falling asleep at night.
   4. The patient states she is anxious about having anesthesia and controlling her pain after surgery.
   5. The patient fractured two ribs several years ago.
8. The nurse reviews the health history of a 48-year-old man and notes that he was started on medications for elevated blood pressure and depression at his last annual physical. He tells the nurse that over the past 6 months he has been having difficulty sustaining an erection. The nurse understands that: (Select all that apply.)
   1. Nurses are not expected to discuss sexual issues with male patients and the physician should address this.
   2. Sexual function can be affected by some medications.
   3. STIs can cause complications such as ED, and screening should be done.
   4. Some men with health issues experience ED.
   5. Medications used to treat hypertension and depression seldom interfere with sexual function.

9. The school nurse is counseling an adolescent male who is returning to school after attempting suicide. He denies substance abuse and has no history of treatment for depression. He says he has no friends or family who understand him. The nurse applies clinical judgment using critical thinking to consider all possibilities for the young man's problems, including which of the following? (Select all that apply.)
   1. Adolescents often explore their sexual identity and expose themselves to complications such as STIs or unplanned pregnancy.
   2. Peer approval and acceptance are not important in this age-group.
   3. Lesbian, gay, bisexual, transgender, queer, questioning, asexual, and others (LGBTQ+) youth often experience stress from identification with a sexual minority group.
   4. Knowledge about normal changes associated with puberty and sexuality can decrease stress and anxiety.
   5. Adolescence is a time of emotional stability and self-acceptance.

10. A 53-year-old woman being treated for breast cancer tells the nurse that she has had no interest in sex since her surgery 2 months ago. The nurse is aware that: (Select all that apply.)
    1. Sexual issues can occur in a woman this age.
    2. Women experience sexual dysfunction more frequently than men.
    3. HSDD occurs in women over 65 years of age.
    4. Medical conditions such as cancer often contribute to HSDD.
    5. Disturbances in self-concept affect sexual functioning.

Answers: 1. 3; **2.** 1, 3, 4; **3.** 3, 4, 5; **6.** 1; **7.** 1, 2, 5; **8.** 2, 4; **9.** 1, 3, 4; **10.** 1, 2, 4, 5

Rationales for Review Questions can be found on the Evolve website.

REFERENCES

American Psychological Association (APA): *APA Dictionary of Psychology*, 2020. https://dictionary.apa.org/. Accessed April 25, 2021.

Annon J: The PLISSIT model: a proposed conceptual scheme for the behavioral treatment of sexual problems, *J Sex Educ Ther* 2(2):1, 1976.

Centers for Disease Control and Prevention (CDC): Estimated HIV incidence and prevalence in the United States, 2010–2016, *HIV Surveill Supplemental Rep* 24(1), 2018.

Centers for Disease Control and Prevention (CDC): *School health profiles*, 2019. https://www.cdc.gov/healthyyouth/data/profiles/index.htm. Accessed April 25, 2021.

Centers for Disease Control and Prevention (CDC): *Medical monitoring project*, 2020a. https://www.cdc.gov/hiv/statistics/systems/mmp/index.html. Accessed August 24, 2020.

Centers for Disease Control and Prevention (CDC): *HIV and youth*, 2020b. https://www.cdc.gov/hiv/group/age/youth/. Accessed April 25, 2021.

Centers for Disease Control and Prevention (CDC): *HIV among people aged 50 and over*, 2020c. https://www.cdc.gov/hiv/group/age/olderamericans/. Accessed April 25, 2021.

Centers for Disease Control and Prevention (CDC): *HPV vaccination information for clinicians*, 2020d. https://www.cdc.gov/vaccines/vpd/hpv/hcp/index.html. Accessed April 25, 2021.

Centers for Disease Control and Prevention (CDC): *STD health equity*, 2020e, https://www.cdc.gov/std/health-disparities/default.htm. Accessed August 18, 2021.

Centers for Disease Control and Prevention (CDC): *HIV basics*, 2021a. https://www.cdc.gov/hiv/basics/index.html. Accessed April 25, 2021

Centers for Disease Control and Prevention (CDC): *Sexually transmitted disease surveillance 2019*, 2021b. https://www.cdc.gov/std/. Accessed April 25, 2021.

Centers for Disease Control and Prevention (CDC): *Sexually transmitted diseases (STDs): syphilis*, 2021c. https://www.cdc.gov/std/syphilis/default.htm. Accessed April 25, 2021.

Centers for Disease Control and Prevention (CDC): *Congenital syphilis – CDC fact sheet*, 2021d. https://www.cdc.gov/std/syphilis/stdfact-congenital-syphilis.htm. Accessed April 25, 2021.

Centers for Disease Control and Prevention (CDC): *HIV Treatment*, 2021e. https://www.cdc.gov/hiv/basics/livingwithhiv/treatment.html. Accessed June 8, 2021.

Davis S, Taylor B: From PLISSIT to Ex-PLISSIT. In Davis S, editor: *Rehabilitation: the use of theories and models in practice*. Edinburgh, 2006, Churchill Livingstone.

Erikson E: *Childhood and society*, ed 2, New York, 1963, W. W. Norton.

HIV.gov: *Overview: Data and Trends: U.S. statistics*, 2021. https://www.hiv.gov/hiv-basics/overview/data-and-trends/statistics. Accessed April 25, 2021.

Johns MM, et al: Strengthening our schools to promote resilience and health among LGBTQ youth: emerging evidence and research priorities from *The State of LGBTQ Youth Health and Wellbeing* symposium, *LGBT Health* 6(4):146–155, 2019. https://www.liebertpub.com/doi/full/10.1089/lgbt.2018.0109. Accessed April 25, 2021.

Kann L, et al: Youth risk behavior surveillance—United States, 2017, *MMWR Surveill Summ* 67(8):1–114, 2018.

Landry J, Kensler P: Providing culturally sensitive care to women who are in the sexual minority or are gender non-conforming, *Nurs Womens Health* 23(2):163–171, 2019.

LeVay S, et al: *Discovering human sexuality*, ed 4, New York, 2019, Oxford University Press.

National Center on the Sexual Behavior of Youth (NCSBY): *Childhood sexual development*, n.d., http://ncsby.org/content/childhood-sexual-development. Accessed August 2021.

Taylor B, Davis S: The Extended PLISSIT Model for addressing the sexual wellbeing of individuals with an acquired disability or chronic illness, *Sex Disabil* 25:135–139, 2007. https://www.researchgate.net/publication/226331562_The_Extended_PLISSIT_Model_for_Addressing_the_Sexual_Wellbeing_of_Individuals_with_an_Acquired_Disability_or_Chronic_Illness/download. Accessed April 25, 2021.

Touhy TA, Jett K: *Ebersole and Hess' gerontological nursing and healthy aging*, ed 6, St. Louis, 2021, Elsevier.

Varcarolis E, Fosbre C: *Essentials of psychiatric-mental health nursing: a communication approach to evidence-based care*, ed 4, St. Louis, 2021, Elsevier.

World Health Organization (WHO): *WHO recommendations on adolescent sexual and reproductive health and rights*, Geneva, 2018, World Health Organization.

World Health Organization (WHO): *Defining sexual health*, 2021. http://www.who.int/reproductivehealth/topics/sexual_health/sh_definitions/en/. Accessed April 25, 2021.

RESEARCH REFERENCES

Bauer M, et al: Organisational enablers and barriers to the recognition of sexuality in aged care: a systematic review, *J Nurs Manag* 27(4):858–868, 2019.

Boothby CA, et al: The effect of cardiac rehabilitation attendance on sexual activity outcomes in cardiovascular disease patients: a systematic review, *Can J Cardiol* 34(12):1590–1599, 2018.

Grossman JM, et al: "We talked about sex." "No, we didn't": exploring adolescent and parent agreement about sexuality communication, *Am J Sex Educ* 12(4):343–357, 2017.

Harder H, et al: Sexual functioning in 4,418 postmenopausal women participating in UKCTOCS: a qualitative free-text analysis, *Menopause* 26(10):1100–1009, 2019.

Komlenac N, et al: Associations between gender role conflict, sexual dysfunctions, and male patients' wish for physician-patient conversations about sexual health, *Psychol Men Masc* 20(3):337–346, 2019.

Lever S, Pryor J: The impact of stroke on female sexuality, *Disabil Rehabil* 39(20):2011–2020, 2017.

Niu Z, et al: Associations of social media use, patient-centered communication, and knowledge with

perceived human papillomavirus vaccine effectiveness, *Am J Health Behav* 44(5):642–651, 2020.

Pachankis JE, et al: Brief online interventions for LGBTQ young adult mental and behavioral health: a randomized controlled trial in a high-stigma, low-resource context, *J Consult Clin Psychol* 88(5):429–444, 2020.

Potts J, Southard E: Teaching it forward: Educating parents about HPV/HPV vaccine, *J Dr Nurs Prac*, 12(1):46–58. 2019 doi: 10.1891/2380-9418.12.1.46. Epub 2019 May 9.

Skałacka K, Gerymski R: Sexual activity and life satisfaction in older adults, *Psychogeriatrics* 19(3):195–201, 2019.

Spiritual Health

OBJECTIVES

- Discuss the influence of spirituality on patients' health practices.
- Explain the relationship among faith, hope, and spiritual well-being.
- Compare the concepts of religion and spirituality.
- Recognize cues when assessing a patient's spirituality and spiritual health.

- Explain the importance of establishing caring relationships with patients to provide spiritual care.
- Use clinical judgment in planning nursing interventions that promote a patient's spiritual health.
- Identify approaches for establishing presence with patients.
- Evaluate patient outcomes related to spiritual health.

KEY TERMS

Agnostic

Atheist

Connectedness

Faith

Holistic

Hope

Inner strength and peace

Meaning and purpose in life

Self-transcendence

Spiritual distress

Spiritual well-being

Spirituality

Transcendence

MEDIA RESOURCES

http://evolve.elsevier.com/Potter/fundamentals/
- Review Questions
- Concept Map Creator
- Case Study with Questions

- Audio Glossary
- Content Updates
- Answers to QSEN Activity and Review Questions

Lisa Owens is a 44-year-old African-American nurse manager, diagnosed 3 months ago with breast cancer. She is married to Joe, an accountant, and she is the mother of two children: Davis, who is 17 years old, and Pamela, who is 15. Lisa describes her family as being close and supportive. Surgeons removed Lisa's cancerous tumor and three involved lymph nodes. Because of the lymphatic involvement, Lisa is at increased risk for the cancer to spread. Now that she has completed her radiation treatments, Lisa is visiting the local cancer clinic with her husband 3 times a week for chemotherapy. Lisa has numerous side effects from her chemotherapy, including nausea, decreased appetite, fatigue, hair loss, and difficulty sleeping. Her husband provides most of her support at home, but this sometimes interferes with his ability to do the work that he brings home. Both Lisa and Joe discuss their concern for their children. Davis and Pamela attend young adult education and prayer meetings weekly. Davis, a senior in high school, is beginning to look at colleges for next year. Davis and Pamela shared with Lisa that they are very worried about her cancer diagnosis and health. The family also has less time to talk together due to fewer family dinners because of Lisa's side effects from the chemotherapy and the children's schedules.

Jeff is a 38-year-old nursing student assigned to the oncology clinic. Jeff's preceptor, a nursing case manager, assigns Jeff to follow Lisa. Jeff is in his last semester at school and hopes to get a position in the clinic after graduation. Lisa's experience is significant for Jeff because he has children who are the same age as Lisa's, and he wonders how his children would react if he or his spouse became ill.

During an earlier clinic visit Lisa and Joe discuss the cancer therapy with Jeff. Joe explains, "We both have a lot of faith in God." Lisa responds, "Even though I know I have cancer, I hope to be able to continue to go to church with my family and my children. My family is supportive, and together I know that we will make it through this experience. But I am worried about my children and what the future holds for me. With God's help I hope that I can help them cope with my illness better."

The word *spirituality* comes from the Latin word *spiritus*, which refers to *breath* or *wind*. The spirit gives life to a person. It signifies whatever is at the center of all aspects of a person's life. Florence Nightingale believed that spirituality was a force that provided energy needed to promote a healthy hospital environment and that caring for a person's spiritual needs was just as essential as caring for that person's physical needs (O'Brien, 2018). Today spirituality is often defined as an awareness of one's inner self and a sense of connection to a higher being, nature, or some purpose greater than oneself (Buchanan, 2021). It includes personal beliefs that help a person maintain hope and get through difficult situations. A person's health depends on a balance of physical, psychological, sociological, cultural, developmental, and spiritual factors. Spirituality helps individuals achieve the balance needed to maintain health and well-being and to cope with changes in their health status.

Too often nurses and other health care providers fail to recognize the spiritual dimension of their patients because spirituality is not scientific enough, it has many definitions, and it is difficult to measure. In addition, there are nurses and health care providers who are uncertain about a supreme God or being and uncomfortable with discussing spirituality, while others claim that they do not have time to address patients' spiritual needs (Chen et al., 2017a; Connerton and Moe, 2018). The concepts of spirituality and religion are often interchanged, but spirituality is a much broader and more unifying concept than religion (Buchanan, 2021, Hodge, 2017). While religion is an organized, institution-related practice that is commonly associated with particular beliefs, spirituality focuses on an individual's connection to a higher being, nature, or some purpose greater than oneself (Caplan, 2021).

The human spirit is powerful, and spirituality has different meanings for different people. Some people do not believe in the existence of God (atheist), or they believe that there is no known ultimate reality (agnostic). Nonetheless, spirituality is important regardless of a person's religious beliefs. Atheists search for meaning in life through their work and their relationships with others. Agnostics discover meaning in what they do or how they live, the "here and now," because they find no ultimate meaning for the way things are. They believe that people bring meaning to what they do.

As a nurse, your personal spiritual health is important to your own values and beliefs and can influence your attitudes toward spiritual care, professional commitment, and caring (Chiang et al., 2016). You need to be aware of your own spirituality to recognize and analyze cues that you gather when assessing patients. This will help you provide appropriate and relevant spiritual care to others. As a nurse, you need to care for the whole person and accept a patient's beliefs and experiences (Connerton and Moe, 2018). Being able to determine the importance that spirituality holds for patients depends on your ability to develop caring relationships (see Chapter 7) and to use clinical judgment to recognize and analyze assessment cues, identify and prioritize problems, and implement patient-centered interventions.

SCIENTIFIC KNOWLEDGE BASE

The relationship between spirituality and healing is not completely understood. However, an individual's intrinsic spirit seems to be an important factor in healing. Healing often takes place because of believing. For example, research shows that spirituality positively affects and enhances physical and psychological health, quality of life, health promotion behaviors, and disease prevention activities (Heo et al., 2018).

Spirituality has a positive impact on the ability to cope with anxiety, stress, and depression in family caregivers (Vitorino et al., 2018), mothers with infants in the neonatal intensive care unit (Alemdar et al., 2018), nursing students (Fabbris et al., 2017), patients living with cancer (Hefner et al., 2017), and patients experiencing infertility (Romeiro et al., 2017). Integrative body-mind techniques that include relaxation, guided imagery, mindfulness training, prayer, and music improve coping and healing (Coats, 2017; Hulett and Armer, 2016). A person's inner beliefs and convictions are powerful resources for healing. When you support the spirituality of patients and their families, you help them achieve desirable health outcomes.

REFLECT NOW

What have you observed as patient outcomes when spiritual care was provided to patients?

NURSING KNOWLEDGE BASE

Nursing research also shows the association between spirituality and health. For example, spiritual well-being can provide a potential protective effect against psychosocial distress at the end of life (Bernard et al., 2017). Research also shows that when patients who have cancer participate in religious and spiritual activities, they remain actively engaged socially and continue to have satisfying relationships (Lee, 2019). More research is needed, but the interest in studying the relationship between spirituality and health is greatly contributing to nursing science.

Current Concepts in Spiritual Health

Spiritual health involves finding a balance between one's values, goals, and beliefs and one's relationships within the self and with others. It is a healthy way of expressing and experiencing one's spirituality. Throughout life our spirituality often grows as we become increasingly aware of the meaning, purpose, and values of life. In times of stress, illness, loss, or recovery, a person who is spiritually healthy will often find ways of responding or adjusting to a situation. Often these coping styles lie within a person's spiritual beliefs.

Spiritual beliefs change as patients grow and develop, potentially developing their spirituality as well (Table 35.1). Spirituality begins as children learn about themselves and their relationships with others, including a higher power. As children mature into adulthood, they experience spiritual growth by entering lifelong relationships with people who share similar values and beliefs.

Beliefs among people vary based on cultural factors such as gender, past experience, religion, ethnicity, and economic status. For example, spiritual health in older adults gives peace and acceptance of the self and is often the result of a lifelong connection with a higher power. Illness and loss sometimes threaten and challenge an individual's spiritual development. Older adults often express their spirituality by turning to important relationships and giving of themselves to others (Touhy and Jett, 2020).

A variety of concepts describing spiritual health are a part of nursing science and professional nursing practice. To provide meaningful and supportive spiritual care, it is important to understand the concepts of spirituality, spiritual well-being, faith, religion, and hope. Each concept offers direction in how to assess patient needs and understand the views that individuals have of life and its value. This level of understanding aids in making clinical judgments about patient needs.

Spirituality. Spirituality is a complex concept that is unique to each individual; it depends on a person's culture, development, life experiences, beliefs, and ideas about life (Connerton and Moe, 2018). It is an inherent human characteristic that exists in all people, regardless of their religious beliefs. Spirituality gives individuals the *energy* needed to discover themselves, cope with difficult situations, and maintain health. Energy generated by spirituality helps patients feel well and guides choices (e.g., type and extent of health care) made throughout life. Spirituality enables a person to love, have faith and hope, seek meaning in life, and nurture relationships with others. Because it is subjective, multidimensional, and personal, researchers and scholars cannot agree on a universal definition of spirituality (Connerton and Moe, 2018). However, five distinct but overlapping constructs define it (Fig. 35.1).

- Self-transcendence—a sense of authentically connecting to one's inner self. This contrasts with transcendence, the belief that a force outside of and greater than the person exists beyond the material world (Rochat et al., 2019). Self-transcendence is a positive force. It allows people to have new experiences and develop new perspectives

TABLE 35.1 Relationship Between Developmental Stage and Spirituality	
Erikson's Developmental Stage	**Spiritual Beliefs**
Trust vs. Mistrust Birth to 18 months	Spiritual well-being provided by parents Trust provides basis for hope Love, affection, security, and a stimulating environment promote spirituality
Autonomy vs. Shame and Doubt 18-36 months	Fascination with magic and mystery Often believes that illness is related to bad behavior Begins to learn the difference between right and wrong Imitates parents' spiritual or religious actions; recites prayers and sings simple religious songs, but does not understand their meanings Interprets meanings literally
Initiative vs. Guilt 3-6 years	Feels guilty when not acting responsibly Influenced by spiritual and religious stories, examples, moods, and actions Models moral behaviors of parents Begins to ask about God or Supreme Beings
Industry vs. Inferiority 6-12 years	Wants to learn about spirituality Has a clear picture of God or Supreme Being, morality, and the difference between right and wrong Sorts fantasy from fact Demands proof of reality and believes literal meanings of spiritual stories
Identity vs. Identity Confusion Adolescence	Reflects on inconsistencies in stories Begins to question spiritual practices, forms own opinions, and occasionally discards parents' beliefs Abstract reasoning leads to exploration of moral issues Spirituality comes from connectedness with family, nature, and God or a Supreme Being
Intimacy vs. Isolation and Loneliness Young adulthood	Establishes self-identity and world view Forms independent beliefs, attitudes, and lifestyles Uses principles to solve problems when individual's and society's rules conflict
Generativity vs. Stagnation Middle-age adulthood	Develops appreciation of past spiritual experiences Embraces people from different faiths and religions Reviews value system during crisis Values others
Ego Identity vs. Despair and Disgust Older adulthood	Values love and interactions with others Focuses on overcoming oppression and violence Beliefs vary based on many factors, such as gender, past experiences, religion, economic status, and ethnic background

Data from Edelman CL, Kudzma EC: *Health promotion throughout the life span*, ed 9, St Louis, 2018, Elsevier; and Hockenberry MJ, et al: *Wong's nursing care of infants and children*, ed 11, St Louis, 2019, Elsevier.

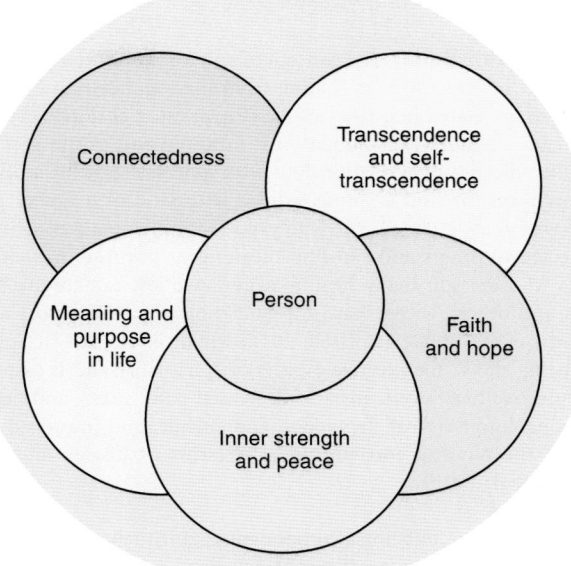

FIG. 35.1 The concept of spirituality has five distinct but overlapping constructs.

that are beyond ordinary physical boundaries. Examples of transcendent moments include the feeling of awe when holding a new baby or looking at a beautiful sunset.

- **Connectedness**—being *intrapersonally* connected within oneself, *interpersonally* connected with others and the environment, and *transpersonally* connected with God or an unseen higher power. Through connectedness patients move beyond the stressors of everyday life and find comfort, faith, hope, and empowerment (Hakanson and Ohlen, 2016).
- **Faith** and **hope**—Faith allows people to have firm beliefs despite lack of physical evidence and enables people to believe in and establish transpersonal connections. Although many people associate faith with religious beliefs, it also exists without them (Christman and Mueller, 2017). For example, one might have faith that all people are good, without being a practitioner of a religion. Hope has several meanings, which vary on the basis of how it is being experienced; it usually refers to an energizing source that has an orientation to future goals and outcomes (Griggs and Walker, 2016).
- **Inner strength and peace**—Spirituality gives people the ability to find a dynamic and creative sense of *inner strength* to use when making difficult decisions. This source of energy helps people stay open to change and life challenges, provides confidence in decision making, and promotes connections with others and a positive outlook on life (Boman et al., 2017). *Inner peace* fosters calm, positive, and peaceful feelings despite life experiences of chaos, fear, and uncertainty. These feelings help people feel comforted, even in times of great distress.
- **Meaning and purpose in life**—Spirituality also helps people find *meaning and purpose* in both positive and negative life events (Dobratz, 2016; Rochat et al., 2019).

Spirituality is an integrating theme to these constructs. A person's spirituality begins in childhood and continues to grow throughout adulthood. It represents the totality of one's being, serving as the overriding perspective that unifies the various aspects of an individual. It spreads through all dimensions of a person's life, whether or not the person acknowledges or develops it.

Spiritual Well-Being. The concept of spiritual well-being is defined as feelings of contentment coming from the inner self and has been shown to be related to quality of life (Phenwan et al., 2019). Spiritual well-being includes four dimensions: meaning and purpose of one's own life, interpersonal relationships with others, a sense of unity with the environment, and a connectedness with God or a higher power (Phenwan et al., 2019). Those who experience spiritual well-being feel connected to others and can find meaning or purpose in their lives. Those who are spiritually healthy experience joy, can forgive themselves and others, accept hardship and mortality, and report an enhanced quality of life (Cottrell, 2016; Khahi et al., 2017). Spiritual well-being shows the positive aspects of spirituality and is associated with positive health outcomes of decreased pain, stress, and negative emotions; lower risk of depression and suicide; and improved tolerance of the physical and emotional stressors of disease and illness (Harrad et al., 2019).

Faith. In addition to being a component of spirituality, the concept of faith has other definitions. It can be described as a cultural or institutional religion such as Judaism, Buddhism, Islam, or Christianity. It is also a relationship with a divinity, higher power, or spirit that incorporates a reasoning faith (belief) and a trusting faith (action). Reasoning faith provides confidence in something for which there is no proof. It is an acceptance of what reasoning cannot explain. Sometimes faith involves a belief in a higher power, spirit guide, God, or Allah. It is also the way a person chooses to live. It gives purpose and meaning to an individual's life, allowing for action.

Religion. Religion is associated with the "state of doing," or a specific system of practices associated with a particular denomination, sect, or form of worship. It is a system of organized beliefs and worship that a person practices to outwardly express spirituality. Many people practice a faith or belief in the doctrines and expressions of a specific religion or sect, such as the Lutheran church or Judaism. People from different religions also view spirituality differently. For example, a Buddhist believes in Four Noble Truths:
1. Life is suffering.
2. Suffering is caused by karma and disturbing emotions.
3. Suffering can be eliminated by eliminating karma and disturbing emotions.
4. To eliminate karma, disturbing emotions, and suffering, one follows an eightfold path (i.e., right understanding, intention, speech, action, livelihood, effort, mindfulness, and concentration) (Rinpoche, 2017).

A Buddhist turns inward, valuing self-control, whereas a Christian looks to the love of God to provide enlightenment and direction in life.

When providing spiritual care, it is important to understand the differences between religion and spirituality. Many people tend to use the terms interchangeably. Although closely associated, they are not synonymous. Religious practices encompass spirituality, but spirituality does not need to include religious practice. Religious care helps patients maintain their faithfulness to their belief systems and worship practices. Spiritual care helps people identify meaning and purpose in life, look beyond the present, and maintain personal relationships and a relationship with a higher being or life force.

Hope. A spiritual person's faith brings hope. When a person has the attitude of something to live for and look forward to, hope is present. It is a multidimensional concept that provides comfort while people endure life-threatening situations, hardships, and other personal challenges. Hope is closely associated with faith; it is energizing and motivates people to achieve goals, such as adopting healthy behaviors. People express hope in all aspects of their lives to help them deal with life stressors. It is a valuable personal resource whenever someone is facing a loss (see Chapter 36) or a difficult challenge (Griggs and Walker, 2016).

Factors Influencing Spirituality

When illness, loss, grief, or a major life change occurs, people often use spiritual resources to help them cope and search for meaning. Spiritual needs and concerns usually develop when people fail to use their spiritual resources during these times. Spiritual distress is "a disruption in the life principle that pervades a person's entire being and transcends the person's biologic and psychosocial nature" (Andrews and Boyle, 2016). It causes people to question their identities and to feel doubt, lose faith, and feel alone or abandoned. Individuals often question their spiritual values or the meaning of life, raising questions about their way of life, purpose for living, and source of meaning (Connerton and Moe, 2018). Spiritual distress also occurs when there is conflict between a patient's beliefs and prescribed health regimens or when patients face the inability to practice usual rituals. An example is the experiences many individuals felt during the COVID-19 pandemic when churches and other religious and community settings were closed.

Acute Illness. Sudden, unexpected illness often creates spiritual distress. For example, both a 50-year-old patient who has a heart attack and a 20-year-old patient who is in a motor vehicle accident face crises that threaten spiritual health. The sudden illness or injury creates an unanticipated scramble to integrate and cope with new realities (e.g., disability). People often look for ways to remain faithful to their beliefs and value systems. Some pray, attend religious services more often, or spend time reflecting on the positive aspects of their lives. Often conflicts develop around a person's beliefs and the meaning of life. Anger is common; sometimes patients express it against God or a higher power, their families, themselves, and their nurses or other health care providers. The strength of patients' spirituality influences their ability to cope with and recover from sudden illness or injury.

Chronic Illness. Many chronic illnesses threaten a person's independence, causing fear, anxiety, and spiritual distress. Dependence on others for routine self-care needs often creates feelings of powerlessness. Powerlessness and the loss of a sense of purpose in life impair the ability to cope with alterations in functioning. Patients often use their spirituality to adapt to and live with chronic illness. Successfully adapting to lifestyle changes strengthens a person spiritually, but it sometimes takes a long-term plan to help a patient with a chronic illness achieve spiritual well-being. Successful adaptation provides spiritual growth. Patients who have a sense of spiritual well-being feel connected with a higher power, are able to find meaning and purpose in life, and are better able to cope with and accept their chronic illness (Larsen, 2019). Exploring the meaning of pain and suffering with patients allows you to provide spiritual support during their illnesses (Harrad et al., 2019).

Terminal Illness. Dying encompasses a patient's physical, social, psychological, and spiritual health (Finocchiaro, 2016). Terminal illness causes fears of physical pain, loss of independence, isolation, the unknown, and dying. It creates an uncertainty about what death means, making patients susceptible to spiritual distress. However, some patients have a spiritual sense of peace that enables them to face death without fear. Spirituality helps these patients find peace in themselves and their death. Individuals experiencing a terminal illness find themselves reviewing life and questioning its meaning. Those who struggle ask common questions, such as "Why is this happening to me?" or "What have I done?" Terminal illness affects family and friends as well. It causes members of the family to ask important questions about its meaning and how it will affect their relationship with the patient (see Chapter 36). When caring for dying patients, help them gain a greater sense of control over their illness, whether they are in a health care setting (e.g., the hospital) or at home.

Near-Death Experience. Some nurses care for patients who have had a near-death experience (NDE). An NDE is a psychological phenomenon of people who either have been close to clinical death or have recovered after being declared dead. It is not associated with a mental disorder. Instead experts agree that NDE describes a powerfully close brush with the physical, emotional, and spiritual experiences of death. For example, people who have an NDE after cardiopulmonary arrest often tell the same story of feeling themselves rising above their bodies and watching caregivers initiate lifesaving measures. Commonly, patients who have had an NDE describe it as feeling totally at peace, having an out-of-body experience, being pulled into a dark tunnel, seeing bright lights, and meeting people who preceded them in death (Martial et al., 2017). Instead of moving toward the light, they learn that it is not time for them to die, and they return to life (Koch, 2020; Rawlings and Devery, 2015). Martone (2019) notes that NDEs are shared across a broad range of cultures and religions so it is unlikely that they are reflections of specific religious expectations. Instead, a commonality suggests that NDEs might reflect changes in how the brain functions as one approaches death.

A recent study compared stories of people experiencing NDEs with stories of patients who had taken psychoactive drugs (Martial et al., 2019). One drug in particular, ketamine, led to experiences similar to NDE. This suggests that an NDE may reflect changes in the same chemical system in the brain that is targeted by drugs like ketamine (Martial et al., 2019).

Patients who have an NDE may be reluctant to discuss it, thinking family or caregivers will not understand. A nurse's acceptance and response to a patient's report of an NDE impacts how much the patient shares about the experience (Rawlings and Devery, 2015). NDEs are often transformational and can be either positive or negative experiences (Koch, 2020). However, individuals experiencing an NDE who discuss it openly with family or caregivers find acceptance and meaning from this powerful experience (Rawlings and Devery, 2015). They are often no longer afraid of death, and they have a decreased desire to achieve material wealth. They also report increased sensitivity to different chemicals such as alcohol and medications. After patients have survived an NDE, promote spiritual well-being by remaining open, giving patients a chance to explore what happened, and supporting them as they share the experience with significant others (Rawlings and Devery, 2015).

Jeff plans for Lisa and Joe's return to the oncology clinic. He spends time learning more about breast cancer, how patients cope with the diagnosis, and Lisa's disease and treatment plan, so he can better assess Lisa's acceptance and how she is coping with her chemotherapy progress. Jeff knows that Joe usually comes to the clinic, and Lisa describes him as a strong source of support. However, Jeff does not know enough about the couple's relationship and wants to explore this further. The role of family members in providing support, particularly regarding decision making, is important for Jeff to understand before he develops a plan of care. As part of this, Jeff wants to learn more about promoting feelings of hope and connectedness as a means for coping with illness. In reviewing information about loss and grieving, Jeff recognizes that Lisa shows acceptance of

her disease because she can discuss cancer and the plan for treatment. Jeff knows that as patients begin to accept the diagnosis of a life-threatening disease, it is important to offer opportunities to share feelings and discuss the future.

CRITICAL THINKING

Successful critical thinking requires a synthesis of knowledge, experience, environmental factors, information gathered from patients, critical thinking attitudes, and intellectual and professional standards. Critical thinking allows a nurse to anticipate what to assess about a patient and to make clinical judgments about the patient's nursing diagnoses so that clinical decisions can be made for planning and providing relevant patient-centered interventions. During assessment, consider all elements that build toward making nursing diagnoses (Fig. 35.2).

The helping role is central to nursing practice. Patients look to nurses for help that is different from the help they seek from other health care professionals. Expert nurses acquire the ability to anticipate personal issues affecting patients and their spiritual well-being. This is based on their knowledge about spirituality concepts as well as the health conditions affecting their patients. For example, knowledge of the course of a terminal disease coupled with an understanding of the factors that contribute to hope and faith can guide a nurse in asking questions that will reveal a patient's coping status.

Critical thinking involves applying knowledge and interpersonal skills that enable nurses to enhance patients' spiritual well-being and health. Nurses who are comfortable with their own spirituality often are more likely to care for their patients' spiritual needs (Harrad et al., 2019). Beliefs of a health care provider affect the discussion of treatment options with patients and ultimately their health care choices. For example, an oncologist might encourage a second round of chemotherapy rather than recommend palliative care. Focusing on patients' spiritual health means advocating for their ability to exercise their beliefs. Spiritual care is a part of holistic practice. When providing spiritual care, do not let your personal biases form wrong conclusions about patient needs. Nurses who foster their own personal, emotional, and spiritual health are resources for their patients if they listen to patients' personal stories and then use their own spirituality as a tool when caring for themselves and their patients.

Use your nursing knowledge about spirituality concepts to anticipate your patients' personal issues and the resulting effect on spiritual well-being. Your knowledge about the concept of spirituality, your understanding of ethics (see Chapter 22), and your knowledge of a patient's faith and belief systems help to provide appropriate spiritual care. Knowledge of a patient's values, beliefs, preferences, and needs provides insight into a person's spiritual practices. Application of therapeutic communication principles (see Chapter 24) and caring principles (see Chapter 7) helps you establish therapeutic trust with patients. An individual's spiritual beliefs are very personal. When you integrate patient preferences, values, and beliefs into spiritual care, you provide patient-centered care with sensitivity and respect for the diversity of human experience (QSEN Institute, 2020).

Personal experience in caring for patients in spiritual distress or who require spiritual care is valuable when assessing a patient's situation and then helping the patient identify coping options. Frequently, your previous clinical experiences in delivering spiritual care for patients will provide you with knowledge of specific religious beliefs and practices. Also, you may have had experiences helping pastoral care or a chaplain meet a patient's need for personal religious practices. Knowing your own spirituality can be beneficial in assisting patients. Nurses who sense a personal faith and hope regarding life may be better able to help their patients. Nurses learn from their personal faith system

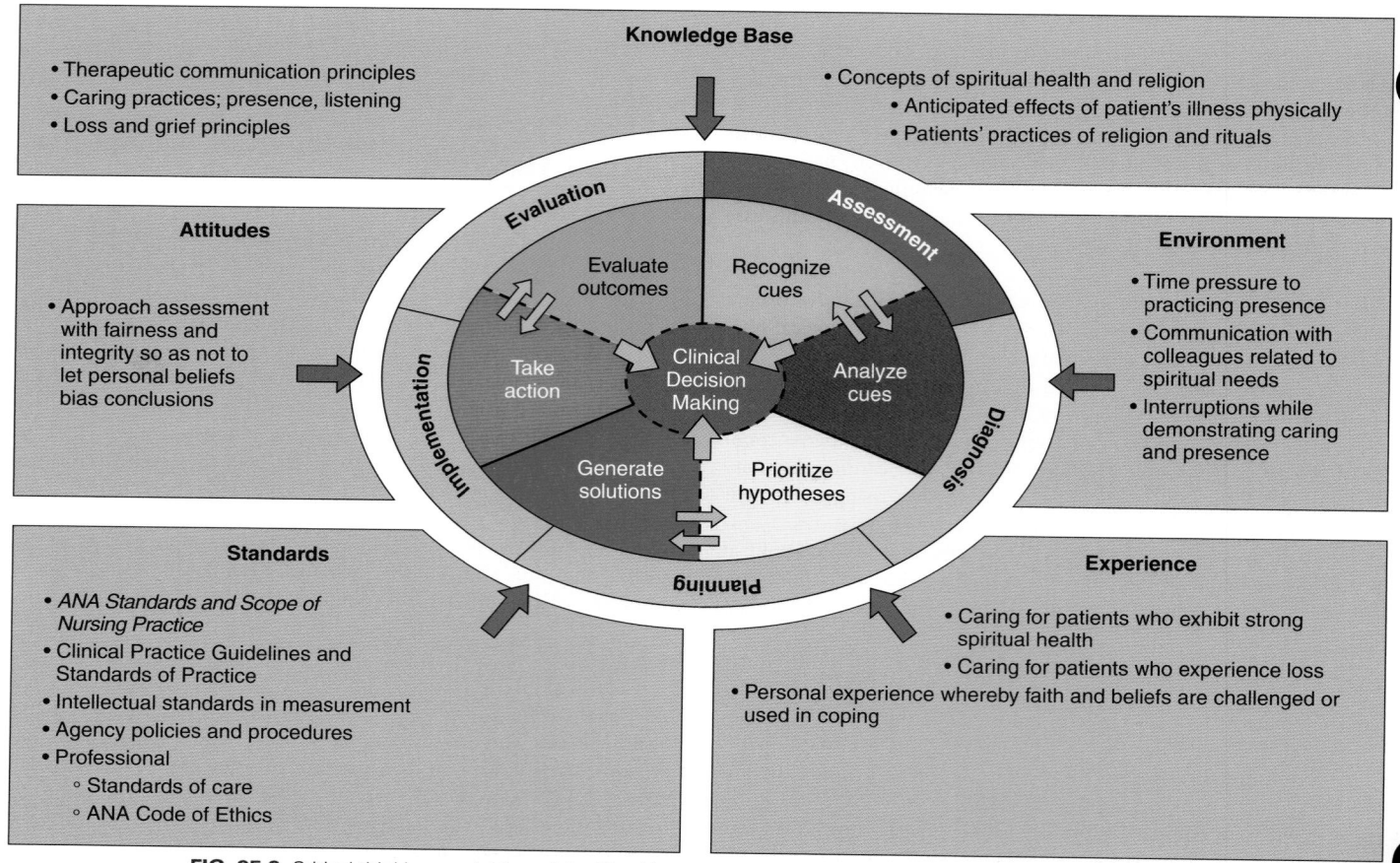

FIG. 35.2 Critical thinking model for spiritual health assessment. *ANA,* American Nurses Association. (Clinical Judgment Measurement Model copyright © NCSBN. All rights reserved.)

and previous professional experiences how to provide spiritual care comfortably (Clarke and Baume, 2019).

Use critical thinking attitudes when assessing each patient's reaction to illness, injury, and loss and determining whether spiritual intervention is necessary. Humility is essential, especially when caring for patients from diverse cultural backgrounds. Recognize personal limitations in knowledge about patients' spiritual beliefs and religious practices. Effective nurses show genuine concern as they assess their patients' beliefs and determine how spirituality influences their patients' health. You demonstrate integrity by refraining from voicing your opinions about religion or spirituality when your beliefs conflict with those of your patients.

Apply intellectual standards to ensure accurate clinical decisions that will help patients find meaningful and logical ways to acquire spiritual wellness. Critical thinking ensures that you obtain significant and relevant information when assessing and making decisions about patients' spiritual needs. Avoid making assumptions about their religion and beliefs. Significance and relevance are standards of critical thinking that allow you to explore the issues that are most meaningful to patients and most likely to affect spiritual well-being.

In setting standards for quality health care, The Joint Commission (TJC) (2020) requires health care organizations to acknowledge patients' rights to spiritual care and to provide for patients' spiritual needs through pastoral care or others who are certified, ordained, or lay individuals. The standards also require that you assess patients' beliefs and spiritual practices. The HealthCare Chaplaincy Network (2021) has developed evidence-based structural and process indicators and outcome metrics for quality spiritual care.

The American Nurses Association *Code of Ethics for Nurses* (2015) requires nurses to practice nursing with compassion and respect for the inherent dignity, worth, and uniqueness of every person. It is essential to promote an environment that respects patients' values, customs, and spiritual beliefs. Routinely implementing standard nursing interventions such as prayer or meditation is coercive and unethical. Therefore, determine which interventions are compatible with your patient's beliefs and values before selecting them based on patient input. An ethic of caring (see Chapter 7) provides a framework for decision making and places the nurse as the patient's advocate.

REFLECT NOW

Consider your own spiritual beliefs and spiritual health. How do your own spiritual beliefs and spiritual health impact the care you provide your patients?

❖ NURSING PROCESS

Apply critical thinking when conducting the nursing process in your care of patients. During each step of the nursing process you will make clinical judgments necessary for clinical decision making. This approach leads to the development and implementation of patient-centered plans for spiritual care. You need a broad perspective and an open mind to understand a patient's spirituality and appropriately identify the level of support and resources a patient requires. As a nurse, you are ethically responsible for meeting the spiritual needs of your patients. People experience the world and find meaning in life differently. Application of the nursing process from the perspective of a patient's spiritual needs is complex. It goes beyond assessing religious practices. Be willing to share and discover your patient's meaning and purpose in life, illness, and health. Identify common values and respect unique commitments and values with your patients by having quiet conversations, listening effectively, and communicating using presence and touch when appropriate (Clarke and Baume, 2019).

◆ Assessment

During the assessment process thoroughly assess each patient and critically analyze findings to ensure that you make patient-centered clinical decisions required for safe nursing care. Because completing a spiritual assessment takes time, conduct an ongoing assessment over the course of a patient's stay in the health care setting if possible. Convey caring in your manner and communication style. Caring is conveyed by knowing your patient's cultural values and beliefs; respecting privacy, diversity, and individual needs; and interacting and listening to the patient and family (Narayan, 2018). Be open to successfully promoting an honest discussion about each patient's spiritual beliefs. Your spiritual assessment will reveal the patient's beliefs about life, health, and a Supreme Being or power.

Through the Patient's Eyes. It is essential to take the time to assess a patient's viewpoints and establish a trusting relationship. Talking about spirituality with a patient helps build a trusting relationship that often leads to conversations about health outcomes (Buchanan, 2021). As you and your patients reach a point of learning together, spiritual caring occurs. Be sure to discuss what is meaningful and relevant to your patients. Encourage them to discuss their personal beliefs and faith traditions. Explore the meaning that their illnesses have in their lives, based on their faith beliefs. Discover the patients' expectations by asking questions such as "How is your illness affecting your health and what is important to you?" "How can we best partner with you to meet your spiritual needs while you are here?" "What is important to you spiritually?" "Are there religious or prayer practices that are important for you to continue while you are in the hospital?" "Are there special practices that help you manage your illness or pain?" or "Is there anyone we can call who is a source of strength, support, or comfort for you?" Assessing a patient's perceptions is therapeutic for you and your patients because it conveys a level of caring and support from the nurse to the patient (ANA, APA, and ISPN, 2014).

Environmental Factors. The health care environment can be noisy and full of interruptions. Assessing a patient's spirituality requires an environment that is quiet, private, and conducive to intimate discussion. Thus you need to determine whether any environmental factors will affect your ability to assess your patient and provide spiritual care. Avoid time conflicts and interruptions by setting aside specific time to be with your patient. Effective assessment requires you to be caring and present and to create an environment that is quiet and free from distractions. Building a trusting relationship and communicating respectfully will help you discover what is most important to your patient and understand the role your patients' spirituality plays in their health and daily life.

Experience With Illness or Disability. Before engaging in a focused spiritual assessment, determine how a patient is responding physically and psychologically to an illness or disability. Is the patient showing improvement? Are there difficult symptoms to expect by the nature of the illness? Having a better understanding of your patients'

BOX 35.1 Nursing Assessment Questions

Spirituality and Spiritual Health
- What experiences with your illness have been most difficult for you?
- What gives you hope during this difficult time?
- In what way has a sense of spirituality been most helpful to you?
- Which aspects of your spirituality would you like to discuss?

Faith, Belief, Fellowship, and Community
- To what or whom do you look as a source of strength, hope, or faith in times of difficulty?
- How does your faith help you cope?
- What can I do to support your religious beliefs or faith commitment? Would you like me to pray with you or perhaps read from the Koran or Bible?
- What gives your life meaning?

Life and Self-Responsibility
- How do you feel about the changes this illness has caused?
- How do these changes affect what you now need to do?

Life Satisfaction
- How happy or satisfied are you with your life?
- Which accomplishments help you feel satisfied with your life?
- What is it that makes you feel dissatisfied?

Connectedness
- What feelings do you have after you pray or meditate?
- Who do you feel is the most important person in your life?

Vocation
- How has your illness affected the way you live your life spiritually at home or where you work?
- In what way has your illness affected your ability to express what is important in life to you?

---

illnesses and conditions helps you support them spiritually (Harrad et al., 2019). Your knowledge about a patient's disease condition and any experience in caring for similar patients helps you anticipate what symptoms they are likely to suffer and the treatments they are likely undergoing. As you listen to their stories about their illness and treatment, you will gain a sense of their coping status and perceptions of their health, including their spiritual health.

Assessment Tools. Listening to a patient's story is an essential method for obtaining a spiritual assessment. You can also assess your patients' spiritual health by using open-ended questions to prompt them to tell their story or by asking them direct questions (Box 35.1). As you determine that spirituality is significant to a patient, focus your assessment on aspects of spirituality most likely to be influenced by the patient's illness and life experiences or events. Does the patient have questions about illness and hospitalization? Asking direct questions requires you to feel comfortable in asking others about their spirituality. Some health care agencies and researchers have created assessment tools to clarify patients' values and to assess their level of spirituality. For example, the spiritual well-being (SWB) scale has 20 questions that assess a patient's relationship with God and sense of life purpose and life satisfaction (Life Advance, 2018). The FICA assessment tool (Borneman et al., 2010; Puchalski and Romer, 2000) evaluates spirituality and is closely correlated to quality of life. FICA stands for the following criteria: F—Faith or belief; I—Importance and Influence, C—Community; A—Address (interventions to address).

Effective assessment tools such as the SWB scale and FICA help you remember important areas to assess. Patient responses to the assessment items on the tools indicate areas that you need to investigate further. *For example, after using the FICA tool with Lisa, Jeff found that Lisa has a strong faith belief, that Lisa's faith is an important part of her life, and that Lisa draws strength from her spirituality and religion. Jeff also discovered that Lisa has a solid support system through her church community.* Remember, when using any spiritual assessment tool, do not impose your personal values on your patient. Be careful about making false assumptions about your patients' beliefs based on your personal values and beliefs. When you understand the overall approach to spiritual assessment, you are able to enter into thoughtful discussions with patients, gain a greater awareness of the personal resources they bring to a situation, and incorporate the resources into an effective plan of care.

Faith/Belief. When assessing a patient's faith, first determine that patient's beliefs, especially those that influence hope. *For example, Jeff asked how Lisa believes a chemotherapy drug will affect her newly diagnosed breast cancer. Jeff also asked Lisa whether she believes in the skill or competence of her physician.* Determine which of your patient's beliefs guide the patient to find meaning in life events and to thus make decisions. Ask your patient whether they are able to live according to their beliefs. Finally, assess to what extent your patient interrelates with self, others, and/or a source of authority. Faith in an authority (such as a health care provider or senior family member) provides a sense of confidence that guides a person in exercising beliefs and experiencing growth. Assess a person's faith in an authority by asking "To whom do you look to for guidance in life?" The patient's response to an open-ended question such as this is likely to open the door for a meaningful discussion. Listen carefully and explore what is meaningful to the patient.

Determine whether a patient has a religious source of guidance that conflicts with medical treatment plans and affects the options that nurses and other health care providers are able to offer patients. For example, if a patient is a Jehovah's Witness, blood products are not an acceptable form of treatment (Jehovah's Witnesses, 2021). Christian Scientists may refuse any medical intervention, believing that their faith heals them. It is also important to understand a patient's philosophy of life. A thorough assessment reveals the basis of a patient's belief system regarding meaning and purpose in life and the patient's spiritual focus. Asking a patient "Describe for me what is most important in your life" or "Tell me what gives your life meaning or purpose" helps to assess the basis of the patient's spiritual belief system. This information often reflects the impact that illness, loss, or disability has on a person's life. Considerable religious diversity exists in the United States. A patient's religious faith and practices, views about health, and the response to illness influence how nurses provide support.

Life and Self-Responsibility. Spiritual well-being includes life and self-responsibility. Individuals who accept change in life, make decisions about their lives, and are able to forgive others in times of difficulty have a higher level of spiritual well-being. During illness patients often are unable to accept limitations or do not know how to regain a functional and meaningful life. However, they often use their spiritual well-being as a resource for adapting to changes and dealing with limitations. Assess the extent to which a patient understands the limitations or threats posed by an illness (e.g., activity restriction, sexual intimacy with a partner, risk of medical complications) and the manner in which the patient chooses to adjust to them. Ask, "Tell me how you feel about the changes caused by your illness" and "How do these changes affect what you now need to do?"

Connectedness. People who are connected to themselves, others, nature, and God or another Supreme Being usually report higher levels of physical and emotional health (Hakanson and Ohlen, 2016). One way patients remain connected is by praying (Fig. 35.3). Prayer is personal communication with one's higher power that provides a sense of hope, strength, security, and well-being; it is a way to exercise one's faith. Patients often use prayer when other treatments are ineffective, when they are experiencing fear or anxiety, or when they feel that they have no control over what is happening to them (Christensen et al., 2018; O'Brien, 2018). Help patients become or remain connected by respecting each patient's unique sense of spirituality. Assess a patient's connectedness by asking open-ended questions: "Whom do you believe is the most important person in your life?" "In what way do you stay connected spiritually?" "Is prayer something helpful to you?" or "What feeling do you have after you pray?"

Life Satisfaction. Spiritual well-being is tied to a person's satisfaction with life and accomplishments, even in the case of children (Dobratz, 2016). When people are satisfied with life and how they are using their abilities, more energy is available to deal with new difficulties and resolve problems. You assess a patient's satisfaction with life by asking questions such as "How happy or satisfied are you with your life?" or "Tell me how satisfied you feel about what you have accomplished in life" or "Describe what makes you feel dissatisfied with your life."

Culture. Spirituality is a personal experience within a cultural context. It is important to know a patient's cultural background and assess a patient's values about the health care problem and impending treatment (see Chapter 9). It is common in many cultures for individuals to believe that they have led a worthwhile and purposeful life. Remaining connected with their cultural heritage often helps patients define their place in the world and express their spirituality. Asking them about their faith and belief systems is a good beginning for understanding the relationship between culture and spirituality (Box 35.2).

Fellowship and Community. Fellowship is one kind of relationship that an individual has with other people, including immediate family, close friends, associates at work or school, fellow members of a place of worship, and neighbors. More specifically, this includes the extent of the community of shared faith between people and their support networks. Many times, social support from faith-based groups helps patients cope with illness and participate in health promotion behaviors (Davis et al., 2018). To assess a patient's supportive community, ask questions such as "Who do you find to be the greatest source of support in times of difficulty?" or "When you have faced difficult times in the past, who has been your greatest resource?"

Explore the extent and nature of a person's support networks and their relationship with the patient. It is unwise to assume that a given network offers the type of support that a patient desires. For example, calling a patient's pastor to request a visit is inappropriate if the patient has little fellowship with the pastor or the pastor's faith community. What level of support does the community or friends give? Do they visit, say prayers, or support the patient's immediate family? Learn whether openness exists between a patient and the people with whom a fellowship has formed.

Ritual and Practice. Assessing the use of rituals and practices that are affected as a result of a patient's illness helps you understand a patient's spirituality. Rituals include participation in worship, prayer, sacraments (e.g., baptism, Holy Eucharist), fasting, singing, meditating, Scripture reading, and making offerings or sacrifices. Different religions have different rituals for life events. For example, Buddhists

FIG. 35.3 Praying keeps individuals connected to their God. (Copyright © iStock/khunpepe; iStock/Goldquest; iStock/palidachan; iStock/Sunshine Seeds.)

🌐 BOX 35.2 CULTURAL ASPECTS OF CARE

Spirituality and Culture

Spirituality and spiritual health vary among cultures. Remember that a person's culture is defined by age, gender, social position, political association, religion, or other variables such as ethnicity and educational background. One's culture influences religious practices as well as beliefs about health and illness. One way to assess a patient's spirituality through a cultural lens is to first understand the patient's definition of health, wellness, and illness. For example, ask questions such as "What do you call your health problem?" "What do you think has caused it?" "What do you think your sickness does to you?" and "How do you find strength to cope with this problem?"

You want to assess how a patient's spirituality is affected by culture. If your focus is on a patient's ethnicity, know the unique characteristics of that ethnic group's spiritual values. Ethnicity impacts culturally significant events such as birth, death, puberty, childbearing, childrearing, and illness and death (Giger and Haddad, 2021). There are often rituals tied to spirituality and religion for events such as weddings and funerals (Giger and Haddad, 2021). Many cultures have treatments for illness and disease that are rooted in folk medicine, holistic care, or spiritual interventions

Implications for Patient-Centered Care
- Explore the spirituality of patients from different cultural backgrounds; assess the meaning of health and how patients achieve balance, peace, or comfort in their lives.
- Offer a universal and holistic approach when assessing patients' needs (see Chapter 9); demonstrate cultural competence and use therapeutic communication techniques.
- During assessment respect patients' human rights, values, customs, and spiritual beliefs (see Chapter 9).
- Include interprofessional health care team members when conducing a spiritual assessment. If you feel uncomfortable with religion or spirituality, respectfully identify whether a patient wishes referral to an appropriate professional chaplain or clergy.
- Avoid use of language that alienates or discriminates among different cultures and belief systems.
- Use a professional interpreter if necessary.

---

practice baptism later in life and find burial or cremation acceptable at death. Followers of Islam practice Salah, the second of the Five Pillars of Islam, requiring all Muslims who have reached puberty to worship five times daily, facing the holy city of Mecca. Orthodox and conservative Jews circumcise their newborn sons 8 days after birth. Determine whether illness or hospitalization has interrupted a patient's ability to

follow usual rituals or practices and what can be done to restore the patient's involvement. If rituals are important to a patient, use them as part of nursing intervention.

Vocation. Individuals express their spirituality on a daily basis in life routines, work, play, and relationships. It is often a part of a person's identity and vocation. Determine whether illness, injury, or hospitalization alters the ability to express some aspect of spirituality as it relates to the person's work or daily activities. Expression of spirituality includes showing an appreciation for life in the variety of things people do, living in the moment and not worrying about tomorrow, appreciating nature, and being productive. When illness or loss prevents patients from expressing their spirituality, understand the implications this has on the patient's identity and vocation, and provide appropriate guidance and support. Questions to ask include "How has your illness affected the way you live your life spiritually at home or where you work?" or "How has your illness affected your ability to express what is important in life for you?"

Jeff's previous experiences with patients who have cancer taught him that when patients express hope, they move forward and cope better with the challenges of their disease. During the last clinic visit Lisa stated that she hoped she would be able to continue to attend religious services at her church. Jeff reflected on that experience and thinks that Lisa and Joe have a strong sense of spiritual well-being that will help them cope with cancer. However, further assessment is necessary.

Jeff also knows that patients' spiritual needs are often associated with their cultural, social, and ethnic background. African-American women generally express a deep relationship with God and strong moral and ethical values. Spirituality for African-Americans often provides a source of healing, coping, and peace. Furthermore, being connected with a caring community environment such as a neighborhood or church is particularly important for African-American women who have breast cancer because caring communities provide great emotional and social support (Davis et al., 2018; Williams, 2019). Jeff applies this information when he assesses Lisa's spiritual needs, validates that this perspective is shared by Lisa, and uses this understanding of breast cancer and spirituality among African-American women to provide patient-centered care for Lisa and her family.

Jeff wants to completely assess Lisa and Joe's level of spiritual health. He begins by asking Lisa and Jeff "What is important in your life?" and "What gives your lives meaning?" Jeff knows it is important to understand how Lisa's breast cancer has impacted their lives, so he asks, "How do the changes caused by Lisa's breast cancer affect what you want or need to do?" Jeff asks if they belong to a church. When Jeff finds out that Lisa and Jeff regularly attend church and get support from their church family, he asks, "Is prayer helpful to you?" When Lisa and Joe tell Jeff that prayer is important to them, Jeff asks Lisa and Jeff if they would like to pray together at this time. As Jeff gathers assessment data, he will begin to analyze the data and look for cues and clusters of data that will help him identify nursing diagnoses for Lisa.

QSEN **Building Competency in Patient-Centered Care** You are caring for Amanda, a 32-year-old who experienced a miscarriage at 14 weeks' gestation. Amanda and her husband have been trying to get pregnant with their second child. They have a 4-year-old son at home. This is the second miscarriage that Amanda has experienced. When you walk into Amanda's room, she is staring out the window and does not turn her head. You can tell that she has been crying. She has a flat affect and states, "I just don't know why God did this to me again. How am I going to go on from here?"

Identify at least three questions you will ask Amanda to assess her spiritual well-being and plan effective, patient-centered care.

Answers to QSEN Activities can be found on the Evolve website.

REFLECT NOW

Consider how your own spiritual and religious beliefs influence your assessment of your patients' spiritual health. In what ways are you most effective? Least effective?

◆ Analysis and Nursing Diagnosis

A spiritual assessment allows a nurse to learn a great deal about a patient and the extent that spirituality plays in the patient's life. Exploring a patient's spirituality sometimes reveals patients have strong resources needed to cope effectively. At other times, assessment reveals responses to health problems that require nursing intervention. You interpret data about your patient's spiritual beliefs and practices, recognizing assessment cues or clusters of data to clearly identify and label a patient's health problems. You form clinical judgments and then select appropriate nursing diagnoses related to spirituality (Box 35.3). In identifying diagnoses, recognize the significance that spirituality has for all types of health problems. Ensure that each negative or problem-focused nursing diagnosis has an accurate related factor to guide the selection of individualized, purposeful, and goal-directed interventions (Herdman and Kamitsuru, 2021).

Decreased Spiritual Distress is based on assessment findings that show a person's ability to experience and integrate meaning and purpose in life through connectedness with self and others. A patient with this nursing diagnosis has effective resources to use when faced with illness or a threat to well-being. The nursing diagnosis *Spiritual Distress* creates a different clinical picture. Assessment findings reveal patterns that reflect sadness, unhappiness, or other emotions related to a poor state of well-being (e.g., expressing lack of hope, meaning, or purpose in life; expressing anger toward God; or verbalizing conflicts about personal beliefs). Patients likely to experience spiritual distress include those who have poor relationships, those who have experienced a recent loss, or those who are suffering from some form of mental or physical illness.

Accurate selection of nursing diagnoses requires critical thinking. Review and analyze all subjective and objective data (e.g., religious rituals and sources of fellowship), your assessment of previous patient experiences, your own spirituality, and your appraisal of the patient's spiritual well-being. Commonly, patients have multiple nursing diagnoses. While there are other possible nursing diagnoses for patients in need of spiritual support and care, the nursing diagnoses in the preceding paragraphs and the following list represent examples of diagnoses commonly associated with spiritual health-related problems:

- Risk for Spiritual Status
- Decreased Spiritual Distress
- Hopelessness
- Powerlessness
- Spiritual Distress

As Jeff analyzes the assessment data gathered from Lisa and Joe, he recognizes cues for three problems leading to nursing diagnoses for Lisa. Jeff recognizes that Lisa has a strong belief in God, attends church when she is able, and draws support from prayer and her church

---

BOX 35.3 **Nursing Diagnostic Process**

Decreased Spiritual Distress

Assessment Activities	Assessment Findings
Ask patient to describe personal source of faith and hope.	Patient expresses inner strength and source of guidance.
Have patient describe level of satisfaction with life.	Life has purpose and meaning; patient finds satisfaction while providing community service as a volunteer.
Determine who provides greatest source of strength and support to patient during times of difficulty.	Patient interacts with friends and family during difficult times.

*family. This leads him to identify **Decreased Spiritual Distress** as the first diagnosis. Jeff also recognizes that Lisa's illness is putting stress on the family by changing the normal family dynamics. Joe and the children are worried and have questions about Lisa's illness and the future. They are spending less time together particularly during their usual family dinner. Lisa is also tired and unable to do as many things right now with Joe and the children. Jeff identifies this as the problem **Impaired Family Process**. Lisa is also showing signs of **Anxiety** as her treatment continues and she worries about the future. She is concerned about the symptoms she is having following the chemotherapy treatments and that Joe is having to take time off work to help her. As Jeff reviews the three problems he identified, he focuses on **Decreased Spiritual Distress** as the priority. Jeff reflects on the data gathered from Lisa's and Joe's statements regarding their strong faith and their connection to their church. Jeff also knows spiritual beliefs and faith are coping mechanisms that are often used by patients with cancer (Davis et al., 2018). Thus Jeff uses his clinical judgment to decide to focus on continuing to decrease the spiritual distress in the family.*

◆ Planning and Outcomes Identification

During the planning step of the nursing process, develop a plan of care for each of a patient's nursing diagnoses. Critical thinking at this step is important as you reflect on knowledge, previous experiences, and environmental factors to recognize the relevance of the diagnoses chosen and consider possible approaches to care. You also apply critical thinking attitudes and standards in selecting the most appropriate nursing interventions (Fig. 35.4). Integrate assessment data with knowledge about resources and therapies available for spiritual care. Match the patient's needs with evidence-based interventions that are supported and recommended in the clinical and research literature. Use a concept map (Fig. 35.5) to organize patient care and show how the patient's medical diagnosis, assessment data, and nursing diagnoses are interrelated.

Prior experience with other patients and your own personal experience are valuable when selecting interventions to support spiritual well-being. For example, you may have prayed with previous patients or helped a patient practice a spiritual ritual. Your previous patient experiences can also help you recognize spiritual practices or dietary restrictions for a select religion. You may have previously worked with patients who have cancer and found that journaling helps them express their feelings about their illness and treatments.

It is also important to recognize environmental factors that impact spiritual health promotion. For example, when you pray with a patient, you want to select a quiet environment and plan for a time when interruptions will not occur. Identify potential interruptions and work to minimize the impact. Also, work with other members of the health care team to respect patient spiritual practices and spiritual care preferences. Consider a patient's culture when planning patient-centered interventions.

Confidence, an important critical thinking attitude, builds trust, enabling you and a patient to enter into a healing relationship together. Attempting to meet or support patients' spiritual needs frequently requires the need of additional resources. Because spiritual care is so personal, standards of autonomy and self-determination are critical in supporting a patient's decisions about the plan of care.

Outcomes. Partner with the patient and family to identify expected outcomes to develop a mutually agreed-on plan of care based on the

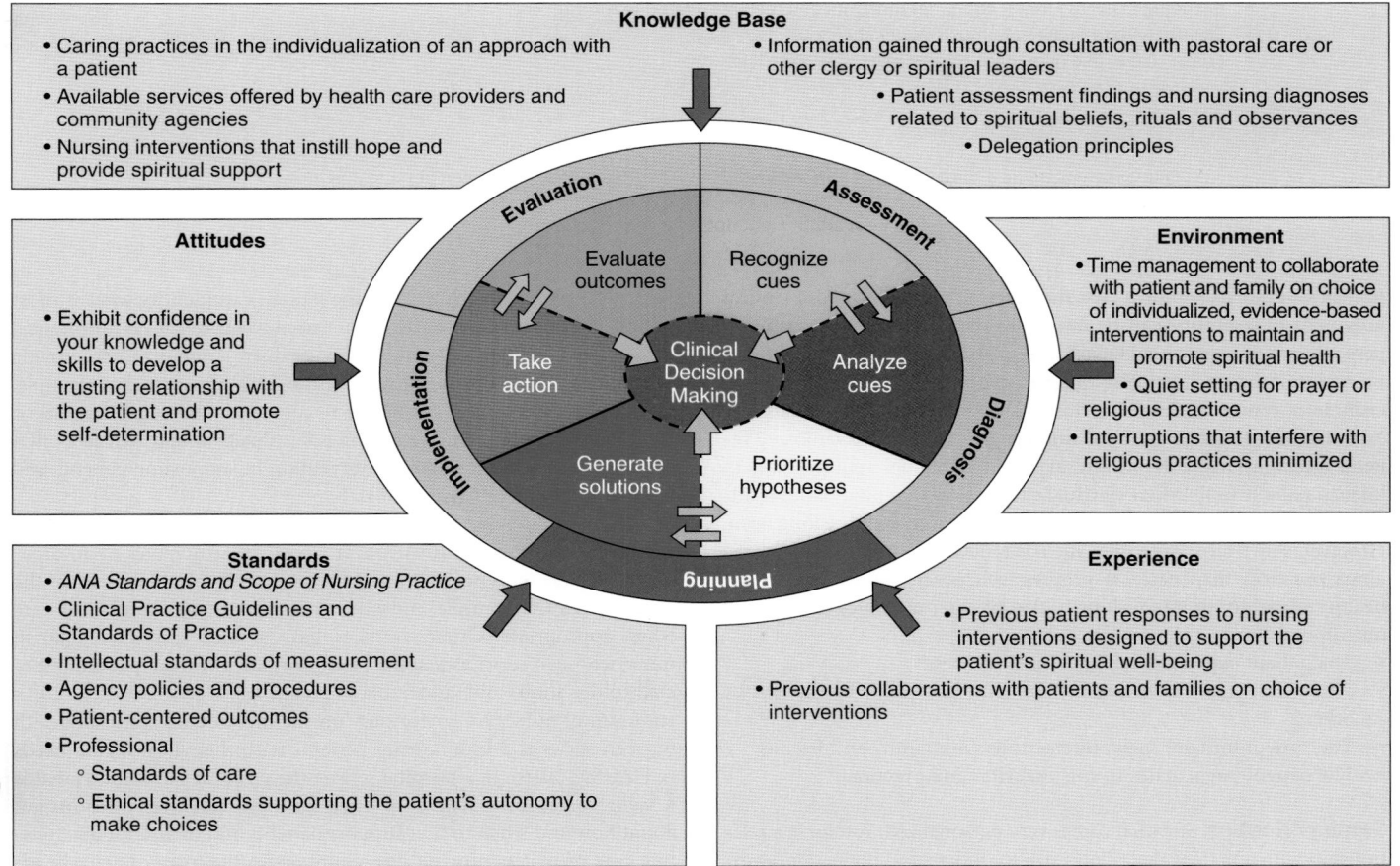

FIG. 35.4 Critical thinking model for spiritual health planning. (Clinical Judgment Measurement Model copyright © NCSBN. All rights reserved.)

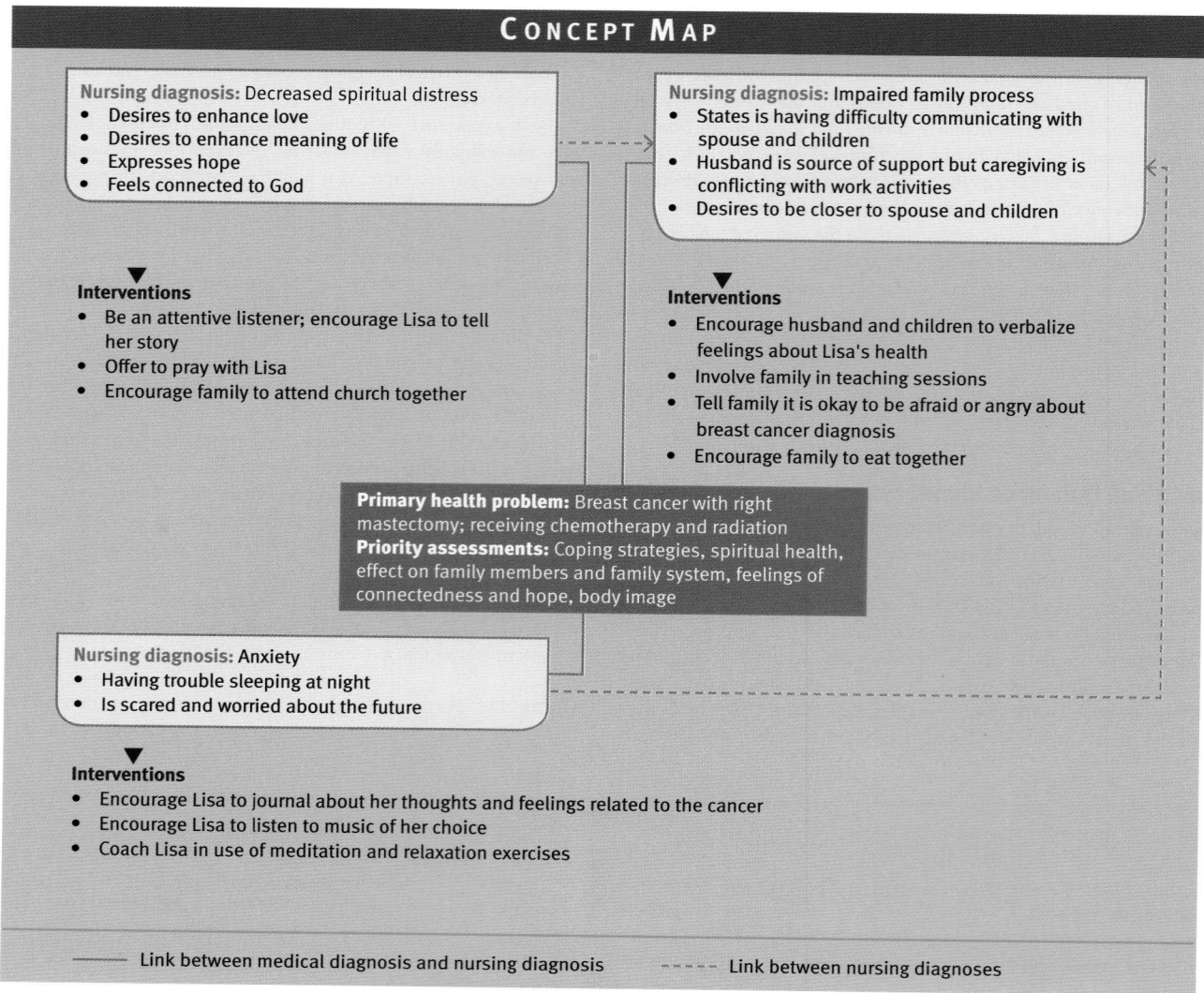

CONCEPT MAP

Nursing diagnosis: Decreased spiritual distress
- Desires to enhance love
- Desires to enhance meaning of life
- Expresses hope
- Feels connected to God

Interventions
- Be an attentive listener; encourage Lisa to tell her story
- Offer to pray with Lisa
- Encourage family to attend church together

Nursing diagnosis: Impaired family process
- States is having difficulty communicating with spouse and children
- Husband is source of support but caregiving is conflicting with work activities
- Desires to be closer to spouse and children

Interventions
- Encourage husband and children to verbalize feelings about Lisa's health
- Involve family in teaching sessions
- Tell family it is okay to be afraid or angry about breast cancer diagnosis
- Encourage family to eat together

Primary health problem: Breast cancer with right mastectomy; receiving chemotherapy and radiation
Priority assessments: Coping strategies, spiritual health, effect on family members and family system, feelings of connectedness and hope, body image

Nursing diagnosis: Anxiety
- Having trouble sleeping at night
- Is scared and worried about the future

Interventions
- Encourage Lisa to journal about her thoughts and feelings related to the cancer
- Encourage Lisa to listen to music of her choice
- Coach Lisa in use of meditation and relaxation exercises

——— Link between medical diagnosis and nursing diagnosis   - - - - Link between nursing diagnoses

FIG. 35.5 Concept map for Lisa Owens.

patient's nursing diagnoses (see the Nursing Care Plan). Use clinical judgment to establish realistic outcomes that align with the patient's personal religious/spiritual beliefs and practices and culture and focus on maintaining or improving the patient's spiritual health. It is especially important to collaborate closely with patients when establishing expected outcomes for spiritual support and growth and choosing related interventions. Establishing expected outcomes requires you to know a patient well. When spiritual care requires helping patients adjust to loss or stressful life situations, expected outcomes are long term. However, short-term outcomes such as renewing participation in religious practices help patients progressively reach a more spiritually healthy situation. In establishing a plan of care, examples of expected outcomes follow:

- The patient expresses feelings of peacefulness.
- The patient reports feelings of connectedness with family and/or others.
- The patient initiates social interactions with family and friends.
- The patient participates in spiritual rites and practices.

Setting Priorities. Spiritual care is very personalized. You form a relationship with a patient that allows you to understand the patient's priorities in the context of their spiritual life. When establishing a mutually

agreed-on plan with the patient, the patient can identify what is most important. Spiritual priorities do not need to be sacrificed for physical care priorities. When a patient is in acute distress, focus care to provide the patient a sense of control to minimize powerlessness. For example, allow the patient to decide whether to complete morning cares now or later in the morning. When a patient is terminally ill, spiritual care often is the most important nursing intervention in supporting patients and families in grief (see Chapter 36).

Teamwork and Collaboration. If a patient participates in an organized religion, with permission of the patient, involve members of the clergy or church, temple, mosque, or synagogue in the plan of care when appropriate. Often churches have a faith community/parish nurse who can serve as a support and resource for the patient, especially older adults and vulnerable populations (CHAUSA, 2016). Faith community nurses focus not only on the individual's spiritual health but can serve as a link helping patients with their health care needs (CHAUSA, 2016). In a hospital setting the pastoral care department is a valuable resource. These spiritual care professionals offer insight about how and when to best support patients and their families. Spiritual care providers provide direct support in the form of actively addressing spiritual or religious needs of a patient and family, having

◎ NURSING CARE PLAN

Decreased Spiritual Distress

ASSESSMENT

Assessment Activities	*Assessment Findings[a]*
Assess Lisa's connections with herself.	Lisa used to feel good about herself. However, since her cancer treatments, she is more tired and feels less positive at times. She states, **"I wish I had more hope about my prognosis."**
Ask Lisa to describe what it is about her cancer that frightens her most.	Lisa explains, "I have found it makes me appreciate what I have with my family. That being said, I worry that I will not see my children grow up, **but I hope the chemotherapy will give me some time and it will make me feel a bit better.**"
Assess Lisa's connections with her family and significant others.	Before Lisa's illness the **children were very close to their parents and shared their faith in God.** However, **now they are struggling with coping with Lisa's illness.** Lisa and Joe **attend their church regularly and hope to continue** doing so even during the chemotherapy. **Members of their church have offered support** by taking Lisa to the clinic if Joe is unable.
Determine Lisa's connections with a power greater than herself.	Lisa **expresses a connectedness with her God,** saying, "I don't feel alone; God is with me. I have a better appreciation of each day God gives me, and I believe God's strength will help me continue to be active in my church."

[a]**Assessment Findings** are shown in bold type.

NURSING DIAGNOSIS: Decreased Spiritual Distress

PLANNING

Expected Outcomes (NOC)[b]

Spiritual Health

By the end of the week, Lisa reports engaging in regular prayer and meditation.
In three weeks, Lisa reports that she and Joe are able to discuss their feelings and fears daily.

[b]Outcome classification labels from Moorhead S, et al: *Nursing Outcomes Classification (NOC)*, ed 6, St Louis, 2018, Elsevier.

INTERVENTIONS (NIC)[c]	*RATIONALE*
Spiritual Growth Facilitation	
Plan discussions with Lisa during treatment and listen, allowing her to sort out concerns she might have about her future.	Listening provides support or comfort in spiritual care (Veloza-Gomez et al., 2017). Building a therapeutic relationship is important to providing spiritual care (Minton et al., 2018).
Encourage Joe to communicate frequently and openly with Lisa so that he can better understand her feelings and to create special times every day to talk about feelings and fears and connect with one another.	Maintaining a sense of connectedness helps improve psychological and mental health (Hakanson and Ohlen, 2016).
Schedule a conference late in the afternoon at the cancer clinic when the children can attend. Provide discussion of their mother's progress. Establish a presence and express a realistic hope of mother's prognosis.	Diagnosis of cancer causes the entire family to grieve. Providing spiritual care and spiritual support has a positive effect on coping and helps the family develop strategies for personal coping (Dobratz, 2016).
Offer to pray with Lisa as she describes what she hopes for.	Individualized spiritual interventions in patients with cancer can improve spiritual well-being and decrease depression (Balboni et al., 2017).
Introduce Lisa to journaling. Encourage her to begin by writing what is meaningful to her about her illness and family	The use of journaling helps individuals facing a crisis deal with the unknown and express their feelings; find meaning and spiritual connection; and physically, emotionally, and spiritually heal (Connerton and Moe, 2018; Neathery, 2018).
Spiritual Support	
Use therapeutic communication to establish presence and trust and demonstrate empathy with Lisa and Joe.	Establishing rapport, active listening, and trust is necessary to connect with patients who have spiritual needs (Harrad et al., 2019).
Discuss with Lisa the likely times that her chemotherapy will affect her most and how she can schedule involvement in church activities around those times.	Chemotherapy can cause severe fatigue. Faith communities such as a church play an important role in fostering belief systems (Davis et al., 2018).
Teach Lisa methods of relaxation, meditation, and guided imagery.	Relaxation methods help promote quality of life and enhance serenity and dignity. Relaxation responses have been associated with improved physiological (blood pressure, exercise capacity, and cardiac symptoms) and psychological (depression and anxiety) outcomes (Heo et al., 2018; Balboni et al., 2017).

[c]Intervention classification labels from Butcher HK, et al: *Nursing Interventions Classification (NIC)*, ed 7, St Louis, 2018, Elsevier.

EVALUATION

Evaluation Activities	*Patient Response*
Ask Lisa to describe in what way meditation exercises have helped her.	Lisa reported using meditation daily after being at clinic. She states, "I feel calm. It allows me to connect with God, and know I have my loving family to help me."
Have Lisa review her discussions with family and/or church members.	Lisa reports, "We have been talking more as a family, but my daily talks with Joe are especially helpful to me. My family knows that I see each day as a blessing. My church really keeps me connected."

discussions about family members' feelings and patient values, and reminiscing with families about a patient (Veloza-Gomez et al., 2017). Significant others such as spouses, siblings, parents, and friends need to be involved in the patient's care as appropriate. This means that you learn from your initial assessment which individuals or groups have formed a relationship with the patient and which ones the patient desires to involve. These individuals sometimes participate in all levels of the plan of care. They often assist in giving physical care, providing emotional comfort, and sharing spiritual support.

*After analyzing the assessment data, Jeff has identified **Decreased Spiritual Distress** as a priority for Lisa. He collaborates with Lisa to identify expected outcomes of Lisa engaging in regular prayer and meditation and Lisa and Joe being able to discuss their feelings and fears daily. Using the identified outcomes, Jeff starts to plan patient-centered personal spiritual care and support for Lisa. He plans to build feelings of hope and to build on the resources that Lisa and Joe have through their church. Jeff determines that Lisa's church has a faith community nurse. With Lisa's permission, he will work with the faith community nurse from their church to enlist church members to help Lisa when Joe or the children cannot. While providing spiritual care, Jeff will also plan interventions that will help decrease Lisa's anxiety and improve the communication and connectedness of the family. Jeff plans on involving Joe and the children in Lisa's plan of care.*

◆ Implementation

Nurses play a key role in helping patients resolve feelings of spiritual distress. Nurses create a healing environment and maximize recovery by enhancing patients' spiritual well-being (Harrad et al., 2019). After establishing a caring relationship with a patient and an individualized plan of care, you can implement a patient-centered care approach. Having a thorough understanding of a patient's spiritual needs enables you to deliver care in a sensitive, creative, and appropriate manner.

Health Promotion. Spiritual care needs to be a central theme in how you promote an individual's overall well-being, leading to improved patient outcomes such as positive coping, decreased stress and anxiety, and lower risk of depression (Harrad et al., 2019). In settings where health promotion activities occur, patients often need information, counseling, and guidance to make the necessary choices to remain healthy.

Establishing Presence. Presence is part of the art of nursing. Benner (1984) explains that presence involves "being with" a patient versus "doing for" a patient. It is being able to offer closeness with a patient physically, psychologically, and spiritually. It helps to prevent emotional and environmental isolation (see Chapter 7). Nurses are present to their patients when they spend time with their patients. Being present contributes to a patient's sense of well-being and provides hope for recovery. Establish presence by sitting with a patient to attentively listen to the patient's feelings and situation, talking with the patient, accepting or supporting the patient's need to cry, and simply offering time. These simple interventions provide a powerful approach to spiritual care (Buchanan, 2021).

When health promotion is the focus of care, your presence gives patients the confidence needed to discuss ways to remain healthy. Show your caring presence by listening to patients' concerns; when appropriate, involve family members in discussions about patients' health. Show self-confidence when providing health instruction, and support patients as they make decisions about their health. The patient who seeks health care is often fearful of experiencing an illness that threatens loss of control and looks for someone to offer competent direction. Encouraging words of support and a calm, decisive approach establish a presence that builds trust and well-being.

Supporting a Healing Relationship. Learn to look beyond isolated patient problems and recognize the broader picture of a patient's holistic needs. For example, do not just look at a patient's back pain as a problem to solve with quick remedies; rather look at how the pain influences the patient's ability to function and achieve goals established in life. A holistic view enables you to establish a helping role and a healing relationship. Three factors are evident when a healing relationship develops between nurse and patient:

1. Realistically mobilizing hope for the nurse and patient
2. Finding an interpretation or understanding of the illness, pain, anxiety, or other stressful emotion that is acceptable to the patient
3. Helping the patient use social, emotional, and spiritual resources (Benner, 1984)

Mobilizing a patient's hope is central to a healing relationship. Hope motivates people to face challenges in life by finding inner strength for coping and acceptance (Gawthorpe, 2018). Help patients find hope. For example, help a patient newly diagnosed with diabetes mellitus learn how to manage the disease in a way that will allow the patient to continue a productive and satisfying way of life. An adult daughter who has decided to become caregiver to her older adult parent hopes to be able to protect the parent from injury or worsening disability. You instruct the daughter on basic care skills so that her hope can be realistic. Hope is future oriented and helps a patient work toward outcomes (Wrigley, 2019). Hope helps patients work toward recovery. To help patients achieve hope, work together to find an explanation for their situation that is acceptable to them. Help a patient realistically exercise hope by supporting positive attitudes toward life or the desire to be informed and make decisions.

Remain aware of a patient's spiritual resources and needs. It is always important to allow patients to express and exercise their beliefs and find spiritual comfort. When life stressors or chronic illness create confusion or uncertainty, recognize the potential effect on a patient's well-being. How do you use and strengthen spiritual resources? Begin by encouraging a patient to discuss the effect that an illness has had on personal beliefs and faith, thus giving the chance to clarify any misconceptions or inaccuracies in information. Having a clear sense of what illness will be like helps an individual apply many resources toward recovery.

Jeff encourages Lisa and her family to strengthen their spiritual health as they continue to cope with Lisa's breast cancer diagnosis and cancer treatment. Jeff asks Lisa, "Are there any communities that you feel connected with?" Lisa responds, "I feel close to the members of my church and my friends at work." Jeff also gets Lisa's permission to share her health problems and concerns with the faith community nurse, who agrees to contact Lisa and arrange a time for them to meet. Jeff determines that Lisa and Joe have used prayer in the past to cope with different stressors. Thus, Jeff prays with Lisa and Joe during their visits to the oncology clinic, encourages them to continue to read the Bible together at home, and encourages Joe to attend church with the children even if Lisa is too ill to attend. Jeff develops a teaching plan for Lisa that focuses on how to do meditation and relaxation exercises to help with her anxiety. Because breast cancer and its treatment often interfere with employment, Jeff helps Lisa explore and plan ways that she can remain connected with her peers at work to help her maintain this important source of support.

Acute Care. Within acute care settings, patients experience multiple stressors that threaten their sense of control. Ongoing assessment of spiritual needs is essential because a patient's needs often change rapidly. Support and enhancement of a patient's spiritual well-being are challenges when the focus of health care seems to be on treatment and cure rather than care. Lack of time, lack of education or training,

BOX 35.4 EVIDENCE-BASED PRACTICE

Spiritual Interventions and Patient Outcomes

PICOT Question: Does the use of spiritual care interventions among adults improve patient outcomes?

Evidence Summary

Nursing care for patients needs to focus on mind, body, and spirit. It is important to include spiritual interventions in a patient's plan of care that will help to relieve spiritual distress and enhance spiritual well-being (Ricci-Allegra, 2018; Fradelos, 2021). Providing spiritual care and spiritual support often helps patients cope with illness and therapies (Davis et al., 2018; Fradelos, 2021). Researchers have found that using spiritual interventions helps to decrease anxiety and reduce depression in patients with cancer and heart failure (Heo et al., 2018; Davis et al., 2018). Both verbal communication and nonverbal communication, such as presence, are useful when providing spiritual care to patients (Minton et al., 2018). The use of a spiritual care board, allowing patients to express their feelings, helped patients cope with their illnesses and feel at peace (Berning et al., 2016). Before providing spiritual care to patients, it is important for nurses to assess for patients' cues to respect patient beliefs and autonomy (Harrad et al., 2019).

Application to Nursing Practice

- Use active listening and therapeutic communication to develop rapport with your patients (Vincensi, 2019).
- Offer to pray or read scripture with patients (Minton et al., 2018).
- Turn on a patient's favorite religious music station or television channel.
- Conduct a spiritual assessment or history from each of your patients (Harrad et al., 2019).
- Be nonjudgmental in your assessment and care of patients, showing respect for each patient's spiritual beliefs (Vincensi, 2019).
- Offer to contact pastoral care or the chaplain for patients (Bone et al., 2018).

TABLE 35.2 Religious Dietary Regulations Affecting Health Care

Religion	Dietary Practices
Hinduism	Some sects are vegetarians. The belief is not to kill *any* living creature.
Buddhism	Some are vegetarians and do not use alcohol. Many fast on Holy Days.
Islam	Consumption of pork and alcohol is *haram* (forbidden). Use of caffeine is *makrooh* (doubtful). Followers fast during the month of Ramadan.
Judaism	Some observe the kosher dietary restrictions (e.g., avoid pork and shellfish; do not prepare and eat milk and meat at same time).
Christianity	Some Baptists, Evangelicals, and Pentecostals discourage use of alcohol and caffeine. Some Roman Catholics fast on Ash Wednesday and Good Friday. Some do not eat meat on Fridays during Lent.
Jehovah's Witnesses	Members avoid food prepared with or containing blood.
Mormonism	Members abstain from alcohol and caffeine.
Russian Orthodox Church	Followers observe fast days and a "no-meat" rule on Wednesdays and Fridays. During Lent all animal products, including dairy products and butter, are forbidden.
Native Americans	Individual tribal beliefs influence food practices.

language barriers, confusion over one's own spirituality, lack of family involvement, and patient privacy are other barriers to spiritual care in acute care settings (Chen et al., 2017a). To meet these challenges, display a soothing presence and supportive touch when providing care. Using your hands artfully, offering encouraging words of support, promoting connectedness, and assuming a calm and decisive approach establish a nursing presence that builds trust. As a nurse, you are in a unique position to help patients reevaluate their lives and achieve spiritual health (Box 35.4).

Support Systems. The use of support systems is important for patients in any health care setting. Support systems can provide patients with the greatest sense of well-being during hospitalization and serve as a human link. For many patients, a part of their caregiving environment is the regular presence of supportive family and friends. Provide privacy during visits, and plan care with the patient and the patient's support network to promote the interpersonal bonding that is needed for recovery. The support system provides a sense of connectedness and is a source of faith and hope and an important resource in conducting meaningful religious rituals.

When patients look to family and friends for support, encourage those family members and friends to visit the patient regularly. Help family members feel comfortable in the health care setting, and use their support and presence to promote the patient's healing. For example, including family members in prayer is a thoughtful gesture if it is appropriate to the patient's religion and if the patient and family members are comfortable with participating together. Having the family bring meaningful spiritual or religious symbols to the patient's bedside offers significant spiritual support.

Collaborate with spiritual advisers or members of the clergy in offering an interprofessional approach to patient care (Bone et al., 2018). Professional spiritual care providers, such as chaplains, have expertise in understanding how an illness influences a person's beliefs and how these beliefs influence the patient's responses to illness, recovery, or preparation for death. When members of the clergy are requested by patients or families, keep clergy informed of any physical, psychosocial, or spiritual concerns affecting the patient. A spiritual care provider is especially helpful in discussing patient and family wishes about end-of-life care (Ruth-Sahd et al., 2018) (see Chapter 36). Respect patients' spiritual values and needs by allowing time for pastoral care members to provide spiritual care and facilitate the administration of sacraments, rites, and rituals.

Diet Therapies. The intake of food satisfies and promotes a sense of comfort. Food and nutrition are important aspects of patient care and often an important component of some religious observances (Table 35.2). Food and the rituals surrounding the preparation and serving of food are sometimes important to a person's spirituality. For example, in the Muslim faith, food is divided into four categories: *halal* (permitted to eat), *haram* (forbidden to eat), *makrooh* (doubtful), and *mashbooh* (suspect) (Huda, 2020; Why Islam, 2018) Consult with a registered dietitian to integrate patients' dietary preferences into daily care. If a health care agency cannot prepare food in the preferred way, ask the family to bring meals that fit into dietary restrictions posed by the patient's condition.

Supporting Rituals. Nurses provide spiritual care by supporting patients' participation in spiritual rituals and activities when possible. Plan care to allow time for religious readings or spiritual visitations, or for participation in religious services. Allow family members to plan a prayer session or an organized reading of scriptures or the Koran on a regular basis. Make arrangements with spiritual care professionals, at

---

BOX 35.5   FOCUS ON OLDER ADULTS
Spirituality and Spiritual Health

- There is an association between an older adult's spirituality and the inner strength and ability to adjust or cope with illness and other life stressors (Chen et al., 2017b; Hodge, 2017).
- Older adults often use prayer as the primary coping mechanism when experiencing illness (Greer and Abel, 2017).
- Encouraging older adults to use prayer, spiritual or scripture readings, meditation, or other religious practices can lead to enhanced wellness and coping (Hodge, 2017).
- Enhance connectedness by helping older patients find meaning and purpose in life by listening actively to concerns and being present (Clarke and Baume, 2019).
- Beliefs in the afterlife increase as adults age. Offer to coordinate visits from clergy, social workers, lawyers, and financial advisers so that patients feel as though they have completed all unfinished business. Leaving a legacy (e.g., oral history, art, photographs) to loved ones prepares an older adult to leave the world with a sense of meaning and maintains a way to continue connection for the one left behind (Touhy and Jett, 2020).
- Greater social support in older adults positively impacts spiritual well-being (Chen et al., 2017b).

BOX 35.6   PATIENT TEACHING
Meditation Techniques

Objective
- The patient will verbalize feelings of relaxation and self-transcendence after meditation.

Teaching Strategies
- Give patient a brief description of information and a printed teaching guide that describes how to meditate.
- Prepare a space: Simple things such as lighting a candle, turning off a cell phone, or sitting in a special quiet room or place that has minimal interruptions can support meditation practice.
- Set an intention or ask a question: This sets a direction for meditation. Have the patient ask an open-ended question such as "What is my purpose?" or "Who/what am I?"
- Explain that peaceful music or the quiet whirring of a fan also blocks out distractions.
- Teach steps of meditation (i.e., sit in a comfortable position with the back straight; breathe slowly; and focus on a sound, prayer, or image).
- Encourage patient to meditate for 10 to 20 minutes twice a day.
- Answer questions and reinforce information as needed.

Evaluation
Use the principles of teach-back to evaluate patient/family caregiver learning:
- How did you feel after meditating?
- What did you learn about yourself while doing meditation?

---

the request of the patient, for the patient and family to participate in religious practices (e.g., receiving sacraments). Clergy from a patient's church often visit patients when they are hospitalized and unable to attend religious services. Taped meditations, classical or religious music, and televised religious services provide other effective options. Always respect the icons, medals, prayer rugs, crosses, or other items that a patient brings to a health care setting, and ensure that they are not accidentally lost, damaged, or misplaced. Supporting spiritual rituals is especially important for older adults (Box 35.5).

Restorative and Continuing Care. Spiritual care often becomes especially important for patients who are recovering from a long-term disability or who are living with a chronic or terminal disease. Many of the nursing interventions applicable in health promotion and acute care apply to this level of health care as well.

Prayer. The act of prayer gives an individual the opportunity to renew personal faith and belief in a higher being in a specific, focused way that is either highly ritualized and formal or quite spontaneous and informal. For example, a patient may choose to say a prayer just before leaving for a surgical procedure. A patient who is a follower of Islam will want to say daily prayers (Salah) five times a day. Prayer is an effective coping resource for physical and psychological symptoms (deAndrade Alvarenga et al., 2017). Patients pray in private or participate in group prayer with family, friends, or clergy. Muslims must be clean before they pray, so offer hygiene measures according to Islam practices (Islamic Supreme Council of America, 2021). Some pray while listening to music. Be supportive of prayer by giving the patient privacy if desired, learning whether the patient wishes to have you participate, and suggesting prayer when you know that it is a coping resource for the patient. You can also be present with the patient through offering to spend several minutes of silence with the patient (Christensen et al., 2018). Alternatives to prayer include listening to calming music or reading a text selected by the patient.

Meditation. Meditation creates a relaxation response that reduces daily stress (see Chapter 32). Patients who meditate often state that they have an increased awareness of their spirituality and of the presence of God or a Supreme Being. Meditation improves symptoms and depression in patients and helps patients move from negative to positive thoughts (Heo et al., 2018). Meditation exercises give patients temporary relief from pain, insomnia, anxiety, and depression and increase coping and the ability to relax (Starkweather, 2021). Meditation involves sitting quietly in a comfortable position with eyes closed and repeating a sound, phrase, or sacred word in rhythm with breathing while disregarding intrusive thoughts. Individuals who meditate regularly (twice a day for 10 or 20 minutes) may experience decreased metabolism and heart rate, easier breathing, and slower brain waves (Box 35.6).

Supporting Grief Work. Patients who experience terminal illness or who have suffered permanent loss of body function because of a disabling disease or injury require a nurse's support in grieving and coping with their loss. Your ability to enter into a caring, therapeutic, and spiritual relationship with patients supports them during times of grief (see Chapter 36).

◆ Evaluation

Through the Patient's Eyes. The evaluation of a patient's spiritual care requires you to think critically in determining whether efforts at restoring or maintaining the patient's spiritual health were successful (Fig. 35.6). This requires including the patient by determining whether expectations were met. Ask patients whether you and the health care team met their expectations of offering spiritual support or whether there was anything else you could have done to enhance their spiritual well-being or to enable them to practice important religious rituals. Additionally, asking a patient, "Have you felt comfortable in saying what you feel is important to you spiritually?" will help determine whether you developed an effective healing relationship. In addition, evaluate any other concerns that arise in the course of the patient's spiritual care and support. Apply critical thinking attitudes and use therapeutic communication techniques to ensure sound nursing judgments.

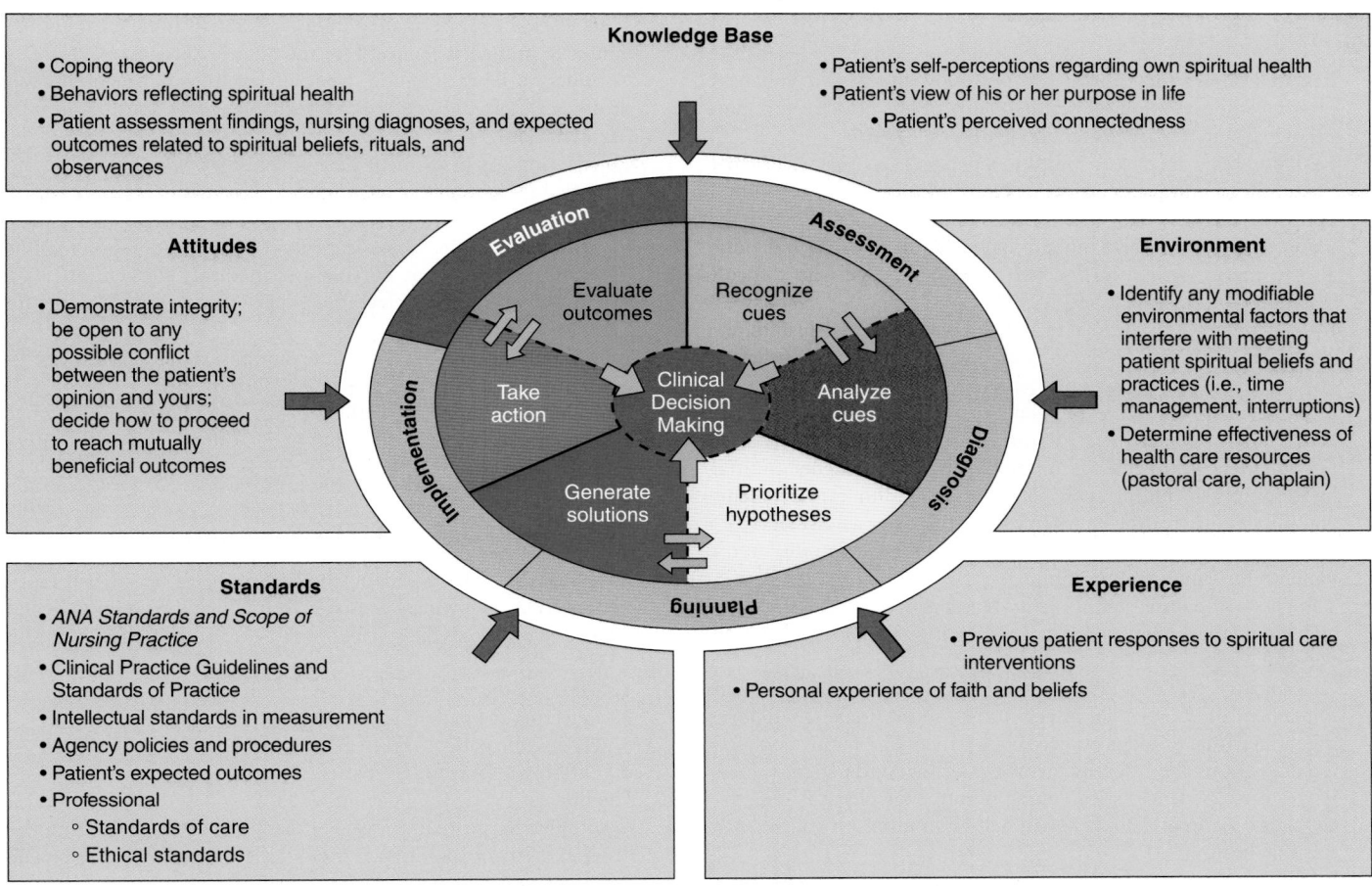

Knowledge Base
- Coping theory
- Behaviors reflecting spiritual health
- Patient assessment findings, nursing diagnoses, and expected outcomes related to spiritual beliefs, rituals, and observances

- Patient's self-perceptions regarding own spiritual health
- Patient's view of his or her purpose in life
- Patient's perceived connectedness

Attitudes
- Demonstrate integrity; be open to any possible conflict between the patient's opinion and yours; decide how to proceed to reach mutually beneficial outcomes

Environment
- Identify any modifiable environmental factors that interfere with meeting patient spiritual beliefs and practices (i.e., time management, interruptions)
- Determine effectiveness of health care resources (pastoral care, chaplain)

Standards
- *ANA Standards and Scope of Nursing Practice*
- Clinical Practice Guidelines and Standards of Practice
- Intellectual standards in measurement
- Agency policies and procedures
- Patient's expected outcomes
- Professional
  - Standards of care
  - Ethical standards

Experience
- Previous patient responses to spiritual care interventions
- Personal experience of faith and beliefs

Evaluation — Assessment — Diagnosis — Planning — Implementation

Evaluate outcomes — Recognize cues — Take action — Clinical Decision Making — Analyze cues — Generate solutions — Prioritize hypotheses

FIG. 35.6 Critical thinking model for spiritual health evaluation. (Clinical Judgment Measurement Model copyright © NCSBN. All rights reserved.)

Lisa returns to the clinic one week after planning to enhance her spiritual health with Jeff. A member of her church accompanies Lisa because Joe is out of town on a business trip. Jeff wants to evaluate whether Lisa continues to feel connected with herself, Joe, her children, and God. Jeff asks, "Tell me, Mrs. Owens, have you had a chance yet to try any of the approaches we talked about last week to give yourself, Joe, and the children a chance to talk about their feelings? If so, what were the results?" Lisa reports, "Yes, I spend at least 10 minutes every morning in prayer while I sit in my garden, and I've been meditating for 10 to 15 minutes every day. Joe and I set aside at least 15 minutes a day to talk in private after the kids go to bed. If he's not in town, we talk on the phone. Joe and I planned a family dinner night last Saturday evening with the kids. We shared lots of funny family stories and began to talk with them about my cancer treatment. The kids really seemed to enjoy being together as a family. They asked many questions, and we talked about what they could do to help me. We also planned for the family to visit two colleges for Davis." Jeff also determines that Lisa has spoken with close friends from her church and they plan to visit her this week. Lisa states that she is going to see the physical therapist today.

Patient Outcomes. Attaining spiritual health is a lifelong process. In evaluating outcomes established during the planning phase, compare a patient's level of spiritual health with the behaviors and perceptions noted in the nursing assessment. Evaluation data related to spiritual health are usually subjective. For example, if during assessment a patient expresses hopelessness, your follow-up evaluation involves asking the patient whether feelings of hope have been restored. Include family and friends, as appropriate, when gathering evaluative information. Successful outcomes reveal the patient developing an increased or restored sense of connectedness with family; maintaining, renewing, or reforming a sense of purpose in life; and for some a confidence and trust in a Supreme Being or power. When outcomes are not met, ask questions to determine appropriate continuing care. Examples of questions to ask include the following:

- Do you feel the need to forgive someone or to be forgiven by someone?
- Which spiritual activities, such as prayer or meditation, were helpful to you?
- Would you like for me to ask a friend, family member, or someone from pastoral care to talk with you?
- What can I do to help you feel more at peace?
- Sometimes people need to give themselves permission to feel hope when they experience difficult events. What can you do to allow yourself to feel hope again?

To evaluate whether the clinic has met Lisa's expectations, Jeff asks, "Your faith is strong, and it is my hope you have felt comfortable in talking about your worries. Do you believe that we have helped you so far with your concerns about your family?" Lisa replies, "The best thing you've done is listen and recognize how important my family is to me. Your suggestions have helped so far; I am truly blessed to have met so many nice people at the clinic."

KEY POINTS

- Research shows that spirituality positively affects and enhances physical and psychological health, quality of life, health promotion behaviors, and disease prevention activities.
- Faith and hope are closely linked to a person's spiritual well-being, providing an inner strength for dealing with illness and disability.
- Spirituality is a much broader and more unifying concept than religion, as it is an inherent human characteristic that gives individuals the energy needed to discover themselves, cope with difficult situations, and maintain health.
- Religion differs from spirituality in that it is an organized, institution-related practice that is commonly associated with particular beliefs.
- During nursing assessment of a patient's spiritual needs, be sure to recognize cues that show problems or distress related to the patient's faith, connectedness, life and self-responsibility, life satisfaction, and fellowship and community. Include the patients' cultural backgrounds, including their values about health care problems and impending treatments when conducting your assessment.
- Learning to practice caring and compassion helps you discover a patient's life values and meaning.
- The personal nature of spirituality requires open communication and the establishment of trust and a caring relationship between you and a patient.
- As a spiritual care provider, you use clinical judgment to plan and implement direct spiritual interventions, addressing and supporting the spiritual or religious needs of a patient and family and having discussions about family members' feelings and patient values.
- Prayer is an evidence-based coping resource for physical and psychological symptoms that is often helpful in promoting a patient's spiritual health.
- Establishing presence involves attentive listening, talking with patients and answering questions, conveying a sense of trust, and simply offering your time.
- During evaluation successful outcomes reveal a patient developing an increased or restored sense of connectedness with family and maintaining, renewing, or reforming a sense of purpose in life.

REFLECTIVE LEARNING

Six years after her initial diagnosis of breast cancer and treatment, Lisa Owens was diagnosed with stage IV breast cancer. At this time, Lisa has undergone three rounds of chemotherapy. She has given up her job as a nurse manager because of the physical strain and pain due to the cancer spread and side effects from the chemotherapy. Lisa has numerous side effects from her advancing disease and chemotherapy. She has ongoing hip pain from the cancer spread to the bone, reduced sensation in her feet, chronic fatigue, and difficulty in sleeping. Joe, her husband, is still working as an accountant and continues to provide support to Lisa. Their two children are adults now and do not live at home. Their daughter is unmarried and lives two miles away. Their son is married; his wife is pregnant, and they live out of town two hours away. Lisa is worried that she will not be alive when her grandchild is born. Her husband provides most of her support at home, but this continues at times to interfere with his ability to do the work that he brings home. The nurse who has been seeing Lisa knows that she regularly attends church with her husband. Lisa is coming to the outpatient chemotherapy infusion center to begin another course of chemotherapy. She tells the nurse, "I am so tired; I am not sure that I can do this next round of chemotherapy. Each round gets harder and harder, and I have more nausea and pain. I am losing hope that the treatment is helping me."

- What assessment information in Lisa's situation is the most important or of immediate concern for the nurse? (Recognize Cues)
- Considering Lisa's situation, what environmental, organizational, or other factors did you see that influence Lisa's spiritual health? (Analyze Cues)
- Considering her assessment data and history, what would be the priority nursing problem in caring for Lisa and her family? (Prioritize Diagnoses)
- Identify two expected outcomes for Lisa. Consider Lisa's situation and describe what nursing and medical interventions that you could utilize to achieve the expected outcomes? (Generate Solutions)
- Which nursing and medical interventions should have priority when implementing Lisa's care plan? (Take Action)
- Considering the implementation of your plan of care for Lisa, what assessment data should you gather to determine whether the interventions were effective? (Evaluate Outcomes)

REVIEW QUESTIONS

1. A nurse is caring for a patient who has just had a near-death experience (NDE) following a cardiac arrest. Which intervention by the nurse best promotes the spiritual well-being of the patient after the NDE?
   1. Allowing the patient to discuss the experience
   2. Referring the patient to pastoral care
   3. Having the patient talk to another patient who had an NDE
   4. Offering to pray for the patient
2. The nurse is caring for a patient who is very depressed and decides to complete a spiritual assessment using the FICA tool. Using the FICA assessment tool, match the criteria on the left with the appropriate assessment question on the right.

   ___1. F—Faith
   ___2. I—Importance of spirituality
   ___3. C—Community
   ___4. A—Interventions to address spiritual needs

   a. Tell me if you have a higher power or authority that helps you act on your beliefs.
   b. Describe which activities give you comfort spiritually.
   c. To whom do you go for support in times of difficulty?
   d. Your illness has kept you from attending church. Is that a problem for you?

3. The nurse is planning spiritual care interventions for an 8-year-old patient. Based on the patient's age, the nurse must consider which growth and development factor when planning the spiritual care?
   1. This age-group's concept of spirituality is provided by parents, and love and affection promote spirituality.
   2. This age-group begins to ask about God or a Supreme Being and is influenced by spiritual and religious stories.
   3. This age-group is fascinated with magic and mystery and often believes illness is related to bad behavior.
   4. This age-group has a clear concept of a higher spiritual being and is interested in learning about spirituality.
4. A nurse is caring for a patient who is Muslim and has diabetes mellitus. Which of the following items does the nurse need to remove from the meal tray when it is delivered to the patient?
   1. Small container of vanilla ice cream
   2. A dozen red grapes
   3. Bacon and eggs
   4. Garden salad with ranch dressing

5. A 44-year-old male patient has just been told that his wife and child were killed in an auto accident while coming to visit him in the hospital. After analyzing the assessment findings, the nurse recognizes that which statements made by the patient support a nursing diagnosis of *Spiritual Distress related to loss of family members*? (Select all that apply.)
   1. "I need to call my sister for support."
   2. "I have nothing to live for now."
   3. "Why would my God do this to me?"
   4. "I need to pray for a miracle."
   5. "I want to be more involved in my church."

6. A patient has just been diagnosed with a malignant brain tumor. She is alone; her family will not be arriving from out of town for an hour. What intervention does the nurse implement that best provides support of the patient's spiritual well-being at this time?
   1. Make a referral to a professional spiritual care adviser.
   2. Sit down and talk with the patient; have her discuss her feelings and listen attentively.
   3. Move the patient's Bible from her bedside cabinet drawer to the top of the over-bed table.
   4. Ask the patient whether she would like to learn more about the implications of having this type of tumor.

7. A nurse is preparing to teach an older adult who has chronic arthritis how to practice meditation. Which of the following teaching strategies are appropriate? (Select all that apply.)
   1. Encourage family members to participate in the exercise.
   2. Have the patient identify a quiet room in the home that has minimal interruptions.
   3. Suggest the use of a quiet fan running in the room.
   4. Explain that it is best to meditate about 5 minutes 4 times a day.
   5. Show the patient how to sit comfortably with the limitation of his arthritis and focus on a prayer.

8. A nursing student is developing a plan of care for a 74-year-old-female patient who has spiritual distress over losing a spouse. As the nurse develops appropriate interventions, which characteristics of older adults should be considered? (Select all that apply.)
   1. Older adults do not routinely use complementary medicine to cope with illness.

2. Older adults dislike discussing the afterlife and what might have happened to people who have passed on.
   3. Older adults achieve spiritual resilience through frequent expressions of gratitude.
   4. Have the patient determine whether her husband left a legacy behind.
   5. Offer the patient her choice of rituals or participation in exercise.

9. A nurse used spiritual rituals as an intervention in a patient's care. Which of the following questions is most appropriate to evaluate the efficacy of the intervention?
   1. Do you feel the need to forgive your wife over your loss?
   2. What can I do to help you feel more at peace?
   3. Did either prayer or meditation prove helpful to you?
   4. Should we plan on having your family try to visit you more often in the hospital?

10. The nurse is caring for a 50-year-old woman visiting the outpatient medicine clinic. The patient has had type 1 diabetes mellitus since age 13. She has numerous complications from her disease, including reduced vision, heart disease, and severe numbness and tingling of the extremities. Knowing that spirituality helps patients cope with chronic illness, which of the following principles should the nurse apply in practice? (Select all that apply.)
   1. Pay attention to the patient's spiritual identity throughout the course of her illness.
   2. Select interventions that you know scientifically support spiritual well-being.
   3. Listen to the patient's story each visit to the clinic, and offer a compassionate presence.
   4. When the patient questions the reason for her longtime suffering, try to provide answers.
   5. Consult with a spiritual care adviser, and have the adviser recommend useful interventions.

Answers: 1.1; 2.1a, 2d, 3c, 4b; 3.4, 4; 5.2, 3; 6.2; 7.2, 3; 8.3, 4, 5; 9.3; 10.1, 3.

Rationales for Review Questions can be found on the Evolve website.

REFERENCES

American Nurses Association (ANA): *Code of ethics for nurses with interpretive statements*, 2015. https://www.nursingworld.org/coe-view-only. Accessed June 13, 2021.

American Nurses Association (ANA), American Psychiatric Nurses Association (APA), International Society of Psychiatric–Mental Health Nurses (ISPN): *Psychiatric–mental health nursing: scope and standards of practice*, ed 2, Washington, DC, 2014, ANA.

Andrews MM, Boyle JS: *Transcultural concepts in nursing care*, ed 7, Philadelphia, 2016, Wolters Kluwer.

Benner P: *From novice to expert*, Menlo Park, CA, 1984, Addison-Wesley.

Buchanan LP: Spirituality. In Giddens JF, editor: *Concepts for nursing practice*, ed 3, St. Louis, 2021, Elsevier.

Caplan S: Culture. In Giddens JF, editor: *Concepts for nursing practice*, ed 3, St. Louis, 2021, Elsevier.

Catholic Health Association of the United States (CHAUSA): *Improving the lives of older adults through faith community partnerships: healing body, mind and spirit*, 2016, Catholic Health Association of the United States. https://www.chausa.org/docs/default-source/eldercare/improving-the-lives-of-older-adults-through-faith-community-partnerships_final-oct-192016.pdf?sfvrsn=0. Accessed June 13, 2021.

Christensen AR, et al: How should clinicians respond to requests from patients to participate in prayer? *AMA J Ethics* 20(7):621, 2018.

Christman SK, Mueller JR: Understanding spiritual care: the faith-hope-love model of spiritual wellness, *J Christ Nurs* 34(1):e1, 2017.

Clarke J, Baume K: Embedding spiritual care into everyday nursing practice, *Nurs Stand* 2019. doi:10.7748/ns.2019.e11354.

Connerton CS, Moe CS: The essence of spiritual care, *Creat Nurs* 24(1):36, 2018.

de Andrade Alvarenga W, et al: The possibilities and challenges in providing pediatric spiritual care, *J Child Health Care* 21(4):435, 2017.

Dobratz MC: Building a middle-range theory of adaptive spirituality, *Nurs Sci Q* 29(2):146, 2016.

Finocchiaro DN: Supporting the patient's spiritual needs at the end of life, *Nursing* 46(5):57, 2016.

Gawthorpe P: *Supporting hope at the end of life*, 2018. https://blogs.bmj.com/ebn/2018/05/07/supporting-hope-at-the-end-of-life/. Accessed June 13, 2021.

Giger JN, Haddad LG: *Transcultural nursing: assessment and intervention*, ed 8, St. Louis, 2021, Elsevier.

Herdman TH, Kamitsuru S, editors: *NANDA International nursing diagnoses: definitions and classification, 2021-2023*, ed 12, New York, 2021, Thieme Publishers.

HealthCare Chaplaincy Network: *What is quality spiritual care in health care and how do you measure it?* 2021, https://www.spiritualcareassociation.org/docs/research/evidence_base/quality_indicators_document_1_7_2021.pdf. Accessed September 3, 2021.

Hodge DR: *Conducting spiritual assessments with older adults*, 2017. https://www.uofazcenteronaging.com/sites/default/files/spiritual_assessment.pdf. Accessed June 13, 2021.

Huda: *Halal and Haram: The Islamic Dietary Laws*, 2020. https://www.learnreligions.com/islamic-dietary-law-2004234. Accessed June 13, 2021.

Islamic Supreme Council of America: *Ritual prayer: its meaning and manner*, 2021. https://wpisca.wpengine.com/?p=117. Accessed June 13, 2021.

Jehovah's Witnesses: *Why don't Jehovah's Witnesses accept blood transfusions?* 2021. https://www.jw.org/en/jehovahs-witnesses/faq/jehovahs-witnesses-why-no-blood-transfusions/. Accessed June 13, 2021.

Koch C: *What near-death experiences reveal about the brain*, 2020. https://www.scientificamerican.com/article/

what-near-death-experiences-reveal-about-the-brain/. Accessed June 13, 2021.

Larsen PD: *Lubkin's chronic illness: impact and intervention*, ed 10, Burlington, MA, 2019, Jones & Bartlett Learning.

Lee Y: Spiritual care for cancer patients, *Asia Pac J Oncol Nurs* 6(2):101, 2019.

Life Advance: *The spiritual well-being scale*, 2018. http://www.lifeadvance.com/spiritual-well-being-scale.html. Accessed June 13, 2021.

Martone R: *New clues found in understanding near-death experiences: research finds parallels to certain psychoactive drugs*, 2019. https://www.scientificamerican.com/article/new-clues-found-in-understanding-near-death-experiences/. Accessed June 13, 2021.

Narayan MC: How to provide "culturally competent care", *Home Healthc Now* 36(1):60, 2018.

Neathery M: Treatment and spiritual care in mental health recovery as a journey, not a destination, *J Christ Nurs* 35(2):86, 2018.

O'Brien ME: *Spirituality in nursing: standing on holy ground*, ed 6, Burlington, MA, 2018, Jones & Bartlett Learning.

QSEN Institute: *QSEN competencies*, 2020. http://qsen.org/competencies/pre-licensure-ksas/. Accessed June 13, 2021.

Rinpoche KT: *The Four Noble Truths and the eightfold path*, 2017. http://www.samyeling.org/buddhism-and-meditation/teaching-archive-2/kenchen-thrangu-rinpoche/the-four-noble-truths-and-the-eightfold-path/. Accessed June 13, 2021.

Rochat E, et al: *Spiritual needs of hospitalized older adults*, 2019. https://www.uofazcenteronaging.com/sites/default/files/spiritual_needs_of_hospitalized_older_adults.pdf. Accessed June 13, 2021.

Ruth-Sahd LA, et al: Collaborating with hospital chaplains to meet the spiritual needs of critical care patients, *Dimens Crit Care Nurs* 37(1):18, 2018.

Starkweather AR: Pain. In Giddens JF, editor: *Concepts for nursing practice*, ed 3, St. Louis, 2021, Elsevier.

The Joint Commission (TJC): *2021 Comprehensive Accreditation Manual*, Oak Brook, IL, 2020, The Joint Commission.

Touhy TA, Jett KF: *Ebersole & Hess' toward health aging: human needs & nursing response*, ed 10 , St. Louis, 2020, Elsevier.

Why Islam: *FAQ's about Muslim dietary restrictions*, 2018. https://www.whyislam.org/faqs/diet/. Accessed June 13, 2021.

Williams EA: *Black women and breast cancer: a cultural theology*, Lanham, MD, 2019, Lexington Books.

Wrigley A: Hope, dying, and solidarity, *Ethical Theory Moral Pract* 22:187, 2019.

RESEARCH REFERENCES

Alemdar DK, et al: The effect of spiritual care on stress levels of mothers in NICU, *West J Nurs Res* 40(7):997, 2018.

Balboni TA, et al: State of the science of spirituality and palliative care research part II: screening, assessment, and interventions, *J Pain Symptom Manage* 54(3):441, 2017.

Bernard M, et al: Relationship between spirituality, meaning in life, psychological distress, wish for hastened death, and their influence on quality of life in palliative care patients, *J Pain Symptom Manage* 54(4):574, 2017.

Berning JN, et al: A novel picture guide to improve spiritual care and reduce anxiety in mechanically ventilated adults in the intensive care unit, *Ann Am Thorac Soc* 13(8):1333, 2016.

Boman E, et al: Inner strength and its relationship to health threats in ageing – a cross-sectional study among community-dwelling older women, *J Adv Nurs* 73:2720, 2017.

Bone N, et al: Critical care nurses' experience with spiritual care: the SPIRIT study, *Am J Crit Care* 27(3):212, 2018.

Borneman T, et al: Evaluation of the FICA tool for spiritual assessment, *J Pain Symptom Manage* 40(2):163, 2010.

Chen SC, et al: Nurses' perceptions of psychosocial care and barriers to its provision: a qualitative study, *J Nurs Res* 25(6):411, 2017a.

Chen Y, et al: The relationship of physiopsychosocial factors and spiritual well-being in elderly residents: implications for evidence-based practice, *Worldviews Evid Based Nurs* 14(6):484, 2017b.

Chiang YC, et al: The impact of nurses' spiritual health on their attitudes toward spiritual care, professional commitment, and caring, *Nurs Outlook* 64(3):215, 2016.

Coats HL: African American elders' psychological-social-spiritual cultural experiences across serious illness: an integrative literature review through a palliative care lens, *Ann Palliat Med* 6(3):253, 2017.

Cottrell L: Joy and happiness: a simultaneous and evolutionary concept analysis, *J Adv Nurs* 72(7):1506, 2016.

Davis CM, et al: Understanding supportive care factors among African American breast cancer survivors, *J Transcult Nurs* 29(1):21, 2018.

Fabbris JL, et al: Anxiety and spiritual well-being in nursing students: a cross-sectional study, *J Holist Nurs* 35(3):261, 2017.

Fradelos EC: Spiritual well-being and associated factors in end-stage renal disease, *Sci World J* 2021:Article ID 6636854, 2021.

Greer DB, Abel WM: Religious/spiritual coping in older African American women, *Qual Rep* 22(1):237, 2017.

Griggs S, Walker RK: The role of hope for adolescents with a chronic illness: an integrative review, *J Pediatr Nurs* 31:404, 2016.

Hakanson C, Ohlen J: Connectedness at the end of life among people admitted to inpatient palliative care, *Am J Hosp Palliat Care* 33(1):47, 2016.

Harrad R, et al: Spiritual care in nursing: an overview of the measures used to assess spiritual care provision and related factors amongst nurses, *Acta Biomed* 90(4):44, 2019.

Hefner J, et al: Adherence and coping strategies in outpatients with chronic myeloid leukemia receiving oral tyrosine kinase inhibitors, *Oncol Nurs Forum* 44(6):e232, 2017.

Heo S, et al: Testing a holistic meditation intervention to address psychosocial distress in patients with heart failure: a pilot study, *J Cardiovasc Nurs* 33(2):126, 2018.

Hulett JM, Armer JM: A systematic review of spiritually based interventions and psychoneuroimmunological outcomes in breast cancer survivorship, *Integr Cancer Ther* 15(4):405, 2016.

Khahi AM, et al: Relationship between self-transcendence and physically-healthy patients under hemodialysis in participating in peer-support group; a randomized clinical trial, *J Renal Inj Prev* 6(4):253, 2017.

Martial C, et al: Temporality of features in near-death experience narratives, *Front Hum Neurosci* 11:311, 2017.

Martial C, et al: Neurochemical models of near-death experiences: a large-scale study based on the semantic similarity of written reports, *Conscious Cogn* 69:52, 2019.

Minton ME, et al: A willingness to go there: nurses and spiritual care, *J Clin Nurs* 27(1-2):173, 2018.

Phenwan T, et al: The meaning of spirituality and spiritual well-being among Thai breast cancer patients: a qualitative study, *Indian J Palliat Care* 25(1):119, 2019.

Puchalski C, Romer AL: Taking a spiritual history allows clinicians to understand patients more fully, *J Palliat Med* 3(1):129, 2000.

Rawlings D, Devery K: Near death experience and nursing practice: lessons from the palliative care literature, *Aust Nurs Midwifery J* 22(8):26, 2015.

Ricci-Allegra P: Spiritual perspective, mindfulness, and spiritual care practice of hospice and palliative nurses, *J Hosp Palliat Nurs* 20(2):172, 2018.

Romeiro J, et al: Spiritual aspects of living with infertility: a synthesis of qualitative studies, *J Clin Nurs* 26(23-24):3917, 2017.

Veloza-Gomez M, et al: The importance of spiritual care in nursing practice, *J Holist Nurs* 35(2):118, 2017.

Vincensi BB: Interconnections: spirituality, spiritual care, and patient-centered care, *Asia Pac J Oncol Nurs* 6:104, 2019.

Vitorino LM, et al: Spiritual/religious coping and depressive symptoms in informal caregivers of hospitalized older adults, *Geriatr Nurs* 39(1):48, 2018.

Loss and Grief

OBJECTIVES

- Identify a nurse's role when caring for patients who are experiencing loss, grief, or death.
- Classify the types of loss experienced throughout life.
- Discuss the process of grief.
- Compare the types of grief.
- Explain how nurses apply grief theory in practice.
- Explain characteristics of a person experiencing grief.
- Assess variables that influence a person's response to grief.

- Develop a nursing care plan for a patient and family experiencing loss and grief.
- Determine ways to collaborate with family members and the interprofessional team to provide palliative care.
- Prioritize interventions for symptom management in patients at the end of life.
- Discuss the criteria for hospice care.
- Summarize care of the body after death.
- Evaluate patient outcomes related to loss and grief.

KEY TERMS

Actual loss
Ambiguous loss
Anticipatory grief
Autopsy
Bereavement
Complicated grief
Disenfranchised grief

Grief
Hope
Hospice
Maturational loss
Mourning
Necessary loss
Normal (uncomplicated) grief

Organ and tissue donation
Palliative care
Postmortem care
Perceived loss
Situational loss

MEDIA RESOURCES

http://evolve.elsevier.com/Potter/fundamentals/
- Review Questions
- Audio Glossary
- Case Study with Questions

- Concept Map Creator
- Content Updates
- Answers to QSEN Activity and Review Questions

Mrs. Allison is an 82-year-old woman who has end-stage heart failure secondary to hypertension and diabetes mellitus. Her quality of life has declined greatly because of shortness of breath, anorexia, fatigue, lack of sleep, and decreased strength. She takes pain medication for severe back pain and frequently has constipation. She was admitted to the hospital 4 times in the past year for heart failure or for care of her venous stasis ulcers. She is now in the intensive care unit with chest pain and heart failure. Tests indicate that her heart function is worsening. Mrs. Allison no longer wants to be hospitalized every time her medical condition deteriorates, and she wants to go home to live out the rest of her life. Mrs. Allison is being evaluated for home hospice care and will temporarily receive home care.

Mrs. Allison lives with her husband of 59 years. Her daughter, Lilly, visits her parents every day. Lilly does not agree with the plan to begin hospice care. She believes that her mother is "giving up" too soon. Mr. Allison does not understand hospice and is not sure if he will be a good caregiver.

Jennifer Brown, a nursing student, will be caring for the Allison family as she learns how to give care in the home. She has never taken care of a person at the end of life in a home setting and feels anxious about her abilities to care for Mrs. Allison. Jennifer will focus on helping Mrs. Allison and her family manage Mrs. Allison's symptoms and physical needs. She also will help Mrs. Allison and her family cope with feelings of loss and grief.

Loss is an inevitable part of life. Accompanying each loss are feelings of grief and sadness. Whether a patient is facing infertility or an amputation, an unwanted diagnosis or impending death, you are in a position to offer both the patient and family support to cope with the loss, and comfort when continued life is not possible. Nurses in all practice settings and specialties provide grief support for the majority of dying patients and their families. Like grief, death is as inescapable in practice as it is in life. There is a trend for an increase in palliative and hospice care for patients with serious chronic illness and for patients with terminal diagnoses. Palliative and hospice care are offered within health care agencies as well as in patients' homes.

Although people agree that death is a part of life, many are hesitant to talk about it because of feelings of fear or uncertainty and not wanting to upset others. Talking openly about death is often uncomfortable, and it usually is not discussed in American society (i.e., in our everyday lives, our language, and even our thinking) (Hess, 2018). An example is our avoidance of the word "died" and instead the use of terms such as "passed away" or "gone." As you gain experience in nursing practice, you will learn how to become comfortable in discussing sensitive topics and in allowing patients to express their desires for care at the end of life. With the Self-Care Determination Act of 1990 (a law requiring that patients be made aware of their medical decision rights), nurses and other health care providers are starting these conversations earlier, but there is more work left to do. You have the opportunity to advocate for patients and the high quality of care deserved at the end of life.

As a nurse you will learn to provide what patients and families need most at the time of a serious loss as well as at the end of life: compassion, attentiveness, and patient-centered care. As with other nursing situations, the more experience you have in caring for individuals who are grieving and dying, the more confident, courageous, and compassionate you will become when caring for patients and families at this intimate and meaningful time. Your knowledge, critical thinking skills, and ability to make clinical judgments and decisions will develop quickly if you have the desire and willingness to learn, be present, and seek the help needed to learn how to give excellent care. Whether it is educating patients and families about advance directives, managing patients' symptoms, or simply holding a hand, nurses care for the grieving and dying and their families every day. It is the caring actions of nurses that help a patient and family during these times (see Chapter 7).

SCIENTIFIC KNOWLEDGE BASE

Loss

Life provides each person with multiple opportunities to grieve a loss or change. Sometimes the change is welcomed (marriage, birth of a child), and sometimes not (divorce, loss of a job, death). Changes related to loss can also be expected (child growing older and moving out of parent's home) or unexpected (sudden accident or death). Losses can be of tangible things, such as a body part or function, a pet, or a possession. Or losses can be intangible, such as the loss of self-esteem, a personal relationship, confidence, or a dream.

The experience of loss starts early in life and continues until death. Children develop independence from the adults who raise them, and as they begin and leave school, change friends, begin careers, and form new relationships, loss is a part of their maturation. From birth to death people form attachments and experience loss. Illness can also be a source of loss. It can change a person's functioning and therefore a person's job, family role, income level, and overall quality of life (Table 36.1). How one grieves depends on cultural norms, belief systems, support systems, and personal faith.

Life changes are normal, expected, and often positive. As people age, they learn that change always involves a necessary loss. They learn to expect that most necessary losses eventually are replaced by something different or better. However, some losses cause them to undergo permanent changes in their lives that threaten their sense of belonging and security. The death of a loved one, divorce, or loss of independence changes life forever and often significantly disrupts a person's physical, psychological, and spiritual health.

A maturational loss is a form of necessary loss and includes all normally expected life changes across the life span. A toddler experiences separation anxiety from a parent when starting preschool. A grade school child may not want to lose a favorite teacher and classroom. A

TABLE 36.1 Types of Loss	
Definition	**Implications of Loss**
Loss of possessions or objects (e.g., theft, deterioration, misplacement, or destruction)	Extent of grieving depends on value of object, sentiment attached to it, or its usefulness.
Loss of known environment (e.g., leaving home, hospitalization, new job, moving out of a rehabilitation unit)	Loss occurs through maturational or situational events or by injury or illness. Loneliness or uncertainty in an unfamiliar setting threatens self-esteem, hopefulness, or belonging.
Loss of a significant other (e.g., divorce, loss of friend, trusted caregiver, or pet)	Close friends, family members, and pets fulfill psychological, safety, love, belonging, and self-esteem needs.
Loss of an aspect of self (e.g., body part, job, psychological or physiological function)	Illness, injury, or developmental changes result in loss of a valued aspect of self, altering personal identity and self-concept.
Loss of life (e.g., death of family member, friend, co-worker, or one's own death)	Those left behind after a death grieve for the loss of life of a loved one. Dying people also feel sadness or fear pain, loss of control, and dependency on others.

college student may not want to leave the campus community. Maturational losses associated with normal life transitions help people develop coping skills to use when they experience unplanned, unwanted, or unexpected loss.

Other losses seem unnecessary and are not part of expected maturation experiences. Sudden, unpredictable external events bring about situational loss. For example, a person in an automobile accident sustains an injury with permanent physical changes that make it impossible to return to work or school, leading to loss of function, income, life goals, and self-esteem.

Losses may be actual or perceived. An actual loss occurs when a person can no longer feel, hear, see, or know a person or object. Examples include the loss of a body part, death of a family member, or loss of a job. Lost valued objects include those that wear out or are misplaced, stolen, or ruined. A perceived loss is uniquely defined by the person experiencing the loss and is less obvious to other people. For example, some people perceive rejection by a friend to be a loss, which creates a loss of confidence or changes an individual's status in the social group. How an individual interprets the meaning of a perceived loss affects the intensity of the grief response. Perceived losses are easy to overlook by others because they are experienced so internally and individually, but they are as painful as an actual loss and grieved in the same way.

Each person responds to loss differently. The type of loss and a person's previous experience with and perception of loss influence the depth and duration of the grief response. For some individuals the loss of an object (e.g., home or treasured gift) generates the same level of distress as the loss of a person, depending on the value the person places on the object. Chronic illnesses, disabilities, and hospitalization produce multiple losses. When entering an institution for care, patients lose access to familiar people and environments, privacy, and control over body functions and daily routines. A chronic illness or disability adds financial hardships for most people and often brings about changes in lifestyle and dependence on others. Even brief illnesses or hospitalizations cause temporary changes in family role functioning, daily activities, and relationships.

Death is the ultimate loss. Although it is an expected part of life, death represents the unknown and can generate anxiety, fear, and uncertainty for many people. It creates a permanent separation of people and can cause fear, sadness, and regret for the dying person, family members, friends, and caregivers. A person's culture, spirituality, personal beliefs, and values; previous experiences with death; and degree of social support influence the way a person approaches death.

Grief

Grief is an individualized response to a loss that is perceived, real, or anticipated by the person experiencing loss (Vacarolis and Fosbre, 2021). It is a complex experience one feels emotionally, cognitively, physically, socially, and spiritually (see Chapters 9 and 35). The grief experience is not a state but a process (Mughal et al., 2020). Grief cannot be prevented. It is very personal. No two people grieve the same loss the same way, nor do they journey through grief in the same way. Grief work is very hard and requires enormous amounts of energy from the griever. It is rarely orderly and predictable. Most individuals recover adequately within a year after a loss; however, some individuals experience an extension of the standard grieving process, described as complicated grief or prolonged grief disorder (Mughal et al., 2020). Because objects, memories, and anniversaries can cause a surge in feelings of loss, grief work is never fully completed. However, grief can diminish, and healing can occur when the pain of loss is less.

Coping with grief involves a period of mourning, all the ways in which an individual outwardly expresses grief and the behaviors taken to manage grief (Vacarolis and Fosbre, 2021). Most mourning rituals are culturally influenced, learned behaviors. For example, the Jewish mourning ritual of *shivah* is a time period when normal life activities come to a stop. Those mourning welcome friends into the home as a way of honoring the dead and receive support during the mourning period.

Grief and mourning occur during the period of bereavement (Vacarolis and Fosbre, 2021). Bereavement refers to the time of sadness after a person experiences a significant loss through death (Vacarolis and Fosbre, 2021). Allow people experiencing bereavement to talk about their loss and sense of grief. Reassure them that their feelings are normal and encourage them to postpone making major decisions. Recognizing that there are different types of grief and processes for coping can help nurses plan and implement appropriate care.

Normal Grief. Normal (uncomplicated) grief is a common and universal reaction characterized by complex emotional, cognitive, social, physical, behavioral, and spiritual responses to loss and death. Some normal feelings of grief are disbelief, yearning, anger, and depression. Although the manner of a person's death (expected, violent, sudden, unexpected) affects a survivor's ability to grieve normally, it does not always determine how an individual will actually grieve. Helpful coping mechanisms for people who are grieving include hardiness and resilience, a personal sense of control, and the ability to make sense of and identify positive possibilities after a loss.

Anticipatory Grief. Often a person experiences anticipatory grief before the actual loss or death occurs, especially in situations of prolonged or predicted loss, such as family members caring for patients diagnosed with dementia or amyotrophic lateral sclerosis (ALS). Family members often grieve the impending death of a loved one because of the impending loss of companionship, control, and sense of freedom and the mental and physical changes experienced by their loved one. Nurses need to recognize anticipatory grief when it occurs and help patients and family members express their feelings. A caregiver support group is often beneficial to helping individuals cope with anticipatory grief (Whitley, 2020).

When grief extends over a long period, people absorb loss gradually and begin to prepare for its inevitability. They may experience intense responses to grief (e.g., shock, denial, and tearfulness) before the actual death occurs and often feel relief when it finally happens. Another way to think about anticipatory grief is that it gives people time to prepare or complete the tasks related to the impending death. Although preparing for death helps some individuals, it increases stress for others, creating an emotional roller coaster of highs and lows.

Disenfranchised Grief. People may experience disenfranchised grief when their relationship to the deceased person is not socially sanctioned, cannot be shared openly, or seems of lesser significance. The person's loss and grief do not meet the norms of grief acknowledged by the person's culture, thereby cutting the grieving person off from social support and the sympathy given to people with more socially acceptable losses. Examples include the death of a former spouse, health care worker, or death from homicide, suicide, or terminated pregnancy (Vacarolis and Fosbre, 2021).

Ambiguous Loss. Sometimes people experience losses that are marked by uncertainty. Ambiguous loss, a type of disenfranchised grief, can occur when the person who is lost is physically present but not psychologically available, as in cases of severe dementia or brain injury. Other times the person is gone (e.g., after a kidnapping, when someone is taken as a prisoner of war, when there is no body found after a disaster such as 9/11, or when someone "goes missing"), but the grieving person maintains an ongoing, intense psychological attachment, never sure of the reality of the situation. Ambiguous losses are particularly difficult to process because of the lack of finality and unknown outcomes (Angle, 2019). Recently, ambiguous loss for parents has become more prevalent as more children identify as transgendered (Coolhart et al., 2018). Nurses also will encounter more refugees and immigrants experiencing ambiguous loss of their homeland (Perez and Arnold-Berkovits, 2018).

Complicated Grief. Some people do not experience a normal grief process. In complicated grief people have a prolonged or significantly difficult time moving forward after a loss. They experience a chronic and disruptive yearning for the deceased; have trouble accepting the death and trusting others; and/or feel excessively bitter, emotionally numb, or anxious about the future. Complicated grief involves prolonged symptoms of painful emotions and sorrow for more than 1 year (Mughal et al., 2020). Complicated grief can also be understood as persistent grief that is so severe that it affects normal functioning and quality of life (Perng and Renz, 2018). Patients show a preoccupation with the deceased and feel inner emptiness, have no interest in life, and sleep poorly (Mughal et al., 2020). Complicated grief occurs more often when a person had a conflicted relationship with the deceased, prior or multiple losses or stressors, mental health issues, or lack of social support. Loss associated with homicide, suicide, sudden accidents, or the death of a child has the potential to become complicated. Specific types of complicated grief include chronic, exaggerated, delayed, and masked grief.

Chronic Grief. A person with chronic grief experiences a normal grief response, except that it extends for a longer period of time. This can include years to decades of intense grieving.

Exaggerated Grief. A person with an exaggerated grief response often exhibits self-destructive or maladaptive behavior, obsessions, or psychiatric disorders. Suicide is a risk for these individuals.

Delayed Grief. In delayed grief a person's grief response is unusually delayed or postponed because the loss is so overwhelming that the person must avoid the full realization of the loss. A delayed grief response is frequently triggered by a second loss, sometimes seemingly not as significant as the first loss—for example, a college student whose parent has died, but the full realization of the loss comes after the family pet dies or the student fails a course.

Masked Grief. With masked grief, a survivor is not aware that their behaviors that interfere with normal functioning are a result of a loss (Petruzzi, 2019). Physical symptoms exhibited by the masked grief could be headaches, heartburn, rashes, or tachycardia.

Theories of Grief and Mourning

Knowledge of grief theories and normal responses to loss and bereavement helps you to better understand these complex experiences and to make clinical judgments about how to help a grieving person. Grief theories describe the physical, psychological, and social reactions to loss. Remember that reactions to grief vary widely. The variety of theories supports the complexity and individuality of grief responses. Although most grief theories describe how people cope with death, they also help to understand responses to other significant losses (Table 36.2).

Early grief theories describe grief as a process in which people move through stages or tasks. (Hamilton, 2016). Newer grief theories suggest that human beings are unique and create their own experiences and truths and make their own meanings when confronted with loss and death. Differences in social and personal context, family structure and meaning of relationships, and thought processes affect an individual's truths and grief experiences. No one's grief follows a set path. Grief is not linear. It is cyclical, with movement forward and backward. Educating grievers about the cyclical pattern of grief work prepares them for difficult days among the better days. Consider a widow several months after the death of her husband. She may have had several weeks of feeling less sad and depressed. If unprepared for the cyclical nature of grief, she may be taken off guard by her strong grief reaction to a phone call for her husband or a commercial advertising his favorite candy. Knowing that these feelings will come and go helps the griever to be prepared for them and allows for the necessary self-care. For example, the widow knows her husband's birthday is approaching and makes plans with her family for dinner that evening so they can share happy memories of their lost loved one.

> **REFLECT NOW**
>
> Reflect on a loss that you experienced. What type of loss was it? How did you experience the cyclical nature of grief related to your loss?

NURSING KNOWLEDGE BASE

Nurses apply their knowledge and nursing experience to develop plans of care to help patients and family members who are experiencing loss, grief, or death. Nurses implement plans of care in all settings based on nursing research, evidence-based practice, assessment findings about patients, and patient and family preferences to care. Extensive nursing education programs and professional standards of care support the improvement of end-of-life care. The End-of-Life Nursing Education Consortium (ELNEC) provides training in palliative care with essential information to practicing nurses and nursing students, including undergraduate and graduate nursing faculty, continuing education providers, staff development educators, specialty nurses, and advanced

TABLE 36.2	Theories of Grief and Mourning
Stages of Dying Kübler-Ross (1969)	**Denial** The person cannot accept the fact of the loss. It is a form of psychological protection from a loss that the person cannot yet bear. **Anger** The person expresses resistance or intense anger at God, other people, or the situation. **Bargaining** The person cushions and postpones awareness of the loss by trying to prevent it from happening. **Depression** The person realizes the full impact of the loss. **Acceptance** The person incorporates the loss into life.
Attachment Theory Bowlby (1980)	**Numbing** Protects the person from the full impact of the loss **Yearning and Searching** Emotional outbursts of tearful sobbing and acute distress; common physical symptoms in this stage: tightness in chest and throat, shortness of breath, a feeling of lethargy, insomnia, and loss of appetite **Disorganization and Despair** Endless examination of how and why the loss occurred or expressions of anger at anyone who seems responsible for the loss **Reorganization** Accepts the change, assumes unfamiliar roles, acquires new skills, builds new relationships, and begins to separate from the lost relationship without feeling that its importance is being lessened
Grief Tasks Model Worden (2008)	Accepts the reality of the loss Experiences the pain of grief Adjusts to a world in which the deceased is missing Emotionally relocates the deceased and moves on with life
Rando's "R" Process Model Rando (1993, 2014)	**Recognize** the loss **React** to the pain of separation **Recollect and reexperience** the relationship with the deceased **Relinquish** old attachments **Readjust** to life after loss **Reinvest** by putting emotional energy into new people
Dual Process Model Stroebe and Schut (1999)	**Loss-oriented** activities: grief work, dwelling on the loss, breaking connections with the deceased person, and resisting activities to move past the grief **Restoration-oriented** activities: attending to life changes, finding new roles or relationships, coping with finances, and participating in distractions, which provide balance to the loss-oriented state

practice nurses (ELNEC, n.d.). The training is designed to prepare nurses with basic and advanced curricula to care for patients and families experiencing loss, grief, death, and bereavement. Evidence-based practice guidelines for managing clinical and ethical issues at the end of life in many health care settings have been published by the American Nurses Association (ANA) in conjunction with the Hospice and Palliative Nurses Association (ANA, 2014), the American Society for Pain Management Nurses (Coyne et al., 2018), and the American Association of Critical-Care Nurses (Jensen et al., 2020).

Factors Influencing Loss and Grief

Multiple factors, such as developmental factors, personal relationships, the nature of the loss, coping strategies, socioeconomic status, and cultural and spiritual influences and beliefs influence the way a person perceives and responds to loss. Nursing research contributes to this knowledge base.

Human Development. Patient age and stage of development affect an individual's grief response. For example, toddlers cannot understand loss or death but often feel anxiety over the loss of objects and separation from parents. Common expressions of grief include changes in eating and sleeping patterns, bowel and bladder disturbances, and increased fussiness. School-age children understand the concepts of permanence and irreversibility but do not always understand the causes of a loss. Some have intense periods of emotional expression, and experience changes in eating, sleeping, and level of social engagement.

Young adults experience many developmental losses related to their evolving future. Illness or death disrupts the young adult's future dreams and establishment of an autonomous sense of self. Midlife adults also experience major life transitions, such as caring for aging parents, dealing with changes in marital status, and adapting to new family roles (McKay and McKay, 2021). For older adults, the aging process leads to expected developmental losses. Some older adults experience age discrimination, especially when they become dependent or are near death, but they show resilience after a loss as a result of their prior experiences and developed coping skills (Box 36.1).

Personal Relationships. When loss involves another person, the quality and meaning of the lost relationship influence the grief response. When a relationship between two people was very rewarding and well connected, the survivor often finds it difficult to move forward after the death. Grief work is hampered by regret and a sense of unfinished business, especially when people are close but did not have a good relationship at the time of death. Social support and the ability to accept help from others are critical variables in recovery from loss and grief. Grievers experience less depression when they have highly satisfying personal relationships and friends to support them in their grief.

Nature of the Loss. Exploring the nature of a loss will help you understand the effect of the loss on a patient's behavior, health, and well-being. Was the loss avoidable? Is it permanent or temporary? Is it actual or imagined? Encouraging patients to share information about their loss will help you better develop appropriate interventions that meet the individualized needs of your patients.

Highly visible losses generally stimulate a helping response from others. For example, the loss of one's home from a tornado often brings community and governmental support. A more private loss such as a miscarriage brings less support from others. A sudden and unexpected death poses challenges different from those of a person in a debilitating chronic illness. When the death is sudden and unexpected, the survivors do not have time to say goodbye. In chronic illness, survivors have

BOX 36.1 FOCUS ON OLDER ADULTS
Grief Considerations in Older Adults

- There is little evidence that grief experiences differ because of age alone. Responses to loss are more likely related to the nature of the specific loss experience and individual differences.
- Increased age increases the likelihood that older adults have faced multiple losses. Older adults residing in communal living situations experience many losses as friends die.
- Older adults may be more encumbered by grief because of the cumulative effect of multiple losses (Perng and Renz, 2018).
- Those with complicated grief are associated with higher mortality, heart disease, and cancer (Perng and Renz, 2018).
- Many older adults exhibit resilience. Others around them can learn from their courage and ability to respond to life challenges.
- Older adults are at risk for complicated grieving as a result of multiple losses, fewer resources, and decreased coping. Complicated grief can lead to cancer, heart disease and higher mortality in this population (Perng and Renz, 2018).
- Physical decline caused by chronic illness sometimes leads to grief over lost health, function, and roles.
- Older adults benefit from the same therapeutic techniques as people in other age-groups. Evidence indicates that positive reappraisal (cognitive restructuring) helps older adults adapt to significant losses (e.g., seeing a cardiac diagnosis as the opportunity to become healthy by eating nutritiously and exercising regularly). Relieving depression and maintaining physical function are therapeutic goals for older adults experiencing grief.

memories of prolonged suffering, pain, and loss of function. Death by violence or suicide or multiple losses by their very nature complicate the grieving process in unique ways (Mayo Clinic, 2020). For example, in the case of suicide, survivors may experience guilt, wondering if there was something that they missed or could have done to prevent the suicide (Mayo Clinic, 2020).

Coping Strategies. The losses that people face when they were children often influence the coping skills they will use when faced with larger and more painful losses in adulthood. These coping strategies such as talking, journaling, and sharing their emotions with others may be healthy and effective. Some strategies, such as using alcohol and drugs or acting out in violence, are unhealthy and ineffective. Nurses support patients by assessing their grief response and coping strategies, providing patient education, and encouraging the use of healthy coping strategies.

Socioeconomic Status. Socioeconomic status influences a person's grief process in direct and indirect ways. For example, a newly widowed mother finds herself changing roles, needs to work several jobs to make ends meet, and does not find time to initiate self-care or grieve the loss of her spouse. With limited resources, activities that support healthy grief work such as buying a tree to plant in honor of the deceased or going to a support group may be unrealistic. Practical implications also exist when there are limited resources. An individual with limited finances may be unable to take time off work to attend a funeral or may be unable to travel to visit a dying family member.

Culture. During times of loss and grief patients and families draw on the social and spiritual practices of their cultures to find comfort, expression, and meaning in the experience (Cancer.Net, 2018). Expressions of grief in one culture do not always make sense to people from a different culture. Try to understand and appreciate each patient's cultural values related to loss, death, and grieving (see Chapter 9). For example, some people are stoic, holding back their public displays of emotion. For others, behaviors such as public wailing and physical demonstrations of grief, including survivor body mutilation, show respect for the dead. Remember, culture extends beyond the geographical location of a person. Consider the influence of sexual and gender orientation, socioeconomic status, and family makeup (blended versus nuclear) when assessing cultural influence on grief practices and death rituals.

Spiritual and Religious Beliefs. Like cultural influences, spirituality and/or religious practices and beliefs provide a framework to navigate, understand, and heal from loss, death, and grief (see Chapter 35). A person's faith often influences the response to an illness, treatment, advanced life-support options, autopsy, organ donation, and what happens to the body and spirit after death. Patients draw on their spiritual beliefs to obtain comfort and seek understanding at times of loss. You must know your own views and beliefs about loss and death while remaining open to other views and beliefs that contrast with your own to best support and care for your patients and their families. Assess your patient's and family's beliefs and practices whenever possible. Encourage patients and families to express their beliefs and practices and draw on their spiritual resources (e.g., faith in a higher power, communities of support, friends, a sense of hope and meaning in life, and religious practices). Spirituality affects a patient's and family members' ability to cope with loss as well. Use a holistic approach when caring for a patient and family to provide them with the best possible individualized care.

Hope, a multidimensional concept considered to be a component of spirituality, energizes and provides comfort to individuals and families experiencing personal challenges. Hope gives a person the ability to see life as long-lasting or having meaning or purpose. With hope a patient moves from feelings of weakness and vulnerability to living as fully as possible. Maintaining a sense of hope depends in part on a person having strong relationships and emotional connectedness to others. On the other hand, spiritual distress often arises from a patient's inability to feel hopeful or to foresee any favorable outcomes. Spirituality and hope play a vital role in a patient's adjustment to loss and death (see Chapter 35).

Before Jennifer meets the Allison family for the first time, she reviews the information needed to complete a thorough assessment. She identifies the key symptoms to look for in a person with end-stage heart failure and chronic pain. Jennifer plans to be sensitive to any embarrassment that Mrs. Allison feels about her constipation and decreased functional abilities. Because of Mrs. Allison's constipation, Jennifer does more reading on the effects of opioids and heart failure on constipation so she can work with Mrs. Allison to develop a plan of care. Jennifer reflects on her own experiences with grief and understands that people experience grief differently, and she recognizes that not all members of the Allison family agree on the plan of care. Therefore Jennifer reads more about grief theories, stages of grief, and signs and symptoms of grieving so she can make appropriate clinical judgments about her patient's and family's needs and develop a plan of care to meet those needs. Jennifer also gathers information about palliative care, hospice, and end-of-life care so she can provide teaching to Mr. Allison and Lilly.

CRITICAL THINKING

To be successful in judging and deciding on a patient's plan of care, you apply critical thinking that requires a synthesis of knowledge, experience, environmental factors, information gathered from patients, critical thinking attitudes, and intellectual and professional standards. Clinical judgment

requires you to reflect on scientific and nursing knowledge, assess information from the patient, analyze the data for cues, and make decisions regarding your patient's care. During assessment consider all elements that build toward making an appropriate nursing diagnosis (Fig. 36.1).

Form assessment questions based on your theoretical and professional knowledge of grief and loss to help you understand a patient's subjective experiences of loss. Be culturally aware and listen carefully to a patient's responses and perceptions when exploring the meaning of grief and loss with a patient.

Personal experience in caring for patients during the grief process is valuable when helping patients and their families identify coping options. Being familiar with commonly experienced responses to loss enables you to better understand a patient's emotions and behaviors. Some patients ignore, lash out, plead with, or withdraw from other people as part of a normal response to loss. You may have taken care of patients in the past who have experienced loss. Draw on these clinical experiences to help you support the patient and family while they are grieving. Think about a time that you experienced a loss and how you responded to and coped with your loss. Your responses to the loss and how you grieved can help you recognize responses to loss in a patient and help you develop an individualized plan of care.

Applying intellectual standards helps you use sound clinical judgment to make accurate clinical decisions and helps patients find meaningful and logical ways to work through their grief. Critical thinking ensures that you obtain significant and relevant information when assessing and making decisions about patients' needs. Use critical thinking to integrate theory, prior experiences, and self-knowledge to respond to your patients with patience and understanding. Avoid making assumptions about how patients should be responding to a loss. Significance and relevance are standards of critical thinking that allow you to explore the issues that are most meaningful to patients and most likely to affect a patient's response to loss and behaviors during grief.

Use professional standards when designing plans of care for patients and families who experience grief and loss. Incorporating standards such as the nursing code of ethics (see Chapter 22), the dying patient's bill of rights (Box 36.2), and the ANA Scope and Standards of Hospice and Palliative Nursing Practice (2014) is often helpful. You may also find the ANA's (2016) position statement on *Nurses' Roles and Responsibilities in Providing Care and Support at the End of Life or* the American Society for Pain Management Nursing and Hospice and Palliative Nurses Association's position statement for pain management at the end of life (Coyne et al., 2018) helpful in supporting patients and families at the end of life.

REFLECT NOW

Remember how you felt after a loss you experienced. What emotions did you feel and what coping strategies worked for you? How does your family/culture typically respond to death and loss?

❖ NURSING PROCESS

Apply the nursing process and critical thinking as you care for patients. The nursing process provides a clinical decision-making approach for you to develop sound clinical judgments so that you can implement an individualized plan of care.

◆ Assessment

During the assessment process thoroughly assess each patient and critically analyze findings to recognize cues to ensure that you use

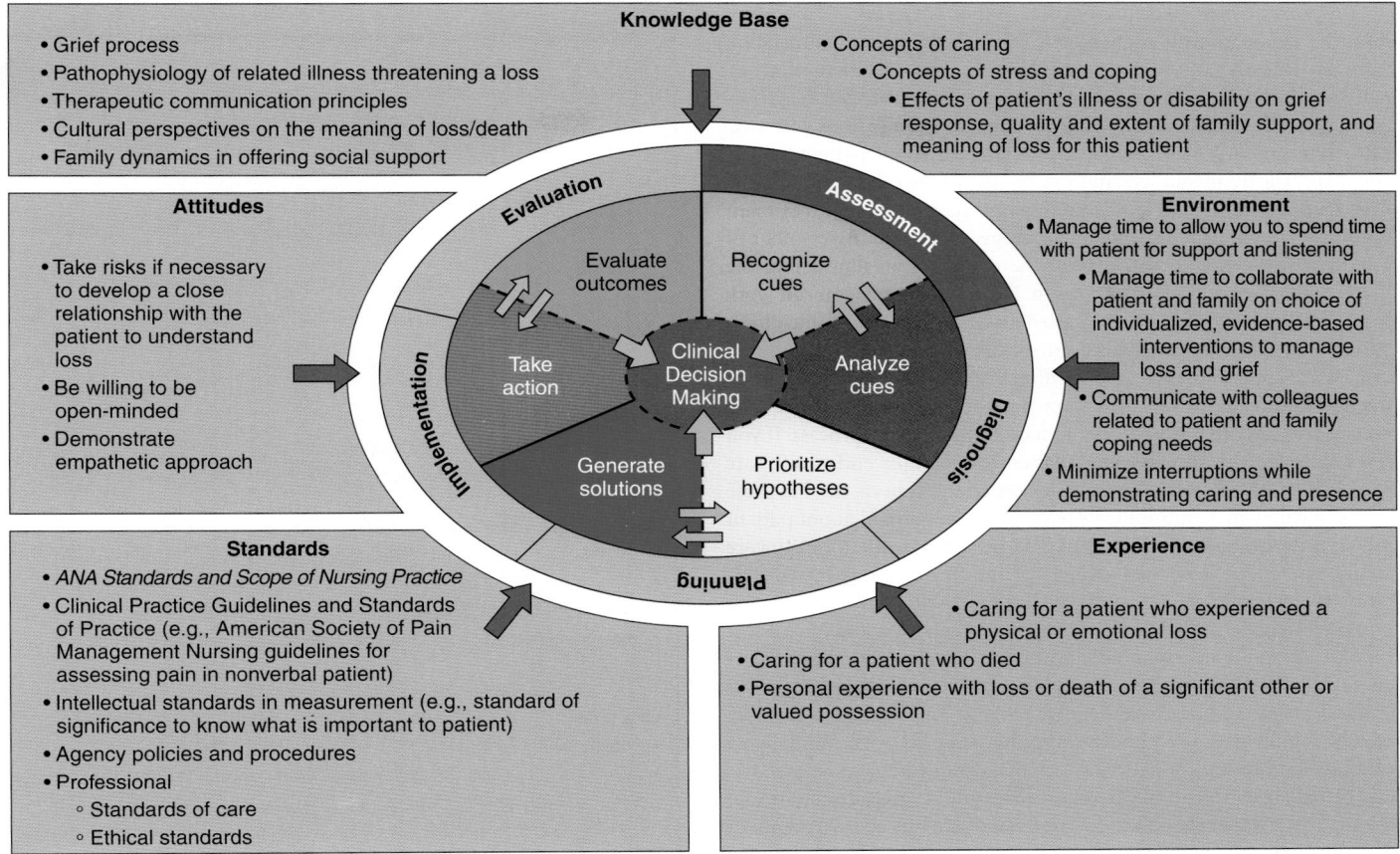

Knowledge Base
- Grief process
- Pathophysiology of related illness threatening a loss
- Therapeutic communication principles
- Cultural perspectives on the meaning of loss/death
- Family dynamics in offering social support

- Concepts of caring
  - Concepts of stress and coping
    - Effects of patient's illness or disability on grief response, quality and extent of family support, and meaning of loss for this patient

Attitudes
- Take risks if necessary to develop a close relationship with the patient to understand loss
- Be willing to be open-minded
- Demonstrate empathetic approach

Environment
- Manage time to allow you to spend time with patient for support and listening
  - Manage time to collaborate with patient and family on choice of individualized, evidence-based interventions to manage loss and grief
  - Communicate with colleagues related to patient and family coping needs
- Minimize interruptions while demonstrating caring and presence

Standards
- *ANA Standards and Scope of Nursing Practice*
- Clinical Practice Guidelines and Standards of Practice (e.g., American Society of Pain Management Nursing guidelines for assessing pain in nonverbal patient)
- Intellectual standards in measurement (e.g., standard of significance to know what is important to patient)
- Agency policies and procedures
- Professional
  - Standards of care
  - Ethical standards

Experience
- Caring for a patient who experienced a physical or emotional loss
- Caring for a patient who died
- Personal experience with loss or death of a significant other or valued possession

Evaluation — Evaluate outcomes — Take action — Implementation
Assessment — Recognize cues — Analyze cues — Diagnosis
Clinical Decision Making
Generate solutions — Prioritize hypotheses — Planning

FIG. 36.1 Critical thinking model for loss, death, and grieving assessment. (Clinical Judgment Measurement Model copyright © NCSBN. All rights reserved.)

BOX 36.2   The Dying Person's Bill of Rights

- I have the right to be treated as a living human until I die.
- I have the right to maintain a sense of hopefulness, however changing its focus may be.
- I have the right to be cared for by those who can maintain a sense of hopefulness, however changing this might be.
- I have the right to express my feelings and emotions about my approaching death in my own way.
- I have the right to participate in decisions concerning my care.
- I have the right to expect continuing medical and nursing attention even though "cure" goals must be changed to "comfort" goals.
- I have the right not to die alone.
- I have the right to be free from pain.
- I have the right to have my questions answered honestly.
- I have the right to retain my individuality and not be judged for my decisions that may be contrary to beliefs of others.
- I have the right to expect that the sanctity of the human body will be respected after death.
- I have the right to be cared for by caring, sensitive, knowledgeable people who will attempt to understand my needs and be able to gain some satisfaction in helping me face my death.

From Betty R. Ferrell, Nessa Coyle: An overview of palliative nursing care, Am J Nurs 102(5):26, 2002. © Wolters Kluwer Health, Inc.

---

sound clinical judgment to make patient-centered clinical decisions required for safe and effective nursing care. A trusting, helping relationship with patients and family members who are grieving is essential to the assessment process. A caring nurse encourages patients to tell their stories. Look for opportunities to invite patients to share their experiences, being aware that attitudes about self-disclosure; sharing of emotions; or talking about illness, fears, and death are shaped by an individual's personality, coping style, and culture. This information is invaluable to understanding the unique and individual needs of each patient.

Through the Patient's Eyes. A nursing priority is to be present for your patients and their families., You establish a trusting relationship with your patients by using the skills of active listening, silence, and therapeutic touch. This trusting relationship allows you to explore your patients' unique responses to grief or their preferences for end-of-life care, which may include advance directives. Patient perceptions and expectations influence your success in understanding patient problems and how you prioritize nursing diagnoses.

Because of the importance of symptom management and priority of comfort in end-of-life care, prioritize your initial assessment to encourage patients to identify any distressing symptoms. Completing a thorough assessment is difficult when patients are in pain, nauseated, anxious, depressed, or short of breath. Offer available measures for symptom relief, determine their efficacy, and then return for your assessment.

To assess patient perceptions, ask, "What is the most important thing I can do for you right now?" You usually gather information from patients first, but with advanced illness and as death approaches, patients often rely on family members to communicate for them. Encourage family members to share their goals and perceptions with you. Most often they provide valuable information about patient preferences and clarify misunderstandings or identify overlooked information. Assess patients' and family members' understanding of treatment options to implement a mutually developed care plan. Assessment of grief responses extends throughout the course of an illness into the bereavement period following a death. During this time you can work to normalize the grief response. Patients with advanced chronic illness and their families eventually face end-of-life care decisions and should discuss the content of any advance directives together. Patients, family members, and the health care team need to discuss end-of-life care preferences early in the assessment phase of the nursing process. If you feel uncomfortable in assessing a patient's wishes for end-of-life care by yourself, ask a health care provider experienced in discussing these issues to help you. Communicate what you have learned about patient preferences during any registered nurse (RN) hand-off, at health care team conferences, in written care plans, and through ongoing consultation (see Chapter 26).

Speak to patients and family members using honest and open communication, remembering that cultural practices and personal preferences influence how much information a patient will share. Ask about cultural beliefs and practices because patients and families will rarely offer this information without prompting. Keep an open mind, listen carefully, and observe a patient's verbal and nonverbal responses. Facial expressions, voice tones, and avoided topics often disclose more than words. Anticipate common grief responses but allow patients to describe their experiences in their own words. Open-ended questions such as "What do you understand about your diagnosis?" or "You seem sad today. Can you tell me more?" may open the door to a patient-centered discussion. Many people find it difficult to talk about loss, fear, death, or grief. The use of pauses, gentle questioning, and silence honors the patient's privacy and readiness to talk. Talk to patients and family members in a private, quiet setting. Consider the culture of the individual and explore what your patients prefer. For example, in some cultures the health care provider is expected to discuss information with the husband or father of a female patient, not directly with her, so that the male can pass the filtered information to the female. Some patients want to have family members present so that everyone hears the same thing and has an opportunity to add to the conversation. However, other patients want their concerns and questions addressed privately. As you gather assessment data, summarize and validate your impressions with the patient or family member. Information from the medical record and from other members of the health care team, including physicians, social workers, and spiritual care providers, contributes to your assessment data.

Grief Variables. Conversations about the meaning of loss to a patient often lead to other important areas of assessment, including the patient's coping style, the nature of family relationships, social support systems, the nature of the loss, cultural and spiritual beliefs, life goals, family grief patterns, self-care, and sources of hope (Box 36.3). Use skills appropriate for assessing a patient's culture, family, self-concept, or spiritual beliefs (see Chapters 9, 10, 33, and 35) to gain a deeper understanding of the loss.

Knowing the commonly experienced reactions to grief and loss and grief theories guides your critical thinking and clinical judgment toward focused assessment skills. A single behavior can occur in all types of grief. If a patient who is grieving describes loneliness and difficulty

---

BOX 36.3 Nursing Assessment Questions

Nature of Relationships
- How long have you known the person who died/who is seriously ill?
- What role did (name person) play in your life?
- Tell me about what your relationship with (name person) meant to you.

Social Support Systems
- In times of loss, who is there for you? Who is absent? Who provides support?
- What do others do for you that is most meaningful or helpful?
- Are family/friends available when needed? Which friends or relatives do you wish were here?

Nature of the Loss
- Tell me what this loss means to you?
- What other losses have you experienced?
- Was this loss expected or unexpected? How has that affected you?

Cultural and Spiritual Beliefs
- What is your belief about death?
- What is your belief about the meaning of life?
- Which rituals/practices are important to you at the end of life?
- How do members of your culture or religious group respond to this type of loss?

Life Goals
- What are your current life goals?
- How have your goals changed because of this experience?
- What will you do in the future?

Family Grief Patterns
- How have you/your family dealt with loss in the past?
- What are your family's strengths?
- How have family relationships changed as a result of your loss?
- What role do you assume in your family during stressful situations?

Self-Care
- Tell me how you're feeling.
- What are you doing to take care of yourself now?
- What helps you when you feel this sad? What doesn't help?
- What can I do for you?

Hope
- What do you hope for right now?
- What helps you to remain hopeful? What causes you to lose hope?

---

in falling asleep, consider all factors surrounding the loss in context. What was the loss? When did it occur? What was the meaning of the loss to the patient? For example, when your patient exhibits signs you expect from a recent loss but you learn that the loss occurred 2 years ago, the patient's response most likely indicates a complicated, chronic grief experience. Focus your assessment on how a patient is reacting to loss or grief and not on how *you* believe that patient should be reacting.

Grief Reactions. Use psychological and physical assessment skills to assess a patient's unique grief responses. Most grieving people show some common outward signs and symptoms (Box 36.4). A patient's culture can also affect the response to grief and the symptoms shown. Analyze assessment data and identify possible related causes for the signs and symptoms that you observe. For example, after a significant loss a person may have a sad affect, withdrawn behaviors, headaches,

BOX 36.4 Common Symptoms of Grief

Feelings
- Sorrow
- Fear
- Anger
- Guilt or self-reproach
- Anxiety
- Loneliness
- Fatigue
- Helplessness/hopelessness
- Yearning
- Relief

Cognitions (Thought Patterns)
- Disbelief
- Confusion or memory problems
- Problems in making decisions
- Inability to concentrate
- Feeling the presence of the deceased

Physical Sensations
- Headaches
- Nausea and appetite disturbances
- Tightness in the chest and throat
- Insomnia
- Oversensitivity to noise
- Sense of depersonalization ("Nothing seems real")
- Feeling short of breath, choking sensation
- Muscle weakness
- Lack of energy
- Dry mouth

Behaviors
- Crying and frequent sighing
- Distancing from people
- Absentmindedness
- Dreams of the deceased
- Keeping the deceased's room intact
- Loss of interest in regular life events
- Wearing objects that belonged to the deceased

setting aside specific time to be with your patient or family. Be sure the patient is comfortable and that any symptoms are managed. Make sure the environment is quiet and free from distractions to allow your patient or family to engage in conversation and express concerns. Being unable to focus on the assessment prevents you from being present and attentive.

At her first home visit 1 week after Mrs. Allison's discharge from the hospital, Jennifer sees that Mrs. Allison has a worried look on her face and she seems distressed. Mrs. Allison cannot independently perform many activities of daily living because of shortness of breath. When Jennifer takes Mrs. Allison's vital signs, she documents blood pressure 92/64 mm Hg; pulse 98; respirations 20; and temperature 36.7°C (98°F). Jennifer also finds that Mrs. Allison has lost an additional 2 lb since leaving the hospital. Mrs. Allison says she does not feel hungry and is only eating small amounts of food at meals. She also reports that she feels very tired all the time and is weak and "wobbly" when walking to the commode. Mrs. Allison rates her back pain as 7 out of 10, telling Jennifer that it is the same pain she has had for many months and it often keeps her awake at night and makes it hard for her to get around the house. She says that she does not like to take too many pain pills for her back pain because they make her constipation worse. Mrs. Allison shares her feelings with Jennifer and asks many questions about dying and what to expect as she nears end of life. While talking about her family, Mrs. Allison states, "My daughter Lilly doesn't know what to do to help me. My husband has been trying to help me, but he's not sure what he should do. I'm just so tired of being sick and not being able to take care of myself. I don't know how I can continue stressing my family like this. I don't want to go back to the hospital again if my heart failure gets bad. I just feel like giving up."

Jennifer worries that she will be asked questions for which she has no answer. She feels more comfortable talking about heart disease than about end-of-life decisions and care. She knows that attitudes of humility and willingness to take risks will help her form helping, trusting relationships. If the family members ask her difficult questions about death or to predict what will happen, Jennifer plans to use open-ended questions to explore their concerns. She knows that she cannot "fix things" for the Allison family, but she can assure them that they will have help. If family members share intense emotions, Jennifer will listen carefully and validate their feelings.

REFLECT NOW

Explore your feelings about entering the sacred space of another's family at the time of an emotionally charged loss. How do you think you would manage your own emotions?

upset stomach, and decreased ability to concentrate. You associate these symptoms with several potential causes, including anxiety, gastrointestinal disturbances, medication side effects, or impaired memory. Careful analysis of the symptoms in context leads you to an accurate nursing diagnosis. Ask: How are the symptoms related to one another when they occur? When did they begin? Were they present before the loss? To what does the person attribute them?

Loss takes place in a social context; therefore family assessment is a vital part of your data gathering. If a father of a young family is dying, he will not be able to fulfill certain roles, causing a change in family structure. When a person develops a disability, the patient and family members change their roles and responsibilities to meet new demands. Family members also experience a variety of physical and psychological symptoms. Assess the family's response to loss and recognize that sometimes they are dealing with grief at a different pace.

Environmental Factors. Determine if any environmental factors will have an impact on your ability to assess a patient or family who is experiencing grief after a loss. Avoid time conflicts and interruptions by

◆ Analysis and Nursing Diagnosis

Apply critical thinking to recognize clusters of assessment data cues, identify emerging patterns, make judgments regarding the patient's actual or potential needs or resources, and identify nursing diagnoses related to loss and grief applicable to the patient's situation (Box 36.5). You cannot make accurate nursing diagnoses based on just one or two assessment findings. Carefully review your patient's assessment data to consider whether more than one diagnosis applies. For example, a dying patient who cries often, has angry outbursts, and reports nightmares gives evidence of several possible nursing diagnoses: *Pain (Acute or Chronic), Dysfunctional Grief,* or *Spiritual Distress.* Examine the available data, validate assumptions with the patient, and look for other validating behaviors and symptoms before making a diagnosis. Further assessment may be necessary. For example, if you think the patient is experiencing dysfunctional grief, clarify if the patient is having pain so that you do not select an inaccurate diagnosis.

BOX 36.5   Nursing Diagnostic Process

Hopelessness Related to Deteriorating Physiological Condition

Assessment Activities	Assessment Findings
Ask patient to discuss her understanding of her health situation.	Patient offers a negative view of her future.
Observe patient's nonverbal behavior.	Patient sighs, keeps eyes closed; decreased verbalization; turns away from health care professionals.
Observe patient's responses to care options.	Patient does not want scheduled test. "There's nothing they can do."
Assess activity level.	Patient states that she has no energy and reports pain; can't sleep, wants to stay in bed.
Observe patient's interactions with others.	Patient shows lack of interest, communicates minimally, and does not want to contact daughter yet.

As part of the diagnostic process, identify the appropriate "related to" factor for each negative or actual nursing diagnosis. Clarification of the related factors ensures that you select appropriate interventions. For example, a nursing diagnosis of *Dysfunctional Grief related to the permanent loss of mobility* requires different interventions than a diagnosis of *Dysfunctional Grief related to infertility after an ectopic pregnancy.*

When identifying nursing diagnoses related to a patient's grief or loss, you sometimes identify other related diagnoses. Some patients experiencing grief or impending death have nursing diagnoses such as *Denial About Illness Severity* or *Impaired Mobility.* A patient entering the phase of active dying often has diagnoses related to physical changes, including *Urinary Incontinence, Bowel Incontinence, Acute Pain, Nausea, Altered Perception,* and *Impaired Breathing.* In addition to numerous diagnoses related to physical symptoms at the end of life, additional nursing diagnoses relevant for patients experiencing grief, loss, or death include:

- Impaired Family Coping
- Death Anxiety
- Pain (Acute or Chronic)
- Dysfunctional Grief
- Anticipatory Grief

Jennifer analyzes the assessment data that she has gathered from her completed assessment of Mrs. Allison. She recognizes that the findings of back pain for several months, inability to sleep, poor appetite, feelings of being tired of being sick, feelings of wanting to give up, and stress about her family caring for her form a cluster of cues that lead Jennifer to the nursing diagnoses of **Hopelessness** *as the priority problem. The cues also lead Jennifer to make an interrelated nursing diagnosis of* **Chronic Pain** *because of Mrs. Allison's persistent back pain. Mrs. Allison's statements about her fatigue and poor appetite coupled with decreased intake lead Jennifer to make a nursing diagnosis of* **Impaired Low Nutritional Intake.** *Mrs. Allison's statements about not wanting to go on, her inability to sleep due to pain, and feeling weak and "wobbly" lead Jennifer to also identify* **Fatigue** *as a problem.*

◆ Planning and Outcomes Identification

Nurses provide patient-centered holistic care to patients experiencing grief, death, or loss. During the planning step of the nursing process, develop a plan of care for each of the patient's nursing diagnoses.

Clinical judgment at this step is important because you reflect on previous experiences and environmental factors and apply knowledge, critical thinking attitudes, and intellectual standards in deciding on the most appropriate nursing interventions. Fig. 36.2 illustrates the interrelatedness of critical thinking factors during the planning phase of the nursing process.

The use of clinical judgment and critical thinking and including patients in the planning process ensures a well-designed care plan that supports a patient's self-esteem and autonomy. Integrate assessment data with knowledge about resources and therapies available for a patient who is grieving loss or dying to develop an individualized plan of care. Match the patient's needs with evidence-based interventions that are supported and recommended in the clinical and research literature. A care plan for a patient who is dying focuses on comfort; preserving dignity and quality of life; and providing family members with emotional, social, and spiritual support.

Your previous patient experiences can help you recognize spiritual needs of the dying patient. You may have previously worked with other patients who experienced a loss, or your own experience with loss can provide insight into behaviors that you might assess in a patient. Prior experience with other patients and your own personal experience with loss and grief are also valuable when selecting interventions to support patients. For example, you may have cared for a patient who was dying and learned interventions that helped with comfort for the patient and supported the family.

It is also important to recognize environmental factors that affect the patient who is dying. For example, when you are providing support to the patient and family, you want to plan a quiet environment and time when interruptions will not occur. Identify potential interruptions and work to minimize their impact. Also, work with other members of the health care team to respect patient wishes and religious practices during the dying process or after the patient has died.

REFLECT NOW

Reflect on your feelings as you plan care for a patient who is terminally ill. How will you feel about engaging in conversations about care while talking about something that causes so many people distress?

Outcomes. Partner with the patient and family to identify expected outcomes to develop a mutually agreed-on plan of care based on the patient's nursing diagnoses (see the Nursing Care Plan). Use clinical judgment to establish realistic outcomes that align with the patient's preferences, beliefs and practices, and culture. The plan needs to focus on meeting the patient's needs during grief or the dying process. During planning establish realistic, mutually agreed-on expected outcomes based on the identified nursing diagnoses. It is especially important to collaborate closely with patients when establishing expected outcomes for a patient who is dying. Consider a patient's own resources, such as physical energy and activity tolerance, family support, and coping style. A nursing diagnosis of *Powerlessness related to experimental cancer therapy* with an expected outcome of "Patient will be able to describe the expected course of disease" is realistic for a patient who frequently asks for clarification about the treatment plan and participates in educational discussions. In contrast, an expected outcome of "Patient will identify a minimum of three effective coping skills" is appropriate for a patient with the same nursing diagnosis who is experiencing depression from feeling powerless about having experimental cancer treatment.

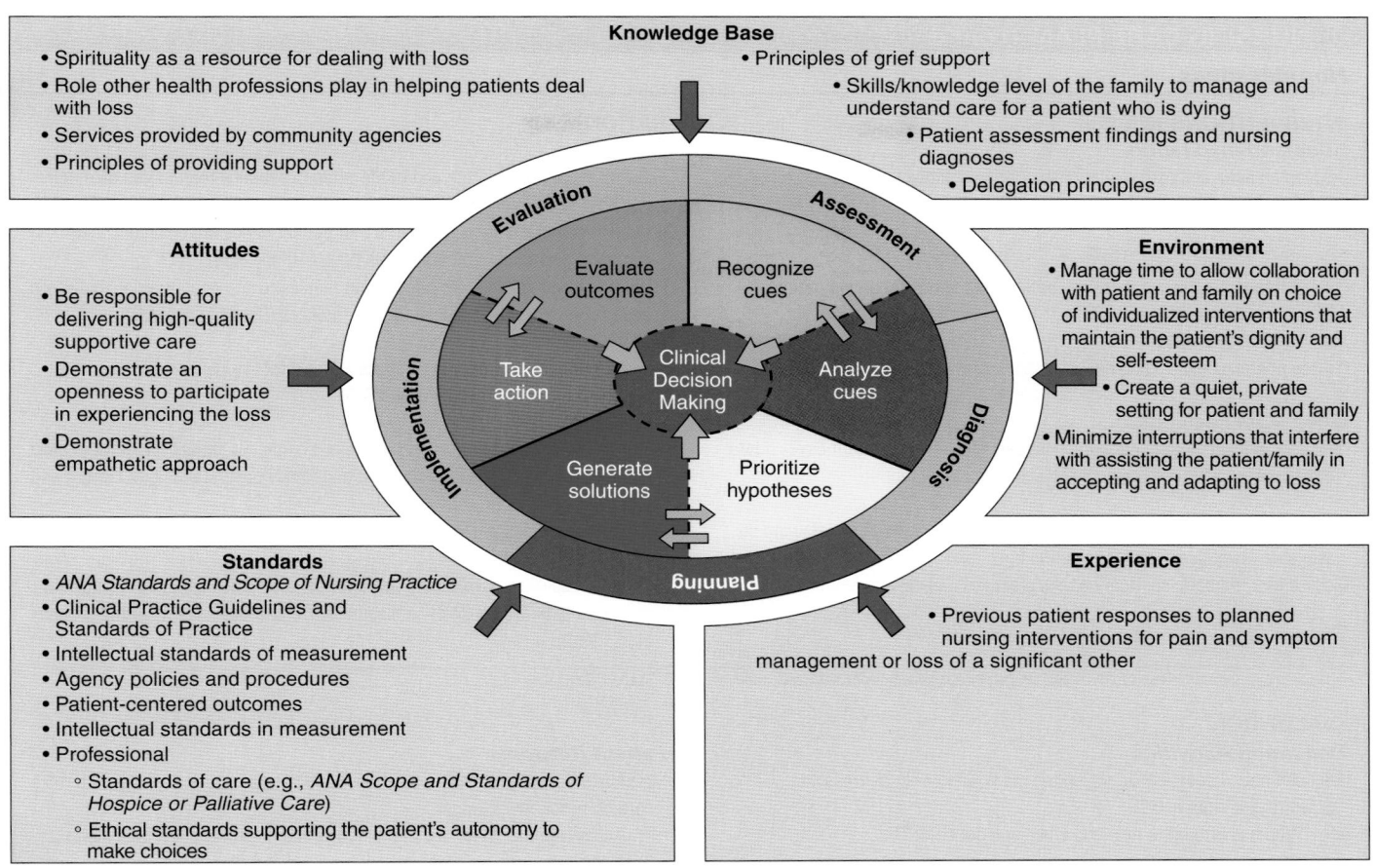

Knowledge Base
- Spirituality as a resource for dealing with loss
- Role other health professions play in helping patients deal with loss
- Services provided by community agencies
- Principles of providing support

- Principles of grief support
  - Skills/knowledge level of the family to manage and understand care for a patient who is dying
    - Patient assessment findings and nursing diagnoses
      - Delegation principles

Attitudes
- Be responsible for delivering high-quality supportive care
- Demonstrate an openness to participate in experiencing the loss
- Demonstrate empathetic approach

Environment
- Manage time to allow collaboration with patient and family on choice of individualized interventions that maintain the patient's dignity and self-esteem
- Create a quiet, private setting for patient and family
- Minimize interruptions that interfere with assisting the patient/family in accepting and adapting to loss

Standards
- *ANA Standards and Scope of Nursing Practice*
- Clinical Practice Guidelines and Standards of Practice
- Intellectual standards of measurement
- Agency policies and procedures
- Patient-centered outcomes
- Intellectual standards in measurement
- Professional
  - Standards of care (e.g., *ANA Scope and Standards of Hospice or Palliative Care*)
  - Ethical standards supporting the patient's autonomy to make choices

Experience
- Previous patient responses to planned nursing interventions for pain and symptom management or loss of a significant other

Inner circle: Evaluation — Evaluate outcomes; Assessment — Recognize cues; Take action; Clinical Decision Making; Analyze cues; Implementation; Diagnosis; Generate solutions; Prioritize hypotheses; Planning

FIG. 36.2 Critical thinking model for loss, death, and grieving planning. (Clinical Judgment Measurement Model copyright © NCSBN. All rights reserved.)

NURSING CARE PLAN

Hopelessness

ASSESSMENT

Assessment Activities	*Assessment Findings[a]*
Ask open-ended questions. "Mrs. Allision, it looks as if you're having a difficult time. What do you understand about your situation right now?"	"The doctors say that **my heart failure is worsening.**" Shrugging her shoulders, she states, "There isn't much more the doctors can do. I feel like everything's out of my control. "
Observe Mrs. Allison's behaviors and nonverbal communication.	Mrs. Allison **appears sad and keeps her eyes closed**. She **cries and sighs frequently.**
Assess Mrs. Allison's pain and energy level.	Mrs. Allison reports **constant back pain.** She has "**no energy for anything.**"
Observe Mrs. Allison's interactions and interest in others.	Mrs. Allison **does not look at people and does not want to talk to her husband or daughter yet.**
Assess meaning of recent events with Mrs. Allison and invite her to talk about her situation.	Mrs. Allison states, "I'm done with life and too tired to keep fighting."

[a] Assessment findings are shown in bold type.

NURSING DIAGNOSIS: Hopelessness related to declining physical condition

PLANNING
Expected Outcomes (NOC)[b]
Hope
Mrs. Allison identifies the concerns causing the greatest amount of suffering or distress.
Mrs. Allison identifies ways she can live at home with the help of others.

[b] Outcome classification labels from Moorhead S, et al: *Nursing Outcomes Classification (NOC): measurement of health outcomes*, ed 6, St Louis, 2018, Elsevier.

Continued

◎ **NURSING CARE PLAN—cont'd**

Hopelessness

INTERVENTIONS (NIC)[c]	RATIONALE
Hope and Inspiration	
Develop an open and caring relationship through active listening and emotional support.	Individuals approaching the end of life often experience fragmented care delivery. Therapeutic communication supports patient- and family-centered care at the end of life and helps to ensure that patient needs are communicated among all health care professionals (Sekse et al., 2018).
Provide frequent conversations with patient and family regarding patient's symptom management and grief.	Frequent conversations with patient and family provide opportunities to discuss end-of-life care values, goals, and preferences (Sekse et al., 2018).
Pain Management	
Provide pharmacological and nonpharmacological relief for chronic back pain.	Anxiety, pain, and suffering are reduced with effective pain management, and quality of life is improved (Paice, 2019).
Grief Work Facilitation	
Help Mrs. Allison identify her personal goals, desires, and priorities. Evaluate effectiveness and promote goal achievement as appropriate.	Allowing the patient to direct care decisions helps the patient and family select priority of care and increases patient and family understanding of current and proposed treatments (Ferrell, 2019).
Help Mrs. Allison identify her desires for advance care planning, drawing on available resources in and outside the hospital.	Provides information and support for the family when making end-of-life decisions (Lai et al., 2018).
Discuss Mrs. Allison's spiritual beliefs, practices, needs, and resources.	Inclusion of spiritual assessment and spiritual care practices at the end of life increases patient's sense of connectedness and overall quality of life (Koper et al., 2019).

[c] Intervention classification labels from Butcher HK, et al: *Nursing Interventions Classification (NIC)*, ed 7, St Louis, 2018, Elsevier.

EVALUATION

Evaluation Activities	Patient Response
Use open-ended question: "Can you tell me what is most distressing or worrisome right now?"	Mrs. Allison explains, "I'm not sure what will happen. I may not be able to take care of myself much longer."
Ask, "Who has offered to help you when you get home?"	Mrs. Allison states, "Well, my Bible study group has offered to take me to appointments if it's too much for my husband and daughter, and the choir members said they'll be happy to bring meals to the house every Tuesday and Thursday."

The expected outcomes for a patient experiencing loss are either short or long term, depending on the nature of the loss and the patient's condition. Some expected outcomes for patients facing loss or death include accommodating grief, accepting the reality of a loss, or maintaining meaningful relationships. In establishing a plan of care for a patient who is dying, examples of expected outcomes are:

- Patient expresses spiritual beliefs about death.
- Patient verbalizes acceptance of the loss.
- Patient participates in planning the funeral service.

Setting Priorities. Encourage patients and family members to share their priorities for care at the end of life. Patients at the end of life or with advanced chronic illness are more likely to want their comfort, social, or spiritual needs met rather than pursuing medical cures. Then prioritize a patient's most urgent physical or psychological needs while also considering the patient's preferences, expectations, and priorities. If a patient's expected outcomes include pain control and promoting self-esteem at the end of life, pain control takes priority when the patient experiences acute physical discomfort. Many terminal conditions can also influence a patient's ability to breathe. Pharmacological approaches are available to relieve dyspnea. When comfort needs have been met, you address other issues important to the patient and family. When it is realistic for the patient to remain independent, strategies that foster a sense of autonomy and ability to function independently take priority. A patient's condition at the end of life often changes quickly; therefore maintain an ongoing assessment to revise the plan of care according to patient needs, preferences, and expectations.

When a patient has multiple nursing diagnoses, it is not possible to address them all simultaneously. Fig. 36.3 illustrates a concept map developed for Mrs. Allison, an older-adult patient in the case study who has a medical diagnosis of advanced heart failure. In conjunction with her recent medical diagnosis, she experiences associated health problems identified in the nursing diagnoses *Chronic Pain, Impaired Low Nutritional Intake, Fatigue,* and *Hopelessness.* In such a situation, determine which of the four diagnoses should take priority. Chronic pain experienced by the patient is often the first focus. Until her pain is under control, it will not be possible for her to feel more energized, eat well, or regain her sense of hopefulness.

Jennifer works with Mrs. Allison to identify agreed-on outcomes and plan patient-centered personal care and support for her and the family. After talking further with Mrs. Allison, Jennifer identifies **Hopelessness** *as a priority for Mrs. Allison. Jennifer needs to reassess Mrs. Allison's eating patterns, dietary intake, and sleep patterns. Mrs. Allison identifies her back pain as a concern for her because it interferes with her ability to walk and sleep. If Mrs. Allison wants comfort interventions and support more than help with her anorexia, Jennifer needs to address Mrs. Allison's hopelessness needs first followed by her comfort and nutrition needs.*

Jennifer will ensure that Mrs. Allison's nutrition, fatigue, and pain are managed before asking about her other priorities for care. A physical therapist came to see Mrs. Allison. She is beginning to feel more secure

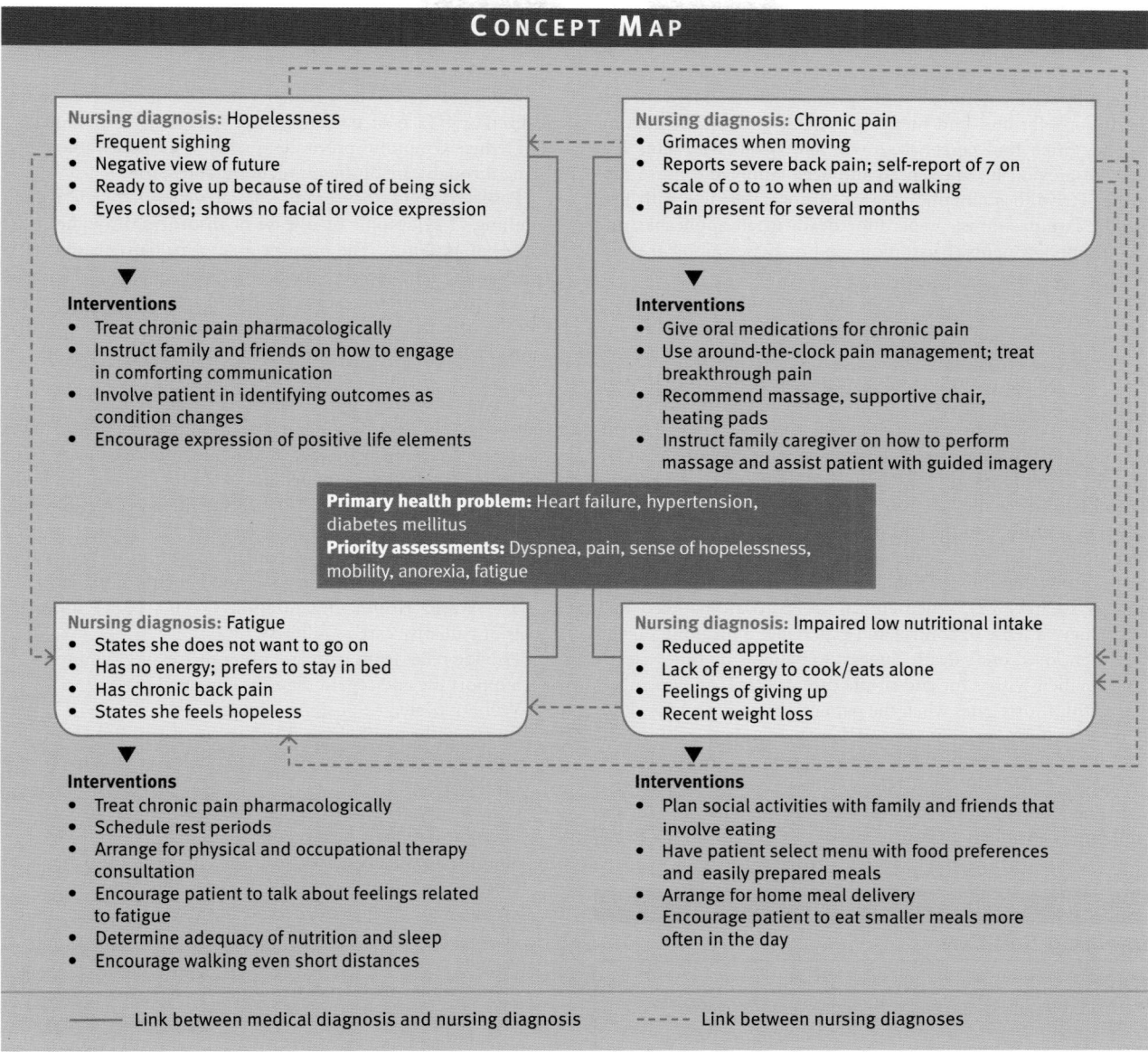

FIG. 36.3 Concept map for Mrs. Allison.

---

using a walker, but she continues to have problems with anorexia and fatigue. Jennifer knows that Mr. Allison and Lilly have never given end-of-life care; therefore she plans to provide teaching for their priority concerns. She anticipates that they will want to learn how to help Mrs. Allison conserve her energy, give medications, help with ambulation, and position her for comfort. Jennifer knows that above all she will honor patient and family preferences, culture, and religious traditions during this meaningful event in the Allison's family history.

Teamwork and Collaboration. As described previously, grief, loss, and death affect people physically, emotionally, spiritually, and culturally. Effectively caring for patients experiencing grief requires a team of nurses, physicians, social workers, spiritual care providers, nutritionists, pharmacists, psychologists, physical and occupational therapists, patients, and family members. Other team members include an advanced practice RN whose focus is on palliative care. Massage or music/art therapists who provide alternative therapies are also sometimes part of the team (see Chapter 32). All health care team members

work together to provide holistic, high-quality palliative, grief, and end-of-life care. As a patient's care needs and priorities change, the roles of team members change as well. Team members communicate with one another on a regular basis to ensure coordination and effectiveness of care.

QSEN **Building Competency in Teamwork and Collaboration**

You are caring for Mrs. Allison, an older patient who has recently been diagnosed with a terminal illness and is preparing for discharge home. She has lost strength as a result of decreased activity, depression, and back pain. Her greatest desire is to be able to attend weekly services at her church, but because of her weakness, pain, and fatigue, she is afraid that she will be unable to do so. She believes that her feelings of depression will improve if she can again participate in church activities. How can you, with the help of the interprofessional team, help Mrs. Allison respond to her spiritual needs and desire to be involved within her faith community?

Answers to QSEN Activities can be found on the Evolve website.

◆ Implementation

Health Promotion. Health promotion in complicated grief, serious chronic illness, or death focuses on facilitating successful coping and optimizing physical, emotional, and spiritual health. Many people continue to look for and find meaning even in difficult life circumstances. They often find personal growth and spiritual insights that they have not previously experienced and need family and nurse support as they strive to maintain a degree of normalcy; live with loss; make health care decisions; prepare for death when applicable; and adjust to disappointments, frustration, and anxieties along the way (Box 36.6).

Assist With End-of-Life Decision Making. Patients and family members often face complex treatment decisions at the end of life. Patients and families must decide which treatments to continue and which to stop; to enroll in hospice or enter palliative care; or to transfer to a nursing home, in-patient unit, or home. Even after the decision to enroll in hospice, questions arise about symptom management, artificial nutrition and hydration (e.g., feeding tube or parenteral nutrition), and the desired location for death. You can support and educate patients and families as they identify, contemplate, and ultimately decide how to best journey to the end of life.

Difficult ethical decisions at the end of life complicate a survivor's grief, create family divisions, or increase family uncertainty at the time of death (see Chapter 22). When ethical decisions are handled well, survivors achieve a sense of control and experience a meaningful conclusion to their loved one's death. Suggest to patients that they clearly communicate their wishes for end-of-life care so that family members can act as faithful surrogates when the patient can no longer speak for himself or herself. Some patients and family members rely on the nurse and other members of the health care team to initiate discussions regarding end-of-life care. Nurses often provide options that family members do not know are available and are advocates for patients and family members making decisions at the end of life in the form of an advance directive. When patients sign consent for a DNR ("do not resuscitate") order, they have improved autonomy as well as increased quality of end-of-life care (Liang et al., 2017).

Palliative Care. Many patients and families benefit from the specialized approach of palliative care. This holistic method to prevent and reduce symptoms promotes quality of life and whole-person well-being through care of the mind, body, and spirit.

Palliative care focuses on the prevention, relief, reduction, or soothing of symptoms of disease or disorders throughout the entire course of an illness. The primary goal of palliative care is to help patients and families achieve the best possible quality of life (Sekse et al., 2017). Patients should receive palliative care as soon as possible when chronic or terminal disease starts creating difficult-to-manage symptoms. Palliative care is appropriate for patients of any age, with any diagnosis, at any time, and in any setting.

A large misconception concerning palliative care is that it is used only when curative treatments are no longer pursued. However, patients still receiving aggressive treatment with hope of achieving a cure and patients who have stopped life-extending treatments both benefit from palliative care (Ferrell, 2019). Sometimes people who might benefit from palliative care refuse it because they do not understand it. Therefore be sure to provide patient education to help patients and their families understand the goals and benefits of palliative care.

The World Health Organization (WHO, 2021) summarizes the goals of palliative care as follows:
- Provide relief from pain and other distressing symptoms.
- Support life and regard dying as a normal process.
- Will not hasten or postpone death.
- Integrate the psychological and spiritual aspects of patient care.
- Offer a support system to help patients live as actively as possible until death.
- Offer a support system to help the family cope during the patient's illness and in their own bereavement.
- Support a team approach to address the needs of patients and their families, including bereavement counseling, if indicated.
- Enhance the quality of life and positively influence the course of illness.
- Provide care early in the course of illness in conjunction with other therapies that are intended to prolong life, such as chemotherapy or radiation therapy, and include investigations needed to better understand and manage distressing clinical complications.

Because the focus of palliative care is comfort and improved quality of life, it is a valuable approach to caring for patients with a complex illness. Palliative care uses a variety of therapies to provide patients with a holistic approach to symptom management and ultimately improved quality of life. Complementary therapies using an integrative approach often have a positive effect on feelings of depression and anxiety (see Chapter 32). For example, fatigue, a common symptom reported by patients receiving palliative care, responds to acupuncture and exercise. Massage helps to reduce the symptoms of pain, anxiety, nausea, shortness of breath, and stress and to increase relaxation and peacefulness.

When the expected outcomes for care change and cure for illnesses becomes less likely, a patient's care ideally shifts from palliative care and transitions to hospice care, a more specialized form of palliative care for the dying.

Hospice Care. Hospice care is a philosophy and model of care that focuses on the care, comfort, and quality of life of a person with a serious illness who is approaching the end of life (National Institute on Aging [NIA], 2021). It gives priority to pain and symptom management, comfort, and quality of life. Hospice strives to meet a patient and family's physical, psychological, social, and spiritual needs. Patients

---

BOX 36.6 PATIENT TEACHING

Maintaining Self-Care

Objective
- The patient will participate in care activities to manage symptoms.

Teaching Strategies
- Identify ways for patient to achieve personal goals.
- Instruct patient on ways to maintain usual daily routines that provide comfort and sense of normalcy.
- Demonstrate forms of complementary therapy that patient can use for symptom management (e.g., meditation, guided imagery).
- Discuss ways that patient can maintain a sense of control over end-of-life planning and maintain a realistic outlook (advance directives, funeral planning, and preferred location of death).
- Discuss patient's needs for the presence of support people or for solitude.
- Include family members and discuss methods to facilitate safety and ease in managing activities of daily living as patient's abilities change (assistive devices, in-home caregivers).

Evaluation
Use the principles of teach-back to evaluate patient/family caregiver learning:
- Tell me what symptom-management methods you use and how effective each method is.
- Show me how you perform guided imagery in symptom management.
- Tell me about the changes that you made in your house that improve your safety.

accepted into a hospice program usually have less than 6 months to live. Hospice services are available in home, hospital, extended care, and nursing home settings.

The cornerstone of hospice care is a trusting relationship between the hospice team and the patient and family. Knowing expectations, desired location of care, and family dynamics helps the hospice team provide individualized care at the end of life. Unlike traditional care, patients are active participants in all aspects of hospice care, and caregivers prioritize care according to patient wishes. Patient care goals are mutually set, and all participants fully understand the patient's care preferences and try to honor them. Hospice programs are built on the following core beliefs and services:

- Patient and family are the unit of care
- Coordinated home care with access to inpatient and nursing home beds when needed
- Symptom management
- Physician-directed services
- Provision of an interprofessional care team
- Medical and nursing services available at all times
- Bereavement follow-up after patient's death
- Use of trained volunteers for visitation and respite support

To be eligible for home hospice services, a patient must have a family caregiver to provide care when the patient is no longer able to function alone. Home care aides offer help with hygienic needs, and a nurse is available to coordinate and manage symptom relief. Nurses providing hospice care use therapeutic communication, offer psychosocial care and expert symptom management, promote patient dignity and self-esteem, maintain a comfortable and peaceful environment, provide spiritual comfort and hope, protect against abandonment or isolation, offer family support, help with ethical decision making, and facilitate mourning. Hospice team members offer 24-hour accessibility and coordinate care between the home and inpatient setting. A patient receiving home hospice care may enter an inpatient hospice unit for stabilization of symptoms or caregiver respite.

When a patient chooses to die at home, family members provide direct care, which is often emotionally stressful and physically exhausting. In the home setting family caregivers benefit from respite care. During respite care a patient temporarily receives care from others so that family members are able to get away to rest and relax. Hospice program benefits include some days of respite care. Inform family members of home care, hospice, and community service options so that they can access the best resources for their situation. As a patient's death comes closer, the hospice team provides intensive support to the patient and family (Hospice Foundation of America, 2018). When the patient dies, family members benefit from the many resources of the health care team. Hospice services provide bereavement visits made by the staff to help the family grieve.

Working with the Allison family, Jennifer implemented the plan of care she and the family developed based on Mrs. Allison's preferences, expectations, and identified outcomes. Jennifer completed the end-of-life care teaching she planned for Mr. Allison and Lilly to help them understand hospice care for Mrs. Allision and better support each other.

Jennifer sat down with Mrs. Allison to talk further about her concerns. During the conversation, Jennifer used therapeutic communication to establish a caring relationship with Mrs. Allison. Mrs. Allison said her biggest concerns were her pain, fatigue, and lack of appetite. She also said that she was concerned about her ability to get around her home. Jennifer verified for Mrs. Allison that physical and occupational therapists would be coming to her home 3 times a week to help her with gaining strength and increasing her mobility, and they discussed how Mr. Allison can help to take care of her during this time.

Therapeutic Communication Approaches. The heart of nursing care is establishing a caring and trusting relationship with your patient. This patient-focused approach allows you to respond to patients rather than react and encourages the sharing of important information. Open-ended questions invite patients to elaborate on their thoughts and encourage them to tell their stories. Patients usually give short answers ("yes" or "no") when you use closed-ended questions, which limits what you can learn about their situation. Use active listening, learn to be comfortable with silence, and use prompts (e.g., "go on," "tell me more") to encourage continued conversation. Empathizing, therapeutic touch, and offering self are also effective ways to therapeutically communicate with patients. Specifically, empathizing allows patients to see that their feelings are normal and that as a nurse you understand. Sometimes questioning a patient feels uncomfortable. Stating an observation, such as "You look worried" or "You didn't eat much lunch," invites patients to respond without feeling pressure to answer (see Chapter 24).

Feelings of sadness, numbness, or anger often make talking about these situations especially difficult. For example, a patient lashes out at caregivers when experiencing anger during grief. Some patients become demanding and accusing. Remain supportive by letting patients and family members know that feelings such as anger are normal by saying, "I see that you're upset right now, and that's understandable. I'm here to talk with you if you want." Encourage patients to share the emotions and concerns of greatest importance to them, and then acknowledge their feelings and concerns in a nonjudgmental manner. If a patient chooses not to share feelings or concerns, express a willingness to be available at any time. Some patients do not discuss emotions for personal or cultural reasons, and others hesitate to express their emotions for fear that people will abandon or judge them. If you are reassuring and respect a patient's privacy, a therapeutic relationship is likely to develop. Sometimes patients need to begin to resolve their grief privately before they discuss their loss with others, especially strangers.

Do not avoid talking about a topic. When you sense that a patient wants to talk about something, make time to do so as soon as possible. This may be particularly challenging if you are in a busy acute care setting; however, it is a necessary part of high-quality nursing care and is a priority. Above all, remember that a patient's emotions are not something you can fix. Instead, view emotional expressions as an essential part of a patient's adjustment to significant life changes and development of effective coping skills. Help family members access other professional resources. Social workers, psychologists, chaplains, and case managers can offer additional information and support to families and patients in grief.

Provide Psychosocial Care. Patients at the end of life experience a range of psychological symptoms, including anxiety, depression, powerlessness, uncertainty, and isolation. They can experience anguish from the unknown surroundings, treatment options, health status, family disruption, and the dying process. Worry or fear is common in many patients and often heightens their perception of discomfort and suffering. You can alleviate some of it by providing information to them about their condition, the course of their disease, and the benefits and burdens of treatment options. Most hospitals have professional psychologists or social workers who can provide counseling.

Manage Symptoms. Managing multiple symptoms commonly experienced when patients are chronically ill or dying is a primary goal of nursing care (Table 36.3). Uncontrolled symptoms cause distress, discomfort, and suffering to patients and families, which often complicates the dying experience. Despite the availability of effective treatment options for pain, many patients experience avoidable pain at the end of life. They refuse aggressive treatment because of misconceptions by nurses or family members (see Chapter 44). Maintain an

TABLE 36.3	Promoting Comfort to the Patient Who Is Terminally Ill	
Symptoms	**Characteristics or Causes**	**Nursing Implications**
Pain	Pain has multiple causes, depending on patient diagnosis.	Collaborate with team members to identify and implement appropriate pharmacological and nonpharmacological interventions to reduce pain and promote comfort (see Chapter 44).
Skin discomfort	Any source of skin irritation increases discomfort.	Keep skin clean, dry, and moisturized. Monitor for incontinence.
Mucous membrane discomfort	Mouth breathing or dehydration leads to dry mucous membranes; tongue and lips become dry or chapped.	Provide oral care at least every 2–4 hours. Apply a light film of lip balm for dryness. Apply topical analgesics to oral lesions as needed.
Corneal irritation	Blinking reflexes diminish near death, causing drying of cornea.	Optical lubricants or artificial tears reduce corneal drying.
Fatigue	Metabolic demands, stress, disease states, decreased oral intake, and heart function cause weakness and fatigue.	Provide periods of rest and educate patient about energy conservation.
Anxiety	Physical, social, or spiritual distress causes anxiety; causes may be situational or event specific.	Provide opportunity for patient to express feelings though active listening. Provide calm, supportive environment. Consult members of the health care team to determine whether pharmacological interventions are appropriate.
Nausea	Nausea is caused by medications, pain, or decreased intestinal blood flow with impending death.	Determine the cause of nausea and work to reduce nausea triggers, such as strong smells. Administer antiemetics or promotility agents. Encourage patients to lie on their right side. Provide oral care at least every 2–4 hours.
Constipation	Opioids, other medications, and immobility slow peristalsis. Lack of bulk in diet or reduced fluid is a cause.	Increase fiber in diet if appropriate. Administer stool softeners or laxatives as needed. If possible, encourage increased liquid intake and regular periods of ambulation.
Diarrhea	Disease processes, treatment or medications, and gastrointestinal (GI) infections are causes.	Consult with members of the health care team to determine the cause and make appropriate changes. Provide skin care and easy accessibility to the toilet or bedside commode.
Urinary incontinence	Progressive disease and decreased level of consciousness are causes.	Provide good skin care and frequent assessment for incontinent urine. Place Foley catheter as appropriate.
Altered nutrition	Medications, depression, decreased activity, and decreased blood flow to GI tract are causes. Nausea produces anorexia.	Encourage patient to eat small, frequent meals of preferred foods. Never force patients to eat.
Dehydration	Patient is less willing or able to maintain oral fluid intake; has fever.	Reduce discomfort from dehydration; give mouth care at least every 2–4 hours; offer ice chips or moist cloth to lips. Keep lips and tongue moist.
Ineffective breathing patterns (e.g., dyspnea, shortness of breath)	Anxiety; fever; pain; increased oxygen demand; disease processes; and anemia, which reduces oxygen-carrying capacity, are causes.	Treat or control underlying cause. Use nonpharmacological interventions such as elevating the head of the bed to promote lung expansion. Provide oxygen as needed. Keeping the air cool provides ease and comfort for the terminal patient. Using morphine or benzodiazepines to treat tachypnea is sometimes appropriate.
Noisy breathing ("death rattle")	Noisy breathing is the sound of secretions moving in the airway during inspiratory and expiratory phases caused by thick secretions, decreased muscle tone, swallow, and cough.	Elevate head to facilitate postural drainage. Turn patient at least every 2 hours. Provide oral care and maintain hydration as tolerated.

ongoing assessment of a patient's pain and evaluate the patient's response to interventions. Reassure the family repeatedly of the need for pain control even if the patient does not appear to be in pain. Discuss pain control with the family frequently and dispel any myths regarding dependence on opioids. You are responsible to advocate for change if the patient does not obtain relief from the prescribed regimen. It is imperative that you assess patients' nonverbal cues because they often are unable to communicate their needs. A patient's renal and liver function decline during the dying process, decreasing metabolism and rate of drug clearance, which might require modification to medication dosages. Also, be aware that advancing disease pathology, anxiety, or delirium sometimes requires the use of higher doses or different drug therapies.

Remain alert to the potential side effects of opioid administration: constipation, nausea, sedation, respiratory depression, or myoclonus. Family members often worry about potential addiction to opioid medications. Not only is the incidence of true addiction very low, but a patient's need for pain relief at the end of life takes priority. Education is necessary to help families understand the need for appropriate use of opioid medications.

Jennifer taught Mrs. Allison meditation and relaxation exercises to use when her pain became more severe. She also taught Mrs. Allison the benefits of taking her pain medications around the clock rather than waiting for the back pain to get severe before taking the medication. Jennifer recommended trying a heating pad in addition to pain medications to help reduce Mrs. Allison's back pain. Jennifer helped the Allisons modify the environment in their home, particularly the bedroom, to make the room more peaceful to improve Mrs. Allison's sleep. She worked with the Allisons to find soothing music that would help them go to sleep. Because Mrs. Allison was still experiencing fatigue, Jennifer encouraged her to take rest periods throughout the day.

Jennifer worked with the Allison family to develop a meal plan that Mrs. Allison found more enticing. Jennifer found out Mrs. Allison's food preferences and incorporated those into the meals. Jennifer also found some simple recipes that Mrs. Allison thought looked good and would be easy for Mr. Allison or Lilly to prepare. She helped the Allisons set a meal schedule so that the couple was eating six small meals a day rather than the three large meals as they had done in the past. Jennifer also encouraged the couple to invite Lilly or one or two friends to dinner for socialization and to encourage Mrs. Allison to eat. Jennifer made a referral to the local meal delivery program for seniors and arranged to have a meal delivered daily during the week to decrease the cooking that Mr. Allison had to do.

Promote Dignity and Self-Esteem. A patient's sense of dignity depends on a positive self-regard and the ability to find meaning in life and feel valued by others. A sense of dignity is reinforced by respectful treatment from caregivers. You promote self-esteem and dignity by respecting patients as a whole person (i.e., as a person with feelings, accomplishments, and passions independent of the illness experience). Respecting and valuing what a patient cares about validates the person and at the same time strengthens communication among the patient, family members, and the nurse. Sharing time with patients as they share their life stories helps you know them and develop individualized interventions.

Attending to the patient's physical appearance also promotes dignity and self-esteem. Cleanliness, absence of body odors, and clean clothing give patients a sense of worth. When caring for a patient's bodily functions, show patience and respect, especially after the patient becomes dependent on others. Remember that patients are directing care at the end of life. Allow them to make decisions such as how and when to administer personal hygiene, diet preferences, and timing of nursing interventions. Keep the patient and family members informed about daily activities, tests, or therapies; their purposes; and anticipated effects. Provide privacy during nursing care procedures and be sensitive to when the patient and family need time alone together.

Maintain a Comfortable and Peaceful Environment. A comfortable, clean, pleasant environment helps patients relax, promotes healthy sleep patterns, and minimizes symptom severity. Keep a patient comfortable through frequent repositioning, making sure that bed linens are dry, and controlling extraneous environmental noise and offensive odors. Pictures, cherished objects, and cards or letters from family members and friends create a familiar and comforting environment for a patient dying in an institutional setting. When possible, allow patients to wear their own pajamas or clothes to promote a sense of comfort and familiarity. Consider nonpharmacological interventions such as massage therapy to increase patient comfort (Paice, 2019). Family members are often able to provide these interventions, which often helps them feel like they are making a positive contribution to the patient's care. Play a patient's preferred music in the background, provide guided-imagery exercises, and dim the lights to provide a soothing environment for the patient and family. Patient-preferred forms of complementary therapies offer noninvasive methods to increase comfort and well-being at the end of life (see Chapter 32).

Promote Spiritual Comfort and Hope. Patients are comforted when they know that some aspect of their lives will transcend death. Therefore helping patients make connections to their spiritual practice or cultural community is often comforting. Draw on the resources of spiritual care providers in an institutional setting or collaborate with a patient's own spiritual or religious leaders and communities. Making an audiotape or videotape for the family, writing letters, or keeping a journal assures patients that a part of their lives will exist after their death.

Feelings of hope frequently have special significance near the end of life. Nursing strategies that promote hope include being present and providing care to the whole person. The love of family and friends, faith, goal setting, positive relationships with professional caregivers, humor, and uplifting memories promote a patient's hope. Abandonment or isolation, uncontrolled symptoms, or being devalued as a person have a negative effect on hope. A patient and family's hope changes over the course of their experience with illness and death. Balance each perspective to provide high-quality patient care at the end of life. Some hope to live for an anniversary, sit outdoors for a meal, see an important person one last time, gain pain relief, or have a peaceful death. Listen for shifts in patients' hopes and find ways to help them meet their desired goals.

Protect Against Abandonment and Isolation. Many patients with terminal illness fear dying alone. Patients with chronic disease often feel socially isolated. However, most patients feel more hopeful when others are near to help them. Nurses in institutional settings need to answer call lights promptly and check on patients often to reassure them that someone is close at hand. If family members always plan to stay with the patient or if you have assessed high privacy needs for the patient and family, a private room is best.

Some family members who have a difficult time accepting a patient's impending death cope by making fewer visits. When family members do visit, inform them of the patient's status and share meaningful insights or encounters that you have had with the patient. Find simple and appropriate care activities for the family to perform, such as offering food, cooling the patient's face, combing hair, or filling out a menu. Nighttime can be particularly lonely for the patient. Suggest that a family member stay through the night if possible. Make exceptions to visiting policies, allowing family members to remain with patients who are dying at any time. Family members appreciate having open access or closeness to their loved one through their experiences at the end of life. Record contact information for them, so you can reach them at any time.

Support the Grieving Family. In palliative and hospice care, patients and family members constitute the unit of care. Family members need special care when a patient becomes debilitated or approaches the end of life. They often describe caregiving at the end of life as unpredictable, frightening, and heartbreaking. Yet many family members find meaning in providing practical and simple care to their loved one. In these extremely intimate and emotionally challenging times, offer holistic, family-centered support, compassion, and education that incorporates the uniqueness of each patient. Often family members face challenging and complex situations long before their loved one is actively dying. Therefore provide support early and consistently to family caregivers throughout the experience of illness and death.

Educate family members in all settings about the symptoms that the patient is likely to experience and the implications for care (see Table 36.3 and Box 36.7). For example, patients in the last days of life often develop anorexia or feel nauseated by food. Illness, excessive respiratory secretions, decreased activity, treatments, and fatigue decrease a patient's caloric needs and appetite. Family members often believe that they need to encourage the patient to eat. Because the goal of palliative care is comfort, do not force the patient to do anything that causes discomfort. Eating in the last days of life often causes pain and discomfort. In addition, as the body shuts down, the nutrients in food cannot be absorbed. Therefore explain to family members that forcing patients to eat can cause more harm than good for the patient. Help families identify other ways they can help the patient at this time.

Family members who have limited experience with death do not know what to expect. They may need personal time with you to share their concerns, ask about treatment options, validate perceived changes in the patient's status, or explore the possible meaning of patient behaviors. Whenever possible, communicate news of a patient's declining

BOX 36.7 EVIDENCE-BASED PRACTICE

Managing Opioid-Induced Constipation

PICOT Question: In patients who are terminally ill, what is the effect of pharmacological interventions to reduce opioid-induced constipation (OIC) compared with nonpharmacological interventions?

Evidence Summary

Most patients at the end of life use opioids to control pain and discomfort. A common side effect of opioids is OIC (Crockett et al., 2019). Patients at higher risk for developing OIC include older adults, those taking other medications that cause constipation, those who have decreased mobility or muscle function, and those who are hospitalized (Keller et al., 2019). This adds to unpleasant and uncomfortable symptoms experienced by the patient. OIC can also decrease the patient's quality of life (Young, 2019). Frequent assessment that leads to early recognition and treatment of OIC reduces its impact on a patient's quality of life (Young, 2019). Patients with OIC often use over-the-counter (OTC) stool softeners or laxatives or make lifestyle and dietary changes to treat OIC (Keller et al., 2019). Commonly used nursing interventions such as ambulation and increasing fiber and fluids to help patients with constipation are sometimes inappropriate for patients at the end of life. In addition to laxatives, stimulants, or stool softeners, several new drugs are available to treat OIC. Research shows that oral peripherally acting selective μ opioid antagonists (e.g., naldemedine, naloxegol) are safe and effective for the treatment of OIC (Crockett et al., 2019; Nee et al., 2018). Methylnaltrexone, a derivative of naltrexone, is a subcutaneous drug that is also effective (Star and Boland, 2018).

Application to Nursing Practice

- For patients who are able to tolerate diets, diet-related management and appropriate fluid intake can be useful (Keller et al., 2019).
- Use the lowest dose possible of the least constipating opioid to control pain—for example, fentanyl instead of oxycodone.
- Try traditional nonpharmacological interventions, if appropriate, and OTC laxatives before trying naldemedine, naloxegol, or methylnaltrexone (Star and Boland, 2018).
- Most common adverse effects associated with prescription medications for OIC are gastrointestinal related (e.g., nausea, diarrhea, abdominal pain, or distention) (Viscusi, 2019).

BOX 36.8 Physical Changes Hours or Days Before Death

- Increased periods of sleeping/unresponsiveness
- Circulatory changes with coolness and color changes in extremities, nose, fingers (cyanosis, pallor, mottling) (see Fig. 36.4)
- Bowel or bladder incontinence
- Decreased urine output; dark-colored urine
- Restlessness, confusion, or disorientation
- Decreased intake of food or fluids; inability to swallow
- Congestion/increased pulmonary secretions; noisy respirations (death rattle)
- Altered breathing (apnea, labored or irregular breathing, Cheyne-Stokes pattern)
- Decreased muscle tone, relaxed jaw muscles, sagging mouth
- Weakness and fatigue

FIG. 36.4 Skin mottling. (From Adams J, et al: *Emergency medicine: clinical essentials,* ed 2, Philadelphia, 2014, Elsevier.)

Depending on agency policies, allow the family the necessary time to be with their loved one.

After death help the family make decisions such as notification of a funeral home, transportation of family members, and collection of the patient's belongings. Nurses are a primary source of family support. Remember that because of differing responses to grief, some family members prefer to be alone at the time of and after the death, whereas others want to be surrounded by a support community. When uncertain about what a family member prefers for support, pose simple questions and offer suggestions for assistance.

Facilitate Mourning. Nurses who work with grieving family members often provide bereavement care after a patient's death. Helpful strategies for assisting grieving persons include the following:

- Help the survivor accept that the loss is real. Discuss how the loss or illness occurred or was discovered and other factual topics to reinforce the reality of the event and put it in perspective.
- Support the survivor's adjustment to the loss. Use a problem-solving approach. Have survivors make a list of their concerns or needs, help them prioritize, and lead them step-by-step through a discussion of how to proceed. Encourage survivors to ask for help.
- Encourage establishment of new relationships. Reassure people that new relationships do not mean that they are replacing the person who has died. Encourage involvement in nonthreatening group social activities (e.g., volunteer activities or church events).
- Allow time to grieve. "Anniversary reactions" (e.g., renewed grief around the time of the loss in subsequent years) are common, along with renewed grief at holidays. A return to sadness or the

condition or impending death when family members are together, so they can support one another. Provide information privately and stay with the family as long as needed or desired. Reduce family member anxiety, stress, or fear by describing what to expect as death approaches. Become familiar with common manifestations of impending death (Box 36.8), remembering that patients usually experience some but not all these changes. Do not try to predict the time of death; instead use your assessments to help family members anticipate what is happening. Be compassionate and sensitive in how you share information. Say "Mottling is an expected sign as a body begins shutting down" instead of "When a person gets closer to death, we see mottling" (Fig. 36.4). Share your observations and use role modeling to encourage a sense of patience, compassion, and comfort throughout the dying process.

Check frequently on families, offering support, information, and, if appropriate, encouragement to continue touching and talking with their loved ones. Determine the family's needs immediately following a patient's death. Some families will want to touch or hold the deceased; others will not. Make the deceased accessible by lowering side rails, leaving hands exposed, and setting a chair close to the bedside.

pain of grief is often worrisome. Openly acknowledge the loss, provide reassurance that the reaction is normal, and encourage the survivor to reminisce.

- Describe behaviors and feelings that survivors frequently experience. Being distractible, having difficulty sleeping or eating, and thinking that they have heard the deceased's voice are common following a loss. These symptoms do not mean that an individual has an emotional problem or is becoming ill. Reinforce that these behaviors are expected and will resolve over time.
- Provide continuing support. Following a loss, survivors need the support of a nurse with whom they have bonded for a time, especially in cases of in-home care or hospice nursing. You play an important role in the deceased's life and death, helping survivors through some very intimate and memorable times. Attachment for a period of time after the death is appropriate and healing for both the survivor and you if you have cared for a patient for an extended time. However, you must always maintain professional boundaries.
- Be alert for signs of ineffective, potentially harmful coping mechanisms, such as alcohol and substance abuse or excessive use of over-the-counter analgesics or sleep aids.

Care After Death. Federal and state laws require institutions to develop policies and procedures for certain events that occur after death, such as requesting organ or tissue donation, performing an autopsy, certifying and documenting the occurrence of a death, and providing safe and appropriate postmortem care. In accordance with federal law, a specially trained professional (e.g., transplant coordinator or social worker) makes requests for organ and tissue donation at the time of every death. The person requesting organ or tissue donation provides information about who can give consent legally, which organs or tissues can be donated, associated costs, and how donation affects burial or cremation.

In extremely stressful circumstances created by the loss of a loved one, grieving survivors usually cannot remember all they were told. Nurses provide support and reinforce or clarify explanations. In addition, understanding the physiology of organ donation is often difficult for family members. Patients who are brain dead remain on life support to provide the vital organs with blood and oxygen before transplant, even though they have been declared dead. The appearance of a live-looking body confuses the family, and they need help to understand that the life support is only preserving the vital organs. Nonvital tissues such as corneas, skin, long bones, and middle ear bones are taken at the time of death without artificially maintaining vital functions. If the deceased has not left behind instructions concerning organ and tissue donation, the family gives or denies consent at the time of death. Review your state organ-retrieval laws and institutional policy and procedure regarding the formal consent process. Be aware that the laws governing whom to approach for organ donation may not be acceptable in other cultures.

Family members give consent for an autopsy (i.e., the surgical dissection of a body after death) to determine the exact cause and circumstances of death or to discover the pathway of a disease (see Chapter 23). In most cases a coroner or medical examiner determines the need to perform an autopsy. Law sometimes requires that an autopsy be performed when death is the result of foul play; homicide; suicide; or accidental causes such as motor vehicle crashes, falls, the ingestion of drugs, or deaths within 24 hours of hospital admission. Follow state and agency requirements regarding removal of lines (e.g., intravenous lines, indwelling urinary catheter) in patients when an autopsy is ordered.

Usually a health care provider asks for autopsy permission while the nurse answers questions and supports the family's choices. Inform family members that an autopsy does not deform the body and that all organs are replaced in the body. Family members are often comforted to know that others may be helped by either the gift of organ and tissue donation or autopsy. Respect and honor family wishes and final decisions.

Documentation provides a legal record of a death. Follow agency policies and procedures carefully to provide an accurate and reliable medical record of all assessments and activities surrounding a death. Physicians or coroners sign some medical forms, such as a request for autopsy, but nurses gather and record much of the remaining information surrounding a death. Nurses also usually witness or delegate the signing of forms (e.g., release of body or personal belongings forms). Nursing documentation becomes relevant in risk management or legal investigations into a death, underscoring the importance of accurate, legal reporting. Documentation also validates success in meeting patient goals or provides justification for changes in treatment or expected outcomes. Box 36.9 lists important documentation elements for end-of-life care.

Family members deserve and expect a clear description of what happened to their loved one, especially in cases of sudden, unusual, or unexpected circumstances. Give *only* factual information in a nonjudgmental, objective manner, and avoid sharing your opinions. State law and agency policy govern the sharing of the written medical record information, which usually involves a written request. Follow legal guidelines for documentation and sharing of medical records (see Chapter 23).

When a patient dies in an institutional or home care setting, nurses provide or delegate postmortem care, the care of a body after death. Above all, a deceased person's body deserves the same respect and dignity as that of a living person and needs to be prepared in a manner consistent with the patient's cultural and religious beliefs. Death produces physical changes in the body quite quickly; therefore you need to perform postmortem care as soon as possible to prevent discoloration, tissue damage, or deformities. Many hospitals have a policy for how many hours the body can stay on the unit before being sent to the morgue. This is important, as this limits the time that family members can spend with the patient immediately after death.

Maintain the integrity of cultural and religious rituals and mourning practices at the time of death to give survivors a sense of fulfilled obligations and promote acceptance of the patient's death (Box 36.10). Encourage and allow families to mourn in a manner consistent with

---

BOX 36.9 Documentation of End-of-Life Care

- Time and date of death and all actions taken to respond to the impending death
- Verification of death according to health care agency policy
- Name of health care provider certifying the death
- People notified of the death (e.g., health care providers, family members, organ request team, morgue, funeral home, spiritual care providers) and person who declared the time of death
- Name of person making request for organ or tissue donation
- Special preparations of the body (e.g., desired or required spiritual, religious, and cultural rituals)
- Medical tubes, devices, or lines left in or on the body
- Personal articles left on and secured to the body
- Personal items given to the family with description, date, time, to whom given
- Location of body identification tags
- Time of body transfer and destination
- Any other relevant information or family requests that help clarify special circumstances

⊕ BOX 36.10 CULTURAL ASPECTS OF CARE

Care of the Body After Death

Loved ones use cultural-specific rituals and mourning practices to achieve a sense of acceptance and inner peace and participate in socially accepted expressions of grief. One's culture greatly influences attitudes, preferences, behaviors, and rituals expected at the end-of-life and at the time of death (Orlovic et al., 2019). Show compassion, maintain privacy and dignity, and respect a patient's and family's cultural beliefs and practices. Allow time for patients and their families to make private and public preparations and to complete unfinished communication. Understanding the uniqueness of cultural expectations at the end of life helps you to know which questions to ask. Culture affects how comfortable the individual or family is with talking to the nurse or health care provider about end of life, and death (American Psychological Association [APA], 2019; Orlovic et al., 2019). As a nurse you can better prepare yourself by recognizing your own cultural biases, treating all people with respect and dignity, communicating with patients and families on their preferences, and providing clear explanations for the care you provide (APA, 2019).

Implications for Patient-Centered Care

Honoring the patient's and the family's cultural and spiritual customs is particularly important when caring for the dying and the dead (Orlovic et al., 2019). Here are some important things to know (or ask) concerning special ways to care for the body during and after death.
- Will there be large extended-family groups, including the church family, coming to be present at the time of death?
- Will the family be having organs donated or an autopsy performed?
- Does the family wish to participate in care for the deceased?
- Do the patient and family believe in an afterlife?
- Should a religious leader be called to the deathbed for a prayer or blessing?
- Does the deceased require special bathing or clothes after death?
- Will family or male members of the religious order need to stay with the deceased while waiting for transport/burial?
- Can only members of the same gender tend to the deceased's body?
- Does the body need to lie with the head facing a certain direction?

their cultural values to help survivors experience some predictability and control in an otherwise uncertain and confusing time. Some cultures consider "family" as more than a nuclear biological unit. You need to understand the makeup of a family network and know which individuals to involve in end-of-life decisions and care.

You will coordinate patient and family care during and after a death. Become familiar with applicable policies and procedures for postmortem care because they vary across settings or institutions. See the procedural guideline (Box 36.11) for standard activities for care of the body after death.

◆ Evaluation

Through the Patient's Eyes. Accuracy in evaluating the outcomes of care is related to how well you know your patient and the family. When you develop a trusting and therapeutic relationship, patients are more likely to share personal expectations or their wishes, especially if encouraged through appropriate questioning. Use the following questions to evaluate if patient expectations were met:
- Tell me if there is anything further we can do for you.
- Are your needs being addressed in a timely manner?
- Are you getting the care for which you hoped?
- Would you like me to help you in a different way?
- Do you have a specific request that I have not met?

Ask the patient and family if they feel the expected outcomes established during the planning phase were met. A patient's responses and perceptions of the effectiveness of nursing interventions help you determine if the existing plan of care is effective or if you need to implement different strategies. Evaluate patients for signs and symptoms of grief when determining how well they are coping with a loss and how they are responding to grief. Clinical judgment and critical thinking ensure that the evaluation process accurately reflects the patient's situation and desired outcomes (Fig. 36.5).

Patient Outcomes. Review the expected outcomes of the plan of care to determine if nursing interventions were successful or if

BOX 36.11 PROCEDURAL GUIDELINES

Care of the Body After Death

Delegation and Collaboration

The skill of care of the body after death can be delegated to assistive personnel (AP). Nurses often find it meaningful to help care for a patient after death and assist the AP whenever possible. Instruct the AP to:
- Contact the nurse for all questions and procedures related to organ/tissue donation and autopsy requests.
- Alert nurse to family members' questions related to manner of death or after-death activities.

Equipment

Bath towels, washcloths, washbasin, scissors, clean disposable gloves, gown (if high risk of exposure to body fluids), shroud kit with name tags, bed linen, documentation forms.

Steps

1. Confirm that the health care provider certified the death and documented the time of death and actions taken.
2. Determine whether the health care provider requested an autopsy. An autopsy is required for deaths that occur under certain circumstances.
3. Validate the status of request for organ or tissue donation. Given the complex and sensitive nature of such requests, only specially trained personnel make

the requests. Maintain sensitivity to personal, spiritual, religious, and cultural beliefs in this process.

4. Identify the patient using two identifiers (e.g., name and birthday or name and medical record number according to agency policy).
5. Perform hand hygiene and apply disposable gloves. Apply gown if risk of exposure to body fluids is high.
6. Provide sensitive and dignified nursing care to the patient and family.
   a. Elevate the head of the bed as soon as possible after death to prevent discoloration of the face.
   b. Collect ordered specimens.
   c. Ask whether the family wishes to participate in preparation of the body. Offer to contact someone to be there to support the family (patient/family religious leader, spiritual care personnel, or bereavement specialist) during body preparation.
   d. Ask about family requests for body preparation, such as wearing special clothing or religious artifacts. Be aware that personal, religious, or cultural practices determine whether to shave male facial hair. Get permission before shaving a beard.
   e. Remove all equipment, tubes, and indwelling lines. Note that autopsy or organ donation often poses exceptions to removal; therefore consult agency policy in these situations.

BOX 36.11   PROCEDURAL GUIDELINES—cont'd

Care of the Body After Death

f. Cleanse the body thoroughly, maintaining safety standards for body fluids and contamination when indicated. Remove gloves and gown (if needed) and perform hand hygiene.

g. Comb patient's hair or apply personal hairpieces.

h. Cover body with a clean sheet, place head on a pillow, and leave arms outside covers if possible. Close eyes by gently holding them shut; leave dentures in the mouth to maintain facial shape; cover any signs of body trauma.

i. Prepare and clean the environment, deodorize room if needed, and lower the lights.

j. Offer family members the option to view the body. Ask whether they want you or other support people to accompany them. Honor and respect individual choices.

k. Encourage grievers to say goodbye in their own way: words, touch, singing, spiritual or religious rituals, or prayers.

l. Provide privacy and a quiet, peaceful atmosphere. Assess family members' need or desire for your presence. If you leave, tell them how to reach you.

m. Determine which personal belongings stay with the body (e.g., wedding ring or religious symbol), and give other personal items to family members. Document time, date, description of the items taken, and who received them. Save any items that are left behind accidentally and contact family for further instructions.

n. Apply identifying name tags and shroud according to agency policy before transporting the body. Perform hand hygiene.

o. Complete documentation in the narrative notes section (see Box 36.9).

p. Maintain privacy and dignity when transporting the body to another location; cover the body or stretcher with a clean sheet.

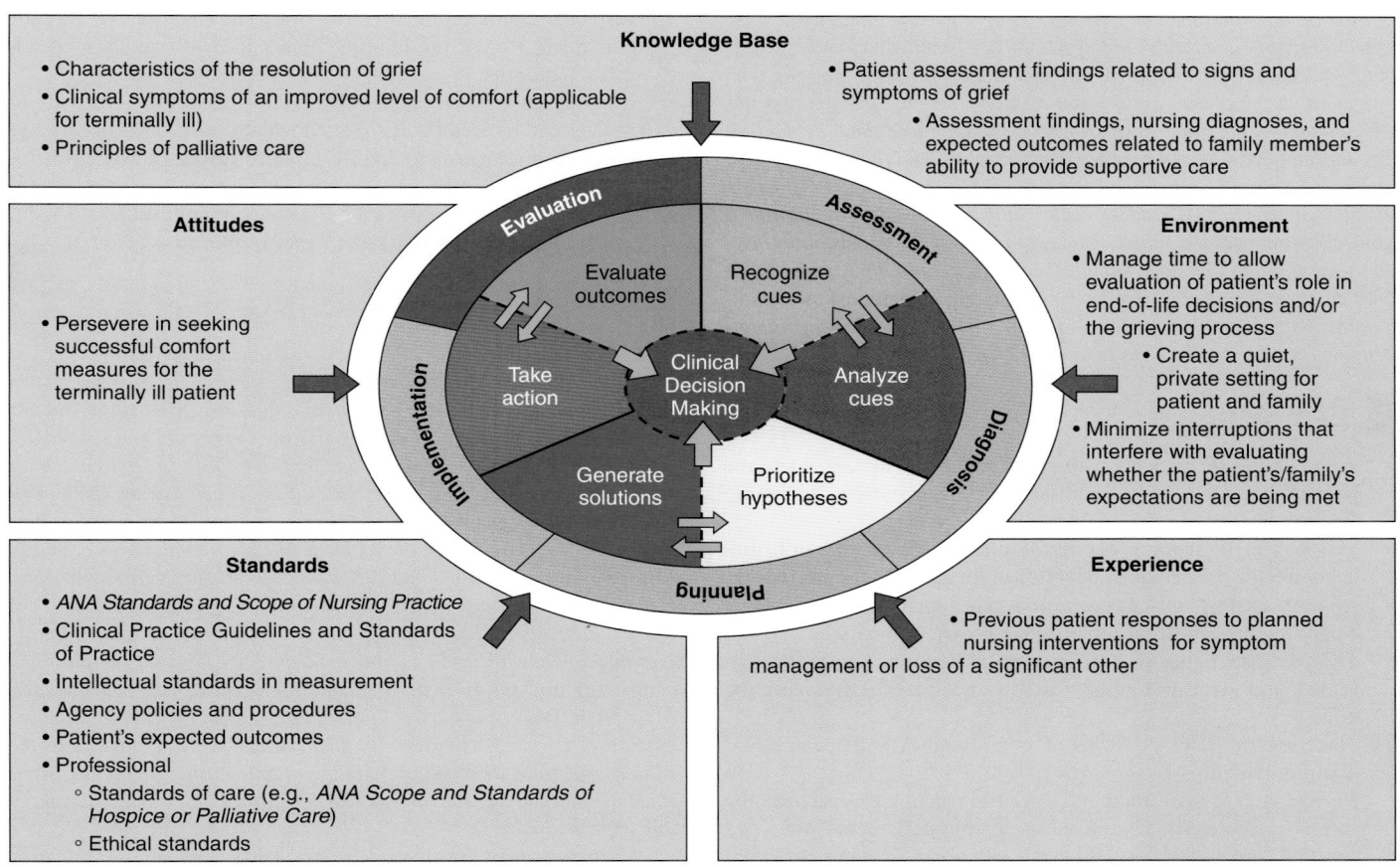

FIG. 36.5 Critical thinking model for loss, death, and grief evaluation. (Clinical Judgment Measurement Model copyright © NCSBN. All rights reserved.)

modifications are needed. For example, if the outcome is to have the patient communicate a sense of hope to family members, evaluate verbal and nonverbal communication and behaviors for cues related to expressions of hope. If the outcome is to achieve a level of comfort, evaluate if the severity of pain has declined and if the patient is able to participate in more self-care activities. Continue to evaluate the pa-

tient's progress, the effectiveness of the interventions, and patient and family interactions.

In home care settings it is critically important to include family members during evaluation. The short- and long-term outcomes that signal a family's recovery from a loss guide your evaluation. Short-term outcomes indicating effectiveness of grief interventions include talking about the loss without feeling overwhelmed, improved energy level, normalized sleep and dietary patterns, reorganization of life patterns, improved ability to make decisions, and finding it easier to be around other people. Long-term achievements include the return of a sense of humor and normal life patterns, renewed or new personal relationships, and decrease of inner pain.

After completing her teaching on end-of-life care for Mr. Allison and Lilly, Jennifer used teach-back to evaluate their learning. Jennifer stated, "I want to be sure I explained end-of-life care in a way that was easy to understand. Please explain to me the difference between hospice care and palliative care." Mr. Allison and Lilly described the differences between hospice and palliative care. Mr. Allison and Lilly expressed their appreciation for the teaching from Jennifer on what to expect at the end of life, end-of-life care, and hospice. They told Jennifer that since they now understand what hospice provides, they are comfortable with the decision for Mrs. Allison to receive hospice care.

Two weeks after discussing her plan of care with the Allison family, Jennifer observes Mr. Allison helping his wife with her bath. He explains that Lilly is "taking a break to catch up on her work." Mr. Allison has obtained a walker, and Mrs. Allison states that she feels less afraid of walking. Walking relieves the back pain that has become worse with bed rest. Mrs. Allison explains that she and Lilly have enjoyed looking through old photo albums together and that yesterday Mr. Allison "wanted to join in the fun, too." Mr. Allison tells Jennifer that his wife still reports some problems with nutrition, but since her pain is better controlled, she has a better appetite. He also told Jennifer that since his wife has talked more about her end-of-life decisions, Mrs. Allison has been more positive about the six small meals during the day and has been able to eat more. He carefully records her pain medication schedule. Mrs. Allison tells Jennifer that the pain medication is controlling her back pain. Taking the pain medication before bedtime helps her sleep through the night. Finally, Mr. Allison and Lilly received information about a support group for family caregivers sponsored by the hospital palliative care service. He tells Jennifer that they are looking into attending meetings to help with caregiver support.

KEY POINTS

- When caring for patients who are experiencing loss, facilitate the grief process by helping them feel the loss, express it, and move through their grief.
- Loss comes in many types based on the values and priorities learned within a person's sphere of influence (i.e., family, friends, religion, society, and culture); these types include loss of known environment, significant other, aspect of self, or life itself.
- The grief experience is a process that is personal, cannot be prevented, and involves a journey that no two people experience the same way.
- There are three major forms of grief: normal, anticipatory, and disenfranchised.
- Normal grief is a common and universal reaction characterized by complex emotional, cognitive, social, physical, behavioral, and spiritual responses to loss and death, whereas anticipatory grief occurs before an actual loss, especially in situations of prolonged or predicted loss.
- Knowledge of grief theories and normal responses to loss helps you to better understand these complex experiences and how to help a grieving person, remembering that reactions to grief vary widely and thus your practice must consider the complexity and individuality of grief responses.
- A person's development, coping strategies, socioeconomic status, personal relationships, nature of loss, and cultural and spiritual

beliefs influence the way a person perceives and responds to loss and grief.
- Assessing a person in grief requires exploration of the person's own unique history, context, and resources to make meaning out of their loss experiences. Listen as patients share the experience in their own way.
- When developing a plan of care for a person facing a loss such as death, include the wishes of a patient and family for end-of-life care, such as the preferred place for death, desired level of intervention, and expectations for pain and symptom management.
- Providing palliative care requires you to establish a caring presence and use effective communication strategies to encourage patients to share feelings to the degree they are comfortable. Collaborate with other members of the health care team to provide holistic care for management of symptoms and to provide a variety of support measures to the patient and family.
- High-quality end-of-life care focuses on improving quality of life through management of symptoms such as pain, anxiety, depression, and nausea. Pain is a common priority requiring you to conduct ongoing assessments of a patient's pain level to evaluate the patient's response to interventions.
- Hospice is a philosophy of family-centered, whole-person care for individuals with a life-limiting illness likely to result in death within 6 months.
- After determining that an autopsy will be performed, the body of the deceased is cared for and treated with the same level of care and compassion, respect, and dignity as when the person was alive.
- During the evaluation of a person in grief, successful outcomes reveal a patient moving through the stages of grief using successful coping mechanisms toward acceptance of the loss.

REFLECTIVE LEARNING

Mrs. Allison's health and mobility have continued to decline over the last 3 months. Although Mr. Allison is at home with his wife; he is not able to provide for all her needs, and he will need respite care. Mrs. Allison has lost strength because of decreased activity, shortness of breath, and severe back pain. She is experiencing weakness and finds it difficult to get around with her walker, spending most of her time either in her recliner chair or in bed. Mrs. Allison has a decreased appetite and no longer wants to help prepare meals. Even though the couple is eating six small meals each day, Mrs. Allison rarely finishes half of her small meal. She continues to drink water regularly throughout the day. Mrs. Allison feels anxious about the changes in her life and impending death and worries about how her family is coping and how they will do after her death. She is genuinely concerned about Lilly and the time she is taking off work to help both her and Mr. Allison. Because of Mrs. Allison's failing health, the couple no longer participate in social activities with their friends. When Jennifer visits the Allisons, she finds Mrs. Allison withdrawn and tearful, saying she is not sure how much longer she can live like this. Mr. Allison is noticeably quiet and appears tired.

- What assessment information in Mrs. Allison's situation is the most important or of immediate concern for the nurse? (Recognize Cues)
- Considering the Allison's situation, what environmental, organizational, or other factors did you see that influence the Allison's grief process? (Analyze Cues)
- Considering the assessment data and history, what is the priority nursing problem in caring for Mrs. Allison and her family? (Prioritize Diagnoses)
- Identify two expected outcomes for Mrs. Allison and her family. Consider Mrs. Allison's situation and describe the nursing and

medical interventions that you could use to achieve the expected outcomes. (Generate Solutions)

- Which nursing and medical interventions should have priority when implementing the care plan for Mrs. Allison and her family? (Take Action)
- Considering the implementation of your plan of care for the Allison family, what data should you gather to determine if the interventions were effective? (Evaluate Outcomes)

■ REVIEW QUESTIONS

1. To best assist a patient in the grieving process, which factors are most important for the nurse to assess? (Select all that apply.)
   1. Previous experiences with grief and loss
   2. Religious affiliation and denomination
   3. Ethnic background and cultural practices
   4. Current financial status
   5. Current medications
2. Which interventions does a nurse implement to help a patient at the end of life maintain autonomy while in a hospital? (Select all that apply.)
   1. Use therapeutic techniques when communicating with the patient.
   2. Allow the patient to determine timing and scheduling of interventions.
   3. Allow patients to have visitors at any time.
   4. Provide the patient with a private room close to the nurses' station.
   5. Encourage the patient to eat when hungry.
3. The nurse recognizes that which factors influence a person's approach to death? (Select all that apply.)
   1. Culture
   2. Spirituality
   3. Personal beliefs
   4. Previous experiences with death
   5. Gender
   6. Level of education
4. A nurse has the responsibility of managing a patient's postmortem care. What is the proper order for completing postmortem care when there is no autopsy ordered?
   1. Bathe the body of the deceased.
   2. Collect any needed specimens.
   3. Remove all tubes and indwelling lines.
   4. Position the body for family viewing.
   5. Speak to the family members about their possible participation.
   6. Ensure that the request for organ/tissue donation and/or autopsy was completed.
   7. Notify support person (e.g., spiritual care provider, bereavement specialist) for the family.
   8. Accurately tag the body, including the identity of the deceased and safety issues regarding infection control.
   9. Elevate the head of the bed.
5. Which comments made by a patient show an understanding of the teaching on palliative care completed by the nurse? (Select all that apply.)
   1. "Even though I'm continuing treatment, palliative care can help manage my symptoms and improve my quality of life."

2. "Palliative care is appropriate for people with any diagnosis."
3. "Only people who are dying can receive palliative care."
4. "Children are able to receive palliative care."
5. "Palliative care is only for people with uncontrolled pain."

6. A patient is receiving palliative care for symptom management related to anxiety and pain. A family member asks whether the patient is dying and now in "hospice." What does the nurse tell the family member about palliative care? (Select all that apply.)
   1. Palliative care and hospice are the same thing.
   2. Palliative care is for any patient, at any time, with any disease, in any setting.
   3. Palliative care strategies are primarily designed to treat the patient's illness.
   4. Palliative care relieves the symptoms of illness and treatment.
   5. Palliative care is started at the end of life.

7. When planning care for a dying patient, which interventions undertaken by the nurse promote the patient's dignity? (Select all that apply.)
   1. Providing respect
   2. Viewing the patient as a whole
   3. Providing symptom management
   4. Showing interest
   5. Being present
   6. Inserting a straight catheter when the patient has difficulty voiding

8. The nurse is caring for a patient who is near death. What assessment finding cues the nurse that death is approaching?
   1. Skin irritation
   2. Mottling
   3. Increased urine output
   4. Weakness

9. The nurse is assessing an older adult who is grieving after the loss of a spouse. What are normal signs of grief that the nurse would expect to find? (Select all that apply)
   1. Loss of interest in attending outside activities
   2. Feeling fatigued
   3. Difficulty making decisions
   4. Problems with remembering things
   5. Change in appetite and eating patterns

10. Which actions implemented by the nurse help grieving families? (Select all that apply.)
    1. Encourage involvement in nonthreatening group social activities.
    2. Follow up with the family to make sure all their questions are answered.
    3. Remind them that feelings of sadness or pain can return around anniversaries.
    4. Encourage survivors to ask for help.
    5. Look for overuse of alcohol, sleeping aids, or street drugs.

Answers: 1. 1, 2, 3, 5; **3.** 1, 2, 3, 4; **3.** 1, 2, 3, 4; **4.** 6, 9, 2, 5, 7, 3, 1, 4, 8; **5.** 1, 2, 4; **6.** 2, 4; **7.** 1, 2, 4, 5; **8.** 2; **9.** 1, 2, 3, 4, 5; **10.** 1, 2, 3, 4, 5.

Rationales for Review Questions can be found on the Evolve website.

REFERENCES

American Nurses Association (ANA): *Scope and standards of hospice and palliative nursing practice*, Atlanta, 2014, ANA.

American Nurses Association (ANA): *Nurses' roles and responsibilities in providing care and support at the end of life*, 2016. https://www.nursingworld.org/,4af078/globalassets/docs/ana/ethics/endoflife-positionstatement.pdf. Accessed July 5, 2020.

American Psychological Association (APA): *Culturally diverse communities and palliative and end-of-life care*, 2019. https://www.apa.org/pi/aging/programs/eol/end-of-life-diversity.pdf. Accessed July 5, 2020.

Angle S: *How to deal with ambiguous loss—the grief you feel when closure isn't an option*, 2019. https://www.wellandgood.com/how-to-deal-with-ambiguous-loss/. Accessed January 23, 2021.

Bowlby J: *Attachment and loss: loss, sadness, and depression* (vol 3), New York, 1980, Basic Books.

Cancer.Net: *Understanding grief within a cultural context*, 2018. https://www.cancer.net/coping-with-cancer/managing-emotions/grief-and-loss/understanding-grief-within-cultural-context. Accessed January 23, 2021.

Coyne P, et al: American Society for Pain Management Nursing and Hospice and Palliative Nurses Association Position Statement: Pain management at the end of life, *Pain Manag Nurs* 19(1):3, 2018.

Crockett SD, et al: American Gastroenterological Association Institute guideline on the medical management of opioid-induced constipation, *Gastroenterology* 156:218, 2019.

End-of-Live Nursing Education Consortium (ELNEC): *HPNA sponsored ELNEC train-the-trainer courses*, n.d. https://advancingexpertcare.org/elnec#:~:text=HPNA%E2%80%99s%20ELNEC%20Train-the-Trainer%20Courses%20provide%20nurses%20with%20education,professionals%20within%20their%20local%20communities%2C%20organizations%2C%20and%20institutions. Accessed June 12, 2021.

Ferrell BR: Introduction to palliative care. In Ferrell BR, Paice JA, editors: *Oxford textbook of palliative nursing*, ed 5, New York, 2019, Oxford University Press.

Hamilton IJ: Understanding grief and bereavement, *Br J Gen Pract* 66(651):523, 2016.

Hess K: *America's death-denying culture*, 2018. https://brightonhospice.com/death-denying-culture/. Accessed January 24, 2021.

Hospice Foundation of America: *Services. What is hospice?* 2018. http://hospicefoundation.org/End-of-Life-Support-and-Resources/Coping-with-Terminal-Illness/Hospice-Services. Accessed July 5, 2020.

Jensen HI, et al: Practice recommendations for end-of-life care in the intensive care unit, *Crit Care Nurse* 40(3):14, 2020.

Kübler-Ross E: *On death and dying*, New York, 1969, Macmillan.

Mayo Clinic: *Suicide grief*, 2020. https://www.mayoclinic.org/healthy-lifestyle/end-of-life/in-depth/suicide/art-20044900. Accessed January 23, 2021.

McKay B, McKay K: *The seasons of a man's life: the mid-life transition*, 2021. https://www.artofmanliness.com/articles/the-seasons-of-a-mans-life-the-mid-life-transition/. Accessed June 12, 2021.

Mughal S, et al: *Grief reaction*, 2020, Stat Pearls. https://www.ncbi.nlm.nih.gov/books/NBK507832/. Accessed June 12, 2021.

National Institute on Aging (NIA): *What are hospice care and palliative care?* 2021. https://www.nia.nih.gov/health/what-are-palliative-care-and-hospice-care. Accessed June 14, 2021.

Paice JA: Pain management. In Ferrell BR, Paice JA, editors: *Oxford textbook of palliative nursing*, ed 5, New York, 2019, Oxford University Press.

Perng A, Renz S: Identifying and treating complicated grief in older adults, *J Nurse Pract* 14(4):289, 2018.

Petruzzi J: *The different forms and reactions of grief and bereavement*, October 2019, Research Gate. https://www.researchgate.net/publication/336926996_The_Different_Forms_and_Reactions_of_Grief_and_Bereavement. Accessed June 12, 2021

Rando T: *Treatment of complicated mourning*, Champaign, IL, 1993, Research Press.

Rando T: *What therapists need to know about traumatic bereavement: what it is and how to approach it*, 2014. http://www.lowcountrymhconference.com/wp-content/uploads/2014/07/drrando_handout.pdf. Accessed July 5, 2020.

Stroebe M, Schut H: The dual process model of coping with bereavement: rationale and description, *Death Stud* 23(3):197, 1999.

Vacarolis EM, Fosbre CD: *Essentials of psychiatric-mental health nursing*, ed 4, St. Louis, 2021, Elsevier.

Viscusi ER: Clinical overview and considerations for the management of opioid-induced constipation in patients with chronic noncancer pain, *Clin J Pain* 35(2):174–188, 2019.

Whitley M: *Anticipatory grief: learning the signs and how to cope*, 2020. https://www.aplaceformom.com/caregiver-resources/articles/anticipatory-grief. Accessed January 23, 2021.

Worden JW: *Grief counseling and grief therapy: a handbook for the mental health practitioner*, ed 4, New York, 2008, Springer.

World Health Organization (WHO): *Definition of palliative care*, 2021. http://www.who.int/cancer/palliative/definition/en/. Accessed June 14, 2021.

RESEARCH REFERENCES

Coolhart D, et al: Experience of ambiguous loss for parents of transgender male youth: a phenomenological exploration, *Contemp Fam Ther* 40:28, 2018.

Keller MS, et al: Patient and provider differences in the treatment of opioid-induced constipation: a qualitative study, *BMC Gastroenterol* 19:182, 2019.

Koper I, et al: Spiritual care at the end of life in the primary care setting: experiences from spiritual caregivers - a mixed methods study, *BMC Palliat Care* 18(98):1, 2019.

Lai XB, et al: The experience of caring for patients at the end-of-life stage in non-palliative care settings: a qualitative study, *BMC Palliat Care* 17:116, 2018.

Liang Y, et al: Do-not-resuscitate consent signed by patients indicates a more favorable quality of end-of-life care for patients with advanced cancer, *Support Care Cancer* 25(2):533, 2017.

Nee J, et al: Efficacy of treatments for opioid-induced constipation: systematic review and meta-analysis, *Clin Gastroenterol Hepatol* 16(10):1569, 2018.

Orlovic M, et al: Racial and ethnic differences in end-of-life care in the United States: evidence from the Health and Retirement Study (HRS), *SSM Popul Health* 7:100331, 2019.

Perez RM, Arnold-Berkovits I: A conceptual framework for understanding Latino immigrant's ambiguous loss of homeland, *Hisp J Behav Sci* 40(2):91, 2018.

Sekse RJT, et al: The nurse's role in palliative care: a qualitative meta-synthesis, *J Clin Nurs* 27:e21, 2018.

Star A, Boland JW: Updates in palliative care – recent advancements in the pharmacological management of symptoms, *Clin Med (Lond)* 18(1):11, 2018.

Young J: An evidence review on managing constipation in palliative care, *Nursing Times* 115(5):28, 2019.

Stress and Coping

OBJECTIVES

- Explain the three stages of the general adaptation syndrome.
- Summarize the characteristics of posttraumatic stress disorder.
- Discuss the integration of stress theory with nursing theories.
- Identify the effects that compassion fatigue can have in the health care workplace.
- Use clinical judgment to choose stress-management techniques that help individuals effectively cope with stress.
- Discuss the process of crisis intervention.
- Develop a care plan for patients who are experiencing stress.
- Discuss how stress in the workplace affects nurses.

KEY TERMS

Adventitious crises
Alarm stage
Allostasis
Allostatic load
Appraisal
Burnout
Compassion fatigue
Coping
Crisis

Crisis intervention
Developmental crises
Ego-defense mechanisms
Exhaustion stage
Fight-or-flight response
Flashbacks
General adaptation syndrome (GAS)
Mindfulness
Posttraumatic stress disorder (PTSD)

Primary appraisal
Resistance stage
Secondary appraisal
Situational crises
Stress
Stressors
Trauma

MEDIA RESOURCES

http://evolve.elsevier.com/Potter/fundamentals/
- Review Questions
- Concept Map Creator
- Case Study with Questions

- Audio Glossary
- Content Updates
- Answers to QSEN Activity and Review Questions

Sandra and John Edwards have been married 3 years and are both 55 years of age. This is the first marriage for both, and they have no children or other family members who live near them. They both are working and are planning their retirement at age 66. Sandra is the manager for a large insurance firm, and John is the vice president of marketing at a large manufacturing company. Last month, John was diagnosed with stage III pancreatic cancer. Presently, John and Sandra are at the Cancer Center to discuss chemotherapy for his cancer. When Matt, the nurse practitioner at the center, greets the couple, he notices that they both look tired; Sandra is disheveled, and John is clean-shaven and well groomed. John states that he is worried about Sandra as she appears "just worn out," and he expresses fear that she will not be able to help him through this medical crisis. Sandra tells Matt that since John's diagnosis, she has felt defeated and hopeless, has no energy, and has difficulty organizing her thoughts. She also reports that she is experiencing headaches and sleep problems and that she has no appetite.

Matt completes his physical and psychological screening on the couple. As Matt interviews Sandra and John, he learns more about the stressors they are facing. Sandra tells Matt that the insurance firm is undergoing a large restructuring and that she has been working late on the project. She is the project manager. Matt knows that Sandra has had hypertension for

7 years. John says it is hard for them because they feel they have no one but each other to talk to during this period. The Edwardses attend church regularly and have a few close friends from church. John also tells Matt that he is unsure whether he will be able to continue to work while receiving his treatments. Currently, the Edwardses have good health insurance coverage through John's employer. Matt recognizes the need to work on a plan to help the Edwardses cope with John's illness.

Stress can impact the physical and mental well-being of patients, as well as entire families and communities. Nurses need to become familiar with stress and consider its effects when delivering patient care. Equally important, health care professionals also experience stressful events during clinical practice and their own lives. Nurses need to consider their own stress by recognizing burnout, compassion fatigue, and second victim syndrome. It is important for nurses to use clinical judgment and critical thinking to recognize assessment findings and analyze cues related to stress. This, along with understanding stress-management techniques, aids their own personal coping and helps the nurse to design a patient-centered stress-management plan with individualized interventions for patients and families.

Stress is described as an actual or alleged hazard to the balance of homeostasis. It is often described as a physical, chemical, or emotional factor that produces tension in the body or the mind (Banasik and Copstead, 2019). Such factors are referred to as stressors. **Stressors** are physical, psychological, or social stimuli that can produce stress and endanger homeostasis (Banasik and Copstead, 2019). Stressors differ in their scope, strength, and duration. A stressor of less intensity can still have a substantial influence if it continues over time. An important element in the perception of a stressor is appraisal. **Appraisal** is how a person interprets the impact of the stressor. It is also a personal evaluation of the meaning of the event to what is happening and a consideration of the resources on hand to help manage the stressor. Stress emerges when an individual considers the event as a threat and the ability to respond to the demands placed on the individual by the event to be overwhelming. Thus, stress can lead to personal growth and development or overwhelm a person and lead to illness or worsening of existing acute or chronic illnesses (Liu et al., 2017).

People experience stress because of daily life events and experiences, such as the loss of a loved one, a change in job responsibilities, or an illness. Stress stimulates their ability to think clearly and stay alert to the environment. How people react to stress depends on how they view and evaluate the impact of the stressor, its effect on their situation and support at the time of the stress, and their usual coping mechanisms. When stress overwhelms existing coping mechanisms, patients lose emotional balance, and a crisis results. If symptoms of stress persist beyond the duration of the stressor, a person experiences a **trauma** (Sacks et al., 2017).

SCIENTIFIC KNOWLEDGE BASE

Hans Selye, a Vienna-born endocrinologist, was the first scientist to single out the physical side effects of stress. While conducting experiments related to hormone production, Selye noticed that his subjects showed a similar set of side effects regardless of the type of life-threatening stimulus that researchers presented. Selye termed this collection of responses the **general adaptation syndrome (GAS)**, a three-stage set of physiological processes that prepare, or adapt, the body for danger so that an individual is more likely to survive when faced with a threat (Selye, 1950).

Selye (1993) identified the three stages of the stress response as (1) initial alarm, (2) resistance as a person attempts to compensate for changes induced by the alarm stage, and (3) a state of exhaustion if the person cannot adapt successfully during the stage of resistance or if stress remains unrelieved. When stress reaches chronic and harmful levels, negative consequences follow. Selye's initial theory has evolved as scientists have learned more about the physiological responses to stress.

General Adaptation Syndrome

The general adaptation syndrome (GAS), the three-stage reaction to stress, describes how the body responds physiologically to stressors (Fig. 37.1). The GAS is triggered either directly by a physical event or indirectly by a psychological event. It involves several body systems, especially the neuroendocrine mechanism, which responds immediately to stress (see Fig. 37.1). When the body encounters a physical demand such as an injury, the pituitary gland initiates the GAS. A fundamental concept underlying this reaction is that the body will attempt to return to a state of balance, a process referred to as **allostasis** (Banasik and Copstead, 2019).

During the **alarm stage** the central nervous system is aroused, and body defenses are mobilized; this is the **fight-or-flight response**. During this stage rising hormone levels result in increased blood volume, blood glucose levels, epinephrine and norepinephrine, heart rate, blood flow to muscles, oxygen intake, and mental alertness. In addition, the pupils of the eyes dilate to produce a greater visual field. If the stressor

poses an extreme threat to life or remains for a long time, the person progresses to the second stage, resistance.

The **resistance stage** also contributes to the fight-or-flight response, and the body stabilizes and responds, attempting to compensate for the changes induced by the alarm stage (Huether et al., 2020). Hormone levels, heart rate, blood pressure, and cardiac output should return to normal, and the body tries to repair any damage that occurred. However, these compensation attempts consume energy and other bodily resources.

In the **exhaustion stage** continuous stress causes progressive breakdown of compensatory mechanisms. This occurs when the body is no longer able to resist the effects of the stressor and has depleted the energy necessary to maintain adaptation. The physiological response has intensified, but the person's ability to adapt to the stressor diminishes (Huether et al., 2020). Even in the face of chronic demands, an ongoing state of chronic activation can occur. This chronic arousal with the presence of powerful hormones causes excessive wear and tear on bodily organs and is called **allostatic load**. A persistent allostatic load can cause long-term physiological problems such as chronic hypertension, depression, sleep deprivation, chronic fatigue syndrome, and autoimmune disorders (Huether et al., 2020).

Immune Response. The physiological interactions between the neuroendocrine stress response and the immune system are complex. The stress response directly influences the immune system (Huether et al., 2020). Stress causes prolonged changes in the immune system, which can result in impaired immune function. As stress increases, the person is more susceptible to changes in health, such as increased risk for infection, high blood pressure, diabetes, and cancer (Casey and Tiaki, 2017).

Reaction to Psychological Stress. Each person responds differently to physiological threats. The same threat can produce different reactions in different people and indirectly activates the GAS. The intensity and duration of the psychological threat and the number of other stressors that occur at the same time affect a person's response. In addition, whether a person anticipated the stressor influences its effect. It is often more difficult to cope with an unexpected stressor. Personal characteristics that influence the response to a stressor include the level of personal control, presence of a social support system, and feelings of competence.

Stress can be viewed as a transaction between a person and the environment. A person appraises or mentally rates an event in terms of its meaning and then experiences stress only if the event or circumstance is considered significant. Evaluating an event in terms of personal meaning is **primary appraisal**. Appraisal of an event or circumstance is an ongoing perceptual process. Stress results when a person identifies an event or circumstance as a harm, loss, threat, or challenge. **Secondary appraisal**, the process by which a person considers possible available coping strategies or resources, occurs at the same time. Stress occurs if the demands placed on the person by the event exceed the ability to cope. Balancing factors contribute to restoring equilibrium. According to crisis theory, because feedback cues lead to reappraisals of the original perception, coping behaviors constantly change as individuals perceive new information. When coping behaviors are ineffective and repeated over and over, a state of stress can result. Stress emerges either when a person views an event as posing a significant risk of harm or when the person is unable to cope with the event's demands.

Coping is a person's cognitive and behavioral efforts to manage a stressor (Buchanan, 2021). It is important to physical and psychological health because stress is associated with a range of psychological and health outcomes (Buchanan, 2021). The effectiveness of coping strategies is influenced by a variety of factors, such as a person's age, cultural

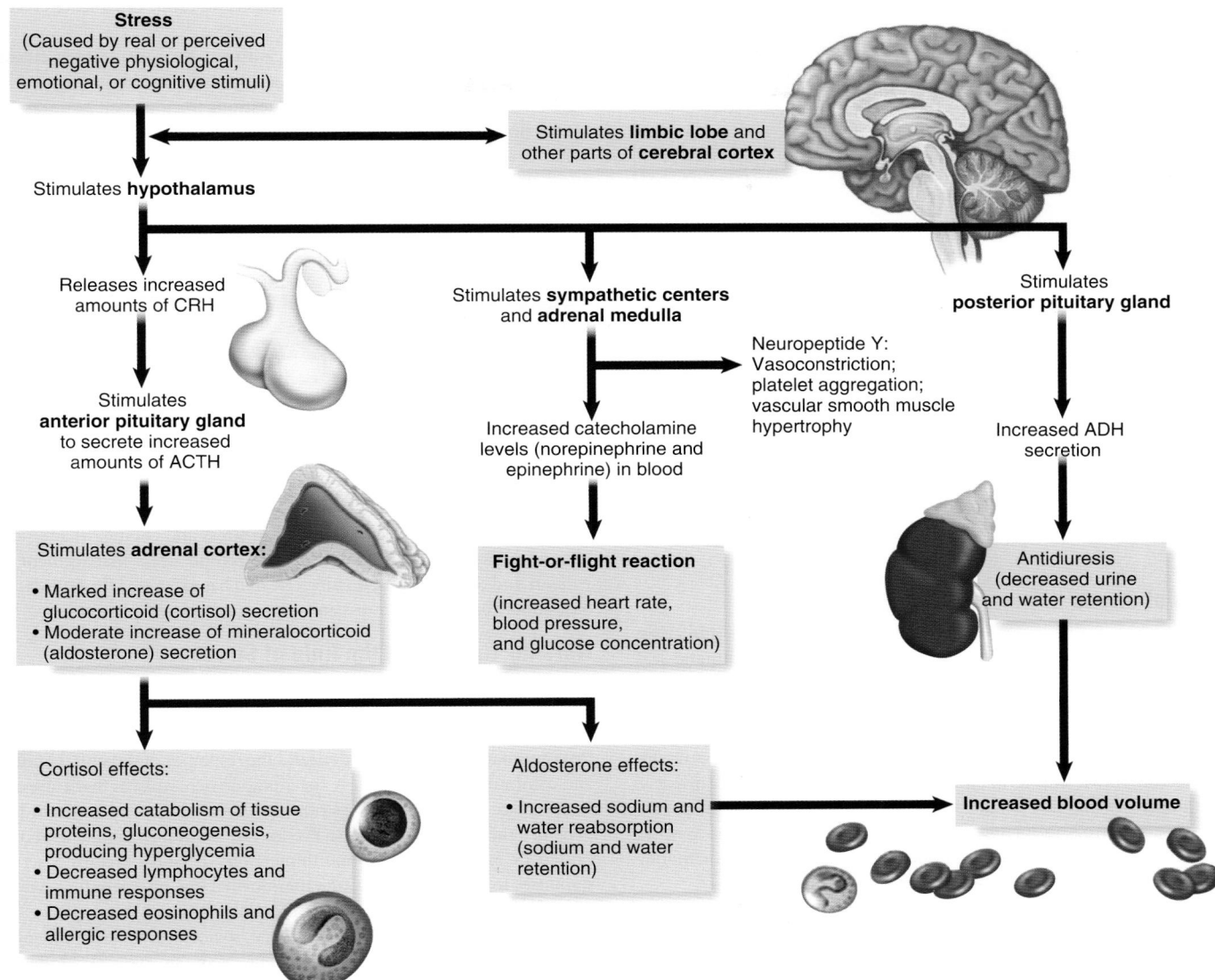

FIG. 37.1 Short-term and long-term stress response. Some effects are immediate, such as the sympathetic fight-or-flight reaction, and some effects are longer-term, such as the hormonal effects. *ACTH,* Adrenocortico-tropic hormone; *ADH,* antidiuretic hormone; *CRH,* corticotropin-releasing hormone. (From Patton KT: *Anatomy & physiology,* ed 10, St Louis, 2019, Elsevier.)

background, individual circumstances, and past use of coping strategies. Thus no single coping strategy works for everyone or for every stressor.

In stressful situations most people use a combination of problem- and emotion-focused coping strategies. In other words, when under stress a person obtains information, takes action to change the situation (problem-focused), and regulates emotions tied to the stress (emotion-focused). In some cases, people avoid thinking about the situation or change the way they think about it without changing the actual situation itself. For example, as a nursing student, you may stop thinking about an examination coming up in a few days to decrease the stress that thinking about the examination causes, yet you continue to study for the exam so that you will do well.

People's goals, their beliefs about themselves and the world, the types of stresses they face, and personal resources determine how people cope with stress (Enns et al., 2018). Personal resources include problem-solving skills, financial status, social skills, support from family and friends, physical attractiveness, health and energy, and personal stress-management techniques such as optimism and mindfulness (Hofmann and Gomez, 2017).

Coping mechanisms include psychological adaptive behaviors. Such behaviors are often task oriented, involving the use of direct problem-solving techniques to cope with threats. Ego-defense mechanisms regulate emotional distress and thus give a person protection from anxiety and stress. They help a person cope with stress indirectly and offer psychological protection from a stressful event. Everyone uses them unconsciously to protect against feelings of worthlessness and anxiety. Occasionally a defense mechanism becomes distorted and no longer helps the person adapt to a stressor. However, people generally find them very helpful in coping and use them spontaneously (Box 37.1). Frequently, short-term stressors activate ego-defense mechanisms. These usually do not result in psychiatric disorders.

BOX 37.1 Examples of Ego-Defense Mechanisms

- Compensation: Making up for a deficiency in one aspect of self-image by strongly emphasizing a feature considered an asset (e.g., a person who is a poor communicator relies on organizational skills)
- Conversion: Unconsciously repressing an anxiety-producing emotional conflict and transforming it into nonorganic symptoms (e.g., difficulty in sleeping, loss of appetite)
- Denial: Avoiding emotional conflicts by refusing to consciously acknowledge anything that causes intolerable emotional pain (e.g., a person refuses to discuss or acknowledge a personal loss)
- Displacement: Transferring emotions, ideas, or wishes from a stressful situation to a less anxiety-producing substitute (e.g., a person transfers anger over an interpersonal conflict to a malfunctioning computer)
- Identification: Patterning behavior after that of another person and assuming that person's qualities, characteristics, and actions
- Dissociation: Experiencing a subjective sense of numbing and a reduced awareness of one's surroundings
- Regression: Coping with a stressor through actions and behaviors associated with an earlier developmental period

Types of Stress

Stress is often caused by work, family, daily hassles, trauma, and crisis. Stress may be acute or chronic. One person looks at a stimulus and sees it as a challenge, leading to mastery and growth. Another sees the same stimulus as a threat, leading to stagnation and loss. The individual with family responsibilities and a full-time job outside the home can experience chronic stress. It occurs in stable conditions and from stressful roles. Living with a long-term illness produces chronic stress. Conversely, time-limited events that threaten a person for a relatively brief period provoke acute stress. Recurrent daily hassles such as commuting to work, maintaining a house, dealing with difficult people, and managing money further complicate chronic or acute stress.

Posttraumatic stress disorder (PTSD) begins when a person experiences or witnesses a traumatic event and responds with intense fear or helplessness. PTSD is common among military personnel, veterans and police. It is particularly seen in soldiers who have been involved in combat or police involved in violent acts. Soldiers often witness or participate in disturbing events, producing dramatic symptoms. Some other examples of traumatic events that lead to PTSD include motor vehicle crashes, natural disasters, or violent personal assault. Anxiety associated with PTSD is sometimes manifested by nightmares and emotional detachment. Some people with PTSD experience flashbacks, or recurrent and intrusive recollections of the event. Depression and PTSD commonly occur together (Halter, 2018).

Secondary traumatic stress is the trauma a person experiences from witnessing other people's suffering. It is a component of compassion fatigue and is common in health care workers and first responders. Secondary traumatic stress results in intrusive symptoms such as nightmares and anxiety. People with this condition begin to avoid interactions and have difficulties in sleeping and relating to friends or family.

A crisis implies that a person is facing a turning point in life. This means that previous ways of coping are ineffective, and the person must change. There are three types of crises: (1) maturational or developmental crises, (2) situational crises, and (3) disasters or adventitious crises (Halter, 2018). A new developmental stage such as marriage or the birth of a child requires new coping styles. Developmental crises occur as a person moves through the stages of life. External sources such as a job change, a motor vehicle crash, or severe illness provoke situational crises.

A major natural disaster, man-made disaster, or crime of violence creates an adventitious crisis.

Patient-centered care offers a context for crisis intervention (SAMHSA, 2020). The view of the person experiencing a crisis is the frame of reference for it. The vital questions for a person in crisis are "What does this mean to you?" and "How is it going to affect your life?" What causes extreme stress for one person is not always stressful to another. The perception of the event, situational supports, and coping mechanisms all influence return of equilibrium. A person either grows or regresses as a result of a crisis, depending on how the person manages the situation (Halter, 2018).

REFLECT NOW

How would a nurse determine that a patient is moving from the alarm stage to the resistance stage of the general adaptation syndrome?

NURSING KNOWLEDGE BASE

Nurses have proposed theories related to stress and coping. In addition, because nurses are taking a more active role in stress management of patients and of themselves, nursing research has expanded the knowledge base about the nature of stress and stress-management alternatives.

Nursing Theory and the Role of Stress

Many nursing theories explain and describe stress. For example, explanation of the concepts of stress and reaction to stress are components of the Betty Neuman Systems Model. The Neuman Systems Model uses a systems approach to help you understand the responses of patients, families, and communities to stressors. A systems approach explains that a stressor at one place in a system affects other parts of the system; a system is a person, family, or community. Events are multidimensional and not caused or affected by only one thing. Every person develops a set of responses to stress that constitute the "normal line of defense" (Lawson, 2018; Neuman and Fawcett, 2011). This line of defense maintains health and wellness. Physiological, psychological, sociocultural, developmental, or spiritual influences buffer stress. The Neuman Systems Model of nursing views a patient, family, or community as constantly changing in response to the environment and stressors.

Callista Roy's Adaptation Model describes how an individual can effectively respond to stressors in the environment. According to Roy's theory, a person has the ability to modify external stimuli to allow adaptation to occur. A nurse assists an individual with modifying and regulating peripheral stimuli to promote a supportive healing environment (Cherry and Jacob, 2019).

On the other hand, Pender's Health Promotion Model (HPM) (see Chapter 6) focuses on promoting health, managing stress, and increasing level of well-being (Murdaugh et al., 2018). In this model people can assess their own abilities and assets and want to live in ways that enable them to be as healthy as possible. Interventions such as increasing physical activity, improving diet and nutrition, and using stress-management strategies help the individual become and remain healthy.

Factors Influencing Stress and Coping

Potential stressors and coping mechanisms vary across the life span (e.g., adolescence, adulthood, and old age bring different stressors). The appraisal of stressors, the amount and type of social support, and coping strategies all depend on previous life experiences and affect how a person reacts to that stressor. Situational and social stressors place people who are vulnerable at higher risk for prolonged stress.

Situational Factors. Different types of situational factors exist. Situational stressors in the health care workplace that affect nurses and other health care professionals include high-acuity patient load, job environment, constant distractions, responsibility, conflicting priorities, and intensity of care (e.g., trauma, emergency, or critical care areas) (Mealer et al., 2017; Ueno et al., 2017). In addition, changing shifts increases fatigue and work-related stress.

Some nurses cope with shift work by knowing their own circadian rhythms. People who function best in the morning have the greatest difficulty with night work and changing shifts. As people age, they tend to become more morning oriented. Morning people need to be counseled about the potentially negative effects of night work for them. In general, people doing shift work need to maintain as consistent a sleep and mealtime schedule as possible (Nena et al., 2018; Solomon et al., 2016).

Adjusting to chronic illness is another type of situational stress. The physical limitations posed by a disease state and the uncertainty associated with treatment and illness trigger stress in patients and family caregivers of all ages. Sometimes illness changes how people manage their stress. For example, Antony et al. (2018) found that caregivers of patients with cancer who were receiving palliative care used both negative and positive coping strategies to deal with the stress of caregiving. Having difficulty in paying for treatment and limited access to health care providers also create stress. Although being a family caregiver for someone with a chronic illness such as Alzheimer disease is stressful, the actions of competent health care providers often help minimize the stress for family caregivers.

Maturational Factors. Stressors vary with life stage. According to Erikson's developmental theory, individuals experience predictable stages of development as particular tasks are accomplished and mastered for each stage. Children who are in the stage of initiative versus guilt identify stressors related to physical appearance, families, friends, and school. During this stage, teaching impulse control and cooperative behaviors is imperative. Preadolescents in the stage of industry versus inferiority experience stress related to self-esteem issues, hospitalizations, or changing family structure because of divorce or death of a parent. Erikson asserts that during this stage, preadolescents can develop a sense of inferiority if they do not receive proper support for learning new skills. In the stage of identity versus role confusion, adolescents search for identity with peer groups and separate from their families. In addition, adolescents face stressful questions about sex, jobs, school, career choices, and using mind-altering substances. During this stage of development, stress can occur because of preoccupation with appearance and body image. Adolescents should strive to develop and accept personal identity.

Stress for younger adults who are in the stages of intimacy versus isolation or for middle-age adults in the stage of generativity versus self-absorption and stagnation centers on major changes in life circumstances. These stressors include many milestones, such as beginning a family and a career, losing parents, seeing children leave home, and accepting physical aging. Social development is important during this stage. In older adults during the stage of integrity versus despair, stressors may include the loss of autonomy and mastery resulting from general frailty or health problems that limit stamina, strength, and cognition (Box 37.2). Nurses and other health care providers need to differentiate signs of stress and crisis in older adults from dementia and acute confusion.

Sociocultural Factors. Environmental and social stressors often lead to developmental problems. Potential stressors that affect any age-group but that are especially stressful for young people include prolonged poverty and physical disability. Children become vulnerable

---

BOX 37.2 FOCUS ON OLDER ADULTS

Understanding Differences in Stress and Coping Among Older Adults

- Ordinary hassles of day-to-day living create a source of stress; older adults have more hassles with home maintenance and health than do younger people.
- Older adults often use more passive, intrapersonal, emotion-focused forms of coping, such as distancing, humor, accepting responsibility, and reappraising the stressor in a positive way (Nieto et al., 2019).
- Life experiences and perspectives of older adults make most problems seem insignificant, especially when older adults have acquired appropriate stress-management techniques (Jackson et al., 2018).
- Older adults' coping improves based on earlier experience with coping with traumatic situations (Jackson et al., 2018).
- Older adults often use prayer and religious practices as coping mechanisms during periods of stress and anxiety (O'Brien et al., 2019).
- Impaired coping affects overall health in older adults more than in younger adults (Touhy and Jett, 2022; 2020).
- Because of the high incidence of depression in older adults, you need to assess for suicidal thoughts and intent.
- Social support and social relationships are important in helping older adults cope with stress (Touhy and Jett, 2022; 2020).

---

when they lose parents and caregivers through divorce, imprisonment, or death or when parents have mental illness or substance-abuse disorders. Living under conditions of continuing violence, disintegrated neighborhoods, or homelessness affects people of any age, especially young people (Murdaugh et al., 2018).

Social isolation and loneliness are common stressors for older adults, especially among those who live in long-term care facilities (Bethell et al., 2019). When an older adult is experiencing social isolation, there may be limited or no social supports or interactions with others (Gardiner et al., 2018). Social isolation frequently leads to loneliness (Gardiner et al., 2018). Gardiner et al. (2018) defined loneliness as a feeling of being alone, not being with others, or as an imbalance between desired social interactions and actual social interactions. Social isolation and loneliness impact the mental and physical health of the individual and can contribute to poor health outcomes, including depression, decreased resistance to infection, poor quality of life, low self-esteem, decreased hope, impaired cognitive function and dementia, impaired functioning in activities of daily living, and cardiovascular disease (Fakoya et al., 2020; O'Rourke et al., 2018). Fakoya et al. (2020) report that risk factors for social isolation and loneliness include family members who live at a distance, decreased income and mobility, the loss of loved ones, and living in communities with lower levels of cohesiveness. Feeling socially connected is important for older adults, and planned interventions should promote social connectedness. For older adults, social connectedness is a subjective feeling. The focus of social connectedness is on being positive and having meaningful and close relationships with individuals, groups, or the community (O'Rourke et al., 2018). These relationships promote a feeling of caring for others, being cared for by others, and a sense of belonging (O'Rourke et al., 2018).

A person's culture also influences stress and coping. Cultural variations produce stress, particularly if a person's values differ from the dominant culture in aspects of gender roles, family relationships, and religious beliefs (Giger and Haddad, 2021, Shavitt et al., 2016). Other aspects of cultural variations begin with language difference, geographical location, family relationships, time orientation, access to health care programs, and disparities in health care (Box 37.3) (see Chapter 9).

BOX 37.3   CULTURAL ASPECTS OF CARE

Cultural Variations in Stress Appraisal and Coping Strategies

A patient's culture defines what is stressful to the person and ways of coping with stress (Giger and Haddad, 2021). Cultural context shapes the types of situations that produce stress. Culture affects how a person leaves the parental home, experiences health crises or chronic illness, cares for the family, or becomes disabled or dependent. Furthermore, how people appraise stress also depends on their culture. What is perceived as a major stressor in one culture is sometimes viewed as a minor problem in another. Cultures may address developmental transitions and turning points in life differently. For example, cultures vary in how birthdays, weddings, or deaths of family members are celebrated or commemorated.

Coping strategies are also influenced by one's cultural background. Cultures vary in their emotion- and problem-focused coping strategies. Some stress that emotions should be controlled, whereas others believe in expressing emotion. Cultures provide different resources for coping with stress (Giger and Haddad, 2021). These include rituals, advice givers or support groups, and a legal system for conflict resolution.

Implications for Patient-Centered Care
- Realize that stressors and coping styles vary with different cultures.
- Reflect on your own perceptions of stress and coping in a cultural context.
- Assess the influence of culture on a patient's appraisal of stress.
- Identify the presence of individualized cultural practices related to stress management.
- Determine resources in a patient's culture that facilitate coping.

Compassion Fatigue

Compassion fatigue is a term used to describe a state of burnout and secondary traumatic stress. Secondary traumatic stress is the stress that health care providers experience when witnessing and caring for others who are suffering. Examples include nurses caring for patients with COVID-19 in an intensive care unit, an oncology nurse who cares for patients undergoing surgery and chemotherapy over the long term for their cancer, or a spouse who witnesses his wife deteriorating over the years from Alzheimer disease. Burnout occurs when perceived demands outweigh perceived resources (Brown et al., 2018). It is a state of physical and mental fatigue and exhaustion that often affects health care providers because of the nature of their work environment. Perceived inadequate staffing, long work shifts, demands of patient acuity, and dysfunctional relationships (patients and other care providers) serve as triggers for ongoing stress. Over time, giving of oneself in often intense caring environments can result in emotional exhaustion, leaving a nurse feeling irritable, restless, and unable to focus and engage with patients. This condition may be viewed as a failure to cope because it often occurs in situations in which the nurse is unable to practice self-care, social support is lacking, and organizational pressures are influencing staffing levels.

Compassion fatigue is a condition that can overwhelm health care providers and cause physical, mental, and emotional health issues (Upton, 2018). During the COVID-19 pandemic, nurses and health care workers faced extreme stress, causing feelings of fear, anxiety, depression, helplessness, and powerlessness because little was known about the virus and how to care for patients extremely ill from the virus (CDC, 2020; Usher et al., 2020). This resulted in stress and compassion fatigue, particularly in critical care nurses (Alharbi et al., 2020). The feelings of fear, hopelessness, and anxiety from compassion fatigue usually result in feelings of inadequacy

and lower self-esteem. These factors can lead to the health care provider using negative coping behaviors, such as lashing out to cope with these feelings and stress (Usher et al., 2020). This can manifest itself as *lateral violence*, which refers to a deliberate and harmful behavior demonstrated in the workplace by one employee toward another. This includes health care providers engaging in bullying and potentially assaultive behaviors toward co-workers (Nolte et al., 2017).

Early recognition of the risk for compassion fatigue is essential. A supportive work environment helps guide a nursing unit in designing communication techniques to identify, prevent, and adapt to potential compassion fatigue situations (Upton, 2018; Wells-English et al., 2019). For example, a nurse-led program on an oncology unit that included education, exercise, and social support was found to be effective in decreasing the nurses' compassion fatigue (Yilmaz et al., 2018). It is also important during stressful times, such as the COVID-19 pandemic, to work at managing your own mental health. Strategies you could use include accessing legitimate information to keep informed, talking about your stressors with co-workers, using social media to stay connected with family and friends, practicing self-care, using deep breathing and relaxation exercises, and maintaining a regular daily exercise routine (CDC, 2020; Wendekier and Kegerreis, 2020).

Second Victim Syndrome

Second victim syndrome affects health care providers when a medical error that results in significant harm to a patient and the patient's family occurs (Hartley, 2018). Often overlooked, nurses who have been involved in such a medical error can sustain complex psychological harm that can lead to detrimental outcomes such as suicide. These fatal errors can haunt nurses throughout their lives, leading to symptoms that are similar to posttraumatic stress disorder. One potential outcome is that nurses "move on" and work on gaining additional knowledge and skills to prevent errors in the future. But in many cases, nurses are reluctant to return to work because of fear of isolation from the organization, loss of confidence, remorse, depression, humiliation, and guilt (Hartley, 2018).

Being aware of the potential for second victim syndrome allows health care agencies to provide support the moment such an event occurs. Health care agencies need to provide support for as long as deemed necessary. Although the care and support of patients and families is a priority, the second victim has a right to be treated with respect and dignity and to be supported by peers and the organization. Proposed rights for second victims include respect, just treatment, understanding and compassion, supportive care, transparency, and the opportunity to contribute (Ozeke et al., 2019).

Before meeting with the Edwardses, Matt reviews John's electronic health record. Matt reads more on the risk factors for pancreatic cancer so that he can answer any questions that John and Sandra have about the progress of the disease. He finds the combination of chemotherapy drugs recommended by the oncologist. Matt researches the drugs to know their actions and expected adverse effects so that he can teach Sandra and John about John's therapy and what to expect. Matt knows that the diagnosis of cancer is causing stress for John, along with the additional stress of the chemotherapy he will receive. Matt is cognizant that situational, maturational, and sociocultural factors are contributing to the Edwardses' stress. He reviews these factors to be able to develop a patient-centered approach to their care. Matt also does additional reading on stress and coping so that he can be aware of early signs of distress in the couple and intervene quickly if needed. Matt recognizes that Sandra may experience additional caregiver stress and reviews interventions that can help Sandra. Matt makes sure to read up on the relationship between stress and hypertension, so he will be able to target interventions to help Sandra keep her blood pressure under control. Because Sandra and John do not have any family locally, Matt is especially concerned about social isolation becoming a problem

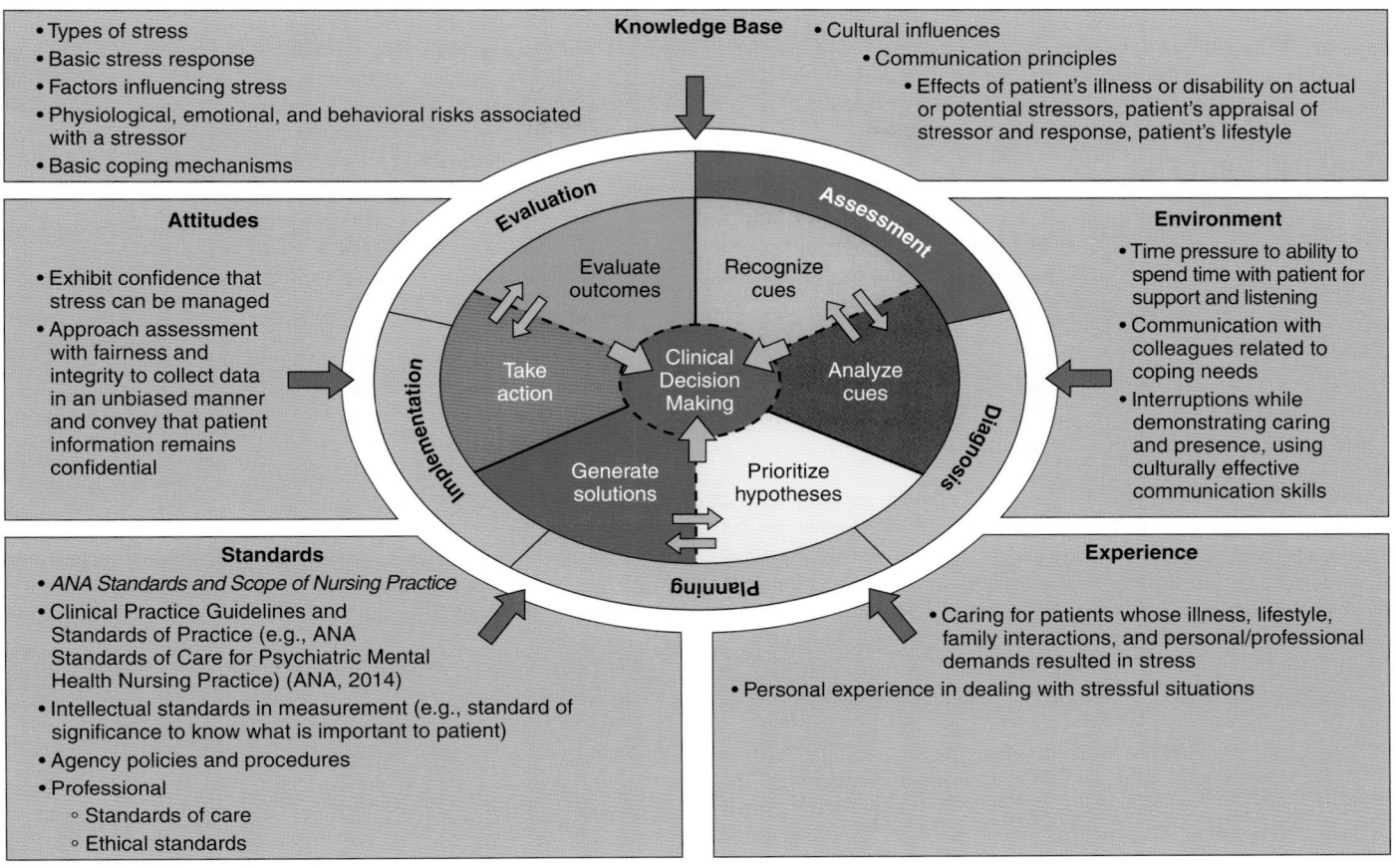

Knowledge Base

- Types of stress
- Basic stress response
- Factors influencing stress
- Physiological, emotional, and behavioral risks associated with a stressor
- Basic coping mechanisms

- Cultural influences
- Communication principles
- Effects of patient's illness or disability on actual or potential stressors, patient's appraisal of stressor and response, patient's lifestyle

Attitudes

- Exhibit confidence that stress can be managed
- Approach assessment with fairness and integrity to collect data in an unbiased manner and convey that patient information remains confidential

Environment

- Time pressure to ability to spend time with patient for support and listening
- Communication with colleagues related to coping needs
- Interruptions while demonstrating caring and presence, using culturally effective communication skills

Standards

- *ANA Standards and Scope of Nursing Practice*
- Clinical Practice Guidelines and Standards of Practice (e.g., ANA Standards of Care for Psychiatric Mental Health Nursing Practice) (ANA, 2014)
- Intellectual standards in measurement (e.g., standard of significance to know what is important to patient)
- Agency policies and procedures
- Professional
  - ◦ Standards of care
  - ◦ Ethical standards

Experience

- Caring for patients whose illness, lifestyle, family interactions, and personal/professional demands resulted in stress
- Personal experience in dealing with stressful situations

Evaluation · Assessment · Diagnosis · Planning · Implementation

Evaluate outcomes · Recognize cues · Clinical Decision Making · Analyze cues · Take action · Generate solutions · Prioritize hypotheses

FIG. 37.2 Critical thinking model for stress and coping assessment. *ANA,* American Nurses Association. (Clinical Judgment Measurement Model copyright © NCSBN. All rights reserved.)

during John's treatments. Matt gathers more information on social isolation and interventions that could be effective for the Edwardses. Matt also researches local support groups that might be of benefit for Sandra and John.

REFLECT NOW

What questions would you ask a patient to determine whether the stress is related to situational, maturational, or sociocultural factors?

CRITICAL THINKING

Successful critical thinking requires a synthesis of knowledge, experience, environmental factors, information gathered from patients, critical thinking attitudes, and intellectual and professional standards. Clinical judgments and critical thinking require you to anticipate information, analyze the data, recognize cues, and make decisions regarding your patient's care (Fig. 37.2). During assessment consider all elements that build toward making an appropriate nursing diagnosis.

Integrate knowledge from nursing and other disciplines, previous experiences, and information gathered from patients to understand stress and its effect on a patient and family. Know the neurophysiological changes that occur in a patient experiencing the alarm reaction, resistance stage, and exhaustion stage of the GAS. In addition, know communication principles that contribute to assessing a patient's behaviors.

Give utmost attention to determining the patient's perception of the situation and ability to cope with the stress. If a patient's usual coping skills have not helped or the support systems have failed, use crisis intervention counseling.

Experience teaches you to understand the patient's unique perspective and to recognize that no two people are alike. Experience with patients also helps you to recognize responses to stress. In addition, personal experiences with stress and coping increase your ability to empathize with a patient temporarily immobilized by stress.

Be confident in the belief that you and your patients can effectively manage stress. Patients who feel overwhelmed and perceive events as beyond their capacity to cope rely on you as an expert. Patients respect your advice and counsel and gain confidence from your belief in their ability to move past the stressful event or illness. Patients overwhelmed by life events are often unable, at least initially, to act on their own behalf and require either direct intervention or guidance. Integrity is an essential attitude that allows you to respect a patient's perception of the stressor. Encourage patients to explain their unique viewpoint and situation.

The practice standards for psychiatric mental health nursing (ANA, 2014) guide assessment of a patient's stress, coping mechanisms, and support system before intervening. The Substance Abuse and Mental Health Services Administration (2020) publishes national guidelines on the behavioral health crisis to help communities deal with crises. Use linguistic and culturally effective communication skills to understand a patient's perception of stress clearly and precisely. Focus on factors relevant to the patient's well-being. In addition, the patient expects you to exhibit confidence and integrity when he or she feels vulnerable. Be especially aware of the ethical responsibility in caring for someone who has reduced autonomy because of stress.

❖ NURSING PROCESS

Apply the nursing process and use sound clinical judgment and a critical thinking approach in your care of patients. The nursing process provides a clinical decision-making approach for you to develop and implement an individualized patient-centered plan of care.

◆ Assessment

During the assessment process, thoroughly assess each patient and critically analyze findings to ensure that you make patient-centered clinical decisions required for safe nursing care.

Through the Patient's Eyes. Assessment of a patient's stress level and coping resources requires that you first establish a trusting nurse-patient relationship because you are asking a patient to share personal and sensitive information. Learn from the patient both by asking questions and by observing nonverbal behavior and the patient's environment. Synthesize the information and adopt a critical thinking attitude while observing and analyzing patient behavior. Often a patient has difficulty in expressing exactly what is most bothersome about a situation until there is an opportunity to discuss it with someone who has time to listen.

Begin your assessment with an open-ended question, such as "What is happening in your life that caused you to come today?" or "What happened in your life that is *different*?" This requires the patient to focus. Next assess the patient's perception of the event, available situational supports, and what the patient usually does when there is an unsolvable problem. Determine whether a person is suicidal or homicidal by asking directly, "Are you thinking of hurting yourself or someone else?" If so, determine in a caring and concerned manner whether the person has a plan and the lethality of the plan (i.e., ingestion of pills versus self-inflicted gunshot wound).

Take time to understand the meaning of the precipitating event to the patient and the ways in which stress is affecting the patient's life. Allow time for the patient to express priorities for coping with stress. For example, in the case of a woman who has just been told that a breast mass was identified on a routine mammogram, it is important to know what the patient wants and needs most from the nurse. Although some women in this situation identify their need for information about biopsy or mastectomy as their personal priority, others need guidance and support in discussing how to share the news with family members.

Stress also occurs in a family or a community. Stress in a family sometimes arises from a critically ill family member, the sudden loss of a job, a move, or becoming homeless. Community stressors include a natural disaster such as a major flood, a sudden outbreak of a pandemic such as COVID-19, or the sudden, unexpected death of a beloved teacher or teenager. To develop appropriate and safe nursing care when caring for families or communities, ensure that you understand the meaning stress has for that group.

Environmental Factors. Create a nonthreatening, quiet environment when assessing a patient's level of stress and coping resources. Sit at the same height as the patient, arranging the interview environment with the chairs at a 90-degree angle or side by side so that you can maintain or avoid eye contact comfortably (Halter, 2018). Set aside sufficient time to talk with the patient, and ensure that your conversation will not be interrupted.

Subjective Findings. Begin to develop a trusting relationship with your patient while you gather information about the patient's health status from his or her perspective. Ask if the patient is experiencing any feelings of loneliness or isolation, or changes in eating or sleeping patterns, mobility levels, or other aspects of health. Use the interview to determine the patient's view of the stress, coping resources, any possible maladaptive coping, and adherence to prescribed medical recommendations such as medication or diet (Box 37.4). If the patient is using denial as a coping mechanism, assess whether the patient is overlooking necessary information. As in all interactions with the patient, respect the confidentiality and sensitivity of the information shared.

Objective Findings. Obtain objective findings related to stress and coping through observation of the appearance and nonverbal behavior of a patient. Observe overall appearance, paying attention to grooming and hygiene, gait, characteristics of the handshake, actions while sitting, quality of speech, eye contact, and the attitude of the patient during the interview. Before the interview begins or at the end of the interview, depending on the anxiety level of the patient, obtain basic vital signs to assess for physiological signs of stress, such as elevated blood pressure, heart rate, or respiratory rate. Make certain to incorporate cultural components of interpreting the patient's nonverbal communication behaviors.

Matt takes time to reflect on his previous experiences with patients experiencing high levels of stress due to a diagnosis of cancer. Many of the patients had physical complaints of stress, including headache, sleep problems, changes in eating habits, and flare-ups of existing medical problems. Previous experience with other patients with cancer has taught Matt the importance of learning about the patient's family, the type of support

---

BOX 37.4 Nursing Assessment Questions

Patient Safety
- Are you having difficulty with sleeping? How long does it take you to fall asleep?
- Are you having trouble staying awake during the day?
- What changes are you having in your eating patterns?
- Have you had any accidents at home, in the car, at school, or on the job?
- Do you have any thoughts of harming yourself or others?

Perception of Stressor
- What do you believe is stressing you right now?
- What impact does this stressor have on your lifestyle?
- How does this stressor impact you now? How will it impact you in the future?

Available Coping Resources
- Which strategies have you used in the past to deal with stress?
- Are you able to talk with friends or family?
- What is relaxing for you?

Maladaptive Coping Used
- Have you started using alcohol or tobacco to deal with your stress?
- Do you use any over-the-counter or herbal medications to manage your stress?
- Do you use any street drugs to cope?

Adherence to Healthy Practices
- How long ago did you see your health care provider?
- What is your exercise routine?
- What type of meals do you eat? Are your meals regular?
- Are you taking your prescribed medications as ordered?

available to the family, and the person's appraisal of the situation. Matt wants to be thorough in assessing the responses and symptoms that Sandra and John are experiencing. During the assessment process, Matt collects a great deal of information regarding the stressors that John and Sandra are experiencing. Through a process of systematic assessment, Matt also identifies the coping strategies and mechanisms that the Edwardses use more frequently. Matt now needs to identify ineffective coping patterns being used and the potential for adverse consequence of stress.

REFLECT NOW

What is the nurse's priority if a patient expresses thoughts of self-harm?

◆ Analysis and Nursing Diagnosis

Analysis of assessment data leads you to cluster data and look for cues that indicate a potential or actual stressor and the patient's response. You cannot make accurate nursing diagnoses based on just one or two assessment findings. Carefully review your patient's assessment data to consider whether more than one diagnosis applies. Clustering data, along with the application of your knowledge and experiences with patients in stress, leads to individualized nursing diagnoses (Box 37.5). For example, an individual who is experiencing stress may have the diagnosis of *Anxiety*, but the individual's stress can also impact the family, causing *Impaired Family Coping*. Examine the available data, validate assumptions with the patient, and look for other behaviors and symptoms before making a diagnosis.

As part of the diagnostic process, identify the appropriate "related to" factor for each negative or actual nursing diagnosis. Clarification of the related factors ensures that you select appropriate interventions. For example, a nursing diagnosis of *Difficulty Coping related to chronic back pain* requires different interventions than a diagnosis of *Difficulty Coping related to loss of spouse*.

Nursing diagnoses for people experiencing stress generally focus on coping. Specifically, major assessment findings of *Difficulty Coping* include verbalization of an inability to cope and an inability to ask for help. To gather assessment data, ask the patient what is of most concern at the time of the interview. It is important to allow patients sufficient

time to answer. Observe for nonverbal signs of anxiety, fear, anger, irritability, and tension, which may indicate ineffective coping. Other assessment findings include the presence of life stress, an inability to meet role expectations and basic needs, alteration in societal participation, self-destructive behavior, change in usual communication patterns, high rate of accidents, excessive food intake, drinking, smoking, and sleep disturbances. Stress or the inability to cope often results in multiple nursing diagnoses. Examples of these diagnoses include but are not limited to the following:

- Anxiety
- Despair
- Difficulty Coping
- Risk for Post Trauma Response
- Stress Overload

Through his assessment, Matt learns more about Sandra's stressors and how she perceives them. Sandra experiences pressures at work and home. This combination of stressors creates continuous intensity. Sandra's stress is affecting all aspects of her life, at work and at home, day and night. Sandra has felt the effects of stress for about 6 weeks. She has problems falling asleep and staying asleep. Sandra admits to having one to two glasses of wine at night to help herself relax and try to sleep. Sandra acknowledges that this is something new for her to do each night. She also reports problems with appetite and eating and feels overwhelmed and hopeless. She told Matt that she has lost 10 pounds over the few weeks since John's diagnosis of cancer. Sandra has multiple stressors. She has stress at home from being John's caregiver as he experiences nausea, vomiting, fatigue, and weakness from his chemotherapy. Sandra feels no control over her husband's illness and chemotherapy. Sandra questions her ability to manage John's care and her ability to complete her work project while caring for John. There is stress from work and the project she is managing. Sandra is telling herself that she is a failure, and she is afraid of losing her job if she cannot keep up with her boss's expectations and the timetable for her project. Sandra reports that she feels as if she does not have anyone to turn to for support currently since they have no family close to them. Matt observes Sandra frequently licking her lips, picking at her fingernails, and being easily startled. Sandra has poor eye contact and then bursts into tears and expresses feelings of being overwhelmed. Her vital signs show changes during the interview: pulse, 120 beats/min; respirations, 24 breaths/min; blood pressure, 168/84 mm Hg.

*As Matt analyzes these assessment findings, the data clusters provide him cues that lead him to identify **Difficulty Coping** as a priority nursing diagnosis for the plan of care. Along with this diagnosis, Matt recognizes that Sandra is also experiencing **Powerlessness** and **Anxiety** related to John's illness. Sandra appears thin and pale and her reports of a lack of appetite, not eating well, and weight loss lead Matt to select **Impaired Low Nutritional Intake: Deficient Food Intake** as another problem for Sandra.*

◆ Planning and Outcomes Identification

During the planning step of the nursing process, develop a plan of care for each of the patient's nursing diagnoses. Clinical judgment and critical thinking at this step are important because you reflect on previous experiences and environmental factors and apply knowledge, critical thinking attitudes, and intellectual standards in selecting the most appropriate nursing interventions.

Prior experience with other patients, your own nursing competence, and personal experience with stress are valuable when selecting interventions to help patients cope with stress. For example, you may have cared for a patient and family during a crisis and used strategies and interventions that helped both the patient and family cope with the stressor. Your competence in dealing with stress and your personal experience with stress provide you with insight on effective coping

---

BOX 37.5 Nursing Diagnostic Process
Difficulty Coping

Assessment Activities	Assessment Findings
Ask patient about change in sleeping patterns.	Sleep disturbance Difficulty falling asleep at night
Ask patient to complete a sleep diary for 2 weeks.	Excessive sleeping Frequent awakenings at night
Observe patient's behavior and response to questions during assessment.	Fatigue Inability to concentrate Inaccurate response to questions Inappropriate laugh or crying
Observe patient's appearance.	Poor grooming Lack of eye contact
Ask patient about changes in eating patterns.	Weight gain or loss Lack of interest in food

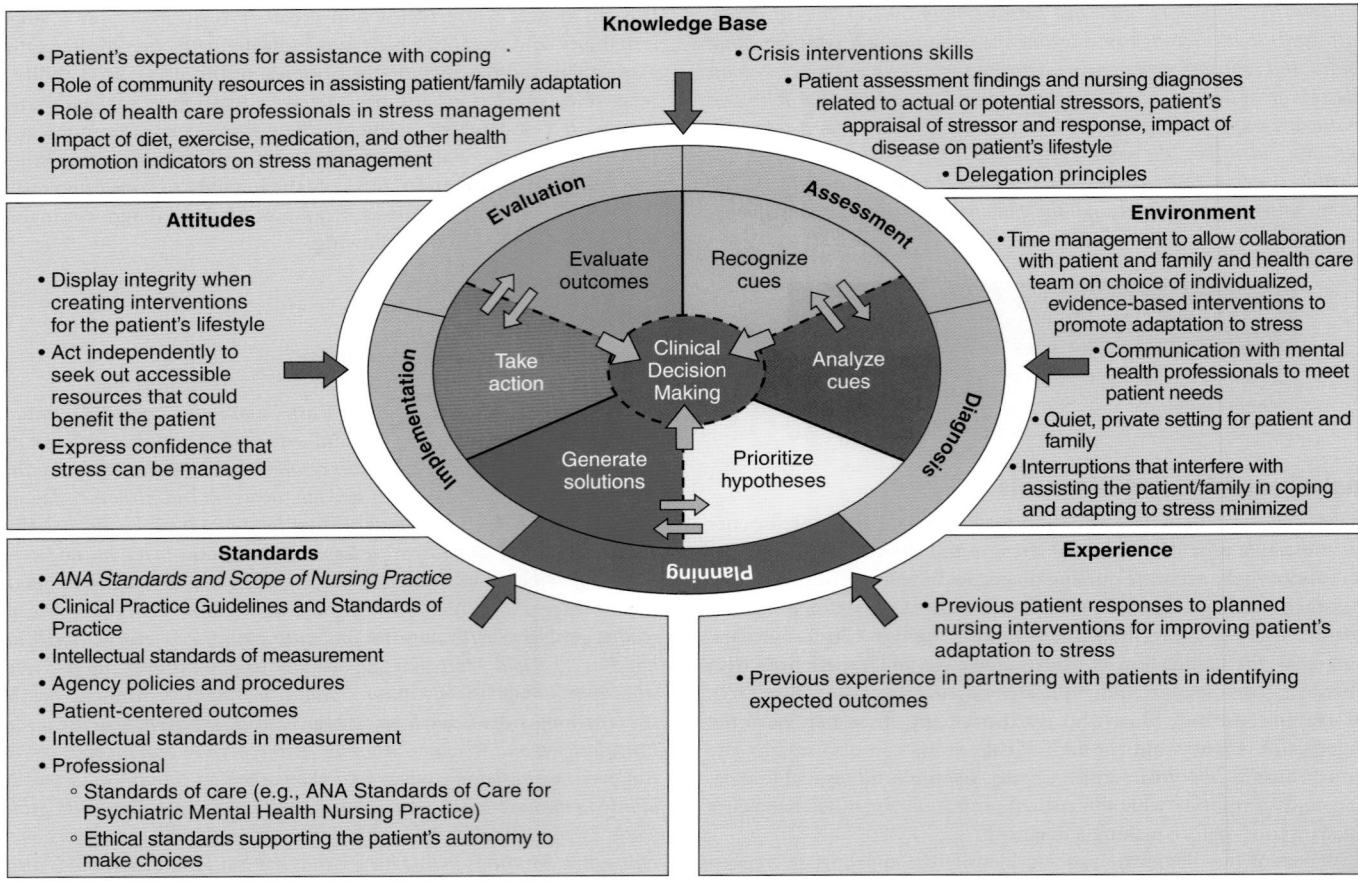

FIG. 37.3 Critical thinking model for stress and coping planning. *ANA,* American Nurses Association. (Clinical Judgment Measurement Model copyright © NCSBN. All rights reserved.)

strategies that can be used with patients and families. When you are helping patients and families deal with stress, make sure the environment is quiet and stress-free.

Outcomes. Planning nursing care for people experiencing stress frequently focuses on identified outcomes of effective coping, family coping, and family caregiver emotional health. The expected outcomes for a patient experiencing stress are either short- or long-term, depending on the nature of the stress and the patient's coping response. Examples of outcomes might include the following: patient engages in a support group, family members are able to discuss loss together, or caregiver participates in respite care. A nurse selects interventions for outcomes of reducing stress and improving coping, such as coping enhancement and crisis intervention. The nurse considers nursing diagnoses and the outcomes identified mutually with the patient when individualizing interventions and selecting resources available to a patient (Fig. 37.3). When developing a patient-centered plan of care, also consider the patient's preferences and culture when selecting interventions.

Nursing interventions for identified outcomes are designed within the framework of primary, secondary, and tertiary prevention. At the primary level of prevention, you direct nursing activities to identify individuals and populations who may be at risk for stress. Nursing interventions at the secondary level include actions directed at symptoms, such as protecting the patient from self-harm. Tertiary-level interventions help a patient re-adapt and can include relaxation training and time-management training. The nurse and patient assess the level and source of the existing stress and

determine the appropriate intervention to reduce it (Murdaugh et al., 2018) (see the Nursing Care Plan).

A concept map is a helpful tool in planning because it identifies multiple nursing diagnoses for a patient from the assessment database and shows how they are related (Fig. 37.4). In this example the nursing diagnoses are linked to the patient's medical diagnosis of depression. In addition, the concept map shows the relationship among the nursing diagnoses *Impaired Low Nutritional Intake: Deficient Food Intake, Difficulty Coping, Anxiety,* and *Powerlessness.* Use of a concept map requires clinical judgment and critical thinking to organize patient data and helps to plan for patient-centered care.

Just as the nursing assessment of a patient's stress and coping depends on the patient's perception of the problem and coping resources, the outcomes and interventions focus on a partnership with the patient and support system, usually the family. In the case of a family or community stressor and impaired family or community coping, the view of the situation and resources is broader.

REFLECT NOW

You are planning care for a patient with two school-age children who is also caring for a sick parent in her home. The patient's three siblings live within a 25-mile radius and refuse to help. A diagnosis of *Stress Overload* is included in the plan of care. Identify two appropriate outcomes for this nursing diagnosis.

⊚ NURSING CARE PLAN

Difficulty Coping

ASSESSMENT

Assessment Activities	*Assessment Findings*[a]
Ask Sandra how she feels about John's diagnosis.	Sandra states, **"I don't know how I feel. I am so tired and overwhelmed. I know I feel very alone."**
Ask John and Sandra about friends and relatives they have for support.	Both are only children and have **no other family**; they moved 1 year ago for new jobs. They work for different companies and state that they have **few close friends**.
Ask Sandra to identify people she can turn to for help.	Sandra **sobs** and **says that she does not have any friends she can rely on.** They are active in their church. On further discussion Sandra mentions a close friend from her hometown.
Ask Sandra about sleep and nutrition patterns.	She **can't get to sleep easily and awakens 3 to 4 times per night.** She states, "My appetite **is poor; I'm just not hungry. I think I've lost weight."**

[a]**Assessment findings** are shown in bold type.

NURSING DIAGNOSIS: Difficulty Coping related to insufficient social support

PLANNING

Expected Outcomes (NOC)[b]

Social Support

Sandra identifies at least one person in her community who can help support her in this crisis.

Sandra participates in a local support group weekly.

[b]Outcome classification labels from Moorhead S, et al: *Nursing Outcomes Classification (NOC),* ed 6, St Louis, 2018, Elsevier.

INTERVENTIONS (NIC)[c]	**RATIONALE**
Support System Enhancement	
Identify community-based cancer support systems for patients and family for Sandra and John.	Support systems for both patient and family are an effective intervention to cope with the stress of a cancer diagnosis and its related therapies and decision making (Meiner and Yeager, 2019).
Help Sandra identify a person who is willing to accompany her to some of John's appointments.	Having another person hear some of the treatment options and treatment procedures provides opportunities to clarify the discussion. During high-stress times social support helps with confidence and building resilience (Buchanan, 2021).
Explore community resources for a short-term educational group for both Sandra and John for self-care tools to reduce stress.	Educational groups help caregivers develop self-care tools to reduce stress, change negative self-talk, communicate more effectively, and make difficult decisions (Oken et al., 2018).

[c]Intervention classification labels from Butcher HK, et al: *Nursing Interventions Classification (NIC),* ed 7, St Louis, 2018, Elsevier.

EVALUATION

Evaluation Activities	*Patient Response*
Ask Sandra for the name of a person she can call for help during a crisis.	Sandra identified two people in her church community. One is a cancer survivor; the second is the spouse of a patient currently receiving cancer treatment.
Ask Sandra whether she attended a support group.	Sandra reports she has attended two sessions and is finding the sessions helpful. She plans on continuing to attend the sessions.

Setting Priorities. Consider the patient's perspective and responses to assessment questions when setting priorities for care (see the Nursing Care Plan). The patient's and family member's physical condition and perception of stressors determine which nursing diagnosis has the greatest priority. As in all areas of nursing, patient safety is the priority.

If suicide or homicide is not an issue, identify whether there are potential threats to the safety of people who are under the care of the patient. Provide for their temporary care or supervision if necessary. Other potential threats to safety include nutritional deficits, insomnia, self-care deficits, and poor judgment and impulsiveness that may lead to unsafe decisions about sex, drugs, money, or personal relationships that the person might later regret. Determine the degree of work, school, home, and family disruption in the person's life. After you have ensured safety, use problem solving with your patient to set priorities.

Based on his analysis of the assessment data, Matt recognizes that Sandra is having trouble coping, is using ineffective coping strategies, and wants to learn how to increase her resistance to stress. He has identified *Difficulty Coping* as the priority for Sandra. Based on this, Matt works with Sandra to identify agreed-on outcomes and to plan patient-centered personal care and support for her and John. The mutually agreed-on outcomes are "Sandra identifies at least one person in her community who can help support her in this crisis, and Sandra verbally identifies two methods to reduce her stress." Matt works to develop a plan that is patient-centered and considers Sandra's preferences.

Matt will ensure that Sandra's nutrition, sleep, and anxiety are managed before asking about her other priorities for care. Matt knows that Sandra has not received any information on support groups for her and John. Matt anticipates that Sandra and John will want to learn how to help John conserve his energy, improve his eating, and control his nausea. Matt knows that above all he will honor patient and family preferences, culture, and religious traditions during this stressful time.

Teamwork and Collaboration. Sometimes nursing practice alone does not meet all the patient's and family's needs. To effectively plan

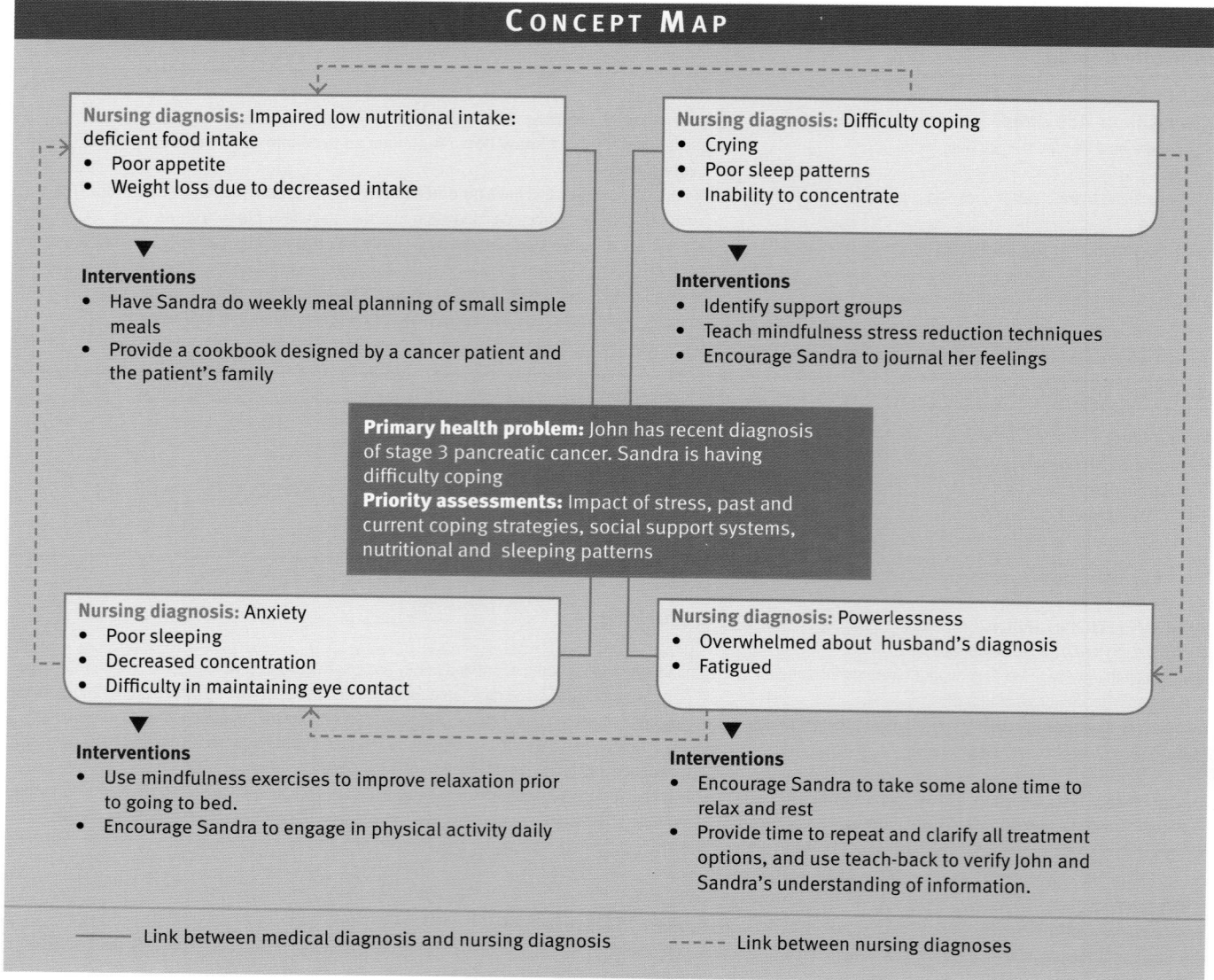

CONCEPT MAP

Nursing diagnosis: Impaired low nutritional intake: deficient food intake
- Poor appetite
- Weight loss due to decreased intake

Interventions
- Have Sandra do weekly meal planning of small simple meals
- Provide a cookbook designed by a cancer patient and the patient's family

Nursing diagnosis: Difficulty coping
- Crying
- Poor sleep patterns
- Inability to concentrate

Interventions
- Identify support groups
- Teach mindfulness stress reduction techniques
- Encourage Sandra to journal her feelings

Primary health problem: John has recent diagnosis of stage 3 pancreatic cancer. Sandra is having difficulty coping
Priority assessments: Impact of stress, past and current coping strategies, social support systems, nutritional and sleeping patterns

Nursing diagnosis: Anxiety
- Poor sleeping
- Decreased concentration
- Difficulty in maintaining eye contact

Interventions
- Use mindfulness exercises to improve relaxation prior to going to bed.
- Encourage Sandra to engage in physical activity daily

Nursing diagnosis: Powerlessness
- Overwhelmed about husband's diagnosis
- Fatigued

Interventions
- Encourage Sandra to take some alone time to relax and rest
- Provide time to repeat and clarify all treatment options, and use teach-back to verify John and Sandra's understanding of information.

——— Link between medical diagnosis and nursing diagnosis   - - - - - Link between nursing diagnoses

FIG. 37.4 Concept map for Sandra.

patient-centered and individualized care, collaborate with occupational therapists, registered dietitians, pastoral care professionals, and health care professionals from other clinical specialties, depending on the patient's situation.

Consulting with advanced practice mental health nurses, psychiatrists, psychologists, or licensed clinical social workers when a patient is experiencing stress from medical conditions or psychiatric disorders is necessary. An interprofessional approach addresses the holistic needs of the patient. Recognize the need for collaboration and consultation; inform the patient about potential resources; and arrange for interventions such as consultations, group sessions, or therapy as needed. A hospital social worker can share ideas for available resources both within the hospital and in the community. A home care nurse knows community services, support groups, and appropriate contacts.

In addition to maximizing the use of available resources for the patient, collaborative care also benefits the nurse. While working with patients experiencing stress, you gain a broad understanding of the multitude of health care disciplines. Work becomes more satisfying. Contacts with other members of the interprofessional team and the

community provide a feeling of contributing to the teamwork of providing holistic care.

◆ Implementation

Health Promotion. Three primary modes of intervention for stress are to decrease stress-producing situations, increase resistance to stress, and learn skills that reduce physiological response to stress (Murdaugh et al., 2018). Educate patients and families about the importance of health promotion (Box 37.6).

Regular Exercise and Rest. A regular exercise program improves muscle tone and posture, controls weight, reduces tension, and promotes relaxation (see Chapter 38). In addition, exercise reduces the risk of cardiovascular disease and improves cardiopulmonary functioning. Patients who have a history of a chronic illness, who are at risk for developing an illness, or are older than 35 years of age should begin a physical exercise program only after discussing the plan with a health care provider (Fig. 37.5).

Regular rest and sleep are also effective in reducing stress and stress-related fatigue. When stressful situations are present, encourage

BOX 37.6 PATIENT TEACHING

Stress Management

Objective
- Patient will report less anxiety, depression, and pain related to chronic health problems.

Teaching Strategies
- Familiarize patient with mind-body therapies that are likely to benefit patient. Refer to a group or specialized practitioner when necessary (Holman et al., 2018; Oken et al., 2018). Therapies include:
  - Meditation
  - Progressive muscle relaxation
  - Guided imagery
  - Hypnosis
  - Yoga
  - Tai chi
- Teach patient how to incorporate 15-30 minutes of exercise into daily activities (Kravitz, 2019).
- Instruct patient to identify and use relaxation techniques. For example:
  - Listen to music that you enjoy.
  - Keep a journal of your thoughts and feelings.
  - Replace unnecessary time-consuming activities with activities that are pleasurable or interesting.

Evaluation
Use the principles of teach-back to evaluate patient/family caregiver learning:
- Tell me how the stress-reduction techniques that we practiced help you to cope.
- Tell me how the mindfulness activities are impacting your anxiety and ability to sleep.
- Show me how you do the progressive muscle relaxation exercises.

FIG. 37.5 Regular exercise helps to cope with stress. (Courtesy Rudolph A. Furtado.)

patients and their family members to establish bedtime and sleep routines and try to stick to the schedule (see Chapter 43). Patients and family members who are well rested can manage stress, problem solve, and maintain a sense of control over the situation (Kravitz, 2019).

QSEN **Building Competency in Evidence-Based Practice** As a nurse educator in a diabetes management clinic, you recognize the value of exercise for patients with diabetes mellitus. However, you know many of your patients have difficulty committing to exercising regularly. You have located current research that supports types of interventions that are effective in promoting physical activity among adults who are chronically ill. Some of these interventions include (1) targeting physical activity exclusively, (2) using behavioral (as opposed to cognitive) strategies, (3) encouraging self-regulation and monitoring, (4) increasing access to exercise facilities, and (5) initially focusing on smaller quantities of physical activity (Phillips et al., 2016; Schwartz et al., 2019).

1. Describe the relationship between an individual's beliefs and that person's intentions for engaging in physical activity.
2. Identify possible barriers that prevent patients from initiating or maintaining an exercise plan. How can you help individuals overcome these barriers?

Answers to QSEN Activities can be found on the Evolve website.

Support Systems. A support system of family, friends, and colleagues who listen, offer advice, and provide emotional support benefits a patient experiencing stress (Sunne and Huntington, 2017). Many support groups are available to individuals (e.g., those sponsored by the American Heart Association, the American Cancer Society, hospitals, churches, and mental health organizations). Recent research shows that cancer survivors who effectively manage their stress make changes in their physical, psychosocial, and preventive health behaviors (Bily, 2017).

Time Management. Time-management techniques include developing lists of prioritized tasks. For example, help patients list tasks that require immediate attention, those that are important, those that can be delayed, and those that are routine and can be accomplished when time becomes available. In many cases setting priorities helps individuals identify tasks that are unnecessary or that can be delegated to someone else.

Guided Imagery and Visualization. Guided imagery is based on the belief that a person significantly reduces stress with imagination. It is a relaxed state in which a person actively uses imagination in a way that allows visualization of a soothing, peaceful setting. Typically, the image created or suggested uses many sensory words to engage the mind and offer distraction and relaxation (see Chapter 32).

Progressive Muscle Relaxation Therapies. In the presence of anxiety-provoking thoughts and events, a common physiological symptom is muscle tension (see Chapter 32). Progressive muscular relaxation diminishes physiological tension through a systematic approach to releasing tension in major muscle groups. Typically, an individual achieves a relaxed state through deep breathing. Once the patient is breathing deeply, direct the patient to alternately tighten and relax muscles in specific groupings (Pangotra et al., 2018; Tsitsi et al., 2017).

Assertiveness Training. Assertiveness includes skills for helping individuals communicate effectively regarding their needs and desires. The ability to resolve conflict with others through assertiveness training reduces their stress. Becoming certified in assertiveness training gives you the chance to teach assertiveness in group settings.

Journal Writing. Journal writing is beneficial for enhancing both psychological and physical health (Pavlacic, 2019). For many people keeping a private, personal journal provides a therapeutic outlet for stress. Suggest that patients keep journals, especially during difficult situations. In a private journal, patients can express a full range of emotion and vent their honest feelings without hurting anyone else's feelings and without concern for how they appear to others.

Mindfulness-Based Stress Reduction. Mindfulness is a moment-to-moment awareness of the present with a nonjudgmental attitude of acceptance and openness. This technique entails focusing on attentiveness on regular activities and truly enjoying pleasant experiences (Parsons et al., 2017). Mindfulness-based stress reduction (MBSR) meditative practices are effective in reducing psychological and physical symptoms or perceptions. They are effective in stress management and symptom control with certain chronic conditions (Box 37.7). Through mindfulness exercises people learn to self-regulate awareness and attention to feeling and to implement effective changes. Patients use cognitive exercises and subjective experiences to process images or feelings (Hofmann and Gomez, 2017). Patients evaluate these feelings as pleasant or unpleasant and learn strategies to enhance the pleasant experiences and replace the unpleasant experiences. Through MBSR patients can control their stress response to illnesses and treatments, employees can manage job-related stress, and students can learn to manage stress anxiety.

BOX 37.7 EVIDENCE-BASED PRACTICE

Impact of Mindfulness on Illness-Related Stressors

PICOT Question: Does the use of a mindfulness-based stress reduction (MBSR) program for adult patients affect their level of anxiety and depression and psychological well-being?

Evidence Summary

Prolonged and recurrent stress is associated with multiple psychological and health outcomes. A person's ability to cope with these stressors impacts physical and psychological health and may result in high rates of morbidity (Greeson et al., 2018; Oken et al., 2018). While conventional medical treatments for common stress-related symptoms may relieve symptoms, they fail to address the underlying causes of stress (Greeson et al., 2018). A participatory medicine approach that incorporates behavioral self-care practices (e.g., yoga, meditation) with conventional care is often beneficial. For example, patients who practiced yoga were effective in decreasing their anxiety and use of pain medication during a procedure (Kartin et al., 2017). Coping skills training in patients with diabetes decreased symptoms of depression and improved quality of life and metabolic control (Edraki et al., 2018). Mindfulness combined with yoga and physical activity has shown to be an effective combination to decrease stress and anxiety (deBruin et al., 2020).

Cognitive therapies, such as mindful meditation, have also been shown to improve subjective, patient-reported outcomes, including symptoms of stress, anxiety, depression, pain, fatigue, and quality of life (Oken et al., 2018; Greeson et al., 2018). Mindfulness is marked by a sense of focused attention, allowing an individual to consciously act versus automatically react to stress (Greeson et al., 2018).

Cognitive therapies such as meditation and MBSR help patients deal with illness-related stressors. Patients who use these therapies often are better at managing the symptoms and psychological distress associated with their chronic conditions (Grensman et al., 2018; Prothero et al., 2018). Individualize these therapies to the patient's needs, the ability to learn the therapy, and the concurrent treatment.

Application to Nursing Practice

- Assess a patient's perception of stress and specific coping strategies to help you identify the stressors and the patient's response to them (Grensman et al., 2018; Edraki et al., 2018).
- Identify priority coping strategies to improve the patient's quality of life and reduce symptoms (Grensman et al., 2018; Edraki et al., 2018).
- Consider a patient's limitations when discussing specific coping strategies to optimize the patient's experience and increase the chance of success (Greeson et al., 2018; Oken et al., 2018).
- When instructing patients about the use of these techniques, reinforce that these stress-management techniques are to be used in an addition to, not instead of, the patient's current treatment.

Stress Management in the Workplace. Stressors such as rapid changes in health care technology, diversity in the workforce, organizational restructuring, and changing work systems place stress on employees. Burnout occurs because of chronic stress. In nursing, burnout results when nurses perceive the demands of their work exceed perceived resources. It is manifested as emotional exhaustion, poor decision making, loss of a sense of personal identity, and feelings of failure.

It is important that nurses participate in self-care practices to help manage their stress. For example, in oncology settings many nurses experience compassion fatigue. Effective strategies for compassion fatigue and how to help nurses deal with this phenomenon are available (see Chapter 1). Health care agencies use mindfulness exercises, resilience training, staff relationship-building activities, and clinical debriefing to manage job-related stress and reduce burnout and nursing staff turnover (Brown et al., 2018). Recognizing the impact of shift work and changes in schedules enables some managers and nurses to use self-scheduling techniques. This reduces job-related stress and improves sleep quality, collaboration, and teamwork (Rizany et al., 2019).

Recognizing the areas over which you have control and can change and those for which you do not have responsibility is a vital insight. Making a clear separation between work and home life is also crucial. Strengthening friendships outside the workplace, participating in creative activities for personal "recharging" of emotional energy, and spending off-duty hours in interesting activities all help reduce compassion fatigue.

Social Isolation and Loneliness Prevention. Decreasing or preventing social isolation and loneliness can improve the health of older adults. Health-promoting goals focus on creating social interaction opportunities, improving the ability to cope with loneliness, and modifying behaviors and skill development to prevent loneliness (Fakoya et al., 2020). In an integrative review of research studies on interventions for the prevention and treatment of social isolation and loneliness, Gardiner et al. (2018) found that strategies could be aligned with one of six categories. The categories were: (1) social facilitation (e.g., participation in social clubs or shared interest topic groups); (2) psychological therapies (e.g., reminiscence therapy, mindfulness therapy); (3) health and social care provision (e.g., enrolling in a formal care program or rehabilitation group); (4) animal interventions (e.g., becoming a pet owner or using animal-assisted therapy); (5) befriending interventions (e.g., telephone interactions or volunteers becoming support persons to older adults); and (6) leisure skill development (e.g., doing volunteer work or joining gardening programs) (Gardiner et al., 2018). O'Rourke et al. (2018) identified similar categories in their integrative review on interventions to promote social connectedness. Research showed varying levels of effectiveness for strategies in each category (Gardiner et al., 2018; O'Rourke et al., 2018).

Working with Sandra and John, Matt implements the plan of care he and Sandra developed based on her preferences, expectations, and identified outcomes. Matt meets with Sandra in a quiet and private setting at a time when Sandra has about 1 hour to talk without interruptions. During this time, Matt encourages Sandra to express her feelings and concerns. Matt suggests that Sandra try to write about her feelings in a personal journal for the next week. Matt takes the time to teach Sandra about two stress-reduction techniques—regular exercise and mindfulness training. He encourages her to use the mindfulness relaxation techniques at bedtime to be able to sleep. Matt also talks to Sandra about trying to incorporate regular exercise into her routine. Matt gives Sandra an exercise log to keep a record of her activities for the upcoming week. Matt also encourages Sandra to take some time for herself, so she can rest and relax. He suggests that Sandra speak with her boss at work to see if she could get some help with her project during this high-stress period. Finally, Matt asks Sandra about any hobbies that she has that might help her relax.

When Matt finds out that Sandra likes to knit, he suggests that knitting might help reduce the stress she is experiencing and help her relax. Matt tells Sandra they will review her records at their next meeting. Matt then scheduled an hour-long follow-up meeting with Sandra for the following week.

Matt set up a meeting for Sandra and John with the registered dietitian (RD) who works at the Cancer Care Center. The RD worked with the couple to evaluate their eating habits. The RD also showed Sandra how to create a weekly meal plan of small healthy meals using the couple's food likes and preferences. Matt also suggested to the Edwardses that they reach out to their close friend from their church to see whether church members would be willing to help provide meals on a temporary basis. Before they left the appointment, Matt gave them a cookbook that was designed by patients who survived cancer and their families to help the Edwardses with meal planning.

Matt implemented interventions in the plan that focused on preventing social isolation for Sandra and John. He explored with them the social support they might find in their church. He encouraged Sandra to reach out to her closest friend at church when she felt a need to talk. Matt provided Sandra and John information on the support group that meets at the Cancer Care Center weekly. He encouraged them to attend the meetings as another source of support. Matt also discussed making a referral to home health services if John's condition should worsen and require nursing supervision and assistance with care at home.

Acute Care

Crisis Intervention. Crisis occurs when stress overwhelms a person's usual coping mechanisms and demands mobilization of all available resources. A crisis creates a turning point in a person's life because it changes the direction of life in some way. The precipitating event usually occurs approximately 1 to 2 weeks before the individual seeks help, but sometimes it has occurred within the past 24 hours. Generally, a person resolves the crisis in some way within approximately 6 weeks. Crisis intervention aims to return the person to a precrisis level of functioning and to promote growth.

Because an individual's or family's usual coping strategies are ineffective in managing the stress of the precipitating event during crisis, the use of new coping mechanisms is necessary. This experience forces the use of unfamiliar strategies and results in either a heightened awareness of previously unrecognized strengths and resources or deterioration in functioning. Thus, a crisis is often referred to as a situation of both danger and opportunity. Some individuals or families emerge from a crisis state functioning more effectively, whereas others find themselves weakened, and still others are completely dysfunctional.

Crisis intervention is a specific type of brief psychotherapy and has two specific goals. The first goal is patient safety. Use external controls to protect the patient and others if the person is suicidal or homicidal. The second goal is anxiety reduction using techniques that put a patient's inner resources into effect. Crisis intervention is more directive than traditional psychotherapy or counseling, and any member of the health care team who has been trained in its techniques can use it. The basic approach is problem solving, and it focuses only on the problem presented by the crisis (Halter, 2018). During crisis intervention, individuals value receiving prompt information to make decisions, being a partner in decision making, having trusting relationships with health care providers, and learning skills to be empowered (Nizum et al., 2020).

As part of this intervention, help patients make the mental connection between stressful events and their reactions to the events. This is crucial because they are sometimes unable to see the whole situation clearly. Help patients explore their feelings and emotions, such as anger, grief, or guilt, to help them reduce feelings of tension. In addition, you can help patients explore coping mechanisms, perhaps identifying new methods of coping. Finally, you help them increase social contacts if they have been isolated and overly self-focused.

Restorative and Continuing Care. A person under stress recovers when the stress is removed or coping strategies are successful; however, a person who has experienced a crisis has changed, and the effects often last for years or for the rest of the person's life. The final stage of adapting to a crisis is acknowledgment of its long-term implications. A person who has coped successfully with a crisis and its consequences becomes more mature and healthier. When a person recovers from a stressful situation, the time is right for introducing stress-management skills to reduce the number and intensity of stressful situations in the future.

◆ Evaluation

Through the Patient's Eyes. A patient recovering from acute stress often spontaneously reports feeling better when the stressor is gone. The recovery from chronic stress occurs more gradually as the patient emerges from the strain. Your evaluation must include the patient's perceptions. Ask the patient about sleep patterns, appetite, and ability to concentrate. Ask how the patient feels about coping strategies that are being used and determine their effectiveness. Ask patients to compare current feelings and behaviors with feelings and behaviors before the patient started to experience stress (e.g., 6 months ago).

An essential part of the evaluation process is to collaborate with patients to determine whether their own expectations from nursing have been met. Any revision in the plan of care includes steps to address patient expectations.

Patient Outcomes. Evaluation involves reassessing any new or recurring stress-related symptoms and whether the expected outcomes in the plan of care were achieved (Fig. 37.6). Remember that coping with stress takes time. Maintain ongoing communication with patients regarding their coping. Patients under severe stress or trauma often experience feelings of powerlessness, vulnerability, and loss of control. Address these feelings by actively involving patients and families in the processes of reexamining problems, prioritizing, identifying outcomes, and revising interventions. Involving patients in these processes gives them an opportunity to direct their energy in a positive way and moves them toward taking greater responsibility for health maintenance and promotion.

Engaging the patient as a partner in health care creates open communication. In such an environment the patient feels comfortable to give important feedback about interventions that are successful and helps you better understand why some interventions fail to meet the expected outcomes and established goals. If a patient reports continued acute stress, assess for safety by asking whether there have been any recent stressors at home or at work. Ask about coping strategies to determine whether the patient is using unsafe, maladaptive strategies. If the patient reports continued chronic stress, ask about perception of the stressor and the coping behaviors used. Discuss the stressor with the patient to determine whether it needs to be redefined. If contact with a patient ends before you have achieved the identified outcomes, it is important to refer the patient to appropriate resources so that progress is not delayed or interrupted.

Matt used teach-back to evaluate Sandra and John's learning. He asked Sandra to bring in her record of exercise and mindfulness activities from the previous week and then reviewed it with her. Matt praised Sandra for her exercising 4 out of 7 days and her use of mindfulness activities each day. Matt continued to monitor Sandra and John's stress levels weekly as they came in for John's chemotherapy appointments.

Three weeks after their initial discussion, Matt has another discussion with John and Sandra about their stress. Sandra expressed to Matt that her expectations for the plan have been met and that she feels as if she is better able to cope with her stress. Matt is relieved to see that Sandra is

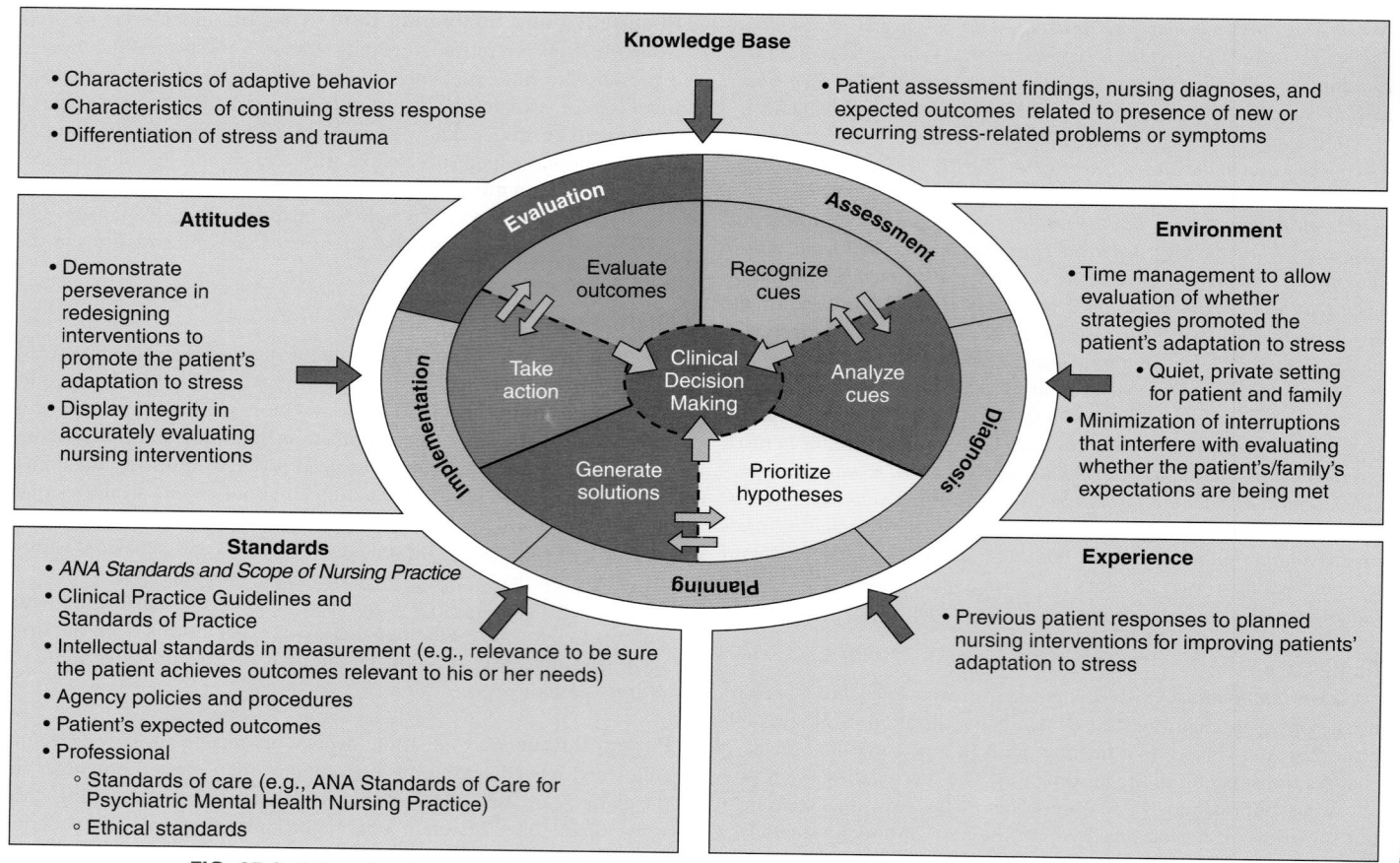

FIG. 37.6 Critical thinking model for stress and coping evaluation. (Clinical Judgment Measurement Model copyright © NCSBN. All rights reserved.)

less anxious and looking better. Her previously assessed nervous behaviors are no longer present. Sandra reports that she feels "more hopeful." Her blood pressure is 134/82 mm Hg, and pulse is 88 beats/min. Sandra says her appetite has improved, she has gained 3 pounds since their first discussion, and that this week she began sleeping through the night. Sandra's friends from church know about their situation and provide meals for John and Sandra two times a week. Sandra and John accept this help by reminding themselves that it is only temporary. Sandra tells Matt that she is going with her husband to a cancer support group meeting held every week at the Cancer Care Center. Although the Edwards family has not yet found full resolution for their stress because of John's ongoing illness and treatments, they are making progress toward achievable outcomes.

▌ KEY POINTS

- The general adaptation syndrome (GAS), an immediate physiological response to stress, has three stages: alarm (fight-or flight response), resistance (body responds to stress and attempts to compensate), and exhaustion (continued stress breaks down compensatory mechanisms) stages.
- Posttraumatic stress disorder begins when a person experiences, witnesses, or is confronted with a traumatic event and responds with intense fear or helplessness. Anxiety associated with PTSD is sometimes manifested by nightmares and emotional detachment.

- Many nursing theories, such as the Neuman Systems Model or Callista Roy's Adaptation Model, explain and describe stress and help you understand how an individual, family, or community effectively responds to stressors in the environment.
- Compassion fatigue is a state of burnout and secondary traumatic stress that can overwhelm health care providers and result in feelings of hopelessness, inadequacy, and anxiety.
- A regular exercise program improves muscle tone and posture, controls weight, reduces tension, and promotes relaxation.
- When personal stress is so severe, the person is unable to cope using any of the means that have worked before is experiencing a crisis. The process of crisis intervention aims to return the person to a precrisis level of functioning and promote growth.
- Assessment of a patient's stress level and coping resources requires that you first establish a trusting nurse-patient relationship because you are asking a patient to share personal and sensitive information.
- Three primary modes of intervention for stress are to decrease stress-producing situations, increase resistance to stress, and learn skills that reduce physiological responses to stress.
- In nursing, burnout results when nurses perceive that the demands of their work exceed perceived resources. It is manifested as emotional exhaustion, poor decision making, loss of a sense of personal identity, and feelings of failure.

REFLECTIVE LEARNING

It has been 9 months since John started his chemotherapy for pancreatic cancer, and Matt is meeting again with John and Sandra. John's most recent scans show that the tumor is not responding to the chemotherapy, and it has metastasized to the liver. The tumor is also obstructing John's common bile duct and partly obstructing his duodenum. He has lost 20 pounds over the last 6 months. John appears jaundiced, gaunt, and fatigued. He states, "I am tired all the time, feel very weak, and can barely get out of bed most mornings. I am having trouble with nausea, don't have any appetite, and food just doesn't taste good to me." John reports that he is having pain of 8 or 9 out of 10, which makes it hard for him to sleep and move around the house. John is on medical leave from his job at the manufacturing company. As John's condition worsens, Sandra is again having difficulty coping with the multiple stressors. To take care of John, Sandra took a leave from her job with the insurance company. When Matt assesses the couple, he once again notices that they both look tired; Sandra is disheveled. John tells Matt, "I am worried about Sandra. She looks so worn out from trying to take care of me. I wonder if she will be able to help me right now." Sandra tells Matt that since they found out about John's recent scan results, she has once again felt defeated, hopeless, and overwhelmed; has no energy; and has difficulty organizing her thoughts. She also reports that she is experiencing headaches, is having problems sleeping again, and that she has no appetite. Sandra appears to have lost weight over the last few months since Matt last saw the couple.

- What assessment information in the Edwardses' situation is the most important or of immediate concern for the nurse? (Recognize Cues)
- Considering the Edwardses' situation, what environmental, organizational, or other factors did you see that influence the Edwardses' stress and coping? (Analyze Cues)
- Considering the assessment data and history, what would be the priority nursing problem in caring for John and Sandra? (Prioritize Diagnoses)
- Identify two expected outcomes for John and Sandra. Consider the Edwardses' situation, and describe the nursing and medical interventions that you could utilize to achieve the expected outcomes. (Generate Solutions)
- Which nursing and medical interventions should have priority when implementing the care plan for John and Sandra? (Take Action)
- Considering the implementation of your plan of care for the Edwards couple, what assessment data should you gather to determine whether the interventions were effective? (Evaluate Outcomes)

REVIEW QUESTIONS

1. The nurse is interviewing a patient in the community clinic and gathers the following information about her: She is intermittently homeless and is a single parent with two children who have developmental delays. She has had asthma since she was a teenager. She does not laugh or smile, does not volunteer any information, and at times appears close to tears. She has no support system and does not work. She is experiencing an allostatic load. As a result, which of the following would be present during a complete patient assessment? (Select all that apply.)
   1. Posttraumatic stress disorder
   2. Rising hormone levels
   3. Chronic illness
   4. Insomnia
   5. Depression

2. A patient who is having difficulty managing his diabetes mellitus responds to the news that his hemoglobin A_{1c}, a measure of blood sugar control over the past 90 days, has increased by saying, "The hemoglobin A_{1c} is wrong. My blood sugar levels have been excellent for the last 6 months." Which defense mechanism is the patient using?
   1. Denial
   2. Conversion
   3. Dissociation
   4. Displacement

3. The nurse is caring for a patient who is suffering from posttraumatic stress disorder (PTSD) after a motor vehicle accident. What assessment findings reported by the patient provide cues to validate the diagnosis of PTSD? (Select all that apply.)
   1. Frequent feelings of anxiety
   2. Need to be around people
   3. Frequent nightmares
   4. Flashbacks to the accident
   5. Feelings of sadness

4. When assessing an older woman who is recently widowed, the nurse suspects that the woman is experiencing a developmental crisis. Which questions provide information about the impact of this crisis? (Select all that apply.)
   1. With whom do you talk on a routine basis?
   2. What do you do when you feel lonely?
   3. Tell me what your husband was like.
   4. I know this must be hard for you. Let me tell you what might help.
   5. Have you experienced any changes in lifestyle habits, such as sleeping, eating, smoking, or drinking?

5. The nurse plans care for a 16-year-old male, taking into consideration that stressors experienced most by adolescents include which of the following? (Select all that apply.)
   1. Loss of autonomy caused by health problems
   2. Physical appearance and body image
   3. Accepting one's personal identity
   4. Separation from family
   5. Taking tests in school

6. A 10-year-old girl was playing on a slide at a playground during a summer camp. She fell and broke her arm. The camp notified the parents and took the child to the emergency department according to the camp protocol for injuries. The parents arrive at the emergency department and are stressed and frantic. The 10-year-old is happy in the treatment room, eating a Popsicle and picking out the color of her cast. List in order of priority what the nurse should say to the parents.
   1. "Can I contact someone to help you?"
   2. "Your daughter is happy in the treatment room, eating a Popsicle and picking out the color of her cast."
   3. "I'll have the doctor come out and talk to you as soon as possible."
   4. "I want to be sure you are OK. Let's talk about what your concerns are about your daughter before we go see her."

7. When assessing an older adult who is showing symptoms of anxiety, insomnia, anorexia, and mild confusion, what is the first assessment the nurse conducts?
   1. The amount of family support
   2. A 3-day diet recall
   3. A thorough physical assessment
   4. Threats to safety in her home

8. A 34-year-old single father who is anxious, tearful, and tired from caring for his three young children tells the nurse that he feels depressed and does not see how he can go on much longer. Which statement would be the nurse's best response?
   1. "Are you thinking of suicide?"
   2. "You've been doing a good job raising your children. You can do it!"
   3. "Is there someone who can help you during the evenings and weekends?"
   4. "Tell me what you mean when you say you can't go on any longer."

9. The nurse is evaluating how well a patient newly diagnosed with multiple sclerosis and psychomotor impairment is coping. Which statements indicate that the patient is beginning to cope with the diagnosis? (Select all that apply.)
   1. "I'm going to learn to drive a car, so I can be more independent."
   2. "My sister says she feels better when she goes shopping, so I'll go shopping."
   3. "I'm going to let the occupational therapist assess my home to improve efficiency."
   4. "I've always felt better when I go for a long walk. I'll do that when I get home."
   5. "I'm going to attend a support group to learn more about multiple sclerosis."

10. A crisis intervention nurse is working with a mother whose child with Down syndrome is hospitalized with pneumonia and who has lost her child's disability payment while the child is hospitalized. The mother worries that her daughter will fall behind in her classes during hospitalization. Which strategies are effective in helping this mother cope with these stressors? (Select all that apply.)
    1. Referral to social service process reestablishing the child's disability payment
    2. Sending the child home in 72 hours and having the child return to school
    3. Coordinating hospital-based and home-based schooling with the child's teacher
    4. Teaching the mother signs and symptoms of a respiratory tract infection
    5. Telling the mother that the stress will decrease in 6 weeks when everything is back to normal

Answers: 1. 3, 4, 5; **2.** 1; **3.** 1, 3, 4, 5; **4.** 1, 2, 5; **5.** 2, 3, 4, 5; **6.** 2, 4, 3; **7.** 3; **8.** 4; **9.** 3, 5; **10.** 1, 3, 4.

Rationales for Review Questions can be found on the Evolve website.

REFERENCES

Alharbi J, et al: The potential for COVID-19 to contribute to compassion fatigue in critical care nurses, *J Clin Nurs* 29(15-16):2762, 2020.

American Nurses Association (ANA): *Psychiatric–mental health nursing: scope and standards of practice*, ed 2, Silver Spring, MD, 2014, ANA.

Banasik JL, Copstead LC: *Pathophysiology*, ed 6, St Louis, 2019, Elsevier.

Buchanan L: Stress and coping. In Giddens JF, editor: *Concepts for nursing practice*, ed 3, St. Louis, 2021, Elsevier.

Centers for Disease Control and Prevention (CDC): *Healthcare personnel and first responders: how to cope with stress and build resilience during the COVID-19 pandemic*, 2020. https://www.cdc.gov/coronavirus/2019-ncov/hcp/mental-health-healthcare.html. Accessed March 9, 2021.

Cherry B, Jacob SR: *Contemporary nursing: issues, trends, & management*, ed 8, St Louis, 2019, Elsevier.

Giger JN, Haddad LG: *Transcultural nursing: assessment and intervention*, ed 8, St Louis, 2021, Elsevier.

Halter MJ: *Varcarolis' foundations of psychiatric mental health nursing: a clinical approach*, ed 6, St Louis, 2018, Elsevier.

Hofmann SG, Gomez AF: Mindfulness-based interventions for anxiety and depression, *Psychiatr Clin North Am* 40(4):739, 2017.

Holman D, et al: Stress management interventions: improving subjective psychological well-being in the workplace. In Diener E, et al., editors: *Handbook of well-being*. Salt Lake City, UT, 2018, DEF Publishers.

Huether SE, et al: *Understanding pathophysiology*, ed 7, St Louis, 2020, Elsevier.

Jackson JS, et al: Social relations, productive activities, and coping with stress in late life. In Stephens MA, et al., editors: *Stress and coping in later-life families (ebook)*, New York, 2018, Taylor & Francis.

Kravitz L: Exercise is good for mental health: but keep in mind that overdoing it does more harm than good. *IDEA Fitness Journal* 16(1):12, 2019.

Lawson TG: Systems model. In Alligood MR, editor: *Nursing theorists and their work*, ed 9, St. Louis, 2018, Elsevier.

Liu JW, et al: Re-conceptualizing stress: shifting views on the consequences of stress and its effects on stress reactivity, *PLoS One*, 12(3):e0173188, 2017. doi: 10.1371/journal.pone.0173188. Accessed July 12, 2020.

Meiner SE, Yeager JJ: *Gerontologic nursing*, ed 6, St Louis, 2019, Elsevier.

Murdaugh CL, et al: *Health promotion and nursing practice*, ed 8, Boston, MA, 2018, Pearson.

Neuman B, Fawcett J, editors: *The Neuman systems model*, ed 5, Upper Saddle River, NJ, 2011, Pearson.

Ozeke O, et al: Second victims in health care: current perspectives, *Adv Med Educ Pract* 10:593, 2019.

Sacks SA, et al: A pilot study of the trauma recovery group for veterans with post traumatic stress disorder and co-occurring serious mental illness, *J Ment Health* 26(3):237, 2017.

Schwartz J, et al: Effectiveness of approaches to increase physical activity behavior to prevent chronic disease in adults: a brief commentary, *J Clin Med* 8(3):295, 2019.

Selye H: Stress and the general adaptation syndrome, *Br Med J* 1(4667):1383, 1950.

Selye H: History of the stress concept. In Goldberger L, Breznitzs, editors: *Handbook of stress: theoretical and clinical aspects*, ed 2, New York, 1993, Free Press.

Substance Abuse and Mental Health Services Administration (SAMHSA): *National guidelines for behavioral health crisis care: best practice toolkit*, 2020, https://www.samhsa.gov/sites/default/files/national-guidelines-for-behavioral-health-crisis-care-02242020.pdf. Accessed July 13, 2020.

Touhy TA, Jett KF: *Ebersole & Hess' toward healthy aging E-Book: human needs and nursing response*, 10 ed, St. Louis, 2020, Elsevier.

Touhy TA, Jett KF: *Ebersole & Hess' gerontological nursing &heathy aging*, 6 ed, St. Louis, 2022, Elsevier.

Usher K, et al: The COVID-19 pandemic and mental health impacts, *Int J Ment Health Nurs* 29:315, 2020.

Wendekier C, Kegerreis K: *Nurse compassion fatigue*, 2020, https://www.chausa.org/publications/health-progress/article/nurses/nurse-compassion-fatigue, Accessed March 9, 2021.

RESEARCH REFERENCES

Antony L, et al: Stress, coping, and lived experiences among caregivers of cancer patients on palliative care: a mixed method research, *Indian J Palliat Care* 24(3):313, 2018.

Bethell J, et al: Social integration and loneliness among long-term care home residents: protocol for a scoping review, *BMJ Open* 9:e033240, 2019.

Bily L: Creative therapeutic activities and support groups benefit all those involved in cancer care, *Am Health Drug Benefits* 10(6), 2017.

Brown S, et al: The impact of resiliency on nurse burnout: an integrative literature review. *Medsurg Nurs* 27(6):349, 2018.

Casey G, Tiaki K: Stress and disease. *Nurs N Z* 23:20, 2017.

deBruin EI, et al: Mindful2Work the next steps: effectiveness of a program combining physical exercise, yoga and mindfulness, adding a wait-list period, measurements up to one year later and qualitative interviews, *Complement Ther Clin Pract* 39:101137, 2020.

Edraki M, et al: The effect of coping skills training on depression, anxiety, stress, and self-efficacy in adolescents with diabetes: a randomized controlled trial, *Int J Community Based Nurs Midwifery* 6(4): 324–333, 2018.

Enns A, et al: Perceived stress, coping strategies, and emotional intelligence: a cross-sectional study of university students in helping disciplines, *Nurse Educ Today* 68:226, 2018.

Fakoya OA, et al: Loneliness and social isolation interventions for older adults: a scoping review of reviews, *BMC Public Health* 20:129, 2020.

Gardiner C, et al: Interventions to reduce social isolation and loneliness among older people: an integrative review, *Health Soc Care Community* 26(2):147, 2018.

Greeson JM, et al: Mindfulness meditation targets transdiagnostic symptoms implicated in stress-related disorders: understanding relationships between changes in mindfulness, sleep quality, and physical symptoms, *Evid Based Complement Alternat Med* 2018: 4505191, 2018.

Grensman A, et al: Effect of traditional yoga, mindfulness-based cognitive therapy, and cognitive behavioral therapy, on health related quality of life: a randomized controlled trial on patients on sick leave because of burnout, *BMC Complement Altern Med* 18(1):80, 2018.

Hartley H: Concept review: second traumatization and the role of a perioperative advanced practice nurse, *ORNAC J* 36(4):37, 2018.

Kartin PT, et al: The effect of meditation and music listening on the anxiety level, operation tolerance and pain perception in people who were performed colonoscopy, *Int J Caring Sci* 10(3):1587, 2017.

Mealer M, et al: Designing a resilience program for critical care nurses, *AACN Adv Crit Care* 28(4):359, 2017.

Nena E, et al: Effect of shift work on Sseep, health, and quality of life of health-care workers, *Indian J Occup Environ Med* 22(1):29, 2018.

Nieto M, et al: Differences in coping strategies between young and older adults: the role of executive functions, *Int J Aging Hum Dev* 90(1):28, 2019.

Nizum N, et al: Nursing interventions for adults following a mental health crisis: a systematic review guided by trauma-informed principles, *Int J Ment Health Nurs* 29(3):348, 2020.

Nolte AGW, et al: Compassion fatigue in nurses: a metasynthesis, *J Clin Nurs* 26:4364, 2017.

O'Brien B, et al: Positive and negative religious coping as predictors of distress among minority older adults, *Geriatric Psychiatry* 34(1):54, 2019.

Oken BS, et al: Predictors of improvements in mental health from mindfulness meditation in stressed older adults, *Altern Ther Health Med* 24(1):48, 2018.

O'Rourke HM, et al: Interventions to address social connectedness and loneliness for older adults: a scoping review, *BMC Geriatrics* 18:214, 2018.

Pangotra A, et al: Effectiveness of progressive muscle relaxation, biofeedback and l-theanine in patients suffering from anxiety disorder, *J Psychosoc Res* 13(1):219, 2018.

Parsons CE, et al: Home practice in mindfulness-based cognitive therapy and mindfulness-based stress reduction: a systematic review and meta-analysis of participants' mindfulness practice and its association with outcomes, *Behav Res Ther* 95(29), 2017.

Pavlacic J, et al: A meta-analysis of expressive writing on posttraumatic stress, posttraumatic growth, and quality of life, *Rev Gen Psychol* 23(2):230, 2019.

Phillips LA, et al: Self-management of chronic illness: the role of 'habit' versus reflective factors in exercise and medication adherence, *J Behav Med* 39(6):1076, 2016.

Prothero L, et al: The evidence base for psychological interventions for rheumatoid arthritis: a systematic review of reviews, *Int J Nurs Stud* 82:20, 2018.

Rizany I, et al: The impact of nurse scheduling management on nurses' job satisfaction in army hospital: a cross-sectional research, *Sage Open* 9(2):1, 2019.

Shavitt S, et al: Culture moderates the relation between perceived stress, social support, and mental and physical health, *J Cross Cult Psychol* 47(7):956, 2016.

Solomon D, et al: Multicenter study of nursing role complexity on environmental stressors and emotional exhaustion, *Appl Nurs Res* 30:52, 2016.

Sunne R, Huntington MK: The 36 hour day, revisited: implementing a caregiver support system into primary care practice, *S D Med* 70(4):173, 2017.

Tsitsi T, et al.: Effectiveness of a relaxation intervention (progressive muscle relaxation and guided imagery techniques) to reduce anxiety and improve mood of parents of hospitalized children with malignancies: A randomized controlled trial in Republic of Cyprus and Greece, *Eur J Oncol Nurs* 26, 9, 2017.

Ueno S, et al: Occupational stress: stressors referred by the nursing team, *J Nurs* 11(4):1632, 2017.

Upton KV: An investigation into compassion fatigue and self-compassion in acute medical care hospital nurses: a mixed methods study, *J Compassionate Health Care* 5:7, 2018.

Wells-English D, et al: Compassion fatigue and satisfaction: Influence on turnover among oncology nurses at an urban cancer center, *Clin J Oncol Nurs* 23(5):487, 2019.

Yilmaz G, et al: Effect of a nurse-led intervention programme on professional quality of life and post-traumatic growth in oncology nurses, *Int J Nurs Pract* 24(6):e12687, 2018.

38

Activity and Exercise

OBJECTIVES

- Discuss the role of the musculoskeletal and nervous systems in the regulation of activity and exercise.
- Examine how exercise and activity maintain and promote health.
- Explain the principles and benefits of safe patient handling.
- Analyze the relationship between clinical judgment and critical thinking in making clinical decisions to improve patients' activity.
- Discuss how to assess patients for level of activity tolerance.
- Explain the approach for assessing a patient's readiness to exercise.
- Select outcomes for patients' nursing diagnoses associated with activity and exercise.

- Explain how sound clinical judgment allows for individualizing interventions for improving an individual's activity tolerance.
- Determine the safe patient-handling techniques to use when transferring a patient from bed to stretcher.
- Explain nurses' responsibility in assisting patients to ambulate safely.
- Evaluate the achievement of patient outcomes following implementation of exercise therapies.

KEY TERMS

Activity tolerance
Activities of daily living
Body alignment
Body mechanics
Cartilaginous joints
Center of gravity

Concentric tension
Crutch gait
Deconditioning
Eccentric tension
Fibrous joints
Isometric contraction

Isotonic contraction
Muscle tone
Proprioception
Stretch reflex
Synovial joints
Unossified

MEDIA RESOURCES

http://evolve.elsevier.com/Potter/fundamentals/
- Review Questions
- Video Clips
- Concept Map Creator
- Case Study with Questions

- Audio Glossary
- Content Updates
- Answers to QSEN Activity and Review Questions
- Skills Performance Checklists

Mrs. Smith is a 52-year-old housewife. She is overweight (admission record shows height and weight as 170 cm and 82.6 kg (5 feet 7 inches and 182 lb) and recently was diagnosed with type 2 diabetes. During a visit to her primary care provider, she tells the nurse practitioner that she always feels tired. Over the last 2 months she has been participating less in family activities involving going outside. Mrs. Smith also has a history of heart failure, which is controlled and treated with medication. She expresses feelings of stress caused by excessive demands on her time at work as a bookkeeper for her husband's small business. She expresses her concerns, saying, "I just feel like a blob. I know I have to do something. I guess I have to start exercising." The nurse practitioner, Beth, will conduct an assessment and apply her knowledge and experience, knowing that Mrs. Smith will benefit from a targeted regular exercise plan.

Regular physical activity and exercise contribute to individuals' physical and emotional well-being. According to the American Heart Association (2018), physical activity:
- Elevates mood and attitude.
- Keeps us physically fit.
- Helps individuals quit smoking and stay tobacco-free.
- Boosts energy level so that individuals can get more done.
- Helps in the management of stress.
- Promotes a better quality of sleep.
- Improves self-image and self-confidence.

Promoting activity and exercise is a principle to apply in the care of patients in all health care settings. It is important to promote activity in a safe and efficient manner, especially for patients who are functionally impaired and in need of your assistance. Patients must have a level of motivation to engage in regular exercise. Your use of critical thinking in clinical judgment will enable you to select activity and exercise strategies that match patients' willingness to participate and benefit their physical and psychosocial health. A program of regular physical activity and exercise has the potential to enhance all aspects of a patient's health.

Frequently patients experience functional decline (the loss of the ability to perform self-care or activities of daily living). Such decline may result not only from illness or adverse treatment effects but also from deconditioning associated with imposed inactivity. You can see the negative effects of deconditioning after very short periods of time, such as hospitalization. Deconditioning involves physiological changes after a period of inactivity (e.g., bed rest or sedentary lifestyle). It is a particular risk for patients who are hospitalized and spend most of their time in bed, even when they are able to walk. Chapter 39 discusses deconditioning in more detail. As a result, nurses play an important role in routinely increasing the overall activity of inpatients to minimize the risk of deconditioning.

Nurses commonly assist patients who are physically dependent. Walking, turning, lifting, and carrying are all common actions used in the delivery of nursing care. These activities pose risks to health care workers, who frequently experience injuries, such as back injuries or overexertion, when moving or lifting patients incorrectly. You will apply safe patient-handling standards and principles to reduce the risk of injury to patients and yourself when assisting patients with activity and exercise.

SCIENTIFIC KNOWLEDGE BASE

Regular physical activity and exercise contribute to physical and emotional well-being. Knowing the physiology and regulation of body movement and exercise and the principles for safe transfer and positioning helps you to understand the impact a patient's health condition has on activity. This knowledge base is essential for the critical thinking needed to recognize and identify a patient's problems and select appropriate activity and exercise interventions.

Nature of Movement

Movement is a complex process that requires coordination between the musculoskeletal and nervous systems. As a nurse you will consider how a patient's physical and psychological conditions affect body movement. Body mechanics is a term that describes the coordinated efforts of the musculoskeletal and nervous systems. Knowing how patients initiate movement and understanding your own movements require a basic grasp of the physics surrounding body mechanics. The body mechanics applied in the lifting techniques historically used in nursing practice often caused debilitating injuries to nurses and other health care staff (Kanaskie and Snyder, 2018; Noble and Sweeney, 2018). Today nurses use evidence-based information about body alignment, balance, gravity, and friction when implementing nursing interventions such as transferring patients, assisting with ambulation, determining the risk of patient falls, and selecting the safest way to move or transfer patients (Kruschke and Butcher, 2017).

Alignment and Balance

The terms body alignment and "posture" are similar and refer to the positioning of the joints, tendons, ligaments, and muscles while standing, sitting, and lying. Body alignment means that an individual's center of gravity is stable. Correct body alignment reduces strain on musculoskeletal structures, aids in maintaining adequate muscle tone, promotes comfort, and contributes to balance and conservation of energy. Without balance control the center of gravity is displaced.

Individuals require balance for maintaining a static position (e.g., sitting) and moving (e.g., transferring or walking). Disease, injury, pain, physical development (e.g., age), and life changes (e.g., pregnancy) compromise the ability to remain balanced. Medications that cause dizziness and prolonged immobility affect balance. Impaired balance is a major threat to mobility and physical safety and contributes to a fear of falling and self-imposed activity restrictions (Dickinson et al., 2018; Musich et al., 2018).

Gravity and Friction

Weight is the force exerted on a body by gravity. The force of weight is always directed downward, which is why an unbalanced object falls. Patients fall if their center of gravity becomes unbalanced because of the gravitational pull on their weight. To lift safely, the lifter has to overcome the weight of the object and know its center of gravity. In symmetrical inanimate objects the center of gravity is at the exact center of the object. However, people are not geometrically perfect; their centers of gravity are usually at 55% to 57% of standing height and are in the midline, which is why using only the principles of body mechanics in lifting patients often leads to injury of a nurse or other health care professional.

Friction is a force that occurs in a direction to oppose movement. The greater the surface area of the object that is moved, the greater is the friction. A larger object produces greater resistance to movement. In addition, the force exerted against the skin while the skin remains stationary and the bony structures move is called shear. Unfortunately, a common example is when the head of a hospital bed is elevated beyond 60 degrees and gravity pulls a patient so that the bony skeleton moves toward the foot of the bed while the skin remains against the sheets. The blood vessels in the underlying tissue are stretched and damaged, resulting in impeded blood flow to the deep tissues. Ultimately pressure injuries often develop within the undermined tissue; the surface tissue appears less affected (see Chapter 39 and 48). To decrease surface area and reduce friction when patients are unable to assist with moving up in bed, nurses use ergonomic assistive devices such as a full-body sling. The sling mechanically lifts a patient off the surface of a bed, thereby preventing friction, tearing, or shearing of the patient's delicate skin; it also protects nurses and other health care staff from injury (Noble and Sweeny, 2018) (see Chapter 39).

Regulation of Movement

Coordinated body movement involves the integrated functioning of the musculoskeletal and nervous systems. Because these systems work together dynamically, they are often considered as a single functional unit.

Skeletal System. The skeletal system provides attachments for muscles and ligaments and the leverage necessary for mobility. Thus, the skeleton is the supporting framework of the body and is made up of four types of bones: long, short, flat, and irregular. Bones are important for movement because they are firm, rigid, and elastic. Some nutritional and disease processes and the aging process have the potential to change the components of bone, which impacts mobility.

Firmness results from inorganic salts such as calcium and phosphate that are in the bone matrix. It is related to the rigidity of the bone, which is necessary to keep long bones straight, and enables bones to withstand weight-bearing. Elasticity and skeletal flexibility change with age. A newborn has a large amount of cartilage and is highly flexible but is unable to support weight. A toddler's bones are more pliable than those of an older person and are better able to withstand traumatic injury. Older adults, especially women, are more susceptible to bone loss (resorption) and osteoporosis, which increases the risk of fractures.

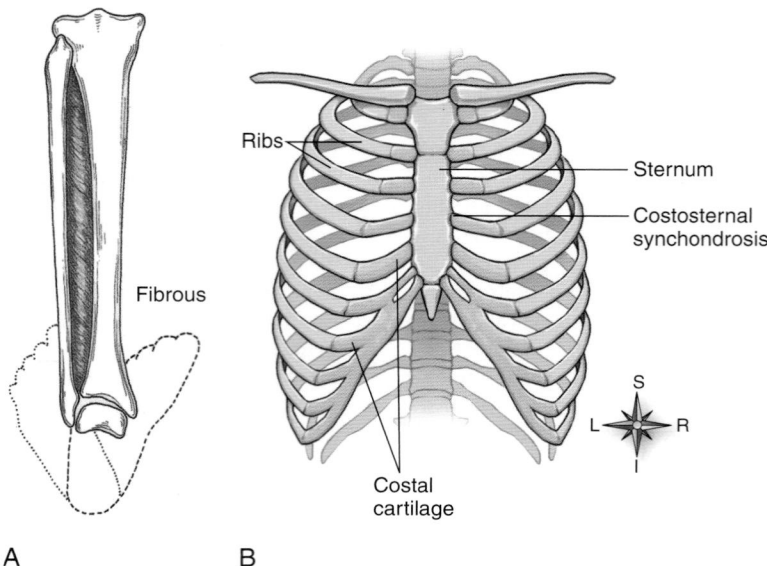

FIG. 38.1 Joint types. (A) Fibrous. (B) Cartilaginous. (B from Patton KT: *Anatomy & physiology*, ed 10, St Louis, 2019, Elsevier.)

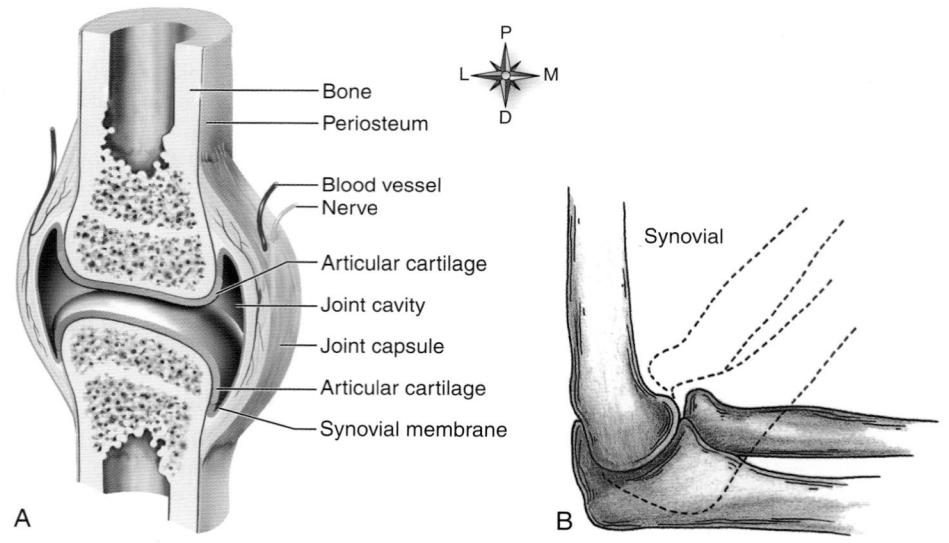

FIG. 38.2 (A) Structure of synovial joint. (B) Synovial joint. (From Patton KT: *Human body in health and disease*, ed 7, St Louis, 2018, Elsevier.)

Joints. The region where two or more bones attach is referred to as a joint. Each joint is classified according to its structure and degree of mobility. There are three classifications of joints: fibrous, cartilaginous, and synovial (McCance and Huether, 2019). **Fibrous joints** fit closely together and are fixed, permitting little if any movement, such as the syndesmosis between the tibia and fibula (Fig. 38.1A). **Cartilaginous joints** have little movement but are elastic and use cartilage to unite separate bony surfaces, such as the synchondrosis that attaches the ribs to the costal cartilage. When bone growth is complete, the joints ossify (see Fig. 38.1B). **Synovial joints**, or true joints, such as the hinge type at the elbow, are freely movable and the most mobile, numerous, and anatomically complex body joints (Fig. 38.2A–B).

Ligaments, Tendons, and Cartilage. Ligaments, tendons, and cartilage support the skeletal system. Ligaments are white, shiny, flexible bands of dense fibrous tissue that bind joints and connect bones and cartilage. A ligament is one type of collagenous fiber that intertwines in irregular, swirling arrangements to form thick connective tissue (Patton, 2019). Ligaments are predominantly elastic fibers and are thus somewhat elastic in nature (Fig. 38.3). Some ligaments serve a protective function. For example, ligaments between the vertebral bodies and the ligamentum flavum prevent damage to the spinal cord during movement of the back.

Tendons are glistening white fibrous bands of tissue that occur in various lengths and thicknesses. Tendons connect muscle to bone and

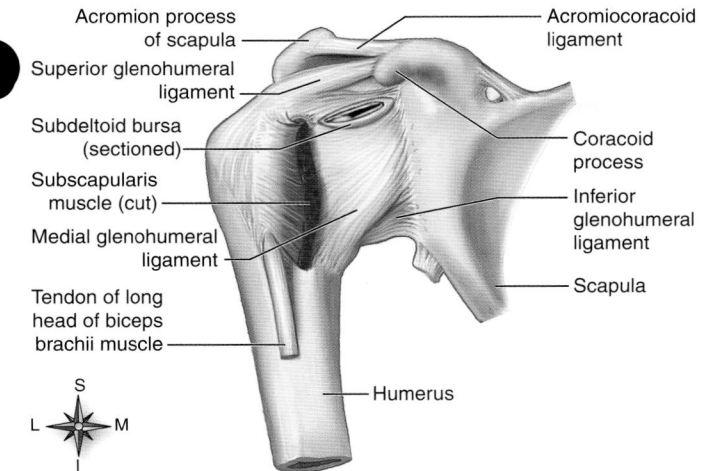

FIG. 38.3 Tendons and ligaments of the shoulder. (From Patton KT: *Anatomy & physiology*, ed 10, St Louis, 2019, Elsevier.)

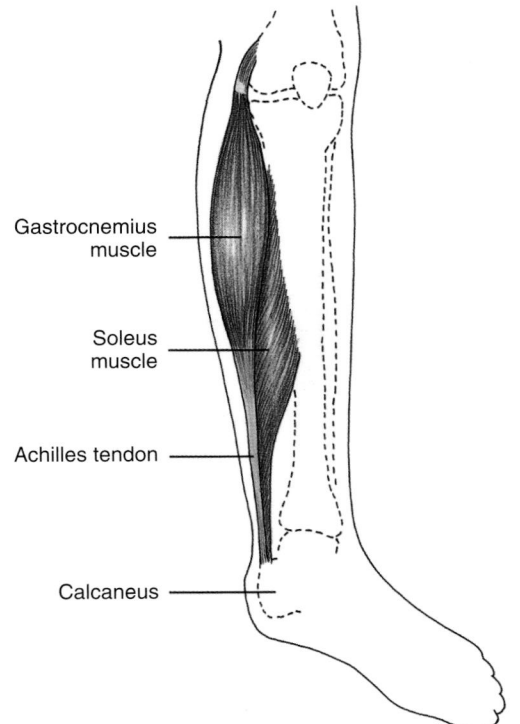

FIG. 38.4 Tendons and muscles of the lower leg.

are strong, flexible, and inelastic. The Achilles tendon is the thickest and strongest tendon in the body. It begins near the midposterior of the leg and attaches the gastrocnemius and soleus muscles in the calf to the calcaneal bone in the back of the foot (Fig. 38.4). Cartilage is nonvascular (without blood vessels), supporting connective tissue located chiefly in the joints and the thorax, trachea, larynx, nose, and ear. It has the flexibility of a firm, plastic material. Because of its gristle-like nature, cartilage sustains weight and serves as a shock absorber between articulating bones. Permanent cartilage is **unossified** (not hardened), except in advanced age and diseases such as osteoarthritis, which impairs mobility.

Strength and flexibility do not result entirely from joints, ligaments, tendons, and cartilage. Adequate skeletal muscle is also necessary.

Skeletal Muscle. Skeletal muscle cells have the ability to be stimulated, or excited, and thus can respond to regulatory mechanisms such as nerve signals (Patton, 2019). Skeletal muscles are composed of bundles of skeletal muscle fibers that generally extend the entire length of the muscle. Muscle fibers contract when stimulated by an electrochemical impulse that travels from the nerve to the muscle across the neuromuscular junction. The electrochemical impulse causes the filaments (predominantly protein molecules of myosin and actin) within the fiber to slide past one another, with the filaments changing length. Continued and efficient use of adenosine triphosphate (ATP), the energy source for muscular contraction, requires glucose and oxygen. Both nutrients reach the muscle fibers through vascular capillaries (Patton, 2019).

Skeletal muscles contract with varying degrees of strength based on the specific task (Patton, 2019). For example, during prolonged inactivity, muscles usually shrink, a condition called disuse atrophy (see Chapter 39) (Patton, 2019). Active use of muscles during exercise can increase muscle size and lead to hypertrophy. Contraction of skeletal muscles allows people to walk, talk, breathe, or participate in any physical activity. There are more than 600 skeletal muscles in the body. In addition to facilitating movement, these muscles determine the form and contour of our bodies. Most of our muscles span at least one joint and attach to both articulating bones. When contraction occurs, one bone is fixed while the other moves. The origin is the point of attachment that remains still; the insertion is the point that moves when the muscle contracts (Patton, 2019).

The amount of load placed on a muscle influences the strength of a skeletal muscle. Generally, the heavier the load, the stronger the contraction. Imagine lifting your hands with palms up in front of you and placing this textbook in your hand. You will feel your arm muscles contract more strongly as the book is placed in your hand because of the **stretch reflex** (Patton, 2019). Your arms and hands will try to maintain constancy of muscle length. The body has a negative feedback response when it detects the increased stretch caused by the load of the textbook. The information is relayed back to the central nervous system, which increases its stimulation of the muscle to counteract the stretch (Patton, 2019). The reflex maintains relatively constant muscle length, but when the load becomes too heavy and threatens injury to the muscle, the body ignores the reflex and causes you to relax and drop the textbook (Patton, 2019).

There are two types of muscle contractions, isotonic and isometric. An isotonic or dynamic contraction is mobilizing, causing the body to move (Patton, 2019). In contrast, an isometric contraction is stabilizing, causing the body to hold a stable position (Patton, 2019). **Isotonic contractions** have two varieties, concentric and eccentric. In **concentric tension**, increased muscle contraction causes muscle shortening, resulting in movement, such as when a patient uses an overhead trapeze to pull up in bed. **Eccentric tension** causes lengthening of a muscle to control the speed and direction of movement. For example, when using an overhead trapeze, a patient slowly lowers himself to the bed. The lowering is controlled when the antagonistic muscles lengthen. Concentric and eccentric muscle actions are necessary for active movement. **Isometric contraction** (static contraction) causes an increase in muscle tension or muscle work but no shortening or active movement of the muscle (e.g., instructing a patient to tighten and relax a muscle group, as in quadriceps set exercises or pelvic floor exercises). Voluntary movement is a combination of isotonic and isometric contractions.

Although isometric contractions do not result in muscle shortening, energy expenditure increases. This type of muscle work is comparable to having a car in neutral with the driver continually depressing the

TABLE 38.1 Functional Classification of Muscle Action

Term	Movement	Example
Prime mover	Muscle that directly performs a specific movement.	Brachialis is a prime mover when flexing the elbow.
Antagonist	Muscle that directly when contracting opposes prime mover or agonist. Relaxes while prime mover contracts. Provides precision and control during contraction of prime mover.	The triceps brachii is an extensor that relaxes when brachialis contracts.
Synergists	Muscle that contracts at same time as prime mover. Facilitates prime mover actions to produce more effective movement.	The deltoid contracts when brachialis contracts.
Fixators	Muscles that stabilize joints, act as type of synergist. Serve to maintain posture and balance.	The deltoid maintains balance of arm when brachialis contracts.

Adapted from Patton KT: *Anatomy & physiology*, ed 10, St Louis, 2019, Elsevier.

FIG. 38.5 Muscle actions. (A) The flexor muscle (brachialis) is the prime mover in flexing the elbow. The extensor muscle (triceps brachii) is the antagonist, relaxing to permit elbow flexion. The pronator teres muscle acts as a synergist by also flexing the elbow. (B) The brachialis is the prime mover of flexion of the elbow. The pronator teres muscle acts as a synergist by also flexing the elbow. To prevent the biceps from also moving, the shoulder strains against the weight; the posterior portion of the deltoid muscle tenses to stabilize the shoulder, thus acting as a fixator muscle. (From Patton KT: *Anatomy & physiology*, ed 10, St Louis, 2019, Elsevier.)

accelerator and racing the engine. The driver is not going anywhere but expends a large amount of energy. It is important to understand the energy expenditure (increased respiratory rate and increased work on the heart) associated with isometric exercises because the exercises are sometimes contraindicated in certain patients' illnesses (e.g., myocardial infarction [MI] or chronic obstructive pulmonary disease [COPD]).

Muscles Concerned With Movement. Skeletal muscles usually act in groups, resulting in movement produced by the coordinated action of several muscles (Patton, 2019). Because some muscles contract while others relax, there is a functional classification of muscles (Table 38.1). These types of muscle actions are important to understand when you use your own muscles to move patients and when you assist patients in independent movement or exercises (Fig. 38.5). Movement is complex. Most muscles function as all the classifications (Patton, 2019). A prime mover during flexion may be an antagonist during extension or a synergist or fixator in rotation.

When muscles shorten to contract, the type and extent of movement are determined by the load or resistance moved, the attachment of the tendons of the muscle to bone, and the type of joint involved (Patton, 2019). The muscles coordinate movement through a system of levers. The lever system makes the work of moving a weight or load easier. It occurs when specific bones such as the humerus, ulna, and radius and the associated joints such as the elbow act as a lever. Thus, the force applied to one end of the bone to lift a weight at another point tends to rotate the bone in the direction opposite that of the applied force. Muscles that attach to bones of leverage provide the necessary strength to move an object.

Muscles Concerned With Posture. Gravity continually pulls on parts of the body; the only way the body is held in position is for muscles to pull on bones in the opposite direction. Muscles accomplish this counterforce by maintaining a low level of sustained contraction. Poor posture places more work on muscles to counteract the force of gravity. This leads to fatigue and eventually interferes with bodily functions and causes deformities.

Posture and movement depend on the skeleton and the shape and development of skeletal muscles. They also contribute to musculoskeletal function and often reflect personality, discomfort, and mood.

For example, a person with a dramatic personality gestures with the hands, a person who is tired or depressed may slouch, and a person with abdominal pain may curl into a fetal-like position. Chapter 39 discusses abnormal types of posture.

Coordination and regulation of different muscle groups depend on muscle tone and activity of antagonistic, synergistic, and antigravity muscles. Muscle tone, or tonus, is the normal state of balanced muscle tension. The body achieves tension by alternating contraction and relaxation without active movement of neighboring fibers of a specific muscle group. Muscle tone helps maintain functional positions such as sitting or standing without excess muscle fatigue and is maintained through continual use of muscles. Activities of daily living (ADLs) require muscle action and help maintain muscle tone. When a patient is immobile or on prolonged bed rest, activity level, activity tolerance, and muscle tone decrease (see Chapter 39).

Nervous System. The nervous system regulates movement and posture. The precentral gyrus, or motor strip, is the major voluntary motor area and is in the cerebral cortex. A majority of motor fibers descend from the motor strip and cross at the level of the medulla. Transmission of impulses from the nervous system to the musculoskeletal system is an electrochemical event and requires a neurotransmitter. Basically, neurotransmitters are chemicals (e.g., acetylcholine) that transfer the electrical impulse from the nerve across the myoneural junction to stimulate the muscle, causing movement. Movement is impaired by disorders that alter neurotransmitter production, transfer of impulses from the nerve to the muscle, or activation of muscle activity. For example, Parkinson disease alters neurotransmitter production, myasthenia gravis disrupts transfer from the neurotransmitter to the muscle, and multiple sclerosis impairs muscle activity (McCance and Huether, 2019).

Proprioception. Proprioception is a muscle sense that makes us aware of the position of the body and its parts, including body movement, orientation in space, and muscle stretch (Patton, 2019). For example, if you close your eyes and bend your elbow, you will know where your hand and lower arm are even if you cannot see them. Stretch receptors associated with muscles, joint capsules, and tendons are classified as proprioceptors (Patton, 2019). Proprioceptors are located within muscle spindles. Rapidly conducting and slower-conducting nerve fibers encircle an area of the muscle spindle found within skeletal muscles. When a muscle stretches, the afferent impulses from sensory neurons pass to the spinal cord and are relayed to the brain, providing a means to monitor changes in muscle length (Patton, 2019). The nervous system regulates posture, which requires coordination of proprioception and balance. As a person carries out ADLs, proprioceptors monitor muscle activity and body position. For example, the proprioceptors on the soles of the feet contribute to correct posture while standing or walking. In standing, pressure is continuous on the bottom of the feet. The proprioceptors monitor the pressure, communicating this information through the nervous system to the antigravity muscles. The standing person remains upright until deciding to change position. As a person walks, the proprioceptors on the bottom of the feet monitor pressure changes. Thus, when the bottom of the moving foot comes in contact with the walking surface, the individual automatically moves the stationary foot forward.

Balance and Alignment. Body balance occurs when a person is properly aligned with a relatively low center of gravity balanced over a wide, stable base of support. In the case of standing, a vertical line falls from the center of gravity through the base of support (see Chapter 39). Adequate balance is necessary to stand, walk, turn, lift, or perform ADLs. Proper posture enhances body balance. The term "posture" means maintaining optimal body position or alignment that favors function. It requires the least muscular work to maintain, and it places the least strain on muscles, ligaments, and bones (McCance and Huether, 2019). Nurses maintain patient alignment when positioning patients and when turning or moving them (see Chapter 39).

The nervous system controls balance specifically through the inner ear, the cerebellum, and vision. The inner ear contains specialized mechanoreceptors or hair cells that are stimulated through sound waves, creating nerve impulses perceived in the brain as either sound or balance (Patton,

2019). These sense organs that are involved in balance are located within the vestibule and semicircular canals of the ear. Together the sense organs function in dynamic equilibrium, a function needed to maintain balance when the head or body rotates or suddenly moves (e.g., when turning in circles or bending over) (Patton, 2019). Normal vision aids balance because visual input from the eyes offers feedback as to whether you or the environment around you is moving.

Normal muscle action involves groups of muscles functioning together as a unit. The cerebellum coordinates patterns of muscle movement with the motor control areas of the cerebrum (Patton, 2019). The cerebellum coordinates action of the prime movers, antagonists, synergists, and fixator muscles to make normal movement smooth, steady, and precise as to the force, rate, and extent of movement (Patton, 2019). These coordinated patterns of movement, such as the sequence of leg movements needed for walking, are learned and stored in the cerebellum (Patton, 2019). Nurses rely on balance to maintain proper body alignment and posture when providing patient care. This reduces strain on musculoskeletal structures and maintains adequate muscle tone. To achieve balance and alignment follow these steps:

- Widen your base of support by separating the feet to a comfortable distance.
- Bring the center of gravity closer to your base of support to increase balance.
- Bend your knees and flex the hips until squatting and maintain proper back alignment to keep the trunk erect.

Nurses apply these techniques in a variety of care activities. For example, you raise the height of a hospital bed when performing a procedure such as changing a dressing to prevent bending too far at the waist and shifting the base of support.

Activity and Exercise

Physical activity (PA) is any movement produced by skeletal muscles that results in energy expenditure (e.g., occupational, sports, conditioning, and household activities). Physical exercise is a subset of PA that is planned, structured, and repetitive and has a final or an intermediate objective, such as the improvement or maintenance of physical fitness (Pinto et al., 2018). Sometimes exercise is also a therapeutic measure, as in the case of rehabilitation following surgery. A patient's individualized exercise program depends on the patient's activity tolerance or the type and amount of exercise or activity that the patient is able to perform. Physiological, emotional, and developmental factors influence a patient's activity tolerance (see below).

An active lifestyle is important for maintaining and promoting health and psychological well-being (Edelman and Kudzma, 2022; CDC, 2021a). The best program of physical activity is a combination of exercises (isotonic, isometric, and resistive) that produce different physiological and psychological benefits. Isotonic exercises (e.g., walking, swimming, jogging, and bicycling) cause muscle contraction and change in muscle length (isotonic contraction). Isotonic exercises enhance circulatory and respiratory functioning; increase muscle mass, tone, and strength; and promote osteoblastic activity that combats osteoporosis. Isometric exercise, which increases muscle tension or muscle work but does not shorten or actively move muscle, is ideal for patients who do not tolerate increased activity, such as a patient who is immobilized in bed (see Chapter 39). The benefits are increased muscle mass, tone, and strength, thus decreasing the potential for muscle wasting; increased circulation to the involved body part; and increased osteoblastic activity.

Resistive isometric exercises are those in which an individual contracts the muscle while pushing against a stationary object or resisting the movement of an object (Kim et al., 2017). A gradual increase in the amount of resistance and the length of time that the muscle contraction is held increases muscle strength and endurance. Examples of resistive isometric exercises are push-ups and hip lifting, in which a patient in a sitting position pushes with the hands against a surface such as a chair seat and raises the hips. Resistive isometric exercises promote muscle strength and provide sufficient stress against bone to promote osteo-blastic activity.

Principles for Transfer and Positioning

Transfer and positioning techniques help patients to be more active. For example, transferring a patient from bed to chair enables the patient to be more participative in self-care activities. Using the principles of bal-ance and alignment aids in safe patient transfer and positioning (see Chapter 39) during routine care activities. Along with safe patient-handling techniques, good balance and alignment decrease work effort and place less strain on musculoskeletal structures (Box 38.1). As a nurse you will teach colleagues and patients' families how to transfer or position patients properly. Teaching a patient's family how to transfer the patient from bed to chair increases and reinforces the family's knowledge about proper transfer and position techniques once the patient returns home. Knowledge of the principles of balance and alignment is crucial. You also incorporate knowledge of physiological and pathological influences on body alignment and mobility.

BOX 38.1   Principles of Safe Patient Transfer and Positioning

- Use mechanical lifts and lift teams when patients are unable to assist.
- When a patient is able to assist, remember these principles:
  - The wider the base of support, the greater the stability of the nurse.
  - The lower the center of gravity, the greater the stability of the nurse.
  - The equilibrium of an object is maintained as long as the line of gravity passes through its base of support.
  - Facing the direction of movement prevents abnormal twisting of the spine.
  - Dividing balanced activity between arms and legs reduces the risk of back injury.
  - Leverage, rolling, turning, or pivoting requires less work than lifting.
  - When friction is reduced between the object to be moved and the surface on which it is moved, less force is required to move it.

Pathological Influences on Body Alignment, Mobility, and Activity. Musculoskeletal conditions are the leading contributor to disability worldwide, with low back pain being the single leading cause of disability across the world (World Health Organization [WHO], 2021). Many pathological conditions affect body alignment and mobility. These conditions include congenital defects; disorders of bones, joints, and muscles; central nervous system disease or injury; and musculoskeletal trauma (Table 38.2) (see Chapter 39). The nature of pathological conditions provides an important source of knowledge when you consider how specific patients are affected and how you must then individualize patient activities. Patients will have a variety of limitations, requiring you to adapt your approaches to care. For example, it is important to understand which type of voluntary and involuntary movement is present after damage to the central nervous system. Does the patient have the ability to move an extremity? Void independently? This information affects the types of interventions you select to maximize your patient's activity level while also keeping the patient safe.

Obesity. Obesity, a chronic health problem, negatively affects the musculoskeletal system, leading to disability. Obesity deserves special consideration because it is a major international public health problem affecting children and adults. The Centers for Disease Control and Prevention (CDC) report that the prevalence of obesity from 2017 to 2018 was 19.3% for children and adolescents aged 2 to 19 years; even more worrisome is the prevalence among 2- to 5-year olds at 13.4% (CDC, 2021b). Researchers in the United States found an upward trend of prevalence in children with the most severe forms of obesity (Klish and Skelton, 2021; Pinto et al., 2016). Risk factors for childhood obesity are numerous; however, poor dietary habits, playing video games with an excess of screen time, and lack of exercise are significant factors. The CDC reported that the age-adjusted prevalence of obesity among all adults was 42.4% and the age-adjusted prevalence of severe obesity in adults was 9.2% from 2017-2018 (CDC, 2020a). Adults are more at risk for obesity due to a lack of healthy diet habits and limited physical activity and exercise.

Obesity impairs an individual's musculoskeletal health because of the increased weight burden on joints and muscles. It has been associated with low back pain, gait disturbances, soft tissue damage, osteoporosis, gout, fibromyalgia, and connective tissue disorders (rheumatoid arthritis)

TABLE 38.2   Pathological Conditions Affecting Body Alignment and Mobility

Condition	Pathological Influence	Examples
Congenital defects	Abnormalities affect the efficiency of the musculoskeletal system in regard to alignment, balance, and appearance.	**Osteogenesis imperfecta**—inherited disorder. Causes bones to be porous, short, bowed, and deformed. As a result, children experience curvature of the spine and shortness of stature. **Scoliosis**—a structural curvature of the spine associated with vertebral rotation. Muscles, ligaments, and other soft tissues become shortened, affecting balance and mobility.
Bone, joint, and muscle disorders	Affect integrity of structures.	**Osteoporosis**—reduction of bone density or mass. The bone remains biochemically normal but has difficulty maintaining integrity and support, leading to fractures.
Inflammatory joint diseases	Cause inflammation or destruction of the synovial membrane and articular cartilage and cause systemic signs of inflammation.	**Arthritis**—changes in articular cartilage combined with overgrowth of bone at the articular ends. Degenerative changes commonly affect weight-bearing joints. **Articular disruption**—trauma to the articular capsules; ranges from mild, such as a tear resulting in a sprain, to severe, such as a separation leading to dislocation.
Central nervous system disorder	Damages part of the central nervous system that regulates voluntary movement and causes impaired body alignment and immobility.	**Traumatic head injury**—damage in the motor strip of the cerebrum. The amount of voluntary motor impairment is directly related to the amount of destruction of the motor strip. **Spinal cord injury**—damage to spinal cord results in loss of function (permanent or temporary) below the level of the injury. A patient's loss of function will depend on level of spinal cord affected.
Musculoskeletal trauma	Results in bruises, contusions, sprains, and/or fractures.	**Bone fracture**—simple or complex disruption of bone tissue continuity; often creates need for temporary immobility of affected body part.

(Onyemaechi et al., 2016; Klish and Skelton, 2021). An association has also been found between obesity and numerous medical conditions, including high blood pressure, atherosclerosis, heart disease, diabetes, high blood cholesterol, cancers, and sleep disorders (National Heart Lung and Blood Institute [NHLBI], n.d.a). Patients who are obese require adaptations in the approaches used to assist with walking, transfer, and positioning. Algorithms are available for the number of staff and the type of assistive device to use when moving, transferring, and ambulating patients who are obese. Obesity directly impacts a patient's quality of life, especially in the ability to perform ADLs effectively. It is a condition that has a major impact on individuals' emotional health as well (NHLBI, n.d.a).

> ### REFLECT NOW
>
> Consider being assigned to a patient who has a history of arthritis affecting the hips. The patient requires assistance with activities of daily living. Reflect on how musculoskeletal system function might be affected and how it will affect ways for planning patient activity.

NURSING KNOWLEDGE BASE

Sound clinical judgment requires application of nursing knowledge about activity and exercise and the pathophysiological effects of any of your patients' diseases when making clinical decisions about patient care. The knowledge allows you to analyze the impact of an illness or disability on patients so that you can accurately identify their holistic needs. A nursing knowledge base for activity and exercise helps you select relevant interventions when patients have a decreased activity tolerance or physical limitation that affects their mobility or ability to exercise.

Safe Patient Handling and Mobility

Nurses are exposed to overexertion and physical injury from the hazards related to moving and transferring patients. This is true in all patient care settings. Providing manual assistance involves excessive physical effort, which is further complicated when tubes and other devices tether a patient to fixed electrical outlets and utilities (Matz, 2019). Manually lifting and transferring patients contributes to a high incidence of work-related musculoskeletal problems and back injuries in nurses and other health care staff. Most care activities related to patient handling involve one or more of the following: lifting with extended arms, lifting when near the floor, lifting when sitting or kneeling, lifting with the trunk twisted or the load off to the side of the body, lifting with one hand or in a restricted space, or pulling or pushing during care (Matz, 2019). The growing trend toward preventing injuries in the health care setting led to important nursing research. Research led by Dr. Audrey Nelson and Andrea Baptiste resulted in the development of safe patient-handling techniques. These techniques are standardized methods for determining how to handle, move, and mobilize patients based on individual patient characteristics and conditions (Matz, 2019; Hilton et al., 2019; Nelson and Baptiste, 2006).

Evidence-based research has shown that safe patient handling and mobility interventions significantly reduce overexertion injuries by replacing manual patient handling with safer methods guided by ergonomic principles (NIOSH, 2013; Matz, 2019). Ergonomics is the design of work tasks to best suit the capabilities of workers. In the case of safe patient handling and mobility (SPHM), it involves improved assessment, the use of mechanical equipment, and safety procedures to lift and move patients. Many states have laws mandating SPHM in health care agencies. Comprehensive SPHM programs include the following (U.S. Department of Veterans Affairs, 2019):

- Standardized assessment tools for identifying a patient's mobility level, such as the Banner Mobility Assessment Tool (BMAT) (Boynton et al., 2014, Matz, 2019)
- An ergonomics assessment of patient rooms and health care environments
- Clinical/patient assessment algorithms to select the right equipment and number of staff for each patient-handling and mobility task
- Right equipment includes assistive devices in the form of ceiling lifts made available in patient rooms. Lifts help care providers transfer patients from beds to stretchers or wheelchairs and can be used to assist patients during walking.
- Portable lifting devices can be moved from room to room. The lifting equipment uses slings or vests to hold patients securely and reduce the risk of slipping, falling, or being dropped when walking.
- Unit peer leaders who function as safe patient-handling experts and staff trainers
- Use of safety huddles to share information among staff members that will keep staff and patients safe
- A minimal-lift policy

The use of SPHM techniques is a standard for best practices in the moving, handling, and transfer of patients. In addition to reducing injuries to health care providers, the use of SPHM techniques improves patient outcomes. OSHA reports that SPHM programs result in patients having fewer falls, skin tears, and pressure injuries (OSHA, 2017).

Factors Influencing Activity and Exercise

Factors influencing activity and exercise include developmental changes, behavior, lifestyle, environmental issues, family and social support, and cultural and ethnic factors. Consider these areas of knowledge and apply this information to develop a patient-centered plan of care whether a patient is seeking health promotion, acute care, or restorative and continuing care.

Developmental Changes. Throughout the life span the appearance and functioning of the body undergo changes affecting movement. Knowledge of growth and development (see Chapters 12 to 14) prepares you to anticipate the types of activities that patients of all ages are capable of performing. For example, the developmental process results in children acquiring independence in daily living by improving their gross motor capacity, as well as manual, intellectual, and communicative functioning (Kim et al., 2017).

A newborn infant's spine is flexed and lacks the anteroposterior curves of an adult. As growth and stability increase, the thoracic spine straightens, and the lumbar spinal curve appears, which allows sitting and standing. As an infant grows, musculoskeletal development permits support of weight for standing and walking, allowing the child to explore its environment. A toddler's posture is awkward because of the slight swayback and protruding abdomen. Toward the end of toddlerhood, posture appears less awkward, curves in the cervical and lumbar vertebrae are accentuated, and foot eversion disappears. From the third year through the beginning of adolescence, the musculoskeletal system continues to grow and develop. Greater coordination enables a child to perform tasks such as washing hands and brushing teeth, which require fine motor skills. Adolescent growth is often sporadic and uneven. As a result, the adolescent appears awkward and uncoordinated. Adolescent girls usually grow and develop earlier than boys. Hips widen, and fat deposits in the upper arms, thighs, and buttocks. The adolescent boy's changes in shape are usually a result of long-bone growth and increased muscle mass.

A middle-age adult should normally have full musculoskeletal function. An adult with correct posture and body alignment feels good, looks

---

BOX 38.2 Common Chronic Health Conditions Among Younger and Older Adults

- Arthritis
- Cancer
- Chronic lung disease
- Dementia
- Diabetes
- Depression
- Chronic kidney disease
- Heart disease
- Hypertension
- Stroke

Data from Adams ML: *Differences between younger and older US adults with multiple chronic conditions,* Centers for Disease Control and Prevention: Preventing Chronic Disease, Volume 14, September 7, 2017, https://www.cdc.gov/pcd/Issues/2017/16_0613.htm. Accessed April 18, 2019; and Centers for Disease Control: CDC's National Center for Chronic Disease Prevention and Health Promotion (NCCDPHP): *Chronic diseases in America,* n.d., https://www.cdc.gov/chronicdisease/pdf/infographics/chronic-disease-H.pdf. Accessed August 24, 2021.

---

good, and generally appears self-confident. A healthy adult also has the necessary musculoskeletal development and coordination to carry out ADLs and physical exercise. However, for people 45 to 64 years of age, the percentage of adults with two or more common chronic conditions increases. Most people with multiple chronic conditions (MCCs) are of working age (Box 38.2). Multiple chronic diseases often create barriers to exercise. Symptoms of one chronic condition (e.g., difficulty in breathing related to asthma) may interfere with another condition (heart failure), preventing the patient from engaging in needed regular exercise. Nurses must consider the burden of MCCs on nonelderly adults, who represent more than 60% of all adults with MCCs (Adams, 2017). Chronic disease significantly affects how to individualize activity and exercise therapy programs. For example, a patient with preexisting heart disease will have different guidelines for the type of exercises to perform and for monitoring exercise tolerance compared with a patient of similar age and no disease.

A progressive loss of total bone mass occurs with older adults. Some of the possible causes of this loss include physical inactivity, hormonal changes, and increased osteoclastic activity (i.e., activity by cells responsible for bone tissue absorption). The effect of bone loss is weaker bones, causing vertebrae to be softer and long shaft bones to be less resistant to bending, making an individual prone to fractures and muscle injuries. Older adults may walk more slowly and incorrectly and appear less coordinated. Many are afraid of falling (Lavidan et al., 2018; Tomita et al., 2018). They often take smaller steps and keep their feet closer together, which decreases the base of support and thus alters body balance. Physical exercise can improve endurance, coordination, and muscle stability and reduce the risk for falls and injuries (see Chapter 14).

Patient Behavior. Intrinsic motivation to adhere to any form of treatment, including an exercise program, is the inherent satisfaction one experiences from physical activity (McArthur et al., 2014). This motivation includes feelings of enjoyment and accomplishment that come from adherence to regular exercise. Understanding how human behavior influences a patient's motivation and willingness to be active and exercise is critical to your success in creating a patient-centered exercise program.

It is important to consider your patients' knowledge of exercise and activity (benefits versus disadvantages), their values and beliefs about exercise and health, perceived barriers to a program of exercise and physical activity, and current exercise behaviors or habits. Patients are more open to developing an exercise program if they are at the stage of readiness to change their behavior (Tsang et al., 2015). A qualitative study

involving middle-age women of Chinese descent found five subthemes to women's motivation to exercise: anticipated positive feelings (physiological or emotional sensations), meaningful exercise, perceived obstacles in the way to avoid exercise, negative or ambivalent feelings about being active, and previous negative experiences with physical performance or emotional upset from an exercise experience (Tsang et al., 2015). Patients' decisions to change behavior and include a daily exercise routine in their lives often occur gradually with repeated information and reinforcement individualized to their personal goals and lifestyle (see Chapter 25).

Lifestyle. An individual's daily lifestyle greatly influences engagement with exercise. A person must be highly motivated to exercise if the lifestyle does not include a convenient time for exercise or if there are frequent interruptions or demands. Individuals who require more than one job for economic security will perceive having little time to exercise. Parents staying at home and caring for multiple children will often have the same perception. When exercise has become a routine part of a person's day, it is of course easier to introduce new exercise options or frequencies. In a study by McArthur et al. (2014), the extent to which middle-age women integrated exercise into their lifestyle routine was characterized by: exercise incorporated into daily structure (established routine), other demands (work or household tasks), being prepared (having necessary equipment and arrangements), and prioritizing (the emphasis women placed on exercise relative to other aspects of their daily lives). Because of the numerous lifestyle conditions that can affect exercise adherence, a nurse must obtain a full picture of a patient's routines, exercise options, and lifestyle conditions.

Cultural Background. Exercise and physical fitness are beneficial to all people. However, there are cultural differences regarding the extent to which people exercise (Box 38.3). The CDC (2021e) reports that 31 million adults (including 28% of adults over age 50) are physically inactive. A study utilizing the American Time Use Surveys has shown that leisure physical activity comprised only about 10% of total nonwork physical activity among adults (Saffer et al., 2013). Individuals with a lower level of education and minority racial/ethnic groups tend to have higher levels of physical activity at work but lower levels of nonwork physical activity. The difference may limit the positive effects of physical activity on an individual's health because the type of nonwork physical activity has a stronger positive association with health relative to work physical activity (Saffer et al., 2013). There are cultures that see exercise as part of a method to optimize health or treat illness (Giger and Haddad, 2021). When developing a physical fitness program for culturally diverse populations, consider their education and beliefs regarding the value of exercise and their access to resources to exercise, and learn about what motivates individuals to exercise and which activities are appropriate and enjoyable.

Environmental Issues.

Home and Work Sites. A common barrier for physical activity is a lack of time needed to engage in a daily exercise program. Some employers help their employees overcome the obstacle of time constraints by offering physical activity opportunities at the work site, reminders, and rewards for those committed to physical fitness. For example, providing a walking path that gives employees the opportunity to walk at work may address barriers such as a lack of time to walk, concerns about their own neighborhood safety, or a lack of social support (CDC, 2021c). Such activity programs improve worker productivity and morale. Reminders within a work site, such as signs that encourage employees to use the stairs instead of elevators, are useful. Rewards such as free parking or discounted parking fees are also effective for employees who park in distant lots and walk.

BOX 38.3 CULTURAL ASPECTS OF CARE

Physical Inactivity Among Ethnic Groups

The Centers for Disease Control and Prevention (Watson et al., 2016) reports that inactivity prevalence among adults 50 years of age and older was significantly higher among women than men, among Hispanics and non-Hispanic Blacks than among non-Hispanic Whites, and among adults who reported ever having one or more chronic diseases than among those not reporting one. The prevalence of inactivity significantly increased with decreasing levels of education and increasing body mass index. When older adults perceive that exercise contributes to independence, participation in exercise is more likely. However, in a study on cultural influences on exercise participation, family traditions and sociocultural norms influenced sedentary behaviors (Rawlings et al., 2019). A systematic review of research studies found many Latino older adults found exercise "not fitting" for older people and "a waste of time" (Jang et al., 2015). This review also found that many Asian, Indian, Latino, and Chinese older adult immigrants found old age as a time to rest or relax. Sedentary behavior is influenced by age, gender, mobility, culture, and socioeconomic status (Rawlings et al., 2019).

Implications for Patient-Centered Care

- Cultural values, beliefs, and perceptions define aging and health and affect an individual's personal meaning of exercise (Jang et al., 2015). Thus you need to assess a patient's feelings about aging and exercise.
- Receiving support and advice from health care providers of the same cultural or language background is often successful in motivating patients to become involved in exercise and other health programs (Jang et al., 2015; Betancourt et al., 2021).
- Ensure that exercise and fall prevention interventions are culturally appropriate and targeted to a patient's values and beliefs.
- Support the promotion of physical activity through formal programs in schools, churches, and governmental agencies.

Depending on where a patient lives, weather patterns affect an individual's willingness and ability to get outdoors for usual exercise. Good weather tends to motivate a person to exercise, while poor weather does the opposite. Some individuals will set up their homes to be able to exercise, using a stationary bike or weight equipment, for example. Exercise needs to be built into an environment where it is safe to participate in activity (Franklin et al., 2021). For example, is riding a bike safe in a particular neighborhood? It is important to know the environmental settings in which patients live and work to understand exercise patterns and to help them choose relevant exercise options.

Schools. Children today are less active, resulting in an increase in childhood obesity. Schools can be very effective in facilitating physical fitness and exercise in children. Strategies to incorporate physical activity early into a child's daily routine often provide a foundation for lifetime commitment to exercise and physical fitness.

Community. Creating or modifying environments to make it easier for people to walk, run, or bike is a strategy that not only increases individuals' physical activity, but also makes communities better places to live (CDC, 2021d). Unfortunately, such resources are unavailable in most poverty-stricken neighborhoods. Communities designed to support physical activity are often called active communities (CDC, 2021d). Community support of physical fitness is instrumental in promoting the health of its members (e.g., providing walking trails and track facilities in parks, maps to guide access, and physical fitness classes). Successful implementation of physical fitness programs requires collaboration among public health agencies, parks and recreational associations, state and local governmental agencies, health care agencies, and the members of the community. You need to include a review of a

patient's community environment and the resources available for safe physical activity when assessing your patients.

Family and Social Support. Social support is one very important motivational tool to encourage and promote exercise and physical fitness. In a systematic review that studied the association between social support and physical activity among older adults, it was found that people with greater social support for physical activity are more likely to do leisure time physical activity, especially when support comes from family members (Smith et al., 2017). This study noted that the physical activity levels of women are more likely than men to be influenced by general social support. An example of the use of social support to influence exercise is to have a friend or significant other engage a patient to participate in a "buddy system" (i.e., they walk together each day at a specified time) or weekly exercise classes. This companionship provides for socialization, increases the enjoyment, and develops a commitment to physical fitness. Parents support their children in engaging in physical activity by providing encouragement, praise, and transportation to sporting events or exercise facilities. Parents also support physical activity by including their children in family outings such as bicycling or a basketball game in the neighborhood schoolyard.

In the case study Beth will reflect on knowledge about the effects of obesity on normal movement and plans on assessing its effects on Mrs. Smith's comfort level, walking gait, and other musculoskeletal conditions. Knowledge of the impact heart failure has on exercise tolerance further informs Beth. Critical thinking involves anticipation of the knowledge that is most relevant to a patient's condition. Beth's knowledge base will help guide patient assessment and further increase Beth's knowledge and understanding of Mrs. Smith's unique condition.

CRITICAL THINKING

Sound clinical judgment is at the core of providing safe and relevant interventions for improving a patient's activity level and tolerance. By applying critical thinking in making sound clinical judgments, nurses recognize and analyze assessment findings, select, and prioritize nursing diagnoses and problems, and respond with appropriate interventions within a variety of contexts (Dickison et al., 2016). Thoughtful evaluation will determine the efficacy of those interventions. Successful critical thinking requires a synthesis of knowledge, experience, environmental factors, critical thinking attitudes, and intellectual and professional standards. Sound clinical judgments require you to anticipate information, analyze the data, and make appropriate clinical decisions regarding patient activity and exercise (Fig. 38.6).

You integrate knowledge from nursing and other disciplines to understand activity tolerance, movement, and physical fitness and their effects on patients. As you conduct the nursing process, consider the relationship among scientific and nursing concepts to provide the best outcome for your patients. For example, begin by understanding the relationship between the musculoskeletal system and your patients' health alterations and how that may create problems with activity and exercise and transferring and moving patients. Professional standards are also a part of your knowledge base and provide valuable guidelines for determining how to promote exercise and physical fitness for patients. One example is the *Physical Activity Guidelines for Americans* issued by the U.S. Department of Health and Human Services (2018); the department's guidelines provide evidence-based recommendations for adults and youth (ages 3 through 17) to safely get the physical activity they need to stay healthy. Another standard is the American Diabetes Association's position statement on physical activity and exercise for individuals with diabetes (Colberg et al., 2016).

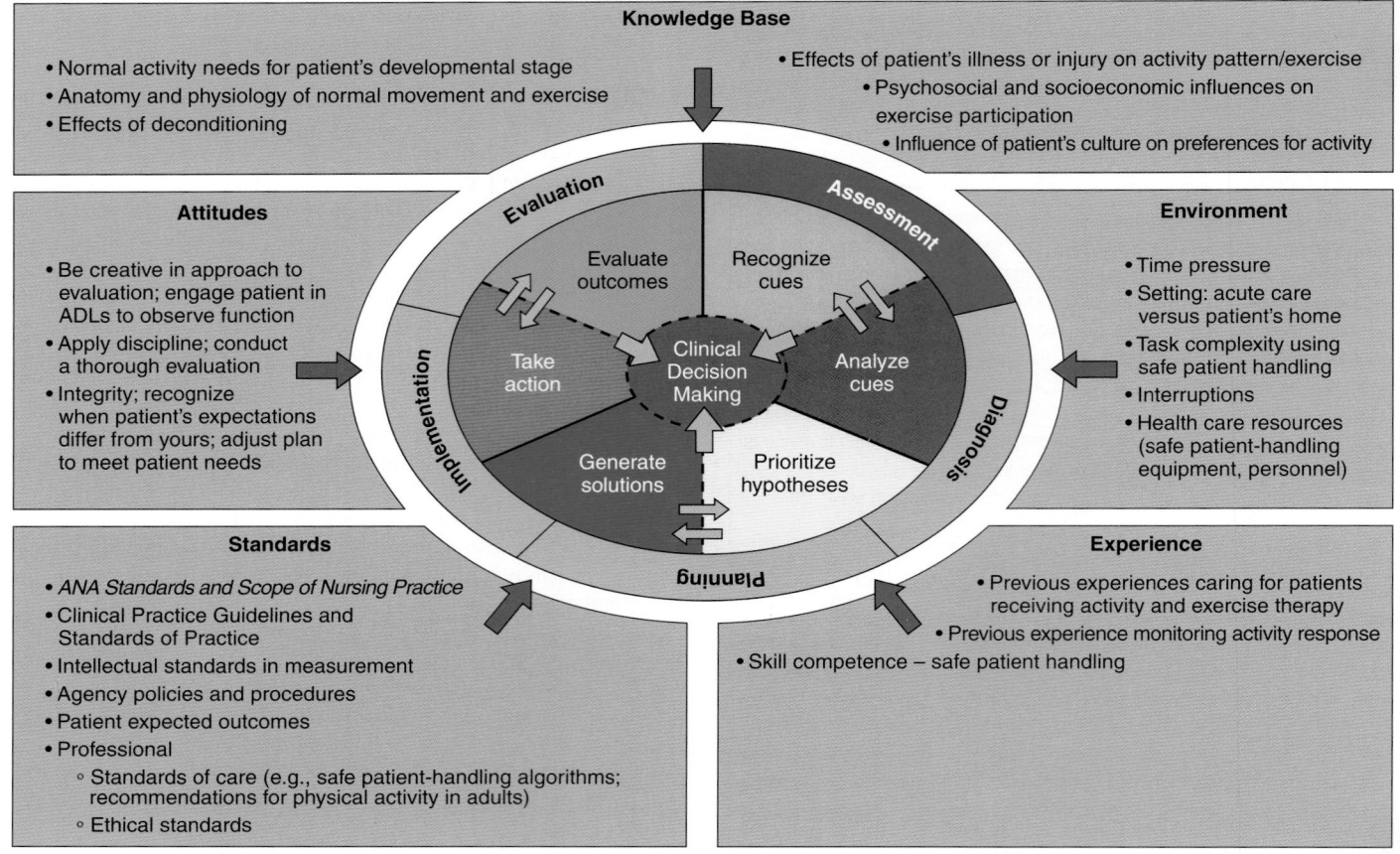

FIG. 38.6 Critical thinking model for assessing activity and exercise. *ADA,* American Diabetes Association; *DHHS,* Department of Health and Human Services. (Clinical Judgment Measurement Model copyright © NCSBN. All rights reserved.)

Your experiences in caring for patients with alterations in their ability to remain active and mobile are valuable. If you work in a home health, clinic, or rehab setting, you will have the opportunity to witness how patients respond over time to activity and exercise recommendations, their adherence, and their attitudes about exercise. This information guides you in making decisions for future patients. With experience comes competency. Many of the skills involving the promotion of movement, such as the use of assistive devices, assistance with ambulation, and the transferring of patients requires consideration of patients' strengths and weaknesses. Your competency in these skills will grow if you collaborate with physical therapists, whose education is focused on these types of skills.

Considering environmental factors is especially important when planning activity and exercise interventions. In acute care and rehabilitation you want an unobstructed walking path for a patient to use. In the home you must accommodate for any barriers that may exist, such as uneven outside walking paths or worn carpets, to ambulate patients safely. You must adapt approaches to patients' environments as well as that of the health care setting. The use of resources such as physical therapy will be pivotal to successful interventions.

Critical thinking attitudes and intellectual standards help guide the problem-solving approach in making clinical judgments during the nursing process. All assessments must be thorough and detailed as you apply critical thinking attitudes in exploring problems with patients. Remember that some patients have the capacity for recovery in spite of the loss of some physical function. Restoration of function begins early in the care

of patients whose ability to perform self-care is disrupted. Creativity, commitment, and perseverance are important intellectual standards to apply for improving patients' activity tolerance and mobility skills.

REFLECT NOW

Think about a patient you cared for; what support systems did he or she have? How did the patient use his or her support system in regard to promoting daily physical activity? How can you incorporate the use of a support system in a patient's exercise program?

❖ NURSING PROCESS

Apply critical thinking in making the necessary clinical judgments to conduct the nursing process successfully. Patient involvement is critical from the beginning. Because patients must have a commitment to initiating activity and maintaining participation in exercise, a patient-centered approach is particularly important.

◆ Assessment

When conducting an assessment to determine a patient's activity and exercise needs, consider scientific and nursing knowledge regarding the patient's condition as it presents itself during assessment. For example, you anticipate assessment findings knowing what is normal about the anatomy and physiology of movement. The patient's presenting medical diagnosis or physical condition then gives clues for what to look for. For example, a patient with osteoarthritis is likely to have pain and tenderness in certain joints. Your experience with similar patients makes it easier to detect a sign—for example, stiffness in a joint. Let your knowledge and experience interact as you conduct your assessment. Know what to look for, but also be thorough, so as not to miss less obvious or more uncommon signs and symptoms. To be thorough, also consider a patient's activity history, developmental status, factors influencing activity and exercise as they relate to the patient, socioeconomic resources, and ability and readiness to exercise. You critically analyze assessment findings to identify nursing diagnoses and problems. The diagnoses will guide you in selecting patient-centered outcomes for achieving safe and effective nursing care. During assessment apply all of the critical thinking elements that help you make sound clinical judgments needed for selecting appropriate nursing diagnoses.

Through the Patient's Eyes. Your ability to provide patient-centered care requires your patient to be willing and ready to participate in any activity or exercise program you plan. This may include your patient getting out of bed and into a chair for the first time or participating in 30-minute daily walks at home. Assess a patient's expectations and understanding of the physical activities necessary for recovery. What are the patient's values, concerns, and beliefs about how activity and exercise affect health? Include a discussion about the patient's perceptions of engaging in activity and exercise at home or in the health care setting. It is also important to assess a patient's perceptions of what activity is acceptable in relationship to any symptoms experienced during exercise. One of the factors affecting physical activity is freedom from pain. When patients experience pain or fatigue following exercise, they often lack commitment to desired interventions. When patients are content with their present physical activity and fitness, they may not perceive a need for improvement.

Readiness to Exercise. Perceived self-efficacy is an individual's belief in the ability to perform different behaviors or perform a task. Self-efficacy affects a person's willingness to engage in an activity such as exercise. The outcomes people anticipate, such as from an exercise program, depend on their judgments of how well they will be able to perform in given situations. The Transtheoretical Model (TTM), which incorporates the concept of self-efficacy, can be applied for tailoring interventions to patients' readiness to change and can enhance patient progress and help patients use therapeutic resources more effectively (LaMorte, 2019). However, individualizing an intervention depends on your accurate assessment of a patient's stage of change (SOC).

The TTM is a model of intentional change that focuses on the decision making of an individual regarding a change in behavior (e.g., starting to exercise, changing a diet, taking medications correctly). The model operates on the assumption that people do not change behaviors quickly and decisively; instead, behavioral change occurs continuously through a cyclical process (LaMorte, 2019). An individual will move back and forth through six stages of change:

- Precontemplation—Individuals do not intend to change their behavior in the next 6 months; they are unaware of the problem behavior or are demoralized by unsuccessful previous attempts to change behavior.
- Contemplation—Individuals are aware they need to change their behavior. They intend to take action within the next 6 months but lack commitment to actually start changing.
- Preparation—Individuals have decided to take action in the immediate future, usually measured as the next month. They often have a concrete plan of action, such as buying an exercise bike, joining a health club, or asking family members to walk with them.

- Action —Individuals have made specific overt changes in their lifestyles within the past 6 months.
- Maintenance—People have shown the desired behavior for over 6 months and are working to prevent relapse.

Your assessment of the stage that best describes your patient's readiness to exercise will influence nursing diagnoses chosen and determine how you plan patient care. Begin by asking to what extent the patient enjoys exercising and the patient's belief in the ability to exercise (Box 38.4). This is a factor positively associated with adult physical activity (Healthy People 2020, n.d.). Ask about the patient's current activity level. If patients tell you that they do not exercise and do not intend to start in the next 6 months, they are in the precontemplation stage. If patients have been thinking about exercising or have tried to exercise but do so inconsistently, they are likely in the contemplation phase. A patient who describes a plan to exercise after discharge from a hospital or rehabilitation center is in the preparation stage. If the patient reports actively being engaged in exercise weekly and for the past several months, the patient is in the action stage. If patients have been exercising but are facing new obstacles that affect the ability to remain active, they are in the maintenance stage. Use your assessment findings related to the patient's readiness for change as cues for nursing diagnoses. The nursing interventions you choose for your patient's plan of care should complement the stage of change and move the patient toward activity engagement.

Cultural and Socioeconomic Factors. An assessment of cultural and socioeconomic resources focuses on those issues that are particularly important to consider for developing a long-term exercise plan. It requires a level of trust for the patient to explore cultural beliefs and attitudes about the value of exercise and how best to include physical activity into a daily schedule. However, this information is vital to your success in developing a relevant plan of care.

It is also important to assess a patient's socioeconomic resources for being able to engage in an activity or exercise plan. Socioeconomic factors affect a patient's readiness or ability to exercise. Studies have shown a correlation between individuals' educational level, income, and ability to pay for fees and equipment and their level of involvement in physical activity (O'Donoghue et al., 2018). Because access to community exercise facilities and programs is positively associated with adult physical activity, ask patients to describe their access to exercise programs and other resources in their community (Office of Disease Prevention and Health Promotion [ODPHP], n.d.). For example, does the patient have access to exercise facilities or public parks and walking areas? Are those areas safe? What time during a typical day does the patient perceive being able to engage in exercise? Will this be impacted by the illness? How many hours in a day does the patient work?

An important resource influencing readiness to exercise is social support. Is there social support available to a patient? Research has shown that among middle-age women, accountability to others or the degree to which a woman feels beholden to others (either through mutual participation or awareness of intent) to keep exercise commitments affects exercise adherence. Available support in the form of another individual, verbal encouragement, or organizational help (e.g., child care), can help women remain active (McArthur et al., 2014).

Physical Health. Assess a patient's physical condition to determine ability and readiness to exercise. This includes status of body alignment, muscle strength and coordination, and integrity of joints and other structures using physical examination techniques (see Chapter 30). Baseline vital signs are essential for later determining exercise tolerance. Assess for the presence of any pain or discomfort in joints or muscles. The presence of pain often limits a person's willingness and ability to move a body part. Remember, never move a painful joint past the position of pain. Also review in the medical record for any chronic diseases

BOX 38.4 Nursing Assessment Questions

Exercise Pattern
- What exercises do you enjoy most?
- How much do you normally exercise each day? Each week? How do you plan for it?
- How long do you exercise at any given time?

Exercise Tolerance
- Tell me how you feel after completing your exercise.
- Describe for me any uncomfortable or disabling symptoms you have when exercising?
- Do you know how to check your pulse before and after exercise?

Patient Values
- Tell me what you believe about how exercise affects your health. Benefits? Disadvantages?
- To what extent do you enjoy exercising?
- How confident are you in being able to perform the exercises your doctor has recommended?

Effects of Exercise
- Tell me about any problems you are having with staying active and exercising regularly.
- Tell me how exercise affects your body.
- How have your exercise habits changed since your illness/injury?
- How has the lack of an exercise routine affected your weight?
- Do you feel more tired since you have been unable to exercise routinely?

Signs and Symptoms
- Tell me about any discomfort you have when you exercise (or after exercising).
- Describe for me the pain or shortness of breath that you feel.
- Do you ever feel chest discomfort or pain during exercise or activity?

Onset and Duration
- Tell me when your discomfort following exercise began. Does it occur each time you exercise?
- How long does it take to resume normal breathing after exercise or an activity?

Severity
- How far do you walk before the pain in your legs begins?
- On a scale of 0 to 10 (10 being the worst discomfort), rate your leg/back pain.
- Do you describe your shortness of breath as minimal, moderate, or severe after activities and/or exercise?

Barriers to Exercise and Activity
- Tell me what prevents you from regularly exercising each day.
- Do you have any health problems (such as asthma, arthritis) that affect your ability to carry out daily activities such as grocery shopping, washing clothes, or daily walking?
- Describe any physical limitations that prevent you from exercising on a daily basis.
- Do you have access to a community walking path and exercise equipment?

or conditions that affect a patient's ability to be mobile and active. Collaborate with a physical therapist about a patient's musculoskeletal status. Apply knowledge of pathological changes so that you can target assessment on expected body systems.

Body Alignment. Help a patient feel at ease when assessing body alignment. Your aim is to not have the patient assume an unnatural or rigid position. You will assess a patient's alignment during standing, sitting, and then lying down as a patient is able. The assessment of body alignment has the following objectives:

- Determining normal physiological changes in body alignment resulting from growth and development for each patient
- Identifying deviations in body alignment caused by incorrect posture
- Providing opportunities for patients to observe their posture
- Identifying learning needs of patients for maintaining correct body alignment
- Identifying trauma, muscle damage, or nerve dysfunction
- Obtaining information concerning other factors that contribute to incorrect alignment, such as fatigue, malnutrition, and psychological problems

Chapter 39 describes in detail how to assess patients' alignment while standing, sitting, and lying supine.

Mobility. The adequacy of a patient's mobility affects coordination and balance while walking, the ability to carry out ADLs, and the ability to participate in an exercise program. The assessment of mobility has five components: sitting, standing, range of motion, gait, and exercise.

Sitting. You may incorporate this assessment into your earlier assessment of sitting alignment. Note whether a patient can sit on the side of the bed or in a chair upright. A patient's ability to sit affects the ability to perform self-care activities. When assessing the ability of patients to sit, allow them to use a side rail (when present). Skill 38.1 describes the Banner Mobility Assessment Tool (BMAT), a validated tool that includes a component for assessment of a patient's mobility while sitting (Boynton et al., 2014, Matz, 2019).

Standing. Do not rely on a patient's self-report of being able to stand independently without support or assistance. This commonly occurs when nurses rush to admit or transfer patients, allowing patients to offer simply "yes" or "no" responses to an admission form question. When you assess a patient's ability to stand, it is appropriate to have the patient use an assistive device for support (if one is typically used). The BMAT (Boynton et al., 2014, Matz, 2019) includes a measure for assessing a patient while standing. A patient should be able to raise the buttocks off the bed and hold for a count of five (Boynton et al., 2014, Matz, 2019). The ability to achieve this maneuver indicates good mobility and balance, which are needed to safely stand and ambulate (see Skill 38.1).

Range of Motion. Observing range of motion (ROM) is one of the first assessment techniques used to determine the degree of limitation or injury to a joint. Assess ROM to clarify the extent of joint stiffness, swelling, pain, limited movement, and unequal movement. Chapter 30 covers a thorough ROM assessment. Limited ROM indicates inflammation such as arthritis, fluid in the joint, altered nerve supply, or contractures. Increased mobility (beyond normal) of a joint indicates connective tissue disorders, ligament tears, and possible joint fractures.

Gait. The term *gait* describes a particular manner or style of walking. It is a coordinated action that requires the integration of sensory function, muscle strength, proprioception, balance, and a properly functioning CNS (vestibular system and cerebellum). A gait cycle begins with the heel strike of one leg and continues to the heel strike of the other leg. Assessing a patient's gait allows you to draw conclusions about balance, posture, and the ability to walk without assistance, all of which affect the risk for falling. Here are a few ways to assess a patient's gait:

1. Observe the patient entering the room, and note speed, stride, and balance.
2. Ask the patient to walk across the room, turn, and come back.
3. Ask the patient to walk heel-to-toe in a straight line. This may be difficult for older patients even in the absence of disease, so stay at the patient's side during the walk.

Chapter 39 reviews gaits characteristic of particular diseases and conditions.

BOX 38.5 Effects of Exercise

Cardiovascular System
- Increased cardiac output
- Improved myocardial contraction, thereby strengthening cardiac muscle
- Decreased resting heart rate
- Improved venous return

Pulmonary System
- Increased respiratory rate and depth followed by a quicker return to resting state
- Improved alveolar ventilation
- Decreased work of breathing
- Improved diaphragmatic excursion

Metabolic System
- Increased basal metabolic rate
- Increased use of glucose and fatty acids
- Increased triglyceride breakdown
- Increased gastric motility
- Increased production of body heat

Musculoskeletal System
- Improved muscle tone
- Increased joint mobility
- Improved muscle tolerance to physical exercise
- Possible increase in muscle mass
- Reduced bone loss

Activity Tolerance
- Improved tolerance
- Decreased fatigue

Psychosocial Factors
- Improved tolerance to stress
- Reports of "feeling better"
- Reports of decrease in illness (e.g., colds, influenza)

Data from McCance KL, Huether SE: *Pathophysiology: the biologic basis for disease in adults and children,* ed 8, St Louis, 2019, Mosby.

BOX 38.6 Factors Influencing Activity Tolerance

Physiological Factors
- Skeletal abnormalities
- Muscular impairments
- Endocrine or metabolic illnesses (e.g., diabetes mellitus, thyroid disease)
- Hypoxemia
- Decreased cardiac function
- Decreased endurance
- Impaired physical stability
- Pain
- Sleep pattern disturbance
- Prior exercise patterns
- Infectious processes and fever

Emotional Factors
- Anxiety
- Depression
- Chemical addictions
- Motivation

Developmental Factors
- Age
- Sex

Pregnancy
- Physical growth and development of muscle and skeletal support

Modified from Harding M, et al: *Lewis's medical-surgical nursing assessment and management of clinical problems,* ed 11, St Louis, 2020, Mosby.

Exercise Pattern. You will assess the patient's daily activity and exercise routine (see Box 38.4), compare with how any illness or injury has changed the routine, and consider the recommendations for exercise made by the patient's health care provider. Also consider standards from the American Heart Association's (2018) *"Recommendations for physical activity in adults and kids,"* and compare those with a patient's actual exercise and activity routine to determine whether exercise is sufficient. Adults need at least 2 hours and 30 minutes (150 minutes) of moderate-intensity aerobic activity (i.e., brisk walking) every week and muscle-strengthening activities on 2 or more days a week that work all major muscle groups (legs, hips, back, abdomen, chest, shoulders, and arms). The activity can be spread across a week.

Determine a patient's preferred form of exercise, level of intensity, and frequency of exercise. Box 38.4 provides examples of questions to ask related to a patient's exercise and activity routines and tolerance. Your assessment of the patient's activity provides baseline information for both exercise and activity tolerance. This baseline information is beneficial when establishing a patient's exercise and rehabilitation plan following an illness or injury. When a person exercises, physiological changes occur in body systems (Box 38.5).

During exercise you improve muscle tone, strength, and size and cardiopulmonary conditioning. As a result, you are able to exercise longer with each strengthening of the muscles. Exercise also enhances joint mobility because the exercise itself requires movement of body parts.

Activity Tolerance. Activity tolerance is the type and amount of exercise or work that a person is able to perform without undue exertion or injury (Box 38.6). Observe patients after ambulation, self-bathing, or sitting in a chair for several hours and assess their verbal report of fatigue and weakness. Do they show difficulty breathing or report being short of breath after exercise? Assess heart rate and blood pressure response to activity by comparing with baseline rates at rest. Both heart rate and blood pressure should increase. When you care for a patient who is relatively healthy and able to exercise regularly, assess what the patient sets

as a target heart rate during exercise. Use this finding to determine whether the patient has set an adequate target rate for exercise training (AHA, 2021; CDC, 2020b).

Environmental Factors. The setting for your practice influences environmental factors to assess when considering a patient's needs for activity and exercise. Is the immediate environment safe for the patient to ambulate? Are there barriers? In the home you will collaborate with a patient or family caregiver on whether any barriers can be altered. In addition, is there space within the home or are the outdoor areas safe so that a patient can build exercise tolerance over time.

As you assess a patient's level of activity and mobility, you will determine the complexity of any task or skill you must perform. You will need to assess the availability of other caregivers to assist with any safe patient-handling techniques as needed. Also assess for the availability of resources (e.g., safe patient-handling equipment).

Factors Influencing Mobility. Assess a patient's development stage and determine whether the condition restricting exercise has a developmental impact on the patient. For example, any major impairment to an older adult's ability to be mobile has serious implications for the ability to normally socialize. Also assess the patient's cultural views about exercise (see Box 38.3). These findings will affect how you approach motivating a patient. The same is true regarding the patient's social support. Take time to determine whether the patient relies on family or friends to become involved in exercise. If not, are there family members or friends who might be recruited to assist or participate in exercise with the patient? Finally, conduct an assessment of the patient's home, work, and school environments to determine to what extent exercise can be performed. Are there community or work areas for exercise? Does the patient feel safe to exercise outdoors? If the patient prefers to do exercises within the home, is there a comfortable space to do so?

Beth begins her assessment by asking Mrs. Smith to describe her normal daily exercise routine. The patient states, "I like to get out and walk, but lately with the problems at my husband's business we both work late, and I have little time to walk."

Beth clarifies, "How far did you walk when you did exercise, and how did it make you feel?"

Mrs. Smith says, "Walking actually makes me feel pretty good, but if I go up the hills in our neighborhood, I sometimes get short of breath and have to take a rest. Sometimes my knees hurt."

Beth responds, "Your knees hurt?"

Mrs. Smith says, "Yes, they just ache if I walk too far."

Beth asks, *"So how many days a week do you walk?"*

Mrs. Smith responds, "I walk about once or twice a week on a good week. When my husband joins me, we tend to walk more often and a bit farther."

"Farther?" Beth asks.

Mrs. Smith says, "Yes, I would say maybe half a mile."

Beth explores by asking, "Are there other exercises you enjoy?"

Mrs. Smith replies, "Not lately, but I have a friend who wants me to try a Pilates class."

To understand Mrs. Smith's beliefs about exercise, Beth says, "Mrs. Smith, you have heart failure and type 2 diabetes. Tell me what you know about how exercise affects your health."

Mrs. Smith responds, "Yes, the doctor tells me I need to exercise regularly. If I do that, he says my diabetes would be better controlled. I worry about how it might affect my heart."

Beth explains, "Exercise is very important for managing diabetes. Let's talk about how we might work together on a plan for exercises that are safe to do."

Beth conducts a cardiopulmonary assessment for the presence of arrhythmias or altered heart sounds, confirming the patient's heart failure. Beth auscultates the patient's heart and hears an extra heart sound. She confirms her finding with notes in the electronic medical record, which identifies that the patient has a mild ventricular gallop associated with her heart failure. The patient's lungs are clear. She measures the patient's resting heart rate at 84 beats/minute and sitting BP at 140/84.

REFLECT NOW

Think about a patient you have cared for who is usually physically active but has been acutely ill. What questions could you ask to assess the patient's current level of physical activity tolerance? What physical assessments would you also measure?

◆ Analysis and Nursing Diagnosis

Sound clinical judgment during the nursing process involves your critical analysis of the cues you gathered during patient assessment and your recognition of data patterns, which leads you to identify accurate nursing diagnoses. Apply your scientific knowledge and experience while you reflect on common findings associated with a patient's condition. Then you mentally compare these findings with actual data gathered from the patient. Sometimes you will need to gather additional data to confirm a pattern. You then identify and analyze familiar clusters of assessment findings to select relevant nursing diagnoses. For example, a patient who is tired and weak following exertion, who exercises less, and who rests more shows cues for the nursing diagnosis of either *Activity Intolerance* or *Fatigue*. Further review of assessment data (e.g., abnormal heart rate and mild shortness of breath after exercise) leads to a definitive diagnosis of *Activity Intolerance*.

Your assessment will also reveal data about the factors contributing to a patient's nursing diagnosis. In the case of negative or problem-focused nursing diagnoses, your assessment should reveal related factors, which are important for correctly directing your choice of nursing interventions. For example, *Activity Intolerance related to excess weight gain* requires very different interventions than if the related factor is prolonged bed rest. Assessment may also reveal risk factors that can be modified for managing risk diagnoses. Box 38.7 provides an example of how the diagnostic process leads to gathering cues for accurate diagnosis selection. The following are examples of nursing diagnoses related to activity and exercise:

- Activity Intolerance
- Risk for Fall-related Injury

BOX 38.7 Nursing Diagnostic Process

Impaired Mobility

Assessment Activities	Assessment Findings
Observe patient's gait.	Shuffled, slow gait Patient looks down while walking
Measure range of joint motion.	Reduced joint motion in lower and/or upper extremities Stiffness in joints
Measure patient's strength.	Has difficulty rising to sitting position or exiting bed

- Impaired Mobility in Bed
- Impaired Mobility
- Acute or Chronic Pain

Beth extends her assessment of Mrs. Smith by asking her to walk down the hallway of the clinic, back and forth 2 times. Beth notices the patient breathes more rapidly when returning. Heart rate decreased from 84 to 78 beats per minute. BP was unchanged. Mrs. Smith reports feeling "a bit short of breath." Beth reviews data and identifies the cues of "always feeling tired," "feeling like a blob," and participating less in outside activities as a pattern for the diagnosis of **Fatigue***. The presence of "shortness of breath," a "reduced heart rate following exercise," a "ventricular gallop," and the patient's report of "fatigue" is a pattern of data revealing the diagnosis of "***Activity Intolerance***." Beth also identifies a diagnostic pattern from Mrs. Smith's comments of "I like to get out and walk, but I have little time," "Walking actually makes me feel pretty good," and "I know I have to do something." She adds the diagnosis of* **Ability to Perform Health Maintenance***.*

◆ Planning and Outcomes Identification

During planning you consider all nursing diagnoses applicable to a patient, prioritize those diagnoses, and then select relevant interventions suited to a patient's ability and willingness to be engaged in exercise and activity (Fig. 38.7). A patient must be engaged, even in circumstances when activity is still limited. Allow the patient to make choices with the type of interventions you choose (e.g., type of exercise, timing of activities). Critical thinking during planning ensures that a patient's plan of care integrates all patient information and is patient centered.

A nurse's previous clinical experiences are highly valuable in planning for activity and exercise interventions. Observing previous patients' performance and responses to exercise helps in selecting realistic and measurable outcomes for subsequent patients. Experience in observing how physical therapists assist patients through activities is also very useful.

The environment is a factor when ensuring patient safety. In acute care, you are responsible for removing and monitoring for any barriers that could create risks when patients begin to ambulate or exercise. For example, when assisting a patient to ambulate down a crowded hallway, think about the route you will take, whether immovable objects are in the way, and whether a chair is close by if the patient needs to stop and rest. Use your resources wisely. Assistive personnel (AP) are trained in assisting with ambulation and transfers. Delegate to AP appropriately when a patient's condition is stable. Always have AP team up with you when transferring patients who meet safe handling weight restrictions.

Professional standards are especially important for developing a plan that is evidence based. These standards follow scientifically supported guidelines for selecting effective nursing interventions (e.g., type and frequency of exercise, level of assistance to provide patients). A concept map is a tool to assist in the planning of care. It shows the

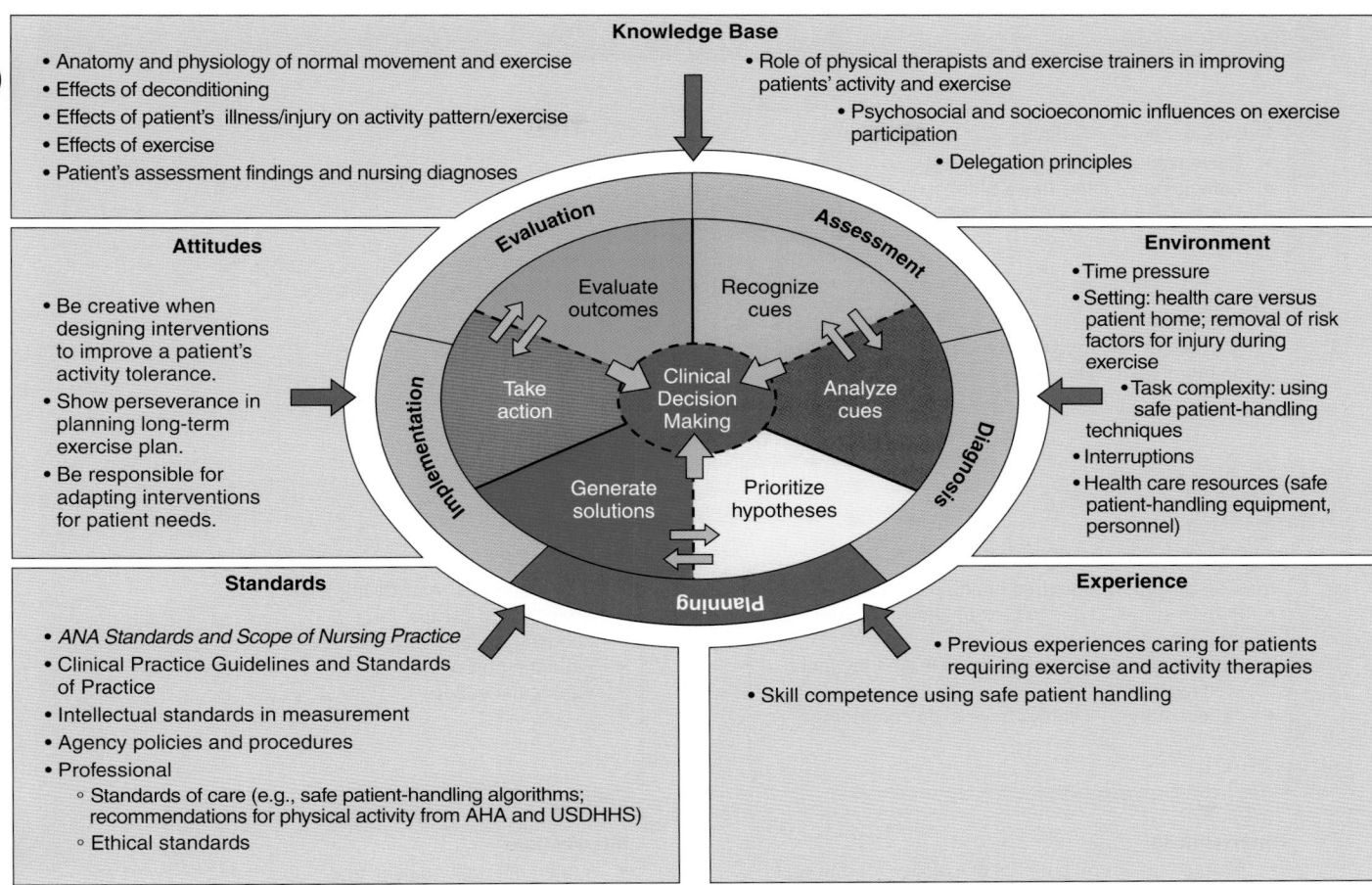

FIG. 38.7 Critical thinking model for planning activity and exercise. *CDC,* Centers for Disease Control and Prevention; *NIOSH,* National Institute for Occupational Safety and Health; *OSHA,* Occupational Safety and Health Administration. (Clinical Judgment Measurement Model copyright © NCSBN. All rights reserved.)

relationship between multiple nursing diagnoses and planned interventions. Fig. 38.8 provides a concept map for Mrs. Smith from the case study.

Outcomes. After identifying appropriate nursing diagnoses, you partner with the patient to set realistic, achievable outcomes to then direct the selection of interventions. Your knowledge of normal versus abnormal physiological responses helps you select outcomes to promote your patients' ability to function and improve or restore their independence. For example, if you know the normal targeted range for the heart rate of an older adult, you know what range to establish as an outcome. The same is true if there are standards for patient education. For example, if you know the guidelines for physical activity in adults, you will know the information a patient must understand to show improvement in knowledge about the activity program. A patient-centered plan includes consideration of any risks for injury to the patient and preexisting health concerns. For example, you will not establish an exercise program with activities that may be too stressful for a certain patient.

It is important to have knowledge of a patient's home environment when planning activity and exercise therapies to maintain or improve activity, body alignment, and mobility. Include the patient's family and/or caregiver in the care plan unless the patient prefers no family involvement. Family caregivers play critical roles in helping to make the home environment safe and in motivating and coaching patients

to stay active and adhere to an exercise plan. Developing a structured plan for regular exercise has been shown to be beneficial in improving adherence and physical conditioning (e.g., weight and blood pressure) (Joseph et al., 2019; Morey, 2021). Outcomes related to exercise and activity aim to improve or maintain a patient's functional status and independence. The following are examples of outcomes for patients with deficits in activity and exercise:

- Takes part in prescribed physical activity while maintaining appropriate heart rate, blood pressure, and breathing rate
- Explains the need to gradually increase activity on the basis of tolerance and symptoms
- Explains how balancing rest and activity will improve health problems
  Beth will identify outcomes for Mrs. Smith's plan of care that will be followed by the health care staff in the primary health care office long term. Beth and the other health care providers will use the outcomes to gauge Mrs. Smith's exercise progression and tolerance to exercise. In addition, Beth will have Mrs. Smith complete an exercise log to track her daily exercise participation. Mrs. Smith chose to use a diary she has at home. After consulting with Mrs. Smith, Beth chooses these outcomes for the nursing diagnosis of **Activity Intolerance***:*
- *Mrs. Smith will take part in the planned moderate exercise program weekly.*
- *Mrs. Smith will demonstrate a 20-pound weight loss in 3 months.*
- *Mrs. Smith will report absence of shortness of breath following a 1-mile walk in 1 month.*

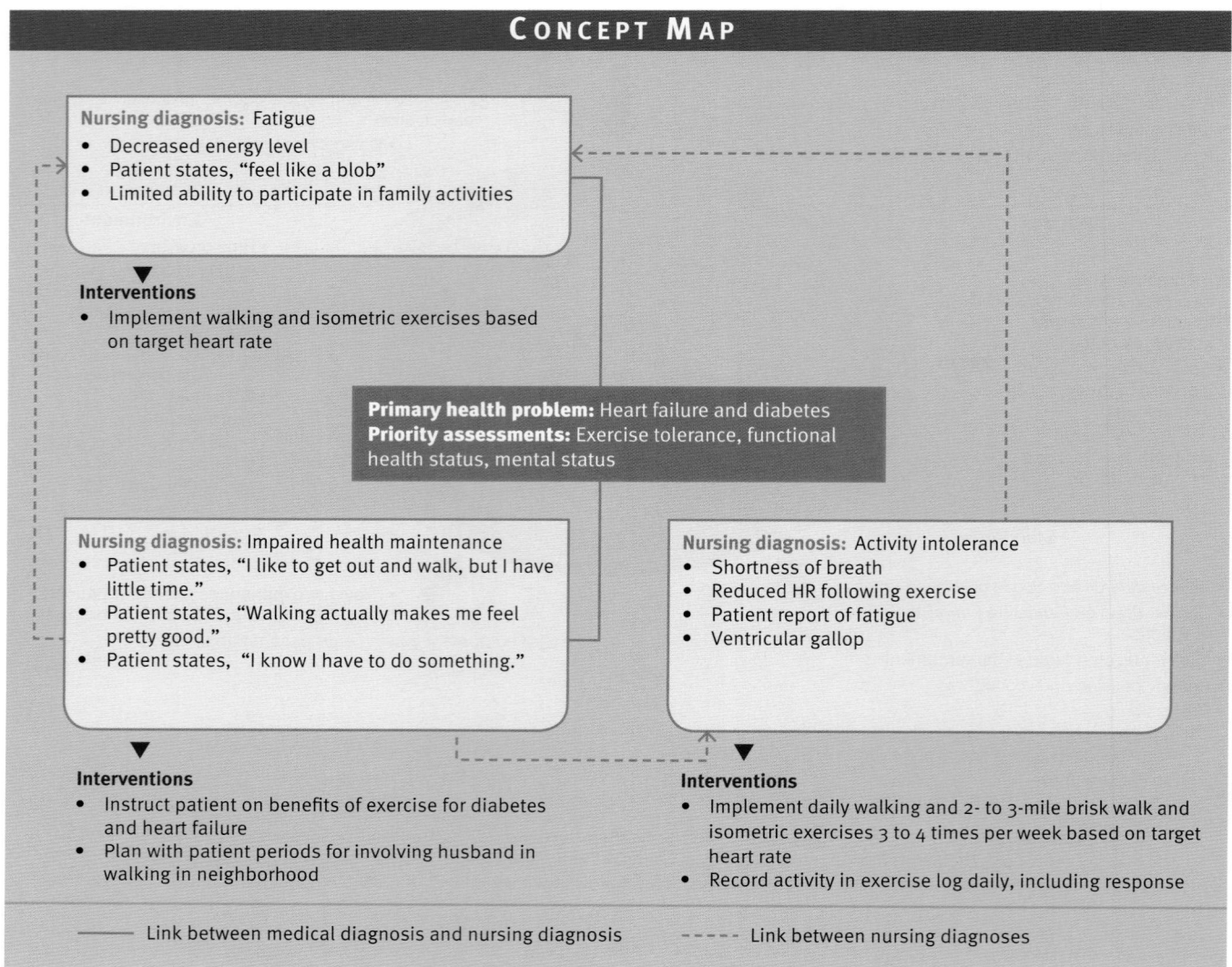

CONCEPT MAP

Nursing diagnosis: Fatigue
- Decreased energy level
- Patient states, "feel like a blob"
- Limited ability to participate in family activities

Interventions
- Implement walking and isometric exercises based on target heart rate

Primary health problem: Heart failure and diabetes
Priority assessments: Exercise tolerance, functional health status, mental status

Nursing diagnosis: Impaired health maintenance
- Patient states, "I like to get out and walk, but I have little time."
- Patient states, "Walking actually makes me feel pretty good."
- Patient states, "I know I have to do something."

Nursing diagnosis: Activity intolerance
- Shortness of breath
- Reduced HR following exercise
- Patient report of fatigue
- Ventricular gallop

Interventions
- Instruct patient on benefits of exercise for diabetes and heart failure
- Plan with patient periods for involving husband in walking in neighborhood

Interventions
- Implement daily walking and 2- to 3-mile brisk walk and isometric exercises 3 to 4 times per week based on target heart rate
- Record activity in exercise log daily, including response

——— Link between medical diagnosis and nursing diagnosis   - - - - Link between nursing diagnoses

FIG. 38.8 Concept map for Mrs. Smith. *ADLs,* Activities of daily living; *ḂP,* blood pressure.

Setting Priorities. Care planning is patient centered, taking into consideration the patient's condition and most immediate needs and preferences. For example, is a patient comfortable enough to participate in exercise, or do acute symptoms require you to delay an exercise session? You determine the immediate urgency of any problem by its effect on the patient's mental and physical health. For example, is it appropriate to ambulate a patient who just learned in the last 15 minutes that cancer therapy is ineffective? Priority setting also includes when to provide patient education. When activity and exercise participation are critical to a patient's recovery, providing information about the importance of activity or exercise must come at a time when a patient is responsive, attentive, and willing to learn. Education is less of a priority when the patient is short of breath or in pain.

Priority setting also involves using sound clinical judgment in the timing of activities and precautions to take. Because of the many common skills associated with the care of patients who have the diagnoses of *Activity Intolerance* and/or *Impaired Mobility,* such as ambulating, positioning, and transferring, it is easy to overlook the complications associated with these health alterations. Therefore, be vigilant in planning for and monitoring the patient and in supervising assistive personnel to carry out activities to prevent complications and potential injury.

Teamwork and Collaboration. Sound clinical judgment involves using the resources needed to maintain a patient's function and independence. For example, it is important to collaborate with health care providers and physical and occupational therapists. Health care providers will prescribe physical and occupational therapy as needed and note any limits or guidelines for activity levels. Physical therapists are best equipped to identify the specific exercises that patients should perform. Occupational therapists assist patients with adaptive devices and techniques to perform ADLs while improving mobility. Sometimes long-term rehabilitation is also necessary. Discharge planning begins when a patient enters the health care system and involves identifying expectations regarding physical activity, readiness and willingness to exercise, and what is planned by the health care team. In addition, always individualize a plan of care directed at meeting the actual or potential needs of the patient (see the Nursing Care Plan).

◆ Implementation

Health Promotion. A sedentary lifestyle contributes to the development of many health-related problems. The U.S. Department of Health

◎ NURSING CARE PLAN

Activity Intolerance

ASSESSMENT

Assessment Activities	*Assessment Findings[a]*
Ask Mrs. Smith her views about participating in regular activity and exercise.	She responds, "I **gained 30 pounds** over the past year. I become easily **fatigued**, and when I get home from work, I don't have the energy to finish my household chores. I used to like to walk—it felt good. But now I don't leave the house for family outings. I just go to work. I know I have to do something."
Ask Mrs. Smith about her routine exercise habits.	She responds, "I once exercised about 4 days a week, walking in the park just down from my house. Sometimes my husband joined me. But recently I have had to stay at work late, and I **have not walked for 2 months**. I just feel tired."
Perform baseline assessment.	Age: 52 years Weight: 82.6 kg (**182 lb**) Blood pressure: **140/84 mm Hg** (at rest) Pulse: 84 beats/min (at rest) Respirations: 20 breaths/min (at rest)

[a]**Assessment findings** are shown in bold type.

NURSING DIAGNOSIS: Activity intolerance related to inactivity and reduced cardiovascular fitness

PLANNING

Expected Outcomes (NOC)[b]

Activity Tolerance

Mrs. Smith will walk 150 minutes a week by the end of 6 weeks.

Mrs. Smith will follow a DASH diet eating plan of 2000 calories a day.

Mrs. Smith will achieve a target heart rate of 60% of maximum heart rate (100 beats per min) after 20 min walking.

Mrs. Smith will self-report a reduced sense of shortness of breath following walking at 1 month.

[b] Outcome classification labels from Moorhead S, et al., editors: *Nursing Outcomes Classification (NOC),* ed 6, St Louis, 2018, Elsevier.

INTERVENTIONS (NIC)[c]	RATIONALE
Exercise Promotion	
Base Mrs. Smith's instruction about beginning an exercise program on her contemplation phase of readiness. Discuss the physiological benefits of how regular exercise can improve her quality of life.	Regular exercise and physical activity are associated with a significantly lower CVD risk. Long-term studies have shown that increased physical activity is associated with a reduction in all-cause mortality and may modestly increase life expectancy (Nystoriak et al., 2018).

Develop a progressive exercise plan:
  Start with warm-up exercises for 3-5 minutes before walking, and perform cool-down exercises for 3-5 minutes after walking.
  Begin walking 20 minutes in neighborhood 4 times a week over the next 2 weeks; then 30 minutes 4 times a week in the third and fourth weeks, increasing to 30 minutes, 7 times weekly by week 6. Exercise within targeted heart rate.
	There is a relationship between greater amounts of physical activity and reduced weight in adults, with some evidence to support that this relationship is most pronounced when physical activity exposure is above 150 minutes per week (USDHHS, 2018). A combination of exercise and nutritional interventions tends to result in greater benefits toward lower weight, BP, and triglycerides than exercise only (Joseph et al., 2019).

Refer to dietitian to begin DASH eating plan. Incorporate patient's daily meal pattern with food preferences in the following groups: • Fresh vegetables, fruits, and whole grains • Fat-free or low-fat dairy products, fish, poultry, beans, nuts, and vegetable oils • Limiting foods that are high in saturated fat • Limiting sugar-sweetened beverages and sweets	DASH is a flexible and balanced eating plan recommended by the National Heart, Lung, and Blood Institute (n.d.b). It helps create a heart-healthy eating style for life, combining it with other lifestyle changes, such as physical activity, to gain control of blood pressure and LDL-cholesterol levels.
Have Mrs. Smith keep daily exercise log. Schedule routine phone calls with Mrs. Smith for follow-up.	Patients are more likely to increase physical activity and adhere to an exercise program if they are counseled by a health care professional (Edelman and Kudzma, 2022).

[c] Intervention classification labels from Butcher HK, et al., editors: *Interventions Classification (NIC),* ed 7, St Louis, 2018, Elsevier.

EVALUATION

Evaluation Activities	*Patient Response*
Review patient's exercise log weekly by phone.	Patient walked 20 minutes on 3 days the first week.
Review dietary log and record weight, blood pressure, and pulse.	Weight after 2 weeks, 80 kg (176 lb); resting heart rate remains between 80 to 90 beats/min; 100 to 110 beats/min after walking; blood pressure, 146/86 mm Hg.
Ask Mrs. Smith how she feels during and after walking.	"That first week or so of walking I felt some shortness of breath. It is not as bad now."

BOX 38.8 Physical Activity Guidelines for Americans (Adults and Older Adults)

Adults

- Move more and sit less throughout the day. Some physical activity is better than none. Adults who sit less and do any amount of moderate-to-vigorous physical activity gain some health benefits.
- Substantial health benefits can be gained for adults who do at least 150 minutes (2 hours and 30 minutes) to 300 minutes (5 hours) a week of moderate-intensity, or 75 minutes (1 hour and 15 minutes) to 150 minutes (2 hours and 30 minutes) a week of vigorous-intensity aerobic physical activity, or an equivalent combination of moderate- and vigorous-intensity aerobic activity. Preferably, aerobic activity should be spread throughout the week.
- Additional health benefits are gained by engaging in physical activity beyond the equivalent of 300 minutes (5 hours) of moderate-intensity physical activity a week.
- Adults should also do muscle-strengthening activities of moderate or greater intensity that involve all major muscle groups on 2 or more days a week, as these activities provide additional health benefits.

Older Adults

Key guidelines for adults also apply. In addition, the following key guidelines apply to older adults:

- As part of weekly physical activity, older adults should do multicomponent physical activity that includes balance training as well as aerobic and muscle-strengthening activities.
- Older adults should determine their level of effort for physical activity relative to their level of fitness (e.g., knowing target heart rate).
- Older adults with chronic conditions should understand whether and how their conditions affect their ability to do regular physical activity safely.
- When older adults cannot do 150 minutes of moderate-intensity aerobic activity a week because of chronic conditions, they should be as physically active as their abilities and conditions allow.

From U.S. Department of Health and Human Services: *Physical activity guidelines for Americans,* ed 2, 2018. https://health.gov/paguidelines/second-edition/pdf/Physical_Activity_Guidelines_2nd_edition.pdf. Accessed July 12, 2020.

and Human Services (USDHHS) has developed guidelines recognizing that physical activity is key to improving the health of the nation. The report, called *Physical Activity Guidelines for Americans,* is based on the latest scientific evidence and is an essential resource for health professionals who make recommendations for how individuals can improve their health through regular physical activity (USDHHS, 2018). There are guidelines for all age-groups, including children, adolescents, adults, older adults, and pregnant women (Box 38.8).

A nurse practicing in a primary care or community setting has a responsibility for partnering with patients to find ways to help them improve their physical activity. For example, community health nurses may work with local governments to find ways to improve access to recreational areas (e.g., parks, walking paths) in a town or city. Participating in health fairs or community walks is a way for nurses to be visible to the community and share information about physical activity with residents.

In primary care a patient-centered approach ensures that individuals set outcomes for activity that allow them to achieve the benefits they value (USDHHS, 2018). A nurse uses clinical judgment, considering the patient's current activity tolerance, the nature of the patient's health condition, and the type of exercise best suited to the patient's needs. Then the nurse uses a patient-centered approach to ensure that elements of the exercise program are relevant and suited to patient preferences and resources (Box 38.9). In setting activity outcomes, people can consider doing a variety of activities that are both indoor and outdoor. For example, a brisk walk in the neighborhood with friends for 45 minutes on 3 days a week and walking to lunch twice a week may be appropriate for someone who wants to increase both physical activity and socializing (USDHHS, 2018). Patients who love gardening might plan regular yard work as part of their aerobic activity. Take a holistic approach to develop and implement a plan that enhances the patient's overall physical fitness.

Before starting an exercise program, be sure the patient has been cleared by the health care provider for regular activity. Then teach patients how to calculate their target heart rate:

- First, subtract the patient's current age in years from 220 (calculates maximum heart rate).

BOX 38.9 PROCEDURAL GUIDELINES

Helping Patients to Exercise

Delegation and Collaboration

The skill of promoting early activity and exercise in the outpatient setting cannot be delegated to assistive personnel (AP).

Equipment

Weights, resistance bands (optional based on physical therapy recommendations)

Procedural Steps

1. Identify patient using at least two identifiers (e.g., name and birthday or name and medical record number) according to agency policy.
2. Measure patient's baseline heart rate or have patient/family caregiver do measurement.
3. Assess patient's or family caregiver's knowledge, experience, and health literacy (CDC, 2021f).
4. Identify patient's activity/exercise history:
   - Which type of regular daily exercise do you perform at home?
   - Do you exercise or play a sport at least 3 times a week?
   - On a scale of 0 to 5, with 0 being no daily exercise and 5 being strenuous regular daily exercise, how would you rate yourself?
   - How long have you been exercising regularly?

5. Ask patient to describe personal beliefs about exercise, including the ability to exercise and if exercise is enjoyable. Does the patient prefer indoor or outdoor activities?
6. Determine whether patient has social support from peers, family, or spouse.
7. Determine whether patient has access to a fitness center or other area to exercise. Is the neighborhood considered safe?
8. Consider assessment findings that may create a barrier to exercise, such as patient's age, income level, time available to exercise, where the patient lives, excess weight, or disability.
9. Have patient rate level of quality of life based on current activity level.
10. Initiate an outpatient exercise program that contains any of the following components:
    - Warm-up (5-10 minutes)—*directs needed blood flow to muscles and prepares body for exercise, helping to prevent injury*
    - Strengthening exercises
    - Endurance exercises
    - Balance exercises
    - Flexibility exercises—*lessen tightness of muscles and improve joint ROM*
    - Cool-down exercises (5-10 minutes)—*help body recover from exercises*

BOX 38.9 PROCEDURAL GUIDELINES—cont'd

Helping Patients to Exercise

11. Consult with physical therapy and evidence-based guidelines, such as the *Physical Activity Guidelines for Americans* available at: https://health.gov/sites/default/files/2019-09/Physical_Activity_Guidelines_2nd_edition.pdf, to help develop a complete exercise program that fits the needs of your patient.

12. Recommend strength training for adults to improve strength and bone density in collaboration with physical therapy.

13. Recommend aerobic exercise for endurance (see Box 38.8). The U.S. Department of Health and Human Services (2018) recommends aerobic exercises to include moderate and vigorous activities (e.g., climbing stairs; playing sports; or walking, jogging, swimming, or biking). Activities such as dancing, yoga, and brisk yard work are beneficial to older adults who prefer what they perceive as less rigorous forms of exercise.

14. Recommend balance exercises for older adults to decrease risk of falls. Ensure patient has something sturdy nearby to hold (e.g., wall or chair) in case the patient becomes unsteady. Perform exercises: standing on one foot, walking heel to toe, balance walking, and standing from a seated position (National Institutes of Health [NIH], 2021).

15. Have patient do strength exercises (lifting weights, carrying groceries, gripping a tennis ball, arm curls) 2 or more days per week, but not on any 2 days in a row (NIH, 2021) .

16. Recommend flexibility exercises (stretching back, inner thigh, back of leg and ankle) (NIH, 2021).

17. Recommend that the patient perform a cool-down (5 to 10 minutes) after exercising: quadriceps stretch; hamstring/calf stretch; chest and arm stretch; neck, upper back, and shoulder stretch.

18. Measure heart rate during and after exercise. Compare with baseline. Stop physical activity when:
    - Heart rate (HR) is above targeted heart rate OR
    - HR is more than a 20% decrease from resting value OR
    - HR is less than 40 beats/min

19. **Use Teach-Back:** "We have talked about doing a warm-up and cool-down as part of your exercise plan. Tell me why each is important." Revise your instruction now or develop a plan for revised patient/family caregiver teaching if patient/family caregiver is not able to teach back correctly.

20. Record in outpatient record the exercises recommended. Record patient response if you see the patient exercising.

- Then have the patient calculate the target heart rate by taking 60% to 90% of the maximum (depending on health care provider recommendations).

Mrs. Smith is 52 years old, and she has a resting heart rate of 84. Her target rate (220-52 × 60%) equals 100 beats/min. Beth sets a target heart rate of 60% to start Mrs. Smith's exercise program and outlines the planned weekly progression. Beth spends some time discussing how exercise can strengthen the patient's heart and improve blood glucose control. The patient was unaware of the effect exercise has on blood glucose and seemed excited about the potential benefits. "I can do this," she said. Beth knows the patient has two factors that call for a gradual increase in Mrs. Smith's level of walking. She has heart failure, meaning the heart has a reduction in stroke volume, decreasing delivery of the blood to cells and tissues. Rigorous exercise can stress the heart. Mrs. Smith has also not been regularly exercising for some time. She is not meeting the standard for 150 minutes of moderate intensive exercise. Gradual exercise progression will place less strain on the heart. Beth teaches Mrs. Smith how to take her pulse at the carotid artery. The two practice together. Then Beth encourages Mrs. Smith to try to include her husband during walking, making the walk an opportunity for both to wind down after work. Beth knows the teaching session has been lengthy. She wants Mrs. Smith to benefit. So, Beth schedules an appointment for the patient to see a dietitian to learn about the DASH diet plan. Beth will monitor Mrs. Smith by checking on her over the next few weeks. If exercise is well tolerated she will direct the patient to increase the time walking and to consider perhaps adding a Pilates class with her friend.

The patient's health care provider should recommend a maximum heart rate. When patients have activity intolerance or are just beginning exercise, it is wise to start on the low end of the target heart rate range and steadily increase the target as exercise tolerance improves.

No matter which exercise prescription is implemented for the patient, include warm-up and cool-down periods in the program (Edelman and Kudzma, 2022). The warm-up period usually lasts about 5 to 10 minutes and frequently includes stretching, calisthenics, and/or the aerobic activity performed at a lower intensity. It prepares the body and decreases the potential for injury. The cool-down period follows the exercise routine and usually lasts about 5 to 10 minutes. It allows the body to readjust gradually to baseline functioning and provides an opportunity to combine movement such as stretching with relaxation-enhancing mind-body awareness. When caring for older adults, special considerations are needed to adapt an exercise plan that ensures patient safety (Box 38.10).

QSEN **Building Competency in Quality Improvement** To assess individualized improvement in a patient's tolerance to activity, you need to use quality measures to understand a patient's performance. Determine the optimal cardiopulmonary response(s) to exercise for a patient who is 45 years old and whose health care provider set a desired 80% of maximum heart rate as a target.

Answers to the QSEN Activities can be found on the Evolve website.

Many patients find it difficult to incorporate an exercise program into their daily lives because of time constraints or lack of resources (e.g., no open parks or walking paths). For these patients it is beneficial to reinforce that they can use ADLs (e.g., gardening, climbing stairs when doing laundry) to accumulate the recommended 30 minutes or more per day of moderate-intensity physical activity. Encourage patients to find sports or activities that they enjoy, then vary their routines to keep them interesting by making activity fun, setting individual goals, and joining family or friends (Mayo Clinic, 2021). Other patients benefit from a prescribed exercise and physical fitness program carefully designed to meet personal goals and expectations. A patient-centered exercise program will include a combination of aerobic exercises, stretching and flexibility exercises, and strengthening and resistance training suited to a patient's home or community environment. Cross-training is recommended for the patient who prefers to exercise every day. For example, the patient runs one day and does yoga the next day.

BOX 38.10   FOCUS ON OLDER ADULTS

Special Considerations for Older Adults in Initiating and Maintaining an Exercise Program

- Encourage older adults to avoid prolonged sitting and get up and stretch. Frequent stretching decreases the risk of developing joint contractures.
- Be sure that the older patient maintains proper body alignment when sitting to minimize joint and muscle stress.
- Caution patients to listen to their bodies: endurance activities (e.g., brisk walking or cycling) should not cause dizziness, chest pain or pressure, or a feeling like heartburn (National Institute on Aging [NIA], 2021).
- Be sure to drink liquids when doing any activity that makes you sweat.
- Participate in exercises that promote endurance, strength, balance, and flexibility (NIA, 2021).
- Provide resources for planned exercise programs. Weight-bearing exercise, such as tai chi, walking, hiking, jogging, climbing stairs, playing tennis, and dancing, and resistance exercises, such as lifting weights, strengthen bones (NIA, 2021).

- Recommend resistance- and agility-training programs. These forms of exercise reduce the fear of falling and increase a sense of well-being in older adults (Kwun et al., 2012).
- Have older adults avoid high-impact programs that can lead to bone fractures (NIH, 2018; NIA, 2021).
- Teach older adults that it is never too late to begin an exercise program (Edelman and Kudzma, 2022). Consult a health care provider before beginning an exercise program, particularly in the presence of heart or lung disease and other chronic illnesses.
- Use assessment data and consult with physical therapy to determine when you need to adjust exercise programs for those of advanced age.
- Encourage older adults who are unable to participate in a formal exercise program to improve joint mobility and enhance circulation by simply stretching and exaggerating movements during the performance of routine activities of daily living.

Stretching and flexibility exercises include active ROM and stretching of all muscle groups and joints. This form of exercise is ideal for warm-up and cool-down periods. Benefits include increased flexibility, improved circulation and posture, and an opportunity for relaxation. Examples of stretching exercises include those performed in tai chi, yoga, and Pilates.

Resistance training increases muscle strength and endurance and is associated with improved performance of ADLs and avoidance of injuries and disability. Formal resistance training includes weight training, but patients can obtain the same benefits by performing ADLs such as pushing a vacuum cleaner, raking leaves, or shoveling snow. Some patients use weight training to bulk up their muscles for the purpose of developing tone and strength and to stimulate and maintain healthy bone.

Acute Care. Because patients in acute care are at risk for deconditioning, a nursing priority is to implement interventions to help patients ambulate and perform stretching and active ROM exercises as soon as possible. The level of exercise allowed will depend on a patient's physical condition. Physical therapists will collaborate on an exercise plan, including progressive walking, walking with assistive devices, and strengthening exercises. If needed, administer ordered analgesics 30 minutes before exercise. This provides patients relief from pain, which will help encourage their participation in their exercise plan. Do not administer an analgesic that makes the patient feel dizzy.

Early Mobility. Recently hospitals have introduced programs to increase inpatients' activity and mobility levels as soon as possible to prevent deconditioning and other complications of immobilization. When patients enter acute care, their activity and mobility often decline immediately. Limited activity and prolonged bed rest creates multiple problems, such as reduced physical function, sleep deprivation, delirium, and altered nutrition. Interprofessional health care teams have come together in many agencies to develop programs that increase patients' activity and mobility levels (Linke et al., 2020) (Box 38.11). Early mobility protocols have been developed and tested for patients who are critically ill (AACN, 2013; Schujmann et al., 2018; Linke et al., 2020), who have orthopedic problems (King et al., 2012), and who are having general surgery or neurosurgery (Walia et al., 2018) (see agency policy). Research shows nurse-facilitated early mobility programs reduce the incidence of delirium, improve muscle strength, increase independent functional status after discharge, and improve overall quality of life in patients who are critically ill (Cain, 2018) (Box 38.12). Early mobility programs need to continue when patients are transferred to general

nursing units. Continuing early mobility programs can be challenging on general nursing units because of staffing limitations, overall patient care demands, access to equipment, or unfamiliarity with transfer skills. To overcome these challenges, some hospitals have designated special mobility teams or mobility assistants to engage patients in early ambulation and activity. Typical early mobility protocols include specific assessment parameters for each level of mobility (e.g., assessing myocardial, oxygenation, and neurological stability), with patients progressing from passive and active assistive ROM exercises to sitting on the side of the bed, transferring to and sitting in a chair, and progressive ambulation (AACN, 2013; Schujmann et al., 2018).

Isotonic and Isometric Exercises. Isometric and isotonic exercises are safe for many patients. They are particularly helpful as an option for patients who are limited in mobility and not yet ambulating (Chapter 39). A physical therapist will typically collaborate with the patient's health care provider in selecting isometric exercises most beneficial for a patient. During isometrics, a patient tightens or contracts a muscle group (such as pushing down on mattress with the thigh) for 10 seconds and then completely relaxes for several seconds without joint involvement (Mayo Clinic, 2020). Patients gradually increase the repetitions for each muscle group until the isometric exercise is repeated 8 to 10 times. The exercise should be performed slowly, with patients increasing repetitions as their physical condition improves. A patient benefits from isometric exercise for quadriceps and gluteal muscle groups, which are used for walking, 4 times a day until the patient is ambulatory.

Isotonic exercises involve moving the joints Examples of isotonic exercise include:

- Palm stretch: Have patient open palm of hand, then extend the fingers for a few seconds. Then, touch the thumb with each finger. Repeat this exercise on the other hand.
- Plantar flexion/Dorsiflexion: As a patient lies supine, have the patient bend and stretch each foot forward for several seconds, and then flex the foot back toward the knee and hold for several seconds.
- Arm lifts: As a patient lies supine, have the patient lift the arm as high as possible and hold it there for 10 seconds. Repeat with the other arm. If the patient is unable to hold the arm up for that long, have the patient place the upper arm on the bed and lift the elbow until it reaches a 90-degree angle.

Your role as a nurse is to support patients in knowing how the exercises are to be performed correctly so that you can observe for any problems or difficulties. For example, an exercise program that includes

BOX 38.11 PROCEDURAL GUIDELINES

Assisting With Ambulation (Without Assist Devices)

Delegation and Collaboration

The skill of assisting patients with ambulation can be delegated to assistive personnel (AP). The nurse directs the AP to:

- Apply safe patient-handling principles when assisting the patient out of bed or chair.
- Review steps to ensure the patient is not having orthostatic hypotension when rising from a lying position in bed to sitting. Check patient's blood pressure before ambulation.
- Immediately return a patient to the bed or chair if patient is nauseated, dizzy, pale, or diaphoretic (Shibao et al., 2013; Frith et al., 2014; Biswas et al., 2019). Report these signs and symptoms to the nurse immediately.
- Apply safe, nonskid shoes/socks and ensure that the environment is free of clutter and that there is no moisture on the floor before ambulating the patient.

Equipment

Gait/transfer belt, nonskid shoes/socks, stethoscope, sphygmomanometer, pulse oximeter (as needed), pedometer *(optional)*

Procedural Steps

1. Identify patient using at least two identifiers (e.g., name and birthday or name and medical record number) according to agency policy (TJC, 2021).
2. Review medical record for patient's most recent activity experience, including distance ambulated, use of assist device, activity tolerance, balance, and gait. Note history of orthostatic hypotension and any medications, chronic illnesses, gait alterations, or a history of falling.
3. Review medical record for patient's most recently recorded weight and any descriptions of patient's ability to stand and bear weight.

   CLINICAL JUDGMENT: Use mechanical lift or transfer aid with minimum of two or three caregivers if a patient has partial weight-bearing with upper body strength or caregiver must lift more than 15.9 kg (35 lb) (Matz, 2019).

4. Review health care provider's order for ambulation; note any mobility, range of motion, or weight-bearing restrictions.
5. Assess patient's or family caregiver's health literacy (CDC, 2021f).
6. Perform hand hygiene. Assess patient's physical readiness to ambulate:
   a. Assess baseline resting heart rate, blood pressure, oxygen saturation (when available), and respirations.
   b. If patient's strength and endurance have been affected by illness or deconditioning, assess range of motion (ROM) and muscle strength (see Chapter 6) of lower extremities while patient in bed.
   c. Ask whether patient feels excessively tired or is currently experiencing any pain. Determine source and severity of pain (using a 0-to-10 pain-rating scale). This may delay ambulation. Offer an analgesic 30 minutes before ambulation to improve patient's tolerance to exercise.

   CLINICAL JUDGMENT: Do not administer an analgesic that could make the patient feel dizzy.

   d. Assess the patient's mobility: ability to sit up on side of bed or chair independently or with assist, ability to stand by using the Banner Mobility Assessment Tool (BMAT) (see Chapter 38) (Matz, 2019).
7. Assess patient's response to commands. Is the patient able to cooperate during ambulation?
8. Refer to patient's mobility status (e.g., BMAT score) and safe-handling algorithm (available in most agencies) to determine whether patient needs to walk with assist of a movable lift (Martin et al., 2016). The BMAT ensures a safe method of ambulation (Innovative Outcomes Management, 2017). Do not start procedure until all required caregivers are available.
9. Assess patient for any hearing or visual deficits (see Chapter 30) to ensure that patient can see the walking path and hear your instructions.
10. Check patient's environment for any barriers or safety risks. When walking, it is helpful within a hospital or rehabilitation center to walk in an area where handrails are on the walls and chairs are nearby.
11. Assess patient's or family caregiver's knowledge and experience regarding ambulation with assistance and patient's goals for ambulating.
12. Determine the best time to ambulate, considering all scheduled activities.
13. If this is the first time ambulating or if patient has been unsteady in past, have a chair or wheelchair positioned close to the path you choose for ambulation. *Option:* The patient can push a wheelchair, using it for stability, or can use a rollator. You want to be able to move the patient quickly into a safe sitting position if patient becomes unstable.
14. Close room door and bedside curtain. Provide privacy. Obtain and organize equipment for ambulation at bedside
15. Remove sequential compression devices (SCDs) from patient's legs if present (exception: may wear mobile compression devices (MCDs) while walking [see Chapter 39]).
16. Explain to patient in simple language how you are going to prepare for ambulation (e.g., gait belt application, use of wheelchair or rollator, distance planned to walk). Discuss benefits of walking and steps you are taking to reduce the chance of falling.
17. If hands became soiled during assessment, perform hand hygiene.
18. Assist patient from supine position to sitting position on edge of bed:
    a. With patient in supine position in bed, raise head of bed 30 to 45 degrees and place bed in low position, level with your hips. Raise upper side rail on side where patient will exit bed. Apply nonskid shoes or socks. If patient is fully mobile, allow to sit up on side of bed independently, using side rail to raise up.
    b. If patient needs assistance to sit on side of bed, turn patient onto side facing you while standing on side of bed where patient will sit.
    c. Stand opposite patient's hips. Turn diagonally to face patient and far corner of foot of bed.
    d. Place your feet apart in wide base of support with foot closer to head of bed in front of other foot.
    e. Place your arm nearer to head of bed under patient's lower shoulder, supporting the patient's head and neck. Place your other arm over and around patient's thighs (see illustration).

STEP 18e Nurse places arm over patient's thighs, other arm under patient's shoulder as patient raises up.

Continued

BOX 38.11   PROCEDURAL GUIDELINES—cont'd

Assisting With Ambulation (Without Assist Devices)

f. Move patient's lower legs and feet over side of bed as patient uses side rail to push and raise the upper body. Pivot weight onto your rear leg as you allow patient's upper legs to swing downward (see illustration). **Do not lift legs.** At same time, continue to shift weight to your rear leg, and guide patient in elevating the trunk into upright position.

STEP 18f Nurse shifts weight to rear leg and guides patient to raise up to sitting position.

19. Allow patient to sit on the side of the bed with feet on floor for 2 to 3 minutes (see illustration). Have patient alternately flex and extend feet and move lower legs up and down without touching floor. Ask whether patient feels dizzy; if so, check blood pressure. Have patient relax and take a few deep breaths until dizziness subsides and balance is gained. If dizziness lasts more than 60 seconds or if systolic BP has dropped at least 20 mm Hg within 3 minutes of sitting upright, return patient to bed (Biswas et al., 2019; Shibao et al., 2013; Frith et al., 2014). Recheck blood pressure.

STEP 19 Patient sits on side of bed.

20. Apply gait belt. Be sure that it completely encircles a patient's waist below the belly button. Belt should fit snugly, being sure two fingers fit between the belt and patient's body Avoid placing belt over any intravenous lines, incisions, or drainage tubes. You may need to adjust belt once patient stands (see illustration).

STEP 20 Application of gait/transfer belt.

21. If patient is alert and can bear weight and balance while standing, allow him/her to stand independently. Assist by holding gait belt to offer balance assistance.

22. If patient cannot bear weight or balance to stand independently but is clear to attempt ambulation, use an ambulation lift or ceiling lift with gait harness if available (see Chapter 39). Patient can walk with support of this mechanical device.

23. Confirm with patient distance to ambulate.

24. If patient has an IV line, place the IV pole on the same side as the site of infusion and instruct patient where to hold and push the pole while ambulating. It is best if another caregiver can push IV pole.

25. If a Foley catheter is present, carry the bag below the level of the bladder and prevent tension on the tubing.

26. For patients with orthopedic problems, stand on patient's unaffected side. For patients with neurological deficits (e.g., stroke), stand on the affected side. *For all other patients requiring assistance to maintain balance while weight bearing, stand on affected side.*

27. Grasp belt firmly with one hand, palm facing up (see illustration). Take a few steps, guiding patient with one hand grasping the gait belt and the other hand placed under the elbow of the patient's flexed arm.

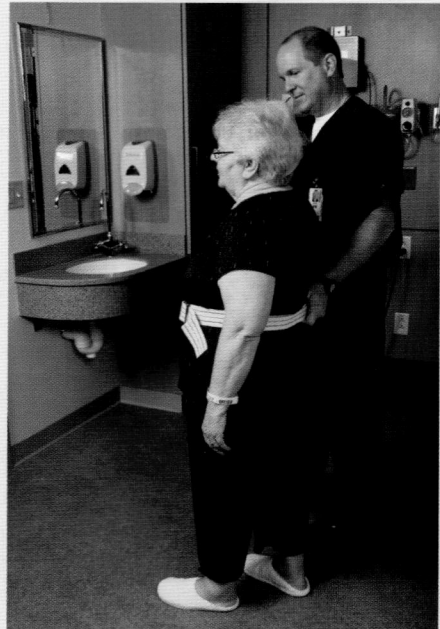

STEP 27 Nurse grasps gait belt firmly.

BOX 38.11 PROCEDURAL GUIDELINES—cont'd

Assisting With Ambulation (Without Assist Devices)

28. When ambulating in a hallway, position patient between yourself and the wall. Encourage patient to use handrails if available (see illustration).

STEP 28 Nurse helps patient by providing support under patient's flexed arm.

29. Observe how patient walks (posture, gait, balance) and determine distance patient can safely continue walking. Measure pulse and respirations as needed. (In patients experiencing deconditioning or those ambulating for the first time, you can also measure oxygen saturation.)

30. Return patient to bed or chair (independent transfer or use of mechanical lift) and assist patient to assume a comfortable position. Place the nurse call system within patient's reach.

31. Raise side rails (as appropriate) and lower bed to lowest position. Perform hand hygiene.

32. Dispose of any contaminated supplies in appropriate receptacle, remove and dispose of gloves, and perform hand hygiene.

33. **Teach-Back**: "Let us review what we discussed about taking steps in your home to have a safe path for walking. Tell me how you can prepare the rooms in your home." Revise your instruction now or develop a plan for revised patient/family caregiver teaching if patient/family caregiver is not able to teach back correctly.

34. Record time or distance ambulated, any changes in vital signs, and patient's tolerance (symptoms such as pain and fatigue) in nurses' notes in electronic health record (EHR) or chart.

35. Hand-off reporting: Report to health care provider any incident of orthostatic hypotension or patient's unexpected intolerance to exercise.

BOX 38.12 EVIDENCE-BASED PRACTICE

Benefits of Early Mobility Protocols

PICOT Question: Do patients who are acutely ill have improved clinical outcomes after participating in early mobility protocols compared with standard postoperative recovery routines while hospitalized?

Evidence Summary

Early mobilization is a complex intervention that requires careful patient assessment and management, as well as interprofessional team cooperation (Hodgson et al., 2018; Schujmann et al., 2018).The reported benefits of early mobilization include reduced ICU-acquired weakness, improved functional recovery within the hospital, reduced time from admission to ambulation, improved overall frequency and walking distance at hospital discharge, and reduced length of hospital stay (Hashem et al., 2016; Tipping et al., 2017; Linke et al., 2020). Outcomes vary depending on patient factors such as physiological instability (hemodynamic, respiratory, neurological), sedation, delirium/agitation, psychological state, and pain (Hodgson et al., 2018). Certain characteristics of the health care team can create barriers to early mobility intervention, including poor work culture, lack of communication, lack of leadership, disengaged team members, and inexperienced staff (Hodgson et al., 2018). Research has shown that unit culture, rather than patient-related factors,

may be the main barrier to early mobilization in ICUs (Hodgson et al., 2015). A study involving interdisciplinary collaboration within three adult ICUs showed that an early mobility protocol increased mobility for ICU patients without the addition of staff resources (Linke et al., 2020).

Application to Nursing Practice

• Having a dedicated mobility team with strong unit leadership facilitates protocol implementation (Hodgson et al., 2018).

• Interprofessional team planning with team meetings and daily goal setting is essential (Linke et al., 2020).

• Be knowledgeable of a patient's current condition and the clinical parameters set for early mobility to begin or proceed, and carefully assess patient response to activity.

• Invasive intravenous lines, endotracheal intubation, and feeding tubes do not contraindicate early mobility (Hashem et al., 2016).

• Variation in the supply and types of treatments available within critical care units may be the main barrier to achieving benefits and standardization with early and progressive mobility programs (Schujmann et al., 2018).

isometric exercises of the biceps and triceps will prepare a patient for crutch walking. Instruct the patient to stop the activity if pain, fatigue, or discomfort is experienced. Review the patient's chart and collaborate with physical therapy and the health care provider if any clinical changes develop (e.g., increased blood pressure, heart irregularity) that might contraindicate isometric exercise.

Range-of-Motion Exercise. The easiest intervention to maintain or improve joint mobility for patients and one that can be coordinated with other activities is the use of ROM exercises (see Chapter 39). There are three types of range-of-motion exercise: active, active assisted, and passive. In active range-of-motion (AROM) exercises patients move specific joints independently based on their muscular weakness and the type of activity that needs strengthening. The exercise moves the joint and soft tissues through the available physiological ranges of motion. AROM exercises are used when a patient is able to voluntarily contract, control, and coordinate a movement when such a movement is not contraindicated. As a nurse you should know the contraindications to AROM, including a healing fracture site, a healing surgical site, severe and acute soft tissue trauma, joint pain, limited joint movement, joint instability, deformity, and contractures. These suggest caution or investigation if you are planning on initiating AROM (Ball et al., 2019).

Walking. Walking increases joint mobility and can be measured by length of time or distance walked, such as down a hospital hallway or actual number of feet walked. Measure distances walked in estimated feet or yards instead of charting "ambulated to nurses' station and back." Some hospital or rehab units will have markers along floorboards designating distances. Illness or trauma usually reduces activity tolerance, resulting in the need for help with walking or the use of assistive devices such as crutches, canes, or walkers. Patients who increase their walking distance before discharge improve their ability to independently perform basic ADLs, increase activity tolerance, and have a faster recovery after surgery (Walia et al., 2018).

Helping a Patient Walk. Helping a patient walk requires preparation. Assess the patient's strength, coordination, baseline vital signs, and balance to determine the type of assistance needed. The procedural guideline for assisting with ambulation (see Box 38.11) describes in detail the approach to use to ensure patient safety. Reflect on your knowledge about the patient's status and physical condition; then judge whether it is safe to ambulate the patient. Postpone walking if you determine that the patient cannot walk safely. Assess the environment for safety before ambulation (e.g., removal of obstacles, a clean and dry floor, and the identification of rest points in case the patient's activity tolerance becomes less than expected or if the patient becomes dizzy). You may require the assistance of AP in case the patient requires a two-person assist.

When you help a patient to a position of sitting at the side of the bed, dangle the legs over the side of the bed for 1 to 2 minutes before standing. This prevents a sudden drop in BP when sitting or standing. Some patients experience orthostatic (postural) hypotension (i.e., a drop in systolic pressure by at least 20 mm Hg or a drop in diastolic pressure by at least 10 mm Hg within 3 minutes of rising to an upright position) (Shibao et al., 2013; Fedorowski and Melander, 2013). Orthostatic hypotension is a manifestation of abnormal BP regulation due to various conditions such as reduced intravascular volume and impaired autonomic reflexes, and not a specific disorder (Kaufmann, 2021). Neurogenic orthostatic hypotension is a sustained reduction in blood pressure (BP) upon standing that is caused by autonomic dysfunction (Biswas et al., 2019)

Patients at higher risk for orthostatic hypotension include patients who are immobilized or on prolonged bed rest, older adults, and patients with chronic illnesses such as diabetes mellitus and cardiovascular disease. Signs and symptoms of orthostatic hypotension include dizziness, light-headedness, nausea, tachycardia, pallor, and even fainting (Kaufmann, 2021). Patients at risk for neurogenic orthostatic hypotension have neurodegenerative disorders such as Parkinson disease and will exhibit similar symptoms.

If dizziness lasts more than 60 seconds or if systolic BP has dropped at least 20 mm Hg within 3 minutes of sitting upright, return a patient to bed immediately (Biswas et al., 2019). Orthostatic hypotension usually stabilizes quickly (Myszenski, 2017). Dangling a patient's legs before standing is an intermediate step that allows you to assess the patient before changing positions to maintain safety and prevent injury. In some instances, you need to take the patient's blood pressure while the patient sits on the side of the bed.

Several methods are used to help a patient ambulate. For those who can bear weight easily, provide support at the waist with a gait belt so that the patient's center of gravity remains midline. The belt helps you to stabilize patients if they lose their balance. A gait belt is *not* to be used in *lifting* or *carrying a patient by the waist.* Place a gait belt around a patient's waist below the belly button, snugly, being sure two fingers fit between the belt and patient's body. Don't place a gait belt over incisions, stitches, tubes, or intravenous lines, and never use one on a patient who is pregnant. When using a gait belt, hold the gait belt behind the patient with your palms facing up, but avoid trying to lift or catch patients by mistake, causing you a back injury. When patients are unable to walk independently or have too high a risk of falls, you need to use something more protective than a gait belt (i.e., motorized sit-to-stand lift, ceiling lift with ambulation sling, or a nonpowered stand-raise aide with ambulation capacity).

If a patient has a fainting (syncope) episode or begins to fall, your natural instinct will be to support or catch the patient. *Trying to stop or minimize a fall can cause you injury.* However, an approach used by physical therapists involves assuming a wide base of support with one foot in front of the other, thus supporting the patient's body weight (Fig. 38.9A). While holding the gait belt, try to extend one leg, let the patient slide against the leg, and gently lower the patient to the floor, protecting the head (Figs. 38.9B–C). Use caution to prevent your own injury, especially if the patient is overweight. When the patient attempts to ambulate again, proceed more slowly, monitoring for reports of dizziness; take the patient's blood pressure before, during, and after ambulation. The key to preventing staff injuries is to focus on reducing the number of preventable patient falls and falls with injury through accurate patient assessments and the use of proper equipment.

Restorative and Continuing Care. Restorative and continuing care involves implementing activity and exercise strategies to help a patient perform ADLs after acute care is no longer needed. Restorative and continuing care also includes activities and exercises that restore and promote optimal functioning in patients with specific chronic illnesses such as coronary heart disease (CHD), hypertension, COPD, and diabetes mellitus.

Assistive Devices for Walking. In collaboration with physical therapists, promote activity and exercise by teaching the proper use of canes, walkers, or crutches, depending on the assistive device most appropriate for the patient's condition. Assistive devices are recommended for patients unable to bear full weight on one or more joints of the lower extremities. Other indications for use are instability, poor balance, or pain in weight bearing. An assistive device can reduce the risk of falls, decrease pain with mobility, and improve balance (Touhy and Jett, 2020). However, the devices can also be a risk factor for falling if used incorrectly. You will collaborate with a physical therapist in selecting the proper device for a patient (Table 38.3).

Walkers. A walker is a lightweight, movable device that stands about waist high and consists of a metal frame with handgrips, four widely placed sturdy legs, and one open side (Fig. 38.10). A walker can be used by a patient who has lower extremity weakness or has problems with balance. Walkers with wheels are useful for patients who have difficulty lifting and advancing the walker as they walk because of limited balance or endurance. However, the disadvantage is that the walker can roll forward when weight is applied A patient uses a walker correctly by holding the handgrips on the upper bars, taking a step, moving the walker forward, and taking another step. A walker requires the patient to lift the device up and forward. The patient should not lean over the walker or walk behind it; otherwise the patient might lose balance and fall. Walkers should not be used on stairs. Teach patients how to use walkers safely and avoid the risk of falling.

FIG. 38.9 How to support a patient who is falling. (A) Stand with feet apart to provide a broad base of support. (B) Extend one leg and let patient slide against it to the floor. (C) Bend knees to lower body as patient slides to the floor.

TABLE 38.3 Types of Assistive Devices

Type of Device	Features	Measurement
Canes: lightweight, easily movable devices approximately waist high, made of wood or metal. Two types: single straight-legged and quad (see Fig. 38.11).	Straight canes provide support and balance for patients who have mild balance or strength impairments. Quad canes are often used for patients who have unilateral weakness from a neurological event/disease (i.e., stroke) and require more support than a straight cane. Patient keeps the cane on the stronger side of the body (Fairchild et al., 2018). Nurse stands on the patient's weak side for support (Fairchild et al., 2018).	Have patient stand upright with arms relaxed down with normal bend at the elbow (15 to 30 degrees). The handle of the cane should be close to the patient's wrist crease. Cane handle should fit comfortably in palm of hand.
Crutches: wooden or metal staff. Two types of crutches: the double adjustable Lofstrand or forearm crutch and the axillary wooden or metal crutch.	Use of crutches is usually temporary (e.g., after ligament damage to the knee). Some patients, such as those with paralysis of the lower extremities, need crutches permanently.	Measurements include the patient's height, the angle of elbow flexion, and the distance between the crutch pad and the axilla. Measure standing: Position crutches with crutch tips at 15 cm (6 inches) laterally to side and 15 cm in front of patient's feet (tripod position). Crutch pads should be 3.75–5 cm (1½–2 inches or 2–3 finger widths) under axilla with the elbows slightly flexed (American College of Foot & Ankle Surgeons, 2021; Fairchild et al., 2018). Height of handgrips must be adjusted so that patient's elbow is slightly flexed or grip sits at approximate height of wrist crease. Both height of crutch and handgrip dimensions are adjustable on a well-made crutch.
Walkers: extremely light, movable devices, approximately waist high and made of metal tubing (see Fig. 38.10). They have four widely placed, sturdy legs. They can also have 2–4 wheels.	Has a wide base of support, providing stability and security when walking.	Have patient step inside walker. When patient relaxes arms at side of body and stands up straight, top of walker should line up with crease on inside of wrist. Elbows should flex about 15 to 30 degrees when standing inside walker, with hands on handgrips (American Academy of Orthopaedist Surgeons, 2015; Fairchild et al., 2018).

FIG. 38.10 Patient using a walker.

FIG. 38.11 Bottom of quad cane.

Canes. Canes provide less support than a walker and are less stable. The most common cane is the straight-legged, the length of which should be equal to the distance between the greater trochanter and the floor (Fairchild et al., 2018). Have the patient keep the cane on the stronger side of the body. For maximum support when walking, the patient places the cane forward 15 to 25 cm (6 to 10 inches), keeping body weight on both legs. The patient moves the weaker leg forward to the cane, so body weight is divided between the cane and the stronger leg. The patient then advances the stronger leg past the cane, so the weaker leg and the body weight are supported by the cane and weaker leg. During walking the patient continually repeats these three steps. The patient needs to learn that two points of support, such as both feet or one foot and the cane, are on the floor at all times.

The quad cane provides the most support and is used when there is partial or complete leg paralysis or some hemiplegia (Fig. 38.11). You teach the patient the same three steps that are used with the straight-legged cane.

Crutches. Crutches are used by people who cannot bear weight on one or both legs because of short-term injury or permanent disability. A crutch is a wooden or metal staff. The forearm crutch has a handgrip and a metal band that fits around the patient's forearm. The metal band and the handgrip are adjusted to fit the patient's height. The more common axillary crutch has a padded curved surface at the top, which fits under the axilla. A handgrip in the form of a crossbar is held at the level of the palms to support the body. It is important to measure crutches for the appropriate length and to teach patients how to use their crutches safely to achieve a stable gait, ascend and descend stairs, and rise from a sitting position. Always begin crutch instruction with guidelines for safe use (Box 38.13).

Measuring for Crutches. Measurement for an axillary crutch includes the patient's height, the angle of elbow flexion, and the distance between the crutch pad and the axilla (see Table 38.3). When crutches are fitted, ensure that the length of the crutch is two to three finger widths from the axilla, and position the tips approximately 2 inches lateral and 4 to 6 inches anterior to the front of the patient's shoes.

Position the handgrips so that the axillae are not supporting the patient's body weight. Pressure on the axillae increases risk to underlying nerves, which sometimes results in partial paralysis of the arm. Determine correct position of the handgrips with the patient upright, supporting weight by the handgrips with the elbows slightly flexed. Elbow flexion (approximately 15 to 30 degrees) may be verified with a goniometer (Fig. 38.12). When you determine the height and placement of the handgrips, verify that the distance between the crutch pad and the patient's axilla is 1½ to 2 inches (two to three finger widths) (Fig. 38.13).

FIG. 38.12 Using the goniometer to verify correct degree of elbow flexion for crutch use.

FIG. 38.13 Verifying correct distance between crutch pads and axilla.

FIG. 38.14 Tripod position, basic crutch stance.

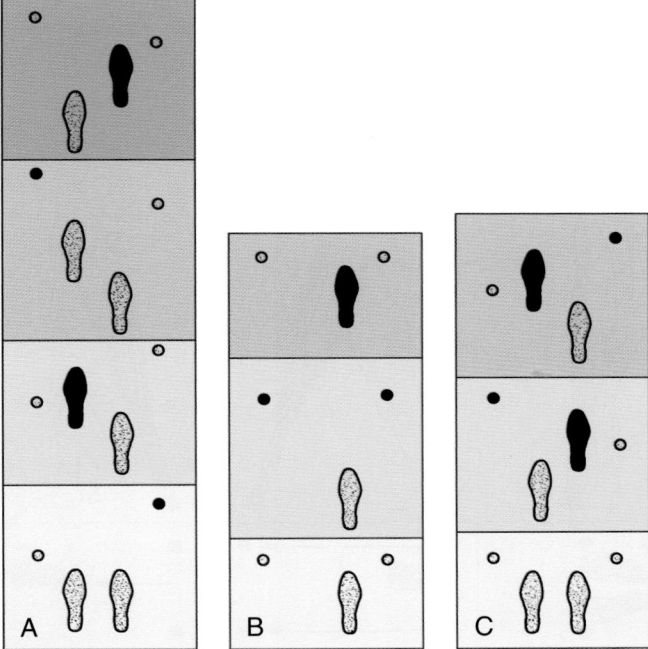

FIG. 38.15 (A) Four-point alternating gait. Solid feet and crutch tips show the order of foot and crutch tip movement in each of the four phases. (Read from bottom to top.) (B) Three-point gait with weight borne on unaffected leg. Solid foot and crutch tips show weight-bearing in each phase. (Read from bottom to top.) (C) Two-point gait with weight borne partially on each foot and each crutch advancing with opposing leg. Solid areas indicate leg and crutch tips bearing weight. (Read from bottom to top.)

Crutch Gait. Patients assume a crutch gait by alternately bearing weight on one or both legs and on the crutches. A physical therapist in collaboration with the health care provider will determine the appropriate gait by assessing the patient's physical and functional abilities and the disease or injury that resulted in the need for crutches. This section summarizes the basic crutch stance and the four standard gaits: four-point alternating gait, three-point alternating gait, two-point gait, and swing-through gait.

The basic crutch stance is the tripod position, formed when the crutches are placed 15 cm (6 inches) in front of and 15 cm (6 inches) to the side of each foot (Fig. 38.14). This position maintains a patient's balance by providing a wider base of support. The body alignment of the patient in the tripod position includes an erect head and neck, straight vertebrae, and extended hips and knees. The axillae should not bear any weight. The patient assumes the tripod position before crutch walking.

Four-point alternating, or four-point, gait gives stability to the patient but requires weight bearing on both legs. Each leg is moved alternately with each opposing crutch so that three points of support are on the floor at all times (Fig. 38.15A).

Three-point alternating, or three-point, gait requires the patient to bear all of the weight on one foot. In a three-point gait the patient bears weight on both crutches and then on the uninvolved leg, repeating the sequence (Fig. 38.15B). The affected leg does not touch the ground during the early phase of the three-point gait. Gradually the patient progresses to touchdown and full weight bearing on the affected leg.

The two-point gait requires at least partial weight bearing on each foot (Fig. 38.15C). The patient moves a crutch at the same time as the opposing leg, so the crutch movements are similar to arm motion during normal walking.

Individuals with paraplegia who wear weight-supporting braces on their legs frequently use the swing-through gait (Fig. 38.16). It is used for full or partial restricted weight bearing on one leg. A patient steps past crutches with the weight-bearing leg; the gait assumes a two-point (see Fig 38.16) or three-point pattern. This gait reduces pressure on the patient's involved leg.

Using Crutches to Ascend and Descend Stairs. Climbing stairs with the use of a railing is the safest way for a patient with crutches to ascend stairs. *Be aware that there is a risk for falling using this technique.* Your responsibility is to monitor a patient's balance carefully. Be sure there are no obstacles on the stairs, such as stacks of magazines or other items. Reassess the patient for any dizziness or sudden weakness. Have the patient hold the handrail for support with one hand (strong leg next to railing). You carry the crutch positioned next to the handrail as the patient places the other crutch under the axilla of the affected side. Have the patient transfer body weight to the crutch while holding the handrail with one hand (Fig. 38.17A). Stay behind the patient, holding on to the gait belt. Then have the patient support the weight evenly between the handrail and crutch. Next, the patient places some weight on crutch and then steps up the first step with

weight-bearing foot (stronger leg) (Fig. 38.17B). Have patient balance by leaning forward with weight on good leg. Then ask the patient to straighten the good knee, push down on crutches and lift body weight, bringing the affected leg and then the crutch up the stair (Fig. 38.17C). Always make sure the crutch tip is completely on the stair (Washington University Physicians, 2017). Repeat sequence for each step, and instruct patient to climb one stair at a time.

A patient remains at risk for falling when descending stairs. Assist the patient using extreme caution. Have the patient stand close to the edge of the top step (Fig. 38.18A). Have the patient hold the handrail with one hand (affected leg next to railing). You carry the crutch positioned next to the handrail as the patient places the other crutch under the axilla of the strong side. Stand above the patient while holding the gait belt. For support, have the patient lower the crutch down to the step below and then move the affected leg down (Fig. 38.18B) (Washington University Physicians, 2017; Webster and Murphy, 2019). The patient then brings the strong leg down the step and supports the weight evenly among handrail, good leg, and crutch (Fig. 38.18C). Be sure that patient has good balance. Always make sure the crutch tip is completely on the stair. Caution the patient not to hop.

Remember, when going up stairs, the patient leads with the stronger leg. When going down stairs, lead with the affected leg. Because in most cases patients need to use crutches for some time, they need to be taught to use them on stairs before discharge. Instruction applies to all patients who are dependent on crutches, not just those who have stairs in their homes.

Sitting in a Chair With Crutches. The procedure for sitting in a chair involves phases and requires the patient to transfer weight (Fig. 38.19). First position the patient at the center front of the chair with the posterior aspect of the legs touching the chair. Then the patient holds both crutches in the hand opposite the affected leg. If both legs are affected, as with a person with paraplegia who wears weight-supporting braces, the patient holds the crutches in the hand on the stronger side. With both crutches in one hand, the patient supports body weight on the unaffected leg and the crutches. While still holding the crutches, the patient grasps the arm of the chair with the remaining hand and lowers the body into it. To stand the procedure is reversed, and the patient, when fully erect, assumes the tripod position before beginning to walk.

Restoration of Activity and Chronic Illness. Nurses deliver patient-centered interventions for increasing activity and exercise in patients

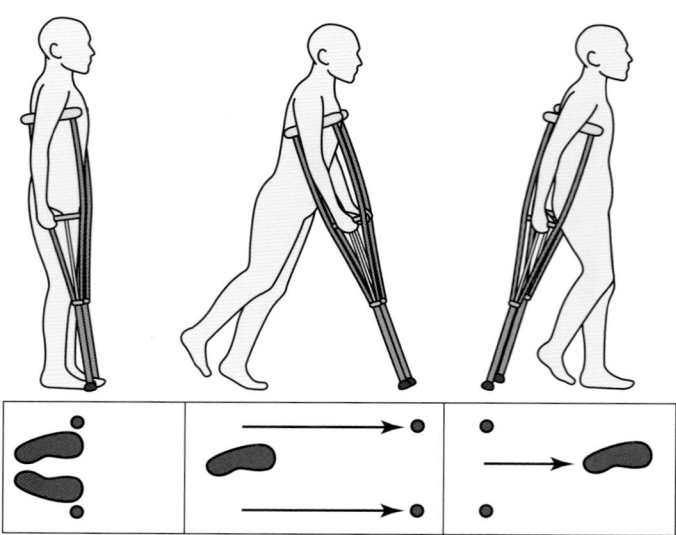

FIG. 38.16 Swing-through crutch walking gait.

A   B   C

FIG 38.17 Ascending stairs with crutches.

with specific disease conditions and chronic illnesses such as coronary artery disease (CAD), hypertension, chronic obstructive pulmonary disease (COPD), and diabetes mellitus.

Coronary Artery Disease. Regular moderate-intensity aerobic exercise has been shown to reduce the risk of sudden cardiac death and acute MI (Wenger et al., 2020). Increasing physical activity is an important modifiable behavior that can reduce the relative risk of CAD events (such as angina and myocardial infarction) because of its systemic benefits (Fig. 38.20). Regular moderate exercise enhances coronary artery

blood flow and reduces incidents of angina by enhancing oxygen delivery to the heart muscle (myocardium). Adherence and access to the necessary resources are often barriers to implementing healthy lifestyle changes in patients with CAD (Wenger et al., 2020). As a nurse you will play a role in discussing with patients how regular exercise specifically improves heart function and reduces development of other complications. Collaborate with home health and community nurses to help patients find resources to participate in cardiac rehab programs. Such programs provide valuable resources that have shown measurable

A   B   C

FIG. 38.18 Descending stairs with crutches.

A   B   C

FIG. 38.19 Sitting in a chair. (A) Both crutches are held in one hand. Patient transfers weight to crutches and unaffected leg. (B) Patient grasps arm of chair with free hand and begins to lower herself into chair. (C) Patient completely lowers herself into chair.

FIG. 38.20 Systemic benefits of regular moderate-intensity exercise. (From *Prog Cardiovasc Dis.* Author manuscript; available in PMC 2016 Mar 1. Published in final edited form as *Prog Cardiovasc Dis.* 2015 Mar-Apr; 57(5): 443–453.)

benefits to patients. Cardiac rehab programs are comprehensive, long-term services involving medical evaluation, supervised exercise, cardiac risk factor modification, education, and counseling (Wenger et al., 2020). Patient participation in cardiac rehabilitation speeds recovery from acute cardiovascular events such as myocardial infarction, myocardial revascularization, or hospitalization for heart failure and improves quality of life (Braun et al., 2021).

Hypertension. In addition to standard antihypertensive medications, the benefits of physical activity on hypertension and cardiovascular disease have been well demonstrated (Hegde and Solomon, 2015; Braun et al., 2021). A number of studies have consistently shown beneficial effects of exercise on hypertension, resulting in reductions in both systolic and diastolic blood pressure with as much as 5 to 7 mm Hg reductions in those with hypertension (Hegde and Solomon, 2015). Encourage patients to participate in low- to moderate-intensity aerobic exercise as it is the most effective in lowering blood pressure. In addition, tai chi exercise programs have shown promise in managing hypertension, although more rigorous research is needed (Wang et al., 2013; Edelman and Kudzma, 2022). Have patients with hypertension measure their BP daily at home, and help them learn how reactions to stress can raise BP. Relaxation exercises are useful in reducing stress reactions.

Chronic Obstructive Pulmonary Disease. Pulmonary rehabilitation helps patients with COPD reach an optimal level of functioning. It is a multidisciplinary program of care for people with chronic respiratory impairment and is individually tailored and designed to each person's physical and social performance and autonomy (National Institute for Health and Care Excellence [NICE], 2019). Exercise training has been shown to significantly improve health-related quality of life, respiratory muscle strength, symptoms (e.g. exertional dyspnea in patients with COPD), and normal exercise capacity (Bennett et al., 2017; Souto-Miranda et al., 2021). Some patients are fearful of participating in exercise because of the potential of worsening dyspnea (difficulty breathing). This aversion to physical activity sets up a progressive deconditioning in which minimal physical exertion results in dyspnea. Pulmonary rehabilitation can help patients gain strength, reduce symptoms of anxiety or depression, and make it easier to manage routine activities, work, and social activities. Patients may have pulmonary rehabilitation in the hospital or a clinic, or they may learn physical therapy

or breathing exercises to do at home. Outpatient pulmonary rehabilitation provides a safe environment for monitoring patients' progress.

Diabetes Mellitus. Along with diet, glucose monitoring, and medication, physical activity and regular exercise are important components in the care of patients with diabetes mellitus. Moderate to high levels of aerobic activity have been found to be associated with substantially lower cardiovascular risk and better glycemic control in both type 1 and type 2 diabetes (McCulloch, 2019). In type 1 diabetes, aerobic exercise increases cardiorespiratory fitness, decreases insulin resistance, and improves lipid levels and endothelial function (Chimen et al., 2012; McCulloch, 2019). In individuals with type 2 diabetes, regular exercise reduces HbA$_{1c}$, triglycerides, blood pressure, and insulin resistance (Colberg et al., 2016; McCulloch, 2019). *This is the case for Mrs. Smith, who might gain the benefit of not having to take an oral hypoglycemic if she is able to adhere to a regular exercise program. This is an incentive Beth can discuss to promote patient participation.*

The recommendations for physical activity and exercise in diabetes from the position statement of the American Diabetes Association (Colberg et al., 2016; ADA, 2020) can be found at the following website: https://care.diabetesjournals.org/content/diacare/39/11/2065.full.pdf. It includes current clinical practice recommendations for diabetes care, treatment goals, and guidelines. Include these recommendations in your teaching plan for patients with all types of diabetes.

◆ Evaluation

Through the Patient's Eyes. For activity and exercise you measure the effectiveness of nursing interventions by evaluating whether the patient's expectations have been reached. The patient is the only one who knows the effectiveness and benefits of activity and exercise on overall well-being. Ask the patient questions such as "How well did you tolerate walking, and is that what you expected?" and "You have been walking regularly for a month now; how has it made you feel?" Continuous evaluation helps to determine whether new or revised therapies are needed and whether new nursing diagnoses have developed.

Patient Outcomes. Sound clinical judgment in patient evaluation involves comparing a patient's baseline mobility and activity tolerance

Knowledge Base

- Normal activity needs for patient's developmental stage
- Effects of patient's illness or injury on activity pattern/exercise

- Patient's assessment findings, nursing diagnoses, and expected outcomes
- Characteristics of improved activity and exercise tolerance
- Anticipated effects of therapies

Attitudes

- Be creative in approach to evaluation; engage patient in ADLs to observe function.
- Apply discipline; conduct a thorough evaluation
- Integrity; recognize when patient's expectations differ from yours; adjust plan to meet patient needs

Evaluation

Evaluate outcomes

Assessment

Recognize cues

Take action

Clinical Decision Making

Analyze cues

Implementation

Diagnosis

Generate solutions

Prioritize hypotheses

Planning

Environment

- Time pressure
- Setting: acute care versus patient home
  - Task complexity using safe patient-handling
  - Interruptions
- Health care resources (safe patient-handling equipment, personnel)

Standards

- *ANA Standards and Scope of Nursing Practice*
- Clinical Practice Guidelines and Standards of Practice
- Intellectual standards in measurement
- Agency policies and procedures
- Patient expected outcomes
- Professional
  - Standards of care (e.g., safe patient-handling algorithms; recommendations for physical activity in adults)
  - Ethical standards

Experience

- Previous experiences caring for patients receiving activity and exercise therapy
- Previous experience monitoring activity response
- Skill competence – safe patient handling

FIG. 38.21 Critical thinking model for activity and exercise evaluation. (Clinical Judgment Measurement Model copyright © NCSBN. All rights reserved.)

measures (e.g., pulse, blood pressure, respirations, strength, self-report of fatigue, and psychological well-being) with expected outcomes and standards for improvement (Fig. 38.21). In cases of patients who have lost muscle tone or those first ambulating after extended bed rest, measuring oxygen saturation can help inform your evaluation of patient outcomes. The comparison of actual outcomes with expected outcomes determines the patient's health status and whether progression has occurred. Standards for physical activity performance (e.g., the ability to reach the target heart rate) are one of the more objective ways to evaluate whether a patient's activity tolerance improves. Also, when evaluating a patient's functional ability to determine whether exercise has improved performance, engage the patient in ADL activities. In this way you will see whether the patient can perform self-care successfully.

Apply critical thinking when you evaluate your findings. Your scientific knowledge and experience will assist in evaluation, especially when there are subtle and less obvious changes. For example, after having a patient perform isotonic exercises over a 3- to 4-day time span, the nurse who has assisted the patient routinely can notice changes in the patient's ability to reach full ROM (dorsiflexion/plantar flexion) or improved muscle strength (able to raise arms over longer time). Because changes in mobility and activity tolerance can be subtle, it is important for nurses to communicate clear and specific measures to other health care providers so that consistent evaluation can occur.

The following is a list of potential questions you might ask when your patients do not meet their expected outcomes:

- The last time we met you planned to walk outside for 20 minutes 3 days a week. However, you report that you are able to walk only twice a week right now. Tell me what you think is preventing you from meeting your goal.

- Your weight is the same this month as it was last month. We were hoping that increasing your activity would lead to a decrease in your weight. Help me understand the factors you believe are preventing you from losing weight right now.
- You state that you experience leg pain after walking short distances. Describe your pain. Which pain-relieving measures have you tried?

It has been three weeks since Beth saw Mrs. Smith in the primary care clinic. She calls Mrs. Smith to follow up on her progress with the exercise plan. Mrs. Smith reports, "I have been filling out my diary, and I feel good about everything so far. The first week I walked 2 times for 20 minutes each; I felt comfortable, and my pulse was 96 to 102 beats/min when I finished. The second week I walked 3 days, and it was for a total of 90 minutes. I pushed myself, I guess, and felt a little short of breath afterward. My husband went with me, and we walked farther. My pulse got to 105 beats/min midway on the third day. I slowed down and stopped as you suggested. Then we walked back. This week I have walked once for 25 minutes, and my pulse was 96 when I finished."

Beth responded, "That is great news. I am so glad you knew to slow down when your pulse got a little high last week. That is a good way to listen to your body. Tell me how walking works with your husband?"

Mrs. Smith replied, "He tends to walk a bit faster than me, but he slows down. You were right. We have used the time to talk about some work issues, and it helps to get it out. But walking also just gives us some quality time."

Beth said, "I want you to continue your walking plan. Now tell me about your progress with your new diet."

Mrs. Smith said, "I saw the dietitian for the first time last week. It will take some adjustment as my husband and I have not regularly eaten lots of vegetables, but we have set a menu for this week. So far, so good."

TABLE 38.4   Preventing Lift Injuries in Health Care Workers

Action	Rationale
When planning to move a patient, arrange for adequate help. If your institution has a lift team, use it as a resource (OSHA, 2017).	A lift team is properly educated in techniques to prevent musculoskeletal injuries.
Use patient-handling equipment and devices such as height-adjustable beds, ceiling-mounted lifts, friction-reducing slide sheets, and air-assisted devices (OSHA, 2017).	These devices reduce the caregiver's muscular strain during patient handling.
Encourage patient to help as much as possible.	This promotes patient's independence and strength while minimizing workload.
Take position close to patient (or object being lifted).	Keeps object in same plane as lifter and close to caregiver's center of gravity. Reduces horizontal reach and stress on caregiver's back.
Tighten abdominal muscles and keep back, neck, pelvis, and feet aligned. Avoid twisting.	Reduces risk of injury to lumbar vertebrae and muscle groups. Twisting increases risk of injury.
Bend at knees; keep feet wide apart.	A broad base of support increases stability. Maintains center of gravity.
Use arms and legs (not back).	Leg muscles are stronger, larger muscles capable of greater work without injury.
Slide patient toward your body using friction-reducing pull sheet or slide board. When transferring patient onto a stretcher or bed, a slide board is more appropriate.	Sliding requires less effort than lifting. Friction-reducing sheet minimizes shearing forces, which can damage patient's skin.
Person with heaviest load coordinates efforts of team involved by counting to three.	Simultaneous lifting minimizes load for any one lifter.
Perform manual lifting as last resort and only if it does not involve lifting most or all of patient's weight.	Lifting is a high-risk activity that causes significant biochemical and postural stressors.

SAFETY GUIDELINES FOR NURSING SKILLS

Ensuring patient safety is an essential role of the professional nurse. Use sound clinical judgment by communicating clearly with members of the health care team, assessing and analyzing the patient's clinical findings, and incorporating the patient's priorities of care and preferences. Use the best evidence, applying professional standards, when selecting interventions to use in patient care delivery. When performing the skills in this chapter, remember the following points to ensure safe, patient-centered care.

- Know a patient's level of mobility and strength to determine the assistance that is required during ambulation and transferring.
- Assess a patient's physical risks for activity intolerance before beginning early mobility.
- Mentally review the transfer steps before beginning the procedure; this ensures both your safety and that of the patient. This is a part of critical thinking—knowing your competency.

- When assisting patients who have orthopedic problems with ambulation, stand on their unaffected side. For all other patients, including those with neurological deficits, stand on their affected side.
- Determine the transfer equipment indicated and the number of personnel needed to safely transfer a patient and prevent harm to health care providers (Table 38.4).
- Raise the side rail on the side of the bed opposite of where you are standing to prevent the patient from falling out of bed on that side.
- Arrange equipment (e.g., intravenous lines, feeding tube, indwelling catheter) so that it does not interfere with the transfer process.
- Evaluate the patient for correct body alignment and pressure risks after a transfer.
- Make sure that all personnel understand how the equipment functions before it is used.

SKILL 38.1   USING SAFE AND EFFECTIVE TRANSFER TECHNIQUES

Delegation and Collaboration

The skill of safe and effective transfer techniques can be delegated to trained assistive personnel (AP). The nurse is responsible for initially assessing a patient's readiness and functional ability to transfer. The nurse directs the AP by:

- Assisting and supervising after patient assessment on how to move patients who are transferred for the first time after prolonged bed rest, extensive surgery, critical illness, or spinal cord trauma.
- Explaining the patient's mobility restrictions, changes in blood pressure to look for, or sensory alterations that may affect safe transfer (e.g., medicated or confused).
- Explaining what to observe and report back to the nurse, such as dizziness or the patient's ability/inability to assist.

Equipment

- Gait belt, sling, or lapboard (as needed)
- Nonskid shoes, bath blankets, and pillows
- Chair with arms or wheelchair (position chair at 45- to 60-degree angle to bed, lock brakes, remove footrests, and lock bed brakes)
- Stretcher (position next to bed, lock brakes on stretcher, lock brakes on bed)
- Lateral transfer device: sliding board or inflatable air-assisted transfer device

- Mechanical/hydraulic lift (use frame, canvas strips or chains, and hammock or canvas strips)
- *Option:* Stand-assist lift device (Fig. 38.22)
- *Option:* Clean gloves (if risk of contacting soiled linen)

FIG. 38.22 Stand-assist lift device.

STEP	RATIONALE

ASSESSMENT

1. Identify patient using at least two identifiers (e.g., name and birthday or name and medical record number) according to agency policy.

Ensures correct patient. Complies with The Joint Commission standards and improves patient safety (TJC, 2021).

2. Refer to medical record for most recent recorded weight and height for patient.

Data determines whether a mechanical transfer device or friction-reducing device is needed for transfer.

3. Review history for previous fall and whether patient has a fear of falling.

Previous fall history is one of the significant fall risk factors (CDC, 2017). Having a fear of falling can alter one's gait and security in walking.

4. Assess previous mode of transferring to bed or chair (if applicable).

Ensures some consistency in how to assist with transfer.

5. Review medical record for presence of neuromuscular deficits, motor weakness or incoordination, calcium loss from bone, cognitive and visual dysfunction, altered balance.

Certain conditions increase risk of tripping, falling, or suffering potential injury during fall.

6. Assess patient and family caregiver health literacy.

Ensures patient has the capacity to obtain, communicate, process, and understand basic health information (CDC, 2021f).

7. Assess patient's cognitive status, including ability to follow verbal instructions, short-term memory, and recognition of physical deficits and limitations to movement.

Determines patient's ability to follow directions during assessment and to learn transfer techniques.

CLINICAL JUDGMENT: *Patients with certain conditions that affect cognition, such as dementia, head trauma, or degenerative neurological disorders, may have perceptual cognitive defects that create safety risks. If the patient has difficulty comprehending, simplify instructions by providing one step at a time and maintaining consistency.*

8. Perform hand hygiene.

Reduces transmission of microorganisms.

9. Assess the patient's mobility: administer the Banner Mobility Assessment Tool (BMAT) (Matz, 2019):

The BMAT is a tool that assesses four functional tasks to identify the level of mobility a patient can achieve (Matz, 2019). The assessment aids in determining a patient's level of mobility and recommends assistive devices needed to safely lift, transfer, and mobilize a patient.

   a. **Sit and Shake:** From a semi-reclined position, ask patient to sit upright and rotate to a seated position at the side of the bed; patient may use the bed rail. Note patient's ability to maintain bedside position. Ask patient to reach out and grab your hand and shake, making sure patient reaches across his/her midline.

     If patient fails to Sit and Shake: Use total lift with sling and/or positioning sheet and/or straps, and/or use lateral transfer devices such as rollboard, friction-reducing (slide sheets/tube) equipment, or air-assisted device.

   b. **Stretch and Point:** With patient in seated position at the side of the bed, have patient place both feet on the floor (or stool) with knees no higher than hips. Ask patient to extend one leg and straighten the knee, then bend the ankle and point the toes. Repeat with the other leg.

     If patient fails Stretch and Point: Use total lift for patient unable to weight-bear on at least one leg; use sit-to-stand lift for patient who can weight-bear on at least one leg.

   c. **Stand:** Ask patient to elevate off the bed or chair (seated to standing) using an assistive device (walker, cane, bed rail). Patient should be able to raise buttocks off bed and hold for a count of five. May repeat once. Note patient's proprioception (awareness of position of body) and balance.

     If patient fails to Stand: Use nonpowered raising/stand aid (default to powered sit-to-stand lift if no stand aid available) or use total lift with ambulation accessories or use assistive device (cane, walker, crutches).

   d. **Walk** (march in place and advance step). Ask patient to march in place at bedside; then ask patient to step forward and back with each foot. Patient should display stability while performing tasks. Assess for stability and safety awareness

     If patient cannot Walk: Use nonpowered raising/stand aid (default to powered sit-to-stand lift if no stand aid available) or use total lift with ambulation accessories or use assistive device (cane, walker, crutches).

CLINICAL JUDGMENT: *Do not rely on self-report from patient or family caregiver as to patient's ability to sit, stand, or ambulate. An objective assessment is needed to accurately determine a patient's capabilities.*

Continued

SKILL 38.1   USING SAFE AND EFFECTIVE TRANSFER TECHNIQUES—cont'd

STEP	RATIONALE
10. While assessing mobility, note any weakness, dizziness, or risk for orthostatic hypotension (OH) (e.g., previously on bed rest, first time arising from supine position after surgical procedure, history of dizziness when arising).	Determines risk of fainting or falling during transfer. Patients have decreased ability of autonomic nervous system to equalize blood supply when they are immobilized. Specifically, after 3 minutes of standing (or 3 minutes of sitting upright), a decrease of $\geq$20 mm Hg in systolic BP or a decrease of $\geq$10 mm Hg in diastolic BP indicates that a patient has OH (Biswas et al., 2019). Neurogenic orthostatic hypotension (nOH) is a sustained reduction in blood pressure (BP) upon standing that is caused by autonomic dysfunction and is common among patients with neurodegenerative disorders (e.g., Parkinson disease). In this situation a systolic BP drop of $\geq$20 mm Hg (or $\geq$10 mm Hg diastolic) upon standing with little or no compensatory increase in heart rate is consistent with neurogenic orthostatic hypotension (Biswas et al., 2019).
11. Assess activity tolerance, noting any fatigue during sitting and standing.	Determines ability of patient to help with transfer.
12. Assess sensory status, including central and peripheral vision, adequacy of hearing, and presence of peripheral sensation loss.	Visual field loss decreases patients' ability to see in direction of transfer and may impact their balance. Peripheral sensation loss decreases proprioception. Patients with visual and hearing losses need transfer techniques and communication methods adapted to their deficits.

CLINICAL JUDGMENT: *Patients with hemiplegia may "neglect" one side of the body (inattention to or unawareness of one side of body or environment), which distorts perception of the visual field. If patient experiences neglect of one side, instruct patient to scan all visual fields when transferring.*

STEP	RATIONALE
13. Assess level of comfort (e.g., joint discomfort, muscle spasm) and measure level of pain using scale of 0 to 10. Offer prescribed analgesic 30 minutes before transfer. (**Note:** Patient will require assistance when analgesic has been given.)	Pain reduces patient's motivation and ability to be mobile. In conditions of chronic pain, deficits in dopamine signaling emerge that impair motivated behavior (Taylor et al., 2016; Czarnecki and Turner, 2018). Pain relief before a transfer enhances patient's ability to participate.
14. Assess patient's level of motivation such as eagerness versus unwillingness to be mobile and perception of value of exercise. Consider age and other cultural factors that influence beliefs.	Will affect patient's desire to engage in activity.
15. Assess previous mode of transfer in home setting (if applicable).	Providing appropriate aids greatly enhances transfer ability at home.
16. Assess patient's vital signs just before transfer.	Baseline measures will determine whether vital sign changes occur during activity, which will indicate activity intolerance (see Chapter 29).
17. Analyze assessment data and refer to mobility status and safe-handling algorithms (e.g., Veterans Affairs Safe Patient Handling App, 2019) available in most agencies, to determine whether a lift device or mechanical transfer device is needed and the number of people needed to help with transfer (Martin et al., 2016) (see illustrations A & B). **Do not start procedure until all required caregivers are available.**	Ensures safe patient handling, reducing risk of injury to patient and caregivers.
18. Assess patient's knowledge, prior experience with transfer, and feelings about procedure.	Reveals need for patient instruction and/or support.
19. Assess patient's goals or preferences for how skill will be performed or what patient expects.	Allows care to be individualized to patient.

PLANNING

1. Perform hand hygiene.	Reduces transmission of microorganisms.
2. Obtain and organize equipment/lift device for transfer at bedside.	Ensures more efficient procedure.
3. Close room door and bedside curtain.	Provides patient privacy.
4. Explain to patient how you are going to prepare for transfer technique and the safety precautions to be used. Explain benefits and reasons for increasing mobility. Do so in a way that matches patient's beliefs and values regarding recovery or maintaining health (Shieh et al., 2015; Carey et al., 2021).	Provides for clearer understanding by patient. Motivates patient to be involved in transfer.

IMPLEMENTATION

1. **Assist patient from lying to sitting position on edge of bed**.	Minimizes strain on your back during patient transfer. Patient can use side rails for lifting upward into sitting position.
a. With patient in supine position in bed, raise head of bed 30-45 degrees and lower bed, level with your hips. Raise upper side rail on side where patient will exit bed. Apply nonskid shoes or socks.	Technique incorporates body mechanics into transfer move to sitting position.
b. If patient is fully mobile, allow to sit up on side of bed independently, using side rail to raise up.	

STEP   **RATIONALE**

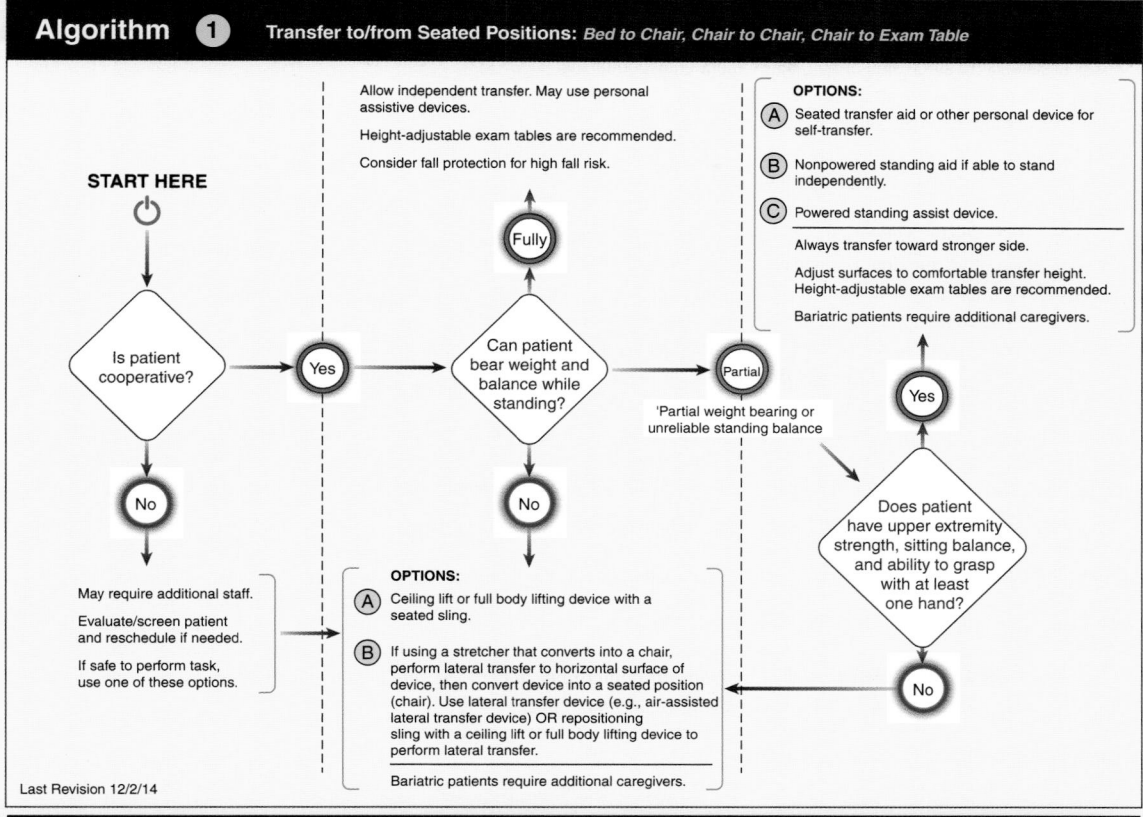

Algorithm 1   Transfer to/from Seated Positions: *Bed to Chair, Chair to Chair, Chair to Exam Table*

Allow independent transfer. May use personal assistive devices.

Height-adjustable exam tables are recommended.

Consider fall protection for high fall risk.

OPTIONS:
- (A) Seated transfer aid or other personal device for self-transfer.
- (B) Nonpowered standing aid if able to stand independently.
- (C) Powered standing assist device.

Always transfer toward stronger side.

Adjust surfaces to comfortable transfer height. Height-adjustable exam tables are recommended.

Bariatric patients require additional caregivers.

START HERE

Is patient cooperative? — Yes → Can patient bear weight and balance while standing? → Fully

No

Partial → 'Partial weight bearing or unreliable standing balance

Does patient have upper extremity strength, sitting balance, and ability to grasp with at least one hand? — Yes / No

May require additional staff.

Evaluate/screen patient and reschedule if needed.

If safe to perform task, use one of these options.

OPTIONS:
- (A) Ceiling lift or full body lifting device with a seated sling.
- (B) If using a stretcher that converts into a chair, perform lateral transfer to horizontal surface of device, then convert device into a seated position (chair). Use lateral transfer device (e.g., air-assisted lateral transfer device) OR repositioning sling with a ceiling lift or full body lifting device to perform lateral transfer.

Bariatric patients require additional caregivers.

A   Last Revision 12/2/14

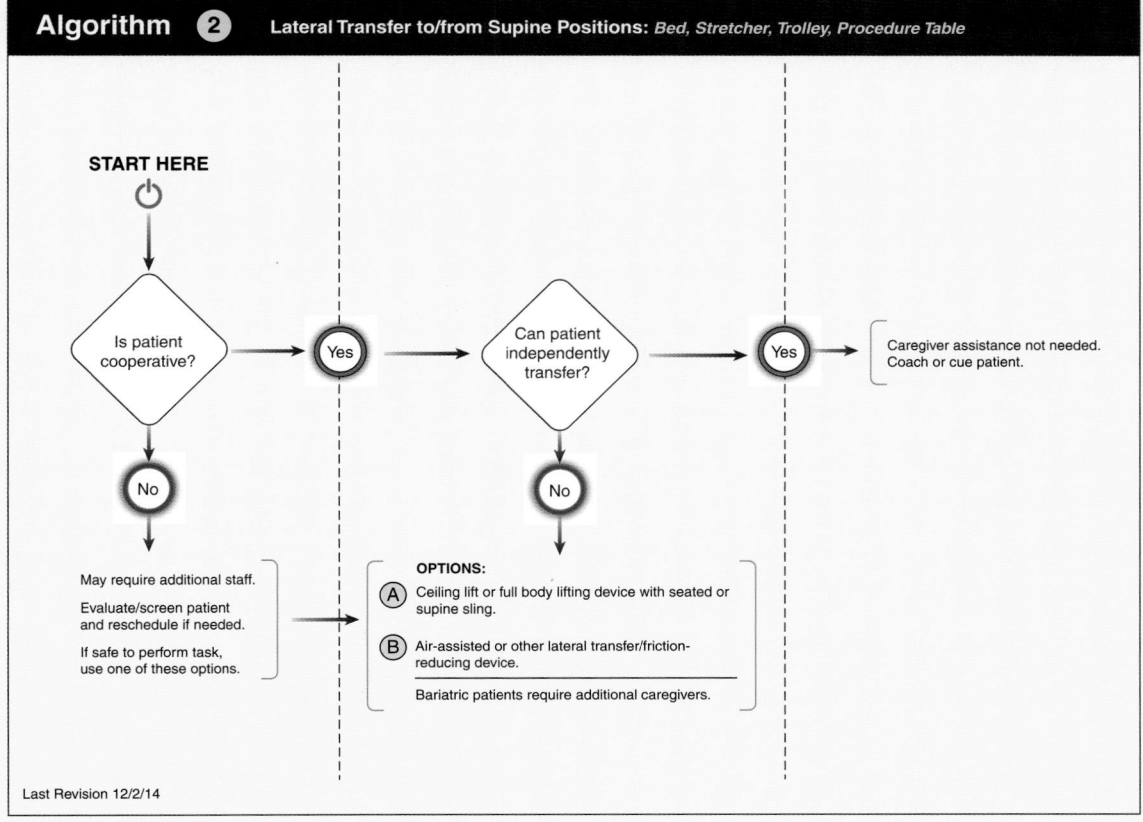

Algorithm 2   Lateral Transfer to/from Supine Positions: *Bed, Stretcher, Trolley, Procedure Table*

START HERE

Is patient cooperative? — Yes → Can patient independently transfer? — Yes → Caregiver assistance not needed. Coach or cue patient.

No

No

May require additional staff.

Evaluate/screen patient and reschedule if needed.

If safe to perform task, use one of these options.

OPTIONS:
- (A) Ceiling lift or full body lifting device with seated or supine sling.
- (B) Air-assisted or other lateral transfer/friction-reducing device.

Bariatric patients require additional caregivers.

B   Last Revision 12/2/14

STEP 17 (A) VHA safe patient handling and mobility algorithm 1. (B) VHA safe patient handling and mobility algorithm 2. (From VHA: *Safe patient handling and mobility algorithms.* 2014 revision.)

Continued

SKILL 38.1   USING SAFE AND EFFECTIVE TRANSFER TECHNIQUES—cont'd

STEP	RATIONALE

c. If patient needs assistance to sit on side of bed, turn patient onto side facing you while standing on side of bed where patient will sit.

d. Stand opposite patient's hips. Turn diagonally to face patient and far corner of foot of bed.

e. Place your feet apart in wide base of support with foot closer to head of bed in front of other foot.

f. Place your arm nearer to head of bed under patient's lower shoulder, supporting the head and neck. Place your other arm over and around patient's thighs (see illustration in Box 38.11, Step 18e).

g. Move patient's lower legs and feet over side of bed as patient uses side rail to push and raise the upper body. Pivot weight onto your rear leg as you allow patient's upper legs to swing downward. **Do not lift legs.** At the same time, continue to shift weight to your rear leg and guide patient in elevating his/her trunk into upright position.

2. Lower bed so that patient can sit on the side of the bed with feet on floor for 2 to 3 minutes. Have patient alternately flex and extend feet and move lower legs up and down without touching floor. Ask whether patient feels dizzy; if so, check blood pressure. Have patient relax and take a few deep breaths until dizziness subsides and balance is gained. If dizziness lasts more than 60 seconds or if systolic BP has dropped at least 20 mm Hg within 3 minutes of sitting upright, return patient to bed. Recheck blood pressure.

Rationale for step 2: Feet placement allows patient to achieve balance while sitting. Exercise promotes circulation and provides range of motion.

Allows patient's circulation to equilibrate to reduce chance of orthostatic hypotension. After 3 minutes of standing (or 3 minutes of sitting upright), a decrease of $\geq$20 mm Hg in systolic BP or a decrease of $\geq$10 mm Hg in diastolic BP indicates orthostatic hypotension (Biswas et al., 2019).

CLINICAL JUDGMENT: *Remain in front of patient until patient regains balance, and continue to provide physical support to weak or cognitively impaired patient.*

---

3. **Transfer patient from bed to chair** (*Option:* Apply clean gloves if bed linen is soiled):

   a. Have chair in position at 45-degree angle with one side against bed, facing foot of bed. — Positions chair with easy access for transfer.

   b. Be sure patient's feet are comfortably flat on the floor with the hip and knees at a 90-degree angle. Help patient apply stable, nonskid shoes/socks. — Provides patient stability when transferring. Shoes/socks prevent slipping on floor.

   c. *Patient can bear weight fully during transfer.* — Key criteria for determining transfer method (Matz, 2019).

   (1) Stand by bedside and allow patient to transfer independently. — Caregiver assistance not needed; stand by for safety as needed.

   d. *Patient has partial weight bearing, is cooperative, and has upper body strength.* — Use stand-and-pivot technique with one caregiver. (*Option:* powered standing assist lift.)

   (1) Apply gait belt. Be sure that it completely encircles a patient's waist. Belt buckle is in front of patient. Belt should fit snugly, being sure two fingers fit between the belt and patient's body. Do not place belt over any intravenous lines, wounds, drains, or tubes. You may need to adjust belt once patient stands. — Transfer belt allows you to maintain stability and balance of patient during transfer and reduces risk for falling (Matz, 2019; OSHA, 2014).

   (2) Place patient's weight-bearing or strong leg under the patient and the weak or non–weight-bearing foot forward. — Patient will stand on stronger, or weight-bearing, leg initially, raising torso.

   (3) Hold the gait belt with both hands and fingers pointing up, along patient's sides. Caregivers should never plan to push, pull, lift, or catch patients with use of gait belt. — Provides patient's stability and allows nurse to direct patient's movement.

   (4) Spread your feet apart. Flex hips and knees, aligning knees with patient's knees (see illustration). — Ensures balance with wide base of support. Flexing knees and hips lowers your center of gravity to object to be raised; aligning knees with those of patient stabilizes knees when patient stands.

   (5) Rock patient up to standing position on count of three while straightening hips and legs and keeping knees slightly flexed (see illustration). While rocking patient in back-and-forth motion, make sure that your body weight is moving in the same direction as patient's to ensure that you and patient are moving in same direction simultaneously. Unless contraindicated, patient may be instructed to use hands to push up if applicable. — Rocking motion gives patient's body momentum and requires less muscular effort to lift.

   (6) Maintain stability of patient's weaker leg with your knee if needed. — Ability to stand can often be maintained in weak limb with support of knee to stabilize.

   (7) Pivot on foot farthest from chair. — Maintains support of patient while allowing adequate space for patient to move.

   (8) Instruct patient to use armrests on chair for support and ease into chair (see illustration). — Increases patient stability.

STEP	RATIONALE

STEP 3d(4) Nurse flexes hips and knees, aligns knees with patient's knee, and grasps transfer belt palms up.

STEP 3d(5) Patient stands up at bedside before pivoting over to chair, bearing weight.

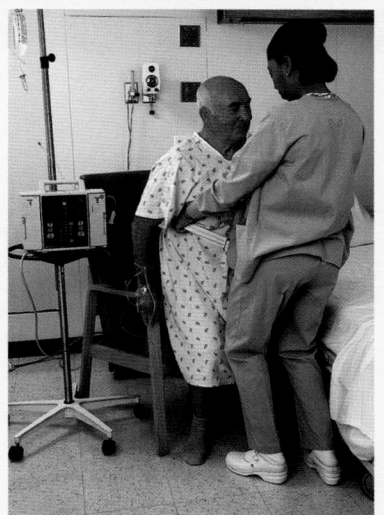

STEP 3d(8) Patient uses armrests to ease into chair.

STEP	RATIONALE
(9) Flex hips and knees while lowering patient into chair.	Prevents injury from poor body mechanics.
(10) Assist patient to assume proper alignment in sitting position. Provide support for weakened extremity (as needed). You can use a sling or lap board to support an injured or flaccid arm.	Prevents injury to patient from poor body alignment.
(11) Proper alignment for sitting position: Head is erect, and vertebrae are in straight alignment. Body weight is evenly distributed on buttocks and thighs. Thighs are parallel and in horizontal plane. Both feet are supported flat on floor, and ankles are comfortably flexed. A 2.5- to 5-cm (1- to 2-inch) space is maintained between edge of seat and popliteal space on posterior surface of knee.	Prevents stress on intravertebral joints. Prevents increased pressure over bony prominences and reduces damage to underlying musculoskeletal system.
e. Return patient to bed. *Patient has partial weight bearing, is cooperative, and has upper body strength.*	
(1) Adjust the height of the bed to the level of the chair when possible.	Lessens physical burden of transferring patient's body weight.
(2) Position chair against the side of the bed midway between the head and foot of the bed, with the chair facing toward the foot of the bed.	Reduces distance of transfer.
(3) Be sure that gait belt is on patient and that it completely circles patient's waist. Be sure that it is snug and not placed over any intravenous lines, incisions, drains, or tubes.	Reduces risk of fall during transfer.
(4) Have patient place hands on arms of chair and stand by as you have patient move to the front of the chair.	Easier to flex knees up from edge of chair compared to when sitting deep in back of chair.
(5) Stand slightly in front of patient.	Guards and protects patient throughout transfer.
(6) Instruct patient to stand at a count of three as you place both hands (palms up) under gait belt while bending your knees.	Ensures coordinated movement to standing position.
(7) Allow patient to stand a few seconds to ensure that patient is not dizzy and has good balance. Pivot with patient. The patient turns to face away from the side of the bed. Then have patient sit on the edge of the mattress. Be sure that patient is firmly sitting and not slipping off the edge of the bed.	Promotes patient safety in the event of a hypotensive response. Firm position on edge of mattress prevents falls.
(8) With patient sitting on the edge of the bed, place your arm nearest the head of the bed under the patient's shoulder while supporting the head and neck. Place your other arm under patient's knees. Bend your knees and keep your back straight.	Prepares you to pivot patient into supine position.
(9) Tell patient to help lift the legs when you begin to move. On a count of three, standing with a wide base of support, raise patient's legs as you pivot the patient's body and lower the shoulders onto the bed. Remember to keep your back straight.	Smooth, coordinated movement reduces risk of injury to patient and caregiver.
(10) Help patient assume comfortable position in bed.	

Continued

SKILL 38.1	USING SAFE AND EFFECTIVE TRANSFER TECHNIQUES—cont'd

STEP	RATIONALE
f. **Transfer patient from bed to chair.** *Patient is limited cognitively, is uncooperative, or has weight-bearing precautions with upper body strength or caregiver must lift more than 15.9 kg (35 lb):* Use a full body sling lift with minimum of two or three caregivers (Matz, 2019). Follow manufacturer lift guidelines to apply correctly.	Research supports use of mechanical lifts to prevent musculoskeletal injuries (Matz, 2019). Use of ceiling-mounted lifts is a popular choice (when available) because of location in each patient's room.

CLINICAL JUDGMENT: *Patient who requires a lift will not initially be assisted to sit on side of bed. Lift will be applied with patient lying supine in bed.*

CLINICAL JUDGMENT: *Patients with new hip replacements who have hip precautions should not be using a Hoyer lift because it may promote hip flex > 90 degrees, which is contraindicated for patients with posterior hip precautions.*

STEP	RATIONALE
(1) Bring mechanical floor lift to bedside or lower ceiling lift and position properly.	Ensures safe elevation of patient off bed.
(2) Be sure chair is available along one side of bed, facing foot of bed. Allow adequate space to maneuver the lift.	Prepares environment for safe use of lift and subsequent transfer of patient into chair.

CLINICAL JUDGMENT: *If patient demonstrates weakness or paralysis of one side of the body, place chair on the patient's strong side.*

STEP	RATIONALE
(3) Raise bed to safe working height with mattress flat. Lower side rail on side near chair.	Allows you to use proper body mechanics.
(4) Have second nurse positioned at opposite side of bed.	Maintains patient safety, preventing fall from bed.
(5) Roll patient on side away from you.	Positions patient for placement of lift sling.
(6) Place hammock or canvas strips under patient to form sling. With two canvas pieces, lower edge fits under patient's knees (wide piece), and upper edge fits under patient's shoulders (narrow piece).	Two types of seats are supplied with mechanical/hydraulic lift: hammock style is better for patients who are flaccid, weak, and need support; canvas strips can be used for patients with normal muscle tone. Be sure hooks face away from patient's skin. Place sling under patient's center of gravity and greatest part of body weight.
(7) Roll patient back toward you as second nurse pulls hammock (straps) through.	Ensures that sling is in proper position before lift.
(8) Return patient to supine position. Be sure that hammock or straps are smooth over bed surface. Sling should extend from shoulders to knees (hammock) to support patient's body weight equally.	Completes positioning of patient on mechanical/hydraulic sling.
(9) Remove patient's glasses if worn.	Swivel bar is close to patient's head and could break eyeglasses.
(10) Roll the horseshoe base of floor lift under patient's bed (on side with chair).	Positions lift efficiently and promotes smooth transfer.
(11) Lower horizontal bar to sling level by following manufacturer directions. Lock valve if required.	Positions hydraulic lift close to patient. Locking valve prevents injury to patient.
(12) Attach hooks on strap (chain) to holes in sling. Short chains or straps hook to top holes of sling; longer chains hook to bottom of sling (see manufacturer's directions).	Secures hydraulic lift to sling.
(13) Elevate head of bed to Fowler's position.	Positions patient in sitting position.
(14) Have patient fold arms over chest.	Prevents injury to patient's arms during transfer.
(15) If the lift is electric, then push the button to raise the patient off the bed. If the lift is nonelectric, then pump the hydraulic handle using long, slow, even strokes until patient is raised off bed (see illustration A). For ceiling lift, turn on control device to move lift (see illustration B).	Ensures safe support of patient during elevation.
(16) Use lift to raise patient off bed, and use steering handle to pull lift from bed as you and another nurse maneuver patient to chair. Have second nurse alongside patient.	Lifts patient off the bed safely; nurse's position reduces any risk of patient falling from sling.
(17) Roll base of lift around chair. Release check valve slowly or push the button down and lower patient into chair (see manufacturer's directions) (see illustration).	Positions lift in front of chair into which patient is to be transferred. Safely guides patient into back of chair as seat descends.
(18) Close check valve, if needed, as soon as patient is down in chair and straps can be released. Newer lifts may not need this step (see manufacturer's directions).	If valve is left open, boom may continue to lower and injure patient.
(19) Remove straps and roll mechanical/hydraulic lift out of patient's path.	Prevents damage to skin and underlying tissues.
(20) Check patient's sitting alignment and correct if necessary.	Prevents injury from poor posture.

STEP	RATIONALE

STEP 3f(15) (A) Patient lifted in hydraulic lift above bed. (B) Ceiling lift. (Courtesy Waverly Glen Systems, a Prism Medical Co.)

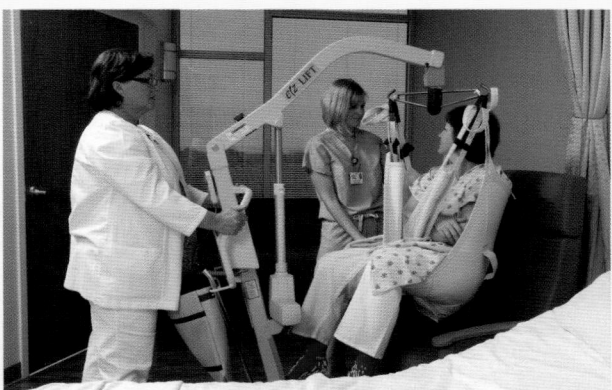

STEP 3f(17) Use of hydraulic lift to lower patient into chair.

4. **Perform lateral transfer from bed to stretcher.** (A number of friction-reducing devices (FRDs) are available to assist with lateral transfers both in and out of beds or stretchers. This skill summarizes the use of friction-reducing slide boards, mechanical lifts, and air-assisted FRDs.)

The three-person lift (using common drawsheet) for horizontal transfer from bed to stretcher is no longer recommended and is discouraged as it is used inappropriately (Matz, 2019; OSHA, 2014). Physical stress can be decreased significantly by using slide board or friction-reducing board positioned under drawsheet beneath patient. In addition, patient is more comfortable using this method.

a. *Patient can assist* (refer to patient's weight last recorded).

Patient's level of strength and weight determine level of help required for safe transfer (Matz, 2019).

    (1) If patient can assist, caregiver is only needed to stand by for safety, with stretcher and bed locked in flat position, as patient moves to stretcher. Surface of stretcher should be ½ inch lower for lateral move.

Promotes patient's independent mobility.

b. If patient is partially or not at all able to assist and is <91 kg (200 lb), use a friction-reducing sheet (see illustration A) and/or lateral transfer board (see illustration B) (Nelson and Baptiste, 2006).

Prevents the need for nurse to lift patient. During any patient transferring task, if any caregiver is required to lift more than 35 lb of a patient's weight, then the patient should be considered to be fully dependent and assistive devices should be used for the transfer (Matz, 2019; OSHA 2014, n.d.).

c. If patient is partially or not at all able to assist and is >91 kg (200 lb), use a ceiling lift (see Step 3f(15)B) with supine sling, a lateral transfer device or air-assisted device with three caregivers (Nelson and Baptiste, 2006).

CLINICAL JUDGMENT: *Air-assisted devices float patients from an air-layered surface directly across to another surface (bed, stretcher). They can also be used for repositioning. Indicated for patients with compromised skin integrity, pressure injuries, multiple trauma, burns, patients experiencing cancer and severe pain, and patients who are obese (Baptiste-McKinney and Halvorson, 2018).*

Continued

SKILL 38.1	USING SAFE AND EFFECTIVE TRANSFER TECHNIQUES—cont'd

STEP	RATIONALE

(1) Lateral transfer FRD (e.g., slide board) or air-assisted device:

    i. Apply clean gloves if there is risk of soiling. Lower head of bed as much as patient can tolerate, then raise bed to comfortable working height. Be sure to lock bed brakes.

    ii. Have patient cross arms on chest.

    iii. Lower side rails. To place transfer device (slide board) or deflated air-assisted mattress under patient, position nurse on side of bed toward which patient will be turned. Position other two nurses on other side of bed.

    iv. Fanfold drawsheet on both sides.

    v. On count of three logroll patient onto side toward the nurse. Turn patient as one unit with smooth, continuous motion.

    vi. Place slide board (or *option:* deflated mattress of air-assisted device) under drawsheet (see illustrations). Spread out deflated mattress on bed under patient as you would a new sheet.

    vii. Advise patient that next step will involve rolling over hard or irregular surface. Ask patient to roll toward the two nurses on other side of bed, staying aligned (see illustration). Gently turn patient.

    viii. Be sure board and mattress are under patient. *Option: Roll out the deflated air mattress so that it is positioned over bed mattress.* Then position patient supine and centered over board or mattress. Secure patient to air-assisted mattress (see illustration).

Maintains alignment of spinal column. Ensures that bed does not move inadvertently.
Reduces transmission of microorganisms. Eases positioning on an FRD. Prevents accidental patient fall during transfer.

Prevents injury to arms during transfer.
Distributes weight equally between nurses.

Provides strong handles to grip drawsheet without slipping.
Maintains body in alignment, preventing stress on any body part.
Positions patient for board or mattress placement.
Prevents friction from contact of skin with board or mattress.

Positions patient onto board or mattress surface.

Centering patient ensures transfer of torso and lower extremities.

STEP 4b (A) Friction-reducing sheet. (From EZ Way, Inc., Clarinda, IA.) (B) Slide board.

STEP 4c(1)vi (A) Two caregivers placing slide board under drawsheet and patient. (B) Two caregivers placing air-assisted device under drawsheet and patient.

STEP	RATIONALE
ix. Line up stretcher so that surface is ½ inch lower than bed mattress. Lock brakes on stretcher. Instruct patient not to move	Ensures that stretcher does not move inadvertently during transfer.
x. *Option:* At this time, inflate the mattress (see illustration).	Provides for smooth transfer with no shear force.
xi. Two nurses position themselves on side of stretcher while third nurse positions self on side of bed without stretcher (see illustration). All three nurses place feet widely apart with one foot slightly in front of the other and grasp friction-reducing device	Promotes easy transfer.

CLINICAL JUDGMENT: *For patients with Stage 3 or 4 pressure injuries, take care to avoid shearing force against skin.*

CLINICAL JUDGMENT: *A nurse may also be positioned at the head of patient's bed to protect and support the head and neck if patient is weak or unable to help.*

STEP	RATIONALE
xii. Holding the edges of slide board or air-inflated mattress and one nurse counting to three, the two nurses slide board or mattress to stretcher, positioning patient onto stretcher (see illustration). The third nurse guides slide board or mattress in place.	Slide board remains stationary, provides slippery surface to reduce friction, and allows patient to transfer easily to stretcher.

CLINICAL JUDGMENT: *Air-assisted devices have a limitation. Once a transfer begins, the friction-reduction capability contributes to an increase in momentum, making it more difficult to stop the transfer. Use caution to be sure the patient does not slide beyond or even off the stretcher or bed to which the patient is being transferred (Baptiste-McKinney and Halvorson, 2018).*

STEP 4c(1)vii Patient rolls to opposite side, while other caregiver unrolls air-assisted device.

STEP 4c(1)viii Secure safety straps over patient on air-assisted device.

STEP 4c(1)x Inflation of air-assisted transfer mattress.

STEP 4c(1)xi Transfer of patient to stretcher using slide board.

Continued

SKILL 38.1	USING SAFE AND EFFECTIVE TRANSFER TECHNIQUES—cont'd

STEP	RATIONALE
xiii. Position patient in center of stretcher. Raise head of stretcher if not contraindicated. Raise stretcher side rails. Cover patient with blanket.	Provides for patient comfort.

CLINICAL JUDGMENT: *An air-assisted device can be left under a patient when deflated. Such a device is waterproof, antibacterial, and anti-stain nylon. Limited evidence exists on whether the presence of the device increases risk for pressure injuries.*

STEP	RATIONALE
d. Bariatric lateral transfer to and from bed or stretcher.	
(1) If patient can fully assist, use minimum of two caregivers.	If a patient who is obese is about to fall, little can be done by a caregiver to prevent the fall. Caregiver should be prepared to move any items out of the way that could cause injury. Try to protect patient's head.
(2) If patient can only partially assist or not assist at all, use a sliding board with slide sheet, mechanical floor-based lift, bariatric ceiling lift with supine sling, or air-assisted FRD with a minimum of three caregivers (see illustration) (Baptiste-Kinney and Halvorson, 2018).	Transfer toward stronger side. Use of mechanical devices ensures patient and caregiver safety.

CLINICAL JUDGMENT: *When used in combination with slide boards, a slide sheet may be of value as the use of a sliding board alone often does not function well due to the high level of friction created by a patient's mass in body size.*

STEP	RATIONALE
5. After transferring patient to bed, chair, or stretcher, be sure patient is positioned comfortably.	Ensures patient safety.
6. Place nurse call system in an accessible location within patient's reach.	
7. Raise side rails (as appropriate) and lower bed to lowest position.	Ensures patient safety.
8. Dispose of all contaminated supplies in appropriate receptacle, remove and dispose of gloves, and perform hand hygiene.	Reduces transmission of microorganisms.

STEP 4c(1)xii Transfer of patient using air-assisted transfer device.

STEP 4d(2) Bariatric lift. (Courtesy MedCare Products, Burnsville, Minn.)

STEP	RATIONALE

EVALUATION

1. Monitor vital signs. Ask whether patient feels dizzy or tired. Ask patient to rate pain on pain scale.

Evaluates patient's response to postural changes and activity.

2. Note patient's behavioral response to transfer.

Reveals level of motivation and self-care potential.

3. Be sure to check condition of patient's skin after next transfer.

Determines whether injury to skin has occurred.

4. **Use Teach-Back:** "I want to be sure I explained the steps we are going to use to transfer you to the chair. Tell me the steps you can take to make the transfer safe." Revise your instruction now or develop a plan for revised patient/family caregiver teaching if patient/family caregiver is not able to teach back correctly.

Teach-back is an evidence-based health literacy intervention that promotes patient engagement, patient safety, adherence, and quality. The goal of teach-back is to ensure that you have explained medical information clearly so that patients and their families understand what you communicated to them (AHRQ, 2020).

UNEXPECTED OUTCOMES AND RELATED INTERVENTIONS

1. Patient is unable to comprehend or is unwilling to follow directions for transfer.
   - Reassess continuity and simplicity of your instruction.
   - If patient is tired or in pain, allow for rest period before transferring.
   - Consider medicating for pain, if indicated.
   - Consider using hydraulic lift.
2. Patient sustains injury on transfer.
   - Evaluate incident that led to injury (e.g., inadequate assessment, change in patient status, improper use of equipment).
   - Complete incident report according to agency policy.
3. Patient is unable to stand for time required to transfer to chair.
   - Consider use of lateral transfer slide board or hydraulic lift.

RECORDING AND REPORTING

- Record procedure, including pertinent observations: weakness, level of pain, ability to follow directions, weight-bearing ability, balance, strength, ability to pivot, length of time to perform activity, number of personnel needed to help, assistive device used, and patient's response in nurses' notes in electronic health record (EHR) or chart.
- Document your evaluation of patient and family caregiver learning.
- Report transfer ability and help needed to next shift or other caregivers.
- Report progress or remission to rehabilitation staff (physical therapist, occupational therapist).

HOME CARE CONSIDERATIONS

- Teach family how to use safe patient-handling equipment if necessary.
- Teach patient and family safety precautions to take while helping patients with mobility.
- Have family caregiver practice and demonstrate transfer of the patient to a chair in the hospital to achieve success before taking patient home. Alternatively, have patient (if living alone) practice transfer skills in bed that will be used at home. Teach patient to transfer to a chair with arms for ease of rising and sitting. Home should be free of hazards (e.g., throw rugs, electrical cords in walkways, slippery floors). If wheelchair is used as a chair, access must be possible through all doors, and space for transfer must be available in bedroom and bathroom.

KEY POINTS

- The musculoskeletal and nervous systems work in coordination to maintain balance, posture, and body alignment during lifting, bending, moving, and activities of daily living.
- Regular physical activity elevates mood, boosts energy level, manages stress, and promotes a better quality of sleep.
- Safe patient handling includes standardized methods for determining how to handle, move, and mobilize patients based on individual patient characteristics and conditions, thereby reducing overexertion injuries to staff and reducing patient falls and injuries.
- Clinical judgment involves applying critical thinking to consider knowledge about the relationship between the musculoskeletal system and a patient's health alterations when deciding on interventions for problems related to activity and exercise.
- To assess a patient's activity tolerance, observe the individual after ambulation, self-bathing, or sitting in a chair for several hours, and obtain a verbal self-report of fatigue, shortness of breath, or weakness. Also assess heart rate and blood pressure response to activity by comparing with baseline rates at rest.

- Assess a patient's readiness to exercise by applying the Transtheoretical Model (TTM). First ask to what extent the patient enjoys exercising and the patient's belief in the ability to exercise, and then compare the patient's responses with the six stages of change to identify patient-centered interventions that will help the patient engage in exercise.
- Outcome selection for patients requiring activity and exercise therapies is focused on improving functional status and independence.
- A nurse uses clinical judgment, considering a patient's current activity tolerance, the nature of the health condition, and the type of exercise best suited to the patient's needs, as part of selecting patient-centered interventions based on patient preferences.
- A nurse will analyze assessment findings and refer to safe patient-handling algorithms to select the transfer technique best suited for the patient's weight, weight-bearing capability, and need for transfer devices and personnel assistance.
- Ensuring that a patient is safe during assisted ambulation requires you to use a gait belt, to stand on the correct side by the patient, and to monitor the patient's tolerance to walking.

- Sound clinical judgment in patient evaluation involves comparing a patient's baseline mobility and activity tolerance measures (e.g., pulse, blood pressure, respirations, strength, self-report of fatigue, and psychological well-being) with expected outcomes and standards for improvement.

REFLECTIVE LEARNING

Mrs. Smith has a resting heart rate of 84 beats/min. Beth set a target heart rate of 100 beats/min (60% of Mrs. Smith's maximum heart rate) to start Mrs. Smith's exercise program. Beth spent time discussing how exercise strengthens the patient's heart and improves blood glucose control. The patient was unaware of the effect exercise has on blood glucose and seemed excited about the potential benefits. She stated a willingness to get serious about exercise. Beth encouraged Mrs. Smith to try to include her husband during walking, making the walk an opportunity for both to wind down after work. At a 3-week follow-up visit Mrs. Smith reported walking twice the first week and 3 times the second week for a total of 90 minutes. The patient felt a little short of breath afterward. When her husband walked with her, they walked farther. Her pulse reached 105 beats/min midway on the third day. She knew to slow down and stopped briefly, as Beth had suggested. Now, 6 weeks after her last clinic visit, Mrs. Smith returns to the primary care clinic for an evaluation of her progress with diabetes management. She has seen the dietitian once. When she sees Beth, Mrs. Smith says, "Oh, Beth, you are going to be a little disappointed in me. I have not walked as much as we had planned."

- What assessment information in this patient situation is the most important and of immediate concern for Beth to consider? (Recognize Cues)

Beth learns that Mrs. Smith has walked an average of 100 minutes each week with good tolerance. Her pulse stays close to the target of 100, except when she walks up hills. She also learns that Mr. Smith dislikes his wife's new diet. Mrs. Smith says, "I think I understand what to include in my diet. I don't mind it really."

Beth asks the patient, "Tell me what is most affecting your progress right now."

- In what way is Beth's question relevant, and how might findings influence her approach to intervention for the patient? (Analyze Cues)
- Which problems affecting Mrs. Smith's adherence to diet and exercise are most likely to be present in this patient situation? Which problems are the most serious or the priority? (Prioritize Diagnoses)

Beth learns that Mrs. Smith can explain the types of food to include in her prescribed DASH diet. Part of the patient's problem is to eat right when at work. Beth also assesses that Mrs. Smith can explain how diet helps manage her blood glucose but that she has difficulty in explaining the benefits of exercise. The patient reports feeling good after walking but is inconsistent in adhering.

- How might Beth adapt/revise the plan of care and more likely achieve the desired outcomes for this patient? (Generate Solutions)
- Are there any actions that would probably be less beneficial? (Take Action)
- What evaluation measures should Beth use to determine whether the new plan for Mrs. Smith is effective? (Evaluate Outcomes)

REVIEW QUESTIONS

1. A nurse is instructing a patient who has decreased leg strength on the left side on how to use a cane. Which actions indicate proper cane use by the patient? (Select all that apply.)
   1. The patient keeps the cane on the left side of the body.
   2. The patient slightly leans to one side while walking.
   3. The patient keeps two points of support on the floor at all times.
   4. After the patient places the cane forward, the patient then moves the right leg forward to the cane.
   5. The patient places the cane forward 15 to 25 cm (6 to 10 inches) with each step.
2. A patient is admitted to a rehabilitation facility for cardiac rehabilitation following open heart surgery. The patient is 72 years old, 4 days postoperative, and reportedly was walking with a one-person assist in the hospital before transfer. The patient has a history of hypertension. His wife accompanies him at the time of transfer. Which of the following assessment data would you collect for this patient? (Select all that apply.)
   1. Condition of surgical wound
   2. Patient's expectations of rehabilitation
   3. Previous hospitalization experience
   4. Vital signs
   5. Ability to sit on side of bed unassisted
   6. Gait and balance
   7. History of recent weight changes
   8. Social support from wife
3. A patient comes to an urgent care clinic with reports of pain in the right lower calf and ankle after participating in a 5K run. Which of the following assessment questions will determine the effects exercise has had on this patient?
   1. Tell me specifically when your pain began.
   2. Describe for me the pain you are having.
   3. In what way has your daily activity changed since you noticed your pain?
   4. How long have you been having the pain?
4. The nurse is caring for an older adult in a long-term care setting. The nurse reviews the medical record to find that the patient has progressive loss of total bone mass. The patient's history and tendency to take smaller steps with feet kept closer together will most likely result in which of the following?
   1. Increase the patient's risk for falls and injuries
   2. Result in less stress on the patient's joints
   3. Decrease the amount of work required for patient movement
   4. Allow for mobility in spite of the aging effects on the patient's joints
5. Place the following steps in the correct order to show how to transfer a patient with partial weight bearing and sufficient upper body strength to a chair.
   1. Spread your feet apart. Flex hips and knees, aligning knees with patient's knees.
   2. Instruct patient to use armrests on chair for support and ease into chair.
   3. Apply gait belt.
   4. Flex hips and knees while lowering patient into chair.
   5. Pivot on foot farthest from chair.
   6. Hold the gait belt with both hands and fingers pointing up.
   7. Maintain stability of patient's weaker leg with your knee if needed.
   8. Rock patient up to standing position on count of three while straightening hips and legs.
6. Before transferring a patient from the bed to a stretcher, which assessment data does the nurse need to gather? (Select all that apply.)
   1. Patient's weight
   2. Patient's activity tolerance
   3. Patient's level of mobility
   4. Recent laboratory values

5. Nutritional intake
6. Safe mobility algorithm
7. Which of the following indicates that additional assistance is needed to transfer a patient from the bed to the stretcher? (Select all that apply.)
   1. The patient is 167.6 cm (5 feet 6 inches) and weighs 54.5 kg (120 lb).
   2. The patient speaks and understands English.
   3. The patient is returning to the unit from the recovery room after a procedure requiring conscious sedation.
   4. The patient has a history of being able to stand independently.
   5. The patient received analgesia for pain 30 minutes ago.
8. Which of the following is the proper sequence for a four-point crutch gait?

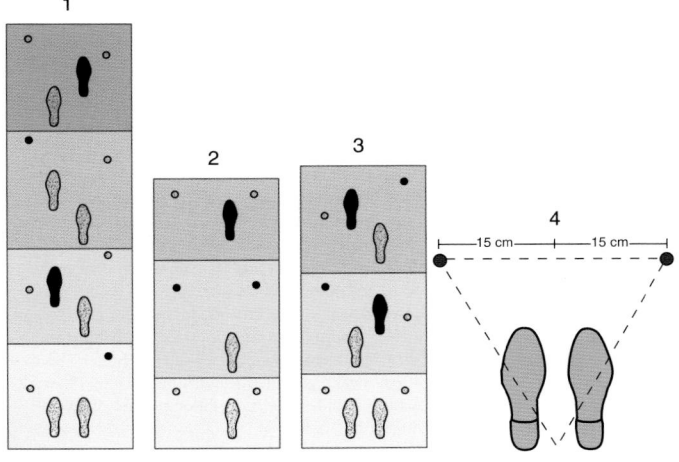

9. A 51-year-old adult comes to a medical clinic for an annual physical exam. The patient is found to be slightly overweight and reports being inactive, walking only 2 to 3 times a week with his wife after work. He has good muscle strength and coordination of lower extremities. Which of the following recommendations from the *Physical Activity Guidelines for Americans* should the nurse suggest? (Select all that apply.)
   1. Move more and sit less throughout the day.
   2. Participate in at least 90 minutes a week of moderate-intensity aerobic physical activity.
   3. Perform muscle-strengthening activities using light weights on 2 or more days a week.
   4. Walk at a vigorous pace with wife at least 150 minutes over five days a week.
   5. Focus on balance training.
10. Family members have asked for a meeting with the nursing staff of an assisted-living residential center to discuss the feasibility of their mother using a walker. The family is worried that her health is declining; they wonder whether she can use the walker safely. Which of the following instructions should the nurse give the family after assessing that it is safe for the woman to use a walker? (Select all that apply.)
   1. A walker is useful for patients who have impaired balance.
   2. The patient uses a walker by pushing the device forward.
   3. Leaning over the walker improves the patient's balance.
   4. Walkers should not be used on stairs.
   5. If the patient has difficulty advancing the walker, a walker with wheels is an option.

Answers: 1. 3, 5; **2.** 1, 2, 4, 5, 6; **3.** 3, 4, 1; **5.** 2, 4; **6.** 1, 2, 3; **7.** 3, 5; **8.** 1; **9.** 1, 3, 4; **10.** 1, 4, 5.

Rationales for Review Questions can be found on the Evolve website.

REFERENCES

Agency for Healthcare Research and Quality (AHRQ): *Health Literacy Universal Precautions Toolkit,* ed 2, Rockville, MD, 2020, Agency for Healthcare Research and Quality. https://www.ahrq.gov/health-literacy/improve/precautions/index.html. Accessed August 15, 2021.

American Academy of Orthopaedist Surgeons: *How to use crutches, canes, and walkers,* 2015. http://orthoinfo.aaos.org/topic.cfm?topic=A00181. Accessed August 15, 2021.

American Association of Critical Care Nurses (AACN): *Early progressive mobility protocol,* 2013. https://www.aacn.org/docs/EventPlanning/WB0007/Mobility-Protocol-szh4mr5a.pdf. Accessed August 15, 2021.

American College of Foot & Ankle Surgeons: *Crutch use,* 2021. https://www.foothealthfacts.org/conditions/crutch-use. Accessed August 15, 2021.

American Diabetes Association (ADA): Improving Care and Promoting Health in Populations: Standards of Medical Care in Diabetes—2020, *Diabetes Care* 43(Suppl 1): S7–S13, 2020.

American Heart Association (AHA): *Target heart rates,* 2021. https://www.heart.org/en/healthy-living/fitness/fitness-basics/target-heart-rates. Accessed August 15, 2021.

American Heart Association (AHA): *American Heart Association recommendations for physical activity in adults and kids,* 2018. https://www.heart.org/en/healthy-living/fitness/fitness-basics/aha-recs-for-physical-activity-in-adults. Accessed August 15, 2021.

Ball J, et al: *Physical examination: an interprofessional approach,* ed 9, St. Louis, 2019, Elsevier.

Baptiste-McKinney A, Halvorson B: The use of friction-reducing devices in a safe patient handling & mobility program, *Int J SPHM* 8(3):132–141, 2018.

Betancourt J, et al: *Cross-cultural care and communication,* 2021, UpToDate. https://www.uptodate.com/contents/cross-cultural-care-and-communication. Accessed August 15, 2021.

Braun L, et al: *Cardiac rehabilitation programs,* 2021, UpToDate. https://www.uptodate.com/contents/cardiac-rehabilitation-programs/print. Accessed August 26, 2021.

Cain C: No time for early mobility? *Am J Crit Care* 27(3):204, 2018.

Carey E, et al: *Cultural aspects of palliative care,* 2021, UpToDate. https://www.uptodate.com/contents/cultural-aspects-of-palliative-care. Accessed August 27, 2021.

Centers for Disease Control and Prevention (CDC): *Benefits of physical activity,* 2021a. https://www.cdc.gov/physicalactivity/basics/pa-health/index.htm. Accessed August 24, 2021.

Centers for Disease Control and Prevention (CDC): *Childhood obesity facts: prevalence of childhood obesity in the United States,* 2021b. https://www.cdc.gov/obesity/data/childhood.html. Accessed August 24, 2021.

Centers for Disease Control and Prevention (CDC): *Worksite physical activity,* 2021c. https://www.cdc.gov/physicalactivity/worksite-pa/index.htm. Accessed August 15, 2021.

Centers for Disease Control and Prevention (CDC): *Physical activity: community strategies,* 2021d. https://www.cdc.gov/physicalactivity/community-strategies/index.htm. Accessed July 12, 2020.

Centers for Disease Control and Prevention (CDC): *Adults need more physical activity,* 2021e. https://www.cdc.gov/physicalactivity/inactivity-among-adults-50plus/index.html. Accessed August 15, 2021.

Centers for Disease Control and Prevention (CDC): *What is health literacy?* 2021f. https://www.cdc.gov/healthliteracy/learn/index.html. Accessed August 15, 2021.

Centers for Disease Control and Prevention (CDC): *Prevalence of obesity and severe obesity in adults: United States 2017-2018,* 2020a. https://www.cdc.gov/nchs/products/databriefs/db360.htm. Accessed August 15, 2021.

Centers for Disease Control and Prevention (CDC): *Target heart rate and estimated maximum heart rate,* 2020b. https://www.cdc.gov/physicalactivity/basics/measuring/heartrate.htm. Accessed August 15, 2021.

Centers for Disease Control and Prevention (CDC): *FACT SHEET: Risk factors for falls,* 2017. https://www.cdc.gov/steadi/pdf/STEADI-FactSheet-RiskFactors-508.pdf. Accessed August 15, 2021.

Colberg S, et al: Physical activity/exercise and diabetes: a position statement of the American Diabetes Association, *Diabetes Care* 39(11):2065–2079, 2016. https://care.diabetesjournals.org/content/39/11/2065. Accessed August 15, 2021.

Czarnecki M, Turner H: *Core curriculum for pain management nursing,* ed 3, St. Louis, 2018, Elsevier.

Dickison P, et al: Assessing higher-order cognitive constructs by using an information-processing framework, *J Appl Test Technol* 17:1–19, 2016.

Edelman CL, Kudzma EC: *Health promotion throughout the life span,* ed 10, St Louis, 2022, Mosby.

Fairchild SL, et al: *Pierson & Fairchild's principles & techniques of patient care,* ed 6, St. Louis, 2018, Elsevier.

Fedorowski A, Melander O: Syndromes of orthostatic intolerance: a hidden danger, *J Intern Med* 273(4): 322, 2013.

Franklin B, et al: *Exercise prescription and guidance for adults*, 2021, UpToDate. https://www.uptodate.com/contents/exercise-prescription-and-guidance-for-adults. Accessed August 24, 2021.

Frith J, et al: Measuring and defining orthostatic hypotension in the older person, *Age Ageing* 43(2):168, 2014.

Giger J, Haddad L: *Transcultural nursing: assessment and intervention*, ed 8, St. Louis, 2021, Elsevier.

Hashem MD: Early mobilization and rehabilitation in the ICU: moving back to the future, *Respir Care* 61(7):971, 2016.

Healthy People 2020 [Internet]: *Physical activity*, Washington, DC, n.d., U.S. Department of Health and Human Services, Office of Disease Prevention and Health. https://www.healthypeople.gov/2020/topics-objectives/topic/physical-activity#:~:text=Healthy%20People%202020%20reflects%20a%20multidisciplinary%20approach%20to,urban%20planning%2C%20recreation%2C%20environmental%20health%2C%20and%20other%20fields. Accessed August 24, 2021.

Hegde SM, Solomon SD: Influence of physical activity on hypertension and cardiac structure and function, *Curr Hypertens Rep* 17(10):77, 2015.

Hilton T, et al: *Safe patient handling and mobility, national program Veterans health administration*, 2019. https://www.cdc.gov/nora/councils/hcsa/pdfs/15-Hilton-508.pdf. Accessed August 15, 2021.

Innovative Outcomes Management: *BMAT implementation workbook*, 2017. https://www.sph-solutions.com/wp-content/uploads/2017/12/BMAT-Implementation-Workbook-2018.pdf. Accessed August 15, 2021.

Kanaskie ML, Snyder C: Nurses and nursing patient handling decision-making regarding use of safe patient handling and mobility technology: a qualitative study, *Appl Nurs Res* 39:141, 2018.

Kaufmann H: *Mechanisms, causes, and evaluation of orthostatic hypotension*, 2021, UpToDate. https://www.uptodate.com/contents/mechanisms-causes-and-evaluation-of-orthostatic-hypotension. Accessed August 15, 2021.

Klish W, Skelton J: *Overview of the health consequences of obesity in children and adolescents*, 2021, UpToDate. https://www.uptodate.com/contents/definition-epidemiology-and-etiology-of-obesity-in-children-and-adolescents. Accessed August 24, 2021.

Kruschke C, Butcher HK: Evidence-based practice guideline: fall prevention for older adults, *J Gerontol Nurs* 3(11):15–21, 2017. doi:10.3928/00989134-20171016-01.

Kwun S, et al: Prevention and treatment of postmenopausal osteoporosis, *Obstet Gynaecol* 14:251, 2012.

LaMorte WW: *Behavioral change models: the Transtheoretical Model (stages of change)*, Boston University School of Public Health, 2019. http://sphweb.bumc.bu.edu/otlt/MPH-Modules/SB/BehavioralChangeTheories/BehavioralChangeTheories6.html. Accessed August 15, 2021.

Martin M, et al: *New and improved VA algorithms*, 2016. https://slidetodoc.com/new-and-improved-va-algorithms-new-sphm-app. Accessed August 15, 2021.

Matz M: *Patient handling and mobility assessments*, ed 2, The Facility Guidelines Institute, 2019. https://fgiguidelines.org/resource/patient-handling-and-movement-assessments/. Accessed August 15, 2021.

Mayo Clinic: *Fitness: tips for staying motivated*, 2021. https://www.mayoclinic.org/healthy-lifestyle/fitness/in-depth/fitness/art-20047624. Accessed August 15, 2021.

Mayo Clinic: *Healthy lifestyle: fitness; are isometric exercises a good way to build strength*, 2020. https://www.mayoclinic.org/healthy-lifestyle/fitness/expert-answers/isometric-exercises/faq-20058186. Accessed August 15, 2021.

McCance KL, Huether SE: *Pathophysiology: the biologic basis for disease in adults and children*, ed 8, St Louis, 2019, Elsevier.

McCulloch D: *Effects of exercise in adults with diabetes mellitus*, UpToDate, 2019. https://www.uptodate.com/contents/effects-of-exercise-in-adults-with-diabetes-mellitus. Accessed August 27, 2021.

Morey M: *Physical activity and exercise in older adults*, UpToDate, 2021. https://www.uptodate.com/contents/physical-activity-and-exercise-in-older-adults. Accessed August 25, 2021.

Myszenski A: *The role of lab values and vital signs in clinical decision making and patient safety for the acutely ill patient*, 2017. https://www.physicaltherapy.com/articles/essential-role-lab-values-and-3637. Accessed August 15, 2021.

National Heart, Lung and Blood Institute (NHLBI): *Overweight and obesity*, n.d.a. https://www.nhlbi.nih.gov/health-topics/overweight-and-obesity. Accessed September 30, 2021.

National Heart, Lung and Blood Institute (NHLBI): *DASH eating plan*, n.d.b. https://www.nhlbi.nih.gov/health-topics/dash-eating-plan. Accessed August 15, 2021.

National Institute for Health and Care Excellence (NICE): *Chronic obstructive pulmonary disease in over 16s: diagnosis and management, NICE guideline [NG115]*. December 05, 2018. https://www.nice.org.uk/guidance/ng115/chapter/Recommendations. Accessed August 26, 2021.

National Institute on Aging (NIA): *Four types of exercise can improve your health and physical activity*, 2021. https://www.nia.nih.gov/health/four-types-exercise-can-improve-your-health-and-physical-ability. Accessed August 15, 2021.

National Institutes of Health (NIH): *Four types of exercise can improve your health and physical ability*, 2021. https://www.nia.nih.gov/health/four-types-exercise-can-improve-your-health-and-physical-ability. Accessed August 25, 2021.

National Institutes of Health (NIH): *Osteoporosis and related bone diseases national resource center: exercise for your bone health*, 2018. https://www.bones.nih.gov/health-info/bone/bone-health/exercise/exercise-your-bone-health. Accessed August 15, 2021.

National Institute for Occupational Safety and Health (NIOSH): *Safe patient handling and mobility (SPHM)*, 2013. http://www.cdc.gov/niosh/topics/safepatient. Accessed August 15, 2021.

Nelson A, Baptiste AS: Evidence-based practices for safe patient handling and movement, *Orthop Nurs* 25(6):366, 2006.

Noble NL, Sweeney NL: Barriers to the use of assistive devices in patient handling, *Workplace Health Saf* 66(1):41–48, 2018.

Nystoriak MA, et al: Cardiovascular effects and benefits of exercise, *Front Cardiovasc Med* 5:135, 2018.

Occupational Safety & Health Association (OSHA): *Safe patient handling—preventing musculoskeletal disorders in nursing homes*, OSHA Publication 3108, 2014, https://www.osha.gov/Publications/OSHA3708.pdf. Accessed August 15, 2021.

Occupational Safety & Health Administration (OSHA): *Worker safety in hospitals*, OSHA Publication, n.d. https://www.osha.gov/dsg/hospitals/. Accessed August 15, 2021.

Occupational Safety & Health Administration (OSHA): *Handling with care: practicing safe patient handling*, 2017. https://www.jcrinc.com/assets/1/7/Pages_from_ECN_20_2017_08-2.pdf. Accessed August 15, 2021.

Office of Disease Prevention and Health Promotion (ODPHP): Physical activity. *Healthy People 2030*, US Department of Health and Human Services, n.d. https://health.gov/healthypeople/objectives-and-data/browse-objectives/physical-activity. Accessed August 15, 2021.

Patton KT: *Anatomy & physiology*, ed 10, St Louis, 2019, Elsevier.

Saffer H, et al: Racial, ethnic, and gender differences in physical activity, *J Hum Cap* 7(4):378, 2013.

Shibao C, et al: Evaluation and treatment of orthostatic hypotension, *J Am Soc Hypertens* 7(4):317, 2013.

Smith GL, et al: The association between social support and physical activity in older adults: a systematic review, *Int J Behav Nutr Phys Act* 14(1):56, 2017.

The Joint Commission (TJC): *2021 National patient safety goals*, Oakbrook Terrace, IL, 2021, The Commission. https://www.jointcommission.org/en/standards/national-patient-safety-goals/. Accessed August 15, 2021.

Touhy T, Jett K: *Ebersole and Hess' toward healthy aging*, ed 10, St Louis, 2020, Elsevier.

U.S. Department of Health and Human Services: *Physical activity guidelines for Americans*, ed 2, Washington, DC, 2018, U.S. Department of Health and Human Services. https://health.gov/sites/default/files/2019-09/Physical_Activity_Guidelines_2nd_edition.pdf. Accessed August 24, 2021.

US Department of Veterans Affairs (USDVA): *Safe patient handling app user manual*, 2019. https://mobile.va.gov/sites/default/files/user-manual-safe-patient-handling-app.pdf. Accessed August 15, 2021.

Washington University Physicians: *How to fit and use crutches*, 2017, Washington University Orthopedics. https://www.ortho.wustl.edu/content/Education/3628/Patient-Education/Educational-Materials/How-to-Fit-and-Use-Crutches.aspx. Accessed August 15, 2021.

Watson KB, et al: Physical inactivity among adults aged 50 years and older — United States, 2014, *MMWR Morb Mortal Wkly Rep* 65(36):954, 2016. https://www.cdc.gov/mmwr/volumes/65/wr/mm6536a3.htm. Accessed August 15, 2021.

Webster JB, Murphy DP, editors: *Atlas of orthoses and assistive devices*, ed 5, Philadelphia, 2019, Elsevier.

Wenger N, et al: *Cardiac rehabilitation: indications, efficacy, and safety in patients with coronary heart disease*, 2020, Up To Date. https://www.uptodate.com/contents/cardiac-rehabilitation-indications-efficacy-and-safety-in-patients-with-coronary-heart-disease/print. Accessed August 15, 2021.

World Health Organization (WHO): *Musculoskeletal conditions*, 2021. https://www.who.int/news-room/fact-sheets/detail/musculoskeletal-conditions. Accessed August 15, 2021.

RESEARCH REFERENCES

Adams ML: *Preventing Chronic Disease: Differences between younger and older US adults with multiple chronic conditions*, vol 14, September 7, 2017, Centers for Disease Control and Prevention. https://www.cdc.gov/pcd/Issues/2017/16_0613.htm. Accessed August 15, 2021.

Bennett D, et al: Outcomes of pulmonary rehabilitation for COPD in older patients: a comparative study, *COPD* 14(2):170–175, 2017.

Biswas D, et al: Role of nurses and nurse practitioners in the recognition, diagnosis, and management of neurogenic orthostatic hypotension: a narrative review, *Int J Gen Med* 12:173–184, 2019.

Boynton T, et al: Banner Mobility Assessment Tool for nurses instrument validation, *Am J SPHM* 4(3):86, 2014.

Chimen M: What are the health benefits of physical activity in type 1 diabetes mellitus? A literature review, *Diabetologia* 55(3):542, 2012.

Dickinson S, et al: Integrating a standardized mobility program and safe patient handling, *Crit Care Nurs Q* 41(3):240, 2018.

Hodgson CL, et al: Early mobilization and recovery in mechanically ventilated patients in the ICU: a bi-national, multi-centre, prospective cohort study, *Crit Care* 19:81, 2015.

Hodgson CL, et al: Early mobilization of patients in intensive care: organization, communication and safety factors that influence translation into clinical practice, *Crit Care* 22(1):77, 2018.

Jang H, et al: Cultural influences on exercise participation and fall prevention: a systematic review and narrative synthesis, *Disabil Rehabil* 38(8):1–9, 2015.

Joseph MS, et al: The impact of structured exercise programs on metabolic syndrome and its components: a systematic review, *Diabetes Metab Syndr Obes* 12:2395–2404, 2019.

Kim K, et al: Relationship between mobility and self-care activity in children with cerebral palsy, *Ann Rehabil Med* 41(2):266, 2017.

King L, et al: Developing a progressive mobility activity protocol, *Orthop Nurs* 31(5):253, 2012.

Lavidan A, et al: Fear of falling in community-dwelling older adults: a cause of falls, a consequence, or both? *PLoS One* 13(5):e0197792, 2018. https://journals.plos.org/plosone/article?id=10.1371/journal.pone.0194967. Accessed August 15, 2021.

Linke CA, et al: Early mobilization in the ICU: a collaborative, integrated approach, *Crit Care Explor* 2(4):e0090. 2020. https://pubmed.ncbi.nlm.nih.gov/32426732/. Accessed August 25, 2021.

McArthur D, et al: Factors influencing adherence to regular exercise in middle-aged women: a qualitative study to inform clinical practice, *BMC Womens Health* 14:49, 2014.

Musich S, et al: The impact of mobility limitations on health outcomes among older adults, *Geriatr Nurs* 39(2):162, 2018.

O'Donoghue G, et al: Socio-economic determinants of physical activity across the life course: a DEterminants of DIet and Physical Activity (DEDIPAC) umbrella literature review, *PLoS One* 13(1):e0190737, 2018.

Onyemaechi N, et al: Impact of overweight and obesity on the musculoskeletal system using lumbosacral angles, *Patient Prefer Adherence* 10:291–296, 2016.

Pinto RM, et al: Basic and genetic aspects of food intake control and obesity: role of dopamine receptor D2 TAQIA polymorphism, *Obes Res Open J* 2:119, 2016.

Pinto RM, et al: Physical activity: benefits for prevention and treatment of childhood obesity, *J Child Obes* 3 (S2-003), 2018.

Rawlings GH, et al. Exploring adults' experiences of sedentary behaviour and participation in non-workplace interventions designed to reduce sedentary behaviour: a thematic synthesis of qualitative studies. *BMC Public Health* 19:1099, 2019.

Schujmann D, et al: Progressive mobility program and technology to increase the level of physical activity and its benefits in respiratory, muscular system, and functionality of ICU patients: study protocol for a randomized controlled trial, *Trials* 19:272, 2018.

Shieh C, et al: Association of self-efficacy and self-regulation with nutrition and exercise behaviors in a community sample of adults, *J Community Health Nurs* 32(4):199, 2015.

Souto-Miranda S, et al: Pulmonary rehabilitation outcomes in individuals with chronic obstructive pulmonary disease: a systematic review, *Ann Phys Rehabil Med* 2021;101564. doi:10.1016/j.rehab.2021.101564. Online ahead of print.

Taylor AMW, et al: Mesolimbic dopamine signaling in acute and chronic pain: implications for motivation, analgesia, and addiction, *Pain* 157(6):1194–1198, 2016.

Tipping CJ, et al: The effects of active mobilisation and rehabilitation in ICU on mortality and function: a systematic review, *Intensive Care Med* 43:171, 2017.

Tomita Y, et al: Prevalence of fear of falling and associated factors among Japanese community-dwelling older adults, *Medicine (Baltimore)* 97(4):e9721, 2018.

Tsang M, et al: Examination of the readiness to learn and the best teaching method regarding health education and promotion within the Chinese elderly population, *Nurs Res* 64(2), 2015.

Walia S, et al: Early mobilization in the ICU: assessing a standardized early mobility protocol on neurological patients, *Neurology* 90(Suppl 15), 2018.

Wang J, et al: Tai chi for essential hypertension, *Evid Based Complement Alternat Med*, 2013, 215254, 2013. https://www.ncbi.nlm.nih.gov/pmc/articles/PMC3748756/. Accessed August 15, 2021.

Immobility

OBJECTIVES

- Discuss physiological and pathological influences on mobility.
- Discuss changes in physiological and psychosocial function associated with immobility.
- Explain the factors associated with sound clinical judgment and critical thinking in caring for patients who are immobile.
- Assess for correct and impaired body alignment and mobility.
- Analyze assessment cues to form appropriate nursing diagnoses for patients with impaired mobility.
- Explain the importance of involving patients and their assessment data in setting priorities regarding a plan of care focused on immobility.
- Discuss a nurse's role in the prevention of deep vein thrombosis (DVT) in patients with reduced mobility.
- Select patient-centered interventions for improving or maintaining patients' mobility.
- Evaluate patient outcomes for improving or maintaining mobility.

KEY TERMS

Atelectasis
Bed rest
Body alignment
Body mechanics
Disuse osteoporosis
Embolus
Foot drop
Friction
Gait
Hemiparesis
Hemiplegia

Hypostatic pneumonia
Immobility
Instrumental activities of daily living (IADLs)
Joint contracture
Mobility
Muscle atrophy
Negative nitrogen balance
Orthostatic hypotension
Osteoporosis
Pathological fractures

Pressure injury
Range of motion (ROM)
Renal calculi
Shear
Thrombus
Trapeze bar
Trochanter roll
Urinary stasis
Venous thromboembolism (VTE)
Virchow triad

MEDIA RESOURCES

http://evolve.elsevier.com/Potter/fundamentals/
- Review Questions
- Audio Glossary
- Case Study with Questions
- Concept Map Creator

- Video Clips
- Content Updates
- Answers to QSEN Activity and Review Questions
- Skills Performance Checklists

Ms. Carnella Cavallo, an 81-year-old patient, is admitted to a skilled care unit for rehabilitation 4 days after recovering from a surgically repaired fractured left hip she injured during a fall. She has a history of smoking but stopped 40 years ago. She has a history of osteoporosis but has no cardiac problems and no hypertension. She describes having "aches" and "stiffness" when lying still in bed, but when she tries to move or turn, she rates her pain a 6 on a pain rating scale. The three small incisions over the left hip are open to air, the edges are approximated, and there is no redness or drainage. Joseph is the nursing case manager for the rehab unit. He is responsible for an initial assessment of Ms. Cavallo and development of her plan of care.

Optimal mobility correlates with positive patient outcomes. People need mobility to work, enjoy their leisure time, and communicate emotions both verbally and nonverbally. Mobility is also essential for self-defense, activities of daily living (ADLs), and recreational activities. Many functions of the body depend on mobility. Intact musculoskeletal

and nervous systems are necessary for optimal physical mobility and functioning (see Chapter 38). When patients lose the ability to remain mobile and active, it is essential for you to apply critical thinking when applying the nursing process to make relevant and accurate clinical judgments regarding interventions necessary to prevent complications and improve existing function.

SCIENTIFIC KNOWLEDGE BASE

Nature of Movement

Chapter 38 describes in detail the nature of movement—how muscles, bones, and the nervous system coordinate together to create movement. As a nurse you need to learn how each patient's physical and psychological conditions affect body movement, including balance, body alignment, posture, and physical activity. Knowing how patients initiate movement and understanding your own movements require a basic understanding of the physics surrounding body mechanics. **Body mechanics** describes the coordinated efforts of the musculoskeletal and nervous systems. The body mechanics applied in the lifting and positioning techniques historically used in nursing practice often caused debilitating injuries to nurses and other health care staff (Kanaskie and Snyder, 2018; Noble and Sweeney, 2018). Today nurses use evidence-based information about body alignment, balance, gravity, and friction when positioning patients, determining patients' risk for falls, and selecting the safest way to move or transfer patients (see Chapter 38).

Changes affecting the normal coordination of the musculoskeletal and nervous systems place patients at risk for numerous health-related problems. Understanding the physiology of these changes prepares you to better anticipate problems, implement prevention strategies, and also intervene proactively when there are problems.

Balance and Alignment.
Correct **body alignment** reduces strain on musculoskeletal structures, aids in maintaining adequate muscle tone, promotes comfort, and contributes to balance and conservation of energy. Without balance control, the center of gravity is displaced. Individuals require balance for maintaining a static position (e.g., sitting) and moving (e.g., walking). Disease, injury, pain, physical development (e.g., age), and life changes (e.g., pregnancy) compromise the ability to remain balanced. Medications that cause dizziness and prolonged immobility affect balance. Impaired balance is a major threat to mobility and physical safety and contributes to a fear of falling and self-imposed activity restrictions (Dickinson et al., 2018; Musich et al., 2018).

Gravity and Friction.
Weight is the force exerted on a body by gravity. The force of weight is always directed downward, which is why an unbalanced object falls. Unsteady patients fall if their center of gravity becomes unbalanced because of the gravitational pull on their weight. Patients who are at risk for being unsteady require the use of safe patient-handling techniques (see Chapter 38).

Patient lifting is now discouraged as a patient care practice. To lift safely, a lifter has to overcome the weight of the object and know its center of gravity. In symmetrical inanimate objects the center of gravity is at the exact center of the object. However, people are not geometrically perfect; their centers of gravity are usually at 55% to 57% of standing height and are in the midline, which is why choosing to use only the principles of body mechanics in lifting patients often leads to injury of a nurse or other health care professional (see Chapter 38).

Friction is a force that occurs in a direction to oppose movement. The greater the surface area of the object that is moved, the greater the friction. A larger object produces greater resistance to movement. For example, a patient who is obese produces greater resistance when moved against a bed surface than a patient who has normal weight. In addition, the force exerted against the skin while the skin remains stationary and the bony structures move is called **shear**. A common example is when the head of a hospital bed is elevated beyond 60 degrees and gravity pulls a patient so that the bony skeleton moves toward the foot of the bed while the skin remains against the sheets. The blood vessels in the underlying tissue are stretched and damaged, resulting in impeded blood flow to the deep tissues. Ultimately pressure injuries often develop within the undermined tissue; the surface tissue appears less affected (see Chapter 48). One way to decrease surface area and reduce friction when patients are unable to assist with moving up in bed is the use of ergonomic assistive devices such as a full-body hydraulic lift. The lift moves a patient off the surface of a bed, thereby preventing friction, tearing, or shearing of delicate skin, and protects you and other health care staff from injury (Noble and Sweeney, 2018).

Skeletal System.
The skeletal system provides attachments for muscles and ligaments and the leverage necessary for mobility. Bones are important for mobilization because they are firm, rigid, and elastic. The aging process, as well as some nutritional and disease processes, have the potential to change the components of bone, which affects mobility.

Firmness in bones results from inorganic salts such as calcium and phosphate that are in the bone matrix. It is related to the rigidity of the bone, which is necessary to keep long bones straight, and enables bones to withstand weight bearing. Elasticity and skeletal flexibility change with age. Chapter 38 describes developmental changes in the musculoskeletal system.

The skeletal system protects vital organs (e.g., the skull around the brain and the ribs around the heart and lungs) and aids in calcium regulation. Bones store calcium and release it into the circulation as needed. Patients who have decreased calcium regulation and metabolism and who are immobile are at risk for developing osteoporosis and **pathological fractures** (fractures caused by weakened bone tissue).

The internal structure of long bones contains bone marrow, participates in red blood cell (RBC) production, and acts as a reservoir for blood. Patients with altered bone marrow function or diminished RBC production tire easily because of reduced hemoglobin and oxygen-carrying ability. This fatigue decreases their mobility and increases the risk for falling.

Joints. The region where two or more bones attach is referred to as a joint. Each joint is classified according to its structure and degree of mobility (see Chapter 38).

Ligaments, Tendons, and Cartilage. Ligaments are white, shiny, flexible bands of fibrous tissue that bind joints together, connect bones and cartilages, and aid joint flexibility and support. Tendons are white, glistening, fibrous bands of tissue that connect muscle to bone and are strong, flexible, and inelastic. Cartilage is nonvascular (without blood vessels) supporting connective tissue located chiefly in the joints and thorax, trachea, larynx, nose, and ear (see Chapter 38). The characteristics of the cartilage change with the aging process, resulting in reduced thickness and calcification.

Skeletal Muscle.
Movement of bones and joints involves active processes that are carefully integrated to achieve coordination. Skeletal muscles, because of their ability to contract and relax, are the working elements of movement. Anatomical structure and attachment to the skeleton enhance contractile elements of the skeletal muscle (see Chapter 38).

Nervous System.
The nervous system regulates movement and posture. The precentral gyrus, or motor strip, is the major voluntary motor area and is in the cerebral cortex. A majority of motor fibers descend from the motor strip and cross at the level of the medulla. Movement is impaired by disorders that alter neurotransmitter production, transfer of impulses from the nerve to the muscle, or activation of muscle activity.

Pathological Influences on Mobility.
Many pathological conditions affect mobility. Knowledge of these conditions is important for you to apply when you assess patients' mobility status to anticipate the health problems they will face, and the interventions required. Although a complete description of each condition is beyond the scope of this chapter, an overview of five pathological influences is presented.

Postural Abnormalities. Disorders of stance or posture result from an inequality of tone in muscle groups, because of a loss of normal postural reflexes, resulting in posturing of the limbs (McCance and Huether, 2019) (Table 39.1). Postural abnormalities can also be congenital, such as scoliosis, or idiopathic (cause unknown). Equilibrium and balance are disrupted. Congenital or acquired postural abnormalities

TABLE 39.1   Postural Disorders

Abnormality	Description	Cause
Lordosis	Exaggeration of anterior convex curve of lumbar spine	Congenital condition; temporary condition (e.g., pregnancy)
Kyphosis	Increased convexity in curvature of thoracic spine	Congenital condition; rickets, osteoporosis; tuberculosis of spine
Scoliosis	Lateral S- or C-shaped spinal column with vertebral rotation, unequal heights of hips and shoulders	Sometimes a consequence of numerous congenital, idiopathic, and neuromuscular disorders
Decorticate posture (hemiplegic posture)	Upper extremities flexed at the elbows and held close to the body; lower extremities externally rotated and extended	Caused by damage between the brain and spinal cord; brainstem is no longer inhibited by the cerebral cortex motor area; seen in cases of cerebral vascular accident
Decerebrate posture	Increased tone in extensor muscles and trunk muscles, with active tonic neck reflexes	Caused by severe injury to the brain and brainstem, resulting in overstimulation of postural righting and vestibular reflexes
Dystonia	Maintenance of an abnormal posture through muscular contractions may last several seconds to weeks; long term, can cause permanent, fixed contractures	Seen in basal ganglia abnormalities; exact pathological cause unknown
Basal ganglion posture	Stooped, hyperflexed posture with a narrow-based, short-stepped gait; due to loss of normal postural reflexes	Common in Parkinson disease (see Fig. 39.1); person loses stability and cannot make postural adjustment to tilting or loss of balance, and falls instead

Adapted from Huether SE, et al: *Understanding pathophysiology,* ed 7, St Louis, 2020, Elsevier.

FIG. 39.1 Stooped posture in Parkinson disease. (From Perkin DG: *Mosby's color atlas and text of neurology,* ed 2, London, 2002, Mosby.)

affect the efficiency of the musculoskeletal system, body alignment, and appearance (Fig. 39.1). Postural abnormalities can cause pain, impair alignment or mobility, or both. Knowledge about the characteristics, causes, and treatment of common postural abnormalities is necessary for safe lifting, transfer, and positioning. Some postural abnormalities limit range of motion (ROM). Nurses intervene to maintain maximum ROM in unaffected joints and collaborate with physical therapists who are expert at designing interventions that strengthen affected muscles

and joints, improve patients' posture, and improve use of affected and unaffected muscle groups.

Muscle Abnormalities. Two types of abnormalities affecting muscles include changes in muscle tone and changes in muscle movement. Normal muscle tone involves a slight resistance to passive joint movement. Normally as a joint moves through its ROM, muscle resistance is smooth, constant, and even (McCance and Huether, 2019). One type of abnormality in muscle tone is hypotonia. It is a decreased muscle tone with little or no resistance during passive muscle movement. It is common in patients with cerebellar damage. Patients with hypotonia tire easily and have difficulty rising from a sitting position, sitting down without support, and walking up and down stairs (McCance and Huether, 2019).

Normal movement also requires a change in the contractility of muscles; muscles must move. Changes in muscle movement occur when there is central nervous system (CNS) dysfunction altering muscle innervation (McCance and Huether, 2019). Some movement disorders (e.g., akinesias) result from too little dopamine to stimulate muscle or too much dopamine (e.g., chorea). There are also movement disorders that are not associated with muscle mass, strength, or tone but are neurological disorders (McCance and Huether, 2019). Conditions such as Parkinson and Huntington disease cause insufficient or excessive movement or involuntary movement.

Damage to the Central Nervous System. Damage to or dysfunction of any component of the CNS that regulates voluntary movement results in impaired body alignment and posture, balance, and mobility. Prolonged bed rest is associated with sensorimotor dysfunction that commonly manifests as postural instability and a dysregulated sense of balance (Yuan et al., 2018). This, together with reduced muscle mass and strength, increases the risk of falls.

Trauma from a head injury, ischemia from a stroke (cerebrovascular accident [CVA]), or bacterial infection such as meningitis can damage the cerebellum or the motor strip in the cerebral cortex. Damage to the cerebellum causes problems with balance, and motor impairment is directly related to the amount of destruction of the motor strip. For example, a person with a right-sided cerebral hemorrhage with necrosis has destruction of the right motor strip that results in left-sided hemiplegia. Trauma to the spinal cord also impairs mobility. For example, a complete transection of the spinal cord results in a bilateral loss of voluntary motor control below the level of the trauma because motor fibers are cut.

Direct Trauma to the Musculoskeletal System. Direct trauma to the musculoskeletal system results in bruises, contusions, tears, sprains, and fractures. A fracture is a disruption of bone tissue continuity. Fractures most commonly result from direct external trauma, but they also occur as a consequence of some deformity of the bone (e.g., pathological fractures of osteoporosis, Paget disease, metastatic cancer, or osteogenesis imperfecta). Young children are usually able to form new bone more easily than adults and, as a result, have few complications after a fracture. Treatment often includes positioning the fractured bone in proper alignment and immobilizing it to promote healing and restore function. Even this temporary immobilization results in some muscle atrophy, loss of muscle tone, and joint stiffness.

Joint Disease. One of the most common pathological influences on mobility comes in the form of joint disease. As the U.S. population ages, the prevalence of arthritis is expected to increase to 44% of the population by the year 2040 (Centers for Disease Control and Prevention [CDC], 2019). Osteoarthritis (OA) is one of the most common causes of chronic disability in adults due to pain and altered joint function, typically affecting knees and hips. The disease was thought to be simply a degenerative "wear and tear" process and therefore often misnamed as degenerative joint disease (Loeser, 2020). However, the pathogenesis of OA is more complex and involves a variety of pathogenic factors, including biomechanical factors, inflammatory factors, and proteases (Loeser, 2020). Rheumatoid arthritis is a chronic, systemic, inflammatory autoimmune disease. Patients have joint swelling, tenderness, and destruction of synovial joints. Joints most commonly affected include the fingers, feet, wrists, elbows, ankles, and knees. Other joints can be affected, as well as tissues of the lungs, heart, and kidneys (Huether et al., 2020). Joint disease creates pain and alters mobility as a result of that pain in addition to pathological bone and cartilage changes. In the acute care setting, nurses care for patients with a variety of conditions who also have a history of joint disease. In addition, nurses care for patients with medical or surgical problems related to a specific joint disorder. An example of this is a patient admitted for a total joint replacement.

REFLECT NOW

As a registered nurse, you are responsible for completing a thorough admission assessment on each of your patients. Given the prevalence of comorbid issues that have the potential to impact mobility, what are five questions you would ask as you begin to explore mobility and immobility issues with your patient?

NURSING KNOWLEDGE BASE

Sound clinical judgment requires the application of a scientific nursing knowledge base. Fully understanding movement and mobility requires more than an overview of the basic science of movement and the physiology and regulation of movement by the musculoskeletal and nervous systems. You also need to know the science of immobility, much of which has been researched by nurses and other health care professionals. Applying the scientific principles of immobility in the clinical setting will help you identify the specific nature of a patient's mobility problems and determine the safest way to move patients and to understand the effect of immobility on the physiological, psychosocial, and developmental aspects of patient care.

The Effects of Immobility

Mobility refers to a person's ability to move about freely, and immobility refers to the inability to do so. Think of mobility as a continuum, with mobility on one end, immobility on the other, and varying degrees of partial immobility between the end points. Some patients move back and forth between mobility and immobility (e.g., short-term arm fracture, progressive amyotrophic lateral sclerosis [ALS]), but for others immobility is absolute and continues indefinitely (e.g., traumatic spinal cord injury). The terms *bed rest* and *impaired physical mobility* are used frequently when discussing patients on the mobility-immobility continuum.

Bed rest is an intervention that restricts patients to bed for therapeutic reasons and is sometimes prescribed for selected patients. The therapeutic reasons for bed rest include decreasing the oxygen needs of the body, reducing cardiac workload and pain, and allowing a patient who is debilitated to rest. Bed rest has many different interpretations among health care professionals. The duration of bed rest depends on the illness or injury and a patient's prior state of health. Patients who are hospitalized do not necessarily have to be on bed rest to be physically inactive. Critically ill patients are often incapable of physical activity. Often older adults limit their activity voluntarily. Nurse researchers have found four reasons for this limited activity: fear of bothering staff, not wanting to further overburden staff, viewing the seeking or receiving of help as something negative, and not wanting to feel dependent on others (Lafrenière et al., 2017).

Immobility has serious consequences. Physical inactivity can have strong deconditioning effects on the human body, in particular on bones, muscles, and the cardiovascular system (Kramer et al., 2017). The effects of muscular deconditioning associated with lack of physical activity are often apparent in a matter of days. An individual of average weight and height without a chronic illness on bed rest loses muscle strength from baseline levels at a rate of about 3% a day (McCance and Huether, 2019). Vulnerable populations, such as older adults, are especially at risk for loss of function during acute illness and hospitalization (Wald et al., 2019). The term *disuse atrophy* describes the pathological reduction in the normal size of muscle fibers after prolonged inactivity resulting from bed rest, trauma, casting of a body part, or local nerve damage (McCance and Huether, 2019).

Periods of immobility due to disability or injury or prolonged bed rest during hospitalization cause major physiological, psychological, and social effects. These effects are gradual or immediate and vary from patient to patient. The greater the extent and the longer the duration of immobility, the more pronounced the consequences. The patient with complete mobility restrictions is continually at risk for the hazards of immobility. When possible, it is imperative that patients, especially older adults, have limited bed rest and begin activity progression as soon as possible. See the early mobility protocol described in Chapter 38. Loss of walking independence increases hospital stays and the need for rehabilitation services or nursing home placement. In addition, the deconditioning related to reduced walking increases the risk for patient falls (American Academy of Nursing [AAN], 2018; Krupp et al., 2018; Kruschke and Butcher, 2017).

Systemic Effects. All body systems work more efficiently with some form of movement. When there is an alteration in mobility, each body system is at risk for impairment. The severity of the impairment depends on a patient's overall health, degree and length of immobility, and age. For example, older adults with chronic illnesses develop pronounced effects of immobility more quickly than do younger patients with the same immobility problem.

Metabolic Changes. Changes in mobility alter endocrine metabolism, calcium resorption, and functioning of the gastrointestinal (GI) system. The endocrine system, composed of hormone-secreting glands, maintains and regulates vital functions such as (1) response to stress and injury; (2) growth and development; (3) reproduction; (4) maintenance of the internal environment; and (5) energy production, use, and storage.

When injury or stress occurs, the endocrine system triggers a series of responses aimed at maintaining blood pressure and preserving life. It is important in maintaining homeostasis. Tissues and cells live in an internal environment that the endocrine system helps regulate through maintenance of sodium, potassium, water, and acid-base balance. It also regulates energy metabolism. Thyroid hormone increases the basal metabolic rate (BMR), and energy becomes available to cells through the integrated action of GI and pancreatic hormones (McCance and Huether, 2019).

Immobility disrupts normal metabolic processes, decreasing the metabolic rate; altering the metabolism of carbohydrates, fats, and proteins; causing fluid, electrolyte, and calcium imbalances; and causing GI disturbances such as decreased appetite and slowing of peristalsis. However, in the presence of an infectious process, immobilization often causes an increased BMR as a result of fever or wound healing because these increase cellular oxygen requirements (McCance and Huether, 2019).

Older adults often experience decreased stamina, reduced appetite, and increased fatigue when they are hospitalized, which may further diminish their capacity to perform ADLs (Mattison, 2021). A deficiency in calories and protein is characteristic of patients with a decreased appetite secondary to immobility. The body is constantly synthesizing proteins and breaking them down into amino acids to form other proteins (see Chapter 45). When a patient is immobile, the body often excretes more nitrogen (the end product of amino acid breakdown) than it ingests in proteins, resulting in negative nitrogen balance. Weight loss, decreased muscle mass, and weakness result from tissue catabolism (tissue breakdown) (McCance and Huether, 2019).

Another metabolic change associated with immobility is calcium resorption (loss) from bones. Immobility causes the release of calcium into the circulation. Normally the kidneys excrete the excess calcium. However, if they are unable to respond appropriately, hypercalcemia results. Pathological fractures may occur if calcium resorption continues as a patient remains on bed rest or continues to be immobile (McCance and Huether, 2019).

Impairments of GI functioning caused by decreased mobility vary. Difficulty in passing stools (constipation) is a common symptom. A condition known as pseudodiarrhea often results from a fecal impaction (accumulation of hardened feces). This finding is not normal diarrhea, but rather liquid stool passing around the area of fecal impaction (see Chapter 47). Left untreated, fecal impaction results in a mechanical bowel obstruction that partly or completely occludes the intestinal lumen, blocking normal propulsion of liquid and gas. The resulting fluid in the intestine produces distention and increases intraluminal pressure. Over time intestinal function becomes depressed, dehydration occurs, absorption ceases, and fluid and electrolyte disturbances worsen.

Respiratory Changes. Lack of movement and exercise places patients at risk for respiratory complications. Patients who are immobile are at high risk for developing pulmonary atelectasis (collapse of alveoli) and hypostatic pneumonia (inflammation of the lung from stasis or pooling of secretions). Both decreased oxygenation and prolonged recovery add to patients' discomfort (Harding et al., 2020). In atelectasis, secretions block a bronchiole or a bronchus, and the distal lung tissue (alveoli) collapses as the existing air is absorbed, producing hypoventilation. The site of the blockage affects the severity of atelectasis. Sometimes an entire lung lobe or a whole lung collapses. At some point in the development of these complications, there is a proportional decline in the patient's ability to cough productively. Ultimately the distribution of mucus in the bronchi increases, particularly when the patient is in the supine, prone, or lateral position. Mucus accumulates in the dependent regions of the airways (Fig. 39.2). Hypostatic pneumonia frequently results because mucus is an excellent place for bacteria to grow.

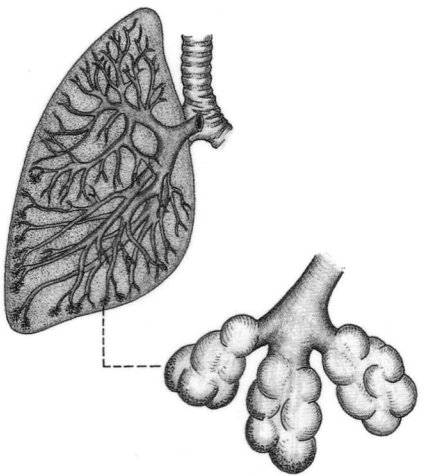

FIG. 39.2 Pooling of secretions in dependent regions of lungs in supine position.

FIG. 39.3 Thrombus formation in a vessel.

Cardiovascular Changes. Immobilization also affects the cardiovascular system, frequently resulting in orthostatic hypotension, increased cardiac workload, and thrombus formation. Orthostatic hypotension is a drop in systolic pressure by at least 20 mm Hg or a drop in diastolic pressure by at least 10 mm Hg within 3 minutes of rising to an upright position (Ball et al., 2019; Biswas et al., 2019). Patients also experience symptoms of dizziness, light-headedness, nausea, tachycardia, pallor, or fainting when changing from the supine to standing position (Ball et al., 2019). When patients are immobilized, decreased circulating fluid volume, pooling of blood in the lower extremities, and decreased autonomic response occur. These are especially evident in the older adult.

As the workload of the heart increases, so does its oxygen consumption. Therefore the heart works harder and less efficiently during periods of prolonged rest. As immobilization increases, cardiac output falls, further decreasing cardiac efficiency and increasing workload.

Patients who are immobile are also at risk for thrombus formation. A thrombus is an accumulation of platelets, fibrin, clotting factors, and the cellular elements of the blood attached to the interior wall of a vein or artery, which sometimes occludes the lumen of the vessel (Fig. 39.3). Three factors contribute to venous thrombus formation:

BOX 39.1 EVIDENCE-BASED PRACTICE

Prevention of Joint Contractures in the Lower Extremities

PICOT Question: Can the use of early alignment, exercises, and mechanical treatment modalities reduce joint contractures in the lower extremities in patients with at-risk conditions compared with patients who do not have any early intervention?

Evidence Summary

Joint contractures are common preventable disorders that can result in significant long-term morbidity and reduced patient independence. Contracture is the shortening of the connective tissue and is an abnormal and possibly permanent condition characterized by decreased range of joint motion and/or fixation of the joint. Contractures occur following prolonged joint positioning (immobility), neurological disorders, and surgical joint manipulation (Odgaard et al., 2018). Evidence shows that early prevention of contractures is essential. Researchers found that nonsurgical approaches, including antispasmodic medications, serial casting, splinting, and physical and occupational therapies such as range-of-motion (ROM) exercises, were helpful in preventing and minimizing this complication of impaired mobility. A systematic review of the efficacy of interventions for preventing contractures showed active stretching programs for healthy older people to be statistically beneficial in improving joint mobility (Saal et al., 2017). However, there is also research that has suggested that passive range of motion (PROM) is not effective for the prevention

and treatment of contractures and that stretch does not prevent or reverse joint contractures in people with neurologic conditions (Seidel et al., 2020). Because many of these clinical trials did not provide a sufficient duration of exercise or did not have combined modalities together, the evidence is unclear. Thus PROM, proper positioning, and stretching are still recommended for treatment and prevention (Seidel et al., 2020). More research is needed to determine the benefit of nursing interventions such as positioning and passive movement (Saal et al., 2017).

Application to Nursing Practice

- In conjunction with an interprofessional health care team, develop an early intervention protocol using prescribed positioning, ROM exercises, and/or splints to reduce the risk of joint deformity and contracture formation (Winterton and Baldwin, 2018).
- Health care agencies need to provide equipment (e.g., splints) and appropriate education for staff to reduce the risk of contractures.
- A collaborative plan of care, including a discharge plan, with a contracture prevention and muscle strengthening protocol must be developed on patient admission.
- Use positioning and ROM and stretching exercises according to the individualized need of the patient and as ordered (Winterton and Baldwin, 2018; Saal et al., 2017).

---

(1) damage to the vessel wall (e.g., injury during surgical procedures), (2) alterations of blood flow (e.g., slow blood flow in calf veins associated with bed rest), and (3) alterations in blood constituents (e.g., a change in clotting factors or increased platelet activity). These three factors are often referred to as the **Virchow triad** (Huether et al., 2020). One of the dangers of a deep vein thrombosis (DVT) is the development of a pulmonary **embolus** (PE). A PE occurs when a part of the thrombus or clot breaks off and travels to the lungs and then blocks the pulmonary artery, altering the blood supply to lung tissue. PE has a variety of presenting features, ranging from no symptoms to shock or sudden death. The most common presenting symptom is dyspnea followed by pleuritic chest pain and cough (Thompson et al., 2021). However, many patients, including those with large PE, have mild or nonspecific symptoms or are asymptomatic (Thompson et al., 2021). As a nurse you will practice in numerous situations in which DVT must be prevented, especially during perioperative care (see Chapter 50).

Musculoskeletal Changes. Immobility causes permanent or temporary impairment of musculoskeletal structures. Because of protein breakdown, a patient loses lean body mass during immobility. The reduced muscle mass makes it difficult for patients to sustain activity without increased fatigue. If immobility continues and a patient does not exercise, there is further loss of muscle mass. Prolonged immobility often leads to disuse atrophy. Loss of endurance, decreased muscle mass and strength, and joint instability place patients at risk for falls (see Chapter 27).

Immobilization also causes two skeletal changes: impaired calcium metabolism and joint abnormalities. Because immobilization results in bone resorption, the bone tissue is less dense or atrophied, and **disuse osteoporosis** results. When disuse osteoporosis occurs, a patient is at risk for pathological fractures.

Osteoporosis is a major health concern in this country. By 2025 it is expected to be responsible for approximately 3 million fractures, with the lifetime risk of an osteoporosis fracture at 50% for women and 20% to 25% for men (Gupta et al., 2018). Although primary osteoporosis is different in origin from the osteoporosis that results from immobility, it is imperative that nurses recognize that patients are at high risk

for accelerated bone loss when they are immobilized and if they have primary osteoporosis.

Immobility can lead to joint contractures. A **joint contracture** is an abnormal and possibly permanent condition characterized by fixation of a joint. It is important to note that flexor muscles for joints are stronger than extensor muscles and therefore contribute to the formation of contractures. Disuse, atrophy, and shortening of the muscle fibers cause joint contractures. When a contracture occurs, the joint cannot achieve full ROM. Contractures sometimes leave a joint or joints in a nonfunctional position, as seen in patients who are permanently curled in a fetal position. Early prevention of contractures is essential (Box 39.1) (Meyers, 2017).

One common and debilitating contracture is foot drop (Fig. 39.4). When **foot drop** occurs, the foot is permanently fixed in plantar flexion. Ambulation is difficult with the foot in this position because the patient cannot dorsiflex the foot. A patient with foot drop is unable to lift the toes off the ground and is at risk of stumbling. Patients who have right- or left-sided paralysis (hemiplegia) because of a nerve injury or a disorder affecting the muscles, nerves, brain, or spinal cord (e.g., compression of the peroneal nerve after hip or knee replacement surgery, CVA, multiple sclerosis) are at risk for foot drop.

Urinary Elimination Changes. Immobility alters a patient's urinary elimination. In the upright position urine flows out of the renal pelvis and into the ureters and bladder because of gravitational forces. When a patient is recumbent or flat, the kidneys and ureters move toward a more level plane. Urine formed by the kidney needs to enter the bladder unaided by gravity. Because the peristaltic contractions of the ureters are insufficient to overcome gravity, the renal pelvis fills before urine enters the ureters. This condition is called **urinary stasis** and increases the risk of urinary tract infection (UTI) and renal calculi (see Chapter 46).

Renal calculi are calcium stones that lodge in the renal pelvis or pass through the ureters. Patients are at risk for calculi when they are immobilized because they frequently have hypercalcemia (McCance and Huether, 2019). As the period of immobility continues, fluid intake often diminishes. When combined with other problems such as fever, the risk for dehydration increases. As a result, urinary output declines on or about

FIG. 39.4 Foot drop. (A) Ankle is fixed in plantar flexion. Normally ankle is able to flex *(dashed line),* which eases walking. (B) Foot drop. (B from Rosenberg RN: *Atlas of clinical neurology,* ed 2, Current Medicine Group, 2009, Springer Science and Business Media.)

Tissue metabolism depends on the supply of oxygen and nutrients to and the elimination of metabolic wastes from the blood. Pressure affects cellular metabolism by decreasing or totally eliminating tissue circulation. When a patient lies in bed or sits in a chair, the weight of the body is on bony prominences. The longer the pressure is applied, the longer the period of ischemia, and therefore the risk of skin breakdown increases (Stephens et al., 2018). The prevalence of pressure injuries is highest in long-term care facilities, whereas the rate of hospital-acquired pressure injuries is the highest in adult intensive care units (Ayello, 2017; Berlowitz, 2020).

Psychosocial Effects. Nursing research shows that immobilization often leads to emotional and behavioral responses, sensory alterations, and changes in coping. Illnesses that result in limited or impaired mobility can cause social isolation and loneliness (Musich et al., 2018). Every patient responds to immobility differently.

Patients with restricted mobility sometimes also experience depression. Depression is an affective disorder characterized by exaggerated feelings of sadness, melancholy, dejection, worthlessness, emptiness, and hopelessness out of proportion to reality. It results from worrying about present and future levels of health, finances, and family needs. Because immobilization removes a patient from a daily routine, the patient has more time to worry about disability. Worrying contributes to depression, causing patients to withdraw and become unable to participate in their own care.

Developmental Changes

Immobility often leads to developmental changes in the very young and in older adults. A young or middle-age adult who is immobile and has been healthy experiences few, if any, developmental changes. However, there are exceptions. For example, a mother with complications following birth may need to go on bed rest and as a result cannot interact with her newborn as expected.

Infants, Toddlers, and Preschoolers. As an infant grows, musculoskeletal development permits support of weight for standing and walking (see Chapter 12). Posture is awkward because the head and upper trunk are carried forward. Because body weight is not distributed evenly along a line of gravity, posture is normally off balance, and falls occur often. When an infant, toddler, or preschooler becomes immobilized, it is usually because of trauma or the need to correct a congenital skeletal abnormality. Prolonged immobilization delays progression of a child's gross-motor skills, intellectual development, and musculoskeletal development.

Adolescents. The adolescent stage usually begins with a tremendous increase in growth (see Chapter 12). When the activity level is reduced because of trauma, illness, or surgery, the adolescent is often behind peers in gaining independence and accomplishing certain skills, such as obtaining a driver's license. Social isolation is a concern for this age-group when immobilization occurs.

Adults. An adult who has correct posture and body alignment feels good, looks good, and generally appears self-confident. The healthy adult also has the necessary musculoskeletal development and coordination to carry out ADLs (see Chapter 13). When periods of prolonged immobility occur, all physiological systems are at risk. In addition, the role of the adult often changes with regard to the family or social structure. Some adults lose their jobs, which affects their self-concept (see Chapter 33).

Older Adults. A progressive loss of total bone mass in older adults results from decreased physical activity, hormonal changes, and bone

the fifth or sixth day after immobilization, and the urine becomes concentrated. Concentrated urine increases the risk for calculi formation and infection. Another cause of UTI, especially in patients who are immobilized, is the use of an indwelling urinary catheter (see Chapter 46).

Integumentary Changes. The changes in metabolism that accompany immobility add to the harmful effect of pressure on the skin. This makes immobility a major risk factor for pressure injuries. Any break in the integrity of the skin is difficult to heal. Preventing a pressure injury is much less expensive than treating one; therefore preventive nursing interventions are imperative (Barnes-Daly et al., 2018; Berlowitz, 2020).

A **pressure injury** is localized damage to the skin and underlying soft tissue, usually over a bony prominence or related to a medical device or other device (Berlowitz, 2020). It develops as a result of prolonged ischemia (decreased blood supply) in tissues aggravated by superficial shear or friction (see Chapter 48). It is characterized initially by inflammation and usually forms over a bony prominence. Ischemia develops when the pressure on the skin is greater than the pressure inside the small peripheral blood vessels supplying blood to the skin (Agency for Healthcare Research and Quality [AHRQ], 2014). Multiple factors in addition to immobility promote formation of pressure injuries, including moisture on the skin (e.g., from diaphoresis or incontinence), poor nutritional intake, and shear and friction on the skin.

BOX 39.2 FOCUS ON OLDER ADULTS

Functional Decline in Older Adults as a Result of Hospitalization and Immobility

For many older adults, admission to a health care agency often results in functional decline despite the treatment for which they were admitted. Some older adults have problems related to mobility and quickly regress to a dependent state (Chase et al., 2018). Usually aging is associated with decreased muscle strength and aerobic capacity, which become exacerbated if a patient's nutritional state is poor.

- Include a nutritional assessment before developing a plan of care for the older adult experiencing immobility.
- Anorexia and insufficient assistance with eating lead to malnutrition, which contributes to the known problems associated with immobility.
- Improved nutrition increases a patient's ability to perform physical reconditioning exercises (Heflin, 2021; Kruschke and Butcher, 2017).
- There is a direct relationship among the success of older adults' rehabilitation, risk for falls, and their nutritional status (Barbour et al., 2017; Heflin, 2021).

resorption. The effect of bone loss is weaker bones. Older adults often walk more slowly, take smaller steps, and appear less coordinated. Prescribed medications often alter their sense of balance or affect their blood pressure when they change position too quickly, increasing their risk for falls and injuries (see Chapter 27). The outcomes of a fall include not only possible injury but also hospitalization, loss of independence, psychological effects, and quite possibly death (Hallford et al., 2017; Musich et al., 2018; Wald et al., 2019).

Older adults often experience functional status changes secondary to hospitalization and altered mobility status (Box 39.2). Immobilization of older adults increases their physical dependence on others and accelerates functional losses (Chase et al., 2018). Immobilization of some older adults results from degenerative diseases, neurological trauma, or chronic illness. In some it occurs gradually and progressively; in others, especially those who have had a stroke, it is sudden. When providing nursing care for an older adult, encourage the patient to perform as many self-care activities as possible, thereby maintaining the highest level of mobility. Sometimes nurses inadvertently contribute to a patient's immobility by providing unnecessary help with activities such as bathing and transferring.

In the case study, Ms. Cavallo has a number of factors contributing to problems from immobility, including her age, restricted activity during hospitalization, the type of surgery, and her osteoporosis. Joseph will reflect on his knowledge of the nature of movement and effects of immobility when applying the nursing process for this patient.

CRITICAL THINKING

Critical thinking in making clinical judgments about the approach to the care of a patient who is immobilized can be complicated. The physical effects of any restrictions in movement caused by a sudden illness or injury coupled with any preexisting health conditions (e.g., heart disease, diabetes, previous injury) require you to consider a broad number of potential complications. The key is anticipation. During the nursing process, always anticipate a patient's potential risks as well as actual risks related to immobility as you gather data, analyze and identify diagnoses, and select and deliver interventions.

Application of scientific knowledge and experience in the care of patients experiencing immobility will promote early recognition of problems. Witnessing the effects of immobility prepares you to identify problems earlier for subsequent patients. Show humility by being willing to involve other health professionals such as physical therapists and registered dietitians, who can give valuable insight as to the nature of immobility problems and appropriate interventional strategies.

There are environmental factors that influence your approach to caring for a patient with limited mobility. Know the availability of assistive personnel (AP) and others who can assist with those tasks requiring moving and positioning patients. Are resources such as special lifts and friction-reducing devices (FRDs) available? Environmental conditions in health care settings will affect your approach. In acute care there is a focus on maintaining mobility and preventing complications, whereas in long-term care the focus is rehabilitation. These factors will influence how you identify problems affecting the patient's long term recovery.

Use of critical thinking attitudes and intellectual standards allows you to be thorough in your assessment and more effective as a problem solver. For example, being disciplined and curious creates a mindset for understanding how immobility affects a patient psychologically and the impact that has in patient participation in the plan of care.

Numerous professional standards incorporating evidence-based approaches exist for the care of patients who are immobilized. Examples include the National Pressure Injury Advisory Panel (NPIAP) recommendations, the Intensive Care Society (ICS)–recommended bundle of interventions for the prevention of ventilator-associated pneumonia, and the Society of Critical Care Medicine (SCCM)/ American Society of Parenteral and Enteral Nutrition (ASPEN) guidelines for early nutritional support of the critically ill.

REFLECT NOW

Three patients are being admitted to an acute care hospital for surgery on their right hip. Patient #1 is a 9-month-old male, patient #2 is a 44-year-old male, and patient #3 is a 75-year-old female. Using foundational nursing knowledge, compare and contrast developmental needs, effects of immobility, and how their plans of care may differ.

❖ NURSING PROCESS

Apply the nursing process and use critical thinking in making sound clinical judgments about your approach to a patient's care. The nursing process provides a clinical decision-making approach for you to develop and implement an individualized plan that will reduce threats posed by immobility and maintain or improve existing physical function. Patients with preexisting mobility impairments and those who are at risk for immobility will greatly benefit from a care plan that improves the patient's functional status, promotes self-care, and maintains psychological well-being.

◆ Assessment

During assessment, consider your patient's normal mobility status, the effects of any diseases or conditions on mobility, and the patient's risks for mobility alterations as a result of treatments (Fig. 39.5). Also consider whether a patient's mobility status poses risks for mobility complications. Critically analyze findings to ensure that you make patient-centered clinical decisions required for safe nursing care.

Through the Patient's Eyes. It is impossible for you to know how a person who is less mobile and suddenly dependent on others feels. Remember that your patient is a full partner in making decisions that contribute to the plan of care. Your assessment must explore how any limitations in mobility are perceived by the patient, as well as expectations of care. Does the patient understand whether a particular disease

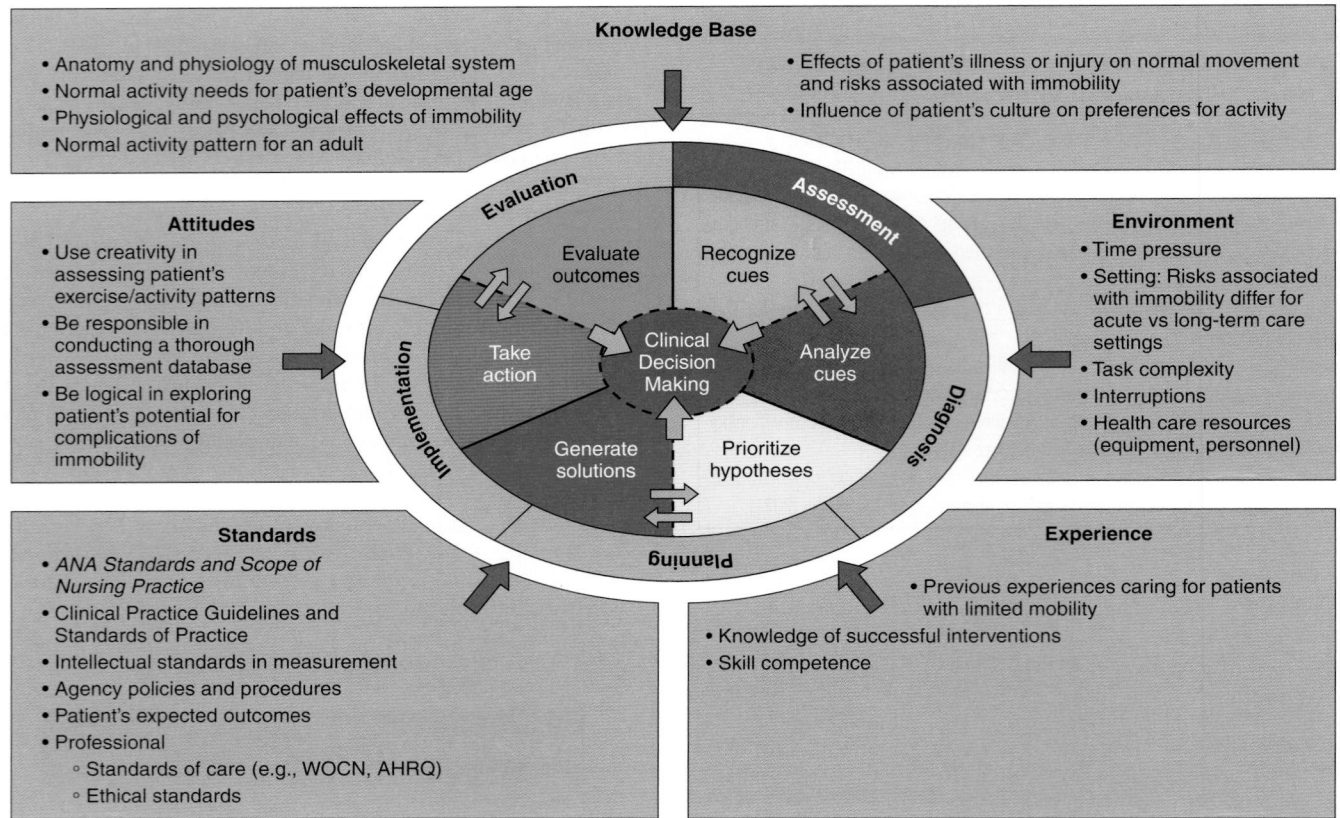

Knowledge Base
- Anatomy and physiology of musculoskeletal system
- Normal activity needs for patient's developmental age
- Physiological and psychological effects of immobility
- Normal activity pattern for an adult

- Effects of patient's illness or injury on normal movement and risks associated with immobility
- Influence of patient's culture on preferences for activity

Attitudes
- Use creativity in assessing patient's exercise/activity patterns
- Be responsible in conducting a thorough assessment database
- Be logical in exploring patient's potential for complications of immobility

Environment
- Time pressure
- Setting: Risks associated with immobility differ for acute vs long-term care settings
- Task complexity
- Interruptions
- Health care resources (equipment, personnel)

Evaluation — Evaluate outcomes — Take action — Clinical Decision Making — *Implementation* — Generate solutions — *Assessment* — Recognize cues — Analyze cues — *Diagnosis* — Prioritize hypotheses — *Planning*

Standards
- *ANA Standards and Scope of Nursing Practice*
- Clinical Practice Guidelines and Standards of Practice
- Intellectual standards in measurement
- Agency policies and procedures
- Patient's expected outcomes
- Professional
  - Standards of care (e.g., WOCN, AHRQ)
  - Ethical standards

Experience
- Previous experiences caring for patients with limited mobility
- Knowledge of successful interventions
- Skill competence

FIG. 39.5 Critical thinking model for assessing impaired mobility. *AHRQ,* Agency for Healthcare Research and Quality; *ANA,* American Nurses Association; *WOCN,* Wound, Ostomy, and Continence Nurses Society. (Clinical Judgment Measurement Model copyright © NCSBN. All rights reserved.)

or condition will likely cause permanent disability? Has the patient had a disability for an extended period, and is the patient well adapted to the use of an assistive device or even a wheelchair? Is the limitation in mobility sudden and unexpected, causing the patient to be fearful or full of questions? Always convey respect for the patient's preferences, values, and needs during assessment and when designing a plan of care (Ackley and Ladwig, 2019).

Joseph knows from experience working in a skilled nursing facility that many patients are apprehensive about their transfer and not knowing what to expect. Hospitals often provide little information to patients about a long-term facility, its services, and standards for quality. Joseph also knows that to engage Ms. Cavallo in a rehab program that will be of benefit will require her full participation. He states, 'Ms. Cavallo, we are happy to have you here. My name is Joseph and I will be the nurse coordinating your care here. Tell me what you know about why you are coming to this facility." Ms. Cavallo responds, "Oh, I so want to be able to go home. The hospital really took my strength out of me. I'm here to get better." Joseph replies, "Yes, you are. We will be planning activities for you to get your strength back. I want to ask you a series of questions to learn more about how we can meet your needs together."

Mobility and Activity Tolerance. Usually you will assess a patient's degree of mobility and immobility during the history interview and physical examination (Box 39.3). When unsure of a patient's abilities, begin assessment of mobility with the patient in the most supported position, and move to higher levels according to the patient's tolerance. Begin the assessment of movement while the patient is lying down, and proceed to assessing the sitting position in bed, ability to transfer to chair, and finally walking. Assess what the patient can do independently.

BOX 39.3   Nursing Assessment Questions

Activity and Mobility
- Describe your normal daily activities including exercise. Explain how this has changed recently.
- Explain for me. Have you experienced any stiffness, swelling of a joint, muscle or joint pain, or difficulty with moving? If so, tell me how this affects your movement and daily activities.
- Tell me about any problems you have when walking. Have you noticed any shortness of breath or pain?
- Do you require the use of a cane or walker to get about inside the home? Outdoors?

Immobility
- How does your current situation, being limited in moving about, make you feel?
- How have your appetite and diet changed since you have had problems moving around? Describe what you eat in a normal day.
- Does your day seem very long?
- Describe for me a typical night's sleep.
- Have you noticed any places on your skin that are reddened or have any open sores?
- Describe any changes you have noticed in urinating and/or having bowel movements.

If assistance is needed, assess the degree of help required. This progression of the assessment promotes the patient's safety.

When a patient is immobile, assessment focuses on the status of the musculoskeletal system and includes ROM, muscle strength, activity tolerance, and posture and alignment. **Range of motion (ROM)** is the maximum amount of movement available at a joint in one of the three planes of the body: sagittal, transverse, or frontal (Fig. 39.6). The sagittal plane is a line that passes through the body from front to back, dividing it into a left and right side. The frontal plane passes through the body from side to side and divides it into front and back. The transverse plane is a horizontal line that divides the body into upper and lower portions.

Ligaments, muscles, and the nature of the joint limit joint mobility in each of the planes. However, some joint movements are specific to each plane. In the sagittal plane, movements are flexion and extension (e.g., fingers and elbows), dorsiflexion and plantar flexion (feet), and extension (e.g., hip). In the frontal plane, movements are abduction and adduction (e.g., arms and legs) and eversion and inversion (feet). In the transverse plane, movements are pronation and supination (hands) and internal and external rotation (hips).

Assessment of ROM is an important baseline measurement that compares and evaluates whether loss in joint mobility is developing or has occurred. Refer to Table 39.2 for normal joint ROM to compare with findings when you assess a patient's ROM. Be sure to assess all joints in the body. Ask questions about and physically examine a patient for stiffness, swelling, pain, or limited movement, and compare sides for unequal movement (see Chapter 30). If a patient has restricted ROM, your information will help you collaborate with physical therapists to select the type of ROM exercise a patient is able to perform, so you can reduce risk of complications (Table 39.3).

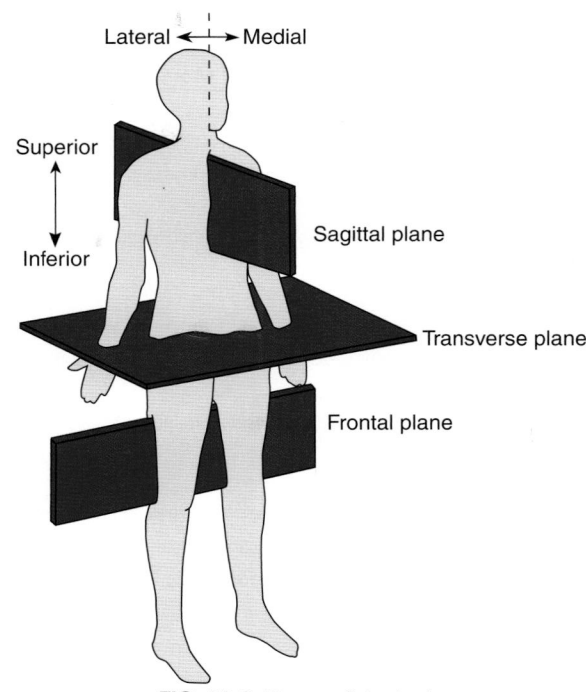

FIG. 39.6 Planes of the body.

TABLE 39.2 Range-of-Motion Exercises

Body Part	Type of Joint	Type of Movement	Range (Degrees)	Primary Muscles
Neck, cervical spine	Pivotal	*Flexion:* Bring chin to rest on chest.	45	Sternocleidomastoid
		Extension: Return head to erect position.	45	Trapezius
		Hyperextension: Bend head back as far as possible.	10	Trapezius
		Lateral flexion: Tilt head as far as possible toward each shoulder.	40–45	Sternocleidomastoid
		Rotation: Turn head as far as possible in circular movement.	180	Sternocleidomastoid, trapezius
Shoulder	Ball and socket	*Flexion:* Raise arm from side position forward to position above head.	45–180	Coracobrachialis, biceps brachii, deltoid, pectoralis major
		Extension: Return arm to position at side of body.	180	Latissimus dorsi, teres major, triceps brachii
		Shoulder extension: Move arm behind body, keeping elbow straight.	0–60	Latissimus dorsi, teres major, deltoid
		Internal rotation: With elbow flexed and shoulder abducted, rotate shoulder by moving arm until thumb is turned inward and toward back.	70–90	Pectoralis major, latissimus dorsi, teres major, subscapularis
		External rotation: With elbow flexed and shoulder abducted, move arm until thumb is upward and lateral to head.	90	Infraspinatus, teres major, deltoid
		Circumduction: Move arm in full circle. (Circumduction is combination of all movements of ball-and-socket joint.)	360	Deltoid, coracobrachialis, latissimus dorsi, teres major
Elbow	Hinge	*Flexion:* Bend elbow so lower arm moves toward its shoulder joint and hand is level with shoulder.	150	Biceps brachii, brachialis, brachioradialis
		Extension: Straighten elbow by lowering hand.	150	Triceps brachii
Forearm	Pivotal	*Supination:* Turn lower arm and hand so palm is up.	70–90	Supinator, biceps brachii
		Pronation: Turn lower arm so palm is down.	70–90	Pronator teres, pronator quadratus

Continued

TABLE 39.2   Range-of-Motion Exercises—cont'd

Body Part	Type of Joint	Type of Movement	Range (Degrees)	Primary Muscles
Wrist	Condyloid	*Flexion:* Move palm toward inner aspect of forearm.	80–90	Flexor carpi ulnaris, flexor carpi radialis
		Extension: Move fingers and hand posterior to midline, bring dorsal surface of hand back as far as possible.	70–80	Extensor carpi radialis brevis, extensor carpi radialis longus, extensor carpi ulnaris
		Radial deviation: Bend wrist medially toward thumb.	Up to 30	Flexor carpi radialis brevis, extensor carpi radialis brevis, extensor carpi radialis longus
		Ulnar deviation: Bend wrist laterally toward fifth finger.	30	Flexor carpi ulnaris, extensor carpi ulnaris
Fingers	Condyloid hinge	*Flexion:* Make fist.	90	Lumbricales, interosseus volaris, interosseus dorsalis
		Extension: Straighten fingers.	90	Extensor digiti quinti proprius, extensor digitorum communis, extensor indicis proprius
		Hyperextension: Bend fingers back as far as possible.	30–60	Extensor digitorum
		Abduction: Spread fingers apart.	30	Interosseus dorsalis
		Adduction: Bring fingers together.	30	Interosseus volaris
Thumb	Saddle	*Flexion:* Move thumb across palmar surface of hand.	0–90	Flexor pollicis brevis
		Extension: Move thumb straight away from hand.	0–90	Extensor pollicis longus, extensor pollicis brevis
		Abduction: Extend thumb laterally (usually done when placing fingers in abduction and adduction).	0–30	Abductor pollicis brevis
		Adduction: Move thumb back toward hand.	0–30	Adductor pollicis obliquus, adductor pollicis transversus
		Opposition: Touch thumb to each finger of same hand.		Opponens pollicis, opponens digiti minimi
Hip	Ball and socket	*Flexion:* Move leg forward and up.	110–120	Psoas major, iliacus, sartorius
		Extension: Move leg back beside other leg.	90–120	Gluteus maximus, semitendinosus, semimembranosus
		Hyperextension: Move leg behind body as far as possible.	30–50	Gluteus maximus, semitendinosus, semimembranosus
		Abduction: Move leg laterally away from body.	30–50	Gluteus medius, gluteus minimus
		Adduction: Move leg back toward medial position and beyond if possible.	20–30	Adductor longus, adductor brevis, adductor magnus
		Internal rotation: Turn foot and leg toward other leg.	0–45	Gluteus medius, gluteus minimus, tensor fasciae latae
		External rotation: Turn foot and leg away from other leg.	0–45	Obturator internus, obturator externus
		Circumduction: Move leg in circle 360 degrees.		Psoas major, gluteus maximus, gluteus medius, adductor magnus
Knee	Hinge	*Flexion:* Bring heel back toward back of thigh.	120–130	Biceps femoris, semitendinosus, semimembranosus, sartorius
		Extension: Return leg to floor.	120–130	Rectus femoris, vastus lateralis, vastus medialis, vastus intermedius
Ankle	Hinge	*Dorsal flexion:* Move foot so toes are pointed upward.	20–30	Tibialis anterior
		Plantar flexion: Move foot so toes are pointed downward.	45–50	Gastrocnemius, soleus
Foot	Gliding	*Inversion:* Turn sole of foot medially.	35 or less	Tibialis anterior, tibialis posterior
		Eversion: Turn sole of foot laterally.	10 or less	Peroneus longus, peroneus brevis
Toes	Condyloid	*Flexion:* Curl toes downward.	30–60	Flexor digitorum, lumbricalis pedis, flexor hallucis brevis
		Extension: Straighten toes.	30–60	Extensor digitorum longus, extensor digitorum brevis, extensor hallucis longus
		Abduction: Spread toes apart.	15 or less	Abductor hallucis, interosseus dorsalis
		Adduction: Bring toes together.	15 or less	Adductor hallucis, interosseus plantaris

TABLE 39.3   Range-of-Motion Alterations

Body Part	Alteration	Assessment Finding(s)
Neck	A patient's neck is permanently flexed with the chin close to or actually touching the chest.	Altered body alignment, changes in the visual field, and decreased level of independent functioning.
Shoulder	The strongest muscle controlling the shoulder is the deltoid. It is in complete elongation in the normal position, but with alteration there is limited elongation.	Difficulty moving the arms.
Elbow	Fixed in full extension.	Difficulty flexing and using arm for self-care activities.
Forearm	Forearm becomes fixed in full supination.	Use of hand is limited, unable to perform self-care activities.
Wrist	Wrist becomes fixed, slightly flexed.	Grasp is weaker.
Fingers and thumb	Digits become more flexed; pain with movement.	Unable to perform fine-motor skills: picking up objects, ADLs, needlework, drawing.
Hip	Contractures often fix the hip in positions of deformity. Excessive abduction makes the affected leg appear too short, whereas excessive adduction makes it appear too long.	Limited ability to move about; walks with limp. Internal and external rotation contractures cause abnormal and unbalanced gait.
Knee	Knees cannot remain stable under weight-bearing conditions unless there is adequate quadriceps power to maintain them in full extension.	Knee is stiff. If fixed in full extension, a person needs to sit with leg out in front. If knee is stiffened in flexed position, person limps while walking.
Ankle and foot	Joint becomes unstable. When the person relaxes as in sleep or coma, the foot relaxes and assumes a position of plantar flexion. As a result, it becomes fixed in plantar flexion (foot drop).	Abnormal gait. Impaired ability to walk independently.
Toes	Excessive flexion of the toes results in clawing. Permanent clawing results in the foot being unable to rest flat on the floor.	Abnormal gait.

ADLs, Activities of daily living.

There are three types of ROM exercises: active, active assisted, and passive (PROM). An example of active assisted ROM is having to provide support for a patient who is weak and assist while the patient performs most of the joint movement. Some patients are able to move some joints actively and independently, whereas you will passively move others. Ligaments, muscles, and the nature of the joint limit patients' mobility, and some joint movements are specific to their location in the body. Abduction and adduction of the arms and legs are an example of this specific type of movement. Abduction is the movement of an extremity away from the midline of the body, and adduction is the movement of an extremity toward the midline of the body.

The major musculoskeletal changes expected during assessment of a patient who is immobilized include decreased muscle strength, loss of muscle tone and mass, and contractures. Patients with musculoskeletal injuries or chronic conditions require careful palpation of joints and extremities to minimize discomfort. Because patients experiencing immobility are weakened, determine whether difficulty in moving joints is the result of fatigue or decreased ROM. Remember that a patient's total musculoskeletal system must be evaluated from the head and neck down to the toes. Any limitation not identified early can result in the patient developing a permanent complication that will affect mobility in the future.

Observing a patient's posture and alignment while sitting and lying in bed determines the type of assistance the patient requires for safe repositioning (i.e., notice which method the patient uses to push up in bed or whether the patient grabs onto objects to steady himself or herself). Aligning patients properly within their own restrictions helps to reduce discomfort and placement of stress on weakened or injured extremities.

Activity Tolerance. Activity tolerance is the type and amount of exercise or work that a person is able to perform without undue exertion or injury. Many patients who have become immobilized may be very limited in their ability to walk or change position in bed. The first step in assessing activity tolerance is to collect a baseline set of heart rate, respirations, and blood pressure. Then if you assess a patient who is mobile initially (such as preoperatively) but who you know will have reduced mobility following treatment (such as postoperatively), have the patient walk a short distance down a hallway or back and forth in a hospital room. Does the patient experience dyspnea, shortness of breath, fatigue, chest pain, and/or a change in heart rate, respirations, or blood pressure? Both heart rate and blood pressure should increase. Chapter 38 further describes how to assess a patient's activity tolerance. Assessment of activity tolerance is necessary when planning activity such as walking, ROM exercises, or ADLs. Use the patient's baseline vital signs to evaluate activity tolerance during subsequent patient encounters. When a patient experiences decreased activity tolerance, carefully assess how much time is needed to recover. Decreasing recovery time indicates improving activity tolerance.

Gait. Gait is the manner or style of walking, including rhythm, cadence, length of stride, and speed. Assessing gait allows for conclusions about balance, posture, and the ability to walk without assistance (see Chapter 38). While a patient walks, look for conformity in use of extremities, a regular, smooth rhythm and symmetry in the length of leg swing; smooth swaying related to the gait phase; and a smooth, symmetrical arm swing (Ball et al., 2019). An abnormal gait is a common risk factor for patient falls.

Exercise Pattern. Exercise is physical activity for conditioning the body, improving health, and maintaining fitness. When a person exercises, beneficial physiological changes occur in numerous body systems. Assess a patient's exercise history by asking what exercise the patient normally engages in and the normal amount of exercise performed daily and weekly. If a patient does not exercise regularly, you will want to focus on assessing activity tolerance. Chapter 38 describes the approach for assessment of a patient's exercise patterns.

People who are depressed, worried, or anxious are frequently unable or unwilling to participate in exercise. Depression often causes patients to withdraw rather than participate. Patients who worry or are frequently anxious expend a tremendous amount of mental energy and often report feeling fatigued. Your assessment should be broad and relevant to the patient: "What type of exercise do you enjoy when you are active?" "Tell me what has led you to exercise less." "You have told me that you feel worried; does that affect your desire to be active?"

Body Alignment. The first step in assessing body alignment is to put patients at ease so that they do not assume unnatural or rigid positions. Observe the appearance and position of your patient's extremities and measure the ROM of your patient's joints during your assessment of body alignment. You will begin with the patient standing and then progress based on the patient's level of mobility. When assessing the body alignment of a patient with reduced mobility or a patient who is unconscious, remove pillows and positioning supports from the bed and place the patient in the supine position.

Standing. During assessment look for characteristics of correct body alignment for the standing patient:
1. The head is erect and midline.
2. When observed posteriorly, the shoulders and hips are straight and parallel.
3. When observed posteriorly, the vertebral column is straight.
4. When observed laterally, the head is erect, and the spinal curves are aligned in a reversed S pattern. The cervical vertebrae are anteriorly convex, the thoracic vertebrae are posteriorly convex, and the lumbar vertebrae are anteriorly convex.
5. When observed laterally, the abdomen is comfortably tucked in, and the knees and ankles are slightly flexed. The person appears comfortable and does not seem conscious of the flexion of knees or ankles.
6. The arms hang comfortably at the sides.
7. The feet are slightly apart to achieve a base of support, and the toes are pointed forward.
8. When viewing the patient from behind, the center of gravity is in the midline, and the line of gravity is from the middle of the forehead to a midpoint between the feet. Laterally the line of gravity runs vertically from the middle of the skull to the posterior third of the foot (Fig. 39.7).

Sitting. Assessment also includes characteristics of correct alignment of the sitting patient:
1. The head is erect, and the neck and vertebral column are in straight alignment.
2. The body weight is distributed evenly on the buttocks and thighs.
3. The thighs are parallel and in a horizontal plane.
4. Both feet are supported on the floor (Fig. 39.8), and the ankles are flexed comfortably. With patients of short stature, use a footstool to ensure that ankles are flexed comfortably.
5. A 2.5- to 5-cm (1- to 2-inch) space is maintained between the edge of the seat and the popliteal space on the posterior surface of the knee. This space ensures that there is no pressure on the popliteal artery or nerve to decrease circulation or impair nerve function.
6. The patient's forearms are supported on the armrest, in the lap, or on a table in front of the chair.

It is particularly important to assess alignment when sitting if the patient has muscle weakness, muscle paralysis, or nerve damage. Patients who have these problems have diminished sensation in the affected area and are unable to perceive pressure or decreased circulation. Proper alignment while sitting reduces the risk of musculoskeletal system damage in such a patient. The patient with severe respiratory disease who has orthopnea sometimes assumes a posture of leaning on the table in front of the chair in an attempt to breathe more easily.

Lying. People who are conscious have voluntary muscle control and normal perception of pressure. As a result, they usually assume a position of comfort when lying down. Because their ROM, sensation, and circulation are within normal limits, they change positions when they perceive muscle strain and decreased circulation.

Assess body alignment for a patient who is immobilized or bedridden with the patient in the lateral position (Fig. 39.9). Remove all positioning

FIG. 39.8 Correct body alignment when sitting.

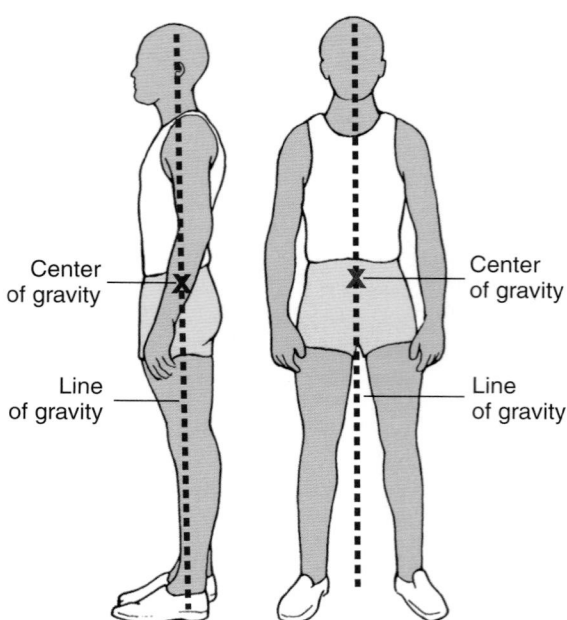

FIG. 39.7 Correct body alignment when standing.

Center of gravity

Center of gravity

Line of gravity

Line of gravity

FIG. 39.9 Correct body alignment when lying down.

supports from the bed except for the pillow under the head. This position allows for full view of the spine and back and helps provide other baseline body alignment data such as whether the patient is able to remain positioned without aid. The vertebrae should normally be aligned, and the position does not cause discomfort. Patients with impaired mobility (e.g., traction or arthritis), decreased sensation (e.g., sensory deficits caused by hemiparesis following a CVA), impaired circulation (e.g., peripheral vascular disease caused by diabetes), and lack of voluntary muscle control (e.g., spinal cord injury) are at risk for skin damage when lying down.

Joseph begins his assessment of Ms. Cavallo by examining her existing mobility and activity level while she is in bed. The patient weighs 77.2 kg (170 lb). She is 167.7 cm (5 feet 6 inches) tall. She shows good eye contact and is attentive to Joseph's questions. She tells Joseph that her favorite activity is gardening. She works on her flower beds by sitting on a stool. "I have trouble bending over very far. I hope this hip won't keep me from gardening when I get home. You know, my fall was in my garden." In addition, Joseph learns that Ms. Cavallo walks about a mile a day with a neighbor without feeling fatigued. Baseline heart rate is 84 beats/min; respirations, 18 breaths/min; and blood pressure, 142/90 mm Hg. She has full extension and flexion of the arms but moves her extremities slowly. Her hand grasps are 3 bilaterally with full ROM against gravity. Ms. Cavallo is able to bend the right knee, extend the right leg, and rotate the right ankle with normal ROM. She can wiggle the toes of her left foot and rotate the foot slowly. She can flex the left hip forward independently only 10 degrees off of the bed surface. Flexion in the knee is only 20 to 30 degrees. Movement of the left leg causes discomfort. Pain with flexion of the knee is 6 on a scale of 0 to 10 at this time. Joseph gets assistance from an assistive personnel and finds that the patient can assist in turning on her side. He notices an area of normal, blanchable erythema over her sacral area and heels. She has no signs of skin breakdown overlying pressure points.

Immobility. A patient who presents with impaired mobility requires you to assess for actual and potential physiological impairments associated with immobility while performing a head-to-toe physical assessment (Table 39.4) (see Chapter 30). As you conduct your assessment consider your knowledge of how immobility affects physiological functioning, specifically in relationship to the patient's health problems. This information will allow you to recognize risks for complications. Be sure your assessment also focuses on the patient's psychosocial and developmental dimensions.

Metabolic System. Measures of height and weight are important when assessing metabolic functioning. Also examine the turgor of the skin. Dehydration and edema increase the rate of skin breakdown in a patient who is immobilized. Review intake and output records for fluid balance. Does intake equal output? Intake and output measurements help to determine whether a fluid imbalance exists (see Chapter 42). Monitoring laboratory data such as levels of electrolytes, serum protein (albumin and total protein), and blood urea nitrogen (BUN) also helps you to determine metabolic functioning.

Monitoring food intake and elimination patterns and assessing wound healing help to determine altered GI functioning and potential metabolic problems. If the patient has a wound, the rate of healing is affected by nutritional intake and nutrient absorption. Chapter 48 describes wound assessment. Normal progression of healing indicates that metabolic needs of injured tissues are being met. Anorexia commonly occurs in patients who are immobilized. Assess the patient's food intake before removing a meal tray to determine the amount of food the patient ate. Assess dietary patterns and food preferences at the onset of immobilization to help prevent nutritional imbalances (see Chapter 45).

Respiratory System. Perform a respiratory assessment at least every 2 hours for patients with restricted activity. Inspect chest wall movements during the full inspiratory-expiratory cycle. If a patient has an atelectatic area, chest movement is often asymmetrical. Auscultate the entire lung region to identify diminished breath sounds, crackles, or wheezes (see Chapter 30). Focus auscultation on the dependent lung fields because pulmonary secretions tend to collect in these lower regions. Assessment findings that indicate pneumonia include productive cough with greenish yellow sputum; fever; pain on breathing; and crackles, wheezes, and dyspnea.

Cardiovascular System. Cardiovascular nursing assessment of a patient who is immobilized includes monitoring blood pressure and heart rate and assessing the arteriovenous system. Because of the risk for orthostatic hypotension, measure blood pressure when a patient moves from lying to a sitting or standing position. Move patients gradually during position changes and monitor them closely for dizziness while assessing blood pressure in each position. These measurements document the patient's tolerance to postural changes and are vital to know when positioning or transferring patients from one position or location to another. The longer the period of immobility,

TABLE 39.4	**Assessment of the Physiological Hazards of Immobility**	
System	**Assessment Techniques**	**Abnormal Findings**
Metabolic	Inspection	Slowed wound healing, abnormal laboratory data
	Inspection	Muscle atrophy
	Palpation	Generalized edema
Respiratory	Inspection	Asymmetrical chest wall movement, dyspnea, increased respiratory rate
	Auscultation	Crackles, wheezes
Cardiovascular	Auscultation	Orthostatic hypotension
	Auscultation, palpation	Increased heart rate, third heart sound, weak peripheral pulses, peripheral edema
Musculoskeletal	Inspection	Decreased range of motion, erythema, increased diameter in calf or thigh
	Palpation	Joint contracture, reduced muscle strength
	Inspection	Activity intolerance, muscle atrophy, joint contracture
Skin	Inspection, palpation	Break in skin integrity, bogginess of tissue, inflammation of skin
Elimination	Inspection	Decreased urine output, cloudy or concentrated urine, decreased frequency of bowel movements
	Palpation	Distended bladder and abdomen
	Auscultation	Decreased bowel sounds

the greater is the risk of orthostatic hypotension when the patient stands (McCance and Huether, 2019).

Assess heart rate, including the apical pulse. Lying down increases cardiac workload and results in an increased pulse rate. In older adults, the heart rate often does not tolerate the added workload, and a form of heart failure may develop. A third heart sound, heard at the apex of the heart, is an early indication of heart failure.

Monitoring peripheral pulses (see Chapter 30) allows you to assess the ability of the heart to pump blood and the condition of the arterial system. Immediately document and report the absence of a peripheral pulse in the lower extremities, especially if the pulse was present previously. Check for capillary refill to determine tissue perfusion. Also note the color of extremities, as changes in venous and arterial function will alter skin color.

Edema sometimes develops in patients who have had tissue injury or whose heart is unable to handle the increased workload of bed rest. Because edema moves to dependent body regions, assessment of the patient experiencing immobility includes inspection of the sacrum, legs, and feet for edema. If the heart is unable to tolerate the increased workload, peripheral body regions such as the hands, feet, nose, and earlobes are colder than central body regions.

Venous thromboembolism (VTE) is a blood clot in a vein and is the third leading vascular diagnosis after heart attack and stroke, affecting between 300,000 and 600,000 Americans each year (American Heart Association [AHA], 2017a). There are two types: DVT (a clot in a deep vein that usually involves the leg or pelvis but can also occur in the arms) and pulmonary embolus (PE; a deep vein clot that breaks free from a vein wall, travels to the lungs, and blocks some or all of the blood supply) (AHA, 2017a). VTE is a hazard of immobility.

Common risk factors for DVT include conditions that influence the Virchow triad: hypercoagulability (e.g., inherited clotting disorders, fever, dehydration); venous wall abnormalities (e.g., major general and orthopedic surgery, varicose veins); and blood flow stasis (e.g., immobility after serious injury, illness, or long-term travel; obesity; and pregnancy) (Cleveland Clinic, 2019; AHA, 2017b). More than 90% of all pulmonary emboli begin in the deep veins of the lower extremities as a DVT (McCance and Huether, 2019).

Signs of a DVT usually occur on one side of the body at a time, including swelling in the affected leg or arm; warm, cyanotic skin; and pain or tenderness in the affected extremity. A patient may complain of cramping or soreness. If a DVT is suspected, keep the patient calm and quiet in bed and notify the health care provider.

Always consider a patient's risk factors for a DVT, especially when the patient is immobile (Box 39.4). The Wells score is an objective and widely used measure for determining a patient's risk for a DVT (Table 39.5) (Wells, 1998; Modi et al., 2016; Shen et al., 2016). Report clinical indicators of a possible DVT to a health care provider immediately and include the Wells score as appropriate. If a patient has antiembolic stockings or a sequential compression device (SCD) or mobile compression device (MCD), remove the stockings or device once every 8 hours or according to agency policy and reassess the calves and thighs.

Measure bilateral calf circumference and record it daily as an alternative assessment for DVT. To do this, mark a point on each calf 10 cm down from the midpatella. Measure the circumference each day, using this mark for placement of the tape measure. Unilateral increases in calf circumference are an early indication of thrombosis (Harding et al., 2020). If a patient has a history of DVT, measure the thighs daily because the upper thigh is also a common site for clot formation. Many health care agencies now order Doppler ultrasound examinations to assess blood flow in arteries and veins to detect presence of clots. There is a high prevalence of asymptomatic DVTs, especially among older-adult patients.

BOX 39.4   Risk Factors for Developing Deep Vein Thrombosis (DVT)

- Major general surgery, major orthopedic surgery
- Fracture of pelvis, hips, or long bones
- Lower extremity paralysis from spinal cord injury
- Long periods of inactivity (bed rest, sitting, long car or airplane trips)
- Cancer (especially metastatic) and cancer therapy
- Past history of DVT
- Family history of venous thromboembolism (VTE)
- Increasing age
- Pregnancy and the 4–6 weeks after giving birth
- Certain illnesses, including heart failure, inflammatory bowel disease, and some kidney disorders
- Autoimmune disease, including systemic lupus erythematosus
- Overweight and obesity
- Smoking
- Oral contraceptives or use of estrogen for menopause
- Having a tube in a main vein (sometimes needed to give medications over a period of time)
- Having thrombophilia, one of several diseases in which the blood does not clot correctly

From American Heart Association (AHA): *Risk factors for venous thromboembolism (VTE)*, 2017a. https://www.heart.org/en/health-topics/venous-thromboembolism/risk-factors-for-venous-thromboembolism-vte. Accessed August 7, 2021; and Bauer KA, Huisman MV: *Clinical presentation and diagnosis of the nonpregnant adult with suspected deep vein thrombosis of the lower extremity, UpToDate,* 2021. https://www.uptodate.com/contents/clinical-presentation-and-diagnosis-of-the-nonpregnant-adult-with-suspected-deep-vein-thrombosis-of-the-lower-extremity. Accessed August 7, 2021.

TABLE 39.5   Wells Score for the Prediction of Deep Vein Thrombosis (DVT)

Parameter	Score
Active cancer (patient receiving treatment for cancer within previous 6 months or currently receiving palliative treatment)	1
Paralysis, paresis, or recent plaster immobilization of lower extremities	1
Recently bedridden for 3 days or more, or major surgery within previous 12 weeks requiring general or regional anesthesia	1
Localized tenderness along distribution of the deep vein system	1
Entire leg swollen	1
Calf swelling at least 3 cm more when compared with asymptomatic leg	1
Pitting edema localized to symptomatic leg	1
Collateral superficial veins	1
Previously documented DVT	1
Alternative diagnosis as likely as or greater than that of DVT	−2

Wells scoring system for DVT: −2 to 0: low probability; 1 to 2 points: moderate probability; 3 to 8 points: high probability.
From Wells PS et al.: Use of a clinical model for safe management of patients with suspected pulmonary embolism. *Ann Intern Med* 129:997, 1998. doi: 10.7326/0003-4819-129-12-199812150-00002; and Modi S, et al: Wells criteria for DVT is a reliable clinical tool to assess the risk of deep venous thrombosis in trauma patients. *World J Emerg Surg* 11:24, 2016. Published online 2016 Jun 8. https://www.ncbi.nlm.nih.gov/pmc/articles/PMC4898382/. Accessed May 12, 2020.

Musculoskeletal System. Major musculoskeletal abnormalities to identify during nursing assessment include decreased muscle tone and strength, loss of muscle mass, reduced ROM, and contractures. During assessment of ROM (described earlier) you can detect muscle tone by asking the patient to relax and then passively moving each limb at several joints to get a feeling for any resistance or rigidity that may be present. You assess for muscle strength by having the patient assume a stable position and then performing maneuvers to demonstrate strength of the major muscle groups (see Chapter 30).

Physical assessment cannot identify disuse osteoporosis. However, patients on prolonged bed rest, women who are postmenopausal, patients taking steroids, and people with increased serum and urine calcium levels have a greater risk for bone demineralization. Consider the risk of disuse osteoporosis when planning nursing interventions. Although some falls result in injury, others occur because of pathological fractures secondary to osteoporosis.

Integumentary System. Continually assess a patient's skin for breakdown and color changes such as pallor or redness, especially in patients who are immobile. Assess skin integrity during any routine patient contact. Consistently use a standardized assessment tool such as the Braden Scale for a baseline measure and then at least daily. The screening tool identifies patients with a high risk for impaired skin integrity or early changes in the condition of patients' skin. Early identification allows for early intervention. When assessing the skin during routine care (e.g., when the patient is turned, during hygiene measures, and when providing for elimination needs) be sure to inspect pressure points after the patient has been lying in one position. Frequent skin assessment, which can be performed as often as every hour and is based on patients' mobility, hydration, and physiological status, is essential to promptly identify changes in the skin and underlying tissues (see Chapter 48).

Elimination System. To determine the effects of immobility on elimination, assess the patient's normal 24-hour intake and output and then compare and monitor total intake and output each shift and every 24 hours. Compare the amounts over time. Determine if the patient is receiving the correct amount and type of fluids orally or parenterally (see Chapter 42). Inadequate intake and output or fluid and electrolyte imbalances increase the risk for renal system impairment, ranging from recurrent infections to kidney failure. Dehydration also increases the risk for constipation.

Immobility impairs GI peristalsis. Assessment of bowel elimination status includes the adequacy of a patient's dietary choices, bowel sounds, passing of flatus, and the frequency and consistency of bowel movements (see Chapter 47). Accurate assessment enables you to intervene before constipation and fecal impaction occur.

Psychosocial Assessment. Because altered mobility can lead to numerous physical complications, some life threatening, it may be difficult for nurses to have the time to complete accurate and thorough assessments of patients' psychosocial responses to being less mobile. However, discipline is an intellectual standard to apply when assessing the psychosocial status of a patient who is immobile. The impact that mobility alterations have on a patient's emotional, social, and economic health is significant.

The ability to be mobile and remain active affects how energetic individuals feel (National Institutes of Health [NIH], 2019). Research shows that mood alterations can influence a person's desire to be physically active, but recent research has shown that physical inactivity may lead to a depressed mood and mood changes (NIH, 2019). Patients who are confined to bed rest often experience a reduction in environmental and psychosocial stimuli because of limited opportunities for interactions outside of their immediate environment (Knight et al., 2018). This restriction is often called sensory deprivation. Restricted mobility in time may lead to restlessness, increased aggression, and insomnia

(Knight et al., 2018). There is also an uncertainty and unpredictability when a person's illness or injury has caused significant reduction in physical activity. This uncertainty and unpredictability may lead to anxiety or hopelessness. As part of your assessment, use a patient-administered screening tool for depression. There has been an increased availability of quick and reliable screening tools for depression (Bienenfeld, 2018). Patients who screen positive for depression must have a follow-up clinical interview by a licensed psychologist or psychiatrist to make the diagnosis of clinical depression.

Psychosocial responses to immobilization can be less serious than depression but still significantly affect a patient's motivation and willingness to participate in recovery from immobilization. Common reactions to immobilization include boredom, anxiety, and feelings of isolation and anger. These patients often experience an intolerance to exercise and thus a potential barrier to recovery. Ask patients to describe how their loss in mobility affects how they feel about themselves. "How does this loss of function in your _____ affect the sense of who you are?" Your acknowledgment of the fact that there are normal emotional reactions to losing mobility may help patients be willing to share their thoughts and feelings.

During your assessment be observant for changes in a patient's emotional responses during interactions and listen carefully to family if they report emotional changes. Examples of behavior change that indicate psychosocial concerns are a patient who suddenly becomes less cooperative or a patient who begins asking for more help than is necessary. Investigate reasons for such alterations. Identifying how a patient usually copes with loss is vital (see Chapters 36 and 37). A change in mobility status, whether permanent or not, causes a grief reaction. Families are a key resource for information about behavioral changes. Because psychosocial changes usually occur gradually, observe the patient's behavior on a daily basis.

Abrupt changes in personality often have a physiological cause such as surgery, a medication reaction, a PE, or an acute infection. For example, the primary symptom of a UTI or fever in older patients is confusion. Identifying confusion is an important component of a nurse's assessment. Acute confusion, or delirium, is a neuropsychiatric syndrome with alterations in arousal, attention, and cognition (American Psychiatric Association [APA], 2013; Francis and Young, 2020). Delirium can be triggered by a wide variety of medical or surgical conditions (Mulkey et al., 2018). Delirium in older adults is not normal, especially after surgery or procedures (see Chapter 50). A thorough nursing assessment is the priority (Chase et al., 2018).

A final element in a psychosocial assessment is determining the social resources available to a patient. Does the patient have visitors while in a health care setting to provide stimulation and reinforcement for recovery? Does the patient live alone at home? Is there a primary family caregiver, and, if so, how does that person provide the patient assistance?

Developmental Assessment. Include a developmental assessment of patients who are immobilized. When caring for a young child, determine whether the child is able to meet developmental tasks and is progressing normally (see Chapter 12). The child's development sometimes regresses or slows because of the immobilization.

Immobilization of a family member changes family functioning. The family's response to this change often leads to relationship problems, stress, and anxieties. When children see parents who are immobile, they sometimes have difficulty understanding and coping with what is occurring. Assess the family's perceptions as to how roles have changed and how they are coping.

Immobility has a significant effect on an older adult's levels of health, independence, and functional status. Focus your assessment on the patient's ability to meet needs independently and to adapt to developmental changes such as declining physical functioning and altered family and peer relationships. A decline in developmental functioning prompts investigation to determine why the change occurred and identification of interventions that can return the patient to an optimal level of functioning as soon as possible. Activities that reduce immobility and promote participation in ADLs are vital to preventing functional decline (Hallford et al., 2017; Musich et al., 2018).

Environmental Factors. A patient's environment in the home or health care setting influences the patient's level of mobility. Assess if there are any barriers to how a patient can remain mobile. For example, in the health care setting is there a clear pathway free of equipment obstacles when you prepare to assist a patient with ambulation. In the home, patients with impaired mobility due to long-term injuries or chronic conditions also need a free path to ambulate and to be able to rise from bed and reach a bathroom. Patients restricted to a wheelchair benefit if they can easily exit their home and then be able to exercise down a driveway or safe street. Chapter 38 details environmental factors to consider for patients living in their communities.

Time and patient assignment load are always issues that nurses who work in acute care and long-term care settings will face. A patient who has limited mobility may have limited acute physical needs, but it is important to not ignore or delay assisting patients with maintaining their movement. Use the time you have at a bedside to encourage ROM as much and as often as possible.

Treatments. Include in your assessment the anticipated effects of treatments for immobility that a patient is currently receiving. For example, if a patient with a leg fracture is going to have an immobilization device or a cast, obtain knowledge about how the treatments work therapeutically and the extent of their impact on mobility. A device applied to an extremity introduces a factor that can cause pressure and friction on the skin, adding to the risk of skin breakdown.

In home health and long-term care settings it is important to assess the extent to which mobility alterations affect patients' ability to self-medicate. Many medications are dispensed in packages or in containers that are difficult to access by individuals with disabilities or impaired mobility of the hands. Other medication administration tasks such as activating an inhaler, applying eyedrops, or administering an injection can be major obstacles to medication adherence. Observe patients preparing medication doses to assess if mobility limitations exist.

Comfort. Chapter 44 provides detail on how to conduct a pain assessment. Patients immobilized or experiencing reduced mobility frequently have discomfort from trauma (physical or surgical), inflammation of muscles and joints, and pulled muscles. Assessing a baseline pain level is important for you to use as a standard in later determining if pain relief measures successfully manage pain. If you cannot manage a patient's pain, it can become difficult to perform many of the procedures the patient requires.

Joseph examines Ms. Cavallo's surgical incision. The incision remains closed with no signs of inflammation. Joseph palpates over the incision; Ms. Cavallo acknowledges tenderness. When Ms. Cavallo lies still, pain from the incision is rated a 3 on a scale of 0 to 10. When Joseph helps Ms. Cavallo lift her left leg, pain over the incisional area is a 6. Joseph knows from previous experience that Ms. Cavallo's rehab plan will involve progressive activities aimed at getting her up in a chair and ambulating before discharge. Ms. Cavallo tells Joseph that she got up in the chair a couple of times in the hospital. He has the assistive personnel help him sit Ms. Cavallo up on the side of the bed to assess her tolerance. The patient helps with turning, and an increase in pain is noticeable as the patient rises to a sitting position. Ms. Cavallo reacts: "Oh, oh! It really hurts!" She grimaces and places her hand over her upper leg. Ms. Cavallo's heart rate increases to 96 beats/min, her blood pressure is 136/84 mm Hg, and her respirations are 20 breaths/min. The nursing team returns Ms. Cavallo to bed. Joseph decides to consult with the health care provider regarding the type of analgesic Ms. Cavallo can receive and how to time a dose before the team gets her up and into a chair this afternoon.

QSEN **Building Competency in Quality Improvement** Ms. Cavallo is a patient on a skilled care unit that is implementing a quality improvement (QI) project on fall prevention. The number of falls on the unit has increased over the past several months. A review of the literature notes that patients who sustained falls in long-term care have common risk factors or characteristics. The nursing team on the unit reviews which of these commonalities are related to alterations in mobility. As a part of the team, you recognize the need to develop a collaborative plan of care that includes all health care professionals who work on the unit, the patients, and their families. How can you best communicate your findings and strategies for fall prevention to all health care providers and family members participating in Ms. Cavallo's care? How do you identify gaps between the unit and best practices? How do you evaluate whether change has taken place?

Answers to QSEN Activities can be found on the Evolve website.

REFLECT NOW

Mr. Brown, a 50-year-old man, is 1 day postop after left shoulder surgery to repair a rotator cuff injury sustained in a fall from a roof. He also has a fractured right tibia and mild concussion. As a nursing student, you know that assessment of mobility focuses on ROM, gait, exercise and activity tolerance, and body alignment. Given the multiple body parts injured in Mr. Brown's fall, reflect on what limitations and physical findings you might encounter. What questions can you ask to gain deeper understanding of what these injuries mean to Mr. Brown?

◆ Analysis and Nursing Diagnosis

Critical analysis of all assessment data, comparing findings with the anticipated effects of mobility alterations, reveals patterns of data indicating nursing diagnoses. There are two diagnoses most directly related to mobility problems: *Impaired Mobility* and *Risk for Disuse Syndrome*. The diagnosis of *Impaired Mobility* applies to a patient who has some limitation but is not completely immobile. The diagnosis of *Risk for Disuse Syndrome* applies to the patient who is immobile and at risk for multisystem problems because of inactivity. There are numerous nursing diagnoses that might apply to patients with mobility limitations because immobility affects multiple body systems. Possible nursing diagnoses include the following:

- Impaired Airway Clearance
- Risk for Impaired Gastrointestinal System Function
- Risk for Constipation
- Social Isolation

Assessment reveals clusters of data that indicate whether a patient is at risk or if a negative or problem-focused diagnosis exists (Box 39.5). The clusters of data reveal at-risk factors or assessment findings that are observable assessment cues to support a diagnostic label. In the case of a negative or problem-focused diagnosis, the assessment data will also reveal a related factor for the diagnosis. Accuracy in selecting related factors or risk factors is important because you will apply clinical judgment in choosing interventions that treat or modify the related factor or risk factors. For example, *Impaired Mobility related to reluctance to initiate movement* requires different interventions than does *Impaired Mobility related to pain in the left shoulder*. The diagnosis that is related to reluctance to initiate movement requires interventions aimed at keeping the patient as mobile as possible and encouraging the patient to perform self-care and ROM. The diagnosis related to pain requires you to assist the patient with pharmacological and nonpharmacological comfort measures (see Chapter 44) so that the patient is then willing and more able to move. In both situations you explain how activity enhances healthy body functioning.

Often the physiological dimension is the major focus of nursing care for patients with impaired mobility. Thus the psychosocial and developmental dimensions are neglected. Yet all dimensions are important to health. During immobilization, some patients experience decreased social interaction and stimuli. These patients frequently use the nurse's call bell to request minor physical attention when their real need is greater socialization. Nursing diagnoses for health needs in developmental areas

BOX 39.5   Nursing Diagnostic Process

Impaired Mobility Related to Left Hip/Leg Pain

Assessment Activities	Assessment Findings
Measure range of motion (ROM) during extension and flexion of the hip.	Patient has limited ROM in left hip or leg.
Observe patient's attempt to move her left leg.	Patient requires support from nurse (support under thigh) to lift her left leg off mattress.
Measure patient's perception of pain.	Patient identifies sharp pain (7 on scale of 0 to 10) in hip and leg when she tries to move them.
Ask patient about endurance and activity tolerance.	Patient reports no muscle strength in left leg. "I really have trouble moving it by myself."

reflect changes from the patient's normal activities. Immobility leads to a developmental crisis if the patient is unable to resolve problems and continue to mature.

Immobility also leads to multiple complications (e.g., renal calculi, DVT, pulmonary emboli, or pneumonia). If these conditions develop, collaborate with the health care provider or nurse practitioner for prescribed therapy to intervene. Be alert for and prevent these potential complications when possible.

*Joseph analyzes data collected on Ms. Cavallo. Findings of left hip pain, tenderness on palpation of incision, restriction of leg movement, and facial grimacing are cues identifying **Acute Pain**. The patient cannot lift her left leg more than 10 degrees off the bed, flexion of the knee is at 20 degrees, there is pain in the left side of the leg, she requires assistance sitting on the side of the bed, and she has increased heart rate and respirations on exertion. These data indicate the nursing diagnosis **Impaired Mobility**. Ms. Cavallo's zimpaired mobility, effects of pain, and body weight also place her at **Risk for Impaired Skin Integrity**. Joseph also considers data regarding Ms. Cavallo's desire to return home, her ability to attend, and her past history of being active for her age. The diagnosis of **Ability to Mobilize** is possible and important for her recovery. He will assess further.*

◆ Planning and Outcomes Identification

During planning, critical thinking and sound clinical judgment will guide you to synthesize what you know about immobility and a patient's condition, the patient's nursing diagnoses, the resources available, environmental conditions, your past clinical experiences, and clinical standards to develop a plan of care (Fig. 39.10). Involving a patient in clinical decisions about your approach to restoring mobility is essential to obtain patient

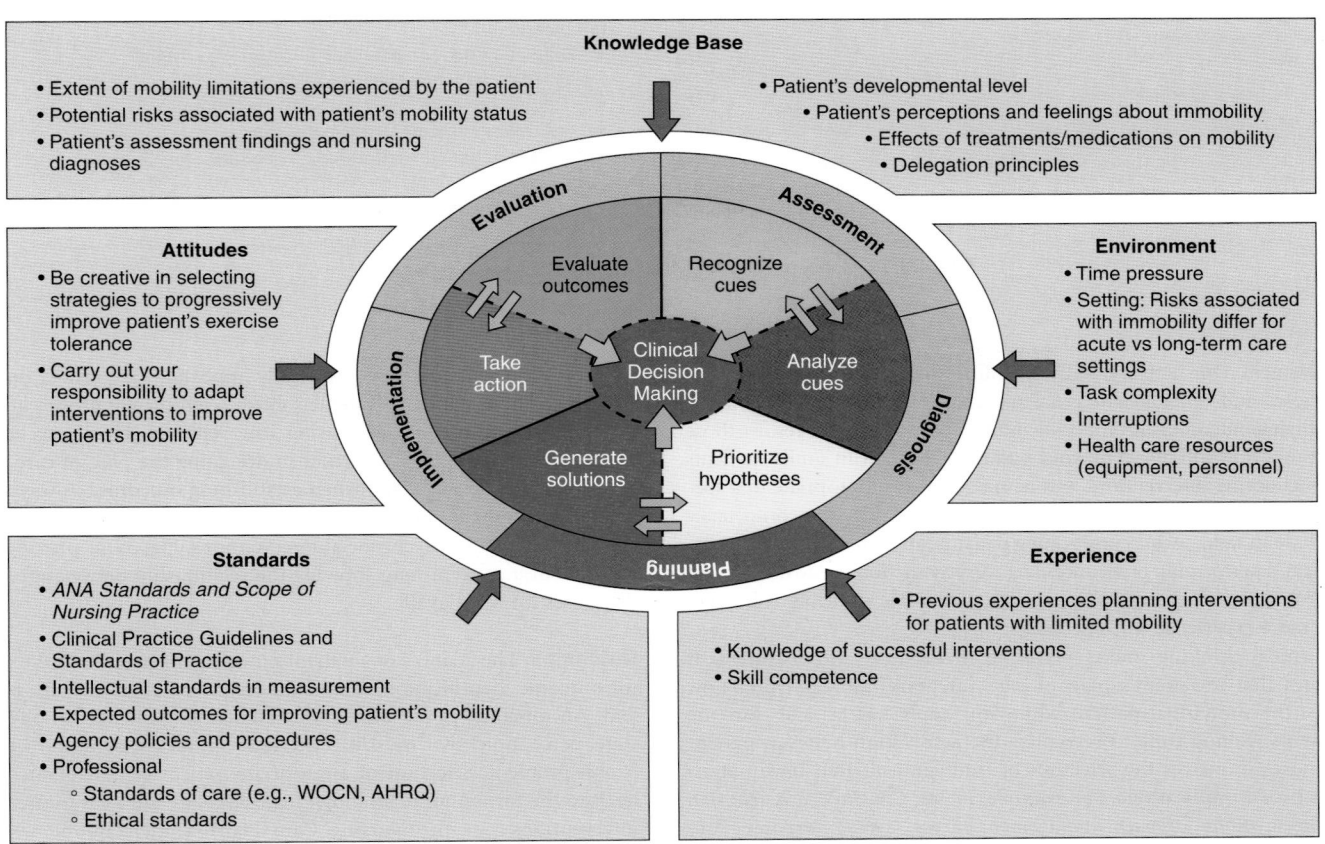

FIG. 39.10 Critical thinking model for planning for impaired mobility. *AHRQ,* Agency for Healthcare Research and Quality; *ANA,* American Nurses Association; *WOCN,* Wound, Ostomy, and Continence Nurses Society. (Clinical Judgment Measurement Model copyright © NCSBN. All rights reserved.)

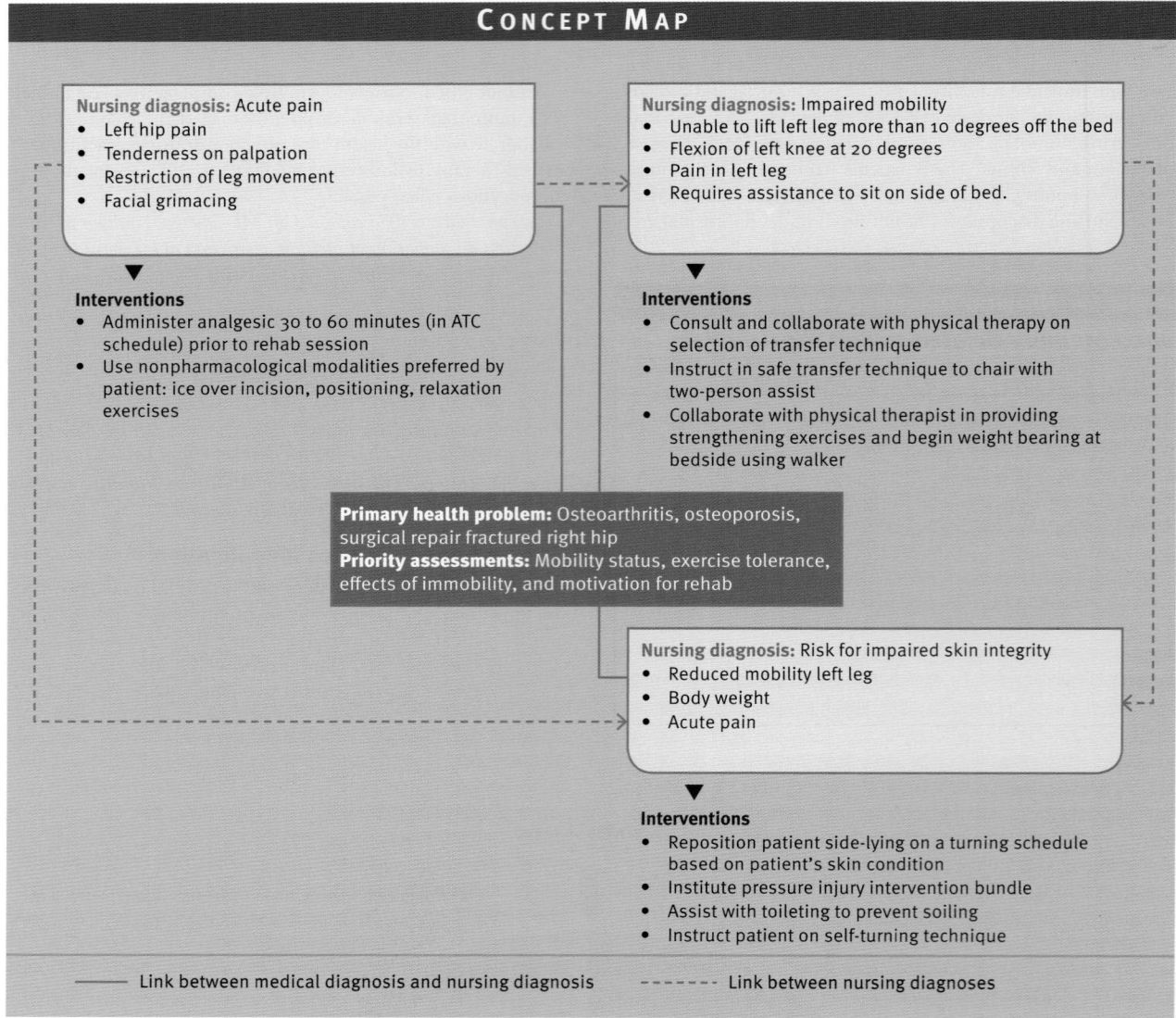

CONCEPT MAP

Nursing diagnosis: Acute pain
- Left hip pain
- Tenderness on palpation
- Restriction of leg movement
- Facial grimacing

Interventions
- Administer analgesic 30 to 60 minutes (in ATC schedule) prior to rehab session
- Use nonpharmacological modalities preferred by patient: ice over incision, positioning, relaxation exercises

Nursing diagnosis: Impaired mobility
- Unable to lift left leg more than 10 degrees off the bed
- Flexion of left knee at 20 degrees
- Pain in left leg
- Requires assistance to sit on side of bed.

Interventions
- Consult and collaborate with physical therapy on selection of transfer technique
- Instruct in safe transfer technique to chair with two-person assist
- Collaborate with physical therapist in providing strengthening exercises and begin weight bearing at bedside using walker

Primary health problem: Osteoarthritis, osteoporosis, surgical repair fractured right hip
Priority assessments: Mobility status, exercise tolerance, effects of immobility, and motivation for rehab

Nursing diagnosis: Risk for impaired skin integrity
- Reduced mobility left leg
- Body weight
- Acute pain

Interventions
- Reposition patient side-lying on a turning schedule based on patient's skin condition
- Institute pressure injury intervention bundle
- Assist with toileting to prevent soiling
- Instruct patient on self-turning technique

——— Link between medical diagnosis and nursing diagnosis   - - - - - Link between nursing diagnoses

FIG. 39.11 Concept map for Mrs. Cavallo. *ATC*, Around-the-clock.

involvement. During planning you confirm the priority level of nursing diagnoses and other health problems and then generate solutions by identifying outcomes and choosing interventions to meet or resolve those outcomes. You will reflect on your past experiences with similar patients when choosing interventions, but be sure they are appropriate to a specific patient. Also, as you plan interventions, consider the competency you have in tasks such as positioning patients, applying compression devices, and performing procedures (e.g., airway suctioning, advanced skin care) to minimize immobility complications. Use available colleagues with more experience when necessary.

Critical thinking makes planning methodical and reasoned. It ensures that a patient's plan of care integrates all that you know about the individual patient while you apply key critical thinking elements. Taking time to recognize the association between patient diagnoses improves the selection of interventions that have potentially broad implications. *For example, in Ms. Cavallo's case, selection of interventions for pain management serves several purposes. Pain management will reduce acute pain, improve the patient's mobility and, as a result, lessen the risk of impaired skin integrity.*

Professional standards are especially important to consider during planning. These standards often establish scientifically proven guidelines for selecting effective nursing interventions. Finally, as stated earlier, the patient is a full partner in designing the plan of care, and this input must be reflected when establishing outcomes. Always stay mindful of how the experience of immobility is affecting a patient, to ensure inclusion of psychosocial interventions. Fig. 39.11 provides an example of a concept map showing the relationship between nursing diagnoses for Ms. Cavallo.

Outcomes. The analysis of a patient's nursing diagnoses sets the stage for outcome identification. A nursing diagnosis labels a health problem. An outcome is the measurable change (e.g., behavior, physical state, perception) that must be achieved to improve or minimize the health problem. Selection of appropriate patient-centered outcomes leads to the formation of an individualized plan with relevant nursing interventions (see the Nursing Care Plan). Understanding what a patient can physically do compared with what the patient potentially and realistically can achieve helps you set realistic outcomes. *In the case*

⊚ NURSING CARE PLAN

Impaired Mobility

ASSESSMENT

Assessment Activities	*Assessment Findings*[a]
Ask Ms. Cavallo to rate her pain on a scale of 0 to 10.	Rates pain as a 3 on a scale of 0 to 10 at rest; **increases to 7** with movement of her left leg.
Assess Ms. Cavallo's ability to transfer.	She is able to assist with turning, requires assistance to sit on side of bed.
Assess range of motion (ROM) of lower extremities.	Can flex the left hip forward independently only 10 degrees off of bed surface. Flexion in the knee is 20 to 30 degrees.

[a] Assessment findings are shown in bold type.

NURSING DIAGNOSIS: Impaired mobility related to musculoskeletal impairment from surgery and pain with movement

PLANNING

Expected Outcomes[b]

Pain Control

Ms. Cavallo's pain is less than 6 when moving left leg in 24 hours.
Body repositioning will be self-initiated in 72 hours.

Transfer

Ms. Cavallo is able to move from her bed to her chair and back again using a walker and two-person assist within 4 days.
Ms. Cavallo is able to transfer from her chair to her bedside commode using her walker within 4 days.

[b] Nursing outcomes classification from Moorhead S, et al., editors: *Nursing Outcomes Classification (NOC),* ed 6, St Louis, 2018, Elsevier.

INTERVENTIONS[c]

Exercise Therapy: Transfer

INTERVENTIONS	RATIONALE
Consult and team with physical therapist on selection of transfer technique.	Ensures safe transfer technique with less risk of patient injury.
Instruct Ms. Cavallo on safe transfer technique to chair in an environment with few distractions. Provide written materials and the use of the teach-back method to reinforce verbal instructions.	Providing instruction in a quiet environment and using the teach-back method enhance learning (Bodenheimer, 2018; Centrella-Nigro and Alexander, 2017).
Collaborate with physical therapist in teaching Ms. Cavallo turning techniques for repositioning and providing strengthening exercises. Begin weight bearing at bedside using walker. Establish realistic increments for activity.	Physiotherapy exercises, physical activity, and setting realistic outcomes for ambulation encourage activity in older adults (Kruschke and Butcher, 2017; Musich et al., 2018).

Pain Management

Administer analgesic on an around-the-clock schedule that includes doses before each planned activity or rehabilitation center visit. Consult with health care provider for order to adjust dose if patient exhibits signs of pain or states pain is not relieved with current regimen.	Obtain analgesic order to adjust (increase or decrease dose) based on a patient's report of pain severity or her ability to perform activities of daily living (ADLs) (Bonkowski et al., 2018).
Introduce nonpharmacological modalities preferred by patient such as ice over incision, positioning, and relaxation exercises to complement pharmacological pain management.	The Joint Commission (TJC) revised its pain mandate to include required addition of evidence-based nonpharmacological therapies for pain as a scorable element of a health care agency's performance (TJC, 2018). Evidence-based nonpharmacological therapies are safe and effective components in postsurgical pain management and have potential to decrease the use of opioids and the related risk for misuse (Tick et al., 2018).

[c] Intervention classification labels from Butcher HK, et al.: *Nursing Interventions Classification (NIC),* ed 7, St Louis, 2018, Elsevier.

EVALUATION

Evaluation Activities	*Patient Response*
Ask Ms. Cavallo to rate her level of pain when moving left leg.	Patient reports pain at 5 when lifting leg, pain at 4 when bending knee.
Observe Ms. Cavallo's ability to turn and reposition in bed.	Patient needs limited assistance to turn onto right side, requires help lifting left leg. Is able to turn halfway onto right side independently.
Observe Ms. Cavallo transfer to chair with two assistive personnel in attendance.	Patient is able to sit on side of bed, requires assistance to stand, able to use walker with assistance to reach edge of chair and sit.
Observe Ms. Cavallo transfer to bedside commode.	Patient requires assistance to reach commode and sit.

of Ms. Cavallo, the patient was mobile prior to her fall and surgery. She was active. At this time, her hip is healing well. Setting outcomes for ultimately being able to ambulate safely by discharge from rehabilitation is realistic. Therefore Joseph establishes outcomes for progressive repositioning (assist to self-turning) and transfer and weight bearing to a chair. He wants to increase frequency of time in the chair, building on what Ms. Cavallo did in the hospital.

Outcomes must be individualized and measurable. Develop outcomes to help patients achieve their highest level of health and mobility as possible and reduce the hazards of immobility. When setting outcomes, include the patient and a family caregiver when possible. The care plan for Ms. Cavallo (see Nursing Care Plan) contains outcomes that reflect measurable improvement in pain, transfer ability, and ambulation. Each outcome has measures easily gathered and relevant to the patient's potential for progress. If you set outcomes for changes in a patient's psychosocial adjustment to being immobile, write clear behavioral responses that can be observed. For example, the outcomes "Patient reports use of support from caregiver for hygiene needs in 3 days" and "Patient discusses outcomes for recovery in 2 days" are suitable for patients who have a diagnosis of *Hopelessness* because of their loss of independence.

Setting Priorities. The effect that problems have on a patient's mental and physical health determines the immediacy of any problems. Set priorities when planning care to ensure that immediate needs are met first. As a patient's condition changes you will reorder the priorities of your diagnoses as well as the interventions you select. This is particularly important when patients have multiple diagnoses. Plan therapies according to severity of risks to the patient, and individualize the plan according to the patient's developmental stage, level of health, and lifestyle.

When setting priorities with patients who are immobilized, it is especially important to make sure that you do not overlook potential complications. Many times, actual problems such as pressure injuries and disuse syndrome are addressed only after they develop. Therefore monitor the patient often, aggressively use prevention techniques, and supervise AP in carrying out activities aimed at preventing complications of impaired mobility.

Teamwork and Collaboration. Care of the patient experiencing alterations in mobility requires a team approach. Nurses often delegate select interventions that are appropriate for AP to perform. For example, in the case of patients who are at risk for respiratory problems from temporary immobility following surgery, AP can encourage the patient to do leg exercises, use the incentive spirometer, and cough and deep breathe (see Chapter 50). When patients have limited mobility as a result of paralysis, AP can turn and position patients and apply elastic stockings. They can also help the nurse measure leg circumferences and height and weight.

Collaborate with other health care team members such as physical or occupational therapists when it is essential to consider mobility needs. Understanding the need for and having open communications with members of the interprofessional care team result in better patient outcomes and hopefully prevent the hazards of immobility. It is through these collaborative efforts and teamwork that patients benefit most. For example, physical therapists are a resource for planning ROM or strengthening exercises, and occupational therapists are a resource for planning new or altered ways to perform ADLs that patients need to learn. Wound care specialists and respiratory therapists are often involved in patient care, especially with patients who are experiencing complications related to their immobility. Consult a registered dietitian when the patient is experiencing nutritional problems; refer the patient to a mental health advanced practice nurse, licensed social worker, or psychologist to assist with coping or other psychosocial issues.

Discharge planning begins when a patient enters the health care system. In anticipation of the patient's discharge from an institution, make appropriate referrals or consult a case manager or a discharge planner to ensure that the patient's needs are met at home. Consider the patient's home environment when planning therapies to maintain or improve body alignment and mobility. Referrals to home care or outpatient therapy are often needed if a patient continues to have mobility limitations when discharged.

◆ Implementation

Health Promotion. Health promotion activities include a variety of interventions such as education, prevention, and early detection to prevent alterations in mobility. These activities apply to health care workers and patients. Examples of health promotion activities that address mobility and immobility include prevention of work-related injury, fall prevention measures, regular daily exercise, and early detection of scoliosis.

Prevention of Health Care Worker Work-Related Musculoskeletal Injuries. The rate of work-related injuries in health care settings has increased in recent years. Nurses stand and move throughout the day, have regular contact with patients, and often are involved in lifting patients. As a result, overexertion and bodily reaction are the most prevalent events leading to occupational injuries and illnesses to registered nurses (RNs), accounting for 45.6% of all cases within the occupation in 2016 (U.S. Bureau of Labor Statistics, 2018) The causes of these events are excessive physical effort, bending, twisting, lifting, and repetitive motion. Back injuries are often the direct result of improper lifting and bending. The most common back injury is strain on the lumbar muscle group, which includes the muscles around the lumbar vertebrae. Injury to these areas affects the ability to bend forward, backward, and from side to side and limits the ability to rotate the hips and lower back. Research has demonstrated that ergonomic programs including safe patient-handling policies in health care agencies are highly effective in reducing injuries to patients and health care workers, costs, and missed workdays (Klein et al., 2018; Noble and Sweeney, 2018; Teeple et al., 2017).

Because of nurses' risk for injury, be aware of agency policies and protocols that protect staff and patients from injury. When lifting, assess the weight of the patient you will lift and determine the assistance you will need. Current safe patient-handling algorithms support that using mechanical or other ergonomic assistive devices is the safest way to reposition and lift patients who are unable to do these activities themselves. Many agencies have developed special patient lift teams and have instituted a minimal lift policy (see Chapter 38).

Exercise. Although many diseases and physical problems cause or contribute to immobility, it is important to remember that exercise programs enhance feelings of well-being and improve endurance, strength, and health. If immobility is an acute event, a patient will be able to recover and return to regular exercise routines. Exercise reduces the risk or worsening of many health problems such as cardiovascular disease, diabetes, and osteoporosis. It is important to give patients options for how to stay active and how to change their behavior if exercise has not been their routine. As a nurse you can encourage all patients to find a type of exercise that meets their lifestyle and particular health-related needs once they recover. For example, a patient with severe arthritis of the knees might benefit from aquatic therapy (exercise in a pool) rather than walking. Encourage patients in the hospital to perform stretching, ROM exercises, and light walking within the limits of their condition (see Chapter 38). Take cultural preferences into consideration when helping patients design exercise plans (Box 39.6).

Bone Health in Patients With Osteoporosis. Patients at risk for or diagnosed with osteoporosis have special health promotion needs. Encourage patients at risk to be screened for osteoporosis regularly,

BOX 39.6 CULTURAL ASPECTS OF CARE

Cultural Influences on Mobility

Culture influences an individual's preferences for activity and exercise. Certain cultures discourage involvement in organized recreational physical activities such as basketball, running, and aerobics. In contrast, ethnic dancing is an effective activity that is acceptable in many cultures. Other cultures emphasize exercise in terms of activities of daily living, such as walking, gardening, and prayer or meditation. A sedentary lifestyle places an individual at risk for being overweight (see Chapter 38). Children from many cultures who live in the United States are becoming more sedentary. Therefore a national health approach is needed for communities to provide social and physical environments that promote healthy choices. Nurses need to include preventive health practices in patient education for patients of all ages.

Implications for Patient-Centered Care

- Assess patterns of daily living and culturally prescribed activities before suggesting specific forms of exercise to patients.
- Help patients plan physical activities that are culturally acceptable.
- Create exercise programs that are flexible and accommodate family and community responsibilities of the culture.
- Encourage culturally specific and individually tailored interventions to facilitate commitment to exercise.
- Educate patients of all ages on the importance of exercise in preserving health, and correct any misconceptions.

BOX 39.7 PATIENT TEACHING

Teaching Patients With Osteoporosis

Objective

- Patient will identify strategies to prevent or limit the severity of osteoporosis.

Teaching Strategies

- Instruct patient and/or family caregiver about common risk factors and how to modify lifestyle (e.g., stop smoking, caffeine, alcohol, or hormone replacement as recommended by health care provider).
- Teach patient and/or caregiver the current recommended dietary allowances for calcium, and review culturally specific foods high in calcium (e.g., milk fortified with vitamin D, leafy green vegetables, yogurt, and cheese).
- Instruct patient and/or caregiver in appropriate types of weight-bearing exercises as recommended by health care provider or physical therapist to prevent injury or fractures.
- Teach patient and/or caregiver about safety, fall prevention, and strategies to create a safe home environment (e.g., remove scatter rugs; ensure that hallways and steps are well lit).
- Instruct patient and/or caregiver in self-administration of prescribed medication used to treat osteoporosis.
- Promote positive self-image in patient by providing realistic yet optimistic and positive feedback about changes in appearance and mobility.

Evaluation

Use the principles of teach-back to evaluate patient/family caregiver learning:

- I want to make sure that you understand the teaching about osteoporosis. Tell me three lifestyle modifications you can make to prevent or limit the severity of osteoporosis.
- Describe for me four foods high in calcium and vitamins to include in your diet.
- Demonstrate for me weight-bearing exercises and tell me your plan for when to do the exercises.
- Describe three safety strategies for your home that will prevent falls.
- Explain the dosage schedule you will follow for your osteoporosis medications and the side effects that you should watch for.

and assess their diets for calcium and vitamin D intake. Patients who have lactose intolerance need dietary teaching about alternative sources of calcium.

For patients diagnosed with osteoporosis, early evaluation and consultation with and referral to health care providers, dietitians, and physical therapists are important interventions, especially when these patients become immobilized. The goal of the patient with osteoporosis is to maintain independence with ADLs. Assistive ambulatory devices, adaptive clothing, and safety bars help patients maintain independence. Patient teaching needs to focus on limiting the severity of the disease through diet and activity (Box 39.7).

Acute Care. Patients in acute care settings who experience altered physical mobility are usually more debilitated than those in outpatient settings. These patients are often at risk for the hazards of immobility such as impaired respiratory status, orthostatic hypotension, DVT, and impaired skin integrity. Therefore design nursing interventions to reduce the impact of immobility on body systems and prepare patients for the restorative phase of care.

Metabolic System. Because the body needs protein to repair injured tissue and rebuild depleted protein stores, consult with a registered dietitian to ensure that patients who are immobilized receive high-protein, high-calorie diets. A high-calorie intake provides sufficient fuel to meet metabolic needs and replace subcutaneous tissue. Also ensure that a patient is taking vitamin B and C supplements when necessary. Supplementation with vitamin C is needed for skin integrity and wound healing, and vitamin B complex assists in energy metabolism. You can offer dietary instruction on important diet elements as you deliver your care.

If the patient is unable to eat, nutrition must be provided parenterally or enterally. Total parenteral nutrition refers to delivery of nutritional supplements through a central or peripheral intravenous (IV) catheter. Enteral feedings include delivery through a nasogastric, gastrostomy, or jejunostomy tube of high-protein, high-calorie solutions with complete requirements of vitamins, minerals, and electrolytes (see Chapter 45).

Respiratory System. Patients who are immobilized and have reduced ventilation benefit from a variety of nursing interventions that promote lung expansion and removal of pulmonary secretions. Patients need to frequently fully expand their lungs to maintain elastic recoil. In addition, secretions accumulate in the dependent areas of the lungs. Often patients with restricted mobility experience weakness, and as this progresses the cough reflex gradually becomes inefficient and patients have less energy to breathe deeply. All of these factors place patients at risk for developing pneumonia. The stasis of secretions in the lungs is life threatening.

Deep-breathing exercises, incentive spirometry, and controlled coughing are among the nursing interventions available to expand the lungs, dislodge and mobilize stagnant secretions, and clear the lungs (see Chapters 41 and 50). All of these interventions help reduce the risk of pneumonia. It is essential to implement pulmonary interventions early in all patients with limited mobility, even those who do not have pneumonia or a nursing diagnosis of an actual respiratory problem. *For example, Joseph and his team will ensure Ms. Cavallo turns laterally to alternate side-lying positions frequently while she is in bed, keep the patient's head of bed elevated to semi-Fowler position, and proceed with assisting the patient to the side of bed and chair. The care team will increase the frequency of Ms Cavallo sitting in the chair as often as possible. All interventions will improve the patient's ventilation.*

Encourage patients who are immobile to deep breathe and cough every 1 to 2 hours. Teach patients to deep breathe or yawn every hour or to use an incentive spirometer (when ordered). Controlled coughing, a common therapy following surgery, involves taking in three deep breaths and then coughing with the third exhalation.

Ensure that patients who are immobile have an adequate fluid intake. Unless there is a medical contraindication, an adult needs to drink at least 1100 to 1400 mL of noncaffeinated fluids daily. This helps keep mucociliary clearance normal. Expect pulmonary secretions to be removed easily with coughing and to appear thin, watery, and clear. Without adequate hydration, pulmonary secretions become thick, tenacious, and difficult to remove. Offering fluids that patients prefer on a regularly timed schedule also helps with bowel and urine elimination and aids in maintaining circulation and skin integrity.

Cardiovascular System. The effects of bed rest or immobilization on the cardiovascular system include orthostatic hypotension, increased cardiac workload, and thrombus formation. Select and individualize nursing therapies to minimize or prevent these alterations.

Reducing Orthostatic Hypotension. When patients who are on bed rest or have been immobile move to a sitting or standing position, they often experience orthostatic hypotension. They have an increased pulse rate, a decreased pulse pressure, and a drop in blood pressure. If symptoms become severe enough, the patient can faint (McCance and Huether, 2019). To prevent injury, implement interventions that reduce or eliminate the effects of orthostatic hypotension. Mobilize the patient as soon as the physical condition allows, even if this only involves dangling legs at the bedside or moving to a chair. This activity maintains muscle tone and increases venous return. Isometric exercises (i.e., activities that involve muscle tension without muscle shortening) have no beneficial effect on preventing orthostatic hypotension, but they improve activity tolerance. When getting a patient who has been immobile up for the first time, assess the situation using a safe patient-handling algorithm (Martin et al., 2016; U.S. Department of Veterans Affairs, n.d.) or another appropriate mobility assessment, screening, or scoring system. This is a precautionary step that protects you and the patient from injury and also allows the patient to do as much of the transfer as possible.

Reducing Cardiac Workload. A nursing intervention that reduces cardiac workload involves instructing patients to avoid using a Valsalva maneuver when moving up in bed, defecating, or lifting household objects. During a Valsalva maneuver a patient holds the breath and strains, which increases intrathoracic pressure and in turn decreases venous return and cardiac output. When the strain is released, venous return and cardiac output immediately increase, and systolic blood pressure and pulse pressure rise. These pressure changes produce a reflex bradycardia and possible decrease in blood pressure that can result in sudden cardiac death in patients with heart disease. Teach patients to breathe out while defecating, lifting, or moving side to side or up in bed and to not hold their breath and strain.

Preventing Thrombus Formation. Well-established clinical standards for the prevention of VTE have been published by the American Society of Hematology (ASH) (Anderson et al., 2019; ASH, 2021). The ASH recommendations include:

- Provision of pharmacological VTE prophylaxis (anticoagulant therapy) in acutely or critically ill inpatients at acceptable bleeding risk
- Use of mechanical prophylaxis (compression stockings, intermittent compression) when bleeding risk is unacceptable
  Conditional recommendations include:
- Not to use VTE prophylaxis routinely in long-term care patients or outpatients with minor VTE risk factors
- Use of graduated compression stockings or low-molecular-weight heparin in long-distance travelers only if they are at high risk for VTE

Nurses play a critical role in promoting mechanical prophylaxis in at-risk patients, including early ambulation, administration of anticoagulants, applying intermittent SCDs or compression stockings, and applying foot pumps (Box 39.8). Mechanical compression of veins facilitates venous emptying by altering pressure gradients and decreasing stasis (Weinberger and Cipolle, 2016; Lip and Hull, 2021). When compression is applied (uniformly or sequentially), the increase in the arterial-venous pressure gradient enables an increase in arterial blood flow and decreases peripheral vascular resistance. Beyond simply overcoming stasis, some forms of mechanical VTE prophylaxis also appear to offer fibrinolytic properties to combat the hypercoagulable component of the Virchow triad (Weinberger and Cipolle, 2016).

All intermittent compression systems, including SCDs and MCDs, pump blood into deep veins, thus removing pooled blood and preventing stasis. On deflation of a compression cuff the veins will refill, and because of the intermittent nature of the system, this will ensure periodic flow of blood through the deep veins as long as there is a supply. Compression stockings appear to function more by preventing distention of veins. An additional benefit of circumferential compression is the increase in hydrostatic pressure on the extracellular interstitial spaces, which may augment blood flow and decrease edema (Weinberger and Cipolle, 2016). The effects of the compression stockings are aided by muscular activity of the limb and may have less efficacy in patients who are immobile. Intermittent pneumatic compression (IPC) devices are preferred over graduated compression stockings owing to their improved efficacy and better patient adherence (Weinberger and Cipolle, 2016). Research has shown that IPC significantly reduces the risk of DVT and improves survival in a variety of patients who are immobile after stroke (Zhang et al., 2018). Using an additional device, such as IPC devices plus graduated compression stockings, offers no additive benefit regarding VTE outcomes.

Another option for mechanical prophylaxis is venous plexus foot pumps designed to promote venous return by pumping blood through compression, mimicking the natural action of walking. The muscles in the foot, however, are much less compressible and the overall blood volume in the plantar venous plexus is much smaller in comparison to the calf, which therefore requires larger compressive forces to obtain similar effects seen with SCDs or compression stockings (Weinberger and Cipolle, 2016). This increased pressure requirement may cause increased pain and discomfort during application of venous foot pumps, and poorer patient adherence.

The SCD and MCD consist of sleeves or stockings made of fabric or plastic that are wrapped around the leg and secured with Velcro (see Box 39.8). Once they are applied, connect the sleeves to a pump that alternately inflates and deflates the stocking around the leg. A typical cycle is inflation for 10 to 15 seconds and deflation for 45 to 60 seconds. Inflation pressures average 40 mm Hg. For optimal use, begin SCD/MCD use as soon as possible (e.g., immediately after major abdominal or joint surgery) and maintain until the patient becomes fully ambulatory. Increasing numbers of IPC devices allow patients to ambulate with the devices in place. This decreases the chance for the device to be removed or turned off during ambulation with a failure to reapply later in a timely manner (Link, 2018).

Elastic stockings (sometimes called *antiembolic stockings*) also aid in maintaining external pressure on the muscles of the lower extremities and thus promote venous return (see Box 39.8). To obtain the correct size, measure the patient's calf, thigh, and leg length accurately. When considering applying graded compression stockings, first assess the patient's suitability for wearing them. Do not apply them if the patient has a local condition affecting the leg (e.g., any skin lesion, gangrenous condition, or recent vein ligation) because application compromises circulation. Apply them properly and remove them at

BOX 39.8   PROCEDURAL GUIDELINES

Applying Sequential Compression Devices and Elastic Stockings

Delegation and Collaboration

The skill of applying and maintaining graduated compression stockings and intermittent sequential compression device (SCDs) and mobile compression devices (MCDs) may be delegated to assistive personnel (AP). The nurse initially determines the size of elastic stockings and assesses the patient's lower extremities for any signs and symptoms of deep vein thrombosis (DVT) or impaired circulation. The nurse directs the AP to:

- Remove SCD sleeves before allowing a patient to get out of bed.
- Report to the nurse if a patient's calf or thigh appears larger than the other or is red, tender, hot, or swollen or if the patient complains of calf pain.
- Report to the nurse if there is redness, itching, or irritation on the legs (signs of allergic reactions to elastic).
- Report to the nurse if the patient is routinely removing the compression device from the legs.

Equipment

Tape measure; powder or cornstarch *(optional)*; graduated compression stockings or Velcro compression device sleeves; SCD/MCD insufflator with air hoses attached; compression device pump; hygiene supplies; *Option:* cotton stockinette with MCD

Procedural Steps

1. Identify patient using at least two identifiers (e.g., name and birthday or name and medical record number) according to agency policy (TJC, 2021).
2. Review medical record for order for SCDs/MCDs or graduated compression stocking.
3. Review medical record to assess patient for risk factors for developing DVT (see Box 39.4). An option is to use the Wells score, an objective and widely used measure for determining a patient's risk for a DVT (Wells et al. 1998; Modi et al., 2016) (see Table 39.5).
4. Perform hand hygiene. (If patient has any skin lesions, apply disposable gloves). Assess for contraindications to use of elastic stockings or compression devices:
   a. Dermatitis or open skin lesions on area to be covered by stockings/sleeves.
   b. Recent skin graft to lower leg.
   c. Decreased arterial circulation in lower extremities as evidenced by cyanotic, cool extremities and/or gangrenous conditions affecting the lower limb(s).
   d. If signs/symptoms of a DVT are present, manipulation could cause a clot in vein within the leg to dislodge.
5. Assess condition of patient's skin and circulation to the legs. Palpate pedal pulses; note any palpable veins, and inspect skin over lower extremities for edema, skin discoloration, warmth, presence of lesions.
6. Assess patient's or family caregiver's health literacy and experience.
7. Assess patient's knowledge regarding elastic compression stockings or compression devices, and feelings about procedure.
8. Assess patient's goals or preferences for how skill is to be performed or what patient expects. Explain procedure and reason for applying elastic stockings/SCD/MCD to prevent DVT.
9. Close room curtains or door to provide privacy. Obtain and organize equipment for application of sequential compression devices and elastic stockings at bedside. Position patient in supine position.
10. Perform hand hygiene. Bathe patient's legs as needed. Dry thoroughly. Perform hand hygiene.
11. **Apply graduated compression stocking:**
    a. Use tape measure to measure patient's leg to determine proper elastic stocking size (follow package directions).
    b. *Option:* Apply a small amount of powder or cornstarch to legs, provided that patient does not have sensitivity.

c. Turn elastic stocking inside out: place one hand into stocking, holding heel of stocking. Take other hand and pull stocking inside out until reaching the heel (see illustration).

d. Place patient's toes into foot of elastic stocking up to the heel, making sure that stocking is smooth (see illustration).

e. Slide remaining portion of stocking over patient's foot, making sure that toes are covered. Make sure that foot fits into toe and heel position of stocking. Stocking will now be right side out (see illustration).

STEP 11c Turn stocking inside out; hold heel and pull through.

STEP 11d Place toes into foot of stocking.

STEP 11e Slide remaining part of stocking over foot.

Continued

BOX 39.8   PROCEDURAL GUIDELINES—cont'd

Applying Sequential Compression Devices and Elastic Stockings

f. Slide stocking up over patient's calf until sock is completely extended. Be sure that stocking is smooth and that no ridges or wrinkles are present (see illustration).

g. Instruct patient not to roll stockings partially down, avoid wrinkles, avoid crossing legs, and elevate legs while sitting.

12. **Apply SCD sleeve(s):**

a. Remove SCD sleeves from plastic cover; unfold and flatten onto bed.

b. Arrange SCD sleeve under patient's leg according to leg position indicated on inner lining of sleeve.

c. Place patient's leg on SCD sleeve. Back of ankle should line up with ankle marking on inner lining of sleeve.

d. Position back of knee with popliteal opening on inner sleeve (see illustration).

e. Wrap SCD sleeve securely around patient's leg. Check fit of SCD sleeve by placing two fingers between patient's leg and sleeve (see illustration).

f. Attach SCD sleeve connector to plug on mechanical unit. Arrows on connector line up with arrows on plug from mechanical unit (see illustration).

g. Turn mechanical unit on. Green light indicates that unit is functioning. Monitor functioning SCD through one full cycle of inflation and deflation.

13. **Apply MCD sleeve:**

a. A cotton stockinette is provided along with the calf sleeves. Apply over patient's calves.

b. Wrap the sleeve smoothly around the patient's calf and fasten it, beginning at the top, moving toward the bottom.

c. Place two fingers between patient's calf and sleeve to be sure it is snug but not too tight (see illustration).

STEP 12e Check fit of sequential compression device (SCD) sleeve.

STEP 11f Slide sock up leg until completely extended.

STEP 12f Align arrows when connecting plug to mechanical unit.

STEP 12d Position back of patient's knee with popliteal opening.

STEP 13c Application of sleeve to calves.

BOX 39.8   PROCEDURAL GUIDELINES—cont'd

Applying Sequential Compression Devices and Elastic Stockings

d. The device has two identical extension tubes (see illustration). Use either end of the extension tube to connect to the sleeve or device pump.

   (1) Connect one end of the extension tube to the sleeve connector. The white arrows should be pointing toward each other.

   (2) Connect the other end of the extension tube to the device pump. The white arrow should be facing upward.

e. Press the power switch located at the back of the device to ON position (see illustration). After turning the device on, the Configuration Setup Screen is shown on the LCD screen and the sleeves should immediately start to inflate, from the bottom to the top.

f. Wait 60 seconds for the automatic operation of the device. The device automatically identifies which sleeves are connected, selects the suitable treatment mode, and will display information on the main LCD screen.

STEP 13d Application of MCD connector hose to pump.

STEP 13e Powering on MCD.

14. Position patient comfortably. Then place nurse call system in accessible location within patient's reach. When wearing MCD sleeves a patient may walk with device in place (see illustration).

   CLINICAL JUDGMENT: Caution patient not to exit bed and walk with SCDs in place. Have patient call for assistance. The patient may walk with MCD in place (see illustration).

15. Raise side rails (as appropriate) and lower bed to lowest position. Perform hand hygiene.

16. Remove compression stockings or SCD/MCD sleeves at least once per shift (e.g., long enough to inspect skin for irritation or breakdown and to determine patient's comfort level).

17. Evaluate skin integrity and circulation to patient's lower extremities as ordered (see agency policy).

18. **Use Teach-Back:** "We have reviewed the signs and symptoms you might have if a clot forms in your leg. Tell me what those symptoms are." Revise your instruction now or develop a plan for revised patient/family caregiver teaching if patient/family caregiver is not able to teach back correctly.

19. Record condition of lower extremities, application of stockings/SCDs/MCDs, patient response to education.

20. Report to health care provider or nurse in charge any signs that may indicate formation of DVT.

⚠ WARNING: Extension tubes may become tangled when walking with the device. Adjust their length to avoid tripping injury or equipment damage.

STEP 14 Walking with MCD.

least once per shift. Be sure to assess circulation at the toes to ensure that the stockings are not too tight.

Proper positioning reduces a patient's risk of thrombus formation because compression of the leg veins is minimized. Therefore when positioning patients, use caution to prevent pressure on the posterior knee and deep veins in the lower extremities. Teach patients to avoid the following: crossing the legs, sitting for prolonged periods of time, wearing clothing that constricts the legs or waist, and massaging the legs. Report suspected DVT or signs of PE immediately to the patient's health care provider. Elevate the leg but avoid pressure on the suspected thrombus area. Instruct the family, patient, and all health care personnel not to massage the area because of the danger of dislodging the thrombus.

ROM exercises and early mobility aid in preventing thrombi. Activity causes contraction of the skeletal muscles, which in turn exerts pressure on the veins to promote venous return, thereby reducing venous stasis. Specific exercises that help prevent thrombophlebitis are ankle pumps, foot circles, and knee flexion. Ankle pumps, sometimes called *calf pumps,* include alternating plantar flexion and dorsiflexion. Foot circles require the patient to rotate the ankle. Encourage patients to make the letters of the alphabet with their feet every 1 to 2 hours. Knee flexion involves alternately extending and flexing the knee. These exercises are sometimes referred to as *antiembolic exercises* and need to be done hourly while awake and are excellent for patients on bed rest.

Maintaining Musculoskeletal Function. Exercises to prevent excessive muscle atrophy and joint contractures help maintain musculoskeletal function. Active ROM should be encouraged for any patient at risk for reduced musculoskeletal strength or functionality by improving joint mobility. When a patient has muscle weakness, fatigue, or pain, active assisted ROM exercises are most appropriate. A patient needs assistance with movement from an external force (e.g., manual support of an extremity, positioning to use the effects of gravity) because of weakness, pain, or changes in muscle tone. Passive ROM exercises are indicated when a patient is not able or permitted to move a body part, as in the case of a paralyzed extremity or healing fracture.

To ensure that patients routinely receive ROM exercises, schedule them at specific times, perhaps during another nursing activity such as the patient's bath. This enables you to systematically reassess mobility while improving the patient's ROM. In addition, bathing usually requires that extremities and joints be put through complete ROM.

Passive ROM exercises begin as soon as a patient's ability to move an extremity or joint is lost. Carry out movements slowly and smoothly, through a prescribed range, just to the point of resistance. ROM exercises should not cause pain. **Never force a joint beyond the point of resistance.** Repeat each joint movement 5 times during a session, with sessions performed 2 to 3 times a day. When performing passive ROM exercises, stand at the side of the bed closest to the joint being exercised. Use a head-to-toe sequence and move from larger to smaller joints. If an extremity is to be moved or lifted, support the joint by holding distal and proximal areas adjacent to the joint (Fig. 39.12). Use a cupped hand to provide support under the joint (Fig. 39.13). See Table 39.2 for detailed ROM for each joint. Patients on bed rest may benefit from having active ROM exercises incorporated into their daily schedules.

Positioning Techniques. Patients with impaired nervous, skeletal, or muscular system functioning, and increased weakness and fatigue often require help from nurses for positioning and maintenance of proper body alignment while in bed or sitting (see Skill 39.1). Several positioning devices are available for positioning and maintaining good body alignment for patients. Friction-reducing sheets and boards are available to make it easier to move patients up in bed or laterally to the side. Use of friction-reducing sheets reduces shear and friction on the skin.

FIG. 39.12 Use cupped hand under joint for support.

FIG. 39.13 Support joint by holding distal and proximal areas adjacent to joint.

Pillows are positioning aids and are sometimes readily available. Before using a pillow, determine whether it is the proper size. A thick pillow under a patient's head increases cervical flexion, which is not desirable. A thin pillow under bony prominences does not protect skin and tissue from damage caused by pressure. When additional pillows are unavailable or if they are an improper size, use folded sheets, blankets, or towels as positioning aids. Patients with severely limited mobility in the feet or who are unwilling to actively move their feet and legs benefit from foot boots. A foot boot prevents foot drop by maintaining a foot in dorsiflexion. Ankle-foot orthotic (AFO) devices also help maintain dorsiflexion. Patients who wear positioning boots or AFOs need to have these removed periodically (e.g., 2 hours on, 2 hours off).

A **trochanter roll** prevents external rotation of the hips when a patient is in a supine position. This is especially useful in patients who have lost the ability to move the lower extremities. To form a trochanter roll, fold a cotton bath blanket lengthwise to a width that extends from the greater trochanter of the femur to the lower border of the popliteal space (Fig. 39.14). Place the blanket under the buttocks and roll it counterclockwise until the thigh is in neutral position or inward rotation. When the hip is aligned correctly, the patella faces directly upward. Use sandbags in place of or in addition to trochanter rolls. Sandbags are sand-filled plastic tubes or bags that are shaped to body contours.

Hand rolls maintain the thumb in slight adduction and in opposition to the fingers, which maintain a functional position. Assess the hand roll positioning to make sure that the hand is indeed in a functional position. Hand rolls are most often used with patients whose arms are paralyzed or who are unconscious. Do not use rolled washcloths as hand rolls because

FIG. 39.14 Trochanter roll.

FIG. 39.15 Patient using trapeze bar. (From Yoost BL, Crawford LR: *Fundamentals of nursing*, ed 3, St Louis, 2023, Elsevier.)

they do not keep the thumb well abducted, especially in patients who have a spastic paralysis. Hand-wrist splints are individually molded for a patient to maintain proper alignment of the thumb (slight adduction) and wrist (slight dorsiflexion). Use splints only on the patient for whom they were made and follow the splint schedule (e.g., wear for 2 hours, remove for 2 hours).

The **trapeze bar** is a triangular device that hangs down from a securely fastened overhead bar that is attached to the bedframe. It allows a patient to pull with the upper extremities to raise the trunk off the bed, assist in transfer from bed to wheelchair, or perform upper-arm exercises (Fig. 39.15). It increases independence, maintains upper-body strength, and decreases the shearing action from sliding across or up and down in bed as the patient raises the hips.

Although each procedure for positioning has specific guidelines, there are universal steps to follow for patients who require positioning assistance. Following the guidelines reduces the risk of injury to the musculoskeletal system when a patient is sitting or lying. When joints are unsupported, their alignment is impaired. Likewise, if joints are not positioned in a slightly flexed position, their mobility is decreased.

During positioning, also assess for pressure points. When actual or potential pressure areas exist, nursing interventions involve removal of the pressure, thus decreasing the risk for development of pressure injuries and further trauma to the musculoskeletal system. In these patients use the 30-degree lateral position (see Chapter 48).

Supported Fowler Position. In the supported Fowler position, the head of the bed is elevated 45 to 60 degrees, and the patient's knees are slightly elevated without pressure to restrict circulation in the lower legs. The patient's illness and overall condition influence the angle of head and knee elevation and the length of time that the patient needs to remain in the supported Fowler position. Supports need to permit flexion of the hips and knees and proper alignment of the normal curves in the cervical, thoracic, and lumbar vertebrae. The following are common trouble areas for a patient in the supported Fowler position:
- Increased cervical flexion because the pillow at the head is too thick and the head thrusts forward
- Extension of the knees, allowing the patient to slide to the foot of the bed
- Pressure on the posterior aspect of the knees, decreasing circulation to the feet
- External rotation of the hips
- Arms hanging unsupported at the patient's sides
- Unsupported feet or pressure on the heels
- Unprotected pressure points at the sacrum and heels
- Increased shearing force on the back and heels when the head of the bed is raised more than 60 degrees

Supine Position. Patients in the supine position rest on their backs. In the supine position the relationship of body parts is essentially the same as in good standing alignment, except that the body is in the horizontal plane. Use pillows, trochanter rolls, and hand rolls or arm splints to increase comfort and reduce injury to the skin or musculoskeletal system. The mattress needs to be firm enough to support the cervical, thoracic, and lumbar vertebrae. Shoulders are supported, and the elbows are slightly flexed to control shoulder rotation. A foot support prevents foot drop and maintains proper alignment. The following are some common trouble areas for patients in the supine position:
- Pillow at the head that is too thick, increasing cervical flexion
- Head flat on the mattress
- Shoulders unsupported and internally rotated
- Elbows extended
- Thumb not in opposition to the fingers
- Hips externally rotated
- Unsupported feet
- Unprotected pressure points at the occipital region of the head, vertebrae, coccyx, elbows, and heels

Prone Position. The prone position is one used rarely because many individuals, especially older adults, are simply uncomfortable in the position. Conditions such as arthritis of the neck and hips make it physically difficult to lie prone. However, the prone position is considered first-line therapy for critically ill patients with severe acute respiratory distress syndrome (ARDS), such as patients with COVID-19, to reduce lung trauma and optimize the ventilation and perfusion to regions of the dependent dorsal lung fields (Bahloul et al., 2021; Makic, 2020). Studies show that lying face-down for up to 16 hours a day can improve oxygenation and decrease mortality in these patients (American Association of Critical-Care Nurses [AACN], 2019).

A patient in the prone position lies face or chest down. Often the head is turned to the side, but if a pillow is under the head, it needs to be thin enough to prevent cervical flexion or extension and maintain alignment of the lumbar spine. Placing a pillow under the lower leg permits dorsiflexion of the ankles and some knee flexion, which promote relaxation. If a pillow is unavailable, the ankles need to be in dorsiflexion over the end of the mattress. Although the prone position is seldom used in practice, consider this as an alternative, especially in patients who normally sleep in this position. Specialty beds that safely position patients who are acutely ill in the prone position are available. Assess for and correct any of the following potential trouble points with patients in the prone position:

- Neck hyperextension
- Hyperextension of the lumbar spine
- Plantar flexion of the ankles
- Unprotected pressure points at the chin, elbows, female breasts, hips, knees, and toes

Side-Lying Position. In the side-lying (or lateral) position a patient rests on the side with the major portion of body weight on the dependent hip and shoulder. A 30-degree lateral position on the side is recommended for patients at risk for pressure injuries (see Chapter 48). Trunk alignment needs to be the same as in standing. The patient needs to maintain the structural curves of the spine, the head needs to be supported in line with the midline of the trunk, and rotation of the spine needs to be avoided.

The following trouble points are common in the side-lying position:

- Lateral flexion of the neck
- Spinal curves out of normal alignment
- Shoulder and hip joints internally rotated, adducted, or unsupported
- Lack of foot support
- Lack of protection for pressure points at the ear, shoulder, anterior iliac spine, trochanter, and ankles
- Excessive lateral flexion of the spine if the patient has large hips and a pillow is not placed superior to the hips at the waist

Lateral Recumbent Position. The lateral recumbent position differs from the side-lying position in the distribution of the patient's weight. In the lateral recumbent position the patient lies on a side with the same hip and lower extremity straight and the opposite hip and knee bent. Trouble points common in this position include the following:

- Lateral flexion of the neck
- Internal rotation, adduction, or lack of support to the shoulders and hips
- Lack of foot support
- Lack of protection for pressure points at the ileum, humerus, clavicle, knees, and ankles

Moving Patients. When moving a patient during repositioning, the priority always is a safe transfer. Patients require various levels of assistance to move up in bed, move to the side-lying position, or sit up at the side of the bed. For example, a young healthy woman may need minimal support as she sits at the side of the bed for the first time after childbirth, whereas an older adult may need help from two or more nurses to sit on the side of the bed after surgery. Transfer devices assist in patient positioning.

Always ask patients to help to their fullest extent possible during positioning. To determine what a patient is able to do alone and how many people are needed to help with positioning or transferring (see Chapter 38), assess the patient to determine whether the illness contradicts exertion (e.g., cardiovascular disease). Is the patient cooperative and capable of moving? Next determine whether the patient comprehends what is expected. For example, a patient recently medicated for postoperative pain is too lethargic to understand instructions; thus, to ensure safety, two nurses are necessary to move the patient. Then determine the patient's comfort level. It is important to assess your personal strength and knowledge of the procedure. Finally, determine whether the patient is too heavy or immobile for you to move alone (Kanaskie and Snyder, 2018; Olinsky and Norton, 2017) (see Chapter 38).

Preventing Injury to the Integumentary System. The major risk to the skin from restricted mobility is the formation of pressure injuries. Early identification of patients at highest risk helps prevent pressure injuries (see Chapter 48). Interventions aimed at prevention include turning and positioning and the use of therapeutic support surfaces and devices (e.g., low-air-loss mattresses, heel boots, flotation mattresses) to relieve pressure. Regular skin care (cleansing of soiled areas and use of moisturizers) aims to maintain the condition of the skin. Change immobilized patients' positions according to their activity level, perceptual ability, treatment protocols, and daily routines. For example, you are caring for one patient who is obese and another who is cachectic, and both patients have bowel incontinence. Both patients will require more frequent turning than standard practice.

Usually the time that a patient sits uninterrupted in a chair is limited to 1 hour. This interval is shortened in patients who are at very high risk for skin breakdown. Reposition patients frequently because uninterrupted pressure causes skin breakdown. Teach patients to shift their weight in a chair every 15 minutes. Patients who are chairbound may benefit from a pressure-relief cushion such as an air, viscous fluid/foam, or gel/foam cushion that reduces pressure.

In Ms. Cavallo's case, Joseph conveys to the rehab team a plan for being sure Ms. Cavallo turns side to side 30 degrees laterally a minimum of every 2 hours while awake. He consults with the physical therapist on the best technique to help Ms. Cavallo learn how to turn independently, given her limited mobility in the left leg. The team also plans to get Ms. Cavallo up into a chair twice this afternoon. Ms. Cavallo's plan also includes pressure injury prevention strategies. Joseph discusses with the patient that because of reddened areas observed on her skin, her limited mobility, and her weight, he will place a pressure-reducing surface on her bed.

Elimination System. The nursing interventions for maintaining optimal urinary functioning are directed at keeping the patient well hydrated and preventing urinary stasis, calculi, and infections without causing bladder distention. Normal hydration (e.g., 800–2000 mL of noncaffeinated fluids daily) helps prevent renal calculi and UTIs. A patient who is well hydrated needs to void large amounts of dilute urine that is approximately equal to fluid intake. Also record the frequency and consistency of bowel movements. Provide a diet rich in fluids, fruits, vegetables, and fiber to facilitate normal peristalsis. If a patient is unable to maintain regular bowel patterns, stool softeners, cathartics, or enemas are sometimes necessary. For patients who are incontinent, modify the care plan to include toileting aids and a hygiene schedule so their urinary or bowel elimination patterns do not cause skin breakdown.

Psychosocial Health. People who have a tendency toward depression, feelings of powerlessness, or mood swings require nursing interventions that maintain normal development and provide physical and psychosocial stimuli. Anticipate changes in a patient's psychosocial status and provide routine and informal socialization. Involve family or significant others when appropriate. Observe the patient's ability to cope with restricted mobility. Does the patient become frustrated when unable to move normally? Does the patient refuse to move? Is anger expressed toward the care team? When these warning signs appear, take time and reassess a patient's feelings and motivation towards managing stress. Focus interventions on what is important to the patient.

In institutional health care settings, try not to schedule nursing care activities between 10:00 p.m. and 7:00 a.m. to minimize sleep interruptions. When care is required, combine activities. For example, administer medications, check an IV infusion, and assess vital signs when you enter the room to turn the patient or provide special skin care. If the nursing care plan is not improving coping patterns, consult a clinical nurse specialist, counselor, social worker, spiritual adviser, or other health care professional. Incorporate their recommendations into the care plan.

Joseph and the team successfully assist Ms. Cavallo to the chair. The analgesic she received 45 minutes ago relieved her pain to a 4 on the pain scale as she sat on the side of the bed. A two-person assist was used to move her from partial weight bearing standing and then to the chair. While Ms. Cavallo is in the chair Joseph takes time to assess further how he can partner with Ms. Cavallo to keep her involved in her rehab. Joseph states, "Ms. Cavallo, you told me what you like to do at home. You are obviously an active person; how can we best help you here in rehab?" Ms. Cavallo responds, "Give me something to do. My hip hurts, but having something to do helps distract me." Joseph then assesses what type of activities Ms. Cavallo enjoys. He learns she likes to read mystery novels and work on crossword puzzles. He decides to get Ms. Cavallo a book and puzzles. Then the two discuss the plan for ambulation training in rehab.

Nurses provide meaningful stimuli to maintain a patient's orientation. Plan nursing activities so that a patient is able to talk and interact with staff. If possible, place the patient in a room with others who are mobile and interactive. If a private room is required, ask staff members to visit throughout the shift to provide meaningful interaction. A daily newspaper helps the patient keep track of events and time. Bedside conversations at appropriate moments familiarize the patient with nursing activities, meals, and visiting hours. Books help occupy the patient while alone. In rehab facilities patients can participate in craft activities. Electronic devices such as television, streaming devices, smartphones, and electronic tablets can also be used to provide stimulation and help pass the time.

Involve patients in their care whenever possible. For example, encourage a patient to determine when the bed should be made and when scheduled ambulation is preferred. Some patients rest better during the night when fresh sheets are put on in the evening rather than in the morning. The patient needs to provide as much self-care as possible. Keep hygiene and grooming articles within easy reach. Encourage patients to wear their glasses or artificial teeth and shave or apply makeup. People use these activities to maintain their body image, thus improving their outlook.

Developmental Health. Ideally a patient who is immobilized for a lengthy period is able to maintain normal developmental processes. Nursing care provides the mental and physical stimulation appropriate to a patient's age and developmental status. In the case of young children, incorporate play activities into the care plan. For example, completing puzzles helps a child to continue developing fine-motor skills, and reading helps with cognitive development. Encourage parents to stay with a child who is hospitalized. Place a child who is immobilized with children of the same age who are not immobilized unless a contagious disease is present. Allow the child to participate in nursing interventions such as dressing changes, cast care, and care of traction. Learn to recognize significant changes from normal behavioral patterns, and consult with a pediatric clinical nurse specialist, counselor, or other health care professional.

Restricted mobility of older patients presents unique nursing problems. Older patients who are frail or have chronic illnesses are often at increased risk for the psychosocial hazards of immobility. Maintaining a calendar and clock with a large dial, conversing about current events and family members, and encouraging visits from significant others reduce the risk of social isolation. Spending time in the room talking and listening to the patient is very beneficial in reducing the risk of social isolation.

Encourage older adults to perform as many ADLs as independently as possible. Patients need to continue to perform personal grooming if they did so before their mobility was restricted. This type of activity preserves the patient's dignity and provides a sense of accomplishment.

Restorative and Continuing Care. The goal of restorative care for the patient who is immobile is to maximize functional mobility and independence and reduce residual functional deficits such as impaired gait and decreased endurance. The focus in restorative care is not only on ADLs that relate to physical self-care but also on instrumental activities of daily living (IADLs). IADLs are activities that are necessary to be independent in society beyond eating, grooming, transferring, and toileting and include such skills as shopping, preparing meals, banking, and taking medications.

Nurses use many of the same interventions as described in the health promotion and acute care sections, but the emphasis is on working collaboratively with patients and their significant others and occupational therapists to facilitate a patient's return to maximal functional ability in both ADLs and IADLs.

Intensive specialized therapy such as occupational or physical therapy is common. Patients in a rehabilitation institution often go to the therapy department 2 to 3 times a day. Your role is to work collaboratively with these professionals and reinforce exercises and teaching. For example, after a stroke a patient is likely to receive gait training from a physical therapist; speech rehabilitation from a speech therapist; and help from an occupational therapist for how to perform household chores or ADLs, such as dressing, bathing, and toileting. The therapy is not always able to restore total functional health, but it often helps the patient adapt to the mobility limitations or complications. Equipment frequently used to help patients adapt to mobility limitations includes walkers, canes, wheelchairs, and assistive devices such as toilet seat extenders, reaching sticks, special utensils and plates, and clothing with Velcro closures.

REFLECT NOW

Mrs. Kline is currently in a rehabilitation facility and uses a walker. Her discharge to home is planned in 2 days. Her husband has participated in her rehabilitation but feels he needs help in the home. Their insurance will provide home physical therapy three times a week for 3 weeks. The first visit will be a home assessment. Which items in the home might need modification following a home visit, and which items might need to be relocated to provide a clear walking path? Which kitchen items may need to be relocated to avoid overreaching?

Walking and Exercise. A patient who is receiving restorative care continues to be involved in an exercise program, including progressive walking. Chapter 38 describes in detail how to assist a patient to ambulate. Any patient getting out of the bed for the first time requires assistance to move to a chair or walk. The same is true for patients with limited weight bearing on one extremity. Patients with hemiplegia (one-sided paralysis) or hemiparesis (one-sided weakness) will need assistance with walking. Many patients initially require assistive devices (e.g., walker, cane, crutch) to provide stability for walking. When helping a patient with an assistive device to ambulate, always have a gait belt on the patient and stand slightly behind and off to the side of the patient (on the weak/affected side or on the strong/unaffected side if the patient has an orthopedic condition) (see Chapter 38). Do not support patients by holding onto their arms because you cannot easily lower patients to the floor if they faint or fall. In addition, if the patient falls with the nurse holding an arm, a shoulder joint may be dislocated.

Psychotherapy. Recovery from a physical disability is difficult. Telerehabilitation is one holistic therapeutic approach that acknowledges the importance of addressing the body and spirit as well as the mind during therapeutic work (Good Therapy, 2016; Capri et al., 2020). Therapists combine physical movement work and psychotherapy techniques to help patients gain greater awareness of their abilities and how to proceed toward recovery. Rehabilitation psychologists support individuals as they cope with the mental and physical challenges their conditions present. They often teach their patients how to adapt and make lifestyle choices that promote good health (American Psychological Association, 2015). A nurse involved in a patient's rehab collaborates with the patient, family, and therapists to provide continuity in psychological support and patient education.

◆ Evaluation

Through the Patient's Eyes. Expert nurses actively involve their patients in all stages of the nursing process. Evaluation is no different

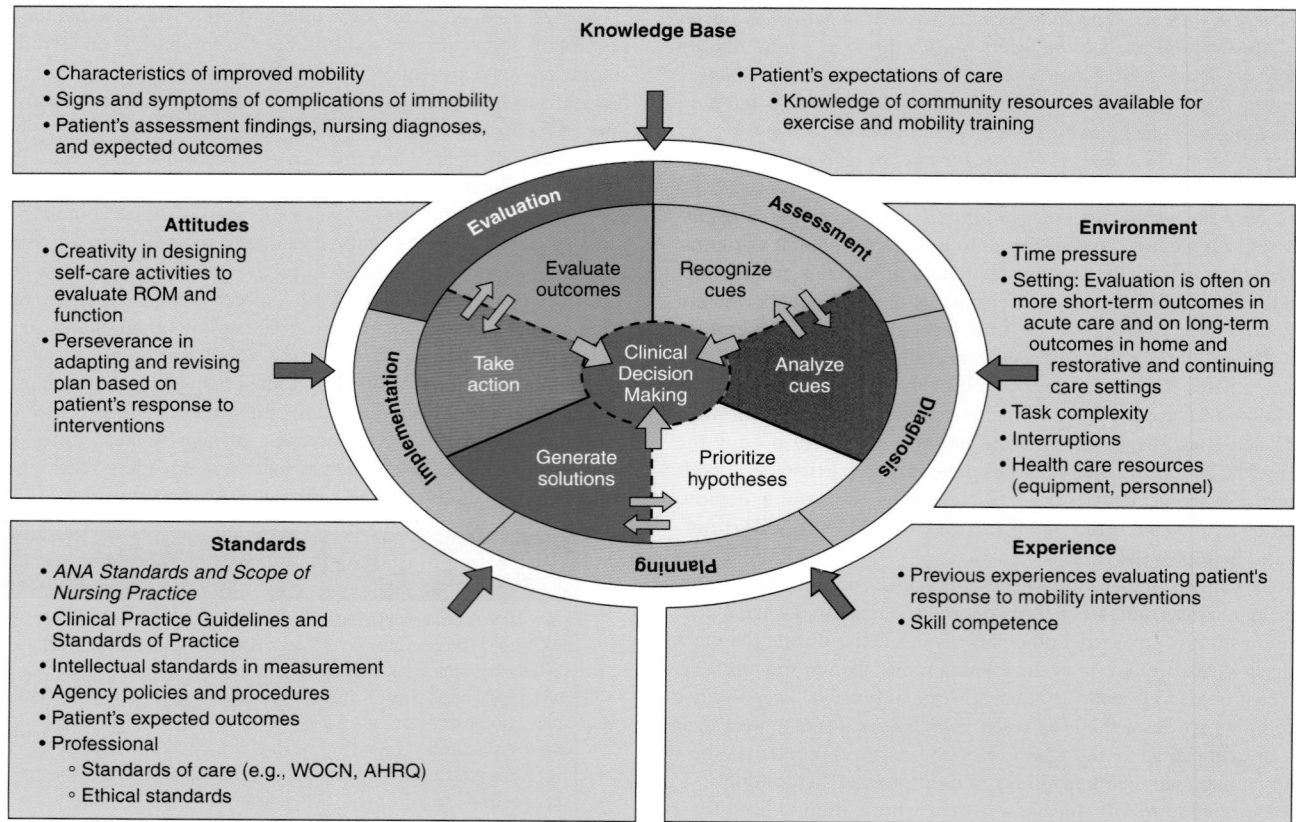

FIG. 39.16 Critical thinking model for evaluation of impaired mobility. *AHRQ*, Agency for Healthcare Research and Quality; *ANA*, American Nurses Association; *ROM*, range of motion; *WOCN*, Wound, Ostomy, and Continence Nurses Society. (Clinical Judgment Measurement Model copyright © NCSBN. All rights reserved.)

(Fig. 39.16). It is essential to ask patients to evaluate their plan of care. Were their expectations met? Were they satisfied with their level of involvement in their care? Questions you can ask patients to evaluate their care include: What are your perceptions of your recovery? Do you feel your mobility is improving? If not, what factors do you believe are preventing your improvement? Determine with the patient and others involved with care whether the outcomes established with and for the patient have indeed been met and whether it is necessary to revise the plan of care. A study involving patients found that patients' intention of becoming independent following a stroke positively affected their motor recovery, and family members' positive attitudes promoted patients' cognitive improvement (Fang et al., 2017). Involvement of patient and family is critical.

Patient Outcomes. As activity is incorporated into the plan of care, monitor a patient's physical tolerance, and reassess for dyspnea, shortness of breath, fatigue, chest pain, and/or a change in heart rate or blood pressure. What are the normal signs and symptoms of improved mobility and what are the presenting signs and symptoms for the patient? The patient who is weak or acutely ill is often unable to sustain even slight changes in activity because of the increased demand for energy. Seemingly simple tasks such as eating and moving in bed often result in extreme fatigue.

When a care plan includes interventions designed to prevent complications of immobility, compare a patient's baseline with the signs and symptoms of complications for which the patient is most at risk. *For example, Ms. Cavallo is at risk for impaired skin integrity, especially over pressure points. Joseph compares her baseline of normal blanchable* *erythema to see if there is a change. Have the reddened areas become nonblanchable; are there more reddened areas?* Sound clinical judgment is very important in tracking and recognizing complications early.

From your perspective as the nurse, you evaluate a patient's response to nursing care to determine if expected outcomes were achieved. Remember, this is when you conduct assessment activities similar to those performed during assessment, to observe for change. Your knowledge base allows you to critically interpret your findings to know if a patient is progressing or not. For example, you evaluate a patient's ability to maintain or improve joint mobility by observing walking or transferring and by measuring ROM, muscle strength and body alignment, posture, and balance. Evaluate the effectiveness of specific interventions designed to promote body alignment, improve mobility, and protect the patient from the hazards of immobility. Evaluate the patient's and family's understanding of all teaching provided as well. The continuous nature of evaluation allows you to determine whether new or revised therapies are required and whether new nursing diagnoses have developed.

When outcomes are not met, consider asking the following questions:
- Are there ways we can help you to increase your activity?
- Which activities are you having trouble completing right now?
- How do you feel about not being able to dress yourself and make your own meals?
- Which exercises do you find most helpful?
- What goals for your activity would you like to set now?

Once you have asked these questions and have addressed the limited mobility and its associated problems through the patient's eyes, you are prepared to adjust the plan of care to address the remaining clinical problems that your patient is experiencing related to immobility.

SAFETY GUIDELINES FOR NURSING SKILLS

Ensuring patient safety is an essential role of the professional nurse. Use sound clinical judgment by communicating clearly with members of the health care team, assessing, and analyzing a patient's clinical findings and incorporating the patient's priorities of care and preferences. Use the best evidence, applying professional standards, when selecting interventions to use in patient care delivery. When performing the skills in this chapter, remember the following points to ensure safe, patient-centered care.

- Determine the amount and type of assistance required for safe positioning, including any transfer equipment and the number of personnel to safely transfer and prevent harm to patient and health care providers.

- During positioning, raise the side rail on the side of the bed opposite of where you are standing to prevent the patient from falling out of bed on that side.
- Arrange equipment (e.g., IV lines, feeding tube, indwelling catheter) so that it does not interfere with the positioning process.
- Evaluate the patient for correct body alignment and pressure risks after repositioning.

SKILL 39.1 MOVING AND POSITIONING PATIENTS IN BED

Delegation and Collaboration

The skills of moving and positioning patients in bed and maintaining correct body alignment can be delegated to assistive personnel (AP). The nurse directs the AP by:

- Explaining about any moving and positioning restrictions (e.g., avoid prone position, patient has one-sided weakness) and type of safe patient-handling devices needed.
- Designating specific times throughout the shift that AP must reposition the patient.
- Providing information regarding patient's individual needs for body alignment (e.g., patient with spinal cord injury or severe contractures), ability to help, and number of other caregivers needed to help.

Equipment

- Pillows, friction-reducing device (FRD)/slide sheet or tube
- Appropriate safe patient-handling assistive device (e.g., FRD such as slide board or slide sheet, ceiling lift, or mechanical floor lift)
- Therapeutic boots or splints (optional)
- Trochanter roll
- Sandbag
- Hand rolls
- Clean gloves

STEPS	RATIONALE

ASSESSMENT

1. Identify patient using at least two identifiers (e.g., name and birthday or name and medical record number) according to agency policy.

Ensures correct patient. Complies with The Joint Commission standards and improves patient safety (TJC, 2021).

2. Refer to medical record for most recent recorded weight and height for patient.

Factors help to determine if mechanical lift, mechanical transfer device, or FRD is needed for moving patient up in bed.

3. Check health care provider's orders for any restrictions in movement before positioning patient, such as spinal cord injury; hip fracture; respiratory difficulties; neurological conditions; presence of incisions, drains, or tubing.

Some positions may be contraindicated to prevent patient injury.

4. Assess patient's health literacy, knowledge, and experience with positioning.

Ensures patient has the capacity to obtain, communicate, process, and understand basic health information (CDC, 2021).

5. Perform hand hygiene.

Reduces transmission of microorganisms.

6. Assess patient's ROM (see Chapter 30) of affected extremities and current body alignment while patient is lying down.

Provides baseline data for later comparisons. Determines ways to improve position and alignment.

7. Examine patient to assess for risk factors that contribute to complications of immobility.

Risk factors require patient to be repositioned more frequently.

   a. *Reduced sensation:* CVA, spinal cord injury, or neuropathy

With reduced sensation a patient has poor awareness of pressure on involved body part. Patient is unable to position body part and protect it from pressure.

   b. *Impaired mobility:* Traction, arthritis, CVA, spinal cord injury, bone fractures, joint surgery, or other contributing disease processes

These diseases and conditions have potential for decreased ROM. Loss of function caused by CVA or spinal injury can lead to contractures.

   c. *Impaired circulation:* Arterial insufficiency

Decreased circulation predisposes patient to pressure injury.

   d. *Age:* Very young, older adult

Premature and young infants require frequent turning because their skin is fragile. Normal physiological changes of aging predispose to greater risks for developing complications of immobility.

8. Assess patient's level of consciousness (see Chapter 30).

Determines need for special aids or devices. Patients with altered levels of consciousness may not understand instructions and may be unable to help with positioning.

9. Assess patient for presence of pain; rate on scale of 0 to 10 (see Chapter 44).

Pain reduces patient's motivation and ability to be mobile. Pain relief before transfer enhances patient participation.

10. Perform a thorough assessment of condition of patient's skin, especially over bony prominences (see Chapter 48). Know patient's Braden Scale score and level of risk for developing a pressure ulcer.

Skin condition and risks for breakdown provide baseline to determine effects of positioning and frequency required. Routine positioning reduces occurrence of pressure injuries.

Continued

SKILL 39.1	MOVING AND POSITIONING PATIENTS IN BED—cont'd

STEPS	RATIONALE

CLINICAL JUDGMENT: *Braden Scale score of 19 indicates patient is not at risk for pressure ulcer development. However, in examining the subscales (see Chapter 48), note whether a patient has very moist skin (moisture subscale of 2) and whether there is a potential problem with friction and shear (subscale score of 2). These two subscales need to be addressed in the plan of care and in determining the frequency of repositioning despite the overall score. The subscales are important indicators of risk (AHRQ, 2014).*

STEPS	RATIONALE
11. Assess patient's vision and hearing (see Chapter 16).	Sensory deficits affect patient's ability to cooperate during repositioning.
12. Perform hand hygiene. Apply clean gloves (as needed) to assess for presence of incisions, drainage tubes, and equipment (e.g., traction). Empty drainage bags before positioning. Remove and dispose of gloves. Perform hand hygiene.	Alters positioning procedure and type of position in which to place patient. Eliminates barriers to moving patient.
13. Assess motivation of patient and ability of family caregivers to participate in moving and positioning if patient is to be discharged home.	Indicates level of instruction needed before discharge.
14. Assess patient's goals or preferences for how skill is to be performed or what patient expects.	Allows care to be individualized to patient.

PLANNING

STEPS	RATIONALE
1. If patient perceives level of pain to be enough to avoid movement, offer an analgesic 30 minutes (if ordered) before repositioning.	Will lessen discomfort when positioning extremities. **Note:** Analgesic administration may not be available as frequently as a patient will require turning.
2. Remove all pillows and any devices used in previous position.	Reduces interference from bedding during positioning procedure.
3. Get additional caregivers and/or necessary lift or transfer device to perform positioning.	Safe-handling algorithms (see agency policy and illustration) determine number of caregivers and type of devices needed to position a patient if lifting is required (Nelson and Baptiste, 2006; Martin et al., 2016).

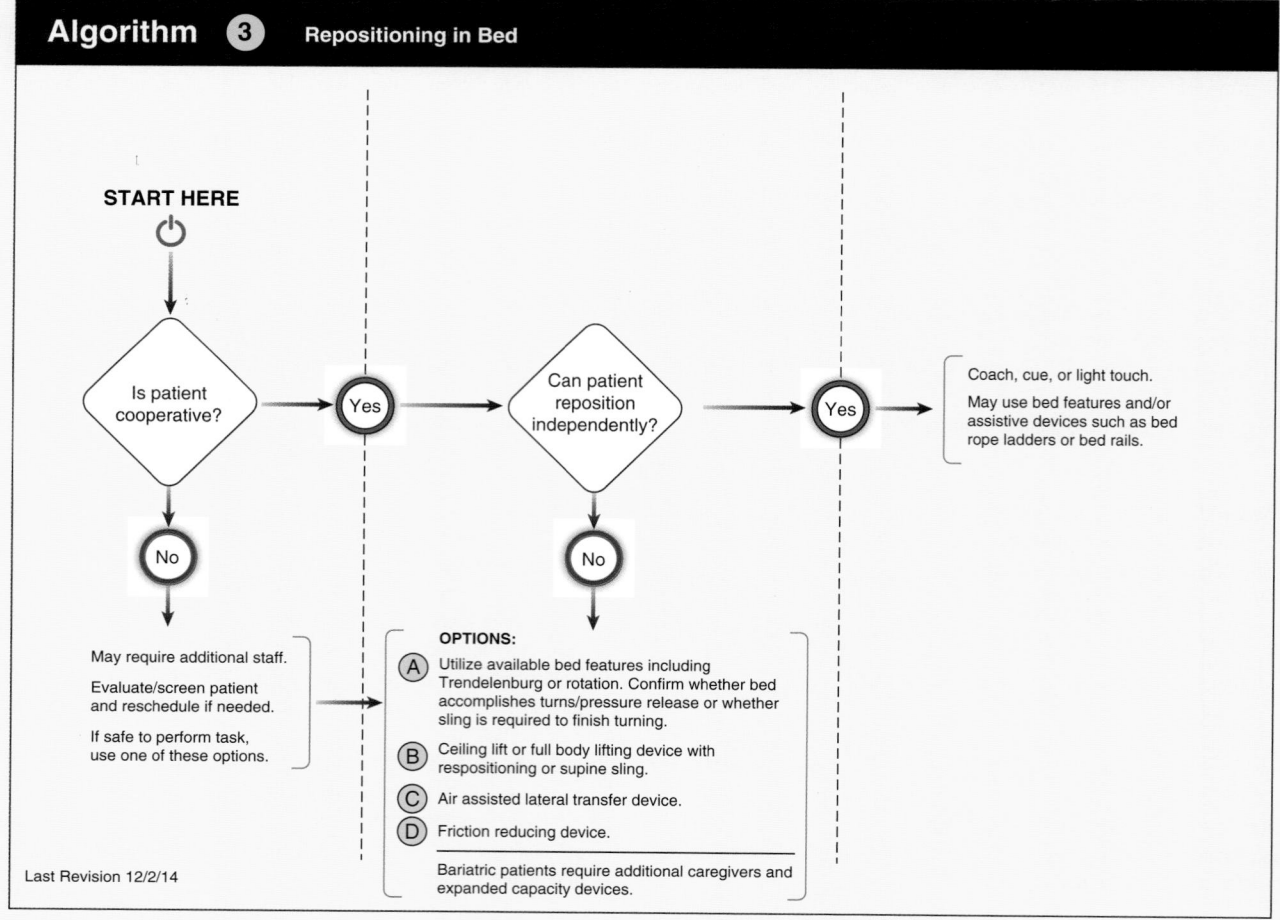

STEP 3 Algorithm for positioning patients in bed. (Courtesy Tampa VA Research and Education Foundation, Inc.)

STEPS	RATIONALE
4. Explain positioning procedure to patient using plain language.	Helps to decrease anxiety and increase cooperation.
5. Close door to room or bedside curtains.	Provides for patient privacy
6. Obtain and organize equipment for positioning at bedside.	Ensures more efficient procedure.

IMPLEMENTATION

1. Perform hand hygiene.	Reduces transmission of microorganisms.
2. Raise level of bed to comfortable working height, level with your elbows.	Raises level of work toward your center of gravity and reduces risk for back injuries.
3. Help patient to move up in bed (see Step 3, Planning).	This is not a one-person task unless patient can help completely (OSHA, n.d.b). Pulling patients who have migrated in bed carries an extremely high risk of caregiver injury (Matz et al., 2019).
a. Patient can fully assist:	Technique promotes patient independence.
(1) Stand at bedside to help with positioning of tubing and equipment as patient moves.	Prevents accidental tube dislodgement.
(2) Have patient place feet flat on mattress, grasp either side rails or overhead trapeze and, on a count of 3, lift hips up and push legs so body moves up in bed.	Technique prevents shear and friction against skin.
(3) Position for comfort.	
b. Patient is partially able to assist:	
(1) Have patient use a repositioning aid such as FRD (slide board or slide sheet).	Repositioning device reduces friction as patient is moved up in bed.
(2) Patient weighs 91 kg (200 lb) or less: use FRD and two to three caregivers.	Reduces musculoskeletal stress on caregivers.
(3) Patient weighs more than 91 kg (200 lb): use FRD (e.g., slide board or slide sheet) and at least three caregivers (Nelson and Baptiste, 2006; Martin et al., 2016).	Reduces musculoskeletal stress on caregivers.
i. Using a slide board with three nurses, position patient supine with head of bed flat. A nurse stands on each side of bed.	Prevents friction from contact of skin with board.
ii. Remove pillow from under head and shoulders and place it at head of bed.	Allows you to move patient freely up to head of bed.
iii. Turn patient side to side to place slide board under drawsheet on bed, with device extending from shoulders to thighs/ankles.	Centering device ensures repositioning of entire trunk and extremities.
iv. Return patient to supine position.	
v. Have the two nurses grasp draw sheet (one on each side of bed) firmly, and have the third nurse hold sliding board at end of bed.	Draw sheet slides upward, reducing friction and shear, allowing patient to move up in bed easily.
vi. Place feet apart with forward-backward stance. Flex knees and hips. On count of 3, shift weight from back to front leg and move patient and drawsheet to desired position up in bed (see Chapter 38).	Positions patient smoothly without exerting shear against skin and without risk of injury to nurses.
c. Patient unable to assist:	
(1) Use three nurses and appropriate safe-handling device (e.g., ceiling lift with supine sling or floor-based lift) to move and position patient (Martin et al., 2016).	Repositioning patients manually is associated with high risk of musculoskeletal injury (Matz et al., 2019; OSHA, n.d.b).

CLINICAL JUDGMENT: *Protect patient's heels from shearing force by having another caregiver lift heels while moving patient up in bed.*

4. Position patient in bed in one of the following positions while ensuring correct body alignment. In all cases protect pressure areas. Follow weight guidelines and level of assistance to determine number of nurses needed to position patient.	Prevents injury to patient's musculoskeletal system and integument. Even positioning patient side to side requires use of safe patient handling and mobility (SPHM) techniques.
a. Determine if patient can assist.	Determines degree of risk in repositioning patient and the technique required to safely help patient.
b. For a patient who can assist fully, begin by having patient lie supine and move up in bed following Steps 3a(1)–(3).	Research supports use of mechanical lifts to prevent musculoskeletal injuries (Matz et al., 2019; OSHA, n.d.a).
For a patient only partially able to assist in assuming supine position, follow Steps 3b(3)i–vi.	
For a patient unable to assist in assuming a supine position, follow Step 3c(1).	
c. **Supported semi-Fowler Position** (see illustration) or **Fowler position**:	
(1) With patient lying supine, elevate head of bed 45 to 60 degrees if not contraindicated.	Increases comfort, improves ventilation, and increases patient's opportunity to socialize or relax.
(2) Rest head against mattress or on small pillow.	Prevents flexion contractures of cervical vertebrae.

Continued

SKILL 39.1   MOVING AND POSITIONING PATIENTS IN BED—cont'd

STEPS	RATIONALE
(3) Use pillows to support arms and hands if patient does not have voluntary control or use of hands and arms.	Prevents shoulder dislocation from effect of downward pull of unsupported arms, promotes circulation by preventing venous pooling, and prevents flexion contractures of arms and wrists.
(4) Position small pillow at lower back.	Supports lumbar vertebrae and decreases flexion of vertebrae.
(5) Place pillows longwise under each leg (midthigh to ankle) to support the knee in slight flexion (avoids hyperextension) and to allow the heels to float.	Prevents hyperextension of knee and occlusion of popliteal artery from pressure from body weight. Heels should not be in contact with bed. Floating heels prevents prolonged pressure of mattress on heels.

d. Patient with hemiplegia placed in supported semi-Fowler or Fowler position:

CLINICAL JUDGMENT: *A patient who has hemiplegia (e.g., from a cerebrovascular accident [CVA] or spinal cord injury) may have problems with muscle tone that could affect your ability to position appropriately. Consider consulting with physical therapist or occupational therapist for special limb braces.*

STEPS	RATIONALE
(1) Elevate head of bed 30 to 60 degrees according to patient's condition. For example, those with increased risk for pressure injury remain at 30-degree angle (see Chapter 48).	Increases comfort, improves ventilation, and increases patient's opportunity to relax.
(2) Position patient in semi-Fowler (Step 4c) or Fowler position as anatomically straight as possible.	Counteracts tendency to slump toward affected side. Improves ventilation and cardiac output; decreases intracranial pressure. Improves patient's ability to swallow and helps prevent aspiration of food, liquids, and gastric secretions.
(3) Position head on small pillow with chin slightly forward. If patient is totally unable to control head movement, avoid hyperextension of neck.	Prevents hyperextension of neck. Too many pillows under head may cause or worsen neck flexion contracture.
(4) Provide support for involved arm and hand by placing arm away from patient's side and supporting elbow with pillow.	Paralyzed muscles do not automatically resist pull of gravity as they do normally. As a result, shoulder subluxation, pain, and edema may occur.
(5) Place rolled blanket (trochanter roll) or pillows firmly alongside patient's legs to help prevent the patient from leaning toward the affected side.	Ensures proper alignment. Prevents external rotation of hips, which contributes to muscle contractures.
(6) Support feet in dorsiflexion with therapeutic boots, splints, or sandbag (see illustration).	Prevents plantar flexion contractures or foot drop by positioning patient's ankle in neutral dorsiflexion. Positions foot so heel is aligned in opening of splint to prevent pressure. Other therapeutic boots or splints are manufactured with thick padding to cushion heel and prevent pressure injury.

e. Supported supine position:

STEPS	RATIONALE
(1) Place patient supine with head of bed flat.	Necessary for properly aligning patient.
(2) Place small rolled towel under lumbar area of back.	Provides support for lumbar spine.
(3) Place pillow under upper shoulders, neck, and head.	Maintains correct alignment and prevents flexion contractures of cervical vertebrae.
(4) Place trochanter rolls or sandbags parallel to lateral surface of patient's thighs.	Reduces external rotation of hip.
(5) Place patient's feet in therapeutic boots or splints.	Maintains feet in dorsiflexion. Prevents plantar flexion contractures or foot drop.
(6) Place pillows under pronated forearms, keeping upper arms parallel to patient's body (see illustration).	Reduces internal rotation of shoulder and prevents extension of elbows. Maintains correct body alignment.
(7) Place hand rolls in patient's hands. Consider physical therapy referral for use of hand splints.	Reduces extension of fingers and abduction of thumb. Maintains thumb slightly adducted and in opposition to fingers.

STEP 4c Supported semi-Fowler position.

STEP 4d(6) Foot boot with lower leg extension.

STEPS	RATIONALE

STEP 4e(6) Supported supine position with pillows in place.

f. Position **patient with hemiplegia in supine position:**

(1) Place head of bed flat.

(2) Place folded towel or small pillow under shoulder of affected side.

(3) Keep affected arm away from body with elbow extended and palm up. Position affected hand in one of recommended positions for flaccid or spastic hand. (Alternative is to place arm out to side, with elbow bent and hand toward head of bed.)

(4) Place folded towel under hip of involved side.

(5) Flex affected knee 30 degrees by supporting it on pillow or folded blanket.

(6) Support feet with soft pillows placed against sole of feet at right angle to leg.

g. Position patient in **30-degree lateral (side-lying) position** (Example using two nurses):

(1) Lower head of bed completely or as low as patient can tolerate. One nurse on each side of bed.

(2) Lower side rails and position patient on side of bed in opposite direction toward which patient is to be turned using an FRD. Move upper trunk, supporting shoulders first; then move lower trunk, supporting hips.

(3) Flex the patient's knee that will not be next to mattress after being turned, and keep that foot on mattress. Nurse on side to which patient is to be turned places one hand on patient's upper bent leg near hip and other hand on patient's shoulder.

(4) Using knee and hip for leverage, nurse rolls patient onto side.

(5) Place pillow under patient's head and neck.

(6) Nurse facing patient's back places hands under patient's dependent shoulder and gently brings shoulder blade forward.

(7) Position both of patient's arms in slightly flexed position. Support upper arm with pillow level with shoulder; position other arm comfortably against chest or abdomen or behind head.

(8) Nurse facing patient's back places hands under dependent hip and brings hip slightly forward so angle from hip to mattress is approximately 30 degrees.

(9) Place small tuck-back pillow behind patient's back. (Make by folding pillow lengthwise. Smooth area is slightly tucked under patient's back.)

(10) Place pillows under semiflexed upper leg level at hip from groin to foot (see illustration).

(11) *Option:* Place pillows or sandbags (if available) parallel against plantar surface of dependent foot. May also use AFO device on feet if available.

RATIONALE

Necessary for positioning in supine position.

Decreases possibility of pain, joint contracture, and subluxation. Maintains mobility in muscles around shoulder to permit normal movement patterns.

Maintains mobility in arm, joints, and shoulder to permit normal movement patterns. (Alternative position counteracts limitation of ability of arm to rotate outward at shoulder [external rotation]. External rotation must be present to raise arm overhead without pain.)

Diminishes effect of spasticity in entire leg by controlling hip position.

Slight flexion breaks up abnormal extension pattern of leg. Extensor spasticity is most severe when patient is supine.

Maintains foot in dorsiflexion and prevents foot drop. Pillows prevent stimulation to ball of foot by hard surface, which has tendency to increase muscle tone in patient with extensor spasticity of lower extremity.

This position is recommended to prevent development of pressure injuries by reducing direct contact of trochanter with support surface (see Chapter 48).

Provides position of comfort for patient and removes pressure from bony prominences on back.

Provides room for patient to turn to side.

Use of leverage makes turning to side easy.

Rolling decreases trauma to tissues. In addition, patient is positioned so leverage on hip makes turning easy.

Maintains alignment. Reduces lateral neck flexion. Decreases strain on sternocleidomastoid muscle.

Prevents patient's weight from resting directly on shoulder joint.

Decreases internal rotation and adduction of shoulder. Supporting both arms in slightly flexed position protects joint. Ventilation improves because chest is able to expand more easily.

The 30-degree lateral position reduces pressure on trochanter; designed to prevent pressure injury.

Provides support to maintain patient on side.

Flexion prevents hyperextension of leg. Maintains leg in correct alignment. Prevents pressure on bony prominences.

Maintains dorsiflexion of foot.

Continued

SKILL 39.1	MOVING AND POSITIONING PATIENTS IN BED—cont'd
STEPS	**RATIONALE**

STEP 4g(10) Thirty-degree lateral position with pillows in place.

h. **Logroll patient** (Example using three nurses):

> **CLINICAL JUDGMENT:** *A registered nurse supervises and helps AP when there is a health care provider's order to logroll a patient. Patients with spinal cord injuries or who are recovering from neck, back, or spinal surgery need to keep the spinal column in straight alignment to prevent further injury.*

STEPS	RATIONALE
(1) Place small pillow between patient's knees.	Prevents tension on spinal column and adduction of hip.
(2) Cross patient's arms on chest.	Prevents injury to arms.
(3) Position two nurses on side toward which patient is to be turned and one nurse on side where pillows are to be placed behind patient's back. This nurse also supports patient's neck as needed (see illustration).	Distributes weight equally between nurses during turning. Prevents lateral flexion of patient's neck if muscles are weakened.
(4) Fanfold drawsheet along backside of patient.	Provides strong handles for nurses to grip drawsheet without slipping.
(5) With one nurse grasping drawsheet at lower hips and thighs and the other nurse grasping drawsheet at patient's shoulders and lower back, roll patient as one unit in a smooth, continuous motion on count of 3 (see illustration).	Maintains proper alignment by moving all body parts at the same time, preventing tension or twisting of spinal column.
(6) Nurse on opposite side of bed places pillows along length of patient for support (see illustration).	Maintains patient in side-lying position.
(7) Gently lean patient as a unit back toward pillows for support (see illustration). Place patient's feet in therapeutic boots or splints.	Ensures continued straight alignment of spinal column, preventing injury. Prevents foot drop.

STEP 4h(3) Preparing patient for logroll.

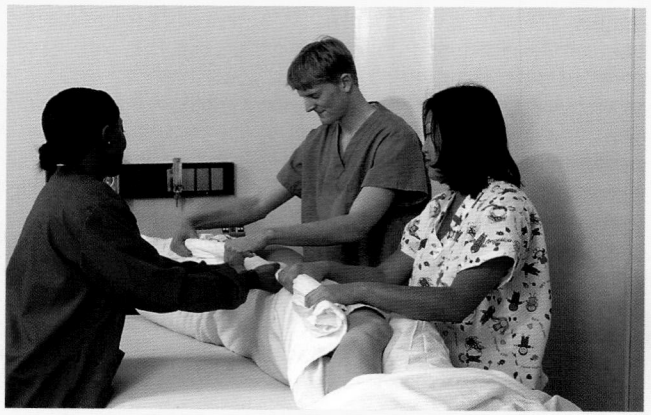

STEP 4h(5) Move patient as a unit, logrolling onto side.

STEPS	RATIONALE

STEP 4h(6) Place pillows along patient's back for support.

STEP 4h(7) As a unit, gently lean patient against pillows.

5. Be sure patient feels comfortable in new position.
6. Place nurse call system in an accessible location within patient's reach.
7. Raise side rails (as appropriate) and lower bed to lowest position.
8. Dispose of any contaminated supplies in appropriate receptacle. Perform hand hygiene.

Gives patient sense of well-being.
Ensures patient can call for assistance if needed.
Promotes patient safety.
Reduces transmission of microorganisms.

EVALUATION

1. Assess patient's respiratory status, body alignment, position, and level of comfort on an ongoing basis. Patient's body should be supported by adequate mattress, and vertebral column should be without observable curves.

Determines effectiveness of positioning and patient's tolerance. Additional supports (e.g., pillows, bath blankets) may be added or removed to promote comfort and correct body alignment.

CLINICAL JUDGMENT: *Ongoing evaluation and patient feedback is critical, as patient is usually in best position to indicate when developing symptoms require repositioning.*

2. Observe for changes in joint ROM.
3. Observe for areas of erythema or breakdown involving skin (see Chapter 48).

Early identification of muscle contracture development is critical.
Provides ongoing observation regarding patient's skin and musculoskeletal systems. Indicates complications of immobility or improper positioning of body part.

4. **Use Teach-Back:** "I want to be sure I explained the steps we are going to use to move and position you in bed. Please repeat the steps you can follow to help us move you up in bed." Revise your instruction now or develop a plan for revised patient or family caregiver teaching if patient or family caregiver is not able to teach back correctly.

Teach-back is an evidence-based health literacy intervention that promotes patient engagement, patient safety, adherence, and quality. The goal of teach-back is to ensure that you have explained medical information clearly so that patients and their families understand what you communicated to them (AHRQ, 2020).

UNEXPECTED OUTCOMES AND RELATED INTERVENTIONS

1. Joint contractures develop or worsen.
   - Increase frequency of ROM exercises to affected and immobilized areas (see Chapter 38).
   - Consider physical therapy consultation for different positioning.
2. Skin shows localized areas of erythema and breakdown.
   - Increase frequency of repositioning.
   - Use a different FRD.
   - Place a turning schedule above patient's bed.
3. Patient avoids moving.
   - Medicate with analgesia as ordered by health care provider to ensure patient's comfort before moving.
   - Allow pain medication to take effect before repositioning.

▌ KEY POINTS

- Injuries or disease processes that affect coordination and regulation of muscle groups pathologically influence mobility.
- Periods of immobility due to disability or injury or prolonged bed rest during hospitalization cause major physiological, psychological, and social effects; the greater the extent and the longer the duration of immobility, the more pronounced the consequences.

- Immobility increases the risk of skin breakdown and is also directly related to the development of deep vein thrombosis (DVT) and pulmonary embolus (PE).
- Immobility can negatively affect the ability to complete daily activities and can lead to boredom and social isolation.
- Clinical judgment in your approach to caring for patients who are immobilized is complicated. Anticipate the physical effects of any restrictions in movement caused by a sudden illness or injury and

apply knowledge of a patient's preexisting health conditions so you can consider a broad number of potential complications.

- Observe the appearance of extremities and measure the range of motion (ROM) of joints in various body positions to assess for correct body alignment and mobility.
- Critical analysis of all assessment data and comparing findings with the anticipated effects of mobility alterations reveal patterns of data indicating nursing diagnoses.
- Understanding what a patient can physically do compared with what the patient potentially and realistically can achieve helps you set realistic patient-centered outcomes for the plan of care.
- Patients with impaired body alignment and mobility require the use of correct positioning techniques.
- Working collaboratively with health care providers, a nurse will identify patient risk factors for DVT and employ nursing interventions that reduce risk, such as early ambulation; leg, foot, and ankle exercises; regularly provided fluids; and frequent position changes.
- When a care plan includes interventions designed to prevent complications of immobility, compare a patient's baseline with the signs and symptoms of complications for which the patient is most at risk.

REFLECTIVE LEARNING

- You are a home health nurse. You are seeing a patient for the first time for a home health visit. You know the patient had a stroke affecting her right side. As you enter the patient's home, your initial assessment finds the patient to be female, age 78, with weakness in both arms and legs on the right side. The patient walks over to her chair in the living room using a walker, and the patient's posture is stooped. The patient tells you she is happy you came to see her and wants you to help her with her medications. What assessment information in this patient situation is the most important and of immediate concern for the patient's safety? (Recognize Cues)
- Regarding your immediate concern for the patient above, what additional information in the case example might you want to further assess and what nursing diagnosis do you see as possibly the most relevant for this patient? (Analyze Cues)
- You further assess the patient and learn that she fell at home 2 weeks ago without sustaining an injury. The patient wears glasses and has some decline in hearing. The patient shows you the five medications she is currently taking. You ask the patient to read the labels and find that she cannot explain when are the best times to take each medication dose. Considering diagnoses for *Risk for Falls* and *Complex Medication Regimen*, which diagnosis is most urgent? In what way are the diagnoses possibly related? (Prioritize Diagnoses)
- Considering the case study patient above, what outcomes might you select for each nursing diagnosis: *Risk for Falls* and *Complex Medication Regimen*? (Generate Solutions)
- Identify interventions to implement for this patient in the case study based on the outcomes you selected. Explain how you chose interventions based on what you know about the patient. Is there a particular intervention that is more of a priority? (Take Action)
- What measures would you use to evaluate whether the patient met the outcomes of care selected? (Evaluate Outcomes)

REVIEW QUESTIONS

1. A patient has been hospitalized with a serious flulike infection and is on bed rest. He is receiving multiple medications through two different IV infusions and is on high-flow oxygen therapy by oxygen mask. Currently the patient's head of bed is elevated to semi-Fowler position. The patient initiates little movement and responds only to being shaken. Vitals signs are temperature, 38.6°C (101.6°F); heart rate, 88 beats/min; blood pressure 140/84 mm Hg; and respirations, 20. Which of the following assessment findings suggest that the patient has a risk for an immobility complication? (Select all that apply.)
   1. High-flow oxygen therapy by mask
   2. Positioned semi-Fowler
   3. Temperature 38.6°C (101.6°F)
   4. Receiving multiple medications
   5. Initiates little movement
   6. Reduced conscious response
   7. Bed rest
2. A nurse is caring for a patient who was in an auto accident and has entered rehab after a 6-day hospitalization. The patient had multiple internal injuries and has nursing diagnoses of *Hopelessness* and *Impaired Mobility* at time of discharge. The nurse's assessment revealed the patient asking nurses to let him stay in bed and the patient having limited involvement in hygiene and a loss of appetite. The patient has a cast on his nondominant left hand and has reduced movement in the right lower leg, which is splinted. The health care provider has ordered the patient to ambulate 3 times a day. Which of the following is a priority for the rehab nurse?
   1. Providing assistance with meals
   2. Teaching patient exercises to strengthen right leg
   3. Making preferred hygiene products available to the patient to use
   4. Setting times to discuss relationship of hopelessness to injuries
3. A patient has been on bed rest for over 5 days. Which of these findings during the nurse's assessment may indicate a complication of immobility?
   1. Decreased peristalsis
   2. Decreased heart rate
   3. Increased blood pressure
   4. Increased urinary output
4. Place the following steps in the correct order for repositioning a patient in the 30-degree lateral side-lying position using two nurses.
   1. Using knee and hip for leverage, nurse rolls patient onto side.
   2. Nurse facing patient's back places hands under patient's dependent shoulder and brings shoulder blade forward.
   3. Place pillows under semiflexed upper leg level at hip from groin to foot.
   4. Flex patient's knee that will not be next to mattress, after being turned. Keep foot on mattress. Nurse places one hand on patient's upper bent leg.
   5. Place hands under dependent hip and bring hip slightly forward so angle from hip to mattress is approximately 30 degrees.
   6. Position patient on side of bed in opposite direction toward which patient is to be turned, then move upper and lower trunk.
   7. Lower head of bed completely or as low as patient can tolerate. One nurse on each side of bed.
5. The effects of immobility on the cardiac system include which of the following? (Select all that apply.)
   1. Thrombus formation
   2. Increased cardiac workload
   3. Weak peripheral pulses
   4. Irregular heartbeat
   5. Orthostatic hypotension

6. A 46-year-old patient is admitted to the emergency department following an automobile accident. The patient has a pelvic fracture and is ordered on bed rest and placed in an immobilization device to limit further injury until the fracture can safely be repaired. Which measures are appropriate for this patient to prevent complications of bed rest? (Select all that apply.)
   1. Administer IV analgesic as ordered.
   2. Have patient perform incentive spirometry.
   3. Support patient in active assisted ROM exercises of upper extremities.
   4. Provide patient a low-calorie diet.
   5. Apply SCDs to legs.

7. A patient has an order for application of compression stockings. Place the following steps for application of the compression stockings in the correct order:
   1. Place patient's toes into foot of stocking up to the heel; keep smooth.
   2. Use tape measure to measure patient's leg for proper stocking size.
   3. Slide stocking up over patient's calf until sock is completely extended.
   4. Turn elastic stocking inside out, keeping hand inside holding heel. Take other hand and pull stocking inside out until reaching the heel.
   5. Slide remaining portion of stocking over patient's foot, covering toes. Be sure foot fits into toe and heel of stocking.

8. An older-adult patient is admitted following a hip fracture and surgical repair. Before ambulating the patient postoperatively on the evening of surgery, which of the following would be most important to assess? (Select all that apply.)
   1. Patient's usual exercise pattern at home
   2. Time and date of the patient's last bowel movement
   3. Preadmission activity tolerance
   4. Baseline heart rate and blood pressure
   5. Patient's home living situation

9. A nurse is helping a patient perform active assisted ROM in the right elbow. Which statement describes the correct technique?
   1. Support elbow by holding distal part of extremity.
   2. Grasp joint with fingers to provide support.
   3. Have patient move joint independently.
   4. Move the joint past the point of resistance.
   5. Perform the exercise three times during the session, and gradually build up to more.

10. A middle-aged adult patient has limited mobility following a total knee arthroplasty. During assessment, the nurse notes that the patient is having difficulty breathing while lying supine. Which assessment data support a pulmonary issue related to immobility? (Select all that apply.)
    1. Oxygen saturation of 89%
    2. Irregular radial pulse
    3. Diminished breath sounds in bilateral bases of lungs
    4. Blood pressure 132/84 mm Hg
    5. Pain reported at 3 on scale of 0 to 10 following medication
    6. Respiratory rate of 26

Answers: 1. 1, 3, 5, 6; **7.** 2, 4; **3.** 1; **4.** 7, 6, 4, 1, 2, 5, 3; **5.** 1, 2, 5; **6.** 1, 2, 5; **2.** 3, 5; **7.** 2, 4, 1, 5, 3; **8.** 3, 4; **9.** 1; **10.** 1, 3, 6.

Rationales for Review Questions can be found on the Evolve website.

REFERENCES

Ackley BJ, Ladwig GB: *Nursing diagnosis handbook: an evidence-based guide to planning care*, ed 12, St Louis, 2019, Elsevier.

Agency for Healthcare Research and Quality (AHRQ): *Health Literacy Universal Precautions Toolkit*, ed 2, Rockville, MD, 2020, Agency for Healthcare Research and Quality. https://www.ahrq.gov/health-literacy/quality-resources/tools/literacy-toolkit/healthlittoolkit2-tool5.html. Accessed August 8, 2021.

American Academy of Nursing (AAN): *Twenty-five things nurses and patients should question*, 2018. https://higherlogicdownload.s3.amazonaws.com/AANNET/c8a8da9e-918c-4dae-b0c6-6d630c46007f/UploadedImages/AAN_Nursing-Choosing-Wisely-List__11_19_18_.pdf. Accessed August 1, 2021.

American Association of Critical-Care Nurses (AACN): *ICUs turn to prone positioning for patients with ARDS*, 2019. https://www.aacn.org/newsroom/icus-turn-to-prone-positioning-for-patients-with-ards. Accessed August 8, 2021.

American Heart Association: *What is venous thromboembolism? VTE?* 2017a. https://www.heart.org/en/health-topics/venous-thromboembolism/what-is-venous-thromboembolism-vte. Accessed August 7, 2021.

American Heart Association (AHA): *Risk factors for venous thromboembolism (VTE)*. 2017b. https://www.heart.org/en/health-topics/venous-thromboembolism/risk-factors-for-venous-thromboembolism-vte. Accessed August 7, 2021.

American Psychiatric Association (APA): *Diagnostic and statistical manual of mental disorders*, ed 5, Arlington, VA, 2013, American Psychiatric Publishing.

American Psychological Association: *Rehabilitation psychology*, 2015. https://www.apa.org/ed/graduate/specialize/rehabilitation. Accessed August 8, 2021.

Ayello EA: CMS MDS 3.0 section M skin conditions in long-term care: pressure ulcers, skin tears, and moisture-associated skin damage data update, *Adv Skin Wound Care* 30(9):415–429, 2017.

Ball JE, et al: *Seidel's guide to physical examination*, ed 9, St Louis, 2019, Elsevier.

Barbour KE, et al: Vital signs: prevalence of doctor-diagnosed arthritis and arthritis-attributable activity limitation—United States, 2013–2015, *MMWR Morb Mortal Wkly Rep* 66(9):246–253, 2017.

Barnes-Daly MA, et al: Improving health care for critically ill patients using an evidence-based collaborative approach to the ABCDEF bundle dissemination and implementation. *Worldviews Evid Based Nurs* 15(3):206–216, 2018.

Bienenfeld D: *Screening tests for depression*, 2018, MedScape. https://emedicine.medscape.com/article/1859039-overview. Accessed August 7, 2021.

Biswas D, et al: Role of nurses and nurse practitioners in the recognition, diagnosis, and management of neurogenic orthostatic hypotension: a narrative review, *Int J Gen Med* 12:173–184, 2019.

Bodenheimer T: Teach-back: a simple technique to enhance patients' understanding, *Fam Pract Manag* 25(4):20–22, 2018. Available at: https://www.aafp.org/fpm/2018/0700/p20.html. Accessed August 7, 2021.

Bonkowski SL, et al: Evaluation of a pain management education program and operational guideline on nursing practice, attitudes, and pain management, *J Contin Educ Nurs* 49(4):178–185, 2018.

Centers for Disease Control and Prevention (CDC): *Disabilities and limitations*, 2019, https://www.cdc.gov/arthritis/data_statistics/disabilities-limitations.htm. Accessed August 8, 2021.

Centers for Disease Control and Prevention (CDC): *What is health literacy*, 2021. https://www.cdc.gov/healthliteracy/learn/index.html. Accessed August 8, 2021.

Centrella-Nigro A, Alexander C: Using the teach-back method in patient education to improve patient satisfaction, *J Contin Educ Nurs* 48(1):47–52, 2017.

Cleveland Clinic: *Deep Vein Thrombosis (DVT)*, 2019. https://my.clevelandclinic.org/health/diseases/16911-deep-vein-thrombosis-dvt. Accessed August 16, 2021.

Dickinson S, et al: Integrating a standardized mobility program and safe patient handling, *Crit Care Nurs Q* 41(3):240–252, 2018.

Good Therapy: *Psycho-physical therapy*, 2016. https://www.goodtherapy.org/learn-about-therapy/types/psycho-physical-therapy. Accessed August 8, 2021.

Gupta MJ, et al: Rush fracture liaison service for capturing "missed opportunities" to treat osteoporosis in patients with fragility fractures. *Osteoporos Int* 29(8):1861–1874, 2018.

Harding MH, et al: *Lewis' medical-surgical nursing*, ed 11, St Louis, 2020, Elsevier.

Huether SE, et al: *Understanding pathophysiology*, ed 7, St. Louis, 2020, Elsevier.

Kruschke C, Butcher HK: Evidence-based practice guideline: fall prevention for older adults. *J Gerontol Nurs* 43(11):15–21, 2017.

Knight J, et al: Effects of bedrest 3: gastrointestinal, endocrine and nervous systems. *Nursing Times* 115:(2):50–53, 2018.

Link T: Guideline implementation: prevention of venous thromboembolism, *AORN J* 107(6):737–748, 2018.

Loeser RF: *Pathogenesis of osteoarthritis*, 2020, Up to Date. https://www.uptodate.com/contents/pathogenesis-of-osteoarthritis. Accessed July 30, 2021.

Makic MBF: Prone position of patients with COVID-19 and acute respiratory distress syndrome, *J Perianesth Nurs* 35(4):437–438, 2020.

Martin M, et al: *New and improved VA algorithms*, 2016. https://view.officeapps.live.com/op/view.aspx?src =https%3A%2F%2Fasphp.org%2Fwp-content%2Fupl oads%2F2016%2F06%2FNew-and-Improved-VA-Algorithms-and-New-SPHM-App-ASPHP-rev-MMM. pptx. Accessed August 17, 2021.

Matz M, et al: *Patient handling and mobility assessments*, ed 2, 2019, The Facility Guidelines Institute. http:// www.fgiguidelines.org/wp-content/uploads/2019/10/ FGI-Patient-Handling-and-Mobility-Assessments_191008. pdf. Accessed August 8, 2021.

McCance KL, Huether SE: *Pathophysiology: the biologic basis for disease in adults and children*, ed 8, St Louis, 2019, Elsevier.

Mulkey MA, et al: Choosing the right delirium assessment tool, *J Neurosci Nurs* 50(6):343–348, 2018.

Musich S, et al: The impact of mobility limitations on health outcomes among older adults, *Geriatr Nurs* 39(2):162–169, 2018.

National Institutes of Health (NIH): *NIH Research Matters - Physical activity may reduce depression symptoms*, 2019. https://www.nih.gov/news-events/nih-research-matters/physical-activity-helps-reduce-depression-symptoms. Accessed August 7, 2021.

Occupational Safety and Health Administration (OSHA): *Safe patient handling*, n.d.a. https://www.osha.gov/ SLTC/healthcarefacilities/safepatienthandling.html. Accessed July 14, 2020.

Occupational Safety and Health Administration (OSHA): *Ergonomics*, n.d.b. https://www.osha.gov/SLTC/etools/ hospital/hazards/ergo/ergo.html#residenthandling program. Accessed August 8, 2021.

Olinsky C, Norton CE: Implementation of a safe patient handling program in a multihospital health system from inception to sustainability, *Workplace Health Saf* 65(11):546–559, 2017.

Seidel BJ, et al: Contractures, 2020, PM & R Knowledge Now. https://now.aapmr.org/contractures/. Accessed August 16, 2021.

Stephens M, et al: Developing the tissue viability seating guidelines, *J Tissue Viability* 27(1):74–79, 2018.

The Joint Commission (TJC): *2021 National patient safety goals*, Oakbrook Terrace, IL, 2021, The Commission. https://www.jointcommission.org/en/ standards/national-patient-safety-goals/. Accessed August 7, 2021.

The Joint Commission (TJC): Non-pharmacologic and non-opioid solutions for pain management, *Quick Safety* (44), 2018. https://www.jointcommission.org/-/ media/tjc/documents/resources/painmanagement/qs_ nonopioid_pain_mgmt_8_15_18_final1.pdf. Accessed August 8, 2021.

Tick H, et al: Evidence-based nonpharmacologic strategies for comprehensive pain care: the Consortium Pain Task Force white paper, *Explore (NY)* 14(3):177–211, 2018.

U.S. Bureau of Labor Statistics: *Monthly Labor Review - Occupational injuries and illnesses among registered nurses*, 2018. https://www.bls.gov/opub/mlr/2018/ article/occupational-injuries-and-illnesses-among-registered-nurses.htm. Accessed August 7, 2021.

U.S. Department Veterans Affairs: *Safe patient handling app*, n.d. https://mobile.va.gov/app/safe-patient-han-dling. Accessed August 7, 2021.

Wald HL, et al: The case for mobility assessment in hospitalized older adults: American Geriatric Society white paper executive summary, *J Am Geriatr Soc* 67(1):11, 2019.

Weinberger J, Cipolle M: Mechanical prophylaxis for post-traumatic VTE: stockings and pumps, *Curr Trauma Rep* 2(1):35–41, 2016.

Winterton MT, Baldwin K: The neuro-orthopedic approach, *Phys Med Rehabil Clin N Am* 29(3):567–591, 2018.

RESEARCH REFERENCES

Agency for Healthcare Research and Quality (AHRQ): *Preventing pressure ulcers in hospitals: a toolkit for improving quality of care*, 2014. https://www.ahrq.gov/ patient-safety/settings/hospital/resource/pressureulcer/ tool/index.html. Accessed August 1, 2021.

American Society of Hematology (ASH): *Clinicians: ASH clinical practice guidelines on venous thromboembolism*, 2021. https://www.hematology.org/education/clinicians/ guidelines-and-quality-care/clinical-practice-guidelines/venous-thromboembolism-guidelines. Accessed August 16, 2021.

Anderson D, et al: American Society of Hematology 2019 guidelines for management of venous thromboembolism: prevention of venous thromboembolism in surgical hospitalized patients, *Blood Adv* 3(23):3898–3944, 2019.

Bahloul M, et al: Impact of prone position on outcomes of COVID-19 patients with spontaneous breathing, *Acute Crit Care* 36:208–214, 2021, doi:10.4266/acc.2021.00500.

Berlowitz D: *Prevention of pressure-induced skin and soft tissue injury*, 2020, UpToDate. https://www.uptodate. com/contents/clinical-staging-and-management-of-pressure-induced-skin-and-soft-tissue-injury. Accessed August 1, 2021.

Capri T, et al: The TCTRS Project: a holistic approach for tele-rehabilitation in Rett syndrome, *Electronics* 9(3):491, 2020.

Chase JD, et al: Identifying factors associated with mobility decline among hospitalized older adults, *Clin Nurs Res* 27(1):81–104, 2018.

Fang Y, et al: Patient and family member factors influencing outcomes of poststroke inpatient rehabilitation, *Arch Phys Med Rehabil* 98(2):249-255.e2, 2017.

Francis J, Young G: *Diagnosis of delirium and confusional states*, 2020, UpToDate. https://www.uptodate.com/ contents/diagnosis-of-delirium-and-confusional-states. Accessed August 7, 2021.

Hallford DJ, et al: The association between anxiety and falls: a meta-analysis, *J Gerontol B Psychol Sci Soc Sci* 72(5):729–741, 2017.

Heflin M: *Geriatric health maintenance*, 2021, UpToDate. https://www.uptodate.com/contents/geriatric-health-maintenance. Accessed August 1, 2021.

Kanaskie ML, Snyder C: Nurses and nursing assistants decision-making regarding use of safe patient handling and mobility technology: a qualitative study, *Appl Nurs Res* 39:141–147, 2018.

Klein LM, et al: Increasing patient mobility through an individualized goal-centered hospital mobility program: a quasi-experimental quality improvement project, *Nurs Outlook* 66(3):254–262, 2018.

Kramer A, et al: How to prevent the detrimental effects of two months of bed-rest on muscle, bone and cardiovascular system: an RCT, *Sci Rep* 7:13177, 2017.

Krupp A, et al: A systematic review evaluating the role of nurses and processes for delivering early mobility interventions in the intensive care unit, *Intensive Crit Care Nurs* 47:30–38, 2018.

Lafrenière S, et al: Strategies used by older patients to prevent functional decline during hospitalization, *Clin Nurs Res* 26(1):6–26, 2017.

Lip GYH, Hull RD: *Overview of the treatment of lower extremity deep vein thrombosis (DVT)*, 2021, UpToDate. https://www.uptodate.com/contents/overview-of-the-treatment-of-lower-extremity-deep-vein-thrombosis-dvt. Accessed August 7, 2021.

Mattison M: *Hospital management of older adults*, 2021, UpToDate. https://www.uptodate.com/contents/ hospital-management-of-older-adults/print. Accessed August 1, 2021.

Meyers T: Prevention of heel pressure injuries and plantar flexion contractures with use of a heel protector in high-risk neurotrauma, medical, and surgical intensive care units: a randomized controlled trial, *J Wound Ostomy Continence Nurs* 44(5):429, 2017.

Modi S, et al: Wells criteria for DVT is a reliable clinical tool to assess the risk of deep venous thrombosis in trauma patients, *World J Emerg Surg* 11:24, 2016.

Nelson A, Baptiste AS: Evidence-based practices for safe patient handling and movement, *Orthop Nurs* 25(6):366, 2006.

Noble NL, Sweeney NL: Barriers to the use of assistive devices in patient handling, *Workplace Health Saf* 66(1):41–48, 2018.

Odgaard L, et al: Nursing sensitive outcomes after severe traumatic brain injury: a nationwide study, *J Neurosci Nurs* 50(3):149–156, 2018.

Saal S, et al: Interventions for the prevention and treatment of disability due to acquired joint contractures in older people: a systematic review, *Age and Ageing* 46(3): 373–382, 2017.

Shen J, et al: Comparison of the Wells score with the revised Geneva score for assessing suspected pulmonary embolism: a systematic review and meta-analysis, *J Thromb Thrombolysis* 41(3):482–492, 2016.

Teeple E, et al: Outcomes of safe patient handling and mobilization programs: a meta-analysis, *Work* 58(2):173–184, 2017.

Thompson BT, et al: *Clinical presentation, evaluation, and diagnosis of the nonpregnant adult with suspected acute pulmonary embolism*, 2021, UpToDate. https://www. uptodate.com/contents/clinical-presentation-evaluation-and-diagnosis-of-the-nonpregnant-adult-with-suspected-acute-pulmonary-embolism?topicRef= 8253&source=see_link. Accessed August 16, 2021.

Wells PS, et al: Use of a clinical model for safe management of patients with suspected pulmonary embolism, *Ann Intern Med* 1998;129:997-1005. doi:10.7326/0003-4819-129-12-199812150-00002.

Yuan P, et al: Vestibular brain changes within 70 days of head down bed rest, *Hum Brain Mapp* 39(7):2753–2763, 2018.

Zhang DZ, et al: Effect of intermittent pneumatic compression on preventing deep vein thrombosis among stroke patients: a systematic review and meta-analysis, *Worldviews Evid Based Nurs* 15(3):189–196, 2018.

Hygiene

OBJECTIVES

- Outline factors that influence personal hygiene practices.
- Discuss how a nurse applies clinical judgment when assessing patients' hygiene problems.
- Assess a patient's total hygiene needs.
- Discuss conditions that place patients at risk for impaired skin integrity.
- Discuss factors that influence the condition of the nails and feet.
- Explain the importance of foot care for the patient with diabetes mellitus.
- Discuss conditions that place patients at risk for impaired oral mucous membranes.
- Summarize common hair and scalp problems and their related interventions.
- Explain how hygiene care for the older adult patient differs from that for the younger patient.
- Explain how clinical judgment is used to implement patient-centered interventions to maintain a patient's comfort and safety during hygiene care.
- Discuss how to adapt hygiene care for a patient who is cognitively impaired.
- Demonstrate hygiene procedures for the care of the skin, perineum, feet and nails, mouth, eyes, ears, and nose.

KEY TERMS

Alopecia

Cerumen

Cheilitis

Complete bed bath

Dental caries

Edentulous

Effleurage

Gingivitis

Glossitis

Halitosis

Maceration

Mucositis

Partial bed bath

Pediculosis capitis

Perineal care

Stomatitis

Xerostomia

MEDIA RESOURCES

http://evolve.elsevier.com/Potter/fundamentals/

- Review Questions
- Video Clips
- Concept Map Creator
- Case Study with Questions

- Skills Performance Checklists
- Audio Glossary
- Content Updates
- Answers to QSEN Activity and Review Questions

Mrs. White is 78 years old and is a resident of an assisted-living facility. She is admitted to the hospital for a colon resection. She also has rheumatoid arthritis, diabetes mellitus, hypertension, and a body mass index (BMI) of 40. The arthritis has resulted in chronic pain and deformity in her hands and knees. The pain and joint deformity have caused Mrs. White to have limited ability to use her hands. She lives alone, but her granddaughter is going to nursing school and has offered to help when her grandmother returns to her residence. Jamie Johnson is a first-semester nursing student assigned to care for Mrs. White.

Personal hygiene influences patients' comfort, safety, and well-being. Hygiene includes cleaning and grooming activities that maintain personal body cleanliness and appearance. A variety of personal, emotional, social, economic, environmental, and cultural factors influence hygiene practices. Because hygiene care requires close contact with your patients, use communication skills (e.g., listening, reflecting, focusing) to promote caring therapeutic relationships (see Chapter 24). When providing hygiene, integrate other nursing activities. For example, perform ongoing patient assessment or interventions such as range-of-motion (ROM) exercises, application of dressings, observation of pressure injuries, or inspection and care of intravenous (IV) sites.

Healthy people are normally able to meet their own hygiene needs. However, physical or cognitive impairments and emotional challenges often cause individuals to need some degree of assistance with hygiene care. In health care agency and home care settings, assess each patient's ability to perform self–hygiene care according to individual needs and preferences. Critical thinking applied with clinical judgment enables you to plan and implement patient-centered hygiene care for your patients. When planning and making adaptations for hygiene interventions and approaches, always ensure privacy, convey respect, and foster a patient's independence, safety, and comfort.

SCIENTIFIC KNOWLEDGE BASE

Proper hygiene care requires an understanding of the anatomy and physiology of the skin, nails, oral cavity, eyes, ears, and nose. The skin and mucosal cells exchange oxygen, nutrients, and fluids with underlying blood vessels. The cells require adequate nutrition, hydration, and circulation to resist injury and disease. Good hygiene techniques promote the normal structure and function of these tissues.

Your knowledge of pathophysiology assists you to provide preventive hygiene care. For example, you can recognize disease states that create changes in the integument, oral cavity, and sensory organs. Diabetes mellitus often results in chronic vascular changes that impair healing of the skin and mucosa. In the early stages of acquired immunodeficiency syndrome (AIDS), fungal infections of the oral cavity are common. Paralysis of the trigeminal nerve (cranial nerve V) eliminates the blink reflex, causing risk of corneal drying. In the presence of conditions such as these, use your clinical judgment to adapt hygiene practices to minimize injury. When implementing hygiene, it is important to use your time with patients as an additional opportunity to completely assess for and identify skin and musculoskeletal abnormalities and any self-care deficits related to hygiene. As a result, you will have sufficient information to establish a plan of care to individualize hygiene interventions designed to prevent further injury to sensitive tissues.

The Skin

The skin serves several functions, including protection, secretion, excretion, body temperature regulation, and cutaneous sensation (Table 40.1). The layers of the skin include the epidermis, the dermis, and the subcutaneous tissue (also known as the *hypodermis*), which shares some of the protective functions of the skin.

The epidermis (outer layer) shields underlying tissues against water loss and injury, prevents entry of disease-producing microorganisms, and generates new cells to replace the dead cells that are continuously shed from the outer surface of the skin. Bacteria (normal flora) commonly reside on the outer epidermis. The resident normal flora do not cause disease but instead inhibit the multiplication of disease-causing microorganisms (see Chapter 28).

Bundles of collagen and elastic fibers form the thicker dermis that underlies and supports the epidermis. Nerve fibers, blood vessels, sweat glands, sebaceous glands, and hair follicles run through the dermal layers. Sebaceous glands secrete sebum, an oily, odorous fluid, into the hair follicles. Sebum softens and lubricates the skin and slows water loss from the skin when the humidity is low. More important, sebum has bactericidal action.

The subcutaneous tissue functions as a heat insulator, supports upper skin layers in withstanding stresses and pressure, and anchors the skin loosely to underlying structures such as muscle. The subcutaneous tissue layer contains blood vessels, nerves, lymph tissue, and loose connective tissue filled with fat cells. Little subcutaneous tissue underlies the oral mucosa.

The skin often reflects a change in physical condition by alterations in color, thickness, texture, turgor, temperature, and hydration (see Chapter 30). If the skin remains intact and healthy, its physiological function remains optimal. Hygiene practices frequently influence skin status and can have beneficial and negative effects on the skin. For example, too-frequent bathing and use of hot water frequently lead to dry, flaky skin and loss of protective oils.

The Feet, Hands, and Nails

The feet, hands, and nails often require special attention to prevent infection, odor, and injury. The condition of a patient's hands and feet

---

TABLE 40.1 Function of the Skin and Implications for Care

Function/Description	Implications for Care
Protection Epidermis is a relatively impermeable layer that prevents entrance of microorganisms. Although microorganisms reside on skin surface and in hair follicles, relative dryness of the surface of skin inhibits bacterial growth. Sebum removes bacteria from hair follicles. Acidic pH of skin further retards bacterial growth.	Weakening of the epidermis occurs by scraping or stripping its surface (e.g., use of dry razors, tape removal, improper turning or positioning techniques). Excessive dryness causes cracks and breaks in skin and mucosa that allow bacteria to enter. Emollients soften skin and prevent moisture loss, and hydrating mucosa prevents dryness. Constant exposure of skin to moisture causes maceration or softening, interrupting dermal integrity and promoting ulcer formation and bacterial growth. Keep bed linen and clothing dry. Misuse of soap, detergents, cosmetics, deodorant, and depilatories causes chemical irritation. Alkaline soaps neutralize the protective acid condition of skin. Cleaning skin removes excess oil, sweat, dead skin cells, and dirt, which promote bacterial growth. Minimize friction to avoid loss of stratum corneum, which increases risk for pressure injuries.
Sensation Skin contains sensory organs for touch, pain, heat, cold, and pressure.	Smooth linen out to remove sources of mechanical irritation. Make sure that bath water is not excessively hot or cold.
Temperature Regulation Radiation, evaporation, conduction, and convection control body temperature.	Factors that interfere with heat loss alter temperature control. Wet bed linen or gowns increase heat loss. Excess blankets or bed coverings conserve heat and interfere with heat loss through radiation and conduction. Coverings promote heat conservation.
Excretion and Secretion Sweat promotes heat loss by evaporation. Sebum lubricates skin and hair.	Perspiration and oil sometimes harbor microorganisms. Bathing removes excess body secretions, but excessive bathing causes dry skin.

influences the ability to perform hygiene care. Without the ability to bear weight, ambulate, or manipulate the hands, a patient is at risk for losing self-care ability.

A wide range of dexterity exists in the hand because of the movement between the thumb and fingers. Any condition (e.g., arthritis, multiple sclerosis, traumatic hand injury) that interferes with hand movement (e.g., superficial or deep pain or joint inflammation) impairs a patient's self-care abilities. Foot pain often changes a patient's gait, causing strain on different joints and muscle groups. Discomfort while standing or walking limits self-care abilities.

The nails are epithelial tissues that grow from the root of the nail bed, located in the skin at the nail groove hidden by a fold of skin called the *cuticle*. A normal healthy nail appears transparent, smooth, and convex, with a pink nail bed and translucent white tip. Inadequate nutrition and disease cause changes in the shape, thickness, and curvature of the nail (see Chapter 30).

The Oral Cavity

The oral cavity consists of the lips surrounding the opening of the mouth, the cheeks running along the sidewalls of the cavity, the tongue and its muscles, and the hard and soft palate. The mucous membrane, continuous with the skin, lines the oral cavity. The floor of the mouth and the undersurface of the tongue are richly supplied with blood vessels. Normal oral mucosa glistens and is pink, soft, moist, smooth, and without lesions. Ulcerations or trauma frequently results in significant bleeding. Several glands within and outside the oral cavity secrete saliva. Saliva cleanses the mouth, dissolves food chemicals to promote taste, moistens food to facilitate bolus formation, and contains enzymes. Medications, exposure to radiation, dehydration, and mouth breathing may impair salivary secretion in the mouth, which increases the patient's risk for **xerostomia**, or dry mouth.

A normal tooth consists of the crown, neck, and root. Healthy teeth appear in a variety of shades of white, smooth, shiny, and aligned. The condition of the oral cavity reflects overall health and indicates oral hygiene needs (see Chapter 30).

Difficulty in chewing develops when surrounding gum tissues become inflamed or infected or when teeth are lost or become loosened. Regular oral hygiene helps to prevent **gingivitis** (i.e., inflammation of the gums) and **dental caries** (i.e., tooth decay produced by interaction of food with bacteria).

The Hair

Hair growth, distribution, and pattern indicate a person's general health status. Special hair-care practices focus on care of the scalp, axilla, and pubic areas. Hormonal changes, nutrition, emotional and physical stress, aging, infection, and some illnesses affect hair characteristics. The hair shaft itself is lifeless, and physiological factors do not affect it directly. However, hormonal and nutrient deficiencies of the hair follicle cause changes in hair color or condition.

The Eyes, Ears, and Nose

When providing hygiene, the eyes, ears, and nose require careful attention because of sensitive anatomical structures. For example, the cornea of the eye contains many nerve endings sensitive to irritants such as soap.

The eyes secrete tears, which contain substances to cleanse and lubricate the eye and protect it from bacteria. Specialized glands in the auditory canal secrete cerumen, which traps foreign bodies and repels insects. Cerumen builds up and becomes impacted in some people. Patients with alterations in one or more of the senses often need help to meet their hygiene needs. Chapter 30 describes the structure and function of these organs.

> ### REFLECT NOW
>
> When you were in your anatomy and physiology classes, you learned about the skin and mucous membranes. Think about the impact of sun on the skin. What types of short- or long-term issues can occur on the skin with sun exposure?

NURSING KNOWLEDGE BASE

A number of factors influence personal preferences for hygiene and the ability to maintain hygiene practices. Since no two individuals perform hygiene care in the same manner, you must individualize care based on assessing for your patient's unique hygiene practices and preferences. Individualized hygiene care requires knowing the patient and using therapeutic communication skills to promote a trusting therapeutic relationship. Use the opportunities provided during hygiene care to assess a patient's health promotion practices, emotional status, and health care education needs and then offer educational interventions. Be aware that developmental changes also influence the need and preferences for types of hygiene care.

Factors Influencing Hygiene

Social Practices. Social practices influence a person's hygiene preferences and practices, including the type of hygiene products used and the nature and frequency of personal care practices. Parents and caregivers perform hygiene care for infants and young children. Family customs play a major role during childhood in determining hygiene practices, such as the frequency of bathing, the time of day bathing is performed, and even whether certain hygiene practices such as brushing the teeth or flossing are performed. As children enter adolescence, peer groups and media often influence hygiene practices, and health education is important. For example, health education impacts adolescent girls' choices related to menstrual hygiene (Kole et al., 2018). Young girls become more interested in their personal appearance and begin to wear makeup. During the adult years, involvement with friends and work groups shapes the expectations that people have about personal appearance. Some individuals' hygiene practices change because of changes in living conditions and available resources. This is common in older adults who have changes in functional status and/or limited finances and in the homeless and people living in poverty.

Personal Preferences. Patients have individual preferences about how and when to perform hygiene and grooming care. Some patients prefer to shower, whereas others prefer to take a bath. Patients select different hygiene and grooming products according to personal preferences. Knowing patients' personal preferences and cultural practices promotes individualized care (Box 40.1) (see Chapter 9). Help a patient develop new hygiene practices when indicated by an illness or condition. For example, you may need to teach a patient with diabetes mellitus proper foot hygiene or a bariatric patient adaptive bathing methods. Safe and effective patient-centered nursing care improves patient satisfaction, health outcomes, adherence to treatments, and reduces costs (Mason et al., 2019).

Body Image. Body image is a person's subjective concept of their body, including physical appearance, structure, or function (see Chapter 33). Body image affects the way in which individuals maintain personal hygiene. If a patient maintains a neatly groomed appearance, be sure to consider the details of grooming when planning care, and consult with the patient before making decisions about

BOX 40.1   CULTURAL ASPECTS OF CARE

Hygiene Practices

It is important to provide your patient with a culturally congruent plan for hygiene care. For many patients, culture influences hygiene practices, and hygiene care may become a potential source of conflict and stress in the caregiving environment (Marion et al., 2017). Patient-centered care mandates that care is aligned with patients' values, needs, practices, and expectations, providing equitable and ethical care, and that care be based on respect for an individual patient's cultural background (Henderson et al., 2018). When delivering hygiene, be aware of other sociocultural factors, such as a patient's educational and developmental levels, the extent of any physical disabilities, and the geographical location of the home.

Implications for Patient-Centered Care

- Maintain privacy, especially for women from cultures that value female modesty, and provide gender-congruent caregivers as requested (Giger and Haddad, 2021).
- Collaborate with community leaders when providing health education for a diverse community (LaFleur et al., 2017).
- Allow family members to participate in care if desired by adapting the schedule of hygiene activities.
- Be aware of cultural practices that may affect the timing of hygiene activities. For example, does bathing need to occur before or after prayers? Are there specific hygiene practices during religious holidays (Giger and Haddad, 2021)?
- Recognize that some cultures prohibit or restrict touching. Incorporate awareness that people from different cultural backgrounds have differing preferences regarding touch and personal space. In some cases, touch is considered magical and healing; others view it as evil or anxiety producing (Giger and Haddad, 2021).
- Recognize cultural hair practices, and do not cut or shave hair without prior discussion with the patient or family (Bowen and O'Brien-Richardson, 2017; O'Brien-Richardson, 2019).
- Be aware that toileting practices vary by culture (Giger and Haddad, 2021).
- Recognize that different cultures have preferences about hot water and cold water and their effects on healing or diseases (Morgan-Consoli and Unzueta, 2018).

---

how to provide hygiene. Patients who appear unkempt or uninterested in hygiene sometimes need further assessment regarding their ability to participate with daily hygiene or additional education about its importance.

Surgery, illness, or a change in emotional or functional status often affects a patient's body image. Discomfort and pain, emotional stress, and fatigue diminish the ability or desire to perform hygiene self-care and require extra effort to promote hygiene and grooming.

Socioeconomic Status. A person's economic resources influence the type and extent of hygiene practices used. Be sensitive in considering that a patient's economic status influences the ability to regularly maintain hygiene. The patient may not be able to afford desired basic supplies such as deodorant, shampoo, and toothpaste. A patient may need to modify the home environment by adding safety devices such as nonskid surfaces and grab bars in the bath to perform hygiene self-care safely. When patients lack socioeconomic resources, it becomes difficult for them to participate and take responsible roles in health promotion activities such as basic hygiene.

Health Beliefs and Motivation. Knowledge about the importance of hygiene and its implications for well-being influences hygiene practices. However, knowledge alone is not enough. Motivation also plays

a key role in a patient's hygiene practices. Motivational interviewing during assessment can assist you in identifying how a patient perceives benefit in performing hygiene and the patient's willingness to change behavior (see Chapter 24). Adapt what you learn about a patient's willingness to change into your patient teaching approach. Provide information that focuses on a patient's personal health-related issues relevant to the desired hygiene care behaviors. Patient perceptions of the benefits of hygiene care and the susceptibility to and seriousness of developing a problem affect the motivation to change behavior. For example, do patients perceive that they are at risk for dental disease, or that dental disease is serious, and that brushing and flossing are effective in reducing risk? When they recognize that there is a risk and that they can take reasonable cost-effective action without negative consequences, they are more likely to be receptive to adopting healthy behaviors (Gomes et al., 2020; Broadbent et al., 2016).

Cultural Variables. Cultural beliefs, religious practices, and personal values influence hygiene care (see Box 40.1). People from diverse cultural backgrounds (e.g., level of education, gender preference, geographic location) frequently follow different self-care practices (see Chapter 9). For example, maintaining cleanliness does not hold the same importance for some ethnic or social groups as it does for others (Giger and Haddad, 2021). In North America many are fortunate to be able to bathe or shower daily and use deodorant to prevent body odors. However, people from some socioeconomic or cultural groups are not sensitive to body odors, prefer to bathe less frequently, and do not use deodorant. Avoid expressing disapproval or forcing changes in hygienic practices unless the practices affect a patient's health. In these situations, use tact, provide information, and allow choices.

Developmental Stage. The normal process of aging affects the condition of body tissues and structures. Apply your knowledge of physical and psychosocial developmental changes as you assess your patients and plan, implement, and evaluate hygiene care. A patient's developmental stage affects the ability of the person to perform hygiene care and the type of care needed.

Skin. The neonate's skin is relatively immature at birth. The epidermis and dermis are bound together loosely, and the skin is very thin. Friction against the skin layers causes bruising. Handle a neonate carefully during bathing. Any break in the skin easily results in an infection.

A toddler's skin layers become more tightly bound together. Thus the child has a greater resistance to infection and skin irritation. However, because of the child's more active play and the absence of established hygiene habits, parents and caregivers need to provide thorough hygiene and teach good hygiene habits.

During adolescence, the growth and maturation of the integument increase. In girls, estrogen secretion causes the skin to become soft, smooth, and thicker, with increased vascularity. In boys, male hormones produce an increased thickness of the skin, with some darkening in color. Sebaceous glands become more active, predisposing adolescents to acne (i.e., active inflammation of the sebaceous glands accompanied by pimples). Sweat glands become fully functional during puberty. Adolescents usually begin to use antiperspirants. More frequent bathing and shampooing also become necessary to reduce body odors and eliminate oily hair.

The condition of the adult's skin depends on bathing practices and exposure to environmental irritants. Normally the skin is elastic, well hydrated, firm, and smooth. When an adult bathes frequently or is exposed to an environment with low humidity, the skin becomes dry and flaky. With aging the rate of epidermal cell replacement slows, and the skin thins and loses resiliency. Moisture leaves the skin, increasing the risk for bruising and other types of injury. As the production of lubricating substances from skin glands decreases, the skin becomes dry and itchy (Touhy and Jett, 2021). These changes warrant caution when bathing, turning, and repositioning older adults. Too-frequent bathing and bathing with hot water or harsh soap cause the skin to become excessively dry (American Academy of Dermatology, 2020).

Feet and Nails. Foot health is a key component to a person's mobility, health, and overall well-being. With aging and continued exposure to the trauma of walking and weight-bearing, a patient is more likely to develop chronic foot problems, compounded as a result of poor foot care, improper fit of footwear, and local abnormalities and systemic disease (Sibbald et al., 2019; Persaud et al., 2018). For example, Morton's neuroma, a common condition in middle-age women, affects health-related quality of life by causing burning, numbness, and pain of the foot on weight-bearing (Park et al., 2018).

Older adults do not always have the strength, flexibility, visual acuity, or manual dexterity to care for their feet and nails. Foot problems may be overlooked and impact a patient's comfort, mobility, and quality of life. Older adults frequently complain of foot pain, and this pain is a source of falls. Modifications in footwear can reduce this risk and improve comfort and safe mobility (Halton and Rome, 2019). Dry feet are the result of a decrease in sebaceous gland secretion and dehydration of epidermal cells. In addition to pain, other common problems of the feet affecting older adults include corns, calluses, bunions, hammertoes, maceration between toes, and fungal infections (Arthritis Foundation, 2017).

The Mouth. At approximately 6 to 8 months of age, infants begin teething. The first permanent (secondary) teeth erupt at about 6 years of age (Hockenberry et al., 2019). From adolescence, when all the permanent teeth are in place, through middle adulthood, the teeth and gums remain healthy if a person follows healthy eating patterns and dental care. Avoiding fermentable carbohydrates and sticky sweets helps to keep the teeth free of dental caries. In addition, regular brushing (twice a day) and flossing reduce caries and periodontal disease.

As a person ages, numerous factors result in poor oral health, including age-related changes of the mouth, changes resulting from chronic disease such as diabetes mellitus, physical disabilities involving hand grasp or strength affecting the ability to perform oral care, lack of attention to oral care, and prescribed medications that have oral side effects. Gums lose vascularity and tissue elasticity, which may cause dentures to fit poorly.

Hair. Throughout life, changes in the growth, distribution, and condition of the hair influence hair hygiene. As males reach adolescence, shaving becomes a part of routine grooming. Young girls who reach puberty often begin to shave their legs and axillae. With aging, as scalp hair becomes thinner and drier, shampooing is usually performed less frequently.

Eyes, Ears, and Nose. Changes in hearing, vision, and olfaction can occur across the life span (see Chapter 49). Alterations in sensory function often require modifications in hygiene care. Hygiene of sensory structures must be provided in a way to prevent injury to sensitive tissues such as the cornea of the eye and the internal ear canal.

Physical Condition. Patients with certain types of functional limitations or disabilities associated with disease and injury lack the physical energy and/or dexterity to perform hygiene self-care safely. A weakened grasp resulting from arthritis, stroke, or muscular disorders makes using a toothbrush, washcloth, or hairbrush difficult or ineffective.

Jamie spent time studying rheumatoid arthritis and the impact of the disease on a person's lifestyle and independence. Mrs. White has rheumatoid arthritis, and when Jamie reviewed her medical record, she noted that Mrs. White has physical changes in her arms and hands, which result in pain and decreased dexterity. Jamie knows that these changes impact

Mrs. White's ability to independently perform personal hygiene. Jamie also notes that Mrs. White wants to return to her assisted-living apartment.

Sensory deficits alter a patient's ability to perform care. However, decreased sensation also places a patient at risk for pressure or thermal injuries. Safety is a priority for a patient with a sensory deficit. For example, a patient with paresthesia who is unable to feel that bath water is too hot can incur a burn injury during bathing.

Chronic illnesses such as cardiac, pulmonary, and neurological diseases; cancer; and some mental health illnesses often exhaust or incapacitate patients. Patients who become tired or short of breath sometimes need to have complete hygiene care provided. Include periods of rest during care to allow patients who are tired the opportunity to participate in their care. Pain often accompanies illness and injury, limiting a patient's ability to tolerate hygiene and grooming activities or perform self-care. Pain frequently limits ROM, resulting in impaired use of the arms or hands or limited ability to move about in the environment, impairing the ability to perform hygiene self-care. When possible, administer an analgesic for pain 30 minutes before hygiene care. However, be aware that sedation and drowsiness associated with analgesics used for pain management may also limit a patient's ability to safely participate in care.

Limited mobility caused by a variety of factors (e.g., obesity, physical injury, weakness, surgery, pain, prolonged inactivity, medication effect, and presence of medical devices [e.g., indwelling catheter, feeding tube, or IV line]) decreases a patient's ability to perform hygiene self-care activities safely. Individualized care considers a patient's ability to perform care, the amount of assistance needed, and the need for assistive and safety devices to facilitate safe hygiene care.

Acute and chronic cognitive impairments resulting from conditions such as stroke, brain injury, psychoses, and dementia often result in the inability to perform self-care independently. Patients with dementia often forget to attend to their basic hygiene needs. When people with cognitive impairments are unaware of their hygiene and grooming needs, they may become fearful and agitated during hygiene care, resulting in aggressive behavior (Mendes, 2018). Safe, effective patient-centered care takes the effect of cognitive impairment on personal care into consideration and provides appropriate modifications (Scales et al., 2018).

CRITICAL THINKING

The care of any patient who requires complete hygiene care is complex. Sound clinical judgment requires critical thinking, the synthesis of knowledge, experience, environmental factors, critical thinking attitudes, and intellectual and professional standards. Sound clinical judgments require you to consider a patient's condition, anticipate any risks or problems, gather thorough assessment data, and then analyze data to form nursing diagnoses. Critical thinking will enable you to make the clinical decisions necessary for identifying appropriate nursing diagnoses (Fig. 40.1).

Integrate nursing knowledge with knowledge from other disciplines. For example, a patient with diabetes mellitus has special needs for nail and foot care to prevent injury and infection. Knowledge about the pathophysiology of diabetes mellitus and its potential effects on a patient's peripheral circulation and sensory status provides the scientific knowledge base needed to implement safe and effective foot care. In addition, integrate knowledge about developmental and cultural influences as you identify and meet hygiene needs.

Think about prior experiences as you help with your patients' hygiene care. Did you help family members or others close to you with their hygiene? Frequently an early clinical experience involves providing or helping with hygiene care for a patient. Also, you may have had experience helping a colleague with providing hygiene care for a complicated patient.

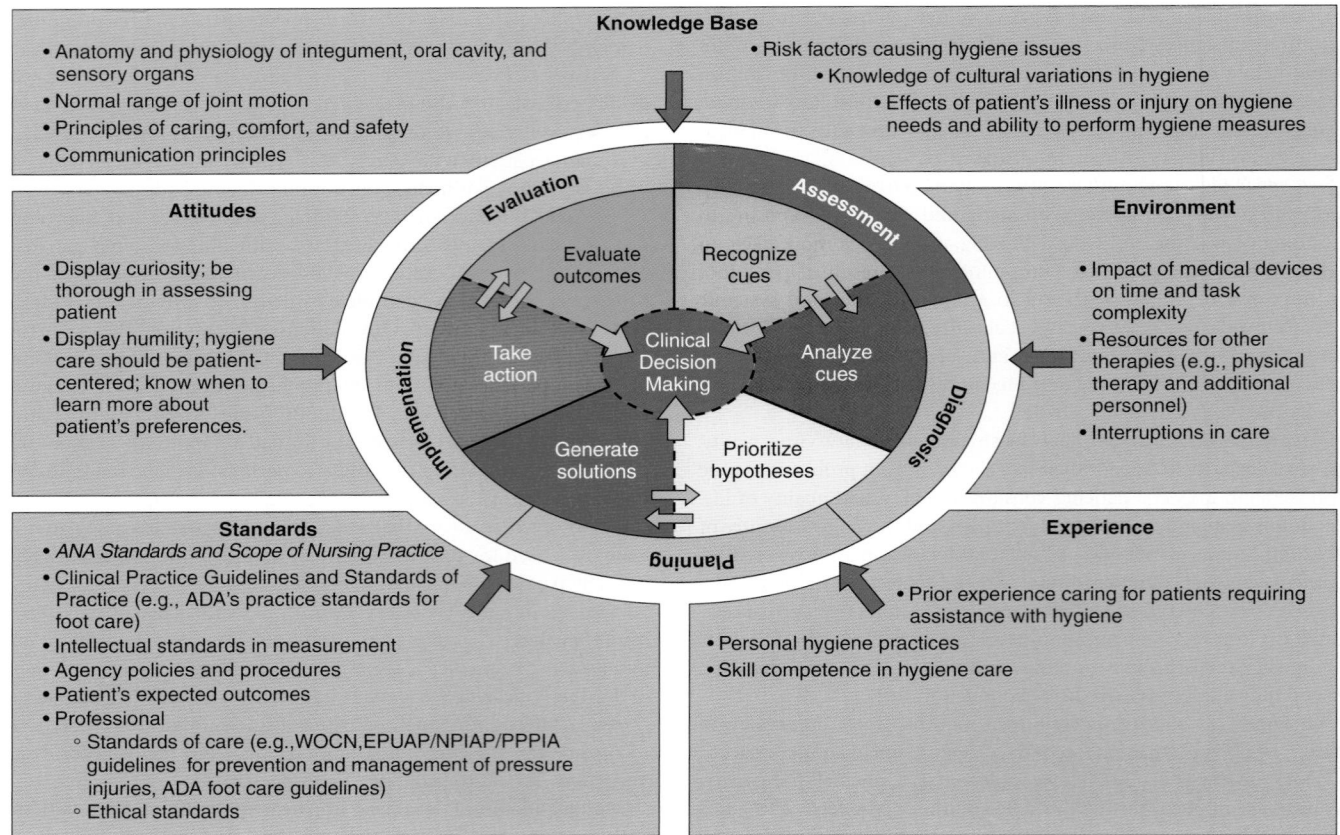

FIG. 40.1 Critical thinking model for hygiene assessment. (Clinical Judgment Measurement Model copyright © NCSBN. All rights reserved.)

Determine whether there are any environmental factors that will impact patient care. For example, does the patient have a roommate who has complicated hygiene needs? Is the patient on a busy hospital unit where interruptions from other health care providers impact care? Identify any environmental factors, and when possible incorporate these into the timing of care.

Prior to assessment, review the patient's medical record for new information—for example, specific skin care practices, mobility restrictions, or new orders for medical equipment, adaptive devices, or therapies. Avoid time conflicts. For example, determine whether additional personnel are needed for certain care activities or whether additional therapies, medical equipment, or devices increase the length of time needed to provide hygiene care.

Be aware of the impact of critical thinking attitudes as you plan and implement care. For example, think creatively to help patients adapt existing hygiene practices or develop new ones when illness, loss of function, or decreased activity tolerance impairs self-care abilities. Be nonjudgmental and confident when providing care. Because of variations in individual patients' physical status and hygiene practices, you need to approach care with an attitude of flexibility. For example, when caring for a patient with decreased activity tolerance, pace activities and plan rest periods during bathing and other hygiene measures.

Finally, rely on professional standards, such as those for skin and foot care from specialty groups (e.g., the Wound Ostomy and Continence Nurses Society [WOCN] and the American Diabetes Association [ADA]), and ethical standards when planning care to meet a patient's hygiene needs. As your experience and knowledge grow, your comfort and expertise in meeting the individualized hygiene needs of your patients increase.

REFLECT NOW

You know that people and cultures differ in their types and frequencies of hygiene practices. Think about how you might address your own personal biases so that you can provide more patient-centered hygiene care in the future.

❖ NURSING PROCESS

Apply the nursing process and use a critical thinking approach as you identify your patient's needs and plan individualized care. The nursing process provides a clinical decision-making approach for you to develop and implement an individualized plan of care.

◆ Assessment

During assessment, use critical thinking to make clinical judgments that apply knowledge about patient comfort and privacy, early risk factors for impaired skin or oral mucosal integrity, and the impact of impaired circulation on skin and nail integrity. Review your past experiences to determine how to completely assess your patient for individual hygiene preferences. Include information from personal hygiene practices and professional experiences, and collaborate with your patient. Hygiene practices are personal and private, and your patient needs to be assured that you will maintain that privacy. Critically analyze your assessment findings to ensure that you make patient-centered clinical decisions required for safe and effective hygiene. Include a review of a patient's medications, medical and surgical history, and the specific risk factors that the patient presents.

Assessment of a patient's hygiene status and self-care abilities requires you to complete a nursing history and perform a physical assessment (see Chapter 30). You do not assess all body regions routinely before providing hygiene. However, conduct a brief history to determine priority areas (e.g., diabetic patient with foot ulcers, an overweight patient's skinfolds, an immobilized patient's skin condition) and to help you plan relevant and individualized care. Assessment of a patient's ability to provide hygiene self-care helps you decide about the type and amount of hygiene care to provide and how much the patient can be encouraged to participate in care.

Through the Patient's Eyes. Because patients have varying expectations, you need to avoid making personal hygiene care a simple routine. Complete a nursing history that not only elicits personal preferences and practices but also addresses the patient's cultural or religious customs and beliefs.

Explore a patient's perspective regarding hygiene care by asking about personal care products desired and preferences such as frequency, time of day, and amount of assistance needed. Also ask questions such as "To make you most comfortable and help you feel at home, how can I best perform your bath and personal care?" Determine the patient's awareness of any hygiene-related problems and the knowledge and ability to perform hygiene care measures (Box 40.2). Learning a patient's expectations and applying them in practice foster a caring relationship. Fully individualizing hygiene care shows your respect for the patient's needs. As you learn what the patient expects, you incorporate this information into a plan of care.

Assessment of Self-Care Ability. Assess a patient's physical ability to perform or assist with hygiene care safely and efficiently; include assessment of the patient's pain and pain control measures, fatigue level, muscle strength, flexibility, balance, visual acuity, and ability to detect thermal and tactile stimuli. Determine your patient's mental status, including orientation and cognitive function (see Chapter 30). A patient with impaired cognitive function may be less able to follow instructions and help with care. Observe the patient performing hygiene care, noting complaints or physical manifestations that suggest activity intolerance. Assess respiratory rate and effort, skin color, and pulse rate. Ask questions to assess the patient for dizziness, weakness, or fatigue. To determine the amount of assistance the patient needs, observe the patient performing care activities such as brushing teeth or combing hair (Fig. 40.2). Patients who have limited upper-extremity mobility and strength, reduced vision, fatigue, or inability to grasp small objects require help. Patients having difficulty with manual dexterity and cognitive function are likely to show deterioration in physical or oral health. Poor oral care increases the risk for aspiration pneumonia in patients recovering from a stroke or who have dementia (Murray and Scholten, 2018). Also note the presence of medical devices such as feeding tubes, intravenous (IV) lines, or urinary catheters. These devices require special, more complex hygiene measures and require more time for care.

When patients have self-care limitations, family caregivers may help with care. Work with the family to design patient-centered care. *Mrs. White's granddaughter has indicated a desire to help her grandmother when she returns to her residence. Jamie will need to involve the granddaughter in some of the care.* Determine how the family can help the patient, how often family members can provide this assistance, and their feelings about being caregivers (Pinkert et al., 2018). In addition, when necessary, assess the home environment and its influence on the patient's hygiene practices. Are there barriers in the home that affect

---

BOX 40.2 Nursing Assessment Questions

Cultural and/or Religious Practices
- Do you have preferences for how you bathe, shampoo your hair, brush your teeth, or care for your feet?
- How comfortable are you with someone helping you with your bathing? Would you prefer a care provider of your same gender?
- In what way can I best help you with your bath, skin and hair care, and nail care?

Tolerance of Hygiene Activities
- Tell me about any symptoms, such as shortness of breath, pain, or fatigue, that you experience during bathing.
- What can I do to minimize these symptoms?
- Which aspects of bathing, toothbrushing, hair care, or foot care cause discomfort or fatigue?
- Is there a particular time of day when hygiene activities may be less fatiguing?

Assistance with Hygiene
- Do you use any aids to help you with your bath, such as grab bars in your tub or shower?
- Which parts of the bath, toothbrushing, and foot care can you do for yourself? With which parts of hygiene care do you need help?

Skin Care
- Which type of bath do you prefer?
- How often and when do you usually bathe?
- Do you have preferences for bath soap or lotion?
- Have you noticed any skin changes or irritation?
- Do you have any known allergies or reactions to soaps, cosmetics, or skin care products?

Mouth Care
- Do you have any mouth pain or toothaches? Have you noticed any sores in your mouth? Do your gums bleed during brushing or flossing?
- Do you wear dentures or a partial plate?

Foot and Nail Care
- How do you usually care for your feet and nails? Do you soak your feet?
- Do you file or trim your own fingernails and toenails?

Hair and Scalp Care
- Have you recently experienced itching of the scalp or noticed flaking or dandruff?
- Have you noticed any changes in the texture or thickness of your hair?

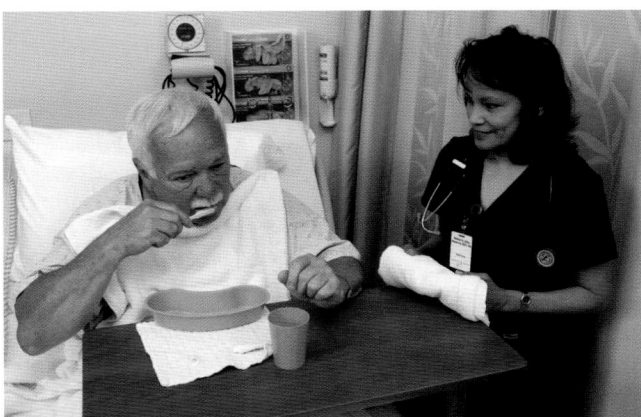

FIG. 40.2 Nurse observes patient brushing teeth. During such observations the nurse can determine how much assistance the patient may need.

the patient's self-care abilities (e.g., water faucets that are too tight to adjust easily, bathtubs with high sides, a bathroom too small to fit a chair in front of a sink, or a lack of an adjustable bed or adaptive equipment available for assisting with bathing)?

Environmental Factors. Determine if any environmental factors will affect patient care and hygiene practices. Review the patient's medical record for information such as new orders for medical equipment or therapies. Avoid time conflicts by determining if additional personnel are needed for certain care activities or if additional therapies, medical equipment, or devices will increase the length of time needed to administer hygiene.

Assessment of the Skin. Perform an assessment of the skin (see Chapter 30), noting color, texture, thickness, turgor, temperature, and hydration. In a healthy person the skin is smooth, warm, and supple with good turgor. Pay special attention to the presence, location, and condition of any lesions. Note dryness indicated by flaking, redness, scaling, and cracking. Also carefully inspect areas of the skin in contact with any medical device at least daily (e.g., skin under an oxygen

cannula or the nasal mucosa under an endotracheal or feeding tube) (EPUAP/NPIAP/PPPIA, 2019a, 2019b; Fumarola et al., 2020) (see Chapter 48). Look for edema under the sites. Discovering manifestations of common skin problems influences how you administer hygiene care and preventive practices (Table 40.2).

Determine a patient's level of cleanliness by observing the appearance of the skin and detecting body odors that can indicate inadequate cleansing or excessive perspiration caused by fever or pain. Inspect less obvious or difficult-to-reach skin surfaces such as under the breasts or scrotum, around the female patient's perineum, or in the groin for redness, excessive moisture, and soiling or debris. Separate skinfolds for observation and palpation. It is important to keep these areas dry, especially in patients who are overweight. A light application of cornstarch may be used to decrease friction and absorb moisture (Dial et al., 2018).

Be attentive to characteristics of skin problems most influenced by hygiene measures. Is the skin dry from too much bathing or from use of hot water or irritating soap? Does the patient have a rash caused by an allergic reaction to a skin care product? Certain conditions place patients at risk for impaired skin integrity (Table 40.3). Because of

---

TABLE 40.2 Common Skin Problems

Characteristics	Implications	Interventions
Dry Skin Flaky, rough texture on exposed areas such as hands, arms, legs, or face	Skin becomes infected if epidermal layer cracks.	Bathe less frequently and use warm, not hot water. Rinse body of all soap because residue left on skin can cause irritation and breakdown. Add moisture to air with use of humidifier. Increase fluid intake when skin is dry. Use moisturizing cream to aid healing. (Cream forms protective barrier and helps maintain fluid within skin.) Use creams to clean skin that is dry or allergic to soaps and detergents.
Acne Inflammatory, papulopustular skin eruption, usually involving bacterial breakdown of sebum; appears on face, neck, shoulders, and back	Infected material within pustule spreads if area is squeezed or picked. Permanent scarring can result.	Wash hair and skin thoroughly each day with warm water and soap to remove oil. Use cosmetics sparingly. Oily cosmetics or creams accumulate in pores and make condition worse. Implement dietary restrictions if necessary. (Eliminate foods that aggravate condition from diet.) Use prescribed topical antibiotics for severe forms of acne.
Skin Rashes Skin eruptions that result from overexposure to sun or moisture or from allergic reaction (flat or raised, localized or systemic, pruritic or nonpruritic)	If skin is scratched continually, inflammation and infection may occur. Rashes also cause discomfort.	Wash area thoroughly and apply antiseptic spray or lotion to prevent further itching and aid in healing process. Apply warm or cold soaks to relieve inflammation if indicated.
Contact Dermatitis Inflammation of skin characterized by abrupt onset with erythema; pruritus; pain; and appearance of scaly, oozing lesions (seen on face, neck, hands, forearms, and genitalia)	Dermatitis is often difficult to eliminate because person is usually in continual contact with substance causing skin reaction. Substance is often hard to identify.	Avoid causative agents (e.g., adhesives, cleansers, and soaps).
Abrasion Scraping or rubbing away of epidermis that results in localized bleeding and later weeping of serous fluid	Infection occurs easily because of loss of protective skin layer.	Remove jewelry and trim fingernails so as not to scratch patient during hygiene care. Wash abrasions with mild soap and water; dry thoroughly and gently. Observe dressing or bandage for retained moisture because it increases risk of infection.

TABLE 40.3 Risk Factors for Hygiene Care

Risks	Hygiene Implications
Oral Problems	
Inability to use upper extremities because of paralysis, weakness, or restriction (e.g., cast, dressing)	Patient lacks upper-extremity strength or dexterity needed to brush teeth (Harding et al., 2020).
Dehydration, inability to take fluids or food by mouth (NPO)	Causes excess drying and fragility of mucosa; increases accumulation of secretions on tongue and gums.
Presence of nasogastric or oxygen tubes; mouth breathers	Tubes cause pressure, friction, and drying of mucosa and/or lips.
Chemotherapeutic drugs	Drugs kill rapidly multiplying cells, including normal cells lining oral cavity. Ulcers and inflammation develop.
Lozenges, cough drops, antacids, and chewable over-the-counter vitamins	Medications contain large amounts of sugar. Repeated use increases sugar or acid content in mouth, causing dental caries.
Radiation therapy to head and neck	Reduces salivary flow and lowers pH of saliva; leads to stomatitis and tooth decay (Harding et al., 2020).
Oral surgery, trauma to mouth, placement of oral airway	These cause trauma to oral cavity with swelling, ulcerations, inflammation, and bleeding.
Immunosuppression; altered blood clotting	Predispose to inflammation and bleeding gums.
Diabetes mellitus	Patients are prone to dryness of mouth, gingivitis, periodontal disease, and loss of teeth.
Endotracheal intubation with mechanical ventilation	Potential for ventilator-associated pneumonia (VAP) exists. Chlorhexidine gluconate (CHG) 0.12% used in oral care has been found in a review of research studies to probably prevent ventilator-assisted pneumonia from developing in very ill patients treated in intensive care units (Zhao et al., 2020).
Dialysis	Oral problems commonly found in these patients include halitosis, xerostomia (dry mouth), gingivitis, stomatitis, tooth decay, tooth loss, and jaw problems. Causes may include micronutrient deficiencies, elevated blood sugar, rheumatoid arthritis, weight control, and smoking (Chapple et al., 2017).
Cognitive impairment	Patients are prone to poor oral health and are at risk for aspiration pneumonia (Murray and Scholten, 2017).
Skin Problems	
Immobilization	Dependent body parts are exposed to pressure from underlying surfaces. The inability to turn or change position increases risk for pressure injuries.
Presence of external medical devices, such as cast, restraint, oxygen mask, nasogastric tube (see Chapter 48).	Devices such as casts, cloth restraints, bandages, tubing, and orthopedic devices exert pressure or friction against surface of skin and increase risk for medical device–related pressure injuries (MDRPI) (EPUAP/NPIAP/PPPIA, 2019a, b).
Presence of medical adhesives to secure ostomy appliances, dressings, tubing, etc. (see Chapter 48).	Medical adhesive–related skin injury (MARSI) is an occurrence in which erythema and/or other manifestations of cutaneous abnormality (including but not limited to vesicle, bulla, erosion, or skin tear) persist 30 minutes or more after removal of a device or adhesive securing the device (Kelly-O'Flynn et al., 2020; Fumarola et al., 2020). Assess for the presence of a MARSI by looking for skin stripping, skin tears, maceration, dermatitis, inflammation, and/or tape burns. These develop from repeated removal of adhesives and application of devices, common around intravenous insertion sites. This is a commonly overlooked and underestimated skin injury.
Bariatric patient	Patient cannot visualize skin properly and keep it clean and dry. Excessive adipose tissue creates pressure from weight, lack of air circulation, and an increase in moisture with poor tissue perfusion (Dial et al., 2018). Increases risk for pressure injuries.
Reduced sensation caused by stroke, spinal cord injury, diabetes, local nerve damage	Patient unable to sense skin injury. Does not receive normal transmission of nerve impulses when applying excessive heat or cold, pressure, friction, or chemical irritants to skin. Increases risk for pressure injuries.
Altered cognition resulting from dementia, psychological disorders, or temporary delirium	Patient unable to verbalize skin care needs. Does not realize effect of pressure or prolonged contact with excretions or secretions, requiring more vigilant assessment.
Limited protein or caloric intake and reduced hydration (e.g., fever, burns, gastrointestinal alterations, poorly fitting dentures)	Predispose to impaired tissue synthesis. Skin becomes thinner, less elastic, and smoother with loss of subcutaneous tissue. Poor wound healing results. Reduced hydration impairs skin turgor.
Excessive secretions or excretions on skin from perspiration, urine, watery fecal material, and wound drainage	Moisture is medium for bacterial growth and causes local skin irritation, softening of epidermal cells, and skin maceration. Increases risk for pressure injuries.
Vascular insufficiency	Arterial blood supply to tissues is inadequate or venous return is impaired, causing decreased circulation to extremities. Tissue ischemia and breakdown often occur. Risk for infection is high.
Foot Problems	
Patient unable to bend over or has reduced visual acuity	Patient is unable to fully visualize entire surface of each foot, impairing ability to adequately assess condition of skin and nails.
Eye Care Problems	
Reduced dexterity and hand coordination	Physical limitations create inability to safely insert or remove contact lenses.

increased risk, be particularly alert when assessing patients with reduced sensation, impaired circulation, nutrition or hydration alterations, body secretions, incontinence, altered cognition, external medical devices, and decreased mobility. Patients may be unaware of skin problems because they are unable to feel pain or pressure or see their skin in some places (e.g., the back or the feet). Carefully assess the skin under orthopedic devices (braces, splints, casts) and beneath items such as antiembolic stockings and tape. Assess the condition and cleanliness of the perineal and anal areas during hygiene care and when the patient requires toileting assistance. When prolonged contact of urine or feces occurs, such as with diarrhea or incontinence, skin breakdown often results. Most people consider these areas private; therefore, be sensitive in your approach (Touhy and Jett, 2021).

When caring for patients with dark skin pigmentation, be aware of assessment techniques and skin characteristics unique to highly pigmented skin (Ball et al., 2019). Several skin conditions are more common in persons with skin of color, including certain atopic dermatitis, melanoma, vitiligo, and hyperpigmentation (melasma) (Espinosa and Lio, 2019). These conditions require special approaches to skin care. Also be very careful in assessing the skin in dark-skinned patients who are at risk for pressure injuries (see Chapter 48).

Assessment of the Feet and Nails.
A variety of common foot and nail problems can be caused by inadequate hygiene and are often detected during hygiene care. Problems sometimes result from abuse or poor care of the feet and hands, such as nail biting, improper nail trimming, exposure to harsh chemicals, and poorly fitting shoes. Question the patient to determine type of footwear and usual foot and nail care practices.

Examine all skin surfaces of the feet, including the areas between the toes and over the entire sole of the foot. Observe for trauma, calluses, ulceration, and foot or toe deformity, which indicate increased risk for diabetic foot ulcers (Woody, 2020). Poorly fitting shoes often irritate the heels, soles, and sides of the feet. Inspection of the feet for lesions includes noting areas of dryness, inflammation, or cracking (Chapman, 2017). Chronic foot problems are common in older adults, who often experience dry feet because of a decrease in sebaceous gland secretion, dehydration, or poor condition of footwear.

People are often unaware of foot or nail problems until pain or discomfort occurs. Assess patients with diseases that affect peripheral circulation and sensation for the adequacy of circulation and sensation of the feet. Diabetic neuropathy and decreased peripheral circulation put people with diabetes mellitus at greater risk for foot problems. Daily inspection and preventive foot care help maintain ulcer-free feet (Chapman, 2017). Inspect a patient's shoes and inspect feet for areas of blistering or abrasion from improper shoes or fit (Jeffcoate et al., 2018). Palpate the dorsalis pedis and posterior tibial pulses, and assess for intact sensation to light touch, pinprick, and temperature (Ball et al., 2019).

Observe a patient's gait. Painful foot disorders or decreased sensation causes limping or an unnatural gait. Ask whether the patient has foot discomfort, and determine factors that aggravate the pain. Foot problems sometimes result from bone or muscular alterations or poorly fitting footwear.

Inspect the condition of the fingernails and toenails, looking for lesions, dryness, inflammation, or cracking, which are often associated with a variety of common foot and nail problems (Table 40.4). The cuticle that surrounds the nail can grow over it and become inflamed if nail care is not performed correctly and periodically. Ask women whether they polish their nails and use polish remover frequently because chemicals in these products cause excessive nail dryness. Disease changes the shape and curvature of the nails (Ball et al., 2019). Inflammatory lesions and fungus of the nail bed cause thickened, horny nails that separate from the nail bed.

Assessment of the Oral Cavity.
The condition of the oral cavity reflects overall health and also indicates oral hygiene needs. Inspect all areas of the mouth carefully for color, hydration, texture, and lesions (see Chapter 30). Patients frequently develop oral problems because of inadequate oral care or disease (e.g., oral malignancy) or as a side effect of treatments such as radiation and chemotherapy. These problems include receding gum tissue, inflamed gums (gingivitis), a coated tongue, glossitis (inflamed tongue), discolored teeth (particularly along gum margins), cheilitis (cracked lips), dental caries, missing teeth, and halitosis (foul-smelling breath). Localized pain and infection commonly accompany oral problems.

Apply clean gloves to palpate any tender areas or lesions. Observe for cleanliness, and use olfaction to detect halitosis. If you identify any oral problems, notify the patient's health care provider. Early identification of poor oral hygiene practices and common oral problems reduces the risk for gum disease and dental caries (USDHHS, 2020). If the older adult becomes edentulous (i.e., without teeth) and wears complete or partial dentures, include an assessment of underlying gums and palate.

Assessment of the Hair.
Assess the condition of a patient's hair and scalp before performing hair care. Findings help determine the frequency and type of care needed. You can anticipate certain patients who might require a more focused assessment, such as a patient who has had head trauma or a homeless patient unable to perform regular hygiene. Normally the hair is clean, shiny, and untangled, and the scalp is clear of lesions. Table 40.5 summarizes hair and scalp problems, with implications and interventions.

Observe a patient's ability to perform hair care. A person's appearance and feeling of well-being often are related to the way the hair looks and feels. Illness, disability, and conditions such as arthritis, fatigue, obesity, and the presence of physical barriers (e.g., cast or IV access) alter a patient's ability to maintain daily hair care.

In community health and home care settings it is particularly important to inspect the hair for lice so that you can provide appropriate hygienic treatment. If you suspect pediculosis capitis (head lice), guard against self-infestation by hand hygiene and the use of gloves or tongue blades to inspect the patient's hair.

The loss of hair (alopecia) results from the effects of chemotherapy medications, hormonal changes, or improper hair care practices. Alopecia often appears as brittle and broken hair in the hair line that progresses to bald patches. If noted, be sure to question the patient about specific hair care practices, especially the use of chemicals and heat application during hair care.

Assessment of the Eyes, Ears, and Nose.
Examine the condition and function of the eyes, ears, and nose (see Chapter 30). The healthy eye is not inflamed and is without drainage. The presence of redness indicates allergic or infectious conjunctivitis, which can be highly contagious. The crusty drainage associated with conjunctivitis easily spreads from one eye to the other. Wear clean gloves to examine the eyes and perform proper hand hygiene before and after the examination. Determine whether a patient wears contact lenses, especially when the patient enters the health care agency in an unresponsive or confused state. To determine whether a contact lens is present, stand to the side of the patient's eyes and observe the corneas for the presence of a soft or rigid lens. Also observe the sclera because the lens may have shifted off the cornea. An undetected contact lens causes corneal injury when left in place too long.

Assessment of the external ear structures includes inspection of the auricle and external ear canal (see Chapter 30). Observe for the presence of accumulated cerumen (earwax) or drainage in the ear canal and local inflammation. Question patients about tenderness on palpation or the presence of pain and ask how they usually clean their ears.

TABLE 40.4 Common Foot and Nail Problems

Problem	Characteristics	Implications	Interventions
Callus	Thickened portion of epidermis, consisting of mass of horny, keratotic cells; usually flat and painless; found on undersurface of foot or on palm of hand; caused by local friction or pressure	Foot calluses often cause discomfort when wearing tight-fitting shoes.	Refer patient to podiatrist; do not self-treat. The use of orthotic devices cushions and redistributes weight to relieve pressure on calluses.
Corns From Weston WL, Lane AT: *Color textbook of pediatric dermatology,* ed 4, St Louis, 2007, Mosby.	Keratosis caused by friction and pressure from shoes; mainly on toes, over bony prominence; usually cone shaped, round, and raised; calluses with painful core	Conical shape compresses underlying dermis, making it thin and tender. Tight shoes aggravate pain. Tissue attaches to bone if allowed to grow. Patient may suffer alteration in gait because of pain.	Refer patient to podiatrist. Avoid use of oval corn pads, which increase pressure on toes. Use wider, softer shoes.
Plantar warts From Zitelli BJ et al: *Zitelli and Davis' Atlas of pediatric physical diagnosis,* ed 7, Philadelphia, 2018, Elsevier.	Fungating lesion that appears on sole of foot; caused by papillomavirus	Warts are sometimes contagious, are painful, and make walking difficult.	Refer patient to podiatrist.
Athlete's foot (tinea pedis)	Fungal infection of foot; scaliness and cracking of skin between toes and on soles of feet; small blisters containing fluid appear, apparently induced by constricting footwear (e.g., sneakers)	Athlete's foot can spread to other body parts, especially hands. It is contagious and often recurs.	Feet should be well ventilated. Drying feet well after bathing and applying powder help prevent infection. Wearing clean socks or stockings reduces incidence. Health care provider orders application of griseofulvin, miconazole nitrate, or tolnaftate.
Ingrown nails From Habif TP: *Clinical dermatology: a color guide to diagnosis and therapy,* ed 2, St Louis, 1990, Mosby.	Toenail or fingernail growing inward into soft tissue around nail; results from improper nail trimming, poor shoe fit, or heredity	Ingrown nails cause localized swelling and pain at the lateral nail; some become infected.	Treatment is frequent warm soaks *(exception: patient with diabetes mellitus or other vascular diseases, such as Buerger's disease)* in antiseptic solution and removal of part of nail that has grown into skin. Teach patient proper nail-trimming techniques. Refer to podiatrist.
Paronychia	Inflammation of tissue between nail fold and nail plate	Area sometimes becomes infected.	Treatment is warm compresses or soaks *(exception: patient with diabetes)* and local application of antibiotic ointments. Paronychia can be prevented by careful manicuring.
Foot odors	Result of excess perspiration promoting microorganism growth; faulty foot hygiene or improper footwear causes foot odor	Odor frequently embarrasses patient.	Frequent washing, use of foot deodorants and powders, and clean footwear prevent or reduce this problem.

TABLE 40.5   Hair and Scalp Problems

Characteristics	Implications	Interventions
Dandruff Scaling of scalp is accompanied by itching. In severe cases dandruff is on eyebrows.	Dandruff causes embarrassment. If it enters eyes, conjunctivitis often develops.	Shampoo regularly with medicated shampoo. In severe cases obtain health care provider's advice.
Ticks Small, gray-brown parasites burrow into skin and suck blood.	Ticks may transmit disease to people, including Rocky Mountain spotted fever, tularemia, and Lyme disease.	Use fine-tipped tweezers to grasp tick as close to the skin's surface as possible. Pull upward with steady, even pressure. Do not twist or jerk the tick; this can cause the mouthparts to break off and remain in the skin. If this happens, remove the mouthparts with tweezers. If you are unable to remove the mouth easily with clean tweezers, leave it alone and let the skin heal. After removing the tick, thoroughly clean the bite areas and your hands with rubbing alcohol and iodine scrub, or soap and water. Dispose of a live tick by putting it in alcohol, placing it in a sealed bag/container, wrapping it tightly in tape, or flushing it down the toilet (CDC, 2019b). **Follow-up:** If you develop a rash or fever within several weeks of tick removal, contact your health care provider and inform about your tick bite.
Pediculosis (Lice) ***Pediculosis Capitis (Head Lice)*** Parasite resides on scalp attached to hair strands. Eggs look like oval particles, similar to dandruff. Bites or pustules may be observed behind ears and at hairline.	Head lice are difficult to remove and spread to furniture and other people if not treated. They do not carry disease, cannot fly or jump, and are carried by animals.	Wearing gloves, check entire scalp by using tongue depressor or special lice comb. Use medicated shampoo for eliminating lice. *Caution against use of products containing lindane because the ingredient is toxic and known to cause adverse reactions* (CDC, 2019a). Check hair for nits and comb with a nit comb for 2 to 3 days until all lice and nits have been removed. Vacuum infested areas of home.
Pediculosis Corporis (Body Lice) Parasites tend to cling to clothing; thus, they are not always easy to see. Body lice suck blood and lay eggs on clothing and furniture.	Patient itches constantly. Scratches seen on skin become infected. Hemorrhagic spots appear on skin where lice are sucking blood.	Bathe or shower thoroughly. After skin is dried, apply recommended pediculicide lotion. After 12 to 24 hours take another bath or shower. Bag infested clothing or linen until laundered in hot water. Vacuum rooms thoroughly and throw away bag after completion.
Pediculosis Pubis (Crab Lice) Parasites are in pubic hair. Crab lice are gray-white with red legs.	Lice spread through bed linen, clothing, or furniture or between people via sexual contact.	Shave hair off affected area. Clean as for body lice. If lice were sexually transmitted, notify partner.
Hair Loss (Alopecia) Alopecia occurs in all races. Balding patches are in periphery of hairline. Hair becomes brittle and broken.	Patches of uneven hair growth and loss alter patient's appearance.	Stop hair-care practices that damage hair (e.g., teasing hair, hair picks, tight braiding, excessive heat when blow-drying).

Inspect the nares for signs of inflammation, discharge, lesions, edema, and deformity (see Chapter 30). The nasal mucosa is normally pink and clear and has little or no discharge. Allergies cause a clear, watery discharge. If patients have any form of tubing exiting the nose (e.g., nasogastric), observe for edema, skin ulceration, localized tenderness, inflammation, drainage, and bleeding where the tubing comes in contact with the nares. Also observe surface of nose if adhesive is used to keep any tubing in place.

Use of Sensory Aids. For patients who wear eyeglasses, contact lenses, artificial eyes, or hearing aids, assess their knowledge and methods used for care, and have them describe the typical approach used in routine care (see Chapter 49). When possible, observe a patient perform care. Compare information gathered from the patient with the proper care technique for these devices. Any difference between a patient's practice and standard practice provides an opportunity for patient education.

Assessment of Hygiene Care Practices. Assessment of hygiene practices reveals a patient's preferences for grooming. For example, a patient chooses to groom the hair in a certain style or trim nails in a certain way. When a patient has a physical disability, special safety precautions are often necessary when grooming. For example, teach patients with loss of sensation to file nails instead of clipping. By observing a patient's performance of hygiene care, you can detect any needed areas of teaching or assistance while maintaining the patient's maximal level of independence.

Assessment of Cultural Influences. Ask what will make a patient feel most comfortable during a bath or other hygiene measures while receiving health care. Because hygiene is very personal, this question may help reveal cultural practices. Perhaps the patient prefers a partial instead of a full bath from a nurse, with a family member completing the bathing of more private body parts.

Some patients also defer hygiene. For example, if you believe that frequent skin care is critical to prevent skin breakdown, take the time to understand the patient's concerns about frequency of hygiene and then explain the rationale using plain language. Many health care agencies are using chlorhexidine gluconate (CHG) for daily bathing. CHG can leave the skin feeling sticky. If patients complain about its use, you need to explain their vulnerability to infection and how CHG helps reduce occurrence of health care–associated infection (HAI). Consider a patient's level of literacy, and be sure that you have adapted your assessment questions to a level the patient can understand (CDC, 2019c).

Patients at Risk for Hygiene Problems. Some patients present risks that require more attentive and rigorous hygiene care (see Table 40.3). These risks may result from side effects of medications or other medical therapy; a lack of knowledge; immobilization; an inability to perform hygiene; or a physical condition that potentially injures the skin, mouth, feet and nails, or hair. Anticipate whether a patient is predisposed to risks and follow through with a complete assessment. For example, if a patient is receiving cancer chemotherapy, there is a risk of the medication producing mouth ulcerations, which are painful and create a risk for infection and impaired nutrition because of reluctance to eat and drink. A patient who receives broad-spectrum antibiotics may develop an opportunistic infection when the normal flora of the mouth is disrupted by the antibiotic. Be thorough and detailed during the oral examination, checking all surfaces of the tongue and mucosa. For a bariatric patient or a patient who is diaphoretic, provide special attention to body areas such as beneath a woman's breasts and in the groin, skinfolds, and perineal area, where moisture collects and irritates skin surfaces, resulting in moisture-associated skin damage (MASD) (Mitchell and Hill, 2020).

This is Mrs. White's second postoperative day. Prior to starting care, Jamie reviewed the medical record and with help from her nursing instructor organized her approach for assessing Mrs. White's needs. Her nursing instructor pointed out some environmental issues, such as the need for adaptive equipment and occupational and physical therapy activities, which have the potential to interrupt some hygiene activities. Jamie and her instructor discussed how to avoid and adjust to some of these interruptions should they occur.

Jamie noted in the medical record that Mrs. White had an abdominal incision and received pain medication before she went to sleep. Because of this information, Mrs. White's comfort level is a priority, and Jamie first assessed Mrs. White's pain. Mrs. White rated her abdominal discomfort as 7/10, and she indicated that the pain medicine last night relieved her discomfort. Today she says that her buttocks, thighs, and breasts feel inflamed. Mrs. White also commented that her arms were "stiff." During review of Mrs. White's medical record, Jamie noted that she was due to have pain medication. She administered an analgesic 30 minutes before the assessment. Jamie organized her assessment and hygiene equipment for smooth progression from the assessment to the bed bath.

Before conducting her assessment, Jamie wanted to determine whether the pain medication had been effective and asked Mrs. White to rate her pain level, which was improved to 2/10. Jamie observed the areas where Mrs. White commented on sensations that the areas were inflamed. Jamie observed redness but intact skin under Mrs. White's buttocks and thighs and the skinfolds underneath her breasts. Mrs. White's range of motion was decreased, and she was unable to grasp objects, such as the washcloth. Mrs. White was crying and upset that she was so dependent and needed so much assistance.

REFLECT NOW

Think about how you would modify your nursing assessment to correctly identify hygiene risks for a patient who is an older adult.

◆ Analysis and Nursing Diagnosis

Clinical judgment requires application of critical thinking to analyze assessment findings. You consider the knowledge you have about a patient's condition and your assessment findings to differentiate normal versus abnormal findings. Your review of data will interpret your patient's hygiene status and self-care abilities and reveal clusters to clearly identify and label the patient's health problems related to hygiene. *Mrs. White has rheumatoid arthritis, and Jamie observed swollen, painful hands and assessed limited ROM.* Closer review of data confirms that your patient has difficulty using a hairbrush, turning in bed, and regulating a water faucet; she is unable to completely wash body parts. The nursing diagnosis of *Self-care Deficit: Impaired Ability to Bath* becomes part of the plan of care. Accurate selection of nursing diagnoses requires critical thinking to identify actual or potential problems. Be thorough in assessment to reveal all appropriate findings or risk factors so that you can make an accurate diagnosis (Box 40.3).

Use a patient's actual alteration (e.g., *Impaired Tissue Integrity*) or one for which the patient is at risk (e.g., *Risk for Infection*) to determine the focus of nursing interventions. When a patient has an actual alteration, such as *Impaired Tissue Integrity*, more thorough skin care is needed. Initiate care more frequently to keep skin surfaces clean and dry and eliminate factors such as moisture or drainage. Also provide care to promote healing of injured tissue and skin surfaces (see Chapter 48). If a patient is at risk for a problem, take preventive measures. For example, if a patient is at risk for developing an infection in the mouth and has the nursing diagnosis *Risk for Infection of Oral Mucous Membrane*, keep the oral mucosa well hydrated, minimize foods irritating to tissues, and provide cleaning that soothes and reduces tissue inflammation.

Completing a nursing diagnosis requires identification of the related factor for a problem-focused or negative diagnosis, which guides you to select nursing interventions. A diagnosis of *Impaired Oral Mucous Membrane related to malnutrition* and a diagnosis of *Impaired Oral Mucous Membrane related to side effects of chemotherapy* require different interventions. When poor nutrition is a causal factor, you consult with a registered dietitian for appropriate dietary supplements and incorporate patient education into the plan. When chemotherapy injures the oral mucosa, you follow cancer nursing guidelines regarding care

BOX 40.3 Nursing Diagnostic Process

Self-Care Deficit: Impaired Ability to Bath

Assessment activities	Assessment findings
Observe patient attempt to bathe self.	Patient is unable to change position to wash lower body, back, or perineal area.
Assess patient's upper-extremity strength and range of motion.	Patient has restricted upper-extremity range of motion in elbows and weakness in hands.
	Patient has difficulty turning in bed by self or reaching items needed.
	Patient is unable to turn water faucets on and off without hand pain.
Observe patient's ability to move from bed to bathroom and maneuver in bathroom.	Patient cannot transfer from bed to chair without assistance, cannot ambulate, relies on wheelchair to move around, is unable to maneuver wheelchair in bathroom without help or to transfer to shower seat unassisted.
	Patient needs lift equipment for transfers.

for oral mucositis (i.e., painful inflammation of oral mucous membranes), including frequent gentle brushing with a soft toothbrush, flossing, rinsing with bland rinse, limiting diet to soft foods, and applying water-based moisturizer to lips (USDHHS, 2020).

While there are other possible nursing diagnoses for patients in need of supportive hygiene care, the nursing diagnoses in the preceding paragraphs and the following list represent examples of diagnoses commonly associated with hygiene-related problems:

- Activity Intolerance
- Impaired Mobility
- Impaired Health Maintenance
- Impaired Skin Integrity
- Low Self Esteem

During assessment Jamie observes Mrs. White's swollen and deformed hands. When she asks Mrs. White to pick up basic hygiene care objects, she observes that her patient is slow to move her hands and is unable to grasp the bathing lotion and the washcloth. These patterns of assessment findings support **Self-Care Deficit: Impaired Ability to Bath.** *Jamie also identifies abnormal skin assessment findings; while the skin is intact, there is redness under Mrs. White's buttocks, thighs, and breasts. The redness was an early cue for pressure injuries and* **Risk for Impaired Skin Integrity.** *From the nursing literature, Jamie knows it is imperative to prevent pressure injuries, and she will need to take nursing measures to reduce this risk.*

Planning and Outcomes Identification

After the nursing diagnoses are identified, use clinical judgment to develop a plan of care to meet your patient's hygiene preferences and needs. During planning, synthesize information from multiple resources (Fig. 40.3). The application of critical thinking ensures that you integrate your experiences and all that you know about the individual patient to form an appropriate patient-centered plan of care. Patients who require assistance with personal hygiene have multiple nursing diagnoses. Use a concept map to help visualize and understand how nursing diagnoses interrelate with one another (Fig. 40.4). Rely on your knowledge, experience, and established standards of care when developing a care plan.

Personal and previous experience and knowledge about the effects of chronic illness and impaired mobility on a patient's skin integrity, overall feelings of comfort and wellness, and functional independence will guide you as you plan hygiene care for your patients. Perhaps you and a colleague gave a complete bed bath to a patient with limited physical mobility. You learned how to safely use adaptive devices and observed how these devices increased a patient's independence. You may have had experience with medical devices, such as oxygen masks or wound drainage systems, and gained an understanding of the risks for medical device–related pressure injuries (MDRPI) and the importance of observing a patient's skin for redness or blistering under such devices.

Previous experience with other patients will also assist in recognizing some environmental factors that impact hygiene care. For example, when you need assistive personnel to help with patient care, communicate what assistance you need, and plan a time so that personnel will be available. Frequently patients who require a complete bath are acutely ill, have limited mobility and/or activity tolerance, or require rehabilitative care. When caring for these patients, recognize that there is a potential

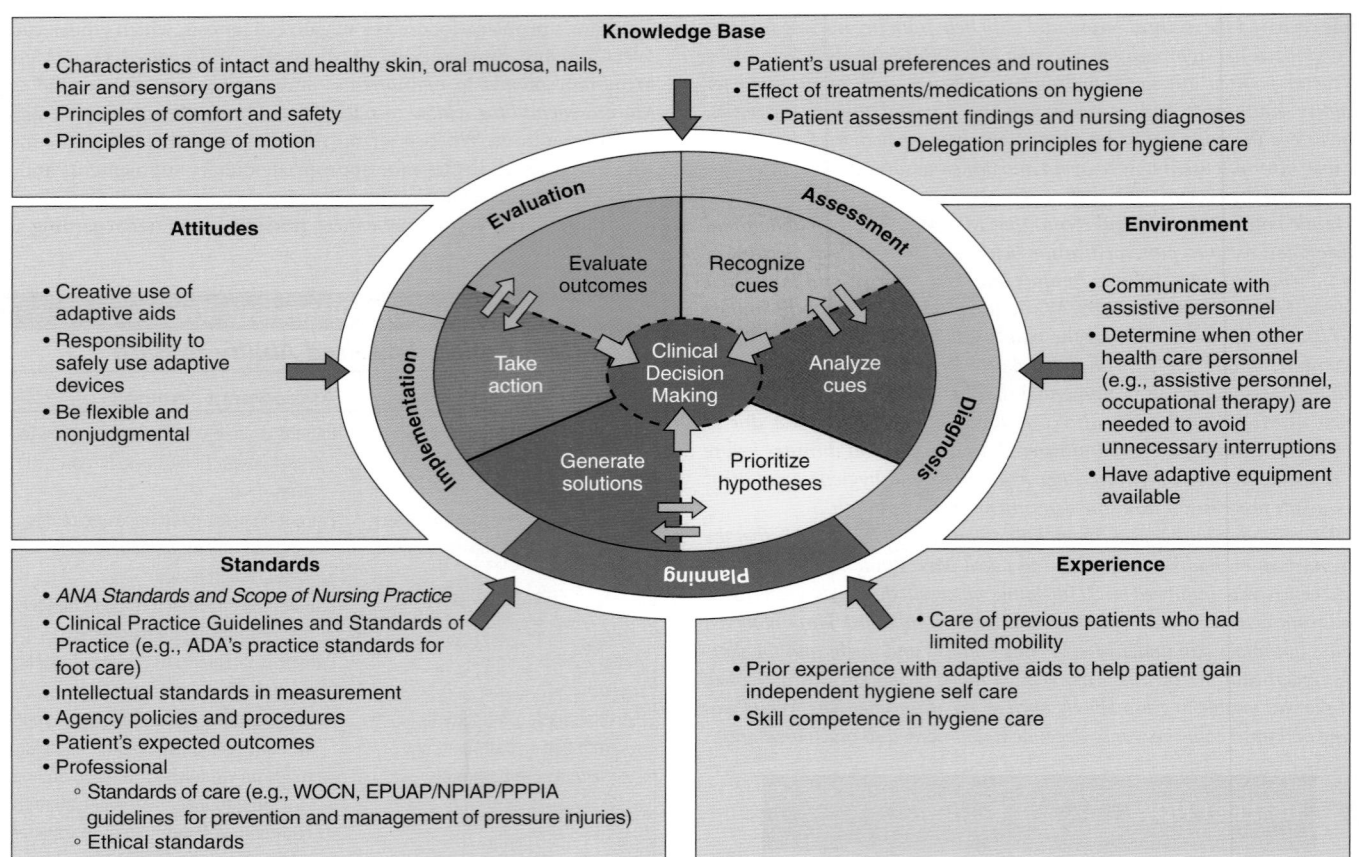

FIG. 40.3 Critical thinking model for hygiene planning. (Clinical Judgment Measurement Model copyright © NCSBN. All rights reserved.)

for interruption in care from health care providers providing therapy, such as physical and occupational therapy. Identify these potential interruptions and determine when these therapies are scheduled and plan hygiene care accordingly to reduce unnecessary interruptions.

Critical thinking attitudes, such as creativity and confidence, are helpful when developing a patient-centered plan for hygiene care. Partner with the patient to identify patient outcomes, set priorities for care, and plan evidence-based interventions. Consider continuity of care, and involve other health care team members (e.g., occupational or physical therapy) when developing the plan.

Professional standards help guide selection of the most effective nursing interventions. These standards are evidence-based guidelines for care. Incorporating these guidelines into your knowledge base and

experiential learning will enhance your clinical judgment as you plan and implement patient-centered hygiene care for each of your patients.

Outcomes. Partner with the patient and family to identify expected outcomes to develop a mutually agreed-on plan of care based on the patient's nursing diagnoses (see the Nursing Care Plan). Use clinical judgment to establish realistic outcomes that align with the patient's preferences, self-care abilities, and resources, and focus on maintaining or improving the patient's overall hygiene. Make outcomes measurable and achievable within patient limitations. In addition, work with the patient to select individualized hygiene measures. For example, a nurse and a patient who has one-sided paralysis following a cerebral vascular accident develop the following outcome: "Patient

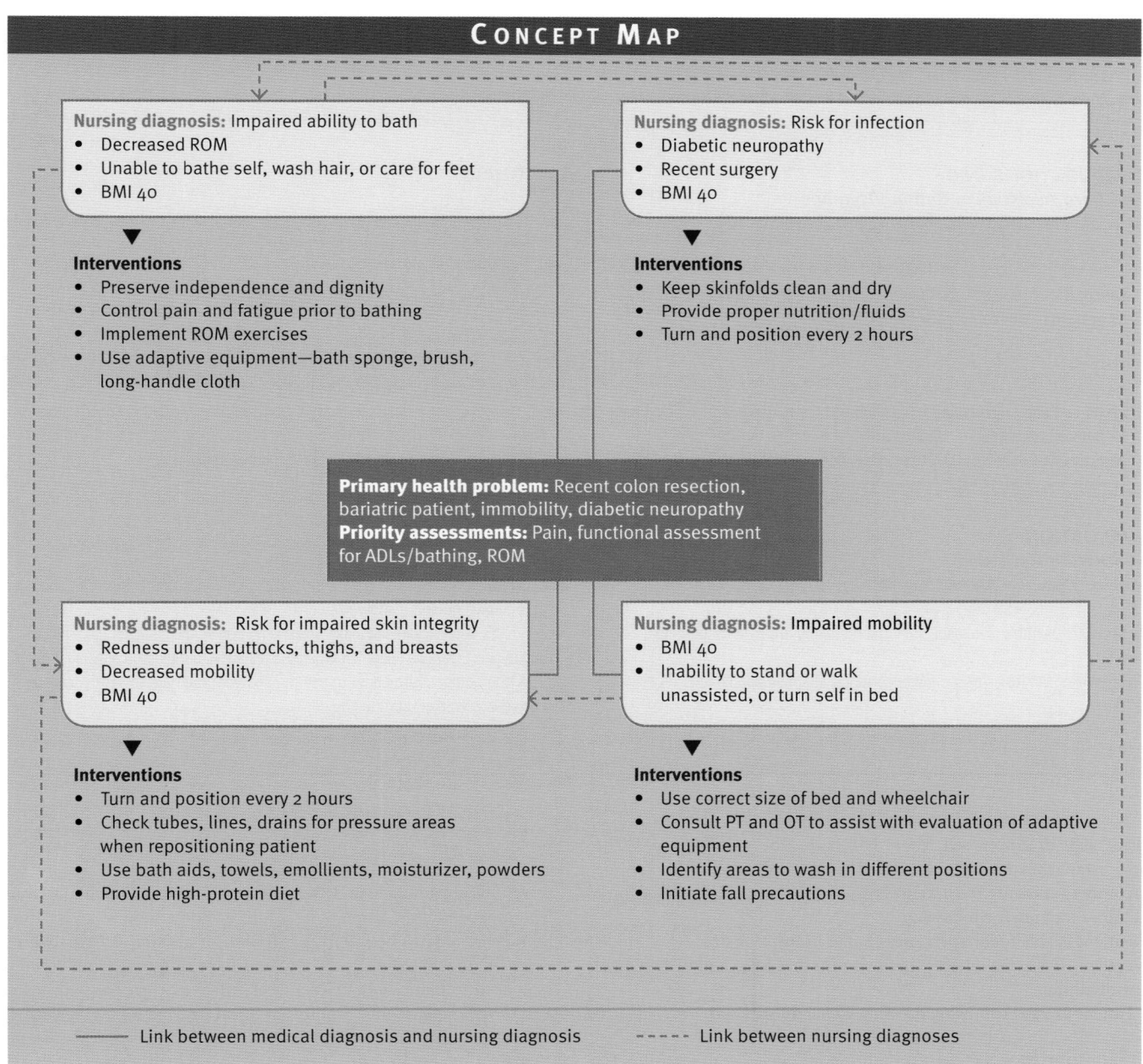

CONCEPT MAP

Nursing diagnosis: Impaired ability to bath
- Decreased ROM
- Unable to bathe self, wash hair, or care for feet
- BMI 40

Interventions
- Preserve independence and dignity
- Control pain and fatigue prior to bathing
- Implement ROM exercises
- Use adaptive equipment—bath sponge, brush, long-handle cloth

Nursing diagnosis: Risk for infection
- Diabetic neuropathy
- Recent surgery
- BMI 40

Interventions
- Keep skinfolds clean and dry
- Provide proper nutrition/fluids
- Turn and position every 2 hours

Primary health problem: Recent colon resection, bariatric patient, immobility, diabetic neuropathy
Priority assessments: Pain, functional assessment for ADLs/bathing, ROM

Nursing diagnosis: Risk for impaired skin integrity
- Redness under buttocks, thighs, and breasts
- Decreased mobility
- BMI 40

Interventions
- Turn and position every 2 hours
- Check tubes, lines, drains for pressure areas when repositioning patient
- Use bath aids, towels, emollients, moisturizer, powders
- Provide high-protein diet

Nursing diagnosis: Impaired mobility
- BMI 40
- Inability to stand or walk unassisted, or turn self in bed

Interventions
- Use correct size of bed and wheelchair
- Consult PT and OT to assist with evaluation of adaptive equipment
- Identify areas to wash in different positions
- Initiate fall precautions

——— Link between medical diagnosis and nursing diagnosis   - - - - - Link between nursing diagnoses

FIG. 40.4 Concept map for Mrs. White. *ADLs,* Activities of daily living; *BMI,* body mass index; *OT,* occupational therapist; *PT,* physical therapist; *ROM,* range of motion.

NURSING CARE PLAN

Self-Care Deficit: Impaired Ability to Bath Related to Deformed Hands and Decreased ROM

ASSESSMENT

Assessment Activities	**Assessment Findings**[a]
Ask Mrs. White what hygiene care is important this morning.	Mrs. White says, "I want to feel comfortable, clean, and smell good."
Assess Mrs. White's skin condition.	On visual inspection reveals redness under buttocks, thighs, and breasts. The abdominal incision is dry and pink, and the suture line is well approximated.
Assess Mrs. White's ability to bathe, including an assessment of her range of motion (ROM) and upper- and lower-extremity strength.	Mrs. White is **unable to gather bath supplies** because of her hand deformity and **limited hand mobility**. Her arms have **decreased ROM** and decreased sensation.

[a]**Assessment Findings** are shown in bold type.

NURSING DIAGNOSIS: Self-care deficit: Impaired ability to bath related to reduced hand mobility and limited ROM

PLANNING

Expected Outcomes (NOC)[b]
Self-Care: Bathing
Mrs. White self-reports feeling comfortable and clean after bathing.
Skin is clean and dry skin without skin breakdown between skinfolds.
Mrs. White is able to demonstrate correct use of adaptive equipment during her bath by discharge.

[b]Outcome classification labels from Moorhead S et al: *Nursing outcomes classification (NOC)*, ed 6, St Louis, 2018, Elsevier.

INTERVENTIONS (NIC)[c]	**RATIONALE**
Self-Care Assistance: Bathing/Hygiene	
Administer prn ordered analgesic before bath; begin bath 20-30 minutes later.	Patient participation in bathing or other self-care activities will improve with pain control. Give prn pain medication before pain is severe (Butcher et al., 2018).
Help patient to the shower, and place her on a shower seat. Demonstrate for patient use of grab bar and how to use wash mitt with soap pocket. Stay close by to prevent an accidental fall.	Proper education on use of shower seats, grab bars in showers/baths, and assistive devices reduce the risk for injuries while bathing (King et al., 2018). Using a wash mitt with a soap pocket or a wall-mounted soap dispenser minimizes difficulty of manipulating soap and a washcloth. A shower seat or bath bench makes it easier for patient to focus on washing rather than on balance required for standing (King et al., 2018).
Teach patient and granddaughter (as needed) how to use adaptive equipment for bathing, safe patient-handling skills, and how to perform skin assessments. Help Mrs. White plan hygiene schedule with granddaughter.	Family members who are taught methods to meet patient's bathing needs increase patient satisfaction, making the experience safe, easy, and successful (King et al., 2018). Appropriate assistive devices encourage independence.

[c]Intervention classification labels from Butcher HK et al: *Nursing interventions classifications (NIC)*, ed 7, St Louis, 2018, Elsevier.

EVALUATION

Evaluation Activities	**Patient Response**
Ask Mrs. White how she feels after bathing.	Mrs. White states that she feels comfortable and clean and enjoys that she was able to give herself a shower.
Inspect Mrs. White's skin, especially the reddened areas, after bathing	Mrs. White's skin is clean and intact; there is no skin erythema under her buttocks and thighs. Erythema under her breasts is resolving, but the skin appears irritated.
Observe Mrs. White using a shower seat and adaptive equipment.	Mrs. White demonstrates how to use the shower grab bars to safely transfer between a walker and the shower seat.
	Mrs. White demonstrates using a soap dispenser and washing mitt while safely sitting on a shower seat.

will be able to groom self (dress and bathe) before discharge." The nurse establishes measurable, realistic, and individualized expected outcomes to measure the patient's response to care. Examples of these outcomes include the following:

- Patient is able to independently bathe in front of sink.
- Patient uses assist devices (bathing mitt and long-handled sponge) for bathing.
- Patient dresses self, using dressing stick and sock aid.

Setting Priorities. A patient's condition influences your priorities for hygiene care. Set priorities based on your assessment of the required assistance needed by the patient, the extent of the hygiene-related problems, and the nature of the patient's nursing diagnoses. For example, a seriously ill patient usually needs a daily bath because body secretions accumulate, and the patient is unable to maintain cleanliness independently. Some older adults at home require a visit from a home care aide to help with a tub bath or shower. Patients who are normally inactive during the day and have skin that tends to be dry may need to bathe only twice a week, whereas a patient with urinary and bowel incontinence requires perineal hygiene following each episode of soiling. Plan to help patients who are weakened or possess poor coordination. For example, a patient who has hemiplegia (paralysis on one side of the body) and has difficulty getting out of a tub needs a tub chair and requires handrails or extra personnel for assistance.

Timing is also important in planning hygiene care. Being interrupted in the middle of a bath often frustrates and embarrasses a patient. Assess for cultural preferences on time of day or who may help patient with hygiene care.

Teamwork and Collaboration. During hospitalization, know a patient's schedule for therapy or diagnostic procedures and plan hygiene care accordingly. Collaborate with other health team members as indicated (e.g., work with physical and occupational therapy to enhance the patient's independence with self-care activities). If a patient is hospitalized, plan care before discharge to home, a rehabilitation center, or extended-care facility. Be sure that family caregivers know any physical or cognitive limitations that will affect their ability to provide safe, effective hygiene care. For example, a patient with reduced sensation in one foot is at risk for burns from hot water; in this case, plan to teach the patient proper foot care and how to safely test the water temperature.

When a patient needs assistance because of a self-care limitation and family caregivers are the ones to provide it, proper education and preparation should be included in the plan of care. *For example, Jamie knows that Mrs. White's granddaughter is willing to assist with care at home, and it is important that Jamie include her in the plan of care and patient teaching.* Give clear directions on how to perform hygiene and how to obtain appropriate adaptive equipment and supplies. Family members also need guidance in providing safety and adapting techniques to fit patient limitations. Be aware of equipment and procedures used in the agency, and support the patient and family to make them knowledgeable about making necessary adaptations. Depending on a patient's limitations, some insurance plans provide home care assistants to help with basic hygiene needs. Explore this option with the patient and family members.

Collaborate with community agencies as needed. For example, a nurse involved in the care of a homeless patient needs to be aware of the locations of distribution centers for clothing and basic hygiene supplies, shelters where bathing facilities are available, and organizations that offer free health care or reduced fees. Partner with social workers or staff in local area churches, not-for-profit organizations, and schools to be sure that patients have the resources they need to maintain hygiene.

Jamie starts to plan patient-centered personal hygiene care while giving attention to Mrs. White's physical and emotional comfort level. Maintaining Mrs. White's pain at less than 5/10 is an outcome of pain control, and Jamie notes that Mrs. White rates her level of pain at 2/10. A second outcome is to increase Mrs. White's hygiene self-care. To begin to achieve this outcome Jamie collaborates with occupational therapy to help plan interventions to assist Mrs. White to correctly use adaptive equipment (e.g., a shower chair and wash mitt). As part of the plan, Jamie includes Mrs. White's granddaughter, who is willing to help her when she returns to her residence.

◆ Implementation

Hygiene is an essential part of basic patient care. When you use caring practices to perform hygiene measures, you reduce the patient's anxiety and promote comfort and relaxation. For example, use a gentle approach when giving patients their baths and changing gowns as you turn and reposition them. A soft, gentle voice when conversing with patients relieves fears or concerns. For patients suffering symptoms such as pain or nausea, administering medications to relieve the symptoms before providing hygiene helps to maintain patient comfort during hygiene procedures.

Consider the stress that hygiene care can cause, and be alert for any cues of embarrassment or anxiety. Some patients fear pain or are frightened about falling or sustaining injury when being assisted to a bathroom.

Implementation also focuses on assisting and preparing patients to perform much of their hygiene care independently. Discuss any signs and symptoms of hygiene problems. Teach patients proper hygiene techniques and how their use is associated with better health. Inform patients about available resources in the community.

Jamie prioritizes two nursing diagnoses: Self-care Deficit: Impaired Ability to Bath related to deformed hands and decreased ROM and Risk for Impaired Skin Integrity related to reddened areas on thighs, buttocks, and underneath the breasts. From previous clinical experience, Jamie knows that patients want and need to provide input about their nursing care. Jamie encourages Mrs. White to make decisions about how to proceed with her hygiene care by engaging her in a therapeutic conversation.

Jamie knows that a priority for Mrs. White is to maintain her independence for hygiene and other activities of daily living, and part of her normal routine is to wash her face and hands and care for her dentures before breakfast. But then she tells Jamie that right now she cannot do these things by herself and that she does not want to be "any trouble." Jamie reassures Mrs. White that assisting her with prebreakfast hygiene is a priority. She also explains to Mrs. White how occupational therapy and the correct use of adaptive devices will improve her independence.

Even at an optimal level of functioning with assistance, Mrs. White is at continued risk for self-care deficits. During hygiene care, Mrs. White starts to ask questions about how to use adaptive shower devices to assist with personal care. Jamie knows that Mrs. White is showing some readiness to learn. Jamie wants to preserve as much of Mrs. White's independence as possible, ensure privacy, and foster physical well-being.

Health Promotion. In primary health care situations educate and counsel patients and family caregivers on why proper hygiene techniques are necessary. For example, a new mother needs to learn how to bathe her newborn to reduce risk of skin irritation and infection, whereas an older adult needs information on the importance of regular ear care to avoid accumulated cerumen and hearing impairment. The hygiene skills described throughout this chapter provide standards for excellent physical care. When caring for patients in primary health care settings, maintain these standards and incorporate adaptations as needed to meet the patient's lifestyle, functional status, living arrangements, and preferences. Key points when teaching patients about hygiene include the following:

- Make any instruction relevant based on your assessment of the patient's knowledge, motivation, preferences, cultural practices, and health beliefs. For example, when teaching a patient who has diabetes mellitus, include risks for impaired foot circulation and how this causes a risk for infection and poor healing, especially when the skin is injured or broken.
- Adapt instruction to a patient's personal bathing facilities and resources. Not all patients have the ideal situation that exists in a health care setting (e.g., easily accessible shower or a bedside table to place over a bed). Adapt available resources so that the patient can reach, and use needed items comfortably and safely. For example, an older adult couple need to adapt their bathtub to accommodate a shower chair.
- Teach patients ways to avoid injury. Almost any hygiene procedure poses risks (e.g., cutting a nail too close to the skin or failing to adjust the water temperature of the bath). Include safety risks and tips with all instructions.
- Reinforce infection control practices. Damage to the skin, mucosa, eyes, or other tissues creates an immediate risk for infection. Determine that a patient understands the relationship among healthy and intact skin and tissues, hand hygiene practices, and the prevention of infection (see Chapter 28).

BOX 40.4 Hygiene Care Schedule in Acute and Long-Term Care Settings

Early Morning Care
Nursing personnel on the night shift may provide basic hygiene to patients getting ready for breakfast, scheduled tests, or early morning surgery. "AM care" includes offering a bedpan or urinal if the patient is not ambulatory, washing the patient's hands and face, and helping with oral care.

Routine Morning Care
After breakfast help by offering a bedpan or urinal to patients confined to bed; provide a full or partial bath or a shower, including perineal care and oral, foot, nail, and hair care; give a back rub; change a patient's gown or pajamas; change the bed linens; and straighten a patient's bedside unit and room. This is often referred to as "complete AM care."

Afternoon Care
Hospitalized patients often undergo many exhausting diagnostic tests or procedures in the morning. In rehabilitation centers patients participate in physical therapy in the morning. Afternoon hygiene care includes washing the hands and face, helping with oral care, offering a bedpan or urinal, and straightening bed linen.

Evening, or Hour-before-Sleep, Care
Before bedtime offer personal hygiene care that helps patients relax and promotes sleep. "PM care" often includes changing soiled bed linens, gowns, or pajamas; helping patients wash the face and hands; providing oral hygiene; giving a back massage; and offering the bedpan or urinal to nonambulatory patients. Some patients enjoy a beverage such as juice; check diet to determine which beverages are allowed.

BOX 40.5 Types of Baths

Complete bed bath: Bath administered to totally dependent patient in bed.

Partial bed bath: Bed bath that consists of bathing only body parts that would cause discomfort if left unbathed, such as the hands, face, axilla, and perineal area. Partial bath also includes washing back and providing back rub. Dependent patients in need of partial hygiene or self-sufficient bedridden patients who are unable to reach all body parts receive a partial bed bath.

Sponge bath at the sink: Involves bathing from a bath basin or sink with patient sitting in a chair. Patient can perform part of the bath independently. Nurse helps with hard-to-reach areas.

Tub bath: Involves immersion in a tub of water that allows more thorough washing and rinsing than a bed bath. Patients may require nurse's help. Some agencies have tubs equipped with lifting devices that facilitate positioning dependent patients in the tub.

Shower: Patient sits or stands under a continuous stream of water. The shower provides more thorough cleaning than a bed bath but can be tiring.

Disposable bed bath/travel bath: The bag bath contains several soft, nonwoven cotton cloths that are premoistened in a solution of no-rinse surfactant cleaner and emollient. The bag bath offers an alternative because of the ease of use, reduced time bathing, and patient comfort

Chlorhexidine gluconate (CHG) bath: Antimicrobial agent used to reduce incidence of hospital-acquired infections on skin, invasive lines, and catheters (Frost et al., 2018; Dray et al., 2019).

Acute, Restorative, and Continuing Care. Nursing knowledge and skills needed for performing hygiene care are consistent across all health care settings. In addition, some of the skills in this section are applicable in areas of health promotion. The variety, frequency, and timing of hygiene measures vary across health care settings and according to individual patient needs. In the acute care setting factors such as frequent diagnostic and treatment plans, patient symptoms, and the need for more extensive hygiene care resulting from acute illness or injury impact timing and frequency of care. In extended-care facilities and nursing homes, bathing may be scheduled less often.

Bathing and Skin Care. The extent, type, and timing or frequency of bathing and the methods used depend on a patient's physical abilities, health problems, personal preferences, and the degree of hygiene required (Box 40.4 and Box 40.5). In addition to cleansing baths, the health care provider may prescribe therapeutic baths, including sitz baths. Medicated baths (e.g., oatmeal, cornstarch, or Aveeno) may be recommended in the home setting. A sitz bath cleans and reduces pain and inflammation of perineal and anal areas (see Chapter 48). Medicated baths relieve skin irritation and create an antibacterial and drying effect.

Chlorhexidine gluconate (CHG) is often added to a patient's bath water to reduce the risk for health care–associated infections (HAIs). HAIs are one of the most common adverse events during hospitalization. While the critically ill might be most susceptible, all hospitalized patients are at risk (Frost et al., 2018). Using this solution in a patient's bath is detailed in a later section.

If a patient is physically dependent or cognitively impaired, increase the frequency of skin assessment and provide skin care directed toward reducing the risk for skin breakdown. When bathing patients with cognitive impairments, consider their special needs and challenges (Sullivan et al., 2018; Wilson, 2018). These patients easily become afraid. Patients with dementia often refuse, withdraw, or fight during a bath or shower. A patient-centered approach better enables you to manage their physical limitations and aggressive behaviors (Box 40.6). Use assessment and communication skills to learn possible triggers that affect participation with hygiene care (Villar et al., 2018; Yevchak et al., 2017). For example, unmanaged pain; being cold; feeling frightened, vulnerable, and exposed; feeling embarrassed; feeling a loss of control; or not understanding what is happening often causes aggressive behavior. Adapt your bathing procedures and the environment to reduce the triggers. For example, administer any ordered analgesic 30 minutes before a bath, and be gentle in your approach. Keep the patient's body as warm as possible with warm towels, and be sure that the room temperature is comfortable. Reduce fear by making sure that all safety devices (e.g., grab bars in a shower, bathmats) are available. Ask for permission to conduct the bath, and give the patient options for making decisions (e.g., choice of soap, timing of when to wash face). Use comforting words during bathing to enhance a patient's relaxation. Collaborate and communicate to teach family members how to communicate with and how to help bathe cognitively impaired patients for optimal outcomes once the patient is discharged (Vaingankar et al., 2016).

Complete Bed Bath. A complete bed bath (see Skill 40.1), tub bath, or shower often exhausts a patient. Turning during a complete bed bath and receiving back care increase oxygen consumption and demand. Getting out of a low tub requires considerable exertion. Assess and be alert for a patient's activity intolerance during hygiene care. Assessing heart rate before, during, and after a bath provides a measure of the patient's physical tolerance. Provide a partial bed bath (see Skill 40.1) to patients who are aging, dependent, in need of only partial hygiene, or bedridden and unable to reach all body parts. Wear clean gloves when there is a risk of coming in contact with body fluids. Control environmental factors that alter skin integrity, including moisture, heat, and external sources of pressure, such as wrinkled bed linen and improperly placed drainage tubing.

BOX 40.6 EVIDENCE-BASED PRACTICE

Improving Hygiene Care for Patients with Cognitive Impairments

PICOT Question: Does implementing a person-centered approach for hygiene care improve patient cooperation and nurse satisfaction in adults with cognitive impairments?

Evidence Summary

Noisy and unfamiliar surroundings are very distressing to patients with cognitive impairments, such as confusion or dementia. In addition, this distress is worsened by the patient's physical illness, pain, dehydration, toileting needs, medications, and stimulation from the hospital environment (Mendes, 2018). A person-centered care approach can work with the family caregiver, the patient, and the health care team to design hygiene measures and routines that are congruent with the patient's usual practices (Shelton et al., 2018). Research supports the use of nurse-facilitated person-centered care interventions when caring for patients with cognitive disorders (Yevchak et al., 2017).

Application to Nursing Practice

- Design person-centered care to meet the individual needs of patients and minimize agency-based constraints on care routines (Pinkert et al., 2018).
- Do not rush, and speak in a low, pleasant voice, giving information before and throughout the bathing process (Rokstad et al., 2017).
- Work with family and patient to determine factors that may trigger anxiety or reduced cooperation. These triggers may vary from person to person and can include (but are not limited to) new nursing staff, a full bladder, the time of day, or too much environmental noise (Hirschman and Hodgson, 2018; Yevchak et al., 2017).
- Avoid incongruent care preferences between the patient and the agency caregiver to reduce patient anxiety (Shelton et al., 2018).
- Involve the patient in the hygiene care plan, and maintain prehospital routines (Villar et al., 2018; Mendes, 2018).
- Communicate the patient's preferences related to hygiene and activities of daily living (ADL) with all agency caregivers to promote patient comfort, reduce patient anxiety, and improve nurse satisfaction (Rokstad et al., 2017; Shelton et al., 2018).

Traditionally, baths have been given using soap and warm water. The question of whether to use bath basins with soap and water is an issue because bath basins provide a reservoir for bacteria and are a possible source of transmission of hospital-acquired infections (HAIs) (Alserehi et al., 2018). Daily bathing with chlorhexidine substantially reduces patients' cutaneous microbial burden, thus reducing a patient's risk for bloodstream HAIs, including methicillin-resistant *Staphylococcus aureus* (MRSA) and vancomycin-resistant *Enterococcus* (VRE) infections (Frost et al., 2018).

There is a link between waterborne pathogens and the development of biofilm (multiple colonies of microorganisms attached to a surface such as a bath basin). The formation of a biofilm combined with transmission of organisms through contact with unwashed hands can create a reservoir of bacteria. The bacteria can be transferred to and maintained in a patient's bath basin. In contrast, the use of chlorhexidine gluconate (CHG) 4% solution in place of standard soap and water in washbasins has been shown to decrease bacterial growth in basins and reduce methicillin-resistant *Staphylococcus aureus* (MRSA) (Dray et al., 2019). It is important to air-dry bath basins completely and not to use a basin for storing supplies.

Another option to using CHG in bath basins is the use of CHG 2% in disposable impregnated washcloths. CHG in the cloths is fast acting, has broad-spectrum microorganism coverage, continues antimicrobial activity up to 24 hours after application, and is rinse free and disposable. The cloths can be used in any setting and for all bathing purposes, including once-a-day full-body bathing, incontinence care, or any reason for additional cleaning (AHRQ, 2013). Research has shown that CHG bathing is particularly effective for ICU patients (Ruiz et al., 2017; Johns Hopkins Medicine, 2021). Daily bathing with 2% CHG-impregnated cloths versus nonantimicrobial washcloths reduces cross-contamination and colonization of multidrug-resistant organisms (MDROs) (Martin et al., 2017; Ruiz et al., 2017). Daily bathing with some form of CHG is becoming more of a standard practice across hospitals. Patients often describe their skin as feeling a bit sticky. Explain to patients the importance of using CHG to protect them against serious infection. When using CHG solution in bath water or impregnated cloths, use a clean CHG washcloth/cloth for each area of the body (see Skill 40.1, Step 26).

There are precautions to follow in using CHG. CHG is safe to use on superficial wounds, abrasions, and rashes (AHRQ, 2013). In the case of open or deep wounds such as Stage 3 or 4 pressure injuries, bathe with CHG around a dressing or wound. Do not use CHG on third- or fourth-degree burns (AHRQ, 2013).

Use a tub bath or shower (see Skill 40.1) to give a more thorough bath than a bed bath. CHG 4% solution can be used in showers, but instruct patients to exit the shower after application, and do not rinse the CHG off. Implement safety measures to prevent fall injuries because the surface of a tub or shower stall is slippery. In some settings a health care provider's order for a shower or tub bath is necessary. Place a chair in the shower for patients with weakness or poor balance. Both tubs and showers need to have grab bars for patients to hold during entry and exit and maneuvering during the bath or shower. Patients vary in how much physical assistance they need from care providers. Regardless of the type of bath a patient receives, use the following guidelines:

- *Provide privacy.* Close the door and/or pull room curtains around the bathing area. While bathing a patient, expose only the areas being bathed by using proper draping.
- *Maintain safety.* Keep side rails up when away from a patient's bedside when patients are dependent or unconscious. **NOTE:** When side rails serve as a restraint, you need a health care provider's order (see agency-specific policy for restraint usage) (see Chapter 27). Place the nurse call system in the patient's reach if leaving the bedside even temporarily.
- *Maintain warmth.* Keep the room warm because the patient is partially uncovered and easily chilled. Wet skin causes an excessive loss of heat through evaporation. Control drafts and keep windows closed. Keep the patient covered. Expose only the body part being washed during the bath.
- *Promote independence.* Encourage the patient to participate in as much of the bathing activities as possible. Offer assistance when needed.
- *Anticipate needs.* Bring a new set of clothing and hygiene products to the bedside or bathroom.

Teach patients to follow a few general rules for skin health. Encourage them to routinely inspect their skin for changes in color or texture and to report abnormalities to their health care provider. Instruct them to handle the skin gently, avoiding excessive rubbing. Patients with excessively dry skin are predisposed to skin impairment. If patients use bar soap at home, recommend that they choose one that contains emollients to hydrate dry skin. Avoid overly hot water because it can dry the skin by removing natural oils. Lubricate the skin with emollient lotions to reduce dryness.

Good skin health requires patients to eat nutritious foods from all food groups, including those rich in vitamins and minerals, and to consume adequate fluids. Stress safety concerns such as failing to adjust or check the water temperature and slipping on wet surfaces. Ensure that patients understand that healthy and intact skin and tissues protect them from infection. Reinforce infection control practices, including proper hand hygiene.

Perineal Care. A patient routinely receives perineal care during a complete bed bath (see Skill 40.1). However, more frequent perineal care is needed for patients at risk for acquiring an infection, such as those who have incontinence-associated dermatitis (IAD), patients with an indwelling Foley catheter, women who are postpartum, or patients recovering from rectal or genital surgery. This is especially important for patients with indwelling Foley catheters in the effort to reduce catheter-associated urinary tract infection (CAUTI) (Galiczewski, 2016; Meddings et al., 2017) (see Chapter 46). In addition, women who are having a menstrual period require perineal care. CHG is safe to use on the perineum and external mucosa for thorough cleansing (AHRQ, 2013).

When the patient's condition allows, encourage the patient to perform perineal care. Sometimes you are embarrassed about providing perineal care, particularly to patients of the opposite sex. Similarly, the patient may feel embarrassed. Do not let embarrassment cause you to overlook the patient's hygiene needs. When staffing levels permit, use a gender-congruent caregiver. A professional, dignified, and sensitive approach reduces embarrassment and helps put the patient at ease.

If a patient performs self-care, various problems such as vaginal and urethral discharge, skin irritation, and unpleasant odors often go unnoticed. Stress the importance of perineal care in preventing skin breakdown and infection. Be alert for complaints of burning during urination or localized soreness, excoriation, or pain in the perineum. Inspect vaginal and perineal areas and the patient's bed linen for signs of discharge, and use your sense of smell to detect abnormal odors. Risk factors for skin breakdown in the perineal area include urinary or fecal incontinence, rectal and perineal surgical dressings, indwelling urinary catheters, and morbid obesity.

Back Rub. A good time to give a back rub or back massage is after a patient's bath. It promotes relaxation, relieves muscular tension, and decreases perception of pain. Effleurage (i.e., long, slow, gliding strokes of a massage) is associated with reduced measured anxiety, heart rate, and respiratory rate. Studies show that slow-stroke back massages of 3 minutes and hand massages of 10 minutes significantly improve both physiological and psychological indicators of relaxation in older people (Touhy and Jett, 2021).

When providing a back rub, enhance relaxation by reducing noise and ensuring that the patient is comfortable. It is important to ask whether a patient would like a back rub, because some individuals dislike physical contact. Consult the medical record for any contraindications to a massage (e.g., fractured ribs, burns, heart surgery). Chapter 44 describes steps for back massage.

Foot and Nail Care. Routine nail and foot care involves soaking the hands and feet to soften cuticles and layers of horny cells, thorough cleaning, drying, and proper nail trimming. The one exception is patients with diabetes mellitus or peripheral vascular disease, who are at risk for tissue ulceration or infection because soaking causes skin softening or maceration of tissue.

When providing nail care, have the patient remain in bed or sit in a chair (see Skill 40.2). In some settings, such as long-term care, or with specific patients, such as a person with diabetes mellitus or peripheral vascular disease, you need a health care provider's order to trim toenails. The risk of accidentally cutting skin around a nail and predisposing a patient to infection is the reason orders are required. Check agency policy to determine whether an order is necessary.

Take time during the procedure to teach the patient and family caregivers proper techniques for cleaning and nail trimming. Stress the importance of how thorough nail care prevents infection and promotes good circulation. All patients must learn to protect the feet from injury, never walk barefoot, keep feet clean and dry, and wear footwear that fits properly. Instruct patients in the proper way to inspect all surfaces of the feet and hands for redness, lesions, dryness, or signs of infection. Teach foot care to family caregivers for patients who need regular foot care and have peripheral vascular disease, visual difficulties, physical constraints that prevent movement, or cognitive problems.

Certain conditions place patients with diabetes mellitus at increased risk for amputation (ADA, 2020). These factors include peripheral neuropathy, limited joint mobility, bony deformity, peripheral vascular disease, and a history of skin ulcers or previous amputation. Observe for changes that indicate peripheral neuropathy or vascular insufficiency (Box 40.7). Advise patients to use the following guidelines in a routine foot and nail care program (ADA, 2020, CDC, 2019c):

- Inspect the feet daily, including the bottoms and tops, heels, and areas between the toes. Use a mirror to help inspect the feet thoroughly, or ask a family member to check daily.
- Wash feet daily in lukewarm water. Dry thoroughly, especially between the toes. Avoid harsh chemicals or long soaks, which can cause skin softening or maceration of tissue, causing ulceration or infection. **Do Not Soak the Feet.**
- Wear well-fitting shoes and clean, dry socks at all times; never go barefoot. Check inside shoes before wearing them for rough areas or objects that may rub against the foot.
- Keep skin soft and smooth by applying an emollient lotion over all surfaces of the feet but not between the toes.
- If you can see and reach your toenails, trim them straight across and square file the edges smooth.
- Keep the blood flowing to your feet by putting them up when sitting and wiggling your toes and moving your ankles up and down for 5 minutes, 2 or 3 times a day. Do not cross your legs for long periods and do not smoke.
- Protect the feet from hot and cold. Do not use heating pads or electric blankets, and always wear shoes at the beach or on hot pavement.

Oral Hygiene. Regular oral hygiene, including brushing, flossing, and rinsing, prevents and controls plaque-associated oral diseases. Brushing cleans the teeth of food particles, plaque, and bacteria. It also massages

BOX 40.7 Signs of Peripheral Neuropathy or Vascular Insufficiency

Peripheral Neuropathy	Vascular Insufficiency
• Muscle wasting of lower extremities	• Decreased hair growth on legs and feet
• Foot deformities	• Absent or decreased pulses
• Soft tissue infection in lower extremities	• Infection of the foot
• Abnormal gait	• Poor wound healing
• Absent or decreased deep tendon reflexes and/or response to vibratory, touch, or painful stimuli	• Thickened nails
	• Shiny appearance of the skin
	• Blanching of skin on elevation

Data from Ball J, et al: *Seidel's guide to physical examination*, ed 9, St Louis, 2019, Mosby.

the gums and relieves discomfort resulting from unpleasant odors and tastes. Daily flossing removes food particles, plaque, and tartar that collect between teeth and at the gum line. Rinsing removes dislodged food particles and excess toothpaste. Complete oral hygiene enhances well-being and comfort and stimulates the appetite.

When patients become ill, many factors influence their need for oral hygiene, such as their ability to take fluids orally, the presence of oral lesions or trauma, and level of consciousness. Patients who are unconscious or have artificial airways, such as a tracheostomy or endotracheal tube, have special precautions for oral care because they do not have a gag reflex. Patients in hospitals or long-term care facilities do not always receive the aggressive oral care they need. Base the frequency of care on the condition of the oral cavity, risk for aspiration of saliva, and the patient's level of comfort. Some patients (e.g., in cases of stroke, trauma to oral cavity, or presence of endotracheal tube) require oral care as often as every 1 to 2 hours.

Brushing. The American Dental Association guidelines (2020) for effective oral hygiene include brushing the teeth at least twice a day with American Dental Association–approved fluoride toothpaste. Fluoride and antimicrobial mouth rinses help prevent tooth decay. Do not use fluoride rinse in children ages 6 or under because of the risk of swallowing the rinse.

Use antimicrobial toothpastes and 0.12% CHG oral rinses for patients with an increased risk for poor oral hygiene (e.g., older adults and patients with cognitive impairments and who are immunocompromised) (Jenson et al., 2018). In critically ill patients, the use of a chlorhexidine gluconate (CHG) oral hygiene protocol as part of daily oral care reduces the incidence of oral infections and ventilator-associated pneumonia (VAP) (de Lacerda Vidal et al., 2017). The Institute for Healthcare Improvement (2020) recommends the use of 0.12% chlorhexidine gluconate (CHG) as part of daily oral care in critically ill patients.

The toothbrush needs to have a straight handle and a brush small enough to reach all areas of the mouth. Rounded soft bristles stimulate the gums without causing abrasion and bleeding. Any patient who has decreased dexterity because of a medical condition or the aging process requires an enlarged handle with an easier grip (Box 40.8).

Brush all tooth surfaces thoroughly (Box 40.9). Commercially made foam swabs are ineffective in removing plaque. Electric or battery-powered toothbrushes improve the quality of cleaning and may be easier to use than manual brushes when nurses provide care for dependent patients. Do not use lemon-glycerin sponges because they dry mucous membranes and erode tooth enamel.

To prevent cross-contamination, teach patients to avoid sharing toothbrushes with family members or drinking directly from a bottle of mouthwash. Disclosure tablets or drops to stain the plaque that collects at the gum line are useful for showing patients how effectively they brush. Instruct patients to obtain a new toothbrush every 3 months or after a cold or upper respiratory infection to minimize the growth of microorganisms on the brush surfaces (American Dental Association, 2020).

Flossing. Dental flossing removes plaque and tartar between teeth and is part of oral health. Flossing involves inserting waxed or unwaxed dental floss between all tooth surfaces, one at a time. The seesaw motion used to pull floss between teeth removes plaque and tartar from tooth enamel. Use unwaxed floss and avoid vigorous flossing near the gum line on patients who are receiving chemotherapy, radiation, or anticoagulant therapy to prevent bleeding. If toothpaste is applied to the teeth before flossing, fluoride comes in direct contact with tooth surfaces, aiding in cavity prevention. According to American Dental Association (2020) recommendations, flossing once a day is sufficient. Flossing a patient's teeth is not realistic or appropriate in all care settings.

Patients With Special Needs. Some patients require special oral hygiene methods. For example, patients with diabetes mellitus or those

---

BOX 40.8 FOCUS ON OLDER ADULTS

Oral Health

- Some patients may lack the manual dexterity needed to perform oral hygiene and may need assistance from family members or in-home care providers.
- Many older adults are edentulous (without teeth), and the teeth that are present are often diseased or decayed (Touhy and Jett, 2021).
- The periodontal membrane weakens with aging, making it more prone to infection. Periodontal disease predisposes older adults to systemic infection.
- Dentures or partial plates do not always fit properly, causing pain and discomfort, which in turn affects chewing, digestive processes, enjoyment of food, and nutritional status.
- An age-related decline in saliva secretion and some medications (e.g., antihypertensives, diuretics, antiinflammatories, antidepressants) cause dry mouth (Touhy and Jett, 2021).
- Changes in oral health and oral hygiene practices also impact nutritional status. Reinforce the need to maintain a healthy diet, and teach patients how to select soft, nutritious foods.
- Financial limitations and the belief that dentures eliminate the need for routine dental care are some of the reasons older adults do not seek dental care (Touhy and Jett, 2021).

---

receiving chemotherapy frequently experience periodontal disease. Therefore, they need to visit a dentist every 3 to 4 months, clean their teeth up to 4 times a day, and handle oral tissues gently with a minimum of trauma. Xerostomia, bruxism, and dental caries may be present with patients who are methamphetamine users. Cravings for sugary sweets may cause decay and gum disease.

Patients may depend on their caregivers for oral care. Being unconscious or having an artificial airway (e.g., endotracheal or tracheal tubes) increases the susceptibility for patients to have drying of salivary secretions because they are unable to eat or drink, unable to swallow, and frequently breathe through the mouth. Unconscious patients often have a reduced gag reflex, or they cannot swallow salivary secretions that accumulate in the mouth. Pooling of salivary secretions in the back of the throat harbors microorganism growth. These secretions often contain gram-negative bacteria that cause pneumonia if aspirated into the lungs. Proper oral hygiene requires keeping the mucosa moist and removing secretions that contribute to infection. While providing hygiene, protect the patient from choking and aspiration and use topical CHG, especially in ventilated patients (see Skill 40.3). Current evidence shows that the use of CHG with oral hygiene reduces the risk for ventilator-associated pneumonia (IHI, 2020).

To provide oral care for these patients, have two nurses provide the care; turn the patient's head toward you and place the bed in semi-Fowler's position. You can delegate assistive personnel to participate. One nurse does the actual cleaning, and the other caregiver removes secretions with suction equipment. Some health care agencies use equipment that combines a mouth swab with the suction device; you can use this equipment safely by yourself. While cleansing the oral cavity, use a small oral airway or a padded tongue blade to hold the mouth open. Never use your fingers to hold a patient's mouth open. A human bite contains multiple pathogenic microorganisms. Even though the patient is not awake or alert, explain the steps of mouth care and the sensations that will be felt. Also tell the patient when the procedure is completed.

Some treatments such as chemotherapy, immunosuppressive agents, head and neck radiation, and nasogastric intubation place patients at higher risk of experiencing stomatitis or inflammation of the oral mucosa. Stomatitis causes burning, pain, and change in food and fluid tolerance. When caring for patients with stomatitis, brush

BOX 40.9   PROCEDURAL GUIDELINES

Providing Oral Hygiene

Delegation and Collaboration

The skill of oral hygiene (including toothbrushing, flossing, and rinsing) can be delegated to assistive personnel (AP). However, the nurse is responsible for assessing the patient's gag reflex to determine whether the patient is at risk for aspiration. The nurse instructs the AP about:

- Types of changes in oral mucosa to report to the nurse.
  - Reporting ulcerations, lesions, open sores, or bleeding of oral mucosa or gums and patient report of pain.
- Positioning the patient to avoid aspiration.
  - Keeping head of bed (HOB) raised 30-45 degrees.
- The need to immediately report to the nurse excessive patient coughing, drooling, or choking during or after oral hygiene.

Equipment

Soft-bristle toothbrush; nonabrasive fluoride toothpaste; chlorhexidine gluconate (CHG) solution (see agency policy); tongue depressor; water glass with cool water, normal saline, or an antiseptic mouth rinse *(optional depending on patient preference)*; moisturizing lubricant for lips *(optional)*; emesis basin; face towel; paper towels; clean gloves; penlight; linen bag or hamper

Procedural Steps

1. Identify patient using at least two identifiers (e.g., name and birthday or name and medical record number) according to agency policy (TJC, 2021).
2. Review medical record and identify presence of common oral hygiene problems.
3. Determine patient's or family caregiver's knowledge, experience, and health literacy.
4. Assess patient's oral hygiene practices, such as frequency of brushing and flossing, type of toothpaste and mouthwash used, last and frequency of dental visits.
5. Perform hand hygiene and apply clean gloves.
6. Using tongue depressor and penlight, inspect integrity of lips, teeth, buccal mucosa, gums, palate, and tongue; also assess for gag reflex and ability to swallow (see Chapter 30). Note presence of dental caries—chalky white discoloration of tooth or presence of brown or black discoloration; gingivitis—inflammation of gums; periodontitis—receding gum lines, inflammation, gaps between teeth; halitosis—bad breath; cheilitis—cracked lips; dry, cracked, and coated tongue.
7. Remove and dispose of gloves and perform hand hygiene.
8. Explain procedure to patient, discussing patient's preferences; assess patient's ability to grasp and manipulate toothbrush and willingness to help with oral care.

9. Place paper towels on over-bed table and arrange other equipment within easy reach.
10. Provide privacy by closing room doors and drawing room divider curtain. Raise bed to comfortable working position.
11. Raise head of bed (if allowed) and lower near side rail. Move patient or help them move closer to side. Place patient in side-lying position if needed (if aspiration risk). Place towel over patient's chest.
12. Apply clean gloves. Apply enough toothpaste to brush to cover length of bristles. Hold brush over emesis basin. Pour small amount of water over toothpaste.
13. Patient may help with brushing. Hold toothbrush bristles at 45-degree angle to gum line (see illustration A). Be sure that tips of bristles rest against and penetrate under gum line. Brush inner and outer surfaces of upper and lower teeth by brushing from gum to crown of each tooth. Clean biting surfaces of teeth by holding top of bristles parallel with teeth and brushing gently back and forth (see illustration B). Brush sides of teeth by moving bristles back and forth (see illustration C).
14. Have patient hold brush at 45-degree angle and lightly brush over surface and sides of tongue. Avoid initiating gag reflex.
15. Allow patient to rinse mouth thoroughly by taking several sips of cool water, swishing water across all tooth surfaces, and spitting into emesis basin. Use this time to observe patient's brushing technique and teach the importance of regular hygiene (see Fig. 40.2).
16. Have patient rinse mouth with antiseptic rinse for 30 seconds. Then have patient spit rinse.
17. Allow patient to rinse mouth thoroughly with cool water and spit into emesis basin. Help wipe the patient's mouth.
18. Inspect oral cavity to determine effectiveness of oral hygiene and rinsing. Ask patient whether mouth feels clean or if there are any sore or tender areas. Remove towel and place in linen bag.
19. Remove and dispose of gloves and perform hand hygiene. Return patient to a comfortable position. Raise side rails (as appropriate), and lower bed to lowest position. Place nurse call system within patient reach.
20. **Use Teach-Back:** "I want to be sure you know how often to floss your teeth. Show me how you will floss your teeth." Revise your instruction now or develop a plan for revised patient/family caregiver teaching if patient/family caregiver is not able to teach back correctly.
21. Record and Report: bleeding, pain, or presence of lesions to nurse in charge or health care provider.

STEP 13 Direction of brushing for tooth brushing.

with a soft toothbrush and floss gently to prevent bleeding of the gums. In some cases, flossing needs to be omitted temporarily from oral care. Advise patients to avoid alcohol and commercial mouthwash and to stop smoking. Normal saline rinses (approximately 30 mL) on awakening in the morning, after each meal, and at bedtime help clean the oral cavity. Patients can increase the rinses to every 2 hours if necessary. Consult with the health care provider to obtain topical or oral analgesics for pain control.

Denture Care. Encourage patients to clean their dentures on a regular basis to avoid gingival infection and irritation. When patients become disabled, someone else assumes responsibility for denture care (Box 40.10). Dentures are a patient's personal property and must

---

BOX 40.10 PROCEDURAL GUIDELINES

Care of Dentures

Delegation and Collaboration

The skill of denture care can be delegated to assistive personnel (AP). The nurse instructs the AP to:

- Not use hot or excessively cold water when caring for dentures.
- Inform the nurse if there are cracks in dentures.
- Inform the nurse if the patient has any oral discomfort or if sores, lesions or bleeding is observed.

Equipment

Soft-bristled toothbrush or denture toothbrush; denture dentifrice or toothpaste; denture adhesive *(optional);* glass of water; emesis basin or sink; 4 × 4–inch gauze; washcloth; denture cup (for storage); clean gloves

Procedural Steps

1. Identify patient using at least two identifiers (e.g., name and birthday or name and medical record number) according to agency policy (TJC, 2021).
2. Assess environment for safety (e.g., check room for spills; make sure that bed is in locked, low position).
3. Determine patient's or family caregiver's knowledge, experience, and health literacy.
4. Perform hand hygiene.
5. Ask patient whether dentures fit and whether there is any gum or mucous membrane tenderness or irritation. Ask patient about denture care and product preferences.
6. Determine whether patient has necessary dexterity to clean dentures independently or requires help.
7. Lower side rail. Position patient comfortably sitting up in bed or help patient walk from bed to chair placed in front of sink.
8. Fill emesis basin with tepid water. (If using sink, place washcloth in bottom of sink and fill sink with approximately 2.5 cm [1 inch] of water.)
9. Perform hand hygiene again and apply clean gloves.
10. Ask patient to remove dentures. If patient is unable to do this independently, grasp upper plate at front with thumb and index finger wrapped in gauze and pull downward. Gently lift lower denture from jaw and rotate one side downward to remove from patient's mouth. Place dentures in emesis basin or sink lined with washcloth and 2.5 cm (1 inch) of water.
11. Inspect oral cavity, paying attention to gums, tongue, and upper palate. Observe for lesions, plaques, and areas of irritation. Palpate areas as needed.

CLINICAL JUDGMENT: Oral mucosal lesions are common in older adults, especially in patients living in long-term care homes. These lesions are associated with local and systemic factors (e.g., ill-fitting dentures, infection). Lesions can occur anywhere in the oral cavity (Yoon et al., 2018).

12. Apply cleaning agent to brush and brush surfaces of dentures (see illustration). Hold dentures close to water. Hold brush horizontally and use back-and-forth motion to clean biting surfaces. Use short strokes from top of denture to biting surfaces to clean outer teeth surfaces. Hold brush vertically and use short strokes to clean inner teeth surfaces. Hold brush

STEP 12 Brushing surface of dentures.

horizontally and use back-and-forth motion to clean undersurface of dentures (see Procedural Guideline Box 40.9).

13. Rinse thoroughly in tepid water. If water is too cold, dentures can crack. If it is too hot, dentures can become warped and no longer fit.
14. When necessary, apply a thin layer of denture adhesive to undersurface before inserting.
15. Reinsert dentures as soon as possible. If patient needs help with inserting dentures, moisten upper denture and press firmly to seal it in place. Insert moistened lower denture (if applicable). Ask whether denture(s) feels comfortable. **NOTE:** It is common for patients to choose not to wear their dentures during an acute illness.
16. Some patients prefer to store their dentures to give gums a rest and reduce risk for infection. Store in tepid water in enclosed, labeled denture cup. Keep denture cup in a secure place labeled with patient's name to prevent loss when not worn (e.g., at night, during surgery).

CLINICAL JUDGMENT: Dentures are expensive. Help prevent the potential loss of dentures by giving them to a family member, when possible (e.g., when a patient goes to surgery). A patient may not always return to the same preoperative room; giving the dentures to a family member helps avoid misplacement of the dentures.

17. **Use Teach-Back:** "I want to be sure I explained clearly how to clean your dentures. Show me how you would brush your lower denture." Revise your instruction now or develop a plan for revised patient/family caregiver teaching if patient/family caregiver is not able to teach back correctly.
18. Dispose of supplies. Remove and discard gloves and perform hand hygiene.
19. Return patient to a comfortable position. Raise side rails (as appropriate), and lower bed to lowest position. Place nurse call system within patient reach.
20. Record and report any abnormalities noted involving oral mucosa.

be handled with care because they break easily. They must be removed at night to rest the gums and prevent bacterial buildup. To prevent warping, keep dentures covered in water when they are not worn, and always store them in an enclosed, labeled cup with the cup placed on the patient's bedside stand. Discourage patients from removing their dentures and placing them on a napkin or tissue because they could easily be thrown away.

Implement measures to prevent denture-induced stomatitis when caring for patients who wear dentures. Poorly fitting dentures, wearing dentures while sleeping, and poor dental hygiene habits contribute to denture-induced stomatitis (Yoon et al., 2018: Maciag et al., 2017). Signs and symptoms range from redness and swelling under the dentures to painful red sores on the roof of the mouth and infection with the yeast *Candida albicans*. Some patients deny pain, and others complain of pain worsened by wearing dentures. To prevent denture-induced stomatitis, rinse the mouth and dentures after meals, clean them carefully and regularly, remove and soak them overnight, brush and floss (if appropriate) any remaining teeth, and visit a dentist regularly for examination (American Dental Association, 2020).

Hair and Scalp Care. A person's appearance and feeling of well-being often depend on the way the hair looks and feels. Illness or disability often prevents a patient from maintaining daily hair care. When patients are immobilized, their hair soon becomes tangled. Some dressings or diagnostic procedures leave sticky residue on the hair. Basic hair and scalp care includes brushing, combing, and shampooing.

Brushing and Combing. Frequent brushing helps keep hair clean and distributes oil evenly along hair shafts. Combing prevents hair from tangling. Encourage patients to maintain routine hair care and provide help for patients with limited mobility or weakness and those who are confused or weakened by illness. Patients in a hospital or extended-care facility appreciate the opportunity to have their hair brushed and combed before being seen by others.

When caring for patients from different cultures, learn as much as possible from them or their family about preferred hair care practices. For example, the hair of some cultures tends to be quite dry. Use special lanolin conditioners for conditioning. Cultural preferences also affect how hair is combed and styled and whether it can be cut.

Long hair becomes matted easily when a patient is confined to bed, even for a short period. When lacerations or incisions involve the scalp, blood and topical medications also cause tangling. Frequent brushing and combing keep long hair neatly groomed. Braiding helps to avoid repeated tangles; however, patients need to unbraid hair periodically and comb it to ensure good hygiene. Braids that are too tight lead to bald patches. Obtain permission from the patient before braiding the hair.

To brush hair, part it into two sections and separate each section into two more sections. Brushing from the scalp toward the hair ends minimizes pulling. Moistening the hair with water or an alcohol-free detangle product makes it easier to comb. Never cut a patient's hair without consent.

Patients who develop head lice require special considerations in the way combing is performed (Box 40.11). The lice are small, about the size of a sesame seed; thus, you need bright light or natural sunlight to see them. If a pediculicidal shampoo is ordered, review pertinent information and instruct the patient and caregiver in its proper use. Use with caution because these shampoos may have severe neurological side effects. Make sure to thoroughly rinse shampoo from hair to avoid itching.

Shampooing. Frequency of shampooing depends on a person's daily routines and the condition of the hair. Remind patients in hospitals or extended-care facilities that increased time in bed, excess perspiration, or treatments that leave blood or solutions in the hair require more frequent shampooing. In some health care agencies you need a health

---

BOX 40.11   Hygiene Care for Head Lice

- Perform hand hygiene and apply disposable gown and gloves.
- Use a grooming comb or hairbrush to remove tangles. Do not use shampoo or conditioner before using lice medicine.
- Apply lice medicine according to instructions on label. Note that medicine may take 8 to 12 hours to work. Medicine is effective when dead or slowly moving lice are observed. **NOTE:** If after 8 to 12 hours of treatment no dead lice are found, the medicine may not be working. Do not retreat without consulting a health care provider (CDC, 2019a).
- Divide patient's hair in sections, and fasten off hair that is not being combed.
- Use the comb (also called a nit comb) that comes with the treatment. Comb out from scalp to the end of the hair. (Special combs are available in drugstores.)
- Dip comb in a cup of water, or use a paper towel to remove lice between each pass with the comb.
- After combing, look through hair carefully for attached lice; you can catch live lice with a tweezers or comb.
- After combing thoroughly, move to next section of hair.
- Soak combs in hot water, at least 130°F, for 5 to 10 minutes (CDC, 2019a). The ideal is to discard the comb after each use, but some patients' financial situations prevent the purchase of multiple combs.
- Instruct patient and family not to rewash hair for 1 to 2 days after treatment.
- Instruct family to comb and screen for lice daily.
- Instruct family to contain patient's clothes, bed linens, and bath towels; wash them in hot water that is at least 130°F; and dry on hot cycle (CDC, 2019a).
- Instruct family to vacuum the floor and furniture and patient's room and immediately empty vacuum bag or bagless collection device.
- Instruct caregivers on how to prevent transmission of lice: Do not share bed linens or hair care products. Avoid placing bare hand on patient's head. Immediately wash hands after providing hair care.

---

care provider's order to shampoo a patient who is dependent, has head and/or neck injuries, or has limited mobility because it is challenging to find ways to safely shampoo the hair without causing injury.

The patient who can shower or tub bathe usually shampoos the hair without difficulty. A shower or tub chair facilitates shampooing for patients who are ambulatory and weight-bearing and become tired or faint. Handheld shower nozzles allow patients to easily wash the hair in the tub or shower. Some patients allowed to sit in a chair choose to be shampooed in front of a sink or over a washbasin; however, certain conditions (e.g., eye surgery or neck injury) limit bending. In these situations, teach the patient and family the degree of bending allowed.

If a patient is unable to sit but can be moved, transfer the patient to a stretcher for transportation to a sink or shower equipped with a handheld nozzle. Use caution when positioning the patient's head and neck, particularly in patients with any form of head or neck injury.

If a patient is unable to sit in a chair or be transferred to a stretcher, shampoo the hair with the patient in bed (Box 40.12). Position a special shampoo trough under the patient's head to catch water and shampoo suds. After shampooing, patients like having their hair styled and dried. Most health care agencies have portable hair dryers. Dry shampoos that reduce the need to wet the patient's hair are also available but are not highly effective. Shampoo caps provide a warm, wet massage to the scalp while cleaning the hair.

Shaving. Shave a patient's facial hair after the bath or shampoo. Some women prefer to shave their legs or axillae while bathing. When helping a patient, take care to avoid cutting the patient with the razor blade. Patients prone to bleeding (e.g., those receiving anticoagulants or high doses of aspirin or those with low platelet counts) must use a

BOX 40.12 PROCEDURAL GUIDELINES

Hair Care: Shampooing and Shaving

Delegation and Collaboration

The skills of combing, shampooing, and shaving can be delegated to assistive personnel (AP). The nurse instructs the AP to:

- Properly position a patient with head or neck mobility restrictions.
- Provide proper care in cases of head lice, stressing steps to take to prevent transmission to other patients.
- Report how the patient tolerated the procedure and any concerns (e.g., neck pain).
- Use an electric razor for any patient at risk for bleeding tendencies.

Equipment

Hair Care

- Bath towels; clean gloves; clean gown *(optional)* (if patient has known head lice); clean comb and brush; wide-tooth comb *(optional)*

Regular Shampoo

- Washcloth; shampoo, hair conditioner *(optional)*, hydrogen peroxide and saline 50/50 mixture *(optional if blood in hair)*; water pitcher with warm water; plastic shampoo board, washbasin; bath blanket, waterproof pad.

Disposable Shampoo

- Disposable shampoo cap product

Shaving with Razor

- New disposable or electric razor; clean gloves; bath towel(s), mirror, washcloth, washbasin; shaving cream or soap, aftershave lotion (if patient desires and not contraindicated)

Mustache Care

- Scissors, brush or comb; bath towel; gooseneck lamp or overhead light

Procedural Steps

1. Identify patient using at least two identifiers (e.g., name and birthday or name and medical record number) according to agency policy (TJC, 2021).
2. Assess whether patient has bleeding tendency. Review medical history, medications, and laboratory values (e.g., platelet count, anticoagulation studies).

   CLINICAL JUDGMENT: Have any patient on anticoagulants or who has low platelets use an electric razor.

3. Review medical record to determine that there are no contraindications to procedure (e.g., position or manipulation of head and neck). Check agency policy for health care provider order as needed. Certain medical conditions place patient at risk for injury.

   CLINICAL JUDGMENT: Certain medical conditions such as head and neck injuries, spinal cord injuries, and arthritis place patient at risk for injury during shampooing because of positioning and manipulation of patient's head and neck. In addition, patients with positional vertigo are not able to tolerate neck hyperextension as it might increase dizziness.

4. Assess environment for safety (e.g., check room for spills; make sure that bed is in locked, low position).
5. Determine patient's or family caregiver's health literacy.
6. Perform hand hygiene. Inspect condition of hair and scalp (this can also be done just before starting shampoo or combing). Inspect for presence of any infestation (e.g., pediculosis). Inspect for drainage from any head wounds. **NOTE:** Apply clean gloves if drainage or infestation is suspected. Apply a gown if infestation is suspected (National Pediculosis Association, 2020).

7. Remove and discard gloves and perform hand hygiene.
8. Assess patient's hair care and shaving product preferences (e.g., shampoo, aftershave lotion, skin conditioner).
9. Assess patient's knowledge, prior experience with hair lice removal, and feelings about procedure.
10. Assess patient's ability to manipulate comb, brush, or razor.
11. Gather equipment and supplies at patient's bedside. Explain your intent to provide hair/beard care. Ask patient to explain during procedure the steps to take when combing hair and/or shaving. Ask patient to indicate if they become uncomfortable during procedure.
12. Position patient sitting in chair or up in bed with head elevated 45 to 90 degrees (as tolerated).
13. Provide privacy; close door or pull curtain. Arrange supplies at bedside table and adjust lighting.
14. Perform hand hygiene.
15. Combing and brushing hair:
    a. Apply clean gloves if necessary. Part hair into two sections and then separate it into two more sections (see illustrations).

A

B

STEP 15a Parting hair. (A) Part hair down the middle and divide it into two main sections. (B) Part main section into two smaller sections.

Continued

BOX 40.12   PROCEDURAL GUIDELINES—cont'd

Hair Care: Shampooing and Shaving

b. Brush or comb from scalp toward hair ends.

c. Moisten hair lightly with water, conditioner, or alcohol-free detangle product before combing.

d. Move fingers through hair to loosen any larger tangles.

e. Using a wide-tooth comb, start on either side of head and insert comb with teeth upward to hair near scalp. Comb through hair in circular motion by turning wrist while lifting up and out. Continue until all hair is combed through, and comb into place to shape and style.

16. Shampooing bed-bound patient with shampoo board:

a. Apply clean gloves. Place waterproof pad under patient's shoulders, neck, and head.

b. Position patient supine with head and shoulders at top edge of bed. Place shampoo board under patient's head and washbasin under end of trough spout (see illustration). Be sure that trough spout extends beyond edge of mattress.

STEP 16b Patient positioned over shampoo board. (Copyright © Mosby's Clinical Skills: Essentials Collection.)

c. Place rolled towel under patient's neck and bath towel over patient's shoulders.

d. Brush and comb patient's hair.

e. Ask patient to hold towel or washcloth over eyes.

f. Test water temperature. Slowly pour water from pitcher over hair until it is completely wet (see illustration). If hair contains matted blood, apply hydrogen peroxide to dissolve clots and rinse with saline. Apply small amount of shampoo.

STEP 16f Nurse pouring water over patient's hair. (Copyright © Mosby's Clinical Skills: Essentials Collection.)

g. Work up lather with both hands. Start at hairline and work toward back of neck. Lift head slightly with one hand to wash back of head. Shampoo sides of head. Massage scalp by applying pressure with fingertips.

h. Rinse hair with water. Make sure that water drains into basin. Repeat rinsing until hair is free of soap. (If you need to refill pitcher, raise side rail when leaving bedside.)

i. Apply conditioner or crème rinse if requested, and rinse hair thoroughly.

j. Wrap patient's head in bath towel. Dry face with cloth used to protect eyes. Dry off any moisture along neck or shoulders.

k. Dry patient's hair and scalp. Use second towel if first one becomes saturated.

l. Comb hair to remove tangles, and dry with dryer if desired.

m. Apply oil preparation or conditioning product to hair if desired by patient.

n. Variation for patients with coarse, curly hair: Condition hair after washing. To untangle hair, use wide teeth of comb. Beginning at nape of neck, comb small subsections of hair, starting at hair ends. Continue to work through small sections until hair is free of tangles.

17. Shampooing with disposable shampoo product:

a. Patient can be sitting on chair or in bed. Apply clean gloves.

b. Comb hair to remove any tangles or debris (see Step 15 above).

c. Open package, apply cap, and secure all hair beneath cap (see illustration).

STEP 17c Patient wearing disposable shampoo cap.

d. Massage head through cap. Check fitting around head to maintain correct fit.

e. Massage 2 to 4 minutes according to directions on package; additional time may be required for longer hair or hair matted with blood.

f. Discard cap in trash; do not dispose of in toilet because it may clog plumbing.

g. If patient desires, towel-dry hair. Brush or comb patient's hair.

18. Shaving with disposable razor:

a. Place bath towel over patient's chest and shoulders.

b. Run warm water in washbasin. Check water temperature.

c. Place washcloth in basin and wring out thoroughly. Apply cloth over patient's entire face for several seconds.

BOX 40.12 PROCEDURAL GUIDELINES—cont'd

Hair Care: Shampooing and Shaving

d. Apply approximately ¼-inch shaving cream or soap to patient's face. Smooth cream evenly over sides of face, on chin, and under nose.

e. Hold razor in dominant hand at 45-degree angle to patient's skin. Begin by shaving across one side of patient's face using short, firm strokes in direction that hair grows (see illustration). Use nondominant hand to gently pull skin taut while shaving. Ask patient whether he feels comfortable.

STEP 18e Shaving patient using short, firm strokes.

f. Dip razor blade in water because shaving cream accumulates on edge of blade.

g. After all facial hair is shaved, rinse face thoroughly with warm, moistened washcloth.

h. Dry face thoroughly and apply aftershave lotion if desired. Remove towel.

19. Shaving with electric razor:
    a. Place bath towel over patient's chest and shoulders.
    b. Apply skin conditioner or preshave preparation.
    c. Turn razor on and begin by shaving across side of face. Gently hold skin taut while shaving over surface of skin. Use gentle downward stroke of razor in direction of hair growth.
    d. After completing shave, turn razor off, remove towel, and apply aftershave lotion as desired unless contraindicated.

20. Mustache and beard care:
    a. Place bath towel over patient's chest and shoulders.
    b. If necessary, gently comb mustache or beard. Offer option for patient to shampoo beard.
    c. Allow patient to use mirror and direct areas to trim with scissors.
    d. After completing, remove towel.

21. Discard soiled linen in dirty laundry bag. Remove and dispose of gloves. Perform hand hygiene.

22. Help patient to comfortable position and raise side rails (as appropriate) and lower bed to lowest position. Place nurse call system in an accessible location within patient's reach.

23. Return reusable equipment to proper place.

24. Inspect condition of hair and scalp, condition of shaved area, and skin underneath beard or mustache. Look for areas of localized bleeding from cuts and areas of dryness.

25. Ask patient whether face feels clean and comfortable.

26. **Use Teach-Back:** "Since you are on a blood thinner, I want to be sure I explained to you the risks of using a regular razor at home, including what type of razor you should use. Tell me the things to watch for with a bleeding tendency." Revise your instruction now or develop a plan for revised patient/family caregiver teaching if patient/family caregiver is not able to teach back correctly.

27. Record or report any lesions or presence of lice to health care provider.

---

personal electric razor. Before using an electric razor, check for frayed cords or other electrical hazards. Use a razor blade on only one patient because of infection control considerations.

When using a razor blade for shaving, soften the skin to prevent pulling, scraping, or cuts. Moisten the skin with lukewarm water and apply shaving cream. Bar soap may leave a film on the blade, resulting in a poorer-quality shave. You need to shave patients when they are unable to shave themselves independently. To avoid causing discomfort or razor cuts, gently pull the skin taut, and use long, firm razor strokes in the direction the hair grows (Fig. 40.5). Short downward strokes work best to remove hair over the upper lip or chin. A patient usually explains the best way to move the razor across the skin.

Facial hair of people of color tends to be curly and becomes ingrown unless shaved close to the skin. However, there are common skin lesions among people of color that require a different shaving technique. An example is the common condition of pseudofolliculitis barbae, commonly referred to as razor bumps and recognized by inflammation of hair follicles and hyperpigmented papules and pustules (Adotama et al., 2017). It typically results from cut hairs penetrating the skin. The idea is to avoid shaving completely to treat this condition. However, when a shave is preferred, use the following techniques for this condition: Avoid a close shave, leaving hair at a length of 0.5 mm to 3 mm; use clippers, a single-blade razor, shave in the direction of hair growth, and do not pull the skin taut while shaving (Adotama et al., 2017).

FIG. 40.5 Shave using short, firm strokes in direction of hair growth.

Mustache and Beard Care. Mustaches or beards require daily grooming, including shampooing. Grooming keeps food particles and mucus from collecting in the hair. If a patient is unable to carry out self-care, do so at the patient's request. Comb out beards gently and obtain the patient's permission before trimming or shaving off a mustache or beard.

Care of the Eyes, Ears, and Nose.
Give special attention to cleaning the eyes, ears, and nose during a routine bath and when drainage or discharge accumulates. This aspect of hygiene not only makes a patient more comfortable but also improves sensory reception (see Chapter 49). Care focuses on preventing infection and maintaining normal sensory function. In addition, care of the eyes, ears, and nose requires approaches that consider the patient's special needs.

Medical Devices. If a patient has oxygen tubing, a feeding tube, or a nasotracheal tube, it is essential that you care for the area of the skin around the nose or ears underlying the device to protect the patient from Medical Device Related Pressure Injuries (MDRPI) (Fumarola et al., 2020). The National Pressure Ulcer Advisory Panel (EPUAP/NPIAP/PPPIA, 2019a; 2019b) recommends the following: cushion and protect the skin with dressings in high-risk areas (e.g., nasal bridge) (see Chapter 48), do not place device(s) over sites of prior or existing pressure injury, and be sure to gently cleanse a potential area of irritation that underlies a device at least daily.

Basic Eye Care. Cleaning the eyes involves simply washing with a clean washcloth moistened in water (see Skill 40.1). Soap may cause burning and irritation. Never apply direct pressure over the eyeball because it causes serious injury. When cleaning a patient's eyes, obtain a clean washcloth and clean from inner to outer canthus. Use a different section of the washcloth for each eye. **NOTE: never use CHG solution or cloths to clean the eyes, ears, or face.**

Unconscious patients require more frequent eye care. A complication of sedation and coma is that some patients are unable to maintain effective eye closure, which results in exposure keratopathy. Thus, these patients lose their natural protective mechanisms to protect the cornea. When unprotected, there is an increased risk of corneal dehydration, abrasion, perforation, and infection (Morris et al., 2018). Normal protective mechanisms include blinking with lubrication of the eye. Blinking provides a mechanical barrier to injury and prevents dehydration. Secretions collect along the lid margins and inner canthus when the blink reflex is absent or when the eye does not close completely. Prompt assessment of impaired blinking is essential to protect your patient's eyes. When an eye does not close completely, you may need to place an eye patch over it to prevent corneal drying and irritation. Apply lubricating eye drops according to the health care provider's orders to assist in preventing corneal damage (Kocacal et al., 2018). When a corneal abrasion or trauma results, topical nonsteroidal antiinflammatory drugs (NSAIDs) are an option for treatment (Kaye et al., 2019).

Eyeglasses. Eyeglasses are expensive. Be careful when cleaning glasses and protect them from breakage or other damage when they are not worn. Put them in a case in a drawer of the bedside table when not in use. Cool water sufficiently cleans glass lenses. Prevent scratching by using a soft cloth for drying; do not use paper towels. Plastic lenses in particular scratch easily; special cleaning solutions and drying tissues are available.

Contact Lenses. A contact lens is a thin, transparent disk that fits directly over the cornea of the eye. Contact lenses correct refractive errors of the eye or abnormalities in the shape of the cornea. In outpatient or home settings instruct patients on the routines to follow for regular cleansing and care (Box 40.13). Explain that all contact lenses must be removed periodically to prevent ocular infection and corneal ulcers or abrasions from infectious agents such as *Pseudomonas aeruginosa* and

staphylococci. Pain, tearing, discomfort, and redness of the conjunctivae indicate excessive lens wear. Encourage patients to report persistence of these symptoms, even after lens removal, to their health care provider.

When patients are admitted to the health care agency in an unresponsive or confused state, determine whether they normally wear contact lenses and whether the lenses are in place. If a patient wears contact lenses and no one detects this, severe corneal injury can result. If you find that your patient is wearing contact lenses and cannot remove them, seek help. Once the lenses are removed, document the removal, the condition of the patient's eyes after removal, and the storage of the lenses.

Ear Care. Routine ear care involves cleaning the outer ear with a washcloth and warm water. Cleanse the outer ear canal with the end of a moistened washcloth rotated gently into the canal. Gentle, downward retraction at the entrance of the ear canal usually causes visible cerumen to loosen and slip out. Instruct patients never to use objects such as bobby pins, toothpicks, paper clips, or cotton-tipped applicators to remove earwax. These objects can injure the ear canal and rupture the tympanic membrane. They may also cause cerumen to become impacted within the ear canal.

Children and older adults commonly have impacted cerumen. You can usually remove excessive or impacted cerumen by irrigation, which requires a health care provider's order. Review the order for type of solution and ear(s) to receive the irrigation. Before irrigation, question the patient for history of perforated eardrum, and inspect the tympanic

---

BOX 40.13   PATIENT TEACHING
Care of Contact Lenses

Objective
- Patient verbalizes and/or demonstrates proper care for contact lenses and common warning signs of problems associated with contact lens wear.

Teaching Strategies
- Instruct patients on the following:
  - Do not use fingernail on lens to remove dirt or debris.
  - Do not use tap water to clean soft lenses.
  - Follow recommendations of the lens manufacturer or eye care practitioner when inserting, cleaning, and disinfecting lenses.
  - Keep lenses moist or wet when not worn.
  - Use fresh solution daily when storing and disinfecting lenses.
  - Thoroughly wash and rinse lens storage case daily. Clean periodically with soap or liquid detergent, rinse thoroughly with warm water, and air-dry.
  - If lens is dropped, moisten finger with cleaning or wetting solution and gently touch lens to pick it up. Then clean, rinse, and disinfect it.
- To avoid mix-up, instruct patient to always start with the same lens when inserting or removing lenses.
- Throw away disposable or planned replacement lenses after prescribed wearing period.
- Encourage patient to remember the acronym RSVP: *R*edness, *S*ensitivity, *V*ision problems, and *P*ain. If one of these problems occurs, remove contact lenses immediately. If problems continue, contact a vision care specialist (Harding et al., 2020).

Evaluation
Use the principles of teach-back to evaluate patient/family caregiver learning:
- Explain to me the warning signs of corneal irritation and eye infection.
- Describe for me the methods of contact lens care that lead to infection.
- I want to make sure that you understand the information on lens cleaning and storage. Show me how you will clean your lenses and store them.

membrane to be sure that it is intact; a perforated tympanic membrane contradicts performing irrigation. Visually inspect the pinna and external meatus for redness, swelling, drainage, and presence of foreign objects. Also determine the patient's ability to hear in the affected ear before irrigation.

To irrigate the ear, have the patient sit or lie on the side with the affected ear up. For adults and children over 3 years of age, gently pull the pinna up and back. In children 3 years of age or younger, the pinna should be pulled down and back. Using a bulb-irrigating syringe, gently wash the ear canal with warm solution (37°C or 98.6°F), being careful not to occlude the canal, which would result in pressure on the tympanic membrane. Direct the fluid slowly and gently toward the superior aspect of the ear canal, maintaining the flow in a steady stream. Periodically during the irrigation ask whether the patient is experiencing pain, nausea, or vertigo. These symptoms indicate that the solution is too hot or too cold or is being instilled with too much pressure. After the canal is clear, wipe off any moisture from the ear with cotton balls and inspect the canal for remaining earwax.

Hearing Aid Care. A hearing aid amplifies sounds in a controlled manner; the aid receives normal low-intensity sound inputs and delivers them to a patient's ear as louder outputs. Hearing aids come in a variety of types. The new class of hearing aids reduces background noise interference. Computer chips placed in the aids allow for fine adjustments to the specific patient's hearing needs. Be sure a patient has stored the aid when not in use. Many require regular recharging.

There are several popular types of hearing aids. A completely-in-canal (CIC) aid (Fig. 40.6, A) is the newest, smallest, and least visible and fits entirely in the ear canal. It is used for patients with moderately severe hearing loss. It has cosmetic appeal, is easy to manipulate and place in the ear, and does not interfere with wearing eyeglasses or using the telephone. The patient can wear it during most physical exercise. However, it requires adequate ear diameter and depth for proper fit. It does not accommodate progressive hearing loss, and it requires manual dexterity to operate, insert, remove, and change batteries. In addition, cerumen tends to plug this model more than the others.

An in-the-ear (ITE, or intraaural) aid (Fig. 40.6, B) fits into the external auditory canal and allows for finer tuning. It is more powerful and stronger and therefore is more useful for mild-to-severe hearing loss than the CIC aid. It is easier to position and adjust and does not interfere with wearing eyeglasses. However, it is more noticeable than the CIC aid and is not for people with moisture or skin problems in the ear canal.

A behind-the-ear (BTE, or postaural) aid (Fig. 40.6, C) hooks around and behind the ear. It is connected by a short, clear, hollow plastic tube to an ear mold inserted into the external auditory canal. A BTE aid allows for fine tuning. It is the largest aid and is useful for patients with mild to profound hearing loss or manual dexterity difficulties or for those who find partial ear occlusion intolerable. The larger size of this type of aid can make the use of eyeglasses and phones difficult; it is more difficult to keep in place during physical exercise.

Digital hearing aids (Fig. 40.6, D) analyze sounds to remove background noise. This aid is beneficial for people with mild to severe hearing loss. Digital hearing aids program for low-frequency and high-frequency sounds and must be programmed and adjusted by a licensed audiologist. Box 40.14 reviews guidelines for the care and cleaning of hearing aids.

Nasal Care. If a patient cannot remove nasal secretions, help by using a wet washcloth or a cotton-tipped applicator moistened in water or saline. Never insert the applicator beyond the length of the cotton tip. You also can remove excessive nasal secretions through gentle nasal suctioning (see Chapter 41).

When nasogastric, feeding, or endotracheal tubes are inserted through a patient's nose, change the tape anchoring the tube at least once a day. When the tape becomes moist from nasal secretions, the

FIG. 40.6 Common types of hearing aids. **A,** Completely-in-canal (CIC) hearing aid. **B,** In-the-ear (ITE) hearing aid. **C,** Behind-the-ear (BTE) hearing aid. **D,** Digital hearing aid.

skin and mucosa can easily become macerated (softened by soaking). Friction from a tube causes tissue injury. Anchor tubing correctly with tape or fixative devices to minimize tension or friction on the nares (see Skill 47.2).

Patient's Room Environment. Attempt to make a patient's room as comfortable as the home. It needs to be safe and large enough to allow the patient and visitors to move about freely. Removal of barriers around the bed and along walkways reduces risk of falls. Control room temperature, ventilation, noise, and odors. Keeping the room neat and orderly also contributes to the patient's sense of well-being.

Maintaining Comfort. What makes a comfortable environment depends on a patient's age, severity of illness, and level of normal daily activity. Depending on age and physical condition, maintain the room temperature between 20°C and 23°C (68°F and 73.4°F). Infants, older adults, and the acutely ill often need a warmer room. However, certain

BOX 40.14   Care and Use of Hearing Aids

- Initially wear hearing aid 15 to 20 minutes; gradually increase time to 10 to 12 hours.
- Once inserted, turn aid slowly to one-third to one-half volume.
- Whistling sound indicates incorrect earmold insertion, improper fit of aid, or buildup of earwax or fluid.
- Adjust volume to comfortable level for talking at distance of 1 yard.
- Do not wear aid under heat lamps or hair dryer or in very wet, cold weather.
- Batteries last 1 week with daily wearing of 10 to 12 hours.
- Remove or disconnect battery when not in use.
- Replace earmolds every 2 or 3 years.
- Routinely check battery compartment: Is it clean? Are batteries inserted properly? Is compartment shut all the way?
- Make sure that dials on hearing aid are clean and easy to rotate, creating no static during adjusting.
- Keep aid clean. See manufacturer's instructions. Aids are usually cleaned with a soft cloth.
- Avoid use of hairspray and perfume while wearing hearing aids, residue from spray causes aid to become oily and greasy.
- Do not submerge in water.
- Routinely check cord or tubing (depending on type of aid) for cracking, fraying, and poor connections.
- Routine follow-up with audiologist is recommended to evaluate effectiveness of current aid.

Data from Touhy T, Jett P: *Ebersole and Hess' gerontological nursing & healthy aging,* ed 5, St Louis, 2018, Elsevier.

FIG. 40.7 Typical hospital room.

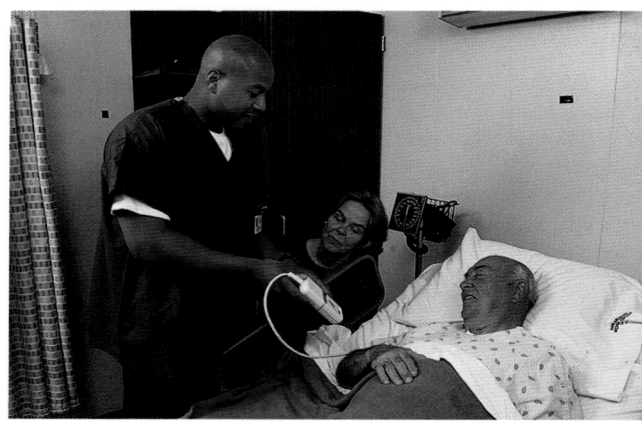

FIG. 40.8 Nurse instructing patient in use of nurse call system and bed controls.

ill patients benefit from cooler room temperatures to lower the metabolic demands of the body.

An effective ventilation system prevents stale air and odors from lingering in the room. Good ventilation reduces lingering odors caused by draining wounds, emesis, bowel movements, and used bedpans and urinals. Always empty and cleanse bedpans and urinals promptly. Room deodorizers help remove many unpleasant odors. Before using room deodorizers, determine that your patient is not allergic or sensitive to the deodorizer itself.

Ill patients seem to be more sensitive to noises and lighting commonly found in health care settings. Try to control the noise level, especially when a patient is trying to sleep. Explain the source of unfamiliar noises such as an IV pump or pulse oximeter alarms.

Proper lighting provides for safety and comfort. A brightly lit room usually stimulates, whereas a darkened room promotes rest and sleep. Adjust room lighting by closing or opening drapes, regulating over-bed and floor lights, and closing or opening room doors. When entering a patient's room at night, refrain from abruptly turning on an overhead light unless necessary.

Room Equipment. Although there are variations across health care settings, a typical hospital room contains the following basic pieces of furniture: over-bed table, bedside stand, chairs, and bed (Fig. 40.7). The over-bed table is an ideal working space for performing procedures. It also serves as a surface for meal trays, toiletry items, and objects that a patient often uses. Clean the top of the over-bed table with an antiseptic cleaner before using it for meals. Do not place a bedpan or urinal on the over-bed table. Use the bedside stand to store a patient's personal possessions and hygiene equipment. Patients often use bedside stands for their telephone, water pitcher, and drinking cup.

Most patient rooms contain a straight-backed chair or an upholstered lounge chair with arms. Armless straight-backed chairs are convenient when temporarily transferring a patient from the bed, such

as during bed making. Upholstered lounge chairs or recliners tend to be more comfortable for patients who can sit for longer times.

Each room usually has an over-bed light and floor-level night lighting. Patients need instructions as to how to access the lighting and other controls via their nurse call system, which may also be integrated into the side rails (Fig. 40.8). Additional portable or built-in examination lighting provides extra light during bedside procedures.

Other equipment usually found in a patient's room includes the nurse call system (often integrated into side rails), a television, a wall-mounted blood pressure gauge, oxygen and vacuum wall outlets, and personal care items. Special equipment designed for comfort or positioning patients includes foot boots and special mattresses (see Chapter 48). Whenever you use comfort and positioning equipment, check agency policy and manufacturer directions before application.

Beds. Seriously ill patients often remain in bed for a long time. Because a bed is the piece of equipment used most by a hospitalized patient, it is designed for comfort, safety, and adaptability for changing positions. A typical hospital bed has a firm mattress on a metal frame that you can raise and lower horizontally. More and more hospitals are converting the standard hospital bed to one in which the mattress surface can be adjusted electronically for safety and comfort. For example, low beds are being used to prevent falls, and beds that regulate pressure in the mattress help to reduce pressure injuries. Different bed positions promote patient comfort, minimize symptoms, promote lung expansion, and improve access during certain procedures (Table 40.6).

TABLE 40.6 Common Bed Positions

Position	Description	Uses
Fowler's	Head of bed raised to angle of 45 to 90 degrees; semi-sitting position; foot of bed may also be raised at knee	While patient is eating During nasogastric tube insertion and nasotracheal suction Promotes lung expansion Eases difficult breathing
Semi-Fowler's	Head of bed raised approximately 30 to 45 degrees; inclination less than Fowler's position; foot of bed may also be raised at knee	Promotes lung expansion, especially with ventilator-assisted patients Used when patients receive oral care and for gastric feedings to reduce regurgitation and risk of aspiration
Trendelenburg's	Entire bedframe tilted with head of bed down	Used for postural drainage Facilitates venous return in patients with poor peripheral perfusion
Reverse Trendelenburg's	Entire bedframe tilted with foot of bed down	Used infrequently Promotes gastric emptying Prevents esophageal reflux

Continued

TABLE 40.6   Common Bed Positions—cont'd

Position	Description	Uses
Flat	Entire bedframe horizontally parallel with floor	Used for patients with vertebral injuries and in cervical traction Used for patients who are hypotensive Patients usually prefer for sleeping

You change the position of a bed by using electrical controls that are either incorporated into the patient's nurse call system or in a panel on the side or foot of the bed (see Fig. 40.8). Know how to use the bed controls. Ease in raising and lowering a bed and changing position of the head and foot eliminates undue musculoskeletal strain. Also instruct patients and family members in the proper use of controls and caution them against raising the bed to a position that causes the patient harm. Maintain the bed height at the lowest horizontal position when a patient is unattended.

Beds contain safety features such as locks on the wheels or casters. Lock wheels when a bed is stationary to prevent accidental movement. Side rails allow patients to move more easily in bed and prevent accidents. Do not use side rails to restrict a patient from moving in bed. *When using side rails as a restraint, you need a health care provider's order* (see Chapter 27). You can remove the headboard and footboard from most beds. This is important when the medical team needs to have easy access to the patient, such as during cardiopulmonary resuscitation.

Bed Making. Keep a patient's bed clean and comfortable. This requires frequent inspection to be sure that linen is clean, dry, and free of wrinkles. When patients are diaphoretic, have draining wounds, or are incontinent, check more frequently for wet or soiled linen.

Usually you make a bed in the morning after patients bathe or while they bathe at a sink or in a shower, while patients are sitting in a chair eating, or when they are out of the room for procedures or tests. Throughout the day straighten linen that is loose or wrinkled. Also check the bed linen for food particles after meals and for wetness or soiling. Change any linen that becomes soiled or wet.

When changing bed linen, follow principles of medical asepsis by keeping soiled linen away from your uniform (Fig. 40.9). Place soiled linen in special linen bags before placing in a hamper. To avoid air currents that spread microorganisms, never shake the linen. To avoid transmitting infection, do not place soiled linen on the floor. If clean linen touches the floor or any unclean surface, immediately place it in the dirty-linen container.

During bed making use safe patient-handling procedures (see Chapter 27). Always raise the bed to the appropriate height before changing linen so that you minimize the extent to which you bend or stretch over the mattress. Move back and forth to opposite sides of the bed while applying new linen. Body mechanics and safe handling are important when turning or repositioning a patient in bed.

When patients are confined to bed, you must make an occupied bed. Organize bed-making activities to conserve time and energy (Box 40.15). The patient's privacy, comfort, and safety are all important when making

FIG. 40.9 Holding linen away from uniform prevents contact with microorganisms.

a bed. Using side rails to aid positioning and turning, keeping nurse call systems within the patient's reach, and maintaining the proper bed position help promote comfort and safety. After making a bed, return it to the lowest horizontal position and verify that the wheels are locked to prevent accidental falls when the patient gets in and out of the bed.

When possible, make the bed while it is unoccupied (Box 40.16). Use clinical judgment to determine the best time for a patient to sit in a chair so that you can make the bed. When making an unoccupied bed, follow the same basic principles as for occupied bed making.

An unoccupied bed can be made as an open or closed bed. In an open bed the top covers are folded back, so it is easy for a patient to get into bed. Draw up the top sheet, blanket, and bedspread to the head of the mattress and place a pillow at the top to make a closed bed. A closed bed is prepared in a hospital room before a new patient is admitted to that room. A surgical, recovery, or postoperative bed is a modified version of the open bed. The top bed linen is arranged for easy transfer of the patient from a stretcher to the bed. The top sheets and spread are not tucked or mitered at the corners. Instead they are folded to one side or to the bottom third of the bed (Fig. 40.10). This makes patient transfer into the bed easier.

Linens. Many health care agencies have "nurse servers" either within or just outside a patient's room to store a daily supply of linen.

BOX 40.15 PROCEDURAL GUIDELINES

Making an Occupied Bed

Delegation and Collaboration

The skill of making an occupied bed can be delegated to assistive personnel (AP). The nurse instructs the AP about:

- Any position or activity restrictions that apply.
- Looking for wound drainage or dislodged equipment that might be found in the bed linens.
- When to obtain help from other caregivers for positioning a patient during linen change and the importance of using safe patient-handling techniques and supporting patient alignment.
- Using special precautions (e.g., aspiration precautions [see Chapter 45] or positioning for tube-feeding infusion [see Chapter 45]) when positioning a patient during bed making.

Equipment

Linen bags: mattress pad (change only when soiled); bottom sheet (flat or fitted); draw sheet *(optional)*; top sheet, blanket, bedspread, pillowcases; waterproof pads *(optional)*; clean gloves (if linen is soiled or there is risk of exposure to body fluids); antiseptic cleanser; washcloth

Equipment for making occupied bed.

Procedural Steps

1. Review medical record, and assess restrictions in mobility/positioning of patient.
2. Organize supplies and close room door or divider curtain to provide privacy.
3. Assess environment for safety (e.g., check room for spills; make sure that equipment is working properly and that bed is in locked position and appropriate number of side rails are raised).
4. Perform hand hygiene. Apply clean gloves if patient has been incontinent or if drainage is present on linen.
5. Explain procedure to patient, noting that patient will be asked to turn over layers of linen.
6. Raise bed to a comfortable working height; lower head of bed (HOB) as tolerated, keeping patient comfortable. Remove nurse call system (if separate from bed rails).

> **CLINICAL JUDGMENT:** If patient is on aspiration precautions or receiving tube feeding, always keep HOB 30 degrees or higher.

7. Lower side rail on side where you are standing. Loosen all top linen. Remove bedspread and blanket separately, leaving patient covered with top sheet. If blanket or spread is soiled, place in linen bag. If to be reused, fold into square and place over back of chair.

8. Cover patient with clean bath blanket by unfolding it over top sheet. Have patient hold top edge of bath blanket or tuck blanket under shoulders. Grasp top sheet under bath blanket at patient's shoulders and bring sheet down to foot of bed. Remove sheet and discard in dirty laundry bag.
9. Position patient on far side of bed, turned onto side and facing away from you. **NOTE:** This is when another caregiver can help you by standing at bedside across from you. Encourage patient to use side rail to turn. Adjust pillow under patient's head.
10. Assess to make sure that there is no tension on any external medical devices.
11. Loosen bottom linens, moving from head to foot. Fanfold or roll any cloth incontinence pads, drawsheet (if present), and bottom sheet (in that order) toward patient. Tuck edges of old linen just under patient's buttocks, back, and shoulders (see illustration). Do not fanfold mattress pad (if it is to be reused). Remove any disposable pads and discard in receptacle.

STEP 11 Tuck all soiled linen from one side of bed alongside patient's back. (From Harkreader H, Hogan MA, Thobaben M: *Fundamentals of nursing: caring and clinical judgment*, ed 3, St Louis, 2007, Elsevier.)

12. Clean, disinfect, and dry mattress surface if it is soiled or has moisture (see agency policy).
13. Apply clean linens to the exposed half of bed in separate layers. When needed, start with a new mattress pad by placing it lengthwise with center crease in middle of bed. Fanfold pad to center of bed alongside patient. Repeat process with bottom sheet.
14. If bottom sheet is fitted, pull corners of new sheet smoothly over mattress corner at top and bottom of bed. Fold remaining portion of sheet across bed surface, toward patient's back.
15. If bottom sheet is flat, place over mattress. Allow edge of sheet closest to you to hang about 25 cm (10 inches) over mattress edge on side and at head of bed (HOB). Be sure that lower hem of bottom sheet lies seam down along bottom edge of mattress. Spread remaining portion of sheet over mattress toward patient's back.
16. For a flat sheet, miter the top corner at HOB.
    a. Face HOB diagonally. Place hand away from HOB under top corner of mattress, near mattress edge, and lift.
    b. With other hand, tuck top edge of bottom sheet smoothly under mattress so that side edges of sheet above and below mattress meet when brought together.
    c. To miter a corner, pick up top edge of sheet at about 45 cm (18 inches) from top end of mattress (see illustration).

Continued

BOX 40.15   PROCEDURAL GUIDELINES—cont'd

Making an Occupied Bed

STEP 16c Top edge of sheet picked up.

d. Lift sheet and lay it on top of mattress to form a neat triangular fold with lower base of triangle even with mattress side edges (see illustration).

STEP 16d Sheet on top of mattress in a triangular fold.

e. Tuck lower edge of sheet, which is hanging free below the mattress, under the mattress. Tuck with palms down, without pulling triangular fold.

f. Hold part of sheet covering side of mattress in place with one hand (see illustrations). With other hand pick up top of triangular linen fold and bring it down over side of mattress. Tuck under mattress with palms down without pulling fold (see illustration).

STEP 16f Triangular fold placed over side of mattress; sheet tucked under mattress.

17. Tuck remaining part of sheet under side of mattress, moving toward foot of bed. Keep linen smooth.

18. Place new drawsheet along middle of bed lengthwise. Fanfold or roll drawsheet on top of clean bottom sheet. Tuck under patient's buttocks and torso without touching old linen.

19. Add waterproof pad (absorbent side up) over drawsheet with seam side down. Fanfold toward patient. Continue to keep clean and soiled linen separate. Also keep linen under patient as flat as possible because patient will need to roll over old and new layers of linen when you are ready to make other side of bed.

20. Advise patient that they will be rolling over a thick layer of linens. Keeping patient covered, ask patient to roll toward you slowly over layers of

STEP 20 Patient begins rolling over layers of linen. (From Harkreader H, Hogan MA, Thobaben M: *Fundamentals of nursing: caring and clinical judgment,* ed 3, St Louis, 2007, Elsevier.)

linen and to not raise the hips (see illustration). Stress the need to roll while staying aligned.

21. You will now raise side rail and move to opposite side of bed. *Option:* The caregiver helping you will help position patient. Have patient roll away from you toward other side of bed, over all of the folds of linen. Again, have patient keep hips still.

22. Lower side rail. Loosen edges of soiled linen from under mattress. Remove soiled linen by folding into a bundle or square.

23. Hold linen away from your body and place it in laundry bag.

24. Clean, disinfect, and dry other half of mattress as needed.

25. Pull clean, fan-folded or rolled mattress pad; sheet; drawsheet; and incontinence pad out from beneath patient toward you. Smooth all linen out over mattress from head to foot of bed. Help patient roll back to supine position and reposition pillow.

26. If bottom sheet is fitted, pull corners over mattress edges. Smooth out sheet.

27. If flat sheet is used, miter top corner of bottom flat sheet (see Steps 16a–f).

28. Facing side of bed, grasp remaining edge of bottom flat sheet. Lean back slightly, keep back straight, and pull while tucking excess linen under mattress from HOB to foot of bed. Avoid lifting mattress during tucking.

29. Smooth fanfolded drawsheet over bottom sheet (tucking is optional). Smooth waterproof incontinence pads, making sure that bed surface is wrinkle free.

30. Place top sheet over patient with vertical centerfold lengthwise down middle of bed and with seam side of hem facing up. Open sheet out from head to foot and unfold over patient. Be sure that top edge of sheet is even with top edge of mattress.

31. Place clean or reused bed blanket on bed over patient. Make sure that top edge is parallel with top edge of sheet and 15 to 20 cm (6 to 8 inches) from edge of top sheet. Raise side rail.

32. Go to other side of bed. Lower side rail. Spread sheet and blanket out evenly.

33. Have patient hold onto sheet and blanket while you remove bath blanket; discard in linen bag.

34. Make cuff by turning edge of top sheet down over top edge of blanket.

35. Make horizontal toe pleat; stand at foot of bed and fanfold in sheet and blanket 5 to 10 cm (2 to 4 inches) across bed. Pull sheet and blanket up from bottom to make fold approximately 15 cm (6 inches) from bottom edge of mattress.

36. Standing at side of bed, tuck in remaining part of sheet and blanket under foot of mattress. Tuck top sheet and blanket together. Be sure that toe pleats are not pulled out.

BOX 40.15 PROCEDURAL GUIDELINES—cont'd

Making an Occupied Bed

37. Make modified mitered corner with top sheet and blanket. (Follow Steps 16a–f.) After making triangular fold, do not tuck tip of triangle (see illustration).

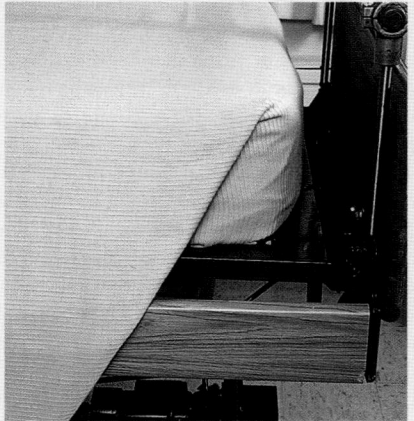

STEP 37 Modified mitered corner.

38. Go to other side of bed. Repeat Steps 35 and 37.
39. Change pillowcase. Have patient raise head. While supporting neck with one hand, remove pillow. Allow patient to lower head. Remove soiled case and place in linen bag. Grasp clean pillowcase at center of closed end. Gather case, turning it inside out over the hand holding it. With the same hand, pick up middle of one end of pillow. Pull pillowcase down over pillow with other hand. Do not hold pillow against your uniform. Be sure that pillow corners fit evenly into corners of case. Reposition pillow under patient's head.
40. Help patient to a comfortable position. Raise side rails (as appropriate), and lower bed to lowest position.
41. Place nurse call system in an accessible location within patient's reach.
42. Place all linen in dirty laundry bag. Remove and dispose of gloves.
43. Arrange and organize patient's room and perform hand hygiene.
44. During procedure inspect skin for areas of irritation. Observe patient for signs of fatigue, dyspnea, pain, or other sources of discomfort.

BOX 40.16 PROCEDURAL GUIDELINES

Making an Unoccupied Bed

Delegation and Collaboration
The skill of making an unoccupied bed can be delegated to assistive personnel (AP).

Equipment
Linen bag, mattress pad (change only when soiled), bottom sheet (flat or fitted), drawsheet *(optional)*, top sheet, blanket, bedspread, waterproof pads *(optional)*, pillowcases, bedside chair or table, clean gloves (if linen is soiled), washcloth or paper towel, and antiseptic cleanser.

Procedural Steps
1. Perform hand hygiene. If patient has been incontinent or if excess drainage is on linen, gloves are necessary.
2. Assess activity orders or restrictions in mobility in planning whether patient can get out of bed for procedure. Help patient to bedside chair or recliner.
3. Lower side rails on both sides of bed, and raise bed to comfortable working position.
4. Remove soiled linen and place in laundry bag. Avoid shaking or fanning linen.
5. Reposition mattress, and wipe off any moisture with a washcloth or paper towel moistened in antiseptic solution. Dry thoroughly.
6. Apply all bottom linen on one side of bed (before moving to opposite side):
   a. To apply a fitted sheet, be sure it is placed smoothly over mattress.
   b. To apply a flat unfitted sheet, allow about 25 cm (10 inches) to hang over sides of mattress edges (along sides and head of bed). Make sure that lower hem of sheet lies seam down, even with bottom edge of mattress. Pull remaining top part of sheet over top edge of mattress.
7. While standing at head of bed, miter top corner of bottom sheet (see Box 40.15, Steps 16a-f).
8. Tuck remaining part of unfitted sheet under mattress from head to foot of bed.
9. *Optional:* Apply drawsheet and waterproof incontinence pad, laying center-folds along middle of bed lengthwise. Smooth drawsheet and pad over mattress and tuck excess edge of drawsheet under mattress, keeping palms down. Center position of pad over bottom sheet.
10. Move to opposite side of bed and spread bottom sheet smoothly over edge of mattress from head to foot of bed.
11. Apply fitted sheet smoothly over each mattress corner. For an unfitted sheet, miter top corner of bottom sheet (see Step 7), making sure that corner is taut.
12. Grasp remaining edge of unfitted bottom sheet and tuck tightly under mattress while moving from head to foot of bed.
13. Smooth folded drawsheet over bottom sheet and tuck under mattress, first at middle, then at top, and then at bottom.
14. If needed, apply single waterproof pad over bottom sheet or drawsheet.
15. Place top sheet over bed with vertical centerfold lengthwise down middle of bed. Open sheet out from head to foot, being sure that top edge of sheet is even with top edge of mattress.
16. Make horizontal toe pleat: stand at foot of bed and make fanfold in sheet 5 to 10 cm (2 to 4 inches) across bed. Pull sheet up from bottom to make fold approximately 15 cm (6 inches) from bottom edge of mattress.
17. Tuck in remaining part of sheet under foot of mattress. Place blanket over bed with top edge parallel to top edge of sheet and 15 to 20 cm (6 to 8 inches) down from edge of sheet. (*Optional:* Apply additional spread over bed.)
18. Make cuff by turning edge of top sheet down over top edge of blanket and spread.
19. Standing on one side at foot of bed, lift mattress corner slightly with one hand; with other hand tuck top sheet, blanket, and spread under mattress. Be sure that toe pleats are not pulled out.
20. Make modified mitered corner with top sheet, blanket, and spread. After making triangular fold, do not tuck tip of triangle (see Box 40.15, Step 37).
21. Go to other side of bed. Spread sheet, blanket, and spread out evenly. Make cuff with top sheet and blanket. Make modified corner at foot of bed.
22. Apply clean pillowcase.
23. Place nurse call system within patient's reach on bedrail or pillow and return bed to low position, allowing for patient transfer. Lock wheels. Help patient to bed.
24. Arrange patient's room. Remove and discard supplies. Perform hand hygiene.

FIG. 40.10 Surgical or recovery bed.

Because of the importance of cost control in health care, avoid bringing excess linen into a patient's room. Once you bring linen into a patient's room, if unused, it must be laundered before being used. Excess linen lying around a patient's room creates clutter and obstacles for patient care activities.

Before making a bed, collect necessary bed linens and the patient's personal items. In this way all equipment is accessible to prepare the bed and room. When fitted sheets are unavailable, flat sheets usually are pressed with a center crease to be placed down the center of the bed. The linens unfold easily to the sides, with creases often fitting over the mattress edge. Apply clean linens whenever there is soiling.

Handle linen properly to minimize the spread of infection (see Chapter 28). Agency policies provide guidelines for the proper way to bag and dispose of soiled linen. After a patient is discharged, all bed linen goes to the laundry, and housekeeping cleans the mattress and bed before clean linen is applied.

◆ Evaluation

Through the Patient's Eyes. During assessment you collected information about a patient's expectations of care. Both during and after hygiene, ask the patient whether care is being provided in an expected and acceptable manner. For example, while bathing a patient, encourage verbalization of any discomfort such as too-cool water or discomfort with movement. To evaluate a patient's satisfaction with your care, ask questions, such as "Do you think your bath helped you feel more comfortable?" "Tell me ways we can make you feel less tired during your bath?" "Were you pleased with how we bathed and cleaned your feet?" Being aware of and addressing a patient's expectations and any concerns foster a caring therapeutic relationship.

Determine whether there were any modifiable environmental factors that promoted or impeded efficient care. For example, did other health care provider interactions coordinate with hygiene care or did they interrupt care. If additional personnel were needed, were they readily available, or did care need to be delayed. Recognizing these factors is important when planning continuing care for patients.

Patient Outcomes. Evaluate patient responses to hygiene measures both during and after each particular hygiene intervention. For example, while bathing a patient, inspect the skin carefully to see whether soiling or drainage is effectively removed. Once a bath is completed, evaluate whether the patient feels more comfortable by asking the level of comfort using a pain scale (see Chapter 44). Frequently it takes time for hygiene care to result in an improvement in a patient's condition.

Evaluate nursing interventions promoting and maintaining personal hygiene by determining the patient's response and comparing with expected outcomes to determine whether the outcomes of care were achieved (Fig. 40.11). The presence of oral lesions, a scalp infestation, or skin excoriation often requires repeated measures and a combination of nursing interventions to fully resolve the problem(s). An ongoing evaluation of the patient's response to hygiene measures determines the effectiveness of the interventions. Your knowledge base and experience provide important perspectives when analyzing evaluation data. For example, frequent observation of the skin helps to determine the effectiveness of hygiene practices. Does a rash clear or a pressure injury show signs of worsening? Is the patient able to complete hygiene care using adaptive equipment?

Use teach-back to evaluate a patient's or family caregiver's ability to perform self-care hygiene measures. For example, say, "I want to be sure you are clear about why foot care is so important for you since you have diabetes. Tell me three things you can do to protect your feet from infection." As another example, say, "We talked about ways to prevent your skin from drying. Describe how you will protect your skin from dryness."

When established outcomes for the care plan are not met, revise the plan. Use clinical judgment when reviewing evaluation findings. Then determine appropriate changes in interventions. Ask yourself questions, such as:

- Are there other skin care measures available to reduce dryness?
- Do I need to consult a skin/wound care specialist for new interventions to protect my patient's skin?

There are also times when you need to involve the patient or family caregiver for changes in care. Examples of questions include:

- What is preventing you from being able to perform your foot care at home?
- Which further measures do you think are necessary to keep your mouth feeling clean?
- What do you think would help you be more independent with your hygiene?

Jamie includes Mrs. White in evaluating her care and the use of adaptive devices to increase her self-care ability. Mrs. White verbally expresses satisfaction with both her involvement in hygiene care planning and with the caregiver's consideration of her preferences and needs. She explains that the use of the adaptive devices was easier than she anticipated and that the shower seat helped to reduce fatigue. Also, the assistive devices made her less fearful of falling during showering.

Jamie tells Mrs. White that the skin under her breasts is still red but that the other areas of redness are resolved. Jamie reminds Mrs. White that increasing her mobility, such as walking and changing positions, will help prevent future redness to her thighs and buttocks. Jamie uses a mirror to show Mrs. White that the redness under the breasts is reduced but that the skin is irritated. During a discussion about measures to decrease the redness and irritation, Mrs. White explained that she had felt this irritation many times before this recent hospitalization but that she was too embarrassed to tell anyone about the problem. Together they modified the care plan to include a consult from a skin/wound care specialist.

QSEN **Building Competency in Patient Safety** Mrs. White is discharged to her home. Her granddaughter and a home care aide will provide care for her over the next few weeks. During evaluation you note that Mrs. White is making progress using the walker and bath-adaptive equipment that have been ordered for home care. Which assessments should be made for her following discharge from the hospital? What teaching needs to be provided to the granddaughter to perform safe hygiene care for her grandmother?

Answers to QSEN Activities can be found on the Evolve website.

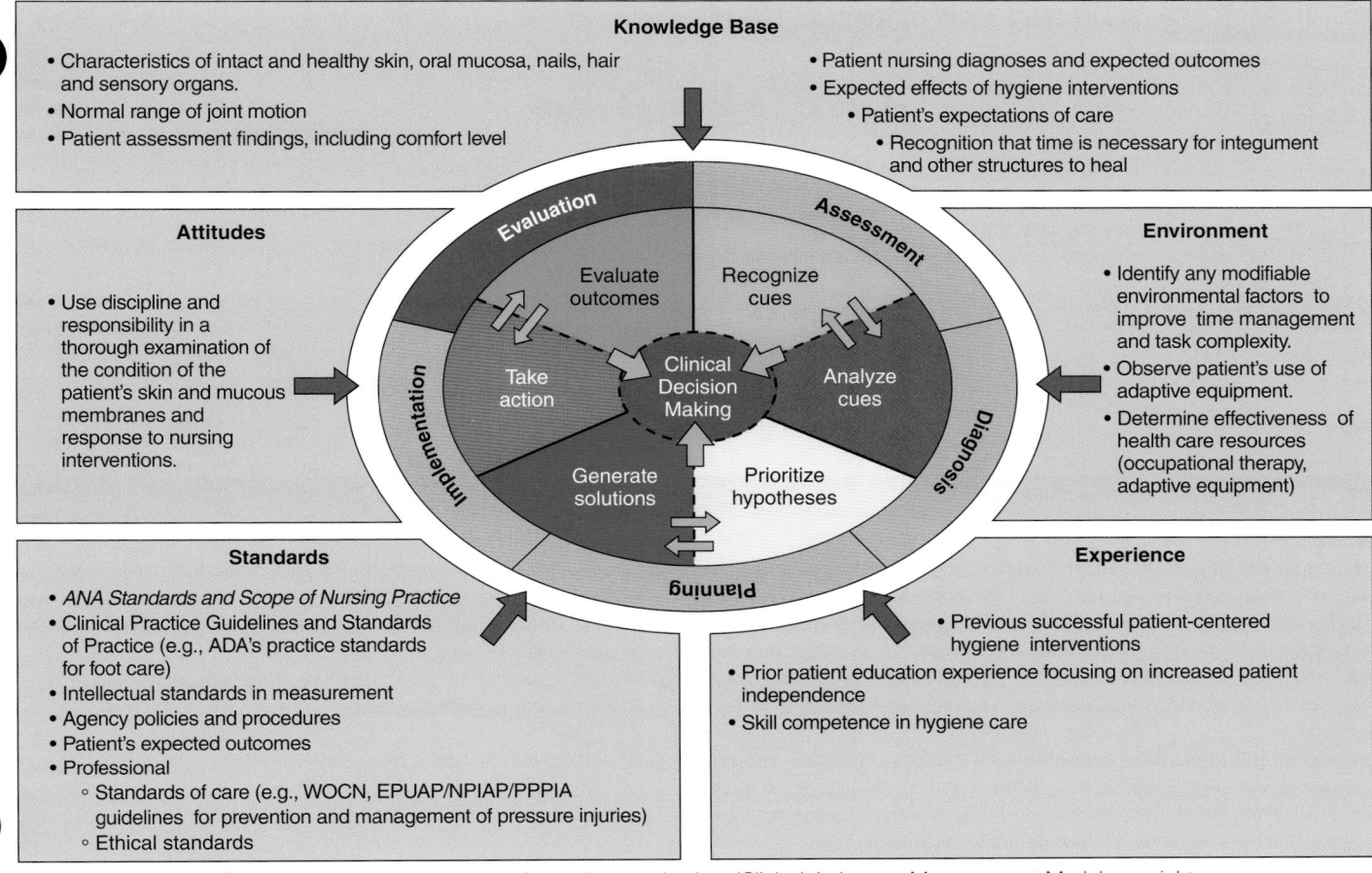

FIG. 40.11 Critical thinking model for hygiene evaluation. (Clinical Judgment Measurement Model copyright © NCSBN. All rights reserved.)

Content of the diagram:

Knowledge Base
- Characteristics of intact and healthy skin, oral mucosa, nails, hair and sensory organs.
- Normal range of joint motion
- Patient assessment findings, including comfort level
- Patient nursing diagnoses and expected outcomes
- Expected effects of hygiene interventions
  - Patient's expectations of care
    - Recognition that time is necessary for integument and other structures to heal

Attitudes
- Use discipline and responsibility in a thorough examination of the condition of the patient's skin and mucous membranes and response to nursing interventions.

Environment
- Identify any modifiable environmental factors to improve time management and task complexity.
- Observe patient's use of adaptive equipment.
- Determine effectiveness of health care resources (occupational therapy, adaptive equipment)

Standards
- *ANA Standards and Scope of Nursing Practice*
- Clinical Practice Guidelines and Standards of Practice (e.g., ADA's practice standards for foot care)
- Intellectual standards in measurement
- Agency policies and procedures
- Patient's expected outcomes
- Professional
  - Standards of care (e.g., WOCN, EPUAP/NPIAP/PPPIA guidelines for prevention and management of pressure injuries)
  - Ethical standards

Experience
- Previous successful patient-centered hygiene interventions
- Prior patient education experience focusing on increased patient independence
- Skill competence in hygiene care

Center wheel: Evaluation (Evaluate outcomes), Assessment (Recognize cues), Implementation (Take action), Diagnosis (Analyze cues), Planning (Generate solutions, Prioritize hypotheses), Clinical Decision Making

SAFETY GUIDELINES FOR NURSING SKILLS

Ensuring patient safety is an essential role of the professional nurse. Use sound clinical judgment by communicating clearly with members of the health care team, assessing and analyzing the patient's clinical findings, and incorporating the patient's priorities of care and preferences. Use the best evidence, applying professional standards, when selecting interventions to use in patient care delivery. When performing the skills in this chapter, remember the following points to ensure safe, patient-centered care.

- Patients who are totally dependent on someone else require help with personal hygiene or must learn or adapt to new hygiene techniques. When providing personal hygiene, important safety principles to follow are prevention of infection and patient injury.
- To reduce the risk of infection, always perform hygiene measures while moving from cleanest to less clean or dirty areas. (**NOTE:** This often requires you to change gloves and perform hand hygiene during care activities.)
- Continence issues in people with impaired cognition or dementia are difficult to manage and pose threats to a patient's skin integrity, increase the risk of falls, and increase social isolation (Wilson, 2018).

- Use clean gloves when you anticipate contact with nonintact skin or mucous membranes or when there is or may likely be contact with drainage, secretions, excretions, or blood. Additional precautions requiring other personal protective equipment (PPE) may be necessary, depending on the patient's condition (see agency policy and Chapter 28).
- When using water or solutions for hygiene care, be sure to test the solution temperature to prevent burn injury. This is especially important for patients with reduced sensation, such as those with diabetes mellitus, peripheral neuropathy, or spinal cord injury.
- Keep all personal hygiene items within a patient's reach. When the head of the bed is raised, the bedside stand is usually not within easy reach and must be moved forward. If a patient must leave the bed to go to the bathroom, be sure that there is a clear pathway to prevent falls.
- To prevent bleeding monitor laboratory findings, such as coagulation studies, before administering oral hygiene or shaving a patient.

Continued

| **SKILL 40.1** | **BATHING AND PERINEAL CARE** | |

Delegation and Collaboration

Assessment of the patient's skin, pain level, and ROM cannot be delegated to assistive personnel (AP). The skill of bathing and perineal care can be delegated to AP. Direct the AP about:

- Not massaging reddened skin areas during bathing (EPUAP/NPIAP/PPPIA, 2019b).
- Contraindications for soaking a patient's feet.
- Reporting any signs of impaired skin integrity to the nurse.
- Properly positioning patients with musculoskeletal limitations and indwelling catheters or intravenous (IV) lines.
- Reporting patient fatigue, shortness of breath, or pain during hygiene care.

Equipment

- Washcloths and bath towels
- Bath blanket
- Bar or liquid soap, or 4-oz bottle of 2% to 4% chlorhexidine gluconate (CHG) (dispensed in a single bath-size bottle) (*option:* 2% CHG bathing cloths)
- Toiletry items (deodorant, lotion). **NOTE**: If using CHG, use an agency-approved lotion.
- Disposable wipes
- Warm water
- Clean hospital gown or patient's own pajamas or gown
- Laundry bag
- Clean gloves
- Washbasin dedicated for bathing only
- Eye patch/shield and nonallergenic tape (for unconscious patient)

STEP	**RATIONALE**

ASSESSMENT

1. Identify patient using at least two identifiers (e.g., name and birthday or name and medical record number) according to agency policy.	Ensures correct patient. Complies with The Joint Commission standards and improves patient safety (TJC, 2021).
2. Review medical record for orders for specific precautions concerning patient's movement or positioning and for whether there is an order for a therapeutic bath.	Prevents accidental injury to patient during bathing activities. Determines level of help that patient needs.
3. Review prior nurses' notes to determine patient's tolerance for bathing: activity tolerance, comfort level, musculoskeletal function, and presence of shortness of breath.	Determines patient's ability to perform or tolerate bathing and type of bath to administer (e.g., tub bath, bed bath).
4. Review EHR to determine patient's risk for developing a medical adhesive–related skin injury (MARSI) using adhesive devices or tape on skin: age, dehydration, malnutrition, exposure to radiation therapy, underlying chronic conditions (e.g., diabetes, immunosuppression) and edema of skin.	Common risk factors for MARSI (Fumarola et al., 2020).
5. Assess room environment for safety (e.g., check room for spills; make sure that equipment is working properly and that bed is in locked, low position).	Identifies safety hazards in patient environment that could cause or potentially lead to harm (QSEN, n.d.).
6. Assess patient's or family caregiver's health literacy.	Ensures that patient or family caregiver has the capacity to obtain, communicate, process, and understand basic health information (CDC, 2021).
7. Perform hand hygiene. Assess patient's fall risk status (if partial bathing out of bed or self-bath is to be performed).	Reduces transmission of microorganisms. Allows you to anticipate needed precautions such as having patient sit on chair in front of basin.
8. Assess patient's tolerance for bathing: activity tolerance, comfort level during movement, cognitive function, musculoskeletal function, and presence of shortness of breath (see Chapter 30).	Determines patient's comfort level and ability to perform or tolerate bathing and level of assistance required (e.g., tub bath, partial bed bath).
9. If cognitive level is reduced, assess patient's cognitive (Mini-Mental State Examination) and functional status (e.g., Barthel's index or the index of activities of daily living [ADLs] to measure self-care ability). For patients with suspected dementia, observe behavior, especially after telling patient it is bath time; does the patient become agitated?	Every person entering a long-term care setting should be formally assessed for cognitive and functional status (Hirschman and Hodgson, 2018; Shelton et al., 2018). Functional status assesses a patient's capacity for self-bathing and how much supervision/help is needed to accomplish daily ADL tasks. Every attempt should be made to avoid bathing people against their will.

CLINICAL JUDGMENT: *Patients with dementia may become agitated and aggressive during bathing activities. Consider using alternative bathing procedures such as bag wipes with these patients (Villar et al., 2018; Scales et al., 2018). Maintain a calm, nonthreatening, quiet environment using therapeutic communication (see Box 40.6).*

10. Assess patient's visual status, ability to sit without support, hand grasp, ROM of extremities.	Determines degree of assistance patient needs for bathing. ROM may be delegated to assistive personnel.
11. Assess for presence and position of external medical device/equipment (e.g., intravenous [IV] line, oxygen tubing, Foley catheter).	Affects how you plan bathing activities and positioning. Helps determine how to set up supplies.
12. Assess patient's bathing preferences: frequency and time of day preferred, type of hygiene products used, and other factors related to preferences.	Allows patient to participate in plan of care. Promotes patient's comfort and willingness to cooperate. Using a patient's established routine may reduce agitation in a patient with dementia (Scales et al., 2018).
13. Ask whether patient has noticed any problems related to condition of skin and genitalia: excess moisture, inflammation, drainage or excretions from lesions or body cavities, rashes, or other skin lesions.	Provides you with information to direct physical assessment of skin and genitalia during bathing. Also influences selection of skin care products.

STEP	RATIONALE
14. Identify risks for skin impairment: older age, immobilization, reduced sensation, nutrition and hydration, excess skin moisture or drainage, shear or friction on skin, vascular insufficiencies, presence of external devices. *Option*: Use a pressure injury assessment tool (e.g., Braden Scale; see Chapter 48).	Risk factors increase the likelihood of injury to the skin because of pressure, impaired tissue synthesis, softening of or friction on tissues, and impaired circulation (EPUAP/NPIAP/PPPIA, 2019b).
15. Before and during bath assess condition of patient's skin. Note presence of dryness, indicated by flaking, redness, scaling, and cracking.	Provides a baseline for comparison over time in determining whether bathing improves condition of skin.
16. Assess patient's comfort on a 0-to-10 pain scale.	Provides baseline measure. Determine whether patient needs pain medication before bathing. A bath can also soothe and comfort patient.
17. Assess patient's knowledge, prior experience with skin hygiene in terms of its importance, preventive measures to take, and common problems.	Reveals need for patient instruction and/or support.
18. Assess patient's goals or preferences for how skill is to be performed or what patient expects.	Allows care to be individualized to patient.

PLANNING

1. Adjust room temperature and ventilation, close room doors and windows, and draw room divider curtain.	Warm room that is free of drafts prevents rapid loss of body heat during bathing. Privacy provides for patient's mental and physical comfort.
2. Explain procedure and ask patient for suggestions on how to prepare supplies. If partial bath, ask how much of bath patient wishes to complete. If using CHG, explain benefit of reducing infection and that solution leaves a sticky feeling on the skin.	Promotes patient's cooperation and participation. Patients who prefer using their own bathing supplies may need to discuss benefits of CHG.
3. Prepare equipment and organize supplies on bedside table. If it is necessary to leave room, be sure that nurse call system is within patient's reach, bed is in low position, and wheels are locked.	Organized work area avoids interrupting procedure or leaving patient unattended to retrieve missing equipment. Provides for patient safety.

CLINICAL JUDGMENT: *Never leave the bedside without ensuring that appropriate number of side rails have been raised (see agency policy). The number of side rails depends on the patient's fall risk assessment; however, having all side rails raised is considered a restraint.*

IMPLEMENTATION

1. Offer patient bedpan or urinal. Apply clean gloves to help patient as needed. Provide toilet tissue and dispose of any excrement properly. Provide patient towel and moist washcloth. Dispose of gloves if applied and perform hand hygiene.	Patient feels more comfortable after voiding. Prevents interruption of bath. Reduces transmission of microorganisms.
2. Raise bed to comfortable working height. Lower side rail closest to you and help patient assume comfortable supine position, maintaining body alignment. Bring patient toward side closest to you (staying supine).	Aids access to patient. Maintains patient's comfort throughout procedure. Uses proper body mechanics, thus minimizing strain on back muscles. If patient is overweight, use other caregiver or lift device for positioning (see Chapter 39).
3. Complete or partial bed bath	
a. If patient has nonintact skin or skin is soiled with drainage, excretions, or body secretions, apply clean gloves. Ensure that patient is not allergic to latex.	Prevents allergic reaction if latex gloves are used.
b. Place bath blanket over patient and loosen and remove top covers without exposing patient. If possible, have patient hold top of bath blanket while you remove linen. Place soiled linen in laundry bag. Take care to not allow linen to touch your uniform. *Optional:* Use top sheet when bath blanket is not available or if patient prefers.	Bath blanket provides warmth and privacy during bath.
4. Remove patient's gown or pajamas.	Provides full exposure of body parts during bathing.
a. If gown with ties or snaps on sleeves, simply untie or unsnap and remove gown without pulling IV line (if present).	
b. If regular gown is used and patient has reduced mobility and IV access, remove gown from *unaffected side first*.	Undressing unaffected side first allows easier manipulation of gown over body part with reduced ROM.
c. If patient has an IV line and gown with no snaps, remove gown from arm *without* IV line first. Then remove gown from arm with IV line (see illustration A). Pause IV fluid infusion by pressing appropriate sensor on IV pump. Remove IV tubing from pump; use regulator to slow IV infusion. Remove IV bag from pole (see illustration B) and slide IV bag and tubing through arm of patient's gown (see illustration C). Rehang IV bag (see illustration D), reconnect tubing to pump, open regulator clamp, and restart IV fluid infusion by pressing appropriate sensor on IV pump. If IV fluids are infusing by gravity, check IV flow rate and regulate if necessary. *Do not disconnect IV tubing to remove gown.*	Manipulation of IV tubing and container may disrupt flow rate. Do **not** delegate regulation of IV flow rate to AP.

Continued

SKILL 40.1   BATHING AND PERINEAL CARE—cont'd

STEP	RATIONALE

STEP 4c (A) Remove patient's gown. (B) Remove IV tubing from pole. (C) Slide IV tubing through arm of patient's gown. (D) Rehang IV bag.

---

5. Raise side rail. Lower bed temporarily to lowest position. Fill washbasin two-thirds full of warm water Place basin and supplies on over-bed table. Raise bed to comfortable working height. Check water temperature and also have patient place fingers in water to test temperature tolerance. Place plastic container of bath lotion in bath water to warm if desired.

   Raising side rail and lowering bed position maintain patient's safety while you leave bedside. Keeping bed at working height during bath prevents back strain. Warm water promotes comfort, relaxes muscles, and prevents unnecessary chilling. CHG is most effective at full strength. Testing temperature prevents accidental burns. Bath water warms lotion for application to patient's skin.

6. Lower side rail, remove pillow if tolerated, and raise head of bed 30 to 45 degrees if allowed. Place bath towel under patient's head. Place second bath towel over patient's chest.

   Removal of pillow makes it easier to wash patient's ears and neck. Placing towels prevents bed linen and bath blanket from getting soiled or wet.

7. Wash face.

CLINICAL JUDGMENT: *Do not use bath water with 4% CHG solution or 2% CHG bathing cloths on the eyes or face. Only use clear water or mild soap and water on the face (AHRQ, 2013).*

---

a. Ask whether patient is wearing contact lenses. You may choose to remove them at this time.

   Prevents accidental injury to eyes.

b. Form a mitt with washcloth (see illustration). Immerse mitt in water and wring thoroughly.

   Mitt retains water and heat better than loosely held washcloth; keeps cold edges from brushing against patient and prevents splashing.

8. Wash patient's eyes with plain warm water. Use different section of mitt for each eye. Move mitt from inner to outer canthus (see illustration). Soak any crusts on eyelid for 2 to 3 minutes with damp cloth before attempting removal. Dry eyes thoroughly but gently.

   Soap irritates eyes. Use of separate sections of mitt reduces infection transmission. Bathing eye from inner to outer canthus prevents secretions from entering nasolacrimal duct. Pressure can cause internal injury.

STEP	RATIONALE

STEP 7b Steps for folding washcloth to form a mitt.

STEP 8 Wash eye from inner to outer canthus. (Copyright © Mosby's Clinical Skills: Essentials Collection.)

9. Ask whether patient prefers to use soap on face. Otherwise wash, rinse, and dry forehead, cheeks, nose, neck, and ears without using soap. (Men may wish to shave at this point or wait until after bath.)

Soap tends to dry face, which is exposed to air more than other body parts.

10. Provide eye care for unconscious patient.

Patients who are unconscious have lost the normal protective corneal reflex of blinking, increasing the risk for corneal drying, abrasions, and eye infection (Kaye et al., 2019; Morris et al., 2018).

   a. Instill eye drops or ointment per health care provider's order (see Chapter 31).

Keeps cornea lubricated.

   b. In the absence of blink reflex, keep eyelids closed. Close eye gently, using back of your fingertip, before placing eye patch or shield. Place tape over patch or shield. Do not tape eyelid.

When blink reflex is absent, patient loses a protective mechanism. Keeping eyelids closed maintains eye moisture and prevents injury (Kocacal et al., 2018).

11. Wash trunk and upper extremities. *Option:* Change bath water at this time. Obtain new 6-quart basin and mix contents of a 4-ounce bottle of 4% CHG with warm water (Dray et al., 2019).

Evidence shows that CHG use in daily bathing can reduce incidence of hospital-acquired infections (Martin et al., 2017; Dray et al., 2019). CHG reduces bacteria for up to 24 hours and prevents infection (AHRQ, 2013).

CLINICAL JUDGMENT: *When using CHG in a bath basin of water, use one washcloth for washing each major body part. Then dispose of cloth and use a new cloth for the next body part (Martin et al., 2017). Dipping cloth back into basin contaminates solution and makes CHG less effective. Do not rinse after bathing with CHG solution. Allow CHG to dry on the skin to achieve antimicrobial effects.*

   a. Remove bath blanket from patient's arm that is closest to you. Place bath towel lengthwise under arm. Bathe arm with soap and water, using long, firm strokes from distal to proximal areas (fingers to axilla).

Towel prevents soiling of bed. Soap lowers surface tension and facilitates removal of debris and bacteria when friction is applied during washing. Long, firm strokes stimulate circulation; moving distal to proximal promotes venous return.

   b. Raise and support arm above head (if possible) to wash, rinse, and dry axilla thoroughly (see illustration). Apply deodorant or powder to underarms if desired or needed.

Movement of arm exposes axilla and exercises normal ROM of joint. Alkaline residue from soap discourages growth of normal skin bacteria. Drying prevents excess moisture, which can cause skin maceration or softening. Respect patient's preference for use of hygiene products.

   c. Move to other side of bed and repeat steps with other arm.

Provides for better access to patient and helps prevent back strain.

   d. Cover patient's chest with bath towel and fold bath blanket down to umbilicus. Bathe chest with long, firm strokes. Take special care with skin under female patient's breasts, lifting breast upward if necessary while bathing underneath breast. Rinse if using soap and water and dry well.

Draping prevents unnecessary exposure of body parts. Towel maintains warmth and privacy. Secretions and dirt collect easily in areas of tight skinfolds. Skin under breasts is vulnerable to excoriation if not kept clean and dry.

12. Wash hands and nails.

   a. Fold bath towel in half and lay it on bed beside patient. Place basin on towel. Immerse patient's hand in water. Allow hand to soak for 2 to 3 minutes before washing hand and fingernails. Remove basin and dry hand well. Repeat for other hand.

Soaking softens cuticles and calluses of hand, loosens debris beneath nails, and enhances feeling of cleanliness. Thorough drying removes moisture between fingers.

Continued

SKILL 40.1	BATHING AND PERINEAL CARE—cont'd

STEP	RATIONALE

STEP 11b Positioning arm to wash axilla. (Copyright © Mosby's Clinical Skills: Essentials Collection.)

CLINICAL JUDGMENT: *Do not soak fingers of patient with diabetes mellitus (CDC, 2019c). Soaking hands of patient with diabetes mellitus can lead to maceration and risk for infection. When a patient has diabetes, gently clear any dirt from under the nails and file across (see Skill 40.2).*

---

13. Check temperature of bath water and change water when cool or soapy. **NOTE:** If using CHG solution in bath water, do not discard water. One bottle of CHG soap is sufficient for a complete bath.	Warm water maintains patient's comfort.

CLINICAL JUDGMENT: *If patient is at risk for falling, be sure that two side rails are up before obtaining fresh water. In addition, lower bed when it is necessary to leave bedside.* NOTE: *Having all side rails raised is considered a restraint. Check agency policy.*

---

14. Wash abdomen.	
a. Place bath towel lengthwise over chest and abdomen. (Two towels may be needed.) Fold bath blanket down to just above pubic region. With one hand lift bath towel. With mitted hand bathe and rinse abdomen, giving special attention to umbilicus and skinfolds of abdomen and groin. Stroke from side to side. Keep abdomen covered between washing and rinsing. Rinse and dry well.	Draping prevents unnecessary exposure of body parts. Towel maintains warmth and privacy. Keeping skinfolds clean and dry helps prevent odor and skin irritation. Moisture and sediment that collect in skinfolds predispose skin to maceration.
b. Apply clean gown or pajama top. If an extremity is injured or immobilized, dress affected side first. (This step may be omitted until completion of bath; gown should not become soiled during remainder of bath.)	Maintains patient's warmth and comfort. Dressing affected side first allows easier manipulation of gown over body part with reduced ROM.

CLINICAL JUDGMENT: *If one extremity is injured or immobilized, always dress affected side first.*

---

15. Wash lower extremities.	
a. Cover chest and abdomen with top of bath blanket. Expose near leg by folding blanket toward midline. Be sure to keep other leg and perineum draped. Place bath towel under leg as you support patient's knee and ankle.	Prevents unnecessary exposure.
b. Wash leg using long, firm strokes from ankle to knee and from knee to thigh (see illustration). Rinse and dry well. Remove and discard towel.	Promotes circulation and venous return. Excess massage of calf could loosen deep vein thrombus. Secretions and moisture may be present between toes, predisposing patient to maceration and breakdown. Do not cut nails of a patient with diabetes. See agency policy for podiatrist care.

CLINICAL JUDGMENT: *When bathing lower extremities, assess for signs of warmth, redness, swelling, tenderness, and pain in the lower extremities because these might be early signs of deep vein thrombosis (DVT).*

---

c. Clean foot, making sure to bathe between toes. Rinse and dry toes and feet completely. Clean and file nails as needed (see Skill 40.2).	Secretions and moisture are often present between toes, predisposing patient to maceration and skin breakdown.

STEP	RATIONALE

d. Raise side rail, move to opposite side of bed, lower side rail, and repeat steps for other leg and foot. If skin is dry, apply moisturizer. When finished, cover patient with bath blanket.

Moisturized skin is less at risk for breakdown. Moisturizers are effective in reducing dry skin; however, in excess they can cause maceration.

e. Cover patient with bath blanket, raise side rail for patient's safety, remove and dispose of soiled gloves, and perform hand hygiene. Change bath water and/or CHG solution and water.

Decreased bath water temperature causes chilling. Clean water reduces microorganism transmission to perineal structures.

16. Provide perineal hygiene.

a. If patient can maneuver and handle washcloth, allow patient to clean perineum on own.

Maintains patient's dignity and self-care ability.

CLINICAL JUDGMENT: *CHG is safe to use on the perineum and external mucosa (AHRQ, 2013). However, cleansing of the urinary meatus is best performed with soap and water (Manojlovich, n.d.)*

---

b. Female patient

(1) Apply pair of clean gloves. Lower side rail. Help patient into dorsal recumbent position. Note restrictions or limitations in patient's positioning. Place waterproof pad under patient's buttocks. Drape patient with bath blanket placed in shape of a diamond. Lift lower edge of bath blanket to expose perineum (see illustration).

Provides full exposure of female genitalia. If patient is totally dependent, provide assistance to support her in side-lying position and raise leg as perineum is bathed. If position causes patient discomfort, reduce degree of abduction in her hips.

(2) Fold lower corner of bath blanket up between patient's legs onto abdomen. Wash and dry patient's upper thighs.

Keeping patient draped until procedure begins minimizes anxiety. Buildup of perineal secretions soils surrounding skin surfaces.

(3) Wash labia majora. Use nondominant hand to gently retract labia from thigh, with dominant hand wash carefully in skinfolds. Wipe in direction from perineum to rectum. Repeat on opposite side with separate section of washcloth. Rinse and dry area thoroughly.

Perineal care involves thorough cleaning of patient's external genitalia and surrounding skin. Skinfolds may contain body secretions that harbor microorganisms. Wiping front to back reduces chance of transmitting fecal organisms to urinary meatus.

(4) Gently separate labia with nondominant hand to expose urethral meatus and vaginal orifice. With dominant hand, wash downward from pubic area toward rectum in one smooth stroke (see illustration). Wash middle and both sides of perineum. Use separate section of cloth for each stroke. Clean thoroughly around labia minora, clitoris, and vaginal orifice. Avoid placing tension on indwelling catheter if present, and clean area around it thoroughly.

Cleansing method reduces transfer of microorganisms to urinary meatus. (For menstruating women or patients with indwelling catheters, clean with cotton balls.)

STEP 15b Washing leg. (Copyright © Mosby's Clinical Skills: Essentials Collection.)

STEP 16b(1) Drape patient for perineal care.

STEP 16b(4) Cleanse from perineum to rectum (front to back).

Continued

SKILL 40.1	BATHING AND PERINEAL CARE—cont'd

STEP	RATIONALE
(5) Provide catheter care as needed per agency requirements (see Chapter 46).	Proper cleansing around periurethral area and catheter reduces the risk for catheter-associated urinary tract infections (CAUTI) (CDC, 2015).
(6) Rinse area thoroughly. May use bedpan and pour warm water over perineal area. Dry thoroughly from front to back.	Rinsing removes soap and microorganisms more effectively than wiping. Retained moisture harbors microorganisms.
(7) Fold lower corner of bath blanket back between patient's legs and over perineum. Ask patient to lower legs and assume comfortable position.	
c. Male patient	
(1) Apply clean gloves. Lower side rail. Help patient to supine position. Note any restriction in mobility.	Provides full exposure of male genitalia. Position patients who are unable to lie supine on their side.
(2) Fold lower half of bath blanket up to expose upper thighs. Wash and dry thighs.	Buildup of perineal secretions soils surrounding skin surfaces.
(3) Cover thighs with bath towels. Raise bath blanket up to expose genitalia. Gently raise penis and place bath towel underneath. Gently grasp shaft of penis. If patient is uncircumcised, retract foreskin (see illustration). If patient has an erection, defer procedure until later.	Draping minimizes patient anxiety. Towel prevents moisture from collecting in inguinal area. Gentle but firm handling of penis reduces chance of an erection. Secretions capable of harboring microorganisms collect underneath foreskin.
(4) Wash tip of penis at urethral meatus first. Using circular motion, clean from meatus outward (see illustration). Discard washcloth and repeat with clean cloth until penis is clean. Rinse and dry gently.	Direction of cleaning moves from area of least contamination to area of most contamination, preventing microorganisms from entering urethra.
(5) Return foreskin to its natural position. This is extremely important in patients with decreased sensation in their lower extremities.	Tightening of foreskin around shaft of penis causes local edema and discomfort. Patients with reduced sensation do not feel tightening of foreskin.
(6) Gently clean shaft of penis and scrotum by having patient abduct legs. Pay special attention to underlying surface of penis. Lift scrotum carefully and wash underlying skinfolds. Rinse and dry thoroughly.	Vigorous massage of penis may cause an erection. Underlying surface of penis is an area where secretions accumulate. Abduction of legs provides easier access to scrotal tissues. Secretions collect easily between skinfolds.
(7) Avoid placing tension on indwelling catheter if present and clean area around it thoroughly. Provide catheter care (see Chapter 46).	Cleaning along catheter from exit site reduces incidence of nosocomial urinary infection.
17. Remove soiled gloves and discard in trash; raise side rail before leaving bedside to dispose of water and obtain fresh water.	Prevents transmission of infection. Protects patient from injury.
18. Wash back. (This follows both female and male perineal care.)	
a. Perform hand hygiene and apply clean gloves. Lower side rail. Help patient into prone or side-lying position (as applicable). Place towel lengthwise along patient's side and keep the patient covered with bath blanket.	Exposes back and buttocks for bathing while limiting exposure.
b. Keep patient draped by sliding bath blanket over shoulders and thighs during bathing. Wash, rinse, and dry back from neck to buttocks using long, firm strokes.	Cleaning back before buttocks and anus prevents contamination of water.
c. Next move from back to buttocks and anus. Have patient remain in prone or side-lying position and keep covered to avoid chilling. Clean anus and buttocks area.	Exposes back and buttocks for bathing while limiting exposure.
d. If fecal material is present, enclose in fold of underpad or toilet tissue and remove with disposable wipes.	Skinfolds near buttocks and anus may contain fecal secretions that harbor microorganisms.
e. Clean buttocks and anus, washing front to back (see illustration). Clean, rinse, and dry area thoroughly. If needed, place a clean absorbent pad under patient's buttocks. Remove contaminated gloves. Raise side rail and perform hand hygiene.	Cleaning motion prevents contamination of perineal area with fecal material or microorganisms.

STEP 16c(3) Retract foreskin.   **STEP 16c(4)** Use circular motion to clean tip of penis.   **STEP 18e** Cleanse buttocks from front to back.

STEP	RATIONALE
19. Return to bed and lower side rail; give a back rub (see Chapter 44).	Promotes patient relaxation. Make sure that back rub is appropriate for your patient. Back rubs are contraindicated in some cardiac patients.
a. Apply additional body lotion or oil to patient's skin as needed. When finished, raise side rail.	Moisturizing lotion prevents dry, chapped skin.
20. Remove soiled linen and place in dirty-linen bag. Clean and replace bathing equipment. Perform hand hygiene.	Reduces transmission of microorganisms.
21. Optional Bathing Methods	
a. Commercial bag bath or CHG cleansing pack:	
(1) A cleansing pack contains six to eight premoistened towels for cleaning. Warm package contents in microwave following package directions. If you are bathing patient using warm commercial or CHG cloth, check temperature of cloth before use. Gloves diminish sense of heat.	Provides warm, soothing heat. CHG has been shown to reduce bacteria for up to 24 hours and prevents infection such as bloodstream infection and multidrug-resistant organisms (Frost et al., 2018; AHRQ, 2013). Checking temperature prevents burn to skin.
(2) Use all six CHG cloths in the following order (see illustration):	Reduces transmission of microorganisms.
• Cloth 1: Neck, shoulders, and chest	
• Cloth 2: Both arms, both hands, web spaces, and axilla	
• Cloth 3: Abdomen and then groin/perineum	
• Cloth 4: Right leg, right foot, and web spaces	
• Cloth 5: Left leg, left foot, and web spaces	
• Cloth 6: Back of neck, back, and buttocks	
(3) Firmly massage skin when using cloth. Allow skin to air-dry for 30 seconds. Do not rinse. It is permissible to lightly cover patient with bath towel to prevent chilling.	Drying skin with towel removes emollient that is left behind after water/cleaner solution evaporates.

CLINICAL JUDGMENT: *If there is excessive soiling (e.g., in perineal region), use an extra cloth or conventional washcloths, soap, water, and towels.*

STEP	RATIONALE
22. Help patient dress. Comb patient's hair. If a woman wants to apply makeup, help as needed.	Promotes patient's body image.
23. Make patient's bed (see Box 40.15 and Box 40.16).	Provides clean, comfortable environment.
24. Check function and position of external devices (e.g., indwelling urethral catheters, nasogastric tubes, IV lines).	Ensures that systems remain functional after bathing activities.
25. Help patient to a comfortable position.	Restores comfort and sense of well-being.
26. Place bed in lowest position. Wheels locked. Side rails up as appropriate.	Maintains patient's safety by decreasing height of bedframe from floor.
27. Replace nurse call system and personal possessions. Leave room as clean and comfortable as possible. Perform hand hygiene.	Prevents transmission of infection. Clean environment promotes patient's comfort. Keeping nurse call system and articles of care within reach promotes patient's safety.

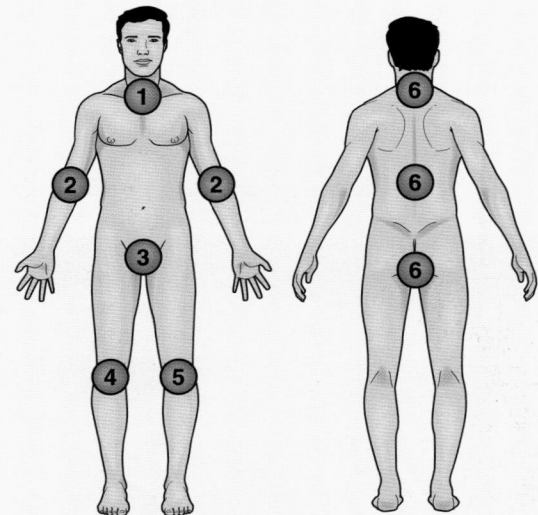

STEP 21a(2) Using CHG bathing cloths. (From Universal ICU decolonization: *An enhanced protocol.* Appendix E: *Training and educational materials,* Rockville, MD, September 2013, Agency for Healthcare Research and Quality.)

Continued

SKILL 40.1	BATHING AND PERINEAL CARE—cont'd

STEP	RATIONALE

28. Tub bath or shower:

STEP	RATIONALE
a. Consider patient's condition and review orders for precautions concerning the patient's movement or positioning.	Prevents accidental injury to patient during bathing.
b. Schedule use of shower or tub.	Prevents unnecessary waiting, which causes fatigue.
c. Check tub or shower for cleanliness. Use cleaning techniques outlined in agency policy. Place rubber mat on tub or shower bottom. Place disposable bathmat or towel on floor in front of tub or shower.	Cleaning prevents transmission of microorganisms. Mats prevent slipping and falling.
d. Collect all hygienic aids, toiletry items, and linens requested by patient. Place within easy reach of tub or shower.	Placing items close at hand prevents possible falls when patient reaches for equipment.
e. Help patient to bathroom if necessary. Have the patient wear robe and slippers.	Assistance prevents accidental falls. Wearing robe and slippers prevents chilling.
f. Demonstrate how to use nurse call system in the bathroom for assistance.	Bathrooms are equipped with signaling devices in case patient feels faint or weak or needs immediate assistance. Patients prefer privacy during bath if safety is not jeopardized.
g. Instruct patient to use safety bars when getting in and out of tub or shower. Caution patient against use of bath oil in tub water.	Prevents slipping and falling. Oil causes tub surfaces to become slippery.

CLINICAL JUDGMENT: *Before leaving patient alone in the tub or shower area, have patient demonstrate how to use the safety bars and nurse call system. It is important that the patient can correctly use these safety devices in case the patient feels weak, faint, or needs immediate assistance*

STEP	RATIONALE
h. Place "occupied" sign on bathroom door.	Maintains patient's privacy.
i. Fill bathtub halfway with warm water. Check temperature of bath water, have patient test water, and adjust temperature if water is too warm. Explain which faucet controls hot water. If patient is taking shower, turn shower on and adjust water temperature before the patient enters shower stall. Use shower seat or tub chair if needed (see illustration).	Adjusting water temperature prevents accidental burns. Older adults and patients with neurological alterations (e.g., diabetes, spinal cord injury) are at high risk for burn because of reduced sensation. Use of assistive devices facilitates bathing and minimizes physical exertion.
j. Instruct patient not to remain in tub longer than 10 or 15 minutes. Check on the patient every 5 minutes.	Prolonged exposure to warm water causes vasodilation and pooling of blood in some patients, leading to light-headedness or dizziness.
k. Return to bathroom when patient signals, and knock before entering.	Provides privacy.
l. For patient who is unsteady, drain tub of water before patient tries to get out. Place bath towel over patient's shoulders. Help patient out of tub as needed and help with drying.	Prevents accidental falls. Patient may become chilled as water drains.

CLINICAL JUDGMENT: *Weak or unstable patients need extra assistance in getting out of a tub. Planning for additional personnel is essential before attempting to help the patient. Lift equipment may be used for transfer. See agency policy.*

STEP	RATIONALE
m. Help patient as needed with getting dressed in clean gown or pajamas, slippers, and robe. (In home setting patient may put on regular clothing.)	Maintains warmth to prevent chilling.
n. Help patient to room and comfortable position in bed or chair.	Maintains relaxation gained from bathing.

STEP 28i Shower seat for patient safety.

STEP	RATIONALE
o. Place nurse call system in an accessible location within patient's reach.	Ensures that patient can call for assistance if needed and promotes safety and prevents falls.
p. Raise side rails (as appropriate) and lower bed to lowest position.	Promotes safety and prevents falls.
q. Clean tub or shower according to agency policy.	Prevents transmission of infection through soiled linen and moisture.
r. Remove soiled linen and place in dirty-linen bag. Discard disposable equipment in proper receptacle. Place "unoccupied" sign on bathroom door. Return supplies to storage area.	Reduces transmission of infection.
s. Perform hand hygiene.	Reduces transfer of microorganisms.

EVALUATION

1. Observe skin, paying particular attention to areas previously soiled, reddened, dry, or showing early signs of pressure injuries.	Techniques used during bathing leave skin clean and clear. Over time dry skin diminishes. If patient shows areas of redness, use Braden scale to measure risk for pressure injury (see Chapter 48).
2. Observe ROM during bath.	Measures joint mobility.
3. Ask patient to rate level of comfort (on a scale of 0-10).	Determines patient's tolerance of bathing activities.
4. Ask patient to rate level of fatigue (on a scale of 0-10).	Determines patient's tolerance of bathing activities.
5. **Use Teach-Back:** "We talked about the importance of keeping your skin clean with these special bathing cloths. Explain to me why we are using bathing cloths for your bath." Revise your instruction now or develop a plan for revised patient/family caregiver teaching if patient/family caregiver is not able to teach back correctly.	Teach-back is an evidence-based health literacy intervention that promotes patient engagement, patient safety, adherence, and quality. The goal of teach-back is to ensure that you have explained medical information clearly so that patients and their families understand what you communicated to them (AHRQ, 2020).

UNEXPECTED OUTCOMES AND RELATED INTERVENTIONS

1. Areas of excessive dryness, rashes, or pressure injuries or MARSI appear on skin.
   - Complete pressure injury assessment (see Chapter 48).
   - Apply moisturizing lotions or topical skin applications per agency policy.
   - Limit frequency of complete baths. It may become necessary (if patient has a sensitivity to CHG) to switch to plain soap and water.
   - Obtain special bed surface if patient is at risk for skin breakdown.
2. Patient becomes excessively tired or is unable to cooperate or participate in bathing.
   - Reschedule bathing to a time when patient is more rested.
   - Provide pillow or elevate head of bed during bath for patient with breathing difficulties.
   - Notify health care provider if this is a change in patient's fatigue level.
   - Perform hygiene measures in stages between scheduled rest periods.
3. The rectum, perineum, or genital area is inflamed or swollen or has foul-smelling odor.
   - Provide frequent perineal care and keep area clean and dry.
   - Obtain an order for a sitz bath.
   - Apply protective barrier ointment or antiinflammatory cream.
   - Report findings to health care provider.

RECORDING AND REPORTING

- Record procedure, amount of assistance provided, patient's participation in care, level of fatigue, and condition of skin. Include any significant findings (e.g., reddened areas, breaks in skin, inflammation, ulcerations).
- Document your evaluation of patient learning.
- Report any skin irritations, breaks in skin, or ulcerations to nurse in charge or health care provider. These are serious in patients with altered circulation to the lower extremities.
- Report intolerance of activity to patient's oncoming nurse.

HOME CARE CONSIDERATIONS

- Assess patient's tub and shower area for need for safety devices (e.g., grab bars, shower chair, handheld shower).
- Assess patient for the need for assistive bathing devices (e.g., long-handle sponge, mirrors, or lift equipment).

Continued

SKILL 40.2   PERFORMING NAIL AND FOOT CARE

Delegation and Collaboration

The skill of nail and foot care of patients *without diabetes mellitus* or *peripheral vascular disease* can be delegated to assistive personnel (AP). The nurse instructs the AP about:

- Not trimming patient's nails (unless permitted by agency or health care provider).
- Special considerations for patient positioning.
- Reporting any breaks in skin, redness, numbness, swelling, or pain to the nurse.

Equipment

- Washbasin
- Emesis basin
- Washcloth and towel
- Nail clippers (check agency policy)
- Soft nail or cuticle brush
- Plastic applicator stick
- Emery board or nail file
- Body lotion
- Disposable bath mat
- Clean gloves

STEP	RATIONALE
ASSESSMENT	
1. Identify patient using at least two identifiers (e.g., name and birthday or name and medical record number) according to agency policy.	Ensures correct patient. Complies with The Joint Commission standards and improves patient safety (TJC, 2021).
2. Review patient's record, including health care provider's order and nurses' notes. Verify health care provider's order for cutting nails (check agency policy).	Patients with diabetes or reduced peripheral circulation are more at risk for infection. Accidental cutting of skin increases risk for infection. A podiatrist should assess and develop a regular schedule for nail care for patients with vascular insufficiency or peripheral neuropathy.
3. Review patient's medical record for foot or nail problems.	Certain conditions increase likelihood of foot or nail problems (e.g., diabetes mellitus, immunocompromised).
a. Older adult	Normal physiological changes such as poor vision, lack of coordination, or inability to bend over contribute to difficulty in performing foot and nail care (Touhy and Jett, 2021). Normal physiological changes of aging can result in brittle nails. Discolored, extremely thickened, and deformed nails can indicate infection, fungus, or disease (Howes-Trammel and Bryant, 2016).
b. Diabetes mellitus	Vascular changes reduce blood flow to peripheral tissues. Break in skin integrity places patient with diabetes mellitus at high risk for skin infection (CDC, 2019c; ADA, 2020).
c. Heart failure, renal disease	Both conditions increase tissue edema, particularly in dependent areas (e.g., feet). Edema reduces blood flow to neighboring tissues.
d. Cerebrovascular accident (stroke)	Presence of residual foot or leg weakness or paralysis results in altered walking patterns. Altered gait pattern causes increased friction and pressure on feet.
e. History of leg pain	Claudicating pain is related to ischemia with diabetic and neuropathic disorders.
4. Assess environment for safety (check room for spills; make sure that equipment is working properly and that bed is in locked, low position).	Reduces risk for falls.
5. Assess patient's or family caregiver's health literacy.	Ensures that patient or family caregiver has the capacity to obtain, communicate, process, and understand basic health information (CDC, 2021).
6. Assess patient's ability to care for feet (vision, musculoskeletal function) and foot and nail care practices. Rule out use of the following practices for existing foot problems:	Identifies patient's self care ability and whether self-care practices place patient at risk for foot injuries. Identifies patient education needs.
a. Use of over-the-counter liquid preparations to remove corns	Liquid preparations cause burns and ulcerations.
b. Cutting corns or calluses with razor blade or scissors	Cutting corns or calluses sometimes results in infection caused by a break in skin integrity. The patient with diabetes or any patient with decreased peripheral circulation should never trim corns or calluses because of the increased risk for infection secondary to a break in skin integrity (CDC, 2019c).
c. Use of oval corn pads	Oval pads exert pressure on toes, thereby decreasing circulation to surrounding tissues.
d. Application of adhesive tape	Skin of older adult is thin and delicate and prone to tearing when adhesive tape is removed (Touhy and Jett, 2021).
7. Ask female patients whether they use nail polish and polish remover frequently.	Chemicals in these products cause excessive dryness.
8. Assess type of footwear worn by patients, including type and cleanliness of socks worn, type and fit of shoes, and whether restrictive garters or knee-high hose are worn.	Types of shoes and footwear predispose patient to foot and nail problems (e.g., infection, areas of friction, ulcerations). These conditions decrease mobility and increase risk for amputation in patient with diabetes (Chapman, 2017).
9. If possible, observe patients walking to assess their gait.	Sores or alterations in bony structures of the foot cause pain, imbalance, and unsteady gait.

STEP	RATIONALE
10. Perform hand hygiene. Apply clean gloves if drainage is present. Inspect all surfaces of fingers, toes, feet, and nails. Pay particular attention to areas of dryness, inflammation, or cracking. Also inspect areas between toes, heels, and soles of feet.	Integrity of feet and nails determines frequency and level of hygiene required. Heels, soles, and sides of feet are prone to irritation from ill-fitting shoes.

CLINICAL JUDGMENT: *Patients with peripheral vascular diseases or diabetes mellitus, older adults, and patients whose immune system is suppressed often require nail care from a specialist to reduce the risk of tissue injury and infection. Defer care other than washing the feet in these cases until patient has been evaluated.*

STEP	RATIONALE
11. Assess color and temperature of toes, feet, and fingers. Assess capillary refill of nails. Palpate radial and ulnar pulse of each hand and dorsalis pedis pulse of each foot; note character of pulses (see Chapter 30). Remove and dispose of gloves. Perform hand hygiene.	Assesses adequacy of blood flow to extremities. Circulatory alterations often change integrity of nails and increase patient's chance of localized infection when break in skin integrity occurs.
12. Assess patient's knowledge, prior experience, and preferences for care of nails or feet.	Determines patient's ability to perform self-care and degree of assistance required from nurse. Reveals need for patient instruction and support.
13. Assess patient's goals for how skill is to be performed or what patient expects.	Allows care to be individualized to patient.

PLANNING

STEP	RATIONALE
1. Collect appropriate equipment and arrange on over-bed table.	Provides easy access to equipment and promotes an organized procedure.
2. Close room door or pull curtain around patient's bed.	Provides privacy.
3. Explain procedure, including need to soak feet, which requires several minutes.	Patient needs to be able to place fingers and feet in basin for 10 to 20 minutes. Some patients may become tired.

IMPLEMENTATION

STEP	RATIONALE
1. Assist ambulatory patient to seated position in bedside chair. Help bed-bound patient to supine position with head of bed elevated. Place disposable bath mat or towel on floor under patient's feet, or place towel on bed.	Sitting in chair facilitates immersion of feet in basin. Bath mat or towel protects feet from exposure to soil or microorganisms on floor; towel lessens chance of splashing water on floor or bed.

CLINICAL JUDGMENT: *Soaking the feet of patients with diabetes mellitus or peripheral vascular disease is not recommended. Soaking may lead to maceration (excessive softening of the skin) and drying of the skin (CDC, 2019c; ADA, 2020), leading to tissue breakdown and infection.*

STEP	RATIONALE
2. Fill washbasin with warm water. Test water temperature. Place basin on floor and lower side rail or place basin on waterproof pad on the mattress. Assist patient to immerse feet.	Warm water softens nails and thickened epidermal cells, reduces inflammation of skin, and promotes local circulation. Proper water temperature prevents burns.
3. Adjust over-bed table to low position and place it over patient's lap. (Patient sits in chair or lies in bed.)	Easy access prevents accidental spills.
4. Instruct patient to place fingers in emesis basin and arms in comfortable position.	Prolonged positioning causes discomfort unless normal anatomical alignment is maintained.
5. Allow patient's feet and fingernails to soak for 10 to 20 minutes. Rewarm water after 10 minutes. **NOTE:** If patient is diabetic or has peripheral vascular disease, skip this step (CDC, 2019c).	Softening corns, calluses, and cuticles ensures easy removal of dead cells and easy manipulation of cuticle. *Do not soak if patient has diabetes.*
6. Perform hand hygiene and apply clean gloves. Clean gently under nails with plastic applicator stick or soft brush while immersing fingers (see illustration).	Removes debris under nails that harbors microorganisms.

STEP 6 Clean under fingernails.

Continued

SKILL 40.2 PERFORMING NAIL AND FOOT CARE—cont'd

STEP	RATIONALE

CLINICAL JUDGMENT: *Check agency policy for appropriate process for cleaning beneath nails. Do not use an orange stick or end of cotton swab; these splinter and can cause injury.*

7. Use soft cuticle brush or nail brush to clean around cuticles to decrease overgrowth.	Nail brush helps prevent inflammation and injury to cuticles. The cuticle grows slowly over the nail and must be pushed back with a soft nail brush regularly.
8. Remove hands from basin and dry thoroughly.	Thorough drying impedes fungal nail growth and prevents maceration of tissues.

CLINICAL JUDGMENT: *Check agency policy on nail care regarding filing and trimming.*

9. File fingernails straight across and even with tops of fingers (CDC, 2019a). If permitted by agency policy, use nail clippers and clip fingernails straight across and even with tops of fingers (see illustration); then smooth nail, using file. Use disposable emery board, and file nail to ensure that there are no sharp corners.	Filing nail straight across to eliminate sharp nail edges minimizes risk that nail can injure the adjacent tissues (Howes-Trammel and Bryant, 2016).
10. Move over-bed table away from patient.	Provides easier access to patient's feet.
11. Perform hand hygiene and apply clean gloves. Begin foot care by scrubbing callused areas of feet with washcloth. Clean between toes with washcloth.	Friction removes dead skin layers. Gloves prevent transmission of fungal infection. Areas between toes harbor debris.
12. Dry feet thoroughly and clean under nails (see Step 6).	Nails harbor debris and dirt and are a source of potential infection from poor care habits (Ball et al., 2019).
13. Trim toenails straight across, and gently smooth any sharp edges with a nail file (CDC, 2019c). **NOTE:** Do not file corners of toenails. Check agency policy for trimming patient's nails.	Smoothing sharp edges prevents damage to tissues surrounding the toes. Shaping corners of toenails damages tissues, which increases the risk for infection (Jeffcoate et al., 2018).
14. Apply lotion to hands and feet. Rub in thoroughly. Do not leave excess lotion between toes.	Lotion lubricates dry skin by helping to retain moisture. Excess lotion can macerate the skin.
15. Help patient to a comfortable position in bed or chair.	Restores comfort and sense of well-being.
16. Place nurse call system in an accessible location within patient's reach.	Ensures that patient can call for assistance if needed; promotes safety and prevents falls.
17. Raise side rails (as appropriate) and lower bed to lowest position.	Promotes safety and prevents falls.
18. Sanitize equipment according to agency policy. Dispose of used equipment, remove and dispose of gloves, and perform hand hygiene.	Reduces transmission of infection.

CLINICAL JUDGMENT: *Instruct patients to report any of the following to their health care provider: any tingling, burning, or pain in the feet; decreased sensation to heat and cold in the feet; changes in the shape of feet; loss of hair on toes or lower legs; abnormalities or changes in the nail, including changes in nail shape or color; bleeding around the nails; thinning or thickening of the nails; and redness, swelling, or pain around the nails (CDC, 2019c).*

EVALUATION

1. Inspect nails, cuticles, and areas between fingers and toes and surrounding skin surfaces.	Inspection enables you to evaluate condition of skin and nails. Allows you to note any remaining rough nail edges.
2. When possible, observe patient walking after foot and nail care. Ask patient whether there is any pain or discomfort.	Evaluates level of comfort and whether nail care removed excess skin or uneven nail surfaces that caused discomfort or problems with mobility.

STEP 9 Trim nails straight across when using nail clipper.

STEP	RATIONALE
3. Use Teach-Back: "I want to be sure you know what problems you can have if you do not trim your nails correctly. Show me how to properly trim your toenails." Revise your instruction now or develop a plan for revised patient/family caregiver teaching if patient/family caregiver is not able to teach back correctly.	Teach-back is an evidence-based health literacy intervention that promotes patient engagement, patient safety, adherence, and quality. The goal of teach-back is to ensure that you have explained medical information clearly so that patients and their families understand what you communicated to them (AHRQ, 2020).

UNEXPECTED OUTCOMES AND RELATED INTERVENTIONS

1. Cuticles and surrounding tissues are inflamed and tender to touch.
   - Repeated soakings are necessary to relieve inflammation and loosen layers of skin cells.
   - Patients with peripheral vascular disease or diabetes often require referral to a podiatrist.
   - Evaluate need for antifungal cream.
2. Localized areas of tenderness occur on feet, with calluses or corns at point of friction.
   - Recommend a change in footwear if necessary.
   - Refer patient to a podiatrist.
3. Tissue injury appears between toes or other pressure areas in foot.
   - Institute wound care policies (see Chapter 48).
   - Consult with wound care specialist and/or podiatrist.
   - Increase frequency of assessment and hygiene.

RECORDING AND REPORTING

- Record procedure and observations of integument (e.g., breaks in skin, inflammation, ulcerations).
- Report any breaks in skin or tissue injury to nurse in charge or physician. These are serious in patients with peripheral vascular disease and illnesses in which patient's circulation is impaired. Special foot-care treatments are often necessary.
- Document your evaluation of patient learning.

HOME CARE CONSIDERATIONS

- Instruct family and patient to remove foot hazards from the home (e.g., throw rugs, objects that block pathways, or uneven flooring).
- Alternative therapies: moleskin applied to areas of feet that are under friction is less likely to cause pressure to tissues; wrapping small pieces of lamb's wool around toes reduces irritation of soft corns between toes.
- Provide contact information for a podiatrist; this is especially important for patients with diabetes or peripheral vascular disease.

SKILL 40.3   PERFORMING MOUTH CARE FOR AN UNCONSCIOUS OR DEBILITATED PATIENT

Delegation and Collaboration

The skill of providing oral hygiene to an unconscious or debilitated patient can be delegated to assistive personnel (AP). The nurse is responsible for assessing a patient's gag reflex. The nurse instructs the AP to:

- Have another AP assist and properly position patient for mouth care.
- Be aware of aspiration precautions.,
- Use an oral suction catheter for clearing oral secretions (see Chapter 41, Skill 41.1).
- Report any signs of impaired oral mucosa integrity, bleeding of mucosa or gums, excessive coughing, or choking to the nurse.

Equipment

- Small pediatric, soft-bristled toothbrush, toothette sponges, or suction toothbrushes for patients for whom brushing is contraindicated
- Antibacterial solution per agency policy (e.g., chlorhexidine gluconate [CHG] 0.12%)
- Fluoride toothpaste
- Water-based mouth moisturizer
- Tongue blade
- Penlight
- Oral suction equipment
- Oral airway (uncooperative patient or patient who shows bite reflex)
- Water-soluble lip lubricant
- Water glass with cool water
- Face and bath towel
- Emesis basin
- Clean gloves

STEP	RATIONALE
ASSESSMENT	
1. Identify patient using at least two identifiers (e.g., name and birthday or name and medical record number) according to agency policy.	Ensures correct patient. Complies with The Joint Commission standards and improves patient safety (TJC, 2021).
2. Assess patient's risk for oral hygiene problems (see Box 40.9).	Certain conditions increase likelihood of alterations in integrity of oral cavity mucosa and structures, necessitating more frequent care.
3. Assess patient's or family caregiver's knowledge, experience, and health literacy.	Assures that patient or family caregiver has the capacity to obtain, communicate, process, and understand basic health information (CDC, 2021).
4. Perform hand hygiene and apply clean gloves.	Reduces transmission of microorganisms in blood or saliva.
5. Assess for presence of gag reflex by placing tongue blade on back half of tongue.	Helps in determining aspiration risk.

Continued

SKILL 40.3	PERFORMING MOUTH CARE FOR AN UNCONSCIOUS OR DEBILITATED PATIENT—cont'd

STEP	RATIONALE

CLINICAL JUDGMENT: *Patients with impaired gag reflex are unable to clear airway secretions and often accumulate secretions in the back of the oral cavity and have a higher risk for aspiration. Keep suction equipment available when caring for patients who are at risk for aspiration.*

6. Inspect condition of oral cavity. Inspect lips, teeth, gums, buccal mucosa, palate, and tongue using tongue depressor and penlight if necessary. Observe for color, moisture, lesions, injury or ulcers, and condition of teeth or dentures (see Chapter 30).	Determines condition of oral cavity and need for hygiene. Establishes baseline to show improvement following oral care.

CLINICAL JUDGMENT: *The critically ill patient with an artificial airway and who is on mechanical ventilation is at risk for ventilator-associated pneumonia (VAP). Once intubated, the artificial airway bypasses normal airway defenses, which also causes a rapid change in the normal oral flora (IHI, 2020; de Lacerda Vidal et al., 2017). Studies have shown use of CHG to significantly reduce incidence of VAP (Kallet, 2019). In a review of studies, CHG was shown to be effective in preventing nosocomial pneumonia among adult populations in cardiothoracic intensive care units (ICUs) (Rabello et al., 2018). In a Cochrane review, oral hygiene with CHG was found to probably prevent VAP from developing in very ill patients treated in ICUs (Zhao et al., 2020).*

7. Assess patient's respirations and/or oxygen saturation *(optional)*.	Assists in early recognition of aspiration.
8. Remove and dispose of gloves. Perform hand hygiene.	Prevents transmission of infection.

PLANNING

1. Ensure safety of environment (e.g., check the room for spills, make sure that suction equipment is working properly, and check that bed is in locked, low position).	Identifies safety hazards in patient environment that could cause or potentially lead to harm.
2. Provide privacy and gather equipment and supplies at bedside.	Avoids interrupting procedure or leaving patient unattended to retrieve missing equipment.
3. Explain procedure to patient or family caregiver if present.	Even debilitated or intubated patients are generally able to hear. Explanation can reduce anxiety.

IMPLEMENTATION

1. Perform hand hygiene and apply clean gloves.	Reduces transfer of microorganisms.
2. Raise bed to appropriate working height; lower side rail closest to you.	Promotes good body mechanics for caregiver.
3. Place towel on over-bed table and arrange equipment. If needed, turn on suction machine and connect tubing to suction catheter.	Prevents soiling of tabletop. Equipment prepared in advance ensures smooth, safe procedure. Supplies within reach create organized workspace.
4. Unless contraindicated (e.g., head injury, neck trauma), position patient in side-lying position. Turn patient's head toward mattress in dependent position with HOB elevated at least 30 degrees.	Position promotes drainage of secretions from mouth instead of collecting behind pharynx. Prevents aspiration.
5. Place second towel under patient's head and emesis basin under chin.	Prevents soiling of bed linen.
6. Remove dentures or partial plates if present.	Allows for thorough cleaning of prosthetics later. Provides clearer access to oral cavity.
7. If patient is uncooperative or having difficulty keeping mouth open, insert an oral airway. Insert upside down and turn airway sideways and over tongue to keep teeth apart. Insert when patient is relaxed if possible. Do not use force.	Prevents patient from biting down on nurse's fingers and provides access to oral cavity.

CLINICAL JUDGMENT: *Never place fingers into the mouth of an unconscious or debilitated patient. This could occlude the airway. Also, the normal patient response is to bite down.*

8. Clean mouth using brush moistened in water. Apply toothpaste or use antibacterial solution first to loosen crusts. Hold toothbrush bristles at 45-degree angle to gum line. Be sure that tips of bristles rest against and penetrate under gum line. Brush inner and outer surfaces of upper and lower teeth by brushing from gum to crown of each tooth; then clean biting surfaces of teeth by holding top of bristles parallel with teeth and brushing gently back and forth (see Box 40.9). Brush sides of teeth by moving bristles back and forth. Use a toothette sponge if patient has a bleeding tendency or if use of toothbrush is contraindicated (see illustration). Suction any accumulated secretions. Moisten brush with clear water or CHG solution to rinse. Use brush or toothette to clean roof of mouth, gums, and inside cheeks. Gently brush tongue but avoid stimulating gag reflex (if present). Repeat rinsing several times and use suction to remove secretions. Use towel to dry off lips.	Brushing action removes food particles between teeth and along chewing surfaces and removes crusts and secretions from mucosa. The use of a chlorhexidine gluconate (CHG) oral hygiene protocol as part of daily oral care reduces the incidence of ventilator-associated pneumonia (VAP) (Jenson et al., 2018; de Lacerda Vidal et al., 2017). The Institute for Healthcare Improvement (2020) recommends the use of 0.12% chlorhexidine gluconate (CHG) as part of daily oral care in critically ill patients. Repeated rinsing removes all debris and aids in moistening mucosa. Suction removes secretions and fluids that collect in posterior pharynx, thus reducing aspiration risk.
9. Apply thin layer of water-soluble moisturizer to lips (see illustration).	Lubricates lips to prevent drying and cracking.
10. Inform patient that procedure is completed. Return the patient to comfortable and safe position.	Provides meaningful stimulation to unconscious or less-responsive patient.

STEP	RATIONALE

STEP 8 Cleaning lips and mucosa around oral airway with toothette.

STEP 9 Application of water-soluble moisturizer to lips.

11. Clean equipment and return to its proper place. Place soiled linen in dirty laundry bag.

Proper disposal of soiled equipment prevents spread of infection.

12. Remove and dispose of gloves in proper receptacle and perform hand hygiene.

Reduces transmission of microorganisms.

13. When suction equipment is used, be sure to have a clean suction catheter ready and attached to the suction source.

In case of an emergency, suction equipment is clean and ready to use to clear patient's airway.

14. Raise side rails (as appropriate), and lower bed to lowest position.

Promotes safety and prevents falls.

15. Place nurse call system in an accessible location within patient's reach.

Ensures that patient can call for assistance if needed and promotes safety and prevents falls.

EVALUATION

1. Apply clean gloves and use tongue blade and penlight to inspect oral cavity.

Determines efficacy of cleaning. Once thick secretions are removed, underlying inflammation or lesions may be revealed.

2. Ask debilitated patient if mouth feels clean.

Evaluates level of comfort.

3. **Use Teach-Back:** "I explained what is needed to reduce your husband's risk of choking on secretions in his throat. Tell me the ways to prevent him from choking." Revise your instruction now or develop a plan for revised patient/family caregiver teaching if family caregiver is not able to teach back correctly.

Teach-back is an evidence-based health literacy intervention that promotes patient engagement, patient safety, adherence, and quality. The goal of teach-back is to ensure that you have explained medical information clearly so that patients and their families understand what you communicated to them (AHRQ, 2020).

UNEXPECTED OUTCOMES AND RELATED INTERVENTIONS

1. Secretions or crusts remain on mucosa, tongue, or gums.
   - Provide more frequent oral hygiene.
2. Localized inflammation or bleeding of gums or mucosa is present.
   - Provide more frequent oral hygiene with toothette sponges.
   - Apply a water-based mouth moisturizer to provide moisture and maintain integrity of oral mucosa.
   - Chemotherapy and radiation can cause mucositis (inflammation of mucous membranes in mouth) because of sloughing of epithelial tissue. Room temperature saline rinses, bicarbonate and sterile water rinses, and oral care with a soft-bristled toothbrush decrease severity and duration of mucositis.
3. Lips are cracked or inflamed.
   - Apply moisturizing gel or water-soluble lubricant to lips more often.
4. Patient aspirates secretions.
   - Suction oral airway to maintain airway patency (see Chapter 41).
   - Elevate patient's HOB to facilitate breathing.
   - If aspiration is suspected, notify health care provider immediately. Prepare patient for chest x-ray examination.

RECORDING AND REPORTING

- Record procedure, appearance of oral cavity before and after procedure, presence of gag reflex, and patient's response to procedure.
- Document your evaluation of patient/family caregiver learning.
- Use agency's standardized hand-off communication to communicate specific patient risks for aspiration and dry mouth. Discuss patient-specific interventions taken.
- Report any unusual findings (e.g., bleeding, ulceration, lesions, choking response) to nurse in charge or health care provider.
- Report immediately to the health care provider if patient aspirates.

Continued

SKILL 40.3	PERFORMING MOUTH CARE FOR AN UNCONSCIOUS OR DEBILITATED PATIENT—cont'd

HOME CARE CONSIDERATIONS

- Irrigate oral cavity with bulb syringe; patient can use a gravy baster to remove secretions.
- Give mouth care at least twice a day.
- Have caregivers demonstrate positioning patient to prevent aspiration.

KEY POINTS

- Various health beliefs, personal, sociocultural, economic, and developmental factors influence patients' hygiene preferences and practices.
- Sound clinical judgment requires you to consider a patient's condition, anticipate any risks or problems, gather thorough assessment data, and then analyze data to form nursing diagnoses.
- Hygiene needs, preferences, and the ability to participate in care change as people age.
- Assess a patient's skin, feet and nails, oral mucosa, hair, and eyes and ears to obtain a complete assessment of the patient's hygiene needs.
- Assess a patient's physical and cognitive ability to perform basic hygiene measures.
- Vascular insufficiency and reduced mobility, cognition, and sensation increase a patient's risk for impaired skin integrity.
- Diabetes mellitus and peripheral vascular diseases increase the patient's risk for foot and nail problems.
- Clinical judgment and critical thinking about a patient's hygiene preferences, needs, and ability to participate in care results in patient-centered hygiene care matching the patient's needs and preferences.
- Administering therapies to relieve symptoms such as pain or nausea before hygiene better prepares patients for any procedure.
- Position patients and make suction available to reduce the risk for aspiration when providing oral care to unconscious patients.
- A patient's environment needs to be comfortable, safe, and large enough to provide care and allow the patient and visitors to move about freely.
- Evaluation of hygiene procedures is based on outcomes of care; a patient's sense of comfort, relaxation, and well-being; and a patient's understanding of hygiene techniques.

REFLECTIVE LEARNING

Providing complete hygiene care must be patient-centered. The case study integrated within this chapter will guide you in addressing the questions that follow. However, if you have had an opportunity to provide complete personal hygiene to a patient with a self-care deficit and a risk for impaired skin integrity, use information you gained from the experience to reflect on these questions.

- Describe assessment data that put Mrs. White at risk for continued impaired self-care ability to perform hygiene as she progresses from hospital to home. (Recognize Cues)
- From the case study, nursing care plan, and concept map identify other assessment data and cues that support additional nursing diagnoses. (Analyze Cues)
- Consider the assessment information in the case study and Mrs. White's nursing care plan to prioritize health care problems or nursing diagnoses. (Prioritize Diagnoses)

- After reviewing the case study information and Mrs. White's nursing care plan, describe other nursing interventions to maintain or improve mobility and prevent pressure injury. (Generate Solutions)
- From the list below identify the priorities when planning and providing hygiene care for Mrs. White. List them in order of priority, with number 1 being the most important. (Take Action)
  1. Skin care
  2. Pain control
  3. Range-of-motion activities
  4. Initiation of consult with skin/wound care specialist
  5. Patient education regarding adaptive aids
- In addition to the information in the care plan identify other factors you would use to determine the effectiveness of your plan of care for Mrs. White. What evaluation findings would indicate the nursing interventions were effective? What evaluation findings would indicate a need to modify the care plan? (Evaluate Outcomes)

REVIEW QUESTIONS

1. What is the proper position to use for an unresponsive patient during oral care to prevent aspiration? (Select all that apply.)
   1. Prone position
   2. Modified left lateral recumbent position
   3. Semi-Fowler's position with head to side
   4. Trendelenburg position
   5. Supine position
2. The student nurse is teaching a family member the importance of foot care for their mother, who has diabetes mellitus. Which safety precautions are important for the family member to know to prevent infection? (Select all that apply.)
   1. Cut nails frequently.
   2. Assess skin for redness, abrasions, and open areas daily.
   3. Soak feet in water at least 10 minutes before nail care.
   4. Apply lotion to feet daily.
   5. Clean between toes after bathing.
3. Which of the following factors directly impairs salivary gland secretion? (Select all that apply.)
   1. Use of cough drops
   2. Immunosuppression
   3. Radiation therapy
   4. Dehydration
   5. Presence of oral airway
4. A nurse is assigned to care for the following patients. Which patient is most at risk for developing skin problems that will require thorough bathing and skin care?
   1. A 44-year-old female patient who has had removal of a breast lesion and is in pain and unwilling to ambulate postoperatively.

2. A 56-year-old male patient who is homeless and admitted to the emergency department with malnutrition and dehydration.

3. A 60-year-old female patient who experienced a stroke with right-sided paralysis and has an orthopedic brace applied to the left leg

4. A 70-year-old patient who has diabetes and dementia and has been incontinent of urine and stool

5. When the nurse is assigned to a patient who has a reduced level of consciousness and requires mouth care, which physical assessment techniques should the nurse perform before the procedure? (Select all that apply.)

   1. Oxygen saturation
   2. Heart rate
   3. Respirations
   4. Gag reflex
   5. Response to painful stimulus

6. The American Dental Association suggests that patients who are at risk for poor hygiene use the following interventions for oral care: (Select all that apply.)

   1. Use fluoride toothpaste.
   2. Brush teeth 4 times a day.
   3. Use 0.12% chlorhexidine gluconate (CHG) oral rinses for high-risk patients.
   4. Use a soft toothbrush for oral care.
   5. Avoid cleaning the gums and tongue.

7. While planning morning care, which of the following patients would have the highest priority to receive a bath first?

   1. A patient who just returned to the nursing unit from a diagnostic test
   2. A patient with a fever who just finished a dose of intravenous antibiotics.
   3. A patient who is experiencing frequent incontinent diarrheal stools and urine
   4. A patient who has been awake all night because of pain 8/10

8. A patient with a malignant brain tumor requires oral care. The patient's level of consciousness has declined, with the patient only being able to respond to voice commands. Place the following steps in the correct order for administration of oral care.

   1. If patient is uncooperative or having difficulty keeping mouth open, insert an oral airway.
   2. Raise bed, lower side rail, and position patient close to side of bed with head of bed raised up to 30 degrees.
   3. Using a brush moistened with chlorhexidine paste, clean chewing and inner tooth surfaces first.
   4. For patients without teeth, use a toothette moistened in chlorhexidine rinse to clean oral cavity.
   5. Remove partial plate or dentures if present.
   6. Gently brush tongue but avoid stimulating gag reflex.

9. The nurse delegates to the assistive personnel hygiene care for an alert older adult patient who had a stroke. Which intervention(s) would be appropriate for the assistive personnel to accomplish during the bath? (Select all that apply.)

   1. Checking distal pulses
   2. Providing range-of-motion (ROM) exercises to extremities
   3. Determining type of treatment for Stage 1 pressure injury
   4. Changing the dressing over an intravenous site
   5. Providing special skin care as indicated by nurse

10. The nurse will delegate hygiene care for two patients of different cultures to the assistive personnel (AP). What cultural information does the nurse need to provide to the AP? (Select all that apply.)

    1. Specific hygiene products
    2. Timing of hygiene care
    3. Socioeconomic status
    4. The need for gender congruent caregiver
    5. Religious practices

Answers: 1. 2, 3; **2.** 2, 4, 5; **3.** 3, 4; **4.** 5; **5.** 1, 3, 4; **6.** 1, 3, 4; **7.** 3; **8.** 2, 5, 1, 3, 6, 4; **9.** 2, 5; **10.** 1, 2, 4, 5.

Rationales for Review Questions can be found on the Evolve website.

REFERENCES

Adotama P, et al: Barber knowledge and recommendations regarding pseudofolliculitis barbae and Acne keloidalis nuchae in an urban setting, *JAMA Dermatology* 153(2):1325, 2017.

Agency for Healthcare Research and Quality (AHRQ): *Health literacy universal precautions toolkit*, ed 2, Rockville, MD, 2020, Agency for Healthcare Research and Quality. https://www.ahrq.gov/health-literacy/quality-resources/tools/literacy-toolkit/healthlittoolkit2-tool5.html. Accessed August 23, 2020.

Agency for Healthcare Research and Quality (AHRQ): *Universal ICU decolonization: an enhanced protocol*, 2013. https://www.ahrq.gov/professionals/systems/hospital/universal_icu_decolonization/universal-icu-overvw.html. Accessed May 2020.

American Academy of Dermatology: *Dermatologists' top tips for relieving dry skin*, 2020. https://www.aad.org/public/skin-hair-nails/skin-care/dry-skin. Accessed May 2020.

American Dental Association: *Mouth healthy: brushing your teeth*, 2020. https://www.mouthhealthy.org/en/az-topics/b/brushing-your-teeth. Accessed May 2020.

American Diabetes Association (ADA): *Foot complications*, 2020. https://www.diabetes.org/diabetes/complications/foot-complications. Accessed May 2020.

Arthritis Foundation: Foot pain, *Arthritis Today* 31(2):36, 2017.

Ball J, et al: *Seidel's guide to physical examination*, ed 8, St Louis, 2019, Elsevier.

Bowen F, O'Brien-Richardson P: Cultural hair practices, physical activity, and obesity among urban African-American girls, *J Am Assoc Nurse Pract* 29(12):754, 2017.

Broadbent JM, et al: Oral health-related beliefs, behaviors, and outcomes through life course, *J Dent Res* 95(7):808, 2016.

Butcher HK, et al: *Nursing interventions classification (NIC)*, ed 7, St. Louis, 2018, Elsevier.

Centers for Disease Control and Prevention (CDC): *Catheter-associated urinary tract infections (CAUTI): guidelines for prevention of CAUTI 2009*, 2015. https://www.cdc.gov/hai/ca_uti/uti.html. Accessed August 23, 2020.

Centers for Disease Control and Prevention (CDC): *Parasites-lice-head lice*, 2019a. http://www.cdc.gov/parasites/lice/head/treatment.html. Accessed September 2020.

Centers for Disease Control and Prevention (CDC): *Tick removal*, 2019b. https://www.cdc.gov/lyme/removal/index.html. Accessed September 2020.

Centers for Disease Control and Prevention (CDC): *Diabetes and your feet*, 2019c. https://www.cdc.gov/diabetes/library/features/healthy-feet.html. Accessed September 16, 2020.

Centers for Disease Control and Prevention (CDC): *What is health literacy*, 2021, https://www.cdc.gov/healthliteracy/learn/index.html. Accessed October 2021.

Chapman S: Foot care for people with diabetes: prevention of complications and treatment, *Br J Community Nurs* 22(5):226, 2017.

Espinosa M, Lio P: Skin and disparity issues that affect patients with skin of color, *Dermatol Times* 40(2):20, 2019.

European Pressure Ulcer Advisory Panel (EPUAP) and National Pressure injury Advisory Panel (NPIAP) and Pan Pacific Pressure Injury Alliance (PPPIA): Treatment of pressure ulcers/injuries: Clinical Practice Guideline. The International Guideline, Emily Haesler (ED). EPUAP/NPIAP/PPPIA, 2019a.

European Pressure Ulcer Advisory Panel (EPUAP) and National Pressure injury Advisory Panel (NPIAP) and Pan Pacific Pressure Injury Alliance (PPPIA): Treatment of pressure ulcers/injuries: Quick Reference Guide, Emily Haesler (ED). EPUAP/NPIAP/PPPIA, 2019b.

Giger J, Haddad LG: *Transcultural nursing: assessment and intervention*, ed 8, St Louis, 2021, Elsevier.

Halton AL, Rome K: Falls, footwear, and podiatric intervention in older adults, *Clin Geriatr Med* 35(2):161, 2019.

Harding MM, et al: *Lewis's medical-surgical nursing: assessment and management of clinical problems*, ed 11, St Louis, 2020, Elsevier.

Hockenberry ML, et al: *Wong's nursing care of infants and children*, ed 11, St Louis, 2019, Elsevier.

Howes-Trammel S, Bryant RA: Foot and nail care. In Bryant RA, Nix DP, editors: *Acute and chronic wounds: current management concepts,* ed 5, St Louis, 2016, Elsevier.

Institute for Healthcare Improvement (IHI): *Ventilator-associated pneumonia,* 2020. http://www.ihi.org/Topics/VAP/Pages/default.aspx. Accessed September 2020.

Jeffcoate WJ, et al: Current challenges and opportunities in the prevention and management of diabetic foot ulcers, *Diabetes Care* 41(4):645, 2018.

Johns Hopkins Medicine: CHG bathing to prevent healthcare-associated infections, 2021, https://www.hopkinsmedicine.org/health/treatment-tests-and-therapies/chg-bathing-to-prevent-healthcareassociated-infections. Accessed November 2021.

Kelly-O'Flynn S, et al: Medical adhesive-related skin injury, *Br J Nurs* 29(6):S20 (Stoma Care Supplement), 2020.

King EC, et al: Care challenges in the bathroom: the views of professional care providers working in clients' homes, *J Appl Gerontol* 37(4):493, 2018.

Manojlovich M: *Indwelling urinary catheter insertion and maintenance,* Centers for Disease Control (CDC),

Health Research and Educational Trust, n.d., https://www.cdc.gov/infectioncontrol/pdf/strive/CAUTI104-508.pdf. Accessed October 2021.

Marion L, et al: Implementing the new ANA Standard 8: culturally congruent practice, *Online J Issues Nurs* 22(1):1, 2017.

Mendes A: Meeting the care needs of a person with dementia who is distressed, *Br J Nurs* 27(4):219, 2018.

Mitchell A, Hill B: Moisture-associated skin damage: an overview of its diagnosis and management, *Br J Community Nurs* 25(3):S12, 2020.

Morgan-Consoli ML, Unzueta E: Female Mexican immigrants in the United States: cultural knowledge and healing, *Women Ther* 41(2):165, 2018.

National Pediculosis Association: *Welcome to headlice.org,* 2020. http://www.headlice.org/index.html. Accessed May 2020.

Quality Safety Education for Nurses (QSEN): *QSEN competencies,* n.d. https://qsen.org/competencies/pre-licensure-ksas/. Accessed September 16, 2020.

Scales K, et al: Evidence-based nonpharmacological practices to address behavior and psychological symptoms of dementia, *Gerontologist* 58:S88, 2018.

Sullivan WF, et al: Primary care of adults with intellectual and developmental disabilities: 2018 Canadian Guidelines, *Can Fam Phys* 64:254, 2018.

The Joint Commission (TJC): *2021 National patient safety goals,* Oakbrook Terrace, IL, 2021, The Commission. https://www.jointcommission.org/en/standards/national-patient-safety-goals/. Accessed August 3, 2021.

Touhy T, Jett P: *Ebersole & Hess' Toward healthy,* ed 10, St Louis, 2021, Elsevier.

US Department of Health and Human Services (USDHHS): *Oral health,* 2020. http://www.healthypeople.gov/2020/topics-objectives/topic/oral-health. Accessed May 2020.

Wilson M: Skin care for older people living with dementia, *Nurs Resid Care* 20(3):151, 2018.

Woody J: Overview of diabetic foot care for the nurse practitioner, *J Nurs Pract* 16(1):28, 2020.

RESEARCH REFERENCES

Alserehi H, et al: Chlorhexidine gluconate bathing practices and skin concentrations in intensive care unit patients, *Am J Infect Control* 46(2):226, 2018.

Chapple ILC, et al: Interaction of lifestyle, behaviour or systemic diseases with dental caries and periodontal diseases: consensus report of group2 of the joint EFP/ORCA workshop on the boundaries between caries and periodontal diseases, *J Clin Periodontol* 44(Suppl 18):S39, 2017.

de Lacerda Vidal CF, et al: Impact of oral hygiene involving toothbrushing versus chlorhexidine irrigation in the prevention of ventilator-associated pneumonia: a randomized study, *BMC Infect Dis* 17(1):112, 2017.

Dial M, et al: "I do the best I can:" Personal care preferences of patients of size, *Appl Nurs Res* 39:259, 2018.

Dray S, et al: What's new in the prevention of health-care associated infections using chlorhexidine gluconate impregnated wash cloths, *Intensive Care Med* 45(2):249, 2019.

Frost SA, et al: Evidence for the effectiveness of chlorhexidine bathing and health care -associated infections among adult intensive care patients: a trial sequential meta-analysis, *BMC Infect Dis* 18(1):1474, 2018.

Fumarola S, et al.: Overlooked and underestimated: medical adhesive-related skin injuries. Best practice consensus document on prevention. *J Wound Care* 29(Suppl 3c):S1, 2020.

Galiczewski JM: Intervention for prevention of catheter associated urinary tract infections in intensive care units: an integrative review, *Intensive Crit Care Nurs* 32:1, 2016.

Gomes AC, et al: Socioeconomic status, social support, oral health beliefs, psychosocial factors, health behaviours and health-related quality of life in adolescents, *Qual Life Res* 29:141, 2020.

Henderson S, et al: Cultural competence in healthcare in the community: a concept analysis, *Health Soc Care Community* 26(4):590, 2018.

Hirschman KB, Hodgson NA: Evidence-based interventions for transitions in care for individuals living with dementia, *Gerontol* 58(Suppl 1):S129, 2018.

Jenson H, et al: Improving oral care in hospitalized non-ventilated patients: standardizing products and protocol, *Medsurg Nurs* 27(1):38, 2018.

Kallet RH: Ventilator bundles in transition: from prevention of ventilator associated pneumonia to

prevention of ventilator associated events, *Respir Care* 64(8):994, 2019.

Kaye AD, et al: Postoperative management of corneal abrasions and clinical implications: a comprehensive review, *Curr Pain Headache Rep* 23(7):1, 2019.

Kocacal G, et al: Nurses can play an active role in the early diagnosis of exposure keratopathy in intensive care patients, *Crit Care Nurs* 15(1):31, 2018.

Kole U, et al: Knowledge in practice regarding menstrual hygiene among female students in selected schools, *Int J Nurs Educ* 10(2):85, 2018.

LaFleur RC, et al: Improving culturally congruent health care for children with disabilities: stakeholder perspectives of cultural competence training in an interdisciplinary training program, *J Transcult Nurs* 29(1):101, 2017.

Maciag J, et al: The effects of treatment of denture-related stomatitis on peripheral T cells and monocytes, *Oral Health Prev Dent* 15(3):259, 2017.

Martin ET, et al: Bathing hospitalized dependent patients with prepackaged disposable washcloths instead of traditional bath basins: a case crossover study, *Am J Infect Control* 45(9):990, 2017.

Mason NR, et al: A patient-centered approach to comparative effectiveness research focused on older adults: lessons from the patient-centered outcomes research institute, *J Am Geriatr Soc* 67(1):22, 2019.

Meddings J, et al: Systematic review of intervention to reduce urinary tract infection in nursing home residents, *J Hosp Med* 12(5):356, 2017.

Morris A, et al: Effectiveness of corneal abrasion prevention interventions for adults undergoing general anesthesia for more than one hour: a systematic review protocol, *JBI Database System Rev Implement Rep* 16(9):1785, 2018.

Murray J, Scholten I: An oral hygiene protocol improves oral health for patients in inpatient stroke rehabilitation, *Gerodontology* 35(1):18, 2018.

O'Brien-Richardson P: The case for hair health in health education: exploring hair and physical activity among urban African American Girls, *AM J Health Educ* 50(2):135, 2019.

Park YH, et al: Risk factors and the associated cutoff values for failure of corticosteroid injection in treatment of Morton's neuroma, *Int Orthop* 42(2):323, 2018.

Persaud R, et al: Validation of the healthy foot screen: a novel assessment tool for common clinical abnormalities, *Adv Skin Wound Care* 31(4):154, 2018.

Pinkert C, et al: Experiences of nurses with care of patients with dementia in acute hospitals: a secondary analysis, *J Clin Nurs* 27:163, 2018.

Rabello F, et al.: Effectiveness of oral chlorhexidine for the prevention of nosocomial pneumonia and ventilator-associated pneumonia in intensive care units: Overview of systematic reviews, *Int J Dent Hyg* 16(4):441, 2018.

Rokstad AMM, et al: The impact of the Dementia ABC educational programme on competence in person-centered dementia care and job satisfaction of care staff, *Int J Older People Nurs* 12(2), n/a N.PAG, 2017.

Ruiz J, et al: Daily bathing strategies and cross-contamination of multidrug-resistant organisms: impact of chlorhexidine-impregnated wipes in a multidrug-resistant gram-negative bacteria endemic intensive care unit, *Am J Infect Control* 45(10):1069, 2017.

Shelton EG, et al: Does it matter if we disagree? The impact of incongruent care preferences on persons with dementia and their care partners, *Gerontologist* 58(3):556, 2018.

Sibbald RG, et al: Validated 60 second general foot screen: a pilot trial and guide to diagnosis and treatment, *Adv Skin Wound Care* 32(11):490, 2019.

Vaingankar JA: Care participation and burden among informal caregivers of older adults with care needs and associations with dementia, *Int Psychogeriatr* 28(2):221, 2016.

Villar F, et al: Involving institutionalised people with dementia in their care-planning meetings: lessons learnt by staff, *Scand J Caring Sci* 32(3):567, 2018.

Yevchak A, et al: Implementing nurse-facilitated person-centered care approaches for patient with delirium superimposed on dementia in the acute care setting, *J Gerontol Nurs* 43(12):21, 2017.

Yoon MN, et al: Oral health status of long-term residents in Canada, *Gerodontology* 35(4):359, 2018.

Zhao T, et al.: Oral hygiene care for critically ill patients to prevent ventilator-associated pneumonia, *Cochrane Review,* 2020, https://www.cochrane.org/CD008367/ORAL_oral-hygiene-care-critically-ill-patients-prevent-ventilator-associated-pneumonia. Accessed October 2021.

Oxygenation

OBJECTIVES

- Describe the structure and function of the cardiopulmonary system.
- Explain the interrelationship among ventilation, perfusion, and exchange of respiratory gases.
- Explain the interrelationship among cardiac output, myocardial blood flow, and systemic circulation.
- Explain the relationship of cardiac output (preload, afterload, contractility, and heart rate) to the process of oxygenation, hypoventilation, and/or hypoxemia.
- Explain the relationship between the cardiac conduction system and mechanical dysfunction of the heart.
- Discuss the effect of a patient's level of health, age, lifestyle, and environment on oxygenation.

- Identify how to assess for the risk factors affecting a patient's oxygenation.
- Identify how clinical judgment in assessment identifies the physical manifestations that occur with alterations in oxygenation.
- Discuss potential clinical outcomes occurring as a result of disturbances in conduction, altered cardiac output, impaired valvular function, myocardial ischemia, and/or impaired tissue perfusion.
- Develop a plan of care for a patient with altered oxygenation.
- Explain how clinical judgment is used to identify nursing diagnoses and interventions to promote oxygenation in the health promotion, acute care, and restorative and continuing care settings.
- Evaluate a patient's responses to nursing interventions to promote oxygenation.

KEY TERMS

Acute coronary syndrome (ACS)
Afterload
Angina pectoris
Bilevel positive airway pressure (BiPAP)
Bronchoscopy
Capnography
Cardiac output
Cardiopulmonary rehabilitation
Cardiopulmonary resuscitation (CPR)
Chest physiotherapy (CPT)
Chest tube
Cheyne-Stokes respiration
Continuous positive airway pressure (CPAP)
Diaphragmatic breathing
Diffusion

Electrocardiogram (ECG)
Endotracheal (ET) tube
Hematemesis
Hemoptysis
Hemothorax
Humidification
Hyperventilation
Hypoventilation
Hypovolemia
Hypoxia
Incentive spirometry
Invasive mechanical ventilation
Kussmaul respiration
Myocardial infarction (MI)
Myocardial ischemia
Nasal cannula

Nebulization
Noninvasive positive-pressure ventilation (NPPV)
Orthopnea
Perfusion
Pneumothorax
Postural drainage
Preload
Pursed-lip breathing
Stroke volume
Tracheostomy
Ventilation
Ventilator-associated pneumonia (VAP)
Ventricular fibrillation
Ventricular tachycardia

MEDIA RESOURCES

http://evolve.elsevier.com/Potter/fundamentals/
- Review Questions
- Video Clips
- Concept Map Creator
- Case Study with Questions

- Skills Performance Checklists
- Audio Glossary
- Content Updates
- Answers to QSEN Activity and Review Questions

Mr. Edwards, age 62, is admitted to the hospital with a 6-day history of chest pain, fatigue, and shortness of breath. The admission physical examination and chest ray confirmed that he has a community-acquired right upper lobe pneumonia with an intermittent productive cough with occasional thick, yellow sputum. Lying flat makes him more short of breath and the cough worse. John Smith, a junior nursing student, is the nurse assigned to Mr. Edwards.

Oxygen is a basic human need. When a patient's oxygen level decreases, the body cannot carry out basic vital functions. Disturbances in oxygenation often result from ineffective gas exchange (lungs) or an ineffective pump (heart). You will use your knowledge about the function and physiology of the cardiopulmonary system to understand how the heart and the lungs work together to provide oxygen to the tissues. Clinical judgment with the application of critical thinking will enable you to identify patient needs, plan evidence-based patient-centered care, and select interventions to effectively improve oxygenation status.

SCIENTIFIC KNOWLEDGE BASE

The cardiac and respiratory systems work together to supply the body with oxygen necessary for carrying out the respiratory and metabolic processes needed to sustain life. Blood is oxygenated through the mechanisms of ventilation, perfusion, and transport of respiratory gases. Neural and chemical regulators control the rate and depth of respiration in response to changing tissue oxygen demands. The cardiovascular system provides the transport mechanisms to distribute oxygen to cells and tissues of the body (McCance and Huether, 2019).

Respiratory Physiology

Respiration is the exchange of oxygen and carbon dioxide during cellular metabolism. It is commonly confused with the act of air moving in and out of the lungs, which is actually ventilation. The airways of the lung transfer oxygen from the atmosphere to the alveoli and the alveolar capillary membrane, where respiratory gases, oxygen and carbon dioxide (CO_2), are exchanged. There are three steps in the process of oxygenation: ventilation, perfusion, and diffusion (McCance and Huether, 2019).

Structure and Function. The respiratory muscles, pleural space, lungs, and alveoli are essential for ventilation, perfusion, and the exchange of respiratory gases. Gases move into and out of the lungs through pressure changes. Intrapleural pressure is negative, or less than atmospheric pressure, which is 760 mm Hg at sea level. For air to flow into the lungs, intrapleural pressure becomes more negative, setting up a pressure gradient between the atmosphere and the alveoli. The diaphragm and external intercostal muscles contract (move downward and outward) to create a negative pleural pressure and increase the size of the thorax for inspiration. Relaxation of the diaphragm and contraction of the internal intercostal muscles allow air to escape from the lungs (Cedar, 2018; McCance and Huether, 2019).

Ventilation is the process of moving gases into and out of the lungs, with air flowing into the lungs during inhalation (inspiration) and out of the lungs during exhalation (expiration). It requires coordination of the muscular and elastic properties of the lungs and thorax. The major inspiratory muscle of respiration is the diaphragm. It is innervated by the phrenic nerve, which exits the spinal cord at the fourth cervical vertebra. Perfusion relates to the ability of the cardiovascular system to pump oxygenated blood to the tissues and return deoxygenated blood to the lungs. Finally, diffusion is responsible for moving the respiratory gases from one area to another by concentration gradients. For the exchange of respiratory gases to occur, the organs, nerves, and muscles of respiration need to be intact, and the central nervous system needs to be able to regulate the respiratory cycle (Cedar, 2018; McCance and Huether, 2019).

Conditions or diseases that change the structure and function of the pulmonary system alter respiration. Some of these conditions include chronic obstructive pulmonary disease (COPD), asthma, lung cancer, and cystic fibrosis. In these conditions, patients may experience increased respiratory rate, decreased oxygen saturation levels, decreased lung expansion, or adventitious lung sounds (McCance and Huether, 2019).

Work of Breathing. Work of breathing (WOB) is the effort required to expand and contract the lungs. In the healthy individual breathing is quiet and accomplished with minimal effort. The amount of energy expended on breathing depends on the rate and depth of breathing, the ease in which the lungs can be expanded (compliance), and airway resistance (McCance and Huether, 2019).

Inspiration is an active process, stimulated by chemoreceptors, which monitor pH, $PaCO_2$, and PaO_2 in the blood. Expiration is a passive process that depends on the elastic recoil properties of the lungs, requiring little or no muscle work. Surfactant is a chemical produced in the lungs to maintain the surface tension of the alveoli and prevent them from collapsing. Patients with advanced COPD lose the elastic recoil of the lungs and thorax. As a result, the patient's work of breathing increases. In addition, patients with certain pulmonary diseases have decreased surfactant production and sometimes develop atelectasis. Atelectasis is a collapse of the alveoli that prevents normal exchange of oxygen and carbon dioxide (McCance and Huether, 2019).

Accessory muscles of respiration (the intercostal muscles in the rib cage and abdominal muscles) can increase lung volume during inspiration. Patients with COPD, especially emphysema, frequently use these muscles to increase lung volume. Prolonged use of the accessory muscles does not promote effective ventilation and eventually causes fatigue. During assessment, a patient's clavicles may elevate during inspiration, which can indicate ventilatory fatigue, air hunger, or decreased lung expansion (McCance and Huether, 2019).

Compliance is the ability of the lungs to distend or expand in response to increased intraalveolar pressure. Compliance decreases in diseases such as pulmonary edema, interstitial and pleural fibrosis, and congenital or traumatic structural abnormalities such as kyphosis or fractured ribs (McCance and Huether, 2019).

Airway resistance is the increase in pressure that occurs as the diameter of the airways decreases from mouth/nose to alveoli. Any further decrease in airway diameter by bronchoconstriction or the presence of excess mucus can increase airway resistance. Diseases causing airway obstruction, such as asthma, tracheal edema, or COPD, increase airway resistance. When airway resistance increases, the amount of oxygen delivered to the alveoli decreases (McCance and Huether, 2019).

Increased use of accessory muscles, decreased lung compliance, and increased airway resistance increase the WOB, resulting in increased energy expenditure. Therefore, the body increases its metabolic rate and the need for more oxygen. The need for elimination of carbon dioxide also increases. This sequence is a vicious cycle for a patient with impaired ventilation, causing further deterioration of respiratory status and the ability to oxygenate adequately (McCance and Huether, 2019).

Lung Volumes. The normal lung volumes are determined by age, gender, and height. Tidal volume is the amount of air exhaled following a normal inspiration. Residual volume is the amount of air left in the alveoli after a full expiration. Forced vital capacity is the maximum amount of air that can be removed from the lungs during forced expiration (McCance and Huether, 2019). Variations in tidal volume and other lung volumes are associated with alterations in patients' health status or activity, such as pregnancy, exercise, obesity, or obstructive and restrictive conditions of the lungs.

Pulmonary Circulation. The primary function of pulmonary circulation is to move blood to and from the alveolar capillary membrane for gas exchange. Pulmonary circulation begins at the pulmonary artery, which receives poorly oxygenated mixed venous blood from the right ventricle. Blood flow through this system depends on the pumping ability of the right ventricle. The flow continues from the pulmonary artery through the pulmonary arterioles to the pulmonary capillaries, where blood comes in contact with the alveolar capillary membrane and the exchange of respiratory gases occurs. The oxygen-rich blood then circulates through the pulmonary venules and pulmonary veins, returning to the left atrium (McCance and Huether, 2019).

Respiratory Gas Exchange. Diffusion is the process for the exchange of respiratory gases in the alveoli of the lungs and the capillaries of the body tissues. Diffusion of respiratory gases occurs at the alveolar capillary membrane (Fig. 41.1). The thickness of the membrane affects the rate of diffusion. Increased thickness of the membrane impedes diffusion because gases take longer to transfer across the membrane. Patients with pulmonary edema, pulmonary infiltrates, or pulmonary effusion have a thickened membrane, resulting in slow diffusion, slow exchange of respiratory gases, and decreased delivery of oxygen to tissues. Chronic diseases (e.g., emphysema), acute diseases (e.g., pneumothorax), and surgical processes (e.g., lobectomy) often alter the amount of alveolar capillary membrane surface area (McCance and Huether, 2019).

Oxygen Transport. The oxygen-transport system consists of the lungs and cardiovascular system. Delivery depends on the amount of oxygen entering the lungs (ventilation), blood flow to the lungs and tissues (perfusion), rate of diffusion, and oxygen-carrying capacity. Three things influence the capacity of the blood to carry oxygen: the amount of dissolved oxygen in the plasma, the amount of hemoglobin, and the ability of hemoglobin to bind with oxygen. Hemoglobin, which is a carrier for oxygen and carbon dioxide, transports most oxygen (approximately 97%). The hemoglobin molecule combines with oxygen to form oxyhemoglobin. The formation of oxyhemoglobin is easily reversible, allowing hemoglobin and oxygen to dissociate (deoxyhemoglobin), which frees oxygen to enter tissues. Patients who are acidotic (pH less than 7.35; seen in patients with sepsis or diabetic ketoacidosis), hypercapnic (elevated $PaCO_2$ levels; seen in patients with COPD), or who have low hemoglobin levels (seen in patients with anemia or excess blood loss) have decreased ability to carry oxygen and therefore to deliver oxygen to the tissues (McCance and Huether, 2019).

Carbon Dioxide Transport. Carbon dioxide, a product of cellular metabolism, diffuses into red blood cells and is rapidly hydrated into carbonic acid (H_2CO_3). The carbonic acid then dissociates into hydrogen (H) and bicarbonate (HCO_3^-) ions. Hemoglobin buffers the hydrogen ion, and the HCO_3^- diffuses into the plasma. Reduced hemoglobin (deoxyhemoglobin) combines with carbon dioxide, and the venous blood transports the majority of carbon dioxide back to the lungs to be exhaled (McCance and Huether, 2019).

Regulation of Ventilation. Regulation of ventilation is necessary to ensure sufficient oxygen intake and carbon dioxide elimination to meet the demands of the body (e.g., during exercise, infection, or pregnancy). Neural and chemical regulators control the process of ventilation. Neural regulation includes the CNS control of respiratory rate, depth, and rhythm. The cerebral cortex regulates the voluntary control of respiration by delivering impulses to the respiratory motor neurons by way of the spinal cord. Chemical regulation maintains the appropriate rate and depth of respirations based on changes in the carbon dioxide (CO_2), oxygen (O_2), and hydrogen ion (H^+) concentration (pH) in the blood. Changes in levels of O_2, CO_2, and H^+ (pH) stimulate the chemoreceptors located in the medulla, aortic body, and carotid body, which in turn stimulate neural regulators to adjust the rate and depth of ventilation to maintain normal arterial blood gas levels (McCance and Huether, 2019).

Cardiovascular Physiology

Cardiopulmonary physiology involves delivery of deoxygenated blood (blood high in carbon dioxide and low in oxygen) to the right side of the heart and then to the lungs, where it is oxygenated. Oxygenated blood (blood high in oxygen and low in carbon dioxide) then travels from the lungs to the left side of the heart and the tissues. The cardiac system delivers oxygen, nutrients, and other substances to the tissues and facilitates the removal of cellular metabolism waste products by way of blood flow through other body systems such as respiratory, digestive, and renal (McCance and Huether, 2019).

Structure and Function. The right ventricle pumps deoxygenated blood through the pulmonary circulation (Fig. 41.2). The left ventricle pumps oxygenated blood through the systemic circulation. As blood passes through the circulatory system, there is an exchange of respiratory

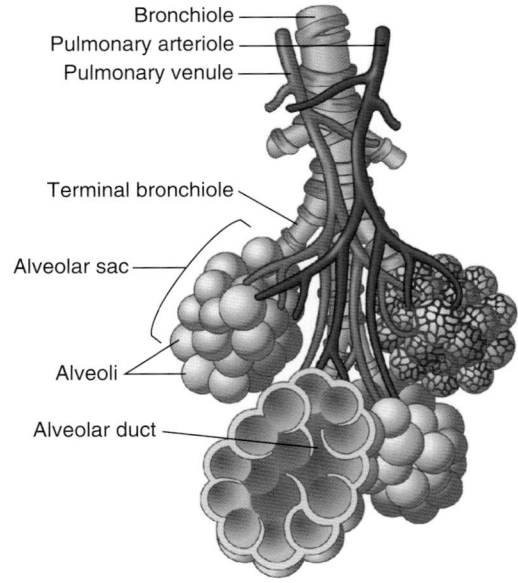

FIG. 41.1 Alveoli at terminal end of lower airway. (From Patton KT, Thibodeau GA: *Human body in health and disease*, ed 7, St Louis, 2018, Elsevier.)

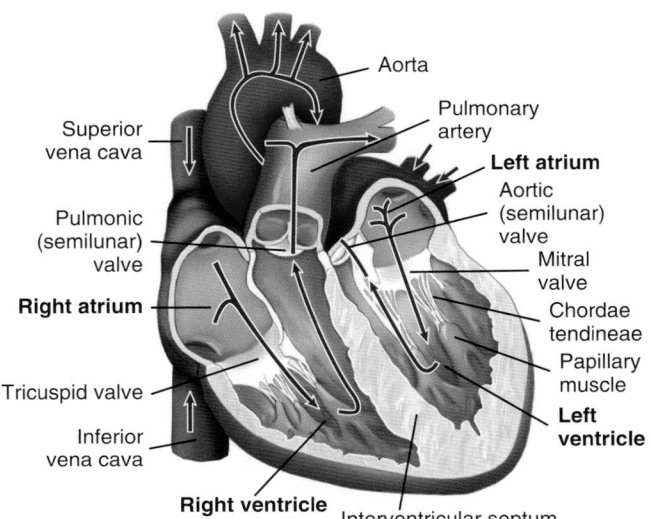

FIG. 41.2 Schematic representation of blood flow through the heart. *Arrows* indicate direction of flow and pulmonary circulation. (Modified from Harding MM et al: *Lewis's Medical-surgical nursing: assessment and management of clinical problems*, ed 11, St Louis, 2020, Elsevier.)

gases, nutrients, and waste products between the blood and the tissues. Alterations in structure and function of the heart can lead to a variety of symptoms, including but not limited to dyspnea, edema, and weak pulses. Nurses hear abnormal heart sounds, such as murmurs or rubs, when the structure of the heart is altered (McCance and Huether, 2019).

Myocardial Pump. The pumping action of the heart is essential to oxygen delivery. There are four cardiac chambers: two atria and two ventricles. The ventricles fill with blood during diastole and empty during systole. The volume of blood ejected from the ventricles during systole is the **stroke volume.** Hemorrhage and dehydration cause a decrease in circulating blood volume and a decrease in stroke volume (McCance and Huether, 2019).

Myocardial fibers have contractile properties that allow them to stretch during cardiac filling. In a healthy heart this stretch is proportionally related to the strength of contraction. As the myocardium stretches, the strength of the subsequent contraction increases; this is known as the *Frank-Starling (Starling's) law of the heart.* In the diseased heart (cardiomyopathy), Starling's law does not apply because the increased stretch of the myocardium is beyond the physiological limits of the heart. The subsequent contractile response results in insufficient stroke volume, and blood begins to "back up" in the pulmonary (left heart failure) or systemic (right heart failure) circulation (McCance and Huether, 2019).

Myocardial Blood Flow. To maintain adequate blood flow to the pulmonary and systemic circulation, myocardial blood flow must supply sufficient oxygen and nutrients to the myocardium itself. Blood flow through the heart is unidirectional. The four heart valves ensure this forward blood flow (see Fig. 41.2). During ventricular diastole the atrioventricular (mitral and tricuspid) valves open, and blood flows from the higher-pressure atria into the relaxed ventricles. As systole begins, ventricular pressure rises and the mitral and tricuspid valves close. Valve closure causes the first heart sound (S_1) (McCance and Huether, 2019) (see Chapter 30).

During the systolic phase, the semilunar (aortic and pulmonic) valves open, and blood flows from the ventricles into the aorta and pulmonary artery. The mitral and tricuspid valves stay closed during systole, so all of the blood is moved forward into the pulmonary artery and aorta. As the ventricles empty, the ventricular pressures decrease, allowing closure of the aortic and pulmonic valves. Valve closure causes the second heart sound (S_2). Some patients with valvular disease have backflow or regurgitation of blood through the incompetent valve, causing a murmur that you can hear on auscultation (McCance and Huether, 2019) (see Chapter 30).

Coronary Artery Circulation. The coronary circulation is the branch of the systemic circulation that supplies the myocardium with oxygen and nutrients and removes waste. The coronary arteries fill during ventricular diastole. The left coronary artery has the most abundant blood supply and feeds the more muscular left ventricular myocardium, which does most of the work of the heart (McCance and Huether, 2019).

Systemic Circulation. The arteries of the systemic circulation deliver nutrients and oxygen to tissues, and the veins remove waste from tissues. Oxygenated blood flows from the left ventricle through the aorta and into large systemic arteries. These arteries branch into smaller arteries; then arterioles; and finally, the smallest vessels, the capillaries. The exchange of respiratory gases occurs at the capillary level, where the tissues are oxygenated. The waste products exit the capillary network through venules that join to form veins. These veins become larger and form the vena cava, which carry deoxygenated blood back to the right side of the heart, where it then returns to the pulmonary circulation (McCance and Huether, 2019).

Blood Flow Regulation. The amount of blood ejected from the left ventricle each minute is the **cardiac output.** The normal cardiac output is 4 to 8 L/min in the healthy adult at rest. The circulating volume of blood changes according to the oxygen and metabolic needs of the body. For example, cardiac output increases during exercise, pregnancy, and fever but decreases during sleep. The following formula represents cardiac output:

$$\text{Cardiac Output} = \text{Stroke Volume (SV)} \times \text{Heart Rate (HR)}$$

Stroke volume is the amount of blood ejected from the ventricle with each contraction. The normal range for a healthy adult is 50 to 75 mL per contraction. Preload, afterload, and myocardial contractility all affect stroke volume. **Preload** is the amount of blood in the left ventricle at the end of diastole before the next contraction. It is often referred to as end-diastolic volume. The ventricles stretch when filling with blood. The more stretch on the ventricular muscle, the greater the contraction and the greater the stroke volume (Starling's law). In certain clinical situations, medical treatment alters preload and subsequent stroke volumes by changing the amount of circulating blood volume. For example, when treating a patient who is hemorrhaging, increased fluid therapy and replacement of blood increase circulating volume, thus increasing the preload and stroke volume, which in turn increases cardiac output. If volume is not replaced, preload, stroke volume, and the subsequent cardiac output decrease (McCance and Huether, 2019).

Afterload is the resistance to the ejection of blood from the left ventricle. The heart works harder to overcome the resistance so that blood can be ejected from the left ventricle. The diastolic aortic pressure is a good clinical measure of afterload. In hypertension, the afterload increases, causing an increase in cardiac workload (McCance and Huether, 2019).

Myocardial contractility is the ability of the heart to squeeze blood from the ventricles. It also affects stroke volume and cardiac output. Poor ventricular contraction decreases the amount of blood ejected. Injury to the myocardial muscle, such as an acute MI, causes a decrease in myocardial contractility (McCance and Huether, 2019). The myocardium in some older adults is stiffer with a slower ventricular filling rate and prolonged contraction time (Touhy and Jett, 2018).

Heart rate affects blood flow because of the relationship between heart rate and diastolic filling time. For example, a sustained heart rate greater than 160 beats/min decreases diastolic filling time, which decreases stroke volume and cardiac output (McCance and Huether, 2019). The heart rate of the older adult is slow to increase under stress, but studies have found that this may be caused more by lack of conditioning than age. Exercise is beneficial in maintaining function at any age (Touhy and Jett, 2018).

Conduction System. The rhythmic relaxation and contraction of the atria and ventricles depend on continuous, organized transmission of electrical impulses. The cardiac conduction system generates and transmits these impulses (Fig. 41.3).

The conduction system of the heart generates the impulses needed to initiate the electrical chain of events for a normal heartbeat. The autonomic nervous system influences the rate of impulse generation and the speed of transmission through the conductive pathway and the strength of atrial and ventricular contractions. Sympathetic and parasympathetic nerve fibers innervate all parts of the atria and ventricles and the sinoatrial (SA) and atrioventricular (AV) nodes. Sympathetic fibers increase the rate of impulse generation and speed of transmission. The parasympathetic fibers originating from the vagus nerve decrease the rate (McCance and Huether, 2019).

The conduction system originates with the SA node, the "pacemaker" of the heart. The SA node is in the right atrium next to the entrance of the superior vena cava. Impulses are initiated at the SA

FIG. 41.3 Conduction system of the heart. *AV,* Atrioventricular; *SA,* sinoatrial. (From Harding MM et al: *Lewis's Medical-surgical nursing: assessment and management of clinical problems,* ed 11, St Louis, 2020, Elsevier.)

node at an intrinsic rate of 60 to 100 cardiac action potentials per minute in an adult at rest. The electrical impulses are transmitted through the atria along intraatrial and internodal pathways to the AV node. The AV node mediates impulses between the atria and the ventricles. It assists atrial emptying by delaying the impulse before transmitting it through the bundle of His and the ventricular Purkinje network. A normal sinus rhythm is necessary to ensure optimal perfusion of the tissues in the body (McCance and Huether, 2019).

An electrocardiogram (ECG) is a measurement of the electrical activity of the conduction system. An ECG monitors the regularity and path of the electrical impulse through the conduction system; however, it does not reflect the muscular work of the heart. The normal sequence on the ECG is called the normal sinus rhythm (NSR) (see Fig. 41.3) (Urden et al., 2020).

NSR implies that the impulse originates at the SA node and follows the normal sequence through the conduction system. The P wave (atrial depolarization) represents the electrical conduction through both atria. Atrial contraction follows the P wave. The PR interval represents the impulse travel time from the SA node through the AV node, through the bundle of His, and to the Purkinje fibers. The normal length for the PR interval is 0.12 to 0.2 seconds. An increase in the time greater than 0.2 seconds indicates a block in the impulse transmission through the AV node, whereas a decrease, less than 0.12 seconds, indicates the initiation of the electrical impulse from a source other than the SA node (Urden et al., 2020).

The QRS complex (ventricular depolarization) indicates that the electrical impulse traveled through the ventricles. Normal QRS duration is 0.06 to 0.1 seconds. An increase in QRS duration indicates a delay in conduction time through the ventricles. Ventricular contraction usually follows the QRS complex (Urden et al., 2020).

The QT interval represents the time needed for ventricular depolarization and repolarization. The normal QT interval is 0.12 to 0.42 seconds. This interval varies inversely with changes in heart rate. Changes in electrolyte values, such as hypocalcemia or hypomagnesemia, or therapy with medications (disopyramide, amiodarone, haloperidol, and azithromycin are examples) increase the QT interval. An increased QT interval increases the person's risk for lethal dysrhythmias (Urden et al., 2020).

Factors Affecting Oxygenation

Four types of factors influence the adequacy of circulation, ventilation, perfusion, and transport of respiratory gases to the tissues: (1) physiological, (2) developmental, (3) lifestyle, and (4) environmental. The physiological factors are discussed here, and the others are discussed in the Nursing Knowledge Base section that follows.

Physiological Factors. Any condition affecting cardiopulmonary functioning directly affects the ability of the body to meet oxygen demands. Respiratory disorders include hyperventilation, hypoventilation, and hypoxia. Cardiac disorders include disturbances in conduction, impaired valvular function, myocardial hypoxia, cardiomyopathy conditions, and peripheral tissue hypoxia. Other physiological processes affecting a patient's oxygenation include alterations affecting the oxygen-carrying capacity of blood (anemia), decreased inspired oxygen concentration, increases in the metabolic demand of the body (fever), and alterations affecting chest wall movement caused by musculoskeletal abnormalities or neuromuscular alterations (muscular dystrophy) (McCance and Huether, 2019; Urden et al., 2020).

Decreased Oxygen-Carrying Capacity. Hemoglobin carries the majority of oxygen to tissues. Anemia and inhalation of toxic substances decrease the oxygen-carrying capacity of blood by reducing the amount of available hemoglobin to transport oxygen. Anemia (e.g., a lower-than-normal hemoglobin level) is a result of decreased hemoglobin production, increased red blood cell destruction, and/or blood loss. Patients have fatigue, decreased activity tolerance, increased breathlessness, increased heart rate, and pallor (especially seen in the conjunctiva of the eye). Oxygenation decreases as a secondary effect with anemia. The physiological response to chronic hypoxemia is the development of increased red blood cells (polycythemia). This is the adaptive response of the body to increase the amount of hemoglobin and the available oxygen-binding sites (Harding et al., 2020; McCance and Huether, 2019).

Carbon monoxide (CO) is a colorless, odorless gas that causes decreased oxygen-carrying capacity of blood. In CO toxicity, hemoglobin strongly binds with CO, creating a functional anemia. Because of the strength of the bond, CO does not easily dissociate from hemoglobin, making hemoglobin unavailable for oxygen transport. People with CO poisoning are often unaware of their exposure to this gas, and the symptoms of CO poisoning (headache, dizziness, nausea, vomiting, and dyspnea) mimic other illnesses (Urden et al., 2020).

Hypovolemia. Conditions such as shock and severe dehydration cause extracellular fluid loss and reduced circulating blood volume, or hypovolemia. Decreased circulating blood volume results in hypoxia to body tissues. With significant fluid loss, the body tries to adapt by peripheral vasoconstriction and by increasing the heart rate to increase the volume of blood returned to the heart, thus increasing the cardiac output (McCance and Huether, 2019).

Decreased Inspired Oxygen Concentration. With the decline of the concentration of inspired oxygen, the oxygen-carrying capacity of the blood decreases. Decreases in the fraction of inspired oxygen concentration (FiO_2) are caused by upper or lower airway obstruction, which limits delivery of inspired oxygen to alveoli; decreased environmental oxygen (at high altitudes); or hypoventilation (occurs in opiate overdoses) (Harding et al., 2020).

Increased Metabolic Rate. Increased metabolic activity increases oxygen demand. An increased metabolic rate is normal in pregnancy, wound healing, and exercise because the body is using energy for building tissue. Most people are able to meet the increased oxygen demand and do not display signs of oxygen deprivation. The level of oxygenation declines when cardiopulmonary systems are unable to meet this demand.

For example, fever increases the tissues' need for oxygen; as a result, carbon dioxide production increases. When fever persists, the metabolic rate remains high, and the body begins to break down protein stores. This causes muscle wasting and decreased muscle mass, including respiratory muscles such as the diaphragm and intercostal muscles. The body attempts to adapt to the increased carbon dioxide levels by increasing the rate and depth of respiration. The patient's WOB increases, and the patient eventually displays signs and symptoms of hypoxemia. Patients with pulmonary diseases are at greater risk for hypoxemia (McCance and Huether, 2019).

Conditions Affecting Chest Wall Movement. Any condition reducing chest wall movement results in decreased ventilation. If the diaphragm does not fully descend with breathing, the volume of inspired air decreases, delivering less oxygen to the alveoli and tissues (McCance and Huether, 2019).

Pregnancy. As the fetus grows during pregnancy, the enlarging uterus pushes abdominal contents upward against the diaphragm. In the last trimester of pregnancy, the inspiratory capacity declines, resulting in dyspnea on exertion and increased fatigue (Ball et al., 2019).

Obesity. Patients who are morbidly obese have reduced lung volumes from the heavy lower thorax and abdomen, particularly when in the recumbent and supine positions; this often causes obstructive sleep apnea. Morbid obesity creates a reduction in a patient's lung and chest wall compliance as a result of encroachment of the abdomen into the chest, increased WOB, and decreased lung volumes. In some patients, an obesity-hypoventilation syndrome develops in which oxygenation is decreased and carbon dioxide is retained. The patient is also susceptible to atelectasis or pneumonia after surgery because

the lungs do not expand fully and the lower lobes retain pulmonary secretions (McCance and Huether, 2019).

Musculoskeletal Abnormalities. Musculoskeletal impairments in the thoracic region reduce oxygenation. Such impairments result from abnormal structural configurations, trauma, muscular diseases, and diseases of the central nervous system. Abnormal structural configurations impairing oxygenation include those affecting the rib cage, such as pectus excavatum, and the vertebral column, such as kyphosis, lordosis, or scoliosis (Ball et al., 2019; McCance and Huether, 2019).

Trauma. Any rib fracture or bruising causes pain and resultant reduced ventilation. Flail chest is a condition in which multiple rib fractures cause chest wall instability. This instability causes the lung under the injured area to contract on inspiration and bulge on expiration, resulting in hypoxia. Patients with thoracic or upper abdominal surgical incisions use shallow respirations to avoid pain, which decreases chest wall movement. Opioids for pain depress the respiratory center, further decreasing respiratory rate and chest wall expansion (Urden et al., 2020).

Neuromuscular Diseases. Neuromuscular diseases affect tissue oxygenation by decreasing a patient's ability to expand and contract the chest wall. Ventilation is impaired, resulting in atelectasis, hypercapnia, and hypoxemia. Examples of conditions causing hypoventilation include myasthenia gravis and Guillain-Barré syndrome (McCance and Huether, 2019).

Central Nervous System Alterations. Diseases or trauma of the medulla oblongata and/or spinal cord result in impaired ventilation. When the medulla oblongata is affected, neural regulation of ventilation is impaired, and abnormal breathing patterns develop. Cervical trauma at C3 to C5 usually results in paralysis of the phrenic nerve. When the phrenic nerve is damaged, the diaphragm does not descend properly, thus reducing inspiratory lung volumes and causing hypoxemia. Spinal cord trauma below the C5 vertebra usually leaves the phrenic nerve intact but damages nerves that innervate the intercostal muscles, preventing anteroposterior chest expansion.

Influences of Chronic Lung Disease. Oxygenation decreases as a direct consequence of chronic lung disease due to alveolar and/or airway alterations. Changes in the anteroposterior diameter of the chest wall (barrel chest) occur because of overuse of accessory muscles and air trapping in COPD or cystic fibrosis. Chronic lung disease results in varying degrees of dyspnea, tachypnea, hypoxemia, and/or hypercapnia (Ball et al., 2019; Harding et al., 2020; McCance and Huether, 2019).

Alterations in Respiratory Functioning

Illnesses and conditions affecting ventilation or oxygen transport alter respiratory functioning. The three primary alterations are hypoventilation, hyperventilation, and hypoxia.

The goal of ventilation is to produce a normal arterial carbon dioxide tension ($PaCO_2$) between 35 and 45 mm Hg and a normal arterial oxygen tension (PaO_2) between 80 and 100 mm Hg. Hypoventilation and hyperventilation are often determined by arterial blood gas analysis (McCance and Huether, 2019). Hypoxemia refers to a decrease in the amount of arterial oxygen. Nurses monitor arterial oxygen saturation (SpO_2) using a pulse oximeter, a noninvasive oxygen saturation monitor. Normally SpO_2 is greater than or equal to 95% (see Chapter 30).

Hypoventilation. Hypoventilation occurs when alveolar ventilation is inadequate to meet the oxygen demand of the body or to eliminate sufficient carbon dioxide. As alveolar ventilation decreases, the body retains carbon dioxide. For example, atelectasis, a collapse of the alveoli, prevents normal exchange of oxygen and carbon dioxide. As more alveoli collapse, less of the lung is ventilated, and hypoventilation occurs.

In patients with COPD, the administration of excessive oxygen can result in hypoventilation. These patients have adapted to a high carbon dioxide level, so their carbon dioxide–sensitive chemoreceptors do not function normally. Their peripheral chemoreceptors of the aortic arch and carotid bodies are primarily sensitive to lower oxygen levels, causing increased ventilation. Because the stimulus to breathe is a decreased arterial oxygen (PaO_2) level (hypoxic drive to breathe), administration of oxygen greater than 24% to 28% (1 to 3 L/min) prevents the PaO_2 from falling to a level (60 mm Hg) that stimulates the peripheral receptors, thus destroying the stimulus to breathe. The resulting hypoventilation causes excessive retention of carbon dioxide, which can lead to respiratory acidosis and respiratory arrest. Signs and symptoms of hypoventilation include mental status changes, dysrhythmias, and potential cardiac arrest. If untreated, the patient's status rapidly declines, leading to convulsions, unconsciousness, and death (McCance and Huether, 2019).

Hyperventilation. Hyperventilation is a state of ventilation in which the lungs remove carbon dioxide faster than it is produced by cellular metabolism. Severe anxiety, infection, drugs, or an acid-base imbalance induces hyperventilation (see Chapter 42). Acute anxiety leads to hyperventilation and exhalation of excessive amounts of carbon dioxide. Increased body temperature (fever) increases the metabolic rate, thereby increasing carbon dioxide production. The increased carbon dioxide level stimulates an increase in the patient's rate and depth of respiration, causing hyperventilation (McCance and Huether, 2019).

Hyperventilation is sometimes chemically induced. For example, salicylate (aspirin) poisoning and amphetamine use result in excess carbon dioxide production, stimulating the respiratory center to compensate by increasing the rate and depth of respiration. It also occurs as the body tries to compensate for metabolic acidosis. For example, the patient with diabetes in ketoacidosis produces large amounts of metabolic acids. The respiratory system tries to correct the acid-base balance by overbreathing. Ventilation increases to reduce the amount of carbon dioxide available to form carbonic acid (see Chapter 42). This can also result in the patient developing respiratory alkalosis. Signs and symptoms of hyperventilation include rapid respirations, sighing breaths, numbness and tingling of hands/feet, light-headedness, and loss of consciousness (McCance and Huether, 2019).

Hypoxia. Hypoxia is inadequate tissue oxygenation at the cellular level. It results from a deficiency in oxygen delivery or oxygen use at the cellular level. It is a life-threatening condition. Untreated, it has the potential to produce fatal cardiac dysrhythmias (McCance and Huether, 2019).

Causes of hypoxia include (1) a decreased hemoglobin level and lowered oxygen-carrying capacity of the blood; (2) a diminished concentration of inspired oxygen, which occurs at high altitudes; (3) the inability of the tissues to extract oxygen from the blood, as with cyanide poisoning; (4) decreased diffusion of oxygen from the alveoli to the blood, as in pneumonia or pulmonary edema; (5) poor tissue perfusion with oxygenated blood, as with shock; and (6) impaired ventilation, as with multiple rib fractures or chest trauma (McCance and Huether, 2019).

The clinical signs and symptoms of hypoxia include apprehension, restlessness (often an early sign), inability to concentrate, decreased level of consciousness, dizziness, and behavioral changes. The patient with hypoxia is unable to lie flat and appears both fatigued and agitated. Vital sign changes include an increased pulse rate and increased rate and depth of respiration. During early stages of hypoxia the blood pressure is elevated unless the condition is caused by shock. As the hypoxia worsens, the respiratory rate declines as a result of respiratory muscle fatigue (Harding et al., 2020).

Cyanosis, blue discoloration of the skin and mucous membranes caused by the presence of desaturated hemoglobin in capillaries, is a late sign of hypoxia. The presence or absence of cyanosis is not a reliable measure of oxygen status. Central cyanosis, observed in the tongue, soft palate, and conjunctiva of the eye where blood flow is high, indicates hypoxemia. Peripheral cyanosis, seen in the extremities, nail beds, and earlobes, is often a result of vasoconstriction and stagnant blood flow (Ball et al., 2019; Harding et al., 2020).

Alterations in Cardiac Functioning

Illnesses and conditions affecting cardiac rhythm, strength of contraction, blood flow through the heart or to the heart muscle, and decreased peripheral circulation alter cardiac function. For example, older adults have structural changes in the heart, including vascular and valve stiffening, increased left ventricular wall thickness, and changes in the conduction system. Chronic heart disease, including heart failure and coronary artery disease, is the number one chronic disease in the United States (CDC, 2021f).

Disturbances in Conduction. Electrical impulses that do not originate from the SA node cause conduction disturbances. These rhythm disturbances are called dysrhythmias, meaning a deviation from the normal sinus heart rhythm. Dysrhythmias occur as a primary conduction disturbance such as in response to ischemia; valvular abnormality; anxiety; drug toxicity; caffeine, alcohol, or tobacco use; or a complication of acid-base or electrolyte imbalance (see Chapter 42).

Dysrhythmias are classified by cardiac response and site of impulse origin. Cardiac response is tachycardia (greater than 100 beats/min), bradycardia (less than 60 beats/min), a premature (early) beat, or a blocked (delayed or absent) beat. Tachydysrhythmias and bradydysrhythmias lower cardiac output and blood pressure. Tachydysrhythmias reduce cardiac output by decreasing diastolic filling time. Bradydysrhythmias lower cardiac output because of the decreased heart rate (McCance and Huether, 2019; Urden et al., 2020).

Atrial fibrillation is a common dysrhythmia in older adults. The electrical impulse in the atria is chaotic and originates from multiple sites. The rhythm is irregular because of the multiple pacemaker sites and the unpredictable conduction to the ventricles. The QRS complex is normal; however, it occurs at irregular intervals. Atrial fibrillation is often described as an irregularly irregular rhythm. It decreases cardiac output by altering preload and contractility (Hartjes, 2018; McCance and Huether, 2019; Urden et al., 2020).

Abnormal impulses originating above the ventricles are supraventricular dysrhythmias. The abnormality on the waveform is the configuration and placement of the P wave. Ventricular conduction usually remains normal, and there is a normal QRS complex. Paroxysmal supraventricular tachycardia is a sudden, rapid onset of tachycardia originating above the AV node. It often begins and ends spontaneously. Sometimes excitement, fatigue, caffeine, smoking, or alcohol use precipitates paroxysmal supraventricular tachycardia (McCance and Huether, 2019; Urden et al., 2020).

Ventricular dysrhythmias represent an ectopic site of impulse formation within the ventricles. They are ectopic in that the impulse originates in the ventricle, not the SA node. The configuration of the QRS complex is usually widened and bizarre. P waves are not always present; often they are buried in the QRS complex. Ventricular tachycardia and ventricular fibrillation are life-threatening rhythms that require immediate intervention. Ventricular tachycardia is a life-threatening dysrhythmia because of the decreased cardiac output and the potential to deteriorate into ventricular fibrillation or sudden cardiac death (Hartjes, 2018; Urden et al., 2020).

Altered Cardiac Output. Failure of the myocardium to eject sufficient volume to the systemic and pulmonary circulations occurs in heart failure. Primary coronary artery disease, cardiomyopathy, valvular disorders, and pulmonary disease lead to myocardial pump failure (McCance and Huether, 2019; Urden et al., 2020).

Left-Sided Heart Failure. Left-sided heart failure is an abnormal condition characterized by decreased functioning of the left ventricle. If left ventricular failure is significant, the amount of blood ejected from the left ventricle drops greatly, resulting in decreased cardiac output. Signs and symptoms include fatigue, breathlessness, dizziness, and confusion as a result of tissue hypoxia from the diminished cardiac output. As the left ventricle continues to fail, blood begins to pool in the pulmonary circulation, causing pulmonary congestion. Clinical findings include crackles in the bases of the lungs on auscultation, hypoxia, shortness of breath on exertion, cough, and paroxysmal nocturnal dyspnea (Hartjes, 2018; McCance and Huether, 2019).

Right-Sided Heart Failure. Right-sided heart failure results from impaired functioning of the right ventricle. It more commonly results from pulmonary disease or as a result of long-term left-sided failure. The primary pathological factor in right-sided failure is elevated pulmonary vascular resistance (PVR). As the PVR continues to rise, the right ventricle works harder, and the oxygen demand of the heart increases. As the failure continues, the amount of blood ejected from the right ventricle declines, and blood begins to "back up" in the systemic circulation. Clinically the patient has systemic symptoms, such as weight gain, distended neck veins, hepatomegaly and splenomegaly, and dependent peripheral edema (Hartjes, 2018; McCance and Huether, 2019).

Impaired Valvular Function. Valvular heart disease is an acquired or congenital disorder of a cardiac valve that causes either hardening (stenosis) or impaired closure (regurgitation) of the valves. When stenosis occurs, the flow of blood through the valves is obstructed. For example, when stenosis occurs in the semilunar valves (aortic and pulmonic valves), the adjacent ventricles have to work harder to move the ventricular blood volume beyond the stenotic valve. Over time the stenosis causes the ventricle to hypertrophy (enlarge), and if the condition is untreated, left- or right-sided heart failure occurs. When regurgitation occurs, there is a backflow of blood into an adjacent chamber. For example, in mitral regurgitation the mitral leaflets do not close completely. When the ventricles contract, blood escapes back into the atria, causing a murmur, or "whooshing" sound (see Chapter 30) (Hartjes, 2018; McCance and Huether, 2019).

Myocardial Ischemia. Myocardial ischemia results when the supply of blood to the myocardium from the coronary arteries is insufficient to meet myocardial oxygen demands. Two common outcomes of this ischemia are angina pectoris and myocardial infarction (Hartjes, 2018; McCance and Huether, 2019).

Angina. Angina pectoris is a transient imbalance between myocardial oxygen supply and demand. The condition results in chest pain that is aching, sharp, tingling, or burning or that feels like pressure. Typically, chest pain is left sided or substernal and often radiates to the left or both arms, the jaw, neck, and back. In some patients, angina pain does not radiate. It usually lasts from 3 to 5 minutes. Patients report that it is often precipitated by activities that increase myocardial oxygen demand (e.g., eating heavy meals, exercise, or stress). It is usually relieved with rest and coronary vasodilators, the most common being a nitroglycerin preparation.

Women have different symptoms or no symptoms at all. Some will also have atypical symptoms, such as palpitations, anxiety, weakness, and fatigue. In addition, many women with angina will have ischemia noted on electrocardiogram, but no evidence of coronary artery disease (McCance and Huether, 2019).

Myocardial Infarction. Myocardial infarction (MI) or acute coronary syndrome (ACS) results from sudden decreases in coronary blood flow or an increase in myocardial oxygen demand without adequate coronary perfusion. Infarction occurs because ischemia is not reversed. Cellular death occurs after 20 minutes of myocardial ischemia (McCance and Huether, 2019).

Chest pain associated with MI in men is usually described as crushing, squeezing, or stabbing. The pain is often in the left chest and sternal area; may be felt in the back; and radiates down the left arm to the neck, jaws, teeth, epigastric area, and back. It occurs at rest or exertion and lasts more than 20 minutes. Rest, position change, or sublingual nitroglycerin administration does not relieve the pain (Hartjes, 2018; McCance and Huether, 2019).

There are differences between men and women in relation to coronary artery disease. As women get older, their risk of heart disease begins to rise, making it the leading cause of death for women in the United States. Women on average have greater blood cholesterol and triglyceride levels than men. Obesity in women is more prevalent, which also increases risk for diabetes and cardiac disease. Women's symptoms differ from those of men. The most common initial symptom in women is angina, but they also present with atypical symptoms such as fatigue, indigestion, shortness of breath, and back or jaw pain. Women have twice the risk of dying within the first year after a heart attack than men (CDC, 2020a; Ball et al., 2019; Harding et al., 2020).

REFLECT NOW

You are caring for a patient who was recently told he has decreased cardiac output due to atrial fibrillation. How would you describe cardiac output, the conduction system, and this dysrhythmia to the patient?

NURSING KNOWLEDGE BASE

Factors Influencing Oxygenation

In addition to physiological factors, multiple developmental, lifestyle, and environmental factors affect patients' oxygenation status. It is important to recognize these as possible risks or factors that impact their health care goals.

Developmental Factors. The developmental stage of a patient and the normal aging process affect tissue oxygenation.

Infants and Toddlers. Healthy full-term infants younger than 3 months of age are presumed to have a lower infection rate because of the protective function of maternal antibodies. The infection rate increases in infants from 3 to 6 months of age. Infants and toddlers are at risk for upper respiratory tract infections, especially when they are exposed to secondhand smoke or other children. Upper respiratory tract infections are usually not dangerous, and infants and toddlers recover with little difficulty. Infants and toddlers are also at risk for airway obstruction because of their anatomically smaller airways and their tendency to place foreign objects in their mouths (Hockenberry et al., 2019).

School-Age Children and Adolescents. School-age children and adolescents are exposed to respiratory infections and respiratory risk factors such as cigarette smoking or secondhand smoke. This age-group is also at risk for experimenting with cigarette smoking and other recreational inhalants. A healthy child usually does not have adverse pulmonary effects from respiratory infections. The CDC (2018a) reported that 5.6% of middle school–age children and 19.6% of high school–age children use tobacco products, with electronic cigarettes being the most commonly used tobacco product among these age-groups. School-age children and adolescents possess other cardiopulmonary disease risk factors such as obesity, inactive lifestyles, unhealthy diets, and excessive use of caffeinated beverages or other energy drinks (Hockenberry et al., 2019).

Young and Middle-Age Adults. Young and middle-age adults are exposed to multiple cardiopulmonary risk factors: an unhealthy diet, lack of exercise, stress, over-the-counter and prescription drugs not used as intended, illegal substances, and smoking. Reducing these modifiable factors decreases a patient's risk for cardiac or pulmonary diseases. This is also the time when individuals establish lifelong habits and lifestyles. It is important to help your patients make good choices and informed decisions about their health care practices. The increased cost of cigarettes plus the states' smoke-free air policies, laws that reduce smoking in public places, and access to cessation programs and medications have proven to be helpful in smoking cessation (CDC, 2018b).

Older Adults. The cardiac and respiratory systems undergo changes throughout the aging process (Box 41.1). The changes are associated with calcification of the heart valves, vascular stiffening and increased left ventricular wall thickness, impaired SA node function, and costal cartilage stiffening. The arterial system develops atherosclerotic plaques.

Osteoporosis leads to changes in the size and shape of the thorax. The trachea and large bronchi become enlarged from calcification of the airways. The alveoli enlarge, decreasing the surface area available for gas exchange. The number of functional cilia is reduced, causing a decrease in the effectiveness of the cough mechanism, putting the older adult at increased risk for respiratory infections (Touhy and Jett, 2018).

Lifestyle Factors. Lifestyle modifications are difficult for patients because they often have to change an enjoyable habit, such as smoking cigarettes or eating certain foods. Risk-factor modification is important and includes smoking cessation, weight reduction, a low-cholesterol

and low-sodium diet, management of hypertension, and moderate exercise (see Chapter 6). Although it is difficult to change long-term behavior, helping patients acquire healthy behaviors reduces the risk for or slows or halts the progression of cardiopulmonary diseases.

Nutrition. Good nutrition affects cardiopulmonary function by supporting normal metabolic functions. A poor diet leads to risk factors affecting the heart and lungs. Without essential nutrients, a patient may experience respiratory muscle wasting, resulting in decreased muscle strength and respiratory excursion. Cough efficiency is reduced secondary to respiratory muscle weakness, putting a patient at risk for retention of pulmonary secretions. A patient with chronic lung disease often requires a diet higher in calories and smaller, more frequent meals due to the increased work of breathing. A diet with a moderate amount of carbohydrates is recommended to prevent an increase in carbon dioxide production. Obesity affects the respiratory and cardiovascular systems. It can lead to a decrease in lung expansion and an increase in oxygen demand to meet metabolic demands (Harding et al., 2020).

Dietary practices also influence the prevalence of cardiovascular diseases (see Chapter 45). Patients with nutritional alterations are at risk for anemia, which reduces the oxygen-carrying capacity of the blood and can alter cardiac output. Cardioprotective nutrition includes diets rich in fiber; whole grains; fresh fruits and vegetables; nuts; antioxidants; lean meats, fish, and chicken; and omega-3 fatty acids. A diet of fruits, vegetables, and low-fat dairy foods that are high in fiber, potassium, calcium, and magnesium and low in saturated and total fat helps prevent and reduce the effects of hypertension (Harding et al., 2020).

Hydration. Fluid intake is essential for cellular health. Fluid volume overload may lead to vascular congestion in patients with heart, kidney, or lung diseases and impair the body's ability to deliver oxygen to the tissues. Dehydration or fluid volume deficit may result in dizziness, fainting, hypotension, or a thickening of respiratory secretions, which makes it difficult for a patient to expectorate secretions (Harding et al., 2020).

Exercise. Exercise increases the metabolic activity and oxygen demand of the body. The rate and depth of respiration increase, enabling the person to inhale more oxygen and exhale excess carbon dioxide. A physical exercise program has many benefits (see Chapter 38). People who exercise for 30 to 60 minutes daily have a lower pulse rate and blood pressure, decreased cholesterol level, increased blood flow, and greater oxygen extraction by working muscles (Harding et al., 2020).

Smoking. Cigarette smoking and secondhand smoke are associated with a number of diseases, including heart disease, COPD, and lung cancer. Cigarette smoking worsens peripheral vascular and coronary artery diseases. Inhaled nicotine causes vasoconstriction of peripheral and coronary blood vessels, increasing blood pressure and decreasing blood flow to peripheral vessels (McCance and Huether, 2019).

Women who take birth control pills and smoke cigarettes have an increased risk for thrombophlebitis and pulmonary emboli. Smoking during pregnancy can result in low-birth-weight babies, preterm delivery, and babies with reduced lung function (CDC, 2020a).

Smoking accounts for approximately 30% of all cancer deaths in the United States, including 80% of all lung cancer deaths. Smoking has been linked to the development of other cancers, including cancers of the mouth, esophagus, liver, bladder, kidney, and cervix, and myeloid leukemia (ACS, 2020a). Nicotine patches, gum, and lozenges are available over the counter, and nicotine nasal spray and inhalers can be obtained by prescription. Prescription drugs such as bupropion and varenicline are also available to help people quit smoking (ACS, 2020b).

Exposure to environmental tobacco smoke (secondhand smoke) increases the risk of lung cancer and cardiovascular disease in the nonsmoker. Children with parents who smoke have a higher incidence of asthma, pneumonia, and ear infections. Infants exposed to secondhand smoke are at higher risk for sudden infant death syndrome (NCI, 2018).

BOX 41.1 FOCUS ON OLDER ADULTS

Cardiopulmonary Implication in Older Adults

- Older patients are at an increased risk for developing tuberculosis (TB) through exposure or reactivation of dormant organisms that were present for decades (CDC, 2019).
- When screening older adults for TB, a two-step process is used. The standard 5-TU Mantoux test is given and repeated or repeated with the 250-TU strength to create a booster effect. If the older patient has a positive reaction, a complete history is necessary to determine any risk factors.
- Cardiac problems differ from other chronic conditions in that when they become acute, symptoms worsen rapidly and necessitate hospitalization, whereas other chronic conditions can be managed in the home (Touhy and Jett, 2018).
- Controlling blood pressure in older adults results in 30% fewer strokes, 64% less heart failure, 23% fewer fatal cardiac events, and 21% fewer cardiac-related deaths (Touhy and Jett, 2018).
- Mental status changes are often the first signs of cardiac and/or respiratory problems and often include forgetfulness and irritability.
- Changes in the older adult's cough mechanism lead to retention of pulmonary secretions, airway occlusion, and atelectasis if patients do not use cough suppressants with caution.
- Age-related changes in the immune system lead to a decline of both cell-mediated and humoral immunity, resulting in an increased risk of respiratory infections (McCance and Huether, 2019).
- Changes in the thorax that occur from ossification of costal cartilage, decreased space between vertebrae, and diminished respiratory muscle strength lead to problems with chest expansion and oxygenation (Touhy and Jett, 2018).

Substance Abuse. Excessive use of alcohol and other illicit drugs impairs tissue oxygenation in two ways. First, the person who chronically abuses substances often has a poor nutritional intake. With the resultant decrease in intake of iron-rich foods, hemoglobin production declines. Second, excessive use of alcohol and certain other drugs depresses the respiratory center, reducing the rate and depth of respiration and the amount of inhaled oxygen. Substance abuse by either smoking or inhaling substances such as crack cocaine or fumes from paint or glue cans causes direct injury to lung tissue that leads to permanent lung damage (McCance and Huether, 2019). The report on inhalant abuse (huffing) by teenagers to get a euphoric effect includes use of a wide variety of substances such as paint thinner, nail polish remover, glue, spray paint, nitrous oxide, and other common household products. Sudden death can occur from cardiac arrhythmias, or chronic abuse can cause damage to heart, lungs, and kidneys (NIDA, 2020).

Stress. Stress is a perceived threat that results in sympathetic stimulation. Continuous stress adversely affects a patient's health and well-being (see Chapter 37). A continuous state of stress increases the metabolic rate and oxygen demand of the body. The body responds to stress with an increased rate and depth of respiration and increased cardiac output. Stress causes an increased release of cortisol, which affects the metabolism of fat and creates a risk for CAD and hypertension. Stressors can be a trigger for asthma exacerbations. Patients with chronic illnesses or life-threatening illnesses cannot tolerate the oxygen demands associated with stress (McCance and Huether 2019).

Environmental Factors. Consider a patient's environment. Rural populations have more COPD-related issues that are not directly related to the environment but rather related to more people smoking, increased exposure to secondhand smoke, less access to smoking cessation programs, and a higher likelihood of rural residents being uninsured (CDC, 2018c). A patient's workplace sometimes increases the risk for pulmonary disease. Occupational pollutants include asbestos, talcum powder, dust, and airborne fibers. For example, farm workers in dry regions of the southwestern United States are at risk for coccidioidomycosis, a fungal disease caused by inhalation of spores of the airborne bacterium *Coccidioides immitis* (CDC, 2020b). Asbestosis is an occupational lung disease that develops after exposure to asbestos. The lung with asbestosis often has diffuse interstitial fibrosis, creating a restrictive lung disease. Patients exposed to asbestos are at risk for developing lung cancer, and this risk increases with exposure to tobacco smoke (McCance and Huether, 2019).

John uses his knowledge of the pulmonary system and the impact of certain risk factors on pulmonary functioning to plan a complete cardiopulmonary assessment for Mr. Edwards. John's prior experience in health assessment and his clinical judgment help him to target important assessment areas without increasing Mr. Edwards' respiratory distress or worsening his fatigue. Before he begins the assessment, he reviews Mr. Edwards' medical record and notes that Mrs. Edwards has a smoking history.

CRITICAL THINKING

Caring for patients with impaired oxygenation can be complex. Clinical judgment in applying the nursing process requires critical thinking, the synthesis of knowledge, experience, environmental factors, data gathered from patients, critical thinking attitudes, and intellectual and professional standards to ensure safe and appropriate care. Clinical judgments and critical thinking require you to anticipate information, analyze the data, recognize cues, and make decisions about your patient's care. During assessment consider all elements that will assist you to make clinical decisions for identifying appropriate nursing diagnoses (Fig. 41.4).

Knowledge of cardiac and respiratory physiology and oxygen supply and demand provides a scientific basis for how you approach an assessment for your patient. As you conduct your assessment, also consider the

pathogenesis and impact on the overall health and function in a patient with cardiopulmonary diseases and the potential effects of underlying diseases. Critical thinking attitudes ensure that you approach patient care in a methodical and logical way. For example, you will assess a patient who has coronary artery disease, chronic lung disease, and diabetes differently from a patient who has pneumonia and diabetes. Assessment will differ by the nature of a patient's condition. A patient with primary heart problems will have a cardiac focus, whereas a condition such as pneumonia has a pulmonary focus. Use clinical judgment to integrate what you learn about your patient, knowledge from nursing and other disciplines, past experience with other patients, and relevant clinical guidelines. The use of professional standards such as those of the American Association for Respiratory Care (AARC) and the American Nurses Association (ANA) provides valuable guidance in the care and management of patients (see Fig. 41.4). Your ability to manage the care of patients with alterations in oxygenation will improve as you gain experience and competency.

> **REFLECT NOW**
>
> You are preparing to teach a group of young adults about lifestyle habits and their relationship to heart and lung diseases. What information would you include in the teaching plan specific to this population? Compare this teaching plan to education that you would provide to a group of middle-age adults. How would it differ? Would content change?

❖ NURSING PROCESS

Apply clinical judgment as you use the nursing process and a critical thinking approach in your care of patients. The nursing process provides a clinical decision-making approach for you to develop and implement a patient-centered, individualized plan of care.

◆ Assessment

During the assessment process, thoroughly assess each patient, critically analyze findings, and identify cues to ensure that you make patient-centered clinical decisions about the nature of a patient's health problems. You will use clinical judgment by assessing a patient's presenting condition and comparing with signs and symptoms anticipated from known medical conditions to identify if physical manifestations of altered oxygenation exist. Nursing assessment includes an in-depth history of a patient's normal and present cardiopulmonary function; past impairments in cardiac, circulatory, or respiratory functioning; and methods that a patient uses to optimize oxygenation. The nursing history includes a review of drug, food, and other allergies. Physical examination of a patient's cardiopulmonary status reveals the extent of existing signs and symptoms (Ball et al., 2019) (see Chapter 30). Utilizing assessment values of pulse oximetry and capnography aids in the assessment of patients with spontaneous breathing, patients who are intubated, and patients requiring oxygen therapy or mechanical ventilation. Pulse oximetry provides instant feedback about the patient's level of oxygenation. Capnography, also known as *end-tidal CO_2 monitoring,* provides instant information about the patient's ventilation (how effectively CO_2 is being eliminated by the pulmonary system), perfusion (how effectively CO_2 is being transported through the vascular system), and how effectively CO_2 is produced by cellular metabolism (Hartjes, 2018; Urden et al., 2020). Capnography is measured near the end of exhalation. Finally, a review of laboratory and diagnostic test results provides valuable assessment data.

Through the Patient's Eyes. As you conduct your assessments, ask patients about their priorities and what they expect from their health care visit. Identifying their expectations regarding their health,

Knowledge Base

- Cardiopulmonary anatomy and physiology
- Cardiopulmonary pathophysiology
- Physiological factors affecting oxygenation
- Pharmacological factors affecting oxygenation
- Environmental factors affecting oxygenation

- Developmental factors affecting oxygenation
- Risk factors for impaired oxygenation
- Signs and symptoms of impaired oxygenation
- Anticipated effects of patient's illness or disability on patient's oxygenation and energy needs

Attitudes

- Display confidence when assessing extent of patient's cardiopulmonary alterations
- Use creativity when assessing cultural factors influencing patient's risk factors and care needs

Environment

- The presence of medical devices that may impact time and complexity when providing care
- Available resources or equipment to improve patient's oxygenation
- Need for additional necessary personnel interventions

Standards

- *ANA Standards and Scope of Nursing Practice*
- Clinical Practice Guidelines and Standards of Practice
- Intellectual standards in measurement
- Agency policies and procedures
- Professional
  - Standards of care (e.g., American Cancer Society, American Heart Association, American Association for Respiratory Care)
  - Ethical standards

Experience

- Experience caring for patients with cardiopulmonary conditions
- Experience observing patient responses to oxygen therapies
- Personal experiences with cardiopulmonary alterations (e.g., respiratory infections, heart disease)

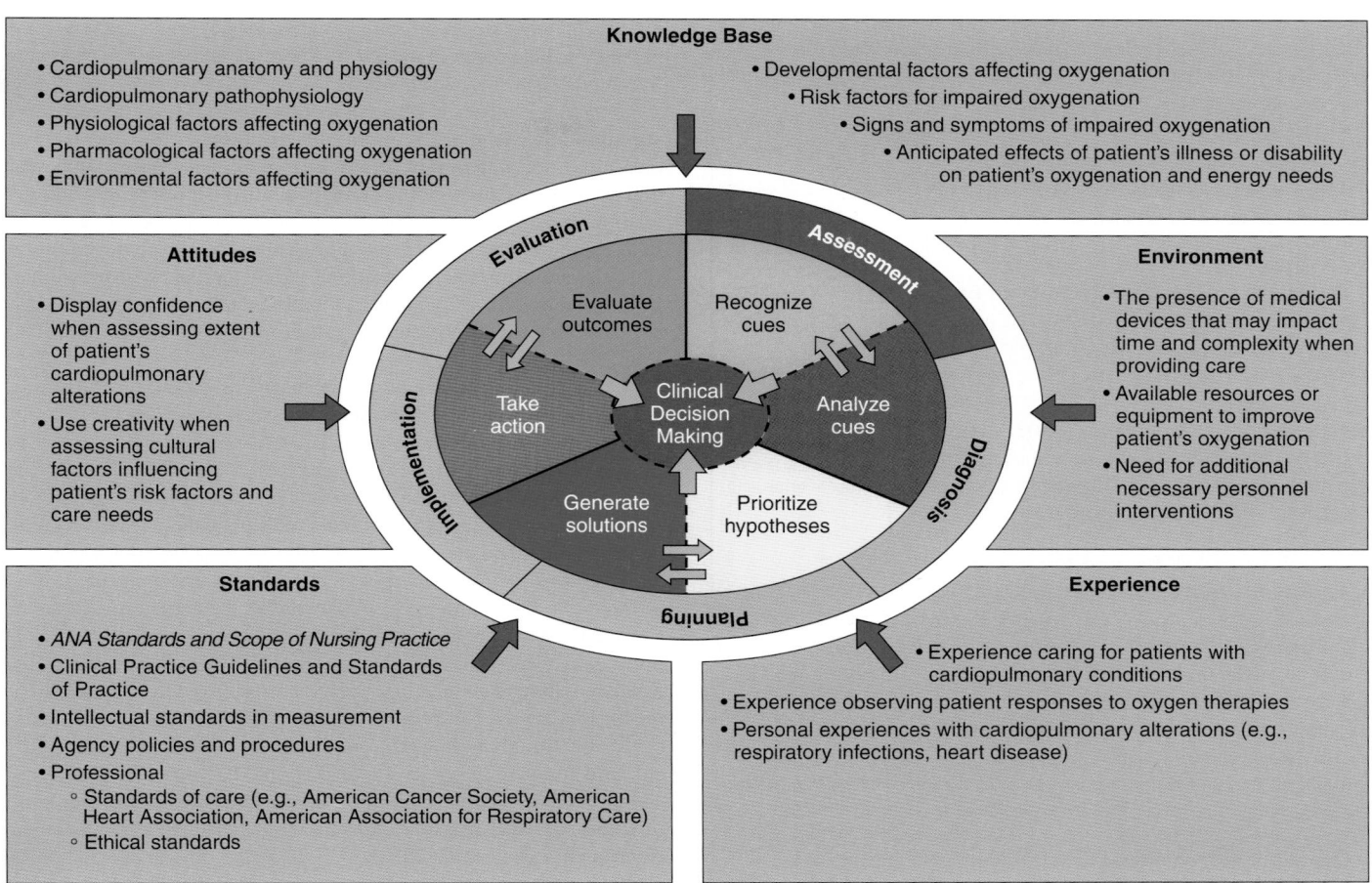

FIG. 41.4 Critical thinking model for oxygenation assessment. (Clinical Judgment Measurement Model copyright © NCSBN. All rights reserved.)

symptoms, and treatment plan ensures you involve patients in the decision-making process, which helps them participate in their care. For example, planning an exercise program for a patient who expresses a desire to improve activity tolerance helps meet the patient's health objectives. In contrast, planning a smoking-cessation program for a patient who is not ready for the change is frustrating for both the patient and you.

Establish realistic short-term outcomes. For example, exercise programs and tobacco-cessation treatments are effective in improving cardiopulmonary functioning, but a patient needs to be willing to participate in the program and may need to use several short-term strategies to be successful. Educating the patient on the opportunities for individual, group, or telephone counseling and identifying a social support system give more individual choices when developing the plan. Various community centers have several exercise programs individualized to a person's specific outcomes. When smoking cessation is a patient priority, there are smoking-cessation programs and various nicotine and non-nicotine medications that can be discussed to identify one that fits the patient's lifestyle. A combination of counseling and medication is more effective than either one alone (CDC, 2018b).

Remember that your outcomes and expectations do not always coincide with those of your patient. By addressing a patient's concerns and expectations, you establish a relationship that addresses how to achieve expected outcomes. Knowing your patients' perspectives and expectations and respecting their wishes go a long way in helping them make significant beneficial lifestyle changes.

Nursing History. The nursing history focuses on the patient's ability to meet oxygen needs and maintain cardiopulmonary health. The nursing history for respiratory function includes ruling out the presence of a cough, shortness of breath, dyspnea, wheezing, pain, environmental exposures, frequency of respiratory tract infections, pulmonary risk factors, past respiratory problems, current medication use, and smoking history or secondhand smoke exposure. The nursing history for cardiac function includes pain and characteristics of pain, fatigue, peripheral circulation, cardiac risk factors, diet, and the presence of past or concurrent cardiac conditions. Assessment data are often similar for respiratory and cardiac health problems. Thus it is important to ask specific questions related to cardiopulmonary disease and to carefully analyze all assessment findings for cues that indicate potential reasons and treatments for a patient's altered oxygenation (Box 41.2).

Health Risks. Determine familial risk factors such as a family history of lung cancer or cardiovascular disease. Documentation includes blood relatives who had cardiopulmonary disease and their present level of health or age at time of death. Assess for an exposure to infectious organisms, such as tuberculosis (TB). Also assess for occupational and environmental risk factors (e.g., asbestos exposure) (Ball et al., 2019; McCance and Huether, 2019).

Pain. The presence of chest pain requires an immediate thorough assessment, including location, duration, radiation, and frequency. In addition, it is important to note any other symptoms associated with chest pain, such as nausea, diaphoresis, extreme fatigue, or weakness. Cardiac pain does not occur with respiratory variations. Chest pain in men is most often on the left side of the chest and radiates to the left arm. Chest

BOX 41.2   Nursing Assessment Questions

Nature of the Cardiopulmonary Problem
- Describe the problem that you're having with your heart.
- Does the problem (e.g., chest pain, rapid heart rate) occur at a specific time of the day, during or after exercise, or all the time?
- Do you notice abnormal beats? Do these occur at a specific time of day or during/after activity? What makes these abnormal beats better or worse?
- Does your problem affect your ability to perform daily activity?

Questions to Ask Associated With Breathing
- Describe the breathing problems you are having.
- How has your breathing pattern changed?
- Do you have a cough? Is the coughing increasing? Is it worse at a certain time of day?
- Describe your cough. Is it dry or moist? Do you have sputum with coughing? Is this different in color, volume, or thickness?
- On a scale of 0 to 10, with 10 being the most severe, rate your shortness of breath. What helps your shortness of breath?

Questions to Ask Related to Chest Pain
- If you are having chest pain, what causes the pain and how long does it last? Is this a different type of pain? What relieves or worsens it? Show me where the pain is located.
- Does the chest pain occur with coughing?
- On a scale of 0 to 10, with 0 being no pain and 10 being the most severe pain, rate your chest pain at its worst. How would you describe your pain? Is the pain different today?
- Do you have any other symptoms, such as nausea, numbness and tingling in your arm, palpitations, or anxiety, when you have chest pain?

Questions to Ask Regarding Predisposing Factors
- Have you been exposed to a cold or flu or other respiratory illnesses?
- Tell me the medications you are taking. Are you taking over-the-counter medications or supplements? If so, what are they?
- Do you smoke? How long have you smoked? How much do you smoke during a day? Have you been exposed to secondhand smoke?
- Have you been doing any unusual exercises?

Questions to Ask Regarding Effect of Symptoms
- Describe for me a typical daily diet.
- Tell me how your symptoms affect your daily activities, appetite, sleeping, and exercise routine.

---

pain in women is much less definitive and often manifests itself as a sensation of breathlessness, jaw or back pain, nausea, and/or fatigue (CDC, 2020a). Pericardial pain results from inflammation of the pericardial sac, occurs on inspiration, and does not usually radiate (Ball et al., 2019).

Pleuritic chest pain results from inflammation of the pleural space of the lungs; the pain is peripheral and radiates to the scapular regions. Inspiratory maneuvers such as coughing, yawning, and sighing worsen pleuritic chest pain. Patients usually describe it as knifelike, lasting from a minute to hours and always in association with inspiration. Musculoskeletal pain is often present following exercise, rib trauma, and prolonged coughing episodes. Inspiration worsens this pain, and patients often confuse it with pleuritic chest pain (Ball et al., 2019).

Fatigue. Fatigue is a subjective sensation in which a patient reports a loss of endurance. Fatigue in the patient with cardiopulmonary alterations is often an early sign of a worsening of the chronic underlying process. To provide an objective measure of fatigue, ask the patient to rate it on a scale of 0 to 10, with 10 being the worst level and 0 representing no fatigue. Ask your patients when they noticed the fatigue, what makes it better or worse, if the onset was sudden or gradual, if it is worse in the morning or later in the day, and how the fatigue affects what they want to do (Ball et al., 2019; Harding et al., 2020).

Dyspnea. Dyspnea is associated with hypoxia. It is the subjective sensation of difficult or uncomfortable breathing or observed labored breathing with shortness of breath. Dyspnea is usually associated with exercise or excitement, but in some patients it is present without any relation to activity or exercise. It is associated with many conditions, such as pulmonary diseases, cardiovascular diseases, neuromuscular conditions, and anemia. In addition, it occurs in the pregnant woman in the final months of pregnancy. Finally, environmental factors such as pollution, cold air, and smoking also cause or worsen dyspnea (Ball et al., 2019).

When gathering information about a patient's sensation of dyspnea, ask the patient when the dyspnea occurs (such as with exertion, stress, or respiratory tract infection) and what improves the dyspnea (e.g., rest, inhaled medication, or position change). Determine whether the patient's dyspnea affects the ability to lie flat. Orthopnea is an abnormal condition in which a patient uses multiple pillows when reclining to breathe easier or sits leaning forward with arms elevated. The number of pillows used usually helps to quantify the orthopnea (e.g., two- or three-pillow orthopnea). Also ask whether the patient must sleep in a recliner chair to breathe easier. Paroxysmal nocturnal dyspnea (PND) occurs when a patient is sleeping. The patient often awakens in a panic, feels a sensation of suffocating, and has a strong need to sit up to relieve the breathlessness (Ball et al., 2019).

Cough. Coughing is a protective reflex to clear the trachea, bronchi, and lungs of irritants and secretions. Patients with a chronic cough tend to deny, underestimate, or minimize their coughing, often because they are so accustomed to it that they are unaware of its frequency (Ball et al., 2019).

If a patient has a cough, determine the onset of the cough, how frequently it occurs, and whether it is productive or nonproductive. Chronic coughs are often a sign of chronic lung disease, whereas acute coughs can be a sign of infection or an inhaled irritant. A nonproductive cough is often associated with allergies or gastroesophageal reflux disease. A productive cough results in sputum production (e.g., material coughed up from the lungs that a patient swallows or expectorates). Sputum contains mucus, cellular debris, microorganisms, and sometimes pus or blood. Collect data about the type and quantity of sputum. Instruct patients to try to cough up some sputum and not to simply clear the throat, which produces only saliva. Have the patient cough into a specimen cup. Inspect the sputum for color (such as green or blood tinged), consistency (such as thin or thick), odor (none or foul), and amount in tablespoons or milliliters (Ball et al., 2019).

If hemoptysis (bloody sputum) is present, determine whether it is associated with coughing and bleeding from the upper respiratory tract, sinus drainage, or the gastrointestinal tract (hematemesis). Hemoptysis has an alkaline pH, and hematemesis has an acidic pH; thus, pH testing of the specimen may help to determine the source (McCance and Huether, 2019). Describe hemoptysis according to amount and color and whether it is mixed with sputum. Note whether the patient is on anticoagulant therapy. When there is bloody or blood-tinged sputum, health care providers frequently perform diagnostic tests such as examination of sputum specimens, chest x-ray examinations, bronchoscopy, and other scans.

Environmental and Occupational Factors. Environmental exposure to inhaled substances, such as smog, dust, silicon, mold, cockroaches, pet dander, and asbestos, is linked with respiratory disease. Investigate exposures in the patient's home, workplace, and recent travel. In addition, determine whether a patient who is a nonsmoker is exposed to secondhand smoke (ATSDR, 2018; McCance and Huether, 2019).

Carbon monoxide (CO) poisoning often results from an improperly vented furnace flue or fireplace. The patient will have vague complaints of general malaise, flulike symptoms, and excessive sleepiness. Patients are particularly at risk in the late fall when they turn the furnace on or begin to use the fireplace again (CDC, 2020c). Ask whether there is a CO detector in the home.

Radon gas is a radioactive substance from the breakdown of uranium in soil, rock, and water that enters homes through the ground or well water. When homes are poorly ventilated, this gas is unable to escape and becomes trapped. If a patient who smokes also lives in a home with a high radon level, the risk for lung cancer is very high (EPA, 2016). Ask whether the patient has any radon detectors in the home.

Smoking. It is important to determine a patient's direct and secondary exposure to tobacco. Ask about any history of smoking; include the number of years smoked and the number of packages smoked per day. This is recorded as pack-year history (packages per day × years smoked). For example, if a patient smoked two packs a day for 20 years, the patient has a 40 pack-year history. Determine exposure to secondhand smoke, because any form of tobacco exposure increases a patient's risk for cardiopulmonary diseases (American Lung Association [ALA], 2020a).

Respiratory Infections. Obtain information about the frequency and duration of a patient's respiratory tract infections. Although everyone occasionally has a self-limiting cold, some people develop bronchitis or pneumonia. On average, patients have four colds per year. Determine if and when a patient has had a pneumococcal or influenza (flu) vaccine. This is especially important when assessing older adults because of their increased risk for respiratory disease (Touhy and Jett, 2018). Ask about any known exposure to tuberculosis (TB) and the date and results of the last tuberculin skin test.

Determine a patient's risk for human immunodeficiency virus (HIV) infection. Patients with a history of intravenous (IV) drug use and multiple unprotected sex partners are at risk of developing HIV infection. Patients do not always display symptoms of HIV infection until they present with *Pneumocystis* or *Mycoplasma* pneumonia. Patients with HIV/AIDS (acquired immunodeficiency syndrome) or other immunocompromised states are at increased risk for respiratory infections (McCance and Huether, 2019).

The COVID-19 pandemic poses increased health risks. While people of any age, even healthy young adults, can get this virus, the risk for severe illness increases with age, with older adults at highest risks. People with underlying medical conditions, such as but not limited to cancer, chronic cardiopulmonary illness, immunosuppression, obesity, diabetes, or Down syndrome, also have an increased risk for severe illness. This is an easily transmissible respiratory infection by respiratory droplets and airborne transmission; it commonly spreads during close contact. Initial symptoms are similar to influenza, but this virus spreads more efficiently than influenzas (CDC, 2021d).

Allergies. Inquire about your patient's exposure to airborne allergens (e.g., pet dander, pollen, or mold). Typical allergy symptoms include watery eyes, sneezing, runny nose, or respiratory symptoms such as cough or wheezing. When obtaining information from the patient, ask specific questions about the type of allergens, response to these allergens, and successful and unsuccessful relief measures. In addition, determine the effect of environmental air quality and secondhand smoke exposure on the patient's allergy and symptoms. Safe nursing practice also includes obtaining information about food, drug, or insect sting allergies on the initial history and physical. However, always double-check this information with the patient on subsequent assessments, especially concerning respiratory allergens (Ball et al., 2019).

Medications. Another component of the nursing history includes determining all the medications that a patient is using. These include prescribed medications, over-the-counter medications, folk medicine, herbal medicines, alternative therapies, and illicit drugs and substances. Some of these preparations have adverse effects by themselves or because of interactions with other drugs (Ball et al., 2019). For example, a person using a prescribed bronchodilator drug may choose to use an over-the-counter inhalant as well. Many of these contain ephedrine or *ma huang,* a natural ephedrine, which acts like epinephrine. This product reacts with the prescribed medication by potentiating or decreasing the effect of the prescribed medication. Patients taking warfarin for blood thinning prolong the prothrombin time (PT)/international normalized ratio (INR) results if they are taking ginkgo biloba, garlic, or ginseng with the anticoagulant. The drug interaction can precipitate life-threatening bleeding, such as gastrointestinal bleeding (Harding et al., 2020).

It is important to determine whether a patient uses illicit drugs. Inhaled opioids, which are often diluted with talcum powder, cause pulmonary disorders resulting from the irritant effect of the powder on lung tissues. Marijuana is usually smoked in the form of a joint or pipe. Marijuana smoke is an irritant to the lungs, putting users at higher risk for respiratory illnesses (NIDA, 2019). Cocaine is snorted through the nose, placed on the gums, smoked, or injected. Cocaine abusers can have acute cardiovascular changes such as constricted blood vessels and increased heart rate and blood pressure. People who use the inhaled form of cocaine often develop respiratory infections such as pneumonia. Cocaine deaths are often caused by heart attack or stroke (NIDA, 2018).

As with all medications, assess a patient's knowledge and ability to self-administer medications correctly (see Chapter 31). It is especially important to assess that your patient understands the potential side effects of medications. Patients need to recognize adverse reactions and be aware of the dangers in combining prescribed medications with over-the-counter drugs.

Physical Examination. The physical examination includes assessment of the cardiopulmonary system (see Chapter 30). Give special consideration when assessing an older adult patient for changes that occur with the aging process (Table 41.1). These changes affect the patient's activity tolerance and level of fatigue or cause transient changes in vital signs and are not always associated with a specific cardiopulmonary disease. Use clinical judgment to ensure appropriate analysis of assessment data.

Inspection. Using inspection techniques, observe the patient from head to toe, assessing the patient's skin and mucous membrane color, general appearance, level of consciousness, adequacy of systemic circulation, breathing patterns, and chest wall movement (Table 41.2). Identify unexpected findings and investigate them further during palpation, percussion, and auscultation.

Inspection includes observing the nails for clubbing (see Chapter 30). Clubbed nails often occur in patients with chronic oxygen deficiency, such as cystic fibrosis and congenital heart defects. Also note the shape of the chest wall. Conditions such as advancing age and chronic obstructive pulmonary disease (COPD) cause the chest to assume a rounded "barrel" shape (Ball et al., 2019; Harding et al., 2020).

Observe chest wall movement for retraction (e.g., sinking in of soft tissues of the chest between the intercostal spaces) and use of accessory muscles. Elevation of a patient's clavicles at rest reveals increased work of breathing. Also observe the patient's breathing pattern and assess for paradoxical breathing (the chest wall contracts during inspiration and expands during exhalation) or asynchronous breathing. At rest, the normal adult respiratory rate is 12 to 20 breaths/min. Bradypnea is less than 12 breaths/min, and tachypnea is greater than 20 breaths/min (see Chapter 29). In some conditions, such as metabolic acidosis, the acidic pH stimulates an increase in rate, usually greater than 35 breaths/min, and depth of respirations (Kussmaul respiration) to compensate by

TABLE 41.1 Effects of Aging on Cardiopulmonary Assessment Findings

Function	Pathophysiological Change	Key Clinical Findings
Heart		
Muscle contraction	Thickening of the ventricular wall, increased collagen, and decreased elastin in the heart muscle	Decreased cardiac output (edema, dyspnea, activity intolerance, inability to lie flat for extended time)
Blood flow	Heart valves become thicker and stiffer, more often in the mitral and aortic valves	Systolic ejection murmur
Conduction system	SA node becomes fibrotic from calcification; decrease in number of pacemaker cells in SA node	Increased P-R, QRS, and Q-T intervals, decreased amplitude of QRS complex; tachycardia more poorly tolerated
Arterial vessel compliance	Calcified vessels, loss of arterial distensibility, decreased elastin in vessel walls, more tortuous vessels	Hypertension with an increase in systolic blood pressure
Lungs		
Breathing mechanics	Decreased chest wall compliance, loss of elastic recoil Decreased respiratory muscle mass/strength	Prolonged exhalation phase Decreased vital capacity Activity intolerance
Oxygenation	Decreased alveolar surface area Decreased carbon dioxide diffusion capacity	Decreased PaO_2 Slightly increased $PaCO_2$
Breathing control/ breathing pattern	Decreased responsiveness of central and peripheral chemoreceptors to hypoxemia and hypercapnia	Increased respiratory rate Decreased tidal volume
Lung defense mechanisms	Decreased number of cilia Decreased IgA production and humoral and cellular immunity Drier mucous membranes	Decreased airway clearance Diminished cough reflex Increased risk for infection
Sleep and breathing	Decreased respiratory drive Decreased tone of upper airway muscles	Increased risk of aspiration and respiratory infection Snoring, obstructive sleep apnea

IgA, Immunoglobulin A; *PaCO₂,* arterial carbon dioxide tension; *PaO₂,* arterial oxygen tension; *SA,* sinoatrial. (Data from Ball JW, et al: *Seidel's guide to physical examination,* ed 9, St Louis, 2019, Elsevier, and Touhy T, Jett K: *Gerontological nursing and healthy aging,* ed 5, St Louis, 2018, Elsevier.)

TABLE 41.2 Inspection of Cardiopulmonary Status

Abnormality	Cause
Eyes	
Xanthelasma (yellow lipid lesions on eyelids)	Hyperlipidemia
Pale conjunctivae	Anemia
Cyanotic conjunctivae	Hypoxemia
Petechiae on conjunctivae	Fat embolus or bacterial endocarditis
Nose	
Flaring nares	Air hunger, dyspnea
Mouth and Lips	
Cyanotic mucous membranes	Decreased oxygenation (hypoxia)
Pursed-lip breathing	Associated with chronic lung disease
Pallor	Anemia
Neck Veins	
Distention	Associated with right-sided heart failure
Chest	
Retractions	Increased work of breathing, dyspnea
Asymmetry	Chest wall injury
Barrel chest	COPD; may be normal in some older adults
Fingertips and Nail Beds	
Cyanosis	Decreased cardiac output or hypoxia
Splinter hemorrhages	Infective endocarditis
Clubbing of nail beds	Chronic hypoxemia
Skin	
Peripheral cyanosis	Vasoconstriction and diminished blood flow; cold environment
Central cyanosis	Hypoxemia
Decreased skin turgor	Dehydration (normal finding in older adults as a result of decreased skin elasticity)
Dependent edema	Associated with right- and left-sided heart failure
Periorbital edema	Associated with kidney disease

From Ball JW et al: *Seidel's Physical examination handbook,* ed 9, St Louis, 2019, Elsevier.

decreasing carbon dioxide levels. Apnea is the absence of respirations for 15 to 20 seconds or longer. **Cheyne-Stokes respiration** occurs when there is decreased blood flow or injury to the brainstem. This type of breathing is an abnormal respiratory pattern, with periods of apnea followed by periods of deep breathing and then shallow breathing followed by more apnea (McCance and Huether, 2019; Harding et al., 2020).

Palpation. Palpation of the chest provides assessment data in several areas. It documents the type and amount of thoracic excursion; elicits any areas of tenderness; and helps to identify tactile fremitus, thrills, heaves, and the cardiac point of maximal impulse (PMI). Palpation of the extremities provides data about the peripheral circulation (e.g., the presence and quality of peripheral pulses, skin temperature, color, and capillary refill) (see Chapter 30).

Palpation of the feet and legs determines the presence or absence of peripheral edema. Patients with alterations in cardiac function, such as those with heart failure or hypertension, often have pedal or lower-extremity edema. Edema is graded from 1+ to 4+, depending on the depth of visible indentation after firm finger pressure (see Chapter 30).

Palpate the pulses in the neck and extremities to assess arterial blood flow (see Chapter 30). Use a scale of 0 (absent pulse) to 4+ (full, bounding pulse) to describe what you feel. The normal pulse is 2+; a weak, thready pulse is 1+. *Never palpate both carotid arteries at the same time as doing so may cause the patient to lose consciousness* (Ball et al., 2019).

Percussion. Percussion detects the presence of abnormal fluid or air in the lungs. It also determines diaphragmatic excursion (see Chapter 30).

TABLE 41.3 Cardiopulmonary Diagnostic Blood Studies

Test and Normal Values	Interpretation
Complete Blood Count Normal values for a complete blood count (CBC) vary with age and gender	A CBC determines the number and type of red and white blood cells per cubic millimeter of blood. White blood cells assess for presence of infection. Red blood cells and hemoglobin assess for presence of anemia and ability of the blood to carry oxygen to the tissues.
Cardiac Enzymes *Creatine kinase (CK-MB):* Cardiospecific enzyme released from cells when myocardial tissue is damaged. If greater than 4%-6% of total CK, then highly indicative of MI; levels increase within 4-6 hours of MI	Providers use cardiac enzymes, along with troponin, to diagnose acute myocardial infarcts.
Cardiac Troponins Plasma cardiac troponin I <0.03 ng/mL	Value elevates as early as 3 hours after myocardial injury.
Plasma cardiac troponin T <0.1 ng/mL	Value often remains elevated for 10-14 days.
Serum Electrolytes Potassium (K+) 3.5-5 mEq/L or 3.5-5 mmol/L	Patients on diuretic therapy are at risk for hypokalemia (low potassium). Patients receiving angiotensin-converting enzyme (ACE) inhibitors are at risk for hyperkalemia (elevated potassium). Since potassium has an effect on cardiac rhythm, it is important to keep this value as close to normal as possible.
Cholesterol Adult <200 mg/dL or <5.2 mmol/L (SI units)	Contributing factors include sedentary lifestyle with intake of saturated fatty acids, familial hypercholesterolemia.
Low-density lipoproteins (LDLs) (bad cholesterol) <130 mg/dL Very low–density lipoproteins (VLDLs) 7-32 mg/dL	High LDL cholesterol (hypercholesterolemia) is caused by excessive intake of saturated fatty acids, dietary cholesterol intake, and obesity. Familial hypercholesterolemia and hyperlipidemia, hypothyroidism, nephrotic syndrome, and diabetes mellitus are also contributing factors. VLDLs are predominant carriers of triglycerides and can be converted to LDL by lipoprotein lipase. Levels in excess of 25%-50% indicate increased risk of cardiac disease.
High-density lipoproteins (HDLs) (good cholesterol) Male: >45 mg/dL; female: >55 mg/dL	Factors such as cigarette smoking, obesity, lack of regular exercise, beta-adrenergic blocking agents, genetic disorders of HDL metabolism, hypertriglyceridemia, and type 2 diabetes cause low HDL cholesterol.
Triglycerides Male: 40-160 mg/dL; female: 35-135 mg/dL	Obesity, excessive alcohol intake, diabetes mellitus, beta-adrenergic blocking agents, and familial hypertriglyceridemia cause hypertriglyceridemia.
Additional Tests Brain natriuretic peptide <100 pg/mL	Increased levels may be used to help determine severity of congestive heart failure.
C-reactive protein <0.1/dL or <10 mg/L	Test used by clinicians to detect inflammation if there is a high suspicion of tissue injury or infection somewhere in the body. It can also be used to evaluate a patient's risk of developing coronary artery disease and stroke. Used to help evaluate patient for sepsis.

Data from Pagana KD et al: *Mosby's diagnostic and laboratory test reference,* ed 15, St Louis, 2021, Elsevier.

Auscultation. Auscultation identifies the presence of normal and abnormal heart and lung sounds (see Chapter 30). Auscultation of the cardiovascular system includes assessing for normal S_1 and S_2 sounds and the presence of abnormal S_3 and S_4 sounds (gallops), murmurs, or rubs. Identify the location, intensity, pitch, and quality of a murmur. Auscultation also identifies any bruits over the carotid, abdominal aorta, and femoral arteries (Ball et al., 2019).

"Adventitious breath sounds" is another term for abnormal breath sounds. They include wheezing, crackles, and rhonchi. Wheezing is a continuous, high-pitched musical sound caused by high-velocity movement of air through a narrowed airway. It is associated with asthma, acute bronchitis, or pneumonia. It occurs during inspiration, expiration, or both. Determine whether there are any precipitating factors, such as respiratory infection, allergens, exercise, or stress. Crackles are discontinuous sounds of various pitch most often heard during inspiration. They are a result of the disruption of the small respiratory passages and cannot be cleared by coughing. They are often heard in patients with pneumonia or emphysema or chronic bronchitis. Rhonchi, or sonorous wheezes, are deeper sounding in pitch than crackles and are often heard during expiration. They reflect the presence of thick secretions or muscle spasms in the airway. Rhonchi can often be cleared by coughing and are most commonly heard in patients with asthma or pneumonia (Ball et al., 2019).

Diagnostic Tests. A variety of diagnostic tests are used to monitor and assess cardiopulmonary function. Some of these tests are noninvasive, while others are more invasive. Diagnostic testing used in the assessment and evaluation of the patient with cardiopulmonary alterations is summarized in Tables 41.3 through 41.5. When reviewing results of pulmonary function studies, be aware of expected variations in patients from different cultures (Box 41.3).

One screening test is TB Mantoux skin testing (Box 41.4). This is a simple test and is recommended for health care workers who care for patients at increased risk for TB. Those patients at greater risk include people from countries where TB is common (most countries in Latin America, Africa, and Asia, for example), prisoners and correctional facility employees, and residents of long-term care facilities (CDC, 2016a).

Invasive diagnostic tests, such as a thoracentesis, are painful. How painful a diagnostic procedure is depends on the patient's tolerance for pain (see Chapter 44). Reduce anxiety by explaining the procedure and telling patients what to expect. Be sure that patients understand the importance of following instructions related to the procedure. For example, a patient undergoing a thoracentesis will need to understand the importance of not coughing during the procedure. Provide appropriate pain management 30 to 60 minutes before procedures, as ordered, to reduce the perception of pain. After any procedure monitor the patient for signs of changes in cardiopulmonary functioning such as sudden shortness of breath, pain, oxygen desaturation, and anxiety.

TABLE 41.4   Cardiac Function Diagnostic Tests

Test	Significance
Holter monitor	Portable ECG worn by a patient at home or work or school. The test produces a continuous ECG tracing over a period of time. Patients use either a diary or smart phone app to note when they experience rapid heartbeats or dizziness. Evaluation of the ECG recording along with the diary provides information about the electrical activity of the heart during activities of daily living.
ECG exercise stress test	ECG is monitored while a patient walks on a treadmill at a specified speed and duration of time. Test evaluates the cardiac response to physical stress. It is not a valuable tool for evaluation of cardiac response in women because of an increased false-positive finding.
Thallium stress test	ECG stress test with the addition of thallium-201 injected intravenously. It determines coronary blood flow changes with increased activity. Often used for people who cannot walk on the treadmill.
Electrophysiological study (EPS)	EPS is an invasive measure of intracardiac electrical pathways. It provides more specific information about difficult-to-treat dysrhythmias and assesses adequacy of antidysrhythmic medication.
Transthoracic echocardiography	This is a noninvasive measure of heart structure and heart wall motion. It graphically demonstrates overall cardiac performance.
Scintigraphy	Scintigraphy is radionuclide angiography; used to evaluate cardiac structure, myocardial perfusion, and contractility.
Cardiac catheterization and angiography	These are used to visualize cardiac chambers, valves, the great vessels, and coronary arteries. Pressures and volumes within the four chambers of the heart are also measured.

ECG, Electrocardiogram.
Data from Pagana KD, et al: *Mosby's diagnostic and laboratory test reference*, ed 15, St Louis, 2021, Elsevier.

TABLE 41.5   Ventilation and Oxygenation Diagnostic Studies

Measurement and Normal Values	Interpretation/Purpose
Arterial Blood Gases pH 7.35-7.45 PCO_2 35-45 mm Hg HCO_3 21-28 mEq/L PO_2 80-100 mm Hg SaO_2 saturation 95%-100% Older adult: 95% Base excess 0 ± 2 mEq/L	Provides important information for assessment of patient's respiratory and metabolic acid/base balance and adequacy of oxygenation (see Chapter 42)
Pulmonary Function Tests Basic ventilation studies (Pulmonary functions vary by ethnic group.)	Determines ability of the lungs to efficiently exchange oxygen and carbon dioxide Used to differentiate pulmonary obstructive from restrictive disease
Peak Expiratory Flow Rate (PEFR) The point of highest flow during maximal expiration (Normal in adults is based on age and body weight.)	Reflects changes in large airway sizes; an excellent predictor of overall airway resistance in a patient with asthma Daily measurement for early detection of asthma exacerbations
Bronchoscopy Normal airways without masses, pus, or foreign bodies	Visual examination of the tracheobronchial tree through a narrow, flexible fiberoptic bronchoscope Performed to obtain fluid, sputum, or biopsy samples; remove mucus plugs or foreign bodies
Lung Scan Normal lung structure without masses	Nuclear scanning test used to identify abnormal masses by size and location Identification of masses used in planning therapy and treatments Also used to find a blood clot preventing normal perfusion or ventilation ($\dot{V}/\dot{Q}$ scan)

TABLE 41.5 Ventilation and Oxygenation Diagnostic Studies—cont'd

Measurement and Normal Values	Interpretation/Purpose
Thoracentesis Surgical perforation of chest wall and pleural space with a needle to aspirate fluid for diagnostic or therapeutic purposes or to remove a specimen for biopsy; performed using aseptic technique and local anesthetic. (Patient usually sits upright with the anterior thorax supported by pillows or an over-bed table.)	Specimen of pleural fluid obtained for cytological examination Results may indicate an infection or neoplastic disease Identification of infection or a type of cancer important in determining a plan of care
Sputum specimens • Normal: negative	Nasal aspirate/swabs for respiratory syncytial virus, influenza; sometimes are obtained while patient expectorates into specimen container; true sputum cultures are obtained via airway suctioning or through bronchoscopy
• Sputum culture and sensitivity	Obtained to identify a specific microorganism or organism growing in sputum Identifies drug resistance and sensitivities to determine appropriate antibiotic therapy
• Sputum for acid-fast bacillus (AFB)	Screens for presence of AFB for detection of tuberculosis by early-morning specimens on 3 consecutive days
• Sputum for cytology	Obtained to identify lung cancer Differentiates type of cancer cells (small cell, oat cell, large cell)

Data from Pagana KD, et al: *Mosby's diagnostic and laboratory test reference,* ed 15, St Louis, 2021, Elsevier.

⊕ BOX 41.3 CULTURAL ASPECTS OF CARE

Cultural Impact on Pulmonary Diseases

The impact of pulmonary diseases on patients and their families varies among cultures. It is important to understand these variations in terms of assessing for and providing care in patients with lung diseases. In 2018, approximately two-thirds of the new cases of TB diagnosed in the United States occurred in people who were not born in the United States. The countries where these patients were most likely to be born were Mexico, the Philippines, India, Vietnam, and China (CDC, 2016a).

The cigarette smoking rate in the United States is highest in American Indian/Alaskan Natives (24.6%), followed by Caucasians (15.3%), African Americans (15.1%), Hispanics (9.9%), and Asians (7.0%). Smoking rates are also higher in those who have less than a high school education (22%) than in those who have a baccalaureate degree or higher (5.8%). Smoking increases the risk for a number of cancer types, chronic obstructive pulmonary disease (COPD), and heart disease (ALA, 2020c).

People of certain ethnic or cultural backgrounds tend to live in the same area, which can affect their exposure to certain environmental pollutants or triggers of respiratory exacerbations. Where they live can also affect their socioeconomic status and their access to health care, which can also have a great impact on their pulmonary health (Celedon et al., 2017).

While ethnic and cultural differences can contribute to overall health, it should be noted that in today's globalization, health care providers should look more at acculturation (cultural exchange of beliefs, values, or behaviors as a result of interacting with people of other cultures) as an influence on a person's or a family's health. For example, smoking rates are higher in females of Mexican descent who have lived in the United States (Celedon et al., 2017).

The American Thoracic Society and the National Heart, Lung, and Blood Institute recommend looking more at the individual person and less at the person's race or ethnicity when trying to develop a plan of care. There is discussion about looking at a person's genetic makeup to develop a plan of care as genetic testing could help determine actual risk of disease and which medications would work best for that particular patient (Celedon et al., 2017).

Implications for Patient-Centered Care
- Ask patients who were born outside the United States if they have had the bacille Calmette-Guérin (BCG) vaccine, which can cause a positive reaction to the TB skin test. Also assess their exposure to people with known TB or other pulmonary infectious diseases (CDC, 2016a, 2016b).
- Immunization clinics should concentrate on the underserved urban and rural communities, especially those with large numbers of older adults. Provide TB skin testing, flu vaccines, and pneumonia vaccines as needed.
- Community health departments need to target at-risk populations for flu and pneumonia vaccine clinics.
- Public health programs for those at highest risk for pulmonary diseases should focus on pollution prevention, immunizations, and smoking-cessation programs.

REFLECT NOW

You are preparing to assess a patient with COPD. What would be important questions to ask this patient when gathering a health history? What are your expected physical assessment findings? What diagnostic tests would you expect the health care provider to order for this patient?

Mr. Edwards' history reveals risk factors (alcohol abuse, sedentary lifestyle) in addition to a 40-year history of smoking 2 packs per day, and he still continues to smoke. John knows that the current increase in

Mr. Edwards' shortness of breath is due to his respiratory infection. The secretions are obstructing his alveolocapillary membrane, preventing oxygenation of blood in some parts of his lung.

Mr. Edwards works as a salesman and lives with his wife. He has a history of chronic obstructive pulmonary disease (COPD) and alcohol abuse but at present is not drinking. Mrs. Edwards has also smoked 2 packs per day for more than 40 years. Mr. Edwards used to help with the housework and states that he loves to tinker in the garden; however, lately he has been unable to participate in any of these activities. His wife states, "All he seems to be able to do is sit in his chair and watch TV."

When John meets Mr. Edwards and performs his morning assessment, he observes Mr. Edwards' breathing; his respiratory rate is 26, and every

BOX 41.4 Tuberculosis Skin Testing

- Skin testing determines whether a person is infected with *Mycobacterium tuberculosis*.
- Tuberculosis (TB) skin testing (TST) is performed by an intradermal injection of 0.1 mL of tuberculin purified protein derivative (PPD) on the inner surface of the forearm (see Chapter 31). The injection produces a pale elevation of the skin (a wheal) 6 to 10 mm in diameter. Afterward the injection site is circled, and the patient is instructed not to wash the circle off.
- Read tuberculin skin tests between 48 and 72 hours after the test. If the site is not read within 72 hours, a patient must have another skin test.
- *Positive results:* A palpable elevated, hardened area around the injection site, caused by edema and inflammation from the antigen-antibody reaction, measured in millimeters. (See Chapter 31 for evaluation of positive results by millimeters.)
- People born outside the United States may have had the bacille Calmette-Guérin (BCG) vaccine for TB disease, which results in a positive reaction to the TST and may complicate the treatment plan. The positive skin reaction does not indicate that the BCG vaccine provided protection against the disease (CDC, 2016a, 2016b).
- Reddened flat areas are *not* positive reactions and are not measured.
- TST is less reliable in older adults (see Box 41.1) and in those with an altered immune function, such as patients with rheumatoid arthritis, human immunodeficiency virus (HIV), or those receiving chemotherapy.

BOX 41.5 Nursing Diagnostic Process

Impaired Gas Exchange Related to Decreased Lung Expansion

Assessment Activities	Assessment Findings
Ask patient or family about patient's mood, attentiveness, memory, and activity level.	Confusion Decreased activity Fatigue Irritability Restlessness Sleepiness
Observe patient's respirations for rate, rhythm, depth.	Dyspnea Nasal flaring Tachypnea Use of accessory muscles
Inspect skin and mucous membranes.	Diaphoresis Pallor Cyanosis
Auscultate chest.	Decreased respiratory excursion Abnormal, distant lung sounds

breath seems to be a struggle. He is tachycardic with a heart rate of 110 beats per minute, his oxygen saturations are 86%, and he is extremely anxious. Mr. Edwards still has chest pain on inspiration; he rates his pain 4/10. There are decreased breath sounds in his right lung and crackles on auscultation. John also notes that the lung sounds do not improve with coughing, and Mr. Edwards has a lot of difficulty managing his respiratory secretions. Mr. Edwards requested John to help him from the bed to the bedside chair. After Mr. Edwards was comfortable in the chair, he commented that "getting out of bed took all my energy."

◆ Analysis and Nursing Diagnosis

Clinical judgment requires the application of critical thinking to analyze assessment findings. Consider the knowledge you have about a patient's condition and assessment findings to differentiate normal versus abnormal findings. Your review and analysis of assessment data will reveal cues and clusters of data to support nursing diagnoses for patients with impaired oxygenation. In addition, use these assessment data, cues, and clusters to reveal information about any related or risk factors (Box 41.5). Carefully reflect on your patient's assessment data and use clinical judgment to identify the most appropriate nursing diagnoses. For example, both *Impaired Gas Exchange* and *Impaired Breathing* involve dyspnea and nasal flaring. A closer analysis of assessment findings and the patient's history will help you select the correct diagnosis. For example, a patient who was in a motor vehicle accident and who has fractured ribs, pain on inspiration, and an increased respiratory rate is more likely to have *Impaired Breathing*. The cues and clustered assessment findings and related factors support a problem or negative nursing diagnosis. If assessment results in the clustering of risk factors, a risk nursing diagnosis will be made.

It is important to remember that a patient's oxygenation status is related to the integrated function of the cardiac and respiratory systems, and an illness in one system affects the other system. For example, when a patient has severe congestive heart failure, the heart is unable to effectively pump blood through the circulation, and fluid accumulates in the lungs, causing pulmonary edema, which decreases oxygenation. If a patient has a pulmonary embolism and the oxygen saturation (SaO_2) drops, the heart rate will increase to meet the patient's oxygen demand.

Additional nursing diagnoses associated with impaired oxygen may include the following examples:
- Impaired Cardiac Output
- Acute Pain
- Activity Intolerance
- Fatigue
- Impaired Cardiac Function

John's analysis of the nursing assessment data for Mr. Edwards identified several problem areas leading to multiple nursing diagnoses. John focused on assessment cues related to Mr. Edwards' respiratory issues and identified two priority nursing diagnoses. John observed Mr. Edwards' difficulty in breathing and clearing his respiratory secretions. John auscultated Mr. Edwards' lungs and noted decreased breath sounds and crackles, which support the nursing diagnosis of **Impaired Airway Clearance**. *His rapid respirations, difficulty with breathing, and reduced oxygen saturation are cues for* **Impaired Gas Exchange**.

◆ Planning and Outcomes Identification

Once nursing diagnoses are identified, use clinical judgment to develop a patient-centered plan of care to improve and maintain a patient's oxygenation status. During planning synthesize information from multiple sources (Fig. 41.5). Critical thinking and clinical judgment ensure that your plan of care is based on knowledge of a patient's assessment findings and expectations of care, and also that it includes how hospital or health care environmental issues impact patient-centered care. For example, frequency of airway suctioning is based on a patient's respiratory assessment, and it is often a complicated procedure. In addition, many patients who need airway suctioning require care from other disciplines, such as physical, occupational, and respiratory therapy. As a result, coordination of care among disciplines is crucial to maintain patient-centered care.

Professional standards and nurse competency are especially important to consider when developing a plan of care. These standards often are the result of scientifically proven guidelines for selecting effective nursing interventions.

Outcomes. Develop an individualized plan of care for each nursing diagnosis (see the Nursing Care Plan). Together with your patient, set realistic expectations and relevant, measurable outcomes of care.

FIG. 41.5 Critical thinking model for oxygenation planning. (Clinical Judgment Measurement Model copyright © NCSBN. All rights reserved.)

◎ NURSING CARE PLAN

Impaired Airway Clearance

ASSESSMENT

Assessment Activities	*Assessment Findings*[a]
Ask Mr. Edwards how long he has been short of breath.	He replies, "I have been **short of breath for 1 week,** and it has **gotten worse, especially when I lie flat.**" His vital signs are pulse rate 110 beats/min; temperature 102°F orally; **respiratory rate 26 breaths per minute;** blood pressure 110/45 mm Hg; and **a SpO2 of 86% on room air.** Mr. Edwards is short of breath as he answers questions.
Ask Mr. Edwards how long he has had his cough and whether it is a productive cough.	"I usually **cough** when I wake up in the morning. Three days ago I noticed that I **was coughing up thick yellow-green mucus** that has not stopped."
Auscultate Mr. Edwards' lung fields.	On auscultation there are **audible expiratory wheezes, crackles, and diminished breath sounds** over right lower lobe.
Ask Mr. Edwards to produce a sputum sample.	**Sputum is thick and discolored (yellow-green).**

[a]**Assessment Findings** are shown in bold type.

NURSING DIAGNOSIS: Impaired airway clearance related to thick pulmonary secretions

---

PLANNING

Expected Outcomes (NOC)[b]

Respiratory Status: Gas Exchange

Adventitious lung sounds will begin to clear within 24 hours.

Respiratory rate will return to normal values within 24 hours.

SpO₂ will be >95% within 24 hours.

[b]Outcome classification labels from Moorhead S, et al., editors: *Nursing outcomes classification (NOC),* ed 6, St. Louis, 2018, Elsevier

Continued

◎ NURSING CARE PLAN—cont'd

Impaired Airway Clearance

INTERVENTIONS (NIC)[c]	RATIONALE
Airway Management	
Position Mr. Edwards with head of bed elevated 30–45 degrees or sitting in a chair.	Increases depth of lung expansion and reduces airway resistance and improves respiratory gas exchange (Elliott and Morrell-Scott, 2017).
Ambulate in room or hall progressively as tolerated at least 2 times a day.	Early mobilization and changes in positioning prevent muscle weakness. Mobilization facilitates expectoration of respiratory secretions (Harding et al., 2020).
Have Mr. Edwards deep-breathe and cough, using huff technique, every 2 hours while awake.	Helps expectorate the sputum; promotes gas exchange. Retained secretions predispose patient to atelectasis and worsening pneumonia. Controlled coughing improves cough effectiveness and removal of airway secretions (Urden et al., 2020).
Encourage Mr. Edwards to increase his fluid intake to at least 2500 mL/24 hours, if not contraindicated.	Fluids help to liquify airway secretions, which helps patient to effectively expectorate secretions. Hydration also relieves oral mucosa and skin dryness (Harding et al., 2020).
Avoid caffeinated beverages and alcohol; recommend water.	Caffeinated and alcoholic beverages promote diuresis and dehydration.

[c] Intervention classification labels from Bulechek GM, et al., editors: *Nursing interventions classification (NIC)*, ed 7, St. Louis, 2018, Elsevier.

EVALUATION

Evaluation Activities	*Patient Response*
Auscultate chest.	Bilateral lung sounds are clear, no crackles. Respiratory rate 18 breaths/min SpO$_2$ 95
Ask Mr. Edwards to keep track of his fluid intake.	Mr. Edwards has completed accurate intake list daily, averaging 2700 mL/day.
Review flow sheet for recent vital signs.	Mr. Edwards' 0600 set of vital signs shows a heart rate of 98 beats/min, respiratory rate of 20 breaths/min, oral temperature of 98.6°F, BP 112/62 mm Hg, and a pulse oximetry of 95% on room air.

Patients with impaired oxygenation require a nursing care plan directed toward meeting actual or potential oxygenation needs. Collaborate with your patient and family caregiver. Develop individual outcomes based on patient expectations and problems. For example, if the priority for the patient is an improved breathing pattern, select specific expected outcomes, such as the following:

- Patient's respiratory rate is between 12 and 20 breaths/minute.
- Patient achieves bilateral lung expansion.
- Patient breathes without the use of accessory muscles.

Often a patient with cardiopulmonary disease has multiple nursing diagnoses (Fig. 41.6). In this case, identify when outcomes apply to more than one diagnosis. The presence of multiple diagnoses also makes priority setting a critical activity.

Setting Priorities. A patient's level of health, age, lifestyle, and environmental risk factors affect tissue oxygenation. Patients with severe impairments in oxygenation have multiple priorities of care. Use your clinical judgment to determine which outcome is the highest priority. For example, in an acute care setting, maintaining a patent airway has a higher priority than improving the patient's exercise tolerance. The need for a patent airway is immediate; as the patient's level of oxygen improves, activity tolerance increases (Urden et al., 2020). In a second example, when caring for a patient who has an abdominal incision, pain control is a priority. In this situation, controlling the patient's pain facilitates coughing and deep breathing and activity (Harding et al., 2020). However, in a community-based or primary care setting, priorities often focus on primary or tertiary health promotion activities, such as smoking cessation, exercise, and/or diet modifications.

Both you and your patient need to focus on the same expected outcomes. In addition to individualizing each outcome, be sure that the outcomes are realistic, have reasonable time frames, and are attainable for the patient. Be sure to respect the patient's preferences for the degree of active engagement in the care process. Some patients will choose to be very active and desire to make day-to-day decisions.

Others may choose to assume a more passive role, preferring that you choose a course of action while keeping them informed (Harding et al., 2020).

Teamwork and Collaboration. The time spent with a patient in any setting is limited. Therefore, collaborate with family members, colleagues, and other health care specialists to achieve the established expected outcomes. Some patients need to improve their exercise and activity tolerance; for other patients, continuing care involves participating in a community-based cardiopulmonary rehabilitation program. Some patients need home physical therapy.

Collaboration with physical therapists, nutritionists, respiratory therapists, and community-based nurses is valuable for patients with heart failure or chronic lung conditions. These professionals work with patients and their caregivers using resources in the community to assist them in attaining and maintaining the highest possible level of wellness. In addition, professionals identify community resources and support systems to help prevent and manage symptoms related to cardiopulmonary diseases. Communication among everyone on the patient's health care team and recognition of everyone's contributions in achieving the health care outcomes for the patient are imperative.

John's priorities of care for Mr. Edwards are to improve his airway clearance and gas exchange. John plans interventions to teach Mr. Edwards effective coughing techniques, to position him in semi-Fowler's to high Fowler's position, to maintain hydration, and to begin ambulation. As Mr. Edwards' airway clearance improves, his gas exchange will improve, and his dyspnea and oxygen saturation will also improve.

John knows that Mr. and Mrs. Edwards' smoking history poses risks for respiratory disease, but Mr. Edwards has the greatest risk. As Mr. Edwards improves, John wants to learn Mr. and Mrs. Edwards' understanding of how smoking affects Mr. Edwards' health. Information about smoking cessation may be useful if they are receptive. He knows from experience that acute care issues need to be resolved before a patient can benefit from patient education.

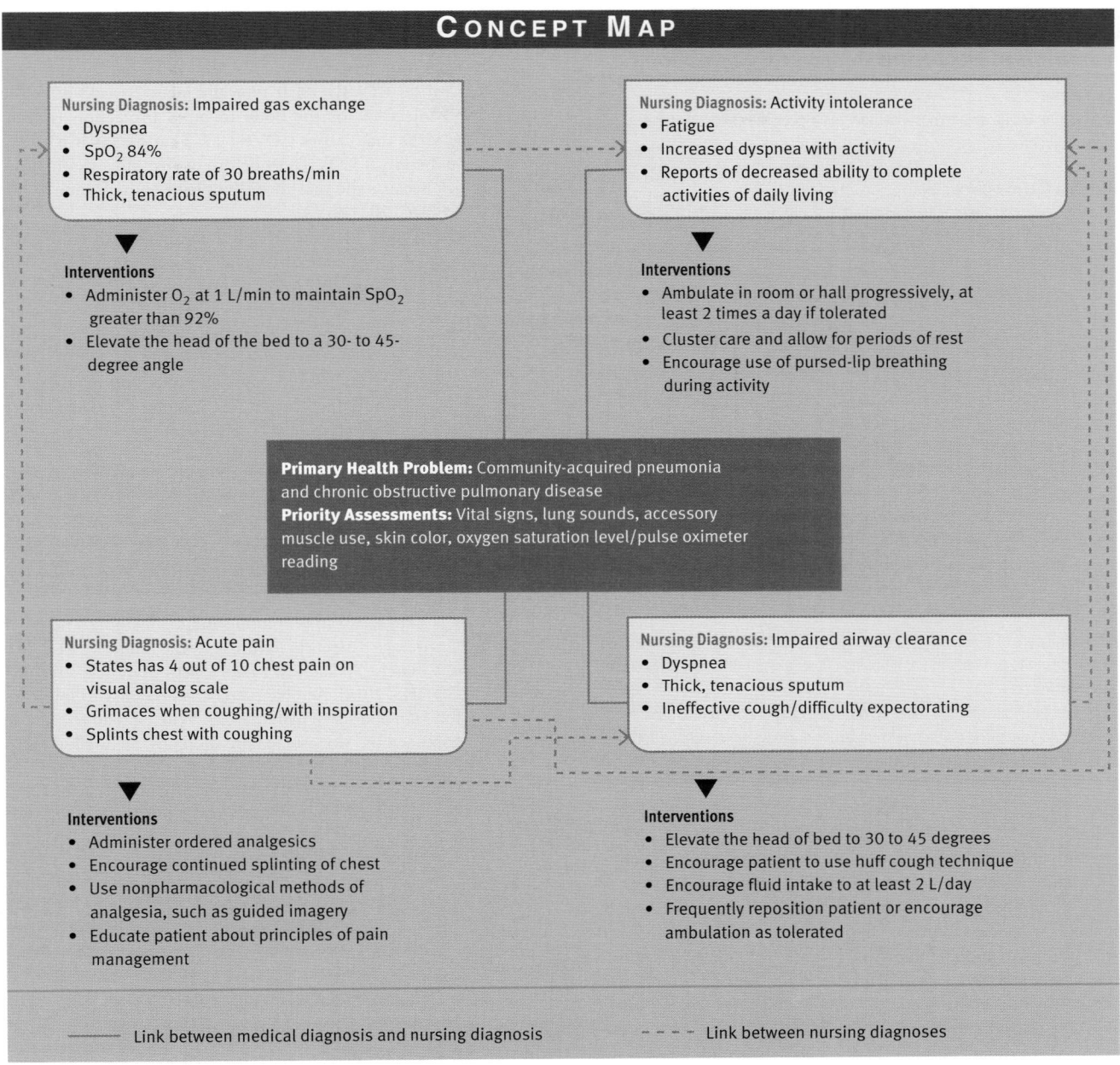

CONCEPT MAP

Nursing Diagnosis: Impaired gas exchange
- Dyspnea
- SpO_2 84%
- Respiratory rate of 30 breaths/min
- Thick, tenacious sputum

Interventions
- Administer O_2 at 1 L/min to maintain SpO_2 greater than 92%
- Elevate the head of the bed to a 30- to 45-degree angle

Nursing Diagnosis: Activity intolerance
- Fatigue
- Increased dyspnea with activity
- Reports of decreased ability to complete activities of daily living

Interventions
- Ambulate in room or hall progressively, at least 2 times a day if tolerated
- Cluster care and allow for periods of rest
- Encourage use of pursed-lip breathing during activity

Primary Health Problem: Community-acquired pneumonia and chronic obstructive pulmonary disease
Priority Assessments: Vital signs, lung sounds, accessory muscle use, skin color, oxygen saturation level/pulse oximeter reading

Nursing Diagnosis: Acute pain
- States has 4 out of 10 chest pain on visual analog scale
- Grimaces when coughing/with inspiration
- Splints chest with coughing

Interventions
- Administer ordered analgesics
- Encourage continued splinting of chest
- Use nonpharmacological methods of analgesia, such as guided imagery
- Educate patient about principles of pain management

Nursing Diagnosis: Impaired airway clearance
- Dyspnea
- Thick, tenacious sputum
- Ineffective cough/difficulty expectorating

Interventions
- Elevate the head of bed to 30 to 45 degrees
- Encourage patient to use huff cough technique
- Encourage fluid intake to at least 2 L/day
- Frequently reposition patient or encourage ambulation as tolerated

——— Link between medical diagnosis and nursing diagnosis - - - - Link between nursing diagnoses

FIG. 41.6 Concept map for Mr. Edwards.

◆ Implementation

There are interventions for promoting and maintaining adequate oxygenation across the continuum of care. As a nurse, you use clinical judgment to determine which interventions are appropriate for your patients. You will be responsible for independent interventions such as positioning, coughing techniques, and health education for disease prevention. In addition, you will provide physician-initiated interventions such as oxygen therapy, lung inflation techniques, and chest physiotherapy.

Health Promotion. Maintaining a patient's optimal level of health reduces the number and/or severity of respiratory symptoms. Prevention of respiratory infections is foremost in maintaining optimal health (Box 41.6). Providing cardiopulmonary-related health information is an important nursing responsibility.

The health information that your patients and their families bring to the situation varies. Some patients have a lot of exposure to health care information and understand their treatment plans. Other families might have a lot of exposure to health care information but are unable to understand and follow treatment plans. Last, you might encounter families who are experiencing their first exposure to health care information and are very unsure of their interpretation of the information. When providing health information, be sure to assess a patient's health literacy level and then individualize findings into an individualized education session (see Chapter 25).

Vaccinations. Seasonal flu vaccine protects against influenza viruses that research indicates will be the most common during that year. The vaccines are formulated annually based on worldwide surveillance data. Annual flu vaccines are recommended for all people 6 months and older.

BOX 41.6 PATIENT TEACHING

Prevention of Recurrent Respiratory Infections

Objective
- The patient will be able to describe how to reduce the risk factors for recurring respiratory infections.

Teaching Strategies
- Adapt teaching strategies to the patient's health literacy, educational background, reading level, and cultural preferences (CDC, 2021a).
- Instruct patient and family about appropriate hand hygiene techniques to reduce transmission of microorganisms.
- Collaborate with patient and family to identify outcomes for reducing risk factors.
- Explain the link between smoking and increased risk for respiratory infections (CDC, 2018a; McCance and Huether, 2019).
- Refer to smoking-cessation programs and discuss appropriate medication to support smoking cessation from the primary health provider (ACS, 2020b).
- If a patient does not smoke, teach the importance of avoiding secondhand smoke and areas of high air pollution.
- Explain to patient and family why annual influenza vaccines and appropriate pneumonia vaccines are needed (CDC, 2020d, 2021b).
- Instruct patient and family about signs and symptoms of respiratory infection that should be reported to health care provider, such as increased coughing, shortness of breath, change of color of sputum, fever, and fatigue.

Evaluation
Use the principles of teach-back to evaluate patient/family caregiver learning:
- Please describe the benefits of smoking cessation and the risks for secondhand smoke.
- Tell me about your family's plans to get your flu and pneumonia vaccines.
- How would you know if you might be experiencing a respiratory infection?
- Describe what symptoms would prompt you to call your health care provider.

Patients with chronic illnesses (heart, lung, kidney, or immunocompromised), infants, older adults, and pregnant women can get very sick; thus, they should be immunized (CDC, 2021b). The vaccine is also recommended for people in close or frequent contact with anyone in the high-risk groups, including infants and health care workers. It is effective in reducing the severity of illness and the risk of serious complications and death. It is important to assess a patient's allergies and any allergic response to vaccines or any components. People with a known hypersensitivity to eggs or other components of the vaccine should consult their physician before being vaccinated (CDC, 2021b). Adults with an acute febrile illness should schedule the vaccination after they have recovered. The live, attenuated nasal spray vaccine is given to healthy people from 2 through 49 years of age if they are not pregnant. The live vaccine is also not indicated in people who are immunocompromised or have certain chronic health conditions such as asthma or heart disease (CDC, 2021b).

Pneumococcal vaccine (PCV13) is routinely given to children younger than 2 years of age and is recommended for patients with certain medical conditions (such as heart disease) who are at risk of complications from pneumococcal disease (CDC, 2020d). Adults over 65 years of age and any adult who smokes may receive the pneumococcal polysaccharide vaccine (PPSV23). These vaccines should not be administered if the patient has had an allergic reaction to the vaccine in the past or while the patient is recovering from a febrile illness. Women should not receive the vaccine while pregnant; instead, they should try to receive the vaccine before pregnancy.

In 2020, COVID-19 caused a global pandemic, and the need for COVID vaccines became a global health priority. Research showed that COVID-19 vaccines were effective in keeping people from getting COVID-19 or becoming seriously ill if infected with COVID-19. These vaccines teach our immune systems how to recognize and fight the virus that causes COVID-19. It typically takes 2 weeks after the last vaccination injection for the body to build protection (immunity) against the virus that causes COVID-19. That means it is possible a person could still get COVID-19 before or just after vaccination and then get sick because the vaccine did not have enough time to provide protection (CDC, 2021e).

Healthy Lifestyle. Identification and elimination of risk factors for cardiopulmonary disease are important parts of primary care. The risk factors for cardiac disease are lower when total cholesterol levels are less than 200 mg/dL, high-density lipoprotein (HDL) levels are greater than 40 mg/dL in men and 50 mg/dL in women, and low-density lipoprotein (LDL) levels are less than 160 mg/dL (Harding et al., 2020). Encourage patients to eat a healthy low-fat, high-fiber diet and maintain a body weight in proportion to their height (see Chapter 45). The Dietary Approaches to Stop Hypertension (DASH) diet, along with exercise, stress reduction, and limiting alcohol intake, has been shown to decrease a patient's risk of hypertension (NHLBI, n.d.a). Eliminating cigarettes and other tobacco use and adequately hydrating are additional healthy behaviors. Encourage patients to examine their habits and make appropriate changes. Patients with cardiopulmonary alterations need to minimize their risk for infection, especially during the winter months (see Box 41.6).

Exercise is a key factor in promoting and maintaining a healthy heart and lungs. Encourage patients to have at least 150 minutes a week of moderate intensity exercise and at least 2 days a week of muscle-strengthening activity (USDHHS, 2018). Aerobic exercise is necessary to improve lung and heart function and strengthen muscles. Walking is an efficient way to achieve a good aerobic workout. Many shopping malls allow people to walk in the enclosed mall before the shops open. During the hot summer months, teach patients to limit activities to early in the day or late in the evening, when temperatures are lower. In addition, teach the importance of maintaining adequate hydration and sodium intake, especially if they are taking diuretics. Caution patients with known cardiac disease and those with multiple risk factors to avoid exertion in cold weather. Shoveling snow is especially risky and often precipitates a cardiac event. Other activities, such as hanging holiday lights and decorations in the extreme cold, can precipitate chest pain and bronchospasm. Please refer to Chapter 38 for further discussion on activity and exercise.

Environmental Pollutants. Avoiding exposure to secondhand smoke is essential to maintaining optimal cardiopulmonary function (ALA, 2020a). Most public places, such as businesses or restaurants, ban smoking or have separate areas designated as smoking areas. Provide counseling and support so that a patient who lives with secondhand smoke in the home understands its effects. If the patient is smoking and wants to quit, encourage the patient's family to support the patient in the attempt to quit.

Help patients develop a plan to avoid environmental hazards in their home or work environments when possible. For example, teach patients who know that pollen triggers an asthma exacerbation to keep windows closed and use air filters when air pollen counts are high (Hockenberry et al., 2019; Harding et al., 2020). Many health care agency dress codes prohibit the use of perfumes or colognes because they often affect patient breathing patterns and allergies. People in some occupations, such as farming, painting, and carpentry, may benefit from the use of particulate filter masks to reduce the inhalation of particles.

Acute Care. Patients with acute pulmonary illnesses require nursing interventions directed toward halting the pathological process (e.g., respiratory tract infection), shortening the duration and severity of an illness (e.g., hospitalization with pneumonia), and preventing complications from the illness or treatments (e.g., hospital-acquired infection resulting from invasive procedures) (Harding et al., 2020; Urden et al., 2020).

Dyspnea Management. Dyspnea is difficult to treat. Health care providers individualize treatments for each patient and usually implement more than one therapy. Treatment of the underlying process causing dyspnea is then followed with other therapies (e.g., pharmacological measures, oxygen therapy, physical techniques, and psychosocial techniques). Pharmacological agents include bronchodilators, inhaled steroids, mucolytics, and low-dose antianxiety medications. Oxygen therapy reduces dyspnea associated with exercise and hypoxemia. Physical and psychological techniques such as cardiopulmonary reconditioning (e.g., exercise, breathing techniques, and cough control), relaxation techniques, biofeedback, and meditation are also beneficial (Harding et al., 2020).

Airway Maintenance. The airway is patent when the trachea, bronchi, and large airways are free from obstructions. Airway maintenance requires adequate hydration to prevent thick, tenacious secretions. Proper coughing techniques remove secretions and keep the airway open. A variety of interventions such as suctioning, chest physiotherapy, and nebulizer therapy assist patients in managing alterations in airway clearance (Urden et al., 2020).

Mobilization of Pulmonary Secretions. The ability of a patient to mobilize pulmonary secretions makes the difference between a short-term illness and an illness involving a long recovery with complications. Nursing interventions promoting removal of pulmonary secretions such as repositioning and suctioning assist in achieving and maintaining a clear airway and help to promote lung expansion and gas exchange (Mendes et al., 2019; Strickland et al., 2013; Strickland, 2015).

Hydration. Maintenance of adequate systemic hydration keeps mucociliary clearance normal. In patients with adequate hydration, pulmonary secretions are thin, white, watery, and easily removable with minimal coughing. Excessive coughing to clear thick, tenacious secretions is fatiguing and energy depleting. It can also cause pain in the chest muscles and ribs, which further decreases the patient's ability to cough and clear secretions. The best way to maintain thin secretions is to provide a fluid intake of 1500 to 2500 mL/day unless contraindicated by cardiac or renal status. The color, consistency, and ease of mucus expectoration determines adequacy of hydration (Harding et al., 2020).

Humidification. Humidification is the process of adding water to gas to keep airways moist. It is necessary for patients receiving oxygen therapy at high flow rates, typically greater than 4 L/minute (see agency protocols). Oxygen humidification via nasal cannula or face mask is achieved by bubbling oxygen through sterile water (see Skill 41.4). Sterile water should be used to decrease the risk of hospital-acquired infection; follow agency protocols to change the solution (Wen et al., 2017).

When caring for pediatric patients, humidity may be applied to all oxygen devices, regardless of flow rates. Infants and children have smaller airways than adults, and secretions are more likely to obstruct airways in the younger population. Humidity is added to help ease the ability of infants and children to clear their airways (ATS, 2019; Walsh and Smallwood, 2017).

Nebulization. Nebulization adds moisture to inspired air by mixing particles of varying sizes with the air. Aerosolization suspends the maximum number of water drops or particles of the desired size in inspired air. When the thin layer of fluid supporting the mucous layer over the cilia dries, the cilia are damaged and unable to adequately clear the airway. Humidification through nebulization enhances mucociliary clearance, the natural mechanism of the body for removing mucus and cellular debris from the respiratory tract. This, in turn, improves the clearance of pulmonary secretions. Nebulization is also a method of administration for certain medications, such as bronchodilators and mucolytic agents (Harding et al., 2020).

Coughing and Deep-Breathing Techniques. Coughing is an effective technique for maintaining a patent airway. Deep-breathing exercise with coughing is an airway clearance maneuver that is effective when spontaneous coughing is inadequate (Hanada et al., 2020; Eltorai et al., 2018). It permits a patient to remove secretions from both the upper and lower airways. The normal series of events in the directed cough is deep inhalation, closure of the glottis, active contraction of the expiratory muscles, and glottis opening. Deep inhalation increases the lung volume and airway diameter, allowing the air to pass through partially obstructing mucous plugs or other foreign matter. Contraction of the expiratory muscles against the closed glottis causes a high intrathoracic pressure to develop. When the glottis opens, a large flow of air is expelled at a high speed, providing momentum for mucus to move to the upper airways, allowing a patient to expectorate or swallow it.

The *huff cough* stimulates a natural cough reflex and is generally used to help move secretions to the larger airways. The patient inhales deeply and then holds the breath for 2 to 3 seconds. While forcefully exhaling, the patient opens the glottis by saying the word *huff*. With practice the patient inhales more air and is able to progress to the cascade cough. When using a cascade cough, the patient takes a slow, deep breath, holds it for 1 to 2 seconds, then opens the mouth and performs a series of coughs throughout exhalation. This technique is often used in patients with large amounts of sputum, such as those with cystic fibrosis (CFF, n.d.b).

The *quad cough,* or *manually assisted cough* technique, is for patients without abdominal muscle control, such as those with spinal cord injuries. While the patient breathes out with a maximal expiratory effort, the patient or nurse pushes inward and upward on the abdominal muscles toward the diaphragm, causing the cough (Chatwin et al., 2018).

Diaphragmatic breathing is a technique that encourages deep nasal inspiration to increase air flow to the lower lungs. The diaphragm descends (belly moves out) when breathing in and ascends (belly sinks in) when breathing out. For patients with COPD, this technique increases the patient's tidal volume and oxygen saturation, reduces dyspnea, and improves exchange of respiratory gases (Mendes et al., 2019).

Encourage patients with chronic pulmonary diseases, upper respiratory tract infections, and lower respiratory tract infections to deep-breathe and cough at least every 2 hours while awake. Encourage patients with a large amount of sputum to cough every hour while awake. After some surgeries, it is recommended that patients perform deep breathing and coughing techniques every 2 to 4 hours while awake to prevent accumulation of secretions. Offer postoperative patients support devices (folded blanket, pillow, or palmed hands) to splint an abdominal or thoracic incision to minimize pain during directed coughing. Cough is a source of droplet transmission of pulmonary pathogens; thus, the health care provider should follow Standard Precautions (Harding et al., 2020).

Chest Physiotherapy. Chest physiotherapy (CPT) is external chest wall manipulation using percussion, vibration, or high-frequency chest wall compression (HFCWC) (Fig. 41.7). It is often used in conjunction with postural drainage and can help mobilize pulmonary secretions in a select group of patients. Box 41.7 describes the guidelines to determine whether CPT is indicated. Because there is no evidence to support its routine use in all patient populations, the American Association for Respiratory Care (AARC) does not support the routine use of CPT with all patients. Instead CPT is used for patients with retained secretions who cannot expectorate those secretions, such as patients with cystic fibrosis (CF) (Strickland, 2015; Strickland et al., 2013).

Postural drainage is a component of pulmonary hygiene; it consists of drainage, positioning, and turning and is sometimes accompanied by

FIG. 41.7 High-frequency chest wall compression (HFCWC). (Copyright © 2019 Hill-Rom Services, Inc. Reprinted with permission. All rights reserved.)

BOX 41.7 Guidelines for Chest Physiotherapy

Nursing and respiratory therapy collaborate with the health care provider to determine whether chest physiotherapy (CPT) is best for a patient. The following guidelines help in physical assessment and subsequent decision making:

- Conduct a complete respiratory assessment to confirm need for CPT, including sputum production, effectiveness of cough, history of pulmonary problems successfully relieved with CPT, abnormal lung sounds, and documented conditions such as atelectasis, complicated pneumonia, vital signs, or changes in oxygenation status (Harding et al., 2020; Strickland et al., 2013).
- Know the patient's medications. Certain medications, particularly diuretics and antihypertensives, cause fluid and hemodynamic changes. These decrease a patient's tolerance to positional changes and postural drainage. Long-term steroid use increases a patient's risk of pathological rib fractures and often contraindicates vibration.
- Know the patient's medical history. Certain conditions such as increased intracranial pressure, spinal cord injuries, and abdominal aneurysm resection contraindicate the positional changes of postural drainage. Thoracic trauma or surgery contraindicates percussion and vibration.
- Know the patient's level of cognitive function. Participation in controlled coughing techniques requires the patient to follow instructions. Congenital or acquired cognitive limitations alter a patient's ability to learn and participate in these techniques.
- Be aware of the patient's exercise tolerance. CPT maneuvers are fatiguing (Strickland, 2015).

---

chest percussion and vibration. It aids in improving secretion clearance and oxygenation. Positioning involves draining affected lung segments (Table 41.6) and helps to drain secretions from those segments of the lungs and bronchi into the trachea. Some patients do not require postural drainage of all lung segments. Clinical assessment is crucial in identifying specific lung segments requiring it. For example, patients with left lower lobe atelectasis require postural drainage of only the affected region, whereas a child with CF often requires postural drainage of all lung segments (CFF, n.d.a; Hockenberry et al., 2019; Harding et al., 2020).

Manual chest percussion involves rhythmically clapping on the chest wall over the area being drained to force secretions into larger airways for expectoration (Strickland et al., 2013). It is commonly performed by respiratory therapists in larger health care settings. Position your hand so that the fingers and thumb touch and the hands are cupped. The cupping makes the hand conform to the chest wall while trapping a cushion of air to soften the intensity of the clapping. The procedure should produce a hollow sound and should not be painful. Perform chest percussion by vigorously striking the chest wall alternately with cupped hands (Fig. 41.8). Perform percussion over a single layer of clothing, not over buttons, snaps, or zippers. The single layer of clothing prevents slapping the patient's skin. Thicker or multiple layers of material dampen the vibrations. Percussion is contraindicated in patients with bleeding disorders, osteoporosis, or fractured ribs. Avoid percussion over burns, open wounds, or skin infections of the thorax. Take caution to percuss the lung fields under the ribs and not over the spine, breastbone, stomach, or lower back or trauma can occur to the spleen, liver, or kidneys. Commercial devices that are shaped similar to cups are also available to use to perform manual chest percussion (CFF, n.d.a).

Vibration is a gentle shaking pressure applied to the chest wall only during exhalation to shake secretions into larger airways. This pressure can be applied either manually or with a commercially available device. Vibration may be tolerated better than percussion. You use vibration most often with patients with CF (CFF, n.d.a).

High-frequency chest wall compression (HFCWC) consists of an inflatable vest that is attached to an air-pulse generator (Fig. 41.9). HFCWC loosens and removes secretions from the airway by delivering high-frequency, small-volume expiratory pulses to a patient's external chest wall. The vest can be worn over clothes. This therapy is beneficial for patients with neuromuscular diseases and for patients with chronic lung diseases with thick sputum, such as CF (Strickland, 2015; Strickland et al., 2013).

Positive Expiratory Pressure. Positive expiratory pressure (PEP) is an airway clearance technique that can be used with and without oscillation. Its use is typically reserved for patients with CF or other lung diseases in which sputum is retained (Franks et al., 2019; Strickland, 2015). The Acapella and Flutter devices are commonly used PEP devices (Fig. 41.10). PEP allows air to be inhaled easily but forces the patient to exhale against resistance. This action helps air get behind the mucus, which then makes it easier to expectorate the mucus (CFF, n.d.c; Franks et al., 2019). Patients must be physically capable of maintaining a seal with their mouth around the device.

Maintenance and Promotion of Lung Expansion. Nursing interventions to maintain or promote lung expansion include noninvasive techniques such as ambulation, positioning, and incentive spirometry.

Ambulation. Immobility is a major factor in developing atelectasis, ventilator-associated pneumonia (VAP), and functional limitations, including muscle weakness and fatigue (Nuwi and Irwan, 2018). This decline in status is often referred to as deconditioning. Early-ambulation studies indicate that the therapeutic benefits of activity include an increase in general strength and lung expansion. Even the patient who requires invasive mechanical ventilation benefits by an early-mobility program. Such mobility programs should include input from both respiratory and physical therapists in the treatment plan. Progressive mobilization from dangling the legs to standing and then walking is safe for intubated patients (Hartjes, 2018) (see Chapter 38).

Positioning. A person who is healthy and completely mobile maintains adequate ventilation and oxygenation by frequent position changes during daily activities. However, when a person's illness or injury restricts mobility, the risk for respiratory impairment increases.

TABLE 41.6 Positions for Postural Drainage

Lung Segment	Position of Patient	Lung Segment	Position of Patient
Adult—Make sure to assess patient prior to positioning. Some patients, such as those with head injuries, heart failure, or pulmonary embolus, should not be placed in the Trendelenburg position (Harding et al., 2020).			
Bilateral	High-Fowler's	Left lower lobe—lateral segment	Right side-lying in Trendelenburg's position
Apical segments	Sitting on side of bed	Right lower lobe—lateral segment	Left side-lying in Trendelenburg's position
Right upper lobe—anterior segment	Supine with head elevated	Right lower lobe—posterior segment	Prone with right side of chest elevated in Trendelenburg's position
Left upper lobe—anterior segment	Supine with head elevated	Right middle lobe—posterior segment	Prone with thorax and abdomen elevated
Right upper lobe—posterior segment	Side-lying with right side of chest elevated on pillows	Both lower lobes—anterior segments	Supine in Trendelenburg's position
Left upper lobe—posterior segment	Side-lying with left side of chest elevated on pillows	Both lower lobes—posterior segments	Prone in Trendelenburg's position
Right middle lobe—anterior segment	Three-fourths supine position with dependent lung in Trendelenburg's position		

FIG. 41.8 Chest wall percussion, alternating hand clapping against patient's chest wall.

FIG. 41.9 High-frequency chest wall oscillation vest for home use. (Copyright © 2012 Hill-Rom Services, Inc. Reprinted with permission. All rights reserved.)

FIG. 41.10 Acapella airway clearance device. (Courtesy Smiths Medical North America.)

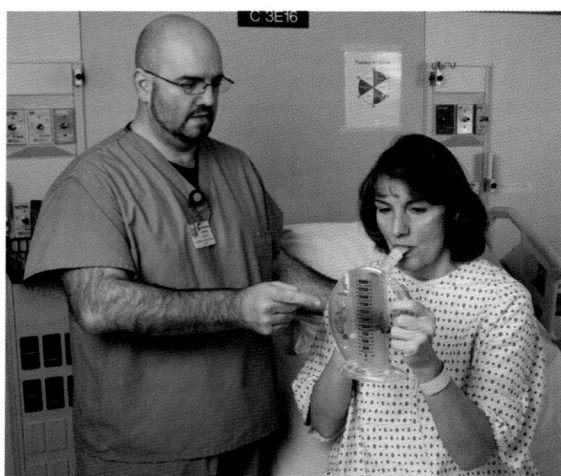

FIG. 41.11 Volume-oriented incentive spirometer.

Frequent changes of position are simple and cost-effective methods for reducing stasis of pulmonary secretions and decreased chest wall expansion, both of which increase the risk of pneumonia.

The 45-degree semi-Fowler's position is the most effective to promote lung expansion and reduce pressure from the abdomen on the diaphragm. When a patient is in this position, be sure that the patient does not slide down in bed, which can reduce lung expansion. Sliding also increases the risk of pressure injuries. Position a patient with unilateral lung disease, such as pneumothorax, atelectasis, or pneumonia of one lung, in a manner to promote perfusion of the healthy lung and improve oxygenation. In most cases, you position the patient with the good lung down. The majority of patients with COVID-19 who develop ARDS and are mechanically ventilated improve their oxygenation in the prone position, likely due to a better ventilation-perfusion matching (Langer et al., 2021). In the presence of pulmonary abscess or hemorrhage, position the patient with the affected lung down to prevent drainage toward the healthy lung.

Incentive Spirometry. Incentive spirometry encourages voluntary deep breathing by providing visual feedback to patients about inspiratory volume. It is a commonly used intervention that promotes deep breathing and is thought to prevent or treat atelectasis in the postoperative patient. Recent evidence suggests that the use of the incentive spirometer is not as effective at preventing postoperative pulmonary complications

as it once was thought to be. The AARC recommends that its use be reserved for patients with existing atelectasis or those with risk factors for developing atelectasis, such as those who have undergone thoracic or abdominal surgery, patients with prolonged bed rest, or patients with neuromuscular disease or spinal cord injuries (Eltorai et al., 2018).

There are two types of incentive spirometers. Flow-oriented incentive spirometers consist of one or more plastic chambers that contain freely moving colored balls. A patient inhales slowly and with an even flow to elevate the balls and keep them floating as long as possible to ensure a maximally sustained inhalation. Volume-oriented incentive spirometry devices have a bellows that is raised to a predetermined volume by an inhaled breath (Fig. 41.11). An achievement light or counter provides visual feedback. Some devices are constructed so the light does not turn on unless the bellows is held at a minimum desired volume for a specified period to enhance lung expansion (see Chapter 50).

The AARC guidelines (2011) recommend 5 to 10 breaths per session every hour while awake. Administration of pain medications before incentive spirometry helps a patient achieve deep breathing by reducing pain and splinting. Use incentive spirometry in combination with other pulmonary measures, such as deep breathing and coughing, and early mobilization in patients who are a risk for atelectasis (Hanada et al., 2020).

Maintenance of Patent Airway. Nursing interventions aimed at maintaining airway patency include artificial airway management and airway suctioning.

Artificial Airways. An artificial airway is for a patient with a decreased level of consciousness or airway obstruction or who is in need of prolonged ventilatory support and aids in removal of tracheobronchial secretions and maintaining a patent airway. The presence of an artificial airway places a patient at high risk for infection and airway injury. Use clean technique for oral airways but use sterile technique in

FIG. 41.12 Artificial oral airways.

FIG. 41.13 Endotracheal tube inserted into trachea. Cuff inflated to maintain position. (Copyright © 2015 Medtronic. All rights reserved. Used with the permission of Medtronic.)

caring for and maintaining endotracheal and tracheal airways to prevent health care–associated infections (HAIs). Artificial airways need to stay in the correct position to prevent airway damage (Urden et al., 2020; Wiegand, 2017) (see Skill 41.2).

Oral Airway. The oral airway, the simplest type of artificial airway, prevents obstruction of the trachea by displacement of the tongue into the oropharynx (Fig. 41.12). The oral airway extends from the teeth to the oropharynx, maintaining the tongue in the normal position. Determine the proper oral airway size by measuring the distance from the corner of the mouth to the angle of the jaw just below the ear. The length is equal to the distance from the flange of the airway to the tip. Use only the correct size airway. If the airway is too small, the tongue does not stay in the anterior portion of the mouth; if the airway is too large, it forces the tongue toward the epiglottis and obstructs the airway (Wiegand, 2017).

Insert the airway upside down, then turn the curve of the airway toward the cheek and place it over the tongue. When the airway is in the oropharynx, turn it so that the opening points downward. Correctly placed, the airway moves the tongue forward away from the oropharynx, and the flange (e.g., the flat portion of the airway) rests against the patient's teeth. Incorrect insertion merely forces the tongue back into the oropharynx (Wiegand, 2017).

Endotracheal and Tracheal Airways. An **endotracheal (ET) tube** is a short-term artificial airway used to administer invasive mechanical ventilation, relieve upper airway obstruction, protect against aspiration, or clear secretions. A physician or specially trained clinician inserts the ET tube. The tube is passed through the patient's mouth, past the pharynx, and into the trachea (Fig. 41.13). It is generally removed within 14 days; however, it is sometimes used for a longer period of time if the patient is still showing progress toward weaning from invasive mechanical ventilation and extubation (removal of the endotracheal tube) (Urden et al., 2020; Wiegand, 2017).

If a patient requires long-term assistance from an artificial airway, a **tracheostomy** is performed with insertion of a tracheostomy tube (TT). A TT is inserted either surgically or percutaneously directly into the trachea through a small incision made in a patient's neck. Reasons for a TT include the need for prolonged mechanical ventilation, upper airway obstruction secondary to trauma or tumor, or difficulties with airway clearance that can occur in conditions such as spinal cord injury or neuromuscular disease (Urden et al., 2020). Most tracheostomy tubes have a small plastic inner tube that fits inside a larger one (the inner cannula). The most common complication of a tracheostomy tube is partial or total airway obstruction caused by buildup of respiratory secretions. If this occurs, the inner tube can

be removed and cleaned or replaced with a temporary spare inner tube that should be kept at the patient's bedside. Keep tracheal dilators at the bedside to have available for emergency tube replacement or reinsertion. Humidification from air humidifiers or humidified oxygen tracheostomy collars can help prevent drying of secretions that cause occlusion. Perform tracheostomy suctioning as necessary to clear secretions. Tracheal suctioning has complications, including hypoxemia, cardiac dysrhythmias, changes in blood pressure (can be either hypertensive or hypotensive), laryngeal or bronchospasm, pain, infection, or bradycardia. Bradycardia is associated with stimulation of the vagus nerve. Respiratory or cardiac arrest can even occur as a result of tracheal suctioning. The majority of patients with a tracheostomy tube cannot speak because the tube is inserted below the vocal cords. It is important to use written or nonverbal communication (lipreading) strategies to help patients communicate. Be sure to assess patients for anxiety caused by the inability to speak. Care and cleaning of the tracheostomy tube is discussed in Skill 41.2 (Urden et al., 2020; Wiegand, 2017).

Open and Closed Airway Suctioning. The two current methods of airway suctioning are the open and closed methods. Suctioning through the nose into the trachea and pharynx and in established long-term tracheostomies is more commonly performed using open suction. When a patient is on a ventilator, open suctioning is performed by introducing the catheter through a port where the endotracheal tube connects to the ventilator. Open suctioning is sometimes necessary with ventilated patients who need to have sputum specimens obtained. Open suctioning involves the use of a new sterile catheter for each suction session (Wiegand, 2017). Wear sterile gloves and follow Standard Precautions during the suction procedure.

Closed suctioning involves the use of a suction catheter system that is included in the ventilatory circuit of a patient on a mechanical ventilator. The reusable sterile suction catheter is encased in a plastic sheath to protect it between suction sessions (see Skill 41.1). Closed suction is used on new artificial airways, endotracheal and tracheal tubes, and allows you to introduce the suction catheter into the airways without disconnecting a patient from the ventilator. Closed suctioning supports a patient's respiratory efforts because it permits continuous delivery of oxygen while suction is performed and reduces the risk of oxygen desaturation. Although sterile gloves are not used in this procedure, nonsterile gloves are recommended to prevent contact with splashes from body fluids (see Skill 41.1). When comparing open versus closed suction, there is a decreased risk of infection for a health care provider from exposure to patient secretions with a closed system and a decrease in the development of late-onset ventilator-associated pneumonia for the patient (Letchford and Bench, 2018; Urden et al., 2020).

Suctioning Techniques. Suctioning of the pharyngeal and tracheal airways is needed when patients are unable to clear respiratory secretions. When secretions are only in the mouth, oropharyngeal suction (Skill 41.1) is indicated. Secretions that are not removed are more likely to be aspirated into the lungs, increasing the risk for infection, ventilator-associated pneumonia (VAP), and respiratory failure. Suctioning techniques include oropharyngeal and nasopharyngeal suctioning, orotracheal and nasotracheal suctioning, and suctioning an artificial airway.

In most cases, use sterile technique for suctioning because the oropharynx and trachea are considered sterile. The mouth is considered only clean, so it requires clean technique. When suctioning both the oral pharynx and the trachea, always suction the trachea (sterile) before the oral pharynx (clean) (Wiegand, 2017).

Each type of suctioning requires the use of a round-tipped, flexible catheter with holes on the sides and end of the catheter. When suctioning, you apply negative pressures (80-150 mm Hg for adults) during withdrawal of the catheter and **never** on insertion (Urden et al., 2020; Wiegand, 2017). Patient assessment determines the frequency of suctioning. It is indicated when rhonchi, gurgling breath sounds, and diminished breath sounds are audible on auscultation or visible secretions are present after other methods to remove airway secretions have failed. You may also use suctioning to obtain a sputum specimen for culture or cytology if the patient is unable to cough productively. There is no evidence to support suctioning on a scheduled basis. Too-frequent suctioning puts patients at risk for development of hypoxemia, hypotension, arrhythmias, and possible trauma to the mucosa of the lungs (Urden et al., 2020; Wiegand, 2017).

Oropharyngeal and Nasopharyngeal Suctioning. Perform oropharyngeal or nasopharyngeal suctioning when a patient is able to cough effectively but is unable to clear secretions by expectorating. Apply suction after a patient has coughed (see Skill 41.1). Once the pulmonary secretions decrease and a patient is less fatigued, the patient is then able to expectorate or swallow the mucus, and suctioning is no longer necessary.

Orotracheal and Nasotracheal Suctioning. Perform orotracheal or nasotracheal suctioning when a patient with pulmonary secretions is unable to manage secretions by coughing and does not have an artificial airway present (see Skill 41.1). You pass a sterile catheter through the mouth or nose into the trachea. The nose is the preferred route because stimulation of the gag reflex is minimal. The procedure is similar to nasopharyngeal suctioning, but you advance the catheter tip farther into the patient's trachea. The entire procedure from catheter passage to its removal is done quickly, lasting no longer than 10 to 15 seconds (Wiegand, 2017). Allow the patient to rest between passes of the catheter. If the patient develops respiratory distress, stop suctioning unless the collection of secretions is causing distress. If the patient is using supplemental oxygen, replace the oxygen cannula or mask during rest periods.

Tracheal Suctioning. Perform tracheal suctioning through an artificial airway such as an ET or TT. Use the smallest catheter possible, but ensure that it is large enough to remove secretions. Never apply suction pressure while inserting the catheter to avoid traumatizing the lung mucosa. Once you insert a catheter the necessary distance, maintain suction pressure between 80 and 120 mm Hg (Wiegand, 2017) as you withdraw. Apply suction intermittently only while withdrawing the catheter. Rotating the catheter enhances removal of secretions that have adhered to the sides of the airway.

The practice of normal saline instillation (NSI) into artificial airways to improve secretion removal may be harmful and is not recommended. Clinical studies comparing the results of suctioning following NSI with standard suctioning have not shown any clinical or significant results (Wang et al., 2017).

REFLECT NOW

You are caring for a patient with cystic fibrosis. When entering the room, you note the patient to be in a supine position and complaining of a frequent, nonproductive cough. What interventions can you perform to help increase the patient's ability to expectorate the sputum?

Maintenance of Ventilation. A variety of conditions either affect a patient's ability to ventilate normally or affect the level of oxygenation and require artificial support for cardiopulmonary gas exchange. Invasive medical interventions, such as mechanical ventilation, noninvasive ventilation, and chest tube insertion and managment assist in restoring the ventilatory capacity of the lungs.

Invasive Mechanical Ventilation. Invasive mechanical ventilation, also referred to as positive-pressure ventilation, is a lifesaving technique used with artificial airways (ET or tracheostomy) for various physiological and clinical indications. Physiological indications for invasive mechanical ventilation include supporting cardiopulmonary gas exchange (alveolar ventilation and arterial oxygenation), increasing lung volume (ventilation), and reducing the work of breathing (Urden et al., 2020). Clinical indications for invasive mechanical ventilation include reversing hypoxia and acute respiratory acidosis; relieving respiratory distress; preventing or reversing atelectasis and respiratory muscle fatigue; allowing for sedation and/or other neuromuscular blockade, thereby decreasing oxygen consumption; and stabilizing the chest wall (Urden et al., 2020). It can be used to either fully or partially replace spontaneous breathing, depending on the need of the patient. Invasive mechanical ventilation also redistributes oxygen demand from working respiratory muscles to other vital organs.

Ventilator-associated pneumonia (VAP) is a common health-associated infection (HAI) in the intensive care unit (ICU). It is associated with increased hospital length of stay, increased mortality, and increased hospital costs of an estimated $40,000 per patient (Alja'afreh et al., 2019; Ferrer and Torres, 2018; Letchford and Bench, 2018). VAP is typically described as pneumonia that develops greater than 48 hours after insertion of artificial airway or initiation of mechanical ventilation and is a type of ventilator-associated event (VAE) (CDC, 2021c; Ferrer and Torres, 2018) (Box 41.8). Hospitals are not reimbursed for costs associated with VAP.

Noninvasive Ventilation. Noninvasive positive-pressure ventilation (NPPV), a form of noninvasive ventilation (NIV), maintains positive airway pressure and improves alveolar ventilation without the need for an artificial airway. There are two types of NPPV: continuous positive airway pressure (CPAP) and bilevel positive airway pressure (BiPAP). BiPAP and CPAP are usually applied via a mask covering the nose or both the mouth and nose, but those who require home CPAP may wear nasal prongs instead (Hill et al., 2019; Rochwerg et al., 2017).

NPPV is used both in acute care settings and increasingly more in home care settings to treat a variety of conditions, including obstructive sleep apnea (OSA), chronic obstructive pulmonary disease (COPD),

BOX 41.8 EVIDENCE-BASED PRACTICE

Effect of Adherence to a Ventilator Care Bundle on Reducing Ventilator-Associated Pneumonia

PICOT Question: In critically ill patients requiring invasive mechanical ventilation, does adhering to an evidence-based ventilator care bundle contribute to a reduction of ventilator-associated pneumonia (VAP)?

Evidence Summary

Ventilator-associated pneumonia (VAP) is a health care–acquired infection (HAI) that develops in a person requiring invasive mechanical ventilation (via endotracheal intubation or tracheostomy tube) for at least 48 hours (Alja'afreh et al., 2019; Ferrer and Torres, 2018). *Pseudomonas, Acinetobacter,* and methicillin-resistant *Staphylococcus aureus* are frequent bacterial causes of VAP (Chacko et al., 2017). Patients with VAP have fever, increased secretions, and pulmonary infiltrates seen on chest radiograph. Over time these infiltrates progressively increase, and the patient's lung functions decline. VAP increases length of stay in the intensive care unit, is associated with increased morbidity and mortality, and increases the patient's cost of hospitalization.

In 2012, the Institute for Healthcare Improvement published an evidence-based how-to guide for the prevention of VAP (IHI, 2012). This guide was the beginning of a series of evidence-based interventions related to ventilator care that, when implemented together, achieve significantly better outcomes than when implemented individually (Bassi et al., 2017). The key components of the VAP bundle include:

- Use of proper hand hygiene measures before and after patient contact
- Elevation of the head of the bed to at least 30 degrees, unless contraindicated
- Oral hygiene care with chlorhexidine at least twice a day (AACN, 2017a; Alja'afreh et al., 2019)
- Peptic ulcer prophylaxis (Virk and Wiersinga, 2019)
- Daily "sedation vacations" and assessment of readiness to extubate
- Venous thromboembolism prophylaxis
- Delirium monitoring

- Use of silver-coated endotracheal tubes when possible (Tokmaji et al., 2018; Rouzé et al., 2017)

The use of probiotics has not been shown to have an effect on VAP rates (Mahmoodpoor et al., 2019). Their safety has not been established for use in critically ill patients (Virk and Wiersinga, 2019).

Application to Nursing Practice

- Implement the VAP bundle when mechanical ventilation is initiated (Anand et al., 2018).
- Avoid prolonged supine positioning. Pulmonary aspiration is increased by supine positioning and pooling of secretions above the ET tube cuff (AACN, 2018).
- Position the patient with head-of-bed (HOB) elevation to 45 degrees or higher significantly reduces gastric reflux and VAP.
- Use orotracheal and orogastric tubes when possible rather than nasal devices to reduce the risk of VAP (Rouzé et al., 2017).
- Initiate early mobilization (Bassi et al., 2017).
- Suction oropharyngeal and subglottic secretions to reduce the risk of early-onset VAP. Utilize subglottic suctioning to decrease the amount of secretions that pool in the oropharyngeal cavity (Bassi et al., 2017; Huang et al., 2018).
- Perform endotracheal and tracheostomy tube suctioning only when indicated by patient assessment findings and not on a scheduled basis.
- Monitor cuff pressure of the endotracheal and tracheostomy tubes frequently to ensure that there is an adequate seal to prevent aspiration of secretions. Maintain airway cuff pressure between 20–30 mm Hg (AACN, 2017b).
- Always drain ventilator circuit condensation away from patient and into the appropriate receptacle. Drain the tubing hourly to prevent accumulation.
- Assess for and treat delirium.
- Change ventilator circuits only when dirty or contaminated and not on a routine basis (AACN, 2017b).

---

cardiogenic pulmonary edema, hypoxic and/or hypercapnic respiratory failure, and neuromuscular disorders. It is commonly used in these conditions to avoid the complications of invasive ventilation strategies, including pneumonia and aspiration. It should not be used in patients who cannot protect their airway or in patients with an inadequate respiratory drive or apnea, and it should be used with caution in patients with asthma, facial injuries, and patients who are uncooperative or hemodynamically unstable (Ghosh and Elliott, 2019; Hill et al., 2019).

The advantages of this type of ventilation versus invasive ventilation include an increased ability to communicate with caregivers and family, better ability to cough and clear secretions, and allowance for eating and drinking, if stable and not at risk for aspiration. There are disadvantages, problems, and concerns to this type of ventilation. The mask must fit tightly and have a good seal to prevent air from leaking. This pressure can cause feelings of claustrophobia and intolerance in patients, which can lead to issues with adherence to therapy. The tight-fitting mask can also lead to medical device–related pressure injuries (MDRPI), particularly on the bridge of the nose (Hill et al., 2019; Jackson et al., 2019; Wiegand, 2017).

Continuous positive airway pressure (CPAP) maintains a steady stream of pressure throughout a patient's breathing cycle. It benefits patients with obstructive sleep apnea (OSA), patients with heart failure, and preterm infants with underdeveloped lungs. In obstructive sleep apnea (OSA), the upper airway collapses, causing obstruction that leads to shallow or absent breathing. Any air moving past the obstruction results in loud snoring. An overnight sleep study may be needed to determine the need and the correct settings for a CPAP

machine (see Chapter 43). Equipment includes a mask (Fig. 41.14) that fits over the nose or both nose and mouth and a CPAP machine that delivers air to the mask. The smallest mask with the proper fit is the most effective. It must be tight enough to form a seal on the face so that the air does not escape but not so tight as to cause pressure injury formation or necrosis where the mask is against the face.

Bilevel positive airway pressure (BiPAP) works by providing assistance during inspiration and preventing alveolar closure during expiration. It provides both inspiratory positive airway pressure (IPAP) and expiratory airway pressure (EPAP), also known as *positive end-expiratory pressure (PEEP)*. During inhalation the positive pressure increases the patient's tidal volume and alveolar ventilation. The pressure support decreases when the patient exhales, allowing for easier exhalation. The overall result of BiPAP is an increased amount of air in the lungs at the end of expiration (functional residual capacity), reduced airway closure, expansion of areas of atelectasis, and improved oxygenation (Hartjes, 2018; Urden et al., 2020).

Complications of noninvasive ventilation include facial and nasal injury and skin breakdown, dry mucous membranes and thick secretions, and aspiration of gastric contents if vomiting occurs (AACN, 2018). Complications avoided by noninvasive ventilation are VAP, sinusitis, and the effects of large-dose sedative agents. Use of noninvasive ventilation results in shorter intensive care unit (ICU) and hospital stays (Ghosh and Elliot, 2019).

Chest Tubes. A **chest tube** (Fig. 41.15) is a catheter inserted through the rib cage into the pleural space to remove air, fluids, or blood; to

FIG. 41.14 CPAP mask. ResMed's AirFit N30™. (© ResMed. All rights reserved.)

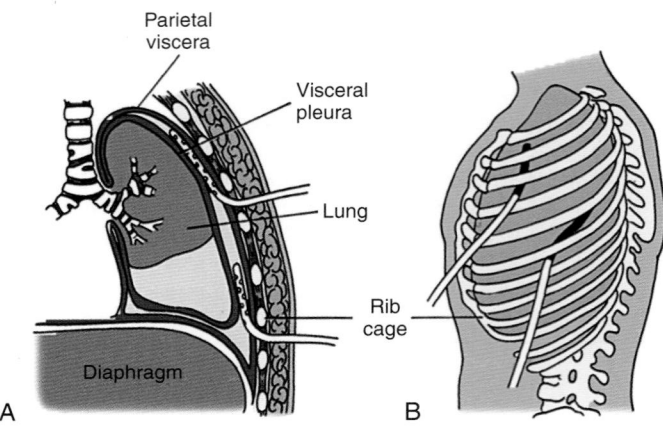

FIG. 41.15 Diagram of sites for chest tube placement. (A) Anatomical drawing of upper tube placement for removal of air and lower tube placement for blood and fluid. (B) View of tubes exiting through intra-costal sites.

prevent air or fluid from reentering the pleural space; or to reestablish normal intrapleural and intrapulmonic pressures after trauma or surgery (Chotai and Mosenifar, 2018). Chest tubes are common after chest surgery and chest trauma and are used for treatment of pneumothorax or hemothorax to promote lung reexpansion (see Skill 41.3).

A **pneumothorax** is a collection of air in the pleural space. The loss of negative intrapleural pressure causes the lung to collapse. There are a variety of causes for a pneumothorax. A pneumothorax can occur as a result of chest trauma (e.g., stabbing, gunshot wound, or rib fracture). Other causes of pneumothorax are the rupture of an emphysematous bleb on the surface of the lung (the destruction caused by emphysema), tearing of the pleura from an invasive procedure such as surgery, insertion of a subclavian IV line, and invasive mechanical ventilation, including PEEP. Spontaneous pneumothorax occurs due to the rupture of small blebs (air-filled sacs). A spontaneous pneumothorax can occur in young, healthy individuals or in patients with a history of lung disease such as COPD or CF (Harding et al., 2020). A patient with a pneumothorax usually feels sharp pain that is pleuritic and worsens on inspiration. Dyspnea is common and worsens as the size of the pneumothorax increases.

A tension pneumothorax is a life-threatening condition in which air enters the pleural space and cannot escape. The accumulation of air eventually leads to compression of the affected lung and pressure on the heart, causing the heart and great vessels to shift to the unaffected side. This shift then leads to compression of the unaffected lung, leading to decreased oxygenation and decreased cardiac output. Clinical manifestations include dyspnea, tachycardia, tracheal deviation laterally, and absent breath sounds on the affected side. A tension pneumothorax is a medical emergency and requires immediate intervention, including needle decompression and chest tube placement (Sasa, 2019; Urden et al., 2020).

A **hemothorax** is an accumulation of blood and fluid in the pleural space, usually as a result of trauma. It produces a counter pressure and prevents the lung from full expansion. A rupture of small blood vessels from inflammatory processes such as pneumonia or TB can cause a hemothorax, as can trauma. In addition to pain and dyspnea, signs and symptoms of shock develop if blood loss is severe (Harding et al., 2020; Urden et al., 2020).

A variety of chest tubes are available to drain air or excess fluid from the pleural space to relieve respiratory distress. Typically, a small-bore chest tube (12 to 20 Fr) is used to remove a small amount of air, and a larger-bore chest tube (greater than 20 Fr) is used to remove large amounts of fluid or blood (Urden et al., 2010; Wiegand, 2017).

After a chest tube is inserted, it is attached to a drainage system. A traditional chest drainage unit (CDU) has three chambers for collection of drainage, water seal, and suction control. This unit can drain a large amount of both fluid and air. Disposable chest drainage systems, such as the Codman, Pleur-evac, or Atrium, allow for more mobility than previous bottle systems and are now more commonly used. The disposable systems also allow for increased ability to maintain sterility of the system (Chotai and Mosenifar, 2018). Patients who are not on ventilators and patients who had thoracoscopic lung surgery or minimally invasive cardiac surgery do well with these mobile chest drains.

Special Considerations. Keep a chest tube drainage system closed and below the chest (see Skill 41.3). The chest tube should be secured to the chest wall. Watch for slow, steady bubbling in the water-seal chamber, and keep it filled with sterile water at the prescribed level. A constant or intermittent bubbling in the water-seal chamber, or new more vigorous bubbling, indicates a leak in the drainage system or another pneumothorax, and you must assess the system and the patient to accurately identify the source of the leak. Watch for fluctuation (tidaling) of the fluid level to ensure that the chest tube and system are working. Mark the level on the outside of the collection chambers every shift. Report any unexpected cloudy or bloody drainage. Avoid kinks and dependent loops in the tubing. Ideally, it should lie horizontally across the bed or chair before dropping vertically into the drainage device. Encourage your patient to cough, breathe deeply, and use the incentive spirometer. Make sure that the patient is in a semi-Fowler's or high Fowler's (45 to 90 degrees) position and is ambulated if not contraindicated. Routinely evaluate respiratory rate, breath sounds, SpO$_2$ levels, and the insertion site for subcutaneous emphysema (Chotai and Mosenifar, 2018). Subcutaneous emphysema is the presence of air under the skin, and crepitus is palpated in the area where it is located (Hartjes, 2018).

Clamping a chest tube is contraindicated when ambulating or transporting a patient. Clamping can result in a tension pneumothorax. Air pressure builds in the pleural space, collapsing the lung and creating a life-threatening event. A chest tube is clamped only when replacing the chest drainage system, assessing for an air leak, or as a trial before removal to assess whether the air leak has stopped. Stripping or milking chest tubes to keep them patent is based on nursing assessment and may be necessary to remove clots in the tube (Chotai and Mosenifar, 2018). Routine milking or stripping of the chest tubes is not recommended as it can cause increased intrathoracic pressure and tissue damage (Wiegand, 2017).

Handle the chest drainage unit carefully and maintain the drainage device below the patient's chest. The drainage unit should always be maintained in an upright position. If it is knocked over, replacement of the unit is needed (Chotai and Mosenifar, 2018).

Removal of chest tubes requires patient preparation. The most frequent sensations reported by patients during chest tube removal include burning, pain, and a pulling sensation. Make sure that the patient receives pain medication at least 30 minutes before removal. Assist the health care provider in removing the chest tube and monitor the dressing placed over the insertion site and the patient's respiratory status after tube removal (Wiegand, 2017). An unplanned removal of the chest tube, such as the tube being accidentally removed while repositioning the patient, requires you to cover the site with a gloved hand and ask for help in retrieving supplies to cover the site. Petrolatum gauze, dry gauze, and tape will be needed to dress the site. If the chest tube becomes disconnected from the drainage system, clamp the tubing with a shodded hemostat or crimp the tubing with a gloved hand to prevent air from entering the pleural space. Ask for someone to get a new chest drainage system and attach it to the chest tube in a sterile manner. Regardless of how the tube comes out, monitor the patient for signs of respiratory distress and auscultate lung sounds (Urden et al., 2020; Muzzy and Butler, 2015).

Maintenance and Promotion of Oxygenation. Promotion of lung expansion, mobilization of secretions, and maintenance of a patent airway assist patients in meeting their oxygenation needs. However, some patients also require oxygen therapy to keep a healthy level of tissue oxygenation.

Oxygen Therapy. Oxygen therapy is widely available and used in a variety of settings to relieve or prevent hypoxia, which can lead to hypoxemia. The goal of oxygen therapy is to prevent or relieve hypoxemia by delivering the lowest amount of oxygen possible to achieve adequate tissue oxygenation (Walsh and Smallwood, 2017). The dosage or concentration of oxygen is monitored continuously. Routinely check the health care provider's orders to verify that the patient is receiving the prescribed oxygen concentration. The seven rights of medication administration also pertain to oxygen administration (see Chapter 31).

Supplemental oxygen therapy offers many benefits to patients with acute and/or chronic cardiopulmonary diseases. This therapy reduces mortality, increases exercise tolerance, decreases pulmonary hypertension, and improves a patient's quality of life (Wen et al., 2017). It is important to explain to your patients why they may require supplemental oxygen in the acute care setting, as well as possible home use (Box 41.9).

Safety Precautions. Oxygen is a highly combustible gas. Although it does not burn spontaneously or cause an explosion, it can easily cause a fire when exposed to a naked flame or electrical spark (Moore, 2019). With increasing use of home oxygen therapy, patients and health care professionals need to be aware of the dangers of oxygen therapy combustion (Moore, 2019). Be cognizant of agency procedures for managing a fire or know the local emergency response phone number (often 911) in case of a fire at a patient's home.

Follow these oxygen safety precautions:

- Oxygen is a therapeutic gas and must be prescribed and adjusted only with a health care provider's order. Distribution must be in accordance with federal, state, and local regulations (Jacobs et al., 2018).
- Oxygen is a combustible substance. Determine that all electrical equipment in the room is functioning correctly and properly grounded (see Chapter 27). An electrical spark in the presence of oxygen can result in a serious fire as oxygen supports combustion.

BOX 41.9 PROCEDURAL GUIDELINES

Applying a Nasal Cannula or Oxygen Mask

Delegation and Collaboration

The skill of applying a nasal cannula or oxygen mask can be delegated to assistive personnel (AP) after the method of delivery and percentage of oxygen needed by a patient is determined. The nurse is responsible for assessing the patient's respiratory system and the response to oxygen therapy. The nurse, in some agencies, may collaborate with the respiratory therapist in the setup of oxygen therapy, including adjustment of oxygen flow rate. The nurse instructs the AP to:

- Safely adjust the device (e.g., loosening the strap on the oxygen cannula or mask) and clarify its correct placement and positioning.
- Inform the nurse immediately about any changes in vital signs; changes in pulse oximetry (SpO_2); changes in level of consciousness (LOC); skin irritation from the cannula, mask, or straps; or patient complaints of pain or shortness of breath.
- Provide extra skin care around patient's ears and nose or other parts of the patient's body that might be irritated by the device.

Equipment

(**NOTE:** If device is used in the home, the home care equipment vendor provides the equipment.)

Oxygen-delivery device as ordered by health care provider; oxygen tubing (consider extension tubing as needed); humidifier, if indicated; sterile water for humidifier; oxygen source; oxygen flowmeter; "Oxygen in use" sign; pulse oximeter; stethoscope; clean gloves; additional personal protective equipment as needed, e.g. face shield, if risk of splash from secretions is present.

Procedural Steps

1. Identify patient using at least two identifiers (e.g., name and birthday or name and medical record number) according to agency policy. Compare identifiers with information on patient's MAR or medical record.
2. Review accuracy of health care provider's order for oxygen, noting delivery method, flow rate, duration of oxygen therapy, and parameters for titration of oxygen settings.
3. Obtain data from patient's electronic health record (vital signs, pulse oximetry, arterial blood gas values).
4. Assess for patient's or family caregiver's knowledge, experience, and health literacy.
5. Perform hand hygiene and apply gloves. Perform respiratory assessment, including symmetry of chest wall expansion, chest wall abnormalities (e.g., kyphosis), temporary conditions (e.g., pregnancy, trauma) affecting ventilation, respiratory rate and depth, sputum production, lung sounds, and signs and symptoms associated with hypoxia.
6. Inspect condition of skin around nose and ears. Note if patient has history of impaired sensation, poor perfusion, altered tissue tolerance, poor nutrition, edema, and the tendency for moisture to develop under device—all known risk factors for medical device–related pressure injury (MDRPI) (Fumarola et al., 2020).
7. Observe for cognitive and/or behavioral changes (e.g., apprehension, anxiety, confusion, decreased ability to concentrate, decreased LOC, fatigue, and dizziness).

Continued

BOX 41.9 PROCEDURAL GUIDELINES—cont'd

Applying a Nasal Cannula or Oxygen Mask

CLINICAL JUDGMENT: Patients with sudden changes in their vital signs, LOC, or behavior may be experiencing profound hypoxia. Patients who demonstrate subtle changes over time may have worsening of a chronic or existing condition or a new medical condition (Harding et al., 2020).

8. Assess airway patency and remove airway secretions by having patient cough and expectorate mucus or by suctioning (see Skill 41.1). **NOTE:** Continue to wear gloves. However, remove and dispose of gloves and perform hand hygiene if there is contact with mucus. Then reapply gloves if contact with mucus is likely.

CLINICAL JUDGMENT: Excessive amounts of secretions, signs of respiratory distress (increased work of breathing, increased respiratory rate), presence of rhonchi on auscultation, excessive coughing, or decrease in oxygen saturation indicate need for suctioning.

9. Apply face shield if risk of exposure to splashing mucus exists.
10. Attach oxygen-delivery device (e.g., cannula, mask) to oxygen tubing, and attach end of tubing to humidified oxygen source adjusted to prescribed flow rate (see illustration).
11. Apply oxygen device and check function:
    a. *Nasal cannula:* Place tips of the cannula into patient's nares. If tips are curved, they should point downward inside nostrils. Then loop cannula

tubing up and over patient's ears. Adjust lanyard so that cannula fits snugly but not too tight and without pressure to patient nares and ears (see illustration). Cannula is positioned properly in nares if oxygen flows through tips.

b. *Partial nonrebreather mask:* Plastic face mask seals tightly around mouth using adjustable straps. It is designed to get hold of the first 150 mL of exhaled air and hold it so that it can be used for the next inhalation. Thus, the reservoir fills on exhalation and almost collapses on inspiration. Reservoir should not collapse completely (see illustration).

c. *Oxygen-conserving cannula (Oximizer):* Fit as for nasal cannula. Reservoir is located under patient's nose and worn as a pendant (see illustration).

d. *Nonrebreather (NRB) mask:* Apply as regular mask. Contains one-way valves with reservoir. It is designed to fill with oxygen and as the oxygen depletes due to the patient's breathing, it gets filled with oxygen from an

STEP 11b Plastic face mask with reservoir bag.

STEP 10 Flowmeter attached to oxygen source.

STEP 11a Nasal cannula adjusted for proper fit.

STEP 11c Oxygen-reserving cannula. (From Lewis S, et al: *Medical-surgical nursing: assessment and management of clinical problems,* ed 9, St Louis, 2014, Mosby.)

BOX 41.9 **PROCEDURAL GUIDELINES—cont'd**

Applying a Nasal Cannula or Oxygen Mask

oxygen source. The exhaled air does not enter reservoir bag. The NRB helps in delivering high oxygen concentrations. It can be combined with nasal cannula to provide higher inspired oxygen concentration (F_iO_2).

 e. *Simple face mask* (see illustration): Used for short-term oxygen delivery.

 f. *Venturi mask* (see illustration): Apply as regular mask. Select appropriate flow rate (see Table 41.7).

STEP 11e Simple face mask.

STEP 11f Venturi mask.

 g. *High-flow nasal cannula* (see illustration): High-flow nasal cannula (HFNC) therapy is an oxygen supply system capable of delivering up to 100% humidified and heated oxygen at a flow rate of up to 60 liters per minute.

12. Verify setting on flowmeter and oxygen source for proper setup and prescribed flow rate.

13. Check cannula/mask every 4 hours or as agency policy indicates. Keep humidification container filled at all times.

CLINICAL JUDGMENT: Pressure from face masks can result in medical device–related pressure injuries (MDRPI). Patients with sensitive skin (e.g., older adults, the critically ill) will need more frequent skin assessments in areas under and around the face mask (see Chapter 48).

14. Post "Oxygen in use" signs on wall behind bed and at entrance to room.

15. Properly dispose of gloves (if used) and perform hand hygiene.

16. Place the nurse call system in an accessible location within the patient's reach.

17. Monitor patient's response to changes in oxygen flow rate with SpO_2. **NOTE:** Monitor arterial blood gases (ABGs) when ordered; however, obtaining ABG measurement is an invasive procedure, and ABGs are not measured frequently.

18. Perform physical assessment, auscultating lung sounds; palpating chest excursion; inspecting color and condition of skin; and observing for decreased anxiety, improved LOC and cognitive abilities, decreased fatigue, and absence of dizziness. Measure vital signs.

19. Assess adequacy of oxygen flow each shift or as agency policy dictates.

20. Observe patient's external ears, bridge of nose, nares, and nasal mucous membranes for evidence of MDRPI.

21. **Use Teach-Back:** "I want to be sure I explained how oxygen will help you. Tell me why oxygen is beneficial for you." Revise your instruction now or develop a plan for revised patient/family caregiver teaching if patient/family caregiver is not able to teach back correctly.

STEP 11g High-flow nasal cannula. (Courtesy Fischer & Paykel Healthcare.)

- Notify the local fire department that oxygen is used in the home (Fields et al., 2020).
- Keep oxygen-delivery systems 10 feet from any open flames.
- Be sure the home has working smoke detectors.
- When using oxygen cylinders, secure them so that they do not fall over. Store them upright and either chained or secured in appropriate holders.
- Check the oxygen level of portable tanks before transporting a patient to ensure that there is enough oxygen in the tank.
- Ensure that patients have adequate oxygen tubing to safely move around their agency or home environment.
- Inform power and phone companies that oxygen is used in the home, so they can prioritize restoring service in the case of a power outage (Fields et al., 2020).

Supply of Oxygen. Oxygen is supplied to a patient's bedside either by oxygen tanks or through a permanent wall-piped system. Oxygen tanks are transported on wide-based carriers that allow the tank to be placed upright at the bedside. Regulators control the amount of oxygen delivered. One common type is an upright flowmeter with a flow adjustment valve at the top. A second type is a cylinder indicator with a flow adjustment handle.

Methods of Oxygen Delivery. The nasal cannula and oxygen masks are the most common devices to deliver oxygen to patients. These devices deliver different levels of oxygen to patients (see Box 41.9; Table 41.7).

NASAL CANNULA. A nasal cannula has two nasal prongs that are slightly curved and inserted in a patient's nostrils. To keep the nasal prongs in place, fit the attached tubing over the patient's ears and secure it under the chin using the sliding connector. Assess patients for skin breakdown over the ears and in the nostrils, which is common when the oxygen tubing is placed tight against the skin. Attach the nasal cannula to an oxygen source with a flow rate of 1 to 6 L/min (24% to 44% oxygen). Flow rates equal to or greater than 4 L/min have a drying effect on the mucosa and thus need to be humidified (Hartjes, 2018). Know which flow rate produces a given percentage of inspired oxygen concentration (FiO_2).

HIGH-FLOW NASAL CANNULA. High-flow nasal cannula (HFNC) is a relatively new method of oxygen delivery. It provides heated, humidified oxygen through a nasal cannula at flow rates as high as 60 L/minute while an air-oxygen blender allows for the titration of the FiO_2. The

TABLE 41.7   Oxygen-Delivery Systems

Delivery System	FiO_2 Delivered	Advantages	Disadvantages
Low-Flow Delivery Devices			
Nasal cannula	1-6 L/min: 24%-44%	Safe and simple Easily tolerated Effective for low concentrations Does not impede eating or talking Inexpensive, disposable	Unable to use with nasal obstruction Drying to mucous membranes Can dislodge easily May cause skin irritation or breakdown around ears or nares Patient's breathing pattern (mouth or nasal) affects exact FiO_2
Oxygen-conserving cannula *(Oxymizer)*	8 L/min: up to 30%-50%	Indicated for long-term O_2 use in the home Allows increased O_2 concentration and lower flow	Cannula cannot be cleaned More expensive than standard cannula
Simple face mask	6-12 L/min: 35%-50%	Useful for short periods such as patient transportation	Contraindicated for patients who retain CO_2 May induce feelings of claustrophobia Therapy interrupted with eating and drinking Increased risk of aspiration
Partial and nonrebreather masks (**NOTE:** Reservoir bag should always remain partially inflated.)	10-15 L/min: 60%-90%	Useful for short periods Delivers increased FiO_2 Easily humidifies O_2 Does not dry mucous membranes	Hot and confining; may irritate skin; tight seal necessary Interferes with eating and talking Bag may twist or kink; should not totally deflate
High-Flow Delivery Devices			
Venturi mask	24%-50%	Provides specific amount of oxygen with humidity added Administers low, constant O_2	Mask and added humidity may irritate skin Therapy interrupted with eating and drinking Specific flow rate must be followed
High-flow nasal cannula	Adjustable FiO_2 (0.21-1) with modifiable flow (up to 60 L/min)	Wide range of FiO_2 Can use on adults, children, and infants	FiO_2 dependent on patient respiratory pattern and input flow Risk for infection (Urden et al., 2020)
Noninvasive Ventilation			
Continuous positive airway pressure (CPAP) and bilevel positive airway pressure (BiPAP)	21%-100%	Avoids the use of an artificial airway in some patients with acute respiratory distress, postextubation respiratory failure, or neuromuscular disorders Successfully treats obstructive sleep apnea	Nasal pillows/face masks can cause skin breakdown May cause claustrophobia in some patients

CO_2, Carbon dioxide; *FiO_2*, fraction of inspired oxygen concentration. FiO_2 delivered may differ by manufacturer, check manufacturer's guidelines. Data for high-flow nasal cannula: Walsh BK, Smallwood CD: Pediatric oxygen therapy: a review and update, *Respir Care* 62(6):645, 2017. Source for noninvasive ventilation: Wiegand D: *AACN procedure manual for high acuity, progressive, and critical care,* ed 7, St Louis, 2017, Elsevier.

cannula is typically larger in diameter than the standard nasal cannula. HFNC is used to treat respiratory failure, and early evidence indicates that there is less need for invasive ventilation in patients who are initially treated with HFNC (Walsh and Smallwood, 2017; Xu et al., 2018).

OXYGEN MASKS. An oxygen mask is a plastic device that fits snugly over the mouth and nose and is secured in place with a strap. It delivers oxygen as the patient breathes through either the mouth or nose by way of a plastic tubing at the base of the mask that is attached to an oxygen source. An adjustable elastic band is attached to either side of the mask that slides over the head to above the ears to hold the mask in place. There are two primary types of oxygen masks: those delivering low concentrations of oxygen and those delivering high concentrations.

The simple face mask is used for short-term oxygen therapy. It fits loosely and delivers oxygen concentrations from 6 to 12 L/min (35% to 50% oxygen). The mask is contraindicated for patients with carbon dioxide retention because retention can be worsened, leading to decreased levels of consciousness. Flow rates should be 6 L or more to avoid rebreathing exhaled carbon dioxide retained in the mask. Be alert to skin breakdown under the mask with long-term use (Hartjes, 2018).

Partial rebreather and nonrebreather masks are simple masks with a reservoir bag that are capable of delivering higher concentrations of oxygen for a short period of time (60% to 90% oxygen at a flow rate of 10 to 15 L/min). Frequently inspect the reservoir bag to make sure that it is inflated. If it is deflated, the patient is breathing large amounts of exhaled carbon dioxide. (Hartjes, 2018; Harding et al., 2020).

The Venturi mask delivers high-flow, more precise oxygen concentrations of 24% to 60% and usually requires oxygen flow rates of 4 to 12 L/min, depending on the flow-control meter selected. Its use is typically reserved for patients with COPD who need low, constant oxygen concentrations (Hartjes, 2018; Harding et al., 2020).

QSEN Building Competency in Safety Mr. Edwards, a 62-year-old man with COPD, is receiving oxygen therapy via nasal cannula. Identify measures to prevent complications from this type of oxygen-delivery device.

Answers to QSEN Activities can be found on the Evolve website.

Restoration of Cardiopulmonary Functioning. Severe and prolonged hypoxia is one cause of cardiac arrest. Other causes include, but are not limited to, hypovolemia, electrolyte and acid-base imbalances, severe trauma, and infection. A cardiac arrest is a sudden cessation of cardiac output and circulation. When this occurs, oxygen is not delivered to tissues, carbon dioxide is not transported from tissues, tissue metabolism becomes anaerobic, and metabolic and respiratory acidosis occurs. Permanent damage to the heart, brain, and other tissue occurs within 4 to 6 minutes.

Cardiopulmonary Resuscitation. During cardiac arrest there is an absence of pulse and respiration. Patients in cardiac arrest require immediate cardiopulmonary resuscitation (CPR), a basic emergency procedure of artificial respiration and manual external cardiac massage. The sequence for CPR is C-A-B: chest compression, early defibrillation, establishing an airway, and rescue breathing (Link et al., 2015).

The American Heart Association (AHA, 2020) continues to analyze and review research related to cardiac arrest treatment and outcomes. In adults (the majority of cardiac arrests) the critical initial elements found to be essential for survival were adequate chest compressions and early defibrillation. Adequate compressions in adults need to occur at a rate of 100 to 120/minute with a depth of at least 2 inches and allow for full chest recoil between compressions. If no artificial airway (e.g., endotracheal/tracheal tube) is in place, maintain

---

BOX 41.10 Automated External Defibrillator

- The automated external defibrillator (AED) is a device used to administer an electrical shock through the chest wall to the heart to stop the abnormal rhythm and restore a normal heart rhythm.
- The AED has built-in computers that assess a patient's heart rhythm and determine whether defibrillation is necessary. New technology has made them user friendly, with audio and visual cues telling users what to do when using them. The AED delivers a shock to the patient after announcing, "Everyone stand clear of patient." A shock is delivered only if the patient needs it (NHLBI, n.d.b).
- Lay rescuer AED programs train lay personnel on the use of the AED (AHA, 2018).
- When used properly, the AED increases the chance of survival. Patients who received a shock from an AED available in the public had a higher survival rate and rate of discharge from the hospital than those who did not (AHA, 2018).
- For witnessed ventricular fibrillation, early cardiopulmonary resuscitation with defibrillation within the first 3 to 5 minutes results in greater survival rates (Harding et al., 2020).

---

a 30:2 compression-ventilation ratio. If an artificial airway is in place, ventilate one breath every 6 seconds (10/minute) (AHA, 2020).

When a patient has a shockable rhythm, such as ventricular fibrillation, defibrillation is effective when administered early in the cardiac arrest. Defibrillation delivers an electrical current to the myocardium that stops all electrical activity and allows the heart's normal pacemaker to resume its normal activity (Wiegand, 2017). It is recommended that defibrillation occur within 5 minutes for an out-of-hospital sudden cardiac arrest and within 3 minutes for a patient in a hospital (AHA, 2020). An automated external defibrillator (AED) (Box 41.10), available in many public places, such as schools, airports, and workplaces, can be used by health care providers and lay individuals alike to defibrillate people with cardiac arrest (AHA, 2018; Neumar et al., 2015).

If a person is choking and has an obstructed airway, perform abdominal thrusts until the person is able to speak and breathe unassisted or becomes unconscious. Then you perform CPR. You may sweep the mouth and remove the foreign body if you can see it (AHA, 2020).

Restorative and Continuing Care. Restorative and continuing care emphasizes cardiopulmonary reconditioning as a structured rehabilitation program. Cardiopulmonary rehabilitation helps patients achieve and maintain an optimal level of health through controlled physical exercise, nutritional counseling, relaxation and stress-management techniques, prescribed medications, and oxygen. As physical reconditioning occurs, a patient's complaints of dyspnea, chest pain, fatigue, and activity intolerance decrease. The patient's anxiety, depression, or somatic concerns often decrease. The patient and the rehabilitation team define the expected outcomes of rehabilitation.

Respiratory Muscle Training. Respiratory muscle training improves muscle strength and endurance, resulting in improved activity tolerance. It typically consists of repetitive breathing exercises performed against some external force or load. Respiratory muscle training prevents respiratory failure in patients with COPD. There are several devices and methods available for this type of training. One method for respiratory muscle training is the incentive spirometer (Mendes et al., 2019; Menzes et al., 2018).

Breathing Exercises. Breathing exercises include techniques to improve ventilation and oxygenation. The three basic techniques are deep-breathing and coughing exercises, pursed-lip breathing, and diaphragmatic breathing. Deep-breathing and coughing exercises, previously discussed, are routine interventions used by postoperative patients (see Chapter 50).

Pursed-Lip Breathing. Pursed-lip breathing involves deep inspiration and prolonged expiration through pursed lips to prevent alveolar collapse. Instruct the patient, while sitting up, to take a deep breath and exhale slowly through pursed lips as if blowing out a candle. Patients need to gain control of the exhalation phase so that it is longer than inhalation. The patient is usually able to perfect this technique by counting the inhalation time and gradually increasing the count during exhalation (COPD Foundation, 2021). In studies using pursed-lip breathing as a method to improve exercise tolerance in patients with COPD, patients were able to demonstrate increases in their exercise tolerance, breathing pattern, and arterial oxygen saturation (Mendes et al., 2019).

Diaphragmatic Breathing. Diaphragmatic breathing is useful for patients with pulmonary disease and dyspnea secondary to heart failure. This type of breathing increases tidal volume and decreases respiratory rate, which leads to an overall improved breathing pattern and quality of life (Mendes et al., 2019.).

Diaphragmatic breathing is more difficult than other breathing methods because it requires a patient to relax intercostal and accessory respiratory muscles while taking deep inspirations, which takes practice. The patient places one hand flat below the breastbone (upper hand) and the other hand (lower hand) flat on the abdomen. Ask the patient to inhale slowly, making the abdomen push out (as the diaphragm flattens, the abdomen should extend out) and moving the lower hand outward. When the patient exhales, the abdomen goes in (the diaphragm ascends and pushes on lungs to help expel trapped air). The patient practices these exercises initially in the supine position and then while sitting and standing. The exercise is often used with the pursed-lip breathing technique.

Home Oxygen Therapy. Indications for home oxygen therapy include an arterial partial pressure (PaO_2) of 55 mm Hg or less or an arterial oxygen saturation (SaO_2) of 88% or less on room air at rest or if during exercise a patient has a decrease in PaO_2 to 55 mm Hg or less and arterial oxygen saturation (SaO_2) of 88% or less (CMS, 2020). Home oxygen therapy is administered via nasal cannula or face mask. Patients with permanent tracheostomies use either a T tube or tracheostomy collar (Wiegand, 2017). Home oxygen therapy has beneficial effects for patients with chronic cardiopulmonary diseases. This therapy improves patients' exercise tolerance and fatigue levels and, in some situations, assists in the management of dyspnea (see Skill 41.4).

There are three types of oxygen-delivery systems: compressed gas cylinders, liquid oxygen, and oxygen concentrators. Before placing a certain delivery system in a home, assess the advantages and disadvantages (Table 41.8) of each type, along with the patient's needs and community resources. In the home the major consideration is the oxygen-delivery source.

Patients and their family caregivers need extensive teaching to be able to manage oxygen therapy efficiently and safely (see Skill 41.4). Teach the patient and family about home oxygen delivery (e.g., oxygen safety, regulation of the amount of oxygen, and how to use the prescribed home oxygen-delivery system) to ensure their ability to maintain the oxygen-delivery system. The home health nurse coordinates the efforts of the patient and family, home respiratory therapist, and home oxygen equipment vendor. The social worker usually assists initially with arranging for the home care nurse and oxygen vendor.

John identifies that a priority of Mr. Edwards' care is airway clearance. To achieve that outcome John teaches him the huff cough technique and encourages him to expectorate secretions. John has Mr. Edwards do this type of cough at least once an hour. In addition, John explains to Mr. Edwards the benefits of sitting up and doing some walking around the hospital unit. Together they decide that a walk after hygiene care and before lunch is beneficial.

Mr. Edwards states, "I should quit smoking." Because of John's experience with patient education, he knows that Mr. Edwards is showing interest in smoking cessation. He tells Mr. Edwards he would like to bring in some materials tomorrow if Mr. Edwards continues to feel better. John knows that he also needs to include Mrs. Edwards in patient education, as she is also a smoker. John knows that it is easier to quit smoking in a house in which no one else smokes. John also knows that sometimes the acute phase is not the best time to educate patients and families about smoking cessation. John knows that he will have to assess both Mr. and Mrs. Edwards to determine their readiness to receive smoking-cessation education and to stop smoking.

TABLE 41.8 Examples of Home Oxygen-Delivery Systems

	Advantages	Disadvantages
Compressed Oxygen Oxygen is stored under pressure in a cylinder equipped with a regulator that controls the flow rate.	An oxygen-conserving device may be attached to the system to avoid waste; device releases gas only on inhalation and cuts it off with exhalation; does not require an electrical source; smaller tanks are available.	Large tanks are heavy and suitable only for stationary use. Patient must know how to read the regulator and understand when to call medical supplier for replacement cylinder.
Liquid Oxygen System Oxygen is stored as a very cold liquid in a vessel similar to a thermos. When released, the liquid converts to a gas and is breathed in just like compressed gas.	Storage method takes up less space than the compressed gas cylinder; it can transfer the liquid to a small, portable vessel at home.	It is more expensive than compressed gas, and the vessel vents when it is not in use. An oxygen-conserving device may be built into the vessel to conserve the oxygen.
Oxygen Concentrator It separates the oxygen out of the air, concentrates it, and stores it.	It does not have to be resupplied, and it is not as costly as liquid oxygen. Extra tubing permits the user to move around with minimal difficulty. Small, portable systems have been developed that afford even greater mobility.	It must have a cylinder of oxygen as a backup in the event of a power failure.

Adapted from American Thoracic Society (ATS): *Oxygen therapy,* updated 2020, http://www.thoracic.org/patients/patient-resources/resources/oxygen-therapy.pdf. Accessed August 2021.

◆ Evaluation

Evaluation of patients with impaired oxygenation requires clinical judgment with the application of critical thinking in evaluating changes in a patient's oxygen status. Evaluate a patient's response to nursing interventions by comparing actual physical and behavioral responses with the patient's expected outcomes and expectations.

Through the Patient's Eyes. It is important to determine a patient's perceptions of care. For example, does the patient and/or family caregiver feel more in control of the patient's health situation? Does the patient feel that enough information and physical therapy was received to improve activity tolerance when discharged? Be aware of the need to change a treatment plan to be culturally sensitive to improve adherence. Focus on evaluating how a disease is affecting day-to-day activities and the patient's perceived response to treatment. For example, does a patient living at home feel that interventions have improved the ability to maintain a more normal lifestyle, or does a patient in the hospital feel more at ease breathing?

Patient Outcomes. Compare the patient's actual progress with the expected outcomes of the nursing care plan to determine the effectiveness of nursing care and the patient's health status (Fig. 41.16). If a patient is not achieving expected outcomes, reflect on the effectiveness of nursing measures to identify those that may be unsuccessful in improving oxygenation status, modify the care plan appropriately, and reevaluate your patient's oxygenation status. Ongoing, continuous evaluation helps to determine whether new or revised therapies are required and whether new nursing diagnoses have developed and require a new plan of care. Do not hesitate to notify the health care provider about a patient's deteriorating oxygenation status. Prompt notification helps avoid an emergency situation or even the need for CPR. Examples of evaluative measures include the following:

- Ask the patient about the degree of breathlessness.
- Observe respiratory rate and use of respiratory muscles before, during, and after any activity or procedure.
- Monitor pulse oximetry and pulse rate before, during, and after any activity or procedure.
- Ask the patient about fatigue during ambulation.
- Ask the patient to rate breathlessness on a scale of 0 to 10, with 0 being no shortness of breath and 10 being severe shortness of breath.
- Ask the patient which interventions help reduce dyspnea.
- Ask the patient about frequency of cough and sputum production, and assess any sputum produced.
- Auscultate lung sounds for improvement in adventitious sounds.
- When needed, monitor arterial blood gas levels, pulmonary function tests, chest x-ray films, ECG tracings, and physical assessment data to provide objective measurement of the success of therapies and treatments.

John cares for Mr. Edwards throughout his hospital stay. Mr. Edwards is afebrile, his oxygen saturation and lab values are within normal limits, and his sputum cultures are negative on his day of discharge. His lung sounds and airways are clear, and he coughs and expectorates thin yellow sputum easily.

While John is observing Mr. Edwards' preparation for discharge, it is evident that Mr. Edwards is using the breathing and coughing techniques that they have worked on together. He is able to go home with improved activities of daily living. He and his wife both state that they are going to try to quit smoking. Mrs. Edwards even appears less anxious and states that she feels as though for the first time they have taken a small step to improve the quality of their lives.

FIG. 41.16 Critical thinking model for oxygenation evaluation. (Clinical Judgment Measurement Model copyright © NCSBN. All rights reserved.)

SAFETY GUIDELINES FOR NURSING SKILLS

Ensuring patient safety is an essential role of the professional nurse. Use sound clinical judgment by communicating clearly with members of the health care team, assessing and analyzing the patient's clinical findings, and incorporating the patient's priorities of care and preferences. Use the best evidence, applying professional standards, when selecting interventions to use in patient care delivery. When performing the skills in this chapter, remember the following points to ensure safe, patient-centered care.

- Know a patient's baseline range of vital signs. Patients with sudden changes in their vital signs, level of consciousness, or behavior are possibly experiencing profound hypoxemia. Patients who demonstrate subtle changes over time have worsening of a chronic or existing condition or a new medical condition (Hartjes, 2018).
- Identify conditions that increase a patient's risk for aspiration of gastric contents into the lung, resulting in airway obstruction or pneumonia. These include the presence of enteral feeding tubes or nasal and oral gastric tubes, a decreased level of consciousness, and a decreased swallowing ability (AACN, 2018).
- Artificial airways alter the patient's ability to communicate, possibly causing feelings of fear, frustration, anxiety, and vulnerability (Leung et al., 2018).
- Perform tracheal suctioning before oropharyngeal suctioning whenever possible. The mouth and pharynx contain more bacteria than the trachea. If there is an abundance of oral secretions present before beginning the procedure, suction mouth with separate oral suction device.

- Use caution when suctioning patients with a head injury. The suction procedure elevates the intracranial pressure (ICP). Reduce this risk by presuctioning hyperventilation, which results in hypocarbia. This in turn induces vasoconstriction, thereby reducing the risk of elevated ICP (Harding et al., 2020; Urden et al., 2020).
- The routine use of normal saline instillation (NSI) into the airway before endotracheal and tracheostomy suctioning is not recommended. Use of NSI is associated with the adverse effects of excessive coughing, bronchospasm, spread of organisms to the lower respiratory tract, and decreased oxygen saturation (Wang et al., 2017). In certain circumstances, if it is necessary to stimulate a cough, normal saline may be indicated. This requires collaboration with the health care team.
- The most serious tracheostomy complication is airway obstruction, which can result in cardiac arrest. Most tracheostomy tubes are designed with a small plastic inner tube/cannula that sits inside the larger one. If the airway becomes occluded, the smaller one can be removed and replaced with a temporary spare. It is important to always have a spare at the bedside for emergency replacement.
- Review agency policy before stripping or milking chest tubes. Most institutions have stopped using this practice because stripping the tube greatly increases intrapleural pressure, which can damage the pleural tissue and cause pneumothorax or worsen an existing pneumothorax.

SKILL 41.1   SUCTIONING

Delegation and Collaboration

The skill of artificial airway suctioning of newly inserted artificial airways cannot be delegated to assistive personnel (AP). When a patient has been assessed by a nurse as stable, you can delegate oropharyngeal and well-established tracheostomy tube suctioning. **NOTE:** Do not delegate oropharyngeal suctioning for patients with oral or neck surgery in the immediate postoperative period. The nurse directs the AP about:

- Any modifications of the skill, such as the need for supplemental oxygen.
- Appropriate suction limits for suctioning nasotracheally and for suctioning ETs and TTs and the risks of applying excessive or inadequate suction pressure.
- Avoiding mouth sutures, applying suction against sensitive tissues, and dislodging tubes in the patient's nose or mouth.
- Reporting any changes in the patient's respiratory status, vital signs, pulse oximetry (SpO_2), pain level, level of consciousness, restlessness, secretion color and amount, and unresolved coughing or gagging.
- Reporting any signs of skin injury around an oral airway (endotracheal tube) or the tracheal stoma and peristomal area (tracheostomy tube).

When appropriate the nurse may collaborate with the respiratory therapist, as respiratory therapists are also allowed to perform this procedure at certain health care agencies.

Equipment
Oropharyngeal Suctioning
- Clean, nonsterile suction catheter or Yankauer suction tip catheter
- Clean gloves
- Clean towel or paper drape
- Mask, goggles, or face shield if indicated; gown as isolation procedures dictate (check agency policy)
- Disposable cup or basin
- Tap water or normal saline (about 100 mL)
- Suction machine or wall suction device with regulator
- Connecting tubing, 182.8 cm (6 feet)
- Stethoscope

- Pulse oximeter
- Oral airway (if indicated)
- Washcloth
- Manual self-inflating resuscitation bag (bag-valve-mask) with oxygen connecting tubing

Nasotracheal Suctioning
- Sterile suction catheter (12 to 16 Fr) (smallest diameter that effectively removes secretions)
- Two sterile gloves or one sterile and one clean glove
- Sterile basin (e.g., sterile disposable cup)
- Sterile water or normal saline (about 100 mL)
- Clean towel or paper drape
- Mask, goggles, or face shield if indicated; gown as isolation procedures dictate (check agency policy)
- Stethoscope
- Pulse oximeter
- Suction machine or wall suction device with regulator
- Connecting tubing, 182.8 cm (6 feet)
- Manual self-inflating resuscitation bag (bag-valve-mask) with oxygen connecting tubing

Endotracheal or Tracheostomy Suctioning
- Stethoscope
- Pulse oximeter (option for artificial airway suction: end-tidal CO_2 monitor)
- Appropriate-size suction catheter, usually 12 to 16 Fr (smallest diameter that will remove secretions effectively, preferably one that is no more than half of the internal diameter of the artificial airway to minimize decrease in PaO_2) (Billington and Luckett, 2019)
- Suction machine or wall suction device with regulator
- Sterile basin and sterile normal saline/sterile water (about 100 mL)
- Clean towel or sterile drape
- Two sterile gloves or one sterile and one clean glove
- Mask, goggles, or face shield if indicated; gown as isolation procedures dictate (check agency policy)

- Small Y-adapter (if catheter does not have a suction control port)
- Manual self-inflating resuscitation bag (bag-valve-mask) with oxygen connecting tubing
- PEEP valve for resuscitation bag

Closed-System or In-Line Suctioning (see Fig. 41.12)
- Closed-system or in-line suction catheter
- 5- to 10-mL normal saline in syringe or vials
- Two clean gloves

- Suction machine or wall suction device with regulator
- Connecting tubing, 182.8 cm (6 feet)
- Oral suction kit/supplies for oropharyngeal suctioning
- Mask, goggles, or face shield if indicated; gown if isolation procedures dictate.
- Pulse oximeter and stethoscope
- Manual self-inflating resuscitation bag (bag-valve-mask) with oxygen connecting tubing, while not necessary for the procedure, is safe to have on hand.

STEP	RATIONALE

ASSESSMENT

1. Identify patient using at least two identifiers (e.g., name and birthday or name and account number) according to agency policy. Compare identifiers with information on patient's MAR or medical record.

Ensures correct patient. Complies with The Joint Commission standards and improves patient safety (TJC, 2021).

2. Review patient's EHR to identify contraindications to nasotracheal suctioning: occluded nasal passages; nasal bleeding; epiglottitis or croup; acute head, facial, or neck injury or surgery; coagulopathy or bleeding disorder; irritable airway; laryngospasm or bronchospasm; gastric surgery with high anastomosis; myocardial infarction (Hockenberry et al., 2019; Wiegand, 2017).

Passage of suction catheter through nasal route causes trauma to existing facial trauma/surgery, increases nasal bleeding, or causes severe bleeding in presence of coagulopathy or bleeding disorders. In presence of epiglottitis or croup, laryngospasm, or irritable airway, passage of suction catheter through the nose causes intractable coughing, hypoxemia, and severe bronchospasm, necessitating emergency intubation or tracheostomy. Hypoxemia could worsen cardiac damage in myocardial infarction (Hockenberry et al., 2019; Wiegand, 2017).

3. Review sputum microbiology data in laboratory report.

Certain bacteria are easier to transmit or require isolation because of virulence or antibiotic resistance.

4. Review patient's EHR: medical history, normal pulse oximeter and end-tidal CO_2 values, vital sign trends, previous response and tolerance to suctioning procedure, and color and quantity of sputum.

Data helps predict or prevent unexpected outcomes. Changes in neurological status and neuromuscular impairment increase likelihood that patient is unable to clear respiratory secretions. Abnormal anatomy or head and neck surgery/trauma and tumors in and around lower airway impair normal secretion clearance. (Urden et al., 2020).

5. Identify contraindications to nasotracheal suctioning: occluded nasal passages; nasal bleeding; epiglottitis or croup; acute head, facial, or neck injury or surgery; coagulopathy or bleeding disorder; irritable airway; laryngospasm or bronchospasm; gastric surgery with high anastomosis; myocardial infarction (Hockenberry et al., 2019; Urden et al., 2020; Wiegand, 2017).

Nasotracheal suctioning is contraindicated in these conditions because the passage of a suction catheter through the nasal route causes trauma to existing facial trauma/surgery, increases nasal bleeding, or causes severe bleeding in presence of coagulopathy or bleeding disorders. In the presence of epiglottitis or croup, laryngospasm, or irritable airway, passage of suction catheter through the nose causes intractable coughing, hypoxemia, and severe bronchospasm, necessitating emergency intubation or tracheostomy. Hypoxemia could worsen cardiac damage in myocardial infarction (Wiegand, 2017; Urden et al., 2020).

CLINICAL JUDGMENT: *Assess the patient's vital signs, pulse oximetry, end-tidal CO_2, ventilator pressures and volumes (if receiving mechanical ventilation), and respiratory status before the procedure and throughout the procedure* (Wiegand, 2017).

6. Assess for patient's or family caregiver's health literacy.

Ensures patient or family caregiver has the capacity to obtain, communicate, process, and understand basic health information (CDC, 2021a).

7. Perform hand hygiene and apply gloves and other personal protective equipment (PPE) if exposure to airway secretions is present.

Prevents transmission of microorganisms.

8. Assess for signs and symptoms of upper and lower airway obstruction requiring suctioning: abnormal respiratory rate, adventitious lung sounds, nasal secretions, gurgling, drooling, restlessness, gastric secretions, or vomitus in mouth, and coughing without clearing airway secretions and/or improving adventitious lung sounds.

Physical signs and symptoms result from secretions in upper and lower airways and decreased oxygen to the tissues. Presuction assessment provides baseline data to identify the need for suctioning and measures the effectiveness of suction procedures (Wiegand, 2017).

9. Auscultate lungs and assess vital signs and oxygen saturation level for for signs and symptoms associated with respiratory distress, hypoxia and hypercapnia: decreased pulse oximetry (SpO_2), increased pulse and blood pressure, bradycardia, tachypnea, decreased breath sounds, pallor, and cyanosis (a late sign of hypoxia). Keep pulse oximeter on patient for continuous assessment of SpO_2.

Physical signs and symptoms resulting from decreased tissue oxygenation. Provides presuction baseline to measure patient tolerance to suctioning and effectiveness of suctioning on SpO_2 levels.

Continued

SKILL 41.1	**SUCTIONING—cont'd**

STEP	RATIONALE
10. Identify patients with an increased risk for ineffective airway clearance (e.g., patients with decreased level of consciousness, impaired mobility, neuromuscular or neurological impairment, or anatomical factors that influence upper or lower airway function, such as recent surgery; head, chest, or neck trauma; tumors), with nasal feeding tube, a decreased cough or gag reflex, or decreased swallowing ability.	Risk factors can impair patient's ability to clear secretions from airway, increase risk for retaining secretions. Changes in neurological status and neuromuscular impairment increase likelihood that patient is unable to clear respiratory secretions. Abnormal anatomy or head and neck surgery/trauma and tumors in and around lower airway impair normal secretion clearance. Accumulating pulmonary secretions impede patient's ability to effectively clear airway through cough mechanism (Urden et al., 2020).
11. Assess for excessive amounts of secretions or secretions visible in the oral cavity or artificial airway, signs of respiratory distress (increased work of breathing, increased respiratory rate), presence of rhonchi on auscultation, excessive coughing, increased peak inspiratory pressures (if on mechanical ventilator), sawtooth pattern on ventilator monitor, or changes in capnography waveform (if patient on mechanical ventilator) or decrease in patient pulse oximeter (Wiegand, 2017).	Perform suctioning based on patient assessment, not on a routine schedule, such as hourly (Harding et al., 2020; Urden et al., 2020).
12. Assess patency of ETT (if present) with capnography/end-tidal carbon dioxide (CO_2) detector.	ETT may become displaced or blocked by secretions. Capnography allows for the detection of secretions by visualizing the sawtooth pattern on the capnography monitor (Wiegand, 2017).
13. Assess for factors that may affect volume and consistency of secretions.	Thickened or copious secretions increase risk for airway obstruction.
a. Fluid balance	Fluid overload increases amount of secretions. Dehydration can cause thicker secretions.
b. Lack of humidity	Environment influences secretion formation and gas exchange. Airway suctioning is needed when patient cannot clear secretions effectively.
c. Infection (e.g., pneumonia)	Patients with respiratory infections are prone to increased secretions that are thicker and sometimes more difficult to expectorate.
14. For endotracheal suctioning, assess patient's peak inspiratory pressure when on volume-controlled ventilation or tidal volume during pressure-controlled ventilation. Remove gloves and perform hand hygiene.	Increased peak inspiratory pressure or decreased tidal volume may indicate airway obstruction (Urden et al., 2020; Wiegand 2017). Prevents transmission of microorganisms.
15. Remove and dispose of gloves. Perform hand hygiene. (Other PPE may be kept on for actual suctioning.)	Reduces transmission of microorganisms.
16. Determine presence of apprehension, anxiety, decreased ability to concentrate, lethargy, decreased level of consciousness (especially acute), increased fatigue, dizziness, behavioral changes (especially irritability), pallor, cyanosis, dyspnea, or use of accessory muscles.	These are behavioral signs and symptoms of hypoxia and/or hypercapnia, which can indicate need for suction. These signs can also help to identify patient's ability to cooperate with procedure.
17. Assess patient's goals or preferences for how suctioning should be performed.	Patient adherence is increased when the patient is involved in the planning of the care. Allows care to be individualized.

PLANNING

1. Prepare and organize equipment. Place towel across patient's chest.	Reduces transmission of microorganisms. Ensures that the nurse has the necessary equipment to implement all interventions that should be completed for the patient.
2. Close room door or pull curtain around bed.	Provides privacy.
3. Assist patient to comfortable position, typically semi-Fowler's or high Fowler's.	Reduces stimulation of gag reflex, promotes patient comfort and secretion drainage, and prevents aspiration.
4. If not already present, place pulse oximeter on patient's finger. Take reading and leave oximeter in place.	Provides continuous SpO_2 value to determine patient's response to suctioning.
5. Explain to patient how procedure will help clear airway and relieve some breathing difficulty. Explain that temporary coughing, sneezing, gagging, or shortness of breath is normal during procedure.	Encourages cooperation and minimizes anxiety and pain of procedure.

IMPLEMENTATION

1. Perform hand hygiene and apply appropriate personal protective equipment if not already applied during assessment (mask with face shield or goggles; gown if necessary).	Reduces transmission of microorganisms.
2. Adjust bed to appropriate height (if not already done), and lower side rail on side nearest you. Check locks on bed wheel.	Minimizes caregiver's muscle strain and prevents injury. Prevents bed from moving.

STEP	**RATIONALE**
3. Connect one end of connecting tubing to wall suction device and place other end in convenient location near patient. Turn suction device on and set suction pressure to as low a level as possible and yet able to effectively clear secretions. This value is typically between 80 and 150 mm Hg (AARC, 2010; Urden et al., 2020; Wiegand, 2017).	Ensures equipment function. Excessive negative pressure damages tracheal mucosa and induces greater hypoxia (Wiegand, 2017).
4. Preparation for open suctioning:	
a. Perform hand hygiene. Using aseptic technique, open suction kit or catheter package. If sterile drape is available, place it across patient's chest or on bedside table. Do not allow suction catheter to touch any nonsterile surfaces. **NOTE**: When performing oropharyngeal suction only, there is no need to place a sterile drape; it is a clean procedure, not sterile.	Prepares catheter, maintains asepsis, and reduces transmission of microorganisms. Provides sterile surface on which to lay catheter between passes.
b. Unwrap or open sterile basin and place on bedside table. Be careful not to touch inside of basin. Fill with about 100 mL sterile normal saline solution or water (see illustration).	Saline or water is used to clean tubing after each suction pass.
c. If performing nasotracheal suctioning, open packet of water-soluble lubricant and apply small amount (about 1 inch) along catheter tip. **NOTE**: *Lubricant is not necessary for artificial airway suctioning.*	Water-soluble lubricant helps avoid lipid aspiration pneumonia. Excessive amount of lubricant occludes catheter.
d. For oropharyngeal suctioning, clean technique using clean gloves is appropriate. For nasotracheal, endotracheal tube, or tracheal tube suctioning, apply sterile gloves to each hand or nonsterile glove to nondominant hand and sterile glove to dominant hand.	Reduces transmission of microorganisms and maintains sterility of suction catheter.
e. Pick up suction catheter or Yankauer suction with dominant hand without touching nonsterile surfaces. Pick up connecting tubing with nondominant hand. Secure catheter to tubing (see illustration).	Maintains catheter sterility. Connects catheter to suction.
f. Place tip of catheter into sterile basin and suction small amount of normal saline solution from basin by occluding suction vent.	Ensures equipment function. Lubricates internal catheter and tubing.
5. Suction airway using open suctioning.	
a. Oropharyngeal suctioning	Removes oral secretions.

CLINICAL JUDGMENT: *In patients who require sterile suctioning of the airways, oropharyngeal suction is performed **after** the sterile suctioning to prevent contamination of the suction catheters or tubing with bacteria present in the oral cavity (Wiegand, 2017).*

---

(1) Remove patient's oxygen mask, if present, but keep it close. Nasal cannula may remain in place.	Allows access to mouth. Reduces chance of hypoxia.

CLINICAL JUDGMENT: *Be prepared to quickly reapply supplemental oxygen if SpO$_2$ value falls below 90% or respiratory distress develops during or at the end of oropharyngeal suctioning. Be prepared to use the bag-valve-mask if patient has serious acute respiratory distress or decline in SpO$_2$.*

STEP 4b Pouring sterile saline into tray.

STEP 4e Attaching suction catheter to suction tubing.

Continued

SKILL 41.1	SUCTIONING—cont'd

STEP	RATIONALE

CLINICAL JUDGMENT: *If patient has been suctioned tracheally prior to oropharyngeal suctioning, the patient may require some recovery from the suctioning procedure before oropharyngeal suctioning is performed. Allow for that recovery to happen by reapplying the oxygen mask until just before oropharyngeal suctioning.*

(2) Insert catheter into mouth along gum line to pharynx. Move Yankauer catheter around mouth until secretions have cleared. Encourage patient to cough. Replace oxygen mask. **NOTE**: If ET is present, be careful when moving the catheter so as not to dislodge the ET.	Movement of catheter prevents suction tip from invaginating oral mucosal surfaces and causing trauma. Coughing moves secretions from lower airway into mouth and upper airway.

CLINICAL JUDGMENT: *Use caution when suctioning a patient who had recent oral or head/neck surgery. Aggressive suctioning and excessive coughing should not be used or encouraged in patients who have undergone throat surgery, such as a tonsillectomy. Aggressive suctioning in these patient populations can aggravate the operative site, increasing the risk of bleeding or infection (Urden, 2020).*

(3) Rinse catheter with water or normal saline in cup or basin until connecting tubing is cleared of secretions. Turn off suction. Place catheter in clean, dry area.	Rinses catheter and reduces probability of transmission of microorganisms. Clean suction tubing enhances delivery of set suction pressure. Catheter may be reused.

b. Nasopharyngeal and nasotracheal suctioning:

(1) Have patient take deep breaths, if able, or increase oxygen flow rate with delivery device through cannula or mask (if ordered).	May help to decrease risks of hypoxemia.
(2) Lightly coat distal 6 to 8 cm (2–3 inches) of catheter with water-soluble lubricant.	Lubricates catheter for easier insertion.
(3) Remove oxygen-delivery device, if applicable, with nondominant hand.	Allows access to nares and catheter.

CLINICAL JUDGMENT: *Be sure to insert catheter during patient inhalation, especially if inserting it into trachea, because epiglottis is open. Do not insert during swallowing or catheter will most likely enter esophagus. **Never apply suction during insertion.** Patient should cough. If patient gags or becomes nauseated, catheter is most likely in esophagus, and you need to remove it (Wiegand, 2017).*

(4) *Nasopharyngeal* (without applying suction): As patient takes deep breath, insert catheter following natural course of naris; slightly slant catheter downward and advance to back of pharynx. Do not force through nares. In adults insert catheter approximately 16 cm (6.5 inches); in older children, 8–12 cm (3–5 inches); in infants and young children, 4–7.5 cm (1.5–3 inches). Rule of thumb is to insert catheter distance from tip of nose (or mouth) to angle of mandible.	Ensure that catheter tip reaches pharynx for suctioning.

CLINICAL JUDGMENT: *If resistance is met during insertion, you may need to try the other naris. Do not force the catheter up the nares because this will cause mucosal damage.*

(5) *Nasotracheal* (without applying suction): As patient takes deep breath, advance catheter following natural course of naris. Advance catheter slightly slanted and downward to just above entrance into larynx and then trachea. While patient takes deep breath, quickly insert catheter: for adults insert approximately 16–20 cm (6–8 inches) into trachea (see illustration). While patient takes a deep breath, quickly insert the catheter. Patient will begin to cough; then pull back catheter 1–2 cm (½ inch) before applying suction. **NOTE**: In older children, insert 16–20 cm (6–8 inches); in infants and young children, 8–14 cm (3–5½ inches).	Ensures that catheter tip reaches trachea for suctioning.

CLINICAL JUDGMENT: *When using the nasal approach, perform tracheal suctioning before oropharyngeal suctioning whenever possible. The mouth and pharynx contain more bacteria than the trachea. If copious oral secretions are present before beginning the procedure, suction mouth with oral suction device first (see Step 5a).*

CLINICAL JUDGMENT: *When there is difficulty passing the catheter, ask patient to cough or say "ahh," or try to advance the catheter during inspiration. Both measures help to open the glottis to permit passage of the catheter into the trachea.*

STEP	RATIONALE

STEP 5b(5) Distance of insertion of nasotracheal catheter.

(a) *Positioning option:* In some instances, turning patient's head helps you suction more effectively. If you feel resistance after insertion of catheter, use caution; it has probably hit the carina. Pull catheter back 1–2 cm (0.4–0.8 inches) before applying suction (Wiegand, 2017).

Turning patient's head to side elevates bronchial passage on opposite side. Turning head to right helps with suctioning of left mainstem bronchus; turning head to left helps you suction right mainstem bronchus. Suctioning too deep may cause tracheal mucosa trauma.

  i. Apply intermittent suction for no more than 10–15 seconds by placing and releasing nondominant thumb over catheter vent. Slowly withdraw catheter while rotating it back and forth between thumb and forefinger.

Intermittent suction of 10–15 seconds safely removes secretions. Suction time greater than 15 seconds increases risk for suction-induced hypoxemia (Urden et al., 2020; Wiegand, 2017). Intermittent suction and rotation of catheter prevent injury to tracheal mucosa. If catheter "grabs" mucosa, remove thumb to release suction.

CLINICAL JUDGMENT: *Monitor patient's vital signs and oxygen saturation throughout suctioning process. Stop suctioning if there is a 20 beats/min change (increase or decrease) in pulse rate or if SpO2 falls below 90% or 5% from baseline.*

(6) Reapply oxygen-delivery device and encourage patient to take some deep breaths, if able.

Helps to decrease risk of hypoxia. Increases patient comfort.

(7) Rinse catheter and connecting tubing with normal saline or water until cleared.

Secretions that remain in suction catheter or connecting tubing decrease suctioning efficiency.

(8) Assess for need to repeat suctioning. Do not perform more than two passes with catheter. Allow patient to rest at least 1 minute. Ask patient to deep-breathe and cough.

Observe for alterations in cardiopulmonary status. Suctioning induces hypoxemia, irregular pulse, laryngospasm, and bronchospasm. Hyperoxygenation is recommended before, during, and after open suctioning to reduce suction-induced hypoxemia (Urden et al., 2020; Wiegand, 2017).

c. Artificial airway suctioning:

(1) With assistance from respiratory therapy when a patient has an artificial airway, hyperoxygenate the patient with 100% oxygen for at least 30 to 60 seconds before suctioning by (1) pressing suction hyperoxygenation button on ventilator OR (2) increasing baseline fraction of inspired oxygen (FiO2) level on mechanical ventilator OR (3) disconnecting ventilator, attaching self-inflating resuscitation bag-valve device to tube with nondominant hand (or have assistant do this), and administering 5 to 6 breaths over 30 seconds (or have assistant do this) (Wiegand, 2017). **NOTE:** Some mechanical ventilators have a button that, when pushed, delivers 100% oxygen for a few minutes, and then resets to previous setting.

Preoxygenation decreases risk of decreased arterial oxygen levels while ventilation or oxygenation is interrupted and volume is lost during suctioning. Some models of resuscitation bags do not deliver 100% oxygen; therefore, this is not the best way to oxygenate patient (Wiegand, 2017).

(2) If patient is receiving mechanical ventilation, open swivel adapter or, if necessary, remove oxygen- or humidity-delivery device with nondominant hand.

Exposes artificial airway.

CLINICAL JUDGMENT: *Suctioning can cause elevations in intracranial pressure (ICP) in patients with head injuries. Reduce this risk by presuction hyperoxygenation, which results in hypocarbia, which in turn induces vasoconstriction. Vasoconstriction reduces the potential for an increase in ICP (Urden et al., 2020).*

Continued

SKILL 41.1	SUCTIONING—cont'd
STEP	**RATIONALE**

CLINICAL JUDGMENT: *Be sure to insert catheter during patient inhalation, especially if inserting it into trachea, because epiglottis is open. Do not insert during swallowing, or catheter will most likely enter esophagus.* ***Never apply suction during insertion.*** *Patient should cough. If patient gags or becomes nauseated, catheter is most likely in esophagus, and you need to remove it (Wiegand, 2017).*

(3) Advise patient that you are about to begin suctioning. Without applying suction, gently but quickly insert catheter into artificial airway using dominant thumb and forefinger (it is best to try to time catheter insertion into artificial airway with inspiration) (see illustration). Advance catheter until patient coughs, which is usually 0.5 to 1 cm below the level of the tube. Then pull back 1 cm (0.4 inch) before applying suction (Billington and Luckett, 2019).

Application of suction pressure while introducing catheter into trachea increases risk for damage to tracheal mucosa and increased hypoxia. Pulling back stimulates cough and removes catheter from mucosal wall so that catheter is not resting against tracheal mucosa during suctioning. Shallow suctioning is recommended to prevent tracheal mucosa trauma (Urden et al., 2020; Wiegand, 2017).

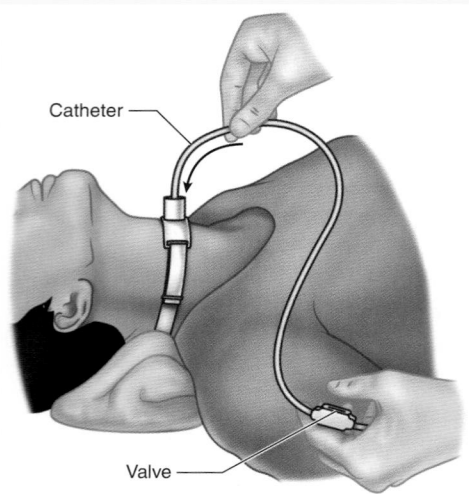

Catheter

Valve

STEP 5c(3) Suctioning tracheostomy.

CLINICAL JUDGMENT: *If unable to insert catheter past the end of the ET, the catheter is probably caught in the Murphy eye (i.e., side hole at the distal end of the ET that allows for collateral airflow in the event of tracheal main-stem intubation). If this happens, rotate the catheter to reposition it away from the Murphy eye or withdraw it slightly and reinsert with the next inhalation. Usually the catheter meets resistance at the carina. One indication that the catheter is at the carina is acute onset of coughing because the carina contains many cough receptors. Pull the catheter back 1 cm (½ inch) (Billington and Luckett, 2019).*

(4) Apply intermittent suction for 10–15 seconds (Wiegand, 2017). Apply intermittent suction by placing and releasing nondominant thumb over vent of catheter; slowly withdraw catheter while rotating it back and forth between dominant thumb and forefinger. Do not use suction for greater than 15 seconds. Encourage patient to cough. Watch for respiratory distress.

Intermittent suction up to 10–15 seconds safely removes pharyngeal secretions. Suction time greater than 15 seconds increases risk for suction-induced hypoxemia (Urden et al., 2020; Wiegand, 2017). Intermittent suction and rotation of catheter prevent injury to tracheal mucosa. If catheter "grabs" mucosa, remove thumb to release suction.

CLINICAL JUDGMENT: *If patient develops respiratory distress during the suction procedure, immediately withdraw catheter and supply additional oxygen and breaths as needed. In an emergency administer oxygen directly through the catheter. Disconnect suction and attach oxygen at prescribed flow rate through the catheter. If the patient does not tolerate the suctioning procedure, you may need to consider switching to closed (in-line) suctioning or allowing longer recovery times. Notify health care provider if patient develops significant cardiopulmonary compromise during suctioning (Urden et al., 2020; Wiegand, 2017).*

(5) If patient is receiving mechanical ventilation, close swivel adapter or replace oxygen-delivery device. Hyperoxygenate patient for 30–60 seconds.

Reestablishes artificial airway. Helps to decrease risks of hypoxia.

(6) Rinse catheter and connecting tubing with normal saline until clear. Use continuous suction.

Removes catheter secretions. Secretions left in tubing decrease suctioning efficiency and provide environment for microorganism growth.

STEP	RATIONALE
(7) Assess patient's vital signs, cardiopulmonary status, and ventilator measures for secretion clearance. Repeat Steps (1) through (6) above once or twice more to clear secretions. Unless the patient is in respiratory distress, allow adequate time (at least 1 full minute) between suction passes (Wiegand, 2017).	Suctioning can induce dysrhythmias, hypoxia, and bronchospasm and impair cerebral circulation or adversely affect hemodynamic stability (Wiegand, 2017).

CLINICAL JUDGMENT: *Base the number of suction passes on patient assessment and presence of secretions. If secretions persist after two passes, reapply oxygen source and allow patient more time to rest and recover before suctioning again (Wiegand, 2017).*

CLINICAL JUDGMENT: *In the past, the practice of instilling normal saline into the artificial airway was performed to try to thin the secretions, making them easier to suction out of the airway. Evidence indicates that this practice should no longer be performed because it causes more damage to the lungs (Larrow and Klich-Heartt, 2016; Wiegand, 2017).*

(8) When trachea is sufficiently cleared of secretions, perform oropharyngeal suctioning (see Step 5a) to clear mouth of secretions. Do not suction nose again after suctioning mouth.	Removes upper airway secretions. More microorganisms generally are present in mouth. Upper airway is considered "clean," and lower airway is considered "sterile." You can use same catheter to suction from sterile to clean areas (e.g., tracheal suctioning to oropharyngeal suctioning) but not from clean to sterile areas.

6. Closed suctioning of artificial airway using in-line suctioning (see illustration)

STEP 6 (A) Closed-system suction catheter attached to endotracheal tube. (B) Closed suction system attached to an endotracheal tube. (B from Rothrock JC, McEwen DR, editors: *Alexander's care of the patient in surgery*, ed 14, St Louis, 2011, Mosby.)

Continued

SKILL 41.1	SUCTIONING—cont'd

STEP	RATIONALE
a. Turn suction device on, set vacuum regulator to appropriate negative pressure (usually 80 to 150 mm Hg), and check pressure. See manufacturer's guidelines for recommended pressure to use with the agency's brand of catheter.	Excessive negative pressure damages tracheal mucosa and induces greater hypoxia (Wiegand, 2017).
b. Attach suction. In many agencies a respiratory therapist attaches the catheter to the mechanical ventilator circuit. If catheter is not already in place, apply sterile gloves or sterile glove for dominant hand and clean glove for nondominant hand (see agency policy). Open suction catheter package using aseptic technique, and attach closed-system suction catheter to ventilator circuit by removing swivel adapter and placing closed-system suction catheter apparatus on endotracheal tube (ET) or tracheostomy tube (TT). Connect mechanical ventilator circuit to closed-system suction catheter with flex tubing.	Maintains surgical asepsis during suctioning.
c. With assistance from respiratory therapy when patient has an artificial airway and is on a ventilator, hyperoxygenate the patient with 100% oxygen for at least 30 to 60 seconds before suctioning by (1) pressing the suction hyperoxygenation button on the ventilator (mechanical ventilators that have this button deliver 100% oxygen for a few minutes and then reset to previous setting) **OR** (2) increasing baseline fraction of inspired oxygen (FiO$_2$) level on mechanical ventilator.	Preoxygenation decreases risk of decreased arterial oxygen levels while ventilation or oxygenation is interrupted and volume is lost during suctioning (AARC, 2010; Wiegand, 2017). Some models of resuscitation bags do not deliver 100% oxygen; therefore, this is not the best way to hyperoxygenate patient (Wiegand, 2017).

CLINICAL JUDGMENT: *Manual resuscitation bags do not always deliver 100% oxygen, and they are not recommended for hyperoxygenation prior to suctioning (Wiegand, 2017).*

CLINICAL JUDGMENT: *Suctioning can cause elevations in intracranial pressure (ICP) in patients with head injuries. Reduce this risk by presuction hyperoxygenation, which results in hypocarbia, which in turn induces vasoconstriction. Vasoconstriction reduces the potential for an increase in ICP (Urden et al., 2020).*

STEP	RATIONALE
d. Unlock suction control mechanism, if required by manufacturer. Open saline port and attach saline syringe or vial.	Allows for suctioning and prepares saline, which allows for irrigation of the catheter lumen.
e. Pick up suction catheter enclosed in plastic sleeve with dominant hand.	
f. Insert catheter: Advise patient that you are about to begin suctioning. Wait until patient inhales to insert catheter. Then insert catheter using a repeating maneuver of pushing catheter and sliding plastic sleeve back between thumb and forefinger until resistance is felt or patient coughs.	Application of suction pressure while introducing catheter into trachea increases risk for damage to tracheal mucosa and increased hypoxia. Pulling back stimulates cough and removes catheter from mucosal wall so that catheter is not resting against tracheal mucosa during suctioning. Shallow suctioning is recommended to prevent tracheal mucosa trauma (Wiegand, 2017).

CLINICAL JUDGMENT: *If unable to insert catheter past the end of the ET, the catheter is probably caught in the Murphy eye (i.e., side hole at the distal end of the ET that allows for collateral airflow in the event of tracheal main-stem intubation). If this happens, rotate the catheter to reposition it away from the Murphy eye or withdraw it slightly and reinsert with the next inhalation. Usually the catheter meets resistance at the carina. One indication that the catheter is at the carina is acute onset of coughing because the carina contains many cough receptors. Pull the catheter back 1 cm (½ inch) (Billington and Luckett, 2019).*

STEP	RATIONALE
g. Pull back 1 cm (0.4 inches) before applying suction to avoid tissue damage to carina. **NOTE:** If patient has a history of bleeding during previous suction procedures, care should be taken to avoid hitting the carina with the suction catheter.	Avoids damage to tracheal carina.
h. Encourage patient to cough, and apply suction by squeezing on suction control mechanism while withdrawing catheter. Be sure to withdraw catheter completely into plastic sheath and past the tip of the airway so that it does not obstruct airflow.	
i. Apply continuous suction for 10 seconds as you remove the suction catheter (AARC, 2010; Wiegand, 2017). Be sure to withdraw the catheter completely into the plastic sheath and past the tip of the airway so that it does not obstruct airflow.	Time for suctioning reduces incidence of oxygen desaturation.
j. Reassess patient's vital signs, cardiopulmonary status, and ventilator measures for secretion clearance. Repeat Steps 6a through 6h above once or twice more to clear secretions. Allow adequate time (at least 1 full minute) between suction passes.	Suctioning can induce dysrhythmias, hypoxia, and bronchospasm and impair cerebral circulation or adversely affect hemodynamic stability (Wiegand, 2017).

STEP	RATIONALE
k. When airway is clear, withdraw catheter completely into sheath. Be sure that colored indicator line on catheter is visible in the sheath. Attach sterile solution lavage container or sterile saline or water syringe to side port of suction catheter. Squeeze vial or push syringe while applying suction to rinse inner lumen of catheter. **NOTE:** Do not let the saline go down the ET or TT. Use at least 5 to 10 mL of saline to rinse the catheter until it is clear of retained secretions, which can cause bacterial growth and increase the risk for infection (Wiegand, 2017).	Cleans the suction catheter, thereby reducing risk of bacterial growth and infection.
l. Hyperoxygenate for at least 30 seconds by following the same technique used to preoxygenate (Wiegand, 2017).	Prevents hypoxemia.
m. If patient requires oral or nasal suctioning, suction the patient with separate Yankauer or standard catheter.	Clears oral and nasal passages of mucous secretions.
n. Lock the suction mechanism, if applicable. Perform oropharyngeal suctioning if patient requires (see Step 5a).	Prevents migration of the suction catheter into the airway, which could lead to obstruction.
7. When the suction procedure is complete, disconnect catheter from connecting tubing. Roll catheter around fingers of dominant hand. Pull off other glove over first glove in same way. Discard in appropriate receptacle. Perform hand hygiene.	Seals contaminants in gloves. Reduces transmission of microorganisms.
8. Remove towel, place in laundry or appropriate receptacle, and reposition patient.	Reduces transmission of microorganisms.
9. If oxygen level was changed during procedure, readjust oxygen to original ordered level because patient's blood oxygen level should have returned to baseline.	Prevents absorption atelectasis (i.e., tendency for airways to collapse if proximally obstructed by secretions). Prevents oxygen toxicity while allowing patient time to reoxygenate blood.
10. Discard remainder of normal saline into appropriate receptacle. If basin is disposable, discard into appropriate receptacle. If basin is reusable, rinse it out and place it in soiled utility room. Perform hand hygiene.	Reduces transmission of microorganisms.
11. Place a new unopened suction kit on suction machine table or at head of bed.	Provides immediate access to suction catheter for next procedure.
12. Apply clean gloves to continue personal care, such as washing the patient's face or performing oral hygiene.	Promotes comfort.
13. Help patient to comfortable position, and provide oral hygiene as needed.	
14. Raise side rails (as appropriate); lower bed to lowest position.	Ensures patient safety.
15. Place the nurse call system in an accessible location within patient's reach.	Ensures patient can call for assistance if needed.
16. Remove personal protective equipment and gloves. Discard into appropriate receptacle. Perform hand hygiene.	Reduces transmission of microorganisms.

EVALUATION

1. Compare patient's vital signs, cardiopulmonary assessments, E_tCO_2 and SpO_2 values before and after suctioning. If on ventilator, compare FiO_2 and tidal volumes and peak inspiratory pressures.	Identifies physiological effects of suction procedure to restore airway patency.
2. Ask patient whether breathing is easier and congestion is decreased.	Provides subjective confirmation that suctioning procedure has relieved airway.
3. Auscultate lungs and compare patient's respiratory assessment before and after suctioning.	Provides objective information about any change in lung sounds.
4. Observe character of airway secretions.	Provides data to document presence or absence of respiratory tract infection or thickened secretions.
5. Use Teach-Back: "I need to suction your father, and I want to be sure that I explained the suctioning procedure and when I need to do it. Please tell me in your own words why suctioning is beneficial." Revise your instruction now or develop a plan for revised patient/family caregiver teaching if patient/family caregiver is not able to teach back correctly.	Teach-back is an evidence-based health literacy intervention that promotes patient engagement, patient safety, adherence, and quality. The goal of teach-back is to ensure that you have explained medical information clearly so that patients and their families understand what you communicated to them (AHRQ, 2020).

UNEXPECTED OUTCOMES AND RELATED INTERVENTIONS

1. Patient has decrease in overall cardiopulmonary status as evidenced by decreased SpO_2, increased E_tCO_2, continued tachypnea, continued increased work of breathing, and cardiac dysrhythmias.
- Limit length of time for suctioning.
- Determine need for more frequent suctioning, possibly of shorter duration.
- Determine need for supplemental or increase in supplemental oxygen. Supply oxygen between suctioning passes.
- Notify health care provider.

2. Bloody secretions are returned during suctioning.
- Determine amount of suction pressure used. May need to be decreased.
- Ensure that suction is completed correctly using intermittent suction and catheter rotation. Do not apply suction until after catheter has been pulled back 1 cm (0.4 inches) to prevent applying suction while catheter is touching carina.

Continued

| **SKILL 41.1** | **SUCTIONING—cont'd** |

- Evaluate suctioning frequency.
- Provide more frequent oral hygiene.

3. Inability to obtain secretions during suction procedure.
- Evaluate patient's fluid status and adequacy of humidification on oxygen-delivery device.
- Assess for signs of infection.
- Determine need for chest physiotherapy.

RECORDING AND REPORTING

- Respiratory assessments (including vital signs, pulse oximetry values, and $EtCO_2$ values, if applicable) before and after suctioning; size of catheter used; suctioning route; amount, consistency, and color of secretions obtained; frequency of suctioning; and oxygen requirement after procedure.
- Note which naris was used/should be used and why for nasopharyngeal/tracheal suctioning.
- Report quantity and quality of sputum obtained during suction procedure, including whether blood was present and any cardiopulmonary abnormalities.
- Document your evaluation of patient learning.

HOME CARE CONSIDERATIONS

- Adhere to best practices for infection control while weighing cost-effectiveness in the presence of a chronic situation. If a patient has an established tracheostomy or requires long-term nasotracheal suctioning and infection is not present, clean suction technique may be appropriate.
- Although most patients with airway clearance problems at home have a tracheostomy, some also require nasal pharyngeal suctioning. Catheters are often used for a 24-hour period and then cleaned and disinfected, or they are cleaned with soapy water after each use and discarded after 24 hours.
- Stress to family caregivers the importance of brief intervals of applying suction pressure. Instruct those performing suction to hold their breath during the application of negative suction pressure to help them remember to not suction too long.
- Instruct patient and family caregiver about infection control practices (e.g., to clean and disinfect or change the secretion collection container every 24 hours according to home care or institutional protocol and to avoid splash when emptying the suction container jar in the toilet). Instruct caregiver to apply mask (shield if available) and gloves and bring the jar as close to the toilet bowl as possible to decrease the risk of splash.
- Ensure that power companies are notified of homes in which there are patients receiving home suction or ventilation. In the event of a power outage, these homes are the priority for receiving power.

| **SKILL 41.2** | **CARE OF AN ARTIFICIAL AIRWAY** | ◉ |

Delegation and Collaboration

This skill of performing endotracheal (ET) care cannot be delegated to assistive personnel (AP). AP may assist the nurse with ET care. Often, the nurse collaborates with a respiratory therapist in performing this care. In some settings, the skill of tracheal tube (TT) care for patients with a well-established TT can be delegated to AP. The nurse directs the AP to:
- Immediately report any signs of respiratory problems or increased airway secretions.
- Immediately report if the ET or TT appears to have moved or become obstructed or dislodged.
- Immediately report changes in patient's mood, level of consciousness, irritability, vital signs, decreased pulse oximetry value, or changes in end-tidal CO_2 values.
- Immediately report any redness, irritation, or injury around the patient's mouth, neck, or lips or naris
- Immediately report abnormal color of the tracheal stoma and drainage.

Equipment

- Towel
- Stethoscope
- Pulse oximeter and end-tidal CO_2 detector
- Personal protective equipment: goggles/mask/face shield; gloves; gown
- Oral and artificial airway suction supplies (see Skill 41.1)
- Oxygen source
- Self-inflating manual resuscitation bag-valve device and appropriate-size mask
- Oral hygiene supplies: soft toothbrush (or suction toothbrush); foam oral swab; cleaning solution: 0.12% to 0.20% chlorhexidine mouthwash (*option*: 1.5% hydrogen peroxide or 0.05% antiseptic solution), mouth moisturizer, or gel

- Face cleanser (e.g., wet washcloth, towel, soap, shaving supplies)
- Communication device—*optional* (letter or picture board, tablet, pen and paper)
- Reintubation equipment at bedside in case of accidental tube dislodgment

Endotracheal Tube Care

- Additional health care team member (two people are needed to safely complete some of the ET care steps)
- Two pairs of clean gloves
- ET stabilization device or 1- to 1½-inch adhesive or waterproof tape
- Adhesive remover swab
- Liquid skin barrier
- Clean 2 × 2–inch gauze
- Oral airway or bite block
- Tongue blade *(optional)*

Tracheostomy Care

- Additional health care team member (two people are needed to safely complete some of the TT care steps)
- Sterile tracheostomy care kit, if available, or:
  - Three sterile 4 × 4–inch gauze pads
  - Sterile cotton-tipped applicators
  - Sterile tracheostomy dressing
  - Sterile basin
  - Small sterile brush (or disposable cannula)
  - Tracheostomy ties (e.g., twill tape, manufactured tracheostomy ties, Velcro tracheostomy ties)
  - Tracheostomy stabilization device *(optional)*
- Sterile normal saline or water

- Scissors
- Pair of sterile and clean gloves
- Disposable inner cannula if patient has one

- Skin barrier product
- Extra sterile tracheostomy kit
- Cuff pressure manometer

STEP	RATIONALE
ASSESSMENT	
1. Identify patient using at least two identifiers (e.g., name and birthday or name and account number) according to agency policy. Compare identifiers with information on patient's MAR or medical record.	Ensures correct patient. Complies with The Joint Commission standards and improves patient safety (TJC, 2021).
2. Review medical record to assess patient's hydration status, humidity delivered to airway/ventilator circuit, status of any existing infection, patient's nutritional status, and ability to cough.	Determines factors that affect amount and consistency of secretions in ET/TT and patient's ability to clear airway.
3. Assess for patient's or family caregiver's health literacy.	Assures patient or family caregiver has the capacity to obtain, communicate, process, and understand basic health information (CDC, 2021a).
4. Perform hand hygiene, and apply gloves and other PPE as determined by patient condition and agency policy.	Reduces transmission of organisms.
5. Perform complete assessment of patient's cardiopulmonary status, including lung sounds, pulse oximetry, E_tCO_2, vital signs, and level of consciousness. Keep pulse oximeter in place.	Provides baseline to determine status of ventilation and patient response to and tolerance of therapy.
6. Observe condition of tissues surrounding ET/TT for impaired skin integrity (e.g., blistering, abrasions, pressure injuries) on nares, lips, cheeks, corner of mouth, or neck; excess nasal or oral secretions; patient moving tube with tongue or biting tube or tongue; or foul-smelling mouth.	Increased risk for developing pressure injuries around ET or TT from impaired circulation as tube is pulled or pressed against oral mucosal tissues. Exposure to medical adhesive can cause medical adhesive–related skin injury (MARSI). Tube impairs ability of patient to swallow oral secretions (Wiegand, 2017).
7. Observe patency of airway: excess peristomal, intratracheal, or endotracheal secretions; diminished airflow; or signs and symptoms of airway obstruction.	Buildup of secretions in ET/TT impairs oxygen delivery and subsequent tissue oxygenation. Excess secretions in the artificial airways may indicate need for suctioning before performing any other airway care.
8. Observe for signs and symptoms of gurgling on expiration, decreased exhaled tidal volume (mechanically ventilated patient), signs and symptoms of inadequate ventilation (rising end-tidal carbon dioxide concentration [E_tCO_2], patient-ventilator desynchrony, or dyspnea), spasmodic coughing, tense test balloon on tube, flaccid test balloon on tube, and ability to speak or vocalize.	Cuff underinflation increases risk for aspiration, allows secretions to enter the trachea, and permits vocalization. Cuff overinflation may cause ischemia or necrosis of tracheal tissue from obstruction of capillary bed, resulting in tracheomalacia or tracheoesophageal fistula (Sanaie et al., 2019; Rouzé et al., 2017). End-tidal carbon dioxide concentration [E_tCO_2] validates the correct placement of the ET by analyzing the exhaled gas for carbon dioxide levels (Wiegand, 2017).

CLINICAL JUDGMENT: *When assessment indicates possible overinflation or underinflation of ET cuff (pressures less than 20 mm Hg or greater than 25 mm Hg), notify respiratory therapy and follow agency policy for correcting cuff pressures (Sanaie et al., 2019; Wiegand, 2017).*

STEP	RATIONALE
9. Observe for factors that increase risk for complications from ET/TT: type and size of tube, movement of tube up and down trachea (in and out), duration of tube placement, presence of facial trauma, malnutrition, and neck or thoracic radiation.	Tube rotating from side to side causes MDRPI. Tube can become dislodged from lower airway (incidental extubation), or it can enter right main-stem bronchus. Longer duration of intubation is associated with increased risk for lower airway complications such as ventilator-associated pneumonia (VAP) (Urden et al., 2020; Wang et al., 2019).
10. **FOR ET:** Determine proper ET depth as noted by centimeters at lip or gum line. This line is marked on tube and recorded in patient's record at time of intubation and every shift. Remove and dispose of gloves. Perform hand hygiene.	Ensures that tube is at proper depth to adequately ventilate both lungs and that it is not too high, which causes vocal cord damage, or too low, which results in right mainstem intubation, in which only the right lung is ventilated. Reduces transmission of microorganisms.
11. Determine when oral and airway care were last performed. Know the health care agency protocols and procedures but be aware of patient-specific needs for more frequent care.	Oral care protocols help to reduce the incidence of ventilator-associated pneumonia (AACN, 2017a; IHI, 2012; Wiegand, 2017).
12. Assess patient's and caregiver's knowledge of and experience with artificial airway care.	Helps to determine how much to teach the patient and family caregiver as well as provides an opportunity to correct any misinformation they may have. Helps to identify their comfort level with the skill. Encourages cooperation, minimizes risks and anxiety.
13. Assess patient's goals or preferences with how the care should be performed.	Patient adherence is increased when patients are involved in the planning of the care. Allows care to be individualized.
PLANNING	
1. Perform hand hygiene. Gather equipment/supplies and arrange at bedside.	Reduces transmission of microorganisms. Ensures the nurse has the necessary equipment to implement all interventions that should be completed for the patient.

Continued

SKILL 41.2	CARE OF AN ARTIFICIAL AIRWAY—cont'd

STEP	RATIONALE
2. Obtain assistance from available staff.	Reduces risk for accidental extubation of ET or dislodgment of the TT.
3. Close room door or curtains around bed.	Provides for patient privacy.
4. Assist patient in assuming comfortable position for both patient and staff. Elevate patient's head to at least 30 degrees, unless contraindicated.	Provides access to site and facilitates completion of procedure. Prepares patient for any suctioning that may be required. Position may decrease risk of aspiration (AACN, 2018).
5. Explain procedure and patient's need to participate, including not biting or moving ET with tongue, trying not to cough when tape or holder is off ET/TT, keeping hands down, and not pulling on tubing.	Reduces anxiety, encourages cooperation, and reduces risk of accidental extubation or tube dislodgment.

CLINICAL JUDGMENT: *Patients with artificial airways are not always able to verbalize their wants, fears, anxieties, or needs. This impaired ability to communicate can lead to increased anxiety and apprehension. While the patient can often understand what is being said, communication aids should be offered to patients to allow them to ask questions or communicate their concerns (Karlsen et al., 2018; Leung et al., 2018; Salem and Ahmad, 2018).*

IMPLEMENTATION

1. Perform hand hygiene. Apply clean gloves and mask, goggles, or face shield if indicated. Have assistant do so as well.	Reduces transmission of microorganisms.
2. Adjust bed to appropriate height and lower side rail on side nearest you. Check locks on bed wheel.	Minimizes caregiver's muscle strain and prevents injury. Prevents bed from moving.
3. Place clean towel across patient's chest.	Reduces soiling of bedclothes and linen.
4. Perform airway suctioning if indicated (see Skill 41.1).	Removes secretions. Diminishes patient's need to cough during procedure.
5. Perform ET care:	
a. Connect Yankauer suction catheter to suction source and have it ready to use. Ensure that suction source/machine for oral suctioning is on and functioning properly.	Need to have functioning equipment to perform oral care appropriately. Prepares suction apparatus.
b. Remove oral airway or bite block, if present, and cleanse with mild soap and water, rinse. Place on towel.	Provides access to and complete observation of patient's oral cavity.

CLINICAL JUDGMENT: *If patient is biting the tube, do not remove bite block until absolutely necessary. This prevents obstruction of the ET and occlusion of the artificial airway. Wait until the new commercial device is in place and partially or completely secured.*

c. Brush teeth with soft toothbrush, using solution or toothpaste that helps to break down plaque buildup on teeth. Suction oropharyngeal secretions, as necessary.	There may be need for pediatric toothbrush, depending on size of patient's oral cavity. It is recommended to brush teeth at least twice a day (AACN, 2017a; Wiegand, 2017).
d. Use 0.12% chlorhexidine solution, 1.5% hydrogen peroxide, or 0.05% antiseptic solution and oral swabs to clean mouth. Suction oropharyngeal secretions as necessary. Apply mouth moisturizer to oral mucosa and lips after each cleaning. Complete this step every 2–4 hours (check agency policy).	The use of chlorhexidine solution is effective in reducing VAP (AACN, 2017a; Alja'afreh et al., 2019; Wiegand, 2017).
e. Perform subglottic secretion drainage (SSD) if not being continuously performed. **NOTE:** Many ventilators have an integrated subglottic secretion mechanism.	SSD allows for the suction of secretions above the cuff of the ET. Its use, whether continuous or intermittent, helps to reduce the incidence of VAP (Letchford and Bench, 2018; Wiegand, 2017).

CLINICAL JUDGMENT: *The ability to perform SSD is not available on every ET or at every institution. Use SSD if the patient is intubated for greater than 48 to 72 hours, but the provider must choose the tube that allows for SSD when intubating (AACN, 2017b; Rouzé et al., 2017). Continuous SSD has been associated with an increased risk of tracheal hemorrhage or necrosis, so those patients should be closely monitored (Huang et al., 2018).*

f. Prepare to secure the ET:	
(1) Open commercially available ET holder package per manufacturer's instructions. Set device aside with head guard in place and Velcro strips open.	Commercial devices are latex free, convenient, disposable, and provide access to oral mucosa for cleansing. Reduces risk of MARSI.

CLINICAL JUDGMENT: *Commercially available ET holders are recommended for use in patients. ETs are usually taped for short-term use, such as a surgical intubation when extubation is expected when the patient awakes from anesthesia or emergently in the emergency department (ED) (Smith and Pietrantonio, 2016; Wiegand, 2017). However, the use of adhesive tape can lead to medical adhesive–related skin injury (MARSI). This injury occurs during removal of tape when the attachment between the skin and an adhesive is stronger than that between the individual cells, causing either the epidermal layers to separate or the epidermis to detach completely from the dermis (mechanical trauma) (Fumarola et al., 2020). The procedure for taping an ET can be found in Box 41.11.*

BOX 41.11 Steps for Securing an ET With Tape

1. Prepare tape by cutting piece of tape long enough to go completely around patient's head from naris to naris plus 15 cm (6 inches). This is typically 30–60 cm (12–24 inches) in total length.
2. Lay tape adhesive-side up on bedside table.

3. Cut and lay 8–15 cm (3–6 inches) of second piece of tape, adhesive sides together, in center of the long strip to prevent tape from sticking to hair. Smaller strip of tape should cover area between ears around back of head (see illustration A).

4. While one person is holding and stabilizing ET, the other person should remove old tape from patient, using adhesive tape remover to remove sticky residue from patient's skin. The tape will also need to be removed from ET itself. Note that if the sticky adhesive residue is not removed, the new adhesive tape will not properly adhere to tube and/or patient's skin.
5. While one person continues to hold and stabilize ET, clean face and shave patient if needed. Apply skin barrier to area where tape is applied.
6. Slip prepared tape under patient's head and neck, adhesive side up. Take care not to twist tape or catch hair. Do not allow tape to stick to itself. Then slide tape under patient's neck. **NOTE:** In some situations, it may help to gently stick end of tape to tongue blade, which serves as guide.
7. Center tape so that double-faced tape extends around back of neck from ear to ear.

8. On one side of face secure tape from ear to naris (nasal ET) or over lip to ET (oral ET).
9. Tear remaining tape in half lengthwise, forming two pieces that are 1–1.5 cm (0.4–0.6 inch) wide.
10. Secure bottom half of tape across upper lip (oral ET) or across top of nose (nasal ET) to opposite ear.
11. Wrap top half of tape around tube and up from bottom (see illustration B). Tape should encircle tube at least 2 times for security.
12. Gently pull other side of tape firmly to pick up slack and secure to opposite side of face and ET same as first piece (see illustration C). **NOTE:** ET is secured.
13. Assistant can release hold.
14. Check depth mark at lips or gum line.

Illustrations A-C from *Wiegand's AACN procedure manual for high acuity, progressive, and acuity care,* St Louis, 2017, Elsevier.

Continued

SKILL 41.2	CARE OF AN ARTIFICIAL AIRWAY—cont'd

STEP	RATIONALE
(2) Remove Velcro strips from ET and remove ET holder from patient.	Velcro adhesive strips hold ET in place and provide marker to measure distance to patient's lips or gums. These devices permit access to patient's mouth and lips for ease in oropharyngeal suctioning, skin assessment, and oral hygiene.
CLINICAL JUDGMENT: *Clean exterior surface of ET tube with soap and water as needed. If adhesive tape was initially used to secure ET,* ***DO NOT*** *apply adhesive tape remover to the ET itself. This action will make it nearly impossible for the new commercial holder to appropriately stick to the ET, which increases risk of tube dislodgment. Do not allow assistant to hold the tube away from the lips or nares. Doing so allows too much movement in the tube and increases the risk for tube movement and accidental extubation. Instruct assistant not to let go of the ET because it could become dislodged.*	
(3) Remove excess secretions or adhesive from patient's face. Clean facial skin with mild soap and water and dry thoroughly. Shave male patient as necessary.	Application of tape adherence product over dry skin is necessary for new device to stay on patient's face (Wiegand, 2017).
CLINICAL JUDGMENT: *Be sure there is an assistant to hold the ET tube in position while shaving the patient. When shaving patients, take great care to keep the cuff inflation port away from the razor. The razor can inadvertently cut or nick the tubing, causing air loss from the cuff and the possible need for reintubation.*	
(4) Note level of ET by looking at mark or noting centimeter value on tube itself. Move oral ET to other side of mouth and ensure that tube marking at lip is unchanged. **Have assistant hold tube firmly; do not advance or pull out the tube.** Perform oral care as needed on side where tube was initially positioned.	The ET should be repositioned at least daily. Changing sides of ET removes pressure and decreases risk of tissue injury at corners of mouth and oral mucosa (Wiegand, 2017).
CLINICAL JUDGMENT: *The cuff of the ET may need to be deflated before changing its position. If this step needs to be performed, deep oral suctioning should be completed before deflating the cuff. Do not perform oral care until the cuff is properly reinflated (Wiegand, 2017).*	
CLINICAL JUDGMENT: *The patient may cough excessively when the tube is being moved. The person who is holding the tube in place should be prepared for this and take extra caution while holding. The assistant needs to continue holding the ET in place until oral care and, if necessary, shaving is completed, and the commercial ET holder is stabilized and secured. In some cases, the patient may need an antianxiety or sedating medication.*	
CLINICAL JUDGMENT: *If a nasotracheal tube is in place, take special care in removing and reapplying tape to secure the tube. The nasotracheal tube is not moved or repositioned. It is out of the scope of nurse practice to move the nasotracheal tube from one naris to another and could cause great harm to the patient.*	

g. Secure tube. (**NOTE:** Assistant must continue to hold ET in place.)

(1) Thread ET through opening designed to secure it. Be sure that pilot balloon is accessible.

Commercially available holders have a slit in front of holder designed to secure ET.

(2) Place strips of ET holder under patient at occipital region of head.

(3) Verify that ET is at established depth using lip or gum line marker as guide.

Ensures that ET remains at correct depth as determined during assessment.

(4) Attach Velcro strips at base of patient's head. Leave 1 cm (0.4 inch) slack in strips.

(5) Verify that tube is secure, that it does not move forward from patient's mouth or backward down into patient's throat, and that there are no pressure areas on oral mucosa or occipital region of head (see illustration).

Tube must be secure so that it remains at correct depth. It can be secured without being tight and causing pressure.

h. For patient who is unconscious, reinsert cleansed oral airway without pushing tongue into oropharynx, and secure with tape.

Prevents patient from biting ET and allows access for oropharyngeal suctioning. An oral airway is not used in a patient who is conscious and cooperative because it causes excessive gagging and pressure areas to mouth and tongue.

i. Ensure proper cuff inflation by using the pressure manometer to keep the pressure between 20 and 25 mm Hg (Larrow and Klich-Heartt, 2016).

Underinflated cuffs lead to an increased risk of VAP, while overinflated cuffs increase risk of tracheal ischemia or damage (Rouzé et al., 2017; Sanaie et al., 2019; Wiegand, 2017).

STEP	RATIONALE

STEP 5g(5) Commercial endotracheal tube holder. (Modified from Sills JR: *Entry-level respiratory therapist exam guide*, St Louis, 2000, Mosby.)

CLINICAL JUDGMENT: *Other methods to check cuff pressure (minimal leak technique and minimal occluding volume) are utilized in agencies without access to manometers. These techniques have been found to not be as accurate and can lead to overinflation or underinflation of the cuff (Sanaie et al., 2019; Stevens et al., 2018).*

j. Clean rest of face and neck with soapy washcloth, rinse, and dry thoroughly.	Promotes patient comfort.

6. Perform tracheostomy tube care:

a. Preoxygenate patient for 30 seconds or ask patient to take 5 to 6 deep breaths. Then suction tracheostomy (see Skill 41.1). Before removing gloves, remove soiled tracheostomy dressing and discard in glove with coiled catheter.

Removes secretions to avoid occluding outer cannula while inner cannula is removed. Reduces need for patient to cough.

b. Perform hand hygiene. Arrange equipment on bedside table.

Allows for smooth, organized completion of tracheostomy care.
Tracheostomy care should be performed every 4 to 8 hours or per agency protocol (Wiegand, 2017).

c. Open sterile tracheostomy kit. Open two 4 × 4–inch gauze packages using aseptic technique and pour normal saline on one package. Leave second package dry. Open two cotton-tipped swab packages and pour normal saline on one package. Do not recap normal saline.

Decreases risk of infection. Prepares equipment and allows for smooth, organized completion of tracheostomy care. Perform tracheostomy care every 4 to 8 hours or per agency protocol (Wiegand, 2017).

d. Open sterile tracheostomy dressing package.

e. Unwrap sterile basin and pour about 0.5–2 cm (0.2–1 inch) of normal saline into it.

f. Open small sterile brush package and place aseptically into sterile basin.

g. Prepare TT fixation device.

   (1) If using twill tape: Prepare length of twill tape long enough to go around patient's neck 2 times, about 60–75 cm (24–30 inches) for an adult. Cut ends on diagonal. Lay aside in dry area.

Cutting ends of tie on diagonal aids in inserting tie through eyelet.

   (2) If using commercially available TT holder, open package according to manufacturer's directions.

h. Open inner cannula package (if new one is to be inserted such as with disposable inner cannulas or if patient does not tolerate being disconnected from oxygen source while cleaning reusable inner cannula).

i. Apply sterile gloves. Keep dominant hand sterile throughout procedure.

Reduces transmission of microorganisms.

j. Remove oxygen source if present.

CLINICAL JUDGMENT: *It is important to stabilize TT at all times during tracheostomy care to prevent injury, unnecessary discomfort, or accidental extubation. Instruct assistant to apply clean gloves and how to stabilize the TT.*

Continued

SKILL 41.2	**CARE OF AN ARTIFICIAL AIRWAY—cont'd**

STEP	**RATIONALE**

k. Care of tracheostomy with reusable inner cannula:

(1) While touching only outer aspect of tube, unlock and remove inner cannula with nondominant hand following line of tracheostomy. Drop inner cannula into normal saline basin. Clean either twice a day or every 8 hours, depending upon agency policy (Billington and Luckett, 2019; Masood et al., 2018).

Removes inner cannula for cleaning. Normal saline loosens secretions from inner cannula.

> **CLINICAL JUDGMENT:** *If patient is receiving mechanical ventilation, instruct assistant to apply clean gloves and to hold and stabilize TT and to remove the ventilator tube from the connection while you remove the inner cannula. This action helps to ensure that the TT itself is not removed accidentally if difficulties removing the ventilator from the TT or removing the inner cannula from the TT occur.*

(2) Place tracheostomy collar, T tube, or ventilator oxygen source over outer cannula. (**NOTE:** May not be able to attach T tube and ventilator oxygen devices to all outer cannulas when inner cannula is removed.)

Maintains supply of oxygen to patient as needed.

> **CLINICAL JUDGMENT:** *If patient is unable to tolerate being disconnected from the ventilator, replace the inner cannula with a clean new one and reattach the ventilator to the tracheostomy. Then proceed with cleaning the original inner cannula as described in the next steps and store it in a sterile container until the next inner cannula change (Wiegand, 2017).*

(3) To prevent oxygen desaturation if patient is affected, quickly pick up inner cannula and use small brush to remove secretions inside and outside inner cannula (see illustration).

Tracheostomy brush provides mechanical force to remove thick or dried secretions.

(4) Hold inner cannula over basin and rinse with sterile normal saline, using nondominant (clean) hand to pour normal saline.

Removes secretions and normal saline from inner cannula.

(5) Remove oxygen source, replace inner cannula (see illustration), and secure "locking" mechanism. Reapply ventilator, tracheostomy collar, or T tube. Hyperoxygenate patient if needed.

Secures inner cannula and reestablishes oxygen supply.

l. Tracheostomy with disposable inner cannula:

(1) Remove new cannula from manufacturer packaging.

Prepares you for change of inner cannula. Should be changed twice a day (Masood et al., 2018).

(2) While touching only outer aspect of tube, withdraw inner cannula and replace with new cannula by inserting it at a 90-degree angle then rotate downward. Lock into position.

Maintains clean, sterile inner cannula for patient.

> **CLINICAL JUDGMENT:** *If patient is receiving mechanical ventilation, instruct assistant to apply clean gloves and to hold and stabilize TT and to remove the ventilator tube from the connection while you remove the inner cannula. This action helps to ensure that the TT itself is not removed accidentally if difficulties removing the ventilator from the TT or removing the inner cannula from the TT occur.*

(3) Dispose of contaminated cannula in appropriate receptacle and reconnect to ventilator or oxygen supply.

Prevents transmission of infection. Restores oxygen delivery.

STEP 6k(3) Cleaning tracheostomy inner cannula.

STEP 6k(5) Reinserting inner cannula.

STEP	RATIONALE

m. Using normal saline-saturated cotton-tipped swabs and 4 × 4–inch gauze, clean exposed outer cannula surfaces and stoma under faceplate extending 5–10 cm (2–4 inches) in all directions from stoma (see illustration). Clean in circular motion from stoma site outward with dominant hand to handle sterile supplies. Do not go over previously cleaned area.

Aseptically removes secretions from stoma site. Moving in outward circle pulls mucus and other contaminants from stoma to periphery (Bolsega and Sole, 2018; Sole et al., 2015).

n. Using dry 4 × 4–inch gauze, pat lightly at skin and exposed outer cannula surfaces.

Dry surfaces prohibit formation of moist environment for microorganism growth and skin excoriation (Wiegand, 2017).

o. Secure tracheostomy.

CLINICAL JUDGMENT: *Some agencies do not recommend changing the securement device for the first 72 hours after insertion of the TT because of risk of stoma closure if the tube were to become dislodged accidentally (Wiegand, 2017).*

(1) Tracheostomy tie/twill tape method:
  (a) Instruct assistant, if available, to apply clean gloves and securely hold TT in place. With assistant holding TT, cut old ties. **Do not cut pilot balloon of cuff.**

Prevents transmission of infection. Secures TT to prevent accidental dislodgment. If pilot balloon is cut, there is no ability to inflate cuff (Wiegand, 2017).

CLINICAL JUDGMENT: *Assistant must not release hold on TT until new ties are firmly tied. If working without an assistant, do not cut old ties until new ties are in place and securely tied (Harding et al., 2020). When ties are off, this is a good time to clean the back of the patient's neck and assess patient's skin under TT flange and under the ties or tube holder, making sure that skin is intact, free of pressure, and dry before applying securement device.*

  (b) Take prepared twill tape, insert one end of tie through faceplate eyelet, and pull ends even (see illustration).

Diagonal cuts ensure ease of threading end of tie through holes of eyelet (Wiegand, 2017).

  (c) Slide both ends of tie behind head and around neck to other eyelet, and insert one tie through second eyelet.
  (d) Pull snugly

Secures TT.

  (e) Tie ends securely in double square knot, allowing space for insertion of only one loose or two snug finger widths between tie and neck (see illustration).

One finger width of slack prevents ties from being too tight when tracheostomy dressing is in place and prevents movement of tracheostomy tube into lower airway (Wiegand, 2017).

  (f) Apply skin barrier on neck where dressing is applied and allow to dry. Insert fresh 4 × 4–inch precut tracheostomy dressing under clean ties and faceplate (see illustration).

Absorbs drainage. Dressing prevents pressure on clavicle heads (Bolsega and Sole, 2018; Wiegand, 2017). However, gauze dressings may retain secretions and keep the area moist, leading to increased risk of skin breakdown. Barrier product helps prevent skin breakdown around the stoma (Karaca and Korkmaz, 2018).

CLINICAL JUDGMENT: *Never cut a 2 × 2–inch or 4 × 4–inch gauze pad because the cut edges fray and increase the risk of infection (Wiegand, 2017).*

(2) Tracheostomy tube holder method:
  (a) Instruct assistant, if available, to apply clean gloves and securely hold TT in place. When an assistant is unavailable, leave old TT holder in place until new device is secure.

Ensures that tracheostomy stays in correct position. Prevents accidental dislodgment of tube.

STEP 6m Cleaning around stoma.

STEP 6o(1)(b) Replacing tracheostomy ties. Do not remove old tracheostomy ties until new ones are secure.

Continued

SKILL 41.2 CARE OF AN ARTIFICIAL AIRWAY—cont'd

STEP	RATIONALE

STEP 6o(1)(e) Tracheostomy ties properly placed. (From Sorrentino SA: *Mosby's textbook for nursing assistants*, ed 8, St Louis, 2013, Mosby.)

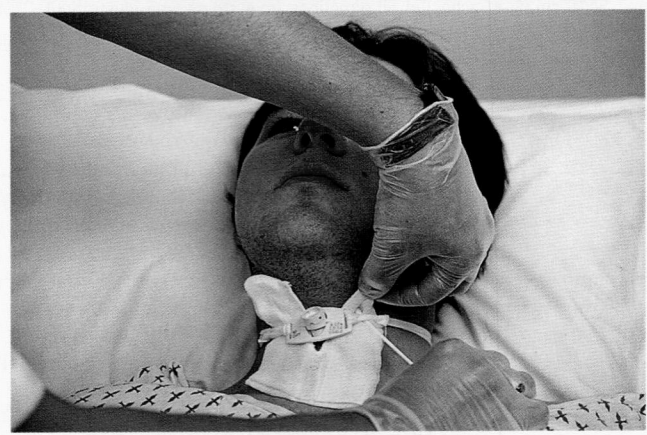

STEP 6o(1)(f) Applying tracheostomy dressing.

STEP	RATIONALE
(b) Align strap under patient's neck. Be sure that Velcro attachments are on either side of TT.	Ensures proper securement of TT.
(c) Place narrow end of ties under and through faceplate eyelets. Pull ends even and secure with Velcro closures (see illustration).	
(d) Verify that there is space for only one loose or two snug finger widths to be inserted under neck strap.	Ensures proper securement of TT without securement device being too tight.
(e) Apply barrier product over skin where dressing is to be applied. Insert fresh 4 × 4–inch precut tracheostomy dressing under clean neck plate (see Step 6o[1][f]).	Absorbs drainage. Dressing prevents pressure on clavicle heads (Bolsega and Sole, 2018; Wiegand, 2017). However, gauze dressings may retain secretions and keep the area moist, leading to increased risk of skin breakdown. Barrier product helps prevent skin breakdown around the stoma (Karaca and Korkmaz, 2018).

CLINICAL JUDGMENT: *Never cut a 2 × 2–inch or 4 × 4–inch gauze pad because the cut edges fray and increase the risk of infection* (Wiegand, 2017).

STEP	RATIONALE
7. Ensure that the tracheostomy tube is midline and that no excess traction is applied.	Prevents the development of complications such as tracheal erosion or skin ulcerations (Wiegand, 2017).
8. Perform oral care with toothbrush or oral swabs and chlorhexidine rinse.	Use of chlorhexidine may decrease patient risk of developing a ventilator-associated event (VAE)/ventilator-associated pneumonia (VAP) and promotes patient comfort (AACN, 2017b; Huang et al., 2018).

STEP 6o(2)(c) Tracheostomy tube holder in place. (Courtesy Dale Medical Products, Plainville, MA.)

STEP	RATIONALE
9. Measure cuff pressure with the manometer; add or remove air/saline/water from cuff to maintain pressure between 20 and 25 mm Hg.	Complete at least once per shift but could be every 2 to 4 hours (follow agency policy). Prevents aspiration of oral secretions. Prevents tracheal damage (Billington and Luckett, 2019; Wiegand, 2017).

CLINICAL JUDGMENT: *Overinflated cuffs (pressure greater than 25 cm H$_2$O) can lead to tracheal stenosis, necrosis, tracheomalacia, and fistula formation. Underinflated cuffs can lead to ineffective mechanical ventilation and increase risk of aspiration (Billington and Luckett, 2019; Wiegand, 2017).*

CLINICAL JUDGMENT: *If cuff is deflated during use of speaking valve, then inflate cuff once the use of the valve is finished and measure cuff pressures. Oral and/or subglottic suctioning should be performed before a cuff is deflated (Pozuelo-Carrascosa et al., 2020).*

STEP	RATIONALE
10. Discard soiled items in appropriate receptacle; remove towel and place in laundry. Remove gloves and mask, goggles, or face shield or gown; discard in receptacle; and perform hand hygiene. (Assistant performs same steps.) Place clean items (e.g., oral care solution, excess swabs) in place of storage.	Reduces transmission of microorganisms. Ensures that contaminated gloves and hands do not touch clean items.
11. Be sure that oxygen- or humidification-delivery sources are in place and set at correct levels.	Humidification provides moisture for airway, makes it easier to suction secretions, and decreases risk of mucous plugs.
12. Reposition patient comfortably, with head of bed elevated at least 30 degrees (unless contraindicated), and assess respiratory status. Raise side rails (as appropriate) and lower bed to lowest position.	Promotes comfort. Some patients require post-tracheostomy care suctioning. Keeping the head of the bed at 30–45 degrees helps to decrease risk of VAP (Wiegand, 2017). Ensures patient safety.
13. Place the nurse call system in an accessible location within patient's reach.	Ensures patient can call for assistance if needed.
14. Replace cap on reusable normal saline bottles. Store reusable liquids, date container, and store unused supplies in appropriate place. Perform hand hygiene.	Once opened, normal saline is considered free of bacteria for 24 hours.

EVALUATION

1. Compare respiratory assessments before and after ET/TT care.	Identifies any physiological changes, including presence and quality of breath sounds after procedure.
2. Observe depth and position of ET according to health care provider recommendation.	Do not alter position of ET.
3. Assess security of tape by *gently* tugging at tube.	Tape should remain attached to face. Patient may cough during tugging.
4. Assess skin around mouth, oral mucous membranes, and/or tracheal stoma for intactness and pressure sores or MARSI.	Tape should not tear skin. Pressure areas (blisters, tears) should be absent.
5. Compare pulse oximeter and E$_t$CO$_2$ values from before and after ET/TT care.	Changes in oxygen saturation and E$_t$CO$_2$ can help identify displacement or dislodgment of ET/TT.
6. Observe for excessive phonation or presence of gastric secretions in airway secretions.	Occurs with inadequate or excessive cuff inflation.
7. **Use Teach-Back:** "I want to be sure I explained why we need to clean your breathing tube routinely. Tell me why the cleaning of your tube is important for your breathing." Revise your instruction now or develop plan for patient/family caregiver teaching if patient/family caregiver is not able to teach back correctly.	Teach-back is an evidence-based health literacy intervention that promotes patient engagement, patient safety, adherence, and quality. The goal of teach-back is to ensure that you have explained medical information clearly so that patients and their families understand what you communicated to them (AHRQ, 2020).

UNEXPECTED OUTCOMES AND RELATED INTERVENTIONS

1. Tube is dislodged or misplaced accidentally, including extubation.
   - Remain with patient while calling for help.
   - Ventilate with bag-valve-mask as needed.
   - Assess patient for airway patency, spontaneous breathing, and vital signs.
   - Prepare for retaping or securing procedure or reintubation.
2. Patient has pressure injury in mouth, lips, nares, or tracheal stoma or MARSI underlying any adhesive.
   - Increase frequency of ET care.
   - Apply antimicrobial ointment per agency protocol.
   - Align oxygen and humidity supply tubing so that they do not pull ET, creating pressure sores.
   - Monitor for infection. If skin tear is present on cheeks or over nose or upper lip, apply protective barrier such as stoma adhesive patch or hydrocolloid dressing and apply tape to it. Consider using commercial fixation device if tape used previously.
3. Cuff leak develops.
   - Verify position of tube, notify respiratory therapy, and follow agency policy.

Continued

SKILL 41.2	CARE OF AN ARTIFICIAL AIRWAY—cont'd

RECORDING AND REPORTING

- Record respiratory assessments before and after tube care, condition of skin and areas underlying tube, depth of ET or type and size of tracheostomy tube, frequency and extent of care, patient tolerance, and any complications related to presence of the tube.
- Document your evaluation of patient learning.
- Report signs of infection or displacement of ET or tracheostomy tube immediately.
- Report time of care and patient tolerance, including vital sign changes or any changes in pulse oximeter, E_tCO_2, or respiratory status, and presence of any areas of impaired skin integrity on face or neck, in the mouth, or around the nares or tracheal stoma.

HOME CARE CONSIDERATIONS

- Instruct family caregivers in how to obtain supplies. Perform routine tracheostomy care at least once a day after discharge from hospital. At home, clean technique with nonsterile gloves is usually used.
- Patients with tracheostomies may need to communicate with others by writing or use of computer. Ensure that they have communication devices that meet their needs.
- Instruct family caregivers in signs and symptoms of respiratory distress, tube dysfunction, and respiratory and stoma infections. Call health care provider if patient feels pain or discomfort longer than a week after insertion, if breathing does not improve after usual method of clearing secretions, or if secretions become thick or mucous plugs are present.
- When outside, use tracheostomy covers to protect from dust or cold air.
- Never remove the outer cannula unless instructed by health care provider to do so.

SKILL 41.3	CARE OF PATIENTS WITH CHEST TUBES

Delegation and Collaboration

The skill of chest tube management cannot be delegated to assistive personnel (AP). The nurse directs the AP about:

- Proper positioning of the patient with chest tubes to facilitate chest tube drainage and optimal functioning of the system.
- Ambulating, repositioning, and transferring patient with chest drainage system in place.
- Reporting changes in vital signs, complaints of chest pain or sudden shortness of breath, or excessive bubbling in water-seal chamber to the nurse immediately.
- Danger of any disconnection of drainage system, change in type and amount of drainage, sudden bleeding, or sudden cessation of bubbling.

Equipment

- Prescribed chest drainage system
- Water-seal system or waterless (dry suction system): sterile water or normal saline per manufacturer's directions
- Suction source and setup
- Sterile skin preparation solution (povidone-iodine or chlorhexidine solutions)
- Clean gloves
- Sterile gauze sponges
- Local anesthetic, if not an emergent procedure
- Chest tube tray (all items are sterile): knife handle (1), knife blade No. 10 or disposable safety scalpel No. 10, chest tube clamp, small sponge forceps, needle holder, size 3-0 silk sutures, tray liner (sterile field), curved 8-inch Kelly clamps (2), 4 × 4–inch sponges (10), suture scissors, hand towels (3), sterile gloves
- Dressings: Petrolatum or Xeroform gauze, split chest-tube dressings, several 4 × 4–inch gauze dressings, large gauze dressings (2), and 4-inch tape
- Personal protective equipment (PPE): head cover, face mask/face shield, sterile gloves
- Two rubber-tipped hemostats (shodded) for each chest tube
- 2.5-cm (1-inch) waterproof adhesive tape or plastic zip ties for securing connections.
- Stethoscope, sphygmomanometer, and pulse oximeter

STEP	RATIONALE

ASSESSMENT

1. Identify patient using at least two identifiers (e.g., name and birthday or name and account number) according to agency policy. Compare identifiers with information on the patient's MAR or medical record.

Ensures correct patient. Complies with The Joint Commission standards and improves patient safety (TJC, 2021).

2. Review health care provider's order for chest tube placement.

Insertion of chest tube requires health care provider order.

3. Assess EHR for significant medical history or report of injury, including chronic lung disease, spontaneous pneumothorax, pulmonary disease, therapeutic procedures, and mechanism of injury (Pickett, 2017).

Medical history or injury may provide the reason for the occurrence of the pneumothorax, hemothorax, empyema, and/or pleural effusion.

4. If nonemergent, assess for patient's or family caregiver's health literacy.

Assures patient or family caregiver has the capacity to obtain, communicate, process, and understand basic health information (CDC, 2021a).

5. Review patient's medication record for anticoagulant therapy, including aspirin, warfarin, heparin, or platelet aggregation inhibitors such as ticlopidine or dipyridamole.

Anticoagulation therapy can increase procedure-related blood loss.

6. Assess patient for known allergies. Ask patient about any history of problems (such as skin sensitivity) with medications, latex, or anything applied to the skin.

Povidone-iodine and chlorhexidine are antiseptic solutions used to clean skin before tube insertion (Huggins et al., 2021; Walters, 2017). Lidocaine is a local anesthetic administered to reduce pain. The chest tube will be held in place with tape and sutures (Wiegand, 2017).

7. Inspect condition of skin around chest. Note if patient is diaphoretic or has history of impaired poor perfusion, altered tissue tolerance, poor nutrition, or edema.

Provides baseline for monitoring development of a medical device–related pressure injury (MDRPI) (Fumarola et al., 2020).

STEP	RATIONALE
8. Review patient's hemoglobin and hematocrit levels.	Parameters reflect whether blood loss is occurring, which may affect oxygenation.
9. Assess patient's comfort level on a scale of 0 to 10.	Provides a baseline to compare after chest tube insertion.

CLINICAL JUDGMENT: *In some situations it may be necessary to administer prescribed analgesics or sedatives during the assessment phase. The medications reduce the patient's discomfort and anxiety and help to facilitate patient cooperation during assessment and the subsequent procedure (Huggins et al., 2021; Pickett, 2017).*

STEP	RATIONALE
10. Perform hand hygiene and perform a complete respiratory assessment, baseline vital signs, and pulse oximetry (SpO_2).	Baseline assessment and vital signs are essential for any invasive procedure. Chest tube insertion often relieves respiratory distress.
a. Assess for signs and symptoms of increased respiratory distress and hypoxia (e.g., decreased breath sounds over affected and unaffected lungs, marked cyanosis, asymmetrical chest movements, displaced trachea, shortness of breath, and confusion).	Signs and symptoms associated with respiratory distress are related to type and size of pneumothorax, hemothorax, or preexisting illness. Signs of hypoxia are related to inadequate oxygen to tissues.
b. Assess for sharp, stabbing chest pain or chest pain on inspiration, hypotension, and tachycardia. If possible, ask patient to rate level of comfort on a scale of 0 to 10.	Sharp, stabbing chest pain with or without decreased blood pressure and increased heart rate may indicate tension pneumothorax. Presence of pneumothorax or hemothorax is painful, frequently causing sharp inspiratory pain. In addition, discomfort is associated with presence of a chest tube, not just with its insertion. Adequate pain control promotes better patient participation in activity (Chotai and Mosenifar, 2018).
11. For patients who have existing chest tubes, observe:	
a. Inspect skin around chest tube dressing and site surrounding tube insertion. Keep a box of sterile 4 × 4–inch gauze pads and petroleum gauze at bedside.	Ensures that dressing is intact and that occlusive seal remains without air or fluid leaks and that area surrounding insertion site is free of drainage or skin irritation (Chotai and Mosenifar, 2018). The 4 × 4–inch gauze pads are used in the event of chest tube(s) dislodgment. Covering the site immediately and taping the dressing on three sides is essential. Notify health care provider immediately.
b. The amount and type of chest tube drainage by marking the drainage level on the outside of the drainage-collection chamber in hourly or shift increments, or in increments established by the health care provider, or the agency's policy.	Marking the container provides reference point for future measurements. Drainage should decrease gradually and change from bloody to pink to straw colored. Sudden flow of dark bloody drainage that occurs with position change is often old blood.
c. Tubing for kinks, dependent loops, or clots.	Maintains a patent, freely draining system, preventing fluid accumulation in chest cavity. When tubing is coiled, looped, or clotted, drainage is impeded, and there is an increased risk for tension pneumothorax or surgical emphysema (Chotai and Mosenifar, 2018; Pickett, 2017).
d. Verify that chest drainage system is upright and below level of tube insertion.	An upright drainage system facilitates drainage and maintains water seal.
12. Remove and dispose of gloves. Perform hand hygiene.	
13. Assess patient's knowledge, prior experience with a chest tube, and feelings about procedure.	Reveals need for patient instruction and/or support.
14. Assess patient's goals or preferences for how skill is to be performed or what patient expects.	Allows care to be individualized to patient.

PLANNING

STEP	RATIONALE
1. Perform hand hygiene. Organize equipment/supplies and arrange at bedside.	Reduces transmission of infection and ensures the necessary equipment is available to implement all interventions that should be completed.
2. Close room curtain or door.	Maintains privacy.
3. Assist patient in assuming supine or a semirecumbent position for insertion of the chest tube. Assist to a position of optimal comfort during other chest tube care.	Appropriate positioning is important for the proper insertion of the chest tube. Position of optimal comfort, once tube is inserted, will allow for increase in physical activity, including deep breathing, coughing, and use of the incentive spirometer.
4. Be available while provider explains insertion procedure to the patient. Once tube is inserted and during normal management, explain the care that you will be providing. If applicable, teach patient how to move with chest tube in place.	Reduces anxiety and encourages cooperation.

IMPLEMENTATION

STEP	RATIONALE
1. Check agency policy and determine whether informed consent is needed. Complete "Time Out" procedure.	Invasive medical procedures typically require informed consent. "Time Out" is completed to determine right patient, procedure, and location of insertion or incision site (Wiegand, 2017).
2. Perform hand hygiene and don appropriate PPE.	Reduces transmission of microorganisms.

Continued

SKILL 41.3   CARE OF PATIENTS WITH CHEST TUBES—cont'd

STEP	RATIONALE
3. Set up water-seal system (or dry system with suction); see manufacturer's guidelines.	The water-seal system contains two or three compartments or chambers. Fluid drains into the first chamber. The second chamber contains the water seal, which allows air to escape because of the force of expiration but not to reenter on inspiration. If suction is needed, a third chamber is used.
a. Prepare chest drainage system. Remove wrappers and prepare to set up two- or three-chamber system.	Maintains sterility of system for use under sterile operating room conditions.
b. While maintaining sterility of drainage tubing, stand system upright and add sterile water or normal saline (NS) to appropriate compartments.	Reduces possibility of contamination.
(1) *Two-chamber system (without suction):* Add sterile solution to water-seal chamber (second chamber), bringing fluid to required level as indicated or ordered by health care provider.	Water-seal chamber acts as one-way valve, so air cannot enter pleural space (Sasa, 2019; Chotai and Mosenifar, 2018).
(2) *Three-chamber system (with suction):* Add sterile solution to water-seal chamber (second chamber). Add amount of sterile solution prescribed by health care provider to suction-control chamber (third chamber), usually -20 cm H_2O pressure. Connect tubing from suction-control chamber to suction source. Tailor length of drainage tube to patient. **NOTE:** Suction control chamber vent must not be occluded when using suction (see illustration).	Depth of fluid level dictates highest amount of negative pressure that can be present within system. For example, 20 cm of water is approximately -20 cm of H_2O pressure. After chest tube is inserted, turn up the wall or portable suction device until water in suction-control bottle exhibits continuous, gentle bubbling.

CLINICAL JUDGMENT: *When increasing suction, remember that increased bubbling does not result in more suction to the chest cavity, but only serves to evaporate the water more quickly. The suction pressure should not exceed -20 cm H_2O because lung tissue damage may occur (Chotai and Mosenifar, 2018).*

---

(3) *Dry suction system:* Fill water-seal chamber with sterile solution. Adjust suction-control dial to prescribed level of suction; suction ranges from -10 to -40 cm of water pressure. Suction-control chamber vent is never occluded when suction is used. **NOTE:** On dry suction system, **DO NOT** obstruct positive-pressure relief valve. This allows air to escape.	Automatic control valve on dry suction-control device adjusts to changes in patient air leaks and fluctuation in suction source and vacuum to deliver prescribed amount of suction.
4. Set up waterless system (see manufacturer's guidelines).	A waterless system is like a water-seal system except that sterile water is not required for suction. The suction-control chamber is replaced by a one-way valve located near the top of the system. The suction-control chamber contains a suction-control float ball that is set by a suction-control dial (between -10 and -40 cm H_2O after the suction is connected and turned on) (Zisis et al., 2015).

STEP 3b(2) *Left,* Pleur-Evac three-chamber drainage system. *Right,* Schematic of drainage device.

STEP	RATIONALE
5. Secure all tubing connections with tape applied in double-spiral fashion using 2.5-cm (1-inch) adhesive tape or zip ties (nylon cable) with a clamp (Pickett, 2017). Check system for patency by: 　**a.** Clamping drainage tubing that will connect to patient's chest tube. 　**b.** Connecting tubing from float ball chamber to suction source. 　**c.** Turning on suction to prescribed level.	Prevents atmospheric air from leaking into system and patient's intrapleural space. Provides chance to ensure airtight system before connection to patient.
6. Turn off suction source and unclamp drainage tubing before connecting patient to system. Suction source is turned on again after patient is connected.	Having patient connected to suction when it is initiated could damage pleural tissues from sudden increase in negative pressure. Tubing that is coiled or looped prevents adequate drainage and may cause tension pneumothorax (Pickett, 2017; Wiegand, 2017).
7. If not administered during assessment, administer procedure medications such as sedatives or analgesics as ordered. (Give medications 30 minutes before procedure.)	Reduces patient anxiety and pain during procedure.

CLINICAL JUDGMENT: *During procedure, carefully monitor patient for changes in level of sedation.*

STEP	RATIONALE
8. Provide psychological support to patient (Kirkwood, 2017). 　**a.** Reinforce preprocedure explanation. 　**b.** Coach and support patient throughout procedure.	Reduces patient anxiety and helps complete procedure efficiently.
9. Perform hand hygiene and apply clean gloves. Check patient position for tube insertion so that side in which tube is to be inserted is accessible to health care provider.	Reduces transmission of microorganisms. For pneumothorax, place patient in lateral supine position. For hemothorax, place patient in semi-Fowler's position (Chotai and Mosenifar, 2018).
10. Assist health care provider with chest tube insertion by providing needed equipment and local analgesic. Health care provider anesthetizes skin over insertion site, makes small skin incision, inserts clamped tube, sutures it in place, and applies occlusive dressing.	Ensures smooth insertion.
11. Help health care provider attach drainage tube to chest tube; remove clamp. Turn on suction to prescribed level.	Connects drainage system and suction (if ordered) to chest tube.
12. Tape or zip-tie all connections between chest tube and drainage tube. (**NOTE:** Chest tube is usually taped by health care provider at time of tube placement; check agency policy.)	Secures chest tube to drainage system and reduces risk for air leak that causes breaks in airtight system (Chotai and Mosenifar, 2018; Wiegand, 2017).
13. Check systems for proper functioning. Health care provider orders chest x-ray film.	Verifies intrapleural placement of tube.
14. After tube placement position patient: 　**a.** Semi-Fowler's or high-Fowler's position to evacuate air (pneumothorax) (Chotai and Mosenifar, 2018) 　**b.** High-Fowler's position to drain fluid (hemothorax) (Chotai and Mosenifar, 2018)	Permits optimum drainage of fluid and/or air.
15. Check patency of air vents in system. 　**a.** Water-seal vent must have no occlusion. 　**b.** Suction-control chamber vent is not occluded when suction is used. 　**c.** Waterless systems have relief valves without caps.	Permits displaced air to pass into atmosphere. Provides safety factor of releasing excess negative pressure into atmosphere. Provides safety factor of releasing excess negative pressure.
16. Position excess tubing horizontally on mattress next to patient. Secure with clamp provided so that it does not obstruct tubing.	Prevents excess tubing from hanging over edge of mattress in dependent loop. Drainage collected in loop can occlude drainage system, which predisposes patient to tension pneumothorax (Pickett, 2017; Wiegand, 2017).
17. Adjust tubing to hang in straight line from chest tube to drainage chamber.	Promotes drainage and prevents fluid or blood from accumulating in pleural cavity.

CLINICAL JUDGMENT: *Frequent gentle lifting of the drain allows gravity to help blood and other viscous material to move to the drainage bottle. Patients with recent chest surgery or trauma need to have the chest drain lifted on the basis of assessment of the amount of drainage; some patients might need chest tube drains lifted every 5 to 10 minutes until drainage volume decreases. However, when coiled or dependent looping of tubing is unavoidable, lift the tubing every 15 minutes at a minimum to promote drainage (Pickett, 2017).*

STEP	RATIONALE
18. Place two rubber-tipped hemostats (for each chest tube) in easily accessible position (e.g., taped to top of patient's headboard). These should remain with patient when ambulating.	Chest tubes are double clamped under specific circumstances: (1) to assess for air leak, (2) to empty or quickly change disposable systems, (3) to assess whether patient is ready to have tube removed, or (4) if chest tube becomes accidentally disconnected from drainage system (Muzzy and Butler, 2015).

CLINICAL JUDGMENT: *In the event of a chest tube disconnection or if the drainage system breaks, submerge the distal part of the tube 2 to 4 cm (1 to 2 inches) below the surface of a 250-mL bottle of sterile water or NS until a new chest tube unit can be set up (Harding et al., 2020).*

STEP	RATIONALE
19. Dispose of sharps in proper container, dispose of used supplies.	Reduces transmission of microorganisms.

Continued

SKILL 41.3	CARE OF PATIENTS WITH CHEST TUBES—cont'd

STEP	RATIONALE

20. Care of patient after chest tube insertion:

a. Perform hand hygiene and apply clean gloves. Assess vital signs; oxygen saturation; skin color; breath sounds; rate, depth, and ease of respirations; and insertion site every 15 minutes for first 2 hours, and then at least every shift (see agency policy).

Provides immediate information about procedure-related complications such as respiratory distress and leakage.

b. For severe pain, administer ordered analgesics and use complementary pain relief measures (e.g., repositioning) as needed.

c. Monitor color, consistency, and amount of chest tube drainage every 15 minutes for first 2 hours after insertion. Indicate level of drainage fluid, date, and time on write-on surface of chamber.

Provides baseline for continuous assessment of type and quantity of drainage. Ensures early detection of complications.

(1) From mediastinal tube, expect less than 100 mL/hr immediately after surgery and no more than 500 mL in first 24 hours.

Sudden gush of drainage may result from coughing or changing patient's position (i.e., releasing pooled/collected blood rather than indicating active bleeding). Acute bleeding indicates hemorrhage. Notify health care provider if there is more than 100–200 mL of bloody drainage in an hour (Harding et al., 2020; Wiegand, 2017).

(2) From posterior chest tube, drainage is grossly bloody during first several hours after surgery and changes to serous (Harding et al., 2020).

Acute bleeding indicates hemorrhage. Notify health care provider if there is more than 200 mL of bloody drainage in an hour (Harding et al., 2020; Pickett, 2017).

(3) Expect little or no output from anterior chest tube that is inserted for a pneumothorax (Wiegand, 2017).

CLINICAL JUDGMENT: *Routine stripping or milking of the chest tube is not a recommended practice. Doing so can result in increased pressure in the thoracic cavity, causing damage to the lungs or the pleural tissues. If there is a visible clot in the tubing, gentle milking of the tubing (manual squeezing and releasing of parts of the tubing) may be indicated, but only if the patient is at risk of further harm from the clot, such as the development of a tension pneumothorax (Wiegand, 2017).*

d. Observe chest dressing for drainage and determine whether it is still occlusive.

Drainage around tube may indicate blockage of the tube. Many health care agencies require the chest tube dressings to be occlusive in nature.

CLINICAL JUDGMENT: *If the dressing is not occlusive or is saturated with drainage, it may need to be changed. There is no standard for how chest tube dressings should be performed, such as a sterile versus a nonsterile dressing change. Know the health care agency standards for this procedure. Some health care agencies require the use of petrolatum gauze around the chest tube while others do not (Gross et al., 2016).*

e. Perform hand hygiene and apply clean gloves. Observe chest dressing for drainage and palpate around tube for swelling and crepitus (subcutaneous emphysema) as noted by crackling.

Indicates presence of air trapping in subcutaneous tissues. Most occurrences of crepitus are minor as small amounts are commonly absorbed. Large amounts are potentially dangerous, and you need to notify the health care provider (Pickett, 2017; Sasa, 2019).

CLINICAL JUDGMENT: *When patients develop subcutaneous emphysema (i.e., a collection of air under the skin after chest tube placement), a crepitus (a crackling sensation) is felt with tactile fremitus on palpation. Subcutaneous emphysema can occur if tubing is blocked or kinked.*

f. Check tubing to ensure that it is free of kinks and dependent loops.

Promotes drainage and prevents the development of a tension pneumothorax.

g. Observe for fluctuation of water-seal chamber and drainage in tubing during inspiration and expiration. Observe for clots or debris in tubing.

If fluctuation or tidaling stops, it means that either the lung is fully expanded or system is obstructed. In patient who is spontaneously breathing, fluid rises in water-seal or diagnostic indicator (waterless system) with inspiration and falls with expiration. The opposite occurs in patient who is mechanically ventilated. This indicates that system is functioning properly (Wiegand, 2017).

h. Keep drainage system upright and below level of patient's chest.

Promotes gravity drainage and prevents backflow of fluid and air into pleural space.

i. Check for air leaks by monitoring bubbling in water-seal chamber. Intermittent bubbling is normal during expiration when air is being evacuated from pleural cavity, but continuous bubbling during both inspiration and expiration indicates leak in system.

Absence of bubbling may indicate that lung is fully expanded in patient with pneumothorax. Check all connections and locate sources of air leak.

21. Instruct patient how to regularly take deep breaths and reposition as often as possible.

Facilitates and maintains lung expansion.

22. Assist patient to semi- or high Fowler's position. Verify that patient is comfortable.

Facilitates lung expansion and chest tube drainage.
Promotes patient comfort and safety.

STEP	RATIONALE
23. Raise side rails (as appropriate) and lower bed to lowest position.	Ensures patient safety.
24. Place the nurse call system in an accessible location within patient's reach.	Ensures patient can call for assistance if needed.
25. Dispose of all contaminated supplies in appropriate receptacle, remove and dispose of gloves, and perform hand hygiene.	Reduces transmission of microorganisms. Use appropriate disposal receptacle if patient is on hazardous drugs (Oncology Nursing Society [ONS], 2018).

EVALUATION

1. Observe patient for decreased respiratory distress and chest pain. Auscultate patient's lungs and observe chest expansion.	Determines status of lung expansion.
2. Monitor vital signs and SpO$_2$.	Determines whether level of oxygenation has improved.
3. Determine patient's level of comfort on scale of 0 to 10, comparing level with comfort before chest tube insertion and/or pain medication administration.	Indicates need for analgesia. Patient with chest tube discomfort hesitates to take deep breaths and as a result is at risk for pneumonia and atelectasis.
4. Observe patient's ability to use deep-breathing exercises and reposition self while maintaining comfort.	Indicates patient's ability to promote lung expansion and prevent complications. Patients need to be repositioned every 2 hours when a chest tube is in place (Wiegand, 2017).
5. Monitor continued functioning of system as indicated by reduction in amount of drainage, resolution of air leak, and complete reexpansion of the lung.	Detects early signs of system complications or indicates possible removal of chest tube.
6. Use Teach-Back: "I want to be sure I explained why you have a chest tube. Explain to me why you have this tube and what we are doing to keep the system functioning." Revise your instruction now or develop a plan for revised patient/family caregiver teaching if patient/family caregiver is not able to teach back correctly.	Teach-back is an evidence-based health literacy intervention that promotes patient engagement, patient safety, adherence, and quality. The goal of teach-back is to ensure that you have explained medical information clearly so that patients and their families understand what you communicated to them (AHRQ, 2020).

UNEXPECTED OUTCOMES AND RELATED INTERVENTIONS

1. Patient develops respiratory distress. Chest pain, decrease in breath sounds over affected and unaffected lungs, marked cyanosis, asymmetrical chest movements, presence of subcutaneous emphysema around tube insertion site or neck, hypotension, tachycardia, and/or mediastinal shift are critical and indicate severe change in patient status, such as excessive blood loss or tension pneumothorax.
   - Notify health care provider immediately.
   - Collect set of vital signs and SpO2.
   - Prepare for chest x-ray film.
   - Provide oxygen as ordered.
   - Be sure patient has head of bed elevated 45 degrees.
2. Air leak is unrelated to patient's respirations.
   - Locate leak by clamping chest tube with two rubber-shodded or toothless clamps close to the chest wall. If bubbling stops, air leak is inside patient's thorax or at the insertion site, and the health care provider should be notified.
   - If bubbling continues with the clamps near the chest wall, gradually move one clamp at a time down the drainage tubing away from the patient and toward the drainage chamber. When the bubbling stops, the leak is in the section of the tubing between the two clamps. If the leak occurs when the clamps are near the drainage system, then the leak is in the drainage system itself. If there is a leak in the tubing or the drainage system, the nurse can replace the tubing or the drainage system (Wiegand, 2017).
3. Chest tube is disconnected/dislodged.
   - Check connections and reattach using sterile technique (Chotai and Mosenifar, 2018).
   - Immediately apply pressure over chest tube insertion site.
   - Have assistant obtain sterile petroleum gauze dressing. Apply as patient exhales. Secure dressing with tight seal. Dressing with tape over three of four sides may allow for escape of air if there is residual pneumothorax.
   - Notify health care provider.

RECORDING AND REPORTING

- Record and report respiratory assessment; amount of suction, if used; amount of drainage since the previous assessment; type and amount of drainage in chest tubing; presence or absence of an air leak, including amount if present; and patient comfort level.
- Record integrity of dressing, presence of drainage on dressing, and condition of skin around dressing and tube insertion site.
- Document your evaluation of patient learning.
- Record and report patient tolerance to new chest tube insertion; comfort level and any analgesia; respiratory assessment before and after insertion; quantity and quality of chest tube drainage.

HOME CARE CONSIDERATIONS

- Patients with chronic conditions (e.g., uncomplicated pneumothorax, effusions, or empyema) that require long-term chest tube therapy may be discharged with smaller mobile drains (Venuta et al., 2017).
- Instruct patient in how to ambulate and remain active with a mobile chest tube drainage system.
- Instruct patient and family caregivers about when to contact health care provider or seek emergency medical care regarding changes in the drainage system (e.g., chest pain, breathlessness, change in color or amount of drainage, leakage on the dressing around the chest tube).

SKILL 41.4	USING HOME OXYGEN EQUIPMENT

Delegation and Collaboration

The skill of administering home oxygen equipment cannot be delegated to assistive personnel (AP). However, in some instances assistive personnel (AP) are in the patient's home to provide hygiene and other care. Therefore, it is important to instruct the home care AP about:

- The unique needs of the patient (e.g., amount of assistance in applying nasal cannula or mask) and any assistance needed in filling liquid canisters.
- The type of equipment the patient should have in the home and the oxygen flow rate.
- Immediately reporting to the nurse concerning an increased rate of breathing, decreased level of consciousness, increased confusion, or pain.
- Reporting to the nurse about potential or actual problems with the home oxygen equipment

Equipment

- Nasal cannula, oxygen mask, or other prescribed delivery device (see Procedural Guidelines Box 41.9 for required equipment)
- Humidification device if oxygen delivery greater than 4 L/min
- Oxygen tubing available in lengths of 50 feet
- Home oxygen-delivery system (compressed oxygen, oxygen concentrator, or liquid oxygen) with all required equipment (varies with supplier and system used)
- "No Smoking/Oxygen in Use" sign for each entrance to the home

STEP	RATIONALE

ASSESSMENT

1. Identify patient using at least two identifiers (e.g., name and birthday or name and account number) according to agency policy. Compare identifiers with information on patient's MAR or medical record.

Ensures correct patient. Complies with The Joint Commission Standards and improves patient safety (TJC, 2021).

2. Review health care provider's order for home oxygen equipment.

A health care provider's order is required for home oxygen use.

3. Review patient's medical record for previous teaching sessions about home oxygen therapy and patient's or family caregiver's response to teaching.

Identifies status of patient teaching and potential concerns of patient and/or family caregiver regarding how to manage oxygen equipment in the home.

4. Assess patient's or family caregiver's health literacy.

Ensures patient or family caregiver has the capacity to obtain, communicate, process, and understand basic health information (CDC, 2021a).

5. While patient is still in the hospital, determine patient's or family caregiver's ability to use oxygen equipment correctly. In home setting, reassess for access to and appropriate use of equipment.

Physical or cognitive impairments necessitate instructing family member or significant other how to operate home oxygen equipment. Ongoing assessment enables you to determine specific components of skill that patient or family can complete easily.

6. Inform the patient/family caregiver that the home oxygen vendor will assess home environment for adequate electrical service if oxygen concentrator is ordered.

Oxygen concentrators require electricity to work. Continuous oxygen therapy must not be interrupted.

7. Complete a risk assessment that includes assessment of the patient's and family members' or visitors' smoking status, and other household risks of fire, falls, or other injuries (Suntharalingam et al., 2018).

NOTE: This may be done with home care nursing services and equipment vendor.

Ensures safe, continuous delivery of home oxygen.

8. Assess patient's and family's knowledge of home oxygen use, their ability to understand safety precautions, and their ability to observe for signs and symptoms of hypoxia: apprehension, anxiety, decreased ability to concentrate, decreased level of consciousness, increased fatigue, dizziness, behavioral changes, increased pulse, increased respiratory rate, pallor, or cyanosis of the mucous membranes.

Hypoxia occurs at home despite use of oxygen therapy. Worsening of patient's physical condition or another underlying condition such as a change in the respiratory status can cause hypoxia.

9. Assess patient's goals or preferences for how skill is to be performed or what patient expects.

Allows care to be individualized to patient.

PLANNING

1. Explain need for and use of home oxygen therapy.

Improves adherence to the treatment regimen. Decreases anxiety and the need for home oxygen.

2. Plan time for patient and family caregiver to meet with home oxygen vendor to determine appropriate resources in community for equipment and assistance, including maintenance and repair services and medical equipment supplier.

Ensures readily available assistance for patients with home oxygen systems. Delivery and setup with basic instruction on how to use and maintain home oxygen equipment must be in accordance with federal, state, and local laws (CMS, 2020; Jacobs et al., 2018).

3. Provide resources to the family to investigate municipal requirements for home medical equipment, especially oxygen.

Many municipalities require that patients with home oxygen equipment notify emergency medical service (EMS) before bringing equipment home. When there is a power outage, EMS calls the home, and in some cases the home is on a priority list for power restoration.

4. Obtain appropriate referrals to determine whether patient meets standards for third-party reimbursement.

Indications for home oxygen therapy include (1) a PaO_2 less than or equal to 55 mm Hg or SaO_2 less than or equal to 88% breathing room air; (2) PaO_2 less than or equal to 56-59 mm Hg or SaO_2 less than or equal to 89% with conditions such as cor pulmonale, heart failure, or hematocrit greater than 56%; or (3) oxygen therapy is needed during activities that cause hypoxia such as ambulation, sleep, or exercise causing an SaO_2 of less than or equal to 88% (CMS, 2020). Providing evidence of inclusion criteria is often necessary for third-party reimbursement.

STEP	RATIONALE

IMPLEMENTATION

1. Perform hand hygiene and teach patient or family caregiver how to perform hand hygiene before handling oxygen equipment.

Reduces transmission of infection.

2. Place oxygen-delivery system in clutter-free environment that is well ventilated; away from walls, drapes, bedding, and combustible materials; and at least 8 feet from heat source.

Prevents injury from improper placement of oxygen equipment (ATS, 2016).

CLINICAL JUDGMENT: *Do not place oxygen-delivery system in a closet. Keep grease, oil, and petroleum away from equipment. Turn off the equipment when not in use (ALA, 2020b).*

---

3. Demonstrate each step for preparation and completion of oxygen therapy.

Teaches psychomotor skills and enables patient to ask questions. When patients and family caregivers are adequately informed about supplemental oxygen therapy, the patient's consistent use of the therapy is enhanced (Harding et al., 2020).

   a. **Compressed oxygen system**

      (1) Turn cylinder valve counterclockwise two or three turns with wrench.

Turns on oxygen.

      (2) Check cylinders by reading amount on pressure gauge.

Verifies adequate oxygen supply for patient use.

      (3) Store wrench with oxygen tank or in other safe place near the tank.

Storing wrench in safe place ensures that it is available whenever needed.

   b. **Oxygen concentrator system**.

Extracts oxygen from other gases in atmospheric air (ATS, 2016).

      (1) Plug concentrator into appropriate outlet.

Provides power source. Make sure that it is in an open area and never in a closet or other closed space.

      (2) Turn on power switch.

Starts concentrator motor.

      (3) Alarm sounds for a few seconds.

Alarm turns off when desired pressure inside concentrator is reached.

   c. **Liquid oxygen systems**

      (1) Check liquid system by depressing button, often located in lower right corner, and reading dial on stationary oxygen reservoir or ambulatory tank.

Verifies amount of oxygen supply for patient use.

      (2) Collaborate with durable medical equipment (DME) vendor to provide instruction in refilling ambulatory tank.

Ensures continuation of home oxygen therapy.

CLINICAL JUDGMENT: *There are numerous options for home oxygen equipment available to patients. In some situations the DME vendor will demonstrate how to refill oxygen tank or make home visits to refill tank. Keep the DME supplier contact number in a visible location for questions about the equipment (Jacobs et al., 2018). Tell neighbors and friends that oxygen is in the home.*

---

      (3) To refill oxygen tank:

        (a) Wipe both filling connectors with clean, dry, lint-free cloth.

Removes dust and moisture from system.

        (b) Turn off flow selector of ambulatory unit.

        (c) Attach ambulatory unit to stationary reservoir by inserting female adapter from ambulatory tank into male adapter of stationary reservoir (see illustration).

Secures connection between oxygen reservoir and ambulatory tank.

        (d) Open fill valve on ambulatory tank (e.g., lever or button), and apply firm pressure to top of stationary reservoir (see illustration). Stay with unit while it is filling. You will hear a loud hissing noise. Tank fills in about 2 minutes.

Prevents leaking of oxygen during filling process. If oxygen leaks during filling process, connection between ambulatory tank and reservoir ices up and valves stick together.

STEP 3c(3)(c) Top view of stationary reservoir.

STEP 3c(3)(d) Fill valve on ambulatory tank is opened while applying firm pressure to top of ambulatory unit.

Continued

SKILL 41.4	USING HOME OXYGEN EQUIPMENT—cont'd

STEP	RATIONALE
(e) Disconnect ambulatory unit from stationary reservoir when hissing noise changes and vapor cloud begins to form from stationary unit.	Overfilling causes ambulatory unit to malfunction, caused by high pressure in tank.

CLINICAL JUDGMENT: *If ambulatory unit does not separate easily, valves from reservoir and ambulatory unit may be frozen together. Wait until valves warm to disengage (about 5 to 10 minutes). Do not touch any frosted areas because contact with skin causes skin damage from frostbite.*

(f) Wipe both filling connectors with clean, dry, lint-free cloth.	Ice sometimes forms during filling. Removes moisture from oxygen system.
4. Connect oxygen-delivery device to oxygen system (see illustration).	Connects oxygen source to delivery system.
5. Adjust to prescribed flow rate (L/min).	Ensures appropriate oxygen prescription.
6. Have patient or family caregiver apply oxygen-delivery device. Ensure that patient knows to have two sets of oxygen-delivery devices and tubing.	Verifies that patient or family caregiver can apply device. Extra set of equipment is necessary for cleaning or in case of equipment malfunction.
7. Instruct patient and family caregiver not to change oxygen flow rate. Also explain rationale.	Exceeding prescribed amount of oxygen is harmful in some patients, such as those with chronic obstructive pulmonary disease (COPD).
8. Have patient or family caregiver perform each step with guidance. Provide written material for reinforcement and review.	Allows you to correct for errors in technique and discuss their implications.
9. Instruct patient or family caregiver to notify health care provider if signs or symptoms of hypoxia occur, including apprehension, anxiety, decreased ability to concentrate, decreased levels of consciousness, increased fatigue, dizziness, behavioral changes, increased pulse, increased respiratory rate, pallor, and cyanosis or respiratory tract infection (e.g., fever, increased sputum, change in color of sputum, foul sputum odor).	Hypoxia sometimes occurs at home when patient uses oxygen. Possible causes of hypoxia include poor tubing connections; use of long oxygen tubing; or worsening of patient's physical problem, with change in respiratory status. Respiratory tract infections increase oxygen demand and often affect oxygen transfer from lungs to blood, creating exacerbation of patient's pulmonary disease.
10. Discuss emergency plan for power loss, natural disaster, and acute respiratory distress. Have patient or family caregiver call 911 and notify health care provider and home care agency.	Ensures appropriate response and prevents worsening of patient's condition. Power companies will often work to supply power to houses requiring oxygen therapy first.
11. Instruct patient and family caregiver in safe home oxygen practices, including placing "No Smoking/Oxygen in Use" signs at each entrance to home, not allowing smoking in house, keeping oxygen tanks 8 feet (2.4 meters) away from open flames, eliminating potential trip hazards related to tubing and cylinders, and storing oxygen tanks upright.	Ensures safe use of oxygen in home and prevents injury to patient and family (Suntharalingam et al., 2018).
12. Instruct patient and family caregiver that home oxygen-delivery equipment must be maintained and serviced routinely according to manufacturer's guidelines (CMS, 2020).	Routine maintenance ensures proper function of equipment.
13. Assist patient to comfortable position.	Ensures comfort and well-being.
14. Remove and dispose of any extraneous supplies. Perform hand hygiene.	Reduces transmission of microorganisms. Patient and family caregiver must be knowledgeable about infection prevention techniques.

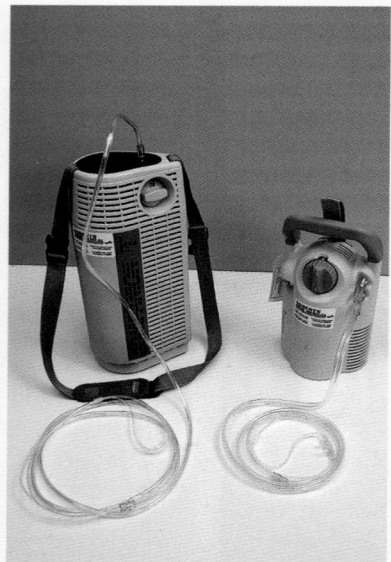

STEP 4 Oxygen-delivery device (nasal cannulas) and tubing attached to ambulatory oxygen tanks.

STEP	RATIONALE

EVALUATION

1. Monitor rate at which oxygen is being delivered at the beginning of each home visit.

2. Ask patient and family caregiver about ease of administering and any problems or concerns with the home oxygen delivery and equipment.

3. Ask patient and family caregiver to state safety guidelines, emergency precautions, and emergency plan.

4. **Use Teach-Back:** "I want to be sure I explained how to administer and use the home oxygen equipment. Show me how to apply your nasal cannula and regulate the oxygen source." Revise your instruction now or develop a plan for revised patient/family caregiver teaching if patient/family caregiver is not able to teach back correctly.

Determines whether patient or family caregiver is regulating oxygen at prescribed rate.

Determines whether patient and family caregivers are able to safely use the equipment and solve minor problems.

Determines patient's knowledge of what to do if power fails, if equipment fails, or if patient's status worsens.

Teach-back is an evidence-based health literacy intervention that promotes patient engagement, patient safety, adherence, and quality. The goal of teach-back is to ensure that you have explained medical information clearly so that patients and their families understand what you communicated to them (AHRQ, 2020).

UNEXPECTED OUTCOMES AND RELATED INTERVENTIONS

1. Patient has signs and symptoms associated with hypoxia.
   - Determine whether oxygen-delivery device and oxygen source are delivering oxygen properly.
   - Determine whether prescribed oxygen flow rate is set properly.
   - Assess patient for change in respiratory status, such as airway plugging, respiratory tract infection, or bronchospasm.
2. Patient or family caregiver uses unsafe practices with oxygen therapy, uses oxygen around fire or cigarette smoking, or sets incorrect flow rate.
   - Reinforce patient education and perform follow-up reassessment.
   - Include caregiver in instruction, and set up problem-solving exercises with patient.
3. Patient or family caregiver is unable to fill ambulatory system.
   - Identify and instruct family caregiver or family friend who can help patient fill ambulatory system.

RECORDING AND REPORTING

- Record teaching plan and describe patient's and family caregiver's ability to safely use home oxygen equipment.
- Record type of home oxygen equipment being used and oxygen flow rate, knowledge of safety guidelines, how to use equipment, unexpected outcomes to observe, and ability to return demonstrate proper use of oxygen-delivery device.

HOME CARE CONSIDERATIONS

- Ensure emergency numbers are programmed into a phone or are readily available for use in case of an emergency. These numbers include health care provider, supplier of medical equipment, and utility company.
- Place emergency numbers next to all phones in the home.
- Power companies should be notified of homes in which there are patients receiving home oxygen. In the event of a power outage, these homes would be the priority for receiving power.

KEY POINTS

- The cardiopulmonary system consisting of the heart, lungs, airways, and blood vessels function to provide and deliver oxygen to the tissues and to remove carbon dioxide from the body.
- Ventilation, diffusion, respiration, and perfusion are processes for providing adequate oxygenation from the alveoli to the blood.
- Cardiac output is determined by the patient's heart rate, strength of contraction, amount of blood in the ventricle, and amount of resistance the heart has to overcome to eject the blood.
- Myocardial blood flow is the path the blood takes to perfuse the muscles of the heart.
- Systemic circulation allows for the perfusion of tissues, delivering oxygen to the tissues and taking carbon dioxide and other waste substances away from the tissues.
- Patients with decreased cardiac output have difficulties in delivering oxygen to the tissues.
- Patients who are hypoxic are at risk for decreased cardiac output.

- Altered level of consciousness, tachypnea, dyspnea, and anxiety are all signs of hypoxemia.
- Abnormal conduction can cause cardiac dysrhythmias and decreased cardiac output, leading to decreased delivery of oxygen to the tissues.
- Myocardial ischemia can damage the cardiac muscle, thereby decreasing cardiac output, which leads to decreased oxygen delivery to the tissues.
- Decreased hemoglobin levels, seen in patients with anemia or blood loss, alter a patient's ability to transport oxygen, causing disturbances in oxygenation.
- Age (both young and the elderly), nutritional intake, hydration status, level of exercise, exposure to smoke or other environmental pollutants, and stress can all have a negative impact on a patient's oxygenation status.
- A nurse uses clinical judgment by assessing a patient's presenting condition and comparing with signs and symptoms anticipated from known medical conditions to identify if physical manifestations of altered oxygenation exist.

- Nurses and health care providers should ask patients about their risk factors for altered oxygenation, such as smoking history, substance abuse, exposure to pollutants and environmental substances, exercise patterns, diet patterns, and chronic illnesses.
- Nursing assessment includes respiratory rate and pattern, presence of cough and/or secretions, fatigue, dyspnea, wheezing, chest pain, oxygen saturation, vital signs, and signs of respiratory infection. In addition, assess for signs of chronic hypoxemia, such as clubbed fingers or barrel chest.
- Nursing plan of care should include positioning, medication administration, oxygen administration, respiratory muscle training, and airway suctioning.
- Oxygen therapy, either by nasal cannula, mask, or mechanical ventilation, helps to improve tissue oxygenation by increasing the amount of oxygen available to the patient.
- Breathing exercises, such as diaphragmatic breathing and pursed-lip breathing, benefit patients with chronic pulmonary disease.
- Chest physiotherapy is reserved for use in patients with thick secretions to help them mobilize those secretions.
- Vaccinations, smoking-cessation programs, exercise programs, and nutritional support are health promotion strategies to utilize when working with patients and their families.
- Mobilization of secretions through positioning and adequate hydration helps to maintain the airway.
- Suctioning may be necessary to maintain airway patency in patients who have difficulties in maintaining their own airway.
- Artificial airways may be used in patients who cannot maintain their own airway.
- Assess breath sounds, SpO_2 levels, breathing rate and patterns, activity tolerance, level of fatigue, and ability to maintain airway to determine a patient's response to therapies.

◼ REFLECTIVE LEARNING

- Describe assessment data that would place Mr. Edwards at risk for worsening **Impaired Airway Clearance** during his hospitalization. (Recognize Cues)
- From the case study and nursing care plan, identify other assessment data and cues that support additional nursing diagnoses for Mr. Edwards. (Analyze Cues)
- Consider all the assessment information in the case study and the additional nursing diagnoses you just identified for Mr. Edwards. Prioritize health care problems or nursing diagnoses. (Prioritize Diagnoses)
- Review the case study information, Mr. Edwards' nursing care plan, and the concept map. Describe other nursing interventions to promote airway clearance and improve respiratory gas exchange. (Generate Solutions)
- Prioritize appropriate nursing actions when planning and providing interventions to improve airway clearance for Mr. Edwards. (Take Action)
- In addition to the information in the care plan, identify measurable/objective factors you would use to determine the effectiveness of your nursing interventions for Mr. Edwards. What evaluation findings would indicate the nursing interventions were effective? What evaluation findings would indicate a need to modify the care plan? (Evaluate Outcomes)

◼ REVIEW QUESTIONS

1. The nurse is preparing to perform nasotracheal suctioning on a patient. Arrange the steps in order.
   1. Apply suction.
   2. Assist patient to semi-Fowler's or high Fowler's position, if able.
   3. Advance catheter through nares and into trachea.
   4. Have patient take deep breaths.
   5. Lubricate catheter with water-soluble lubricant.
   6. Apply sterile gloves.
   7. Perform hand hygiene.
   8. Withdraw catheter.
2. Which skills can the nurse delegate to assistive personnel (AP)? (Select all that apply.)
   1. Initiate oxygen therapy via nasal cannula.
   2. Perform nasotracheal suctioning of a patient.
   3. Educate the patient about the use of an incentive spirometer.
   4. Assist with care of an established tracheostomy tube.
   5. Reposition a patient with a chest tube.
3. The nurse is caring for a patient with pneumonia. On entering the room, the nurse finds the patient lying in bed, coughing, and unable to clear secretions. What should the nurse do first?
   1. Start oxygen at 2 L/min via nasal cannula.
   2. Elevate the head of the bed to 45 degrees.
   3. Encourage the patient to use the incentive spirometer.
   4. Notify the health care provider.
4. The nurse is performing discharge teaching for a patient with chronic obstructive pulmonary disease (COPD). What statement, made by the patient, indicates the need for further teaching?
   1. "Pursed-lip breathing is like exercise for my lungs and will help me strengthen my breathing muscles."
   2. "When I am sick, I should limit the amount of fluids I drink so that I don't produce excess mucus."
   3. "I will ensure that I receive an influenza vaccine every year, preferably in the fall."
   4. "I will look for a smoking-cessation support group in my neighborhood."
5. Which assessment findings indicate that the patient is experiencing an acute disturbance in oxygenation and requires immediate intervention? (Select all that apply.)
   1. SpO_2 value of 95%
   2. Chest retractions
   3. Respiratory rate of 28 breaths per minute
   4. Nasal flaring
   5. Clubbing of fingers
6. The nurse is caring for a patient with an artificial airway. What are reasons to suction the patient? (Select all that apply.)
   1. The patient has visible secretions in the airway.
   2. There is a sawtooth pattern on the patient's E_tCO_2 monitor.
   3. The patient has clear breath sounds.
   4. It has been 3 hours since the patient was last suctioned.
   5. The patient has excessive coughing.
7. The nurse is caring for a patient with a chest tube for treatment of a right pneumothorax. Which assessment finding necessitates immediate notification of the health care provider?
   1. New, vigorous bubbling in the water-seal chamber.
   2. Scant amount of sanguineous drainage noted on the dressing.

3. Clear but slightly diminished breath sounds on the right side of the chest.

4. Pain score of 2 one hour after the administration of the prescribed analgesic.

8. The nurse has just witnessed her patient go into cardiac arrest. The family is in the patient's room at the time the cardiac arrest occurs. What priority interventions should the nurse perform at this time? (Select all that apply.)

   1. Perform chest compressions.
   2. Ask someone to bring the automatic external defibrillator (AED) to the room for immediate defibrillation.
   3. Apply oxygen via nasal cannula.
   4. Place the patient supine.
   5. Educate the family about the need for CPR.

9. The nurse is performing tracheostomy care on a patient. What finding would indicate that the tracheostomy tube has become dislodged?

   1. Clear breath sounds
   2. Patient speaking to nurse
   3. SpO$_2$ reading of 96%
   4. Respiratory rate of 18 breaths/minute

10. Which number corresponds to the spot where you would assess for an air leak in the patient with a chest tube?

Answers: 1. 7, 2, 6, 4, 5, 3, 1, 8; **2.** 4, 5; **3.** 4, 2, 5, 3, 2, 3, 4; **6.** 1, 2, 5; **7.** 1; **8.** 1, 2, 4; **9.** 2; **10.** 1.

Rationales for Review Questions can be found on the Evolve website.

REFERENCES

Agency for Healthcare Research and Quality (AHRQ): *Teach-Back: Intervention. Quick Start Guide Full Page*, Rockville, MD, 2020, Agency for Healthcare Research and Quality. https://www.ahrq.gov/health-literacy/quality-resources/tools/literacy-toolkit/healthlittoolkit2-tool5.html. Accessed August 2021.

Agency for Toxic Substances and Disease Registry (ATSDR): *Environmental triggers of asthma*, 2018. https://www.atsdr.cdc.gov/csem/asthma/overview_of_asthma.html. Accessed August 2021.

American Association of Critical Care Nurses (AACN): *AACN practice alert: prevention of aspiration*, 2018. http://www.aacn.org/wd/practice/content/practicealerts/aspiration-practice-alert.pcms?menu=practice. Accessed August 2021.

American Association of Critical Care Nurses (AACN): AACN practice alert: oral care for acutely and critically ill patients, *Crit Care Nurse* 37(3):e19, 2017a.

American Association of Critical Care Nurses (AACN): *AACN practice alert: prevention of ventilator-associated pneumonia in adults*, 2017b. https://www.aacn.org/clinical-resources/practice-alerts/ventilator-associated-pneumonia-vap. Accessed August 2021.

American Association of Respiratory Care (AARC): AARC clinical practice guideline, endotracheal suctioning of mechanically ventilated patients with artificial airways—2010 update, *Respir Care* 55(60):758, 2010.

American Association of Respiratory Care (AARC): Clinical practice guideline: incentive spirometry, *Respir Care* 56(10):1600, 2011.

American Cancer Society (ACS): *Health risks of smoking tobacco*, 2020a. https://www.cancer.org/cancer/cancer-causes/tobacco-and-cancer/health-risks-of-smoking-tobacco.html. Accessed March 2021.

American Cancer Society (ACS): *Prescription drugs to help you quit tobacco*, 2020b. https://www.cancer.org/healthy/stay-away-from-tobacco/guide-quitting-smoking/prescription-drugs-to-help-you-quit-smoking.html. Accessed March 2021.

American Heart Association (AHA): *Cardiac arrest survival greatly increases when bystanders use an automated external defibrillator*, 2018. http://newsroom.heart.org/news/cardiac-arrest-survival-greatly-increases-when-bystanders-use-an-automated-external-defibrillator. Accessed March 2021.

American Heart Association (AHA): *Highlights of the 2020 American Heart Association guidelines update for CPR and ECC*, 2020. https://cpr.heart.org/-/media/cpr-files/cpr-guidelines-files/highlights/hghlghts_2020_ecc_guidelines_english.pdf?la=en. Accessed March 2021.

American Lung Association (ALA): *Health effects of secondhand smoke*, 2020a. https://www.lung.org/stop-smoking/smoking-facts/health-effects-of-secondhand-smoke.html. Accessed March 2021.

American Lung Association (ALA): *Using oxygen at home*, 2020b. https://www.lung.org/lung-health-and-diseases/lung-procedures-and-tests/oxygen-therapy/using-oxygen-at-home.html. Accessed August 2021.

American Lung Association (ALA): *Health effects of smoking*, 2020c. https://www.lung.org/quit-smoking/smoking-facts/health-effects/smoking. Accessed March 2021.

American Thoracic Society: *ATS publishes new clinical guideline on home oxygen for children*, 2019. https://www.thoracic.org/about/newsroom/press-releases/journal/2019/ats-publishes-new-clinical-guideline-on-home-oxygen-for-children.php. Accessed August 2021.

American Thoracic Society (ATS): *Oxygen therapy*, 2016. http://www.thoracic.org/patients/patient-resources/resources/oxygen-therapy.pdf. Accessed August 2021.

Ball J, et al: *Seidel's guide to physical examination*, ed 9, St. Louis, 2019, Elsevier.

Billington J, Luckett A: Care of the critically ill patient with a tracheostomy, *Nurs Stand* 34(2):59, 2019.

Bolsega T, Sole M: Tracheostomy care practices in a simulated setting: an exploratory study, *Clin Nurse Spec* 32(4):182, 2018.

Cedar SH: Every breath you take: the process of breathing explained, *Nurs Times* 114(1):47, 2018.

Centers for Disease Control and Prevention (CDC): *What is health literacy?* 2021a. https://www.cdc.gov/healthliteracy/learn/index.html. Accessed March 2021.

Centers for Disease Control and Prevention (CDC): *Who should do it, who should not, and who should take precautions*, 2021b. https://www.cdc.gov/flu/prevent/whoshouldvax.htm. Accessed March 2021.

Centers for Disease Control and Prevention (CDC): *Ventilator-associated event (VAE)*, 2021c. https://www.cdc.gov/nhsn/PDFs/pscManual/10-VAE_FINAL.pdf, Accessed March 2021.

Centers for Disease Control and Prevention (CDC): *How COVID-19 spreads*, 2021d. https://www.cdc.gov/coronavirus/2019-ncov/prevent-getting-sick/how-covid-spreads.html. Accessed March 2021.

Centers for Disease Control and Prevention (CDC): *Key things to know about COVID-19 vaccines*, 2021e. https://www.cdc.gov/coronavirus/2019-ncov/vaccines/keythingstoknow.html. Accessed March 2021.

Centers for Disease Control and Prevention: *National Center for Chronic Disease Prevention and Health Promotion*, 2021f, https://www.cdc.gov/chronicdisease/resources/infographic/chronic-diseases.htm.

Centers for Disease Control and Prevention (CDC): *Women and heart disease*, 2020a. https://www.cdc.gov/heartdisease/women.htm. Accessed March 2021.

Centers for Disease Control and Prevention (CDC): *Valley fever: coccidioidomycosis*, 2020b. https://www.cdc.gov/fungal/diseases/coccidioidomycosis/index.html. Accessed March 2021.

Centers for Disease Control and Prevention (CDC): *Carbon monoxide poisoning*, 2020c, https://www.cdc.gov/co/faqs.htm. Accessed March 2021.

Centers for Disease Control and Prevention (CDC): *Pneumococcal vaccination: what everyone should know*, 2020d. https://www.cdc.gov/vaccines/vpd/pneumo/public/index.html. Accessed March 2021.

Centers for Disease Control and Prevention (CDC): Tuberculosis – United States, 2018, *MMWR Morb Mortal Wkly Rep* 68(11):257, 2019. https://www.cdc.gov/mmwr/volumes/68/wr/pdfs/mm6811-H.pdf. Accessed March 2021.

Centers for Disease Control and Prevention (CDC): Tobacco product use among middle and high school students — United States, 2011–2017, *MMWR Morb Mortal Wkly Rep* 67(22):629–633, 2018a. https://www.cdc.gov/mmwr/volumes/67/wr/mm6722a3.htm. Accessed March 2021.

Centers for Disease Control and Prevention (CDC): Current cigarette smoking among adults — United States, 2016, *MMWR Morb Mortal Wkly Rep* 67(2):53, 2018b. https://www.cdc.gov/mmwr/volumes/67/wr/mm6702a1.htm. Accessed March 2021.

Centers for Disease Control and Prevention (CDC): *Urban-rural differences in chronic obstructive pulmonary disease (COPD)*, 2018c. https://www.cdc.gov/ruralhealth/copd/; https://www.cdc.gov/ruralhealth/copd/index.html. Accessed March 2021.

Centers for Disease Control and Prevention (CDC): *Tuberculosis: who should be tested*, 2016a. https://www.cdc.gov/tb/topic/testing/whobetested.htm. Accessed March 2021.

Centers for Disease Control and Prevention (CDC): *Tuberculosis: basic TB facts*, 2016b. https://www.cdc.gov/tb/topic/basics/default.htm. Accessed March 2021.

Centers for Medicare and Medicaid Services (CMS): *Home oxygen therapy*, 2020. https://www.cms.gov/Research-Statistics-Data-and-Systems/Computer-Data-and-Systems/Electronic-Clinical-Templates/DMEPOS-Templates/DMEPOS-Home-Oxygen-Therapy. Accessed March 2021.

Chotai P, Mosenifar Z: *Tube thoracostomy management*, 2018. https://emedicine.medscape.com/article/1503275-overview. Accessed August 2021.

COPD Foundation: *Breathing exercises and techniques for COPD*, 2021. https://www.copdfoundation.org/Learn-More/I-am-a-Person-with-COPD/Breathing-Techniques.aspx. Accessed August 2021.

Cystic Fibrosis Foundation (CFF): *Basics of postural drainage and percussion*, n.d.a. https://www.cff.org/Life-With-CF/Treatments-and-Therapies/Airway-Clearance/Basics-of-Postural-Drainage-and-Percussion/. Accessed August 2021.

Cystic Fibrosis Foundation (CFF): *Coughing and huffing*, n.d.b. https://www.cff.org/Life-With-CF/Treatments-and-Therapies/Airway-Clearance/Coughing-and-Huffing/. Accessed August 2021.

Cystic Fibrosis Foundation (CFF): *Positive expiratory pressure*, n.d.c. https://www.cff.org/Life-With-CF/Treatments-and-Therapies/Airway-Clearance/Positive-Expiratory-Pressure/. Accessed August 2021.

Environmental Protection Agency (EPA): *A citizen's guide to radon: the guide to protecting yourself and your family from radon*, 2016. https://www.epa.gov/sites/production/files/2016-12/documents/2016_a_citizens_guide_to_radon.pdf. Accessed March 2021.

Fields BE, et al: Home oxygen therapy, *Am J Nurs*, 120(11):51, 2020.

Franks LJ, et al: Comparing the performance characteristics of different positive expiratory pressure devices, *Respir Care* 64(4):434, 2019.

Fumarola S, et al.: Overlooked and underestimated: medical adhesive-related skin injuries. Best practice consensus document on prevention. *J Wound Care* 29(Suppl 3c):S1–S24, 2020.

Ghosh D, Elliott M: Acute non-invasive ventilation – getting it right on the acute medical take, *Clin Med J* 19(3):237, 2019.

Harding MM, et al: *Medical surgical nursing, assessment and management of clinical problems*, ed 11, St. Louis, 2020, Elsevier.

Hartjes TM: *AACN core curriculum for high acuity, progressive, and critical care nursing*, ed 7, St. Louis, 2018, Elsevier.

Hill N, et al: Noninvasive ventilatory support for acute hypercapnic respiratory failure, *Respir Care* 64(6):647, 2019.

Hockenberry MJ, et al: *Wong's nursing care of infants and children*, ed 11, St. Louis, 2019, Elsevier.

Huang X, et al: Influence of subglottic secretion drainage on the microorganisms of ventilator associated pneumonia, *Medicine* 97(28):1, 2018.

Huggins J, et al: *Placement and management of thoracostomy tubes and catheters in adults and children*, 2021. https://www.uptodate.com/contents/placement-and-management-of-thoracostomy-tubes-and-catheters-in-adults-and-children. Accessed August 2021.

Institute for Healthcare Improvement (IHI): *How-to guide: prevent ventilator-associated pneumonia*, 2012. http://www.ihi.org/resources/Pages/Tools/HowtoGuidePreventVAP.aspx. Accessed March 2021.

Jacobs SS, et al: Optimizing home oxygen therapy: an official American Thoracic Society workshop report, *Ann Am Thorac Soc* 15(12):1369, 2018.

Karlsen M, et al: Communication with patients in intensive care units: a scoping review, *Nurs Crit Care* 24(3):115, 2019.

Kirkwood P: Chest tube removal (assist). In Wiegand D, editor: *AACN procedure manual for critical care*, ed 7, St. Louis, 2017, Elsevier.

Larrow V, Klich-Heartt EI: Prevention of ventilator-associated pneumonia in the intensive care unit: beyond the basics, *J Neurosci Nurs* 48(3):160, 2016.

Letchford E, Bench S: Ventilator-associated pneumonia and suction: a review of the literature, *Br J Nurs* 27(1):13, 2018.

Leung C, et al: Exploring the scope of communication content of mechanically ventilated patients, *J Crit Care* 44:136, 2018.

Link M, et al: Part 7: Adult advanced cardiovascular life support: 2015 American Heart Association guidelines update for cardiopulmonary resuscitation and emergency cardiovascular care, *Circulation* 132(18 Suppl 2):S444, 2015.

Masood M, et al: Association of standardized tracheostomy care protocol implementation and reinforcement with the prevention of life-threatening respiratory events, *JAMA Otolaryngol Head Neck Surg*, 144(6):527, 2018.

McCance KL, Huether SE: *Pathophysiology: the biologic basis for disease in adults and children*, ed 8, St. Louis, 2019, Elsevier.

Menzes KKP, et al: A review on respiratory muscle training devices, *J Pulm Respir Med* 8(2):451, 2018.

Moore D: Home oxygen therapy in patients with COPD: safety issues for nurse prescribers, *Br J Nurs*, 28(14):912, 2019.

Muzzy AC, Butler AK: Managing chest tubes: air leaks and unplanned tube removal, *Am Nurse Today* 10(5), 2015.

National Cancer Institute (NCI): *Secondhand smoke and cancer*, 2018. https://www.cancer.gov/about-cancer/causes-prevention/risk/tobacco/second-hand-smoke-fact-sheet. Accessed March 2021.

National Heart Lung and Blood Institute (NHLBI): *DASH eating plan*, n.d.a, National Institutes of Health. https://www.nhlbi.nih.gov/health-topics/dash-eating-plan. Accessed March 2021.

National Heart Lung and Blood Institute (NHLBI): *Defibrillators*, n.d.b, National Institutes of Health. https://www.nhlbi.nih.gov/health-topics/defibrillators. Accessed March 2021.

National Institute on Drug Abuse (NIDA): *Marijuana* DrugFacts, 2019, National Institutes of Health. https://www.drugabuse.gov/publications/drugfacts/marijuana. Accessed March 2021.

National Institute on Drug Abuse (NIDA): *Cocaine* DrugFacts, 2018, National Institutes of Health. https://www.drugabuse.gov/publications/drugfacts/cocaine. Accessed March 2021.

National Institute on Drug Abuse (NIDA): Inhalants *DrugFacts*, 2020, National Institutes of Health. https://www.drugabuse.gov/publications/drugfacts/inhalants. Accessed March 2021.

Neumar RW, et al: Part 1: Executive summary 2015 American Heart Association guidelines update for cardiopulmonary resuscitation and emergency cardiovascular care, *Circulation* 132(18 Suppl 2):S315, 2015.

Oncology Nursing Society (ONS): *Toolkit for safe handling of hazardous drugs for nursing in oncology*, 2018. https://www.ons.org/sites/default/files/2018-06/ONS_Safe_Handling_Toolkit_0.pdf. Accessed August 2021.

Pickett J: Closed chest-drainage system. In Wiegand D, editor: *AACN procedure manual for critical care*, ed 7, St. Louis, 2017, Elsevier.

Rochwerg B, et al: Official ERS/ATS clinical practice guidelines: noninvasive ventilation for acute respiratory failure, *Eur Respir J* 50:1, 2017.

Rouzé A, et al: Tracheal tube design and ventilator-associated pneumonia, *Respir Care* 62(10):1316, 2017.

Sasa R: Evidence-based update on chest tube management: Is your practice current? *Am Nurse Today*, 14(4):10, 2019.

Smith SG, Pietrantonio T: Best method for securing an endotracheal tube, *Crit Care Nurs* 36(2):78, 2016.

Sole ML, et al: Clinical indicators for endotracheal suctioning in adult patients receiving mechanical ventilation, *Am J Crit Care* 24(4):318, 2015.

Stevens G, et al: Intraoperative endotracheal cuff pressure study: how education and availability of manometers help guide safer pressure, *Mil Med* 183:e416, 2018.

Strickland SL: Year in review 2014: airway clearance, *Respir Care* 60(4):603, 2015.

Strickland SL, et al: AARC clinical practice guideline: effectiveness of nonpharmacologic airway clearance techniques in hospitalized patients, *Respir Care* 58(12):2187, 2013.

Suntharalingam J, et al: British Thoracic Society quality standards for home oxygen use in adults, *BMJ Open Respir Res* 18:4(1):e000223, 2018.

The Joint Commission (TJC): *2021* National Patient Safety Goals, Oakbrook Terrace, IL, 2021, The Commission. http://www.jointcommission.org/en/standards/national-patient-safety-goals/. Accessed August 2021.

Tokmaji G, et al: Silver-coated endotracheal tubes for prevention of ventilator-associated pneumonia in critically ill patients (review), *Cochrane Database Syst Rev* 2015(8):1, 2018.

Touhy T, Jett K: *Gerontological nursing and healthy aging*, ed 5, St. Louis, 2018, Elsevier.

Urden LD, et al: *Priorities in critical care nursing*, ed 8, St. Louis, 2020, Elsevier.

US Department of Health and Human Services (USDHHS): *Physical activity guidelines for Americans*, ed 2, 2018. https://health.gov/paguidelines/second-edition/pdf/Physical_Activity_Guidelines_2nd_edition.pdf. Accessed March 2021.

Venuta F, et al: Chest tubes: generalities, *Thorac Surg Clin* 27(1):1, 2017.

Walsh BK, Smallwood CD: Pediatric oxygen therapy: a review and update, *Respir Care* 62(6):645, 2017.

Walters J: Chest tube placement (assist): In Wiegand D, editor: *AACN procedure manual for high acuity, progressive, and critical care*, ed 7, St. Louis, 2017, Elsevier.

Wiegand D: *AACN procedure manual for high acuity, progressive, and critical care*, ed 7, St. Louis, 2017, Elsevier.

Virk H, Wiersinga J: Current place of probiotics for VAP, *Crit Care* 23:46, 2019.

Zisis C, et al: Chest drainage systems in use, *Ann Transl Med* 3(3):43, 2015.

RESEARCH REFERENCES

Alja'afreh M, et al: The effects of oral care protocol on the incidence of ventilator-associated pneumonia in selected intensive care units in Jordan, *Dimens Crit Care Nurs* 38(1):5, 2019.

Anand T, et al: Results from a quality improvement project to decrease infection-related ventilator events in trauma patients at a community teaching hospital, *Am Surg* 84(10):1701, 2018.

Bassi GL, et al: Prevention of ventilator-associated pneumonia, *Curr Opin Infect Dis* 30(2):214, 2017.

Celedon JC, et al: An American Thoracic Society/National Heart, Lung, and Blood Institute workshop report: addressing respiratory health equality in the United States, *Ann Am Thorac Soc* 14(5):814, 2017.

Chacko R, et al: Oral decontamination techniques and ventilator-associated pneumonia, *Br J Nurs* 26(11):594, 2017.

Chatwin M, et al: Airway clearance techniques in neuromuscular disorders: a state of the art review, *Respir Med* 136:98, 2018.

Elliott S, Morrell-Scott N: Care of patients undergoing weaning from mechanical ventilation in critical care, *Nurs Stand* 32(13):41, 2017.

Eltorai AE, et al: Perspectives on incentive spirometry utility and patient protocols, *Respir Care* 63(5):519, 2018.

Ferrer M, Torres A: Epidemiology of ICU-acquired pneumonia, *Curr Opin Crit Care* 24(5):325, 2018.

Fumarola S, et al: Overlooked and underestimated: medical adhesive-related skin injuries. Best practice consensus document on prevention. *J Wound Care* 29(Suppl 3c): S1–S24, 2020.

Gross SL, et al: Comparison of three practices for dressing chest tube insertion sites: a randomized controlled trial, *Medsurg Nurs* 25(4):229, 2016.

Hanada M, et al: Aerobic and breathing exercises improve dyspnea, exercise capacity and quality of life in idiopathic pulmonary fibrosis patients: a systematic review and meta-analysis, *J Thorac Dis* 12(3):1041, 2020.

Jackson D, et al: Medical device-related pressure ulcers: a systematic review and meta-analysis, *Int J Nurs Stud* 92:109, 2019.

Karaca T, Korkmaz F: A quasi-experimental study to explore the effect of barrier cream on the peristomal skin of patients with a tracheostomy, *Ostomy Wound Manage* 64(3):32, 2018.

Langer T, et al.: Prone position in intubated, mechanically ventilated patients with COVID-19: a multi-centric study of more than 1000 patients *Crit Care* 25:128, 2021. Published online 2021 Apr 6. doi: 10.1186/s13054-021-03552-2

Mahmoodpoor A, et al: Effect of a probiotic preparation on ventilator-associated pneumonia in critically ill patients admitted to the intensive care unit: a prospective double-blind randomized controlled trial, *Nutr Clin Pract* 34(1):156, 2018.

Mendes LPA, et al: Effects of diaphragmatic breathing with and without pursed-lips breathing in subjects with COPD, *Respir Care* 64(2):136, 2019.

Nuwi D, Irwan AM: Effect of active mobilization on patients in the intensive care unit: a systematic review, *Int J Caring Sci* 11(3):1942, 2018.

Pozuelo-Carrascosa DP, et al: Subglottic secretion drainage for preventing ventilator associated pneumonia: an overview of systematic reviews and an updated meta-analysis, *Eur Respir Rev* 29(155), 2020.

Salem A, Ahmad M: Communication with invasive mechanically ventilated patients and the use of alternative devices: integrative review, *J Res Nurs* 23(7):614, 2018.

Sanaie S, et al: Comparison of tracheal tube cuff pressure with two techniques: fixed volume and minimal leak test techniques, *J Cardiovasc Thorac Res* 11(1):48, 2019.

Wang R, et al: The impact of tracheotomy timing in critically ill patients undergoing mechanical ventilation: a meta-analysis of randomized controlled clinical trials with trial sequential analysis, *Heart Lung* 48:46, 2019.

Wang CH, et al: Normal saline instillation before suctioning: a meta-analysis of randomized controlled trials, *Aust Crit Care* 30(5):260, 2017.

Wen Z, et al: Is humidified better than non-humidified low-flow oxygen therapy? A systematic review and meta-analysis, *J Adv Nurs* 73(11):2522, 2017.

Xu Z, et al: High-flow nasal cannula in adults with acute respiratory failure and after extubation: a systematic review and meta-analysis, *Respir Res* 19(1):202, 2018.

Fluid, Electrolyte, and Acid-Base Balance

Mrs. Mendoza, age 77, fell at home after having vomiting and diarrhea for 24 hours. She was admitted to the hospital for oral and intravenous (IV) fluid therapy after x-rays indicated no fractured bones. Mrs. Mendoza lives alone in an apartment and has no chronic illnesses except osteoarthritis of her hands.

Robert is a nursing student assigned to Mrs. Mendoza. He has cared for other patients with gastrointestinal (GI) disorders but none with fluid and electrolyte imbalances. Robert plans his care by reviewing Mrs. Mendoza's electronic health record (EHR) and health care provider's orders.

Fluid is internal to and surrounds all the cells in the body. Cellular fluids contain electrolytes such as sodium and potassium and also have a degree of acidity. Fluid, electrolyte, and acid-base balances within the body maintain the health and function of all body systems. The characteristics of body fluids influence body system function because of their effects on cell function. These characteristics include the fluid amount (volume), concentration (osmolality), composition (electrolyte concentration), and degree of acidity (pH). All of these characteristics have regulatory mechanisms that keep them in balance for normal cellular function. It is important to understand how the body normally maintains fluid, electrolyte, and acid-base balance. You also need to understand how imbalances develop; how various fluid, electrolyte, and acid-base imbalances affect patients; and ways to help patients maintain or restore balance safely.

SCIENTIFIC KNOWLEDGE BASE

This section provides the foundation of scientific knowledge for your clinical judgment and clinical decisions regarding patients who have or are at risk of having fluid, electrolyte, or acid-base imbalances.

Location and Movement of Water and Electrolytes

Water comprises a substantial proportion of body weight. In fact, about 60% of the body weight of an adult man is water. This proportion decreases with age; approximately 50% of an older man's weight is water. Women typically have less water content than men. People who are obese have less water in their bodies than people who are lean because fat contains less water than muscle (Huether et al., 2020). The term **fluid** means water that contains dissolved or suspended substances such as glucose, mineral salts, and proteins.

Fluid Distribution. Body fluids are located in two distinct compartments: **extracellular fluid (ECF)** outside the cells and **intracellular fluid (ICF)** inside the cells (Fig. 42.1). In adults, ICF comprises approximately two-thirds of total body water. ECF makes up approximately one-third of total body water. ECF has two major divisions (**intravascular fluid** and **interstitial fluid**) and a minor division (transcellular fluids). Intravascular fluid is the liquid part of the blood (i.e., the plasma). Interstitial fluid is located between the cells and outside the blood vessels. Transcellular fluids such as cerebrospinal, pleural, peritoneal, and synovial fluids are secreted by epithelial cells (Huether et al., 2020).

Composition of Body Fluids. Fluid in the body compartments contains mineral salts known technically as electrolytes. An electrolyte is a compound that separates into ions (charged particles) when it dissolves in water. Ions that are positively charged are called cations; ions that are negatively charged are called anions. Cations in body fluids are sodium (Na^+), potassium (K^+), calcium (Ca^{2+}), and magnesium (Mg^{2+}) ions. Anions in body fluids are chloride (Cl^-) and bicarbonate (HCO_3^-). Anions and cations combine to make salts. If you put table salt (NaCl) in water, it separates into Na^+ and Cl^-. Other combinations of anions and cations do the same. Clinical laboratories usually report electrolyte measurements in milliequivalents per liter (mEq/L) or millimoles per liter (mmol/L), which are two different units of concentration (Table 42.1). Millimoles per liter represent the number of milligrams of the electrolyte divided by its molecular weight that are contained in a liter of the fluid being measured (usually blood plasma or serum). Milliequivalents per liter are the millimoles per liter multiplied by the electrolyte charge (e.g., 1 for Na^+, 2 for Ca^{2+}). One milliequivalent of one electrolyte can combine with one milliequivalent of another electrolyte, which is why this measurement unit is used.

Fluid that contains a large number of dissolved particles is more concentrated than the same amount of fluid that contains only a few particles. **Osmolality** of a fluid is a measure of the number of particles per kilogram of water. Some particles (e.g., urea) pass easily through cell membranes; others such as Na^+ cannot cross easily. The particles that cannot cross cell membranes easily determine the tonicity (effective concentration) of a fluid. A fluid with the same tonicity as normal blood is called **isotonic**. A **hypotonic** solution is more dilute than the blood, and a **hypertonic** solution is more concentrated than normal blood (Fig. 42.2).

Movement of Water and Electrolytes. Active transport, diffusion, osmosis, and filtration are processes that move water and electrolytes

FIG. 42.1 Body fluid compartments. (From Hall JE, Hall ME: *Guyton and Hall textbook of medical physiology,* ed 14, Philadelphia, 2021, Elsevier.)

TABLE 42.1	Normal Laboratory Values for Adults
Item Measured	**Normal Value in Serum or Blood**
Osmolality	285–295 mOsm/kg H_2O (285–295 mmol/kg H_2O)
Electrolytes	
Sodium (Na^+)	136–145 mEq/L (136–145 mmol/L)
Potassium (K^+)	3.5–5.0 mEq/L (3.5–5 mmol/L)
Chloride (Cl^-)	98–106 mEq/L (98–106 mmol/L)
Total CO_2 (CO_2 total content)	22–30 mEq/L (22–30 mmol/L)
Bicarbonate (HCO_3^-)	Arterial 21–28 mEq/L (21–28 mmol/L)
	Venous 24–30 mEq/L (24–30 mmol/L)
Total calcium (Ca^{2+})	9.0–10.5 mg/dL (2.25–2.62 mmol/L)
Ionized calcium (Ca^{2+})	4.5–5.6 mg/dL (1.05–1.3 mmol/L)
Magnesium (Mg^{2+})	1.3–2.1 mEq/L (0.65–1.05 mmol/L)
Phosphate	3.0–4.5 mg/dL (0.97–1.45 mmol/L)
Anion gap	6+/ −4 mEq/L (6+/ −4 mmol/L)
Arterial Blood Gases	
pH	7.35–7.45
$PaCO_2$	35–45 mm Hg (4.7–6 kPa)
PaO_2	80–100 mm Hg (10.7–13.3 kPa)
O_2 saturation	95%–100% (0.95–1.00)
Base excess	−2 to +2 mm Eq/L (mmol/L)

between body compartments. These processes maintain equal osmolality in all compartments while allowing for different electrolyte concentrations.

Active Transport. Fluids in different body compartments have different concentrations of electrolytes that are necessary for normal function. For example, concentrations of Na^+, Cl^-, and HCO_3^- are higher in the ECF, whereas concentrations of K^+, Mg^{2+}, and phosphate are higher in the ICF. Cells maintain their high intracellular electrolyte concentration by active transport. Active transport requires energy in the form of adenosine triphosphate (ATP) to move electrolytes across cell membranes against the concentration gradient (from areas of lower concentration to areas of higher concentration). One example of active transport is the sodium-potassium pump, which moves Na^+ out of a cell and K^+ into it, keeping the ICF lower in Na^+ and higher in K^+ than the ECF.

Diffusion. Diffusion is passive movement of electrolytes or other particles down a concentration gradient (from areas of higher concentration to areas of lower concentration). Within a body compartment

electrolytes diffuse easily by random movements until the concentration is the same in all areas. However, diffusion of electrolytes across cell membranes requires proteins that serve as ion channels. For example, when a sodium channel in a cell membrane is open, Na^+ diffuses passively across the cell membrane into the ICF because concentration is lower in the ICF. Opening of ion channels is tightly controlled and plays an important part in muscle and nerve function.

Osmosis. Water moves across cell membranes by osmosis, a process by which water moves through a membrane that separates fluids with different particle concentrations (Fig. 42.3). Cell membranes are semipermeable, which means that water crosses them easily, but they are not freely permeable to many types of particles, including electrolytes such as sodium and potassium. These semipermeable cell membranes separate interstitial fluid from ICF. The fluid in each of these compartments exerts osmotic pressure, an inward-pulling force caused by particles in the fluid. The particles already inside the cell exert ICF osmotic pressure, which tends to pull water into the cell. The particles in the interstitial fluid exert interstitial fluid osmotic pressure, which tends to pull water out of the cell. Water moves into the compartment that has a higher osmotic pressure (inward-pulling force) until the particle concentration is equal in the two compartments.

If the particle concentration in the interstitial compartment changes, osmosis occurs rapidly and moves water into or out of cells to equalize the osmotic pressures. For example, when a hypotonic solution (more dilute than normal body fluids) is administered intravenously, it dilutes the interstitial fluid, decreasing its osmotic pressure below intracellular osmotic pressure. Water moves rapidly into cells until the two osmotic pressures are equal again. On the other hand, infusion of a hypertonic IV solution (more concentrated than normal body fluids) causes water to leave cells by osmosis to equalize the osmolality between interstitial and intracellular compartments.

Filtration. Fluid moves into and out of capillaries (between the vascular and interstitial compartments) by the process of filtration (Fig. 42.4). Filtration is the net effect of four forces, two that tend to move fluid out of capillaries and small venules and two that tend to move fluid back into them. Hydrostatic pressure is the force of the fluid pressing outward against a surface. Similarly, capillary hydrostatic pressure is a relatively strong outward-pushing force that helps move fluid from capillaries into the interstitial area. Interstitial fluid hydrostatic pressure is a weaker opposing force that tends to push fluid back into capillaries (Huether et al., 2020).

Blood contains albumin and other proteins known as colloids. These proteins are much larger than electrolytes, glucose, and other molecules

FIG. 42.2 Effects of isotonic (A), hypertonic (B), and hypotonic (C) solutions. (From Hall JE, Hall ME: *Guyton and Hall textbook of medical physiology*, ed 14, Philadelphia, 2021, Elsevier.)

FIG. 42.3 Osmosis moves water through semipermeable membrane. (From Patton KT, Thibodeau GA: *The human body in health and disease*, ed 7, St Louis, 2018, Elsevier.)

FIG. 42.4 Capillary filtration moves fluid between vascular and interstitial compartments. (From Banasik JL, Copstead LC: *Pathophysiology*, ed 6, St Louis, 2019, Saunders.)

that dissolve easily. Most colloids are too large to leave capillaries in the fluid that is filtered; therefore they remain in the blood. Because they are particles, colloids exert osmotic pressure. Blood colloid osmotic pressure, also called oncotic pressure, is an inward-pulling force caused by blood proteins that helps move fluid from the interstitial area back into capillaries. Interstitial fluid colloid osmotic pressure normally is a very small opposing force.

Capillary hydrostatic pressure is strongest at the arterial end of a normal capillary. Fluid moves from the capillary into the interstitial area, bringing nutrients to cells. At the venous end, capillary hydrostatic pressure is weaker and the colloid osmotic pressure of the blood is stronger. Thus fluid moves into the capillary at the venous end, removing waste products from cellular metabolism. Lymph vessels remove any extra fluid and proteins that have leaked into the interstitial fluid.

Disease processes and other factors that alter these forces may cause accumulation of excess fluid in the interstitial space, known as *edema*. For example, people with heart failure often develop edema. In this situation, venous congestion from a weakened heart that no longer pumps effectively increases capillary hydrostatic pressure, causing edema by moving excessive fluid into the interstitial space. Inflammation is another cause of edema. It increases capillary blood flow and allows capillaries to leak colloids into the interstitial space. The resulting increased capillary hydrostatic pressure and increased interstitial colloid osmotic pressure produce localized edema in the inflamed tissues.

Fluid Balance

Fluid homeostasis is the dynamic interplay of three processes: fluid intake and absorption, fluid distribution, and fluid output (Felver, 2021c). To maintain fluid balance, fluid intake must equal output. Because some of the normal daily fluid output (e.g., urine, sweat) is a hypotonic salt solution, people must have an equivalent fluid intake of hypotonic sodium-containing fluid (or water plus foods with some salt) to maintain fluid balance (intake equal to output).

Fluid Intake. Fluid intake occurs orally through drinking but also through eating because most foods contain some water. Food metabolism creates additional water. Average fluid intake from these routes for healthy adults is about 2300 mL, although this amount can vary widely, depending on exercise habits, preferences, and the environment (Table 42.2). Other routes of fluid intake include IV, rectal (e.g., enemas), and irrigation of body cavities that can absorb fluid.

Although you might think that the major regulator of oral fluid intake is thirst, habit and social reasons also play major roles in fluid intake. Thirst, the conscious desire for water, is an important regulator of fluid

TABLE 42.2 Healthy Adult Average Fluid Intake and Output

	Normal (per Day)	Prolonged Heavy Exercise (per Hour)
Fluid Intake		
Fluids ingested, oral	1100–1400 mL	280–1100 mL/hr
Foods	800–1000 mL	Highly variable
Metabolism	300 mL	16–50 mL/hr
Total	2200–2700 mL	300–1150 mL/hr
Fluid Output		
Skin (insensible and sweat)	500–600 mL	300–2100 mL/hr
Insensible lungs	400 mL	20 mL/h
Gastrointestinal	100–200 mL	Negligible, unless diarrhea during exercise
Urine	1200–1500 mL	20–1000 mL/hr, depending on hydration status
Total	2200–2700 mL	340–3120 mL/hr Rehydration with Na^+-containing fluid necessary after prolonged vigorous exercise

Data from Hall JE: *Guyton and Hall textbook of medical physiology*, ed 14, Philadelphia, 2020, Saunders.

intake when plasma osmolality increases (osmoreceptor-mediated thirst) or the blood volume decreases (baroreceptor-mediated thirst and angiotensin II– and III–mediated thirst) (Gizowski and Bourgue, 2018). The thirst-control mechanism is located within the hypothalamus in the brain (Fig. 42.5). Osmoreceptors continually monitor plasma osmolality; when it increases, they cause thirst by stimulating neurons in the hypothalamus. People who are alert can obtain fluid or communicate their thirst to others, and fluid intake restores fluid balance. Infants, patients with neurological or psychological problems, and some older adults who are unable to perceive or communicate their thirst are at risk for dehydration.

Fluid Distribution. The term *fluid distribution* means the movement of fluid among its various compartments. Fluid distribution between the extracellular and intracellular compartments occurs by osmosis.

Fluid distribution between the vascular and interstitial parts of the ECF occurs by filtration.

Fluid Output. Fluid output normally occurs through four organs: the skin, lungs, GI tract, and kidneys. Examples of abnormal fluid output include vomiting, wound drainage, or hemorrhage (Felver, 2021c). Table 42.2 shows average amounts of fluid excretion for healthy adults, although urine output varies greatly, depending on fluid intake. Insensible (not visible) water loss through the skin and lungs is continuous. It increases when a person has a fever or a recent burn to the skin (Kamel and Halperin, 2017; Sterns, 2021). Sweat, which is visible and contains sodium, occurs intermittently, and increases fluid output substantially. The GI tract plays a vital role in fluid balance. Approximately 3 to 6 L of fluid moves into the GI tract

daily and returns to the ECF. The average adult normally excretes only 100 mL of fluid each day through feces. However, diarrhea causes a large fluid output from the GI tract (Kear, 2017; Sterns, 2021).

The kidneys are the major regulator of fluid output because they respond to hormones that influence urine production. When healthy adults drink more water, they increase urine production to maintain fluid balance. If they drink less water, sweat a lot, or lose fluid by vomiting, their urine volume decreases to maintain fluid balance. These adjustments primarily are caused by the actions of antidiuretic hormone (ADH), the renin-angiotensin-aldosterone system (RAAS), and atrial natriuretic peptides (ANPs) (Huether et al., 2020) (Fig. 42.6).

Antidiuretic Hormone. ADH regulates the osmolality of the body fluids by influencing how much water is excreted in urine. It is synthesized by neurons in the hypothalamus that release it from the posterior pituitary gland. ADH circulates in the blood to the kidneys, where it acts on the collecting ducts (Huether et al., 2020). Its name—antidiuretic hormone—tells you what it does. It causes renal cells to resorb water, taking water from the renal tubular fluid and putting it back in the blood. This action decreases urine volume, concentrating the urine while diluting the blood by adding water to it (see Fig. 42.6A).

People normally have some ADH release to maintain fluid balance. More ADH is released if body fluids become more concentrated. Factors that increase ADH levels include severely decreased blood volume (e.g., dehydration, hemorrhage), pain, stressors, and some medications.

ADH levels decrease if body fluids become too dilute. This allows more water to be excreted in urine, creating a larger volume of dilute urine, and concentrating the body fluids back to normal osmolality.

Renin-Angiotensin-Aldosterone System. The RAAS regulates ECF volume by influencing how much sodium and water are excreted in urine. It also contributes to regulation of blood pressure (BP). Specialized cells in the kidneys release the enzyme renin, which acts on angiotensinogen, an inactive protein secreted by the liver that circulates in the blood. Renin converts angiotensinogen to angiotensin I, which is

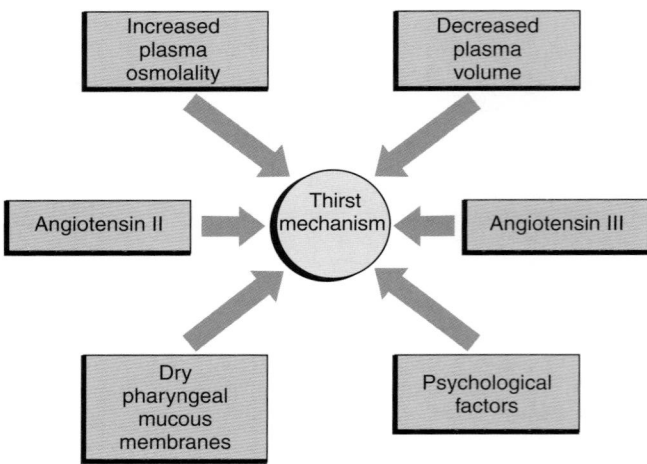

FIG. 42.5 Stimuli affecting thirst mechanism.

FIG. 42.6 Major hormones that influence renal fluid excretion. (A) Antidiuretic hormone *(ADH)*. (B) Aldosterone. (C) Atrial natriuretic peptide *(ANP)*.

converted to angiotensin II by other enzymes in the lung capillaries (Huether et al., 2020). Angiotensin II has several functions, one of which is vasoconstriction in some vascular beds. The important fluid homeostasis functions of angiotensin II include stimulation of aldosterone release from the adrenal cortex.

Aldosterone circulates to the kidneys, where it causes resorption of sodium and water in isotonic proportion in the distal renal tubules. Removing sodium and water from the renal tubules and returning it to the blood increases the volume of the ECF (see Fig. 42.6B). Aldosterone also contributes to electrolyte and acid-base balance by increasing urinary excretion of potassium and hydrogen ions.

To maintain fluid balance, normally some action of the RAAS occurs. Certain stimuli increase or decrease the activity of this system to restore fluid balance. For example, if hemorrhage or vomiting decreases the extracellular fluid volume (ECV), blood flow decreases through the renal arteries, and more renin is released. This increased RAAS activity causes more sodium and water retention, helping to restore ECV.

Atrial Natriuretic Peptide. ANP also regulates ECV by influencing how much sodium and water are excreted in urine. Cells in the atria of the heart release ANP when they are stretched (e.g., by an increased ECV). ANP is a weak hormone that increases the loss of sodium and water in the urine (see Fig. 42.6C). Thus ANP opposes the effect of aldosterone (Huether et al., 2020).

Fluid Imbalances

If disease processes, medications, or other factors disrupt fluid intake or output, imbalances sometimes occur (Felver, 2021c). For example, with diarrhea there is an increase in fluid output, and a fluid imbalance (dehydration) occurs if fluid intake does not increase appropriately. There are two major types of fluid imbalances: volume imbalances and osmolality imbalances (Fig. 42.7). Volume imbalances are disturbances of the *amount of fluid in the extracellular compartment.* Osmolality imbalances are disturbances of the *concentration of body fluids.* Volume and osmolality imbalances occur separately or in combination.

Extracellular Fluid Volume Imbalances. In an ECV imbalance there is either too little (ECV deficit) or too much (ECV excess) isotonic fluid. **Extracellular volume deficit** is present when there is insufficient isotonic fluid in the extracellular compartment. Remember that there is a lot of sodium in normal ECF. With ECV deficit, output of

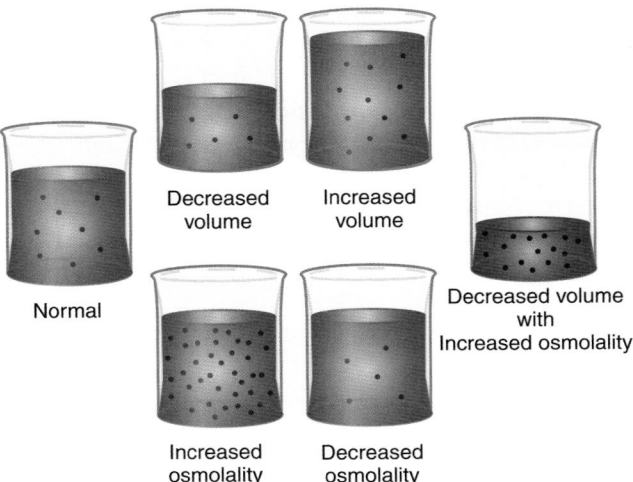

FIG. 42.7 Fluid volume and osmolality imbalances. (From Banasik JL, Copstead LC: *Pathophysiology online for pathophysiology,* ed 6, St Louis, 2019, Elsevier.)

isotonic fluid exceeds intake of sodium-containing fluid. Because ECF is both vascular and interstitial, signs and symptoms arise from lack of volume in both of these compartments. Table 42.3 lists specific causes and signs and symptoms of ECV deficit. The term **hypovolemia** means decreased vascular volume and often is used when discussing ECV deficit (Huether et al., 2020).

Extracellular volume excess occurs when there is too much isotonic fluid in the extracellular compartment. Intake of sodium-containing isotonic fluid has exceeded fluid output. For example, when you eat more salty foods than usual and drink water, you may notice that your ankles swell or rings on your fingers feel tight and you gain 1 kg (2 lb) or more overnight. These are manifestations of mild ECV excess. See Table 42.3 for other specific causes and signs and symptoms.

Osmolality Imbalances. In an osmolality imbalance body fluid becomes hypertonic or hypotonic, which causes osmotic shifts of water across cell membranes. The osmolality imbalances are called *hypernatremia* and *hyponatremia.*

Hypernatremia, also called *water deficit,* is a hypertonic condition. Two general causes make body fluids too concentrated: loss of relatively more water than salt, or gain of relatively more salt than water (Felver, 2021c). Table 42.3 lists specific causes under these categories. When the interstitial fluid becomes hypertonic, water leaves cells by osmosis, and they shrivel. Signs and symptoms of hypernatremia are those of cerebral dysfunction, which arise when brain cells shrivel. Hypernatremia may occur in combination with ECV deficit; this combined disorder is called *clinical dehydration.*

Hyponatremia, also called *water excess* or *water intoxication,* is a hypotonic condition. It arises from gain of relatively more water than salt or loss of relatively more salt than water (Felver, 2021c) (see Table 42.3). The excessively dilute condition of interstitial fluid causes water to enter cells by osmosis, causing the cells to swell. Signs and symptoms of cerebral dysfunction occur when brain cells swell (Hoorn et al., 2017; Sterns, 2021).

Clinical Dehydration. ECV deficit and hypernatremia often occur at the same time; this combination is called *clinical dehydration.* The ECV is too low, and the body fluids are too concentrated. Clinical dehydration is common with gastroenteritis or other causes of severe vomiting and diarrhea when people are unable to replace their fluid output with enough intake of dilute sodium-containing fluids. Signs and symptoms of clinical dehydration are those of both ECV deficit and hypernatremia (see Table 42.3).

Electrolyte Balance

You can best understand electrolyte balance by considering the three processes involved in electrolyte homeostasis: electrolyte intake and absorption, electrolyte distribution, and electrolyte output (Table 42.4) (Felver, 2021c). Although sodium is an electrolyte, it is not included here because serum sodium imbalances are the osmolality imbalances discussed previously.

Electrolyte distribution is an important issue. Plasma concentrations of K^+, Ca^{2+}, Mg^{2+}, and phosphate are very low compared with their concentrations in cells and bone (Huether et al., 2020). These concentration differences are necessary for normal muscle and nerve function. The electrolyte values that you review from laboratory reports are measured in blood serum and do not measure intracellular levels.

Electrolyte output occurs through normal excretion in urine, feces, and sweat. Output also occurs through vomiting, drainage tubes, or fistulas. When electrolyte output increases, electrolyte intake must increase to maintain electrolyte balance. Similarly, if electrolyte output decreases such as with oliguria, electrolyte intake must also decrease to maintain balance (Felver, 2021b).

TABLE 42.3 Fluid Imbalances

Imbalance and Related Causes	Signs and Symptoms
Isotonic Imbalances—Water and Sodium Lost or Gained in Equal or Isotonic Proportions	
Extracellular Fluid Volume Deficit—Body Fluids Have Decreased Volume but Normal Osmolality	
Sodium and Water Intake Less Than Output, Causing Isotonic Loss: Severely decreased oral intake of water and salt Increased GI output: vomiting, diarrhea, laxative overuse, drainage from fistulas or tubes Increased renal output: use of diuretics, adrenal insufficiency (deficit of cortisol and aldosterone) Loss of blood or plasma: hemorrhage, burns Massive sweating without water and salt intake	*Physical examination:* Sudden weight loss (overnight), postural hypotension, tachycardia, thready pulse, dry mucous membranes, poor skin turgor, slow vein filling, flat neck veins when supine, dark yellow urine If severe: Thirst, restlessness, confusion, hypotension; oliguria (urine output ***below*** 30 mL/hr); cold, clammy skin; hypovolemic shock *Laboratory findings:* Increased hematocrit; increased BUN ***above*** 20 mg/dL (7.1 mmol/L) (hemoconcentration); urine specific gravity usually ***above*** 1.030, unless renal cause
Extracellular Fluid Volume Excess—Body Fluids Have Increased Volume but Normal Osmolality	
Sodium and Water Intake Greater Than Output, Causing Isotonic Gain: Excessive administration of Na$^+$-containing isotonic IV fluids or oral intake of salty foods and water Renal retention of Na$^+$ and water: Heart failure, cirrhosis, aldosterone or glucocorticoid excess, acute or chronic oliguric renal disease	*Physical examination:* Sudden weight gain (overnight), edema (especially in dependent areas), full neck veins when upright or semi-upright, crackles in lungs If severe: Confusion, pulmonary edema *Laboratory findings:* Decreased hematocrit, decreased BUN ***below*** 10 mg/dL (3.6 mmol/L) (hemodilution)
Osmolality Imbalances	
Hypernatremia (Water Deficit; Hyperosmolar Imbalance)—Body Fluids Too Concentrated	
Loss of Relatively More Water Than Salt: Diabetes insipidus (ADH deficiency) Osmotic diuresis Large insensible perspiration and respiratory water output without increased water intake **Gain of Relatively More Salt Than Water:** Administration of tube feedings, hypertonic parenteral fluids, or salt tablets Lack of access to water, deliberate water deprivation, inability to respond to thirst (e.g., immobility, aphasia) Dysfunction of osmoreceptor-driven thirst drive	*Physical examination:* Decreased level of consciousness (confusion, lethargy, coma), perhaps thirst, seizures if develops rapidly or is very severe *Laboratory findings:* Serum Na$^+$ level ***above*** 145 mEq/L (145 mmol/L), serum osmolality ***above*** 295 mOsm/kg (295 mmol/kg)
Hyponatremia (Water Excess; Water Intoxication; Hypoosmolar Imbalance)—Body Fluids Too Dilute	
Gain of Relatively More Water Than Salt: Excessive ADH (SIADH) Psychogenic polydipsia or forced excessive water intake Excessive IV administration of D$_5$W Use of hypotonic irrigating solutions Tap-water enemas **Loss of Relatively More Salt Than Water:** Replacement of large body fluid output (e.g., diarrhea, vomiting) with water but no salt	*Physical examination:* Decreased level of consciousness (confusion, lethargy, coma), seizures if develops rapidly or is very severe *Laboratory findings:* Serum Na$^+$ level ***below*** 136 mEq/L (136 mmol/L), serum osmolality ***below*** 285 mOsm/kg (285 mmol/kg)
Combined Volume and Osmolality Imbalance	
Clinical Dehydration (ECV Deficit Plus Hypernatremia)—Body Fluids Have Decreased Volume and Are Too Concentrated	
Sodium and Water Intake Less Than Output, With Loss of Relatively More Water Than Salt: All of the causes of ECV deficit (see previous causes) plus poor or no water intake, often with fever causing increased insensible water output	*Physical examination and laboratory findings:* Combination of those for ECV deficit plus those for hypernatremia (see previous signs)

ADH, Antidiuretic hormone; *BUN,* blood urea nitrogen; *D$_5$W,* 5% dextrose in water; *ECV,* extracellular fluid volume; *GI,* gastrointestinal; *IV,* intravenous; *SIADH,* syndrome of inappropriate secretion of antidiuretic hormone.

Electrolyte Imbalances

Factors such as diarrhea, endocrine disorders, and medications that disrupt electrolyte homeostasis cause electrolyte imbalances. Electrolyte intake greater than electrolyte output or a shift of electrolytes from cells or bone into the ECF causes plasma electrolyte excess. Electrolyte intake less than electrolyte output or shift of electrolyte from the ECF into cells or bone causes plasma electrolyte deficit (Felver, 2021b).

Potassium Imbalances. Hypokalemia is abnormally low potassium concentration in the blood. It results from decreased potassium intake and absorption, a shift of potassium from the ECF into cells, and an

TABLE 42.4 Electrolyte Intake and Absorption, Distribution, and Output

Electrolyte	Intake and Absorption	Distribution	Output/Loss	Important Function
Potassium (K⁺)	Fruits Potatoes Instant coffee Molasses Brazil nuts Absorbs easily	Low in ECF, high in ICF. Insulin, epinephrine, and alkalosis shift K⁺ into cells. Some types of acidosis shift K⁺ out of cells.	Aldosterone, black licorice, hypomagnesemia, and polyuria increase renal excretion; oliguria decreases renal excretion. Acute or chronic diarrhea increases fecal excretion.	Maintains resting membrane potential of skeletal, smooth, and cardiac muscle, allowing normal muscle function
Calcium (Ca²⁺)	Dairy products Canned fish with bones Broccoli Oranges Requires vitamin D for best absorption Undigested fat prevents absorption	Ca²⁺ is low in ECF, mostly in bones and intracellular. Some Ca²⁺ in blood is bound and inactive; only ionized Ca²⁺ is active. Parathyroid hormone shifts Ca²⁺ out of bone; calcitonin shifts Ca²⁺ into bone. Ca²⁺ decreases in blood if phosphate rises and vice versa.	Thiazide diuretics decrease renal excretion. Chronic diarrhea and undigested fat increase fecal excretion.	Influences excitability of nerve and muscle cells; necessary for muscle contraction
Magnesium (Mg²⁺)	Dark green leafy vegetables Whole grains Mg²⁺-containing laxatives and antacids Undigested fat prevents absorption	Mg²⁺ is low in ECF, mostly in bones and intracellular. Some Mg²⁺ in blood is bound and inactive; only free Mg²⁺ is active.	Rising blood ethanol increases renal excretion; oliguria decreases renal excretion. Chronic diarrhea and undigested fat increase fecal excretion.	Influences function of neuromuscular junctions; is a cofactor for numerous enzymes
Phosphate	Milk Processed foods Aluminum antacids prevent absorption	Phosphate is low in ECF; it is higher in ICF and in bones. Insulin and epinephrine shift phosphate into cells. Decreases in blood if calcium rises and vice versa.	Oliguria and elevated fibroblast growth factor 23 (FGF-23) decrease renal excretion.	Necessary for production of ATP, the energy source for cellular metabolism

ATP, Adenosine triphosphate; *ECF,* extracellular fluid volume; *ICF,* intracellular fluid.

increased potassium output (Table 42.5). Common causes of hypokalemia from increased potassium output include diarrhea, repeated vomiting, and use of potassium-wasting diuretics (Kovesdy et al., 2017; Mount, 2019). People who have these conditions need to increase their potassium intake to reduce their risk of hypokalemia. Hypokalemia causes muscle weakness, which becomes life threatening if it includes respiratory muscles. It can also cause potentially life-threatening cardiac dysrhythmias.

Hyperkalemia is abnormally high potassium ion concentration in the blood. Its general causes are increased potassium intake and absorption, shift of potassium from cells into the ECF, and decreased potassium output (see Table 42.5). People who have oliguria (decreased urine output) are at high risk of hyperkalemia from the resultant decreased potassium output unless their potassium intake also decreases substantially. Understanding this principle helps you remember to check urine output before you administer IV solutions containing potassium. Hyperkalemia can cause muscle weakness, potentially life-threatening cardiac dysrhythmias, and cardiac arrest (Heckle et al., 2018).

Calcium Imbalances. Hypocalcemia is abnormally low calcium concentration in the blood (see Table 42.5). The physiologically active form of calcium in the blood is ionized calcium. Total blood calcium also contains inactive forms that are bound to plasma proteins and small anions such as citrate. Factors that cause too much ionized calcium to shift to the bound forms cause symptomatic *ionized hypocalcemia* (Kyle et al., 2018). People who have acute pancreatitis frequently develop hypocalcemia because calcium binds to undigested fat in their feces and is excreted. This process decreases absorption of dietary calcium and

also increases calcium output by preventing reabsorption of calcium contained in GI fluids. Hypocalcemia increases neuromuscular excitability, the basis for its signs and symptoms.

Hypercalcemia is abnormally high calcium concentration in the blood. Hypercalcemia results from increased calcium intake and absorption, shift of calcium from bones into the ECF, and decreased calcium output (see Table 42.5). Patients with some types of cancers such as lung and breast cancers often develop hypercalcemia because some cancer cells secrete chemicals into the blood that are related to parathyroid hormone. When these chemicals reach the bones, they cause shift of calcium from bones into the ECF. This weakens bones, and the person sometimes develops pathological fractures (i.e., bone breakage caused by forces that would not break a healthy bone). Hypercalcemia decreases neuromuscular excitability, the basis for its other signs and symptoms, the most common of which is lethargy (Huether et al., 2020).

Magnesium Imbalances. Hypomagnesemia is abnormally low magnesium concentration in the blood. Its general causes are decreased magnesium intake and absorption, shift of plasma magnesium to its inactive bound form, and increased magnesium output (see Table 42.5). Signs and symptoms are similar to those of hypocalcemia because hypomagnesemia also increases neuromuscular excitability (Huether et al., 2020).

Hypermagnesemia is abnormally high magnesium concentration in the blood (see Table 42.5). End-stage renal disease causes hypermagnesemia unless the person decreases magnesium intake to match the decreased output. Signs and symptoms are caused by decreased

TABLE 42.5 Electrolyte Imbalances

Imbalance and Related Causes	Signs and Symptoms
Hypokalemia—Low Serum Potassium (K⁺) Concentration **Decreased K⁺ Intake:** Excessive use of K⁺-free IV solutions **Shift of K⁺ Into Cells:** Alkalosis; treatment of diabetic ketoacidosis with insulin **Increased K⁺ Output:** Acute or chronic diarrhea; vomiting; other GI losses (e.g., nasogastric or fistula drainage); use of potassium-wasting diuretics; aldosterone excess; polyuria; glucocorticoid therapy	*Physical examination:* Bilateral muscle weakness that begins in quadriceps and may ascend to respiratory muscles, abdominal distention, decreased bowel sounds, constipation, dysrhythmias *Laboratory findings:* Serum K⁺ level ***below*** 3.5 mEq/L (3.5 mmol/L) ECG abnormalities: U waves; flattened or inverted T waves; ST segment depression
Hyperkalemia—High Serum Potassium (K⁺) Concentration **Increased K⁺ Intake:** Iatrogenic administration of large amounts of IV K⁺; rapid infusion of stored blood; excess ingestion of K⁺ salt substitutes **Shift of K⁺ out of Cells:** Massive cellular damage (e.g., crushing trauma, cytotoxic chemotherapy); insufficient insulin (e.g., diabetic ketoacidosis); some types of acidosis **Decreased K⁺ Output:** Acute or chronic oliguria (e.g., severe ECV deficit, end-stage renal disease); use of potassium-sparing diuretics; adrenal insufficiency (deficit of cortisol and aldosterone)	*Physical examination:* Bilateral muscle weakness in quadriceps, transient abdominal cramps, diarrhea, dysrhythmias, cardiac arrest if severe *Laboratory findings:* Serum K⁺ level ***above*** 5 mEq/L (5 mmol/L) ECG abnormalities: Peaked T waves; widened QRS complex; PR prolongation; terminal sine-wave pattern
Hypocalcemia—Low Serum Calcium (Ca²⁺) Concentration **Decreased Ca²⁺ Intake and Absorption**: Calcium-deficient diet; vitamin D deficiency (includes end-stage renal disease); chronic diarrhea; laxative misuse; steatorrhea **Shift of Ca²⁺ Into Bone or Inactive Form:** Hypoparathyroidism; rapid administration of citrated blood; hypoalbuminemia; alkalosis; pancreatitis; hyperphosphatemia (includes end-stage renal disease) **Increased Ca²⁺ Output:** Chronic diarrhea; steatorrhea	*Physical examination:* Numbness and tingling of fingers, toes, and circumoral (around mouth) region, positive Chvostek sign (contraction of facial muscles when facial nerve is tapped), hyperactive reflexes, muscle twitching and cramping; carpal and pedal spasms, tetany, seizures, laryngospasm, dysrhythmias *Laboratory findings:* Total serum Ca²⁺ level ***below*** 9.0 mg/dL (2.25 mmol/L) or serum ionized Ca²⁺ level ***below*** 4.5 mg/dL (1.05 mmol/L) ECG abnormalities: Prolonged ST segments
Hypercalcemia—High Serum Calcium (Ca²⁺) Concentration **Increased Ca²⁺ Intake and Absorption:** Milk-alkali syndrome **Shift of Ca²⁺ out of Bone:** Prolonged immobilization; hyperparathyroidism; bone tumors; nonosseous cancers that secrete bone-resorbing factors **Decreased Ca²⁺ Output:** Use of thiazide diuretics	*Physical examination:* Anorexia, nausea and vomiting, constipation, fatigue, diminished reflexes, lethargy, decreased level of consciousness, confusion, personality change, cardiac arrest if severe *Laboratory findings:* Total serum Ca²⁺ level ***above*** 10.5 mg/dL (2.62 mmol/L) or serum ionized Ca²⁺ level ***above*** 5.6 mg/dL (1.3 mmol/L) ECG abnormalities: Heart block, shortened ST segments
Hypomagnesemia—Low Serum Magnesium (Mg²⁺) Concentration **Decreased Mg²⁺ Intake and Absorption:** Malnutrition; chronic alcoholism; chronic diarrhea; laxative misuse; steatorrhea **Shift of Mg²⁺ Into Inactive Form:** Rapid administration of citrated blood **Increased Mg²⁺ Output:** Chronic diarrhea; steatorrhea; other GI losses (e.g., vomiting, nasogastric or fistula drainage); use of thiazide or loop diuretics; aldosterone excess	*Physical examination:* Positive Chvostek sign, hyperactive deep tendon reflexes, muscle cramps and twitching, grimacing, dysphagia, tetany, seizures, insomnia, tachycardia, hypertension, dysrhythmias *Laboratory findings:* Serum Mg²⁺ level ***below*** 1.3 mEq/L (0.65 mmol/L) ECG abnormalities: Prolonged QT interval
Hypermagnesemia—High Serum Magnesium (Mg²⁺) Concentration **Increased Mg²⁺ Intake and Absorption:** Excessive use of Mg²⁺-containing laxatives and antacids; parenteral overload of magnesium **Decreased Mg²⁺ Output:** Oliguric end-stage renal disease; adrenal insufficiency	*Physical examination:* Lethargy, hypoactive deep tendon reflexes, bradycardia, hypotension Acute elevation in Mg²⁺ levels: Flushing, sensation of warmth Severe acute hypermagnesemia: Decreased rate and depth of respirations, dysrhythmias, cardiac arrest *Laboratory findings:* Serum Mg²⁺ level ***above*** 2.1 mEq/L (1.05 mmol/L) ECG abnormalities: Prolonged PR interval

ECG, Electrocardiogram, *ECV,* extracellular fluid volume, *GI,* gastrointestinal, *IV,* intravenous.

Data from Felver L: Fluid and electrolyte homeostasis and imbalances. In Banasik JL, Copstead LC, editors: *Pathophysiology,* ed 6, St Louis, 2019, Elsevier.

TABLE 42.6   Arterial Blood Gas Measures

Laboratory Measure	Normal Range in Adult Arterial Blood	Definition and Interpretation
pH	7.35–7.45	pH is a negative logarithm of the free H^+ concentration, a measure of the blood's acidity or alkalinity. Values below 7.35 indicate abnormally acid; above 7.45 they indicate abnormally alkaline. Small changes in pH denote large changes in H^+ concentration and are clinically important.
$PaCO_2$	35–45 mm Hg (4.7–6 kPa)	$PaCO_2$ is partial pressure of carbon dioxide (CO_2), a measure of how well the lungs are excreting CO_2 produced by cells. Increased $PaCO_2$ indicates CO_2 accumulation in blood (more carbonic acid) caused by hypoventilation; decreased $PaCO_2$ indicates excessive CO_2 excretion (less carbonic acid) through hyperventilation.
HCO_3^-	21–28 mEq/L (21–28 mmol/L)	HCO_3^- is concentration of the base (alkaline substance) bicarbonate, a measure of how well the kidneys are excreting metabolic acids. Increased HCO_3^- indicates that the blood has too few metabolic acids; decreased HCO_3^- indicates that the blood has too many metabolic acids.
PaO_2	80–100 mm Hg (10.7–13.3 kPa)	PaO_2 is partial pressure of oxygen (O_2), a measure of how well gas exchange is occurring in the alveoli of the lungs. Values below normal indicate poor oxygenation of the blood.
SaO_2	95%–100%	SaO_2 is oxygen saturation, the percentage of hemoglobin that is carrying as much O_2 as possible. It is influenced by pH, $PaCO_2$, and body temperature. It drops rapidly when PaO_2 falls below 60 mm Hg (8 kPa).
Base excess	−2 to +2 mEq/L (mmol/L)	Base excess is observed buffering capacity minus the normal buffering capacity, a measure of how well the blood buffers are managing metabolic acids. Values below −2 (negative base excess) indicate excessive metabolic acids; values above +2 indicate excessive amounts of bicarbonate.

neuromuscular excitability, with lethargy and decreased deep tendon reflexes being most common (Kala and Abudayyeh, 2017; Huether et al., 2020).

Acid-Base Balance

For optimal cell function the body maintains a balance between acids and bases. Acid-base homeostasis is the dynamic interplay of three processes: acid production, acid buffering, and acid excretion (Felver, 2021a). Normal acid-base balance is maintained with acid excretion equal to acid production. Acids release hydrogen (H^+) ions; bases (alkaline substances) take up H^+ ions. The more H^+ ions that are present, the more acidic is a solution.

The degree of acidity in blood and other body fluids is reported from the clinical laboratory as pH. The pH scale goes from 1.0 (very acid) to 14.0 (very alkaline; basic). A pH of 7.0 is considered neutral. The normal pH range of adult arterial blood is 7.35 to 7.45. Maintaining pH within this normal range is very important for optimal cell function. If the pH goes outside the normal range, enzymes within cells do not function properly, hemoglobin does not manage oxygen properly, and serious physiological problems occur, including death. Laboratory tests of a sample of arterial blood called **arterial blood gases (ABGs)** are used to monitor a patient's acid-base balance (Felver, 2021a) (Table 42.6).

Acid Production. Cellular metabolism constantly creates two types of acids: carbonic acid and metabolic acids (Fig. 42.8). As shown in the formula below, cells produce carbon dioxide (CO_2), which combines with water to produce carbonic acid (H_2CO_3). The carbonic acid (H_2CO_3) can then separate to a hydrogen ion (H^+) and a bicarbonate ion (HCO_3^-):

$$CO_2 + H_2O \leftrightarrow H_2CO_3 \leftrightarrow H^+ + HCO_3^-$$

Carbon dioxide + Water ↔ Carbonic acid ↔ Hydrogen ion + Bicarbonate

Metabolic acids are any acids that are not carbonic acid. They include citric acid, lactic acid, and many others.

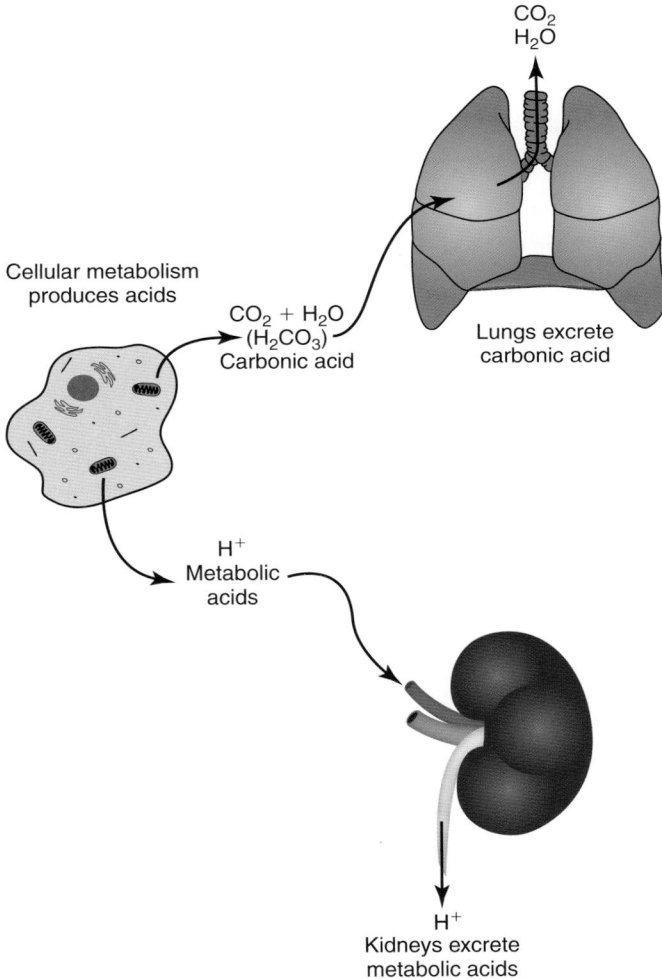

FIG. 42.8 Acid production and excretion.

Acid Buffering. Buffers are pairs of chemicals that work together to maintain normal pH of body fluids. If there are too many free H^+ ions, a buffer takes them up so that they no longer are free. If there are too few, a buffer can release H^+ ions to prevent an acid-base imbalance. Buffers work rapidly, within seconds.

All body fluids contain buffers. The major buffer in the ECF is the bicarbonate (HCO_3^-) buffer system, which buffers metabolic acids. It consists of a lot of bicarbonate and a small amount of carbonic acid (normally a 20:1 ratio). Addition of H^+ released by a metabolic acid to a bicarbonate ion makes more carbonic acid. Now the H^+ is no longer free and will not decrease the blood pH:

$$HCO_3^- + H^+ \leftrightarrow H_2CO_3$$

Bicarbonate ion + Hydrogen ion ↔ Carbonic acid

If there are too few H^+ ions, the carbonic acid part of the buffer pair releases some, increasing the bicarbonate, again returning pH to normal.

$$H_2CO_3 \leftrightarrow HCO_3^- + H^+$$

Carbonic acid ↔ Bicarbonate ion + Hydrogen ion

Other buffers include hemoglobin, protein buffers, and phosphate buffers. Cellular and bone buffers also contribute to acid-base balance. Buffers normally keep the blood from becoming too acid when acids that are produced by cells circulate to the lungs and kidneys for excretion.

Acid Excretion. The body has two acid-excretion systems: lungs and kidneys. The lungs excrete carbonic acid; the kidneys excrete metabolic acids (see Fig. 42.8).

Excretion of Carbonic Acid. When you exhale, you excrete carbonic acid in the form of CO_2 and water. If the $PaCO_2$ (i.e., level of CO_2 in the blood) rises, the chemoreceptors trigger faster and deeper respirations to excrete the excess. If the $PaCO_2$ falls, the chemoreceptors trigger slower and shallower respirations so that more of the CO_2 produced by cells remains in the blood and makes up the deficit. These alterations in respiratory rate and depth maintain the carbonic acid part of acid-base balance (Kamel and Halperin, 2017; Huether et al., 2020). People who have respiratory disease may be unable to excrete enough carbonic acid, which causes the blood to become more acidic and blood CO_2 to increase. If an increased respiratory rate is unable to correct the problem, the kidneys begin some compensatory excretion of metabolic acid.

Excretion of Metabolic Acids. The kidneys excrete all acids except carbonic acid. They secrete H^+ into the renal tubular fluid, putting HCO_3^- back into the blood at the same time. If there are too many H^+ ions in the blood, renal cells move more H^+ ions into the renal tubules for excretion, retaining more HCO_3^- in the process. If there are too few H^+ ions in the blood, renal cells excrete fewer H^+ ions.

Phosphate buffers in the renal tubular fluid keep the urine from becoming too acidic when the kidneys excrete H^+ ions. If the kidneys need to excrete a lot of H^+, renal tubular cells secrete ammonia, which combines with the H^+ ions in the tubules to make NH_4^+, ammonium ions. Buffering by phosphate and the creation of NH_4^+ turn free H^+ ions into other molecules in the renal tubular fluid (Kamel and Halperin, 2017; Huether et al., 2020). This process enables metabolic acid excretion in urine without making urine too acidic. People who have oliguric kidney disease often are unable to excrete metabolic acids normally, and these acids accumulate, making the blood too acidic (Nagami and Hamm, 2017). If the kidneys are unable to correct this problem, respiratory rate and depth increase, causing compensatory excretion of carbonic acid.

Acid-Base Imbalances

People develop acid-base imbalances when their normal homeostatic mechanisms are dysfunctional or overwhelmed. The term acidosis describes a condition that tends to make the blood relatively too acidic. Because our cells produce two types of acid, there are two different types of acidosis: respiratory acidosis and metabolic acidosis. The term alkalosis describes a condition that tends to make the blood relatively too basic (alkaline). There are two types of alkalosis: respiratory alkalosis and metabolic alkalosis.

The body has compensatory mechanisms that limit the extent of pH change with acid-base imbalances (Kamel and Halperin, 2017; Huether et al., 2020). Compensation involves physiological changes that help normalize the pH but do not correct the cause of the problem. If the problem is a respiratory acid-base imbalance, only the lungs can correct the problem, but the kidneys can compensate by changing the amount of metabolic acid in the blood. If the problem is a metabolic acid-base imbalance, only the kidneys can correct the problem, but the lungs can compensate by changing the amount of carbonic acid in the blood. Thus the kidneys compensate for respiratory acid-base imbalances, and the respiratory system compensates for metabolic acid-base imbalances. These compensatory mechanisms do not correct the problem, but they help the body survive by moving the blood pH toward normal. However, if the underlying condition is not corrected, these compensatory mechanisms eventually will fail.

Respiratory Acidosis. Respiratory acidosis arises from alveolar hypoventilation; the lungs are unable to excrete enough CO_2. The $PaCO_2$ rises, creating an excess of carbonic acid in the blood, which decreases pH (Table 42.7). The kidneys compensate by increasing excretion of metabolic acids in the urine, which increases blood bicarbonate. This compensatory process is slow, often taking 24 hours to show clinical effect and 3 to 5 days to reach steady state. Decreased cerebrospinal fluid (CSF) pH and intracellular pH of brain cells cause decreased level of consciousness.

Respiratory Alkalosis. Respiratory alkalosis arises from alveolar hyperventilation; the lungs excrete too much carbonic acid (CO_2 and water). The $PaCO_2$ falls, creating a deficit of carbonic acid in the blood, which increases pH (see Table 42.7). Respiratory alkalosis usually is short lived; therefore the kidneys do not have time to compensate. When the pH of blood, CSF, and ICF increases acutely, cell membrane excitability also increases, which can cause neurological symptoms such as excitement, confusion, and paresthesia. If the pH rises high enough, central nervous system (CNS) depression can occur.

Metabolic Acidosis. Metabolic acidosis occurs from an increase of metabolic acid or a decrease of base (bicarbonate). The kidneys are unable to excrete enough metabolic acids, which accumulate in the blood, or bicarbonate is removed from the body directly as with diarrhea (see Table 42.7). In either case the blood HCO_3^- decreases, and the pH falls (Ferrari et al., 2017; Huether et al., 2020). With an increase of metabolic acids, blood HCO_3^- decreases because it buffers metabolic acids. Similarly, when patients have conditions that cause the removal of HCO_3^-, the amount of HCO_3^- in the blood decreases. To help identify the specific cause, health care providers and the laboratory calculate the anion gap, a reflection of unmeasured anions in plasma. You calculate anion gap by subtracting the sum of plasma concentrations of the anions Cl^- and HCO_3^- from the plasma concentration of the cation Na^+ (Kamel and Halperin, 2017; Emmett and Hoorn, 2020). When reviewing laboratory reports, check the reference values from the laboratory that measured the electrolyte concentrations (Table 42.8).

TABLE 42.7 Acid-Base Imbalances

Imbalance and Related Causes	Signs and Symptoms
Respiratory Acidosis—Excessive Carbonic Acid Caused by Alveolar Hypoventilation	
Impaired Gas Exchange: Type B COPD (chronic bronchitis) or end-stage type A COPD (emphysema) Bacterial pneumonia Airway obstruction Extensive atelectasis (collapsed alveoli) Severe acute asthma episode **Impaired Neuromuscular Function:** Respiratory muscle weakness or paralysis from hypokalemia or neurological dysfunction Respiratory muscle fatigue, respiratory failure Chest wall injury or surgery causing pain with respiration **Dysfunction of Brainstem Respiratory Control:** Drug overdose with a respiratory depressant Some types of head injury	*Physical examination:* Headache, light-headedness, decreased level of consciousness (confusion, lethargy, coma), dysrhythmias *Laboratory findings:* Arterial blood gas alterations: pH *below* 7.35, PaCO$_2$ *above* 45 mm Hg (6 kPa), HCO$_3^-$ level normal if uncompensated or *above* 28 mEq/L (28 mmol/L) if compensated
Respiratory Alkalosis—Deficient Carbonic Acid Caused by Alveolar Hyperventilation	
Hypoxemia from any cause (e.g., initial part of asthma episode, pneumonia) Acute pain Anxiety, psychological distress, sobbing Inappropriate mechanical ventilator settings Stimulation of brainstem respiratory control (e.g., meningitis, gram-negative sepsis, head injury, aspirin overdose)	*Physical examination:* Light-headedness, numbness and tingling of fingers, toes, and circumoral region, increased rate and depth of respirations, excitement and confusion possibly followed by decreased level of consciousness, dysrhythmias *Laboratory findings:* Arterial blood gas alterations: pH *above* 7.45, PaCO$_2$ *below* 35 mm Hg (4.7 kPa), HCO$_3^-$ level normal if short lived or uncompensated or *below* 21 mEq/L (21 mmol/L) if compensated
Metabolic Acidosis—Excessive Metabolic Acids	
Increase of Metabolic Acids (High Anion Gap): Ketoacidosis (diabetes, starvation, alcoholism) Hypermetabolic state (severe hyperthyroidism, burns, severe infection) Oliguric renal disease (acute kidney injury, end-stage renal disease) Circulatory shock (lactic acidosis) Ingestion of acid or acid precursors (e.g., methanol, ethylene glycol, boric acid) **Loss of Bicarbonate (Normal Anion Gap):** Diarrhea Pancreatic fistula or intestinal decompression Renal tubular acidosis	*Physical examination:* Decreased level of consciousness (lethargy, confusion, coma), abdominal pain, dysrhythmias, increased rate and depth of respirations (compensatory hyperventilation) *Laboratory findings:* Arterial blood gas alterations: pH *below* 7.35, PaCO$_2$ normal if uncompensated or *below* 35 mm Hg (4.7 kPa) if compensated, HCO$_3^-$ level *below* 21 mEq/L (21 mmol/L)
Metabolic Alkalosis—Deficient Metabolic Acids	
Increase of Bicarbonate: Excessive administration of sodium bicarbonate Massive blood transfusion (liver converts citrate to HCO$_3^-$) Mild or moderate ECV deficit (contraction alkalosis) **Loss of Metabolic Acid:** Excessive vomiting or gastric suctioning Hypokalemia Excess aldosterone	*Physical examination:* Light-headedness, numbness and tingling of fingers, toes, and circumoral region; muscle cramps; possible excitement and confusion followed by decreased level of consciousness, dysrhythmias (may be caused by concurrent hypokalemia) *Laboratory findings:* Arterial blood gas alterations: pH *above* 7.45, PaCO$_2$ normal if uncompensated or *above* 45 mm Hg (6.0 kPa) if compensated, HCO$_3^-$ *above* 28 mEq/L (28 mmol/L)

Data from Felver L: Acid-base homeostasis and imbalances. In Banasik JL, Copstead LC, editors: *Pathophysiology,* ed 6, St Louis, 2019, Saunders. *COPD,* Chronic obstructive pulmonary disease, *ECV,* extracellular fluid volume.

The abnormally low pH in metabolic acidosis stimulates the chemoreceptors, so the respiratory system compensates for the acidosis by hyperventilation. Compensatory hyperventilation begins in a few minutes and removes carbonic acid from the body. This process does not correct the problem, but it helps limit the pH decrease. Metabolic acidosis decreases a person's level of consciousness (see Table 42.7).

Metabolic Alkalosis. Metabolic alkalosis occurs from a direct increase of base HCO$_3^-$ or a decrease of metabolic acid, which increases blood HCO$_3^-$ by releasing it from its buffering function. Common causes include vomiting and gastric suction (see Table 42.7). The respiratory compensation for metabolic alkalosis is hypoventilation. The decreased rate and depth of respiration allow carbonic acid to increase in the blood, as seen by an increased PaCO$_2$. The need for oxygen may limit the degree of respiratory compensation for metabolic alkalosis. Because HCO$_3^-$ crosses the blood-brain barrier with difficulty, neurological signs and symptoms are less severe or even absent with metabolic alkalosis (Kamel and Halperin, 2017; Huether et al., 2020).

TABLE 42.8	Anion Gap in Metabolic Acidosis	
Anion Gap Type	**Values (Without K⁺)**	**Causes**
Normal anion gap	6+ / −4 mEq/L (6+ / −4 mmol/L) Varies, depending on laboratory	*Excess output of bicarbonate:* Diarrhea, pancreatic fistula, intestinal decompression, renal tubular acidosis *Increase of chloride-containing acid:* Parenteral HCl therapy
High anion gap	Greater than 5 mEq/L (5 mmol/L) above the laboratory reference range	*Increase of any acid except HCl:* Ketoacids (DKA, starvation, alcoholism), lactic acid (circulatory shock, extreme exercise), excessive normal metabolic acids (oliguric acute kidney injury, end-stage renal disease, severe hyperthyroidism, burns, severe infection), unusual organic acids (salicylate overdose, acids metabolized from methanol, ethylene glycol, paraldehyde)

Data from Kamel K, Halperin M: *Fluid, electrolyte, and acid–base physiology*, ed 5, St Louis, 2017, Elsevier.
DKA, Diabetic ketoacidosis.

REFLECT NOW

Think about the risk for specific fluid, electrolyte, and acid-base imbalances when caring for a patient with chronic diarrhea. What types of imbalances is the patient likely to have?

NURSING KNOWLEDGE BASE

You will apply knowledge about fluid, electrolyte, and acid-base imbalance when you work in the clinical setting. In addition to scientific knowledge, there is a nursing knowledge base established from research and nursing practice, such as the Infusion Nurses Society (INS) standards of practice. Nursing knowledge also includes risk factors for fluid imbalances. An example of using this knowledge when making clinical judgments is incorporating the knowledge along with the physiology of normal aging when assessing older adults, knowing that this age-group has high risk of fluid imbalances (Touhy and Jett, 2021). *Robert knows that Mrs. Mendoza is 77 years old and that this may put her at additional risk for fluid imbalances. He plans his assessment to incorporate how this factor may contribute to the other risks she has for fluid and electrolyte imbalance.*

Your nursing knowledge helps you formulate assessment questions to determine patients' risk factors for fluid, electrolyte, and acid-base imbalances; assess for signs and symptoms of these imbalances; and implement nursing and collaborative interventions to maintain or restore fluid and electrolyte and acid-base balance (Felver, 2021a; Felver, 2021b; Felver, 2021c). *Robert has reviewed Mrs. Mendoza's EHR and knows that she has been vomiting and has had diarrhea for 24 hours, so he uses his knowledge of fluid and electrolyte balance and all of the patient's risk factors to identify areas to assess and lab results to review.*

CRITICAL THINKING

Successful clinical judgment requires critical thinking with a synthesis of knowledge, experience, environmental factors, critical thinking attitudes, and intellectual and professional standards. Clinical judgments require you to anticipate the information necessary to analyze the data and make decisions regarding patient care. During assessment consider all elements that build toward making an appropriate nursing diagnosis (Fig. 42.9).

Determine if any environment factors will impact how you deliver patient care. Prior to assessment review the patient's medical record for new information—for example, specific fluid and electrolyte practices, new orders for IV equipment, or therapies. Avoid time and resource problems; for example, determine if additional personnel are needed for certain care activities or if additional medical equipment or devices need to be obtained for you to manage the patient's fluid and electrolyte alterations.

In the case of fluid, electrolyte, and acid-base balance, you integrate knowledge of physiology, pathophysiology, and pharmacology and previous experiences and information gathered from patients. Critical analysis of data enables an understanding of how fluid, electrolyte, and acid-base imbalances affect a specific patient and family. In addition, critical thinking attitudes such as accountability, discipline, and integrity, applied during assessment, help you identify appropriate nursing diagnoses and plan successful interventions. Professional standards such as the INS standards of practice (Gorski et al., 2021) provide evidence-based guidance for appropriate assessment.

REFLECT NOW

You are preparing to care for a patient with dehydration. What scientific concepts and standards will guide you in obtaining accurate assessment data regarding a patient's fluid, electrolyte, and acid-base status?

❖ NURSING PROCESS

Use clinical judgment while applying critical thinking to the nursing process. The nursing process provides a clinical decision-making approach for you to identify patient problems, develop and implement an individualized patient-centered plan of care, and evaluate that plan. For patients at high risk for fluid, electrolyte, and/or acid-base imbalances or those who already have these imbalances, an individualized approach is the foundation for safe and effective patient-centered nursing care.

◆ Assessment

During the assessment process thoroughly assess each patient and critically analyze findings to ensure that you make patient-centered clinical decisions required for safe nursing care. Using a systematic approach in assessment enables you to identify patient problems correctly so that you can help patients maintain or restore fluid, electrolyte, and acid-base balances safely (see Fig. 42.9).

Robert begins his assessment of Mrs. Mendoza using his knowledge of fluid and electrolytes to determine her hydration status with its related assessments. Health care provider orders include IV infusion of 0.9% saline at 125 mL/hr, intake and output (I&O) recordings, vital signs every 4 hours, and daily weights. His assessment reveals her current vital signs: temperature, 37.6°C (99.6°F); pulse, 110 beats/min and regular; supine BP, 90/58 mm Hg with no changes when standing; respirations, 18 breaths/min. Her vital signs show findings of ECV deficit.

FIG. 42.9 Critical thinking model for fluid, electrolyte, and acid-base balance assessment. *IV,* Intravenous. (Clinical Judgment Measurement Model copyright © NCSBN. All rights reserved.)

Through the Patient's Eyes. A patient's fluid, electrolyte, or acid-base imbalance is sometimes so severe that it is difficult to determine a patient's needs, values, and preferences. However, when a patient is alert enough to discuss care, be sure to assess the patient's perceptions of the illness. For example, for a patient who is hospitalized for clinical dehydration from diarrhea, ask about any previous experiences with dehydration and assess the patient's interpretation of the signs and symptoms experienced and possible causes. Consider therapies the patient might have received. Did the patient require IV therapy in the past? If so, what was that like? Also ask how the person managed diarrhea at home to assess an understanding of how to prevent the imbalances from occurring in the future. Assess potential barriers to rehydration, such as concerns regarding IV therapy. Ask about the patient's greatest concerns regarding fluid status to build the basis for active partnership in planning, implementing, and evaluating patient-centered care.

Nursing History. Clinical assessment begins with a patient history designed to reveal risk factors that cause or contribute to fluid, electrolyte, and acid-base imbalances (Table 42.9). Ask specific, focused questions to identify factors that contribute to a patient's potential imbalances (Box 42.1).

Age. First consider a patient's age. An infant's proportion of total body water (70%–80% total body weight) is greater than that of children or adults. Infants and young children have greater water needs and immature kidneys (Hockenberry et al., 2019; Huether et al., 2020). They are at greater risk for ECV deficit and hypernatremia because body water loss is proportionately greater per kilogram of weight (Box 42.2).

Children who are between the ages of 2 and 12 frequently respond to illnesses with fevers of higher temperatures and longer duration than those of adults (Hockenberry et al., 2019). At any age fever increases the rate of insensible water loss. Adolescents have increased metabolism and water production because of their rapid growth changes. Fluctuations in fluid balance are greater in adolescent girls because of hormonal changes associated with the menstrual cycle.

Older adults experience a number of age-related changes that potentially affect fluid, electrolyte, and acid-base balances (see Box 42.2). They often have more difficulty recovering from imbalances resulting from the combined effects of normal aging, various disease conditions, and multiple medications (Kear, 2017; Touhy and Jett, 2021).

Environment. Hot environments increase fluid output through sweating. Sweat is a hypotonic sodium-containing fluid. Excessive sweating without adequate replacement of salt and water can lead to ECV deficit, hypernatremia, or clinical dehydration (McDermott et al., 2017; Sterns, 2020). Ask patients about their normal level of physical work and whether they engage in vigorous exercise in hot environments. Do the patients have fluid replacements containing salt available during exercise and activity?

Dietary Intake. Assess dietary intake of fluids; salt; and foods rich in potassium, calcium, and magnesium (see Table 42.4). Ask patients if they follow weight-loss diets as these pose risks. Starvation diets or those with high fat and no carbohydrate content often lead to metabolic acidosis (see Table 42.7). In addition, assess a patient's ability to chew and swallow,

TABLE 42.9 Risk Factors for Fluid, Electrolyte, and Acid-Base Imbalances

Age	*Very young:* ECV deficit, osmolality imbalances, clinical dehydration *Very old:* ECV excess or deficit, osmolality imbalances
Environment	*Sodium-rich diet:* ECV excess *Electrolyte-poor diet:* Electrolyte deficits *Hot weather:* Clinical dehydration
Gastrointestinal output	*Diarrhea:* ECV deficit, clinical dehydration, hypokalemia, hypocalcemia (if chronic), hypomagnesemia (if chronic), metabolic acidosis *Drainage (e.g., nasogastric suctioning, fistulas):* ECV deficit, hypokalemia; metabolic acidosis if intestinal or pancreatic drainage *Vomiting:* ECV deficit, clinical dehydration, hypokalemia, hypomagnesemia, metabolic alkalosis
Chronic diseases	*Cancer:* Hypercalcemia; with tumor lysis syndrome: hyperkalemia, hypocalcemia, hyperphosphatemia; other imbalances, depending on side effects of therapy *Chronic obstructive pulmonary disease:* Respiratory acidosis *Cirrhosis:* ECV excess, hypokalemia *Heart failure:* ECV excess; other imbalances, depending on therapy *Oliguric renal disease:* ECV excess, hyperkalemia, hypermagnesemia, hyperphosphatemia, metabolic acidosis
Trauma	*Burns:* ECV deficit, metabolic acidosis *Crush injuries:* Hyperkalemia *Head injuries:* Hyponatremia or hypernatremia, depending on ADH response *Hemorrhage:* ECV deficit, hyperkalemia if circulatory shock
Therapies	Diuretics and other medications (see Box 42.3) *IV therapy:* ECV excess, osmolality imbalances, electrolyte excesses *PN:* Any fluid or electrolyte imbalance, depending on components of solution

ADH, Antidiuretic hormone; *ECV*, extracellular fluid volume; *IV*, intravenous; *PN*, parenteral nutrition.

BOX 42.1 Nursing Assessment Questions

Environment
- Tell me what type of environment you work in. Is it a hot environment?
- If so, what do you do to manage the heat?

Dietary Intake
- About how many glasses of fluids do you usually drink every day? What type of fluids do you normally drink?
- Tell me what you usually eat in a day.
- In the past month, was there any day when you went hungry because you did not have enough money for food?
- Which snacks do you usually eat?
- Are you on a special diet because of a medical problem? How does that work for you?
- Are you following any weight-loss program?
- Do you use a salt substitute?
- Do you take calcium, magnesium, or potassium supplements? If so, how often?
- Do you have any difficulties chewing or swallowing?

Lifestyle
- How much alcohol do you drink in a typical week?

Gastrointestinal Output
- Have you had recent vomiting or diarrhea? If so, for how long? How many times per day?

Medications and Other Therapies
- Which medicines, including over-the-counter and herbal remedies, do you use regularly? Occasionally?
- Do you take diuretics? Drugs for high blood pressure?
- Do you use antacids? If so, which ones? How often? Do you ever use baking soda as an antacid? Do you use fizzy (effervescent) medications for colds?
- Do you use laxatives? If so, how often? Which type of stool do you get when you use them?
- What do you use for an upset stomach?

Signs and Symptoms
- If you weigh yourself every day, how has your weight changed over the past few days?
- Do you get light-headed when you stand up?
- Do you feel thirsty, have a dry mouth, or notice a lack of tears?
- Have you noticed a change in your urine output: decreased volume, dark color, or concentrated appearance?
- Are you experiencing swelling of your fingers, feet, or ankles?
- Do you have difficulty breathing when you lie down at night?
- Are you having difficulty concentrating, or do you feel confused? What is normal for you?
- Are you having more difficulty than usual standing up from a sofa or soft chair? Do your legs feel unusually heavy when you climb stairs? Do you have muscle weakness that is unusual for you?
- Have you noticed any muscle cramps or unusual sensations such as numbness or tingling fingers?

which, if altered, interferes with adequate intake of electrolyte-rich foods and fluids.

Alcohol Intake. Assess your patient's alcohol intake. How many days does a person have an alcoholic drink each week, and how many drinks does the person have at any one time? Chronic alcohol abuse commonly causes hypomagnesemia, in part because it increases renal magnesium excretion (Huether et al., 2020; Palmer and Clegg, 2017).

Medications. Obtain a complete list of your patient's current medications, including over-the-counter (OTC) and herbal preparations, to assess the risk for fluid, electrolyte, and acid-base imbalances (Box 42.3). Use a drug reference book or reputable online database to check the potential effects of other medications. Ask specifically about the use of baking soda as an antacid; it can cause ECV excess because of its high sodium content that holds water in the extracellular compartments. For an individual who uses laxatives, ask about the type of laxative, the frequency of use, and the consistency and frequency of stools. Multiple loose stools remove fluid and electrolytes from the body, thus causing numerous imbalances.

Medical History

Recent Surgery. Surgery causes a physiological stress response, which increases with extensive surgery and blood loss. In the first 24 to 48 hours after surgery, increased secretion of aldosterone, glucocorticoids, and ADH cause increased ECV, decreased osmolality, and increased potassium excretion (Harding et al., 2020). In otherwise healthy patients these imbalances resolve without difficulty, but patients who

BOX 42.2 FOCUS ON OLDER ADULTS

Factors Affecting Fluid, Electrolyte, and Acid-Base Balance

- During aging, body composition changes, causing a decreased percentage of body weight as water (50%), which increases risk of extracellular fluid volume (ECV) deficit and dehydration (Felver, 2021c).
- The combined effects of age (neonates, infants, and older adults), chronic diseases, and multiple medications often pose challenges to maintaining fluid and electrolyte balance.
- Patients with impaired mobility or bladder-control issues may restrict fluid intake, which increases the risk of hypernatremia and ECV deficit.
- Decreased thirst sensation increases risk of hypernatremia and dehydration; do not rely on thirst to assess hypernatremia, ECV deficit, or dehydration in patients who are confused, patients with altered level of consciousness, the very young, and older adults.
- Severe dehydration can result in postural hypotension; have patients, especially older adults, arise slowly when you take orthostatic blood pressure measurements.
- Cardiovascular illnesses can decrease the body's ability to adapt to a sudden increase in vascular volume, increasing risk of pulmonary edema with rapid infusion of isotonic intravenous fluids.
- Chronic renal disease results in a decrease in the kidneys' ability to concentrate urine, thus increasing the risk for hypernatremia, ECV deficit, and dehydration.
- Kidney changes of normal aging make it more difficult to excrete a large acid load, increasing the risk of metabolic acidosis (Touhy and Jett, 2021).

BOX 42.3 Commonly Used Medications That Cause Fluid, Electrolyte, and Acid-Base Imbalances

- ACE inhibitors (e.g., captopril) and angiotensin II receptor blockers (e.g., losartan): Hyperkalemia
- Antidepressants, SSRI (e.g., fluoxetine [Prozac]): Hyponatremia
- Calcium carbonate antacids: Hypercalcemia, mild metabolic alkalosis
- Corticosteroids (e.g., prednisone): Hypokalemia, metabolic alkalosis
- Diuretics, potassium-wasting (e.g., furosemide [Lasix], thiazides): ECV deficit, hyponatremia (thiazides), hypokalemia, hypomagnesemia, mild metabolic alkalosis
- Diuretics, potassium-sparing (e.g., spironolactone): Hyperkalemia, mild metabolic acidosis
- Effervescent (fizzy) antacids and cold medications (high Na$^+$ content): ECV excess
- Laxatives: ECV deficit, hypokalemia, hypocalcemia, hypomagnesemia, metabolic acidosis
- Magnesium hydroxide (e.g., Milk of Magnesia): Hypermagnesemia
- Nonsteroidal antiinflammatory drugs (e.g., ibuprofen): Mild ECV excess, hyponatremia
- Penicillins, high-dose (e.g., carbenicillin): Hypokalemia, metabolic alkalosis; hyperkalemia with penicillin G (contains K$^+$)

Data from Burchum JR, Rosenthal LD: *Lehne's pharmacology for nursing care*, ed 10, St Louis, 2019, Elsevier.
ACE, Angiotensin-converting enzyme; *ECV*, extracellular fluid volume; *SSRI*, selective serotonin reuptake inhibitor.

have preexisting illnesses or additional risk factors often need treatment during this period.

Gastrointestinal Output. Increased output of fluid through the GI tract is a common and important cause of fluid, electrolyte, and acid-base imbalances and requires accurate measurement and assessment. Always note the volume and appearance of any output. Vomiting and diarrhea, either acute or chronic, can cause ECV deficit, hypernatremia, clinical dehydration, and hypokalemia by increasing the output of fluid, Na$^+$, and K$^+$. In addition, chronic diarrhea can cause hypocalcemia and hypomagnesemia by decreasing electrolyte absorption. Removal of gastric acid from the body through vomiting or nasogastric suction can cause metabolic alkalosis. In contrast, removal of the bicarbonate-rich intestinal or pancreatic fluids through diarrhea, intestinal suction, or fistula can cause metabolic acidosis (Ferrari et al., 2017).

Acute Illness or Trauma. Acute conditions that place patients at high risk for fluid, electrolyte, and acid-base alterations include respiratory diseases, burns, trauma, GI alterations, and acute oliguric renal disease.

Respiratory Disorders. Many acute respiratory disorders predispose patients to respiratory acidosis. For example, bacterial pneumonia causes alveoli to fill with exudate that impairs gas exchange, causing the patient to retain carbon dioxide, which leads to increased PaCO$_2$ and respiratory acidosis. Measure respirations accurately and auscultate lung sounds.

Burns. Burns place patients at high risk for ECV deficit from numerous mechanisms, including plasma-to-interstitial fluid shift and increased evaporative and exudate output. Fluid loss increases with the percentage of body surface burned (Harding et al., 2020). Patients with burns have cellular damage that releases potassium into the blood, and they may become hyperkalemic. In addition, these patients often develop metabolic acidosis because of greatly increased cellular metabolism, which produces more metabolic acids than their kidneys are able to excrete. Your assessment will include the depth of tissue injury (e.g., superficial, superficial partial-thickness, deep partial-thickness, full-thickness, and fourth degree for the most severe) and the extent of the body surface affected. Burn wounds are dynamic and can progress, thus a precise assessment of the depth of the burn wound may be difficult initially (Rice and Orgill, 2021). It may require several days for a final determination.

Trauma. When a patient experiences trauma, consider the cause and potential effects. Hemorrhage from any type of trauma causes ECV deficit from blood loss. Some types of trauma create additional risks. For example, crush injuries destroy cellular structure, causing hyperkalemia by massive release of intracellular K$^+$ into the blood.

Head injury typically alters ADH secretion. It may cause diabetes insipidus (deficit of ADH), in which patients excrete large volumes of very dilute urine and develop hypernatremia. In contrast, head injury may cause the syndrome of inappropriate antidiuretic hormone (SIADH), in which excess secretion of ADH causes hyponatremia by retaining too much water and concentrating the urine (Harding et al., 2020).

Chronic Illness. Many chronic diseases create ongoing risk of fluid, electrolyte, and acid-base imbalances. For example, type B chronic obstructive pulmonary disease (COPD) often causes chronic respiratory acidosis. In addition, the treatment regimens for chronic disease often cause imbalances. Assess patients for the presence of these conditions and signs or symptoms suggesting fluid and electrolyte imbalances (see Box 42.2).

Cancer. The specific fluid and electrolyte imbalances that occur with cancer depend on the type and progression of the cancer and the treatment regimen. Many patients with cancer develop hypercalcemia when their cancer cells secrete chemicals that circulate to bones and cause calcium to enter the blood. Other fluid and electrolyte imbalances occur in cancer because some types of tumors cause metabolic and endocrine abnormalities (Wagner and Arora, 2017). In addition, patients with cancer are at risk for fluid and electrolyte imbalances as a result of the side effects (e.g., anorexia, diarrhea) of chemotherapy, biological response modifiers, or radiation (Harding et al., 2020).

Heart Failure. Patients who have chronic heart failure have diminished cardiac output, which reduces kidney perfusion and activates the RAAS. The action of aldosterone on the kidneys causes ECV excess and risk of hypokalemia. Most diuretics used to treat heart failure increase the risk of hypokalemia while reducing the ECV excess. Dietary sodium restriction is important with heart failure because Na^+ holds water in the ECF, making the ECV excess worse. In severe heart failure a restriction of both fluid and sodium may be prescribed to decrease the workload of the heart by reducing excess circulating fluid volume (Harding et al., 2020).

Oliguric Renal Disease. Oliguria occurs when the kidneys have a reduced capacity to make urine. Some conditions such as acute nephritis cause sudden onset of oliguria, whereas other problems such as chronic kidney disease lead to chronic oliguria. Oliguric renal disease prevents normal excretion of fluid, electrolytes, and metabolic acids, resulting in ECV excess, hyperkalemia, hypermagnesemia, hyperphosphatemia, and metabolic acidosis. The severity of these imbalances is proportional to the degree of renal failure. Although chronic kidney disease is progressive, successful management of imbalances is possible with dietary restriction of sodium and other electrolytes, fluid restriction in severe cases, and eventually dialysis or renal transplant (Harding et al., 2020).

Physical Assessment. Data gathered through a focused physical assessment validate and extend the information collected in the patient history. Table 42.10 summarizes focused assessments for patients with fluid, electrolyte, and acid-base imbalances. Use your clinical judgment to focus your assessment on the areas pertinent to each patient situation. For example, for patients at risk of fluid imbalances, focus your assessment on body weight changes, clinical markers of vascular and interstitial volume, thirst, behavioral changes, and level of consciousness. Additional focused assessments for patients at high risk of electrolyte and acid-base imbalances include specific cardiac, respiratory, neuromuscular, and GI markers. Grouping your assessments under these categories helps you know which assessments to prioritize and enables you to assess effectively.

Daily Weights and Fluid Intake and Output Measurement. Daily weights are an important indicator of fluid status (Felver, 2021c). Each kilogram (2.2 lb) of weight gained or lost overnight is equal to 1 L of fluid retained or lost. These fluid gains or losses indicate changes in the amount of total body fluid, usually ECF, but do not indicate shift between body compartments. Weigh patients with heart failure and those who are at high risk for or actually have ECV excess daily. Daily weights are also useful for patients with clinical dehydration or other causes or risks for ECV deficit. Have the patient void and weigh the patient at the same time each day with the same scale. Calibrate the scale each day or routinely. The patient needs to wear the same clothes or clothes that weigh the same; if using a bed scale, use the same number of sheets on the scale with each weighing. Compare the weight of each day with that of the previous day to determine fluid gains or losses. Look at the weights over several days to recognize trends. Interpretation of daily weights guides medical therapy and nursing care.

Teach patients with heart failure to take and record their daily weights at home and to contact their health care provider if their weight increases suddenly by a set amount (obtain parameters from their health care providers). Recognizing trends in daily weights taken at home is important (Horwitz and Krumholz, 2020; Park et al., 2017). Patients who are hospitalized for decompensated heart failure often experience steady increases in daily weights during the week before hospitalization.

Measuring and recording all liquid I&O during a 24-hour period is an important aspect of fluid balance assessment. Compare a patient's 24-hour intake with the 24-hour output. The two measures should be approximately equal if the person has normal fluid balance (Felver, 2021c). To interpret situations in which I&O are substantially different, consider the individual patient. For example, if intake is substantially greater than output, there are two possibilities: the patient may be gaining excessive fluid or returning to normal fluid status by replacing

fluid lost previously from the body. Similarly, if intake is substantially smaller than output, there are also two possibilities: the patient may be losing needed fluid from the body and developing ECV deficit and/or hypernatremia or returning to normal fluid status by excreting excessive fluid gained previously.

In most health care settings, I&O measurement is a nursing assessment. Some agencies require a health care provider's order for I&O. If you want to measure I&O for a patient with compromised fluid status, check your agency's policies to determine whether you can set it up or if you need a health care provider's order.

Fluid intake includes all liquids that a person eats (e.g., gelatin, ice cream, soup), drinks (e.g., water, coffee, juice), or receives through nasogastric or jejunostomy feeding tubes (see Chapter 45). IV fluids (continuous infusions and intermittent IV piggybacks) and blood components also are sources of intake. Water swallowed while taking pills and liquid medications counts as intake. A patient receiving tube feedings often receives numerous liquid medications and water to flush the tube before and/or after medications. Over a 24-hour period these liquids amount to significant intake and always are recorded on an I&O record. Ask patients who are alert and oriented to help with measuring their oral intake and explain to families why they should not eat or drink from the patient's meal trays or water pitcher.

Fluid output includes urine, diarrhea, vomitus, gastric suction, and drainage from postsurgical wounds or other tubes (see Chapter 50). Record a patient's urinary output after each voiding. Instruct patients who are alert, oriented, and ambulatory to save their urine in a urinal or a calibrated insert, which attaches to the rim of the toilet bowl (Fig. 42.10). Teach patients and families the purpose of I&O measurements. Also teach them to notify the nurse or assistive personnel (AP) to empty any container with voided fluid or how to measure and empty the container themselves and report the result appropriately. Patients need to have good vision and motor skills to perform these measurements. Active involvement of patient and family is an aspect of patient-centered care that is essential to maintaining accurate I&O measurements. When a patient has an indwelling urinary catheter, drainage tube, or suction, record output (e.g., at the end of each nursing shift or every hour) as the patient's condition requires.

You can delegate parts of I&O measurement and recording to AP with competent skills in measurement. Actual measurement of fluid volumes is more accurate than visual estimates. In many institutions AP record oral intake but not intake through feeding or IV tubes, which are nursing responsibilities. Similarly, AP often record urine, diarrhea, and vomitus output but not drainage through tubes. The responsible registered nurse (RN) or licensed practical nurse/licensed vocational nurse (LPN/LVN) and the AP work as a team to record measurements in the designated location in the EHR, often on a flow sheet with other information. The EHR program usually calculates the 24-hour totals. If an EHR is not used, record I&O on paper forms attached to the bedside chart or room door. You or the AP calculates the 24-hour totals (see agency policy). Accurate I&O facilitates ongoing evaluation of a patient's hydration status.

Laboratory Values. Review the patient's laboratory test results and compare them with the normal ranges to obtain further objective data about fluid, electrolyte, and acid-base balances. Normal and abnormal test results are summarized in Tables 42.1, 42.3, and 42.5 to 42.7. The frequency of electrolyte level measurements depends on the severity of a patient's illness. Analyzing a patient's laboratory results requires you to be thorough and to apply extensive scientific and nursing knowledge, especially if a person develops an acute imbalance while also having a chronic disease. Serum electrolyte tests usually are performed routinely on patients entering a hospital to screen for imbalances and serve as a baseline for future comparisons.

TABLE 42.10 Focused Nursing Assessments for Patients With Fluid, Electrolyte, and Acid-Base Imbalances

Assessment	Imbalances
Body Weight Changes From Previous Day	
Loss of 1 kg (2.2 lb) or more in 24 hours for adults	ECV deficit
Gain of 2.2 lb (1 kg) or more in 24 hours for adults	ECV excess
Clinical Markers of Vascular Volume	
Blood pressure:	
Hypotension or orthostatic hypotension	ECV deficit
Light-headedness on sitting upright or standing	ECV deficit
Pulse rate and character:	
Rapid, thready	ECV deficit
Bounding	ECV excess
Fullness of neck veins:	
Flat or collapsing with inhalation when supine	ECV deficit
Full or distended when upright or semi-upright	ECV excess
Other assessments of vascular volume:	
Capillary refill: Sluggish	ECV deficit
Lung auscultation, dependent lobe: Crackles or rhonchi with progressive dyspnea	ECV excess
Urine output: Small volume of dark yellow urine	ECV deficit
Clinical Markers of Interstitial Volume	
Inspection and Palpation	
Presence of edema: Present in dependent areas (ankles or sacrum) and possibly fingers or around eyes	ECV excess
Mucous membranes: Dry between cheek and gum, decreased or absent tearing	ECV deficit
Skin turgor: Pinched skin fails to return to normal position within 3 seconds	ECV deficit
Presence of thirst: Thirst present	Hypernatremia, severe ECV deficit
Behavior and level of consciousness:	
Restlessness and mild confusion	Severe ECV deficit
Decreased level of consciousness (lethargy, confusion, coma)	Hyponatremia, hypernatremia, hypercalcemia, acid-base imbalances
Cardiac and Respiratory Signs of Electrolyte or Acid-Base Imbalances	
Pulse rhythm and ECG: Irregular pulse and ECG changes	K^+, Ca^{2+}, Mg^{2+}, and/or acid-base imbalances
Rate and depth of respirations:	
Increased rate and depth	Metabolic acidosis (compensatory mechanism); respiratory alkalosis (cause)
Decreased rate and depth	Metabolic alkalosis (compensatory mechanism); respiratory acidosis (cause)
Neuromuscular Markers of Electrolyte or Acid-Base Imbalances	
Muscle strength bilaterally, especially quadriceps muscles:	
Muscle weakness	Hypokalemia, hyperkalemia
Reflexes and sensations:	
Decreased deep tendon reflexes	Hypercalcemia, hypermagnesemia
Hyperactive reflexes, muscle twitching and cramps, tetany	Hypocalcemia, hypomagnesemia
Numbness, tingling in fingertips, around mouth	Hypocalcemia, hypomagnesemia, respiratory alkalosis
Muscle cramps, tetany	Hypocalcemia, hypomagnesemia, respiratory alkalosis
Tremors	Hypomagnesemia
Gastrointestinal Signs of Electrolyte Imbalances	
Inspection and auscultation:	
Abdominal distention	Hypokalemia, third-spacing of fluid
Decreased bowel sounds	Hypokalemia
Motility: Constipation	Hypokalemia, hypercalcemia

ECG, Electrocardiogram; *ECV,* extracellular fluid volume.

FIG. 42.10 Containers for measuring urine output.

REFLECT NOW

How would your assessments related to fluid, electrolyte, and acid-base imbalances differ between patients with acute illness and patients with chronic illnesses?

◆ **Analysis and Nursing Diagnosis**

When caring for patients with suspected fluid, electrolyte, and acid-base imbalances, it is particularly important to use critical thinking to formulate nursing diagnoses. The assessment data that establish the risk for or the actual presence of a nursing diagnosis may be subtle, and patterns and trends emerge only when there has been astute assessment. Multiple body systems often are involved; careful clustering of assessment findings leads to selection of the appropriate diagnoses (Box 42.4).

In addition to the accurate clustering of assessment data, an important part of formulating nursing diagnoses is identifying the relevant causative or related factor (when a diagnosis is negative, or problem focused) or risk factors (when a diagnosis is a risk diagnosis). You choose interventions that treat or modify the specific related factor or risk for the diagnosis to be resolved. For example, *Dehydration related to loss of GI fluids from vomiting* requires therapies that manage the patient's emesis and restore fluid volume with IV therapy. In contrast, the diagnosis of *Fluid Imbalance related to elevated body temperature* requires therapies to lower the patient's body temperature and replace lost body fluids through oral fluid replacement or possibly IV therapy. Possible nursing diagnoses for patients with fluid, electrolyte, and acid-base alterations include the following:

- Fluid Imbalance
- Dehydration
- Electrolyte Imbalance
- Acid Base Imbalance
- Lack of Knowledge of Fluid Regimen

*Robert's assessments reveal that Mrs. Mendoza has had vomiting and diarrhea for the past 6 days, has lost weight, has dizziness and increased heart rate on standing, and has postural hypotension. Robert also notes that Mrs. Mendoza had three brown, watery stools this morning, as well as hypoactive bowel sounds with abdominal cramping. He also noted a 3 cm area of redness on the perineum with intact skin and decreased skin turgor. As Robert analyzes these assessment findings, the data clusters provide him cues that lead him to identify **Dehydration** as a priority nursing diagnosis for the plan of care. Along with this diagnosis, Ryan recognizes that Mrs. Mendoza is also experiencing **Nausea**, stating that she is currently "slightly nauseated," and **Diarrhea** because of the persistent brown, watery diarrhea, including more than 6 stools yesterday. Robert recognizes that Mrs. Mendoza has **Risk for Impaired Skin Integrity** because of the persistent diarrhea.*

BOX 42.4 Nursing Diagnostic Process

Dehydration Related to Loss of Gastrointestinal Fluids via Vomiting

Assessment Activities	Assessment Findings
Obtain postural blood pressure and pulse.	Patient has postural hypotension with increased heart rate; pulse is weak.
Inspect oral mucous membranes for degree of moisture.	Oral mucous membranes between cheek and gum are dry.
Obtain daily weight measurements.	Adult patient loses 1 kg (2.2 lb) or more in 24 hours.
Measure urine output and observe color; if possible, measure specific gravity of urine.	Patient produces small volume of dark yellow urine; urine specific gravity is increased.
Test skin turgor (not reliable for older adults).	Decreased skin turgor noted.

◆ **Planning and Outcomes Identification**

During the planning process, apply clinical judgment to synthesize information from multiple resources so that relevant outcomes and interventions are chosen (Fig. 42.11). Ensure that a patient's plan of care integrates both scientific and nursing knowledge and all of the information that you collected about the individual patient.

As a nurse, your personal and previous experience about fluid, electrolyte, and acid-base balance and imbalances will be your guide in the care of patients. Your experience with laboratory data and IV equipment (e.g., pumps, electronic infusion devices [EIDs], IV fluids) will assist in the management of patients with alterations in fluid, electrolyte, and acid-base status.

It is also important to recognize environmental factors that affect fluid, electrolyte, and acid-base balance issues such as when you can use AP in patient care. It is essential to identify the patient's needs and plan care around these needs.

Outcomes. Establish an individual patient plan of care for each nursing diagnosis (see the Nursing Care Plan) that includes mutually established expected outcomes for each diagnosis. Collaborate with and inform patients as you individualize realistic, measurable expected outcomes. For example, with a nursing diagnosis of *Dehydration,* the following outcomes are appropriate for a patient to achieve normal hydration status at discharge:

- The patient is free of complications associated with the IV device throughout the duration of IV therapy.
- The patient demonstrates balanced I&O measurements within 48 hours.

In the nursing care plan, Robert sets outcomes for improving Mrs. Mendoza's fluid status. The interventions chosen for delivering care will focus on one or more outcomes. After interventions are delivered, Robert will decide if the outcomes have been met (e.g., by monitoring the outcome of focused assessments and I&O). Each outcome needs a time frame for achievement.

Setting Priorities. The patient's clinical condition determines which of the nursing diagnoses takes the greatest priority. Many nursing diagnoses in the area of fluid, electrolyte, and acid-base alterations are of highest priority because the consequences for the patient can be serious or even life threatening. For example, in the concept map (Fig. 42.12) for Mrs. Mendoza, the occurrence of vomiting and diarrhea created a high-priority nursing diagnosis of *Dehydration.* The priority for Mrs. Mendoza is to restore her fluid balance. To achieve this priority, her vomiting and diarrhea must be controlled and resolved, and her fluid volume replaced. If these outcomes are unmet, Mrs. Mendoza's fluid imbalance is likely to worsen.

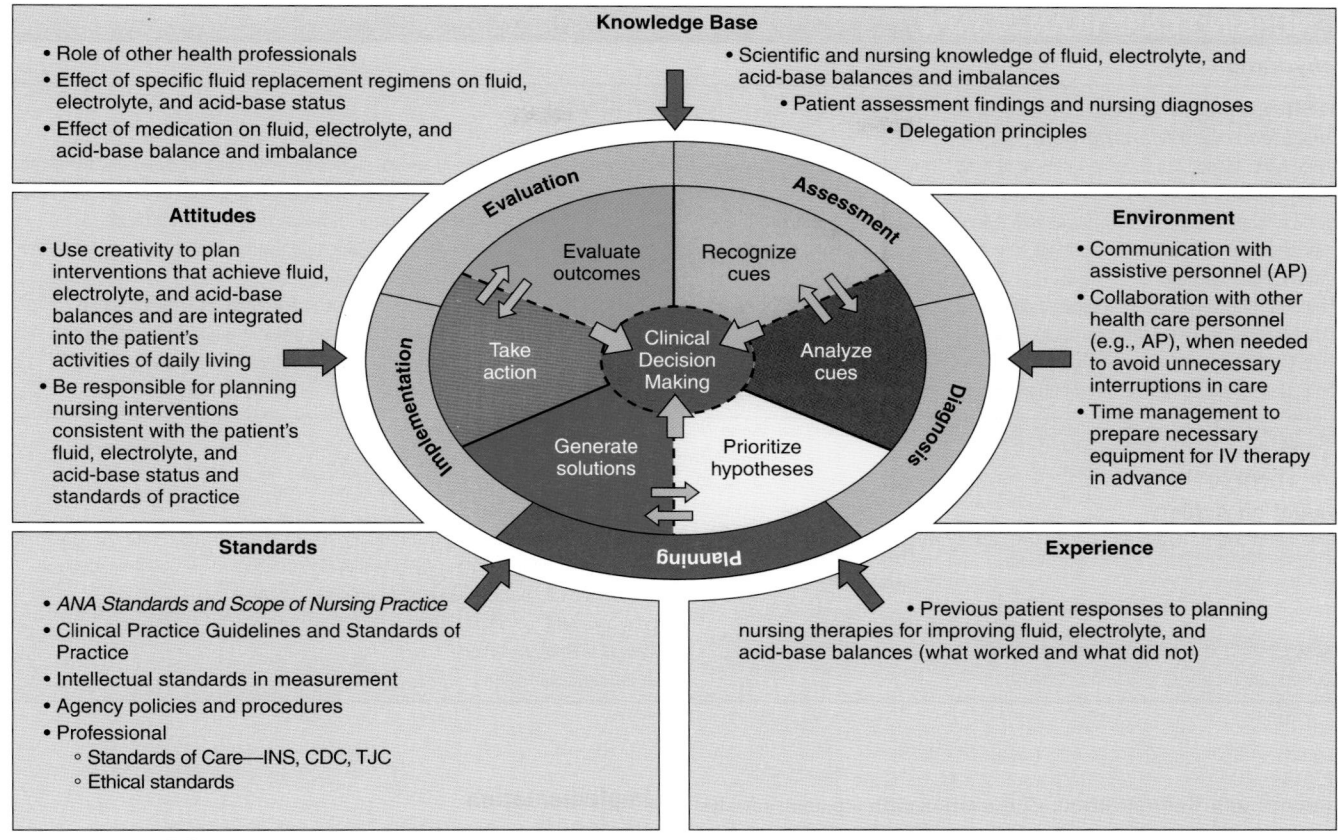

FIG. 42.11 Critical thinking model for fluid, electrolyte, and acid-base balance planning. *CDC,* Centers for Disease Control and Prevention; *INS,* Infusion Nurses Society; *TJC,* The Joint Commission. (Clinical Judgment Measurement Model copyright © NCSBN. All rights reserved.)

◎ NURSING CARE PLAN

Dehydration

ASSESSMENT

Assessment Activities

Ask Mrs. Mendoza to describe when her vomiting and diarrhea began and any accompanying signs and symptoms.

Ask her about current status of vomiting and diarrhea.

Assess Mrs. Mendoza's vital signs.

Evaluate physical signs of extracellular fluid volume (ECV).

Weigh Mrs. Mendoza using a bed scale.

Assessment Findings[a]

Gastrointestinal (GI) problems began suddenly yesterday. Reports **getting weak and light-headed when she stands or sits upright.**

Says she was vomiting earlier this morning but not in the past 3 hours. Had three episodes of watery diarrhea this morning and more than six yesterday.

Heart rate, 110 beats/min; regular, **weak pulse; supine blood pressure (BP) 90/58 mm Hg.** Temperature and respirations within normal limits. Postural BP measurement omitted for patient safety.

Neck veins flat when supine; 100 mL of dark yellow urine in past 4 hours; dry mucous membranes between cheek and gum; prolonged capillary refill time of 5 seconds.

Weight 54.5 kg (120 lb). States usual weight at home is 57.7 kg (127 lb) **(3.17-kg [7-lb] weight loss).**

[a] Assessment findings are shown in bold type.

NURSING DIAGNOSIS: Dehydration related to prolonged vomiting and diarrhea

PLANNING

Expected Outcomes (NOC)[b]

Fluid Balance

• Mrs. Mendoza will deny light-headedness when sitting or standing within 24 hours.
• Daily output of light yellow urine equals intake of at least 1500 mL by discharge.
• Vomiting and diarrhea are absent within 48 hours.

[b] Outcome classification labels from Moorhead S, et al: *Nursing Outcomes Classification (NOC),* ed 6, St Louis, 2018, Elsevier.

Continued

⊚ **NURSING CARE PLAN—cont'd**

Dehydration

INTERVENTIONS[c] (NIC)	RATIONALE
Fluid/Electrolyte Management	
Provide Mrs. Mendoza's favorite fluids at her preferred temperature.	Patient-centered care takes individual preferences into account; types and temperature of oral fluids can influence oral intake (Giger and Haddad, 2021; Rong et al., 2017).
Provide pitcher and glass of water at Mrs. Mendoza's preferred temperature at her bedside; ensure that she can access and pour from it easily; provide straw if she wishes.	Chronic disease such as osteoarthritis of hands may make it difficult to manipulate a full water pitcher. Make fluid available in form that is easy for patient to access (Felver, 2021c).
Administer intravenous (IV) therapy as prescribed, monitoring closely for early side effects of complications.	IV fluid replacement augments oral replacement when ECV deficit exists. Age-appropriate care is needed because of older adult's anatomical and physiological changes that affect volume delivery (Touhy and Jett, 2021).
Administer medications (antidiarrheal) as ordered for vomiting and diarrhea.	Management of cause of gastroenteritis necessary to reduce fluid loss.

[c] Intervention classification labels from Butcher HK, et al: *Nursing Interventions Classification (NIC)*, ed 7, St Louis, 2018, Elsevier.

EVALUATION

Evaluation Activity	*Patient Response*
Monitor vital signs, intake and output (I&O), daily weight, and postural BP.	Temperature, 37°C (98.6°F); respirations, 10 breaths/min; heart rate, 72 beats/min; BP, 120/78 mm Hg sitting, 122/78 mm Hg standing; denies light-headedness
	Intake 2000 mL, output 2000 mL of light yellow urine
	Today's weight: 58.5 kg (129 lb)
Assess intake and output and mucous membranes.	Mucous membranes moist.
Question patient about sensation of nausea.	Patient denies nausea.

Teamwork and Collaboration. Consultation with a patient's health care provider helps to set realistic time frames for the outcomes of care, particularly when a patient's physiological status is unstable. Ongoing communication and consultation are important because the patient's condition can change quickly. Collaboration with the patient and family and other members of the interprofessional health care team such as IV therapists and pharmacists helps in achieving patient outcomes. Patients and family members are very helpful in identifying approaches for successful therapies such as ways to increase fluid intake. Incorporate patient preferences and resources into the plan of care. Do not delegate administration of IV fluid and hemodynamic assessment to AP. When the patient is stable, you can delegate daily weights, I&O, and direct physical care to AP (Gorski et al., 2021).

Begin discharge planning early for patients with acute or chronic fluid and electrolyte disturbances by anticipating the needs of the patient and family as they transition to another setting. In the hospital, collaboration with other members of the health care team ensures that care will continue in the home or long-term care setting with few disruptions. You ensure that therapeutic regimens established in one setting continue through completion at the next setting. For example, for a patient who is discharged on IV therapy, you assess the knowledge and skills of the family member or friend who will assume caregiving responsibilities and initiate a referral to home IV therapy as soon as possible. Close collaboration with members of the health care team such as the patient's health care provider, registered dietitian, and pharmacist is essential to ensure positive patient outcomes. A registered dietitian is a valuable resource in recommending food sources to increase or reduce intake of specific electrolytes, incorporating the patient's preferences when possible (see Chapter 45). A pharmacist helps identify medications or combinations of medications likely to cause electrolyte or acid-base disturbances and offers information regarding patient education about side effects to anticipate for prescribed drugs. The patient's health care provider directs the treatment of fluid, electrolyte, or acid-base imbalances.

◆ **Implementation**

Health Promotion. Health promotion activities focus primarily on patient education, which you provide based on a patient's and family's health literacy. Use plain language to teach patients and caregivers to recognize risk factors for developing fluid and electrolyte imbalances and implement appropriate preventive measures. For example, parents of infants need to understand that GI losses quickly lead to serious imbalances; therefore when vomiting or diarrhea occurs in an infant, parents need to promptly rehydrate with sodium-containing fluid or seek health care to restore normal balance. People of any age need to learn to replace body fluid losses with sodium-containing fluid and water, especially during exercise or while spending time outside in hot weather.

Patients with chronic health alterations need to understand their own risk factors and the measures they need to take to avoid fluid and electrolyte imbalances. For example, patients with end-stage renal disease often need to restrict intake of fluid, sodium, potassium, magnesium, and phosphate (Berns, 2020; Norton et al., 2017). Through diet education these patients learn the types of foods to avoid and the suitable volume of fluid that they are permitted daily (see Chapter 45). Teach patients with chronic diseases and their family caregivers the early signs and symptoms of the fluid, electrolyte, and acid-base imbalances for which they are at risk and what to do if these occur.

REFLECT NOW

What should you teach an older adult who has frequent diarrhea about how to replace fluids to avoid dehydration?

Acute Care. Although fluid, electrolyte, and acid-base imbalances occur in all settings, they are common in acute care. Acute care nurses administer medications and oral and IV fluids to replace fluid and

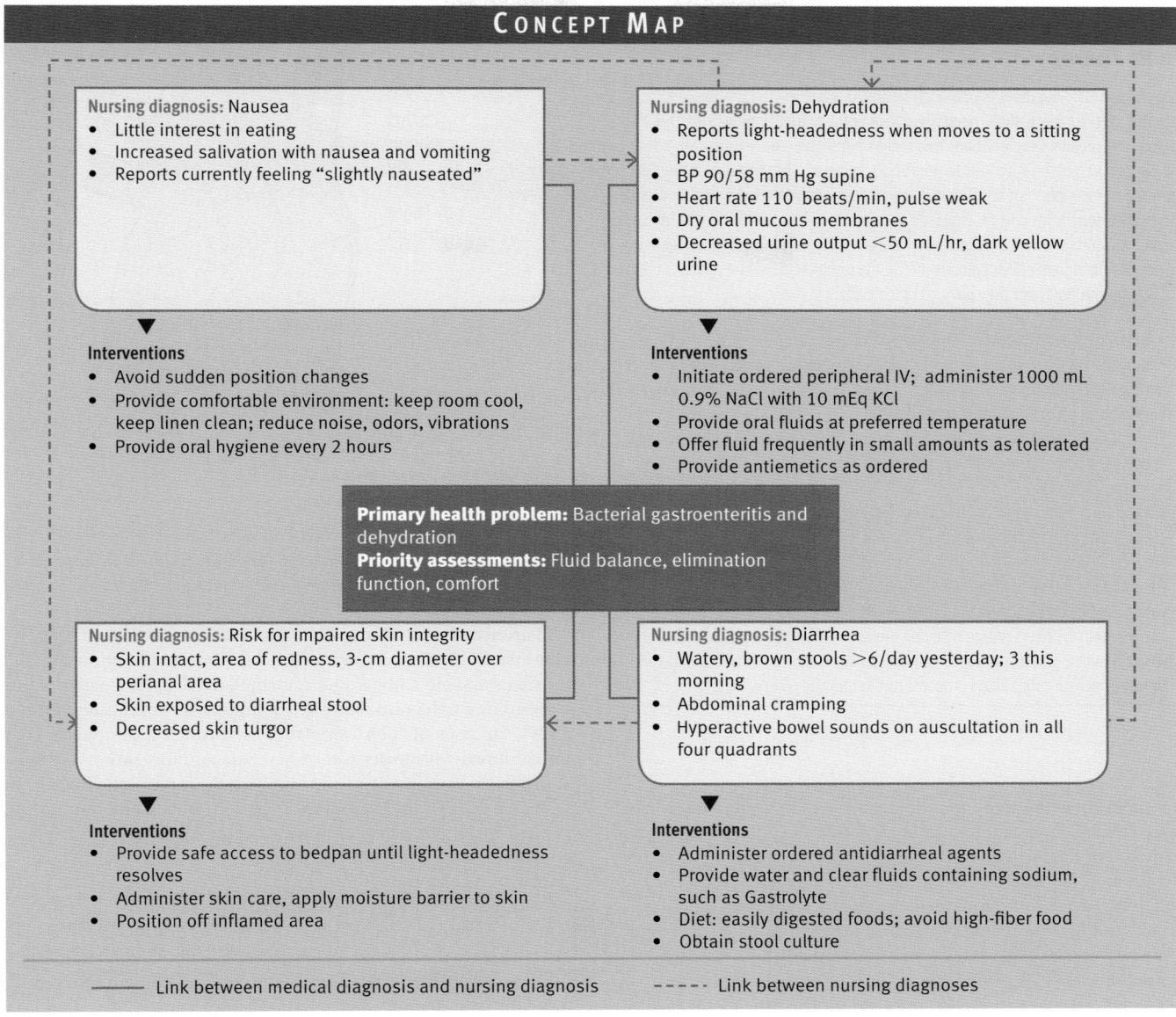

CONCEPT MAP

Nursing diagnosis: Nausea
- Little interest in eating
- Increased salivation with nausea and vomiting
- Reports currently feeling "slightly nauseated"

Interventions
- Avoid sudden position changes
- Provide comfortable environment: keep room cool, keep linen clean; reduce noise, odors, vibrations
- Provide oral hygiene every 2 hours

Nursing diagnosis: Dehydration
- Reports light-headedness when moves to a sitting position
- BP 90/58 mm Hg supine
- Heart rate 110 beats/min, pulse weak
- Dry oral mucous membranes
- Decreased urine output <50 mL/hr, dark yellow urine

Interventions
- Initiate ordered peripheral IV; administer 1000 mL 0.9% NaCl with 10 mEq KCl
- Provide oral fluids at preferred temperature
- Offer fluid frequently in small amounts as tolerated
- Provide antiemetics as ordered

Primary health problem: Bacterial gastroenteritis and dehydration
Priority assessments: Fluid balance, elimination function, comfort

Nursing diagnosis: Risk for impaired skin integrity
- Skin intact, area of redness, 3-cm diameter over perianal area
- Skin exposed to diarrheal stool
- Decreased skin turgor

Interventions
- Provide safe access to bedpan until light-headedness resolves
- Administer skin care, apply moisture barrier to skin
- Position off inflamed area

Nursing diagnosis: Diarrhea
- Watery, brown stools >6/day yesterday; 3 this morning
- Abdominal cramping
- Hyperactive bowel sounds on auscultation in all four quadrants

Interventions
- Administer ordered antidiarrheal agents
- Provide water and clear fluids containing sodium, such as Gastrolyte
- Diet: easily digested foods; avoid high-fiber food
- Obtain stool culture

—— Link between medical diagnosis and nursing diagnosis   - - - - Link between nursing diagnoses

FIG. 42.12 Concept map for Mrs. Mendoza. *BP,* Blood pressure; *IV,* intravenous infusion.

electrolyte deficits or maintain normal homeostasis; they also help with restricting intake as part of therapy for fluid excesses.

Enteral Replacement of Fluids. Oral replacement of fluids and electrolytes is appropriate as long as the patient is not so physiologically unstable that they cannot be replaced rapidly enough (Carson et al., 2017; Heuschkel and Duggan, 2019). Oral replacement of fluids is contraindicated when a patient has a mechanical obstruction of the GI tract, has severe nausea, is at high risk for aspiration, or has impaired swallowing. Some patients unable to tolerate solid foods are still able to ingest fluids. Strategies to encourage fluid intake include offering frequent small sips of fluid, popsicles, and ice chips. Record one-half the volume of the ice chips in I&O measurement. For example, if a patient ingests 240 mL of ice chips, you record 120 mL of intake. Encourage patients to keep their own record of intake to involve them actively. Family members who are properly instructed can also help. Pay attention to each patient's preferred temperature of oral fluids. Cultural beliefs regarding appropriate fluids and fluid temperature may become

a barrier to achieving adequate fluid intake unless the fluid with the preferred temperature is available (Box 42.5).

When replacing fluids by mouth in a patient with ECV deficit, choose fluids that contain sodium (e.g., Pedialyte and Gastrolyte). Liquids that contain lactose or have a low sodium content are inappropriate when a patient has diarrhea.

A feeding tube is appropriate when a patient's GI tract is healthy but oral fluids cannot be ingested (e.g., after oral surgery or with impaired swallowing). Options for administering fluids include gastrostomy or jejunostomy instillations or infusions through small-bore nasogastric feeding tubes (see Chapter 45).

Restriction of Fluids. Patients who have hyponatremia usually require restricted water intake. Patients who have very severe ECV excess sometimes have both sodium and fluid restrictions. Fluid restriction often is difficult for patients, particularly if they take medications that dry the oral mucous membranes or if they are mouth breathers. Explain the reason that fluids are restricted. Make sure that the patient, family,

⊕ BOX 42.5 CULTURAL ASPECTS OF CARE

Fluid Therapy

Cultural and religious beliefs influence how you manage fluid therapy and how patients communicate their needs. For example, a family elder may be the person who receives explanations and makes health care decisions, rather than the patient. A person may refuse therapies because of cultural and religious beliefs. For example, hot-cold beliefs cause some patients to refuse cold oral fluids when they have certain illnesses because they believe that hot fluids are needed to restore balance (Giger and Haddad, 2021). Religious practices may require modifications of intravenous (IV) tubing length (e.g., when patients need to kneel on the floor and pray several times daily).

Implications for Patient-Centered Care

- Establish communication; a professional interpreter may be necessary. If appropriate, determine who makes decisions for the patient and explain fluid restriction or IV therapy procedures.
- Elicit patient/family values and preferences in your clinical interview. Ask specifically about preferred temperature of oral fluids and provide (if oral intake is allowed).
- Determine needed length of IV tubing and incorporate one or more segments of long extension tubing into the IV setup if patient kneels on the floor to pray.
- Determine acceptance of or abstinence from therapeutic regimens and respect patient/family choices regarding therapy (Boucher et al., 2017).
- Know patient's beliefs regarding blood therapy. Although some patients refuse whole blood or packed red blood cells because of religious or personal beliefs, they may accept other blood products or alternatives (Tingle, 2017).

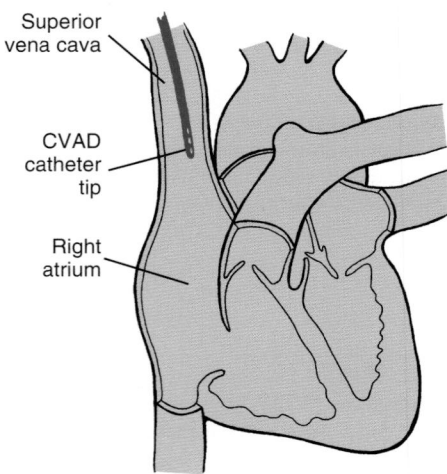

FIG. 42.13 Central venous lines deliver intravenous fluid into superior vena cava near heart. *CVAD,* Central venous access device.

her IV therapy. When Robert checks the policy and procedures at his agency for an IV therapy protocol, he applies professional standards in practice. He reviews the standards for initiating and maintaining IV sites to be familiar with the procedures.

Parenteral Nutrition. PN, also called *total PN (TPN),* is IV administration of a complex, highly concentrated solution containing nutrients and electrolytes that is formulated to meet a patient's needs. Depending on the osmolality, PN solutions are administered through a CVC in cases of high osmolality or through a peripheral IV line for solutions with lower osmolality. Safe administration depends on appropriate assessment of nutrition needs, meticulous management of the CVC or IV line to prevent infection, and careful monitoring to prevent metabolic complications. Chapter 45 reviews principles and guidelines for PN administration, which is used when patients are unable to receive enough nutrition orally or through enteral feeding.

Intravenous Therapy (Crystalloids). The goal of IV fluid administration is to correct or prevent fluid and electrolyte disturbances. It allows for direct access to the vascular system, permitting the continuous infusion of fluids over a period of time. IV therapy requires a health care provider's order for type, amount, and speed of administration of a solution. You regulate IV fluid therapy continuously because of ongoing changes in a patient's fluid and electrolyte balance and cardiovascular status. To provide safe and appropriate therapy to patients who require IV fluids, apply knowledge of the correct ordered solution, the reason the solution was ordered, the equipment needed, the procedures required to initiate an infusion, how to regulate the infusion rate and maintain the system, how to identify and correct problems, and how to discontinue the infusion.

Types of Solutions. Many prepared IV solutions are available for use (Table 42.11). An IV solution is isotonic, hypotonic, or hypertonic. Isotonic solutions have the same effective osmolality as body fluids. Sodium-containing isotonic solutions such as normal saline are indicated for ECV replacement to prevent or treat ECV deficit. Hypotonic solutions have an effective osmolality less than body fluids, thus decreasing osmolality by diluting body fluids and moving water into cells. Hypertonic solutions have an effective osmolality greater than body fluids. If they are hypertonic sodium-containing solutions, they increase osmolality rapidly and pull water out of cells, causing them to shrivel (Huether et al., 2020). The decision to use a hypotonic or hypertonic solution is made on the basis of a patient's specific fluid and electrolyte imbalance. For example, a patient with hypernatremia that cannot be treated with oral water generally receives a hypotonic IV solution to dilute the ECF and rehydrate cells.

and visitors know the amount of fluid permitted orally and understand that ice chips, gelatin, and ice cream are fluids. Help the patient decide the amount of fluid to drink with each meal, between meals, before bed, and with medications. It is important to allow patients to choose preferred fluids unless contraindicated. Frequently patients on fluid restriction can swallow a number of pills with as little as 1 oz (30 mL) of liquid.

In acute care settings fluid restrictions usually allot half the total oral fluids between 7 a.m. and 3 p.m. (i.e., the period when patients are more active, receive two meals, and take most of their oral medications). Offer the remainder of the fluids during the evening and night shifts. Patients on fluid restriction need frequent mouth care to moisten mucous membranes, decrease the chance of mucosal drying and cracking, and maintain comfort (see Chapter 40).

Parenteral Replacement of Fluids and Electrolytes. Fluids and electrolytes may be replaced through infusion of fluids directly into veins (intravenously) rather than via the digestive system. Parenteral replacement includes parenteral nutrition (PN), IV fluid and electrolyte therapy (crystalloids), and blood and blood component (colloids) administration. IV devices are called *peripheral IVs* when the catheter tip lies in a vein in one of the extremities; they are called *central venous catheters (CVCs) or IVs* when the catheter tip lies in the central circulatory system (e.g., in the vena cava close to the right atrium of the heart) (Fig. 42.13).

Practice standard body fluid precautions and infection control when preparing and administering parenteral fluids (see Chapter 28) to minimize your own risk for exposure to bloodborne pathogens. Read and understand the policy and procedures for parenteral infusions at the agency for which you work.

Robert knows that Mrs. Mendoza will require careful monitoring of I&O and stabilization of GI function, including management and monitoring of

TABLE 42.11 Intravenous Solutions

Solution	Concentration in IV Container and at Tip of VAD	Effective Concentration in Body	Comments
Dextrose (Glucose) in Water Solutions			
Dextrose 5% in water (D_5W)	Isotonic	Hypotonic	Isotonic when first enters vein; dextrose enters cells rapidly, leaving free water, which dilutes ECF; most of the water then enters cells by osmosis.
Dextrose 10% in water ($D_{10}W$)	Hypertonic	Hypotonic	Hypertonic when first enters vein; dextrose enters cells rapidly, leaving free water, which dilutes ECF; most of the water then enters cells by osmosis.
Saline (Sodium Chloride [NaCl] in Water) Solutions			
0.225% NaCl (¼ NS)	Hypotonic	Hypotonic	Expands ECV (vascular and interstitial) and rehydrates cells.
0.45% NaCl (½ NS)	Hypotonic	Hypotonic	Expands ECV (vascular and interstitial) and rehydrates cells.
0.9% NaCl (NS)	Isotonic	Isotonic	Expands ECV (vascular and interstitial); does not enter cells.
3% or 5% NaCl (hypertonic saline; 3% or 5% NaCl)	Hypertonic	Hypertonic	Draws water from cells into ECF by osmosis.
Dextrose in Saline Solutions			
Dextrose 5% in 0.45% NaCl (½ NS; $D_5$0.45% NaCl)	Hypertonic	Hypotonic	Dextrose enters cells rapidly, leaving 0.45% NaCl.
Dextrose 5% in 0.9% NaCl (D_5NS; $D_5$0.9% NaCl)	Hypertonic	Isotonic	Dextrose enters cells rapidly, leaving 0.9% NaCl.
Multiple Electrolyte Solutions			
Lactated Ringer (LR) solution	Isotonic	Isotonic	LR contains Na^+, K^+, Ca^{2+}, Cl^-, and lactate, which liver metabolizes to HCO_3^-; expands ECV (vascular and interstitial); does not enter cells.
Dextrose 5% in LR (D_5LR)	Hypertonic	Isotonic	Dextrose enters cells rapidly, leaving LR.

ECF, Extracellular fluid; *ECV,* extracellular fluid volume; *IV,* intravenous; *NS,* normal saline; *VAD,* vascular access device.

Too-rapid or excessive infusion of any IV fluid has the potential to cause serious patient problems.

Additives such as potassium chloride (KCl) are common in IV solutions (e.g., 1000 mL D_5 ½NS with 20 mEq KCl at 125 mL/hr). Administer KCl carefully because hyperkalemia can cause fatal cardiac dysrhythmias. **Under no circumstances should KCl be administered by IV push (directly through a port in IV tubing).** Verify that a patient has adequate kidney function and urine output before administering an IV solution containing potassium. Patients with normal renal function who are receiving nothing by mouth should have potassium added to IV solutions. The body cannot conserve potassium, and the kidneys continue to excrete it even when the plasma level falls. Without potassium intake, hypokalemia develops quickly.

Vascular Access Devices. Vascular access devices (VADs) are catheters or infusion ports designed for repeated access to the vascular system. Peripheral catheters are for short-term use (e.g., fluid restoration after surgery and short-term antibiotic administration). Devices for long-term use include central catheters and implanted ports, which empty into a central vein. Remember that the term *central* applies to the location of the catheter tip, not to the insertion site. Peripherally inserted central catheter (PICC) lines enter a peripheral arm vein and extend through the venous system to the superior vena cava, where they end. Other central lines enter a central vein such as the subclavian or jugular vein or are tunneled through subcutaneous tissue before entering a central vein. Central lines are more effective than peripheral catheters for administering large volumes of fluid,

PN, and medications or fluids that irritate veins. Proper care of central line insertion sites is critical for the prevention of central line–associated bloodstream infection (CLABSI) (Box 42.6) (Centers for Disease Control and Prevention [CDC], 2020; Gorski et al., 2021; Wei et al., 2019). Nurses and health care providers must have specialized education regarding care of CVCs and implanted infusion ports (The Joint Commission [TJC], 2021b). Nursing responsibilities for central lines include careful monitoring, flushing to keep the line patent, and site care and dressing changes to prevent CLABSIs (Gorski et al., 2021; Layne and Anderson, 2019).

Equipment. Correct selection and preparation of IV equipment helps in safe and rapid placement of an IV line. Because fluids infuse directly into the bloodstream, aseptic technique is necessary. Organize all equipment at the bedside for an efficient insertion. IV equipment includes VADs; tourniquet; clean gloves; dressings; IV fluid containers; various types of tubing; and EIDs, also called *electronic infusion pumps*. VADs that are short peripheral IV catheters are available in a variety of gauges, such as the commonly used 20 and 22 gauges. A larger gauge indicates a smaller-diameter catheter. A peripheral VAD is called an over-the-needle catheter; it consists of a small plastic tube or catheter threaded over a sharp stylet (needle). Once you insert a stylet and advance the catheter into the vein, you withdraw the stylet, leaving the catheter in place. These devices have a safety mechanism that covers the sharp stylet when withdrawing it to reduce the risk of needlestick injury (Fig. 42.14). Needleless systems allow you to make connections without using needles, which reduces needlestick injuries.

Preventing Central Line–Associated Bloodstream Infection (CLABSI)

PICOT Question: In patients who are hospitalized, do bundled interventions compared with routine central line site care alone prevent central line–associated bloodstream infection (CLABSI)?

Evidence Summary

CLABSI is a serious complication of intravenous (IV) therapy that increases morbidity, hospital length of stay, and health care costs. Research shows that effective strategies for prevention of CLABSI include the use of several evidence-based practices combined as a multicomponent "bundle" (Biasucci et al., 2018; Layne and Anderson, 2019). Such bundles have been found to be effective in reducing CLABSIs at the time of insertion of central lines and also during their maintenance (Biasucci et al., 2018; Layne and Anderson, 2019). The Infusion Nursing Society standards of practice (Gorski et al., 2021) and The Joint Commission (TJC, 2021b) specify a central line bundle: hand hygiene; maximum sterile barrier precautions; chlorhexidine skin antisepsis using chlorhexidine (>0.5%) in alcohol; avoidance of the femoral vein for central venous access for adults; and placement under planned controlled conditions. Effective reduction of CLABSIs requires ongoing staff education to promote consistent adherence to bundle components and attention to institutional support and culture in addition to the use of bundled central line insertion and maintenance practices (Hawes and Lee, 2018; TJC, 2021b).

Application to Nursing Practice

• Verify and use all of the components of the CLABSI prevention bundle (Biasucci et al., 2018; Hawes and Lee, 2018).

• Work with a practice or infection control committee to perform an audit of adherence to CLABSI prevention practices in your unit (Gorski et al., 2021; TJC, 2021b).

• If your agency does not have a multidisciplinary CLABSI prevention program, collaborate with infection control personnel and medical and nursing administration to establish one that includes institutional support for education, competency demonstration, use of insertion and maintenance bundles, and daily line audits with feedback to nurses (TJC, 2021b).

• Clinical factors that may reduce CLABSI include catheter choice, catheter site selection, insertion technique, and proper catheter maintenance (Layne and Anderson, 2019).

The main IV fluid used in a continuous infusion flows through tubing called the *primary line*. The primary line connects to the IV catheter. Injectable medications such as antibiotics are usually added to a small IV solution bag and "piggybacked" as a secondary set into the primary line or as a primary intermittent infusion to be administered over a 30- to 60-minute period (Thoele et al., 2018). The type and amount of solution are prescribed by the patient's health care provider and depend on the medication added and the patient's physiological status. If an IV infusion is connected to an EID, use the tubing designated for that EID. For gravity-flow IVs (not using an EID), select tubing as described in the equipment list of Skill 42.1. Add IV extension tubing to increase the length of the primary line, which reduces pulling of the tubing and increases a patient's mobility when changing positions.

Inserting the Intravenous Line. The Infusion Nurses Society (INS) now recommends the use of standard Aseptic Non-Touch Technique (ANTT®) for the insertion and maintenance of VADs. ANTT® is a combination of standard precautions and an approach of protecting any VAD site and any part of the procedure equipment that, if contaminated, is likely to contaminate the patient (e.g., during insertion of syringe tip or needle or spiking of infusion set) (Gorski et al., 2021). Standard ANTT® involves Standard Precautions, use of appropriate personal protective equipment (PPE), management of the sterile field during insertion, use of a non-touch technique, and use of sterilized supplies. If it becomes necessary to directly touch the VAD site or equipment parts, then sterile gloves must be used (Gorski et al., 2021). To achieve standard ANTT®, use appropriate skin antisepsis and maintain asepsis during VAD dwell time by the use and management of sterile dressings and appropriate securement devices (Gorski et al., 2021).

After you collect the equipment at the patient's bedside, prepare to insert the IV line by assessing the patient for a venipuncture site (see Skill 42.1). The most common IV sites are on the inner arm (Fig. 42.15). Do not use hand veins on older adults or patients who are ambulatory. IV insertion in a foot vein is common with children, but avoid these sites in adults because of the increased risk of thrombophlebitis (Gorski, 2018; Gorski et al., 2021). Consider using vascular visualization technology (e.g., near-infrared, ultrasound) if available to increase success for patients with difficult IV access (Gorski et al., 2021).

As you assess a patient for potential venipuncture sites, consider conditions that exclude certain sites. Venipuncture is contraindicated in a site that has signs of infection, infiltration, or thrombosis. An infected site is red, tender, swollen, and possibly warm to the touch.

FIG. 42.14 Over-the-needle catheter for venipuncture.

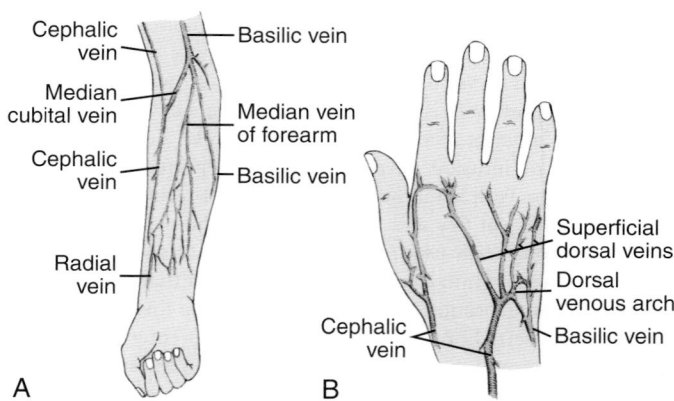

FIG. 42.15 Cephalic, basilic, and median cubital veins are best for intravenous placement in adults.

Exudate may be present. Do not use an infected site because of the danger of introducing bacteria from the skin surface into the bloodstream. Avoid using an extremity with a vascular (dialysis) graft/fistula or on the same side as a mastectomy. Do not use visible veins of the chest, breast, abdomen, or other locations on the trunk of the body as there is no evidence supporting their safe outcomes (Gorski et al., 2021). Avoid areas of flexion if possible and veins that are compromised (Gorski et al., 2021).

Venipuncture is a technique in which a vein is punctured through the skin by a sharp rigid stylet (e.g., metal stylet). The stylet is partially covered either with a plastic catheter or a needle attached to a syringe. General purposes of venipuncture are to collect a blood specimen, start an IV infusion, provide vascular access for later use, instill a medication, or inject a radiopaque or other tracer for special diagnostic examinations. Skill 42.1 describes venipuncture for peripheral IV fluid infusion, incorporating INS standards of practice (Gorski et al., 2021). It takes practice to become proficient in venipuncture. Gorski et al. (2021) recommends that after a nurse makes two unsuccessful attempts at venipuncture, the clinician should escalate the insertion with a higher skill level and/or consider alternate routes of administration. Only experienced practitioners should perform it for patients whose veins are fragile or easily collapse, such as older adults. Box 42.7 describes principles to follow for venipuncture in older adults.

Nurses require specialized knowledge and education to place PICCs. Some central lines and implanted ports require insertion by physicians or advanced practice nurses. Both types of central catheters require close monitoring and maintenance. This chapter focuses on peripheral catheters.

BOX 42.7 FOCUS ON OLDER ADULTS

Protection of Skin and Veins During Intravenous Therapy

- Use the smallest-gauge catheter or needle possible (e.g., 22–24 gauge). Veins are very fragile, and a smaller gauge allows better blood flow to provide increased hemodilution of the intravenous (IV) fluids or medications (Gorski et al., 2021).
- Avoid the back of the hand, which may compromise a patient's need for independence and mobility.
- Avoid placement of an IV line in veins that are easily bumped because older adults have less subcutaneous support tissue (Touhy and Jett, 2021).
- Avoid vigorous friction while cleaning a site, to prevent tearing fragile skin.
- If a patient has fragile skin and veins, use minimal or no tourniquet pressure (Gorski et al., 2021).
- If using a tourniquet, place it over the patient's sleeve or use a blood pressure cuff.
- With loss of supportive tissue, veins tend to lie more superficially; lower the insertion angle for venipuncture to 10 to 15 degrees after penetrating the skin.
- Veins roll away from the needle easily because of loss of subcutaneous tissue. To stabilize a vein, apply traction to the skin below the projected insertion site.
- Secure IV site with a catheter stabilization device, avoiding excessive use of tape on fragile skin; consider covering the site additionally with surgical stretch mesh.
- Numerous medications and supplements (e.g., anticoagulants, antibiotics, glucocorticoids, and garlic) increase the likelihood of bruising and bleeding (Burchum and Rosenthal, 2019).

Regulating the Infusion Flow Rate. After initiating a peripheral IV infusion and checking it for patency, regulate the rate of infusion according to the health care provider's orders (see Skill 42.2). For patient safety avoid the uncontrolled flow of IV fluid into a patient. You are responsible for calculating the flow rate (mL/hr) that delivers the IV fluid in the prescribed time frame. The correct IV infusion rate ensures patient safety by preventing too-slow or too-rapid administration of IV fluids. An infusion rate that is too slow often leads to further physiological compromise in a patient who is dehydrated, in circulatory shock, or critically ill. An infusion rate that is too rapid overloads the patient with IV fluid, causing fluid and electrolyte imbalances and cardiac complications in vulnerable patients (e.g., older adults or patients with preexisting heart disease).

EIDs, also called IV pumps or infusion pumps, deliver an accurate hourly IV infusion rate. An EID uses positive pressure to maintain correct flow rates and catheter patency to deliver a measured amount of fluid over a prescribed period of time (e.g., 100 mL/hr). Infusion pumps are needed for patients who require low hourly rates, are at risk for volume overload, have impaired renal function, or are receiving solutions or medications that require a specific hourly volume. EIDs use an electronic sensor and an alarm that signals if pressure in the system changes and the desired flow rate changes. Many EIDs have operating and programming capabilities that allow for infusions of single or multiple solutions at different rates. Familiarize yourself with the brand of EID in use at your agency so that you are able to set the flow rate accurately. Electronic detectors and alarms respond to air in IV lines, occlusion, completion of infusion, high and low pressure, and low battery power.

When you open a roller clamp or other type of clamp on an infusion tubing that is not yet properly inserted in an EID or on a gravity-flow IV system, the IV fluid infuses very rapidly. When variation in flow rate is not critical (such as a keep-vein-open infusion), consider using a manual flow regulator in lieu of the roller clamp to allow for easier regulation and more consistent flow (Gorski et al., 2021). To avoid rapid infusions, nonelectronic volume-control devices are used occasionally with an IV solution infused by gravity to prevent accidental infusion of a large fluid volume. These devices are more commonly used with children. The volume-controlled flow regulator uses gravity to deliver only a limited amount of solution and is placed between the IV container and the insertion spike and drip chamber of an administration set. Mechanical infusion devices (e.g., elastomeric devices, piston-driven pumps) regulate infusion rates with no outside power source.

Patency of an IV catheter means that IV fluid flows easily through it. For patency there must be no clots at the tip of the catheter, and the catheter tip must not be against the vein wall. An occluded catheter slows or stops the rate of infusion of the IV fluids. A catheter may become occluded for the following reasons: bent catheter, positional catheter (catheter resting against catheter wall), kink or knot in infusion tubing, external pressure on tubing, clot formation, or precipitate formation from administration of incompatible medications or solutions (Gorski, 2018). IV flow rate also can also be slowed by infiltration and vasospasm. If the flow decreases or stops and the EID is working correctly, inspect the tubing. Sometimes the patient is lying or sitting on it. The tubing may be kinked or caught in or under equipment. Also inspect the area around the insertion site for anything that obstructs the flow of IV fluids. For gravity flow, the height of the container influences flow rate. Raising the container usually increases the rate because of increased driving pressure.

Joint stabilization devices promote infusion of the IV fluid and maintain function of the VAD; however, their use should be avoided if possible so as to not restrict movement of the body part (Gorski et al., 2021).

Flexion of an extremity, particularly at the hand and wrist or elbow, can decrease IV flow rate by compressing the vein. When joint stabilization becomes necessary, the INS standards specify use of a hand or arm joint stabilization device to protect the IV site by keeping the joint extended (Gorski et al., 2021). The device should be applied in a manner that permits visual inspection and assessment of the VAD site and vascular pathway and does not exert pressure that will cause circulatory constriction, pressure injury, or nerve damage in the area of flexion or under the device (Gorski et al., 2021). Use padding with arm boards because they may cause skin or nerve damage from pressure. Starting an infusion in a new location rather than relying on a site that causes problems may be more comfortable for a patient. Before discontinuing the current infusion, choose another site and start the infusion to verify that the patient has other accessible veins.

Maintaining the System. After placing an IV line and regulating the flow rate, maintain the IV system. Line maintenance involves (1) using standard ANTT® to keep the system sterile and intact; (2) using standard ANTT® to change IV fluid containers, tubing, and contaminated site dressings; (3) helping a patient with self-care activities so as not to disrupt the system; and (4) monitoring for complications of IV therapy. The frequency and options for maintaining the system are identified in agency policies.

An important component of patient care is maintaining the integrity of an IV line to prevent infection. Potential sites for contamination of a VAD are shown in Fig. 42.16. Inserting an IV line under appropriate aseptic technique reduces the chances of contamination from a patient's skin. After insertion, prevent infection by the conscientious use of infection control principles such as thorough hand hygiene before and after handling any part of the IV system and maintaining sterility of the system during tubing and fluid container changes.

Always maintain the integrity of an IV system. Never disconnect tubing because it becomes tangled or it might seem more convenient for positioning or moving a patient or applying a gown. If a patient needs more room to maneuver, use aseptic technique to add extension tubing to an IV line. However, keep the use of extension tubing to a minimum because each connection of tubing provides opportunity for contamination. *Never let IV tubing touch the floor. Do not use stopcocks* for connecting more than one solution to a single IV site because they are sources of contamination (Hadaway, 2018; Gorski et al., 2021). IV tubing contains needleless injection ports through which syringes or

other adaptors can be inserted for medication administration. Clean an injection port thoroughly with alcohol-based 2% chlorhexidine (preferred), 70% alcohol, or povidone-iodine solution and let it dry before accessing the system (Gorski et al., 2021; Jacob and Gaynes, 2021).

Gorski et al. (2021) recommends a securement device in addition to the primary dressing to stabilize and secure VADs. There are two types of devices for short peripheral VADs: (1) an adhesive securement device (ASD), which is an adhesive-backed device that adheres to the skin with a mechanism to hold the VAD in place (Fig. 42.17) (both the dressing and ASD must be removed and replaced at specific intervals during the VAD dwell time), and (2) an integrated securement device (ISD), which is a device that combines a dressing with securement functions (transparent, semipermeable dressing and a bordered fabric collar with built-in securement technology). If you choose to use an ASD, carefully monitor a patient for development of a medical device–related pressure injury (MDRPI). These devices are designed to prevent movement or accidental dislodgment of a VAD. Avoid the use of nonsterile tape as an option (Gorski et al., 2021). Use of securement devices is a patient safety issue. Movement of the VAD in a vein can cause phlebitis and infiltration; VAD dislodgment requires using another VAD at a new IV infusion site.

Changing Intravenous Fluid Containers, Tubing, and Dressings. Patients receiving IV therapy over several days require periodic changes of IV fluid containers (Skill 42.3). It is important to organize tasks so that you can change containers rapidly before a thrombus forms in a catheter.

The changing of IV tubing requires the use of standard ANTT® practices. The frequency of a change is based on a patient's condition and the type, rate, and frequency of solution administered, as well as immediately upon suspected line contamination or insertion of a new VAD (Gorski et al., 2021). Replace primary and secondary *continuous* administration sets used for crystalloid solutions and medications *no more frequently* than every 96 hours but at least every 7 days (unless otherwise stated in manufacturers' directions (Gorski et al., 2021).

In contrast, change tubing for *intermittent* infusions every 24 hours because of the increased risk of contamination from opening the IV system (Gorski et al., 2021). Blood, blood components, and lipids are likely to promote bacterial growth in tubing. INS standards (Gorski et al., 2021) specify tubing changes every 4 hours for blood and blood components and every 24 hours for continuous IV lipids. For lipids

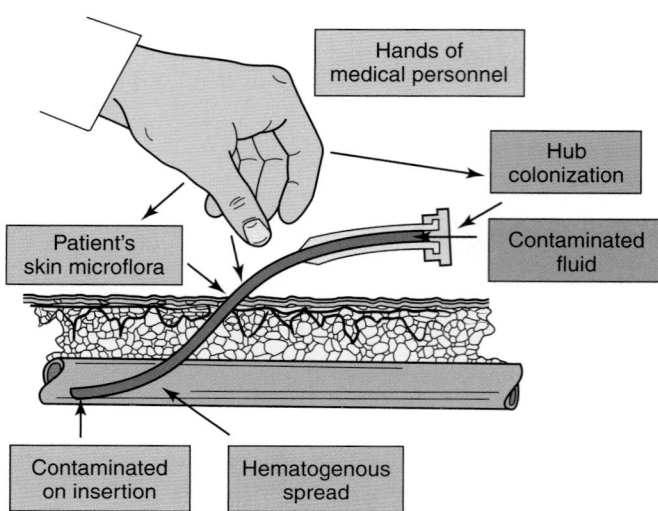

FIG. 42.16 Potential sites for contamination of vascular access device.

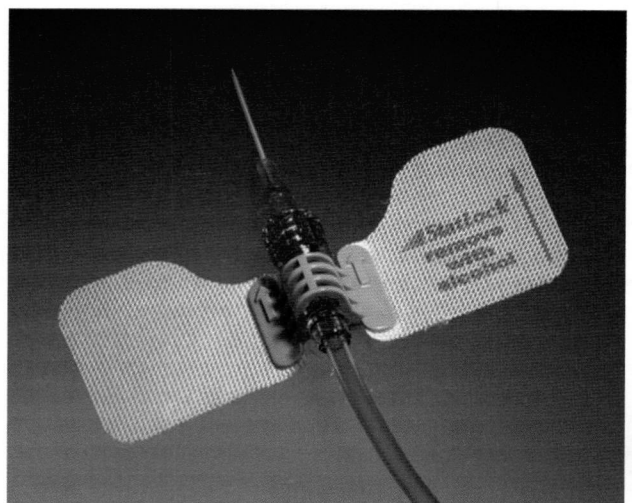

FIG. 42.17 Catheter stabilization device. (Copyright © C.R. Bard, Inc. Used with permission.)

use tubing that is free of diethylhexyl phthalate (DEHP), a toxin that leaches into lipid solutions (Gorski et al., 2021). Whenever possible, schedule tubing changes when it is time to hang a new IV container to decrease risk of infection. To prevent entry of bacteria into the bloodstream, maintain sterility using standard ANTT® practices during tubing and IV fluid container changes.

A sterile dressing over an IV site reduces the entrance of bacteria into the insertion site. Transparent dressings, the most common type, help secure the VAD, allow continuous visual inspection of the IV site, and are less easily soiled or moistened than gauze dressings. Change transparent semipermeable membrane (TSM) dressings at least every 7 days (except neonatal patients) or immediately if dressing integrity is disrupted (e.g., lifted/detached on any border edge or within transparent portion of dressing, visibly soiled, presence of moisture, drainage, or blood) or if skin integrity is compromised under the dressing (Gorski et al., 2021). If a gauze dressing is used, change the dressing every 48 hours at the time of an inspection or if dressing integrity is disrupted (e.g., if damp, loosened, or visibly soiled) (Gorski et al., 2021) (see Skill 42.4).

A complication directly related to an IV site dressing is a medical adhesive–related skin injury (MARSI). Such injuries can occur from any adhesive (e.g., tape, device adhesive) that results in mechanical injury (skin stripping, blistering, skin tears), dermatitis (irritation in response to the adhesive), and other complications (maceration and folliculitis) (Fumarola et al., 2020). Use of skin barriers during application of any adhesive device and the use of sterile adhesive removers are recommended for the prevention of MARSI (Fumarola et al., 2020).

Helping Patients to Protect Intravenous Integrity. To prevent the accidental disruption of an IV system, a patient often needs help with hygiene, comfort measures, meals, and ambulation. Changing gowns is difficult for a patient with an IV in the arm. Teach AP and patients that they must not break the integrity of an IV line to change a gown because it leads to contamination. It helps to use a gown with snaps along the top sleeve seam to facilitate changing the gown without disturbing the venipuncture site. Change regular gowns by following these steps for maximum speed and arm mobility (see also Skill 40.1 in Chapter 40 for photos):

1. *To remove a gown,* remove the sleeve of the gown from the arm without the IV line, maintaining the patient's privacy.
2. Remove the sleeve of the gown from the arm with the IV line.
3. Remove the IV solution container from its stand and pass it and the tubing through the sleeve. (If this involves removing the tubing from an EID, use the roller clamp to slow the infusion to prevent the accidental infusion of a large volume of solution or medication.)
4. *To apply a gown,* place the IV solution container and tubing through the sleeve of the clean gown and hang it on its stand. (If the IV line is controlled by an EID, reassemble, turn on the pump, and open the roller clamp.)
5. Place the arm with the IV line through the gown sleeve.
6. Place the arm without the IV line through the other gown sleeve.

A patient with an arm or a hand infusion is able to walk unless contraindicated. Offer a rolling IV pole on wheels. Help the patient get out of bed and place the IV pole next to the involved arm. Teach the patient to hold the pole with the involved hand and push it while walking. Check that the IV container is at the proper height, there is no tension on the tubing, and the flow rate is correct. Infusion pumps connect to IV poles and can be used during ambulation because they will function on battery power during the time the patient walks. Instruct the patient to report any blood in the tubing, a stoppage in the flow, or increased discomfort. Once patient returns to a bed or chair, plug in the infusion pump.

Complications of Intravenous Therapy. Carefully assess and monitor your patient's response to IV therapy (Table 42.12). A severe complication

is circulatory overload, which occurs when a patient receives too-rapid administration or an excessive amount of fluids. Assessment findings depend on the type of IV solution that infuses in excess. The signs and symptoms of circulatory overload and other complications often arise rapidly, which highlights the importance of frequent assessment of patients receiving IV therapy.

The other most common complications of IV therapy involve phlebitis and infiltration. Prevention of these complications requires frequent assessment of the peripheral VAD site to see if replacement of a VAD is clinically indicated. Gorski et al. (2021) standards recommend the following:

1. Assess a VAD site, an entire infusion system, and a patient for signs of complications at a frequency dependent on patient factors, such as age, clinical condition, and cognition; type/frequency of infusion solution; and health care setting.
2. Palpate and inspect the VAD site, including catheter pathway in vein, for integrity of skin, dressing, and securement device.
3. In acute care and nursing facilities, assess the VAD site at least daily.
4. In outpatient or home care settings, assess the VAD site at every visit. Teach the patient or caregiver to check the VAD site with each infusion or at least daily or, for continuous PICC infusions, every 4 hours during waking hours.

QSEN **Building Competency in Safety** A patient who has a peripheral intravenous (IV) infusion wants to wear a special shirt rather than a hospital gown when family members come to celebrate a birthday later today. How can you assist the patient while maintaining patient safety in this situation?

Answers to QSEN Activities can be found on the Evolve website.

Infiltration occurs when an IV catheter becomes dislodged or a vein ruptures and IV fluids inadvertently enter subcutaneous tissue around the venipuncture site (Helm, 2019). When the IV fluid contains additives that damage tissue, **extravasation** occurs (Helm, 2019; Matsui et al., 2017). Infiltration and extravasation cause coolness, paleness, and swelling of the area. When infiltration occurs, immediately assess for any additives in the infiltrated fluid to determine the type of action necessary to prevent local tissue damage and sloughing. Vasoconstrictors, high-dose potassium, and other IV additives in subcutaneous tissue need different treatments from those needed for an infiltrated additive-free IV (see Table 42.12). Although the INS does not include an infiltration scale for adults in its 2021 standards, the society does recommend using a standardized scale for documentation (Gorski et al., 2021).

Phlebitis (i.e., inflammation of a vein) results from chemical, transient mechanical, infectious, or postinfusion causes (Helm, 2019; Gorski et al., 2021). Risk factors for phlebitis include acidic or hypertonic IV solutions; rapid IV rate; IV drugs such as KCl, vancomycin, and penicillin; VAD inserted in area of flexion; poorly secured catheter; poor hand hygiene; and lack of aseptic technique. The typical signs of inflammation (i.e., heat, erythema [redness], tenderness) occur along the course of a vein. Table 42.13 offers a widely used scale for assessing severity of phlebitis; however, further study is recommended for a valid and reliable assessment tool (Gorski et al., 2021). When a patient has dark skin, these signs may be less obvious; assess carefully for subtle color changes at the VAD site that might indicate phlebitis.

Phlebitis is dangerous because the inflammation of the vein wall can lead to associated blood clots (thrombophlebitis). Clots form along the vein and in some cases cause emboli, which can break off and enter the circulation. This may permanently damage veins. Frequent changes of peripheral IV catheters to reduce infection are not recommended (Gorski et al., 2021).

TABLE 42.12   Complications of Intravenous Therapy With Nursing Interventions

Complication	Description	Assessment Findings	Nursing Interventions
Circulatory overload of IV solution	IV solution infused too rapidly or in too great an amount	Depends on type of solution ECV excess with Na$^+$-containing isotonic fluid (crackles in dependent parts of lungs, shortness of breath, dependent edema) Hyponatremia with hypotonic fluid (confusion, seizures) Hypernatremia with Na$^+$-containing hypertonic fluid (confusion, seizures) Hyperkalemia from K$^+$-containing fluid (cardiac dysrhythmias, muscle weakness, abdominal distention)	If symptoms appear, reduce IV flow rate and notify patient's health care provider. With ECV excess, raise head of bed; administer oxygen and diuretics if ordered. Monitor vital signs and laboratory reports of serum levels. Health care provider may adjust additives in IV solution or type of IV fluid; watch for and implement order.
Infiltration and extravasation	IV fluid entering subcutaneous tissue around venipuncture site Extravasation: technical term used when a vesicant (tissue-damaging) drug (e.g., chemotherapy) enters tissues	Skin around catheter site taut, blanched, cool to touch, edematous; may be painful as infiltration or extravasation increases; infusion may slow or stop	Use standard scale for assessing and documenting infiltration (Gorski et al., 2021). Stop infusion. Discontinue IV infusion if no vesicant drug (see Skill 42.3). If vesicant drug, disconnect IV tubing and aspirate drug from catheter. Agency policy and procedures may require delivery of antidote through catheter before removal. Elevate affected extremity. Avoid applying pressure over site; can force solution into contact with more tissue. Contact health care provider if solution contained KCl, a vasoconstrictor, or other potential vesicant. Apply warm, moist, or cold compress according to procedure for type of solution infiltrated. Start new IV line in other extremity.
Phlebitis	Inflammation of inner layer of a vein	Redness, tenderness, pain, warmth along course of vein starting at access site; possible red streak and/or palpable cord along vein	Use standard scale for assessing and documenting phlebitis (Gorski et al., 2021). Stop infusion and discontinue IV line (see Skill 42.3). Start new IV line in other extremity or proximal to previous insertion site if continued IV therapy is necessary. Apply warm, moist compress or contact IV therapy team or health care provider if area needs additional treatment. Elevate affected extremity. Document phlebitis using a standardized scale, including nursing interventions per agency policy and procedure.
Local infection	Infection at catheter-skin entry point during infusion or after removal of IV catheter	Redness, heat, swelling at catheter-skin entry point; possible purulent drainage	Culture any drainage (if ordered). Clean skin with alcohol; remove catheter and save for culture; apply sterile dressing. Notify health care provider. Start new IV line in other extremity. Initiate appropriate wound care (see Chapter 48) if needed.
Air embolism	Air in the vein from unpurged syringe or tubing	Sudden onset of dyspnea, coughing, chest pain, hypotension, tachycardia, decreased level of consciousness, possible signs of stroke	Prevent further air from entering the system by clamping or covering the leak. Place patient on left side, preferably with head of bed raised, to trap air in the lower portion of the left ventricle. Call emergency support team and notify patient's health care provider.
Bleeding at venipuncture site	Oozing or slow, continuous seepage of blood from venipuncture site	Fresh blood evident at venipuncture site, sometimes pooling under extremity	Assess whether IV system is intact. If catheter is within vein, apply pressure dressing over site or change dressing. Start new IV line in other extremity or proximal to previous insertion site if VAD is dislodged, IV is disconnected, or bleeding from site does not stop.

ECV, Extracellular volume; *IV,* intravenous; *VAD,* vascular access device.

TABLE 42.13 Phlebitis Scale

Grade	Clinical Criteria
0	No symptoms
1	Erythema at access site with or without pain
2	Pain at access site with erythema and/or edema
3	Pain at access site with erythema; streak formation; palpable venous cord
4	Pain at access site with erythema; streak formation; palpable venous cord >2.54 cm (1 inch) in length; purulent drainage

Visual Infusion Phlebitis Scale

Score	Observation
0	IV site appears healthy
1	One of the following signs is evident: • Slight pain near IV site *or* slight redness near IV site
2	Two of the following signs are evident: • Pain at IV site • Erythema • Swelling
3	All of the following signs are evident: • Pain along the path of cannula • Induration
4	All of the following signs are evident and extensive: • Pain along the path of cannula • Erythema • Induration • Palpable venous cord
5	All of the following signs are evident and extensive: • Pain along the path of cannula • Erythema • Induration • Palpable venous cord • Pyrexia

From Gorski LA, et al. *Infusion therapy standards of practice,* ed 8, *J Infus Nurs* 44(Suppl 1):S1, 2021.

In the absence of phlebitis, local infection at the venipuncture site is usually caused by poor aseptic technique during catheter insertion, daily monitoring, or catheter removal. Early recognition of local infection and treatment is important to prevent bacteria from entering the bloodstream (see Table 42.12). Bloodstream infections may arise from short peripheral IV catheter sites.

Air embolism occurs when air is present inside syringes, IV tubing is not primed with fluid, or connectors are not removed before use and cause air to enter a patient's vein. It also can occur if the VAD is not clamped before changing the tubing or if the IV tubing is punctured inadvertently (Gorski et al., 2021; Mattox, 2017).

Bleeding can occur around the venipuncture site during the infusion or through the catheter or tubing if these become disconnected inadvertently (see Table 42.12). Bleeding is more common in patients who receive heparin or other anticoagulants or who have a bleeding disorder (e.g., hemophilia or thrombocytopenia).

Discontinuing Peripheral Intravenous Access. Discontinue IV access after infusion of the prescribed amount of fluid; when infiltration, phlebitis, or local infection occurs; or if the IV infusion slows or stops, indicating the catheter has developed a thrombus at its tip. Skill 42.3 presents the steps for discontinuing peripheral IV access. Help patients and families understand that moving from IV infusion to oral fluid intake is a sign of progress toward recovery.

Blood Transfusion. Blood transfusion, or blood component therapy, is the IV administration of whole blood or a blood component such as packed red blood cells (RBCs), platelets, or plasma. Objectives for administering blood transfusions include (1) increasing circulating blood volume after surgery, trauma, or hemorrhage; (2) increasing the number of RBCs and maintaining hemoglobin levels in patients with severe anemia; and (3) providing selected cellular components as replacement therapy (e.g., clotting factors, platelets, albumin).

Caring for patients receiving blood or blood-product transfusion is a nursing responsibility. You must be thorough in patient assessment, checking the blood product against prescriber's orders, checking it against patient identifiers, and monitoring for any adverse reactions. Blood transfusions are never regarded as routine; overlooking any minor detail can have dangerous and life-threatening events for a patient (American Association of Blood Banks [AABB], 2020a; AABB, 2020b).

Blood Groups and Types. Blood transfusions must be matched to each patient to avoid incompatibility. RBCs have antigens in their membranes; the plasma contains antibodies against specific RBC antigens. If incompatible blood is transfused (i.e., a patient's RBC antigens differ from those transfused), the patient's antibodies trigger RBC destruction in a potentially dangerous transfusion reaction (i.e., an immune response to the transfused blood components).

The most important grouping for transfusion purposes is the ABO system, which identifies A, B, O, and AB blood types. Determination of blood type is made on the basis of the presence or absence of A and B RBC antigens. Individuals with type A blood have A antigens on their RBCs and anti-B antibodies in their plasma. Individuals with type B blood have B antigens on their RBCs and anti-A antibodies in their plasma. A person who has type AB blood has both A and B antigens on the RBCs and no antibodies against either antigen in the plasma. A type O individual has neither A nor B antigens on RBCs but has both anti-A and anti-B antibodies in the plasma (Gorski, 2018). Table 42.14 shows the compatibilities between blood types of donors and recipients. People with type O-negative blood are considered *universal blood donors* because they can donate packed RBCs and platelets to people with any ABO blood type. People with type AB-positive blood are called *universal blood recipients* because they can receive packed RBCs and platelets of any ABO type.

Another consideration when matching blood components for transfusions is the Rh factor, which refers to another antigen in RBC membranes. Most people have this antigen and are Rh positive; a person without it is Rh negative. People who are Rh negative receive only Rh-negative blood components.

Autologous Transfusion. Autologous transfusion (autotransfusion) is the collection and reinfusion of a patient's own blood. Blood for an autologous transfusion most commonly is obtained by preoperative donation up to 6 weeks before a scheduled operation (e.g., heart, orthopedic, plastic, or gynecological). A patient can donate several units of blood, depending on the type of surgery and the patient's ability to maintain an acceptable hematocrit. Blood for autologous transfusion is also obtained at the time of surgery or through blood salvage (e.g., during surgery for liver transplantation, trauma, or vascular and orthopedic conditions). After surgery blood is salvaged from the drainage from chest tubes or joint cavities. Autologous transfusions are safer for patients because they decrease the risk of mismatched blood and exposure to bloodborne infectious agents (AABB, 2020a; Gorski, 2018).

Transfusing Blood. Transfusion of blood or blood components is a nursing procedure that requires an order from a health care provider. Patient safety is a nursing priority, and patient assessment, verification of

TABLE 42.14 ABO Compatibilities for Transfusion Therapy

Component	Compatibilities	
Whole blood	Give type-specific blood only	
Packed red cells (stored, washed, or frozen/washed)	Donor	Recipient
	0	0, A, B, AB
	A	A, AB
	B	B, AB
	AB	AB
Fresh-frozen plasma	Donor	Recipient
	0	0
	A	A, 0
	B	B, 0
	AB	AB, B, A, 0
Platelets	RBC: ABO and Rh compatible *preferred*	
	Donor	Recipient
	0	0, A, B, AB
	A	A, AB
	B	B, AB
	AB	AB

ABO, Blood group consisting of groups A, AB, B, and O.

FIG. 42.18 Filling tubing for blood administration.

the health care provider's order, and verification of correct blood products for the correct patient are imperative (AABB, 2020a; AABB, 2020b).

Perform a thorough patient assessment before initiating a transfusion and monitor carefully during and after the transfusion. Assessment is critical because of the risk of transfusion reactions. Pretransfusion assessment includes establishing whether a patient knows the reason for the blood transfusion and whether the patient has ever had a previous transfusion or transfusion reaction. A patient who has had a transfusion reaction is usually at no greater risk for a reaction with a subsequent transfusion but may be anxious about the transfusion, requiring nursing intervention. Before beginning a transfusion, explain the procedure and instruct the patient (if alert) to report any side effects (e.g., chills, dizziness, or fever) once the transfusion begins. Have a professional translator available if the patient does not speak English. Ensure that the patient has signed an informed consent form. Patients with certain cultural or religious backgrounds may refuse blood transfusions (see Box 42.5).

Because of the danger of transfusion reactions and fluid volume overload, your baseline pretransfusion assessment always includes the patient's vital signs, lung assessment, identification of conditions that may increase the risk of transfusion-related adverse reactions (e.g., current fever, heart failure, renal disease, and the patient's risk of fluid volume excess [FVE]), the presence of an appropriate and patent VAD, and current laboratory values (Gorski et al., 2021). The measurement of physiological data allows you to identify when vital sign changes occur as a result of a transfusion reaction.

Always follow agency policy and procedures before initiating any blood therapy. For patient safety always verify three things: (1) that blood components delivered are the ones that were ordered, (2) that blood delivered to a patient is compatible with the blood type listed in the medical record, and (3) that the right patient receives the blood. Together two RNs or one RN and an LPN (check agency policy and procedures) must check the label on the blood product against the medical record and the patient's identification number,

blood group, and complete name. If even a minor discrepancy exists, do not give the blood; notify the blood bank immediately to prevent infusion errors.

When administering a transfusion, you need an appropriate-size IV catheter and blood administration tubing that has a special in-line filter (Fig. 42.18). Adults require a large catheter (e.g., 20 to 24 gauge based on vein size and patient preference), or use a large-size catheter gauge when rapid transfusion is required (e.g., 18 to 20 gauge) because blood is more viscous than crystalloid IV fluids (Gorski et al., 2021). CVADs can be used for blood transfusion. Children with small veins need a smaller catheter; thus use the umbilical vein (neonates) or a vein large enough for a 22- to 24-gauge catheter (Gorski et al., 2021). Prime the tubing with 0.9% sodium chloride (normal saline) to prevent hemolysis or breakdown of RBCs.

The transfusion rate usually is specified in the health care provider's orders. Ideally a unit of whole blood or packed RBCs is transfused in 2 hours. This time can be lengthened to 4 hours if the patient is at risk for ECV excess. Beyond 4 hours there is a risk for bacterial contamination of the blood.

Initiate a nonemergent transfusion slowly to allow for the early detection of a transfusion reaction. Remain near the patient; major reactions usually appear before the first 50 mL have been transfused (Gorski et al., 2021). Increase the infusion rate after 15 minutes when there are no signs of a reaction and to ensure the completion of the unit within 4 hours (Gorski et al., 2021). Always have a second IV infusion bag containing 0.9% sodium chloride on standby in case it becomes necessary to stop the blood infusion. Maintain the ordered blood infusion rate, monitor for side effects, assess vital signs, and promptly record all findings per agency policy. If a transfusion reaction is anticipated or suspected, obtain vital signs more frequently (Table 42.15). Monitor patients for transfusion reactions for at least 4 to 6 hours to detect febrile or pulmonary reactions associated with the transfusion (Gorski et al., 2021).

TABLE 42.15   Transfusion Reactions

Reaction	Etiology	Onset	Signs and Symptoms	Prevention	Nursing Intervention
Acute Immediate (<24 Hours)					
Febrile, nonhemolytic	Most common type of transfusion reaction; caused by WBC antigen-antibody reaction	May begin early in transfusion or as long as several hours after completion	Temperature increase of >1°C (2°F) or more above baseline, chills, headache, vomiting	Premedicate as ordered with antipyretics if prior history of reaction. Use leukocyte-reduced blood products.	**Stop the transfusion.** Change administration set and administer 0.9% sodium chloride at rate to maintain patent IV access. Institute transfusion reaction protocol. Administer antipyretics as ordered to treat fever. Document clinical symptoms, when transfusion was stopped, notification of health care provider and blood bank, nursing interventions and response to interventions, and patient teaching.
Acute hemolytic transfusion reaction (AHTR)	Transfusion of ABO incompatible red cells in blood; usually caused by misidentification or improper labeling	Within minutes of transfusion initiation	Fever with or without chills; tachycardia; hypotension; abdominal, chest, back, and flank pain; dyspnea; red or dark urine; shock	Use extreme care during the entire patient identification process; proper labeling of blood sample; meticulous verification of ABO/Rh compatibility between donor and recipient before administration; start transfusion slowly and monitor carefully for the first 15 minutes.	**Stop the transfusion.** Get help immediately. Change administration set and administer 0.9% sodium chloride at rate to maintain patent IV access. Notify health care provider and blood bank. Treat shock. Maintain blood pressure and renal perfusion. Insert Foley catheter. Monitor intake and output hourly. Dialysis may be required. Obtain blood and urine samples and send to laboratory with unused part of unit of blood. Document reaction according to agency policy.
Allergic reaction (mild to moderate)	Caused by recipient sensitivity to allergens in the blood components	Within minutes of transfusion initiation	Urticaria, pruritus, facial flushing, mild wheezing	May administer antihistamines 30 minutes before transfusion if prescribed.	**Stop the transfusion.** Change administration set and administer 0.9% sodium chloride at rate to maintain patent IV access. Notify health care provider and blood bank. Administer antihistamines as ordered. Monitor and document vital signs every 15 min. Transfusion may be restarted if fever, dyspnea, and wheezing are not present.
Severe allergic reaction (anaphylaxis)	Caused by recipient allergy to a donor antigen (usually IgA) Agglutination of RBCs obstructing capillaries and blocking blood flow, causing symptoms to all major organ systems	Within minutes of transfusion initiation	Hypotension, tachycardia, urticaria, bronchospasm, anxiety, shock, nausea, vomiting, diarrhea, abdominal pain	Use autologous blood or blood from donors that are IgA deficient. Transfusion of saline-washed or leukocyte-depleted RBCs.	**Stop the transfusion.** Change administration set and administer 0.9% sodium chloride at rate to maintain patent IV access. Notify health care provider and blood bank. Administer antihistamines, corticosteroids, epinephrine, and antipyretics as ordered. Monitor and document vital signs until stable. Initiate cardiopulmonary resuscitation if necessary.
Transfusion-related acute lung injury (TRALI)	Presence of WBC antibodies from donor who has a WBC-activating agent in blood. Leading cause of transfusion-related death.	During or within 6 hours of transfusion	Fever, respiratory failure, hypoxemia, hypotension, pulmonary edema	Currently there is no method to identify patients at risk.	**Stop the transfusion.** Provide respiratory support, administer oxygen; frequently mechanical ventilation is required; administer vasopressor agents.

Continued

TABLE 42.15 Transfusion Reactions—cont'd

Reaction	Etiology	Onset	Signs and Symptoms	Prevention	Nursing Intervention
Transfusion-associated circulatory overload (TACO)	Related to volume overload. Patients older than 70 years and infants are at highest risk	Usually occurs during or within 6 hours of transfusion	Dyspnea, orthopnea, cyanosis, tachycardia, jugular vein distention (JVD), hypertension, cough	Frequent patient monitoring is required for those at high risk, including slowing infusion rate.	**Stop the transfusion.** Place patient in high-Fowler position, notify health care provider, and administer oxygen and diuretics.
Delayed Transfusion Reactions					
Transfusion-associated graft-versus-host disease (TA-GVHD)	Usually rare, but fatal. Donor lymphocytes destroyed by recipient's immune system. In immunocompromised patients the donor lymphocytes are identified as foreign; however, patient's immune system is not capable of destroying, and in turn patient's lymphocytes are destroyed	8–10 days after transfusion	Maculopapular rash, watery diarrhea, fever, jaundice caused by liver dysfunction, bone marrow suppression (pancytopenia)	Administration of irradiated blood and leukocyte-depleted RBC products as prescribed.	No effective therapy. Treatment of symptoms.
Iron overload	Iron from donated blood binds to protein and is not eliminated	Usually occurs when multiple units (>100 units of PRBCs) are transfused	Cardiac dysfunction, organ failure, arrhythmias, heart failure symptoms, increased serum transferrin, increased liver enzymes, jaundice	Iron chelation, phlebotomy, monitoring of serum iron levels.	No effective therapy. Iron chelation therapy. Monitor patient for heart failure, cardiac disorder, liver disorder, serum transferrin.
Infection-Related Complications					
Bacterial contamination	Microorganism contamination of infused product during donation or in preparing component for infusion. Highest risk when administering platelets	Occurs at time of donation. Symptoms may appear during transfusion or within 4 hours of completion	High fever, severe chills, hypotension, flushed skin, shock, hemoglobinuria, renal failure, DIC	Use good skin antisepsis prior to venipuncture. Inspect blood unit carefully and do not administer if clots, bubbles, bag leaks, or discoloration of unit noted.	**Stop the transfusion.** Treat shock, and administer ordered steroids and antibiotics. Culture patient's blood, blood component, and all intravenous solutions.

Data adapted from American Association of Blood Banks (AABB): *Technical manual of the American Association of Blood Banks,* ed 19, Bethesda, MD, 2020, American Association of Blood Banks; and Gorski L: *Phillip's manual of IV therapeutics: evidence-based practice for infusion therapy,* ed 7, Philadelphia, 2018, FA Davis.

DIC, Disseminated intravascular coagulation; *IgA,* immunoglobulin A; *IV,* intravenous; *PRBCs,* packed red blood cells; *RBC,* red blood cell; *WBC,* white blood cell.

When patients have a severe blood loss such as with hemorrhage, they often receive rapid transfusions through a CVC. A blood-warming device often is necessary because the tip of the CVC lies in the superior vena cava, above the right atrium. Rapid administration of cold blood can cause cardiac dysrhythmias. Patients who receive large-volume transfusion of citrated blood have a high risk of hyperkalemia, hypocalcemia, hypomagnesemia, and metabolic alkalosis; therefore they need careful monitoring (Lim et al., 2017; Teruya, 2021).

Transfusion Reactions. A transfusion reaction is an adverse event that occurs from transfusion of a blood product (DeLisle, 2018). Many transfusion reactions involve immune system reaction to the transfusion that ranges from a mild response to severe anaphylactic shock or acute intravascular hemolysis, both of which can be fatal. Table 42.15 presents the causes, manifestations, management, and prevention of the most common acute transfusion reactions. Prompt intervention when a transfusion reaction occurs maintains or restores a patient's physiological stability. When you suspect acute intravascular hemolysis, do the following (DeLisle, 2018):

- **Stop the transfusion immediately.**
- Keep the IV line open by replacing the IV tubing down to the catheter hub with new tubing and running 0.9% sodium chloride (normal saline) at a slow rate.
- *Do not* turn off the blood and simply turn on the 0.9% sodium chloride (normal saline) that is connected to the Y-tubing infusion set. This would cause blood remaining in the IV tubing to infuse into the patient. Even a small amount of additional blood can make the situation worse. **You must change out all the IV tubing.**
- Immediately notify the health care provider or emergency response team.
- Remain with the patient, observing signs and symptoms and monitoring vital signs as often as every 5 minutes.
- Prepare to administer emergency drugs such as antihistamines, vasopressors, fluids, and corticosteroids per health care provider order or protocol.
- Prepare to perform cardiopulmonary resuscitation.
- Save the blood container, tubing, attached labels, and transfusion record for return to the blood bank.
- Obtain blood and urine specimens per health care provider order or protocol.

Acute transfusion reactions that do not involve an immune response to the blood components also can occur (see Table 42.15). Transfusion-associated circulatory overload (TACO) is a risk when a patient receives massive whole blood or packed RBC transfusions for massive hemorrhagic shock or when a patient with normal blood volume receives blood. Patients particularly at risk for circulatory overload are older adults and those with cardiopulmonary diseases. Transfusion of blood components that are contaminated with bacteria, especially gram-negative bacteria, can cause sepsis.

Blood from infected donors who are asymptomatic can transmit diseases. Symptoms of these conditions may arise long after a transfusion. Diseases transmitted through transfusions include hepatitis B and C, human immunodeficiency virus (HIV) infection and acquired immunodeficiency syndrome (AIDS), Chagas disease, and cytomegalovirus infection. In the United States all units of blood for blood banks undergo screening for HIV, hepatitis B and C viruses, syphilis, and West Nile and Zika virus, which reduces the risk of acquiring these bloodborne infections (CDC, 2020).

Interventions for Electrolyte Imbalances. In addition to the administration of prescribed medical therapies, nursing interventions preserve or restore electrolyte imbalance (Felver, 2021c). For example, people who have hypokalemia or hypercalcemia often need bowel management for constipation. Patient safety interventions to prevent falls are vital for patients who become lethargic from hypercalcemia and those with muscle weakness. Patients who have hypercalcemia need an increased fluid intake to prevent renal damage; nurses can help them meet the oral fluid intake goals. Teach patients the reasons for their therapies and the importance of balancing electrolyte I&O to prevent imbalances in the future.

Interventions for Acid-Base Imbalances. Nursing interventions to promote acid-base balance support prescribed medical therapies and aim at reversing the existing acid-base imbalance while providing for patient safety (Felver, 2021b). When these imbalances are life threatening, they require rapid treatment. Maintain a functional IV line and check the health care provider's orders frequently for new medications or fluids. Give fluid and electrolyte replacement and prescribed drugs such as insulin promptly. In addition, monitor patients closely for changes in their status. Use protective measures such as placing patients in the side-lying position and implementing fall prevention protocols for patients with decreased level of consciousness. Support compensatory hyperventilation for patients with metabolic acidosis by keeping their oral mucous membranes moist and positioning them to facilitate chest expansion. Chapter 41 reviews appropriate therapies for patients with respiratory acidosis. Patients with acid-base imbalances often require repeated ABG analysis.

Arterial Blood Gases. Determination of a patient's acid-base status requires obtaining a sample of arterial blood for laboratory testing. ABG analysis reveals acid-base status and the adequacy of ventilation and oxygenation. A qualified RN or other health care provider draws arterial blood from a peripheral artery (usually the radial) or from an existing arterial line (see agency policy and procedures). Before an arterial blood draw, perform an Allen test, which assesses arterial circulation in the hand (Pagana et al., 2021). When performing the Allen test, apply pressure to both the ulnar and radial arteries in the selected hand. The fingers to the hand should be pale and blanched, indicating a lack of arterial blood flow. Release the pressure on the ulnar artery and observe for color to return to the fingers and hand, which indicates that there is adequate collateral circulation to the hand and fingers via the ulnar artery. The Allen test ensures that a patient will have adequate blood flow to the hand if the radial artery is damaged. If color does not return, do not perform radial artery puncture on that arm. After the ABG puncture, apply pressure to the puncture site for at least 5 minutes to reduce the risk of hematoma formation. A longer time is necessary if the patient takes anticoagulant medications. Reassess the radial pulse after removing the pressure. After obtaining the specimen, take care to prevent air from entering the syringe because this alters the blood gas values. To reduce oxygen usage by blood cells, submerge the syringe in crushed ice and transport it immediately to the laboratory.

Restorative Care. After experiencing acute alterations in fluid, electrolyte, or acid-base balance, patients often require ongoing maintenance to prevent a recurrence of health alterations. Older adults require special considerations to prevent complications from developing (see Box 42.2).

Home Intravenous Therapy. IV therapy often continues in the home setting for patients requiring long-term hydration, PN, or long-term medication administration. Initiate patient referral for discharge planning to social services, counselors, or a home care coordinator for assessment of patient and community resources. A home IV therapy nurse works closely with a patient to ensure that a sterile IV system is maintained and that complications can be avoided or recognized promptly. Box 42.8 summarizes patient education guidelines for home IV therapy.

Nutritional Support. Most patients who have had electrolyte disorders or metabolic acid-base imbalances require ongoing nutritional support. Depending on the type of disorder, fluid or food intake may be encouraged or restricted (see Chapter 45). Patients or family members who are responsible for meal preparation need to learn to understand nutritional content of foods and read the labels of commercially prepared foods. Patients who are more seriously ill may receive total parenteral nutrition in the home. This again requires involvement of home IV therapy. The European Society for Clinical Nutrition and Metabolism (ESPEN) offers guidelines on home parenteral nutrition (Pironi et al., 2020).

Medication Safety. Numerous medications, OTC drugs, and herbal preparations contain components or create potential side effects that can alter fluid and electrolyte balance. Patients with chronic

---

BOX 42.8   PATIENT TEACHING

Home Intravenous Therapy

Objective

- The patient and/or family caregiver will demonstrate competence with administering intravenous (IV) therapy safely in the home.

Teaching Strategies

- Explain the importance of IV therapy in maintaining hydration and access for the delivery of medications.
- Emphasize the risks involved when the IV system is not kept sterile.
- Be sure that the patient and/or family caregiver is able to manipulate the required equipment.
- Instruct in aseptic technique and hand hygiene in the handling of all IV equipment.
- Teach how to change IV solutions, tubing, and dressing when they become soiled or dislodged (Gorski et al., 2021). (**NOTE:** As the home care nurse, you may be able to visit frequently enough to perform scheduled tubing changes.)
- Teach procedures for safe disposal in appropriate containers of all sharps and IV materials exposed to blood. Check with the patient's local trash removal services or health department to see which disposal methods are available in the community (U.S. Food and Drug Administration, 2021). Options include:
  - Drop box or supervised collection sites: Located at appropriate collection sites such as doctors' offices, hospitals, pharmacies, health departments, medical waste facilities, and police or fire stations. Services may be free or have a nominal fee.
  - Household hazardous waste collection sites: Located at local public household hazardous waste collection sites. These are sites that also commonly accept hazardous materials such as household cleaners, paints, and motor oil.

- Mail-back programs: You may be able to mail certain FDA-cleared sharps disposal containers to a collection site for proper disposal, usually for a fee.
- Keep sharps containers away from children (see Chapter 28).
- Instruct to apply pressure with sterile gauze if catheter falls out and, if patient is on anticoagulants, to tape pieces of sterile gauze in place for at least 20 minutes with pressure or until bleeding stops.
- Instruct about signs and symptoms of infiltration, phlebitis, and infection; their significance; and the need to report symptoms immediately.
- Instruct patient and/or family caregiver to report if the infusion slows or stops or if blood is seen in the tubing.
- Teach patient with family caregiver's assistance how to ambulate, perform hygiene, and participate in other activities of daily living without dislodging or disconnecting catheter and tubing:
  - For showering, protect the IV site and dressing from getting wet by covering it completely with plastic. If using an electronic infusion device, unplug around water.
  - Wear clothes that avoid pressure on the IV site, and avoid trauma to the site when changing clothes.
  - Have patient avoid strenuous exercise of the arm with the IV line.

Evaluation

Use the principles of teach-back to evaluate patient/family caregiver learning:

- I want to be sure I explained how to care for your IV correctly. Please tell and/or show me how you will start and stop your infusion, and change the IV container, tubing, and dressing.
- Describe what you would do if your IV infusion stops flowing.
- What would you see if the skin around your IV site becomes red and swollen? What might that mean? What would you do next?

---

disease who are receiving multiple medications and those with renal disorders are at significant risk for imbalances. Once patients return to restorative care settings, whether in the home, long-term care, or other setting, drug safety is very important. Patient and family education regarding potential side effects and drug interactions that can alter fluid, electrolyte, or acid-base balance is essential. Review all medications with patients and encourage them to consult with their local pharmacist, especially if they wish to try a new OTC drug or herbal preparation (Chapter 32).

◆ Evaluation

Through the Patient's Eyes. Review with patients and family caregivers (as appropriate) how well their major concerns and expectations regarding fluid, electrolyte, or acid-base management were alleviated or addressed. For example, for a person admitted with dehydration who was concerned about falling because of light-headedness, say, "Tell me if you feel we took the precautions necessary to reduce your risk of falling." If the patient's concern was feeling uncomfortable with a very dry mouth, ask, "How does your mouth feel now? Do you feel we made you comfortable?" If the patient had a concern about better understanding a chronic health problem, focus evaluation on the patient's knowledge and ability to apply knowledge to home care needs. A patient's perspectives regarding care often depend in part on involvement of family and friends. If patients have concerns about returning home or to a different

care setting, it is important to evaluate how well prepared they feel for the transition from acute care. When the patient receives home care, ask family caregivers if they feel comfortable and competent to perform home IV therapy; when evaluating outcomes, have them demonstrate their skills.

Patient Outcomes. Clinical judgment during evaluation involves application of critical thinking as you consider knowledge of the patient's condition and then compare assessment findings with outcome measures. This comparison will reveal the effectiveness of interventions for the patient's nursing diagnoses. For example, a patient with the nursing diagnosis of *Electrolyte Imbalance* with hypokalemia demonstrates improvement when the serum potassium is increasing toward normal and the physical signs and symptoms of hypokalemia begin to disappear or lessen in intensity. Specifically, the patient's quadriceps muscles become stronger, normal bowel function returns, and heart rhythm becomes more regular. Evaluation of a patient's clinical status is especially important if acute fluid, electrolyte, and/or acid-base imbalances exist. A patient's condition can change very quickly, and it is important to recognize impending problems by integrating information about the presenting risk factors, clinical status, effects of the present treatment regimen, and potential causative agent. When making clinical decisions during evaluation, apply knowledge of how various pathophysiological conditions affect fluid, electrolyte, and acid-base balance;

FIG. 42.19 Critical thinking model for fluid, electrolyte, and acid-base balance evaluation. (Clinical Judgment Measurement Model copyright © NCSBN. All rights reserved.)

the effects of medications and fluids; and the patient's presenting clinical status (Fig. 42.19).

Robert continues to care for Mrs. Mendoza 2 days after her admission. He asks her how she feels and prepares to conduct a brief physical assessment. Mrs. Mendoza remarks, "I feel much better. I have had no nausea since early yesterday and no diarrhea since late yesterday afternoon." The IV infusion of 0.9% sodium chloride (normal saline) still is in place in the right forearm, infusing now at 100 mL/hr. The IV site has no redness, tenderness, or inflammation. Because Mrs. Mendoza is tolerating oral fluids, her health care provider just ordered to reduce the IV infusion rate to 40 mL/hr. During examination Robert notices that her skin turgor has returned to normal, but her oral mucosa is still slightly dry. Mrs. Mendoza's vital signs are BP, 100/58 mm Hg; pulse, 80 beats/min; and respirations, 18 breaths/min.

Robert is encouraged by Mrs. Mendoza's progress. He brings her breakfast meal tray, which includes the first soft food that she has had since being hospitalized. Robert sits down and discusses with Mrs. Mendoza the need for ongoing IV fluids to fully restore her fluid and electrolyte balance. Robert says, "Now that you are beginning to feel better, tell me why it is important to increase your oral fluids so we can remove the IV." Mrs. Mendoza identifies three reasons why she will drink more fluids so that the IV line can be removed.

For patients with less acute alterations, evaluation is likely to occur over a longer period. In this situation evaluation may be more focused on

behavioral changes (e.g., the patient's adherence to dietary restrictions and medication schedules). Another important element of evaluation is the family's ability to anticipate alterations and prevent a recurrence of problems.

The patient's level of progress determines whether the plan of care needs to continue or be revised. If outcomes are not met, you may need to consult a health care provider to discuss additional methods, such as increasing the frequency of an intervention (e.g., providing more fluids to a patient experiencing dehydration), introducing a new therapy (e.g., initiating insertion of an IV line), or discontinuing a therapy. Once outcomes are met, the nursing diagnosis is resolved and you are able to focus on other priorities, including maintaining normal fluid, electrolyte, and acid-base balance. If established outcomes are not achieved, explore factors that contributed to why the planned outcomes were not met. Modification of the care plan occurs after this evaluation. If outcomes are not achieved, the questions you ask may include the following:

- "What difficulties are you having with measuring your I&O daily and keeping a record?"
- "What barriers are preventing you from obtaining the potassium-rich foods you need?"
- "Are you continuing to have frequent loose stools or diarrhea?"
- "Have you purchased an antacid, or are you still using baking soda as an antacid?"

SAFETY GUIDELINES FOR NURSING SKILLS

Ensuring patient safety is an essential role of the professional nurse. Use sound clinical judgment by communicating clearly with members of the health care team; assessing and analyzing the patient's clinical findings; and incorporating the patient's priorities of care and preferences. Use the best evidence, applying professional standards, when selecting interventions to use in patient care delivery. When performing the skills in this chapter, remember the following points to ensure safe, patient-centered care:

- Check that you have the necessary information, a health care provider's order if required, and equipment available for the procedure before beginning.
- Before initiation of therapy, check patient identification using two patient identifiers (TJC, 2021a) and assess the appropriate route and rate of infusion and potential incompatibilities between infusing fluids and medications (Gorski et al., 2021).
- Determine whether the patient has a latex allergy, such as children with birth defects/diseases requiring multiple surgeries/indwelling urinary catheters, patients with myelomeningocele and multiple surgeries, and patients with an allergy to tropical fruits (e.g., avocado, banana, chestnut, kiwi) who have a high cross-reactivity to latex as such fruits contain proteins with allergenic similarities to latex (Gorski et al., 2021). Use nonpowdered, nonlatex gloves and nonlatex supplies if a latex allergy is present (Gorski et al., 2021).

- Conduct a complete history and physical assessment, including vital signs, and review laboratory findings before initiating any solutions or medications.
- Know the indications for prescribed therapy before initiating IV therapy. Obtain and review the health care provider's order to ensure appropriateness of the prescribed solution of medications (Gorski et al., 2021).
- Use special designated tubing for the brand of EID and for blood transfusions and some medications.
- Review the steps of the procedure mentally before entering a patient's room (i.e., consider modifications that you may need to make for this specific patient and verify that the type of IV solution is appropriate for this patient).
- Maintain standard ANTT® guidelines, which include Standard Precautions, use of appropriate PPE, and no touch or strict sterile techniques when handling connections with tubing and VAD device and handling infusion system (Gorski et al., 2021).
- If you contaminate a sterile object during the procedure, do not use it. Use a new sterile one.
- Place all disposable blood-contaminated items and sharp items in designated puncture-resistant biohazard containers.

SKILL 42.1   INSERTION OF A SHORT-PERIPHERAL INTRAVENOUS DEVICE

Delegation and Collaboration

The skill of inserting a short-peripheral IV access device cannot be delegated to assistive personnel (AP). Delegation to licensed practical nurses (LPNs) varies by state nurse practice act. Instruct the AP to:

- Notify the nurse if the patient complains of any IV site–related complications such as redness, pain, tenderness, swelling, bleeding, drainage, or leaking from under dressing.
- Notify the nurse if the patient's IV dressing becomes wet or loose.
- Notify the nurse if the level of fluid in the IV bag is low or the EID is alarming.

Equipment

- Short-peripheral IV start kit supplies (available in some agencies): single-use tourniquet, tape (**NOTE:** Plastic tape preferable for short-term use), transparent semipermeable membrane (TSM) dressing or sterile gauze and sterile tape, antiseptic wipes (alcohol-based 2% chlorhexidine gluconate [CHG] solution preferred, povidone-iodine, or 70% alcohol), 2 × 2–inch gauze pads, and label
  - Smallest-gauge catheter (with safety mechanism) for short-peripheral IV that will accommodate the prescribed therapy and patient need (Gorski et al., 2021):
    - Adults: 20- to 24-gauge catheter
    - Neonates, children, and older adults, and adult patients with limited venous options to minimize insertion-related trauma: 22- to 26-gauge catheter
    - Select a large-gauge catheter (e.g., 20-gauge catheter) for adult and pediatric patients when rapid fluid replacement is required
- Clean gloves (powderless and latex free for patients with latex allergy); sterile gloves are needed if palpating the site after skin antisepsis (Gorski et al., 2021)
- Single-use hair clippers or scissors for hair removal if indicated

- Short extension tubing with fused needleless connector or separate needleless connector (also called *injection cap, saline lock, heparin lock, IV plug, buff cap, buffalo cap,* or *PRN adapter*)
- 10-mL syringe prefilled with preservative-free 0.9% sodium chloride (normal saline [NS])
- Alcohol-based 2% chlorhexidine swabs or, if sensitivity exists, use 70% alcohol or povidone iodine antiseptic swabs
- Sterile, alcohol-free skin barrier product, compatible with skin antiseptic agent
- Engineered catheter securement device (if available) and polymer-based skin protectant swab
- *Option:* IV site protection device
- Prescribed IV solution or medication
- IV administration set (IV tubing), either macrodrip or microdrip, depending on prescribed rate; if using EID, appropriate administration set
- 0.2-micron filter for nonlipid (fat emulsions) solutions (may be incorporated into the infusion set)
- Additional personal protective equipment (PPE): goggles and mask (*optional* based on agency policy)
- EID and IV pole
- Vein visualization device (*optional* based on agency policy)
- Stethoscope
- Watch with second hand to calculate drip rate
- Special patient gown with snaps at shoulder seams if available
- Needle disposal container (sharps container or biohazard container)
- *Option:* Hand or arm joint stabilization device

STEPS	RATIONALE

ASSESSMENT

1. Review accuracy of health care provider's order: date and time, IV solution, route of administration, volume, rate, duration, and signature of ordering health care provider (Gorski, 2018). Follow the seven rights of medication administration (see Chapter 31).

Before IV therapy, an order from a health care provider is needed (Gorski et al., 2021). Verification that order is complete prevents medication errors.

   a. Check approved online database, drug reference book, or pharmacist about IV solution composition, purpose, potential incompatibilities, adverse reactions, and side effects.

Ensures safe and correct administration of IV therapy and appropriate selection of VAD.

STEPS	RATIONALE
2. Assess patient's level of health literacy.	Ensures patient or family caregiver has the capacity to obtain, communicate, process, and understand basic health information (CDC, 2021).
3. Perform hand hygiene. Obtain data from patient's EHR or perform physical examination of clinical factors/conditions that will respond to or be affected by administration of IV solutions.	Reduces transmission of microorganisms during physical measurements. Provides baseline to determine effectiveness of prescribed therapy. A systems approach is recommended to assess for fluid and electrolyte imbalances (Gorski, 2018).
a. Body weight	Changes in body weight can be an indication of fluid loss or gain (Gorski, 2018).
b. Clinical markers of vascular volume:	
(1) Urine output (decreased, dark yellow)	Kidneys respond to ECV deficit by reducing urine production and concentrating urine. Kidney disease can also cause oliguria.
(2) Vital signs: BP, respirations, pulse, temperature	Changes in BP may be associated with fluid volume status (fluid volume deficit [FVD]) seen in postural hypotension.
	Respirations can be altered in presence of acid-base imbalances.
	Temperature elevations increase need for fluid requirements (temperatures of 38.3°C [101°F] to 39.4°C [103°F] necessitate at least 500 mL of fluid replacement within a 24-hr period) (Gorski, 2018).
(3) Distended jugular neck veins (normally veins are full when person is supine and flat when person is upright)	Indicator of fluid volume status: flat or collapsing with inhalation when supine with ECV deficit; full when upright or semi-upright with ECV excess.
(4) Auscultation of lungs	Crackles or rhonchi in dependent parts of lung may signal fluid buildup caused by ECV excess.
(5) Capillary refill	Indirect measure of tissue perfusion (sluggish with ECV deficit).
c. Clinical markers of interstitial volume:	
(1) Skin turgor (pinch skin over sternum or inside of forearm)	Failure of skin to return to normal position after several seconds indicates FVD (Gorski, 2018).
(2) Dependent edema (pitting or nonpitting)	Edema is not usually apparent until 2 to 4 kg (4.4–8.8 lb) of fluid is retained. A weight gain of 1 kg (2.2 lb) is equivalent to the retention of 1 L of body water (Gorski, 2018).
(3) Oral mucous membrane between cheek and gum	More reliable indicator than dry lips or skin. Dry between cheek and gums indicates ECV deficit.
d. Thirst	Occurs with hypernatremia and severe ECV deficit. Not a reliable indicator for older adults (Gorski, 2018; Kear, 2017).
e. Behavior and level of consciousness	
(1) Restlessness and mild confusion	Occurs with FVD or acid-base imbalance.
(2) Decreased level of consciousness (lethargy, confusion, coma)	Occurs with severe ECV deficit. May occur with osmolality, fluid and electrolyte, and acid-base imbalances.
4. Review with interprofessional team the medications that should or should not be given through a peripheral IV.	Allows collaboration with an interprofessional team to identify medications that should and should not be given through peripheral veins (Gorski et al., 2021).
5. Determine whether patient is to undergo any planned operations or procedures.	Allows anticipation and placement of appropriate VAD for infusion and avoids placement in an area that will interfere with medical procedures (Gorski et al., 2021).
6. Assess available laboratory data (e.g., hematocrit, serum electrolytes, ABGs, and kidney functions [blood urea nitrogen, urine specific gravity, and urine osmolality]).	Helps determine priority assessments and establishes baseline for determining whether therapy is effective. Laboratory values are an assessment of hydration status (Gorski, 2018).
7. Ask patient to describe history of allergies: known type of allergies, and type of allergic reaction. Focus on allergy or sensitivity to latex, adhesive, and medications. Check patient's allergy wristband.	Early identification of allergies prevents allergic reaction.
8. Assess patient's or family caregiver's knowledge and previous experience with IV therapy.	Determines level of instruction necessary and patient's familiarity with how to participate in procedure.
9. Assess patient's feelings about procedure, such as concern about pain of procedure.	Reveals need for patient support. Steps can be taken to minimize pain of insertion (Gorski et al., 2021).
10. Assess patient's goals or preferences for how skill is to be performed or what patient expects.	Allows care to be individualized to patient.
11. Assess patient's preference for site for placement of IV.	Provides patient-centered care. Discuss site selection with the patient and/or caregiver, including recommendations to use sites on the nondominant side (Gorski et al., 2021).

PLANNING

1. Close room door or bedside curtains. Remove clutter from the over-bed or bedside table.	Providing privacy and preparing the environment ensure patient comfort and organize procedure.
2. Perform hand hygiene. Collect and organize equipment on clean bedside table. Verify that you have the correct infusion set for the EID that will be used.	Reduces transmission of microorganisms. Easy access to equipment improves efficiency. Ensures patient safety.

Continued

SKILL 42.1   INSERTION OF A SHORT-PERIPHERAL INTRAVENOUS DEVICE—cont'd

STEPS	RATIONALE
3. Select appropriate-sized catheter; open and prepare sterile packages using sterile aseptic technique (see Chapter 28).	Use smallest-gauge peripheral catheter that will accommodate prescribed therapy and patient needs (Gorski et al., 2021).
4. Help patient to comfortable sitting or supine position. Change patient's gown to one more easily removed with snaps at shoulder if available. Provide adequate lighting.	Promotes comfort and relaxation for patient. Use of this type of gown decreases risk of accidental dislodgment of catheter or administration set. Aids in successful vein location.
5. Explain/instruct patient about rationale for infusion, including solution and medications ordered, procedure for IV insertion, and signs and symptoms of complications (e.g., bleeding, tenderness, and swelling) to watch out for.	Provides patient with information about procedure and promotes adherence (Gorski et al., 2021). May minimize anxiety.

IMPLEMENTATION

1. Identify patient using at least two identifiers (e.g., name and birthday or name and medical record number) according to agency policy. Compare identifiers with information on patient's medication administration record (MAR) or medical record.	Ensures correct patient. Complies with The Joint Commission standards and improves patient safety (TJC, 2021a).
2. *Option:* Perform hand hygiene. Use a local anesthetic agent to reduce pain in all adult and pediatric populations before inserting IV: vapocoolant, topical transdermal agent, jet injection of pressure-accelerated lidocaine (needle-free method), intradermal lidocaine (to be avoided in pregnancy). Also plan using distraction measures during insertion.	May decrease pain during insertion although studies are inconclusive (Gorski et al., 2021).

CLINICAL JUDGMENT: *Local anesthetic may reduce discomfort associated with insertion of a VAD. Both topical and injectable drugs require a health care provider's order. Apply topical local anesthetic to intended IV site 30 minutes before procedure. Follow manufacturer recommendations and monitor for allergic reaction (Gorski et al., 2021).*

3. Perform hand hygiene. Prepare short extension tubing with fused needleless connector or separate needleless connector (injection cap) to attach to catheter hub.	Injection cap facilitates intermittent infusion of solutions and medications. The primary purpose of needleless connectors is to eliminate the use of needles when connecting administration sets and/or syringes to the VAD or injection sites and reduce subsequent needlestick injuries and exposure to bloodborne pathogens (Gorski et al., 2021).

CLINICAL JUDGMENT: *Avoid using a needleless connector for red blood cell (RBC) transfusion and when continuous infusion of rapid flow rates of crystalloid solutions is required. Needleless connectors have been shown to reduce flow rates through large-bore catheters. Negative clinical outcomes might result when therapies with rapid flow rates are impeded (Gorski et al., 2021).*

a. Remove protective cap from needleless connector and attach syringe with 1 to 3 mL 0.9% sodium chloride (normal saline [NS]), maintaining sterility. Slowly inject enough saline to prime (fill) short extension tubing and connector, removing all air. Leave syringe attached to tubing.	Replaces air with NS, preventing air from entering patient's vein later during VAD insertion.
b. Adhere to standard ANTT®, maintaining sterility of end of connector by reapplying end caps, and set aside for attaching to catheter hub after successful venipuncture. Do not overtighten end caps.	Prevents touch contamination, which allows microorganisms to enter infusion equipment and bloodstream. Overtightening end caps will make it difficult to remove them.

CLINICAL JUDGMENT: *Short extension sets may be used on short-peripheral catheters. Reduces catheter manipulation. For patient safety, all connections should be of Luer-Lok type (Gorski et al., 2021). Luer-Lok connections prevent accidental disconnection and leaks (Gorski et al., 2021). Many agencies use short extension tubing for continuous infusions and stand-alone saline locks (capped catheters).*

4. Prepare IV tubing and solution for continuous infusion, Adhere to principles of standard ANTT®.	Follows standard of INS (Gorski et al., 2021).
a. Check IV solution using seven rights of medication administration (see Chapter 31) and review label for name and concentration of solution, type and concentration of any additives, volume, beyond-use and expiration dates, and sterility state. If using bar code, scan code on patient's wristband and then on IV fluid container. Be sure that prescribed additives such as potassium and vitamins have been added. Check solution for color and clarity. Check bag for leaks.	Reviewing label for accuracy reduces risk for medication errors (Gorski et al., 2021). Risk for medication errors can be reduced with safe medication practices, including (Gorski et al., 2021): • Do not add medications to infusing containers of IV solutions. • Do not use IV solutions that are discolored, contain precipitates, or are expired.
b. Open IV infusion set, maintaining sterility. **NOTE:** EIDs sometimes have a dedicated administration set; follow manufacturer's instructions.	Prevents touch contamination, which allows microorganisms to enter infusion equipment and bloodstream.

STEPS	**RATIONALE**
c. Place roller clamp (see illustration A) about 2 to 5 cm (1–2 inches) below drip chamber and move roller clamp to "off" position (see illustration B).	Close proximity of roller clamp to drip chamber allows more accurate regulation of flow rate. Moving clamp to "off" prevents accidental spillage of IV solution during priming.
d. Remove protective sheath over IV tubing port on plastic IV solution bag (see illustration) or top of IV solution bottle while maintaining sterility.	Provides access for insertion of IV tubing spike into solution using sterile technique.
e. Remove protective cover from IV tubing spike while maintaining sterility of spike. Insert spike into port of IV bag using a twisting motion (see illustration). If solution container is glass bottle, clean rubber stopper on glass-bottled solution with antiseptic swab and insert spike into rubber stopper of IV bottle. Bottles require vented tubing.	Flat surface on top of bottled solution may contain contaminants, whereas opening to plastic bag is recessed. Prevents contamination of bottled solution during insertion of spike. If sterility of spike is compromised, discard IV tubing, and obtain new one.

CLINICAL JUDGMENT: *If solution container is glass bottle, clean rubber stopper on glass-bottled solution with antiseptic swab and insert spike into rubber stopper of IV bottle. Bottles require vented tubing.* Rationale: *Prevents contamination of bottled solution during insertion of spike. If sterility of spike is compromised, discard IV tubing and obtain new one.*

---

f. Compress drip chamber and release, allowing it to fill one-third to one-half full (see illustration).	Compression creates suction effect; fluid enters drip chamber to prevent air from entering tubing.

 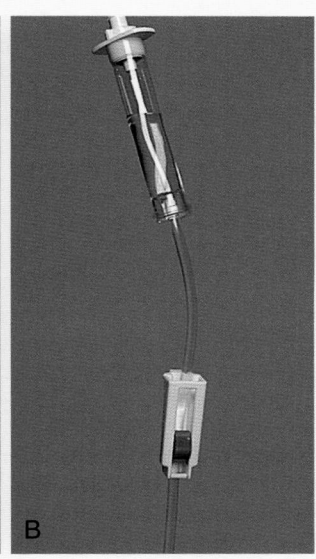

STEP 4c (A) Roller clamp in open position. (B) Roller clamp in closed position.

STEP 4d Removing protective sheath from intravenous tubing port.

STEP 4e Inserting spike into intravenous bag.

STEP 4f Squeezing drip chamber to fill with fluid one-third to one-half full.

Continued

SKILL 42.1   INSERTION OF A SHORT-PERIPHERAL INTRAVENOUS DEVICE—cont'd

STEPS	RATIONALE
g. Prime air out of IV tubing by filling with IV solution: Remove protective cover on end of IV tubing (some tubing can be primed without removing protective cover) and slowly open roller clamp to allow fluid to flow from drip chamber to distal end of IV tubing. If tubing has a Y connector, invert Y connector when fluid reaches it to displace air. Return roller clamp to "off" position after priming tubing (filled with IV fluid). Replace protective cover on distal end of tubing. Label IV tubing with date according to agency policy and procedure.	Priming ensures that IV tubing is clear of air and filled with IV solution before connecting to VAD. Slowly filling tubing decreases turbulence and chance of bubble formation. Closing clamp prevents accidental loss of fluid. Maintains sterility. Labeling IV tubing allows for recognition of length of time that tubing has been in use and when to change it.
h. Be certain that IV tubing is clear of air and air bubbles. To remove small air bubbles, firmly tap tubing where they are located. Air bubbles will ascend to drip chamber. Check entire length of tubing to ensure that all air bubbles are removed (see illustration).	Large air bubbles act as emboli and should be avoided (Gorski, 2018; Mattox, 2017).
i. If using optional long extension tubing, remove protective cover and attach it to distal end of IV tubing, maintaining sterility. Then prime long extension tubing with IV solution. Insert IV tubing into EID with power off.	Priming removes air from long extension tubing so that it does not enter patient's vascular system. Facilitates starting infusion as soon as IV site is ready.
5. Perform hand hygiene.	Decreases potential risk of microbial contamination and cross-contamination.

CLINICAL JUDGMENT: *Gloves are not necessary to locate vein but must be applied for VAD insertion using standard ANTT® no-touch technique in which the site is not palpated after skin antisepsis (Gorski et al., 2021).*

---

6. Apply tourniquet around upper arm about 10 to 15 cm (4–6 inches) above proposed insertion site (see illustration). Do not apply tourniquet too tightly. Check for presence of pulse distal to tourniquet. *Option A:* Apply tourniquet on top of thin layer of clothing such as gown sleeve to protect fragile or hairy skin. *Option B:* BP cuff may be used in place of tourniquet: activate cuff and hold at approximately 50 mm Hg.	Tourniquet should be tight enough to impede venous flow while maintaining arterial circulation. Reduces trauma to skin.
7. Select a venous site most likely to last the full length of the prescribed therapy (Gorski et al., 2021) (see Fig. 42.15). Discuss the preference for VAD site selection with the patient. *Option:* Use vascular visualization technology. Veins on dorsal and ventral surfaces of arms (e.g., metacarpal, cephalic, basilic, or median) are preferred in adults.	The most appropriate vein and insertion site is selected to best accommodate the VAD required for the prescribed infusion therapy (Gorski et al., 2021). Ensures adequate vein that is easy to puncture and less likely to rupture.
a. Use most distal site in nondominant arm if possible.	Patients with VAD placement in their dominant hand have decreased ability to perform self-care.

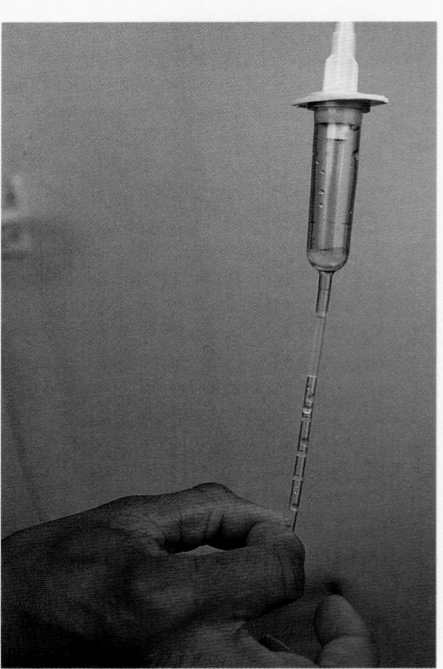

STEP 4h Removing air bubbles from tubing.

STEP 6 Tourniquet placed on arm for initial vein selection.

STEPS	RATIONALE
b. With your fingertip, palpate vein at intended insertion site by pressing downward. Note resilient, soft, bouncy feeling while releasing pressure (see illustration).	Fingertip is more sensitive and better for assessing vein location and condition.
c. Select well-dilated vein. Methods to improve vascular distention:	Increased volume of blood in vein at venipuncture site makes vein more visible. Use of gravity promotes vascular distention (Gorski et al., 2021).
(1) Position extremity lower than heart, have patient open and close fist slowly, and lightly stroke vein downward.	
(2) Apply dry heat to extremity for several minutes.	Dry heat has been found to promote vein dilation and increase successful peripheral catheter insertion (Gorski et al., 2021).

CLINICAL JUDGMENT: *Vigorous friction, slapping, or hard tapping of a vein, especially in older adults, can cause venous constriction and/or bruising and hematoma (Gorski, 2018).*

STEPS	RATIONALE
8. When selecting a vein:	
a. Avoid vein selection in:	Aids in selecting a vein that will prolong the dwell time, increase the likelihood of the IV catheter lasting the full length of the prescribed therapy, decrease pain during dwell time, promote self-care, and prevent accidental removal and occlusions (Gorski et al., 2021). Most commonly used veins are found on the dorsal and ventral surfaces of the upper extremities, including the metacarpal, cephalic, basilic, and median veins (Gorski et al., 2021).
(1) Area of joint flexion (e.g., wrist, antecubital fossa)	
(2) Area with pain on palpation	
(3) Site distal to previous venipuncture site, sclerosed or hardened veins, previous infiltrations or extravasations, areas of venous valves, or phlebitic vessels	
(4) Compromised skin and sites distal to these areas (e.g., areas with open wounds, extremities with an infection)	
(5) Location that interferes with planned procedures	
(6) Veins that are compromised (upper extremity on side of breast surgery with axillary node dissection or lymphedema or after radiation, arteriovenous [AV] fistulas/grafts, or affected extremity from cerebrovascular accident [CVA])	
(7) Fragile dorsal veins in older adults	
b. Choose site that will not interfere with patient's activities of daily living (ADLs), use of assist devices, or planned procedures.	Keeps patient as mobile as possible.
9. Release tourniquet temporarily.	Restores blood flow and prevents venospasm when preparing for venipuncture.

CLINICAL JUDGMENT: *Remove excess hair at the insertion site if needed to facilitate application of VAD dressings. Use single-patient-use scissors or disposable-head surgical clippers; do not shave as this may increase the risk for infection (Gorski et al., 2021).*

STEPS	RATIONALE
10. Perform hand hygiene and apply clean gloves. Wear eye protection and mask (see agency policy) if splash or spray of blood is possible.	Standard ANTT® decreases potential risk of microbial contamination and cross-contamination (Gorski et al., 2021).
11. Place adapter end of short extension set (prepared in Step 3) or needleless connector (injection cap) for saline lock nearby in sterile package.	Permits smooth, quick connection of infusion to short-peripheral catheter once vein is accessed. Keeps items sterile.
12. If area of insertion is visibly soiled, clean site with antiseptic soap and water first and dry. Perform skin antisepsis with alcohol-based 2% chlorhexidine solution using friction in back-and-forth motion (see illustration) for 30 seconds and allow to dry completely. If using plain alcohol or povidone-iodine, clean in concentric circle, moving from insertion site outward with swab. Allow drying time between agents if agents are used in combination (alcohol and povidone-iodine).	Mechanical friction in this pattern allows penetration of antiseptic solution to epidermal layer of skin. Reduces incidence of catheter-related infections. Follow manufacturers' directions for use to determine appropriate product application and dry times (usually at least 30 seconds); always allow product to dry naturally for complete antisepsis (Gorski et al., 2021).

STEP 7b Palpate vein.

STEP 12 Clean site with antiseptic swab (alcoholic chlorhexidine solution preferred, 70% alcohol, or povidone-iodine).

Continued

SKILL 42.1	INSERTION OF A SHORT-PERIPHERAL INTRAVENOUS DEVICE—cont'd
STEPS	**RATIONALE**

CLINICAL JUDGMENT: *If vein palpation is necessary after performing skin antisepsis, use sterile gloves for palpation or perform skin antisepsis again because touching cleaned area introduces microorganisms from your finger to site (Gorski et al., 2021).*

13. Reapply tourniquet 10 to 15 cm (4–6 inches) above anticipated insertion site. If vein is not distended, use gravity (keeping hand and arm in dependent position). Check for presence of pulse distal to tourniquet.	Pressure of tourniquet and dependent position promote vein distention. Diminished arterial flow prevents venous filling. Do not apply warming at this time as it will contaminate antiseptic insertion site.
14. Perform venipuncture. Anchor vein below anticipated insertion site by placing thumb over vein 4 to 5 cm (1½–2 inches) distal to site (see illustration) and gently stretching skin against direction of insertion. Instruct patient to relax hand or arm.	Stabilizes vein for needle insertion, prevents vein from rolling, and stretches skin taut, decreasing drag during insertion. Some devices require loosening needle (stylet) from catheter before venipuncture. Follow manufacturer directions for use.
a. Warn patient of a sharp stick.	Accessing vein at an angle reduces risk of puncturing posterior vein wall.
b. Hold VAD with needle bevel up. Align catheter on top of vein at 10- to 30-degree angle. Puncture skin and anterior vein wall (see illustration).	Superficial veins require smaller angle. Deeper veins require greater angle.

CLINICAL JUDGMENT: *Use each catheter only once for each insertion attempt.*

15. Observe for blood return in catheter or flashback chamber of catheter, indicating that bevel of needle has entered vein (see illustration A). Advance VAD approximately ¼ inch (0.6 cm) into vein and loosen stylet (needle) of the catheter. Continue to hold skin taut while stabilizing VAD and, with index finger on push-off tab of VAD, advance catheter off needle into vein until hub rests at venipuncture site (see illustration B). *Do not reinsert stylet into catheter once catheter has been advanced into vein.* Advance catheter while safety device automatically retracts stylet (techniques for retracting stylet vary with different VADs). Place stylet directly into sharps container.	Increased venous pressure from tourniquet causes backflow of blood into catheter and/or flashback chamber. Some VADs have a notch in the stylet, allowing flash of blood into catheter. Stabilizing VAD allows for placement of catheter into vein and advancement of catheter off stylet. Advancing entire stylet into vein may penetrate wall of vein, resulting in hematoma. Advancing catheter with finger on open hub causes contamination. Reinsertion of stylet can cause catheter to shear off and embolize into vein. Devices with safety mechanisms and proper sharps disposal prevent needlestick injuries (Occupational Safety and Health Administration [OSHA], n.d.).

STEP 14 Stabilize vein below insertion site.

STEP 14b Puncture skin with catheter at 10- to 30-degree angle.

STEP 15 (A) Observe for blood return in catheter and/or flashback chamber. (B) Advance catheter into vein until hub rests at venipuncture site.

STEPS	RATIONALE

CLINICAL JUDGMENT: *A single clinician should not make more than two unsuccessful attempts at initiating IV access. Limit total attempts (Gorski et al., 2021). Multiple unsuccessful attempts cause pain to the patient, delay treatment, limit future vascular access, increase cost, and increase the risk for complications (Gorski et al., 2021).*

16. Stabilize VAD with nondominant hand and release tourniquet or BP cuff with other. Apply gentle but firm pressure with middle finger of nondominant hand 3 cm (1¼ inches) above insertion site. Keep catheter stable with index finger.	Permits venous flow and reduces backflow of blood. Digital pressure minimizes blood loss and allows attachment of extension set or needleless connector.
17. Quickly connect Luer-Lok end of short extension tubing with needleless connector to end of catheter hub. Secure connection. Avoid touching sterile connection ends. *Option:* IV tubing can be attached directly to catheter hub in place of short extension tubing or needleless connector.	Prompt connection maintains patency of vein, minimizes blood loss, and prevents risk of exposure to blood. Maintains sterility.
18. Take the previously attached 10-mL prefilled syringe that contains 0.9% sodium chloride (normal saline [NS]) and is connected to short extension set. Aspirate by pulling back on syringe to remove air and assess blood return. Then, slowly inject NS from syringe into VAD (see illustration A). Remove syringe and discard. *Option:* To begin primary infusion, swab needleless connector with antiseptic swab and attach Luer-Lok end of IV tubing to needleless connector (see illustration B). Open roller clamp of IV tubing, turn on EID, and program it. Begin infusion at correct rate. If using gravity flow instead of EID, begin infusion by slowly opening roller clamp to regulate rate.	Aspirating air prevents air embolism. Blood return that is color and consistency of whole blood confirms placement of catheter in vein (Gorski et al., 2021). Flushing prevents reflux of blood into catheter and occlusion (Gorski et al., 2021). Initiates flow of fluid through IV catheter, preventing clotting of device. Swelling indicates infiltration, and catheter would need to be removed. Initiates flow of fluid through IV catheter, preventing clotting of VAD.

CLINICAL JUDGMENT: *Needleless connectors protect health care workers and decrease risk for needlestick injuries. They have different internal mechanisms for fluid displacement (e.g., negative or positive displacement, neutral, or antireflux). Follow manufacturer's directions for use for flushing, clamping, and disconnection (Gorski et al., 2021). In the absence of manufacturer's directions, consider the reported reflux volume for each type and use the following sequence:*
- *Negative displacement: flush, clamp, disconnect*
- *Positive displacement: flush, disconnect, clamp*
- *Neutral and antireflux: no specific sequence required*

19. Observe insertion site for swelling.	Swelling indicates infiltration, which necessitates immediate catheter removal.
20. *Option:* Secure IV catheter using engineered securement device (follow manufacturer directions and agency policy). (Example described in steps and shown in illustration is an adhesive securement device.)	Use of engineered securement devices that allow visual inspection of insertion site can reduce risk of VAD complications (i.e., phlebitis, infection, migration) and unintentional loss of access (Gorski et al., 2021).

CLINICAL JUDGMENT: *Adhesive securement devices are contraindicated in patients with known adhesive sensitivity or allergy.*

a. Once IV catheter is in place, apply the small strip of sterile tape provided with device across catheter hub.	Temporarily secures catheter.

STEP 18 (A) Flush short extension set after aspirating air and assessing blood return. (B) Connect intravenous tubing to the short extension set that is attached to the catheter.

Continued

SKILL 42.1	INSERTION OF A SHORT-PERIPHERAL INTRAVENOUS DEVICE—cont'd
STEPS	**RATIONALE**

STEP 20a Place sterile tape over catheter hub.

STEPS	RATIONALE
b. Apply alcohol swab to cleanse and degrease the skin. Allow to dry completely.	Will allow adhesive-backed devices to adhere to skin.
c. Apply polymer-based skin protectant (skin barrier) to area of skin around IV site using cream or wipe) and allow to dry completely.	Risk for medical adhesive–related skin injury (MARSI) is increased as result of age, joint movement, and edema; use of skin protectant can decrease risk (Gorski et al., 2021).
d. Align anchoring pads of device with directional arrow pointing to insertion site. Press device retainer over top of Luer-Lok connection while supporting underneath connection.	Holds IV catheter in place.
e. Stabilize and secure catheter, peel off one side of liner, and press to adhere to skin. Repeat on other side.	Secures IV in place

21. Apply sterile dressing over site.

a. If engineered stabilization device is in place, then skin has already been prepped with adhesive and grease remover and skin barrier protectant.
If engineered stabilization device is not in place:

(1) Apply alcohol swab to cleanse and degrease the skin. Allow to dry completely.

Will allow adhesive-backed devices to adhere to skin.

(2) Apply polymer-based skin protectant (skin barrier) to area of skin around IV site (using cream or wipe) and allow to dry completely.

Skin barrier prevents skin tears, blistering, and erythema—all forms of MARSI (Gorski et al., 2021). TSM dressing allows for full visualization of IV site without disrupting dressing and allows for fewer dressing changes (Gorski et al., 2021).

b. TSM dressing:

(1) **NOTE:** *If stabilization device has been applied, place TSM over stabilization device unless a TSM dressing is incorporated in device.* Patients with at-risk skin include older adults/neonates; Black patients; and patients at risk for MARSI (e.g., malnutrition; dehydration; dermatologic conditions; edema; diabetes mellitus; renal insufficiency; immunosuppression; hematologic malignancies; low/high humidity; radiation therapy; medications such as antineoplastic agents, antiinflammatories, long-term corticosteroid use, anticoagulants; and use of an adhesive-based securement method).

(2) Continue to hold hub of catheter with nondominant hand or stabilization device to secure catheter. Remove adherent backing of dressing. Apply one edge of dressing and gently smooth over IV insertion site and securement device. Do not apply with tension or stretching. Leave the Luer-Lok connection between tubing and catheter hub uncovered. Apply in the correct orientation to allow for stretching of body part if movement or swelling is anticipated. Smooth into place without gaps or wrinkles. Remove outer covering and smooth dressing gently over site (see illustrations).

TSM dressing protects catheter insertion site and minimizes risk for infection (Gorski, 2018). Allows visualization of insertion site and surrounding area for complications (Gorski et al., 2021). Access to Luer-Lok connection between tubing and catheter hub facilitates changing tubing if necessary. Steps of application follow evidence-based guidelines for prevention of medical adhesive–related skin injuries (MARSI) (Fumarola et al., 2020).

c. Sterile gauze dressing:

(1) Be sure skin barrier is dry. Place 5-cm (2-inch) piece of sterile tape over catheter hub (see illustration Step 20a). **NOTE:** Plastic tape is preferred over other tapes for short-term wear to prevent MARSI (Fumarola et al, 2020).

Moisture reduces effectiveness of adhesion (Fumarola et al, 2020). Stabilizes catheter under gauze dressing.

(2) Place 2 × 2–inch gauze pad over insertion site and edge of catheter hub. Secure all edges with tape. Do not place tape over insertion site. Do not cover connection between IV tubing and catheter hub (see illustration).

Use gauze dressings when there is site drainage, excessive perspiration, or sensitivity/allergic reactions to TSM dressings (Gorski et al., 2021; Gorski, 2018).

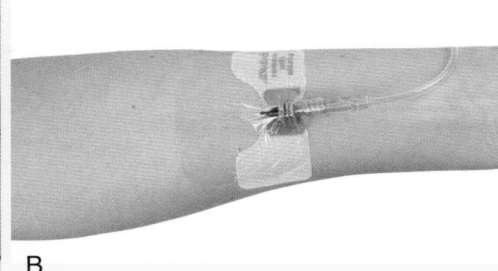

STEP 21b(2) (A) Transparent membrane dressing applied without engineered stabilization device. (B) Engineered stabilization device with transparent semipermeable membrane. (B courtesy C.R. Bard, Inc. All rights reserved.)

(3) Fold 2 × 2–inch gauze in half and cover with 1 inch–wide tape so about an inch extends on each side. Place under Luer-Lok connection (see illustration). Secure Luer-Lok connection and tubing to tape on folded gauze with 2.5-cm (1-inch) piece of tape. Avoid applying tape or gauze around arm. Do not use rolled bandages with or without elastic to secure VAD. Taping Luer-Lok connection can be eliminated if engineered stabilization device is to be used.

Tape on top of gauze makes it easier to access hub/tubing junction. Gauze pad elevates hub off skin to prevent pressure area.
Prevents back-and-forth motion of catheter.
Rolled bandages do not secure VAD adequately, can impair circulation or flow of infusion, and obscure visualization for complications.

22. *Option:* Apply site protection device (e.g., I.V. House Ultra Dressing).

Reduces risk of VAD dislodgement (Gorski et al., 2021).

23. Loop extension or short IV tubing alongside dressing on arm and secure with second piece of tape directly over tubing (see illustration).

Securing tubing further reduces risk for dislodging catheter if IV tubing is pulled (i.e., loop comes apart before catheter dislodges).

24. For continuous infusion, verify ordered rate of infusion and be sure EID is programmed correctly. If infusing by gravity drip, adjust flow rate to correct drops per minute.

Ensures prescribed rate of infusion.

25. Label dressing per agency policy. Include date and time of IV insertion, VAD gauge size and length, and your initials (see illustration).

Allows for recognition of type of device and length of time that device has been in place.

STEP 21c(2) Place 2 × 2–inch gauze over insertion site and catheter hub.

STEP 21c(3) Apply 2 × 2–inch gauze dressing under tubing junction.

STEP 23 Loop and secure tubing.

STEP 25 Label intravenous dressing.

Continued

SKILL 42.1	INSERTION OF A SHORT-PERIPHERAL INTRAVENOUS DEVICE—cont'd

STEPS	RATIONALE
26. Dispose of any remaining sharps in appropriate sharps container. Discard supplies.	Prevents accidental needlestick injuries (OSHA, n.d.).
27. Dispose of all contaminated supplies in appropriate receptacle, remove and dispose of gloves, and perform hand hygiene.	Reduces transmission of microorganisms. Use appropriate disposal receptacle if patient is on hazardous drugs. The National Institute for Occupational Safety and Health (NIOSH) provides an updated list of antineoplastic, nonantineoplastic, other drug categories, and biologic agents that meet the definition of hazardous drugs (Gorski et al., 2021).
28. Help patient to a comfortable position and instruct on how to move and turn without dislodging VAD.	Restores comfort and sense of well-being. Instruction prevents accidental dislodgment of catheter and minimizes risk for falls.
29. Raise side rails (as appropriate) and lower bed to lowest position.	Promotes safety and prevents falls.
30. Place nurse call system in an accessible location within patient's reach. Instruct patient in its use.	Ensures patient can call for assistance if needed and promotes safety and prevents falls.

EVALUATION

1. Observe patient every 1 to 2 hours, or at established intervals per agency policy and procedure, for function, intactness, and patency of IV system and for correct infusion rate and accurate type/amount of IV solution infused by observing level in IV container.	Ensures delivery of prescribed volume over prescribed time and decreases risk for fluid and electrolyte imbalance.
2. Evaluate patient to determine response to therapy (e.g., laboratory values, I&O), weights, vital signs, postprocedure assessments).	Early recognition of complications leads to prompt treatment.
3. Evaluate insertion site at least every 4 hours, or every 1 to 2 hours for patients who are critically ill or sedated or who have cognitive deficits (Gorski et al., 2021). Evaluate the VAD catheter-skin junction site and surrounding area by visually inspecting and palpating through the intact dressing for redness, tenderness, swelling, drainage, and signs of catheter-related complications.	Identifies complications that compromise integrity of VAD or cause inaccurate IV solution flow rate.
4. Inspect skin around insertion site for signs of MARSI (e.g., formation of vesicle, bulla, erosion, or skin tear).	MARSI is a term used to define any skin damage related to the use of medical adhesive products or devices such as tapes, wound dressings, stoma products, securement devices, electrodes, medication patches, and wound closure strips (Fumarola et al., 2020).

CLINICAL JUDGMENT: *If IV infusion is positional, fluid will run slowly or stop, depending on position of patient's arm; if this continues, you may have to restart IV line.*

5. **Use Teach-Back:** "I want to make sure that I explained the problems that can happen with your IV. Tell me the signs or symptoms that you should tell me or the other nurses about." Revise your instruction now or develop a plan for revised patient/family caregiver teaching if patient/family caregiver is not able to teach back correctly.	Teach-back is an evidence-based health literacy intervention that promotes patient engagement, patient safety, adherence, and quality. The goal of teach-back is to ensure that you have explained medical information clearly so that patients and their families understand what you communicated to them (AHRQ, 2020).

UNEXPECTED OUTCOMES AND RELATED INTERVENTIONS

1. Fluid and electrolyte imbalances, including FVD, FVE, and abnormal serum electrolyte levels.
   - Notify health care provider.
   - Readjust infusion rate based on health care provider order.
   - Adjust additives in type of IV fluid as ordered.
2. IV-related complications including infiltration, phlebitis, local infection, air embolus, and bleeding.
   - See Table 42.12.
3. Catheter occlusion.
   - Determine cause and consider catheter removal.
   - Positional catheters can be repositioned to improve IV flow.
   - Remove occluded IV catheter. Occluded catheters should not be flushed because an embolus can result from dislodging a clot (Gorski, 2018).
4. Catheter-related infection can present as erythema extending at least 1 cm from the insertion site, induration, exudate, fever with no other obvious source of infection, or the patient reports any pain or tenderness associated with the catheter (Gorski et al., 2021).
   - Notify health care provider. Obtain order to culture drainage (Gorski et al., 2021).
   - Remove IV catheter and culture purulent drainage from around IV site (see Chapter 48) (Gorski et al., 2021).

RECORDING AND REPORTING

- Record number of attempts at insertion; date and time of insertion; type of solution and additives infusing; precise description of insertion site; catheter gauge, type, length and brand; rate and method of infusion (e.g., gravity or name of EID); purpose of infusion; patient's response to insertion (e.g., what the patient reports); and when infusion was started. Always complete entry with full signature and credentials.
- After each regular assessment of the insertion site, record condition of the site, dressing, type of catheter securement, dressing change, site care, patient report of discomfort/pain, and changes related to the VAD or access site (Gorski et al., 2021).

- Record and report signs or symptoms of observed or patient-reported IV-related complications (e.g., redness, tenderness, swelling, drainage, leaking from under dressing, change in flow rate, or infection).
- Document your evaluation of patient learning.
- Report to health care provider any adverse events occurring on VAD placement (e.g., persistent pain or suspected nerve damage, hematoma formation, or arterial puncture).
- Report to health care provider any signs or symptoms of complications.

HOME CARE CONSIDERATIONS

- Ensure that patient is able and willing to self-administer IV therapy or that a reliable family caregiver is willing to provide IV therapy at home.
- Teach patient and family caregiver information needed to administer IV therapy safely (see Box 42.8). Consider their cultural norms (e.g., health beliefs and comfort with caregivers using touch).

| **SKILL 42.2** | **REGULATING INTRAVENOUS FLOW RATE** | |

Delegation and Collaboration

The skill of regulating IV flow rates cannot be delegated to assistive personnel (AP). Delegation to licensed practical nurses (LPNs) varies by state nurse practice act. The nurse instructs the AP to:
- Inform the nurse when the EID alarm signals.
- Inform the nurse when the fluid container is near completion.
- Report any patient complaints of discomfort related to infusion such as pain, burning at IV site, bleeding, or swelling.

Equipment
- Watch with a second hand
- Calculator, paper, and pencil/pen
- Label
- IV solution bag and appropriate administration set
- EID, IV regulating device
- Clean gloves

STEPS	**RATIONALE**

ASSESSMENT

1. Review accuracy and completeness of health care provider order in patient's medical record for patient name; type and volume of IV fluid; additives; infusion rate; and duration of IV therapy. Follow seven rights of medication administration.

  Ensures administration of correct IV fluid at proper rate. IV fluids are medications. The seven rights prevent medication administration error.

2. Review medical record and identify patient risk for fluid and electrolyte imbalance given type of IV solution (e.g., neonate, history of cardiac or renal disease).

  Helps prioritize assessments. Volume control needs to be strict. Guides choice of infusion device.

3. Perform hand hygiene and apply clean gloves.

  Reduces risk of contamination using standard ANTT® (Gorski et al, 2021).

4. Assess patient's and family caregiver's health literacy.

  Ensures patient or family caregiver has the capacity to obtain, communicate, process, and understand basic health information (CDC, 2021).

5. Check infusion system from solution container down to VAD insertion site for integrity.

  Identifies complications that can compromise integrity of VAD and patient safety.

   a. Assess IV container for discoloration, cloudiness, leakage, and expiration date.

   Incompatibility of solutions or medications compromises integrity of VAD and patient safety (Gorski, 2018).

   b. Assess IV tubing for puncture, contamination, or occlusion.

   Compromised tubing results in fluid leakage and bacterial contamination.

6. Assess the integrity, patency, and functioning of the existing VAD (according to agency policy). Assess the VAD catheter-skin junction site and surrounding area for catheter-related complications by visually inspecting and palpating through the intact dressing. Inspect for redness, swelling, and drainage. Ask patient if tenderness is present on palpation.

  Identifies complications that compromise integrity of VAD and necessitate replacement of VAD.

7. Remove and dispose of gloves and perform hand hygiene.

  Reduces risk of contamination.

8. Assess patient's knowledge, prior experience with IV therapy, and feelings about procedure.

  Reveals need for patient instruction and/or support.

9. Assess patient's goals or preferences for how skill is to be performed or what patient expects.

  Allows care to be individualized to patient.

PLANNING

1. Prepare and organize equipment

   a. Gather paper and pencil or calculator to calculate flow rate.

   Calculating hourly flow rates ensures that the prescribed amount of fluid to be infused over the prescribed time frame is correct.

   b. Check medical order to see how long each liter of fluid should infuse. If hourly rate (mL/hr) is not provided in order, calculate it by dividing volume by hours. For example:

   Basis of calculation to ensure infusion of solution over prescribed hourly rate.

$$mL/hr = \frac{\text{Total infusion volume (mL)}}{\text{Hours of infusion}}$$

1000 mL/8 hr = 125 mL/hr

or if 3 L is ordered for 24 hours,

3000 mL/24 hr = 125 mL/hr

Continued

SKILL 42.2	REGULATING INTRAVENOUS FLOW RATE—cont'd

STEPS	RATIONALE

CLINICAL JUDGMENT: *It is common for health care providers to write an abbreviated IV order such as "D₅W with 20 mEq KCl 125 mL/hr continuous." This order implies that IV infusion should be maintained at this rate until an order has been written for IV infusion to be discontinued or changed to another order.*

c. If keep-vein-open (KVO) rate is ordered, check agency policy regarding flow rate.

Prevents catheter clotting, thus preserving venous access while infusing a minimal amount of fluid. An order for KVO rate must specify an infusion rate as required by the seven rights of medication administration (see Chapter 31). Rates may vary from 0.5 mL/hr to 30 mL/hr based of type of VAD, patient-specific therapy, and method of infusion (gravity or EID).

d. Use hourly rate to program EID (see Implementation) or, if gravity-flow infusion, use minute flow rate (drops per minute [gtt/min]).

EID automatically delivers correct minute flow rate. Gravity infusion requires calculation of gtt/min.

e. Know calibration (drop factor) in drops per milliliter (gtt/mL) of infusion set used by agency.

Drop factor for macrodrip tubing varies with manufacturer.

  (1) *Microdrip:* 60 gtt/mL: used to deliver rates less than 100 mL/hr.

Microdrip tubing universally delivers 60 gtt/mL. Used when small or precise volumes are ordered.

  (2) *Macrodrip:* 10 or 15 gtt/mL: used to deliver rates greater than 100 mL/hr.

These are different commercial parenteral administration sets for macrodrip tubing. Used when large volumes or fast rates are necessary. **Know drip factor for tubing being used.**

f. Select one of the following formulas to calculate minute flow rate (drops/min) based on drop factor of infusion set:

Formulas compute correct flow rate over 1 minute.

  (1) mL/hr/60 min = mL/min

Drop factor × mL/min = gtt/min

Or

  (2) mL/hr × drop factor/60 min = gtt/min

Calculate minute flow rate for a bag of 1000 mL with 20 mEq of KCl at 125 mL/hr:

Once you determine hourly rate, these formulas compute the correct flow rate.

Microdrip:

When using microdrip, mL/hr always equals gtt/min.

125 mL/hr × 60 gtt/mL = 7500 gtt/hr

7500 gtt ÷ 60 minutes = 125 gtt/min

Macrodrip:

Multiply hourly rate (mL/hr) by drop factor and divide product by 60 to convert hours to minutes.

125 mL/hr × 15 gtt/mL = 1875 gtt/hr

1875 gtt ÷ 60 minutes = 31−32 gtt/min

2. Prepare patient and family caregiver by explaining procedure, its purpose, and what is expected of patient.

Provides patient and family caregiver with information about procedure and promotes adherence (Gorski et al., 2021).

IMPLEMENTATION

1. Identify patient using at least two identifiers (e.g., name and birthday or name and medical record number) according to agency policy. Compare identifiers with information on patient's MAR or medical record.

Ensures correct patient. Complies with The Joint Commission standards and improves patient safety (TJC, 2021a).

CLINICAL JUDGMENT: *Manual and mechanical flow-control devices may be used for low-risk infusions in which some variation in flow rate is not critical (Gorski et al., 2021). Consider the use of a manual flow regulator in lieu of a roller clamp (e.g., allows for setting the infusion rate in milliliters per hour) to allow for easier regulation and more consistent flow (Gorski et al., 2021). Fluids run by gravity are adjusted through use of a flow control/regulator. Manual flow regulators (i.e., roller clamp, dial, or barrel-shaped) are not recommended for use in infants and children because accuracy cannot be guaranteed (Gorski, 2018) and can be affected by mechanical and patient factors.*

2. Regulate gravity infusion:

  a. Ensure that IV container is at least 76.2 cm (30 inches) above IV site for adults, and increase height for more viscous fluids.

Pressure caused by gravity is necessary to overcome venous pressure and resistance from tubing and catheter.

  b. Slowly open roller clamp on tubing until you can see drops in drip chamber. Hold a watch with second hand at same level as drip chamber and count drip rate for 1 minute (see illustration). Adjust roller clamp to increase or decrease rate of infusion.

Regulates flow to prescribed rate.

  c. Monitor drip rate at least hourly.

Many factors influence drip rate; frequent monitoring ensures IV fluid administration as prescribed.

STEPS	**RATIONALE**

CLINICAL JUDGMENT: *Various detectors and alarms respond to air in IV lines, completion of infusion, high and low pressure, low battery power, occlusion, and the inability to deliver at a preset rate. The use of an EID still requires you to check to ensure that the pump is functioning and infusing at the prescribed rate.*

3. Regulate EID (infusion pump or smart pump): Follow manufacturer guidelines for setup of EID. Be sure you are using infusion tubing compatible with EID.

Smart pumps with medication safety software are designed for administration of IV fluids that contain medications.

   a. Close roller clamp on primed IV infusion tubing. Roller clamp on IV tubing goes between EID and patient.

Prevents fluid leakage.

   b. Insert infusion tubing into chamber of control mechanism (see manufacturer directions) (see illustration).

Most EIDs use positive pressure to infuse. Infusion pumps propel fluid through tubing by compressing and milking IV tubing.

   c. Secure part of IV tubing through "air in line" alarm system. Close door (see illustration A) and turn on power button, select required drops per minute or volume per hour, close door to control chamber, and press start button (see illustration B). If infusing medication, access the smart pump drug library of medications and set appropriate rate and dose limits. If smart pump alarms immediately and shuts down, your settings were outside unit parameters.

Ensures safe administration of ordered flow rate or medication dose. Smart pumps require additional information such as patient unit and medication. Computer matches pump setting against a drug database, and dose error reduction systems (DERSs) provide a means for decreasing IV medication administration errors (Wolf and Hughes, 2019).

CLINICAL JUDGMENT: *An anti–free-flow safeguard (preventing bolus infusion in the event of machine malfunction or when tubing is removed from machine) is an important element of an EID and is required. Always check and follow manufacturer recommendations for specific device features (Gorski, 2018).*

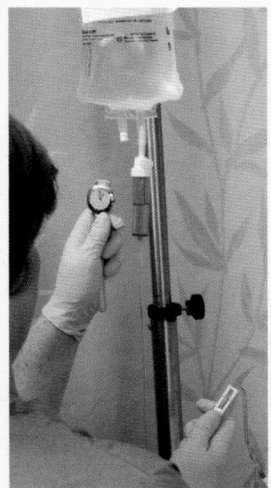

STEP 2b Nurse counting drip rate on gravity infusion.

STEP 3b Insert intravenous tubing into chamber of control mechanism.

STEP 3c (A) Close door of control mechanism. (B) Select rate and volume to be infused and press start button.

Continued

SKILL 42.2	REGULATING INTRAVENOUS FLOW RATE—cont'd

STEPS	RATIONALE
d. Open roller clamp on infusion tubing to wide open while EID is in use.	Ensures that pump freely regulates infusion rate.
e. Monitor infusion rate and IV site for complications according to agency policy. Use watch to verify rate of infusion, even when using EID (Gorski et al., 2021).	Flow controllers and pumps do not replace frequent, accurate nursing evaluation. EIDs can continue to infuse IV solutions after a complication has developed.

CLINICAL JUDGMENT: *Recognize the problem of alarm and alert fatigue with multiple electronic monitoring and therapeutic devices. Implement evidence-based recommendations (e.g., alarm parameter settings, pump/infusate height) from professional agencies and device manufacturers through collaboration with the health care team (Gorski et al., 2021).*

STEPS	RATIONALE
f. Assess IV system from container to VAD insertion site when alarm signals.	Alarm indicates situation that requires attention. Empty solution container, tubing kinks, closed clamp, infiltration, clotted catheter, air in tubing, and/or low battery can trigger EID alarm.
4. Attach label to IV solution container with date and time container is changed (check agency policy).	Provides reference to determine next time for container change, especially with keep-vein-open (KVO) rate that contains a specific infusion rate as ordered by health care provider.
5. Teach patient purpose of EID if infusion therapy is delivered by EID, purpose of alarms, to avoid raising hand or arm that affects flow rate, and to avoid touching control clamp.	Information allows patient to protect IV site and informs patient about rationale for not altering control rate.
6. Dispose of all contaminated supplies in appropriate receptacle, remove and dispose of gloves, and perform hand hygiene.	Reduces transmission of microorganisms. Use appropriate disposal receptacle if patient is on hazardous drugs.
7. Help patient to a comfortable position and instruct on how to move and turn without dislodging VAD.	Restores comfort and sense of well-being. Instruction prevents accidental dislodgment of catheter and minimizes risk for falls.
8. Raise side rails (as appropriate) and lower bed to lowest position.	Promotes safety and prevents falls.
9. Place nurse call system in an accessible location within patient's reach. Instruct patient in its use.	Ensures patient can call for assistance if needed and promotes safety and prevents falls.

EVALUATION

1. Evaluate the entire infusion system through visual inspection, from the solution container, progressing down the administration set to the patient and VAD insertion site with each infusion intervention and per agency policy. Note volume of IV fluid infused and rate of infusion. Assess manually regulated infusion sets at regular intervals; verify flow by counting drops and monitoring the infusion volume infused (Gorski et al., 2021).	Ensures delivery of prescribed volume over prescribed time and decreases risk for fluid and electrolyte imbalance.
2. Evaluate patient's response to therapy (e.g., laboratory values, input, and output [I&O], weights, vital signs, postprocedure assessments).	Provides ongoing evaluation of patient's fluid status, including monitoring for FVE or FVD. Early recognition of complications leads to prompt treatment.
3. Evaluate the IV insertion site at least every 4 hours, every 1 to 2 hours for patients who are critically ill/sedated or have cognitive deficits, and more often in patients receiving vesicants (Gorski et al., 2021). Evaluate IV site for signs and symptoms of IV-related complications, especially infiltration or extravasation.	Prevents complications that compromise integrity of VAD or cause inaccurate IV solution flow rate. EIDs do not detect infiltration or extravasation (Gorski et al., 2021).
4. Use Teach-Back: "I want to be sure that I explained the importance of your IV fluids running on time at the rate ordered. Tell me what you think may cause the pump to alarm and what you would do." Revise your instruction now or develop a plan for revised patient/family caregiver teaching if patient/family caregiver is not able to teach back correctly.	Teach-back is an evidence-based health literacy intervention that promotes patient engagement, patient safety, adherence, and quality. The goal of teach-back is to ensure that you have explained medical information clearly so that patients and their families understand what you communicated to them (AHRQ, 2020).

UNEXPECTED OUTCOMES AND RELATED INTERVENTIONS

1. Solution does not infuse at prescribed rate.
  a. Sudden infusion of large volume of solution occurs; patient develops dyspnea, crackles in lung, dependent edema (edema in legs), and increased urine output, indicating FVE.
  - Slow infusion rate: KVO rates must have specific rate ordered by health care provider.
  - Notify health care provider immediately.
  - Place patient in high-Fowler position.
  - Anticipate new IV orders.
  - Anticipate administration of oxygen per order.
  - Administer diuretics if ordered.
  b. IV solution runs slower than ordered.
  - Check for factors that may cause occlusion (e.g., positional change that affects rate, height of IV container, kinking or obstruction of tubing).
  - Check VAD site for complications.
  - Consult health care provider for new order to provide necessary fluid volume.

2. IV is no longer patent.
  - Discontinue present IV infusion and restart new short-peripheral catheter in new site.

RECORDING AND REPORTING

- Record type and rate of infusion in milliliters per hour (drops per minute in gravity flow) in patient's medical record and any ordered change in fluid rates, rate of infusion, and volume left in infusion. At end of shift, complete I&O record. Document use of EID.
- Document your evaluation of patient learning.
- Report at end of shift current IV flow rate and status of IV site.
- Report to provider any signs or symptoms of IV rate–related complication (e.g., fluid and electrolyte imbalances).

HOME CARE CONSIDERATIONS

- Ensure that patient or family caregiver is able and willing to operate infusion pump and administer IV therapy. Assess for any visual or physical limitations with ability to connect and disconnect infusion therapy and problem solve infusion pump malfunction.
- Home care nurse should be in the home during initiation of infusion therapy to ensure correct pump settings for solution, rate, time, and alarms. The nurse ensures that EID functions properly before use and that patient's electrical outlets are properly grounded.
- Provide a 24-hour access telephone number for patient to call for assistance.

SKILL 42.3   MAINTENANCE OF AN INTRAVENOUS SYSTEM

Delegation and Collaboration

The skill of changing an IV fluid container and tubing and discontinuing an IV cannot be delegated to assistive personnel (AP). Delegation to licensed practical nurses (LPNs) varies by state nurse practice act. The nurse instructs the AP to:

- Inform the nurse when an IV container is near completion.
- Report any leakage from or around the IV tubing and any cloudiness or precipitate in the IV solution.
- Report any alarm sounding on EID.
- Report any patient complaints of discomfort related to infusion such as pain, burning at site, bleeding, or swelling.
- Report if tubing has become contaminated (lying on the floor).
- Protect the IV dressing during hygiene and activities of daily living (ADLs).

Equipment

- Handheld bar-code scanner if using bar-code system to charge supplies

Changing Intravenous Container

- Correct volume and type of solution (with additives if indicated) as ordered by health care provider
- Time tape
- Pen

Changing Infusion Tubing

- Clean gloves
- Antiseptic swabs (alcohol-based 2% chlorhexidine solution preferred, 70% alcohol, or povidone-iodine)
- Tubing label
- Sterile 2 × 2–inch gauze pads *(optional)*

Continuous IV Infusion

- Microdrip or macrodrip administration set as appropriate
- Add-on device as necessary (e.g., filters, extension set, needleless connector)

Intermittent Extension Set

- Syringe prefilled with preservative-free 0.9% sodium chloride (normal saline [NS]) (Gorski et al., 2021)
- Short extension tubing (if necessary), injection cap

Discontinuing Peripheral IV Access

- Clean gloves
- Sterile 2 × 2– or 4 × 4–inch gauze pad
- Antiseptic swab (alcohol-based 2% chlorhexidine solution preferred) (Gorski et al., 2021)
- Tape

STEPS	RATIONALE

ASSESSMENT

1. Review accuracy and completeness of health care provider's order in patient's medical record for patient name and correct solution: type, volume, additives, rate, and duration of IV therapy. Follow seven rights of medication administration.

   Ensures delivery of correct IV solution and prescribed volume over prescribed time (Gorski et al., 2021).

2. Check medical record for pertinent laboratory data such as potassium level.

   Compare data with baseline to determine ongoing response to IV solution administration.

3. For discontinuation of IV, check EHR for medical order.

   Order is required.

4. For discontinuation, assess if patient is receiving an anticoagulant or has a history of a coagulopathy.

   Factors can increase bleeding at IV site once catheter is removed.

5. Determine compatibility of all IV solutions and additives by consulting approved online database, drug reference, or pharmacist.

   Incompatibilities cause physical, chemical, and therapeutic changes with adverse patient outcomes (Gorski, 2018).

6. Perform hand hygiene and apply clean gloves.

   Reduces risk of contamination and cross-contamination.

7. Note labels on tubing for date and time when IV tubing was last changed.

   Ensures correct timing of tubing changes. Decreases risk for infection.

Continued

SKILL 42.3	MAINTENANCE OF AN INTRAVENOUS SYSTEM—cont'd

STEPS	RATIONALE
8. Check infusion system from solution container down to VAD insertion site for integrity, including patency and functioning of system.	Identifies complications that can compromise integrity of VAD and patient safety. Administration set changes are performed at a frequency based on factors such as patient condition; type, rate, and frequency of solution administered; immediately upon suspected contamination; when the integrity of the product or system has been compromised; and when a new VAD is placed (Gorski et al., 2021).
a. Assess IV container for discoloration, cloudiness, leakage, and expiration date.	Incompatibility of solutions or medications compromises integrity of VAD and patient safety (Gorski, 2018).
b. Assess IV tubing for puncture, contamination, or occlusion.	Compromised tubing results in fluid leakage and bacterial contamination.

CLINICAL JUDGMENT: *If the tubing and/or IV bag becomes damaged, is leaking, or becomes contaminated, it must be changed, regardless of the tubing change schedule. If there has been a break in the integrity of the solution container, a new container is needed (Gorski, 2018).*

STEPS	RATIONALE
9. Determine when dressing on VAD was last changed. Ensure label includes date and time applied, size and type of VAD, and insertion date.	Provides information regarding length of time dressing has been in place and allows planning for dressing change (see Skill 42.1).
10. Assess the VAD catheter-skin junction site and surrounding area for catheter-related complications by visually inspecting and palpating through the intact dressing for redness, tenderness, swelling, and drainage.	Identifies complications that compromise integrity of VAD and necessitate replacement of VAD.
11. Remove and dispose of gloves and perform hand hygiene.	Reduces risk of contamination.
12. Assess patient's and family caregiver's knowledge, health literacy, and experience regarding protection of IV site, need to change tubing, or reason for discontinuing IV.	Ensures patient and family caregiver have the capacity to obtain, communicate, process, and understand basic health information (CDC, 2021). Determines need for patient instruction.
13. Assess patient's goals or preferences for how skill is to be performed or what patient expects.	Allows care to be individualized to patient.

PLANNING

STEPS	RATIONALE
1. Close room door or bedside curtains. Remove clutter from the over-bed or bedside table.	Provides privacy. Prepares the setting for the procedure.
2. Perform hand hygiene. Collect and organize equipment on clean, over-bed or bedside table.	Reduces transmission of microorganisms. Keeps procedure organized and provides patient safety.
a. Have next solution prepared at least 1 hour before needed. If prepared in pharmacy, ensure that it has been delivered to patient care unit. Check that solution is correct and properly labeled. Allow solution to warm to room temperature if refrigerated. Follow seven rights of medication administration and verify solution expiration date. Observe for precipitate, discoloration, and leakage.	Adequate planning for changing solution reduces risk of clot formation at catheter tip caused by lack of flow from an empty IV container. Checking that a solution is correct prevents medication error (Gorski et al., 2021).
b. Verify correct administration set for the type of infusion and the EID. Coordinate IV tubing changes with solution changes when possible (Gorski et al., 2021). Replace primary continuous infusion tubing to administer solutions other than lipid, blood, or blood products no more frequently than every 96 hours but at least every 7 days (Gorski et al., 2021).	Ensures patient safety. Decreasing the number of times the system is open reduces the transmission of infection and contamination of equipment.
3. Help patient to a comfortable position.	Promotes comfort and relaxation.
4. Explain to patient/family member procedure, its purpose, and what is expected of patient.	Provides patient and family caregiver with information about procedure and promotes adherence (Gorski et al., 2021). May also minimize anxiety.
a. *For discontinuing peripheral IV access:* Explain that patient must hold extremity still; that a burning sensation may be felt when you remove catheter; and that procedure will take about 5 minutes.	

IMPLEMENTATION

STEPS	RATIONALE
1. Identify patient using at least two identifiers (e.g., name and birthday or name and medical record number) according to agency policy. Compare identifiers with information on patient's MAR or medical record.	Ensures correct patient. Complies with The Joint Commission standards and improves patient safety (TJC, 2021a).
2. Changing IV fluid container	Patients receiving IV therapy periodically require changes of IV solutions or containers depending on the rate of infusion, volume in the container, and stability of the solution or medication (Gorski et al., 2021). It becomes clinically appropriate to change the type of solution, depending on a patient's fluid and electrolyte balance, response to therapy (e.g., therapeutic drug monitoring), and goals of therapy.

STEPS	RATIONALE
a. Change solution when fluid remains only in neck of container (about 50 mL) or when new type of solution has been ordered.	Prevents waste of solution.

CLINICAL JUDGMENT: *The maximum hang time for routine replacement of IV containers is established by agency policy and procedure. Maximum hang time is based on factors such as the use of strict standard ANTT®, whether the system remains closed without injection ports or add-on tubing, stability of the solution or medication being infused, and how long the solution in the IV container will last (Gorski, 2018; Gorski et al., 2021). Solution and medication containers on ambulatory infusion devices may remain longer than 24 hours if aseptic technique is used, the system remains closed without injection ports or add-on tubing, and the medication is stable for the anticipated infusion time (Gorski, 2018).*

STEPS	RATIONALE
b. Perform hand hygiene.	Reduces transmission of microorganisms.
c. Prepare new solution for changing. If using plastic bag, hang on IV pole and remove protective cover from IV tubing port. If using glass bottle, remove metal cap and metal and rubber disks.	Solution and medication containers include plastic bags, plastic bottles, and glass bottles. Permits quick, smooth, organized change from old to new container.
d. Close roller clamp on existing solution to stop flow rate. Remove IV tubing from EID (if used). Then remove old IV solution container from IV pole. Hold container with tubing port pointing upward.	Prevents solution remaining in drip chamber from emptying while changing solutions. Prevents solution in bag from spilling.
e. Quickly remove spike from old solution container and, without touching tip, insert spike into new container (see illustrations).	Reduces risk for solution in drip chamber becoming empty and maintains sterility.

CLINICAL JUDGMENT: *If spike becomes contaminated by touching an unsterile object, you will need a new IV tubing set.*

STEPS	RATIONALE
f. Hang new container of solution on IV pole.	Gravity helps with delivery of fluid into drip chamber.
g. Check for air in IV tubing. If air bubbles have formed, remove them by closing roller clamp, stretching tubing downward, and tapping tubing with finger (bubbles rise in fluid to drip chamber) (see Skill 42.1, Step 4h).	Reduces risk of air entering tubing. Use of an air-eliminating filter also reduces risk.
h. Make sure that drip chamber is one-third to one-half full. If drip chamber is too full, level can be decreased by removing bag from IV pole, pinching off IV tubing below drip chamber, inverting container, squeezing drip chamber (see illustration), releasing and turning solution container upright, and releasing pinch on tubing.	Reduces risk for air entering IV tubing. If chamber is filled, you cannot observe or regulate drip rate.
i. Regulate flow to ordered rate by opening and adjusting roller clamp on IV tubing or by opening roller clamp and programming and turning on EID.	Maintains measures to restore fluid balance and deliver IV solution as ordered.
j. Place time label on side of container and label with time hung, time of completion, and appropriate intervals. If using plastic bags, mark only on label and not container.	Provides visual comparison of volume infused compared with prescribed rate of infusion.
k. Instruct patient on purpose of new IV solution, additives, flow rate, potential side effects, how to avoid occluding tubing, and what to report.	Information informs patient about purpose for continued IV therapy and what to report and protects VAD patency.

STEP 2e (A) Remove spike from old solution container. (B) Without touching tip, insert spike into new container.

STEP 2h Squeeze drip chamber to fill with fluid. Be sure to leave chamber one-third to one-half full.

Continued

SKILL 42.3	**MAINTENANCE OF AN INTRAVENOUS SYSTEM—cont'd**

STEPS	**RATIONALE**

3. Changing infusion tubing

CLINICAL JUDGMENT: *Administration sets are the primary method to carry a solution or medication to a patient. These administration sets are considered the primary set. In addition, patients may have add-on devices (e.g., filters, extension sets), which you connect to the primary set as indicated by the prescribed therapy. Secondary sets may be used as a method to administer additional medications in conjunction with the primary infusion (e.g., antibiotics). Follow agency policy and procedures for specific requirements.*

a. Perform hand hygiene. Open new infusion set and connect add-on pieces (e.g., filters, extension tubing) using aseptic technique. Keep protective coverings over infusion spike and distal adapter. Place roller clamp about 2 to 2.5 cm (1–2 inches) below drip chamber and move roller clamp to "off" position. Secure all connections.	Close proximity of roller clamp to drip chamber allows more accurate regulation of flow rate. Securing connections reduces risk later of air emboli and infection. Protective covers reduce entrance of microorganisms. All connections should be of Luer-Lok type (Gorski et al., 2021).
b. Apply clean gloves. If patient's IV cannula hub is not visible, remove IV dressing as described in Skill 42.4. **Do not** remove tape securing cannula to skin.	Cannula hub must be visible to provide smooth transition when removing old and inserting new tubing.
c. To prepare IV tubing with new IV infusion bag (see Skill 42.1, Step 4), use standard ANTT® technique.	Prevents contamination of infusion system.
d. To prepare IV tubing with existing continuous IV infusion bag:	
(1) Move roller clamp on new IV tubing to "off" position.	Prevents fluid spillage.
(2) Slow rate of infusion through old tubing to keep-vein-open (KVO) rate using EID or roller clamp.	Prevents occlusion of VAD.
(3) Compress and fill drip chamber of old tubing.	Ensures that drip chamber remains full until new tubing is changed.
(4) Invert container and remove old tubing. Keep spike sterile and upright.	Solution in drip chamber will continue to run and maintain catheter patency.
(5) Insert spike of new infusion tubing into solution container. Hang solution bag on IV pole, compress drip chamber on new tubing, and release, allowing it to fill one-third to one-half full.	Permits drip chamber to fill and promotes rapid, smooth flow of solution through tubing.
(6) Prime air out of IV tubing by filling with IV solution: Remove protective cover on end of tubing and slowly open roller clamp to allow solution to flow from drip chamber to distal end of IV tubing. If tubing has Y connector, invert Y connector when solution reaches it to displace air. Return roller clamp to "off" position after priming tubing (filled with IV solution). Replace protective cover on end of IV tubing. Place end of adapter near patient's IV site.	Priming ensures that IV tubing is clear of air before connection with VAD and filled with IV solution. Slow fill of tubing decreases turbulence and chance of bubble formation. Closing clamp prevents accidental loss of fluid. Maintains sterility. Equipment is positioned for quick connection of new tubing.
(7) Stop EID or turn roller clamp on old tubing to "off" position.	Prevents fluid spillage. Prepares EID for insertion of new tubing.
e. Prepare tubing with extension set or saline lock.	Placement of a short extension tubing or loop between a catheter hub and injection cap allows manipulation of the injection cap without moving the catheter.

CLINICAL JUDGMENT: *The extension tubing remains attached to the short-peripheral catheter and is changed when the catheter is changed.*

(1) If short extension tubing is needed, use standard ANTT® technique to connect new injection cap to new extension set or IV tubing (Gorski et al., 2021).	Prepares extension set for connecting with IV.
(2) Scrub injection cap with antiseptic swab for at least 15 seconds and allow to dry completely. Attach syringe with 3 to 5 mL of NS flush solution and inject through injection cap into extension set.	Ensures effective disinfection. Maintains patency of catheter.
f. Reestablish infusion.	
(1) Gently disconnect old tubing from extension tubing (or from IV catheter hub) and quickly insert Luer-Lok end of new tubing or saline lock into extension tubing connection (or IV catheter hub) (see illustrations for example of connecting tubing to short extension set).	Allows smooth transition from old to new tubing, minimizing time that system is open.
(2) For continuous infusion, open roller clamp on new tubing and regulate drip rate using roller clamp, or insert tubing into EID, program to desired rate, and push the power button on.	Ensures catheter patency and prevents occlusion.
(3) Attach piece of tape or preprinted label with date and time of IV tubing change onto tubing below drip chamber.	Provides reference to determine next time for tubing change.
(4) Form loop of tubing and secure it to patient's arm with strip of tape.	Avoids accidental pulling against site and stabilizes catheter.
(5) If necessary, apply new dressing (see Skill 42.4).	Maintains integrity of VAD site.

STEPS	RATIONALE

STEP 3f(1) (A) Disconnect old tubing. (B) Insert adapter of new tubing.

CLINICAL JUDGMENT: *You may need to assist patients with many aspects of hygiene (e.g., gown changes, bathing) while patients are receiving IV therapy. Never disconnect infusion tubing to change a gown or any article of clothing. Coordinate care so that bathing or hygiene activities are done after discontinuing an IV site and before another venipuncture is performed. If infusion cannot be discontinued, use special "IV gowns" if available.*

4. Discontinuing peripheral IV access

a. Perform hand hygiene. Apply clean gloves.	Reduces transmission of microorganisms.
b. Observe existing IV site for signs and symptoms of IV-related complications (redness, pain, tenderness at site, swelling, bleeding, drainage, or leaking from under dressing). Palpate catheter site through intact dressing.	Identifies the need for postprocedure interventions, such as warm compress to site. Remove peripheral IV catheter when IV is discontinued or clinically indicated based on findings from site assessment and/or clinical signs and symptoms of phlebitis, infiltration, or systemic complications (Gorski et al., 2021).
c. Turn off EID and close roller clamp or, if no EID, close roller clamp that controls rate.	Prevents spillage of IV fluid.
d. Remove IV site dressing and catheter engineered stabilization device (see Skill 42.4). Do not use scissors. Avoid tearing patient's skin.	Exposes catheter with minimal discomfort. Scissors might accidentally damage catheter or injure patient (Gorski et al., 2021).
e. Stabilize IV catheter hub and clean site with antiseptic swab. Allow to dry completely.	Removes secretions around skin puncture site.
f. Place clean sterile gauze above insertion site and, using dominant hand, withdraw catheter using a slow, steady motion, keeping the hub parallel to the skin (see illustration). Do not raise or lift catheter before it is completely out of vein. Inspect end of catheter, being sure it is intact after removal.	Dry pad causes less irritation to puncture site. Removal technique avoids trauma to vein or hematoma formation. Inspection determines whether catheter tip is intact. Tip of catheter can break off and embolize, which is an emergency situation.
g. Keep gauze in place and apply continuous pressure to site for at least 30 seconds or until bleeding has stopped.	Controls bleeding and hematoma formation. Pressure should be applied until hemostasis occurs (Gorski, 2018).

CLINICAL JUDGMENT: *If patient receives anticoagulants or platelet inhibitors (e.g., low-dose aspirin, warfarin sodium, heparin) or has a low platelet count, apply steady pressure longer (for 5–10 minutes) and assess bleeding.*

h. Apply sterile folded gauze dressing over insertion site and secure with tape.	Maintains pressure to prevent bleeding and reduces bacterial entry into puncture site.

STEP 4f Remove intravenous catheter slowly, keeping catheter parallel to vein.

Continued

| **SKILL 42.3** | **MAINTENANCE OF AN INTRAVENOUS SYSTEM—cont'd** |

STEPS	**RATIONALE**
5. Dispose of all contaminated supplies in appropriate receptacle, remove and dispose of gloves, and perform hand hygiene.	Reduces transmission of microorganisms. Use appropriate disposal receptacle if patient is on hazardous drugs.
6. Help patient to a comfortable position and instruct on how to move and turn properly with VAD.	Restores comfort and sense of well-being. Instruction prevents accidental dislodgment of IV catheter.
7. Raise side rails (as appropriate) and lower bed to lowest position.	Promotes safety and prevents falls.
8. Place nurse call system in an accessible location within patient's reach. Instruct patient in its use.	Ensures patient can call for assistance if needed and promotes safety and prevents falls.

EVALUATION

1. Observe patient with a short-peripheral IV at least every 4 hours, or every 1 to 2 hours for patients who are critically ill, are sedated, or have cognitive deficits, or at established intervals per agency policy and procedure for:	Ensures delivery of infusion therapy as ordered.
a. Correct type and amount of solution infused and appearance of solution.	Ensures delivery of prescribed volume over prescribed time and decreases risk for fluid and electrolyte imbalance. Solution that becomes cloudy could be contaminated.
b. Leaking at connection sites	Minimizes risk of infection caused by breach in system integrity.
c. Function, intactness, and patency of IV system	Validates that IV line is patent and infusing correctly. Manipulation of catheter and tubing may affect rate of infusion.
d. IV-related complications by visually inspecting and gently palpating skin around and above IV site through the intact dressing	Identifies complications that compromise integrity of VAD or cause inaccurate IV solution flow rate.
2. Evaluate patient to determine response to therapy (e.g., laboratory values, I&O, weights, vital signs, postprocedure assessments).	Provides ongoing evaluation of patient's fluid status.
3. Monitor patient for signs of ECV excess, ECV deficit, or signs and symptoms of electrolyte imbalances.	Early recognition of complications leads to prompt treatment.
4. **Use Teach-Back:** "We talked about the importance of your IV solutions running as prescribed. I want to be sure I explained this clearly. Tell me in your own words what you should do if you notice that the IV is not dripping or you notice leaking." Revise your instruction now or develop a plan for revised patient/family caregiver teaching if patient/family caregiver is not able to teach back correctly.	Teach-back is an evidence-based health literacy intervention that promotes patient engagement, patient safety, adherence, and quality. The goal of teach-back is to ensure that you have explained medical information clearly so that patients and their families understand what you communicated to them (AHRQ, 2020).
5. For discontinuing short-peripheral IV access:	
a. Observe site for bleeding soon after procedure and redness, tenderness at site, drainage, or swelling during a later evaluation.	Detects bleeding after catheter removal. Detects local infection or postinfusion phlebitis (Gorski et al., 2021).
b. **Use Teach-Back:** "I want to be sure I explained why I removed the IV. Please tell me why you no longer need an IV." Revise your instruction now or develop a plan for revised patient/family caregiver teaching if patient/family caregiver is not able to teach back correctly.	Teach-back is an evidence-based health literacy intervention that promotes patient engagement, patient safety, adherence, and quality. The goal of teach-back is to ensure that you have explained medical information clearly so that patients and their families understand what you communicated to them (AHRQ, 2020).

UNEXPECTED OUTCOMES AND RELATED INTERVENTIONS

1. Flow rate is incorrect; patient receives too little or too much solution.
   - Notify health care provider if patient's anticipated infusion is 100 to 200 mL less than or greater than anticipated (per agency policy and procedure).
   - Evaluate patient for signs and symptoms of adverse effects of infusion (e.g., ECV excess or deficit).
   - Consult health care provider for new order to provide necessary fluid volume.
   - Check for positional IV site and reposition catheter; apply new dressing if necessary.
   - Check IV catheter for loss of patency or dislodgment; catheter may require replacement.
   - Check VAD site for complications.
2. Leaking occurs at IV connection.
   - Determine site of leaking and secure connection aseptically.
   - Apply new dressing if necessary (see Skill 42.4).
3. IV catheter is removed or dislodged accidentally.
   - Restart new short-peripheral IV line in other extremity or above previous insertion site if continued therapy is necessary (see Skill 42.1).
4. Catheter tip is missing after withdrawal.
   - Apply tourniquet high on extremity to restrict mobility of catheter embolus.
   - Immediately notify health care provider.

RECORDING AND REPORTING

- Record solution and tubing changes, type of infusion solution including any additives, volume of container, and rate of infusion. Record time of discontinuing solution or IV medication.
- When discontinuing a peripheral VAD, document condition of site, condition of the VAD (e.g., length of the catheter compared to length documented at insertion), reason for device removal, interventions during removal, dressing applied, date/time of removal, and any necessary continuing management for complications (Gorski et al., 2021).
- Document your evaluation of patient learning.
- Report details of tubing and or equipment change or discontinuing of IV. Report any complications, treatments; report any changes in IV catheter, tubing, and IV fluid type and rate.
- Notify the health care team of signs and symptoms of suspected catheter-related bloodstream infection and discuss the need for obtaining cultures before removing a peripheral IV catheter (Gorski et al., 2021).

HOME CARE CONSIDERATIONS

- Ensure that patient is able and willing to self-manage IV therapy (including changing IV containers) or that reliable family caregiver is at home and willing to provide IV care.
- Instruct patient or family caregiver in procedure for performing an IV solution and tubing change. Consider their cultural norms (e.g., health beliefs and comfort with caregivers using touch).
- Instruct patient or caregiver to notify health care provider if bleeding or drainage is noted at insertion site or if pain or tenderness occurs up to 4 days after catheter removal.

SKILL 42.4   CHANGING A SHORT-PERIPHERAL INTRAVENOUS DRESSING

Delegation and Collaboration

The skill of changing a short-peripheral IV dressing cannot be delegated to assistive personnel (AP). Delegation to licensed practical nurses (LPNs) varies by state nurse practice act. The nurse instructs the AP to:

- Report to the nurse if a patient indicates moistness or loosening of an IV dressing.
- Protect the IV dressing during hygiene and activities of daily living (ADLs).

Equipment

- Clean gloves
- Antiseptic swabs (alcohol-based 2% chlorhexidine gluconate [CHG] solution preferred, povidone-iodine, or 70% alcohol)
- Sterile adhesive remover
- Skin barrier protectant (film, cream, swab, or wipe)
- Engineered stabilization device or precut strips sterile tape
- Commercially available IV site protection device *(optional)*
- Sterile transparent semipermeable membrane (TSM) dressing or sterile 2 × 2– or 4 × 4–inch gauze pad

---

STEPS	RATIONALE
ASSESSMENT	
1. Determine agency policy regarding peripheral IV dressing changes. Transparent (TSM) dressings should be changed at least every 7 days (except neonatal patients) or immediately if dressing integrity is disrupted (e.g., lifted/detached on any border edge or within transparent portion of dressing, visibly soiled, presence of moisture, drainage, or blood) or if compromised skin integrity is present under the dressing (Gorski et al., 2021). Gauze dressings may be changed every 2 days or sooner if dressing is compromised (Gorski et al., 2021).	Dressing change increases risk of catheter displacement and is performed only if dressing is compromised.
2. Review EHR to determine patient's risk for developing a medical adhesive–related skin injury (MARSI) using adhesive devices or tape: age, dehydration, malnutrition, exposure to radiation therapy, underlying chronic conditions (e.g., diabetes, immunosuppression), and edema of extremity.	Common risk factors for MARSI (Fumarola et al., 2020).
3. Assess patient's and family caregiver's knowledge, experience, and health literacy regarding the need for continued IV therapy.	Ensures patient and family caregiver have the capacity to obtain, communicate, process, and understand basic health information (CDC, 2021).
4. Ask patient to describe history of allergies: known type of allergies and normal allergic reaction. Focus on latex, antiseptics, and adhesives. Check patient's allergy wristband.	Communication of patient allergies is essential for safe medication administration.
5. Perform hand hygiene and apply clean gloves. Observe present dressing for moisture and intactness. Determine whether moisture is from site leakage or external source.	Moisture is a medium for bacterial growth and contaminates dressing. Loose dressing increases risk for bacterial contamination of venipuncture site or displacement of VAD.
6. Inspect and gently palpate skin around and above IV site over dressing. Assess VAD for patency and signs and symptoms of IV-related complications (e.g., infiltration, occlusion of VAD, phlebitis, infection, patient complaints of pain, or leaking under dressing).	Unexplained decrease in flow rate requires investigating VAD placement and patency. Pain is associated with both phlebitis and infiltration.

Continued

SKILL 42.4	CHANGING A SHORT-PERIPHERAL INTRAVENOUS DRESSING—cont'd

STEPS	RATIONALE
7. Assess skin around dressing for temperature, color, moisture level, turgor, fragility, and integrity. Observe for local signs of irritation or skin damage at the site where any adhesive has been or will be applied.	Signs and symptoms of MARSI (Fumarola et al., 2020).
8. Remove and discard gloves in appropriate receptacle and perform hand hygiene.	Reduces transmission of infection.
9. Assess patient's goals or preferences for how skill is to be performed or what patient expects.	Allows care to be individualized to patient.

PLANNING

1. Close room curtains or door. Prepare environment by removing clutter from bedside and over-bed table.	Provides privacy. Prepares environment for efficient procedure.
2. Perform hand hygiene. Collect and organize equipment on clean over-bed or bedside table.	Reduces transmission of microorganisms. Keeps procedure organized and provides patient safety.
3. Explain procedure and purpose to patient and family. Explain that patient must hold affected extremity still and how long procedure will take.	Decreases anxiety, promotes cooperation, and gives patient time frame around which to plan personal activities.

IMPLEMENTATION

1. Identify patient using at least two identifiers (e.g., name and birthday or name and medical record number) according to agency policy. Compare identifiers with information on patient's MAR or medical record.	Ensures correct patient. Complies with The Joint Commission standards and improves patient safety (TJC, 2021a).
2. Perform hand hygiene and apply clean gloves.	Reduces transmission of microorganisms.
3. Remove existing dressing:	
a. For TSM dressing:	Technique minimizes discomfort during removal. Use of sterile adhesive remover on TSM dressing next to patient's skin loosens dressing without pulling. (Fumarola et al., 2020).
(1) Stabilize catheter with nondominant hand.	
(2) Loosen the edges of the TSM dressing with the fingers of the dominant hand by pushing the skin down and away from the TSM dressing.	
(3) With fingers of the dominant hand, loosen a corner of the dressing and stretch it horizontally in the opposite direction of the IV site (stretch-and-relax technique) (see illustration). Walk your fingers under the dressing to continue stretching it. One hand should continuously support the skin adhered to the TSM dressing.	
(4) This process can be repeated around the dressing. Use medical adhesive remover if needed to loosen the adhesive bond. Follow the manufacturer's instructions for use.	
b. For gauze dressing:	Guidelines for MARSI prevention (Fumarola et al., 2020).
(1) Stabilize catheter hub.	
(2) Remove tape strips by slowly lifting and removing each side toward the center of dressing. When both sides are completely loosened, lift the strip up from the center of the dressing.	
(3) Remove old dressing one layer at a time by pulling toward insertion site. Be cautious if tubing becomes tangled between two layers of dressing. Use medical adhesive remover if needed to loosen the adhesive bond of tape.	

STEP 3a(3) Remove transparent semipermeable membrane (TSM) dressing by pulling side laterally. (Courtesy I.V. House, St Louis, MO.)

STEPS	**RATIONALE**
4. Assess exposed VAD insertion site again for signs and symptoms of IV-related complications (Tables 42.12 to 42.14) or skin damage. If complication exists, determine whether VAD requires removal. Remove catheter if ordered by health care provider (see Skill 42.3).	Presence of complication may require VAD removal.
5. If catheter is to remain in place, assess integrity of engineered stabilization device. Continue to stabilize catheter and remove as recommended by manufacturer directions for use. Inspect for adhesive residue or signs of MARSI. Attach a new stabilization device (see Skill 42.1, Step 20). **Note:** Some stabilization devices are designed to remain in place for length of time VAD is in as long as adequate stabilization is evident.	Removing stabilization device allows for appropriate skin antisepsis before applying dressing and new stabilization device (Gorski et al., 2021). Stabilization prevents accidental dislodgement of VAD.

CLINICAL JUDGMENT: *Keep one finger stabilizing VAD at all times until stabilization device or dressing secures catheter hub. This requires careful planning regarding placing and opening supplies and how to work with one hand. If patient is restless or uncooperative, it is helpful to have another staff member help with procedure.*

6. While continuing to stabilize IV catheter, use adhesive remover to remove adhesive residue if needed. Then perform skin antisepsis to insertion site with antiseptic wipe using friction in back-and-forth motion for 30 seconds; allow to dry completely. If using alcohol or povidone-iodine, clean in concentric circle, moving from insertion site outward with the swab (see illustration). Allow antiseptic solution to dry completely.	Adhesive residue decreases ability of new tape to adhere securely to skin. Skin antisepsis reduces incidence of catheter-related infections (Gorski, 2018). Allow any skin antiseptic agent to fully dry for complete antisepsis (Gorski et al., 2021).
7. Apply skin protectant to area where you will apply tape, dressing, or engineered stabilization device. Allow to dry.	Coats skin with protective solution to maintain skin integrity, prevents irritation from adhesive, prevents MARSI, and promotes adherence of dressing (Fumarola et al., 2020).
8. While stabilizing VAD, apply new sterile dressing over site (procedures differ; follow agency policy).	Prevents accidental dislodgment of catheter and protects site from infection (Gorski et al., 2021).

CLINICAL JUDGMENT: *Because adhesive Band-Aids are not occlusive and nonsterile tape increases the risk for insertion site infection, do not use either over catheter insertion points.*

a. *TSM dressing:* Apply as directed in Skill 42.1, Step 21b.	Occlusive dressing protects site from bacterial contamination.
b. Gauze *dressing:* Apply as directed in Skill 42.1, Step 21c.	Less frequently used than transparent dressing.
9. *Option:* Apply protective device (e.g., I.V. House) over area if patient may pick at or bump dressing (see illustration).	Site-protection devices include vented plastic or stretch netting coverings and mitts for hands. Designed to reduce risk of phlebitis, infiltration, or catheter displacement from mechanical motion.
10. Anchor extension tubing or IV tubing alongside dressing on arm, and secure with tape directly over tubing. When using TSM dressing, avoid placing tape over dressing.	Prevents accidental dislodgment of VAD or tubing. More frequent dressing changes due to dislodgment are associated with greater risk of infection (Gorski et al., 2021).
11. Label dressing per agency policy. Label information should include date and time of original IV insertion, VAD gauge and length, and your initials.	Communicates type of device and time interval for dressing change.
12. Dispose of all contaminated supplies in appropriate receptacle, remove and dispose of gloves, and perform hand hygiene.	Reduces transmission of microorganisms. Use appropriate disposal receptacle if patient is on hazardous drugs.

STEP 6 Cleanse peripheral insertion site with antiseptic swab.

STEP 9 I.V. House protective device.

Continued

SKILL 42.4	CHANGING A SHORT-PERIPHERAL INTRAVENOUS DRESSING—cont'd

STEPS	RATIONALE
13. Help patient to a comfortable position and instruct on how to move and turn properly with VAD.	Restores comfort and sense of well-being. Instruction prevents accidental dislodgment of IV catheter.
14. Raise side rails (as appropriate) and lower bed to lowest position.	Promotes safety and prevents falls.
15. Place nurse call system in an accessible location within patient's reach. Instruct patient in its use.	Ensures patient can call for assistance if needed and promotes safety and prevents falls.

EVALUATION

1. Observe new dressing to be sure that it is applied, taped, and labeled properly. Continue routine monitoring of infusion system, IV site and dressing.	Validates quality of completed dressing change.
2. Ensure that flow rate is accurate.	Validates that IV line is patent and functioning correctly. Manipulation of catheter and tubing may affect rate of infusion.
3. **Use Teach-Back:** "I want to be sure I explained why I changed your IV dressing. Tell me why I needed to change your dressing." Revise your instruction now or develop a plan for revised patient/family caregiver teaching if patient/family caregiver is not able to teach back correctly.	Teach-back is an evidence-based health literacy intervention that promotes patient engagement, patient safety, adherence, and quality. The goal of teach-back is to ensure that you have explained medical information clearly so that patients and their families understand what you communicated to them (AHRQ, 2020).

UNEXPECTED OUTCOMES AND RELATED INTERVENTIONS

1. VAD is accidentally dislodged or removed.
   - Start new IV line in other extremity or proximal to previous insertion site if continued therapy is necessary.

2. IV site develops infiltration, phlebitis, MARSI, or local infection.
   - See Table 42.12.

RECORDING AND REPORTING

- Record time that peripheral dressing was changed, reason for change, type of dressing material used, patency of system and IV infusion rate, and description of venipuncture site.
- Document any complication of VAD.
- Document your evaluation of patient learning.
- Report to charge nurse or oncoming nursing shift that dressing was changed and any significant information about integrity of system.
- Report any complications to health care provider.

KEY POINTS

- Body fluids containing water, Na$^+$, and other electrolytes are distributed between extracellular fluid (ECF) and intracellular fluid (ICF) compartments by the processes of active transport, diffusion, osmosis, and filtration.
- The interplay of fluid intake (thirst, habit, social aspects, nonoral routes), fluid distribution (filtration and osmosis), and fluid output (skin, lungs, gastrointestinal [GI] tract, kidneys) determines the location, volume, and osmolality of body fluid.
- Fluid moves between blood vessels and interstitial fluid by filtration; water moves between ECF and ICF by osmosis; both processes maintain fluid and electrolyte balance.
- The relationship of electrolyte intake and absorption; electrolyte distribution between plasma, cells, and bones; and electrolyte output determines the plasma concentrations of potassium, calcium, magnesium, and phosphate ions.
- Acid-base homeostasis is the dynamic interplay of three processes—acid production, acid buffering, and acid excretion—regulated by metabolism and normal function of the kidneys and lungs.
- Extracellular fluid volume (ECV) deficit and excess are abnormal volumes of isotonic fluid in the vascular and interstitial compartments.
- Plasma electrolyte imbalances (e.g., potassium, sodium, calcium, and magnesium) affect body electrolyte content and/or abnormal distribution of electrolytes.
- Risk factors for fluid, electrolyte, and acid-base imbalances include factors that alter the regulatory mechanisms, such as age (very young or very old), environmental factors, increases in GI output, chronic diseases, trauma, and therapies such as medications or intravenous (IV) infusions.
- Clinical judgment in selecting nursing interventions requires the synthesis of knowledge about normal fluid and electrolyte balance, a patient's clinical condition and presenting signs, and the treatments ordered for a patient.
- The osmolality imbalances hyponatremia and hypernatremia manifest with decreased level of consciousness and abnormal serum Na$^+$ levels.
- Potassium imbalances manifest with bilateral muscle weakness, cardiac dysrhythmias, and abnormal serum K$^+$ levels.
- Calcium and magnesium imbalances manifest with altered neuromuscular excitability and abnormal serum Ca^{2+} or Mg^{2+} levels.
- Acid-base imbalances manifest with changes in level of consciousness, abnormal breathing patterns, and abnormalities of PaCO$_2$, HCO$_3^-$, and pH.
- Clinical assessments for ECV imbalances include sudden changes in body weight and markers of vascular and interstitial volume.
- During initiation and maintenance of IV therapy, nurses prevent infection by maintaining sterility and patency of the system by following safety guidelines and making clinical decisions regarding assessment findings, organized planning with appropriate

equipment, skillful implementation of procedural steps, evaluation of outcomes, and careful recording and reporting.

- Nurses monitor and take immediate action for complications of IV therapy, which include circulatory overload of the IV solution, infiltration and extravasation, phlebitis, local infection, air embolism, and bleeding at the insertion site.
- Actions to reduce phlebitis and infiltration include ensuring the IV catheter is secure and that standard ANTT® precautions are used to prevent infection during dressing and tubing changes.
- Blood and blood products must be matched to each patient to avoid incompatibility. Administration involves patient safety steps and use of special equipment, careful monitoring, and rapid knowledgeable action in case of transfusion reaction or other acute adverse events.
- Evaluation of interventions for specific fluid, electrolyte, and acid-base imbalances requires comparison of current clinical signs and symptoms and laboratory status with previous findings, discussion of patient concerns and expectations, and evaluation of patient learning about prevention and treatment of fluid, electrolyte, or acid-base imbalances.

REFLECTIVE LEARNING

- Think about Mrs. Mendoza and describe assessment data that put her at risk for fluid, electrolyte, and acid-base imbalances. (Recognize Cues)
- Considering the hospital setting, what environmental, organizational, or other factors did you see that influence Mrs. Mendoza's intake or output of fluid and electrolytes? (Analyze Cues)
- Considering her assessment data and history, what would be the priority clinical issues in caring for Mrs. Mendoza? (Prioritize Diagnoses)
- Consider Mrs. Mendoza's clinical situation and describe what nursing and medical interventions for management of fluid, electrolyte, and acid-base imbalances you could use. (Generate Solutions)
- Which nursing and medical interventions should have priority when implementing Mrs. Mendoza's care plan? (Take Action)
- Considering the implementation of Mrs. Mendoza's health care provider's orders, how would you determine if they were effective based on current assessment data? (Evaluate Outcomes)

REVIEW QUESTIONS

1. An IV fluid is infusing more slowly than ordered. The infusion pump is set correctly. Which factors could cause this slowing? (Select all that apply.)
   1. Infiltration at VAD site
   2. Patient lying on tubing
   3. Roller clamp wide open
   4. Tubing kinked in bedrails
   5. Circulatory overload
2. The nurse assesses pain and redness at a VAD site. Which action is taken first?
   1. Apply a warm, moist compress.
   2. Aspirate the infusing fluid from the VAD.
   3. Report the situation to the health care provider.
   4. Discontinue the IV infusion.
3. When delegating I&O measurement to assistive personnel, the nurse instructs them to record what information for ice chips?
   1. Two-thirds of the volume
   2. One-half of the volume
   3. One-quarter of the volume
   4. Two times the volume

4. What assessments does a nurse make before hanging an IV fluid that contains potassium? (Select all that apply.)
   1. Urine output
   2. ABGs
   3. Fullness of neck veins
   4. Serum potassium laboratory value in EHR
   5. Level of consciousness
5. The health care provider's order is 500 mL 0.9% NaCl intravenously over 4 hours. Which rate does the nurse program into the infusion pump?
   1. 100 mL/hr
   2. 125 mL/hr
   3. 167 mL/hr
   4. 200 mL/hr
6. Which of the following steps are necessary when inserting a short-peripheral IV? (Select all that apply.)
   1. Apply tourniquet to arm 10 to 15 cm (4–6 inches) above the intended insertion site.
   2. Cleanse skin using an approved antiseptic agent such as alcohol-based 2% chlorhexidine and allow to dry thoroughly.
   3. Stabilize the vein by placing the thumb proximal to the insertion site, stretching the skin in the direction of insertion.
   4. Use the smallest-gauge, shortest catheter available and insert with the bevel up at a 10- to 15-degree angle.
   5. Observe for blood in the flashback chamber of the catheter and advance the catheter off the needle into the vein.
   6. Release the tourniquet once the catheter has been secured and the dressing has been applied.
7. Place the following steps for discontinuing IV access in the correct order:
   1. Perform hand hygiene and apply gloves.
   2. Explain procedure to patient.
   3. Remove IV site dressing and tape.
   4. Use two identifiers to ensure correct patient.
   5. Stop the infusion and clamp the tubing.
   6. Carefully check the health care provider's order.
   7. Clean the site, withdraw the catheter, and apply pressure.
8. A patient has hypokalemia with stable cardiac function. What are the priority nursing interventions? (Select all that apply.)
   1. Fall prevention interventions
   2. Teaching regarding sodium restriction
   3. Encouraging increased fluid intake
   4. Monitoring for constipation
   5. Explaining how to take daily weights
9. A patient is admitted to the hospital with severe dyspnea and wheezing. ABG levels on admission are pH 7.26; PaO_2, 68 mm Hg; $PaCO_2$, 55 mm Hg; and HCO_3^-, 24. How does the nurse interpret these laboratory values?
   1. Metabolic acidosis
   2. Metabolic alkalosis
   3. Respiratory acidosis
   4. Respiratory alkalosis
10. Which assessment does the nurse use as a clinical marker of vascular volume in a patient at high risk of ECV deficit?
   1. Dryness of mucous membranes
   2. Skin turgor
   3. Fullness of neck veins when supine
   4. Fullness of neck veins when upright

Answers: 1. 1, 2, 4; **2.** 4; **3.** 2; **4.** 1, 4; **5.** 2; **6.** 1, 2, 4, 5; **7.** 6, 4, 2, 1, 5, 3, 7; **8.** 1, 4; **9.** 3; **10.** 3.

Rationales for Review Questions can be found on the Evolve website.

REFERENCES

Agency for Healthcare Research and Quality (AHRQ): *Health Literacy Universal Precautions Toolkit*, ed 2, Rockville, MD, 2020, Agency for Healthcare Research and Quality. https://www.ahrq.gov/health-literacy/quality-resources/tools/literacy-toolkit/healthlittoolkit2-tool5.html. Accessed May 2020.

American Association of Blood Banks (AABB): *Standards for blood banks and transfusion services*, ed 32, Bethesda, MD, 2020a, AABB.

American Association of Blood Banks (AABB): *Technical manual of the American Association of blood banks*, ed 19, Bethesda, MD, 2020b, AABB.

Berns J: *Patient education: hemodialysis (beyond the basics)*, 2020, UpToDate. https://www.uptodate.com/contents/hemodialysis-beyond-the-basics/print.

Boucher N, et al: Supporting Muslim patients during advanced illness, *Perm J* 21:16, 2017.

Burchum JR, Rosenthal LD: *Lehne's pharmacology for nursing care*, ed 10, St. Louis, 2019, Elsevier.

Centers for Disease Control and Prevention (CDC): *Blood safety basics*, 2020. https://www.cdc.gov/bloodsafety/basics.html. Accessed August 2, 2020.

Centers for Disease Control and Prevention (CDC): *What is health literacy?* 2021. https://www.cdc.gov/healthliteracy/learn/index.html. Accessed August 28, 2021.

DeLisle J: Is this a blood transfusion reaction? Don't hesitate; check it out, *J Infus Nurs* 41(1):42, 2018.

Emmett M, Hoorn E: *Serum anion gap in conditions other than metabolic acidosis*, 2020, UpToDate, 2020. https://www.uptodate.com/contents/serum-anion-gap-in-conditions-other-than-metabolic-acidosis.

European Pressure Ulcer Advisory Panel (EPUAP) and National Pressure Injury Advisory Panel (NPIAP) and Pan Pacific Pressure Injury Alliance: *Treatment of pressure ulcers/injuries: Clinical Practice Guideline. The International Guideline*, Emily Haesler (ED). EPUAP/NPIAP/PPPIA, 2019.

Felver L: Acid-base balance. In Giddens JF, editor: *Concepts for nursing practice*, ed 3, St. Louis, 2021a, Mosby.

Felver L: Fluid and electrolyte balance. In Giddens JF, editor: *Concepts for nursing practice*, ed 3, St. Louis, 2021b, Mosby.

Felver L: Fluid and electrolyte homeostasis and imbalances. In Banasik JL, Copstead LC, editors: *Pathophysiology*, ed 6, St. Louis, 2021c, Saunders.

Ferrari MC, et al: Watery stools and metabolic acidosis, *Intern Emerg Med* 12(4):487, 2017.

Giger JN, Haddad L: *Transcultural nursing: assessment and intervention*, ed 8, St. Louis, 2021, Elsevier.

Gizowski C, Bourque CW: The neural basis of homeostatic and anticipatory thirst, *Nat Rev Nephrol* 14(1):11, 2018.

Gorski L: *Manual of IV therapeutics: evidence-based practice for infusion therapy*, ed 7, Philadelphia, 2018, FA Davis.

Gorski LA, et al. *Infusion therapy standards of practice*, ed 8, *J Infus Nurs* 44(Suppl 1):S1–S224, 2021. doi:10.1097/NAN.0000000000000396.

Hadaway L: Stopcocks for infusion therapy: evidence and experience, *J Infus Nurs* 41(1):24, 2018.

Harding M, et al: *Lewis's medical-surgical nursing: assessment and management of clinical problems*, ed 11, St. Louis, 2020, Elsevier.

Heckle M, et al: ST elevations in the setting of hyperkalemia, *JAMA Intern Med* 178:133, 2018.

Heuschkel R, Duggan C: *Enteral feeding: gastric versus post-pyloric*, 2019, UpToDate. https://www.uptodate.com/contents/enteral-feeding-gastric-versus-post-pyloric.

Hockenberry MJ, et al: *Wong's nursing care of infants and children*, ed 11, St. Louis, 2019, Elsevier.

Hoorn EJ, et al: Diagnosis and treatment of hyponatremia: compilation of the guidelines, *J Am Soc Nephrol* 28(5):1340, 2017.

Huether S, et al: *Understanding pathophysiology*, ed 7, St. Louis, 2020, Elsevier.

Infusion Nurses Society (INS): *Policy and procedures for infusion therapy*, ed 5, Norwood, MA, 2016, Author.

Jacob J, Gaynes R: *Intravascular catheter-related infection: prevention*, 2021, UpToDate. https://www.uptodate.com/contents/intravascular-catheter-related-infection-prevention.

Kala J, Abudayyeh A: Magnesium: an overlooked electrolyte, *J Emerg Med* 52(5):741, 2017.

Kamel K, Halperin M: *Fluid, electrolyte, and acid–base physiology*, ed 5, St. Louis, 2017, Elsevier.

Kear TM: Fluid and electrolyte management across the age continuum, *Nephrol Nurs J* 44(6):491, 2017.

Kovesdy CP, et al: Potassium homeostasis in health and disease: a scientific workshop cosponsored by the National Kidney Foundation and the American Society of Hypertension, *Am J Kidney Dis* 70:844, 2017.

Lim F, et al: Managing hypocalcemia in massive blood transfusion, *Nursing* 47(5):26, 2017.

Mattox EA: Complications of peripheral venous access devices: prevention, detection, and recovery strategies, *Crit Care Nurs* 37(2):e1, 2017.

McDermott BP, et al: National athletic trainers' association position statement: fluid replacement for the physically active, *J Athl Train* 52(9):877, 2017.

Mount D: *Clinical manifestations and treatment of hypokalemia in adults*, 2019, UpToDate. https://www.uptodate.com/contents/clinical-manifestations-and-treatment-of-hypokalemia-in-adults.

Nagami GT, Hamm LL: Regulation of acid-base balance in chronic kidney disease, *Adv Chronic Kidney Dis* 24(5):274, 2017.

Norton JM, et al: Improving outcomes for patients with chronic kidney disease: part 1, *Am J Nurs* 117(2):22, 2017.

Occupational Safety and Health Administration (OSHA): *Bloodborne pathogens standard*, n.d., US Department of Labor. https://www.osha.gov/laws-regs/regulations/standardnumber/1910/1910.1030. Accessed August 2, 2020.

Pagana KD, et al: *Mosby's manual of diagnostic and laboratory tests*, ed 7, St. Louis, 2021, Elsevier.

Palmer BF, Clegg DJ: Electrolyte disturbances in patients with chronic alcohol-use disorder, *N Engl J Med* 377(14):1368, 2017.

Rice PL, Orgill DP: *Assessment and classification of burn injury*, 2021, Up To Date. https://www.uptodate.com/contents/assessment-and-classification-of-burn-injury#:~:text=1%20A%20burn%20is%20defined%20as%20a%20traumatic,the%20epidermal%20layer%20of%20skin.%20More%20items...%20. Accessed August 30, 2021.

Rong X, et al: Cultural factors influencing dietary and fluid restriction behaviour: perceptions of older Chinese patients with heart failure, *J Clin Nurs* 26(5/6):717, 2017.

Sterns R: *Etiology, clinical manifestations, and diagnosis of volume depletion in adults*, 2020, UpToDate. https://www.uptodate.com/contents/etiology-clinical-manifestations-and-diagnosis-of-volume-depletion-in-adults.

Sterns R: *Maintenance and replacement fluid therapy in adults*, 2021, UpToDate. https://www.uptodate.com/contents/maintenance-and-replacement-fluid-therapy-in-adults.

Teruya J: *Red blood cell transfusion in infants and children: selection of blood products*, 2020, UpToDate. https://www.uptodate.com/contents/red-blood-cell-transfusion-in-infants-and-children-indications.

The Joint Commission (TJC): *2021 National Patient Safety Goals*, Oakbrook Terrace, IL, 2021a, The Commission. https://www.jointcommission.org/en/standards/national-patient-safety-goals/. Accessed August 2, 2021.

The Joint Commission (TJC): *CLABSI Toolkit – Introduction Central Line-Associated Bloodstream Infection Introduction*, 2021b. https://www.jointcommission.org/resources/patient-safety-topics/infection-prevention-and-control/central-line-associated-bloodstream-infections-toolkit-and-monograph/clabsi-toolkit-–-introduction/. Accessed August 2, 2020.

Tingle J: Patient consent and conscientious objection, *Brit J Nurs* 26(2):118, 2017.

Touhy TA, Jett KF: *Ebersole and Hess' gerontological nursing & healthy aging*, ed 6, St. Louis, 2021, Elsevier.

US Food and Drug Administration: *Best way to get rid of used needles and other sharps*, 2021 https://www.fda.gov/medical-devices/safely-using-sharps-needles-and-syringes-home-work-and-travel/best-way-get-rid-used-needles-and-other-sharps. Accessed August 31, 2021.

Wagner J, Arora S: Oncologic metabolic emergencies, *Hematol Oncol Clin North Am* 31:941, 2017.

Wolf Z, Hughes R: Best practices to decrease infusion-associated medication errors, *J Infus Nurs* 42(4):183, 2019.

RESEARCH REFERENCES

Biasucci DG, et al: Targeting zero catheter-related bloodstream infections in pediatric intensive care unit: a retrospective matched case-control study, *J Vasc Access* 19(2):119, 2018.

Carson RA, et al: Evaluation of a nurse-initiated acute gastroenteritis pathway in the pediatric emergency department, *J Emerg Nurs* 43(5):406, 2017.

Fumarola S, et al: Overlooked and underestimated: medical adhesive-related skin injuries. Best practice consensus document on prevention, *J Wound Care* 29(Suppl 3c):S1, 2020.

Hawes JA, Lee KS: Reduction in central line-associated bloodstream infections in a NICU: practical lessons for its achievement and sustainability, *J Neonatal Netw* 37(2):105, 2018.

Helm R: Accepted but unacceptable: peripheral IV catheter failure, *J Infus Nurs* 42(3):149, 2019.

Horwitz L, Krumholz H: *Heart failure self-management*, 2020, UpToDate. https://www.uptodate.com/contents/heart-failure-self-management.

Kyle T, et al: Ionised calcium levels in major trauma patients who received blood en route to a military medical treatment facility, *Emerg Med J* 35(3):176, 2018.

Layne D, Anderson T: A collaborative approach to reducing central line-associated bloodstream infections, *J Nurs Care Qual* 34(4):285, 2019.

Matsui Y, et al: Evaluation of the predictive validity of thermography in identifying extravasation with intravenous chemotherapy infusions, *J Infus Nurs* 40(6):367, 2017.

Park LG, et al: Symptom diary use and improved survival for patients with heart failure, *Circ Heart Fail* 10:e003874, 2017.

Pironi L, et al: ESPEN guideline on home parenteral nutrition, *Clin Nutr* 39:1645–1666, 2020. https://www.espen.org/files/ESPEN-Guidelines/ESPEN_guideline_on_home_parenteral_nutrition.pdf. Accessed September 1, 2021.

Thoele K, et al: Optimizing drug delivery of small-volume infusions, *J Infus Nurs* 41(2):113, 2018.

Wei L, et al.: Chlorhexidine-impregnated dressing for the prophylaxis of central venous catheter-related complications: a systematic review and meta-analysis. *BMC Infect Dis* 19:429, 2019.

Sleep

OBJECTIVES

- Explain the effects that the 24-hour sleep-wake cycle has on biological function.
- Summarize mechanisms that regulate sleep.
- Outline the stages of a normal sleep cycle.
- Explain the functions of sleep.
- Compare and contrast the sleep requirements of different age-groups.
- Identify factors that normally promote and disrupt sleep.
- Compare and contrast characteristics of common sleep disorders.
- Interview a patient to conduct a sleep history.
- Select nursing interventions designed to promote normal sleep cycles for patients of all ages.
- Evaluate the effectiveness of sleep therapies.

KEY TERMS

Biological clocks

Cataplexy

Circadian rhythm

Excessive daytime sleepiness (EDS)

Hypersomnolence

Hypnotics

Insomnia

Narcolepsy

Nocturia

Nonrapid eye movement (NREM) sleep

Polysomnogram

Rapid eye movement (REM) sleep

Rest

Sedatives

Sleep

Sleep apnea

Sleep deprivation

Sleep hygiene

MEDIA RESOURCES

http://evolve.elsevier.com/Potter/fundamentals/

- Review Questions
- Concept Map Creator
- Case Study with Questions
- Audio Glossary
- Content Updates
- Answers to QSEN Activity and Review Questions

Susan, a newly hired family nurse practitioner at the health clinic, is getting ready to see her first patient of the day, Julie Arnold, a 51-year-old attorney. During her chart review, Susan notes that Julie was diagnosed with depression last year and takes an antidepressant. When Susan asks Julie how she is doing, Julie tells Susan that she is having difficulty sleeping. Julie is married and has two children in high school. Julie's husband, Blake, is an attorney with another law firm. He works long hours and often does not get home until late in the evening.

As Susan questions Julie further about her difficulty sleeping, Julie explains that she wakes up once or twice a night. She states, "I feel tired when I wake up, and I have trouble concentrating at work in the afternoon." Julie reports that because of her heavy work schedule, she has stopped her routine of walking 1 to 2 miles daily. She reports that she has no time for any exercise when she gets home because she needs to fix dinner for the family, care for her mother, and help the children with homework. Julie reports that she is going to bed between 12 a.m. and 1 a.m., which is 2 hours later than her usual bedtime. It takes her an hour to fall asleep. She says that she used to get 7 to 8 hours of sleep a night and now it is more like 5 to 6 hours. She drinks two to three cups of coffee after dinner while she is working on her cases before bedtime.

Julie also tells Susan that her 80-year-old mother, Louise, moved in with them 2 weeks ago. Louise was just discharged from a skilled nursing facility where she underwent rehabilitation after a hip fracture repair

from a fall at home. Louise has a history of hypertension, heart failure, diabetes mellitus, and osteoarthritis. Julie expresses concern about her mother, how she appears to be doing, and how Julie must take care of her in addition to her other work and home responsibilities. The plan is for Louise to stay with Julie and her family until she is strong enough to return to her own home. Julie helps her mother with her personal hygiene and other matters after dinner in the evening. Julie is concerned that her mother is having sleep problems, too, because she can hear Louise moving about at night and she looks very tired during the day. Julie says that taking care of her mother delays her getting started on the work that she brings home to review. Julie says to Susan, "I don't know how I can continue caring for everyone at home and working at the pace I have been keeping."

Proper rest and sleep are as important to health as good nutrition and adequate exercise. Physical and emotional health depend on the ability to fulfill these basic human needs. Individuals need different amounts of sleep and rest. Without proper sleep and rest, the ability to concentrate, make judgments, and participate in daily activities decreases, and irritability increases.

As a nurse, you will use critical thinking and clinical judgment to identify and treat patients' sleep pattern disturbances. To help patients you need to understand the nature of sleep, the factors influencing it, and patients' sleep habits. This understanding will help you gather and analyze assessment data to identify a patient's priority sleep problem. Patients require individualized approaches based on their personal habits, preferences, patterns of sleep, and the problems influencing sleep. A patient-centered nursing care plan with individualized nursing interventions is often effective in resolving short- and long-term sleep disturbances.

Sleep provides healing and restoration (Huether et al., 2020). Achieving the best possible sleep quality is important for the promotion of good health and recovery from illness. Patients who are ill often require more sleep and rest than patients who are healthy. However, the nature of illness often prevents some patients from getting adequate rest and sleep. The environment of a health care agency or long-term care facility and the activities of health care personnel often make sleep difficult. Some patients have preexisting sleep disturbances; others develop sleep problems because of an illness or hospitalization.

SCIENTIFIC KNOWLEDGE BASE

Physiology of Sleep

Sleep is a cyclical physiological process that alternates with longer periods of wakefulness. The sleep-wake cycle influences and regulates physiological function and behavioral responses.

Circadian Rhythms. People experience cyclical rhythms as part of their everyday lives. The most familiar rhythm is the 24-hour, day-night cycle known as the diurnal or circadian rhythm (derived from Latin: *circa*, "about," and *dies*, "day"). The suprachiasmatic nucleus (SCN) nerve cells in the hypothalamus control the rhythm of the sleep-wake cycle and coordinate this cycle with other circadian rhythms (Huether et al., 2020). Circadian rhythms influence the pattern of major biological and behavioral functions. The predictable changing of body temperature, heart rate, blood pressure, hormone secretion, sensory acuity, and mood depend on the maintenance of the 24-hour circadian cycle (Kryger et al., 2017).

Factors such as light, temperature, social activities, and work routines affect circadian rhythms and daily sleep-wake cycles. All people have biological clocks that synchronize their sleep cycles. This explains why some people fall asleep at 8 p.m., whereas others go to bed at midnight or early in the morning. Different people also function best at different times of the day.

Health care agencies or extended-care centers usually do not adapt care to an individual's sleep-wake cycle preferences. Typical hospital routines interrupt sleep or prevent patients from falling asleep at their usual time. Poor quality of sleep results when a person's sleep-wake cycle changes. Reversals in the sleep-wake cycle, such as when a person who is normally awake during the day falls asleep during the day, sometimes indicate a serious illness.

The biological rhythm of sleep frequently becomes synchronized with other body functions. For example, changes in body temperature correlate with sleep patterns. Normally, body temperature peaks in the afternoon, decreases gradually, and drops sharply after a person falls asleep. When the sleep-wake cycle becomes disrupted (e.g., by working rotating shifts), other physiological functions usually change as well. For example, a new nurse who starts working the night shift experiences a decreased appetite and loses weight. Anxiety, restlessness, irritability, and impaired judgment are other common symptoms of sleep cycle disturbances. Failure to maintain an individual's usual sleep-wake cycle negatively influences a patient's overall health.

Sleep Regulation. Sleep involves a sequence of physiological states maintained by highly integrated central nervous system (CNS) activity. It is associated with changes in the peripheral nervous, endocrine,

cardiovascular, respiratory, and muscular systems (Huether et al., 2020). Specific physiological responses and patterns of brain activity identify each sequence. Instruments such as the electroencephalogram (EEG), which measures electrical activity in the cerebral cortex; the electromyogram (EMG), which measures muscle tone; and the electrooculogram (EOG), which measures eye movements, provide information about some structural physiological aspects of sleep.

The major sleep center in the body is the hypothalamus (Chen et al., 2018). It secretes hypocretins (orexins) that promote wakefulness and rapid eye movement (REM) sleep. Prostaglandin D_2, L-tryptophan, and growth factors control sleep (Huether et al., 2020).

Researchers believe that the ascending reticular activating system (RAS) located in the upper brainstem contains special cells that maintain alertness and wakefulness. The RAS receives visual, auditory, pain, and tactile sensory stimuli. Activity from the cerebral cortex (e.g., emotions or thought processes) also stimulates the RAS. Arousal, wakefulness, and maintenance of consciousness result from neurons in the RAS releasing catecholamines such as norepinephrine (Kryger et al., 2017).

Current evidence suggests that two processes help to regulate sleep/wake cycles. The homeostatic process (Process S), which primarily regulates the length and depth of sleep; and the circadian rhythms (Process C: "biological time clocks"), which influence the internal organization of sleep and the timing and duration of sleep-wake cycles, operate simultaneously to regulate sleep and wakefulness (Kryger et al., 2017). Time of wake-up is defined by the intersection of Process S and Process C (Fig. 43.1).

Stages of Sleep. There are two sleep phases: nonrapid eye movement (NREM) sleep and rapid eye movement (REM) sleep (Box 43.1). In the classical definition of NREM sleep, people progress through four stages during a typical 90-minute sleep cycle. The American Academy of Sleep Medicine defines three stages in NREM sleep, combining stages 3 and 4 (Kryger et al., 2017). The quality of sleep from stage 1 through stage 3 becomes increasingly deep. Lighter sleep is characteristic of stages 1 and 2, when a person is more easily arousable. Stage 3 (formerly stages 3 and 4) involves a deeper sleep called slow-wave sleep, from which a person is more difficult to arouse (Kryger et al., 2017). REM sleep is the phase at the end of each 90-minute sleep cycle. During REM sleep there is

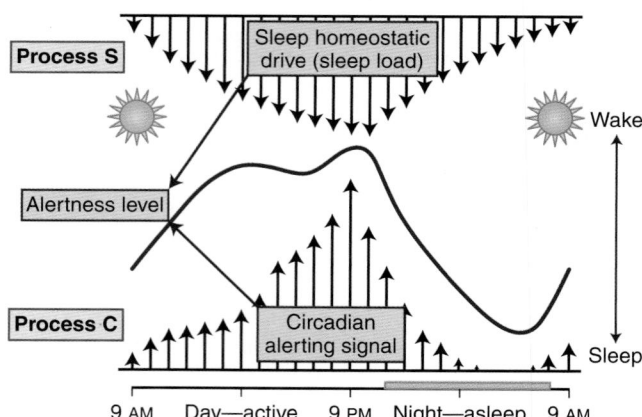

FIG. 43.1 Two-process model of sleep regulation shows the time course of the homeostatic process *(Process S)* and the circadian process *(Process C)*. Process S rises during waking and declines during sleep. The intersection of Process S and Process C defines the time of wake-up. (From Jankovic J, et al: *Bradley and Daroff's neurology in clinical practice*, ed 8, Philadelphia, 2022, Elsevier.)

BOX 43.1 Stages of the Sleep Cycle

NREM Sleep (75% of Night)

N1 (Formerly Stage 1)
- Stage of lightest level of sleep, lasting a few minutes.
- Decreased physiological activity begins with gradual fall in vital signs and metabolism.
- Sensory stimuli such as noise easily arouse sleeper.
- If awakened, person feels as though daydreaming has occurred.

N2 (Formerly Stage 2)
- Stage of sound sleep during which relaxation progresses.
- Arousal is still relatively easy.
- Brain and muscle activity continue to slow.

N3 (Formerly Stages 3 and 4)
- Called slow-wave sleep.
- Deepest stage of sleep.
- Sleeper is difficult to arouse and rarely moves.
- Brain and muscle activity are significantly decreased.
- Vital signs are lower than during waking hours.

REM Sleep (25% of Night)
- Vivid, full-color dreaming occurs.
- Stage usually begins about 90 minutes after sleep has begun.
- Stage is typified by autonomic response of rapidly moving eyes, fluctuating heart and respiratory rates, and increased or fluctuating blood pressure.
- Loss of skeletal muscle tone occurs.
- Gastric secretions increase.
- It is very difficult to arouse sleeper.
- Duration of REM sleep increases with each cycle and averages 20 minutes.

NREM, Nonrapid eye movement; *REM,* rapid eye movement.
Data from American Sleep Association: *What is sleep?* 2020, https://sleepassociation.org/patients-general-public/what-is-sleep, accessed July 18, 2020.; Kryger M, et al: *Principles and practice of sleep medicine,* 6e, St Louis, 2017, Elsevier; National Sleep Foundation: *What happens when you sleep?* 2020, https://sleepfoundation.org/how-sleep-works/what-happens-when-you-sleep, accessed July 18, 2020.

increased brain activity associated with rapid eye movements and muscle atonia.

Sleep Cycle. Normally an adult's routine sleep pattern begins with a presleep period during which the person is aware only of a gradually developing sleepiness. This period normally lasts 10 to 30 minutes. Individuals who have trouble falling asleep often remain in this stage for an hour or more. Once asleep a person usually passes through four to six complete sleep cycles, each cycle consisting of three stages of NREM sleep and a period of REM sleep, for a total of 90 to 110 minutes (Huether et al., 2020).

With each successive cycle, stage 3 of NREM sleep shortens, and REM sleep lengthens. REM sleep lasts up to 60 minutes during the last sleep cycle. Not all people progress consistently through the usual stages of sleep. For example, a sleeper fluctuates back and forth for short intervals between NREM stages 2 and 3 before entering REM sleep. The amount of time spent in each stage varies. The number of sleep cycles depends on the total amount of time that the person spends sleeping.

Functions of Sleep

Sleep functions as a time of restoration, memory consolidation, and preparation for the next period of wakefulness (Huether et al., 2020).

During NREM sleep biological functions slow. A healthy adult's heart rate decreases from a normal average of 70 to 80 beats/min to 60 beats/min or less during sleep, thus preserving cardiac function. Other biological functions that decrease during sleep are respirations, temperature, blood pressure, and muscle tone (Kryger et al., 2017).

Sleep restores biological processes. During NREM stage 3 sleep, the body releases human growth hormone for the repair and renewal of epithelial and specialized cells such as brain cells (Huether et al., 2020). Protein synthesis and cell division for the renewal of tissues also occur during rest and sleep. The basal metabolic rate lowers during sleep, which conserves the energy supply of the body (Huether et al., 2020).

REM sleep appears to be important for early brain development, cognition, and memory. Researchers associate REM sleep with changes in the brain, including cerebral blood flow and increased cortical activity. In addition, there is increased oxygen consumption and epinephrine release. These changes are associated with memory storage and learning (Huether et al., 2020).

The benefits of sleep often go unnoticed until a person develops a problem resulting from sleep deprivation. Current estimates show that 50 million to 70 million adults in the United States have some type of sleep disorder (American Sleep Association, 2020). Sleep deprivation affects immune function, metabolism, nitrogen balance, and protein catabolism. A loss of REM sleep often leads to confusion and suspicion. Prolonged sleep loss alters various body functions (e.g., mood, motor performance, memory, equilibrium) (National Sleep Foundation, 2020b). Individuals with sleep problems are also more likely to have chronic diseases such as hypertension, cardiovascular disease, diabetes mellitus, obesity, and depression (Jike et al., 2018; Tan et al., 2018). In addition, they may experience poorer quality of life and productivity (Jike et al., 2018). Millions of health care dollars are spent on indirect costs related to sleep deprivation, such as motor vehicle and industrial accidents, litigation, property damage, hospitalization, medical errors, and death (Hillman et al., 2018; Sleep Advisor, 2020).

Dreams. Although dreams occur during both NREM and REM sleep, the dreams of REM sleep are more vivid and elaborate, and some believe that they are functionally important to learning, memory processing, and adaptation to stress (Kryger et al., 2017). REM dreams progress in content throughout the night from dreams about current events to emotional dreams of childhood or the past. Personality influences the quality of dreams (e.g., a creative person has elaborate and complex dreams, whereas a depressed person dreams of helplessness).

Most people dream about immediate concerns such as an argument with a spouse or worries over work. Sometimes a person is unaware of fears represented in bizarre dreams. Clinical psychologists try to analyze the symbolic nature of dreams as part of a patient's psychotherapy. The ability to describe a dream and interpret its significance sometimes helps resolve personal concerns or fears.

Another theory suggests that dreams erase certain fantasies or nonsensical memories. Most people forget their dreams, and few have dream recall or do not believe they dream at all. To remember a dream, a person has to consciously think about it on awakening. People who recall dreams vividly usually awaken just after a period of REM sleep.

Physical Illness

Any illness that causes pain, physical discomfort, or mood problems such as anxiety or depression often results in sleep problems. People with such alterations frequently have trouble falling or staying asleep. Illnesses also force patients to sleep in unfamiliar positions. For example, it is difficult for a patient with an arm or leg in traction to rest comfortably.

Respiratory disease also interferes with sleep. Patients with chronic lung disease such as emphysema are short of breath and frequently cannot sleep without two or three pillows to raise their heads. Asthma, bronchitis, and allergic rhinitis alter the rhythm of breathing and disturb sleep. A person with a common cold has nasal congestion, sinus drainage, and a sore throat, which impair breathing and the ability to relax.

Connections among heart disease, sleep, and sleep disorders exist. Sleep-related breathing disorders are linked to increased incidence of nocturnal angina (chest pain), increased heart rate, electrocardiogram changes, high blood pressure, and risk of heart diseases and stroke (Huether et al., 2020). Hypertension often causes early-morning awakening and fatigue. Research also identifies an increased risk of sudden cardiac death in the first hours after awakening. Sleep disruptions and frequent arousals occur in people with heart failure because of the apnea, hypercapnia, and hypoxemia that develop as the disease progresses (Kryger et al., 2017). Hypothyroidism decreases the last sleep stage, whereas hyperthyroidism causes people to take more time to fall asleep.

Nocturia, or urination during the night, disrupts sleep and the sleep cycle, often leading to excessive daytime sleepiness or fatigue (Morris et al., 2021). After repeated awakenings to urinate, returning to sleep is difficult, and the sleep cycle is incomplete. Although this condition is most common in older adults with reduced bladder tone or in people with cardiac disease, diabetes mellitus, urethritis, or prostatic disease, it also occurs in a significant number of younger people (Cleveland Clinic, 2020).

Many people experience restless legs syndrome (RLS), which occurs before sleep onset. More common in women, older adults, and those with iron deficiency anemia, RLS symptoms include recurrent, rhythmical movements of the feet and legs. Severity of RLS in adults has been associated with vitamin D deficiency (Wali et al., 2018). Patients feel an itching sensation deep in the muscles. Relief comes only from moving the legs, which prevents relaxation and subsequent sleep. RLS is sometimes a relatively benign condition, depending on how severely sleep is disrupted. Primary RLS is a CNS disorder. Researchers believe early-onset RLS could be transmitted as an autosomal-dominant trait. Late-onset RLS may occur in those with anemia, pregnancy, uremia, renal failure, stress, or as a side effect of drugs (Chaiard and Weaver, 2019b). Late-onset RLS typically occurs in persons over 45 years of age and has a more rapid progression with more severe symptoms (Chaiard and Weaver, 2019b).

Researchers have found a relationship between sleep and gastrointestinal diseases. People with peptic ulcer disease often awaken in the middle of the night. Studies showing a relationship between gastric acid secretion and the stages of sleep are conflicting. One consistent finding is that people with duodenal ulcers fail to suppress acid secretion in the first 2 hours of sleep (Kryger et al., 2017). The challenge to researchers is to determine whether sleep disruption impacts gastrointestinal problems such as gastroesophageal reflux and irritable bowel disease or whether the diseases disrupt the sleep cycle (Parekh et al., 2018).

Sleep Disorders

Sleep disorders are conditions that, if untreated, generally cause disturbed nighttime sleep that results in one of three problems: insomnia, abnormal movements or sensation during sleep or when waking up at night, or excessive daytime sleepiness (EDS) (Kryger et al., 2017). Many adults in the United States have significant sleep problems from inadequacies in either the quantity or quality of their nighttime sleep and experience hypersomnolence daily (National Sleep Foundation, 2020c). Sleep disorders are more common in children and adolescents with either neurological conditions or neurodevelopmental disabilities (Maski and Owens, 2018). The American Academy of Sleep Medicine developed the International Classification of Sleep Disorders version 2 (ICSD-2), which classifies sleep disorders into eight major categories (Box 43.2).

BOX 43.2 Classification of Select Sleep Disorders

Insomnias
- Adjustment sleep disorder (acute insomnia)
- Inadequate sleep hygiene
- Behavioral insomnia of childhood
- Insomnia caused by medical condition

Sleep-Related Breathing Disorder
Central Sleep Apnea Syndromes
- Primary central sleep apnea
- Central sleep apnea caused by medical condition
- Obstructive sleep apnea syndromes

Hypersomnias of Central Origin (Not Caused by a Sleep-Related Breathing Disorder)
- Narcolepsy (four specified types)
- Menstrual-related hypersomnia
- Hypersomnia caused by a medical condition

Parasomnias
Disorders of Arousal
- Sleepwalking
- Sleep terrors

Parasomnias Usually Associated With REM Sleep
- Nightmare disorder
- REM sleep-behavior disorder

Other Parasomnias
- Sleep-related hallucinations
- Sleep-related eating disorder
- Sleep-related enuresis (bed-wetting)

Circadian Rhythm Sleep Disorders
Primary Circadian Rhythm Sleep Disorders
- Delayed–sleep phase type
- Advanced–sleep phase type

Behaviorally Induced Circadian Rhythm Sleep Disorders
- Jet lag type
- Shift work type
- Drug or substance use

Sleep-Related Movement Disorders
- Restless legs syndrome
- Periodic limb movements
- Sleep-related bruxism (teeth grinding)

Isolated Symptoms, Apparently Normal Variants, and Unresolved Issues
- Long sleeper
- Short sleeper
- Sleep talking

Other Sleep Disorders
- Physiological (organic) sleep disorders
- Environmental sleep disorder

Data from American Academy of Sleep Medicine: International classes of diseases and international classification of sleep disorders. In Kryger HM, et al: *Principles and practice of sleep medicine*, ed 6, St Louis, 2017, Saunders; and Thorpy MJ: Classification of sleep disorders, *Neurotherap 9* (4): 687, 2012.

Insomnia disorders are related to difficulty in falling asleep, frequent awakenings from sleep, short periods of sleep, or sleep that is nonrestorative (Kryger et al., 2017). Individuals with sleep-related breathing disorders have changes in respirations during sleep. Hypersomnias are sleep disturbances that result in daytime sleepiness and are not caused by disturbed sleep or alterations in circadian rhythms (Kryger et al., 2017). The circadian rhythm sleep disorders are caused by a misalignment between the timing of sleep and individual desires or the societal norm. The parasomnias are undesirable behaviors that occur usually during sleep. Sleep and wake disturbances are associated with many medical and psychiatric sleep disorders, including psychiatric, neurological, or other medical disorders. In sleep-related movement disorders the person experiences simple stereotyped movements that disturb sleep. The category of "isolated symptoms, apparently normal variants, and unresolved issues" includes sleep-related symptoms that fall between normal and abnormal sleep. The "other sleep disorders" category contains sleep problems that do not fit into other categories.

Sleep laboratory studies diagnose sleep disorders. A **polysomnogram** involves the use of EEG, EMG, and EOG to monitor stages of sleep and wakefulness during nighttime sleep. The Multiple Sleep Latency Test (MSLT) provides objective information about sleepiness and selected aspects of sleep structure by measuring eye movements, muscle-tone changes, and brain electrical activity during at least four napping opportunities spread throughout the day. The MSLT takes 8 to 10 hours to complete. Patients wear an Actigraph device on the wrist to measure sleep-wake patterns over an extended period of time, such as one week. Actigraphy data provide information about sleep time, sleep efficiency, number and duration of awakenings, and levels of activity and rest. An increasingly popular alternative, particularly among younger adults, is the use of technology in the form of sleep apps for smartphones (Adams et al., 2017). Further study of these sleep apps needs to be conducted to validate the accuracy of measurement of sleep (Lorenz and Williams, 2017).

Insomnia.
Insomnia is a symptom that patients experience when they have chronic difficulty in falling asleep, frequent awakenings from sleep, and/or a short sleep or nonrestorative sleep (Kryger et al., 2017). It is the most common sleep-related complaint, with up to 30% of adults suffering from the problem (American Sleep Association, 2020). It is commonly experienced by individuals diagnosed with depression (Hedges and Gotelli, 2019). People with insomnia experience EDS and insufficient sleep quantity and quality. However, frequently a patient gets more sleep than is realized. Insomnia often signals an underlying physical or psychological disorder. It occurs more frequently in and is the most common sleep problem for women.

People experience transient insomnia because of situational stresses such as family, work, or school problems; jet lag; illness; or loss of a loved one. Insomnia sometimes recurs, but between episodes a patient is able to sleep well. However, a temporary case of insomnia caused by a stressful situation can lead to chronic difficulty in getting enough sleep, perhaps because of the worry and anxiety that develop about getting sleep.

Insomnia is often associated with poor sleep hygiene, or practices that a patient associates with sleep (Hedges and Gotelli, 2019). If the condition continues, the fear of not being able to sleep is enough to cause wakefulness. During the day people with chronic insomnia feel sleepy, fatigued, depressed, and anxious. Treatment is symptomatic, including improved sleep-hygiene measures, biofeedback, cognitive techniques, and relaxation techniques (Hedges and Gotelli, 2019; Rash et al., 2019). Behavioral and cognitive therapies have few adverse effects and show evidence of sustained improvement in sleep over time (Haynes et al., 2018).

Sleep Apnea.
Sleep apnea is a disorder in which an individual is unable to breathe and sleep at the same time. There is a lack of airflow through the nose and mouth for periods from 10 seconds to 1 to 2 minutes in length. There are three types of sleep apnea: obstructive; central; and mixed apnea, which has both an obstructive and a central component.

The most common form is obstructive sleep apnea (OSA), which is a cessation or stopping of airflow despite the effort to breathe. It occurs when muscles or soft structures of the oral cavity or throat relax during sleep. The upper airway becomes partially or completely blocked, and nasal airflow diminishes (hypopnea) or stops (apnea). The person tries to breathe because chest and abdominal movements continue, which often results in loud snoring sounds. When breathing is partially or completely diminished, the person becomes sufficiently hypoxic and must awaken to breathe. Structural abnormalities such as a deviated septum, nasal polyps, narrow lower jaw, or enlarged tonsils sometimes predispose a patient to OSA. It is estimated that 9% to 21% of women and 24% to 31% of men in the United States are affected by OSA (American Sleep Association, 2020). However, a large majority of people are undiagnosed and untreated (Kryger et al., 2017).

Obesity and hypertension are major factors in OSA. Smoking, increasing age (greater than 65 years old), heart failure, alcohol, nasopharyngeal structural abnormalities, large neck circumferences, and menopause are increased risks for OSA (American Thoracic Society, 2017; Chaiard and Weaver, 2019a). Some research indicates that there may be a link between OSA and occupations in which the individual is exposed to and breathes in solvents (Schwartz et al., 2017).

Central sleep apnea (CSA) involves dysfunction in the respiratory control center of the brain. The impulse to breathe fails temporarily, and nasal airflow and chest wall movement cease. The oxygen saturation of the blood falls. The condition is common in patients with brainstem injury, stroke, obesity, muscular dystrophy, and encephalitis. Less than 10% of sleep apnea is predominantly central in origin. People with CSA tend to awaken during sleep and therefore complain of insomnia and EDS. Mild and intermittent snoring is also present.

Excessive daytime sleepiness (EDS) is a common complaint in people experiencing OSA and CSA. Other common symptoms of OSA include fatigue, morning headaches, irritability, depression, difficulty in concentrating, and a decrease in sex drive (Kryger et al., 2017). Untreated sleep apnea increases the risk of hypertension, diabetes mellitus, heart disease, and heart failure. Lifestyle changes, including a weight-reduction program in people who are obese, improved sleep hygiene, bilevel positive airway pressure (BPAP or BiPAP), continuous positive airway pressure (CPAP), surgery, hypoglossal nerve stimulation, and oral repositioning devices for the jaw and tongue, are treatment options for OSA (Chaiard and Weaver, 2019a).

OSA causes a serious decline in arterial oxygen saturation level. Patients are at risk for cardiac dysrhythmias, right-sided heart failure, pulmonary hypertension, angina attacks, stroke, and hypertension.

Patients with sleep apnea rarely achieve deep sleep. OSA affects quality-of-life issues such as concentration, social interactions, libido, and sexual activity and often is an embarrassment to a patient (Chaiard and Weaver, 2019a). Treatment includes therapy for underlying cardiac or respiratory complications and any emotional problems that occur because of the symptoms of this disorder.

Narcolepsy.
Narcolepsy is a dysfunction of the processes that regulate sleep and wake states. Excessive daytime sleepiness is the most common complaint associated with this disorder. During the day a person suddenly feels an overwhelming wave of sleepiness and falls asleep; REM sleep occurs within 15 minutes of falling asleep. Cataplexy, or sudden muscle weakness during intense emotions such as anger, sadness, or laughter that occurs at any time during the day, is

a symptom of narcolepsy type 1, differentiating it from narcolepsy type 2 (Chaiard and Weaver 2019b; Maski and Owens, 2018). Cataplexy usually lasts only a few seconds, but if the cataplectic attack is severe, a patient loses voluntary muscle control and falls to the floor (Maski and Owens, 2018). A person with narcolepsy often has vivid dreams that occur while falling asleep. These dreams are difficult to distinguish from reality. Sleep paralysis, or the feeling of being unable to move or talk just before waking or falling asleep, is another symptom. Some studies show a genetic link for narcolepsy (Chaiard and Weaver, 2019b).

A person with narcolepsy falls asleep uncontrollably at inappropriate times. When individuals do not understand this disorder, a sleep attack is easily mistaken for laziness, lack of interest in activities, or drunkenness. Typically, the symptoms first begin to appear in adolescence and are often confused with the EDS that commonly occurs in adolescents. Patients diagnosed with narcolepsy are treated with stimulants or wakefulness-promoting agents such as modafinil, armodafinil, methylphenidate, or sodium oxybate, which only partially increase wakefulness and reduce sleep attacks (Chaiard and Weaver, 2019b; Maski and Owens, 2018). Patients also receive antidepressant medications that suppress cataplexy and the other REM-related symptoms. Brief daytime naps no longer than 20 minutes help reduce subjective feelings of sleepiness. Other management methods that help are following a regular exercise program, practicing good sleep habits, avoiding shifts in sleep, strategically timing daytime naps if possible, eating light meals high in protein, practicing deep breathing, chewing gum, and taking vitamins (Kryger et al., 2017). Patients with narcolepsy need to avoid factors that increase drowsiness (e.g., alcohol, heavy meals, exhausting activities, long-distance driving, and long periods of sitting in hot, stuffy rooms).

Sleep Deprivation. Many patients experience sleep deprivation because of a sleep disorder. It can be acute or chronic and results from insufficient or disrupted sleep. Causes include illness (e.g., fever, difficulty breathing, or pain), emotional stress, medications, environmental disturbances (e.g., frequent interruptions in sleep during nursing care, noisy neighbors or pets), and variability in the timing of sleep as a result of shift work. Sleep disorders such as sleep apnea or insomnia can cause sleep deprivation.

With sleep deprivation, there is a decrease in the quantity or quality of sleep and/or an inconsistency in the timing of sleep. When sleep becomes interrupted or fragmented, changes in the normal sequencing of the sleep cycles occur. Cumulative sleep deprivation develops over time.

Individuals respond to sleep deprivation differently. Patients experience a variety of physiological and psychological symptoms (Box 43.3). The severity of symptoms is often related to the duration of sleep deprivation. The most effective treatment for sleep deprivation is to eliminate or correct the environmental factors and patient care activities that disrupt the sleep pattern. Nurses play an important role in identifying treatable sleep-deprivation problems. Evidence suggests that both chronic sleep deprivation and long sleep duration are associated with obesity, type 2 diabetes mellitus, poor memory, depression, digestive problems, and the development of cardiovascular disease (Jike et al., 2018).

Parasomnias. The parasomnias are sleep problems that are more common in children than adults and occur during non-REM or REM sleep (Maski and Owens, 2018). Some have hypothesized that sudden infant death syndrome (SIDS) is thought to be related to apnea, hypoxia, and cardiac arrhythmias caused by abnormalities in the autonomic nervous system that are manifested during sleep (Kryger et al., 2017). Because of an association between the prone position and the occurrence of SIDS, the American Academy of Pediatrics (AAP) recommends that parents place infants in the supine position during sleep to reduce the risk of sudden infant death syndrome (AAP, 2016).

Parasomnias that occur among older children include confusional arousals, somnambulism (sleepwalking), night terrors, nightmares, nocturnal enuresis (bed-wetting), body rocking, and bruxism (teeth grinding). Parasomnias in children are usually benign and the child will "outgrow" the problem (Maski and Owens, 2018). When adults have these problems, it often indicates more serious disorders. Specific treatment varies. However, in all cases it is important to support patients and maintain their safety.

REFLECT NOW

Interview a patient with chronic respiratory, renal, or cardiac disease. Discuss how the disease affects the patient's ability to sleep.

NURSING KNOWLEDGE BASE

Sleep and Rest

When people are at **rest**, they usually feel mentally relaxed, free from anxiety, and physically calm. Rest does not imply inactivity, although everyone often thinks of it as settling down in a comfortable chair or lying in bed. When people are at rest, they are in a state of mental, physical, and spiritual activity that leaves them feeling refreshed, rejuvenated, and ready to resume the activities of the day. People have their own habits for obtaining rest and can find ways to adjust to new environments or conditions that affect the ability to rest. They rest by reading a book, practicing a relaxation exercise, listening to music, taking a long walk, or sitting quietly.

Illness and unfamiliar health care routines easily affect the usual rest and sleep patterns of people entering a hospital or other health care setting. Nurses frequently care for patients who are on bed rest to reduce physical and psychological demands on the body in a variety of health care settings. However, patients on bed rest do not necessarily feel rested. Some experience emotional distress that prevents complete relaxation. For example, concern over physical limitations or a fear of being unable to return to their usual lifestyle causes such patients to feel stressed and unable to relax. You must always be aware of a patient's need for rest. A lack of rest for long periods causes illness or worsening of existing illness.

Normal Sleep Requirements and Patterns

Sleep duration and quality vary among people of all age-groups. For example, one person feels adequately rested with 4 hours of sleep, whereas another requires 10 hours. Nurses play an important role in identifying treatable sleep-deprivation problems.

BOX 43.3 Sleep-Deprivation Symptoms

Physiological Symptoms	Psychological Symptoms
• Ptosis, blurred vision	• Confused and disoriented
• Fine-motor clumsiness	• Increased sensitivity to pain
• Decreased reflexes	• Irritable, withdrawn, apathetic
• Slowed response time	• Agitated
• Decreased reasoning and judgment	• Hyperactive
• Decreased auditory and visual alertness	• Decreased motivation
• Cardiac arrhythmias	• Excessive sleepiness

Neonates. The neonate up to the age of 3 months averages about 16 hours of sleep a day, sleeping almost constantly during the first week. The sleep cycle is generally 40 to 50 minutes with wakening occurring after one to two sleep cycles. Approximately 50% of this sleep is REM sleep, which stimulates the higher brain centers. This is essential for development because the neonate is not awake long enough for significant external stimulation (Hockenberry et al., 2019).

Infants. Infants usually develop a nighttime pattern of sleep by 3 months of age. The infant normally takes several naps during the day but usually sleeps an average of 8 to 10 hours during the night for a total daily sleep time of 15 hours. About 30% of sleep time is in the REM cycle. (Hockenberry et al., 2019). Awakening commonly occurs early in the morning, although it is not unusual for an infant to wake up during the night.

Toddlers. By 2 years of age children usually sleep through the night and take daily naps. Total sleep averages 12 hours a day. After 3 years of age children often give up daytime naps (Hockenberry et al., 2019). It is common for toddlers to awaken during the night. The percentage of REM sleep continues to fall. During this period toddlers may be unwilling to go to bed at night because they need autonomy or fear separation from their parents.

Preschoolers. On average a preschooler sleeps about 12 hours a night (about 20% is REM). By 5 years of age children rarely take daytime naps except in cultures in which a siesta is the custom (Hockenberry et al., 2019). The preschooler usually has difficulty relaxing or quieting down after long, active days and has bedtime fears, awakens during the night, or has nightmares. Partial awakening followed by normal return to sleep is frequent (Hockenberry et al., 2019). In the awake period the child exhibits brief crying, walking around, unintelligible speech, sleepwalking, or bed-wetting.

School-Age Children. The amount of sleep needed varies during the school years. A 6-year-old averages 11 to 12 hours of sleep nightly, whereas an 11-year-old sleeps about 9 to 10 hours (Hockenberry et al., 2019). The 6- or 7-year-old usually goes to bed with some encouragement or by doing quiet activities. The older child often resists sleeping because the child is unaware of fatigue or has a need to be independent. When children experience sleep problems, it often causes sleep disruption in parents (Meltzer and Pugliese, 2017).

Adolescents. On average most adolescents get about 7 hours or less of sleep per night, although the recommended requirement is 8 to 10 hours (Jakobsson et al., 2020; National Sleep Foundation, 2018). The typical adolescent is subject to many changes, such as school demands, after-school social activities, and part-time jobs, which reduce the time spent sleeping (Bruce et al., 2017). Adolescents perceived additional causes of poor sleep to be stress, technology use, poor sleep habits and routines, worry about relationships and the future, and feelings of anxiety and depression (Jakobsson et al., 2020). Adolescents typically have electronic devices such as televisions, computers, smartphones, or video games in their rooms, which further contributes to sleep disruption, poor sleep quality, and decreased amount of sleep (Bruce et al., 2017; Shimura et al., 2018). Shortened sleep time often results in EDS, which frequently leads to reduced performance and failures in school, obesity, vulnerability to accidents, and increased use of alcohol (Litsfeldt et al., 2020; National Sleep Foundation, 2020d). Adolescents' mood and behavior are affected by duration of sleep. Less sleep is associated with mood changes such as depression, anger, and anxiety (Short et al., 2020).

Young Adults. Most young adults average 6 to 8½ hours of sleep a night. Approximately 20% of sleep time is REM sleep, which remains consistent throughout life. It is common for the stresses of jobs, family relationships, and social activities to lead to insomnia, and some may use medication to help them sleep. Daytime sleepiness contributes to an increased number of accidents, decreased productivity, and interpersonal problems in this age-group.

Pregnancy increases the need for sleep and rest. However, a majority of pregnant women describe variations in sleep habits (Christian et al., 2019). Sleep disruption occurs due to pregnancy-related hormone changes and the anatomical and physiological changes that occur in the body to maintain the pregnancy (Christian et al., 2019). First-trimester sleep disturbances include a reduction in overall sleep time and quality. Daytime drowsiness, insomnia, and nighttime awakenings also increase because of frequent nocturnal voiding. These disturbances level off in the second trimester. Insomnia, periodic limb movements, RLS, and sleep-disordered breathing are common problems during the third trimester of pregnancy (Kryger et al., 2017). Sleep quality is improved in pregnant women who regularly exercise (Yang et al., 2020).

Middle Adults. The recommended sleep requirement for adults is 7 to 9 hours per night (National Sleep Foundation, 2020c). During middle adulthood the total time spent sleeping at night begins to decline. The amount of stage 4 sleep begins to fall, a decline that continues with advancing age. Insomnia is particularly common, probably because of the changes and stresses of middle age. Anxiety, depression, or certain physical illnesses cause sleep disturbances. Women experiencing menopausal symptoms often experience insomnia.

Older Adults. Sleeping difficulties increase with age. Approximately 40% of older adults report problems with sleep (Kryger et al., 2017; National Sleep Foundation, 2020a). Older adults spend more time in stage 1 and less time in stages 3 and 4 (NREM sleep); some older adults have almost no NREM stage 4 or deep sleep. Episodes of REM sleep tend to shorten. Older adults experience fewer episodes of deep sleep and more episodes of lighter sleep (Miner and Kryger, 2020). They tend to awaken more often during the night, and it takes more time for them to fall asleep. To compensate they increase the number of naps taken during the day. Older adults often experience excessive daytime sleepiness, which can lead to decreased physical abilities and falls (Miner and Kryger, 2020).

Older adults who have a chronic illness often experience sleep disturbances. For example, an older adult with arthritis frequently has difficulty sleeping because of painful joints. Changes in sleep patterns are often caused by changes in the CNS that affect the regulation of sleep. Many older adults with insomnia have co-morbid mental health or medical conditions, take medications that disrupt sleep patterns, or use drugs or alcohol. Sensory impairment reduces an older person's sensitivity to time cues that maintain circadian rhythms.

Factors Influencing Sleep

Many factors affect the quantity and quality of sleep. Often a single factor is not the only cause for a sleep problem. Physiological, psychological, and environmental factors frequently alter the quality and quantity of sleep.

Drugs and Substances. Sleepiness, insomnia, and fatigue often result as a direct effect of commonly prescribed medications (Box 43.4). These medications alter sleep and weaken daytime alertness, which is problematic (Kryger et al., 2017). Medications prescribed for sleep often cause more problems than benefits. Older adults take a variety of drugs to control or treat chronic illness, and the combined effects of

BOX 43.4 Drugs and Their Effects on Sleep

Hypnotics
- Interfere with reaching deeper sleep stages
- Provide only temporary (1-week) increase in quantity of sleep
- Eventually cause "hangover" during day; excess drowsiness, confusion, decreased energy
- Sometimes worsen sleep apnea in older adults

Antidepressants and Stimulants
- Suppress REM sleep
- Decrease total sleep time

Alcohol
- Speeds onset of sleep
- Reduces REM sleep
- Awakens person during night and causes difficulty returning to sleep

Caffeine
- Prevents person from falling asleep
- Causes person to awaken during night
- Interferes with REM sleep

Diuretics
- Nighttime awakenings caused by nocturia

Beta-Adrenergic Blockers
- Cause nightmares
- Cause insomnia
- Cause awakening from sleep

Benzodiazepines
- Alter REM sleep
- Increase sleep time
- Increase daytime sleepiness

Nicotine
- Decreases total sleep time
- Decreases REM sleep time
- Causes awakening from sleep
- Causes difficulty staying asleep

Opiates
- Suppress REM sleep
- Cause increased daytime drowsiness

Anticonvulsants
- Decrease REM sleep time
- Cause daytime drowsiness

their drugs often seriously disrupt sleep. Some substances such as L-tryptophan, a natural protein found in foods such as milk, cheese, and meats, promote sleep.

Lifestyle. A person's daily routine influences sleep patterns. An individual working a rotating shift (e.g., 2 weeks of days followed by a week of nights) often has difficulty adjusting to the altered sleep schedule. For example, the body's internal clock is set at 11 p.m., but the work schedule forces sleep at 9 a.m. instead. The individual can sleep only 3 or 4 hours because the body clock perceives that it is time to be awake and active. Difficulties maintaining alertness during work time result in decreased and even hazardous performance. After several weeks of working a night shift, a person's biological clock usually does adjust. Other alterations in routines that disrupt sleep patterns include performing unaccustomed heavy work, engaging in late-night social activities, and changing evening mealtime.

Usual Sleep Patterns. In the past century the amount of sleep obtained nightly by U.S. citizens has decreased, causing many Americans to be sleep deprived and to experience excessive sleepiness during the day. Sleepiness becomes pathological when it occurs at times when individuals need or want to be awake. People who experience temporary sleep deprivation because of an active social evening or lengthened work schedule usually feel sleepy the next day. However, they are able to overcome these feelings even though they have difficulty performing tasks and remaining attentive. Chronic lack of sleep is much more serious and causes serious alterations in the ability to perform daily functions. Sleepiness tends to be most difficult to overcome during sedentary (inactive) tasks such as driving. An increasingly common contributor to EDS is the use of technology close to bedtime, such as watching television, talking or texting on a cell phone, or reading information on electronic devices.

Emotional Stress. Worry over personal problems or a situation frequently disrupts sleep. Emotional stress causes a person to be tense and often leads to frustration when sleep does not occur. Stress also causes a person to try too hard to fall asleep, to awaken frequently during the sleep cycle, or to oversleep. Continued stress causes poor sleep habits.

Older adults frequently experience losses that lead to emotional stress, such as retirement, physical impairment, or the death of a loved one. Older adults and other individuals who experience depressive mood problems experience delays in falling asleep, earlier appearance of REM sleep, frequent or early waking, feelings of sleeping poorly, and daytime sleepiness.

Environment. The physical environment in which a person sleeps significantly influences the ability to fall asleep and remain asleep. Good ventilation is essential for restful sleep. The size, firmness, and position of the bed affect the quality of sleep. If a person usually sleeps with another individual, sleeping alone often causes wakefulness. On the other hand, sleeping with a restless or snoring bed partner disrupts sleep.

In hospitals and other inpatient agencies, noise creates a problem for patients. Noise in hospitals is usually new or strange and often loud. Thus, patients wake easily. This problem is greatest the first night of hospitalization, when patients often experience increased total wake time, increased awakenings, and decreased REM sleep and total sleep time. People-induced noises (e.g., nursing activities) are sources of increased sound levels. ICUs are often louder because of staff, monitor alarms, and equipment. Close proximity of patients, noise from confused and ill patients, ringing alarm systems and telephones, and disturbances caused by emergencies make the environment unpleasant. Noise causes increased agitation, delayed healing, impaired immune function, and increased blood pressure, heart rate, and stress (Patel et al., 2018).

Light levels affect the ability to fall asleep. Some patients prefer a dark room, whereas others such as children or older adults prefer keeping a soft light on during sleep. Patients also have trouble sleeping because of the room temperature. A room that is too warm or too cold often causes a patient to become restless.

Exercise and Fatigue. A person who is moderately fatigued usually achieves restful sleep, especially if the fatigue is the result of enjoyable work or exercise. Exercising 2 hours or more before bedtime allows the body to cool down and maintain a state of fatigue that promotes relaxation. However, excess fatigue resulting from exhausting or stressful work makes falling asleep difficult. This is often seen in grade-school children and adolescents who keep long, stressful schedules because of school, social activities, and work.

Food and Caloric Intake. Good eating habits are important for proper sleep. Eating a large, heavy, and/or spicy meal at night often results in indigestion that interferes with sleep. Caffeine, alcohol, and nicotine consumed in the evening produce insomnia. Coffee, tea, cola, and chocolate contain caffeine and xanthines, which cause sleeplessness. Thus, drastically reducing or avoiding these substances can improve sleep. Some food allergies cause insomnia. A milk allergy sometimes causes nighttime waking and crying or colic in infants.

Weight loss or gain influences sleep patterns. Weight gain contributes to OSA because of increased size of the soft tissue structures in the upper airway (Kryger et al., 2017). Weight loss caused by semistarvation diets sometimes causes sleep disorders such as reduced sleep and insomnia.

Susan reviewed Julie's electronic health record before their first meeting. After talking with Julie, Susan recognizes that both Julie and Louise are experiencing sleep problems. She identifies the need to review information on the mechanisms of sleep, the sleep cycle, changes in sleep that happen with aging, and evidence-based research on best strategies to promote sleep. Susan pays attention to literature that discusses the relationship between sleep problems and depression. Susan recognizes that Julie is experiencing caregiver stress. Susan also searches the literature for information on caregiver stress and effective coping strategies. Susan plans to gather information on sleep in older adults to help Julie resolve Louise's sleep problems. Susan reviews information about hip fracture recovery and how Louise's chronic illnesses could affect her recovery so that she can answer Julie's questions about her mother. Susan also gathers information to share with Julie on fall prevention of older adults in the home so that home modifications can be made to permit Louise to safely return to her own home.

CRITICAL THINKING

Successful critical thinking requires a synthesis of knowledge, experience, environmental factors, critical thinking attitudes, and intellectual and professional standards. Sound clinical judgments require you to anticipate the information, analyze the data, and make decisions regarding your patient's care. During assessment consider all elements to build toward making an appropriate nursing diagnosis.

Integrate knowledge from nursing and other disciplines such as pharmacology and psychology, previous experiences, and information gathered from patients to understand sleep problems and their effect on a patient. Know the neurophysiological changes that occur in a patient through the sleep cycle. In addition, use communication principles that contribute to assessing a patient's behaviors that arise from lack of sleep. Give attention to determining the patient's perception of the situation and ability to resolve the sleep problem.

Personal experience with a sleep problem and experience with patients prepares you to know effective forms of sleep therapies. Experience teaches you to understand the patient's perspective and to recognize that no two people are alike. Experience with patients also helps you to recognize responses to sleep deprivation. In addition, personal experiences with sleep problems help you better understand a patient experiencing adverse effects from sleep problems.

You use critical thinking attitudes such as perseverance, confidence, and discipline to complete a comprehensive assessment and develop a patient-centered, individualized plan of care to successfully manage the sleep problem. Patients experiencing sleep problems are often overwhelmed and look to you as the expert to help them resolve their sleep issues.

Professional standards such as the *Nursing Scope and Standards of Practice* (American Nurses Association, 2021), *Clinical Practice Guidelines for the Pharmacologic Treatment of Chronic Insomnia in Adults: An American Academy of Sleep Medicine Clinical Practice Guideline* (Sateia et al., 2017), and "Sleep Disorders in the Older Adult" in *Evidence-based Geriatrics Nursing Protocols for Best Practice* (Morris et al., 2021) provide valuable guidelines to assess and address the needs of patients with sleep disorders.

REFLECT NOW

Consider your lifestyle choices. What factors contribute to promoting or disrupting your sleep? What changes can you make that will improve your sleep?

❖ NURSING PROCESS

Apply the nursing process and use sound clinical judgment and a critical thinking approach in your care of patients. The nursing process provides a clinical decision-making approach for you to develop and implement an individualized patient-centered plan of care.

◆ Assessment

During the assessment process, thoroughly assess each patient and critically analyze findings to ensure that you make patient-centered clinical decisions required for safe nursing care (Fig. 43.2).

Through the Patient's Eyes. Sleep is a subjective experience. Only the patient can report whether it is sufficient and restful. If the patient is satisfied with the quantity and quality of sleep received, you consider it normal, and the nursing history that you will collect is brief. If a patient admits to or suspects a sleep problem, you will need a detailed history and assessment. If a patient has an obvious sleep problem, consider asking whether the patient's sleep partner can be approached for further assessment data.

A poor night's sleep for a patient often starts a vicious cycle of anticipatory anxiety. The patient fears that sleep will again be disturbed while trying harder and harder to sleep. Use a skilled and caring approach to assess the patient's sleep needs. A caring nurse individualizes care for each patient. Always ask patients what they expect regarding sleep. This includes asking about the interventions that they currently use and how successful they are. It is important to understand patients' expectations regarding their sleep pattern. When they ask for help because of sleep disturbances, they typically expect a nurse to respond promptly to help them improve the quantity and quality of their sleep.

Sleep Assessment. Most people can provide a reasonably accurate estimate of their sleep patterns, particularly if any changes have occurred. Aim your assessment at first understanding the characteristics of the patient's sleep problem and usual sleep habits so that you incorporate ways for promoting sleep into nursing care. For example, if the nursing history reveals that a patient always reads before falling asleep, it makes sense to offer reading material at bedtime.

Sources for Sleep Assessment. Usually patients are the best resource for describing sleep problems and how they are a change from their usual sleep and waking patterns. Often the patient knows the cause for sleep problems, such as a noisy environment or worry over a relationship.

In addition, bed partners can provide information about patients' sleep patterns that help reveal the nature of certain sleep disorders. For example, partners of patients with sleep apnea often complain that the patients' snoring disturbs their sleep. Ask bed partners (if the patient agrees) whether patients have breathing pauses during sleep and how frequently the apneic attacks occur. Some partners mention becoming fearful when patients apparently stop breathing for periods.

When caring for children, seek information about sleep patterns from parents or guardians because they are usually a reliable source of information. Hunger, excessive warmth, and separation anxiety often contribute to an infant's difficulty in going to sleep or frequent awakenings during the night. Parents of infants need to keep a 24-hour log of their infant's waking and sleeping behavior for several days to determine the cause of the problem. Describing the infant's eating pattern and sleeping environment in the log will help identify which factors are influencing the baby's sleeping behavior. Older children often are able to relate fears or worries that inhibit their ability to fall asleep. If children frequently awaken in the middle of bad dreams, parents are able to identify the problem but perhaps do not understand the meaning of

FIG. 43.2 Critical thinking model for sleep assessment. (Clinical Judgment Measurement Model copyright © NCSBN. All rights reserved.)

the dreams. Ask parents to describe the typical behavior patterns that foster or impair sleep. For example, excessive stimulation from active play or visiting friends predictably impairs sleep. With chronic sleep problems, parents need to relate the duration of the problem, its progression, and children's responses.

Tools for Sleep Assessment. Two effective subjective measures of sleep are the Epworth Sleepiness Scale and the Pittsburgh Sleep Quality Index. The Epworth Sleepiness Scale contains eight questions about the likeliness of a patient being sleepy during certain activities (e.g., watching television, reading, sitting and talking with someone) on a scale of 0 (would never doze or sleep) to 3 (high chance of dozing or sleeping). A score of 0 to 5 indicates lower normal daytime sleepiness; 6 to 10 is considered higher than normal daytime sleepiness; a score of 11 or 12 is mild excessive daytime sleepiness; 13 to 15 is moderate excessive daytime sleepiness; and a score of 16 to 24 is severe excessive daytime sleepiness (Johns, n.d.). The scale is available at http://epworthsleepinessscale.com/about-the-ess/. The second tool, the Pittsburgh Sleep Quality Index, assesses sleep quality and patterns (Mollayeva et al., 2016). This scale is available at https://www.opapc.com/uploads/documents/PSQI.pdf.

Another brief, effective method for assessing sleep quality is the use of a visual analog scale. Draw a straight horizontal line 100 mm (4 inches) long. Opposing statements such as "best night's sleep" and "worst night's sleep" are at opposite ends of the line. Ask patients to place a mark on the horizontal line at the point corresponding to their perceptions of the previous night's sleep. Measuring the distances of the mark along the line in millimeters offers a numerical value for

satisfaction with sleep. Use the scale repeatedly to show change over time. Such a scale is useful to assess an individual patient, not to compare patients.

Another brief, subjective method to assess sleep is a numeric scale with a 0-to-10 sleep rating. Ask individuals to separately rate the quantity and quality of their sleep on the scale. Instruct them to indicate with a number between 0 and 10 their sleep quantity and then their quality of sleep, with 0 being the worst sleep and 10 being the best.

Sleep History. When you suspect a patient has a sleep problem, assess the quality and characteristics of sleep in greater depth by asking the patient to describe the problem. This includes recent changes in sleep patterns, sleep symptoms experienced during waking hours, the use of prescribed or over-the-counter sleep medications, diet and intake of substances such as caffeine or alcohol that influence sleep, and recent life events that have affected the patient's mental and emotional status.

Description of Sleeping Problems. Conduct a more detailed history when a patient has a persistent or what appears to be a serious sleep problem. Open-ended questions help a patient describe a problem more fully. A general description of the problem followed by more focused questions usually reveals specific characteristics that are useful in planning therapies. To begin, you need to understand the nature of the sleep problem, its signs and symptoms, its onset and duration, its severity, any predisposing factors or causes, and the overall effect on the patient. Ask specific questions related to the sleep problem (Box 43.5).

Proper questioning helps to determine the type of sleep disturbance and the nature of the problem. Box 43.6 provides examples of

BOX 43.5   Nursing Assessment Questions

Nature of the Problem
- Describe the type of sleep problem you're having.
- Why do you think you are not getting enough sleep?
- Describe a recent night's sleep. Is this similar to your usual sleep? How is this sleep different from your usual sleep?

Signs and Symptoms
- Do you have difficulty falling asleep, staying asleep, or waking up?
- Have you been told that you snore loudly?
- Do you have headaches when awakening?

Onset and Duration of Signs and Symptoms
- When did you notice the problem?
- What do you do to relieve the symptom?
- How long has this problem lasted?

Severity
- How long does it take you to fall asleep?
- How often during the week do you have trouble falling asleep?
- On average, how many hours of sleep a night did you get this week?
- How does this compare to your usual amount of sleep?
- What do you do when you awaken during the night or too early in the morning?

Predisposing Factors
- What do you do just before you go to bed?
- Have you recently had any changes at work or at home?
- How is your mood? Have you noticed any changes recently?
- Which medications or recreational drugs do you take on a regular basis?
- Are you taking any new prescriptions or over-the-counter medications?
- Do you eat food (spicy or greasy foods) or drink substances (alcohol or caffeinated beverages) that affect your sleep?
- Do you have a physical illness that affects your sleep?
- Does anyone in your family have a history of sleep problems?

Effect on Patient
- How has the loss of sleep affected you?
- Do you feel excessively sleepy or irritable or have trouble concentrating during waking hours?
- Do you have trouble staying awake? Have you fallen asleep at the wrong times (e.g., while driving, sitting quietly in a meeting)?

BOX 43.6   Questions to Ask to Assess for Specific Sleep Disorders

Impaired Sleep
- How easily do you fall asleep?
- Do you fall asleep and have difficulty staying asleep? How many times do you awaken? Do you awaken at the same time?
- What time do you awaken in the morning? What causes you to awaken early?
- What do you do to prepare for sleep? To improve your sleep?
- What do you think about as you try to fall asleep?
- How often do you have trouble sleeping?

Sleep Apnea
- Do you snore loudly? Does anyone else in your family snore loudly?
- Has anyone ever told you that you often stop breathing for short periods during sleep? (Spouse or bed partner/roommate may report this.)
- Do you experience headaches after awakening?
- Do you have difficulty staying awake during the day?

Narcolepsy
- Do you fall asleep at the wrong times? (Friends or relatives may report this.)
- Do you have episodes of losing muscle control or falling to the floor?
- Have you ever had the feeling of being unable to move or talk just before waking or falling asleep?
- Do you have vivid, lifelike dreams when going to sleep or awakening?

additional questions for you to ask a patient when you suspect specific sleep disorders. The STOP-BANG sleep assessment tool is a reliable evidence-based tool used to screen for OSA and is frequently used in preanesthesia and/or preoperative assessments (see Chapter 50) (Chung et al., 2016; Kawada, 2019). The questions help to select specific sleep therapies and the best time for implementation.

To add to the sleep history, have the patient and bed partner keep a sleep-wake log for 1 to 4 weeks. The patient completes the sleep-wake log daily to provide information on day-to-day variations in sleep-wake patterns over extended periods. Entries in the log often include 24-hour information about various waking and sleeping health behaviors such as physical activities, mealtimes, type and amount of intake (alcohol and caffeine), time and length of daytime naps, evening and bedtime routines, the time the patient tries to fall asleep, nighttime awakenings, and the time of morning awakening. A partner helps record the estimated times the patient falls asleep or awakens. Although the log is helpful, the patient needs to be motivated to participate in its completion.

Usual Sleep Pattern. Normal sleep is difficult to define because individuals vary in their perception of adequate quantity and quality of sleep. However, it is important to have patients describe their usual sleep pattern to determine the significance of the changes caused by a sleep disorder. Knowing a patient's usual, preferred sleep pattern allows you to try to match sleeping conditions in the health care setting with those in the home. Ask the following questions to determine a patient's sleep pattern:

1. What time do you usually get in bed each night?
2. How much time does it usually take to fall asleep? Do you do anything special to help you fall asleep?
3. How many times do you wake up during the night? What do you think is the cause?
4. What time do you typically wake up in the morning?

Compare patient data with their pattern before the sleep problem or with the predominant pattern usually found for other patients of the same age. Use this comparison to assess for identifiable patterns such as insomnia. Patients with sleep problems frequently report sleep patterns that are drastically different from their normal patterns, or sometimes the change is relatively minor. Patients in the hospital usually need or want more sleep as a result of illness. However, some require less sleep because they are less active. Some patients who are ill think that it is important to try to sleep more than usual, eventually making sleeping difficult.

Physical and Psychological Illness. Determine whether the patient has any preexisting health problems that interfere with sleep. Chronic diseases such as chronic obstructive pulmonary disease (COPD) and painful disorders such as arthritis interfere with sleep. Also assess the patient's medication history, including a description of over-the-counter and prescribed drugs. Assess individuals for polypharmacy, especially older adults, because polypharmacy can cause sleep problems (Miner and Kryger, 2020). A history of psychiatric problems also makes a difference. For example, a patient who is living with bipolar disorder sleeps more when depressed than when manic. A patient who is depressed often experiences an inadequate amount of fragmented sleep. If a patient takes medications to aid sleep, gather information about the type and amount of medication and the frequency of its use. Also assess the patient's daily caffeine intake.

If a patient has recently undergone surgery with general anesthesia, expect that patient to experience some sleep disturbance. Patients usually awaken frequently during the first night after surgery and receive little deep or REM sleep. Depending on the type of anesthesia, it takes several days to months for a normal sleep cycle to return.

Current Life Events. In your assessment learn whether the patient is experiencing any changes in lifestyle that disrupt sleep. A person's occupation often offers a clue to the nature of the sleep problem. Changes in job responsibilities, rotating shifts, or long hours contribute to a sleep disturbance. Questions about social activities, recent travel, or mealtime schedules help clarify the assessment.

Emotional and Mental Status. A patient's emotions and mental status affect the ability to sleep. For example, a patient who is experiencing anxiety, emotional stress related to illness, or situational crises such as loss of job or a loved one often experiences insomnia. Ask whether the individual is a caregiver because caregiver stress, physical strain, and irregular schedules of caregivers often contribute to sleep disruption (Miner and Kryger, 2020). When a sleep disturbance is related to an emotional problem, the key is to treat the primary problem; its resolution often improves sleep (Murawski et al., 2018; Miner and Kryger, 2020). Patients with mental illnesses may need mild sedation for adequate rest. Assess the effectiveness of any medication and its effect on daytime function.

Bedtime Routines. Ask patients what they do to prepare for sleep. For example, some patients drink a glass of milk, take a sleeping pill, eat a snack, or watch television. Assess habits that are beneficial compared with those that disturb sleep. For example, watching television promotes sleep for one person, whereas it stimulates another to stay awake. Sometimes pointing out that a habit is interfering with sleep helps patients find ways to change or eliminate habits that are disrupting sleep.

Pay special attention to a child's bedtime rituals. For example, the parents need to report whether it is necessary to read a bedtime story, rock the child to sleep, or engage in quiet play. Some young children need a special blanket or stuffed animal when going to sleep.

Bedtime Environment. During assessment ask the patient to describe preferred bedroom conditions, including preferences for lighting in the room, music or television in the background, or needing to have the door open versus closed. Include questions about the presence of electronic devices in the bedroom (e.g., phones, televisions), all of which have small lights that remain on or have a light that blinks when the battery is low. Patients are often surprised by how many of these devices are in the sleeping environment.

In addition, some children need the company of a parent to fall asleep. Environmental distractions in a health care setting such as a roommate's television, an electronic monitor in the hallway, a noisy nurses' station, or another patient who cries out at night often interfere with sleep. Modify the environment whenever possible to promote sleep.

Behaviors of Sleep Deprivation. Some patients are unaware of how their sleep problems affect their behavior. Observe for behaviors such as irritability, disorientation (similar to a drunken state), frequent yawning, and slurred speech. If sleep deprivation has lasted a long time, psychotic behavior such as delusions and paranoia sometimes develops. For example, a patient reports seeing strange objects or colors in the room or acts afraid when the nurse enters the room.

As Susan prepares to assess Julie, she knows that it is important to consider sleep alterations in adults. She knows that in adulthood total time spent sleeping begins to decline and sleep problems often occur. She also recognizes that depression can cause sleep problems, as can menopause; Julie had reported she was having menopausal symptoms. Susan completes a sleep history on Julie. As part of the history, Susan asks Julie to describe her bedtime routine. Julie reports that her bedtime varies and that her total amount of sleep is decreasing. She reports that she drinks coffee late into the evening and then has a glass of wine just before bedtime to help her relax. Julie tells Susan that when she gets in bed and it takes her an hour to fall asleep, she is worrying about her cases from work and her mother's recovery from her fractured hip. During the examination Susan notes that Julie has dark circles under her eyes; she shifts her position in the chair multiple times and yawns frequently. She admits to fatigue. She tells Susan, "I am not sure how much longer I can continue this way. I am caring for everyone else and feel as if I don't have any time for myself."*

As Susan prepares to share with Julie suggestions that she found in the literature to improve her mother's sleep, Susan also draws from her experience in a skilled nursing facility, where she worked with older adults. She knows that older adults' sleep is often fragmented and that they experience problems with sleep. Furthermore, Susan has read journal articles that cite multiple factors in affecting sleep in older adults, including physical illness, dementia, depression, high prevalence of sleep-disordered breathing, circadian rhythm disturbances, and the noise and lighting of the environment. She wants to be sure that her proposed plan for Louise considers all potential factors influencing her sleep pattern. Susan asks Julie about Louise's sleep patterns before her fall so that she can make a comparison and develop an individualized plan of care for Louise.

REFLECT NOW

Take either the Epworth Sleepiness Scale or Pittsburgh Sleep Quality Index. After analyzing your results, what does the instrument tell you about your sleep quality?

❖ Analysis and Nursing Diagnosis

Review your assessment, looking for clusters of data that provide cues that the patient is experiencing a sleep pattern disturbance or other health problem. You cannot make accurate nursing diagnoses based on just one or two assessment findings. Carefully review your patient's assessment data to consider whether more than one diagnosis applies. For example, an individual who is experiencing a sleep disturbance may have the diagnosis of *Impaired Sleep,* but the individual's sleep problems can also cause *Fatigue.* If you identify a sleep problem, specify the condition, such as insomnia or sleep deprivation. By specifying the sleep disturbance diagnosis, you can design more effective interventions. For example, you choose different therapies for patients with *Impaired Sleep related to chronic pain* than for a patient with *Impaired Sleep related to unfamiliar environment of the hospital.* Box 43.7 demonstrates how to use nursing assessment activities to identify and cluster assessment findings to make an accurate nursing diagnosis.

Assessment also identifies the related factor or probable cause of a sleep disturbance such as a noisy environment or a high intake of caffeinated beverages in the evening. These causes become the focus of interventions for minimizing or eliminating a negative or problem-focused diagnosis. For example, if a patient is experiencing insomnia because of a noisy health care environment, offer some basic recommendations for helping sleep, such as controlling the noise of hospital equipment, reducing interruptions, or keeping doors closed. If the insomnia is related to anxiety or stress over a threatened marital separation, introduce coping strategies and create an environment for sleep. If you incorrectly define the probable cause or related factors, the patient does not benefit from care.

BOX 43.7 Nursing Diagnostic Process

Impaired Sleep

Assessment Activities	Assessment Findings
Ask patient to explain nature of sleep problem.	Patient reports difficulty falling asleep, taking up to 1 hour. Patient reports waking up two to three times nightly with difficulty returning to sleep.
Observe patient's behavior and ask spouse whether patient is experiencing behavioral changes.	Patient admits to not feeling well rested. Spouse describes times when patient was lethargic and irritable.
Determine whether patient has had recent lifestyle changes.	Spouse reports that patient recently lost job and is concerned about finding new position.

Sleep problems affect patients in other ways. For example, you find that a patient with sleep apnea has problems with a spouse who is tired and frustrated over the patient's snoring. In addition, the spouse is concerned that the patient is breathing improperly and thus is in danger. Examples of nursing diagnoses for patients with sleep problems include the following:

- Adequate Sleep
- Fatigue
- Impaired Sleep
- Impaired Alertness
- Sleep Deprivation

Through her assessment, Susan learns more about Julie's sleep patterns, bedtime routines, and sleep difficulties and how she perceives them. Susan also recognizes that Julie is anxious and stressed about her mother's condition and recovery and about providing care for her mother. Julie experiences pressures both at work and home. This combination of stressors creates sleep problems for Julie. Julie's sleep difficulty is affecting all aspects of her life, both at work and at home. Julie has felt the effects of stress and sleep problems for about 4 weeks. Julie reports she has problems falling asleep and staying asleep. She admits to having multiple cups of coffee after dinner to be able to review her work cases and then a glass of wine just before bed to help herself relax and try to sleep. Julie acknowledges that this is something new for her to do each night. Julie also is going to bed 2 hours past her normal bedtime, and it takes her an hour to fall asleep. During this time, she is worrying about work and her mother. Julie is beginning to feel stress about being a caregiver since her mother's discharge from the skilled nursing facility. Julie questions her ability to continue to manage her mother's care and her ability to complete her legal case work while also caring for her children. Julie also reports that she quit walking because she does not have time to walk anymore. Susan observes Julie during the visit and notes the signs of fatigue and stress Julie is showing. During the visit, Julie has poor eye contact and then bursts into tears and expresses feelings of being tired and starting to feel overwhelmed. Her vital signs show changes during the interview: pulse, 108 beats/min; respirations, 20 breaths/min; blood pressure, 152/84 mm Hg.

As Susan analyzes these assessment findings, the data clusters provide her cues that lead her to identify Impaired Sleep as a priority nursing diagnosis for the plan of care. Along with this diagnosis, Susan recognizes that Julie is also experiencing Fatigue and Caregiver Stress related to her mother's illness. Julie's stopping of her exercise and other healthy behaviors leads Susan to identify Impaired Health Maintenance as another problem for Julie.

❖ Planning and Outcomes Identification

Outcomes. During the planning step of the nursing process, develop a plan of care for each of the patient's nursing diagnoses. Clinical judgment and critical thinking at this step are important because you reflect on previous experiences and environmental factors and apply knowledge, critical thinking attitudes, and professional and intellectual standards to develop an individualized, patient-centered plan of care (Fig. 43.3) (see the Nursing Care Plan). When developing a patient-centered plan of care, also consider a patient's preferences and culture when selecting interventions.

Professional standards are especially important to consider in developing a care plan. These standards often offer evidence-based guidelines for effective nursing interventions. For example, in *Evidence-Based Geriatrics Nursing Protocols for Best Practice,* the chapter titled "Disorders of Sleep in the Older Adult" (Morris et al., 2021) recommends individualized nursing interventions that maintain and support an older adult's normal sleep pattern and bedtime ritual. It is important for a plan of care for sleep promotion to include strategies appropriate to the patient's sleep routines, living environment, and lifestyle.

Prior experience with other patients with sleep disturbances and your own personal experience with sleep problems are valuable when selecting interventions to help patients improve sleep. For example, you may have cared for a patient who was experiencing sleep problems due to chronic pain and used strategies and interventions that helped the patient better manage the pain so that sleep was improved. Your own personal experience with sleep disturbances provides you with insight on effective strategies that can be used with patients and families.

As you plan care for a patient with sleep disturbances, creation of a concept map is another method for developing holistic patient-centered care (Fig. 43.4). Create the map after identifying relevant nursing diagnoses from the assessment database. In this example the nursing diagnoses are linked to the patient's medical diagnosis of depression and situational stress. The concept map shows the relationships among the nursing diagnoses *Impaired Sleep, Caregiver Stress, Fatigue,* and *Impaired Health Maintenance.* This approach to planning care helps you recognize relationships among planned interventions. For this patient, interventions and successful outcomes for one nursing diagnosis affect the resolution of another. When developing outcomes, it is important to collaborate with your patients. As a result, you are more likely to set realistic goals and measurable outcomes with your patients. An effective plan includes outcomes established over a realistic time frame that focus on improving the quantity and quality of sleep in the home. Often family members are helpful in contributing to the plan. A sleep-promotion plan frequently requires many weeks to accomplish. The following are examples of outcomes that you might use for a patient with a sleep disturbance:

- Patient will express feeling rested after sleep.
- Patient reports fewer awakenings during the night.
- Patient falls asleep within 30 minutes of going to bed.
- Patient reports sleeping 8 hours each night.

REFLECT NOW

Analyze the results of your sleep quality using one of the instruments described in the assessment section. Based on the results, develop one goal and two outcomes for yourself that focus on improving your sleep quality or sleep-hygiene habits.

Setting Priorities. Work with patients to establish priority outcomes and interventions. Frequently, sleep disturbances are the result of other

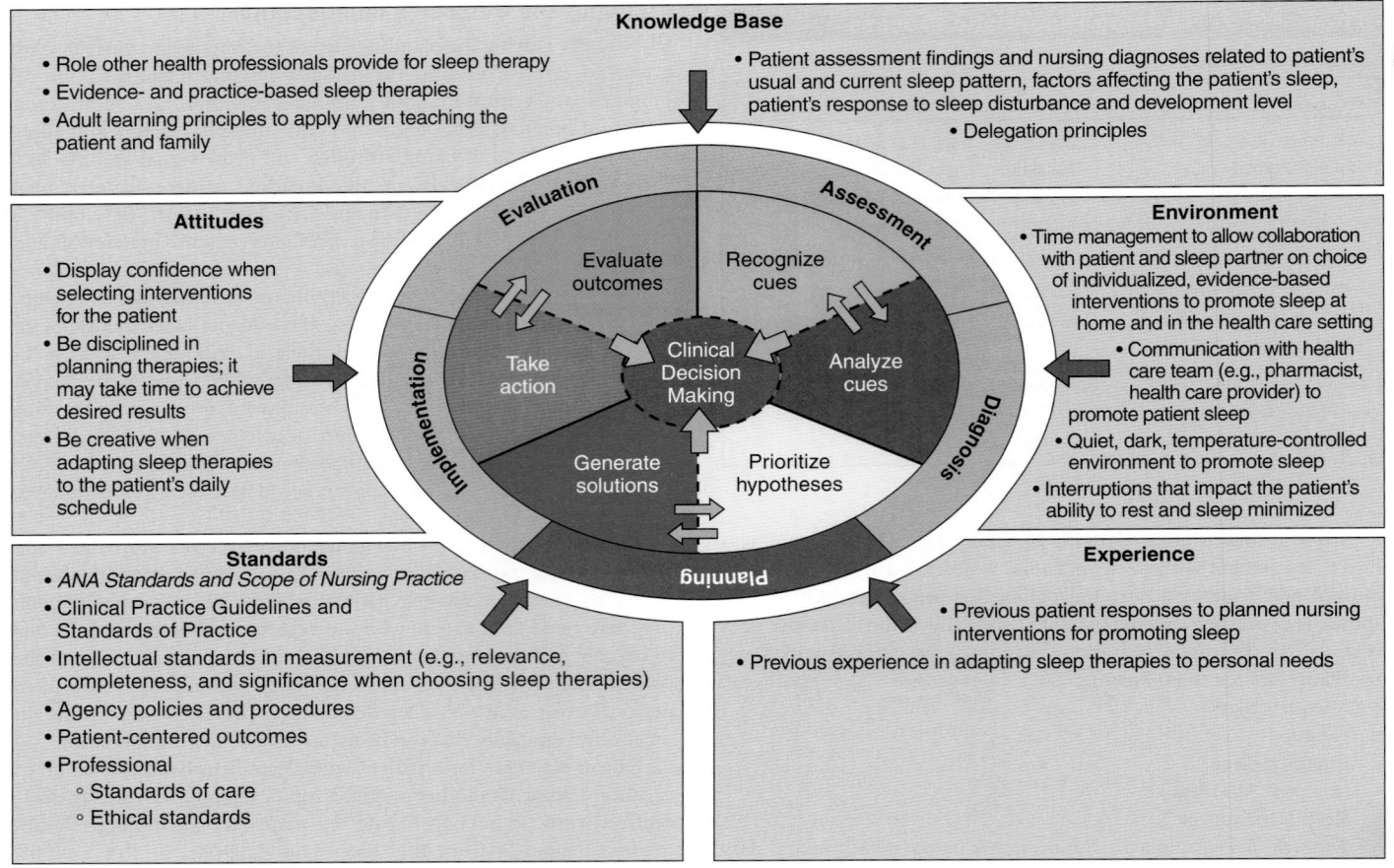

FIG. 43.3 Critical thinking model for sleep planning. (Clinical Judgment Measurement Model copyright © NCSBN. All rights reserved.)

health problems. For example, when physical symptoms interfere with sleep, managing the physical symptoms is your priority. After symptoms are relieved, focus on sleep therapies. Patients are a helpful resource in determining which interventions hold priority. For example, once patients understand the factors that disrupt sleep, they make choices about the types of changes they would like to make in their lifestyle or sleeping environment.

Teamwork and Collaboration. Partner closely with the patient and sleep partner to ensure that any therapies such as a change in the sleep schedule or changes to the bedroom environment are realistic and achievable. In a health care setting, plan treatments or routines so that the patient can rest. For example, in the ICU use available electronic monitors to track trends in vital signs without waking a patient each hour. Other staff members need to be aware of the care plan so that they can cluster activities at certain times to reduce awakenings. In a skilled nursing facility the focus of the plan involves better planning of rest periods around the activities of the other residents. Roommates often have quite different care and sleep schedules.

When patients have chronic sleep problems, the initial referral for a patient is often to a comprehensive sleep center for assessment of the problem. The nature of the sleep disturbance then determines whether referrals to additional health care providers are necessary. For example, if a sleep problem is related to a situational crisis or emotional problem, refer the patient to a mental health clinical nurse specialist or clinical psychologist for counseling. If the nurse works

in an inpatient setting and the patient needs a referral for continued care after discharge, offering information about the sleep problem is useful to the home care nurse. The success of sleep therapy depends on an approach that fits the patient's lifestyle and the nature of the sleep disorder.

*Based on her analysis of the assessment data, Susan recognizes that Julie is having trouble sleeping, is using poor sleep-hygiene practices, is experiencing stress related to her mother's care, and wants to improve her sleep. Susan recognizes that she needs to plan care to help Julie improve her sleep and deal with her stress, along with giving Julie suggestions to help her mother improve her sleep. Susan has identified **Impaired Sleep** as the priority for Julie. Based on this, Susan works with Julie to identify agreed-on outcomes and plan patient-centered personal care and support for her and the family. The mutually agreed-on outcomes are "Julie reports waking up less frequently during the night and feeling rested within 4 weeks" and "Julie verbalizes adherence to a regular bedtime routine within 4 weeks." Susan works to develop a plan that is patient-centered and considers Julie's preferences.*

*Susan will ensure that Julie's **Fatigue, Caregiver Stress,** and **Impaired Health Maintenance** are managed before asking about her other priorities for care. Susan knows that Julie is worried about her mother and her problems sleeping, so she asks Julie questions about her mother and the environment in her mother's room. Susan then includes teaching for Julie to help her mother improve her sleep. Susan knows that above all she will honor patient and family preferences, culture, and religious traditions while planning care.*

◎ NURSING CARE PLAN

Impaired Sleep

ASSESSMENT

Assessment Activities	*Assessment Findings[a]*
Ask Julie to explain the nature of her sleep problem.	Julie explains that she **wakes up two or three times a night.** She states, **"I feel tired when I wake up, and I have trouble concentrating at work in the afternoon."**
Ask Julie if there have been any recent changes in her life.	Julie reports that because of her heavy work schedule, she has stopped her routine of walking 1 to 2 miles daily. She reports that she has no time for any exercise when she gets home because **she needs to take care of her mother and the children.**
Ask Julie to describe her bedtime routine.	Julie responds that she is **going to bed** between midnight and 1 a.m., which is **2 hours later than her usual bedtime. It takes her an hour to fall asleep.** She says that she used to get 7 to 8 hours of sleep a night and now **it is more like 5 to 6 hours.** She drinks two to three cups of coffee after dinner while she is working on her cases before bedtime.
Assess Julie for physical signs of sleep problems.	During the examination you note that Julie has dark circles under her eyes; she shifts her position in the chair multiple times and yawns frequently. She admits to **fatigue.**

[a]**Assessment findings** are shown in bold type.

NURSING DIAGNOSIS: Impaired Sleep

PLANNING

Expected Outcomes (NOC)[b]

Sleep

Patient reports waking up less frequently during the night and feeling rested within 4 weeks.

Patient verbalizes adherence to a regular bedtime routine within 4 weeks.

[b]Outcome classification labels from Moorhead S, et al: *Nursing outcomes classification (NOC),* ed 6, St Louis, 2018, Elsevier.

INTERVENTIONS (NIC)[c]

	RATIONALE
Sleep Enhancement	
Encourage patient to establish a bedtime routine and a regular sleep pattern.	Maintaining a consistent schedule helps induce sleep (Hedges and Gotelli, 2019).
Instruct patient to avoid caffeine and nicotine before bedtime.	Caffeine and nicotine are stimulants and cause difficulty in falling asleep (Hedges and Gotelli, 2019).
Help patient identify ways to eliminate stressful concerns about work before bedtime (e.g., taking time before actual sleep to read a light novel).	Excess worry and intense activities before bedtime stimulate patient and prevent sleep (MacLeod et al., 2018).
Adjust environment; have patient control noise, temperature, and light in the bedroom.	Creates an environment conducive to sleep (Patel et al., 2018).
Relaxation Therapy	
Teach patient how to perform muscle relaxation before bedtime; include demonstration.	Relaxation reduces anxiety, which interferes with sleep (National Sleep Foundation, 2020b; Patel et al., 2018).

[c]Intervention classification labels from Butcher HK, et al: *Nursing interventions classification (NIC),* ed 7, St Louis, 2018, Elsevier.

EVALUATION

Evaluation Activities	*Patient Response*
Ask Julie to describe her sleep and her waking behaviors at work and home.	Julie responds that she has been sleeping better at night and wakes up only one time during the night. She reports that she has completed her cases at work and feels less pressure. She has restarted her walking routine and is better able to cope with her children. She can concentrate at work more. Julie sits in the chair without shifting position. She does not yawn during the conversation. The dark circles under her eyes are almost gone.
Ask Julie to describe her bedtime routine over the last 2 weeks.	Julie reports that she is now consistently going to bed at 10:30 p.m. each night. She has lowered her bedroom temperature and uses quiet music to fall asleep. Julies says that she no longer does work while sitting in her bed. She has stopped drinking coffee after dinner.

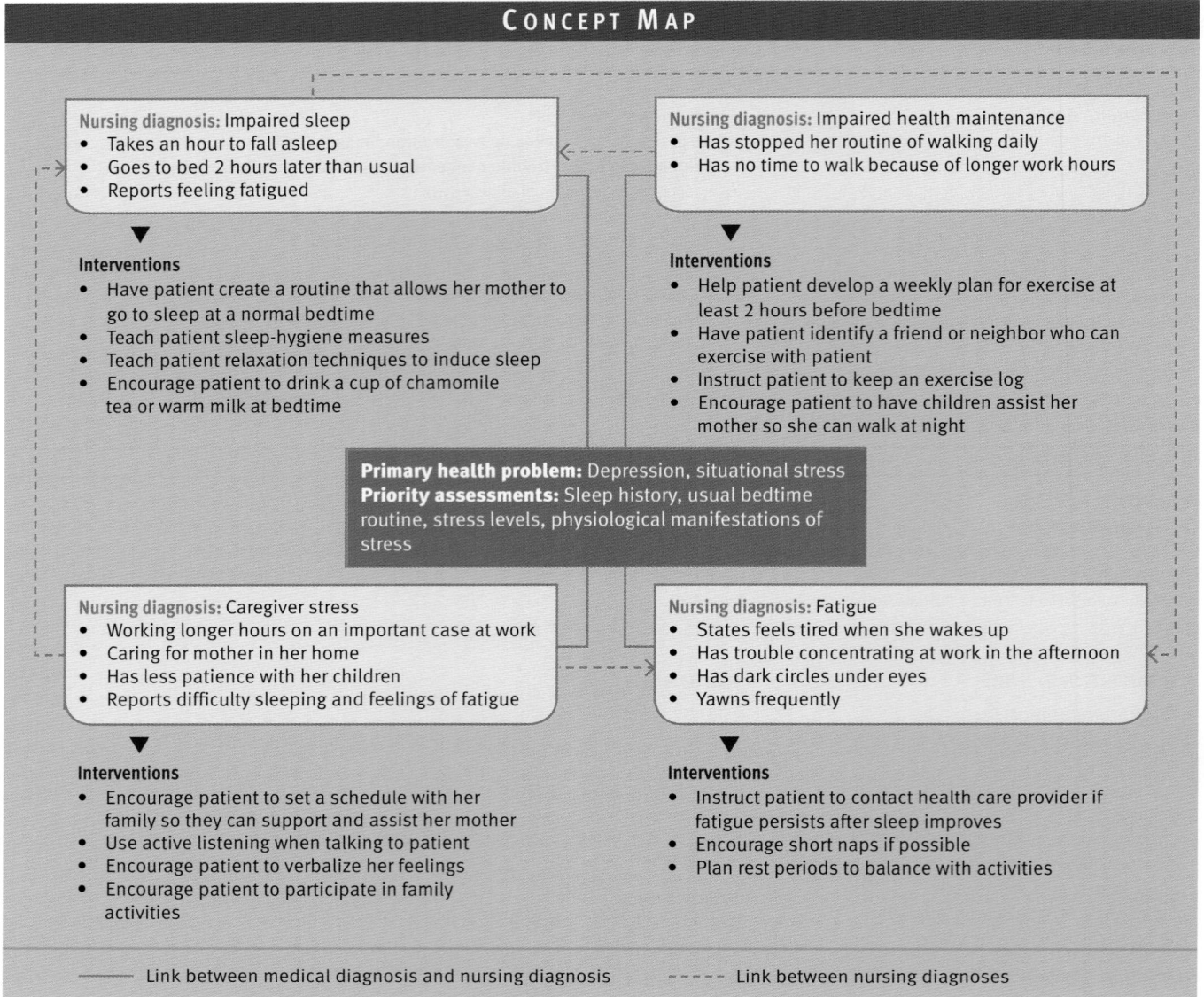

CONCEPT MAP

Nursing diagnosis: Impaired sleep
- Takes an hour to fall asleep
- Goes to bed 2 hours later than usual
- Reports feeling fatigued

Interventions
- Have patient create a routine that allows her mother to go to sleep at a normal bedtime
- Teach patient sleep-hygiene measures
- Teach patient relaxation techniques to induce sleep
- Encourage patient to drink a cup of chamomile tea or warm milk at bedtime

Nursing diagnosis: Impaired health maintenance
- Has stopped her routine of walking daily
- Has no time to walk because of longer work hours

Interventions
- Help patient develop a weekly plan for exercise at least 2 hours before bedtime
- Have patient identify a friend or neighbor who can exercise with patient
- Instruct patient to keep an exercise log
- Encourage patient to have children assist her mother so she can walk at night

Primary health problem: Depression, situational stress
Priority assessments: Sleep history, usual bedtime routine, stress levels, physiological manifestations of stress

Nursing diagnosis: Caregiver stress
- Working longer hours on an important case at work
- Caring for mother in her home
- Has less patience with her children
- Reports difficulty sleeping and feelings of fatigue

Interventions
- Encourage patient to set a schedule with her family so they can support and assist her mother
- Use active listening when talking to patient
- Encourage patient to verbalize her feelings
- Encourage patient to participate in family activities

Nursing diagnosis: Fatigue
- States feels tired when she wakes up
- Has trouble concentrating at work in the afternoon
- Has dark circles under eyes
- Yawns frequently

Interventions
- Instruct patient to contact health care provider if fatigue persists after sleep improves
- Encourage short naps if possible
- Plan rest periods to balance with activities

——— Link between medical diagnosis and nursing diagnosis   - - - - Link between nursing diagnoses

FIG. 43.4 Concept map for Julie Arnold.

❖ Implementation

Nursing interventions designed to improve the quality of a person's rest and sleep are largely focused on health promotion. Patients need adequate sleep and rest to maintain active and productive lifestyles. During times of illness, rest and sleep promotion are important for recovery. Nursing care in an acute, restorative, or continuing care setting differs from that provided in a patient's home. The primary differences are in the environment and the nurse's ability to support normal rest and sleep habits. A patient's age also influences the types of therapies that are most effective. Box 43.8 provides principles for promoting sleep in older adults.

Health Promotion. In community health and home settings help patients develop behaviors conducive to rest and relaxation. To develop good sleep habits at home, patients and their bed partners need to learn techniques that promote sleep and the conditions that interfere with it (Kryger et al., 2017) (Box 43.9). Parents also learn how to promote good sleep habits for their children. Patients benefit most

from instructions based on information about their homes and lifestyles, such as which types of activities promote sleep when a person must work during the night shift or how to make the home environment more conducive to sleep. Patients are more likely to apply information that they find useful and valuable.

Environmental Controls. All patients require a sleeping environment with a comfortable room temperature and proper ventilation, minimal sources of noise, a comfortable bed, and proper lighting (Patel et al., 2018). Children and adults vary in regard to comfortable room temperature. Instruct parents to place infants on mattresses that are covered by a fitted sheet that meets current safety standards; to clothe babies in sleepers for warmth; to keep cribs free of pillows, quilts, toys, or anything else; and to position cribs away from open windows or drafts (AAP, 2016; Gaw et al., 2017). Older adults often require extra blankets or covers.

Eliminate distracting noise so that the bedroom is as quiet as possible. In the home the television, telephone, or intermittent chiming of a clock often disrupts a patient's sleep. Involve the family in identifying

BOX 43.8 FOCUS ON OLDER ADULTS
Promoting Sleep

Sleep-Wake Pattern
- Maintain a regular bedtime and wake-up schedule (Hedges and Gotelli, 2019).
- Eliminate naps unless they are a routine part of the schedule.
- If naps are taken, limit to 30 minutes and time them early in the day (Morris et al., 2021).
- Go to bed when sleepy.
- Use warm bath and relaxation techniques (Touhy and Jett, 2020).
- If unable to sleep in 15 to 30 minutes, do a relaxing activity such as reading (Haynes et al., 2018).
- Avoid stimulating activities such as exercise or watching television before bedtime (Morris et al., 2021).

Environment
- Sleep where you sleep best.
- Keep noise to a minimum; use soft music to mask it if necessary.
- Use night-light and keep path to bathroom free of obstacles.
- Set room temperature to preference; use socks to promote warmth.
- Listen to relaxing music (Touhy and Jett, 2020).
- Sit in natural sunlight upon awakening if possible (Morris et al., 2021).

Medications
- Use sedatives and hypnotics with caution as last resort and then only short term if necessary (Hedges and Gotelli, 2019).
- Adjust medications being taken for other conditions and assess for drug interactions that may cause insomnia or excessive daytime sleepiness.

Diet
- Limit caffeine and nicotine in late afternoon and evening (Hedges and Gotelli, 2019).
- Avoid large meals and alcohol close to bedtime (Hedges and Gotelli, 2019)
- Consume carbohydrates or milk as a light snack before bedtime (Touhy and Jett, 2020).
- Decrease fluids 2 to 4 hours before sleep (Touhy and Jett, 2020).

Physiological/Illness Factors
- Elevate head of bed and provide extra pillows as preferred.
- Use analgesics 30 minutes before bed to ease aches and pains.
- Use therapeutics to control symptoms of chronic conditions as prescribed (Morris et al., 2021).

BOX 43.9 PATIENT TEACHING
Sleep-Hygiene Habits

Objective
- Patient will follow proper sleep-hygiene habits at home.

Teaching Strategies
- Instruct patient to try to exercise daily, preferably in the morning or afternoon, and to avoid vigorous exercise in the evening within 2 hours of bedtime.
- Caution patient against sleeping long hours during weekends or holidays to prevent disturbance of normal sleep-wake cycle.
- Explain that, if possible, patients should not use the bedroom for intensive studying, snacking, television watching, or other nonsleep activity besides sex.
- Encourage patients to try to avoid worrisome thinking when going to bed and to use relaxation exercises.
- If patient does not fall asleep within 30 minutes of going to bed, advise to get out of bed and do some quiet activity until feeling sleepy enough to go back to bed.
- Recommend that patients limit caffeine to morning coffee and limit alcohol intake (more than one to two drinks a day interrupts sleep cycle).
- Recommend that patients discontinue use of electronic devices about 30 minutes before going to bed.
- Ask patient to examine environment. Instruct that use of earplugs and eyeshades may be helpful.
- Instruct patient to avoid heavy meals 3 hours before bedtime; a light snack may help.

Evaluation
Use the principles of teach-back to evaluate patient/family caregiver learning:
- "I want to be sure I explained the important information you need to include in your sleep-wake log. Explain the information you are going to include in your log for the next week."
- "Tell me about three of the approaches we planned to help you sleep at home."

approaches for reducing noise in the home, especially if there are several family members, all with different sleep schedules. It is also important to remember that some patients sleep with familiar inside noises such as the hum of a fan. Some patients benefit from using commercial products that produce a soothing noise, such as the sounds of ocean waves or rainfall, to create an environment for sleep.

A bed and mattress need to provide support and comfortable firmness. Bed boards placed under mattresses add support. Sometimes extra pillows are important to help a person position comfortably in bed. The position of the bed in the room also makes a difference for some patients.

Patients vary regarding the amount of light that they prefer at night. Infants and older adults sleep best in softly lit rooms. Light should not shine directly on their eyes. Small table lamps prevent total darkness. For older adults, light reduces the chance of confusion and prevents falls when walking to the bathroom. If streetlights shine through windows or when patients nap during the day, heavy shades, drapes, or slatted blinds are helpful.

Avoid excessive use of smartphones, tablets, and computers in the bedroom. Electronic devices and some smart televisions emit a blue light that affects sleep and circadian rhythms in some patients (Gronil et al., 2016). These devices increase sleep deprivation in all age-groups, with the greatest impact in children and adolescents (Glauser, 2018; Jakobsson et al., 2020). Encourage patients to avoid the use of their electronic devices in bed and, whenever possible, to discontinue use about 30 minutes before sleep.

Promoting Bedtime Routines. Bedtime routines and sleep-hygiene measures relax patients in preparation for sleep. It is always important for people to go to sleep when they feel tired or sleepy. Going to bed while fully awake and thinking about other things often causes insomnia and interferes with the bed as a stimulus for sleep. Newborns and infants sleep through so much of the day that a specific routine is not necessary. However, quiet activities such as holding them snugly in blankets, singing or talking softly, and gentle rocking help them fall asleep.

A bedtime routine (e.g., same hour for bedtime, snack, bathing, cuddling, rocking, or quiet activity) used consistently helps young children avoid delaying sleep (Mindell and Williamson, 2018). Parents need to reinforce patterns of preparing for bedtime. Quiet activities such as reading stories, coloring, allowing children to sit in a parent's lap while listening to music or listening to a prayer are routines that are often associated with preparing for bed. Lack of education is often the reason that parents do not follow good sleep-hygiene practices with infants (Ordway et al., 2020). Therefore, it is important to provide education to parents on best practices for sleep in children.

Adults need to avoid excessive mental stimulation just before bedtime. Reading a light novel or listening to music helps a person relax. Relaxation exercises such as slow, deep breathing for 1 or 2 minutes relieve tension and prepare the body for rest (see Chapter 44). Guided imagery and praying also promote sleep for some patients.

At home discourage patients from trying to finish office work or resolve family problems before bedtime. The bedroom is not a place to work, and patients need to always associate it with sleep. Working toward a consistent time for sleep and awakening helps most patients gain a healthy sleep pattern and strengthens the rhythm of the sleep-wake cycle.

Promoting Safety. For any patient prone to confusion or falls, safety is critical. A small night-light helps a patient orient to the room environment before going to the bathroom. Beds set lower to the floor can lessen the chance of a person falling when first standing. Instruct patients to remove clutter and throw rugs from the path used to walk from the bed to the bathroom. If a patient needs help to ambulate from a bed to the bathroom, place a small bell at the bedside to call family members. Sleepwalkers are unaware of their surroundings and are slow to react, increasing the risk of falls. Do not startle sleepwalkers but instead gently wake them and lead them back to beds.

Infants' beds need to be safe. To reduce the chance of suffocation, do not place pillows, stuffed toys, or the ends of loose blankets in cribs (AAP, 2016). Loose-fitting plastic mattress covers are dangerous because infants pull them over their faces and suffocate.

Promoting Comfort. People fall asleep only after feeling comfortable and relaxed. Minor irritants often keep patients awake. Soft cotton nightclothes keep infants or small children warm and comfortable. Instruct patients to wear loose-fitting nightwear. An extra blanket is sometimes all that is necessary to prevent a person from feeling chilled and being unable to fall asleep. Patients need to void before going to bed so that they are not kept awake by a full bladder.

Promoting Activity. In the home encourage patients to stay physically active during the day so that they are more likely to sleep at night. Increasing daytime activity lessens problems with falling asleep. Always plan rigorous exercise at least 2 to 3 hours before bedtime because exercise just before bed acts as a stimulant (Markwald et al., 2018). Research indicates that exercise is beneficial, particularly for older adults, to improve nighttime sleep. General recommendations include increasing daytime activity or exercise (Meiner and Yeager, 2019). However, older adults with chronic diseases that influence their functional abilities are likely to have limited activity (Touhy and Jett, 2020). Recommend activities that are safe for older adults to perform. Walking, swimming, wheelchair propulsion, and cycling on a stationary bike are excellent for patients with limited physical impairment. Weight lifting using light weights (e.g., 2 to 5 lb) builds upper body strength and endurance. Activity and exercise often prove to be beneficial by improving activity endurance, mobility, and sense of well-being. Plan quiet activities for children before bedtime (e.g., listening to music, reading a book) (Ordway et al., 2020).

Stress Reduction. The inability to sleep because of emotional stress also makes a person feel irritable and tense. When patients are emotionally upset, encourage them to try not to force sleep. Otherwise, insomnia frequently develops, and soon bedtime is associated with the inability to relax. Encourage a patient who has difficulty in falling asleep to get up and pursue a relaxing activity such as sewing or reading rather than staying in bed and thinking about sleep.

Preschoolers have bedtime fears (fear of the dark or strange noises), awaken during the night, or have nightmares. After nightmares, encourage the parent to enter the child's room immediately and talk to the child briefly about fears to provide a cooling-down period. One approach is to comfort children and leave them in their own beds so that their fears are not used as excuses to delay bedtime. Keeping a light on in the room also helps some children. Cultural tradition causes families to approach sleep practices differently (Box 43.10). Always respect those practices that differ from traditional recommendations.

Bedtime Snacks. Some people enjoy bedtime snacks, whereas others cannot sleep after eating. A dairy product such as warm milk or cocoa that contains L-tryptophan is often helpful in promoting sleep. A full meal before bedtime often causes gastrointestinal upset or reflux and interferes with the ability to fall asleep.

Warn patients against drinking or eating foods high in sugar or with caffeine before bedtime. Coffee, tea, colas, and chocolate act as stimulants, causing a person to stay awake or to awaken throughout

---

🌐 BOX 43.10 CULTURAL ASPECTS OF CARE

Co-sleeping/Bed-sharing

Practices and patterns of sleep and rest vary among cultures. Culture and biology influence the development of sleep problems in children. Sleep patterns, bedtime routines, sleep aids, and sleep arrangements are components of cultural practices related to the use of space and interaction distances (Giger and Haddad, 2021). Traditionally, experts recommend having infants and children sleep in their own beds. Co-sleeping or bed-sharing, in which infants and children sleep with their parents, is a culturally preferred habit that varies among cultures (Barry, 2019). In the United States, bed-sharing is more common in mothers who are younger and less educated (Bombard et al., 2018; Stiffler et al., 2018). Reasons for bed-sharing practices relate to breastfeeding, comfort, tradition, better or more sleep, attachment and bonding with the infant, and protection for an infant (i.e., to protect against the cold) (Marinelli et al., 2019; Barry, 2019). Health care providers in the United States discourage it because of safety issues. One belief is that co-sleeping does not promote independence (Barry, 2019). Research results indicate that co-sleeping or bed-sharing is a risk factor for sudden infant death syndrome (SIDS) (Carlin and Moon, 2017). Research does not show that using a device to make bed-sharing safe reduces infant suffocation or SIDS (AAP, 2016). Bed-sharing is not recommended for infants who were born prematurely or with parents who use alcohol or drugs or smoke because of the increased risk for SIDS (Mitchell et al., 2017; Carlin and Moon, 2017). Bed-sharing is often related to infant sleep problems such as frequent awakenings, nighttime crying, increased time spent awake at night and less nighttime sleep (Mindell et al., 2017). As a nurse, be culturally sensitive when discussing co-sleeping practices with parents and developing sleeping plans for children.

Implications for Patient-Centered Care
- Complete a thorough sleep assessment of the child and family.
- Discuss the risks of co-sleeping with parents. During the discussion remain culturally sensitive and respectful of the parents' views (Barry, 2019).
- Instruct parents who practice co-sleeping to avoid using alcohol or drugs that impair arousal. Decreased arousal prevents the parents from waking if the child is having problems (Mitchell et al., 2017).
- Recommend to parents that they share a room but not the bed with their infant (Bombard et al., 2018).
- Encourage parents to use light sleeping clothes, to keep room temperature comfortable, and to avoid bundling the child tightly or in too many clothes.
- Remove pillows and blankets from the infant's bed (Gaw et al., 2017).

the night. Caffeinated foods and liquids and alcohol act as diuretics and cause a person to awaken in the night to void.

Infants require special measures to minimize nighttime awakenings for feeding. It is common for children to need middle-of-the-night bottle-feeding or breastfeeding. Hockenberry et al. (2019) recommend offering the last feeding as late as possible. Tell parents not to give infants bottles in bed. Providing a bottle or juice to the infant or child at bedtime is related to dental caries formation (Ordway et al., 2020).

> **QSEN** **Building Competency in Evidence-Based Practice** At her annual checkup, Julie Arnold tells you that she continues to have trouble falling asleep, so she drinks 1 to 2 glasses of wine before bedtime to make her sleepy. Based on the current evidence, what is your best response?
>
> Answers to QSEN Activities can be found on the Evolve website.

Pharmacological Approaches. Melatonin is a neurohormone produced in the brain that helps control circadian rhythms and promote sleep (Kryger et al., 2017). It is a popular nutritional supplement that is found to be helpful in improving sleep efficiency and decreasing nighttime awakenings. The recommended dose is 0.3 to 3 mg taken 2 hours before bedtime. Older adults who have decreased levels of melatonin find it beneficial as a sleep aid (Kryger et al., 2017). Short-term use of melatonin has been found to be safe, with mild, infrequent side effects of nausea, headache, and dizziness. A melatonin receptor agonist, such as ramelteon or tasimelteon, is well tolerated and appears to be effective in improving sleep by improving the circadian rhythm and shortening the time needed for sleep onset (Avidan and Neubauer, 2017; Patel et al., 2018). It is safe for long- and short-term use, particularly in older adults. Common side effects include diarrhea, drowsiness, tiredness and dizziness.

Several other herbal products help in sleep. Valerian has been shown to be effective in mild insomnia by reducing the time to fall asleep and improving quality of sleep. Typically, individuals who use valerian do not experience morning grogginess (WebMD, 2019). Lavender essential oil may improve sleep quality (O'Malley, 2017). Passionflower (maypop) has mild sedative effects and is used as a natural sleep aid (WebMD, 2019). Chamomile, an herbal tea, has a mild sedative effect that may be beneficial in promoting sleep (WebMD, 2019). Caution patients about the dosage and use of herbal compounds because the U.S. Food and Drug Administration (FDA) does not regulate them. Herbal compounds may interact with prescribed medications, and patients need to avoid using these together (Meiner and Yeager, 2019).

The use of nonprescription sleeping medications is not recommended. Patients need to learn the risks of such drugs. Over the long term these drugs lead to further sleep disruption, even when they initially seemed effective. Caution older adults about using over-the-counter antihistamines because of their long duration of action, which can cause confusion, constipation, urinary retention, and an increased risk of falls (Stewart et al., 2018). Help patients use behavioral and proper sleep-hygiene measures to establish sleep patterns that do not require the use of drugs.

Susan implements the plan of care she and Julie developed based on Julie's preferences, expectations, and identified outcomes. Susan starts by discussing with Julie the need to practice good sleep-hygiene habits. Susan cautions Julie against delaying bedtime or sleeping long hours during weekends or holidays so that Julie can maintain her normal sleep-wake cycle. Susan tells Julie that she should select a reasonable bedtime for her

schedule and try to go to bed at the same time each night. Susan explains to Julie not to use the bedroom, especially the bed, for watching television, snacking, or other nonsleep activity. Susan suggests that Julie take a warm bath before bedtime to relax. Susan also encourages Julie to start walking again and to try to walk for at least 30 minutes every morning. Susan includes in the plan instructions to play soft, relaxing music at bedtime to help Julie fall asleep. Susan demonstrates relaxation techniques to Julie that could help her relax and asks Julie to practice the techniques before leaving. Susan stresses that if Julie does not fall asleep within 20 minutes, she needs to get out of bed and do some quiet activity until feeling sleepy enough to go back to bed. Susan instructs Julie to avoid heavy meals, caffeine, and alcohol for 3 hours before bedtime, suggesting a light snack, including protein and carbohydrates, if Julie is hungry before bedtime. Susan asks Julie about the temperature and lighting in her bedroom, suggesting that a cooler temperature is more conducive to sleep. Susan also suggests that Julie keep a log of her walking and sleeping so that she can see her progress.

Julie tells Susan she plans to speak with her boss at work to see whether someone could help with her caseload during this stressful time with her mother. Susan suggests to Julie that the soft music and relaxation techniques might help her mother sleep better, too. Susan also tells Julie to check the temperature, lighting, and noise levels around her mother's room to make sure the environment is not contributing to Louise's sleep troubles. Susan also tells Julie it is all right if her mother takes short naps during the day, as long as the naps are no longer than 30 minutes. Susan and Julie discuss the concerns Julie has about caring for her mother at her house and her concern that her mother may be unable to return to her own home. Susan provides information on a caregiver support group that meets weekly at a local church. Susan also provides information on home health services that might be able to help with care of her mother. At the end of the teaching session, Susan answers Julie's questions about her mother's sleep problems. Susan tells Julie they will review her records at their next meeting. Susan then schedules a follow-up appointment with Julie in 4 weeks.

Acute Care. Patients in acute care settings have their normal rest and sleep routine disrupted, which generally leads to sleep problems. In this setting nursing interventions focus on controlling factors in the environment that disrupt sleep, relieving physiological or psychological disruptions to sleep, and providing for uninterrupted rest and sleep periods for patients. "Disorders of Sleep in the Older Adult" in the *Evidence-based Geriatric Nursing Protocols for Best Practice* is based on the principle that nurses need to individualize an effective strategy based on patient needs and that sleep medications are a last-resort intervention (Morris et al., 2021).

Environmental Controls. In a hospital you control the environment in several ways (Box 43.11). For example, nurses close the curtains between patients in semiprivate rooms and dim lights on a hospital nursing unit at night. One of the biggest problems for patients in the hospital is noise. Important ways to reduce noise are to conduct conversations and reports in a private area away from patient rooms and to keep necessary conversations to a minimum, especially at night. Provide patients with ear plugs or eye masks to decrease noise and light stimulation (Litton et al., 2016; Sanjanwala et al., 2020). Additional ways to control noise in the hospital are listed in Box 43.12.

Promoting Comfort. Make the patient more comfortable by providing personal hygiene before bedtime. A warm bath or shower is very relaxing. Offer patients restricted to bed the opportunity to wash their face and hands. Tooth brushing and care of dentures also help to prepare the patient for sleep. Have patients void before going to bed so that they are not kept awake by a full bladder. While a patient prepares

BOX 43.11 EVIDENCE-BASED PRACTICE

Sleep Hygiene in Hospitalized Patients

PICOT Question: Does the use of a sleep-hygiene protocol versus routine care in patients in the intensive care unit decrease delirium related to decreased sleep?

Evidence Summary

Sleep disruption commonly occurs in patients in the intensive care unit because of disruption of normal routines, anxiety and stress, noise, pain, medical treatments, and environmental factors (Martinez et al., 2017; Owens et al., 2017). Sleep deprivation impacts physical and psychological healing and often causes delirium (Pavone et al., 2020). Maintenance of a normal sleep-wake pattern helps to decreases delirium due to sleep deprivation (Sanjanwala et al., 2020). Implementation of nurse-driven sleep-hygiene protocols has been shown to be effective in improving sleep in patients in the intensive care unit (Martinez et al., 2017; Smithburger et al., 2017). Effective strategies in the protocols focused on education of staff nurses on protocol and interventions to decrease environmental stimuli and limit patient disruptions, pain management, avoidance of the use of restraints, early mobility, and family involvement (Martinez et al., 2017; Smithburger et al., 2017). Implementing these strategies improved patient sleep and decreased delirium (Ding et al., 2017; Martinez et al., 2017).

Application to Nursing Practice

- Work with nurses on the unit to develop a sleep-hygiene protocol.
- Cluster nursing activities to provide uninterrupted periods of sleep (Martinez et al., 2017).
- Maintain the patient's sleep-wake cycle as much as possible (Sanjanwala et al., 2020).
- Provide early physical therapy and mobility for patients (Martinez et al., 2017).
- Reduce lighting, telephone volumes, and staff conversations in the halls during quiet time and nighttime (McGovern et al., 2018).
- Use sleep-hygiene measures with patients, such as personal hygiene, adjusting room temperature, and relaxation methods.
- Educate and involve family in implementing strategies (Smithburger et al., 2017).

BOX 43.12 Control of Noise in the Hospital

- Close doors to patients' room when possible.
- Keep doors to work areas on unit closed when in use.
- Reduce volume of nearby telephone and paging equipment.
- Wear rubber-soled shoes. Avoid clogs.
- Turn off bedside oxygen and other equipment that is not in use.
- Turn down alarms and beeps on bedside monitoring equipment.
- Turn off room television and radio unless patient prefers soft music.
- Avoid abrupt loud noise such as flushing a toilet or moving a bed.
- Keep necessary conversations at low levels, particularly at night.
- Designate a time during the day for "quiet time" for patients.

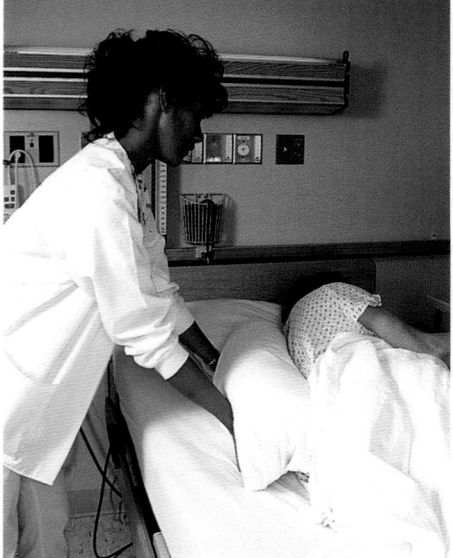

FIG. 43.5 Positioning patient for sleep.

Establishing Periods of Rest and Sleep. In a hospital or extended-care setting it is difficult to provide patients with the time needed to rest and sleep. The most effective treatment for sleep disturbances is to eliminate factors that disrupt the sleep pattern. You need to plan care to avoid waking patients for nonessential tasks. Do this by scheduling assessments, treatments, procedures, and routines for times when patients are awake. For example, if a patient's physical condition has been stable, avoid waking the patient to check vital signs, unless ordered. Allow patients to determine the timing and methods of delivery of basic care measures to promote rest. Do not give baths and routine hygiene measures during the night for nursing convenience. Draw blood samples at a time when the patient is awake. Unless maintaining the therapeutic blood level of a drug is essential, give medications during waking hours. Work with the radiology department and other support services to schedule diagnostic studies and therapies at intervals that allow patients time for rest. Always try to provide the patient with 2 to 3 hours of uninterrupted sleep during the night.

When a patient's condition demands more frequent monitoring, plan activities to allow extended rest periods. A nurse instructs assistive personnel in the coordination of patient care to reduce patient disturbances. This means planning activities so that the patient has as long as an hour or more to rest quietly rather than having a nurse or other personnel return to the room every few minutes. For example, if a patient needs frequent dressing changes, is receiving intravenous therapy, and has drainage tubes from several sites, do not make a separate trip into the room to check each problem. Instead use a single visit to perform all three tasks. Become the patient's advocate for promoting optimal sleep. This means becoming a gatekeeper by postponing or rescheduling visits by family or by questioning the frequency of certain procedures.

Promoting Safety. Patients with OSA are at risk for complications while in the hospital. Surgery and anesthesia disrupt normal sleep patterns (see Chapter 50). After surgery, patients reach deep levels of REM sleep. This deep sleep causes muscle relaxation that leads to OSA. Patients with OSA who are given opioid analgesics after surgery have an increased risk of developing airway obstruction because the medications suppress normal arousal mechanisms. These patients often need ventilator support in the postoperative period because of the increased risk of respiratory complications. Monitor a patient's airway, respiratory rate and depth, and breath sounds frequently after surgery.

for bed, help to position the patient off any potential pressure sites (Fig. 43.5). Offering a back rub or massage helps relax the patient.

Removal of irritating stimuli is another way to improve a patient's comfort for a restful sleep. Changing or removing moist dressings, repositioning drainage tubing, reapplying wrinkled thromboembolic hose, and changing tape on nasogastric tubes eliminate constant irritants to a patient's skin. Cleanse the perineal or anal area thoroughly for patients who are incontinent. Patients who are diaphoretic benefit from a cool bath and dry clothes or linens.

Recommend lifestyle changes to patients with OSA, changes such as sleep hygiene, alcohol moderation, smoking cessation, and a weight-loss program (McNicholas, 2017). Teach the patient to elevate the head of the bed and use a side or prone position for sleep. Use pillows to prevent a supine position.

If patients normally use a continuous positive airway pressure (CPAP) machine at home because of sleep apnea, it is important that they bring their home equipment with them to the hospital and use it every night. Check to make sure the mask fits snugly and is put on correctly so that the positive pressure is maintained (Chaiard and Weaver, 2019a). In patients with sleep apnea who have surgery and receive general anesthesia, the anesthesia in combination with pain medications used after surgery reduces the patient's defenses against airway obstruction. After surgery the patient achieves very deep levels of REM sleep that lead to muscle relaxation and airway obstruction. Use pain medication carefully in these patients. These patients need ventilator support in the postoperative period because OSA is linked to increased postoperative respiratory complications. Monitor the patient's breathing and oxygen saturation levels regularly (see Chapter 29). Notify the health care provider immediately if a patient is difficult to arouse or is having trouble breathing.

Patients who experience EDS can fall asleep while sitting up in a chair or wheelchair. Position patients so that they do not fall out of the chair when sleeping. Elevating their feet on an ottoman or small bench may help to position them safely. A pillow placed in the patient's lap offers some support. If a patient enjoys leaning over an over-bed table while sitting in a chair, be sure that the table is locked and secure. Do not use safety belts because they are considered restraints (see Chapter 27).

Stress Reduction. Patients who are hospitalized for extensive diagnostic testing often have difficulty resting or sleeping because of uncertainty about their health. Giving patients control over their health care minimizes uncertainty and anxiety. Providing information about the purpose of procedures and routines and answering questions gives patients the peace of mind needed to rest or fall asleep. Take time to sit and talk with your patients who are unable to sleep to determine the factors keeping them awake. Providing comfort measures such as back rubs also help patients relax more thoroughly. If a sedative is indicated, confer with the patient's health care provider to be sure that the lowest dose is used initially. Discontinuing a sedative as soon as possible prevents a dependence that seriously disrupts the normal sleep cycle. Older adults' metabolism of drugs is slow, making them more vulnerable to the side effects of sedatives, hypnotics, antianxiety drugs, or analgesics.

Restorative or Continuing Care. The nursing interventions implemented in the acute care setting are also used in the restorative or continuing care environment. Controlling the environment, especially noise; establishing periods of rest and sleep; and promoting comfort are important considerations. Nursing interventions related to stress reduction and controlling physiological disturbances are also implemented in these settings. Helping a patient achieve restful sleep in this environment sometimes takes time.

Maintaining Activity. Limit the time residents spend in bed whenever possible. In long-term care settings, serve meals in the resident dining area. Make sure residents are up in a chair for meals and for personal hygiene activities. It is also important to keep the residents involved in planned social activities (e.g., card playing or arts and crafts). Regular exercise keeps people active and stimulated. It is also ideal to limit daytime napping to 30 minutes or less. Short naps taken in the midafternoon increase alertness and cognitive ability. Research has shown that exposure to natural sunlight for 2 hours a day improved the sleep quality of residents in a nursing home (Duzgun and Akyol, 2017).

Residents with dementia often have disrupted sleep-wake cycles. They often become easily fatigued and experience periods of insomnia (Meiner and Yeager, 2019). In this situation shorten activities and visits to allow patients to maintain an adequate energy level. If a patient wakes up during the night, keeping the lights at a low level and using soothing techniques such as quiet music or a back rub promote returning to sleep.

Controlling Physiological Disturbances. As a nurse you learn to control symptoms of physical illness that disrupt sleep. For example, a patient with respiratory abnormalities sleeps with two pillows or in a semi-sitting position to ease the effort to breathe. The patient benefits from taking prescribed bronchodilators before sleep to prevent airway obstruction. A patient with a hiatal hernia also needs special care. After meals the patient often experiences a burning sensation because of gastric reflux. To prevent sleep disturbances, have the patient eat a small meal several hours before bedtime and sleep in a semi-sitting position. Time medications to relieve pain, nausea, or other recurrent symptoms so that the drug takes effect at bedtime. Remove or change any irritants against the patient's skin such as moist dressings or drainage tubes.

Pharmacological Approaches. The liberal use of drugs to manage insomnia is quite common in American culture. CNS stimulants such as amphetamines, caffeine, nicotine, terbutaline, theophylline, and modafinil need to be used sparingly and under medical management (Burchum and Rosenthal, 2019). In addition, withdrawal from CNS depressants such as alcohol, barbiturates, tricyclic antidepressants (amitriptyline, imipramine, and doxepin), and triazolam causes insomnia. Consult with pharmacists and health care providers about managing doses.

Medications that induce sleep are called **hypnotics**. **Sedatives** are medications that produce a calming or soothing effect (Burchum and Rosenthal, 2019). A patient who takes sleep medications needs to know about their proper use and their risks and possible side effects. Long-term use of antianxiety, sedative, or hypnotic agents disrupts sleep and leads to more serious problems. The FDA requires that the product labels of all sleep medications contain safety information related to the potential adverse effects of severe allergic reactions; severe facial swelling; and complex sleep behaviors such as sleep-driving, making phone calls, and preparing and eating food while asleep (USFDA, 2019).

Benzodiazepines and benzodiazepine-like drugs are commonly used to treat sleep problems and are intended for short-term use (Avidan and Neubauer, 2017). The benzodiazepine-like drugs are the treatment of choice for insomnia because of improved efficacy and safety of use (Burchum and Rosenthal, 2019). Experts recommend a low dose of a short-acting medication such as zolpidem for short-term use (no longer than 2 to 3 weeks) (Burchum and Rosenthal, 2019). These drugs cause fewer problems with dependence and abuse and fewer rebound insomnia and hangover effects than benzodiazepines.

The benzodiazepines cause relaxation, antianxiety, and hypnotic effects by facilitating the action of neurons in the CNS that suppress responsiveness to stimulation, thereby decreasing levels of arousal (Burchum and Rosenthal, 2019). Short-acting benzodiazepines (e.g., oxazepam, lorazepam, or temazepam) at the lowest possible dose for short-term treatment of insomnia are recommended. Initial doses are small, and increments are added gradually, based on patient response, for a limited time. Warn patients not to take more than the prescribed dose, especially if the medication seems to become less effective after initial use. The use of benzodiazepines in older adults is potentially dangerous because of the tendency of the drugs to remain active in the body for a longer time. As a result, they also cause respiratory depression; next-day sedation; amnesia; rebound insomnia; and impaired motor functioning and coordination, which leads to an increased risk of falls (Picton et al., 2018). If older patients who were recently continent, ambulatory, and alert become incontinent or confused and/or demonstrate impaired mobility, consider the use of benzodiazepines as a possible cause.

Administer benzodiazepines cautiously to children under 12 years of age. These medications are contraindicated in infants less than 6 months old. Patients who are pregnant need to avoid them because their use is associated with risk of congenital anomalies. Mothers who are breastfeeding do not receive the drugs because they are excreted in breast milk. Raise these issues with patients' health care providers if you are concerned about the safety of a prescribed medication.

Trazodone is a serotonin antagonist and reuptake inhibitor (SARI) antidepressant often used in patients with depression or anxiety and insomnia. The most common side effects are daytime grogginess and orthostatic hypotension. Low-dose trazodone is often used as an alternative to benzodiazepines, especially in older patients.

Regular use of any sleep medication often leads to tolerance and withdrawal. Rebound insomnia is a problem after stopping a medication, particularly the benzodiazepines (Avidan and Neubauer, 2017). Immediately administering a sleeping medication when a hospitalized patient is unable to sleep does the patient more harm than good. Consider alternative approaches to promote sleep first. Routine monitoring of patient response to sleeping medications is important.

◆ **Evaluation**

Through the Patient's Eyes. The patient is the source for evaluating whether expectations about sleep are met. Each patient has a unique need for sleep and rest. The patient is the only one who knows whether sleep problems are improved and which interventions or therapies are most successful in promoting sleep (Fig. 43.6). It is important to ask the patient whether sleep needs have been met. For example, ask the patient, "Are you feeling more rested?" or "Can you tell me if you believe that we've done all we can to help improve your sleep?" or "Which interventions have been most effective in helping you sleep?" If expectations have not been met, you need to spend more time trying to understand the patient's needs and preferences. Working closely with the patient and bed partner enables you to redefine expectations that can be met realistically within the limits of the patient's condition and treatment.

Patient Outcomes. To evaluate the effectiveness of your nursing care, make comparisons with baseline assessment data to evaluate whether your patient's sleep has improved. Determine whether expected outcomes have been met. Use evaluative measures shortly after a therapy has been implemented (e.g., observing whether a patient falls asleep after reducing noise and darkening a room). Use other evaluative measures after a patient wakes from sleep (e.g., asking the patient to describe the number of awakenings during the previous night). The patient and bed partner usually provide accurate evaluative information. Over longer periods use assessment tools such as the visual analog or sleep-rating scale to determine whether sleep has progressively improved or changed.

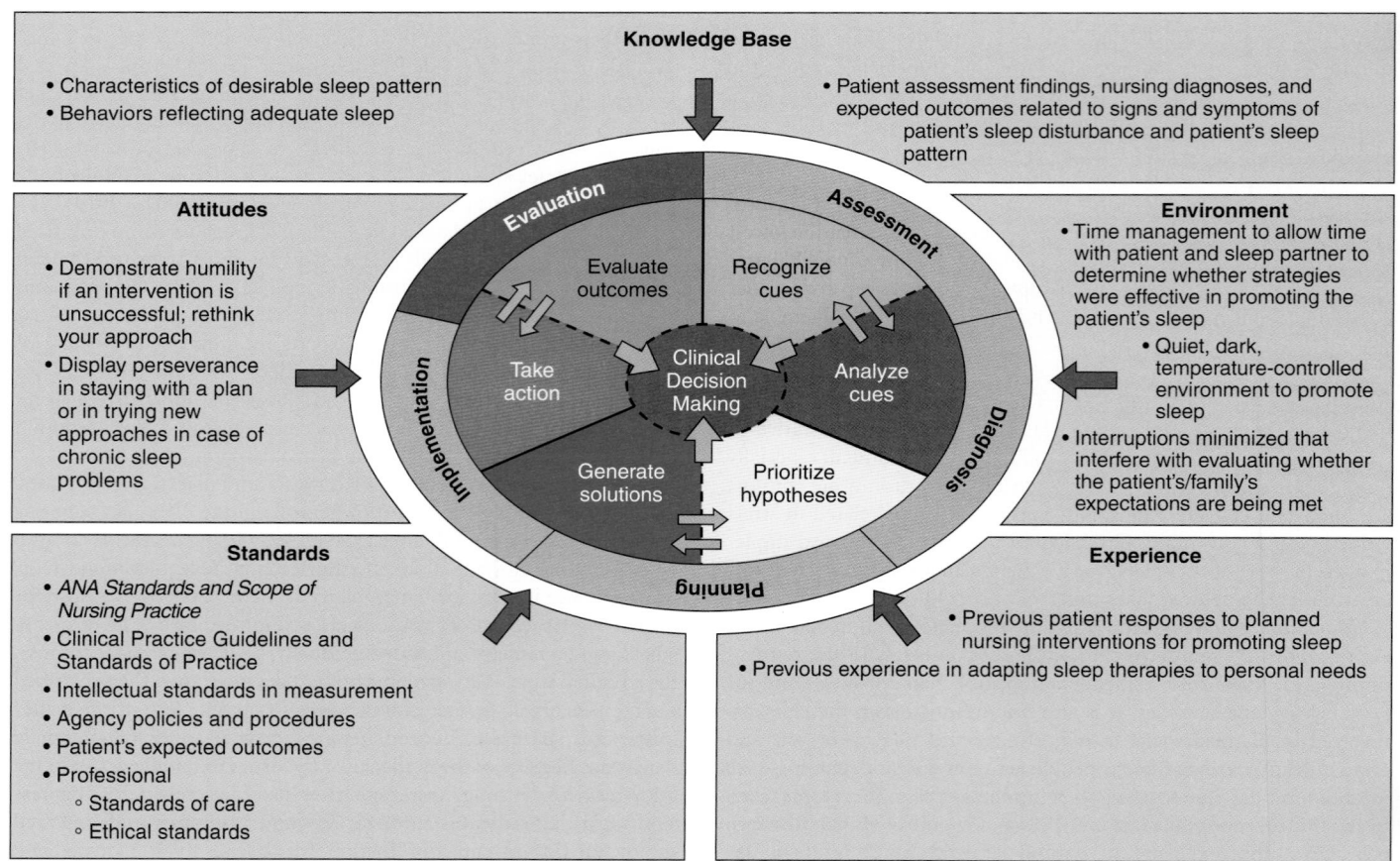

FIG. 43.6 Critical thinking model for sleep evaluation. (Clinical Judgment Measurement Model copyright © NCSBN. All rights reserved.)

Also use teach-back to evaluate the level of understanding that patients or family caregivers gain after receiving instruction in sleep habits. You measure adherence to these practices during a home visit while observing the environment. When expected outcomes are not met, revise the nursing measures or expected outcomes based on the patient's needs or preferences. When outcomes are not met, ask questions such as:

- Are you able to fall asleep within 20 minutes of getting in bed?
- Describe how well you sleep when you exercise.
- Does the use of quiet music at bedtime help you to relax?
- Do you feel rested when you wake up?

If you have successfully developed a good relationship with a patient and a therapeutic plan of care, subtle behaviors often indicate the level of the patient's satisfaction. Note the absence of signs of sleep problems such as lethargy, frequent yawning, or position changes in the patient. You are effective in promoting rest and sleep if the patient's outcomes and expectations are met.

At the end of her appointment with Julie, Susan uses the principles of teach-back to evaluate Julie's learning. She asks Julie:

- *Tell me three sleep-hygiene habits that we discussed to improve your sleep.*
- *Demonstrate a relaxation technique you learned that promotes sleep.*
- *Tell me the benefits of listening to soothing music at bedtime.*

Julie tells Susan three sleep-hygiene practices that she plans to implement: going to bed at the same time each night, increasing her daytime exercise, and decreasing her caffeine and alcohol within 3 hours of bedtime. Julie demonstrates one of the relaxation techniques that Susan had demonstrated earlier. Julie also relates the benefits of listening to soothing music at bedtime and discusses how she is going to get earbuds for listening to the music so that she will not disturb her husband.

When Julie returns for her follow-up appointment, Susan wants to know Julie's level of satisfaction with her care. She asks, "Are you satisfied with the care you have received? Have I met your expectations so far? If not, tell me how I can better help you." Julie replies, "You've been great. You gave me so many suggestions to help me improve my sleep. Keeping the log of exercise and sleep was beneficial. I am enjoying walking again, and I feel so much more rested when I wake up." Julie reports that since she has followed the sleep-hygiene practices and goes to bed at the same time each night, she falls asleep within 20 minutes, only wakens once during the night, and is back to getting about 7 hours of sleep a night. Julie's blood pressure is 126/82 mm Hg, and pulse is 78 beats/min. Susan reviews Julie's log of walking and sleep. Susan praises Julie for the changes she has made and the progress she has shown in achieving her identified outcomes. Julie also thanks Susan for the suggestions that she gave her to help her mother. Julie reports that she got her mother earbuds and soothing music and that she is sleeping much better. Julie feels less stressed and better prepared to care for her. Julie contacted a home care agency for help for her mother. A home care aide comes three times a week to help her mother with bathing, which relieves some stress from Julie at night. Julie tells Susan that she has investigated the caregiver support meetings and is considering attending them now that things are more settled at home. Susan instructs Julie to continue to monitor her exercise and sleep and encourages her to make another appointment if her sleep problems return or do not fully resolve.

KEY POINTS

- The 24-hour sleep-wake cycle is a circadian rhythm that influences physiological function and behavior.

- The control and regulation of sleep depend on a balance among regulators within the CNS.
- During a typical night's sleep, a person passes through four to five complete sleep cycles. Each sleep cycle contains three NREM stages of sleep and a period of REM sleep; time in each stage varies.
- Sleep provides physiological and psychological restoration.
- Sleep requirements vary by age, with neonates sleeping on average 16 hours a day and older adults needing 7 to 8 hours of sleep a night.
- The hectic pace of a person's lifestyle, emotional and psychological stress, and alcohol ingestion frequently disrupt the sleep pattern.
- An environment with a darkened room, reduced noise, comfortable bed, and good ventilation promotes sleep.
- A regular bedtime routine of relaxing activities prepares a person physically and mentally for sleep.
- The most common type of sleep disorder is insomnia. Characteristics of insomnia include the inability to fall asleep, to remain asleep during the night, or to go back to sleep after waking up earlier than desired.
- If a patient's sleep is adequate, assess the usual bedtime, normal bedtime ritual, preferred environment for sleeping, and usual preferred rising time.
- When planning interventions to promote sleep, consider the usual characteristics of the patient's home environment and normal lifestyle.
- Important nursing interventions for promoting sleep in the hospitalized patient are to establish periods for uninterrupted sleep and rest and to control noise levels.
- Use your patient's self-report to determine whether sleep was restful.

REFLECTIVE LEARNING

Julie returns to the clinic with her husband, Blake, to see Susan. Julie is concerned about Blake because he is also having sleep problems, which are making him feel fatigued during the day. Blake is 55 years old. He has a history of hypertension for 6 years and smokes a half-pack of cigarettes a day. Over the last year, he has gained 30 pounds because he quit walking due to work responsibilities. Susan weighs Blake and finds his weight is 108.9 kg (240 pounds). He is 6 feet (1.83 m) tall. Susan calculates Blake's BMI at 32.5. Blake's vital signs at the appointment are BP 168/94, P 102, R 20, T. 36.8°C (98.2°F). Susan reports that she is frequently awakened by Blake's snoring. Blake says that he wakes up several times during the night and is having a hard time staying awake in the afternoon. He also reports that he frequently has headaches when he wakes up in the morning and that he is having difficulty concentrating on his cases at work. Julie tells Susan that Blake is more irritable at home and has less patience with their children.

- What assessment information in Blake's situation is the most important or of immediate concern for the nurse? (Recognize Cues)
- Considering Blake's situation, what environmental, organizational, or other factors did you see that influence Blake's sleep? (Analyze Cues)
- Considering the assessment data and history, what is the priority nursing problem in caring for Blake? (Prioritize Diagnoses)
- Identify two expected outcomes for Blake. Consider Blake's situation and describe the nursing and medical interventions that you could utilize to achieve the expected outcomes. (Generate Solutions)
- Which nursing and medical interventions have priority when implementing the care plan for Blake? (Take Action)
- Considering the implementation of your plan of care for Blake, what assessment data should you gather to determine whether the interventions were effective? (Evaluate Outcomes)

REVIEW QUESTIONS

1. A nurse is developing a plan for a patient who was diagnosed with narcolepsy. Which interventions should the nurse include on the plan? (Select all that apply.)
   1. Take brief naps, no longer than 20 minutes, no more than twice a day.
   2. Drink a glass of wine with dinner.
   3. Eat a large meal at lunch rather than dinner.
   4. Establish a regular exercise program.
   5. Teach the patient about the side effects of modafinil.

2. The nurse recognizes that which statements made by a patient indicate an understanding of behaviors that will promote sleep? (Select all that apply.)
   1. "I will not watch television in bed."
   2. "I will not drink caffeine later in the day."
   3. "A short nap late in the evening will lead to a more restful night of sleep."
   4. "I am going to start eating dinner closer to my bedtime."
   5. "I will start to exercise regularly during the day."

3. A 72-year-old patient asks the nurse about using an over-the-counter antihistamine as a sleeping pill to help her get to sleep. What is the nurse's best response?
   1. "Antihistamines are better than prescription medications because prescription medications can cause a lot of problems."
   2. "Antihistamines should not be used because they can cause confusion and increase your risk of falls."
   3. "Antihistamines are effective sleep aids because they do not have many side effects."
   4. "Over-the-counter medications when combined with sleep-hygiene measures are a good plan for sleep."

4. Which nursing interventions best promote effective sleep in an older adult? (Select all that apply.)
   1. Limit fluids 2 to 4 hours before sleep.
   2. Ensure that the room is completely dark.
   3. Ensure that the room temperature is comfortably cool.
   4. Provide warm covers.
   5. Encourage walking an hour before going to bed.

5. The nurse recognizes that which statement made by the patient indicates an understanding of sleep-hygiene practices?
   1. "I usually drink a cup of warm milk in the evening to help me sleep."
   2. "If I exercise right before bedtime, I will be tired and fall asleep faster."
   3. "I know it does not matter what time I go to bed as long as I am tired."
   4. "If I use hypnotics for a long time, my insomnia will be cured."

6. Which nursing interventions are appropriate to include in a plan of care to promote sleep for patients who are hospitalized? (Select all that apply.)
   1. Give patients a cup of coffee 1 hour before bedtime.
   2. Plan vital signs to be taken before the patients are asleep.
   3. Turn television on 15 minutes before bedtime.
   4. Have patients follow at-home bedtime schedule.
   5. Close the door to patients' rooms at bedtime.

7. The nurse is contacting the health care provider about a patient's sleep problem. Place the steps of the SBAR (situation, background, assessment, recommendation) in the correct order.
   1. Mrs. Dodd, 46 years old, was admitted 3 days ago following a motor vehicle accident. She is in balanced skeletal traction for a fractured left femur. She is having difficulty falling asleep.
   2. "Dr. Smithson, this is Pam, the nurse caring for Mrs. Dodd. I'm calling because Mrs. Dodd is having difficulty sleeping."
   3. "I'm calling to ask if you would order a hypnotic such as zolpidem to use on a prn basis."
   4. Mrs. Dodd is taking her pain medication every 4 hours as ordered and rates her pain as 2 out of 10. Last night she was still awake at 0100. She states that she is comfortable but just can't fall asleep. Her vital signs are BP 124/76, P 78, R 12 and T 37.1°C (98.8°F).

8. A mother brings her 4-year-old son into the health clinic for a checkup and tells the nurse practitioner that he is having sleep problems. The nurse practitioner provides teaching on sleep hygiene for toddlers. Which statement made by the mother indicates a need for further teaching?
   1. "I will make sure he has his favorite blanket when he gets in bed."
   2. "We will play hide and seek just before bed to wear him out."
   3. "I can read him one of his favorite books before bed."
   4. "I will work on getting him into bed at the same time each night."

9. A nurse is taking a sleep history from a patient. The nurse recognizes that which statement made by the patient needs further follow-up?
   1. "I feel refreshed when I wake up in the morning."
   2. "I use soft music at night to help me relax."
   3. "It takes me about 45 to 60 minutes to fall asleep."
   4. "I take the pain medication for my leg pain about 30 minutes before I go to bed."

10. Which sleep-hygiene actions at bedtime can the nurse delegate to assistive personnel? (Select all that apply.)
    1. Giving the patient a back rub
    2. Turning on quiet music
    3. Dimming the lights in the patient's room
    4. Giving a patient a cup of coffee
    5. Monitoring for the effect of the sleeping medication that was given

Answers: 1. 1, 4, 5; **2.** 1, 2, 5; **3.** 2, 4, 1, 3, 4; **5.** 1; **6.** 2, 4, 5; **7.** 2, 1, 4, 3; **8.** 2; **9.** 3; **10.** 1, 2, 3.

Rationales for Review Questions can be found on the Evolve website.

REFERENCES

Adams SK, et al: Technology as a tool to encourage young adults to sleep and eat healthy, *ACSMs Health Fit J* 21(4):4, 2017.

American Academy of Pediatrics: *SIDS and other sleep-related infant deaths: updated 2016 recommendations for a safe infant sleeping environment*, 2016. http://pediatrics.aappublications.org/content/138/5/e20162938. Accessed July 18, 2020.

American Nurses Association: *Nursing scope and standards of practice*, ed 4, Silver Springs, MD, 2021, The Association.

American Sleep Association: *Sleep and sleep disorder statistics*, 2020. https://www.sleepassociation.org/about-sleep/sleep-statistics/. Accessed July 18, 2020.

American Thoracic Society: What is obstructive sleep apnea in adults? *Am J Respir Crit Care Med* 196:P1, 2017.

Avidan AY, Neubauer DN: Chronic insomnia disorder, *Continuum (Minneap Minn)* 23(4):1064, 2017.

Bruce ES, et al: Sleep in adolescents and young adults, *Clin Med (Lond)* 17(5):424, 2017.

Burchum JR, Rosenthal LD: Lehne's pharmacology for nurses, ed 10, St. Louis, 2019, Elsevier.

Cleveland Clinic: Nocturia, 2020. https://my.clevelandclinic.org/health/diseases/14510-nocturia. Accessed July 19, 2020.

Giger JN, Haddad LG: *Transcultural nursing: assessment and intervention,* ed 8, St Louis, 2021, Elsevier.

Glauser W: Overscheduled and glued to screens: children are sleeping less than ever before, *CMAJ* 190(48):E1428, 2018.

Haynes J, et al: Cognitive behavioral therapy in the treatment of insomnia, *South Med J* 111(20):75, 2018.

Hedges C, Gotelli J: Managing insomnia in older adults, *Nurse Pract* 44(9):16, 2019.

Hockenberry MJ, et al: *Wong's nursing care of infants and children,* ed 11, St Louis, 2019, Elsevier.

Huether SE, et al: *Understanding pathophysiology,* ed 7, St Louis, 2020, Elsevier.

Johns M: About the ESS, n.d. http://epworthsleepinessscale.com/about-the-ess/. Accessed July 18, 2020.

Kawada T: Screening ability of STOP-Bang questionnaire for obstructive sleep apnea, *Anesth Analg* 128(3):e48, 2019.

Kryger MH, et al: *Principles and practice of sleep medicine,* ed 6, St Louis, 2017, Elsevier.

Lorenz CP, Williams AJ: Sleep apps: what role do they play in clinical medicine? *Curr Opin Pulm Med* 23(6):512, 2017.

Markwald RR, et al: Behavioral strategies, including exercise, for addressing insomnia, *ACSMs Health Fit J* 22(2):23, 2018.

Maski K, Owens J: Pediatric sleep disorders , *Continuum (Minneap Minn)* 24(1):210, 2018.

Meiner SE, Yeager JJ: *Gerontologic nursing,* ed 6, St Louis, 2019, Mosby.

McGovern C, et al: Pain, agitation and delirium in the intensive care unit, *Anaesth Intensive Care Med* 19(12):634, 2018.

Mindell JA, Williamson AA: Benefits of a bedtime routine in young children: sleep, development, and beyond, *Sleep Med Rev* 40:93, 2018.

Miner B, Kryger MH: Sleep in the aging population, *Sleep Med Clin* 15:311, 2020.

Morris JL, et al: Disorders of sleep in the older adult. In Boltz M, et al., editors: *Evidence-based geriatric nursing protocols for best practice,* ed 6, New York, 2021, Springer Publishing Company.

National Sleep Foundation: *National Sleep Foundation's 2018 Sleep in America® poll shows Americans failing to prioritize sleep,* Washington, DC, 2018. https://www.sleepfoundation.org/media-center/press-release/2018-sleep-in-america-poll-shows. Accessed July 18, 2020.

National Sleep Foundation: *Aging and sleep,* Washington, DC, 2020a. http://www.sleepfoundation.org/article/sleep-topics/aging-and-sleep. Accessed July 18, 2020.

National Sleep Foundation: *Depression and sleep,* 2020b. https://www.sleepfoundation.org/articles/depression-and-sleep. Accessed July 18, 2020.

National Sleep Foundation: *How much sleep do we really need?* Washington, DC, 2020c. https://www.sleepfoundation.org/articles/how-much-sleep-do-we-really-need. Accessed July 18, 2020.

National Sleep Foundation: *Teens and sleep,* Washington, DC, 2020d. https://www.sleepfoundation.org/articles/teens-and-sleep. Accessed July 19, 2020.

O'Malley PA: Lavender for sleep, rest, and pain: evidence for practice and research, *Clin Nurse Spec* 31(2):74, 2017.

Owens RL, et al: Sleep in the intensive care unit in a model of family-centered care, *AACN Adv Crit Care* 28(2):171, 2017.

Parekh PJ, et al: The effects of sleep on the commensal microbiota: eyes wide open? *J Clin Gastroenterol* 52(3):204, 2018.

Picton JD, et al: Benzodiazepine use and cognitive decline in the elderly, *Am J Health Syst Pharm* 75(1):e6, 2018.

Sanjanwala R, et al: Delirium prevention in postcardiac surgical critical care, *Crit Care Clin* 36:675, 2020.

Sateia MJ, et al: Clinical practice guideline for the pharmacologic treatment of chronic insomnia in adults: an American Academy of Sleep Medicine clinical practice guideline, *J Clin Sleep Med* 13(2):307, 2017.

Sleep Advisor: *ZZZs to dollars: how much does sleep deprivation cost?* 2020. https://www.sleepadvisor.org/sleep-deprivation-cost/. Accessed July 22, 2020.

Stewart NH, et al: Sleep in hospitalized older adults, *Sleep Med Clin* 13:127, 2018.

Touhy TA, Jett KF: *Ebersole and Hess' toward health aging: human needs & nursing response,* ed 10, St Louis, 2020, Elsevier.

US Food and Drug Administration (USFDA): *Sleep problems,* 2019. https://www.fda.gov/forconsumers/byaudience/forwomen/ucm118563.htm. Accessed July 18, 2020.

WebMD: *Natural sleep aids and remedies,* 2019. https://www.webmd.com/women/natural-sleep-remedies#1. Accessed July 18, 2020.

RESEARCH REFERENCES

Barry ES: Co-sleeping as a proximal context for infant development: the importance of physical touch, *Infant Behav Dev* 57:101385, 2019.

Bombard JM, et al: Vital signs: trends and disparities in infant safe sleep practices, United States, 2009-2015, *MMWR Morb Mortal Wkly Rep* 67(1):39, 2018.

Carlin RF, Moon RY: Risk factors, protective factors, and current recommendations to reduce sudden infant death syndrome: a review, *JAMA Pediatr* 171(2):175, 2017.

Chaiard J, Weaver TE: Update on research and practices in major sleep disorders: part I. obstructive sleep apnea syndrome, *J Nurs Scholarsh* 51(5):500, 2019a.

Chaiard J, Weaver TE: Update on research and practices in major sleep disorders: part II—insomnia, Willis-Ekbom Disease (restless leg syndrome), and narcolepsy, *J Nurs Scholarsh* 51(6):624, 2019b.

Chen KS, et al: A hypothalamic switch for REM and Non-REM sleep, *Neuron* 97:1168, 2018.

Christian LM, et al: Sleep quality across pregnancy and postpartum: effects of parity and race, *Sleep Health* 5:327, 2019.

Chung F, et al: STOP-Bang questionnaire: a practical approach to screen for obstructive sleep apnea, *Chest* 149(3):631, 2016.

Ding Q, et al: Factors influencing patients' sleep in the intensive care unit: patient and clinical staff perceptions, *Am J Crit Care* 26(4):278, 2017.

Duzgun G, Akyol AD: Effect of natural sunlight on sleep problems and sleep quality of the elderly staying in the nursing home, *Holist Nurs Pract* 31(5):295, 2017.

Gaw CE, et al: Types of objects in the sleep environment associated with infant suffocation and strangulation, *Acad Pediatr* 17(8):893, 2017.

Gronil J, et al: Reading from an iPad or book in bed: the impact on human sleep. A randomized crossover trial, *Sleep Med* 21:86, 2016.

Hillman D, et al: The economic cost of inadequate sleep, *Sleep* 41(8):1, 2018.

Jakobsson M, et al: Reasons for sleeping difficulties as perceived by adolescents: a content analysis, *Scand J Caring Sci* 34(2):464, 2020.

Jike M, et al: Long sleep duration and health outcomes: a systematic review, meta-analysis and meta-regression, *Sleep Med Rev* 39:25, 2018.

Litsfeldt S, et al: Association between sleep duration, obesity, and school failure among adolescents, *J Sch Nurs,* 36:458–463, 2020. doi:10.1177/1059840520901335.

Litton E, et al: The efficacy of earplugs as a sleep hygiene strategy for reducing delirium in the ICU: a systematic review and meta-analysis, *Crit Care Med* 44(5):992, 2016.

MacLeod S, et al: Practical non-pharmacological intervention approaches for sleep problems among older adults, *Geriatr Nurs* 39:506, 2018.

Marinelli KA, et al: An integrated analysis of maternal-infant sleep, breastfeeding, and sudden infant death syndrome research: supporting a balanced discourse, *J Hum Lact* 35(3):510, 2019.

Martinez F, et al: Implementing a multicomponent intervention to prevent delirium among critically ill patients, *Crit Care Nurse* 37(6):36, 2017.

McNicholas WT: Obstructive sleep apnoea of mild severity: should it be treated? *Curr Opin Pulm Med* 23(6):506, 2017.

Meltzer LJ, Pugliese CE: Sleep in young children with asthma and their parents, *J Child Health Care* 21(3):301, 2017.

Mindell JA, et al: Sleep location and parent-perceived sleep outcomes in older infants, *Sleep Med* 39:1–7, 2017.

Mitchell EA, et al: The combination of bed sharing and maternal smoking leads to a greatly increased risk of sudden unexpected death in infancy: the New Zealand SUDI Nationwide Case Control Study, *N Z Med J* 130(1456):52, 2017.

Mollayeva T, et al: The Pittsburgh sleep quality index as a screening tool for sleep dysfunction in clinical and non-clinical samples: a systematic review and meta-analysis, *Sleep Med Rev* 25:52, 2016.

Murawski B, et al: A systematic review and meta-analysis of cognitive and behavioral interventions to improve sleep health in adults without sleep disorders, *Sleep Med Rev* 40:160, 2018.

Ordway MR, et al: Sleep health in young children living with socioeconomic adversity, *Res Nurs Health* 43:329, 2020.

Patel R, et al: Innovations in insomnia management: a review of current approaches and novel targets including orexin receptor antagonists, *Am J Ther* 25:e28, 2018.

Pavone KJ, et al: Evaluating delirium outcomes among older adults in the surgical intensive care unit, *Heart Lung* 49:578, 2020.

Rash JA, et al: A meta-analysis of mindfulness-based therapies for insomnia and sleep disturbance: moving towards processes of change, *Sleep Med Clin* 14:209, 2019.

Schwartz DA, et al: Occupation and obstructive sleep apnea: a meta-analysis, *J Occup Environ Med* 59(6):502, 2017.

Shimura A, et al: Comprehensive assessment of the impact of life habits on sleep disturbance, chronotype, and daytime sleepiness among high-school students, *Sleep Med* 44(12), 2018.

Short MA, et al: The relationship between sleep duration and mood in adolescents: a systematic review and meta-analysis, *Sleep Med Rev* 52:101311, 2020.

Smithburger PL, et al: Perceptions of family members, nurses, and physicians on involving patients' families in delirium prevention, *Crit Care Nurse* 37(6):48, 2017.

Stiffler D, et al: Sudden infant death and sleep practices in the Black community, *J Spec Pediatr Nurs* 23(2):e12213, 2018.

Tan X, et al: Association between long sleep duration and increased risk of obesity and type 2 diabetes: a review of possible mechanisms, *Sleep Med Rev* 40:127, 2018.

Wali S, et al: The association between vitamin D level and restless legs syndrome: a population-based case-control study, *J Clin Sleep Med* 14(4):557, 2018.

Yang S, et al: Effects of exercise on sleep quality in pregnant women: a systematic review and meta-analysis of randomized controlled trials, *Asian Nurs Res* 14:1, 2020.

Pain Management

OBJECTIVES

- Describe the physiology of nociceptive pain.
- Recognize patient cues to differentiate categories of pain.
- Identify the various factors that influence pain.
- Explain how cultural factors influence the pain experience.
- Apply clinical judgment in assessing a patient experiencing pain.
- Contrast the characteristics of acute pain with those of chronic pain.

- Explain the nursing guidelines for administering analgesics safely.
- Explain how clinical judgment guides selection of various nonpharmacological versus pharmacological approaches to treating pain.
- Identify environmental and individual factors that create barriers to effective pain management.
- Evaluate a patient's response to pain interventions.

KEY TERMS

Acupressure
Acute pain
Addiction
Adjuvants
Analgesics
Biofeedback
Breakthrough cancer pain
Chronic pain
Cutaneous stimulation
Drug tolerance
Epidural analgesia

Guided imagery
Idiopathic pain
Local anesthesia
Modulation
Multimodal analgesia
Nociception
Opioids
Pain threshold
Pain tolerance
Patient-controlled analgesia (PCA)
Perineural infusions

Physical dependence
Placebos
Pseudoaddiction
Regional anesthesia
Relaxation
Transcutaneous electrical nerve stimulation (TENS)
Transduction
Transmission

MEDIA RESOURCES

http://evolve.elsevier.com/Potter/fundamentals/
- Review Questions
- Video Clips
- Concept Map Creator
- Case Study with Questions

- Skills Performance Checklists
- Audio Glossary
- Content Updates
- Answers to QSEN Activity and Review Questions

Mrs. Mays, 72 years old, has osteoarthritis, hypertension, and diabetes mellitus. She was recently hospitalized because she developed pneumonia, and her blood glucose levels were very high because of her acute illness. Currently, her pneumonia is resolving, and her blood glucose is more stable. She is preparing to go home in the next 24 hours. She lives at home with her husband, who helps her with her activities of daily living (ADLs).

Matt is a nursing student assigned to care for Mrs. Mays and prepare her for discharge home. Matt asks Mrs. Mays, "What is your main concern about going home?" Mrs. Mays responds, "My pneumonia is getting better, and I know how to manage my diabetes. The pain in my hips, knees, and hands is so bad right now, I am not sure how I am going to get around the house and take care of myself. My pain is so severe I have only been able to walk short distances and the pain wakes me up two or three times a night while I sleep."

Pain is experienced by everyone. However, every individual who has pain has a unique pain experience. You will encounter patients who have pain in all health care settings. It is the most common reason patients

seek health care, yet it is often underrecognized, misunderstood, and inadequately treated. A person in pain often feels distress or suffering and seeks relief. One of the major challenges of pain is that as a nurse you cannot see or feel a patient's pain. It is purely subjective. No two people experience pain in the same way, and no two painful events create identical responses or feelings in a person. The International Association for the Study of Pain (IASP) defines pain as "an unpleasant, subjective sensory and emotional experience associated with, or resembling that associated with, actual or potential tissue damage" (IASP, 2020). In the Declaration of Montreal, the IASP declared that access to pain management is a fundamental human right (IASP, 2018a).

Nurses are legally and ethically responsible for assessing and managing pain (American Nurses Association, 2018). The Institute of Medicine's 2011 report, *Relieving Pain in America,* called for increased coordination of pain research and pain management across the United States in response to several issues, including that pain is a public health problem. The opioid crisis adds another dimension to the urgency in identifying ways to effectively reduce pain while protecting patients from harm (CDC, 2021a). With the aim of enhancing pain research efforts and promoting collaboration across governmental agencies, a federal advisory committee, the Interagency Pain Research Coordinating Committee (IPRCC), was commissioned by the Department of Health and Human Services (IPRCC, 2021a). The National Pain Strategy is a broad-ranging plan that aims to change how the nation perceives and manages pain (IPRCC, 2021a). The Federal Pain Research Strategy provides a long-term strategic plan to guide federal agencies that support pain research and advance the science to better understand pain and improve pain care (IPRCC, 2021b). Many of the recommendations directly address the need to improve systems of care for pain management and increase resources to prevent and treat substance use disorders, which disproportionately affect patients with chronic pain conditions.

It is important to apply clinical judgment when caring for patients who are in pain. Pain management needs to be patient-centered, requiring the recognition that pain can and should be relieved. Thus, you need to be prepared to practice patient advocacy, empowerment, compassion, and respect. Effective communication among the patient, family, and professional caregivers is essential to assess a patient's pain effectively and achieve adequate pain management. Recognize cues related to the subjective nature of pain, and respect your patients who are in pain. Remember that "pain is whatever the experiencing person says it is, existing whenever he says it does" (Pasero and McCaffery, 2011).

Effectively managing your patient's pain requires clinical judgment and sound clinical decision making. Your ability to recognize and analyze cues, identify the nature of pain, generate solutions, take action, and evaluate the outcomes of your care will help your patients experience improved quality of life and reduced physical discomfort. Effective pain management results in earlier mobilization, improvement in activity levels, fewer hospital and clinic visits, decreased hospital lengths of stay, and lower health care costs.

SCIENTIFIC KNOWLEDGE BASE

Nature of Pain

Pain is more than a single physiological sensation caused by a specific stimulus. It is subjective and highly individualized. Only the patient knows whether pain is present and how the experience feels. Pain is a physiological mechanism that protects an individual from a harmful stimulus. However, it also has physical, emotional, and cognitive components. It reduces a person's energy and often causes fatigue. It interferes with interpersonal relationships and influences a patient's quality of life. Left untreated, it may lead to serious physical, psychological, social, and financial consequences.

Physiology of Pain

Although pain is a subjective perception, nociception is an observable activity in the nervous system that allows people to detect pain (Treede, 2018). Normal or nociceptive pain is the protective physiological series of events that brings awareness of actual or potential tissue damage. There are four physiological processes of nociception: transduction, transmission, perception, and modulation (Huether and McCance, 2019). A patient in pain cannot discriminate among the processes. Understanding each process helps you recognize factors that cause pain, symptoms that accompany it, and the rationale for selected therapies.

Transduction. A thermal, mechanical, or chemical stimulus usually activates a pain event. Transduction converts energy produced by these noxious stimuli into electrical impulses. The process begins in

BOX 44.1 Neurophysiology of Pain: Neuroregulators

Neurotransmitters (Excitatory)

Prostaglandins
- Generated from the breakdown of phospholipids in cell membranes
- Thought to increase sensitivity to pain

Bradykinin
- Released from plasma that leaks from surrounding blood vessels at the site of tissue injury
- Binds to receptors on peripheral nerves, increasing pain stimuli
- Binds to cells that cause the chain reaction producing prostaglandins

Substance P
- Found in pain neurons of dorsal horn (excitatory peptide)
- Needed to transmit pain impulses from periphery to higher brain centers
- Causes vasodilation and edema

Histamine
- Produced by mast cells, causing capillary dilation and increased capillary permeability

Serotonin
- Released from the brainstem and dorsal horn to inhibit pain transmission

Neuromodulators (Inhibitory)
- Are the natural supply of morphine-like substances in the body
- Activated by stress and pain
- Located within the brain, spinal cord, and gastrointestinal tract
- Cause analgesia when they attach to opiate receptors in the brain
- Present in higher levels in people who have less pain than others with a similar injury

the periphery when the pain-producing stimulus sends an impulse across a sensory peripheral pain nerve fiber, known as a nociceptor. Nociceptors are classified by the type of stimuli they respond to; some nociceptors respond to multiple types of stimuli (polymodal nociceptors). Once transduction is complete, transmission of the nociceptive impulse begins (Huether and McCance, 2019).

Inflammation caused by disease processes or cellular damage resulting from thermal, mechanical, or chemical stimuli cause the release of vasoactive and pronociceptive mediators such as prostaglandins, bradykinin, substance P, and histamine (Box 44.1). These substances directly affect the nerve fibers, lowering the threshold required to activate nociceptors and generating action potentials across the synaptic cleft, a process known as peripheral sensitization (Iyer and Lee, 2021; O'Leary et al., 2017) (Fig. 44.1). Peripheral sensitization, which lowers the threshold for causing an action potential within the peripheral afferent neurons, can also result from changes in receptors, ion channels, and the amount of neurotransmitters released.

Transmission. Each nociceptor has an axon composed of peripheral afferent nerve fibers that are either myelinated (A-delta fibers) or unmyelinated (C fibers). The nociceptive impulses are transmitted from the periphery to the spinal cord via the peripheral afferent fibers to the dorsal root ganglia and the superficial lamina I/II of the dorsal horn of the spinal cord. The fast-transmitting myelinated A-delta fibers transmit sharp, localized nociceptive information, whereas the smaller-diameter unmyelinated C fibers relay impulses that are dull, achy, and poorly localized (Iyer and Lee, 2021). For example, after stepping on a nail,

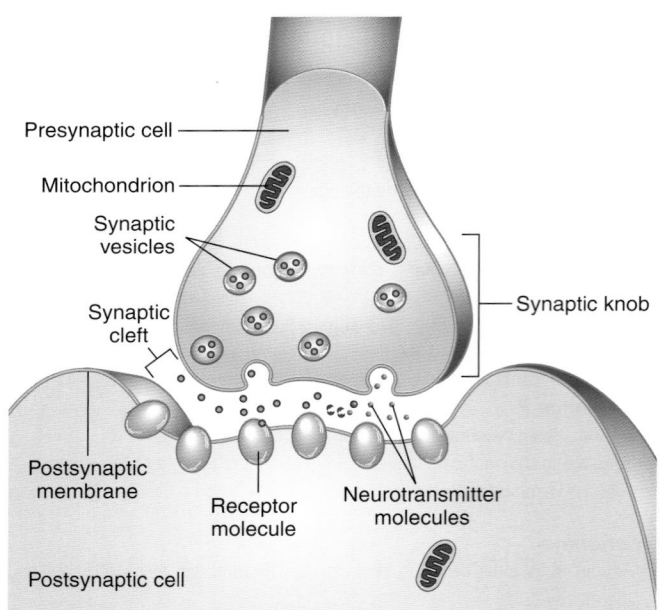

FIG. 44.1 Chemical synapses involve transmitter chemicals (neurotransmitters) that signal postsynaptic cells. (From Patton KT, Thibodeau GA: *Anatomy & physiology*, ed 9, St Louis, 2016, Elsevier.)

a person initially feels a sharp, localized pain, which is a result of A-delta fiber transmission, or first pain. Within a few seconds the whole foot aches from C-fiber transmission, or second pain.

The A-delta fibers transmit nociceptive impulses from the dorsal horn to the interior deeper laminae (III-IV) of the spinal cord and higher centers of the brain by way of the spinothalamic tracts (Fig. 44.2). Dorsal horn neurons carrying nociceptive input include projection neurons, local interneurons, and propriospinal neurons. Many of the projection neurons have axons that cross the midline and ascend to multiple areas of the brain, including the thalamus, gray matter of the cerebral cortex, the pons, and parts of the medullary reticular formation. It is this cellular system of communication (action potentials carrying nociceptive input) that allows pain, arising from any area of the body including the nerve or areas of the brain itself, to be perceived by an individual.

Perception. Once a pain stimulus reaches the cerebral cortex, the brain interprets the quality of the pain and processes information from past experiences, knowledge, and cultural associations in the perception of the pain (Iyer and Lee, 2021; O'Leary et al., 2017). Perception is the point at which a person is aware of nociceptive impulses and perceives pain. The somatosensory cortex identifies the location and intensity of pain, whereas the association cortex, primarily the limbic system, determines how a person feels about it. There is no single pain center.

As a person becomes aware of pain, a complex reaction occurs. Psychological and cognitive factors interact with neurophysiological ones. Perception gives awareness and meaning to pain, resulting in a reaction. The reaction to pain includes the physiological and behavioral responses that occur after an individual perceives pain (Iyer and Lee, 2021; O'Leary et al., 2017).

Modulation. The fourth and final phase of the normal pain process is known as modulation (Pasero and McCaffery, 2011). When a person perceives a harmful impulse, projection neurons activate endogenous descending inhibitory mediators (see Box 44.1), such as endorphins (endogenous opioids), serotonin, norepinephrine, and gamma-aminobutyric acid (GABA), to help produce an analgesic effect. These mediators hinder

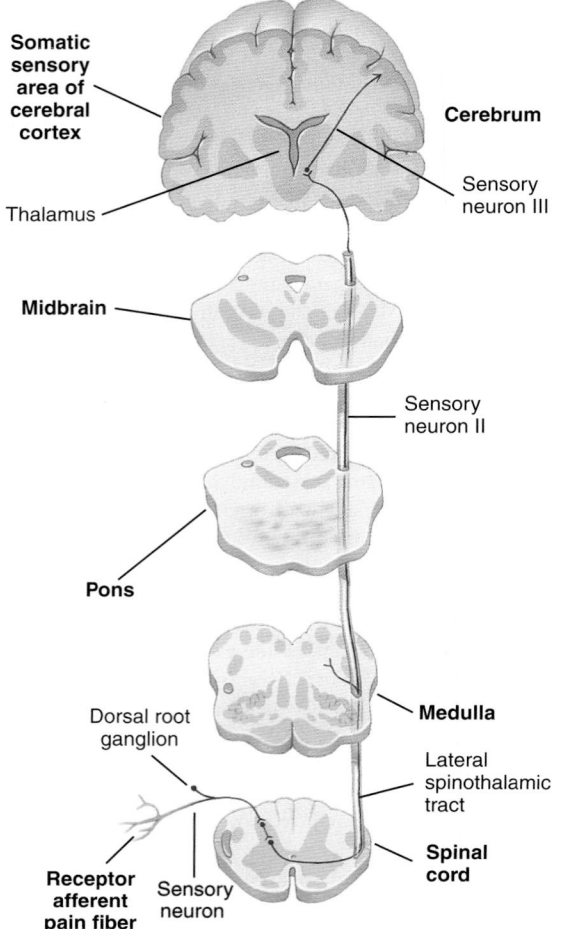

FIG. 44.2 Spinothalamic pathway that conducts pain stimuli to the brain.

the transmission of nociceptive impulses in the dorsal horn neurons. Modulation can also occur through peripheral and/or central sensitization, resulting in increased perception of pain (Huether and McCance, 2019; Iyer and Lee, 2021). Afferent nerve fibers sensitized by vasoactive and pronociceptive mediators lower the threshold of activation and result in continuous nociceptive input to dorsal horn neurons and central sensitization. Clinical manifestations of central sensitization include expansion of the pain beyond the initial location, exaggerated response to noxious stimuli known as hyperalgesia, and pain in response to normally nonnoxious stimuli, also called allodynia.

A protective reflex response also occurs with pain (Fig. 44.3). A-delta fibers send sensory impulses to the spinal cord, where they synapse with spinal motor neurons. The motor impulses travel via a reflex arc along efferent (motor) nerve fibers back to a peripheral muscle near the site of stimulation, thus bypassing the brain. Contraction of the muscle leads to a protective withdrawal from the source of pain. For example, when you accidentally touch a hot iron, you feel a burning sensation, but your hand also reflexively withdraws from the surface of the iron. Pain perception requires consciousness and an intact central nervous system. Common factors that disrupt the pain process include trauma, drugs, tumor growth, and metabolic disorders.

Gate-Control Theory of Pain

Melzack and Wall's gate-control theory (1965) was the first to suggest that pain has emotional and cognitive components in addition to

TABLE 44.1 Physiological Reactions to Pain

Response	Cause or Effect
Sympathetic Stimulation[a]	
Dilation of bronchial tubes and increased respiratory rate	Provides increased oxygen intake
Increased heart rate	Provides increased oxygen transport
Peripheral vasoconstriction (pallor, elevation in blood pressure)	Elevates blood pressure with shift of blood supply from periphery and viscera to skeletal muscles and brain
Increased blood glucose level	Provides additional energy
Increased cortisol level (short term)	Heightened memory functions, a burst of increased immunity, and lower sensitivity to pain
Diaphoresis	Controls body temperature during stress
Increased muscle tension	Prepares muscles for action
Dilation of pupils	Affords better vision
Decreased gastrointestinal motility	Frees energy for more immediate activity
Parasympathetic Stimulation[b]	
Pallor	Causes blood supply to shift away from periphery
Nausea and vomiting	Vagus nerve sends impulses to chemoreceptor trigger zone in the brain
Decreased heart rate and blood pressure	Results from vagal stimulation
Rapid, irregular breathing	Causes body defenses to fail under prolonged stress of pain

[a] Pain of low-to-moderate intensity and superficial pain.
[b] Severe or deep pain.

FIG. 44.3 Protective reflex to pain stimulus.

physical sensations. The theory explains how rubbing an injured area can reduce pain. The small-diameter fibers activated by noxious stimuli open the gate to pain transmission, and the large-diameter fibers have inhibitory effects to shut the gate. Rubbing the injured area promotes proprioceptive large-diameter fiber input and therefore inhibits further transmission of pain signals from small-diameter nerves to the brain. Melzack (1999) later proposed the neuromatrix theory of pain, which suggests that each individual possesses a genetically determined neural matrix that develops and is modulated by sensory input, making pain perception unique to each individual.

Physiological Responses. As pain impulses ascend the spinal cord toward the brainstem and thalamus, the stress response stimulates the autonomic nervous system (ANS). Pain of low-to-moderate intensity and superficial pain elicit the fight-or-flight reaction of the general adaptation syndrome (see Chapter 37). Stimulation of the sympathetic

branch of the ANS results in physiological responses (Table 44.1). Continuous, severe, or deep pain typically involving the visceral organs (e.g., with a myocardial infarction or colic from gallbladder or renal stones) activates the parasympathetic nervous system. Except in cases of severe traumatic pain, which cause a person to go into shock, most people adapt to their pain reflexively, and their physical signs return to normal baseline. Note that normal is not the same for everyone. Thus, patients in pain do *not* always have changes in their vital signs (Laures et al., 2020). Changes in vital signs more often indicate problems other than pain (Manocha and Taneja, 2016).

Behavioral Responses. The behavioral response to pain is also complex, influenced by a person's culture, pain experiences, perception of pain, and ability to manage stress. If left untreated or unrelieved, pain significantly alters quality of life with physical and psychological consequences; this phenomenon is referred to as high-impact pain (Dahlhamer et al., 2018). Effective pain management is essential. Some patients choose not to report pain if they believe that it inconveniences others or if it signals loss of self-control. Others endure severe pain without asking for assistance. Clenching the teeth, facial grimacing, holding or guarding the painful part, and bent posture are common indications of acute pain. Chronic pain can affect a patient's activity (eating, sleeping, socialization), thinking (confusion, forgetfulness), emotions (anger, depression, irritability), quality of life, and productivity (IOM, 2011). Nurses often recognize patterns of behavior that reflect pain even when patients do not or cannot report it verbally (e.g., patients with dementia or other cognitive changes) (Laures et al., 2020).

Assessing the success of pain-management therapies requires you to recognize a patient's unique response to pain. Be open to how your patient expresses pain; do not ignore a person's need, for example, to cry out or be verbally expressive. Encourage your patients to accept pain-relieving measures so that they remain active and continue to maintain daily activities. A patient's ability to tolerate pain significantly influences your perceptions of the degree of discomfort. Patients who have a low **pain tolerance** (level of pain a person is willing to accept) are sometimes inaccurately perceived as complainers. Teach patients the importance of reporting their pain when it occurs to facilitate better control and optimal functional status.

Acute and Chronic Pain

Pain is categorized by duration (acute or chronic) or pathological condition (e.g., cancer or neuropathic). The two types of pain that you observe in patients are acute (transient) and chronic (persistent), which includes cancer and noncancer pain.

Acute/Transient Pain. Acute pain is protective, usually has an identifiable cause, is of short duration, and has limited tissue damage and emotional response. It is common after acute injury, disease, or surgery. Acute pain is protective because it warns people of injury or disease. It eventually resolves, with or without treatment, after an injured area heals. Patients in acute pain are often frightened and anxious and expect relief quickly. It is self-limiting. Because acute pain has a predictable ending (healing) and an identifiable cause, health team members are usually willing to treat it aggressively, and patients understand that their pain will eventually go away.

Acute pain often slows recovery because it interferes with a patient's ability to become active and involved in self-care. Patients who cannot care for themselves often experience prolonged hospitalization and recovery from complications such as physical and emotional exhaustion, immobility, sleep deprivation, and pulmonary complications. Patients often focus all their energy on pain relief, delaying physical and psychological progress. Patient teaching and motivating a patient toward self-care are often hampered until pain is successfully managed. If not adequately controlled, unrelieved acute pain can progress to chronic pain. When acute pain is relieved, a patient can direct full attention toward recovery.

Chronic/Persistent Noncancer Pain. Chronic pain affects more than 50 million American adults, and among those affected, nearly 20 million live with high-impact chronic pain (Dahlhamer et al., 2018). Unlike acute pain, chronic pain is not protective. It is prolonged, varies in intensity, and usually lasts longer than 3 to 6 months and beyond the expected or predicted healing time (ACPA & Stanford Medicine, 2021; Huether and McCance, 2019). Chronic pain does not always have an identifiable cause. Examples of chronic noncancer pain include arthritis, low back pain, headache, fibromyalgia, and peripheral neuropathy. It may result from an initial injury such as a back sprain, or there may be an ongoing cause such as illness. Chronic noncancer pain may be viewed as a disease since it has a distinct pathology that causes changes throughout the nervous system that may worsen over time. It has significant psychological and cognitive effects and is sometimes considered a serious, distinct disease. Chronic noncancer pain is usually non–life threatening. In some cases an injured area healed long ago, yet the pain is ongoing and does not respond to treatment.

The possible unknown cause of chronic pain, combined with ineffective treatments and the unrelenting nature and uncertainty of its duration, frustrates a patient, which can lead to psychological depression and even suicide. Chronic pain is a major cause of psychological and physical disability, leading to problems such as job loss, inability to perform simple daily activities, sexual dysfunction, and social isolation.

A person with chronic noncancer pain often experiences pain that may not have the same physiological response as acute pain; however, the subjective reports and interference with activities of daily living (ADLs), socialization, and ability to perform work duties are very real. Over time, patients often experience physical and mental exhaustion. Symptoms associated with chronic pain include fatigue, insomnia, anorexia, weight loss, apathy, hopelessness, depression, and anger.

Chronic pain creates the uncertainty of how one will feel from day to day. A person with chronic noncancer pain often does not show obvious symptoms and does not adapt to the pain. A person with chronic pain who consults with numerous health care providers is sometimes labeled a drug seeker when that person is actually seeking adequate pain relief. Nurses need to discourage patients from having multiple health care providers for treating pain and instead refer them to specialists. Pain centers specialize in diagnostic testing and take a holistic approach to pain management, which may include a variety of pharmacological, nonpharmacological, noninvasive, and invasive treatments (Pasero and McCaffery, 2011).

Chronic Episodic Pain. Pain that occurs sporadically over an extended period of time is episodic pain. Pain episodes last for hours, days, or weeks. Examples of chronic episodic pain include migraine headaches and pain related to sickle cell crisis.

Cancer Pain. Not all patients with cancer experience pain. For patients who do have pain, 90% are able to manage their pain with simple interventions (Burchum and Rosenthal, 2019). Some patients with cancer experience acute and/or chronic pain. Nociceptive pain is more common, resulting from tissue injury. Neuropathic pain results from peripheral nerve injury (Table 44.2). Cancer pain is usually caused by tumor progression and related pathological processes, invasive procedures, toxicities of chemotherapy, infection, and physical limitations. A patient senses pain at the actual site of the tumor or distant to the site, called *referred pain*. Always assess reports of new pain by a patient with existing pain. Although the treatment of cancer pain has greatly improved, undertreatment of cancer pain still occurs (Burchum and Rosenthal, 2019). Inadequate education of health care providers, fear of addiction, cultural and religious beliefs, and health care agency barriers (e.g., lack of communication, time constraints, short staffing) often lead to undertreatment of cancer pain (Burchum and Rosenthal, 2019; Gerber et al., 2021).

Idiopathic Pain. Idiopathic pain is chronic pain that either does not have an identifiable physical or psychological cause or is perceived as excessive for the extent of an organic pathological condition. An example of idiopathic pain is complex regional pain syndrome (CRPS). Research is needed to better identify the causes of idiopathic pain to identify more effective treatments.

> **REFLECT NOW**
>
> A nurse is caring for one patient who is experiencing acute abdominal pain related to appendicitis and another patient who is experiencing abdominal pain related to ovarian cancer. Compare the pain of these two patients. How might the patients' pain be similar? How might it be different?

NURSING KNOWLEDGE BASE

Nursing knowledge of pain mechanisms and interventions continues to grow through nursing research. This section explores factors that influence the pain experience.

Knowledge, Attitudes, and Beliefs

The knowledge, attitudes and beliefs of nurses and other health care providers affect their approach to pain management. Preconceptions about patients in pain often exist. Some believe that patients are experiencing

TABLE 44.2 Classification of Pain by Inferred Pathology

Nociceptive Pain	Neuropathic Pain

I. *Nociceptive pain:* Normal stimulation of special peripheral nerve endings—called *nociceptors;* usually responsive to nonopioids and/or opioids.
  A. *Somatic pain:* Comes from bone, joint, muscle, skin, or connective tissue; is usually aching or throbbing in quality and well localized
  B. *Visceral pain:* Arises from visceral organs such as the gastrointestinal tract and pancreas; is sometimes subdivided:
    1. Tumor involvement of organ capsule that causes aching and fairly well-localized pain.
    2. Obstruction of hollow viscus, which causes intermittent cramping and poorly localized pain.
	I. *Neuropathic pain:* Pain caused by a lesion or disease of the somatosensory nervous system; treatment usually includes adjuvant analgesics.
	  A. Centrally generated pain
	    1. *Deafferentation pain:* Injury to either the peripheral or central nervous system.
	    Examples: Phantom pain indicates injury to the peripheral nervous system; burning pain below the level of a spinal cord lesion reflects injury to the central nervous system.
	    2. *Sympathetically maintained pain:* Associated with impaired regulation of the autonomic nervous system.
	    Examples: Pain is associated with complex regional pain syndrome, type I, type II.
	  B. Peripherally generated pain
	    1. *Painful polyneuropathies:* Pain felt along the distribution of many peripheral nerves.
	    Examples: Diabetic neuropathy, alcohol-nutritional neuropathy, and Guillain-Barré syndrome.
	    2. *Painful mononeuropathies:* Usually associated with a known peripheral nerve injury; pain is felt at least partly along the distribution of the damaged nerve.
	    Examples: Nerve root compression, nerve entrapment, trigeminal neuralgia.

From Pasero C, McCaffery M: *Pain assessment and pharmacologic management,* St Louis, 2011, Mosby.

pain only when they show objective signs of pain. Thus, when there is no obvious source of pain (e.g., the patient with chronic low back pain or neuropathies), these health care providers stereotype patients with pain as malingerers, complainers, or difficult patients. This belief about patients in pain negatively influences pain assessment and seriously limits interventions offered to relieve pain.

Studies of nurses' attitudes regarding pain management show that pain assessment and resultant titration of pain medication doses are often affected by a nurse's opinion about a patient's self-report of pain. A nurse's assessment of pain intensity often underestimates a patient's report of pain (Shen et al., 2017). Nurses have also been shown to significantly underrate the beliefs patients have about pain management (Dequeker, 2018). Some nurses only use information about how a patient's pain is treated to determine a patient's cues about pain severity and to make clinical judgments about a patient's symptoms, which leads to underestimation and overestimation of pain (Dekel et al., 2016). Patients with a high self-report of pain, even when nurses are aware of their pain experience and analgesic treatment, are vulnerable to underestimation and hence to pain undertreatment (Dekel et al., 2016). Patients with a low self-report of pain are subject to overestimation and thus are exposed to overtreatment with potential treatment hazards. Many nurse and patient variables (e.g., culture, gender, age, education, knowledge, patient diagnosis) contribute to differences in pain ratings. A study showed that patients experience better quality of care when they are treated by nurses who receive continuing education about pain management and who have greater autonomy in modifying pain-treatment protocols (Tomaszek and Debska, 2018).

Nurses' assumptions and biases about patients in pain seriously limit their ability to offer pain relief (Box 44.2). Too often nurses allow misconceptions about pain to affect their willingness to provide pain relief. While some nurses believe patients' reports of pain only if the patients appear to be in pain, other nurses avoid acknowledging patients' pain because of fear of contributing to medication addiction. These beliefs and fears lead to mistrust, increased patient recovery time, complications, mortality, psychological problems, and increased health care costs (Pasero and McCaffery, 2011). Nurses are entitled to their personal beliefs, but they must accept patients' reports of pain; act according to professional guidelines, standards, and

BOX 44.2 Common Biases and Misconceptions About Pain

The following statements are *false:*
- Patients who abuse substances (e.g., use drugs or alcohol) overreact to discomfort.
- Patients with minor illnesses have less pain than those with severe physical alteration.
- Administering analgesics regularly leads to drug addiction.
- The amount of tissue damage in an injury accurately indicates pain intensity.
- Health care personnel are the best authorities on the nature of a patient's pain.
- Psychogenic pain is not real.
- Chronic pain is psychological.
- Patients who are hospitalized experience pain.
- Patients who cannot speak do not feel pain.

position statements; individualize appropriate policies, procedures, and protocols; and provide evidence-based care (American Nurses Association, 2018).

To help a patient gain pain relief, it is important to view the experience through the patient's eyes. Acknowledging personal values and beliefs about pain and pain management and recognizing that patient expectations influence outcomes related to pain management are essential to patient-centered care (QSEN, 2020). Nurses who are knowledgeable about the concepts of pain can more objectively analyze a patient's pain experience and make clinical judgments to provide effective treatment that recognizes a patient's preferences, values, and needs.

Factors Influencing Pain

Because each individual's pain experience is different, you need to consider an array of factors to ensure you take a holistic approach in assessing and caring for a patient in pain. Some of these factors are modifiable and can be changed, while others are nonmodifiable, such as age. Nursing interventions target the modifiable factors, such as attention, fear, and anxiety, by providing patients and families with the knowledge and skills to cope with pain.

Physiological Factors.

Age. Age influences the pain experience. It is important to consider how a painful event affects a patient developmentally. For example, pain may prevent an adolescent from engaging socially with friends. A middle-aged adult may be unable to continue work in cases when pain is severe. It is particularly important to recognize how developmental differences affect how infants and older adults react to pain. It is necessary to address misconceptions about pain management in the very young and in older adults before intervening for a patient (Tables 44.3 and 44.4).

Young children have trouble understanding pain, its meaning, and the procedures that cause it. If they have not developed full vocabularies, they have difficulty with verbally describing and expressing pain to parents or caregivers. Toddlers and preschoolers are unable to recall explanations about pain or to associate it with experiences that may be unrelated to the painful condition. With these developmental considerations in mind, it is necessary to adapt approaches for assessing a child's pain (e.g., type of assessment tool to use, what to ask, including what to ask parents) and to learn which behaviors to observe and how to prepare a child for a painful medical procedure.

TABLE 44.3 Misconceptions About Pain in Infants

Misconception	Correction
Infants cannot feel pain.	Infants have the anatomical and functional requirements for pain processing by mid- to late gestation.
Infants are less sensitive to pain than older children and adults.	Term neonates have the same sensitivity to pain as older infants and children. Preterm neonates have a greater sensitivity to pain than term neonates or older children.
Infants cannot express pain.	Although infants cannot verbalize pain, they respond with behavioral cues and physiological indicators that are observable.
Infants must learn about pain from previous painful experiences.	Pain requires no prior experience; infants do not need to learn it from earlier painful experience. It occurs with the first pain experience.
You cannot accurately assess pain in infants.	You use behavioral cues (e.g., facial expressions, cry, body movements) and physiological indicators of pain (e.g., changes in vital signs) to assess pain reliably and validly in infants.
You cannot safely give analgesics and anesthetics to infants and neonates because of their immature capacity to metabolize and eliminate drugs and their sensitivity to opioid-induced respiratory depression.	Infants are very sensitive to drugs. Response to drugs is often intense and prolonged. Absorption is faster than expected. Dosages of drugs excreted by the kidneys need to be reduced (Burchum and Rosenthal, 2019). Prescribers carefully select the medication, dosage, administration route, and time. Nurses monitor frequently for desired and undesired effects. They also follow medication orders to titrate and wean medications to minimize adverse effects.

TABLE 44.4 Misconceptions About Pain in Older Adults

Misconception	Correction
Pain is a natural outcome of growing old.	Older adults are at greater risk (as much as twofold) than younger adults for many painful conditions; however, pain is not an inevitable result of aging.
Pain perception, or sensitivity, decreases with age.	This assumption is unsafe. Although there is evidence that emotional suffering specifically related to pain may be less in older than in younger patients, no scientific basis exists for the claim that a decrease in perception of pain occurs with age or that age dulls sensitivity to pain.
If the older patient does not report pain, the patient does not have pain.	Older patients commonly underreport pain. Reasons include expecting to have pain with increasing age; not wanting to alarm loved ones; being fearful of losing their independence; not wanting to distract, anger, or bother caregivers; and believing that caregivers know they have pain and are doing all they can to relieve it. The absence of a report of pain does not mean the absence of pain.
If an older patient appears to be occupied, asleep, or otherwise distracted from pain, the patient does not have pain.	Older patients often believe that it is unacceptable to show pain and have learned to use a variety of ways to cope with it (e.g., many patients use distraction successfully for short periods of time). Sleeping is sometimes a coping strategy; alternately, it indicates exhaustion, not pain relief. Do not make assumptions about the presence or absence of pain solely based on a patient's behavior.
The potential side effects of opioids make them too dangerous to use to relieve pain in older adults.	In most cases nonopioids are preferred to opioids for noncancer pain, but opioids can be used safely for older adults with moderate to severe cancer pain. Although an older adult who is opioid-naïve is usually more sensitive to opioids, this does not justify withholding their use in pain management. Initiate analgesics at the lowest effective dose and titrate to achieve pain control with minimal adverse effects; this requires frequent reassessment of patients for pain relief and side effects as doses are adjusted (Touhy and Jett, 2020).
Patients with Alzheimer disease and other cognitive impairments do not feel pain, and their reports of pain are most likely invalid.	No evidence exists that older adults who are cognitively impaired experience less pain or that their reports of pain are less valid than those of individuals with intact cognitive function (Horgas, 2020). Patients with dementia or other deficits of cognition most likely suffer significant unrelieved pain and discomfort. The best approach to assessment is to accept a patient's report of pain and use relevant pain assessment tools.
Older patients report more pain as they age.	Even though older patients experience a higher incidence of painful conditions such as arthritis, osteoporosis, peripheral vascular disease, and cancer than younger patients, studies show that they underreport pain. Many older adults grew up valuing the ability to "grin and bear it" (Pasero and McCaffery, 2011).

Pain is not an inevitable part of aging. Likewise, pain perception does not decrease with age. However, older adults have a greater likelihood of developing pathological conditions, which are accompanied by acute and chronic pain. Persistent pain may be associated with impaired physical function, falls, diminished appetite, impaired sleep, depression, anxiety, agitation, delirium, and reduced cognitive function. In addition, age-related changes and increased frailty may lead to a less predictable response to analgesics, increased sensitivity to medications, and potentially harmful drug effects (O'Sullivan et al., 2017). Serious impairment of functional status often accompanies pain in older patients. It often reduces mobility and activity tolerance and impairs the ability to perform ADLs and be involved in social and physical activities. Pain in an older adult requires aggressive assessment, diagnosis, and management (Box 44.3).

Some older patients have difficulty interpreting their pain, especially when they have multiple diseases with symptoms that are similar or that affect similar parts of the body. For example, chest pain can indicate a heart attack, arthritis of the spine, or an abdominal disorder. A thorough assessment is especially needed in these cases to determine the source of pain. When older adults experience cognitive impairment and confusion, they often have difficulty recalling pain experiences and providing detailed explanations of their pain (Pasero and McCaffery, 2011).

Fatigue. Fatigue heightens the perception of pain and decreases coping abilities. A patient's perception of pain is even greater when fatigue is accompanied with sleeplessness. Pain is often experienced less after a restful sleep than at the end of a long day.

Genes. Research on healthy human subjects suggests that genetic information passed on by parents possibly increases or decreases a person's sensitivity to pain and determines pain threshold or tolerance. Current evidence shows that slight changes in deoxyribonucleic acid (DNA) or in the expression of genes can partly explain individual differences in pain. Some studies have identified genetic risk factors for patients with migraines and musculoskeletal disorders such as osteoarthritis and degenerative disc disease (de Boer et al., 2019; Narusyte et al., 2020). Genetic influences may also help explain a patient's sensitivity to pain as well as metabolism of pain medications (e.g., opioids)

BOX 44.3 FOCUS ON OLDER ADULTS
Factors Influencing Pain in Older Adults

- With aging, muscle mass decreases, body fat increases, and percentage of body water decreases. This increases the concentration of water-soluble drugs such as morphine given in normal doses. The volume of distribution for fat-soluble drugs such as fentanyl increases (Burchum and Rosenthal, 2019).
- Some older adults eat poorly, resulting in low serum albumin levels. Many analgesics are highly protein bound. When serum albumin is low, less of the medication is bound to proteins, resulting in the availability of higher levels of the active medication ("free" drug), which increases the risk for side effects or toxic effects (Burchum and Rosenthal, 2019).
- Liver and renal function naturally decline as a person ages. This results in reduced metabolism and excretion of drugs. Thus, older adults often experience a greater peak effect and longer duration of analgesics (Touhy and Jett, 2020).
- Pain is common in the advanced stages of many chronic diseases, including heart failure, end-stage renal disease, and chronic obstructive pulmonary disease. In addition, a significant number of patients undergoing joint replacement procedures (e.g., knee joint replacement) report chronic pain following surgery (Wluka et al., 2020; Khalid et al., 2021).
- Age-related changes in the skin such as thinning and loss of elasticity affect the absorption rate of topical analgesics.

(Bugada et al., 2020). Thus, it may be helpful to encourage patients who have persistent pain syndromes to seek genetic counseling.

Neurological Function. A patient's neurological function influences the pain experience. Any factor that interrupts or influences normal pain reception or perception (e.g., spinal cord injury, peripheral neuropathy, or neurological disease) affects a patient's awareness of and response to pain. Some pharmacological agents (analgesics, sedatives, and anesthetics) influence pain perception and response because of their effect on the nervous system.

Social Factors.
Previous Experience. Each person learns from painful experiences. Prior experience does not mean that a person accepts pain more easily in the future. Previous frequent episodes of pain without relief or bouts of severe pain cause anxiety or fear. In contrast, if a person repeatedly experiences the same type of pain that was relieved successfully in the past, the person finds it easier to interpret the pain sensation. As a result, the patient is better prepared to take necessary actions to relieve the pain.

When a patient has no experience with a painful condition, the first perception of pain often impairs the ability to cope. For example, patients often experience severe incisional pain for several days after abdominal surgery. Unless a patient knows that this is a common occurrence following surgery, the onset of pain seems like a serious complication. In the preoperative and anticipatory phase of the pain experience, you prepare the patient with a clear explanation of the type of pain to expect and methods available to reduce it. Patient education on pain management can help reduce a patient's perception of pain and ability to participate in activities, such as postoperative breathing exercises to reduce postoperative complications (see Chapter 50).

Family and Social Network. People in pain often depend on family members or close friends for support, assistance, or protection. Although pain still exists, the presence of family or friends can often make the experience less stressful. Conversation with family is a useful distraction. The presence of parents is especially important for children experiencing pain.

Spiritual Factors. Spirituality is an active search for meaning in situations (see Chapter 35). Spiritual beliefs affect the way patients view or cope with pain. Evidence shows that interventions that address spirituality have benefits for individuals' physical and emotional health, including the relief of pain (Ferreira-Valente et al., 2020).

Patients often ask spiritually based questions, such as "Why has this happened to me?" or "Why am I suffering?" Spiritual pain goes beyond what we can see. "Why has God done this to me?" "Is this suffering teaching me something?" Other spiritual concerns include loss of independence and becoming a burden to family. Recall that pain is an experience that has physical *and* emotional components. Patients who deal with persistent pain using positive spiritual coping practices such as looking to a higher being for strength and support adjust better to pain and have significantly better mental health (Ferreira-Valente et al., 2020). Providing support for patients to utilize their spiritual practices is essential for pain management.

Psychological Factors.
Attention. The degree to which a patient focuses attention on pain influences the patient's perception. Increased attention is associated with increased pain, whereas distraction is associated with a diminished pain response. Nurses apply this concept in various pain-relief interventions such as relaxation, guided imagery, and massage. By focusing patients' attention and concentration on other stimuli, their perception of pain declines (see Chapter 32).

Anxiety and Fear. A person perceives pain differently if it suggests a threat, loss, punishment, or challenge. For example, a woman in labor perceives pain differently than a woman with a history of cancer who is experiencing a new pain and fearing recurrence. In addition, the meaning of pain is influenced by a patient's perception of the degree and quality of the pain. The relationship between pain and anxiety and fear is complex. Anxiety and fear often increase the perception of pain, and pain causes feelings of anxiety and fear. It is difficult to separate the two sensations.

Patients who are critically ill or injured often perceive a lack of control over their environment and their care, which can cause anxiety. This anxiety leads to serious pain-management problems. Pharmacological and nonpharmacological approaches to the management of anxiety are appropriate; however, anxiolytic medications are not a substitute for analgesia (Pasero and McCaffery, 2011).

Coping Style. Pain is a lonely experience that often causes patients to feel a loss of control. Coping style influences the ability to deal with pain (see Chapter 37). People with internal loci of control perceive themselves as having control over events in their lives and the outcomes such as pain. They ask questions, desire information, and make choices about treatment. In contrast, people with external loci of control perceive that other factors in their lives, such as nurses, are responsible for the outcome of events. These patients follow directions and are more passive in managing their pain. Learn to understand patients' coping resources during painful experiences so that you can incorporate these into your plan of care. For example, a patient who does not ask for pain medication but shows behavioral signs of discomfort might require you to be more responsive in offering as-needed (prn) medications on time.

Cultural Factors.
The meaning that a person associates with pain affects the experience of pain and how one adapts to it. This is often closely associated with a person's cultural background, including age, education, race, and familial factors. Cultural beliefs and values affect how individuals cope with pain. They learn what is expected and accepted by their culture, including how to react to pain.

Health care providers often mistakenly assume that everyone responds to pain in the same way. Different meanings and attitudes are associated with pain across various cultural groups. An understanding of the cultural meaning of pain helps you design culturally sensitive care for people with pain.

Culture affects pain expression. In general, most Americans use facial expressions as a part of nonverbal communication. However, facial expressions vary with culture. Some people use facial features to help communicate that they are in pain, while others use less facial expression and are generally less responsive, especially with people they do not know. In some cultures, negative emotions, such as pain, may be concealed by smiling (Giger and Haddad, 2021).

As a nurse, explore the impact of culture on a patient's pain experience and how the patient expresses pain. Then adjust the plan of care appropriately (Box 44.4). Ask a patient about previous experiences with pain and pain management. Work with a patient and family to learn their cultural beliefs, values, and preferences to adequately assess and manage pain (see Chapter 9). Use a culturally appropriate pain assessment tool, and communicate the use of that tool to other health care providers in an effort to provide culturally sensitive care.

Factors Impacted By Pain.
Quality of Life. Pain affects a patient's daily activities and quality of life. Pain affects an individual's ability to provide self-care, work, perform at school, and interact socially with friends and family. Chronic pain is a major public health problem, producing significant economic and social burdens that affect the patient, family, and social circles (Dueñas et al., 2016; IPRCC, 2021a). The biopsychosocial model for chronic pain offers a valuable framework for understanding how a variety of factors can contribute to chronic pain and ultimately affect an individual's quality of life.

Self-Care. Pain can limit a person's ability to perform activities of self-care, including ADLs and instrumental activities of daily living (IADLs) (e.g., shopping and house cleaning). Research shows a strong correlation between chronic pain and reduced physical activity and increased disability (Narusyte et al., 2020; Geneen et al., 2017). For example, individuals who experience chronic pain often experience limitations that affect the ability to exercise, walk, complete household chores (e.g., vacuum, washing dishes), participate in social activities, and maintain an independent lifestyle (Dueñas et al., 2016).

⊕ BOX 44.4 CULTURAL ASPECTS OF CARE

Assessing Pain in Culturally Diverse Patients

Pain is a biopsychosocial phenomenon. Culture shapes the experience of pain, including its expression and a patient's behaviors, or coping responses. For example, an individual from a higher socioeconomic group may have more resources for managing pain and is more likely to adapt behaviors that will lessen pain. Several research studies have shown that people in the lowest as compared with the highest socioeconomic class are more likely to feel disabled because of their pain (Dahlhamer et al., 2018). A recent literature review demonstrated that Hispanic Americans often face numerous barriers to seeking and receiving pain care, including financial limitations, lack of insurance, language barriers, and immigration status (Hollingshead et al., 2016). Culture also affects a person's choice of lay remedies, help-seeking activities, and receptivity to medical treatment. Some health care providers undertreat pain because they do not understand the cultural effects on the perception of pain intensity. Nurses care for patients with pain from a variety of cultural backgrounds; thus you need to develop strategies to assess and manage pain in culturally diverse patients.

Implications for Patient-Centered Care
- Use culturally appropriate assessment tools, such as the Wong-Baker FACES® Pain Rating Scale, to assess pain (Givler et al., 2020; Wong-Baker FACES Foundation, 2016).
- Assess a patient's health literacy because this affects your ability to provide appropriate education about pain management and therapies (CDC, 2021b). Spanish-speaking Hispanic-American patients often report difficulty in describing their pain experiences to providers and report better pain control when a Spanish-language translator is present (Hollingshead et al., 2016).
- Recognize variations in subjective responses to pain. Undertreatment, overtreatment, or lack of trust in the health care provider might occur if members of the health care team are unaware of the cultural norms associated with pain and pain expression, since pain is subjective (Givler et al., 2020).
- Be sensitive to variations in communication styles. Some cultures believe that nonverbal expression of pain is sufficient to describe the pain experience, whereas others assume that if pain medication is appropriate, the nurse will bring it; thus, asking for pain medication is inappropriate (Giger and Haddad, 2021).
- Understand that expression of pain is unacceptable within certain cultures. Some patients believe that asking for help indicates a lack of respect, whereas others believe acknowledging pain is a sign of weakness (Giger and Haddad, 2021).
- Pain is personal and related to religious beliefs. Some cultures consider suffering a part of life to be endured to enter heaven.
- Use knowledge of biological variations of pain. Significant differences in drug metabolism, dosing requirements, therapeutic response, and adverse effects occur in cultural groups. A wide range of responses is also possible within cultural groups. Therefore, assess each patient's response to pain medication carefully (Burchum and Rosenthal, 2019).
- Develop a personal awareness of your own values and beliefs that affect your responses to patients' reports of pain (QSEN, 2020).

Work and School. Acute and chronic pain affect how a person performs at work or school. Children with chronic pain have higher levels of absenteeism in school (Allison et al., 2019). Likewise, pain affects attendance at work. Individuals who work often need to change their occupational duties or positions and may end up losing their jobs because of their pain symptoms (Narusyte et al., 2020). When a person is unable to perform as expected, the threatened loss can result in loss of sleep, change in eating habits, depression, and fear of loss of independence.

Social Support. Support from family and friends is critical for a patient who is experiencing pain. But when a person has pain, the members of the family are also affected. Pain often restricts an individual's leisure activities and social contacts. Social isolation becomes a common problem. The negative emotions, irritability, and feelings of anger that affect patients in pain have a negative impact on interpersonal relationships and the levels of stress in families and social connections. The quality of life for a family caregiver can be negatively affected when the caregiver is involved in the care of a patient with chronic pain (Rouhi et al., 2020).

As Matt is preparing to care for Mrs. Mays, he reflects on what he understands about osteoarthritis and its effect on Mrs. Mays. Matt understands that Mrs. Mays is experiencing chronic noncancer pain in her hips, knees, and hands. Matt considers his knowledge of the physiology of pain and his understanding about the gate-control theory of pain. He knows that the pain caused by the osteoarthritis most likely will have emotional, cognitive, and physical effects on Mrs. Mays and

her husband. Knowing that chronic pain is a major cause of psychological and physical disability, Matt begins to wonder how Mrs. Mays' pain affects her ability to move and to perform ADLs, as well as her emotional and spiritual well-being. This knowledge will help direct Matt's assessment.

REFLECT NOW

Modifiable and nonmodifiable factors can influence pain. Helping the patient and the patient's family to understand that mood, coping strategies, and the social environment can all have positive and negative influences on pain and functional outcomes is important. What types of modifiable and nonmodifiable factors that affect pain can you identify in a family member who had pain or in a patient for whom you have provided care?

CRITICAL THINKING

Sound clinical judgment is essential to providing a patient effective pain management. You will apply critical thinking as you synthesize the scientific knowledge pertinent to a patient's condition, the information gathered from patient assessment, your previous experience in pain management, environmental factors influencing your care approaches, your critical thinking attitudes, and intellectual and professional standards (Fig. 44.4).

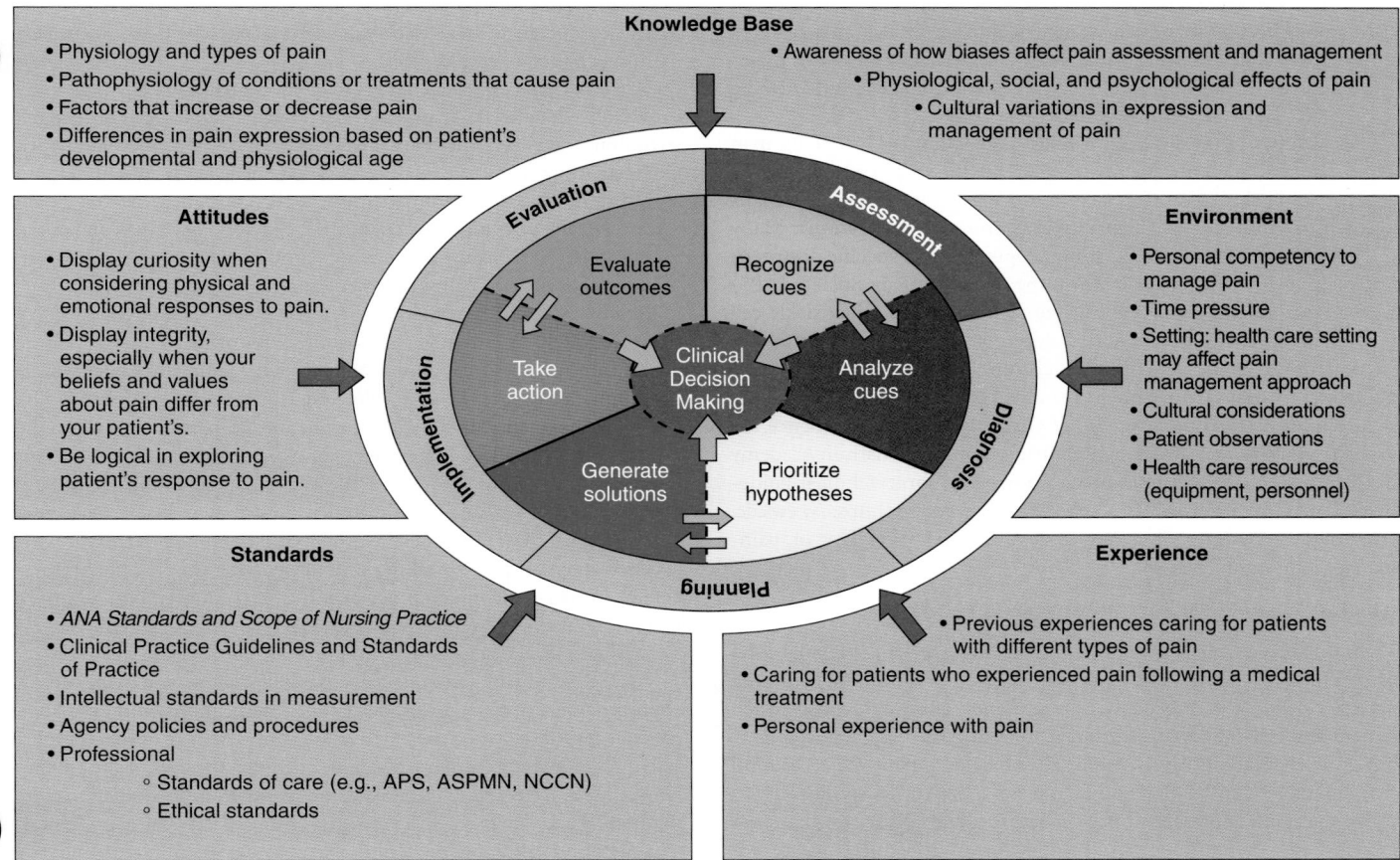

FIG. 44.4 Critical thinking model for pain assessment. *APS,* American Pain Society; *ASPMN,* American Society for Pain Management Nursing; *NCCN,* National Comprehensive Cancer Network. (Clinical Judgment Measurement Model copyright © NCSBN. All rights reserved.)

You anticipate a patient's pain based on the patient's clinical condition along with anticipated pain your patient may experience from surgical and/or medical treatments. To make timely clinical judgments, you anticipate the information you need, analyze the data, and make decisions regarding patient care. A patient's condition or situation is always changing. During assessment consider all critical thinking elements that lead to appropriate nursing diagnoses.

Knowledge of pain physiology and the many factors that influence pain promotes early recognition of patient problems. Similarly, understanding how a patient's illness or condition causes pain offers a perspective of what to expect when you examine a patient. Previous experience in caring for patients with pain sharpens your assessment skills and ability to choose effective therapies. Environmental conditions within a health care setting will influence the resources you have to assess and manage pain. Critical thinking attitudes and intellectual standards ensure the aggressive assessment, creative planning, and thorough evaluation needed to obtain an acceptable level of patient pain relief while balancing treatment benefits with treatment-associated risks. Successful pain management does not necessarily mean pain elimination but rather attainment of a mutually agreed-on pain-relief goal that allows patients to control their pain instead of the pain controlling them.

❖ NURSING PROCESS

Apply the nursing process, and use a critical thinking approach in making the sound clinical judgments necessary to develop and implement an individualized plan of care. Nurses use critical thinking and approach pain management systematically to understand and treat a patient's pain. Successful management of pain depends on establishing a relationship of trust among health care providers, patient, and family. Pain management includes relieving a patient's pain, identifying ways to improve or maintain a patient's quality of life and ability to work productively, and helping patients to enjoy recreation and function normally.

According to the American Nurses Association (ANA, 2018), pain assessment and pain management are within the scope of every nurse's practice. Thus the ANA offers a certification examination in pain management to staff nurses (http://www.aspmn.org/certification). Many clinical guidelines are available for managing pain in specific disorders. For example, guidelines available on the American Pain Society (APS) website include managing pain in the primary care setting; sickle cell pain; cancer pain in adults and children; and pain in osteoarthritis, rheumatoid arthritis, and juvenile chronic arthritis. Evidence-based guidelines for pain management for older adults originally developed by the John A. Hartford Centers of Geriatric Nursing Excellence are available at https://geriatricpain.org/. In addition, the American Academy of Pain Medicine (http://www.painmed.org/library/clinical-guidelines/) and Centers for Disease Control and Prevention (https://www.cdc.gov/drugoverdose/prescribing/guideline.html) post a variety of pain-management guidelines.

◆ Assessment

During the assessment process, consider your patient's normal level of comfort, the painful effects of any diseases or conditions, and the patient's risks for pain because of treatments. Thoroughly assess each patient and critically analyze findings to ensure that you make patient-centered clinical decisions required for safe nursing care. Careful assessment is essential. Remember, it is not a patient's responsibility to prove that pain is present; it is your responsibility to accept that pain exists when a patient reports it. Pain itself cannot be measured objectively; it is a subjective experience. A comprehensive assessment of pain aims to gather information about the cause of a person's pain and determine its effect on the patient and family.

Through the Patient's Eyes. Many people view pain as a part of life. Some patients experience it for hours or days before seeking health care assistance. Others experience pain while in the care of health care personnel. Patients often expect and even accept a certain amount of pain while being hospitalized. It is important to learn a patient's own values and beliefs about the management of pain and recognize that patient expectations will influence your ability to achieve outcomes in its management (QSEN, 2020). Asking patients to tell their personal story about their pain is your first step in being able to identify their pain problems. Assess how this pain experience is affecting a patient and determine the patient's tolerable level of pain. One of your aims is to help a patient regain pain control. Assessing previous pain experiences and effective home interventions provides foundational information. Patients expect nurses to accept their reports of pain and be prompt in meeting their pain needs.

When assessing pain, be sensitive to the level of discomfort and determine which level will allow your patient to function. For example, when caring for a patient with pain, ask, "Which level of pain will allow you to walk down the hall?" The patient answers that walking is possible when pain is at a level of 2 on a scale of 0 to 10, with 0 being no pain and 10 being the worst pain imaginable. You then plan therapies to decrease the patient's pain to that level. Be sure that you partner with your patient when making decisions about the best approaches for managing pain.

Another aspect of assessing pain through the patient's eyes is to determine health literacy. People who struggle to find a range of words to talk about their pain lack the ability to use language for symptom relief. Patients who have a large vocabulary with which to describe pain symptoms are often better able to manage pain and reduce distress. Many health care agencies use assessment tools to help you accurately identify a patient's literacy skills.

Some patients experiencing acute or severe pain will have difficulty providing a detailed description. Thus, during an episode of acute pain, streamline your assessment and assess its location, severity, and quality. Collect a more detailed acute pain assessment when a patient is more comfortable (Box 44.5). For patients with chronic pain, a thorough pain assessment includes affective, cognitive, behavioral, spiritual, and social dimensions. In the home care setting, family members can assess pain by using the ABCs of pain assessment and management (Box 44.6).

Pain is dynamic; it can change frequently. Thus, you need to assess pain accurately on a regular basis along with other vital signs. Some health care agencies treat pain as the fifth vital sign. Pain assessment is *not* simply a number. Relying solely on a number fails to capture the multidimensionality of pain and may be unsafe, particularly when the number fails to reflect the entire pain experience or when a patient does not understand the use of the selected pain-rating scale. Pain assessment is a nursing responsibility. However, assistive personnel (AP), physical therapists, social workers, and other health care providers also screen for pain by asking patients whether they are uncomfortable or in pain. Encourage other health care team members to notify you immediately when pain is noted so that you can thoroughly assess the patient's level of discomfort and provide appropriate treatment.

Factual, timely, and accurate pain assessment allows you to identify an appropriate nursing diagnosis, determine interventions, and evaluate a patient's response (outcomes) to interventions. The core of this complex activity is to explore the pain experience through the eyes of the patient. Nurses use a variety of tools to assess nociceptive and neuropathic pain. In selecting a tool to use with a patient, be aware of the clinical usefulness, reliability, and validity of the tool in that specific patient population. For example, a tool that has been validated for use with children who are not old enough to describe their pain may not have validity or reliability for use with adults. Assessment tools (or scales) are available for use with

BOX 44.5   Nursing Assessment Questions

Current Pain: (Modify Assessment for Patient's Age, Cognitive Ability, Culture, Language, and Other Factors)

Palliative or Provocative factors: What makes your pain worse? What makes it better?

Quality: Describe your pain for me.

Relief measures: What do you take at home to gain pain relief? What makes your pain go away?

Region (location): Show me where you hurt.

Severity: On a scale of 0 to 10, how bad is your pain now?
- What is the worst pain you have had in the past 24 hours?
- What is the average pain you have had in the past 24 hours?

Timing: Do you have pain all of the time, only at certain times, or only on certain days?

U: Effect of pain: Describe what you cannot do because of your pain.
- With whom do you live, and how do they help you when you have pain?

Current Medications
- Which medications/herbs are you taking now?
- Tell me how these medications and herbs affect your pain?
- What approaches other than medications have you tried to relieve the pain?
- Have you ever used recreational drugs or alcohol to alleviate pain?

Activity
- What level of daily exercise can you maintain with your pain?
- Which type of movement increases or relieves your pain?
- Which types of activities do you now avoid because of your pain?

BOX 44.6   Routine Clinical Approach to Pain Assessment and Management: ABCDE

A: **Ask** about pain regularly. Assess pain systematically.

B: **Believe** patient and family in their report of pain and what relieves it.

C: **Choose** pain control options appropriate for the patient, family, and setting.

D: **Deliver** interventions in a timely, logical, and coordinated fashion.

E: **Empower** patients and their families. Enable them to control their course to the greatest extent possible.

From Jacox A, et al: *Management of cancer pain,* Clinical Practice Guideline No. 9, AHCPR Publication No. 94-0592, Rockville, MD, 1994, Agency for Health Care Policy and Research, Public Health Service, U.S. Department of Health and Human Services.

BOX 44.7   Possible Sources for Error in Pain Assessment

- Bias, which causes nurses to consistently overestimate or underestimate the pain that patients experience
- Vague, closed-ended, or unclear assessment questions, which lead to unreliable assessment data
- Use of pain assessment tools that are not evidence based or validated for a specific patient population
- Use of medical terms that patients with low health literacy cannot understand
- Patients who do not always provide complete, relevant, and accurate pain information
- Patients who are cognitively impaired and unable to use pain scales

response. Maintain a calm and nonjudgmental environment during your assessment. Do not rush the patient. If patients sense that you doubt their pain exists or that you are unwilling to listen to them, they may share little information about their pain experience or minimize their report of pain.

Ensure that the environment protects a patient's privacy and is free from interruptions. Simple measures, such as sitting when talking to patients about pain, let them know that you are sincerely concerned about their pain.

Physical Examination. When a patient is in pain, conduct a focused physical examination and observe for nonverbal responses to pain (e.g., grimacing, rigid body posture, limping, frowning, or crying) (see Chapter 30). Examine painful areas to see whether palpation or manipulation of the site increases pain. Determine whether movement affects the pain. Assess the effects pain has on a patient's mobility/balance, especially in older adults with persistent pain (Heden et al., 2020). Mobility assessment is critical because of the potential effect of pain and some analgesics on the risk for falling. Patients with chest or back pain may have a decrease in chest excursion. A neurological assessment includes determining whether the pain is also associated with changes in sensation and level of a patient's responsiveness.

Patients unable to communicate effectively often require special attention during assessment. For example, patients who are critically ill and have a clouded sensorium or the presence of nasogastric tubes or artificial airways require specific questions that they can answer with a nod of the head or by writing out a response. Patients with cognitive impairments require insightful assessment approaches involving close observation of vocal response, facial movements (e.g., grimacing, clenched teeth), and body movements (e.g., restlessness, pacing). Assess social interaction (e.g., does the patient avoid conversation?). You will need to use different approaches with infants and children, people who are developmentally delayed, patients who are psychotic, a patient who is critically ill or at the end of life, patients with dementia, and patients who are aphasic or do not speak English.

Follow clinical practice recommendations and use behavior-assessment pain tools with patients who are cognitively impaired (Box 44.8). These tools identify the presence of pain but do not determine its intensity. Thus, the number obtained when using a pain-behavior scale is a behavior score, not a pain-intensity rating (Pasero and McCaffery, 2011). If a patient speaks a different language, pain assessment requires the assistance of a professional interpreter.

Characteristics of Pain. Assessing the characteristics of pain allows you to understand the type of pain, its pattern, and the types of interventions that bring relief. Assessment tools to quantify the extent and degree of pain require your patient to be cognitively alert enough to be able to understand and follow instructions.

different patient populations, including critically ill adults, young children, or adults with advanced dementia. These tools identify how much pain exists, not how much pain a patient tolerates.

Be aware of possible errors in pain assessment (Box 44.7). Using the right tools and methods helps to avoid errors and ensures the selection of effective pain interventions. Failure of clinicians to accurately assess a patient's pain, accept the findings, and treat the report is a common cause of unrelieved pain and suffering.

Environmental Factors. A patient's self-report of pain is the single most reliable indicator of its existence and intensity (Pasero and McCaffery, 2011). Pain is unique. Many patients fail to report or discuss discomfort. At the same time many nurses believe that patients report pain if they have it. Thus, it is essential to maintain a therapeutic relationship that fosters open communication and creates an environment that conveys respect. Be alert for a patient's emotional responses, such as signs of anxiety, and be prepared to pause your assessment based on your patient's

BOX 44.8 EVIDENCE-BASED PRACTICE

Pain Assessment in Patients Who Are Nonverbal

PICOT Question: In adult patients who are nonverbal, which pain-assessment tool is most effective in determining presence of pain?

Evidence Summary

A common misconception is that individuals who are nonverbal because of dementia or cognitive impairments do not experience pain. These patients often present with atypical symptoms of pain, such as fearful expressions, combativeness, and resistance to care caused by pathophysiological changes in the brain (Atee et al., 2017). An evidence-based position statement and clinical practice recommendations for pain assessment in patients who are nonverbal were developed by the Hartford Institute for Geriatric Nursing and the Alzheimer's Association (Horgas, 2020). No single assessment strategy, such as interpretation of behaviors, pathology, or estimates of pain by others, will accurately indicate the presence of pain in a patient who is unable to communicate. However, initial assessment can be performed by using self-assessment with a numeric rating scale or verbal descriptor scale (Horgas, 2017).

Several tools assess for the presence of pain in adults who are cognitively impaired. Although research shows that these tools can be used to determine the presence of pain, there has been little evidence to determine whether they can be used to identify pain intensity. Commonly used instruments include the Abbey Pain Scale, Pain Assessment in Advanced Dementia Scale (PAINAD), and Noncommunicative Patient's Pain Assessment Instrument (NOPPAIN) to recognize the presence or absence of pain and provide a rating of pain severity in older people with impaired cognition. An electronic pain assessment tool (ePAT) is a point-of-care app that provides facial recognition technology for detecting facial microexpressions that indicate pain, as well as the presence of pain-related behaviors under five additional domains (voice, movement, behavior, activity, and body) (Atee, 2017). An analysis revealed a sensitivity of 96.1% and accuracy of 95% (Hoti et al., 2018). This assessment supports the clinical usefulness of the ePAT for identifying pain in patients with moderate to severe dementia.

A qualitative study found that critical care nurses experience challenges when using pain scales with patients who are nonverbal. Nursing challenges were categorized as "forgotten priority," "organizational barriers," "attitudinal barriers," and "barriers to knowledge" (Deldar et al., 2018). Findings suggest the need for better education and mentoring on how to use pain scales and the nature of pain in patients who are nonverbal to empower nurses to use nonverbal pain scales.

Application to Nursing Practice

- Ask patients to self-report pain using simple yes/no responses or vocalizations or a numerical rating scale (Chow et al., 2016).
- Search for potential causes of pain (Horgas, 2017). Examples include pain associated with intravenous insertion site infiltrations, abdominal cramping and fullness, urinary retention, or prolonged pressure on body parts associated with immobility.
- Assume that pain is present after ruling out other problems (infection, constipation) that cause pain.
- Identify pathological conditions or procedures that cause pain.
- Observe patient behaviors and list behaviors (e.g., facial expressions, vocalizations, body movements, changes in interactions or mental status) that indicate pain (Horgas, 2017).
- Ask family members, parents, or caregivers for a surrogate report (Horgas, 2020).
- Use standardized evidence-based behavioral pain assessment tools to ensure appropriate pain assessment (Horgas, 2020).
- Use the PAINAD to assess pain in patients with advanced dementia (Horgas, 2017).

Timing (Onset, Duration, and Pattern). Ask questions to determine the onset, duration, and time sequence of pain. When did it begin? How long has it lasted? Does it occur at the same time each day? Is it intermittent, constant, or a combination? How often does it recur? It is sometimes easier to diagnose the nature of pain by identifying time factors. Knowing the time cycle or pattern of pain helps you intervene before the pain occurs or worsens (see Box 44.5).

Location. Ask a patient to describe or point to all areas of discomfort to assess pain location. To localize the pain specifically, have the patient trace the area from the most severe point outward. This is difficult to do if pain is diffuse or involves several sites or parts of the body. Do not assume that your patient's pain always occurs in the same location. When describing pain location to other health care providers, use anatomical landmarks and descriptive terminology. The statement "Pain is localized in the upper right abdominal quadrant" is more specific than "The patient states the pain is in the abdomen." Pain classified by location can be further classified as superficial or cutaneous, deep or visceral, referred, or radiating (Table 44.5).

Severity. One of the most subjective and therefore most useful characteristics for reporting pain is its severity. Nurses teach patients how to use pain scales to help them communicate pain severity or intensity. Many scales are available in several languages to aid nurses when a professional interpreter is not present. The purpose of using a pain scale is to identify a patient's perception of pain intensity over time so that the effectiveness of interventions can be evaluated. It is important to select the scale that is appropriate for a patient's age, language, condition, and ability and to ensure that the patient understands how to use it (Karcioglu et al., 2018; Zielinski et al., 2020).

Pain Scales. Use a scale to measure the current severity of a patient's pain. Also ask patients to rate their average pain and the worst pain they have had in the past 24 hours. This information allows you to see trends in pain severity. An effective pain scale is easy to use, understandable, not time consuming, and provides an accurate pain description. If patients use a hearing aid or glasses, be sure that they are using them when answering pain-assessment questions or marking a pain scale. Once you determine which scale works best for a patient, be sure to use it consistently. Do not use a pain scale to compare the pain of one patient with that of another.

There are three types of pain scales: numerical rating scale, verbal descriptive scale, and visual analog scale. In a systematic review of the efficacy of pain scales, all three scales were found to be valid, reliable, and appropriate for use in clinical practice, although the visual analog scale has more difficulties than the others (Karcioglu et al., 2018).

A numerical rating scale (NRS) requires patients to rate pain on an 11-point line of 0 to 10, with 0 representing no pain and 10 representing the worst pain the patient can imagine (Fig. 44.5A). The scale has been found to be very effective in many populations, including youth with disabilities (Miró et al., 2016). This scale is also used to assess pain intensity before and after therapeutic interventions. A verbal descriptive scale (VDS) consists of a line with two- to six-word descriptors equally spaced along the line (Fig. 44.5B). Ask a patient to look at the scale and choose the descriptor that best represents the severity of pain. A visual analog scale (VAS) consists of a straight line without labeled subdivisions (Fig. 44.5C). The straight line shows a continuum of intensity and has labeled end points. A patient indicates pain by marking the appropriate point on the line.

TABLE 44.5 Classification of Pain By Location

Location	Characteristics	Examples of Causes
Superficial or Cutaneous Pain resulting from stimulation of skin	Pain is of short duration and localized. It usually is a sharp sensation.	Needlestick; small cut or laceration
Deep or Visceral Pain resulting from stimulation of internal organs	Pain is diffuse and radiates in several directions. Duration varies, but it usually lasts longer than superficial pain. Pain is sharp, dull, or unique to organ involved.	Crushing sensation (e.g., angina pectoris); burning sensation (e.g., gastric ulcer)
Referred Common in visceral pain because many organs themselves have no pain receptors (The entrance of sensory neurons from affected organ into same spinal cord segment as neurons from areas where individual feels pain causes perception of pain in unaffected areas.)	Pain is in part of body separate from source of pain and assumes any characteristic.	Myocardial infarction, which causes referred pain to the jaw, left arm, and left shoulder; kidney stones, which refer pain to groin
Radiating Sensation of pain extending from initial site of injury to another body part	Pain feels as though it travels down or along body part. It is intermittent or constant.	Low back pain from ruptured intravertebral disk accompanied by pain radiating down leg from sciatic nerve irritation

FIG. 44.5 Sample pain scales. (A) Numerical. (B) Verbal descriptive. (C) Visual analog.

Assessing a child's pain sometimes requires a different approach, especially with younger children. Young children do not always know what the word *pain* means. Therefore, use words a child may understand (e.g., *owie, boo-boo, hurt*) when assessing a child's pain. You can also use a pain scale designed specifically for children to assess their pain. These self-report measures of pain are most often used for children older than 3 to 4 years, but even 2-year-olds can report pain (Hockenberry and Wilson, 2019). As children develop, newer cognitive skills such as measurement and classification mature so that school-age children can use the NRS to assess pain (Hockenberry and Wilson, 2019). Current evidence also shows that tools originally created for children may be useful in adults who have difficulty verbalizing their pain (Pathak et al., 2018).

The Wong-Baker Faces Pain Rating Scale (FPS-revised), originally developed to be used with children, provides a pictorial representation of pain intensity (Fig. 44.6) (Wong and Baker, 1988; IASP, 2018b). Current evidence supports the reliability and validity of this internationally used scale in measuring pain severity (Wong-Baker FACES Foundation, 2016). Another pain scale shown to be valid and reliable with children is the Oucher pain scale (0-10) (Beyer et al., 1992). It uses a series of

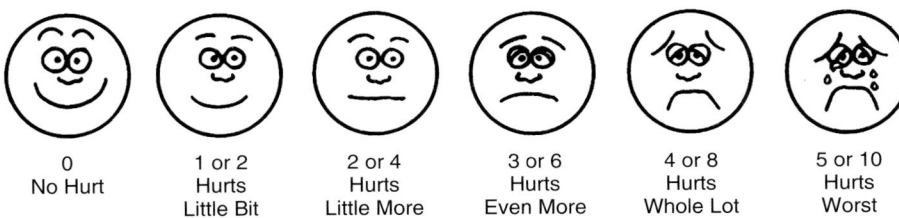

Brief word instructions: Point to each face using the words to describe the pain intensity. Ask the child to choose face that best describes own pain and record the appropriate number.

FIG. 44.6 Wong-Baker FACES® Pain Scale-Revised. (From Hockenberry MJ, et al: *Wong's nursing care of infants and children,* ed 11, St Louis, 2019, Elsevier.)

photographic images of faces in varying degrees of distress (Fig. 44.7). A child points to a face on the tool, thus simplifying the task of describing the pain. Different forms of the Oucher pain scale have been developed for specific ethnic groups, including Asian, Hispanic, and African American.

Quality. People use a variety of words to describe the quality of their pain (e.g., pain, ache). Ask patients to describe their discomfort using their own words whenever possible; then use these words consistently to obtain an accurate report. For example, say, "Tell me what your discomfort feels like. What do you call it?" The patient may describe the pain as aching, crushing, throbbing, sharp, or dull. If the patient reports the pain as dull, ask if it is still "dull" or if it has changed when you return to assess the patient's pain.

There is some consistency in the way people describe certain types of pain. The pain associated with a myocardial infarction is often described as crushing or viselike, whereas the pain of a surgical incision is often described as dull, aching, and throbbing, indicating nociceptive pain. Neuropathic pain is usually pricking pain, burning, electric-like, or numbness (Colloca et al., 2017). When a patient's descriptions fit the pattern forming in the assessment, you then make a clearer analysis of the nature and type of pain. This leads to more appropriate pain management because you treat nociceptive and neuropathic pain differently.

Aggravating and Precipitating Factors. Various factors or conditions bring on or make pain worse. Ask a patient to describe activities that cause or aggravate pain, such as physical movement, positions, drinking coffee or alcohol, urination, swallowing, eating food, or psychological stress. Also ask them to demonstrate actions that cause a painful response, such as coughing or turning a certain way. Some symptoms (depression, anxiety, fatigue, sedation, anorexia, sleep disruption, spiritual distress, and guilt) cause the pain to get worse. Likewise, pain can also make these symptoms worse. Assess for associated symptoms, and evaluate their effects on the patient's pain perception. After identifying specific aggravating or precipitating factors, it is easier to plan interventions to avoid worsening the pain.

Relief Measures. Ask patients how they relieve their pain, such as changing position, using ritualistic behavior (pacing, rocking, or rubbing), eating, meditating, praying, or applying heat or cold to a painful site. Encourage patients to continue to use their own pain-relieving measures if they are effective and appropriate to the cause of pain. Patients gain trust when they know that nurses are willing to try their relief measures, especially in the home setting. Patients gain a sense of control over the pain instead of the pain controlling them. Identify all the patient's health care providers (e.g., internist, orthopedist, acupuncturist, chiropractor, or dentist) in addition to assessing relief measures.

Effects of Pain on the Patient. Pain alters a person's lifestyle and psychological well-being. For example, chronic/persistent pain causes suffering, loss of control, loneliness, exhaustion, and an impaired quality of life. To understand a pain experience, ask patients what the pain prevents them from doing.

Behavioral Effects. When a patient has pain, assess verbalization, vocal response, facial and body movements, and social interaction. A verbal report of pain is a vital part of assessment. You need to be willing to listen and understand. When a patient is unable to communicate pain, it is especially important for you to be alert for behaviors that indicate it (Box 44.9).

The nonverbal expression of pain provides valuable information. If a woman in labor reports that her labor pains are occurring more frequently and if she begins to massage her abdomen more often, this confirms her report. If a patient reports severe abdominal pain but continues to grasp the chest, a more detailed assessment is probably needed.

Influence on Activities of Daily Living. Patients who live with daily pain or have prolonged pain are often less able to participate in routine activities, which results in physical deconditioning. This deconditioning can slow a patient's recovery (see Chapter 38). Assessment of these changes reveals the extent of patients' disabilities and the adjustments

Oucher®

10 ——
9 ——
8 ——
7 ——
6 ——
5 ——
4 ——
3 ——
2 ——
1 ——
0 ——

FIG. 44.7 Asian girl version of the Oucher pain scale. (The Asian versions of the Oucher scale [male and female] were developed and copyrighted in 2003 by CH Yeh [University of Pittsburgh] and CH Wang, Taiwan.)

BOX 44.9   Behavioral Indicators of Effects of Pain

Vocalizations
- Moaning
- Crying
- Gasping
- Grunting

Facial Expressions
- Grimace
- Clenched teeth
- Wrinkled forehead
- Tightly closed or widely opened eyes or mouth
- Lip biting

Body Movement
- Restlessness
- Immobilization

- Muscle tension
- Increased hand and finger movements
- Pacing activities
- Rhythmic or rubbing motions
- Protective movement of body parts
- Grabbing or holding a body part

Social Interaction
- Avoidance of conversation
- Focus only on activities for pain relief
- Avoidance of social contacts
- Reduced attention span
- Reduced interaction with environment

necessary to help them participate in self-care. A primary nursing focus is to help your patients improve their functioning.

Ask a patient whether pain interferes with sleep. Some patients have trouble falling asleep and/or staying asleep. The pain may awaken the patient during the night and make it hard to fall back to sleep.

Depending on the location of the pain, some patients have difficulty independently performing ADLs. For example, some pain restricts mobility to the point at which a patient is no longer able to bathe in a bathtub or get dressed. Some patients with severe arthritis find it painful to grasp eating utensils or lower themselves to a toilet seat. Assess a patient's need for help with self-care activities, determine whether a family caregiver provides assistance at home, and collaborate with members of the health care team (e.g., physical and occupational therapy).

Pain sometimes impairs the ability to maintain normal sexual relations. Physical conditions such as arthritis or back pain may prevent patients from assuming usual positions during intercourse. Pain or fatigue may reduce a patient's desire for sex. Include the extent to which pain affects the patient's usual sexual activity (i.e., physically unable or reduced desire) in your assessment.

Pain can affect a person's ability to work. The more physical activity required in a job, the greater the risk of discomfort when the pain is associated with movement. Pain related to emotional stress increases in individuals whose jobs involve stressful decision making. Assess the work that patients do and their ability to function in their jobs. Assess the daily activities of homemakers in the same manner as the duties involved in jobs outside the home. Also assess whether it is necessary for patients to stop activities because of pain, and help them to select ways to minimize or control it so that they are able to remain productive.

Include an assessment of the effect of pain on social activities. Some pain is so debilitating that the patient becomes too exhausted to socialize. Identify a patient's normal social activities, the extent to which activities have been disrupted, and the desire to participate in these activities.

Concomitant Symptoms. Concomitant symptoms occur with pain and usually increase a patient's pain severity. Examples include nausea, headache, dizziness, urge to urinate, constipation, depression, and restlessness. Certain types of pain have predictable concomitant symptoms. For example, severe rectal pain often leads to constipation. These symptoms are as much a problem to a patient as the pain itself.

REFLECT NOW

Consider a patient you recently cared for in a clinical experience or consider a time when you experienced a painful condition. In what way did pain limit your daily activities/the activities of the patient? How did you or the patient adapt to those limitations?

To prepare to ask Mrs. Mays questions to assess her pain, Matt reflects on his knowledge about the pathophysiology of osteoarthritis as well as his experience in caring for other patients with osteoarthritis. Matt successfully used an NRS to assess the severity of pain with his previous patients. On a personal level, Matt's grandfather has pain in his knees because of osteoarthritis. Matt knows that his grandfather has trouble moving around when his knees start to ache and that the pain in his knees disturbs his sleep. Matt has also seen the effect that this chronic pain has on his grandmother. Matt begins to assess Mrs. Mays based on his knowledge and experience.

Matt asks Mrs. Mays, "Please rate your pain from your arthritis for me on a scale of 0 to 10, with 0 being no pain and 10 being the worst pain possible."

Mrs. Mays responds, "Usually my pain ranges from 2 to 3; right now, it is a 4. My knees hurt more than my hands and hips right now."

Matt responds, "Can you please describe your pain and how it affects your ability to move around and take care of yourself?"

Mrs. Mays responds, "My knees, hips, and hands just ache. They even hurt when I touch them. It makes it hard to walk and to do things with my hands, such as open my medication bottles, cook our meals, and get dressed. The pain is worse in the morning. It gets better after I get up and start moving."

Matt then asks, "Some patients I have taken care of have told me their arthritis pain sometimes wakes them up at night. Does that ever happen to you?"

Mrs. Mays responds, "I can't tell you how long it has been since I've had a good night's sleep. My knees will start to ache so much, they wake me up, and then I end up waking my husband because I can't seem to get comfortable."

◆ **Analysis and Nursing Diagnosis**

The development of accurate nursing diagnoses for a patient in pain requires you to perform a complete assessment and use your clinical judgment to recognize cues and analyze the data you collected. During your analysis, look for patterns of data to help you identify individualized nursing diagnoses or collaborative problems (Box 44.10). Careful assessment reveals the presence of or a potential for pain. Be sure that your assessment considers what you know about the patient's history of recent procedures or preexisting painful conditions, and the nature of those conditions. Much of your analysis involves recognizing patterns of data and comparing what you normally would find for a certain diagnosis or problem.

A nursing diagnosis focuses on the specific nature of a patient's pain to identify the most relevant types of interventions for alleviating pain and improving function. For example, *Acute Pain related to physical trauma* and *Acute Pain related to natural childbirth processes* require very different nursing interventions. Accurate identification of related factors for problem-focused or negative nursing diagnoses helps you choose appropriate nursing interventions. You will sometimes use this information to identify interventions that treat or modify the related factor *or risk* for the diagnosis to be resolved. For example, interventions for *Acute Pain related to physical trauma* usually require pharmacological intervention, whereas *Acute Pain related to natural childbirth processes* is sometimes managed with nonpharmacological interventions, such as controlled breathing techniques.

BOX 44.10 Nursing Diagnostic Process

Chronic Pain

Assessment Activities	Assessment Findings
Have patient describe pain intensity.	Verbally reports 4 on a scale of 0 to 10
Assess onset and location of pain.	Present in hips, knees, and hands. Pain is constant; worse in the morning and awakens patient at night
Observe patient behaviors.	Grimaces when gets up to move; rubs knees after walking and frequently rubs fingers of one hand in the palm of the other
Assess effect of pain on activities of daily living (ADLs).	Is tired; wakens spouse at night; difficulty opening containers, cooking, and dressing
Review medical history.	Osteoarthritis, hypertension, and diabetes mellitus; osteoarthritis is currently affecting quality of life

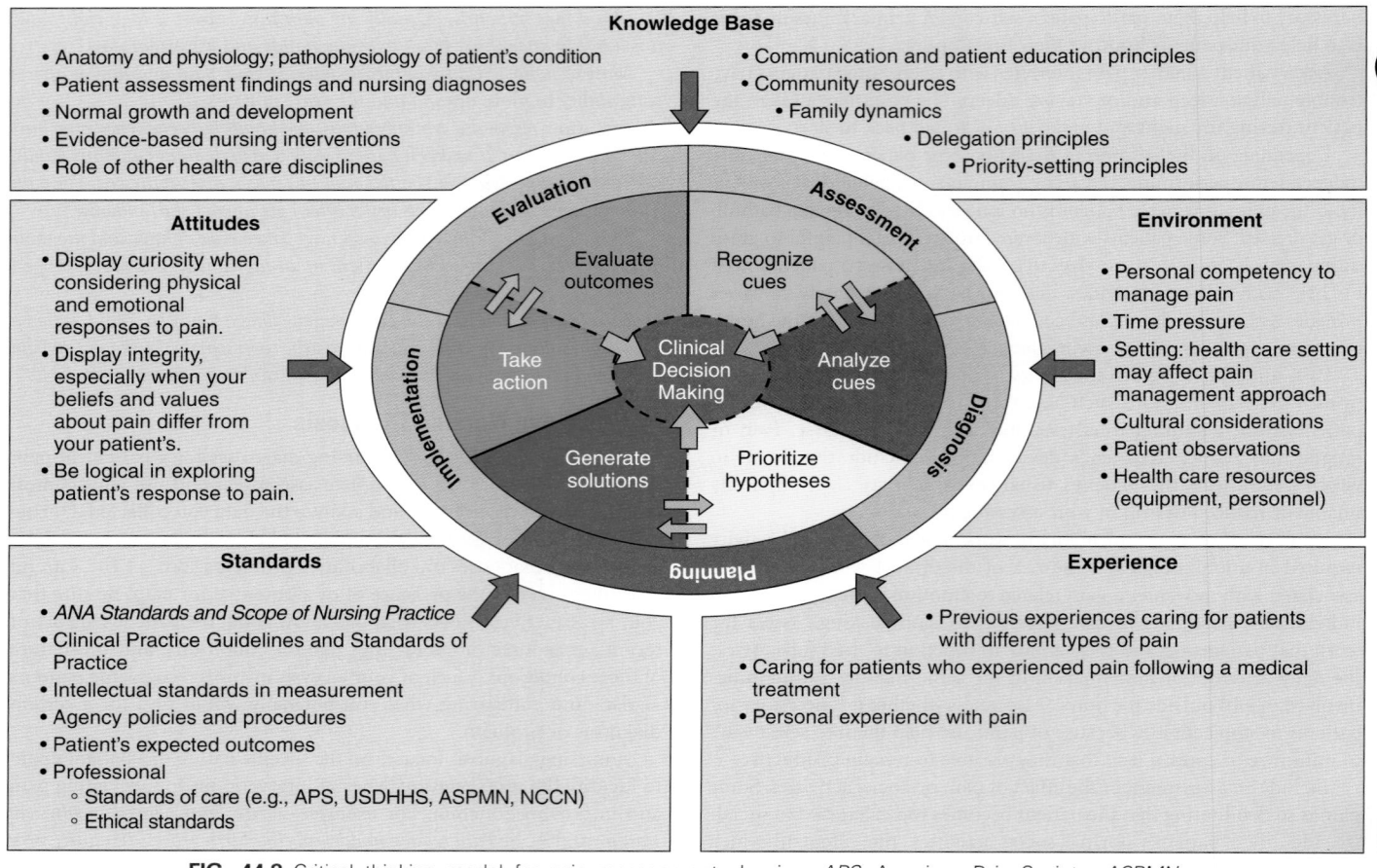

FIG. 44.8 Critical thinking model for pain management planning. *APS,* American Pain Society; *ASPMN,* American Society for Pain Management Nursing; *NCCN,* National Comprehensive Cancer Network; *USDHHS,* U.S. Department of Health and Human Services. (Clinical Judgment Measurement Model copyright © NCSBN. All rights reserved.)

A pain assessment often directs you to identify additional diagnoses other than that of *Acute* or *Chronic Pain.* The extent to which pain affects a patient's function and general state of health determines whether other nursing diagnoses are relevant. For example, you are caring for a patient who has a 3-year medical history of rheumatoid arthritis with persistent discomfort and weakness of the upper extremities. Your assessment reveals that the patient reports having pain of the hands and shoulders and has difficulty removing or fastening necessary items of clothing. The nursing diagnoses for this patient are *Self-Care Deficit* and *Arthritis Pain.* The diagnosis of *Self-Care Deficit* requires involvement by members of the interprofessional health care team to provide the patient with assistive devices for performing self-care. Examples of other diagnoses that may be related to pain follow:
- Difficulty Coping With Pain
- Inadequate Pain Control
- Fatigue
- Impaired Mobility
- Impaired Sleep
- Social Isolation

Matt analyzes the data he gathered from Mrs. Mays' assessment. As he reflects on her responses to his questions, he uses his clinical judgment and identifies cues to develop nursing diagnoses to help guide her care as she prepares to go home. Because she reports that her pain from her osteoarthritis is constant (she currently rates it at a 4, but it usually ranges from

2 to 3) and it affects many aspects of her daily life, he determines that **Arthritis Pain related to stiffened joints** *is her priority nursing diagnosis. Matt also considers Mrs. Mays' comments about her difficulty in caring for herself and trouble sleeping to identify* **Self-Care Deficit related to difficulty in dressing self, cooking, and opening containers** *and* **Fatigue related to frequent awakening at night** *as other important nursing diagnoses he will need to address to help Mrs. Mays improve her quality of life.*

◆ Planning and Outcomes Identification

During planning, critical thinking and sound clinical judgment will guide you to synthesize what you know about pain and a patient's condition, the patient's nursing diagnoses, the resources available, environmental conditions, your past clinical experiences, and clinical standards to develop a plan of care (Fig. 44.8). Recognize your own knowledge, biases, and competency in addressing concerns related to pain. Include evidence-based professional standards regarding pain management to help you select effective nursing interventions (see Nursing Care Plan). Professional standards of care are available as agency policies or through professional organizations such as the American Society for Pain Management Nursing (ASPMN). Consider the health care environment in which you provide care. Are there other professional resources available, such as physical therapists, pain-management specialists, or registered dietitians, to collaborate with your plan?

⊚ NURSING CARE PLAN

Chronic Pain

ASSESSMENT

Assessment Activities	Assessment Findings[a]
Ask Mrs. Mays to describe the pain she is having now.	Pain is **constant; knees, hands, and hips "ache"**
Ask Mrs. Mays to rate her pain on a scale of 0 to 10.	**Pain usually ranges from 2 to 3, but she currently rates pain at a 4** on a scale of 0 to 10.
Ask Mrs. Mays what has helped and worsened her pain.	Pain is worse with activity (e.g., walking, completing ADLs); pain is also worse in the morning and whenever being still (e.g., sleeping); stretching, moving, and ibuprofen make it better.
Observe Mrs. Mays' nonverbal behavior.	**Grimaces when she walks;** she **rubs her hands and fingers together** while watching television and during meals.

[a] **Assessment findings** are shown in bold type.

NURSING DIAGNOSIS: Arthritis pain related to stiffened joints

PLANNING

Expected Outcomes (NOC)[b]

Pain Control

Mrs. Mays reports joint pain at tolerable level of 3 or below.

Pain: Disruptive Effects

Mrs. Mays reports sleeping for 5 to 6 hours without interruption from pain.

[b] Outcome classification labels from Moorhead S, et al: *Nursing Outcomes Classification (NOC)*, ed 6, St Louis, 2018, Elsevier.

INTERVENTIONS (NIC)[c]	RATIONALE
Pain Management: Chronic	
Encourage to take medications as ordered by health care provider.	Some patients with arthritis have difficulty taking their medications as prescribed, which can lead to further pain and limit mobility (Arthritis Foundation, n.d.).
Have patient select nonpharmacological interventions that have relieved her pain in the past (e.g., distraction, music, simple relaxation therapy, warm or cool compresses) or that are acceptable to her.	Nonpharmacological approaches augment pharmacological therapy and help patients improve quality of life and decrease anxiety and depression (Tick et al., 2018).
Teach spouse how to perform slow-stroke back massage; instruct to perform massage at night before bedtime.	Slow-stroke back massage is easy to do, takes a short time, and induces relaxation (Tick et al., 2018).

[c] Intervention classification labels from Bulechek GM, et al: *Nursing Interventions Classification (NIC)*, ed 7, St Louis, 2018, Elsevier.

EVALUATION

Evaluation Activities	Patient Response
Ask Mrs. Mays if she has attained her pain-relief goal most of the time.	She responds, "My pain is back to a 2 to 3 most of the time as long as I take my medications and do my stretching exercises."
Ask Mrs. Mays if her pain is continuing to interrupt her sleep.	Mrs. Mays states that her pain is better controlled at night but that she is able to sleep uninterrupted for only about 4 hours.
Ask Mr. Mays if he was able to give his wife a back rub before bedtime.	Mr. Mays reported that he was able to perform slow-stroke massage without difficulty; Mrs. Mays stated, "It helped me relax and fall asleep."

Another strategy for planning care is to use a concept map. Patients who are in pain frequently have interrelated problems. As one problem gets worse, other aspects of a patient's level of health are affected. A concept map helps you determine how the nursing diagnoses are interrelated with one another and linked to the patient's health problems. This eventually allows you to also see how interventions are related for different diagnoses. See the example for Mrs. Mays' plan of care (Fig. 44.9). Identifying the relationships between diagnoses and interventions helps you develop a holistic and patient-centered plan of care.

Outcomes. Because the pain experience is so closely connected to a patient's perceptions, beliefs, and attitudes, it is essential that you include your patient when setting outcomes of care. A patient-centered plan will manage pain effectively and promote optimal function. Partner with the patient to determine relevant and realistic expectations for pain relief. Decide on a mutually acceptable level of pain that allows return of function. Make sure that patients understand that complete pain relief may not be possible but that every effort will be made to allow them to safely reach a pain level that allows for maximum function.

It is important to remember that a successful plan of care requires an ongoing therapeutic relationship with a patient and family to focus on relevant pain-management therapies and patient education. You help by listening to a patient's concerns, needs, and understanding of available pain-relief measures. Patients know the most about their pain and are important partners in selecting successful pain therapies.

An indication of the success of a plan of care is determined through attainment of outcomes. When complete pain relief is not achievable,

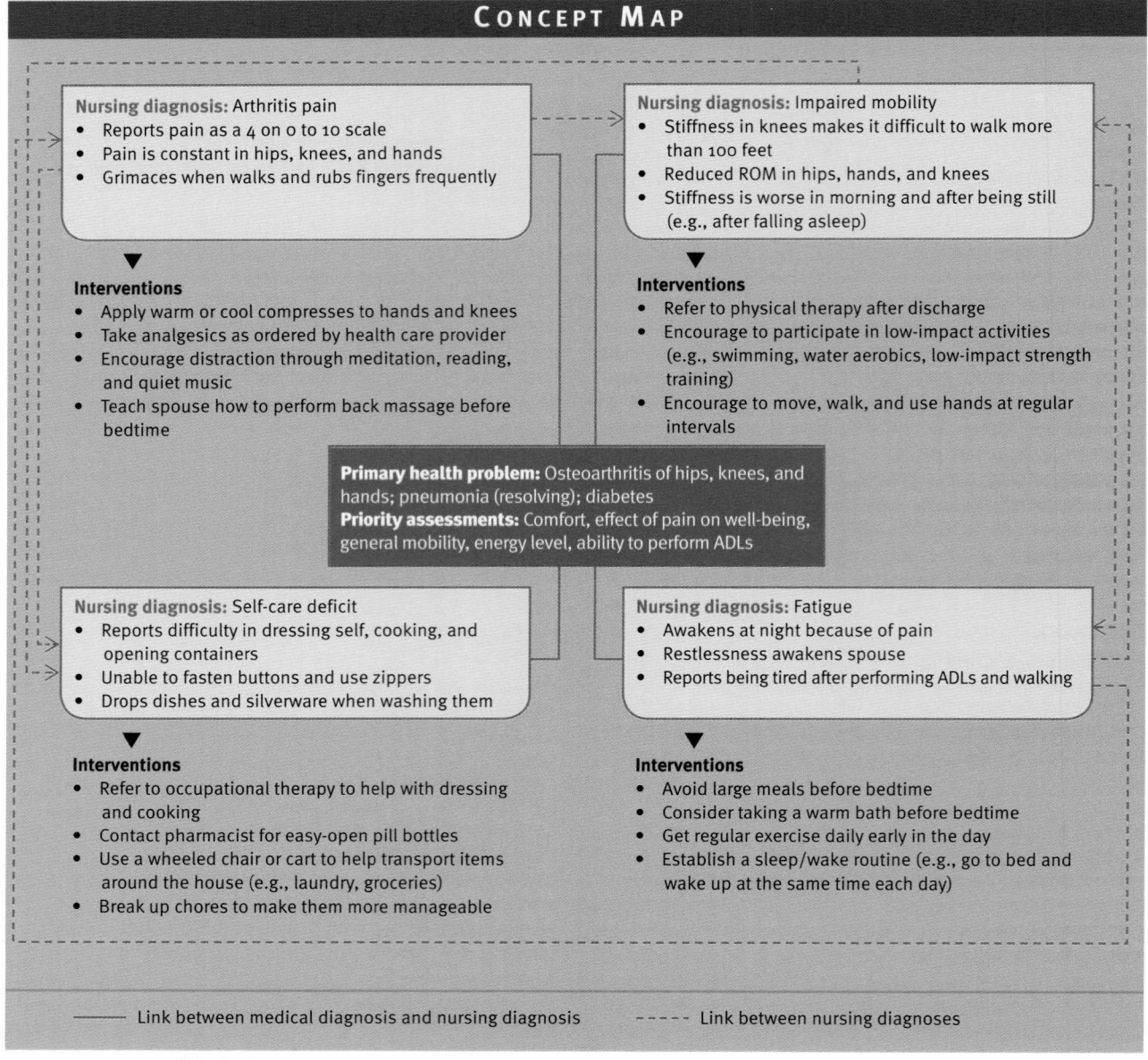

FIG. 44.9 Concept map for Mrs. Mays. *ADLs,* activities of daily living; *ROM,* range of motion.

reducing pain to a tolerable level is a realistic outcome. For example, the following are possible outcomes:

- Reports that pain is at a tolerable level of 3 or less on a scale of 0 to 10
- Modifies activities that intensify pain
- Uses pain-relief measures safely
- Is able to complete ADLs independently

REFLECT NOW

In addition to identifying outcomes for reducing pain intensity, outcomes should be set with patients concerning their physiological, affective, cognitive, behavioral, spiritual, and social functioning with the use of pharmacological and nonpharmacological management strategies. Why is it important to address these other domains of pain rather than just focusing on reducing pain intensity?

Setting Priorities. You need to use clinical judgment to effectively determine your patient's priorities in pain management. Priorities change as a patient's pain experience changes. Consider the type of pain a patient is experiencing and the effect that it has on function and quality of life. Any episode of acute pain is a priority because of its potential effects on physical and psychological function. In addition, acute pain may cause the interruption or delay of other important therapies (e.g., ambulation, physical therapy, or a planned diagnostic procedure).

For chronic pain, work with the patient to select interventions that are appropriate, relevant, and within the patient's financial means. The primary focus with patients experiencing chronic pain often is to decrease pain to a level that will allow the patient to participate in disease management, restore or improve function in performing daily activities, and prevent complications. For example, if a nonsteroidal antiinflammatory medication is relieving chronic pain to an acceptable level for your patient, turn your attention to how the pain is affecting the patient's activity, appetite, and sleep. What other nonpharmacological therapies can you provide to help manage the effects of pain on your patient?

Teamwork and Collaboration. A comprehensive plan requires collaboration of all the members from the health care team, including advanced practice nurses, pharmacists (PharmDs), physical therapists, occupational therapists, physicians, social workers, psychologists, and clergy. An oncology or pain clinical nurse specialist is very familiar with pharmacological and nonpharmacological interventions that are most effective for chronic/persistent pain. PharmDs are knowledgeable about pharmacological treatments of pain. Physical therapists plan exercises and provide therapies that strengthen muscle groups and lessen pain in affected areas. Occupational therapists devise splints to support painful body parts and plan approaches for performing ADLs. Physicians are familiar with pharmacological interventions, and some are skilled in interventional pain procedures such as nerve blocks and spinal cord stimulator implantations. Social workers and psychologists may offer cognitive behavioral therapy or mindfulness training for pain relief. Clergy members help patients focus on spiritual health by helping patients find the meaning of their pain. It is important to also involve family caregivers in the plan of care. They will often administer care in the home after discharge. If the pain-management plan is unsuccessful in achieving the identified pain-relief goal(s), collaborate with the patient and the health care team about appropriate revisions to the plan. Consulting with a pain expert is sometimes necessary.

When patients require hands-on assistance from family caregivers or when a family caregiver lives with a patient, be sure that the family caregiver understands the patient's drug regimen and other treatment measures to help promote adherence. The family caregiver can be very useful to all other members of the health care team when making adaptations within the home that aid in pain management.

Matt knows that pain can affect a patient in many ways. Helping Mrs. Mays manage her pain will help improve her mobility and will help her sleep better. Thus, Matt identifies **Arthritis Pain** *as the priority nursing diagnosis. He then collaborates with Mrs. Mays to identify appropriate outcomes and begins to explore pain-management techniques she is willing to try. Matt also uses his personal experience as well as his knowledge about evidence-based pain-management guidelines to identify interventions to help Mrs. Mays manage her pain. Matt knows that he needs to establish a trusting relationship and provide as much privacy as possible before exploring pain-management options and providing patient education.*

◆ Implementation

Pain therapy requires an individualized patient-centered approach, perhaps more so than any other patient problem (USDHHS, 2019). The patient and frequently the family are partners in pain management with the entire health care team. Your clinical judgment is important in knowing the best approaches for pain management, when to deliver them, and how to make any adjustments. Effective pain management requires patience and the ability to be flexible in choosing interventions. You are responsible for administering and monitoring therapies ordered by health care providers for pain relief and for independently providing interventions that complement those prescribed. Usually you will try the least invasive or safest therapy first along with previously used successful patient strategies. If you question a medical therapy, consult with the health care provider.

The Pain Management Best Practices Inter-Agency Task Force of the U.S. Department of Health and Human Services (USDHHS) (2019) recommends the following for an effective pain treatment plan:

- **Acute pain**—A multimodal approach that includes medications, nerve blocks, physical therapy, and other nonpharmacological modalities should be considered for acute pain conditions.

- **Chronic pain**—An interprofessional approach across various disciplines is needed, using one or more treatment modalities. These include the following five broad treatment categories, which have been reviewed for best practices:
  - Medications: Various classes of medications, including nonopioids and opioids, should be considered for use. The choice of medication should be based on the pain diagnosis, the mechanisms of pain, and related co-morbidities following a thorough history, physical exam, other relevant diagnostic procedures, and a risk-benefit assessment. The goal is to limit adverse outcomes.
  - Restorative therapies, including those implemented by physical therapists and occupational therapists (e.g., physiotherapy, therapeutic exercise, and other movement modalities), are valuable components of multidisciplinary, multimodal acute and chronic pain care.
  - Interventional approaches, including image-guided and minimally invasive procedures (e.g., trigger point injections, neuromodulation), are available as diagnostic and therapeutic treatment modalities for acute, acute on chronic, and chronic pain when clinically indicated.
  - Behavioral approaches for psychological, cognitive, emotional, behavioral, and social aspects of pain can have a significant impact on treatment outcomes.
  - Complementary and integrative health, including treatment modalities such as acupuncture, massage, movement therapies (e.g., yoga, tai chi), and spirituality, should be considered when clinically indicated.

Your ability to show compassionate care toward patients has the potential for maximizing their pain control. You can help a patient minimize pain through caring behaviors such as listening, offering a gentle touch, and responding promptly to a pain request.

Health Promotion. When providing pain-relief measures, apply these guidelines for individualizing pain therapy:
- Use different types of pain-relief measures. Persistent pain is multifactorial, requiring an approach that addresses a variety of etiologies and includes pharmacological and nonpharmacological strategies (Heden et al., 2020).
- Be willing to use more than one type of pain-relief measure as appropriate.
- Use measures that the patient believes are effective (Auxier et al., 2020).
- Keep an open mind about ways to relieve pain.
- Keep trying. When efforts at pain relief fail, do not abandon the patient but reassess the situation (Auxier et al., 2020). Persistent pain is treatable, with improvement anticipated, but it is not always curable.
- When pain is not totally eliminated, strive for improvement in function.

Maintaining Wellness. Patients are better prepared to handle almost any situation when they understand it. The experience of pain and its related therapies is no exception. However, patients with moderate to severe pain are not always able to participate in decision making or attend to patient education until the pain is controlled at an acceptable level.

Pain often affects a patient's ability to sleep and remain asleep. Consider consulting with a health care provider on appropriate medications for the patient and try nonpharmacological interventions to promote sleep (see Chapter 43). Instruct patients to not use medications that promote sleep as a substitute for pain relief.

Health literacy significantly affects a patient's pain experience and understanding of pain-management strategies. Low health literacy poses significant barriers to optimal pain management. In a study of patients with chronic pain, patients with low health literacy were more likely to misuse and have a higher dependence on opioids, to report severe pain, and to experience disability related to their pain (Rogers et al., 2020).

Adapt educational materials and approaches so that they are suited for patients with low health literacy. In addition, combat any cultural norms that may stop patients from talking about pain. Stoicism (suffering without verbalizing complaint) often prevents people from admitting they have pain or describing their pain accurately, which ultimately can prevent you from providing essential care. For example, reporting chest pain is essential to the treatment of patients experiencing a myocardial infarction (MI). If a patient who is having an MI fails to report chest pain, the patient will not receive appropriate treatment and could die from not reporting it. Help patients understand the importance of reporting their pain and find words to describe their pain when they are having trouble explaining it on their own (Pasero and McCaffery, 2011). Because pain affects physical and mental functioning, holistic health approaches are important interventions.

Encourage patients to actively participate in their own well-being whenever possible. When you provide holistic health, you care for the whole person: body, mind, spirit, and emotions. Assist your patients in finding balance of all aspects of their health to help them achieve optimal health and well-being. Common holistic health approaches include wellness education, regular exercise, rest, relaxation techniques (see Chapter 32), attention to good hygiene practices and nutrition, and management of interpersonal relationships.

Nonpharmacological Pain-Relief Interventions. When a person develops pain, offer nonpharmacological strategies when appropriate. Nonpharmacological interventions can be used alone or in combination with pharmacological measures. Some require an order from a health care provider while others are nurse-initiated. In the case of moderate to severe acute pain, nonpharmacological therapies should be used with pharmacological therapies.

Evidence-based nonpharmacological therapies include acupuncture, massage, osteopathic and chiropractic manipulation, cognitive-behavioral intervention, meditative movement and mind-body interventions, and dietary and self-management approaches to pain management (see Chapter 32) (Tick et al., 2018). Use evidence-based nonpharmacological interventions routinely to provide a comprehensive plan for pain management. Tailor nonpharmacological techniques to the individual and use cognitive behavioral strategies cautiously in patients who are cognitively impaired. The effectiveness of the interventions often varies depending on the type of pain the patient is experiencing and the patient's belief in the therapy. Both active (physical movement) and passive nonpharmacological strategies target different pathways for pain relief while increasing physical functioning. For example, cognitive-behavioral interventions change patients' perceptions of pain, alter pain behavior, and provide patients with a greater sense of control. Distraction, prayer, mindfulness, relaxation, guided imagery, music, and **biofeedback** are examples of therapies frequently initiated by nurses (U.S. Department of Veterans Affairs, 2017).

Physical therapies (e.g., applying hot or cold compresses, massage, exercise, transcutaneous electrical nerve stimulation [TENS]) treat pain by improving physical function, altering physiological responses, and reducing pain-related immobility. Complementary and alternative medicine (CAM) therapies such as therapeutic touch and mindfulness meditation also help to alleviate pain in some patients (see Chapter 32).

Relaxation and Guided Imagery. Relaxation and **guided imagery** allow patients to alter affective-motivational and cognitive pain perception. **Relaxation** is mental and physical freedom from tension or stress that provides individuals a sense of self-control. You use relaxation techniques at any phase of health or illness. Physiological and behavioral changes associated with relaxation include decreased pulse, blood pressure, and respirations; heightened awareness; decreased oxygen

consumption; a sense of peace; and decreased muscle tension and metabolic rate (Tick et al., 2018). Relaxation techniques include meditation, yoga, mindfulness, guided imagery, and progressive relaxation exercises (see Chapter 32). For effective relaxation, teach techniques only when a patient is comfortable. Sometimes a combination of these techniques is needed to achieve optimal pain relief. With practice the patient performs relaxation exercises independently.

Distraction. The reticular activating system inhibits painful stimuli if a person receives sufficient or excessive sensory input. With sufficient sensory stimuli, a person ignores or becomes unaware of pain. People who are bored or in isolation have only their pain to think about and thus perceive it more acutely. Distraction directs a patient's attention to something other than pain and thus reduces awareness of it. A disadvantage of distraction is that, if it works, health care providers or family members may question the existence or severity of the pain. Distraction works best for short, intense pain lasting a few minutes such as during an invasive procedure or while waiting for an analgesic to work. Use activities enjoyed by the patient as distractions (e.g., singing, praying, listening to music, or playing games).

Music. Music therapy may be useful in treating acute or chronic pain, stress, anxiety, fatigue, and depression (Lin et al., 2020; American Music Therapy Association [AMTA], 2021). It diverts a person's attention away from the pain and creates a relaxation response. Music creates positive changes in mood and emotional states and allows patients to actively participate in treatment. It can be used with relaxation to help patients cue positive visual imagery. Music therapy uses all kinds of music. It is important to let patients select the types of music they prefer. Music produces an altered state of consciousness through sound, silence, space, and time. Therapeutic sessions usually last 20 to 30 minutes (Tick et al., 2018). Patients may use earphones to enhance their concentration on the music. This allows them to adjust the volume without interrupting other patients or staff. Evidence shows that music provides pain relief and sometimes decreases the amount of pain medication (e.g., analgesics) required to manage pain (Ames et al., 2017; Tick et al., 2018).

Cutaneous Stimulation. Although **cutaneous stimulation** of the skin through a massage, warm bath, cold application, or **transcutaneous electrical nerve stimulation (TENS)** reduces pain perception in some patients, how it works remains unclear. One suggestion is that it causes release of endorphins, thus blocking the transmission of painful stimuli. The gate-control theory suggests that cutaneous stimulation activates larger, faster-transmitting A-beta sensory nerve fibers. This closes the gate, thus decreasing pain transmission through small-diameter C fibers (Melzack and Wall, 1965).

Cutaneous stimulation gives patients and families some control over pain symptoms and treatment in the home. Using it properly helps to reduce muscle tension, resulting in less pain. When using cutaneous stimulation, eliminate sources of environmental noise, help the patient to assume a comfortable position, and explain the purpose of the therapy. Do not use it directly on sensitive skin areas (e.g., burns, bruises, skin rashes, inflammation, and underlying bone fractures).

Massage produces physical and mental relaxation, reduces pain, and enhances the effectiveness of pain medication. Massaging the back, shoulders, hands, and/or feet for 3 to 5 minutes relaxes muscles and promotes sleep and comfort (Tick et al., 2018). Massages communicate caring and are easy for family members or other health care personnel to learn (Box 44.11).

Cold and heat applications (see Chapter 48) relieve pain and promote healing. The selection of heat-versus-cold interventions varies with patients' conditions and the physiological effects of the two modalities (Tick et al., 2018). For example, moist heat helps to relieve the pain from a tension headache, and cold applications reduce the acute pain from

BOX 44.11 PROCEDURAL GUIDELINES
Massage

Delegation and Collaboration

Assessment of a patient's pain cannot be delegated to assistive personnel (AP). The skill of massage can be delegated to AP. The nurse directs the AP by:
- Identifying and explaining when massage can work best for a patient.
- Explaining how to adapt use of massage to patient restrictions (e.g., massage in side-lying versus prone position).
- Instructing to report worsening of a patient's pain.

Equipment

Lotion or oil (consider lavender aromatherapy lotion [non–alcohol-based]), sheet, bath towel

Procedural Steps
1. Identify patient using at least two identifiers (e.g., name and birthday or name and medical record number) according to agency policy.
2. Assess patient's health literacy.
3. Perform hand hygiene. Perform complete pain assessment.
4. Assess character of patient's respirations.
5. Review health care provider's orders for pain relief (if required by agency).
6. Review medical record for any restrictions in patient's mobility or positioning.
7. Assess patient's and/or family caregiver's knowledge and experience with massage.
8. Assess values patient has regarding alternative pain-relief approaches. Identify descriptive terms that you will use when guiding patient through relaxation during massage.
9. Dim room lights and/or turn on soft music according to patient preference.

   CLINICAL JUDGMENT: Massage is contraindicated in cases of muscle, bone, or joint injury; bruised, swollen, or inflamed areas.

10. Place patient in comfortable position such as prone or side-lying. Have patients with difficulty breathing lie on side of bed with head of bed elevated.
11. Adjust bed to comfortable position for you; lower upper side rail on side where you are standing. Drape patient to expose only area that you will massage.
12. Ensure that patient is not allergic to lotion. Warm lotion in hands or place bottle in basin of warm water. **Note:** If you massage head and scalp, delay use of lotion until completed.
13. Choose stroke technique based on desired effect or body part.

    CLINICAL JUDGMENT: Use very gentle massage with patients who are unable to communicate and monitor nonverbal behavior because they cannot tell you if massage becomes uncomfortable.

    a. Effleurage: massaging upward and outward from vertebral column and back again (see illustration). Smooths and extends muscles; improves lymph and venous circulation.
    b. Pétrissage: kneading tense muscle groups (see illustration). Promotes relaxation and stimulates local circulation.
    c. Friction: strong circular strokes bring blood to skin surface. Increases local circulation and loosens tight muscles.
14. Encourage patient to breathe deeply and relax during massage.
15. Standing behind patient, stimulate scalp and temples.
16. Supporting patient's head, use friction to rub muscles at base of head.
17. Reposition if needed. With patient in supine position, massage hands and arms as appropriate.
    a. Support hand and apply friction to palm using both thumbs.
    b. Support base of finger and work each finger in corkscrew-like motion.
    c. Complete hand massage using effleurage strokes from fingertips to wrist.
    d. Knead muscles of forearm and upper arm between thumb and forefinger.

STEP 13a Effleurage.

STEP 13b Pétrissage.

18. After determining that patient has no neck injury or condition that contraindicates neck manipulation, offer to massage neck as appropriate:
    a. Place patient prone unless contraindicated.
    b. Knead each neck muscle between thumb and forefinger.
    c. Gently stretch neck by placing one hand on top of shoulders and other at base of head. Gently move hands away from one another.
19. Massage back as appropriate:
    a. Assist patient to prone position unless contraindicated; side-lying position is an option.
    b. Do not allow hands to leave patient's skin.
    c. Apply hands first to sacral area; massage in circular motion. Stroke upward from buttocks to shoulders. Massage over scapulae with smooth, firm stroke. Continue in one smooth stroke to upper arms and laterally along sides of back down to iliac crest (see illustration). Continue massage pattern for 3 minutes.
    d. Use effleurage along muscles of spine in upward and outward motion.
    e. Use pétrissage on muscles of each shoulder toward front of patient.
    f. Use palms in upward and outward circular motion from lower buttocks to neck.
    g. Knead muscles of upper back and shoulder between thumb and forefinger.
    h. Use both hands to knead muscles up one side of back and then the other.
    i. End massage with long, stroking effleurage movements.

Continued

BOX 44.11   **PROCEDURAL GUIDELINES—cont'd**

Massage

STEP 19c Circular massage of the back.

20. Massage feet as appropriate:
    a. Place patient in supine position.
    b. Hold foot firmly. Support ankle with one hand or support sides of foot with each hand while performing massage.
    c. Make circular motions with thumb and fingers around bones of ankle and top of foot.

d. Trace space between tendons with firm finger pressure, moving from toe to ankle.
e. Massage sides and top of each toe.
f. Use top of fist to make circular motions on bottom of foot.
g. Knead sides of foot between index finger and thumb.
h. Conclude with firm, sweeping motions over top and bottom of foot.

21. Tell patient that you are ending massage.
22. When procedure is complete, instruct patient to relax and inhale deeply and exhale slowly. Caution the patient to move slowly after resting a few minutes.
23. Wipe excess lotion or oil from patient's body with bath towel.
24. Help patient to a comfortable position.
25. Place nurse call system in an accessible location within patient's reach.
26. Raise side rails (as appropriate) and lower bed to lowest position.
27. Observe character of respirations, body position, facial expression, tone of voice, mood, mannerisms, verbalization of discomfort.
28. Ask patient to use pain rating scale to rate comfort level; compare with patient's goal.
29. Observe patient perform pain-control measures.
30. Perform teach-back: "I want to ensure you know how to perform massage for your husband. Show me how you would massage his back and feet."
31. Record in EHR or printed record the patient's response to massage.

---

inflamed joints. When using any form of heat or cold application, instruct a patient to avoid injury to the skin by checking the temperature and not applying cold or heat directly to the skin. Especially at risk for injury are patients with neuropathies (e.g., diabetic neuropathy, peripheral neuropathy), patients with spinal cord or other neurological disorders, older adults, and patients who are confused.

Ice massage is effective for acute pain relief. It involves the use of a large ice cube or a small paper cup filled with water and frozen (water rises out of the cup as it freezes to create a smooth surface of ice for massage). Patients can implement their own ice massage if they can reach the site. When using ice massage, cover the ice with a lightweight cloth and then apply the ice with firm pressure to the skin. Massage the area slowly and steadily in a circular pattern. Apply cold within a 15 cm (6-inch) circular area near the pain site or on the opposite side of the body corresponding to the pain site. Limit application to 5 minutes or until the patient feels numbness. Application near the actual site of pain tends to work best, and it can be applied several times each hour to help reduce pain (Tick et al., 2018). Cold is effective for tooth or mouth pain when you place the ice on the web of the hand between the thumb and index finger. This point on the hand is an acupressure point that influences nerve pathways to the face and head.

Heat application is often more effective for patients with chronic pain. Chapter 48 discusses in detail the types of heat devices (e.g., warm compresses and commercial heat packs) that are safe to use. Never place a heat application in a microwave unless it is directed by the manufacturer. Then follow directions carefully. Teach patients to check the temperature of a compress carefully and not to lie on the heating element because burning can occur.

TENS stimulates the skin with a mild electrical current passed through external electrodes. A TENS unit consists of a battery-powered transmitter, lead wires, and electrodes. TENS therapy is thought to work in two ways. It stimulates nerve cells to block the transmission of

pain, and it increases the level of endorphins released by the body to block the perception of pain (Tick et al., 2018). TENS is applied at various frequencies ($<$10 Hz to $>$50 Hz) and intensities (sensory versus motor). A TENS unit requires a health care provider's order that identifies the site for the TENS electrode placement. Remove any hair or skin preparations before attaching the electrodes. Then place the electrodes directly over or near the pain site. Turn the transmitter on to the ordered level when the patient feels pain. The TENS creates a buzzing or tingling sensation. After assessing tolerance, the patient can then turn on the transmitter and adjust the intensity and quality of skin stimulation until pain relief occurs. Recent review of the evidence found that it cannot be confidently stated whether TENS is effective in relieving pain in people with chronic pain (Gibson et al., 2019). Some patients experience relief of pain while others do not. TENS seems to be most effective for acute, emergent, and postsurgical and procedural pain control (Tick et al., 2018).

Herbals. Many patients use herbal and dietary supplements such as echinacea, ginseng, ginkgo biloba, and garlic despite conflicting research evidence supporting their use in pain relief. Significant attention has been paid to the potential benefits of glucosamine and chondroitin in the treatment of pain from osteoarthritis. Current evidence-based guidelines do not support the use of glucosamine in patients with osteoarthritis in the knee, hip, or hand. Chondroitin is conditionally recommended only for patients with osteoarthritis in the hand (Kolasinski et al., 2020). Herbal supplements may interact with prescribed analgesics and condition-specific medications. For example, glucosamine and chondroitin supplements may interact with the anticoagulant drug warfarin and increase the risk of bleeding. Thus it is important to ask patients to report to their health care provider any type of herbal or dietary supplements taken to relieve pain (see Chapter 32).

Reducing Pain Perception and Reception. One simple way to promote comfort is to remove or prevent painful stimuli (Box 44.12).

BOX 44.12 Controlling Painful Stimuli in Patient's Environment

- Tighten and smooth wrinkled bed linen.
- Reposition patient anatomically to relieve any pressure points according to individual preferences or requirements.
- Reposition patient to avoid lying on tubing (e.g., intravenous tubing, chest tubes).
- Loosen constricting bandages (unless specifically applied as a pressure dressing).
- Change wet dressings and linens.
- Check temperature of hot or cold applications, including bath water.
- Lift patient in bed—do not pull. Use safe patient-handling lift devices and techniques.
- Position patient correctly on a bedpan.
- Avoid exposing skin or mucous membranes to irritants (e.g., urine, stool, wound drainage).
- Keep patients clean, dry, and turned if needed. Use urinary incontinence pads if indicated.
- Prevent urinary retention by keeping Foley catheters patent and free flowing if in use, while also monitoring urinary output.
- Prevent constipation with fluids, diet, exercise, and stimulant laxatives if needed.

This is especially important for patients who are immobilized or who have difficulty expressing themselves. For example, your patient becomes constipated and has abdominal distention and cramping. You intervene to ensure that the normal elimination process continues by increasing fluids, ambulating the patient, and/or requesting stool softeners or laxatives. Another example involves reducing pain perception during procedures using techniques such as proper patient positioning and coaching to perform progressive muscle relaxation. Always consider the patient's condition, aspects of the procedure that are uncomfortable, and techniques to avoid causing pain. In a patient with severe arthritic knee pain who has discomfort while flexing the knee, take precautions before walking the patient to the bathroom. The patient may benefit from using a walker or an elevated toilet seat to help with mobility and reduce discomfort.

*As Matt begins to care for Mrs. Mays, he decides to implement interventions to address her priority diagnosis of **Arthritis Pain** first. He knows that patients often experience reduced pain when they take their prescribed analgesics and use different types of distraction techniques. He begins by teaching Mrs. Mays about her pain medications and encouraging her to take them as prescribed while he is administering her medications. Later in the day, he helps Mrs. Mays with her bath. After her bath is complete, Matt begins discussing different distraction techniques such as meditation, reading, and quiet music. He also includes information to address her impaired mobility, such as how important it is for Mrs. Mays to keep moving and to participate in low-impact activities such as swimming and strength training, as well as information to address her fatigue. While Matt is explaining the importance of exercising early in the day and establishing a sleep/wake routine that includes taking a warm bath before bedtime, a housekeeper suddenly enters to clean the room. Matt asks Mrs. Mays, "Would you like to continue our discussion while your room is being cleaned, or would you prefer for me to come back later?"*

Mrs. Mays responds, "It's okay with me if we keep talking. Can you tell me a little more about meditation? Also, I would love it if you could teach my husband how to do a back massage."

Acute Care. Nurses often care for patients who have acute pain resulting from invasive procedures (e.g., surgery) or trauma. Many professional organizations such as the APS, American Society of Anesthesiologists (2010), the ANA and ASPMN (ANA, 2016), and the Pain Management Best Practices Inter-Agency Task Force (USDHHS, 2019) have published guidelines and position papers related to pain management. The key to success is ongoing pain assessment and evaluation of the efficacy of interventions. Does the patient feel relief? Are there any unacceptable side effects from therapies? It is the responsibility of the health care team to collaborate to find the combination of therapy that works best for a patient.

Pharmacological Pain Therapies. A multimodal approach is recommended for acute and chronic pain relief (USDHHS, 2019). Your judgment in the use and management of analgesics with or without other pain therapies ensures the best pain relief possible. Unfortunately, the ideal analgesic (i.e., one that provides highly effective pain relief without significant risks or side effects) has yet to be developed.

Analgesics. Analgesics are the most common and effective method of pain relief. Use your knowledge of a medication, including its indications for use, desired effects, adverse effects, and risks for addiction, to safely administer it. Reassure patients that treating pain is necessary to aid recovery and that nonpharmacological strategies can be used to enhance the effectiveness of analgesics.

There are three types of analgesics: (1) nonopioids, including acetaminophen and nonsteroidal antiinflammatory drugs (NSAIDs); (2) opioids (traditionally called *narcotics*); and (3) adjuvants or coanalgesics, a variety of medications that enhance analgesics or have analgesic properties (U.S. Department of Veterans Affairs, 2017).

Nonopioids. Acetaminophen, considered one of the most tolerated and safest analgesics available, is available orally by itself or in combination with other medications (e.g., in cold and flu remedies). You can also administer it rectally and intravenously (IV) (see Chapter 31). Although acetaminophen was first prepared in the late 1800s and is used frequently to manage pain today, scientists are still unsure how it works. Some believe it affects the central nervous system by selectively inhibiting cyclooxygenase (COX), an enzyme needed to make prostaglandins (Burchum and Rosenthal, 2019). Although acetaminophen reduces pain and fever, it has limited effects on the peripheral nervous system, and it does not reduce inflammation (Burchum and Rosenthal, 2019). IV acetaminophen crosses the blood-brain barrier rapidly, thus providing nonopioid analgesia for patients after surgery. Acetaminophen is often combined with opioids (e.g., oxycodone, hydrocodone, tramadol) because it reduces the dose of opioid needed to achieve successful pain control. When acetaminophen is combined with an opioid, it is important to recognize the abbreviations that describe the contents of the product. The order and package label often include the name and dose of the opioid along with acetaminophen, which is sometimes abbreviated as APAP. For example, a medication labeled "oxycodone/APAP 5/325" indicates that each tablet contains 5 mg of oxycodone and 325 mg of acetaminophen. Similar abbreviations are used for combination products of hydrocodone and tramadol.

The maximum 24-hour dose is 4 g for adults (the same limitation as aspirin). The major adverse effect of acetaminophen is hepatotoxicity. Because of the wide use of acetaminophen and its potential to cause severe liver failure, the Food and Drug Administration limits the amount of acetaminophen contained in prescription combination products to 325 mg per tablet, capsule, or other dosage unit (USFDA, 2018). Acetaminophen is available in higher doses in over-the-counter (OTC) products, but the products are required to include dosage labeling information about safety risks (e.g., liver injury, serious skin rashes). Administer reduced doses in patients with limited liver function, and carefully assess how many milligrams of acetaminophen your patients take in a 24-hour period to reduce the chance of accidental overdose. Dangerous hepatotoxic overdoses of acetaminophen are treated with acetylcysteine (Burchum and Rosenthal, 2019).

Nonselective NSAIDs such as aspirin, ibuprofen, and naproxen relieve mild to moderate acute intermittent pain such as that from headache or muscle strain. Treatment of mild to moderate postoperative pain begins with an NSAID unless contraindicated. NSAIDs act by inhibiting COX, the enzyme that synthesizes prostaglandins and related compounds (Burchum and Rosenthal, 2019). The drugs inhibit cellular responses to inflammation. Most NSAIDs act on peripheral nerve receptors to reduce transmission of pain stimuli and inflammation. Unlike opioids, NSAIDs do not depress the central nervous system, nor do they interfere with bowel or bladder function. However, because COX normally synthesizes the prostaglandins that protect gastric mucosa, NSAIDs can cause gastrointestinal irritation. NSAIDs may reduce renal blood flow since COX causes vasodilation to maintain renal blood flow (Burchum and Rosenthal, 2019). Thus NSAID use in older patients is not recommended because it is associated with more frequent adverse effects (gastrointestinal bleeding as well as renal insufficiency) (American Geriatrics Society Beers Criteria Expert Panel, 2019). Mild to moderate musculoskeletal pain in older adults is managed effectively with acetaminophen. Some patients with asthma or an allergy to aspirin are also allergic to NSAIDs. As with all OTC medications, advise patients to discuss their use of NSAIDs and their pain with their health care provider (Burchum and Rosenthal, 2019).

Opioids. Opioids play an important role in pain management and are used to manage moderate to severe pain (e.g., acute pain, cancer pain). They act on higher centers of the brain and spinal cord by binding with opiate receptors to modify perceptions of pain. Examples of opioids include morphine, codeine, hydromorphone, fentanyl, oxycodone, and hydrocodone. Some are available in IV and oral preparations (morphine and hydromorphone), whereas others are available only in oral formulations (oxycodone and hydrocodone). Most are available in a short-acting form, which provides relief for about 4 hours; some are also available in longer-acting preparations (oral morphine, oxycodone, hydromorphone, and a transdermal fentanyl patch).

The goal of opioid therapy is a reduction in pain intensity to a level of acceptable comfort. In both types of pain, progress toward pain relief is often measured by changes in pain-intensity scores. Opioid doses often need to be adjusted up or down according to individual patient circumstances and conditions. A prescriber must carefully individualize drug selection, dosing, and schedule.

Because of the wide variability in patient response to analgesics, health care providers commonly prescribe as-needed (prn) range orders for opioids (e.g., "morphine 2 to 6 mg IV q2h prn for pain"). Range orders are medication orders in which a dose varies over a prescribed range to provide flexibility in dosing depending on a patient's condition or situation (Drew et al., 2018). The Joint Commission requires health care agencies to have range-order policies in place to guide nurses in selecting the most appropriate dose of a medication. Chapter 31 describes principles of range orders. A proper range order offers specifics (e.g., a patient's pain severity score) for when a range of doses can be given and gives nurses the flexibility needed to treat patients' pain in a timely way while allowing for differences in patient response to pain and analgesia. Nurses base decisions about the administration of range orders on a thorough pain assessment and knowledge of the drug to be administered (Drew et al., 2018). Safe and effective range orders consider the patient's age, pain intensity, pain tolerance, pharmacogenetic profile, renal and liver function, and co-morbidities and prescribe a maximum dose that ranges to 2 to 3 times the lower or minimum dose (Drew et al., 2018).

BOX 44.13 Common Opioid Side Effects

Central Nervous System (CNS) Toxicity
- Thought and memory impairment
- Drowsiness, sedation, and sleep disturbance
- Confusion
- Hallucinations, potential for diminished psychomotor performance
- Delirium
- Depression
- Dizziness and seizures

Ocular
- Pupil constriction

Respiratory
- Bradypnea
- Hypoventilation

Cardiac
- Hypotension
- Bradycardia
- Peripheral edema

Gastrointestinal
- Constipation
- Nausea and vomiting
- Delayed gastric emptying

Genitourinary
- Urinary retention

Endocrine
- Hormonal and sexual dysfunction
- Hypoglycemia—reported with tramadol and methadone

Skin
- Pruritus

Immunological
- Immune system impairment possible with chronic use

Musculoskeletal
- Muscle rigidity and contractions
- Osteoporosis

Pregnancy and Breastfeeding
- When at all possible, avoid opioid use during pregnancy to prevent fetal risks

Tolerance
- Over time, increased doses needed to obtain analgesic effect

Withdrawal Syndrome
- Rapid or sudden cessation or marked dose reduction may cause rhinitis, chills, pupil dilation, diarrhea, "gooseflesh"

Adapted from American Chronic Pain Association (ACPA) & Standford Medicine: *ACPA and Standford Resource Guide to Chronic Pain Management*, 2021. https://www.theacpa.org/resources/acpa-resource-guide/. Accessed October 25, 2021.

Short-term use of opioid medications (3 to 5 days) is relatively safe. However, many patients experience at least one adverse event/effect, especially when they begin taking opioids (Box 44.13). Some patients are at higher risk for experiencing side effects than others (Box 44.14). The most common side effects of opioids include nausea, vomiting, constipation, and memory and thought changes (ACPA & Stanford Medicine, 2021). Except for constipation and central nervous system changes, patients usually become tolerant to many of the opioid side effects. To reduce side effects, give patients the lowest dose of an opioid needed to manage pain. For example, if a prescriber initially orders oxycodone 10 mg PO every 4 hours but the patient has nausea and is very drowsy, you might suggest that the prescriber reduce the dose to 5 mg. After administration, reassess a patient for the effect of the lowered dose on pain level and side effects. If reducing a dose does not relieve a side effect, confer with the prescriber about a change in the type of opioid. If side effects persist, it may be necessary to prevent or treat them by administering other medications (antihistamines, stool softeners, antiemetics, stimulants). Always anticipate that your patients will experience constipation. Help patients prevent constipation through diet changes, adequate hydration, and the use of stool softeners and stimulants as needed.

All patients who take opioids are at risk for respiratory depression, a common and serious adverse effect. Patients most at risk include those

BOX 44.14 Patient Characteristics Associated with Higher Risk for Opioid-Related Adverse Drug Events

- Snoring and sleep apnea or sleep-disordered breathing
- Morbid obesity with high risk of sleep apnea
- Older age
- Significant co-morbidities (cardiac, pulmonary, or major organ failure)
- No recent opioid use
- Increased opioid dose requirement
- Receiving other sedating medications (e.g., antihistamines, antipsychotics)
- Recent surgery, especially thoracic or upper abdominal
- Prolonged general anesthesia
- Smoker

Modified from The Joint Commission: *Sentinel Event Alert: safe use of opioids in hospitals*, Issue 49; August 8, 2012. http://www.jointcommission.org/assets/1/18/SEA_49_opioids_8_2_12_final.pdf. Accessed May 5, 2021.

who are opioid naïve (patients who have taken opioids around-the-clock [ATC] *less* than 1 week), who have a history or show signs of obstructive sleep disorder, who are on high-dose opioids, or who are taking opioids with other sedative medications (U.S. Department of Veterans Affairs, 2017). Assess your patients thoroughly when administering opioids. Obtain a complete opioid medication history, including dose, frequency, and duration of use to identify patients who are opioid naïve or tolerant. Sedation always occurs before a patient experiences respiratory depression. Thus, closely monitor patients for sedation when they are taking opioids. Respiratory depression is clinically significant when a patient's rate and depth of respirations are lower than what they were on initial assessment. If an adult patient experiences respiratory depression, administer naloxone (0.4 mg diluted with 9 mL saline) IV push (IVP) at a rate prescribed by health care provider. Once respiratory depression has been reversed, you can use intramuscular (IM) or subcutaneous routes. Administering naloxone too fast may cause severe pain and serious complications such as hypotension, hypertension, cardiac arrhythmias, dyspnea, and pulmonary edema. Naloxone's duration of action is often less than that of the opioid. Thus, you need to evaluate patients who receive naloxone every 15 minutes for 2 hours for respiratory depression following administration (Burchum and Rosenthal, 2019).

One way to maximize pain relief while potentially decreasing opioid use is to administer analgesics around the clock (ATC) or at scheduled times rather than a prn basis. This approach ensures a more constant therapeutic blood level of an analgesic. There are also a variety of extended- or controlled-release oral opioid formulations (dosing intervals of 8, 10, 12, or 24 hours) and transdermal patches (72 hours). These formulations maintain constant serum opioid concentration, minimizing toxic and subtherapeutic concentrations (Burchum and Rosenthal, 2019). An ATC medication lessens the severity of end-of-dose pain, allowing a patient to sleep through the night and reduce "clock watching" for the next dose.

Critical thinking, clinical judgment, and careful assessment are required to safely administer analgesics (Box 44.15). The current pharmacological approach to acute and chronic pain management is to provide **multimodal analgesia**. Multimodal analgesia combines drugs with at least two different mechanisms of action to optimize pain control. Medications are combined to target different sites in the peripheral or central pain pathways (Fig. 44.10). The use of different agents allows for lower-than-usual doses of each medication, which is a benefit of multimodal analgesia. A multimodal regimen lowers the risk of side

BOX 44.15 Nursing Principles for Administering Analgesics

Know Patient's Previous Response to Analgesics
- Determine whether patient has sensitivities or allergies.
- Know whether patient is at risk for using NSAIDs (e.g., history of GI bleeding or renal insufficiency) or opioids (e.g., history of obstructive or central sleep apnea).
- Identify previous doses and routes of analgesic administration to avoid undertreatment.
- Determine whether patient obtained relief.
- Ask whether a nonopioid was as effective as an opioid.

Select Proper Medications When More Than One Is Ordered
- Consult with health care provider to use nonopioid analgesics or opioid combination drugs for mild to moderate pain.
- Recommend opioids with nonopioids to provide a multimodal analgesia approach.
- Avoid using multiple opioids with the same duration and mechanism of action.
- Intravenous medications act more quickly and usually relieve severe, acute pain within 1 hour, whereas oral medications take as long as 2 hours to relieve pain.
- Avoid intramuscular analgesics, especially in older adults.
- Recommend use of an opioid with a nonopioid analgesic for severe pain because such combinations treat pain peripherally and centrally.
- For chronic pain give sustained-release oral formulations ATC.

Know Accurate Dosage
- Recall that 4 g is considered the maximum 24-hour dosage for acetaminophen and acetylsalicylic acid; 3200 mg for ibuprofen.
- Adjust doses as appropriate for children and older patients.
- Large doses of opioids are acceptable in opioid-tolerant patients but not in opioid-naïve patients.
- When titrating an opioid, it is important to titrate to effect or to uncontrollable side effects.

Assess Right Time and Interval for Administration
- Administer analgesics as soon as pain occurs and before it increases in severity.
- An ATC administration schedule is usually best.
- Give analgesics before pain-producing procedures or activities.
- Know the average duration of action for a drug and the time of administration so that the peak effect occurs when the pain is most intense.
- Use extended-release opioid formulations to treat chronic pain.
- Avoid stopping opioids abruptly in patients who are opioid tolerant.

ATC, Around the clock; *GI*, gastrointestinal; *NSAIDs*, nonsteroidal antiinflammatory drugs.
Modified from Centers for Disease Control and Prevention: CDC guideline for prescribing opioids for chronic pain—United States, 2016, *MMWR* 65(1):1-49, 2016.

effects while providing pain relief that is as good as or even better than could be obtained from each of the medications alone.

A person's response to an analgesic is highly individualized. If the pain is caused by inflammation, an NSAID is sometimes as effective as, or more effective than, an opioid. An orally administered analgesic usually has a longer onset and duration of action than an injectable form. In addition, for pain that persists for most of the day, controlled- or extended-release opioid formulations (morphine sulfate extended release, oxycodone sustained/extended release, and methadone) are available for administration every 8 to 12 hours ATC; they are not ordered prn.

Gray matter
White matter
Nerve tracts

Opioids[1]
α_2 – agonists[1]
Acetaminophen[2][3]
NMDA antagonists[3]

Local anesthetics[1]
Opioids[1]
α_2 – agonists[1]
NMDA antagonists[3]

Local anesthetics[1]
NSAIDs[1]
COXIB[1]
Ice

FIG. 44.10 Multimodal analgesia sites of action. (© Elsevier collections.) *COXIB,* Cox-2 inhibitor; *NMDA, N*-methyl-d-aspartate; *NSAID,* nonsteroidal antiinflammatory drug. 1. Gottschalk A, Smith DS. New concepts in acute pain therapy: preemptive analgesia. *Am Fam Physician* 63(10):1979-1984, 2001. (http://www.aafp.org/afp/2001/0515/p1979.html). 2. Smith HS. Potential analgesic mechanisms of acetaminophen. *Pain Physician* 12:269-280, 2009. (http://www.painphysicianjournal.com/current/pdf?article=MTE4NA%3D%3D&journal=47). 3. Sinatra RS, Jahr JS, editors. *The essence of analgesia and analgesics.* New York, 2011, Cambridge University Press.

Morphine is inactivated by hepatic metabolism as it passes through the liver on its way to the systemic circulation. Thus, when taken orally, much of the oral dose is inactivated during the first pass through the liver. A drug can be completely inactivated on its first pass through the liver, with minimal or no therapeutic effects (Burchum and Rosenthal, 2019). As a result, oral doses need to be substantially larger than parenteral doses to achieve equivalent analgesic effects (Burchum and Rosenthal, 2019). Know the comparative potencies of analgesics in oral and injectable form. In addition, know the route of administration most effective for a patient so that controlled, sustained pain relief is achieved. The IM and subcutaneous routes are painful and the absorption is unreliable; thus these routes are generally avoided (Burchum and Rosenthal, 2019). When comparing opioids, refer to equianalgesic charts (i.e., charts converting one opioid to another, or parenteral forms of opioids to oral forms [e.g., morphine to hydromorphone] or vice versa) or contact the pharmacy staff. Check agency policy before using a smartphone app for opioid-dosing conversions.

Age-related changes and increased frailty lead to less predictable drug responses in older adults, including increased drug sensitivity and severity of side effects. Prescribers should follow a "start-low" (dose) and "go-slow" (upward dose titration) philosophy to minimize risks associated with opioid therapy (Burchum and Rosenthal, 2019). Combining smaller doses of more than one medication may minimize the dose-limiting adverse effects of using a single drug (ACPA & Stanford Medicine, 2021).

BOX 44.16 Key Steps for Safe Opioid Use

- Fill opioid prescriptions from only one health care provider.
- Notify all health care providers about your opioid use. Alert your opioid prescriber about any new medications.
- Inform your health care provider about current/past history of alcohol or substance abuse.
- Follow directions for taking opioids carefully. Do not crush, break, or dissolve pills.
- Reduce the risk of drug interactions. Do not mix opioids with alcohol, antihistamines, barbiturates, benzodiazepines, other sedatives, or muscle relaxants.
- Prevent theft, diversion, and child access to opioids. Keep opioids in a locked box.
- Keep track of when refills are needed to prevent going without medications, which can lead to withdrawal.

Adapted from American Chronic Pain Association (ACPA) & Standford Medicine: *ACPA and Standford Resource Guide to Chronic Pain Management,* 2021. https://www.theacpa.org/resources/acpa-resource-guide/. Accessed October 25, 2021.

Dizziness, confusion, and changes in vision are opioid-related side effects that place the older adult at increased risk for falls and other injuries. Take special care to ensure that the environment is safe, and provide appropriate patient education about injury prevention. Avoid unintentional medication overdoses in the home by helping an older adult with memory problems create a safe plan for taking medication (ACPA & Stanford Medicine, 2021). Appropriate interventions may include help from family caregivers, home care medication reconciliation, or using time-of-day labeled pillboxes (that are also kept in a locked safe).

Many older adults have multiple co-morbidities and require various medications, placing them at risk for polypharmacy and drug-drug interactions. Morphine-like drugs can interact unfavorably when taken with other medications, such as CNS depressants, anticholinergic drugs, hypotensives, and monoamine oxidase inhibitors (Burchum and Rosenthal, 2019). Thus, you need to take a thorough medication history when caring for older adults and determine the potential for dangerous drug-drug interactions.

The misuse and improper prescribing of opioids has led to a crisis in the United States. Among patients who use opioids for more than 8 days, 13.5% will be on opioids at 1 year; in addition, 30% of people who take opioids for more than 31 days remain on them 1 year later (ACPA & Stanford Medicine, 2021). Nurses play a key role in monitoring patient response when opioids are being used and in detecting potential misuse or prolonged unnecessary use. Some patients who use opioids for an extended time experience increased adverse effects, have reduced function, and need to take multiple other medications to treat their side effects. Long-term use is also associated with the development of opioid tolerance, which results in patients needing increased doses of opioids to control their pain over time (ACPA & Stanford Medicine, 2021). Because of the risks of tolerance and addiction, you need to be knowledgeable of the effects of opioids and implications for patient monitoring and management.

Because of the risks, it is important to educate patients about how to take opioids safely. Because of widespread media reports about the dangers of opioids, many patients who can benefit from opioids will be reluctant to take the medications. Carefully selected opioids and doses, along with patient education and monitoring, are important in providing safe and effective pain management for patients of all ages (Box 44.16).

Adjuvants. Coanalgesics or adjuvants are drugs originally developed to treat conditions other than pain but that also have analgesic properties. For example, tricyclic antidepressants (e.g., nortriptyline), anticonvulsants (e.g., gabapentin), and infusional lidocaine successfully treat chronic pain, especially neuropathic pain. Corticosteroids relieve the pain from

FIG. 44.11 Patient-controlled analgesia pump with cassette. (Courtesy Smiths Medical ASD, Inc., St Paul, MN.)

inflammation and bone metastasis. Other examples of coanalgesics are bisphosphonates and calcitonin for bone pain. Adjuvants have analgesic properties, enhance pain control, or relieve other symptoms associated with neuropathic pain. You give adjuvants alone or with analgesics. Sedatives, antianxiety agents, and muscle relaxants have *no* analgesic effect, although they may be effective for their specific indications.

Patient-Controlled Analgesia. When patients depend on nurses for prn analgesia, an erratic cycle of alternating pain and analgesia often occurs. A patient feels pain and asks for medication, but the patient first must be assessed, and then the medication must be obtained and prepared. Under this circumstance analgesia finally occurs in about an hour, but pain relief may last only 30 minutes. Gradually the patient again feels discomfort, and the cycle begins again. The patient is constantly going in and out of analgesic therapeutic range.

A drug delivery system called **patient-controlled analgesia (PCA)** is a method for pain management that many patients prefer (see Skill 44.1). It is a drug delivery system that allows patients to self-administer opioids (usually morphine, hydromorphone, or fentanyl) with minimal risk of overdose. The goal is to maintain a constant plasma level of analgesic to avoid the problems of prn dosing. Systemic PCA traditionally involves IV or subcutaneous drug administration; however, a controlled analgesia device for oral medications is available. This device allows patients access to their own oral prn medications, including opioids and other analgesics, antiemetics, and anxiolytics, at the bedside.

PCA infusion pumps are portable and computerized and contain a chamber for a syringe or bag that delivers a small, preset dose of opioid (Fig. 44.11). To receive a demand dose, a patient pushes a button attached to the PCA device. The PCA infusion pumps deliver a specific dose, which is programmed to be available at specific time intervals (usually in the range of 8 to 15 minutes) when the patient activates the delivery button. A limit on the number of doses per hour or a 4-hour interval may also be set. To reduce the risk for oversedation and respiratory depression

in opioid-naïve patients, do not increase the demand or basal dose *and* shorten the interval time simultaneously.

Most pumps have locked safety systems that prevent tampering by patients or family members and are generally safe to be managed in the home. For patients who are opioid tolerant, such as those with cancer pain, a low-dose continuous infusion (basal rate) is sometimes programmed to deliver a steady dose of continuous medication. PCA basal doses are *not* recommended for opioid-naïve patients following surgery because of the possibility for respiratory depression.

There are many benefits to PCA use. The patient gains control over pain, and pain relief does not depend on nurse availability. Patients also have access to medication when they need it. This decreases anxiety and leads to decreased medication use. Small doses of medications are delivered at short intervals, stabilizing serum drug concentrations for sustained pain relief.

Patient preparation and teaching are critical to the safe and effective use of PCA devices (Box 44.17). A patient needs to understand the PCA and be physically able to locate and press the button to deliver a dose. Family members and visitors must be instructed not to "push the button" for the patient (a dangerous action known as "PCA by proxy"), because this action bypasses the safety feature of PCA, which requires an awake patient to activate the device. When patients are unable to activate the PCA device, a carefully selected family member or nurse may be authorized to activate the device based on specific criteria and authorized agent–controlled analgesia (AACA) guidelines (Cooney et al., 2013). The use of agent-controlled analgesia has been shown effective in the critically ill population (Benjenk et al., 2020).

Programming the settings usually requires independent verification by two nurses to ensure accuracy. Even though patients control administration of analgesics, a nurse's diligence is needed to prevent errors related to programmable PCA devices. Document drug dosages and track medication wastes according to agency policy.

Topical and Transdermal Analgesics. Topical analgesics include prescription and OTC creams, gels, sprays, liquids, patches, or rubs applied on the skin over painful muscles or joints and for peripheral neuropathy (ACPA & Stanford Medicine, 2021) Commonly used topical agents include NSAID products (ketoprofen patch) and capsaicin and local anesthetics such as lidocaine, prilocaine, and diclofenac (ACPA & Stanford Medicine, 2021). The medications are effective in chronic pain management. Topical agents work locally, have few side effects, and must be applied directly over the painful area.

Transdermal drugs are also applied directly to the skin but have systemic effects and work when applied away from the area of pain (ACPA & Stanford Medicine, 2021). Transdermal medication in a patch is absorbed through the skin by the bloodstream over time. Examples of analgesic transdermal medications are fentanyl, buprenorphine, and clonidine. Chapter 31 describes the administration of topical and transdermal medications.

The lidocaine patch is a topical analgesic effective for cutaneous neuropathic pain such as postherpetic neuralgia in adults. Up to three patches can be used. Cut each patch to the size and shape needed to cover the painful area using a 12-hour on, 12-hour off schedule (U.S. National Library of Medicine, 2016). Products such as ELA-Max/LMX (topical lidocaine) and eutectic mixture of local anesthetics (EMLA) are available for children. Apply EMLA via a disk or thick cream to the skin 30 to 60 minutes before minor procedures (e.g., IV start, intramuscular injection) or anesthetic infiltration of soft tissue.

Do not place topical or transdermal analgesics on wounds, damaged skin, or the face. Pruritus, redness, swelling, or burning of the skin or a localized rash is common after topical applications. Application of a topical analgesic to vascular mucous membranes increases the chance of systemic effects such as a change in heart rate. Wear disposable gloves when removing and applying transdermal patches. Lastly, after application, wash your hands thoroughly to avoid getting these products in sensitive areas such as the eyes (ACPA & Stanford Medicine, 2021).

Local Anesthesia via Injection. Local anesthesia is the local infiltration of an anesthetic medication to induce loss of sensation to a body part. Health care providers often use local anesthesia during brief surgical procedures such as removing a skin lesion or suturing a wound by applying local anesthetics topically on skin and mucous membranes or injecting them subcutaneously or intradermally to anesthetize a body part. Regional anesthesia is the injection or infusion of local anesthetics to block a group of sensory nerve fibers. The anesthetics produce temporary loss of sensation by inhibiting nerve conduction. Local anesthetics also block motor and autonomic functions, depending on the amount used and the location and depth of administration. Smaller sensory nerve fibers are more sensitive to local anesthetics than are large motor fibers. As a result, the patient loses sensation before losing motor function; conversely, motor activity returns before sensation.

Perineural Local Anesthetic Infusion. Perineural injections and infusions of local anesthetic agents are used for a variety of inpatient and outpatient adult and pediatric surgical procedures to relieve pain. A surgeon places the tip of an unsutured catheter near a nerve or groups of nerves, and the catheter exits from the surgical wound. Infusions of local anesthetics (bupivacaine or ropivacaine) administered regionally may be run on a pump similar to those used for IV infusions, on ambulatory pumps, or on disposable systems (e.g., On-Q). The pump may be set on demand or continuous mode, and the catheter is usually left in place for 48 hours. Some patients have pump systems that are left in place after discharge. Patients learn how to discontinue the pump at home and bring the catheter to the next health care provider visit. Some patients still need oral analgesics, but perineural infusions often reduce the total dosage (von Plato et al., 2019).

Local anesthetics cause side effects, depending on their absorption into the circulation. The use of local anesthetics in peripheral nerve and epidural infusions (see following paragraph) may block both motor nerves and sensory nerves. This effect resolves within hours of the reduction or discontinuation of an infusion.

Epidural Analgesia. Another pain therapy that often involves the administration of anesthetic agents is epidural analgesia, a form of regional anesthesia. Preservative-free opioids are often administered as

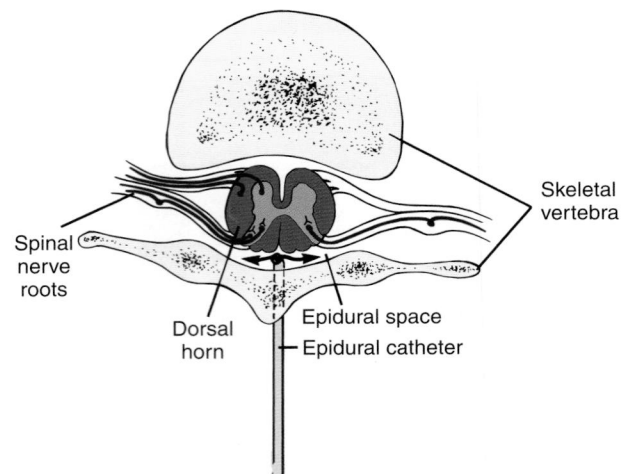

FIG. 44.12 Anatomical drawing of epidural space.

single agents or in combination with local anesthetics into a patient's epidural space. Epidural analgesia effectively treats acute postoperative pain, rib fracture pain, labor and delivery pain, and chronic cancer pain. It often reduces a patient's overall opioid requirement, thus minimizing adverse effects such as constipation and hypotension (Baeriswyl et al., 2018). It is short or long term, depending on a patient's condition and life expectancy.

Health care providers administer epidural analgesia into the spinal epidural space (Fig. 44.12) by inserting a blunt-tip needle into the level of the vertebral interspace nearest to the area requiring analgesia. They advance the catheter into the epidural space, remove the needle, and secure the remainder of the catheter with a dressing while ensuring that the catheter is taped securely. The end of the catheter is capped or, if a continuous infusion is prescribed, it is connected to special tubing and an infusion pump that is designated for epidural infusion. Nurse anesthetists, anesthesiologists, and certified nurses control epidural analgesia, depending on agency policy. Some patients are able to use a technique known as *patient-controlled epidural analgesia (PCEA),* which allows them to self-administer demand doses of epidural solution when connected to a special administration pump (Koh et al., 2017).

One of the concerns related to the use of peripheral and epidural anesthetic techniques is the risk of bleeding and subsequent hematoma formation near the injection/insertion site. Although relatively uncommon, the risk is increased when patients receive anticoagulant or antiplatelet medications. Thus, safe placement or removal of these injections and catheters is made based on a patient's coagulation status and when the patient takes anticoagulant or antiplatelet medications. Guidelines for the use of anticoagulation in patients with regional anesthesia are available (Narouze et al., 2018) Because the epidural space is a highly vascular area, patients with epidural catheters are at risk for the development of epidural hematomas, which may lead to ischemia of the spinal cord and, if left unaddressed, serious neurological complications.

Nursing Implications for Local and Regional Anesthesia. Provide emotional support to patients receiving local or regional anesthesia by explaining the insertion technique and warning patients that they will temporarily lose sensory function within minutes of injection. Motor and autonomic (bowel and bladder control) function may also be lost quickly, depending on the area anesthetized. It is common for patients to fear paralysis because epidural and spinal injections come close to the spinal cord. To reassure the patient, explain that numbness, tingling, and coldness are common. Catheter insertion should be comfortable because the health care provider should first numb the injection site, but prepare patients for possible discomfort. Before a patient receives an analgesic, check for allergies. Also check to be sure that the drugs (e.g., morphine injection and fentanyl citrate) administered via the epidural catheter are free of potentially neurotoxic substances such as preservatives and additives. Assess vital signs to monitor systemic effects.

After administration of a local or regional anesthetic, protect the patient from injury and educate about necessary precautions until full sensory and motor function return. Patients are at risk for injuring an anesthetized body part without knowing it. For patients with topical anesthesia, do not apply heat or cold to numb areas. After an injection into the knee joint, warn the patient to avoid standing without assistance because there is a high risk of falling. With peripheral nerve or epidural local anesthetics, patients may experience sensory loss along with significant motor weakness. Assess patients for sensory and motor nerve blockade, and notify the prescriber when motor blockade is unintended. During and after epidural anesthesia a patient stays in bed until motor function returns. Help patients the first time they try to get out of bed.

When managing epidural infusions, if agency policy allows, connect the catheter to an infusion pump, a port, or a reservoir or cap it off for bolus injections. Because of the catheter location, use surgical asepsis to prevent a serious and potentially fatal infection. To reduce the risk of accidental epidural injection of drugs intended for IV use, clearly label the catheter *epidural catheter*. Always administer continuous infusions through appropriately labeled electronic infusion devices for proper control. Notify a patient's health care provider immediately of any signs or symptoms of infection or pain at the insertion site. Thorough hygiene is necessary during nursing procedures to keep the catheter system clean and dry. Maintain a closed system and prevent catheter disconnection by ensuring tight connections.

Nursing implications for managing epidural analgesia are numerous (Table 44.6). Do not administer supplemental doses of opioids or sedative/hypnotics because of possible additive central nervous system adverse effects. Monitoring for effects of medications differs, depending on the medication being administered and whether infusions are intermittent or continuous. Complications of epidural opioid use include nausea and vomiting, hypotension, urinary retention, constipation, respiratory depression, and pruritus. When patients receive epidural analgesia, initially monitor them as often as every 15 minutes, including assessment of vital signs, respiratory effort, and skin color. Once stabilized, monitor patients every hour in the first 12 to 24 hours and then with less frequency if the patient is stable (refer to agency policy).

To minimize bleeding risks and the potential for hematoma formation, do not administer anticoagulant and antiplatelet medications until a pain specialist can verify safe use. Notify the health care provider or pain specialist if the patient develops severe pain at the epidural insertion site or unexplained sensory or motor loss, which are signs and symptoms of a possible epidural hematoma. Also notify the health care provider who performs the procedure when patients with peripheral nerve injections/catheter have similar signs and symptoms.

Provide patient education about epidural analgesia in terms of the action of the medication and its advantages and disadvantages. Instruct patients about the potential for side effects, and advise them to notify you if side effects develop. If the patient requires long-term epidural use, the health care provider tunnels a permanent catheter through the skin. The catheter exits at the patient's side. Teach a patient on long-term therapy how to safely administer home infusions with minimal ongoing nursing intervention, which signs and symptoms need to be reported to the health care provider, and to coordinate with the case manager or social worker to ensure that appropriate home care services are provided.

TABLE 44.6 Nursing Care for Patients With Epidural Infusions

Outcome	Actions
Prevent catheter displacement.	Secure catheter (if not connected to implanted reservoir) carefully to outside skin.
Maintain catheter function.	Check external dressing around catheter site for dampness or discharge. (Leakage of epidural solution may occur if catheter is dislodged.) Use transparent dressing to secure catheter and aid inspection. Inspect catheter for breaks.
Prevent infection.	Use strict aseptic technique when caring for catheter (see Chapter 28). Do not change dressing routinely over site. Inspect insertions site for signs of infection. Follow agency policies for tubing change.
Monitor for respiratory depression.	Monitor vital signs, especially respirations, and level of consciousness per agency policy. Use pulse oximetry, end-tidal carbon dioxide, and apnea monitoring.
Prevent undesirable complications.	Assess for hypotension: <ul><li>Ensure adequate hydration and administer prescribed intravenous fluids.</li><li>Notify health care provider if significant change in vital signs occurs, and reduce or stop epidural infusion.</li><li>Anticipate need for change in epidural solution.</li></ul> Assess for pruritus (itching) and nausea and vomiting associated with use of epidural opioids: <ul><li>Notify health care provider for dose reduction or epidural solution change.</li><li>Administer antihistamines and antiemetics as ordered.</li></ul> Assess sensation and motor strength; notify health care provider if deviation from baseline.
Maintain urinary and bowel function.	Monitor intake and output. Assess for bladder and bowel distention. Assess for discomfort, frequency, and urgency.

Invasive Interventions for Pain Relief. When severe pain persists despite medical treatment, available invasive interventions include intrathecal implantable pumps or injections, spinal cord and deep brain stimulation, neuroablative procedures (cordotomy, rhizotomy), trigger point injections, cryoablation, and intraspinal medications (e.g., opioids, steroids, local anesthetics). These techniques are used to treat chronic pain. It is unacceptable to tell a patient with severe unrelieved pain that there is "nothing more we can do for you." Refer patients with severe chronic pain to comprehensive pain-management programs whenever possible. These programs offer many different interventional strategies, pharmacological options, physical medicine, and rehabilitation therapies to address the complex needs of patients with chronic pain. When comprehensive pain programs are unavailable, refer patients to a chronic pain-management program.

Pain Management for Procedures. Diagnostic and treatment procedures potentially produce pain and anxiety, both of which should be assessed and treated before a procedure begins. Barriers to successful pain control include numerous patient-specific factors. However, a major barrier occurs when health care providers do not recognize that pain may occur during or after a procedure. This is especially true when administering an intervention to a patient who is nonverbal (e.g., an intubated patient) or a patient with a reduced level of consciousness. Many types of routine procedures can cause pain, especially in patients who are critically ill, including turning, wound drain removal, femoral catheter removal, placement of a central line or feeding tube, and changing wound dressings. Common pharmacological agents for managing procedural comfort include local anesthetics, NSAIDs, acetaminophen, opioids, anxiolytics, and sedatives. Premedicating patients before painful procedures allows them to cooperate more fully and reduces the experience of pain. Using nonpharmacological therapies such as relaxation techniques, meditation, imagery, and music, in addition to medications, has also been effective in select situations (Wren et al., 2019). When you premedicate a patient before a procedure, keep in mind how long it takes for the onset and peak effect of the analgesic to occur so that you can properly time the beginning of the painful procedure to coincide with the medication's peak effect.

Cancer Pain and Chronic Noncancer Pain Management. Cancer pain varies among patients and can be either chronic or acute. Pain is commonly experienced in patients with metastatic, advanced, or terminal cancer; patients receiving cancer treatment; and patients following their treatment. Organizations such as the APS and the National Comprehensive Cancer Network (NCCN) have published guidelines for assessing and treating cancer-related pain. The guidelines support comprehensive and aggressive treatment, including many options for pain relief. The best choice of pain treatment often changes as a patient's condition and the characteristics of pain change. Use multimodal pharmacological strategies and nonpharmacological interventions to optimize pain management (ACPA & Stanford Medicine, 2021).

Many patients with cancer experience breakthrough cancer pain (BTCP), a temporary increase in pain in someone who has relatively stable and an adequately controlled level of baseline pain (ACPA & Stanford Medicine, 2021). It occurs either spontaneously or in relation to a specific predictable or unpredictable trigger (Scarborough and Smith, 2018). BTCP is a challenging aspect of cancer because, even though it is self-limiting in nature, its presence has a significant, negative impact on the quality of life of patients and family caregivers (Scarborough and Smith, 2018). Individualized assessment is critical for understanding how BTCP affects a patient's life. A holistic approach to care is often needed (Box 44.18).

BOX 44.18 Types of Breakthrough Pain and Treatment

Types of Breakthrough Pain

Incident pain: Pain that is predictable and elicited by specific behaviors or triggers, such as a voluntary act (walking), involuntary act (coughing), or treatments (e.g., wound dressing changes)

End-of-dose failure pain: Pain that occurs toward the end of the usual dosing interval of a regularly scheduled analgesic

Spontaneous pain: Pain that is unpredictable and not associated with any activity or event

Treatment

- Lifestyle changes
- Management of reversible causes
- Modification of pathological processes
- Nonpharmacological management
- Pharmacological management—rescue dose of medication
- Interventional techniques

From Scarborough BM, Smith CB: Optimal pain management for patients with cancer in the modern era, *CA Cancer J Clin* 68(3):182-196, 2018.

Always use opioids judiciously. The benefits from the use of opioids for chronic pain are measured by an increase in the person's level of functioning; a reduction or elimination of reports of pain; a more positive, hopeful attitude; and minimal or controllable side effects (ACPA & Stanford Medicine, 2021). The use of opioid therapy in patients with chronic pain requires careful patient selection and consideration of the risks and benefits of opioids. For example, to determine whether opioids may be beneficial, it is necessary to assess a patient's opioid addiction risk, level of participation in ADLs, physical function, family activities, and work-related requirements (CDC, 2016). Family members are often included in office visits to provide input about a patient's functional level. Use of opioids can increase adverse events and lead to polypharmacy when medications are added to treat side effects of the opioids (ACPA & Stanford Medicine, 2021). It is recommended that each person with chronic noncancer pain be medically managed individually; medication use should be determined by weighing benefit compared with other alternatives, cost, potential side effects, and the person's other medical problems (ACPA & Stanford Medicine, 2021).

The World Health Organization (WHO) in 1986 introduced the WHO three-step analgesic ladder as a recommended approach for the slow introduction and upward titration of analgesics for managing pain. This approach has been used worldwide and has been praised for its simplicity and ease of use. However, the ladder has been the object of criticism because of the absence of nonpharmacological therapies in providing analgesia, with modifications suggested in subsequent iterations (U.S. Department of Veterans Affairs, 2017) (Fig. 44.13). The original three-step approach recommended that therapy begin at the first step with the use of nonopioid analgesics and/or adjuvants and progress to the next higher step, using opioids as pain intensity increases.

Different modifications attempt to provide more holistic, simple, and effective guidelines, which include (Anekar and Cascella, 2020):

- Around-the-clock (ATC) administration rather than on-demand administration of medications.
- Thorough clinical assessments of the pain to allow providers to prescribe the appropriate analgesics based on the patient's pain severity.
- Individualized therapy, including the dosage of medications as there is no standardized dosage that treats pain for all patients.
- The use of nonpharmacological approaches (e.g., yoga, acupuncture, psychotherapy) and addressing psychosocial aspects of a patient's pain.

Long-acting or controlled-release medications may provide relief for cancer pain but are not recommended for the initial treatment of noncancer pain (CDC, 2016). These controlled-release medications (e.g., morphine sulfate extended release and oxycodone HCl) relieve pain for 8 to 12 hours. Long-acting or sustained-release opioids are dosed on a scheduled basis, not prn or "as needed." Transdermal fentanyl, which is 100 times more potent than morphine, is available for patients who are opioid tolerant with cancer or chronic pain. It delivers predetermined doses that provide analgesia for up to 72 hours. The transdermal route is useful when patients are unable to take drugs orally. Patients find the transdermal patch easy to use because it allows for continuous opioid administration without needles or pumps. Self-adhesive patches release the medication slowly over time, achieving effective analgesia. Transdermal fentanyl is not for adult patients who weigh less than 45.5 kg (100 lb) (too little subcutaneous tissue for absorption) or who are hyperthermic (increases drug absorption). Guidelines for the use of transdermal fentanyl patches include: *Do not expose the patch to direct heat (e.g., heating pads, electric blankets, hot baths, or through sunbathing), instruct patients to avoid physical activity that causes them to get hot, and monitor patients who have fevers closely; also, never cut a patch* (U.S. National Library of Medicine, 2021). To dispose of a patch, fold in half, adhesive side onto itself, and flush down the toilet.

FIG. 44.13 Adaptation of the WHO analgesic ladder. *NSAID,* Nonsteroidal antiinflammatory drug; *PCA,* patient-controlled analgesia. (From Vargas-Schaffer G: Is the WHO analgesic ladder still valid?: twenty-four years of experience, *Can Fam Physician* 56:514, 2010.)

All patients on chronic opioid therapy require monitoring and follow-up. Side effects should be anticipated, prevented when possible, and treated when necessary. Over time, patients develop tolerance to the analgesic effect of opioids, requiring higher doses to achieve pain relief. The higher opioid dose is usually not lethal because patients also develop a tolerance to respiratory depression. Less commonly, chronic opioid use may lead to hyperalgesia (increased pain sensitivity). Especially in the case of noncancer pain, monitor patients closely for signs of aberrant opioid-related behaviors, such as misuse, abuse, and addiction.

A transmucosal fentanyl "unit" treats breakthrough pain in patients who are opioid tolerant. Patients take the medication by placing an opened transmucosal package in their mouth between the buccal mucosa and gums and actively sucking on the medicine. Patients need to let it dissolve in the mouth. Teach patients not to chew it and to allow it to absorb over a 15-minute period, delaying swallowing as long as possible and avoiding drinking water or other liquid. A patient should not use more than 1 unit of oral transmucosal fentanyl citrate at a time and no more than 2 units of oral transmucosal fentanyl citrate during each episode of breakthrough cancer pain. If a patient has more than four episodes of breakthrough cancer pain per day, tell the patient to contact the health care provider.

Many patients, family members, and health care providers have concerns about the risks of addiction associated with opioid use. The estimated prevalence of prescription opioid misuse in patients with chronic pain ranges from 21% to 29%, and it is estimated that between 8% and 12% of people who use opioids to manage their chronic pain will develop an opioid use disorder (NIHNIDA, 2021). Patients who consult with numerous health care providers are often labeled as drug seekers when they actually may be seeking adequate pain relief. This situation may be associated with behaviors that are indicative of **pseudoaddiction**. Discourage patients from "doctor shopping" and going to multiple health care providers for treating pain. Refer them to pain specialists when effective management cannot be obtained through their general health care providers.

As with constant acute pain, you need to administer analgesics to patients with chronic pain on a regular basis, using the oral route of administration as the first choice (CDC, 2016). The patient with chronic pain may need to take an analgesic ATC, as regular administration maintains therapeutic drug blood levels for ongoing pain control.

However, the need for continuation of analgesics needs to be assessed routinely by the health care provider (CDC, 2016).

Administer analgesics rectally when patients are unable to swallow, have nausea or vomiting, or are near death. This route is contraindicated for patients with diarrhea or cancerous lesions involving the anus or rectum. Morphine, hydromorphone, and oxymorphone are available in suppositories.

Some patients use PCA devices to treat severe cancer pain in the home. PCA devices provide improved, uniform pain control with fewer peaks and valleys in plasma concentration, more effective drug action, and lower drug dosages overall. Patients who usually benefit from continuous infusions include those with severe pain for whom oral and injectable medications provide minimal relief, those with severe nausea and vomiting, and those unable to swallow oral medications.

When a patient receives opioids intravenously, ensure that the IV access is patent and without complications (see Chapter 42). A central venous catheter, an implanted venous access port, or a peripherally inserted central catheter (PICC) is usually best for long-term IV infusion. When IV access is poor, the subcutaneous route with a concentrated dose is possible. When an infusion begins, monitor a patient's sedation level and respiratory status closely during the first 24 hours and with any increases in the infusion rate (follow agency policy). Patients who are placed on continuous analgesic infusions are usually opioid tolerant; thus respiratory depression is rare.

QSEN **Building Competency in Patient-Centered Care** You are assigned to make home visits to a 68-year-old female patient who was discharged from the hospital 1 day ago. The patient has diabetes mellitus and had a wound debridement of the left leg while hospitalized. When you arrive, the patient describes the pain around the wound as "throbbing" and "never gets much better." The patient tells you that the NSAID prescribed for wound pain has not worked very well. She states, "I have been taking this medication that I had left over from my surgery last year to help with my pain since this new medication isn't working." You note that the medication the patient has been taking is hydrocodone, an oral opioid. What options do you have in helping this patient achieve a realistic and effective approach to managing her pain?

Answers to QSEN Activities can be found on the Evolve website.

BOX 44.19   Barriers to Effective Pain Management

Patient Barriers
- Fear of addiction
- Worry about side effects
- Fear of tolerance (will not be there when I need it)
- Takes too many pills already
- Concern about not being a "good" patient
- Does not want to worry family and friends
- May need more tests
- Suffering in silence is expected and needs to suffer to be cured
- Inadequate education
- Reluctance to discuss pain
- Belief that pain is inevitable
- Belief that pain is a part of aging
- Fear of disease progression
- Believes health care providers and nurses are doing all they can
- Forgets to take analgesics
- Fear of distracting health care providers from treating illness
- Believes health care providers have more important or sicker patients to see

Health Care Provider Barriers
- Inadequate pain-assessment skills
- No pain-management protocols available
- Concern with addiction or accidental overdose

- Concern with co-morbid mental health conditions
- Opiophobia, fear of opioids
- Fear of legal repercussions
- Patient shows no visible cause of pain
- Belief that patients need to learn to live with pain
- Reluctance to deal with side effects of analgesics
- Not believing patient's report of pain
- Fear that giving a dose will kill patient
- Time constraints
- Inadequate reimbursement
- Belief that opioids "mask" symptoms
- Belief that pain is part of aging
- Overestimation of rates of respiratory depression

Health Care System Barriers
- Concern with creating "addicts"
- Difficulty in filling prescriptions
- Limitation on reimbursement for prescriptions
- Mail-order pharmacy restrictions
- Advanced practice nurses not used efficiently
- Poor pain policies and procedures regarding pain management
- Inadequate access to pain clinics
- Poor understanding of economic impact of unrelieved pain

Barriers to Effective Pain Management. Barriers to effective pain management are complex and often involve the patient, the patient's family caregivers, health care providers, and the health care system (Box 44.19). Lack of knowledge and misconceptions about pain and appropriate pain management present significant barriers. Various cultural beliefs about the meaning of pain and pain interventions also pose challenges to effective pain management. Lack of pain-management protocols and limited access to health care pose further barriers, particularly for patients with chronic noncancer pain.

Patients and health care providers often do not understand the differences among physical dependence, addiction, and drug tolerance (Box 44.20). Experiencing a physical dependency does not imply addiction, and drug tolerance in and of itself is not the same as addiction. That is not to say that addiction does not occur or that patients who are addicted should not be treated for pain. Treat patients with addiction and pain with the same amount of dignity and respect as all other patients. Safety and monitoring are priority concerns. An interprofessional team approach ensures a more effective pain-management plan for a patient with acute pain who lives with addiction. Nurses and health care providers need to avoid labeling patients as *drug seeking* because this term is poorly defined and can cause bias and prejudice. Voice concerns about opioid abuse to the patient and the patient's health care provider. Many patients on long-term opioid medications enter into "pain contracts" that state the expected responsibilities of both the patient and health care provider. If the patient violates the agreement or if assessment data indicate potential violation of the contract, help to identify additional resources to aid the patient in addressing the addictive illness.

Placebos. Placebos are pharmacologically inactive preparations or procedures that produce no beneficial or therapeutic effect. Many professional organizations discourage the use of placebos to treat pain. The ethics of therapeutic placebo use is highly controversial. Deceptive placebo use jeopardizes the trust between patients and their caregivers. If a placebo is ordered without a patient's understanding of its purpose,

---

BOX 44.20   Definitions Related to the Use of Opioids in Pain Treatment[a]

Physical Dependence
A state of adaptation that is manifested by a drug class–specific withdrawal syndrome produced by abrupt cessation, rapid dose reduction, decreasing blood level of the drug, and/or administration of an antagonist. Common symptoms of opioid withdrawal include shaking, chills, abdominal cramps, excessive yawning, and joint pain.

Addiction
A primary chronic neurobiological disease with genetic, psychosocial, and environmental factors influencing its development and manifestations. Addictive behaviors include one or more of the following: impaired control over drug use, compulsive use, continued use despite harm, and craving.

Drug Tolerance
A state of adaptation in which exposure to a drug induces changes that result in a diminution of one or more effects of the drug over time.

[a]Approved by the Boards of Directors of the American Academy of Pain Medicine, the American Pain Society, and the American Society of Addiction Medicine, February 2001 (American Pain Society, 2011).

---

question the order. Many health care agencies have policies that limit the use of placebos to only research.

Restorative and Continuing Care. Health professionals recognize pain as a significant health problem. The number of pain centers, palliative care departments, and hospices designed to manage pain and suffering has increased. The Commission on Accreditation of Rehabilitation Facilities (CARF) accredits chronic pain treatment programs and sets standards for chronic pain management. A comprehensive pain center treats people on an inpatient or outpatient basis. Staff members representing all

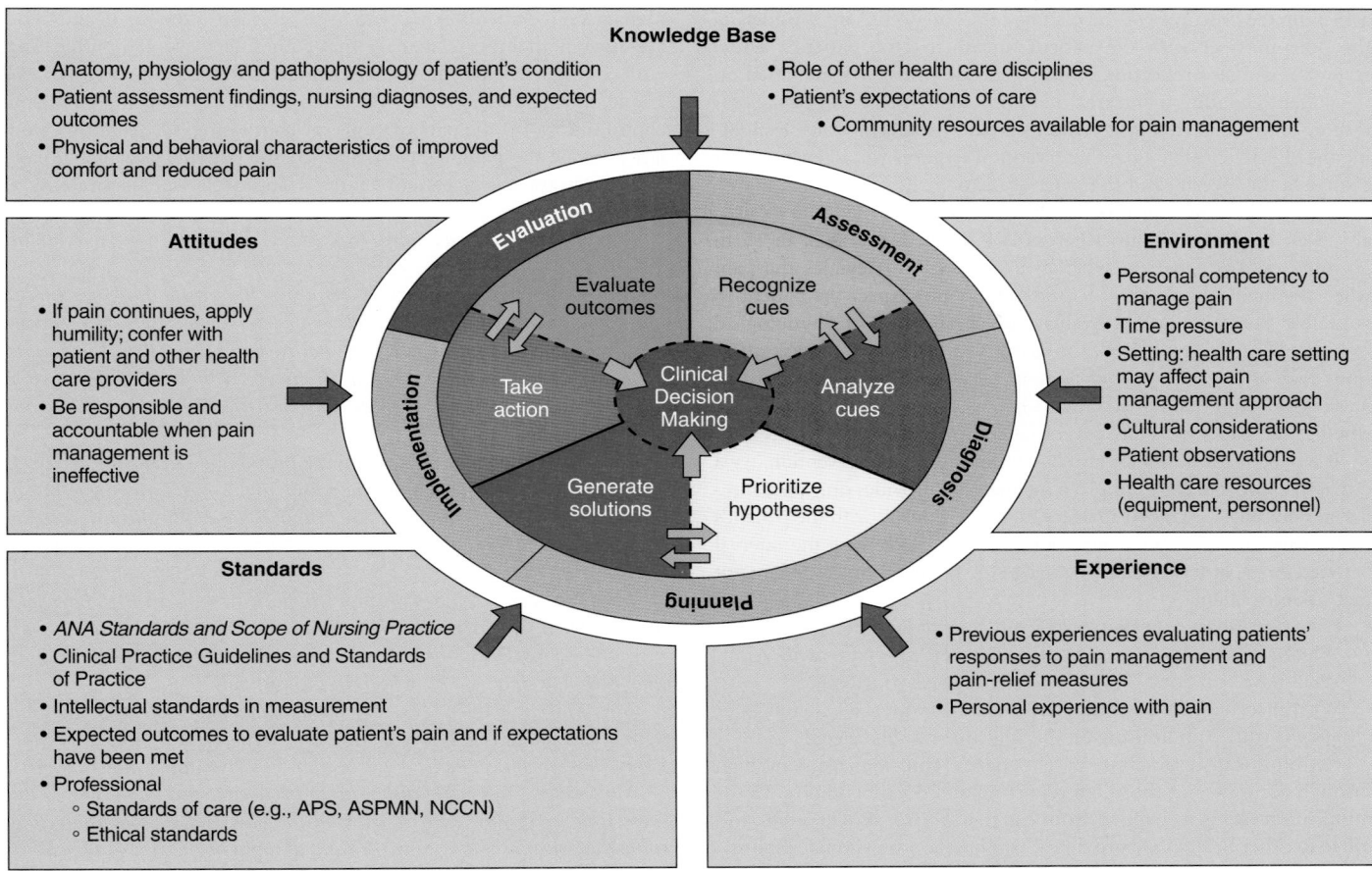

Knowledge Base

- Anatomy, physiology and pathophysiology of patient's condition
- Patient assessment findings, nursing diagnoses, and expected outcomes
- Physical and behavioral characteristics of improved comfort and reduced pain

- Role of other health care disciplines
- Patient's expectations of care
- Community resources available for pain management

Attitudes

- If pain continues, apply humility; confer with patient and other health care providers
- Be responsible and accountable when pain management is ineffective

Environment

- Personal competency to manage pain
- Time pressure
- Setting: health care setting may affect pain management approach
- Cultural considerations
- Patient observations
- Health care resources (equipment, personnel)

Standards

- *ANA Standards and Scope of Nursing Practice*
- Clinical Practice Guidelines and Standards of Practice
- Intellectual standards in measurement
- Expected outcomes to evaluate patient's pain and if expectations have been met
- Professional
  - Standards of care (e.g., APS, ASPMN, NCCN)
  - Ethical standards

Experience

- Previous experiences evaluating patients' responses to pain management and pain-relief measures
- Personal experience with pain

Evaluation — Evaluate outcomes — Take action — Clinical Decision Making — Analyze cues — Recognize cues — Assessment — Diagnosis — Prioritize hypotheses — Generate solutions — Planning — Implementation

FIG. 44.14 Critical thinking model for pain-management evaluation. *APS,* American Pain Society; *ASPMN,* American Society for Pain Management Nursing; *NCCN,* National Comprehensive Cancer Network. (Clinical Judgment Measurement Model copyright © NCSBN. All rights reserved.)

health care disciplines work with patients to find the most effective pain-relief measures. A comprehensive clinic provides diverse therapies and research into new treatments and training for professionals.

Many hospitals have palliative-care departments to help patients and their family members successfully manage their life-limiting conditions. The goal of palliative care is to help patients manage disease-related symptoms while living life fully with an incurable condition (see Chapter 36). Patients and their family members need ongoing assistance in managing pain at home. Teaching pain management during discharge and ensuring the continuation of pain management after discharge are essential.

Hospice programs care for patients at the end of life (see Chapter 36). Hospice care focuses on the quality of life for patients and their family caregivers who are experiencing an advanced, life-limiting illness. Hospice care provides compassionate care for people in the last phases of incurable disease so that they may live as fully and comfortably as possible (American Cancer Society, 2019). It helps patients who are nearing the end of life to continue to live at home or in a health care setting in comfort and privacy. Pain control is a priority for hospices. Under the guidance of hospice nurses, families learn to monitor patients' symptoms and become the primary caregivers. Some patients in hospice become hospitalized, such as in the event of a brief acute care crisis or family problem.

Hospice program practices can help nurses overcome their fear of contributing to a patient's death when administering large doses of opioids. The ANA supports aggressive treatment of pain and suffering even if it hastens a patient's death through the ethical principle of double effect (Fowler, 2015). The use of opioids to treat pain is acceptable, despite the risk that it may hasten a patient's death.

◆ **Evaluation**

Through the Patient's Eyes. Evaluate patients' perceptions of the effectiveness of interventions used to relieve pain. Patients help decide the best times to attempt pain treatments, and they are the best judge of whether a pain-relief intervention works. Often the family is another valuable resource, particularly in the case of a patient with pain who is unable to express discomfort. For patients with chronic pain, consider the effect of the pain intervention on the patient's function when evaluating the patient's response to treatment. You determine the pain intervention is successful if the patient reports the ability to better participate in self-care activities or activities such as physical therapy. Also ask patients about tolerance to therapy and the overall amount of relief obtained. If patients state that an intervention is unhelpful or even makes the pain worse, stop it immediately and seek an alternative. Time and patience are necessary to maximize the effectiveness of pain management. Educate patients about what to expect. For a patient in acute pain, provide reassurance that you will check back frequently to assess for changes in pain level.

Patient Outcomes. Evaluating the effectiveness of pain management is one of many nursing responsibilities that require effective critical thinking and clinical judgment (Fig. 44.14). Evaluate your success in achieving the outcomes of the plan of care. You do this by considering the outcomes set with the patient, measuring the patient's actual response, and also reflecting on the response you anticipate based on the patient's condition and treatment provided. A patient's behavioral responses to pain-relief interventions are not always obvious. Evaluating the effectiveness of a pain intervention requires you to evaluate for change in the severity and character of the pain. Also be sure to schedule your evaluation appropriately. For instance, oral medications usually peak in about 1 hour, whereas IVP medications peak in 15 to 30 minutes. Ask a patient whether a medication alleviates the pain when the medication's effect is peaking. Do not expect the patient to volunteer the information. Evaluate psychological and physiological responses to pain (e.g., check for changes in vital signs and ask questions such as "Please rate your pain on a scale of 0 to 10 now that you have taken your pain medicine"). It is also important to evaluate whether the patient has any adverse effects from pain therapies.

If a patient continues to have discomfort after an intervention, try a different approach. For example, if an analgesic provides only partial relief, add massage or guided-imagery exercises. Consult with the patient's health care provider about increasing the dose, decreasing the interval between doses, or trying different analgesics. If patient outcomes are not met, ask the patient:

- How far away is your pain level from your pain target?
- Which side effects are you experiencing from your pain medication?
- What have you done that successfully reduces your pain?
- What effect has your uncontrolled pain had on your ability to function?
- How is your pain limiting or altering your rest and sleep?

Communicate evaluation of a patient's pain-management plan through accurate and thorough reporting and documentation. Communication needs to happen from nurse to nurse, shift to shift, and nurse to other health care providers. You have a professional responsibility to report the effectiveness of interventions for managing the patient's pain and evaluating patient outcomes. A variety of tools such as a pain flow sheet or diary help centralize information about pain

management. Patients expect you to be sensitive to their pain and to be attentive in attempts to manage that pain. Effectively communicating with colleagues helps your patient achieve optimal pain relief. For example, during a hand-off report for a patient experiencing pain, you communicate (1) the patient's current pain rating, (2) what time you last assessed the patient's pain, and (3) the patient's acceptable pain rating. Always use a patient-centered approach when evaluating a pain-management plan.

As Matt prepares to discharge Mrs. Mays to home, he needs to evaluate the effectiveness of her pain-management plan to determine what to include in her discharge instructions. Matt uses his critical thinking, clinical judgment, and communication skills while interviewing Mrs. Mays about her perceptions and satisfaction with her current plan of care. Matt starts by saying, "I know we have tried a variety of techniques to manage your pain. What have you found to be the most effective and what has not worked so well?"

Mrs. Mays responds, "If I take my medications, do stretching exercises, and move around frequently, my pain stays at a 2 or 3. Listening to music has made me less nervous, but I don't think it has really affected my pain much. And I still can only sleep for about 4 hours at night before my pain wakes me up again."

Matt then says, "Some of my previous patients with arthritis have told me they often feel fatigued. I noticed in your chart that you take a nap most afternoons. Have you been able to go to bed and wake up at the same time each day since you have been in the hospital?"

Mrs. Mays responds, "No, they always wake me up to take my vital signs after I fall asleep; I have a hard time falling back to sleep after that. I hope that when I get home, I will be able to sleep without interruptions."

Matt states, "You might also want to try to go to bed and get up at the same time every day, exercise early in the day, and do something that calms you, such as taking a warm bath, at night before you go to bed."

Mrs. Mays smiles and says, "Those are wonderful ideas. We just remodeled our bathroom and I have a new bathtub. I can't wait to take a bath tonight and see if that helps."

SAFETY GUIDELINES FOR NURSING SKILLS

Ensuring patient safety is an essential role of the professional nurse. Use sound clinical judgment by communicating clearly with members of the health care team, assessing and analyzing the patient's clinical findings, and incorporating the patient's priorities of care and preferences. Use the best evidence, applying professional standards, when selecting interventions to use in patient care delivery. When performing the skill in this chapter, remember the following points to ensure safe patient-centered care.

- The patient is the only person who should press a PCA button to administer the pain medication.

- Monitor the patient for signs and symptoms of oversedation and respiratory depression.
- Monitor for potential side effects of opioid analgesics.

SKILL 44.1 PATIENT-CONTROLLED ANALGESIA

Delegation and Collaboration

The skill of PCA administration cannot be delegated to assistive personnel (AP). The nurse directs the AP to:

- Notify the nurse if the patient expresses a change in status (e.g., unrelieved pain) or has difficulty awakening.
- Notify the nurse if the patient has questions about the PCA process or equipment.
- Never administer a PCA dose for the patient and to notify the nurse if anyone other than the patient is observed administering a dose for the patient.

Equipment

- PCA pump system and tubing
- Analgesic cartridge or syringe with identification label and time tape (may already be attached and completed by pharmacy)
- Needleless connector
- Antiseptic swab
- Adhesive tape
- Clean gloves (when applicable)
- Opioid reversal agent (e.g., naloxone)
- Equipment for vital signs, pulse oximetry, and capnography
- Medication administration record (MAR)

STEP	RATIONALE

ASSESSMENT

1. Check accuracy and completeness of each MAR or computer printout with health care provider's written medication order. Check patient's name, medication name and dosage, route of administration, lockout period, and frequency of medication (demand, continuous, or both). Recopy or reprint any portion of MAR that is difficult to read. Clarify incomplete or unclear orders with health care provider before administration.

The order sheet is the most reliable source and only legal record of medications that the patient is to receive. Ensures that patient receives the correct medications (Palese et al., 2019). Illegible MARs and transcription errors are a source of medication errors (Palese et al., 2019).

2. Assess electronic health record (EHR) for patient's medical and medication history, including drug allergies.

Determines need for medication or possible contraindications for medication administration.

CLINICAL JUDGMENT: *When assessing allergies, be aware that nausea is not an allergic reaction and that it can be treated; pruritus alone is not an allergic reaction and is common with opioid use. Pruritus is treatable and does not contraindicate the use of PCA (Masato et al., 2017).*

3. Review medication information in drug reference manual or consult with pharmacist if uncertain about any PCA medications to be administered.

Understanding medications before administering them prevents medication errors (Pasero et al., 2015).

4. Assess patient's health literacy.

Assures patient or family caregiver has the capacity to obtain, communicate, process, and understand basic health information (CDC, 2021b).

5. Perform hand hygiene. Perform a complete assessment of pain. Measure vital signs.

Reduces transmission of microorganisms. Provides baseline for type and nature of pain condition for determination of efficacy of PCA.

6. Ask patient to describe history of allergies: known allergies and allergic response.

Confirms patient's allergies.

7. Assess environment for factors that could contribute to pain (e.g., noise, room temperature).

Eliminating irritating stimuli may help to reduce pain perception.

8. Assess for conditions that predispose patients to adverse effects from opioids. For example, assess for obstructive sleep apnea syndrome (OSAS) before surgery by anesthesia using the STOP-BANG questionnaire (see Chapter 50) (Gokay et al., 2016) (see agency policy).

Use assessment data to prevent adverse effects from opioids. For example, known, untreated, or unknown OSAS poses a significant risk for respiratory depression, especially when receiving anesthesia (Gokay et al., 2016). Identification allows treatment teams (surgeon, respiratory therapy, anesthesia) to take appropriate precautions, such as making continuous positive airway pressure or bilevel positive airway pressure ventilation devices available.

9. Apply clean gloves. Assess patency of intravenous (IV) access and surrounding tissue for inflammation or swelling (see Chapter 42).

IV line needs to be patent and functioning for safe administration of pain medication.

10. If patient has had surgery, inspect incision, continuing to wear clean gloves. Gently palpate around area for tenderness. Use sterile gloves if necessary to place hand directly on incision. Remove and dispose of gloves and perform hand hygiene.

Unusual incisional pain, swelling, redness, and/or discharge may indicate infection. Reduces transmission of infection.

11. Assess patient's ability to manipulate PCA control and cognitive status for ability to understand purpose of PCA and how to use control device.

Determines patient's competency and ability to use PCA safely and correctly.

12. Assess patient's knowledge and understanding of perceived effectiveness of previous pain-management strategies, especially previous PCA use.

Response to pain-control strategies helps identify learning needs and affects patient's willingness to try therapy.

PLANNING

1. Perform hand hygiene.

Reduces transmission of microorganisms.

2. Collect and bring appropriate supplies to the patient's bedside.

Ensures an organized approach.

3. Provide privacy and prepare bedside environment for patient safety.

Promotes patient comfort and safety.

4. Assist patient into a comfortable position.

Maintains patient comfort and removes barriers that may interfere with procedure.

IMPLEMENTATION

1. Follow "seven rights" for administration of medications (see Chapter 31). Obtain PCA analgesic in module prepared by pharmacy. Check label of medication 2 times—when removed from storage and when preparing for assembly.

Ensures safe and appropriate medication administration. *This is the first and second check for accuracy.*

2. At bedside identify patient using at least two identifiers (e.g., name and birthday or name and medical record number) according to agency policy. Compare identifiers with information on patient's MAR or medical record.

Ensures correct patient. Complies with The Joint Commission standards and improves patient safety (TJC, 2021).

3. At bedside compare MAR or computer printout with name of medication on drug cartridge. Have second registered nurse (RN) confirm health care provider's order and correct setup of PCA. Second RN should check order and the device independently and not just look at existing setup.

Ensures that correct patient receives right medication. *This is the third check for accuracy.*

Continued

SKILL 44.1	PATIENT-CONTROLLED ANALGESIA—cont'd

STEP	RATIONALE
4. Before initiating analgesia, demonstrate function of PCA to patient and family caregiver. Include education about the use of PCA and verbal and written instruction warning against anyone other than the patient pressing the PCA button (Cooney et al., 2013; Pasero, 2015).	It is important that the patient and family members understand how to use PCA safely. Allows for patient-centered care and improved patient outcomes with pain control (Shindul-Rothschild, 2017).
a. Explain type of medication in device.	Informs patient of therapy to be received.

CLINICAL JUDGMENT: *Background basal infusion opioids have been associated with increased risk of nausea, vomiting, and respiratory depression. However, in patients with opioid tolerance, a background basal infusion may be necessary due to the potential for undertreatment and possible opioid withdrawal (Chou et al., 2016).*

STEP	RATIONALE
b. If a background basal rate is used, explain that device safely administers continuous medication; however, self-initiated small but frequent amounts of medication can be administered for unrelieved pain by using the PCA button.	A background basal infusion delivers a continuous dose of analgesic medication. The PCA pump is programmed to allow additional patient-controlled doses for pain that is not relieved by the continuous infusion (breakthrough pain) (Pasero, 2015).
c. Explain that self-dosing aids in pain control for repositioning, walking, coughing, and deep breathing.	Promotes patient's participation in care.
d. Explain that device is programmed to deliver ordered type and dose of pain medication, lockout interval, and 1- to 4-hour dosage limits. Explain how lockout time prevents overdose.	Relieves anxiety in patients who might be concerned about overdosing.
e. Demonstrate to patient how to push medication demand button (see illustrations). *Instruct family caregiver or visitor not to push PCA button to give medication* (Cooney et al., 2013).	Administration by proxy is not recommended in adults (Chou et al., 2016; TJC, 2020).
f. Instruct patient to notify a nurse for possible side effects, problems in gaining pain relief, changes in severity or location of pain, alarm sounding, or questions.	Engages patient as partner in care.
5. Apply clean gloves. Check infuser and patient-control module for accurate labeling or evidence of leaking.	Avoids medication error and injury to patient.
6. Reposition patient to be sure that venipuncture or central line site is accessible.	Ensures unimpeded flow of infusion.
7. Insert drug cartridge into infusion device (see illustration) and prime tubing.	Locks system and prevents air from infusing into IV tubing.
8. Attach needleless adapter to tubing adapter of patient-controlled module.	Needed to connect with IV line.
9. Wipe injection port of maintenance IV line vigorously with antiseptic swab for 15 seconds and allow to dry.	Minimizes entry of surface microorganisms during needle insertion, reducing risk of catheter-related bloodstream infection.
10. Insert needleless adapter into injection port nearest patient (at Y-site of peripheral IV or central line or connect to its own IV site). There should not be a chance to use PCA tubing for administering IV push with another drug.	Establishes route for medication to enter main IV line. Needleless systems prevent needlestick injuries. Prevents medication interaction and incompatibility.
11. Secure connection and anchor PCA tubing with tape. Label PCA tubing.	Prevents dislodging of needleless adapter from port. Facilitates patient's ability to ambulate. Label prevents error from connecting tubing from different device to PCA.
12. Program computerized PCA pump as ordered to deliver prescribed medication dose and lockout interval. Have second nurse check setting. (**NOTE:** Recheck with oncoming RN during shift hand-off to ensure line reconciliation.)	Ensures safe, therapeutic drug administration. With appropriate dose intervals (e.g., 10 min), patient usually experiences an analgesic effect and/or mild sedation before being able to access the next dose; thus, there is lower chance for oversedation and respiratory depression. A second nurse check reduces risk for medication error (Kane-Gill et al., 2017).
13. Administer loading dose of analgesia as prescribed. Manually give 1-time dose or turn on pump and program dose into pump.	Establishes initial level of analgesia.

STEP 4e Patient learns how to press PCA device button.

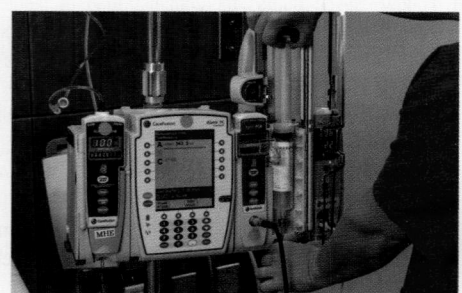

STEP 7 Nurse inserting drug cartridge into PCA device.

STEP	RATIONALE
14. Remove and discard gloves and used supplies in appropriate containers. Dispose of empty cassette or syringe to adhere to agency policy. Perform hand hygiene.	Reduces transmission of microorganisms. The Federal Controlled Substances Act regulates control and dispensation of opioids for all health care agencies.
15. If patient is experiencing pain, have patient demonstrate use of PCA system; if not, have patient repeat instructions given earlier.	Repeating instructions reinforces learning. Checking a patient's understanding through return demonstration helps you determine patient's level of understanding and ability to manipulate device.
16. Be sure that venipuncture or central line site is protected and recheck infusion rate before leaving patient.	Ensures patency of IV line.
17. Help patient into comfortable position.	Restores comfort and sense of well-being
18. Raise side rails (as appropriate) and lower bed to lowest position.	Promotes safety and prevents falls.
19. Place nurse call system in an accessible location within patient's reach.	Ensures patient can call for assistance if needed and promotes safety and prevents falls.
20. To discontinue PCA:	
a. Check health care provider order for discontinuation. Obtain necessary PCA information from pump for documentation; note date, time, amount infused, amount of drug wasted, and reason for wastage.	Ensures correct documentation of a schedule II drug. Two RNs must witness wastage of opioids (narcotics) and sign record to meet requirements of the Controlled Substances Act for scheduled drugs.
b. Perform hand hygiene and apply clean gloves. Turn off pump. Disconnect PCA tubing from primary IV line but maintain IV access.	Reduces transmission of microorganisms. Follow health care provider order for maintenance of IV site.
c. Dispose of empty cartridge, tubing, and gloves according to agency policy. Remove and dispose of gloves and perform hand hygiene.	Reduces transmission of microorganisms.
d. Follow Steps 17-19.	Promotes patient comfort.

EVALUATION

1. Use pain rating scale to evaluate patient's pain intensity following treatments and procedures according to agency policy.	Determines response to PCA dosing. Documenting "PCA in use" or "PCA effective" is not an adequate record of patient's pain level.
2. Observe patient for nausea or pruritus.	Common treatable side effects of opioids.
3. Monitor patient's level of sedation. It is recommended that the Pasero Opioid Sedation Scale (POSS) be used to monitor for unintended patient sedation (Davis et al., 2017; TJC, 2020). Use vital signs, pulse oximetry, and capnography for monitoring. Study findings report nurse observation and administration of the POSS as superior in earlier identification of respiratory depression and oversedation (Chou, et al., 2016). Monitoring should be frequent per agency policy and health care provider order (e.g., every 1 to 2 hours for first 12 hours for the first 24-hour period after surgery). Monitor more often at start, during first 24 hours, and at night when hypoventilation and hypoxia tend to occur during sleep.	Patient is at highest risk for oversedation and respiratory distress (OSRD) during the first 24 hours of PCA administration. Although there is low sensitivity for detecting hypoventilation with pulse oximetry when supplemental oxygen is used and evidence is insufficient to firmly recommend capnography (Chou et al., 2016), these interventions are used in monitoring for OSRD and provide important clinical information in your assessment. Excess sedation (difficult to arouse) precedes respiratory depression. Differences in ventilation are observed between wakefulness and sleep, which correlates with states of brain arousal. Opioid-induced respiratory depression is also regulated by sleep-wake mechanisms (Nagappa et al., 2017).
4. Have patient demonstrate dose delivery.	Evaluates skill in use of PCA.
5. According to agency policy, evaluate number of attempts (number of times patient pushed button), delivery of demand doses (number of times drug actually given and total amount of medication delivered in particular time frame), and basal dose if ordered.	Helps to evaluate effectiveness of PCA dose and frequency in relieving pain. Maintains compliance with Controlled Substances Act.
6. Observe patient initiate self-care.	Demonstrates pain relief.
7. Use Teach-Back: "I want to be sure I explained how the PCA will help with your pain and how you should use the device. Tell me the steps you will use to activate the PCA." Revise your instruction now or develop a plan for revised patient/family caregiver teaching if patient/family caregiver is not able to teach back correctly.	Teach-back is an evidence-based health literacy intervention that promotes patient engagement, patient safety, adherence, and quality. The goal of teach-back is to ensure that you have explained medical information clearly so that patients and their families understand what you communicated to them (AHRQ, 2020).

UNEXPECTED OUTCOMES AND RELATED INTERVENTIONS

1. Patient verbalizes continued or worsening discomfort or displays nonverbal behaviors indicative of pain, suggesting that underlying condition has changed or that patient is undermedicated.
- Perform complete pain reassessment.
- Assess for possible complications.
- Inspect IV site for possible catheter occlusion or infiltration.
- Evaluate number of attempts and deliveries initiated by patient.
- Check that maintenance of IV fluid is running continuously.
- Evaluate pump for operational problems.
- Consult with health care provider.

2. Patient is sedated and not easily aroused.
- Stop PCA. Notify health care provider immediately.
- Elevate head of bed 30 degrees unless contraindicated.
- Instruct patient to take deep breaths.
- Apply oxygen at 2 L/min per nasal cannula (if ordered).
- Assess vital signs, oxygen saturation, and/or capnography. Monitor frequently.

Continued

SKILL 44.1   PATIENT-CONTROLLED ANALGESIA—cont'd

UNEXPECTED OUTCOMES AND RELATED INTERVENTIONS—cont'd

- • Evaluate amount of opioid delivered within the past 4 to 8 hours.
- • Ask family members if they pressed button without patient's knowledge.
- • Review MAR for other possible sedating drugs.
- • Prepare to administer naloxone if signs or symptoms of respiratory depression are noted.

3. Patient unable to manipulate PCA device to maintain pain control.
- • Consult with health care provider regarding alternative medication route or possibly a basal (continuous) dose.

RECORDING AND REPORTING

- • Record appropriate drug, concentration, dose (basal and demand), time started, lockout time, and amount of solution infused and remaining per agency policy immediately after administration, not before. Many agencies have a separate flow sheet for PCA documentation.
- • Record assessment of patient's response to analgesic on PCA medication form, narrative notes, or patient assessment flow sheet (see agency policy), including vital signs, oximetry and capnography results, sedation status, pain rating, and status of vascular access device.
- • Calculate infused dose: add demand and continuous dose together. Record on PCA flow sheet.
- • Document your evaluation of patient learning.
- • During hand-off report, the oncoming and outgoing nurses should inspect and agree with PCA pump programming as a means of medication reconciliation (Kane-Gill, 2017).
- • Hand-off report should include detailed information regarding vital signs, pulse oximetry and capnography, pain assessment scores, STOP-BANG score for OSAS if done, POSS sedation scores, level of consciousness, and activity level (Chou et al., 2016; Cooney, 2016; Meisenberg et al., 2017).
- • Use "safety priming" during hand-off report by using words to activate a mental construct to prompt nursing safety-oriented behavior (Groves et al., 2017). An example of safety priming during hand-off report may include the nurse's words to express concern of what may happen (e.g., excess opioid infusion) because of certain behaviors, instead of reporting only factual information.

KEY POINTS

- • Nociceptive pain provides a protective physiological series of events that allows individuals to become aware of events that may cause tissue damage.
- • Understanding the four physiological processes of nociceptive pain (transduction, transmission, perception, and modulation) helps you recognize factors that cause pain, the accompanying symptoms, and the rationale for selecting therapies to treat or manage pain.
- • Use assessment data and identify cues from your patient to categorize pain based on its duration (acute or chronic) or pathological condition (e.g., cancer or noncancer).
- • Individual, physiological, psychological, social, cultural, and environmental factors influence pain and make each person's pain experience different.
- • Cultural beliefs affect how individuals express, react to, and cope with pain.
- • To make timely clinical judgments while assessing pain, you consider a patient's typical comfort level, the potential for pain based on a patient's health status, and the effects of the associated treatment. Analyze assessment data and patient cues thoroughly before making decisions regarding a patient's care and pain-management plan.
- • Cues for acute pain include an identifiable cause, a sudden onset, and a short duration. In contrast, chronic pain is not protective, may not have an identifiable cause, and has a dramatic effect on a person's quality of life; it varies in intensity, and usually lasts longer than 3 to 6 months, beyond the expected or predicted healing time.
- • Multimodal analgesia provides for safe analgesic administration because it combines drugs with at least two different mechanisms of action to optimize pain control, which allows for lower-than-usual doses of each medication. Thus, an individualized multimodal regimen lowers the risk of side effects while providing pain relief that is as good as or even better than could be obtained if each of the medications were administered alone.

- • Use your clinical judgment when selecting different nonpharmacological and pharmacological approaches to pain management. For example, if you are caring for a patient experiencing moderate to severe acute pain, you use a combination of nonpharmacological therapies with pharmacological therapies to help relieve the pain.
- • Significant individual and environmental factors create barriers to pain management. These factors include a lack of knowledge or misconceptions about pain and appropriate pain management in patients, caregivers and health care providers; cultural beliefs; lack of pain-management protocols; and poor access to care.
- • To evaluate the response to pain treatment, you ask patients to describe how effective they believe their pain management has been. You also evaluate the patient's pain intensity, as well as side effects, behavior, and functional outcomes.

REFLECTIVE LEARNING

Diya, who is 55 years old, is in the emergency department with severe pain in the upper right quadrant of her abdomen, just below her sternum. She has a medical history of diabetes mellitus, hypertension, and obesity. She began walking for about 45 minutes a day 3 months ago and has lost 13.6 kg (30 pounds) since she started regular exercise. She is grimacing and holding her abdomen. She rates her pain as an 8 on a 0-10 numerical rating scale. Diya is also experiencing nausea and vomiting. Her health care provider is working her up for possible gallstones.

- • What assessment data are the most important for you to collect at this time? What cues support your answer? How would you assess her pain? Give examples of questions you could ask Diya to determine this information. (Recognize Cues)
- • What conditions and concerns are consistent with Diya's pain? (Analyze Cues)
- • What do you believe are Diya's current health concerns? Which one is of greatest priority? Is there additional information you require to determine her priority? (Prioritize Diagnoses)

- What might be appropriate outcomes of Diya's care? Which nursing actions and interventions might help Diya achieve these outcomes? Which actions would you plan to avoid because they are irrelevant or potentially harmful? (Generate Solutions)
- Which nursing actions are most appropriate to address Diya's pain? Describe how you would implement them and place them in order of the highest priority to the lowest priority. (Take Action)
- What evaluative statements made by Diya would indicate that your actions to manage her pain were effective? Describe what you would do if Diya did not indicate that she met her outcomes of care. (Evaluate Outcomes)

REVIEW QUESTIONS

1. Which of the following signs or symptoms in a patient who is opioid naïve is of greatest concern to the nurse when assessing the patient 1 hour after administering an opioid?
   1. Oxygen saturation of 95%
   2. Difficulty arousing the patient
   3. Respiratory rate of 12 breaths/min
   4. Pain intensity rating of 5 on a scale of 0 to 10
2. A health care provider writes the following order for a patient who is opioid naïve who returned from the operating room after a total hip replacement: "Fentanyl patch 100 mcg; change every 3 days." On the basis of this order, the nurse takes the following action:
   1. Calls the health care provider and questions the order
   2. Applies the patch the third postoperative day
   3. Applies the patch as soon as the patient reports pain
   4. Places the patch as close to the hip dressing as possible
3. A patient is being discharged home on an around-the-clock (ATC) opioid for postoperative pain. Because of this order, the nurse anticipates an additional order for which class of medication?
   1. Opioid antagonists
   2. Antiemetics
   3. Stool softeners
   4. Muscle relaxants
4. A new medical resident writes an order for oxycodone hydrochloride controlled release (CR) 10 mg PO q2h prn. Which part of the order does the nurse question?
   1. The drug
   2. The time interval
   3. The dose
   4. The route
5. The nurse reviews a patient's medical administration record (MAR) and finds that the patient has received oxycodone/acetaminophen (5/325), two tablets PO every 3 hours for the past 3 days. What concerns the nurse the most?
   1. The patient's level of pain
   2. The potential for addiction
   3. The amount of daily acetaminophen
   4. The risk for gastrointestinal bleeding
6. When using ice massage for pain relief, which of the following is correct? (Select all that apply.)
   1. Apply ice using firm pressure over the skin.
   2. Apply ice for 5 minutes or until numbness occurs.
   3. Apply ice no more than 3 times a day.
   4. Limit application of ice to no longer than 10 minutes.
   5. Use a slow, circular steady massage.

7. A patient with a 3-day history of a stroke that left her confused and unable to communicate returns from interventional radiology following placement of a gastrostomy tube. The patient had been taking hydrocodone/APAP 5/325 up to four tablets/day before her stroke for the past year to manage her arthritic pain. The health care provider's order reads as follows: "Hydrocodone/APAP 5/325 1 tab, per gastrostomy tube, q4h, prn." Which action by the nurse is most appropriate?
   1. No action is required by the nurse because the order is appropriate.
   2. Request to have the order changed to around the clock (ATC) for the first 48 hours.
   3. Ask for a change of medication to meperidine 50 mg IVP, q3h, prn.
   4. Begin the hydrocodone/APAP when the patient shows nonverbal symptoms of pain.
8. Place the following steps in the correct order for administration of patient-controlled analgesia:
   1. Insert drug cartridge into infusion device and prime tubing.
   2. Wipe injection port of maintenance IV line vigorously with antiseptic swab for 15 seconds and allow to dry.
   3. Demonstrate to patient how to push medication demand button.
   4. Secure connection and anchor PCA tubing with tape.
   5. Instruct patient to notify a nurse for possible side effects or changes in the severity or location of pain.
   6. Insert needleless adapter into injection port nearest patient.
   7. Apply clean gloves. Check infuser and patient-control module for accurate labeling or evidence of leaking.
   8. Program computerized PCA pump as ordered to deliver prescribed medication dose and lockout interval.
   9. Attach needleless adapter to tubing adapter of patient-controlled module.
9. When teaching a patient about transcutaneous electrical nerve stimulation (TENS), which of the following represent an accurate description of the nonpharmacological therapy? (Select all that apply.)
   1. Turn TENS on before patient feels discomfort.
   2. TENS works peripherally and centrally on nerve receptors.
   3. TENS does not require a health care provider order.
   4. Remove any skin preparations before attaching TENS electrodes.
   5. Placing electrodes directly over or near the pain site works best.
10. Match the characteristics on the left with the appropriate pain category on the right.

	Acute Pain	Chronic Pain
A. Has a protective effect		
B. Lasts more than 3 to 6 months		
C. Usually has identifiable cause		
D. Dramatically affects quality of life		
E. Viewed as a disease		
F. Eventually resolves with or without treatment		

Answers: 1. 2; **3.** 3; **4.** 2; **5.** 3; **6.** 1, 2, 5; **7.** 2; **8.** 3, 5, 7, 1, 9, 2, 6, 4, 8; **9.** 2, 4, 5; **10.** Acute pain: A, C, F; Chronic pain: B, D, E.

Rationales for Review Questions can be found on the Evolve website.

REFERENCES

Agency for Healthcare Research and Quality (AHRQ): *Health Literacy Universal Precautions Toolkit 2nd edition*, Rockville, MD, 2020, Agency for Healthcare Research and Quality. https://www.ahrq.gov/health-literacy/quality-resources/tools/literacy-toolkit/healthlittoolkit2-tool5.html. Accessed May 7, 2021.

Allison MA, et al: The link between school attendance and good health, *Pediatrics* 143(2), 2019. https://pediatrics.aappublications.org/content/143/2/e20183648. Accessed May 1, 2021.

American Cancer Society: *What is hospice care?* 2019. https://www.cancer.org/treatment/end-of-life-care/hospice-care/what-is-hospice-care.html. Accessed May 7, 2021.

American Chronic Pain Association (ACPA) & Stanford Medicine: *ACPA and Standford Resource Guide to Chronic Pain Management*, 2021. https://www.theacpa.org/resources/acpa-resource-guide/. Accessed October 25, 2021.

American Geriatrics Society Beers Criteria Update Expert Panel: American Geriatrics Society 2019 updated AGS Beers Criteria® for potentially inappropriate medication use in older adults, *JAGS* 67:674, 2019.

American Music Therapy Association (AMTA): *Music therapy with specific populations: fact sheets, resources & bibliographies*, 2021. https://www.musictherapy.org/research/factsheets/. Accessed May 5, 2021.

American Nurses Association (ANA): *The ethical responsibility to manage pain and the suffering it causes*, Silver Spring, MD, 2018, The Association. https://www.nursingworld.org/~495e9b/globalassets/docs/ana/ethics/theethicalresponsibilitytomanagepainandthesufferingitcauses2018.pdf. Accessed May 1, 2021.

American Nurses Association: *ANA and American Society for Pain Management Nursing (ASPMN): Scope and standards of practice: pain management nursing*, ed 2, Silver Spring, MD, 2016, The Association.

American Society of Anesthesiologists (ASA): Practice guidelines for chronic pain management, *Anesthesiology* 112:1, 2010.

Anekar AA, Cascella M: WHO analgesic ladder. In *StatPearls* [Internet]. Treasure Island, FL, 2020, StatPearls Publishing. https://www.ncbi.nlm.nih.gov/books/NBK554435/. Accessed May 5, 2021.

Arthritis Foundation: *Osteoarthritis*, n.d. https://www.arthritis.org/diseases/osteoarthritis. Accessed May 1, 2021.

Atee M, et al: Pain assessment in dementia: evaluation of a point-of-care technological solution, *J Alzheimers Dis* 60(1):137, 2017.

Burchum JR, Rosenthal LD: *Lehne's pharmacology for nursing care*, ed 10, St. Louis, 2019, Elsevier.

Centers for Disease Control and Prevention: CDC guideline for prescribing opioids for chronic pain – United States, *MMWR* 65(1):1–49, 2016. https://www.cdc.gov/mmwr/volumes/65/rr/rr6501e1.htm?CDC_AA_refVal=https%3A%2F%2Fwww.cdc.gov%2Fmmwr%2Fvolumes%2F65%2Frr%2Frr6501e1er.htm. Accessed May 5, 2021.

Centers for Disease Control and Prevention (CDC): *Opioid overdose: understanding the epidemic*, 2021a. https://www.cdc.gov/drugoverdose/epidemic/index.html. Accessed May 1, 2021.

Centers for Disease Control and Prevention (CDC): *What is health literacy?* 2021b. https://www.cdc.gov/healthliteracy/learn/index.html. Accessed May 1, 2021.

Chow S, et al: Pain assessment tools for older adults with dementia in long-term care facilities: a systematic review, *Neurodegener Dis Manag* 6(6):525, 2016.

Colloca L, et al: Neuropathic pain, *Nat Rev Dis Primers* 16(3):17002, 2017.

Cooney MF: Postoperative pain management: clinical practice guidelines, *J Perianesth Nurs* 31(5):445, 2016.

Cooney MF, et al: American Society for Pain Management Nursing position statement with clinical practice guidelines: authorized agent–controlled analgesia, *Pain Manag Nurs* 14(3):178, 2013.

Dahlhamer J, et al: Prevalence of chronic pain and high-impact chronic pain among adults—United States, *MMWR Morb Mortal Wkly Rep* 67(36):1001, 2018. https://www.cdc.gov/mmwr/volumes/67/wr/mm6736a2.htm#suggestedcitation. Accessed May 1, 2021.

Davis C, et al: A multisite retrospective study evaluating the implementation of the Pasero Opioid-Induced Sedation Scale (POSS) and its effect on patient safety outcomes, *Pain Manag Nurs* 18(4):193, 2017.

de Boer I, et al: Advance in genetics of migraine, *Curr Opin Neurol* 32(3):413, 2019. doi:10.1097/WCO.0000000000000687. https://journals.lww.com/co-neurology/fulltext/2019/06000/advance_in_genetics_of_migraine.14.aspx#:~:text=adequate%20genetic%20counseling.-,Specific%20clinical%20features%20of%20common%20migraine%20seem%20to%20be%20determined,genetic%20variant%20risks%20with%20depression. Accessed May 2, 2021.

Drew DJ, et al: "As-needed" range orders for opioid analgesics in the management of pain: a consensus statement of the American Society for Pain Management Nursing and the American Pain Society, *Pain Manag Nurs* 19(3):207, 2018.

Fowler MDM: *Guide to the code of ethics for nurses with interpretive statements*, ed 2, Silver Spring, MD, 2015, American Nurses Association.

Giger JN, Haddad LG: *Transcultural nursing: assessment and intervention*, ed 8, St. Louis, 2021, Elsevier.

Givler A, et al: The importance of cultural competence in pain and palliative care. In *StatPearls* [Internet], 2020. https://www.ncbi.nlm.nih.gov/books/NBK493154/. Accessed May 2, 2021.

Gokay P, et al: Is there a difference between the STOP-BANG and the Berlin Obstructive Sleep Apnoea Syndrome questionnaires for determining respiratory complications during the perioperative period? *J Clin Nurs* 25(9/10):1238, 2016.

Hockenberry MJ, Wilson D: *Wong's nursing care of infants and children*, ed 11, St. Louis, 2019, Elsevier.

Horgas A: *Assessing pain in older adults with dementia*, 2020, Hartford Institute for Geriatric Nursing. https://hign.org/consultgeri/try-this-series/assessing-pain-older-adults-dementia. Accessed May 1, 2021.

Horgas AL: Pain assessment in older adults, *Nurs Clin North Am* 52(3):375, 2017.

Hoti K, et al: Clinimetric properties of the electronic Pain Assessment Tool (ePAT) for aged-care residents with moderate to severe dementia, *J Pain Res* 11:1037, 2018.

Huether S, McCance K: *Pathophysiology: the biologic basis for disease in adults and children*, ed 8, St. Louis, 2019, Elsevier.

Institute of Medicine (IOM): *Relieving pain in America: a blueprint for transforming prevention, care, education, and research*, Washington, DC, 2011, National Academies Press. https://www.ncbi.nlm.nih.gov/books/NBK91497/. Accessed May 1, 2021.

Interagency Pain Research Coordinating Committee (IPRCC): *National pain strategy report*, 2021a. https://www.iprcc.nih.gov/national-pain-strategy-overview/national-pain-strategy-report. Accessed May 1, 2021.

Interagency Pain Research Coordinating Committee (IPRCC): *Federal pain research strategy overview*, 2021b. https://www.iprcc.nih.gov/federal-pain-research-strategy-overview. Accessed May 1, 2021.

International Association for the Study of Pain (IASP): *IASP terminology*, 2020. https://www.iasp-pain.org/publications/iasp-news/iasp-announces-revised-definition-of-pain/. Accessed August 25, 2021.

International Association for the Study of Pain (IASP): *Declaration of Montreal*, 2018a. http://www.iasp-pain.org/DeclarationofMontreal. Accessed May 1, 2021.

International Association for the Study of Pain (IASP): *Faces pain scale—revised home*, 2018b. http://www.iasp-pain.org/Education/Content.aspx?ItemNumber=1519. Accessed May 4, 2021.

Iyer P, Lee YC: Why it hurts: the mechanisms of pain in rheumatoid arthritis, *Rheum Dis Clin North Am* 47(2021):229, 2021.

Kane-Gill S, et al: Clinical practice guideline: safe medication use in the ICU, *Crit Care Med* 45(9):e877, 2017.

Laures EL, et al: Pediatric pain assessment in the intensive care unit: an evidence-based algorithm. *Pain Manag Nurs* 2020. https://doi.org/10.1016/j.pmn.2020.10.005.

Manocha S, Taneja N: Assessment of paediatric pain: a critical review, *J Basic Clin Physiol Pharmacol* 27(4):1, 2016.

Masato H, et al: Prophylactic pentazocine reduces the incidence of pruritus after cesarean delivery under spinal anesthesia with opioids: a prospective randomized clinical trial, *Anesth Analg* 124(6):1930, 2017.

Meisenberg B, et al: Implementation of solutions to reduce opioid-induced oversedation and respiratory depression, *Am J Health Syst Pharm* 74(3):162, 2017.

Melzack R: From the gate to the neuromatrix, *Pain* 6(Suppl):S121, 1999.

Melzack R, Wall PD: Pain mechanisms: a new theory, *Science* 150:971, 1965.

Nagappa M, et al: Opioids, respiratory depression, and sleep-disordered breathing, *Best Pract Res Clin Anaesthesiol* 31(4):469, 2017.

National Institutes of Health: *National Institute on Drug Abuse (NIHNIDA): Opioid overdose crisis*, 2021. https://www.drugabuse.gov/drug-topics/opioids/opioid-overdose-crisis. Accessed May 5, 2021.

Narouze S, et al: Interventional spine and pain procedures in patients on antiplatelet and anticoagulant medications (second edition): guidelines from The American Society of Regional Anesthesia and Pain Medicine, The European Society of Regional Anaesthesia and Pain Therapy, The American Academy of Pain Medicine, The International Neuromodulation Society, The North American Neuromodulation Society, and The World Institute of Pain, *Reg Anesth Pain Med* 43(3):225, 2018.

O'Sullivan K, et al: Understanding pain among older persons: part 1 – the development of novel pain profiles and their association with disability and quality of life, *Age Ageing* 46(1):46, 2017.

Palese A, et al: "I am administering medication – please do not interrupt me": red tabards preventing interruptions as perceived by surgical patients, *J Patient Saf* 15:30, 2019.

Pasero C: Unconventional use of a PCA pump: nurse-activated dosing, *J Perianesth Nurs* 30(1):68, 2015.

Pasero C, McCaffery M: *Pain assessment and pharmacologic management*, St. Louis, 2011, Mosby.

QSEN Institute (QSEN): *QSEN Institute Competencies*, 2020. http://qsen.org/competencies/pre-licensure-ksas/. Accessed May 1, 2021

Scarborough BM, Smith CB: Optimal pain management for patients with cancer in the modern era, *CA Cancer J Clin* 68(3):182, 2018.

Shindul-Rothschild J, et al: Beyond the pain scale: provider communication and staffing predictive of patients' satisfaction with pain control, *Pain Manag Nurs* 18(6):401, 2017.

The Joint Commission (TJC): *Pain management standards for accredited organizations*, Oakbrook Terrace, IL, 2020, Author. https://www.jointcommission.org/resources/patient-safety-topics/pain-management-standards-for-accredited-organizations/. Accessed December 5, 2020.

The Joint Commission (TJC): *2021 National Patient Safety Goals*, Oakbrook Terrace, IL, 2021, The Commission. https://www.jointcommission.org/en/standards/national-patient-safety-goals/. Accessed May 1, 2021

Touhy T, Jett K: *Ebersole & Hess' toward healthy aging*, ed 10, St. Louis, 2020, Elsevier.

Treede RD: The International Association for the Study of Pain definition of pain: as valid in 2018 as in 1979, but in need of regularly updated footnotes, *Pain Rep* 3(2): e643, 2018.

US Food and Drug Administration (USFDA): *FDA drug safety communication: prescription acetaminophen products to be limited to 325 mg per dosage unit; boxed warning will highlight potential for severe liver failure*, 2018. http://www.fda.gov/Drugs/DrugSafety/ucm239821.htm. Accessed May 5, 2021.

US National Library of Medicine: *Medline Plus - Lidocaine transdermal patch*, 2016, Lidocaine Transdermal Patch: MedlinePlus Drug Information. https://medlineplus.gov/druginfo/meds/a603026.html. Accessed May 5, 2021.

US National Library of Medicine: *Medline Plus – Fentanyl transdermal patch*, 2021, https://medlineplus.gov/druginfo/meds/a601202.html. Accessed May 5, 2021.

Wong-Baker FACES Foundation: *Wong-Baker FACES® pain rating scale*, 2016. https://wongbakerfaces.org/. Accessed May 1, 2021.

Wong DL, Baker CM: Pain in children: comparison of assessment scales, *Okla Nurse* 33(1):8, 1988.

RESEARCH REFERENCES

Ames N, et al: Music listening among postoperative patients in the intensive care unit: a randomized controlled trial with mixed-methods analysis, *Integr Med Insights* 12:1, 2017.

Auxier JN, et al: An appreciative inquiry into older adults' pain experience in long term care facilities: a pain education perspective, *Int Pract Dev J* 10(1):1, 2020.

Benjenk I, et al: Authorized Agent–Controlled analgesia for pain management in critically ill adult patients, *Crit Care Nurse* 40(3):31, 2020.

Baeriswyl M, et al: The analgesic efficacy of transverse abdominis plane block versus epidural analgesia: a systematic review with meta-analysis, *Medicine* 97(26): e11261, 2018. doi:10.1097/MD.0000000000011261.

Beyer JE, et al: The creation, validation, and continuing development of the Oucher: a measure of pain intensity in children, *J Pediatr Nurs* 7(5):335, 1992.

Bugada D, et al: Genetics and opioids: towards more appropriate prescription in cancer pain, *Cancers* 12(7):1951, 2020.

Chou R, et al: Management of postoperative pain: a clinical practice guideline from the American Pain Society, the American Society of Regional Anesthesia and Pain Medicine, and the American Society of Anesthesiologists' Committee on Regional Anesthesia, Executive Committee, and Administrative Council, *J Pain* 17(2):131, 2016.

Dekel BGS, et al: Medical evidence influence on inpatients and nurses pain ratings agreement, *Pain Res Manag* 2016:9267536, 2016. https://www.hindawi.com/journals/prm/2016/9267536/. Accessed May 1, 2021.

Deldar K, et al: Challenges faced by nurses in using pain assessment scale in patients unable to communicate: a qualitative study, *BMC Nurs* 17(11), 2018.

Dequeker S, et al: Hospitalized patients' vs. nurses' assessments of pain intensity and barriers to pain management, *J Adv Nurs* 74(1):160, 2018.

Dueñas M, et al: A review of chronic pain impact on patients, their social environment and the health care system, *J Pain Res* 9:457, 2016.

Ferreira-Valente A, et al: The role of spirituality in pain, function, and coping in individuals with chronic pain, *Pain Med* 21(3):448, 2020. https://academic.oup.com/painmedicine/article/21/3/448/5482550?login=true. Accessed May 2, 2021.

Geneen LJ, et al: Physical activity and exercise for chronic pain in adults: an overview of Cochrane Reviews, *Cochrane Database Syst Rev* 14;1(1), 2017.

Gerber K, et al: Barriers to adequate pain and symptom relief at the end of life: a qualitative study capturing nurses' perspectives, 2021, *Collegian*. https://doi.org/10.1016/j.colegn.2021.02.008.

Gibson W, et al: *Transcutaneous electrical nerve stimulation (TENS) for chronic pain - an overview of Cochrane Reviews*, 2019, Cochrane. https://www.cochrane.org/CD011890/SYMPT_transcutaneous-electrical-nerve-stimulation-tens-chronic-pain-overview-cochrane-reviews#:~:text=TENS%20is%20a%20common%20treatment%20for%20pain%20conditions,previously%20investigated%20by%20a%20number%20of%20Cochrane%20Reviews. Accessed May 5, 2021.

Groves PS, et al: Priming patient safety through nursing handoff communication: a simulation pilot study, *West J Nurs Res* 39(11):1394, 2017.

Heden L, et al: Effects of the intervention "reflective STRENGTH-giving dialogues" for older adults living with long-term pain: a pilot study, *J Aging Res* 7597524, 2020.

Hollingshead NA, et al: The pain experience of Hispanic Americans: a critical literature review and conceptual model, *J Pain* 17(5):513, 2016.

Karcioglu O, et al: A systematic review of the pain scales in adults: Which to use? *J Emerg Med* 36(4):707, 2018.

Khalid S, et al: Post-operative determinants of chronic pain after primary knee replacement surgery: analysis of data on 258,386 patients from the National Joint Registry for England (NJR), *Osteoarthr Cartilage Open*, 3(1): 100139. https://www.sciencedirect.com/science/article/pii/S2665913121000029. Accessed May 1, 2021.

Koh JC, et al: Postoperative pain and patient-controlled epidural analgesia-related adverse effects in young and elderly patients: a retrospective analysis of 2435 patients, *J Pain Res* 10:897, 2017. https://www.ncbi.nlm.nih.gov/pmc/articles/PMC5396922/. Accessed May 5, 2021.

Kolasinski SL, et al: *2019 American College of Rheumatology/Arthritis Foundation guideline for the management of osteoarthritis of the hand, hip, and knee*, 2020. https://onlinelibrary.wiley.com/doi/full/10.1002/art.41142. Accessed May 5, 2021.

Lin CL, et al: Effect of music therapy on pain after orthopedic surgery – a systematic review and meta-analysis, *Pain Pract* 20(4):422, 2020.

Miró J, et al: Validity of three rating scales for measuring pain intensity in youths with physical disabilities, *Eur J Pain* 20(1):130, 2016.

Narusyte J, et al: Shared liability to pain, common mental disorders, and long-term work disability differs among women and men, *Pain* 161(5):1005, 2020. https://www.ncbi.nlm.nih.gov/pmc/articles/PMC7170444/. Accessed May 2, 2021.

O'Leary, et al: Nervous system sensitization as a predictor of outcome in the treatment of peripheral musculoskeletal conditions: a systematic review, *Pain Pract* 17(2):249, 2017.

Pathak A, et al: The utility and validity of pain intensity rating scales for use in developing countries, *Pain Rep* 3(5):e672, 2018.

Rogers AH, et al: Health literacy, opioid misuse, and pain experience among adults with chronic pain, *Pain Med* 21(4):670, 2020.

Rouhi S, et al: New model for couple therapy for patients with chronic pain and their caregivers: an attempt to improve quality of life and reduce pain, *Clin Pract Epidemiol Ment Health* 16:53, 2020. https://www.ncbi.nlm.nih.gov/pmc/articles/PMC7324868/. Accessed May 2, 2021.

Shen J, et al: Evaluation of nurse accuracy in rating procedural pain among pediatric burn patients using the Face, Legs, Activity, Cry, Consolability (FLACC) Scale, *Burns* 43(1):114, 2017.

Tick H, et al: Pain Task Force of the Academic Consortium for Integrative Medicine and Health: Evidence-based nonpharmacologic strategies for comprehensive pain care: The Consortium Pain Task Force White Paper, *Explore (NY)* 14(3):177, 2018.

Tomaszek L, Dębska G: Knowledge, compliance with good clinical practices and barriers to effective control of postoperative pain among nurses from hospitals with and without a "Hospital without Pain" certificate, *J Clin Nurs* 27(7-8):1641, 2018.

US Department of Veterans Affairs: *Acute pain management: meeting the challenges, P#96864*, July 2017. https://www.pbm.va.gov/PBM/AcademicDetailingService/Documents/Academic_Detailing_Educational_Material_Catalog/Pain_Provider_AcutePainProviderEducational Guide_IB10998.pdf. Accessed May 5, 2021.

U.S. Department of Health and Human Services (USDHHS): *Report on pain management best practices: updates, gaps, inconsistencies, and recommendations*, 2019. https://www.hhs.gov/sites/default/files/pmtf-final-report-2019-05-23.pdf.

von Plato H, et al: Combination of perineural and wound infusion after above knee amputation: a randomized, controlled multicenter study, *ACTA* 63(10):1406, 2019.

Wluka AE, et al: Does preoperative neuropathic-like pain and central sensitization affect the post-operative outcome of knee joint replacement for osteoarthritis? A systematic review and meta analysis, *Osteoarthritis Cartilage* 28(2020):1403, 2020.

Wren AA, et al: Multidisciplinary pain management for pediatric patients with acute and chronic pain: a foundational treatment approach when prescribing opioids, *Children* 6(2):33, 2019, https://doi.org/10.3390/children6020033. Accessed May 5, 2021.

Zielinski J, et al: Pain assessment and management in children in the postoperative period: a review of the most commonly used postoperative pain assessment tools, new diagnostic methods and the latest guidelines for postoperative pain therapy in children, *Adv Clin Exp Med* 29(3):365, 2020. doi:10.17219/acem/112600.

Nutrition

OBJECTIVES

- Explain the effects of a well-balanced diet on the body throughout the life span.
- Summarize the process of digestion and absorption.
- Explain the MyPlate program and its value in planning meals for healthy nutrition.
- List the current dietary guidelines for the general population.
- Explain the variance in nutritional requirements throughout the life span.
- Identify risk factors that put patients at high risk for aspiration.

- Categorize the major methods of nutritional assessment.
- Explain the nursing management of enteral feedings.
- Explain the approaches for preventing complications of parenteral nutrition (PN).
- Identify medical nutrition therapy (MNT) in relation to the medical condition of cardiovascular disease.
- Propose how to implement diet counseling and patient teaching in relation to patient expectations.

KEY TERMS

Albumin
Anabolism
Anorexia nervosa
Anthropometry
Basal metabolic rate (BMR)
Body mass index (BMI)
Bulimia nervosa
Carbohydrates
Catabolism
Chyme
Daily values
Dietary reference intakes (DRIs)
Dispensable amino acids
Dysphagia
Enteral nutrition (EN)

Fat-soluble vitamins
Fiber
Food security
Hypervitaminosis
Ideal body weight (IBW)
Indispensable amino acids
Insulin
Intravenous fat emulsions
Ketones
Kilocalories (kcal)
Lipids
Macrominerals
Malabsorption
Malnutrition
Medical nutrition therapy (MNT)

Metabolism
Minerals
Nitrogen balance
Nutrient density
Nutrients
Parenteral nutrition (PN)
Peristalsis
Resting energy expenditure (REE)
Simple carbohydrate
Trace elements
Triglycerides
Vegetarianism
Vitamins
Water-soluble vitamins

MEDIA RESOURCES

http://evolve.elsevier.com/Potter/fundamentals/
- Review Questions
- Audio Glossary
- Case Study with Questions
- Concept Map Creator

- Video Clips
- Skills Performance Checklists
- Content Updates
- Answers to QSEN Activity and Review Questions

Ryan Carnes is a family nurse practitioner (FNP) at the health clinic located at the local senior center. The senior center offers daily social activities and lunch Monday through Friday. Mrs. Cooper, who is 72 years old and has a history of diabetes mellitus (DM), hypertension, and heart failure with atrial fibrillation, is a patient at the senior center health clinic. When Mrs. Cooper comes in for her appointment with Ryan to have her blood pressure checked, she reports that she has lost weight and she is not sure why. When Ryan asks Mrs. Cooper about her eating, she says that she drinks some juice in the morning and two or three cups of coffee. In addition, she often has a sandwich in the late afternoon and skips dinner. She states, "I'm just

not interested in food. It has no taste." Three months ago she started taking an antidepressant medication for depression related to the loss of her husband earlier in the year. She no longer participates in her monthly quilting club, which meets as the senior center. She also tells Ryan that she has stopped going to church regularly and does not participate in any of the other activities or outings planned by the senior center. When Ryan asks Mrs. Cooper about her financial situation, Mrs. Cooper responds by saying that it is tight living on a small pension and Social Security but that she has been able to manage. She is currently living in a small apartment in a senior high-rise apartment building near the senior center. Mrs. Cooper has a *daughter and two teenage grandchildren who live in another town about 100 miles away. She sees her family about once a month because the teenagers are busy with school and sports.*

Ryan knows that based on Mrs. Cooper's comments, he will need to complete a thorough nutritional assessment on her. He schedules a longer appointment for Mrs. Cooper later in the week.

Nutrition is a basic component of health and is essential for normal growth and development, tissue maintenance and repair, cellular metabolism, and organ function. Adequate access to nutrition is imperative to attain and maintain this component of health. In 2018 more than 37 million Americans lived in a household that lacked access to proper nutrition (Hunger + Health, 2021). **Food security** is critical for all members of a household. This term means that all household members have access to sufficient, safe, and nutritious food to maintain a healthy lifestyle. Household members should have sufficient food available on a consistent basis and the resources to obtain appropriate food for a nutritious diet. The importance of food security is supported by the U.S. Department of Agriculture (USDA), which found that many children in this country live in a home that lacks the access to enough high-quality food to maintain an active healthy life (USDA, 2020). Decreased food security or access to healthy nutrition can result in poor patient outcomes such as longer hospital admissions due to delayed healing or adverse effects on health conditions (Giddens, 2021). Therefore nutrition and health are interrelated and represent an important concept in nursing practice.

Medical nutrition therapy (MNT) uses nutrition therapy and counseling to manage diseases (Healthline, 2020). In some illnesses such as type 1 diabetes mellitus (DM) or mild hypertension, diet therapy is often the major treatment for disease control (American Diabetes Association [ADA], 2019). Other conditions such as severe inflammatory bowel disease require specialized nutrition support such as enteral nutrition (EN) or parenteral nutrition (PN). Current standards of care promote optimal nutrition in all patients, including a low-fat diet and limiting red meat specifically (American Cancer Society [ACS], 2021; American Heart Association [AHA], 2017).

The U.S. Department of Health and Human Services (USDHHS) and the Office of Disease Prevention and Health Promotion (ODPHP) have published *Healthy People* nutritional goals since 2000 and recently released *Healthy People 2030* (ODPHP, n.d.; USDHHS, 2020) (Box 45.1). These objectives have continued through review and revision of *Healthy People* every 10 years. The overall goals for *Healthy People 2030* are promoting health and healthy behaviors and reducing chronic disease (ODPHP, n.d.). All objectives related to nutrition and healthy eating include baseline data from which progress is measured. The challenge remains to motivate consumers to put these dietary recommendations into practice to reduce the risk of chronic disease and improve overall health.

As a nurse, you use clinical judgment and critical thinking to identify and treat patients' nutritional problems. To help patients you need to understand the process of digestion and absorption, the body's requirements for nutrients, and patients' nutritional needs. Use this knowledge to help you gather and analyze assessment data to identify a patient's priority nutritional problem(s). Patients with nutritional concerns require individualized approaches based on their personal habits, preferences, and nutrition habits, and the cause of their problem. A patient-centered nursing care plan with individualized nursing interventions is often effective in resolving short- and long-term nutritional problems.

SCIENTIFIC KNOWLEDGE BASE

Nutrients: The Biochemical Units of Nutrition

The body requires fuel to provide energy for cellular metabolism and repair, organ function, growth, and body movement. The **basal metabolic**

BOX 45.1 Examples of Nutrition and Healthy Eating Objectives for *Healthy People 2030*

Overweight and Obesity
- Reduce the proportion of adults who are obese.
- Increase the proportion of physician office visits made by adult patients with obesity that include counseling or education related to weight reduction, nutrition, or physical activity.

Nutrition and Healthy Eating
- Increase the consumption of fruits, vegetables, and whole grains by persons aged 2 years and over. Reduce the consumption of added sugars, saturated fats, and sodium by persons aged 2 years and over. Increase the consumption of calcium, potassium, and vitamin D by persons aged 2 years and over.
- Reduce iron deficiency among children who are 1 to 2 years of age.
- Increase the proportion of schools that do not sell less healthy foods and beverages.
- Eliminate very low food security among children.
- Reduce household food insecurity and in doing so reduce hunger.

Heart Disease and Stroke
- Reduce the proportion of adults with high blood pressure.
- Reduce the mean total blood cholesterol level among adults.

Infants, Children, and Adolescents
- Increase the proportion of infants who are breastfed exclusively through 6 months of age.
- Increase the proportion of infants who are breastfed at 1 year.
- Increase the proportion of students participating in the School Breakfast Program.
- Increase the proportion of eligible students participating in the U.S. Department of Agriculture (USDA) Summer Food Service program.

Women
- Increase the proportion of women of childbearing age who have optimal red blood cell folate concentrations.
- Reduce iron deficiency among females aged 12 to 49 years.

Workplace
- Increase the proportion of worksites that offer a nutrition program as part of an employee health promotion program.

Data from U.S. Department of Health and Human Services and Office of Disease Prevention and Health Promotion (ODPHP): *Healthy People 2030*, n.d. https://health.gov/healthypeople/objectives-and-data/browse-objectives/nutrition-and-healthy-eating. Accessed April 7, 2021.

---

rate (BMR) is the energy needed at rest to maintain life-sustaining activities (breathing, circulation, heart rate, and temperature) for a specific amount of time. Factors such as age, body mass, gender, fever, starvation, menstruation, illness, injury, infection, activity level, and thyroid function affect energy requirements. The **resting energy expenditure (REE)**, or resting metabolic rate, is the amount of energy you need to consume over a 24-hour period for your body to maintain its internal working activities while at rest. Factors that affect metabolism include illness, pregnancy, lactation, and activity level.

When the **kilocalories (kcal)** of the food we eat meet our energy requirements, our weight does not change (Grodner et al., 2020). When the kilocalories ingested exceed our energy demands, we gain weight. Likewise, if the kilocalories ingested fail to meet our energy requirements, we lose weight.

Nutrients are the elements necessary for the normal function of numerous body processes. We meet energy needs through the intake of a variety of nutrients: carbohydrates, proteins, fats, water, vitamins, and minerals. The **nutrient density** of food refers to the proportion of essential nutrients to the number of kilocalories. High–nutrient dense foods such as fruits and vegetables provide a large number of nutrients in relationship to kilocalories. Low–nutrient dense foods such as alcohol or sugar are high in kilocalories but nutrient poor.

Carbohydrates. **Carbohydrates**, composed of carbon, hydrogen, and oxygen, are the main source of energy in the diet. Each gram of carbohydrate produces 4 kcal/g, and carbohydrates serve as the main source of fuel (glucose) for the brain, skeletal muscles during exercise, erythrocyte and leukocyte production, and cell function of the renal medulla. We obtain carbohydrates primarily from plant foods, except for lactose (milk sugar). Classification of carbohydrates occurs according to their carbohydrate units, or saccharides.

Monosaccharides such as glucose (dextrose) or fructose do not break down into a more basic carbohydrate unit. Disaccharides such as sucrose, lactose, and maltose are composed of two monosaccharides and water. Simple carbohydrate is the classification for both monosaccharides and disaccharides; they are found primarily in sugars. Polysaccharides such as glycogen also make up carbohydrate units (i.e., complex carbohydrates). They are insoluble in water and digested in varying degrees. Starches are polysaccharides.

The body is unable to digest some polysaccharides because we do not have enzymes capable of breaking them down. **Fiber**, a polysaccharide, is the structural part of plants that is not broken down by our digestive enzymes. Insoluble fibers, including cellulose, hemicellulose, and lignin, are not digestible. The inability to break down fiber means that it does not contribute calories to the diet. Soluble fibers dissolve in water and include barley, cereal grains, cornmeal, and oats.

Proteins. Proteins provide a source of energy (4 kcal/g); they are essential for the growth, maintenance, and repair of body tissue. Collagen, hormones, enzymes, immune cells, deoxyribonucleic acid (DNA), and ribonucleic acid (RNA) are all made of protein. In addition, blood clotting, fluid regulation, and acid-base balance require proteins. Proteins transport nutrients and many drugs in the blood. Ingestion of proteins maintains nitrogen balance.

The simplest form of protein is the amino acid, consisting of hydrogen, oxygen, carbon, and nitrogen. Because the body does not synthesize **indispensable amino acids**, these need to be provided in our diet. Examples of indispensable amino acids are histidine, lysine, and phenylalanine. The body synthesizes **dispensable amino acids**. Examples of amino acids synthesized in the body are alanine, asparagine, and glutamic acid. Amino acids can link together. **Albumin** and **insulin** are simple proteins because they contain only amino acids or their derivatives. The combination of a simple protein with a nonprotein substance produces a complex protein such as lipoprotein, formed by a combination of a lipid and a simple protein.

A complete protein, also called a *high-quality protein,* contains all essential amino acids in sufficient quantity to support growth and maintain nitrogen balance. Most complete proteins come from animal sources, such as fish, poultry, beef, milk, cheese, and eggs, but they can also come from plant sources, such as soy. Incomplete proteins are missing one or more of the nine indispensable amino acids and include grains, seeds and nuts, legumes, and vegetables. Complementary proteins are pairs of incomplete proteins that, when combined, supply the total amount of protein provided by complete protein sources.

Nitrogen is a byproduct of protein catabolism. Achieving **nitrogen balance** means that the intake and output of nitrogen are equal. When the intake of nitrogen is greater than the output, the body is in positive nitrogen balance. Positive nitrogen balance is required for growth, normal pregnancy, maintenance of lean muscle mass and vital organs, and wound healing. The body uses nitrogen to build, repair, and replace body tissues. Negative nitrogen balance occurs when the body loses more nitrogen than it gains (e.g., with infection, burns, fever, starvation, head injury, and trauma). The increased nitrogen loss is the result of body tissue destruction or loss of nitrogen-containing body fluids. Nutrition during this period needs to provide nutrients to put patients into positive balance for healing.

Protein provides energy, but because its essential role is to promote growth, maintenance, and repair, a diet needs to provide adequate kilocalories from nonprotein sources. When there is sufficient carbohydrate in the diet to meet the energy needs of the body, protein is spared as an energy source.

Fats. Fats (**lipids**) are the most calorie-dense nutrient, providing 9 kcal/g. Fats are composed of triglycerides and fatty acids. **Triglycerides** circulate in the blood and are composed of three fatty acids attached to a glycerol. Fatty acids are composed of chains of carbon and hydrogen atoms with an acid group on one end of the chain and a methyl group at the other. Fatty acids can be *saturated,* in which each carbon in the chain has two attached hydrogen atoms, or *unsaturated,* in which an unequal number of hydrogen atoms are attached, and the carbon atoms attach to one another with a double bond. Monounsaturated fatty acids have one double bond, whereas polyunsaturated fatty acids have two or more double carbon bonds. The various types of fatty acids referred to in the dietary guidelines have significance for health and the incidence of disease.

Fatty acids are also classified as essential or nonessential. Linoleic acid, an unsaturated fatty acid, is the only essential fatty acid in humans. Linolenic acid and arachidonic acid, other types of unsaturated fatty acids, are important for metabolic processes. The body manufactures them when linoleic acid is available. Deficiency occurs when fat intake falls below 10% of daily nutrition. Most animal fats have high proportions of saturated fatty acids, whereas vegetable fats have higher amounts of unsaturated and polyunsaturated fatty acids.

Water. Water is critical because cell function depends on a fluid environment. Water makes up 60% to 70% of total body weight. People who are lean have a greater percent of total body water than those who are obese because muscle contains more water than any other tissue except blood. Infants have the greatest percentage of total body water because of greater surface area, and older people have the least. When deprived of water, a person usually cannot survive for more than a few days.

We meet our fluid needs by drinking liquids and eating solid foods high in water content such as fresh fruits and vegetables. Digestion produces fluid during food oxidation. In a healthy individual fluid intake from all sources equals fluid output through elimination, respiration, and sweating (see Chapters 41 and 46). People who are ill have an increased need for fluid (e.g., with fever or gastrointestinal [GI] losses). By contrast, they also have a decreased ability to excrete fluid (e.g., with cardiopulmonary or renal disease), which often leads to the need for fluid restriction.

Vitamins. **Vitamins** are organic substances present in small amounts in foods that are essential to normal metabolism. They are chemicals that act as catalysts in biochemical reactions. When there is enough of any specific vitamin to meet the catalytic demands of the body, the rest of the vitamin supply acts as a free chemical and is often toxic to the body. Certain vitamins are currently of interest in their role as antioxidants. These vitamins neutralize substances called *free radicals,* which produce oxidative damage to body cells and tissues. Researchers think that oxidative damage increases a person's risk for various cancers. Antioxidant vitamins include beta-carotene and vitamins A, C, and E (Grodner et al., 2020).

The body is unable to synthesize vitamins in the required amounts. Vitamin synthesis depends on dietary intake. Vitamin content is usually highest in fresh foods that have minimal exposure to heat, air, or water before their use. Vitamin classifications include fat soluble or water soluble.

Fat-Soluble Vitamins. The fat-soluble vitamins (A, D, E, and K) are stored in the fatty compartments of the body. People acquire vitamins primarily through dietary intake, although vitamin D also comes from the sun. The body has a high storage capacity for fat-soluble vitamins. As a result, toxicity is possible when a person takes large doses of them. Hypervitaminosis of fat-soluble vitamins results from megadoses (intentional or unintentional) of supplemental vitamins, excessive amounts in fortified food, and large intake of fish oils.

Water-Soluble Vitamins. The water-soluble vitamins are vitamin C and the B complex (which is eight vitamins). The body does not store water-soluble vitamins; therefore we need them provided in our daily food intake. Water-soluble vitamins are absorbed easily from the GI tract. Although they are not stored, toxicity can still occur.

Minerals. Minerals are inorganic elements essential to the body as catalysts in biochemical reactions. They are classified as macrominerals when the daily requirement is 100 mg or more and microminerals or trace elements when less than 100 mg is needed daily. Macrominerals help to balance the pH of the body, and specific amounts are necessary in the blood and cells to promote acid-base balance. Interactions occur among trace minerals. For example, excess of one trace mineral sometimes causes deficiency of another. Selenium is a trace element that also has antioxidant properties. Silicon, vanadium, nickel, tin, cadmium, arsenic, aluminum, and boron are trace elements. Arsenic, aluminum, and cadmium can have toxic effects.

Anatomy and Physiology of the Digestive System

Digestion. Digestion of food is the mechanical breakdown that results from chewing, churning, and mixing with fluid and chemical reactions in which food is reduced to its simplest form (Grodner et al., 2020). Each part of the GI system has an important digestive or absorptive function (Fig. 45.1). Enzymes are the protein-like substances that act as catalysts to speed up chemical reactions. They are an essential part of the chemistry of digestion.

Most enzymes have one specific function. Each enzyme works best at a specific pH. For example, the enzyme amylase in the saliva breaks down starches into sugars. The secretions of the GI tract have very different pH levels. Saliva is relatively neutral, gastric juice is highly acidic, and the secretions of the small intestine are alkaline.

The mechanical, chemical, and hormonal activities of digestion are interdependent. Enzyme activity depends on the mechanical breakdown of food to increase its surface area for chemical action. Hormones regulate the flow of digestive secretions needed for enzyme supply. Physical, chemical, and hormonal factors regulate the secretion of digestive juices and the motility of the GI tract. Nerve stimulation from the parasympathetic nervous system (e.g., the vagus nerve) increases GI tract action (Grodner et al., 2020).

Digestion begins in the mouth, where chewing mechanically breaks down food. The food mixes with saliva, which contains ptyalin (salivary amylase), an enzyme that acts on cooked starch to begin its conversion to maltose. The longer an individual chews food, the more starch digestion occurs in the mouth. Proteins and fats are broken down physically but remain unchanged chemically because enzymes in the mouth do not react with these nutrients. Chewing reduces food particles to a size suitable for swallowing, and saliva provides lubrication to ease swallowing of the food. The epiglottis is a flap of skin that closes over the trachea to prevent aspiration as a person swallows. Swallowed food enters the esophagus, and wavelike muscular contractions (peristalsis) move the food to the base of the esophagus, above the cardiac sphincter. Pressure from a bolus of food at the cardiac sphincter causes it to relax, allowing the food to enter the fundus, or uppermost part, of the stomach.

The chief cells in the stomach secrete pepsinogen, and the pyloric glands secrete gastrin, a hormone that triggers parietal cells to secrete hydrochloric acid (HCl). The parietal cells also secrete HCl and intrinsic factor (IF), which is necessary for absorption of vitamin B_{12} in the ileum. HCl turns pepsinogen into pepsin, a protein-splitting enzyme. The body produces gastric lipase and amylase to begin fat and starch digestion, respectively. A thick layer of mucus protects the lining of the stomach from autodigestion. Alcohol and aspirin are two substances directly absorbed through the lining of the stomach. The stomach acts as a reservoir where food remains for approximately 3 hours, with a range of 1 to 7 hours.

Food leaves the antrum, or distal stomach, through the pyloric sphincter and enters the duodenum. Food is now an acidic, liquefied mass called chyme. Chyme flows into the duodenum and quickly mixes with bile, intestinal juices, and pancreatic secretions. The small intestine secretes the hormones secretin and cholecystokinin (CCK). Secretin activates release of bicarbonate from the pancreas, raising the pH of chyme. CCK inhibits further gastrin secretion and initiates release of additional digestive enzymes from the pancreas and gallbladder.

Bile, manufactured in the liver, is then concentrated and stored in the gallbladder. It acts as a detergent because it emulsifies fat to permit enzyme action while suspending fatty acids in solution. Pancreatic secretions contain six enzymes: amylase to digest starch; lipase to break down emulsified fats; and trypsin, elastase, chymotrypsin, and carboxypeptidase to break down proteins.

Peristalsis continues in the small intestine, mixing the secretions with chyme. The mixture becomes increasingly alkaline, inhibiting the action of the gastric enzymes and promoting the action of the duodenal secretions. Epithelial cells in the small intestinal villi secrete enzymes (e.g., sucrase, lactase, maltase, lipase, and peptidase) to facilitate digestion. The major part of digestion occurs in the small intestine, producing glucose, fructose, and galactose from carbohydrates; amino acids and dipeptides from proteins; and fatty acids, glycerides, and glycerol from lipids. Peristalsis usually takes approximately 5 hours to pass food through the small intestine.

Absorption. The small intestine, lined with fingerlike projections called *villi*, is the primary absorption site for nutrients. Villi increase the surface area available for absorption. The body absorbs nutrients by means of passive diffusion, osmosis, active transport, and pinocytosis (Table 45.1).

Absorption of carbohydrates, protein, minerals, and water-soluble vitamins occurs in the small intestine. Then the nutrients are processed in the liver and released into the portal vein circulation. Fatty acids are absorbed in the lymphatic circulatory systems through lacteal ducts at the center of each microvilli in the small intestine.

Approximately 85% to 90% of water is absorbed in the small intestine (Huether et al., 2020). The GI tract manages approximately 8.5 L of GI secretions and 1.5 L of oral intake daily. The small intestine resorbs 9.5 L, and the colon absorbs approximately 0.4 L. Elimination of the remaining 0.1 L occurs via feces. In addition, electrolytes and minerals are absorbed in the colon, and bacteria synthesize vitamin K and some B-complex vitamins. Finally, feces form for elimination.

Metabolism and Storage of Nutrients. Metabolism refers to all the biochemical reactions within the cells of the body. Metabolic processes are

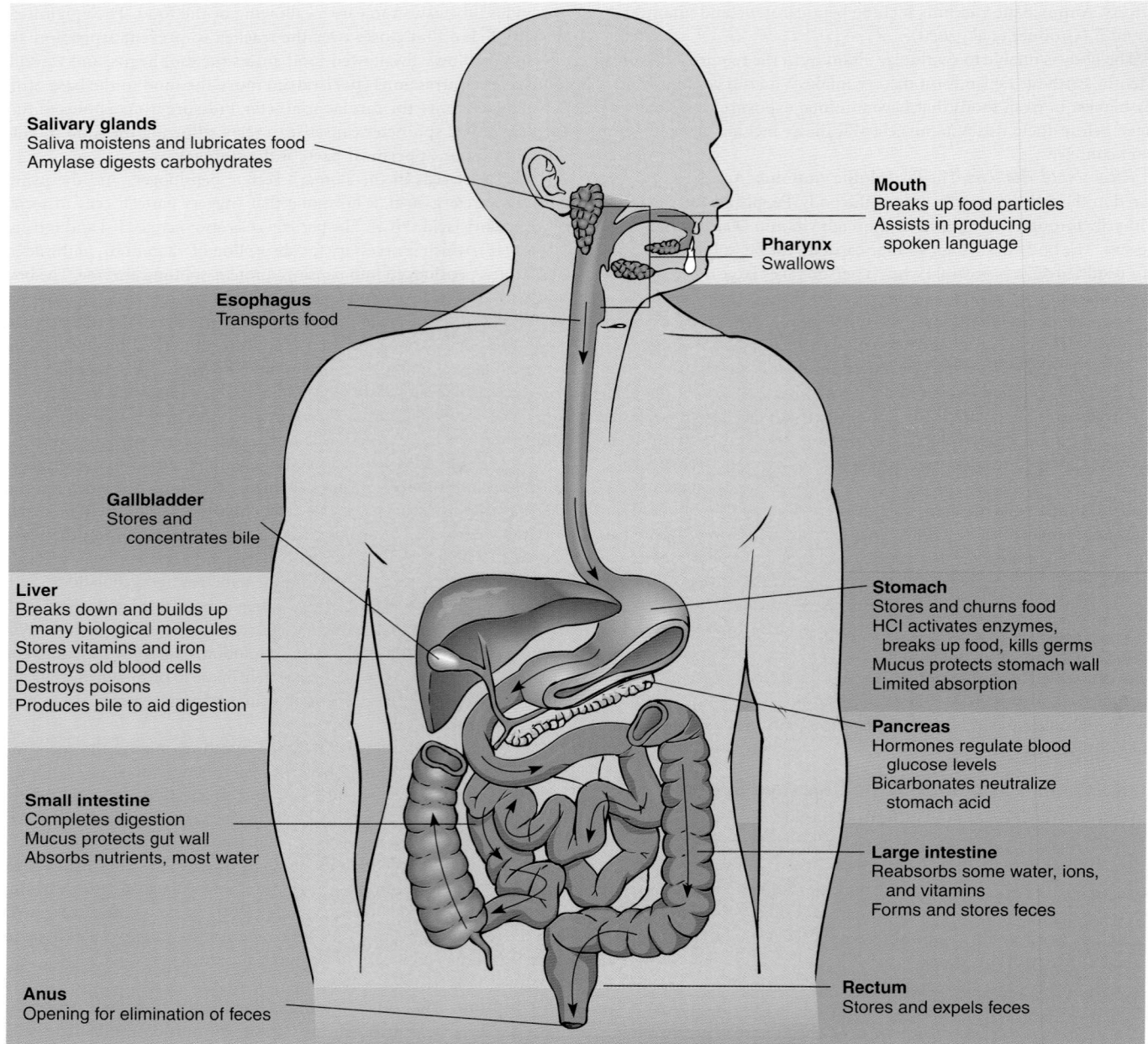

Salivary glands
Saliva moistens and lubricates food
Amylase digests carbohydrates

Mouth
Breaks up food particles
Assists in producing
    spoken language

Pharynx
Swallows

Esophagus
Transports food

Gallbladder
Stores and
    concentrates bile

Liver
Breaks down and builds up
    many biological molecules
Stores vitamins and iron
Destroys old blood cells
Destroys poisons
Produces bile to aid digestion

Stomach
Stores and churns food
HCl activates enzymes,
    breaks up food, kills germs
Mucus protects stomach wall
Limited absorption

Pancreas
Hormones regulate blood
    glucose levels
Bicarbonates neutralize
    stomach acid

Small intestine
Completes digestion
Mucus protects gut wall
Absorbs nutrients, most water

Large intestine
Reabsorbs some water, ions,
    and vitamins
Forms and stores feces

Anus
Opening for elimination of feces

Rectum
Stores and expels feces

FIG. 45.1 Summary of digestive system anatomy/organ function. *HCl,* Hydrochloric acid.

anabolic (building) or catabolic (breaking down). Anabolism is the building of more complex biochemical substances by synthesis of nutrients. It occurs when an individual adds lean muscle through diet and exercise. Amino acids are anabolized into tissues, hormones, and enzymes. Normal metabolism and anabolism are physiologically possible when the body is in positive nitrogen balance. Catabolism is the breakdown of biochemical substances into simpler substances and occurs during physiological states of negative nitrogen balance. Starvation is an example of catabolism when wasting of body tissues occurs.

Nutrients absorbed in the intestines, including water, travel through the circulatory system to the body tissues. Through the chemical changes of metabolism, the body converts nutrients into several required substances. Carbohydrates, protein, and fat metabolism produce chemical energy and maintain a balance between anabolism and catabolism.

To carry out the work of the body, the chemical energy produced by metabolism converts to other types of energy by different tissues. Muscle contraction involves mechanical energy, nervous system function involves electrical energy, and the mechanisms of heat production involve thermal energy.

Some of the nutrients required by the body are stored in tissues. The major form of body reserve energy is fat, stored as adipose tissue. Protein is stored in muscle mass. When the energy requirements of the body exceed the energy supplied by ingested nutrients, stored energy is used. Monoglycerides from the digested part of fats are converted to glucose by gluconeogenesis. Amino acids are also converted to fat and stored or catabolized into energy through gluconeogenesis. All body cells except red blood cells and neurons oxidize fatty acids into ketones for energy when dietary carbohydrates (glucose) are not adequate. Glycogen,

TABLE 45.1   Mechanisms for Intestinal Absorption of Nutrients

Mechanism	Definition
Active transport	An energy-dependent process, typically driven by adenosine triphosphate (ATP). During the process particles move from an area of lower concentration to an area of greater concentration (against the concentration gradient).
Passive diffusion	The force by which particles move outward from an area of greater concentration to one of lesser concentration. The particles do not need a special "carrier" to move outward in all directions.
Facilitated diffusion	Movement of molecule occurs when the molecule, despite positive pressure flow, moves through a membrane pore aided by another particle or molecule.
Osmosis	Movement of water through a semipermeable membrane that separates solutions of different concentrations. Water moves to equalize the concentration pressures on both sides of the membrane.
Pinocytosis	Engulfing of large molecules of nutrients by the absorbing cell when the molecule attaches to the absorbing cell membrane.

Data from Grodner M et al: Nutritional foundations and clinical application, ed 7, St Louis, 2020, Elsevier.

synthesized from glucose, provides energy during brief periods of fasting (e.g., during sleep). It is stored in small reserves in liver and muscle tissue. Nutrient metabolism consists of three main processes:

1. Catabolism of glycogen into glucose, carbon dioxide, and water (glycogenolysis)
2. Anabolism of glucose into glycogen for storage (glycogenesis)
3. Catabolism of amino acids and glycerol into glucose for energy (gluconeogenesis)

Elimination. Chyme moves by peristaltic action through the ileocecal valve into the large intestine, where it becomes feces (see Chapter 47). Water is absorbed in the mucosa as feces move toward the rectum. The longer the material stays in the large intestine, the more water is absorbed, causing the feces to become firmer. Exercise and fiber stimulate peristalsis, and water maintains consistency. Feces contain cellulose and similar indigestible substances, sloughed epithelial cells from the GI tract, digestive secretions, water, and microbes.

Dietary Guidelines

Dietary Reference Intakes. Dietary reference intakes (DRIs) present evidence-based criteria for an acceptable range of amounts of vitamins and nutrients for each gender and age-group (National Institutes of Health [NIH], n.d.a; USDHHS, 2020). There are four components to the DRIs. The estimated average requirement (EAR) is the recommended amount of a nutrient that appears sufficient to maintain a specific body function for 50% of the population based on age and gender. The recommended dietary allowance (RDA) represents the average needs of 98% of the population, not the exact needs of the individual. The adequate intake (AI) is the suggested intake for individuals based on observed or experimentally determined estimates of nutrient intakes and is used when there is not enough evidence to set the RDA. The tolerable upper intake level (UL) is the highest level that likely poses no risk of adverse health events. It is not a recommended level of intake (NIH, n.d.b).

BOX 45.2   2020–2025 Dietary Guidelines for Americans: Key Guidelines and Recommendations for the General Population

Follow a Healthy Dietary Pattern at Every Life Stage
- Meet nutritional needs primarily from nutrient-dense foods and beverages.
- Choose a variety of options from each food group in recommended amounts and within calorie limits.
- Pay attention to portion size.

Customize and Enjoy Food and Beverage Choices to Reflect Personal Preferences, Cultural Traditions, and Budgetary Considerations
- Start food planning with consideration of personal preferences.
- Incorporate cultural traditions by choosing nutrient-dense, culturally relevant foods from all food groups.
- Meet budgetary considerations by doing advance meal planning; considering regional and seasonal food availability; and incorporating a variety of fresh, frozen, dried, and canned options.

Focus on Meeting Food Group Needs With Nutrient-Dense Foods and Beverages, and Stay Within Calorie Limits
- Eat an appropriate mix of foods from the food groups and subgroups that is within the appropriate calorie level to promote health at each life stage.
- Eat a variety of nutrient dense vegetables from each of the vegetable subgroups—dark green; red and orange; beans, peas, and lentils; starchy; and other.
- Eat a variety of whole fruits (fresh, canned, frozen, dried) and 100% fruit juice.
- Whole grains should make up at least half of the grains eaten; limit the amount of refined grains.
- Eat a variety of protein foods in nutrient-dense forms that includes proteins from both animal and plant sources, and includes subgroups of meats, poultry, and eggs; seafood; and nuts, seeds, and soy products.
- Practice food safety to prevent bacterial foodborne illness. Use food-safety principles of *Clean, Separate, Cook,* and *Chill.*

Limit Foods and Beverages Higher in Added Sugars, Saturated Fat, and Sodium, and Limit Alcoholic Beverages
- Eighty-five percent of daily required calories should be met through the requirements from each of the food groups in the form of nutrient dense foods.
- Limit saturated fats and *trans* fats; consume less than 10% of calories per day from saturated fats.
- Limit added sugar or sweeteners so that less than 10% of calories comes from added sugars.
- Consume less than 2300 milligrams (mg) of sodium per day.
- Overall calorie intake should not exceed recommended intake to maintain or achieve a healthy weight.
- Read Nutrition Facts labels on food products to make informed and healthy food decisions.

Data from U.S. Department of Health and Human Services and U.S. Department of Agriculture: *Dietary guidelines for Americans 2020–2025,* ed 9. https://www.dietaryguidelines.gov/sites/default/files/2020-.12/Dietary_Guidelines_for_Americans_2020-2025.pdf. Accessed April 7, 2021.

Food Guidelines. The USDA and the USDHHS (2020) published the *Dietary Guidelines for Americans 2020–2025.* The updated guidelines were revised for Americans from infancy through older-adult years and include a special section for women who are pregnant or lactating. There are four major guidelines providing the foundation for the recommendations for healthy dietary patterns for health promotion and quantitative guidance on foods throughout the life span (Box 45.2).

FIG. 45.2 MyPlate. (From U.S. Department of Agriculture: What is MyPlate?, n.d. https://www.myplate.gov/eat-healthy/what-is-myplate. Accessed April 5, 2021.)

When planning care, consider your patients' food preferences and food access, which are affected by their culture and socioeconomic resources. The USDA developed the MyPlate program to replace the My Food Pyramid program. MyPlate provides a basic guide for making food choices for a healthy lifestyle (Fig. 45.2). It includes guidelines for balancing calories; decreasing portion size; increasing healthy foods; increasing water consumption; and decreasing fats, sodium, and sugars (USDA, n.d.a).

Daily Values. The U.S. Food and Drug Administration (FDA) created daily values for food labels in response to the 1990 Nutrition Labeling and Education Act (NLEA). The FDA first established two sets of reference values. The referenced daily intakes (RDIs) are the first set, comprising protein, vitamins, and minerals based on the RDA. The daily reference values (DRVs) make up the second set and consist of nutrients such as total fat, saturated fat, cholesterol, carbohydrates, fiber, sodium, and potassium. Combined, both sets make up the daily values used on food labels. Daily values did not replace RDAs but provided a separate, more understandable format for the public. Daily values are based on percentages of a diet consisting of 2000 kcal/day for adults and children 4 years or older.

> **REFLECT NOW**
>
> In your geographical area, identify a population at risk for poor nutrition. What is the population, and what nutritional deficiencies do you believe they are most at risk for having and why?

NURSING KNOWLEDGE BASE

There are many sociological and psychological factors associated with eating and drinking in all societies. We celebrate holidays and events with food, bring it to those who are grieving, and use it for medicinal purposes. We incorporate food into family traditions and rituals and often associate food with eating behaviors. You need to understand patients' values, beliefs, preferences, and attitudes about food and how these values affect food purchase, preparation, and intake to affect eating patterns.

Nutritional requirements depend on many factors. Individual caloric and nutrient requirements vary by stage of development, body composition, activity levels, pregnancy and lactation, and the presence of disease. Registered dietitians (RDs) use predictive equations that consider some of these factors to estimate patients' nutritional requirements.

Factors Influencing Nutrition

Environmental Factors. Environmental factors beyond the control of individuals contribute to the development of obesity. Obesity is an epidemic in the United States. Presently 68.7% of Americans are overweight or obese (Centers for Disease Control and Prevention [CDC], 2021a). Overweight is defined as having a body mass index (BMI) of 25 to 29, and obesity is defined as a BMI of 30 or greater (CDC, 2021a). Obesity is often associated with several factors, such as sedentary lifestyle, overeating, and genetics (Giddens, 2021). Environmental factors can limit a person's likelihood of healthy eating and participation in exercise or other activities of healthy living. Lack of access to full-service grocery stores, high cost of healthy food, widespread availability of less healthy foods in fast-food restaurants, widespread advertising of less healthy food, and lack of access to safe places to play and exercise are environmental factors that contribute to obesity (Katmarzyk et al., 2019).

Developmental Needs

Infants Through School-Age. Rapid growth and high protein, vitamin, mineral, and energy requirements mark the developmental stage of infancy. The average birth weight of an American baby is 7 to 7½ lb (3.2–3.4 kg). An infant usually doubles birth weight at 4 to 5 months and triples it at 1 year. A healthy infant from birth to 1 year needs an energy intake of approximately 100 kcal/kg of body weight per day, with neonates needing 100 to 135 kcal/kg per day (Patel and Rouster, 2020). The nutritional needs of premature infants vary with gestational age and stage of growth, but typically these infants require higher amounts of energy to promote growth (Patel and Rouster, 2020). Commercial formulas and human breast milk both provide approximately 20 kcal/oz. A full-term newborn can digest and absorb simple carbohydrates, proteins, and a moderate amount of emulsified fat. Infants need about 100 to 120 mL/kg/day of fluid because a large part of total body weight is water.

Breastfeeding. The American Academy of Pediatrics (AAP) strongly supports breastfeeding for the first 6 months of life and breastfeeding with complementary foods from 6 to 12 months (AAP, 2017). Breastfeeding has multiple benefits for both infant and mother, including fewer food allergies and intolerances; fewer infant infections; easier digestion; convenience, availability, and freshness; milk temperature always correct; economical because it is less expensive than formula; and increased time for mother and infant interaction.

Formula. Infant formulas contain the approximate nutrient composition of human milk. Protein in the formula is typically whey, soy, cow's milk base, casein hydrolysate, or elemental amino acids. Infants with allergies or an intolerance to cow's milk should consume hydrolyzed protein–based or amino acid–based formulas instead (Patel and Rouster, 2020).

Infants should not have regular cow's milk during the first year of life. It is too concentrated for an infant's kidneys to manage, increases the risk of milk-product allergies, and is a poor source of iron and vitamins C and E (Grodner et al., 2020). Furthermore, children under 1 year of age should never ingest honey and corn syrup products because they are potential sources of the botulism toxin, which increases the risk of infant death.

Introduction to Solid Food. Breast milk or formula provides sufficient nutrition for the first 4 to 6 months of life. The development of fine-motor skills of the hand and fingers parallels an infant's interest in food and self-feeding. Iron-fortified cereals are typically the first semisolid food to be introduced. For infants 4 to 11 months, cereals are the most important nonmilk source of protein (Hockenberry et al., 2019).

Adding foods to an infant's diet depends on the infant's nutrient needs, physical readiness to handle different forms of foods, and the need to detect and control allergic reactions. Introducing foods that have a high incidence of causing allergic reactions such as wheat, egg white, nuts, citrus juice, and chocolate should happen later in the infant's life (American Academy of Allergy Asthma, and Immunology [AAAAI], 2020). In addition, caregivers should introduce new foods one at a time, approximately 4 to 7 days apart, to identify allergies. It is best to introduce new foods before milk or other foods to avoid satiety (Hockenberry et al., 2019).

The growth rate slows during toddler years (1–3 years). A toddler needs fewer kilocalories but an increased amount of protein in relation to body weight; consequently appetite often decreases at 18 months of age. Toddlers exhibit strong food preferences and become picky eaters. Small, frequent meals consisting of breakfast, lunch, and dinner with three interspersed high–nutrient-dense snacks help improve nutritional intake (Hockenberry et al., 2019). Calcium and phosphorus are important for healthy bone growth.

Toddlers who consume more than 24 ounces of milk daily in place of other foods sometimes develop milk anemia because milk is a poor source of iron. Toddlers need to drink whole milk until the age of 2 years to make sure that there is adequate intake of fatty acids necessary for brain and neurological development. Avoid certain foods such as hot dogs, hard candy, nuts, grapes, raw vegetables, and popcorn because they present a choking hazard. Dietary requirements for preschoolers (3–5 years) are similar to those for toddlers. They consume slightly more than toddlers, and nutrient density is more important than quantity.

School-age children, 6 to 12 years old, grow at a slower and steadier rate, with a gradual decline in energy requirements per unit of body weight. Despite better appetites and more varied food intake, you need to assess school-age children's diets carefully for adequate protein and vitamins A and C. They often fail to eat a proper breakfast and have unsupervised intake at school. Diets high in fat, sugar, and salt result from too-liberal intake of snack foods. Physical activity level decreases consistently, and consumption of high-calorie, readily available food increases, leading to an increase in childhood obesity (Katmarzyk et al., 2019).

Although the rate of childhood obesity slowed from 2004 through 2016 and the rate of obesity in children from kindergarten through third grade declined, the obesity rate still increased to 18.5% in 2016 (Anderson et al., 2019). A combination of factors contributes to the childhood obesity problem, including a diet rich in high-calorie foods, food advertising targeting children, inactivity, genetic predisposition, use of food as a coping mechanism for stress or boredom or as a reward or celebration, and family and socioeconomic factors (Hockenberry et al., 2019). Childhood obesity contributes to medical problems related to the cardiovascular system, endocrine system, and mental health. With the increase in obesity, the incidence of type 2 diabetes in children is also increasing. Prevention of childhood obesity is critical because of its long-term effects. The CDC (2021b) reports that, building on previous childhood obesity research demonstration (CORD) projects, CORD 3.0 research teams are now focusing on adapting, testing, and packaging effective programs to reduce obesity among children from lower-income families. As a nurse, family education is an important nursing intervention to assist in decreasing the prevalence of this problem. Promote healthy food choices and eating in moderation along with increased physical activity.

Adolescents. During adolescence physiological age is a better guide to nutritional needs than chronological age. Energy needs increase to meet greater metabolic demands of growth. Daily requirement of protein also increases. Calcium is essential for the rapid bone growth of adolescence, and girls need a continuous source of iron to replace menstrual losses. Boys also need adequate iron for muscle development. Iodine supports increased thyroid activity, and the use of iodized table salt ensures availability. B-complex vitamins are necessary to support heightened metabolic activity.

Many factors other than nutritional needs influence the adolescent's diet, including concern about body image and appearance, desire for independence, eating at fast-food restaurants, peer pressure, and fad diets. Nutritional deficiencies often occur in adolescent girls because of dieting and use of oral contraceptives. An adolescent boy's diet is often inadequate in total kilocalories, protein, iron, folic acid, B vitamins, and iodine. Snacks provide approximately 25% of a teenager's total dietary intake. Fast food, particularly value-size or super-size meals, is common and adds extra salt, fat, and kilocalories. Skipping meals or eating meals with unhealthy choices of snacks contributes to nutrient deficiency and obesity (Hockenberry et al., 2019). Research on adolescents in school lunch programs has shown that they eat healthier lunches but that, overall, the 24-hour dietary intake of the adolescents in the school lunch program was similar to that in adolescents not participating in school lunch programs (Gearan et al., 2021).

Fortified foods (nutrients added) are important sources of vitamins and minerals. Snack food from the dairy, fruit, and vegetable groups are good choices. To counter obesity, increasing physical activity is often more important than curbing intake. The onset of eating disorders such as anorexia nervosa or bulimia nervosa often occurs during adolescence. Recognition of eating disorders is essential for early intervention (Box 45.3).

Sports and regular moderate to intense exercise necessitate dietary modification to meet increased energy needs for adolescents. Carbohydrates, both simple and complex, are the main source of energy, providing

---

BOX 45.3 Diagnostic Criteria for Eating Disorders

Anorexia Nervosa
- Restriction of energy intake relative to requirements, leading to a significantly low body weight in relation to age, sex, developmental trajectory, and physical health
- Intense fear of gaining weight or of becoming fat, or persistent behavior that interferes with weight gain, even though at a significantly low weight
- Disturbance in the way in which one's body weight, size, or shape is experienced; undue influence of body weight or shape on self-evaluation; or persistent lack of recognition of the seriousness of the current low body weight (e.g., the person claims to "feel fat" even when emaciated, believes that one area of the body is "too fat" even when person is obviously underweight)

Bulimia Nervosa
- Recurrent episodes of binge eating (rapid consumption of a large amount of food in a discrete time period)
- A feeling of lack of control over eating behavior during eating binges
- Recurrent inappropriate compensatory behaviors to prevent weight gain, such as self-induced vomiting, use of laxatives or diuretics, strict dieting or fasting, or vigorous exercise
- Binge eating and inappropriate compensatory behaviors that both occur, on average, at least once a week for 3 months
- Self-evaluation unduly influenced by body shape and weight

Reprinted with permission from the *Diagnostic and Statistical Manual of Mental Disorders,* Fifth Edition, Text Revision (Copyright © 2013), American Psychiatric Association.

55% to 60% of total daily kilocalories. Protein needs increase to 1 to 1.5 g/kg/day. Fat needs do not increase. Adequate hydration is very important. Adolescents need to ingest water before and after exercise to prevent dehydration, especially in hot, humid environments. Vitamin and mineral supplements are not required, but intake of iron-rich foods is required to prevent anemia.

Parents have more influence on adolescents' diets than they believe. Effective strategies include limiting the amount of unhealthy food choices kept at home; encouraging smart snacks such as fruits, vegetables, or string cheese; and enhancing the appearance and taste of healthy foods (Mayo Clinic, 2021a). Some ways to promote healthy eating include making healthy food choices more convenient at home and at fast-food restaurants and discouraging adolescents from eating while watching television or using the computer.

Pregnancy occurring within 4 years of menarche places a mother and fetus at risk because of anatomical and physiological immaturity. Malnutrition at the time of conception increases risk to the adolescent and her fetus. Most teenage girls do not want to gain weight. Counseling related to nutritional needs of pregnancy is often difficult, and teens tolerate suggestions better than rigid directions. The diet of pregnant adolescents is often deficient in calcium, iron, and vitamins A and C. The American College of Obstetricians and Gynecologists (ACOG) recommends prenatal vitamin and mineral supplements (ACOG, 2021).

Young and Middle Adults. There is a reduction in nutrient demands as the growth period ends. Mature adults need nutrients for energy, maintenance, and repair. Energy needs usually decline over the years. Obesity becomes a problem because of decreased physical exercise, dining out more often, and increased ability to afford more luxury foods. Adult women who use oral contraceptives often need extra vitamins. Iron and calcium intake continue to be important.

Pregnancy. Poor nutrition during pregnancy causes low birth weight in infants and decreases chances of survival. In general, meeting the needs of a fetus is at the expense of the mother. However, if nutrient sources are unavailable, both suffer. The nutritional status of the mother at the time of conception is important. Significant aspects of fetal growth and development often occur before the mother suspects the pregnancy. The energy requirements of pregnancy relate to the mother's body weight and activity. The quality of nutrition during pregnancy is important, and food intake in the first trimester includes balanced parts of essential nutrients with emphasis on quality. Protein intake throughout pregnancy needs to increase to 60 g daily. Calcium intake is especially critical in the third trimester, when fetal bones mineralize. Providing iron supplements to meet the mother's increased blood volume, fetal blood storage, and blood loss during delivery is important.

Folic acid intake is particularly important for DNA synthesis and the growth of red blood cells. Inadequate intake can lead to fetal neural tube defects, anencephaly, or maternal megaloblastic anemia (Grodner et al., 2020). Women of childbearing age need to consume 400 mcg of folic acid daily, increasing to 600 mcg daily during pregnancy. Prenatal care usually includes vitamin and mineral supplementation to ensure daily intakes; however, pregnant women should not take additional supplements beyond prescribed amounts.

Lactation. Women who are lactating need 500 kcal/day above the usual allowance because the production of milk increases energy requirements. Protein requirements during lactation are greater than those required during pregnancy. The need for calcium remains the same as during pregnancy. There is an increased need for vitamins A and C. Daily intake of water-soluble vitamins (B and C) is necessary to ensure adequate levels in breast milk. Fluid intake needs to be adequate but not excessive. Excretion of caffeine, alcohol, and drugs occurs through breast milk. Therefore mothers who are lactating need to avoid their ingestion.

BOX 45.4 FOCUS ON OLDER ADULTS

Factors Affecting Nutritional Status

- Age-related gastrointestinal changes that affect digestion of food and maintenance of nutrition include changes in the teeth and gums, reduced saliva production, atrophy of oral mucosal epithelial cells, increased taste threshold, decreased thirst sensation, reduced gag reflex, and decreased esophageal and colonic peristalsis (Touhy and Jett, 2018).
- The presence of chronic illnesses (e.g., diabetes mellitus, end-stage renal disease, cancer) often affects nutrition intake.
- Adequate nutrition in older adults is affected by multiple causes, such as life-long eating habits, culture, socialization, income, educational level, physical functional level to meet activities of daily living (ADLs), loss, dentition, and transportation (Meiner and Yeager, 2019).
- Adverse effects of medications cause problems such as anorexia, gastrointestinal bleeding, xerostomia, early satiety, and impaired smell and taste perception (Burchum and Rosenthal, 2019).
- Cognitive impairments such as delirium, dementia, and depression affect ability to obtain, prepare, and eat healthy foods.

Older Adults. Adults 65 years and older have a decreased need for energy because their metabolic rate slows with age. However, vitamin and mineral requirements remain unchanged from middle adulthood. Numerous factors influence the nutritional status of the older adult (Box 45.4). Age-related changes in appetite, taste, smell, and the digestive system affect nutrition (Touhy and Jett, 2018). For example, older adults often experience a decrease in taste cells that alters food flavor and may decrease intake. Multiple factors contribute to the risk of food insecurity in the older adult. Income is significant because living on a fixed income often reduces the amount of money available to buy food. Health is another important influence that affects a person's desire and ability to eat. Lack of transportation or ability to get to the grocery store because of mobility problems contributes to inability to purchase adequate and nutritious food. Often availability of nutritionally adequate and safe foods is limited or uncertain.

Maintaining good oral health is significant throughout adulthood, particularly as an individual ages. Difficulty in chewing, missing teeth, having teeth in poor condition, and oral pain result from poor oral health. These often contribute to malnutrition and dehydration in older adults (Touhy and Jett, 2018). Poor oral hygiene and periodontal disease are potential risk factors for systemic diseases such as joint infections, ischemic stroke, cardiovascular disease, DM, and aspiration pneumonia (Touhy and Jett, 2018).

The older adult is often on a therapeutic diet; has difficulty eating because of physical symptoms, lack of teeth, or dentures; or is at risk for drug-nutrient interactions (Table 45.2). Caution older adults to avoid grapefruit and grapefruit juice because they alter absorption of many drugs. Thirst sensation diminishes, leading to inadequate fluid intake or dehydration (see Chapter 42). Symptoms of dehydration in older adults include confusion; weakness; hot, dry skin; furrowed tongue; rapid pulse; and high urinary sodium. Some older adults avoid meats because of cost or because they are difficult to chew. Cream soups and meat-based vegetable soups are nutrient-dense sources of protein. Cheese, eggs, and peanut butter are also useful high-protein alternatives. Foods rich in calcium, such as dairy products, green leafy vegetables, soy, nuts, fish (canned sardines and salmon with bones), and fortified grains, help protect against osteoporosis (a decrease of bone mass density) (National Osteoporosis Foundation [NOF], 2021). Screening and treatment are necessary for both older men and women.

TABLE 45.2 Sample of Drug-Nutrient Interactions[a]

Drug	Effect	Drug	Effect
Analgesic		**Antihypertensive**	
Acetaminophen	Decreased drug absorption with food; overdose associated with liver failure	Captopril	Taste alteration, anorexia
Aspirin	Absorbed directly through stomach; decreased drug absorption with food; decreased folic acid, vitamins C and K, and iron absorption	Hydralazine	Enhanced drug absorption with food, decreased vitamin B_6
		Labetalol	Taste alteration (weight gain for all beta blockers)
Antacid		Methyldopa	Decreased vitamin B_{12}, folic acid, iron
Aluminum hydroxide	Decreased phosphate absorption	**Antiinflammatory**	
Sodium bicarbonate	Decreased folic acid absorption	All steroids	Increased appetite and weight, increased folic acid, decreased calcium (osteoporosis with long-term use); promotes gluconeogenesis of protein
Antiarrhythmic			
Amiodarone	Taste alteration	**Antiparkinson**	
Digitalis	Anorexia, decreased renal clearance in older people	Levodopa	Taste alteration, decreased vitamin B_6 and drug absorption with food
Antibiotic		**Antipsychotic**	
Penicillin	Decreased drug absorption with food, taste alteration	Chlorpromazine	Increased appetite
Cephalosporin	Decreased vitamin K	Thiothixene	Decreased riboflavin, increased need
Rifampin	Decreased vitamin B_6, niacin, vitamin D	**Bronchodilator**	
Tetracycline	Decreased drug absorption with milk and antacids; decreased nutrient absorption of calcium, riboflavin, vitamin C caused by binding	Albuterol sulfate	Appetite stimulant
		Theophylline	Anorexia
Trimethoprim/ sulfamethoxazole	Decreased folic acid	**Cholesterol Lowering**	
		Cholestyramine	Decreased fat-soluble vitamins (A, D, E, K), vitamin B_{12}, iron
Anticoagulant		**Diuretic**	
Warfarin	Acts as antagonist to vitamin K	Furosemide	Decreased drug absorption with food
Anticonvulsant		Spironolactone	Increased drug absorption with food
Carbamazepine	Increased drug absorption with food	Thiazides	Decreased magnesium, zinc, and potassium
Phenytoin	Decreased calcium absorption; decreased vitamins D and K and folic acid; taste alteration; decreased drug absorption with food	**Laxative**	
		Mineral oil	Decreased absorption of fat-soluble vitamins (A, D, E, K), carotene
Antidepressant		**Platelet Aggregate Inhibitor**	
Amitriptyline	Appetite stimulant	Dipyridamole	Decreased drug absorption with food
Clomipramine	Taste alteration, appetite stimulant	**Potassium Replacement**	
Fluoxetine (selective serotonin reuptake inhibitor [SSRI])	Taste alteration, anorexia	Potassium chloride	Decreased vitamin B_{12}
		Tranquilizer	
		Benzodiazepines	Increased appetite

Data from Hermann J: *Nutrient and drug interactions*, 2019. http://pods.dasnr.okstate.edu/docushare/dsweb/Get/Document-2458/T-3120web.pdf. Accessed March 29, 2021; and Burchum JR, Rosenthal LD: *Lehne's pharmacology for nursing care*, ed 10, St Louis, 2019, Elsevier.
[a]Not intended to be an exhaustive or all-inclusive list. Always check pharmacology references before administering medications.

Vitamin D supplements are important for improving strength and balance, strengthening bone health, and preventing bone fractures and falls. The diet of older adults needs to contain choices from all food groups and often requires a vitamin and mineral supplement. MyPlate for Older Adults addresses the specific nutritional needs for older adults and encourages physical activity (USDA, n.d.a).

The USDHHS Administration on Aging (AOA) requires states to provide nutritional screening services to older adults who benefit from home-delivered or congregate meal services. This program requires meals to provide at least one-third of the DRI for an older adult and meet the Dietary Guidelines for Americans (Academy of Nutrition and Dietetics, 2021). Older adults who are homebound and have chronic illnesses have additional nutritional risks. They frequently live alone with few or no social or financial resources to help obtain or prepare nutritionally sound meals, contributing to the risk for food insecurity. Food insecurity in older adults is more prevalent if the individual is living with a disability, is living in southern or western states, or is a member of a racial or ethnic minority (National Council on Aging, 2021b). Increased nutritional screening by nurses results in early recognition and treatment of nutritional deficiencies. Undernourishment of older adults often results in health problems that lead to admission to acute care hospitals or long-term care facilities.

Alternative Food Patterns

Long before the FDA issued recommended allowances and guidelines, many people followed special patterns of food intake on the basis of religion (Table 45.3), cultural background (Box 45.5), health beliefs, personal preference, or concern for the efficient use of land to produce food. Such special diets are not necessarily more or less nutritious than diets based on the MyPlate or other nutritional guidelines because good nutrition depends on a balanced intake of all required nutrients.

Vegetarian Diet. A common alternative dietary pattern is the vegetarian diet. Vegetarianism is the consumption of a diet consisting predominantly of plant foods. Some vegetarians are ovolactovegetarian (avoid meat, fish, and poultry but eat eggs and milk), lactovegetarians (drink milk but avoid eggs), or vegans (consume only plant foods). Through careful selection of foods, individuals following a vegetarian diet can meet recommendations for proteins and essential nutrients (Grodner et al., 2020). Children who follow a vegetarian diet are especially at risk for

TABLE 45.3	Examples of Religious Dietary Restrictions					
Muslim	**Christianity**	**Hinduism**	**Judaism**	**Church of Jesus Christ of Latter-Day Saints (Mormons)**	**Seventh-Day Adventists Church**
Pork	Some faiths such as	All meats	Pork	Alcohol	Pork
Alcohol	Baptists allow	Fish, shellfish	Predatory fowl	Tobacco	Shellfish
Ramadan fasting	minimal or no	with some	Shellfish (eat only fish with scales)	Caffeine such as in teas,	Fish
sunrise to sunset	alcohol	restrictions	Rare meats	coffees, and sodas	Alcohol
for a month	Some meatless	Alcohol	Blood (e.g., blood sausage)		Caffeine
Ritualized methods	days may be		Mixing of milk or dairy products with meat		Vegetarian or
of animal	observed during		dishes		ovolactovegetarian
slaughter	the calendar year,		Must adhere to kosher food preparation		diets encouraged
required for	commonly during		methods		
meat ingestion	Lent		24 hr of fasting on Yom Kippur, a day of		
			atonement		
			No leavened bread eaten during Passover		
			(8 days)		
			No cooking on the Sabbath from sundown		
			Friday to sundown Saturday		

🌐 BOX 45.5 CULTURAL ASPECTS OF CARE

Nutrition

Food patterns developed as a child, habits, and culture interact to influence food intake. Culture also influences the meaning of food not related to nutrition. Eating is associated with sentiments and feelings such as "good" and "bad." For example, children are often rewarded for "being good" with a treat such as candy. They then associate candy with "being good." Food frequently enhances interpersonal relationships and demonstrates love and caring.

Sometimes certain ethnic groups develop genetically related conditions. For example, lactose intolerance, a deficiency of the intestinal enzyme lactase, can be found among individuals of Asian-Pacific, African and African American, Native American, Mexican American, Middle Eastern, and Caucasian descent. Lactose intolerance affects nutrient absorption. Calcium deficiency often results, causing decreased bone mass density.

The theory of hot and cold foods predominates in many cultures. The origin appears to be from Hippocratic beliefs concerning health and the four humors. Arabs were keepers of this knowledge during the Dark Ages and later influenced the Spanish to adopt this belief system in the later Middle Ages. The foundation of the theory is keeping harmony with nature by balancing "cold," "hot," "wet," and "dry." Some cultures believe that hot is warmth, strength, and reassurance, whereas cold is menacing and weak. Classification has nothing to do with spiciness but is a symbolic representation of temperature (Giger and Haddad, 2021).

Different cultures also have beliefs about food and special dishes that should be eaten when sick (e.g., chicken soup during illness).

Implications for Patient-Centered Care

- Ask patient or family caregiver to identify the meaning that they have for the types of food they commonly eat.
- Lactose and other food intolerances unique to specific cultures require diet adaptation to meet nutrient, mineral, and vitamin daily intake requirements.
- When patients use hot and cold foods as part of their cultural health practices, dietary modifications are necessary. Hot foods include rice, grain cereals, alcohol, beef, lamb, chili peppers, chocolate, cheese, temperate zone fruits, eggs, peas, goat's milk, cornhusks, oils, onions, pork, radishes, and tamales. By contrast, cold foods are beans, citrus fruits, tropical fruits, dairy products, most vegetables, honey, raisins, chicken, fish, and goat.
- Ask patient or family caregiver if there are:
  - Specific conditions such as menstruation, cancer, pneumonia, earache, colds, paralysis, headache, or rheumatism, which are cold illnesses and require hot foods
  - Other conditions such as pregnancy, fever, infections, diarrhea, rashes, ulcers, liver problems, constipation, kidney problems, or sore throats, which are hot conditions and require cold foods

protein and vitamin deficiencies, such as a lack of vitamin B₁₂. Careful planning helps to ensure a balanced, healthy diet.

Prior to his next appointment with Mrs. Cooper, Ryan reviews Mrs. Cooper's electronic health record, so he is prepared to work with her on her nutrition and depression problems. He found that she is taking metoprolol 25 mg twice a day, glipizide 10 mg daily, and warfarin 2.5 mg daily. Ryan reviews her medications and the effects that they might have on appetite and nutritional status. After talking with Mrs. Cooper, Ryan recognizes that she has been experiencing nutritional problems along with depression and coping problems. As Ryan prepares to assess Mrs. Cooper, he recalls information about nutrition and older adults, especially the importance of adequate calorie, protein, and fluid intake in patients who have DM, hypertension, and heart failure. Ryan goes over the components of a nutritional assessment to ensure that he gathers as much assessment data from Mrs. Cooper as possible so that he can develop an individualized plan. He knows that preferences, finances, culture, and religion can impact food choice and meal planning. Ryan completes reading on how DM, hypertension, and heart failure affect nutrition, especially in older adults. He also reviews typical diet therapy related to Mrs. Cooper's three chronic health problems, knowing how important it is for her to watch her sodium, cholesterol, carbohydrate, and sugar intake. Also, because she is taking warfarin, Mrs. Cooper needs to watch her intake of green leafy vegetables. Ryan recognizes that Mrs. Cooper is depressed and continues to grieve the loss of her husband, so he reviewed the literature regarding the relationship between eating patterns and depression. Ryan suspects that Mrs. Cooper is experiencing social isolation because she has stopped interacting regularly with friends and attending social activities. He knows that this is common in older adults and reads about strategies to help Mrs. Cooper. He wants to be able to develop a plan that addresses this problem because of its impact on her overall nutritional status.

CRITICAL THINKING

Successful clinical judgment requires critical thinking that involves a synthesis of knowledge, experience, environmental factors, critical thinking attitudes, and intellectual and professional standards. Sound clinical judgments require you to anticipate information, analyze the data, and make clinical decisions regarding your patient's care. During assessment consider all elements that build toward making an appropriate nursing diagnosis (Fig. 45.3).

Integrate knowledge from nursing and other disciplines such as dietetics, pharmacology, and psychology; previous experiences; and assessment information gathered from a patient and the patient's diet history to understand the patient's nutritional problem and its effects. Knowing how digestion and absorption work aids in understanding the rationale for a patient's nutritional problems. In addition, communication principles allow you to effectively assess a patient's behaviors and problems that arise from lack of nutrition. Give patients time to describe their perception of the situation and their ability to resolve the nutritional problem. It is important to consider a patient's preferences, culture, socioeconomic status, environment, and religious practices when developing meal plans to meet the patient's nutritional needs.

FIG. 45.3 Critical thinking model for nutrition assessment. (Clinical Judgment Measurement Model copyright © NCSBN. All rights reserved.)

Personal experience with a nutritional problem and experience with patients prepares you to know effective forms of nutritional therapies. Experience teaches you to understand the patient's unique perspective and recognize that no two people are exactly alike. Experience with patients also helps you to recognize responses to poor nutrition or digestion and absorption problems. In addition, personal experiences with good nutritional practices helps you better understand a patient who is experiencing inadequate nutrition.

Use critical thinking attitudes such as open-mindedness, confidence, creativity, and discipline to complete a comprehensive assessment and develop a patient-centered, individualized plan of care to provide successful management of the nutritional problem. Patients experiencing nutritional problems are often overwhelmed and look to you as the expert to help them resolve their food and nutrition issues.

Professional standards such as the DRIs, the USDA MyPlate dietary guidelines, and *Healthy People 2030* objectives provide guidelines to assess and maintain patients' nutritional status. Other professional standards and guidelines from the AHA (2017), the ADA (2021b), the ACS (2021), and the American Society for Parenteral and Enteral Nutrition (ASPEN, 2021) are available. These standards are evidence based and regularly updated for optimal patient care.

REFLECT NOW

What assessment findings in an adolescent child would be indicative of altered nutrition? What are risk factors that lead to altered nutritional status in this age-group?

❖ NURSING PROCESS

Use clinical judgment while applying critical thinking to the nursing process. The nursing process provides a clinical decision-making approach for you to identify patient problems, develop and implement an individualized patient-centered plan of care, and evaluate that plan.

◆ Assessment

During the assessment process thoroughly assess each patient and critically analyze findings to recognize patterns of data and then identify accurate and relevant nursing diagnoses. This ensures a patient-centered approach for safe nursing care. Early recognition of patients who are malnourished or at risk has a strong positive influence on both short- and long-term health outcomes. Studies demonstrate a link between malnutrition in adult hospitalized patients and readmission rates, higher mortality rates, and increased cost (Reed Mangels, 2018). Patients who are malnourished on admission are at greater risk of significant complications such as arrhythmia, skin breakdown, sepsis, or hemorrhage during hospitalization.

Through the Patient's Eyes. Close contact with patients and their families enables you to observe physical status, food intake, food preferences, weight changes, and cultural practices in eating. Always ask patients about their food preferences, values regarding nutrition, and expectations from nutritional therapy. For example, does a patient want to learn about a diet? In attempting to affect eating patterns, you need to understand patients' preferences, values, beliefs, and attitudes about food. Assess family traditions and rituals related to food, cultural values and beliefs, and nutritional needs. Determine how these factors affect the patient's ability to purchase and prepare food and the patient's food intake.

Screening. Gather a patient's nursing history to collect information about factors that usually influence nutrition. You are in an excellent position to consider the patient's condition, anticipate signs or symptoms related to that condition, and then recognize signs of poor nutrition that the patient presents. These findings lead you to additional questions to ask beyond screening. Nutrition screening is an essential part of an initial assessment. Screening a patient is a quick method of identifying malnutrition or risk of malnutrition using simple tools (McEvilly, 2017). Nutrition screening tools gather data on a patient's response to the current condition and typically include objective measures such as height, weight, weight change, primary diagnosis, and the presence of other comorbidities (McEvilly, 2017). Combine multiple objective measures with subjective measures related to nutrition to adequately screen for nutritional problems. Identification of risk factors such as unintentional weight loss, presence of a modified diet, or the presence of altered nutritional symptoms (i.e., nausea, vomiting, diarrhea, and constipation) requires nutritional consultation.

Several standardized nutritional screening tools are available for use in outpatient and inpatient settings. The Subjective Global Assessment (SGA) uses the patient history, weight, and physical assessment data to assess nutritional status (Wittenaar and Ottery, 2017). The SGA is a simple, inexpensive technique that predicts nutrition-related complications. The Mini Nutritional Assessment (MNA) (Fig. 45.4) screens older adults receiving care in their homes, nursing homes, and hospitals. The tool has 18 items divided into screening and assessment. If a patient scores 11 or lower on the screening part, the health care provider completes the assessment part. The MNA has been used successfully to screen for frailty in older adults (Soysal et al., 2019). Malnutrition screening tools (MSTs), such as the MNA or the DETERMINE checklist, are an effective way to measure nutritional problems for patients in a variety of health care settings (Dodd, 2020).

Assess patients for malnutrition when they have conditions that interfere with their ability to ingest, digest, or absorb adequate nutrients. Use standardized tools to assess nutritional risks when possible and identify factors that place your patients at risk for nutritional problems. For example, congenital anomalies and surgical revisions of the GI tract are risk factors because they interfere with normal function. Patients receiving only an intravenous (IV) infusion of 5% or 10% dextrose are at risk for nutritional deficiencies because of lack of proteins and fats in the infusions. Chronic diseases or altered metabolic requirements, such as kidney disease or DM, are risk factors for development of nutritional problems. Infants and older adults are at greatest risk.

Anthropometry. Anthropometry is a systematic method of measuring the size and makeup of the body. Nurses obtain height and weight for each patient on hospital admission or entry into any health care setting. If you are unable to measure height with the patient standing, position the patient lying flat in bed as straight as possible with arms folded on the chest and measure the patient lengthwise. Serial measures of weight over time provide more useful information than one measurement. Weigh the patient at the same time each day, on the same scale, and with the same type of clothing or linen. Document the patient's actual weight and compare height and weight with standards for height-weight relationships. An ideal body weight (IBW) provides an estimate of what a person should weigh.

Rapid weight gain or loss is important to note because it usually reflects fluid shifts. One pint or 500 mL of fluid equals 1 lb (0.45 kg). For example, for a patient with renal failure, a weight increase of 2 lb (0.90 kg) in 24 hours is significant because it usually indicates that the patient has retained 1 L (1000 mL) of fluid.

Mini Nutritional Assessment
MNA®

Last name:		First name:		
Sex:	Age:	Weight, kg:	Height, cm:	Date:

Complete the screen by filling in the boxes with the appropriate numbers. Total the numbers for the final screening score.

Screening

A Has food intake declined over the past 3 months due to loss of appetite, digestive problems, chewing or swallowing difficulties?
0 = severe decrease in food intake
1 = moderate decrease in food intake
2 = no decrease in food intake ☐

B Weight loss during the last 3 months
0 = weight loss greater than 3 kg (6.6 lbs)
1 = does not know
2 = weight loss between 1 and 3 kg (2.2 and 6.6 lbs)
3 = no weight loss ☐

C Mobility
0 = bed or chair bound
1 = able to get out of bed / chair but does not go out
2 = goes out ☐

D Has suffered psychological stress or acute disease in the past 3 months?
0 = yes   2 = no ☐

E Neuropsychological problems
0 = severe dementia or depression
1 = mild dementia
2 = no psychological problems ☐

F1 Body Mass Index (BMI) (weight in kg) / (height in m^2)
0 = BMI less than 19
1 = BMI 19 to less than 21
2 = BMI 21 to less than 23
3 = BMI 23 or greater ☐

IF BMI IS NOT AVAILABLE, REPLACE QUESTION F1 WITH QUESTION F2.
DO NOT ANSWER QUESTION F2 IF QUESTION F1 IS ALREADY COMPLETED.

F2 Calf circumference (CC) in cm
0 = CC less than 31
3 = CC 31 or greater ☐

Screening score ☐☐
(max. 14 points)

12-14 points:	Normal nutritional status
8-11 points:	At risk of malnutrition
0-7 points:	Malnourished

Ref.   Vellas B, Villars H, Abellan G, et al. *Overview of the MNA® - Its History and Challenges.* J Nutr Health Aging 2006;10:456-465.

Rubenstein LZ, Harker JO, Salva A, Guigoz Y, Vellas B. *Screening for Undernutrition in Geriatric Practice: Developing the Short-Form Mini Nutritional Assessment (MNA-SF).* J. Geront 2001;56A: M366-377.

Guigoz Y. *The Mini-Nutritional Assessment (MNA®) Review of the Literature - What does it tell us?* J Nutr Health Aging 2006; 10:466-487.

Kaiser MJ, Bauer JM, Ramsch C, et al. *Validation of the Mini Nutritional Assessment Short-Form (MNA®-SF): A practical tool for identification of nutritional status.* J Nutr Health Aging 2009; 13:782-788.

® Société des Produits Nestlé, S.A., Vevey, Switzerland, Trademark Owners

© Nestlé, 1994, Revision 2009. N67200 12/99 10M

For more information: www.mna-elderly.com

FIG. 45.4 Mini Nutritional Assessment (MNA). (Copyright © Nestlé, 1994, Revision 2009. N67200 12/99 10M.)

Other anthropometric measurements often obtained by RDs help identify nutritional problems. These include the ratio of height-to-wrist circumference, mid–upper arm circumference (MAC), triceps skinfold (TSF), and mid–upper arm muscle circumference (MAMC). An RD compares values for MAC, TSF, and MAMC to standards and calculates them as a percentage of the standard. Changes in values for an individual over weeks to months are of greater significance than isolated measurements (Grodner et al., 2020).

Body mass index (BMI) measures weight corrected for height and serves as an alternative to traditional height-weight relationships. Calculate BMI by dividing a patient's weight in kilograms by height in meters squared: weight (kg) divided by height^2 (m^2). For example, a patient who weighs 165 lb (75 kg) and is 1.8 m (5 feet 9 inches) tall has a BMI of 23.15 ($75 \div 1.8^2 = 23.15$). The website for the National Heart, Lung, and Blood Institute (https://www.nhlbi.nih.gov/health/educational/lose_wt/BMI/bmicalc.htm) provides an easy way to calculate BMI. Patients are overweight if their BMI is 25 to 30. Obesity, defined by a BMI of greater than 30, places a patient at higher medical risk of coronary heart disease, some cancers, DM, and hypertension.

Laboratory and Biochemical Tests. Multiple laboratory and biochemical tests are used to diagnose malnutrition. Factors that frequently alter test results include fluid balance, liver function, kidney function, and the presence of disease. Common laboratory tests used to study nutritional status include measures of plasma proteins such as albumin, transferrin, prealbumin, retinol-binding protein, total iron-binding capacity, and hemoglobin. After feeding, the response time for changes in these proteins ranges from hours to weeks. The metabolic half-life of albumin is 21 days, transferrin is 8 days, prealbumin is 2 days, and retinol-binding protein is 12 hours. Use this information to determine the most effective measure of plasma proteins for your patients. Factors that affect serum albumin levels include hydration; hemorrhage; renal and hepatic disease; drainage from wounds, drains, burns, or the GI tract; steroid administration; exogenous albumin infusions; age; trauma; burns; stress; or surgery. Albumin level is a better indicator of malnutrition in patients with long-term chronic illnesses, whereas prealbumin level is preferred for short-term changes in acute conditions (Grodner et al., 2020).

Nitrogen balance is important in determining serum protein status (see discussion of protein in this chapter). To determine a patient's nitrogen balance, you need to know how many grams of protein your patient ingests in a 24-hour period as well as the results from a 24-hour urine urea nitrogen (UUN) test, which measures nitrogen output. Calculate nitrogen balance by dividing 6.25 into the total grams of protein ingested in a day (24 hours). Use laboratory analysis of a 24-hour UUN to determine nitrogen output. For patients with diarrhea or fistula drainage, estimate a further addition of 2 to 4 g of nitrogen output. Nitrogen balance is calculated by subtracting the nitrogen output from the nitrogen intake. A positive 2- to 3-g nitrogen balance is necessary for anabolism. By contrast, negative nitrogen balance is present when catabolic states exist.

Diet History and Health History. After gathering data in a general nursing history, focus assessment on a more specific diet history to assess a patient's actual or potential nutritional needs. Box 45.6 lists some specific assessment questions to ask in the diet history. The diet history includes an assessment of a patient's knowledge about any therapeutic diet that has been prescribed and about general nutritional health. If a patient is on a therapeutic diet, ask for examples of the patient's typical food choices. What is a patient's normal daily intake of food and liquids? The diet history also focuses on a patient's food preferences, allergies, and other relevant areas such as the patient's ability to

---

BOX 45.6 Nursing Assessment Questions

Dietary Intake and Food Preferences
- What type of food do you like?
- How many meals a day do you eat?
- What times do you normally eat meals and snacks?
- What portion sizes do you eat at each meal?
- Describe any special diet that you follow for a medical problem.
- Tell me about your dietary religious or cultural food preferences.
- Who prepares the food at home?
- Who purchases the food?
- How do you cook your food (e.g., fried, broiled, baked, grilled)?

Unpleasant Symptoms
- Which foods cause indigestion, gas, or heartburn?
- How often does this occur?
- What relieves the symptoms?

Allergies
- Are you allergic to any foods?
- Which types of problems do you have when you eat these foods?
- How are these food allergies treated (e.g., EpiPen, oral antihistamines)?

Taste, Chewing, and Swallowing
- Have you noticed any changes in taste?
- Did these changes occur with medications or following an illness?
- Do you wear dentures? Are the dentures comfortable?
- Do you have any mouth pain or sores (e.g., cold sore, canker sores)?
- Do you have difficulty swallowing?
- Do you cough or gag when you swallow?

Appetite and Weight
- Tell me about any recent change in appetite.
- Tell me about any recent change in your weight.
- Was this change anticipated (e.g., were you on a weight-reduction diet)?

Use of Medications
- Which medications do you take?
- Describe any over-the-counter medications you take that your doctor does not prescribe.
- Do you take any nutritional or herbal supplements?

---

obtain food. Gather information about the patient's illness and activity level to determine energy needs and compare food intake. Your nursing assessment of nutrition also includes health status; age; cultural background (see Box 45.5); religious food patterns (see Table 45.3); socioeconomic status; psychological factors; use of alcohol or illegal drugs; and a complete medication history (see Table 45.2).

In an outpatient setting, have a patient keep a 3- to 7-day food diary if you suspect nutritional problems. This allows you to calculate nutritional intake and to compare it with DRI to see whether the patient's dietary habits are adequate. Use food questionnaires to establish patterns over time. In a health care setting, nurses collaborate with RDs to complete calorie counts for patients.

Environment. Assessment of the individual's home environment is an important component in nutritional assessment. Environment includes where you eat, how you eat, who you eat with, social media and advertising, and your grocery store (Team Legion, 2021). "How you eat" is affected by portion sizes. "Who you eat with" includes eating habits through socialization and peer pressure. For older adults, eating with someone can improve eating habits (National Council on Aging, 2021a). Social media and advertising can convince individuals to purchase foods that are not healthy and are not normally in their diet. At the grocery store, the layout of the aisles and the size of the cart that you use can influence purchases (Team Legion, 2021). To avoid problems at the grocery store, have patients make a list before they go and stick with the list. It is important to explore with individuals how their environment affects their eating habits and food choices so that individuals can avoid making poor decisions related to dietary habits (Team Legion, 2021).

Physical Examination. A physical examination is one of the most important aspects of a nutritional assessment. Because improper nutrition affects all body systems, observe for malnutrition during physical assessment (see Chapter 30). Complete the general physical assessment of body systems and review relevant areas to assess a patient's nutritional status. The clinical signs of alterations in nutritional status (Table 45.4) serve as guidelines for observation during physical assessment.

Dysphagia. Dysphagia refers to difficulty swallowing. There are a variety of causes and complications of dysphagia (Box 45.7). Complications include aspiration pneumonia, dehydration, decreased nutritional status, and weight loss. Dysphagia leads to disability or decreased functional status, increased length of stay and health care costs, increased likelihood of discharge to institutionalized care, and increased mortality (Yang et al., 2017).

Be aware of warning signs for dysphagia. They include cough during eating; change in voice tone or quality after swallowing; abnormal movements of the mouth, tongue, or lips; and slow, weak, imprecise, or uncoordinated speech. Abnormal gag, delayed swallowing, incomplete oral clearance or pocketing, regurgitation, pharyngeal pooling, delayed or absent trigger of swallow, and inability to speak consistently are other signs of dysphagia. Patients with dysphagia often do not show overt signs such as coughing when food enters the airway. *Silent aspiration* is aspiration that occurs in patients with neurological problems that leads to decreased sensation. It often occurs without a cough, and symptoms (e.g., adventitious breath sounds, slight fever) usually do not appear for 24 hours. Silent aspiration is common in patients with dysphagia following stroke (Yang et al., 2017).

Dysphagia often leads to an inadequate amount of food intake, which results in malnutrition. Frequently patients with dysphagia become frustrated with eating and show changes in skinfold thickness and albumin. During the rehabilitation period patients experience longer adjustment periods regarding new dietary restrictions. Furthermore, malnutrition significantly slows swallowing recovery and may increase mortality (Grodner et al., 2020).

Dysphagia screening quickly identifies problems with swallowing and helps you initiate referrals for more in-depth assessment by an RD or a speech-language pathologist (SLP) (see Skill 45.1). Early and ongoing assessment of patients with dysphagia using a valid dysphagia-screening tool increases quality of care and decreases incidence of aspiration pneumonia (Suiter et al., 2020). Dysphagia screening includes medical record review; observation of a patient at a meal for change in voice quality, posture, and head control; percentage of meal consumed; eating time; drooling or leakage of liquids and solids; cough during or after a swallow; facial or tongue weakness; palatal movement; difficulty with secretions; pocketing; choking; and a spontaneous dry cough. Several validated screening tools are available, such as the Bedside Swallowing Assessment, Burke Dysphagia Screening Test, Acute Stroke Dysphagia Screen, and Standardized Swallowing Assessment (Dong et al., 2016). The Acute Stroke Dysphagia Screen is an easily administered and reliable tool for health care professionals who are not SLPs. Screening for and treatment

TABLE 45.4 Physical Signs of Alterations in Nutritional Status

Body Area	Indicators of Malnutrition
General appearance	Easily fatigued, no energy, falls asleep easily; looks tired, apathetic, cachectic
Weight	Overweight, obese, or underweight (special concern for underweight); unplanned weight loss over period of time
Posture	Poor posture, sagging shoulders, sunken chest, humped back
Muscles	Flaccid, weak, poor tone, tender; "wasted" appearance; impaired mobility
Mental status	Inattentive, irritable, confused
Neurological function	Burning and tingling of hands and feet (paresthesia), loss of position and vibratory sense, decrease or loss of ankle and knee reflexes
Gastrointestinal function	Anorexia, indigestion, constipation or diarrhea, symptoms of malabsorption, liver or spleen enlargement, abdominal distention
Cardiovascular function	Tachycardia, abnormal rhythm, elevated blood pressure
Hair	Stringy, dull, brittle, dry, thin and sparse, depigmented
Skin (general)	Rough, dry, scaly, pale, pigmented, irritated, bruises, petechiae
Face and neck	Swollen, skin dark over cheeks and under eyes
Lips	Dry, scaly, swollen; redness and swelling at the corners of the mouth (cheilosis); angular lesions at corners of mouth, fissures, or scars (stomatitis)
Mouth, oral mucous membranes	Swollen, deep red oral mucous membranes; oral lesions
Gums	Spongy, bleed easily, inflamed, receding
Tongue	Swelling, scarlet and raw, magenta color, beefy (glossitis)
Teeth	Missing teeth, broken teeth
Eyes	Eye membranes pale (pale conjunctivae), redness of membrane (conjunctival injection), dryness or infection
Nails	Spoon-shaped (koilonychia), brittle, ridged
Legs and feet	Edema, tender calf, tingling, weakness, lesions
Skeleton	Bowlegs, knock-knees, chest deformity at diaphragm, beaded ribs, prominent scapulas

Data from Ball JW et al: *Seidel's guide to physical examination: an interprofessional approach,* ed 9, St Louis, 2019, Elsevier; Grodner M, et al: *Nutritional foundations and clinical applications,* ed 7, St Louis, 2020, Elsevier; Jensen GL, et al: GLIM criteria for the diagnosis of malnutrition: a consensus report from the Global Clinical Nutrition Community, *JPEN J Ent Parent Nutr* 43(1):32, 2019; and World Health Organization (WHO): *Malnutrition,* 2020. https://www.who.int/news-room/fact-sheets/detail/malnutrition. Accessed August 1, 2020.

of dysphagia requires an interprofessional team approach of nurses, RDs, health care providers, and SLPs (American Speech-Language-Hearing Association [ASHA], 2021b).

As Ryan prepares to assess Mrs. Cooper, he knows that it is important to consider nutrition changes that occur in older adults. He knows that with aging, changes in digestion and absorption and nutrition needs occur. He also recognizes that depression can cause eating problems. Ryan completes a nutrition assessment on Mrs. Cooper. Mrs. Cooper's vital signs are blood

BOX 45.7   Causes of Dysphagia

Myogenic
- Myasthenia gravis
- Aging
- Muscular dystrophy
- Polymyositis

Neurogenic
- Stroke
- Cerebral palsy
- Guillain-Barré syndrome
- Multiple sclerosis
- Amyotrophic lateral sclerosis (Lou Gehrig disease)
- Diabetic neuropathy
- Parkinson disease

Obstructive
- Benign peptic stricture
- Lower esophageal ring
- Candidiasis
- Head and neck cancer
- Inflammatory masses
- Trauma/surgical resection
- Anterior mediastinal masses
- Cervical spondylosis

Other
- Gastrointestinal or esophageal resection
- Rheumatological disorders
- Connective tissue disorders
- Vagotomy

BOX 45.8   Nursing Diagnostic Process

Impaired Low Nutritional Intake

Assessment Activities	Assessment Findings
Changes in weight	72-year-old woman 24-lb (10.8-kg) weight loss Weight is 20% below her ideal body weight
Body mass index (BMI)	BMI = 17
24-hour food and fluid history	Does not eat breakfast Frequently skips dinner Eats sandwich in afternoon Caloric intake is less than daily requirement Fluid intake is juice and coffee
Physical assessment	Poor muscle tone Fatigue Hair loss Dry, scaly skin Pale conjunctiva and mucous membranes
Medication history	Takes antidepressant for depression
Social	Husband died 9 months ago Has quit attending monthly quilting club Started counseling 3 months ago

pressure, 144/88 mm Hg; pulse, 92 beats/min and irregular; and respirations, 14 breaths/min. Mrs. Cooper's international normalized ratio (INR) from the previous week was 2.2. As part of the nutrition history, Ryan asks Mrs. Cooper to describe her normal eating habits over a period of 3 days. She responds that she drinks some juice in the morning and two or three cups of coffee. In addition, she often has a sandwich in the late afternoon and skips dinner. "Recently, I'm just not interested in food. It has no taste." Ryan's assessment also reveals that Mrs. Cooper's weight is 20% below her IBW and her BMI is 17. Mrs. Cooper has lost 24 lb over the past 9 months. Ryan also notes that Mrs. Cooper's posture is stooped when she walks and sits. Other assessment findings include that Mrs. Cooper is experiencing hair loss and has sore mucous membranes and pale mucous membranes. She also reports feelings of fatigue and appears to be frail. Ryan knows that Mrs. Cooper's husband died 9 months ago and that 3 months ago she started taking an antidepressant medication. When Ryan questions Mrs. Cooper about how she is feeling, Mrs. Cooper complains of loneliness and says that she does not get out much. Her friends at church call her to come back to meetings, but she is just not ready, and she has stopped attending weekly services. She says that since she feels tired all the time, she no longer attends the monthly meetings of her quilt club at the senior center. Ryan recognizes that Mrs. Cooper's behavior is representative of social isolation.

As Ryan prepares to develop a plan with Mrs. Cooper to improve her nutrition and social isolation, he draws from his experience working with older adults. He knows that older adults often experience decreased appetite, and socialization helps improve appetite and eating. Ryan also knows that physical and financial problems can alter meal planning. Ryan has read evidence-based journal articles on nutrition, social isolation in older adults, and depression. He wants to be sure that the proposed plan for Mrs. Cooper considers all potential factors influencing her nutrition, social isolation, and depression. Ryan asks Mrs. Cooper about nutrition and social activities prior to her husband's death so he can make a comparison and develop an individualized plan of care for Mrs. Cooper.

REFLECT NOW

Consider a patient you recently cared for during a clinical experience and who had risks for nutritional alterations. What assessments did you make of his or her nutritional status? What are some risk factors that potentially put your patient at risk for malnutrition?

◆ Analysis and Nursing Diagnosis

Review your assessment data, looking for clusters of data that provide cues that reveal the type of health problems exhibited by your patient (Box 45.8). A nutritional problem occurs when overall intake is significantly decreased or increased or when one or more nutrients are not ingested, completely digested, or completely absorbed. Carefully review your patient's assessment data to consider whether more than one diagnosis applies. For example, an individual who is experiencing *Impaired Low Nutritional Intake* may also have a nursing diagnosis of *Fatigue* due to the poor nutrition. However, be sure that assessment cues are present or if you need more information. When assessment data analysis identifies a negative or problem-focused nursing diagnosis, you select the appropriate related factors (e.g., inability to digest food or reduced daily activity). Related factors need to be accurate, so you select the right interventions. For example, *Impaired Low Nutritional Intake* related to economic disadvantage will require vastly different interventions than *Impaired Low Nutritional Intake* related to an inability to ingest food. These related factors become the focus of interventions for minimizing or eliminating a negative or problem-focused diagnosis.

A patient will have a risk nursing diagnosis when assessment reveals risk factors instead of an actual nutritional problem. For example, *Risk for Nutritional Excess* can be identified by the presence of risk factors such as excessive alcohol consumption or high frequency of eating restaurant food and adult BMI approaching 25 kg/m². Be specific so that you can direct interventions toward risk factors.

Assessment findings may also point to a health promotion diagnosis such as *Health-Seeking Behavior*. The following are examples of nursing diagnoses applicable to nutritional problems:
- Risk for Aspiration
- Overweight
- Impaired Low Nutritional Intake
- Impaired Self-Feeding
- Impaired Swallowing

CONCEPT MAP

Nursing diagnosis: Impaired low nutritional intake
- States lack of interest in food
- Recent weight loss of 24 lb
- Body weight more than 20% under ideal weight
- Lonely and tires easily

Interventions
- Teach Mrs. Cooper about dietary guidelines for older adults
- Encourage Mrs. Cooper to eat small, well-balanced meals and nutritious snacks
- Encourage Mrs. Cooper to increase protein in her diet
- Assist Mrs. Cooper in a 3-day meal plan that increases fluid and fiber intake

Nursing diagnosis: Impaired socialisation
- States, "I am having trouble connecting with my friends since my husband died"
- Friend reports that relationship with patient has become "strained" since Mrs. Cooper's husband died

Interventions
- Encourage Mrs. Cooper to call a friend and attend a church meeting
- Recommend that Mrs. Cooper begin attending her quilting group meetings
- Encourage Mrs. Cooper to eat lunch at the senior center 5 times per week

Primary health problem: Heart failure, depression
Priority assessments: Diet history, medication history, nutritional screening, anthropometric measures, food security

Nursing diagnosis: Fatigue
- Difficulty paying attention and concentrating during patient teaching
- States, "I am so tired; even after I wake up, I can hardly get out of bed"
- Inability to maintain usual routines (e.g., make dinner, clean the house)

Interventions
- Instruct Mrs. Cooper to rest for 30 minutes before meals
- Teach Mrs. Cooper how to balance her activities with rest periods
- Encourage Mrs. Cooper to take a short afternoon nap
- Encourage Mrs. Cooper to contact a friend and take a walk daily

Nursing diagnosis: Difficulty coping
- Fatigue and inability to sleep through the night
- States, "I cannot seem to do anything right without my husband around"
- Recent change in appearance; disheveled; wearing dirty clothes; states, "I really don't care how I look anymore"

Interventions
- Encourage Mrs. Cooper to verbalize her feelings and fears
- Use a calm, reassuring, active listening approach when talking with Mrs. Cooper
- Refer Mrs. Cooper to a counselor for help with her grief
- Encourage Mrs. Cooper to attend the local grief support group

——— Link between medical diagnosis and nursing diagnosis   - - - - - Link between nursing diagnoses

FIG. 45.5 Concept map for Mrs. Cooper.

In addition, there are clinical situations in which patients have multiple related nursing diagnoses. The concept map in Fig. 45.5 that contains Mrs. Cooper's nursing diagnoses is one tool to show the relationship among numerous identified nursing diagnoses.

Through his assessment, Ryan learns more about Mrs. Cooper's food preferences, eating habits, and knowledge about nutrition. Ryan also recognizes that Mrs. Cooper is experiencing grief and depression from the loss of her husband and is becoming more socially isolated. This combination of stressors contributes to Mrs. Cooper's nutritional problems, affecting all aspects of her life and leading to her weight loss and fatigue. Mrs. Cooper

provides her eating history for the last 3 days, she reports not eating breakfast except for juice and coffee, having a sandwich for a late lunch, and often skipping the evening meal. She tells Ryan that she does not have an appetite, and nothing sounds appealing to her for meals. Mrs. Cooper has been grieving her husband's loss for the past 9 months. She started her antidepressant for depression 3 months ago. Mrs. Cooper reports she has problems falling asleep and staying asleep. Along with her weight loss, Mrs. Cooper reports feeling tired all the time and withdrawing from all her activities such as making dinner, cleaning the house, and going to church and her quilting club. During her appointment with Ryan, Mrs. Cooper becomes teary eyed when talking about her husband and states, "I miss him so much and am so lonely without him. We were together for 48 years and enjoyed our travels and friends. Now I don't feel like going out with our friends anymore. I hardly call my friends these days." Ryan notes the physical changes that Mrs. Cooper has due to her poor nutrition. He assesses Mrs. Cooper's mucous membranes and finds that they are pale with sores. Mrs. Cooper's skin is pale and she has a stooped posture. Mrs. Cooper does not maintain eye contact when talking with Ryan. She appears to have difficulty paying attention and concentrating during the conversation. Ryan also notes that Mrs. Cooper's appearance is disheveled.

As Ryan analyzes these assessment findings, the data clusters provide him cues that lead him to identify **Impaired Low Nutritional Intake** as a priority nursing diagnosis for the plan of care. Along with this diagnosis, Ryan recognizes that Mrs. Cooper is also experiencing **Fatigue** related to her impaired nutrition and **Difficulty Coping** related to her husband's death. Mrs. Cooper's stopping of her visits to the senior center, church activities, and quilt club leads Ryan to identify **Impaired Socialisation** as another problem for Mrs. Cooper.

◆ Planning and Outcomes Identification

During the planning step of the nursing process, develop a plan of care for each of the patient's nursing diagnoses. Planning to maintain patients' optimal nutritional status requires a higher level of care than simply correcting day-to-day nutritional problems. Often there is a need for patients to make long-term changes for nutrition to improve.

Clinical judgment and critical thinking at this step are important because you reflect on previous experiences and environmental factors and apply knowledge, critical thinking attitudes, and professional and intellectual standards to create an individualized approach of care that is relevant to a patient's needs and situation (Fig. 45.6). Apply clinical judgment and critical thinking to ensure that you consider all data sources in developing a patient's plan of care. What you learn about a patient not only builds the database from which you identify nursing diagnoses, but it also provides data on how interventions might be best individualized based on patient condition, food preferences, and medical treatment plan. Thinking about your prior experiences with patients with nutritional problems can provide you with insight into appropriate interventions for nursing diagnoses. Accurately identifying nursing diagnoses related to patients' nutritional problems results in a care plan that is patient centered, relevant, and appropriate (see the Nursing Care Plan). Referring to professional standards for nutrition is important during this step because scientific findings support current published standards.

Outcomes. Outcomes of care reflect a patient's physiological, therapeutic, and individualized needs. Consider what behaviors or physical changes would most benefit your patient as a result of your interventions. If an outcome is to improve patient's knowledge, nutritional education and counseling are important to prepare a patient to know how to prevent disease and promote health. Plan to educate your patients

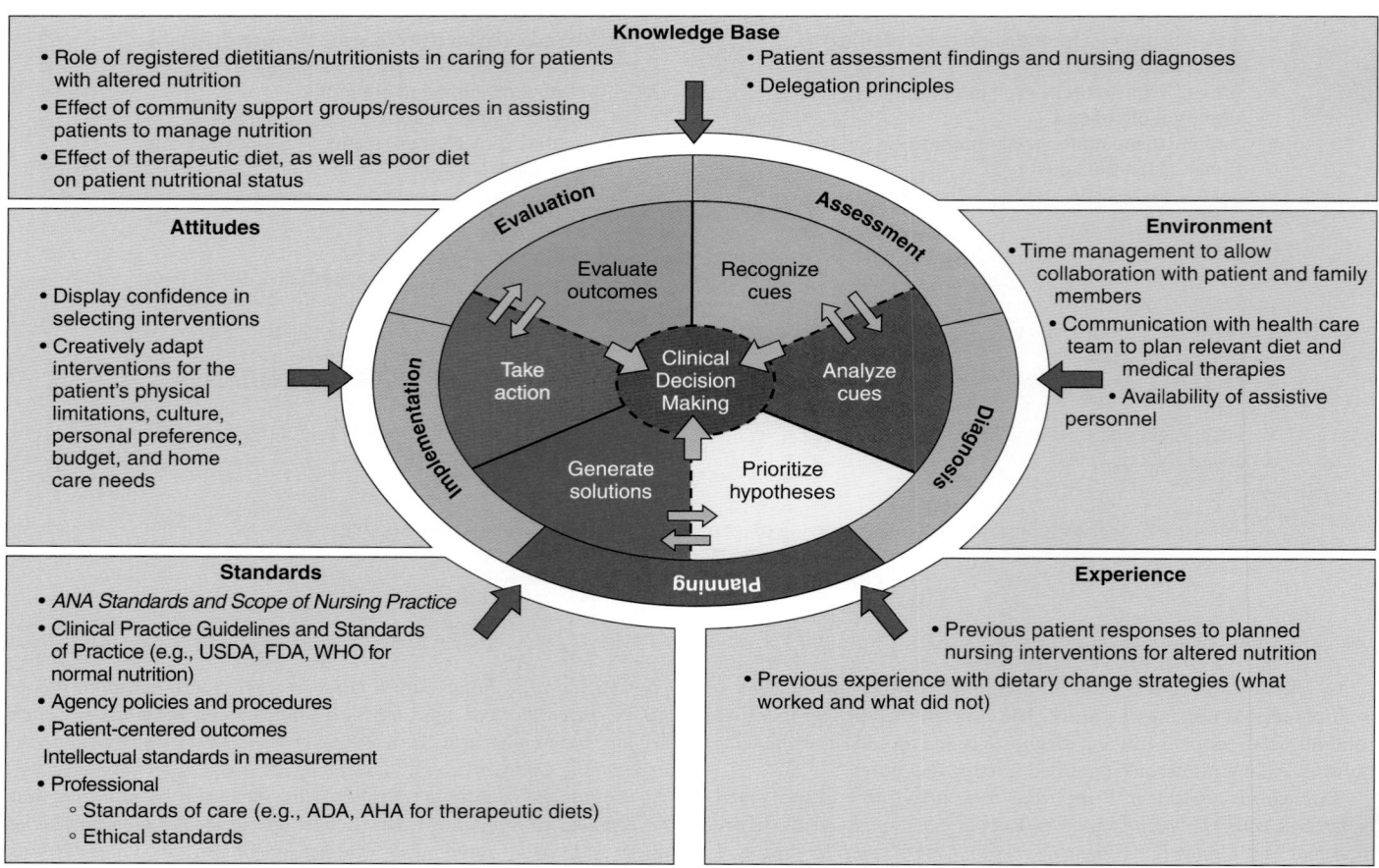

FIG. 45.6 Critical thinking model for nutrition planning. *ADA,* American Diabetes Association; *AHA,* American Heart Association; *FDA,* U.S. Food and Drug Administration; *USDA,* U.S. Department of Agriculture; *WHO,* World Health Organization. (Clinical Judgment Measurement Model copyright © NCSBN. All rights reserved.)

◎ NURSING CARE PLAN

Impaired Low Nutritional Intake

ASSESSMENT

Assessment Activities	*Assessment Findings[a]*
Ask Mrs. Cooper about her food intake during the past 3 days.	She responds that she drinks some juice in the morning and two or three cups of coffee. In addition, she often has a sandwich in the late afternoon. She often **skips dinner**. "I'm just not interested in food. It has no taste."
Ask Mrs. Cooper about social interaction.	Mrs. Cooper **states she is lonely** and does not get out much. Her friends at church call her to come back to meetings, but she is just not ready.
	She says that she **tires easily** and no longer attends the monthly meetings of her quilt club.
Weigh patient and assess posture.	Her weight is 20% below her ideal body weight (IBW) and her body mass index (BMI) is 17. This weight loss has happened over the past 6 months, and she has **lost 24 lb.** She has stooped posture.
Observe Mrs. Cooper for signs of poor nutrition.	Hair loss
	Sores on oral mucous membranes
	Pale mucous membranes

[a]Assessment findings are shown in bold type.

NURSING DIAGNOSIS: Impaired low nutritional intake related to a decreased ability to ingest food as a result of depression and insufficient intake

PLANNING

Expected Outcomes (NOC)[b]

Weight Gain Behavior

Mrs. Cooper will gain 1 to 2 lb per month until reaching a target weight of 130 lb.

Mrs. Cooper will commit to a healthy eating plan.

[b]Outcome classification labels from Moorhead S, et al: *Nursing Outcomes Classification (NOC),* ed 6, St Louis, 2018, Elsevier.

INTERVENTIONS (NIC)[c]	RATIONALE
Nutritional Counseling	
Coordinate plan of care with health care provider, psychologist, Mrs. Cooper, and registered dietitian.	Successful nutrition care planning requires an interprofessional approach throughout the continuum of care (Ukleja et al., 2018).
Individualize menu plans according to Mrs. Cooper's preferences.	Incorporating food preferences into the meal plans encourages the patient to eat (Meiner and Yeager, 2019).
Teach Mrs. Cooper about MyPlate for Older Adults.	MyPlate for Older Adults is adapted to meet the nutritional requirements for older adults (USDA, n.d.b).
Nutritional Management	
Encourage Mrs. Cooper to eat small nutritious meals and snacks and to increase dietary intake to help offset anorexia secondary to sertraline.	Sertraline is a selective serotonin reuptake inhibitor (SSRI) antidepressant medication that causes diminished taste and anorexia. Frequent small nutritious meals and snacks help to reduce anorexia-associated weight loss (Mayo Clinic, 2021b).
Encourage fluid intake of eight 8-oz glasses daily.	Older adults need eight 8-oz (240 mL) glasses per day of fluid from beverage and food sources. Concentrating intake in the morning and early afternoon is acceptable to prevent nocturia (Meiner and Yeager, 2019).
Encourage fiber intake.	Prevents constipation and enhances appetite.
Encourage Mrs. Cooper to eat lunch at the senior center 5 times per week.	Eating with others encourages good nutrition and promotes socialization with peers (National Council on Aging, 2021a).

[c]Intervention classification labels from Butcher HK, et al: *Nursing Interventions Classification (NIC),* ed 7, St Louis, 2018, Elsevier.

EVALUATION

Evaluation Activities	*Patient Response*
Monitor Mrs. Cooper monthly for weight gain and changes in physical appearance.	After 2 weeks Mrs. Cooper has gained 3 lb, her mucous membranes are less pale, and her hair appears to be in better condition and styled.
Ask Mrs. Cooper to describe changes in her food choices.	Mrs. Cooper responds that she eats lunch at the senior center 3 to 4 days a week now. She reports that on days on which she eats at the senior center her appetite seems better and she "wants to do more things." She will continue to follow her plan for preparing small evening meals at home.

about prescribed therapeutic diets, specifically how diet choices affect their illnesses and how to begin to make dietary modifications if needed. This is important for long-term diet adherence. When planning care, be aware of all factors that influence a patient's food intake. For example, patients with heart failure often experience decreased hunger, dietary restrictions, fatigue, shortness of breath, and sadness, which influence their food intake.

Prior experience with other patients with nutritional problems and your own personal experience with nutrition and health are valuable when selecting interventions to help patients improve nutrition. For example, you may have cared for a patient with poor nutritional intake due to chronic illness and used strategies and interventions that helped the patient better manage the illness so that nutrition was improved. Your own personal experience with good nutrition practices provides you with insight on effective strategies that can be used with patients and families.

Individualized planning is essential. Incorporate what you learn about a patient's preferences, feelings about food, weight, diet, and medical condition to identify realistic and achievable outcomes. Mutually planned outcomes negotiated among the patient, RD, health care provider, and nurse ensure success. For example, for Mrs. Cooper in the case study, the following outcomes will help her meet her nutritional needs:

- Patient's daily nutritional intake meets the minimal DRIs.
- Patient will eat well-balanced meals and healthy snacks every day.
- Patient will increase daily protein intake.

Meeting nutritional outcomes requires input from the patient and the interprofessional team. You need to understand the role of each discipline in providing nutritional support to maximize your patients' nutritional outcomes. For example, collaborating with an RD helps develop appropriate nutritional treatment plans. Calorie counts are frequently ordered, and help is necessary to obtain accurate data. An effective patient-centered plan of care requires accurate exchange of information among disciplines.

Setting Priorities. Analyzing cues helps you focus on what cues from your patient assessment are most important. Based on this, you can identify the nursing diagnoses for the patients and consider the urgency of each of the identified problems. Identify your priorities by considering which problems are most likely and most serious and why (Ignatavicius, 2021). After identifying and prioritizing patients' nursing diagnoses, use the priorities to plan timely and successful interventions. For example, managing a patient's oral pain will be a priority over the intervention of diet education to improve nutrition if the patient's paint makes it difficult to swallow and maintain adequate food intake. *Lack of Knowledge* regarding diet therapy will become a priority if it is necessary to promote long-term and effective weight loss for a patient being discharged from a hospital.

Food intake varies during the perioperative period. The priority of care is to provide optimal preoperative nutritional support for surgical patients. The priority to resume food intake after surgery depends on the return of bowel function, the extent of the surgical procedure, and the presence of any complications (see Chapter 50). For example, when patients have oral and throat surgery, they chew and swallow food in the presence of excision sites, sutures, or tissue manipulated during surgery. The priority of care is to first provide comfort and pain control. Then address nutritional priorities and plan care to maintain nutrition that does not cause pain or injury to the healing tissues.

Collaborate with the patient and family while planning care and setting priorities. This is important because food preferences, purchases, and preparation involve the entire family. The plan of care cannot succeed without their commitment to, involvement in, and understanding of the nutritional priorities.

Teamwork and Collaboration. Patient care often extends beyond the acute hospital setting, requiring continued collaboration among members of the health care team after discharge. It is important to include nutritional interventions in discharge planning as patients return to their homes or extended-care settings. Communication of patient outcomes and planned interventions to all team members helps to achieve the established patient outcomes. In addition, consult with an SLP, RD, pharmacist, and/or occupational therapist about patients with dysphagia and those who need ongoing nutritional assessment and interventions to meet their nutritional needs.

Occupational therapists work with patients and their families to identify assistive devices when patients have difficulty in feeding themselves. Devices such as utensils with large handles and plates with elevated sides help a patient with self-feeding. An SLP helps a patient with swallowing exercises and techniques to reduce the risk of aspiration. Occupational therapists also help patients maintain function in the home setting by rearranging food preparation areas to maximize a patient's functional capacity. The RD is an important partner in helping patients modify diets in response to illness.

*Ryan recognizes that Mrs. Cooper is experiencing nutritional problems with poor eating habits and has an unplanned weight loss leading to ongoing fatigue. Ryan has identified **Impaired Low Nutritional Intake** as the priority for Mrs. Cooper. Ryan works with Mrs. Cooper to develop a plan of care to improve her eating habits and overall nutritional status. During the plan development, Ryan and Mrs. Cooper identify agreed-on outcomes and a patient-centered personal plan of care for her. The mutually agreed-on outcomes are "Mrs. Cooper gains 1 to 2 lb per month until reaching a target weight of 130 lb" and "Mrs. Cooper is able to create a healthy eating plan in a week." Ryan works to develop a teaching plan that is patient centered and considers Mrs. Cooper's preferences and finances. He recognizes the need to include an RD to help with Mrs. Cooper's meal planning. Ryan knows that he will need to teach in short sessions because of Mrs. Cooper's fatigue and difficulty paying attention and concentrating during longer conversations.*

*Ryan will ensure that Mrs. Cooper's **Fatigue, Difficulty Coping,** and **Impaired Socialisation** are managed before asking about her other priorities for care. Ryan knows that Mrs. Cooper does not get out of her apartment very much and seems to have stopped all her social activities owing to her fatigue and depression. He knows that he needs a plan to address these problems because of their impact on eating and nutrition. Ryan knows that above all he will honor Mrs. Cooper's preferences, culture, and religious traditions while planning care.*

REFLECT NOW

Identify nursing interventions that you would use on clinical to assist a patient with dysphagia to improve his or her nutritional status.

◆ **Implementation**

The focus of health promotion is to educate patients and family caregivers about balanced nutrition and to help them obtain resources to eat high-quality meals. Diet therapies are numerous and chosen based on a patient's overall health status, ability to eat and digest normally, and long-term nutritional needs. In acute care your role as a nurse is to manage acute conditions that alter patients' nutritional status and to help in ways that promote their appetite and ability to take in nutrients. Patients who are ill or debilitated often have poor appetites (anorexia). Anorexia has many causes (e.g., pain, fatigue, and the effects of medications). Help patients understand the factors that cause anorexia and use creative approaches to stimulate appetite. In the restorative care setting you help patients learn how to follow the therapeutic diets necessary for recovery and treatment of chronic health conditions.

Health Promotion. As a nurse you are in a key position to educate patients about healthy food choices and good nutrition. Helping patients incorporate knowledge of nutrition into their preferences and lifestyles often prevents the development or worsening of diseases or complications from diseases. Outpatient, home, and community-based settings are optimal locations for you to provide education about good nutritional practices. Your interactions with patients will reveal if serious, previously unidentified problems exist. For example, you may have a chance to watch a patient eat or prepare food. Similarly, patients with nutritional problems such as obesity often require help in planning menus and adopting strategies that enhance adherence to healthy dietary behaviors. Your role as educator includes confirming a patient's and family's health literacy (i.e., how much do they understand regarding their nutritional needs) and providing nutritional education and information about community resources. Telephone numbers of an RD or nurse for follow-up questions are always a part of counseling.

Meal planning considers a family's budget and different preferences of family members. Help patients choose specific foods based on the dietary prescription and recommended food groups. For families on limited budgets, use substitutes. For example, bean or cheese dishes often replace meat in a meal, and using evaporated milk or powdered milk when cooking is a low-cost nutritional supplement. Have patients modify the method of preparation when it is necessary to minimize certain substances. For example, baking rather than frying reduces fat intake, and patients can use lemon juice or spices to add flavor to low-sodium diets.

Planning menus a week in advance has several benefits. It helps ensure good nutrition or adherence to a specific diet and helps families stay within their allotted budgets. Nurses or RDs need to check menus created by patients for content. Often a simple tip, such as avoiding grocery shopping when hungry, prevents impulsive purchases of more expensive or less nutritious foods that are not included in meal plans. The USDA (n.d.c) provides sample weekly meal-planning services for a range of budgets on its website.

Support individuals who are interested in losing weight. A high percentage of those who attempt to lose weight are unsuccessful, regaining lost weight over time. Adherence to diet and exercise affect success with weight loss. Information on weight loss is available from multiple sources. Help patients develop a successful weight-loss plan that considers their preferences and resources and includes awareness of portion sizes and knowledge of energy content of food (AHA, 2017).

Food safety is an important public health issue. Foodborne bacteria can occur from improper food cleaning, preparation, or poor hygiene practices of food workers. Health care professionals not only need to be aware of the factors related to food safety but also should provide patient education to reduce the risks for foodborne illnesses (Table 45.5; Box 45.9).

TABLE 45.5 Food Safety

Foodborne Disease	Organism	Food Source	Symptoms[a]
Botulism	Clostridium botulinum	Improperly home-canned foods, smoked and salted fish, ham, sausage, shellfish	Symptoms vary from mild discomfort to death in 24 hours; initially nausea, vomiting, dizziness, and weakness progressing to motor (respiratory) paralysis
Campylobacteriosis	Campylobacter jejuni	Raw and undercooked poultry, unpasteurized milk, contaminated water	Diarrhea, cramps, fever, and vomiting. Diarrhea may be bloody; appears 2–5 days after eating contaminated food; lasts 2–10 days
Escherichia coli	E. coli	Undercooked meat (ground beef)	Severe cramps, nausea, vomiting, diarrhea (may be bloody), renal failure; symptoms appear 1–8 days after eating; last 1–7 days
Listeriosis	Listeria / Listeria monocytogenes	Soft cheese, meat (hot dogs, pâté, lunch meats), unpasteurized milk, poultry, seafood	Severe diarrhea, fever, headache, pneumonia, meningitis, endocarditis; symptoms appear 3–21 days after infection; duration is variable
Norovirus	Norovirus	Contaminated foods and surfaces, uncooked shellfish from contaminated waters; person-to-person spread	Diarrhea, vomiting, nausea, stomach cramping or pain, fever, headache; usually appear 1–2 days after ingestion but can occur within 12 hours; last 12 hours to 5 days
Perfringens enteritis	Clostridium / Clostridium perfringens	Cooked meats, meat dishes held at room or warm temperature	Mild diarrhea, vomiting; appear 8–24 hours after eating; last 1–2 days
Salmonellosis	Salmonella / Salmonella typhi / Salmonella paratyphi	Milk, custards, egg dishes, salad dressings, sandwich fillings, polluted shellfish	Mild to severe diarrhea, cramps, vomiting; appear up to 72 hours after ingestion; last 4–7 days
Shigellosis	Shigella / Shigella dysenteriae	Milk, milk products, seafood, salads	Cramps, diarrhea to fatal dysentery; appear 12–50 hours after ingestion; last 3–14 days
Staphylococcus	Staphylococcus / Staphylococcus aureus	Custards, cream fillings, processed meats, ham, cheese, ice cream, potato salad, sauces, casseroles	Severe abdominal cramps, pain, vomiting, diarrhea, perspiration, headache, fever, prostration; appear 1–6 hours after ingestion; last 1–2 days

From Centers for Disease Control and Prevention (CDC): *Foodborne germs and illnesses*, 2020. https://www.cdc.gov/foodsafety/foodborne-germs.html. Accessed April 14, 2021; and U.S. Food and Drug Administration (FDA): *Foodborne illness causing organisms in the U.S.: what you need to know*, n.d. https://www.fda.gov/media/77727/download. Accessed April 14, 2021.
[a] Symptoms are generally most severe for youngest and oldest age-groups.

BOX 45.9 PATIENT TEACHING

Food Safety

Objective
- Patient verbalizes measures to prevent foodborne illness.

Teaching Strategies
- Explain that food safety is an important public health issue. Populations particularly at risk are older adults, children, and individuals who are immunosuppressed.
- Instruct patients using the following four principles:

1. CLEAN
   - Wash hands with warm, soapy water before touching or eating food.
   - Wash fresh fruits and vegetables thoroughly.
   - Clean the inside of refrigerator and microwave regularly to prevent microbial growth.
   - Clean cutting surfaces after each use.
   - When possible, use separate surfaces for fruit, meat, poultry, and fish.

2. SEPARATE
   - Wash cooking utensils and cutting boards with hot, soapy water.
   - Wash hands after handling foods, especially meats, poultry, and eggs.
   - Clean vegetables and lettuce used in salads thoroughly.
   - Wash dishrags, towels, and sponges regularly or use paper towels.

3. COOK
   - Use a food thermometer to verify that meat, poultry, and fish are cooked properly.
   - Do not eat raw meats or unpasteurized milk.

4. CHILL
   - Keep foods properly refrigerated at 40°F (4.4°C) and frozen at 0°F (−17.8°C).
   - Do not save leftovers for more than 2 days in refrigerator.

Evaluation
Use the principles of teach-back to evaluate patient/family caregiver learning:
- Tell me what you do to prevent foodborne illnesses while you are preparing meals.
- Please show me what you do while cooking to ensure that your food will be safe to eat.

Data from U.S. Department of Agriculture: *Keep food safe! Food safety basics,* 2016. https://www.fsis.usda.gov/food-safety/safe-food-handling-and-preparation/food-safety-basics/steps-keep-food-safe. Accessed April 5, 2021.

QSEN **Building Competency in Teamwork and Collaboration**
You are the nurse in charge of developing an interprofessional team to help patients with Crohn disease, an inflammatory bowel disease, manage their diets at home. Knowing that patients with Crohn disease must adhere to a diet that is low in fiber and high in calories and protein, you bring your nursing knowledge to the team. What strengths and limitations do you bring to the team? What other members of the team would you need to help prepare the plan of care for patients with Crohn disease? How would you promote effective teamwork?

Answers to QSEN Activities can be found on the Evolve website.

Acute Care. The nutritional care of patients who are acutely ill requires you to consider a variety of factors that influence nutritional intake. Diagnostic testing and procedures in the acute care setting often disrupt food intake. Sometimes patients must refrain from eating or drinking anything by mouth (NPO) as they prepare for or recover from a diagnostic test. Patients are often too ill to eat solid food due to nausea, vomiting, or gastrointestinal alterations. Frequent interruptions during mealtimes occur in the health care setting, and some patients have poor appetites. Patients often are too tired or uncomfortable to eat. It is important to continuously analyze cues when assessing a patient's nutritional status and to adopt interventions that promote normal intake, digestion, and metabolism of nutrients. Patients who are NPO and receive only standard IV fluids for more than 5 to 7 days are at high nutritional risk.

Advancing Diets. Acute and chronic conditions affect a patient's immune system and nutritional status. Patients with decreased immune function (e.g., from cancer, chemotherapy, human immunodeficiency virus/acquired immunodeficiency syndrome [HIV/AIDS], or organ transplants) require special diets that decrease exposure to microorganisms and are higher in selected nutrients. Table 45.6 provides an overview of the immune system, the impact of malnutrition, and beneficial nutrients. In addition, patients who are ill, who have had surgical procedures, or who were NPO for an extended time have specialized dietary needs. Health care providers order a gradual progression of dietary intake or therapeutic diet to manage patients' illnesses (Box 45.10).

Promoting Appetite. Providing an environment that promotes nutritional intake includes keeping a patient's environment free of odors, providing oral hygiene as needed to remove unpleasant tastes, and maintaining patient comfort. Offering smaller, more frequent

TABLE 45.6 Nutrition and the Immune System

Immune/Physiological Component	Malnutrition Effect	Vital Nutrients
Antibodies	Decreased amount	Protein; vitamins A, B₆, B₁₂, C; folic acid; thiamin; biotin; riboflavin, niacin
GI tract	Systemic movement of bacteria	Arginine, glutamine, omega-3 fatty acids
Granulocytes and macrocytes	Longer time for phagocytosis kill time and lymphocyte activation	Protein; vitamins A, B₆, B₁₂, C; folic acid; thiamin; riboflavin; niacin; zinc; iron
Mucus	Flat microvilli in GI tract, decreased antibody secretion	Vitamins B₆, B₁₂, C; biotin
Skin	Integrity compromised, density reduced, wound healing slowed	Protein, vitamins A, B₁₂, C; niacin; copper; zinc
T lymphocytes	Depressed T-cell distribution	Protein; arginine; iron; zinc; omega-3 fatty acids; vitamins A, B₆, B₁₂; folic acid; thiamin; riboflavin; niacin; pantothenic acid

Modified from Grodner M, et al: *Nutritional foundations and clinical applications of nutrition: a nursing approach,* ed 7, St Louis, 2020, Elsevier. *GI,* Gastrointestinal.

BOX 45.10 Diet Progression and Therapeutic Diets

Clear Liquid

Clear fat-free broth, bouillon, coffee, tea, carbonated beverages, clear fruit juices, gelatin, fruit ices, popsicles

Full Liquid

Same as clear liquid, with addition of smooth-textured dairy products (e.g., ice cream), strained or blended cream soups, custards, refined cooked cereals, vegetable juice, pureed vegetables, all fruit juices, sherbets, puddings, frozen yogurt

Dysphagia Stages, Thickened Liquids, Pureed

As for clear and full liquid, with addition of scrambled eggs; pureed meats, vegetables, and fruits; mashed potatoes and gravy

Mechanical Soft

As for clear and full liquid and pureed, with addition of all cream soups, ground or finely diced meats, flaked fish, cottage cheese, cheese, rice, potatoes, pancakes, light breads, cooked vegetables, cooked or canned fruits, bananas, soups, peanut butter, eggs (not fried)

Soft/Low Residue

Addition of low-fiber, easily digested foods such as pastas, casseroles, moist tender meats, and canned cooked fruits and vegetables; desserts, cakes, and cookies without nuts or coconut

High Fiber

Addition of fresh uncooked fruits, steamed vegetables, bran, oatmeal, and dried fruits

Low Sodium

4-g (no added salt), 2-g, 1-g, or 500-mg sodium diets; vary from no added salt to severe sodium restriction (500-mg sodium diet), which requires selective food purchases

Low Cholesterol

300 mg/day cholesterol, in keeping with American Heart Association guidelines for serum lipid reduction

Diabetic

Nutrition recommendations by the American Diabetes Association: focus on total energy, nutrient and food distribution; include a balanced intake of carbohydrates, fats, and proteins; varied caloric recommendations to accommodate patient's metabolic demands

Gluten Free

Eliminates wheat, oats, rye, barley, and their derivatives

Regular

No restrictions unless specified

---

to manage symptoms that interfere with nutrition requires health care provider consultation.

Mealtime is usually a social activity. If appropriate, encourage visitors to eat with a patient. When patients experience anorexia, encourage other nurses or care providers to converse and engage them in conversation. Mealtime is also an excellent opportunity for any patient education topic. Instruct a patient about any therapeutic diets, medications, energy conservation measures, or adaptive devices to help with independent feeding.

Assisting Patients With Oral Feeding. When a patient needs help, it is important to protect the patient's safety, independence, and dignity. Clear the table or over-bed tray of clutter. Assess the patient's risk of aspiration (see Skill 45.1). A patient at high risk for aspiration has a decreased level of alertness, decreased gag and/or cough reflexes, and difficulty managing saliva (see Assessment section of this chapter).

Patients with dysphagia are at risk for aspiration and need more help with feeding and swallowing. An SLP identifies patients at risk and provides recommendations for therapy (Pietsch et al., 2018). Provide a 30-minute rest period before eating and position the patient in an upright, seated position in a chair or raise the head of the bed to 90 degrees. Have the patient flex the head slightly to a chin-down position to help prevent aspiration. Teach patients with unilateral weakness and their caregivers to place food in the stronger side of the mouth. With the help of an SLP, determine the viscosity of foods that a patient tolerates best by using trials of different consistencies of foods and fluids. Thicker fluids are generally easier to swallow. According to ASHA (2021b), there are four levels of diet: dysphagia puree, dysphagia mechanically altered, dysphagia advanced, and regular. The four levels of liquid include thin liquids (low viscosity), nectarlike liquids (medium viscosity), honeylike liquids (viscosity of honey), and spoon-thick liquids (viscosity of pudding).

Feed patients with dysphagia slowly, providing smaller-size bites. Allow them to chew thoroughly and swallow the bite before taking another. More frequent chewing and swallowing assessments throughout the meal are necessary. Allow the patient time to empty the mouth after each spoonful, matching the speed of feeding to the patient's readiness (see Skill 45.1). If a patient begins to cough or choke, remove the food immediately. Sometimes it is necessary to have oral suction equipment available at the patient's bedside.

Provide opportunities for patients to direct the order in which they want to eat the food items and how fast they wish to eat. Determine a patient's food preferences and, unless contraindicated, try to have these items included on the dietary tray. Ask the patient whether the food is the right temperature. These seem like small acts, but they go a long way in maintaining a patient's sense of independence and control.

Patients with visual deficits also need special assistance. Patients with decreased vision are able to feed themselves when given adequate information. For example, identify the food location on a meal plate as if it were a clock (e.g., meat at 9 o'clock and vegetable at 3 o'clock). Tell the patient where the beverages are located in relation to the plate. Be sure that other care providers set the meal tray and plate in the same manner. Patients with impaired vision and those with decreased motor skills are more independent during mealtimes with the use of large-handled adaptive utensils (Fig. 45.7). These are easier to grip and manipulate.

Enteral Tube Feeding. Enteral nutrition (EN) provides nutrients into the GI tract. It is the preferred method of meeting nutritional needs if a patient is unable to swallow or take in nutrients orally yet has a functioning GI tract. EN provides physiological, safe, and economical nutritional support. Patients with enteral feedings receive formula via the nasoenteral route (nasogastric, nasoduodenal, and nasojejunal) or through gastric tubes inserted into the stomach (gastrostomy) or jejunum (jejunostomy). The route selected to provide nutrition support therapy is appropriate to

---

meals often helps. In addition, certain medications affect dietary intake and nutrient use. For example, medications such as insulin, glucocorticoids, and thyroid hormones affect metabolism. Other medications such as antifungal agents frequently affect taste. Some of the psychotropic medications affect appetite, cause nausea, and alter taste. You and the RD help patients select foods that reduce the altered taste sensations or nausea. Consult with an RD regarding using seasonings that improve food taste. In other situations, medications need to be changed. Assessing patients for the need for pharmacological agents to stimulate appetite such as cyproheptadine, megestrol, or dronabinol or the patient's clinical status or condition and is periodically assessed for appropriateness and for its adequacy in meeting the goals of the nutrition care plan (Ukleja et al., 2018). Patients with a low risk of gastric reflux receive gastric feedings; however, if there is a risk of gastric reflux, which leads to aspiration, jejunal feeding is preferred. Box 45.11 lists indications for enteral tube feeding. Either a nurse or a family caregiver can administer enteral tube feedings in the home setting. After insertion of an enteral tube, it is initially necessary to verify tube placement by x-ray film examination. Confirmation of placement is needed before a patient receives the first enteral feeding (see Skill 45.2).

FIG. 45.7 Adaptive equipment. Clockwise from upper left: Two-handled cup with lid, plate with plate guard, utensils with splints, and utensils with enlarged handles.

An enteral formula is usually one of four types. Polymeric (1–2 kcal/mL) includes milk-based blenderized foods prepared by hospital dietary staff or in a patient's home. The polymeric classification also includes commercially prepared whole-nutrient formulas. For this type of formula to be effective, a patient's GI tract needs to be able to absorb whole nutrients. The second type, modular formulas (3.8–4 kcal/mL), consists of single macronutrient (e.g., protein, glucose, polymers, or lipids) preparations and is not nutritionally complete. You can add this type of formula to other foods to meet your patient's individual nutritional needs. The third type, elemental formulas (1–3 kcal/mL), contains predigested nutrients that are easier for a partially dysfunctional GI tract to absorb. Finally, specialty formulas (1–2 kcal/mL) are designed to meet specific nutritional needs in certain illnesses (e.g., liver failure, pulmonary disease, or HIV infection).

Typically tube feedings are delivered intermittently or continuously. A systematic review was conducted as part of the ASPEN guidelines to investigate whether intermittent bolus enteral nutrition has an advantage over continuously administered enteral feedings. The review showed that there is a significant reduction in diarrhea with continuous versus bolus administration; however, there were no differences in gastric residual volume, rates of aspiration, or pneumonia (Lambell et al., 2020). Currently continuous feedings remain the most common therapy. A feeding usually starts at full strength at slow rates (see Skill 45.3; Box 45.12). Increase the hourly rate every 8 to 12 hours per health care provider's order if no signs of intolerance appear (high gastric residuals, nausea, cramping, vomiting, or diarrhea). Implement evidence-based guidelines when caring for patients receiving tube feedings (Box 45.13). Studies have demonstrated a beneficial

---

BOX 45.11 Indications for Enteral and Parenteral Nutrition

Enteral Nutrition
(Used with patients who have a functional gastrointestinal tract)
- Cancer
  - Head and neck
  - Upper GI
- Critical illness/trauma
- Neurological and muscular disorders
  - Brain neoplasm
  - Cerebrovascular accident
  - Dementia
  - Myopathy
  - Parkinson disease
- GI disorders
  - Enterocutaneous fistula
  - Inflammatory bowel disease
  - Mild pancreatitis
- Respiratory failure with prolonged intubation
- Inadequate oral intake
  - Anorexia nervosa
  - Difficulty chewing, swallowing
  - Severe depression

Parenteral Nutrition
- Nonfunctional GI tract
  - Massive small bowel resection, GI surgery, or massive GI bleed
  - Paralytic ileus
  - Intestinal obstruction
  - Trauma to abdomen, head, or neck
  - Severe malabsorption
  - Intolerance to enteral feeding (established by trial)
  - Chemotherapy, radiation therapy, bone marrow transplantation
- Extended bowel rest
  - Enterocutaneous fistula
  - Inflammatory bowel disease exacerbation
  - Severe diarrhea
  - Moderate to severe pancreatitis
- Preoperative total parenteral nutrition
  - Preoperative bowel rest
  - Treatment for comorbid severe malnutrition in patients with nonfunctional GI tract
- Severely catabolic patients when GI tract not usable for more than 4 to 5 days

GI, Gastrointestinal.

BOX 45.12 Advancing the Rate of Tube Feeding

Protocols for advancing tube feedings are commonly institution specific. There does not appear to be a benefit to slow initiation of enteral nutrition over days. Most patients are able to tolerate feeding 24 to 48 hours after initiation. Do not dilute formulas with water; this increases the risk of bacterial contamination (Harding et al., 2020). The common delivery options for enteral feedings are continuous, intermittent via a pump or gravity, and cyclical. Usually patients who are more critically ill receive continuous feedings (Harding et al., 2020). Patients who are stable or are getting feedings in the home frequently receive intermittent feedings (Harding et al., 2020). Cyclical feedings are used when patients begin to eat a normal diet but still need additional nutritional support (Harding et al., 2020).

Intermittent
1. Start formula at full strength for isotonic formulas (300–400 mOsm) or at ordered concentration.
2. Infuse bolus of formula over at least 20 to 30 minutes via syringe or feeding container.
3. Begin feedings with a volume of 2.5 to 5 mL/kg 5 to 8 times per day. Increase by 60 to 120 mL per feeding every 8 to 12 hours to achieve needed volume and calories in four to six feedings (Stewart, 2014).

Continuous
1. Start formula at full strength for isotonic formulas (300–400 mOsm) or at ordered concentration.
2. Begin infusion rate at designated rate, typically at 10 to 40 mL/h (Stewart, 2014).
3. Advance rate slowly (e.g., 10–20 mL/h every 8–12 hours) to target rate if tolerated (tolerance indicated by absence of nausea and diarrhea and low gastric residuals) (Stewart, 2014).

BOX 45.13 EVIDENCE-BASED PRACTICE

Reducing Malnutrition and Risk of Aspiration With Enteral Feedings

PICOT Question: In adult patients who are receiving enteral feedings, does use of an evidence-based nutrition bundle reduce malnutrition and the risk of aspiration?

Evidence Summary

Enteral feedings provide calories, preserve a patient's immune system, preserve the integrity of the gut, and reduce the severity of disease (Jordan and Moore, 2020; VanBlarcom and McCoy, 2018).

In collaboration with a registered dietitian, the nurse works to prevent undernutrition and aspiration, two common complications associated with enteral feedings that can lead to pneumonia. Proactive interventions involve use of an evidence-based nutrition bundle. An essential element of the bundle is a regular nutritional assessment in adult patients who are receiving enteral feedings. The assessment focuses on risk factors, and patients are considered malnourished if they exhibit two of the following six characteristics: insufficient protein intake, weight loss, loss of muscle mass, loss of subcutaneous fat, localized or generalized fluid accumulation, and diminished functional status measured by handgrip strength (ASPEN, 2021). Ongoing interprofessional nutritional assessment of a patient leads to an appropriate individualized nutrition plan (Ukleja et al., 2018).

According to VanBlarcom and McCoy (2018), one cause of undernutrition in patients in critical care units is interrupted enteral feedings. Each time the head of the bed is lowered below 30 degrees (e.g., for hygiene care, dressing changes, moving the patient), the nurse pauses a patient's feeding to prevent aspiration. However, this interruption in enteral feedings can contribute to poor nutrition.

To reduce the risk for aspiration, nurses follow several evidence-based practices, such as keeping the head of bed elevated at 30 to 45 degrees, reducing the use of sedatives, assessing placement of the enteral access device and tolerance to the enteral feeding every 4 hours, and ensuring adequate bowel function (Ukleja et al., 2018; VanBlarcom and McCoy, 2018). Patients diagnosed with pancreatitis, gastric outlet obstruction, gastroparesis, and a history of aspiration are at an increased risk for aspiration with an enteral feeding and may benefit from a small-bore feeding tube placed into the duodenum (VanBlarcom and McCoy, 2018).

A nutrition bundle also includes assessment of a patient's tolerance to enteral feedings to reduce risk of aspiration. New guidelines from ASPEN (2021) limit the use of measuring gastric residual volumes as an assessment tool to determine the patient's tolerance to enteral feeding. The current literature indicates that there is no correlation between gastric residual volumes and gastric emptying and that these are poor indicators of intolerance to enteral feedings (VanBlarcom and McCoy, 2018). In addition, measuring gastric residual volumes may clog the enteral access device and inappropriately stop the enteral feeding, which also places the patient at an increased risk for undernutrition.

Application to Nursing Practice

- Implement an evidence-based nutrition bundle to reduce malnutrition and reduce the risk of aspiration, such as the one created by ASPEN in conjunction with the Society of Critical Care Medicine (VanBlarcom and McCoy, 2018).
- Assess patients for malnutrition. Registered dietitians will perform assessment by using the gold standard of indirect calorimetry to estimate protein/energy needs (ASPEN, 2021).
- Implement and maintain enteral feeding using evidence-based and institution-specific protocols.
- Initiate parenteral feeding when enteral nutrition is not appropriate.
- Administer a prokinetic agent, especially in patients with high gastric residual volumes, as ordered to further reduce the risk of aspiration (Tatsumi, 2019; VanBlarcom and McCoy, 2018).

ASPEN, American Society for Parenteral and Enteral Nutrition.

effect of enteral feedings compared with parenteral nutrition (PN). Feeding by the enteral route reduces sepsis, minimizes the hypermetabolic response to trauma, decreases hospital mortality, and maintains intestinal structure and function (Jordan and Moore, 2020). EN is successful within 24 to 48 hours after surgery or trauma to provide fluids, electrolytes, and nutritional support. Patients who develop a gastric ileus cannot receive nasogastric (NG) feedings. Nasointestinal or jejunal tubes allow successful postpyloric feeding because the formula is instilled directly into the small intestine or jejunum, which is beyond the pyloric sphincter of the stomach (Ukleja et al., 2018).

A serious complication associated with enteral feedings is aspiration of formula into the tracheobronchial tree. Aspiration of enteral formula into the lungs irritates the bronchial mucosa, resulting in decreased blood supply to affected pulmonary tissue (Huether et al., 2020). This leads to necrotizing infection, pneumonia, and potential abscess formation. The high glucose content of a feeding serves as a bacterial medium for growth, promoting infection. Acute respiratory distress syndrome (ARDS) is also an outcome frequently associated with pulmonary aspiration. Some of the common conditions that increase the risk of aspiration include coughing, gastroesophageal reflux disease (GERD), cerebrovascular accident (CVA), Parkinson disease, nasotracheal suctioning, an artificial airway, decreased level of consciousness, and lying flat. Prokinetic medications such as metoclopramide, erythromycin, or cisapride promote gastric emptying and decrease the risk of aspiration (Tatsumi, 2019). Keep the head of the bed elevated a minimum of 30 degrees, preferably 45 degrees, unless medically contraindicated, during feedings and for 30 to 60 minutes after feeding (Metheny, 2018). Many institutional policies still require you to measure gastric residual volumes (GRVs) every 4 to 6 hours in patients receiving continuous feedings and immediately before the feeding in patients receiving intermittent feedings (Boullata et al., 2017). A GRV of between 250 and 500 mL could indicate delayed gastric emptying and may require you to implement measures to reduce the risk of aspiration (Boullata et al., 2017). A literature review found that enteral feedings were typically not held if the GRV was 500 mL or less (Jordan and Moore, 2020); however, follow your institution's policy. The North American Summit on Aspiration in the Critically Ill Patient recommends the following: (1) stop feedings immediately if aspiration occurs; (2) withhold feedings and reassess patient tolerance to feedings if GRV is over 500 mL; (3) routinely evaluate the patient for aspiration; and (4) use nursing measures to reduce the risk of aspiration if GRV is between 250 and 500 mL (Boullata et al., 2017).

Enteral Access Tubes. Enteral tube feedings are used with patients who are unable to ingest food but maintain the ability to digest and absorb nutrients. Feeding tubes are inserted through the nose (NG or nasointestinal), surgically (gastrostomy or jejunostomy), or endoscopically (percutaneous endoscopic gastrostomy or jejunostomy [PEG or PEJ]). NG or nasoduodenal or nasojejunal feeding tubes may be used if a patient is expected to need EN therapy for fewer than 4 weeks. Surgically or endoscopically placed tubes are preferred for long-term feeding (more than 6 weeks) to reduce the discomfort of a nasal tube and provide a more secure, reliable access (Ukleja et al., 2018). Some patients such as those with gastroparesis (decreased or absent innervation to the stomach that results in delayed gastric emptying), esophageal reflux, or a history of aspiration pneumonia require placement of tubes beyond the stomach into the intestine (Harding et al., 2020).

Most health care settings use small-bore feeding tubes because they create less discomfort for a patient (Fig. 45.8A). Adult patients typically have an 8- to 12-Fr tube that is 36 to 44 inches (90–110 cm) long. These flexible tubes come with a stylet, which makes the tube stiffer and is used when the tube is inserted. The stylet is removed after correct tube location is confirmed and before feedings are started. **Never reinsert the**

FIG. 45.8 (A) Enteral tubes, small bore. (B) Enteral-only connector (ENFit) tubing.

stylet in the tube. It is now becoming standard to use an enteral-only connector (ENFit) designed for the specific enteral tube. BioSphere announced the phase-out of all existing legacy feeding devices and transition adaptors starting July 1, 2020, in order to comply with ENFit implementation (BioSphere, 2019). This phase-out is supported by the U.S. Food and Drug Administration (FDA), The Joint Commission, and Centers for Medicare & Medicaid Services (CMS) to reduce medical tubing misconnections; however, specific regulations have not been established. Standardization of connector tubing improves patient safety (Fig. 45.8B). Tubing standards are designed to reduce tubing misconnections that result in patient injury (The Joint Commission [TJC], 2014). Skill 45.3 describes the procedure for initiating NG, gastrostomy, and jejunostomy enteral feedings.

Historically nurses confirmed placement of feeding tubes by injecting air into the tube while auscultating the stomach for a bubbling or gurgling sound or by asking the patient to speak. *Current evidence shows that these methods are ineffective in verifying tube placement.* Currently, the most accurate method for verification of tube placement is x-ray film examination. At the bedside, nurses test the pH of secretions withdrawn from the feeding tube to confirm tube location on an ongoing basis (Box 45.14).

Table 45.7 outlines major complications of EN. Of special note, patients who are severely malnourished are at risk for electrolyte disturbances from refeeding syndrome during EN or PN therapy. In refeeding syndrome, potassium, magnesium, and phosphate move intracellularly, resulting in low serum (extracellular) levels and edema. These changes may cause cardiac dysrhythmias, heart failure, respiratory distress, convulsions, coma, or death.

Parenteral Nutrition. Parenteral nutrition (PN) is a form of specialized nutritional support provided intravenously. Patients who are unable to digest or absorb EN benefit from PN. Patients in highly stressed physiological states such as sepsis, head injury, or burns are candidates for PN therapy (see Box 45.11). A basic PN formula is a combination of crystalline amino acids, hypertonic dextrose, electrolytes, vitamins, and trace elements. Total PN (TPN), administered through a central line, is a 2-in-1 formula in which administration of fat emulsions occurs separately from the protein and dextrose solution (Grodner et al., 2020). Safe administration depends on appropriate assessment of nutritional needs, meticulous management of the central venous catheter (CVC), and careful monitoring to prevent or treat metabolic complications. Administration of PN happens in a variety of settings, including a patient's home. Regardless of the setting, adhere to principles of asepsis and infusion management to ensure safe nutritional support.

PN therapy requires clinical and laboratory monitoring by an interprofessional team. Consistent reevaluation for the continuation of PN

is required. The goal is to make PN short-term and to move toward enteral or oral feedings so that use of the GI tract is constant (Ukleja et al., 2018). Disuse of the GI tract has been associated with villus atrophy and generalized cell shrinkage. Furthermore, the disuse of the GI tract may cause bacteria to move from the unused gut into the bloodstream, resulting in gram-negative septicemia.

Sometimes adding intravenous fat emulsions to PN supports a patient's need for supplemental kilocalories to prevent essential fatty-acid deficiencies and help control hyperglycemia during periods of stress (Phillips, 2018). Administer these emulsions through a separate peripheral line, through the central line by using Y-connector tubing (see Chapter 42), or as an admixture to the PN solution. The addition of fat emulsion to a PN solution is called a *3-in-1 admixture* or *total nutrient admixture.* The patient receives it over a 24-hour period. Do not use the admixture if you observe oil droplets or an oily or creamy layer on the surface of the admixture. This observation indicates that the emulsion has broken into large lipid droplets that cause fat emboli if administered. IV fat emulsions are white and opaque. Take care to avoid confusing enteral formula with parenteral lipids.

Initiating Parenteral Nutrition. Patients with short-term nutritional needs often receive IV solutions of less than 10% dextrose via a peripheral vein in combination with amino acids and lipids. TPN is more calorically dense than peripheral solutions; peripheral solutions are therefore usually temporary. PN with greater than 10% dextrose requires a CVC that a health care provider places into a high-flow central vein such as the superior vena cava under sterile conditions (see Chapter 42). If you are using a CVC that has multiple lumens, use a port exclusively dedicated for the TPN. Label the port for TPN and do not infuse other solutions or medications through it (Harding et al., 2020). Nurses with special training insert peripherally inserted central catheters (PICCs) that start in a vein of the arm and then thread into the subclavian or superior vena cava vein.

After catheter placement, wait to flush and use the catheter until radiology confirms its position. The health care provider secures the CVC with a securement device and covers the site with a sterile bio-occlusive dressing. Before applying the sterile dressing, stabilize the PICC with sterile strips of tape, and follow the institution's central line infection prevention protocol (Harding et al., 2020).

Before beginning any PN infusion, verify the health care provider's order and inspect the solution for particulate matter or a break in the fat emulsion. Always use an infusion pump to deliver a constant rate. The initial rate delivers no more than 50% of estimated needs for the first 24 to 48 hours and gradually increases the rate until a patient's complete nutritional needs are supplied. Patients receiving PN at home frequently administer the entire daily solution over 12 hours at night.

BOX 45.14 PROCEDURAL GUIDELINES

Obtaining Gastrointestinal Aspirate for pH Measurement and Large-Bore, and Small-Bore Feeding Tubes: Intermittent and Continuous Feeding

Delegation and Collaboration

The skill of verifying tube placement and irrigating a feeding tube is the responsibility of the nurse and cannot be delegated to assistive personnel (AP). The nurse directs the AP to:

- Immediately inform the nurse if patient's respirations change or patient complains of shortness of breath, coughing, or choking.
- Immediately inform the nurse if the patient vomits or the AP notices vomitus in patient's mouth during oral hygiene.
- Immediately inform the nurse if nasal skin irritation or excoriation is present.
- Immediately inform the nurse if a change in the external length of the tube occurs, which could indicate displacement of the tube.
- Report when a continuous tube feeding stops infusing.

Equipment

60-mL ENFit syringe; water (tap water or sterile [see agency policy], dated and initialed container at patient's bedside); towel; stethoscope; clean gloves; pH indicator strip (scale of 1.0–11.0); small medication cup; measuring tape/device; pulse oximeter

Procedural Steps

1. Review agency policy and procedures for frequency of irrigation and frequency and method of checking tube placement. **Do not insufflate air into tube to check placement.**
2. Identify patient using at least two identifiers (e.g., name and birthday or name and medical record number) according to agency policy (TJC, 2021).
3. Review patient's medication record for orders for enteral feeding, a gastric acid inhibitor (e.g., ranitidine, famotidine, nizatidine), or a proton pump inhibitor (e.g., omeprazole).
4. Review patient's medical record for history of prior tube displacement.
5. Observe for signs and symptoms of respiratory distress during feeding: coughing, choking, or reduced oxygen saturation.
6. Identify conditions that increase risk for spontaneous tube migration or dislocation: altered level of consciousness, agitation; retching; vomiting; nasotracheal suction.
7. Perform hand hygiene. Assess bowel sounds and perform abdominal examination.
8. Obtain pulse oximetry reading.
9. Note ease with which previous tube feedings infuse through tubing. Monitor volume of continuous enteral formula administered during shift and compare with ordered amount.
10. Assess patient's or family caregiver's knowledge, experience, and health literacy.
11. Perform hand hygiene and apply clean gloves. Be sure pulse oximeter is in place.
12. Verify tube placement.

   CLINICAL JUDGMENT: Listening for insufflated air instilled through tube to check tube tip position is unreliable (Boullata et al., 2017; Metheny et al., 2019).

   a. Check tube placement at following times:

   (1) For patients receiving intermittent tube feedings, test placement immediately before each feeding (usually a period of at least 4 hours will have elapsed since previous feeding) and before medications.

   (2) Follow agency policy regarding when to test pH for patients receiving continuous tube feedings. AACN (2016) recommends stopping continuous feedings for several hours to obtain reliable pH readings. However, this is not always appropriate for a patient's therapeutic plan of care.

   (3) Wait to verify placement at least 1 hour after medication administration by tube or mouth.

   (4) Measure length of tube extending from nares.

   b. If tube feeding is infusing, turn off or place tube feeding on hold. Clamp or kink feeding tube and disconnect from end of infusion bag tubing. For intermittent feedings, remove plug at end of feeding tube. Draw up 30 mL of air into a 60-mL ENFit syringe. Place tip of syringe into end of gastric or small bowel feeding tube. Flush with air before attempting to aspirate fluid. Repositioning patient from side to side is helpful. In some cases, more than one bolus of air is necessary.

   c. Draw back on syringe slowly and obtain 5 to 10 mL of gastric aspirate (see illustration). Observe appearance of aspirate. Aspirates from gastric tubes of patients receiving continuous tube feedings often look like curdled enteral formula. Gastric aspirates from patients receiving intermittent feedings typically are not bile stained (unless intestinal fluid has refluxed into stomach) (AACN, 2016).

STEP 12c Obtain gastric aspirate.

   d. Gently mix aspirate in syringe. Expel a few drops into clean medicine cup. Note color of aspirate. Measure pH of aspirated GI contents by dipping pH strip into fluid or applying a few drops of fluid to strip. Compare color of strip with color on chart (see illustration) provided by manufacturer.

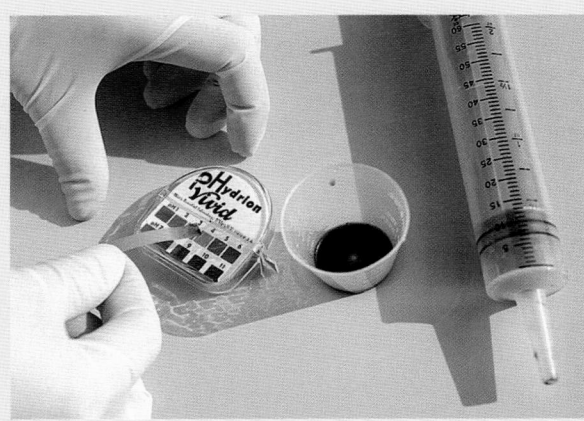

STEP 12d Compare color on test strip with color on pH chart.

Continued

BOX 45.14 PROCEDURAL GUIDELINES—cont'd

Obtaining Gastrointestinal Aspirate for pH Measurement and Large-Bore, and Small-Bore Feeding Tubes: Intermittent and Continuous Feeding

(1) Gastric fluid from patient who has fasted for at least 4 hours usually has pH range of 5.0 or less.

(2) Fluid from tube in small intestine of patient who is fasting usually has pH greater than 6.0 (Metheny et al., 2019).

(3) The pH of pleural fluid from the tracheobronchial tree is generally greater than 6.0.

13. If after repeated attempts it is not possible to aspirate fluid from tube that was confirmed by x-ray film to be in desired position and if (1) there are no risk factors for tube dislocation, (2) tube has remained in original taped position, and (3) patient is not in respiratory distress, assume that tube is correctly placed. Continue with irrigation (AACN, 2016; Fan et al., 2017).

14. Irrigate tube.

   a. Irrigate routinely before, between, and after final medication (before feedings are reinstituted), and before an intermittent feeding is administered.

   b. Draw up 30 mL of water in ENFit syringe. Do not use irrigation fluids from bottles that are used on other patients. Patient should have individual bottle of solution.

   CLINICAL JUDGMENT: Do not use cola or fruit juices for flushing tubing, as these liquids can clog tube.

   c. Change irrigation bottle every 24 hours. Irrigation trays, which hold both irrigation fluid and syringe, are considered open systems and may be more easily contaminated than sterile water bottles. **NOTE:** Be sure that syringe in tray has ENFit adapter.

   d. Kink feeding tube while disconnecting it from infusion tubing (continuous feeding) or while removing plug at end of tube (intermittent feeding).

   e. Insert tip of ENFit syringe into end of feeding tube. Release kink and slowly instill irrigation solution.

   f. If unable to instill fluid, reposition patient on left side and try again.

   g. When water or sterile saline has been instilled, remove syringe. Reinstitute tube feeding or administer medication as ordered. Then flush each medication completely through tube (see Chapter 31).

15. Help patient assume comfortable position. Raise side rails as appropriate and lower bed to lowest position. Remove and discard gloves; dispose of supplies in appropriate receptacle and perform hand hygiene.

16. Place nurse call system in an accessible location within patient's reach. Instruct patient in its use.

17. Observe patient for respiratory distress: persistent gagging, paroxysms of coughing, drop in oxygen (O_2) saturation, or respiratory patterns (e.g., rate and depth) that are inconsistent with baseline measures.

18. Verify that external length of tube, pH, and appearance of aspirate are consistent with initial tube placement.

19. Observe ease with which tube feeding instills through tubing.

20. Monitor patient's caloric intake.

21. **Use Teach-Back:** "I want to go over what I explained earlier. Tell me why it is important for me to test the gastric pH and the color of the gastric secretions in your stomach before feedings." Revise your instruction now or develop a plan for revised patient/family caregiver teaching if patient/family caregiver is not able to teach back correctly.

This allows the patient to disconnect from the infusion each morning, flush the central line, and have independent mobility during the day.

Preventing Complications. Complications of PN include catheter-related problems and metabolic alterations (Table 45.8). Pneumothorax results from an initial puncture during catheter insertion and CVC placement when the tip of the catheter accidentally enters the pleural space. This results in the accumulation of air in the pleural cavity with subsequent collapse of the lung and impaired breathing. The clinical symptoms of a pneumothorax include sudden sharp chest pain, dyspnea, and coughing. Monitor a patient with a CVC for the first 24 hours for signs and symptoms of pulmonary distress.

An air embolus that enters intravenously can occur during insertion of the catheter or when changing the tubing or cap. Turn the patient into a left lateral decubitus position and have the patient perform a Valsalva maneuver (holding the breath and "bearing down") during catheter insertion to help prevent air embolus. The increased venous pressure created by the maneuver prevents air from entering the bloodstream. Maintaining integrity of the closed IV system also helps prevent air embolus.

Catheter occlusion is present when there is sluggish or no flow through the catheter. Temporarily stop the infusion and flush with saline or per protocol orders. If this is unsuccessful, attempt to aspirate a clot. If still unsuccessful, follow institution protocol for use of a thrombolytic agent (e.g., urokinase).

Suspect catheter sepsis if a patient develops fever, chills, or glucose intolerance and has a positive blood culture. To prevent infection, change the TPN administration set infusion tubing with inline and add-on filters (with or without lipids) every 24 hours or with each new PN container (Gorski et al., 2021). Do not hang a single container of PN for more than 24 hours or lipids more than 12 hours.

During any administration set change, manipulation of the tubing, or CVC dressing change, always use the Infusion Nurses Society's (INS) recommended standard Aseptic Non-Touch Technique (ANTT®) practices (Gorski et al., 2021). This is a specific and comprehensively defined type of aseptic technique for any handling of IV site or connectors on IV devices. It integrates Standard Precautions such as hand hygiene and personal protective equipment with appropriate aseptic field management, nontouch technique, and sterilized supplies (Gorski et al., 2021) (see Chapter 42). Change the CVC dressing per institution policy and any time it becomes wet, disrupted, or contaminated. Use either 2% alcohol-based chlorhexidine gluconate (preferred), 70% alcohol, or povidone iodine to clean the injection port or catheter hub 15 seconds before and after each time it is used. Use a 1.2-micron filter for 3-in-1 formulas and an inline 0.22-micron filter for PN solutions that do not include IV fat emulsions.

PN solutions contain most of the major electrolytes, vitamins, and minerals. Patients also need supplemental vitamin K as ordered throughout therapy. Synthesis of vitamin K occurs by the microflora found in the jejunum and ileum with normal use of the GI tract; however, because PN circumvents GI use, patients need to receive exogenous vitamin K.

Electrolyte and mineral imbalances often occur. Administration of concentrated glucose accompanies an increase in endogenous insulin production, which causes cations (potassium, magnesium, and phosphorus) to move intracellularly. Monitor blood glucose levels every 6 hours to assess for hyperglycemia, and administer supplemental insulin as ordered (Harding et al., 2020) (see Skill 45.4).

TABLE 45.7 Enteral Tube-Feeding Complications

Problem	Possible Cause	Intervention[a]
Pulmonary aspiration	Regurgitation of formula	Verify tube placement. Place patient in high-Fowler position or elevate head of bed a minimum of 30 (preferably 45) degrees during feedings and for 2 hours afterward.
	Feeding tube displaced	Reposition tube and verify tube placement by ordered x-ray.
	Deficient gag reflex	Reassess for return of normal gag reflex; until then, place patient on aspiration precautions and in semi-Fowler position.
	Delayed gastric emptying	See delayed gastric emptying below.
Diarrhea	Hyperosmolar formula or medications	Deliver formula continuously, lower rate, dilute, or change to isotonic enteral nutrition.
	Antibiotic therapy	Antibiotics destroy normal intestinal flora; consult with health care provider to consider changing medication; treat symptoms with antidiarrheal agents; culture stool for *Clostridium difficile.*
	Bacterial contamination	Do not hang formula longer than 4–8 hours in bag, wash bag out well when refilling, change tube-feeding bags and tubing every 24 hours, and use aseptic practices. Check expiration dates.
	Malabsorption	Check for pancreatic insufficiency; use low-fat, lactose-free formula and continuous feedings.
Constipation	Lack of fiber	Consult with a dietitian to select a formula containing fiber.
	Lack of free water	Add water during tube flushes.[a]
	Inactivity	Monitor patient's ability to ambulate; collaborate with health care provider and/or physical therapist for activity order.
Tube occlusion	Pulverized medications given per tube	Irrigate with 30 mL of water before and after each medication per tube.[a] Use liquid medications when available. Completely dissolve crushed medications in liquid if liquid medication is unavailable.
	Sedimentation of formula	Shake cans well before administering (read label).
	Reaction of incompatible medications or formula	Read pharmacological information on compatibility of drugs and formula.
Tube displacement	Coughing, vomiting	Replace tube and confirm placement before restarting tube feeding.
	Not taped securely	With placement verification, check that tape is secure (nasoenteric).
Abdominal cramping, nausea/vomiting	High osmolality of formula	Suggest an isotonic formula or dilution of current formula to health care provider.
	Rapid increase in rate/volume	Lower rate of delivery to increase tolerance. Maintain head of bed at least 45 degrees.
	Lactose intolerance	Suggest use of lactose-free formula.
	Intestinal obstruction	Stop feeding with GI obstruction.
	High-fat formula used	Use greater proportion of carbohydrate.
	Cold formula used	Warm formula to room temperature.
Delayed gastric emptying	Diabetic gastroparesis	Consult with health care provider regarding prokinetic medication for increasing gastric motility.
	Serious illnesses	Consult health care provider regarding advancing tube to intestinal placement.
	Inactivity	Monitor medications and pathological conditions that affect GI motility.
Serum electrolyte imbalance	Excess GI losses Dehydration Presence of disease states such as cirrhosis, renal insufficiency, heart failure, or diabetes mellitus	Monitor serum electrolyte levels daily. Provide free water per registered dietitian recommendation.
Fluid overload	Refeeding syndrome in malnutrition	Restrict fluids if necessary and use either a specialized formula or a diluted enteral formula at first.
	Excess free water or diluted (hypotonic) formula	Monitor levels of serum proteins and electrolytes. Use more concentrated formula with fluid volume excess without risk of refeeding syndrome.
Hyperosmolar dehydration	Hypertonic formula with insufficient free water	Slow rate of delivery, dilute, or change to isotonic formula.

[a]First, check for fluid-restricted conditions that affect how much water can be given safely.
GI, Gastrointestinal.

TABLE 45.8   Metabolic Complications of Parenteral Nutrition

Problem	Signs/Symptoms	Intervention
Electrolyte imbalance	See Chapter 42 for signs of deficiency or toxicity	Check TPN for supplemental electrolyte levels. Notify health care provider of imbalances. Maintain steady rate of infusion. Monitor intake and output.
Hypercapnia	Increased oxygen consumption, CO_2, respiratory quotient (>1), and minute ventilation	Patients who are dependent on a ventilator are at risk; provide 30% to 60% of energy requirements per health care provider's order.
Hypoglycemia	Diaphoresis, shakiness, confusion, loss of consciousness	To prevent hypoglycemia, do not abruptly discontinue TPN but taper rate down to within 10% of infusion rate 1 to 2 hours before stopping. If you suspect hypoglycemia, test blood glucose and administer IV bolus of 50% dextrose or glucagon per order or protocol if necessary.
Hyperglycemia	Thirst, headache, lethargy, increased urination	Monitor blood glucose level every 6 hours. Initiate TPN slowly and taper up to maximal infusion rate to prevent hyperglycemia. Additional insulin may be required during therapy if problem persists or patient has diabetes mellitus.
Hyperglycemic hyperosmolar nonketotic coma (HHNKC) or hyperosmolar hyperglycemic nonketotic syndrome (HHNS)	Hyperglycemia (>500 mg/dL), glycosuria, serum osmolarity >350 mOsm/L, confusion, azotemia, headache, severe signs of dehydration (see Chapter 42), hypernatremia, metabolic acidosis, convulsions, coma	Monitor blood glucose, BUN, serum osmolarity, glucose in urine, and fluid losses; administer insulin as ordered; replace fluids as ordered; maintain constant infusion rate; and provide 30% of daily energy needs as fat. Patients at risk are those receiving steroids; older adults diagnosed with diabetes who have impaired renal or pancreatic function or increased metabolism or who are septic.

BUN, Blood urea nitrogen; *IV,* intravenous; *TPN,* total parenteral nutrition.

Too-rapid administration of hypertonic dextrose can result in an osmotic diuresis and dehydration (see Chapter 42). If an infusion falls behind schedule, do not increase the rate in an attempt to catch up. Sudden discontinuation of a solution can cause hypoglycemia. Usually it is recommended to infuse 10% dextrose when discontinuing PN solution suddenly. Patients with diabetes are more at risk.

The goal is to move patients from PN to EN and/or oral feeding. Once patients are meeting one-third to one-half of their kilocalorie needs per day, health care providers usually decrease PN by half the original volume and increase EN feedings to meet the patient's nutritional needs. Patients who make the transition from PN to oral feedings typically have early satiety and decreased appetite. Consult with an RD about decreasing PN in response to increased oral intake. If oral intake is inadequate, small frequent meals are helpful. Recommend calorie/protein counts when patients begin taking soft foods. When meeting 75% of nutritional needs by enteral feedings or reliable dietary intake, it is usually safe to discontinue PN therapy. Discontinuation of PN may also happen if complications occur or the health care provider determines that it is not benefiting the patient (Harding et al., 2020).

Restorative and Continuing Care. Patients discharged from a hospital with diet prescriptions often need dietary education to plan meals that meet specific therapeutic requirements. Restorative care includes both immediate postsurgical care and routine medical care and therefore includes patients in the hospital and at home. The following sections address nutritional interventions for some common disease states.

Medical Nutrition Therapy. Optimal nutrition is just as important in illness as it is in health. As a result, dietary modifications and intake are often needed to maintain the nutritional requirements of patients with certain illnesses. Medical nutrition therapy (MNT) is the use of specific nutritional therapies to treat an illness, injury, or condition. It is necessary to help the body metabolize certain nutrients, correct nutritional deficiencies related to a disease, and eliminate foods that may exacerbate disease symptoms. It is most effective using a team approach that promotes collaboration between the health care team and an RD (CDC, 2021c; Healthline, 2020).

Gastrointestinal Diseases. Control peptic ulcers with regular meals and ordered medications such as histamine receptor antagonists that block secretion of HCl or proton pump inhibitors. *Helicobacter pylori,* a bacterium that causes peptic ulcers, is confirmed by laboratory tests or a biopsy during endoscopy (Grodner et al., 2020). Antibiotics treat and control the bacterial infection. Stress and overproduction of gastric HCl also irritate a preexisting ulcer. Encourage patients to avoid foods that increase stomach acidity and pain such as caffeine, decaffeinated coffee, frequent milk intake, citric acid juices, and certain seasonings (hot chili peppers, chili powder, black pepper). Discourage smoking, alcohol, aspirin, and nonsteroidal antiinflammatory drugs (NSAIDs). Teach patients to eat a well-balanced, healthy diet; avoid eating large meals and foods that cause symptoms; and eat three regular meals (or several small meals) without snacks, especially at bedtime (Grodner et al., 2020; Ignatavicius et al., 2021). Family members of the patient with *H. pylori* infection also need to be tested and, if indicated, treated.

Inflammatory bowel disease includes Crohn disease and idiopathic ulcerative colitis. Treatment of acute inflammatory bowel disease includes elemental diets (formula with the nutrients in their simplest form ready for absorption) or PN when symptoms such as diarrhea and weight loss are prevalent. In the chronic stage of the disease, a regular highly nourishing diet is appropriate. Vitamins and iron supplements are often required to correct or prevent anemia. Patients manage inflammatory bowel syndrome by decreasing fiber, reducing fat, avoiding large meals, and avoiding lactose or sorbitol-containing foods for susceptible individuals.

The treatment of malabsorption syndromes such as celiac disease includes a gluten-free diet. Gluten is present in wheat, rye, and barley. Short-bowel syndrome results from extensive resection of the bowel, after which patients have malabsorption caused by lack of intestinal surface area. These patients require lifetime feeding with either elemental enteral formulas or PN.

Diverticulitis is a condition that results from an inflammation of diverticula, which are abnormal but common pouchlike herniations that occur in the bowel lining. Nutritional treatment for diverticulitis includes a moderate- or low-residue diet until the infection subsides. Afterward, a high-fiber diet for chronic diverticula problems is prescribed.

Diabetes Mellitus. Type 1 DM requires both insulin and dietary management for optimal control, with treatment beginning at diagnosis (CDC, 2021c). By contrast, patients often control type 2 DM initially with exercise and diet therapy. If these measures prove ineffective, it is common to add oral medications. Insulin injections often follow if type 2 DM worsens or fails to respond to these initial interventions.

Individualize the diet according to a patient's age, build, weight, and activity level. Maintaining a prescribed carbohydrate intake is the key in diabetes management. A diet that includes fruits and nonstarchy vegetables, lean meat and plant-based proteins, less added sugar, and foods that are less processed is recommended (ADA, 2021a). Monitoring carbohydrate consumption is a key strategy in achieving glycemic control (ADA, 2019). Limit saturated fat to less than 7% of the total calories and cholesterol intake to less than 200 mg/day. In addition, varieties of foods containing fiber are recommended. Patients can substitute sucrose-containing foods for carbohydrates but need to make sure to avoid excess energy intake. Patients with diabetes can eat sugar alcohols and nonnutritive sweeteners if they follow the recommended daily intake level (ADA, 2019). Patients with diabetes and normal renal function should continue to consume usual amounts of protein (15%–20% of energy) (ADA, 2019).

The goal of MNT treatment is to have glycemic levels that are normal or as close to normal as safely possible; lipid and lipoprotein profiles that decrease the risk of microvascular (e.g., renal and eye disease), cardiovascular, neurological, and peripheral vascular complications; and blood pressure in the normal or near-normal range (ADA, 2019). Be aware of signs and symptoms of hypoglycemia and hyperglycemia.

Cardiovascular Diseases. The goal of the AHA dietary guidelines (AHA, 2017) is to reduce risk factors for the development of hypertension and coronary artery disease. Diet therapy for reducing the risk of cardiovascular disease includes balancing calorie intake with exercise to maintain a healthy body weight; eating a diet high in fruits, vegetables, and whole-grain high-fiber foods; eating fish at least 2 times per week; and limiting food and beverages that are high in added sugar and salt. The AHA guidelines also recommend limiting saturated fat to less than 7%, *trans* fat to less than 1%, and cholesterol to less than 300 mg/day. To accomplish this goal, patients choose lean meats and vegetables, use fat-free dairy products, and limit intake of fats and sodium.

Cancer and Cancer Treatment. Malignant cells compete with normal cells for nutrients, increasing a patient's metabolic needs. Most cancer treatments cause nutritional problems. Patients with cancer often experience anorexia, nausea, vomiting, and taste distortions. The goal of nutritional therapy is to meet the metabolic needs of the patient through interprofessional collaboration of health care providers (Cotogni et al., 2019). Malnutrition in cancer is associated with increased morbidity and mortality. Enhanced nutritional status often improves a patient's quality of life.

Radiation therapy destroys rapidly dividing malignant cells; however, normal rapidly dividing cells such as the epithelial lining of the GI tract are often affected. Radiation therapy causes anorexia, stomatitis, severe diarrhea, strictures of the intestine, and pain. Radiation treatment of the head and neck region causes taste and smell disturbances, decreased salivation, and dysphagia. Nutritional management of a patient with cancer focuses on maximizing intake of nutrients and fluids. Individualize diet choices to a patient's needs, symptoms, and situation. Use creative approaches to manage alterations in taste and smell. For example, patients with altered taste often prefer chilled foods or foods that are spicy. Encourage patients to eat small frequent meals and snacks that are nutritious and easy to digest.

Human Immunodeficiency Virus/Acquired Immunodeficiency Syndrome. Patients with HIV/AIDS typically experience body wasting and severe weight loss related to anorexia, stomatitis, oral thrush infection, nausea, or recurrent vomiting, all resulting in inadequate intake. Factors associated with weight loss and malnutrition include severe diarrhea, GI malabsorption, and altered metabolism of nutrients. Systemic infection results in hypermetabolism from cytokine elevation. The medications that treat HIV infection often cause side effects that alter patients' nutritional status.

Restorative care of malnutrition resulting from AIDS focuses on maximizing kilocalories and nutrients. Address each cause of nutritional depletion in the care plan. The progression of individually tailored nutritional support begins with administering oral nutrition, to EN, and finally to PN. Good hand hygiene and food safety are essential because of a patient's reduced resistance to infection. For example, minimization of exposure to *Cryptosporidium* in drinking water, lakes, or swimming pools is important. Small, frequent, nutrient-dense meals that limit fatty and overly sweet foods are easier to tolerate. Patients benefit from eating cold foods and lean, low-fat protein sources, and limiting foods with high sugar content (Robinson, 2019).

Ryan implemented the plan of care by first discussing with Mrs. Cooper the need to improve her nutritional status through improving her eating habits. Ryan reviewed with Mrs. Cooper a balanced nutrition plan for her to meet her identified outcome of weight gain to meet a target weight, but the plan also considered her own food preferences and her diabetes, hypertension, and heart failure. Ryan scheduled the RD to come to this appointment with Mrs. Cooper. Together, the three planned meals that were nutritious and within Mrs. Cooper's budget. The RD recommended that Mrs. Cooper try eating six small meals through the day rather than three large meals. The RD also recommended healthy snacks for Mrs. Cooper and encouraged her to drink more water during the day. Prior to leaving, the RD gave Mrs. Cooper healthy recipes that are not hard or expensive to make. Ryan gave Mrs. Cooper a journal in which she could record her food intake over the next 4 weeks. Ryan reviewed Mrs. Cooper's medications with her, emphasizing any food-drug and drug-drug interactions that she needs to avoid so that she does not develop adverse effects from the medications.

Ryan, concerned about Mrs. Cooper's depression and social isolation, developed a plan with her to address both problems. Ryan shared with Mrs. Cooper the name of a counselor and suggested that she might want to talk to the counselor to help her move through her grieving process. He also provided Mrs. Cooper with information on the grief support group that meets weekly at Mrs. Cooper's church. Ryan encouraged Mrs. Cooper to consider attending a meeting over the next few weeks. He also encouraged Mrs. Cooper to begin attending the senior center 1 to 2 times per week for lunch. He recognized that for older adults, socializing at mealtimes helps to improve appetite and eating. Together, they added to the plan that Mrs. Cooper would reach out and call one of her church friends within the next 2 weeks.

Ryan scheduled a follow-up appointment with Mrs. Cooper in 4 weeks. He asked that she bring the food journal with her to her next appointment in 4 weeks. At this appointment he wants to follow up on her meal planning, eating habits, and follow-through with activities to help with her social isolation.

◆ Evaluation

Through the Patient's Eyes. Patients expect competent, timely, and accurate care. Patients also expect nurses to determine when nutritional therapies do not result in successful outcomes and alter the plan of care accordingly. Expectations and health care values held by nurses frequently differ from those held by patients. Successful interventions and outcomes require nurses to know what patients expect when a plan of care is developed. Evaluation of that plan involves incorporating nursing knowledge and skill. Work closely with your patients to confirm their expectations and talk with them about their concerns if their expectations are not realistic. Consider the limits of your patients' conditions and treatment, their dietary preferences, and their cultural beliefs when evaluating outcomes.

Patient Outcomes. Patient-centered care plans should reflect achievable outcomes. Evaluate the actual outcomes of nursing actions and compare them with expected outcomes to determine whether the outcomes were met (Fig. 45.9). Interprofessional collaboration remains essential in providing nutritional support (Ukleja et al., 2018). Nutritional therapy does not always produce rapid results. Evaluate a patient's current weight in comparison with the baseline weight, serum albumin or prealbumin, and protein and kilocalorie intake routinely. If your patient does not gain weight gradually or continues to lose weight, evaluate the dietary EN prescription, and determine whether the patient is experiencing any adverse effects from medications that are affecting nutritional status. Changes in condition also indicate a need to change the nutritional plan of care. Consult with all members of the health care team to better individualize this plan. The patient is an active participant whenever possible. In the end a patient's ability to incorporate dietary changes into lifestyle activities with the least amount of stress or disruption facilitates attainment of outcome measures. Failing to meet expected outcomes requires revising the nursing interventions or expected outcomes based on the patient's most current nursing diagnoses. When outcomes are unmet, ask questions such as "How has your appetite been?" "Have you noticed a change in your weight?" "How much would you like to weigh?" "Have you

been trying to lose/gain weight?" or "Have you changed your exercise pattern?" At times a reassessment will reveal new nursing diagnoses.

After completing his teaching session with Mrs. Cooper, Ryan used the principles of teach-back to evaluate Mrs. Cooper's learning. He says to Mrs. Cooper:

- *Tell me three foods that are high in protein that you will include in your diet.*
- *Explain to me one food-medication interaction that you will avoid.*
- *Discuss with me two ways you will begin that will decrease your social isolation.*

Mrs. Cooper was able to tell Ryan three sources of protein that she was going to add to her diet. Mrs. Cooper told Ryan that she would avoid green leafy vegetables and OTC medications that contain aspirin so she does not have interactions that would interfere with her warfarin. Mrs. Cooper also tells Ryan that she is going to call one of her church friends within 2 weeks to see if they can get together for lunch and that she will call the counselor and set up an appointment. She says that she feels that talking with a counselor could help her cope better with her grief and depression.

When Mrs. Cooper returns for her follow-up appointment, Ryan notes that Mrs. Cooper's appearance is better. She has more color, she seems more alert and focused on their conversation, her posture is less stooped, and her clothing is neat and clean. Ryan wants to know Mrs. Cooper's level of satisfaction with her care and the plan they developed. He asks, "Are you satisfied with the care you have received? Is the plan we developed working to your satisfaction? Have I met your expectations so far? If not, tell me how I can better help you." Mrs. Cooper replies, "I'm happy with the plan that we developed. I've cooked three of the recipes the RD gave me. They

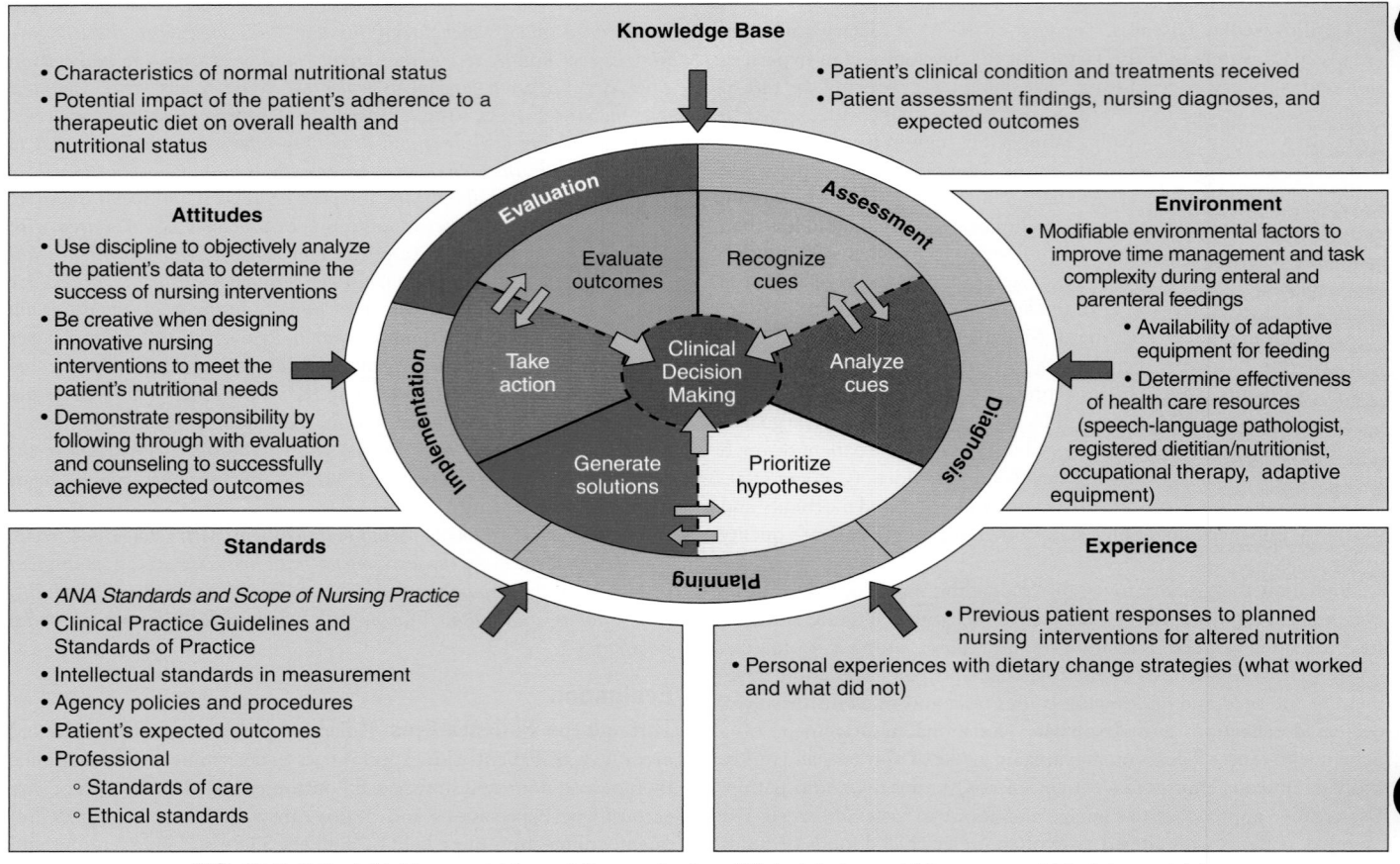

FIG. 45.9 Critical thinking model for nutrition evaluation. (Clinical Judgment Measurement Model copyright © NCSBN. All rights reserved.)

were easy to make and tasted good. My appetite seems to be getting better. I also started meeting my church friend at the senior center for lunch 1 or 2 times a week. It feels good to get out of the apartment again. I'm thinking of going back to my quilting club next month. The counselor that you recommended is extremely easy to talk with, and I feel like I'm making progress with my grief." Ryan weighs Mrs. Cooper and finds that she has gained 1 lb over the last 4 weeks. Mrs. Cooper's blood pressure is 130/82 mm Hg, her pulse is 82 beats/min, and her respirations are 14 breaths/min. The INR drawn the week before was 2.3. Ryan reviews Mrs. Cooper's food log. Ryan sees that Mrs. Cooper's eating habits have

improved. Most days she had at least three meals, and on some days she had six smaller meals. He also notes that Mrs. Cooper has increased her protein along with eating more fruits and vegetables. Mrs. Cooper reports to Ryan that she has been visiting the local farmer's market and is able to get the fruits and vegetables at a good price for her budget. Ryan praises Mrs. Cooper for the changes she has made and the progress she has shown in achieving her identified outcomes. Ryan instructs Mrs. Cooper to continue to monitor her food intake and meal planning and encourages her to make another appointment if her nutritional problems do not fully resolve or if she feels that she is having more difficulty coping.

SAFETY GUIDELINES FOR NURSING SKILLS

Ensuring patient safety is an essential role of the professional nurse. Use sound clinical judgment by communicating clearly with members of the health care team, assessing and analyzing patient's clinical findings, and incorporating the patient's priorities of care and preferences. Use the best evidence, applying professional standards, when selecting interventions to use in patient care delivery. When performing the skills in this chapter, remember the following points to ensure safe, patient-centered care:

- All candidates for NG or nasointestinal tube placement require an assessment of their coagulation status. Anticoagulation and bleeding disorders pose a risk for epistaxis during nasal tube placement.
- Nasal tubes are associated with sinusitis, otitis, vocal cord paralysis, and medical device–related pressure injuries (MDRPIs) to the nose.
- Use ENFit connectors for all enteral nutrition sets, syringes, and feeding tubes to prevent instillation of feeding into a different device (e.g., IV or drainage tube). Verify connector with each administration of tube feeding (TFC, 2014).
- Use aseptic technique when preparing and delivering enteral feedings. Check agency policy for wearing gloves when handling feedings (Harding et al., 2020).
- Label enteral equipment with patient name and room number; formula name, rate, and date and time of initiation; and nurse initials (Ukleja et al., 2018).
- Practice "right patient, right formula, right tube, right ENFit adapter" by matching formula and rate to feeding order and verifying that the enteral tubing set connects formula to a feeding tube (Harding et al., 2020).

- Position the patient upright or elevate the head of the bed a minimum of 30 (preferably 45) degrees unless medically contraindicated for patients receiving enteral feedings (Ukleja et al., 2018; ASPEN 2021).
- Trace all lines and tubing back to the patient to ensure only enteral-to-enteral connections (Ukleja et al., 2018).
- Do not add food coloring or dye to EN because the use of dye has been linked to hypotension, metabolic acidosis, and death (Harding et al., 2020).
- Refer to manufacturer guidelines to determine hang time for enteral feedings. Maximum hang time for formula is 8 hours in an open system and 24 to 48 hours in a closed, ready-to-hang system (if it remains closed). There is increased risk of bacterial growth in feedings that exceed the recommended hang time.
- Follow standard ANTT® practices when manipulating parts of the IV infusion for PN.
- Always use the appropriate type of infusion pump for continuous enteral feedings and PN.
- Be alert for signs of aspiration during oral feedings as well as when EN is administered.
- Clean and disinfect a point-of-care (POC) blood glucose testing meter after each patient use.

SKILL 45.1   ASPIRATION PRECAUTIONS

Delegation and Collaboration

The skill of following aspiration precautions while feeding a patient can be delegated to assistive personnel (AP). However, the nurse is responsible for the ongoing assessment of a patient's risk for aspiration and determination of positioning and any special feeding techniques. The nurse directs the AP to:

- Position patient upright (45–90 degrees preferred) or according to medical restrictions during and after feeding.
- Use aspiration precautions while feeding patients who need help and explain feeding techniques that are successful for specific patients.
- Immediately report any onset of coughing, gagging, or a wet voice or pocketing of food to the nurse.

Equipment

- Chair or bed that allows patient to sit upright
- Thickening agents as ordered by SLP (rice, cereal, yogurt, gelatin, commercial thickener)
- Tongue blade
- Penlight
- Oral hygiene supplies (see Chapter 40)
- Suction equipment (see Chapter 41)
- Clean gloves
- *Option:* Pulse oximeter

STEPS | RATIONALE

ASSESSMENT

1. Identify patient using at least two identifiers (e.g., name and birthday or name and medical record number) according to agency policy.

   Ensures correct patient. Complies with The Joint Commission standards and improves patient safety (TJC, 2021).

2. Review patient's medical history, nutritional risks, and results of nutritional screening in medical record. Assess for presence of conditions that cause dysphagia (see Box 45.7). Note patient's weight. Consult with SLP and/or RD.

   Reveals patient risk patterns for altered nutrition and dysphagia. Weight provides baseline for determining change in nutritional status.

3. Assess patient's current medications for use of sedatives, hypnotics, or other agents that may impair cough or swallowing reflex and for any medications that dry oral secretions (e.g., calcium channel blockers, diuretics) (Tan et al., 2018).

   Medication side effects may increase risk of developing dysphagia.

Continued

SKILL 45.1	ASPIRATION PRECAUTIONS—cont'd

STEPS	RATIONALE
4. Perform hand hygiene. Assess patient for signs and symptoms of dysphagia. Use a screening tool if agency recommended. Refer to SLP or RD if findings are positive for dysphagia.	Patient symptoms aid in determining whether further swallow evaluation is needed and approach to feeding.
5. Assess patient's or family caregiver's health literacy.	Ensures patient has the capacity to obtain, communicate, process, and understand basic health information (CDC, 2021d).
6. Assess patient's mental status: alertness, orientation, and ability to follow simple commands (e.g., open your mouth; stick out your tongue).	Disorientation and inability to follow commands present higher risk for dysphagia. Patients with progressive dementia develop dysphagia.
7. Apply gloves. Assess patient's oral cavity, level of dental hygiene, missing teeth, or poorly fitting dentures. Remove and dispose of gloves.	Poorly fitting dentures and absence of teeth can cause chewing and swallowing difficulties, increasing aspiration risk. Poor oral hygiene and periodontal disease can result in growth of bacteria in oropharynx, which if aspirated can lead to pneumonia (Makhnevich et al., 2019). Findings indicate level of oral hygiene needed and diet selection needed.
8. *Option:* Apply pulse oximeter to obtain baseline assessment of oxygen saturation. Keep oximeter in place. A decline in SpO_2 ≥2% has been regarded as a possible marker of aspiration (Marian et al., 2017). Perform hand hygiene.	Despite its clinical use, research findings question whether oximetry can reliably detect aspiration (ASHA, 2021a; Marian et al., 2017). Monitoring of SpO_2 during feeding may detect developing problem.
9. Prepare to observe patient during mealtime for signs of dysphagia. Observe patient attempt to feed self; note type of food consistencies and liquids able to swallow. Note during and at end of meal if patient tires.	Detects abnormal eating patterns such as frequent clearing of throat or prolonged eating time. Chewing and sitting up for feeding bring on onset of fatigue (Meiner and Yeager, 2019). Provides data for future planning of meal assistance.
10. Indicate in patient's health record that dysphagia/aspiration risk is present. *Option:* Some agencies use different-colored meal trays to signify patients at risk for aspiration.	Identifying patients with dysphagia reduces risk that they will receive improperly prepared oral nutrition without supervision.
11. Assess patient's or family caregiver's knowledge of and experience with dysphagia risk, diet options, and aspiration precautions.	Reveals need for patient instruction and/or support.
12. Assess patient's goals or preferences for how you should provide assistance with eating. Ask for patient or family caregiver's commitment to plan.	Matching your approach with patient outcomes will likely improve patient's participation. Initial commitment from a learner is critical. The learner processes information just collected from the assessment and articulates own plan (Chinai et al., 2018).

PLANNING

1. Provide patient 30-minute rest time before meals.	Some practitioners recommend rest time before meals (Metheny, 2018). Muscle weakness and fatigue may increase risk of aspiration.
2. Explain to patient why you are observing him or her while eating. Discuss signs and symptoms of aspiration. Teach patient how to perform aspiration precautions as appropriate.	Reduces anxiety and promotes cooperation. Signs or symptoms associated with aspiration indicate need for further swallowing evaluation such as fluoroscopic examination. Self-care supports patient's sense of autonomy.
3. Explain to patient and family caregiver about the aspiration precautions you are implementing.	Increases patient cooperation and prepares family caregiver for being able to assist.
4. Close room door and bedside curtain.	Provides patient privacy.
5. Obtain and organize equipment for aspiration prevention.	Ensures more efficient procedure.

IMPLEMENTATION

1. Perform hand hygiene and have patient or family caregiver (if going to help with feeding) perform hand hygiene.	Prevents transmission of microorganisms. Educates patient and family caregiver about need to maintain infection control practices.
2. Apply clean gloves. Use penlight and tongue blade to gently inspect mouth for pockets of food.	Pockets of food found inside cheeks occur when patient has difficulty moving food from mouth into pharynx; may lead to aspiration (Zupec-Kania and O'Flaherty, 2017). Patient is usually unaware of pocketing.
3. Provide thorough oral hygiene, including brushing tongue, before meal (see Chapter 40). Remove and dispose of gloves; perform hand hygiene.	Risk for aspiration pneumonia has been associated with poor oral hygiene (Makhnevich et al., 2019).
4. Position patient upright (90 degrees) in chair or elevate head of patient's bed to a 90-degree angle or highest position allowed by medical condition during meal. *Option:* Position patient in the side-lying position if patient cannot have head elevated.	Position facilitates safe swallowing and enhances esophageal motility (Metheny, 2018; Thomas et al., 2019).
5. Have oximeter in position to monitor during feeding.	Pulse oximetry continues to be used in many agencies in an effort to predict aspiration, but recent research questions its efficacy (ASHA, 2021a; Marian et al., 2017).
6. Provide appropriate thickness of liquids per SLP and RD assessment (International Dysphagia Diet Standardisation Initiative, 2021). Encourage patient to feed self.	Thin liquids are difficult to control in mouth and pharynx and are more easily aspirated.

STEPS	RATIONALE
7. Have patient assume chin-down position. Remind patient to not tilt head backward when eating or while drinking.	Chin-down position may help reduce aspiration (Metheny, 2018). One study suggests a head-turn-plus-chin-down maneuver may be more successful (Nagy et al., 2016).
8. Adjust the rate of feeding and size of bites to match the patient's tolerance. If patient unable to feed self, place ½ to 1 teaspoon of food on unaffected side of mouth, allowing utensil to touch mouth or tongue (Metheny, 2018).	Small bites help patient swallow (Metheny, 2018). Provides tactile cue to food being eaten; avoids pocketing of food on weaker side.
9. Provide verbal coaching: remind patient to chew and think about swallowing with comments such as the ones that follow: • Open your mouth. • Feel the food in your mouth. • Chew and taste the food. • Raise your tongue to the roof of your mouth. • Think about swallowing. • Close your mouth and swallow. • Swallow again. • Cough to clear your airway.	Verbal cueing keeps patient focused on normal swallowing (Metheny, 2018). Positive reinforcement enhances patient's confidence in ability to swallow.
10. Avoid mixing foods of different textures in same mouthful. Alternate liquids and bites of food (Metheny, 2018). Refer to RD for next meal if patient has difficulty with particular consistency.	Gradual increase in types and textures combined with constant monitoring helps patient to eat more safely. Single textures are easier to swallow than multiple textures. Alternating solids with liquids removes food residue in mouth.
11. During the meal explain to patient and family caregiver the techniques being used to promote swallowing.	Enhances patient and family caregiver's ability to use techniques in the home.
12. Monitor swallowing and observe for any respiratory difficulty. Observe for throat clearing, coughing, choking, gagging, and drooling of food; suction airway as needed (see Chapter 41).	These are indications that suggest dysphagia and thus pose risk for aspiration (American Stroke Association, 2018).
13. Minimize distractions, do not talk, and do not rush patient (Metheny, 2018). Allow time for adequate chewing and swallowing. Provide rest periods as needed during meal.	Environmental distractions and conversations during mealtime increase risk for aspiration. Avoiding fatigue reduces aspiration risk.

CLINICAL JUDGMENT: *If patient remains stable without difficulty, this is a good time to delegate continued feeding to AP so that you can attend to other patients and assigned priorities.*

14. Use sauces, condiments, and gravies (if part of dysphagia diet) to facilitate cohesive food bolus formation.	Cohesive food bolus helps to prevent pocketing or small food particles from entering the airway.
15. Ask patient to remain sitting upright for at least 30 to 60 minutes after a meal.	Remaining upright after meals or snacks reduces chance of aspiration by allowing food particles remaining in pharynx to clear (Metheny, 2018).
16. Apply gloves. Provide thorough oral hygiene after meal (see Chapter 40).	Rigorous oral hygiene reduces plaque and secretions containing bacteria, with studies showing reduction in incidence of pneumonia (Makhnevich et al., 2019; Metheny, 2018).
17. Return patient's meal tray to appropriate place. Remove and dispose of gloves.	Reduces spread of microorganisms.
18. Be sure patient is comfortable in upright position.	Promotes patient comfort and safety.
19. Place nurse call system in an accessible location within patient's reach.	Ensures patient can call for assistance if needed.
20. Raise side rails (as appropriate) and lower bed to lowest position. Perform hand hygiene.	Promotes patient safety. Reduces transmission of microorganisms.

EVALUATION

1. Observe patient's ability to swallow food and fluids of various textures and thickness without choking.	Indicates whether there is ease with swallowing and absence of signs related to aspiration.
2. Monitor pulse oximetry readings (if ordered) for high-risk patients during eating.	Deteriorating oxygen saturation levels may indicate aspiration, but current research questions predictive accuracy of oximetry.
3. Monitor patient's intake and output (I&O), calorie count, and food intake.	Helps to detect malnutrition and dehydration resulting from dysphagia.
4. Weigh patient daily or weekly.	Determines whether weight is stable and reflects nutritional status.
5. Observe patient's oral cavity after meal.	Determines presence of food pockets after meal that has included foods of various textures.
6. **Use Teach-Back:** "We talked about why your husband is at risk to aspirate and choke on his food. Tell me the things to observe for that will tell you if he is having trouble swallowing. What should you do if these things happen during a meal?" Revise your instruction now or develop a plan for revised patient/family caregiver teaching if patient/family caregiver is not able to teach back correctly.	Teach-back is an evidence-based health literacy intervention that promotes patient engagement, patient safety, adherence, and quality. The goal of teach-back is to ensure that you have explained medical information clearly so that patients and their families understand what you communicated to them (AHRQ, 2020).

Continued

SKILL 45.1	ASPIRATION PRECAUTIONS—cont'd

UNEXPECTED OUTCOMES AND RELATED INTERVENTIONS

1. Patient coughs, gags, complains of food "stuck in throat," and has wet quality to voice when eating.
- Stop feeding immediately and place patient on NPO.
- Notify health care provider and suction as needed (see Chapter 41).
- Anticipate consultation with SLP for swallowing exercises and techniques to improve swallowing.

2. Patient experiences weight loss over next several days or weeks.
- Discuss findings with health care provider and RD. Determine whether increasing frequency or quality of foods is needed.
- Nutritional supplements may be needed.

RECORDING AND REPORTING

- Record patient's diet, tolerance of liquids and food textures, amount of assistance required, response to instruction, position during meal, absence or presence of any symptoms of dysphagia, oxygen saturation (if measured), fluid intake, and amount of food eaten.
- Document your evaluation of patient learning.
- Report patient's tolerance to diet and degree of assistance required during hand-off report.
- Report any coughing, gagging, choking, or swallowing difficulties to nurse in charge or health care provider immediately.

HOME CARE CONSIDERATIONS

- Teach the patient and family the importance of frequent small meals with small bites and balancing with MNT.
- Teach patient and family how to recognize problems in swallowing.
- Teach patient and family about when to seek medical attention and what to report to the health care provider.

SKILL 45.2	INSERTING AND REMOVING A SMALL-BORE NASOENTERIC TUBE FOR ENTERAL FEEDINGS

Delegation and Collaboration
The skill of feeding tube insertion cannot be delegated to assistive personnel (AP). However, AP may help with patient positioning and comfort measures during tube insertion.

Equipment
Insertion
- Small-bore feeding tube with or without stylet (select the smallest diameter possible to enhance patient comfort)
- 60-mL ENFit syringe
- Stethoscope, pulse oximeter, capnography *(optional)*
- Hypoallergenic tape, semipermeable (transparent) dressing, or tube fixation device
- Liquid barrier spray or wipe
- pH indicator strip (scale 1.0–11.0)
- Cup of water and straw or ice chips (for patients able to swallow)
- Water-soluble lubricant

- Emesis basin
- Towel or disposable pad
- Facial tissues
- Clean gloves
- Suction equipment in case of aspiration
- Penlight to check placement in nasopharynx
- Tongue blade
- Oral hygiene supplies
- Measuring tape

Removal
- Disposable pad
- Tissues
- Clean gloves
- Disposable plastic bag
- Towel

STEPS	RATIONALE

ASSESSMENT

1. Verify health care provider's order for type of tube and EN feeding schedule. Also check order to determine whether health care provider wants prokinetic agent (e.g., metoclopramide) given before tube placement.

Health care provider's order is needed to insert feeding tube. Prokinetic agent given before tube placement may help advance tube (if it is to be advanced into intestine).

2. Identify patient using at least two identifiers (e.g., name and birthday or name and medical record number) according to agency policy.

Ensures correct patient. Complies with The Joint Commission standards and improves patient safety (TJC, 2021).

3. Review patient's medical history (e.g., for basilar skull fracture, nasal problems, nosebleeds, facial trauma, nasal-facial surgery, deviated septum, anticoagulant therapy, coagulopathy).

History of these problems requires you to consult with health care provider to change route of nutritional support. Passage of tube intracranially can cause neurological injury.

STEPS	RATIONALE

CLINICAL JUDGMENT: *If a patient is at risk for intracranial passage of the tube, avoid the nasal route. Oral placement or placement under medical supervision using fluoroscopic direct visualization is preferable. Insertion of a gastrostomy or jejunostomy tube is another alternative.*

STEPS	RATIONALE
4. Review medical record to determine patient's risk for developing a medical adhesive–related skin injury (MARSI) using adhesive devices or tape: Age, dehydration, malnutrition, exposure to radiation therapy, underlying chronic conditions (e.g., diabetes, immunosuppression), and edema of extremity.	These are common risk factors for MARSI (Fumarola et al., 2020).
5. Assess patient's or family caregiver's health literacy.	Ensures patient or family caregiver has the capacity to obtain, communicate, process, and understand basic health information (CDC, 2021d).
6. Ask patient to describe history of allergies: known type of allergies and normal allergic reaction. Focus on foods and adhesives. Check patient's allergy wristband.	Communication of patient allergies is essential for safe patient care. If medical adhesive is used to anchor enteral tube to nose, patient is at risk for MARSI (Fumarola et al., 2020).
7. Assess patient's height, weight, hydration status, electrolyte balance, caloric needs, and I&O.	Provides baseline information to measure nutritional improvement after enteral feedings.
8. Perform hand hygiene. Have patient close each nostril alternately and breathe. Examine each naris for patency and skin breakdown (apply clean gloves if drainage present). If patient previously had NG tube, check for medical device–related pressure injury (MDRPI) (see illustration).	Reduces transmission of microorganisms. Nares can sometimes be obstructed or irritated, or septal defect or facial fractures may be present. Place tube in more patent naris.
9. Perform physical assessment of abdomen (see Chapter 30). Remove and dispose of gloves (if worn). Perform hand hygiene.	Absent bowel sounds, abdominal pain, tenderness, or distention may indicate medical problem contraindicating feedings. Reduces transmission of microorganisms.
10. Assess patient's mental status (ability to cooperate with procedure, level of sedation), presence of cough and gag reflex, ability to swallow, critical illness, and presence of artificial airway.	These are risk factors for inadvertent tube placement into tracheobronchial tree (Metheny, 2018). Sedation impairs the ability of the patient to clear contents in the pharynx, thus increasing the risk of aspiration (Boullata et al., 2017).
11. Assess patient's knowledge, prior experience with small-bore feeding tube insertion, and feelings about the procedure.	Reveals need for patient instruction and/or support.
12. Assess patient's goals or preferences for how skill is to be performed or what patient expects.	Allows care to be individualized.

CLINICAL JUDGMENT: *Recognize situations in which blind placement of a feeding tube poses an unacceptable risk for placement. Devices designed to detect pulmonary intubation such as CO_2 sensors or electromagnetic tracking devices enhance patient safety. Alternatively, to avoid insertion complications from blind placement in high-risk situations, clinicians trained in the use of visualization or imaging techniques should place tubes (Metheny and Meert, 2017; Metheny et al., 2019).*

PLANNING

1. Explain procedure to patient, including sensations that will be felt during insertion (burning in nasal passages).	Increases patient's cooperation with procedure and helps lessen anxiety.
2. Explain to patient how to communicate during intubation by raising index finger to indicate gagging or discomfort.	Patient must have a way of communicating to alleviate stress and enhance cooperation.
3. Close room door and bedside curtain.	Provides patient privacy.
4. Obtain and organize equipment needed for insertion of small-bore feeding tube at the bedside.	Ensures more efficient procedure.

STEP 8 Medical device–related pressure injury under nose.

Continued

SKILL 45.2	INSERTING AND REMOVING A SMALL-BORE NASOENTERIC TUBE FOR ENTERAL FEEDINGS—cont'd

STEPS	RATIONALE

IMPLEMENTATION

1. Perform hand hygiene. Stand on same side of bed as naris chosen for insertion and position patient upright in high-Fowler position (unless contraindicated). If patient is comatose, raise head of bed as tolerated in semi-Fowler position with head tipped forward, using a pillow chin to chest. If necessary, have an AP help with positioning of confused or comatose patients. If patient is forced to lie supine, place in reverse Trendelenburg position.	Reduces transmission of microorganisms. Allows for easier manipulation of tube. Fowler position reduces risk of aspiration and promotes effective swallowing. Forward head position helps with closure of airway and passage of tube into esophagus.
2. Apply pulse oximeter/capnograph and measure vital signs. Maintain oximetry or capnography continuously.	Provides baseline for objective assessment of respiratory status during tube insertion and throughout time a tube is in place. Lowered oxygen saturation or increased end-tidal CO_2 can indicate tube being misplaced into the lungs or moving out of the stomach into lungs (Metheny et al., 2019).

CLINICAL JUDGMENT: *If patient has increase in end-tidal carbon dioxide or decrease in oxygen saturation, do **not** insert tube until you determine patient stability.*

3. Place bath towel over patient's chest. Keep facial tissues within reach.	Prevents soiling of gown. Insertion of tube frequently produces tearing.
4. Determine length of tube to be inserted and mark location with tape or indelible ink. Some tubes have centimeter markings.	Ensures organized procedure and estimation of the proper length of tube to insert into patient.
a. *Option, Adult:* Measure distance from tip of nose to earlobe to xyphoid process (NEX) of sternum (see illustration). Mark this distance on tube with tape.	Most traditional method. Length approximates distance from nose to stomach. Research has shown that this method may be least effective compared with others, although additional research is needed (Hodin and Bordeianou, 2019).
b. *Option, Adult:* A nose to earlobe to mid-umbilicus (NEMU) method to estimate appropriate NG tube placement has been recommended.	Promotes placement of the tube end holes in or closer to the gastric fluid pool (Boullata et al., 2017).
c. *Option, Adult:* Measure distance from xyphoid process to earlobe to nose (XEN) + 10 cm.	Provides best estimate of NG insertion length (Monica et al., 2019).
d. *Option, Child:* Use NEMU option.	Estimates proper length of tube insertion for pediatric patient.
e. Add 20 to 30 cm (8–12 inches) for postpyloric tubes.	Length approximates distance from nose to jejunum.

CLINICAL JUDGMENT: *Tip of prepyloric tubes must reach stomach to avoid the risk for pulmonary aspiration, which occurs when tubes end instead in the esophagus. Research has mixed findings regarding the best technique for estimating tube length (Santos et al., 2016). Confirmation of placement via x-ray immediately after completed insertion is still needed.*

5. Prepare tube for intubation. **NOTE: Do not ice tubes**.	Iced tube becomes stiff and inflexible, causing trauma to nasal mucosa.
a. Obtain order for stylet tube and check agency policy for trained clinician to insert tube.	The practice of inserting a tube requires great care and attention to practice guidelines.

STEP 4a Measure to determine length of tube to insert. (Copyright © Mosby's Clinical Skills: Essentials Collection.)

STEPS	RATIONALE
b. If tube has guidewire or stylet, inject 10 mL of water from ENFit syringe into tube.	Aids in guidewire or stylet removal. Activates lubrication of tube for easier passage and ensures that tube is patent. ENFit devices are not compatible with Luer connection or any other type of small-bore medical connector, thus preventing misadministration of an enteral feeding (Boullata et al., 2017; Institute for Safe Medication Practices [ISMP], 2020).
c. If using stylet, make certain that it is positioned securely within tube. Inject 10 mL of water from ENFit syringe into tube.	Promotes smooth passage of tube into GI tract. Improperly positioned stylet can cause tube to kink or injure patient. Ensures that tube is patent and aids in stylet removal. Once tube insertion is confirmed, have trained clinician remove stylet.
6. Prepare tube fixation materials (e.g., membrane dressing, tube fixation device, or precut piece of hypoallergenic tape, 10 cm [4 inches] long).	Used to secure tubing after insertion. Fixation devices allow tube to float free of nares, thus reducing pressure on nares and preventing medical device–related pressure injury (MDRPI).
7. Apply clean gloves.	Reduces transmission of microorganisms.
8. *Option:* Dip tube with surface lubricant into glass of room-temperature water or apply water-soluble lubricant (see manufacturer directions).	Activates lubricant to facilitate passage of tube into naris and GI tract.
9. Offer patient a cup of water with straw (if alert and able to swallow).	Patient will be asked to swallow water to facilitate tube passage.
10. **Tube Insertion**. Explain next steps and gently insert tube through nostril to back of throat (posterior nasopharynx). This may cause patient to gag. Aim back and down toward ear (see illustration).	Natural contours facilitate passage of tube into GI tract.
11. Have patient take deep breath, relax, and flex head toward chest after tube has passed through nasopharynx.	Closes off glottis and reduces risk for tube entering trachea.
12. Encourage patient to swallow small sips of water. Advance tube as patient swallows. Rotate tube gently 180 degrees while inserting.	Swallowing water lubricates and facilitates passage of tube into esophagus. Distinct tug may be felt as patient swallows, indicating that tube is following expected path. Tube rotation redirects the tip of tube away from glottis.
13. Emphasize need to mouth breathe and swallow during insertion.	Helps facilitate passage of tube and alleviates patient's fears during procedure.
14. Do not advance tube during inspiration or coughing because it is more likely to enter respiratory tract. Monitor oximetry and capnography at this time.	Can cause tube to inadvertently enter patient's airway, which will be reflected in changes in oxygen saturation and/or capnography.
15. Advance tube each time patient swallows until desired length has been reached (see illustration).	Reduces discomfort and trauma to patient. Helps facilitate tube passage.

CLINICAL JUDGMENT: *Do not force the tube or push against resistance. If patient starts to cough, experiences a drop in oxygen saturation or rise in end-tidal CO_2, or shows other signs of respiratory distress, withdraw the tube into the posterior nasopharynx until normal breathing resumes.*

STEPS	RATIONALE
16. Check for position of tube in back of throat using penlight and tongue blade.	Tube may be coiled, kinked, or entering trachea.
17. Temporarily anchor tube to nose with small piece of hypoallergenic tape.	Movement of tube stimulates gagging. Temporary anchoring of tube allows for assessment of general tube position before anchoring tube more securely.
18. Keep tube secure and check its placement by aspirating stomach contents to measure gastric pH (see Box 45.14). Also measure amount, color, and quality of return.	Provides baseline for appearance and pH of aspirate at initial location before x-ray confirmation.

CLINICAL JUDGMENT: *Insufflation of air into tube while auscultating abdomen is not a reliable means to determine position of feeding tube tip (Metheny et al., 2019).*

STEP 10 Insert tube through nostril to back of throat.

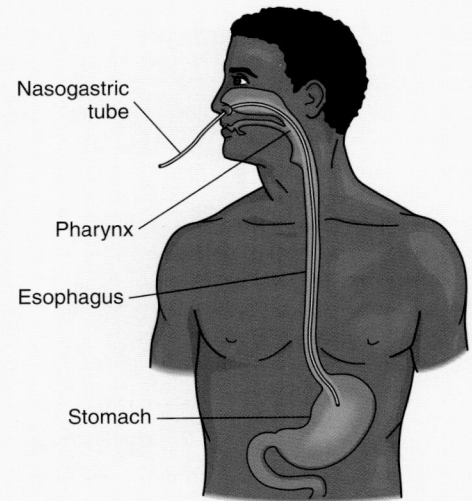

STEP 15 Nasogastric tube inserted through nasopharynx and esophagus into stomach.

Nasogastric tube

Pharynx

Esophagus

Stomach

Continued

SKILL 45.2   **INSERTING AND REMOVING A SMALL-BORE NASOENTERIC TUBE FOR ENTERAL FEEDINGS—cont'd**

STEPS	RATIONALE
19. Anchor tube to patient's nose, avoiding pressure on nares. Mark exit site on tube with indelible ink. Be sure skin over nose is clean and dry. Apply liquid barrier spray or wipe on bridge of patient's nose and allow it to dry completely. Select one of the following options for anchoring.	Movement of tube mark can alert nurses to possible displacement of tube. Properly secured tube allows patient more mobility and prevents trauma to nasal mucosa. Skin should be protected with a barrier product before an adhesive medical device is applied (Fumarola et al., 2020).
a. Membrane dressing:	
(1) Apply additional skin protectant to patient's cheek and area of tube to be secured.	Reduces risk of MARSI (Fumarola et al., 2020).
(2) Place tube against patient's cheek and secure tube with membrane dressing, out of patient's line of vision.	Eliminates application of tape around naris. Decreases risk for patient's inadvertent extubation.
b. Tube fixation device:	Secures tube and reduces friction on naris.
(1) Apply wide end of patch to bridge of nose (see illustration).	
(2) Slip connector around feeding tube as it exits nose (see illustration).	

> **CLINICAL JUDGMENT:** *Adhesive fixation materials create high risk for MARSI (Fumarola et al., 2020). If possible, use product with least adhesive content.*

STEPS	RATIONALE
c. Apply a strip of 4-inch tape:	Prevents pulling of tube. May require frequent change if tape becomes soiled.
(1) Remove gloves and tear two horizontal slits on each side of tape at ¹/₃ and ²/₃ length. Do not split tape. Fold middle sections forward.	Creates a gap in tape that, once secured, will allow tube to float and exert less pressure on naris.
(2) Tear vertical strip at bottom of tape. Print date and time on nasal part of tape.	Secures tube firmly and provides date of insertion.
(3) Place intact end of tape over bridge of patient's nose. Wrap each strip around tube as it exits (see illustrations).	Tube is free floating in the naris with this taping method, resulting in movement of tube in pharynx. Securing tape to naris in this method reduces pressure on naris and risk for medical device–related pressure injury (MDRPI) (Zakaria et al., 2018).

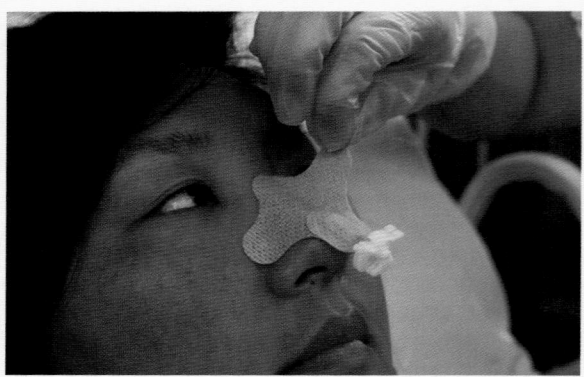

STEP 19b(1)   Apply tube fixation device to bridge of nose.

STEP 19b(2)   Slip connector around feeding tube.

A   B

STEP 19c(3)   (A) Applying tape to anchor nasoenteral tube. (B) Naris is free of pressure from tape and tube.

STEPS	RATIONALE
20. Fasten end of tube to patient's gown using clip (see illustration) or piece of tape. Do not use safety pins to secure tube to gown.	Reduces traction on naris if tube moves, which can cause medical device–related pressure injury (MDRPI). Safety pins become unfastened and cause injury to patients.
21. Help patient to comfortable position but keep head of the bed elevated at least 30 degrees (preferably 45 degrees) unless contraindicated (Metheny et al., 2019). For intestinal tube placement, place patient on right side when possible until radiographic confirmation of correct placement is made.	Promotes patient comfort and safety and lowers risk of aspiration for patients receiving tube feedings. Placing patient on right side promotes passage of nasal intestinal tube into small intestine.
22. Remove gloves and perform hand hygiene.	Reduces transmission of microorganisms.

CLINICAL JUDGMENT: *Leave stylet in place until correct position is verified by x-ray film. Never reinsert a partially or fully removed stylet while feeding tube is in place. This can cause perforation of tube and injure patient. Contact the health care provider if problems arise with feeding tube.*

STEPS	RATIONALE
23. Contact radiology department to obtain x-ray film of chest/abdomen.	Radiographic examination is most accurate method to determine feeding-tube placement (Metheny et al., 2019).
24. Perform hand hygiene. Apply clean gloves and administer oral hygiene (see Chapter 40). Clean tubing at nostril with washcloth dampened in mild soap and water.	Promotes patient comfort and integrity of oral mucous membranes. Reduces transmission of microorganisms.
25. Place nurse call system in an accessible location within patient's reach. Instruct patient in its use.	Ensures patient can call for assistance if needed.
26. Raise side rails (as appropriate) and lower bed to lowest position.	Promotes patient safety.
27. Dispose of all contaminated supplies in appropriate receptacle, remove and dispose of gloves, and perform hand hygiene.	Reduces transmission of microorganisms. Use appropriate disposal receptacle if patient is on hazardous drugs.
28. **Tube removal**	
a. Verify health care provider's order for tube removal.	Health care provider's order is needed to remove feeding tube.
b. Gather equipment.	Ensures organized procedure.
c. Explain procedure to patient.	Encourages cooperation, reduces anxiety, and minimizes risks. Identifies teaching needs.
d. Perform hand hygiene. Apply clean gloves.	Reduces transmission of microorganisms.
e. Position patient in high-Fowler position unless contraindicated.	Reduces risk for pulmonary aspiration in event patient should vomit.
f. Place disposable pad or towel over patient's chest.	Prevents mucus and gastric secretions from soiling patient's clothing.
g. Disconnect tube from feeding administration set (if present), and clamp or cap end.	Prevents formula from spilling from tube as it is removed.
h. Remove tape or tube fixation device from patient's nose. Unclip tube from patient's gown.	Allows tube to be removed easily.
i. Instruct patient to take deep breath and hold it. Then as you kink end of tube securely (folding it over on itself), completely withdraw tube by pulling it out steadily and smoothly onto towel or disposable bag. Dispose of it in appropriate receptacle.	Prevents inadvertent aspiration of gastric contents while tube is removed. Kinking prevents leakage of fluid from tube. Promotes patient comfort. Reduces transmission of microorganisms.
j. Offer tissues to patient to blow nose.	Clears nasal passages of remaining secretions.
k. Offer mouth care.	Promotes patient's comfort.
l. Help patient to comfortable position.	Promotes patient comfort and safety.
m. Place nurse call system in an accessible location within patient's reach.	Ensures patient can call for assistance if needed.
n. Raise side rails (as appropriate) and lower bed to lowest position.	Promotes patient safety.
o. Dispose of all contaminated supplies in appropriate receptacle, remove and dispose of gloves; perform hand hygiene.	Reduces transmission of microorganisms. Use appropriate disposal receptacle if patient is on hazardous drugs.

STEP 20 Fasten feeding tube to patient's gown.

Continued

SKILL 45.2	**INSERTING AND REMOVING A SMALL-BORE NASOENTERIC TUBE FOR ENTERAL FEEDINGS—cont'd**

STEPS	**RATIONALE**

EVALUATION

1. Observe patient's response to tube placement. Assess lung sounds; have patient speak; check vital signs; note any coughing, dyspnea, cyanosis, or decrease in oxygen saturation or increase in end-tidal CO_2.

Symptoms may indicate placement in respiratory tract. Auscultation of crackles, wheezes, dyspnea, or fever may be delayed response to aspiration. Lowered oxygen saturation or increased end-tidal CO_2 may detect tip of tube is in trachea or lung.

2. Confirm radiographic film results with health care provider.

Verifies position of tube before initiating enteral feeding.

3. Remove stylet after x-ray film verification of correct placement. Review agency policy regarding requirement of trained clinician for insertion.

If placement needs adjustment and stylet is still in place, contact health care provider.

4. Routinely observe condition of nares, location of external exit site marking on tube, and color and pH of fluid aspirated from tube.

Routine evaluation helps to prevent MDRPI and MARSI and verifies correct placement of tube.

5. Assess patient's level of comfort after removal.

Provides for continued comfort of patient.

6. **Use Teach-Back:** "I want to be sure that I explained to you what you can do while I insert the feeding tube into your stomach so that you can communicate with me. Tell me how you are going to communicate with me during tube insertion." Revise your instruction now or develop a plan for revised patient/family caregiver teaching if patient/family caregiver is not able to teach back correctly.

Teach-back is an evidence-based health literacy intervention that promotes patient engagement, patient safety, adherence, and quality. The goal of teach-back is to ensure that you have explained medical information clearly so that patients and their families understand what you communicated to them (AHRQ, 2020).

UNEXPECTED OUTCOMES AND RELATED INTERVENTIONS

1. Aspiration of stomach contents into respiratory tract (delayed response or small-volume aspiration), evidenced by auscultation of crackles or wheezes, dyspnea, or fever.
   - Report change in patient condition to health care provider immediately; if there has not been a recent chest x-ray film, suggest ordering one.
   - Position patient on side to protect airway.
   - Suction nasotracheally and orotracheally (Chapter 41).
   - Prepare for possible initiation of antibiotics.
2. Displacement of feeding tube to another site (e.g., from duodenum to stomach), which possibly occurs when patient coughs or vomits.
   - Aspirate GI contents and measure pH.
   - Remove displaced tube and insert and verify placement of new tube.
   - If there is question of aspiration, obtain chest x-ray film.
3. Erosion of skin at tube exit site or skin tear, blistering and redness around skin of nose (signs of MDRPI or MARSI) (Fumarola et al., 2020).
   - Avoid washing skin too much.
   - Use a pH-balanced soap to avoid drying of skin.
   - Be sure patient is hydrated.
   - If enteral tube is likely needed long term, consider reinsertion into other naris. Consult with health care provider.

RECORDING AND REPORTING

- Tube insertion: Record procedure and report type and size of tube placed; location of distal tip of tube; patient's tolerance of procedure; confirmation of tube position by x-ray film examination; length of tube that extends from nostril; color, pH, and amount of aspirate; condition of nares and surrounding skin; and securing device.
- Tube removal: Record procedure and patient's level of comfort and condition of naris.
- Report any type of unexpected outcome and the interventions performed to health care provider.
- During hand-off report, include tube placement, when confirmation of placement was received, and condition of patient's nares.

SKILL 45.3	**ADMINISTERING ENTERAL FEEDINGS VIA NASOENTERIC, GASTROSTOMY, OR JEJUNOSTOMY TUBES**

Delegation and Collaboration

The skill of administration of nasoenteric tube feeding can be delegated to assistive personnel (AP) (refer to agency policy). A registered nurse (RN) or licensed practical nurse (LPN) must first verify tube placement and patency. The nurse directs the AP to:

- Elevate head of bed to 30 to 45 degrees or sit patient up in bed or a chair unless contraindicated.
- Maintain the feeding rate (do not adjust it), to infuse the feeding as ordered.
- Report any difficulty in infusing the feeding or any discomfort voiced by the patient.
- Report any gagging, vomiting, paroxysms of coughing, or choking.
- Provide frequent oral hygiene.

Equipment

- Disposable feeding bag, tubing, or ready-to-hang system
- 60-mL or larger ENFit syringe
- Stethoscope
- Enteral infusion pump for continuous feedings
- pH indicator strip (scale 1.0–11.0)
- Water for flushing tube; sterile or purified water as indicated
- Prescribed enteral formula based on patient's disease process (Ukleja et al., 2018)
- Clean gloves
- ENFit connector

STEPS	RATIONALE

ASSESSMENT

1. Identify patient using at least two identifiers (e.g., name and birthday or name and medical record number) according to agency policy.

   Ensures correct patient. Complies with The Joint Commission standards and improves patient safety (TJC, 2021).

2. Verify health care provider's order for type of tube feeding formula, rate, route, and frequency.

   Ensures that correct formula will be administered in appropriate volume. Enteral formulas are not interchangeable.

3. Assess patient's or family caregiver's health literacy.

   Ensures patient has the capacity to obtain, communicate, process, and understand basic health information (CDC, 2021d).

4. Ask patient to describe history of allergies: known type of allergies, and normal allergic reaction. Focus on foods. Check patient's allergy wristband.

   Do not administer tube feeding formula if there is a known patient allergy. Communication of patient allergies is essential for safe patient care.

5. Review medical record for risk factors of malnutrition and current clinical characteristics of malnutrition (see Table 45.4). Consult with nutritional support team and health care provider.

   Determines patient's risk for malnutrition and potential need for early initiation of EN (Meehan et al., 2016; Ukleja et al., 2018).

6. Assess patient for factors that increase risk for aspiration: sedation, mechanical ventilation, nasotracheal suctioning, neurological compromise, lying flat, and sepsis (Eglseer et al., 2018).

   Identifies patients at high risk for aspiration so that decision may be made based on safety of gastric versus intestinal feeding (Ukleja et al., 2018).

7. Perform hand hygiene. Perform physical assessment of abdomen, including auscultation for bowel sounds, before feeding (see Chapter 30). Report findings to health care provider to determine whether tube feeding can proceed safely (Harding et al., 2020).

   Objective measures for assessing tolerance include changes in bowel sounds, expanding girth, tenderness and firmness on palpation, increasing NG output, and vomiting (Tatsumi, 2019).

8. Obtain baseline weight and review serum electrolytes and blood glucose measurement (see Skill 45.4). Assess patient for fluid volume excess or deficit, electrolyte abnormalities, and metabolic abnormalities (e.g., hyperglycemia).

   The goal of enteral feedings is to restore or maintain patient's nutritional status. Measures provide objective data and baseline to determine selection of formula and measure effectiveness of feedings.

9. Collaborate with RD to determine patient's caloric and protein requirements. Then set goal for delivery of EN (Ukleja et al., 2018).

   Sets objective measure for determining percent of prescribed calories and protein delivered.

10. Assess patient' knowledge, prior experience with enteral feedings, and feelings about the procedure.

    Reveals need for patient instruction and/or support.

11. Assess patient's goals or preferences for how skill is to be performed or what patient expects.

    Allows care to be individualized to patient.

PLANNING

1. Explain enteral feeding administration procedure to patient and/or caregiver. Discuss need for and procedure related to EN. If applicable, teach patient or family caregiver how to perform enteral feedings.

   Reduces anxiety and promotes cooperation.

2. Close room door and bedside curtain.

   Provides patient privacy.

3. Obtain and organize equipment for enteral feeding administration.

   Ensures more efficient procedure.

IMPLEMENTATION

1. Perform hand hygiene. Apply clean gloves.

   Reduces transmission of microorganisms and potential contamination of enteral formula.

2. Reverify correct formula and check expiration date second time; note integrity of container and appearance of formula.

   Ensures that correct therapy is to be administered and checks integrity of formula.

   a. Prepare formula for administration, following manufacturer guidelines.

CLINICAL JUDGMENT: *Discard unused reconstituted and refrigerated formulas within 24 hours of preparation (Boullata et al., 2017).*

---

   b. Have formula at room temperature.

   Cold formula causes gastric cramping and discomfort because liquid is not warmed by mouth and esophagus.

   c. Use aseptic technique to connect administration set tubing to container as needed. Use proper ENFit connecter and avoid handling feeding system or touching can tops, container openings, spike, and spike port.

   Bag, connections, and tubing must be free of contamination to prevent bacterial growth. The use of a closed system lowers the risk of infections due to bacterial contamination (Boullata et al., 2017).

   d. Shake formula container well. Clean top of canned formula with alcohol swab before opening it.

   Ensures integrity of formula; prevents transmission of microorganisms.

   e. For closed systems, connect administration tubing to container. If using open system, pour formula from brick pack or can into administration bag (see illustration).

   Formulas are available in closed-system containers that contain a 24- to 48-hour supply of formula or in an open system, in which formula must be transferred from brick packs or cans to a bag before administration.

3. Open roller clamp and allow administration tubing to fill. Clamp off tubing with roller clamp. Hang container on IV pole.

   Prevents introduction of air into stomach once feeding begins.

Continued

SKILL 45.3   ADMINISTERING ENTERAL FEEDINGS VIA NASOENTERIC, GASTROSTOMY, OR JEJUNOSTOMY TUBES—cont'd

STEPS	RATIONALE

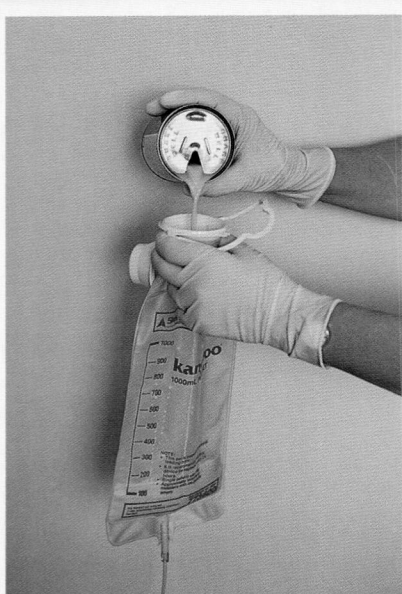

STEP 2e Pour formula into open feeding container.

4. Keep patient in high-Fowler position or elevate head of bed at least 30 degrees (45 degrees recommended). For patient forced to remain supine, place in reverse Trendelenburg position, which raises head.

Elevation of head of bed helps prevent pulmonary aspiration (Boullata et al., 2017; ASPEN, 2021). Researchers recommend head-of-bed elevation of 45 degrees for patients receiving EN who require mechanical ventilation or are heavily sedated, but lowering the head of bed to 30 degrees might be done periodically for patient comfort and in patients at risk for developing pressure injury (MDRPI) (Schallom et al., 2015; Metheny et al., 2019).

5. Verify tube placement (see Skill 45.2). Observe appearance of aspirate, measure the length of the tube extending from the nares and compare to the insertion length, and note pH.

Verifies whether tip of tube is in stomach, intestine, or lung based on pH value (<5.0) (Fan et al., 2017; Ni et al., 2017).

   a. *Nasoenteric and gastrostomy tube:* Attach ENFit syringe to end of enteral feeding tube and aspirate gastric or intestinal contents.

Gastric fluid for patient who has fasted for at least 4 hours usually has pH of 1.0 to 4.0 (if not receiving gastric acid inhibitor, then pH of <5.0) (Fan et al., 2017). If continuous feedings into stomach or intestine, check pH if feedings held for at least 1 hour for diagnostic reason (stomach pH <5.0; intestinal pH >6.0) (Fan et al., 2017).

   b. *Jejunostomy tube:* Attach ENFit syringe to end of tube and aspirate intestinal secretions. Observe appearance; if significant amounts are returned or resemble gastric secretions, check pH.

Presence of intestinal fluid at pH greater than 6.0 indicates that end of tube is in small intestine. If fluid tests acidic on pH test or looks like gastric fluid, tube may be displaced into stomach.

6. Check GRV per agency policy. Routine use is no longer recommended (Boullata et al., 2017), and GRV should not be used as a single measure of tolerance.

GRV has poor correlation with pneumonia, regurgitation, and aspiration. Frequent checking may delay feeding. However, if other signs of intolerance (e.g., abdominal distention, vomiting, or pain) are present, GRV of 250 to 500 mL may indicate the need to take measures to prevent aspiration or hold feeding completely (Boullata et al., 2017). Intestinal residual is usually very small. If residual volume is greater than 10 mL, displacement of intestinal tube into stomach may have occurred.

CLINICAL JUDGMENT: *Limit gastric residual checks to recommended standard intervals, as acidic gastric contents may cause protein in enteral formulas to precipitate within the lumen of the tube, creating risk for obstruction (Boullata et al., 2017). Use of GRVs leads to increased tube clogging, inappropriate cessation of EN, consumption of nursing time, and allocation of health care resources and may adversely affect outcome through reduced volume of EN delivered (Boullata et al., 2017).*

---

   a. Draw up 10 to 30 mL air into ENFit syringe and connect to end of feeding tube. Inject air slowly into tube. Pull back slowly and aspirate total amount of gastric contents you can aspirate.

GRV may not be easy to obtain from small-bore feeding tube. A 60-mL syringe prevents gastric tube collapse.

STEPS	RATIONALE
b. Return aspirated contents to stomach slowly. Refer to agency policy for any cutoff to hold aspirated contents instead (Boullata et al., 2017).	Prevents loss of nutrients and electrolytes in discarded fluid. Some questions exist regarding safety of returning high volumes of fluid into stomach.
c. GRVs in range of 200 to 500 mL may raise concern and lead to implementation of measures to reduce risk of aspiration. Automatic cessation of feeding should not occur for GRV less than 500 mL in absence of other signs of intolerance (Boullata et al., 2017; Jordan and Moore, 2020).	Raising cutoff value for GRV from lower number to higher number does not increase risk for regurgitation, aspiration, or pneumonia (Boullata et al., 2017).
d. Flush feeding tube with 30 mL water.	Prevents clogging of tubing and ensures that complete feeding is administered.

CLINICAL JUDGMENT: *Minimize the use of sedatives in patients receiving continuous feeding because airway clearance is reduced in patients when they are sedated (Boullata et al., 2017).*

7. Intermittent feeding (administered at certain times during the day):	
a. Pinch proximal end of feeding tube and remove cap. Connect distal end of administration set tubing to ENFit device on feeding tube and release tubing.	Prevents excessive air from entering patient's stomach and leakage of gastric contents. Ensures that feeding will be administered into correct tubing (Boullata et al., 2017).
b. Set rate by adjusting roller clamp on tubing or attach tubing to feeding pump (see illustration). Allow bag to empty gradually over 30 to 45 minutes (length of time of a comfortable meal). Bag label should include patient identifiers, formula type, enteral delivery site (route and access), administration method and type, and volume and frequency of water flushes (Ukleja et al., 2018). Also include a label with date, time, and initials when hanging a feeding.	Gradual emptying of tube feeding reduces risk for abdominal discomfort, vomiting, or diarrhea induced by intermittent bolus or too-rapid infusion of tube feedings. Critical elements for an EN order should be on EN label (Ukleja et al., 2018). Labeling indicates when to change administration set and confirms that right patient is receiving feeding.

CLINICAL JUDGMENT: *Use pumps designated for tube feeding, not IV fluids.*

c. Immediately follow feeding with prescribed amount of water (per health care provider's orders or agency policy). Cover end of feeding tube with cap when not in use. Keep bag as clean as possible. Change administration set every 24 hours.	Prevents tube from clogging. Prevents air from entering stomach between feedings and limits microbial contamination of system.
8. Continuous infusion method:	Method delivers prescribed hourly rate of feeding and reduces risk for abdominal discomfort.
a. Remove cap on tubing and connect distal end of administration set tubing to feeding tube using ENFit connector as in Step 7a.	Prevents excess air from entering patient's stomach and leakage of gastric contents.
b. Thread tubing through feeding pump; set rate on pump and turn on (see illustration).	Delivers continuous feeding at steady rate and pressure. Feeding pump alarms for increased resistance.
c. Advance rate of tube feeding (and concentration of feeding) gradually, as ordered.	Tube feeding can usually begin with full-strength formula. Conservative initiation and advancement of EN nutrition depend on patient's age, medical condition, nutritional status, and expected patient tolerance (Grodner et al., 2020).

CLINICAL JUDGMENT: *Limit infusion time for open EN feeding systems to 4 to 8 hours maximum (12 hours in the home setting) (Boullata et al., 2017). Follow the manufacturer's recommendations for duration of infusion through an intact closed delivery device (Boullata et al., 2017).*

STEP 7b Administer intermittent feeding.

STEP 8b Connect tubing through infusion pump. (Kangaroo ePump © 2018 Courtesy of Cardinal Health UK Ltd.)

Continued

STEPS	RATIONALE
9. After feeding, flush tubing with 30 mL water every 4 hours during continuous feeding (see agency policy) or before and after an intermittent feeding. Have RD recommend total free-water requirement per day and obtain health care provider's order.	Provides patient with source of water to help maintain fluid and electrolyte balance. Clears tubing of formula and helps maintain tube patency.
10. Rinse bag and tubing with warm water whenever feedings are interrupted. Use new administration set every 24 hours.	Rinsing bag and tubing with warm water clears old tube feedings and reduces bacterial growth.
11. Be sure patient is comfortable and remains in position with head of elevated 30 to 45 degrees.	Promotes patient comfort and safety. Reduces risk of aspiration.
12. Place nurse call system in an accessible location within patient's reach.	Ensures patient can call for assistance if needed.
13. Raise side rails (as appropriate) and lower bed to lowest position.	Promotes patient safety.
14. Dispose of all contaminated supplies in appropriate receptacle, remove and dispose of gloves, and perform hand hygiene.	Reduces transmission of microorganisms. Use appropriate disposal receptacle if patient is on hazardous drugs.

EVALUATION

1. Monitor patient's tolerance to feeding by assessing for abdominal distention, firmness, feeling of fullness, or nausea (Boullata et al., 2017). GRV checks should be limited and done per policy.	Symptoms are warnings that patient may have gastric reflux, leading to aspiration. Bowel sounds indicate whether peristalsis is present.
2. Monitor I&O at least every 8 hours and calculate daily totals every 24 hours.	Intake and output are indications of fluid balance, which can indicate fluid volume excess or deficit.
3. Weigh patient daily until maximum administration rate is reached and maintained for 24 hours; then weigh patient 3 times per week.	Slow weight gain is indicator of improved nutritional status; however, sudden gain of more than 2 lb (0.9 kg) in 24 hours usually indicates fluid retention.
4. Monitor patient for appropriate feeding tube placement at least every 4 hours or per agency protocol. Monitor visible length of tubing or marking at tube exit site (naris or stoma); check placement when a deviation is noted (Boullata et al., 2017).	Accidental displacement of tip of tube could lead to aspiration.
5. Monitor laboratory values as ordered by health care provider.	Determines correct administration of formula rate and strength.
6. Observe patient's respiratory status for coughing, dyspnea, tachypnea, change in oxygen saturation, hoarseness, crackles in lungs.	Change in respiratory status may indicate aspiration of tube feeding into respiratory tract.
7. Inspect site of gastrostomy or jejunostomy tube for signs of impaired skin integrity and symptoms of infection, injury, or tightness of tube.	Enteral tubes often cause pressure and excoriation at insertion site.
8. Inspect point of tube insertion and securement at least daily for MDRPI or MARSI: skin irritation, abrasion, inflammation, tenderness, edema.	Enteral tubes often cause pressure and excoriation at insertion site. If adhesive secures tubing, patient is also at risk for MARSI.
9. **Use Teach-Back:** "I want to be sure that I explained to you what you need to look for that may tell us you are not tolerating your tube feeding. Tell me two things that may tell us that you are not tolerating your tube feedings." Revise your instruction now or develop a plan for revised patient/family caregiver teaching if patient/family caregiver is not able to teach back correctly.	Teach-back is an evidence-based health literacy intervention that promotes patient engagement, patient safety, adherence, and quality. The goal of teach-back is to ensure that you have explained medical information clearly so that patients and their families understand what you communicated to them (AHRQ, 2020).

UNEXPECTED OUTCOMES AND RELATED INTERVENTIONS

1. Feeding tube becomes clogged.
   - Attempt to flush tube with water.
   - Special products are available for unclogging feeding tubes; **do not** use carbonated beverages or juices.
   - Hold feeding and notify health care provider.
   - Maintain patient in semi-Fowler position.
   - Contact pharmacist to change medications to liquid form and flush before and after intermittent feedings and medications.
2. Patient develops more than three loose stools in 24 hours.
   - Notify health care provider.
   - Consult dietitian about need to change formula to prevent malabsorption.
   - Identify and treat underlying medical/surgical issues and infections.
   - Provide perianal skin care after each stool.
   - Determine other causes of diarrhea (e.g., *Clostridium difficile* infection, contaminated tube feeding, medication containing sorbitol).
3. Patient has an enteral tube misconnection (e.g., connecting an enteral tube to an IV site or ventilator in-line suction catheter).
   - Infusion of enteral feeding into vein or directly into lung is a medical emergency.
   - Call health care provider and rapid response team immediately.
4. Patient aspirates formula, indicated by sudden appearance of respiratory symptoms (such as severe coughing, dyspnea, and cyanosis) associated with eating, drinking, or regurgitation of gastric contents. Auscultation of lungs reveals crackles or wheezes.
   - Immediately position patient on side with head of bed elevated.
   - Report change in condition to health care provider.
   - Suction nasotracheally or orotracheally.

CLINICAL JUDGMENT: *Small-volume aspirations that produce no overt symptoms are common and are often not discovered until the condition progresses to aspiration pneumonia (Eglseer et al., 2018).*

RECORDING AND REPORTING

- Record placement checks (length of tube; GRV type, pH, and amount), findings on abdominal assessment, amount and type of feeding, infusion rate (continuous feeding) or time for infusion (intermittent method), patient's response to tube feeding, patency of tube, and condition of skin at tube site.
- Document your evaluation of patient learning.
- Record volume of formula and any additional water on I&O form.
- Report adverse outcomes to health care provider.
- During a hand-off report note the type of feeding, infusion rate and volume infused during shift, status of feeding tube placement, and patient's tolerance, and trace the administration set tubing to the enteral tube connection point to ensure the feeding is being infused enterally (Ukleja et al., 2018).

HOME CARE CONSIDERATIONS

- Teach patient or family caregiver how to determine correct placement of feeding tube.
- Inform patient or family caregiver of signs associated with pulmonary aspiration, delayed gastric emptying.
- Reinforce signs and symptoms associated with feeding tube complications and when to call health care provider.
- Explain and demonstrate how to do skin care around gastrostomy or jejunostomy tube and explain signs and symptoms of infection at the insertion site.

SKILL 45.4 BLOOD GLUCOSE MONITORING

Delegation and Collaboration

During an acute illness, assessment of a patient's blood glucose cannot be delegated to assistive personnel (AP). When the patient's condition is stable, the skill of obtaining and testing for blood glucose level can be delegated to AP. The nurse informs the AP by:

- Explaining appropriate sites to use for puncture and when to obtain glucose levels.
- Instructing AP to report all glucose levels to RN.

Equipment

- Antiseptic swab
- Cotton ball
- Lancet device, either self-activating or button activated
- Blood glucose meter (e.g., Accucheck III, OneTouch) (Fig. 45.10)
- Blood glucose test strips appropriate for meter brand used
- Clean gloves
- Paper towel

FIG. 45.10 Blood glucose monitor. (Courtesy LifeScan, Inc., Milpitas, CA.)

Continued

SKILL 45.4	**BLOOD GLUCOSE MONITORING—cont'd**

STEPS	**RATIONALE**

ASSESSMENT

1. Identify patient using at least two identifiers (e.g., name and birthday or name and medical record number) according to agency policy.

Ensures correct patient. Complies with The Joint Commission standards and improves patient safety (TJC, 2021).

2. Review health care provider's order for time or frequency of measurement.

Health care provider determines test schedule on basis of patient's physiological status and risk for glucose imbalance.

> **CLINICAL JUDGMENT:** *For some critically ill patients, handheld point-of-care (POC) glucometers yield inconsistent results when the patient has low hematocrit levels or is hypotensive; when the patient is taking vasopressors, ascorbic acid, or other medications; or when capillary blood specimens as opposed to arterial or venous blood samples are used. These factors can potentially lead to incorrect insulin dosing. For the most accurate results use arterial or venous blood samples (Isbell, 2017).*

3. Determine whether specific conditions need to be met before or after sample collection (e.g., fasting, postprandial, after certain medications, before insulin doses).

Dietary intake of carbohydrates and ingestion of concentrated glucose preparations alter blood glucose levels.

4. Determine whether risks exist for performing skin puncture (e.g., low platelet count, anticoagulant therapy, bleeding disorders).

Abnormal clotting mechanisms increase risk for local ecchymosis and bleeding.

5. Perform hand hygiene. Assess area of skin to be used as puncture site. Inspect fingers or forearms for edema, inflammation, cuts, or sores. Avoid areas of bruising, recently punctured areas, and open lesions. Avoid using hand on side of mastectomy. Sides of fingers are commonly selected because they have fewer nerve endings.

Recently punctured sites are avoided because these factors cause increased interstitial fluid and blood to mix and increase risk for infection.

6. Assess patient's or family caregiver's health literacy.

Ensures patient or family caregiver has the capacity to obtain, communicate, process, and understand basic health information (CDC, 2021d).

7. Assess patient's knowledge, prior experience with blood glucose testing, and feelings about the procedure.

Reveals need for patient instruction and/or support.

8. Assess patient's goals or preferences for how skill is to be performed or what patient expects.

Allows care to be individualized to patient.

PLANNING

1. Explain procedure and purpose to patient and family. Offer patient and family opportunity to practice testing procedure. Provide resources and teaching aids for patient and family.

Promotes understanding of the procedure and cooperation.

2. Close room door and bedside curtain.

Provides patient privacy.

3. Obtain and organize equipment needed for blood glucose monitoring.

Ensures more efficient procedure.

IMPLEMENTATION

1. Perform hand hygiene. Instruct adult to perform hand hygiene, including forearm (if applicable), with soap and warm water. Rinse and dry.

Promotes skin cleansing and vasodilation at selected puncture site. Reduces transmission of microorganisms.

2. Position patient comfortably in chair or in semi-Fowler position in bed.

Ensures easy accessibility to puncture site. Patient assumes position when self-testing.

3. Remove reagent strip from vial and tightly seal cap. Check code on test strip vial. Use only test strips recommended for glucose meter. Some newer meters do not require code and/or have disk or drum with 10 or more test strips.

Protects strips from accidental discoloration caused by exposure to air or light. Code on test strip vial must match code entered into glucose meter.

4. Insert strip into meter (refer to manufacturer directions (see illustration). Do not bend strip. Meter turns on automatically.

Some machines must be calibrated; others require zeroing of timer. Each meter is adjusted differently.

STEP 4 Load test strip into meter. (Courtesy Accu-Chek Glucometer.)

STEPS	**RATIONALE**
5. Remove unused reagent strip from meter and place on paper towel or clean, dry surface with test pad facing up (see manufacturer directions).	Moisture on strip can alter accuracy of final test results.
6. Meter displays code on screen that must match code from test strip vial. Press proper button on meter to confirm matching codes. Meter is ready for use.	Codes must match for meter to operate. Meters have different messages that confirm that meter is ready for testing and blood can be applied.
7. Perform hand hygiene and apply clean gloves. Prepare single-use lancet or multiple-use lancet device. **NOTE:** For some meters, it is recommended that this step be completed before preparing test strip. Remove cap from lancet device; insert new lancet. Some lancet devices have disk or cylinder that rotates to new lancet.	Reduces transmission of microorganisms. Never reuse a lancet, because of risk of infection.
a. Twist off protective cover on tip of lancet. Replace cap of lancet device.	
b. Cock lancet device, adjusting for proper puncture depth.	Each patient varies as to depth of insertion needed for lancet to produce blood drop.
8. Obtain blood sample.	
a. Wipe patient's finger or forearm lightly with antiseptic swab and allow to dry. Choose vascular area for puncture site. In stable adults select lateral side of finger. Avoid central tip of finger, which has denser nerve supply (Pagana et al., 2019).	Removes microorganisms from skin surface. Side of finger is less sensitive to pain.
b. Hold area to be punctured in dependent position. Do not milk or massage finger site.	Increases blood flow to area before puncture. Milking may hemolyze specimen and introduce excess tissue fluid (Pagana et al., 2019).
c. Hold tip of lancet device against area of skin chosen for test site (see illustration). Press release button on device. Some devices allow you to see blood sample forming. Remove device.	Placement ensures that lancet enters skin properly.
d. With some devices, a blood sample begins to appear. Otherwise gently squeeze or massage fingertip until round drop of blood forms (see illustration).	Adequate-size blood sample is needed to test glucose.
9. Obtain test results.	Exposure of blood to test strip for prescribed time ensures proper results.
a. Be sure that meter is still on. Bring test strip in meter to drop of blood. Blood will be wicked onto test strip (see illustration). Follow specific meter instructions to be sure that you obtain adequate sample.	Blood enters strip, and glucose device shows message on screen to signal that enough blood is obtained.

CLINICAL JUDGMENT: *Do not scrape blood onto the test strips or apply it to wrong side of test strip. This results in an inaccurate glucose measurement.*

---

b. Blood glucose test result will appear on screen (see illustration). Some devices "beep" when completed.	
10. Turn meter off. Some meters turn off automatically. Dispose of test strip, lancet, and gloves in proper receptacles.	Meter is battery powered. Proper disposal reduces risk for needlestick injury and spread of infection.

CLINICAL JUDGMENT: *POC blood glucose testing meters must be cleaned and disinfected after each patient use.*

---

11. Perform hand hygiene.	Reduces transmission of microorganisms.

STEP 8c Prick side of finger with lancet. (Courtesy Accu-Chek Glucometer.)

STEP 8d Gently squeeze puncture site until drop of blood forms.

STEP 9a Touch test strip to blood drop. Blood wicks into test strip. (Courtesy Accu-Chek Glucometer.)

Continued

SKILL 45.4	BLOOD GLUCOSE MONITORING—cont'd
STEPS	**RATIONALE**

STEP 9b Results appear on meter screen. (Courtesy Accu-Chek Glucometer.)

12. Discuss test results with patient and encourage questions and eventual participation in care if this is a new DM diagnosis.	Promotes participation and adherence to therapy.
13. Help patient to comfortable position as needed.	Promotes patient comfort and safety.
14. Place nurse call system in an accessible location within patient's reach (if appropriate).	Ensures patient can call for assistance if needed.
15. Raise side rails (as appropriate) and lower bed to lowest position, if applicable.	Promotes patient safety.

EVALUATION

1. Inspect puncture site for bleeding or tissue injury.	Site can be source of discomfort and infection.
2. Compare glucose meter reading with normal blood glucose levels and previous test results.	Determines whether glucose level is normal.
3. **Use Teach-Back:** "I want to be sure I explained the way to obtain a blood glucose reading. Show me the steps you will use to obtain your blood glucose measurement." Revise your instruction now or develop a plan for revised patient/family caregiver teaching if patient/family caregiver is not able to teach back correctly.	Teach-back is an evidence-based health literacy intervention that promotes patient engagement, patient safety, adherence, and quality. The goal of teach-back is to ensure that you have explained medical information clearly so that patients and their families understand what you communicated to them (AHRQ, 2020).

UNEXPECTED OUTCOMES AND RELATED INTERVENTIONS

1. Puncture site is bruised or continues to bleed.
   - Apply pressure.
   - Notify health care provider if bleeding continues.
2. Blood glucose level is above or below target range.
   - Continue to monitor patient.
   - Check for any medication orders for deviations in glucose level.
   - Notify health care provider.
   - Administer insulin or carbohydrate source as ordered, depending on glucose level.
3. Glucose meter malfunctions.
   - Review instructions for troubleshooting glucose meter.
   - Repeat test.

RECORDING AND REPORTING

- Record glucose results on appropriate flow sheet and describe response, including presence or absence of pain or excessive oozing of blood at puncture site.
- Document your evaluation of patient learning
- Report blood glucose levels out of target range and the action taken for hypoglycemia or hyperglycemia.
- Report patient response to treatment for out-of-range blood glucose levels.

KEY POINTS

- Ingestion of a diet balanced with carbohydrates, fats, proteins, and vitamins and minerals provides the essential nutrients to carry out the normal physiological functioning of the body across the life span.
- Through digestion food is broken down into its simplest form for absorption by chewing, churning, and mixing with fluid and chemical reactions.
- Absorption is the movement of nutrients into the body through the processes of passive diffusion, osmosis, active transport, and pinocytosis.
- The MyPlate program provides guidelines for a heart-healthy lifestyle. The guidelines are focused on ways to balance calories; decrease portion size; increase healthy foods; increase water intake; and decrease fats, sodium, and sugars.
- Guidelines for dietary change for the general population recommend reduced fat, saturated fats, sodium, refined sugar, and cholesterol and increased intake of complex carbohydrates and fiber.
- Breastfeeding is recommended for infants for the first 6 months of life with supplemental food added for infants 6 to 12 months old.
- Dietary requirements for preschool-age children (3–5 years) are similar to those for toddlers. They consume slightly more than toddlers, and nutrient density is more important than quantity.
- School age-children grow at a slower and steadier rate, with a gradual decline in energy requirements per unit of body weight; however, they still require adequate protein and vitamins A and C.
- There is a reduction in nutrient demands as the growth period ends. Mature adults need nutrients for energy, maintenance, and repair.
- Patients with alterations in chewing and swallowing (e.g., patients with reduced consciousness, mouth surgery, or stroke) are at risk for aspiration.
- Conducting a thorough dietary and health history along with taking anthropometric measurements, reviewing pertinent laboratory data, and completing a physical examination will provide the nurse with assessment data to identify a patient's nutritional problem(s).
- One of the most important responsibilities of a nurse administering enteral feedings is to take precautions to prevent patients from aspirating the feeding.
- The most important responsibility of the nurse monitoring parenteral nutrition (PN) is to implement interventions per agency protocol and take precautions to prevent patients from developing a catheter-related infection, hyperglycemia, or fluid overload.
- Medical nutrition therapy (MNT) is a recognized treatment modality for both acute and chronic disease states, including cardiovascular conditions; the focus of MNT is on balancing calorie intake of lean meats and vegetables, fat-free dairy products, and limited fats and sodium with exercise to maintain a healthy body weight.
- Plan and provide patient teaching on specialized diets based on patient health problems and nutritional needs, and consider patient preferences, culture, and budget.

REFLECTIVE LEARNING

A year after Mrs. Cooper started working with Ryan, she arrives at the emergency department with slurred speech, right facial droop, and weakness in her upper and lower right-side extremities. Mrs. Cooper's vital signs are blood pressure, 162/94 mm Hg; pulse, 102 beats/min; and respirations, 18 breaths/min. Her lab data show that her INR is 3.6. She is admitted to the hospital with a diagnosis of acute hemorrhagic stroke. Currently Mrs. Cooper is awake and alert in her hospital room but continues to have slurred speech, drooping of the right side of her mouth, and weakness in her arm and leg. When she speaks her voice
sounds wet, and Mrs. Cooper is demonstrating difficulty clearing her airway when she coughs. She also continues to experience right-sided weakness in her arm and leg. When the SLP tries to give Mrs. Cooper liquids, she has difficulty swallowing. Mrs. Cooper starts coughing and she becomes very anxious and says that she feels like she cannot catch her breath.

- What assessment information in Mrs. Cooper's situation is the most important or of immediate concern for the nurse? (Recognize Cues)
- Considering Mrs. Cooper's situation, what are the variety of problems that she might be experiencing? (Analyze Cues)
- Considering the assessment data and history, what would be the priority nursing problem in caring for Mrs. Cooper? (Prioritize Diagnoses)
- Identify two expected outcomes for Mrs. Cooper. Consider Mrs. Cooper's situation and describe the nursing and medical interventions that you could use to achieve the expected outcomes. (Generate Solutions)
- Which nursing and medical interventions should have priority when implementing the nutritional care plan for Mrs. Cooper? (Take Action)
- Considering the implementation of your plan of care for Mrs. Cooper, what assessment data should you gather to determine if the interventions were effective? (Evaluate Outcomes)

REVIEW QUESTIONS

1. The nurse is caring for a patient with pneumonia, who has severe malnutrition. The patient's condition places her at risk for which of the following life-threatening complications during hospitalization? (Select all that apply.)
   1. Heart disease
   2. Sepsis
   3. Hemorrhage
   4. Skin breakdown
   5. Diarrhea

2. The nurse is preparing to perform a blood glucose monitoring test on a patient. Place the steps for performing the procedure in the correct sequence.
   1. Press button on meter to confirm match codes.
   2. Bringing meter to test strip, allow blood drop to wick onto test strip.
   3. Instruct patient to perform hand hygiene with soap and water.
   4. Clean patient finger with antiseptic swab.
   5. Interpret results and document.
   6. Check code on test strip vial.
   7. Holding lancet to finger, press release button on machine.
   8. Perform hand hygiene and put on clean gloves.

3. The nurse is caring for a patient with dysphagia and is feeding her a pureed chicken diet. Suddenly the patient begins to choke. What is the priority nursing intervention?
   1. Suction her mouth and throat.
   2. Turn her on her side.
   3. Put on oxygen at 2 L nasal cannula.
   4. Stop feeding her.

4. The nurse is changing the PN tubing. What action should the nurse take to prevent an air embolus?
   1. Have the patient turn on the left side and perform a Valsalva maneuver.
   2. Have the patient cough vigorously when tubing is disconnected.
   3. Have the patient take a deep breath and hold it.
   4. Place patient in supine position with head of bed elevated 90 degrees.

5. A patient is receiving both PN and EN. When would the nurse collaborate with the health care provider and request a discontinuation of PN?
   1. When 25% of the patient's nutritional needs are met by the tube feedings
   2. When bowel sounds return
   3. When the central line has been in for 10 days
   4. When 75% of the patient's nutritional needs are met by the tube feedings

6. A patient is receiving an enteral feeding at 65 mL/h. The GRV in 4 hours was 125 mL. What is the priority nursing intervention?
   1. Assess bowel sounds.
   2. Raise the head of the bed to at least 45 degrees.
   3. Continue the feedings; this is normal gastric residual for this feeding.
   4. Hold the feeding until you talk to the primary care provider.

7. Which action can a nurse delegate to AP?
   1. Performing glucose monitoring every 6 hours on a stable patient
   2. Teaching the patient about the need for enteral feeding
   3. Administering enteral feeding bolus after tube placement has been verified
   4. Evaluating the patient's tolerance of the enteral feeding

8. Which statement made by the parents of a 2-month-old infant requires further education by the nurse?
   1. "I'll continue to use formula for the baby until he is at least a year old."
   2. "I'll make sure that I purchase iron-fortified formula."
   3. "I'll start feeding the baby cereal at 4 months."
   4. "I'm going to alternate formula with whole milk, starting next month."

9. A nurse sees an AP perform the following interventions for a patient receiving continuous enteral feedings. Which action would require immediate attention by the nurse?
   1. Fastening tube to the gown with new tape
   2. Placing patient supine while giving a bath
   3. Monitoring the patient's weight as ordered
   4. Ambulating patient with enteral feedings still infusing

10. A patient is receiving total parenteral nutrition (TPN). What are the primary interventions the nurse should follow to prevent a central line infection? (Select all that apply.)
    1. Change the dressing using sterile technique.
    2. Change TPN containers every 48 hours.
    3. Change the TPN tubing every 24 hours.
    4. Monitor glucose levels to watch and assess for glucose intolerance.
    5. Elevate head of the bed 45 degrees to prevent aspiration.

Answers: 1. 2, 3, 4; **2.** 3, 6, 1, 8, 4, 7, 2, 5; **3.** 4, 1; **5.** 4; **6.** 3; **7.** 1; **8.** 4; **9.** 2; **10.** 1, 3.

Rationales for Review Questions can be found on the Evolve website.

REFERENCES

Academy of Nutrition and Dietetics: *Food insecurity and health,* 2021. https://www.eatright.org/health/weight-loss/overweight-and-obesity/food-insecurity-and-health. Accessed September 11, 2021.

Agency for Healthcare Research and Quality (AHRQ): *Health literacy universal precautions toolkit 2nd edition,* Rockville, MD, March 2020, Agency for Healthcare Research and Quality. https://www.ahrq.gov/health-literacy/quality-resources/tools/literacy-toolkit/healthlittoolkit2-tool5.html. Accessed April 3, 2021.

American Academy of Allergy Asthma, and Immunology (AAAAI): *Prevention of allergies and asthma in children,* 2020. https://www.aaaai.org/conditions-and-treatments/library/allergy-library/prevention-of-allergies-and-asthma-in-children#:,:text5Solid%20foods%20should%20be%20introduced,baby's%20risk%20of%20developing%20allergies. Accessed April 14, 2021.

American Academy of Pediatrics (AAP): Policy statement: breast feeding and the use of human milk, *Pediatrics* 129(3):496, 2017.

American Association of Critical-Care Nurses (AACN): AACN practice alerts: initial and ongoing verification of feeding tube placement in adults, *Crit Care Nurse* 36(2):e8, 2016.

American Cancer Society (ACS): *American Cancer Society guideline for diet and physical activity for cancer prevention,* 2021. http://www.cancer.org/healthy/eathealthygetactive/acsguidelinesonnutritionphysicalactivityforcancerprevention/acs-guidelines-on-nutrition-and-physical-activity-for-cancer-prevention-intro. Accessed March 29, 2021.

American Diabetes Association (ADA): Management of hyperglycemia in type 2 diabetes: a patient-centered approach, *Diabetes Care* 35(6):1364, 2019.

American Diabetes Association (ADA): *Eat good to feel good,* 2021a. https://www.diabetes.org/healthy-living/recipes-nutrition/eating-well. Accessed April 9, 2021.

American Diabetes Association (ADA): Standards of medical care in diabetes-2021, *Diabetes Care* 44(Suppl 1), 2021b. https://care.diabetesjournals.org/content/diacare/suppl/2020/12/09/44.Supplement_1.DC1/DC_44_S1_final_copyright_stamped.pdf. Accessed April 8, 2021.

American Heart Association (AHA): *Diet and lifestyle recommendations,* 2017. https://www.heart.org/en/healthy-living/healthy-eating/eat-smart/nutrition-basics/aha-diet-and-lifestyle-recommendations. Accessed March 29, 2021.

American Society for Parenteral and Enteral Nutrition (ASPEN): *Standards,* 2021. https://www.nutritioncare.org/Guidelines_and_Clinical_Resources/Clinical_Practice_Library/Standards/. Accessed April 8, 2021.

American Speech-Language-Hearing Association (ASHA): *Adult dysphagia,* 2021a. https://www.asha.org/practice-portal/clinical-topics/adult-dysphagia/#collapse_6. Accessed September 2021.

American Speech-Language-Hearing Association (ASHA): *Dysphagia diets,* 2021b. https://www.asha.org/SLP/clinical/dysphagia/Dysphagia-Diets/. Accessed March 29, 2021.

American Stroke Association: *Trouble swallowing after stroke (dysphasia),* 2021. https://www.stroke.org/en/about-stroke/effects-of-stroke/cognitive-and-communication-effects-of-stroke/difficulty-swallowing-after-stroke--dysphagia, Accessed October 27, 2021.

BioSpace: ENFit® Connector Conversion Schedule for the U.S., July 2019. https://www.biospace.com/article/releases/enfit-connector-conversion-schedule-for-the-u-s-/. Accessed October 27, 2021.

Boullata J, et al: ASPEN safe practices for enteral nutrition therapy, *JPEN J Parenter Enteral Nutr* 41(1):15, 2017.

Burchum JR, Rosenthal LD: *Lehne's pharmacology for nursing care,* ed 10, St. Louis, 2019, Elsevier.

Centers for Disease Control and Prevention (CDC): *Childhood obesity facts,* 2021a. https://www.cdc.gov/obesity/data/childhood.html. Accessed March 29, 2021.

Centers for Disease Control and Prevention (CDC): *Childhood Obesity Research Demonstration (CORD) 3.0,* 2021b. https://www.cdc.gov/obesity/strategies/healthcare/cord3.html.

Centers for Disease Control and Prevention (CDC): *Medical nutrition therapy,* 2021c. https://www.cdc.gov/diabetes/dsmes-toolkit/reimbursement/medical-nutrition-therapy.html. Accessed April 8, 2021.

Centers for Disease Control and Prevention (CDC): *What is health literacy,* 2021d. https://www.cdc.gov/healthliteracy/learn/index.html. Accessed March 29, 2021.

Chinai SA, et al: Taking advantage of the teachable moment: a review of learner-centered clinical teaching models, *West J Emerg Med* 19(1);28, 2018.

Cotogni P, et al: Nutritional therapy in cancer patients receiving chemoradiotherapy: should we need stronger recommendations to act for improving outcomes? *J Cancer* 10(18):4318, 2019.

Dodd K: *Which malnutrition screening tool is best?* 2020. https://www.thegeriatricdietitian.com/malnutrition-screening-tool/. Accessed April 9, 2021.

Eglseer D, et al: Dysphagia in hospitalized older patients: associated factors and nutritional interventions, *J Nutr Health Aging* 22(1):103, 2018.

Fan EMP, et al: Nasogastric tube placement confirmation: where we are and where we should be heading, *Proc Singapore Healthc* 26(3):189, 2017.

Fumarola S, et al: Overlooked and underestimated: medical adhesive-related skin injuries: best practice consensus document on prevention. *J Wound Care* 29(Suppl 3c): S1–S24, 2020.

Giddens J: *Concepts for nursing practice,* ed 3, St. Louis, 2021, Elsevier.

Giger JN, Haddad LG: *Transcultural nursing: assessment and intervention,* ed 8, St. Louis, 2021, Elsevier.

Gorski LA, Hadaway L, Hagle ME, et al. Infusion therapy standards of practice, 8th ed, *J Infus Nurs* 44(Suppl 1):S1, 2021. doi:10.1097/NAN.0000000000000396.

Grodner M, et al: *Nutritional foundations and clinical applications: a nursing approach*, ed 7, St. Louis, 2020, Elsevier.

Harding M, et al: *Lewis's medical-surgical nursing: assessment and management of clinical problems*, ed 11, St. Louis, 2020, Elsevier.

Healthline: *What is medical nutrition therapy? All you need to know*, 2020. https://www.healthline.com/nutrition/nutrition-therapy. Accessed April 8, 2021.

Hockenberry MJ, et al: *Wong's nursing care of infants and children*, ed 11, St. Louis, 2019, Elsevier.

Hodin R, Bordeianou L: *Inpatient placement and management of nasogastric and nasoenteric tubes in adults*, 2019, UpToDate. https://www.uptodate.com/contents/inpatient-placement-and-management-of-nasogastric-and-nasoenteric-tubes-in-adults. Accessed September 14, 2021.

Huether SE, et al: *Understanding pathophysiology*, ed 7, St. Louis, 2020, Elsevier.

Hunger + Health: *Understand food insecurity: what is food insecurity?* 2021. https://hungerandhealth.feedingamerica.org/understand-food-insecurity/. Accessed March 29, 2021.

Ignatavicius DD: *Developing clinical judgment for professional nursing and next-generation NCLEX-RN examination*, St. Louis, 2021, Elsevier.

Ignatavicius DD, et al: *Medical-surgical nursing: concepts for interprofessional collaborative care*, ed 10, St. Louis, 2021, Elsevier.

Institute for Safe Medication Practices (ISMP): *2020–2021 targeted medication safety best practices for hospitals*, 2020. https://www.ismp.org/sites/default/files/attachments/2020-02/2020-2021%20TMSBP-%20FINAL_1.pdf. Accessed April 15, 2021.

International Dysphagia Diet Standardisation Initiative: *IDDSI framework*, 2021 https://iddsi.org/Framework. Accessed April 5, 2021.

Isbell TS: Bedside blood glucose testing in critically ill patients, *Med Lib Observ* 49(4):8, 2017.

Makhnevich A, et al: Aspiration pneumonia in older adults, *J Hosp Med* 14(7):429, 2019.

Mayo Clinic: *Childhood obesity*, 2021a. https://www.mayoclinic.org/diseases-conditions/childhood-obesity/symptoms-causes/syc-20354827. Accessed September 11, 2021.

Mayo Clinic: *Selective serotonin reuptake inhibitors (SSRIs)*, 2021b. https://www.mayoclinic.org/diseases-conditions/depression/in-depth/ssris/art-20044825. Accessed April 9, 2021.

McEvilly A: Causes of malnutrition in older adults and what can be done to prevent it, *Br J Community Nurs* 22(10):474, 2017.

Meehan A, et al: Health system quality improvement: impact of prompt nutrition care on patient outcomes and health care costs, *J Nurs Care Qual* 31(3):217, 2016.

Meiner SE, Yeager JJ: *Gerontologic nursing*, ed 6, St. Louis, 2019, Elsevier.

Metheny NA, Meert KL: Update on effectiveness of an electromagnetic feeding tube-placement device in detecting respiratory placements, *Am J Crit Care* 26(2):157, 2017.

Metheny N: Preventing aspiration in older adults with dysphagia, *Try This: Best Practices in Nursing Care to Older Adults Issue No 20*, 2018. https://hign.org/sites/default/files/2020-06/Try_This_General_Assessment_20.pdf, Accessed March 29, 2021.

National Council on Aging: *Facts and benefits about senior centers you probably didn't know*, 2021a. https://www.ncoa.org/article/facts-and-benefits-about-senior-centers-you-probably-didnt-know. Accessed April 8, 2021.

National Council on Aging: *Get the facts on SNAP and senior hunger*, 2021b. https://www.ncoa.org/article/get-the-facts-on-snap-and-senior-hunger. Accessed April 8, 2021.

National Institutes of Health (NIH): *Nutrient recommendations: Dietary reference intakes (DRI)*, n.d.a. https://ods.od.nih.gov/HealthInformation/Dietary_Reference_Intakes.aspx. Accessed April 5, 2021.

National Institutes of Health (NIH): *Tolerable upper-level intake*, n.d.b. http://ods.od.nih.gov/pubs/conferences/tolerable_upper_intake.pdf. Accessed March 29, 2021.

National Osteoporosis Foundation (NOF): *Nutrition: food and your bones – osteoporosis nutrition guidelines*, 2021. https://www.nof.org/patients/treatment/nutrition/. Accessed March 29, 2021.

Office of Disease Prevention and Health Promotion (ODPHP): *Healthy People 2030*, n.d., U.S. Department of Health and Human Services. https://health.gov/healthypeople. Accessed April 5, 2021.

Pagana KD, et al: *Mosby's diagnostic and laboratory test reference*, ed 14, St. Louis, 2019, Elsevier.

Patel JK, Rouster AS: *Infant nutrition requirements and options*, 2020. https://www.ncbi.nlm.nih.gov/books/NBK560758/. Accessed April 14, 2021.

Phillips LD: *Manual of IV therapeutics: evidence-based practice for infusion therapy*, ed 7, Philadelphia, 2018, FA Davis.

Pietsch K, et al: Rehabilitation in patients with dysphonia. Speech Language Pathology Rehabilitation, *Med Clin* 102(6):1121, 2018.

Robinson J: *Nutrition and HIV/AIDS*, 2019. https://www.webmd.com/hiv-aids/guide/nutrition-hiv-aids-enhancing-quality-life. Accessed April 15, 2021.

Tatsumi H: Enteral tolerance in critically ill patients, *J Intensive Care* 7:30, 2019.

Team Legion: *5 ways your environment influences what you eat*, 2021. https://legionathletics.com/ways-your-environment-influences-what-you-eat/. Accessed April 9, 2021.

The American College of Obstetricians and Gynecologists (ACOG): *Nutrition during pregnancy*, 2021. https://www.acog.org/womens-health/faqs/nutrition-during-pregnancy. Accessed September 2021.

The Joint Commission (TJC): *Sentinel event alert 53: managing risk during transition to new ISO tubing connector standards*, 2014. https://www.jointcommission.org/resources/patient-safety-topics/sentinel-event/sentinel-event-alert-newsletters/sentinel-event-alert-53-managing-risk-during-transition-to-new-iso-tubing-connector-standards/. Accessed October 27, 2021.

The Joint Commission (TJC): *2021 National Patient Safety Goals*, Oakbrook Terrace, IL, 2021, The Commission. https://www.jointcommission.org/en/standards/national-patient-safety-goals/. Accessed March 29, 2021.

Thomas L, et al: Aspiration prevention: a matter of life and breath, *Nursing* 49(3):64, 2019.

Touhy TA, Jett KF: *Ebersole and Hess' gerontological nursing healthy aging*, ed 5, St. Louis, 2018, Elsevier.

Ukleja A, et al: Standards for nutrition support: adult hospitalized patients, *JPEN J Parenter Enteral Nutr* 33(6):906, 2018.

U.S. Department of Agriculture (USDA): *MyPlate*, n.d.a. https://www.myplate.gov/. Accessed March 29, 2021.

U.S. Department of Agriculture (USDA): *MyPlate: older adults*, n.d.b. https://www.myplate.gov/life-stages/older-adults. Accessed April 3, 2021.

U.S. Department of Agriculture (USDA): *MyPlate kitchen*, n.d.c. https://www.myplate.gov/myplate-kitchen. Accessed April 3, 2021.

U.S. Department of Agriculture (USDA): *National school lunch program*, 2020. https://www.ers.usda.gov/topics/food-nutrition-assistance/child-nutrition-programs/national-school-lunch-program/. Accessed March 29, 2021.

U.S. Department of Agriculture and U.S. Department of Health and Human Services (USDA and USDHHS): *Dietary Guidelines for Americans*, 2020-2025, ed 9, 2020. https://www.dietaryguidelines.gov/sites/default/files/2021-03/Dietary_Guidelines_for_Americans-2020-2025.pdf. Accessed September 2021.

U.S. Department of Health and Human Services (USDHHS): *Dietary reference intakes (DRI)*, 2020. https://health.gov/our-work/food-nutrition/dietary-reference-intakes-dris. Accessed April 5, 2021.

VanBlarcom A, McCoy MA: New nutrition guidelines: promoting enteral nutrition via a nutrition bundle, *Crit Care Nurse* 38(3):46, 2018.

Zupec-Kania B, O'Flaherty T: Medical nutrition therapy for neurologic disorders. In Mahan LK, Raymond JL, editors: *Krause's food nutrition and the nutrition care process*, ed 14, Philadelphia, 2017, Elsevier.

RESEARCH REFERENCES

Anderson PM, et al: Understanding recent trends in childhood obesity in the United States, *Econ Hum Biol* 34:16, 2019.

Dong Y, et al: Clinical application of ICF key codes to evaluate patients with dysphagia following stroke, *Medicine (Baltimore)* 95(38):e4479, 2016.

Gearan EC, et al: Adolescent participants in the school lunch program consume more nutritious lunches but their 24-hour diets are similar to nonparticipants, *J Adolesc Health* 69(2): 308, 2021.

Jordan EA, Moore SC: Enteral nutrition in critically ill adults: literature review of protocols, *Nurs Crit Care* 25:24, 2020.

Katmarzyk PT, et al: International study of childhood obesity, lifestyle and the environment (ISCOLE): contributions to understanding the global obesity epidemic, *Nutrients* 11(4):848, 2019.

Lambell KJ, et al: Nutrition therapy in critical illness: a review of the literature for clinicians, *Crit Care* 24:35, 2020. https://www.ncbi.nlm.nih.gov/pmc/articles/PMC6998073/. Accessed September 14, 2021.

Marian T, et al: Measurement of oxygen desaturation is not useful for the detection of aspiration in dysphagic stroke patients, *Cerebrovasc Dis Extra* 7(1):44, 2017.

Metheny NA, et al: A review of guidelines to distinguish between gastric and pulmonary placement of nasogastric tubes, *Heart Lung* 48:226, 2019.

Monica FPJ, et al: Adequacy of different measurement methods in determining nasogastric tube insertion lengths: an observational study, *Int J Nurs Stud* 92:73, 2019.

Nagy A, et al: The effectiveness of the head-turn-plus-chin-down maneuver for eliminating vallecular residue, *Codas* 28(2):113, 2016.

Ni MA, et al: Selecting pH cut-offs for the safe verification of nasogastric feeding tube placement: a decision analytical modelling approach, *BMJ Open* 7(11):e018128, 2017.

Reed Mangels A: Malnutrition in older adults: an evidence-based review of risk factors, assessment, and intervention, *Am J Nurs* 118(3):34, 2018.

Santos SC, et al: Methods to determine the internal length of nasogastric feeding tubes: an integrative review, *Int J Nurs Stud* 61:95, 2016.

Schallom M, et al: Head-of-bed elevation and early outcomes of gastric reflux, aspiration, and pressure ulcers; a feasibility study, *Am J Crit Care* 24(1):57, 2015.

Soysal P, et al: Mini Nutritional Assessment Scale-Short Form can be useful for frailty screening in older adults, *Clin Interv Aging* 14:693, 2019.

Stewart ML: Interruptions in enteral nutrition delivery in the critically ill patients and recommendations for clinical practice, *Crit Care Nurse* 34(4):14, 2014.

Suiter DM, et al: Swallowing screening: purposefully different from an assessment sensitivity and specificity related to clinical yield, interprofessional roles, and patient selection, *Am J Speech Lang Pathol* 29(2S):979, 2020.

Tan ECK, et al: Medications that cause dry mouth as an adverse effect in older people: a systematic review and meta-analysis, *J Am Geriatr Soc* 66(1):76, 2018.

Wittenaar H, Ottery F: Assessing nutritional status in cancer: role of the Patient-Generated Subjective Global Assessment, *Curr Opin Clin Nutr Metab Care* 20(5):322, 2017.

Yang W, et al: Research progress on nurses' ability to identify and manage dysphagia in stroke patients, *Chin Nurs Res* 31(36):4602, 2017.

Zakaria A, et al: Impact of a suggested nursing protocol on the occurrence of medical device-related pressure ulcers in critically ill patients, *J Nurs Midwifery* 9(4):924, 2018.

Urinary Elimination

OBJECTIVES

- Explain the function and role of urinary system structures in urine elimination.
- Identify factors that commonly affect urinary elimination.
- Compare common alterations associated with urinary elimination.
- Compile a nursing history from a patient with an alteration in urinary elimination.
- Demonstrate a physical assessment focused on urinary elimination.
- Interpret features of normal and abnormal urine.
- Appraise nursing implications of common diagnostic tests of the urinary system.
- Select nursing diagnoses associated with alterations in urinary elimination.
- Discuss nursing interventions to promote normal urinary elimination.
- Discuss nursing interventions to reduce risk for urinary tract infections (UTIs).
- Summarize nursing interventions that prevent catheter-associated urinary tract infections (CAUTIs).
- Describe nursing interventions for patients with urinary incontinence (UI).
- Demonstrate safety skills using clinical judgment associated with assessment and promotion of urinary elimination.

KEY TERMS

Bacteremia

Bacteriuria

Catheter-associated urinary tract infection (CAUTI)

Catheterization

Cystitis

Dysuria

Hematuria

Micturition

Nephrostomy

Pelvic floor muscle training

Postvoid residual (PVR)

Proteinuria

Pyelonephritis

Suprapubic catheter

Ureterostomy

Urinary incontinence (UI)

Urinary retention

MEDIA RESOURCES

http://evolve.elsevier.com/Potter/fundamentals/
- Review Questions
- Audio Glossary
- Case Study with Questions
- Concept Map Creator

- Video Clips
- Skills Performance Checklists
- Content Updates
- Answers to QSEN Activity and Review Questions

Mrs. Grayson is 65 years old and the mother of five adult children. Her husband died 6 months ago; before her husband's death she was his primary caregiver for 4 years. She has a 2-year history of type 2 diabetes mellitus. She is 165 cm (5 feet, 5 inches) in height and currently weighs 90.9 kg (200 lb). She has a recent history of a urinary tract infection that was treated with antibiotics. She is preparing for retirement and would like to travel. For the past 2 years she has noticed an increase in urinary incontinence (UI) when she sneezes, laughs, coughs, or exercises. In addition, she has noted dribbling of urine throughout the day. She feels the weight she gained while caring for her husband made the incontinence worse.

Carly is a new graduate nurse assigned to Mrs. Grayson. She has cared for other patients with urinary disorders but none with UI. Carly plans her care by reviewing Mrs. Grayson's electronic health record (EHR) and health care provider's orders.

Urinary elimination is a basic human function that can be compromised by a variety of illnesses and conditions. Nurses are key members of the health care team when treating patients with urinary problems.

You will assess patients' urinary tract function and use clinical judgment to identify and treat patients experiencing alterations in urinary elimination. During acute illness, a patient may require urinary catheterization for close monitoring of urine output or to facilitate bladder emptying when bladder function is impaired. Some patients require long-term indwelling urethral or suprapubic catheters when the bladder fails to empty effectively. You will analyze assessment data and identify cues when planning care and implementing measures to minimize risk for infection when bladder function is impaired or urinary drainage tubes are required. Nurses in all health care settings play an important role in teaching patients about bladder health and in supporting them to improve or obtain continence.

SCIENTIFIC KNOWLEDGE BASE

Urinary elimination is the last step in the removal and elimination of excess water and by-products of body metabolism. Adequate elimination

FIG. 46.1 Organs of urinary system.

depends on the coordinated function of the kidneys, ureters, bladder, and urethra (Fig. 46.1). The kidneys filter waste products of metabolism from the blood. The ureters transport urine from the kidneys to the bladder. The bladder holds urine until the volume in the bladder triggers a sensation of urge, indicating the need to pass urine. **Micturition** occurs when the brain triggers the bladder to empty, the bladder contracts, the urinary sphincter relaxes, and urine leaves the body through the urethra.

Kidneys

The kidneys lie retroperitoneally on either side of the vertebral column behind the peritoneum and against the deep muscles of the back. Normally the left kidney is higher than the right because of the anatomical position of the liver.

Nephrons, the functional unit of the kidneys, remove waste products from the blood and play a major role in the regulation of fluid and electrolyte balance. Each nephron contains a cluster of capillaries called the *glomerulus*. The glomerulus filters water, glucose, amino acids, urea, uric acid, creatinine, and major electrolytes. Large proteins and blood cells do not normally filter through the glomerulus. Suspect glomerular injury when protein (**proteinuria**) or blood (**hematuria**) is found in the urine.

Not all glomerular filtrate is excreted as urine. Approximately 99% is resorbed into the plasma by the proximal convoluted tubule of the nephron, the loop of Henle, and the distal tubule. The remaining 1% is excreted as urine. It is the resorption process that maintains the delicate balance of fluid and electrolytes. The normal range of urine production is 1 to 2 L/day (Huether et al., 2020). Many factors can influence the production of urine such as fluid intake and body temperature (Box 46.1).

The kidneys have essential functions other than elimination of body wastes. Erythropoietin, produced by the kidneys, stimulates red blood cell production and maturation in bone marrow. Patients with chronic kidney conditions cannot produce sufficient quantities of this hormone; therefore they often experience anemia. The kidneys play an important role in blood pressure control via the renin-angiotensin system (i.e., release of aldosterone and prostacyclin) (Huether et al., 2020). In times of renal ischemia (decreased blood supply), renin is released from juxtaglomerular cells. Renin functions as an enzyme to convert angiotensinogen (a substance synthesized by the liver) into angiotensin I. Angiotensin I is converted to angiotensin II in the lungs. Angiotensin II causes vasoconstriction and stimulates aldosterone

release from the adrenal cortex. Aldosterone causes retention of water, which increases blood volume and blood pressure. The kidneys also produce prostaglandin E_2 and prostacyclin, which help maintain renal blood flow through vasodilation. These mechanisms increase arterial blood pressure and renal blood flow (Huether et al., 2020).

The kidneys produce a hormone that converts vitamin D into its active form. This affects calcium and phosphate regulation and can cause low vitamin D levels. Patients with kidney impairment can have problems such as anemia, hypertension, and electrolyte imbalances.

Ureters

A ureter is attached to each kidney pelvis and carries urinary waste to the bladder. Urine draining from the ureters to the bladder is sterile. Peristaltic waves cause the urine to enter the bladder in spurts rather than steadily. Contractions of the bladder during micturition compress the lower part of the ureters to prevent urine from backflowing into the ureters (Huether et al., 2020). Obstruction of urine flow through the ureters such as by a kidney stone can cause a backflow of urine (urinary reflux) into the ureters and pelvis of the kidney, causing distention (hydroureter/hydronephrosis) and in some cases permanent damage to sensitive kidney structures and function.

Bladder

The urinary bladder is a hollow, distensible, muscular organ that holds urine. When empty, the bladder lies in the pelvic cavity behind the symphysis pubis. In males the bladder rests against the rectum, and in females it rests against the anterior wall of the uterus and vagina. The bladder has two parts: a fixed base called the *trigone* and a distensible body called the *detrusor*. The bladder expands as it fills with urine. Normally the pressure in the bladder during filling remains low, preventing the dangerous backward flow of urine into the ureters and kidneys. Backflow can cause infection. In a woman who is pregnant, the developing fetus pushes against the bladder, reducing capacity and causing a feeling of fullness.

Urethra

Urine travels from the bladder through the urethra and passes to the outside of the body through the urethral meatus. The urethra passes through a thick layer of skeletal muscles called the *pelvic floor muscles*. These muscles stabilize the urethra and contribute to urinary continence. The external urethral sphincter, made up of striated muscles, contributes to voluntary control over the flow of urine. The female urethra is approximately 3 to 4 cm (1–1½ inches) long, and the male urethra is about 18 to 20 cm (7–8 inches) long. The shorter length of the female urethra increases risk for urinary tract infection (UTI) because of close access to the bacteria-contaminated perineal area (Huether et al., 2020).

Act of Urination

Urination, micturition, and *voiding* are all terms that describe the process of bladder emptying. Micturition is a complex interaction among the bladder, urinary sphincter, and central nervous system. Several areas in the brain are involved in bladder control: cerebral cortex, thalamus, hypothalamus, and brainstem. There are two micturition centers in the spinal cord: one coordinates inhibition of bladder contraction; the other coordinates bladder contractility. As the bladder fills and stretches, bladder contractions are inhibited by sympathetic stimulation from the thoracic micturition center. When the bladder fills to approximately 400 to 600 mL, most people experience a strong sensation of urgency. When in the appropriate place to void, the central nervous system sends a message to the micturition centers, stopping sympathetic stimulation and starting parasympathetic stimulation from the sacral micturition center. The urinary sphincter relaxes, and the bladder contracts. When the time

BOX 46.1 Factors Influencing Urinary Elimination

Growth and Development

- Children cannot voluntarily control voiding until age 18 to 24 months.
- Readiness for toilet training includes the ability to recognize the feeling of bladder fullness, hold urine for 1 to 2 hours, and communicate the sense of urgency.
- Older adults may experience a decrease in bladder capacity, increased bladder irritability, and an increased frequency of bladder contractions during bladder filling.
- In older adults the ability to hold urine between the initial desire to void and an urgent need to void decreases.
- Older adults are at increased risk for urinary incontinence because of chronic illnesses and factors that interfere with mobility, cognition, and manual dexterity.

Sociocultural Factors

- Cultural and gender norms vary. Some cultures expect toilet facilities to be private, whereas some cultures accept communal toilet facilities.
- Religious or cultural norms may dictate who is acceptable to help with elimination practices.
- Social expectations (e.g., school recesses, work breaks) can interfere with timely voiding.

Psychological Factors

- Anxiety and stress sometimes affect a sense of urgency and increase the frequency of voiding.
- Anxiety can impact bladder emptying because of inadequate relaxation of the pelvic floor muscles and urinary sphincter.
- Depression can decrease the desire for urinary continence.

Personal Habits

- The need for privacy and adequate time to void can influence the ability to empty the bladder adequately.

Fluid Intake

- If fluids, electrolytes, and solutes are balanced, increased fluid intake increases urine production.
- Alcohol decreases the release of antidiuretic hormones, thus increasing urine production.

- Fluids containing caffeine and other bladder irritants can cause bladder contractions, resulting in frequency, urgency, and incontinence.

Pathological Conditions

- Diabetes mellitus, multiple sclerosis, and stroke can alter bladder contractility and the ability to sense bladder filling. Patients experience either bladder overactivity or deficient bladder emptying.
- Arthritis, Parkinson disease, dementia, and chronic pain syndromes can interfere with timely access to a toilet.
- Spinal cord injury or intervertebral disk disease (above S1) can cause the loss of urine control because of bladder overactivity and impaired coordination between the contracting bladder and urinary sphincter.
- Prostatic enlargement (e.g., benign prostatic hyperplasia [BPH]) can cause obstruction of the bladder outlet, causing urinary retention.

Surgical Procedures

- Local trauma during lower abdominal and pelvic surgery sometimes obstructs urine flow, requiring temporary use of an indwelling urinary catheter.
- Urinary retention in the postoperative period has two main causes—one is mechanical obstruction of the lower urinary tract; the other is altered neural control of the bladder and detrusor mechanism, most commonly due to analgesic drugs (Glick, 2020).

Medications

- Diuretics increase urinary output by preventing resorption of water and certain electrolytes.
- Some drugs change the color of urine (e.g., phenazopyridine–orange, riboflavin—intense yellow).
- Anticholinergics (e.g., atropine, overactive agents) may increase the risk for urinary retention by inhibiting bladder contractility (Burchum and Rosenthal, 2019).
- Hypnotics and sedatives (e.g., analgesics, antianxiety agents) may reduce the ability to recognize and act on the urge to void.

Diagnostic Examinations

- Cystoscopy may cause localized trauma of the urethra, resulting in transient (1–2 days) dysuria and hematuria.
- Whenever the sterile urinary tract is catheterized, there is a risk for infection.

---

and place are inappropriate, the brain sends messages to the micturition centers to contract the urinary sphincter and relax the bladder muscle.

Factors Influencing Urination. Physiological factors, psychosocial conditions, and diagnostic or treatment-induced factors can all affect normal urinary elimination (see Box 46.1). Knowledge of these factors enables you to anticipate possible elimination problems and intervene when problems develop.

Common Urinary Elimination Problems. The most common urinary elimination problems involve the inability to store urine or fully empty urine from the bladder. Problems can result from infection; irritable or overactive bladder; obstruction of urine flow; impaired bladder contractility; or issues that impair innervation to the bladder, resulting in sensory or motor dysfunction.

Urinary Retention. Urinary retention is the inability to empty the bladder partially or completely. Acute or rapid-onset urinary retention stretches the bladder, causing feelings of pressure, discomfort/pain, tenderness over the symphysis pubis, restlessness, and sometimes diaphoresis. Patients may have no urine output over several hours and in some cases experience frequency, urgency, small-volume voiding, or incontinence of small volumes of urine. Chronic urinary retention has a slow, gradual onset during which patients may experience a decrease

in voiding volumes, straining to void, frequency, urgency, incontinence, and sensations of incomplete emptying. **Postvoid residual (PVR)** is the amount of urine left in the bladder after voiding and is measured with either ultrasonography or straight catheterization. Incontinence caused by urinary retention is called *overflow incontinence* or *incontinence associated with chronic retention of urine*. The pressure in the bladder exceeds the ability of the sphincter to prevent the passage of urine, and the patient will dribble urine (Table 46.1).

Urinary Tract Infections. Urinary tract infections (UTIs) are the fifth most common type of health care–associated infection, virtually all caused by instrumentation of the urinary tract (Centers for Disease Control and Prevention [CDC], 2020). *Escherichia coli,* a bacterium commonly found in the colon, is the most common causative pathogen (Fekete, 2020). The risk for a UTI increases in the presence of an indwelling catheter, any instrumentation of the urinary tract, urinary retention, urinary and fecal incontinence, and poor perineal hygiene practices.

UTIs are characterized by location (i.e., upper urinary tract [kidney] or lower urinary tract [bladder, urethra]) and have signs and symptoms of infection. **Bacteriuria**, or bacteria in the urine, does not always mean that there is a UTI. In the absence of symptoms, the presence of bacteria in the urine as found on a urine culture is called *asymptomatic bacteriuria* and is not considered an infection and should not be treated with

TABLE 46.1　Urinary Incontinence

Definition	Characteristics	Selected Nursing Interventions
Transient Incontinence		
Incontinence caused by medical conditions that in many cases are treatable and reversible	Common reversible causes include: • Delirium and/or acute confusion • Inflammation (e.g., urinary tract infection [UTI], urethritis) • Medications (e.g., diuretics) (Burchum and Rosenthal, 2019) • Excessive urine output (e.g., hyperglycemia, congestive heart failure) • Mobility impairment from any cause • Fecal impaction • Depression • Acute urinary retention	With new-onset or increased incontinence, look for reversible causes Notify health care provider of any suspected reversible causes
Functional Incontinence		
Loss of continence because of causes outside the urinary tract Usually related to functional deficits such as altered mobility and manual dexterity, cognitive impairment, poor motivation, or environmental barriers Direct result of caregivers not responding in a timely manner to requests for help with toileting	Toilet access restricted by: • Sensory impairments (e.g., vision) • Cognitive impairments (e.g., delirium, dementia, severe retardation) • Altered mobility (e.g., hip fracture, arthritis, chronic pain, spastic paralysis associated with multiple sclerosis, slow movements associated with Parkinson disease, hemiparesis) • Altered manual dexterity (e.g., arthritis, upper extremity fracture) • Environmental barriers (e.g., caregiver not available to help with transfers, pathway to bathroom not maneuverable with a walker, tight clothing that is difficult to remove, incontinence briefs)	Adequate lighting in the bathroom Individualized toileting program designed for the degree of cognitive impairment: habit training program, scheduled toileting program, prompted voiding program Mobility aides (e.g., raised toilet seats, toilet grab bars) Toilet area cleared to allow access for a walker or wheelchair Elastic-waist pants without buttons or zippers Nurse call system always within reach Use of incontinence containment product patient can easily remove, such as a pull-up–type pant or a pad that can be moved aside easily for voiding
Urinary Incontinence Associated With Chronic Retention of Urine (Overflow Urinary Incontinence)		
Involuntary loss of urine caused by an overdistended bladder often related to bladder outlet obstruction or poor bladder emptying because of weak or absent bladder contractions	Distended bladder on palpation High postvoid residual Frequency Involuntary leakage of small volumes of urine Nocturia	Interventions individualized related to the severity of the urinary retention, ability of bladder to contract, existing kidney damage Mild retention with some bladder function: • Timed voiding • Double voiding • Monitor postvoid residual per health care provider's direction • Intermittent catheterization Severe retention, no bladder function: • Intermittent catheterization • Indwelling catheterization
Stress Urinary Incontinence		
Involuntary leakage of small volumes of urine associated with increased intraabdominal pressure related to either urethral hypermobility or an incompetent urinary sphincter (e.g., weak pelvic floor muscles, trauma after childbirth, radical prostatectomy) Result of weakness or injury to the urinary sphincter or pelvic floor muscles Underlying result: urethra cannot stay closed as pressure increases in the bladder because of increased abdominal pressure (e.g., a sneeze or cough)	Small-volume loss of urine with coughing, laughing, exercise, walking, getting up from a chair Usually does not leak urine at night when sleeping	As directed by the health care provider, instruct patient in pelvic muscle exercises

TABLE 46.1	Urinary Incontinence—cont'd	
Definition	**Characteristics**	**Selected Nursing Interventions**
Urge or Urgency Urinary Incontinence		
Involuntary passage of urine often associated with strong sense of urgency related to an overactive bladder caused by neurological problems, bladder inflammation, or bladder outlet obstruction In many cases bladder overactivity is idiopathic; cause is not known Caused by involuntary contractions of the bladder associated with an urge to void that causes leakage of urine	May experience one or all of the following symptoms: • Urgency • Frequency • Nocturia • Difficulty or inability to hold urine once the urge to void occurs • Leaks on the way to the bathroom • Leaks larger volumes of urine, sometimes enough to wet outer clothing • Dribbles small amounts on the way to the bathroom • Strong urge/leaks when one hears water running, washes hands, drinks fluids	Ask patient about symptoms of a UTI Avoid bladder irritants (e.g., caffeine, artificial sweeteners, alcohol) As directed by the health care provider, instruct patient in pelvic muscle exercises, in urge-inhibition exercises, and/or in bladder training If ordered by the health care provider, monitor patient symptoms and for the presence of side effects of antimuscarinic medications
Reflex Urinary Incontinence		
Involuntary loss of urine occurring at somewhat predictable intervals when patient reaches specific bladder volume related to spinal cord damage between C1 and S2	Diminished or absent awareness of bladder filling and the urge to void Leakage of urine without awareness May not completely empty the bladder because of dyssynergia of the urinary sphincter—inappropriate contraction of the sphincter when the bladder contracts, causing obstruction to urine flow **CAUTION:** At risk for developing autonomic dysreflexia, a life-threatening condition that causes severe elevation of blood pressure and pulse rate and diaphoresis	Follow the prescribed schedule for emptying the bladder either through voiding or by intermittent catheterization Supply urine-containment products: condom catheter, undergarments, pads, briefs Monitor for signs and symptoms of urinary retention and UTI Monitor for autonomic dysreflexia—a medical emergency requiring immediate intervention; notify health care provider immediately

antibiotics (Duncan, 2019). Symptomatic infection of the bladder can lead to a serious upper UTI (**pyelonephritis**) and life-threatening bloodstream infection (**bacteremia** or urosepsis) and should be treated with antibiotics. Symptoms of a lower UTI (bladder) can include burning or pain with urination (**dysuria**); irritation of the bladder (**cystitis**) characterized by urgency, frequency, incontinence, or suprapubic tenderness; and foul-smelling cloudy urine. Older adults who develop infections, including UTIs, often have nonspecific symptoms such as delirium, confusion, fatigue, loss of appetite, decline in function, mental status changes, incontinence, falls, or subnormal temperature (Touhy and Jett, 2020).

UTIs are the most common hospital-acquired infection, accounting for up to 40% of infections reported by acute care hospitals. The major risk factors for **catheter-associated urinary tract infection (CAUTI)** are the presence of an indwelling urinary catheter and the duration of its use. Because CAUTIs are common, costly, and believed to be reasonably preventable, as of October 1, 2008, the Centers for Medicare and Medicaid Services (CMS) chose it as one of the complications for which hospitals no longer receive additional payment to compensate for the extra cost of treatment. Consequently, there has been a shift in clinical care practices from the traditional focus on early recognition and prompt treatment to one of prevention. Effective prevention strategies that must be implemented to reduce the risk of CAUTIs include training and education of health care providers focused on increasing their awareness regarding basic infection control knowledge, optimal hand hygiene practices, and methods for handling indwelling catheter and urine collecting systems appropriately; securing catheters properly; and maintaining unobstructed urine flow and

a closed sterile drainage system using sterile technique properly (Assadi, 2018; Lawrence et al., 2019).

Urinary Incontinence. Urinary incontinence (UI) is defined as the "complaint of any involuntary loss of urine" (Lukacz, 2020; Vethanayagam et al., 2017) (see Table 46.1). Common forms are urge or urgency UI (involuntary leakage associated with urgency), stress UI (involuntary loss of urine associated with effort or exertion on sneezing or coughing), and overflow UI (continuous dribbling or leakage) (Fekete, 2020). Mixed UI is when stress- and urgency-type symptoms are both present. Overactive bladder is defined as urinary urgency, often accompanied by increased urinary frequency and nocturia that may or may not be associated with urgency incontinence and is present without obvious bladder pathology or infection. UI associated with chronic retention of urine (formally called *overflow UI*) is urine leakage caused by an overfull bladder. Functional UI is caused by factors that prohibit or interfere with a patient's access to the toilet or other acceptable receptacle for urine. In most cases there is no bladder pathology. It is a significant problem for older adults who experience problems with mobility or the dexterity to manage their clothing and toileting behaviors. A recently added category of incontinence is identified as multifactorial incontinence. This describes incontinence that has multiple interacting risk factors, some within the urinary tract and others not, such as multiple chronic illnesses, medications, age-related factors, and environmental factors (Saito et al., 2017).

Urinary Diversions. Patients who have had the bladder removed (cystectomy) because of cancer or significant bladder dysfunction related to radiation injury or neurogenic dysfunction with frequent UTI require surgical procedures that divert urine to the outside of the body through an opening in the abdominal wall called a *stoma*. Urinary diversions are

FIG. 46.2 Types of urinary diversions. (A) Continent urinary reservoir. (B) Ureterostomy (ileal conduit).

constructed from a section of intestine to create a storage reservoir or conduit for urine. Diversions can be either temporary or permanent and either continent or incontinent.

There are two types of continent urinary diversions. The first is called a *continent urinary reservoir* (Fig. 46.2A), which is created from a distal part of the ileum and proximal part of the colon. The ureters are embedded into the reservoir. This reservoir is situated under the abdominal wall and has a narrow ileal segment brought out through the abdominal wall to form a small stoma. The ileocecal valve creates a one-way valve in the pouch through which a catheter is inserted through the stoma to empty the urine from the pouch. Patients must be willing and able to catheterize the pouch 4 to 6 times a day for the rest of their lives.

The second type of continent urinary diversion is called an *orthotopic neobladder*, which uses an ileal pouch to replace the bladder. Anatomically the pouch is in the same position as the bladder was before removal, allowing a patient to void through the urethra using a Valsalva technique.

A **ureterostomy** or ileal conduit is a permanent incontinent urinary diversion created by transplanting the ureters into a closed-off part of the intestinal ileum and bringing the other end out onto the abdominal wall, forming a stoma (see Fig. 46.2B). The patient has no sensation or control over the continuous flow of urine through the ileal conduit, requiring the effluent (drainage) to be collected in a pouch.

Nephrostomy tubes are small tubes that are tunneled through the skin into the renal pelvis. These tubes are placed to drain the renal pelvis when the ureter is obstructed. Patients go home with these tubes and need careful teaching about site care and signs of infection (Fig. 46.3).

Bilateral nephrostomy tubes inserted into renal pelvis; catheters exit through an incision on each flank, or there may be just one kidney

FIG. 46.3 Nephrostomy tubes. (From Harding MM et al: *Medical-surgical nursing,* ed 11, St Louis, 2020, Elsevier.)

REFLECT NOW

You recently cared for a young woman with recurrent urinary tract infections (UTIs). Think about how these affect her lifestyle.

NURSING KNOWLEDGE BASE

Urinary elimination is a basic body function and carries with it a variety of psychological and physiological needs. When illness or disability interferes with meeting these needs, nursing care that addresses both

the physiological and the psychological needs is essential. You need an understanding beyond anatomy and physiology of the urinary system to give appropriate care.

Infection Control and Hygiene

The urinary tract is sterile. Use infection control principles to help prevent the development and spread of UTIs. You need to follow the principles of medical and surgical asepsis when carrying out procedures involving the urinary tract or external genitalia. Perineal hygiene is an essential component of care (see Chapter 40) when there is an alteration in the usual pattern of urinary elimination. Perineal care or examination of the genitalia requires medical asepsis, including proper hand hygiene. Any invasive procedure such as catheterization requires sterile aseptic technique.

Growth and Development

It is important to apply knowledge of normal growth and development when caring for the patient with urinary problems. A patient's ability to control micturition changes during the life span. The neurological system is not well developed until 2 to 3 years of age. Until this stage of development, the small child is unable to associate the sensation of filling and urge with urination. When the child recognizes feelings of urge, can hold urine for 1 to 2 hours, and is able to communicate needs, toilet training becomes successful. Continence starts during daytime hours. Children who wet the bed at night without waking from sleep have what is called *nocturnal enuresis*. In some cases, they can experience this nighttime incontinence until late in childhood. Infants and young children cannot effectively concentrate urine. Their urine appears light yellow or clear. In relation to their small body size, infants and children excrete large volumes of urine. For example, a 6-month-old infant who weighs 13 to 18 lb (6–8 kg) excretes 400 to 500 mL of urine daily.

Pregnancy causes many changes in the body, including the urinary tract. In early and late pregnancy urinary frequency is common. Hormonal changes and the pressure of the growing fetus on the bladder cause increased urine production and shrinking bladder capacity.

Normal aging causes changes in the urinary tract and the rest of the body. These changes are not the cause of bladder dysfunction, but age does increase risk and incidence (Box 46.2).

Psychosocial Implications

Self-concept, culture, and sexuality are all closely related concepts that are affected when patients have elimination problems. Self-concept changes over one's life span and includes body image, self-esteem, roles, and identity (see Chapters 33 and 34). When children begin to achieve bladder control and learn appropriate toileting skills, they sometimes resist urinating on the toilet and associate their urine and feces as extensions of self and thus do not want to flush them away. The process of micturition is often a culturally private event and requires you to be sensitive to a need for privacy. Incontinence can be devastating to self-image and self-esteem. When your patient asks for help for such a private and personal activity, it can be perceived as embarrassing or as being treated like a child, or it may threaten the patient's sense of self-determination. When a patient has a urinary diversion, it will influence the sense of body image, resulting in a perceived threat in being able to maintain a healthy sexual relationship with a partner. As a nurse, be aware of how elimination disorders affect patients psychosocially so that you can understand the full impact of the patient's elimination problem.

Carly has a knowledge base of the urinary system and factors that impact urination and incontinence. She knows that Mrs. Grayson has a history of UTI and urinary incontinence. Based on her assessment of Mrs. Grayson, Carly identified multiple factors that may be contributing to the current incontinence issues. Carly has reviewed Mrs. Grayson's EHR and knows she has had five children, is obese, and has a history of type 2 diabetes mellitus, so Carly uses her knowledge of urinary elimination to identify areas to assess and labs results to review.

CRITICAL THINKING

Successful critical thinking requires synthesis of knowledge, experience, environmental factors, critical thinking attitudes, and intellectual and professional standards. Clinical judgment requires you to anticipate and collect necessary information, analyze data, identify cues, and make decisions regarding your patient's care. During assessment consider all elements that build toward making an appropriate nursing diagnosis (Fig. 46.4).

When applying the nursing process, take into consideration the knowledge you have learned about the urinary system. Use critical thinking to integrate knowledge from nursing and other disciplines, previous experiences, and patients to understand the process of urinary

BOX 46.2 FOCUS ON OLDER ADULTS

Urinary Incontinence

Urinary incontinence is caused by anatomical and functional deficits, including an inappropriately functioning lower urinary tract, physical problems, cognitive decline, functional impairment comorbidities, and medications. The most common type of urinary incontinence is urgency urinary incontinence in elderly men and women. The most common reasons for urgency urinary incontinence in men and women are prostate hypertrophy and atrophic urethral mucosa, respectively. Age-related urinary incontinence often remains untreated in the elderly because the condition is considered a part of normal aging (Eshkoor et al., 2017; Ignatavicius et al., 2018). Older adults have a decreased ability to delay voiding, an increased incidence of overactive bladder, and potentially a loss of bladder contractility, increasing the risk for urinary retention. Older women have a decrease in estrogenization of perineal tissue, which increases the risk of urinary tract infection (Lukacz, 2020). The use of multiple medications, called *polypharmacy,* is more common in older adults (Touhy and Jett, 2020). Many of these medications have the potential to impact normal elimination by affecting the ability of the bladder to hold urine or adequately empty (antihypertensives, cholinesterase inhibitors, antidepressants, sedatives) (Burchum and Rosenthal, 2019).

Implications for Practice

- Remind older adults with cognitive impairment to void more frequently to improve continence.
- Evaluate all possible causes of new-onset incontinence, which include new medications that can affect cognition, alertness, mobility, or voiding.
- Carefully assess older adults newly started on an antimuscarinic medication for mental status changes. This class of medications has the potential to cause cognitive impairment in older adults (American Geriatrics Society, 2018).
- Implement interventions to maximize self-care and continence (e.g., toileting program, mobility aids, help with hygiene) when caring for older adults with impaired mobility and incontinence.
- Teach older women with stress incontinence about pelvic muscle exercises. There is no age limit on their effectiveness.
- The sensation of thirst decreases with aging. Adequate hydration promotes bladder health. Thus encourage older adults to drink adequate amounts of water (Touhy and Jett, 2020).
- To decrease nocturia, instruct patients to restrict fluid intake for 2 hours before bedtime.
- Assess older men with voiding pattern changes (e.g., urgency, frequency, slow stream, decreased output, dribbling) for urinary retention because of age-related prostate enlargement.

elimination and the impact on a patient and family. The urinary system is affected by many factors, both as part of and outside the urinary tract. As a result, you can identify the unique impact of these problems on patients and families. For example, men after prostate cancer surgery may experience stress UI because of trauma to the urinary sphincter, people with high caffeine intake or those who take a diuretic may experience increased urinary urgency and frequency, and patients who are normally continent and become immobile may become incontinent.

Urinary elimination problems are common in all health care settings. Reflect on previous and personal experiences to help you determine a patient's elimination needs. If you have personally had a UTI, the experience helps you to understand a patient's frustration and embarrassment as a result of frequency, urgency, and dysuria. Caring for older adults with functional disabilities helps you to anticipate patient needs related to toileting.

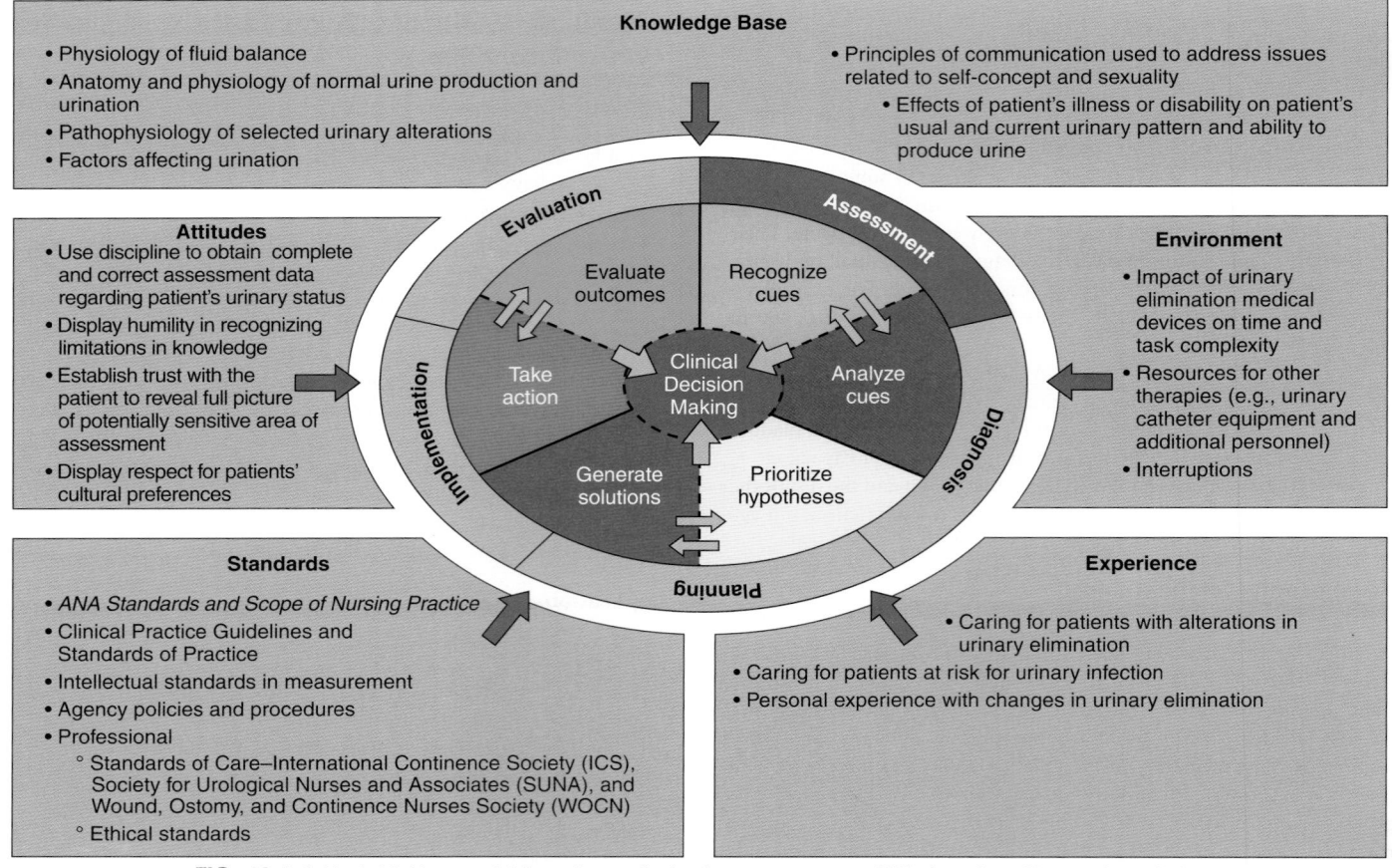

FIG. 46.4 Critical thinking model for urinary elimination assessment. *ANA*, American Nurses Association. (Clinical Judgment Measurement Model copyright © NCSBN. All rights reserved.)

In addition, use critical thinking attitudes such as perseverance to create a plan leading to the successful management of urinary elimination problems. Professional standards also provide valuable directions. You are in a key position to serve as a patient advocate by suggesting noninvasive alternatives to catheterization use (e.g., using a bladder scanner to evaluate urine volume without invasive instrumentation, or starting a voiding schedule for a patient who is incontinent).

Refer to practice standards and guidelines prepared by nursing specialty organizations and national and international professional organizations when critically assessing patient problems and developing a plan of care. Box 46.3 lists some of these resources. Incorporate these evidence-based guidelines into a patient's plan of care.

REFLECT NOW

Your patient assignment includes an 85-year-old male with a history of urinary retention. Describe the toileting needs you anticipate this patient might have.

❖ NURSING PROCESS

Apply the nursing process and use a critical thinking approach in the care of patients. The nursing process provides a clinical judgment approach for you to develop and implement an individualized plan of care.

BOX 46.3   Resources for Urology/Continence Nurses

- Centers for Disease Control and Prevention (CDC, 2020)—Catheter-associated urinary tract infection (CAUTI) and non–catheter-associated urinary tract infection (UTI) and other urinary system infection (USI) events: https://www.cdc.gov/nhsn/PDFs/pscManual/7pscCAUTIcurrent.pdf
- European Association of Urology Nurses (EAUN): https://nurses.uroweb.org/
- International Continence Society (ICS): http://www.ics.org/
- National Association for Continence (NAFC): http://www.nafc.org/
- Society of Urologic Nurses and Associates (SUNA): https://www.suna.org/
- The Simon Foundation for Continence: http://www.simonfoundation.org/index.html
- Wound, Ostomy, and Continence Nurses Society (WOCN): http://www.wocn.org/

◆ Assessment

During the assessment process, thoroughly assess each patient and critically analyze assessment findings to ensure that you make patient-centered clinical judgments required for safe nursing care.

Carly begins her assessment of Mrs. Grayson by using her knowledge of the urinary system and her past experience with patients with urinary alterations. She continues to collect data on Mrs. Grayson's urinary patterns, how she currently manages these issues, and how she feels these are affecting her life. Mrs. Grayson reports she currently has to change her undergarments frequently. She also avoids activities that cause her dribbling to worsen.

Through the Patient's Eyes. Throughout the nursing assessment it is important for you to consider a patient's frame of reference related to the illness or urinary problem. Assess the patient's understanding of the urinary problem and expectations of treatment. Because urination is a private matter, some patients find it difficult to talk about UI or their voiding habits. Approach patients in a professional manner and assure them that their problems will be kept confidential. Postoperative patients or patients receiving medications that affect bladder function may become concerned that something is wrong when you assess voiding amount and frequency. Patients receiving intravenous (IV) fluids do not always realize that they have an increased need for urination. Sensitivity to patient misconceptions allows you to quickly identify areas for patient education. Always ask what the patient expects from care. For example, does the patient expect that the UTI will be resolved? Does the patient expect the ureterostomy to be temporary?

Self-Care Ability. It is important to thoroughly assess a patient's ability to perform necessary behaviors associated with voiding. Investigate which activities a patient can complete independently as well as the patient's expectations of nursing care. Do not assume that a patient with a diagnosis of cognitive impairment cannot understand or participate in care. Balancing patient safety and supporting self-care are sometimes challenging and need to be discussed with the patient. For example, a patient with poor balance needs assistance with transfers to a toilet and requires continued supervision while on the toilet, something the patient may find embarrassing or demeaning.

Cultural Considerations. Assess cultural and gender differences related to the very private act of voiding and how they affect nursing assessment and care. Be sensitive and ask questions in a straightforward manner. Be aware of gender preferences in positioning for urination: most men stand to void, whereas women sit. This makes a difference in how you will assist patients unable to use a bathroom. There are gender-linked urinary alterations such as prostate enlargement in men and pelvic organ prolapse in women. Culture often dictates gender-specific roles when it comes to care of elimination issues. It may be inappropriate for a male to touch or even talk about elimination matters with a woman (Box 46.4).

Environmental Factors. Determine if any environmental factors will affect urinary elimination and patient care. Prior to assessment, review the patient's medical record for new information—for example, specific elimination practices, or new orders for medical equipment or therapies. Avoid time conflicts; determine if additional personnel are needed for certain care activities or if additional therapies, medical equipment, or devices increase the length of time needed to manage urinary elimination needs.

Patients in a health care setting may have difficulty urinating in a bedpan or bedside commode. Provide a private environment for urination by closing the door or curtains around the bed. If allowed, ambulate the patient into the bathroom and ensure the patient can call for assistance if needed.

Nursing History. Before gathering a history, assess your patient's health literacy to be sure you communicate clearly and can understand the patient's problems. The nursing history includes a review of the patient's elimination patterns, symptoms of urinary alterations, and assessment of factors that are affecting the ability to urinate normally. Box 46.5 lists nursing history questions that will help direct the patient to focus on urinary problems.

Pattern of Urination. Ask the patient about daily voiding patterns, including frequency and times of day, normal volume at each voiding,

---

BOX 46.4   CULTURAL ASPECTS OF CARE

Urinary Elimination

Urinary elimination is private. It is important when caring for patients from diverse cultures and religions to incorporate into the plan of care sensitivity and awareness of factors that may have an impact on care when dealing with urinary elimination problems. Some cultures may have specific beliefs and practices related to elimination, privacy, and gender-specific care. Because of the personal nature and cultural practices surrounding elimination, urinary problems such as incontinence often are not discussed with medical professionals (Giger and Haddad, 2021; Lai et al., 2017). Variations within a cultural group are common; therefore assess and care for each patient as an individual.

Implications for Patient-Centered Care

- Each patient is unique. As a professional nurse you must determine the extent to which a patient's cultural background, age-group, geographical location, ethnicity, or race, affects individual elimination problems.
- Whenever possible, provide for a same-gender caregiver for individuals whose cultural preferences emphasize female modesty and prohibit nonrelated males and females from touching (Jarvis, 2020).
- Privacy is important in many cultures; therefore careful attention to closing doors, bedside curtains, and draping is important (Lai et al., 2017).
- Ensure the patient understands patient education when English is not the primary language. If available, provide written materials in the patient's primary language. Provide a professional interpreter as needed.
- Certain cultures may observe meticulous hygiene practices that designate the left hand to perform unclean procedures, such as genitourinary hygiene. Ask patient or family caregivers about their practice preferences.
- Some cultures may continue to practice female genital circumcision, leaving only a small opening for urine and menses. Long-term consequences include recurrent urinary tract infections, incontinence, pelvic infections, fistulas, scarring, and sexual dysfunction (Malik et al., 2018).
- Cultural practices dictate the level of involvement of family in a patient's care. This source of strength is important to the health of the patient, and family must be included in the plan of care.

---

and history of recent changes. Frequency of voiding varies among individuals depending on fluid intake, medications such as diuretics, and the intake of bladder irritants such as caffeine or other caffeinated beverages. The common times for urination are on awakening, after meals, and before bedtime. Most people void an average of 5 or more times a day. Be sure to ask whether the patient is awakened from sleep with an urge to void and how many times this occurs. It is normal for patients who wake at night because of noise, pain, or nighttime treatments to experience an urge to void. Information about the pattern of urination is necessary to establish a baseline for comparison.

Symptoms of Urinary Alterations. Certain symptoms specific to urinary alterations may occur in more than one type of disorder. During assessment ask the patient about the presence of symptoms related to urination (Table 46.2). Also determine whether the patient is aware of conditions or factors that precipitate or aggravate the symptoms and determine what the patient does if any of these symptoms occur.

Physical Assessment. A physical examination (see Chapter 30) provides you with data to determine the presence and severity of urinary elimination problems. The primary areas to assess include the kidneys, bladder, external genitalia, urethral meatus, and perineal skin. Fluid intake, voiding pattern, and amounts provide additional objective data.

BOX 46.5 Nursing Assessment Questions

Nature of the Problem
- Which problems are you having with passing urine?

Signs and Symptoms
- Does it hurt or burn when you pass your urine?
- Are you having abdominal pain/flank pain/fevers/chills?
- Has there been a change in the color or odor of your urine? Please describe that change.
- Do you feel like you are emptying your bladder completely?
- Are you passing urine more frequently than normal during the day?
- Do you need to strain and/or wait before your urine stream starts?
- Do you need to get up at night to pass urine?
- Do you leak urine when feeling a strong desire to void?
- Do you ever leak urine when you cough, sneeze, and/or exercise?
- Are you ever wet with urine and do not know when it happened?
- Do you dribble urine before you void, after you void, or at other times?

Onset and Duration
- When did you first notice a problem?
- How long has this problem lasted?

Severity
- How many times a day do you pass urine?
- How many times a day and how many times at night do you leak urine?
- How many times are you wet or must change a pad in a day and at night?
- How often are you awakened with the urge to void and get up to use the bathroom?
- How does this pattern compare with the pattern you last remember?

Predisposing Factors
- Have you noticed any patterns to your urinary problem?
- Tell me what you usually eat/drink in a day. Does it include such things as caffeinated beverages, chocolate, citrus, or alcohol?
- Which medicines do you take routinely, and have any recently changed?
- Have you been hospitalized or diagnosed with a new medical problem recently?

Effect on Patient
- How have these symptoms affected your life?
- Tell me how your urinary problem affects any of your usual activities.
- Have you ever tried any treatment for this problem (self-help, complementary therapies, over-the-counter remedies, medical professional, or specialist)?

Kidneys. When the kidneys become infected or inflamed, they can become tender, resulting in flank pain. You assess for tenderness by gently percussing the costovertebral angle (the angle formed by the spine and twelfth rib). Auscultation with the bell of the stethoscope is sometimes performed to detect the presence of a renal artery bruit (sound resulting from turbulent blood flow through a narrowed artery), but this skill is usually performed by an advanced practice nurse.

Bladder. In adults the bladder rests below the symphysis pubis. When distended with urine, the bladder will rise above the symphysis pubis along the midline of the abdomen. A very full bladder can extend as far as the umbilicus. On inspection you may observe a swelling or convex curvature of the lower abdomen. On gentle palpation of the lower abdomen, a full bladder may be felt as a smooth and rounded mass. When a full bladder is palpated, patients report a sensation of urinary urge tenderness or even pain. If an overfull bladder is suspected, further assessment with an ultrasound device or a bladder scanner is recommended if available.

External Genitalia and Urethral Meatus. Careful and sensitive inspection of the external genitalia and urethral meatus yields important data that may indicate inflammation and infection. Normally there should be no drainage or inflammation. To best examine the female patient, position her in the dorsal recumbent position to provide full exposure of the genitalia. Observe the labia majora for swelling, redness, tenderness, rashes, lesions, or evidence of scratching. Using a gloved hand, retract the labial folds. The labia minora is normally pink and moist. The urethral meatus will appear as an irregular or slitlike opening below the clitoris and above the vaginal opening. Look for drainage and lesions and ask the patient whether there is discomfort. If there is drainage, note the color and consistency and any odor. The vaginal tissue of a postmenopausal woman may be drier and less pink than that of younger women.

For the male patient, examine the penis. Look for any redness or irritation. If the man is uncircumcised, retract the foreskin or ask the patient to do so. The foreskin should move back easily to expose the glans penis. In some cases, the foreskin will become tight and cannot be retracted (phimosis), increasing risk for inflammation and infection. The urethral meatus is a slitlike opening just below the tip of the penis. Inspect the glans penis and meatus for discharge, lesions, and inflammation. Following inspection, return the foreskin to the unretracted position. Retracted foreskins can cause dangerous swelling (paraphimosis) of the penis (Ball et al., 2019).

Assess the urinary meatus when your patient has an indwelling catheter. Identify any catheter-related damage. Assess for the presence of inflammation and discharge that can indicate infection. Pulling and traction on catheters can damage the urinary meatus by creating pressure on the urethra and meatus. Catheter-related damage can result in pressure injury near the external meatus and adjacent tissues (see Chapter 48). This injury is a medical device–related pressure injury (MDRPI). In some severe cases the catheter will erode through the meatus to the vagina in women or through the glans and shaft of the penis in men. Early detection of trauma means that a plan for prevention of further damage can be implemented.

Perineal Skin. Assessment of skin exposed to moisture, especially urine, needs to occur at least daily (and more often if incontinence is ongoing) to pick up early signs of skin damage related to the moisture (see Chapter 40). Patients at risk for acquiring an infection need more frequent perineal care, such as those who have incontinence-associated dermatitis (IAD), who have an indwelling Foley catheter, who are postpartum, or who are recovering from rectal or genital surgery. This is especially important for patients with indwelling Foley catheters in the effort to reduce the incidence of CAUTIs (Fekete, 2020; Goldner and Fransway, 2020). Observe for erythema in areas exposed to moisture and skin erosion. Ask patients if they are experiencing burning, itching, or pain in the perineal area.

Assessment of Urine. The assessment of urine includes measuring the patient's fluid intake and urinary output (I&O) and observing the characteristics of the urine.

Intake and Output. Assessment of I&O is a way to evaluate bladder emptying, renal function, and fluid and electrolyte balance. Although often written as part of a health care provider's order, placing a patient on I&O is also a nursing judgment. Obtaining accurate I&O measurement often requires cooperation and assistance from the patient and family. Intake measurements need to include all oral liquids and semi-liquids, enteral feedings, and any parenteral fluids (see Chapter 42). Output measurement includes not only urine but any fluid that leaves the body that can be measured, such as vomitus, gastric drainage tube contents, and fluids from wound drains.

Urinary output is a key indicator of kidney and bladder function. A change in urine volume can be a significant indicator of fluid imbalance,

TABLE 46.2 Common Symptoms of Urinary Alterations

Description	Common Causes	Description	Common Causes
Urgency An immediate and strong desire to void that is not easily deferred	Full bladder Urinary tract infection Inflammation or irritation of the bladder Overactive bladder	**Nocturia** Awakened from sleep because of the urge to void	Excess intake of fluids (especially coffee or alcohol before bedtime) Bladder outlet obstruction (e.g., prostate enlargement) Overactive bladder Medications (e.g., diuretic taken in the evening) Cardiovascular disease (e.g., hypertension) Urinary tract infection
Dysuria Pain or discomfort associated with voiding	Urinary tract infection Inflammation of the prostate Urethritis Trauma to the lower urinary tract Urinary tract tumors	**Dribbling** Leakage of small amounts of urine despite voluntary control of micturition	Bladder outlet obstruction (e.g., prostatic enlargement) Incomplete bladder emptying Stress incontinence
Frequency Voiding more than 8 times during waking hours and/or at decreased intervals, such as less than every 2 hours	High volumes of fluid intake Bladder irritants (e.g., caffeine) Urinary tract infection Increased pressure on bladder (e.g., pregnancy) Bladder outlet obstruction (e.g., prostate enlargement, pelvic organ prolapse) Overactive bladder	**Hematuria** Presence of blood in urine Gross hematuria (blood is easily seen in urine) Microscopic hematuria (blood not visualized but measured on urinalysis)	Tumors (e.g., kidney, bladder) Infection (e.g., glomerular nephritis, cystitis) Urinary tract calculi Trauma to the urinary tract
Hesitancy Delay in start of urinary stream when voiding	Anxiety (e.g., voiding in public restroom) Bladder outlet obstruction (e.g., prostate enlargement, urethral stricture)	**Retention** Acute retention: Suddenly unable to void when bladder is adequately full or overfull Chronic retention: Bladder does not empty completely during voiding, and urine is retained in the bladder	Bladder outlet obstruction (e.g., prostatic enlargement, urethral obstruction) Absent or weak bladder contractility (e.g., neurological dysfunction such as caused by diabetes, multiple sclerosis, lower spinal cord injury) Side effects of certain medications (e.g., anesthesia, anticholinergics, antispasmodics, antidepressants)
Polyuria Voiding excessive amounts of urine	High volumes of fluid intake Uncontrolled diabetes mellitus Diabetes insipidus Diuretic therapy		
Oliguria Diminished urinary output in relation to fluid intake	Fluid and electrolyte imbalance (e.g., dehydration) Kidney dysfunction or failure Increased secretion of antidiuretic hormone (ADH) Urinary tract obstruction		

kidney dysfunction, or decreased blood volume. For example, using an indwelling catheter to measure a patient's hourly urinary output following surgery provides an indirect measure of circulating blood volume. If the urinary output falls below 30 mL/h, the nurse should immediately assess for signs of blood loss and notify the health care provider. Urinary output is also an indicator of bladder function. Patients who have not voided for longer than 3 to 6 hours and have had fluid intake recorded should be evaluated for urinary retention. Just helping some patients to a normal position to void prompts voiding. Assess for any extreme increase or decrease in urine volume. Urine output of less than 30 mL/h for more than 2 consecutive hours or excessive urine output (polyuria) is a cause for concern and should prompt further assessment and notification of the health care provider.

Urine volume is measured using receptacles with volume-measurement markings. After voiding in a bedside commode, bedpan, or urinal, or when urine is emptied from a catheter drainage bag, urine can be measured using a graduated measuring container. For patients who void in a toilet, a urine hat (Fig. 46.5) collects urine, allowing for patient privacy in the bathroom. Some catheters have a specialized drainage bag with a urometer (Fig. 46.6) attached between the drainage tubing and drainage bag that allows for accurate hourly urine measurement. When emptying catheter drainage bags, follow Standard Precautions and infection control practices (Chapter 28), and make sure that the drainage tube is reclamped and secured. Each patient needs to have a graduated receptacle for individual use to prevent potential cross-contamination. Label each container with the patient's name or other identifiers according to agency policy. Rinse the container after each use to minimize odor and bacterial growth.

Characteristics of Urine. Inspect a patient's urine for color, clarity, and odor. Monitor and document any changes.

Color. Normal urine ranges in color from a pale straw to amber, depending on its concentration. Urine is usually more concentrated in

FIG. 46.5 Urine hat.

FIG. 46.6 Urometer. (Courtesy Michael Gallagher, RN, BSN, OSF Saint Francis Medical Center, Peoria, IL.)

the morning or with fluid volume deficits. As the patient drinks more fluids, urine becomes less concentrated, and the color lightens. Patients taking diuretics commonly void dilute urine while the medication is active.

Blood in the urine (hematuria) is never a normal finding. Bleeding from the kidneys or ureters usually causes urine to become dark red; bleeding from the bladder or urethra usually causes bright red urine. Hematuria and blood clots are a common cause of urinary catheter blockage.

Various medications and foods change the color of the urine. For example, patients taking phenazopyridine, a urinary analgesic, void urine that is bright orange. Eating beets, rhubarb, or blackberries causes red urine. The kidneys excrete special dyes used in IV diagnostic studies, and this discolors the urine. Dark amber urine is the result of high concentrations of bilirubin (urobilinogen) in patients with liver disease. Report unexpected color changes to the health care provider.

Clarity. Normal urine appears transparent at the time of voiding. Urine that stands several minutes in a container becomes cloudy. In patients with renal disease, freshly voided urine appears cloudy because of protein concentration. Urine may also appear thick and cloudy because of bacteria and white blood cells. Early-morning voided urine may be cloudy because of urine held in the bladder overnight but will be clear on the next voiding.

Odor. Urine has a characteristic ammonia odor. The more concentrated the urine, the stronger the odor. As urine remains standing (e.g., in a collection device), more ammonia breakdown occurs, and the odor becomes stronger. A foul odor may indicate a UTI. Some foods such as asparagus and garlic can change the odor of urine.

Laboratory and Diagnostic Testing. You are often responsible for collecting urine specimens for laboratory testing. The type of test determines the method of collection. Label all specimens with the patient's name, date, time, and type of collection. Most urine specimens need to reach the laboratory within 2 hours of collection or must be preserved according to the laboratory protocol (Pagana et al., 2021). Urine that stands in a container at room temperature without the required preservative will grow bacteria, resulting in changes that will affect the accuracy of the test. Agency infection control policies require adherence to Standard Precautions during the handling of urine specimens (see Chapter 28). To obtain urine that is fresh or new, you need to ask the patient to double void. The second voided specimen is the one sent to the laboratory. To obtain urine as free of bacterial contamination as possible, a midstream clean-catch urine specimen may be required. Table 46.3 describes nursing considerations for a variety of common tests. Table 46.4 describes the components of the most common of the urinary tests, urinalysis.

Diagnostic Examinations. The urinary system is one of the few organ systems accessible for accurate diagnostic study by means of radiographic techniques. Studies can be simple and noninvasive or complex and invasive. See Table 46.5 for a review of some common diagnostic testing of the urinary tract.

Many of the nursing responsibilities related to diagnostic testing of the urinary tract are common to most studies. Those responsibilities before testing include the following:

- Ensure that a signed consent form is completed (check agency policy).
- Assess the patient for any iodinated dye allergies and any experience of a previous reaction to a contrast agent (Pagana et al., 2021).
- Administer agency bowel-cleansing protocol to ensure that kidneys can be visualized (check agency policy).
- Ensure that the patient adheres to the appropriate pretest diet (clear liquids) or nothing by mouth (NPO).

Responsibilities after testing include:

- Assessing I&O.
- Assessing voiding and urine (color, clarity, presence of blood, dysuria, problems with emptying).
- Encouraging fluid intake, especially if using radiopaque dye.

Carly has completed her initial assessment of Mrs. Grayson and is gathering her data cues into clusters that will lead her into the planning of her care. Mrs. Grayson's vital signs remain stable during the interview: pulse, 88 beats/min; respirations, 18 breaths/min; blood pressure, 132/804 mm Hg. Current orders include a midstream urine sample, intake and output (I&O) recordings, and a bladder scan for PVR. Carly asks Mrs. Grayson some additional history questions regarding her current experience with incontinence.

REFLECT NOW

In providing care for a patient with urinary incontinence, what are some physical assessment findings to expect?

TABLE 46.3 Urine Testing

Collection Type/Use of Specimen	Nursing Considerations
Random (routine urinalysis) Includes a number of tests that are used for screening and are diagnostic for fluid and electrolyte disturbances, urinary tract infection, presence of blood and other metabolic problems	Collect during normal voiding or from an indwelling catheter or urinary diversion collection bag. Use a clean specimen cup. In some health care settings, you may be responsible for testing urine with reagent strips. Follow manufacturer instructions when performing and reading the strips. Dip the reagent strip into fresh urine, then observe color changes on the strip. Compare the color on the strip with the color chart on the reagent strip container. Examine each color at the exact time indicated on the container.
Clean-voided or midstream (culture and sensitivity)	Urine may be collected by the patient after detailed instruction on proper cleansing and collection technique (see Skill 46.1). Always use a sterile specimen cup.
Sterile specimen for culture and sensitivity Determines the presence of bacteria and to which antibiotic the bacteria are sensitive	If the patient has an indwelling catheter, collect a specimen by using sterile aseptic technique through the special sampling port (see Fig. 46.12) found on the side of the catheter. Never collect the specimen from the drainage bag. Clamp the tubing below the port, allowing fresh, uncontaminated urine to collect in the tube. After wiping the port with an antimicrobial swab, insert a sterile syringe hub and withdraw at least 3–5 mL of urine (check agency policy). Using sterile aseptic technique, transfer the urine to a sterile container (see Chapter 28). Patients with a urinary diversion need to have the stoma catheterized to obtain an accurate specimen. A preliminary report will be available in 24 hours, but usually 48–72 hours is needed for bacterial growth and sensitivity testing.
Timed urine specimens Measure bodily substances that may be excreted at higher levels at specific times of the day or over a specific time period	Requires urine collection and testing either at a specific time of day or urine collected over a specific time period (e.g., 2-, 12-, or 24-h collections). The timed period begins after the patient urinates and ends with a final voiding at the end of the time period. In most 24-hour specimen collections, discard the first voided specimen and then start collecting urine. Patient voids into a clean receptacle, and the urine is transferred to the special collection container, which often contains special preservatives. Depending on the test, the urine container may need to be kept cool by setting it in a container of ice. Each specimen must be free of feces and toilet tissue. Missed specimens make the whole collection inaccurate. Check with agency policy and the laboratory for specific instructions. Patients' education should include an explanation of the test, an emphasis on the need to collect all urine voided during the prescribed time period, and urine collection procedure.

TABLE 46.4 Routine Urinalysis

Measurement (Normal Value)	Interpretation
pH (4.6–8.0)	pH level indicates acid-base balance. Acid pH helps protect against bacterial growth. Urine that stands for several hours becomes alkaline from bacterial growth.
Protein (up to 8 mg/100 mL)	Protein is normally not present in urine. The presence of protein is a very sensitive indicator of kidney function. Damage to the glomerular membrane (such as in glomerulonephritis) allows for the filtration of larger molecules such as protein to seep through.
Glucose (not normally present)	Patients with poorly controlled diabetes have glucose in the urine because of inability of tubules to resorb high serum glucose concentrations ($>$180 mg/100 mL). Ingestion of high concentrations of glucose causes some to appear in urine of healthy people.
Ketones (not normally present)	With poor control of type 1 diabetes, patients experience breakdown of fatty acids. End products of fatty acid metabolism are ketones. Patients with dehydration, starvation, or excessive aspirin ingestion may also have ketonuria.
Specific gravity (1.005–1.030)	Specific gravity tests measure concentration of particles in urine. High specific gravity reflects concentrated urine, and low specific gravity reflects diluted urine. Dehydration, reduced renal blood flow, and increase in ADH secretion elevate specific gravity. Overhydration, early renal disease, and inadequate ADH secretion reduce specific gravity.
Microscopic examination RBCs (up to 2)	Damage to glomeruli or tubules allows RBCs to enter the urine. Trauma, disease, presence of urethral catheters, or surgery of the lower urinary tract also causes RBCs to be present.
WBCs (0–4 per low-power field)	Elevated numbers indicate inflammation or infection.
Bacteria (not normally present)	Bacteria in the urine can mean infection or colonization (if the patient shows no symptoms).
Casts (cylindrical bodies not normally present, the shapes of which take on the likeness of objects within the renal tubule)	Types include hyaline, WBCs, RBCs, granular cells, and epithelial cells. Their presence indicates renal disease.
Crystals (not normally present)	Crystals indicate increased risk for the development of renal calculi (stone). Patients with high uric acid levels (gout) may develop uric acid crystals.

Data from Pagana KD, et al: *Mosby's diagnostic and laboratory test reference,* ed 15, St Louis, 2021, Elsevier.
ADH, Antidiuretic hormone; *RBC,* red blood cell; *WBC,* white blood cell.

TABLE 46.5   Common Diagnostic Tests of Urinary Tract

Procedure	Description	Special Nursing Considerations
Noninvasive Procedures		
Abdominal roentgenogram (plain film; kidney, ureter, bladder [KUB] or flat plate)	X-ray film of the abdomen to determine the size, shape, symmetry, and location of the structures of the lower urinary tract. Common uses: Detect and measure the size of urinary calculi.	No special preparation.
Computed tomography of abdomen and pelvis (CT)	Detailed imagery of the abdominal structures provided by computerized reconstruction of cross-sectional images. Common uses: Identify anatomical abnormalities, renal tumors and cysts, calculi, and obstruction of the ureters.	**Preparation:** Explain procedure to patient. Assess for presence of allergies and previous reaction to contrast iodinated dye. All patients with allergies are at increased risk for anaphylactoid reactions to radiocontrast. NPO: Restrict food and fluid up to 4 hours before test (see agency or health care provider protocol). **After procedure:** Encourage fluids to promote dye excretion. Assess for delayed hypersensitivity reaction to the contrast media. **Patient teaching:** Explain that the patient will be placed on a special bed that will move through a tunnel-like imaging chamber. The patient will need to lie still when instructed by the technician; some patients may feel claustrophobic.
Intravenous pyelogram (IVP)	Imaging of the urinary tract that views the collecting ducts and renal pelvis and outlines the ureters, bladder, and urethra. (After intravenous injection of contrast medium [iodine based that converts to a dye], a series of x-ray films are taken to observe the passage of urine from the renal pelvis to the bladder.) Common uses: Detect and measure urinary calculi, tumors, hematuria, obstruction of the urinary tract.	**Preparation:** Assess for allergies to iodinated dyes and shellfish. Assess for dehydration. Follow agency bowel cleansing protocol. Follow agency food and fluid restriction protocol. **After procedure:** Assess for delayed hypersensitivity to the contrast medium. Encourage fluids after the test to dilute and flush dye from the patient. Assess urine output. Less than 30 mL/h increases risk for contrast-induced nephropathy. **Patient teaching:** Facial flushing is a normal response during dye injection, and patients may feel dizzy or warm or feel some nausea.
Ultrasound: Renal bladder	Imaging of the kidneys, ureters, and bladder using sound waves. Identifies gross structural abnormalities and estimates the volume of urine in the bladder. Common uses: Detect masses, obstruction, presence of hydronephrosis or hydroureter, abnormalities of the bladder wall, and calculi; measure postvoid residual.	Patients may be instructed to void before scan or come with a full bladder; verify preprocedure order for patient. Do not schedule within 24 hours after IVP.
Invasive Procedures		
Cystoscopy	Introduction of a cystoscope through the urethra into the bladder to provide direct visualization, specimen collection, and/or treatment of the bladder and urethra. (In most cases the procedure is performed using local anesthesia, but under certain circumstances general anesthesia or conscious sedation may be used.) Common uses: Microscopic hematuria, detect bladder tumors and obstruction of the bladder outlet and urethra.	Follow agency bowel cleansing protocol. Obtain informed consent. Patients may be requested to drink fluids before procedure. Maintain NPO status as ordered. Encourage fluids after procedure. **Patient teaching:** Urine may be pink tinged after the test; signs and symptoms of urinary tract infection.

Data from Pagana KD, et al: *Mosby's diagnostic and laboratory test reference*, ed 15, St Louis, 2021, Elsevier.
NPO, Nothing by mouth.

◆ Analysis and Nursing Diagnosis

A thorough assessment of a patient's urinary elimination function reveals patterns of data cues that allow you to make relevant and accurate nursing diagnoses. Use clinical judgment to reflect on your knowledge of previous patients, apply knowledge of urinary function and the effects of disorders, review assessment findings, and make a specific nursing diagnosis. Analyzing your patient's cues about the urinary system is important in identifying nursing diagnoses.

Carly's assessment reveals that Mrs. Grayson has a history of five pregnancies, type 2 diabetes mellitus, and a recent UTI. Mrs. Grayson is obese, and she experiences leakage of urine on exertion, laughing, and sneezing. She is unable to hold her urine when she needs to void. Carly knows that

BOX 46.6 Nursing Diagnostic Process

Urge Incontinence of Urine Related to Bladder Infection

Assessment Activities	Assessment Findings
Ask patient to describe voiding problems/incontinence.	Patient states urine leakage associated with a strong urge to void, coughing, sneezing, or laughing.
Assess patient's voiding pattern.	Bladder record shows episodes of urinary incontinence. Patient describes or is observed to leak urine on the way to or at the toilet. Patient describes or is observed to rush or hurry to the toilet.

Mrs. Grayson may have weakened pelvic muscles from her multiple pregnancies that may contribute to her current issue with incontinence. As Carly begins to analyze these assessment findings, the data clusters provide cues that lead her to identify **Stress Incontinence of Urine** *as a priority nursing diagnosis for the plan of care. Along with this diagnosis, Carly recognizes that Mrs. Grayson is also experiencing* **Risk for Urinary Infection** *and* **Risk for Impaired Skin Integrity** *related to her incontinence.*

The diagnosis focuses on a specific urinary elimination alteration or an associated problem such as *Impaired Tissue Integrity related to urinary incontinence.* Identification of assessment findings leads to selection of an appropriate negative or problem-focused diagnosis. Identification of risk factors leads to selection of a risk diagnosis (see Chapter 17).

An important part of formulating negative or problem-focused nursing diagnoses lies in identifying the relevant causative or related factor. In the case of risk diagnoses, you select correct risk factors. You will choose interventions that treat or modify the related factor or risk factor for the diagnosis to be resolved. Specifying related factors for a diagnosis allows selection of individualized nursing interventions. For example, *Stress Incontinence of Urine related to weakened pelvic muscles* guides the selection of nursing interventions that remove barriers to urination. *Impaired Self Toileting related to cognitive impairment* guides the selection of nursing interventions such as a prompted voiding program or habit training program. Box 46.6 provides an example of diagnostic reasoning. Some nursing diagnoses common to patients with urinary elimination problems include the following:

- Incontinence of Urine: Functional; Overflow; Reflex; Stress; Urge
- Urinary Tract Infection
- Impaired Self Toileting
- Impaired Skin Integrity
- Urinary Retention

◆ Planning and Outcomes Identification

During the planning step of the nursing process, develop an individualized plan of care for each of the patient's nursing diagnoses by integrating knowledge from assessment and information about available resources and therapies (see the Nursing Care Plan). Clinical judgment and critical thinking at this step in the planning process are important because you reflect on previous experiences and environmental factors and apply knowledge, critical thinking attitudes, and professional and intellectual standards to develop a patient-centered plan of care. Match the patient's needs with clinical and professional standards recommended in the literature (Fig. 46.7). Building a relationship of trust with patients is important because the implementation of care involves interaction of a very personal nature.

As the nurse your personal and previous experience with urinary elimination and alterations will be your guide in identifying interventions to help in the care of patients. Your experience with laboratory data and urinary equipment (e.g., bladder scanner, Foley, straight catheterization) will assist in the management of patients with alterations in urinary elimination.

It is also important to recognize environmental factors that affect urinary elimination issues, such as when you can use assistive personnel (AP) in patient care. It is essential to identify the patient's needs and plan care around these needs.

Outcomes. The plan of care for urinary elimination alterations must include realistic and individualized expected outcomes. A concept map helps you develop patient-centered care (Fig. 46.8). You develop a concept map after identifying a patient's nursing diagnoses. For Mrs. Grayson, the nursing diagnoses are linked to her issues related to urinary incontinence. The concept map demonstrates the relationships among her nursing diagnoses of *Stress Incontinence of Urine, Risk for Impaired Skin Integrity, Risk for Infection,* and *Lack of Knowledge of Treatment Regime.*

Using a systematic approach to planning care helps you recognize relationships among planned interventions. For Mrs. Grayson, interventions and successful outcomes for one nursing diagnosis may impact the resolution of a different diagnosis. For example, if the diagnosis of *Stress Incontinence of Urine* is resolved, then the diagnosis related to *Risk for Impaired Skin Integrity* is resolved. You collaborate with your patients to set realistic outcomes and select appropriate nursing interventions. An effective plan includes individualized patient-centered outcomes established over a realistic time frame that focus on improving urinary incontinence.

For example, a realistic outcome for a patient with *Impaired Self Toileting related to impaired mobility status* is that the patient will independently use the toilet. You set another outcome that the "patient will safely transfer to the toilet." To achieve this outcome, you identify interventions such as ensuring that the nurse call system is within reach, providing assistive devices such as a raised toilet seat, and providing easy access to the urinal when in bed. Conversely, a patient with stress incontinence often has a long-term outcome that depends on weeks of pelvic floor muscle exercise to improve urinary control: "Patient will experience normal continence." Another outcome would be "Patient will decrease the number of incontinence pads used daily by 1 to 2 within 8 weeks." Make sure that the outcomes are reasonably achievable and relevant to the patient's situation (see Box 46.8).

Setting Priorities. It is important to establish priorities of care on the basis of a patient's immediate physical and safety needs, patient expectations, and readiness to perform self-care activities. Establish a relationship with the patient that allows discussion and intervention. While you are collaborating with the patient, priorities become apparent, enhancing patient understanding of the expected outcomes of care. When a patient has multiple nursing diagnoses, it is important to recognize the primary health problem and its influence on other problems. For example, a patient with a long-term indwelling catheter is admitted to acute care with a severe UTI. The patient expects to resume self-care of the catheter. However, because of the severity of the infection and the patient's condition, the nurse will perform all care for the patient's catheter. In this case the priorities are to treat the infection, prevent reinfection, and teach the patient how to resume care of the catheter using techniques to prevent infection.

Teamwork and Collaboration. When planning individualized care, it is essential to include the patient, family caregivers, and the health

◎ NURSING CARE PLAN

Stress Incontinence of Urine

ASSESSMENT

Assessment Activities	*Assessment Findings[a]*
Ask Mrs. Grayson about the effects of her urinary symptoms on her daily life.	She responds, "I am embarrassed and frustrated for **losing control. I dribble** when I'm on the way to the bathroom. I'm afraid to cough, sneeze, or laugh because I **leak urine.** I don't go places and stay away from other people because I'm afraid I smell bad."
Ask her about any interventions she has tried to help with the incontinence.	She states, "I've been **wearing a pad and will go to the bathroom** every hour just in case. I try to limit the amount of water I drink, so I will not have to go to the bathroom."
Ask Mrs. Grayson about any other effects caused by her leakage.	She begins to cry and states, "I don't even like to go to the movies or visit my grandchildren. It's safer to stay home."
Observe Mrs. Grayson's behavior.	She appears **anxious and sad.**
Conduct a focused nursing history addressing urinary leakage and other lower urinary tract symptoms.	Mrs. Grayson's report of **urine leakage on physical exertion, sneezing, coughing, and laughing** and leakage on the way to the bathroom increases the likelihood of a diagnosis of mixed incontinence. Her risk factors for this condition include **five pregnancies,** being **postmenopausal,** and being **overweight.** The history helps to define the proper interventions.

[a] Assessment findings are shown in bold type.

NURSING DIAGNOSIS: Stress incontinence of urine related to weakened pelvic musculature

---

PLANNING

Expected Outcomes (NOC)[b]

Urinary Continence

Patient reports fewer than two episodes of daily incontinence.

Patient reports less incontinence during coughing or sneezing.

Patient states decreased anxiety about her incontinence.

[b] Outcome classification labels from Moorhead S, et al: *Nursing Outcomes Classification (NOC)*, ed 6, St Louis, 2018, Elsevier.

INTERVENTIONS (NIC)[c]	RATIONALE
Urinary Incontinence Care	
Teach Mrs. Grayson measures to reduce intraabdominal pressure by:	These measures reduce intraabdominal and bladder pressure, which increase leakage.
• Losing weight	
• Avoiding heavy lifting	
Teach Mrs. Grayson about how to keep her bladder healthy (see Box 46.7):	Fluids that contain caffeine and other irritants can prompt unwanted bladder contractions, resulting in frequency, urgency, and incontinence.
• Avoid bladder irritants (e.g., caffeine).	
• Drink adequate amounts of water; avoid drinking large amounts at one time.	
Pelvic Muscle Exercise	
Teach Mrs. Grayson how to perform pelvic muscle exercises (see Box 46.8):	Pelvic muscle training is effective in treating stress urinary incontinence (Fekete, 2020).
• Instruct her how to identify and contract the muscle.	
• Help her set up a daily schedule for performing the exercises.	
Bladder Retraining (Behavioral Therapy)	
• Instruct her how to inhibit strong sensations of urinary urgency by taking slow and deep breaths to relax and performing five to six quick, strong pelvic muscle exercises (flicks) in quick succession, followed by focusing the attention away from the bladder sensations.	Bladder training and pelvic floor muscle exercises progressively reestablish voluntary control over micturition (Fekete, 2020).
• Once successful with inhibiting the urge to void and avoiding incontinence, instruct her to gradually increase the time between trips to the bathroom.	

[c] Intervention classification labels from Butcher HK, et al: *Nursing Interventions Classifications (NIC)*, ed 7, St Louis, 2018, Elsevier.

EVALUATION

Evaluation Activities	*Patient Response*
Ask Mrs. Grayson about frequency of incontinence.	She responds, "I'm dry most of the time now. I'm now babysitting my grandchildren and have returned to my volunteer job."
Ask Mrs. Grayson to keep a 3-day bladder diary.	Bladder diary revealed one small-volume loss of urine with a strong cough and voiding every 3 to 4 hours.
Ask Mrs. Grayson if she feels less anxious about her urinary incontinence.	She responds, "I feel so much better now that I know how to manage my incontinence."

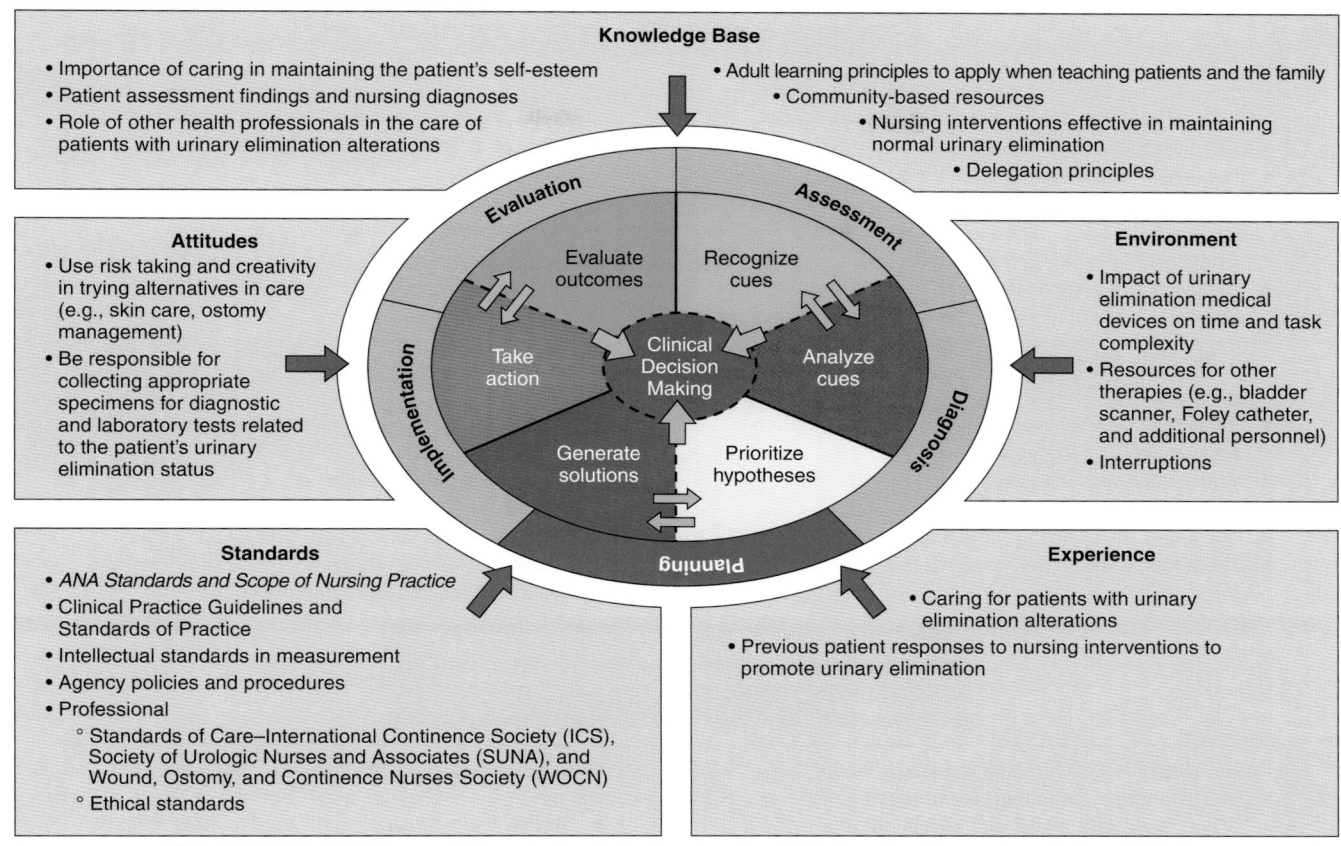

FIG. 46.7 Critical thinking model for urinary elimination planning. *ANA,* American Nurses Association. (Clinical Judgment Measurement Model copyright © NCSBN. All rights reserved.)

care team. For example, when planning care for a patient with urge UI, incorporate the expertise of a continence nurse specialist to help the patient learn techniques to inhibit the urinary urge, strengthen pelvic floor muscles, and learn fluid and food modifications. Have the occupational therapist help the patient learn efficient and safe toilet transfers; the physical therapist help with strengthening exercises of the lower extremities; and the social worker facilitate obtaining assistive devices in the home that are covered by insurance. Input from the patient and family caregiver help determine which assistive devices will be appropriate for home use. When a patient requires an indwelling urinary catheter because of acute illness and a need to measure accurate urinary output, the nurse is a key member of the team by monitoring patient progress and ensuring that the catheter is removed in a timely manner. Your active and thoughtful role in planning these interventions will result in the patient's progress toward improved urinary elimination.

Based on her analysis of the assessment data, Carly identifies that Mrs. Grayson is having incontinence issues, is not knowledgeable about how to manage these issues, and is at risk for infection and impaired skin integrity. Carly needs to plan care for Mrs. Grayson that improves her urinary incontinence, prevents skin breakdown, and improves her knowledge of managing the incontinence. Carly identifies **Stress Incontinence of Urine** *as Mrs. Grayson's priority. Carly consults with Mrs. Grayson to ensure that the outcomes in the plan of care are individualized, patient-centered, and include Mrs. Grayson's preferences, including her cultural and religious traditions. Carly also ensures the outcomes are measurable, realistic, and include a reasonable time frame for achievement.*

After talking with Mrs. Grayson, Carly sets the following patient-centered outcomes: "Mrs. Grayson will report a decrease in incontinence episodes during the day within 6 weeks" and "Mrs. Grayson will verbalize methods to improve pelvic muscle strength within 6 weeks." Carly will ensure that the outcomes in the plan of care are individualized and patient-centered to include patient and family preferences, cultural, and religious traditions.

Carly plans to select nursing interventions to help Mrs. Grayson achieve these outcomes. The nursing interventions will help Mrs. Grayson better manage and improve her incontinence. Later, Carly will evaluate whether Mrs. Grayson's urinary incontinence has improved by monitoring the outcome of focused assessments and I&O.

◆ Implementation

Use clinical judgment and critical thinking to select and implement independent and collaborative interventions that will help a patient achieve the desired outcomes of care. You implement some independent interventions, such as providing patient education about self-care activities. Dependent activities are those prescribed by the health care provider and carried out by the nurse, such as medication administration.

Health Promotion. Health promotion helps the patient understand and participate in self-care practices to preserve and protect healthy urinary system function (Box 46.7). You can achieve this focus using several means.

Patient Education. Success of therapies aimed at eliminating or minimizing urinary elimination problems depends in part on successful patient education (see Box 46.7). Although many patients need to learn

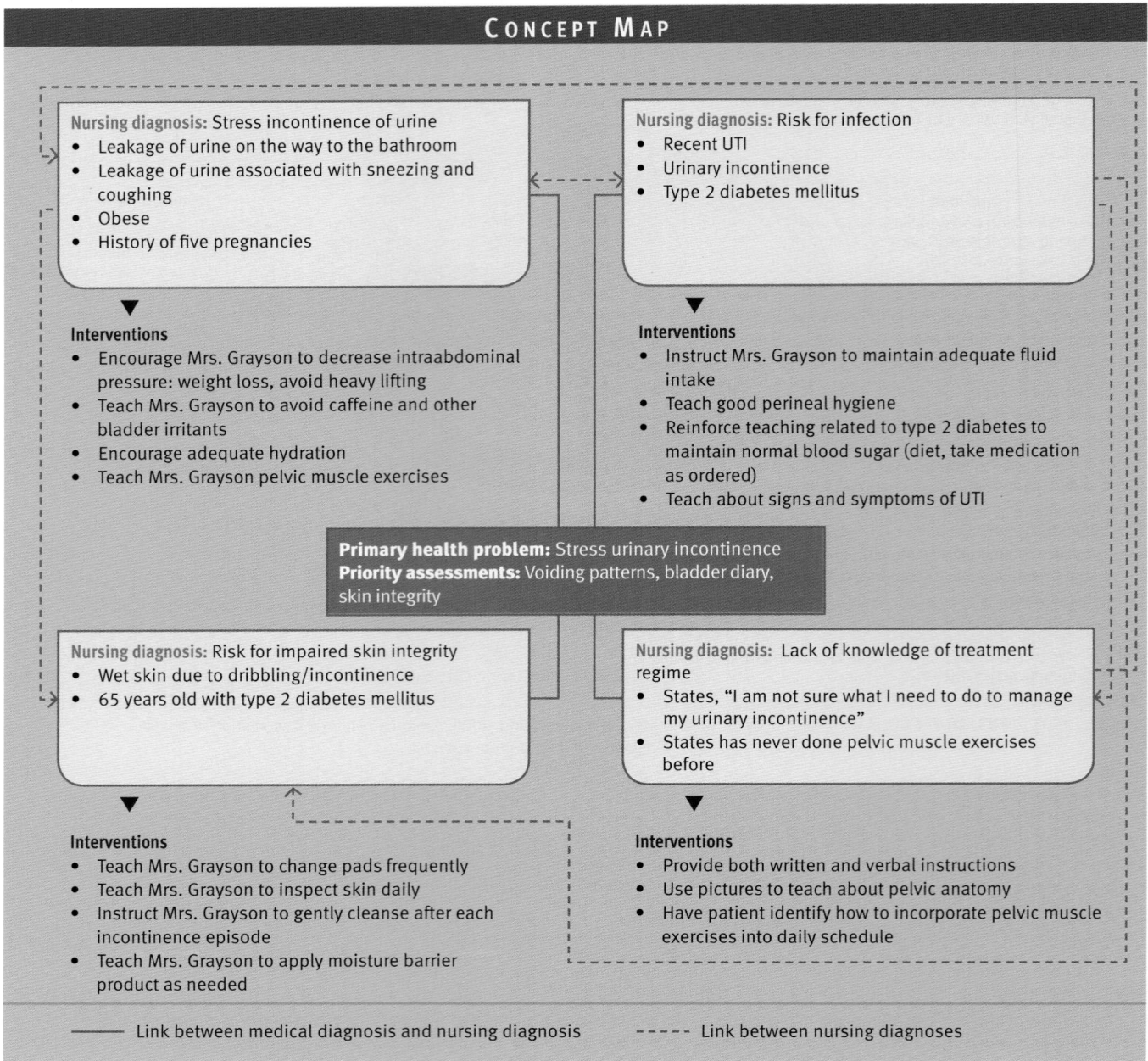

CONCEPT MAP

Nursing diagnosis: Stress incontinence of urine
- Leakage of urine on the way to the bathroom
- Leakage of urine associated with sneezing and coughing
- Obese
- History of five pregnancies

Nursing diagnosis: Risk for infection
- Recent UTI
- Urinary incontinence
- Type 2 diabetes mellitus

Interventions
- Encourage Mrs. Grayson to decrease intraabdominal pressure: weight loss, avoid heavy lifting
- Teach Mrs. Grayson to avoid caffeine and other bladder irritants
- Encourage adequate hydration
- Teach Mrs. Grayson pelvic muscle exercises

Interventions
- Instruct Mrs. Grayson to maintain adequate fluid intake
- Teach good perineal hygiene
- Reinforce teaching related to type 2 diabetes to maintain normal blood sugar (diet, take medication as ordered)
- Teach about signs and symptoms of UTI

Primary health problem: Stress urinary incontinence
Priority assessments: Voiding patterns, bladder diary, skin integrity

Nursing diagnosis: Risk for impaired skin integrity
- Wet skin due to dribbling/incontinence
- 65 years old with type 2 diabetes mellitus

Nursing diagnosis: Lack of knowledge of treatment regime
- States, "I am not sure what I need to do to manage my urinary incontinence"
- States has never done pelvic muscle exercises before

Interventions
- Teach Mrs. Grayson to change pads frequently
- Teach Mrs. Grayson to inspect skin daily
- Instruct Mrs. Grayson to gently cleanse after each incontinence episode
- Teach Mrs. Grayson to apply moisture barrier product as needed

Interventions
- Provide both written and verbal instructions
- Use pictures to teach about pelvic anatomy
- Have patient identify how to incorporate pelvic muscle exercises into daily schedule

——— Link between medical diagnosis and nursing diagnosis   - - - - Link between nursing diagnoses

FIG. 46.8 Concept map for Mrs. Grayson. *UTI,* Urinary tract infection.

about all aspects of healthy urinary elimination, it is best to focus on a specific elimination problem first. For example, a patient who presents with a UTI would greatly benefit from learning about symptoms of UTI and measures to prevent recurring UTIs. Incorporate teaching when giving nursing care. For example, teach about common bladder irritants such as caffeine while assisting a patient with a meal tray. Include in any teaching an awareness of the patient's health literacy. Pictures are helpful when teaching about urinary tract anatomy and the relationship with UTI. If a patient speaks a different language, involve a professional interpreter.

Promoting Normal Micturition. Maintaining normal urinary micturition helps to prevent many problems. Many measures that promote normal voiding are independent nursing interventions.

Maintaining Elimination Habits. Many patients follow routines to promote normal voiding. When in a hospital or long-term care setting, institutional routines often conflict with those of the patient. Integrating a patient's habits into the care plan fosters a more normal voiding pattern. Elimination is a very private act. Create as much privacy as possible by closing the door and bedside curtain; asking visitors to leave a room when a bedside commode, bedpan, or urinal is used; and masking the sounds of voiding with running water. Respond to requests for help with toileting as quickly as possible. Embarrassing accidents are easily avoided when help comes in time. Avoid the use of incontinence-containment products unless needed for uncontrolled urine leakage. Some containment products may be difficult to remove and interfere with prompt toilet access.

BOX 46.7 Health Promotion/Restoration: Patient Education for a Healthy Bladder

1. Maintain adequate hydration.
   - Drink six to eight glasses of water a day. Spread it out evenly throughout the day.
   - Avoid or limit drinking beverages that contain caffeine (coffee, tea, chocolate drinks, soft drinks).
   - To decrease nocturia, avoid drinking fluids 2 hours before bedtime.
   - Do not limit fluids if you experience incontinence. Concentrated urine may irritate the bladder and increase bladder symptoms.
2. Maintain good voiding habits.
   - Women: Sit well back on the toilet seat, avoid "hovering" over the toilet, and make sure that the feet are flat on the floor.
   - Void at regular intervals, usually every 3 to 4 hours, depending on fluid intake.
   - Avoid straining when voiding or moving the bowels.
   - Take enough time to empty the bladder completely.
3. Keep the bowels regular. A rectum full of stool may irritate the bladder, causing urgency and frequency.
4. Prevent urinary tract infections.
   - Women: Cleanse the perineum from front to back after each voiding and bowel movement; wear cotton undergarments.
   - Drink enough water to pass pale yellow urine.
   - Shower or bathe regularly.
5. Stop smoking to reduce your risk for bladder cancer and reduce the risk of developing a cough, which can contribute to stress urinary incontinence.
6. Report to your health care provider any changes in bladder habits, frequency, urgency, pain when voiding, or blood in the urine.

FIG. 46.9 Male urinals.

that accommodates her food preferences and lifestyle. She suggests that Mrs. Grayson practice toileting at regular intervals and to void as soon as she recognizes the urge. Carly demonstrates methods to strengthen pelvic muscles and reduce intraabdominal pressure and allows Mrs. Grayson time to demonstrate these exercises. Carly also teaches Mrs. Grayson to avoid caffeine and other bladder irritants such as carbonated beverages. She suggests Mrs. Grayson hydrate with her favorite beverages throughout the day.

To address Mrs. Grayson's diagnoses of **Risk for Impaired Skin Integrity** and **Risk for Infection,** Carly encourages and reinforces education about diabetes. To prevent skin breakdown, Carly teaches Mrs. Grayson the need for frequent perineal hygiene, changing her perineal pad frequently, how to cleanse her perineal area, and how to inspect her skin for breakdown. She suggests Mrs. Grayson obtain a skin barrier cream to use in between perineal care. Finally, Carly teaches Mrs. Grayson the signs and symptoms of a urinary tract infection and what to do if she suspects she has developed one.

Carly also knows that Mrs. Grayson will need her bladder scanned to determine her PVR. Carly applies the critical thinking attitude of discipline by completing a thorough examination and assessment. The attitude of curiosity is important when a clinical sign or symptom may be unclear and further information is needed. When Carly checks the policy and procedures at her agency for urinary elimination practices, including bladder scanning, she applies professional standards in practice. She reviews the standards for bladder scanning to be familiar with the procedures.

A strategy to promote relaxation and stimulate bladder contractions is to help patients assume the normal position for voiding. The normal anatomical position for female voiding is in the squatting position. Women empty the bladder better when sitting on the toilet or bedside commode with the feet on the floor. If the patient cannot use a toilet, position her on a bedpan (see Chapter 47). After bedpan use, help the patient perform perineal hygiene (see Chapter 40). A man voids more easily in the standing position. If the patient is unable to reach a toilet, have him stand at the bedside and void into a urinal (a plastic or metal receptacle for urine) (Fig. 46.9).

Always assess mobility status and determine whether the male patient can stand safely. At times it is necessary for one or more nurses to help a male patient stand. If the patient is unable to stand at the bedside, you will need to help him use the urinal in bed. Some patients need the nurse to position the penis completely within the urinal and hold the urinal in place or help them hold the urinal. Once the patient has finished voiding, carefully remove the urinal, and perform perineal hygiene (see Chapter 40).

There are specially designed urinals for women. The female urinal has a larger opening at the top with a defined rim, which helps position the urinal closely against the genitalia.

There are other measures that improve bladder emptying. To promote relaxation and stimulate bladder contractions, use sensory stimuli

Maintaining Adequate Fluid Intake. A simple method to promote normal micturition is to maintain optimal fluid intake. A patient with normal renal function who does not have heart disease or alterations requiring fluid restriction should have approximately 2300 mL of fluid in a 24-hour period. Adequate fluid intake helps flush out solutes or particles that collect in the urinary system and decreases bladder irritability. Help patients change their fluid intake by teaching the importance of adequate hydration. If a patient needs to increase fluid intake, set a schedule for drinking extra fluids, identify fluid preferences, increase high-fluid foods such as fruits, and encourage fluid intake in small volumes frequently. Patients need to avoid excessive fluid intake as well. To prevent nocturia, suggest that the patient avoid drinking fluids 2 hours before bedtime.

Promoting Complete Bladder Emptying. It is normal for a small volume of urine to remain in the bladder after micturition. When the bladder does not empty completely and residual urine volumes are high, there is risk for incontinence and dangerous urinary retention. Urinary retention increases the risk for UTI and damage to the kidneys. Adequate bladder emptying depends on feeling an urge to urinate, contraction of the bladder, and the ability to relax the urethral sphincter.

*Carly implements the plan of care that she developed. The plan of care incorporates Mrs. Grayson's preferences and expectations. To address Mrs. Grayson's **Lack of Knowledge of Treatment Regime,** Carly knows that Mrs. Grayson will require education on improving her urinary incontinence, including bladder retraining, pelvic muscle exercises, and measures to reduce intraabdominal pressure. Keeping these needs in mind, Carly begins by discussing with Mrs. Grayson the need to learn to use interventions that will improve her pelvic muscle strength. Carly encourages Mrs. Grayson to begin to identify methods to lose weight and to avoid heavy lifting. Carly suggests Mrs. Grayson find a weight loss plan*

BOX 46.8 PATIENT TEACHING

Teaching Patients About Pelvic Muscle Exercises (Kegel Exercises)

Objective
- Patient will verbalize and/or demonstrate how to perform pelvic muscle exercises (Kegel exercises).

Teaching Strategies
- Use pictures and plain language to teach the patient pelvic anatomy and the location of the pelvic muscles (see Fig. 46.16).
- Teach patient how to identify and contract the correct muscle.
  - Women: Instruct the patient to squeeze the anus as if to hold in gas or to insert a finger into the vagina and feel the muscle squeeze around her finger. The woman can also observe the perineum pulling in by using a mirror.
  - Men: Instruct the patient to stand in front of a mirror, squeeze the anus as if to hold in gas, and watch to see if the penis moves up and down as he contracts the pelvic floor muscles.
  - Instruct to not contract the abdomen, buttocks, or thighs when contracting the pelvic muscles.
- Teach patients pelvic muscle contraction exercises.
  - Quick flicks: Squeeze the muscle for 2 to 3 seconds and relax.
  - Sustained contractions: Squeeze the muscle for 10 seconds and relax after each contraction for 10 seconds.
  - Counting out loud prevents breath holding during exercises.
- Teach patient to maintain a daily exercise schedule.
  - Perform three to five quick flicks followed by 10 sustained contractions.
  - Do these exercises 3 to 4 times a day.

Evaluation
Use the principles of teach-back to evaluate patient/family caregiver learning:
- Describe how you would correctly identify the pelvic floor muscles.
- Explain how you would perform pelvic muscle exercises.

REFLECT NOW

Think about health promotion for your next assigned patient. What strategies would improve this patient's urinary elimination?

Acute Care. Patients with acute illness, surgery, or impaired function of the urinary tract may require more invasive interventions that support urinary elimination.

Catheterization. Urinary catheterization is the placement of a tube through the urethra into the bladder to drain urine (see Skill 46.2). There is a risk for CAUTIs, which are the fourth leading cause of health care–associated infections in acute care hospitals (Ferguson, 2018). The ANA developed an evidenced-based tool, the *ANA CAUTI Prevention Tool*, to guide the decision making of the health care team regarding indwelling catheter insertion and care, maintenance of sterile technique, and best practices for timely catheter removal (ANA, n.d.).

Urinary catheterization can be intermittent (one-time catheterization for bladder emptying) or indwelling (remains in place over a period of time). Indwelling catheterization may be short term (2 weeks or less) or long term (more than 1 month) (Taylor, 2018). Accurately monitor a patient's intake and output when a short- or long-term urinary catheter is used. Patients commonly need a catheter when they have urological or gynecological procedures or when their bladder inadequately empties due to an obstruction or a neurological condition. Excessive accumulation of urine in the bladder is painful for a patient, increases the risk for UTI, and can cause backward flow of urine up the ureters, increasing risk for kidney damage. For some patients, the only method of managing their bladder dysfunction is through a catheter. Intermittent catheterization is used to measure PVR when ultrasound or a bladder scanner is unavailable or as a way to manage chronic urinary retention.

Types of Catheters. The difference among urinary catheters is related to the number of catheter lumens, the presence of a balloon to keep the indwelling catheter in place, the shape of the catheter, and a closed drainage system. Urinary catheters are made with one to three lumens. Single-lumen catheters (Fig. 46.10A) are used for intermittent/straight catheterization. Double-lumen catheters, designed for indwelling catheters, provide one lumen for urinary drainage while a second lumen is used to inflate a balloon that keeps the catheter in place (see Fig. 46.10B). Triple-lumen catheters (see Fig. 46.10C) are used for continuous bladder irrigation (CBI) or when it becomes necessary to instill medications into the bladder. One lumen drains the bladder, a second lumen is used to inflate the balloon, and a third lumen delivers irrigation fluid into the bladder.

A health care provider chooses a catheter based on factors such as latex allergy, history of catheter encrustation, anatomical factors, and susceptibility to infection. Indwelling catheters are made of latex or silicone. Latex catheters with special coatings reduce urethral irritation. All silicone catheters have a larger internal diameter and may be helpful in patients who require frequent catheter changes as a result of encrustation. Intermittent/straight catheters are made of rubber (softer and more flexible) or polyvinyl chloride (PVC). Patients who self-catheterize have a large selection of catheters, some with special coatings that do not require lubrication and others that are self-contained systems consisting of a prelubricated catheter and packaged with a preconnected drainage bag. Catheter shape can differ; shape chosen is based on anatomical differences in patients. One such catheter is a Coudé-tip catheter. This catheter has a curvature at the end that helps it maneuver through the prostatic urethra in the presence of a large prostate. Nurses need special training to use this type of catheter.

(e.g., turning on running water, putting a patient's hand in a pan of warm water) and provide privacy. In addition, bladder exercises help to improve pelvic muscles, which reduces stress incontinence and improves bladder emptying (Box 46.8).

To improve bladder emptying, encourage patients to wait until the urine flow completely stops when voiding and encourage them to attempt a second void (double voiding). Timed voiding is voiding according to the clock, not the urge to void, and is a helpful strategy when the bladder does not fully empty. The Credé method or manual compression of the bladder (i.e., placing the hands over the bladder and compressing it to help in emptying) should not be implemented until consultation with the health care provider. In the presence of high PVRs or a complete inability of the bladder to empty, urinary catheterization, either intermittent or indwelling, is needed.

Preventing Infection. UTIs are the fifth most common type of health care–associated infection (CDC, 2020). It is important to implement evidence-based practices to avoid this common and potentially dangerous infection. Some key interventions include promoting adequate fluid intake, promoting perineal hygiene, and having patients void at regular intervals. Encourage women to wipe front to back after voiding and defecation and teach them to avoid perfumed perineal washes and sprays, bubble baths, and tight clothing. If a patient has a problem with urine leakage, perineal hygiene should be especially stressed. Patients should use containment products that are designed for urine and wick wetness away from the body. Prolonged periods of urine wetness should be avoided.

A **Straight catheter (cross section)**

Catheter tip

5- to 10-mL inflated balloon

Balloon inflation

Urine drainage

B **Indwelling retention catheter (cross section)**

30-mL inflated balloon

Balloon inflation

Urine drainage flows out

Irrigation solution flows in

C **Triple-lumen catheter (cross section)**

FIG. 46.10 (A) Straight catheter (cross section). (B) Indwelling (Foley) retention catheter (cross section). (C) Triple-lumen catheter (cross section).

FIG. 46.11 Size of catheter and balloon printed on catheter.

Catheter Sizes. The size of a urinary catheter is based on the French (Fr) scale, which reflects the internal diameter of the catheter. Most adults with an indwelling catheter need a size 14 to 16 Fr for short-term use and 20 to 24 Fr if there is hematuria or clots (Harding et al., 2021; Schaeffer, 2020a). Although larger catheter diameters increase the risk for urethral trauma, larger catheters are used in special circumstances, such as after urological surgery or in the presence of gross hematuria. Smaller sizes are needed for children, such as a 5 to 6 Fr for infants, 8 to 10 Fr for children, and 12 Fr for young girls.

Indwelling catheters come in a variety of balloon sizes—from 3 mL (for a child) to 30 mL for CBI. The size of the balloon is usually printed on the catheter port (Fig. 46.11). The recommended balloon size for an adult is a 5-mL balloon (the balloon is 5 mL and requires 10 mL to fill completely) (Harding et al., 2021). Long-term use of larger balloons (30 mL) has been associated with increased patient discomfort, irritation and trauma to the urethra, increased risk of catheter expulsion, and incomplete emptying of the bladder resulting from urine that pools below the level of the catheter drainage eyes.

FIG. 46.12 Urine specimen collection: aspiration from a collection port in drainage tubing of indwelling catheter (needleless technique). (Courtesy and © Becton, Dickinson and Company.)

Catheter Changes. Use clinical indicators, such as obstruction, poor drainage, malfunction of the catheter, or encrustation to determine when to change long-term indwelling catheters and drainage bags (Schaeffer, 2020a). When long-term catheterization is required, the catheter will need to be changed every 4 to 6 weeks. Whenever possible, avoid the use of long-term catheterization to reduce the risk for CAUTI.

Closed Drainage Systems. An indwelling catheter is attached to a urinary drainage bag to collect the continuous flow of urine. This is a closed drainage system, and tubing connections should not be separated to avoid introducing pathogens. In patients with indwelling catheters, specimens are collected without opening the drainage system by using a special port in the tubing (Fig. 46.12). Always hang the drainage bag below the level of the bladder on the bedframe or a chair so that urine will drain down out of the bladder. The bag should never touch the floor to prevent accidental contamination during emptying. When a patient ambulates, carry the bag below the level of the patient's bladder. Ambulatory patients may use a leg bag. This is a bag that attaches to the leg with straps. Leg bags are usually worn during the day and replaced at night with a standard drainage bag. The only drainage bag that does not need to be kept dependent to the bladder is a specially designed drainage bag (belly bag) that is worn across the abdomen. A one-way valve prevents the backflow of urine into the bladder. To keep the drainage system patent, check for kinks or bends in the tubing, avoid positioning the patient on drainage tubing, prevent tubing from becoming dependent, and observe for clots or sediment that may block the catheter or tubing.

Routine Catheter Care. Patients with indwelling catheters require regular perineal hygiene, especially after a bowel movement, to reduce the risk for CAUTI (CDC, 2020; Schaeffer, 2020a). In many health care agencies patients receive catheter care every 8 hours as the minimal standard of care. See Chapter 40 for routine perineal care and Skill 46.3 for catheter care. Empty drainage bags when they are half full (Fig. 46.13). An overfull drainage bag can create tension and pull on the catheter, resulting in trauma to the urethra and/or urinary meatus and increasing risk for CAUTI (CDC, 2020). Expect continuous drainage of urine into the drainage bag. In the presence of no urine drainage, first check to make sure that there are no kinks or obvious occlusion of the drainage tubing or catheter.

Preventing Catheter-Associated Urinary Tract Infection. A critical part of routine catheter care is reducing the risk for CAUTI (Box 46.9).

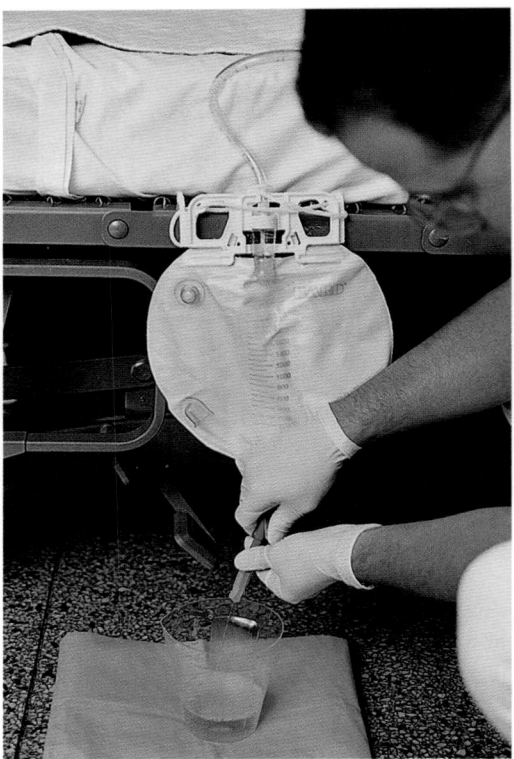

FIG. 46.13 Urine drainage bag.

In addition, there are specific CDC (2020) guidelines and interventions (Box 46.10). A key intervention to prevent infection is to maintain a closed urinary drainage system. Portals for entry of bacteria into the system are illustrated in Fig. 46.14. Another key intervention is prevention of urine backflow from the tubing and bag into the bladder. Many urine drainage systems are equipped with an antireflux valve, but you should monitor the system to prevent pooling of urine within the tubing and to keep the drainage bag below the level of the bladder.

> **QSEN** **Building Competency in Evidence-Based Practice** A nursing unit is experiencing an increase in catheter-associated urinary tract infections (CAUTIs). A team of staff nurses is investigating this problem and discovers that some nurses are resistant to implementing new evidence-based practice (EBP) guidelines in CAUTI prevention. What can you do to decrease resistance and enhance EBP care on this unit?
>
> Answers to QSEN Activities can be found on the Evolve website.

Catheter Irrigations and Instillations. To maintain the patency of indwelling urinary catheters, it is sometimes necessary to irrigate or flush a catheter with sterile solution. However, irrigation poses the risk of causing a UTI and thus must be done maintaining a closed urinary drainage system. In general, if a catheter becomes occluded, it is best to change it rather than risk flushing debris into the bladder. In some instances, the health care provider will determine that irrigations are needed to keep a catheter patent, such as after genitourinary surgery when there is high risk for catheter occlusion from blood clots. Bladder instillations are used to instill medication into the bladder. Refer to specific instructions for these medications in terms of how long the medication needs to stay in the bladder.

BOX 46.9 EVIDENCE-BASED PRACTICE

Preventions of Catheter-Associated Urinary Tract Infection (CAUTI)

PICOT Question: Does the use of evidence-based nursing protocols reduce the occurrence of catheter-associated urinary tract infection (CAUTI) in hospitalized patients with an indwelling catheter?

Evidence Summary

Approximately 12% to 16% of adult hospital inpatients will have an indwelling urinary catheter at some time during their hospitalization, and each day the indwelling urinary catheter remains, a patient has a 3% to 7% increased risk of acquiring a catheter-associated urinary tract infection (CAUTI) (CDC, 2020). Measures to reduce CAUTI are organized into five areas: appropriate catheter use, proper insertion and maintenance techniques, quality improvement programs, ongoing surveillance for CAUTI, and related causative factors (CDC, 2020; TJC, 2021). Nurse-led interventions reduced the duration of indwelling catheter use and incidence of CAUTI (Graham et al., 2020). In addition, a hospital-wide strategy that included reeducation of nurses about CAUTI prevention and infusing best practice into current-practice nursing care also decreased CAUTI rates (Cartwright, 2018). Best practices, staff education, data reporting, and the use of an electronic health record as a catheter reminder decreased the CAUTI rates (Fekete, 2020; Ferguson, 2018; Lawrence et al., 2019; Schaeffer, 2020a).

Application to Nursing Practice

- Become familiar with guidelines related to CAUTI prevention and care (see Box 46.10).
- Be aware of indications for catheter insertion and advocate for a patient if the indications do not meet accepted guidelines (Ferguson, 2018).
- Collaborate with health care providers to remove catheters early when medical indications no longer exist.
- Develop or use evidence-based nurse-driven protocols for CAUTI prevention (Ferguson, 2018; Graham et al., 2020).
- Use only trained dedicated personnel to insert urinary catheters.
- Quality improvement/surveillance programs should be in place that alert providers that a catheter is in place and include regular educational programming about catheter care.

Closed catheter irrigation provides intermittent or continuous irrigation of a urinary catheter without disrupting the sterile connection between the catheter and the drainage system (see Skill 46.4). CBI is an example of a continuous infusion of a sterile solution into the bladder, usually using a three-way irrigation closed system with a triple-lumen catheter. CBI is frequently used following genitourinary surgery to keep the bladder clear and free of blood clots or sediment.

Removal of Indwelling Catheter. The CMS identified CAUTI as a never event (CDC, 2020; CMS, 2020). Prompt removal of an indwelling catheter after it is no longer needed is a key intervention that has proven to decrease the incidence and prevalence of hospital-acquired urinary tract infections (HAUTIs) (see Skill 46.2). Monitor patient's voiding after catheter removal for at least 24 to 48 hours by using a voiding record or bladder diary. The bladder diary records the time and amount of each voiding, including any incontinence. The use of ultrasonography or a bladder scanner can monitor bladder function by measuring PVR volume (Box 46.11). The first few times a patient voids after catheter removal may be accompanied by some discomfort, but continued painful urination indicates possible infection. Abdominal pain and distention, a sensation of incomplete emptying, incontinence, constant dribbling of urine, and voiding in very small amounts can indicate inadequate bladder emptying requiring intervention.

BOX 46.10 Preventing Catheter-Associated Urinary Tract Infection (CAUTI)

- Prevention of CAUTI often requires use of an evidence-based "bundle" to perform all elements of care at one time along with completion of a checklist to ensure that each element is included in that care. Know the policies of your institution to determine which components are in a care bundle (American Association of Colleges of Nursing [AACN] Clinical Practice Alert, 2018; Graham et al., 2020).
- Use aseptic catheter insertion using sterile equipment (Fekete, 2020; TJC, 2021).
- Patients in need of long-term catheterization should be managed with intermittent catherization (Fekete, 2020; Schaeffer, 2020b).
- Use only trained dedicated personnel to insert urinary catheters.
- Use smallest catheter possible and individualize the size to the patient (Schaeffer, 2020b).
- Remove catheter as soon as possible. If patient had surgery, removal in recovery room is ideal (Schaeffer, 2020b).
- Secure indwelling catheters to prevent movement and pulling on the catheter.
- Maintain a sterile, closed urinary drainage system (Schaeffer et al., 2020a).
- Maintain an unobstructed flow of urine through the catheter, drainage tubing, and drainage bag.
- Always keep the urinary drainage bag below the level of the bladder.
- When emptying the urinary drainage bag, use a separate measuring receptacle for each patient. Do not let the drainage spigot touch the receptacle.
- Perform routine perineal hygiene daily and after soiling.

Data from Centers for Disease Control and Prevention (CDC): Urinary tract infection (catheter-associated urinary tract infection [CAUTI] and non–catheter-associated urinary tract infection [UTI]) and other urinary system infection [USI] events, 2020. http://www.cdc.gov/nhsn/PDFs/pscManual/7pscCAUTIcurrent.pdf. Accessed July 2021.

FIG. 46.14 Potential sites for introduction of infectious organisms into the urinary drainage system.

Alternative to Urethral Catheterization. To avoid the risks associated with urethral catheters, two alternatives are available for urinary drainage.

Suprapubic Catheterization. A suprapubic catheter is a urinary drainage tube inserted surgically into the bladder through the abdominal wall above the symphysis pubis (Fig. 46.15). The catheter may be sutured to the skin, secured with an adhesive material, or retained in the bladder with a fluid-filled balloon in the same way as an indwelling catheter. Suprapubic catheters are placed when there is blockage of the urethra (e.g., enlarged prostate, urethral stricture, after urological surgery) and in situations in which a long-term urethral catheter causes irritation or discomfort or interferes with sexual functioning.

Care of a suprapubic catheter involves daily cleansing of the insertion site and catheter. The same care for the tubing and drainage bag for a urethral catheter applies to a suprapubic catheter. Thus assess the insertion site for signs of inflammation and the growth of overgranulation tissue. If insertion is new, slight inflammation may be expected as part of normal wound healing, but it can also indicate infection. Overgranulation tissue can develop at the insertion site as a reaction to the catheter. In some instances, intervention is needed. Use the principles of applying a dry dressing when providing site care; institutional policy will indicate whether aseptic or sterile technique is required (see Chapter 48).

External Catheter. The external catheter, also called a *condom catheter* or *penile sheath,* is a soft, pliable condom-like sheath that fits over the penis, providing a safe and noninvasive way to contain urine. Most external catheters are made of soft silicone to reduce friction and are clear to allow for easy visualization of skin under the catheter. Latex catheters are still available and used by some patients. It is important to verify that a patient does not have a latex allergy before applying this type of catheter. Condom-type external catheters are held in place by an adhesive coating of the internal lining of the sheath, a double-sided self-adhesive strip, brush-on adhesive applied to the penile shaft, or in rare cases an external strap or tape. They may be attached to a small-volume (leg) drainage bag or a large-volume (bedside) urinary drainage bag, both of which need to be kept lower than the level of the bladder. The condom-type external catheter is suitable for patients who are incontinent and have complete and spontaneous bladder emptying. Condom-type external catheters come in a variety of styles and sizes. Refer to manufacturer guidelines to determine the best fit and correct application. See Box 46.12 for the steps in applying a condom catheter. Condom-type external catheters are associated with less risk for UTI than indwelling catheters; thus they are an excellent option for the male with UI. For men who cannot be fitted for a condom-type external catheter, there are other externally applied catheters.

Urinary Diversions. Immediately after surgery the patient with an incontinent urinary diversion must wear a pouch to collect the effluent (drainage). The pouch keeps the patient clean and dry, protects the skin from damage, and provides a barrier against odor. Urinary pouches with an antireflux flap can be opaque or clear, drainable one-piece or two-piece pouches, with cut-to-fit or precut wafers. Change the pouch every 4 to 6 days. Each pouch may be connected to a bedside drainage bag for use at night.

When changing a pouch, gently cleanse the skin surrounding the stoma with warm tap water using a washcloth and pat dry. Do not use soap because it can leave a residue on the skin. Measure the stoma and cut the opening in the pouch. Then apply the pouch after removing the protective backing from the adhesive surface. Press firmly into place over the stoma. Observe the appearance of the stoma and surrounding skin. The stoma is normally red and moist and is located in the right lower quadrant of the abdomen. It is important for the patient to have

BOX 46.11 PROCEDURAL GUIDELINES

Using a Bladder Scanner to Measure Postvoid Residual (PVR)

Delegation and Collaboration

The skill of measuring bladder volume by bladder scan can be delegated to assistive personnel (AP). The nurse must first determine the timing and frequency of the bladder scan measurement and interpret the measurements obtained. The nurse also assesses the patient's ability to toilet before measuring postvoid residual (PVR) and the abdomen for distention if urinary retention is suspected. The nurse directs the AP to:

- Follow manufacturer recommendations for the use of the device.
- Measure PVR volumes within 5 to 15 minutes after helping the patient to void.
- Report and record bladder scan volumes.

Equipment

Bladder scanner, ultrasound gel, cleansing agent (e.g., alcohol pad) for scanner head, urethral catheterization tray for single-use catheter/intermittent (see Skill 46.2), paper towel or washcloth

Procedural Steps

1. Identify patient using at least two identifiers (e.g., name and birthday or name and medical record number) according to agency policy (TJC, 2021).
2. Review electronic health record (EHR), and assess urinary pattern and ability to empty bladder effectively.
3. Assess intake and output (I&O) record to determine urine output trends and whether patient has voided since surgery; check the plan of care to verify correct timing of the bladder scan measurement.

   CLINICAL JUDGMENT: Failure to measure PVR 5 to 15 minutes after a patient voids can result in an inaccurate bladder scan.

4. Assess patient's or family caregiver's knowledge, experience, and health literacy.
5. Assess patient's knowledge, prior experience with bladder scanning, and feelings about procedure.
6. Assess patient's goals or preferences for how skill is to be performed or what patient expects.
7. Provide privacy by closing room door and bedside curtain.
8. Help patient to supine position with head slightly elevated. Raise bed to appropriate working height. If side rails are raised, lower side rail on working side.
9. Perform hand hygiene and apply clean gloves.
10. Discuss procedure with patient. If measurement is for PVR, ask patient to void, and measure volume retained in bladder with scanner within 5 to 15 minutes of voiding:
    a. Pull back sheet to expose patient's lower abdomen.
    b. Turn on scanner per manufacturer guidelines.
    c. Set gender designation per manufacturer guidelines. Designate women who have had a hysterectomy as male.
    d. Wipe scanner head with alcohol pad or other cleaner and allow to air-dry.
    e. Palpate patient's symphysis pubis (pubic bone). Apply generous amount of ultrasound gel (or if available a bladder scan gel pad) to midline abdomen 2.5 to 4 cm (1–1½ inches) above symphysis pubis.

f. Place scanner head on gel, ensuring that scanner head is oriented per manufacturer guidelines.
g. Apply light pressure, keep scanner head steady, and point it slightly downward toward bladder. Press and release the scan button.
h. Verify accurate aim (refer to manufacturer guidelines). Complete scan and print image (if needed) (see illustration).

STEP 10h Bladder scanner with image. (Courtesy Verathon, Inc.)

11. Remove ultrasound gel from patient's abdomen with paper towel or moist cloth.
12. Remove ultrasound gel from scanner head and wipe with alcohol pad or other cleaner; allow to air-dry.
13. Help patient to comfortable position.
14. Raise side rails (as appropriate) and lower bed to lowest position.
15. Place nurse call system in an accessible location within patient's reach.
16. Remove and dispose of gloves and perform hand hygiene.
17. Compare PVR results with prevoiding scan (if available); urine volume should be less. Or if first-time scan, PVR should be <100 mL urine.
18. Review health care provider's order to determine how often to assess residual urine or whether catheterization is ordered.
19. Review I&O record to determine urine output trends.
20. Record findings of scan, PVR, and patient tolerance of procedure.

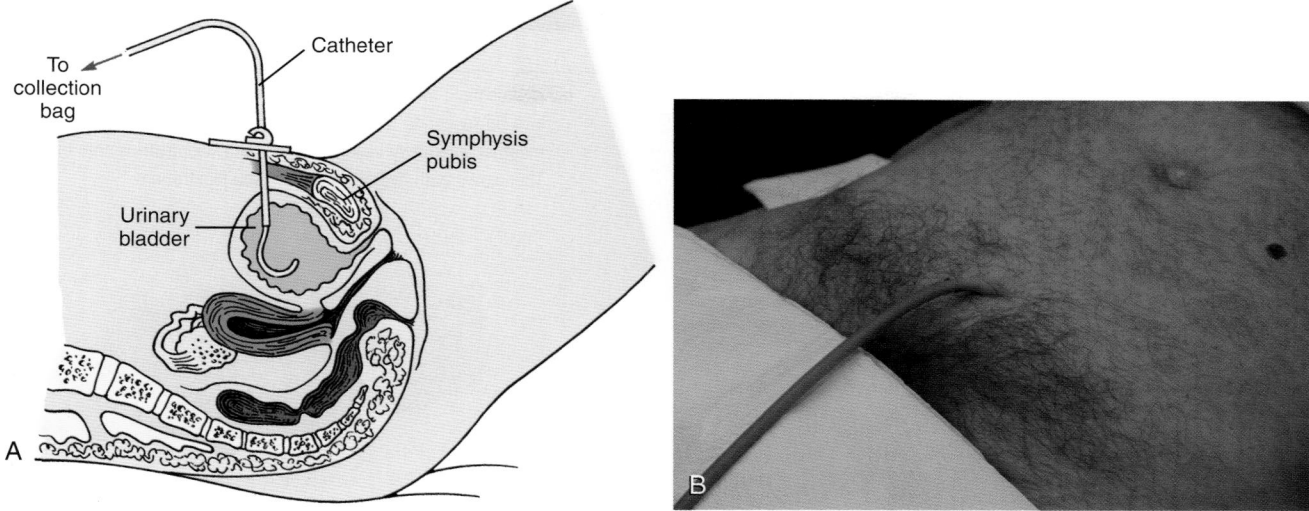

FIG. 46.15 (A) Placement of suprapubic catheter above symphysis pubis. (B) Suprapubic catheter without a dressing.

BOX 46.12 PROCEDURAL GUIDELINES

Applying a Male Incontinence Device

Delegation and Collaboration

Assessment of the skin of a patient's penile shaft and determination of a latex allergy are done by a registered nurse before catheter application. The skill of applying a condom catheter can be delegated to assistive personnel (AP), depending on agency policy. The nurse directs the AP to:

• Follow manufacturer directions for applying the condom catheter and securing device.
• Monitor intake and output (I&O) and record if applicable.
• Immediately report any redness, swelling, or skin irritation or breakdown of glans penis or penile shaft.

Equipment

Condom catheter kit—condom sheath of appropriate size, securing device (internal adhesive, strap), skin preparation solution (per manufacturer's recommendations). *Option:* hydrocolloid incontinence device; urinary collection bag with drainage tubing or leg bag and straps; basin with warm water and soap; towels, washcloth, bath blanket; clean gloves; scissors, hair guard, or paper towel

Procedural Steps

1. Identify patient using at least two identifiers (e.g., name and birthday or name and medical record number) according to agency policy (TJC, 2021).
2. Review electronic health record (EHR), and assess urinary pattern, ability to empty bladder effectively, and degree of urinary continence.
3. Assess patient's or family caregiver's knowledge, experience, and health literacy.
4. Review EHR for history of allergy to rubber or latex. Confirm with patient if possible. Check patient's allergy wristband.
5. Assess patient's or family caregiver's mental status, knowledge of and experience with condom-type catheter, and ability to apply device.
6. Assess patient's goals or preferences for how skill is to be performed or what patient expects.
7. Perform hand hygiene. Assess integrity of penile tissue. Verify patient's size and type of condom catheter from plan of care, or use manufacturer measuring guide to measure length and diameter of penis in flaccid state (apply gloves for measurement). Perform hand hygiene.

CLINICAL JUDGMENT: Apply condom catheters only when the skin on the penile surface is intact.

8. Provide privacy by closing room door or curtain. Organize and set up equipment needed.
9. Raise bed to appropriate working height. Lower side rail on working side.
10. Explain procedure to patient.
11. Perform hand hygiene.
12. Prepare urinary drainage collection bag and tubing (large-volume drainage bag or leg bag). Clamp off drainage bag port. Place bag nearby ready to attach to condom after applied.
13. Help patient to supine or sitting position.
14. Place bath blanket over upper torso. Fold sheets so that only penis is exposed.
15. Apply clean gloves. Provide perineal care (see Chapter 40). Dry thoroughly before applying device. If the patient is uncircumcised, ensure that foreskin has been replaced to normal position before applying condom catheter. Do not apply barrier cream.
16. Remove and dispose of gloves. Perform hand hygiene.
17. Apply clean gloves. Assess skin of penis for rashes, erythema, and/or open areas.
18. Clip hair at base of penis as necessary before application of condom sheath. Some manufacturers provide hair guard that is placed over penis before applying device. Remove hair guard after applying catheter. An alternative to hair guard is to tear a hole in a paper towel, place it over penis, and remove after application of device.

CLINICAL JUDGMENT: Do not shave the pubic area because any microabrasions in skin increase risk for skin irritation and infection.

19. Apply incontinence device.
    a. **Condom catheter.** With nondominant hand, grasp penis along shaft. With dominant hand, hold rolled condom sheath at tip of penis with head of penis in cone. Smoothly roll sheath onto penis. Allow 2.5 to 5 cm (1–2 inches) of space between tip of glans penis and end of condom catheter (see illustration).

Continued

BOX 46.12 PROCEDURAL GUIDELINES—cont'd

Applying a Male Incontinence Device

STEP 19a Condom catheter.

2.5 to 5 cm
(1 to 2 in)

b. **Hydrocolloid device.** One size fits all. Place the device onto the tip of the penis, not the shaft (see manufacturer's directions).
20. Apply appropriate securement device as indicated in manufacturer guidelines.
   a. Self-adhesive condom catheters: After application, apply gentle pressure on penile shaft for 10 to 15 seconds.
   b. Outer securing strip-type condom catheters: Spiral wrap penile shaft with strip of supplied elastic adhesive. Strip should not overlap itself. Elastic strip should be snug, not tight (see illustration).

CLINICAL JUDGMENT: Never use regular adhesive tape to secure a condom catheter. Constriction from tape can reduce blood flow to tissues.

Elastic adhesive strip

STEP 20b Spiral application of adhesive strip.

c. Hydrocolloid incontinence device: Remove release papers from adhesive on faceplate of device. Center faceplate over opening of urinary meatus. Smooth hydrocolloid adhesive backing strips onto tip of penis. Then cover with hydrocolloid seal (see illustration).

STEP 20c Men's Liberty acute male incontinence device. (Courtesy BioDerm, Inc., Largo, FL.)

21. Remove hair guard or paper towel (if used). Connect drainage tubing to end of incontinence device. Be sure that a condom catheter is not twisted. If using large drainage bag, place excess tubing on bed and secure to bottom sheet.
22. Help patient to safe, comfortable position.
23. Raise side rails (as appropriate) and lower bed to lowest position.
24. Place nurse call system in an accessible location within patient's reach.
25. Dispose of contaminated supplies, remove and dispose of gloves, and perform hand hygiene.
26. Remove and reapply daily following the previous steps unless an extended-wear device is used. To remove condom, wash penis with warm, soapy water and gently roll sheath and adhesive off penile shaft.
27. Observe urinary drainage.
28. Inspect penis with condom catheter in place within 15 to 30 minutes after application. Assess for swelling and discoloration and ask patient whether there is any discomfort.
29. Inspect skin on penile shaft for signs of breakdown or irritation at least daily, when performing hygiene, and before reapplying condom or incontinence device.
30. Record condition of penis, type of external device applied, patient's response to procedure, and patient's level of understanding of purpose of device.

the correct type and fit of an ostomy pouch. A specialty ostomy nurse is an essential resource when selecting the right appliance so that the pouch fits snugly against the surface of the skin around the stoma, preventing damaging leakage of urine (see Chapter 47).

Patients with continent urinary diversions do not have to wear an external pouch. However, teach a patient with a continent urinary reservoir how to intermittently catheterize the pouch. Patients need to be able and willing to do these 4 to 6 times a day for the rest of their lives. After creation of an orthotopic neobladder, patients will have frequent episodes of incontinence until the neobladder slowly stretches and the urinary sphincter is strong enough to contain the urine. To achieve continence the patient will need to follow a bladder-training schedule and perform pelvic muscle exercises (Lukacz, 2020). The postoperative care of patients having continent urinary diversions varies widely with

the surgical techniques used; it is important to learn the surgeon's preferred routine or health care agency procedures before caring for these patients.

Medications. A small number of medications, antimuscarinics (e.g., oxybutynin and trospium), are used to treat urinary urgency. Another medication, mirabegron, is in a class of medications called beta$_3$-adrenergic agonists. It relaxes the bladder muscles to prevent urgent, or uncontrolled, urination. The most common adverse effects of antimuscarinics are dry mouth, constipation, and blurred vision. In some cases, these medications can cause a change in mental status in older adults (Burchum and Rosenthal, 2019). Patients taking mirabegron should have their blood pressure monitored because of possible increases. There are no medications, other than off-label use of vaginal estrogen in postmenopausal women, to treat stress UI (Lukacz, 2020).

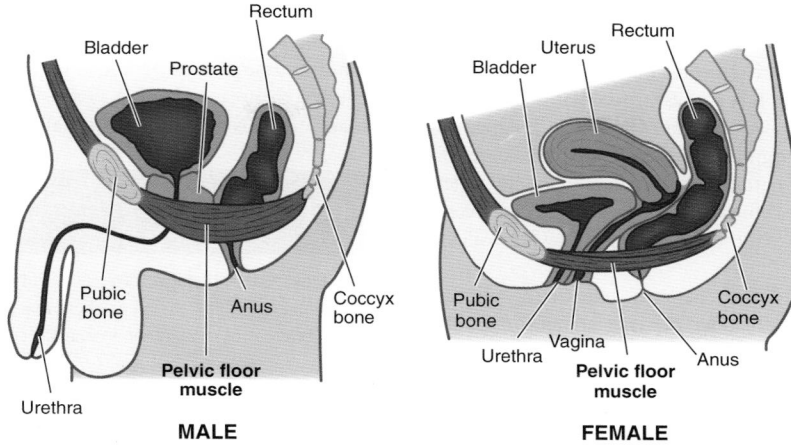

FIG. 46.16 Pelvic floor muscles. (From Harding MM et al: *Medical-surgical nursing,* ed 11, St Louis, 2020, Elsevier.)

Urinary retention is sometimes treated with bethanechol. Men with outlet obstruction caused by an enlarged prostate are treated with agents that relax the smooth muscle of the prostatic urethra, such as tamsulosin and silodosin, and agents that shrink the prostate, such as finasteride and dutasteride. Know the medications and indications for all medications your patient is taking.

When a patient starts taking an antimuscarinic, monitor for effectiveness, including a decrease in urgency, frequency, and incontinence episodes. A bladder diary is one of the best ways to do this. In addition, regularly assess the patient for side effects such as constipation by monitoring the bowel movement record. Watch for a decrease in bowel movement frequency, straining at bowel movements, and changes in stool consistency.

UTIs are treated with antibiotics. Patients with painful urination are sometimes prescribed urinary analgesics that act on the urethral and bladder mucosa (e.g., phenazopyridine). Patients taking drugs with phenazopyridine need to be aware that their urine will be orange. They must drink large amounts of fluids to prevent toxicity from the sulfonamides and maintain optimal flow through the urinary system (Burchum and Rosenthal, 2019).

Continuing and Restorative Care. There are techniques that can improve control over bladder emptying and restore some degree of urinary continence. These techniques are commonly referred to as behavioral therapy and are considered first-line treatment for stress, urge, and mixed incontinence (Lukacz, 2020). They include lifestyle changes, **pelvic floor muscle training** (PFMT), bladder retraining, and a variety of toileting schedules (see Table 46.1). In some cases, when the bladder does not empty, patients or caregivers learn to intermittently catheterize. Whenever there is a risk for urine leakage, skin care is an essential component of the plan of care. Adequate urine containment and skin protection promote patient comfort and dignity.

Lifestyle Changes. Lifestyle modifications can improve bladder function and decrease incontinence. In addition to interventions listed earlier in this chapter under health promotion and in Box 46.7, you can teach patients about foods and fluids that cause bladder irritation and increase symptoms, such as frequency, urgency, and incontinence. Teach patients to avoid common irritants such as artificial sweeteners, spicy foods, citrus products, and especially caffeine (Bykoviene et al., 2018). Discourage patients from drinking large volumes of fluid at one time. Constipation can also affect bladder symptoms. Thus you need to implement measures to promote bowel regularity (see Chapter 47). Encourage patients

with edema to elevate the feet for a minimum of a few hours in the afternoon to help diminish nighttime voiding frequency.

Pelvic Floor Muscle Training. Evidence has shown that patients with urgency, stress, and mixed UI experience improvement and can eventually achieve continence when treated with PFMT (Bykoviene et al., 2018; Lukacz, 2020). PFMT involves teaching patients how to identify and contract the pelvic floor muscles in a structured exercise program. This exercise program is commonly called *Kegel exercises* and is based on therapy first developed by obstetrician-gynecologist Dr. Arnold Kegel in the 1940s. The exercises work by increasing the pressure within the urethra by strengthening the pelvic floor muscles and inhibiting unwanted bladder contractions (Fig. 46.16). Many patients benefit from verbal instructions on how to do the exercises (see Box 46.8). Refer patients who have difficulty correctly identifying and contracting the pelvic floor muscles to a continence specialist for biofeedback. Biofeedback involves intensive instruction augmented by computerized measurement of muscle activity that is displayed on a monitor. The visual feedback helps the patient learn to contract the muscles correctly.

Bladder Retraining. Bladder retraining is a behavioral therapy designed to help patients control bothersome urinary urgency and frequency. Patients are taught about their bladder and techniques to suppress urgency. They are given a schedule of toileting based on their diary of voiding and leaking; the schedule is designed to slowly increase the interval between voiding. Successful bladder retraining requires that patients get regular support and positive reinforcement. Patients are taught to inhibit the urge to void by taking slow, deep breaths to relax, performing five to six quick, strong pelvic muscle exercises (flicks) in quick succession, followed by distracting attention from bladder sensations. Instruct the patient to go to the bathroom to void after the urge to void lessens or subsides. Only patients who are highly motivated and cognitively intact are candidates for this therapy. If a patient is in such a program, you can provide support by reinforcing the schedule and providing emotional encouragement.

Toileting Schedules. A key component to any treatment plan for UI is regular toilet access. Individualize toileting schedules based on the type of incontinence and functional disability (e.g., cognitive impairment). Toileting can be implemented in any care setting and should be the first plan of action when you assess a patient to be incontinent. Timed voiding or scheduled toileting is toileting based on a fixed schedule, not the patient's urge to void. The schedule may be set by a time interval, such as every 2 to 3 hours, or at times of day, such as before and after meals. Using timed voiding or scheduled toileting is effective when caring for patients who are cognitively impaired or who are experiencing impaired mobility. Habit training is a toileting schedule based on the patient's usual voiding pattern. With use of a bladder diary, the usual times a patient voids are identified. It is at these times that the patient is then toileted. Prompted voiding is a program of toileting designed for patients with mild or moderate cognitive impairment. Patients are toileted based on their usual voiding pattern. This is a very successful toileting program; however, it requires a consistent and motivated caregiver, a cooperative patient, and evidence that the patient will void when toileted at least 50% of the time or more.

Intermittent Catheterization. Some patients experience chronic inability to completely empty the bladder because of neuromuscular damage related to multiple sclerosis, diabetes, spinal cord injury, and urinary retention caused by outlet obstruction. To minimize the risk of UTI, patients or family caregivers are taught to catheterize the bladder. It is important that they follow the principles of asepsis as discussed earlier in the chapter. Teach patients and caregivers about the importance of adequate fluid intake, signs of infection, and their individualized catheterization schedule. The goal for intermittent catheterization is drainage of 400 mL of urine, with the schedule individualized to meet this goal.

Skin Care. Moisture-associated skin damage (MASD) presents as inflammation of the skin with or without erosion to the affected area (Werth and Justice, 2019). MASD has many causes. Usually MASD is mainly caused by moisture from incontinence, so preventing incontinence or having a good management plan when a patient is incontinent is imperative. The *do's* for effective management include identification and treatment, use of skin risk assessment tools, use of appropriate barrier products, and ensuring adequate hydration (Werth and Justice, 2019). Keep the patient's sheets clean and dry, and do not double pad the bed. Also remember that incontinence is not an expected or normal finding in most adults. Thus, do **not** assume that incontinence is inevitable, especially in older adults (Yates, 2018).

◆ Evaluation

Through the Patient's Eyes. The patient is the best source of evaluation of outcomes and responses to nursing care. Include patients in the revision of the care plan based on their perception of its success. It is important to remember that urinary problems affect the patient not only physically but also emotionally, psychologically, spiritually, and socially. Carefully assess the patient's self-image, social interactions, sexuality, and emotional status as impacted by the urinary problem (Fig. 46.17).

Patient Outcomes. To evaluate the care plan, use the expected outcomes developed during planning to determine whether interventions were effective. This evaluation process is dynamic. Information gathered is used to modify the plan of care to meet expected outcomes. Evaluate

FIG. 46.17 Critical thinking model for urinary elimination evaluation. *ANA,* American Nurses Association. (Clinical Judgment Measurement Model copyright © NCSBN. All rights reserved.)

for changes in the patient's voiding pattern and/or presence of symptoms such as dysuria, urinary retention, and UI. If a behavioral plan is in effect, evaluate patient/caregiver adherence to the plan, such as toileting according to the schedule, or determine the number of incontinent episodes. Actual outcomes are compared with expected outcomes to determine success or partial success in achieving these outcomes. Examples of questions to ask for evaluation include:

- "Tell me, how frequently are you voiding now?" "How many times are you awakened from sleep with a strong urge to void?"
- "Do you continue to experience that sensation of urgency or need to rush to the toilet?"
- "How many episodes of urine leakage have you experienced over the past week?"
- "Do you have pain or burning when you pass urine?"

The effectiveness of an intervention may take place within a day or two, or it may take weeks or months to fully evaluate effectiveness. Evaluate initial adherence to dietary changes, understanding of instructions for pelvic muscle exercise, or effectiveness of antibiotic treatment for UTI in 1 to 2 days. Evaluation of the effectiveness of pelvic muscle exercises in decreasing urgency and incontinence will need to be weeks or months after therapy is started. Continuous evaluation, when possible, allows you to determine progress toward goals, encourage adherence, and revise the diagnosis and/or plan as needed.

After Carly finished teaching Mrs. Grayson about her urinary incontinence regimen, she wanted to evaluate Mrs. Grayson's understanding. She asks Mrs. Grayson, "I want to be sure I explained how you can improve your urinary continence at home. Can you please describe three things you can do at home to manage and improve your urinary continence?" Mrs. Grayson states she is going to do her pelvic muscle exercises, she is going to use the toilet every 2 to 3 hours, and she is going to stop drinking fluids 2 hours before she goes to bed. Mrs. Grayson also describes how she will prevent skin breakdown in her perineal area.

Carly continues to care for Mrs. Grayson 2 days later. While making rounds, Carly talks with Mrs. Grayson, who states she has been practicing her pelvic muscle exercises and that she has only "dribbled" urine. She is worried and states, "I thought this was all under control." Carly notifies the health care provider of her current assessment findings. A bladder scan reveals 100 mL of retained urine. Mrs. Grayson is encouraged that there is only a small amount of urine retained on the bladder scan.

Carly is encouraged by Mrs. Grayson's progress. Carly sits down and discusses with Mrs. Grayson the need for ongoing bladder retraining and pelvic muscle exercise. Carly says, "Now that you are beginning to feel better, tell me why it is important to continue with these bladder exercises." Mrs. Grayson identifies four reasons why she will continue her bladder exercises.

SAFETY GUIDELINES FOR NURSING SKILLS

Ensuring patient safety is an essential role of the professional nurse. Use sound clinical judgment by communicating clearly with members of the health care team, assessing and analyzing patient's clinical findings, and incorporating the patient's priorities of care and preferences. Use the best evidence, applying professional standards, when selecting interventions to use in patient care delivery. When performing the skills in this chapter, remember the following points to ensure safe, patient-centered care:

- Follow principles of surgical and medical asepsis as indicated when performing catheterizations, handling urine specimens, or helping patients with their toileting needs.

- Identify patients at risk for latex allergies (i.e., patient history of hay fever; asthma; and allergies to certain foods such as bananas, grapes, apricots, kiwifruit, and hazelnuts).
- Identify patients with allergies to povidone-iodine. Provide alternatives such as chlorhexidine.

SKILL 46.1 COLLECTING MIDSTREAM (CLEAN-VOIDED) URINE SPECIMEN

Delegation and Collaboration

The skill of collecting urine specimens can be delegated to assistive personnel (AP). The nurse instructs the AP to:

- Obtain the specimens at a specified time when appropriate.
- Position patient as necessary when mobility restrictions are present.
- Report to the nurse if the urine is not clear (e.g., contains blood, cloudiness, or excess sediment).
- Report to the nurse when a patient is unable to initiate a stream or has pain or burning on urination.

Equipment

- Completed identification labels with appropriate patient identifiers
- Completed laboratory requisition, including patient identification, date, time, name of test, and source of culture
- Biohazard bag or container for delivery of specimen to laboratory (as specified by agency)

Clean-Voided Urine Specimen

- Commercial kit (Fig. 46.18) for clean-voided urine, containing:
  - Sterile cotton balls or antiseptic towelettes
  - Antiseptic solution (chlorhexidine or povidone-iodine solution)
  - Sterile water or normal saline
  - Sterile specimen container
  - Urine cup
- Clean gloves
- Soap, water, washcloth, and towel
- Bedpan (for nonambulatory patient), urine hat (for ambulatory patient)

Sterile Urine Specimen From Urinary Catheter

- 20-mL Luer-Lok for routine urinalysis or 3-mL safety Luer-Lok syringe for culture
- Alcohol, chlorhexidine, or another disinfectant swab
- Clamp or rubber band
- Specimen container (nonsterile for routine urinalysis; sterile for culture)
- Clean gloves

Continued

SKILL 46.1   **COLLECTING MIDSTREAM (CLEAN-VOIDED) URINE SPECIMEN—cont'd**

FIG. 46.18 Commercial midstream urine collection kit.

STEP	RATIONALE

ASSESSMENT

1. Identify patient using at least two identifiers (e.g., name and birthday or name and medical record number) according to agency policy.

   Ensures correct patient. Complies with The Joint Commission standards and improves patient safety (TJC, 2021).

2. Review patient's EHR, including health care provider's order and nurses' notes. Note previous midstream collections, including patient response.

   Ensures accurate testing of specimen; order is needed to perform test.

3. Refer to agency procedures for specimen collection methods.

   Agency policies may vary regarding collection and/or handling of specimens.

4. Assess patient's or family caregiver's knowledge, experience, and health literacy.

   Ensures patient or family caregiver has the capacity to obtain, communicate, process, and understand basic health information (CDC, 2021).

5. Assess patient's knowledge, prior experience with midstream urine collection, and feelings about procedure.

   Reveals need for patient instruction and/or support.

6. Assess patient's goals or preferences for how skill is to be performed or what patient expects.

   Allows care to be individualized to patient.

7. Assess patient's ability to help with urine specimen collection; able to position self and hold container.

   Determines degree of help patient requires.

8. Assess for signs and symptoms of UTI (frequency, urgency, dysuria, hematuria, flank pain, fever; cloudy malodorous urine).

   May indicate need for health care provider intervention.

PLANNING

1. Perform hand hygiene. Close room door or bedside curtains around bed.

   Reduces transmission of microorganisms. Provides privacy.

2. Organize equipment needed for procedure (see Fig. 46.18).

   Facilitates organized completion of procedure.

3. Explain the procedure and what is required of the patient. **NOTE:** Patients who are mobile may be able to collect a clean-voided specimen in the bathroom.

   Patients often prefer to obtain their own clean voided specimen but need appropriate education to correctly collect the sample.

IMPLEMENTATION

1. Check labels and verify complete laboratory requisition for specimen container.

   Organizes procedure.

2. **Collect clean-voided urine specimen.**

   a. Perform hand hygiene and apply clean gloves. Give patient cleaning towelette or towel, washcloth, and soap to clean perineum or help with cleaning perineum. Help patient who cannot get out of bed onto bedpan to facilitate access to perineum. Remove and dispose of gloves and perform hand hygiene.

      Reduces transfer of microorganisms. Patients prefer to wash their own perineal areas when possible. Cleaning prevents contamination of specimen from skin and surface bacteria after urine passes from urethra.

   b. Using aseptic technique, open outer package of commercial specimen kit.

      Maintains sterility of equipment.

   c. Apply clean gloves.

      Prevents contact of microorganisms on your hands.

   d. Pour antiseptic solution over cotton balls (unless kit contains prepared antiseptic towelettes).

      Cotton ball or towelette is used to clean perineum.

   e. Open specimen container, maintaining sterility of inside specimen container, and place cap with sterile inside up. Do not touch inside of cap or container.

      Contaminated specimen is most frequent reason for inaccurate reporting of urine culture and sensitivity (C&S).

STEP	RATIONALE
f. Use aseptic technique to help patient or allow patient to independently clean perineum and collect specimen. Amount of help needed varies with each patient. Inform patient that antiseptic solution will feel cold.	Maintains patient's dignity and comfort.

(1) *Male:*

(a) Hold penis with one hand; using circular motion and antiseptic towelette, clean meatus, moving from center to outside 3 times with 3 different towelettes (see illustration). If patient is not circumcised, retract foreskin for effective cleaning of urinary meatus and keep retracted during voiding. Return foreskin when done.

Reduces number of microorganisms at urethral meatus and moves from areas of least to most contamination. Return of foreskin prevents stricture of penis.

(b) If agency procedure indicates, rinse area with sterile water and dry with cotton balls or gauze pad.

Prevents contamination of specimen with antiseptic solution.

(c) After patient initiates urine stream into toilet, urinal, or bedpan, have him pass urine specimen container into stream and collect 90 to 120 mL of urine (Pagana et al., 2021) (see illustration).

Initial urine flushes out microorganisms that normally accumulate at urinary meatus and prevents transfer into specimen.

(2) *Female:*

(a) Either nurse or patient spreads labia minora with fingers of nondominant hand.

Provides access to urethral meatus.

(b) With dominant hand clean urethral area with antiseptic swab (cotton ball or gauze). Move from front (above urethral orifice) to back (toward anus). Use fresh swab each time; clean 3 times; begin with labial fold farthest from you, then labial fold closest, and then down center (see illustration).

Prevents contamination of urinary meatus with fecal material. Cleaning down center last decreases contamination from labia.

(c) If agency procedure indicates, rinse area with sterile water and dry with cotton ball.

Prevents contamination of specimen with antiseptic solution.

(d) While continuing to hold labia apart, patient initiates urine stream into toilet or bedpan; after stream is achieved, pass specimen container into stream, and collect 90 to 120 mL of urine (Pagana et al., 2021) (see illustration).

Initial stream flushes out resident microorganisms that accumulate at urethral meatus and prevents transfer into specimen.

STEP 2f(1)(a) Cleaning technique (male).

STEP 2f(1)(c) Collecting midstream urine specimen (male).

STEP 2f(2)(b) Clean from front to back, holding labia apart (female).

STEP 2f(2)(d) Collecting midstream urine specimen (female).

Continued

| SKILL 46.1 | COLLECTING MIDSTREAM (CLEAN-VOIDED) URINE SPECIMEN—cont'd |

STEP	RATIONALE

g. Remove specimen container before flow of urine stops and before releasing labia or penis. Patient finishes voiding into bedpan or toilet. Offer to help with personal hygiene as appropriate.

Prevents contamination of specimen with skin flora. Prevents sediment from bladder getting into specimen.

h. Replace cap securely on specimen container, touching only outside.

Retains sterility of inside of container and prevents spillage of urine.

i. Clean urine from exterior surface of container.

Prevents transfer of microorganisms to others.

3. Collect urine from indwelling urinary catheter.

a. Explain that you will use syringe without needle to remove urine through catheter port and that patient will not experience any discomfort.

Minimizes anxiety when you manipulate catheter and aspirate urine with syringe from catheter port.

b. Explain that you will need to clamp catheter for 10 to 15 minutes before obtaining urine specimen and that urine cannot be obtained from drainage bag.

Allows urine to accumulate in catheter. Urine in drainage bag is not considered sterile.

c. Perform hand hygiene and apply clean gloves. Clamp drainage tubing with clamp or rubber band for as long as 15 minutes below site chosen for withdrawal (see illustration).

Permits collection of fresh sterile urine in catheter tubing rather than draining into bag.

d. After 15 minutes, position patient so that catheter sampling port is easily accessible. Location of port is where catheter attaches to drainage bag tube (see Fig. 46.12). Clean port for 15 seconds with disinfectant swab and allow to dry.

Prevents entry of microorganisms into catheter.

e. Attach needleless Luer-Lok syringe to built-in catheter sampling port (see illustration). Some needleless ports use blunt plastic valve or slip-tip syringe inserted into port diaphragm.

Guideline recommends use of Luer-Lok needleless system. Needleless system prevents injury by needlestick.

f. Withdraw 3 mL for culture or 20 mL for routine urinalysis.

Allows collection of urine without contamination. Proper volume is needed to perform test.

g. Transfer urine from syringe into clean urine container for routine urinalysis or into sterile urine container for culture.

Prevents contamination of urine during transfer procedure.

h. Place lid tightly on container.

Prevents contamination of specimen by air and loss by spillage.

i. Unclamp catheter and allow urine to flow into drainage bag. Ensure that urine flows freely.

Allows urine to drain by gravity and prevents stasis of urine in bladder.

4. Securely attach label to container (not lid). If patient is female, indicate if she is menstruating. In presence of patient, complete label (two identifiers, specimen source, collection date and time) and attach to container. Attach completed laboratory requisition to container. Enclose specimen in a biohazard bag and send immediately to laboratory.

Incorrect patient identification could lead to diagnostic or therapeutic error (TJC, 2021). Bacteria multiply quickly. Specimen should be analyzed promptly for accurate results.

5. Dispose of all contaminated supplies in appropriate receptacle, remove and dispose of gloves, and perform hand hygiene.

Reduces transmission of microorganisms. Use appropriate disposal receptacle if patient is on hazardous drugs.

6. Offer patient hand hygiene or provide time to wash hands.

Reduces transmission of microorganisms

7. Assist patient to comfortable position.

Restores comfort and sense of well-being.

8. Place nurse call system in an accessible location within patient's reach.

Ensures patient can call for assistance if needed and promotes safety and prevents falls.

STEP 3c Rubber band used to clamp drainage tube.

STEP 3e Access urinary catheter port with Luer-Lok syringe or syringe with blunt plastic valve.

STEP	RATIONALE
9. Raise side rails (as appropriate) and lower bed to lowest position.	Promotes patient safety and prevents falls.
10. Send specimen and completed requisition to laboratory within 20 minutes. Refrigerate specimen if delay cannot be avoided.	Delay of analysis may significantly alter test results (Pagana et al., 2021).

EVALUATION

1. Inspect clean-voided specimen for contamination with toilet paper or stool.	Contaminants prevent specimen from being used.
2. Evaluate patient's urine C&S report for bacterial growth.	Routine cultures identify organism(s), and sensitivity study identifies antimicrobial medications that may be effective against pathogen.
3. Observe urinary drainage system in catheterized patient to ensure that it is intact and patent.	System must remain closed to remain sterile.
4. Use Teach-Back: "I want to be sure I explained the way to obtain a clean-voided specimen. Please repeat the steps back to me." Revise your instruction now or develop a plan for revised patient/family caregiver teaching if patient/family caregiver is not able to teach back correctly.	Teach-back is an evidence-based health literacy intervention that promotes patient engagement, patient safety, adherence, and quality. The goal of teach-back is to ensure that you have explained medical information clearly so that patients and their families understand what you communicated to them (Agency for Healthcare Research and Quality [AHRQ], 2020).

UNEXPECTED OUTCOMES AND RELATED INTERVENTIONS

1. Urine specimen is contaminated with stool or toilet paper.
   - Repeat patient instruction and specimen collection. If unable to obtain specimen through clean voiding, patient may need catheterization (see Skill 46.2).
2. Urine culture reveals bacterial growth (determined by colony count of more than 10,000 organisms per milliliter).
   - Report findings to health care provider.
   - Administer medications as ordered.
   - Monitor patient for fever and dysuria.
3. Lumen leading to balloon that holds catheter in place is punctured.
   - Notify health care provider.
   - Prepare for removal of existing catheter and insertion of new catheter.

RECORDING AND REPORTING

- Record method used to obtain specimen, date and time collected, type of test ordered, laboratory receiving specimen, characteristics of specimen, and patient's tolerance to procedure of specimen collection.
- Document your evaluation of patient learning.
- Report any abnormal findings to health care provider, the type of urinalysis, and when specimen was sent to laboratory.

HOME CARE CONSIDERATIONS

- If patient is to collect specimen as an outpatient, a clean technique may be used. Provide instruction for collection and appropriate equipment.
- Provide information about storing specimen until time for delivery to health care provider's office or hospital laboratory.

SKILL 46.2 INSERTING A STRAIGHT (INTERMITTENT) OR INDWELLING CATHETER

Delegation and Collaboration

The skill of inserting a straight or indwelling urinary catheter cannot be delegated to assistive personnel (AP). The nurse directs the AP to:

- Assist the nurse with patient positioning, focus lighting for the procedure, maintain privacy, empty urine from collection bag, and help with perineal care.
- Report postprocedure patient discomfort or fever to the nurse.
- Report abnormal color, odor, or amount of urine in drainage bag and whether the catheter is leaking or causes pain.

Equipment

- Catheter kit containing sterile items (**NOTE:** Catheter kits vary.)
  - Straight catheterization kit: single-lumen catheter (12–14 Fr), drapes (one fenestrated—has an opening in the center), sterile gloves, lubricant, cleansing solution incorporated in an applicator or to be added to cotton balls, and specimen container and label.
  - Indwelling catheterization kit (Fig. 46.19): double-lumen catheter, drapes (one fenestrated—has an opening in the center), sterile gloves, lubricant, antiseptic cleansing solution incorporated in an applicator or to be added to cotton balls, specimen container and label, and a prefilled syringe with sterile water or normal saline (to inflate balloon). **NOTE:** Some kits contain a catheter with attached drainage bag; others contain only a catheter; others have no catheter.
- Sterile drainage tubing and bag (if not included in indwelling catheter insertion kit)
- Device to secure catheter (catheter strap or other device)
- Extra sterile gloves and catheter *(optional)*
- Clean gloves
- Basin with warm water, washcloth, towel, and soap for perineal care
- Flashlight or other additional light source
- Bath blanket, waterproof absorbent pad
- Measuring container for urine

Continued

SKILL 46.2   **INSERTING A STRAIGHT (INTERMITTENT) OR INDWELLING CATHETER—cont'd**

FIG. 46.19 Indwelling catheterization kit. (Image used with permission of Medline Industries. All rights reserved.)

STEP	RATIONALE

ASSESSMENT

1. Identify patient using at least two identifiers (e.g., name and birthday or name and medical record number) according to agency policy. Compare identifiers with information on patient's MAR or medical record.

   Ensures correct patient. Complies with The Joint Commission standards and improves patient safety (TJC, 2021).

2. Review patient's EHR, including health care provider's order and nurses' notes. Note previous catheterization, including catheter size, response of patient, and time of catheterization.

   Identifies purpose of inserting catheter (such as for measurement of PVR, preparation for surgery, or specimen collection) and potential difficulty with catheter insertion.

3. Review EHR for any pathological conditions that may impair passage of catheter (e.g., enlarged prostate gland in men, urethral strictures).

   Obstruction of urethra may prevent passage of catheter into bladder.

4. Assess patient's gender and age.

   Assists with selection of catheter size.

5. Assess patient's or family caregiver's knowledge, experience, and health literacy.

   Ensures patient or family caregiver has the capacity to obtain, communicate, process, and understand basic health information (CDC, 2021).

6. Ask patient and check EHR for history of allergies. Check allergy bracelet.

   Catheter made of different material is needed if patient has latex allergy.

7. Perform hand hygiene. Assess patient's weight, level of consciousness, developmental level, ability to cooperate, and mobility.

   Determines positioning to use for catheterization; indicates how much help is needed to properly position patient, ability of patient to cooperate during procedure, and level of explanation needed.

8. Assess for pain and bladder fullness. Palpate bladder over symphysis pubis or use bladder scanner (if available) (see Box 46.11).

   Palpation of full bladder causes pain and/or urge to void, indicating full or overfull bladder.

9. Apply clean gloves. Inspect perineal region, observing for perineal anatomical landmarks, erythema, drainage or discharge, and odor. Remove and dispose of gloves and perform hand hygiene.

   Assessment of perineum (especially female perineal landmarks) improves accuracy and speed of catheter insertion. Reduces transmission of microorganisms.

10. Assess patient's knowledge, prior experience with catheterization, and feelings about procedure.

    Reveals need for patient instruction and/or support.

11. Assess patient's goals or preferences for how skill is to be performed or what patient expects.

    Allows care to be individualized to patient.

PLANNING

1. Close room door or curtains around bed.

   Provides privacy.

2. Organize and set up any equipment needed to perform the procedure.

   Organization ensures efficiency in completing the skill.

CLINICAL JUDGMENT: *Some patients may be unable to assume positioning independently. Arrange for extra assistance before initiating the procedure.*

3. Explain procedure to patient.

   Reduces patient anxiety and promotes cooperation.

IMPLEMENTATION

1. Check patient's plan of care for size and type of catheter (if this is a reinsertion). Use smallest-size catheter possible. Size 14 to 16 Fr most common for adults; older adults (12–14 Fr); larger sizes (20–24 Fr) are needed in special circumstances, such as after urological surgery or in the presence of gross hematuria.

   Ensures that patient receives correct size and type of catheter. Larger catheter diameters increase the risk for urethral trauma. Small catheter allows for adequate drainage of periurethral glands.

STEP	RATIONALE
2. Perform hand hygiene.	Reduces transmission of microorganisms.
3. Raise bed to appropriate working height. If side rails are in use, raise side rail on opposite side of bed and lower side rail on working side.	Promotes good body mechanics. Use of side rails in this manner promotes patient safety.
4. Place waterproof pad under patient.	Prevents soiling bed linen.
5. Position patient:	
a. *Female patient:*	
(1) Help to dorsal recumbent position (on back with knees flexed). Ask patient to relax thighs so that you can rotate hips.	Exposes perineum and allows hip joints to be externally rotated.
(2) Alternate female position: Position in side-lying position with upper leg flexed at knee and hip. Support patient with pillows, if necessary, to maintain position.	Alternate position is more comfortable if patient cannot abduct leg at hip joint (e.g., patient has arthritic joints or contractures).
b. *Male patient:*	
(1) Position supine with legs extended and thighs slightly abducted.	Comfortable position for patient and aids in visualization of penis.
6. Drape patient:	
a. *Female:*	
(1) Drape with bath blanket. Place blanket diamond fashion over patient, with one corner at patient's midsections, side corners over each thigh and abdomen, and last corner over perineum (see illustration).	
b. *Male:*	
(1) Drape patient by covering upper part of body with small sheet or towel; drape with separate sheet or bath blanket so that only perineum is exposed (see illustration).	
7. Apply clean gloves. Clean perineal area with soap and water, rinse, and dry (see Chapter 40). Use gloves to examine patient and identify urinary meatus. Remove and discard gloves. Perform hand hygiene.	Hygiene before initiating aseptic catheter insertion removes secretions, urine, and feces that could contaminate sterile field and increase risk for CAUTI. Perform hand hygiene immediately before catheter insertion (Gould et al., 2019).
8. Position portable light to illuminate genitals or have assistant available to hold light.	Adequate visualization of urinary meatus assists with accuracy of catheter insertion.
9. Open outer wrapping of catheterization kit. Place inner wrapped catheter kit tray on clean, accessible surface such as bedside table or, if possible, between patient's open legs. Patient size and positioning dictate exact placement.	Provides easy access to supplies during catheter insertion.

STEP 6a(1) Female patient draped and in dorsal recumbent position.

STEP 6b(1) Drape male patient with blankets.

Continued

| SKILL 46.2 | INSERTING A STRAIGHT (INTERMITTENT) OR INDWELLING CATHETER—cont'd |

STEP	RATIONALE
10. Open inner sterile wrap covering tray containing catheterization supplies using sterile technique (see Chapter 28). Fold back each flap of sterile covering with first flap opened away from you, next two flaps open to each side one at a time, and last flap opened toward patient.	Sterile wrap serves as sterile field. Sequence prevents you from reaching over sterile field.
a. Indwelling catheterization open system: Open separate package containing drainage bag, check to make sure that clamp on drainage port is closed, and place drainage bag and tubing in easily accessible location. Open outer package of sterile catheter, maintaining sterility of inner wrapper (see Chapter 28).	Open drainage bag systems have separate sterile packaging for sterile catheter, drainage bag and tubing, and insertion kit.
b. Indwelling catheterization closed system: All supplies are in sterile tray and arranged in sequence of use.	Closed drainage bag systems have catheter preattached to drainage tubing and bag.
c. Straight catheterization: All needed supplies are in sterile tray that contains supplies and can be used for urine collection.	
11. Apply sterile gloves.	Maintains surgical asepsis.
12. *Option:* Apply sterile drape with ungloved hands when drape is packed as first item. Touch only 2.5 cm (1 inch) edges of drape. Then apply sterile gloves.	Maintains surgical asepsis.
13. Drape perineum, keeping gloves and working surface of drape sterile.	Sterile drapes provide sterile field over which you will work during catheterization.
a. *Drape female:*	
(1) Pick up square sterile drape, touching only edges (2.5 cm [1 inch]).	
(2) Allow drape to unfold without touching unsterile surfaces. Allow top edge of drape (2.5 to 5 cm [1–2 inches]) to form cuff over both hands.	When creating cuff over sterile gloved hands, sterility of gloves and workspace is maintained.
(3) Place drape with shiny side down on bed between patient's thighs. Slip cuffed edge just under buttocks as you ask patient to lift hips. Take care not to touch contaminated surfaces or patient's thighs with sterile gloves. If gloves are contaminated, remove, and apply clean gloves.	
(4) Pick up fenestrated sterile drape out of tray. Allow drape to unfold without touching unsterile surfaces. Allow top edge of drape to form cuff over both hands. Apply drape over perineum so that opening is over exposed labia (see illustration).	Opening in drape creates sterile field around labia.
b. *Drape male:*	
(1) Use of square drape is optional; you may apply fenestrated drape instead.	
(2) Pick up edges of square drape and allow to unfold without touching unsterile surfaces. Place over thighs, with shiny side down, just below penis. Take care not to touch contaminated surfaces with sterile gloves.	
(3) Place fenestrated drape with opening centered over penis (see illustration).	

STEP 13a(4) Place sterile fenestrated drape (with opening in center) over female's perineum.

STEP 13b(3) Drape male with fenestrated drape.

STEP	**RATIONALE**
14. Move tray closer to patient. Arrange remaining supplies on sterile field, maintaining sterility of gloves. Place sterile tray with cleaning solution (premoistened swab sticks or cotton balls, forceps, and solution), lubricant, catheter, and prefilled syringe for inflating balloon (indwelling catheterization only) on sterile drape.	Provides easy access to supplies during catheter insertion and helps to maintain aseptic technique. Appropriate placement is determined by size of patient and position during catheterization.
a. If kit contains sterile cotton balls, open package of sterile antiseptic solution and pour over cotton balls. Some kits contain package of premoistened swab sticks. Open end of package for easy access (see illustration).	Use of sterile supplies and antiseptic solution reduces risk of CAUTI (Gould et al., 2019).
b. Open sterile specimen container if specimen is to be obtained (see Skill 46.1).	Makes container accessible to receive urine from catheter if specimen is needed.
c. For indwelling catheterization, open sterile inner wrapper of catheter and leave catheter on sterile field. If part of closed system kit, remove tray with catheter and preattached drainage bag and place on sterile drape. Make sure that clamp on drainage port of bag is closed. If needed and if part of sterile tray, attach catheter to drainage tubing.	Indwelling catheterization trays vary. Some have preattached catheters; others need to be attached but are part of the sterile tray; others do not have catheter or drainage system as part of tray.
d. Open packet of lubricant and squeeze out on sterile field. Lubricate catheter tip by dipping it into water-soluble gel 2.5 to 5 cm (1–2 inches) for women and 12.5 to 17.5 cm (5–7 inches) for men (see illustration).	Lubrication minimizes trauma to urethra and discomfort during catheter insertion. Male catheter needs enough lubricant to cover length of catheter inserted.

CLINICAL JUDGMENT: *Pretesting a balloon on an indwelling catheter by injecting fluid from the prefilled sterile normal saline syringe into the balloon port is **no longer recommended**. Testing the balloon may distort and stretch it and lead to damage, causing increased trauma on insertion.*

---

15. Clean urethral meatus:	
a. *Female patient:*	
(1) Separate labia with fingers of nondominant hand (now contaminated) to fully expose urethral meatus.	Optimal visualization of urethral meatus is possible.
(2) Maintain position of nondominant hand throughout procedure.	Closure of labia during cleaning means that area is contaminated and requires cleaning procedure to be repeated.
(3) Holding forceps in dominant hand, pick up one moistened cotton ball or pick up one swab stick at a time. Clean labia and urinary meatus from clitoris toward anus. Use new cotton ball or swab for each area that you clean. Clean by wiping far labial fold, near labial fold, and last, directly over center of urethral meatus (see illustration).	Front-to-back cleaning moves from area of least contamination toward highly contaminated area. Follows principles of medical asepsis (see Chapter 28). Dominant gloved hand remains sterile.
b. *Male patient:*	
(1) With nondominant hand (now contaminated) retract foreskin (if uncircumcised) and gently grasp penis at shaft just below glans. Hold shaft of penis at right angle to body. This hand remains in this position for remainder of procedure.	When grasping shaft of penis, avoid pressure on dorsal surface to prevent compression of urethra. Losing grasp during cleaning means that area is contaminated and requires cleaning procedure to be repeated.
(2) Using uncontaminated dominant hand, clean meatus with cotton balls/swab sticks, using circular strokes, beginning at meatus, and working outward in spiral motion.	Circular cleaning pattern follows principles of medical asepsis (see Chapter 28).
(3) Repeat cleaning 3 times using clean cotton ball/swab stick each time (see illustration).	

STEP 14a Sterile kit includes antiseptic swabs.

STEP 14d Lubricate catheter.

Continued

SKILL 46.2	INSERTING A STRAIGHT (INTERMITTENT) OR INDWELLING CATHETER—cont'd
STEP	**RATIONALE**

STEP 15a(3) Clean female perineum.

STEP 15b(3) Clean male urinary meatus.

16. Pick up and hold catheter 7.5 to 10 cm (3–4 inches) from catheter tip with catheter loosely coiled in palm of hand. If catheter is not attached to drainage bag, make sure to position urine tray so that end of catheter can be placed there once insertion begins.

Holding catheter near tip allows for its easier manipulation during insertion. Coiling catheter in palm prevents distal end from striking nonsterile surface.

17. Insert catheter. Explain to patient that feeling of discomfort or pressure may be experienced as catheter is inserted into urethra. This sensation is normal and will go away quickly.

Helps to minimize patient anxiety.

   a. *Female patient:*

     (1) Ask patient to bear down gently, and slowly insert catheter through urethral meatus (see illustration).

Bearing down may help visualize urinary meatus and promotes relaxation of external urinary sphincter, aiding in catheter insertion.

     (2) Advance catheter total of 5 to 7.5 cm (2–3 inches) or until urine flows out of catheter. When urine appears, advance catheter another 2.5 to 5 cm (1–2 inches). Do not use force to insert catheter.

Urine flow indicates that catheter tip is in bladder or lower urethra.

     (3) Release labia and hold catheter securely with nondominant hand.

Prevents accidental expulsion of catheter from the patient's bladder.

STEP 17a(1) Insert catheter into female urinary meatus.

STEP	RATIONALE

b. *Male patient:*

(1) Lift penis to position perpendicular (90 degrees) to patient's body and apply gentle upward traction.

Straightens urethra to ease catheter insertion.

(2) Ask patient to bear down as if to void, and slowly insert catheter through urethral meatus (see illustration).

Relaxation of external sphincter aids in insertion of catheter.

(3) Advance catheter 17 to 22.5 cm (7–9 inches) or until urine flows out of catheter.

Length of male urethra varies. Flow of urine indicates that tip of catheter is in bladder or urethra but not necessarily that balloon part of indwelling catheter is in bladder.

(4) Stop advancing with straight catheter. When urine appears in indwelling catheter, advance it to bifurcation (inflation and deflation ports exposed) (see illustration).

Further advancement of catheter to bifurcation of drainage and balloon inflation port ensures that balloon part of catheter is not still in prostatic urethra.

(5) Lower penis and hold catheter securely in nondominant hand.

Prevents accidental expulsion of catheter from the patient's bladder.

18. Allow bladder to empty fully unless agency policy restricts maximum volume of urine drained (see agency policy).

There is no definitive evidence regarding whether there is benefit in limiting maximal volume drained.

19. Collect urine specimen as needed (see Skill 46.1). Fill specimen container to 20 to 30 mL by holding end of catheter over cup. Set aside. Keep end of catheter sterile.

Sterile specimen for culture analysis can be obtained.

20. *Option for straight catheterization*: When urine stops flowing, withdraw catheter slowly and smoothly until removed.

Minimizes trauma to urethra.

21. Inflate indwelling catheter balloon with amount of fluid designated by manufacturer.

Indwelling catheter balloon should not be underinflated. Underinflation causes balloon distortion and potential bladder damage.

a. Continue to hold catheter with nondominant hand.

Holding catheter before inflating balloon prevents expulsion of catheter from urethra.

b. With free dominant hand, connect prefilled syringe to injection port at end of catheter.

c. Slowly inject total amount of solution (see illustration).

Full amount of solution needed to inflate balloon properly.

STEP 17b(2) Insert catheter into male urinary meatus.

STEP 17b(4) Male anatomy with correct catheter insertion to bifurcation.

STEP 21c Inflate balloon (indwelling catheter).

Continued

SKILL 46.2   INSERTING A STRAIGHT (INTERMITTENT) OR INDWELLING CATHETER—cont'd

STEP	RATIONALE

CLINICAL JUDGMENT: *If patient reports sudden pain during inflation of a catheter balloon or when resistance is felt when inflating the balloon, stop inflation, allow the fluid from the balloon to flow back into the syringe, advance catheter farther, and reinflate balloon. The balloon may have been inflating in the urethra. If pain continues, remove catheter, and notify the health care provider.*

d. After inflating catheter balloon, release catheter from nondominant hand. *Gently* pull catheter until resistance is felt. Then advance catheter slightly.

By moving catheter slightly back into bladder, pressure on bladder neck is avoided.

e. Connect drainage tubing to catheter if it is not already preconnected.

22. Secure indwelling catheter with catheter strap or other securement device. Leave enough slack to allow leg movement. Attach securement device at tubing just above catheter bifurcation.

Securing catheter reduces risk of movement, urethral erosion, CAUTI, or accidental catheter removal (Gould et al., 2019; McNeill, 2017). Attachment of securement device at catheter bifurcation prevents occlusion of catheter.

  a. *Female patient:*

  (1) Secure catheter tubing to inner thigh, allowing enough slack to prevent tension (see illustration).

  b. *Male patient:*

  (1) Secure catheter tubing to upper thigh (see illustration) or lower abdomen (with penis directed toward chest). Allow slack in catheter so that movement does not create tension on catheter.

Anchoring catheter reduces traction on urethra and minimizes urethral injury (Gould et al., 2019; McNeill, 2017).

  (2) If retracted, replace foreskin over glans penis.

Leaving foreskin retracted can cause discomfort and dangerous edema.

23. Clip drainage tubing to edge of mattress. Position drainage bag below level of bladder by attaching to bedframe (Gould et al., 2019). Do not attach to side rails of bed, and do not rest on floor (see illustration).

Keeping the collection bag below the level of the bladder at all times prevents backflow into bladder, which can cause risk for CAUTI (Gould et al., 2019). Bags attached to movable objects such as side rails increase risk for urethral trauma because of pulling or accidental dislodgment.

STEP 22a(1) Secure indwelling catheter on female with adhesive securement device.

STEP 22b(1) Secure indwelling catheter on male.

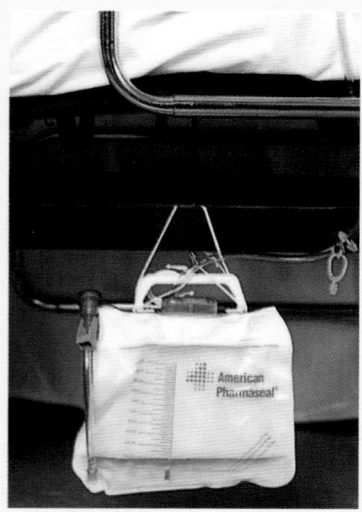

STEP 23 Drainage bag below level of bladder.

STEP	RATIONALE
24. Check to ensure that there is no obstruction to urine flow. Coil excess tubing on bed and fasten to bottom sheet with clip or other securement device.	Keeping the catheter and collecting tube free from kinking may reduce risk of CAUTI (Gould et al., 2019).
25. Provide perineal hygiene as needed. Help patient to comfortable position.	Restores comfort and sense of well-being.
26. Dispose of supplies in appropriate receptacles.	Reduces transmission of microorganisms.
27. If ordered, label and bag specimen according to agency policy. Label specimen in front of patient. Send to laboratory as soon as possible.	Fresh urine specimen ensures more accurate findings. Labeling ensures that diagnostic results will be connected to correct patient (TJC, 2021).
28. Measure urine and record.	Provides baseline for urine output.
29. Dispose of all contaminated supplies in appropriate receptacle, remove and dispose of gloves, and perform hand hygiene.	Reduces transmission of microorganisms. Use appropriate disposal receptacle if patient is on hazardous drugs.
30. Place nurse call system in an accessible location within patient's reach.	Ensures patient can call for assistance if needed and promotes safety and prevents falls.
31. Raise side rails (as appropriate) and lower bed to lowest position.	Promotes patient safety and prevents falls.

EVALUATION

1. Palpate bladder for distention or use bladder scan (see Box 46.11) as per agency protocol.	Determines whether distention is relieved.
2. Ask patient to describe level of comfort.	Determines whether patient's sensation of discomfort or fullness has been relieved.
3. Indwelling catheter: Observe character and amount of urine in drainage system.	Determines whether urine is flowing adequately.
4. Indwelling catheter: Determine that there is no urine leaking from catheter or tubing connections.	Prevents injury to patient's skin and ensures closed sterile system.
5. **Use Teach-Back:** "I want to be sure I explained clearly about your urinary catheter and some things you can do to ensure the urine flows out of the catheter. Tell me what you can do to keep the urine flowing." Revise your instruction now or develop a plan for revised patient/family caregiver teaching if patient/family caregiver is not able to teach back correctly.	Teach-back is an evidence-based health literacy intervention that promotes patient engagement, patient safety, adherence, and quality. The goal of teach-back is to ensure that you have explained medical information clearly so that patients and their families understand what you communicated to them (AHRQ, 2020).

UNEXPECTED OUTCOMES AND RELATED INTERVENTIONS

1. Catheter goes into vagina.
   - Leave first catheter in vagina so that you can correctly identify the urinary meatus.
   - Clean urinary meatus again. Using **another** catheter kit, reinsert sterile catheter into meatus (check agency policy). **Note:** If gloves become contaminated, start procedure again.
   - Remove first catheter that was left in vagina after successful insertion of second catheter.
2. Sterility is broken during catheterization by nurse or patient.
   - Replace gloves if contaminated and start over.
   - If patient touches sterile field but equipment and supplies remain sterile, avoid touching that part of sterile field.
   - If equipment and/or supplies become contaminated, replace with sterile items, or start over with new sterile kit.
3. Patient reports bladder discomfort, and catheter is patent as evidenced by adequate urine flow.
   - Check catheter to ensure that there is no traction on it.
   - Notify health care provider. Patient may be experiencing bladder spasms or symptoms of UTI.
   - Monitor catheter output for color, clarity, odor, and amount.

RECORDING AND RECORDING

- Record reason for catheterization, type and size of catheter inserted, amount of fluid used to inflate balloon, specimen collection (if applicable), characteristics and amount of urine, patient's response to procedure, and evaluation of patient learning.
- Record I&O on flow sheet record.
- Report at change of shift reason for catheterization, type and size of catheter inserted, amount of fluid used to inflate balloon, specimen collection (if applicable), characteristics and amount of urine, patient's response to procedure, and any education.
- Report to health care provider persistent catheter-related pain and discomfort.

HOME CARE CONSIDERATIONS

- Patients who are at home may use a leg bag during the day and switch to a larger-volume bag at night. If a patient changes from a large-volume bag to a leg bag, instruct in the importance of handwashing and cleansing the connection ports with alcohol before changing bags.
- Teach patients and family caregivers how to properly position the drainage bag, empty a urinary drainage bag, and observe urine color, clarity, odor, and amount.
- Educate patients and/or caregivers about the signs of UTI and troubleshooting techniques for a leaking catheter.
- Arrange for home delivery of catheter supplies, always ensuring that there is at least one extra catheter, insertion kit, and drainage bag in the home.

SKILL 46.3	CARE AND REMOVAL OF AN INDWELLING CATHETER

Delegation and Collaboration

The skill of performing routine catheter care can be delegated to assistive personnel (AP). Depending on agency policy, the skill of removing an indwelling catheter may be delegated to AP; however, a nurse must first assess a patient's status and verify the order. The nurse directs the AP to:

- Report characteristics of the urine (color, clarity, odor, and amount) before and after removal.
- Report the condition of the patient's genital area (e.g., color, rashes, open areas, odor, soiling from fecal incontinence, trauma to tissues around urinary meatus).
- If allowed to remove catheter per agency policy, check size of balloon and syringe needed to deflate balloon; report if balloon does not deflate and if there is bleeding after removal.
- Report time and amount of first voiding after catheter is removed.
- Report if patient experiences fever, chills, change in mental status, burning, flank or back pain, and/or hematuria (signs of UTI); dysuria after catheter removal.

Equipment

Catheter Care
- Clean gloves
- Waterproof pad
- Bath blanket
- Basin with warm water, washcloth, towel, and soap for perineal care

Catheter Removal
- Clean gloves
- 10-mL syringe or larger without a needle (size depends on volume of solution used to inflate the balloon)
- Graduated cylinder to measure urine
- Waterproof pad
- Toilet, bedside commode, urine "hat," urinal, or bedpan
- Bladder scanner (as indicated)

STEP	RATIONALE

ASSESSMENT

1. Identify patient using at least two identifiers (e.g., name and birthday or name and medical record number) according to agency policy.

Ensures correct patient. Complies with The Joint Commission standards and improves patient safety (TJC, 2021).

2. Perform hand hygiene. Apply clean gloves.

Reduces transmission of microorganisms.

3. Assess patient's or family caregiver's knowledge, health literacy, and prior experience with catheter care and/or catheter removal.

Ensures patient has the capacity to obtain, communicate, process, and understand basic health information (CDC, 2021).

4. **Assess need for catheter care:**

   a. Observe urinary output and urine characteristics.

   Sudden decrease in urine output may indicate occlusion of catheter. Cloudy, foul-smelling urine associated with other systemic symptoms may indicate CAUTI.

   b. Assess for history or presence of bowel incontinence.

   Most common bacteria to cause CAUTI are *E. coli,* a major colonizer of the bowel; thus fecal incontinence increases risk for CAUTI (Fekete, 2020).

   c. Position patient; retract labia or foreskin to observe for any discharge, redness, bleeding, or presence of tissue trauma around urethral meatus (this may be deferred until catheter care).

   Indicates inflammatory process, possible infection, or erosion of catheter through urethra.

   d. Remove and dispose of gloves; perform hand hygiene.

   Reduces transmission of microorganisms.

5. **Assess need for catheter removal:**

   a. Review patient's EHR, including health care provider's order and nurses' notes. Note length of time catheter has been in place.

   Catheters in place for more than a few days cause higher risk for catheter encrustation and UTI.

   b. Perform hand hygiene and apply clean gloves. Assess urine color, clarity, odor, and amount. Note any urethral discharge, irritation of genital region, or trauma to urinary meatus (this may be deferred until just before removal). Remove and dispose of gloves. Perform hand hygiene.

   May be indicator of inflammation or UTI and source of discomfort during catheter removal. Reduces transmission of microorganisms.

   c. Determine size of catheter inflation balloon by looking at balloon inflation valve.

   Determines size of syringe needed to deflate balloon and amount of fluid expected in syringe after deflation.

6. Assess patient's knowledge, prior experience with catheter care and removal, and feelings about procedure.

Reveals need for patient instruction and/or support.

7. Assess patient's goals or preferences for how skill is to be performed or what patient expects.

Allows care to be individualized to patient.

PLANNING

1. Close room door and bedside curtain

Provides privacy.

2. Obtain and organize equipment for perineal care/catheter removal at bedside.

Ensures more efficient procedure.

3. Explain procedure to patient. Discuss signs and symptoms of UTI. If applicable, teach patient or family caregiver how to perform catheter hygiene.

Reduces anxiety and promotes cooperation. Self-care supports patient's sense of autonomy.

IMPLEMENTATION

1. Perform hand hygiene.

Reduces transmission of microorganisms.

2. Raise bed to appropriate working height. If side rails are raised, lower side rail on working side.

Promotes use of proper body mechanics. Position provides access to catheter.

STEP	RATIONALE

3. Position patient with waterproof pad under buttocks and cover with bath blanket, exposing only genital area and catheter (see Skill 46.2).
   a. Female in dorsal recumbent position.
   b. Male in supine position.
	Shows respect for patient dignity by exposing only genital area and catheter.

4. Apply clean gloves.	Reduces transmission of microorganisms.
5. Remove catheter securement device while maintaining connection with drainage tubing.	Provides ability to easily clean around catheter and to remove it.
6. Catheter care:	
a. *Female:* Use nondominant hand to gently separate labia to fully expose urethral meatus and catheter. Maintain hand position throughout procedure.	Provides full visualization of urethral meatus. Full separation of labia prevents contamination of meatus during cleaning.
b. *Male:* Use nondominant hand to retract foreskin if not circumcised and hold penis at shaft just below glans. Maintain hand position throughout procedure.	Retraction of foreskin provides full visualization of urethral meatus.
c. Grasp catheter with two fingers of nondominant hand to stabilize it.	Prevents unnecessary traction on catheter. Pulling on catheter is cause of discomfort for patient and can damage urethra and bladder neck.
d. If not performed earlier, assess urethral meatus and surrounding tissues for inflammation, swelling, discharge, or tissue trauma, and ask patient if burning or discomfort is present.	Determines frequency and type of ongoing care required. Indicates possibility of CAUTI or catheter erosion through urethra.
e. Provide perineal hygiene using mild soap and warm water (see Chapter 40). *Option:* Use chlorhexidine gluconate (CHG) 2% cloth.	Antiseptic cleaners have not been shown to definitively decrease CAUTI; mild soap and water are appropriate (Schaeffer, 2020b). Although CHG 2% cloth can be used, there is no clear scientific evidence for use of antiseptics versus nonantiseptics to reduce rates of CAUTI (Fasugba et al., 2017; Rea et al., 2018).
f. Using clean washcloth or CHG 2% cloth, clean catheter. **(1)** Starting close to urinary meatus, clean catheter in circular motion along its length for about 10 cm (4 inches), moving away from body (see illustration). Remove all traces of soap. *For male patients:* Reduce or reposition foreskin after care.	Reduces presence of secretions or drainage on outside catheter surface.
g. Reapply catheter securement device. Allow slack in catheter so that movement does not create tension on it.	Securing indwelling catheter reduces risk of urethral trauma, urethral erosion, CAUTI, or accidental removal (Gould et al., 2019; Lawrence et al., 2019; Rea et al., 2018).

7. Routinely check drainage tubing and bag.
   a. Catheter is secured to upper thigh.
   b. Tubing is coiled and secured onto bed linen.
   c. Tubing is not looped or positioned above level of bladder.
   d. Tubing is not kinked or clamped.
	Maintains unobstructed flow of urine out of bladder (Gould et al., 2019; Rea et al., 2018).

STEP 6f(1) Clean catheter starting at meatus and moving downward while holding it securely.

Continued

STEP	RATIONALE
e. Drainage bag is positioned below level of bladder with urine flowing freely into bag.	
f. Drainage bag is not overfull. Empty drainage bag when ½ full.	Overfull drainage bag creates tension and pulls on catheter, resulting in trauma to urethra and/or urinary meatus. Facilitates unobstructed flow of urine (Gould et al., 2019).
8. Catheter removal: (Perform catheter care; see Step 6 before catheter removal.)	
a. With clean gloves still on, move syringe plunger up and down to loosen and then pull it back to 0.5 mL. Insert hub of syringe into inflation valve (balloon port). Allow balloon fluid to drain into syringe automatically by itself. Syringe should fill. Make sure that entire amount of fluid is removed by comparing removed amount to volume needed for inflation.	Partially inflated balloon can traumatize urethral wall during removal. Passive drainage of catheter balloon prevents formation of ridges in balloon. These ridges can cause discomfort or trauma during removal.
b. Pull catheter out smoothly and slowly. Examine it to ensure that it is whole. Catheter should slide out easily. Do not use force. If you note any resistance, repeat Step 8a to remove remaining inflation fluid.	A nonwhole catheter means that pieces of catheter may still be in bladder. Notify health care provider immediately.
c. Wrap contaminated catheter in waterproof pad. Unhook collection bag and drainage tubing from bed.	Promotes safety and reduces the risk for transmission of microorganisms.
d. Empty, measure, and record urine present in drainage bag.	Documents urinary output.
e. Encourage patient to maintain or increase fluid intake (unless contraindicated by restrictions).	Maintains normal urine output.
f. Initiate voiding record or bladder diary. Instruct patient to tell you when need to empty bladder occurs, and that all urine needs to be measured. Make sure that patient understands how to use collection container.	Evaluates bladder function.
g. Explain that many patients experience mild burning, discomfort, or small-volume voiding with first voiding, which soon subsides.	Burning results from urethral irritation.
h. Measure PVR volume (if ordered) (see Box 46.11) within 5 to 15 minutes after helping the patient to void.	Provides the most reliable PVR reading (Huether et al., 2020).
i. Inform patient to report any signs of UTI.	Promotes patient safety.
j. Ensure easy access to toilet, commode, bedpan, or urinal. Place urine "hat" on toilet seat if patient is using toilet. Place nurse call system within easy reach.	Reduces incidence of falls during toileting. Urine hat collects first voided urine.
9. Provide patient personal hygiene as needed.	Promotes patient comfort and safety. Reduces transmission of microorganisms.
10. Dispose of all contaminated supplies in appropriate receptacle, remove and dispose of gloves, and perform hand hygiene.	Reduces transmission of microorganisms. Use appropriate disposal receptacle if patient is on hazardous drugs.
11. Help patient to comfortable position.	Restores comfort and sense of well-being.
12. Place nurse call system in an accessible location within patient's reach.	Ensures patient can call for assistance if needed and promotes safety and prevents falls.
13. Raise side rails (as appropriate) and lower bed to lowest position.	Promotes safety and prevents falls.

EVALUATION

1. Inspect catheter and genital area for soiling, irritation, and skin breakdown. Ask patient about discomfort.	Determines whether area is cleaned properly and/or if patient has any irritation.
2. Observe time and measure amount of first voiding after catheter removal.	Indicates return of bladder function after catheter removal.
3. Evaluate patient for signs and symptoms of UTI.	Any patient who has a catheter or has had a catheter removed recently is at risk for UTI.
4. Use Teach-Back: "I want to be sure I clearly explained the signs of a UTI and some things you should do to prevent infection. Tell me about some ways in which you can prevent a urinary tract infection." Revise your instruction now or develop a plan for revised patient/family caregiver teaching if patient/family caregiver is not able to teach back correctly.	Teach-back is an evidence-based health literacy intervention that promotes patient engagement, patient safety, adherence, and quality. The goal of teach-back is to ensure that you have explained medical information clearly so that patients and their families understand what you communicated to them (AHRQ, 2020).

UNEXPECTED OUTCOMES AND RELATED INTERVENTIONS

1. Normal saline from inflation balloon does not return into syringe.
- Reposition patient; ensure that catheter is not pinched or kinked.
- Remove syringe. Attach new syringe and allow enough time for passive emptying.
- Attempt to empty balloon by gently pulling back on syringe plunger.
- If catheter balloon does not deflate, *do not* cut balloon inflation valve to drain fluid. Notify health care provider.

2. Patient has cloudy foul-smelling urine, fever, chills, dysuria, flank pain, back pain, hematuria, urgency, frequency, lower abdominal pain, change in mental status, and lethargy.
- Assess for bladder distention and tenderness.
- Monitor vital signs and urine output.
- Report findings to health care provider; signs and symptoms may indicate UTI.
- Consult with health care provider for order to remove catheter.

3. Patient is unable to void within 6 to 8 hours after catheter removal, has sensation of not emptying, strains to void, or experiences small voiding amounts with increasing frequency.
   - Assess for bladder distention. Perform bladder scan (see Box 46.11)
   - Help to normal position for voiding and provide privacy.
   - If patient is unable to void within 6 to 8 hours of catheter removal and/or experiences abdominal pain, notify health care provider.

RECORDING AND REPORTING

- Record time catheter was removed; teaching related to increasing fluid intake and signs and symptoms of UTI; and time, amount, and characteristics of first voiding.
- Record intake and voiding times and amounts on voiding record or bladder diary as indicated.
- Record patient symptoms experienced on and after catheter removal.
- Document your evaluation of patient learning.
- Report hematuria, dysuria, inability or difficulty voiding, and any new incontinence after a catheter is removed to health care provider.

HOME CARE CONSIDERATIONS

- If patient is discharged with indwelling catheter, teach patient and family catheter care and signs and symptoms to report to nurse or health care provider.

SKILL 46.4   CLOSED CATHETER IRRIGATION

Delegation and Collaboration

The skill of catheter irrigation cannot be delegated to assistive personnel (AP). The nurse directs the AP to:

- Report if the patient has concerns of pain, discomfort, or leakage of fluid around the catheter.
- Monitor and record intake and output (I&O) and to report immediately any decrease in urine output to the nurse.
- Report any change in the color of the urine, especially if blood clots are noted.

Equipment

- Clean gloves
- Antiseptic swabs
- Container of sterile irrigation solution at room temperature as prescribed
- IV pole (closed continuous or intermittent)

Closed Intermittent Irrigation

- Sterile 50-mL syringe to access system: Luer-Lok syringe for needleless access port (per manufacturer's instructions)
- Screw clamp or rubber band (used to occlude catheter temporarily as irrigant is instilled)

Closed Continuous Irrigation

- Sterile irrigation tubing with clamp to regulate irrigation flow rate
- Y connector *(optional)* to connect irrigation tubing to triple-lumen catheter

---

STEP	RATIONALE
ASSESSMENT	
1. Identify patient using at least two identifiers (e.g., name and birthday or name and medical record number), according to agency policy. Compare identifiers with information on patient's MAR or medical record.	Ensures correct patient. Complies with The Joint Commission standards and improves patient safety (TJC, 2021).
2. Verify in EHR:	
a. Order for irrigation method (continuous or intermittent), solution type (sterile saline or medicated solution), and amount of irrigant.	Health care provider's order is required to initiate therapy. Frequency and volume of solution used for irrigation may be in the order or standardized as part of agency policy.
b. Type of catheter in place (see Fig. 46.10).	Triple-lumen catheters are used for intermittent and continuous closed irrigation.
3. Assess patient's or family caregiver's knowledge, health literacy, and prior experience with catheter care and/or catheter removal.	Ensures patient has the capacity to obtain, communicate, process, and understand basic health information (CDC, 2021).
4. Perform hand hygiene. Palpate bladder for distention and tenderness or use bladder scan (see Box 46.11).	Reduces transmission of microorganisms. Bladder distention indicates that flow of urine may be blocked from draining.
5. Assess patient for abdominal pain or spasms, sensation of bladder fullness, or catheter bypassing (leaking). (Wear clean gloves if risk of coming in contact with urine.)	May indicate overdistention of bladder caused by catheter blockage. Offers baseline to determine whether therapy is successful.
6. Observe urine for color, amount, clarity, and presence of mucus, clots, or sediment. Remove and dispose of gloves (if worn), perform hand hygiene.	Indicates if patient is bleeding or sloughing tissue, which would require increased irrigation rate or frequency of catheter irrigation.
7. Monitor I&O. If CBI is being used, amount of fluid draining from bladder should exceed amount of fluid infused into bladder.	If output does not exceed irrigant infused, catheter obstruction (i.e., blood clots, kinked tubing) should be suspected, irrigation stopped, and prescriber notified (Ignatavicius et al., 2018).
8. Assess patient's knowledge, prior experience with catheter irrigation, and feelings about procedure.	Reveals need for patient instruction and/or support.
9. Assess patient's goals or preferences for how skill is to be performed or what patient expects.	Allows care to be individualized to patient.

Continued

SKILL 46.4	CLOSED CATHETER IRRIGATION—cont'd

STEP	RATIONALE

PLANNING

1. Close room door and bedside curtains.	Provides privacy.
2. Obtain supplies and set up at bedside.	Ensures efficient procedure.
3. Raise bed to an appropriate working height. If side rails are raised, lower side rail on working side.	Promotes good body mechanics. Position provides access to catheter.
4. Explain procedure to patient.	Reduces anxiety and promotes cooperation.

IMPLEMENTATION

1. Perform hand hygiene.	Reduces transmission of microorganisms.
2. Position patient supine and expose catheter junctions (catheter and drainage tubing).	Position provides access to catheter and promotes patient dignity as much as possible.
3. Remove catheter securement device.	Eases access to catheter parts.
4. Organize supplies according to type of irrigation prescribed. Apply clean gloves.	Ensures an efficient procedure.
5. **Closed continuous irrigation:**	
a. Close clamp on new irrigation tubing and hang bag of irrigating solution on IV pole. Insert (spike) tip of sterile irrigation tubing into designated port of irrigation solution bag using aseptic technique (see illustration).	Prevents air from entering tubing. Air can cause bladder spasms. Technique prevents transmission of microorganisms.
b. Fill drip chamber half full by squeezing chamber. Remove cap at end of tubing, and then open clamp and allow solution to flow (prime) through tubing, keeping end of tubing sterile. Once fluid has completely filled tubing, close clamp, and recap end of tubing.	Priming tubing with fluid prevents introduction of air into bladder.
c. Using aseptic technique, remove cap and connect end of tubing securely to port for infusing irrigation fluid into double/triple–lumen catheter.	Reduces transmission of microorganisms.
d. Adjust clamp on irrigation tubing to begin flow of solution into bladder. If set volume rate is ordered, calculate drip rate, and adjust rate at roller clamp (see Chapter 42). If urine is bright red or has clots, increase irrigation rate until drainage appears pink (according to ordered rate or agency protocol).	Continuous drainage is expected. It helps to prevent clotting in presence of active bleeding in bladder and flushes clots out of bladder.
e. Observe for outflow of fluid into drainage bag. Empty catheter drainage bag as needed.	Discomfort, bladder distention, and possible injury can occur from overdistention of bladder when bladder irrigant cannot adequately flow from bladder. Bag will fill rapidly and may need to be emptied every 1 to 2 hours.
6. **Closed intermittent irrigation:**	Fluid is instilled through catheter in a bolus, flushing system. Fluid drains out after irrigation is complete.
a. Pour prescribed sterile irrigation solution into sterile container.	

STEP 5a Spiking bag of sterile irrigation solution for continuous bladder irrigation.

STEP	RATIONALE
b. Draw prescribed volume of irrigant (usually 30–50 mL) into sterile syringe, using aseptic technique. Place sterile cap on tip of needleless syringe.	Ensures sterility of irrigating fluid.
c. Clamp catheter tubing below soft injection port with screw clamp (or fold catheter tubing onto itself and secure with rubber band).	Occluding catheter tubing below point of injection allows irrigating solution to enter catheter and flow into bladder.
d. Using circular motion, clean catheter port (specimen port) with antiseptic swab. Allow to dry.	Reduces transmission of microorganisms.
e. Insert tip of needleless syringe using twisting motion into port.	Ensures that catheter tip enters lumen of catheter.
f. Inject solution using slow, even pressure.	Gentle instillation of solution minimizes trauma to bladder mucosa.
g. Remove syringe and clamp (or rubber band), allowing solution to drain into urinary drainage bag. (**NOTE:** Some medicated irrigants may need to dwell in bladder for prescribed period, requiring catheter to be clamped temporarily before being allowed to drain.)	Allows drainage to flow out by gravity. Medications must be instilled long enough to be absorbed by lining of bladder. Clamped drainage tubing and bag should not be left unattended.
7. Anchor catheter with catheter securement device (see Skill 46.2).	Prevents trauma to urethral tissue caused by pulling catheter.
8. Help patient to safe and comfortable position.	Restores comfort and sense of well-being.
9. Place nurse call system in an accessible location within patient's reach.	Ensures patient can call for assistance if needed and promotes safety and prevents falls.
10. Raise side rails (as appropriate) and lower bed to lowest position.	Promotes safety and prevents falls.
11. Dispose of all contaminated supplies in appropriate receptacle, remove and dispose of gloves, and perform hand hygiene.	Reduces transmission of microorganisms. Use appropriate disposal receptacle if patient is on hazardous drugs.

EVALUATION

1. Measure actual urine output by subtracting total amount of irrigation fluid infused from total volume drained into collection bag or basin.	Determines accurate urinary output.
2. Review I&O documentation to verify that hourly output into drainage bag is in appropriate proportion to irrigating solution entering bladder. Expect more output than fluid instilled because of urine production.	Determines urinary output in relation to irrigation.
3. Inspect urine for blood clots and sediment and be sure that tubing is not kinked or occluded.	Decrease in blood clots means that therapy is successful in maintaining catheter patency. System is patent.
4. Evaluate patient's comfort level.	Indicates catheter patency by absence of symptoms of bladder distention.
5. Monitor for signs and symptoms of infection.	Patients with indwelling catheters remain at risk for infection.
6. **Use Teach-Back:** "I want to be sure I explained clearly about why we are irrigating your catheter. Tell me in your own words the reason we are doing the irrigation." Revise your instruction now or develop a plan for revised patient/family caregiver teaching if patient/family caregiver is not able to teach back correctly.	Teach-back is an evidence-based health literacy intervention that promotes patient engagement, patient safety, adherence, and quality. The goal of teach-back is to ensure that you have explained medical information clearly so that patients and their families understand what you communicated to them (AHRQ, 2020).

UNEXPECTED OUTCOMES AND RELATED INTERVENTIONS

1. Drainage output is less than amount of irrigation solution infused.
- Examine drainage tubing for clots, sediment, or kinks.
- Inspect urine for presence of or increase in blood clots and sediment.
- Evaluate patient for pain and distended bladder.
- Notify health care provider.

2. Bright-red bleeding with the irrigation (CBI) infusion wide open.
- Assess for hypovolemic shock (vital signs, skin color and moisture, anxiety level).
- Leave irrigation infusion wide open and notify health care provider.

3. Patient experiences pain with irrigation.
- Examine drainage tubing for clots, sediment, or kinks.
- Evaluate urine for presence of or increase in blood clots and sediment.
- Evaluate for distended bladder.
- Notify health care provider.

RECORDING AND REPORTING

- Record irrigation method, amount of and type of irrigation solution, amount returned as drainage, characteristics of output, and urine output.
- Record I&O.
- Document your evaluation of patient learning.
- Report catheter occlusion, sudden bleeding, infection, or increased pain.

HOME CARE CONSIDERATIONS

- Patients and/or family caregivers can be taught to perform catheter irrigations with adequate support, demonstration/return demonstration, and written instructions.
- Teach patients and/or family caregivers to observe urine color, clarity, odor, and amount and to observe for signs of catheter obstruction and UTI.
- Arrange for home delivery and storage of catheter/irrigation supplies.

KEY POINTS

- Micturition involves complex interactions among the central nervous system, bladder, and urinary sphincter.
- Multiple factors affect urinary function such as fluid intake, medications, functional ability, environment, medical problems outside the urinary tract, and dysfunction within the urinary tract.
- Common urinary tract symptoms include urgency, dysuria, frequency, hesitancy, polyuria, oliguria, nocturia, dribbling, hematuria, and urinary retention.
- The presence or recent history of an indwelling catheter increases risk for a urinary tract infection (UTI).
- To minimize the risk for infection when caring for a patient with a closed bladder drainage system, nursing care must include careful attention to aseptic technique.
- Planning care for a patient who is incontinent requires selecting interventions specific to the type of incontinence.
- Inserting a catheter using aseptic technique, maintaining a closed urinary drainage system, and removing an indwelling catheter as soon as it is no longer needed are essential in preventing CAUTIs.
- Integrating a patient's typical voiding habits into the plan of care and ensuring patient privacy foster a patient's normal urinary elimination.
- Interventions that prevent UTIs include promoting adequate fluid intake, promoting perineal hygiene, and encouraging patients to void at regular intervals.
- Prevention of catheter-associated urinary tract infection (CAUTI) requires use of an evidence-based "bundle" to perform all elements of care at one time.

REFLECTIVE LEARNING

- Think about Mrs. Grayson and describe assessment data that put her at risk for alterations in urinary elimination. (Recognize Cues)
- What priority collaborative problems support or contradict Mrs. Grayson's UI issues? (Analyze Cues)
- Considering her assessment data and history, what would be the priority clinical issues in caring for Mrs. Grayson? (Prioritize Diagnoses)
- Consider Mrs. Grayson's clinical situation and describe what nursing and medical interventions for management of UI that you could use. (Generate Solutions)
- Which nursing and medical interventions should have priority when implementing Mrs. Grayson's care plan? (Take Action)
- Considering the implementation of Mrs. Grayson's health care provider's orders, how would you determine if they were effective based on current assessment data? (Evaluate Outcomes)

REVIEW QUESTIONS

1. A patient is scheduled to have an intravenous pyelogram (IVP) tomorrow morning. Which nursing measures should be implemented before the test? (Select all that apply.)
   1. Ask the patient about any allergies and reactions.
   2. Instruct the patient that a full bladder is required for the test.
   3. Instruct the patient to save all urine in a special container.
   4. Ensure that informed consent has been obtained.
   5. Instruct the patient that facial flushing can occur when the contrast medium is given.
2. What is a critical step when inserting an indwelling catheter into a male patient?
   1. Slowly inflate the catheter balloon with sterile saline.
   2. Secure the catheter drainage tubing to the bedsheets.
   3. Advance the catheter to the bifurcation of the drainage and balloon ports.
   4. Advance the catheter until urine flows, then insert ¼ inch more.
3. Which instruction should the nurse give the assistive personnel (AP) concerning a patient who has had an indwelling urinary catheter removed that day?
   1. Limit oral fluid intake to avoid possible UI.
   2. Expect patient complaints of suprapubic fullness and discomfort.
   3. Report the time and amount of first voiding.
   4. Instruct patient to stay in bed and use a urinal or bedpan.
4. A patient with a three-way indwelling urinary catheter and CBI complains of lower abdominal pain and distention after surgery. What should be the nurse's *initial* intervention(s)? (Select all that apply.)
   1. Increase the rate of the CBI.
   2. Assess the patency of the drainage system.
   3. Measure urine output.
   4. Assess vital signs.
   5. Administer ordered pain medication.
5. After abdominal surgery, the patient is on the surgical unit with an indwelling urinary catheter placed. What aspects of care for this patient can be delegated to the assistive personnel (AP)? (Select all that apply.)
   1. Assessing the patient for any postoperative issues with the indwelling catheter
   2. Assisting the nurse with patient positioning and maintaining privacy during catheter care
   3. Teaching the patient signs and symptoms of a UTI
   4. Reporting to the nurse any patient discomfort or fever
   5. Reporting any abnormal color, odor, or amount of urine in the drainage bag
6. What should the nurse teach a young woman with a history of UTIs about UTI prevention? (Select all that apply.)
   1. Maintain regular bowel elimination.
   2. Limit water intake to 1 to 2 glasses a day.
   3. Wear cotton underwear.
   4. Cleanse the perineum from front to back.
   5. Practice pelvic muscle exercises (Kegel) daily.
7. Place the following steps for insertion of an indwelling catheter in a female patient in appropriate order.
   1. Insert and advance catheter.
   2. Lubricate catheter.
   3. Inflate catheter balloon.
   4. Cleanse urethral meatus with antiseptic solution.
   5. Drape patient with the sterile square and fenestrated drapes.
   6. When urine appears, advance another 2.5 to 5 cm.
   7. Prepare sterile field and supplies.
   8. Gently pull catheter until resistance is felt.
   9. Attach drainage tubing.
8. Which nursing interventions should a nurse implement when removing an indwelling urinary catheter in an adult patient? (Select all that apply.)
   1. Attach a 3-mL syringe to the inflation port.
   2. Allow the balloon to drain into the syringe by gravity.
   3. Initiate a voiding record/bladder diary.
   4. Pull the catheter quickly.
   5. Clamp the catheter before removal.
9. Which nursing intervention decreases the risk for CAUTI?
   1. Cleansing the urinary meatus 3 to 4 times daily with antiseptic solution
   2. Hanging the urinary drainage bag below the level of the bladder

3. Emptying the urinary drainage bag daily

4. Irrigating the urinary catheter with sterile water

10. The nurse is inserting a urinary catheter for a female patient, and after the catheter has been inserted 3 inches, no urine is returned. What should the nurse do next?

    1. Remove the catheter and start all over with a new kit and catheter.

    2. Leave the catheter there and start over with a new catheter.

3. Pull the catheter back and reinsert at a different angle.

4. Ask the patient to bear down and insert the catheter farther.

Answers: 1. 1, 4, 5; **2.** 3, 3; **4.** 2, 3; **5.** 2, 4, 5; **6.** 1, 3, 4; **7.** 5, 7, 2, 4, 1, 6, 3, 8, 9; **8.** 2, 3; **9.** 2; **10.** 2.

Answers to Review Questions can be found on the Evolve website.

REFERENCES

AACN Clinical Practice Alert: Prevention of catheter-associated urinary tract infections in adults, *Crit Care Nurse* 38(1):84, 2018.

Agency for Healthcare Research and Quality (AHRQ): *Health literacy universal precautions toolkit*, ed 2, Rockville, MD, March 2020, Agency for Healthcare Research and Quality. https://www.ahrq.gov/health-literacy/quality-resources/tools/literacy-toolkit/healthlittoolkit2-tool5.html. Accessed July 2021.

American Geriatrics Society: *Updated Beers Criteria for potentially inappropriate medication use in older adults*, 2018. https://www.americangeriatrics.org/media-center/news/draft-ags-updated-2018-beers-criterian-potentially-inappropriate-medication-use. Accessed July 2021.

American Nurses Association (ANA): *Streamlined evidence-based RN tool: catheter associated urinary tract infection (CAUTI) prevention*, n.d. https://www.nursingworld.org/~4aede8/globalassets/practiceandpolicy/innovation—evidence/clinical-practice-material/cauti-prevention-tool/anacautipreventiontool-final-19dec2014.pdf. Accessed July 2021.

Assadi F: Strategies for preventing catheter-associated urinary tract infection, *Int J Prev Med* 9:50, 2018.

Ball JW, et al: *Seidel's guide to physical examination*, ed 9, St. Louis, 2019, Elsevier.

Burchum JR, Rosenthal LD: *Lehne's Pharmacology for nursing care*, ed 10, St. Louis, 2019, Elsevier.

Bykoviene L, et al: Pelvic floor muscle training with or without tibial nerve stimulation and lifestyle changes have comparable effects on the overactive bladder: a randomized clinical trial, *Urol J* 15(4):186, 2018.

Cartwright A: Reducing catheter-associated urinary infections: standardizing practice, *Br J Nurs* 27(1):7, 2018.

Centers for Disease Control and Prevention (CDC): *Urinary tract infection (catheter-associated urinary tract infection [CAUTI] and non-catheter-associated urinary tract infection [UTI]) and other urinary system infection [USI] events*, 2020. https://www.cdc.gov/nhsn/pdfs/pscManual/7pscCAUTIcurrent.pdf. Accessed July 2021.

Centers for Disease Control and Prevention (CDC): *What is health literacy*, 2021. https://www.cdc.gov/healthliteracy/learn/index.html. Accessed October 2021.

Centers for Medicare & Medicaid (CMS): *2020 hospital-acquired condition (HAC) reduction program*, 2020. https://www.cms.gov/Medicare/Quality-Initiatives-Patient-Assessment-Instruments/Value-Based-Programs/HAC/Hospital-Acquired-Conditions. Accessed July 2021.

Duncan D: Alternative to antibiotics for managing asymptomatic and non-symptomatic bacteriuria in older persons: a review, *Br J Community Nurs* 24(3):116, 2019.

Eshkoor S, et al: Factors related to urinary incontinence among the Malaysian elderly, *J Nutr Health Aging* 21(2):220, 2017.

Fekete T: *Catheter-associated urinary tract infection in adults*, UpToDate, 2020. https://www.uptodate.com/contents/catheter-associated-urinary-tract-infection-in-adults. Accessed July 2021.

Fransway AF, Reeder MJ: *Irritant contact dermatitis in adults*, UpToDate, 2020. https://www.uptodate.com/contents/irritant-contact-dermatitis-in-adults. Accessed July 2021.

Giger J, Haddad L: *Transcultural nursing: assessment and intervention*, ed 8, St. Louis, 2021, Elsevier.

Glick D: *Overview of post-anesthetic care for adult patients*, UpToDate, 2020. https://www.uptodate.com/contents/overview-of-post-anesthetic-care-for-adult-patients. Accessed July 2021.

Gould CV, et al: *Guideline for prevention of catheter-associated urinary tract infections 2009*, Healthcare Infection Control Practices Advisory Committee, Centers for Disease Control and Prevention, June 2019. https://www.cdc.gov/infectioncontrol/pdf/guidelines/cauti-guidelines-H.pdf. Accessed July 2021.

Harding MM, et al: *Medical-surgical nursing*, ed 11, St. Louis, 2021, Elsevier.

Huether SE, et al: *Understanding pathophysiology*, ed 7, St. Louis, 2020, Mosby.

Ignatavicius D, et al: *Medical-surgical nursing: concepts for interprofessional collaborative care*, ed 9, St. Louis, 2018, Elsevier.

Jarvis C: *Physical examination & health assessment*, ed 8, St. Louis, 2020, Elsevier.

Lai D, et al: Mediating effect of social participation on the relationship between incontinence and depressive symptoms in older Chinese women, *Health Soc Work* 42(2):e94, 2017.

Lawrence K, et al: The CAUTI prevention tool kit: A professional and collaborative project of the Wound, Ostomy and Continence nurses, *J Wound Ostomy Continence Nurs* 46(2):154, 2019.

Lukacz E: *Evaluation of females with urinary incontinence*, UpToDate, 2020. https://www.uptodate.com/contents/evaluation-of-females-with-urinary-incontinence. Accessed July 2021.

Malik Y, et al: Mandatory reporting of female genital mutilation in children in the UK, *Br J Nurs* 26(6):377, 2018.

McNeill L: Back to basics: how evidence-based nursing practice can prevent catheter-associated urinary tract infections, *Urol Nurs* 37(4):204, 2017.

Pagana KD, et al: *Mosby's diagnostic and laboratory test reference*, ed 15, St. Louis, 2021, Elsevier.

Saito M, et al: No association of caffeinated beverage or caffeine intake with prevalence of urinary incontinence among middle-aged Japanese women: a multicenter cross-sectional study, *J Womens Health* 26(8):860, 2017.

Schaeffer A: *Placement and management of urinary bladder catheters in adults*, UpToDate, 2020a. https://www.uptodate.com/contents/placement-and-management-of-urinary-bladder-catheters-in-adults. Accessed July 2021.

Schaeffer A: *Complications of urinary bladder catheters and preventive strategies*, UpToDate, 2020b. https://www.uptodate.com/contents/complications-of-urinary-bladder-catheters-and-preventive-strategies. Accessed July 2021.

Taylor J: Reducing the incidence of inappropriate indwelling urinary catheterization, *J Community Nurs* 32(3):50, 2018.

The Joint Commission (TJC): *2021 National Patient Safety Goals*, Oakbrook Terrace, IL, 2021, The Commission. https://www.jointcommission.org/en/standards/national-patient-safety-goals/. Accessed July 2021.

Touhy TA, Jett KF: *Ebersole and Hess' toward healthy aging*, ed 10, St. Louis, 2020, Elsevier.

Vethanayagam N, et al: Understanding help-seeking in older people with urinary incontinence: an interview study, *Health Soc Care Community* 25(3):1061, 2017.

Yates A: Incontinence-associated dermatitis in older people: prevention and management, *Br J Community Nurs* 23(5):218, 2018.

RESEARCH REFERENCES

Fasugba O, et al: Systematic review and meta-analysis of the effectiveness of antiseptic agents for meatal cleaning in the prevention of catheter-associated urinary tract infections, *J Hosp Infect* 95(3):233, 2017.

Ferguson A: Implementing a CAUTI prevention program in an acute care hospital setting, *Urol Nurs* 38(6):273, 2018.

Graham G, et al: Implementation of a multifaceted nurse led intervention to reduce indwelling urinary catheter use in four Australian hospitals: a pre- and postintervention study, *J Clin Nurs* 29(5-6):872, 2020.

Rea K, et al: A technology intervention for nurses engaged in preventing catheter-associated urinary tract infection, *Comput Inform Nurs* 36(6):305, 2018.

Werth S, Justice R: Prevalence of moisture-associated skin damage in an acute care setting outcome from a quality improvement project, *J Wound Ostomy Continence Nurs* 46(1):51, 2019.

Bowel Elimination

OBJECTIVES

- Discuss the role of gastrointestinal organs and their physiological function in digestion and elimination.
- Discuss how psychological and physiological factors may alter the elimination process.
- Recognize cues that help you to assess patients' elimination patterns.
- Describe nursing implications for common diagnostic examinations of the gastrointestinal tract.

- Select individualized nursing interventions using your clinical judgment that promote normal elimination in your patients.
- Prioritize nursing interventions for patients with intestinal diversions.
- Describe nursing procedures related to bowel elimination.
- Use critical thinking and clinical decision making when providing care to patients with alterations in bowel elimination.

KEY TERMS

Bowel training
Cathartics
Chyme
Clostridium difficile
Colonoscopy
Colostomy
Constipation
Diarrhea

Effluent
Enemas
Fecal immunochemical test (FIT)
Fecal occult blood test (FOBT)
Flatulence
Hemorrhoid
Ileostomy
Ileus

Impaction
Incontinence
Laxatives
Polyps
Stoma
Wound, ostomy, and continence nurse (WOCN)

MEDIA RESOURCES

http://evolve.elsevier.com/Potter/fundamentals/
- Review Questions
- Video Clips
- Concept Map Creator
- Case Study with Questions

- Skills Performance Checklists
- Audio Glossary
- Content Updates
- Answers to QSEN Activity and Review Questions

Chavela Josefa Rivas Mendez is 78 years old and has been widowed for 10 years. She lives in a first-floor condominium that is in a community for active older adults. The community has a shared garden, offers regular game nights, and organizes trips to local grocery stores, markets, restaurants, museums, and libraries. Chavela's niece, Ana, lives in the same town; the rest of her family is scattered across the country and Mexico.

Sergio is a home health nurse visiting Chavela, who was discharged to home following a left knee replacement. Chavela has hypertension, osteoarthritis, and frequent constipation. Sergio's priority is to determine how well Chavela is recovering from her surgery and to assess her ability to perform her activities of daily living (ADLs).

Regular elimination of bowel waste products is essential for normal body functioning. Alterations in bowel elimination are often early signs or symptoms of problems within either the gastrointestinal (GI) tract or other body systems. Because bowel function depends on the interaction among several different factors, elimination patterns and habits vary among individuals.

Understanding normal bowel elimination and factors that promote, slow down, or cause alterations in elimination help you manage patients' elimination problems. Supportive nursing care respects a patient's privacy and emotional needs. Measures designed to promote normal elimination also need to minimize a patient's discomfort and embarrassment.

SCIENTIFIC KNOWLEDGE BASE

The GI tract consists of the alimentary canal and its accessory organs. The alimentary canal is a single tube that extends from the mouth to the anus and includes the mouth, esophagus, stomach, and intestines. The accessory organs include the teeth, tongue, salivary glands, liver, pancreas, and gallbladder. These organs absorb fluid and nutrients, prepare food for absorption and use by body cells, and provide for temporary storage of feces (Fig. 47.1). The GI tract absorbs high volumes of fluids, making fluid and electrolyte balance a key function of the GI system. In addition to ingested fluids and foods, the GI tract also receives secretions from the gallbladder and pancreas.

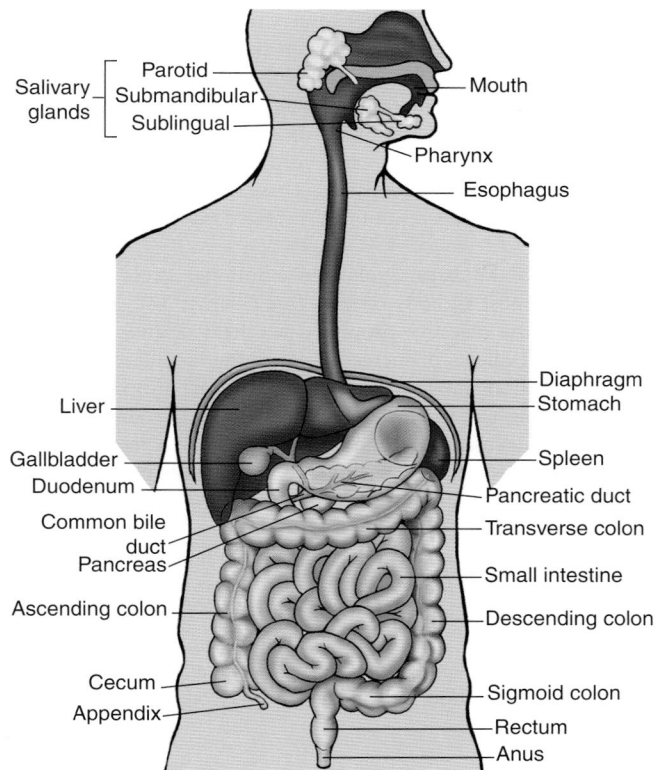

FIG. 47.1 Organs of gastrointestinal tract. (From Monahan FD, Neighbors M: *Medical-surgical nursing,* ed 2, Philadelphia, 1998, Saunders.)

Mouth

The mouth mechanically and chemically breaks down nutrients into usable size and form. The teeth chew food, breaking it down into a size suitable for swallowing. Saliva, produced by the salivary glands in the mouth, dilutes and softens the food in the mouth for easier swallowing.

Esophagus

As food enters the upper esophagus, it passes through the upper esophageal sphincter, a circular muscle that prevents air from entering the esophagus and food from refluxing into the throat. The bolus of food travels down the esophagus with the aid of *peristalsis*, which is a contraction that propels food through the length of the GI tract. The food moves down the esophagus and reaches the cardiac sphincter, which lies between the esophagus and the upper end of the stomach. The sphincter prevents reflux of stomach contents back into the esophagus.

Stomach

The stomach performs three tasks: storage of swallowed food and liquid, mixing of food with digestive juices into a substance called chyme, and regulated emptying of its contents into the small intestine. The stomach produces and secretes hydrochloric acid (HCl), mucus, the enzyme pepsin, and intrinsic factor. Pepsin and HCl help to digest protein. Mucus protects the stomach mucosa from acidity and enzyme activity. Intrinsic factor is essential in the absorption of vitamin B_{12}.

Small Intestine

Movement within the small intestine, occurring by peristalsis, facilitates both digestion and absorption. Chyme comes into the small intestine as a liquid material and mixes with digestive enzymes. Resorption in the small intestine is so efficient that by the time the fluid reaches the end of the small intestine it is a thick liquid with some semisolid particles. The small intestine is divided into three sections: the duodenum, the jejunum, and the ileum.

The duodenum is approximately 20 to 28 cm (8 to 11 inches) long and continues to process fluid from the stomach. The second section, the jejunum, is approximately 2.5 m (8 feet) long and absorbs carbohydrates and proteins. The ileum is approximately 3.7 m (12 feet) long and absorbs water, fats, and bile salts. The duodenum and jejunum absorb most nutrients and electrolytes in the small intestine. The ileum absorbs certain vitamins, iron, and bile salts. Digestive enzymes and bile enter the small intestine from the pancreas and the liver to further break down nutrients into a form usable by the body.

The digestive process is greatly altered when small intestine function is impaired. Conditions such as inflammation, infection, surgical resection, or obstruction disrupt peristalsis, reduce absorption, or block the passage of fluid, resulting in electrolyte and nutrient deficiencies.

Large Intestine

The lower GI tract is called the *large intestine* or *colon* because it is larger in diameter than the small intestine. However, its length, 1.5 to 1.8 m (5 to 6 feet), is much shorter. The large intestine is divided into the cecum, ascending colon, transverse colon, descending colon, sigmoid colon, and rectum. The large intestine is the primary organ of bowel elimination.

Digestive fluid enters the large intestine by waves of peristalsis through the ileocecal valve (i.e., a circular muscle layer that prevents regurgitation back into the small intestine). The muscular tissue of the colon allows it to accommodate and eliminate large quantities of waste and gas (flatus). The colon has three functions: absorption, secretion, and elimination. The colon resorbs a large volume of water (up to 1.5 L) and significant amounts of sodium and chloride daily. The amount of water absorbed depends on the speed at which colonic contents move. Normally the fecal matter becomes a soft, formed solid or semisolid mass. If peristalsis is abnormally fast, there is less time for water to be absorbed, and the stool will be watery. If peristaltic contractions slow down, water continues to be absorbed, and a hard mass of stool forms, resulting in constipation.

Peristaltic contractions move contents through the colon. Mass peristalsis pushes undigested food toward the rectum. These mass movements occur only 3 or 4 times daily, with the strongest during the hour after mealtime.

The rectum is the final part of the large intestine. Normally the rectum is empty of fecal matter until just before defecation. It contains vertical and transverse folds of tissue that help to control expulsion of fecal contents during defecation. Each fold contains veins that can become distended from pressure during straining. This distention results in hemorrhoid formation.

Anus

The body expels feces and flatus from the rectum through the anus. Contraction and relaxation of the internal and external sphincters, which are innervated by sympathetic and parasympathetic nerves, aid in the control of defecation. The anal canal contains a rich supply of sensory nerves that allow people to tell when there is solid, liquid, or gas that needs to be expelled and aids in maintaining continence.

Defecation

The physiological factors essential to bowel function and defecation include normal GI tract function, sensory awareness of rectal distention and rectal contents, voluntary sphincter control, and adequate rectal capacity and compliance. Normal defecation begins with movement in the left colon, moving stool toward the anus. When stool reaches the rectum, the distention causes relaxation of the internal sphincter and an awareness of the need to defecate. At the time of defecation, the external sphincter relaxes, and abdominal muscles contract, increasing intrarectal pressure and forcing the stool out. Normally defecation is painless, resulting in the passage of soft, formed stool. Straining while having a bowel movement indicates that the patient may need changes in diet or fluid intake or that there is an underlying disorder in GI function.

REFLECT NOW

The digestive system is a complex group of organs that allow the body to transport and digest food and fluids and eliminate waste products. Each part of the system plays an important role, yet illness or surgery can cause significant changes in digestive function. Consider symptoms patients may experience as a result of these changes and how their quality of life may be affected.

NURSING KNOWLEDGE BASE

Factors Influencing Bowel Elimination

Many factors influence the process of bowel elimination. Knowledge of these factors helps to anticipate measures required to maintain a normal elimination pattern.

Age. Infants have a smaller stomach capacity, less secretion of digestive enzymes, and more rapid intestinal peristalsis. The ability to control defecation does not occur until 2 to 3 years of age. Adolescents experience rapid growth and increased metabolic rate. There is also rapid growth of the large intestine and increased secretion of gastric acids to digest food fibers and act as a bactericide against swallowed organisms. Older adults may have decreased chewing ability. Partially chewed food is not digested as easily. Peristalsis declines, and esophageal emptying slows. This impairs absorption by the intestinal mucosa. Muscle tone in the perineal floor and anal sphincter weakens, which sometimes causes difficulty in controlling defecation (NIH, n.d.a).

Diet. Regular daily food intake helps maintain a regular pattern of peristalsis in the colon. Fiber in the diet provides the bulk in the fecal material. Bulk-forming foods such as whole grains, fresh fruits, and vegetables help remove the fats and waste products from the body with more efficiency. Some of these foods such as cabbage, broccoli, or beans may also produce gas, which distends the intestinal walls and increases colonic motility. The bowel walls stretch, creating peristalsis and initiating the defecation reflex.

Fluid Intake. Although individual fluid needs vary with the person, a fluid intake of 3.7 L per day for men and 2.7 L per day for women is recommended (Mayo Clinic, 2020). You meet some fluid needs by drinking fluids, but you also ingest fluid when you eat some foods, such as fruits and vegetables. The character of feces is affected when individuals do not drink enough fluid or experience disturbances resulting in fluid loss (such as vomiting). The fiber a patient eats absorbs fluid, which liquefies intestinal contents and creates a larger, softer stool mass. This increases peristalsis and promotes movement of stool through the colon. Reduced fluid and fiber intake slows the passage of food through the intestine and results in hardening of stool contents, causing constipation.

Physical Activity. Physical activity promotes peristalsis, whereas immobilization slows it. Encourage early ambulation as illness begins to

resolve or as soon as possible after surgery to promote normal peristalsis and elimination. Maintaining tone of skeletal muscles used during defecation is important. Weakened abdominal and pelvic floor muscles impair the ability to increase intraabdominal pressure and control the external sphincter. Muscle tone is sometimes weakened or lost because of long-term illness, spinal cord injury, or neurological diseases that impair nerve transmission. These changes in the abdominal and pelvic floor muscles result in an increased risk for constipation.

Psychological Factors. Prolonged emotional stress impairs the function of almost all body systems (see Chapter 37). During emotional stress, the digestive process is accelerated, and peristalsis is increased. Side effects of increased peristalsis include diarrhea and gaseous distention. Several diseases of the GI tract are exacerbated by stress, including ulcerative colitis, irritable bowel syndrome, certain gastric and duodenal ulcers, and Crohn's disease. If a person becomes depressed, the autonomic nervous system may slow impulses, which slows peristalsis, resulting in constipation.

Personal Habits. Personal elimination habits influence bowel function. Most people benefit from being able to use their own toilet facilities at a time that is most effective and convenient for them. A busy work schedule sometimes prevents an individual from responding appropriately to the urge to defecate, disrupting regular habits and causing possible alterations, such as constipation. Individuals need to recognize the best time for elimination.

Position During Defecation. Squatting is the normal position during defecation. Modern toilets facilitate this posture, allowing a person to lean forward, exert intraabdominal pressure, and contract the gluteal muscles. For a patient immobilized in bed, defecation is often difficult. In a supine position it is hard to effectively contract the muscles used during defecation. If a patient's condition permits, raise the head of the bed to a more normal sitting position on a bedpan, enhancing the ability to defecate.

Pain. Normally the act of defecation is painless. However, several conditions such as hemorrhoids; rectal surgery; anal fissures, which are painful linear splits in the perianal area; and abdominal surgery result in discomfort. In these instances, the patient often suppresses the urge to defecate to avoid pain, contributing to the development of constipation.

Pregnancy. As pregnancy advances, the size of the fetus increases, and pressure is exerted on the rectum. A temporary obstruction created by the fetus impairs passage of feces. Slowing of peristalsis during the third trimester often leads to constipation. A pregnant woman's frequent straining during defecation or delivery may result in the formation of hemorrhoids.

Surgery and Anesthesia. General anesthetic agents used during surgery cause temporary cessation of peristalsis (see Chapter 50). Inhaled anesthetic agents block parasympathetic impulses to the intestinal musculature. The action of the anesthetic slows or stops peristaltic waves. A patient who receives a local or regional anesthetic is less at risk for elimination alterations because this type of anesthesia generally affects bowel activity minimally or not at all.

Any surgery that involves direct manipulation of the bowel temporarily stops peristalsis. This condition, called an **ileus**, usually lasts about 24 to 48 hours. If a patient remains inactive or is unable to eat after surgery, return of normal bowel elimination is further delayed.

Medications. Many medications prescribed for acute and chronic conditions have secondary effects on a patient's bowel elimination patterns. For example, opioid analgesics slow peristalsis and contractions, often resulting in constipation, and antibiotics decrease intestinal bacterial flora, often resulting in diarrhea (Burchum and Rosenthal, 2021). It is important for you and your patients to be aware of these possible side effects and use appropriate measures to promote healthy bowel elimination. Some medications are used primarily for their action on the bowel and may promote defecation (e.g., laxatives or cathartics) or control diarrhea. Fiber laxatives are used first when a patient needs to take a laxative for regular evacuation of the rectum. An osmotic laxative is used next if fiber laxatives do not relieve constipation. Patients need to avoid regular use of a stimulant laxative because the intestine often becomes dependent on it.

Diagnostic Tests. Diagnostic examinations involving visualization of GI structures often require a prescribed bowel preparation (e.g., laxatives and/or enemas) to ensure that the bowel is empty. Usually, patients cannot eat or drink several hours before examinations such as an endoscopy, colonoscopy, or other testing that requires visualization of the GI tract. Following the diagnostic procedure, changes in elimination such as increased gas or loose stools often occur until the patient resumes a normal eating pattern.

Common Bowel Elimination Problems

You will frequently care for patients who have or are at risk for elimination problems because of physiological changes in the GI tract, such as abdominal surgery, inflammatory diseases, medications, emotional stress, environmental factors, or disorders impairing defecation.

Constipation. Constipation is a symptom, not a disease. There are many possible causes (e.g., improper diet, reduced fluid intake, lack of exercise, certain medications) (Box 47.1). For example, patients receiving opioids for pain after surgery often require a stool softener or laxative to prevent constipation. Female gender and older age are other risk factors for constipation (NIH, n.d.b). Signs of constipation include infrequent bowel movements (fewer than three per week) and hard, dry stools that are difficult to pass (NIH, n.d.b). When intestinal motility slows, the fecal mass becomes exposed to the intestinal walls over time, and most of the fecal water content is absorbed. Little water is left to soften and lubricate the stool. Passage of a dry, hard stool often causes rectal pain. Constipation is a significant source of discomfort. You need to assess patients and provide appropriate interventions to prevent painful defecation and fecal impactions.

Impaction. Fecal impaction results when a patient has unrelieved constipation and is unable to expel the hardened feces retained in the rectum. In cases of severe impaction, the mass extends up into the sigmoid colon. If not resolved or removed, severe impaction results in intestinal obstruction. Patients who are debilitated, confused, or unconscious are most at risk for impaction. They are dehydrated or too weak or unaware of the need to defecate, and the stool becomes too hard and dry to pass.

An obvious sign of impaction is the inability to pass a stool for several days, despite the repeated urge to defecate. Suspect an impaction when a continuous oozing of liquid stool occurs. The liquid part of feces located higher in the colon seeps around the impacted mass. Loss of appetite (anorexia), nausea and/or vomiting, abdominal distention and cramping, and rectal pain may accompany the condition. If you suspect an impaction, gently perform a digital examination of the rectum and palpate for the impacted mass (Setya et al., 2020).

Diarrhea. Diarrhea is an increase in the number of stools and the passage of liquid, unformed feces. It is associated with disorders affecting digestion, absorption, and secretion in the GI tract. Intestinal contents pass through the small and large intestine too quickly to allow for the usual absorption of fluid and nutrients. Irritation within the colon results in an increased secretion of mucus. As a result, feces become watery, and the patient often has difficulty controlling the urge to defecate.

Excess loss of colonic fluid results in dehydration (Box 47.2), with fluid and electrolyte or acid-base imbalances if the fluid is not replaced. Infants and older adults are particularly susceptible to associated complications (see Chapter 42). Because repeated passage of diarrhea stools exposes the skin of the perineum and buttocks to irritating intestinal contents, meticulous skin care and containment of fecal drainage is necessary to prevent skin breakdown (see Chapter 48).

Incontinence. Fecal incontinence is the inability to control the passage of feces and gas from the anus. Incontinence harms a patient's body image (see Chapter 33). The embarrassment of soiling clothes often leads to social isolation. Physical conditions that impair anal sphincter function or create large-volume liquid stools (e.g., diarrhea) often cause incontinence. Impaired cognitive function often leads to incontinence of both urine and stool.

Many conditions cause diarrhea and/or fecal incontinence. You need to identify precipitating conditions and refer patients to health care providers for medication management. Antibiotic use alters the normal flora in the GI tract. A common causative agent of diarrhea is *Clostridium difficile (C. difficile)*, which produces symptoms ranging from mild diarrhea to severe colitis. The Infectious Diseases Society of America (IDSA) identified *C. difficile* as the most common health care–related infection in America. Patients acquire *C. difficile* infection

---

BOX 47.1 Common Causes of Constipation

- Irregular bowel habits and ignoring the urge to defecate
- Chronic illnesses (e.g., Parkinson's disease, multiple sclerosis, rheumatoid arthritis, chronic bowel diseases, depression, eating disorders)
- Low-fiber diet high in animal fats (e.g., meats and carbohydrates); low fluid intake
- Stress (e.g., illness of a family member, death of a loved one, divorce)
- Physical inactivity
- Medications, especially use of opiates
- Changes in life or routine, such as pregnancy, aging, and travel
- Neurological conditions that block nerve impulses to the colon (e.g., stroke, spinal cord injury, tumor)
- Chronic bowel dysfunction (e.g., colonic inertia, irritable bowel)

BOX 47.2 Signs of Dehydration

- Signs of dehydration in adults include:
  - Thirst
  - Less frequent urination than usual
  - Dark-colored urine
  - Dry skin
  - Fatigue
  - Dizziness
  - Light-headedness
- Signs of dehydration in infants and young children include:
  - Dry mouth and tongue
  - No tears when crying
  - No wet diapers for 3 hours or more
  - Sunken eyes or cheeks or soft spot in the skull
  - High fever
  - Listlessness or irritability

in one of two ways: by antibiotic therapy that causes an overgrowth of *C. difficile* and by contact with the *C. difficile* organism. Patients are exposed to the organism from a health care worker's hands or direct contact with environmental surfaces contaminated with it. Only hand hygiene with soap and water is effective to physically remove *C. difficile* spores from the hands. Older adult patients are especially vulnerable to *C. difficile* infection when exposed to antibiotics, and higher mortality and morbidity are observed in this age-group (McDonald et al., 2018). The 2017 IDSA guidelines recommend using an evidence-based algorithm which includes a NAAT (nucleic acid amplification test) to identify the presence of *C. difficile* in the stool (McDonald et al., 2018). To decrease the spread of infection, patients with *C. difficile* are placed on contact/enteric isolation precautions. A private room with a dedicated toilet is preferred to help prevent transmission to other patients.

Communicable foodborne pathogens also cause diarrhea. Hand hygiene following the use of the bathroom, before and after preparing foods, and when cleaning and storing fresh produce and meats greatly reduces the risk of foodborne illnesses. When diarrhea results from a foodborne pathogen, the goal usually is to rid the GI system of the pathogen rather than to slow peristalsis.

Surgeries or diagnostic testing of the lower GI tract may also cause diarrhea. Patients receiving enteral nutrition are also at risk for diarrhea and need a dietary consult to find the right formula for the feeding (see Chapter 45). Food intolerances can increase peristalsis and cause diarrhea, cramps, or flatulence within a few hours after an individual ingests the food. For example, people who lack the enzyme needed to digest the milk sugar lactase and are lactose intolerant will often experience abdominal pain, nausea, bloating, gas, and diarrhea after drinking cow's milk. Another condition called *celiac disease* is an immune disease in which patients experience damage to the small intestine when they eat gluten. Food allergies create an immune system reaction after people eat a certain food. Some food allergies are life threatening and lead to anaphylaxis. The U.S. Food and Drug Administration (USFDA) enforces the Food Allergen Labeling and Consumer Protection Act of 2004, which requires accurate food labels. People with food intolerances and allergies need to read food labels carefully to ensure that they do not ingest foods that they are intolerant or allergic to (USFDA, 2021).

Flatulence. As gas accumulates in the lumen of the intestines, the bowel wall stretches and distends. Flatulence is a common cause of abdominal fullness, pain, and cramping. Normally intestinal gas escapes through the mouth (belching) or the anus (passing of flatus). However, flatulence causes abdominal distention and severe, sharp pain if intestinal motility is reduced because of opiates, general anesthetics, abdominal surgery, or immobilization.

Hemorrhoids. Hemorrhoids are dilated, engorged veins in the lining of the rectum. They are either external or internal. External hemorrhoids are clearly visible as protrusions of skin. There is usually a purplish discoloration (thrombosis) if the underlying vein is hardened. This causes increased pain and sometimes requires excision. Internal hemorrhoids occur in the anal canal and may be inflamed and distended. Increased venous pressure from straining at defecation, pregnancy, heart failure, and chronic liver disease frequently cause hemorrhoids.

Bowel Diversions

Certain diseases or surgical alterations make the normal passage of intestinal contents throughout the small and large intestine difficult or inadvisable. When these conditions are present, a temporary or permanent opening (stoma) is created surgically by bringing part of the intestine out through the abdominal wall. These surgical openings are

FIG. 47.2 Sigmoid colostomy.

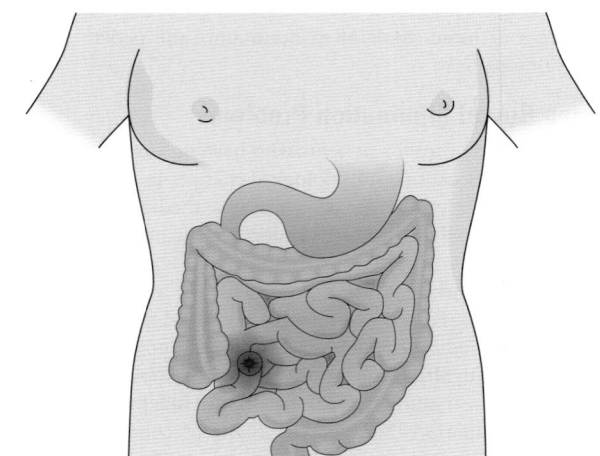

FIG. 47.3 Ileostomy.

called an ileostomy or colostomy, depending on which part of the intestinal tract is used to create the stoma (Figs. 47.2 and 47.3). Newer surgical techniques allow more patients to have parts of their small and large intestine removed and the remaining parts reconnected; these techniques enable patients to continue to defecate through the anal canal.

Ostomies. The location of an ostomy determines stool consistency. A person with a sigmoid colostomy will have a more formed stool. The output from a transverse colostomy will be thick liquid to soft consistency. These ostomies are the easiest to perform surgically and are done as a temporary means to divert stool from an area of trauma or perianal wounds. They may also be a palliative diversion if obstruction from a tumor is present. With an ileostomy the fecal effluent leaves the body before it enters the colon, creating frequent, liquid stools.

Loop colostomies are reversible stomas that a surgeon constructs in the ileum or the colon. The surgeon pulls a loop of intestine onto the abdomen and often places a plastic rod, bridge, or rubber catheter temporarily under the bowel loop to keep it from slipping back. The surgeon then opens the bowel and sutures it to the skin of the abdomen. The loop ostomy has two openings through the stoma. The proximal end drains fecal effluent, and the distal part drains mucus.

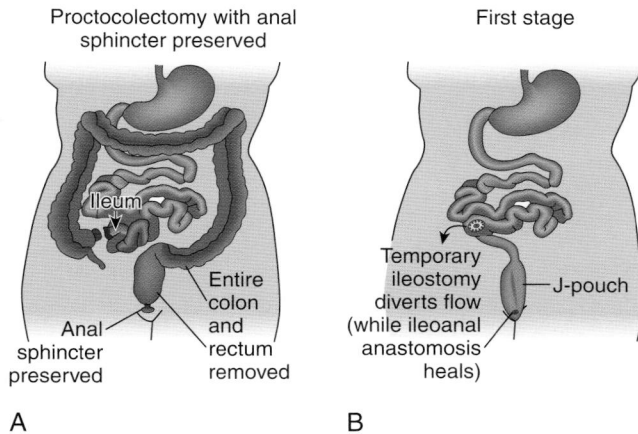

Proctocolectomy with anal
sphincter preserved

First stage

Ileum

Entire
colon
and
rectum
removed

Anal
sphincter
preserved

Temporary
ileostomy
diverts flow
(while ileoanal
anastomosis
heals)

J-pouch

A

B

FIG. 47.4 Ileoanal pouch anastomosis.

The end colostomy consists of a stoma formed by bringing a piece of intestine out through a surgically created opening in the abdominal wall, turning it down like a turtleneck and suturing it to the abdominal wall. The intestine distal to the stoma is either removed or sewn closed (called *Hartmann's pouch;* see Fig. 47.2) and left in the abdominal cavity. End ostomies are permanent or reversible. The rectum is either left intact or removed.

Other Procedures.

Ileoanal Pouch Anastomosis. The ileoanal pouch anastomosis is a surgical procedure for patients who need to have a colectomy for treatment of ulcerative colitis or familial adenopolyposis (FAP) (Mayo Clinic, 2021). In this procedure the surgeon removes the colon, creates a pouch from the end of the small intestine, and attaches the pouch to the patient's anus (Fig. 47.4). The pouch provides for the collection of fecal material, which simulates the function of the rectum. The patient is continent of stool because stool is evacuated via the anus. When the ileal pouch is created, the patient has a temporary ileostomy to divert the effluent and allow the suture lines in the pouch to heal.

A continent ileostomy involves creating a pouch from the small intestine. The pouch has a continent stoma on the abdomen created with a valve that can be drained only when the patient places a large catheter into the stoma. The patient empties the pouch several times a day. This procedure is rarely performed now.

Children with fecal soiling associated with neuropathic or structural abnormalities of the anal sphincter sometimes have an antegrade continence enema (ACE) procedure. The surgeon uses the child's appendix or cecum to create a continence valve on the abdomen. This allows the patient or family caregiver to insert a tube and administer an enema that comes out through the anus. Colonic evacuation begins about 10 to 20 minutes after a patient receives the enema fluid.

Before Sergio meets Chavela for the first time, he reviews the information he will need to complete a thorough assessment. Sergio uses his knowledge from caring for other patients following surgery to identify the key symptoms to look for in patients following a knee replacement. Sergio plans to assess Chavela's pain, mobility, and functional status. He also plans to review her medication list. Because Sergio knows that many pain medications cause constipation and that Chavela has a history of constipation, Sergio recognizes it is a priority to assess how often she is having a bowel movement and the quality of her stools. He also plans to assess her level of mobility, check her nutritional status and fluid intake, and identify foods she typically eats.

CRITICAL THINKING

Successful critical thinking requires a synthesis of knowledge, experience, environmental factors, critical thinking attitudes, and intellectual and professional standards. Sound clinical judgments require you to anticipate the information, analyze the data, and make decisions regarding your patient's care. During assessment consider all elements that build toward making an appropriate nursing diagnosis (Fig. 47.5).

In the case of bowel elimination, integrate knowledge from nursing and other disciplines to understand a patient's response to bowel elimination alterations. Experience in caring for patients with elimination alterations helps you provide an appropriate plan of care. Use critical thinking attitudes such as fairness, confidence, and discipline when listening to and exploring a patient's nursing history. Apply relevant standards of practice, such as the Wound, Ostomy, and Continence Nurses Society (WOCN) Clinical Practice Guidelines, when selecting nursing measures.

> ### REFLECT NOW
>
> Consider the social stigma of impaired bowel function and try to understand your personal attitudes toward caring for patients who may suffer from odor, soiling, and embarrassment when they lose control of this important bodily function.

❖ NURSING PROCESS

Apply the nursing process and use a critical thinking approach in your care of patients. The nursing process provides a clinical decision-making approach for you to develop sound clinical judgments so that you can implement an individualized plan of care. Nurses use critical thinking and complete a thorough assessment to understand and treat alterations in bowel elimination. Successful management depends on establishing a relationship of trust among health care providers, patient, and family.

◆ Assessment

Assessment for bowel elimination patterns and alterations in bowel elimination includes a nursing history, physical assessment of the abdomen, inspection of fecal characteristics, and review of relevant test results. In addition, determine a patient's medical history, pattern and types of fluid and food intake, mobility, chewing ability, medications, recent illnesses and/or stressors, and environmental situation.

Through the Patient's Eyes. Patients expect nurses to answer their questions regarding diagnostic tests and the preparation for these tests. Patients often experience concern regarding their abdominal discomfort and exposure of their perineal area. Bowel problems are often a source of embarrassment for patients and their families. Fecal and urinary incontinence in older adults is often a reason for admission to a long-term care agency. Admission to a long-term care agency is also a risk factor for fecal incontinence (Massirfufulay et al., 2019). Some older adults who fail to recognize their elimination needs require monitoring for elimination patterns to prevent complications related to altered elimination patterns. Remember that each patient has a unique situation and a perception of what is "right or normal." Patients expect a knowledgeable nurse with the ability to teach how to promote and maintain normal bowel elimination patterns or manage altered elimination. Encourage the patient and/or family caregiver to describe cultural practices, and use this information when providing care to enhance the patient's comfort.

Knowledge Base

- Normal gastrointestinal anatomy and physiology
- Factors that influence bowel elimination
- Common intestinal alterations
- The effect of a patient's developmental stage on bowel elimination

- Patient responses to alterations in elimination
  - Effects of patient's illness or disability, diet, medications, and activity level on elimination
    - Knowledge of caring principles

Attitudes

- Be creative when planning interventions to achieve normal bowel elimination patterns
- Display independence when integrating interventions from other disciplines in the patient's plan of care
- Act responsibly by ensuring interventions are consistent within standards

Evaluation

Assessment

Evaluate outcomes

Recognize cues

Take action

Clinical Decision Making

Analyze cues

Implementation

Diagnosis

Generate solutions

Prioritize hypotheses

Planning

Environment

- Time pressure
- Setting: The patient's experiences with and responses to alterations in bowel elimination may differ in acute versus long-term care versus home settings.
- Task complexity
- Interruptions
- Health care resources (equipment, personnel)

Standards

- *ANA Standards and Scope of Nursing Practice*
- Clinical Practice Guidelines and Standards of Practice (e.g., Clinical Practice Guidelines for *Clostridium difficile* infection in adults and children)
- Intellectual standards in measurement
- Agency policies and procedures
- Patient's expected outcomes
- Professional
  - Standards of care (e.g., WOCN ostomy care standards to assess stoma site and output)
  - Ethical standards

Experience

- Previous experiences caring for patients with alterations in bowel elimination
- Personal experience with the effects of stress, dietary changes, and medications on elimination patterns
- Knowledge of successful interventions
- Skill competence

FIG. 47.5 Critical thinking model for elimination assessment. *WOCN,* Wound, Ostomy and Continence Nurses Society. (Clinical Judgment Measurement Model copyright © NCSBN. All rights reserved.)

Nursing History. The nursing history provides information about a patient's usual bowel pattern and habits. What a patient describes as normal or abnormal is sometimes different from factors and conditions that tend to promote normal elimination. Identifying normal and abnormal patterns, habits, and the patient's perception of normal and abnormal bowel elimination helps you analyze cues and allows you to better determine a patient's problems. Organize the nursing history around factors that affect elimination.

- *Determine a patient's usual elimination pattern:* Include frequency and time of day. Having a patient or family caregiver complete a bowel elimination diary provides an accurate assessment of a patient's current bowel elimination pattern.
- *Patient's description of usual stool characteristics:* Determine whether the stool is normally watery or formed, soft or hard, and the typical color. Ask the patient to describe the shape of a normal stool and the number of stools per day. Use a scale such as the Bristol Stool Form Scale to get an objective measure of stool characteristics (Fig. 47.6).
- *Identify the routines followed to promote bowel elimination:* Examples include drinking hot liquids, eating specific foods, taking time to defecate during a certain part of the day, or using laxatives, enemas, or bulk-forming fiber additives.
- *Presence and status of bowel diversions:* If a patient has an ostomy, assess frequency of emptying the ostomy pouch, character of feces, appearance, and condition of the stoma (color, height at or above skin level), condition of peristomal skin, type of pouching system device used, and methods used to maintain the function of the ostomy.

Type 1	Separate hard lumps like nuts (difficult to pass)
Type 2	Sausage shaped but lumpy
Type 3	Like a sausage but with cracks on surface
Type 4	Like a sausage or snake, smooth and soft
Type 5	Soft blobs with clear-cut edges (passed easily)
Type 6	Fluffy pieces with ragged edges, a mushy stool
Type 7	Watery, no solid pieces (entirely liquid)

FIG. 47.6 Bristol Stool Form Scale. (Used with permission. Bristol Stool Form Guideline. https://www.webmd.com/digestive-disorders/poop-chart-bristol-stool-scale.)

- *Changes in appetite:* Include changes in eating patterns and a change in weight (amount of loss or gain). If a loss of weight is present, ask whether the patient intended to lose weight (e.g., a diet or exercise routine) or whether it happened unexpectedly.
- *Diet history:* Determine the patient's dietary preferences. Determine the intake of fruits, vegetables, and whole grains and whether mealtimes are regular or irregular.
- *Description of daily fluid intake:* This includes the type and amount of fluid. Patients often estimate the amount using common household measurements.
- *History of surgery or illnesses affecting the GI tract:* This information helps explain symptoms, the potential for maintaining or restoring normal bowel elimination pattern, and whether there is a family history of GI cancer.
- *Medication history:* Ask patients for a list of all the medications they take, and assess whether they take medications such as laxatives, antacids, iron supplements, and analgesics that alter defecation or fecal characteristics.
- *Emotional state:* A patient's emotional status may alter frequency of defecation. Ask the patient about any experiences of unusual stress and, if so, whether the patient thinks that these experiences may have caused a change in bowel movements.
- *History of exercise:* Ask the patient to specifically describe the type and amount of daily exercise.
- *History of pain or discomfort:* Ask the patient whether there is a history of abdominal or anal pain. The type, frequency, and location of pain help identify the source of the problem. For instance, cramping pain, nausea, and the absence of bowel movements sometimes indicate the presence of an intestinal obstruction.

- *Social history:* Patients have many different living arrangements. Where patients live affects their toileting habits. If the patient lives with other people, ask how many bathrooms there are in the setting. Find out whether the patient must share a bathroom, creating a need to adjust the time that the bathroom is used to accommodate others. If the patient lives alone, can the patient ambulate to the toilet safely? When patients are not independent in bowel management, determine who helps them and how.
- *Mobility and dexterity:* Evaluate patients' mobility and dexterity to determine whether they need assistive devices or help from personnel. See Box 47.3 for a summary of the types of assessment questions to use for gathering a detailed nursing history.

Environmental Factors. It is also important to recognize environmental factors that affect a patient's bowel elimination patterns. Patients usually feel most comfortable with their bowel elimination routine in their own homes. When patients are not at home, they can easily become uncomfortable and self-conscious about alterations or problems with their bowels. Environmental factors such as noise, interruptions, and lack of privacy greatly affect a patient's comfort level and willingness to discuss problems associated with bowel elimination. Be sure that the environment is quiet and ensure privacy when assessing your patients' bowel status. Identify and minimize potential interruptions, especially during physical assessment and when asking assessment questions the patient may consider embarrassing or very personal.

Physical Assessment. Conduct a physical assessment of body systems and functions likely to be influenced by the presence of elimination problems (see Chapter 30).

BOX 47.3 Nursing Assessment Questions

Signs and Symptoms
Nausea or Vomiting: Onset, Duration, Associated Symptoms, Character, Exposures
- When did the nausea/vomiting start?
- Is it related to particular stimuli (odors, after eating specific food)?
- How does the emesis look (mucus, blood, coffee-ground appearance, undigested food), and what is the color?
- Do you have other symptoms such as fever, dizziness, headaches, abdominal pain, or weight loss?
- Do you have family members who are experiencing the same symptoms?

Indigestion: Onset, Character, Location, Associated Symptoms, Alleviating Factors
- Is the indigestion related to meals, types or quantity of food, time of day or night?
- Does the discomfort from indigestion radiate to the shoulders or arms?
- Do you feel bloated after eating?
- Do you have any other symptoms (vomiting, headaches, diarrhea, belching, flatulence, heartburn, or pain)?
- Does the indigestion respond to antacids or other self-care measures?

Diarrhea: Onset, Duration, Character, Associated Symptoms, Alleviating Factors, Exposure
- When did the diarrhea start? Was it gradual or sudden?
- How many stools do you have per day? Is it watery or explosive? What is the color and consistency?
- Have you had fever, chills, weight loss, or abdominal pain?
- Have you taken antibiotics recently?
- Have you been under stress?

- What have you used to try to alleviate the diarrhea? Was it successful?
- Have you been out of the country recently?

Constipation: Onset, Character, Symptoms, Alleviating Factors
- When was your last bowel movement? How many bowel movements do you have in a typical week?
- Is this a recent occurrence or a long-standing problem?
- Describe your bowel movements.
- Do you have to strain to have a bowel movement?
- Do you have abdominal or rectal pain when you have a bowel movement?
- Do you feel as though your bowel movements are incomplete?
- Have you recently changed your diet or fluid intake?
- Have you recently taken any opioid medications?
- Do you use stool softeners, laxatives, or enemas?
- Has it ever been necessary to manually remove the bowel movements?

Medical History
- Do you have a previous history of gastrointestinal problems or disease? If yes, explain.
- Have you had abdominal surgery or trauma?
- Do you have a history of major illnesses such as cancer; arthritis; or respiratory, kidney, or cardiac disease?
- Which medications do you take?

Effect on the Patient
- How do these symptoms affect you?
- Have you missed work or social engagements because of these symptoms?

Mouth. Inspect the patient's teeth, tongue, and gums. Poor dentition or poorly fitting dentures influence the ability to chew. Sores in the mouth make eating not only difficult but also painful.

Abdomen. Inspect all four abdominal quadrants for contour, shape, symmetry, and skin color. Note masses, peristaltic waves, scars, venous patterns, stomas, and lesions. Normally you do not see peristaltic waves. Observable peristalsis is often a sign of intestinal obstruction

Abdominal distention appears as an overall outward protuberance of the abdomen. Intestinal gas, large tumors, or fluid in the peritoneal cavity causes distention. A distended abdomen feels tight like a drum; the skin is taut and appears stretched.

Normal bowel sounds occur every 5 to 15 seconds and last a second to several seconds. Absent (no auscultated bowel sounds) or hypoactive sounds occur with an ileus, such as after abdominal surgery, but may also mean that you did not capture the bowel sounds when you were assessing them. High-pitched and hyperactive bowel sounds occur with small intestine obstruction and inflammatory disorders.

Although auscultating bowel sounds with a stethoscope during assessment is standard nursing practice, some current studies question its validity. A systematic review of the literature on bowel sound auscultation in ICU patients concluded that there is a low sensitivity, low positive predictive value, and poor inter- and intra-observer agreement in auscultating bowel sounds. The results suggest that bowel sounds were not sufficiently accurate for clinical decision making and questioned the usefulness of the practice (Van Bree et al., 2018).

Percussion identifies underlying abdominal structures and detects lesions, fluid, or gas within the abdomen. Gas or flatulence creates a tympanic note. Masses, tumors, and fluid are dull to percussion.

Gently palpate the abdomen for masses or areas of tenderness. It is important for your patient to relax. Tensing abdominal muscles interferes with palpating underlying organs or masses.

Rectum. Inspect the area around the anus for lesions, discoloration, inflammation, and hemorrhoids. Pain results when hemorrhoid tissues are irritated. The primary goal for a patient with hemorrhoids is to have soft-formed, painless bowel movements. Proper diet, fluids, and regular exercise improve the likelihood of stools being soft. If the patient becomes constipated, passage of hard stools causes bleeding and irritation. An ice pack or a warm sitz bath (see Chapter 48) provides temporary relief of swollen hemorrhoids. A health care provider sometimes prescribes topical medication to relieve the swelling and pain.

Laboratory Tests. There are no blood tests to specifically diagnose most GI disorders, but hemoglobin and hematocrit help determine whether anemia from GI bleeding is present. Other laboratory tests often ordered by the health care provider include liver function tests, serum amylase, and serum lipase, which are used to assess for hepatobiliary diseases and pancreatitis.

Fecal Specimens. You need to ensure that specimens are obtained accurately, labeled properly in appropriate containers, and transported to the laboratory on time. Laboratories provide special containers for fecal specimens. Some tests require that specimens are placed in chemical preservatives, and some require that they are refrigerated or placed on ice after collection and before delivery to the laboratory. Use medical aseptic technique during collection of stool specimens (see Chapter 28).

Hand hygiene is necessary for anyone who comes in contact with the specimen. Often the patient is able to obtain the specimen if properly instructed. Teach the patient to avoid mixing feces with urine or water. The patient defecates into a clean, dry bedpan or a special container under the toilet seat. Observe the stool characteristics when collecting a specimen (Table 47.1).

Tests performed by the laboratory for occult (microscopic) blood in the stool and stool cultures require only a small sample. Collect about a 3-cm (1.18-inch) mass of formed stool or 15 to 30 mL of liquid stool. Tests for measuring the output of fecal fat require a 3- to 5-day collection of stool. You need to save all fecal material throughout the test period.

After obtaining a specimen, label and tightly seal the container and complete all laboratory requisition forms. Record specimen collections in the patient's medical record. It is important to avoid delays in sending

TABLE 47.1   Fecal Characteristics

Characteristic	Normal	Abnormal	Abnormal Cause
Color	Infant: yellow; adult: brown	White or clay	Absence of bile
		Black or tarry (melena)	Iron ingestion or gastrointestinal (GI) bleeding
		Red	GI bleeding, hemorrhoids, ingestion of beets
		Pale and oily	Malabsorption of fat
Odor	Malodorous; may be affected by certain foods	Noxious change	Blood in feces or infection
Consistency	Soft, formed	Liquid	Diarrhea, reduced absorption
		Hard	Constipation
Frequency	Varies: infant 4 to 6 times daily (breastfed) or 1 to 3 times daily (bottle-fed); adult twice daily to 3 times a week	Infant more than 6 times daily or less than once every 1 to 2 days; adult more than 3 times a day or less than once a week	Hypermotility or hypomotility
Shape	Resembles diameter of rectum	Narrow, pencil shaped	Obstruction, increased peristalsis
Constituents	Undigested food, dead bacteria, fat, bile pigment, cells lining intestinal mucosa, water	Blood, pus, foreign bodies, mucus, worms	Internal bleeding, infection, swallowed objects, irritation, inflammation, infestation of parasites
		Oily stool	Malabsorption syndrome, enteritis, pancreatic disease, surgical resection of intestine
		Mucus	Intestinal irritation, inflammation, infection, or injury

specimens to the laboratory. Some tests, such as measurement for ova and parasites, require the stool to be warm. When stool specimens remain at room temperature, bacteriological changes that alter test results occur.

A common stool test is the fecal occult blood test (FOBT), which measures microscopic amounts of blood in the feces. It is a useful screening test for colon cancer as recommended by the American Cancer Society. There are two types of tests, the guaiac fecal occult blood test (gFOBT) and the fecal immunochemical test (FIT). The FIT test requires no preparation or dietary restrictions and is a more sensitive test, but it is more expensive; thus, the gFOBT is more commonly used. The nurse or the patient needs to repeat the test at least 3 times on three separate bowel movements. The FOBT is done in a patient's home or health care provider's office (Box 47.4). All positive tests are followed up with flexible sigmoidoscopy or colonoscopy (ACS, 2021).

When your patients are going to have a gFOBT, it is important to instruct them to avoid eating red meat for 3 days before testing. If there are no contraindications and it is approved by the health care provider,

---

BOX 47.4 PROCEDURAL GUIDELINES

Performing a Guaiac Fecal Occult Blood Test

Delegation and Collaboration

The skill of fecal occult blood test (FOBT) can be delegated to assistive personnel (AP). However, the nurse is responsible for assessing the significance of the findings. You may need to send the specimen to the laboratory. Refer to your agency policies. The nurse instructs the AP to:

- Notify the nurse if frank bleeding occurs after obtaining the sample.

Equipment

Hemoccult test paper, Hemoccult developer, wooden applicator, and clean gloves. (Check the expiration dates on the developer and the test paper before using.)

Procedural Steps

1. Identify patient using at least two identifiers (e.g., name and birthday or name and account number) according to agency policy.
2. Explain purpose of test and ways patient can help. Patient can collect own specimen if possible.
3. Perform hand hygiene and apply clean gloves.
4. Use tip of wooden applicator (see illustration) to obtain a small part of stool specimen. Be sure that specimen is free of toilet paper and not contaminated with urine.

STEP 4 Equipment needed for fecal occult blood testing.

5. Perform Hemoccult slide test:
   a. Open flap of slide and, using a wooden applicator, thinly smear stool in first box of the guaiac paper. Apply a second fecal specimen from a different part of the stool to second box of slide (see illustration).
   b. Close slide cover and turn the packet over to reverse side (see illustration). After waiting 3 to 5 minutes, open cardboard flap and apply 2 drops of developing solution on each box of guaiac paper. A blue color indicates a positive guaiac or presence of fecal occult blood.

STEP 5a Application of fecal specimen on guaiac paper.

STEP 5b Application of Hemoccult developing solution on guaiac paper on reverse side of test kit.

   c. Interpret the color of the guaiac paper after 30 to 60 seconds.
   d. After determining whether the patient's specimen is positive or negative, apply 1 drop of developer to the quality control section and interpret within 10 seconds.
   e. Dispose of test slide in proper receptacle.
6. Wrap wooden applicator in paper towel, remove gloves, and discard in proper receptacle.
7. Perform hand hygiene.
8. Record results of test; note any unusual fecal characteristics. (Submit only one sample per day.)

BOX 47.5 Radiological and Diagnostic Tests

Direct Visualization

Endoscopy

- Examinations such as a gastroscopy or colonoscopy use a lighted fiberoptic tube to gain direct visualization of the upper gastrointestinal (GI) tract (upper endoscopy) or large intestine (colonoscopy). The fiberoptic tube contains a lens, forceps, and brushes for biopsy. If an endoscopy identifies a lesion such as a polyp, the polyp can be removed, and a biopsy will be done.
- These tests are done under sedation, usually in outpatient centers.
- Patients receive instruction about the preparation needed for the tests at the time they are scheduled for the procedure. Patients are usually on a clear liquid diet the day before the test. Bowel preparation is necessary before a colonoscopy can be performed successfully.

Indirect Visualization

Anorectal Manometry

- Measures the pressure activity of internal and external anal sphincters and reflexes during rectal distention, relaxation during straining, and rectal sensation.

Plain Film of Abdomen/Kidneys, Ureter, Bladder (KUB)

- A simple x-ray film of the abdomen requiring no preparation.

Barium Swallow/Enema

- An x-ray film examination using an opaque contrast medium (barium, which is swallowed) to examine the structure and motility of the upper GI tract, including pharynx, esophagus, and stomach. Barium instilled through the anal opening via an enema provides visualization of the structures of the lower GI tract.
- Preparation required varies by health care provider and agency doing the procedure but usually includes a clear liquid diet, laxatives the day before the procedure, and in some instances enemas to empty out any remaining stool particles.

Ultrasound Imaging

- A technique that uses high-frequency sound waves to echo off body organs, creating a picture of the GI tract

Computed Tomography Scan (Virtual Colonoscopy)

- An x-ray examination of the body from many angles using a scanner analyzed by a computer. An oral contrast solution for the patient to drink may be ordered before the test. Intravenous contrast solution may be injected during the test to improve visualization. If contrast is used, patient should not have food or fluids for 4 to 6 hours before the examination.
- Virtual colonoscopy or computerized tomography (CT) colonography requires bowel preparation before the test. This does not replace the colonoscopy because it does not allow for removal of **polyps** and for biopsies to be obtained.

Colonic Transit Study

- The patient swallows a capsule containing radiopaque markers.
- The patient maintains a normal diet and fluid intake for 5 days and refrains from medications that affect bowel function. On the fifth day x-ray film examination is performed.

Magnetic Resonance Imaging

- A noninvasive examination that uses magnet and radio waves to produce a picture of the inside of the body.
- Preparation is NPO 4 to 6 hours before examination.
- The patient needs to lie very still. If claustrophobia is a problem, light sedation may be ordered.
- No metallic objects, including metal objects on clothes, are allowed in the room. A patient with a pacemaker or metal implanted in the body may not be able to have magnetic resonance imaging (MRI).

---

instruct your patient to stop taking aspirin, ibuprofen, naproxen, or other nonsteroidal antiinflammatory drugs for 7 days because these could cause a false-positive test result. Patients also need to avoid vitamin C supplements and citrus fruits and juices for 3 days before the test because they can cause a false-negative result (ACS, 2021).

Diagnostic Examinations. For patients experiencing alterations in the GI system, various radiological and diagnostic examinations such as a colonoscopy require bowel preparation (bowel prep) for the test to be completed successfully. A bowel-cleansing program is sometimes difficult or unpleasant for patients. You provide education and support to ensure an optimal test result (Box 47.5).

REFLECT NOW

The assessment of the body and fecal matter related to bowel elimination requires questions and procedures that are very private to many patients. What actions can you take while conducting this assessment that promote patients' comfort and decrease their embarrassment?

Sergio visits Chavela at her home 3 days after her discharge from the hospital. Sergio notices that Chavela seems to be uncomfortable. She frequently rubs both her knee at her surgical site and her abdomen. Chavela's vital signs are BP 132/84, P 86, R 20, and T 36.7°C (98°F). Sergio weighs Chavela and finds that she has lost 0.68 kg (1.5 pounds) since leaving the hospital. Chavela says she does not feel hungry because her abdomen feels bloated and tight. When asked, Chavela states her bowels have not

moved since she has been home. She states that her pain from her surgery ranges from a 3 to a 6 out of 10, which is affecting her ability to walk and move about her house. Chavela states, "I am taking the oxycodone pain pills my doctor gave me. I am afraid to not take them right now. I feel so tired and I can't remember all the exercises the physical therapist told me to do when I got home."

Sergio asks Chavela, "How many glasses of water or other fluids are you drinking now?"

Chavela responds, "I don't drink that much because I don't want to have to go to the bathroom too often. I am afraid I won't make it to the toilet in time because I can't walk as fast as I used to. I also don't have any fresh fruits or vegetables in my house right now because I can't go shopping yet."

Sergio then asks Chavela what she ate regularly before her surgery.

Chavela answers, "Oh I used to love to cook, especially when my niece came to visit. I used to eat flour tortillas, beans, tomatoes, and rice. I usually have eggs with tortillas for breakfast; a salad and chicken, rice, beans, and corn tortillas for lunch; and tacos or tamales for dinner."

◆ **Analysis and Nursing Diagnosis**

Nursing assessment of a patient's bowel function sometimes reveals data that indicate an actual or potential elimination problem or a problem resulting from elimination alterations. The development of accurate nursing diagnoses for a patient with changes in bowel elimination requires you to perform a complete assessment, think critically, and use your clinical judgment to recognize cues and analyze the data you collected. Be sure that your assessment considers what you know about a patient's health status and related factors that potentially affect bowel elimination patterns. During your analysis, look for patterns of data to help you identify individualized nursing diagnoses or collaborative problems.

Use your critical thinking to recognize clusters of assessment data cues, identify emerging patterns, make clinical judgments, and draw conclusions regarding a patient's actual or potential bowel elimination problems. Accurate nursing diagnosis requires that you analyze all assessment findings to identify a patient's priority problems. For example, if you are caring for a patient who is starting to take an antibiotic, one of the patient's nursing diagnoses might be *Risk for Diarrhea*. A patient who is experiencing immobility following a spinal cord injury on the other hand has a nursing diagnosis of *Risk for Constipation*. Examples of nursing diagnoses that apply to patients with elimination problems include the following:

- Bowel Incontinence
- Constipation
- Faecal Impaction
- Lack of Knowledge of Dietary Regime
- Impaired Defaecation

Associated problems such as age, body-image changes, or skin breakdown require interventions unrelated to bowel function impairment. It is important to establish the correct "related to" factor for a diagnosis. This depends on the thoroughness of your assessment and your recognition of the assessment findings and factors that impair elimination (Box 47.6). For example, with the diagnosis of *Constipation* you distinguish between related factors of *nutritional imbalance, exercise, medications,* and *emotional problems*. Selection of the correct related factors for each diagnosis ensures that you will implement the appropriate nursing interventions.

After completing his assessment, Sergio analyzes the data and clusters the assessment cues he gathered during his visit with Chavela. He identifies **Constipation related to opiate-containing pain medication, decreased mobility, and decreased food and fluid intake** *as the priority nursing diagnosis based on the following assessment cues: Chavela is taking only opioid pain medications, she is not eating fresh fruits or vegetables, she has reduced her fluid intake, she has reduced mobility, she states that she feels bloated, and she has not had a bowel movement since discharge (3 days). Sergio identifies* **Impaired Mobility related to pain and lack of knowledge about postsurgical exercises** *as another diagnosis, based on Chavela's statement that she cannot remember the exercises she is supposed to do and her statement that she is unable to walk around the house much because of the pain from her*

surgery. He also identifies **Impaired Ability to Manage Regime** *as Chavela stated she could not remember exercises and is not drinking water due to fear of not getting to the toilet on time. Finally, Sergio determines that Chavela also has a nursing diagnosis of* **Acute Pain related to left knee surgery,** *based on her nonverbal behavior (rubbing her knee), her taking the opioid pain medication as ordered, and her rating of pain as a 3-6/10 on the pain scale.*

◆ Planning and Outcomes Identification

When planning care, use critical thinking to synthesize information from multiple resources (Fig. 47.7). Critical thinking and clinical judgment ensure that the plan of care integrates everything you know about a patient, including current clinical problems. During planning, you develop a plan of care for each of your patient's nursing diagnoses. Reflect on your previous experiences in caring for patients with bowel elimination problems, and consider how they responded to different nursing therapies. Also consider the effect the environment is having or will likely have on your patient. Remember that a quiet environment free from interruptions and that ensures privacy will allow you to create a trusting therapeutic relationship with your patient that is critical for meeting bowel elimination needs. Include your patients and use professional standards when planning individualized care. For example, when caring for a patient with a colorectal disorder, use the *American College of Gastroenterology Rome IV Criteria for Colorectal Disorders* (Simren et al., 2017). For a patient with a fecal diversion, referring to *Clinical Guideline: Management of the Adult with a Fecal or Urinary Ostomy* (WOCN, 2018) may be helpful. Match a patient's needs with evidence-based interventions, focusing on helping patients resume normal bowel elimination patterns when possible or adapt to altered patterns when indicated.

Outcomes. Help patients establish goals and outcomes by incorporating their elimination habits or routines as much as possible and reinforcing the routines that promote health (see the Nursing Care Plan). In addition, consider preexisting health concerns. For example, if a patient's diet, activity, and irregular bowel habits caused the elimination problem, help the patient learn to make lifestyle changes to improve bowel function. Returning a patient to a normal bowel elimination pattern includes the following outcomes:

- Patient establishes a regular defecation schedule
- Patient lists proper fluid and food intake needed to soften stool and promote regular bowel elimination
- Patient implements a regular exercise program
- Patient reports daily passage of soft, formed brown stool
- Patient does not report straining or discomfort associated with defecation

---

BOX 47.6 Nursing Diagnostic Process

Constipation

Assessment Activities	Assessment Findings
Ask patient about bowel elimination patterns.	Patient reports no bowel movement since discharge to home.
Ask patient about other gastrointestinal symptoms.	Patient is experiencing abdominal cramping, bloating, and loss of appetite.
Ask patient to describe recent food and fluid intake.	Patient reports a reduction in fluid and nutritional intake since surgery; she is not eating fresh fruits and vegetables and does not have the energy to cook right now.
Palpate abdomen.	Patient reports feeling of fullness. Left lower quadrant is firm.

QSEN Building Competency in Patient-Centered Care

Chavela started to take a stool softener every day to treat her constipation. She drank more fluids, especially water, and began to add more fruits and vegetables to her diet. She began to have daily bowel movements with soft, formed stool. Now it is 2 weeks later. She is still taking her stool softener, but she has not continued with the fluid and dietary modifications that were recommended. The physical therapist is ready to discharge her from home care but asks Sergio to make another visit because Chavela states that she is starting to have trouble moving her bowels again. Which assessment questions and teaching strategies, approaches, and tools can Sergio use to enhance Chavela's learning and ability to prevent constipation?

Answers to QSEN Activities can be found on the Evolve website.

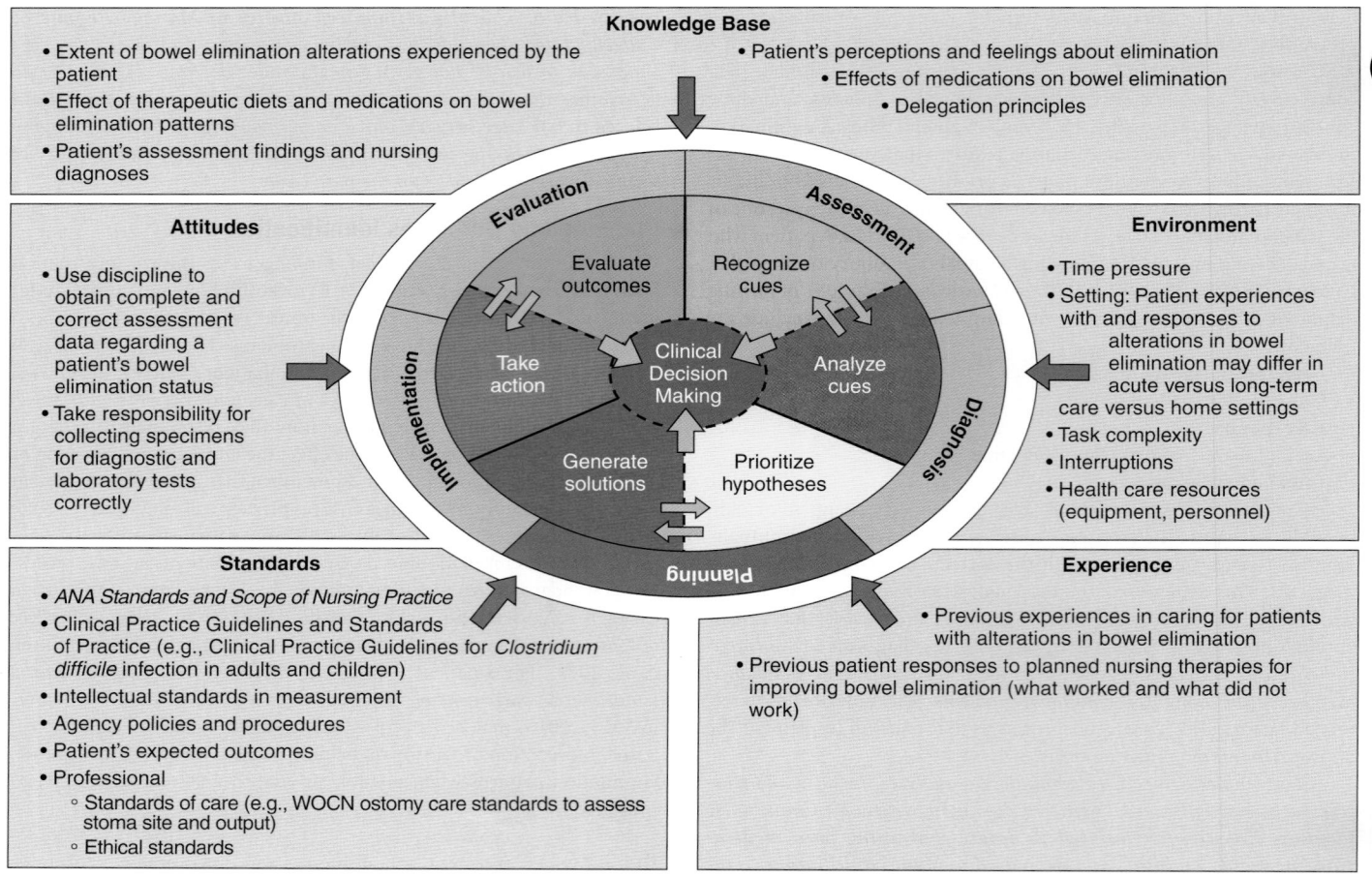

FIG. 47.7 Critical thinking model for planning for bowel elimination. *WOCN,* Wound, Ostomy and Continence Nurses Society. (Clinical Judgment Measurement Model copyright © NCSBN. All rights reserved.)

Setting Priorities. Defecation patterns vary among individuals. For this reason, a nurse and patient work together closely to plan effective interventions. Patients often have multiple diagnoses. The concept map (Fig. 47.8) shows an example of how the nursing diagnosis of constipation is related to three other diagnoses and their respective interventions. A realistic time frame to establish a normal defecation pattern for one patient is sometimes very different for another. Consider which of the nursing diagnoses are your patient's priorities. Your patient's priority needs will help you meet your patients' needs safely, effectively, and efficiently. Your ability to prioritize nursing diagnoses and generate appropriate nursing interventions will improve as you have more clinical experience (Dickison et al., 2019). For example, if you are caring for a patient with recent abdominal surgery, the priorities of pain management and preventing constipation through increasing fluids in the diet and encouraging early ambulation help in the recovery process. Although teaching about foods high in fiber is also helpful, if a patient's pain is not controlled, the patient will not be ready to learn about important nutritional modifications needed to make at home.

Teamwork and Collaboration. When patients are disabled or debilitated by illness, you need to include the family in the plan of care. In some situations, family members have the same ineffective elimination habits as the patient. Thus, teaching both the patient and the family is an important part of the care plan. Other health team members such as registered dietitians and WOCNs are often valuable resources. You coordinate activities of the interprofessional health care team.

A patient with alterations in bowel elimination sometimes requires intervention from several members of the health care team. Certain tasks such as assisting patients onto the bedpan or bedside commode are appropriate to delegate to assistive personnel (AP). It is important to remind the AP to report any abnormal findings or difficulties encountered during the elimination process. Many of the diagnostic tests for evaluation of the GI system are performed by nonnursing personnel. Maintaining ongoing communication with these caregivers will ensure that you provide safe and effective patient-centered care and address a patient's needs, wants, and concerns.

After identifying Chavela's nursing diagnoses, Sergio begins to identify and prioritize patient-centered outcomes and interventions. For the diagnosis of **Constipation**, *Sergio determines that Chavela should increase her consumption of fluids and fiber in her diet and hopes that she will have a soft, formed stool within the next 24 hours. Sergio helps Chavela come up with a plan to drink at least 2000 mL every day and helps her identify foods high in fiber that she likes and can easily add to her diet. He also knows that immobility is a risk factor for constipation, so he consults with a physical therapist and encourages Chavela to be more active, performing range of motion regularly and going for brief walks around her house once an hour while she is awake.*

⊚ NURSING CARE PLAN

Constipation

ASSESSMENT

Assessment Activities	Assessment Findings[a]
Ask Chavela about her bowel elimination patterns since surgery.	Chavela states that **she has not had a bowel movement since she has been home (for 3 days).**
Review patient's medication.	Chavela says she is taking her blood pressure medication, a daily multivitamin with **iron**, a stool softener once a day, and 1 or 2 **oxycodone** 4 times a day (Burchum and Rosenthal, 2021).
Review dietary and fluid intake over last day.	Diet included toast for breakfast; a sandwich for lunch; and a frozen dinner in the evening, which had a small serving of meat, potatoes, and green beans. She says she is **not drinking a lot of fluids** due to fears of not being able to make it to the bathroom on time.
Assess which foods and fluids Chavela likes, can obtain, and will prepare.	Chavela is eating frozen dinners right now because she is unable to get to the grocery store. She used to eat **rice, beans, tomatoes, and other fresh fruits and vegetables.**
Determine frequency of postoperative exercises and ambulation.	Chavela is not doing her exercises because she cannot remember them and does not frequently walk around the house.
Palpate abdomen.	While palpating Chavela's abdomen, she says, "It really **feels full**," and she **winces** with very little pressure applied. **Abdomen feels taut and mildly distended**.

[a] **Assessment findings** are shown in bold type.

NURSING DIAGNOSIS: Constipation related to opiate-containing pain medication, decreased mobility, and decreased food and fluid intake

PLANNING

Expected Outcomes (NOC)[b]

Bowel Elimination

Chavela reports passage of soft, formed stool without straining in next 24 hours.

Nutritional Status: Food and Fluid Intake

Chavela drinks at least 2000 mL of water every day.

Chavela increases the fiber content of her diet by eating bran cereal and an apple at breakfast, lettuce and tomato at lunch, and beans with her dinner.

[b] Outcome classification labels from Moorhead S, et al: *Nursing Outcomes Classification (NOC)*, ed 6, St Louis, 2018, Elsevier.

INTERVENTIONS (NIC)[c]	RATIONALE
Constipation/Impaction Management	
Encourage fluid intake of appropriate fluids, fruit juice, and water.	Adequate fluid intake helps to soften the stool. Women need about 2700 mL fluid intake (about 2000 mL from drinks and 700 mL from food) daily (Mayo Clinic, 2020).
Encourage activity within patient's mobility regimen.	Minimal activity (such as leg lifts) increases peristalsis (Harding et al., 2020).
Instruct to eat more fruits and vegetables and have a bran cereal for breakfast.	Added fiber in food relieves constipation (NIH, n.d.b).
Provide stimulant laxative and stool softeners as ordered.	Stimulant laxatives increase peristalsis and are an effective way to relieve constipation and promote normal bowel function when used on a short-term basis (Burchum and Rosenthal, 2021).
Encourage to try to have a bowel movement at the same time each day.	A regular time for bowel movements encourages normal bowel function (Harding et al., 2020).

[c] Intervention classification labels from Butcher HK, et al: *Nursing Interventions Classification (NIC)*, ed 7, St Louis, 2018, Elsevier.

EVALUATION

Evaluation Activities	Patient Response
Ask Chavela to identify foods high in fiber and fluid intake.	Able to state appropriate foods and fluids but still has little appetite and feels full soon after eating.
Ask Chavela to record how much water she drinks in the next 24 hours.	Chavela drank 1 cup (240 mL) of water every hour she was awake, which equaled a total of 2400 mL of water in 24 hours.
Inquire about bowel movements.	Chavela had a formed, soft bowel movement on Day 4 after returning home.

To help Chavela with her nursing diagnosis of **Impaired Mobility**, Sergio works with Chavela and her physical therapist to set an outcome for Chavela to stand up and walk for at least 5 minutes every hour she is awake. Sergio arranges for the physical therapist to come visit Chavela to teach her the exercises she is to do every day.

To address the nursing diagnosis of **Acute Pain**, Sergio works with Chavela to identify an acceptable level of pain. Together they determine that they want Chavela's pain to stay at a level of 3 or less. Because of the side effects of opioid pain medications, Sergio teaches Chavela about using acetaminophen to help control her pain. Chavela states that ice packs seemed to help reduce her pain in the hospital, so she is going to try to continue to use cool compresses on her knee to help reduce the pain. Sergio also plans to teach Chavela some nonpharmacological ways to help control her pain, such as listening to music and meditating, during his next visit.

CONCEPT MAP

Nursing diagnosis: Acute pain
- Reports pain ranges from 3 – 6 on 0 – 10 scale
- Pain is at left knee surgical site and abdomen
- Grimaces when walks and rubs knee frequently

Interventions
- Apply cold compresses to knee
- Take nonopioid analgesics as ordered by health care provider
- Encourage distraction through meditation, reading, and quiet music

Nursing diagnosis: Impaired mobility
- States she is not walking around the house much right now due to pain
- Reduced ROM in knee
- Cannot remember all postsurgical exercises

Interventions
- Refer to physical therapy
- Encourage to move and walk at regular intervals

Primary health problem: Osteoarthritis with recent left knee replacement, hypertension, constipation
Priority assessments: Comfort, effect of surgery on function and well-being, general mobility, bowel elimination patterns

Nursing diagnosis: Constipation
- Taking only opioid pain medications
- Limited intake of fluids, fruits, and vegetables
- Reduced mobility
- No bowel movement for 3 days
- Feels "bloated"

Interventions
- Suggest to begin using nonopioid pain medications
- Encourage to increase fluid intake – try drinking 1 cup of water every hour while awake
- Encourage to increase ambulation and exercises as ordered
- Collaborate with family and friends to help with cooking and purchasing groceries

Nursing diagnosis: Impaired ability to manage regime
- Reports being unable to go grocery shopping and cook
- Cannot remember exercises
- Reports being afraid of getting to the toilet in time

Interventions
- Identify family members or friends to help with ADLs as needed
- Consult with physical therapist to provide education on exercises and help with ambulation
- Ensure path to bathroom is clear; remove throw rugs
- Have elevated toilet seat with safety bars installed

——— Link between medical diagnosis and nursing diagnosis   - - - - - Link between nursing diagnoses

FIG. 47.8 Concept map for Chavela Josefa Rivas Mendez.

◆ Implementation

Successfully caring for patients with alterations in bowel elimination requires a patient-centered approach. Every patient's perception, experience, needs, and preferences regarding bowel elimination problems are unique. Successful nursing care requires you to partner with the patient, family caregivers, and other members of the health care team, such as a wound, ostomy, and continence nurse (WOCN) or registered dietitian (WOCN, 2018). Use your clinical judgment to determine the best approach and interventions to manage a patient's bowel elimination needs, to determine when to deliver the interventions, and to decide when adjustments are needed. Effective management requires patience and the ability to be flexible in choosing interventions. Patient education focuses on helping patients and family caregivers improve their understanding of bowel elimination. Teach patients and their families about proper

diet, adequate fluid intake, and factors that stimulate or slow peristalsis, such as emotional stress. Patients also need to learn the importance of establishing regular bowel routines, exercising regularly, and taking appropriate measures when elimination problems develop. Consult with other appropriate members of the health care team if you have questions or need assistance in caring for your patients.

Health Promotion. Health promotion interventions focus on keeping the gastrointestinal track healthy. Because bowel elimination affects so many aspects of an individual's life and adopting a healthy lifestyle contributes to maintaining gastrointestinal health, helping patients change health behaviors when indicated is a priority nursing focus. Elimination patterns differ from person to person, and many people are embarrassed to discuss issues surrounding elimination. Providing individualized nursing care is essential; this would include patient education regarding the promotion of normal defecation and how to reduce the risk of colorectal cancer.

Promotion of Normal Defecation. Patients of all ages often experience alterations in bowel elimination that greatly affect quality of life (Edelman and Kudzma, 2018). Thus, you will frequently provide health education to promote normal defecation. Several interventions (e.g., eating a high-fiber diet that includes whole grains and an adequate daily fluid intake) stimulate the defecation reflex, affect the character of feces, or increase peristalsis to help patients evacuate bowel contents normally and without discomfort.

One of the most important habits to teach regarding bowel habits is to take time for defecation. To establish regular bowel habits, a patient needs to know when the urge to defecate normally occurs. Advise a patient to begin to establish a routine during a time when defecation is most likely to occur, usually an hour after a meal. When patients are restricted to bed or need help to ambulate, offer a bedpan or help them reach the bathroom in a timely manner.

The normal position for defecation is to sit or squat. If a patient has difficulty sitting because of pain, muscular weakness, or mobility problems, place an elevated seat on the toilet or bedside commode. These seats require patients to use less effort to sit or stand and help promote normal defecation.

Colorectal Cancer Risk Reduction. Because colorectal cancer is the third most common cancer in the United States and the second most common cause of cancer death, promoting colon health to reduce the risk of colorectal cancer is essential (ACS, 2021). Begin by teaching patients about modifications they can make to reduce the risk of developing colon cancer, such as getting regular exercise, maintaining a healthy weight, and not smoking. Healthy diet choices are also important in promoting a healthy colon. Teach patients to eat a diet high in fiber, reduce the amount of red meat and processed meats (e.g., hot dogs, bacon, sausage), reduce sugar intake, and limit alcohol intake.

Colon cancer screening is also important because it often allows for the early detection of colorectal cancer. When found early, the 5-year relative survival rate of colorectal cancer is 90% (ACS, 2021). Following the guidelines for prevention and screening, knowing the early symptoms, and seeking medical help if these symptoms occur are the most effective ways to prevent death from this disease (Box 47.7). Despite the evidence supporting regular colorectal cancer screening, some populations, especially those affected by the social determinants of health, are less likely to be screened than others for a variety of reasons (Coughlin, 2020; Grywacz, 2018). Establish a therapeutic relationship, provide tailored patient education, and take time to discuss the importance of colorectal screening, especially with patients from these populations (Box 47.8).

Acute Care. Some acute illnesses affect the GI system. Changes in a patient's fluid status, mobility patterns, nutrition, and sleep cycle affect regular bowel habits when patients experience an acute illness. Surgical interventions on the GI tract and on other systems (e.g., musculoskeletal and cardiovascular) also affect bowel elimination.

Patients who are chronically ill or hospitalized are not always able to maintain privacy during defecation. In a hospital or extended-care setting, patients sometimes share bathroom facilities with a roommate. In addition, chronic illness may limit a patient's mobility and activity tolerance and require the use of a bedpan or bedside commode. The sights, sounds, and odors associated with sharing toilet facilities or using bedpans are often embarrassing. This embarrassment often causes patients to ignore the urge to defecate, which leads to constipation and discomfort. Remain sensitive to patients' elimination needs, detect cues that indicate patients are experiencing problems related to

---

BOX 47.7 Screening for Colorectal Cancer

Risk Factors
- Age: Over 50
- Personal history: Colorectal cancer or colorectal polyps, inflammatory bowel disease (IBD)
- Family history: Colorectal cancer, familial adenomatous polyposis, hereditary nonpolyposis colon cancer (Lynch syndrome)
- Racial and ethnic background: African Americans have the highest colon cancer incidence and mortality rates in the United States, and Jews of Eastern European descent (Ashkenazi Jews) have one of the highest risks when compared with other ethnic groups in the world
- Diet: High intake of red meat and processed meats such as lunch meats or hot dogs
- Obesity and physical inactivity
- Smoking and heavy alcohol consumption

Warning Signs
- Change in bowel habits (e.g., diarrhea, constipation, narrowing of stool lasting more than few days)
- Rectal bleeding or blood in stool
- Sensation of incomplete evacuation
- Unexplained abdominal or back pain

American Cancer Society Screening Guidelines for the Early Detection of Colorectal Cancer in Average-Risk Asymptomatic People
- People who are 45 years old should begin regular screening using one of the options listed below.
- People should continue screening through the age of 75 if they are in good health and have an expected life expectancy of more than 10 years.
- Screening decisions for people from 76 to 85 years old are based on a person's preferences, life expectancy, overall health status, and previous screening results.
- Screening is not indicated for people over 85 years of age.

Test	Frequency
Guaiac fecal occult blood test (gFOBT) done on multiple samples at home	Annual
Fecal immunochemical test (FIT) done on multiple samples at home	Annual
Flexible sigmoidoscopy	Every 5 years
DNA stool test	Every 3 years
Computed tomography, colonography	Every 5 years
Colonoscopy	Every 10 years

These procedures will be ordered by a health care provider, depending on availability of resources and patient needs. If positive findings result from the flexible sigmoidoscopy or colonography, follow-up with a colonoscopy should be done. Those with higher risk of colorectal cancer due to personal or family history may be advised to have earlier or more frequent screening.

Data from NIH National Cancer Institute: *Colorectal cancer,* https://www.cancer.gov/types/colorectal, n.d., accessed May 12, 2021; American Cancer Society: *Colorectal cancer,* https://www.cancer.org/cancer/colon-rectal-cancer.html, 2021, accessed May 12, 2021.

---

bowel elimination, and intervene to help patients maintain bowel elimination habits that are as normal as possible.

Positioning Patients on a Bedpan. Patients restricted to bed use bedpans for defecation. Women use bedpans to pass both urine and feces, whereas men use bedpans only for defecation. Sitting on a bedpan is uncomfortable. Help position patients comfortably. Two types

⊕ BOX 47.8 CULTURAL ASPECTS OF CARE

Variables Influencing Colorectal Cancer Screening in African Americans

There has been a decline in the incidence and mortality rates for colorectal cancer in the United States over the past 10 years. However, colorectal cancer rates are frequently correlated with social determinants of health such as low socioeconomic status, lack of education, and race (Coughlin, 2020). For example, African Americans have a higher incidence of colorectal cancer and have a higher rate of death from the cancer. However, in 2019 the American Cancer Society reported that the death rate from colorectal cancer is dropping faster in the African-American population than in whites (ACS, 2019). Patient factors that contribute to disparities in screening include poor knowledge of benefits of colorectal cancer screening, limited access to health care, limited health literacy, and lack of insurance, along with fear and anxiety. Experts anticipate that screening for colorectal cancer starting at age 45 instead of 50 will lead to earlier detection across all racial and ethnic groups in the United States (ACS, 2021).

Implications for Patient-Centered Care

- Lack of routine visits to a primary care provider is one of the strongest predictors for inadequate colorectal cancer (CRC) screening and advanced stage at presentation (Grzywacz et al., 2018).
- Patients who do not have health insurance frequently do not seek CRC screening (Grzywacz et al., 2018).
- Patients are more likely to seek and receive CRC screening when they have in-depth discussions about the importance of screening with their health care provider and understand the importance of screening (Earl et al., 2021).
- Patients who have positive social support networks (e.g., family support, church affiliation) are also more likely to seek and receive timely CRC screening (Coughlin, 2020; Earl et al., 2021).
- Removing barriers of safety, quality, and cost-effectiveness; providing patient education; and involving a patient's social support network improves the involvement of patients in CRC screening (ACS, 2021; Coughlin, 2020; Earl et al., 2021).

FIG. 47.9 Types of bedpans. From left, regular bedpan and fracture bedpan.

FIG. 47.10 Improper positioning of patient on bedpan.

FIG. 47.11 Proper position reduces patient's back strain.

of bedpans are available (Fig. 47.9). The regular bedpan, made of plastic, has a curved smooth upper end and a sharper-edged lower end and is about 5 cm (2 inches) deep. The smaller fracture pan, designed for patients with lower-extremity fractures, has a shallow upper end about 2.5 cm (1 inch) deep. The shallow end of the pan fits under the buttocks toward the sacrum; the deeper end, which has a handle, goes just under the upper thighs. The pan needs to be high enough that feces enter it.

When positioning a patient, it is important to prevent muscle strain and discomfort. Never try to lift a patient onto a bedpan. Never place a patient on a bedpan and then leave with the bed flat unless activity restrictions demand it because it forces the patient to hyperextend the back to lift the hips on the pan. The proper position for the patient on a bedpan is to elevate the head of the bed 30 to 45 degrees (Figs. 47.10 and 47.11). When patients are immobile or it is unsafe to allow them to raise their hips, it is safest for both caregivers and patients to roll them onto the bedpan (Box 47.9). Always wear gloves when handling a bedpan.

Medications. Some patients require medications to initiate and facilitate stool passage, while other patients need medications to treat diarrhea or provide symptomatic relief from diarrhea. Be aware that some patients may overuse these medications. Misuse often occurs when patients do not understand normal bowel function (Burchum and Rosenthal, 2021). Thus, in addition to providing patients information about their medications, it is important that you also provide patient education about the gastrointestinal system, including what is typically considered normal and what constitutes symptoms that need to be reported to a health care provider.

Cathartics and Laxatives. Cathartics and laxatives empty the bowel for patients experiencing constipation. They are also used to cleanse the bowel for patients undergoing GI tests and abdominal surgery. Although the terms *laxative* and *cathartic* are often used interchangeably, cathartics generally have a stronger and more rapid effect on the intestines. Teach patients about the potential harmful effects of overuse of laxatives such as impaired bowel motility and decreased response to sensory stimulus. Make sure patients understand that laxatives are not to be used long term for maintenance of bowel function.

Although patients usually take medications orally, laxatives prepared as suppositories may act more quickly because of their stimulant effect on the rectal mucosa. Suppositories such as bisacodyl act within 30 minutes. Give the suppository shortly before a patient's usual time to defecate or immediately after a meal.

Laxatives are classified by the method by which the agent promotes defecation (Table 47.2). Some prescriptions drugs (e.g., prucalopride, linaclotide, naloxegol) are used for chronic constipation, motility disorders, or irritable bowel syndrome. These medications are not used for the relief of occasional constipation.

Antidiarrheal Agents. Antidiarrheal agents fall into two groups. The specific antidiarrheal drugs treat the cause of diarrhea, while the nonspecific antidiarrheal drugs provide symptomatic relief by acting on or within the bowel (Burchum and Rosenthal, 2021). Health care providers need to determine the cause of diarrhea before they can order effective treatment. For example, if a patient's diarrhea is caused by

BOX 47.9 PROCEDURAL GUIDELINES

Assisting Patient On and Off a Bedpan

Delegation and Collaboration

The skill of providing a bedpan can be delegated to assistive personnel (AP). The nurse instructs the AP to:

- Correctly position patients with mobility restrictions or those who have therapeutic equipment such as wound drains, intravenous (IV) catheters, or traction.
- Provide perineal and hand hygiene for patient as necessary after using a bedpan.

Equipment

Clean gloves; bedpan (regular or fracture) (Fig. 47.9); bedpan cover; toilet tissue or premoisturized perineal wipes; specimen container (if necessary); plastic bag clearly labeled with date, patient's name, and identification number; basin; washcloths; towels; soap; waterproof, absorbent pads (if necessary); clean drawsheet (if necessary); stethoscope.

Procedural Steps

1. Assess patient's normal bowel elimination habits: routine pattern, character of stool, effect of certain foods/fluids and eating habits on bowel elimination, effect of stress and level of activity on normal bowel elimination patterns, current medications, and normal fluid intake.
2. Determine need for stool specimen before bedpan use.
3. Perform hand hygiene.

   CLINICAL JUDGMENT: If patient had surgery or has a gastrointestinal illness, auscultate for bowel sounds and palpate abdomen for distention.

4. Assess patient to determine level of mobility, including ability to sit upright and lift hips or turn.
5. Assess patient's level of comfort. Ask about presence of rectal or abdominal pain, presence of hemorrhoids, or irritation of skin surrounding anus.
6. Apply clean gloves. Inspect condition of perianal and perineal skin. Remove and dispose of gloves and perform hand hygiene.
7. For patient comfort prepare metal bedpan by running warm water over it for a few minutes.

   CLINICAL JUDGMENT: Use a fracture pan if the patient had a total hip replacement. An abduction pillow must be placed between the legs when turning patient to prevent dislocation of new joint.

8. Provide privacy by closing curtains around bed or door of room.
9. Raise side rail on opposite side of bed.
10. Raise bed horizontally according to your height.
11. Assist patient to the supine position.
12. Place patient who can assist on bedpan.
    a. Perform hand hygiene and apply clean gloves. Raise head of patient's bed 30 to 60 degrees.
    b. Remove upper bed linens so that they are out of the way but do not expose patient.
    c. Have patient flex knees and lift hips upward.
    d. Place hand closest to patient's head palm up under patient's sacrum to help lift. Ask patient to bend knees and raise hips. As patient raises hips, use other hand to slip bedpan under patient (see illustration). Be sure that open rim of bedpan is facing toward foot of bed. Do not force pan under patient's hips (see Fig. 47.11). (*Optional:* Have patient use overhead trapeze frame to raise hips.)
    e. *Optional:* If using fracture pan, slip it under patient as hips are raised (see illustration). Be sure that deep, open, lower end of bedpan is facing toward the foot of the bed.
13. Place patient who is immobile or has mobility restrictions on bedpan.
    a. Perform hand hygiene and apply clean gloves. Lower head of bed flat or raise head slightly (if tolerated by medical condition).

STEP 12d Placing bedpan under patient's hips.

STEP 12e Patient lifts hips as fracture pan is positioned.

    b. Remove top linens as necessary to turn patient while minimizing exposure.
    c. Assist patient to roll onto side with back toward you. Place bedpan firmly against patient's buttocks and down into mattress. Be sure that open rim of bedpan is facing toward foot of bed (see illustrations).
    d. Keep one hand against bedpan; place other around far hip of patient. Assist patient to roll back onto bedpan, flat in bed. Do not force pan under patient.
    e. Raise patient's head 30 degrees or to a comfortable level (unless contraindicated).
    f. Have patient bend knees (unless contraindicated).
14. Maintain patient's comfort, privacy, and safety. Cover patient for warmth. Place small pillow or rolled towel under lumbar curve of back. Leave room but stay close by.
15. Place nurse call system and toilet tissue within reach for patient.
16. Ensure that bed is in lowest position and raise upper side rails.
17. Remove and discard gloves and perform hand hygiene.
18. Allow patient to be alone, but monitor status and respond promptly.
19. Perform hand hygiene and apply clean gloves.
20. Remove bedpan:
    a. Perform hand hygiene and apply clean gloves. Place patient's bedside chair close to working side of bed.
    b. Maintain privacy; determine if patient can wipe own perineal area. If you clean perineal area, apply clean gloves and use several layers of toilet tissue or disposable washcloths. For female patients clean from mons pubis toward rectal area.
    c. Deposit contaminated tissue in bedpan if no specimen or intake and output (I&O) is needed. Remove and dispose of gloves and perform hand hygiene.

Continued

BOX 47.9   PROCEDURAL GUIDELINES—cont'd

Assisting Patient On and Off a Bedpan

A   B   C

STEP 13c A, Position patient on one side and place bedpan firmly against buttocks. B, Push down on bedpan and toward patient. C, Nurse places bedpan in position. (A and B from Sorrentino SA, Remmert LA: *Mosby's textbook for nursing assistants*, ed 10, St Louis, 2021, Elsevier.)

d. **For patient who is mobile:** Ask patient to flex knees, placing body weight on lower legs, feet, and upper torso; lift buttocks up from bedpan. At same time place hand farthest from patient on side of bedpan to support it (prevent spillage) and place other hand (closest to patient) under sacrum to help lift. Have patient lift and remove bedpan. Place bedpan on draped bedside chair and cover.

e. **For patient who is immobile:** Apply clean gloves. Lower head of bed. Help patient roll onto side away from you and off bedpan. Hold bedpan flat and steady while patient is rolling off; otherwise, spillage will occur. Place bedpan on draped bedside chair and cover.

f. Assist patient with hand and perineal hygiene as needed.

21. Change soiled linens, remove and dispose of gloves, and return patient to comfortable position.

22. Place bed in its lowest position. Ensure that nurse call system, drinking water, and desired personal items (e.g., books) are within easy access. *Option:* Obtain stool specimen as ordered. Wear clean gloves when emptying contents of bedpan into toilet or in special receptacle in utility room. Use spray faucet attached to most agency toilets to rinse bedpan thoroughly. Use disinfectant if required by agency; store pan. Remove and dispose of gloves.

23. Perform hand hygiene and apply clean gloves. Assess characteristics of stool. Note color, odor, consistency, frequency, amount, shape, and constituents. Assess characteristics of urine if patient voided in bedpan.

24. Evaluate patient's ability to use bedpan.

25. Inspect patient's perianal area and surrounding skin while removing bedpan.

26. **Use Teach-Back:** "Since your leg is immobilized, I want to make sure you are comfortable getting off and on the bedpan by using the trapeze to pull your torso off the bed. Show me how you use the trapeze to move your torso." Revise your instruction now or develop a plan for revised patient/family caregiver teaching if patient/family caregiver is not able to teach back correctly.

---

an infection, a specific antidiarrheal drug, such as an antibiotic may be used for treatment. A patient with a severe flare-up of ulcerative colitis, an inflammatory bowel disease, may require a steroid.

The nonspecific antidiarrheal drugs decrease intestinal motility to slow the passage of feces. As a result, the body absorbs more water through the intestinal walls, which reduces the fluidity and volume of stools. The opioids are the most effective nonspecific antidiarrheal agents (e.g., loperamide, diphenoxylate with atropine). Codeine or tincture of opium may be used for management of chronic severe diarrhea in patients with diseases such as Crohn's disease, ulcerative colitis, and acquired immunodeficiency syndrome (AIDS). Patients need to use antidiarrheal agents that contain opiates with caution because opiates are habit forming.

Enemas. An enema is the instillation of a solution into the rectum and sigmoid colon. The primary reason for an enema is to promote defecation by stimulating peristalsis. The volume of fluid instilled breaks up the fecal mass, stretches the rectal wall, and initiates the defecation reflex. Enemas are also a vehicle for medications that exert a local effect on rectal mucosa. They are used most to provide immediate relief of constipation, to empty the bowel before diagnostic tests or surgery, or to begin a program of bowel training.

Cleansing Enemas. Cleansing enemas promote the complete evacuation of feces from the colon. They act by stimulating peristalsis through the infusion of a large volume of solution or through local irritation of the mucosa of the colon. They include tap water, normal saline, soapsuds solution, and low-volume hypertonic saline. Each solution has a different osmotic effect, influencing the movement of fluids between the colon and interstitial spaces beyond the intestinal wall. Infants and children receive only normal saline because they are at greater risk for fluid imbalance.

Tap Water. Tap water is hypotonic and exerts an osmotic pressure lower than fluid in interstitial spaces. After infusion into the colon, tap water escapes from the bowel lumen into interstitial spaces. The net movement of water is low. The infused volume stimulates defecation before large amounts of water leave the bowel. Use caution if ordered to repeat tap-water enemas because water toxicity or circulatory overload develops if the body absorbs large amounts of water.

Normal Saline. Physiologically normal saline is the safest solution to use because it exerts the same osmotic pressure as fluids in interstitial spaces surrounding the bowel. The volume of infused saline stimulates peristalsis. Giving saline enemas lessens the danger of excess fluid absorption.

Hypertonic Solutions. Hypertonic solutions infused into the bowel exert osmotic pressure that pulls fluids out of interstitial spaces. The colon fills with fluid, and the resultant distention promotes defecation. Patients unable to tolerate large volumes of fluid benefit most from this type of enema, which is by design low volume. This type of enema is contraindicated for patients who are dehydrated and in young infants. A hypertonic solution of 120 to 180 mL (4 to 6 ounces) is usually effective. The commercially prepared Fleet enema is the most common.

TABLE 47.2 Common Types of Laxatives and Cathartics

Agent/Brand Name	Action	Indications	Risks
Bulk Forming Methylcellulose (Citrucel) Psyllium (Metamucil, Naturacil) Polycarbophil (Fibercon)	High-fiber content absorbs water and increases solid intestinal bulk, which will stretch intestinal wall to stimulate peristalsis. Passage of stool will occur in 12 to 24 hours. These agents must be taken with water and should be used with patients who have an adequate food and fluid intake. Patients may note increased gas formation and flatus when they first start taking these laxatives, but this will decrease after 4-5 days.	Agents are least irritating, most natural, and safest type of laxatives. Agents are drugs of choice for chronic constipation (e.g., pregnancy, low-residue diet). They also relieve mild diarrhea. If treating diarrhea, administer less water.	Agents that are in powder form could cause constipation if not mixed with at least 240 mL of water or juice and swallowed quickly. Caution is necessary with bulk-forming laxatives that also contain stimulants. Agents are not for patients for whom large fluid intake is contraindicated.
Emollient or Wetting Docusate sodium (Colace) Docusate calcium (Surfak) Docusate potassium (Dialose)	Stool softeners are detergents that lower surface tension of feces, allowing water and fat to penetrate. They increase secretion of water by intestine.	Agents are for short-term therapy to relieve straining on defecation (e.g., hemorrhoids, perianal surgery, pregnancy, recovery from myocardial infarction).	Agents are of little value for treatment of chronic constipation.
Osmotic Saline-based Magnesium citrate or citrate of magnesia Magnesium hydroxide (Milk of Magnesia) Sodium phosphate (Fleet Phospho-Soda) Polyethylene glycol (MiraLax, GlycoLax, Peglax) Lactulose (Constulose, Enulose)	Osmotic effect increases pressure in bowel to act as stimulant for peristalsis. Osmotic laxatives are any agents that pull fluid into the bowel to soften the stool and distend the bowel to stimulate peristalsis.	Saline-based agents are only for acute emptying of bowel (e.g., endoscopic examination, suspected poisoning, acute constipation). Agents may be used to treat chronic constipation.	Saline-based agents are not for long-term management of constipation or for patients with kidney dysfunction. They may cause toxic buildup of magnesium. Phosphate salts are not recommended for patients on fluid restriction.
Stimulant Cathartics Bisacodyl (Dulcolax) Castor oil Casanthranol (Peri-Colace) Correctol Senna (Ex-Lax, Senokot)	Agents cause local irritation to the intestinal mucosa, increase intestinal motility, and inhibit resorption of water in the large intestine. The rapid movement of feces causes retention of water in the stool. The drugs cause formation of a soft-to-liquid stool in 6 to 8 hours and usually contain bisacodyl or senna. These laxatives should be used occasionally because regular use of a stimulant laxative can lead to dependence on the stimulus for defecation.	Agents prepare bowel for diagnostic procedures or may be needed for those with constipation from frequent opioid use	Agents cause severe cramping. Agents are not for long-term use. Chronic use could cause fluid and electrolyte imbalances.

Soapsuds. You add soapsuds to tap water or saline to create the effect of intestinal irritation to stimulate peristalsis. Use only pure castile soap that comes in a liquid form, included in most soapsuds enema kits. Use soapsuds enemas with caution in pregnant women and older adults because they could cause electrolyte imbalance or damage to the intestinal mucosa.

A health care provider sometimes orders a high- or low-cleansing enema. The terms *high* and *low* refer to the height from which, and hence the pressure with which, the fluid is delivered. High enemas cleanse more of the colon. After the enema is infused, ask the patient to turn from the left lateral to the dorsal recumbent, over to the right lateral position. The position change ensures that fluid reaches the large intestine. A low enema cleanses only the rectum and sigmoid colon.

Oil Retention. Oil-retention enemas lubricate the feces in the rectum and colon. The feces absorb the oil and become softer and easier to pass. To enhance action of the oil, the patient retains the enema for several hours if possible.

Other Types of Enemas. Carminative enemas provide relief from gaseous distention. They improve the ability to pass flatus. An example of a carminative enema is MGW solution, which contains 30 mL of magnesium, 60 mL of glycerin, and 90 mL of water.

Medicated enemas contain drugs. An example is sodium polystyrene sulfonate (Kayexalate), used to treat patients with dangerously high serum potassium levels. This drug contains a resin that exchanges sodium ions for potassium ions in the large intestine. Another medicated enema is neomycin solution, an antibiotic used to reduce bacteria in the colon before bowel surgery. An enema containing steroid medication may be used for acute inflammation in the lower colon.

Enema Administration. Enemas are available in commercially packaged, disposable units or with reusable equipment prepared before use. Sterile technique is unnecessary because the colon normally contains bacteria. However, you need to wear gloves to prevent the transmission of fecal microorganisms.

Explain the procedure, including the position to assume, precautions to take to avoid discomfort, and length of time necessary to retain the solution before defecation. If a patient needs to take the enema at home, explain the procedure to a family member.

Giving an enema to a patient who is unable to contract the external sphincter poses difficulties. Give the enema with the patient positioned on the bedpan. Giving the enema with a patient sitting on the toilet is unsafe because the position of the rectal tubing could injure the rectal wall. Skill 47.1 outlines the steps for an enema administration.

Digital Removal of Stool. For a patient with an impaction, the fecal mass is sometimes too large to pass voluntarily. If a digital rectal examination reveals a hard stool mass in the rectum, it may be necessary to manually remove it by breaking it up and bringing out a section at a time. Digital removal is the last resort in the management of severe constipation, but it may be necessary if the fecal mass is too large to pass through the anal canal. The procedure (Box 47.10) is very uncomfortable for the patient. Excess rectal manipulation causes irritation to the mucosa, bleeding, and stimulation of the vagus nerve, which sometimes results in a reflex slowing of the heart rate (Huether et al., 2020).

Inserting and Maintaining a Nasogastric Tube. A patient's condition or situation sometimes requires special interventions to decompress the GI tract. These conditions include surgery (see Chapter 50), absence of peristalsis, trauma to the GI tract, or obstruction of the GI tract, often caused by tumors,

A nasogastric (NG) tube is a pliable hollow tube that is inserted through the patient's nasopharynx into the stomach. NG intubation has several purposes (Table 47.3). There are two main categories of NG tubes: fine- or small-bore tubes and large-bore tubes. Small-bore tubes are frequently used for medication administration and enteral feedings (see Chapter 45 for enteral feedings). Large-bore tubes, 12-Fr and above, are usually used for gastric decompression or removal of gastric secretions. The Levin and Salem sump tubes are the most common for stomach decompression. The Levin tube is a single-lumen tube with holes near the tip. It is connected to a drainage bag or an intermittent suction device to drain stomach secretions.

The Salem sump tube is preferable for stomach decompression. The tube has two lumina: one for removal of gastric contents and one to provide an air vent. A blue "pigtail" is the air vent that connects with the second lumen. When the main lumen of the sump tube is connected to suction, the air vent permits free, continuous drainage of secretions. Do not clamp off the air vent if the tube is connected to suction.

BOX 47.10 PROCEDURAL GUIDELINES
Digital Removal of Stool

Delegation and Collaboration

The skill of digitally removing stool cannot be delegated to assistive personnel (AP). In some agencies only health care providers perform this procedure. The nurse instructs the AP:

- To provide perineal care and other necessary hygiene following each bowel movement.
- To observe any evacuated stool for color and consistency.

Equipment

Bedpan, waterproof pad, water-soluble lubricant, washcloths, towels, soap, and clean gloves

Procedural Steps

1. Identify patient using at least two identifiers (e.g., name and birthday or name and medical record number) according to agency policy.
2. Perform hand hygiene, pull curtains around bed, obtain patient's baseline vital signs and assess level of comfort, auscultate bowel sounds, and palpate for abdominal distention before the procedure.
3. Explain the procedure and help patient lie on left side with knees flexed and back toward you.
4. Drape trunk and lower extremities with a bath blanket, and place a waterproof pad under buttocks. Keep a bedpan next to patient.
5. Perform hand hygiene and apply clean gloves; lubricate index finger of dominant hand with water-soluble lubricant.
6. Instruct patient to take slow, deep breaths. Gradually and gently insert index finger into the rectum and advance the finger slowly along the rectal wall.
7. Gently loosen the fecal mass by massaging around it. Work the finger into the hardened mass.
8. Work the feces downward toward the end of the rectum. Remove small pieces one at a time and discard into bedpan.
9. Periodically reassess patient's pulse and level of comfort and look for signs of fatigue. Stop the procedure if pulse rate drops significantly (check agency policy) or rhythm changes.
10. Continue to clear rectum of feces and allow patient to rest at intervals.
11. After completion, wash and dry buttocks and anal area.
12. Remove bedpan; inspect feces for color and consistency. Dispose of feces. Remove gloves by turning them inside out and then discard.
13. Help patient to toilet or on a bedpan if urge to defecate develops.
14. Perform hand hygiene. Record results of procedure by describing fecal characteristics and amount.
15. Follow procedure with enemas or cathartics as ordered by health care provider.
16. Reassess patient's vital signs and level of comfort, auscultate bowel sounds, and observe status of abdominal distention.
17. Place nurse call system in an accessible location within patient's reach.
18. Raise side rails (as appropriate) and lower bed to lowest position.

TABLE 47.3 Purposes of Nasogastric Intubation

Purpose	Description	Type of Tube
Decompression	Removal of secretions and gaseous substances from gastrointestinal (GI) tract; prevention or relief of abdominal distention (Harding et al., 2020)	Salem sump, Levin, Miller-Abbott
Enteral feeding (see Chapter 45)	Instillation of liquid nutritional supplements or feedings into stomach or small intestine for patients with impaired swallowing (Harding et al., 2020)	Duo, Dobhoff, Levin
Compression	Internal application of pressure by means of inflated balloon to prevent internal esophageal or GI hemorrhage (Harding et al., 2020)	Sengstaken-Blakemore
Lavage	Irrigation of stomach in cases of active bleeding, poisoning, or gastric dilation (Harding et al., 2020)	Levin, Ewald, Salem sump

You use clean technique when inserting an NG tube; this is not a sterile procedure. The procedure is uncomfortable. Patients experience a burning sensation as the tube passes through the sensitive nasal mucosa. When it reaches the back of the pharynx, patients sometimes begin to gag. Help them relax to make tube insertion easier. Some agencies allow the use of Xylocaine jelly or atomized lidocaine when inserting the tube because it decreases patient discomfort during the procedure. The procedure for inserting an NG tube is described in Skill 47.2.

One of the greatest needs for a patient with an NG tube is to maintain comfort. Because the tube irritates the nasal and pharyngeal mucosa, you assess the condition of the patient's nares and throat for inflammation. The tape or fixation device used to anchor the tube often becomes soiled or loosened. Change it as needed to prevent migration of the tube. Frequent lubrication of the nares may minimize discomfort. With one nostril occluded, the patient breathes through the mouth, and a dry mouth often occurs. Frequent mouth care helps minimize discomfort from a dry mouth. Water-moistened swabs or lozenges for the patient to suck may provide some relief of mouth and throat dryness. Often patients complain of a sore throat. A health care provider may order gargles with topical Xylocaine jelly to minimize the irritation.

The patency of the tube can become blocked. For example, this sometimes occurs when the tip of the tubing rests against the stomach wall or when the tube becomes blocked with thick secretions. Thus, maintaining the tube's patency is a priority. Irrigate the tube regularly with a catheter-tipped syringe filled with normal saline or warm water to prevent blockage of the tube. If an NG tube does not drain properly after irrigating, reposition it by advancing or withdrawing it slightly. A change in tube position sometimes requires a health care provider order for imaging to verify correct placement in the patient's GI tract. Consult agency policy and/or provider preferences as necessary.

Management of the Patient With Fecal Incontinence or Diarrhea. You may apply a fecal collector around the anal opening if a patient is having very frequent liquid stools and if the skin is intact. Fecal collectors can be difficult to apply when there is a deep fold between the buttocks and there is hair in the area. There are also fecal-management systems available for short-term use with high-volume diarrhea. They are intended for use primarily in acute care settings. The devices have an intra-anal soft silicone catheter with a retention balloon much like a Foley catheter for insertion into the rectal vault to divert liquid stool away from the skin in patients who are immobilized. The catheter is connected to a drainage bag for collection of the liquid fecal effluent. Refer to package insertion instructions and agency policies for appropriate use.

Continuing and Restorative Care. Regular elimination patterns should begin before a patient goes home or to an extended-care setting. With a new ostomy, a patient or a family caregiver needs to learn to manage the care that is required (Box 47.11). Other patients require bowel retraining. It is important to remember that you initiate ostomy care and bowel retraining in acute care settings. However, because these are long-term care needs, teaching usually continues in restorative care or home settings.

Care of Patients with Ostomies. Patients with temporary or permanent bowel diversions have unique elimination needs. An individual with an ostomy wears a pouch to collect effluent or output from the stoma. The pouches are odor-proof and have a protective skin barrier surrounding the stoma. Empty the pouch when it is one-third to one-half full. Change the pouching system approximately every 3 to 7 days, depending on a patient's individual needs (WOCN, 2018; Howson, 2019). Assess the stoma color. It should be pink or red. You observe the skin at each pouch change for signs of irritation or skin breakdown.

BOX 47.11   PATIENT TEACHING

Teaching Patients How to Provide Ostomy Care

Objective
- Patient/family caregiver will demonstrate how to empty and change an ostomy pouch.

Teaching Strategies
- Provide a comprehensive list of the products needed to care for the ostomy.
- Provide patient/family caregiver with supplies to last 1 to 2 weeks, including at least five ostomy appliances and accessories needed to go with them, and the contact number information for a medical supply company (Stetzer, 2021).
- Show patient/family caregiver the step-by-step approach for changing an ostomy pouch (Howson, 2019).
- Provide at least one opportunity for patient/family caregiver to empty and change the ostomy pouch while patient is in the hospital (Stetzer, 2021).
- Provide detailed instructions for diet and fluids; peristomal skin care; restrictions on lifting; resuming exercise and intimacy; and when to contact the health care provider.
- Arrange follow-up with an ostomy nurse if possible.

Evaluation
Use the principles of teach-back to evaluate patient/family caregiver learning:
- I want to be sure I explained this procedure so that you can understand it. Please show me how you will change your ostomy pouch.
- Tell me three important points about your diet and fluid intake that you need to follow now that you have an ostomy.

Skin protection is important because the effluent has digestive enzymes that cause irritant dermatitis if there is leakage on the peristomal skin. Other peristomal skin problems are fungal rashes, folliculitis, or ulcerations. Refer patients with these problems to an ostomy care nurse (WOCN, 2018) (Box 47.12).

Irrigating a Colostomy. Although this practice is not as common because of improved odor-proof pouches, some patients irrigate their sigmoid colostomies to regulate colon emptying. This process takes about an hour a day to complete but usually means that a patient wears only a mini-pouch afterward to absorb mucus from the stoma and contain gas. Specific equipment designed for ostomies is used. The equipment has a silicone cone attached by plastic tubing to a bag that will hold the irrigation fluid, which is usually warm water. Follow the routine that the patient has established for this care. Occasionally a patient with a colostomy who has constipation will have an irrigation or enema ordered. Use equipment that is designed specifically for the irrigation rather than an enema administration set used by patients without a stoma.

Pouching Ostomies. An ostomy requires a pouch to collect fecal material. An effective pouching system protects the skin, contains fecal material, remains odor free, and is comfortable and inconspicuous. A person wearing a pouch needs to feel secure enough to participate in any activity (WOCN, 2018).

Many pouching systems are available. To ensure that a pouch fits well and meets a patient's needs, consider the location of the ostomy, type and size of the stoma, type and amount of ostomy drainage, size and contour of the abdomen, condition of the skin around the stoma, physical activities of the patient, patient's personal preference, age and dexterity, and cost of equipment. A wound, ostomy, and continence nurse (WOCN) is a nurse specially educated to care for ostomy patients. A WOCN collaborates with staff nurses and patients to be sure that the patients have the best pouching system for their individual needs.

BOX 47.12   EVIDENCE-BASED PRACTICE

Recognition of Peristomal Skin Problems

PICOT Question: In patients with ostomies, what is the effect of patient knowledge and education on the prevention of peristomal skin breakdown?

Evidence Summary

Patients with an ostomy are at risk for development of peristomal skin problems, many of which are preventable (Salvadalena et al., 2020; Taneja et al., 2019). Maintaining healthy peristomal skin, with the skin around the stoma being clean, dry, and intact, is a priority following ostomy surgery (WOCN, 2018; Salvadalena et al., 2020). Patients with ileostomies and peristomal skin creases or folds are particularly at risk (Salvadalena et al., 2020). The most common cause of peristomal skin disorders is effluent, which causes skin irritation, ulceration, or erosion (Voegeli et al., 2020). Reasons for effluent leakage include poor-fitting stoma pouches, poor adhesive adherence, peristomal hernia, and surgical complications. With shorter postoperative hospital stays, it is challenging for nurses to provide the extensive patient education on pouching systems, ostomy care, and problem-solving techniques needed to prevent peristomal skin problems (WOCN, 2018). One study found that approximately 36% of patients developed a peristomal skin disorder within 90 days following their ostomy surgery, which greatly increased the likelihood of hospital readmission (Taneja et al., 2019). Patient education is an important factor in preventing complications, reducing health care costs, and helping patients return to active lives following ostomy surgery (Maculotti et al., 2019; Taneja et al., 2019).

Application to Nursing Practice

- Evaluate patients' knowledge and ability to assess their peristomal skin changes for early recognition and treatment of skin disorders.
- Provide patient education about signs and symptoms of skin disorders to ensure early identification of skin problems (Taneja et al., 2019).
- Refer patients to an ostomy nurse if assistance is needed to manage the ostomy (WOCN, 2018).
- Ensure that patients receive follow-up care and education after they transition to home to help improve outcomes and reduce health care costs (Taneja et al., 2019; Voegeli et al., 2020).

FIG. 47.12 Ostomy pouches and skin barriers. (A) One-piece pouch with Velcro closure. (B) Two-piece pouching system with separate skin barrier and attachable pouch. **NOTE:** Skin barriers need to be custom cut according to stoma size. (Courtesy Coloplast, Minneapolis, MN.)

popcorn, raw mushrooms, fresh pineapple, and Chinese cabbage can cause this problem. However, if patients eat these foods in small quantities, drink fluids with the food, and chew the food well, they are unlikely to experience any difficulty.

Psychological Considerations. After ostomy surgery patients face a variety of anxieties and concerns, from learning how to manage their stoma to coping with conflicts of self-esteem, body image, and sexuality. Provide emotional support before and after surgery (WOCN, 2018). Adjustment to a stoma takes time and is very individual. Important factors affecting adjustment to the stoma include the ability to successfully assume care of the ostomy, including emptying the pouch and changing the pouching system so that unexpected odor and leakage of stool does not occur. Inability to resume self-care sometimes causes a loss of self-esteem. The aging process often affects the ability to manage stomas, even in people who have had them for years. You need to recognize and intervene when problems resulting from advanced age such as skin changes, weight loss or gain, visual impairments, or changes in diet occur. If possible, consult with an ostomy nurse. The Wound, Ostomy and Continence Nurses Society (http://www.wocn.org) provides information and helps patients locate a WOCN. Consider referral to local ostomy groups such as those affiliated with the United Ostomy Associations of America at http://www.ostomy.org.

A pouching system consists of a pouch and skin barrier (Fig. 47.12). Pouches come in one- and two-piece systems and are flat or convex. Some pouches have the opening precut by the manufacturer; others require the stoma opening to be custom cut to a patient's specific stoma size. Newer pouches have an integrated closure; older ones use a clip to close the pouch. One of the first skills to teach a patient with a new ostomy is how to open and close the pouch. Skill 47.3 describes steps for applying an ostomy pouch.

Nutritional Considerations. After surgery it usually takes a few days for patients with new ostomies to feel that their appetite has returned to normal. Small servings of soft foods are typically more appetizing, as they would be for any patient who has had an abdominal surgery.

Patients with colostomies have no diet restrictions other than the diet discussed for normal healthy bowel function, with adequate fiber and fluid to keep the stool softly formed. Patients with ileostomies digest their food completely but lose both fluid and salt through their stoma and need to be sure to replace them to avoid dehydration. A good reminder for patients is to encourage drinking an 8-ounce glass of fluid when they empty their pouch. This helps them remember that they have greater fluid needs than they did before having an ileostomy. A condition that occurs infrequently with people with ileostomies is called a *food blockage*. Foods with indigestible fiber such as sweet corn,

REFLECT NOW

When patients have a new ostomy, they are experiencing a significant change in body image. Consider how you can help them, the family members, and other nurses to demonstrate acceptance of this change so that the patients feel less isolated and ashamed of their ostomy.

Bowel Training. A patient with chronic constipation or fecal incontinence secondary to cognitive impairment may benefit from **bowel training**, also called *habit training* (NIH, n.d.a). The training program involves setting up a daily routine. By attempting to defecate at the same time each day and using measures that promote defecation, a patient may establish a normal defecation pattern. The program requires time, patience, and consistency. A patient with cognitive impairment needs to have a family caregiver able to devote the time to the training program. A successful program includes the following:

- Assessing the normal elimination pattern and recording times when a patient is incontinent
- Incorporating principles of gerontological nursing when providing bowel retraining programs for an older adult (Box 47.13)
- Choosing a time based on the patient's pattern to initiate defecation-control measures
- Offering a hot drink (hot tea) or fruit juice (prune juice) (or whatever fluids normally stimulate peristalsis for the patient) before the defecation time
- Helping the patient to the toilet at the designated time
- Providing privacy
- Instructing the patient to lean forward at the hips while sitting on the toilet, apply manual pressure with the hands over the abdomen, and bear down but not strain to stimulate colon emptying
- An unhurried environment and a nonjudgmental caregiver
- Maintaining normal exercise within the patient's physical ability

Maintenance of Proper Fluid and Food Intake. Nutrition is especially important in helping patients maintain normal elimination patterns in continuing and restorative care settings. In choosing a diet for promoting normal elimination, consider the frequency of defecation, characteristics of feces, and types of foods that impair or promote defecation. A well-balanced diet with whole grains, legumes, fresh fruits, and vegetables promotes normal elimination. Fiber adds bulk to the stool, eliminates excess fluids, and promotes more frequent and regular movements. It is important to teach patients to drink enough fluid (about 3.7 L per day for men; about 2.7 L per day for women) along with increasing their fiber. If fluid intake is inadequate, the stool becomes hard because less water is retained in the large intestine to soften it. The amount of fiber and fluids necessary for optimal bowel function varies among individuals. Consult with a registered dietitian if a patient has chronic problems with constipation.

BOX 47.13 FOCUS ON OLDER ADULTS

Bowel Retraining

- Older age is a risk factor for having constipation. It is estimated that 55% to 67% of older people who live in nursing homes use laxatives to treat their constipation (Gustafsson et al., 2019).
- Increase fiber in diet with whole grains, legumes, fruits, and vegetables.
- A minimum of 1500 mL of fluid per day reduces the risk of constipation, with increased fluid needs during summer months and for those on diuretics with stable cardiovascular status.
- If holding a drinking cup is a problem, consider using a lighter plastic cup and filling half full, refilling frequently.
- Encourage regular exercise within the limitations imposed by other conditions.
- Ensure that patients are comfortable and safe on toilet or commode. If needed, obtain a raised toilet seat with safety bars.
- Patients need to feel at ease during elimination. Lack of privacy leads a patient to ignore the urge to defecate.
- Review all medications with a patient's health care provider to substitute medications that are less likely to cause constipation whenever possible.
- Behavioral interventions such as timed toileting help establish a scheduled time for bowel elimination. Try to maintain the same schedule each day for toileting.
- Other interventions, such as abdominal massage, reflexology, and probiotics, may help manage constipation in older adults (Baran et al., 2019; Cevik & Zaybak, 2018; Ghafar et al., 2020).

When a patient has diarrhea, low-residue foods such as white rice, potatoes, bread, bananas, and cooked cereals are recommended until the diarrhea is controlled. Discourage foods that typically cause gastric upset or abdominal cramping. Diarrhea caused by illness is sometimes debilitating. If a patient cannot tolerate foods or liquids orally, intravenous therapy with electrolyte replacement is necessary. The patient returns to a normal diet slowly, often beginning with fluids.

Sergio has been visiting Chavela for the past 3 weeks, implementing the plan of care he developed with input from Chavela. During his visit today, Chavela states that her pain is well controlled with acetaminophen and that she no longer is taking her opioid medications. She also has been working with physical therapy twice a week. However, she continues to have some problems with constipation. Thus, Sergio switches the priority of Chavela's care from pain management and identifies that helping Chavela manage her bowel elimination pattern is the priority. Chavela states that she is eating beans, tomatoes, and a salad every day. However, she sometimes forgets to drink her fluids as directed. Sergio creates a food diary for Chavela to use to track the food and fluids she takes in every day. He also works with her to identify other foods high in fiber she could add to her diet.

Chavela states, "Okay, I think I can try adding prune juice, broccoli, blueberries, avocados, corn, and popcorn this week. I also will switch from white to whole-grain bread and tortillas. My niece is going shopping with me tomorrow. I'll be sure to add all this to my grocery list."

Promotion of Regular Exercise. A daily exercise program helps prevent elimination problems. Walking, riding a stationary bicycle, or swimming stimulates peristalsis. It is recommended by the American Heart Association (2018) that adults get at least 150 minutes of exercise each week. For a patient who is temporarily immobilized, attempt ambulation as soon as possible. If the condition permits, help the patient walk to a chair on the evening of the day of surgery, and encourage the patient to walk a little more each day. Collaborate with physical therapists as needed to help patients maintain their activity level.

Maintenance of Skin Integrity. A patient with diarrhea, fecal incontinence, or an ileostomy is at risk for skin breakdown when fecal contents remain on the skin. Liquid stool usually contains digestive enzymes, which cause rapid skin breakdown. Irritation from repeated wiping with toilet tissue or frequent ostomy pouch changes further irritate the skin. Meticulous perianal skin care and frequent removal of fecal drainage is necessary to prevent skin breakdown (see Chapter 48). Clean the skin with a no-rinse cleanser and apply a barrier ointment after each episode of diarrhea. If a patient is incontinent, check on the patient frequently and change absorbent products immediately after providing thorough but gentle skin cleansing. Patients with ostomies are often unaware of the skin irritation under their ostomy wafer or think that this is a normal part of having an ostomy. Education about skin breakdown and its management are important roles for the ostomy nurse (see Box 47.12).

◆ Evaluation

Through the Patient's Eyes. The effectiveness of care depends on success in meeting the expected outcomes of self-care. Accuracy in evaluating patient outcomes is related to how well you know your patient. Optimally a patient will be able to have regular, pain-free defecation of soft, formed stools or the patient will be able to manage alterations in bowel elimination independently. The patient or family caregiver is the only one able to determine whether bowel elimination problems have been relieved and which therapies were the most effective (Fig. 47.13). This information will help you determine whether the plan of care is effective or whether you need to modify it. Use

FIG. 47.13 Critical thinking model for evaluation of bowel elimination. *WOCN*, Wound, Ostomy and Continence Nurses Society. (Clinical Judgment Measurement Model copyright © NCSBN. All rights reserved.)

critical thinking and clinical judgment to ensure that your evaluation accurately reflects the current patient situation and to determine whether the desired outcomes have been met.

Patient Outcomes. When you establish a therapeutic relationship with a patient, the patient feels comfortable to discuss the intimate details often associated with bowel elimination. Patients are less embarrassed as you help them with elimination needs. Patients relate feelings of comfort and freedom from pain as elimination needs are met within the limits of their condition and treatment. Evaluate a patient's level of knowledge regarding the establishment of a normal elimination pattern, the ability to care for an ostomy, and the promotion of skin integrity. Also determine the extent to which a patient accomplishes normal defecation. Ask the patient to describe changes in diet, fluid intake, and activity to promote bowel health. Ask the following questions when the patient's expected outcome has not been achieved:

- Do you use medications such as laxatives or enemas to help you defecate? How often?
- Which barriers prevent you from eating a diet high in fiber and participating in regular exercise?
- How much fluid do you drink in a typical day? Which types of fluids do you normally drink?
- What challenges do you encounter when you change your ostomy pouch?

Sergio is ready to evaluate the outcomes of Chavela's plan of care. Sergio begins by asking, "Where would you rate your pain over the last 24 hours?"

Chavela states, "My pain in my knee has gotten so much better. I only need to take acetaminophen first thing in the morning and right before I go to bed. I sometimes use ice packs after I walk. I'm so glad I had this surgery. It has really helped improved my pain."

Sergio then asks Chavela, "How are you doing with your activity level?"

Chavela states, "I only have to see my physical therapist once a week now. I can walk for 15 to 20 minutes without pain, and I do my exercises 2 or 3 times a day. I am getting so much stronger!"

Sergio then turns his evaluation to Chavela's bowel elimination patterns. Sergio states, "I know you have been having problems with your constipation. It sometimes takes patients a while to get their bowels to move regularly after having surgery. What changes in your diet have you been able to make and how often are your bowels moving now?"

Chavela responds, "I have been researching on the Internet different foods that are high in fiber. In addition to the foods we talked about last week, I have started eating sweet potatoes, and I have added sunflower seeds and almonds to my salads. I didn't realize how good food high in fiber can taste! My bowels are moving more regularly. Writing down how many glasses of water a day I drink really helps. My niece got me a little white board that I use to track how many glasses of water I drink. Thank you so much for taking such good care of me and for helping me learn how to stay healthy."

SAFETY GUIDELINES FOR NURSING SKILLS

Ensuring patient safety is an essential role of the professional nurse. Use sound clinical judgment by communicating clearly with members of the health care team, assessing and analyzing patient's clinical findings and incorporating the patient's priorities of care and preferences. Use the best evidence, applying professional standards, when selecting interventions to use in patient care delivery. When performing the skills in this chapter, remember the following points to ensure safe, patient-centered care:

- Instruct patients who self-administer enemas to use the side-lying position. Tell them not to self-administer an enema while sitting on the toilet because this position results in the rectal tubing causing friction that could injure the rectal wall.
- If a patient has cardiac disease or is taking cardiac or hypertensive medication, obtain a pulse rate, because manipulation of rectal tissue stimulates the vagus nerve and sometimes causes a sudden decline in pulse rate, which increases the patient's risk of fainting while on the bedpan, bedside commode, or toilet

SKILL 47.1   ADMINISTERING A CLEANSING ENEMA

Delegation and Collaboration

The skill of administering an enema can be delegated to assistive personnel (AP). **NOTE:** If a medicated enema is ordered, then it must be administered by a nurse. The nurse instructs the AP about:

- How to properly position patients who have mobility restrictions or therapeutic equipment such as drains, intravenous (IV) catheters, or traction.
- Informing the nurse immediately about patient's new abdominal pain (*exception:* a patient reports cramping) or rectal bleeding.
- Informing the nurse immediately about the presence of blood in the stool or around the rectal area or any change in vital signs.

Equipment

- Clean gloves
- Water-soluble local anesthetic lubricant (**NOTE:** Some agencies require use of water-soluble lubricant without anesthetic when nurse performs procedure.)
- Waterproof, absorbent pads
- Bedpan

- Bedpan cover *(optional, if available)*
- Bath blanket
- Washbasin, washcloths, towels, and soap
- Stethoscope

Enema Bag Administration

- Enema container
- IV pole
- Tubing and clamp (if not already attached to container)
- Appropriate-size rectal tube (adult, 22 to 30 Fr; child, 12 to 18 Fr)
- Correct volume of warmed (tepid) solution (adult, 750 to 1000 mL; adolescent, 500 to 700 mL; school-age child, 300 to 500 mL; toddler, 250 to 350 mL; infant, 150 to 250 mL)

Prepackaged Enema

- Prepackaged enema container with lubricated rectal tip (Fig. 47.14)

STEP	RATIONALE

ASSESSMENT

1. Identify patient using at least two identifiers (e.g., name and birthday or name and medical record number) according to agency policy.

Ensures correct patient. Complies with The Joint Commission standards and improves patient safety (TJC, 2021).

2. Review health care provider's order for enema and clarify reason for administration.

Order by health care provider is usually required for hospitalized patient. Order states which type of enema patient will receive.

3. Review medical record and assess last bowel movement, normal versus most recent bowel pattern, presence of hemorrhoids, and presence of abdominal pain or cramping.

Determines need for enema and type of enema used. Also establishes baseline for bowel function. Hemorrhoids may obscure rectal opening and cause discomfort or bleeding during evacuation.

4. Assess patient's mobility and ability to turn and position on side.

Determines whether assistance is needed for positioning patient.

FIG. 47.14 Prepackaged enema container with rectal tip.

Continued

SKILL 47.1	ADMINISTERING A CLEANSING ENEMA—cont'd

STEP	RATIONALE
5. Assess patient for allergy to any active ingredients of the ordered enema (e.g., Fleet enema).	Reduces risk for allergic reaction.
6. Inspect and palpate abdomen for presence of distention, and auscultate for bowel sounds.	Establishes assessment baseline before enema administration.
7. Assess patient's or family caregiver's knowledge, experience, and health literacy.	Ensures patient or family caregiver has the capacity to obtain, communicate, process, and understand basic health information (Centers for Disease Control and Prevention [CDC], 2021).
8. Assess patient's goals or preferences for how skill is to be performed or what patient expects.	Allows care to be individualized to patient.

CLINICAL JUDGMENT: *When "enemas until clear" is ordered, the water expelled may be tinted but should not contain solid fecal material. It is essential to observe contents of solution passed. Check agency policy, but a patient should receive only three consecutive enemas to prevent fluid and electrolyte imbalance.*

PLANNING

1. Perform hand hygiene.	Reduces transmission of microorganisms.
2. Prepare and organize enema equipment at bedside.	Ensures organized approach to enema administration.
3. Provide privacy by closing curtains around bed or closing door, and prepare bedside environment for patient safety.	Respects patient's right to privacy. Preparing the environment helps the nurse think about the steps needed; removing clutter from over-bed table removes barriers to completing procedure.
4. Place bedpan or bedside commode in easily accessible position. If patient will be expelling contents in toilet, ensure that the toilet is available and place patient's nonskid slippers and bathrobe in easily accessible position.	Bedpan is used if patient is unable to get out of bed. Nonskid slippers help to prevent falls when moving from bed to bathroom.
5. Explain enema administration procedure to patient and/or family caregiver.	Decreases patient anxiety and promotes patient cooperation.

IMPLEMENTATION

1. Check accuracy and completeness of each medication administration record (MAR) with health care provider's written order. Check patient's name, type of enema, and time for administration. Compare MAR with label of enema solution. **NOTE:** If enema is medicated, the skill may not be delegated to AP (see agency policy).	The health care provider's order is the most reliable source and only legal record of drugs or procedure that patient is to receive. Ensures that patient receives correct enema.
2. Perform hand hygiene.	Reduces transmission of microorganisms.
3. With side rail raised on patient's right side and bed raised to appropriate working height, help patient turn onto left side-lying position with right knee flexed. Determine that patient is comfortable and encourage patient to remain in position until procedure is complete. **NOTE:** Place a child in the dorsal recumbent position.	Allows enema solution to flow downward by gravity along natural curve of sigmoid colon and rectum, thus improving retention of solution.

CLINICAL JUDGMENT: *Patients with poor sphincter control require placement of a bedpan under the buttocks. Administering enema with patient sitting on toilet is unsafe because curved rectal tubing can abrade rectal wall.*

4. Apply clean gloves and place waterproof pad, absorbent side up, under hips and buttocks. Cover patient with bath blanket, exposing only rectal area, clearly visualizing anus.	Pad prevents soiling of linen. Blanket provides warmth, reduces exposure of body parts, and allows patient to feel more relaxed and comfortable.
5. Separate buttocks and examine perianal region for abnormalities, including hemorrhoids, anal fissure, and rectal prolapse.	Findings influence approach for inserting enema tip. Prolapse contraindicates enema.
6. Administer enema.	
a. Administer prepackaged disposable enema:	
(1) Remove plastic cap from tip of container. Tip may already be lubricated. Apply more water-soluble lubricant as needed. (see Fig. 47.14).	Lubrication provides for smooth insertion of rectal tube without causing rectal irritation or trauma. With presence of hemorrhoids, extra lubricant provides added comfort.
(2) Gently separate buttocks and locate anus. Instruct patient to relax by breathing out slowly through mouth.	Breathing out promotes relaxation of external rectal sphincter.
(3) Hold container upright and expel any air from enema container.	Introducing air into colon causes further distention and discomfort.
(4) Insert lubricated tip of container gently into anal canal toward umbilicus (see illustration). *Adult:* 7.5–10 cm (3–4 inches) *Adolescent:* 7.5 cm–10 cm (3–4 inches) *Child:* 5–7.5 cm (2–3 inches) *Infant:* 2.5–3.75 cm (1–1½ inches)	Gentle insertion prevents trauma to rectal mucosa.

STEP	RATIONALE

CLINICAL JUDGMENT: *If pain occurs or you feel resistance at any time during procedure, stop and discuss with health care provider. Do not force insertion.*

(5) Squeeze and roll plastic bottle from bottom to tip until all of solution has entered rectum and colon. Instruct patient to retain solution until urge to defecate occurs, usually 2 to 5 minutes.

Prevents instillation of air into colon and ensures that all content enters rectum. Hypertonic solutions require only small volumes to stimulate defecation.

b. Administer enema in standard enema bag:

(1) Add warmed prescribed type of solution and amount to enema bag. Warm tap water as it flows from faucet. Place saline container in basin of warm water before adding saline to enema bag. Check temperature of solution by pouring small amount of solution over inner wrist.

Hot water burns intestinal mucosa. Cold water causes abdominal cramping and is difficult to retain.

(2) If soapsuds enema (SSE) is ordered, add castile soap after water.

Reduces suds in enema bag.

(3) Raise container, release clamp, and allow solution to flow long enough to fill tubing.

Removes air from tubing.

(4) Reclamp tubing.

Prevents further loss of solution.

(5) Lubricate 6–8 cm (2½–3 inches) of tip of rectal tube with lubricant.

Allows smooth insertion of rectal tube without risk for irritation or trauma to mucosa.

(6) Gently separate buttocks and locate anus. Instruct patient to relax by breathing out slowly through mouth. Touch patient's skin next to anus with tip of rectal tube.

Breathing out and touching skin with tube promotes relaxation of external anal sphincter.

(7) Insert tip of rectal tube slowly by pointing it in direction of patient's umbilicus. Length of insertion varies (see Step 6a [4]).

Careful insertion prevents trauma to rectal mucosa from accidental lodging of tube against rectal wall. Insertion beyond proper limit can cause bowel perforation.

CLINICAL JUDGMENT: *If tube does not pass easily, do not force. Consider allowing a small amount of fluid to infuse and then try to reinsert the tube slowly. The instillation of fluid relaxes the sphincter and provides additional lubrication. If fecal impaction is present, remove it before administering the enema (see Box 47.10).*

(8) Hold tubing in rectum constantly until end of fluid instillation.

Prevents expulsion of rectal tube during bowel contractions.

(9) Open regulating clamp and allow solution to enter slowly with container at patient's hip level.

Rapid infusion stimulates evacuation of tubing and can cause cramping.

(10) Raise height of enema container slowly to appropriate level: 12 inches above anus and 18 inches above mattress. (see illustration). Instillation time varies with volume of solution administered (e.g., 1 L may take 10 minutes). You may use an IV pole to hold an enema bag once you establish a slow flow of fluid.

Allows for continuous, slow instillation of solution. Raising container too high causes rapid instillation and possible painful distention of colon. High pressure can result in bowel rupture.

STEP 6a(4) With patient in left lateral position, insert tip of commercial enema into rectum. (From Sorrentino SA, Remmert LA: *Mosby's textbook for nursing assistants*, ed 10, St Louis, 2021, Elsevier.)

STEP 6b(10) IV pole is positioned so that the enema bag is 12 inches above the anus and 18 inches above the mattress. (From Sorrentino SA, Remmert LA: *Mosby's textbook for nursing assistants*, ed 10, St Louis, 2021, Elsevier.)

Continued

SKILL 47.1	ADMINISTERING A CLEANSING ENEMA—cont'd
STEP	**RATIONALE**

CLINICAL JUDGMENT: *Temporary cessation of infusion minimizes cramping and promotes ability to retain solution. Lower container or clamp tubing if patient complains of cramping or if fluid escapes around rectal tube.*

(11) Instill all solution and clamp tubing. Tell patient that procedure is completed and that you will remove tubing.	Prevents entrance of air into rectum. Patients may misinterpret sensation of removing tube as loss of control.
7. Place layers of toilet tissue around tube at anus and gently withdraw rectal tube and tip.	Provides for patient's comfort and cleanliness.
8. Explain to patient that some distention and abdominal cramping are normal. Ask the patient to retain solution as long as possible until urge to defecate occurs. This usually takes a few minutes. Stay at bedside. Have patient lie quietly in bed if possible. (For infant or young child gently hold buttocks together for a few minutes.)	Solution distends bowel. Length of retention varies with type of enema and patient's ability to contract rectal sphincter. Longer retention promotes stimulation of peristalsis and defecation.
9. Discard enema container or disposable bag and tubing in proper receptacle. Remove and dispose of gloves and perform hand hygiene.	Reduces transmission and growth of microorganisms.
10. Help patient to bathroom or commode if possible. If using bedpan, apply clean gloves and help patient to as near a normal position for evacuation as possible (see Box 47.9).	Normal squatting position promotes defecation.
11. Observe character of stool and solution (instruct patient not to flush toilet before inspection).	Determines whether enema was effective.
12. Help patient as needed to wash anal area with warm soap and water (use gloves for perineal care).	Fecal contents irritate skin. Hygiene promotes patient's comfort.
13. Remove and discard gloves and perform hand hygiene.	Reduces transmission of microorganisms.
14. Help patient to comfortable position.	Restores comfort and sense of well-being.
15. Raise side rails (as appropriate) and lower bed to lowest position.	Promotes safety and prevents falls.
16. Place nurse call system in an accessible location within patient's reach.	Ensures patient can call for assistance if needed and promotes safety and prevents falls.

EVALUATION

1. Inspect color, consistency, and amount of stool; odor; and fluid passed.	Determines whether stool is evacuated or fluid is retained. Note abnormalities such as presence of blood or mucus.
2. Palpate for abdominal distention.	Determines whether distention is relieved.
3. Use Teach-Back: "I want to be sure I explained clearly how to position yourself in bed if you need to self-administer a Fleet enema. Show me how you would position yourself." Revise your instruction now or develop a plan for revised patient/family caregiver teaching if patient/family caregiver is not able to teach back correctly.	Teach-back is an evidence-based health literacy intervention that promotes patient engagement, patient safety, adherence, and quality. The goal of teach-back is to ensure that you have explained medical information clearly so that patients and their families understand what you communicated to them (AHRQ, 2020).

UNEXPECTED OUTCOMES AND RELATED INTERVENTIONS

1. Severe abdominal cramping, bleeding, or sudden abdominal pain develops and is unrelieved by temporarily stopping or slowing flow of solution.
- Stop enema.
- Notify health care provider.
- Obtain vital signs.

2. Patient is unable to hold enema solution.
- If this occurs during installation, slow rate of infusion.

RECORDING AND REPORTING

- Record the time, type, and volume of enema administered; patient's signs and symptoms; response to enema; and results, including color, amount, and appearance of stool.
- Report to health care provider failure of patient to defecate or any adverse reactions.

HOME CARE CONSIDERATIONS

- For patients who require enemas at home, instruct family caregiver not to exceed recommended fluid volume levels or number of enemas. Instruct family caregiver about need for slow administration of warmed fluid.
- Place waterproof padding on the bed.
- Instruct family caregiver not to give the enema on the toilet.

SKILL 47.2 INSERTING AND MAINTAINING A NASOGASTRIC TUBE FOR GASTRIC DECOMPRESSION

Delegation and Collaboration

The skill of inserting and maintaining an NG tube cannot be delegated to assistive personnel (AP). The nurse instructs the AP to:

- Measure and record the drainage from an NG tube.
- Provide oral and nasal hygiene measures.
- Perform selected comfort measures such as positioning or offering ice chips if allowed.
- Anchor the tube to patient's gown during routine care to prevent accidental displacement.
- Immediately report to the nurse any patient complaints of burning or signs of redness or irritation to nares.

Equipment

- 14 Fr or 16 Fr NG tube (smaller-lumen catheters are not used for decompression in adults because they must be able to remove thick secretions)
- Water-soluble lubricating jelly
- pH test strips 1.0 to 11.0 or higher (measure gastric aspirate acidity)
- Tongue blade

- Clean gloves
- Flashlight
- Emesis basin
- Asepto bulb or catheter-tipped syringe
- Commercial fixation device or 2.5 cm (1 inch)–wide hypoallergenic tape (*option:* Bridle nasal tube system)
- Rubber band and plastic clip to attach tube to gown
- Clamp, drainage bag, or suction machine or pressure gauge if wall suction is to be used
- Towel
- Glass of water with straw
- Facial tissues
- Normal saline
- Tincture of benzoin *(optional)*
- Gastric suction equipment
- Stethoscope
- Pulse oximeter

STEP	RATIONALE
ASSESSMENT	
1. Identify patient using at least two identifiers (e.g., name and birthday or name and medical record number) according to agency policy.	Ensures correct patient. Complies with The Joint Commission standards and improves patient safety (TJC, 2021).
2. Verify health care provider order for type of NG tube to be placed and whether tube is to be attached to suction or drainage bag.	Requires order from health care provider. Adequate decompression depends on NG suction.
3. Perform hand hygiene (apply clean gloves if risk of body fluid exposure). Inspect condition of skin integrity around patient's nares and nasal and oral cavity.	Provides baseline data on the condition of the patient's skin before NG tube insertion. All patients with any medical device are at risk for pressure injury (Delmore and Ayello, 2017).
4. Assess patient's or family caregiver's knowledge, experience, and health literacy.	Ensures patient or family caregiver has the capacity to obtain, communicate, process, and understand basic health information (CDC, 2021).
5. Ask whether patient has history of nasal surgery or congestion and allergies, and note whether deviated nasal septum is present.	Alerts nurse to potential obstruction. Insert tube into uninvolved nasal passage. Procedure may be contraindicated if surgery is recent.
6. Auscultate for bowel sounds. Palpate patient's abdomen for distention, pain, and rigidity. Remove and discard gloves if applied and perform hand hygiene.	In presence of diminished or absent bowel sounds, auscultate abdomen in all four quadrants (Ball et al., 2019). Documents baseline for any abdominal distention, gastrointestinal (GI) ileus, and general GI function, which later serves as comparison once tube is inserted.
7. Assess patient's level of consciousness and ability to follow instructions.	Determines patient's ability to help in procedure.

CLINICAL JUDGMENT: *If patient is confused, disoriented, or unable to follow commands, get help from another staff member to insert the tube.*

STEP	RATIONALE
8. Assess patient's knowledge and previous experience with NG tube and, if so, determine which naris was used.	Reveals need for patient instruction and/or support. Patient's previous experience complements any explanations and prepares patient for NG tube placement.
9. Assess patient's goals or preferences for how skill to be performed or what patient expects.	Allows care to be individualized to patient.

STEP	RATIONALE
PLANNING	
1. Perform hand hygiene.	Reduces transmission of microorganisms.
2. Prepare and organize NG tube equipment at bedside.	Ensures organized approach to NG tube insertion. Preparing the environment helps the nurse think about the steps needed; removing clutter from over-bed table removes barriers to completing procedure.
3. Provide privacy by closing curtains around bed or closing door and prepare bedside environment for patient safety.	Respects patient's right to privacy.
4. Explain NG tube insertion procedure to patient and/or family caregiver. Inform patient that procedure may cause gagging and that there may be a burning sensation in nasopharynx as tube is passed. Develop hand signal with patient if too much discomfort occurs.	Decreases patient anxiety and promotes patient cooperation. If patient is too uncomfortable or unable to tolerate procedure, the use of a hand signal will alert the nurse.

Continued

SKILL 47.2	INSERTING AND MAINTAINING A NASOGASTRIC TUBE FOR GASTRIC DECOMPRESSION—cont'd

STEP	RATIONALE

IMPLEMENTATION

STEP	RATIONALE
1. Raise the bed to working height. Position patient upright in high-Fowler's position unless contraindicated. If patient is comatose, raise head of bed as tolerated in semi-Fowler's position with head tipped forward, chin to chest.	Promotes patient's ability to swallow during procedure. Good body mechanics prevent injury to you or patient.
2. Perform hand hygiene and place bath towel over patient's chest; give facial tissues to patient. Allow to blow nose if necessary. Place emesis basin within reach.	Prevents soiling of patient's gown. Tube insertion through nasal passages may cause tearing and coughing with increased salivation.
3. Wash bridge of nose with soap and water or alcohol swab. Dry thoroughly.	Removes oils from nose to allow fixation devices to adhere completely.
4. Stand on patient's right side if right-handed, left side if left-handed. Lower side rail.	Allows easiest manipulation of tubing.
5. Instruct patient to relax and breathe normally while occluding one naris. Then repeat this action for other naris. Select nostril with greater airflow.	Tube passes more easily through naris that is more patent.

CLINICAL JUDGMENT: *Insertion of a nasogastric tube is a painful procedure. Research provides evidence that in some instances, topical lidocaine, either as a gel or spray, significantly reduces pain (Solomon and Jurica, 2017).*

STEP	RATIONALE
6. Determine length of tube to be inserted, and mark location with tape or indelible ink.	Ensures organized procedure and estimation of the proper length of tube to insert into patient.
a. *Option for adults:* Measure distance from tip of nose to earlobe to xyphoid process (NEX) of sternum (see illustration). Mark this distance on tube with tape.	Most traditional method. Length approximates distance from nose to stomach. Research has shown this method may be least effective compared with others, though more research is needed (Irving et al., 2018).
b. *Option for adults and children:* Measure distance from tip of nose to earlobe to mid-umbilicus (NEMU).	Promotes placement of the tube end holes in or closer to the gastric fluid pool (Boullata et al., 2017). Estimates proper length of tube insertion for the pediatric patient (Hockenberry et al., 2019).
c. *Option for adults:* Measure distance from xyphoid process to earlobe to nose (XEN) + 10 cm (Fan et al., 2019).	Shown to be more accurate than NEX (Fan et al., 2019).

CLINICAL JUDGMENT: *Tip of NG tube must reach stomach to avoid the risk for pulmonary aspiration, which occurs when tubes terminate in the esophagus. Research has mixed findings in regard to the best technique for estimating tube length (Fan et al., 2019). Confirmation of placement via x-ray immediately after completed insertion is still needed.*

STEP	RATIONALE
7. With small piece of tape placed around tube, mark length that will be inserted.	Indicates length of tube you will insert.
8. Prepare materials for tube fixation. Tear off a 7.5- to 10-cm (3- to 4-inch) length of hypoallergenic tape or open membrane dressing or, when available, use another fixation device (see Step 22a and b).	Fixation devices allow tube to float free of nares, thus reducing pressure on nares and preventing medical device–related pressure injuries (MDRPI) (Coyer et al., 2020).
9. Perform hand hygiene and apply clean gloves.	Reduces transmission of infection.
10. Apply pulse oximetry/capnography device and measure vital signs. Monitor oximetry/capnography during insertion.	Provides objective assessment of respiratory status before and during tube insertion.

STEP 6a Determine length of tube to be inserted.

STEP	RATIONALE
11. *Option:* Dip tube with surface lubricant into glass of room temperature water or lubricate 7.5 to 10 cm (3-4 inches) of end of tube with water-soluble lubricant (see manufacturer's directions).	*Water activates lubricant, minimizes friction against nasal mucosa, and aids in insertion of tube. Water-soluble lubricant is less toxic than oil-based lubricant if aspirated.*
12. Hand patient who is alert a cup of water if able to hold cup and swallow. Explain that you are about to insert tube.	Swallowing water facilitates tube passage. Explanation decreases patient anxiety and increases patient cooperation.
13. Explain next steps. Insert tube gently and slowly through naris to back of throat (posterior nasopharynx). Aim back and down toward patient's ear.	Natural contour facilitates passage of tube into GI tract and reduces gagging.
14. Have patient relax and flex head toward chest after tube is passed through nasopharynx.	Closes off glottis and reduces risk of tube entering trachea.
15. Encourage patient to swallow by taking small sips of water when possible. Advance tube as patient swallows. Rotate tube gently 180 degrees while inserting.	Swallowing facilitates passage of tube past oropharynx. A tug may be felt as patient swallows, indicating that tube is following desired path.
16. Emphasize need to mouth breathe during procedure.	Helps facilitate passage of tube and alleviates patient's anxiety and fear during procedure.
17. Do not advance tube during inspiration or coughing because it is likely to enter respiratory tract. Monitor oximetry/capnography.	When tube inadvertently enters airway, changes in oxygen saturation or end-tidal CO_2 (capnography) occur (Judd, 2020).
18. Advance tube each time patient swallows until you reach desired length.	Reduces discomfort and trauma to patient.

CLINICAL JUDGMENT: *Do not force NG tube. If patient starts to cough or has a drop in O_2 saturation or an increased CO_2, withdraw tube into the posterior nasopharynx until normal breathing resumes.*

19. Using penlight and tongue blade, check to be sure that tube is not positioned or coiled in back of throat.	Tube could become coiled, kinked, or enter trachea.
20. Temporarily anchor tube to nose with small piece of tape.	Securing tube prevents movement of tube and subsequent gagging. Allows for verification of tube placement.
21. Verify tube placement. Check agency policy for recommended methods of checking tube placement.	
a. Follow order for bedside x-ray film and notify radiology for examination of chest and abdomen.	Radiography remains the gold standard for verification of initial placement of tube (Irving et al., 2018; Judd, 2020; Metheny et al., 2019). This must be done before any medication or liquid is administered (ENA, 2019).
b. While waiting for x-ray film to be performed, follow these procedures: Attach Asepto or catheter-tipped syringe to end of tube. Aspirate gently back on syringe to obtain gastric contents, observing amount, color, and quality of return.	Observation of gastric contents is useful to determine initial tube placement. Gastric contents are usually green but are sometimes off-white, tan, bloody, or brown in color. Other common aspirate colors include yellow or bile stained (duodenal placement) or possibly saliva-appearing (esophagus) (Metheny et al., 2019).
c. Use pH test paper to measure aspirate for pH with color-coded pH paper. Be sure that paper range of pH is at least from 1.0 to 11.0 (see illustration).	Evidence supports pH test to be used as indicator for placement (Irving et al., 2018; Metheny et al., 2019). A pH of 1.0 to 5.0 is a good indicator of gastric placement (Judd, 2020).

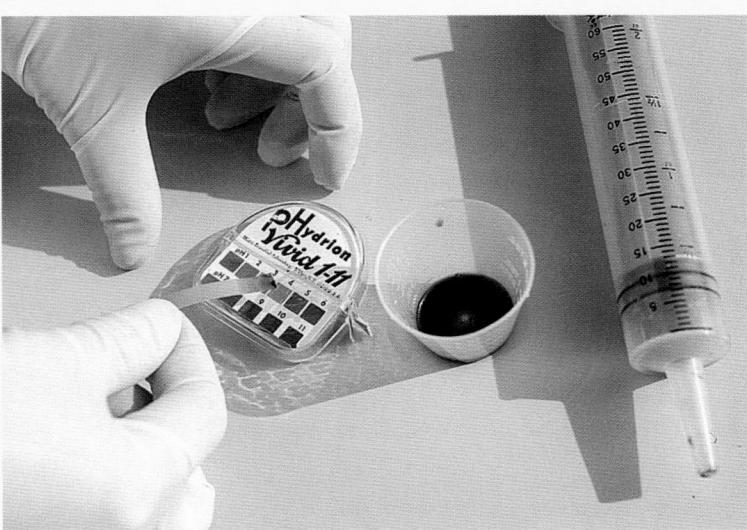

STEP 21c Checking pH of gastric aspirate.

Continued

SKILL 47.2	**INSERTING AND MAINTAINING A NASOGASTRIC TUBE FOR GASTRIC DECOMPRESSION—cont'd**

STEP	RATIONALE
22. After tube is properly inserted and positioned, either clamp end or connect it to drainage bag or suction source. Anchor tube with a fixation device, avoiding pressure on the nares. Select one of the following fixation methods.	Drainage bag is used for gravity drainage. Intermittent low suction is most effective for decompression. Proper anchoring and marking of tube help prevent migration of tube and pressure injury formation.
a. Apply tape.	
(1) Apply tincture of benzoin or other skin adhesive on bridge of patient's nose and allow it to become "tacky."	Helps tape adhere better. Protects underlying skin.
(2) Tear small horizontal slits at one-third and two-thirds length of tape without splitting tape (see illustration). Fold middle sections toward one another to form a closed strip.	The strip holds tubing to lessen rubbing against soft palate and naris.
(3) Print date and time on tape and place top end of tape over bridge of patient's nose.	
(4) Wrap bottom end of tape around tube as it exits nose (see illustration).	

STEP 22a(2) Taping method. (A) Start with piece of tape. (B) Make two slits on both sides of tape. (C) Fold middle section inward. (D) Tear a new slit in bottom of tape. Top part (a) should attach to patient's nose; bottom part (b) should be wrapped around tube.

STEP 22a(4) **A,** Tape applied to anchor nasogastric tube. **B,** Nares are free of pressure from tape and tube.

STEP	RATIONALE
b. Apply tube fixation device using shaped adhesive patch (see manufacturer directions). **(1)** Apply wide end of patch to bridge of nose (see illustration). **(2)** Slip connector around tube as it exits nose (see illustration).	Secures tube and reduces friction on nares, and decreases risk for MDRPI (Coyer, 2020).

CLINICAL JUDGMENT: *Assess at least twice daily the condition of the naris and mucosa for inflammation, blistering, excoriation, or any type of skin or tissue injury. Injury can develop for many reasons: rigidity of device rubbing against mucosa, difficulty in securing or adjusting the device to the body, increased moisture surrounding the tubing, tight securement of the device, and poor positioning or fixation of the device (Delmore and Ayello, 2017).*

STEP	RATIONALE
23. Fasten end of nasogastric tube to patient's gown with piece of tape (see illustration). Do not use safety pins to fasten tube to gown.	Anchors tubing to prevent pulling on nose.
24. Keep head of bed elevated 30 to 45 degrees (preferably 45 degrees) unless contraindicated (AACN, 2017).	Patients receiving nasogastric tube feedings have an increased risk for aspiration. Head-of-bed elevation reduces risk for aspiration of stomach contents (AACN, 2017).

CLINICAL JUDGMENT: *If inserting a Salem sump tube, keep the blue "pigtail" of the tube above level of the stomach. This prevents a siphoning action that clogs the tube. The blue "pigtail" is the air vent that connects with the second lumen When the main lumen of the sump tube is connected to suction, the air vent permits free, continuous drainage of secretions. Never clamp off the air vent, connect to suction, or use for irrigation.*

STEP	RATIONALE
25. Assist radiology as needed in obtaining ordered x-ray film of chest and abdomen.	X-ray verification is the gold standard for NG tube verification (ENA, 2019; Metheny et al., 2019; Irving et al., 2018).
26. Remove and dispose of gloves, perform hand hygiene, and help patient to comfortable position.	Reduces transmission of microorganisms.
27. Once placement is confirmed, measure amount of tube that is external and mark exit of tube at nares with indelible marker as guide for any tube displacement. Record this information in nurses' notes in electronic health record (EHR) or chart.	The mark alerts nurses and other health care providers to possible tube displacement, which will require confirmation of tube placement.

CLINICAL JUDGMENT: *Never reposition an NG tube of a patient who has had gastric surgery since positioning can rupture the suture line.*

STEP	RATIONALE
28. Attach NG tube to suction as ordered.	Suction setting is usually ordered low intermittent, which decreases gastric irritation from NG tube.

CLINICAL JUDGMENT: *If lumen of tube is narrow and secretions are thick, NG will not drain as desired. Irrigate tube (see Step 29). Consult with health care provider for higher suction setting if unable to irrigate tube because of thick secretions.*

STEP	RATIONALE
29. NG tube irrigation: **a.** Perform hand hygiene and apply clean gloves. **b.** Check tube placement in stomach by disconnecting NG tube, connecting irrigating syringe, and aspirating contents (see Step 21b). Temporarily clamp NG tube or reconnect to connecting tube and remove syringe.	Reduces transmission of microorganisms. A gastric pH of less than 5.0 is a good indication that the NG tube is in the stomach to help prevent accidental entrance of irrigating solution into lungs (Judd, 2020; Metheny et al., 2019). Verify pH values with agency policy.

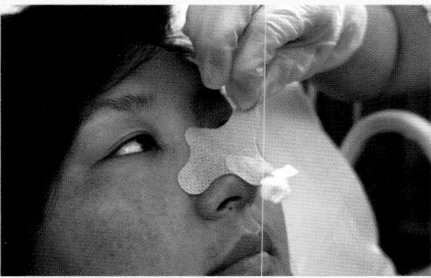

STEP 22b(1) Apply patch to bridge of nose.

STEP 22b(2) Slip connector around naso-gastric tube.

STEP 23 Fasten nasogastric tube to patient gown.

Continued

SKILL 47.2	INSERTING AND MAINTAINING A NASOGASTRIC TUBE FOR GASTRIC DECOMPRESSION—cont'd

STEP	RATIONALE
c. Empty syringe of aspirate and use it to draw up 30 mL of normal saline.	Use of saline minimizes loss of electrolytes from stomach fluids.
d. Disconnect NG from connecting tubing and lay end of connection tubing on towel.	Reduces soiling of patient's gown and bed linen.
e. Insert tip of irrigating syringe into end of NG tube. Remove clamp. Hold syringe with tip pointed at floor and inject saline slowly and evenly. Do not force solution.	Position of syringe prevents introduction of air into vent tubing, which causes gastric distention. Solution introduced under pressure causes gastric trauma.

CLINICAL JUDGMENT: *Do not introduce saline through blue "pigtail" air vent of Salem sump tube.*

STEP	RATIONALE
f. If resistance occurs, check for kinks in tubing. Turn patient onto left side. Repeated resistance should be reported to health care provider.	Tip of tube may lie against stomach lining. Repositioning on left side may dislodge tube away from stomach lining. Buildup of secretions causes distention.
g. After instilling saline, immediately aspirate or pull back slowly on syringe to withdraw fluid. If amount aspirated is greater than amount instilled, record difference as output. If amount aspirated is less than amount instilled, record difference as intake.	Irrigation clears tubing, so stomach should remain empty. Measure and document amount of irrigant fluid inserted in tube as intake.
h. Use an Asepto syringe to place 10 mL of air into blue pigtail.	Ensures patency of air vent.
i. Reconnect NG tube to drainage or suction. (Repeat irrigation if solution does not return.)	Reestablishes drainage collection; may repeat irrigation or repositioning of tube until NG tube drains properly.
30. Removal of NG tube:	
a. Verify order to remove NG tube.	A health care provider order is required for procedure.
b. Per agency policy, auscultate abdomen for presence of bowel sounds or clamp the tube for a short period of time, assessing for nausea or discomfort.	Verifies return of peristalsis. Early removal of the NG tube helps to restore normal anatomy and physiology of the GI system (Goudar et al., 2017).
c. Explain procedure to patient and reassure that removal is less distressing than insertion.	Minimizes anxiety and increases cooperation. Tube passes out smoothly.
d. Perform hand hygiene and apply clean gloves.	Reduces transmission of microorganisms.
e. Turn off suction and disconnect NG tube from drainage bag or suction. With irrigating syringe, insert 20 mL of air into lumen of NG tube. Remove tape or fixation device from bridge of nose and patient's gown.	Have tube free of connections before removal. Clears gastric fluids from tube to prevent aspiration of contents or soiling of clothing and bedding.
f. Hand patient facial tissue; place clean towel across chest. Instruct patient to take and hold breath as tube is removed.	Some patients wish to blow nose after tube is removed. Towel keeps gown from soiling. Temporary airway obstruction occurs during tube removal.
g. Clamp or kink tubing securely and pull tube out steadily and smoothly into towel held in other hand while patient holds breath.	Clamping prevents tube contents from draining into oropharynx. Reduces trauma to mucosa and minimizes patient's discomfort. Towel covers tube, which is an unpleasant sight. Holding breath helps to prevent aspiration.
h. Inspect intactness of tube.	
i. Measure amount of drainage and note character of content. Dispose of tube and drainage equipment into proper container.	Provides accurate measure of fluid output. Reduces transfer of microorganisms.
j. Clean nares and provide mouth care.	Promotes comfort.
k. Position patient comfortably and explain procedure for drinking fluids if not contraindicated. Instruct patient to notify you if nausea occurs.	Sometimes patients are not allowed anything by mouth (NPO) for up to 24 hours. When fluids are allowed, orders usually begin with small amount of ice chips each hour and increase as patient is able to tolerate more.
31. Remove and discard gloves and perform hand hygiene.	Reduces transmission of microorganisms.
32. Raise side rails (as appropriate) and lower bed to lowest position	Promotes safety and prevents falls.
33. Place nurse call system in an accessible location within patient's reach.	Ensures patient can call for assistance if needed and promotes safety and prevents falls.
34. For all procedures, clean equipment and return to proper place. Place soiled linen in utility room or proper receptacle.	Reduces transmission of microorganisms.

EVALUATION

1. Observe amount and character of contents draining from NG tube. Ask whether patient feels nauseated.	Determines whether tube is decompressing the stomach of contents.
2. Auscultate for presence of bowel sounds. Turn off suction while auscultating. Assess for nausea and patient discomfort if tube is clamped for short trial period.	Sound of suction apparatus is sometimes misinterpreted as bowel sounds. Nausea and discomfort will occur if peristalsis is not returned.
3. Palpate patient's abdomen periodically. Note any distention, pain, and rigidity.	Determines success of abdominal decompression and return of peristalsis.
4. Inspect condition of nares, nose, and all skin and tissue around NG tubing.	Evaluates onset of skin and tissue irritation.
5. Observe position of tubing.	Prevents tension applied to nasal structures.
6. Explain that it is normal if patient feels sore throat or irritation in pharynx.	Result of tube irritation.
7. **Use Teach-Back:** "I need to be sure I explained the importance of letting me know if you are nauseated. Tell me why it is important for me to know if you feel nauseated." Revise your instruction now or develop a plan for revised patient/family caregiver teaching if patient/family caregiver is not able to teach back correctly.	Teach-back is an evidence-based health literacy intervention that promotes patient engagement, patient safety, adherence, and quality. The goal of teach-back is to ensure that you have explained medical information clearly so that patients and their families understand what you communicated to them (AHRQ, 2020).

UNEXPECTED OUTCOMES AND RELATED INTERVENTIONS

1. Patient complains of nausea, or patient's abdomen is distended and painful.
   - Assess patency of tube. NG tube may be occluded or no longer in stomach.
   - Irrigate tube.
   - Verify that suction is on as ordered.
   - Notify health care provider if distention is unrelieved.
2. Patient develops irritation or erosion of skin around naris.
   - Provide frequent skin care to area.
   - Use taping method designed to reduce MDRPI (see taping methods, Step 22).
   - Consider switching tube to other naris.
3. Patient develops signs and symptoms of pulmonary aspiration: fever, shortness of breath, or pulmonary congestion.
   - Perform complete respiratory assessment.
   - Notify health care provider.
   - Obtain chest x-ray film examination as ordered.

RECORDING AND REPORTING

- Record length, size, type of gastric tube inserted, and naris in which tube was introduced. Also record patient's tolerance of procedure, confirmation of tube placement, character and pH of gastric contents, results of x-ray film, whether the tube is clamped or connected to drainage bag or to suction, and amount of suction supplied.
- Document your evaluation of patient learning.
- When irrigating NG tube, record difference between amount of normal saline instilled and amount of gastric aspirate removed on I&O sheet. Record amount and character of contents draining from NG tube every shift in nurses' notes or flow sheet.
- Record removal of tube "intact," patient's tolerance to procedure, and final amount and character of drainage.
- Report occurrence of abdominal distention, unexpected increase or sudden stoppage in gastric drainage, and patient complaining of gastric distress to health care provider.

| SKILL 47.3 | POUCHING AN OSTOMY | ▶ |

Delegation and Collaboration

The skill of pouching a new ostomy should not be delegated to assistive personnel (AP). In some agencies care of an established ostomy (4 to 6 weeks or more after surgery) can be delegated to AP. The nurse directs the AP about:

- The expected amount, color, and consistency of drainage from an ostomy
- The expected appearance of the stoma
- Special equipment needed to complete a particular patient's pouching
- The changes in a patient's stoma and surrounding skin integrity that should be reported

Equipment

- Pouch: drainable one-piece or two-piece, cut-to-fit, precut size, or moldable
- Pouch closure device, such as a clip, if needed
- Measuring guide
- Adhesive releaser *(optional)*
- Clean gloves
- Washcloth
- Towel or disposable waterproof barrier
- Basin with warm tap water
- Scissors
- Waterproof bag for disposal of pouch
- Gown and goggles (if there is a risk of splashing when emptying the pouch)

STEP	RATIONALE

ASSESSMENT

1. Identify patient using at least two identifiers (e.g., name and birthday or name and medical record number) according to agency policy.	Ensures correct patient. Complies with The Joint Commission standards and improves patient safety (TJC, 2021).
2. Perform hand hygiene and apply clean gloves.	Reduces transmission of microorganisms.
3. Observe existing skin barrier and pouch for leakage and length of time in place. Pouch should be changed every 3 to 7 days, not daily (Carmel et al., 2021). If an opaque pouch is being used, remove it to fully observe stoma. Dispose of such a pouch in proper receptacle.	Assesses effectiveness of pouching system and detects potential for problems. To minimize skin irritation, avoid unnecessary changing of entire pouching system. When pouch leaks, skin damage from effluent causes more skin trauma than early removal of wafer.

CLINICAL JUDGMENT: *Repeated leaking may indicate need for different type of pouch or addition of accessory products such as rings, seals, or paste. If the pouch is leaking, change it. Taping or patching it to contain effluent leaves the skin exposed to chemical or enzymatic irritation.*

4. Remove used pouch and skin barrier gently and observe amount of effluent. Empty the effluent if it is more than one-third to one-half full by opening the pouch and draining it into a container for measurement of output. Note consistency of effluent, and record intake and output.	Weight of pouch may disrupt seal of adhesive on skin. Monitors fluid balance and bowel function after surgery. Normal colostomy effluent is soft or formed stool, whereas normal ileostomy effluent is liquid.
5. Observe stoma for type, location, color, swelling, presence of sutures, trauma, and healing or irritation of peristomal skin (see illustrations).	Stoma characteristics influence selection of an appropriate pouching system. Convexity in skin barrier is often necessary with a flush or retracted stoma.

Continued

SKILL 47.3	POUCHING AN OSTOMY—cont'd

STEP	RATIONALE

STEP 5 (A) Budded stoma. (B) Retracted stoma. (Courtesy Jane Fellows.)

6. Observe placement of stoma in relation to abdominal contours and presence of scars or incisions. Remove and dispose of gloves; perform hand hygiene.	Determines whether current pouching system is effective or new selection is needed. Abdominal contours, scars, or incisions affect type of system and adhesion to skin surface. Reduces transmission of microorganisms.
7. Assess patient's or family caregiver's knowledge, experience, and health literacy.	Ensures patient or family caregiver has the capacity to obtain, communicate, process, and understand basic health information (CDC, 2021).
8. Explore patient's attitudes, perceptions, knowledge, and acceptance of stoma; discuss interest in learning self-care. Identify others who will be helping patient after leaving hospital.	Determines patient's willingness to learn. Facilitates teaching plan and timing of care to coincide with availability of family caregivers.
9. Assess patient's knowledge, prior experience with ostomy pouching, and feelings about procedure.	Reveals need for patient instruction and/or support.
10. Assess patient's goals or preferences for how skill will be performed or what patient expects.	Allows care to be individualized to patient.

PLANNING

1. Perform hand hygiene.	Reduces transmission of microorganisms.
2. Prepare and organize ostomy pouching equipment at bedside.	Ensures organized approach to changing the ostomy pouch.
3. Provide privacy by closing curtains around bed or closing door, and prepare bedside environment for patient safety.	Respects patient right to privacy. Preparing the environment helps the nurse think about the steps needed; removing clutter from over-bed table removes barriers to completing procedure.
4. Explain ostomy pouching procedure to patient and/or family caregiver.	Decreases patient anxiety and promotes patient cooperation.

IMPLEMENTATION

1. Have patient assume semi-reclining or supine position (same position assumed during assessment and pouching). (**Note:** Some patients with established ostomies prefer to stand.) If possible, provide patient with mirror for observation.	When patient is semi-reclining, there are fewer skinfolds, which allows for ease of application of pouching system.
2. Perform hand hygiene and apply clean gloves. Place towel or disposable waterproof barrier under patient and across patient's lower abdomen.	Reduces transmission of organisms. Protects bed linen; maintains patient's dignity.
3. If not done during assessment, remove used pouch and skin barrier gently by pushing skin away from barrier. Use adhesive releaser to facilitate removal of skin barrier. Empty pouch and dispose of it in an appropriate receptacle. Measure output if needed. **Note:** There may be no output at time of first pouch change.	Reduces skin trauma. Improper removal of pouch and barrier can cause peristomal skin irritation or breakdown.
4. Clean peristomal skin gently with warm tap water using washcloth; do not scrub skin. If you touch stoma, minor bleeding is normal. Pat skin dry. Have washcloth handy for additional cleaning if there is output from the stoma while preparing pouch.	Soap leaves residue on skin, which may irritate skin. Pouch does not adhere to wet skin. Ileostomies have frequent output, especially after eating.
5. Measure stoma (see illustration). Expect size of stoma to change for first 4 to 6 weeks after surgery.	Allows for proper fit of pouch that will protect peristomal skin.
6. Trace pattern of stoma measurement on pouch backing or skin barrier (see illustration).	Prepares for cutting opening in pouch.
7. Cut opening on backing or skin barrier wafer (see illustration). If using moldable or shape to fit barrier, use fingers to mold shape to fit stoma.	Customizes pouch to provide appropriate fit over stoma.
8. Remove protective backing from adhesive backing or wafer (see illustration).	Prepares skin barrier for placement.

STEP	RATIONALE

STEP 5 Patient measuring stoma. (Courtesy Coloplast, Minneapolis, MN.)

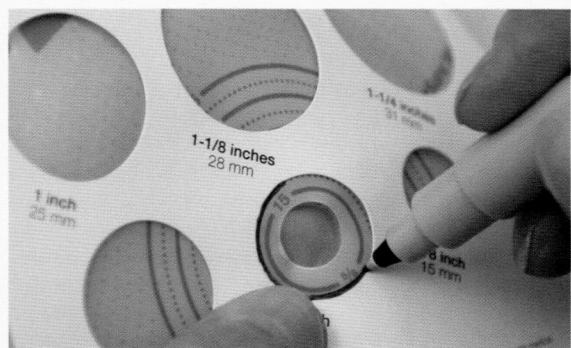

STEP 6 Trace measurement on skin barrier. (Courtesy Coloplast, Minneapolis, MN.)

STEP 7 Cut opening in wafer. (Courtesy Coloplast, Minneapolis, MN.)

STEP 8 Patient removing protective backing. (Courtesy Coloplast, Minneapolis, MN.)

STEP 9 Patient applying pouch over stoma. (Courtesy Coloplast, Minneapolis, MN.)

STEP	RATIONALE
9. Apply pouch over stoma (see illustration). Press firmly into place around stoma and outside edges. Have patient hold hand over pouch to apply heat to secure seal.	Pouch adhesives are heat and pressure sensitive and hold more securely at body temperature.
10. Close end of pouch with clip or integrated closure. Remove drape from patient. Help patient to assume comfortable position.	Ensures that pouch is secure. Contains effluent. Gives patient sense of well-being.
11. Remove and dispose of gloves and other disposables. Perform hand hygiene.	Reduces transmission of microorganisms.
12. Help patient to comfortable position.	Restores comfort and sense of well-being.
13. Raise side rails (as appropriate) and lower bed to lowest position.	Promotes safety and prevents falls.
14. Place nurse call system in an accessible location within patient's reach.	Ensures patient can call for assistance if needed and promotes safety and prevents falls.

Continued

SKILL 47.3   POUCHING AN OSTOMY—cont'd

STEP	RATIONALE

EVALUATION

1. Observe condition of skin barrier and adherence of pouch to abdominal surface

   Determines presence of leaks.

2. Observe appearance of stoma, peristomal skin, abdominal contours, suture line, and presence of any flatus during pouch change.

   Determines condition of stoma and peristomal skin and progress of wound healing.

3. Note whether there is presence of any flatus during pouch change.

   Determines whether peristalsis is returning.

4. Observe patient's and family caregiver's willingness to view stoma and ask questions about procedure.

   Determines level of adjustment and understanding of stoma care and pouch application. Allows planning for future education needs and progress toward acceptance of altered body image.

5. **Use Teach-Back:** "I want to be sure you understand what is involved in changing your ostomy pouch. Tell me what you should do to prevent your skin from becoming irritated and the frequency with which you should empty your pouch." Revise your instruction now or develop a plan for revised patient/family caregiver teaching if patient/family caregiver is not able to teach back correctly.

   Teach-back is an evidence-based health literacy intervention that promotes patient engagement, patient safety, adherence, and quality. The goal of teach-back is to ensure that you have explained medical information clearly so that patients and their families understand what you communicated to them (AHRQ, 2020).

UNEXPECTED OUTCOMES AND RELATED INTERVENTIONS

1. Skin around stoma is irritated, blistered, or bleeding or a rash is noted. May be caused by undermining of pouch seal by fecal contents, causing irritant dermatitis, or by adhesive removal, causing skin stripping or fungal or other skin eruption.
   - Remove pouch more carefully.
   - Change pouch more frequently or use different type of pouching system.
   - Consult ostomy care nurse.
2. Necrotic stoma is manifested by purple or black color, dry instead of moist texture, failure to bleed when washed gently, or tissue sloughing.
   - Report to nurse in charge or health care provider.
   - Document appearance.
3. Patient refuses to view stoma or participate in care.
   - Obtain referral for ostomy care nurse.
   - Allow patient to express feelings.
   - Encourage family support.

RECORDING AND REPORTING

- Record type of pouch and skin barrier applied, amount and appearance of effluent in pouch, size and appearance of stoma, and condition of peristomal skin. Record what patient and family caregivers are able to demonstrate and level of participation.
- Document your evaluation of patient learning.
- Record abnormal appearance of stoma, suture line, or peristomal skin or change in volume, consistency, or color of output.
- Record whether pouch change was done.
- Record patient's response to pouch change and participation in process.

HOME CARE CONSIDERATIONS

- Evaluate patient's home toileting facilities and help patient develop an ostomy care routine that is compatible with available facilities. Ostomy pouches are not flushable.
- Encourage patient to stand in front of a mirror when changing pouch to increase visibility and avoid abdominal creases that might be present in the sitting position.

▌ KEY POINTS

- The GI tract consists of the alimentary canal, which extends from the mouth to the anus, and its accessory organs.
- The GI tract and organs work together to absorb high volumes of fluids and to help maintain fluid and electrolyte balance.
- The interaction among multiple physiological and psychological factors (e.g., age, diet, stress, physical activity, health status, and medications) affects a patient's elimination patterns. For example, stress, exercise, and increased fiber and fluid intake usually increase peristalsis.
- Listening carefully to patients and their family caregivers, completing a thorough physical assessment, and using clinical judgment to recognize and analyze cues are necessary to determine the appropriate plan of care for patients with alterations in their usual elimination patterns.

- When preparing patients for gastrointestinal diagnostic and/or screening procedures, use your clinical judgment to identify a patient's educational needs. Provide timely patient education about the diagnostic or screening procedure, preparation needed (e.g., bowel prep, NPO status), and what to expect following the procedure.
- Select patient-centered nursing interventions to promote normal bowel elimination, including lifestyle changes, medications, and procedures that patients need to learn to improve bodily function and quality of life. Your clinical judgment helps you determine the best approach, when to deliver the interventions, and when adjustments are needed.
- A patient with a new ostomy has a unique combination of physical, emotional, and educational needs. Begin teaching patients early during their hospital stay to prepare them for discharge, and ensure

that they have appropriate follow-up care after discharge, which includes a referral to a nurse with specialized ostomy training.

- Nurses need to be proficient in the skills needed to relieve physical and psychological discomfort from altered bowel elimination. This proficiency ensures that the skills are delivered safely and effectively to patients and that the nurses meet the patients' individualized needs.
- Every patient has bowel elimination needs regardless of age, care setting, diagnosis, and co-morbid conditions. You use critical thinking and clinical decision making to promote normal bowel elimination and provide safe and effective nursing care to patients with altered bowel elimination.

■ REFLECTIVE LEARNING

While Sergio is completing his home visit with Chavela, her niece, Lucia, who is 28 years old, comes to visit. Lucia is tearful. Chavela asks Lucia, "Why are you so sad today?"

Lucia responds, "I just found out my Crohn's disease is getting worse, and I need to have surgery next month to get an ileostomy. I know that this will help relieve the pain I've been having for a long time, but I'm just so scared. I don't know how my boyfriend will react, and what will my friends think? Sergio, can you help me?"

- What assessment information in Lucia's situation is the most important or of immediate concern for the nurse? (Recognize Cues)
- Considering Lucia's situation, what environmental, organizational, or other factors are most relevant at this time? (Analyze Cues)
- Which nursing problems will Lucia most likely experience in this situation? Which are the most serious or the priority? (Prioritize Diagnoses)
- Identify two expected outcomes for Lucia. Consider Lucia's situation and describe the nursing and medical interventions that you could utilize to achieve the expected outcomes. Which actions should be avoided, are irrelevant, or are potentially harmful? (Generate Solutions)
- Which actions are the most appropriate and how should they be implemented? In what priority order should they be implemented? (Take Action)
- Considering the implementation of your plan of care for Lucia, what data should you gather to determine whether the interventions were effective? (Evaluate Outcomes)

■ REVIEW QUESTIONS

1. Which nursing actions does the nurse take when placing a bedpan under a patient who is immobilized? (Select all that apply.)
   1. Lift the patient's hips off the bed and slide the bedpan under the patient.
   2. After positioning the patient on the bedpan, elevate the head of the bed to a 45-degree angle.
   3. Adjust the head of the bed so that it is lower than the feet and use gentle but firm pressure to push the bedpan under the patient.
   4. Have the patient stand beside the bed, and then have the patient sit on the bedpan on the edge of the bed.
   5. Make sure the patient has a nurse call system in reach to notify the nurse when ready to have the bedpan removed.
2. During the administration of a warm tap-water enema, a patient starts to have cramping abdominal pain that he rates a 6 out of 10. What nursing action should the nurse take first?
   1. Stop the instillation.
   2. Ask the patient to take deep breaths to decrease the pain.

3. Tell the patient to bear down as he would when having a bowel movement.
   4. Continue the instillation; then administer a pain medication.
3. Which instructions does the nurse include when educating a person with chronic constipation? (Select all that apply.)
   1. Increase fiber and fluids in the diet.
   2. Use a low-volume enema daily.
   3. Avoid gluten in the diet.
   4. Take laxatives twice a day.
   5. Exercise for 30 minutes every day.
   6. Schedule time to use the toilet at the same time every day.
   7. Take probiotics 5 times a week.
4. Which skills does the nurse teach a patient with a new colostomy before discharge from the health care agency? (Select all that apply.)
   1. How to change the pouch
   2. How to empty the pouch
   3. How to open and close the pouch
   4. How to irrigate the colostomy
   5. How to determine whether the ostomy is healing appropriately
5. Place the steps for an ileostomy pouch change in the correct order.
   1. Close the end of the pouch.
   2. Measure the stoma.
   3. Cut the hole in the wafer to fit around the stoma and not leave skin exposed to the effluent.
   4. Press the pouch in place over the stoma.
   5. Remove the old pouch.
   6. Trace the correct measurement onto the back of the wafer.
   7. Assess the stoma and the skin around it.
   8. Cleanse and dry the peristomal skin.
6. A nurse is teaching a patient about the warning signs of possible colorectal cancer according to the American Cancer Society guidelines. Which statements reflect that the patient understands the teaching? (Select all that apply.)
   1. "I need to let my doctor know if my bowel habits start to change."
   2. "Blood in the stool is one warning sign I need to look for."
   3. "Muscle aches are common in people with colorectal cancer."
   4. "It is not normal to see food particles in the stool."
   5. "Some people with colorectal cancer have unexplained abdominal or back pain."
7. A nurse is teaching a patient to obtain a specimen for fecal occult blood testing using fecal immunochemical testing (FIT) at home. How does the nurse instruct the patient to collect the specimen?
   1. Get three fecal smears from one bowel movement.
   2. Obtain one fecal smear from an early-morning bowel movement.
   3. Collect one fecal smear from three separate bowel movements.
   4. Get three fecal smears when you see blood in your bowel movement.
8. What should the nurse teach family caregivers when a patient has fecal incontinence because of cognitive impairment?
   1. Cleanse the skin with antibacterial soap and apply talcum powder to the buttocks.
   2. Initiate a bowel or habit training program to promote continence.
   3. Help the patient go to the toilet once every hour.
   4. Use sanitary pads in the patient's underwear.
9. The patient states, "I have diarrhea and cramping every time I have ice cream. I am sure this is because the food is cold." Based on this assessment data, which health problem does the nurse suspect?
   1. A food allergy
   2. Irritable bowel syndrome
   3. Increased peristalsis
   4. Lactose intolerance

10. A nurse is caring for a patient with a new ileostomy and is preparing to change the pouch for the first time postoperatively. For each assessment finding listed, indicate whether it is expected or unexpected and whether follow-up is required.

Assessment Finding	Expected	Unexpected	Follow-Up Needed?	
			YES	NO
1. An experienced AP is beginning to pouch the ostomy.				
2. The patient's last name is spelled incorrectly on the armband.				
3. Effluent is leaking around the wafer of the ostomy pouch.				
4. The stoma is pink-red and moist.				
5. The patient is having trouble attending to patient education regarding how to change the ostomy bag.				
6. The patient states, "I can't watch you change this bag."				

Answers: 1. 2, 5; **2.** 1; **3.** 1, 5, 6; **4.** 1, 2, 3, 5; **5.** 5, 8, 7, 2, 6, 3, 4, 1; **6.** 1, 2, 5; 7. 3; **8.** 2; **9.** 4; **10.** See Evolve.

Rationales for Review Questions can be found on the Evolve website.

REFERENCES

Agency for Healthcare Research and Quality (AHRQ): *Health Literacy Universal Precautions Toolkit 2nd edition*, Rockville, MD, 2020. Agency for Healthcare Research and Quality. https://www.ahrq.gov/health-literacy/quality-resources/tools/literacy-toolkit/healthlittoolkit2-tool5.html. Accessed September 18, 2021.

American Association of Critical-Care Nurses (AACN): AACN practice alert: prevention of aspiration in adults, *Crit Care Nurse* 37(3):88, 2017.

American Cancer Society (ACS): *Colorectal cancer*, 2021. http://www.cancer.org/Cancer/ColonandRectumCancer/DetailedGuide/index. Accessed May 10, 2021.

American Cancer Society (ACS): *Gap in cancer death rates between blacks and whites narrows*, 2019. https://www.cancer.org/latest-news/gap-in-cancer-death-rates-between-blacks-and-whites-narrows.html. Accessed May 12, 2021.

American Heart Association: *American Heart Association recommendations for physical activity in adults and kids*, 2018. https://www.heart.org/en/healthy-living/fitness/fitness-basics/aha-recs-for-physical-activity-in-adults. Accessed May 12, 2021.

Ball J, et al: *Seidel's guide to physical examination*, ed 9, St. Louis, 2019, Elsevier.

Boullata J, et al: ASPEN safe practices for enteral nutrition therapy. *J Parenter Enteral Nutr* 41(1):15, 2017.

Burchum JR, Rosenthal LD: *Lehne's pharmacology for nursing care*, ed 11, St. Louis, 2021, Elsevier.

Carmel JE, et al: *Wound, ostomy, and continence nurses Society: core curriculum ostomy management*, ed 2, Philadelphia, 2021, Wolters Kluwer.

Centers for Disease Control and Prevention (CDC): *What is health literacy?* 2021. https://www.cdc.gov/healthliteracy/learn/index.html. Accessed September 18, 2021.

Delmore BA, Ayello EA: Pressure injuries caused by medical devices and other objects: a clinical update, *Am J Nurs* 117(12):36, 2017.

Dickison P, et al: Integrating the National Council of State Boards of Nursing Clinical Judgment Model into nursing educational frameworks, *J Nurs Educ* 58(2):72, 2019.

Edelman CL, Kudzma EC: *Health promotion throughout the lifespan*, ed 9, St. Louis, 2018, Elsevier.

ENA Clinical Practice Guideline Committee (ENA): *Clinical practice guideline: gastric tube placement verification*, *J Emerg Nurs* 45(3):306.e1–306.e19, 2019. doi:10.1016/j.jen.2019.03.011.

Harding MM, et al: *Lewis's medical-surgical nursing: assessment and management of clinical problems*, ed 11, St. Louis, 2020, Elsevier.

Hockenberry ML, et al: *Wong's nursing care of infants and children*, ed 11, St. Louis, 2019, Elsevier.

Howson R: Stoma education for the older person is about keeping it as simple as 1, 2, 3, *J Stomal Ther* 39(3):20, 2019.

Huether SE, et al: *Understanding pathophysiology*, ed 7, St. Louis, 2020, Elsevier.

Judd M: Confirming nasogastric tube placement in adults. *Nursing* 50(4): 43, 2020.

Mayo Clinic: *Water: how much should you drink every day?* 2020. http://www.mayoclinic.org/healthy-living/nutrition-and-healthy-eating/in-depth/water/art-20044256. Accessed May 9, 2021.

Mayo Clinic: *Illeoanal anastomosis (J-pouch) surgery*, 2021. https://www.mayoclinic.org/tests-procedures/j-pouch-surgery/about/pac-20385069. Accessed May 9, 2021.

McDonald L, et al: Clinical practice guidelines for *Clostridium difficile* infection in adults and children, *Clin Infect Dis* 66(7):1, 2018. https://www.idsociety.org/practice-guideline/clostridium-difficile/. Accessed May 9, 2021.

National Institutes of Health (NIH): *Bowel control problems (fecal incontinence)*, n.d.a. https://www.niddk.nih.gov/health-information/digestive-diseases/bowel-control-problems-fecal-incontinence. Accessed May 9, 2021.

National Institutes of Health (NIH): *Constipation*, n.d.b. https://www.niddk.nih.gov/health-information/digestive-diseases/constipation. Accessed May 9, 2021.

Setya A, et al: *Fecal impaction*, Treasure Island, FL, 2020, StatPearls Publishing. https://www.ncbi.nlm.nih.gov/books/NBK448094/. Accessed May 9, 2021.

Simren M, et al: Update on Rome IV Criteria for colorectal disorders: implications for clinical practice, *Curr Gastroenterol Rep* 19(4):15, 2017.

Solomon R, Jurica K: Closing the research-practice gap: increasing evidence-based practice for nasogastric tube insertion using education and an electronic order set, *J Emerg Nurs* 43(2):133, 2017.

Stetzer MN: Essential ostomy knowledge for nurses: promoting adaptation in children with new ostomy and their caregivers, *Pediatr Nurs* 47(2):71, 2021.

The Joint Commission (TJC): *2021 National Patient Safety Goals*, Oakbrook Terrace, IL, 2021, The Commission. https://www.jointcommission.org/en/standards/national-patient-safety-goals/. Accessed May 12, 2021.

US Food and Drug Administration (USFDA): *Food allergies*, 2021. https://www.fda.gov/food/food-labeling-nutrition/food-allergies. Accessed May 9, 2021.

Wound, Ostomy and Continence Nurses Society (WOCN): Management of the adult patient with a fecal or urinary ostomy – an executive summary, *J Wound Ostomy Continence Nurs* 45(1):50, 2018.

RESEARCH REFERENCES

Baran A, et al: The effects of abdominal massage in the management of constipation in elderly people: a randomized controlled trial, *Top Geriatr Rehabil* 35(2):134, 2019.

Cevik K, Zaybak A: The effect of reflexology on constipation in the elderly, *Int J Caring Sci* 11:309, 2018.

Coughlin SS: Social determinants of colorectal cancer risk, stage, and survival: a systematic review, *Int J Colorectal Dis* 35(6):985, 2020.

Coyer F, et al: Securement to prevent device-related pressure injuries in the intensive care unit: a randomised controlled feasibility study, *Int Wound J* 17(6):1566, 2020.

Earl V, et al: Barriers and facilitators to colorectal cancer screening in African-American men, *Dig Dis Sci* 2021. https://doi.org/10.1007/s10620-021-06960-0.

Fan PEM, et al: Adequacy of different measurement methods in determining nasogastric tube insertion lengths: an observational study, *Int J Nurs Stud* 92:73, 2019.

Ghafar MYA, et al: Evaluation of the efficacy of probiotics (MCP® BCMC® Strains) treating constipation in elderly patients with multiple chronic co-morbidities: a randomized controlled trial, *J Nutr Health Aging* 24(10):1066, 2020.

Goudar BV, et al: Early removal versus conventional removal of nasogastric tube after abdominal surgery: a prospective randomized controlled study, *Int Surg J* 4(1):229, 2017.

Grzywacz V, et al: Racial disparities and factors affecting Michigan colorectal cancer screening, *J Racial Ethn Health Disparities* 5:901, 2018.

Gustafsson M, et al: Constipation and laxative use among people living in nursing homes in 2007 and 2013, *BMC Geriatr* 38, 2019. https://doi.org/10.1186/s12877-019-1054-x. Accessed May 12, 2021.

Irving SY, et al: Pediatric nasogastric tube placement and verification: best practice recommendations from the NOVEL Project, *Nutr Clin Pract* 33(6):921, 2018.

Maculotti D, et al: Sport and physical activity after stoma surgery: a survey of patient experiences, *Gastrointest Nurs* 17(Suppl 9):S30, 2019.

Massirfufulay KM, et al: The prevalence, incidence, and correlates of fecal incontinence among older people residing in care homes: a systematic review, *J Am Med Dir Assoc* 20(8):956, 2019.

Metheny NA, et al: A review of guidelines to distinguish between gastric and pulmonary placement of nasogastric tubes, *Heart Lung* 48:226, 2019.

Salvadalena G, et al: Lessons learned about peristomal skin complications: secondary analysis of the ADVOCATE Trial, *J Wound Ostomy Continence Nurs* 47(4):357, 2020.

Taneja C, et al: Risk and economic burden of peristomal skin complications following ostomy surgery, *J Wound Ostomy Continence Nurs* 46(2):143, 2019.

Van Bree SHW, et al: Auscultation for bowel sounds in patients with ileus: an outdated practice in the ICU? *Neth J Crit Care* 26(4): 142, 2018.

Voegeli D, et al: Factors influencing the incidence of peristomal skin complications: evidence from a multinational survey on living with a stoma, *Gastrointest Nurs* 18(Suppl 4):S31, 2020.

Skin Integrity and Wound Care

OBJECTIVES

- Examine risk factors that contribute to pressure injury formation.
- Explain the pressure injury staging system.
- Discuss the normal process of wound healing.
- Contrast the differences in wound healing by primary and secondary intention.
- Summarize factors that impede or promote wound healing.
- Explain the differences in nursing care with acute and chronic wounds.
- Assess a patient with impaired skin integrity.
- Develop a nursing care plan for a patient with impaired skin integrity.
- Apply clinical judgment when providing care to patients at risk for or with actual impaired skin integrity.

KEY TERMS

Abrasion
Approximated
Blanchable hyperemia
Blanching
Debridement
Dehiscence
Epithelialization
Eschar
Evisceration
Exudate
Fluctuance
Friction
Granulation tissue

Hemostasis
Induration
Laceration
Medical adhesive–related skin injury (MARSI)
Medical device–related pressure injury (MDRPI)
Negative-pressure wound therapy (NPWT)
Nonblanchable erythema
Pressure injury
Primary intention
Puncture wound

Purulent
Reactive hyperemia
Sanguineous
Secondary intention
Serosanguineous
Serous
Shearing force
Slough
Tissue ischemia
Vacuum-assisted closure (V.A.C.)
Wound
Wound drainage evacuators

MEDIA RESOURCES

http://evolve.elsevier.com/Potter/fundamentals/
- Review Questions
- Audio Glossary
- Case Study with Questions
- Concept Map Creator

- Video Clips
- Skills Performance Checklists
- Content Updates
- Answers to QSEN Activity and Review Questions

Kelly Johnson is a first-year nursing student assigned to care for Mrs. Stein. Mrs. Stein, an 86-year-old patient, fell at her assisted-living residence and fractured her left hip. Prior to this fall she was independent in activities of daily living, enjoyed congregate meals at her facility, and participated in social activities. She had hip replacement surgery 2 days ago, and her postoperative physical therapy activities are progressing slowly. She is reluctant to move or participate in physical therapy because of pain and fear of falling. When asked to participate in repositioning, she slides her body up and down in bed while protecting her hip. She does not like the staff to reposition her in bed and is fearful of assisting because of pain. Her significant medical problems include heart failure, hypertension, and diabetes mellitus Type 2. She becomes slightly diaphoretic when moving, causing her to sweat on movement. Kelly notes drainage on her gown over the area of the left hip.

Kelly reviews Mrs. Stein's electronic health record (EHR). The nurses' notes describe Mrs. Stein's reluctance to reposition or actively participate in rehabilitation activities in physical therapy. Although Mrs. Stein has orders for pain medication, she rarely takes it because she is "afraid of addiction." The night nurse documented a red, blistered area on the right hip and reddened area on the sacral region.

Skin, the largest organ in the body, is a protective barrier against disease-causing organisms and a sensory organ for pain, temperature, and touch; it also synthesizes vitamin D. Injury to the skin poses risks to an individual's safety. Wound healing is a complex cellular and biochemical process, and it is affected by systemic and local factors such as underlying disease processes (e.g., diabetes mellitus), the cause of the wound (e.g., chemical versus penetrating wounds), and condition of the wound (Calis et al., 2019). Your clinical judgment must integrate scientific and nursing knowledge to thoroughly assess and monitor skin integrity and identify patient risks for or with actual impaired skin integrity. A critical thinking approach to this process will yield clinical decisions for how to plan, implement, and evaluate interventions to maintain skin integrity or improve wound healing.

SCIENTIFIC KNOWLEDGE BASE

Skin

The skin has two layers: the epidermis and the dermis (Fig. 48.1). They are separated by a membrane, often referred to as the *dermal-epidermal junction.* The epidermis, or the top layer, has several layers. The stratum corneum is the thin outermost layer of the epidermis. It consists of flattened, dead, keratinized cells. The cells originate from the innermost epidermal layer, commonly called the *basal layer.* Cells in the basal layer divide, proliferate, and migrate toward the epidermal surface. After they reach the stratum corneum, they flatten and die. This constant movement ensures replacement of surface cells sloughed during normal desquamation or shedding. The thin stratum corneum protects underlying cells and tissues from dehydration and prevents entrance of certain chemical agents. The stratum corneum allows evaporation of water from the skin and permits absorption of certain topical medications.

The dermis, the inner layer of the skin, provides tensile strength; mechanical support; and protection for the underlying muscles, bones, and organs. It differs from the epidermis in that it contains mostly connective tissue and few skin cells. Collagen (a tough, fibrous protein), blood vessels, and nerves are found in the dermal layer. Fibroblasts, which are responsible for collagen formation, are the only distinctive cell type within the dermis.

Understanding skin structure helps you understand the risks for impaired skin integrity and promote wound healing. Intact skin protects patients from chemical and mechanical injury. When the skin is injured, the epidermis functions to resurface the wound and restore the barrier against invading organisms, and the dermis responds to restore the structural integrity (collagen) and the physical properties of the skin. The normal aging process alters skin characteristics and makes skin more vulnerable to damage (Box 48.1).

Pressure Injuries

Pressure injury, pressure ulcer, decubitus ulcer, and *bedsore* are terms used to describe impaired skin integrity related to unrelieved, prolonged pressure. The most current terminology is **pressure injury** (Fig. 48.2), which is consistent with the recommendations of the National Pressure Ulcer Advisory Panel (Edsberg et al., 2016). A pressure injury is localized damage to the skin and underlying soft tissue, usually developing over a bony prominence or related to pressure from a medical device or other device. The injury can present as intact skin, a blister, or an open ulcer and may be painful. The injury occurs because of intense and/or prolonged pressure or pressure in combination with shear. The tolerance of soft tissue for pressure and shear may also be affected by microclimate

---

BOX 48.1 FOCUS ON OLDER ADULTS

Skin-Associated Issues

When caring for the older adult, there are several skin-related issues to consider when assessing skin and risk for skin breakdown. Age-related changes such as reduced skin elasticity, decreased collagen, and thinning of underlying muscle and tissues cause the older adult's skin to be easily torn in response to mechanical trauma, especially shearing forces. The attachment between the epidermis and dermis becomes flattened in older adults, allowing the skin to be easily torn in response to mechanical trauma (e.g., tape removal) (Meiner and Yeager, 2019). Existing medical conditions and polypharmacy are factors that interfere with wound healing. Aging causes a diminished inflammatory response, resulting in slow epithelialization and wound healing (Doughty and Sparks, 2016).

Implications for Practice

- There is a decreased barrier function and less protection from excessive moisture, shear, friction, and pressure.
- Aging skin has decreased epidermal turnover, and healing requires more time (Meiner and Yeager, 2019).
- Comorbidities (e.g., dementia, hemiplegia) increase the risk for incontinence and subsequent skin and tissue injury in frail older adults (Ferris and Harding, 2019).
- When removing any adhesive dressings or tape, gently release the skin from the tape; do not pull the tape away from the skin. Release the skin from the adhesive by gently pushing the skin from the adhesive.
- Decreased subcutaneous tissue reduces padding protection over bony prominences and increases patients' risk of skin injury related to shear (Huether et al., 2020).
- There is a decrease in subcutaneous padding over bony prominences, where impaired skin integrity and injury to other tissues are most likely to occur (Wysocki, 2016).

Stratum corneum
Stratum lucidum
Stratum granulosum
Epidermis
Stratum spinosum
Melanocyte
Stratum basale

Papillae
Dermis
Papillary region
Reticular region

FIG. 48.1 Layers of skin. (From Applegate E: *The anatomy and physiology learning system,* ed 4, St Louis, 2011, Saunders.)

FIG. 48.2 Pressure injury with tissue necrosis.

(skin temperature, humidity, and airflow next to the skin), nutrition, perfusion, comorbidities, and condition of the soft tissue (European Pressure Ulcer Advisory Panel [EPUAP]/National Pressure Injury Advisory Panel [NPIAP]/Pan Pacific Pressure Injury Alliance [PPPIA], 2019a).

A number of contributing factors are associated with pressure injuries. Any patient experiencing decreased mobility, decreased sensory perception, fecal or urinary incontinence, and/or poor nutrition is at risk for pressure injury development. Examples of patients who are at risk for the development of pressure injuries include the following (EPUAP/NPIAP/PPPIA, 2019a):

- Older adults
- Individuals who have experienced trauma
- Individuals with spinal cord injuries (SCIs)
- Individuals who have sustained a fractured hip
- Individuals in long-term homes or community care, the acutely ill, or those in a hospice setting
- Individuals with diabetes mellitus
- Patients in critical care settings

Pathogenesis of Pressure Injuries. Pressure is the major element in the cause of pressure injuries. Tissue receives oxygen and nutrients and eliminates metabolic wastes via the blood. Pressure or other factors that interfere with blood flow in turn interfere with cellular metabolism and the function or life of the cells. Prolonged, intense pressure affects cellular metabolism by decreasing or obliterating blood flow, resulting in tissue ischemia and ultimately tissue death.

Current theory suggests that skin and soft tissue damage can begin at the surface and progress inward or begin at the muscle and progress outward, depending on causation (Wound, Ostomy, and Continence Nurses Society [WOCN], 2016). Top-down damage (superficial) is thought to be caused by superficial shear or friction, presenting as red skin (Stage 1 pressure injury). Bottom-up (deep) damage is believed to be caused by several pressure-related factors: (1) pressure intensity, (2) pressure duration, and (3) tissue tolerance.

Pressure Intensity. A classic research study identified capillary closing pressure as the minimal amount of pressure required to collapse a capillary (e.g., when the pressure exceeds the normal capillary pressure range of 15–32 mm Hg) (Burton and Yamada, 1951). Therefore, when the pressure applied over a capillary exceeds the normal capillary pressure and the vessel is occluded for a prolonged period, **tissue ischemia** occurs. If the patient has reduced sensation and cannot respond to the discomfort of the ischemia, tissue ischemia and tissue death result.

The clinical presentation of obstructed blood flow occurs when evaluating areas of pressure. After a period of tissue ischemia, if the pressure is relieved and the blood flow returns, the skin turns red. The effect of this redness is vasodilation (blood vessel expansion), called *hyperemia* (redness). You assess an area of hyperemia by pressing a finger over the affected area. If it blanches (turns lighter in color) and the erythema returns when you remove your finger, the hyperemia is transient and is an attempt to overcome the ischemic episode, thus called **blanchable hyperemia**. However, if the erythematous area does not blanch (**nonblanchable erythema**) when you apply pressure, deep tissue damage is probable.

Blanching occurs when the normal red tones of the light-skinned patient are absent. When checking for pressure injuries in patients with darkly pigmented skin, dark skin may not show the blanch response (Box 48.2). Inspect suspected pressure-related skin alterations with an adjacent or opposite area of the body for comparison. Skin inspection should include assessment of changes in skin tissue, consistency (firm versus boggy [less than normal stiffness or mushy] when palpated), sensation (pain), edema, and warmer or cooler temperature (EPUAP/NPIAP/PPPIA, 2019a; EPUAP/NPIAP/PPPIA, 2019b; Bryant and Nix, 2016a).

Pressure Duration. Low pressure over a prolonged period and high-intensity pressure over a short period are two concerns related to duration of pressure. Both types of pressure cause tissue damage. Extended pressure occludes blood flow and nutrients and contributes to cell death (Pieper, 2016). Clinical implications of pressure duration include evaluating the amount of pressure (checking skin for nonblanching hyperemia) and determining the amount of time for which a patient tolerates pressure (checking to be sure after relieving pressure that the affected area blanches).

Tissue Tolerance. The ability of tissue to endure pressure depends on the integrity of the tissue and the supporting structures. The extrinsic

---

BOX 48.2   CULTURAL ASPECTS OF CARE

Skin Assessment of Pressure Injuries in Patients With Darkly Pigmented Skin

There is evidence that Stage 1 pressure injuries are underdetected in individuals with darkly pigmented skin. Clinical judgment and clinical decision making are essential when assessing for and detecting cyanosis and other changes in skin color, and assessment is more of a challenge in patients with darkly pigmented skin (EPUAP/NPIAP/PPPIA, 2019a). Patients with darkly pigmented skin cannot be assessed for pressure injury risk by examining only skin color. Skin temperature and skin moisture must also be assessed (WOCN, 2016). Areas of redness are more difficult to assess on darkly pigmented skin. Color differentiation of cyanosis varies according to skin pigmentation. In patients with darkly pigmented skin, you need to know the individual's baseline skin tone. For example, for patients of different cultures with darkly pigmented skin, do not confuse the normal hyperpigmentation of Mongolian spots that are seen on the sacrum with cyanosis.

Implications for Patient-Centered Care
- Use natural lighting.
- When assessing darkly pigmented skin, assess skin temperature and sub-epidermal moisture. Slight moistening of the skin aids in detection of early pressure injury (EPUAP/NPIAP/PPPIA, 2019a).
- Carefully inspect any discoloration over pressure areas and surrounding skin for temperature changes, edema, change in tissue consistency, and pain (EPUAP/NPIAP/PPPIA, 2019a). Assess localized skin color changes. Any of the following may appear:
  - Color remains unchanged when pressure is applied.
  - Color changes occur at site of pressure, which differ from patient's usual skin color.
  - If patient previously had a pressure injury, that area of skin may be lighter than original color.
  - Localized area of skin may be purple/blue or violet instead of red. Purple or maroon discoloration may indicate deep tissue injury (WOCN, 2016).
- Assessment of skin temperature changes: Circumscribed area of intact skin may be warm to touch. As tissue changes color, intact skin will feel cool to touch. **Note:** Gloves may decrease sensitivity to changes in skin temperature (WOCN, 2016; EPUAP/NPIAP/PPPIA, 2019a).
- Localized heat (inflammation) is detected by making comparisons with surrounding skin. Localized area of warmth eventually will be replaced by area of coolness, which is a sign of tissue devitalization.
- Edema may occur with induration of more than 15 mm in diameter and may appear taut and shiny.
- Palpate tissue consistency in surrounding tissues to identify any changes in tissue consistency between area of injury and normal tissue (EPUAP/NPIAP/PPPIA, 2019a).
- Patient complains of discomfort at a site that is predisposed to pressure injury development (e.g., bony prominence, under medical devices).

factors of shear, friction, and moisture affect the ability of the skin to tolerate pressure: the greater the degree to which the factors of shear, friction, and moisture are present, the more susceptible the skin will be to damage from pressure. The second factor related to tissue tolerance is the ability of the underlying skin structures (blood vessels, collagen) to help redistribute pressure. Systemic factors such as poor nutrition, aging, hydration status, and low blood pressure affect the tolerance of the tissue to externally applied pressure.

Risk Factors for Pressure Injury Development.

The goal in preventing the development of pressure injuries is early identification of an at-risk patient and the implementation of prevention strategies. The *Prevention and Treatment of Pressure Ulcers/Injuries: Quick Reference Guide 2019* (EPUAP/NPIAP/PPPIA, 2019b) represents findings from an extensive literature review on the prevention and management of pressure injuries. A variety of factors predispose a patient to pressure injury formation. These factors may be related to a disease (e.g., reduced peripheral circulation from diabetes mellitus), or they may be secondary to an illness (e.g., decreased sensation following a cerebrovascular accident).

Impaired Sensory Perception. Patients with altered sensory perception for pain and pressure are more at risk for impaired skin integrity. They are unable to feel when a part of their body undergoes increased, prolonged pressure or pain. Thus a patient who cannot feel or sense that there is pain or pressure is at risk for the development of pressure injuries.

Impaired Mobility. Patients who are unable to independently change positions are at risk for pressure injury. For example, a patient who is seriously ill will be weakened and less likely to turn independently. A patient who has had a traumatic injury or surgery on an extremity will be limited in the ability to easily reposition the affected limb. Patients with SCIs have decreased or absent motor and sensory function and are unable to reposition off bony prominences.

Alteration in Level of Consciousness. Patients who are comatose, confused, or disoriented; those who have expressive aphasia or the inability to verbalize; and those with changing levels of consciousness are unable to protect themselves from pressure injury. Also, patients who are confused or disoriented may be able to feel pressure but are not always able to understand how to relieve it or communicate their discomfort. A patient in a coma cannot perceive pressure and is unable to move voluntarily to relieve pressure.

Shear. Shear force is the sliding movement of skin and subcutaneous tissue while the underlying muscle and bone are stationary (Bryant, 2016). Shear force occurs when the head of the bed is elevated, and the sliding of the skeleton starts but the skin is fixed because of friction with the bed (Fig. 48.3). It also occurs when transferring a patient from bed to stretcher when a patient's skin is pulled across the bed. (This can be avoided using friction-relief devices during safe patient handling.) When shear is present, the skin and subcutaneous layers adhere to the surface of the bed, and the layers of muscle and the bones slide in the direction of body movement. The damage that shear causes occurs at the deeper fascial level of the tissues over the bony prominence (Cooper et al., 2020; Pieper, 2016). The underlying tissue capillaries are stretched and angulated by the shear force. As a result, necrosis occurs deep within the tissue layers. The tissue damage is deep in the tissues and causes undermining of the dermis and is a cause of pressure injury development.

Friction. The force of two surfaces moving across one another such as the mechanical force exerted when skin is dragged across a coarse surface such as bed linens is called **friction** (WOCN, 2016). Unlike shear injuries, friction injuries affect the epidermis or top layer of the skin (superficial skin loss). The denuded skin appears red and painful

FIG. 48.3 Shear exerted in sacral area.

and is sometimes referred to as a *sheet burn*. A friction injury occurs in patients who are restless, in those who have uncontrollable movements such as spastic conditions, and in those whose skin is dragged rather than lifted from the bed surface during position changes or transfer to a stretcher. This type of injury should not be classified as a pressure injury (EPUAP/NPIAP/PPPIA, 2019b). In addition, friction and shear result when a medical device is used for a prolonged period of time. Friction can cause impaired sensation and reduced circulation, and it can alter the skin's microclimate, which is the heat and humidity at the skin-device interface from moisture (Cooper et al., 2020).

Moisture. The presence and duration of moisture on the skin increase the risk of pressure injury. Moisture reduces the resistance of the skin to other physical factors such as pressure, friction, or shear. Prolonged moisture softens skin, making it more susceptible to damage. The term *moisture-associated skin damage* (MASD) is defined as inflammation and erosion to the skin caused by prolonged exposure to various sources of moisture, including wound drainage, urine or stool, perspiration, wound exudate, mucus, or saliva (Francis, 2020).

Classification of Pressure Injuries

A staging system exists for classifying pressure injuries. Accurate staging requires knowledge of the skin layers. A major drawback of a staging system is that you cannot stage an injury when it is covered with necrotic tissue because the necrotic tissue is covering the depth of the injury. In serious wounds with necrotic tissue, the wound must be debrided or removed (if appropriate to the overall treatment plan) to expose the wound base to allow for assessment. The benefit of a staging system is that each stage indicates the type of topical treatments and pressure-relieving surfaces that will most likely promote healing.

Pressure injury staging describes the pressure injury depth at the time of assessment. Once you stage the pressure injury, the stage endures even as it heals. For example, a Stage 3 pressure injury does not progress from a Stage 3 to a Stage 1. A Stage 3 pressure injury demonstrating signs of healing is described as a healing Stage 3 pressure injury. In 2016 the NPIAP changed the terminology from "pressure ulcer" to "pressure injury" and refined the classification and staging system, which was reviewed in 2019 (EPUAP/NPIAP/PPPIA, 2019b; Edsberg et al., 2016):

- **Stage 1 pressure injury:** Intact skin with a localized area of non-blanchable erythema, which may appear differently in darkly pigmented skin (Fig. 48.4A).
  - Presence of blanchable erythema or changes in sensation, temperature, or firmness may precede visual changes. Color changes do not include purple or maroon discoloration; these may indicate deep tissue pressure injury.
- **Stage 2 pressure injury:** Partial-thickness skin loss with exposed dermis
  - Partial-thickness loss of skin with exposed dermis (see Fig. 48.4B). The wound bed is viable, pink or red, and moist and may also

Lightly Pigmented   Darkly Pigmented

Dark Eschar   Slough Eschar

FIG. 48.4 Diagram of pressure injury stages. (A) Stage 1 pressure injury. (B) Stage 2 pressure injury. (C) Stage 3 pressure injury. (D) Stage 4 pressure injury. (E) Deep tissue injury. (F) Unstageable pressure injury. (Used with permission of the European Pressure Ulcer Advisory Panel [EPUAP], National Pressure Injury Advisory Panel [NPIAP], and Pan Pacific Pressure Injury Alliance [PPPIA]. Haesler E, ed. *Treatment of pressure ulcers/injuries: quick reference guide*, 2019, EPUAP/NPIAP/PPPIA.)

present as an intact or ruptured serum-filled blister. Adipose tissue (fat) is not visible, and deeper tissues are not visible. Granulation tissue, slough, and eschar are not present. These injuries commonly result from adverse microclimate and shear in the skin over the pelvis and shear in the heel. This stage should not be used to describe MASD, including incontinence-associated dermatitis (IAD), intertriginous dermatitis (ITD), medical adhesive–related skin injury (MARSI), or traumatic wounds (skin tears, burns, abrasions).

- **Stage 3 pressure injury:** Full-thickness skin loss
  - Full-thickness loss of skin, in which adipose tissue (fat) is visible in the ulcer and granulation tissue and epibole (rolled wound edges) are often present (see Fig. 48.4C). Slough and/or eschar may be visible. The depth of tissue damage varies by anatomical location; areas of significant adiposity can develop in deep wounds. Undermining and tunneling may occur. Fascia, muscle, tendon, ligament, cartilage, and/or bone are not exposed. If

slough or eschar obscures the extent of tissue loss, this is classified as an unstageable pressure injury.

- **Stage 4 pressure injury:**
  - Full-thickness skin and tissue loss with exposed or directly palpable fascia, muscle, tendon, ligament, cartilage, or bone in the ulcer (see Fig. 48.4D). Slough and/or eschar may be visible. Epibole (rolled edges), undermining, and/or tunneling often occurs. Depth varies by anatomical location. If slough or eschar obscures the extent of tissue loss, this is classified as an unstageable pressure injury.

- **Unstageable pressure injury:** Obscured full-thickness skin and tissue loss
  - Full-thickness skin and tissue loss in which the extent of tissue damage within the ulcer cannot be confirmed because it is obscured by slough or eschar (see Fig. 48.4F). If slough or eschar is removed, a Stage 3 or Stage 4 pressure injury will be revealed. Stable eschar (i.e., dry, adherent, intact without erythema or

fluctuance) on the heel or ischemic limb should not be softened or removed.

- **Deep-tissue pressure injury:**
  - Intact or nonintact skin with localized area of persistent non-blanchable deep red, maroon, purple discoloration, or epidermal separation revealing a dark wound bed or blood-filled blister (see Fig. 48.4E). Pain and temperature change often precede skin color changes. Discoloration may appear differently in darkly pigmented skin. This injury results from intense and/or prolonged pressure and shear forces at the bone-muscle interface. The wound may evolve rapidly to reveal the actual extent of tissue injury or may resolve without tissue loss. If necrotic tissue, subcutaneous tissue, granulation tissue, fascia, muscle, or other underlying structures are visible, this indicates a full-thickness pressure injury (classified as unstageable, Stage 3, or Stage 4). Do not use the category *deep-tissue pressure injury* to describe vascular, traumatic, neuropathic, or dermatological conditions.

The EPUAP/NPIAP/PPPIA (2019a, 2019b) guidelines suggest that when conducting a skin assessment for staging, carefully inspect an individual with darkly pigmented skin. Note any discoloration over pressure areas, and surrounding skin should be assessed more closely for temperature changes, edema, and changes in tissue consistency and pain. For additional aspects of assessing darkly pigmented skin, see Box 48.2.

Medical Device–Related Pressure Injuries

A medical device–related pressure injury (MDRPI) occurs when the skin or underlying tissues are subjected to sustained pressure or shear from medical devices or equipment (Jackson et al., 2019). MDRPI can result "from the use of devices designed and applied for diagnostic or therapeutic purposes. The resultant pressure injury generally conforms to the pattern or shape of the device" (EPUAP/NPIAP/PPPIA, 2019a). Critically ill patients and neonates are particularly vulnerable to MDRPI (Cooper et al., 2020; Maklebust and Magnan, 2016). Because MDRPIs form faster than a Stage 1 or 2 pressure injury, proactive assessment and prevention measures are critical.

Most MDRPIs occur at the face and head region, and the ears specifically (Cooper et al., 2020; Kayser et al., 2018; Pittman et al., 2015). The most common devices linked with MDRPIs are oxygen tubing and masks. Additional at-risk devices include nasal cannulas, cervical collars, indwelling urinary (Foley) catheters and bedside collection tubing, braces, endotracheal tubes, and pulse oximetry devices (see Table 48.1). It is important to be aware of devices, as well as medical adhesives that may secure the devices, that are used for patient care that could damage edematous tissue and to plan care to cushion or redistribute pressure away from susceptible skin and prevent injury.

When you care for patients with medical devices, observe the area of the skin either covered by the device or under the device. For example, inspect the nares and ears of a patient with an oxygen catheter. Inspect areas where a patient has lain on top of a wound drainage tube. Pressure can develop under casts, braces, medical collars, and other orthopedic devices (Table 48.1). Also be aware that even a standard bed mattress can cause an MDRPI (Fig. 48.5). Individualize the frequency of pressure checks for each patient and base your assessment on the response of the skin to the external pressure. Consider adults with medical devices (e.g., tubes, drainage systems, and oxygen devices) to be at greater risk for pressure injuries (Black and Kalowes, 2016).

Medical Adhesive–Related Skin Injury

Tape and other medical adhesives, such as those used to secure ostomy devices, can cause skin injury. Medical adhesive–related skin injury (MARSI) is an occurrence in which erythema and/or other manifestation

of cutaneous abnormality (including but not limited to vesicle, bulla, erosion, or skin tear) persists 30 minutes or more after removal of a device or adhesive securing the device (Kelly-O'Flynn et al., 2020; EPUAP/NPIAP/PPPIA, 2019a). It occurs when the attachment between the skin and an adhesive is stronger than the skin cells, causing the surface epidermal to detach from the underlying layers.

Assess for the presence of an MARSI by looking for skin stripping or tape burns. These develop from repeated removal of adhesives and application of devices, common around intravenous insertion sites. This is a common overlooked and underestimated skin injury. Thus care is needed in removing adhesives, and following removal there must be a comprehensive assessment of skin exposed to adhesive tape or other adhesive devices (Fumarola et al., 2020; McNichol et al., 2013).

Wounds

A wound is a disruption of the integrity and function of tissues in the body (Baranoski et al., 2016). A wound may result from trauma to the skin causing laceration or puncture or from surgical intervention. The two major types of wounds are open and closed. In a closed wound the surface of the skin remains intact, but the underlying tissues may be damaged. Examples of closed wounds are contusions, hematomas, or Stage 1 pressure injuries. With open wounds the skin is split, incised, or cracked, and the underlying tissues are exposed to the outside environment. Open wounds create a significant risk for infection to develop. All wounds require specific treatments based on a thorough assessment of the wound and a patient's overall condition and the goal of treatment. Understanding the etiology of a wound is important because the treatment will vary depending on the underlying disease process.

Wound Classifications. There are many ways to classify surgical and traumatic wounds. Wound classification systems describe onset and duration of healing process (e.g., the status of skin integrity, cause of the wound, or severity or extent of tissue injury or damage) (Table 48.2) and descriptive qualities of the pressure injury or wound tissue such as color (Fig. 48.6). Wound classification enables you to understand the risks associated with a wound and implications for healing.

Process of Wound Healing. Wound healing involves integrated physiological processes. The tissue layers involved and their capacity for regeneration determine the mechanism for repair for any wound (Calis et al., 2019; Doughty and Sparks, 2016). Table 48.2 reviews the classification of wounds by onset and duration and healing process. Wounds can also be classified by the extent of tissue loss: partial-thickness wounds that involve only a partial loss of skin layers (the epidermis and superficial dermal layers) and full-thickness wounds that involve total loss of the skin layers (epidermis and dermis) (Doughty and Sparks, 2016). Partial-thickness wounds are shallow in depth, moist, and painful, and the wound base generally appears red. A full-thickness wound extends into the subcutaneous layer and can be painful, and the depth and tissue type vary depending on body location. The significance of determining whether an injury is a partial- or full-thickness wound lies in the mechanism of healing. A partial-thickness wound heals by regeneration, and a full-thickness wound heals by forming new tissue, a process that can take longer than the healing of a partial-thickness wound.

A clean surgical incision is an example of a wound with little tissue loss. The surgical incision heals by primary intention (Fig. 48.7A). The skin edges are approximated, or closed, and the risk of infection is low. Healing occurs quickly, with minimal scar formation, if infection and secondary breakdown are prevented (Doughty and Sparks, 2016). In contrast, a wound involving loss of tissue such as a burn, Stage 2 pressure injury, or severe laceration heals by secondary intention. The wound is left open until it becomes filled by scar tissue. It takes longer

TABLE 48.1   Strategies to Prevent Medical Device–Related Pressure Injuries

Device	Pressure Areas	Prevention Strategies[a]
Feeding tubes and nasogastric tubes	Nares Skin on nasal bridge	Secure tube using pressure-relieving techniques, which direct the pressure from the tube away from the nares (see Chapters 45 and 47). Reposition tube.
Endotracheal tubes	Lips Tongue	Tubes should be moved laterally to relieve pressure over different portions of the lips and tongue (EPUAP/NPIAP/PPPIA, 2019a). Ensure that the depth of the endotracheal tube depth does not change when moving the tube laterally (EPUAP/NPIAP/PPPIA, 2019a). See Chapter 41.
Nasotracheal tubes	Nose, nasal bridge Nares	Remove securing device daily and inspect for pressure injury (Camacho-Del Rio, 2018) (see Chapter 41). Reposition.
Tracheostomy tubes	Front of neck and stoma site	Remove securing device daily. Increase stoma care (see Chapter 41).
Oxygen cannula and tubing	Ears Nose	Apply dressing to external ear. Periodically remove cannula to relieve pressure and inspect for pressure injury (Cox et al., 2020; Schallom et al., 2015) (see Chapter 41).
Noninvasive positive pressure ventilation (NIPPV)/bilevel positive airway pressure (BiPAP)	Forehead Nose, nasal bridge	Apply protective dressing or liquid skin barrier to bridge of nose or forehead before application of device. If appropriate, remove mask periodically for a few minutes (Cox et al., 2020).
Wound drainage tubing	Area immediately next to drainage tube Adjacent area during patient position changes	Apply appropriate dressing around drainage tube insertion site. Check tubing placement with each position change. Instruct patient not to lie on the tubing (Cooper et al., 2020; Pittman et al., 2015).
Indwelling urinary catheter	Thighs Female: urethra, labia Male: tip of penis	Provide meticulous perineal care (see Chapter 40). Anchor and secure catheter to reduce pressure (see Chapter 46).
Orthopedic devices	All areas where device (e.g., cast or brace) comes in contact with patient's skin and tissues	When possible and not contraindicated, inspect under the device.
Neck collar	Neck and occipital region Scalp	Remove hard collars as soon as possible and replace with softer collar (Cooper et al., 2020; Black et al., 2015). Inspect scalp daily.
Compression stockings	Calf Behind knee Heel Toes	Verify proper fit. To reduce pressure and risk of injury to skin and underlying tissue, remove stockings twice daily for at least 1 hour (Black et al., 2015) (see Chapter 39).
Immobilization devices	Wrists Ankles	Apply dressing between immobilizer and patient's skin (Black et al., 2015). Verify that there is some space between immobilizer and patient's skin. With assistive personnel present, remove restraints one at a time to inspect skin (see Chapter 27).

[a] In addition to routine inspection and cleaning of skin under and around medical device.

for a wound to heal by secondary intention; therefore the chance of infection is greater. If scarring from secondary intention is severe, loss of tissue function is often permanent (see Fig. 48.7B).

The best environment for wound healing is moist and free of necrotic tissue and infection. No specific studies demonstrate the benefit of using one cleaner over another for pressure injuries. In most cases water or saline is sufficient for cleansing a clean wound (WOCN, 2016). Hydrogen peroxide was once widely used but is now known to cause tissue damage. When any wound is contaminated with debris, necrotic tissue, or heavy drainage, use a cleaner that is noncytotoxic to healthy tissue. If the tissue in the wound is devitalized, consult with a patient's health care provider to consider debridement, which is the removal of devitalized tissue. Debridement is accomplished by the choice of dressing and the use of enzyme preparations or surgical or

laser techniques (see Skills 48.2 and 48.3). The choice of the type of debridement depends on a patient's overall condition, the condition of the wound, and the type of devitalized tissue (WOCN, 2016).

Wound Repair. The wound repair process differs depending on whether a wound is partial or full thickness. Partial-thickness wounds are shallow, involving loss of epidermis and possible loss of dermis. Full-thickness wounds extend into the dermis and heal by scar formation because deeper structures do not regenerate. Stage 3 and Stage 4 pressure injuries are examples of full-thickness wounds.

Partial-Thickness Wound Repair. Three components are involved in the healing process of a partial-thickness wound: inflammatory response, epithelial proliferation (reproduction) and migration, and reestablishment of the epidermal layers. Tissue trauma causes the *inflammatory response,*

TABLE 48.2   Wound Classification

Description	Causes	Implications for Healing
Onset and Duration		
Acute		
Wound that proceeds through an orderly and timely reparative process that results in sustained restoration of anatomical and functional integrity	Trauma Surgical incision	Wound edges are clean and intact.
Chronic		
Wound that fails to proceed through an orderly and timely process to produce anatomical and functional integrity	Vascular compromise, chronic inflammation, or repetitive insults to tissue (Doughty and Sparks, 2016)	Continued exposure to insult impedes wound healing.
Healing Process		
Primary Intention		
Wound that is closed	Hematoma, surgical incision that is sutured or stapled	Healing occurs by epithelialization; heals quickly with minimal scar formation.
Secondary Intention		
Wound edges not closed or approximated	Surgical wounds that have tissue loss or contamination	Wound heals by granulation tissue formation, wound contraction, and epithelialization.
Tertiary Intention		
Wound that is left open for several days; then wound edges are approximated (see Fig. 48.4C)	Wounds that are contaminated and require observation for signs of inflammation	Closure of wound is delayed until risk of infection is resolved (Doughty and Sparks, 2016).

FIG. 48.5 Formation of pressure injury on heel resulting from external pressure from bed mattress. (Courtesy Janice Colwell, RN, MS, CWOCN, FAAN, Clinical Nurse Specialist, University of Chicago Medicine.)

which in turn causes redness and swelling to the area with a moderate amount of serous exudate. This response generally is limited to the first 24 hours after wounding. The epithelial cells begin to regenerate, providing new cells to replace the lost cells. The *epithelial proliferation and migration* start at both the wound edges and the epidermal cells lining the epidermal appendages, allowing for quick resurfacing. Epithelial cells begin to migrate across a wound bed soon after the wound occurs. A wound that is kept moist can resurface in 4 days, whereas one left open to air can resurface within 6 to 7 days. The difference in the healing rate is related to the fact that epidermal cells migrate only across a moist surface. In a dry wound the cells migrate down into a moist level before migration can occur (Huether et al., 2020; Doughty and Sparks, 2016). New epithelium is only a few cells thick and must undergo *reestablishment of the epidermal layers*. The cells slowly reestablish normal thickness and appear as dry pink tissue.

Full-Thickness Wound Repair. The four phases involved in the healing process of a full-thickness wound are hemostasis (coagulation), the inflammatory phase, proliferation and new tissue formation, and remodeling and maturation (Huether et al., 2020).

Hemostasis. Hemostasis involves a series of physiological events designed to control blood loss, establish bacterial control, and seal the defect that occurs when there is an injury. During hemostasis injured blood vessels constrict and platelets gather to stop bleeding. Clots form a fibrin matrix that later provides a framework for cellular repair. Hemostasis is impaired when patients are on anticoagulants or have specific diseases that affect platelet production or blood clotting.

Inflammatory Phase. In the inflammatory phase damaged tissue and mast cells secrete histamine, resulting in vasodilation of surrounding capillaries and movement or migration of serum and white blood cells (WBCs) into the damaged tissues. This results in localized redness, edema, warmth, and throbbing. The inflammatory response is beneficial, and there is no value in attempting to cool the area or reduce the swelling unless the swelling occurs within a closed compartment (e.g., SCI, ankle, or neck) (Kelechi et al., 2017).

Leukocytes (WBCs) reach a wound within a few hours. The primary-acting WBC is the neutrophil, which begins to ingest bacteria and small debris. The second important leukocyte is the monocyte; these cells transform into macrophages. The macrophages are the "garbage cells" that clean a wound of bacteria, dead cells, and debris by phagocytosis. Macrophages continue the process of clearing a wound of debris and release growth factors that attract fibroblasts, the cells that synthesize collagen (connective tissue). Collagen appears as early as the second day and is the main component of scar tissue (Huether et al., 2020).

In a clean wound the inflammatory phase establishes a clean wound bed. The inflammatory phase is prolonged if too little inflammation occurs, as in a debilitating disease such as cancer or after administration

FIG. 48.6 Wounds classified by color assessment. (A) Black wound. (B) Yellow wound. (C) Red wound. (D) Mixed-color wound. (A and D courtesy Scott Health Care—A Mölnlycke Company, Philadelphia, PA; B and C from Bryant RA, Nix DP, editors: *Acute and chronic wounds: current management concepts,* ed 5, St Louis, 2016, Elsevier.)

FIG. 48.7 (A) Wound healing by primary intention such as a surgical incision. Edges of wound are pulled together and approximated with sutures or staples, and healing occurs by connective tissue deposition. (B) Wound healing by secondary intention. Wound edges are not approximated, and healing occurs by granulation tissue formation and contraction of the wound edges. (From Black JM, Hawks JH: *Medical-surgical nursing: clinical management for positive outcomes,* ed 8, St Louis, 2009, Mosby.)

of steroids. Too much inflammation also prolongs healing because arriving cells compete for available nutrients. An example is a wound infection in which the increased metabolic energy requirements present in an infected wound compete for the available calorie intake.

Proliferation and New Tissue Formation Phase. With the appearance of new blood vessels as reconstruction progresses, the proliferative and new tissue formation phase begins 3 to 4 days after injury and can last as long as 2 weeks (Huether et al., 2020). The main activities during this phase are the filling of a wound with granulation tissue, wound contraction, and wound resurfacing by means of epithelialization. Fibroblasts are present in this phase and are the cells that synthesize collagen, providing the matrix for granulation. Collagen mixes with the granulation tissue to form a matrix that supports the reepithelialization. Collagen provides strength and structural integrity to a wound. During this period, a wound contracts to reduce the area that requires healing. Finally, the epithelial cells migrate from the wound edges to resurface. In a clean wound the proliferative phase accomplishes the following: the vascular bed is reestablished (granulation tissue), the area is filled with replacement tissue (collagen, contraction, and granulation tissue), and the surface is repaired (epithelialization). Impairment of healing during this stage usually results from systemic factors such as age, anemia, hypoproteinemia, and zinc deficiency.

Remodeling and Maturation. Remodeling and maturation, the final phase of wound healing, begin several weeks after injury and continues for more than a year, depending on the depth and extent of the wound (Huether et al., 2020). The collagen scar continues to reorganize and gain strength for several months. However, a healed wound usually does not have the tensile strength of the tissue it replaces. Collagen fibers undergo remodeling or reorganization before assuming their normal appearance. Usually scar tissue contains fewer pigmented cells (melanocytes) and has a lighter color than normal skin. In individuals with darkly pigmented skin, the scar tissue may be more highly pigmented than surrounding skin.

Complications of Wound Healing

Hemorrhage. Hemorrhage, or bleeding from a wound site, is normal during and immediately after initial trauma. However, hemostasis occurs within several minutes unless large blood vessels are involved or a patient has poor clotting function. Hemorrhage occurring after hemostasis indicates a dislodged surgical suture, a clot, infection, or erosion of a blood vessel by a foreign object (e.g., a drain). Hemorrhage may occur externally or internally. For example, if a surgical suture is dislodged from a blood vessel, bleeding occurs internally within the tissues, and there may not be visible signs of blood unless a surgical drain is present. A surgical drain may be inserted into tissues beneath a wound to remove fluid that collects in underlying tissues.

You detect internal hemorrhaging by looking for distention or swelling of the affected body part, a change in the type and amount of drainage from a surgical drain, or signs of hypovolemic shock. A hematoma is a localized collection of blood underneath the tissues. It appears as swelling and a change in color, sensation, or warmth and often takes on a bluish discoloration. A hematoma near a major artery or vein is dangerous because pressure from the expanding hematoma obstructs blood flow.

External hemorrhaging is obvious. You examine dressings covering a wound for bloody drainage, and you observe for blood underneath the body. If bleeding is extensive, the dressing soon becomes saturated, and frequently blood drains from under the dressing and pools beneath the patient. Observe all wounds closely, particularly surgical wounds, in which the risk of hemorrhage is great during the first 24 to 48 hours after surgery or injury.

Infection. Wound infection is one of the most common health care–associated infections (see Chapter 28). In acute care settings, surgical site infections (SSIs) are a significant problem. Approximately 27 million surgical procedures are performed in the United States each year, with up to 5% resulting in SSIs. An SSI is associated with substantial morbidity that can endanger a patient's life, increase the number of days in the hospital, and increase health care costs (Darouiche, 2017). Microorganisms infect a surgical wound through various forms of contact, such as from the touch of a contaminated health care provider or surgical instrument, through the air, or through contact on or in a person's body and then spread into the wound. Incidence of SSIs is tracked by the Centers for Disease Control and Prevention (CDC) National Healthcare Safety Network (NHSN) (CDC, 2020).

All wounds have some level of bacterial burden; however, few wounds become infected (Stotts, 2016b). Wound infection develops when microorganisms invade the wound tissues. The local clinical signs of wound infection include erythema; increased amount of wound drainage; change in appearance of a wound drainage (thick, color change, presence of odor); and periwound warmth, pain, or edema. A patient may have a fever and an increase in WBC count. Laboratory tests such as a wound culture or tissue biopsy assist in determining presence of wound infection and the causative microorganism.

Some contaminated or traumatic wounds show signs of infection early, within 2 to 3 days. SSIs occur within 30 days of surgery; risk factors include hyperglycemia, smoking, untreated peripheral vascular disease, cancer, obesity, age, and emergency and abdominal surgery (Burden and Thornton, 2018; Johns Hopkins Medicine, 2021). If an SSI occurs, the patient will have a fever, tenderness, and pain at the wound site and an elevated WBC count (Stryja, 2018). The edges of the wound will appear inflamed. If drainage is present, it is odorous and purulent, which causes a yellow, green, or brown color, depending on the causative organism (Table 48.3).

Dehiscence. When a surgical incision fails to heal properly, the layers of skin and tissue separate. This most commonly occurs before collagen formation (3–11 days after injury). Dehiscence is the partial or total separation of wound layers. A patient who is at risk for poor wound healing (e.g., poor nutritional status, infection, or underlying diseases such as diabetes mellitus or peripheral vascular disease) is at risk for dehiscence. It can occur 5 to 12 days after suturing, at a time when wound repair is at its peak. Approximately half of dehiscence occurrences are associated with wound infection. Obesity is another risk because of the constant strain placed on the wounds and the poor healing qualities of adipose tissue (Huether et al., 2020). Dehiscence can happen in abdominal surgical wounds and occurs after a sudden strain such as coughing, vomiting, or sitting up in bed. Patients often report feeling as though something has "given way." When there is an increase in serosanguineous drainage from a wound in the first few days after surgery, be alert for the potential for dehiscence.

Evisceration. With total separation of wound layers, evisceration (protrusion of visceral organs through a wound opening) occurs. The condition is an emergency that requires surgical repair. When evisceration occurs, place sterile gauze soaked in sterile saline over the extruding tissues to reduce chances of bacterial invasion and drying of the tissues. If the organs protrude through the wound, blood supply to the tissues can be compromised. Then contact the surgical team, do not allow the patient anything by mouth (NPO), observe for signs and symptoms of shock, and prepare the patient for emergency surgery.

TABLE 48.3	Types of Wound Drainage
Type	**Appearance**
Serous	Clear, watery plasma
Purulent	Thick, yellow, green, tan, or brown
Serosanguineous	Pale, pink, watery; mixture of clear and red fluid
Sanguineous	Bright red; indicates active bleeding

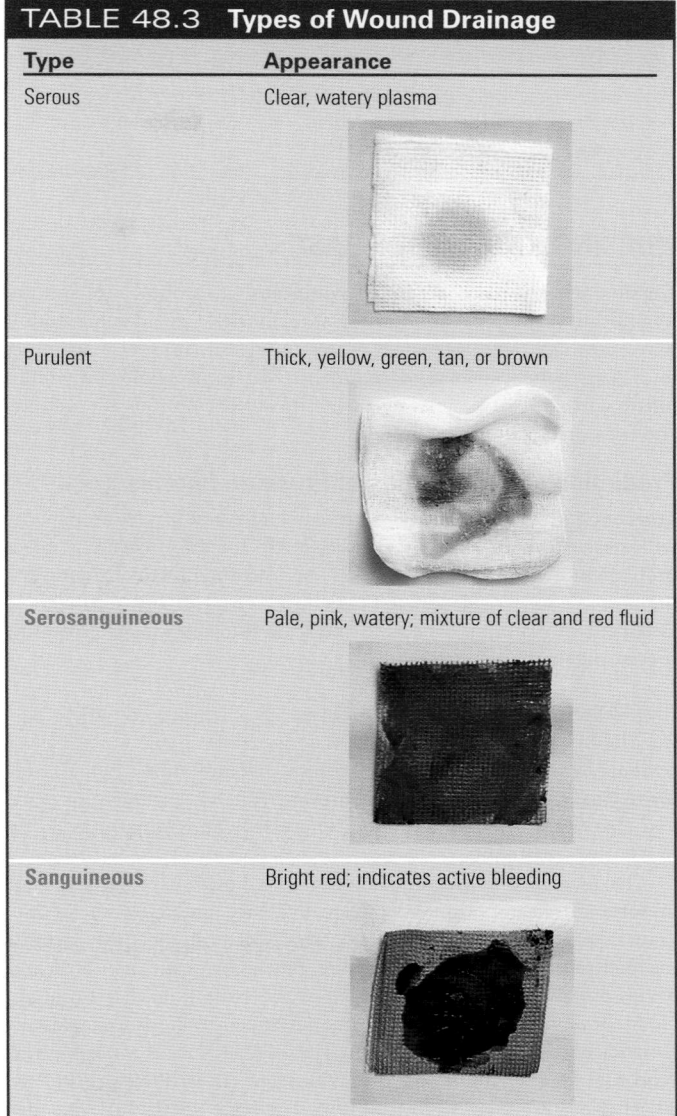

NURSING KNOWLEDGE BASE

Nursing research has contributed significantly to wound care and the identification and prevention of pressure injuries. Considerable studies have examined causative factors related to pressure injuries in an effort to discover beneficial forms of treatment. Nurses are significantly more informed than two decades ago when treatment options for wounds and pressure injuries were limited.

Prediction and Prevention of Pressure Injuries

Preventing pressure injuries is a priority and is not limited to patients with restrictions in mobility. Impaired skin integrity usually is not a problem in healthy individuals but is a serious and potentially devastating problem in ill or debilitated patients (WOCN, 2016). Your clinical judgment in planning consistent skin-care interventions is critical to preventing pressure injuries.

Risk Assessment. Risk assessment varies according to patient status (Table 48.4). Several assessment tools are available for assessing patients who are at risk for developing a pressure injury. By identifying at-risk patients, you can put preventive interventions into place and also spare low-risk patients unnecessary and sometimes costly preventive treatments.

The incidence of pressure injuries in a health care agency is an important indicator of quality of care. Evidence documents that a program of prevention guided by risk assessment simultaneously reduces the institutional incidence of pressure injuries by as much as 60% and brings down the costs of prevention at the same time (Martin et al., 2017). Several risk assessment scales developed by nurses enable systematic risk assessment of patients. The Braden Scale is a reliable and valid tool for pressure injury risk assessment (EPUAP/NPIAP/PPPIA, 2019a; EPUAP/NPIAP/PPPIA, 2019b). The scale (Table 48.5) was developed based on risk factors in a nursing home population (Braden and Bergstrom, 1994) and is widely used on general patient care units

in hospitals and long-term care. The Braden Scale contains six subscales: sensory perception, moisture, activity, mobility, nutrition, and friction/shear. The total score ranges from 6 to 23; a lower total score indicates a higher risk for pressure injury development (Braden and Bergstrom, 1989). The cutoff score for patients not at risk for pressure injury in the general adult population is ≤16 (Ayello et al., 2016).

However, the Braden Scale has shown insufficient predictive validity and poor accuracy in discriminating intensive care patients at risk for developing pressure injuries (Han et al., 2018). Research has shown that in some intensive care patients, the cutoff score for onset of risk is ≤14 (Alderden et al., 2017). Newer research on pressure injury risk in intensive care patients notes that there are unique risk factors including age, cardiovascular disease, use of vasopressor medications, hemodialysis, and hypotension. Norepinephrine is a vasopressor medication that is a potent vasoconstrictor and a strong predictor of pressure injury formation (Cox et al., 2020). In addition, critical care patients are at greater risk for MDRPIs and MARSIs because of the aforementioned risks and their overall physiological status (Cooper et al., 2020).

There has been recent research examining risk factors for pressure injuries during the perioperative period (Bulfone et al., 2018) (see Chapter 50). A scientific review of studies has shown that using a pressure injury risk assessment tool is recommended, and it is very important to assess risk factors throughout the preoperative period and over time. Perioperatively, patients most at risk are older adults and patients with a high anesthesia risk score (American Society of Anesthesiologists [ASA] score), comorbidities, a hematocrit less than 35%, or a probable time on the operating table greater than 6.15 hours (Bulfone et al., 2018).

Economic Consequences of Pressure Injuries. Pressure injuries are a continual problem in acute and restorative care settings, especially in patients age 65 years and older (WOCN, 2016). Paralysis and SCI are common preexisting conditions among younger adults with primary diagnosis of pressure injuries. Older adults admitted to acute and long-term agencies are a vulnerable population. Although the cost to provide pressure injury prevention to patients at risk can affect health care services' budgets, the costs to treat a severe pressure injury are substantially higher (EPUAP/NPIAP/PPPIA, 2019a).

When a pressure injury occurs, the length of stay in a health care agency and the overall cost of health care increase. These injuries are also costly to patients in terms of disability, pain, and suffering. More than 1.6 million patients each year in acute care settings develop pressure injuries, representing an increase in cost of billions of dollars to the health care systems (EPUAP/NPIAP/PPPIA, 2019a). The Centers for Medicare and Medicaid Services (CMS, 2020) no longer reimburses hospitals for care related to Stage 3 and Stage 4 pressure injuries that occur during a hospitalization. Guidelines such as those from the WOCN (2016) help reduce or eliminate the occurrence of pressure injuries and prevent the expenses that will not be reimbursed.

Factors Influencing Pressure Injury Formation and Wound Healing

In addition to previously discussed risk factors of impaired sensation, impaired mobility, shear, friction, and moisture, a patient's nutrition, tissue perfusion, infection, or age may increase the risk for pressure injury and poor wound healing.

Nutrition. Normal wound healing requires proper nutrition (Table 48.6). Deficiencies in any of the nutrients result in impaired or delayed healing (Stotts, 2016a). Physiological processes of wound healing depend on the availability of protein, vitamins (especially A and C), and the trace minerals zinc and copper. Collagen is a protein formed from amino acids

TABLE 48.4 Guidelines for Pressure Injury Risk Assessment		
Level of Care	**Initial**	**Reassessment**
Acute care	Within 8 hours of admission (EPUAP/NPIAP/PPPIA, 2019a; EPUAP/NPIAP/PPPIA, 2019b)	On a defined schedule (e.g., every 24–48 hours) Whenever major change in patient's condition occurs
Critical care	On admission	Every 24 hours
Long-term care	On admission	Weekly for first 4 weeks after admission Routinely on quarterly basis Whenever patient's condition changes or deteriorates
Home care	On admission	Every registered nurse visit

TABLE 48.5   Braden Scale for Predicting Pressure Ulcer Risk

Sensory Perception
Ability to respond appropriately to pressure-related discomfort

1. Completely limited:
Unresponsive (does not moan, flinch, or grasp) to painful stimuli caused by diminished level of consciousness or sedation
or
Limited ability to feel pain over most of body surface

2. Very limited:
Responds only to painful stimuli. Cannot communicate discomfort except by moaning or restlessness
or
Has sensory impairment that limits ability to feel pain or discomfort over half of body

3. Slightly limited:
Responds to verbal commands but cannot always communicate discomfort or need to be turned
or
Has some sensory impairment that limits ability to feel pain or discomfort in one or two extremities

4. No impairment:
Responds to verbal commands
Has no sensory deficit that would limit ability to feel or voice pain or discomfort

Moisture
Degree to which skin is exposed to moisture

1. Constantly moist:
Skin kept moist almost constantly by bodily elimination such as perspiration or urine
Dampness detected every time patient is moved or turned

2. Very moist:
Skin often, but not always, moist
Necessary to change linen at least once a shift

3. Occasionally moist:
Skin occasionally moist, requiring an extra linen change approximately once a day

4. Rarely moist:
Skin usually dry
Required linen changing only at routine intervals

Activity
Degree of physical activity

1. Bedfast:
Confined to bed

2. Chairfast:
Ability to walk severely limited or nonexistent
Cannot bear own weight and/or must be helped into chair or wheelchair

3. Walks occasionally:
Walks occasionally during day but for very short distances, with or without assistance
Spends majority of each shift in bed or chair

4. Walks frequently:
Walks outside room at least twice a day and inside room at least once every 2 hours during waking hours

Mobility
Ability to change and control body position

1. Completely immobile:
Does not make even slight changes in body or extremity position without assistance

2. Very limited:
Makes occasional slight changes in body or extremity position but unable to make frequent or significant changes independently

3. Slightly limited:
Makes frequent, though slight, changes in body or extremity position independently

4. No limitations:
Makes major and frequent changes in position without assistance

Nutrition
Usual food intake pattern

1. Very poor:
Never eats a complete meal; rarely eats more than one-third of any food offered; eats two servings or less of protein (meat or dairy products) per day
Takes fluids poorly
Does not take a liquid dietary supplement
or
Is NPO and/or maintained on clear liquids or IV infusion for more than 5 days

2. Probably inadequate:
Rarely eats a complete meal and generally eats only about one-half of any food offered
Protein intake includes only three servings of meat or dairy products per day
Occasionally takes a dietary supplement
or
Receives less than optimum amount of liquid diet or tube feeding

3. Adequate:
Eats over half of most meals
Eats a total of four servings of protein (meat, dairy products) each day
Occasionally refuses a meal but usually takes a supplement if offered
or
Is on tube feeding or TPN regimen that probably meets most of nutritional needs

4. Excellent:
Eats most of every meal; never refuses a meal; usually eats a total of four or more servings of meat and dairy products
Occasionally eats between meals
Does not require supplementation

Friction and Shear

1. Problem:
Requires moderate to maximum help to move; complete lifting without sliding against sheets impossible
Frequently slides down in bed or chair, requiring frequent repositioning with maximum assistance
Spasticity, contractures, or agitation leads to almost constant friction

2. Potential problem:
Moves feebly or requires minimum assistance; during a move skin probably slides to some extent against sheets, chair, restraints, or other devices
Maintains relatively good position in chair or bed most of the time but occasionally slides down

3. No apparent problem:
Moves in bed and in chair independently and has sufficient muscle strength to sit up completely during move
Maintains good position in bed or chair at all times

Instructions: *Score patient in each of the six subscales. Maximum score is 23, indicating little or no risk. A score of ≤16 indicates "at risk"; ≤9 indicates very high risk.

TABLE 48.6 Role of Selected Nutrients in Wound Healing

Nutrient	Role in Healing	Recommendations	Sources
Calories	Fuel for cell energy "Protein protection"	30–35 kcal/kg/day (Individuals who are underweight or have significant unintentional weight loss may need additional calories.)	Protein smoothies, whole milk, nuts, beans, salmon
Protein	Fibroplasia, angiogenesis, collagen formation and wound remodeling, immune function	1.25–1.5 g protein/kg body weight	Poultry, fish, eggs, beef, milk
Vitamin C (ascorbic acid)	Collagen synthesis, capillary wall integrity, fibroblast function, immunological function, antioxidant	1000 mg/day	Citrus fruits, tomatoes, potatoes, fortified fruit juices
Vitamin A	Epithelialization, wound closure, inflammatory response, angiogenesis, collagen formation Can reverse steroid effects on skin and delayed healing	1600–2000 retinol equivalents per day	Green leafy vegetables (spinach), broccoli, carrots, sweet potatoes, liver
Zinc	Collagen formation, protein synthesis, cell membrane and host defenses	15–30 mg Correct deficiencies No improvement in wound healing with supplementation unless zinc deficient Use with caution—large doses can be toxic May inhibit copper metabolism and impair immune function	Vegetables, meats, legumes
Fluid	Essential fluid environment for all cell function	30–35 mL/kg/day	Use noncaffeinated, nonalcoholic fluids without sugar Water is best; six to eight glasses per day

Adapted from Stotts NA: Nutritional assessment and support. In Bryant RA, Nix DP, editors: *Acute and chronic wounds: current management concepts*, ed 5, St Louis, 2016, Elsevier.

acquired by fibroblasts from protein ingested in food. Vitamin C is necessary for synthesis of collagen. Vitamin A reduces the negative effects of steroids on wound healing. Trace elements are also necessary (i.e., zinc for epithelialization and collagen synthesis and copper for collagen fiber linking).

Calories provide the energy source needed to support the cellular activity of wound healing. Protein needs especially are increased and are essential for tissue repair and growth. A balanced intake of various nutrients is critical to support wound healing. Consult with a nutritional team for dietary prescriptions individualized for the caloric needs of patients who are assessed as being at risk of malnutrition (EPUAP/NPIAP/PPPIA, 2019a).

Serum proteins are biochemical indicators of malnutrition (Stotts, 2016a). Serum albumin is probably the most frequently measured of these laboratory parameters. Albumin alone is not sensitive to rapid changes in nutritional status. The best measure of nutritional status is prealbumin because it reflects not only what the patient has recently ingested but also what the body has absorbed, digested, and metabolized (EPUAP/NPIAP/PPPIA, 2019a; Stotts, 2016a).

Tissue Perfusion. Oxygen fuels the cellular functions essential to the healing process; therefore the ability to perfuse the tissues with adequate amounts of oxygenated blood is critical to wound healing (Doughty and Sparks, 2016). Patients with diabetes mellitus and peripheral vascular disease are at risk for poor tissue perfusion because of poor circulation. Oxygen requirements depend on the phase of wound healing (e.g., chronic tissue hypoxia is associated with impaired collagen synthesis and reduced tissue resistance to infection).

Infection. A major goal of wound management is prevention of infection (Allegranzi et al., 2016). Wound infection prolongs the inflammatory

phase; delays collagen synthesis; prevents epithelialization; and increases the production of proinflammatory cytokines, which leads to additional tissue destruction (Stotts, 2016b). Indications that a wound infection is present include the presence of purulent drainage; change in odor, volume, or character of wound drainage; redness in the surrounding tissue; fever; or pain.

Age. The physiological changes associated with aging affect all phases of wound healing. A decrease in the functioning of macrophages leads to a delayed inflammatory response, delayed collagen synthesis, and slower epithelialization.

Psychosocial Impact of Wounds. The psychosocial impact of wounds on the physiological process of healing is unknown. However, the psychosocial impact can be significant. Body image changes resulting from a wound often impose a great stress on a patient's adaptive mechanisms. They also influence self-concept (see Chapter 33) and sexuality (see Chapter 34). Factors that affect a patient's perception of a wound include location; the presence of scars, stitches, or drains (often needed for weeks or months); odor from drainage; and temporary or permanent prosthetic devices.

Kelly recognizes the importance of reviewing postoperative care guidelines for a fractured hip and information about Mrs. Stein's other medical problems. The information will provide a background for understanding Mrs. Stein's risks for wound-healing problems and assist in directing the assessment. However, she also knows that the risks to Mrs. Stein's skin integrity are a priority problem. Kelly works as an assistive personnel in a skilled nursing facility and has cared for patients with pressure injuries. From this experience she knows the costly and debilitating effects of pressure injuries and that prevention is a priority. Kelly reviews the current literature, professional guidelines, and risk assessment tools about pressure injuries. She suspects that the blistered and reddened area is a Stage 1 injury and can progress to Stage 2. If that occurs, Mrs. Stein's length of hospital stay and subsequent admission to a rehabilitation facility may increase, which may ultimately affect her independence. She wants to work with Mrs. Stein to help improve her pain control and increase her confidence and participation in physical therapy and as a result prevent further injury to her skin and underlying tissues.

REFLECT NOW

Think about the information in the Braden Scale. How will this impact your knowledge about identifying risks for pressure injuries and potential interventions?

CRITICAL THINKING

The care of any patient with an existing wound or who is at risk for developing a wound can be complex. Successful critical thinking requires a synthesis of knowledge, experience, environmental factors, critical thinking attitudes, and intellectual and professional standards. Sound clinical judgments require you to anticipate information, analyze the data, and make clinical decisions regarding your patient's care. During assessment (Fig. 48.8) consider all critical thinking elements that will enable you to make the clinical decisions necessary for identifying appropriate nursing diagnoses.

Knowledge of normal integument and musculoskeletal physiology, the pathogenesis of pressure injuries, pressure injury stages, normal wound healing, and the pathophysiology of underlying diseases provides a scientific basis for how you approach an assessment of a specific patient. For example, you will assess a patient who has a history of diabetes mellitus differently than a patient who has been lying in bed with skeletal traction of the leg. The WOCN (2016) has guidelines for assessment of risk for impaired skin integrity. The same guidelines will provide options for prevention measures, and interventions to promote wound healing based on your assessment. Past experience with patients at risk for impaired skin integrity or patients with wounds increases your experiential knowledge base, helping you to make relevant assessments and identify nursing diagnoses. Examining a wound and observing how healing occurs will help you recognize abnormalities. Your knowledge base, application of clinical guidelines, and previous experience all support your clinical judgments during patient assessment and, as a result, you obtain comprehensive and correct data. With relevant and appropriate nursing diagnoses you will also need to be creative in planning and implementing patient-centered care. Last, because chronic wounds are difficult to heal, be diligent in evaluating nursing interventions and in determining which interventions are effective and which need modification.

FIG. 48.8 Critical thinking model for skin integrity and wound care assessment. *ANA,* American Nurses Association; *EPUAP,* European Pressure Ulcer Advisory Panel; *NPIAP,* National Pressure Injury Advisory Panel; *PPPIA,* Pan Pacific Pressure Injury Alliance; *WOCN,* Wound, Ostomy, and Continence Nurses Society. (Clinical Judgment Measurement Model copyright © NCSBN. All rights reserved.)

❖ NURSING PROCESS

Use clinical judgment while applying critical thinking to the nursing process. The nursing process provides a clinical decision-making approach for you to identify patient problems, develop and implement an individualized patient-centered plan of care, and evaluate that plan.

◆ Assessment

During the assessment process, use critical thinking when making clinical judgments necessary to thoroughly assess a patient's skin integrity and determine that assessment data are accurate and complete. When you detect abnormalities, you may benefit from having a registered nurse (RN) or faculty member confirm your findings. Chapter 50 offers details on assessment of surgical wounds. If the knowledge you have about a patient suggests the patient is at risk for a pressure injury, be sure to focus on the specific factors that create risk for pressure injuries such as a patient's level of sensation, presence of medical devices, presence of medical adhesives, independent or assisted movement, and nutritional and continence status (Box 48.3). These findings will guide you in selecting interventions Comprehensive skin integrity data ensure that you make patient-centered clinical decisions for effective, safe nursing care. Following analysis of baseline skin assessment data, use critical thinking and clinical judgment to determine the frequency of future skin

assessments. An obese patient, for example, may require more frequent monitoring. Baseline and ongoing assessment data provide critical information about any changes in a patient's skin integrity and increased risk for pressure injury development.

Through the Patient's Eyes. When patients have acute surgical or traumatic wounds, the wounds sometimes heal promptly and without complications. However, when pressure injuries or chronic wounds develop, the course of treatments is lengthy and costly. Because a patient and family need to be involved with wound care management, it is important to know a patient's expectations. Does the patient expect to have home care? Is there the expectation the patient's wound will heal to allow a quick return to work? A patient who has realistic expectations and is informed about the length of time for wound healing is more likely to adhere to the specific therapies designed to promote healing and prevent further skin breakdown. In addition, the patient and family caregiver have a better idea of what is expected as they manage the wound and dressing changes at home. Therefore assess each patient's perception of proposed wound treatment and what is occurring once wound-healing interventions begin. For example, why are certain dressings being used and how do they work? Determine a patient's and family's understanding of wound assessment; wound interventions; and supportive interventions such as positioning, nutrition, and ambulation.

Environment. Be aware of environmental factors in the health care setting that have the potential to affect your ability to assess a patient's skin integrity. Often patients require frequent turning or assistance with position changes. Assess the level of coordination needed to ensure you have sufficient personnel to help. Also be sure that necessary equipment, such as positioning or lifting devices, is available. Use the time during positioning to conduct ongoing skin and pressure injury risk assessments.

Interruptions occur frequently in a health care setting. Often, hospitalized patients who have impaired skin integrity or complicated wounds receive care from other specialists, such as respiratory, occupational, or physical therapists or wound specialists, and infection control. Often these bedside visits are unplanned and can interrupt nursing care. In addition, care providers from other specialties may not be aware of positioning schedules or may not correctly reposition the patient in a pressure-reduction position. Therefore you need to anticipate interruptions and be aware of the need to reassess your patient's skin integrity and position following care from providers in other disciplines.

Patients with complicated, nonhealing wounds have complex dressing changes. Assess when visitors or other health care personnel are at the patient's bedside or room. You need to plan to perform wound assessments and dressing changes when there are no extra people in the room or at the bedside. This maintains patient privacy, but also controls for transmission of infection to the wound from others.

Skin. Perform skin assessment of a patient when you initiate care and then at a minimum of once a shift (see agency policies). Inspect the skin for signs of skin breakdown and/or injury (see Skill 48.1). Carefully inspect dependent areas of the skin, such as the sacral area when a patient lies flat or the bottoms of the heels when a patient lies supine (Fig. 48.9). For example, when a patient lies in bed or sits in a chair, body weight is placed heavily on certain bony prominences. Turn the patient in bed to inspect the skin and, once you return a patient to bed from a chair, look at all areas exposed to pressure. Body surfaces subjected to the greatest weight or pressure are at greatest risk for pressure injury formation. High-risk patients—including those who are neurologically impaired, are chronically ill, or have altered mental status; those in the intensive care unit (ICU), oncology units, hospice, or orthopedic units; and patients

---

BOX 48.3 Nursing Assessment Questions

Sensation
- Do you have tingling, a change in or decreased feeling, or absent feeling in your extremities?
- Can you feel pressure when sitting or lying down? Has that sensation changed?
- Is your skin sensitive to moderate heat or cold?

Mobility
- Do you have any physical limitations, injury, or paralysis that limits your ability to move on your own?
- Can you change your position by yourself easily?
- Tell me about any pain you have when you walk, sit down, or move about your home.

Nutrition
- Have you had any changes in your appetite? If so, what are the changes?
- Do you have access to groceries or food delivery services? Are you able to shop?
- Does someone prepare your meals or are you able to prepare your meals?

Continence
- Do you have any problems or accidents leaking urine or stool?
- What help do you need when using the toilet? In what way?
- How often do you need to use the toilet? During the day? At night?

Presence of Wound
- What do you believe caused your wound?
- When did the wound occur? Where is it located?
- When did you last receive a tetanus shot?
- What has changed with this wound since it occurred? What were the changes and what caused them?
- What have you done to treat the wound? Which treatments, activities, or care have slowed or helped the wound to heal?
- Do you have any pain, itching, or other symptoms with the wound? How are you managing the itching, and what works best for you?
- Who helps you care for your wound?

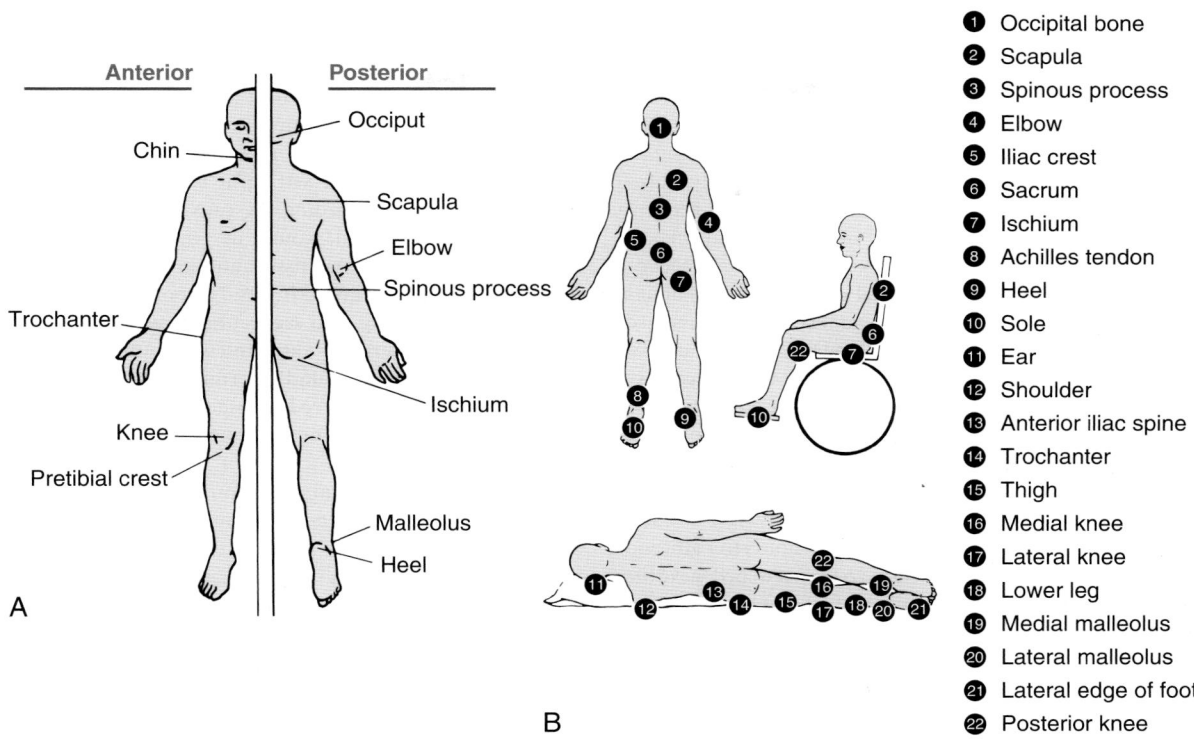

Pressure ulcer sites

1. Occipital bone
2. Scapula
3. Spinous process
4. Elbow
5. Iliac crest
6. Sacrum
7. Ischium
8. Achilles tendon
9. Heel
10. Sole
11. Ear
12. Shoulder
13. Anterior iliac spine
14. Trochanter
15. Thigh
16. Medial knee
17. Lateral knee
18. Lower leg
19. Medial malleolus
20. Lateral malleolus
21. Lateral edge of foot
22. Posterior knee

FIG. 48.9 (A) Bony prominences most frequently underlying pressure injury. (B) Pressure injury sites. (Adapted from Trelease CC: Developing standards for wound care, *Ostomy Wound Manage* 20:46, 1988.)

with medical devices—need more frequent skin assessments, sometimes as often as every 4 hours (see agency policy).

Assessment for tissue pressure damage includes visual and tactile inspection of the skin (see Chapter 30). Perform a baseline assessment to determine a patient's normal skin characteristics and any actual or potential areas of breakdown (Nix, 2016). Use factors such as skin tone, age, underlying comorbidities, and prior pressure injury to individualize your assessment of a patient's skin (EPUAP/NPIAP/PPPIA, 2019a; EPUAP/NPIAP/PPPIA, 2019b). Accurate assessment of patients with darker skin pigmentation is an essential skill for all health care providers (see Box 48.2).

When you note hyperemia of the skin, gently palpate the reddened tissue; differentiate whether the skin redness is blanchable or non-blanchable. Blanchable erythema is visible skin redness that becomes pale or white when pressure is applied and reddens when pressure is relieved. It may result from normal reactive hyperemia that should disappear within several hours or from inflammatory erythema with an intact capillary bed. Nonblanchable erythema is visible skin redness that persists with the application of pressure. It indicates structural damage to the capillary bed and microcirculation. This is an indication for a Stage 1 pressure injury (EPUAP/NPIAP/PPPIA, 2019a).

REFLECT NOW

Think about a patient you have recently cared for who had a medical device, such as a urinary catheter, oxygen mask, or feeding tube. What were the patient's risks for skin breakdown? How did you assess the patient for a medical device–related pressure injury?

Wounds and Pressure Injuries. When you identify the presence of a skin wound or pressure injury, closer assessment is required. Assess the type of tissue in the wound base and the factors influencing the patient's risks for poor healing so that you can plan appropriate interventions. The assessment includes the amount (percentage) and appearance (color) of viable and nonviable tissue. Granulation tissue is red, moist tissue composed of new blood vessels, the presence of which indicates progression toward healing. Soft yellow or white tissue is characteristic of slough (stringy substance attached to wound bed), and it must eventually be removed by a qualified health care provider or by means of an appropriate wound dressing before the wound is able to heal. Black, brown, tan, or necrotic tissue is eschar, which also needs to be removed before healing can occur.

Measurement of the wound size provides information on overall changes in dimensions, which is an indicator for wound-healing progress (Nix, 2016). This includes measuring the length and width of a wound, as well as determining its depth (see Skill 48.2). Use a disposable wound-measuring device to measure wound width and length. This approach offers a uniform, consistent method for measuring meaningful comparisons of wound status across time (EPUAP/NPIAP/PPPIA, 2019b). Measure depth by using a cotton-tipped applicator in the wound bed (see Skill 48.2). Note that if a deep laceration exists it will likely require suturing by a qualified health care provider.

Assessment of wound exudate should describe the amount, color, consistency, and odor of wound drainage. Normally a closed surgical wound has minimal serosanguineous drainage immediately after surgery (see Chapter 50). Excessive exudate indicates the presence of infection. Wound pain, including the location, distribution, type, quality, and intensity, and any aggravating or relieving factors also should be assessed (Krasner, 2016) (see Chapter 44). Examine the skin around a wound (periwound) for redness, warmth, and signs of maceration, and palpate the area for signs of pain or induration. The presence of any of these factors on the periwound skin indicates wound deterioration.

Predictive Measures. On admission to acute care, rehabilitation hospitals, nursing homes, home care, and other health care agencies, patients are assessed for risk of pressure injury development (see Table 48.3) (WOCN, 2016). Assessment for pressure injury risk includes using an appropriate predictive measure and assessing a patient's mobility, nutrition, presence of body fluids, and comfort level (see Skill 48.1). Perform pressure injury risk assessment systematically using an assessment tool such as the Braden Scale (see Table 48.4) or a tool selected by your agency. The interpretation of the meaning of the total numerical scores differs with each risk assessment scale relevant to the population being assessed by the agency. Lower numerical scores on the Braden Scale indicate that the patient is at high risk for skin breakdown. A benefit of the predictive instruments is an increased early detection of patients at greater risk for injury development (WOCN, 2016). Perform reassessment for pressure injury risk on a scheduled basis (see agency policy).

Mobility. Assessment includes noting the baseline level of mobility and the potential effects of impaired mobility on skin integrity. Assess the patient's ability to move the extremities, and note strength and muscle tone (see Chapter 30). If the patient is restricted to bed, have the patient turn or move up in bed independently (as appropriate). For example, determine whether the patient can lift any weight off the sacral area and roll the body to a side-lying position. Some patients have inadequate strength or range of motion to move independently into a more protective position. Finally, assess a patient's activity tolerance to determine whether the patient can be transferred to a chair or ambulated more often to relieve pressure from lying down (see Chapter 39).

Nutritional Status. An assessment of a patient's nutritional status is an integral part of the initial assessment data for any patient, especially one at risk for impaired skin integrity (Stotts, 2016a). The Joint Commission (TJC, 2020) requires nutritional screening assessment within 24 hours of admission. Weigh the patient and perform this measure more often for at-risk patients. A loss of 5% of usual weight, weight less than 90% of ideal body weight, and a decrease of 4.54 kg (10 lb) in a brief period are all signs of actual or potential nutritional problems (Stotts, 2016a). Assess the patient's mouth and teeth for oral sores and ill-fitting dentures that affect nutritional intake (see Chapter 45).

Body Fluids. It is important to prevent and reduce a patient's exposure to body fluids; when exposure occurs, provide meticulous hygiene and skin care (see Chapter 40). Continual exposure of the skin to moisture increases a patient's risk for skin breakdown and pressure injury formation. Some body fluids such as saliva and serosanguineous drainage are not as caustic, and the risk of skin breakdown from exposure to these fluids is low. However, exposure to urine, bile, stool, ascitic fluid, and purulent wound exudate carries a moderate risk for skin breakdown, especially in patients who have other risk factors such as chronic illness or poor nutrition (Francis, 2020). Frequent exposure to urine and fecal contents increases patients' risk for IAD (Francis, 2020; McNichol et al., 2018). In addition, exposure to gastric and pancreatic drainage has the highest risk for skin breakdown. These fluids have digestive qualities that can irritate and break down the skin quickly.

Pain. Significant research has been conducted on the study of pain in surgical patients with wounds. The routine assessment of pain in surgical patients is critical to selecting appropriate pain management therapies and to determine a patient's ability to progress toward recovery (see Chapter 50). The WOCN (2016) has recommended that assessment and management of pain also be included in the care of patients with pressure injuries (EPUAP/NPIAP/PPPIA, 2019b). Use standard pain assessment tools to measure pain acuity and be thorough in assessing

the character of a patient's pain (see Chapter 44). Maintaining adequate pain control and patient comfort increases the patient's willingness and ability to increase mobility, which in turn reduces pressure injury risk.

Surgical and Traumatic Wounds. Assess wounds at the time of injury or postoperatively, during wound care, when a patient's overall condition changes, and on a regularly scheduled basis (see agency policy). Regardless of the setting, it is important that you initially obtain information regarding the cause and history of the wound, treatment of the wound, wound description (location, dimensions, quality of the wound base tissue, and presence of odor, warmth, or redness on the periwound skin), and response to therapy.

Emergency Setting. You see traumatic wounds in any setting, including clinics, emergency departments, youth camps, or your own backyard. The type of wound determines the criteria for inspection. For example, you do not need to inspect for signs of internal bleeding after an abrasion, but you must assess for internal bleeding in the event of a puncture wound.

After a traumatic wound, when you judge a patient's condition to be stable because of the presence of spontaneous breathing, a clear airway, and a strong carotid pulse (see Chapters 30 and 41), inspect the wound for bleeding. An abrasion is superficial with little bleeding and is considered a partial-thickness wound. The wound often appears "weepy" because of plasma leakage from damaged capillaries. A laceration sometimes may bleed more profusely (especially if the patient is taking anticoagulants or other blood thinners), depending on the depth and location of the wound. For example, minor scalp lacerations tend to bleed profusely because of the rich blood supply to the scalp. Lacerations greater than 5 cm (2 inches) long or 2.5 cm (1 inch) deep cause serious bleeding. Puncture wounds bleed in relation to the depth, size, and location of the wound (e.g., a nail puncture does not cause as much bleeding as a knife wound). A puncture wound is usually a small, circular wound with the edges coming together toward the center. The primary dangers of puncture wounds are internal bleeding and infection.

Inspect traumatic wounds for foreign bodies or contaminant material. Most traumatic wounds are dirty. Soil, broken glass, shreds of cloth, and foreign substances clinging to penetrating objects sometimes become embedded in a wound. Next, assess the size and depth of a wound (see Skill 48.2).

When an injury is a result of trauma from a dirty penetrating object, determine when the patient last received a tetanus toxoid injection. Tetanus bacteria reside in soil and in the gut of humans and animals.

Stable Setting. When a patient's condition is stabilized (e.g., after surgery or treatment), assess the wound to determine progress toward healing. If the wound is covered by a dressing and the health care provider has not ordered it changed, do not inspect it directly unless you suspect serious complications such as a large volume of bright red bleeding, excessive odor, or severe pain under the dressing. In such a situation inspect only the dressing and any external drains. If the health care provider prefers to change the dressing, the health care provider should assess the wound at least daily. When removing dressings, remove one dressing layer at a time to avoid accidental removal or displacement of underlying drains. Because removal of dressings can be painful, consider giving an analgesic at least 30 minutes before exposing a wound.

Wound Appearance. A surgical incision healing by primary intention should have clean, well-approximated edges. There may be some redness at the edges of the incision that can be present for the first few days after surgery. Crusts often form along wound edges from exudate. If a wound is open, the edges are separated, and you inspect the condition of tissue at the wound base. The outer edges of a wound normally appear inflamed for the first 2 to 3 days, but this slowly disappears.

TABLE 48.7 Assessment of Abnormal Healing in Primary and Secondary Intention Wounds

Primary Intention Wounds	Secondary Intention Wounds
Incision line poorly approximated	Pale or fragile granulation tissue, hypergranulation tissue present
Drainage present more than 3 days after closure	Wound exudate is purulent
Inflammation increased in first 3–5 days after injury	Nonviable tissues such as necrotic tissue or slough in wound base
No healing ridge by day 9	Fruity, earthy, or putrid odor present after wound base is cleansed
	Presence of fistula(s), tunneling, undermining

Adapted from Nix D: Skin and wound inspection and assessment. In Bryant RA, Nix DP, editors: *Acute and chronic wounds: current management concepts*, ed 5, St Louis, 2016, Elsevier.

FIG. 48.10 (A) Penrose drain with dressing. (B) Penrose drain with safety pin.

Within 7 to 10 days a normally healing wound resurfaces with epithelial cells, and edges close. Table 48.7 lists assessment characteristics for abnormal wound healing in primary and secondary intention wounds. If infection develops, the area directly surrounding the wound becomes brightly inflamed and swollen.

Skin discoloration usually results from bruising of interstitial tissues or hematoma formation. Blood collecting beneath the skin first takes on a bluish or purplish appearance. Gradually, as the clotted blood is broken down, shades of brown and yellow appear.

Character of Wound Drainage. Note the amount, color, odor, and consistency of wound drainage (see Table 48.3). The amount of drainage depends on the type of wound. For example, drainage is minimal after a simple appendectomy. In contrast, drainage is moderate for 1 to 2 days after drainage of a large abscess. When you need an accurate measurement of the amount of drainage within a dressing, weigh the dressing and compare it with the weight of the same dressing that is clean and dry. The general rule is that 1 g of drainage equals 1 mL of volume of drainage. Another method of quantifying wound drainage is to chart the number of dressings used and the frequency of change. An increase or decrease in the number or frequency of dressings indicates a relative increase or decrease in wound drainage. If the drainage has a pungent or strong odor, you should suspect an infection. Describe the appearance of the wound according to characteristics observed, the type of closures used, and the dressing changes performed.

Palpation of Wound. When inspecting a wound, observe for swelling or separation of wound edges. While wearing clean gloves, lightly press the wound edges, detecting localized areas of tenderness or drainage collection. If pressure causes fluid to be expressed, note the characteristics of the drainage. The patient is normally sensitive to palpation of wound edges. Extreme tenderness may indicate infection.

Drains. Drains provide a means for fluid or blood that accumulates within a wound bed to drain out of the body. A surgeon inserts a drain into or near a surgical wound if there is a large amount of drainage (Fig. 48.10A). A drain can also be placed by an interventional radiologist to drain an area found after or before surgery. Some drains are sutured in place. The purpose of a surgical drain is to remove excess wound fluid and promote wound healing in the wound bed. As a result, the wound heals from the inside out.

Exercise caution when changing a dressing around drains that are not sutured in place; this prevents accidental removal. A Penrose drain lies under a dressing; at the time of placement a pin or clip is placed through the drain to prevent it from slipping farther into a wound (see Fig. 48.10B).

One dressing is split and placed around the drain and another over the drain to collect drainage. When removing the dressings, remove one dressing at a time to prevent accidental dislodgement of the drain. It is usually the health care provider's responsibility to pull or advance the drain as drainage decreases to permit healing deep within the drain site.

Assess the number and type of drains, drain placement, character of drainage (determine if the drainage is within expected guidelines for volume or color), and condition of collecting equipment. Observe the security of the drain and its location with respect to the wound. Next note the character of drainage. If there is a collecting device, measure the drainage volume. Because a drainage system needs to be patent, look for drainage flow through and around the tubing. A sudden decrease in drainage through the tubing may indicate a blocked drain, and you need to notify the health care provider. When a drain is connected to suction, assess the system to be sure that the pressure ordered is being exerted. Evacuator units such as a Hemovac or Jackson-Pratt (Fig. 48.11) exert a constant low pressure if the suction device is fully compressed. When the evacuator device is unable to maintain a vacuum on its own, notify the surgeon, who then orders a secondary vacuum system (such as wall suction). If fluid accumulates within the tissues, wound healing does not progress at an optimal rate, and this increases the risk of infection.

Wound Closures. Surgical wounds are closed with staples, sutures, or wound adhesives. A frequently used skin closure is the stainless-steel staple. The staple provides more strength than nylon or silk sutures and tends to cause less irritation to tissue. Look for irritation with redness around staple or suture sites and note whether closures are intact. Normally for the first 2 to 3 days after surgery the skin around sutures or staples is edematous because of the normal inflammatory response.

Surgical glue (cyanoacrylate glue) is a liquid tissue adhesive that forms a strong waterproof barrier across approximated wound edges, allowing normal healing to occur below. It is transparent and the wound is easier to inspect, and it reduces time associated with dressing changes. There is some clinical evidence that surgical glue has antimicrobial properties against gram-positive bacteria, which are common SSI pathogens (Machin et al., 2019). It can be used to replace small

FIG. 48.11 Jackson-Pratt drainage device. Drainage tube and reservoir.

sutures for incisional repair. The wound edges are held (approximated) together until the solution dries, providing an adhesive closure.

Wound Cultures. If you detect purulent or suspicious-looking drainage, report to the health care provider because a specimen of the drainage may need to be obtained for culture. Never collect a wound culture sample from old drainage. Resident colonies of bacterial flora from the skin grow within exudate and are not always the true causative organisms of a wound infection. Clean a wound first with normal saline to remove skin flora. Aerobic organisms grow in superficial wounds exposed to the air, and anaerobic organisms tend to grow within body cavities. Use a different method of specimen collection for each type of organism per agency policy (Box 48.4).

Gram stains of drainage are often performed as well. This test allows a health care provider to order appropriate treatment, such as antibiotics, earlier than when only cultures are done. No additional specimens are usually required. The microbiology laboratory needs only to be notified to perform the additional test. The gold standard of wound culture is tissue biopsy. A health care provider or wound care specialist with special training obtains the biopsy specimen (Stotts, 2016b).

Psychosocial. Assess how a wound is influencing a patient's self-perception and socialization. Ask the patient to describe how the wound affects the view of self. Does the patient have unwarranted fears that the wound will not heal? Does a chronic wound interfere with the patient's willingness to participate in social activities at home? Does it affect the patient's ability to continue working? Make sure that the patient's personal and social resources for adaptation are a part of your assessment. Is there a family caregiver who is able to assist with wound care in the home?

This is Mrs. Stein's second postoperative day. Prior to starting care, Kelly reviews the electronic health record and organizes her plan for assessment. Kelly sees that Mrs. Stein had one dose of pain medication 10 hours ago, as "patient is afraid of addiction and did not request any pain medication" was noted in the record. Kelly asks Mrs. Stein to rate her pain level. Mrs. Stein describes her pain as an 8 out of 10. Before Kelly performs any assessment activities, she discusses pain control with Mrs. Stein and lets Mrs. Stein further describe her fear of addiction. Kelly discusses the fear of addiction and why Mrs. Stein might be more comfortable and better able to participate in physical therapy if she receives something for pain, and Mrs. Stein agrees. Kelly administers the ordered analgesic and

---

BOX 48.4   Recommendations for Standardized Techniques for Wound Cultures

Needle Aspiration Procedure (Anaerobic Organisms)
- Obtain an anaerobic culture tube for specimen (Pagana et al., 2021).
- Clean intact skin with povidone-iodine and allow to dry for 60 seconds to remove skin flora. Then wipe the skin with alcohol and allow to dry, which reduces the possibility that the specimen will be altered by the iodine on the skin surface.
- Use a sterile 10-mL disposable syringe with a 22-gauge needle, pulling 0.5 mL of air into the syringe.
- Insert the needle through intact skin next to the wound; withdraw plunger and apply suction to the 10-mL mark.
- Move the needle back and forward at different angles for two to four explorations. The plunger is then released back to the 0.5 mL mark, the needle is withdrawn, and the syringe is capped and sent to the lab or contents are injected into an anerobic culture tube (check agency policy).

Quantitative Swab Procedure (Aerobic Organisms)
- Clean the wound surface with an antiseptic solution. Allow to dry.
- Use a sterile cotton swab from a culturette tube (Fig. 48.12).
- Identify a 1-cm area of the wound that is free from necrotic tissue. Place the sterile cotton swab into the center of the area to obtain fluid from the wound tissue (Pagana et al., 2021).
- Insert the tip of the swab into the appropriate sterile container, label, and transport to the laboratory.

FIG. 48.12 Wound culturette tube.

tells Mrs. Stein she will leave her alone for 30 minutes to allow the medication to reach its peak effect.

Kelly returns to Mrs. Stein's bedside. A skin assessment reveals that the reddened, blistered area on Mrs. Stein's right hip is 2.5 cm (1 inch) in diameter. The area is not draining, but the underlying skin is not intact. Kelly recognizes this as a Stage 2 pressure injury. Kelly also assesses nonblanchable erythema in the periwound area about 2.5 cm (1 inch) around the wound. On palpation Kelly notes that the periwound underlying tissue has nonblanchable erythema. These findings indicate structural damage to the capillary bed and microcirculation and support the conclusion that a Stage 2 pressure injury is present. On the sacrum there is a 4.0-cm (approximately 2-inch) area of redness. When Kelly applies pressure to this area it blanches and becomes pale, and it reddens when the pressure is relieved. She knows this is blanchable erythema (normal reactive hyperemia) and indicates that the underlying capillary bed is intact. The underlying skin and tissue are normal on palpation. However, although the assessment findings in the sacral area are not abnormal, the redness, Mrs. Stein's mobility and activity status, and pain are all risks for continued pressure to the sacral region and a risk for further impaired skin integrity.

Kelly conducts a wound assessment. She notes drainage on the left side of Mrs. Stein's gown. On wound inspection Kelly notes wound drainage and small openings between staples. The periwound area is warm and tender to palpation. Kelly notifies the charge nurse. Because all patients on this nursing unit have a standing order for a wound culture when assessment findings indicate a possible wound infection, the charge nurse tells Kelly to obtain a specimen for wound culture. Kelly's faculty provides guidance and observes Kelly obtaining the culture specimen.

Kelly assesses Mrs. Stein's mobility status. Mrs. Stein is unable to assist using a bedpan, is refusing to use a bedside commode, and has episodes of incontinence. Kelly observed today's physical therapy session and noted that Mrs. Stein did become diaphoretic, but she was able to complete all activities. The physical therapist told Mrs. Stein that this was perhaps her best session, and Mrs. Stein mentioned that the therapy was not as painful as before.

◆ Analysis and Nursing Diagnosis

Clinical judgment requires application of critical thinking to analyze assessment findings. You consider the knowledge you have about a patient's condition and assessment findings to differentiate normal versus abnormal findings. Your review of data will reveal clusters of data to support a problem-focused or negative diagnosis such as *Impaired Skin Integrity* or a risk diagnosis of *Risk for Impaired Skin Integrity*. In addition, review your assessment data to identify information about any related factors. For example, a postoperative patient has purulent drainage from a surgical wound and reports tenderness around the area of the wound. These data support a nursing diagnosis of *Impaired Skin Integrity* related to infection (Box 48.5). A morbidly obese patient who has limited turning ability, is diaphoretic, and shows evidence of a Stage 1 sacral pressure injury presents data to support *Impaired Skin Integrity* related to moisture and pressure over the sacral prominence. The related factors will guide your selection of interventions. After completing an assessment of a patient's skin and any existing wound, identify nursing diagnoses to direct the most relevant interventions to support wound healing and prevent complications.

BOX 48.5 Nursing Diagnostic Process

Impaired Skin Integrity Related to Infection

Assessment Activities	Assessment Findings
Inspect surface of wound and periwound skin.	Break in skin integrity Serous drainage from wound Edges of wound red and warm, not approximated Macerated periwound area
Inspect wound for signs of healing.	Brown-red or beige drainage 5 days after surgery Edges of wound not approximated
Palpate wound and ask patient if there is tenderness.	Patient expresses pain on palpation; rates pain as a 5 on scale of 0 to 10 Periwound edema
Obtain patient's temperature, heart rate, white blood cell count.	Patient febrile, heart rate 125 beats/min, leukocyte (white blood cell) count 12,000/mm³

Additional nursing diagnoses associated with impaired skin integrity and wounds include:

- Risk for Infection
- Acute or Chronic Pain
- Impaired Mobility
- Impaired Peripheral Tissue Perfusion

Some patients are at risk for poor wound healing because of the presence of previously defined conditions that impair healing. Thus even though a patient's wound appears normal, the nursing diagnoses of *Impaired Nutritional Intake* or *Ineffective Tissue Perfusion* have implications for directing nursing care toward support of wound repair.

The nature of a wound can cause problems unrelated to wound healing. An alteration in comfort and the diagnoses of *Acute Pain* and *Impaired Mobility* has implications for a patient's eventual recovery. For example, a large abdominal incision may cause enough pain to interfere with early mobility or the patient's ability to turn in bed effectively, making the patient at risk for impaired skin integrity.

*Kelly reviews assessment findings and uses her clinical judgment to analyze patterns of data to individualize nursing diagnoses for Mrs. Stein. The Stage 2 pressure injury, the open blistered (2.5-cm [1-inch] in diameter) area on the right hip, and the reddened (4.0-cm [approximately 2-inch]) sacral area identified in assessment support the nursing diagnosis of **Impaired Skin Integrity** related to pressure and shear. The small openings between staples, serous drainage, and redness and tenderness in the periwound region support the nursing diagnosis of **Risk for Infection** related to open surgical wound. Once the wound culture is examined, this nursing diagnosis will probably change to **Infection** related to open surgical wound. Mrs. Stein's level of pain affects her willingness to participate in activity, and as a result there are two nursing diagnoses: **Acute Pain** related to incisional pain and **Impaired Mobility** related to incisional pain.*

◆ Planning and Outcomes Identification

Once the nursing diagnoses have been identified, use clinical judgment to develop a plan of care to promote wound healing and prevent complications of any existing wounds. During planning synthesize information from multiple resources (Fig. 48.13). Critical thinking ensures that you integrate your experiences and all that you know about the individual patient to form an appropriate patient-centered plan of care. Professional standards are especially important to consider when you select strategies for a plan of care, including measures to prevent pressure injuries and specific wound therapies. Last, use critical thinking to evaluate your knowledge and skill competencies regarding the planned wound care interventions. What additional resources might you require?

Patients who have large chronic wounds or infected wounds have multiple nursing care needs. A concept map helps to individualize care for a patient who has multiple health problems and related nursing diagnoses (Fig. 48.14). Use critical thinking as you organize complex patient assessment data into related nursing diagnoses with a patient's chief medical diagnosis. As you identify links between the nursing diagnoses and the chief medical diagnosis, you will also recognize links between potential interventions that apply to the patient's multiple health care problems.

Outcomes. Nursing care is based on a patient's identified nursing diagnoses and collaborative problems. Identify expected outcomes for each diagnosis and plan individualized interventions according to the risk for pressure injuries or the type and severity of an existing wound. As you select interventions, consider the presence of any complications such as infection, poor nutrition, peripheral vascular diseases, or immunosuppression that can affect wound healing (see the Nursing Care Plan).

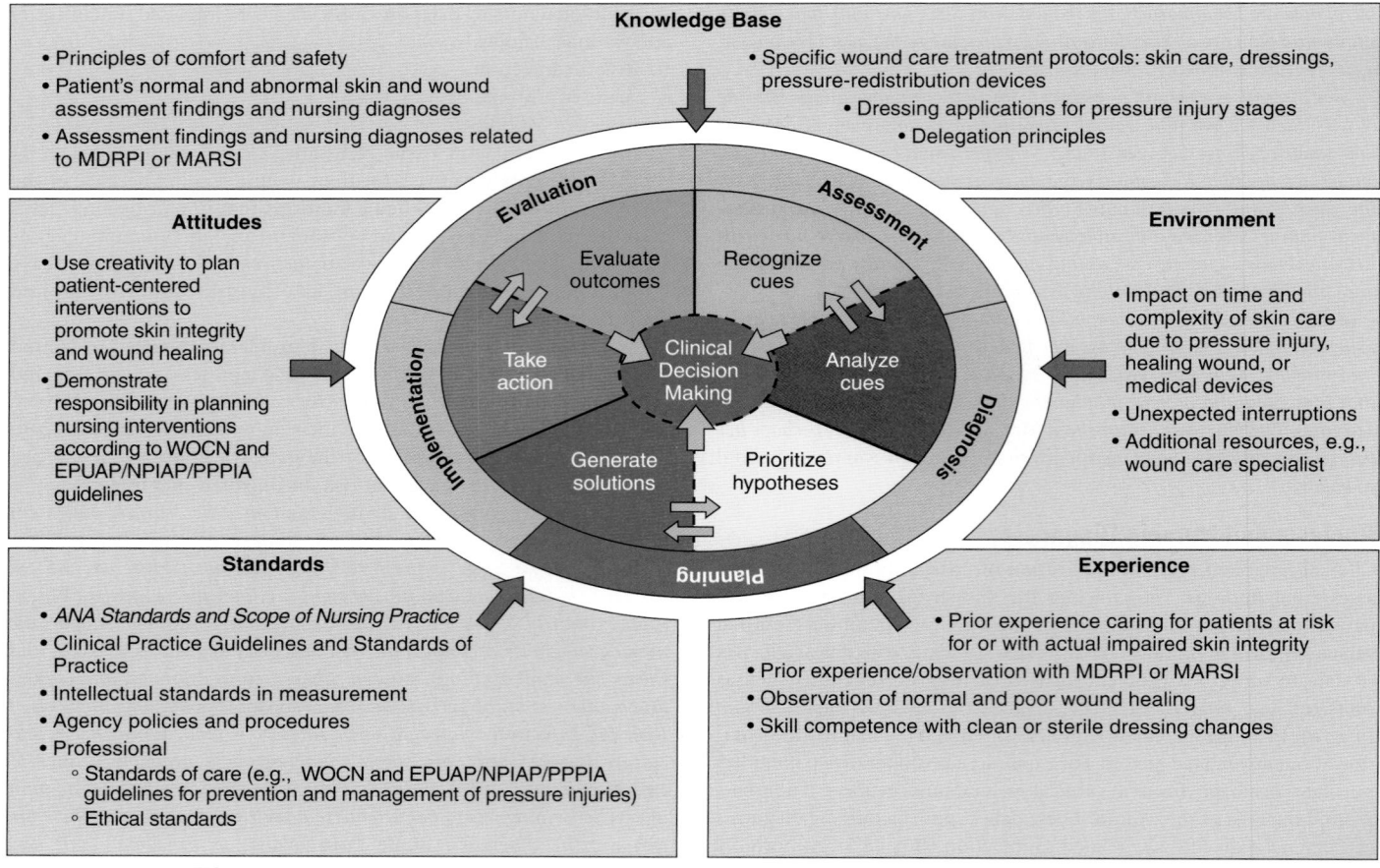

Knowledge Base
- Principles of comfort and safety
- Patient's normal and abnormal skin and wound assessment findings and nursing diagnoses
- Assessment findings and nursing diagnoses related to MDRPI or MARSI

- Specific wound care treatment protocols: skin care, dressings, pressure-redistribution devices
  - Dressing applications for pressure injury stages
  - Delegation principles

Attitudes
- Use creativity to plan patient-centered interventions to promote skin integrity and wound healing
- Demonstrate responsibility in planning nursing interventions according to WOCN and EPUAP/NPIAP/PPPIA guidelines

Environment
- Impact on time and complexity of skin care due to pressure injury, healing wound, or medical devices
- Unexpected interruptions
- Additional resources, e.g., wound care specialist

Evaluation — Assessment — Diagnosis — Planning — Implementation

Evaluate outcomes — Recognize cues — Clinical Decision Making — Analyze cues — Take action — Generate solutions — Prioritize hypotheses

Standards
- *ANA Standards and Scope of Nursing Practice*
- Clinical Practice Guidelines and Standards of Practice
- Intellectual standards in measurement
- Agency policies and procedures
- Professional
  - Standards of care (e.g., WOCN and EPUAP/NPIAP/PPPIA guidelines for prevention and management of pressure injuries)
  - Ethical standards

Experience
- Prior experience caring for patients at risk for or with actual impaired skin integrity
- Prior experience/observation with MDRPI or MARSI
- Observation of normal and poor wound healing
- Skill competence with clean or sterile dressing changes

FIG. 48.13 Critical thinking model for skin integrity and wound care planning. *ANA,* American Nurses Association; *EPUAP,* European Pressure Ulcer Advisory Panel; *MARSI,* medical adhesive–related skin injury; *MDRPI,* medical device–related pressure injury; *NPIAP,* National Pressure Injury Advisory Panel; *PPPIA,* Pan Pacific Pressure Injury Alliance; *WOCN,* Wound, Ostomy, and Continence Nurses Society. (Clinical Judgment Measurement Model copyright © NCSBN. All rights reserved.)

An outcome allows you to target specific interventions. The following are examples of outcomes associated with preventing or reducing risk for pressure injuries and wound healing:

- Increase in the percentage of granulation tissue in the wound base
- No wound erythema or tenderness to palpation
- No further skin breakdown
- Increase in caloric intake by 10%

With every wound it is important to plan care to promote wound hemostasis, prevent infection, promote wound healing, maintain skin integrity, improve comfort, and promote health.

Setting Priorities. Establish nursing care priorities in wound care based on the nursing diagnoses identified and the outcomes of care. These priorities also depend on whether the patient's condition is stable or emergent. Collaborate with the patient, when possible, with regard to when to perform wound care. The management of pain, for example, may be a priority over performing a wound irrigation. When there is a risk for pressure injury development, preventive interventions such as skin-care practices, elimination of risks, and positioning are high priorities. An acute wound needs immediate intervention, whereas in the presence of a chronic, stable wound, the patient's hygiene and education on wound care are more important. Promotion of wound healing and the type of wound care administered depend on the type, size, and location of the wound and overall treatment goals.

Other patient factors to consider when establishing priorities include patient preferences, planning around daily activities, and family caregiver factors. If a family caregiver is required when a patient is discharged home, education of the family caregiver will be essential. These factors are important, regardless of the setting for health care.

Teamwork and Collaboration. Patients with wounds or pressure injuries will often benefit from the expertise of a skin-care specialist or wound care team when available. A patient with a high risk for pressure injury development will also benefit from these resources. These clinicians help you plan specific interventions to manage poorly healing wounds and pressure injuries and to identify strategies for reducing the risk for pressure injuries. When you care for a patient with a chronic complex wound, contact the wound care team if you note a change in the volume and/or consistency of the drainage, a presence of a strong odor in the drainage, and change in wound-healing status. It is also important to plan a dressing change with the wound care team to assess the wound together to determine effectiveness of the treatment plan and if the wound is showing progress toward healing.

With early discharge from health care settings, it is important to consider a patient's plan for discharge as soon as a patient is admitted to an agency. A skin care or wound care specialist can help with anticipating the patient's discharge wound care needs and related equipment and health care resources. For example, referral to a home care agency or

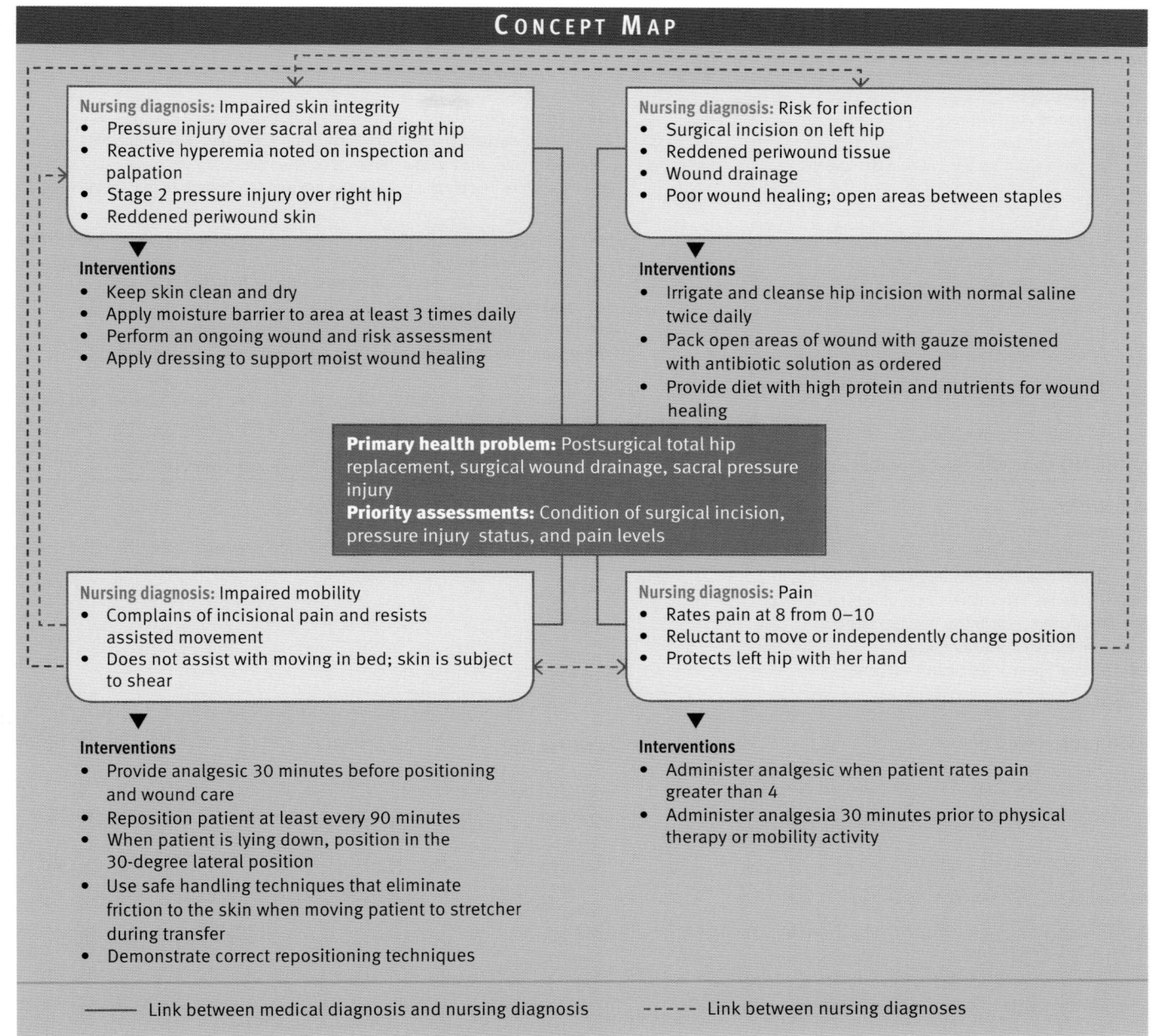

FIG. 48.14 Concept map for Mrs. Stein.

outpatient wound care clinic helps by offering interventions to improve not only wound healing but also the patient's level of independence. A registered dietitian can help develop an appropriate nutrition plan that provides the nutrients needed for wound healing for the patient. Patients and their family caregivers often need to continue the objectives of wound management after discharge. Carefully consider the ability of a family caregiver and the amount of time needed to change a particular dressing when selecting a dressing for the patient to use after discharge. For example, in the home setting a patient's spouse may choose more expensive dressing materials to reduce the frequency of dressing changes (Box 48.6).

As part of planning, Kelly takes time to talk to Mrs. Stein about the risks associated with reduced activity and movement. She explains how the injuries to her skin can worsen and what that will mean to Mrs. Stein's independence

and return to her residence. She tells Mrs. Stein she wants her to be informed about the potential and worsening skin and surgical wound problems. She explains the benefits of activity and the physical therapy session and how that will reduce the risks to her skin and improve her mobility. She explains to Mrs. Stein that the outcome of the activity and movement intervention is improved skin integrity on the right hip and sacral region. Kelly also includes the physical therapist and activities in the plan so that hygiene measures, wound care therapies, and pain control are coordinated with physical therapy sessions.

Kelly collaborates with Mrs. Stein about pain and comfort measures. They agree on the pain-control outcome of a pain rating of 4 or less on a 10-point scale. She mentions to Mrs. Stein and the physical therapist that her tolerance and participation in therapy will be improved with adequate pain control.

◎ NURSING CARE PLAN

Impaired Skin Integrity

ASSESSMENT

Assessment Activities	*Assessment Findings[a]*
Ask Mrs. Stein to move from side to side.	She has incisional pain and soreness in her left hip, **limiting movement**; her lower left leg is also sore, and the pain increases on movement.
Ask Mrs. Stein about her level of pain on movement.	She tells you that she prefers to **keep the hip and leg immobile** to keep the pain level down.
	Position of comfort is right hip and supine, and Mrs. Stein **resists position changes.**
Ask Mrs. Stein to rate her level of pain.	Mrs. Stein rates her **pain 8** out of 10.
Observe and palpate right hip.	There is a partial-thickness injury, **blistered area on right hip is 2.5 cm (1 inch) in diameter**.
	Nonblanchable erythema noted on palpation of periwound area.
Observe and palpate sacral area.	**4.0-cm (approximately 2-inch) blanchable erythema.**
	Incontinent of urine.
Assess left hip, surgical incision.	Small openings between staples oozing serous fluid. **Periwound area red and warm.**

[a]Assessment findings are shown in bold type.

NURSING DIAGNOSIS: Impaired skin integrity related to pressure, friction, and shearing forces over left hip and sacral bony prominence

PLANNING

Expected Outcomes (NOC)[b]

Tissue Integrity: Skin and Mucous Membranes

Skin remains intact over unaffected sacral region.

Stage 2 pressure injury shows signs of healing.

Skin remains intact over other pressure points.

Healing of left hip incisional wound.

Patient reports pain at less than 4 out of 10.

[b]Outcome classification labels from Moorhead S, et al: *Nursing Outcomes Classification (NOC)*, ed 6, St Louis, 2018, Elsevier.

INTERVENTIONS (NIC)[c]	RATIONALE
Skin Surveillance	
Place an order for a pressure-reduction mattress per agency's protocol, and place on bed.	Reduces the duration and magnitude of pressure over vulnerable areas of the body and contributes to comfort, hygiene, dignity, and functional ability (Bryant and Nix, 2016a).
Assist with repositioning every 90 minutes as patient condition allows. Use a friction-reducing sheet or device when helping to reposition.	Repositioning is still required for pressure redistribution and comfort when a support surface is in use. A lift or transfer sheet minimizes friction and/or shear (EPUAP/NPIAP/PPPIA, 2019a).
Elevate head of bed no more than 30 degrees (EPUAP/NPIAP/PPPIA, 2019a; EPUAP/NPIAP/PPPIA, 2019b). **NOTE:** Some hip replacement patients may not be allowed to turn in to 30-degree lateral position.	A slouched position places pressure and shear on the sacrum and coccyx (EPUAP/NPIAP/PPPIA, 2019a).
Keep skin dry and clean; avoid rubbing or massaging around the open area (McNichol et al., 2018).	The presence of skin damage from moisture/maceration contributes to the development of pressure injuries (Francis, 2020; EPUAP/NPIAP/PPPIA, 2019a). Rubbing or massaging areas of nonblanching erythema can cause further tissue damage (EPUAP/NPIAP/PPPIA, 2019a; EPUAP/NPIAP/PPPIA, 2019b; WOCN, 2016).
Use moisture barrier ointment over the injury at least 3 times a day to decrease friction and provide moisture to the open tissue.	Moisture barriers protect the skin by providing a barrier to the effluent (urine, stool, or wound drainage). Skin barriers protect the wound from further damage and promote healing. They may be petroleum, dimethicone, or zinc oxide based (Francis, 2020).

[c]Intervention classification labels from Butcher HK, et al: *Nursing Interventions Classification (NIC)*, ed 7, St Louis, 2018, Elsevier.

EVALUATION

Evaluation Activity	*Patient Response*
Perform daily total body skin and wound assessments.	Intact skin and decreased redness in the sacral region.
	Presence of reepithelialization in right hip pressure injury.
Palpate periwound area on right hip.	Area shows reactive hyperemia and blanching following palpation; no new break in epidermis.
Assess left hip surgical wound.	Nontender, decreased redness, no drainage.
Ask Mrs. Stein to rate her level of pain.	Reports pain as 2 to 3 on a scale of 10.

BOX 48.6   Home Care Recommendations

Injury or Wound Assessment

Assessment and documentation of a pressure injury or wound needs to occur at least weekly unless there is evidence of deterioration, in which case the home health nurse needs to reassess both the pressure injury and the patient's overall management immediately. In the home setting this requires the help of the patient and family caregiver because weekly assessment is not always feasible. Wound assessment in the home is the same as in a health care agency; see Skills 48.1 and 48.2 for specific assessment parameters.

- Consider family caregiver time and ability when selecting a dressing.
- In the home setting some family caregivers choose dressing materials manufactured to reduce the frequency of dressing changes.
- Clean dressings, as opposed to sterile ones, are recommended for home use until research demonstrates otherwise. This recommendation is in keeping with principles regarding nosocomial infections and with past success of clean urinary catheterization in the home setting, and it considers the expense of sterile dressings and the dexterity required for application. The family caregiver can use the "no-touch" technique for dressing changes. This technique is a method of changing surface dressings without touching the wound or the surface of any dressing that might be in contact with the wound. Adherent dressings should be grasped by the corner and removed slowly, whereas gauze dressings can be pinched in the center and lifted off.
- Contaminated dressings in the home should be disposed of in a manner consistent with local regulations. The Environmental Protection Agency recommends placing soiled dressings in securely fastened plastic bags before adding them to other household trash. However, local regulations vary, and home care agencies and patients need to follow procedures that are consistent with local laws.

Data from European Pressure Ulcer Advisory Panel (EPUAP), National Pressure Injury Advisory Panel (NPIAP), and Pan Pacific Pressure Injury Alliance (PPPIA); Haesler E, editor: *Treatment of pressure ulcers/injuries: clinical practice guideline,* EPUAP/NPIAP/PPPIA, 2019; and EPUAP, NPIAP, and PPPIA; Haesler E, editor: *Treatment of pressure ulcers/injuries: quick reference guide,* EPUAP/NPIAP/PPPIA, 2019.

◆ Implementation

Health Promotion. The major health promotion activities regarding skin integrity are prevention of pressure injuries and promotion of normal wound healing. Patients with any type of wounds require nutritional support, proper positioning, and skin care. Prompt identification of patients at high risk for pressure injuries or for impaired wound healing requires timely and appropriate preventive measures (WOCN, 2016).

Nutrition. Patients with existing wounds or those at risk for pressure injury will need extra protein, calories, and nutrients. The Cleveland Clinic (2017) guideline is patient and family caregiver oriented and recommends these daily nutrients to improve and promote wound healing:
- Protein (5–8 servings daily). Eat the protein portion of meals first in case the patient becomes too full.
- Whole grains for higher protein content (5 servings daily).
- Vegetables (2 servings daily). Add to fruit smoothies for an extra boost without a bitter taste.
- Fruit (3 servings daily). Use as toppings for cooked cereals, yogurt, and ice cream. Choose fruit for dessert.
- Dairy (3 servings daily). Substitute milk for water in recipes; add powdered milk or yogurt to shakes, smoothies, and cooked cereals. Top soups with cheese or Greek yogurt.

Prevention of Pressure Injuries. Nursing interventions for patients who are immobile or have other risk factors for pressure injuries focus on prevention (Table 48.8). Prevention minimizes the impact that risk

TABLE 48.8   Quick Guide to Pressure Injury Prevention

Risk Factor	Nursing Interventions
Decreased sensory perception	Provide a support pressure-redistribution surface (Gruccio and Ashton, 2018).
Medical device	Protect pressure points from medical devices such as oxygen tubing, feeding tubes, and casts (Cooper et al., 2020; Kayser et al., 2018).
Moisture	Following each incontinence episode, clean area with no-rinse perineal cleaner and protect skin with moisture barrier ointment (Ferris and Harding, 2020; McNichol et al., 2018). Keep skin dry and free of maceration (Collier, 2016).
Friction and shear	Reposition patient using drawsheet or a transfer board surface. Provide trapeze to facilitate movement in bed. Position patient at a 30-degree lateral turn and limit head elevation to 30 degrees (see Fig. 48.15).
Decreased activity or mobility	Establish and post individualized turning schedule. Turn patient off at-risk areas often (EPUAP/NPIAP/PPPIA, 2019b).
Poor nutrition	Provide adequate nutritional and fluid intake; help with intake as necessary (Stotts, 2016a). Consult registered dietitian for nutritional assessment and recommended nutrients.

factors or contributing factors have on pressure injury development. Three major areas of nursing interventions for prevention of pressure injuries are (1) skin care and management of incontinence; (2) mechanical loading and support devices, which include proper positioning and the use of therapeutic surfaces; and (3) education (EPUAP/NPIAP/PPPIA, 2019a; WOCN, 2016).

Topical Skin Care and Incontinence Management. When you clean the skin, avoid soap and hot water as they increase skin dryness. Use cleaners with nonionic surfactants that are gentle to the skin (WOCN, 2016). Many types of products are available for skin care, and you need to match their use to the specific needs of a patient (e.g., dry skin or skin exposed to incontinent fluids). After you clean the skin and make sure that it is completely dry, apply moisturizer to keep the epidermis well lubricated but not oversaturated.

Make an effort to control, contain, or correct incontinence, perspiration, or wound drainage (see Chapters 46 and 47). Patients who have fecal incontinence and who are also receiving enteral tube feeding provide a management challenge. Often the feedings result in diarrhea. While caring for at-risk patients, it is helpful to use the expertise of an advanced practice nurse with a focus on wound care or management of incontinence. Methods for controlling or containing incontinence vary. Bowel incontinence can sometimes be better managed with proper diet and medications. Urinary incontinence is treated with behavioral techniques, medication, and surgery. Behavioral techniques help patients learn ways to control their bladder and sphincter muscles.

When patients have an incontinence episode, gently clean the area, dry, and apply a thick layer of moisture barrier to the exposed areas. A moisture barrier protects the skin from excessive moisture and from bacteria found in the urine or stool (McNichol et al., 2018).

Although controversial, specialized absorbent products, such as absorptive underpads and garments, are sometimes part of the treatment plan for an incontinent patient. A skin-care specialist is the best resource

FIG. 48.15 Thirty-degree lateral position at which pressure points are avoided. (Adapted from Bryant RA, Nix DP, editors: *Acute and chronic wounds: current management concepts,* ed 5, St Louis, 2016, Elsevier.)

to determine the safest and most efficient absorbent products and pads that wick moisture away from the patient's skin (WOCN, 2016).

Positioning. Repositioning (turning) patients is a consistent element of evidence-based pressure injury prevention (EPUAP/NPIAP/PPPIA, 2019a). The twofold aim of repositioning should be to reduce or relieve pressure at the interface between a bony prominence and support surface (bed or chair) and to limit the amount of time for which the tissue is exposed to pressure (Maklebust and Magnan, 2016). The WOCN guidelines (WOCN, 2016) recommend a 30-degree lateral position (Fig. 48.15), which should prevent positioning directly over the bony prominence of the hip. To prevent shear and friction injuries, use a transfer device to lift rather than drag a patient when changing positions in bed (see Chapter 39). Elevating the head of the bed to 30 degrees or less also decreases the chance of pressure injury development from shearing forces (WOCN, 2016). Change the immobilized patient's position according to tissue tolerance, level of activity and mobility, general medical condition, overall treatment objectives, skin condition, and comfort (EPUAP/NPIAP/PPPIA, 2019a). Repositioning intervals must be based on patient assessment; a standard turning interval of 1.5 to 2 hours does not always prevent pressure injury development. Some patients may need more frequent position changes, whereas other patients can tolerate every-2-hour position changes without tissue injury. When repositioning, use positioning devices to protect bony prominences (WOCN, 2016).

> **QSEN** **Building Competency in Evidence-Based Practice** The nurses on a neurology unit are concerned about patients who develop skin breakdown during recovery from a stroke. The nurses would like to implement a new evidence-based positioning protocol using safe patient handling with the goal of preventing pressure injury development. What is the nurses' PICOT question, and what topics should the nurses include in the evidence-based literature review?
>
> Answers to QSEN Activities can be found on the Evolve website.

For patients at risk for skin breakdown who can sit in a chair, limit the amount of time they sit to 2 hours or less at any given time. In the sitting position the pressure on the ischial tuberosities is greater than in the supine position. In addition, teach the patient to shift weight every 15 minutes while sitting. Shifting weight provides short-term

relief on the ischial tuberosities. Also have the patient sit on foam, gel, or an air cushion to redistribute weight away from the ischial areas. Rigid and donut-shaped cushions are contraindicated because they reduce blood supply to the area, resulting in wider areas of ischemia (EPUAP/NPIAP/PPPIA, 2019b; WOCN, 2016).

After repositioning a patient, inspect the skin that was in the dependent position. Remember to use caution when evaluating early signs of tissue ischemia in darkly pigmented skin. For patients with light-toned skin, observe for reactive hyperemia and blanching. Never massage reddened areas. Massaging reddened areas increases the breakdown of the capillaries in the underlying tissues and leads to the risk of tissue injury and pressure injury formation (WOCN, 2016).

Support Surfaces (Therapeutic Beds and Mattresses). Support surfaces are specialized devices (e.g., mattress overlays, mattress replacements, integrated bed systems, seat cushions, or seat cushion overlays) that redistribute pressure and are designed for management of tissue loads, microclimate, shear, and/or other therapeutic functions (EPUAP/NPIAP/PPPIA, 2019a). Microclimate is the mean skin temperature and skin moisture between the patient's skin and the support surface (WOCN, 2016).

Support surfaces redistribute tissue loads by immersion (depth of penetration or sinking into the support surface by the patient's body) and envelopment (deforment around the body), thus evenly distributing pressure across the entire body surface (Morgan, 2020; Maklebust and Magnan, 2016). Support surfaces reduce the hazards of immobility to the skin and musculoskeletal system. However, none eliminates the need for meticulous skin assessment, skin care, and scheduled repositioning. No single device completely eliminates the effects of pressure on the skin.

When selecting support surfaces, use clinical judgment by considering the patient's risks for skin breakdown, underlying condition, and treatments being administered. This knowledge will allow you to understand a patient's unique needs and make the clinical decision necessary to select the support-surface with the appropriate characteristics (Table 48.9). In selecting a support surface, a flow chart that includes patient risks and the purpose for support surfaces can often be helpful. If your agency has a wound care nurse specialist, consult with the specialist on choice of support surface. Teach patients and families the reason for and proper use of the devices (Box 48.7). When used correctly, these support surfaces help redistribute pressure to the skin of patients who are at risk for or have skin breakdown.

Some common errors with support surfaces are placing the wrong side of the support surface toward the patient, not plugging powered

TABLE 48.9 Support Surfaces

Category and Mechanism of Action	Indications for Use	Advantages	Disadvantages
Support Surfaces and Overlays			
Foam Overlay (Available as an Overlay or in a Full Mattress)			
Reduces pressure; the cover (top) can reduce friction and shear Base height of 7.5–10 cm (3–4 inches); see manufacturer guidelines regarding amount of body weight supported	Use for moderate- to high-risk patients	Onetime charge No setup fee Cannot be punctured Available in various sizes (e.g., bed, chair, operating room table) Little maintenance Does not need electricity	Elevated body temperature Hot and may trap moisture Limited life span Plastic protective sheet needed for incontinent patients or patients with draining wounds Not indicated for those with existing Stage 3 or 4 pressure injuries
Water Overlay (Available as an Overlay or in a Full Mattress)			
Redistributes pressure and pressure points because surface provides flotation by redistributing patient's weight evenly over entire support surface	Use for high-risk patients	Readily available Some control over motion sensations Easy to clean	Easily punctured Heavy Fluid motion may make procedures (e.g., dressing changes, CPR) difficult Maintenance needed to prevent microorganism growth Patient transfers out of bed are difficult Difficult to raise and lower head of bed
Gel Overlay			
Redistributes pressure because surface provides flotation by redistributing patient's weight evenly over entire support surface	Use for moderate- to high-risk patients Use for patients who are wheelchair dependent	Low maintenance Easy to clean Multiple-patient use Impermeable to needle punctures	Heavy Expensive Lacks airflow for moisture control Variable friction control
Nonpowered Air-Filled Overlay			
Redistributes pressure by lowering mean interface pressure between patient's tissue and overlay	Use for moderate- to high-risk patients Use for patients who can reposition themselves	Easy to clean Multiple-patient use Low maintenance Potential repair of some air-filled products Durable	Damaged by punctures from needles and sharps Requires routine monitoring to determine adequate inflation pressure Patient transfers out of bed can be difficult
Low–Air-Loss Overlay (Available as an Overlay or in a Full Mattress)			
Maintains constant and slight air movement against patient's skin; redistributes pressure; assists in managing the heat and humidity (microclimate) of the skin	Use for moderate- to high-risk patients	Easy to clean Maintains constant inflation Deflates to facilitate transfer and CPR Moisture control Fabric covering overlay is air permeable, bacteria impermeable, and waterproof Reduces shear and friction Setup provided by manufacturer	Damaged by needles and sharps Can be noisy Requires electricity, some are available with short backup battery In home may need to purchase backup generator in case of loss of electrical power
Specialty Beds			
Air-Fluidized Bed			
Bedframe contains silicone-coated beads and provides pressure redistribution by the fluidlike medium that is created by forcing air through beads, resulting in immersion and envelopment of the patient	Use for high-risk patients Use for patients with Stage 3 or 4 pressure injuries or burns	Less frequent turning or repositioning Improved patient comfort Becomes firm for CPR or other treatments when device is turned off Reduces shear, friction, and edema to site May facilitate management of copious wound drainage or incontinence Setup provided by manufacturer	Continuous circulation of warm, dry air may increase patient risk for dehydration Possible increase in room temperature Patient may experience disorientation Patient transfer difficult Heavy Expensive May not be wide enough for use with obese patients or patients with contractures Patient cannot lie prone because of risk of suffocation

Continued

TABLE 48.9 Support Surfaces—cont'd

Category and Mechanism of Action	Indications for Use	Advantages	Disadvantages
Low–Air-Loss Bed Bedframe with series of connected air-filled pillows Flow of air controls the amount of pressure in each pillow and assists in managing the heat and humidity (microclimate) of the patient's skin Redistributes pressure	Use for patients who need pressure redistribution, those who cannot be repositioned frequently, or those who have skin breakdown on more than one surface Contraindicated in patients with unstable spinal column	Can raise and lower head and foot of bed Easy transfer in and out of bed Setup provided by manufacturer	Portable motor can be noisy Bed surface material slippery; patients can easily slide down mattress or out of bed when being transferred
Kinetic Therapy Provides continuous passive motion to promote mobilization of pulmonary secretions and low air loss and provides pressure redistribution	Used primarily to facilitate pulmonary hygiene in patients with acute respiratory conditions Should not be used when the patient is hemodynamically unstable	Reduces pulmonary complications associated with restricted mobility	Does not reduce shear or moisture Cannot be used with cervical or skeletal traction Possible motion sickness initially

Data from Doughty D, McNichol L: *Wound, Ostomy, and Continence Nurses Society (WOCN): Core curriculum: wound management,* Philadelphia, 2016, Wound, Ostomy, and Continence Society; and Wound, Ostomy, and Continence Nurses Society (WOCN): *Guideline for prevention and management of pressure ulcers, WOCN clinical practice guideline series,* ed 2, Mt Laurel, NJ, 2016, WOCN.
CPR, Cardiopulmonary resuscitation.

BOX 48.7 PATIENT TEACHING

Pressure-Redistribution Surfaces

Objective
- Patient and family caregiver will describe the purposes and basic operations of the pressure-redistribution surface.

Teaching Strategies
- Explain the reasons for the pressure-redistribution surface.
- Explain the need to maintain proper body mechanics while using the pressure-redistribution surface. Demonstrate technique.
- Discuss possible patient sensations associated with the device.
- Instruct that minimal layers of linens should be placed over the pressure-redistribution surface.
- Educate in the use and care of the pressure-redistribution surface (based on manufacturer guidelines).
- Explain common errors in the use of support surfaces.
- Explain additional pressure-redistribution measures (e.g., safe patient handling during turning, avoidance of friction, 30-degree lateral position) (WOCN, 2016).

Evaluation
Use the principles of teach-back to evaluate patient/family caregiver learning:
- Now that we have discussed the use of the pressure-redistribution surface, explain to me the purpose for using the device.
- Describe to me the possible sensations that you might experience while using the support surface.
- Show me how you will correctly position yourself on the pressure-redistribution surface.

---

support surfaces into the electrical source, not turning on the power source for powered support surfaces, using several layers of sheets and pads between the patient and the surface, and improperly inflating some support surfaces. In addition, the hand checks to assess for "bottoming out" on an air mattress may be used incorrectly. Bottoming out makes the support surface ineffective because the weight of the individual, as well as the weight distribution and shape, may cause support surface deformation, causing the body to sink too deeply into the surface; effective pressure distribution is lost. Hand checks are a satisfactory but subjective method for assessing for bottoming out for air mattress overlays and chair cushions. To use the hand check method, the nurse slides the hand, palm side up, at the interface of the overlay and the mattress just under the patient's sacrum. If the nurse can feel the patient's sacrum resting in the palm of the hand or is not able to feel at least 2.5 cm (1 inch) of the inflated surface between the palm of the hand and the patient's sacrum, the patient is said to be bottoming out (NPUAP, 2015). The hand check method is inappropriate for replacement mattresses and integrated bed systems (bedframe and support surfaces) (EPUAP/NPIAP/PPPIA, 2019a).

Kelly prioritizes two nursing diagnoses: **Impaired Skin Integrity** *related to pressure and shear and* **Impaired Mobility** *related to incisional pain. From previous clinical experiences and postclinical conferences, Kelly knows that postoperative care is more than just pain control and that, in the case of Mrs. Stein, Kelly needs interventions to protect her skin to prevent further pressure injuries and progression of the Stage 2 pressure injury on her right hip. An important aspect to resolving impaired skin integrity issues is maintaining and improving mobility. Mrs. Stein is postoperative; comfort measures and pain control are essential to improving mobility and keeping Mrs. Stein off her sacral and right hip areas. Kelly and Mrs. Stein work together, and Kelly reinforces that managing acute pain often provides patients with physical and emotional energy for care. She explains the pain-control plan from Mrs. Stein's surgeon. She also lets Mrs. Stein know that she also has nonopioid pain medications that she may want to try and that are safe and nonaddictive. Kelly gives Mrs. Stein a written schedule for when she can have pain medication and the different types of medications ordered by her surgeon.*

Acute Care. An acute event involving wound care includes emergency first aid for traumatic wounds and aggressive management of stable acute and chronic wounds. In all cases, principles of infection control and protection of a wound must be followed. Wound care, principles of infection control, and protection of a wound are the same whether you are caring for a patient in an acute care, restorative care, or continuing care agency.

First Aid for Wounds. Use first-aid measures for wound protection and management in an emergency situation. When a patient sustains a traumatic wound, first-aid interventions include stabilizing cardiopulmonary function (see Chapter 41), promoting hemostasis, cleaning the wound, and protecting it from further injury.

Hemostasis. After assessing the type and extent of a wound, control bleeding by applying direct pressure with a sterile or clean dressing such as a washcloth. After bleeding subsides, an adhesive bandage or gauze dressing taped over the laceration allows skin edges to close and a blood clot to form. If a dressing becomes saturated with blood, add another layer of dressing, continue to apply pressure, and elevate the affected part. Avoid further disruption of skin layers. Serious lacerations need to be sutured by a health care provider. Pressure dressings used during the first 24 to 48 hours after trauma help maintain hemostasis.

Normally allow a puncture wound to bleed to remove dirt and other contaminants, such as saliva from a dog bite. When a penetrating object such as a knife blade is present, do not remove the object. The presence of the object provides pressure and controls some bleeding. Removal causes massive, uncontrolled bleeding. Except for skull injuries, apply pressure around the penetrating object but not on it, and transport the patient to an emergency department.

Cleaning. The process of cleaning a wound involves selecting an appropriate cleaning solution and using a mechanical means of delivering that solution without causing injury to the healing wound tissue (WOCN, 2016). Gently cleaning a wound removes contaminants that serve as sources of infection. However, vigorous cleaning using a method with too much mechanical force causes bleeding or further injury. For abrasions, minor lacerations, and small puncture wounds, first rinse the wound with normal saline and lightly cover the area with a dressing. When a laceration is bleeding profusely, only brush away surface contaminants and concentrate on hemostasis until the patient can be cared for in a clinic or hospital.

According to the WOCN guidelines (WOCN, 2016), normal saline is the preferred cleaning agent. It is physiologically neutral and does not harm tissue. Normal saline keeps the wound surface moist to promote the development and migration of epithelial tissue. Gentle cleansing with normal saline and application of moist saline dressings are commonly used for healing wounds.

Protection. Regardless of whether bleeding has stopped, protect a traumatic wound from further injury by applying sterile or clean dressings and immobilizing the body part. A light dressing applied over minor wounds prevents entrance of microorganisms.

Management of Pressure Injuries. Treatment of patients with pressure injuries requires a holistic approach that uses interprofessional expertise (EPUAP/NPIAP/PPPIA, 2019a; WOCN, 2016). Others who are involved, in addition to the nurse, include the health care provider, wound care nurse specialist, physical therapist, occupational therapist, nutritionist, and pharmacist. Aspects of pressure injury treatment include local care of the wound and continuation of supportive measures such as adequate nutrition, skin care, and redistribution of pressure using positioning and support surfaces (see Skill 48.2).

Before treating a pressure injury, reassess the wound for location, stage, size, tissue type and amount, exudate, and surrounding skin condition (see Skill 48.1) (Nix, 2016). Acute wounds require close monitoring (every 4–8 hours; check agency policy). Chronic wound assessment occurs less frequently. Depending on the topical management system, evaluate the wound with every dressing change, usually not more than once a day.

The use and documentation of a systematic approach to monitor progress of an actual pressure injury leads to better decision making

and optimal outcomes (Nix, 2016). Several healing and documentation tools are available to document wound assessments over time. Using a tool helps link assessment to outcomes so that an evaluation of the plan of care follows objective criteria (Nix, 2016). For example, the Bates-Jensen Wound Assessment Tool (BWAT) (Bates-Jensen, 2016; Bates-Jensen et al., 2019) addresses 15 wound characteristics. You score individual items and calculate the total, providing an overall indication of wound status. The scoring helps to evaluate whether the goals of the wound management are effective.

Wound Management. Maintenance of a physiological local wound environment is the goal of effective wound management (Bryant and Nix, 2016b). To maintain a healthy wound environment, you need to address the following objectives: prevent and manage infection, clean the wound, remove nonviable tissue, maintain the wound in a moist environment, eliminate dead space, control odor, eliminate or minimize pain, and protect the wound and periwound skin (Ramundo, 2016).

A wound does not move through the phases of healing if infected. Preventing wound infection includes cleaning and removing nonviable tissue. Clean pressure injuries *only with noncytotoxic wound cleaners* such as normal saline or commercial wound cleaners. Noncytotoxic cleaners do not damage or kill fibroblasts and healing tissue (Bryant and Nix, 2016b). Some commonly used cytotoxic solutions are Dakin solution (sodium hypochlorite solution), acetic acid, and povidone-iodine. These are not to be used in clean, granulating wounds.

Irrigation is a common method of delivering a wound-cleansing solution to the wound. Wound irrigation cleans and debrides necrotic tissue with pressure that can remove debris from the wound bed without damaging healthy tissue (Ramundo, 2016). One method to ensure an irrigation pressure within the correct range is to use a 19-gauge angiocatheter and a 35-mL syringe, which delivers saline to a pressure injury at 8 psi (Fig. 48.16).

Debridement is the removal of nonviable, necrotic tissue. Removal of necrotic tissue is necessary to rid the wound of a source of infection, enable visualization of the wound bed, and provide a clean base necessary for healing. The method of debridement depends on which is most appropriate for a patient's condition and outcomes of care (WOCN, 2016). It is important to remember that during the debridement process some normal wound observations include an increase in wound exudate, odor, and size. You need to assess and prevent or effectively manage pain that occurs with debridement (WOCN, 2016). Plan to administer an ordered analgesic 30 minutes before debridement.

Methods of debridement include mechanical, autolytic, chemical, and sharp/surgical. Autolytic debridement is the removal of dead tissue via lysis of necrotic tissue by the WBCs and natural enzymes of the

FIG. 48.16 Wound irrigation.

body (Ramundo, 2016). You accomplish this by using dressings that support moisture at the wound surface. If the wound base is dry, use a dressing that adds moisture; if there is excessive exudate, use a dressing that absorbs the excessive moisture while maintaining moisture at the wound bed. Some examples of these dressings are transparent film and hydrocolloid dressings.

You can accomplish chemical debridement with the use of a topical enzyme preparation, Dakin solution, or sterile maggots. Topical enzymes induce changes in the substrate, resulting in the breakdown of necrotic tissue (Ramundo, 2016). Depending on the type of enzyme used, the preparation either digests or dissolves the tissue. These preparations require a health care provider's order. Dakin solution breaks down and loosens dead tissue in a wound. Apply the solution to gauze and apply to the wound. Sterile maggots are used in a wound because it is thought that they ingest the dead tissue.

Surgical debridement is the removal of devitalized tissue with a scalpel, scissors, or other sharp instrument. Physicians and, in some states, trained advanced practice nurses perform surgical debridement of an injury or wound. Nurses should check the nurse practice act for their state to see whether surgical debridement is a nursing function. It is the quickest method of debridement. It is usually indicated when the patient has signs of cellulitis or sepsis. Other methods of mechanical debridement are wound irrigation (high-pressure irrigation and pulsatile high-pressure lavage) and whirlpool treatments (Ramundo, 2016).

A moist environment supports the movement of epithelial cells and facilitates wound closure. A wound that has excessive exudate (drainage) provides an environment that supports bacterial growth, macerates the periwound skin, and slows the healing process (EPUAP/NPIAP/PPPIA, 2019a). If excessive wound exudate is present, evaluate the volume, consistency, and odor of the drainage to determine whether an infection is present.

Remember, the wound will not heal unless the contributory factors are controlled or eliminated. Therefore it is critically important for you to address the causative factors (e.g., shear, friction, pressure, and moisture), or it is unlikely that the wound will heal despite topical therapy (Bryant and Nix, 2016b).

Use clinical judgment and ongoing wound assessments to make necessary clinical decisions to modify the treatment plan as a wound heals. For example, a transparent film dressing is used initially to autolytically debride (liquefy the tissue using body moisture) a necrotic wound. Once the wound is cleaned of necrotic tissue, discontinue the transparent film dressing and, based on the wound base characteristics, choose a new dressing. A wound with excessive drainage requires a dressing with a high absorptive capacity. Continued reassessment is key to supporting the wound as it moves through the phases of wound healing.

Protection. Protecting a wound from further injury is a priority. A strategy to prevent surgical wound dehiscence is to place a folded thin blanket or pillow over an abdominal wound so that a patient can splint the area during coughing (see Chapter 50). Because coughing increases the intraabdominal pressure, the patient applies light but firm pressure over the wound when coughing to support the healing tissue. A patient may also wear an abdominal binder to make movement less uncomfortable and to provide support for the abdomen and surgical site. Teach the patient this technique and keep the splint within hand's reach.

Education. Education of the patient and family caregivers is an important nursing function (Bryant and Nix, 2016a). Your approach to teaching will depend on what you assess about a patient and the family caregiver's readiness, willingness, and motivation to learn (see Chapter 25). If patients or family caregivers have low health literacy, you must select an educational approach that adapts to their limitations. A recent study of community-based patients and their family caregivers indicated that despite information leaflets broadly meeting required production and content guidelines, patients appeared to poorly engage with these materials and demonstrated limited health literacy in relation to pressure injury (Durrant et al., 2019). Although health care agencies may attempt to improve readability of materials, emphasis should remain on high-quality patient–health care professional relationships. Such relationships enable you to tailor patient education that can enhance awareness and engagement with treatment and prevention interventions (Durrant et al., 2019).

A variety of educational tools, including videos and written materials, are available for you to use when teaching patients and family caregivers how to prevent and treat pressure injuries and care for wounds. The U.S. National Library of Medicine (2020) has a patient-centered website with information on the prevention of pressure injuries.

Understanding and assessing the experience of the patient and support person are important dimensions in the treatment of people with wounds and pressure injuries (WOCN, 2016). Clinicians are only just now exploring through research the caregiver's perspective of the concerns and issues faced by frail older spouses caring for their loved ones with pressure injuries. Plan interventions to meet the identified psychosocial needs of patients and their support people (WOCN, 2016).

Nutritional Status. Nutritional support of a patient with a wound is based on the appreciation that nutrition is fundamental to normal cellular integrity and tissue repair (Stotts, 2016a). Early intervention is necessary to correct inadequate nutrition and support healing. Refer patients with pressure injuries to a registered dietitian for early intervention involving therapeutic diets or enteral or parenteral nutrition (see Chapter 45). Your patient will need 30 to 35 calories per kilogram of body weight if a pressure injury is present and the patient is assessed to be at risk for malnutrition (EPUAP/NPIAP/PPPIA, 2019a). Increased caloric intake helps replace subcutaneous tissue. Patients will also receive vitamin and mineral supplements if suspected or known deficiencies exist. Vitamin C promotes collagen synthesis, capillary wall integrity, fibroblast function, and immunological function.

Patients with pressure injuries who are underweight or losing weight need enhanced protein supplementation (WOCN, 2016). A patient can lose as much as 50 g of protein per day from an open, high–exudative pressure injury. Although the recommended intake of protein for adults is 0.8 g/kg/day, a higher intake up to 1.8 g/kg/day is necessary for healing. Increased protein intake helps rebuild epidermal tissue (EPUAP/NPIAP/PPPIA, 2019a). Weight, laboratory values, and skin parameters reflect changes in status and effects of nutritional interventions (Stotts, 2016a).

Dressings. The use of dressings requires an understanding of wound healing. A variety of dressing materials are available commercially. The correct dressing selection facilitates wound healing (Bryant and Nix, 2016b). The dressing type depends on the assessment of a wound and the phase of wound healing. When you identify the objectives for wound care, the dressing choice becomes clear. A wound that requires infection management requires a different set of dressings than one requiring the removal of nonviable tissue.

Purposes of Dressings. A dressing serves several purposes:
- Protects a wound from microorganism contamination
- Aids in hemostasis
- Promotes healing by maintaining wound moisture
- Promotes healing by absorbing drainage and debriding a wound
- Supports or splints a wound site
- Promotes thermal insulation of a wound surface

When the skin is broken, a dressing helps reduce exposure to microorganisms. However, when drainage is minimal, the healing process by primary intention forms a natural fibrin seal that eliminates the need for a dressing. A wound that is healing by secondary intention needs the support of a moist wound environment. A moist wound base facilitates the movement of epithelialization, thus allowing the wound to resurface as quickly as possible. Wounds with extensive tissue loss always need a dressing.

The functions of a dressing on a healing wound are to provide protection, deliver medication, and absorb drainage. These dressings can be dry or moist. Gauze dressings come in various types, including gauze sponges, used to pack wounds with depth and drainage; gauze placed over a shallow healing wound as a topper dressing; or gauze placed over a wound to wick the wound drainage. A problem occurs if wound drainage dries, causing the dressing to stick to the suture line. Improperly removing a dressing disrupts the healing epidermal surface. If a gauze dressing sticks to a surgical incision, lightly moisten it with saline solution before removal. This saturates the dressing and loosens it from the incisional area, thus preventing trauma to the incisional area during removal.

The dressing choice and technique vary, depending on the outcome of the treatment plan for a wound. For example, if the expected outcome is to maintain a moist environment to promote wound healing, a saline-moistened gauze dressing must remain moist and not become dry and stick to the wound. This is in direct contrast to the moist-to-dry dressing technique that mechanically debrides a wound. When wounds such as a necrotic wound require debriding, a moist-to-dry dressing technique or dressings can be considered (see Skill 48.3). Also, foam and alginate dressings are used for wounds with large amounts of exudate and are designed to absorb drainage.

Pressure dressings promote hemostasis for bleeding wounds. Applied with elastic bandages, a pressure dressing exerts localized downward pressure over an actual or potential bleeding site. It eliminates dead space in underlying tissues so that wound healing progresses normally. Check pressure dressings to be sure that they do not interfere with circulation to a body part by assessing skin color, pulses in distal extremities, the patient's comfort, and changes in sensation. Pressure dressings are not removed routinely.

Dressings applied to a draining wound require frequent changing to prevent microorganism growth and skin breakdown. Bacteria grow readily in the dark, warm, moist environment under a dressing. The periwound area can become macerated and irritated. Minimize periwound skin breakdown by keeping the skin clean and dry and reducing the use of tape. The inner layer of an absorbent dressing serves as a reservoir for secretions. The wicking action of woven gauze dressings pulls excess drainage into the dressing and away from the wound. The final outer layer of the dressing (usually an ABD pad that has an outer layer that prevents strike-through) helps prevent bacteria and other external contaminants from reaching the wound surface. Apply adhesives to this layer to secure the dressings.

The more extensive a wound, the larger the dressing required. For example, a bulky dressing applied with pressure minimizes movement of underlying tissues and helps immobilize the entire body part. A bandage or cloth wrapped around a penetrating object should immobilize it adequately.

Alternative dressings are available to cover and protect certain types of wounds such as large wounds, wounds with drainage tubes or suction catheters in the wound, and wounds that need frequent changing because of excessive drainage. In the home setting a clean towel or diaper is often the best secondary dressing. Pouches or special wound collection systems cover wounds with excessive drainage and collect the drainage. Some of the collection systems have a plastic window on the front of the wound pouch, allowing you to change the packing without removing the pouch from the skin.

For many surgical wounds, dressings are no longer used (see Chapter 50). However, when a surgical wound has a dressing, its purpose is to promote wound healing by primary intention. Thus it is common to remove surgical dressings as soon as drainage stops. In

---

BOX 48.8 Dressing Considerations

- Clean the wound and periwound area at each dressing change, minimizing trauma to the wound (WOCN, 2016).
- Use a dressing that continuously provides a moist environment.
- Perform wound care using topical dressings as determined by a thorough assessment.
- No specific studies have proven an optimal dressing type for pressure injuries (EPUAP/NPIAP/PPPIA, 2019a; WOCN, 2016).
- Choose a dressing that keeps the periwound skin dry while keeping the injury bed moist.
- Choose a dressing that controls exudate but does not desiccate the injury bed.
- The type of dressing may change over time as the pressure injury heals or deteriorates. The wound should be monitored at every dressing change and regularly assessed to determine whether modifications in the dressing type are needed (WOCN, 2016).
- Consider family caregiver time, ease of use, availability, and cost when selecting a dressing.

---

contrast, when dressing a wound healing by secondary intention, the dressing material becomes a means for providing moisture to the wound or helping in debridement.

Types of Dressings. Dressings vary by type of material and mode of application (moist or dry) (see Skill 48.3). They need to be easy to apply, comfortable, and made of materials that promote wound healing. The WOCN guidelines (WOCN, 2016) are helpful when selecting dressings based on the expected outcomes of wound treatment (Box 48.8). To avoid causing damage to the periwound skin, it is important that the dressing technique that you use to treat pressure injuries and other wounds not be excessively moist.

Most pressure injuries require dressings. The type of dressing is usually based on the stage of the pressure injury, the type of tissue in the wound, and the function of the dressing (Table 48.10). Before placing a dressing on a pressure injury, it is important, based on the nursing diagnosis, to understand the expected outcome of the treatment, the mechanism of action of the dressing, and principles of wound care. It is difficult to sometimes impossible to apply any dressing to an MDRPI injury. Therefore it is important to prevent injury and protect the site from injury (Box 48.9).

Gauze sponges are the oldest and most common dressing. They are absorbent and are especially useful in wounds to wick away wound exudate. Gauze is available in different textures and various lengths and sizes; 4 × 4 inches is the most common size. Gauze can be saturated with solutions and used to clean and pack a wound. When used to pack a wound, the gauze is saturated with the solution (usually normal saline), wrung out (leaving the gauze only moist), unfolded, and lightly packed into the wound. Unfolding the dressing allows easy wicking action. The purpose of this type of dressing is to provide moisture to the wound yet to allow wound drainage to be wicked into the dry cover gauze pad.

Another type of dressing is a self-adhesive, transparent film that traps moisture over a wound, providing a moist environment to encourage epithelial cell growth (Fig. 48.17). A transparent dressing adheres to undamaged skin, does not need a secondary dressing, and permits viewing of the wound. It is ideal for small superficial wounds such as a Stage 1 pressure injury or a partial-thickness wound. Use a film dressing as a secondary dressing and for autolytic debridement of small wounds. It serves as a barrier to external fluids and bacteria but still allows the wound surface to "breathe" because oxygen passes through the transparent dressing (McNichol et al., 2018). This dressing promotes a moist environment to encourage epithelial cell growth.

TABLE 48.10 Dressings by Pressure Injury Stage

Pressure Injury Stage	Pressure Injury Status	Dressing	Comments[a]	Expected Change	Adjuvants
1	Intact	None Transparent dressing Hydrocolloid	Allows visual assessment. Protects from shear. Do not use transparent dressing in presence of excessive moisture. Hydrocolloid does not allow visual assessment.	Resolves slowly without epidermal loss over 7–14 days	Turning schedule. Support hydration. Nutritional support. Use pressure-redistribution bed or chair cushion.
2	Clean	Composite film Hydrocolloid Hydrogel covered with foam or gauze dressing	Limits shear. Change when seal of dressing breaks; maximal wear time 7 days. Provides moist environment.	Heals through reepithelialization	See previous stage. Manage incontinence.
3	Clean	Hydrocolloid Hydrogel covered with foam dressing	Change when seal of dressing breaks; maximum wear time 7 days. Apply over wound to protect and absorb moisture.	Heals through granulation and reepithelialization	See previous stages. Evaluate pressure-redistribution needs.
		Calcium alginate	Use when there is significant exudate. Cover with secondary dressing.		
		Gauze	Use with normal saline or other prescribed solution. Wring out excess solution; unfold to make contact with wound. Cover with dry dressing tape in place.		
		Growth factors	Use with gauze per manufacturer instructions.		
4	Clean	Hydrogel covered with foam dressing	See Stage 3: clean.	Heals through granulation, scar tissue development, and reepithelialization	Surgical consultation may be necessary for closure. See Stages 1, 2, and 3.
		Calcium alginate	Used with significant exudate; must cover with secondary dressing.		
		Gauze	See Stage 3: clean.		
Unstageable	Wound covered with eschar	Adherent film	Facilitates softening of eschar.	Eschar lifts at edges as healing progresses	See previous stages. Surgical consultation may be considered for debridement.
		Gauze plus ordered solution	Delivers solution and may soften the eschar.		May be considered for slow debridement.
		Enzymes	Breaks down eschar, providing debridement.	Eschar loosens over time	
		None	If eschar is dry and intact and debridement is not part of the plan of care, no dressing is used, allowing eschar to act as physiological cover.		

[a]As with *all* occlusive dressings, wounds should not be clinically infected.

It adheres to undamaged skin, does not need a secondary dressing, and permits viewing of the wound.

Hydrocolloid dressings are dressings with complex formulations of colloids and adhesive components. They are adhesive and occlusive. The wound contact layer of this dressing forms a gel as wound exudate is absorbed and maintains a moist healing environment. Hydrocolloids support healing in clean granulating wounds and autolytically debride necrotic wounds; they are available in a variety of sizes and shapes. This type of dressing absorbs drainage through exudate absorbers within the dressing; maintains wound moisture; slowly liquefies necrotic debris; and can be left in place for 3 to 5 days. In addition, hydrocolloid dressings are impermeable to bacteria and other contaminants, act as a preventive dressing for high-risk friction areas, and are self-adhesive and mold to the wound.

The hydrocolloid dressing is useful on shallow to moderately deep dermal injuries. Hydrocolloid dressings cannot absorb drainage from heavily draining wounds, and some are contraindicated for use in full-thickness and infected wounds. Most hydrocolloids leave a residue in the wound bed that is easy to confuse with purulent drainage.

Hydrogel dressings are gauze or sheet dressings impregnated with water or glycerin-based amorphous gel. This type of dressing hydrates wounds and absorbs small amounts of exudate. Hydrogel dressings are

BOX 48.9 EVIDENCE-BASED PRACTICE

Medical Device–Related Pressure Injuries

PICOT Question: In hospitalized patients, which interventions prevent or reduce the risk of medical device–related pressure injuries (MDRPIs)?

Evidence Summary

MDRPIs are becoming more common across all health care settings and in multiple patient age-groups (da Silva Galetto et al., 2019; Kayser et al., 2018). Assessment under, around, and at the edges of medical devices is critical for prevention of and early intervention for these injuries. Use assessment findings to determine the frequency for routine assessment of skin underneath device for edema, risks for potential for skin breakdown, and early signs of skin breakdown (da Silva Galetto et al., 2019; EPUAP/NPIAP/PPPIA, 2019a). Use assessment findings to choose interventions to prevent or reduce the risk of MDRPIs.

Application to Nursing Practice

- Choose the correct size of medical device(s) to fit the individual, especially endotracheal tubes and oxygen equipment (Cox et al., 2020).
- Cushion and protect the skin with dressings in high-risk areas (e.g., nasal bridge) (Kayser et al., 2018).
- Remove or move removable devices to assess skin at least daily (EPUAP/NPIAP/PPPIA, 2019a).
- Carefully remove medical adhesive and assess underlying skin for redness, tears, blistering (Kelly-O'Flynn et al., 2020).
- Avoid placement of device(s) over sites of prior or existing pressure injury.
- Consider interventions such as foam padding to reduce or eliminate the pressure injury (EPUAP/NPIAP/PPPIA, 2019a; Black and Kalowes, 2016).
- Confirm that devices are not placed directly under an individual who is bedridden or immobile.

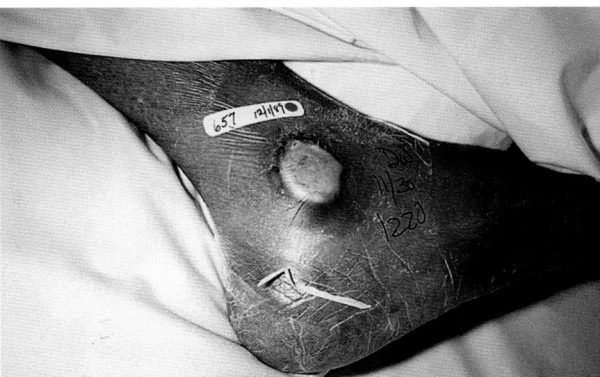

FIG. 48.17 Transparent film dressing.

indicated for use in partial-thickness and full-thickness wounds, deep wounds with some exudate, necrotic wounds, burns, and radiation-damaged skin. They debride necrotic tissue by softening the necrotic area. They can be very useful in painful wounds because they are soothing and do not adhere to the wound bed and thus cause little pain during removal. A disadvantage is that some hydrogels require a secondary dressing, and you must take care to prevent periwound maceration. Hydrogels also come in a tube; thus you are able to apply the gel directly into the wound base.

Many other types of dressings are available. Foam and alginate dressings are for wounds with large amounts of exudate and those that need packing. Foam dressings are also used around drainage tubes to absorb drainage. Calcium alginate dressings are manufactured from seaweed and come in sheet and rope form. The alginate forms a soft gel when in contact with wound fluid. These highly absorbent dressings are for wounds with an excessive amount of drainage and do not cause trauma when removed from the wound. *Do not use these in dry wounds, and they require a secondary dressing.* Several manufacturers produce composite dressings, which combine two different dressing types into one dressing.

Changing Dressings. A health care provider's order for wound care indicates the dressing type, the frequency of changing, and any solutions or ointments to be applied to the wound. An order to "reinforce dressing prn" (add dressings without removing the original one) is common right after surgery, when the health care provider does not want accidental disruption of the suture line or bleeding. Thoroughly review the medical or operating room record because it indicates whether drains are present, the location of the drain, and the type of drainage.

When changing a dressing, always have at hand all the supplies needed. Poor preparation results in disorganized care and can cause a break in aseptic technique (see Chapter 28), accidental pulling of wound tissue, or dislodgement of a drain. Use clinical judgment to modify a dressing change procedure, particularly if the character of a wound changes. Notifying the health care provider of any change is essential.

Sometimes (e.g., with chronic nonsurgical wounds) you will use clean medical aseptic technique for a dressing change. *Clean* refers to the fact that the nurse maintains medical instead of sterile asepsis (see Chapter 28). You wear clean gloves, but the dressing materials are in sterile packages and are carefully placed over the wound. Deep wounds that require irrigation are usually irrigated with a sterile solution. A complete patient and wound history is essential in determining when a clean dressing technique is appropriate. For example, chronic pressure injury wounds require clean technique. On the other hand, a fresh surgical wound may require sterile technique, which involves the use of sterile gloves to prevent the introduction of microorganisms into a healing wound. After the first dressing change, verify that the location of drains and the types of dressing materials and solutions to use are in the patient's care plan.

Often it is necessary to teach patients and family caregivers how to change dressings in preparation for home care. In this situation, demonstrate dressing changes to a patient and/or family caregiver early enough that you can also provide an opportunity for practice. Usually, wound healing has progressed to the point that risks of complications such as dehiscence or evisceration are minimal. When dressing changes are required after a patient returns to the home setting, a patient or family caregiver must be able to demonstrate safe and correct dressing change before discharge and have the resources at home to perform care (e.g., supplies and running water). Contaminated dressings in the home should be disposed of in a manner consistent with local regulations. Skill 48.3 outlines the steps for changing dry and moist dressings.

Packing a Wound. The first step in packing a wound is to assess its size, depth, and shape. These characteristics are important in determining the size and type of dressing used to pack a wound. The dressing needs to be flexible and must make contact with the entire wound surface. Make sure that the type of material used to pack the wound is appropriate. If gauze is the appropriate dressing material, saturate with the prescribed solution, wring out, unfold, and lightly pack into the wound. The entire wound surface needs to be in contact with part of the moist gauze dressing (see Skill 48.3).

Do not pack wounds too tightly, as overpacking causes pressure on the wound bed tissue. Pack the wound only until the packing material

FIG. 48.18 (A) Dehisced wound before wound vacuum-assisted closure (V.A.C.) therapy. (B) Dehisced wound after wound V.A.C. therapy. (Courtesy Kinetic Concepts [KCI], San Antonio, TX.)

reaches the surface of the wound; there should never be so much packing material that it extends higher than the wound surface. Packing that overlaps onto the wound edges causes periwound skin maceration.

Negative-Pressure Wound Therapy. Another treatment for wounds is negative-pressure wound therapy (NPWT) or vacuum-assisted closure (one brand name is V.A.C.). NPWT is the application of subatmospheric (negative) pressure to a wound through suction to facilitate healing and collect wound fluid (Netsch et al., 2016). The vacuum-assisted closure (V.A.C.) is a device that helps in wound closure by applying localized negative pressure to draw the edges of a wound together (Fig. 48.18). NPWT supports wound healing by removing wound exudates and reducing edema, macrodeformation and wound contraction, and microdeformation and mechanical stretch perfusion (see Skill 48.4). Secondary effects include angiogenesis, granulation tissue formation, and reduction in bacterial bioburden (Netsch et al., 2016) (Fig. 48.19). The V.A.C. Instill system allows intermittent instillation of fluids into a wound and liquefies infectious material and wound debris, especially in wounds not responding to traditional NPWT (Fernandez et al., 2019).

Indications for NPWT include chronic, acute, traumatic, subacute, and dehisced wounds; partial-thickness burns; injuries (e.g., diabetic and pressure); flaps and grafts once nonviable tissue is removed; and select high-risk postoperative surgical incisions (e.g., orthopedic, sternal). NPWT is also used in wounds with tunnels, undermining, or sinus tracts if the wound filler can fill the dead space and is easily retrieved (Netsch et al., 2016). Research also supports instillation of wound-rinsing agents to facilitate healing in some chronic wounds (Matiasek et al., 2018). The schedule for changing NPWT dressings varies, depending on the type of wound and amount of drainage. Wear time for the dressing is anywhere from 24 hours to 5 days. As a wound heals, granulation tissue lines its surface. The wound has a stippled or granulated appearance. The surface area sometimes increases or decreases, depending on wound location and the amount of drainage removed by the NPWT system. NPWT also enhances the adherence of split-thickness skin grafts. It is placed over a graft intraoperatively, decreasing the ability of the graft to shift and evacuating fluids that build up under it (Netsch et al., 2016). An airtight seal must be maintained (Box 48.10).

Contraindications to NPWT include necrotic tissue with eschar present; untreated osteomyelitis; nonenteric and unexplored fistulas; malignancy in the wound; exposed vasculature; and exposed nerves,

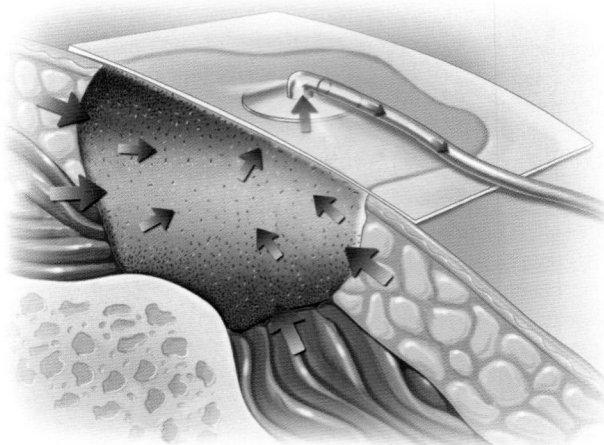

FIG. 48.19 Vacuum-assisted closure (V.A.C.) system using negative pressure to remove fluid from area surrounding wound, reducing edema and improving circulation to area. (Courtesy Kinetic Concepts [KCI], San Antonio, TX.)

anastomotic site, or organs. Other safety precautions to consider are patients at high risk for bleeding or hemorrhage (e.g., patients taking anticoagulants) and patients requiring magnetic resonance imaging (MRI), hyperbaric chamber, or defibrillation (Netsch et al., 2016).

There are different NPWT systems, some of which are gauze or foam based; some are designed for acute care settings or for outpatient care (Netsch, 2016). NPWT can be delivered intermittently or continuously. Review of evidence shows improved microvascular blood flow and granulation tissue formation with intermittent versus continuous therapy delivered at 125 mm Hg (WOCN, 2016). However, for patients with severe pain, lower levels of pressure (75–80 mm Hg) can be used to reduce pain and discomfort without compromising effectiveness (EPUAP/NPIAP/PPPIA, 2019a,b; Netsch et al., 2016).

Securing Dressings. Use tape, ties, or a secondary dressing to secure a dressing over a wound site. The choice of anchoring depends on the wound size and location, the presence of drainage, the frequency of dressing changes, and the patient's level of activity.

BOX 48.10 Negative-Pressure Wound Therapy: Maintaining an Airtight Seal

To avoid loss of suction (negative pressure), the wound and dressing must stay sealed after therapy is initiated. Problem seal areas include wounds around joints; near skin creases and folds; and near moisture such as diaphoresis, wound drainage, and urine or stool. The following points may help to maintain an airtight seal:

- Clip hair on skin around wound (check agency policy).
- Fill uneven skin surfaces with a skin barrier product such as paste or strips.
- Make sure that periwound skin surface is dry.
- Cut transparent film to extend 2.5 to 5 cm (1–2 inches) beyond wound perimeter.
- Frame periwound area with liquid skin barrier, solid skin barrier, or hydrocolloid dressing.
- Cut or mold transparent dressing to fit wound.
- Avoid wrinkles when applying transparent film.
- Identify any air leaks with a stethoscope and repair them with a sealant dressing (e.g., transparent dressing).
- Use only one or two additional layers for large leaks. Multiple layers reduce moisture vapor transmission and cause maceration of wound.
- If an adhesive remover is used, be sure to cleanse periwound well because it leaves a residue that can hinder film adherence.

Data from Netsch DS: Refractory wounds. In Wound, Ostomy, and Continence Nurses Society (WOCN): *Core curriculum: wound management,* Philadelphia, 2016, Wolters Kluwer; and Netsch DS, et al: Negative-pressure wound therapy. In Bryant RA, Nix DP, editors: *Acute and chronic wounds: current management concepts,* ed 5, St Louis, 2016, Mosby.

FIG. 48.20 Montgomery ties. (A) Each tie is placed at side of dressing. (B) Securing ties encloses dressing.

You will most often use strips of tape to secure dressings. Nonallergenic paper and silicone tapes minimize skin reactions. Common adhesive tape adheres well to the surface of the skin, whereas elastic adhesive tape compresses closely around pressure bandages and permits more movement of a body part. Skin sensitive to adhesive tape becomes severely inflamed and denuded and, in some cases, even sloughs when the tape is removed. It is important to assess the condition of the skin under tape at each dressing change.

Tape is available in various widths such as 1.3, 2.5, 5, and 7.5 cm (½, 1, 2, and 3 inches). Choose the size that secures a dressing sufficiently. For example, a large abdominal wound dressing needs to remain secure over a large area despite frequent stress from movement, respiratory effort, and possibly abdominal distention. Strips of 7.5-cm (3-inch) adhesive stabilize such a large dressing, so it does not continually slip off. When applying tape, ensure that it adheres to several inches of skin on both sides of the dressing and that it is placed across the middle of the dressing. When securing a dressing, press the tape gently to the skin and the topper dressing. Never apply tape over irritated or broken skin. Protect irritated skin by using a solid skin barrier and applying the tape over the barrier.

Use of tape and other medical adhesives can cause MARSI, with resultant mechanical injuries (skin stripping, blistering, and tears), dermatitis (skin irritation, pain, and itching), skin maceration, and folliculitis (Fumarola et al., 2020). To remove tape safely, assess the dressing and determine if an adhesive remover is necessary to initially loosen tape from the skin. Gently loosen the ends of the tape and gently pull the outer end parallel with the skin surface toward the wound. Gently move the skin away from the wound as the tape is loosened and removed. If tape covers an area of hair growth, a patient experiences less discomfort if you pull the tape in the direction of the hair growth.

Use Montgomery ties to secure dressings; this will avoid repeated removal of tape from sensitive skin, especially in older adults and individuals with chronic illnesses (Fumarola et al., 2020). Montgomery ties consist of multiple ties, and each section consists of a long strip; half contains an adhesive backing to apply to the skin one time, and the other half folds back and contains a cloth tie or a safety pin/rubber band combination that you fasten across a dressing and untie at dressing changes (Fig. 48.20). A large, bulky dressing often requires two or more sets of Montgomery ties. Another method to protect the surrounding skin on wounds that need frequent dressing changes is to place strips of hydrocolloid dressings on either side of the wound edges, cover the wound with a dressing, and apply the tape to the dressing. To provide even support to a wound and immobilize a body part, apply elastic gauze, elastic stretch net, or binders over a dressing.

Comfort Measures. A wound is often painful, depending on the extent of tissue injury, and wound care often requires the use of well-timed analgesia before any wound procedure (Krasner, 2016). Administer analgesic medications 30 to 60 minutes before dressing changes, depending on the time of peak action of a drug. In addition, several techniques are useful in minimizing discomfort during wound care. Carefully removing tape, gently cleaning wound edges, and carefully manipulating dressings and drains minimize stress on sensitive tissues. Careful turning and positioning also reduce strain on a wound.

Cleaning Skin and Drain Sites. A moderate amount of wound exudate promotes epithelial cell growth. However, the skin around a wound or drain site needs cleaning when a dressing does not absorb drainage properly or if an open drain deposits drainage onto the skin. Wound cleaning requires good hand hygiene and aseptic techniques (see Chapter 28). Unless this is a sterile wound you can clean this area with a nontoxic solution (e.g., water or normal saline). If it is a sterile wound, you need an order for sterile water or normal saline. You can use irrigation to remove debris from a wound (see Skill 48.5).

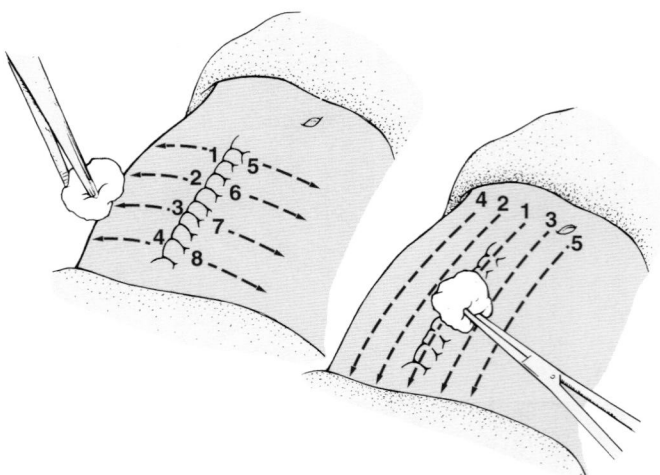

FIG. 48.21 Methods for cleaning wound site.

FIG. 48.22 Cleaning drain site.

Basic Skin Cleaning. Clean sterile surgical or traumatic wounds by applying noncytotoxic solutions with sterile gauze or by irrigation. The following three principles are important when cleaning an incision or the area surrounding a drain:

1. Clean in a direction from the least contaminated area, such as from a wound or incision to the surrounding skin (Fig. 48.21) or from an isolated drain site to the surrounding skin (Fig. 48.22).
2. Use gentle friction when applying solutions locally to the skin.
3. When irrigating, allow the solution to flow from the least to most contaminated area (see Skill 48.5).

After applying a solution to sterile gauze, clean away from the wound. Never use the same piece of gauze to clean across an incision or wound twice.

Drain sites are a source of contamination because moist drainage harbors microorganisms. If a wound has a dry incisional area and a moist drain site, cleaning moves from the incisional area toward the drain. Use two separate swabs or gauze pads: one to clean from the top of the incision toward the drain, and one to clean from the bottom of the incision toward the drain. To clean the area of an isolated drain site, clean around the drain, moving in circular rotations outward from a point closest to the drain. In this situation the skin near the site is more contaminated than the site itself. To clean circular wounds, use the same technique as in cleaning around a drain.

Irrigation. Irrigation is a way of cleaning wounds. Use an irrigation syringe to flush the wound with a constant low-pressure flow of solution. The gentle washing action of the irrigation cleanses a wound of exudate and debris. Irrigation is particularly useful for open, deep wounds; wounds involving an inaccessible body part such as the ear canal; or when cleaning sensitive body parts such as the conjunctival lining of the eye.

Irrigation of an open wound requires sterile technique. Use a 35-mL syringe with a 19-gauge soft angiocatheter (Ramundo, 2016) to deliver the solution. This irrigation system has a safe pressure and does not damage healing wound tissue. It is important to never occlude a wound opening with a syringe because this results in the introduction of irrigating fluid into a closed space. The pressure of the fluid causes tissue damage and discomfort and possibly forces infection or debris into the wound bed. Always irrigate a wound with the syringe tip over but not in the drainage site. Make sure that fluid flows directly into the wound and not over a contaminated area before entering the wound (see Skill 48.5).

Skin Closures. A surgeon closes a wound by bringing the wound edges as close together as possible to reduce scar formation. Proper wound closure involves minimal trauma and tension to tissues with control of bleeding.

Skin glue (cyanoacrylate glue) is a clear gel or paste applied to the edges of clean small wounds to hold the edges of the wound together. It takes only a few minutes for the glue to set, and it usually peels off in 5 to 7 days (U.K. National Health Service [NHS], 2021). Patients will go home with the skin glue in place. Instruct them to avoid touching the glue for 24 hours, to try to keep the wound dry for the first 5 days, that showers are preferable to baths to avoid soaking the wound, to use a shower cap if the wound is on the head, and to pat (not rub) the wound dry if it gets wet (NHS, 2018). Skin glue is not used over joints, the hand, or the groin area. A systematic review of the use of glue compared with traditional sutures showed that medical glues appear to be a viable alternative to staples in select types of surgeries and often are associated with less pain when compared with staples (NHS, 2018).

Sutures are threads or metal used to sew body tissues together (Fig. 48.23). They are available in a variety of materials, including silk, steel, cotton, linen, wire, nylon, and Dacron. Sutures such as polydioxanone (PDS), Vicryl, and Monocryl can be absorbed; others, such as nylon, silk, and steel, are nonabsorbable and must be removed. A patient's history of wound healing, the site of surgery, the tissues involved, and the purpose of the sutures determine the suture material used. For example, if a patient has had repeated surgery for an abdominal hernia, the health care provider can choose wire sutures to provide greater strength for wound closure. In contrast, a small laceration of the face calls for the use of very fine Dacron (polyester) sutures to minimize scar formation.

Sutures are placed within tissue layers in deep wounds and superficially for wound closure. Deep sutures are usually composed of an

FIG. 48.23 Incision closed with metal staples.

FIG. 48.24 Staple remover.

FIG. 48.25 Examples of suturing methods. (A) Intermittent. (B) Continuous. (C) Blanket continuous. (D) Retention.

absorbable material that disappears over time. Sutures are foreign bodies and thus can cause local inflammation. A surgeon tries to minimize tissue injury by using the finest suture possible and the smallest number necessary.

Policies vary within agencies regarding who can remove sutures. If it is appropriate that the nurse remove them, a health care provider's order is required. An order for suture removal is not written until the health care provider believes that the wound has closed (usually in 7 days). Special scissors with curved cutting tips, scissors and pickups from a sterile suture removal kit, or special staple removers slide under the skin closures for suture removal. The health care provider usually specifies the number of sutures or staples to remove. If the suture line appears to be healing in certain locations better than in others, some health care providers choose to have only some sutures removed (e.g., every other one).

To remove staples, insert the tips of the staple remover under each wire staple. While slowly closing the ends of the staple remover together, squeeze the center of the staple with the tips, freeing it from the skin, and gently lift up and out of the skin (Fig. 48.24).

To remove sutures, first check the type of suturing used (Fig. 48.25). With intermittent suturing the surgeon ties each individual suture made in the skin. Continuous suturing, as the name implies, is a series of sutures with only two knots, one at the beginning and one at the end of the suture line. Retention sutures are placed more deeply than skin sutures, and nurses may or may not remove them, depending on agency policy. The way the suture crosses and penetrates the skin determines the method for removal. *Never pull the visible part of a suture through underlying tissue.* Sutures on the surface of the skin harbor microorganisms and debris. The part of the suture beneath the skin is sterile. Pulling the contaminated part of the suture through tissues can lead to infection. Before taking out the sutures, cleanse the suture line with normal saline. Clip suture materials as close to the skin edge on one side as possible and pull the suture through from the other side (Fig. 48.26).

Drainage Evacuation. When drainage interferes with healing, evacuation of the drainage is achieved by using either a drain alone or a drain connected to a drainage tube with continuous suction. You may apply special skin barriers, including hydrocolloid dressings similar to those used with ostomies (see Chapter 47), around drain sites with significant drainage for skin protection. The skin barriers are soft material applied to the skin with adhesive. Drainage flows on the barrier but not directly on the skin. Wound drainage evacuators (Fig. 48.27) are convenient portable units that connect to tubular drains lying within a wound bed and exert a safe, constant low-pressure vacuum to remove and collect drainage. Ensure that suction is exerted and that connection points between the evacuator and tubing are intact. The evacuator collects drainage. Assess for volume and character of drainage every shift and as needed. Measure output by emptying the contents into a graduated cylinder, immediately reset the evacuator to apply suction, and record the output.

Bandages, Binders, and Slings. A simple gauze dressing is often not enough to immobilize or provide support to a wound, and a larger dressing or bandage is required. Binders are made of large pieces of material, usually elastic or cotton, to fit a specific body part (Box 48.11). The most common type is an abdominal binder (Fig. 48.28). Breast binders are also available.

An abdominal binder supports large abdominal incisions that are vulnerable to tension or stress as a patient moves or coughs. Binders support underlying muscles and large incisions, lessening muscle stress, which helps a patient move more freely without additional discomfort. Abdominal binders provide a noninvasive intervention for promoting early ambulation, controlling pain, and improving recovery experience following major abdominal surgery (Gallagher, 2016). Studies involving postoperative patients after major abdominal surgery found that an abdominal binder increased patient mobility soon after surgery, and there was a measurable reduction in pain in patients who used an abdominal binder after any exercise or activity (Arici et al., 2016). Because abdominal binders facilitate early ambulation, patients have fewer postoperative complications related to lack of exercise (e.g., postoperative pneumonia, deep vein thrombosis [DVT]) (Mizell et al., 2020). For some patients, abdominal binders support underlying muscles and

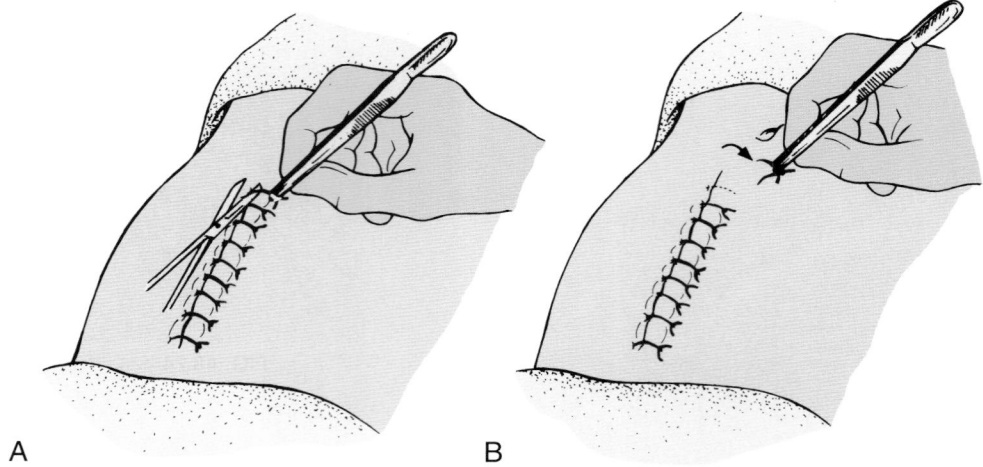

A   B

FIG. 48.26 Removal of intermittent suture. (A) Cut suture as close to skin as possible, away from knot. (B) Remove suture and never pull contaminated stitch through tissues.

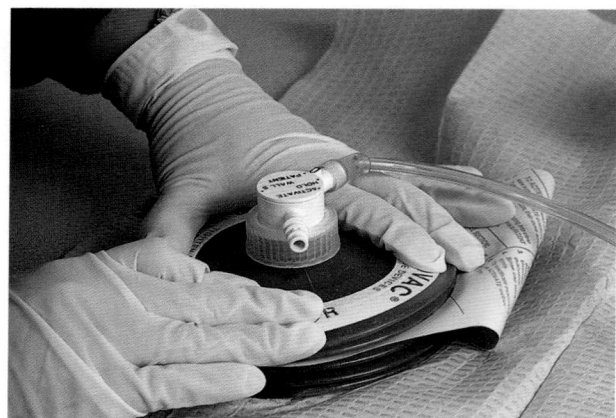

FIG. 48.27 Setting suction on drainage evacuator. *1,* With drainage port open, raise level on diaphragm. *2,* Push straight down on lever to lower diaphragm. *3,* Closure of port prevents escape of air and creates vacuum pressure.

large incisions, thus lessening muscle stress, which helps a patient move more freely without additional discomfort (Giller et al., 2016). Correctly applied bandages and binders do not cause injury to underlying and nearby body parts or create discomfort for a patient. For example, a chest binder should not be so tight as to restrict chest wall expansion.

Binders and bandages applied over or around dressings provide extra protection and therapeutic benefits by the following:

1. Creating pressure over a body part (e.g., an elastic pressure bandage applied over an arterial puncture site)
2. Immobilizing a body part (e.g., an elastic bandage applied around a sprained ankle)
3. Supporting a wound (e.g., an abdominal binder applied over a large abdominal incision and dressing)
4. Reducing or preventing edema (e.g., a stretch pressure bandage applied to the lower leg)
5. Securing a splint (e.g., a bandage applied around hand splints for correction of deformities)
6. Securing dressings (e.g., elastic webbing applied around leg dressings after a vein stripping)

Bandages are available in rolls of various widths and materials, including gauze, elasticized knit, elastic webbing, flannel, and muslin. Gauze bandages are lightweight and inexpensive, mold easily around contours of the body, and permit air circulation to prevent skin maceration. Elastic bandages conform well to body parts but are also for exerting pressure.

After applying a bandage or binder, you assess, document, and immediately report changes in circulation, skin integrity, comfort level, and body function (e.g., ventilation or movement). You may loosen or readjust as necessary based on the patient's response. A health care provider's order is necessary before loosening or removing a bandage applied by the health care provider. The nurse explains to the patient that any bandage or binder feels relatively firm or tight. Carefully assess a bandage to be sure that it is applied properly and providing therapeutic benefit, and replace any soiled bandages.

Slings. Slings support arms with muscular sprains or fractures. A commercially manufactured sling consists of a long sleeve that extends above the elbow with a strap that fits around the neck. In the home patients can use a large triangular piece of cloth. The patient sits or lies supine during sling application (Fig. 48.29). Instruct the patient to bend the affected arm, bringing the forearm straight across the chest. The open sling fits under the patient's arm and over the chest, with the base of the triangle under the wrist and the point of the triangle at the elbow. One end of the sling fits around the back of the patient's neck. Bring the other end up and over the affected arm while supporting the extremity. Tie the two ends at the side of the neck so that the knot does not press against the cervical spine. Fold the loose material at the elbow evenly around the elbow and then pin to secure. Always support the lower arm and hand at a level above the elbow to prevent the formation of dependent edema.

Roll Bandage Application. Rolls of bandage secure or support dressings over irregularly shaped body parts. Each roll has a free outer end and a terminal end at the center of the roll. The rolled part of the bandage is its body, and its outer surface is placed against the patient's skin or dressing. Use a variety of bandage turns, depending on the body part to be bandaged (see Skill 48.6).

Heat and Cold Therapy. Moist heat applications are therapeutically beneficial in increasing muscle and ligament flexibility; promoting relaxation and healing; and relieving spasm, joint stiffness, and pain. Moist heat has many indications; however, it most commonly is used

BOX 48.11 PROCEDURAL GUIDELINES

Applying a Binder

Delegation and Collaboration

The skill of applying a binder can be delegated to assistive personnel (AP). However, the nurse must first assess the condition of any incision, the skin, and patient's ability to breathe before binder application. The nurse directs the AP about:

- How to modify the skill, such as special wrapping or manner of securing the binder.
- Reporting patient's complaint of pain, numbness, tingling, or difficulty breathing after applying abdominal binder or any changes in patient's skin color or temperature.

Equipment

Clean gloves if wound drainage present; gauze bandage as needed; correct type and size of binder; closures for cloth binder

Procedural Steps

1. Identify patient using at least two identifiers (e.g., name and birthday or name and medical record number) according to agency policy (TJC, 2021).
2. Review electronic health record for order for binder (check agency policy).
3. Review electronic health record and nurses' notes to identify data regarding size of patient and appropriate binder to use (see manufacturer guidelines) to ensure proper fit.
4. Assess patient's or family caregiver's knowledge, experience, and health literacy.
5. Observe patient who needs support of thorax or abdomen; observe ability to breathe deeply, cough effectively, and turn or move independently.
6. Perform hand hygiene, apply clean gloves as needed. Inspect skin for actual or potential alterations in integrity. Observe for irritation, abrasion, and skin surfaces that rub against one another.
7. Assess the skin of underlying areas that will be distal to the bandage for signs of circulatory impairment (coolness, pallor or cyanosis, diminished or absent pulses, swelling, numbness, and tingling) to provide a means for comparing changes in circulation after bandage application.
8. Inspect any surgical dressing for intactness, presence of drainage, and coverage of incision. Change any soiled dressing before applying binder (using clean gloves). Dispose of soiled dressings in appropriate container, remove and dispose of gloves, and perform hand hygiene.
9. Determine patient's level of comfort using scale of 0 to 10.

   CLINICAL JUDGMENT: *If patient reports increased pain, administer prescribed analgesic 30 minutes before binder application.*

10. Determine patient's knowledge of purpose of binder.
11. Close curtains or room door. Prepare supplies at bedside.
12. Perform hand hygiene and apply clean gloves (if likely to contact wound drainage).

13. Apply abdominal binder:
    a. Position patient in supine position with head slightly elevated and knees slightly flexed.
    b. Help patient roll on side away from you toward raised side rail while firmly supporting abdominal incision and dressing with hands. Fanfold far side of binder toward midline of binder.
    c. Place binder flat on bed, right side up. Fanfold far side of binder toward midline of binder so patient can roll over with minimal effort.
    d. Place fanfolded ends of binder under patient.
    e. Instruct or assist patient to roll over the folded binder. For overweight patients consider asking nurse colleague to help.
    f. Unfold and stretch ends out smoothly on far side of bed. Then stretch out ends on near side of bed.
    g. Instruct patient to roll back into supine position.
    h. Adjust binder so supine patient is centered over binder, using symphysis pubis and costal margins as lower and upper landmarks.
    i. If patient is very thin, pad iliac prominences with gauze bandage.
    j. Close binder. Pull one end of binder over center of patient's abdomen. While maintaining tension on that end of binder, pull opposite end of binder over center and secure with Velcro closure tabs or metal fasteners. Provides continuous wound support and comfort.

    CLINICAL JUDGMENT: *After binder is in place, assess patient's ability to breathe deeply and cough effectively. When applied correctly, an abdominal binder over midline abdominal incisions should not have any effect on the patient's pulmonary function.*

14. Assess patient's comfort level and adjust binder as necessary. Ask patient to rate pain on scale of 0 to 10.
15. Remove and dispose of gloves and perform hand hygiene.
16. Help patient to a comfortable position. Raise siderails (as appropriate), and lower bed to lowest position.
17. Place nurse call system in an accessible location within patient's reach.
18. Remove binder and surgical dressing to assess skin and wound characteristics at least every 8 hours.
19. Evaluate patient's ability to ventilate properly, including deep breathing and coughing, every 4 hours to determine presence of impaired ventilation and potential pulmonary complications.
20. Record baseline and postbinder condition of skin, circulation, integrity of underlying dressing, and patient's comfort level in nurses' notes in the electronic health record (EHR) or chart.
21. Report any complications (e.g., pain, skin irritation, impaired ventilation) to nurse in charge. Report reduced ventilation (e.g., pulse oximetry) to health care provider immediately.

---

following the acute phase of a musculoskeletal injury and during and after childbirth, surgery, and superficial thrombophlebitis (Petrofsky et al., 2017; Szekeres et al., 2017). Moist heat applications include warm compresses and commercial moist heat packs, warm baths, soaks, and sitz baths. There are also digital moist heat applications that allow patients to control temperature of the heat application. Dry heat is also used to reduce pain and increase healing by increasing blood flow in tissues and can be used at a low level for a longer period with little chance of tissue injury (Petrofsky et al., 2016).

Cold therapy refers to the superficial application of cold to the surface of the skin, with or without compression and with or without a mechanical recirculating device to maintain cold temperatures (Chou et al.,

2016). Cold therapy is designed to treat the localized inflammatory response of an injured body part that presents as edema, hemorrhage, muscle spasm, or pain. Improvement to joint mobility following cold therapy is related to reducing pain and swelling, inhibiting muscle spasm, and reducing muscle tension (Chatterjee, 2017; Quinlan et al., 2017). Cold therapy most commonly is used immediately after soft tissue and musculoskeletal injuries such as sprains or strains; however, it has been used in the postoperative setting with patients who have undergone orthopedic surgeries, spinal fusion, and lumbar discectomy (Quinlan et al., 2017). Research trials of cold therapy have been inconsistent and frequently found no differences compared with no cold therapy in postoperative pain or analgesic use (Chou et al., 2016).

FIG. 48.28 Securing abdominal binder with Velcro.

FIG. 48.29 Application of sling.

Bodily Responses to Heat and Cold. Exposure to heat and cold causes systemic and local responses. Systemic responses occur through heat-loss mechanisms (sweating and vasodilation) or mechanisms promoting heat conservation (vasoconstriction and piloerection) and heat production (shivering) (see Chapter 30). Local responses to heat and cold occur through stimulation of temperature-sensitive nerve endings within the skin. This stimulation sends impulses from the periphery to the hypothalamus, which becomes aware of local temperature sensations and triggers adaptive responses for maintenance of normal body temperature. If alterations occur along temperature sensation pathways, the reception and eventual perception of stimuli are altered.

The body can tolerate wide variations in temperature. The normal temperature of the surface of the skin is 34°C (93.2°F), but temperature receptors usually adapt quickly to local temperatures between 15°C and 45°C (59°F and 113°F). Pain develops when local temperatures exceed this range. Excessive heat causes a burning sensation. Cold produces a numbing sensation before pain.

The adaptive ability of the body creates the major problem in protecting patients from injury resulting from temperature extremes. A person initially feels an extreme change in temperature but within a short time hardly notices it. This is dangerous because a person insensitive to heat and cold extremes can sustain serious tissue injury. You need to recognize patients most at risk for injuries from heat and cold applications (Table 48.11). Heat and cold stimuli create different physiological responses. The choice of heat or cold therapy depends on local responses desired for wound healing.

Assessment for Temperature Tolerance. Before applying heat or cold therapies, assess a patient's physical condition for signs of potential intolerance to heat and cold. First observe the area to be treated. Assess the skin, looking for any open areas such as alterations in skin integrity (e.g., abrasions, open wounds, edema, bruising, bleeding, or localized areas of inflammation) that increase a patient's risk for injury. Because a health care provider commonly orders heat and cold applications for traumatized areas, the baseline skin assessment provides a guide for evaluating skin changes that can occur during therapy. Assess neurological function, testing for sensation to light touch, pinprick, and mild temperature variations (see Chapter 30). Sensory status reveals the ability of a patient to recognize when heat or cold becomes excessive. Assess a patient's mental status to be sure that the patient can correctly communicate any issues with the hot or cold therapy. Level of consciousness influences the ability to perceive heat, cold, and pain. If a patient is confused or unresponsive, make frequent observations of skin integrity after therapy begins.

TABLE 48.11	Conditions That Increase Risk of Injury From Heat and Cold Application
Condition	**Risk Factors**
Very young or older patients	Thinner skin layers in children increase risk of burns. Older patients have reduced sensitivity to pain and may not perceive any pain associated with heat or cold applications.
Open wounds, broken skin, stomas	Subcutaneous and visceral tissues are more sensitive to temperature variations. They also contain no temperature and fewer pain receptors.
Areas of edema or scar formation	Reduced sensation to temperature stimuli occurs because of thickening of skin layers from fluid buildup or scar formation.
Peripheral vascular disease (e.g., diabetes mellitus, arteriosclerosis)	As a result of decreased peripheral circulation, extremities are less sensitive to temperature and pain stimuli because of circulatory impairment and local tissue injury. Cold application further compromises blood flow.
Confusion or unconsciousness	Reduced perception of sensory or painful stimuli. Patient may be unable to move away from or to indicate discomfort from the heat or cold application.
Spinal cord injury	Alterations in nerve pathways prevent reception of sensory or painful stimuli.
Abscessed tooth or appendix	Infection is highly localized. Application of heat causes rupture, with spread of microorganisms systemically.

Assess for conditions that contraindicate heat or cold therapy. Do not cover an active area of bleeding with a warm application because bleeding will continue. Warm applications are contraindicated when a patient has an acute, localized inflammation such as appendicitis because the heat could cause the appendix to rupture. If a patient has cardiovascular problems, it is unwise to apply heat to large parts of the body because the resulting massive vasodilation disrupts blood supply to vital organs.

Cold is contraindicated if the site of injury is already edematous. It further retards circulation to the area and prevents absorption of the interstitial fluid. If a patient has impaired circulation (e.g., arteriosclerosis), it further reduces blood supply to the affected area. Cold therapy is also contraindicated in the presence of neuropathy because the patient is unable to perceive temperature change and damage resulting from temperature extremes. One other contraindication for cold therapy is shivering. Cold applications sometimes intensify shivering and dangerously increase body temperature.

If a patient has peripheral vascular disease, pay particular attention to the integrity of extremities. For example, if the health care provider's order is to apply a cold compress to a lower extremity, assess circulation to the leg by assessing for capillary refill; observing skin color; and palpating skin temperatures, distal pulses, and edematous areas. If signs of circulatory inadequacy are present, it is important for you to question the order.

When applying heat or cold pads, check electrical equipment for cracked cords, frayed wires, damaged insulation, and exposed heating components. Make sure that equipment containing circulating fluids does not have leaks. Check equipment for evenness of temperature distribution.

Local Effects of Heat and Cold Applications. Heat and cold stimuli create different physiological responses. The choice of heat or cold therapy depends on the desired local response for wound healing (Table 48.12).

Effects of Heat Application. In general, heat is quite therapeutic, improving blood flow to an injured part. However, if it is applied for 1 hour or more, the body reduces blood flow by means of a reflex vasoconstriction to control heat loss from the area. Periodic removal and reapplication of local heat restores vasodilation. Continuous

exposure to heat damages epithelial cells, causing redness, localized tenderness, and even blistering.

Effects of Cold Application. The application of cold initially diminishes swelling and pain. Prolonged exposure of the skin to cold results in a reflex vasodilation. The inability of the cells to receive adequate blood flow and nutrients results in tissue ischemia. The skin initially takes on a reddened appearance, followed by a bluish-purple mottling, with numbness and a burning type of pain. Skin tissues freeze from exposure to extreme cold.

Factors Influencing Heat and Cold Tolerance. The response of the body to heat and cold therapies depends on the following factors:
- A person is better able to tolerate short exposure to temperature extremes than prolonged exposure.
- Exposed skin layers and certain areas of the skin (e.g., the neck, inner aspect of the wrist and forearm, and perineal region) are more sensitive to temperature variations. The foot and palm of the hand are less sensitive.
- The body responds best to minor temperature adjustments. If a body part is cool and a hot stimulus touches the skin, the response is greater than if the skin were already warm.
- A person has less tolerance to temperature changes to which a large area of the body is exposed.
- Tolerance to temperature variations changes with age. Patients who are very young or old are most sensitive to heat and cold.
- If a patient's physical condition reduces the reception or perception of sensory stimuli, tolerance to temperature extremes is high, but the risk of injury is also high.
- Uneven temperature distribution suggests that the equipment is functioning improperly.

Application of Heat and Cold Therapies. A prerequisite to using any heat or cold application is a health care provider's order, which includes the body site to be treated and the type, frequency, and duration of application. Safety guidelines for the use of heat and cold are summarized in Box 48.12. Consult agency procedure manual for correct temperatures to use.

You can administer heat and cold applications in dry or moist forms. The type of wound or injury, the location of the body part, and the presence of drainage or inflammation are factors to consider in

TABLE 48.12 Therapeutic Effects of Heat and Cold Applications

Physiological Response	Therapeutic Benefit	Examples of Conditions Treated
Heat Therapy		
Vasodilation	Improves blood flow to injured body part	Arthritis or degenerative joint disease
Reduced blood viscosity	Promotes delivery of nutrients and removal of wastes	Localized joint pain or muscle strains
Reduced muscle tension	Improves delivery of leukocytes and antibiotics to wound site	Low back pain
Increased tissue metabolism	Promotes muscle relaxation	Menstrual cramping
Increased capillary permeability	Reduces pain from spasm or stiffness	Hemorrhoid, perianal, and vaginal inflammation
	Increases blood flow	Local skin abscesses
	Provides local warmth	
	Promotes movement of waste products and nutrients	
Cold Therapy		
Vasoconstriction	Reduces blood flow to injured site, preventing edema formation	Immediately after direct trauma (e.g., sprains, strains, fractures, muscle spasms)
Local anesthesia	Reduces inflammation	Superficial laceration or puncture wound
Reduced cell metabolism	Reduces localized pain	Minor burn
Increased blood viscosity	Reduces oxygen needs of tissues	After injections
Decreased muscle tension	Promotes blood coagulation at injury site	Chronic pain from arthritis, joint trauma, or delayed-onset muscle soreness, inflammation
	Relieves pain	

selecting dry or moist applications. Box 48.13 summarizes advantages and disadvantages of both.

Warm, Moist Compresses. Warm, moist compresses improve circulation, relieve edema, and promote consolidation of purulent drainage. A compress is a piece of gauze dressing moistened in a prescribed warmed solution. Heat from warm compresses dissipates quickly. To maintain a constant temperature, you need to change the compress often. You can use a layer of plastic wrap or a dry towel to insulate the compress and retain heat. Moist heat promotes vasodilation and evaporation of heat from the surface of the skin. For this reason, a patient can feel chilly. Always try to control drafts within the room, and keep the patient covered with a blanket or robe.

BOX 48.12 Safety Suggestions for Applying Heat or Cold Therapy

- *Explain* to patient sensations to be felt during the procedure.
- *Prevention:* Injuries from heat and cold therapies are preventable.
- *Instruct* patient that exposed layers of skin are more sensitive to heat and cold application than intact skin. Therefore instruct patient and family to protect skin when applying heat or cold therapy.
- *Instruct* patient to report changes in sensation or discomfort immediately.
- *Provide* a timer, clock, or watch so that patient can help the nurse time the application.
- *Check* patient and skin every 20 minutes during therapy. Observe for excess redness, pain, tingling.
- *Place* nurse call system within patient's reach.
- *Refer* to the policy and procedure manual of the institution for safe temperatures.
- *Do not* allow patient to adjust temperature settings.
- *Do not* allow patient to move an application or place hands on the wound site.
- *Do not* place patient in a position that prevents movement away from the temperature source.
- *Do not* leave unattended a patient who is unable to sense temperature changes or move from the temperature source.

BOX 48.13 Choice of Moist or Dry Thermal Applications

Advantages
Moist Applications
- Moist application reduces drying of skin and softens wound exudate.
- Moist compresses conform well to most body areas.
- Moist heat penetrates deeply into tissue layers.
- Warm, moist heat does not promote sweating and insensible fluid loss.

Dry Applications
- Dry heat has less risk of burns to skin than moist applications.
- Dry application does not cause skin maceration.
- Dry heat retains temperature longer because evaporation does not occur.

Disadvantages
Moist Applications
- Prolonged exposure causes maceration of skin.
- Moist heat cools rapidly because of moisture evaporation.
- Moist heat creates greater risk for burns to skin because moisture conducts heat.

Dry Applications
- Dry heat increases body fluid loss through sweating.
- Dry applications do not penetrate deep into tissues.
- Dry heat causes increased drying of skin.

Warm Soaks. Immersion of a body part in a warmed solution promotes circulation, lessens edema, increases muscle relaxation, and provides a means to apply medicated solution. Sometimes a soak is also accompanied by wrapping the body part in dressings and saturating them with the warmed solution.

Position the patient comfortably, place waterproof pads under the area to be treated, and heat the solution to about 40.5°C to 43°C (105°F–110°F). Pour solution into a clean or sterile basin or container, then immerse the body part. Cover the container and extremity with a towel to reduce heat loss. It is usually necessary to remove the cooled solution and add heated solution after about 10 minutes. The challenge is to keep the solution at a constant temperature. Never add a hotter solution while the body part remains immersed. After any soak, dry the body part thoroughly to prevent maceration.

Sitz Baths. A patient who has had rectal surgery, an episiotomy during childbirth, painful hemorrhoids, or vaginal inflammation benefits from a sitz bath, a bath in which only the pelvic area is immersed in warm or, in some situations, cool fluid. The patient sits in a special tub or chair or a basin that fits on the toilet seat, so the legs and feet remain out of the water. Immersing the entire body causes widespread vasodilation and nullifies the effect of local heat application to the pelvic area.

The desired temperature for a sitz bath depends on whether the purpose is to promote relaxation or to clean a wound. It is often necessary to add warm or cool water during the procedure to maintain a constant temperature, which normally lasts 20 minutes. Agency procedure manuals recommend safe water temperatures. A disposable sitz basin contains an attachment resembling an enema bag that allows gradual introduction of additional water.

Prevent overexposure of patients by draping bath blankets around their shoulders and thighs and controlling drafts. A patient should be able to sit in the basin or tub with feet flat on the floor and without pressure on the sacrum or thighs. Because exposure of a large part of the body to heat causes extensive vasodilation, assess the pulse, and observe facial color and ask whether the patient feels light-headed or nauseated.

Commercial Heat and Cold Packs. Commercially prepared disposable heat packs apply warm, dry heat to an injured area. The chemicals mix and release heat when you strike, knead, or squeeze the pack. Package directions recommend the time for heat application.

Commercially prepared cold packs that are like the disposable heat packs for dry applications are available. They come in various shapes and sizes to fit different body parts. When using cold compresses, observe for adverse reactions such as burning or numbness, mottling of the skin, redness, extreme paleness, and a bluish skin discoloration.

Cold, Moist, and Dry Compresses. The procedure for applying cold, moist compresses is the same as that for warm compresses. Apply cold compresses for 20 minutes at a temperature of 15°C (59°F) to relieve inflammation and swelling. You can use clean or sterile compresses.

Cold Soaks. The procedure for preparing cold soaks and immersing a body part is the same as for warm soaks. The desired temperature for a 20-minute cold soak is 15°C (59°F). Control drafts and use outer coverings to protect the patient from chilling. It is often necessary to add cold water during the procedure to maintain a constant temperature.

Ice Bags or Collars. For a patient who has a muscle sprain, localized hemorrhage, or hematoma or who has undergone dental surgery, an ice bag is ideal to prevent edema formation, control bleeding, and anesthetize the body part. Proper use of the bag requires the following steps:

1. Fill the bag with water, secure the cap, invert to check for leaks, and pour out the water.
2. Fill the bag two-thirds full with crushed ice, so you are able to easily mold it over a body part.

3. Release any air from the bag by squeezing its sides before securing the cap because excess air interferes with conduction of cold.
4. Wipe off excess moisture.
5. Cover the bag with a flannel cover, towel, or pillowcase.
6. Apply the bag to the injury site for 30 minutes; you can reapply the bag in an hour.

◆ Evaluation

Evaluation of patients who have wounds requires application of critical thinking in making clinical judgments to evaluate change in the healing process. Careful evaluation will allow you to determine the effectiveness of nursing interventions for reducing and treating pressure injuries and other wounds. Application of critical thinking during evaluation ensures a comprehensive and thorough look at a patient's response to nursing therapies and whether outcomes are achieved. As noted earlier in the chapter, the optimal outcomes are to prevent injury to the skin, to reduce further injury to the skin and underlying tissues, and to promote wound healing with restoration of skin integrity.

Through the Patient's Eyes. Collaborate with the patient and family caregiver in the evaluation process. Review whether their expectations of care were met. For example, is the patient satisfied with the comfort measures used during wound care? Chronic wounds such as pressure injuries take time to heal, so home care is likely. Do the patient and family caregiver feel that the education on home wound care provided them with the confidence and knowledge to care for the wound at home? Do the patient and family caregiver feel that they have the information needed to know when to report a problem with a wound? Ask the patient and family caregiver if there are any unmet expectations. If patient and family caregiver expectations are unmet, again apply critical thinking based on what you know about the patient and revise your plan of care to select the best ways to support and reeducate.

Patient Outcomes. The outcomes selected for a patient in the plan of care are the milestones you hope the patient will achieve. Each patient will have unique outcomes depending on preexisting conditions and whether the patient has an actual wound or is at risk to develop a wound. Evaluate nursing interventions for reducing and treating pressure injuries by determining the patient's response and comparing with expected outcomes to determine whether the patient achieved each outcome (Fig. 48.30).

Kelly includes Mrs. Stein in evaluating the outcomes of her care. Mrs. Stein notes that her incisional and hip pain are reduced, and she reports her pain as 2 or 3 on the 0-to-10 scale and is very happy to be using nonopioid medication. Mrs. Stein can change position in bed and is more active in physical therapy. Kelly tells Mrs. Stein that the increase in activity helped reduce the redness on her sacrum and helped to improve the status of the Stage 2 pressure injury. Kelly takes time to

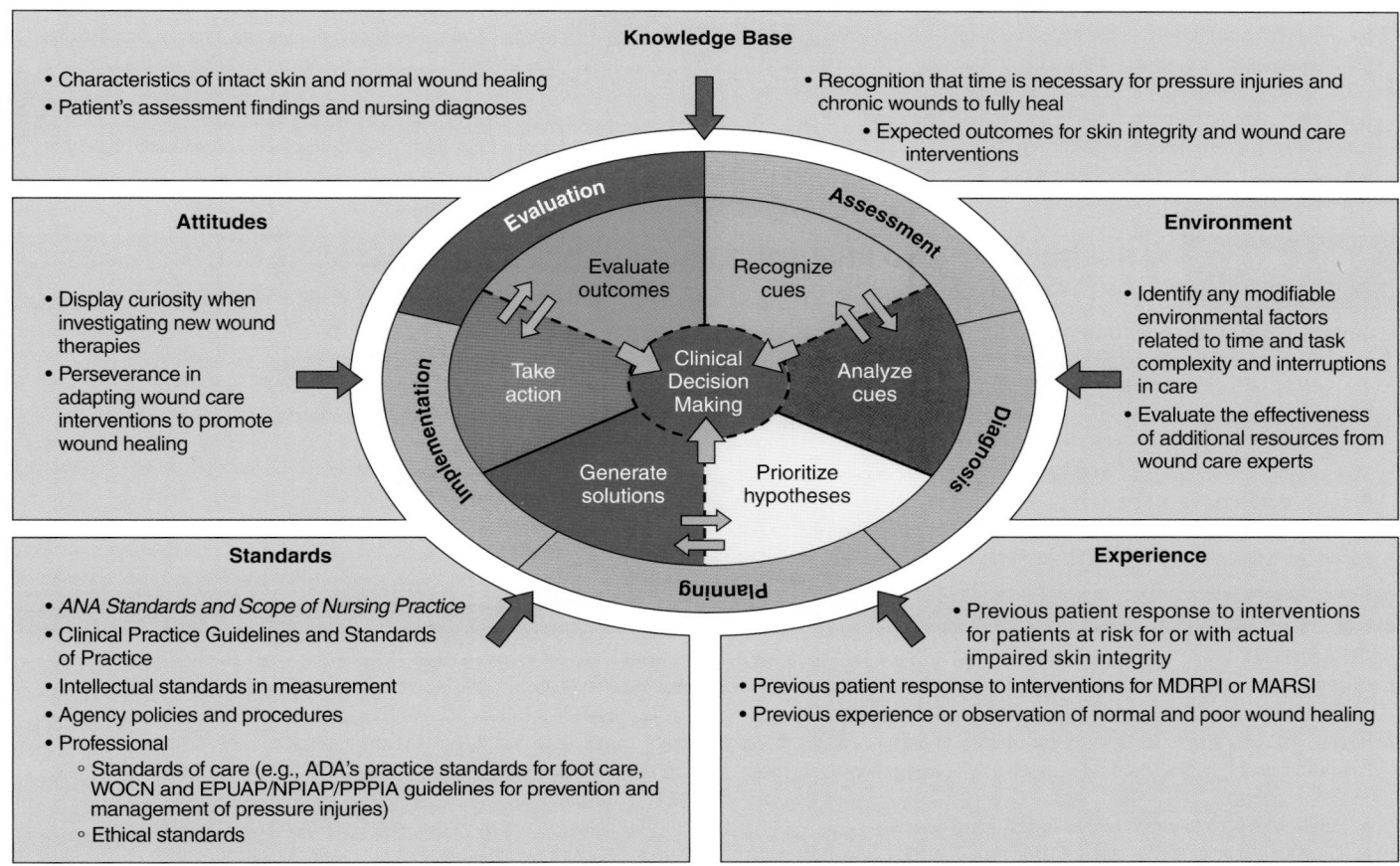

FIG. 48.30 Critical thinking model for skin integrity and wound care evaluation. *ADA,* American Diabetes Association; *ANA,* American Nurses Association; *EPUAP,* European Pressure Ulcer Advisory Panel; *MARSI,* medical adhesive–related skin injury; *MDRPI,* medical device–related pressure injury; *NPIAP,* National Pressure Injury Advisory Panel; *PPPIA,* Pan Pacific Pressure Injury Alliance; *WOCN,* Wound, Ostomy, and Continence Nurses Society. (Clinical Judgment Measurement Model copyright © NCSBN. All rights reserved.)

reinforce patient education regarding pain control and mobility and ask Mrs. Stein when she will take any pain medication and how she will handle her mobility activity.

You will evaluate patients with impaired skin integrity on an ongoing basis by conducting the same skin assessments performed earlier to detect skin breakdown and wound status. For example, during direct patient contact, if a patient continues to be diaphoretic or incontinent, inspect the condition of the skin and repeat any validated predictive measures to determine the current condition of the skin and decide whether additional therapies are needed to treat a patient's skin moisture. Use a validated wound assessment tool when appropriate. Evaluation provides information regarding the patient's progress toward wound healing, whether new risks for impaired skin integrity exist, and the current maintenance of skin integrity.

If the identified outcomes are not met for a patient with impaired skin integrity, questions to ask include the following:
- Was the etiology of the skin impairment addressed? Were the pressure, friction, shear, and moisture components identified, and did the plan of care decrease the contribution of each of these components?
- Was wound healing supported by providing the wound with a moist protected environment?
- Was nutrition assessed and a plan of care developed that provided the patient with food preferences containing the calories needed to support healing?

Finally, evaluate the need for additional referrals to other experts in wound care and pressure injuries, such as a wound care specialist or the wound care team. Care of patients with a pressure injury or wound requires an interprofessional team approach.

SAFETY GUIDELINES FOR NURSING SKILLS

Ensuring patient safety is an essential role of the professional nurse. Use sound clinical judgment by communicating clearly with members of the health care team, assessing and analyzing patient's clinical findings, and incorporating the patient's priorities of care and preferences. Use the best evidence, applying professional standards, when selecting interventions to use in patient care delivery. When performing the skills in this chapter, remember the following points to ensure safe, patient-centered care.
- When changing wound dressings, follow proper aseptic technique. Keep a plastic bag within reach to discard dressing and prevent cross-contamination. Keep extra gloves within reach in case of contamination or additional wound assessment.
- Perform pressure injury risk assessment on all patients who have one or more risk factors when admitted to an acute care setting, home care, hospice, or extended-care facility (EPUAP/NPIAP/PPPIA, 2019b, WOCN, 2016). Use a risk assessment tool; the Braden Scale is one of the most widely used and researched scales (Bryant and Nix, 2016a).

- Inspect skin at least daily or according to agency policy and note and document all pressure points. Modify frequency of skin and wound assessment and frequency of skin-care practices based on patient's risk factors and/or wound condition.
- Use approaches to minimize friction and shear. Use friction-reducing lift sheets when repositioning patients to reduce rubbing skin against sheets. Raise the head of the bed no more than 30 degrees (unless medically contraindicated) to prevent sliding and shear injury (WOCN, 2016).
- When a patient has a previous history of pressure injury or skin damage, the healed area presents a greater risk for skin breakdown than healthy, unwounded skin.
- Chronic diseases, especially vascular disease and diabetes mellitus, increase a patient's risk for pressure injury development and impede wound healing.

SKILL 48.1   ASSESSMENT AND PREVENTION STRATEGIES FOR PRESSURE INJURY DEVELOPMENT

Delegation and Collaboration
The skill of pressure injury risk assessment cannot be delegated to assistive personnel (AP). Instruct the AP to:
- Frequently change patient's position, and use specific positions individualized for the patient.
- Keep patient's skin dry and provide hygiene following fecal or urinary incontinence or exposure of skin to wound drainage.
- Report any changes in patient's skin, such as redness or break in the patient's skin.
- Report any redness and/or abrasion from medical devices.

Equipment
- Risk assessment tool (use agency-approved tool; see agency policy)
- Documentation record
- Pressure-redistribution mattresses, bed, or chair cushion as needed
- Positioning aids
- Clean gloves

STEPS	RATIONALE
ASSESSMENT	
1. Identify patient using at least two identifiers (e.g., name and birthday or name and account number) according to agency policy.	Ensures correct patient. Complies with The Joint Commission standards and improves patient safety (TJC, 2021).
2. Review patient's electronic health record (EHR), including health provider's orders and nurses' notes, to assess patient's risk for pressure injury formation:	Identifies specific factors that place patient at risk and need to administer preventive care (Haesler, 2017; EPUAP/NPIAP/PPPIA, 2019a; EPUAP/NPIAP/PPPIA, 2019b).
a. Paralysis or immobilization caused by restrictive devices	Patient is unable to turn or reposition independently to relieve pressure.
b. Presence of medical device such as nasogastric (NG) tube, oxygen equipment, artificial airways, drainage tubing, or mechanical devices (Doughty and McNichol, 2016)	Medical devices have potential to exert pressure on patient's nares or ears or on tissue adjacent to devices such as artificial airways and drainage tubes (da Silva Galetto et al., 2019; Pittman et al., 2015).
(1) If not medically contraindicated, remove medical device to assess skin and tissues under and around each medical device at least every 12 hours. When possible, reposition device (Cooper et al., 2020).	These devices are often made of rigid plastic to maintain the functionality of the device (e.g., oxygen masks). Pressure area assumes same configuration as medical device (Cooper et al., 2020; WOCN, 2016).

STEPS	RATIONALE

CLINICAL JUDGMENT: *Perform more frequent assessments when patients have fluid shifts, edema, or diaphoresis (Cooper et al., 2020).*

STEPS	RATIONALE
c. Sensory loss (e.g., hemiplegia, SCI)	Patient is unable to feel discomfort from pressure and does not independently change position.
d. Circulatory disorders (e.g., peripheral vascular diseases, vascular changes from diabetes mellitus, neuropathy)	Reduce perfusion of tissue layers of skin.
e. Fever	Increases metabolic demands of tissues. Accompanying diaphoresis leaves skin moist.
f. Anemia	Decreased hemoglobin level reduces oxygen-carrying capacity of blood and amount of oxygen available to tissues.
g. Malnutrition: weight loss, loss of muscle mass, and/or subcutaneous fat	Inadequate nutrition leads to weight loss, muscle atrophy, and reduced tissue mass. Nutrient deficiencies result in impaired or delayed healing (Stotts, 2016a).
h. Fecal or urinary incontinence	Skin exposed to prolonged moisture develops MASD, and such exposure increases the risk for pressure injury (Francis, 2020). Excessive moisture macerates skin (McNichol et al., 2018; Ayello, 2017).
i. Heavy sedation and anesthesia	Sedation alters sensory perception, and patient does not perceive pressure and change position.
j. Age	Neonates and very young children are at high risk, with the head being most common site of pressure injury occurrence (WOCN, 2016). There is loss of dermal thickness in older adults, impairing ability to distribute pressure (Pieper, 2016).
k. Dehydration	Results in decreased skin elasticity and turgor.
l. Edema	Edematous tissues are less tolerant of pressure, friction, and shear.
m. Existing pressure injuries	Limit surfaces available for position changes, placing available tissues at increased risk.
n. History of pressure injury	Tensile strength of skin from previously healed pressure injury is 80% or less; therefore this area cannot tolerate pressure as much as undamaged skin (Doughty and Sparks, 2016).
3. Assess patient's or family caregiver's knowledge, experience, and health literacy.	Ensures patient and family caregiver has the capacity to obtain, communicate, process, and understand basic health information (CDC, 2021).
4. Assess patient's level of comfort on pain scale of 0 to 10. If patient is in pain, administer prescribed analgesic 30 minutes before assessment.	Patients in pain will not be able to comfortably change positions or tolerate a full skin assessment.
5. Select agency-approved risk assessment tool such as the Braden Scale or Norton Scale. Perform risk assessment when patient enters health care setting and repeat on regularly scheduled basis or when there is significant change in patient's condition (see agency policy) (WOCN, 2016).	Valid and reliable risk assessment tools evaluate patient's risk for developing a pressure injury. Identifying risk factors that contribute to the potential for skin breakdown allows you to target specific interventions for decreasing risk.

CLINICAL JUDGMENT: *In acute care settings, perform initial assessment within 8 hours of admission and reassess every 24 hours or as patient condition changes; in critical care areas, perform assessment on admission and reassess every 24 hours or as patient condition changes; and in long-term and home care settings, perform assessment on admission. In long-term care settings reassess weekly and then according to agency standards or when patient condition changes. In home care setting reassess every RN visit (see Table 48.4).*

STEPS	RATIONALE
6. Obtain risk score (see Table 48.5) and evaluate its meaning based on patient's unique characteristics. Research identified Braden Scale scores in specific patient populations: intensive care patients ≤14, older adults ≤14 (Alderden et al., 2017).	Risk cutoff score depends on instrument used. Score involves identifying risk factors that contributed to it and minimizing these specific deficits (Alderden et al., 2017; Ayello, 2017).
7. Close room or pull curtains around bed.	Maintains patient privacy.
8. Perform hand hygiene. Assess condition of patient's skin, focusing on pressure points (see Fig. 48.9). Apply gloves as needed with open and/or draining wounds.	Body weight against bony prominences places underlying skin at risk for the development of skin injuries.
a. Inspect for skin discoloration (see Box 48.2 for patients with darkly pigmented skin); note any redness.	Patients with darkly pigmented skin must also have their skin temperature and moisture assessed (WOCN, 2016).
b. Inspect for pallor and mottling.	Persistent hypoxia in tissues that were under pressure; an abnormal physiological response.
c. Inspect for absence of superficial skin layers.	Represents early pressure injury formation, usually a partial-thickness wound that may have resulted from friction and/or shear.
d. Inspect for changes in skin temperature, edema, and tissue consistency, especially in individuals with darkly pigmented skin (EPUAP/NPIAP/PPPIA, 2019a).	Localized heat, edema, and induration have been identified as warning signs for pressure injury development. Because it is not always possible to observe changes in skin color on darkly pigmented skin, these additional signs should be considered in assessment (EPUAP/NPIAP/PPPIA, 2019a).

Continued

SKILL 48.1	ASSESSMENT AND PREVENTION STRATEGIES FOR PRESSURE INJURY DEVELOPMENT—cont'd

STEPS	RATIONALE
e. Inspect for wound drainage.	Wound drainage increases risk for skin breakdown because it is caustic to skin and underlying tissues. Tubing from drainage devices (e.g., Jackson-Pratt, Hemovac) causes pressure under device and on adjacent skin (EPUAP/NPIAP/PPPIA, 2019a).
f. Palpate for tissue consistency (firm or boggy feel) and/or palpate for abnormal sensations (Nix, 2016).	
g. Use your fingertips to palpate discolored area of the skin and under and around medical devices. Release your fingertips and look for blanching. If on palpation an area of redness blanches (lightens in color), this indicates reactive hyperemia (which is a normal response); tissue is not at risk for the development of an injury. If area does not blanch, suspect tissue injury, and recheck in 1 hour.	Tissue that does not blanch when palpated indicates abnormal reactive hyperemia, an indication of possible ischemic injury.
9. Assess skin and tissue around and beneath medical devices every nursing shift for additional areas of potential pressure injury resulting from medical devices (Black and Kalowes, 2016) (see Table 48.1).	Patients at high risk need more frequent assessments and have multiple sites for pressure necrosis from medical devices in areas other than bony prominences (Chaboyer et al., 2017). Patients at higher risk of MDRPI are individuals who require mechanical ventilation or individuals who are vulnerable to fluid shifts and/or edema (EPUAP/NPIAP/PPPIA, 2019a). Pressure points around medical devices (e.g., oxygen cannula and masks, drainage tubing) can cause pressure injury to underlying tissue, which can become full-thickness pressure injuries (EPUAP/NPIAP/PPPIA, 2019a). Typically the MDRPI conforms to the same size and shape as the medical device that caused the injury (EPUAP/NPIAP/PPPIA, 2019a).
a. Nares: NG tube, feeding tube, oxygen cannula	Pressure to nares occurs from tape and other materials used to secure NG tube.
b. Ears: oxygen cannula, pillow	Oxygen equipment is a significant risk for pressure injuries (Padula et al., 2017). Patients' ears and tips of nares are at risk for pressure injuries from nasal cannula (Black et al., 2015; Schallom et al., 2015).
c. Tongue and lips: oral airway, endotracheal (ET) tube	Pressure can result from artificial airway and materials used to secure airway (Padula et al., 2017; Black et al., 2015).
d. Forehead: pulse oximetry device	Adhesive can cause skin blistering.
e. Drainage or other tubing	Stress and pressure against tissue at exit site or from tubing lying under any part of patient's body can cause skin injury (Black et al., 2015).
f. Indwelling urethral (Foley) catheter	In female patients, catheter can place pressure on labia, especially when edematous. In male patients, pressure from catheter not properly anchored can put pressure on tip of penis and urethra (Black et al., 2015).
g. Orthopedic and positioning devices such as casts, neck collars, splints	Applied devices have potential to cause pressure to underlying and adjacent skin and tissue (Black et al., 2015).
h. Compression stockings	Compression stockings have potential to cause pressure, especially if they fit poorly or are rolled down (Black et al., 2015).

CLINICAL JUDGMENT: *Compression stockings must be completely removed to adequately assess the feet, heels, and legs.*

STEPS	RATIONALE
i. Immobilization device and restraints	Pressure points can occur if the device is too tight or poorly placed or if the patient strains against the device.
10. Remove and dispose of gloves and perform hand hygiene.	Reduces transmission of microorganisms.
11. Observe patient for preferred positions when in bed or chair.	Preferred positions result in weight of body being placed on certain bony prominences. Presence of contractures may result in pressure exerted in unexpected places.
12. Observe ability of patient to initiate and help with position changes.	Potential for friction and shear increases when patient is completely dependent on others for position changes.
13. Assess knowledge and experience of patient with pressure injury prevention techniques.	Reveals need for patient instruction and/or support.
14. Assess patient's goals or preferences for how repositioning will be performed or what the patient expects.	Allows care to be individualized to patient.

PLANNING

1. Close room door or pull the curtain around the bed and position the patient so that only the area currently being examined is exposed.	Provides privacy and exposed area for assessment.

STEPS	RATIONALE
2. Prepare and organize equipment. Be sure you have correct risk assessment tool at bedside.	Preparing equipment before the procedure helps to ensure a clean and distraction-free area for organizing procedure-related equipment.
3. Explain procedure(s) and purpose to patient and family caregiver.	Relieves anxiety and provides opportunity for education.

IMPLEMENTATION

STEPS	RATIONALE
1. Perform hand hygiene. If patient has open, draining wounds, apply clean gloves.	Reduces transmission of microorganisms.
2. Implement prevention guidelines adapted from WOCN *Guideline for Prevention and Management of Pressure Ulcers* (WOCN, 2016).	Reduces patient's risk for developing pressure injury.
3. Following initial assessment, continue to inspect skin at least once a day or as per agency policy.	
a. Observe patient's skin; pay particular attention to bony prominences and areas around and under medical devices and tubes. If you find reddened area, gently press area with gloved finger to check for blanching. If area does not blanch, suspect tissue injury, and recheck in 1 hour. Any discoloration may vary from pink to a deep red.	Routine skin inspection is fundamental to risk assessment and in selecting interventions to reduce risk (WOCN, 2016). Persistent redness when lightly pigmented skin is pressed can indicate tissue injury. If area of redness blanches (lightens in color), it indicates that skin is not at risk for breakdown.

CLINICAL JUDGMENT: *Do not massage reddened areas because doing so may cause additional tissue trauma. Reddened areas indicate blood vessel damage, and massaging has the potential to damage underlying tissues (EPUAP/NPIAP/PPPIA, 2019a; Bryant and Nix, 2016b).*

STEPS	RATIONALE
b. If patient has darkly pigmented skin, look for color changes that differ from the patient's normal skin color.	Darkly pigmented skin may not blanch. A change in color may occur at the site of pressure; this change in color differs from patient's usual skin color (EPUAP/NPIAP/PPPIA, 2019a; EPUAP/NPIAP/PPPIA, 2019b) (see Box 48.2).
4. Each shift, check all medical treatment and assistive devices for potential pressure points.	Pressure from these devices increases risk on bony prominences and other areas.
a. Verify that device is correctly sized, positioned, and secured.	Incorrect size, placement, and securing of medical device can cause excessive pressure and rubbing by device on underlying skin (Cooper et al., 2020).
b. Consider protecting underlying at-risk skin with a protective dressing (silicone, hydrocolloid).	Dressings absorb moisture from body and cushion underlying skin from pressure (Cooper et al., 2020; Black et al., 2015).

CLINICAL JUDGMENT: *Inspect skin around and beneath orthopedic devices (e.g., cervical collar, braces, or cast). Note any abrasions or warmth in areas where devices can rub against the skin. In addition, a medical device can result in an altered microclimate at the skin-device interface, thus increasing the risks for injury (EPUAP/NPIAP/PPPIA, 2019a; WOCN, 2016).*

STEPS	RATIONALE
5. Remove and dispose of gloves; perform hand hygiene. Reapply gloves if exposure to body fluids is anticipated during interventions.	Reduces transmission of microorganisms.
6. Review patient's pressure injury risk assessment score. Adapt interventions based on those risks (WOCN, 2016).	Risk scores aid in identifying interventions to lessen or eliminate present risk factors.
7. If immobility, inactivity, or poor sensory perception is a risk factor for patient, consider one of the following interventions (WOCN, 2016):	Immobility and inactivity reduce patient's ability or desire to independently change position. Poor sensory perception decreases patient's ability to feel sensation of pressure or discomfort.
a. Educate patient and family regarding specific pressure injury risk factors and prevention measures.	Helps patients and family understand and adhere to interventions designed to reduce pressure injury risk (Berlowitz, 2020).
b. Reposition patient on a scheduled basis; when repositioning, reassess individual's skin condition to help identify early signs of pressure damage. If skin changes occur, reevaluate the plan.	Reduces duration and intensity of pressure. Some patients may require more frequent repositioning (EPUAP/NPIAP/PPPIA, 2019a; WOCN, 2016).
c. When patient is in side-lying position in bed, use 30-degree lateral position (see Fig. 48.15). Avoid 90-degree lateral position.	Reduces direct contact of trochanter with support surface.
d. Place patient (when lying in bed) on pressure-redistribution surface.	Reduces amount of pressure exerted on tissues.
e. Place patient (when in chair) on pressure-redistribution device and shift points under pressure at least every hour (WOCN, 2016).	Reduces amount of pressure on sacral and ischial areas.
8. If friction and shear are identified as risk factors, consider the following interventions:	Friction and shear damage underlying skin.
a. Chair-bound patient	Relief of pressure by changing from lying to sitting position is insufficient if sitting lasts a prolonged time. The maximum amount of time a patient can sit before there is a need to reposition is unknown (WOCN, 2016).
(1) Tilt patient's chair seat to prevent sliding forward, and support arms, legs, and feet to maintain proper posture (EPUAP/NPIAP/PPPIA, 2019a).	Proper repositioning of patient prevents creating shear from dragging patient along sheets. Slide board provides slippery surface to reduce friction. Use lift team as needed to reposition patient.

Continued

| **SKILL 48.1** | **ASSESSMENT AND PREVENTION STRATEGIES FOR PRESSURE INJURY DEVELOPMENT—cont'd** |

STEPS	**RATIONALE**
(2) Limit the amount of time patient spends without pressure redistribution.	Relieves pressure on sacrum and ischial tuberosities.
(3) For patients who can reposition themselves while sitting, encourage pressure redistribution every 15 minutes using chair push-ups, forward lean, or side-to-side movement (WOCN, 2016).	
b. Ensure that heels are free from surface of bed by using a pillow under calves to elevate heels or use a heel-suspension device; knees should be in 5- to 10-degree flexion (WOCN, 2016; Baath et al., 2015).	"Floating" heels from bed surface offload the heel completely and redistribute the weight of the leg along the calf without applying pressure on the Achilles tendon (Baath et al., 2015).
c. Maintain head of the bed at 30 degrees or lower or at the lowest degree of elevation consistent with patient's condition (do not lower head of bed if patient is at risk for aspiration) (WOCN, 2016).	Decreases potential for patient to slide toward foot of bed and incur shear injury.
9. If patient receives low score on moisture subscale, consider one of the following interventions:	Continual exposure of body fluids on patient's skin increases risk for skin breakdown and pressure injury development.
a. Apply clean gloves. Clean and dry the skin as soon as possible after each incontinence episode (Francis, 2020). Then apply moisture barrier ointment to perineum and surrounding skin.	Protects skin from fecal or urinary incontinence. Friction and shear are enhanced in the presence of moisture (Francis, 2020; McNichol et al., 2018).
b. If skin is denuded, use protective moisture barrier paste after each incontinence episode.	Protects the skin by providing a barrier to the effluent (stool/urine), allowing for healing (Francis, 2020).
c. If moisture source is from wound drainage, consider more frequent dressing changes, skin protection with protective barriers, or collection devices.	Removes frequent exposure to wound drainage from skin.
10. Help patient to comfortable position.	Restores comfort and sense of well-being.
11. Remove gloves (if worn) and discard in appropriate receptacle. Perform hand hygiene.	Reduces transmission of microorganisms.
12. Raise side rails (as appropriate) and lower bed to lowest position	Promotes safety and prevents falls.
13. Place nurse call system in an accessible location within patient's reach.	Ensures patient can call for assistance if needed and promotes safety and prevents falls.

EVALUATION

1. Continually observe patient's skin for areas at risk for tissue damage, noting change in color, presence of warmth, or change in texture. Compare with previous assessments.	Enables you to evaluate success of prevention techniques. Determines status of wound healing.
2. Observe tolerance of patient for position change by asking patient to rate level of pain on pain scale.	Position changes sometimes interfere with patient's sleep and rest pattern.
3. Compare subsequent risk assessment scores.	Provides ongoing comparison of patient's risk level to facilitate appropriateness of plan of care.
4. **Use Teach-Back:** "I want you to understand why we need to assess your skin on an ongoing basis. Tell me in your own words why we will be checking your skin on a regular basis." Revise your instruction now or develop a plan for revised patient/family caregiver teaching if patient/family caregiver is not able to teach back correctly.	Teach-back is an evidence-based health literacy intervention that promotes patient engagement, patient safety, adherence, and quality. The goal of teach-back is to ensure that you have explained medical information clearly so that patients and their families understand what you communicated to them (Agency for Healthcare Research and Quality [AHRQ], 2020).

UNEXPECTED OUTCOMES AND RELATED INTERVENTIONS

1. Skin becomes mottled, reddened, purplish, or bluish.
   - Refer patient to wound, ostomy, continence nurse; registered dietitian; clinical nurse specialist (CNS); nurse practitioner (NP); and/or physical therapist, as necessary. Reevaluate position changes and bed surface.
2. Areas under pressure develop persistent discoloration, induration, or temperature changes.
   - Refer patient to wound, ostomy, continence nurse (WOCN), registered dietitian, advanced practice nurse, and/or physical therapist, as necessary.
   - Modify patient's positioning and turning schedule.

RECORDING AND REPORTING

- Record patient's risk score and skin assessments, turning intervals, pressure-redistribution support surface, care of medical devices, and moisture protection interventions in electronic health record (EHR) or chart.
- Report need for additional consultations (if indicated) for high-risk patient.
- Document your evaluation of patient learning.

HOME CARE CONSIDERATIONS

- Identify community resources such as neighbors and relatives to provide help if patient needs help with position changes.
- Instruct family caregiver in use of the 30-degree lateral position and how to assist patient into the position.
- Remind patient and family caregiver that position changes need to occur even while a patient is sitting in a chair. Small shifts such as moving or repositioning the legs redistributes pressure over bony prominences (WOCN, 2016).
- Closely monitor home care patients for pressure injury development if they have any of the following risk factors: wheelchair or bed dependence, incontinence, anemia, fracture, and/or skin drainage.

SKILL 48.2   TREATING PRESSURE INJURIES AND WOUNDS

Delegation and Collaboration

The skill of treating pressure injuries and wounds cannot be delegated to assistive personnel (AP). Instruct the AP to:

- Report immediately to the nurse pain, fever, or any wound drainage.
- Report immediately to the nurse any change in skin integrity.
- Report any potential contamination to existing dressing, such as patient incontinence or dislodgement of the dressing.

Equipment

- Protective equipment: clean gloves, goggles, cover gown (if splash is a risk)
- Sterile gloves *(optional)*
- Plastic bag for dressing disposal
- Wound-measuring device
- Sterile cotton-tipped applicators (check agency policy for use of sterile applicators)
- Normal saline or cleansing agent (as ordered)
- Topical agent or solution (as ordered)
- Dressing of choice based on patient wound characteristics (see Table 48.10)
- Hypoallergenic tape (if needed)
- Irrigation syringe *(optional)*
- Scale for assessing wound healing

STEPS	RATIONALE
ASSESSMENT	
1. Identify patient using at least two identifiers (e.g., name and birthday or name and account number) according to agency policy. Compare identifiers with information on patient's medication administration record (MAR) or medical record.	Ensures correct patient. Complies with The Joint Commission standards and improves patient safety (TJC, 2021).
2. Review patient's electronic health record (EHR), including health care provider's orders and nurses' notes. Note previous dressing change for the following: wound assessment findings, types of topical medications, types of analgesia if needed, and wound care supplies.	Identifies purpose of treatment of pressure injury. Ensures continuity in administration of proper medications and treatments for specific wound care needs.

> **CLINICAL JUDGMENT:** *Determine if the order is consistent with established wound care guidelines and outcomes for a patient. If the order is not consistent with guidelines or varies from the identified outcome for a patient, review with the health care team.*

STEPS	RATIONALE
3. Assess patient's/family caregiver's knowledge, experience, and health literacy level.	Ensures patient and family caregiver has the capacity to obtain, communicate, process, and understand basic health information (CDC, 2021).
4. Assess patient's level of comfort on pain scale of 0 to 10. If patient is in pain, determine whether prn pain medication has been ordered and administer 30 minutes before dressing change.	Dressing change should not be traumatic for patient; assess wound pain before change, then evaluate during and after wound care management (Hopf et al., 2016).
5. Determine whether patient has allergies to topical agents.	Topical agents could contain elements that cause localized skin reactions.
6. Close room door or bedside curtains.	Provides privacy.
7. Perform hand hygiene. Position patient to allow dressing removal and position biohazard bag for dressing disposal. **NOTE:** This step can also be done during implementation, just before dressing change.	Reduces transmission of microorganisms. Provides an accessible area for dressing change. Proper disposal of old dressing promotes proper handling of contaminated waste.
8. Apply clean gloves. Remove and discard old dressing.	Reduces transmission of microorganisms and prevents accidental exposure to body fluids.
9. Assess patient's wounds using wound parameters and continue ongoing wound assessment per agency policy. **NOTE:** This may be done during wound care procedure.	Provides baseline or comparison with previous dressing changes for condition of wound and effectiveness of wound care (WOCN, 2016).
a. *Wound location:* Describe body site where wound is located.	
b. *Stage/classification of wound:* Describe extent of tissue destruction using wound classification for surgical and traumatic wounds and stage of a pressure injury.	Staging is way of assessing a pressure injury based on depth of tissue destruction. Wounds are documented as unstageable if wound base is not visible (EPUAP/NPIAP/PPPIA, 2019a). Classification of a wound provides guideline for type of dressing to apply.
c. *Wound size:* Measure length, width, and depth of wound per agency protocol. Use disposable measuring guide for length and width. Use cotton-tipped applicator to assess depth (see illustration).	Injury size changes as healing progresses; therefore longest and widest areas of wound change over time. Measuring width and length by measuring consistent areas provides consistent measurement (Nix, 2016).
d. *Presence of undermining, sinus tracts, or tunnels:* Use sterile cotton-tipped applicator to measure depth and, if needed, a gloved finger to examine wound edges.	Wound depth determines amount of tissue loss.
e. *Condition of wound bed:* Describe type and percentage of tissue in wound bed.	Approximate percentage of each type of tissue in wound provides critical information on progress of wound healing and choice of dressing. Wound with high percentage of black tissue may require debridement; yellow tissue or slough tissue may indicate presence of infection or colonization; and granulation tissue indicates that wound is moving toward healing (EPUAP/NPIAP/PPPIA, 2019a).
f. *Volume of exudate:* Describe amount, characteristics, odor, and color.	Amount and type of drainage or exudate may indicate type and frequency of dressing changes (Bates-Jensen, 2016).

Continued

SKILL 48.2   TREATING PRESSURE INJURIES AND WOUNDS—cont'd

STEPS	RATIONALE

 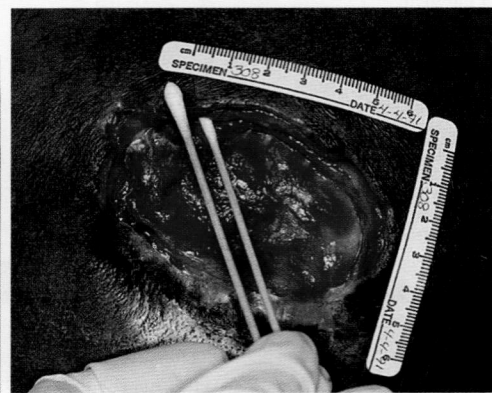

STEP 9c Measuring wound width, length, and undermining of skin. (*Left image* from Bryant RA, Nix DP, editors: *Acute and chronic wounds: current management concepts,* ed 5, St Louis, 2016, Elsevier.)

g. *Condition of periwound skin:* Examine skin for breaks, dryness, maceration, and presence of rash, swelling, redness, or warmth. Modify assessment based on patient's skin color (see Box 48.2).	Impaired periwound skin indicates progressive tissue damage (EPUAP/NPIAP/PPPIA, 2019a). Maceration on periwound skin shows need to alter choice of wound dressing.
h. *Wound edges:* With a gloved finger examine wound edges for condition of tissue.	Provides information regarding epithelialization, chronicity, and etiology.
i. Assess periwound skin; check for maceration, redness, denuded tissue.	Periwound skin is fragile and must be protected from further injury; skin condition determines if skin barrier is needed (EPUAP/NPIAP/PPPIA, 2019a).
10. Remove gloves and discard in appropriate receptacle. Perform hand hygiene.	Reduces transmission of microorganisms.

CLINICAL JUDGMENT: *Repeated hand hygiene is necessary as you assess other wounds or pressure areas. Different organisms contaminate different wounds.*

11. Assess for factors affecting wound healing: poor perfusion, immunosuppression, or preexisting infection.	Factors affect treatment and wound healing.
12. Assess patient's nutritional status (see Chapter 45). Clinically significant malnutrition is present if (1) serum albumin level is less than 3.5 g/dL, (2) lymphocyte count is less than 1800/mm^3, or (3) body weight decreases more than 15% (WOCN, 2016).	Delayed wound healing occurs in poorly nourished patients (Stotts, 2016a; EPUAP/NPIAP/PPPIA, 2019a).

CLINICAL JUDGMENT: *When you suspect malnutrition, obtain a nutritional consultation to modify patient's diet to promote wound healing.*

13. Assess patient's and family caregiver's knowledge, prior experience with prevention, treatment, and factors contributing to recurrence of pressure injuries (WOCN, 2016).	Patient and family caregiver need to partner with health care providers to provide wound care at home as needed to prevent further skin breakdown.
14. Assess patient's goals or preferences for how skill is to be performed or what patient expects.	Allows care to be individualized to patient.

PLANNING

1. Provide privacy by pulling the curtain around the patient and position the patient so that only the area currently being examined is exposed; use sheet to cover rest of the body. Instruct patient not to touch wound or sterile supplies.	Providing privacy and preparing equipment before the procedure help to ensure a clean and distraction-free area for organizing procedure-related equipment. Prevents accidental contamination of sterile supplies.
2. Explain procedure to patient before starting.	Reduces anxiety and provides opportunity for patient/family caregiver education.
3. Organize and prepare the following equipment and supplies.	Ensures more efficient procedure.
a. Wash basin, warm water, equipment, and supplies	
b. Normal saline or other wound-cleaning agent in sterile solution container	Cleanses injury surface before application of topical agents and new dressing.

CLINICAL JUDGMENT: *Use only noncytotoxic agents to clean pressure injuries.*

c. Prescribed topical agent	
(1) Enzyme debriding agents. (Follow specific manufacturer directions for frequency of application.)	Enzymes debride dead tissue to clean injury surface. Enzymes are not applied to healthy tissue.
(2) Topical antibiotics	Topical antibiotics decrease bioburden of wound and should be considered for use if no healing is noted after 2 to 4 weeks of optimal care (WOCN, 2016).

STEPS	RATIONALE
d. Select appropriate dressing based on pressure injury characteristics, principles of wound management, and patient care setting. Dressing options include (see Table 48.10):	Dressing should maintain moist environment for wound while keeping surrounding skin dry (Bryant & Nix, 2016b).
(1) Gauze—Apply as moist dressing, a dry cover dressing when using enzymes or topical antibiotics, or a means to deliver solution to wound.	Gauze delivers moisture to wound and is absorptive.
(2) Transparent film dressing—Apply over superficial injuries with minimal or no exudate and skin subjected to friction	Maintains moist environment and offers intact skin protection.
(3) Hydrocolloid dressing	Maintains moist environment to facilitate wound healing while protecting wound base.
(4) Hydrogel—available in sheet or in tube	Maintains moist environment to facilitate wound healing.
(5) Calcium alginate	Highly absorbent of wound exudate in heavily draining wounds.
(6) Foam dressings	Protective and prevents wound dehydration; also absorbs moderate to large amounts of drainage.
(7) Silver-impregnated dressings/gels	Controls bacterial burden in wound.
(8) Wound fillers	Fills shallow wounds, hydrates, and absorbs.
e. Obtain hypoallergenic tape or adhesive dressing sheet.	Used to secure nonadherent dressing. Prevents skin irritation and tearing.

IMPLEMENTATION

STEPS	RATIONALE
1. Assemble supplies at bedside.	Ensures organized procedure.
2. Perform hand hygiene and apply clean gloves. Open sterile packages and topical solution containers (see Chapter 28). Keep dressings sterile. Wear goggles, mask, and moisture-proof cover gown if potential for contamination from spray exists when cleaning wound.	Reduces transmission of microorganisms.
3. Remove bed linen and arrange patient's gown to expose wound and surrounding skin. Keep remaining body parts draped.	Prevents unnecessary exposure of body parts.
4. Moisten gauze in cleaning solution. Clean wound thoroughly with normal saline or prescribed wound-cleaning agent from least contaminated to most contaminated area. For deep injuries or wounds, clean with saline delivered with irrigating syringe as ordered (see Skill 48.5). Dry skin around wound thoroughly using clean gauze. Remove gloves and discard.	Cleaning wound removes wound exudate, unwanted substances from the skin's surface, and/or dressing residue and reduces surface bacteria (EPUAP/NPIAP/PPPIA, 2019a).
5. Perform hand hygiene and apply clean or sterile gloves. (Refer to agency policy.)	Maintains aseptic technique while cleaning, measuring, and applying dressings.
6. Apply topical agents to wound using cotton-tipped applicators or gauze as ordered:	
a. Enzymes	Follow manufacturer directions for method and frequency of application. Be aware of which solutions inactivate enzymes and avoid their use in wound cleaning.
(1) Apply small amount of enzyme debridement ointment directly to necrotic areas in the pressure injury. *Do not apply enzyme to surrounding healthy skin.*	Thin layer absorbs and acts more effectively than thick layer. Excess medication irritates surrounding healthy skin (Bryant and Nix, 2016b; Rolstad et al., 2016). Proper distribution of ointment ensures effective action.

CLINICAL JUDGMENT: *If using an enzymatic debriding agent, do not use wound-cleaning agents with metals.*

STEPS	RATIONALE
(2) Place moist gauze dressing directly over wound followed by a dry dressing. Follow specific manufacturer recommendation for type of dressing material to use to cover a pressure injury when using enzymes. Tape dressing in place.	Protects wound and prevents removal of ointment during turning or repositioning.
b. *Antibacterials* (e.g., bacitracin, metronidazole, and silver sulfadiazine). Apply evenly over wound surface.	Reduces bacterial growth.
7. Apply prescribed wound dressing:	
a. *Hydrogel:*	Hydrogel dressings are designed to hydrate and bring moisture to wound (Bryant and Nix, 2016b; Rolstad et al., 2016). Hydrogel dressings also promote wound healing and alleviate wound pain (Zhang et al., 2019).
(1) Lightly pack wound with alginate using sterile cotton-tipped applicator or gloved finger.	The dressing swells and increases in size; tight packing can compromise blood flow to the tissues.
(2) Apply secondary dressing, such as dry gauze; tape in place.	Holds hydrogel against wound surface because amorphous hydrogel (in tube) or sheet form does not adhere to wound and requires secondary dressing to hold it in place.
(3) If using impregnated gauze, pack loosely into wound; cover with secondary gauze dressing and tape.	A loosely packed dressing delivers gel to wound base and allows any wound debris to be trapped in gauze.

Continued

SKILL 48.2	TREATING PRESSURE INJURIES AND WOUNDS—cont'd

STEPS	RATIONALE
b. *Calcium alginate:*	Alginate dressings absorb serous fluid or exudate, forming a nonadhesive hydrophilic gel, which conforms to shape of wound (Bryant and Nix, 2016b). Use in heavily draining wounds.
(1) Lightly pack wound with alginate using sterile cotton-tipped applicator or gloved finger.	The dressing swells and increases in size; tight packing can compromise blood flow to the tissues.
(2) Apply secondary dressing and tape in place.	
c. *Transparent film dressing:*	
(1) Be sure skin around wound is thoroughly dry.	Moisture prevents transparent dressing from adhering.
(2) Remove paper backing, taking care not to allow adhesive areas to touch one another. *Do not stretch a film dressing, and avoid wrinkles.*	Ensures smooth application.
(3) Place film smoothly over wound and use your fingers to smooth and adhere dressing over skin.	Ensures occlusive application.
(4) Label dressing with date, your initials, and time of dressing change.	Provides guideline for timing of next dressing change.

CLINICAL JUDGMENT: *Use transparent dressings for minor cuts or abrasions and for autolytic debridement of noninfected superficial pressure injuries. A hydrocolloid dressing protects skin from friction and/or provides moisture to a wound. Some brands have custom shapes available for specific anatomical parts such as heels, elbows, and sacrum.*

STEPS	RATIONALE
d. *Hydrocolloid dressing:*	
(1) Select proper size wafer, allowing dressing to extend onto intact periwound skin at least 2.5 cm (1 inch). *Do not stretch dressing, and avoid wrinkles.*	Dressing prevents shear and friction from loosening edges and circumvents need for tape along dressing borders (Bryant and Nix, 2016b).
(2) For deep wounds, apply hydrocolloid granules, impregnated gauze, or paste before the wafer.	Functions as filler material to ensure contact with all wound surfaces. Cushions wound for pain reduction and protection.
(3) Remove paper backing from adhesive side and place over wound. Do not stretch and avoid wrinkles or tenting. Hold dressing in place for 30 to 60 seconds after application.	Molds dressing at body temperature (Bryant and Nix, 2016b).
(4) If cut from large piece of wafer, tape edges with nonallergenic tape.	Avoids rolling of edges of dressing or adherence to clothing.
e. *Foam dressing:*	
(1) Refer to manufacturer guidelines for removal and application characteristics of specific foam dressing brand.	Foam dressings collect moderate to heavy wound exudate; however, some contain an antimicrobial substance to reduce risk for bacterial colonization in wounds.
(2) Apply a skin barrier wipe to surrounding skin that will come in contact with the thin foam dressing adhesive.	Protects skin from maceration or irritation of adhesive.
(3) Cut foam sheet to extend 2.5 cm (1 inch) out onto intact periwound skin. (Verify which side of foam dressing should be placed toward wound bed and which side should face away from it; see product instructions.)	Ensures proper absorption and keeps wound exudate away from wound (Bryant and Nix, 2016b).
(4) Cover with secondary dressing as needed.	Protects dressing.
8. Reposition patient comfortably off pressure injury.	Prevents pressure to injury.
9. Remove and dispose of gloves. Dispose of soiled supplies in appropriate receptacle. Perform hand hygiene.	Reduces transmission of microorganisms.
10. Help patient to comfortable position.	Restores comfort and sense of well-being.
11. Raise side rails (as appropriate) and lower bed to lowest position	Promotes safety and prevents falls.
12. Place nurse call system in an accessible location within patient's reach.	Ensures patient can call for assistance if needed and promotes safety and prevents falls.

EVALUATION

1. Observe skin surrounding injury for inflammation, edema, and tenderness.	Determines progress of wound healing.
2. Inspect dressings and exposed injuries, observing for drainage, foul odor, and tissue necrosis. Monitor patient for signs and symptoms of infection: fever and elevated WBC count.	Pressure injuries can become infected (Stotts, 2016b).
3. Compare subsequent injury measurements by using one of the scales designed to measure wound healing such as Pressure Ulcer Scale for Healing (PUSH Tool) or BWAT.	Allows comparison of serial measurements to evaluate wound healing. Provides standard method of data collection that demonstrates wound progress or lack thereof.
4. **Use Teach-Back:** "I want to be sure that you understand why we measure and assess your pressure injury on an ongoing basis. Tell me why we measure the injury and look at the tissue and surrounding skin." Revise your instruction now or develop a plan for revised patient/family caregiver teaching if patient/family caregiver is not able to teach back correctly.	Teach-back is an evidence-based health literacy intervention that promotes patient engagement, patient safety, adherence, and quality. The goal of teach-back is to ensure that you have explained medical information clearly so that patients and their families understand what you communicated to them (AHRQ, 2020).

UNEXPECTED OUTCOMES AND RELATED INTERVENTIONS

1. Skin surrounding injury becomes macerated.
   - Reduce exposure of surrounding skin to topical agents and moisture.
   - Select dressing that has increased moisture-absorbing capacity.
2. Wound becomes deeper with increased drainage and/or development of necrotic tissue.
   - Review current wound care management.
   - Consult with interprofessional team regarding changes in wound care regimen.
   - Obtain wound cultures.
3. Pressure injury extends beyond original margins.
   - Monitor for systemic signs and symptoms of poor wound healing such as abnormal laboratory results (WBC count, levels of hemoglobin/hematocrit, serum albumin, serum prealbumin, total proteins), weight loss, and fluid imbalances.
   - Assess and revise current turning schedule.
   - Consider alternate pressure-redistribution devices.

RECORDING AND REPORTING

- Record in electronic health record (EHR) or chart the appearance and condition of the wound or pressure injury, type of topical agent or dressing used, presence of pain and how treated, and patient's response.
- Document your evaluation of patient learning.
- Report any deterioration in wound appearance.
- Describe the location of the wound; type and percentage of wound tissue; presence or absence of wound drainage, odor; type and quantity of dressings used and the location of the dressings (for the next dressing change); and patient's response.

HOME CARE CONSIDERATIONS

- Clean dressings are often used in the home care setting.
- Consider family caregiver time when selecting a dressing. In the home care setting caregivers may sometimes choose more expensive dressing materials to reduce the frequency of dressing changes.
- Teach patients how to dispose of contaminated dressings in the home in a manner consistent with local regulations for contaminated waste.
- Discuss need for home pressure-redistribution surface or bed. Identify adaptive equipment needed to care for patient at home.
- Teach patient and family caregiver about the signs of wound infection.

SKILL 48.3 APPLYING DRY AND MOIST DRESSINGS

Delegation and Collaboration

The skill of applying dry and damp-to-dry dressings can be delegated to assistive personnel (AP) if the wound is chronic (see agency policy and nurse practice act). However, the nurse must first assess the wound and is responsible for the care of acute new wounds, wound care requiring sterile technique, and evaluation of wound healing. Instruct the AP about:

- Any unique modifications of the dressing change such as the need for use of special tape or taping techniques to secure the dressing.
- Reporting pain, fever, bleeding, or wound drainage to the nurse immediately.
- Reporting any potential contamination to existing dressing (e.g., patient incontinence or other body fluids, a dressing that becomes dislodged).

Equipment

- Personal protective equipment (PPE) (i.e., gown, goggles, mask) if needed
- Clean and sterile gloves
- Sterile dressing set including scissors and forceps (check agency policy)

- Sterile drape *(optional)*
- Necessary dressings: fine-mesh gauze, 4 × 4–inch gauze, abdominal pads (ABDs)
- Sterile basin *(optional)*
- Antiseptic ointment (as prescribed)
- Wound cleanser (as prescribed)
- Sterile normal saline (or prescribed solution)
- Debriding gel as ordered
- Tape (include nonallergenic tape as necessary), Montgomery ties, or bandages as needed
- Skin barrier *(optional* if using Montgomery ties)
- Measuring device: cotton-tipped applicator, measuring guide, camera
- Adhesive remover, scissors, or hair clipper *(optional)*
- Protective waterproof underpad
- Biohazard bag
- Additional lighting if needed (e.g., flashlight, treatment light)

STEPS	RATIONALE
ASSESSMENT	
1. Identify patient using at least two identifiers (e.g., name and birthday or name and account number) according to agency policy. Compare identifiers with information on patient's MAR or medical record.	Ensures correct patient. Complies with The Joint Commission standards and improves patient safety (TJC, 2021).
2. Review patient's EHR, including health care provider's order and nurses' notes. Note previous dressing change, including equipment used and patient response.	Verifies dressing orders and any prior dressing change issues.
3. Assess patient's/family caregiver's knowledge, experience, and health literacy level.	Ensures patient/family caregiver has the capacity to obtain, communicate, and understand basic health information (CDC, 2021).

Continued

SKILL 48.3   APPLYING DRY AND MOIST DRESSINGS—cont'd

STEPS	RATIONALE
4. Assess patient for allergies, especially to antiseptics, tape, or latex.	Reduces risk for localized or systemic allergic reactions to these supplies.
5. Ask patient to rate level of pain using a pain scale of 0 to 10 and to assess character of pain. Administer prescribed analgesic as needed 30 minutes before dressing change.	Superficial wounds with multiple exposed nerves may be intensely painful, whereas deeper wounds with destruction of dermis should be less painful (Krasner, 2016). A comfortable patient is less likely to move suddenly, causing contamination to wound or supplies. Serves as baseline to measure response to dressing therapy.
6. Review electronic health record to identify patient's risk for wound-healing problems, including aging, premature infant, obesity, diabetes mellitus, circulation disorders, nutritional deficit, immunosuppression, radiation therapy, high levels of stress, and use of steroids.	Physiological changes resulting from aging, chronic illness, poor nutrition, medications that affect wound healing, and cancer treatments have potential to affect wound healing (Doughty and Sparks, 2016).
7. Perform hand hygiene and apply gloves as needed.	Reduces transmission of microorganisms.
8. Assess condition of skin around wound and existing dressing (see Skill 48.2). Remove and dispose of gloves if worn and perform hand hygiene.	Provides baseline for comparison with previous dressing changes for condition of skin around wound. Helps to plan for proper dressing type and securement of supplies needed and for whether help is needed during dressing procedure.
9. Assess patient's and family caregiver's knowledge and prior experience with dressing change.	Identifies areas for patient education to prepare patient or family caregiver if dressing must be changed at home.
10. Assess patient's goals or preferences for how skill is to be performed or what patient expects.	Allows care to be individualized to patient.

PLANNING

1. Close room door or bedside curtains. Gather all necessary supplies.	Provides privacy and ensures organized procedure.
2. Organize workspace at bedside.	Facilitates a smooth and organized dressing change.
3. Explain procedure to patient and/or family caregiver.	Decreases patient's anxiety.
4. Place biohazard bag within reach of work area (see illustration).	Ensures easy disposal of soiled dressings.
5. Position patient comfortably and drape to expose only wound site. Instruct patient not to touch wound or sterile supplies.	Draping provides access to wound while minimizing exposure. Dressing supplies become contaminated when touched by patient's hand.

IMPLEMENTATION

1. Perform hand hygiene and apply gloves. Apply additional PPE: gown, goggles, and mask if risk for splash exists (check agency policy).	Hand hygiene and use of PPE reduce transmission of microorganisms.
2. Gently remove tape, bandages, or ties from existing dressing. Use nondominant hand to support dressing and with your dominant hand pull tape parallel to skin and toward dressing. If dressing is over hairy area, remove in direction of hair growth. Get patient permission to clip or shave area (check agency policy). Remove any adhesive from skin.	Pulling tape toward dressing reduces stress on suture line or wound edges, irritation, and discomfort.

STEP 4 Disposable waterproof bag placed near dressing site.

STEPS	**RATIONALE**

CLINICAL JUDGMENT: *If surgical glue was used to close the wound, assess that the glue is intact. Do not remove the glue. Replace only the top dressing as necessary.*

3. With gloved hand or forceps remove dressing one layer at a time, observing appearance and drainage of dressing. Carefully remove outer secondary dressing first; then remove inner primary dressing that is in contact with wound bed. If drains are present, slowly and carefully remove dressings (see Fig. 48.10) and avoid tension on any drainage devices. Keep soiled undersurface from patient's sight.

Purpose of primary dressing is to remove necrotic tissue and exudate. Appearance of drainage may be upsetting to patient. Avoids accidental removal of drain.

   a. If bottom layer of damp-to-dry dressing adheres to wound, gently free dressing and alert patient of discomfort.

   Damp-to-dry dressing should debride wound (Bryant and Nix, 2016b; WOCN, 2016).

   b. If dry dressing adheres to wound that is not to be debrided, moisten with normal saline, wait 1 to 2 minutes, and remove.

   Prevents injury to wound surface and periwound during dressing removal.

4. Inspect wound and periwound for appearance, color, size (length, width, and depth), drainage, edema, presence and condition of drains, approximation (wound edges are together), granulation tissue, or odor. Use measuring guide or ruler to measure size of wound (see Skill 48.2). Gently palpate wound edges for bogginess or patient report of increased pain.

Assesses wound and periwound condition. Indicates status of healing.

CLINICAL JUDGMENT: *If drainage is observed or when there is an odor from the wound, verify with health care provider about obtaining a wound culture.*

5. Fold dressings with drainage contained inside and remove gloves inside out. With small dressings remove gloves inside out over dressing (see illustrations). Dispose of gloves and soiled dressing according to agency policy. Cover wound lightly with sterile gauze pad and perform hand hygiene.

Contains soiled dressings, prevents contact of nurse's hands with drainage, and reduces cross-contamination and transmission of microorganisms.

6. Describe appearance of wound and any indicators of wound healing to patient.

Wounds may be unsettling and frightening to patients. It helps patient to know that wound appearance is as expected and whether healing is taking place.

7. Create sterile field with sterile dressing tray or individually wrapped sterile supplies on over-bed table (see Chapter 28). Pour any prescribed solution into sterile basin.

Sterile dressings remain sterile while on or within sterile surface. Preparation of all supplies before dressing change prevents break in technique during dressing change.

8. Clean wound:

   a. Perform hand hygiene and apply clean gloves. Use gauze or cotton ball moistened in saline or antiseptic swab (per health care provider order) for each cleaning stroke, or spray wound surface with wound cleaner.

   Prevents transfer of organisms from previously cleaned area.

   b. Clean from least to most contaminated area (see Fig. 48.21).

   Cleaning in this direction prevents introduction of organisms into wound.

   c. Clean around any drain (if present), using circular strokes starting near drain and moving outward and away from insertion site (see Fig. 48.22).

   Correct aseptic technique in cleaning prevents contamination.

STEP 5 Dispose of soiled dressings by (A) placing in gloved hand and (B) pulling glove off over dressing and then off hand.

Continued

SKILL 48.3	APPLYING DRY AND MOIST DRESSINGS—cont'd

STEPS	RATIONALE
9. Use sterile dry gauze to blot wound bed.	Drying reduces excess moisture, which could eventually harbor microorganisms.
10. Apply antiseptic ointment (if ordered) with sterile cotton-tipped applicator or gauze, using same technique to apply as for cleaning. Remove and dispose of gloves. Perform hand hygiene.	Helps reduce growth of microorganisms.
11. Apply dressing (see agency policy):	
a. Dry sterile dressing:	

CLINICAL JUDGMENT: *Dry dressings are inappropriate for debriding wounds. In the presence of drainage, a dry dressing may adhere to the wound bed and surrounding tissue, causing pain and trauma on removal. Dry dressings have the disadvantage of moisture evaporating quickly, which can cause a dressing to dry out. As a result, frequent dressing changes are usually needed, and there is an increase in infection rate when compared with semiocclusive dressings (Bryant and Nix, 2016b).*

STEPS	RATIONALE
(1) Apply clean gloves (see agency policy).	Some agencies or condition of wounds may require sterile gloves.
(2) Apply loose woven gauze as contact layer (see illustration).	Promotes proper absorption of drainage.
(3) If drain is present, apply precut, split 4 × 4–inch gauze around drain.	Secures drain and promotes drainage absorption at site.
(4) Apply additional layers of gauze as needed.	Ensures proper coverage and optimal absorption.
(5) Apply thicker woven pad (e.g., Surgipad, abdominal [ABD] pad) for the outermost dressing (see illustration).	This dressing is used on postoperative wounds when there is excessive drainage.
b. Damp-to-dry dressing:	A damp-to-dry dressing is a moist primary dressing that brings moisture to the wound surface. The moistened gauze increases the absorptive ability of the dressing to collect exudate and wound debris while providing the wound base with moisture to facilitate healing.
(1) Apply sterile gloves (see agency policy).	Reduces transmission of infection.
(2) Place fine-mesh or loose 4 × 4–inch gauze in container of prescribed sterile solution. Wring out excess solution.	Damp gauze absorbs drainage and, when allowed to dry, traps debris.

CLINICAL JUDGMENT: *When using "packing strips," use sterile scissors to cut the amount of dressing that you will use to pack the wound. Do not let the packing strip touch the side of the bottle. Place packing strip in container of prescribed sterile solution. Wring out excess solution.*

STEPS	RATIONALE
(3) Apply damp fine-mesh or open-weave gauze as single layer directly onto wound surface. If wound is deep, gently pack gauze into wound with sterile gloved hand or forceps until all wound surfaces are in contact with moist gauze, including dead spaces from sinus tracts, tunnels, and undermining (see illustration A). Be sure that gauze does not touch periwound skin (see illustration B).	Inner gauze should be damp, not dripping wet, to absorb drainage and adhere to debris. When packing a wound, gauze should conform to base and side of wound (Bryant and Nix, 2016b). Wound is loosely packed to facilitate wicking of drainage into absorbent outer layer of dressing. Moisture that escapes dressing often macerates the periwound area.

CLINICAL JUDGMENT: *Count and record the number of pieces of gauze that are packed in the wound, especially deep wounds. This ensures that all gauze pieces are removed from the wound with each dressing change.*

CLINICAL JUDGMENT: *When packing the wound, do not overpack or underpack (Bryant and Nix, 2016b). Packing should fill the wound but should not be above the level of the skin.*

STEP 11a(2) Placing dry gauze dressing over simple wound.

STEP 11a(5) Placing abdominal pad over gauze dressing.

STEPS	RATIONALE

A   B

STEP 11b(3) (A) Packing wound with fine-mesh gauze. (B) Cross section of deep wound packed loosely with gauze roll.

  (4) Apply dry sterile 4 × 4–inch gauze over moist gauze.

Dry layer pulls moisture from wound.

  (5) Cover with ABD pad, Surgipad, or gauze.

Protects wound from entrance of microorganisms.

12. Secure dressing:

 a. *Tape:* Apply tape 2.5 to 5 cm (1–2 inches) beyond dressing. Use nonallergenic tape when necessary.

Supports wound and ensures placement and stability of dressing.

 b. *Montgomery ties:* See Fig. 48.20.

Prevents skin irritation. Ties allow for repeated dressing changes without removal of tape, which can cause tissue injury.

  (1) Be sure that skin is clean. Application of skin barrier is recommended (see Skill 48.2).

Skin barrier (a hydrocolloid, e.g., Stomahesive) protects intact skin from stretch and tension of adhesive tape.

  (2) Expose adhesive surface of tape ends.

  (3) Place ties on opposite sides of dressing over skin or skin barrier.

  (4) Secure dressing by lacing ties across dressing snugly enough to hold it secure but without placing pressure on skin.

 c. For protective window:

A protective window is an alternative to Montgomery ties for smaller wounds. There is less skin irritation when tape is placed on window strips.

  (1) Cut strip of Stomahesive or hydrocolloid pad into 1-cm (½-inch) strips.

  (2) Wipe areas of skin where strips will be applied

Skin must be clean for Stomahesive or hydrocolloid pad to adhere.

  (3) Apply hydrocolloid dressing strips to frame a "window" around the wound using four strips, one on each side, one on the top, and one on the bottom of the dressing material (see illustrations).

  (4) Apply dressing; secure tape ends to adhesive strips (see illustration).

 d. For dressing extremity, secure with roller gauze (see illustration) or elastic net (see also Skill 48.6).

Roller gauze conforms to contour of foot or hand.

A   B

STEP 12c(3) Apply adhesive strips to frame a "window" around wound using four strips.

Continued

SKILL 48.3	**APPLYING DRY AND MOIST DRESSINGS—cont'd**

STEPS	**RATIONALE**

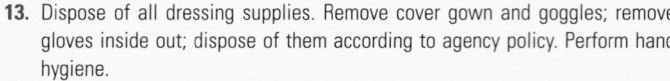

STEP 12c(4) Apply dressing; secure tape ends to adhesive strips.

STEP 12d Wrap roller gauze around extremity to secure dressing.

13. Dispose of all dressing supplies. Remove cover gown and goggles; remove gloves inside out; dispose of them according to agency policy. Perform hand hygiene.	Reduces transmission of microorganisms. Clean environment enhances patient comfort.
14. Label tape over dressing with your initials and date dressing is changed.	Provides timeline for when next dressing change is to be scheduled.
15. Help patient to comfortable position.	Restores comfort and sense of well-being.
16. Raise side rails (as appropriate) and lower bed to lowest position.	Promotes safety and prevents falls.
17. Place nurse call system in an accessible location within patient's reach.	Ensures patient can call for assistance if needed and promotes safety and prevents falls.

EVALUATION

1. Compare observations of the wound with previous assessment and observe appearance of wound for healing: measure size of wound; observe amount, color, and type of drainage and periwound erythema or swelling.	Determines rate of healing.
2. Ask patient to rate pain using a scale of 0 to 10.	Increased pain is often indication of wound complications such as infection or result of dressing pulling tissue.
3. Inspect condition of dressing at least every shift.	Determines status of wound drainage.
4. **Use Teach-Back:** "I want to be sure I explained why and how often you need to continue these dressing changes when you go home tomorrow. Tell me why it is important to change your dressing and when and how often you will do this." Revise your instruction now or develop a plan for revised patient/family caregiver teaching if patient/family caregiver is not able to teach back correctly.	Teach-back is an evidence-based health literacy intervention that promotes patient engagement, patient safety, adherence, and quality. The goal of teach-back is to ensure that you have explained medical information clearly so that patients and their families understand what you communicated to them (AHRQ, 2020).

UNEXPECTED OUTCOMES AND RELATED INTERVENTIONS

1. Wound appears inflamed and tender, drainage is evident, and/or odor is present.
   - Monitor patient for signs of infection (e.g., fever, increased WBC count).
   - Notify health care provider.
   - Obtain wound cultures as ordered.
   - If there is yellow, tan, or brown necrotic tissue, notify health care provider to determine need for debridement (see Table 48.3).
2. Wound bleeds during dressing change.
   - Observe color and amount of bloody drainage. If excessive, may need to apply direct dressing.
   - Inspect area along dressing and directly underneath patient to determine amount of bleeding.
   - Obtain vital signs as needed.
   - Notify health care provider.
3. Patient reports sensation that "something has given way under the dressing."
   - Observe wound for increased drainage or dehiscence (partial or total separation of wound layers) or evisceration (total separation of wound layers and protrusion of viscera through wound opening).
   - If dehiscence or evisceration occurs, protect wound. Cover with sterile saline–moistened dressing.
   - If evisceration is present, do not move patient. Prepare to transfer patient to surgery in patient's bed.
   - Instruct patient to lie still.
   - Stay with patient to monitor vital signs.
   - Notify health care provider.

RECORDING AND REPORTING

- Record appearance and size of wound, characteristics of drainage, presence of necrotic tissue, type of dressings applied, response to dressing change, and level of comfort in electronic health record (EHR) or chart.
- Document your evaluation of patient learning.
- Report any unexpected appearance of wound drainage or bright red bleeding.
- Report any change in wound integrity (e.g., dehiscence or evisceration).

HOME CARE CONSIDERATIONS

- Clean dressings may also be used in the home setting.
- Consider resources within the home, ability of a family caregiver, and the amount of time needed to change a particular dressing when selecting a dressing procedure in the home setting. More expensive dressings may be used to decrease frequency of dressing changes.
- When the patient needs the same type of dressing while at home, be sure to educate the patient and family caregiver on the proper techniques for disposing of medical waste.
- Be sure patient has a family caregiver able to assist with and/or apply dressing, and instruct caregiver on dressing procedure, signs of infection, and when to notify physician.

SKILL 48.4	IMPLEMENTATION OF NEGATIVE-PRESSURE WOUND THERAPY (NPWT)

Delegation and Collaboration

The skill of NPWT cannot be delegated to assistive personnel (AP). Instruct the AP to:

- Use caution in positioning or turning patient to avoid tubing displacement.
- Report any change in dressing shape or integrity to the nurse.
- Report any change in patient's temperature or comfort level to the nurse.
- Report any wound fluid leakage around the edges of the adhesive drape.
- Report any alarms on the NPWT system.

Equipment

- Personal protective equipment (PPE): gown, mask, goggles (used when splashing from wound is a risk)
- Waterproof biohazard bag for disposal

- NPWT unit (requires health care provider's order) (For this skill the vacuum-assisted closure [V.A.C.] unit is used for illustration; several other systems are available, and their applications may differ. See manufacturer instructions.)
- NPWT dressing (gauze or foam [see manufacturer recommendations], transparent dressing, adhesive drape)
- NPWT suction device
- Supplies for wound irrigation if needed (see Skill 48.5)
- Tubing for connection between NPWT unit and NPWT dressing
- Three pairs of gloves, clean and sterile (as needed)
- Scissors, sterile
- Skin preparation, skin barrier protectant, hydrocolloid dressing, or skin barrier
- Adhesive remover (if needed)

STEPS	RATIONALE

ASSESSMENT

1. Identify patient using at least two identifiers (e.g., name and birthday or name and account number) according to agency policy. Compare identifiers with information on patient's MAR or medical record.

Ensures correct patient. Complies with The Joint Commission standards and improves patient safety (TJC, 2021).

2. Review patient's EHR, including health care provider's order and nurses' notes for frequency of dressing change, amount of negative pressure, type of foam or gauze to use, and pressure cycle (intermittent or continuous).

Determines frequency of dressing change, negative-pressure setting, and special instructions. Health care provider's order is also necessary for reimbursement.

3. Review electronic record for signs and symptoms related to condition of patient's wound.

Provides baseline to compare your findings with previous dressing change assessments and reflects wound-healing progress.

4. Assess patient's/family caregiver's knowledge, experience, and health literacy level.

Ensures that patient and family caregiver has the capacity to obtain, communicate, process, and understand basic health information (CDC, 2021).

5. Assess patient's level of comfort on pain scale of 0 to 10.

Serves as baseline to measure patient's level of comfort during and after wound therapy.

6. Perform hand hygiene. Apply clean gloves. Assess condition of wound and status of NPWT dressing (see Skill 48.2). Remove and dispose of gloves. Perform hand hygiene.

Provides information regarding condition of skin around wound and existing dressing, presence of complications, and proper type of supplies and help needed.

7. Assess patient's and family caregiver's knowledge of purpose of dressing and whether they will participate in dressing wound.

Identifies patient's learning needs. Prepares patient and family caregiver if dressing will need to be changed at home.

8. Assess patient's goals or preferences for how NPWT will be performed or what the patient expects.

Allows care to be individualized to patient.

PLANNING

1. Close room door or bed curtains. Position the patient so that only the area currently being examined is exposed; use sheet to cover rest of the body.

Provides privacy and comfort.

2. Administer prescribed analgesic as needed 30 minutes before dressing change.

Comfortable patient will be less likely to move suddenly, causing contamination to wound or supplies.

Continued

SKILL 48.4	IMPLEMENTATION OF NEGATIVE-PRESSURE WOUND THERAPY (NPWT)—cont'd

STEPS	RATIONALE
3. Organize dressing supplies at bedside.	Facilitates a smooth and organized procedure.
4. Explain procedure to patient and family caregiver, instructing not to touch wound or sterile supplies.	Relieves anxiety and promotes understanding of healing process. Prevents contamination of sterile supplies.

IMPLEMENTATION

STEPS	RATIONALE
1. Cuff top of disposable waterproof biohazard bag and place within reach of work area.	Cuff prevents accidental contamination of top of outer bag.
2. Perform hand hygiene and apply clean gloves. If risk for spray exists, apply PPE (e.g., protective gown, goggles, mask) as per agency policy.	Reduces transmission of microorganisms from soiled dressings to nurse's hands.
3. Follow manufacturer directions for removal and replacement of dressing because each NPWT unit varies slightly with approach. Turn off NPWT unit by pushing therapy on/off button.	Deactivates therapy and allows for proper drainage of fluid in drainage tubing.
a. Keeping tube connectors attached to NPWT unit, raise tubing connectors; disconnect tubes from one another and drain fluids into drainage collector.	Prevents backflow of any drainage in tubing back into wound.
b. Before draining, tighten clamp on canister tube and disconnect canister and dressing tubing at connection points.	Prevents drainage from exiting tubing when removed.
4. Remove transparent film by gently stretching, and slowly pull away from skin.	Prevents injury to wound tissue. Protects periwound skin breakdown from transparent adhesive.
5. Remove old dressing one layer at a time and discard in bag. Observe drainage on dressing. Use caution to avoid tension on any drains that are present near the wound or surrounding area. Remove and dispose of gloves.	Determines type and number of dressings needed for replacement. Prevents accidental removal of drains.
6. Perform hand hygiene and conduct a wound assessment. Observe surface area and tissue type, color, odor, and drainage within wound. Measure length, width, and depth of wound as ordered (see Skill 48.2).	Measurement of wound is necessary to assess wound-healing progression and to justify continuation of NPWT for third-party payers (Netsch et al., 2016). Determines condition of wound and need for replacement of dressing.

CLINICAL JUDGMENT: *This is a time when a wound care nurse or physician might debride the wound. Debridement of eschar or slough, if present, should be performed for removal of devitalized tissue to prepare the wound bed (Netsch, 2016).*

STEPS	RATIONALE
7. Remove and discard gloves and perform hand hygiene. Avoid having patient see old dressing because sight of wound drainage may be upsetting.	Reduces transmission of microorganisms. Lessens patient anxiety during procedure.
8. Clean wound.	
a. Perform hand hygiene and apply sterile or clean gloves, depending on agency policy and wound status.	Cleaning periwound is essential for airtight seal.
b. If ordered, irrigate wound with normal saline or other solution ordered by health care provider (see Skill 48.5). Gently blot periwound with gauze to dry thoroughly.	Irrigation removes wound debris and cleans wound bed. Cleaning and removing infectious material has been shown to reduce infection and improve healing (EPUAP/NPIAP/PPPIA, 2019a; Fernandez et al., 2019).

CLINICAL JUDGMENT: *Health care providers may order wound cultures routinely. However, obtain wound culture when drainage is more copious, looks purulent, or has a foul odor. This may be an indication that NPWT may need to be discontinued.*

CLINICAL JUDGMENT: *Health care providers may use normal saline instillation with large, complex wounds. NPWT with instillation in wounds that needed cleaning and removal of infectious material has been shown to reduce infection and improve wound healing (Fernandez et al., 2019).*

STEPS	RATIONALE
9. Apply skin protectant, barrier film, solid skin barrier sheet, or hydrocolloid dressing to periwound skin.	Maintains airtight seal needed for NPWT wound therapy. Protects periwound skin from MASD (Netsch et al., 2016).
10. Fill any uneven skin surfaces (e.g., creases, scars, and skinfolds) with skin barrier product (e.g., paste, strip).	Further helps to maintain airtight seal (Netsch et al., 2016).
11. Remove and discard gloves. Perform hand hygiene.	Prevents transmission of microorganisms.
12. Depending on type of wound, apply sterile or new clean gloves (see agency policy).	Fresh sterile wounds require sterile gloves. Chronic wounds require clean technique (WOCN, 2016).
13. Apply NPWT.	
a. Prepare NPWT filler dressing. Consult with wound care expert for appropriate type.	Filler dressing depends on NPWT used and can include foam or gauze dressings with or without antimicrobials such as silver. Type of dressing may be adjusted based on undermining, tunneling, or sinus tracts present (Netsch et al., 2016).
(1) Measure wound and select appropriate-size dressing.	Black polyurethane (PU) foam has larger pores and is most effective in stimulating granulation tissue and wound contraction. White soft foam is denser with smaller pores and is used when growth of granulation tissue needs to be restricted (Netsch et al., 2016; Panayi et al., 2017).

STEPS	RATIONALE
(2) Using sterile scissors, cut filler gauze dressing or foam to wound size, making sure to fit exact size and shape of wound, including tunnels and undermined areas.	Proper size of dressing maintains negative pressure to entire wound (Netsch et al., 2016).

CLINICAL JUDGMENT: *In some instances, an antimicrobial product such as silver-impregnated gauze or topical antibiotic is in order. These products help reduce the bioburden of the wound.*

b. Place filler dressing in wound following manufacturer instructions. Be sure that filler dressing is in contact with entire wound base, margins, and tunneled and undermined areas. Count number of filler dressings, and document in patient's chart.	Maintains negative pressure to entire wound. Edges of dressing must be in direct contact with patient's skin. Dressing count provides the number of filler dressings that should be removed at the next dressing change.
c. Place suction device per manufacturer instructions.	
d. Apply NPWT transparent dressing over foam or gauze filler dressing.	
(1) Trim dressing to cover wound and dressing so it will extend onto periwound skin approximately 2.5 to 5 cm (1–2 inches).	Prepares dressing for appropriate size of the wound.
(2) Apply transparent dressing, keeping it airtight and wrinkle free (see illustration).	Dressing should be airtight with no wrinkles or tunnels to maintain a negative-pressure environment. A snug and tight application of the dressing must be applied to ensure an airtight seal (see Box 48.10).
(3) Secure tubing to transparent film, aligning drainage holes to ensure occlusive seal. Do not apply tension.	Excessive tension may compress foam dressing and impede wound healing. It also produces shear force on periwound area (Netsch, 2016).
(4) Secure tubing several centimeters away from dressing, avoiding pressure points.	Drainage tubes over bony pressure prominences can cause MDRPIs (Netsch et al., 2016; Netsch, 2016; Pittman et al., 2015).
14. After wound is completely covered, connect tubing from dressing to tubing from canister and NPWT unit and set at ordered suction level.	Intermittent or continuous negative pressure varies from 75 mm Hg to 125 mm Hg, depending on the device and the characteristics of the wound (Netsch et al., 2016; WOCN, 2016).
a. Remove canister from sterile packing and push unit until you hear click. **NOTE:** An alarm sounds if canister is not properly engaged.	
b. Connect dressing tubing to canister tubing (follow manufacturers' instructions). Make sure that both clamps are open.	
c. Place on level surface or hang from foot of bed. **NOTE:** Unit alarms and deactivates therapy if it is tilted beyond 45 degrees.	
d. Press power button (commonly this is a green-lit button) and set pressure as ordered.	
15. Remove and dispose of gloves. Perform hand hygiene.	Reduces transmission of microorganisms.
16. Inspect NPWT system.	
a. Verify that the system is on. This is different for each type of NPWT unit. For example, on some units the display screen shows "Therapy On." Check agency policy and procedure for specific information.	
b. Verify that all clamps are open and that all tubing is patent.	
c. Examine system to be sure that seal is intact and therapy is working.	Negative pressure is achieved when a tight seal is present (Netsch et al., 2016).
d. If a leak is present, perform hand hygiene and apply gloves. Use strips of transparent dressing to patch areas around edges of wound.	
17. Record initials, date, and time on new dressing.	Provides reference for next dressing change.
18. Discard gloves and dispose of any dressing material. Perform hand hygiene.	Prevents transmission of microorganisms.

STEP 13d(2) Foam wound filler; transparent dressing over existing wound. (Courtesy Kinetic Concepts, Inc [KCI], San Antonio, Texas.)

Continued

SKILL 48.4 | IMPLEMENTATION OF NEGATIVE-PRESSURE WOUND THERAPY (NPWT)—cont'd

STEPS	RATIONALE
19. Help patient to comfortable position. Patients may ambulate with NPWT.	Restores comfort and sense of well-being.
20. Raise side rails (as appropriate) and lower bed to lowest position.	Promotes safety and prevents falls.
21. Place nurse call system in an accessible location within patient's reach.	Ensures patient can call for assistance if needed and promotes safety and prevents falls.

EVALUATION

1. Inspect condition of wound and wound bed on an ongoing basis; note drainage and odor.	Determines status of wound healing.
2. Ask patient to rate pain using scale of 0 to 10.	Determines patient's level of comfort following procedure.
3. Verify airtight dressing seal and correct negative-pressure setting.	Determines effective negative pressure being applied.
4. Measure wound drainage output in canister on regular basis.	Monitors fluid balance and wound drainage.
5. **Use Teach-Back:** "I want to be sure I explained clearly what the function of NPWT is. Explain to me how NPWT helps your wound heal and what your wound should look like as it is healing." Revise your instruction now or develop a plan for revised patient/family caregiver teaching if patient/family caregiver is not able to teach back correctly.	Teach-back is an evidence-based health literacy intervention that promotes patient engagement, patient safety, adherence, and quality. The goal of teach-back is to ensure that you have explained medical information clearly so that patients and their families understand what you communicated to them (AHRQ, 2020).

UNEXPECTED OUTCOMES AND RELATED INTERVENTIONS

1. Wound appears inflamed and tender, wound hemorrhages, drainage has increased, and odor is present.
   - Notify health care provider.
   - Obtain wound culture.
   - Increase frequency of dressing changes.
2. Patient reports increase in pain.
   - Consult with health care provider about changing analgesia.
   - Instill normal saline to moisten foam and other filler dressings to allow them to loosen from granulation tissue.
   - Decrease pressure setting.
   - Change from intermittent to continuous cycling.
   - Change type of NPWT system.
3. Negative-pressure seal has broken.
   - Take preventive measures (see Box 48.10).

RECORDING AND REPORTING

- Record appearance of wound (characteristics of wound bed and drainage), placement of NPWT, negative-pressure setting, and patient's response in electronic health record (EHR) or chart.
- Report brisk, bright bleeding; evidence of poor wound healing; and possible wound infection to health care provider.
- Report on location of NPWT, time of dressing change if done, and any interventions, such as reinforcement of dressing.
- Discuss whether the patient or family caregiver is participating in changing the NPWT dressing.
- Document your evaluation of patient learning.

HOME CARE CONSIDERATIONS

- Be sure that patient and family caregiver understand the importance of maintaining a seal on the NPWT dressing and that they have been educated on how to seal the dressing and know whom to call if the alarm alerts them to a leak in the system that they are unable to seal.
- Review how to attach the device to a wall outlet to recharge the battery.
- Instruct the patient and family members on the schedule for the NPWT change.
- Instruct patient and family how to correctly dispose of contaminated dressings according to local health department requirements.

SKILL 48.5 | PERFORMING WOUND IRRIGATION

Delegation and Collaboration

The skill of wound irrigation cannot be delegated to assistive personnel (AP) unless it is a chronic wound (see agency policy). It is the nurse's responsibility to assess and document wound characteristics. Instruct the AP to:

- Notify the nurse when the wound is exposed, so an assessment can be completed.
- Report to the nurse the patient's pain, presence of blood, drainage.

Equipment

- Personal protective equipment (PPE): sterile gloves, gown, and goggles if splash or spray risk exists (check agency policy)

- Irrigation/cleansing solution per order (volume 1.5–2 times the estimated wound volume)
- Irrigation delivery system (per order), depending on amount of desired pressure: sterile irrigation 35-mL syringe with sterile soft angiocatheter or 19-gauge needle (WOCN, 2016) or handheld shower
- Waterproof underpad if needed
- Dressing supplies (see Skills 48.2 and 48.3)
- Disposable waterproof biohazard bag
- Wound assessment supplies (see Skill 48.1)

STEPS	RATIONALE

ASSESSMENT

1. Identify patient using at least two identifiers (e.g., name and birthday or name and account number) according to agency policy. Compare identifiers with information on patient's MAR or medical record.

Ensures correct patient. Complies with The Joint Commission standards and improves patient safety (TJC, 2021).

2. Review patient's EHR, including health care provider's order and nurses' notes. Note status of open wound and type of solution to be used.

Open-wound irrigation requires medical order, including type of solution(s) to use.

3. Review EHR for signs and symptoms related to patient's open wound.

    a. Extent of impairment of skin integrity, including size of wound.

Provides ongoing data to indicate change in wound status (Nix, 2016).

    b. Verify number of drains present.

Awareness of drain position facilitates safe dressing removal and determines need for special dressings.

    c. Drainage, including amount, color, consistency, and any odor noted.

Ongoing data: drainage should decrease in healing wound. When drainage increases, it is often related to infection (Doughty and Sparks et al., 2016).

    d. Wound tissue color.

Color represents balance between necrotic and new scar tissue. Proper selection of wound care products on basis of wound color facilitates removal of necrotic tissue and promotes new tissue growth (Nix, 2016).

    e. Culture reports. Infected wound is colonized with bacteria.

Culture reports identify type of bacteria and proper treatment. Ongoing wound cultures document resolution of infectious process (Stotts, 2016b).

4. Assess patient's/family caregiver's knowledge, experience, and health literacy level.

Ensures patient has the capacity to obtain, communicate, process, and understand basic health information (CDC, 2021).

5. Assess patient's level of comfort using pain scale of 0 to 10.

Serves as baseline to measure patient's level of comfort before wound irrigation.

6. Assess patient for history of allergies to antiseptics, solutions, medications, tapes, latex, or dressing material.

Known allergies suggest applying sample of prescribed wound treatment as skin test before flushing wound with large volume of solution or selecting different tape or dressing material. Latex allergies require the use of "latex-free" gloves and wound care products.

7. Assess patient's and family caregiver's understanding of need for irrigation and of signs of wound infection.

Determines extent of instruction required.

8. Assess patient's goals or preferences for how irrigation will be performed or what the patient expects.

Allows care to be individualized to patient.

PLANNING

1. Perform hand hygiene and administer prescribed analgesic as needed 30 minutes before dressing change.

Promotes pain control and permits patient to move more easily and be positioned to facilitate wound irrigation (Krasner, 2016). A patient who is comfortable will be less likely to move suddenly, causing contamination of wound or supplies.

2. Gather appropriate supplies for wound irrigation and dressing.

Ensures an organized procedure.

3. Explain procedure to patient and family caregiver, instructing not to touch wound or sterile supplies.

Relieves anxiety and promotes understanding of healing process. Prevents contamination of sterile supplies.

4. Close room door or bedside curtains, perform hand hygiene, and position patient.

Maintains privacy.

    a. Position patient comfortably to permit gravitational flow of irrigating solution over wound and into collection receptacle (see illustration).

Directing solution from top to bottom of wound and from cleanest to contaminated area prevents further infection. Position also avoids fluid retention in the wound as the flow of the irrigant moves away from the wound.

    b. Ensure that irrigant is at room temperature, and position patient so that wound is vertical to collection basin.

Room temperature solution increases comfort and reduces vasoconstriction response in tissues.

    c. Place padding or extra towel on bed under area where irrigation will take place.

Protects bedding from becoming wet.

STEP 4a Patient position for wound irrigation.

Continued

SKILL 48.5	PERFORMING WOUND IRRIGATION—cont'd

STEPS	RATIONALE

IMPLEMENTATION

STEPS	RATIONALE
1. Perform hand hygiene.	Reduces transmission of microorganisms.
2. Form cuff on waterproof biohazard bag and place near bed.	Cuffing helps to maintain large opening, thereby permitting placement of contaminated dressings without touching bag itself.
3. Apply PPE: gown, mask, goggles as indicated; apply clean gloves and remove old dressing. Clean wound (see Skill 48.2).	Reduces transmission of microorganisms. Protects from splashes or sprays of blood and body fluids. While cleaning wound, use meticulous hand hygiene and proper infection control procedures before and after removing soiled dressings to limit risk for health care–acquired infection (Jaszarowski and Murphree, 2016).
4. Remove and discard old dressing and gloves in biohazard bag. Perform hand hygiene.	Reduces transmission of microorganisms.
5. Apply clean or sterile gloves (check agency policy). Expose area near wound only and perform wound assessment and examine recent charted assessment of patient's open wound (see Skill 48.2).	Provides privacy and prevents chilling of patient. Provides ongoing wound-healing data. Use sterile precautions when sterile gloves are needed.
6. Irrigate wound with wide opening:	The cleansing solution is introduced directly into the wound with a syringe, a syringe and catheter, or a pulsed lavage device.
a. Fill 35-mL syringe with irrigation solution.	Irrigating wound uses mechanical force, which helps with separation and removal of necrotic debris and surface bacteria (Jaszarowski and Murphree, 2016). Flushing wound helps remove debris and facilitates healing by secondary intention.
b. Attach 19-gauge angiocatheter.	Catheter lumen delivers ideal pressure for cleaning and removing debris with minimal risk for tissue injury (Ramundo, 2016). Mechanical debridement is achieved with irrigation pressures delivered between 4 and 15 psi (WOCN, 2016).

CLINICAL JUDGMENT: *Pulsatile high-pressure lavage is an alternative to using the 35-mL syringe and the 19-gauge angiocatheter. A pulsatile lavage machine combines intermittent high-pressure lavage with suction to loosen necrotic tissue and facilitate removal by other methods of debridement (Ramundo, 2016).*

STEPS	RATIONALE
c. Hold syringe tip 2.5 cm (1 inch) above upper end of wound and over area being cleaned.	Prevents syringe contamination. Careful placement of syringe prevents unsafe pressure of flowing solution.
d. Using continuous pressure, flush wound; repeat Steps 6a to 6d until solution draining into basin is clear.	Flushing wound helps to remove debris; clear solution indicates removal of all debris.
7. Irrigate deep wound with very small opening:	
a. Attach soft catheter to filled irrigation syringe.	Catheter permits direct flow of irrigant into wound. Expect wound to take longer to empty when opening is small.
b. Gently insert tip of catheter into opening about 1.3 cm (½ inch).	Prevents tip from touching fragile inner wall of wound.

CLINICAL JUDGMENT: *Do not force catheter into the wound because this will cause tissue damage.*

STEPS	RATIONALE
c. Using slow, continuous pressure, flush wound.	Use of slow mechanical force of stream of solution loosens particulate matter on wound surface and promotes healing (Ramundo, 2016).

CLINICAL JUDGMENT: *Pulsatile high-pressure lavage is often the irrigation method of choice for necrotic wounds. Pressure settings should be set per provider order, usually between 4 and 15 psi, and should not be used on skin grafts, exposed blood vessels, muscle, tendon, or bone. Use with caution if patient has coagulation disorder or is taking anticoagulants (Ramundo, 2016).*

STEPS	RATIONALE
d. While keeping catheter in place, pinch it off just below syringe.	Avoids contamination of sterile solution.
e. Remove and refill syringe. Reconnect to catheter and repeat until solution draining into basin is clear.	
8. Clean wound with handheld shower:	
a. With patient seated comfortably in shower chair or standing if condition allows, adjust spray to gentle flow; make sure that water is warm.	Useful for patients able to shower with help or independently. May be accomplished at home.
b. Shower for 5 to 10 minutes with shower head 30 cm (12 inches) from wound.	Ensures that wound is cleaned thoroughly.
9. When indicated, obtain cultures after cleaning with nonbacteriostatic saline.	WOCN (2016) recommends using quantitative bacterial cultures (tissue biopsy or swab cultures). Most common types of wound cultures are swab technique, aspirated wound fluid, or tissue biopsy (Stotts, 2016b).

CLINICAL JUDGMENT: *Obtain a wound culture if indicated by the presence of inflammation around the wound, purulent odor or drainage, new drainage, or a febrile patient.*

STEPS	RATIONALE
10. Dry wound edges with gauze; dry patient after shower.	Prevents maceration of surrounding tissue from excess moisture.

STEPS	RATIONALE
11. Remove and dispose of gloves. Perform hand hygiene. Apply clean or sterile gloves (see agency policy). Apply appropriate dressing and label with time, date, and nurse's initials.	Reduces transmission of microorganisms. Maintains protective barrier and healing environment for wound. Provides timeline for when next dressing change is to be scheduled.
12. Remove PPE: mask, goggles, and gown.	Prevents transfer of microorganisms.
13. Dispose of equipment and soiled supplies; remove and dispose of gloves. Perform hand hygiene.	Reduces transmission of microorganisms.
14. Help patient to comfortable position.	Restores comfort and sense of well-being.
15. Raise side rails (as appropriate) and lower bed to lowest position.	Promotes safety and prevents falls.
16. Place nurse call system within reach; instruct patient in use.	Ensures patient can call for assistance if needed and promotes safety and prevents falls.

EVALUATION

1. Have patient rate level of comfort on scale of 0 to 10.	Patient's pain should not increase as a result of wound irrigation.
2. Monitor type of tissue in wound bed.	Identifies wound-healing progress and determines type of wound cleaning and dressing needed.
3. Inspect dressing periodically (see agency policy).	Determines patient's response to wound irrigation and need to modify plan of care.
4. Evaluate periwound skin integrity.	Determines whether extension of wound has occurred or signs of infection are present (warm red periwound skin).
5. Observe for presence of retained irrigant.	Retained irrigant is medium for bacterial growth and subsequent infection.
6. **Use Teach-Back:** "I want to be sure that I explained how to irrigate your wound. Since you are going to be doing this at home; please show me how you will irrigate the wound with this syringe." Revise your instruction now or develop a plan for revised patient/family caregiver teaching if patient/family caregiver is not able to teach back correctly.	Teach-back is an evidence-based health literacy intervention that promotes patient engagement, patient safety, adherence, and quality. The goal of teach-back is to ensure that you have explained medical information clearly so that patients and their families understand what you communicated to them (AHRQ, 2020).

UNEXPECTED OUTCOMES AND RELATED INTERVENTIONS

1. Bleeding or serosanguineous drainage appears.
   - Flush wound during next irrigation using less pressure.
   - Notify health care provider of bleeding.
2. Increased pain or discomfort occurs.
   - Decrease force of pressure during wound irrigation.
   - Assess patient for need for additional analgesia before wound care.
3. Suture line opening extends.
   - Notify health care provider.
   - Reevaluate amount of pressure to use for next wound irrigation.

RECORDING AND REPORTING

- Record wound assessment before and after irrigation, amount and type of solution used, irrigation device used, patient tolerance of the procedure, and type of dressing applied after irrigation in electronic health record (EHR) or chart.
- Document your evaluation of patient learning.
- Report the location of the wound irrigated; discuss the type of solution used, the quality of the return irrigation, and the last time the wound was irrigated.
- Immediately report to the attending health care provider any evidence of fresh bleeding, sharp increase in pain, retention of irrigant, or signs of shock.

HOME CARE CONSIDERATIONS

- Assess patient's home environment to determine adequacy of resources for performing wound care; check especially for adequate lighting, running water, and storage of supplies.
- Solutions to use for irrigation in the home include potable tap water, distilled water, cooled boiled water, and normal saline (WOCN, 2016). Teach patient and family caregiver how to make normal saline by using 8 teaspoons of salt in 1 gallon of distilled water; can keep refrigerated for 1 month. The saline solution should be allowed to reach room temperature before use.
- Instruct the family caregiver on irrigation technique, and have the caregiver demonstrate.
- Be sure the patient and family know signs of infection and when to notify the health care provider.

| **SKILL 48.6** | **APPLYING ROLL GAUZE OR ELASTIC BANDAGE** |

Delegation and Collaboration

The skill of applying a roll gauze or an elastic bandage for compression cannot be delegated to assistive personnel (AP). A nurse assesses the condition of any wound or dressing before applying a bandage. The skill of applying bandages to secure nonsterile dressings can be delegated to AP (refer to agency policy). Instruct the AP about:

- Modifying the bandage application, such as with special taping.
- Reviewing what to observe and report back to the nurse (e.g., patient's complaint of pain, numbness, or tingling after application, or changes in patient's skin color or temperature).

Equipment

- Correct width and number of roll gauze or elastic bandages
- Clips or adhesive tape
- Clean gloves if wound drainage is present
- *Option:* Pillow

STEPS	**RATIONALE**
ASSESSMENT	
1. Identify patient using at least two identifiers (e.g., name and birthday or name and account number) according to agency policy.	Ensures correct patient. Complies with The Joint Commission standards and improves patient safety (TJC, 2021).
2. Review patient's EHR or medical record for specific orders related to application of roll gauze or elastic bandage. Note area to be covered, type of bandage required, frequency of change, and previous response to treatment.	Ensures use of correct products.
3. Assess patient's or family caregiver's knowledge, experience, and health literacy.	Ensures patient or family caregiver has the capacity to obtain, communicate, process, and understand basic health information (CDC, 2021).
4. Assess patient's level of comfort (pain scale of 0 to 10).	Serves as baseline to measure patient's level of comfort when dressing change is performed.
5. Perform hand hygiene. Observe adequacy of circulation to extremity by palpating temperature of skin and pulses, presence of edema, and sensation (distal to area to be bandaged). Observe skin color and movement of body part to be wrapped.	Assesses status of circulation to extremity. Impaired circulation from constricting bandage may delay wound healing. Detection of change to circulation requires frequent observation.

CLINICAL JUDGMENT: *Impaired circulation may result in pain, coolness to touch when compared with the opposite side of the body, cyanosis or pallor of skin, diminished or absent pulses, edema or localized pooling, and numbness and/or tingling of body part.*

6. Apply clean gloves (if drainage or break in skin is present). Inspect skin of area to be bandaged for alterations in integrity as indicated by presence of abrasion, discoloration, or chafing. Pay close attention to areas over bony prominences and areas around medical devices.	It is important to determine whether any new skin alterations are present so that the plan of care can be altered as needed. Bony prominences and pressure areas from medical devices are areas at high risk for skin injury.
7. Inspect the condition of any wound for appearance, size, and presence and character of drainage, and be sure that it is covered with a proper dressing. If not, reapply dressing (check agency policy for type of gloves to use). Remove and dispose of gloves and perform hand hygiene.	An ongoing wound assessment is necessary to judge the progress or lack of progress of the wound toward healing and to plan the appropriate interventions.
8. Assess for size of bandage:	
a. *Roll gauze or basic elastic bandage to secure a dressing:* Assess size of area to be covered. Each successive roll of gauze/elastic should overlap previous layer. Use smaller widths for upper extremities, larger widths for lower extremities.	A bandage too small or too large for the area may not provide the necessary support to stabilize underlying dressings.
b. Elastic bandage to provide simple *compression:* Assess circumference of lower extremity before or shortly after patient gets out of bed in the morning or after patient has been in bed for at least 15 minutes. Select width that will cover and overlap without bulkiness.	An elastic bandage that is too large may not provide sufficient support to immobilize and protect an injured extremity. An elastic bandage that is too small may compromise circulation to the distal extremity.
9. Assess patient's and family caregiver's knowledge of purpose of dressing and ability to manipulate bandage if bandaging will be continued at home.	Identifies patient's learning needs. Prepares patient and family caregiver if dressing will need to be changed at home.
PLANNING	
1. Close room door and pull curtain around the patient's bed. Position patient so that only the affected wound or extremity is exposed; use sheet to cover rest of the body.	Provides privacy and places patient in a position of comfort.
2. Perform hand hygiene and administer prescribed analgesic as needed 30 minutes before applying bandage.	Comfortable patient will be less likely to move suddenly, causing wound or supply contamination or extremity pain.
3. Gather and organize equipment at bedside.	Ensures a clean and distraction-free procedure.
4. Explain procedure to patient before starting.	Reduces anxiety and provides opportunity for patient/family caregiver education.

STEPS	RATIONALE

IMPLEMENTATION

1. Perform hand hygiene and apply clean gloves if drainage is present.

Reduces transmission of microorganisms.

2. Apply roll gauze or elastic bandage to secure dressings:

   a. Elevate dependent extremity for 15 minutes before applying bandage.

   Promotes venous return and decreases swelling.

   b. Make sure that primary dressing over wound is securely in place.

   Wound needs to remain protected once bandage in place.

   c. Hold roll of bandage in your dominant hand and use other hand to lightly hold beginning layer.

   Maintains appropriate and consistent bandage tension.

   d. Begin bandage application at the distal point toward proximal boundary. Apply even tension during application and begin with two circular turns to anchor bandage. Continue to maintain even tension and transfer roll to dominant hand as you wrap bandage, using appropriate turns to cover various shapes of body parts.

   Even tension ensures that bandage exerts even pressure, conforms evenly to body part, and promotes venous return. Spiral and figure-eight dressings are two examples for elastic bandage wrap.

   (1) Spiral dressing is often used to cover cylindrical body parts, such as a wrist. Roll gauze, overlapping each layer by one-half to two-thirds the width of the bandage (see illustration).

   (2) Use figure-eight dressing to cover joint because a snug fit provides support and immobilization to an injured joint. To apply overlap turns, alternate ascending and descending over bandaged part, each turn crossing previous one to form a figure-eight pattern.

CLINICAL JUDGMENT: *Double-check your tension and ensure that bandage is snug but not tight and that primary dressing or splint is positioned correctly. A tight bandage may cause numbness and tingling from impaired circulation and/or pressure on peripheral nerves.*

---

   (3) Unroll and very slightly stretch bandage.

   Maintains bandage tension.

   (4) Overlap turns by one-half to two-thirds width of bandage roll.

   Prevents uneven bandage tension and circulatory impairment.

   (5) Secure bandage with clip before applying additional rolls.

   (6) End bandage with two circular turns; secure end of gauze or elastic bandage to outside layer of bandage, not skin, with tape or clips (see illustration).

CLINICAL JUDGMENT: *Keep toes or fingertips uncovered and visible for follow-up circulatory assessment, except in cases in which toes or fingers are treated because of wounds.*

---

3. Apply elastic bandage over amputated stump (see illustrations):

   a. Elevate stump with pillow or support it with the help of another person.

   Elevation promotes venous return. Bandage turns are designed for uniform bandage tension.

   b. Secure bandage by wrapping it twice around proximal end of stump or person's waist (depending on size of stump)

   c. Make half turn with bandage perpendicular to its edge.

   d. Bring body of bandage over distal end of stump.

   e. Continue to fold bandage over stump, wrapping from distal to proximal points.

   f. Secure with metal clips, Velcro if provided, or tape.

STEP 2d(1) Apply bandage from distal to proximal.

STEP 2d(6) Secure with tape or closure device.

Continued

SKILL 48.6	APPLYING ROLL GAUZE OR ELASTIC BANDAGE—cont'd

STEPS	RATIONALE

STEP 3 *Top,* Correct method for bandaging midthigh amputation stump. Note that bandage must be anchored around patient's waist. *Bottom,* Correct method for bandaging midcalf amputation stump. Note that bandage need not be anchored around waist. (From Monahan F, et al: *Phipps' medical-surgical nursing: health and illness perspectives,* ed 8, St Louis, 2006, Mosby.)

4. Remove and dispose of gloves if worn and perform hand hygiene.	Reduces transmission of microorganisms.
5. Help patient to comfortable position.	Restores comfort and sense of well-being.
6. Raise side rails (as appropriate) and lower bed to lowest position.	Promotes safety and prevents falls.
7. Place nurse call system in an accessible location within patient's reach.	Ensures patient can call for assistance if needed and promotes safety and prevents falls.

EVALUATION

1. Assess degree of tightness of bandage and presence of wrinkles, looseness, and drainage.	Identifies any pressure areas that may cause tissue injury.
2. When bandage application is complete, at least twice during next 8 hours, and then at least every shift assess distal extremity circulation.	Early detection of circulatory impairment promotes neurovascular functioning.
a. Observe skin color for pallor or cyanosis and palpate skin for warmth.	Pallor and cyanosis and cool skin as compared to other extremity indicate diminished blood flow.
b. Palpate distal pulses and compare bilaterally.	Documents status of circulatory flow.
c. Ask patient to rate any pain on scale of 0 to 10 and to describe any numbness, tingling, or other discomfort to evaluate for neurological and vascular changes.	Signs of neurovascular changes that indicate impaired venous return.
3. Observe mobility of extremity.	Determines whether bandage is too tight, which restricts movement, or if joint immobilization is attained.
4. Use Teach-Back: "I want to be sure I explained how to apply the elastic roll to your sprained ankle. Show me how you would apply this elastic roll to your ankle." Revise your instruction now or develop a plan for revised patient/family caregiver teaching if patient/family caregiver is not able to teach back correctly.	Teach-back is an evidence-based health literacy intervention that promotes patient engagement, patient safety, adherence, and quality. The goal of teach-back is to ensure that you have explained medical information clearly so that patients and their families understand what you communicated to them (AHRQ, 2020).

UNEXPECTED OUTCOMES AND RELATED INTERVENTIONS

1. Patient complains of pain or numbness in extremity.
- Assess circulation distal to elastic bandage.
- Release bandage.
- Palpate extremity and assess pulse, temperature, and capillary refill. **NOTE**: If abnormal, notify health care provider.
- Reapply bandage with less pressure.
- If complaints continue, notify health care provider.

RECORDING AND REPORTING

- Record patient's level of comfort, circulation status, type of bandage applied, presence of swelling, and range of motion at baseline and after bandage application on flow sheet in nurses' notes in electronic health record (EHR) or chart.
- Document your evaluation of patient learning.
- Report any changes in neurological or circulatory status to health care provider.

HOME CARE CONSIDERATIONS

- Demonstrate to patient or family caregiver how to correctly apply bandage so that it is not too tight.
- Instruct patient or family caregiver about the signs of impaired circulation.
- Elastic bandages that reduce swelling are best applied to the feet and ankles in the morning, before getting out of bed.
- Instruct patient and family caregiver to remove an elastic bandage daily and inspect skin beneath it twice daily.

■ KEY POINTS

- To plan interventions to reduce or eliminate risk factors and prevent pressure injury formation, it is important to understand and examine how risk factors contribute to pressure injury formation in at-risk patients,.
- Pressure injury Stages 1 through 4 describe the depth of tissue injury, which will guide treatment.
- Acute wounds are usually traumatic or surgical and should move predictably through the normal wound-healing process.
- Chronic wounds are caused by vascular compromise, reinjury, or chronic inflammation and fail to close or heal in a timely fashion.
- In primary intention wound healing, the skin edges are approximated, or closed, and the risk of infection is low. Healing occurs quickly, with minimal scar formation, if infection and secondary breakdown are prevented.
- In secondary intention wound healing, the wound is left open until it becomes filled by scar tissue. It takes longer for a wound to heal by secondary intention; therefore the chance of infection is greater. If scarring from secondary intention is severe, loss of tissue function is often permanent.
- Clinical judgment is important when assessing for and planning interventions for patients with impaired skin integrity and wound care.
- Assessment of the patient with a wound will include the systemic and local complications that affect wound healing and must be addressed with the appropriate interventions that address those complications.
- Use valid and reliable risk assessment tools to assess a patient's risk for developing a pressure injury; these are completed on admission to a health care agency and on a regularly scheduled basis.
- Factors that promote wound healing include adequate protein and nutritional intake, normal circulation, clean dry periwound skin, adequate hydration, and normal hemoglobin.
- Factors that impede wound healing include poor tissue perfusion as with hypovolemic shock, poor circulation as in peripheral vascular disease or diabetes mellitus, incontinence, immunosuppression, and preexisting infection.
- A wound assessment provides the foundation for developing a care plan, revealing data that aid in identification of nursing diagnoses and the selection of wound therapies best targeted for the condition of the patient's wound.
- Exposure to heat and cold causes normal systemic and local responses but can also cause injury to the skin if applied too long or incorrectly.
- An elastic bandage applied too tightly can result in circulatory impairment.

■ REFLECTIVE LEARNING

The case study integrated throughout this chapter focuses on Mrs. Stein's postoperative course for a repair of a fractured hip. Summary assessment data indicate that she is reluctant to move, and she rates her incisional hip pain as an 8 on a 10-point scale; however, following analgesia she rates her pain at 3 or 4. She is reluctant to reposition in bed, transfer to a chair, or participate in physical therapy and as a result her postoperative rehabilitation is moving slowly. Mrs. Stein is unable to assist in using a bedpan and refuses to use a bedside commode and has episodes of incontinence. **Skin assessment** *reveals that the previously reddened, blistered area on Mrs. Stein's right hip is now 2.5 cm (1 inch) in diameter. The area is not draining, but the underlying skin is not intact; this is a Stage 2 pressure injury. There is also nonblanchable erythema in the periwound area about 2.5 cm (1 inch) around the wound. On palpation the nurse, Kelly, notes that the periwound underlying tissue has nonblanchable erythema. These findings indicate structural damage to the capillary bed and microcirculation and support the diagnosis that a Stage 2 pressure injury is present.* **Wound assessment** *reveals wound serous drainage and small openings between staples. The periwound area is warm and tender to palpation.*

- What assessment information in Mrs. Stein's case study is of immediate concern to identify additional risk factors for impaired skin integrity? (Recognize Cues)
- Considering Mrs. Stein's postoperative care, what environmental factors might affect her skin integrity? (Analyze Cues)
- Reviewing the assessment data and postoperative progression, what would be additional priority nursing diagnoses **that are not** in the care plan for Mrs. Stein? (Prioritize Diagnoses)
- If Mrs. Stein's right hip pressure injury does not heal or the sacral redness progresses to a Stage 1 pressure injury, identify two expected outcomes and describe appropriate nursing interventions and appropriate resources to achieve the expected outcomes. (Generate Solutions)
- A wound care specialist assessed Mrs. Stein's wound and recommended NPWT. What nursing interventions would have priority to prevent an MDRPI? (Take Action)
- Evaluate the plan of care; what criteria support achievement of expected outcomes or support revision of treatment and the nursing care plan? (Evaluate Outcomes)

■ REVIEW QUESTIONS

1. When repositioning an immobile patient, the nurse notices redness over the hip bone. What is indicated when a reddened area blanches on fingertip touch?
   1. A local skin infection requiring antibiotics
   2. Sensitive skin that requires special bed linen
   3. A Stage 3 pressure injury needing the appropriate dressing
   4. Blanching hyperemia, indicating the attempt by the body to overcome the ischemic episode

2. Match the pressure injury stages with the correct definition.

____ 1. Stage 1
____ 2. Stage 2
____ 3. Stage 3
____ 4. Stage 4
____ 5. Unstageable pressure injury

a. Partial-thickness loss of skin with exposed dermis. The wound bed is viable, pink or red, and moist, and may also present as an intact or ruptured serum-filled blister. Adipose tissue (fat) and deeper tissues are not visible. Granulation tissue, slough, and eschar are not present. These injuries commonly result from adverse microclimate and shear in the skin over the pelvis and shear in the heel. This stage should not be used to describe moisture-associated skin damage (MASD), including incontinence-associated dermatitis (IAD), intertriginous dermatitis (ITD), medical adhesive–related skin injury (MARSI), or traumatic wounds (skin tears, burns, abrasions).

b. Intact skin with a localized area of non-blanchable erythema, which may appear differently in darkly pigmented skin. Presence of blanchable erythema or changes in sensation, temperature, or firmness may precede visual changes. Color changes do not include purple or maroon discoloration; these may indicate deep-tissue pressure injury.

c. Full-thickness skin and tissue loss with exposed or directly palpable fascia, muscle, tendon, ligament, cartilage, or bone in the ulcer. Slough and/or eschar may be visible. Epibole (rolled edges), undermining, and/or tunneling often occurs. Depth varies by anatomical location. If slough or eschar obscures the extent of tissue loss, this is an Unstageable pressure injury.

d. Full-thickness loss of skin, in which adipose tissue (fat) is visible in the ulcer, and granulation tissue and epibole (rolled wound edges) are often present. Slough and/or eschar may be visible. The depth of tissue damage varies by anatomical location; areas of significant adiposity can develop deep wounds. Undermining and tunneling may occur. Fascia, muscle, tendon, ligament, cartilage, and bone are not exposed. If slough or eschar obscures the extent of tissue loss, this is an unstageable pressure injury.

e. Full-thickness skin and tissue loss in which the extent of tissue damage within the injury cannot be confirmed because it is obscured by slough or eschar. If slough or eschar is removed, a Stage 3 or Stage 4 pressure injury will be revealed. Stable eschar (i.e., dry, adherent, intact, without erythema or fluctuance) on the heel or ischemic limb should not be softened or removed.

3. After surgery the patient with a closed abdominal wound reports a sudden "pop" after coughing. When the nurse examines the surgical wound site, the sutures are open, and small bowel sections are observed at the bottom of the now-opened wound. Which are the priority nursing interventions? (Select all that apply.)
   1. Notify the health care provider.
   2. Allow the area to be exposed to air until all drainage has stopped.
   3. Place several cold packs over the area, protecting the skin around the wound.
   4. Cover the area with sterile, saline-soaked towels immediately.
   5. Cover the area with sterile gauze and apply an abdominal binder.

4. Place the steps when performing wound irrigation of a large open wound in the correct sequence.
   1. Use slow, continuous pressure to irrigate wound.
   2. Attach 19-gauge angiocatheter to syringe.
   3. Fill syringe with irrigation fluid.
   4. Place biohazard bag near bed.
   5. Position angiocatheter over wound.

5. Which skin-care measures are used to manage a patient who is experiencing fecal and/or urinary incontinence? (Select all that apply.)
   1. Frequent position changes
   2. Keeping the buttocks exposed to air at all times
   3. Using a large absorbent diaper, changing when saturated
   4. Using an incontinence cleaner
   5. Applying a moisture barrier ointment

6. Which of the following are measures to reduce tissue damage from shear? (Select all that apply.)
   1. Use a transfer device (e.g., transfer board).
   2. Have head of bed elevated when transferring patient.
   3. Have head of bed flat when repositioning patient.
   4. Raise head of bed 60 degrees when patient is positioned supine.
   5. Raise head of bed 30 degrees when patient is positioned supine.

7. Which of the following is an indication for a binder to be placed around a surgical patient with a new abdominal wound? (Select all that apply.)
   1. Collection of wound drainage
   2. Provision of support to abdominal tissues when coughing or walking
   3. Reduction of abdominal swelling
   4. Reduction of stress on the abdominal incision
   5. Stimulation of peristalsis (return of bowel function) from direct pressure

8. Medical adhesives, such as tape securing a wound dressing, cause MARSI. Which of the following interventions reduce the risk for MARSI?
   1. Gently loosen the ends of the tape and gently pull the outer end parallel with the skin surface toward the wound.
   2. Change dressing only when saturated.
   3. Apply adhesive remover.
   4. Use Montgomery ties to secure the dressing.
   5. Immobilize area of wound.

9. What is the removal of devitalized tissue from a wound called?
   1. Debridement
   2. Pressure distribution
   3. Negative-pressure wound therapy
   4. Sanitization

10. Which of the following nursing activities apply to an MDRPI? (Select all that apply.)
    1. Assess skin under devices every 2 hours.
    2. Cushion at risk areas (e.g., ears, nose with foam or protective dressing).

3. Choose correct size of device.
4. Observe for erythema or irritation that conforms to pattern or shape of device.
5. Observe under casts and splints.

Rationales for Review Questions can be found on the Evolve website.

REFERENCES

Agency for Healthcare Research and Quality (AHRQ): *Teach-Back: Intervention. Quick Start Guide Full Page*, Rockville, MD, 2020, Agency for Healthcare Research and Quality. https://www.ahrq.gov/health-literacy/quality-resources/tools/literacy-toolkit/healthlittoolkit2-tool5.html. Accessed August 2020.

Ayello EA, et al: Pressure ulcers. In Baranoski S, Ayello AE, editors: *Wound care essentials: practice principles*, ed 4, Philadelphia, 2016, Lippincott Williams & Wilkins.

Ayello EA: CMS MDS 3.0 Section M skin conditions in long-term care: pressure ulcers, skin tears, and moisture-associated skin damage data update, *Adv Skin Wound Care* 30(9):415, 2017.

Baranoski S, et al: Wound assessment. In Baranoski S, Ayello AE, editors: *Wound care essentials: practice principles*, ed 4, Philadelphia, 2016, Lippincott Williams & Wilkins.

Bates-Jensen BM: Assessment of the patient with a wound. In *Core curriculum: wound management*, Philadelphia, 2016, Wolters Kluwer.

Berlowitz D: *Epidemiology, pathogenesis, and risk assessment of pressure-induced skin and soft tissue injury*, 2020, UpToDate. https://uptodate.com/contents/epidemiology-pathogenesis-and-risk-assessment-of-pressure-induced-skin-and-soft-tissue-injury. Accessed September 2021.

Black J, et al: Use of wound dressings to enhance prevention of pressure ulcers caused by medical devices, *Int Wound J* 12:322, 2015.

Bryant RA: Types of skin damage and differential diagnosis. In Bryant RA, Nix DP, editors: *Acute and chronic wounds: current management concepts*, ed 5, St. Louis, 2016, Elsevier.

Bryant RA, Nix DP: Developing and maintaining a pressure ulcer prevention program. In Bryant RA, Nix DP, editors: *Acute and chronic wounds: current management concepts*, ed 5, St. Louis, 2016a, Elsevier.

Bryant RA, Nix DP: Principles of wound healing and topical management. In Bryant RA, Nix DP, editors: *Acute and chronic wounds: current management concepts*, ed 5, St. Louis, 2016b, Elsevier.

Burden M, Thornton M: Reducing the risks of surgical site infection: the importance of the multidisciplinary team, *Br J Nurs* 27(17):976, 2018.

Calis H, et al: Non-healing wounds: can it take different diagnosis? *Int Wound J* 17:443, 2019.

Centers for Disease Control and Prevention (CDC): *Healthcare-associated infections: current HAI progress report - 2019 National and State Healthcare-Associated Infections Progress Report*, 2020. https://www.cdc.gov/hai/data/portal/progress-report.html. Accessed September 2021.

Centers for Disease Control and Prevention: *What is health literacy?* 2021. https://www.cdc.gov/healthliteracy/learn/index.html. Accessed September 2021.

Centers for Medicare and Medicaid Services (CMS): *Hospital-acquired conditions*, 2020. https://www.cms.gov/Medicare/Medicare-Fee-for-Service-Payment/HospitalAcqCond/Hospital-Acquired_Conditions. Accessed September 2021.

Camacho-Del Rio, G: Evidence-based practice: medical device–related pressure injury prevention, *Am Nurse Today* 13(10):50, 2018.

Chatterjee R: Elbow pain: the 10-minute assessment, *Co-Kinetic J* 73:18, 2017.

Chou R, et al: Management of postoperative pain: a clinical practice guideline from the American Pain Society, the American Society of Regional Anesthesia and Pain Medicine, and the American Society of Anesthesiologists' Committee on Regional Anesthesia, Executive Committee, and Administrative Council, *J Pain* 17(2):131, 2016.

Cleveland Clinic: *Nutrition guidelines to improve wound healing*, 2017. https://my.clevelandclinic.org/health/articles/11111-nutrition-guidelines-to-improve-wound-healing. Accessed September 2021.

Collier M: Protecting vulnerable skin from moisture-associated skin damage, *Br J Nurs* 25(20):S26, 2016.

Darouiche R: *Hospital infection control: surgical site infections*, 2017, Infectious Disease Advisor. https://www.infectiousdiseaseadvisor.com/home/decision-support-in-medicine/hospital-infection-control/surgical-site-infections/. Accessed September 2021.

Doughty D, McNichol L: *Wound, Ostomy, and Continence Nurses Society (WOCN) core curriculum: wound management*, Philadelphia, 2016, Wound, Ostomy, and Continence Nurses Society.

Doughty DB, Sparks B: Wound-healing physiology and factors that affect the repair process. In Bryant RA, Nix DP, editors: *Acute and chronic wounds: current management concepts*, ed 6, St. Louis, 2016, Elsevier.

Edsberg LE, et al: Revised National Pressure Ulcer Advisory Panel pressure injury staging system, *J Wound Ostomy Continence Nurs* 43(6):585, 2016.

European Pressure Ulcer Advisory Panel (EPUAP), National Pressure injury Advisory Panel (NPIAP), and Pan Pacific Pressure Injury Alliance (PPPIA): *Treatment of pressure ulcers/injuries: Clinical Practice Guideline*. The International Guideline, Emily Haesler (ed.), 2019a, EPUAP/NPIAP/PPPIA.

European Pressure Ulcer Advisory Panel (EPUAP), National Pressure injury Advisory Panel (NPIAP), and Pan Pacific Pressure Injury Alliance (PPPIA): *Treatment of pressure ulcers/injuries: Quick Reference Guide*, Emily Haesler (ed.), 2019b, EPUAP/NPIAP/PPPIA.

Ferris A, Harding K: Wound healing in frail elderly patients, *Wounds UK* 15(2):16, 2019.

Francis K: Damage control: differentiating incontinence-associated dermatitis from pressure injury, *Nursing2019 Critical Care*, 14(6):28, 2020.

Gallagher S: Skin care needs of obese patient. In Bryant RA, Nix DP, editors: *Acute and chronic wounds: current management concepts*, ed 5, St. Louis, 2016, Mosby.

Gruccio P, Ashton K: Support surface technology: an essential component of pressure injury prevention, *J Leg Nurse Consult* 29(1):30, 2018.

Haesler E: Evidence summary: pressure injuries: preventing medical device related pressure injuries, *Wound Pract Res* 25(4):214, 2017.

Hopf H, et al: Managing wound pain. In Bryant RA, Nix DP, editors: *Acute and chronic wounds: current management concepts*, ed 5, St. Louis, 2016, Elsevier.

Huether SE, et al: *Understanding pathophysiology*, ed 7, St. Louis, 2020, Elsevier

Jackson D, et al: Medical device-related pressure ulcers: a systematic review and meta-analysis, *Int J Nurs Stud* 92:109, 2019.

Jaszarowski KA, Murphree RW: Wound cleansing and dressing selection. In *Wound, Ostomy, and Continence Nurses Society, core curriculum: wound management*, Philadelphia, 2016, Wolters Kluwer.

Johns Hopkins Medicine: *Surgical site infections*, 2021. https://www.hopkinsmedicine.org/health/conditions-and-diseases/surgical-site-infections. Accessed September 2021.

Kelly-O'Flynn, et al: Medical adhesive–related skin injury, *Br J Nurs* 29(6):S20 (Stoma Care Supplement), 2020.

Krasner DL: Wound pain: impact and assessment. In Bryant RA, Nix DP, editors: *Acute and chronic wounds: nursing management*, ed 5, St. Louis, 2016, Elsevier.

Maklebust J, Magnan MA: Pressure ulcer prevention: specific measures and agency-wide strategies. In Doughty DB, McNichol LL, editors: *Core curriculum wound management*, Philadelphia, 2016, Wolters Kluwer.

Meiner SE, Yeager JJ: *Gerontologic nursing*, ed 6, St. Louis, 2019, Elsevier.

McNichol L, et al: Medical adhesives and patient safety: state of the science: consensus statements for the assessment, prevention, and treatment of adhesive-related skin injuries, *J Wound Ostomy Continence Nurs* 40(4):365, 2013.

Mizell J, et al: *Complications of abdominal surgical incisions*, 2020, UpToDate. https://www.uptodate.com/contents/complications-of-abdominal-surgical-incisions#!. Accessed September 2021.

Morgan N: *Support surfaces*, 2020, Wound Care Advisor. https://woundcareadvisor.com/support-surfaces/. Accessed September 2021.

National Health Service (United Kingdom): *How do I care for a wound treated with skin glue?* 2021. https://www.nhs.uk/common-health-questions/accidents-first-aid-and-treatments/how-do-i-care-for-a-wound-treated-with-skin-glue/. Accessed September 2021.

National Pressure Ulcer Advisory Panel (NPUAP): Hand check method: is it an effective method to monitor for bottoming out? A National Pressure Ulcer Advisory Panel Position Statement, 2015. https://cdn.ymaws.com/npuap.site-ym.com/resource/resmgr/position_statements/hand-check-position-statemen.pdf. Accessed September 2021.

Netsch DS: Refractory wounds. In *Wound, Ostomy, and Continence Nurses Society, core curriculum: wound management*, Philadelphia, 2016, Wolters Kluwer.

Netsch DS, et al: Negative-pressure wound therapy. In Bryant RA, Nix DP, editors: *Acute and chronic wounds: current management concepts*, ed 5, St. Louis, 2016, Elsevier.

Nix D: Skin and wound inspection and assessment. In Bryant RA, Nix DP, editors: *Acute and chronic wounds: current management concepts*, ed 5, St. Louis, 2016, Elsevier.

Padula CA, et al: Prevention of medical device-related pressure injuries associated with respiratory equipment use in a critical care unit, *J Wound Ostomy Continence Nurs* 44(2):138, 2017.

Pagana KD, et al: *Mosby's diagnostic & laboratory test reference*, ed 15, St. Louis, 2021, Elsevier.

Pieper B: Pressure ulcers: impact, etiology, and classification. In Bryant RA, Nix DP, editors: *Acute and chronic wounds: current management concepts*, ed 5, St. Louis, 2016, Elsevier.

Pittman J, et al: Medical device–related hospital-acquired pressure ulcers, *J Wound Ostomy Continence Nurs* 42(2):151, 2015.

Ramundo JM: Wound debridement. In Bryant RA, Nix DP, editors: *Acute and chronic wounds: current management concepts*, ed 5, St. Louis, 2016, Elsevier.

Rolstad BS, et al: Topical management. In Bryant RA, Nix DP, editors: *Acute and chronic wounds: current management concepts*, ed 5, St. Louis, 2016, Mosby.

Stotts NA: Nutritional assessment and support. In Bryant RA, Nix DP, editors: *Acute and chronic wounds: current management concepts*, ed 5, St. Louis, 2016a, Elsevier.

Stotts NA: Wound infection: diagnosis and management. In Bryant RA, Nix DP, editors: *Acute and chronic wounds: current management concepts*, ed 5, St. Louis, 2016b, Elsevier.

Stryja J: Ten top tips: prevention of surgical site infections, *Wounds Int* 9(2):16, 2018.

The Joint Commission (TJC): *Nutritional and functional screening-requirement,* 2020. https://www.jointcommission.org/en/standards/standard-faqs/critical-access-hospital/provision-of-care-treatment-and-services-pc/000001652/. Accessed September 2021.

The Joint Commission (TJC): *2021 National patient safety goals*, Oakbrook Terrace, IL, 2021, The Commission.

https://www.jointcommission.org/en/standards/national-patient-safety-goals/. Accessed September 2021.

US National Library of Medicine: *Preventing pressure ulcers*, 2020. https://medlineplus.gov/ency/patient instructions/000147.htm. Accessed September 2021.

Wound, Ostomy, and Continence Nurses Society (WOCN): *Guideline for prevention and management of pressure ulcers (injuries), WOCN clinical practice guideline series*, Mount Laurel, NJ, 2016, The Society.

Wysocki AB: Wound-healing physiology. In Bryant RA, Nix DP, editors: *Acute and chronic wounds: current management concepts*, ed 5, St. Louis, 2016, Elsevier.

RESEARCH REFERENCES

Alderden J, et al: Midrange Braden subscale scores are associated with increased risk for pressure injury development among critical care patients, *J Wound Ostomy Continence Nurs* 44(5):420, 2017.

Allegranzi B, et al. New WHO recommendations on intraoperative and postoperative measures for surgical site infection prevention: an evidence based global perspective, *Lancet* (16), e288, 2016.

Arici A, et al: The effect of using an abdominal binder on postoperative gastrointestinal function, mobilization, pulmonary function, and pain in patients undergoing major abdominal surgery: a randomized controlled trial, *Int J Nurs Stud* 62:108, 2016.

Baath C, et al: Prevention of heel pressure ulcers among older patients—from ambulance care to hospital discharge: a multi-centre randomized controlled trial, *Appl Nurs Res* 30:170, 2015.

Bates Jensen BM, et al: Reliability of the Bates-Jensen wound assessment tool for pressure injury assessment: the pressure ulcer detection study, *Wound Repair Regen* 27(4):386–395, 2019.

Black J, Kalowes P: Medical device–related pressure ulcers, *Chronic Wound Care Manag Res* 3:91, 2016.

Braden BJ, Bergstrom N: Clinical utility of the Braden Scale for predicting pressure sore risk, *Decubitus* 2(3):50, 1989.

Braden BJ, Bergstrom N: Predictive validity of the Braden Scale for pressure sore risk in a nursing home population, *Res Nurs Health* 17(6):459, 1994.

Bulfone G, et al: Perioperative pressure injuries: a systematic literature review, *Adv Skin Wound Care* 31(12):556–564, 2018

Burton AC, Yamada S: Relation between blood pressure and flow in the human forearm, *J Appl Physiol* 4(5):329, 1951.

Chaboyer W, et al: Adherence to evidence-based pressure injury prevention guidelines in routine clinical practice: a longitudinal study, *Int Wound J* 14(6):1290, 2017.

Cooper KD, et al: Prevention and treatment of device-related hospital-acquired pressure injuries, *Am J Crit Care*, 29(2):150, 2020.

Cox J, et al: Identifying risk factors for pressure injury in adult critical care patients, *Am J Crit Care*, 29(3):204, 2020.

da Silva Galetto et al: Medical device-related pressure injuries: an integrative literature review, *Rev Bras Enferm* 72(2):505, 2019.

Durrant LA, et al: Health literacy in pressure injury: findings from a mixed methods study of community-based patients and carers, *Nurs Health Sci* 21(1):37, 2019.

Fernandez L, et al: Use of negative pressure wound therapy with instillation in the management of complex wounds in critically ill patients, *Wounds* 31(1):E1, 2019.

Fumarola S: International consensus document: Overlooked and underestimated medical adhesive–related skin injuries, *J Wound Care*, 29(Suppl 3c):S1, 2020.

Giller CM, et al: A randomized controlled trial of abdominal binders for the management of postoperative pain and distress after cesarean delivery, *Int J Gynaecol Obstet* 133(2):188, 2016.

Han Y, et al: Usefulness of the Braden Scale in intensive care units: a study based on electronic health record data, *J Nurs Care Qual* 33(3):238, 2018.

Jackson D, et al: Medical device–related pressure ulcers: a systematic review and meta-analysis, *Int J Nurs Stud*, 92:109, 2019.

Kayser SA, et al: Prevalence and analysis of medical device-related pressure injuries: results from the international pressure prevalence survey, *Adv Skin Wound Care* 31(6):276, 2018.

Kelechi TJ, et al: Does cryotherapy improve circulation compared with compression and elevation in preventing venous leg ulcers, *Int Wound J* 14(4):641, 2017.

Machin M, et al: Systematic review of the use of cyanoacrylate glue in addition to standard wound closure in the prevention of surgical site infection, *Int Wound J*, 16:387, 2019.

Martin D, et al: Healthy skin wins: a glowing pressure ulcer prevention program that can guide evidence-based practice, *Worldviews Evid Based Nurs* 14(6):473, 2017.

Matiasek J, et al: Negative pressure wound therapy with instillation: effects on healing of category 4 pressure ulcers, *Plast Aesthet Res* 5(9):36, 2018. https://doi.org/10.20517/2347-9264.2018.50.

McNichol LL, et al: Incontinence-associated dermatitis: state of the science and knowledge translation, *Adv Skin Wound Care* 31(11):502, 2018.

Panayi AC, Leavitt T, Orgill DP: Evidence based review of negative pressure wound therapy, *World J Dermatol*, 6(1):1, 2017. https://doi.org/10.5314/wjd.v6.i1.1.

Petrofsky J, et al: Use of low level of continuous heat as an adjunct to physical therapy improves knee pain recovery and the compliance for home exercise in patients with chronic knee pain: a randomized controlled trial, *J Strength Cond Res* 30(11):3107, 2016.

Petrofsky J, et al: The efficacy of sustained heat treatment on delayed-onset muscle soreness, *Clin J Sport Med* 27(4):329, 2017.

Quinlan P, et al: Effects of localized cold therapy on pain in postoperative spinal fusion patients: a randomized control trial, *Orthop Nurs* 36(5):344, 2017.

Schallom M, et al: Pressure ulcer incidence in patients wearing nasal-oral versus full-face noninvasive ventilation masks, *Am J Crit Care* 24(4):349, 2015.

Szekeres M, et al: The short-term effects of hot packs vs therapeutic whirlpool on active wrist range of motion for patients with distal radius fracture: a randomized controlled trial, *J Hand Ther*. Published online September 8, 2017.

Zhang L, et al: A systematic review and meta-analysis of clinical effectiveness and safety of hydrogel dressings in the management of skin wounds, *Front Bioeng Biotechnol* 7:342, 2019.

Sensory Alterations

OBJECTIVES

- Differentiate among the processes of reception, perception, and reaction to sensory stimuli.
- Compare and contrast sensory deficits, sensory deprivation, and sensory overload.
- Explain factors that influence sensory function.
- Determine how altered sensory function affects an individual's level of wellness.
- Discuss the components that make up assessment of the sensory system.
- Discuss process of clinical judgment and critical thinking in assessment of patients with signs and symptoms of sensory alterations.
- Explain how clinical judgment enables you to identify appropriate nursing diagnoses and collaborative problems in patients with alterations in sensation.
- Prioritize nursing diagnoses and outcomes relevant to patients with sensory alterations.
- Discuss health promotion strategies for normal sensory function.
- Use clinical judgment to plan and implement nursing interventions for patients with sensory deficits, sensory deprivation, and sensory overload.
- Recommend strategies to maintain a safe environment for patients with altered sensation.
- Evaluate a patient's response to interventions that address alterations in sensation.

KEY TERMS

Aphasia
Audiologist
Auditory
Conductive hearing loss
Expressive aphasia
Global aphasia
Gustatory
Hyperesthesia

Kinesthetic
Olfactory
Otolaryngologist
Ototoxic
Proprioceptive
Receptive aphasia
Refractive error
Sensory deficit

Sensory deprivation
Sensory overload
Stereognosis
Strabismus
Tactile
Visual

MEDIA RESOURCES

http://evolve.elsevier.com/Potter/fundamentals/
- Review Questions
- Audio Glossary
- Case Study with Questions

- Concept Map Creator
- Content Updates
- Answers to QSEN Activity and Review Questions

Ms. Long is a 70-year-old retired widow who lives in a one-level home with her daughter, Vivian, and son, Antonio. Their home has a walkout basement. Ms. Long enjoys reading and sewing, but she is experiencing reduced vision in her left eye because of a cataract that has not been surgically corrected. Her impaired vision affects her ability to participate in these activities. She is also fearful of falling and visited an ophthalmologist a year ago.

Dilyana is a nursing student who is in her last year of nursing school. She is doing a community health rotation and is assigned to see Ms. Long in the community clinic. Dilyana's grandmother, whom she helps care for at home, recently had cataract surgery in both eyes. Dilyana will draw on her knowledge of sensory alterations along with her personal experiences with her grandmother to better understand the effects of the visual disturbances on Ms. Long and develop an individualized, safe, and effective plan of care.

Imagine the world without sight, hearing, the ability to feel objects, or the ability to sense aromas around you. People rely on a variety of sensory stimuli to give meaning and order to events occurring in their environment. The senses form the perceptual base of our world. Stimulation comes from many sources in and outside the body, particularly through the senses of sight (**visual**), hearing (**auditory**), touch (**tactile**), smell (**olfactory**), and taste (**gustatory**). The body also has a **kinesthetic** sense that enables a person to be aware of the position and movement of body parts without seeing them. **Stereognosis** is a sense that allows a person to recognize the size, shape, and texture of an object. Although the ability to speak is not a sense, it is similar because sometimes patients lose the ability to interact meaningfully with other human beings. Meaningful stimuli allow a person to learn about the environment and are necessary for healthy functioning and normal development. When sensory function is altered, you need to use clinical judgment to understand if a person is able to relate to and safely function within the environment.

Many patients seeking health care have preexisting sensory alterations. Others develop them because of medical treatment (e.g., hearing loss from antibiotic use or hearing or visual loss from brain tumor removal) or hospitalization. In addition, consider that there are many factors in the health care environment that possibly affect your patients. Many health care environments have unfamiliar sights, sounds, and smells. Some patients have minimal contact with family and friends, especially when they are admitted to an acute care or long-term care setting. When patients feel depersonalized and are unable to receive meaningful stimuli, serious sensory alterations sometimes develop.

As a nurse you use clinical judgment and critical thinking to identify and meet the needs of patients with existing or potential sensory alterations. You will recognize cues from your patients' assessment data to identify those at risk for developing sensory problems. Consider characteristics of a patient's environment, adapt therapies based on a patient's sensory alterations, and involve family caregivers. An individualized plan of care helps patients with partial or complete loss of a major sense to function safely within their environment.

SCIENTIFIC KNOWLEDGE BASE

Normal Sensation

The nervous system continually receives thousands of stimuli from sensory nerve organs, relays the information through appropriate neurological channels, and integrates the information into a meaningful response. Sensory stimuli reach the sensory organs to elicit an immediate reaction or store information in the brain for future use. The nervous system must be intact for sensory stimuli to reach appropriate brain centers and for an individual to perceive the sensation. After interpreting the significance of a sensation, the person is then able to react to the stimulus. Table 49.1 summarizes normal hearing and vision.

Reception, perception, and reaction are the three components of any sensory experience. Reception begins with stimulation of a nerve cell called a *receptor*, which is usually for only one type of stimulus such as light, touch, taste, or sound. In the case of special senses, the receptors are grouped close together or located in specialized organs such as the taste buds of the tongue or the retina of the eye. When a nerve impulse is created, it travels along pathways to the spinal cord or directly to the brain. For example, sound waves stimulate hair cell receptors within the organ of Corti in the ear, which causes impulses to travel along the eighth cranial nerve to the acoustic area of the temporal lobe. Sensory nerve pathways usually cross over to send stimuli to opposite sides of the brain.

The actual perception or awareness of unique sensations depends on the receiving region of the cerebral cortex, where specialized neurons interpret the quality and nature of sensory stimuli. When a person becomes conscious of a stimulus and receives the information, perception takes place. Perception includes integration and interpretation of stimuli based on a person's experiences. A person's level of consciousness influences perception and interpretation of stimuli. Any factors that lower consciousness impair sensory perception. If sensation is incomplete, such as blurred vision, or if past experience is inadequate for understanding stimuli such as pain, the person can react inappropriately to the sensory stimulus.

It is impossible to react to all stimuli entering the nervous system. The brain prevents sensory bombardment by discarding or storing sensory information. A person usually reacts to stimuli that are most meaningful or significant at the time. After continued reception of the same stimulus, a person stops responding, and the sensory experience goes unnoticed. For example, a person concentrating on reading a good book is not aware of background music. This adaptability phenomenon occurs with most sensory stimuli except for those of pain.

The balance between sensory stimuli entering the brain and those actually reaching a person's conscious awareness maintains a person's well-being. Sensory alterations occur when an individual attempts to react to every stimulus within the environment or if the variety and quality of stimuli are insufficient.

Sensory Alterations

The most common sensory alterations are sensory deficits, sensory deprivation, and sensory overload. A patient's ability to function and

TABLE 49.1	Normal Hearing and Vision
Function	**Anatomy and Physiology**
Ear	
Transmits to the brain a pattern of all sounds received from the environment, the relative intensity of these sounds, and the direction from which they originate	Two ears provide stereophonic hearing to judge sound direction.
	The external ear canal shelters the eardrum and maintains relatively constant temperature and humidity to maintain elasticity.
	The middle ear is an air-containing space between the eardrum and oval window. It contains three small bones (ossicles).
	The eardrum and ossicles transfer sound to the fluid-filled inner ear.
	Movement of the stapes in the oval window creates vibrations in the fluid that bathes the membranous labyrinth, which contains the end organs of hearing and balance.
	The union of the vestibular (balance) and cochlear (hearing) parts of the labyrinth explains the combination of hearing and balance symptoms that occur with inner ear disorders.
	Vibration of the eardrum transmits through the bony ossicles. Vibrations at the oval window transmit in perilymph within the inner ear to stimulate hair cells that send impulses along the eighth cranial nerve to the brain.
Eye	
Transmits to the brain a pattern of light that is reflected from solid objects in the environment and becomes transformed into color and hue	Light rays enter the convex cornea and begin to converge.
	An adjustment of light rays occurs as they pass through the pupil and lens.
	Change in the shape of the lens focuses light on the retina.
	The retina has a pigmented layer of cells to enhance visual acuity.
	The sensory retina contains the rods and cones (i.e., photoreceptor cells sensitive to stimulation from light).
	Photoreceptor cells send electrical potentials by way of the optic nerve to the brain.

BOX 49.1   Common Sensory Deficits

Visual Deficits

- *Presbyopia:* A gradual decline in the ability of the lens to accommodate or focus on close objects. Individual is unable to see near objects clearly.
- *Cataract:* Cloudy or opaque areas in part of the lens or the entire lens that interfere with passage of light through the lens, causing problems with glare and blurred vision. Cataracts usually develop gradually, without pain, redness, or tearing in the eye.
- *Computer vision syndrome or digital eyestrain:* Describes a group of eye and vision-related problems that result from prolonged computer, tablet, e-reader, and cell phone use. Most commonly causes eyestrain, headaches, blurred vision, and dry eyes.
- *Dry eyes:* Result when tear glands produce too few tears, resulting in itching, burning, or even reduced vision.
- *Glaucoma:* A slowly progressive increase in intraocular pressure that, if left untreated, causes progressive pressure against the optic nerve, resulting in peripheral visual loss, decreased visual acuity with difficulty adapting to darkness, and a halo effect around lights.
- *Diabetic retinopathy:* Pathological changes occur in the blood vessels of the retina, resulting in decreased vision or vision loss caused by hemorrhage and macular edema.
- *Macular degeneration:* Condition in which the macula (specialized part of the retina responsible for central vision) loses its ability to function efficiently. First signs include blurring of reading matter, distortion or loss of central vision, and distortion of vertical lines.

Hearing Deficits

- *Presbycusis:* A common progressive hearing disorder in older adults.
- *Cerumen accumulation:* Buildup of earwax in the external auditory canal. Cerumen becomes hard and collects in the canal and causes conduction deafness.

Balance Deficit

- *Dizziness and disequilibrium:* Common condition in older adulthood, usually resulting from vestibular dysfunction. Frequently a change in position of the head precipitates an episode of vertigo or disequilibrium.

Taste Deficit

- *Xerostomia:* Decrease in salivary production that leads to thicker mucus and a dry mouth. Often interferes with the ability to eat and leads to appetite and nutritional problems.

Neurological Deficits

- *Peripheral neuropathy:* Disorder of the peripheral nervous system, characterized by symptoms that include numbness and tingling of the affected area and stumbling gait.
- *Stroke:* Cerebrovascular accident caused by clot, hemorrhage, or emboli disrupting blood flow to the brain. Creates altered proprioception (body position) with marked incoordination and imbalance. Loss of sensation and motor function in extremities controlled by the affected area of the brain also occurs. A stroke affecting the left hemisphere of the brain results in symptoms on the right side, such as difficulty with speech. A stroke affecting the right hemisphere causes symptoms on the left side, which may include visual spatial alterations, such as loss of half of a visual field or inattention and neglect, especially to the left side.

relate effectively within the environment is seriously impaired when the patient has more than one sensory alteration.

Sensory Deficits. A deficit in the normal function of sensory reception and perception is a **sensory deficit**. When visual or hearing acuity change or decline, a person may withdraw by avoiding communication or socialization with others to cope with the sensory loss. It becomes difficult for the person to interact safely with the environment until new skills are learned. When a deficit develops gradually or when considerable time has passed since the onset of an acute sensory loss, a person learns to rely on unaffected senses. Some senses may even become more acute to compensate for an alteration. For example, a patient who is blind develops an acute sense of hearing to compensate for visual loss.

Patients with sensory deficits often change behavior in adaptive or maladaptive ways. For example, a patient with a hearing impairment turns the unaffected ear toward the speaker to hear better, whereas another patient avoids people because of embarrassment about not being able to understand what other people say. Box 49.1 summarizes common sensory deficits and their influence on those affected.

Sensory Deprivation. The reticular activating system in the brainstem mediates all sensory stimuli to the cerebral cortex; thus patients are able to receive stimuli even while sleeping deeply. Sensory stimulation must be of sufficient quality and quantity to maintain a person's awareness. Three types of **sensory deprivation** are reduced sensory input (sensory deficit from visual or hearing loss), the elimination of patterns or meaning from input (e.g., exposure to strange environments), and restrictive environments (e.g., bed rest) that produce monotony and boredom (Touhy and Jett, 2022).

There are many effects of sensory deprivation (Box 49.2). In adults the symptoms are similar to those of mental illness, confusion, severe

BOX 49.2   Effects of Sensory Deprivation

Cognitive

- Reduced capacity to learn
- Inability to think or problem solve
- Poor task performance
- Disorientation/confusion
- Bizarre thinking
- Increased need for socialization, altered mechanisms of attention

Affective

- Boredom
- Restlessness
- Increased anxiety
- Emotional lability

- Depression
- Panic
- Increased need for physical stimulation

Perceptual

- Changes in visual/motor coordination
- Reduced color perception
- Less tactile accuracy
- Changes in ability to perceive size and shape
- Changes in spatial and time judgment

electrolyte imbalance, or the influence of psychotropic drugs. Therefore always be aware of a patient's existing sensory function and the quality of stimuli within the environment.

Sensory Overload. When a person receives multiple sensory stimuli and cannot perceptually disregard or selectively ignore some stimuli, **sensory overload** occurs. Excessive sensory stimulation prevents the brain from responding appropriately to or ignoring certain stimuli. Because of the multitude of stimuli leading to overload, a person no longer perceives the environment in a way that makes sense. Overload prevents meaningful response by the brain. A patient's thoughts race, attention scatters in many directions, and anxiety and restlessness occur. As a result, overload causes a state similar to sensory deprivation. However, in contrast to deprivation, overload is individualized. The number of stimuli necessary for healthy function varies with each individual. People are often subject to environmental overload more at one time than another. A person's tolerance to sensory overload varies with level of fatigue, attitude, and emotional and physical well-being.

Patients who are acutely ill, especially those in a critical care unit (CCU), easily experience sensory overload. Patients who are in constant pain or require frequent monitoring of vital signs are also at risk. Multiple stimuli combine to cause overload even if you offer a comforting word or provide a gentle back rub. Some patients do not benefit from nursing intervention because their attention and energy are focused on stressful stimuli. In a CCU, where the activity is constant, the lights are frequently on. Patients can hear sounds from monitoring equipment, staff conversations, equipment alarms, and the activities of people entering the unit.

It is easy to confuse the behavioral changes associated with sensory overload with mood swings or simple disorientation. Look for symptoms such as racing thoughts, scattered attention, restlessness, and anxiety. Some patients constantly play with tubes and dressings. Constant reorientation and control of excessive stimuli become an important part of a patient's care.

REFLECT NOW

Compare and contrast the symptoms of patients who have sensory deprivation with those of patients who experience sensory overload. How might you intervene differently?

NURSING KNOWLEDGE BASE

Factors That Influence Sensory Function

Many factors influence the capacity to receive or perceive stimuli. You will consider the influence these conditions or factors have on patients' sensation when delivering patient care.

Age. Infants and children are at risk for visual and hearing impairment because of several genetic, prenatal, and postnatal conditions. Early intense visual and auditory stimulation can adversely affect visual and auditory pathways and alter the development of other sensory organs in high-risk neonates (Hockenberry et al., 2019). Visual changes during adulthood include presbyopia and the need for glasses for reading. These changes usually occur from ages 40 to 50. In addition, the cornea, which assists with light refraction to the retina, becomes flatter and thicker, which often leads to astigmatism. Pigment is lost from the iris, and collagen fibers build up in the anterior chamber, which increases the risk of glaucoma by decreasing the resorption of intraocular fluid. Other normal visual changes associated with aging include reduced visual fields, increased glare sensitivity, impaired night vision, reduced depth perception, and reduced color discrimination.

Hearing changes begin at the age of 30. Changes associated with aging include decreased hearing acuity, speech intelligibility, and pitch discrimination. Low-pitched sounds are easiest to hear, but it is difficult to hear conversation over background noise. It is also difficult to discriminate the consonants (z, t, f, g) and high-frequency sounds (s, sh, ph, k). Vowels that have a low pitch are easiest to hear. Speech sounds are distorted, and there is a delayed reception and reaction to speech. A concern with normal age-related sensory changes is that older adults with a deficit are sometimes inappropriately diagnosed with dementia (Touhy and Jett, 2022).

Gustatory and olfactory changes begin around age 50 and include a decrease in the number of taste buds and sensory cells in the nasal lining. Reduced taste discrimination and sensitivity to odors are common.

Proprioceptive changes are common after age 60 due to changes in both the peripheral and central nervous system. Proprioceptive changes include increased difficulty with balance, spatial orientation, and coordination, which alone or in combination increase the risk of falling. In addition, the person cannot avoid obstacles as quickly, and the automatic response to protect and brace oneself when falling is decreased (Touhy and Jett, 2022). There are also tactile changes, including declining sensitivity to pain, pressure, and temperature secondary to peripheral vascular disease and neuropathies.

Meaningful Stimuli. Meaningful stimuli reduce the incidence of sensory deprivation. In the home meaningful stimuli include pets, music, television, pictures of family members, and a calendar and clock. The same stimuli need to be present in health care settings. Note whether patients have roommates or visitors. The presence of others offers positive stimulation. However, a roommate who constantly watches television, persistently tries to talk, or continuously keeps lights on contributes to sensory overload. The presence or absence of meaningful stimuli influences alertness and the ability to participate in care.

Amount of Stimuli. Excessive stimuli in an environment cause sensory overload. The frequency of observations and the number of procedures performed in an acute health care setting are often stressful. If a patient is in pain or restricted by a cast or traction, overstimulation frequently is a problem. In addition, a room that is near repetitive or loud noises (e.g., an elevator, stairwell, or nurses' station) contributes to sensory overload.

Social Interaction. The amount and quality of social contact with supportive family members and significant others influence sensory function. The absence of visitors during hospitalization or residency in extended-care settings influences the degree of isolation a patient feels. This also is a common problem in hospital intensive care settings, where visiting is often restricted. The ability to discuss concerns with loved ones is an important coping mechanism for most people. Therefore the absence of meaningful conversation results in feelings of isolation, loneliness, anxiety, and depression for a patient. Often this is not apparent until behavioral changes occur.

Environmental Factors. A person's occupation can carry a risk for hearing, visual, and peripheral nerve alterations. Individuals who have occupations involving exposure to high noise levels (e.g., factory or airport workers) are at risk for noise-induced hearing loss and need to be screened for hearing impairments. Hazardous loud noise is common in work settings and recreational activities. Noisy recreational activities that weaken hearing ability include target shooting, hunting, woodworking, and listening to loud music.

Individuals who have occupations involving risk of exposure to chemicals or flying objects (e.g., welders) are at risk for eye injuries and need to be screened for visual impairments. Sports activities and consumer fireworks also place individuals at risk for eye injuries.

Occupations that involve repetitive wrist or finger movements (e.g., heavy assembly line work, long periods of computer use) cause pressure on the median nerve, which runs from the forearm into the palm of the hand, resulting in carpal tunnel syndrome. Carpal tunnel syndrome alters tactile sensation and is one of the most common industrial or work-related injuries.

A patient who is hospitalized is sometimes at risk for sensory alterations because of exposure to environmental stimuli or a change in sensory input. Patients who are immobilized by bed rest or who have a chronic disability are unable to experience all the normal sensations of free movement. Another group at risk includes patients who are isolated in a health care setting or at home because of medical conditions due to immunocompromise (e.g., bone marrow transplant) or infections (e.g., active tuberculosis or other respiratory or wound infections) (see Chapter 28). These patients are in private rooms and are often unable to enjoy normal interactions with visitors.

Cultural Factors. Some sensory alterations occur more commonly in select cultural groups. Analysis of data from the National Health Interview Survey (NHIS), Centers for Disease Control and Prevention (CDC), and National Center for Health Statistics showed that African Americans had a higher prevalence of visual impairment due to glaucoma than Hispanics and non-Hispanic Whites. Children and adolescents who are African American or from two different races also have higher rates of blindness and visual impairment than those from other ethnicities (U.S. Department of Health and Human Services [USDHHS], 2020). Cultural disparities in vision impairment are significant, in part because visual impairment is associated with a decrease in physical and mental health and quality of life (Box 49.3) (Tseng et al., 2018). Changes in hearing and visual acuity also affect a person's health literacy and ability to understand medications,

---

⊕ BOX 49.3 CULTURAL ASPECTS OF CARE

Disparities in Eye Care

In estimates from the 2018 National Health Interview Survey (NHIS), 32.2 million American adults 18 years of age and older indicated they were experiencing vision loss. The survey participants reported the following racial identities: about 24.7 million were White; 4.8 million were Black or African American; 1.4 million identified as Asian; 622,000 identified as American Indian or Alaskan Native; and 759,000 reported multiple or other races (American Foundation for the Blind [AFB], 2020]). Even though vision loss is common among Americans, some do not receive the vision services necessary to improve their quality of life. Findings from the National Health and Aging Trends Survey reveal that Medicare beneficiaries who are older and non-White are less likely to report the use of eyeglasses. People with lower socioeconomic and educational levels are also less likely to report the use of eyeglasses (Otte et al., 2018). A disparity also exists between patients with Medicaid and those with private health care insurance. Individuals with Medicaid are often less successful in obtaining eye care appointments (Yoon et al., 2018). These findings are critical because the early diagnosis of visual impairments allows for early intervention to help prevent irreversible causes of vision loss (Burton et al., 2021).

Implications for Patient-Centered Care

- Encourage patients to discuss changes in visual acuity or other eye or vision issues by asking focused assessment questions.
- Educate patients on age-related eye diseases and conditions, eye care services, and the importance of taking care of their eyes and managing underlying illnesses as well as their health (Ghasemi et al., 2018).
- Collaborate with family caregivers and the interprofessional team to help improve access to eye care services (National Association of School Nurses [NASN], 2021).
- Follow up with patients to reiterate important points and to check on their progress (Ghasemi et al., 2018).
- Provide written eye care instructions in type that uses large fonts (14-point type or larger) and sharp contrast to improve readability.
- Participate in creating and supporting innovative public policy to address disparities among people with visual problems (Otte et al., 2018; Yoon et al., 2018).

---

procedures, and restorative and home care interventions, which are further complicated when English is a patient's second language.

As Dilyana prepares to care for Ms. Long, she reflects on what she understands about cataracts and considers their effect on Ms. Long's vision. Dilyana anticipates that Ms. Long is experiencing blurry vision and will have difficulty doing activities that require close vision such as reading, sewing, and cooking. Dilyana considers her knowledge of sensory deficits and her understanding about how a person's age influences overall sensory function. She knows that the visual impairment caused by cataracts most likely will have emotional, cognitive, and physical effects on Ms. Long and her family. Dilyana uses her attitude of curiosity as she considers how to assess Ms. Long's visual deficit, its effects on her ability to perform activities of daily living (ADLs), her safety, and her well-being.

CRITICAL THINKING

Successful clinical judgment requires application of critical thinking and the synthesis of knowledge, experience, environmental factors, critical thinking attitudes, and intellectual and professional standards. Clinical judgment requires you to anticipate the information you need to gather about a patient, analyze the data, and make decisions regarding your patient's care.

Patients' conditions are always changing. During assessment consider all critical thinking elements that help you make appropriate nursing diagnoses (Fig. 49.1). In the case of sensory alterations, integrate knowledge of the pathophysiology of sensory deficits, factors that affect sensory function, and therapeutic communication principles. This knowledge enables you to make clinical judgments about a patient's sensory problems by anticipating expected signs and symptoms and matching with data you gather from a patient. For example, knowing the typical symptoms caused by a cataract helps you recognize the pattern of visual changes that a patient with cataracts reports.

Use critical thinking to consider internal and environmental contextual factors as you assess, identify health care needs, and plan care for your patients (Dickinson et al., 2019). Internal factors include your previous experiences in caring for patients with sensory deficits. Your experience helps you recognize limitations in a patient's functioning and how these limitations affect the ability to carry out daily activities. As you care for more patients with sensory alterations, your competence in providing safe nursing care improves. For example, after caring for one patient with a hearing impairment, you can conduct a more effective assessment of the next patient by using previously successful approaches that promote the patient's ability to hear your questions.

External factors, such as your observations of a patient, the physical environment, and available resources, also play a part in your nursing care of patients with sensory deficits. For example, if you are caring for a toddler who was born with a hearing deficit and is living at home with his parents, you focus on helping the parents and the child adapt to safety risks in their home environment and ensure the toddler's safety as he becomes more mobile and independent. On the other hand, if you are caring for an older adult who is experiencing new-onset hearing loss related to aging, you focus on helping the older adult accept the need to start wearing hearing aids and help the patient determine the financial aspects of purchasing them (e.g., are they covered by Medicare or health insurance or will the patient have to pay for them out of pocket?).

When you apply critical thinking attitudes and standards during assessment, you establish a thorough and accurate database from which to make clinical judgments and decisions. For example, perseverance is necessary to learn details about how visual changes influence a patient's ability to socialize. Evidence-based standards of care and practice such as those from the American Academy of Ophthalmology and the American Speech-Language-Hearing Association provide

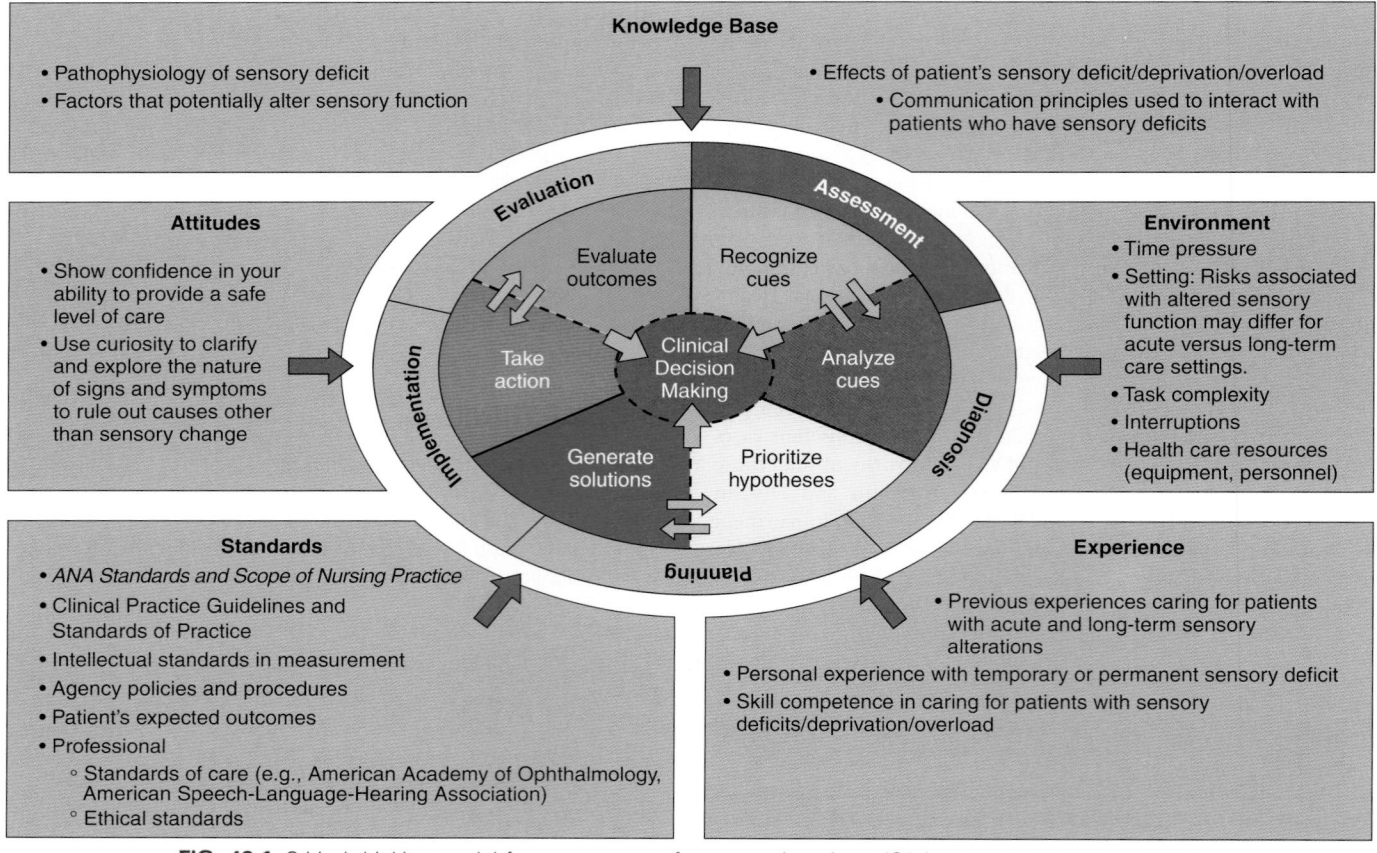

Knowledge Base
- Pathophysiology of sensory deficit
- Factors that potentially alter sensory function

- Effects of patient's sensory deficit/deprivation/overload
- Communication principles used to interact with patients who have sensory deficits

Attitudes
- Show confidence in your ability to provide a safe level of care
- Use curiosity to clarify and explore the nature of signs and symptoms to rule out causes other than sensory change

Environment
- Time pressure
- Setting: Risks associated with altered sensory function may differ for acute versus long-term care settings.
- Task complexity
- Interruptions
- Health care resources (equipment, personnel)

Evaluation
Assessment
Evaluate outcomes
Recognize cues
Take action
Clinical Decision Making
Analyze cues
Implementation
Diagnosis
Generate solutions
Prioritize hypotheses
Planning

Standards
- *ANA Standards and Scope of Nursing Practice*
- Clinical Practice Guidelines and Standards of Practice
- Intellectual standards in measurement
- Agency policies and procedures
- Patient's expected outcomes
- Professional
  ○ Standards of care (e.g., American Academy of Ophthalmology, American Speech-Language-Hearing Association)
  ○ Ethical standards

Experience
- Previous experiences caring for patients with acute and long-term sensory alterations
- Personal experience with temporary or permanent sensory deficit
- Skill competence in caring for patients with sensory deficits/deprivation/overload

FIG. 49.1 Critical thinking model for assessment of sensory alterations. (Clinical Judgment Measurement Model copyright © NCSBN. All rights reserved.)

criteria for screening sensory problems and establishing standards for competent, safe, effective care and practice. Use clinical judgment to conduct a thorough assessment; then plan, implement, and evaluate care that enables a patient to function safely and effectively.

REFLECT NOW

The parents of a toddler share with you their plan to take the toddler to a fireworks show. What recommendations would you share with the parents, and why?

❖ NURSING PROCESS

Clinical judgment during the nursing process applies critical thinking in your patient care. The nursing process provides a clinical decision-making approach for you to develop and implement an individualized plan of care. Use critical thinking and a systematic approach to understand a patient's sensory needs. Because patients may feel embarrassed by or uncomfortable discussing the effects of their sensory dysfunction, be sure you establish a therapeutic relationship with your patients. Consider involving family caregivers and consider referrals to other members of the health care team to create a safe and effective plan of care.

◆ Assessment

During the assessment process, thoroughly assess each patient and critically analyze findings to ensure that you make appropriate and

relevant nursing diagnoses and patient-centered clinical decisions required for safe nursing care.

Through the Patient's Eyes. When conducting an assessment, value the patient as a full partner. Engaging a patient while being thorough during assessment provides the data you will use to identify health care needs and to plan, implement, and evaluate care. Patients are often hesitant to admit sensory losses. Therefore start gathering information by establishing a therapeutic rapport with the patient. Elicit your patients' values, preferences, and expectations regarding their sensory impairment.

Many patients have a definite plan as to how they want their care delivered. Some patients expect caregivers to recognize and appropriately manage and adjust their environment to meet their sensory needs. This includes helping the family and patient ultimately learn and adapt to a changed lifestyle based on the patient's sensory impairment. Determine from the patient any previous interventions that were helpful or did not help in managing limitations. Assess the expertise a patient has in managing personal health and any related problems. Many patients with sensory alterations have strengthened their other senses and expect caregivers to anticipate their needs (e.g., for safety and security).

People at Risk. When assessing a patient with or at risk for sensory alteration, first consider the pathophysiology of existing deficits and the factors influencing sensory function to anticipate how to approach your assessment. For example, if a patient has a hearing disorder, adjust your communication style and focus your assessment on relevant criteria related to hearing deficits. Collect a history that also assesses the patient's current sensory status and the degree to which a sensory deficit affects the patient's lifestyle, psychosocial adjustment, developmental status, self-care ability, health promotion habits, and safety. Also focus the assessment on the quality and quantity of stimuli within the patient's environment.

Older adults are a high-risk group because of normal physiological changes involving sensory organs. However, be careful not to automatically assume that a patient's sensory problem is related to advancing age. For example, adult sensorineural hearing loss is often caused by exposure to excessive and prolonged noise or metabolic, vascular, and other systemic alterations. Some patients benefit from a referral to an audiologist or otolaryngologist when serious hearing problems are identified during assessment.

Other individuals at risk for sensory alterations include those living in a confined environment such as a long-term care agency. For example, an individual with poor hearing who is confined to a wheelchair, has decreased energy, and avoids contact with others is at significant risk for sensory deprivation. High-quality long-term care agencies offer meaningful stimulation through group activities, environmental design, and mealtime gatherings to better manage sensory alterations in their residents.

Patients with balance or proprioceptive changes, such as peripheral neuropathy, are at increased risk for falls. These patients lose the self-awareness of their body position, which can intensify in a new environment. For example, a patient with impaired balance may need a longer period of time to adjust from a sitting to standing position or a patient with peripheral neuropathy may be unaware of an uneven walking surface (Touhy and Jett, 2022).

Patients who are acutely ill are also at risk because of an unfamiliar and unresponsive environment. This does not mean that all patients in the hospital have sensory alterations. However, you need to carefully assess patients exposed to continued sensory stimulation (e.g., intensive care unit (ICU) settings, long-term hospitalization, or multiple therapies). Assess a patient's environment within both the health care setting and the home, looking for factors that pose risks or need adjustment to provide safety and more appropriate sensory stimulation.

Sensory Alterations History. The nursing history includes assessment of the nature and characteristics of sensory alterations and any problem related to an alteration (Box 49.4). When taking the history, consider the ethnic background of the patient because the rates of certain alterations are higher in some groups.

During the history it is useful to have a patient self-rate the sensory deficit by saying "Rate your hearing as excellent, good, fair, poor, or bad." Then, based on the patient's self-rating, explore this perception of a sensory loss more fully. This provides an in-depth look at how the sensory loss influences the patient's quality of life. In the case of hearing problems, a screening tool such as the Hearing Handicap Inventory for the Elderly–Screening Version (HHIE-S) effectively identifies patients needing audiological intervention (Servidoni et al., 2018). The HHIE-S is a 5-minute, 10-item questionnaire that assesses how an individual perceives the social and emotional effects of hearing loss. The higher the HHIE-S score, the greater the handicapping effect of a hearing impairment.

A nursing history also reveals any recent changes in a patient's behavior. Frequently friends or family members are the best resources for this information. Ask a family member the following questions:
- Has your family member shown any recent mood swings (e.g., outbursts of anger, nervousness, fear, or irritability)?
- Have you noticed the family member avoiding social activities?

BOX 49.4 Nursing Assessment Questions

Nature of the Problem
- Describe the problem you are having with your vision/hearing.
- What have you tried to correct your vision/hearing difficulty?
- Do you use any devices to improve your vision/hearing?
- How effective are your glasses or hearing aids? If you are having problems, describe them for me.

Signs and Symptoms
- Ask a patient with visual alterations: Do you require books with large print or on audiotape? Are you able to prepare a meal or write a check? Do you notice any eye irritation or drainage?
- Ask a patient with hearing alterations: Which types of sounds or tones do you have difficulty hearing? Do people tell you that they have to "shout" for you to hear them? Do people ask you not to talk so loudly? Do you have a ringing, crackling, or buzzing in your ears? Is there pain: sharp, dull, burning, itching? Have you noticed any redness, swelling, or drainage?

Onset and Duration
- When did you notice the problem? How long has it lasted?
- Does it come and go, or is it constant?
- What makes the problem better or worse?

Predisposing Factors
- Do you work or participate in any activities that have the potential for vision/hearing injury? If so, how do you protect your hearing and vision?
- Do you have a family history of cataracts, glaucoma, macular degeneration, or hearing loss?
- When was your last vision/hearing examination?

Effect on Patient
- What effect has your vision/hearing problem had on your work, family, or social life?
- Have changes in your vision/hearing affected your feelings of independence?
- How does your vision/hearing problem make you feel about yourself?
- Do you have problems with routine care of glasses, contact lenses, or hearing aids?

Mental Status. Assessment of mental status is valuable when you suspect sensory deprivation or overload. Observation of a patient during history taking, during the physical examination (see Chapter 30), and while providing nursing care offers valuable data about a patient's behaviors and mental status (e.g., ability to hear conversation or respond to questions). Observe a patient's physical appearance and behavior, measure cognitive ability, and assess the patient's emotional status. Use the Mini-Mental State Examination (MMSE) if you suspect disorientation, change in problem-solving abilities, and altered conceptualization and abstract thinking (see Chapter 30). For example, a patient with severe sensory deprivation is not always able to carry on a conversation, remain attentive, or display recent or past memory. An important step toward preventing cognition-related disability is education by nurses about disease process, available services, and assistive devices.

Physical Assessment. To identify sensory deficits and their severity, use physical assessment techniques to assess vision; hearing; olfaction; taste; and the ability to discriminate light touch, temperature, pain, and proprioception (body position) (see Chapter 30). Table 49.2 summarizes specific assessment techniques for identifying sensory deficits. You gather more accurate data when the examination room is private, quiet, and comfortable for the patient. In addition, rely on personal observation to

TABLE 49.2 Assessment of Sensory Function

Assessment Activities	Behavior Indicating Deficit (Children)	Behavior Indicating Deficit (Adults)
Vision Ask patient to read newspaper, magazine, or lettering on menu. Ask patient to identify colors on color chart or crayons. Observe patients performing ADLs.	Self-stimulation, including eye rubbing, body rocking, sniffing or smelling, arm twirling; hitching (using legs to propel while in sitting position) instead of crawling	Poor coordination, squinting, underreaching or overreaching for objects, persistent repositioning of objects, impaired night vision, accidental falls
Hearing Assess patient's hearing acuity (see Chapter 30) using spoken word. Assess for history of tinnitus. Observe patient conversing with others. Inspect ear canal for hardened cerumen. Observe patient behaviors in a group.	Frightened when unfamiliar people approach, no reflex or purposeful response to sounds, failure to be awakened by loud noise, slow or absent development of speech, greater response to movement than to sound, avoidance of social interaction with other children	Blank looks, decreased attention span, lack of reaction to loud noises, increased volume of speech, positioning of head toward sound, smiling and nodding of head in approval when someone speaks, use of other means of communication such as lipreading or writing, complaints of ringing in ears
Touch Check patient's ability to discriminate between sharp and dull stimuli. Assess whether patient is able to distinguish objects (coin or safety pin) in the hand with eyes closed. Ask whether patient feels unusual sensations.	Inability to perform developmental tasks related to grasping objects or drawing, repeated injury from handling of harmful objects (e.g., hot stove, sharp knife)	Clumsiness, overreaction or underreaction to painful stimulus, failure to respond when touched, avoidance of touch, sensation of pins and needles, numbness Unable to identify object placed in hand
Assess patients at risk for carpal tunnel syndrome for numbness, tingling, weakness, and pain in hands.		Decreased grip strength may make it difficult to form a fist, grasp small objects, or perform other manual tasks. Usually starts gradually, with frequent burning, tingling, or itching numbness in the palm of the hand and the fingers, especially the thumb and the index and middle fingers (National Institute of Neurological Disorders and Stroke [NINDS, 2020])
Smell Have patient close eyes and identify several nonirritating odors (e.g., coffee, vanilla).	Difficulty in discriminating noxious odors; difficult to assess until child is 6 or 7 years old	Failure to react to noxious or strong odor, increased body odor, decreased sensitivity to odors
Taste Ask patient to sample and distinguish different tastes (e.g., lemon, sugar, salt). (Have patient drink or sip water and wait 1 minute between each taste.)	Inability to tell whether food is salty or sweet; possible ingestion of strange-tasting things	Change in appetite, excessive use of seasoning and sugar, complaints about taste of food, weight change

ADLs, Activities of daily living.

detect sensory alterations. Patients with a hearing impairment may seem inattentive to others, respond with inappropriate anger when spoken to, believe people are talking about them, answer questions inappropriately, have trouble following clear directions, and have a monotonous voice quality or speak unusually loudly or softly.

Ability to Perform Self-Care. Assess patients' functional abilities in their home environment or health care setting, including the ability to perform feeding, dressing, grooming, and toileting activities. For example, assess whether a patient with altered vision is able to find items on a meal tray and read directions on a prescription. Can a patient recovering from a stroke manipulate buttons or zippers for dressing? Also determine a patient's ability to perform instrumental activities of daily living (IADLs) such as reading bills and writing checks, differentiating money denominations, and driving a vehicle at night. If a patient seems to have a sensory deficit, does the patient show concern for grooming? Does a patient's loss of balance prevent rising from a toilet seat safely? If a sensory alteration impairs a patient's functional ability, providing resources within the home is a necessary part of discharge planning. Your findings may indicate the need for an occupational therapy consultation.

Health Promotion Habits. Assess the daily routines that patients follow to maintain sensory function. Which type of eye and ear care is a part of a patient's daily hygiene? For individuals who participate in sports (e.g., ice hockey, lacrosse) or recreational activities (e.g., motorcycle riding) or who work in a setting in which ear or eye injury is a possibility (e.g., chemical exposure, welding, glass or stone polishing, or constant exposure to loud noise), determine whether they wear safety glasses or hearing-protective devices (HPDs).

It is also important to assess a patient's adherence to routine health screening. When was the last time the patient had an eye examination or hearing evaluation? For adults, routine screening of visual and hearing function is imperative to detect problems early. This is especially true in the case of glaucoma, which if undetected leads to permanent vision loss. Recommended screening guidelines usually are based on age. When a patient begins to show a hearing deficit, incorporate routine screening in regular examinations.

Environmental Factors. Environmental factors play a significant role in the safety of patients with sensory deficits. Thoroughly assess a patient's environment to identify potential safety hazards. Patients with sensory alterations are at risk for injury if their home environments are unsafe. For example, a patient with reduced vision cannot see potential hazards clearly. A patient with proprioceptive problems loses balance easily. A patient with reduced sensation cannot perceive hot versus cold temperatures. The condition of the home, the rooms, and the front and back entrances is often problematic to the patient with sensory alterations. Assess a patient's home for common hazards, including the following:

- Uneven, cracked walkways leading to front and/or back door
- Extension and phone cords in the main route of walking traffic
- Loose area rugs and runners placed over carpeting
- Bathrooms without shower or tub grab bars
- Water faucets unmarked to designate hot and cold
- Unlit stairways, lack of handrails
- Poor lighting in stairways and halls and at entrance doors

In an inpatient or hospital environment caregivers often forget to rearrange furniture and equipment to keep pathways from the bed and chair to the bathroom and entrance clear. It is helpful to walk into a patient's room and look for safety hazards:

- Is the nurse call system within easy, safe reach?
- Are intravenous (IV) poles on wheels and easy to move?
- Are suction machines, IV pumps, or drainage bags positioned so that a patient can rise from a bed or chair easily?
- Are bedside tables and areas clutter free?

An additional problem faced by patients who are visually impaired is the inability to read medication labels and syringe markings. Ask the patient to read a label to determine whether the patient is able to read the dosage and frequency. When a patient needs to self-administer an injection, such as insulin, ask the patient to draw up the medication into a syringe to determine the ability to correctly read the syringe markings. If a patient has a hearing impairment, check to see whether the sounds of a doorbell, telephone, smoke alarm, and alarm clock are easy to discriminate.

Communication Methods. To understand the nature of a communication problem, you need to know whether a patient has trouble speaking, understanding, naming, reading, or writing. Patients with existing sensory deficits often develop alternate ways of communicating. To interact with a patient and promote interaction with others, understand the patient's method of communication. Vision becomes almost a primary sense for people with hearing impairments. As a result, face-to-face communication is essential (Fig. 49.2).

Patients with visual impairments are unable to observe facial expressions and other nonverbal behaviors to clarify the content of spoken communication. Instead they rely on voice tones and inflections to detect the emotional tone of communication. Some patients with visual deficits learn to read Braille. Patients with aphasia have varied degrees of inability to speak, interpret, or understand language. Expressive aphasia, a motor type of aphasia, is the inability to name common objects or express simple ideas in words or writing. For example, a patient understands a question but is unable to express an answer. Sensory or receptive aphasia is the inability to understand written or spoken language. A patient is able to express words but is unable to understand the questions or comments of others. Global aphasia is the inability to understand language or communicate orally.

The temporary or permanent loss of the ability to speak is extremely traumatic to an individual. Assess for alternate communication methods and whether they cause anxiety. Patients who have undergone laryngectomies often write notes, use communication boards or laptop computers, speak with mechanical vibrators, or use esophageal speech. Patients with endotracheal or tracheostomy tubes have a temporary loss of speech. Most use a notepad to write their questions and requests. However, some patients are unable to write messages. Determine whether the patient has developed a sign-language system or symbols to communicate needs.

Social Support. Determine whether a patient lives alone and how often family or friends visit. Assess the patient's social skills and level of satisfaction with the support given by family and friends. Is the patient satisfied with the support available? Is the patient able to solve problems with family members? Is there a family caregiver who offers support when the patient requires assistance because of a sensory loss? The long-term effects of sensory alterations influence family dynamics and a patient's willingness to remain active in society.

Use of Assistive Devices. Assess the use of assistive devices (e.g., use of a hearing aid or glasses) and whether they currently are in working order. Assess whether the patient thinks that these devices are beneficial. This includes learning how often the patient uses the devices, the patient's or family caregiver's method of caring for and cleaning the devices routinely (see Chapter 40), and the patient's knowledge of what to do when a problem develops. When you identify that a patient has an assistive device, remember that just because the individual has a device, it does not mean that it works or that the patient uses it or benefits from it.

Other Factors That Affect Perception. Factors other than sensory deprivation or overload can cause impaired perception (e.g., medications or pain). Assess a patient's medication history, which includes prescribed and over-the-counter (OTC) medications and herbal products. Also gather information regarding the frequency, dose, method of administration, and last time the patient took the medications. Some antibiotics (e.g., streptomycin, gentamicin, and tobramycin) are ototoxic and permanently damage the auditory nerve, whereas chloramphenicol sometimes irritates the optic nerve. Opioid analgesics, sedatives, and antidepressant medications often alter the perception of stimuli. Conduct a thorough pain assessment when you suspect that pain is causing perceptual problems (see Chapter 44).

FIG. 49.2 Nurse sits at eye level so that patient with hearing impairment can communicate.

REFLECT NOW

How would you assess a patient who has recently become confused and is having hallucinations for sensory alterations?

Dilyana considers her knowledge about the effects of cataracts, as well as her personal experience in caring for other patients in other health care settings who experienced visual difficulties, while preparing to assess Ms. Long. Dilyana also reflects on her personal experience with her grandmother who had cataracts before her surgery a year ago. Dilyana organizes her assessment and identifies key questions to ask Ms. Long based on her knowledge and experience.

Dilyana begins by assessing Ms. Long's visual acuity. Ms. Long has difficulty reading a paragraph out of a book she has just started. Ms. Long states, "The words are just really blurry. I also have trouble seeing long distances, especially at night. In order to read I need the light to be really bright. Things are quite a blur these days." Dilyana responds, "Sometimes people who have trouble with their vision are worried about their safety. Do you have any similar concerns?" Ms. Long replies, "Well, I'm really afraid that I might fall down the stairs at my home because I cannot see the edges of the steps very well. And I am really embarrassed by my bad vision. I find that I have a hard time concentrating when people talk with me and I am so scared of what might happen if I lose my vision forever. I can't sleep and I'm starting to get really tired." Dilyana notices that during their conversation, Ms. Long is having trouble maintaining eye contact and she is very restless.

As Dilyana assesses Ms. Long, she asks, "Tell me about how you have your home set up and arranged. Because of your visual difficulty, I want to be sure you are able to move around your house safely." Ms. Long responds, My home has been in our family for such a long time. We love our house. It's full of great memories!" Dilyana remembers that her grandmother had a lot of throw rugs that they had to remove to prevent her from falling and that they had to install brighter light bulbs in her grandmother's kitchen. As Ms. Long describes her house, Dilyana identifies some potential safety hazards. Like her grandmother, Ms. Long has several throw rugs in her house. Mrs. Long admits the carpet in the living room is worn and the edges are curled up. The lighting in the bedrooms, hallways, and basement stairwells is dim, as are the lights on the front porch.

◆ Analysis and Nursing Diagnosis

After assessment, review all available data and analyze cues, looking critically for patterns and trends that reveal nursing diagnoses reflective of alterations in the patient's ability to function (Box 49.5). Using clinical judgment, validate findings to identify and ensure accuracy of nursing diagnoses and collaborative problems. Determine the main factors that likely caused or are creating a patient's health problem. The etiology or related factor of a problem-focused or negative nursing diagnosis is a condition that nursing interventions can affect. The etiology needs to be accurate to ensure nursing therapies

BOX 49.5　Nursing Diagnostic Process

Risk for Injury

Assessment Activities	Assessment Findings
Assess patient's visual acuity.	Reduced ability to see objects clearly; needs brighter light to read; has trouble distinguishing edges of stairs
Have patient describe the home setting, or visit the home setting and assess for hazards that pose risks to patient.	Lighting in rooms, hallways, and stairwells very dim; carpet in living room old, edges curled up; steps leading up to front entrance of home
Review medical record from clinic visit.	Cataract in left eye

are targeted and effective. Similarly, risk factors for any at risk diagnoses need to be accurate.

In some cases the specific sensory alteration is the etiology or risk factor for a diagnosis such as *Risk for Injury*. You select nursing diagnoses by recognizing the way in which the sensory alteration affects a patient's ability to function (e.g., *Self-Care Deficit*). In addition, most patients present themselves to health care professionals with multiple diagnoses. Create a concept map to help you recognize patterns of data that reveal health problems created by a patient's sensory alteration as well as the interrelationships among the diagnoses (Fig. 49.3). Examples of nursing diagnoses that apply to patients with sensory alterations include the following:

- Risk for Injury
- Risk for Fall
- Impaired Verbal Communication
- Impaired Socialization
- Impaired Mobility

Dilyana analyzes the data she gathered during Ms. Long's assessment. As she reflects on Ms. Long's responses to her questions and her assessment findings, Dilyana begins to analyze data to formulate individualized nursing diagnoses. She uses her clinical judgment to identify Ms. Long's priority needs.

Because Ms. Long has a cataract in her left eye that is causing blurred vision and difficulty reading, the first nursing diagnosis Dilyana identifies is **Risk for Injury**. *Dilyana also identifies* **Risk for Fall** *as a nursing diagnosis because of Ms. Long's age, her cataract causing blurry vision, the multiple throw rugs in the home, and the dim lighting in the hallways, stairwells, and bedrooms. Dilyana adds the diagnosis of* **Fear** *to the concept map. Ms. Long expresses that she is fearful to go up and down her stairs and she is afraid of what will happen if she loses her eyesight permanently. Dilyana then adds* **Anxiety** *as her last diagnosis because Ms. Long is restless and makes poor eye contact during their conversations, and she states she is having difficulty concentrating and sleeping, which are all signs of anxiety.*

◆ Planning and Outcomes Identification

During planning, synthesize information from multiple resources (Fig. 49.4). Reflect on information gained from the assessment and knowledge of how sensory deficits affect normal functioning. This approach allows you to recognize the extent of a patient's deficit and know the types of interventions most likely to be helpful. Also consider the patient's environment and role that other health professionals play in planning care and available community resources that will be useful. Previous experience in caring for patients with sensory alterations is invaluable.

When applying critical thinking to planning care, professional standards are particularly useful. These standards recommend evidence-based interventions for a patient's condition. For example, patients who have visual deficits and are hospitalized are often placed on an evidence-based fall prevention protocol to ensure patient safety.

Outcomes. During planning, develop an individualized plan of care for each nursing diagnosis (see the Nursing Care Plan). Partner with your patient to develop a realistic plan that incorporates what you know about the patient's sensory problems and the extent to which sensory function can be maintained or improved. Outcomes need to be realistic and measurable. Examples of outcomes include the following:

- The patient and family report using communication techniques to send and receive messages within 2 days.
- The patient successfully demonstrates correct technique for cleaning a hearing aid within 1 week.
- The patient self-reports improved hearing acuity.

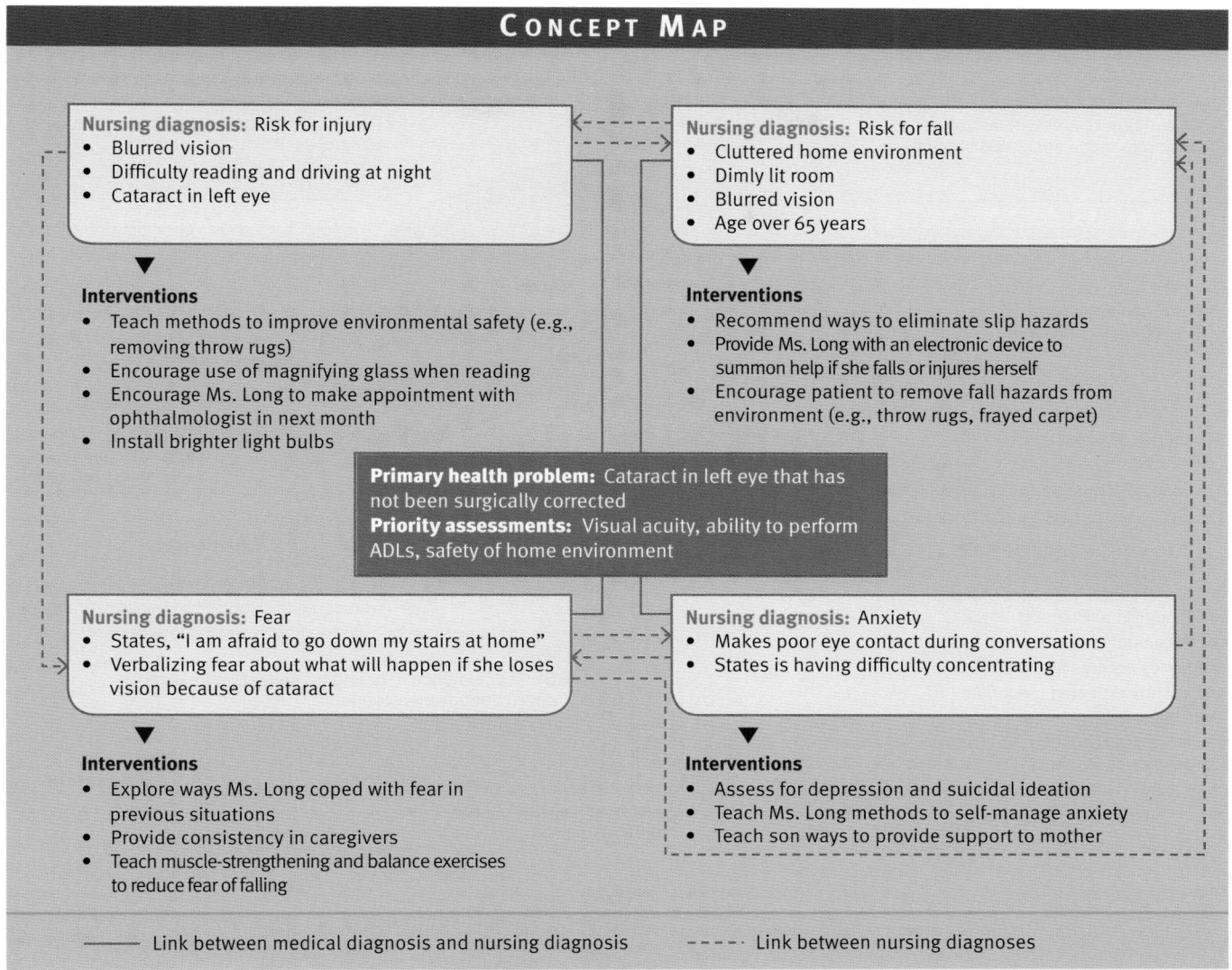

CONCEPT MAP

Nursing diagnosis: Risk for injury
- Blurred vision
- Difficulty reading and driving at night
- Cataract in left eye

Interventions
- Teach methods to improve environmental safety (e.g., removing throw rugs)
- Encourage use of magnifying glass when reading
- Encourage Ms. Long to make appointment with ophthalmologist in next month
- Install brighter light bulbs

Nursing diagnosis: Risk for fall
- Cluttered home environment
- Dimly lit room
- Blurred vision
- Age over 65 years

Interventions
- Recommend ways to eliminate slip hazards
- Provide Ms. Long with an electronic device to summon help if she falls or injures herself
- Encourage patient to remove fall hazards from environment (e.g., throw rugs, frayed carpet)

Primary health problem: Cataract in left eye that has not been surgically corrected
Priority assessments: Visual acuity, ability to perform ADLs, safety of home environment

Nursing diagnosis: Fear
- States, "I am afraid to go down my stairs at home"
- Verbalizing fear about what will happen if she loses vision because of cataract

Interventions
- Explore ways Ms. Long coped with fear in previous situations
- Provide consistency in caregivers
- Teach muscle-strengthening and balance exercises to reduce fear of falling

Nursing diagnosis: Anxiety
- Makes poor eye contact during conversations
- States is having difficulty concentrating

Interventions
- Assess for depression and suicidal ideation
- Teach Ms. Long methods to self-manage anxiety
- Teach son ways to provide support to mother

——— Link between medical diagnosis and nursing diagnosis   - - - - Link between nursing diagnoses

FIG. 49.3 Concept map for Ms. Long.

Setting Priorities. Your ability to recognize and analyze cues to help you prioritize your patient's care will improve as you care for more patients with sensory alterations (Dickinson et al., 2019). Consider the type and extent of sensory alteration affecting a patient when determining priorities of care. For example, a patient who enters the emergency department after experiencing eye trauma has priorities of reducing anxiety and preventing further injury to the eye. In contrast, a patient who is being discharged from an outpatient surgery department following cataract removal has the priority of learning about self-care restrictions. Safety is always a top priority. The patient also helps prioritize aspects of care—for example, a patient might wish to learn ways to communicate more effectively or to participate in favorite hobbies given the patient's limitation.

Some sensory alterations are short term (e.g., a patient experiencing sensory overload in an ICU). Appropriate interventions are therefore likely to be temporary (e.g., frequent reorientation or introduction of pleasant stimuli such as a back rub). Some sensory alterations such as permanent visual loss require long-term goals of care for patients to adapt. Patients who have sensory alterations at the time of entering a health care setting are usually most informed about how to adapt interventions to their lifestyles. For example, allow patients who are

blind to control whichever parts of their care they can. Sometimes it becomes necessary for a patient to make major changes in self-care activities, communication, and socialization to ensure safe and effective nursing care.

> **QSEN** **Building Competency in Safety** Ms. Long's church asks Dilyana to provide a presentation on fall prevention for older-adult members of the congregation. Many members also have impaired vision. How should Dilyana develop a program to educate this population of older adults and communicate observations or concerns related to fall hazards to them?

Teamwork and Collaboration. When developing a plan of care, consider all resources available to patients. The family plays a key role in providing meaningful stimulation by learning ways to help the patient adjust to any limitations. Engaging the family or designated surrogate is a fundamental skill of patient-centered care (Institute for Patient- and Family-Centered Care, 2016). You also refer patients to other health care professionals when appropriate. For example, if a patient has a significant loss of sensory function and is also unable to manage medical needs such

FIG. 49.4 Critical thinking model for sensory alterations planning. (Clinical Judgment Measurement Model copyright © NCSBN. All rights reserved.)

as medication self-administration or dressing changes, you make a referral to home care. Valuing interprofessional collaboration is an essential nurse competency that results in better patient health outcomes and greater patient and family satisfaction (Interprofessional Education Collaborative Expert Panel, 2016). Numerous community-based resources (e.g., local chapter of the Society for the Blind and Visually Impaired and the Area Agency on Aging) are also available. Try to arrange for a volunteer to visit a patient or have printed materials made available that describe ways to cope with sensory problems.

After talking further with Ms. Long, Dilyana identifies Risk for Injury *and* Risk for Fall *as two related priority nursing diagnoses because they directly affect Ms. Long's safety. Other nursing-applicable nursing diagnoses include* Fear *and* Anxiety. *Dilyana works with Ms. Long to identify appropriate and attainable outcomes and plan patient-centered care. Ms. Long tells Dilyana she wants to be able to stay in her home for as long as she possibly can. To address Ms. Long's care holistically, Dilyana knows that if she can make the home environment safer, Ms. Long's fear and anxiety may also improve, which will ultimately allow Ms. Long to continue to live independently at home. Therefore Dilyana starts by asking Ms. Long for input that will lead to outcomes focusing on improving safety in the home. She also begins to consider various community resources available to help patients experiencing changes in their vision.*

◆ **Implementation**

Nursing interventions involve patients and their families so that patients are able to maintain a safe, pleasant, and stimulating sensory environment. Use your clinical judgment to select the interventions that will enable patients with sensory alterations to function safely with their existing deficits and continue a normal lifestyle. Patients can learn to adjust to sensory impairments at any age with the proper support and resources. Use measures to maintain a patient's sensory function at the highest level possible.

Health Promotion. Good sensory function begins with prevention. When a patient seeks health care, provide education about relevant interventions that reduce the patient's risk for sensory losses, including relevant visual and hearing guidelines. Remember to assess a patient's capacity to process and understand the health information to ensure that the patient makes appropriate decisions regarding health.

Screening. According to the World Health Organization (2021), at least 2.2 billion people around the world have a near or distance vision impairment. In at least 1 billion or half of these cases, vision impairment could have been prevented or is yet to be addressed. This raises questions about the etiology of vision impairments, as well as strategies to improve access to early screening programs. The prevalence of distance vision impairment in low- and middle-income regions is about four times higher than in high-income regions (WHO, 2021). Preventable blindness is a worldwide health issue that begins with children and requires appropriate screening. Four recommended interventions are (1) screening for rubella, syphilis, chlamydia, and gonorrhea in women who are considering pregnancy; (2) advocating for adequate prenatal care to prevent premature birth (with the danger of exposure of the

◎ NURSING CARE PLAN

Risk for Injury

ASSESSMENT

Assessment Activities	Assessment Findings[a]
Ask Ms. Long to describe her visual acuity and vision changes.	Ms. Long states, "My left eye has a film over it that makes my **vision blurred.** I am having **difficulty reading, and driving at night.**"
Ask Ms. Long to describe life changes that have occurred since the change in vision.	Ms. Long states, "**I'm afraid to use the stairs at home because I can't judge steps clearly.**"
Ask Ms. Long about the results of the visit to the ophthalmologist.	Ms. Long states, "I was told I had a **cataract of the left eye,** and surgery was recommended."
Conduct a home hazard assessment.	There is **clutter in the home, dim lighting,** and stairs with **poor lighting and a broken handrail.**

[a]Assessment findings are shown in bold type.

NURSING DIAGNOSIS: Risk for injury

PLANNING

Expected Outcomes (NOC)[b]

Safe Home Environment

Ms. Long and her son make recommended changes in lighting, repair the broken handrail, and reduce clutter in the home environment within 2 weeks.

Ms. Long reports an increased sense of home safety and independence within 4 weeks.

[b]Outcome classification labels from Moorhead S, et al: *Nursing Outcomes Classification (NOC),* ed 6, St Louis, 2018, Elsevier.

INTERVENTIONS (NIC)[c]	RATIONALE
Environmental Management	
Teach Ms. Long and her son methods to improve environmental safety, such as installing handrails along stairs, raising toilet seats, removing throw rugs, and painting stairs.	Home environmental and health-related factors place a patient at risk for falls. Environmental safety modifications reduce the risk of falls and injury (Powell-Cope et al., 2018).
Teach Ms. Long to use a light over the shoulder for reading and sewing.	Warm incandescent lighting helps reduce eyestrain and increase enjoyment (Touhy and Jett, 2020).
Explain use of a pocket magnifier, and offer list of locations where Ms. Long can purchase one.	Magnifier enlarges visual images when reading or doing close work (Touhy and Jett, 2022, 2020).
Have Ms. Long make appointment with ophthalmologist within the next 4 weeks.	Adults over the age of 60 need a routine eye examination yearly (AOA, n.d.a).
Emotional Support	
Encourage Ms. Long to discuss with family and friends how a loss of vision affects her independence and lifestyle.	Visual impairments are associated with mobility and activity limitations, social restrictions, and reduced quality of life (Nael et al., 2017; Tseng et al., 2018).

[c]Intervention classification labels from Butcher HK, et al: *Nursing Interventions Classification (NIC),* ed 7, St Louis, 2018, Elsevier.

EVALUATION

Evaluation Activities	Patient Response
Ask Ms. Long and her son to describe the changes made in the home to reduce environmental hazards.	Ms. Long and her son respond that they removed the throw rugs and placed handrails at the entryway. She also placed lighting behind her chair, and there are 100-watt lights in the living room. She has a specific craft light that provides additional "over-the-shoulder" lighting.
Ask Ms. Long whether she is able to maintain a degree of independence with the environmental and lifestyle modifications.	Ms. Long states, "I'm more independent at home, and I'm able to enjoy my hobbies. Until surgery I don't mind having someone drive for me."

infant to excessive oxygen); (3) administering eye prophylaxis in the form of erythromycin ointment approximately 1 hour after an infant's birth; and (4) periodic screening of all children, especially newborns through preschoolers, for congenital blindness and visual impairment caused by refractive errors and strabismus (Hockenberry et al., 2019).

Visual impairments are common during childhood. The most common visual problem is a refractive error such as nearsightedness. The nurse's role is one of detection, education, and referral. Parents need to know the signs of visual impairment (e.g., failure to react to light and reduced eye contact from the infant). Instruct parents to report these signs to their health care provider immediately. When follow-up is available, vision screening of school-age children and adolescents can detect early visual impairments (Rodriguez et al., 2018). School nurses are usually responsible for vision testing.

In the United States glaucoma is the second leading cause of blindness in the general population and the primary cause of blindness in African Americans. If left undetected and untreated, it leads to permanent vision loss. The CDC (2020) recommends that people with diabetes mellitus have a dilated eye examination every year. Individuals who are at a higher risk for glaucoma should have a dilated eye examination every 2 years. Individuals at higher risk include the following: African Americans age 40 years and older and all adults older than 60; those with a family history of glaucoma; and those taking corticosteroids. Individuals who have other problems with their eyes or who have other health concerns or conditions (e.g., diabetes mellitus, hypertension, and heart disease) are also at risk for the development of glaucoma (American Optometric Association [AOA], n.d.b).

Hearing impairment is one of the most common disabilities in the United States. Deafness or hearing impairment affects people across the lifespan. Children at risk include those with a family history of childhood hearing impairment, perinatal infection (rubella, herpes, or cytomegalovirus), low birth weight, chronic ear infection, and Down syndrome. Advise women who are pregnant of the importance of early prenatal care, avoidance of ototoxic drugs, and testing for syphilis or rubella.

Children with chronic middle ear infections, a common cause of impaired hearing, need to receive periodic auditory testing. Warn parents of the risks and to seek medical care when a child has symptoms of earache or respiratory infection.

The prevalence of hearing loss is nearly 50% in those older than 75 years of age (National Institute on Deafness and Other Communication Disorders [NIDCD], 2018). Because aging is associated with degenerative changes in the ear, patients need to have hearing screenings at least every decade through age 50 and every 3 years thereafter (American Speech-Language-Hearing Association, 1997–2021). Once a patient reports a hearing loss, regular testing also becomes necessary. In addition, a patient who works or lives in a high–noise level environment requires annual screening. Occupational health nurses play a key role in the assessment of the auditory system and the initiation of prompt referrals. The early identification and treatment of problems help older adults be more active and healthier.

Preventive Measures. Trauma is a common cause of blindness in children. Penetrating injury from propulsive objects such as firecrackers or thrown rocks or from penetrating wounds from sticks, scissors, or sharp toys are just a few examples. Provide patient education to parents and children about ways to avoid eye trauma, such as avoiding the use of toys with long, pointed projections and instructing children not to walk or run while carrying pointed objects. Instruct patients that they can find safety equipment in most sports shops and large department stores.

Adults are at risk for eye injury while playing sports and working in jobs involving exposure to chemicals or flying objects. The Occupational Safety and Health Administration (OSHA, n.d.) has guidelines for workplace safety. Employers are required to have eyewash stations and to have employees wear eye goggles and/or use equipment such as hearing protection devices (HPDs) to reduce the risk of injury.

Noise-induced hearing loss (NIHL) occurs from continuous exposure to loud and/or long-lasting sounds. The loss can be immediate or occur over time. Risks for NIHL include listening to loud music through headphones or earbuds; repeated exposure to loud bursts of sound, such as explosions, fireworks, or sonic booms in air shows; or occupational sound exposure (NIDCD, 2019). *Healthy People 2030* (Office of Disease Prevention and Health Promotion [ODPHP], n.d.) identifies goals that include reducing new cases of work-related hearing loss. Occupational health nurses reinforce the use of devices. In addition, occupational health nurses routinely assess patients for noise exposure and provide hearing conservation classes for teachers, students, and patients.

Another means of prevention involves regular immunization of children against diseases capable of causing hearing loss (e.g., rubella, mumps, and measles). Nurses who work in health care providers' offices, schools, and community clinics instruct patients about the importance of early and timely immunization. Use caution when administering ototoxic drugs in all populations.

BOX 49.6   Preventing Computer or Digital Eyestrain

Eye Care
- Encourage patients to ask their optometrist or ophthalmologist if they can benefit from glasses prescribed specifically for computer use.
- Persons already wearing glasses may find their current prescription does not provide optimal vision for viewing a computer screen.
- Special lens designs, lens powers, or lens tints or coatings may help to maximize visual abilities and comfort.
- Vision therapy may be needed. Vision therapy, also called visual training, is a prescribed program of visual activities to improve visual abilities. It trains the eyes and brain to work together more effectively.

Computer Viewing
- Improve the conditions for using computers.
- Optimally, place a computer screen 15 to 20 degrees below eye level 1.57 to 2 cm (about 4 or 5 inches) as measured from the center of the screen and 7.8 to 9.8 cm (20 to 28 inches) from the eyes.
- Place reference materials above the keyboard and below the monitor. If such placement is not possible, use a document holder placed next to the monitor.
- Position the computer screen to avoid glare, particularly from overhead lighting or windows. Use blinds or drapes on windows and use lower wattage light bulbs in desk lamps.
- If there is no way to minimize glare from light sources, consider using an antiglare screen filter.
- Chairs should be comfortably padded and conform to the body. Chair height should be adjusted so that the feet rest flat on the floor. If a chair has arms, adjust armrests to provide support while typing. The wrists should not rest on the keyboard.
- Rest the eyes when using the computer for long periods—15 minutes for every 2 hours of continuous computer use. In addition, for every 20 minutes of computer viewing, look into the distance for 20 seconds to allow the eyes to refocus.

Adapted from American Optometric Association (AOA): Computer vision syndrome, n.d.c. https://www.aoa.org/patients-and-public/caring-for-your-vision/protecting-your-vision/computer-vision-syndrome

---

The average American worker spends 7 hours a day on the computer either in the office or working from home. To help prevent or alleviate digital eyestrain, the AOA (n.d.c) recommends following the 20-20-20 rule: take a 20-second break to view something 20 feet away every 20 minutes. Educate patients at risk for computer eyestrain to adopt preventive eye care and computer-viewing practices (Box 49.6).

Use of Assistive Devices. Patients who wear corrective contact lenses, eyeglasses, or hearing aids need to make sure that they are clean, accessible, and functional. It is helpful to have a family member or caregiver who also knows how to care for and clean an assistive aid. People who wear contact lenses must clean their lenses regularly with the appropriate solutions for cleaning and disinfection. Contact lenses increase the risk for serious eye infections caused by infrequent lens disinfection, contamination of lens storage cases or contact lens solutions, and use of homemade saline. Swimming while wearing lenses also creates a serious risk of infection. Reinforce proper lens care in any health maintenance discussion (see Chapter 40).

Older adults are often reluctant to use hearing aids. Reasons cited most often include cost, appearance, insufficient knowledge about hearing aids, amplification of competing noise, and unrealistic expectations. Neuromuscular changes in the older adult such as stiff fingers, enlarged joints, and decreased sensory perception also make the handling and care of a hearing aid difficult. Fortunately, today there are multiple types

BOX 49.7 PATIENT TEACHING

Effective Use of a Hearing Aid

Objective
- Patient and family caregiver will describe the steps to take for correct care and use of a hearing aid.

Teaching Strategies
- Show locations on hearing aid device where damage (e.g., cracks, fraying) is likely to occur: earmold or case, earphone, dials, cord, and connection plugs.
- Instruct on how to assess the integrity of the aid each day.
- Demonstrate battery replacement: Have an extra set of unused batteries available.
- Instruct to store batteries in a dry, secure place away from pets and children.
- Instruct to clean ear canal daily.
- Instruct not to use hair spray or other hair products when hearing aid is in place.
- Review method to check volume: Turn dial to maximum gain and check. Is voice clear?
- Review factors to report to hearing aid laboratory: static, distortion of sound, poor volume quality.

Evaluation
Use the principles of teach-back to evaluate patient/family caregiver learning:
- Tell me what we discussed about storage of your hearing aid.
- Tell me how you check the volume of your hearing aid.
- Tell me what we discussed about ways to clean and protect your hearing aid.
- Tell me what we discussed about battery removal and cleaning of your hearing aid.

of hearing aids that are specific to a person's hearing impairment, are cosmetically acceptable, and are easily used for people with manual dexterity issues (see Chapter 40).

Acknowledging a need to improve hearing is a person's first step. Give patients useful information on the benefits of hearing aid use. A person who understands the need for clear hearing will likely be open to wearing hearing aids. It is also important to have a family caregiver available to assist with hearing aid adjustment (Box 49.7). Federal regulations require a medical examination before hearing aids are purchased for patients younger than 18 years. A medical evaluation by a licensed health care provider is not required but is highly recommended in patients 18 years of age and older (U.S. Food and Drug Administration [FDA], 2018). Hearing aid providers should have prospective users consult their health care provider or an otolaryngologist for the following conditions: visible congenital or traumatic deformity of the ear, active drainage in the last 90 days, sudden or progressive hearing loss within the last 90 days, acute or chronic dizziness, unilateral sudden hearing loss within the last 90 days, visible cerumen accumulation or a foreign body in the ear canal, pain or discomfort in the ear, or an audiometric air-bone gap of 15 decibels or greater (FDA, 2020).

Promoting Meaningful Stimulation. Life becomes more enriching and satisfying when meaningful and pleasant stimuli exist within the environment. You can help patients adjust to their environment in many ways to make it more stimulating. You do this by considering the normal physiological changes that accompany sensory deficits.

Vision. The pupil's ability to adjust to light diminishes because of the normal changes of aging; thus, older adults are often very sensitive to glare. Suggest the use of yellow or amber lenses and shades or blinds on windows to minimize glare. Wearing sunglasses outside obviously reduces the glare of direct sunlight. Other interventions to enhance vision for patients with visual impairment include warm incandescent lighting and colors with sharp contrast and intensity.

The ability to read is important. Therefore allow patients to use their glasses whenever possible (e.g., during procedures and instruction). Some patients with reduced visual acuity need more than corrective lenses. A pocket magnifier helps a patient read most printed material. Telescopic-lens eyeglasses are smaller, are easier to focus, and have a greater range. Many books and other publications are available in large-print formats. If a patient has a legal document or other important document to read, standard copying machines have enlarging capabilities. In addition, low-vision optical devices are available and assist patients in medication self-management and leisure and daily activities. Software is also available that converts text into artificial voice output (Touhy and Jett, 2020).

With aging a person experiences a change in color perception. Perception of the colors blue, violet, and green usually declines. Brighter colors such as red, orange, and yellow are easier to see. Offer suggestions of ways to decorate a room and paint hallways or stairwells so the patient is able to differentiate surfaces and objects in a room.

Hearing. To maximize residual hearing function, work closely with a patient to suggest ways to modify the environment. For example, patients can amplify the sound of telephones and televisions. An innovative way to enrich the lives of patients with hearing impairments is recorded music. Some patients with severe hearing loss are able to hear music recorded in the low-frequency sound cycles.

One way to help an individual with a hearing loss is to ensure that the problem is not impacted cerumen. With aging, cerumen thickens and builds up in the ear canal. Excessive cerumen occluding the ear canal causes **conductive hearing loss**. Wax-removal medication such as carbamide peroxide (Debrox Earwax Removal Kit, Murine Ear Wax Removal System) can be effective. Because these drops can irritate the delicate skin of the eardrum and ear canal, use them only as directed (Mayo Clinic, 1998–2021). In the home setting, suggest patients use an eyedropper to apply a few drops of baby oil, mineral oil, glycerin, or hydrogen peroxide in the ear canal to soften the cerumen (Mayo Clinic, 1998–2021).

Taste and Smell. Promote the sense of taste by using measures to enhance remaining taste perception. Good oral hygiene keeps the taste buds well hydrated. Well-seasoned, differently textured food eaten separately heightens taste perception. Flavored vinegar or lemon juice adds tartness to food. Always ask a patient which foods are most appealing. Improving taste perception improves food intake and appetite.

Stimulation of the sense of smell with aromas such as brewed coffee, cooked garlic, and baked bread heightens taste sensation. Patients need to avoid blending or mixing foods because these actions make it difficult to identify tastes. Older people need to chew food thoroughly to allow more food to contact remaining taste buds.

Improve smell by strengthening pleasant olfactory stimulation. Make a patient's environment more pleasant with smells such as cologne, mild room deodorizers, fragrant flowers, and sachets. Note that some patients develop headaches from fragrances. Consult with patients to find out which scents they can tolerate. The removal of unpleasant odors (e.g., bedpans) also improves the quality of a patient's environment.

Touch. Patients with reduced tactile sensation usually have the impairment over a limited part of their bodies. Providing touch therapy stimulates existing function. If a patient is willing to be touched, hair brushing and combing, a back rub, and touching the arms or shoulders are ways to increase tactile contact. When sensation is reduced, a firm pressure is often necessary for a patient to feel a nurse's hand. Turning and repositioning also improve the quality of tactile sensation.

If a patient is overly sensitive to tactile stimuli (**hyperesthesia**), minimize irritating stimuli. Keeping bed linens loose to minimize direct contact with a patient and protecting the skin from exposure to irritants are helpful measures. Physical therapists can recommend special wrist splints for patients to wear to dorsiflex their wrists and relieve nerve pressure when they have numbness and tingling or pain in the hands, as with carpal tunnel syndrome. For patients who use computers, special keyboards and wrist pads are available to decrease the pressure on the median nerve, aid in pain relief, and promote healing.

Establishing Safe Environments. When sensory function becomes impaired, individuals become less secure within their home and workplace. Security is necessary for a person to feel independent. Make recommendations for improving safety within a patient's living environment without restricting independence. During a home visit or while completing an examination in the clinic, offer several useful suggestions for home safety. The nature of the actual or potential sensory loss determines the safety precautions you take.

Adaptations for Visual Loss. Safety is a concern when a patient experiences a decrease in visual acuity, peripheral vision, adaptation to the dark, or depth perception. With reduced peripheral vision a patient cannot see panoramically because the outer visual field is less discrete. With reduced depth perception a person is unable to judge how far away objects are located. This is a special danger when walking on uneven surfaces (e.g., stairways, cracked sidewalks).

Driving is a particular safety hazard for people with visual alterations. Reduced peripheral vision prevents a driver from seeing a car in an adjacent lane. A sensitivity to glare creates a problem for driving at night with headlights. Although vision is a primary consideration for safety, be alert to other factors that affect a patient's safety. In the case of older adults, decreased reaction time, reduced hearing, and decreased strength in the legs and arms further compromise driving skills. Some safety tips to share with those who continue to drive include the following: drive in familiar areas, do not drive during rush hour, avoid interstate highways for local drives, do not use a mobile phone while driving, drive defensively, use rear-view and side-view mirrors when changing lanes, avoid driving at dusk or night, go slowly but not too slowly, keep the car in good working condition, and carry a preprogrammed cellular phone.

The presence of visual alterations makes it difficult for a person to conduct normal ADLs within the home. Because of reduced depth perception, patients can trip on throw rugs, runners, or the edge of stairs. Teach patients and family members to keep all flooring in good condition and advise them to use low-pile carpeting. Thresholds between rooms need to be level with the floor. Recommend that patients and family members remove clutter to ensure clear pathways for walking and arrange furniture so that a patient can move about easily without fear of tripping or running into objects. Suggest that stairwells have a securely fastened banister or handrail extending the full length of the stairs.

Front and back entrances to the home, work areas, and stairwells need to be lighted properly. Light fixtures need high-wattage bulbs with wider illumination. Stairwells need a light switch at both the top and bottom of the stairs. It is also important to be sure that lighting on the stairs does not cast shadows. Have a family member paint the edge of steps (preferably bright yellow) so that the patient can see each step, especially the first and last, clearly. When possible, have patients replace steps inside and outside the home with ramps.

An added consideration is to administer eye medications safely (see Chapter 31). Patients need to closely adhere to regular medication schedules for conditions such as glaucoma. Labels on medication containers need to be in large print. Make sure that a family caregiver is familiar with dosage schedules in case a patient is unable to self-administer a medication. Patients with visual impairments often have difficulty manipulating eyedroppers.

Adaptations for Reduced Hearing. Patients hear important environmental sounds (e.g., doorbells and alarm clocks) best if they are amplified or changed to a lower-pitched, buzzer-like sound. Lamps designed to turn on in response to sounds such as doorbells, burglar alarms, smoke detectors, and babies crying are also available. Family members or anyone else who calls the patient regularly needs to learn to let the phone ring for a longer period. Amplified receivers for telephones and telephone communication devices (TCDs) that use a computer and printer to transfer words over the telephone for people with a hearing impairment are available. Both sender and receiver need to have the special device to complete a call.

Adaptations for Reduced Olfaction. A patient with a reduced sensitivity to odors is often unable to smell leaking gas, a smoldering cigarette, fire, or spoiled food. Advise patients to use smoke detectors and take precautions such as checking ashtrays or placing cigarette butts in water. In addition, teach patients to check food package expiration dates, inspect the appearance of food, and keep leftovers in labeled containers with the preparation date. Pilot gas flames need to be checked visually.

Adaptations for Reduced Tactile Sensation. When patients have reduced sensation in their extremities, they are at risk for impaired skin integrity and injury from exposure to temperature extremes. Always caution these patients about the use of heating and cooling devices (see Chapter 48). The temperature setting on the home's water heater should be no higher than 48.8°C (120°F). If a patient also has a visual impairment, it is important to be sure that water faucets are clearly marked "hot" and "cold" or use color codes (i.e., red for hot and blue for cold). Discourage the use of heating pads in this population.

Communication. A sensory deficit often causes a person to feel isolated because of an inability to communicate with others. It is important for individuals to be able to interact with people around them. The nature of the sensory loss influences the methods and styles of communication that nurses use during interactions with patients (Box 49.8). Teach family members and significant others about how to use communication methods effectively.

For patients with visual deficits or blindness, speak normally, not from a distance, and be sure to have sufficient lighting. If possible, when describing objects have the person touch the object.

The patient with a hearing impairment is often able to speak normally. To hear more clearly what a person communicates, family and friends need to learn to move away from background noise, avoid dropping their voice at the end of a sentence, speak slightly slower, rephrase rather than repeat sentences, be positive, and have patience. In a group setting it is better to form a semicircle in front of the patient so that the patient can see who is speaking next; this helps foster group involvement. On the other hand, some patients who are deaf have serious speech alterations. Some use sign language or lipreading, wear special hearing aids, write with a pad and pencil, or learn to use a computer for communication. Special communication boards that contain common terms (e.g., *pain, bathroom, dizzy,* or *walk*) help patients express their needs.

Patient education is one aspect of communication. Teaching booklets are available in large print for patients with visual loss. The patient who is blind often requires more frequent and detailed verbal descriptions of information. This is particularly true if there are no instructional booklets written in Braille. Patients with visual impairments can also learn by listening to audiotapes or the sound part of a televised teaching session. Patients with hearing impairments often benefit from written instructional materials and visual teaching aids (e.g., posters and graphs). Demonstrations by the nurse are very useful. Health care agencies are required to make professional interpreters available to read sign language for patients who are deaf.

BOX 49.8 Communication Methods

Patients With Aphasia
- Listen to the patient and provide sufficient time to communicate.
- Do not shout or speak loudly (hearing loss is not the problem).
- If patient has problems with comprehension, use simple, short questions and facial gestures to give additional clues.
- Speak of things familiar and of interest to patient.
- If patient has problems speaking, ask questions that require simple yes-or-no answers or blinking of the eyes. Offer pictures or a communication board so patient can point.
- Speak slowly and give patient time to understand; be calm and patient; do not pressure or tire the patient.
- Avoid patronizing and childish phrases.

Patients With an Artificial Airway
- Use pictures, objects, or word cards so patient can point.
- Offer a pad and pencil or Magic Slate for patient to write messages.
- Do not shout or speak loudly.
- Give patient time to write messages because patients tire easily.
- Provide an artificial voice box (vibrator) for patient with a laryngectomy to use to speak.

Patients With Hearing Impairment
- Get patient's attention. Do not startle the patient when entering the room. Do not approach patient from behind. Be sure patient knows that you want to speak.
- Face patient and stand or sit on the same level. Be sure that your face and lips are illuminated to promote lipreading. Keep hands away from mouth.
- Be sure that the environment is not noisy.
- Be sure that patients keep eyeglasses clean, so they are able to see your gestures and face.
- If patient wears a hearing aid, make sure that it is in place and working.
- Speak slowly and articulate clearly. Sometimes people with hearing loss take longer to process verbal messages.
- Use a normal tone of voice and inflections of speech. Do not speak with something in your mouth.
- When you are not understood, rephrase rather than repeat the conversation.
- Use visible expressions. Speak with your hands, face, and eyes.
- Do not shout. Loud sounds are usually higher pitched and often impede hearing by accentuating vowel sounds and concealing consonants. If you need to raise your voice, speak in lower tones.
- Talk toward patient's better or normal ear.
- Use written information to enhance the spoken word.
- Do not restrict the hands of patient who is deaf. Never have intravenous lines in both of patient's hands if the preferred method of communication is sign language.
- Avoid eating, chewing, or smoking while speaking.
- Avoid speaking from another room or while walking away.

Acute Care. You will use different approaches to maximize existing sensory function when caring for patients who are admitted to acute care settings for therapeutic management of sensory deficits. Sometimes patients experience sensory deficits because of a traumatic injury. Safety is an obvious priority until a patient's sensory status is either stabilized or improved. For example, patients with sensory deficits have a high risk for falls in the acute care environment. It is very important to know the extent of any existing sensory impairment before the acute episode of illness so that you are able to reinforce what the patient already knows about self-care or to plan for more instruction before and after discharge.

Orientation to the Environment. A patient with a sensory impairment requires a complete orientation to the immediate environment. Provide reorientation as needed to their environment by ensuring that name tags on uniforms are visible, addressing the patient by name, explaining where the patient is (especially if patients are transported to different areas for treatment), and using conversational cues to time or location. Reduce the tendency for patients to become confused by offering short, simple, repeated explanations and reassurance. Encourage family members and visitors to help orient patients to the agency's surroundings.

Patients with serious visual impairment need to feel safe and comfortable in knowing the boundaries of the immediate environment. Normally people see physical boundaries within a room. Patients who are blind or severely visually impaired often touch the boundaries or objects to gain a sense of their surroundings. The patient needs to walk through a room and feel the walls to establish a sense of direction. Help patients by explaining objects within the hospital room such as furniture or equipment. It takes time for a patient to absorb room arrangement. The patient often needs to reorient again as you explain the location of key items (e.g., nurse call system, telephone, and chair). Remember to approach from the front to avoid startling the patient.

It is important to keep all objects in the same position and place. After an object is moved even a short distance, it no longer exists for a person who is blind. Simply moving a chair creates a safety hazard. Ask the patient whether any item needs to be rearranged to make ambulation easier. Clear traffic patterns to the bathroom. Give the patient extra time to perform tasks. The patient moves slowly to remain safe and needs a detailed description of how to perform an activity.

Patients confined to bed are at risk for sensory deprivation. Normally, movement gives an awareness of self through vestibular and tactile stimulation. Movement patterns influence sensory perception. The limited movement of bed rest changes how a person interprets the environment; surroundings seem different, and objects seem to assume shapes different from normal. A person who is on bed rest requires routine stimulation through range-of-motion exercises, positioning, and participation in self-care activities (as appropriate). Comfort measures, such as washing the face and hands and providing back rubs, improve the quality of stimulation and lessen the chance of sensory deprivation. Planning time to talk with patients is also essential. Explain unfamiliar environmental noises and sensations. A calm, unhurried approach gives you quality time to help reorient and familiarize the patient with care activities. The patient who is well enough to read will benefit from a variety of reading materials.

Communication. The most common language disorder following a stroke is aphasia. Depending on the type of aphasia, the inability to communicate is often frustrating and frightening (see Box 49.8). Initially you need to establish very basic communication and recognize that it does not indicate intellectual impairment or a change in the patient's personality. Patients with aphasia are usually able to understand what is said to them. Therefore explain situations and treatments that are pertinent to the patient. Because a stroke often causes partial or complete paralysis of one side of a patient's body, some patients need special assistive devices. A variety of communication boards for different levels of disability are available. Sensitive pressure switches activated by the touch of an ear, nose, or chin control electronic communication boards (Touhy and Jett, 2022). Recommend to health care providers referrals to speech therapists to develop appropriate rehabilitation plans.

In acute care or long-term care agencies, nurses often care for patients with artificial airways (such as an endotracheal tube) (see Chapter 41). The placement of an endotracheal tube prevents a patient from speaking. In this case the nurse uses special communication methods to facilitate the patient's ability to express needs. The patient is sometimes completely alert and able to hear and see the nurse normally. Giving the patient time to convey any needs or requests is very important. Use creative communication techniques (e.g., a communication board or electronic tablet) to foster and strengthen the patient's interactions with health care personnel, family, and friends.

Controlling Sensory Stimuli. Hospitalized patients require time for rest and freedom from stress caused by frequent monitoring and repeated tests. Reduce sensory overload by organizing the patient's care. Combine activities such as dressing changes, bathing, and vital sign measurements in one visit to conserve a patient's energy and prevent fatigue. Schedule time for rest and quiet if possible. Planning for rest periods often requires cooperation from family, visitors, and health care colleagues. Coordination with laboratory and radiology departments minimizes the number of interruptions for procedures. A creative solution to decrease excessive environmental stimuli that prevents restful, healing sleep is to institute "quiet time" in ICUs. Quiet time means implementing dimming the lights throughout the unit, closing the shades, and shutting the doors. Data collected from one hospital showed that implementing a quiet time protocol in the ICU improved the patients' sleep quality and decreased the incidence of sleep disorders (Lim, 2018; Tabas et al., 2019) (Box 49.9).

When patients experience sensory overload or deprivation, their behavior is often difficult for family or friends to accept. Encourage the family not to argue with or contradict the patient but to calmly explain location, identity, and time of day. Engaging a patient in a normal discussion about familiar topics helps in reorientation. Anticipating patient needs such as voiding helps reduce uncomfortable stimuli.

Try to control extraneous noise in and around a patient's room. It is often necessary to ask a roommate to lower the volume on a television or to move the patient to a quieter room. Keep equipment noise to a minimum. Turn off bedside equipment not in use such as suction and oxygen equipment. Avoid making abrupt loud noises such as dropping objects or causing the over-bed table to suddenly adjust to the lowest level. Nursing staff also need to control laughter or conversation outside patients' rooms. Allow patients to close their room doors.

When a patient leaves an acute care setting for the home environment, communicate with colleagues in the home care setting about the patient's existing sensory deficits and the interventions that helped the patient adapt to sensory problems. You achieve continuity of care when the patient has to make only minimal changes in the home setting.

Safety Measures. A patient with recent visual impairment often requires help with walking. The presence of an eye patch, frequently instilled eyedrops, and the swelling of eyelid structures following surgery are just a few factors that cause a patient to need more help than usual. Nurses provide ambulatory assistance in health care settings. A "sighted guide" (such as a family member trained in ambulation techniques) is a resource for home care patients. A sighted guide gives confidence to patients with visual impairments and ensures safe mobility. Bosma Enterprises (2021) lists several suggestions for a sighted guide:

1. To ambulate a patient safely, offer your assistance and hold out your arm. Tap the back of your hand against the patient's hand. The person will then grasp your arm directly above the elbow (Fig. 49.5).
2. Walk one step ahead of the person you are guiding, except at the top and bottom of stairs and streets. At these places pause and stand alongside the person. Be sure that the person has a strong grasp on your arm. Relax and walk at a comfortable pace.
3. While walking with a patient, describe the surroundings and ensure that obstacles have been removed. Never leave a patient with a visual impairment standing alone in an unfamiliar area.
4. To guide a person to a seat, place the person's hand on the back of the seat. The person you are guiding will find the seat by following along your arm.

Nursing staff need to ensure that the patient knows the location of the nurse call system before leaving the patient alone. Place necessary

---

BOX 49.9 EVIDENCE-BASED PRACTICE

Quiet Time and Improved Patient Well-Being

PICOT Question: Does a "quiet time" intervention compared with routine intensive care unit (ICU) practices improve sleep quality and satisfaction with care in critically ill hospitalized patients?

Evidence Summary

A quiet environment promotes rest and healing, but many factors contribute to a noisy health care environment. The number of patient rooms and design of the unit, as well as admissions and discharges throughout the day, influence noise levels in health care settings. One strategy suggested to reduce noise to recommended levels is a "quiet time" intervention. "Quiet time" is observed in a number of different ways, but current evidence supports that limiting conversations, eliminating environmental noise, and dimming the lights effectively reduces noise (Goeren et al., 2018; Zauche et al., 2021). Although it can be challenging to create a daily period without distractions, current evidence shows that "quiet time" interventions have improved patients' sleep quality, well-being, restfulness, and satisfaction with care (Tabas et al., 2019; McGough et al., 2018; Lim, 2018).

Application to Nursing Practice

- Encourage visitors to take breaks to allow patients time to rest (Church, 2020).
- Designate areas away from patient rooms for phone conversations and for the health care team to conduct student teaching sessions (Goeren et al., 2018; Zauche et al., 2021).
- Collaborate with the interprofessional team to provide "quiet time" for patients (Sarkar et al., 2021; Goeren et al., 2018).
- Review alarm parameters and adjust the default settings as appropriate (Goeren et al., 2018; Lim, 2018).
- Establish a unit-based "noise reduction program" to modify health care team workflow (e.g., change of shift, health care team rounding) to establish a restful environment for patients during "quiet time" (Sarkar et al., 2021).

FIG. 49.5 Nurse helps to ambulate patient with visual impairment. (From Sorrentino SA, Remmert LN: *Mosby's essentials for nursing assistants*, ed 6, St Louis, 2019, Elsevier.)

objects in front of the patient to prevent falls caused by reaching over the bedside. Appropriate use of side rails is also an option.

Nurses often rely on patients in health care settings to report unusual sounds such as a suction apparatus running improperly or an IV pump alarm. However, a patient with a hearing loss does not always hear these sounds and thus requires more frequent visits by nurses. The patient also benefits from learning to use vision to discover sources of danger. It is wise to note on the intercom system at the nurse's station and in the medical record if the patient is deaf and/or blind. A patient lacking the ability to speak cannot call out for assistance. Patients need to have message boards and nurse call system close at hand.

Patients with reduced tactile sensation risk injury when their conditions confine them to bed because they are unable to sense pressure on bony prominences or the need to change position. These patients rely on nurses for timely repositioning, moving tubes or devices on which the patient is lying, and turning to avoid skin breakdown. When a patient is less able to sense temperature variations, use extra caution in applying heat and cold therapies (see Chapter 48) and preparing bathwater. Check the condition of the patient's skin frequently.

Restorative and Continuing Care

Maintaining Healthy Lifestyles. After a patient has experienced a sensory loss, it becomes important to understand the implications of the loss and make adjustments needed to continue a normal lifestyle. Sensory impairments do not need to prevent a person from leading an active, rewarding life. Many of the interventions applicable to health promotion such as adapting the home environment are useful after a patient leaves an acute care setting.

Understanding Sensory Loss. Help patients who have experienced a recent sensory loss understand how to adapt so that their living environments are safe and appropriately stimulating. All family members need to understand how a patient's sensory impairment affects normal daily activities. Family and friends are more supportive when they understand sensory deficits and factors that worsen or lessen sensory problems. For example, explain how they can communicate with someone who has a hearing loss. Community resources are available to provide information to help patients with personal management needs. The American Foundation for the Blind, American Red Cross, and National Association for Speech and Hearing offer resource materials and product information.

Socialization. The ability to communicate is gratifying. It tests a person's intellect, opens opportunities, and allows an opportunity to exchange the feelings the person has about others. When sensory alterations hinder interactions, a person feels ineffective and loses self-esteem. When patients feel socially unaccepted, they perceive sensory losses as seriously impairing their quality of life.

Interacting with others becomes a burden for many patients with sensory alterations. They lose the motivation to engage in social situations, resulting in a deep sense of loneliness. Use therapies to reduce loneliness, particularly in older adults (Box 49.10). These principles support the *Healthy People 2030* (ODPHP, n.d.) objective to increase the proportion of adults with disabilities reporting sufficient emotional support. In addition, family members need to learn to focus on a person's ability to interact rather than on the disability. For example, do not assume that a person who is hard of hearing does not want to speak. A person who is blind can still enjoy a walk through a park with a companion who is describing the sights around them.

Promoting Self-Care. The ability to perform self-care is essential for self-esteem. Frequently family members and nurses believe that people with sensory impairments require assistance, when in fact they are able

---

BOX 49.10 FOCUS ON OLDER ADULTS

Principles for Reducing Loneliness in Patients With Sensory Impairments

- Spend time with a person in silence or conversation.
- When it is culturally appropriate, use physical contact (e.g., holding a hand, embracing a shoulder) to convey caring.
- Recommend alterations in living arrangements if physical isolation is a factor.
- Help patients maintain contact with people important to them.
- Provide information about support groups or groups that provide assistive services.
- Arrange for security escort services as needed.
- Introduce the idea of bringing a companion such as a pet into the home when appropriate.
- Link a person with organizations attuned to the social needs of older adults.

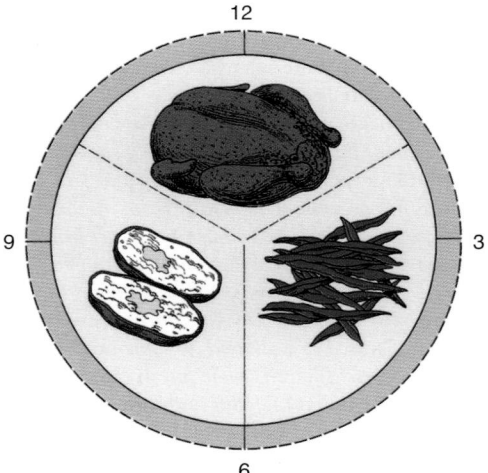

FIG. 49.6 Location of food using clock as frame of reference.

to help themselves. To help with meals, arrange food on the plate and condiments, salad, or drinks according to numbers on the face of a clock (Fig. 49.6). A patient can also use this method to place personal care items on the bedside or on the bathroom vanity. It is easy for a patient to become oriented to the items after you or a family member explains the location of each item. Low-vision optical devices are beneficial for a visually impaired person. These devices are grouped into two categories: "near" activities such as reading and hobbies, or "distance" activities such as reading street signs and going to the movies (Touhy and Jett, 2022).

Help patients reach toilet facilities safely. Safety bars need to be installed near the toilet. It is often helpful when the bar is a different color than the wall for easier visibility. Never place towels on a safety bar because they interfere with a person's grasp. Have the patient keep toilet paper within easy reach. Sharply contrasting colors within the room help people who are partially sighted and promote functional independence. General principles for promoting self-care in older adults also include the assurance of adequate lighting and the control of glare by using shades and blinds (Touhy and Jett, 2020).

If the sense of touch is diminished, a patient can dress more easily with zippers or Velcro strips, pullover sweaters or blouses, and elasticized waists. A patient with partial paralysis and reduced sensation dresses the affected side first. Encourage family members responsible for selecting clothing for patients with visual impairments to follow the patient's preferences. Any sensory impairment has a significant influence on body image; therefore it is important for a patient to feel well-groomed and attractive. Some patients need assistance with basic grooming such as brushing, combing, and shampooing hair. Others need assistance with medication administration, clothing identification, and learning to manage routine procedures such as blood pressure and glucose monitoring. An assortment of low-vision devices is now available. It is important for you to make appropriate referrals to allow patients to maintain a maximum degree of independence.

Patients with proprioceptive problems often lose their balance easily. Make sure that bathrooms have nonskid surfaces in the tub and shower. Install grab bars either vertically or horizontally in tubs and showers, depending on how a patient is able to grasp or hold onto the bar. Instruct family members to supervise ambulation and sitting, make frequent checks to prevent falls, and caution the patient against leaning forward.

Dilyana knows that visual changes affect patients differently. She also knows that some of the interventions she selects will require the assistance of Ms. Long's family. **Risk for Injury** *and* **Risk for Fall** *are priority nursing diagnoses because they are related to her safety. Other applicable nursing diagnoses include* **Fear** *and* **Anxiety.**

Dilyana plans a home visit to facilitate care plan measures. Antonio, Ms. Long's son, is home during the home health visit. Dilyana explains to Ms. Long and Antonio some of the environmental trip hazards in the home and asks if they are willing to modify them. Antonio states that he can pick up the throw rugs and he will arrange to get brighter light bulbs to install in the hallways, stairwell, and front porch. Dilyana asks Ms. Long, "One way to prevent yourself from falling is to make sure you are maintaining your strength. Do you do any exercises regularly?" Ms. Long responds, "I used to walk and do some exercises, but since my eyesight has gotten worse, I haven't done any of that. It makes me really uncomfortable. I'm afraid that I'll fall if I exercise." Dilyana says, "Sometimes when people experience reduced eyesight, they have a hard time concentrating. Have you experienced this at all?" Antonio laughs and says, "Mom, maybe this is why you've been having trouble remembering things lately." Ms. Long responds, "And all this time I thought it was because I was getting old!"

After Dilyana leaves Ms. Long's house, she reflects on her visit with Ms. Long and Antonio. She plans to contact Antonio later and ask if he was able to make all the modifications to the home that they discussed. She also realizes that helping Ms. Long manage her anxiety and fear is becoming a higher priority. Therefore Dilyana plans to start teaching some strength-training exercises, explore how Ms. Long has dealt with fear and anxiety in the past, and teach some healthy options to help Ms. Long manage anxiety and fear during her next visit.

◆ Evaluation

Through the Patient's Eyes. It is important to evaluate whether patients perceive that their care maintained or improved their ability to interact and function within the environment. The patient is the source for evaluating whether expectations were met. Only patients can tell you if their sensory abilities are improving and which interventions or therapies are most successful in facilitating a change in their performance. Ask patients, for example, "Have we been able to meet your expectation of keeping you safe given your vision losses?" or "Tell me how we can improve ways to communicate with you."

If you have developed a positive relationship with a patient, note subtle behaviors that often indicate the level of the patient's satisfaction. You may notice that the patient responds appropriately, such as by smiling. However, it is important for you to ask the patient whether the sensory needs have been met. For example, ask, "Have we done all we can do to help improve your ability to hear?" If the patient's expectations have not been met, ask, "How can the health care team better meet your needs?" Working closely with the patient and family enables you to redefine expectations that can be met realistically within the limits of the patient's condition and therapies. Your care has been effective when the patient's goals and expectations have been met.

Patient Outcomes. To evaluate the effectiveness of specific nursing interventions, use clinical judgment and make comparisons with baseline sensory assessment data to evaluate if sensory alterations have changed (Fig. 49.7). It is your responsibility to determine whether expected outcomes have been met. For example, use evaluative data to determine whether your care improved or maintained a patient's ability to interact and function within the environment. The nature of a patient's sensory alterations influences how you evaluate the outcome of care. When caring for a patient with a hearing deficit, use proper communication techniques and then evaluate whether the patient gained the ability to hear or interact more effectively. When expected outcomes have not been achieved, there is a need to change interventions or alter the patient's environment. If outcomes are unmet, it is important to ask questions such as "How are you feeling emotionally?" or "Do you feel that you are at risk for injury?" Collaborate with family members to determine whether a patient's ability to function within the home has improved.

If you have directed nursing care at improving or maintaining sensory acuity, evaluate the integrity of the sensory organs and the patient's ability to perceive stimuli. Evaluate interventions designed to relieve problems associated with sensory alterations based on a patient's ability to function normally without injury. When you directly or indirectly (through education) alter a patient's environment, evaluate by observing whether the patient makes environmental changes. When designing patient teaching to improve sensory function, it is important to determine whether the patient is following recommended therapies and meeting mutually set goals. Asking a patient to explain or demonstrate self-care skills is an effective evaluative measure. It is often necessary to reinforce previous instruction if learning has not taken place. If outcomes are unmet, these are examples of questions to ask:

- "How often do you wear your hearing aids/corrective lenses?"
- "Are you able to participate in a small group discussion?"
- "Are you able to read (the newspaper, computer screen, your smart phone screen, and so on) without squinting?"

The results of your evaluation will determine whether to continue the existing plan of care, make modifications, or end the use of select interventions.

Dilyana returns to Ms. Long's home to evaluate the outcomes of her care. She will use this information to determine what interventions she will provide next. Dilyana asks Ms. Long and Antonio, "I see that you have removed quite a few of your throw rugs. Can you please describe the other changes you have made to your home since my last visit?" Antonio responds, "We got all the light bulbs changed. Boy, we didn't realize how dark it was in here until we did that. It's so much brighter in here!" Dilyana then asks Ms. Long, "Have you fallen, or have you been afraid of falling since I was here last?" Ms. Long responds, "No, I haven't fallen since you were here last. Getting rid of those rugs and changing the light bulbs has made a huge difference for me. I've really been looking forward to learning about some of those exercises you talked about the last time you were here. Are you ready for our workout?" Dilyana smiles and responds, "Yes, I am ready. Let's get started."

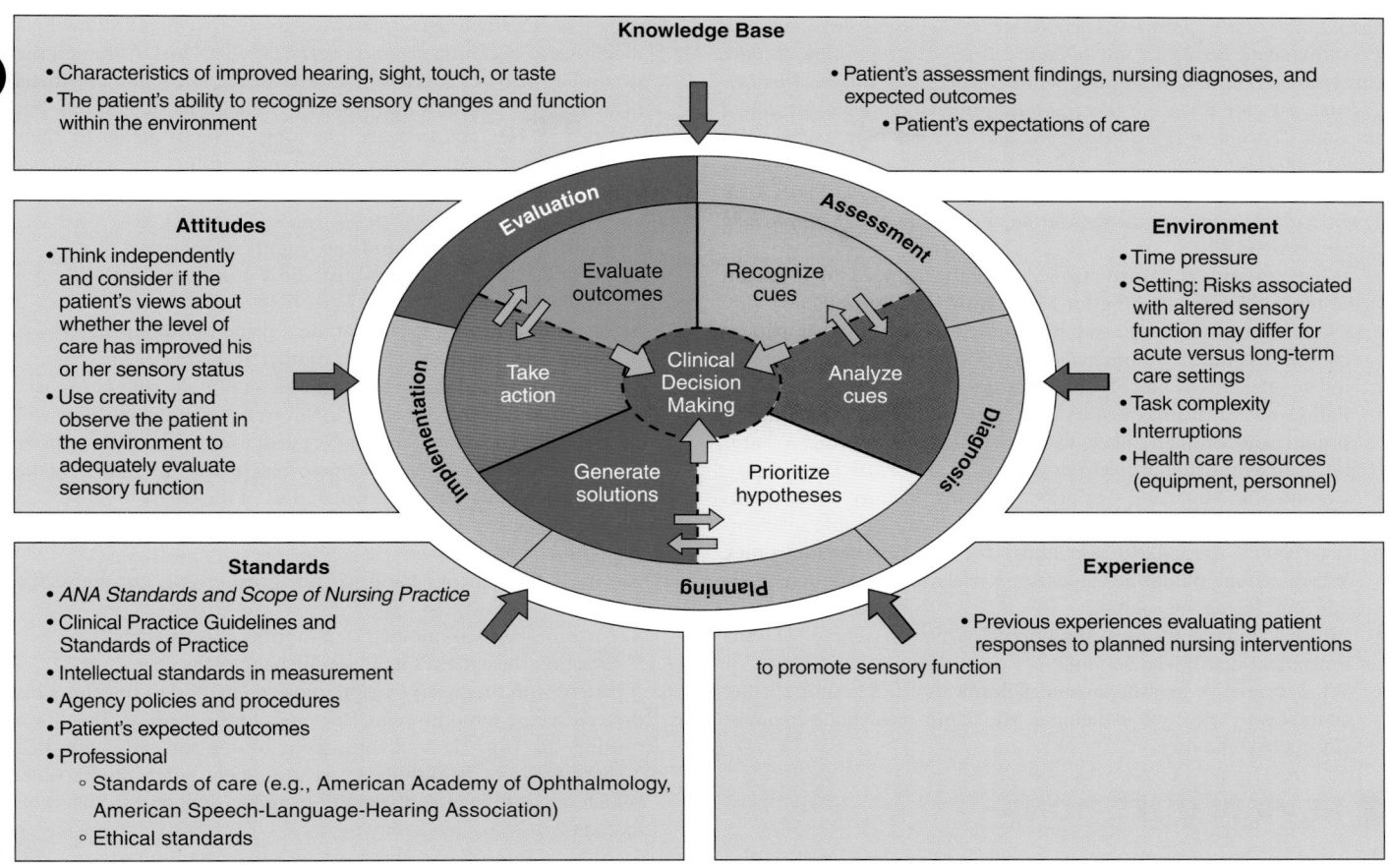

FIG. 49.7 Critical thinking model for sensory alterations evaluation. (Clinical Judgment Measurement Model copyright © NCSBN. All rights reserved.)

KEY POINTS

- Reception, perception, and reaction are the three components of any sensory experience. Your senses receive information from your environment. Perception occurs when you become conscious of a stimulus. You usually react to stimuli that are the most meaningful or significant.
- Sensory alterations occur when a person has difficulty receiving or perceiving stimuli (sensory deficits), when external stimuli are meaningless or deficient (sensory deprivation), or when there is excessive stimulation (sensory overload).
- Many factors affect sensory function. For example, aging results in a gradual decline of acuity in all senses, and excessive environmental stimuli cause sensory overload.
- Sensory alterations can affect a patient's well-being and limit the ability to interact and function within the environment.
- A thorough assessment of the sensory system, which includes components such as assessment of a patient's mental status, a physical assessment, and a survey of environmental hazards, allows you to develop and implement an individualized plan of care.
- You make clinical judgments about a patient's sensory problems by using critical thinking, anticipating expected signs and symptoms of a sensory condition, and matching with data you gather from a patient.
- While assessing a patient's sensory alteration, consider the pathophysiology of the patient's deficit and the degree to which the deficit affects the patient's lifestyle, health, and safety.

- Select nursing diagnoses after reviewing patterns of assessment findings that reveal alterations in the patient's ability to function.
- Involve your patient to develop a realistic plan and prioritize nursing diagnoses and outcomes after taking time to recognize and analyze cues that indicate what is important to your patient and how your patient is affected by sensory deficits.
- Preventive actions and the early identification of sensory alterations require periodic health screenings.
- Involve patients and their families to create effective individualized plans of care that help patients adapt to alterations in sensory function.
- Analyze hazards in the environment when recommending and implementing strategies to reduce the risk of injury in patients with sensory deficits.
- When evaluating care, include your patient's perceptions and use evaluative data to determine if your care improved or maintained your patient's ability to interact and function in the environment.

REFLECTIVE LEARNING

Dilyana is now assigned to care for Elmer Bland, a 75-year-old man who has type 2 diabetes. He is experiencing numbness in his fingers and toes due to diabetic peripheral neuropathy. He also is hard of hearing and wears hearing aids. Mr. Bland is married to Martha, and his daughter, Jessie, lives three blocks down the street with her family. Mr. and Mrs. Bland watch their three grandchildren when they get out of school until Jessie and her husband come home. Dilyana plans to assess the home, paying special attention to potential safety hazards. She begins her home visit by introducing herself to the Blands. During the beginning of their conversation, Dilyana notices that Mr. Bland has difficulty hearing her. Dilyana asks the Blands to identify their primary concerns. Mr. Bland responds, "I want to stay in my home and keep my independence. It's really important for me to be able to take care of my grandkids too. They're here every day after school. I just need to know what I need to do to make sure our house is safe for Martha, the kids, and me. Can you help us figure this out?"

- What assessment information does Dilyana need to focus on immediately while caring for Mr. Bland? (Recognize Cues)
- Considering Mr. Bland and his family's situation, what patient conditions and environmental factors will affect Mr. Bland's ability to live safely in his home? (Analyze Cues)
- Reflect on Mr. Bland's history and assessment data. Which health problems is Mr. Bland likely to be currently experiencing? What is his priority nursing problem or diagnosis? (Prioritize Diagnoses)
- Considering Mr. Bland's priority problems, identify two patient-centered outcomes and describe what actions or nursing interventions would most likely help him achieve the desired outcomes. Which actions should be avoided, are irrelevant, or are potentially harmful? (Generate Solutions)
- Which actions are the most appropriate? Which ones should Dilyana implement first? (Take Action)
- What evaluative measures could Dilyana use to determine if her actions were effective in helping Mr. Bland meet his outcomes? (Evaluate Outcomes)

■ REVIEW QUESTIONS

1. A patient has been on contact isolation for 4 days because of a hospital-acquired infection. He has had few visitors and few opportunities to leave his room. His ambulation is also still limited. Which are the correct nursing interventions to reduce sensory deprivation? (Select all that apply.)
   1. Encourage him to participate in activities he can do in his room such as reading and doing crossword puzzles.
   2. Move him to a room away from the nurses' station.
   3. Turn on the lights and open the room blinds.
   4. Sit down when talking with him and listen to his feelings and perceptions.
   5. Provide auditory stimulation for the patient by keeping the television on continuously.
2. A home care nurse is planning care for a patient with a visual impairment. Which strategies does the nurse plan to implement? (Select all that apply.)
   1. Use of fluorescent lighting
   2. Use of warm incandescent lighting
   3. Use of yellow or amber lenses to decrease glare
   4. Use of adjustable blinds, sheer curtains, or draperies
   5. Use of indirect lighting to reduce glare
3. An older-adult patient with bilateral hearing loss wears a hearing aid in her left ear. Which of the following approaches best facilitates communication with her? (Select all that apply.)
   1. Talk to the patient at a distance so she can read your lips.
   2. Keep your arms at your side; speak directly into the patient's left ear.
   3. Face the patient when speaking; demonstrate ideas you wish to convey.
   4. Position the patient so that the light is on her face when speaking.
   5. Verify that the information that has been given has been clearly understood.

4. A patient is returning to an assisted-living apartment following a diagnosis of declining vision/progressive visual loss. Although she is familiar with her apartment and residence, she reports feeling a little uncertain about walking alone. There is one step up into her apartment. Her children are planning to be available to their mother for the next 2 weeks. Which of the following approaches will you teach the children to assist ambulation? (Select all that apply.)
   1. Walk one-half step behind and slightly to her side.
   2. Have her grasp your arm just above the elbow and walk at a comfortable pace.
   3. Stand next to your mother at the top and bottom of stairs.
   4. Stand one step ahead of your mother at the top of the stairs.
   5. Place yourself alongside your mother and hold onto her waist.
5. A new nurse is going to help a patient walk down the corridor and sit in a chair. The patient has an eye patch over the left eye and poor vision in the right eye. What is the correct order of steps to help the patient safely walk down the hall and sit in the chair?
   1. Tell the patient when you are approaching the chair.
   2. Walk at a relaxed pace.
   3. Guide the patient's hand to your arm, resting just above the elbow.
   4. Position yourself one-half step in front of the patient.
   5. Position the patient's hand on the back of the chair.
6. A patient with progressive vision impairments had to surrender his driver's license 6 months ago. He comes to the medical clinic for a routine checkup. He is accompanied by his son. His wife died 2 years ago, and he admits to feeling lonely much of the time. Which of the following interventions reduce loneliness? (Select all that apply.)
   1. Sharing information about senior transportation services
   2. Reassuring the patient that loneliness is a normal part of aging
   3. Maintaining distance while talking to avoid overstimulating the patient
   4. Providing information about local social groups in the patient's neighborhood
   5. Recommending that the patient consider making living arrangements that will put him closer to family or friends
7. A nurse is performing an assessment on a patient admitted to the unit following treatment in the emergency department for severe bilateral eye trauma. During patient admission the nurse's priority interventions include which of the following? (Select all that apply.)
   1. Conducting a home-safety assessment and identifying hazards in the patient's living environment
   2. Reinforcing eye safety at work and in activities that place the patient at risk for eye injury
   3. Placing necessary objects such as the nurse call system and water in front of the patient to prevent falls caused by reaching
   4. Orienting the patient to the environment to reduce anxiety and prevent further injury to the eyes
   5. Alerting other nurses and health care providers about patient's visual status during hand-off reports
8. An older adult with pneumonia is admitted from a skilled nursing home to a medical unit. A review of the medical record reveals that he had a stroke affecting the right hemisphere of the brain 6 months ago and was placed in the skilled nursing home because he was unable to care for himself. Which of these assessment findings does the nurse expect to find? (Select all that apply.)
   1. Slow, cautious behavioral style
   2. Inattention and neglect, especially to the left side
   3. Cloudy or opaque areas in part of the lens or the entire lens

4. Visual spatial alterations such as loss of half of a visual field
5. Loss of sensation and motor function on the right side of the body
9. A nurse is performing a home care assessment on a patient with a hearing impairment. The patient reports, "I think my hearing aid is broken. I can't hear anything." After determining that the patient's hearing aid works and that the patient is having trouble managing the hearing aid at home, which of the following teaching strategies does the nurse implement? (Select all that apply.)
   1. Demonstrate hearing aid battery replacement.
   2. Review method to check volume on hearing aid.
   3. Demonstrate how to wash the earmold and microphone with hot water.
   4. Discuss the importance of having wax buildup in the ear canal removed.
   5. Recommend a chemical cleaner to remove difficult buildup.
10. A nurse is caring for a patient who has lost the feeling on one side of his body. For each intervention listed, indicate with an **X** whether the intervention would be effective, ineffective, or unrelated to the person's problem.

Intervention	Effective	Ineffective	Unrelated
1. Test bath water with the hand or foot on the side of the body that has lost sensation.			
2. Instruct the patient to wear shoes that fit well.			
3. Teach the patient and family how to check the pulse before going on a walk.			
4. Shift weight or stand up and move every hour.			
5. Teach the patient to use heating pads or hot water bottles on the affected side to bring the feeling back.			

Answers: 1. 1, 3, 4; **2.** 2, 3, 4; **3.** 3, 5; **4.** 2, 3; **5.** 4, 2, 3; **6.** 1, 5; **7.** 3, 4, 5; **8.** 2, 4; **9.** 1, 2, 4; **10.** See Evolve.

Rationales for Review Questions can be found on the Evolve website.

REFERENCES

American Foundation for the Blind (AFB): *Facts and figures on adults with vision loss*, 2020. https://www.afb.org/research-and-initiatives/statistics/adults. Accessed April 7, 2021.

American Optometric Association (AOA): *Senior vision: over 60 years of age*, n.d.a. https://www.aoa.org/healthy-eyes/eye-health-for-life/senior-vision?sso=y. Accessed April 11, 2021.

American Optometric Association (AOA): *Glaucoma*, n.d.b. https://www.aoa.org/healthy-eyes/eye-and-vision-conditions/glaucoma?sso=y Accessed April 11, 2021.

American Optometric Association: *Computer vision syndrome*, n.d.c. https://www.aoa.org/patients-and-public/caring-for-your-vision/protecting-your-vision/computer-vision-syndrome. Accessed April 11, 2021.

American Speech-Language-Hearing Association: *Hearing screening*, 1997-2021. https://www.asha.org/public/hearing/Hearing-Screening/. Accessed April 11, 2021.

Bosma Enterprises: *Human guide techniques*, 2021. https://www.bosma.org/Navigating-Blindness/Sighted-Guide-Techniques. Accessed April 11, 2021.

Burton MJ, et al: *The Lancet Global Health Commission on global eye health: vision beyond 2020*, 2021. https://www.thelancet.com/journals/langlo/article/PIIS2214-109X(20)30488-5/fulltext?utm_source=miragenews&utm_medium=miragenews&utm_campaign=news#seccestitle410. Accessed April 7, 2021.

Centers for Disease Control and Prevention (CDC): *Keep an eye on your vision health*, 2020. https://www.cdc.gov/visionhealth/resources/features/keep-eye-on-vision-health.html. Accessed April 11, 2021.

Church L: Quiet time during postpartum hospitalization can improve rest, bonding, and breastfeeding, *Nurs Womens Health* 24(3):197–201, 2020.

Dickinson P, et al: Integrating the National Council of State Boards of Nursing Clinical Judgment Model into nursing educational frameworks, *J Nurs Educ* 58(2): 72–78, 2019.

Hockenberry MJ, et al: *Wong's nursing care of infants and children*, ed 11, St. Louis, 2019, Elsevier.

Institute for Patient- and Family-Centered Care: *Advancing the practice of patient- and family-centered care in primary care and other ambulatory settings*, 2016. http://www.ipfcc.org/resources/GettingStarted-Ambulatory Care.pdf. Accessed April 11, 2021.

Interprofessional Education Collaborative Expert Panel: *Core competencies for interprofessional collaborative practice: 2016 update*, 2016. https://nebula.wsimg.com/2f68a39520b03336b41038c370497473?AccessKeyId=DC06780E69ED19E2B3A5&disposition=0&alloworigin=1. Accessed April 11, 2021.

Mayo Clinic: *Earwax blockage*, 1998-2021. https://www.mayoclinic.org/diseases-conditions/earwax-blockage/diagnosis-treatment/drc-20353007. Accessed April 11, 2021.

National Association of School Nurses (NASN): *Vision and eye health*, 2021. https://www.nasn.org/nasn-resources/practice-topics/vision-health. Accessed April 7, 2021.

National Institute of Neurological Disorders and Stroke (NINDS): *Carpal tunnel syndrome fact sheet*, 2020. https://www.ninds.nih.gov/Disorders/Patient-Caregiver-Education/Fact-Sheets/Carpal-Tunnel-Syndrome-Fact-Sheet. Accessed April 11, 2021.

National Institute on Deafness and Other Communication Disorders (NIDCD): *Hearing loss and older adults*, 2018. https://www.nidcd.nih.gov/health/hearing-loss-older-adults. Accessed February 8, 2021.

National Institute on Deafness and Other Communication Disorders (NIDCD): *Noise-induced hearing loss*, 2019.

https://www.nidcd.nih.gov/health/noise-induced-hearing-loss. Accessed June 19, 2021.

Occupational Safety and Health Administration (OSHA): *Eye and face protection*, n.d. https://www.osha.gov/SLTC/eyefaceprotection/standards.html. Accessed April 11, 2021.

Office of Disease Prevention and Health Promotion (ODPHP): *Healthy People 2030*, n.d., US Department of Health and Human Services. https://health.gov/healthypeople. Accessed April 11, 2021.

Powell-Cope G, et al: Preventing falls and fall-related injuries at home, *Am J Nurs* 118(1):58, 2018.

Touhy T, Jett P: *Ebersole and Hess' gerontological nursing & healthy aging*, ed 6, St. Louis, 2022, Elsevier.

Touhy T, Jett P: *Ebersole and Hess' toward healthy aging: human needs & nursing response*, ed 10, St. Louis, 2020, Elsevier.

U.S. Department of Health and Human Services (USDHHS): *Vision*, 2020. https://www.healthypeople.gov/2020/topics-objectives/topic/vision/national-snapshot. Accessed April 11, 2021.

U.S. Food and Drug Administration (FDA): *CFR code of federal regulations title 21*, 2020. http://www.accessdata.fda.gov/scripts/cdrh/cfdocs/cfcfr/CFRSearch.cfm?fr=801.420. Accessed April 11, 2021.

U.S. Food and Drug Administration (FDA): *How to get hearing aids*, 2018. http://www.fda.gov/MedicalDevices/ProductsandMedicalProcedures/HomeHealthandConsumer/ConsumerProducts/HearingAids/ucm181479.htm. Accessed April 11, 2021.

World Health Organization (WHO): Blindness and vision impairment: key facts, 2021, https://www.who.int/news-room/fact-sheets/detail/blindness-and-visual-impairment. Accessed October 2021.

RESEARCH REFERENCES

Ghasemi A, et al: Effect of self-management educational program on vision-related quality of life among elderly with visual impairment, *J Evid Based Care* 8(1): 35–44, 2018.

Goeren D, et al: Quiet time: a noise reduction initiative in a neurosurgical intensive care unit, *Crit Care Nurse* 38(4):38, 2018.

Lim R: Benefits of quiet time interventions in the intensive care unit: a literature review, *Nurs Stand* 32(30):41, 2018.

McGough N, et al: Noise reduction in progressive care units, *J Nurs Care Qual* 33(2):166, 2018.

Nael V, et al: Visual impairment, uncorrected refractive errors, and activity limitations in older adults: findings from the three-city Alienor study, *Invest Ophthalmol Vis Sci* 58(4):2359, 2017.

Otte B, et al: Self-reported eyeglass use by US Medicare beneficiaries aged 65 years or older, *JAMA Ophthalmol* 136(9):1047, 2018.

Rodriguez E, et al: Increasing screening follow-up for vulnerable children: a partnership with schools, *Int J Environ Res Public Health* 15(8):1572, 2018.

Sarkar M, et al: Increased patient satisfaction in the post-anesthesia care unit with the implementation of a controlled noise reduction program, *J Perianesth Nurs* 36(1):3, 2021.

Servidoni AB, et al: Hearing loss in the elderly: is the Hearing Handicap Inventory for the elderly: screening version effective in diagnosis when compared to the audiometric test? *Int Arch Otorhinolaryngol* 22(1):1, 2018.

Tabas EE, et al: Effect of eye masks, earplugs, and quiet time protocol on sleep quality of patients admitted to the cardiac care unit: a clinical trial study, *Med Surg Nurs J* 8(3):1–6, 2019.

Tseng YC, et al: Quality of life in older adults with sensory impairments: a systematic review. *Qual Life Res* 27(8): 1957, 2018.

Varma R, et al: Visual impairment and blindness in adults in the United States: demographic and geographic variations from 2015 to 2050, *JAMA Ophthalmol* 134(7):802–809, 2016. doi:10.1001/jamaophthalmol. 2016.1284.

Yoon H, et al: Comparison of access to eye care appointments between patients with Medicaid and those with private insurance, *JAMA Ophthalmol* 136(6):622, 2018.

Zauche LH, et al: Influence of quiet time on the auditory environment of infants in the NICU, *J Obstet Gynecol Neonatal Nurs* 50(1):68–77, 2021.

Perioperative Nursing Care

OBJECTIVES

- Discuss the three phases of perioperative nursing.
- Explain the rationale for a nursing assessment of a patient's surgical risk factors.
- Identify co-morbid conditions that increase patient risks for postoperative complications.
- Explain the approach for assessing a patient's potential psychological response to impending surgery.
- Explain the influence a preoperative teaching plan can have on a patient's surgical recovery.
- Explain the rationale for postoperative exercises.
- Identify the benefits of early ambulation for the postoperative patient.
- Illustrate how a nurse uses sound clinical judgment when making an intraoperative assessment and how it promotes patient safety.
- Explain the differences between postoperative phases.
- Outline the components of SBAR communication for perioperative hand-off.
- Identify nursing care priorities for postoperative patients.
- List the principles for providing education to surgical patients during the restorative phase of recovery

KEY TERMS

Ambulatory surgery
American Society of Anesthesiologists (ASA)
American Society of PeriAnesthesia Nurses (ASPAN)
Association of periOperative Registered Nurses (AORN)
Atelectasis
Bariatric
Circulating nurse
Co-morbid

Conscious sedation
Enhanced Recovery After Surgery (ERAS)
General anesthesia
Informed consent
Intermittent pneumatic compression (IPC) stockings
Laparoscopy
Latex sensitivity
Local anesthesia
Malignant hyperthermia
Moribund

Never event
Obstructive sleep apnea (OSA)
Oxygen desaturation
Paralytic ileus
Perioperative nursing
Postoperative nausea and vomiting (PONV)
Postoperative urinary retention (POUR)
Preanesthesia care unit (PCU)
Preoperative teaching plan
Regional anesthesia
Scrub nurse

MEDIA RESOURCES

http://evolve.elsevier.com/Potter/fundamentals/
- Review Questions
- Video Clips
- Concept Map Creator
- Case Study with Questions

- Skills Performance Checklists
- Audio Glossary
- Content Updates
- Answers to QSEN Activity and Review Questions

Mr. Cooper is a 72-year-old patient scheduled for admission in 5 days for a bowel resection to remove a cancerous tumor. Jeff is the nurse in the preadmission center assigned to Mr. Cooper for his preoperative screening and preparation. Jeff has worked in the center for 2 years. During his initial encounter with Mr. Cooper, Jeff learns that the patient is alert and oriented to person, place, and time. He is attentive and answers questions appropriately. His vision and hearing are normal. The patient has not had major surgery before. He lives at home with his wife, to whom he has been married 42 years.

Jeff provides Mr. Cooper with an explanation of what has to be done before surgery, including bowel prep, diet restrictions, and what time to present at the hospital the day of surgery. Jeff also provides Mr. Cooper with a brief explanation of what to expect with his surgery.

Perioperative nursing includes a registered nurse's planned patient-centered approach in providing care to patients preoperatively, intraoperatively, and postoperatively. Through the application of national practice standards, the registered nurse's role in providing quality patient care before, during, and after surgery is crucial in maintaining patient safety. Perioperative nurses apply sound clinical judgment in the use of the nursing process to guide the delivery of care to patients in hospitals, surgical centers, and/or health care providers' offices. Nursing goals in the preoperative area are based on the following:
- Quality improvement and evidence-based practices through the application of current research and the generation of ideas for new research knowledge
- Patient safety through high-quality care

- Teamwork and collaboration
- Effective communication and interactions with a patient, the patient's family members, and the surgical team, fostering shared decision making
- The nursing process to conduct timely assessment and deliver interventions in all phases of surgery
- Advocacy for a patient and the patient's family
- Cost containment

Perioperative nursing includes multiple intersecting processes guided by theoretical knowledge, ethical principles, ongoing research, specialized clinical skills, and caring practices (Association of periOperative Registered Nurses, 2020a). A nurse working within the perioperative setting responds to complex and fluctuating clinical needs during a crucial period of a patient's surgical experience. A nurse who works in any perioperative setting relies on clinical reasoning skills to maintain strict infection control measures, monitor the patient's physical and psychological response to the surgical experience, communicate effectively with members of the surgical team, and emphasize patient safety in each phase of surgery. Effective teaching and discharge planning involving patients and their family members prevent or minimize complications and contribute to quality outcomes. A patient's smooth transition from admission into the health care system through recovery is the aim of quality perioperative care.

The surgical care of patients is evolving as a result of advancements in technology, which often result in less invasive surgeries and shortened lengths of stay. Surgery takes place in a variety of settings, including hospitals, ambulatory surgery centers, health care providers' offices, and even mobile units. The principles of caring for perioperative patients are basically the same, regardless of the setting, except for the timing and extent of therapy.

SCIENTIFIC KNOWLEDGE BASE

Classification of Surgery

The types of surgical procedures are classified according to seriousness, urgency, and purpose (Table 50.1). Although surgeries are classified as major or minor, any procedure can be considered major from the perspective of the patient and/or the family. Some procedures fall into more than one classification. For example, a colon resection to remove a malignant tumor is major in seriousness, urgent in urgency, and ablative in purpose. In many instances, the classifications intersect. Urgent procedures are major in seriousness. Frequently, the same procedure is performed for different reasons on different patients. For example, a gastrectomy may be performed as an emergency procedure to resect a bleeding ulcer or as an urgent procedure to remove a malignant tumor. Knowing the classifications assists in planning appropriate perioperative care.

Another type of surgical classification describes the condition of a patient facing impending surgery. The American Society of

---

TABLE 50.1 Classification of Surgical Procedures

Classification Type	Description	Example
Seriousness		
Major	Involves extensive reconstruction or alteration in body parts; poses great risks to well-being	Coronary artery bypass, colon resection, removal of larynx, resection of lung lobe
Minor	Involves minimal alteration in body parts; designed to correct deformities; involves minimal risks to well-being	Cataract extraction, facial plastic surgery, tooth extraction
Urgency		
Elective	Performed on basis of patient's choice; is not essential and is not always necessary for health	Bunionectomy; facial plastic surgery; hernia repair; breast reconstruction
Urgent	Necessary for patient's health; often prevents development of additional problems (e.g., tissue destruction or impaired organ function); not necessarily emergency	Excision of cancerous tumor; removal of gallbladder for stones; vascular repair for obstructed artery (e.g., coronary artery bypass)
Emergency	Must be done immediately to save life or preserve function of body part	Repair of perforated appendix or traumatic amputation; control of internal hemorrhaging
Purpose		
Diagnostic	Surgical exploration performed to confirm diagnosis; often involves removal of tissue for further diagnostic testing	Exploratory laparotomy (incision into peritoneal cavity to inspect abdominal organs); breast mass biopsy
Ablative	Excision or removal of diseased body part	Amputation; removal of appendix or an organ such as gallbladder (cholecystectomy)
Palliative	Relieves or reduces intensity of disease symptoms; does not produce cure	Colostomy; debridement of necrotic tissue; resection of nerve roots
Reconstructive/restorative	Restores function or appearance to traumatized or malfunctioning tissues	Internal fixation of fractures; scar revision
Procurement for transplant	Removal of organs and/or tissues from a person pronounced brain dead or from living donors for transplantation into another person	Kidney, heart, or liver transplant
Constructive	Restores function lost or reduced as result of congenital anomalies	Repair of cleft palate; closure of atrial septal defect in heart
Cosmetic	Performed to improve personal appearance	Blepharoplasty for eyelid deformities; rhinoplasty to reshape nose

Anesthesiologists (ASA, 2020) assigns classification on the basis of a patient's physiological condition independent of the proposed surgical procedure (Table 50.2). The classification is a risk assessment that allows surgeons and anesthesia providers to consider factors that influence how surgery will be performed. Anesthesia involves risks even in healthy patients; however, some patients, including but not limited to those with metabolic and cardiac dysfunction, are at higher risk.

Surgical Risk Factors

Numerous factors create risks for patients planning surgery. Risk factors can affect patients in any phase of the perioperative experience. One common risk factor for all patients is the surgical stress response. Physiologically, the stress of surgery causes activation of the endocrine system, resulting in the release of hormones and catecholamines, which increases blood pressure, heart rate, and respiration. Platelet aggregation also occurs, along with many other physiological responses. All patients will be affected physiologically by the stress response. Understanding the physiology of the stress response (Chapter 37) and risk factors that affect patients' responses to surgery is necessary to anticipate patient needs and the types of preparation required preoperatively.

Smoking. Surgical patients who smoke are at a higher risk for developing pneumonia, atelectasis, and delayed wound healing (Smetana, 2020a). Chronic smoking increases the amount and thickness of airway secretions, thus increasing the risk of aspiration. After surgery, a patient who smokes has greater difficulty clearing the airways of mucus, thus contributing to the development of pneumonia. Smoking decreases the amount of oxygen that reaches the cells in the surgical wound. As a result, the wound may heal more slowly and is more likely to become infected (Pachter et al., 2020). Current research suggests that surgical patients who use electronic cigarettes, a practice known as "vaping," are at risk for delayed wound healing and vascular necrosis (Arndt et al., 2020). Although decades of research correlate cigarette smoking to poor patient outcomes in all phases of the perioperative experience, some preoperative patients are unaware of the surgical risks associated with smoking. Recent studies suggest the need for health care providers to implement systematic and planned measures targeted at educating preoperative patients on the surgical risks of smoking all forms of cigarettes (Arndt et al., 2020; Fracol et al., 2017).

Age. Very young and older patients are at greater surgical risk. Both age-groups frequently present problems in temperature control during surgery. General anesthetics inhibit shivering and cause vasodilation, which results in heat loss. These anesthetic changes coupled with age-related physiological factors increase the risk for unintended hypothermia (Barnett, 2020; Black and Maxwell, 2020). Infants also have difficulty in maintaining normal circulatory blood volume, causing risks for dehydration and overhydration. A healthy older adult has reduced physiological reserve, and organ systems may be compromised during illness and/or surgical stress, creating a surgical risk (Barnett, 2020).

Older adults account for the majority of surgeries performed in the United States (Barnett, 2020). Their risks are significant. Among persons age 65 and over, chronic health conditions (co-morbidities) such as hypertension, heart disease, cancer, and diabetes are surgical risk factors (Barnett, 2020). Older patients often experience diminished cardiac, pulmonary, and renal function, which decreases older adults' ability to maintain homeostasis perioperatively (Table 50.3). Baroreceptor function, which regulates blood pressure, may be insufficient and cause postural hypotension and dizziness, increasing fall risks. Decreased respiratory function, impaired functional reserve of the pulmonary system, and decreased cough reflex increase the risk for aspiration, infection, and bronchospasm. Further, dehydration and fluid imbalance present a need for hydration if the patient is unable to drink before surgery (Barnett, 2020).

Nutrition. Tissue repair and resistance to infection depend on adequate nutrition. Surgery increases the need for nutrients (Weimann et al., 2017). Patients who are thin or obese are often deficient in protein and vitamins, putting them at greater risk for complications following surgery (Harding et al., 2020). After surgery, a patient requires at least 1500 kcal/day to maintain energy reserves. This intake is difficult to attain when a patient's food and/or fluid intake is limited after surgery or if a patient develops postoperative nausea and vomiting (PONV). Postoperatively, patients gradually increase their dietary intake (once gastrointestinal activity returns) over 1 to 2 days or 3 to 5 days after surgery until they can tolerate normal meals. Patients who enter surgery malnourished are more likely to have poor tolerance for anesthesia, negative nitrogen balance, delayed postoperative recovery, infection, and delayed wound healing. Current recommendations suggest the use

TABLE 50.2 ASA Physical Status (PS) Classification

ASA PS Classification	Definition	Characteristics
ASA I	A normal healthy patient	Healthy, nonsmoking; no or minimal alcohol use
ASA II	A patient with mild systemic disease	Mild disease only without substantive functional changes (e.g., current smoker, social alcohol drinker, pregnancy, obesity [BMI 30-40], well-controlled DM/HTN, mild lung disease)
ASA III	A patient with severe systemic disease	Substantive functional changes with one or more moderate-to-severe diseases (e.g., poorly controlled DM or HTN, COPD, morbid obesity [BMI 40 or greater], active hepatitis, alcohol dependence or abuse, implanted pacemaker, or moderate reduction of cardiac ejection fraction)
ASA IV	A patient with severe systemic disease that is a constant threat to life	Examples include recent (less than 3 months) MI, CVA, TIA, ongoing cardiac ischemia or severe valve dysfunction, sepsis, disseminated intravascular coagulation, end-stage renal disease not undergoing regularly scheduled dialysis
ASA V	A moribund patient who is not expected to survive without the operation	Examples include ruptured abdominal/thoracic aneurysm, massive trauma, intracranial bleed with mass effect, ischemic bowel with significant cardiac pathology
ASA VI	A patient who has been declared brain dead whose organs are being removed for donor purpose	Wide variety of dysfunctions that are being managed to optimize blood flow to the heart and organs (e.g., aggressive fluid replacement and blood pressure medications)

Modified from American Society of Anesthesiologists: *ASA Physical Status Classification System,* December 13, 2020, https://www.asahq.org/standards-and-guidelines/asa-physical-status-classification-system. Accessed September 27, 2021.

TABLE 50.3   Physiological Factors That Place the Older Adult at Risk During Surgery

Alterations	Risks	Nursing Implications
Cardiovascular System		
Degenerative change in myocardium and valves	Decreased cardiac reserve puts older adults at risk for decreased cardiac output, especially during times of stress (Rosenthal, 2019; Rothrock, 2019)	Assess baseline vital signs for tachycardia, fatigue, and arrhythmias (Rosenthal, 2019). A complete, comprehensive cardiac workup according to agency policy should be completed before surgery.
Rigidity of arterial walls and reduction in sympathetic and parasympathetic innervation to the heart	Alterations predispose patient to postoperative hemorrhage and rise in systolic and diastolic blood pressure	Maintain adequate fluid balance to minimize stress to the heart. Ensure that blood pressure level is adequate to meet circulatory demands.
Increased calcium and cholesterol deposits within small arteries; thickened arterial walls	Predispose patient to clot formation in lower extremities	Instruct patient in techniques of leg exercises and proper turning. Apply elastic stockings or intermittent pneumatic compression (IPC) devices. Administer anticoagulants as ordered by health care provider. Provide education regarding effects, side effects, and dietary considerations.
Integumentary System		
Decreased subcutaneous tissue and increased fragility of skin	Prone to pressure injuries and skin tears	Select appropriate surface for OR table. Assess skin every 4 hours; pad all bony prominences during surgery. Turn or reposition at least every 2 hours.
Pulmonary System		
Decreased respiratory muscle strength and cough reflex (Rothrock, 2019)	Increased risk for atelectasis	Assess risk factors for postoperative pulmonary complications (Rothrock, 2019). Instruct patient in proper technique for coughing, deep breathing, and use of spirometer. Ensure adequate pain control to allow for participation in exercises.
Reduced range of movement in diaphragm	Residual capacity (volume of air left in lung after normal breath) increased, reducing amount of new air brought into lungs with each inspiration	When possible, have patient ambulate and sit in chair frequently.
Stiffened lung tissue and enlarged air spaces	Blood oxygenation reduced	Obtain baseline oxygen saturation; measure throughout perioperative period.
Gastrointestinal System		
Gastric emptying delayed Saliva production decreased (Rothrock, 2019)	Increases risk for reflux and indigestion and constipation (Rothrock, 2019)	Assess nutritional status and implement preventive measures in high-risk patients (Rothrock, 2019). Position patient with head of bed elevated at least 45 degrees. Reduce size of meals in accordance with ordered diet.
Renal System		
Decreased renal function, with reduced blood flow to kidneys	Increased risk of shock when blood loss occurs; increased risk for fluid and electrolyte imbalance	For patients hospitalized before surgery, determine baseline urinary output for 24 hours.
Reduced glomerular filtration rate and excretory times	Limited ability to eliminate drugs or toxic substances	Assess for adverse response to drugs.
Reduced bladder capacity (Rothrock, 2019)	Increased risk for urgency, incontinence, and urinary tract infections. Increased risk for postoperative urinary retention (Rothrock, 2019)	Instruct patient to notify nurse immediately when sensation of bladder fullness develops. Keep nurse call system and bedpan within easy reach. Toilet every 2 hours or more frequently if indicated.
Neurological System		
Sensory losses, including reduced tactile sense and increased pain tolerance	Decreased ability to respond to early warning signs of surgical complications	Inspect bony prominences for signs of pressure that patient is unable to sense. Orient patient to surrounding environment. Observe for nonverbal signs of pain.
Febrile response during surgery (Rosenthal, 2019; Rothrock, 2019)	Increased risk of undiagnosed infection and hypothermia (Rothrock, 2019)	Ensure careful, close monitoring of patient temperature; provide warm blankets; monitor heart function; warm intravenous fluids. Goals are to prevent heat loss (Rosenthal, 2019). Maintain normothermia intraoperatively (Rothrock, 2019).
Decreased reaction time	Confusion and delirium after anesthesia; increased risk for falls	Allow adequate time to respond, process information, and perform tasks. Perform fall-risk screening and institute fall precautions. Screen for delirium with validated tools. Orient frequently to reality and surroundings.

TABLE 50.3 **Physiological Factors That Place the Older Adult at Risk During Surgery—cont'd**

Alterations	Risks	Nursing Implications
Metabolic System		
Lower basal metabolic rate	Reduced total oxygen consumption	Ensure adequate nutritional intake when diet is resumed but avoid intake of excess calories.
Reduced number of red blood cells and hemoglobin levels	Reduced ability to carry adequate oxygen to tissues	Administer necessary blood products as needed. Monitor blood test results and oxygen saturation.
Change in total amounts of body potassium and water volume	Greater risk for fluid or electrolyte imbalance	Monitor electrolyte levels and supplement as necessary. Provide cardiac monitoring (telemetry) as needed.

Rosenthal L, Association of periOperative Registered Nurses (AORN): *Perioperative assessment of the older adult.* The Hartford Institute for Geriatric Nursing, NYU Rory Meyers College of Nursing, 2019; Rothrock JC: *Alexander's care of the patient in surgery,* ed 16, St Louis, 2019, Elsevier.

of immune-enhancing nutritional supplements as needed to address deficiencies before scheduled surgery (Askari, 2020; Weimann et al., 2017). Some studies indicate that recovery can also be enhanced by regulating the metabolic status of a patient before surgery (e.g., minimizing metabolic stress and insulin resistance by giving carbohydrate-based drinks and fluid loading) and after surgery (e.g., early oral feeding and giving prokinetic medications to enhance gastric motility, resulting in improved enteral feeding tolerance) (Kim et al., 2018; Weimann et al., 2017).

Obesity. According to the World Health Organization (WHO) there are approximately 650 million obese adults and 42 million obese children under the age of 5 years. In the United States, 35% of adults and 17% of children are obese (Lim, 2020). As weight increases, a patient's ventilatory and cardiac function diminish, increasing the risk for postoperative atelectasis, pneumonia, and death. Obstructive sleep apnea (OSA), hypertension, coronary artery disease, diabetes mellitus, and heart failure are co-morbid conditions in the bariatric population. Patients who are obese often have difficulty resuming normal physical activity after surgery because of the pain and fatigue caused by surgery in addition to preexisting impaired physical mobility. This combination of factors increases the risk of developing venous thromboembolism (VTE). Obesity is also a significant risk factor for wound infections, surgical blood loss, and pulmonary embolism (Inge, 2020).

Excess weight placed on skin over bony prominences restricts blood flow and poses risks for pressure injuries to form when patients lie on operating tables. Obesity also increases the risk of poor wound healing, wound infection, dehiscence, and evisceration because fatty tissue contains a poor blood supply, slowing the delivery of essential nutrients and antibodies needed for wound healing (see Chapter 48). In addition, surgeons often have difficulty closing surgical wounds because of the thick adipose layer.

Obstructive Sleep Apnea. Obstructive sleep apnea (OSA) is a chronic sleep disorder characterized by periodic episodes of narrowing or collapse of the upper airway (Kline, 2020). It occurs when muscles in the throat relax during sleep, causing soft tissue in the back of the throat to collapse and block the upper airway. These structural and neuromuscular changes can cause OSA, which results in pauses in breathing (apnea) that last at least 10 seconds during sleep. Most apneic episodes last from 10 to 30 seconds, but some may continue for 1 minute or longer, leading to significant oxygen desaturation. During an episode of apnea there is increasing negative intrathoracic pressure (down to −80 mm Hg), which makes it difficult for the heart to pump effectively; thus cardiac output decreases. In response to the oxygen desaturation, there is an arousal, which ends the apnea. The arousal is accompanied by a huge increase in sympathetic output, which causes a significant increase in blood pressure (Wickramasinghe, 2019).

Patients with OSA who are to undergo surgery present a significant risk. Receiving sedatives, opioid analgesics, and general anesthesia causes relaxation of the upper airway and may worsen OSA. The risk is higher when a patient is sedated and lying on the back. Patients have experienced severe apnea and hypoxemia, leading to death after surgical and diagnostic procedures under conscious sedation. Careful screening of patients at risk or symptomatic for OSA is essential before surgery (Olson et al., 2020a).

Patients with OSA often have co-morbid conditions such as asthma, atherosclerosis, myocardial infarction, heart failure, hypertension, atrial fibrillation, chronic kidney disease, and behavioral disorders, such as decreases in attention, vigilance, concentration, motor skills, and verbal and visuospatial memory (Kline, 2020; National Institute of Health, n.d.). Some evidence suggests that the lack of sleep (for various reasons) may play a role in some older adults' mental decline (National Institute of Health, n.d.). The disorder hinders daily functioning because of chronic fatigue and sleepiness and adversely affects health and longevity. Patients who suffer from OSA develop numerous complications, including hypertension, heart disease, vascular disease, neurological disease, and type 2 diabetes (Kline, 2020).

Immunosuppression. Patients with conditions that alter immune function (e.g., primary immune deficiency, acquired immunodeficiency syndrome [AIDS], cancer, bone marrow alterations, and organ transplants) are at an increased risk for developing infection after surgery. The risk for infection increases when patients receive radiation or chemotherapy for cancer treatment, take immunosuppressive medications, or require steroids to treat a variety of inflammatory or autoimmune conditions (Anderson and Sexton, 2020a). Radiation sometimes is given before surgery to reduce the size of a cancerous tumor so that it can be removed surgically. Ideally, a surgeon waits to perform surgery until 4 to 6 weeks after the completion of radiation treatments because of the unavoidable effects that radiation has on normal tissue. Radiation thins the layers of the skin, destroys collagen, and impairs tissue perfusion. Otherwise, the patient may face serious wound-healing problems.

Fluid and Electrolyte Imbalance. The body responds to surgery as a form of trauma. Severe protein breakdown causes a negative nitrogen balance (see Chapter 45) and hyperglycemia. Both of these effects decrease tissue healing and increase the risk of infection. As a result of the adrenocortical stress response, the body retains sodium and water and loses potassium in the first 2 to 5 days after surgery. The severity of the stress response influences the degree of fluid and electrolyte imbalance.

Extensive surgery results in a greater stress response. A patient who is hypovolemic before surgery or who has serious electrolyte alterations is at significant risk during and after surgery. For example, an excess or depletion of potassium increases the chance of dysrhythmias during or after surgery. The risk of fluid and electrolyte alterations is even greater in patients with preexisting diabetes mellitus, renal disease, or gastrointestinal (GI) or cardiovascular abnormalities (see Chapter 42).

Risks for Postoperative Nausea and Vomiting (PONV). The experience of having nausea and vomiting after surgery is uncomfortable and often immobilizing. PONV affects approximately 30% of patients in recovery rooms after surgery (Feinleib et al., 2020). It can lead to serious complications, including pulmonary aspiration, dehydration, and arrhythmias resulting from fluid and electrolyte imbalance. A patient who vomits frequently after surgery runs the risk of dehiscing surgical sutures. Patients at risk for developing PONV are women, individuals with a history of PONV or motion sickness, nonsmoking status, and younger age. Anesthesia-related risk factors include the use of volatile anesthetics (e.g., nitrous oxide), duration of anesthesia, and perioperative opioid use. Certain types of surgery (e.g., abdominal procedures [cholecystectomies] and gynecological surgery) are also associated with PONV (Feinleib, 2020). Ambulatory surgery patients generally have less PONV. However, nausea and vomiting may occur after an ambulatory patient has left a surgical setting. This post-discharge nausea and/or vomiting (PDNV) may be particularly hazardous for ambulatory surgery patients because they no longer have immediate access to fast-onset intravenous antiemetic medications (Feinleib, 2020). Screening for PONV is crucial for nurses to be able to take precautions needed to prevent PONV and possible pulmonary aspiration. Patients with four or more risk factors have a higher incidence of PONV (Rothrock, 2019). Management of PONV begins before surgery.

Risks for Postoperative Urinary Retention (POUR). Postoperative urinary retention (POUR) is common following anesthesia, affecting up to 70% of patients. Usually the inability to void is temporary, but it may be prolonged in some patients. Common risk factors are (Glick, 2020):

- **Patient-specific:** Older age, male gender, history of POUR, neurological disease, or prior pelvic surgery.
- **Procedure-specific:** Anorectal surgery, joint arthroplasty, hernia repair, or incontinence surgery.
- **Anesthesia-specific:** Excessive intraoperative fluid administration, medication-related (e.g., use of opioids, anticholinergic agents, sympathomimetics), prolonged anesthesia, or type of anesthesia.

Patients who are unable to void in the postanesthesia care unit (PACU) may not complain of bladder fullness, and physical assessment may fail to detect an overdistended bladder. Bladder scanning is noninvasive and can usually confirm an overdistended bladder. Bladder scanning is used when a patient has risk factors for POUR or is unable to void 4 hours postoperatively.

A single-time catheterization is recommended when >600 mL of urine is measured on bladder scan. A patient in ambulatory surgery may not spontaneously void prior to discharge. Ambulatory surgery patients should be instructed to seek medical assistance if they are still unable to void 8 hours after discharge.

Risks for Venous Thromboembolism (VTE). In 2008, the Centers for Medicare and Medicaid Services ruled that deep vein thrombosis (DVT) (clot formed in the deep veins) after total knee and hip surgery is a **never event** and thus refused to pay medical expenses for hospital-acquired DVTs (AHRQ, 2019; CMS, 2020). In addition, the CDC found that between 2007 and 2009 over 550,000 patients had a discharge diagnosis of VTE (CDC, 2020a). If a patient develops a DVT

after surgery, Medicare and some private insurance companies withhold payment to the hospital for the costs associated with treating DVT because DVTs are typically preventable. The Joint Commission (2020) has an updated set of accountability measures (i.e., quality measures that produce the greatest positive impact on patient outcomes when hospitals demonstrate improvement in them). One of the accountability measures is treatment and prevention of venous thromboembolism (VTE). Some VTEs are subclinical (without symptoms), whereas others present as sudden pulmonary embolus or symptomatic DVT. Patients most at risk for developing VTE are those who undergo surgical procedures with a general anesthetic and undergo a surgical time of more than 90 minutes, or 60 minutes if the surgery involves the pelvis or lower limb; acute surgical admissions with inflammatory or intraabdominal conditions; and those expected to have significant reduction in mobility after surgery. In addition, patients are at higher risk if they have one or more risk factors (Bauer and Lip, 2020):

- Active cancer or cancer treatment
- Age over 55 years
- Prior venous thromboembolism
- Recent surgery
- Dehydration
- Known clotting disorders
- Obesity (body mass index [BMI] of 40 kg/m^2 or greater)

REFLECT NOW

A nurse conducts a preoperative assessment for an 85-year-old patient who is accompanied by a caregiver. The patient's caregiver assists the patient with ambulation and answers the nurse's questions. A review of the patient's medical record reveals recent episodes of sleep apnea. What questions should the nurse ask to assess this patient's risks for surgical complications? Which risk factors place this patient at risk for surgical complications?

NURSING KNOWLEDGE BASE

Perioperative Communication

Continuity of care is important when caring for surgical patients. In most cases a different nurse cares for a patient during each surgical phase, which requires clear and accurate communication between nurses. However, based on the delivery of care model utilized in the perioperative setting, some nurses may follow patients through the preoperative and intraoperative phases of surgery. In some instances, perioperative nurses follow patients through the postanesthesia care unit (PACU), assessing a patient's health status before surgery, identifying specific patient needs, providing teaching and counseling, preparing for the operating room (OR), and following a patient's recovery. Other health care providers such as respiratory therapists and physical therapists also care for patients during each phase of the surgical experience. A smooth communication "hand-off" between caregivers is needed to ensure continuity of care and reduce risk of medical errors (Rothrock, 2019). Transitions from one care provider to another place patients at risk for injuries, missed care, and errors in translating information. The World Health Organization (WHO, n.d.) offers a Surgical Safety Checklist that ensures effective communication and safe practices during three perioperative periods: prior to administration of anesthesia, prior to skin incision, and prior to the patient leaving the operative area. Hospitals and surgical outpatient centers can modify or add to the checklist based on their practice guidelines. TJC National Patient Safety

Goals address the importance of accurate patient identification and communication (TJC, 2021).

Glycemic Control and Infection Prevention

Perioperative nurses play a key role in monitoring patients throughout the perioperative experience. When a patient has diabetes or prediabetes, monitoring of blood glucose levels is imperative. Evidence supports a relationship between wound and tissue infection and surgical patients' blood glucose levels. Poor control of blood glucose levels (specifically hyperglycemia) during and after surgery increases patients' risks for adverse outcomes, such as wound infection and mortality. Controlling blood sugars perioperatively reduces mortality in patients with or without diabetes who have general surgery and in patients who have cardiac surgery (van den Boom et al., 2018). Perioperative assessment of patients coupled with appropriate insulin administration is a critical standard of care.

Pressure Injury Prevention

Patients who have surgery pose a unique challenge in pressure injury prevention (Joseph et al., 2019). Nursing research reveals that patients are at risk intraoperatively for pressure injuries as a result of intrinsic, extrinsic, and specific OR risk factors (EPUAP, NPIAP, PPPIA, 2019):

- **Intrinsic risks** (patient's tolerance to a pressure injury insult)—altered nutrition (albumin levels <3 g/dL), decreased mobility, older age, decreased mental status, infection, incontinence, impaired sensory perception, and co-morbidities such as diabetes, malnutrition, and weight (Kim et al., 2017; Saghaleini et al., 2018).
- **Extrinsic risks** (variables that increase tissue susceptibility to sustain external pressure)—temperature, friction and shearing forces, and moisture.
- **OR risk factors**—length and type of surgery, position on OR table, positioning devices used, warming devices, anesthetic agents, intraoperative hemodynamics, and length of time on the OR bed.

Although there are numerous potential risk factors, more research is needed to determine which type(s) of surgery contribute to the development of pressure injuries and which clinical condition(s) most likely contribute to the development of pressure injuries in the postoperative period (Bulfone et al., 2018).

A preoperative assessment should include screening for these risk factors. Registered nurses assist in preventing pressure injuries intraoperatively by carefully positioning patients and using pressure-relieving surfaces. Positioning is a shared responsibility among the surgeon, the anesthesia provider, and OR nurses. The optimal position often involves a compromise between the best position for surgical access and the position a patient can tolerate (Welch, 2020). After surgery, perform a careful skin assessment and use appropriate pressure-reduction strategies (see Chapter 48).

Jeff reviews his knowledge of the surgical process and knows that Mr. Cooper has never undergone surgery before this admission. Jeff uses his previous knowledge of surgery and surgical risk factors to identify areas to assess and lab results to review. He also knows that Mr. Cooper has been calling the surgical center with questions, so Jeff wants to ensure that he allows time to answer all of Mr. Cooper's questions.

Preoperative Education

Preoperative education has been linked through research to improved patient outcomes in the postoperative phase of care (Koivisto et al., 2020). Current evidence suggests that patients who receive preoperative education demonstrate reduced anxiety levels and more realistic postoperative expectations (Burgess et al., 2019). In addition, education allows for preoperative collaborative decision making that allows the patient to make better choices (Burgess et al., 2019).

Several methods have been suggested to provide preoperative education. The use of videos allows the patient to reflect on an upcoming surgery, but videos are less effective than verbal communication. Verbal communication allows the patient to ask questions and clarify concerns about the surgical process. Other commonly used methods include preadmission group classes, booklets and brochures, and individual preoperative meetings with a nurse (Burgess et al., 2019).

Current evidence demonstrates improved patient outcomes from preoperative education, including a reduced length of stay, a decrease in anxiety, and a reduced risk for postoperative complications (Burgess et al., 2019; Iqbal et al., 2019). In addition, preoperative education has been shown to lessen postoperative pain, reduce agency costs, and lessen postoperative depression (Burgess et al., 2019). Education about the surgical experience increases patient satisfaction and knowledge, speeds up the recovery process, and facilitates a return to functioning (Harding et al., 2020).

CRITICAL THINKING

Successful critical thinking applied with nursing judgment requires a synthesis of knowledge, experience, environmental conditions, critical thinking attitudes, and intellectual and professional standards. Clinical judgment requires you to reflect on the knowledge you have in order to anticipate what to assess about a patient, such as knowing common surgical risk factors, the type of surgery, and what questions should patients address preoperatively. Clinical judgment involves analyzing patient assessment findings, recognizing patterns of data, forming accurate nursing diagnoses, and then planning and delivering a patient-centered plan of care. During assessment, consider all elements that build toward making an appropriate nursing diagnosis (Fig. 50.1).

When caring for a surgical patient, integrate your knowledge regarding the patient's specific clinical situation and type of surgery along with your previous experiences in caring for surgical patients. This enables you to form questions to ask about the patient's expectations and familiarity with the surgery. Apply this knowledge using a patient-centered care approach, partnering with your patient to make clinical decisions. Using critical thinking attitudes (see Chapter 15) ensures that your assessment and plan of care are comprehensive and incorporates evidence-based principles for successful perioperative care. A key attitude for a perioperative nurse is responsibility (i.e., being responsible not only for standards of care but being a patient advocate as well). Professional perioperative standards developed by the **Association of periOperative Registered Nurses** (AORN, 2020a) (http://www.aorn.org) and the **American Society of PeriAnesthesia Nurses** (ASPAN, 2019) (http://www.aspan.org/) provide valuable guidelines for perioperative management and the evaluation of process and outcomes. TJC Hospital National Patient Safety Goals include two sets of recommendations for perioperative care—to prevent infection and to prevent mistakes in surgery (TJC, 2021). Always review these guidelines within the context of emerging evidence-based practice, agency policies, and the scope of practice of the state in which you practice.

REFLECT NOW

Think about a patient you cared for during his or her surgical experience. Develop a communication hand-off for your patient that you would use to report to the nurse on the next shift.

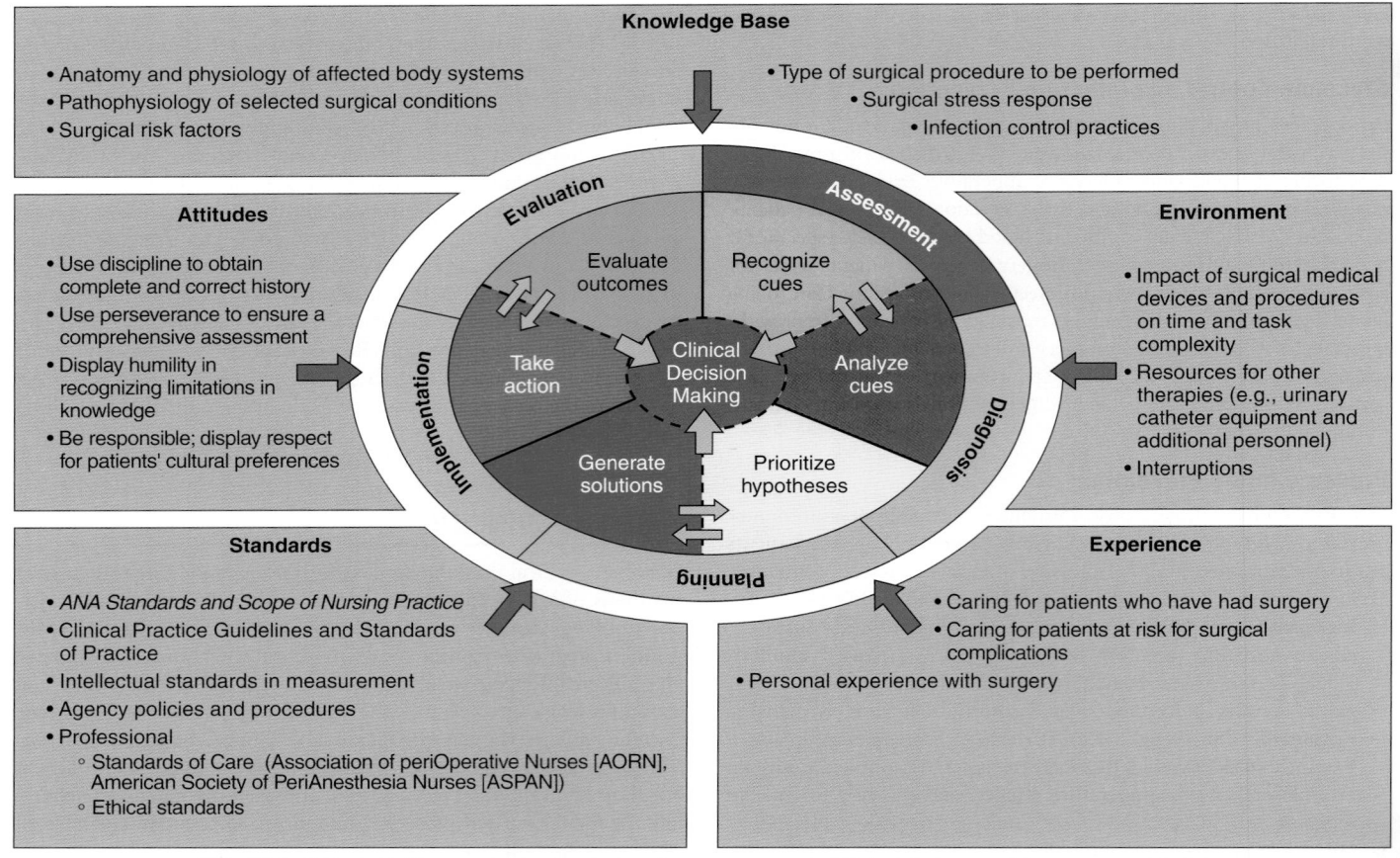

FIG. 50.1 Critical thinking model for surgical patient assessment. (Clinical Judgment Measurement Model copyright © NCSBN. All rights reserved.)

PREOPERATIVE SURGICAL PHASE

❖ NURSING PROCESS

The nursing process provides a clinical decision-making approach that involves the application of critical thinking and sound clinical judgment. Patients having surgery enter the health care setting in different levels of health. For example, a patient may enter the hospital or ambulatory surgery center (ASC) on a predetermined day feeling relatively healthy and prepared to face elective surgery, while another person in a motor vehicle crash will face emergency surgery with no time to prepare. The ability to establish rapport and maintain a professional relationship with a patient and the patient's family is essential during the preoperative phase. Patients having surgery meet many health care personnel, including surgeons, nurse anesthetists, anesthesiologists, surgical technologists, and nurses. All play a role in a patient's care and recovery. Family members attempt to provide support through their presence but face many of the same stressors as the patient. As a nurse you need to form a caring relationship (see Chapter 7) and effectively communicate (see Chapter 24) with the patient and family to gain the patient's trust. This helps you to assess in-depth the information needed to accurately identify nursing diagnoses and problems and provide a patient-centered plan of care. Cultural sensitivity is equally important in developing a patient-centered plan of care reflecting the patient's physical, psychological, emotional, sociocultural, and spiritual well-being (see Chapter 9). You will learn to recognize a patient's degree of surgical risk, coordinate diagnostic tests, identify nursing diagnoses and

nursing interventions, and establish outcomes in collaboration with patients and their families. It is a nurse's responsibility to communicate pertinent data and the plan of care to surgical team members.

Many hospitals have developed Enhanced Recovery After Surgery (ERAS) protocols that are implemented in the preoperative, intraoperative, and postoperative phases of care (Ricciardi et al., 2020). The protocols are interprofessional and based on published scientific evidence. Elements of an ERAS protocol might include minimally invasive surgical approaches instead of large incisions, management of fluids to seek fluid balance rather than large volumes of intravenous fluids, avoidance of or early removal of drains and tubes, early mobilization, and the serving of drinks and food the day of an operation (Ljungqvist et al., 2017; Ricciardi et al., 2020). An ERAS protocol will include evidence-based standards for preoperative and postoperative care as well as clinical guidelines established by an agency. Clinical judgment is needed even when a patient is placed on an ERAS protocol. The appropriateness of the various components of an ERAS protocol and any unexpected clinical changes a patient might experience need to be monitored to make clinical decisions about completing interventions.

◆ Assessment

During the assessment process, thoroughly assess each patient and critically analyze findings to ensure that you make patient-centered clinical decisions required for safe nursing care. The goal of the preoperative assessment is to consider what is normal for a planned surgical procedure, including the anticipated physiological effects, and to compare with a patient's baseline preoperative status. Your assessment will also reveal the presence of any surgical risks so that you can recognize, prevent, and minimize possible postoperative complications. The extent of a nurse's assessment depends on the patient's condition, the surgical setting (outpatient versus inpatient), the time the nurse has with a patient, and the urgency of a procedure. Ambulatory and same-day surgical programs offer challenges in gathering a complete assessment in a short time. In these settings, an interprofessional team approach is essential. Patients are admitted only hours before surgery; consequently, it is important for a nurse to organize and verify data obtained before surgery and implement a perioperative plan of care. This occurs both in ASCs and with patients who require a hospital stay.

Most surgical assessments begin before admission in the health care provider's office, a preadmission clinic, an anesthesia clinic, or by telephone. Some patients answer a self-report inventory before arriving at a center. Other times a health care provider performs a physical examination or orders laboratory tests. Nurses begin to teach, answer questions, and complete paperwork before surgery to streamline patient care on the day of surgery. When surgery is emergent with little time available, you prioritize an assessment based on the patient's presenting clinical condition and risk factors.

Through the Patient's Eyes. When possible, it is important to determine a patient's expectations of surgery and recovery. Ask a patient what is hoped to be gained as a result of surgery. Explore with questions such as "Tell me the type of surgery you are having in your own words" or "Do you understand the expected care and how long you will stay in the hospital after surgery? If not, what do you want to know?" or "Do you expect full pain relief or simply to have your pain reduced after surgery?" and "Do you expect to be independent immediately after surgery, or do you expect to be fully dependent on the nurse or your family?" These are only a few of the questions to ask to establish a plan of care that matches a patient's needs and expectations. Listen to the patient's explanation, be attentive, and explain expectations of surgery. Form a relationship with each patient to foster collaboration and shared decision making. Assessing patient expectations gives you a better understanding of the patient's health and health care needs.

As Jeff begins his assessment of Mr. Cooper, he uses knowledge of the surgical process, including knowledge of cancer and the gastrointestinal system. He always includes his past experience with patients with surgical procedures. When Jeff talks with Mr. Cooper, he finds out that Mr. Cooper has talked with his surgeon and learned that he is going to need a colostomy. Jeff asks Mr. Cooper additional history questions regarding what he understands about his preoperative preparations and any concerns he might have about his impending surgery.

Nursing History. A preoperative nursing history includes information about all body systems, similar to that described in Chapter 30. If a patient is unable to relay all of the necessary information, rely on family members (if appropriate) as resources. As with any admission to a health care agency, include information about advance directives. Ask whether a patient has a durable power of attorney for health care or a living will (see Chapter 23), and include a copy in the patient's medical record. Often directives are modified before surgery but are reestablished after postoperative stabilization. To help ensure a thorough and accurate nursing assessment, electronic health records (EHRs) provide standardized documentation forms for data. Be sure to use all drop-down menus to portray a patient's history most clearly, but also be willing to enter full-text descriptions as needed.

Medical History. A review of a patient's medical history includes past illnesses and surgeries and the primary reason for seeking medical care. The medical history screens surgical candidates for major

medical conditions that increase the risk of complications during or after surgery (Table 50.4). This information allows you to anticipate what some of the preliminary treatments will be before surgery. For example, a patient who has a history of heart failure is at risk for a further decline in cardiac function during and after surgery. The patient with heart failure in the preoperative period often requires beta-blocker medications, intravenous (IV) fluids infused at a slower rate, or administration of a diuretic after blood transfusions. Box 50.1 provides a list of assessment questions for a patient with a cardiac history. If a patient has surgical risks from medical conditions, surgery as an outpatient may be inadvisable, or special precautions will be necessary. In addition, the history includes questions about a family history of anesthetic complications such as malignant hyperthermia (an inherited disorder and life-threatening condition) that may occur during surgery.

Surgical History. A review of a patient's past experience with surgery reveals physical and potential psychological responses that may occur during the planned procedure. Complications such as anaphylaxis or malignant hyperthermia during previous surgeries alert you to the need for preventive measures and the availability of appropriate emergency equipment. For example, if a patient experienced an allergic reaction to latex during a previous surgery, you would document the patient's history and ensure that a latex-free environment is provided for the patient during hospitalization.

A history of postoperative complications such as persistent vomiting or uncontrolled pain will lead to the selection of more appropriate medications (as ordered by the medical team). Reports of severe anxiety before a previous surgery identify the need for additional emotional support, medications, and preoperative teaching. Always inform the surgeon and/or anesthesiologist of these findings, especially when medications may be indicated.

Risk Factors. Knowledge of potential surgical risk factors and risk factors for complications (e.g., pressure injuries) provides focus for the preoperative assessment. The assessment data from careful screening of patients will contain information useful for necessary precautions in planning perioperative care. Consider any risk factors described earlier that may contribute to negative outcomes, and collaborate closely with the health care provider to identify necessary therapies.

A patient's risk for developing pressure injuries intraoperatively cannot be adequately assessed using the standard Braden Scale, as the Braden was not developed to target intraoperative risk factors. The Munro Pressure Ulcer Risk Assessment Scale for Perioperative Patients and the Scott Triggers Risk Assessment Tool are two scales recommended by AORN (n.d.). The Munro Scale is a cumulative scale that assesses risk factors present in each of the different operative phases (Munro, 2019). The preoperative scale includes mobility, nutritional state, weight loss, BMI, and co-morbidities (Munro, 2019). The intraoperative scale includes physical status classification according to the American Society of Anesthesiologists (ASA) scale, type of anesthesia, moisture, surface/motion, hypotension, and body temperature (Munro, 2019). The postoperative component of the scale includes length of the surgical procedure and occurrence of hemorrhage (AORN, n.d.). The benefit of the Munro tool is that it allows nurses to complete the tool at each surgical phase, increasing the frequency of risk assessments. The Scott Triggers tool is a single preoperative measure that assesses a patient's age, albumin or BMI values, ASA classification, and estimated duration of the surgery (Park et al., 2019).

Preoperatively, some patients need to stop taking medications (e.g., anticoagulants) that may affect surgical outcomes and medications that may pose risks based on a potential for drug-to-drug interaction

TABLE 50.4 Medical Conditions That Increase Risks of Surgery

Type of Condition	Reason for Risk
Bleeding disorders (thrombocytopenia, hemophilia)	Increases risk of hemorrhage during and after surgery.
Diabetes mellitus	Increases susceptibility to infection and impairs wound healing from altered glucose metabolism and associated circulatory impairment. Stress of surgery often results in hyperglycemia (Harding et al., 2020).
Heart disease (recent myocardial infarction, dysrhythmias, heart failure) and peripheral vascular disease	Stress of surgery causes increased demands on myocardium to maintain cardiac output. General anesthetic agents depress cardiac function.
Hypertension	Increases risk for cardiovascular complications during anesthesia (e.g., stroke, inadequate tissue oxygenation).
Obstructive sleep apnea	Administration of opioids increases risk of airway obstruction after surgery. Patients desaturate as revealed by drop in oxygen saturation by pulse oximetry.
Upper respiratory infection	Increases risk of respiratory complications during anesthesia (e.g., pneumonia and spasm of laryngeal muscles).
Renal disease	Alters excretion of anesthetic drugs and their metabolites, increasing risk for acid-base imbalance and other complications.
Liver disease	Alters metabolism and elimination of drugs administered during surgery and impairs wound healing and clotting time because of alterations in protein metabolism.
Fever	Predisposes patient to fluid and electrolyte imbalances and sometimes indicates underlying infection.
Chronic respiratory disease (emphysema, bronchitis, asthma)	Reduces patient's means to compensate for acid-base alterations (see Chapter 42). Anesthetic agents reduce respiratory function, increasing risk for severe hypoventilation.
Immunological disorders (leukemia, acquired immunodeficiency syndrome [AIDS], bone marrow depression, and use of chemotherapeutic drugs or immunosuppressive agents)	Increases risk of infection and delayed wound healing after surgery.
Abuse of alcohol, opioid addiction	Alcohol abuse is associated with liver dysfunction and may interfere with the effects of anesthesia. Opioid addiction may result in health care and self-care neglect. Consequently, patients may have underlying diseases that may affect wound healing.
Chronic pain	Regular use of pain medications often results in higher tolerance. Increased doses of analgesics are sometimes necessary to achieve postoperative pain control.

Data from Mohabir PK: Preoperative evaluation, 2021, *Merck manual professional version.* https://www.merckmanuals.com/professional/special-subjects/care-of-the-surgical-patient/preoperative-evaluation. Last revised November 2020. Accessed September 2021; and Harding M, et al: *Lewis's medical-surgical nursing: assessment and management of clinical problems,* ed 11, St Louis, 2020, Elsevier.

BOX 50.1 Nursing Assessment Questions: Cardiac History

Nature of the Problem
- Do you have a history of heart attack, heart failure, angina (chest pain), irregular heartbeat, or valve disease?
- Which medications do you take?
- Tell me about any vitamins or other supplements you are taking.
- Have you had any recent medical testing or procedures on your heart (e.g., cardiac catheterization or echocardiogram)?
- Do you smoke cigarettes, including e-cigarettes? If so, how often and how many per day?

Signs and Symptoms
- Are you having any chest pain?
- How do you sleep at night (position, use of pillows, awakened with chest pain)?
- Do your feet swell?
- Are you short of breath, or do you have any difficulty breathing?

Onset and Duration
- How often do you have chest pain, when does it start, how long does it last, what alleviates it?

- When do your feet swell (all the time, end of the day, only after a busy day)?
- When do you become short of breath?

Severity
- On a scale of 0 to 10 (with 0 being no pain and 10 the worst pain), what number do you give your chest pain?
- Describe your usual activity level. Can you climb stairs; can you do housework?
- Describe the amount of physical activity you have daily. Tell me about the types of exercise you perform.

Self-Management and Culture
- Have you changed your activity level, sleep patterns, diet, or fluid intake recently?
- Are you taking any herbal or over-the-counter medications?

Through the Patient's Eyes
- How are you feeling about your upcoming surgery? Has it affected your symptoms?
- Are you currently having any additional stress?

BOX 50.2   The STOP-BANG Questionnaire

To determine whether a patient has obstructive sleep apnea (OSA) many agencies use the STOP-Bang assessment tool (below). **(Any question answered *Yes* is a risk factor.)**

STOP
- Do you SNORE loudly (louder than talking or loud enough to be heard through closed doors)?
- Do you often feel TIRED, fatigued, or sleepy during the daytime?
- Has anyone OBSERVED you stop breathing during your sleep?
- Do you have or are you being treated for high blood PRESSURE?

BANG
- BMI greater than 35 kg/m²
- AGE over 50 years old
- NECK circumference >40 cm (16 inches)
- GENDER: Male

Modified from Kawada T: Screening ability of STOP-Bang questionnaire for obstructive sleep apnea, *Anesthesia & Analgesia* 128(3): e48, 2019; Olson E, et al: Surgical risk and the preoperative evaluation and management of adults with obstructive sleep apnea, *UpToDate*, 2020a, https://www.uptodate.com/contents/surgical-risk-and-the-preoperative-evaluation-and-management-of-adults-with-obstructive-sleep-apnea.

(Muluk et al., 2020). Carefully screen patients who have signs and symptoms of suspected OSA. Include the patient's sleeping partner as appropriate to assess for signs of OSA such as snoring. Also, determine the patient's use of continuous positive airway pressure (CPAP), non-invasive positive-pressure ventilation (NIPPV), or apnea monitoring at home. Instruct a patient who uses CPAP or NIPPV to bring the machine to the hospital or surgery center. Many health care agencies are now making OSA screening mandatory, using evidence-based tools such as the STOP-Bang sleep apnea assessment tool (Box 50.2) (Kawada, 2019; Olson et al., 2020a). If the STOP-Bang is unavailable, screen patients with simple questions regarding snoring, apnea during sleep, frequent arousals during sleep, morning headaches, daytime somnolence, and chronic fatigue (Kawada, 2019).

Some patients need a detailed nutritional assessment to determine surgical risk. If a patient presents with signs of malnutrition, perform a nutritional screening using your agency's tool, or confer with a registered dietitian (see Chapter 45).

Medications. Review a patient's medications to determine whether any medications may increase the risk for surgical complications (Table 50.5). Include all prescribed, OTC, and herbal medications in your assessment. Many medications interact unpredictably with anesthetic agents during surgery (Burchum and Rosenthal, 2019). Sometimes surgeons temporarily discontinue or adjust doses of a patient's prescription, over-the-counter (OTC) medications, and/or herbal supplements before surgery. For example, there are various medical opinions about when to hold an oral anticoagulant and whether to continue therapy through certain surgical procedures (Douketis and Lip, 2020). Nurses in an outpatient setting should verify with surgeons which, if any, medications patients should take or withhold on the morning of surgery. Often preprinted instruction sheets given to patients in physician offices contain this information. When working in an acute care setting, confirm with the surgeon all discontinued medications. If a patient is having inpatient surgery, all prescription medications taken before surgery are discontinued

TABLE 50.5   Medications With Special Implications for the Surgical Patient

Drug Class	Effects During Surgery
Antibiotics	Potentiate (enhance action of) anesthetic agents. If taken within 2 weeks before surgery, aminoglycosides (gentamicin, neomycin, tobramycin) may cause mild respiratory depression from depressed neuromuscular transmission.
Antidysrhythmics	Medications (e.g., beta blockers) can reduce cardiac contractility and impair cardiac conduction during anesthesia.
Anticoagulants	Medications such as warfarin or aspirin alter normal clotting factors and thus increase risk of hemorrhaging. Discontinue at least 48 hours before surgery.
Anticonvulsants	Long-term use of certain anticonvulsants (e.g., phenytoin and phenobarbital) alters metabolism of anesthetic agents.
Antihypertensives	Medications such as beta blockers and calcium channel blockers interact with anesthetic agents to cause bradycardia, hypotension, and impaired circulation. They inhibit synthesis and storage of norepinephrine in sympathetic nerve endings.
Corticosteroids	With prolonged use, corticosteroids cause adrenal atrophy, reducing the ability of the body to withstand stress. Before and during surgery, dosages are often increased temporarily.
Insulin	A patient's insulin requirements fluctuate after surgery. For example, some patients need increased doses due to the stress response from surgery. Other patients need less insulin due to decreased nutritional intake following surgery.
Diuretics	Diuretics such as furosemide potentiate electrolyte imbalances (particularly potassium) after surgery.
Nonsteroidal antiinflammatory drugs (NSAIDs)	NSAIDs (e.g., ibuprofen) inhibit platelet aggregation and prolong bleeding time, increasing susceptibility to postoperative bleeding.
Herbal therapies: ginger, ginkgo, ginseng	These herbal therapies have the ability to affect platelet activity and increase susceptibility to postoperative bleeding. Ginseng increases hypoglycemia with insulin therapy.

Data from Kuwajerwala K: *Perioperative medication management*, 2021, *Merck manual professional version*. https://www.merckmanuals.com/professional/special-subjects/care-of-the-surgical-patient/preoperative-evaluation. Last reviewed November 2020. Accessed September 27, 2021; Muluk V, et al.: Perioperative medication management, *UpToDate*, 2020, https://www.uptodate.com/contents/perioperative-medication-management.

automatically after surgery unless reordered. It is important that as a patient moves through different areas (e.g., from the holding area to the OR), a complete list of medications is communicated accurately during the hand-off report (TJC, 2021).

Allergies. Allergies to medications, latex, and topical agents used to prepare the skin for surgery create significant risks for patients and staff during surgery. An allergic response to any agent is potentially fatal, depending on severity. Latex allergies affect 8% to 12% of the health care workforce (OSHA, n.d.). Patients most at risk for a latex allergy include people with a genetic predisposition to latex allergy, children with spina bifida, patients with urogenital abnormalities or spinal cord injury (because of a long history of urinary catheter use), patients with a history of multiple surgeries, health care professionals, and workers who manufacture rubber products. Patients with an allergy to certain foods such as bananas, chestnuts, kiwifruit, avocados, potatoes, tomatoes, and wheat often have a cross-sensitivity to latex (Hamilton, 2020). Symptoms of a latex allergy vary in severity (e.g., contact dermatitis with redness, inflammation, and blisters; contact urticaria with pruritus, redness, and swelling; hay fever–like symptoms; and anaphylaxis). When you identify a patient allergy, provide an allergy identification band at the time of admission that remains on until discharge. List all allergies in the patient's medical record. It is also common to list allergies on the front of paper charts.

Smoking Habits. Screen all patients for a history of smoking, including cigarettes, cigars, electronic cigarettes, and pipes. This is usually included in the nursing health history. Use "pack-years" as a guide to determine the number of cigarette packs smoked per day and the number of years the patient has smoked. In addition, ask the patient about the use and frequency of other nicotine products such as snuff and chewing tobacco. Use this information to plan for aggressive pulmonary hygiene, including more frequent turning, deep breathing, coughing, and the use of incentive spirometry after surgery.

Alcohol Ingestion and Substance Use and Abuse. Habitual use of alcohol or illegal drugs and the misuse of prescription drugs predispose patients to adverse reactions to anesthetic agents. Some patients experience a cross-tolerance to anesthetic agents and analgesics, resulting in the need for higher-than-usual doses. Patients with a history of excessive alcohol ingestion are often malnourished, which delays wound healing. These patients are also at risk for liver disease, portal hypertension, and esophageal varices (which increase the risk of bleeding). A patient who habitually uses alcohol and is required to remain in the hospital longer than 24 hours is also at risk for acute alcohol withdrawal and its more severe form, delirium tremens (DTs).

It is important to assess all age-groups because there is a high prevalence of at-risk drinking and binge drinking in adults ages 18 years and older (CDC, 2019). It is common for patients to not disclose their use of alcohol or illegal drug use. Begin the assessment by asking the patient about the consumption of wine, beer, whiskey, or other forms of alcohol. Assess the number of drinks the patient has during a typical day or week. Also ask about the use of illegal drugs and the use of prescription drugs, including the type, frequency, and method of delivery. Some health care agencies require the use of screening tools such as the Alcohol, Smoking and Substance Involvement Screening Test (ASSIST) to assess a patient's use of illegal drugs, smoking, and/or misuse of prescription drugs or the Alcohol Use Disorders Identification Test (AUDIT) to screen for alcohol use problems (National Institute on Alcohol Abuse and Alcoholism, n.d.; Saitz, 2020). Your findings will help in the planning of anesthetic and pain management. In addition, it is important postoperatively to consider opportunities to counsel those patients whose use of alcohol or illicit drugs is excessive.

Pregnancy. During preoperative assessment, routinely ask women of childbearing age who are scheduled for surgery about their last menstrual period and whether it was "typical" for them. Also ask whether they have had unprotected sex in the past month. Because many women do not know they are pregnant early in the first trimester, many institutions require a pregnancy test when a patient is scheduled for surgery. If a woman is pregnant, the perioperative plan of care addresses not one, but two patients: the mother and the developing fetus. A pregnant patient has surgery only on an emergent or urgent basis. Because all of a mother's major systems are affected during pregnancy, the risk for intraoperative complications increases. General anesthesia is administered with caution because of the increased risk of fetal death and preterm labor. Regional anesthesia is used in preference to general anesthesia when appropriate (Sviggum, 2020). Psychological assessment of mother and family is also essential.

Perceptions and Knowledge Regarding Surgery. A patient's past experience with surgery influences potential physical and psychological responses to a procedure. Assess the patient's previous experiences with surgery as a foundation for anticipating and identifying needs and selecting appropriate interventions, including teaching, addressing fears, and clarifying concerns. Ask the patient to discuss the previous type of surgery, level of discomfort, extent of disability, and overall level of care required. Review any past medical records, if available, for surgical complications. Address any complications that the patient experienced. Prior anesthesia records are also a useful source of information if previous surgical problems occurred.

The surgical experience affects the family unit as a whole. Understanding a patient's and family's knowledge and expectations (following discharge) allows you to plan teaching and provide individualized emotional support measures. In many instances, patients fear surgery. Some fears are the result of past hospital experiences, warnings from friends and family, or lack of knowledge. Assess the patient's understanding of planned surgery, its implications, and planned postoperative activities. Ask questions, such as "Tell me what you think will happen before and after surgery" or "Explain what you know about surgery." Nurses face ethical dilemmas when patients are misinformed or unaware of the reason for surgery. Confer with the surgeon if a patient has an inaccurate perception of the surgical procedure before the patient is sent to the surgical suite. Further, determine whether the health care provider explained routine preoperative and postoperative procedures, and assess the patient's readiness and willingness to learn. Reinforce the patient's knowledge of the surgical procedure and postoperative expectations.

Support Sources. Have your assessment include the identification of the patient's primary family caregiver or family support person. The patient usually cannot immediately assume the same level of physical activity enjoyed before surgery. With **ambulatory surgery,** patients and/or family caregivers assume responsibility for postoperative care immediately. The family caregiver is an important resource for a patient with physical limitations and provides the emotional support needed to motivate the patient to return to the previous state of health. Ask the family caregiver about the type of support provided. Is it sufficient to meet the patient's needs? What level of instruction or support is required?

Sometimes the family caregiver remembers preoperative and postoperative teaching better than the patient. Patients having ambulatory surgery will receive a postdischarge phone call to evaluate their recovery. Sometimes patients, especially older adults, are unable to hear or reach a phone after surgery. Ask whether a family member will be staying with the patient to answer the phone. The nurse's responsibility is to fully prepare a patient and any family caregiver for patient self-care if the patient returns home. This includes providing information that allows the patient to anticipate any problems, know the activity level to assume, and be able to perform care measures (e.g., medication administration, dressing changes, prescribed exercises). Often a family member becomes the patient's coach, offering valuable support after surgery when a patient's participation in care is vital.

Occupation. Surgery often results in physical changes and restrictions that prevent a person from immediately returning to work. Assess the patient's occupational history to anticipate the possible effects of surgery on recovery, the time it will take to return to work, and eventual work performance. Knowing the type of surgery, anticipate the postoperative restrictions that will be set by the health care provider (e.g., limits on lifting or walking), and assess the patient's perceptions of the extent this will affect the ability to return to work. This will help establish realistic expectations for the patient postoperatively.

Preoperative Pain Assessment. Surgical manipulation of tissues, treatments, and positioning on the OR table contribute to postoperative pain. However, patients also often present preoperatively with painful conditions. Conduct a comprehensive pain assessment before surgery (see Chapter 44), including the character of any existing pain and the patient's and family's expectations for pain management after surgery. Ask patients to describe their perceived tolerance to pain, past experiences, and prior successful interventions, especially nonpharmacological therapies.

Review of Emotional Health. Surgery is psychologically stressful and creates anxiety in patients and their families. Patients often feel powerless over their situation. Potential disruptions in lifestyle, a lengthy recovery period at home, and uncertainty about the long-term effects of surgery on a patient's life place stress on patients and their families. When a patient has a chronic illness, the family is either fearful that surgery will result in further disability or hopeful that it will improve the patient's lifestyle. To understand the effect of surgery on a patient's and family's emotional health, assess the patient's feelings about surgery, self-concept, body image, and coping resources.

It is difficult to assess a patient's feelings thoroughly when ambulatory surgery is scheduled because a nurse does not have much time to establish a therapeutic relationship with a patient. You can address these concerns initially with the patient during a home visit or on the telephone before surgery. In a hospital room, choose a private time for discussion after completing admitting procedures or diagnostic tests. Explain that it is normal to have fears and concerns. A patient's ability to share feelings partially depends on your willingness to listen, be supportive, and clarify misconceptions. Assure patients of their right to ask questions and seek information.

Self-Concept. Patients with a positive self-concept are more likely to approach surgical experiences with optimism. A person's personal and social identity coupled with a sense of competence in meeting one's own basic needs is a powerful resource for coping with the stress of surgery. Assess self-concept by asking patients to identify personal strengths and weaknesses (see Chapter 33). Patients who quickly criticize or scorn their own personal characteristics may have little self-regard or may be testing your opinion of their character. If the patient is testing your opinion of their character, focus on the facts and remain positive. Poor self-concept hinders the ability to adapt to the stress of surgery and may aggravate feelings of guilt or inadequacy.

Body Image. Surgery or surgical removal of any body part often leaves permanent scars, alteration in body function, or concern over mutilation. Change in or loss of body functions (e.g., with a colostomy or amputation) compounds a patient's fears. Assess patients' perceptions of anticipated body image alterations from surgery. Individuals respond differently, depending on their culture, self-concept, and self-esteem (see Chapter 33).

Some surgeries, such as removal of a breast, an ostomy, or removal of the prostate gland, may change the physical or psychological aspects of a patient's sexuality. In addition, some surgeries, such as a hernia repair, require patients to temporarily refrain from sexual intercourse until they return to normal physical activity. Encourage patients to express concerns about their sexuality. A patient facing even temporary

sexual dysfunction requires understanding and support. Hold discussions about the patient's sexuality with the patient's sexual partner so that the partner gains a shared understanding of how to cope with limitations in sexual function (see Chapter 34).

Coping Resources. Assessment of patients' feelings and self-concept reveals whether they have the ability to cope with the stress of surgery. Thus, ask a patient about perceptions of the upcoming surgery and whether there are other sources of stress in the patient's life. How is the stress affecting life currently? How does the patient typically deal with stressful situations? If your patient has limited coping resources, your assessment findings will guide you in planning for stress management postoperatively by offering healthy coping strategies (see Chapters 32 and 37), initiating more frequent or comprehensive discussions about surgery, knowing how to involve family, and involving social work or clergy as needed.

Cultural and Spiritual Factors. Culture is a system of beliefs and values developed over time and passed on through many generations (see Chapter 9). Each patient is unique in perceptions and reactions to the surgical experience. If you do not acknowledge and plan for cultural and spiritual differences in the perioperative plan of care, your patient may not achieve desired surgical outcomes (Box 50.3). To bridge cultural differences, listen to a patient's story, and explore and respect the patient's beliefs as well as their meaning of illness, preferences, and needs. Understanding a patient's cultural and ethnic heritage helps the nurse care for a patient having surgery. Although it is important

---

⊕ **BOX 50.3 CULTURAL ASPECTS OF CARE**

Providing Culturally Sensitive Care for the Patient Having Surgery

Patients' cultures and religions influence their health care beliefs (Giger and Haddad, 2021). A nurse's approach to perioperative care should respect patients' cultural values and involve partnering with the patient to provide a patient-centered care plan. The use of a wide variety of resources within a health care agency, in the literature, and from the Internet helps complement the data needed for nurses to provide culturally sensitive care.

Implications for Patient-Centered Care
- It takes time to gather a comprehensive culturally based nursing history. Time for assessment preoperatively will be limited. A cultural assessment for preoperative patients can be focused, including questions related to the patient's primary language, feelings regarding surgery and pain, pain-management expectations, support system, and feelings toward self-care with postoperative implications (e.g., Does the patient relate to the concept of pain? Does the patient have feelings about gender of caregiver? Does the patient follow a custom of giving family members control over decisions? Does the patient have religious convictions that affect perioperative care, such as opposition to the administration of blood products?).
- Use sensitivity if a professional interpreter is needed to communicate with non–English-speaking patients because some patients may have difficulty sharing personal health information with people who are younger or of a specific gender.
- Use materials and teaching techniques that are culturally relevant and language-appropriate to communicate and assess the non–English-speaking patient for factors such as pain, general comfort, temperature, and need to void.
- Provide assessment tools and preoperative and postoperative educational materials in a variety of languages.

to recognize and plan for differences on the basis of culture, it is also necessary to recognize that members of the same culture are individuals and do not always hold these shared beliefs.

Physical Examination. Conduct a partial or complete physical examination, depending on the amount of time available and the patient's preoperative condition. Chapter 30 describes physical assessment techniques. Assessment focuses on a patient's medical history and on body systems that the surgery is likely to affect. While completing a nursing assessment, you validate existing information, reinforce basic preoperative teaching, and review standard discharge instructions. Individualized instruction occurs after all assessment data are collected.

General Survey. Observe a patient's gestures and body movements (gait, posture, purposeful movement), which may reflect decreased energy or weakness caused by illness. Height, body weight, and history of recent weight loss are important indicators of nutritional status and are used to calculate medication dosages. Preoperative vital signs, including pulse oximetry and blood pressure while sitting and standing, provide important baseline data with which to compare alterations that occur during and after surgery, including response to anesthetics and medications and fluid and electrolyte abnormalities (see Chapter 42). An elevated temperature is cause for concern. If a patient has an underlying infection, elective surgery is often postponed until the infection is treated or resolved. An elevated body temperature also alters drug metabolism and increases the risk for fluid and electrolyte changes. Notify the surgeon immediately if a patient has an elevated temperature.

Head and Neck. To determine whether a patient is dehydrated, assess the patient's oral mucous membranes. Dehydration increases the risk for serious fluid and electrolyte imbalances during surgery. Inspect the area between the gums and cheek, the soft palate, and the nasal sinuses. Sinus drainage that is yellow or greenish may indicate respiratory or sinus infection.

During the examination of the oral mucosa, identify any loose or capped teeth because they can become dislodged during endotracheal intubation. Note the presence of dentures, prosthetic devices, or piercings so that they can be removed before surgery, especially if the patient receives general anesthesia.

Integument. The overall condition of the skin reveals a patient's level of hydration. Carefully inspect the skin, especially over bony prominences such as the heels, elbows, sacrum, back of head, and scapula. In patients who are obese, separate the body folds to ensure that you examine the skin thoroughly. Pay particular attention to older adults, who are at high risk for alteration in skin integrity from thinning of the epidermis, positioning (pressure forces) for a prolonged time, and repositioning on the OR table (shearing forces) (see Table 50.3). During surgery, patients often lie in a fixed position for several hours, placing them at increased risk for pressure injuries (see Chapter 48). Although physiological blood and lymphatic flow rates vary among patients, capillary pressures may increase to as much as 150 mm Hg during prolonged, unrelieved pressure without a position change. When the intensity of pressure exerted on capillaries exceeds 10.5 to 22.5 mm Hg, ischemic injury can develop (Sterns, 2020). Consider the type of surgery a patient will undergo and the position that is required on the OR table (Fig. 50.2) to identify areas at risk for pressure injury formation. Identify the presence of any current alterations in the skin such as lesions or wounds.

Current evidence shows that using a pressure injury risk assessment instrument is recommended and that it is important to assess risk factors throughout the preoperative period and over time (Bulfone et al., 2018). Older patients, those with a high ASA score, those with co-morbidities, and those with a hematocrit level less than 35% should be monitored carefully, as well as those with a probable time on the operating table greater than 6.15 hours (Bulfone et al., 2018).

Thorax and Lungs. Assess a patient's breathing pattern and chest excursion to detect the presence of a decline in ventilation. When ventilation is reduced, a patient is at increased risk for respiratory complications (e.g., atelectasis) after surgery. Auscultation of breath sounds indicates whether the patient has pulmonary congestion or narrowing of airways, which can postpone a surgery. Breath sounds provide an important baseline for a patient's condition. Certain anesthetics potentially cause laryngeal muscle spasm. If you auscultate wheezing in the airways before surgery, a patient is at risk for further airway narrowing during surgery and after extubation (removal of the endotracheal tube). Notify the health care provider of any abnormalities noted during the assessment, especially if a decline in function is noted.

Heart and Vascular System. If a patient has a history of heart disease, assess the character of the apical pulse, and listen to heart sounds. Assessment of peripheral pulses, capillary refill, and color and temperature of extremities is particularly important for all patients undergoing vascular or orthopedic surgery and for patients who will have constricting bandages or casts on an extremity after surgery. Screen a patient for causative factors of DVT formation as verified in coagulation laboratory tests (AORN, 2020a). If peripheral pulses are not palpable, use a Doppler instrument for assessment of

FIG. 50.2 Examples of lithotomy positions used during surgery. (A) Low. (B) Standard. (C) High. (D) Exaggerated. (From Rothrock J: *Alexander's care of the patient in surgery*, ed 16, St Louis, 2019, Elsevier.)

their presence (McLendon et al., 2021). Acceptable capillary refill occurs in less than 2 seconds. Postoperative changes in circulatory status in a patient who had adequate circulation before surgery indicate impaired circulation.

Abdomen. Alterations in GI function after surgery often result in decreased or absent bowel sounds and abdominal distention. Assess the patient's usual abdominal anatomy for size, shape, symmetry, and presence of distention before surgery. Ask how often the patient has bowel movements, and inquire about the color and consistency of stools. Auscultate bowel sounds over all four abdominal quadrants.

Neurological Status. A surgical patient's level of consciousness changes as a result of anesthesia, sedatives, and complications that may develop during surgery. Preoperative assessment of baseline neurological status is important for all patients. The baseline neurological status helps with the assessment of ascent (awakening) from anesthesia. Patients should normally regain consciousness and return to normal preop states. However, it is also critical to assess neurological status to readily identify when patients develop delirium postoperatively. Delirium is an acute confusional state—not a degenerative process, but rather one linked with a specific medical condition that has caused changes to an individual's normal homeostasis and bodily function (Francis and Young, 2020; Koutoukidis et al., 2017).

Observe a patient's level of orientation, alertness, mood, and ease of speech, noting whether the patient answers questions appropriately and is able to recall recent and past events. Patients who are having surgery for neurological disease (e.g., brain tumor or aneurysm) may demonstrate an impaired level of consciousness or altered behavior.

If a patient is scheduled for spinal or regional anesthesia, preoperative assessment of gross motor function and strength is important. Spinal anesthesia causes temporary paralysis of the lower extremities (see Chapter 44). Be aware of a patient entering surgery with weakness or impaired mobility of the lower extremities, and communicate this to the perioperative team so that care providers do not become alarmed when full motor function does not return as the anesthetic wears off.

Diagnostic Screening. Patients often undergo diagnostic tests and procedures for preexisting abnormalities before surgery. Patients scheduled for elective or ambulatory surgery usually have tests done several days before surgery. Testing done the day of surgery is usually limited to tests designed to rule out or monitor potential problems, such as glucose monitoring for a patient with diabetes or an electrocardiogram (ECG) for patients with heart disease. If tests reveal severe problems, a surgeon or anesthesiologist will postpone surgery until the condition stabilizes. As a preoperative nurse you coordinate the completion of tests and verify that a patient is properly prepared. Be familiar with the purpose of diagnostic tests, know a patient's results, and alert a surgeon or anesthesiologist when findings are abnormal.

A patient's medical history, physical assessment findings, and surgical procedure determine the types of tests ordered. For example, a type and cross-match for blood are indicated before surgery for procedures in which blood loss is expected (e.g., hip replacements) in case a patient needs a blood transfusion during surgery. The surgeon designates the number of blood units to have available during surgery. Table 50.6 gives the purpose and normal values for common blood tests.

TABLE 50.6 Common Laboratory Tests for Surgical Patients

Test	Normal Values[a]	Low	High
Complete Blood Count (CBC)		**SIGNIFICANCE**	
Hemoglobin (Hgb)	Female: 12-16 g/dL; male: 14-18 g/dL	Anemia	Polycythemia (elevated red blood cell count)
Hematocrit (Hct)	Female: 36%-47%; male: 40%-52%	Fluid overload	Dehydration
Platelet count	150,000-400,000/mm^3	Decreased clotting	Increased risk of blood clot
White blood cell count	5000-10,000/mm^3	Decreased ability to fight infection	Infection
Blood Chemistry			
Sodium (Na)	136-145 mEq/L	Fluid overload	Dehydration
Potassium (K)	3.5-5.0 mEq/L	Cardiac rhythm irregularities	Cardiac rhythm irregularities
Chloride (Cl)	98-106 mEq/L	Follows shifts in sodium blood levels	Follows shifts in sodium blood levels
Carbon dioxide (CO_2)	23-30 mEq/L	Affects acid-base balance in blood	Affects acid-base balance in blood
Blood urea nitrogen (BUN)	10-20 mg/dL	Liver disease/fluid overload	Renal disease/dehydration
Glucose	74-106 mg/dL fasting	Insulin reaction, inadequate glucose intake	Diabetes mellitus and stress of surgery
Creatinine	0.5-1.1 mg/dL	Malnutrition	Renal disease
Coagulation Studies			
International Normalized Ratio (INR)	0.8-1.1	Risk of clot	Risk of bleeding
Prothrombin time (PT)	11-12.5 sec; 85%-100%	Risk of clot	Risk of bleeding
Partial thromboplastin time (PTT)	60-70 sec	Risk of clot	Risk of bleeding
Activated PTT	30-40 sec	Risk of clot	Excess heparin; risk of spontaneous bleeding (activated PTT)

[a] Normal ranges vary slightly among laboratories.
From Pagana KD, et al.: *Mosby's diagnostic and laboratory test reference,* ed 15, St Louis, 2021, Elsevier.

Maintenance of circulating blood volume is critical for any patient undergoing surgery and is accomplished with administration of whole blood or blood components. Patients undergoing elective surgery who will most likely need blood products will have a pretransfusion type and screen sample taken 1 to 7 days before surgery (see agency policy) (Rothrock, 2019). This test ensures blood compatibility (if a transfusion is needed) and avoids antibodies that may emerge in response to exposure through transfusions or a patient's disease. Autotransfusion (i.e., the reinfusion of a patient's own blood intraoperatively) is more common today (Rothrock, 2019). During intraoperative autotransfusion (cell salvage), blood is collected as it is lost during the surgery and reinfused to the patient after it is filtered and washed. Predated (up to 1 month before surgery) autologous blood donation is in decreasing use (Rothrock, 2019).

REFLECT NOW

In preparing a preoperative patient for surgery, what are three questions you should ask to identify the patient's religious and cultural preferences for surgery? If you have cared for a surgical patient, consider any specific patient behaviors that demonstrated religious and/or cultural practices.

◆ Analysis and Nursing Diagnosis

Following assessment, you analyze data for cues and clusters of data to recognize patterns reflecting nursing diagnoses relevant for a surgical patient (Box 50.4). Your knowledge and previous experience, coupled with what you learn about the patient, strengthen your ability to make the clinical judgment needed to identify relevant diagnoses. The patient's data are critical. Although there are nursing diagnoses routinely identified preoperatively (e.g., *Risk for Infection* or *Impaired Airway Clearance*), each patient will have unique risk factors and related factors pertinent to a diagnosis. A patient with preexisting health problems is likely to have a variety of risk diagnoses. For example, a patient with type 2 diabetes mellitus who has fasting glucose levels exceeding 110 mg/dL could be at *Risk for Impaired Skin Integrity*. The nature of the surgery and assessment of the patient's health status provide assessment findings and risk factors for a number of nursing diagnoses. For example, because a patient will have a surgical incision and an intravenous (IV) infusion, there is a risk for developing infection at the surgical site, in the bloodstream (sepsis), or phlebitis (at the IV site). A diagnosis of *Risk for Infection* requires the nurse's attention from admission through recovery.

BOX 50.4 Nursing Diagnostic Process

Fear Related to Insufficient Knowledge and Previous Surgical Experience

Assessment Activities	Assessment Findings
Ask patient to describe previous surgical experiences.	Apprehension over anesthesia and postoperative pain
Ask patient about understanding of preoperative education/ preparation before admission.	Expresses feeling of dread, worry over complications that may result; unaware of preoperative testing
Observe patient's nonverbal behavior, including body movements.	Maintains poor eye contact, wrings hands when discussing surgery

---

The related factors for problem-focused or negative diagnoses establish directions for the nursing care that is provided during one or all surgical phases. For example, the diagnosis of *Impaired Mobility related to incisional pain* requires different interventions than the diagnosis of *Impaired Mobility related to decreased muscle strength*. Preoperative nursing diagnoses allow nursing staff to take precautions and implement interventions so that the care provided during the intraoperative and postoperative phases is consistent with the patient's needs.

Nursing diagnoses made before surgery may focus on the potential risks a patient may experience after surgery.

Jeff's assessments reveal that Mr. Cooper has a great deal of anxiety about his surgery and its outcomes. He is concerned about his future and his ability to manage a colostomy. Jeff identifies areas from his preoperative assessment of Mr. Cooper that he can utilize to address his anxiety and questions. Jeff considers an interprofessional consultation with a wound, ostomy, and continence nurse (WOCN) to address any questions about the colostomy. Jeff inquires how Mr. Cooper has handled anxiety in the past. Jeff identifies **Anxiety related to insufficient information about surgery** *as Mr. Cooper's primary nursing diagnosis.*

Preventive care is essential to manage the surgical patient effectively. The following are common nursing diagnoses relevant to the patient having surgery:

- Impaired Airway Clearance
- Anxiety
- Impaired Skin Integrity
- Risk for Infection
- Acute Pain

◆ Planning and Outcomes Identification

During the planning phase, synthesize information to establish a plan of care based on a patient's nursing diagnoses (see the Nursing Care Plan). Apply critical thinking when making the sound clinical judgments needed to select nursing interventions (Fig. 50.3). For example, apply knowledge of adult learning principles, the patient's type of surgery, standards for preoperative education (AORN, 2020a), a patient's unique learning needs, and the patient's anticipated needs after discharge to formulate a well-designed preoperative teaching plan for the diagnosis of *Anxiety*. Critical thinking ensures that a patient's plan of care integrates your knowledge, previous experiences, environmental factors, established standards of practice, and critical thinking attitudes. Use professional standards when selecting interventions for the nursing plan of care. These standards often use evidence-based guidelines for preferred nursing interventions.

Successful planning requires a patient-centered approach involving the patient and family to set realistic expectations for care, especially postoperatively. Early involvement of a patient and family caregiver when developing the surgical care plan minimizes surgical risks and postoperative complications and improves the transition of care through discharge. A patient informed about the planned surgical experience is less likely to be fearful and is better able to participate in the postoperative recovery phase so that expected outcomes are met.

Previous experience in caring for surgical patients helps to establish approaches to patient care (e.g., measures to prevent complications and how to anticipate and reduce a patient's anxiety). For example, when you have seen effective ways to help patients perform preoperative exercises, this will allow you to individualize an approach when your patient has similar needs. Your personal and previous experience with the surgical process and all phases of patient care will assist in the selection of interventions, as well as prepare you to recognize ongoing patient problems. Your experience in interpreting laboratory data and in using pre- and postoperative equipment (e.g., IPC, bladder scanner) will also assist in the management of a patient's surgical needs.

◎ NURSING CARE PLAN

Anxiety

ASSESSMENT

Assessment Activities	*Assessment Findings*[a]
Ask Mr. Cooper what he understands about his surgical procedure.	He learned from his surgeon that he will have an incision down the middle of his abdomen that will take approximately 6 to 9 weeks to heal. Mr. Cooper states, **"I probably will need a colostomy; however, I am worried about how one works and what it will look like. Will I be able to take care of myself?"**
Ask Mr. Cooper about his knowledge of preoperative preparation and what he expects after surgery.	He correctly verbalizes understanding of medicines to take the morning of surgery and NPO status before surgery. Mr. Cooper indicated he is unsure about the length of time he will remain hospitalized, his diet after surgery, and plans for bowel elimination.
Assess Mr. Cooper's concerns about surgery.	He appears slightly anxious, with **reduced eye contact**. His **heart rate is 106 beats per minute** and his **blood pressure is 150/90 mm Hg** (normal for patient 82 to 86 beats per minute, BP 130/78). **He states, "This surgery will change my entire life. It is serious."**

[a] **Assessment Findings** are shown in bold type.

NURSING DIAGNOSIS: Anxiety related to insufficient information about surgery

PLANNING

Expected Outcomes

Anxiety Level

Patient will maintain eye contact during instructions.

Patient will verbalize anxiety over the change an ostomy will have on body function.

Knowledge: Treatment Procedures

Mr. Cooper describes the importance of and demonstrates postoperative exercises by the morning of surgery.

Mr. Cooper describes the need for a colostomy and progression of diet immediately after surgery.

Mr. Cooper will explain location and expected output of colostomy.

Mr. Cooper will discuss plans for ostomy pouching and skin care by day two after surgery.

[b] Outcome classification labels from Moorhead S, et al: *Nursing Outcomes Classification (NOC)*, ed 6, St Louis, 2018, Elsevier.

INTERVENTIONS (NIC)[c]	RATIONALE
Anxiety Reduction	
Encourage verbalization of fears and concerns. Help patient identify specific aspects of surgery that cause him to be anxious.	Minimizing apprehension over relevant concerns helps to relieve patient anxiety and allows for focusing instruction on those concerns.
Refer patient to ostomy specialist in ambulatory care center to reinforce factual information about diagnosis and ostomy care.	Specialist plays an active role in helping patients perform self-care for their ostomy and adjust to it psychologically (Francone, 2020; Heideman, 2017).
Preoperative Teaching	
Provide Mr. Cooper, for home viewing, a compact disc (CD) program that explains a colostomy and the preoperative and postoperative routines to expect. Make a follow-up call 24 hours before surgery to the patient, encouraging him to ask questions and express concerns.	Preoperative education is effective in reducing patients' postoperative anxiety and in improving their knowledge (Francone, 2020; Ramesh et al., 2017; Rothrock, 2019).
Explain purpose of and demonstrate to Mr. Cooper how to perform postoperative exercises.	Demonstration is an effective method to reinforce instruction. Use of teach-back is an effective education strategy (Alper et al., 2020).
Ostomy specialist will schedule visit the morning of surgery to discuss with patient the location of the ostomy and expected progress and output of colostomy and plans for postop ostomy care.	Assists patient in having a realistic sense of postoperative condition and expectations for his involvement in care (Butcher et al., 2018)

[c] Intervention classification labels from Butcher HK, et al: *Nursing Interventions Classification (NIC)*, ed 7, St Louis, 2018, Elsevier.

EVALUATION

Evaluation Activity	*Patient Response*
Observe Mr. Cooper's nonverbal behavior and ask how he feels about surgery during instructional time.	Patient has numerous questions but maintains eye contact. At end of discussion states, "I am still a bit uneasy, but I think I am understanding more what to expect."
Ask Mr. Cooper to describe postoperative activities to expect.	He verbalizes understanding of purpose for postoperative exercises ("helps me to breath and be active") after surgery.
Observe Mr. Cooper demonstrate postoperative exercises.	He correctly demonstrates leg exercises and turning, coughing, and deep breathing (TCDB). Is having difficulty using incentive spirometer unassisted.
Ostomy specialist asks Mr. Cooper to describe location and expected function of colostomy.	Patient describes area on abdomen where colostomy is to be located and type of stool that will be collected in ostomy pouch.

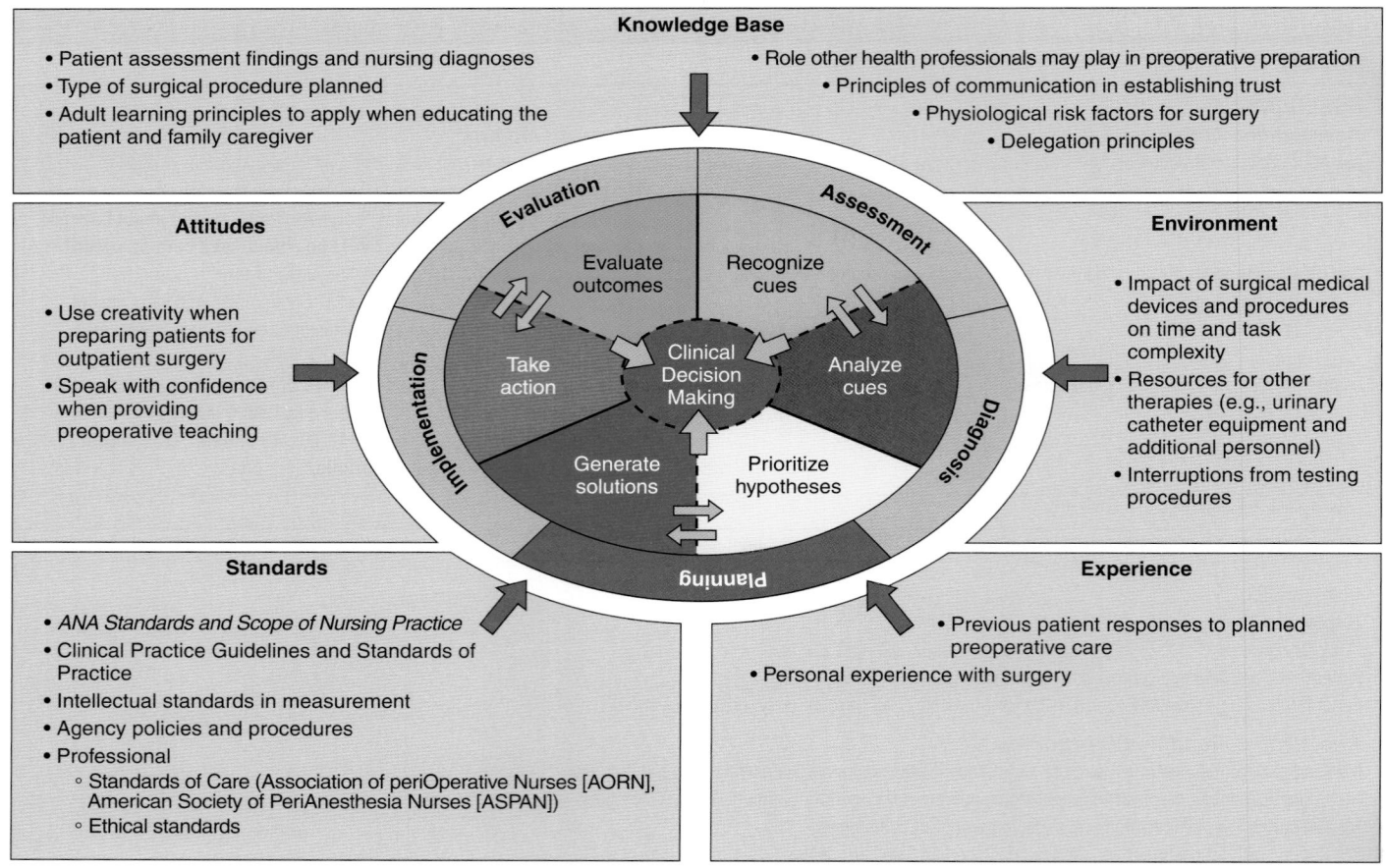

FIG. 50.3 Critical thinking model for surgical patient planning. (Clinical Judgment Measurement Model copyright © NCSBN. All rights reserved.)

It is also important to recognize environmental factors that will affect your care of a surgical patient. When is it best to delegate care to assistive personnel (AP) and what activities are they best prepared to perform for a select patient? Are you able to provide essential preoperative teaching amid interruptions from other health care personnel assessing the patient? The challenge in planning preoperative care is to prepare the patient safely and appropriately for impending surgery.

Outcomes. Establish outcomes of care based on the individualized nursing diagnoses. Perioperative nurses will review and modify the plan during the intraoperative and postoperative periods. Preoperative outcomes focus on preparing the patient for surgery. Outcomes provide measurable evidence to gauge a patient's surgical progress.

In the nursing care plan, Jeff wants to improve Mr. Cooper's ability to manage his anxiety about surgery. Jeff asks Mr. Cooper to explain what he currently understands about his surgery. Later, Jeff determines whether these plans are met (e.g., by monitoring the outcome of focused assessments and postoperative issues). Each outcome needs a time frame for achievement. For Mr. Cooper, the time frame for the outcome of reducing his anxiety is to be met both preoperatively and postoperatively.

Examples of expected outcomes relevant to surgical patients include:
- Patient remains free of pressure injury 24 hours after surgery.
- Patient performs deep-breathing and coughing exercises on awakening from anesthesia.
- Patient performs postoperative leg exercises and early ambulation 12 hours after surgery.

- Patient performs incentive spirometry on return to patient care unit after surgery.
- Patient verbalizes rationale for early ambulation 24 hours after surgery.

Setting Priorities. Use sound clinical judgment to prioritize nursing diagnoses and interventions based on the unique needs of each patient. Patients requiring emergent surgery often experience changes in their physiological status that require urgent reprioritizations. For example, if a patient's blood pressure begins to drop, hemodynamic stabilization becomes a priority over education and stress management. Ensure that the approach to each patient is thorough and reflects an understanding of the implications of a patient's age, physical and psychological health, educational level and ability to learn, cultural and religious practices, and stated or written wishes concerning advance medical directives.

Teamwork and Collaboration. For patients having surgery, the health care team needs to collaborate to ensure continuity of care. Preoperative planning ideally occurs days before admission to a hospital or surgical center. The collaboration between the health care provider's office and the surgical center or hospital is crucial to prepare a patient for a procedure. Preoperative instruction gives patients time to think about their surgical experience, make necessary physical preparations (e.g., altering diet or discontinuing medication use), and ask questions about postoperative procedures. A patient having ambulatory surgery usually returns home on the day of surgery. Thus well-planned preoperative care ensures that the patient is well informed and able to be an active participant during recovery. The family or significant others also play an active supportive role for a patient. For some procedures, such as major joint replacements, physical therapists will provide exercise plans preoperatively over several days to improve patients' exercise tolerance postop.

Collaboration of the health care team is especially important for patients who have special problems or risks (e.g., morbid obesity or advanced lung disease). Health care providers will know precautions to take to avoid intraoperative complications. In collaborative planning nurses can anticipate expected interventions from all members of the health care team (e.g., respiratory and physical therapy) who will be taking part in the patient's care. The need for and implications for inpatient care are discussed with the patient and family before the surgery. Planning might include the use of an ERAS protocol. The postoperative plan of care for inpatients will focus on preventing postoperative complications but will also include interventions to inhibit exacerbations of co-morbid conditions. Postoperative care involves an interprofessional team whose members focus on patients' early recovery.

◆ Implementation

Preoperative nursing interventions provide patients (and families) with a complete understanding of the surgery and anticipated postoperative activities. During this time, you prepare patients physically and psychologically for surgical intervention and recovery.

Informed Consent. Except in emergencies, surgery cannot be performed legally or ethically until a patient fully understands a surgical procedure and all implications. Surgical procedures are not performed without documentation of a patient's informed consent in the medical record. In some instances, the patient's medical power of attorney may give consent if the patient is unable to do so. Persons with only general power of attorney cannot sign surgical consents. When a consent is obtained preoperatively, it must be done before a patient receives any form of sedation to ensure a clear level of consciousness at the time of signing. Chapter 23 discusses a nurse's responsibilities for informed consent. It is the surgeon's responsibility to explain the procedure, associated risks, benefits, alternatives, and possible complications before obtaining the patient's oral and documented informed consent (TJC, 2020). The patient also needs to know who will perform the procedure. To ensure that a patient understands the information about the surgery, TJC (2021) recommends that consent materials be written at a fifth-grade or lower reading level. After the patient or power of attorney signs the consent form, place it in the medical record. The record goes to the OR with the patient. If you have concerns about a patient's understanding of surgery, report these concerns to the operating surgeon or anesthesia provider before the patient goes to surgery (Ryan and Sinha, 2020).

Privacy and Social Media. Although patients can now access their medical records electronically, confidentiality risks exist. Inappropriate discussions of a patient and any planned surgery in elevators, cafeterias, or social settings may end up being communicated "worldwide" (NCSBN, 2018). Nurses have the obligation to protect every patient's privacy by avoiding inappropriate discussions and not using social media to convey patient information. Posting patient information and photos on websites is prohibited; 26 state boards of nursing have taken disciplinary action against nurses who practiced such behaviors (Rothrock, 2019), which are direct violations of federal and state patient privacy laws.

Health Promotion. Health promotion activities during the preoperative phase focus on health maintenance, patient safety, prevention of complications, and anticipation of the continued care needed after surgery.

Preoperative Teaching. Patient education is an important aspect of a patient's surgical experience (see Chapter 25). The topics and principles discussed depend on the type of surgery scheduled, whether a procedure is inpatient or outpatient, and the ability of a patient to attend to and learn the content provided. Providing patient education about pain reduces a patient's preoperative anxiety, which is frequently associated with postoperative pain (Joshi, 2020). Structured teaching throughout the perioperative period influences the following:

- *Ventilatory function*: Teaching improves the ability and willingness to deep-breathe and cough effectively.
- *Physical functional capacity*: Teaching increases understanding and willingness to ambulate and resume activities of daily living.
- *Sense of well-being*: Patients who are prepared for surgery have less anxiety and report a greater sense of psychological well-being (Joshi, 2020).
- *Length of hospital stay*: Being informed reduces a patient's length of hospital stay by preventing or minimizing complications.
- *Anxiety about pain and its management*: Patients who learn about pain and ways to relieve it before surgery are less anxious about it, ask for what they need, and require less analgesia after surgery.

The health care provider's office or hospital often provides preoperative information and instructions by telephone calls and home mailings. Instructions are available as preprinted teaching guidelines and checklists or in the form of videotapes or educational websites. The American College of Surgeons developed a patient education website titled *Surgical Patient Education Program*, which provides patient information and educational materials on types of surgeries, health resources, insurance information, and even some home care skills training (American College of Surgeons, 2020). When a patient is scheduled for surgery (outpatient or inpatient), preadmission nurses call patients up to 1 week before the surgery to clarify questions and reinforce explanations (Rothrock, 2019). For example, they:

- Describe the time for a patient to arrive at the hospital or surgical center and the time of surgery (approximately).
- Explain the extent and purpose of food and fluid restrictions.
- Teach about physical preparation (e.g., bowel preparation, bathing or showering with antiseptic).
- Explain procedures performed in preanesthesia (holding area) just before transport to the OR (IV line insertion, preoperative medications).

Including family members in preoperative instruction is advisable. Often a family member is the coach for postoperative exercises when a patient returns from surgery. A family often has better retention of preoperative teaching and will be with the patient and able to help in recovery. If anxious relatives do not understand routine postoperative events, it is likely that their anxiety heightens the patient's fear and concerns. Preoperative preparation of family members lessens anxiety and misunderstanding. For example, a patient needs to know how recommended care activities (e.g., regular antibiotics, wound care) in the home will prevent wound infection, avoid wound-healing complications (e.g., activity restrictions prevent wound stress), and maintain a level of health (e.g., diet and progressive exercise allowed). Patients having surgery also need to know the signs of complications and when to call their surgeon.

Jeff plans for time after completion of Mr. Cooper's assessment to discuss the planned surgery with him and his wife. Jeff begins by asking Mr. Cooper to describe what he thinks the procedure will involve, to share any concerns, and to identify the type of information he wants to understand. Jeff offers Mr. Cooper, for home viewing, a compact disc (CD) program that explains the preoperative and postoperative routines to expect. He also plans a teaching session prior to surgery so that Mr. Cooper will understand what to expect in all phases of his procedure (e.g., application of IPC, intraoperative processes, and PACU expectations).

Patients are better prepared to participate in their recovery when they receive rationale for preoperative and postoperative procedures. Patients who undergo surgery need to learn how to promote a healthy recovery and prevent complications, which will allow them to return to a normal lifestyle as soon as possible.

Patients who have inpatient surgery need to additionally understand what is required to facilitate their recovery, including pain control, early ambulation, diet progression, wound care, and postoperative exercises (e.g., diaphragmatic breathing, incentive spirometry, coughing, turning, and leg exercises). Postoperative exercises and early ambulation help to prevent pulmonary and vascular complications and deconditioning (see Skill 50.1). Ideally, instruction begins before surgery. After you explain each exercise, demonstrate it for the patient and use teach-back to confirm understanding. Guide the patient through each exercise. Ask the patient to perform a return demonstration of the skill, if possible, to reinforce it and increase the confidence in performing it.

Changes in the circulatory system, a patient's immobility during surgery, and a patient's underlying health condition create risks for the development of DVT. Patients need to know which precautions to take after surgery to avoid DVT (e.g., leg exercises and use of compression hose or intermittent pneumatic compression [IPC] devices). Teach about the purposes and the specific nursing care associated with the devices (see Chapter 39).

Preoperative Routines. Explain the preoperative routines that a patient can expect. Knowing which tests and procedures are planned and why they are planned increases a patient's sense of control. Explain that an anesthesiologist will visit to complete a preanesthesia assessment either during the preoperative admission process or in the presurgical care unit of a hospital or surgical center.

Patients typically do not consume food or fluids by mouth for several hours before surgery to reduce the risk of vomiting and aspirating emesis during surgery. Instruct patients to eat and drink sufficient amounts during the week before surgery to ensure adequate fluid and nutrient intake. This is especially important for older adults living in long-term care settings, who often do not stay adequately hydrated. Recommend foods high in protein with sufficient amounts of carbohydrates, fat, and vitamins. Explain to patients and their families the importance of following oral intake instructions for food and liquids before surgery.

Surgical Procedure. After the surgeon explains the basic purpose of a surgical procedure and its steps, some patients may ask additional questions. First, clarify the information the patient discussed with the surgeon. Avoid using technical medical terms because this adds to a patient's confusion. Avoid saying anything that contradicts the surgeon's explanation. If a patient has little or no understanding about the surgery, notify the surgeon that the patient requires further explanation.

Time of Surgery. The scheduled operative time is only an anticipated time. Unanticipated delays occur for many reasons that often have nothing to do with the patient. Emphasize that the scheduled time is a rough estimate and that the actual time can be sooner or later. Make the family aware that delays occur for various reasons and do not necessarily indicate a problem. Communicate excessive delays when they do occur.

Postoperative Unit and Location of Family During Surgery and Recovery. Few patients are admitted to a hospital unit before surgery unless their case is emergent or a complication develops before the scheduled surgery. Even then it is common for patients to be assigned to a different room after surgery. When surgery is elective, patients and families will come to the surgical center admission area first. During the admission process, the patient and family will find out which patient care unit the patient most likely will be admitted to after surgery. Be sure to explain where the family can wait and where the surgeon will come to find family members after surgery. In many institutions, the circulating nurse gives periodic reports to the family in the waiting room for surgeries that are expected to be prolonged. Many hospitals use pagers to inform family through text messages about patient progress. If a patient will be taken to a special unit, it helps to orient the patient and family members to the environment of the unit before surgery.

Anticipated Postoperative Monitoring and Therapies. Inform a patient and family about routine postoperative monitoring and therapies (e.g., frequency of vital signs, IV therapy, dressings, drains, planned activity, and physical therapy). If they understand the frequency of anticipated monitoring and procedures, they are less apprehensive when nurses perform care activities. Try not to overprepare or underprepare a patient. It is easier to prepare a patient appropriately in elective cases when a surgeon has care guidelines such as an ERAS protocol for a specific procedure and you have adequate time for patient education. You cannot predict all of a patient's care requirements. Contradictions between your explanations and reality cause anxiety for a patient.

Sensory Preparation. Provide patients with information about the sensations typically experienced after surgery. Preparatory information helps them anticipate the steps of a procedure and thus form realistic images of the surgical experience. For example, warn that the OR is very bright and cold. Patients often undergo prewarming or are given warm blankets. A patient will have a cuff for a noninvasive blood pressure monitor placed around the arm. The monitor makes a hum and a beep, and the cuff tightens to take a reading. Informing a patient about these and other sensations in the OR reduces anxiety before the patient is anesthetized, which helps reduce the amount of anesthetic needed for induction. Postoperative sensations include blurred vision from ophthalmic ointment in the eyes, expected pain at the surgical site and in areas of the body affected by prolonged positioning, the tightness of dressings, dryness of the mouth, and the sensation of a sore throat resulting from an endotracheal tube (when one is inserted).

Postoperative Activity Resumption. The type of surgery determines how quickly patients can resume normal physical activity and regular eating habits. Explain what to expect after surgery. It is normal in most surgical cases for patients to progress their diet gradually. Many hospitals implement early mobility protocols to prevent hospital-acquired deconditioning and resultant postoperative complications (Grass et al., 2018; Pai and Douketis, 2020; Smetana, 2020a) (see Chapter 38). Mobility promotes circulation, lung expansion, and peristalsis. Postural hypotension is caused by sudden position changes.

Pain-Relief Measures. Pain following surgery is one of a patient's most common fears. Even in local procedures (e.g., laparoscopy), air inflation into the abdomen causes significant discomfort in the area of surgery. The family is also concerned for the patient's comfort. Pain after surgery is expected. Inform the patient and family of the likely characteristics and course of pain (as it relates to type of surgery). Explain the need to manage pain and the types of therapies likely to be used so that patients can resume activity quickly, knowing they will receive pain relief (e.g., relaxation exercises and splinting). Teach patients before surgery how to use a pain scale so that they are prepared to rate their pain after surgery (see Chapter 44). Patient-controlled analgesia (PCA) may be ordered for inpatients to help them gain control over pain. Explain and demonstrate to a patient how to operate a PCA device and the importance of administering medication as soon as pain becomes persistent (see Chapter 44). Patients who receive epidural analgesia need a thorough understanding of how it will affect their movement and sensation after surgery.

Some patients avoid taking pain-relief drugs after surgery for fear of the negative side effects or of becoming dependent on the drugs. Listen to their concerns and encourage patients to use analgesics as ordered. Unless pain is controlled, it is difficult for a patient to participate in postoperative therapy. Because of the well-publicized problem of opioid addiction, many patients are reluctant to take opioids even for short, appropriate time frames. Some states in the United States are passing legislation that would create a "nonopioid directive" that patients can place in their medical files, formally notifying health care professionals that they do not want to be prescribed or administered opioid medications. When it is anticipated that patients will suffer from severe pain postoperatively, have a serious discussion about how health care providers will gradually reduce the dose of opioids and switch to less addictive medication as patients progress.

Encourage patients to take pain medications at ordered intervals. Optimal pain management is based on patient assessment data throughout the perioperative experience and customized based on assessment findings and the surgical procedure involved, with follow-up evaluation and adjustments as needed.

Multimodal approaches to postoperative pain management vary, depending on the patient, setting, and surgical procedure (Mariano, 2020). Multimodal approaches include opioids and one or more additional pain-management methods, such as a peripheral nerve block, acetaminophen, gabapentin, nonsteroidal antiinflammatory drugs (NSAIDs), cyclooxygenase-2 (COX-2) inhibitors, or ketamine (ASA, 2018). Pain-control regimens should be individualized to the needs of the patient, considering age, medical and physical condition, level of fear/anxiety, personal preferences, type of surgical procedure, and individual patient response. An optimal plan for perioperative pain control should include a multimodal approach to minimize the need for opioids (Mariano, 2020).

When pain is not addressed regularly, it often becomes excruciating, and analgesics do not provide relief at the dose ordered. When educating patients, explain the length of time it takes for pain medications to take effect. Information from a preoperative pain assessment is helpful when teaching about nonpharmacological pain-relief measures (such as positioning and splinting). Remember that pain is subjective, and you must accept patients' perception of pain.

Rest. Rest is essential for normal healing. Anxiety about surgery interferes with the ability to relax and sleep. Meet each patient's individual needs. If a patient is in the hospital, make the environment as quiet and comfortable as possible. The surgeon may order a sedative-hypnotic or antianxiety agent for the night before surgery. Sedative-hypnotics promote sleep. Antianxiety agents (e.g., alprazolam) act on the cerebral cortex and limbic system to relieve anxiety. The advantage of ambulatory surgery is that a patient can sleep at home or in a nearby hotel (for out-of-towners) the night before surgery.

Feelings Regarding Surgery. Some patients feel like part of an assembly line before surgery as a result of frequent staff visits and physical preparation for surgery. The patient has few opportunities to reflect on the experience. Recognize the patient as a unique individual. The patient and family need time to express feelings and concerns about surgery and to ask questions. The patient's level of anxiety influences the frequency of discussions. While delivering preoperative instruction, encourage expression of concerns, be patient, and listen attentively. The family may wish to discuss concerns without the patient present so that their fears do not frighten the patient and vice versa. Establishing a trusting and therapeutic relationship with a patient and family allows this process to happen.

Acute Care. Acute care activities in the preoperative phase focus on the physical preparation of a patient on the morning of surgery or before an emergent surgery.

Minimizing Risk for Surgical Wound Infection. A surgical site infection (SSI) is one of the National Quality Forum (NQF) incidents that hospitals report (NQF, 2019) and that the CMS classifies as a "never event," a serious adverse event that occurs within a hospital and that is usually preventable (AHRQ, 2019). As of 2008, the CMS (Centers for Medicaid and Medicare Services, 2020) no longer pays for the costs associated with "never events," including treatment and hospital days associated with the event. Thus, there is great emphasis within hospitals on preventing the occurrence of SSIs. Antibiotics are sometimes ordered in the preoperative period. A reduction in wound infection rates occurs when an antibiotic is administered 60 minutes before the surgical incision is made and the antibiotics are stopped within 24 hours after surgery (Anderson and Sexton, 2020b; Berríos-Torres et al., 2017). The surgeon orders a specific time before surgery for the patient to have an oral or IV antibiotic.

Preoperative care involves skin antisepsis (i.e., removing soil and transient microorganisms at the surgical site) to reduce the risk of a patient developing an SSI (Berríos-Torres et al., 2017). It is not performed for all surgeries, but it is routine before surgeries involving the chest or abdomen or with major joint replacements. Routine components of skin antisepsis include preoperative bathing (showers or baths) and hair management, both of which reduce the number of microorganisms on the skin. Most patients requiring skin antisepsis bathe the evening before surgery or that morning (George et al., 2017).

Due to a lack of definitive research findings, there is no one antiseptic agent found to be most effective (Anderson and Sexton, 2020b; George et al., 2017), but 2% chlorhexidine (CHG) in 70% alcohol is becoming the preferred antiseptic, with povidone-iodine as an alternative when CHG is contraindicated (Anderson and Sexton, 2020a; George et al., 2017). Patients who undergo head and neck surgery typically shampoo the hair before surgery to reduce resident flora on the scalp.

The AORN (2020a) recommends that the nurse remove the hair at the surgical site only in select clinical situations. The current evidence supports leaving hair at the surgical site in place unless it interferes with exposure, closure, or dressing of the surgical site. When hair removal is required, clipping it is likely to result in less SSI than removal with a razor (Anderson and Sexton, 2020b; AORN, 2020a). Razors cause micro nicks in the skin. Use single-use clipper heads for each patient, and remove hair as close to the time of surgery as possible.

Maintaining Normal Fluid and Electrolyte Balance. A patient having surgery is vulnerable to fluid and electrolyte imbalance as a result of the stress of surgery, inadequate preoperative intake, and the potential for excessive fluid losses during surgery (see Chapter 42). The American Society of Anesthesiologists (ASA) has recommendations for fluid and food intake before nonemergent procedures requiring general and regional anesthesia or sedation/analgesia. These recommendations include fasting from intake of clear liquids for 2 or more hours, breast milk for 4 hours, formula and nonhuman milk for 6 hours, and a light meal of toast and clear liquids for 6 hours. A patient also cannot have any meat or fried foods 8 hours before surgery, unless explicitly specified by the anesthesiologist or surgeon (ASA, 2017; Crowley, 2020). When a patient is hospitalized before surgery, remove all fluids and solid foods as ordered from the bedside and post a sign over the bed to alert personnel to fasting restrictions.

Despite the ASA standards, many surgeons still have patients maintain nothing by mouth after midnight. Ensure that you follow the health care provider's orders. During general anesthesia, the muscles relax, and gastric contents can reflux into the esophagus. The anesthetic reduces the patient's gag reflex. Therefore, a patient is at risk for aspiration of food or fluids from the stomach into the lungs. The surgeon's orders will provide additional guidance for routine procedures (e.g., IV line placement and preoperative medications). Some patients are allowed to take specific medications (e.g., anticoagulants, cardiovascular medications, anticonvulsants, and antibiotics) with a sip of water as ordered by their health care providers. Allow patients time to rinse their mouths with water or mouthwash and brush their teeth immediately before surgery as long as they do not swallow water. Notify the surgeon and anesthesia provider if a patient eats or drinks during the fasting period.

If a patient cannot eat because of GI alterations or impairments in consciousness, the health care provider may order intravenous fluids. The health care provider assesses serum electrolyte levels to determine the type of IV fluids and electrolyte additives to administer before and during surgery. Patients with severe nutritional imbalances sometimes require supplements with concentrated protein and glucose such as total parenteral nutrition (see Chapter 45).

Preventing Bowel Incontinence and Contamination. Some patients receive a bowel preparation (e.g., a cathartic or enema) if the surgery involves the lower GI system. Manipulation of parts of the GI tract during surgery results in absence of peristalsis for 24 hours and sometimes longer. Enemas and cathartics (see Chapter 47) such as a polyethylene glycol electrolyte solution clean the GI tract to prevent intraoperative incontinence. An empty bowel reduces risk of injury to the intestines and minimizes contamination of the operative wound if colon surgery is planned or a part of the bowel is incised or opened accidentally. In addition, bowel cleansing reduces postoperative constipation. If a surgeon's order reads "give enemas until clear," this means that a nurse administers enemas until the enema return solution contains no solid fecal material. Too many enemas given over a short time can cause serious fluid and electrolyte imbalances (see Chapter 42). Most agencies limit the number of enemas (usually three) that a nurse may administer successively. Verify a patient's potassium level following bowel preparation. Diarrhea may cause hypokalemia.

Preparation on the Day of Surgery. You will commonly complete several routine procedures before releasing patients for surgery.

Hygiene. Basic hygiene measures provide additional comfort before surgery. If a patient is unwilling to take a complete bath, a partial bath is refreshing and removes irritating secretions or drainage from the skin. Provide a clean hospital gown as a patient cannot wear personal nightwear to the OR because it is restrictive and is a flammable hazard. When a patient is NPO for hours before surgery, the mouth is often very dry. Offer the patient nonalcohol-based mouthwash and toothpaste, again cautioning the patient not to swallow water.

Preparation of Hair and Removal of Cosmetics. During major surgery, an anesthesiologist positions a patient's head to place an endotracheal tube into the airway (see Chapter 41). This involves manipulation of the hair and scalp. To avoid injury, ask the patient to remove hairpins or clips before leaving for surgery. Electrocautery is frequently used during surgery. Hairpins and clips can become an exit source for the electricity and cause burns. Remove hairpieces or wigs as well. Patients can braid long hair. Disposable caps are made available to patients to contain hair before entering the OR.

During and after surgery, the anesthesia provider and nurse assess skin and mucous membranes to determine a patient's level of oxygenation, circulation, and fluid balance. A pulse oximeter is often applied to a finger to monitor oxygen saturation (see Chapter 30). Anesthesia providers also use end-tidal carbon dioxide, by way of capnography, to assess patients' physical status. When using a pulse oximeter, have patients remove all makeup (lipstick, powder, blush, nail polish) and at least one artificial fingernail to expose normal skin and nail color. Anything in or around the eye irritates or injures the eye during surgery. Have patients remove contact lenses, false eyelashes, and eye makeup. Give the patient's eyeglasses to the family immediately before the patient leaves for the OR. Document all valuables per agency policy.

Removal of Prostheses. It is easy for any type of prosthetic device to become lost or damaged during surgery. Have patients remove all removable prosthetics (e.g., artificial limbs, partial or complete dentures, artificial eyes, and hearing aids) for safekeeping just before leaving for surgery. If a patient has a brace or splint, check with the health care provider to determine whether it should remain in place. For many patients it is embarrassing to remove dentures, wigs, or other devices that enhance personal appearance. Offer privacy as a patient removes personal items. Patients are sometimes allowed to keep these until they reach the preoperative holding area. Place dentures in special containers labeled with the patient's name and other identification required by the agency for safekeeping to prevent loss or breakage. In many agencies, the nurse completes an inventory of all prosthetic devices or personal items and places them in a secured area. It is also common practice for nurses to give prostheses to family members. Document these actions in the appropriate portion of the medical record per agency policy.

Safeguarding Valuables. If a patient has valuables, give them to family members or place in a secure designated location. Hospitals require patients to sign a release to free the facilities of responsibility for lost valuables. Prepare a list with a clear description of items, place a copy with a patient's medical record (see agency policy), and give a copy to a designated family member. Describe any jewelry, including color of stones or metal. For example, if the patient is wearing a silver ring with a red stone, document the ring as silver with a red stone and not as a ruby. There have been instances in which patients claim loss of a diamond, for example, when the actual stone was not a diamond. Patients are often reluctant to remove wedding rings or religious medals. A wedding band can be taped in place, but this is not the preferred practice. If there is a risk that a patient will experience swelling of the hand or fingers (mastectomy, hand surgery, fluid shifts), remove the band. Many hospitals allow patients to pin religious medals to their gowns, although the risk of loss increases. Remove other metal items such as piercings to reduce the risk of burns.

Preparing the Bowel and Bladder. For some patients an enema or cathartic agent is administered at least 1 hour before the patient leaves for surgery, allowing time for defecation without rushing. Instruct a patient to urinate just before leaving for the OR and before giving preoperative medications. An empty bladder reduces discomfort and the risk of incontinence during surgery and makes abdominal organs more accessible to the surgeon. If a patient is unable to void, record this information on the preoperative checklist. The surgeon may order insertion of an indwelling catheter if the surgery is to be lengthy or the incision is in the lower abdomen (see Chapter 46).

Vital Signs. Monitor preoperative vital signs before surgery. The anesthesia provider uses these values as a baseline for intraoperative vital signs. If preoperative vital signs are abnormal, surgery is sometimes postponed. Notify the surgeon of any abnormalities before sending a patient to surgery. In addition, assess the patient for the presence and character of pain (see Chapter 44). Many patients have pain before surgery caused by the condition requiring surgery.

Prevention of Deep Vein Thrombosis—Antiembolism Devices. Preventing DVTs is a priority quality measure. The AORN (2020a) recommends that each health care organization implement a DVT prevention protocol (see Chapter 39). A patient's condition and type of surgery determine the preventive measures taken before surgery. For example, patients who have cardiac, GI, genitourinary (GU), gynecological (GYN), neurological, and orthopedic surgeries will likely have mechanical VTE prophylaxis implemented the morning of surgery. This includes application of one of the following devices: antiembolism stockings (thigh or knee length), foot-impulse devices, or intermittent pneumatic compression (IPC devices: thigh or knee length) (Kozek-Langenecker, 2018; Rothrock, 2019). In addition, some patients receive pharmacological VTE prophylaxis, which includes medications such as low-molecular-weight heparin (LMWH) (Pai and Douketis, 2020). The health care provider will screen patients carefully for the risk of bleeding before ordering pharmacological VTE prophylaxis.

When correctly sized and applied, antiembolism devices reduce the risk for DVT. Antiembolic stockings maintain compression of small veins and capillaries of the legs. The constant compression forces blood into larger vessels, thus promoting venous return and preventing venous stasis. The nurse attaches intermittent pneumatic compression (IPC) stockings to an air pump that inflates and deflates the stockings, allowing intermittent pressure sequentially from the ankle to the knee and alternating calves, mimicking normal venous return when walking (see Chapter 39). Foot-inflation devices simulate natural walking by compressing the plantar venous plexus (AORN, 2020a). Do not use antiembolism devices when patients have an allergy to the material (e.g., latex) or an unusual leg size or shape or a history of peripheral arterial disease, peripheral arterial bypass grafting, or peripheral neuropathy.

Administering Preoperative Medications. The increase in ambulatory surgeries has reduced the use of preoperative medications. However, the anesthesia provider or surgeon may order preanesthetic drugs ("on-call medications," "preops") to reduce patient anxiety, the amount of general anesthesia required, respiratory tract secretions, and the risk of nausea, vomiting, and possible aspiration. Typically, the nurse administers preoperative medications before a patient leaves for the OR. Complete all additional nursing care measures first. Preoperative drugs such as benzodiazepines, opioids, antiemetics, and anticholinergics usually cause dry mouth, drowsiness, and dizziness but do not induce sleep. To maintain patient safety, keep side rails in the up position, the bed in the low position, and the call light within easy reach. Instruct the patient to stay in bed until the surgical nursing assistant or transporter arrives. If the patient needs to get out of bed to void, explain the importance of using the call light to ask for assistance. A patient can easily fall, thinking nothing is wrong. Be sure that the patient has signed surgical consent before administering drugs that will alter consciousness.

Documentation and Hand-Off. Before a patient goes to the OR, an accurate medical record is essential to ensure safe and appropriate patient care. Check the contents of the medical record for the presence of ordered laboratory and imaging test results, accuracy and completeness of consent forms, and the preoperative checklist that agencies use as a tool to document all preoperative preparation activities. Carefully document surgical preparatory interventions and the patient's response to care. Once a patient is ready to go to the OR, a written (or electronic) record is inadequate to communicate information to the receiving health care team. The transfer of information about the patient from one health care provider to another requires an effective hand-off (AORN, 2020a). Box 50.5 lists critical elements for hand-offs from preoperative to intraoperative providers. The AORN (2020a) and TJC (2020, 2021) recommend that hand-off reports occur in person to ensure that the right patient receives the right surgery at the right surgical site.

Eliminating Wrong Site and Wrong Procedure Surgery. Because of errors made in the past with patients undergoing the wrong surgery or having surgery performed on the wrong site, TJC instituted Universal Protocol guidelines for preventing such mishaps. The Universal Protocol is part of TJC's ongoing National Patient Safety Goals (TJC, 2021). The preoperative-to-intraoperative hand-off described previously is an example of part of the protocol. Implement the Universal Protocol whenever an invasive surgical procedure is to be performed no matter the location (e.g., hospital, ASC, or health care provider office). The three principles of the protocol are (1) a preoperative verification ensuring that all relevant documents (e.g., consent forms, allergies, medical history, physical assessment findings) and the results of laboratory tests and diagnostic studies are available before the start of the

procedure and that the type of surgery scheduled is consistent with the patient's expectations; (2) marking the operative site with indelible ink to mark left and right distinction, multiple structures (e.g., fingers), and levels of the spine; and (3) a "time-out" just before starting the procedure for final verification of the correct patient, procedure, site, and any implants (TJC, 2021). The marking and "time-out" most commonly occur in the holding area, just before the patient enters the OR. The individual who is performing the surgery and who is accountable for it must personally mark the site and involve the patient if possible (TJC, 2021). All members of the surgical/procedure team perform the time-out. This protocol includes the patient or a legally designated representative in the entire process. If the patient refuses a mark, document this on the procedure checklist.

BOX 50.5 **Preoperative-to-Intraoperative Hand-Off Using SBAR Communication**

Situation
- Name of patient, date of birth
- Name of operative procedure to be performed, including site and modifiers
- Pertinent documents (e.g., consent, test results) present and consistent

Background
- Elements of patient history pertinent to surgery
- Medical clearance
- Patient allergies and NPO status
- Patient's vital signs and pain level
- Medication profile and medications taken today; laboratory results; imaging results
- Code status of patient

Assessment
- Patient's current level of understanding of the surgery
- Special patient needs, risks, or precautions
- Pertinent cultural or emotional factors
- Anesthesia requests

Recommendations
- State whether the patient has been seen before surgery by a surgeon and anesthesia care provider.
- Determine whether the patient is ready for surgery.
- Allow a chance for all staff members to ask questions and voice concerns.

Adapted from Amato-Vealey EJ, et al: Hand-off communication: a requisite for patient safety, *AORN J* 88(5):766, 2008.

QSEN **Building Competency in Evidence-Based Practice** You are a nurse in a surgical preoperative area. A patient asks, "After a previous surgery on my colon, I got an infection in the incision. What is the chance that I will get an infection or another complication after this surgery?" The patient verified that the previous surgery was uneventful but that within 48 hours after surgery the patient developed a fever of 39.7° C (103.6° F). The patient's question poses an important practice issue. Use the PICOT evidence-based practice framework, and identify the question that will guide your inquiry of the evidence.

Answers to QSEN Activities can be found on the Evolve website.

◆ **Evaluation**

The nurse caring for a patient in the preoperative area evaluates the patient's expectations and initial patient outcomes (e.g., outcomes

Knowledge Base
- Behaviors that demonstrate learning
- Patient assessment findings, nursing diagnoses, and expected outcomes
- Characteristics of anxiety and/or fear
  - Signs and symptoms of conditions that may contraindicate surgery

Attitudes
- Demonstrate perseverance when patients have difficulty performing postoperative exercises
- Display curiosity when a clinical change occurs preoperatively

Environment
- Impact of surgical medical devices and procedures on time and task complexity
- Resources for other therapies (e.g., urinary catheter equipment and additional personnel)
- Interruptions

Standards
- *ANA Standards and Scope of Nursing Practice*
- Clinical Practice Guidelines and Standards of Practice
- Intellectual standards in measurement
- Agency policies and procedures
- Professional
  - Standards of Care (Association of periOperative Nurses [AORN], American Society of PeriAnesthesia Nurses [ASPAN])
  - Ethical standards

Experience
- Previous patient responses to planned preoperative care
- Personal experience with surgery

Inside the model:
Evaluation — Evaluate outcomes
Assessment — Recognize cues
Analyze cues
Diagnosis — Prioritize hypotheses
Planning — Generate solutions
Implementation — Take action
Clinical Decision Making

FIG. 50.4 Critical thinking model for surgical patient evaluation. (Clinical Judgment Measurement Model copyright © NCSBN. All rights reserved.)

expected from education and risk reduction) (Fig. 50.4). There is limited time available to evaluate outcomes before surgery; however, if a patient's condition changes preoperatively, be sure that outcomes are current, and determine whether new or revised interventions and/or nursing diagnoses need to be implemented intraoperatively.

Through the Patient's Eyes. Evaluate whether the patient's expectations were met with respect to surgical preparation. For example, ask patients if they require additional information, if they desire to have their family members more involved, and if they have any unidentified needs. During evaluation, include a discussion of any misunderstandings so that patient concerns can be clarified. When patients have expectations about pain control, this is a good time to reinforce how it will be managed after surgery.

On the day of surgery, Jeff provides a follow-up with Mr. Cooper and his wife about any ongoing concerns, including his anxiety about this surgery. Jeff asks Mr. Cooper about his preoperative preparations (e.g., enemas, special bathing) and determines that these were all completed. Jeff asks Mr. Cooper to demonstrate the use of an incentive spirometer. He ensures that the informed consent was signed.

Patient Outcomes. Evaluate a patient's response to interventions designed for preoperative nursing diagnoses such as *Lack of Knowledge* and *Anxiety*. For example, ask the patient to describe the reason for postoperative exercises and the type of care activities to expect after returning from surgery. Observe the patient's behaviors, and discuss concerns to see whether anxiety remains. Your evaluation is comprehensive to determine

whether further instruction or emotional support is needed after surgery. Interventions continue during and after surgery; thus, the evaluation of outcomes does not occur until after surgery.

TRANSPORT TO THE OPERATING ROOM

Personnel in the OR notify the nursing unit or ambulatory surgery area when it is time for surgery. Inpatient facilities have transporters who bring stretchers to deliver patients to the preoperative care unit. In ambulatory care a patient simply walks into the preop suite if able and not medicated. A transporter or nurse in the holding area checks the patient's identification bracelet for two identifiers (name, birthday, or hospital number) (refer to institutional or agency policy) against the patient's medical record to ensure that the correct person is going to surgery. Because some patients receive preoperative sedatives, the nurses, AP, and transporter help the patient transfer from bed to stretcher to prevent falls. Provide the family an opportunity to visit before the patient is transported to the OR; then direct the family to the appropriate waiting area.

PREANESTHESIA CARE UNIT

In most surgical settings, a patient enters a **preanesthesia care unit** (PCU) or presurgical care unit (PSCU) (sometimes called the *holding area*) outside the OR where preoperative preparations are completed. Nurses in the PCU are members of the OR staff and wear surgical scrub suits, hats, and footwear in accordance with infection control policies. In some ambulatory surgical settings, a perioperative primary nurse admits the patient, circulates during the operative procedure, and manages the patient's recovery and discharge.

If an IV catheter is not present already, a nurse or anesthesia provider inserts one into a vein to establish a route for fluid replacement, IV drugs, or blood products. The nurse also administers preoperative medications at this time and monitors vital signs, including pulse oximetry. The anesthesia provider usually performs a patient assessment. If the patient received preoperative medications, explain why the patient may begin to feel drowsy. The temperature in the PCU and adjacent OR suites is usually cool; therefore, offer the patient an extra blanket or warming blanket. The patient will stay in the PCU only briefly.

INTRAOPERATIVE SURGICAL PHASE

Care of a patient intraoperatively requires careful preparation, knowledge of the events that occur during surgery, and use of stringent safety practices. The OR environment poses unique risks resulting from the procedures followed. Members of the surgical team can suffer injury from skin sticks or cuts (e.g., needle or scalpel) or mucous membrane exposure (splashing of irrigated fluids) to contaminated body fluids. Proper use of personal protective equipment (PPE) is critical. When nurses participate in laser surgical procedures, they use special safety precautions (e.g., use of laser protective eyewear or shields) to prevent injury to the eyes and skin.

NURSING ROLES DURING SURGERY

There are two traditional nursing roles in the OR: circulating nurse and scrub nurse (Fig. 50.5). The **circulating nurse** is an RN who does not scrub in and uses the nursing process in the management of patient care activities in the OR suite. The circulating nurse monitors the surgery closely and also manages patient positioning, antimicrobial skin preparation, medications, implants, placement and function of IPC devices, specimens, warming devices, and surgical counts of instruments and dressings (AORN, 2020a). The circulating nurse does not wear an OR gown. The **scrub nurse** is either an RN or surgical technologist who is often certified (CST). Scrub nurses must have a thorough knowledge of each step of a surgical procedure because they work in the surgical field with the surgeon. The scrub nurse must be able to anticipate each instrument and supply item needed by the surgeons (Rothrock, 2019). A circulating nurse and scrub nurse partner together to ensure patient safety

FIG. 50.5 Nurses in the operating room. (© 2011 Jupiterimages Corporation.)

by minimizing risk of error. The team also works together to ensure cost-efficient use of supplies.

A new role in the OR includes the RN first assistant (RNFA). This is an expanded role that requires formal academic education (AORN, 2020b). The RNFA collaborates with the surgeon by handling and cutting tissue, using instruments and medical devices, providing exposure of the surgical area and hemostasis, and suturing (Rothrock, 2019).

❖ NURSING PROCESS

Apply the nursing process and use a critical thinking approach in your care of patients intraoperatively. If you assume the role of a circulating nurse, your observations and resultant sound clinical judgment can make a difference in surgical outcomes.

◆ Assessment

The circulating nurse in the OR applies sound clinical judgment by thoroughly reassessing a patient and critically analyzing findings to confirm existing nursing diagnoses and problems and to identify any new diagnoses. The nurse uses knowledge of the surgical procedure and any risks the patient presents to make patient-centered clinical decisions required for safe nursing care. For example, assessment focuses on a patient's immediate clinical status, skin integrity (over surgical site and dependent areas where patient will lie on operating table bed), and joint function (when unusual positions on the OR table are required). This involves using clinical judgment so that the nurse can identify risk factors or recognize actual problems that predispose the patient to injury if positioned on the OR table incorrectly. Because patients are unable to speak for themselves while under general anesthesia, this assessment in the OR is very important for their safety. As the nurse, review the preoperative care plan to establish or revise the intraoperative care plan as indicated.

> **REFLECT NOW**
>
> One of the goals of preoperative nursing care is to prevent intraoperative and postoperative complications. Consider the surgical risk factors discussed in preoperative assessment and identify their relationship to potential complications that operating room nurses must prevent.

◆ Analysis and Nursing Diagnosis

Review preoperative nursing diagnoses and modify them to individualize the care plan in the OR. The following are common nursing diagnoses relevant to the patient intraoperatively:

- Impaired Airway Clearance
- Risk for Deep Vein Thrombosis
- Risk for Perioperative Positioning Injury
- Risk for Impaired Skin Integrity
- Risk for Latex Allergy

◆ Planning and Outcomes Identification

Outcomes. Patient-centered outcomes of preoperative nursing diagnoses extend into the intraoperative phase. For example, for the nursing diagnosis of *Impaired Airway Clearance* an expected outcome is: The patient will maintain a clear, open airway as evidenced by clear breath sounds, a respiratory rate of 12 to 20 breaths/minute, and the ability to effectively cough up secretions. How the patient responds during surgery will influence whether outcomes need to be adjusted.

Setting Priorities. The circulating nurse uses clinical judgment to provide a safe operative experience for the patient. Ensuring an aseptic environment, conducting instrument and sponge counts according to policy, managing tissue and specimens correctly, and ensuring the proper use of equipment and instruments are top priorities. A circulating nurse who observes an unsafe practice (e.g., break in sterility, inaccurate sponge count) will notify the circulating team immediately. The circulating nurse is integral in ensuring the safety of the patient and operative personnel.

Teamwork and Collaboration. For optimal patient safety the preoperative health care team communicates assessment findings and patient problems via a formal hand-off with the surgical team to ensure a smooth transition in care (see Box 50.5). For example, alerting the operative team of a latex allergy or risk factors for complications during surgery (smoker) requires collaboration and timely communication among all team members. TJC, AORN, and WHO all recommend a standard or formal hand-off. At a minimum, hand-off should include (Rothrock, 2019):

- Patient name and date of birth
- Operative procedure, including the site
- Patient history relevant to this surgery
- Allergies and nothing by mouth status
- Vital signs and pain level
- Laboratory data and code status
- Current medications taken the day of surgery
- Patient's level of surgical understanding
- Cultural implications
- Whether the patient has seen the surgeon and anesthesiologist

The intraoperative team collaborates after receiving hand-off information to ensure patient-centered approaches are used to ensure safe care.

◆ Implementation

A primary focus of intraoperative care is to prevent injury and complications related to anesthesia, surgery, positioning, and equipment use. A perioperative nurse is an advocate for the patient during surgery and always protects the patient's dignity and rights.

Acute Care.

Physical Preparation. A patient is usually still awake and notices health care providers in their surgical attire and masks when entering the OR. The staff members transfer a patient to the OR bed by being sure that the stretcher and bed are locked in place. Explain to the patient all the activities that will be performed before implementing the activities. Remember that a patient may be partially sedated as a result of medications; use caution. After safely positioning the patient and securing the patient on the OR table with safety straps, the circulating nurse applies monitoring devices such as continuous ECG electrodes, a pulse oximeter sensor, and a blood pressure cuff. For ECG, place electrodes on the chest and extremities correctly to record electrical activity of the heart accurately. The anesthesia provider will use the cuff to monitor the patient's blood pressure. An electronic monitor in the OR will display the patient's heart rate, vital signs, and pulse oximetry continuously. Capnography is also used frequently to measure the patient's ongoing end-tidal carbon dioxide values. Now is also the time to apply antiembolism devices. The nurse also assists with the insertion of temperature probes via the bladder, esophagus, or rectum if required to continuously measure a patient's body temperature.

If a patient is to have a surgical procedure that uses a high-frequency electric current to heat biological tissue to cut or coagulate the tissue, a disposable or reusable grounding pad must be placed on the patient's skin. The grounding pad, adhered to the patient's skin away from the surgical site, is intended to safely return the electrical current from the patient back to the generator through a cord or cable. Correct placement of the pad prevents burns to the skin.

Intraoperative Warming. The unplanned occurrence of perioperative hypothermia is now minimized with the use of active intraoperative warming. Evidence suggests that the prevention of hypothermia (core temperature less than 36° C [96.8° F]) by prewarming helps to reduce complications such as shivering, cardiac arrest, blood loss, SSI, pressure injuries, and mortality (Becerra et al., 2019; Sessler, 2020). The nurse in the OR applies warm cotton blankets, forced-air warmers, or circulating-water mattresses to patients. Forced-air warmers tend to be effective when used before surgery or intraoperatively.

Latex Sensitivity/Allergy. As the incidence and prevalence of latex sensitivity and allergy increase, the need for recognition of potential sources of latex is extremely critical. All medical supplies contain a label notifying the consumer of the latex content. The OR and PCU have many products that contain latex (e.g., gloves, IV tubing, syringes, and rubber stoppers on bottles and vials). It is also present in common objects such as adhesive tape, disposable electrodes, endotracheal tube cuffs, protective sheets, and ventilator equipment. Signs and symptoms of a latex reaction include local effects ranging from urticaria and flat or raised red patches to vesicular, scaling, or bleeding eruptions. Acute dermatitis is sometimes present. Rhinitis and/or rhinorrhea are other common reactions to mild and severe latex allergy. Immediate hypersensitivity reactions are life threatening, with the patient exhibiting focal or generalized urticaria and edema, bronchospasm, and mucous hypersecretion, all of which can compromise respiratory status. Vasodilation compounded by increased capillary permeability sometimes leads to circulatory collapse and eventual death. The draping of a patient during surgery blocks the ability to visualize the skin. Thus, be prepared to investigate any unexplained acute deterioration in a previously healthy patient for possible latex allergy.

A latex-free cart is available in an OR to create a latex-safe environment. All of the contents must be latex free. The Association of Surgical Technologists (AST) recommends that when facilities are not latex safe, nurses need to take steps to prepare an OR the night before to avoid the release of latex particles (AST, 2018). Any patient with a latex allergy should receive scheduling priority and be the first case in the morning. It is important to know that patients may develop anaphylaxis 30 to 60 minutes after being exposed to latex. Box 50.6 lists latex precautions.

Introduction of Anesthesia. The nature and extent of a patient's surgery and current physical status influence the type of anesthesia administered during surgery. Know the complications to anticipate after surgery for each type (Table 50.7).

General Anesthesia. Under general anesthesia a patient loses all sensation, consciousness, and reflexes, including gag and blink reflexes. The patient's muscles relax and the patient experiences amnesia. Amnesia is a protective measure that allows patients to forget any unpleasant events of the procedure. An anesthesia provider gives general anesthetics by IV infusion and inhalation routes through the three phases of anesthesia: induction, maintenance, and emergence. Surgery requiring general anesthesia involves major procedures with extensive tissue manipulation. During emergence, anesthetics are decreased, and the patient begins to awaken. Because of the short half-life of today's medications, emergence often occurs in the OR. The duration of anesthesia depends on the length of surgery.

Regional Anesthesia. Regional anesthesia results in loss of sensation in an area of the body by anesthetizing sensory pathways. This type of anesthesia is accomplished by injecting a local anesthetic along the pathway of a nerve from the spinal cord. A patient requires careful monitoring during and immediately after regional anesthesia for return of sensation and movement distal to the point of anesthetic injection. The circulating nurse protects the patient's limbs from injury until sensation returns. Serious complications such as respiratory paralysis occur if the level of anesthesia rises, moving upward in the spinal cord.

BOX 50.6 Latex Avoidance Precautions

- Health care workers can transmit the allergen by hand to patients after touching any object with latex. *Caution:* Keep the powder from the gloves away from patients because the powder acts as a carrier for the latex protein. Do not snap gloves on and off.
- Identify patients who are latex sensitive. The operating room (OR) needs to be labeled latex free to prevent personnel from bringing rubber products (e.g., wristbands, chart labels) into the room.
- Develop programs to educate health care workers in the care of latex-sensitive patients.

Recommendations for Patient Care (Patients with Latex Allergy or Latex Risk)
The Operating Room
- Notify the OR of patients who have potential latex allergies. Remove all latex products from the OR and bring a latex-free cart (if available) into the room.
- Use a latex-free reservoir bag, airways and endotracheal tubes, and laryngeal mask airways.
- Use a nonlatex anesthesia breathing circuit with plastic mask and bag.
- Place all monitoring devices and cords/tubes (oximeter, blood pressure, electrocardiograph wires) in stockinette and secure with tape to prevent direct skin contact. Rinse items sterilized in ethylene oxide before use. Residual ethylene oxide reacts and can cause an allergic response in a patient with a latex allergy.

Intravenous Line Preparation
- Use intravenous (IV) tubing without latex ports; use stopcocks if available.
- If unable to obtain IV tubing without latex ports, cover latex ports with tape.
- Cover all rubber injection ports on IV bags with tape, and label as follows: *Do not inject or withdraw fluid through the latex port.* **NOTE:** *Pulmonary artery catheters (especially the balloon), central venous catheters, and arterial lines may contain latex components.*

Operating Room Patient Care
- Use nonlatex gloves. (*Caution:* Not all substitutes are equally impermeable to bloodborne pathogens; ensure that substitute gloves provide appropriate protection.)
- Use nonlatex tourniquets and examination gloves, and use polyvinyl chloride tubing. Draw medication directly from opened multidose vials (remove stoppers) if medications are not available in ampules.
- The rubber allergen can possibly move from the plunger of a syringe into the medication, which sometimes causes an allergic reaction. The intensity of this reaction increases over time. Therefore, nurses draw up medications immediately before the beginning of the surgery or just before administration.
- Use latex-free or glass syringes.
- Use stopcocks rather than latex ports to inject drugs.
- Notify pharmacy and central supply that your patient is latex sensitive so that these departments can use appropriate procedures when preparing medications and instruments. Also, notify radiology, respiratory therapy, housekeeping, food service, and postoperative care units so that they will take appropriate precautions to protect the patient.
- Place clear and readily visible signs on the doors of the OR to inform all who enter that the patient has a latex allergy.

Modified from Association of Surgical Technologists (AST): *Guidelines for best practices for the natural rubber latex allergic patient,* http://www.ast.org/uploadedFiles/Main_Site/Content/About_Us/Guideline_Latex_Allergy.pdf, 2018. Accessed September 27, 2021.

TABLE 50.7 Complications of Anesthesia

Type	Complications
General	Hypotension; changes in heart rate or rhythm; lowered body temperature; respiratory depression; emergence delirium in the form of shivering, trembling, confusion, or hallucinations
Spinal	Headache, hypotension, decreased cardiac output, cyanosis, difficulty breathing
Neuromuscular blocking drugs (NMBDs)	Intraocular pressure, intracranial pressure
Local	Skin rash; allergic reaction with edema of the face, lips, mouth, or throat; restlessness; bradycardia; hypotension; ischemic necrosis at injection site
Moderate (conscious) sedation	Respiratory depression, bradycardia, hypotension, nausea, and vomiting
Epidural	Cyanosis, breathing difficulties, decreased heart rate, irregular heart rate, pale skin color, nausea, and vomiting

Elevation of the upper body helps prevents respiratory paralysis. Some patients have a sudden fall in blood pressure, which results from extensive vasodilation caused by the anesthetic blocking sympathetic vasomotor nerves and pain and motor nerve fibers. Remember that grounding pad burns and other trauma can occur on the anesthetized part of the body without the patient being aware of the injury. It is necessary to observe frequently the position of the extremities and the condition of the skin.

Local Anesthesia. Local anesthesia involves loss of sensation at the desired site (e.g., a skin growth or the cornea of the eye) by inhibiting peripheral nerve conduction. It is commonly used in ambulatory surgery. A local can also be used in addition to general or regional anesthesia. The anesthetic agent (e.g., lidocaine) inhibits nerve conduction until the drug diffuses into the circulation. It is injected locally or applied topically. The patient experiences a loss in pain and touch sensation in the area of injection. Patients are at risk for having drug interactions and allergic effects. It is necessary to monitor patients continually during a local procedure. The frequency of observation and monitoring of patients is tailored to the patient, procedure, and the medications used.

Moderate (Conscious) Sedation. IV moderate sedation (i.e., conscious sedation) is used routinely for short-term surgical, diagnostic, and therapeutic procedures that do not require complete anesthesia but rather a depressed level of consciousness. A patient maintains spontaneous ventilation and a patent airway and requires no interventions during conscious sedation (Rothrock, 2019). In addition, the patient responds appropriately to physical (light touch) and verbal stimuli. The preferred sedative for conscious sedation is short-acting IV sedatives such as midazolam.

Advantages of conscious sedation include adequate sedation, reduction of fear and anxiety, amnesia, relief of pain and noxious stimuli, elevation of pain threshold, enhanced patient cooperation, stable vital signs, and rapid recovery. Nurses assisting with the administration of conscious sedation need to demonstrate competency in the care of these patients. Knowledge of anatomy, physiology, cardiac dysrhythmias, procedural complications, and pharmacological principles related to the administration of individual agents is essential. The nurse needs to assess, diagnose, and intervene in the event of unexpected reactions, such as an adverse reaction to a medication, and demonstrate skill in airway management and oxygen delivery. Resuscitation equipment must be readily available when using conscious sedation.

Positioning the Patient for Surgery. A patient will be placed on an operating room table in a position that offers access to the surgical site. Prevention of positioning injuries requires anticipation of the position and surgical approach to be used, the positioning equipment available to be used, and whether a patient has conditions causing risk for injury (AORN, 2020a). When possible, the position during surgery should be one that would be comfortable with the patient fully awake. Patients should be questioned about limited range of motion and their ability to lie comfortably in the expected position prior to induction of general anesthesia. If questions arise, the patient should be placed in the anticipated position as a trial before sedation or induction of anesthesia. If the operating table will be tilted either top to bottom, side to side, or moved into the sitting position (e.g., during breast reconstruction) during surgery, the anticipated position should be practiced before skin preparation and draping to make sure that supports and straps are secure and that the patient tolerates the position physiologically.

During general anesthesia, the nursing personnel and surgeon often wait to position a patient until the full stage of relaxation so that an injury is less likely to be caused by moving and lifting the patient's body parts. As a circulating nurse you can recommend the type of bed surface and positioning devices to use, depending on patient risk factors for pressure injury. A variety of bed surfaces such as the Micro-Pulse air mattress, viscoelastic dry polymer mattress covers, air-inflated static seat cushions, and gel pads are available (de Assunção Peixoto et al., 2019; Park et al., 2019). OR positioning devices and padding are also available. However, caution must be used as pressure injuries can develop from incorrectly placed foam devices (Fife, 2019). When a patient is placed on an OR bed, the perioperative team uses the best devices and bed surfaces available for providing stability and pressure redistribution (Teleten et al., 2019).

Ideally, a patient's position provides clear access to the operative site; sustains adequate circulatory and respiratory function; and ensures the patient's safety, comfort, and skin integrity. If a patient has conditions such as morbid obesity, malnourishment, existing pressure injuries, or chronic disease, special considerations are needed in positioning. It is important for the circulating nurse to assess circulatory, respiratory, integumentary, musculoskeletal, and neurological structures during surgery (AORN, 2020a).

An alert person maintains normal range of joint motion by pain and pressure receptors. If a joint is extended too far, pain stimuli provide a warning that muscle and joint strain is too great. In a patient who is anesthetized, normal defense mechanisms cannot guard against joint damage, muscle stretch, and strain. The muscles are so relaxed that it is relatively easy to place a patient in a position that the individual normally could not assume while awake. The patient often remains in a given position for several hours. Although it is sometimes necessary to place a patient in an unusual position, try to maintain correct alignment and protect skin from pressure, abrasion, and other injuries. Positioning should not impede normal movement of the diaphragm or interfere with circulation to body parts. If restraints are necessary, pad the skin to prevent trauma.

Documentation of Intraoperative Care. Throughout the surgical procedure, the circulating nurse keeps an accurate record of patient care activities and procedures performed by OR personnel (e.g., surgical sponge and instrument count status, special equipment, IV and irrigation fluids, specimens, and medications). A standardized documentation format helps practitioners ensure continuity of information from the OR to the postanesthesia care unit (PACU) or recovery area (AORN, 2020a). The AORN recommends the use of verbal and standardized forms to transfer patient information between care providers.

◆ Evaluation

The circulating nurse conducts an ongoing evaluation to ensure that interventions such as patient position are implemented correctly during the intraoperative phase of surgery.

Through the Patient's Eyes. While a patient is undergoing surgery, it is important to keep the family informed. Pagers are used in some settings to text updates to family members. Agencies vary on their policies for when and how often families are given updates of the patient's condition. Families expect an estimate of when surgery begins, how the surgery is progressing, and the length of time it will probably last. When you give an update to family members, ask whether they have further questions or concerns and whether their needs are being met.

Patient Outcomes. During surgery, the anesthesia provider continuously monitors vital signs. The circulating nurse monitors and records intake and output (I&O), specimens obtained, medications and irrigations, type of dressing packing, and other treatments. Measurement of the patient's body temperature during and at completion of the surgery provides data to achieve the goal of keeping the patient normothermic. The circulating nurse will inspect the skin under the grounding pad and at areas where positioning exerts pressure.

POSTOPERATIVE SURGICAL PHASE

There are three phases of anesthesia recovery. Phase I (Immediate Anesthesia Recovery) begins when a patient leaves the operating room (OR). It extends from the time a patient leaves the OR to the time the patient is stabilized in the PACU or ambulatory recovery area, meets discharge criteria, and is transferred to a nursing unit or other location. During phase I close monitoring is required; for the first 1 to 2 hours the focus is on assessing for the aftereffects of anesthesia, including airway clearance, cardiovascular complications, fluid management, temperature control, and neurological function. A patient's condition can change rapidly; assessments must be timely, knowledgeable, and accurate. A patient who has progressed beyond these elements of care can move to phase II (early postoperative) anesthesia recovery, a level of care in which plans of care are provided to progress the patient home (ASPAN, 2019; Schick and Windle, 2020). When a patient has had ambulatory surgery, this may be in the same physical location as phase I care. Many PACUs provide blended levels of care, in which both levels of care are provided in the same location (ASPAN, 2019).

Phase III (convalescent) anesthesia recovery focuses on providing ongoing care for patients who are hospitalized and require extended observation or intervention after transfer from phase I or phase II. Interventions are directed toward preparing the patient for self-care or care by family members. Phases of recovery are not locations but levels of care (ASPAN, 2019).

The type of anesthesia, nature of surgery, and a patient's previous condition determine the phases of recovery and the length of time spent on an acute care nursing unit. Typically, at the end of surgery the anesthesia provider and the circulating nurse accompany the patient to the PACU and provide a thorough hand-off report to the nursing staff.

IMMEDIATE POSTOPERATIVE RECOVERY (PHASE I)

When a PACU nurse receives a patient during hand-off, the nurse obtains data from the surgical team to prepare for proper support of a patient's recovery status. This includes anticipating potential clinical problems based on assessment and being sure that special equipment needed for nursing care is available. Careful planning allows the nursing staff to consider the placement of patients within the

PACU. For example, patients who undergo spinal anesthesia are aware of their surroundings and benefit from being in a quieter part of the PACU, away from patients needing frequent monitoring. The nurse isolates patients with serious infections, such as tuberculosis, from other patients. Use Standard Precautions for infection control (see Chapter 28) for all patients.

When a patient is admitted to phase I recovery, personnel notify the nurses on the acute care nursing unit of the patient's arrival. This allows the nursing staff to inform family members. Family members usually remain in the designated waiting area so that they are accessible when the surgeon arrives to explain the patient's condition. *It is the surgeon's responsibility* to describe the patient's status, the results of surgery, and any complications that occurred. The nurse is a valuable resource to the family for clarifying explanations if complications occur in the operative phase.

When a patient enters the PACU, the nurse and members of the surgical team discuss the patient's status. A standardized approach or tool for "hand-off" communications helps to provide accurate information about a patient's care, treatment and services, current condition, and any recent or anticipated changes (Rothrock, 2019). The hand-off is interactive, interprofessional, and done at the patient's bedside, allowing for a communication exchange that gives caregivers the chance to dialogue and ask questions. The surgical team's report includes topics such as the type of anesthesia provided, vital sign trends, intraoperative medications, IV fluids, estimated blood and urine loss, and pertinent information about the surgical wound (e.g., dressings, tubes, drains) (Rothrock, 2019). The information obtained from the hand-off report allows a recovery nurse to anticipate how quickly a patient should regain consciousness, any likely complications, and what the analgesic needs will be. A report on IV fluids or blood products administered during surgery from the anesthesia provider or perfusionist alerts the nurse to the patient's fluid and electrolyte balance. The surgeon or anesthesia provider often reports special concerns (e.g., whether the patient is at risk for hemorrhaging or infection) and whether there were complications during surgery such as excessive blood loss or cardiac irregularities. The circulating nurse also reports intraoperative patient positioning and condition of the skin. Frequently, this report takes place while PACU nurses are admitting the patient. The PACU nurse attaches the patient to monitoring equipment such as the noninvasive blood pressure monitor, ECG monitor, and pulse oximeter. Patients often receive some form of oxygen in this immediate recovery period.

After receiving hand-off communication from the OR, the PACU nurse conducts a complete systems assessment during the first few minutes of PACU care (Box 50.7). The nurse applies critical thinking, comparing a patient's baseline (within the OR) to expected physiological changes during recovery to clinically judge a patient's response. Patients will begin to gradually awaken while in the PACU. Try to arouse a patient by calling the patient's name in a moderate tone of voice. If that is unsuccessful, awaken the patient by using touch or gently moving a body part. If painful stimulation is needed to arouse a patient, notify anesthesia immediately. Perform assessments at least every 15 minutes or more frequently, depending on the patient's condition and unit policy. This assessment continues until discharge from the PACU. Perform assessments quickly and thoroughly and target them to a patient's unique needs and type of surgery.

As patients awaken, they expectorate the oral airway, or the nurse asks the patient to expectorate the airway. The ability to do so signifies the return of a normal gag reflex. Before removing an artificial airway (or before the patient removes it), suction the back of the airway so that secretions are not retained. Be alert for nausea and vomiting, which may precipitate regurgitation. Avoid any rapid movement of the patient, and keep the patient's head elevated while lying on the side.

BOX 50.7 Initial Postanesthesia Care Assessment: Parameters to Assess

Initial assessment in the PACU includes the following:

- Integration of data received at hand-off for transfer of care
- Vital signs
- Respiratory status—airway patency, breath sounds, type of artificial airway, mechanical ventilator settings, oxygen saturation, and end-tidal CO_2 values
- Intake and output
- Pain/sedation/comfort assessment (including psychoemotional status), presence of nausea or vomiting
- Neurological function: level of consciousness (may use Glasgow Coma scale), pupillary response (if indicated)
- Position of the patient
- Condition and color of skin, status of any suspected pressure areas
- Patient safety needs (positioning to prevent aspiration)
- Neurovascular status: peripheral pulses and sensation of extremity or extremities
- Condition of surgical dressings or suture line, drains, tubes, receptacles
- Amount, appearance, and type of drainage
- Muscular response and strength/mobility
- Fluid therapy—location of intravenous (IV) lines, patency of IV lines, amount and type of solution (crystalloids or blood products) infused, next fluid to be administered
- Procedure-specific assessments, such as expected drainage amount, specific positioning aids for orthopedic surgery

Adapted from Glick D: Overview of post-anesthetic care for adult patients, *UpToDate*, 2020, https://www.uptodate.com/contents/overview-of-post-anesthetic-care-for-adult-patients; Rothrock JC: *Alexander's care of the patient in surgery,* ed 16, St Louis, 2019, Elsevier.

One of the greatest concerns immediately postoperatively is airway obstruction. A number of factors contribute to obstruction, including history of OSA; weak pharyngeal/laryngeal muscle tone from anesthetics; secretions in the pharynx, bronchial tree, or trachea; and laryngeal or subglottic edema. After anesthesia, a patient's tongue causes the majority of airway obstructions. Ongoing assessment of airway patency is crucial even during phase III recovery. Patients remain in a side-lying position until airways are clear. Continue to assess respiratory status and breath sounds. Older patients, smokers, and patients with a history of respiratory disease are prone to developing complications such as atelectasis or pneumonia. Patients with OSA are often required to have continuous pulse oximetry while receiving IV opioids to detect oxygen desaturation quickly. Use of the Pasero Opioid-Induced Sedation Scale (POSS) in the PACU helps assess patients more accurately and meets the pain needs of the patient while preventing oversedation (Dunwoody and Jungquist, 2020).

Normally a patient who received general anesthesia does not drink fluids in the PACU because of reduced peristalsis, risk of nausea and vomiting, and grogginess from general anesthesia. In the case of ambulatory surgery, once a patient awakens in the recovery area and feels no nausea, ice chips or clear liquids in small amounts will be given. For patients at high risk for the development of nausea and vomiting or those who must not vomit, the nurse administers a combination of antiemetics, as ordered by the surgeon, to block multiple receptors. A combination of antiemetic medications is often more effective than a single agent (Feinleib et al., 2020). If a patient has an NG tube, keep it patent by irrigating it as ordered (see Chapter 47). Occlusion of an NG tube results in an accumulation of gastric contents within the stomach, increasing the risk of regurgitation and aspiration.

You will determine a patient's status and eventual readiness for discharge from the PACU by comparing baseline vital signs with intraoperative and preoperative data. Other outcomes for discharge include body temperature control, good ventilation and oxygenation status, orientation to surroundings, absence of complications, minimal pain and nausea, controlled wound drainage, adequate urine output, and fluid and electrolyte balance. Patients with more extensive surgery requiring anesthesia of longer duration usually recover more slowly.

It is common for hospitals and ambulatory care centers to use objective scoring systems such as the Efficacy Safety Score to identify when patients are ready for discharge (Skraastad et al., 2017). Other standard tools include The Aldrete score and the Postanesthetic Discharge Scoring System (PADSS) for assessment. The PADSS scale uses parameters of activity, respiration, circulation, consciousness, and oxygen saturation. A score of greater than 9 indicates the patient may be discharged to home or to an alternate setting (ASPAN, 2019; Glick, 2020). Health care providers use forms of both tools. Each assessment tool has criteria assessed at select time intervals (e.g., 5, 15, 30, 45, and 60 minutes) and on discharge from the PACU (see agency policy). A patient must receive a predetermined score before discharge from the PACU. If the patient's condition is still poor after 2 or 3 hours or if the stay lengthens, the surgeon may transfer the patient to an intensive care unit (ICU).

When a patient is discharged from the PACU and requires continued monitoring and care, another hand-off communication occurs at the patient's bedside between the PACU nurse and the nurse in the ambulatory care phase II area, acute nursing unit, or in an ICU. The nurses verify the patient's identification using two identifiers. The hand-off includes review of vital signs, the type of surgery and anesthesia performed, blood loss, level of consciousness, general physical condition, medications administered during surgery and in the PACU, and the presence of IV lines, drainage tubes, and dressings. The PACU nurse's report helps the receiving nurse anticipate special patient needs and obtain necessary equipment. It is important to have uninterrupted time to review the recent pertinent events and ask questions. It is also important at this time for the patient's family members to be informed as soon as possible of the patient's transfer plan.

The PACU staff transport the patient to either the final recovery phase II area in an ambulatory setting or on a stretcher to an inpatient nursing unit. Staff members from the unit help to safely transfer the patient (see Chapter 38). The PACU nurse shows the receiving nurse the recovery room record and reviews the patient's condition and course of care. The PACU nurse also reviews the surgeon's orders that require attention. *Before the PACU nurse leaves the acute care area, the staff nurse assuming care for the patient takes a complete set of vital signs to compare with PACU findings.* Minor vital sign variations normally occur after transporting the patient.

RECOVERY IN AMBULATORY SURGERY (PHASE II)

After patients stabilize and no longer require close monitoring, phase II recovery begins. This may occur in the same recovery area of the PACU for ambulatory patients or a different nearby location. With new anesthetic agents and minimally invasive surgical techniques, *fast-track surgery* is becoming more common, with patients experiencing a more rapid awakening in the OR, quicker recovery, and reduced morbidity. Because of this, many ambulatory surgery patients can bypass phase I and immediately enter phase II in the recovery area.

In ambulatory surgery, phase II recovery is performed in a room equipped with medical recliner chairs, side tables, and footrests. Kitchen facilities for preparing light snacks and beverages are usually located in the area, along with bathrooms. The phase II environment promotes a patient's and family's comfort and well-being until discharge. Nurses continue to monitor patients' vital signs and level of

---

Postoperative Instructions for an Ambulatory Surgical Patient

Objective
- Patient will describe signs and symptoms of postoperative problems to report to health care provider.

Teaching Strategies
- Give instruction sheet with contact information, including health care provider's telephone number, telephone number of surgery center, and follow-up appointment date and time. Provide an instruction sheet with clear, focused explanations.
- Allow patient and family to ask questions.
- Individualize standard instructions to patient's specific needs, particularly matching restrictions with any routines or physical limitations patient has reported.
- Explain signs and symptoms of infection to family members.
- Explain name, dose, schedule, and purpose of medications and possible side effects. Provide printed drug information.
- Explain activity restrictions, diet progression, wound care guidelines, and the signs of any associated problems.

Evaluation
Use the principles of teach-back to evaluate patient/family caregiver learning:
- Patient explains when and how to call health care provider with problems.
- Patient recites date for follow-up appointment.
- Patient and family member describe signs and symptoms of infection.
- Patient verbalizes name of drug, dose, when to take, and common side effects.
- Patient demonstrates proper activity/movement and wound care.

---

responsiveness but not at the same intensity as during phase I. In phase II recovery, you will initiate postoperative teaching with patients and family members (Box 50.8).

Patients are discharged to home following ambulatory surgery after they meet certain criteria, such as a designated score on the Postanesthetic Discharge Scoring System (PADSS). Patients with known OSA or at high risk for the condition are not discharged from the recovery area to home until they are no longer at risk for postoperative respiratory depression, which may require a longer stay (Olson et al., 2020b). Postoperative nausea and vomiting (PONV) sometimes occur once the patient is home, even if the symptoms were not present in the surgery center. Options for therapy include the transcutaneous AccuPoint electrical stimulation or the prophylactic use of drugs such as ondansetron, aprepitant, dolasetron, or a transdermal scopolamine patch (Rothrock, 2019).

Review written postoperative instructions and prescriptions with the patient and family caregiver before releasing the patient, and ensure that they verbalize understanding of these instructions. Always discharge the patient to a responsible adult who can drive the patient home.

RECOVERY OF INPATIENTS: POSTOPERATIVE RECOVERY AND CONVALESCENCE

Inpatients remain in the PACU until their condition stabilizes; they then return to the postoperative nursing unit for either continuing phase II or phase III convalescence. Nursing care focuses on returning the patient to a relatively functional level of wellness as soon as possible. The speed of recovery depends on the type or extent of surgery, risk factors, pain management, and postoperative complications.

❖ NURSING PROCESS

The critical application of the nursing process continues during postoperative recovery and convalescence. Sound clinical judgment originates from a nurse's knowledge of surgical procedures and intended effects along with clinical experience in caring for surgical patients. Assessment is a critical step of the nursing process postoperatively as the nurse spends the most time at the bedside, gathering data about the patient and judging the clinical course. Once a surgical patient is transferred to an acute care nursing unit, ongoing postoperative care is essential to support recovery.

◆ Assessment

During the assessment process, thoroughly assess each patient and critically analyze findings to ensure that you make patient-centered clinical decisions required for safe postoperative nursing care. Apply critical thinking while you synthesize information from the preoperative nursing assessment, knowledge regarding the surgical procedure performed, and assessment data and events occurring during surgery and phase I recovery. A variation from the patient's norm possibly indicates the onset of surgically related complications.

Before a patient arrives on the nursing unit, have AP prepare the bed and room for the patient's arrival. In some cases, a patient returns to the same nursing unit. The nurse is better prepared to care for the patient after surgery if the room is readied before the patient's return. A postoperative bedside unit includes the following:

1. Sphygmomanometer and/or automated noninvasive blood pressure monitor, stethoscope, and thermometer
2. Emesis basin
3. Incentive spirometer
4. Clean gown, washcloth, towel, and facial tissues
5. IV pole and infusion pump (if needed)
6. Suction equipment (if needed)
7. Oxygen equipment and oximetry monitor (if needed)
8. Extra pillows for positioning the patient comfortably
9. Bed pads to protect bed linen from drainage
10. Bed raised to stretcher height with bed linens pulled back and furniture moved to accommodate the stretcher and equipment (such as IV lines)

When a patient arrives on the acute care unit, monitor vital signs according to institution policy. Generally, you check vital signs every 15 minutes twice, every 30 minutes twice, hourly for 2 hours, and then every 4 hours or per orders. As the patient's condition stabilizes, the nurses usually assess the patient at least once a shift until discharge. Always base the frequency of assessment on a patient's current condition. *Do not assume that further monitoring is unnecessary if the patient appears normal during the initial assessment.* A patient's condition can change rapidly, especially during the postoperative period.

Thoroughly document the initial nursing assessment findings. Enter patient data into the medical record on flow sheets, surgical assessment drop-down menus, or written progress notes. The initial findings provide a baseline for comparing postoperative changes.

Through the Patient's Eyes. When a patient initially returns to the acute care nursing unit, the family and patient have expectations of receiving prompt and attentive care. There is also the expectation that you will explain the patient's immediate status and the plan of care for the next few hours. Seeing the patient return from surgery is a relief in many ways, but if the patient has had complications or is not responding well, anxiety easily returns. As a patient stabilizes, it is important to assess the patient's and family's expectations for recovery and convalescence after returning home. Be sure to review their expectations for management of pain and other symptoms. What do they expect from staff during the hospitalization? What are their expectations after the patient is discharged from the hospital? Who is the primary family caregiver, and is that family caregiver prepared to assume care at discharge? Make the patient and family partners in your assessment so that you can gather information necessary to develop a relevant plan of care. For example, ask the patient's caregivers to share their work schedules (if applicable) to determine whether the patient will have someone to provide transportation for follow-up appointments and outpatient rehabilitation (if prescribed), prepare meals, and assist with medication administration (if necessary).

Airway and Respiration. The priority in the care of a patient during phase III recovery is to maintain a patent airway. Assess airway patency, respiratory rate, rhythm, depth of ventilation, symmetry of chest wall movement, breath sounds, and color of mucous membranes and compare findings with data from the PACU (see Chapters 30 and 41). Be aware that certain anesthetic agents can still cause respiratory depression during this phase. A patient may present with snoring, little or no air movement on auscultation of the lungs, retraction of intercostal muscles, and decreased oxygen saturation. Be alert for shallow, slow breathing and a weak cough. If breathing is unusually shallow, place your hand near the patient's nose or mouth to feel exhaled air. Normal pulse oximetry values range between 92% and 100% saturation. Postoperative confusion is frequently secondary to hypoxia, especially in older adults. When a patient is responsive, assess the initial ability to use an incentive spirometer and note the volume achieved.

Circulation. The patient is at risk for cardiovascular complications resulting from actual or potential blood loss from the surgical site, side effects of anesthesia, electrolyte imbalances, and depression of normal circulatory-regulating mechanisms and ischemia. Careful assessment of heart rate and rhythm, along with blood pressure, reveals a patient's cardiovascular status. Compare vital signs from preoperative condition and phase I recovery with postoperative values during phase III. If a patient's blood pressure drops progressively with each check or if the heart rate changes or becomes irregular, notify the health care provider. An ECG rhythm strip of the heart is obtained after surgery, compared with preoperative ECG tracings, and placed in the medical record.

Assess circulatory perfusion by noting capillary refill, pulses, and the color and temperature of the nail beds and skin. If a patient had vascular surgery or has casts or constricting devices that may impair circulation, assess peripheral pulses and capillary refill distal to the site of surgery. For example, after surgery to the femoral artery, assess posterior tibial and dorsalis pedis pulses. In addition, compare pulses in the affected extremity with those in the unaffected extremity.

A common early circulatory problem is bleeding or hemorrhage. Blood loss may occur internally or externally through a drain or incision. Either type of hemorrhage results in a fall in blood pressure; elevated heart and respiratory rates; thready pulse; cool, clammy, pale skin; and restlessness. Notify the surgeon if these changes occur. Maintain IV fluid infusion. Monitor the patient's vital signs every 15 minutes or more frequently until the patient's condition stabilizes. Continue oxygen therapy. The surgeon may consider medications or volume replacement and order blood counts and coagulation studies.

Temperature Control. When patients begin to awaken more fully, they often complain of feeling cold and uncomfortable. Older adults and pediatric patients are at higher risk for developing problems associated with postoperative hypothermia (temperature less than 36° C [96.8° F]). Also, closely assess the body temperature of other at-risk patients, including those of female gender, patients with burns, patients who received general anesthesia, patients who are cachexic or had low temperatures intraoperatively, and those whose surgery involved the use of cold irrigants (Rothrock, 2019).

In rare instances a genetic disorder known as **malignant hyperthermia** (MH), a life-threatening complication of anesthesia, develops. It is a hypermetabolic state occurring within skeletal muscle cells that become triggered by anesthesia. It results in an increase in intracellular calcium ion concentration. It is a potentially lethal condition that can occur in patients receiving various inhaled anesthetic agents and succinylcholine. The hyperthermic condition results in high carbon dioxide levels, metabolic and respiratory acidosis, increased oxygen consumption, production of heat, activation of the sympathetic nervous system, high serum potassium levels, and multiple organ dysfunction and failure. Early signs of malignant hyperthermia include tachypnea, tachycardia, heart arrhythmias, hyperkalemia, hypercarbia, and muscular rigidity. Later signs include elevated temperature, myoglobinuria, and multiple organ failure (AANA, 2018; Litman, 2020). In nearly all cases, the first signs and symptoms of MH occur in the operating room during induction of anesthesia; however, MH may also occur in the early postoperative period or after repeated exposures to anesthesia (Litman, 2020; Sinha et al., 2017). Without prompt detection and treatment, it is potentially fatal.

Monitor temperature closely in the acute care area. Because an elevated temperature may be the first indication of an infection, assess the patient for a potential source of infection, including the IV site (if present), the surgical incision/wound, and the respiratory and urinary tracts. Notify the health care provider because further evaluation is often necessary.

Fluid and Electrolyte Balance. Because of the risk for fluid and electrolyte abnormalities after surgery, assess a patient's hydration status and monitor for signs of electrolyte alterations (see Chapter 42). Monitor and compare laboratory test results with the patient's baseline and normal values. Maintain the patency of IV infusions. The patient's only source of fluid intake immediately after surgery is through IV catheters until the gag reflex and bowel sounds resume. Inspect the patient's catheter insertion site to ensure that the catheter is properly positioned within a vein, fluid flows freely, and the site is free of phlebitis or infiltration (see Chapter 42). Accurate recording of I&O assesses renal and circulatory function. Measure all sources of output, including urine, drainage from surgically placed drains, and gastric and wound drainage; note any insensible loss from diaphoresis. Assess daily weight for the first several days after surgery and compare with the preoperative weight. If the patient has a known cardiac history such as heart failure, continue daily weights. It is important to use a consistent scale, amount of clothing, and time of day to obtain accurate weight measurement.

Neurological Functions. After leaving the PACU a patient will still be drowsy. As anesthetic agents begin to metabolize, the patient's reflexes return, muscle strength is regained, and a normal level of orientation returns. Monitor neurological status routinely by assessing whether the patient is oriented to self and the hospital and responds to questions appropriately. Assess pupil and gag reflexes, hand grips, and movement of extremities (see Chapter 30). If a patient had surgery involving part of the neurological system, conduct a more thorough neurological assessment. For example, if the patient had low-back surgery, assess leg movement, sensation, and strength. It is not uncommon for there to be a brief period of delirium when emerging from general anesthesia. Assessments may find postoperative agitation, crying, restlessness, and mental confusion (Mahanna-Gabrielli and Eckenhoff, 2020). Older adults are at increased risk for persistent postoperative delirium.

Patients with regional anesthesia experience a return in motor function before tactile sensation returns. Typically, patients will have remained in the PACU until sensation and voluntary movement of the lower extremities return. Check the patient's sensation to touch (see Chapter 30). Knowing where regional anesthesia was introduced helps you check the distribution of the spinal nerves affected. Typically assess sensation by touching the patient bilaterally in the same area (e.g., lower arm on both sides or leg on both sides), noting where the patient feels touch. Test the sense of touch by using hand pressure or a gentle pinch of the skin. Extremity strength assessment continues to be important if a patient had spinal or epidural anesthesia.

Skin Integrity and Condition of the Wound. During recovery and acute postoperative care, assess the condition of the skin, noting areas of redness or pressure areas, rashes, petechiae, abrasions, or burns. Assessment for pressure injuries must continue during a patient's hospital stay as postoperative pressure injuries often do not appear for 48 hours or more (Hong-Lin et al., 2019). Check any perioperative risk assessment for pressure injuries, and consider what factors might still apply to the patient.

Inspect the skin for lesions. A rash often indicates a drug sensitivity or allergy. Abrasions or petechiae sometimes result from a clotting disorder or inappropriate positioning or restraining that injures skin layers. Burns may indicate that an electrical cautery grounding pad was placed incorrectly on the patient's skin. Document burns or serious injury to the skin on an occurrence or adverse-event report according to agency policy (see Chapter 23). Note whether the patient is complaining of any burning or pain in the eye, which could indicate a corneal abrasion.

After surgery, a patient may have only butterfly tape, skin staples, or even glue to close small wounds (see Chapter 48). Look at the incision carefully, and notice any drainage or swelling. Most surgical wounds that are larger have dressings that protect the wound site and collect drainage. Observe the amount, color, odor, and consistency of drainage on dressings. It is most common to see serosanguineous drainage immediately after surgery. Estimate the amount of drainage by noting the number of saturated gauze sponges. If drainage appears on the outer surface of a dressing, another way of assessing it is to mark the outer perimeter of the drainage with tape or to mark and date it with the time noted. This way the nurse can easily note whether drainage is increasing (see Chapter 48). However, this is not the most accurate measure of volume of fluid lost. Reinforce the dressing as needed and call the surgeon if wound drainage is leaking through the dressing.

Many surgeons prefer to change surgical dressings the first time so that they can inspect the incisional area. This applies to both outpatients and inpatients. You have the opportunity on the acute care nursing unit to view and thoroughly assess and document the status of the incision/wound at the time of this initial dressing change. Assess whether wound edges are approximated and whether bleeding or drainage is present. It is also important to assess the patient's mobility level. If the patient is unable or unwilling to turn because of pain from the incisional area, pressure injury development is a concern. Postoperatively, if no specific pressure injury assessment scale for the surgical patient has been used, you may use the Braden Scale to assess current postoperative risk factors.

Metabolism. Research over the past decade shows that postoperative hyperglycemia (blood glucose greater than 180 mg/dL) is associated with surgical wound infection and longer hospital stays in surgical patients. Maintaining normoglycemia or a glucose level of less than 180 mg/dL and reducing blood glucose variability are recommended as an evidence-based practice for safe and effective patient management (Wahr, 2020).

It is important to know the signs of hypo- and hyperglycemia when managing surgical patients, especially those who have diabetes. Nurses need to monitor blood glucose levels routinely based on surgeon order or hospital policy.

Genitourinary Function. Depending on the surgery, some patients do not regain voluntary control over urinary function for 6 to 8 hours after anesthesia. An epidural or spinal anesthetic often prevents a patient from feeling bladder fullness. Palpate the lower abdomen just above the symphysis pubis for bladder distention. Another option is to use a bladder scan or ultrasound to assess bladder volume. If the patient has a urinary catheter, there should be a continuous flow of urine of approximately 30 to 50 mL/hr in adults (see agency policy). Observe the color and odor of urine. Surgery involving parts of the urinary tract normally causes bloody urine for at least 12 to 24 hours, depending on the type of surgery. A urine output of less than 0.5 mL/kg/hr is reported to the surgeon or health care provider (Harding et al., 2020).

Gastrointestinal Function. General anesthetics slow GI motility and often cause nausea. In addition, manipulation of the intestines during abdominal surgery further impairs peristalsis. Faint or absent bowel sounds are typical immediately after surgery. Normally patients who undergo abdominal or pelvic surgery have decreased peristalsis for at least 24 hours or longer (Rothrock, 2019). Paralytic ileus (i.e., loss of function of the intestine), which causes abdominal distention, is always possible after surgery. Auscultate bowel sounds in all four quadrants, noting faint or absent bowel sounds. Inspect the abdomen for distention caused by accumulation of gas. Ask whether a patient is passing flatus, an important sign indicating return of normal bowel function. The return of flatus is usually more indicative of normal bowel function return than the return of bowel sounds (Rothrock, 2019). If a nasogastric (NG) tube is in place for decompression, assess the patency of the tube and the color and amount of drainage (see Chapter 47).

Mobility. Early postoperative mobility is necessary to promote respiratory, circulatory, and gastrointestinal function. Immobility may result in deconditioning and increase the patient's risk for hospital-acquired conditions (e.g., pressure injuries) and falls (Mattison, 2020). Current research concludes that the use of an early mobilization protocol improves outcomes for patients recovering from major surgery (Rupich et al., 2018). Assess the patient's range of motion, ability to move in the bed and sit on the side of the bed, ability to bear weight, gait, and balance.

Comfort and Sleep. As patients awaken from general anesthesia, the sensation of pain becomes prominent. They perceive pain before regaining full consciousness. Acute incisional pain causes them to become restless and is often responsible for temporary changes in vital signs. It is difficult for patients to begin coughing and deep-breathing exercises when they experience incisional pain. The patient who had regional or local anesthesia usually does not experience pain initially because the incisional area is still anesthetized. Ongoing assessment of the patient's discomfort and the evaluation of pain-relief therapies (pharmacological and nonpharmacological) are essential throughout the postoperative course (Box 50.9). Use a pain scale for assessing postoperative pain, evaluating the response to analgesics, and objectively documenting pain severity (see Chapter 44). Using preoperative pain assessments as a baseline, evaluate the effectiveness of interventions throughout the patient's recovery.

Postoperatively, it is common for patients to experience sleep disturbances, often resulting from preoperative co-morbidity, type of anesthesia, severity of surgical trauma, postoperative pain, and environmental stress (Su and Wang, 2017). In addition, noise that occurs in the hospital

BOX 50.9 EVIDENCE-BASED PRACTICE

Prevention of Acute Pain in the Postsurgical Patient

PICOT Question: In postoperative patients, how effective is preoperative education/pain-management planning, compared to traditional/as-needed pain-management approaches in controlling postoperative pain?

Evidence Summary

Evidence suggests postoperative pain is managed inadequately in more than 80% of patients (García-Monasterio et al., 2019). However, the type of surgery performed, analgesics/anesthetic interventions prescribed, and time elapsed after surgery influence postoperative pain. Correlation exists between poorly controlled acute postoperative pain and increased morbidity, length of stay, and functional and quality-of-life impairments (García-Monasterio et al., 2019; Mariano, 2020). More effective analgesic/anesthetic measures in the perioperative period are needed to prevent the progression to persistent pain (García-Monasterio et al., 2019; Mariano, 2020). Studies suggest local anesthetics and nonopioid analgesics are beneficial as preventive interventions (Mariano, 2020). Current best practices for pain management are based on the principal that optimal management starts in the preoperative period with assessment of the patient and development of a patient-centered plan (García-Monasterio et al., 2019; Mariano, 2020).

Application to Nursing Practice

- Provide individualized education for surgical patients and their caregivers about treatment options for postoperative pain management.
- Conduct preoperative evaluations of patients.
- Use a validated assessment tool to determine patients' responses and to guide the treatment plan.
- Use multimodal analgesia to manage postoperative pain, including pharmacological and nonpharmacological options.
- Tailor pain-control measures to the needs of the patient, considering the patient's age, medical and physical condition, level of fear/anxiety, personal preferences, type of surgical procedure, and response.

prevents patients from sleeping (Auckley, 2020). Implement nonpharmacological and pharmacological measures (as prescribed) to promote a patient's postoperative sleep.

Some studies have shown that postoperative patients who experience sleep disorders are at higher risk for experiencing delirium, pain sensitivity, cardiovascular issues, and delayed recovery.

◆ Analysis and Nursing Diagnosis

Determine the status of preoperative nursing diagnoses by clustering new postoperative assessment data. Then either revise or resolve preoperative diagnoses and identify relevant new diagnoses after surgery. A previously identified potential diagnosis such as *Risk for Infection* may now be a new postoperative problem. It is common to identify new nursing diagnoses after surgery because of the risks or problems associated with it. Also consider the assessed needs of a patient's family when you identify nursing diagnoses. In the formulation of nursing diagnoses, be accurate in identifying a related factor (when appropriate). For example, *Risk for Hypovolemia related to fluid losses* compared with *Acute Pain related to altered skin integrity* requires different nursing interventions. Potential nursing diagnoses for the postoperative patient include the following:

- Impaired Airway Clearance
- Risk for Infection
- Impaired Mobility
- Impaired Skin Integrity
- Acute Pain

◆ Planning and Outcomes Identification

During the recovery phase, use the most current nursing diagnoses and any collaborative problems to plan the patient's care. Previous experience is again valuable in anticipating how patients typically respond during recovery compared with how your assigned patient responds. The surgeon's postoperative orders and surgical team's report of the patient's operative condition also provide valuable data. In many health care agencies, Enhanced Recovery After Surgery (ERAS) protocols are being used, incorporating standard postoperative orders for care activities. Typical postoperative orders include:

- Frequency of vital signs monitoring and special assessments.
- Types of IV fluids and rates of infusion.
- Postoperative medications (especially those for pain and nausea).
- Resumption of preoperative medications as condition allows (some oral medications are converted to the IV route with appropriate dose adjustment).
- Fluids and food allowed by mouth.
- Level of activity that the patient can resume, including progressive mobility protocols.
- Measures to prevent deep vein thrombosis (e.g., sequential compression devices).
- Position that the patient is to maintain while in bed.
- I&O and daily weights.
- Laboratory tests and x-ray film studies.
- Special directions (e.g., surgical drains to suction, tube irrigations, dressing changes).

Outcomes. Review current nursing diagnoses when establishing relevant expected outcomes and interventions for your patient's postoperative care. Measurable outcomes provide specific guidelines for determining a patient's progress toward recovery from surgery. For example, a patient recovering from knee replacement surgery with the diagnosis of *Impaired Mobility related to pain and lower-extremity weakness* has specific outcomes that include targeted ambulation (e.g., steps to take and distance down hallway), pain relief, and improved range of joint movement. After meeting each outcome, the patient in this example ultimately achieves independent ambulation at a preoperative level or better. At times, outcomes extend from the recovery period into the home setting. An example might be one of "Patient able to change surgical dressing" or "Patient resumes normal diet." *Risk for Infection,* a common preoperative nursing diagnosis, will continue postoperatively because a patient has a surgical wound, is still undergoing the stress response, and may still have an IV site. Expected outcomes for the diagnosis *Risk for Infection* include:

- Patient's incision remains closed and intact by discharge.
- Patient's incision remains free of infectious drainage by discharge.
- Patient remains afebrile.

Setting Priorities. During the convalescent phase of recovery from general anesthesia, priorities for the first 24 hours include maintenance of respiratory, circulatory, and neurological status; wound management; pain control; and early mobility. Most surgeons are aggressive in increasing a patient's activity as soon as possible. If a patient is to be placed on an early mobility protocol, patients and families need to understand that the patient is not being rushed unnecessarily but that early mobility prevents hospital-acquired deconditioning. Encourage a patient to be a partner in care. Active patient participation postoperatively improves outcomes. As a patient progresses, focus priorities on the advancement of patient activity (e.g., mobility, diet tolerance) to return the patient to preoperative functioning or better. A patient generally has multiple nursing diagnoses postoperatively (Fig. 50.6). Reestablish priorities as the status of the patient's health problems change.

Teamwork and Collaboration. During Phase III recovery collaborate on the plan of care with respiratory therapy, physical therapy, occupational therapy, dietary, social work, home care, and others. Include family caregivers as much as possible, especially if they will be assuming care responsibilities in the home. The goal of an interprofessional approach to care is to help the patient return to the best possible level of functioning with a smooth transition to home, rehabilitation, or long-term care. Acute care settings often have a nurse or social worker in a case-manager role to coordinate interprofessional care so that the most appropriate resources are available to patients.

◆ Implementation

Acute Care. Primary causes for postoperative complications include impaired healing of the surgical wound, the effects of prolonged immobilization during surgery and recovery, and the influence of anesthesia and analgesics. If a patient had surgical risks before surgery, the likelihood of complications is greater (Box 50.10). Your aim is to direct postoperative nursing interventions at preventing complications so that the patient returns to the highest level of functioning possible. Failure of a patient to become actively involved in recovery adds to the risk of complications (Table 50.8). Virtually any body system can be affected. Consider the interrelationship of all systems and therapies provided.

Health care agencies have instituted purposeful hourly rounds to improve nurse responsiveness and patient satisfaction. Purposeful rounds include the 4 *Ps* (i.e., *p*ain, *p*otty, *p*ositioning, and *p*eriphery). Nursing staff usually conduct hourly rounds and ask patients about their pain and whether they need to toilet; then the patients are positioned for comfort, and an environmental check is done of the periphery to ensure that possessions such as a phone and nurse call system are in reach (Zadvinskis et al., 2019). The AP may alternate hourly rounding with the nursing staff. However, some patient care providers have expanded the 4 *Ps* model to 7 *Ps*, adding *p*lan, *p*ersonal needs, and *p*resence to the care model. The three additional activities in the 7 *Ps* model include the patient's daily priorities and personal needs and the nurse's accessibility to the patient. The implementation of purposeful rounding improves patient safety by decreasing the occurrence of patient preventable events and proactively addresses problems before they occur (Zadvinskis et al., 2019).

Maintaining Respiratory Function. To prevent respiratory complications, begin pulmonary interventions early. The benefits of thorough preoperative teaching are reached when patients can participate actively in postoperative exercises. When patients awaken from anesthesia, help them maintain a patent airway. Position the patient on one side with the face downward and the neck slightly extended to facilitate a forward movement of the tongue and the flow of mucous secretions out of the mouth. A small folded towel supports the head. Another positioning technique to promote a patent airway involves elevating the head of the bed slightly and extending the patient's neck slightly, with the head turned to the side. In the PACU, the nurse may need to perform a jaw-thrust maneuver and/or chin lift continuously to maintain the patient's airway. Never position a patient with arms over or across the chest because this reduces maximum chest expansion.

Place patients with known OSA or at risk for OSA in the lateral, prone, or upright position, never the supine position, throughout the perioperative period (Olson et al., 2020a). Suction artificial airways and the oral cavity for secretions of mucus (see Chapter 41). Avoid continually eliciting the gag reflex, which might cause vomiting. The following interventions promote expansion of the lungs:

- Encourage diaphragmatic breathing exercises every hour while patients are awake.
- Administer CPAP or NIPPV to patients who use this modality at home (Olson et al., 2020b).

CONCEPT MAP

Nursing diagnosis: Acute pain
- Patient describes severity of incision pain as a 6 on a scale of 0 to 10
- Refused first PT session on postoperative day 1 due to pain
- Grimaces and splints abdomen when repositioning

▼

Interventions
- Monitor patient's use of PCA morphine infusion; encourage to use routinely until pain is controlled
- Have patient self-administer PCA before PT session
- Have two nurses reposition patient routinely
- Teach patient relaxation exercises

Nursing diagnosis: Risk for hypovolemia
- NG tube to low intermittent suction
- IV fluids infusing
- Urinary catheter in place
- Remains NPO

▼

Interventions
- Maintain strict intake and output
- Maintain IV access
- Infuse IV solution
- Monitor laboratory data (e.g., electrolytes)

Primary health problem: Postoperative day 1 from a right colectomy (right-sided large bowel resection) for tumor
Priority assessments: Comfort level, risk for deficient fluid volume, risk for infection

Nursing diagnosis: Risk for infection
- 18-cm midline abdominal incision
- IV catheter in right arm
- 72 years old
- Currently afebrile

▼

Interventions
- Change abdominal dressing as ordered
- Provide incision care as ordered
- Monitor condition of IV site every shift
- Keep IV dressing dry and intact

Nursing diagnosis: Self-care deficit: impaired self toileting, impaired ability to bath and dress
- Has difficulty reaching bathing supplies
- Cannot reach back and legs to wash or dry
- Activity restrictions limit ability to care for self

▼

Interventions
- Refer to occupational therapy to learn use of assistive devices for bathing
- Teach wife how to assist with bathing/dressing

——— Link between medical diagnosis and nursing diagnoses   - - - - - Link between nursing diagnoses

FIG. 50.6 Concept map for Mr. Cooper. *IV,* Intravenous; *NG,* nasogastric; *PCA,* patient-controlled analgesia; *PT,* physical therapy.

BOX 50.10   FOCUS ON OLDER ADULTS

Care of the Older Adult After Surgery

- Decreased cardiac reserve decreases cardiac output during physiological stress, which may result in a delay in recovery from tachycardia and the inability to tolerate fluid depletion (Rothrock, 2019).
- Preexisting medical conditions combined with reduction in physiological reserve are predictors for poor postoperative outcomes in older adults.
- During the perioperative period, assess for changes that occur as a result of infection, hemorrhage, alterations in blood pressure, and fluid/electrolyte abnormalities. Ongoing, focused assessments are necessary.
- Older patients are at greater risk for postoperative delirium associated with an acute onset. Reduced level of consciousness, reduced ability to maintain attention, perceptual disturbances, and memory impairment characterize the typical presentation (Barnett, 2020; Meiner and Yeager, 2019).

- Implement individualized measures to help the older adult achieve rest, sleep, and orientation in the postoperative period to reduce the risk of delirium development.
- Altered and unexpected drug responses are often related to different pharmacokinetics in the older adult. The possibility of high risk for adverse medication events with the administration of anesthetic agents and postoperative analgesics, especially narcotics, is likely (Barnett, 2020). "Start low and go slow" is the guiding principle when medicating older adults because of their slow drug-clearance capability.

TABLE 50.8   Postoperative Complications

Complication	Cause
Respiratory System	
Atelectasis: Collapse of alveoli with retained mucous secretions. Signs and symptoms include elevated respiratory rate, dyspnea, fever, crackles auscultated over involved lobes of lungs, and productive cough.	Inadequate lung expansion. Anesthesia, analgesia, and immobilized position prevent full lung expansion. There is greater risk in patients with upper abdominal surgery who have pain during inspiration and repress deep breathing.
Pneumonia: Inflammation of alveoli involving one or several lobes of lung. Development in lower dependent lobes of lung is common in patient who is immobilized after surgery. Signs and symptoms include fever, chills, productive cough, chest pain, purulent mucus, and dyspnea.	Poor lung expansion with retained secretions or aspirated secretions. Common resident bacterium in respiratory tract is *Diplococcus pneumoniae,* which causes most cases of pneumonia.
Hypoxemia: Inadequate concentration of oxygen in arterial blood. Signs and symptoms include restlessness, confusion, dyspnea, hypertension or hypotension, tachycardia or bradycardia, diaphoresis, and cyanosis.	Anesthetics and analgesics depress respirations. Increased retention of mucus with impaired ventilation occurs because of pain or poor positioning. Patients with obstructive sleep apnea are at increased risk for hypoxemia.
Pulmonary embolism: Embolus blocking pulmonary arterial blood flow to one or more lobes of lung. Signs and symptoms include dyspnea, sudden chest pain, cyanosis, tachycardia, and drop in blood pressure.	Same factors lead to formation of thrombus or embolus. Patients with preexisting circulatory or coagulation disorders and patients who are immobile are at risk.
Circulatory System	
Hemorrhage: Loss of large amount of blood externally or internally in short period of time. Signs and symptoms include hypotension, weak and rapid pulse, cool and clammy skin, rapid breathing, restlessness, and reduced urine output.	Slipping of suture or dislodged clot at incisional site. Patients with coagulation disorders are at greater risk.
Hypovolemic shock: Inadequate perfusion of tissues and cells from loss of circulatory fluid volume. Signs and symptoms are same as for hemorrhage.	Hemorrhage usually causes hypovolemic shock after surgery.
Thrombophlebitis: Inflammation of vein often accompanied by clot formation. Veins in legs are most commonly affected. Signs and symptoms include swelling and inflammation of involved site and aching or cramping pain. Vein feels hard, cordlike, and sensitive to touch.	Prolonged sitting or immobilization aggravates venous stasis. Trauma to vessel wall and hypercoagulability of blood increase risk of vessel inflammation.
Thrombus: Formation of clot attached to interior wall of a vein or artery, which can occlude the vessel lumen. Symptoms include localized tenderness along distribution of the venous system, swollen calf or thigh, calf swelling >3 cm (1.2 inches) compared to asymptomatic leg, pitting edema in symptomatic leg, and decrease in pulse below location of thrombus (if arterial).	Venous stasis (see discussion of thrombophlebitis) and vessel trauma. Venous injury is common after surgery of hips and legs, abdomen, pelvis, and major vessels. Patients with pelvic and abdominal cancer or traumatic injuries to the pelvis or lower extremities are at high risk for thrombus formation.
Embolus: Piece of thrombus that has dislodged and circulates in bloodstream until it lodges in another vessel (commonly lungs, heart, brain, or mesentery).	Thrombi form from increased coagulability of blood (e.g., polycythemia and use of birth-control pills containing estrogen).
Musculoskeletal System	
Hospital-associated deconditioning (HAD): Deficits in physical function secondary to immobilization during an acute hospitalization are collectively defined as hospital-associated deconditioning (HAD).	Older adults are particularly vulnerable. Prolonged immobility is associated with declines in muscle strength and muscle mass and with reduced cognitive function, muscle protein synthesis, and physical function (Mattison, 2020).
Gastrointestinal System	
Paralytic ileus: Nonmechanical obstruction of the bowel caused by physiological, neurogenic, or chemical imbalance associated with decreased peristalsis. Common in initial hours after abdominal surgery.	Handling of intestines during surgery leads to loss of peristalsis for a few hours to several days.
Abdominal distention: Retention of air within intestines and abdominal cavity during gastrointestinal surgery. Signs and symptoms include increased abdominal girth, patient complaints of fullness, and "gas pains."	Slowed peristalsis from anesthesia, bowel manipulation, or immobilization. During laparoscopic surgeries influx of air for procedure causes distention and pain up to shoulders.
Nausea and vomiting: Symptoms of improper gastric emptying or chemical stimulation of vomiting center. Patient complains of gagging or feeling full or sick to stomach.	Abdominal distention, fear, severe pain, medications, eating or drinking before peristalsis returns, and initiation of gag reflex.
Genitourinary System	
Urinary retention: Involuntary accumulation of urine in bladder as result of loss of muscle tone. Signs and symptoms include inability to void, restlessness, and bladder distention. It appears 6-8 hours after surgery.	Effects of anesthesia and narcotic analgesics. Local manipulation of tissues surrounding bladder and edema interfere with bladder tone. Poor positioning of patient impairs voiding reflexes.
Urinary tract infection: Infection of the urinary tract as a result of bacterial or yeast contamination. Signs and symptoms include dysuria, itching, abdominal pain, possible fever, cloudy urine, presence of white blood cells, and leukocyte esterase positive on urinalysis.	Most frequently a result of catheterization of the bladder.

TABLE 50.8 Postoperative Complications—cont'd

Complication	Cause
Integumentary System	
Wound infection: Invasion of deep or superficial wound tissues by pathogenic microorganisms; signs and symptoms include warm, red, and tender skin around incision; fever and chills; purulent material exiting from drains or from separated wound edges. Infection usually appears 3-6 days after surgery.	Infection is caused by poor aseptic technique or contaminated wound or surgical site before surgical exploration. For example, with a bowel perforation patient is at increased risk for a wound infection because of bacterial contamination from the large intestine.
Wound dehiscence: Separation of wound edges at suture line. Signs and symptoms include increased drainage and appearance of underlying tissues. This usually occurs 6-8 days after surgery.	Malnutrition, obesity, preoperative radiation to surgical site, old age, poor circulation to tissues, and unusual strain on suture line from coughing or positioning.
Wound evisceration: Protrusion of internal organs and tissues through incision. Incidence usually occurs 6-8 days after surgery.	See discussion of wound dehiscence. Patient with dehiscence is at risk for developing evisceration.
Skin breakdown: Result of pressure or shearing forces. Patients are at increased risk if alterations in nutrition and circulation are present, resulting in edema and delayed healing.	Prolonged periods on the operating room (OR) table and in bed after surgery lead to pressure breakdown. Skin breakdown results from shearing during positioning on the OR table and improperly pulling patient up in bed.
Nervous System	
Intractable pain: Pain that is not amenable to analgesics and pain-alleviating interventions.	Intractable pain may be related to the wound or dressing, anxiety, or positioning.
Malignant hyperthermia: Severe hypermetabolic state and rigidity of the skeletal muscles caused by an increase in intracellular calcium ion concentration.	Rare genetic condition triggered with exposure to inhaled anesthetic agents and the depolarizing muscle relaxant succinylcholine.

- Instruct patients to use an incentive spirometer for maximum inspiration. The patient should try to reach the inspiratory target volume achieved before surgery on the spirometer.
- Encourage early ambulation. Walking causes patients to assume a position that does not restrict chest wall expansion and stimulates an increased respiratory rate. Ambulation increases peristalsis.
- Help patients who are restricted to bed to turn on their side every 1 to 2 hours while awake and to sit on the side of the bed when possible.
- Keep the patient comfortable. A patient who is comfortable can participate in deep breathing and coughing. Administer analgesics on time so that pain does not become severe.

The following measures promote removal of pulmonary secretions if they are present:

- Encourage coughing exercises every 1 to 2 hours while patients are awake, and maintain pain control to promote a deep, productive cough. *For patients who have had eye, intracranial, or spinal surgery, coughing may be contraindicated because of the potential increase in intraocular or intracranial pressure.*
- Provide oral hygiene to facilitate expectoration of mucus. The oral mucosa becomes dry when patients are NPO or placed on limited fluid intake.
- Initiate orotracheal or nasotracheal suction for patients who are too weak or unable to cough (see Chapter 41).
- Administer oxygen as ordered and monitor oxygen saturation with a pulse oximeter. Continue to monitor oxygen saturation for patients at risk for respiratory compromise from OSA (Olson et al., 2020b). Administer oxygen to patients at risk for or diagnosed with OSA until they can maintain their baseline oxygen saturation while breathing room air.

Preventing Circulatory Complications. Some patients are at greater risk of venous stasis because of the nature of their surgery or medical history. The following interventions promote normal venous return and circulatory blood flow:

- Provide pain medications as prescribed and nonpharmacological therapies to ensure that patients ambulate early. Early ambulation promotes venous return and circulatory blood flow.

- Encourage patients to perform leg exercises (Skill 50.1) at least every hour while awake. Exercise may be contraindicated in an extremity with a vascular repair or realignment of fractured bones and torn cartilage.
- Apply graded compression stockings, sequential compression device (SCD), or IPC stockings as ordered by the health care provider (Chapter 39). Remove the stockings or device at least once per shift. Perform a thorough reassessment of the skin of the lower extremities at this time.
- Encourage early ambulation. Most patients ambulate after surgery, depending on the severity of surgery and their conditions. Early ambulation protocols require patients to ambulate sometimes within hours of having surgery (Grass et al., 2018; Pai and Douketis, 2020). The degree of activity allowed progresses as the patient's condition improves. Encourage ambulation even if a patient has an epidural catheter or PCA device.
- Before ambulation, assess the patient's vital signs at rest. Abnormalities such as hypotension or certain arrhythmias may contraindicate ambulation. If vital signs are at baseline, first help the patient sit on the side of the bed. A patient's complaint of dizziness is a sign of postural hypotension. A recheck of blood pressure determines whether ambulation is safe. Assist with ambulation by standing on the patient's strong side and making sure the patient is able to walk steadily. Patients may be able to walk only a few feet the first few times out of bed. This usually improves each time. Assess a patient's tolerance to activity by periodically assessing the response to exercise. Using the baseline resting heart rate, compare it with the heart rate as the patient ambulates. Also note the heart rhythm. You can assess exercise tolerance by knowing the patient's maximum heart rate and then calculate an appropriate target rate. Often this is determined by the patient's health care provider. One simple method to calculate a targeted maximum heart rate is by using this formula (CDC, 2020b):

220 – Patient's age = Predicted maximum heart rate

The predicted maximum heart rate should then be multiplied by 64% to 76%, depending on the patient's condition and progress with exercise, to obtain a target rate.

Example: A 70-year-old patient has an average resting heart rate of 84 beats/min. The patient's predicted maximum heart rate equals:

$$220 - 70 = 150 \text{ beats/min}$$

The patient's target heart rate will range from 64% to 76% of the maximum heart rate, or in this example:

$$96 \text{ to } 114 \text{ beats/min}$$

By comparing resting rate with the patient's actual rate during exercise, you can determine whether it is in a safe target range. Remember that a patient's acute surgical condition may not allow a target rate to be reached. *Confer with the patient's surgeon or physical therapist about a safe heart rate target.* Always ask patients how they feel during exercise and whether they note chest pain or shortness of breath.

- Avoid positioning patients in a manner that interrupts blood flow to extremities. Do not place pillows or rolled blankets under a patient's knees while in bed. Compression of the popliteal vessels can cause thrombi. When patients sit in chairs, elevate their legs on footstools. Never allow a patient to sit with one leg crossed over the other.
- Administer anticoagulant drugs as ordered. Patients at greatest risk for thrombus formation often receive prophylactic doses of anticoagulants such as LMWH (e.g., enoxaparin) or low-dose unfractionated heparin (LDUH) for anticoagulation.
- Promote adequate fluid intake orally or intravenously (IV). Adequate hydration prevents concentrated accumulation of formed blood elements such as platelets and red blood cells. When the plasma volume is low, these elements gather and form small clots within blood vessels.

Promoting Early Mobility. Many surgical postoperative protocols now include early mobility guidelines, which are designed to minimize or prevent hospital-acquired deconditioning (see Chapter 38). Using early mobility protocols is associated with improved outcomes, such as reduced deep vein thrombosis, reduced length of stay in patients with community-acquired pneumonia, and maintained or improved functional status from admission to discharge in the elderly and patients who undergo major surgery (Grass et al., 2018; Pai and Douketis, 2019). Explain to patients and family members how quickly patients will begin activities such as range-of-motion exercises, sitting on the side of the bed, and assisted ambulation, and the projected distance for walking independently. Activities will typically begin within 12 hours of a patient's return to the inpatient nursing unit. Also assure patients that appropriate mobility aids will be used and that assistance by nursing staff or physical therapists will ensure their safety. There are patients who will not be able to initiate early mobility until their conditions have stabilized. Explain that it is normal for a patient to progress gradually in activity. If a patient tolerates activity, activity levels progress more quickly.

Achieving Rest and Comfort. Pain control is a priority to facilitate a patient's recovery. Without pain control, a patient will not move or ambulate as readily or as early. A patient who receives general anesthesia will be less likely to initiate coughing exercises after surgery if the patient has pain. The anesthesia provider orders medications for pain management in the PACU. IV opioid analgesics such as morphine sulfate are the drugs of choice immediately postoperative for inpatients. Advances have been made in the use of multimodal analgesia (more than one analgesic), which combines different drug classes delivered through various routes, including the use of local anesthetics alone or in combination with other nerve blocks or therapies such as PCA. The goal is to enhance the efficacy of pain control while minimizing the side effects of each modality (Mariano, 2020).

A patient's pain increases after surgery as the effects of anesthesia diminish. The patient becomes more aware of the surroundings and more perceptive of discomfort. The incisional area is only one source of pain. Irritation from drainage tubes, tight dressings, or casts and the muscular strains caused from positioning on the OR table also cause discomfort.

After assessing that a patient is in discomfort, check to be sure whether the ordered dose of analgesic is within the recommended range. Patients have the most surgical pain in the first 24 to 48 hours after surgery. IV PCA or epidural analgesia may be ordered. A PCA device delivers analgesic medications by IV or subcutaneous infusion. The PCA system allows patients to administer their own IV analgesics from a specially prepared pump (see Chapter 44). If patients gain a sense of control over their pain, they usually have fewer postoperative problems.

Many patients receive regional analgesia, such as epidural analgesia, continuously throughout the recovery period, especially for thoracic and abdominal surgery. Studies show that continuous epidural analgesia provides superior pain relief in terms of less analgesic use, better postoperative pain relief (especially in the first 24 hours), less sedation, and faster return of GI function (Cummings et al., 2018; Hwang et al., 2018; Mariano, 2020). Epidural techniques are especially useful in patients with OSA, who are at an increased risk for airway compromise and postoperative complications with the use of systemic opioids after surgery. Nonsteroidal antiinflammatory agents are an alternative to systemic opioids in patients (Mariano, 2020). Monitor patients closely for side effects, and educate them and family caregivers regarding the pain-management therapy and expected response.

As the patient who received general anesthesia begins to tolerate oral fluids, surgical protocols usually include changing pain medication from IV or epidural to oral administration. Do not overlook the importance of nonpharmacological interventions (see Chapter 44). Assess which care routines contribute to pain, and use nonpharmacological measures to address this pain. An example is to lower the head of the bed and use a pillow for incisional splinting while turning a patient with recent abdominal surgery. Other methods to promote pain relief include positioning, back rubs, distraction, or imagery. Remember, *do not assume that a patient's pain is incisional.* When a patient without PCA or an epidural analgesic asks for pain medication, obtain orders to provide analgesics as often as allowed around-the-clock (ATC) in the first 24 to 48 hours after surgery to improve pain control. If pain medications are not relieving discomfort, notify the health care provider for additional orders. Nurses need to recognize potential complications of analgesics and know what to do if they occur.

Temperature Regulation. Unless intraoperative warming is used, patients are usually still cool when arriving in the surgical unit. Provide warmed blankets or heated air blankets if no other warming device is available. Increasing a patient's body temperature raises metabolism and improves circulatory and respiratory function.

Sometimes shivering is a side effect of certain anesthetic agents instead of hypothermia. Clonidine in small increments can decrease shivering as prescribed by the health care provider. When this happens, encourage your patient to use deep breathing and coughing to help to expel retained anesthetic gases.

If a patient develops signs or symptoms of malignant hyperthermia, recognize this as a potential emergency. Be prepared to administer dantrolene sodium as ordered by the health care provider (Litman, 2020). The medication is administered to prevent muscle stiffness and spasms caused by the rapid rise in body temperature and severe muscle contractions that accompany malignant hyperthermia.

Preventing Infection. Patients are at risk for infection after surgery for various reasons. If a patient becomes febrile, be aggressive in providing routine postoperative nursing interventions. For example, deep breathing and coughing, early ambulation, prompt removal of indwelling urinary catheter (if appropriate), and aseptic care of the surgical wound decrease the risk of postoperative infections. If a patient no longer requires intravenous fluids, prompt removal of IV catheters also reduces infection rates. Since microorganisms require time to incubate, infections are rare within the first 48 hours after surgery. A health care provider who suspects an infection will order wound and or blood cultures.

Maintaining Neurological Function. Deep breathing and coughing expel retained anesthetic gases and facilitate a patient's return to consciousness. Continue monitoring the patient's level of consciousness and responsiveness to questions. When patients are elderly, know the status of their renal function because delayed renal clearance of operatively administered anesthetic agents slows awakening. As a patient regains consciousness, orientation to the environment is important in maintaining the patient's mental status. Reorient the patient, explain that surgery is completed, and describe procedures and nursing measures.

Maintaining Fluid and Electrolyte Balance. Immediately after surgery, patients receive fluids only intravenously. It is important to maintain the patency of IV infusions postoperatively (see Chapter 42). The nurse typically removes an IV catheter once a patient awakens after ambulatory surgery and can tolerate water without GI upset. A more seriously ill patient on a surgical unit requires IV fluids for a longer period to achieve hydration and electrolyte balance and sometimes to receive antibiotics. Some patients require blood products after surgery, depending on the amount of blood loss during surgery. A surgeon orders a prescribed solution and rate for each IV infusion. As a patient begins to take and tolerate oral fluids, the nurse decreases the IV rate as ordered by the surgeon. When patients no longer need a continuous IV infusion, the nurse will most likely saline lock the IV line (as ordered by the surgeon) to preserve the site for the administration of medications such as antibiotics or other types of intravenous therapy (see Chapter 42). In order to continuously monitor fluid status, measure the contents of the urinary catheter, NG tube, or wound drainage collection devices every 8 hours for output recording. Measure and empty wound drainage devices more often if drainage is excessive.

Promoting Normal Gastrointestinal Function and Adequate Nutrition. A patient probably will begin to take ice chips or sips of fluids when arriving on an acute surgical care unit. If fluids are tolerated, the diet progresses with clear liquids next. Interventions for preventing GI complications promote the return of normal elimination and faster return of normal nutritional intake. It takes several days for a patient who has had GI surgery (e.g., a colon resection) to resume a normal diet. Normal peristalsis often does not return for 2 to 3 days. In contrast, the patient whose GI tract is unaffected directly by surgery can resume dietary intake after recovering from the effects of anesthesia. The following measures promote the return of normal elimination:

- Advance a patient's dietary intake gradually. Most surgeons rely on the return of flatus or bowel sounds to order a normal diet. Use patient assessment data to determine how quickly to advance the patient's diet. For example, provide clear liquids such as water, apple juice, broth, or tea after nausea subsides. Ingesting large amounts of fluids leads to distention and vomiting. If a patient tolerates liquids without nausea, advance the diet as ordered. Patients who undergo abdominal surgery are usually NPO the first 24 to 48 hours. As flatus and peristalsis return, provide clear liquids, followed by full liquids, a light diet of solid foods, and finally a patient's usual diet. Encourage intake of foods high in protein and vitamin C.
- Promote ambulation and exercise. Physical activity stimulates a return of peristalsis. A patient who has abdominal distention and "gas pain" may obtain relief when walking.

- Maintain an adequate fluid intake. Fluids keep fecal material soft for easy passage. Fruit juices and warm liquids are especially effective.
- Promote adequate food intake by stimulating a patient's appetite; remove sources of noxious odors, and provide small servings of nonspicy foods.
- Avoid moving a patient suddenly to minimize nausea.
- Help the patient get into a comfortable position during mealtime. If possible, have the patient sit to minimize pressure on the abdomen.
- Provide frequent oral hygiene. Adequate hydration and cleaning of the oral cavity eliminate dryness and bad tastes.
- Administer fiber supplements, stool softeners, and rectal suppositories as ordered. If constipation or distention develops, the health care provider orders cathartics or enemas to stimulate peristalsis.
- Provide meals when the patient is rested and free from pain. Often a patient loses interest in eating if mealtime follows exhausting activities such as ambulation, coughing and deep-breathing exercises, or extensive dressing changes. When a patient has pain, the associated nausea often causes a loss of appetite.

Promoting Urinary Elimination. The depressant effects of anesthetics and analgesics impair the sensation of bladder fullness. A full bladder is painful and causes a patient awakening from surgery to be restless or agitated. Up to 70% of surgical patients may develop postoperative urinary retention (POUR), but it is usually transient (Glick, 2020). Patients who have abdominal surgery or surgery of the urinary system often have indwelling catheters inserted until voluntary urination returns. Patients without a catheter need to void within 4 to 8 hours after surgery; otherwise it is sometimes necessary to insert a straight catheter. If a patient has an indwelling urinary catheter, the goal is to remove it as soon as possible because of the high risk for the development of a catheter-associated urinary tract infection (CAUTI). The evidence suggests that in operative patients who have an indication for an indwelling catheter, the catheter should be removed as soon as possible postoperatively, preferably within 24 hours, unless there are appropriate indications for continued use (Kranz et al., 2020). The following measures promote normal urinary elimination (see Chapter 46):

- Help patients assume their normal position to void if possible.
- Check a patient frequently for the need to void when a catheter is not in place. The feeling of bladder fullness is often sudden, and you need to respond promptly when a patient calls for assistance.
- Assess for bladder distention. If a patient does not void within 8 to 12 hours of surgery or if bladder distention is present, you will insert a straight urinary catheter if you have an order from a health care provider. Continued difficulty in voiding sometimes requires an indwelling catheter, which increases the risk for a UTI. Although the evidence is inconclusive, some agencies use bladder ultrasound to assess bladder volume and assist in the decision to place a urinary catheter.
- Monitor I&O. If a patient has an indwelling catheter, expect an output of about 30 to 50 mL/hr. Another way to gauge adequacy of output is by determining a patient's weight. An accepted level of urinary output is at least 0.5 mL/kg/hr to 1 mL/kg/hr for adults (Harding et al., 2020). If the urine is dark, concentrated, and low in volume, notify a health care provider. Patients easily become dehydrated as a result of fluid loss from surgical wounds and inadequate fluid intake. Measure I&O for several days after surgery until a patient achieves normal fluid intake and urinary output.

Providing Skin and Wound Care. Wound healing is complicated by impaired circulation, inadequate nutrition, and metabolic alterations (see Chapter 48). All of these factors can affect rate of healing and risk for infection. A wound also undergoes considerable physical stress on the suture line and wound bed. Strain on sutures from coughing, vomiting, distention, and movement of body parts can disrupt wound layers. Protecting a wound promotes healing. A critical time for wound healing is 24 to 72 hours after surgery, after which a seal is established. Monitor surgical patients on an ongoing basis for fever, tenderness at a wound site, and presence of local drainage on dressings (i.e., yellow, green, or brown, and odorous). A clean surgical wound usually does not regain strength against normal stress for 15 to 20 days after surgery.

Surgical dressings (if present) remain in place the first 24 hours after surgery to reduce the risk of infection. During this time, add an extra layer of gauze on top of the original dressing if drainage develops. After that, use aseptic technique during dressing changes and wound care (see Chapter 48). Time any dressing change to begin 5 to 30 minutes after giving a patient pain medication (depending on route—5 minutes IV, 30 minutes oral). Keep surgical drains patent so that accumulated secretions can escape from the wound bed.

If infection of a clean surgical wound occurs, you will usually find symptoms of infection 4 to 5 days after surgery. Prepare a patient and family caregiver by explaining the signs to look for in a wound infection. Most patients will have returned home by the time the risk for infection is greatest.

Maintaining/Enhancing Self-Concept. The appearance of wounds, bulky dressings, drains, and tubes threatens a patient's self-concept. Some patients show revulsion toward their appearance by refusing to look at incisions, carefully covering dressings with bedclothes, or refusing to get out of bed because of tubes and devices. The fear of being unable to return to a functional family role causes some patients to avoid participation in the plan of care. Show compassion by maintaining eye contact with a patient and respecting the patient's privacy.

A family often plays an important role in efforts to improve a patient's self-concept. Explain the patient's appearance to the family and ways to avoid nonverbal expressions of revulsion or surprise. Encourage the family to accept the patient's needs and support the patient's independence. The following measures help to maintain a patient's self-concept:

- Provide privacy during dressing changes or inspection of the wound. Keep room curtains closed around the bed and drape the patient to expose only the dressing or incisional area.
- Maintain the patient's hygiene. Wound drainage and antiseptic solutions from the surgical skin preparation dry on the surface of the skin, causing foul odor and skin irritation. A complete bath the first day after surgery renews the patient. Offer a clean gown and washcloth. Keep the patient's hair neatly combed, and offer oral hygiene every 2 hours while awake, especially if the patient is NPO.
- Prevent drainage devices from overflowing.
- Maintain a pleasant environment. Being in pleasant, comfortable surroundings heightens self-concept. Store or remove unused supplies. Keep the patient's bedside orderly and clean.
- Offer opportunities for the patient to discuss feelings about appearance. A patient who avoids looking at an incision possibly needs to discuss fears or concerns. A patient having surgery for the first time is often more anxious than one who has had multiple surgeries. When a patient looks at an incision for the first time, make sure that the area is clean. Eventually the patient will be able to care for the incision site by applying simple dressings or bathing the affected area.
- Provide the family with opportunities to discuss ways to promote the patient's self-concept. Encouraging independence for the patient is sometimes difficult for a family member who has a strong desire to help the patient in any way. Family members are more able to be supportive during dressing changes when they know about the appearance of a wound or incision. Help family members know when it is appropriate to discuss future plans. This allows the patient and family to discuss realistic plans for a patient's return home.

Restorative and Continuing Care. Preparing a patient for discharge requires an interprofessional effort. All members of the health care team must understand the patient's current status, discharge destination, and implications for an efficient transition in care. In order for an inpatient to be deemed safe and ready for discharge to home or to a nonacute environment, a health care provider must consider the following medical determinants (Alper et al., 2020):

- Patient's cognitive status
- Patient's activity level and functional status
- The nature of the patient's current home and its suitability for the patient's condition (e.g., presence of stairways, cleanliness)
- Availability of family or companion support
- Ability to obtain medications and services
- Availability of transportation from hospital to home and for follow-up visits
- Availability of services in the community to assist the patient with ongoing care

As a nurse you are in a unique position to gather information about the patient's psychological status, perceived readiness for discharge, and home resources. You collaborate with the health care provider, social worker, and other therapists to confirm the most appropriate discharge plan.

Surgical recovery is slowed if patients are deconditioned and then fail to exercise regularly. It is important to keep frail older adults active after surgery by offering assistive devices and referral to rehabilitation. A person is considered frail if exhibiting three of the following: unintentional weight loss, low physical activity, slowed motor performance, weakness, and fatigue or exercise intolerance. Aerobic exercise and physical resistance training sometimes improve patients' gait speed and ability to perform ADLs. Collaborate with physical and occupational therapists in finding strategies to help patients adhere to recommended exercise and active ADL programs. Involve family caregivers in the patient's exercise program.

Patients having surgery performed in ambulatory surgery centers must be accompanied by a responsible family member or friend to allow for discharge after the procedure. The requirements for discharge after ambulatory surgery include:

- All postanesthesia care unit (PACU) discharge criteria met
- No intravenous (IV) narcotics for last 30 minutes; pain controlled
- Minimal nausea and vomiting
- Voided (if appropriate to surgical procedure/orders)
- Able to ambulate if age appropriate and not contraindicated
- Discharge instructions given and understood using teach-back

During the postoperative period, you will apply critical thinking by matching interventions with what you know about a patient's discharge restrictions, willingness to assume self-care, and the home environment. This enables you to make patient teaching relevant. For example, if a patient is required to follow activity restrictions and limit lifting, you consider the routine activities the patient performs at home and explain to the patient what adjustments are needed (e.g., lifting groceries, pets, young children) to meet those restrictions. Patients often must continue wound care, follow activity or diet restrictions, continue medication therapy, and observe for signs and symptoms of complications at home. Education for the preparation of patients to assume self-care is an ongoing process throughout hospitalization. It is important to provide a document that includes language- and literacy-appropriate instructions and patient education materials to help in a successful transition from the hospital (Alper et al., 2020). For example, offer materials with more pictures and illustrations for patients who do not speak English or who have limited reading ability. Ensure that all materials are sensitive to various cultures and religions. This gives patients and family caregivers a simple but accurate resource to use to enhance care of the patient at home. Patients receive a copy of signed discharge instructions, and one copy remains in the medical or electronic record.

Some patients need home care assistance after discharge. For example, nurses make referrals to home care for skilled nursing requirements when patients need ongoing wound care, IV therapy, or drain management. In addition, patients who are more physically dependent often require assistance from assistive personnel to provide bathing and hygiene needs. The case coordinator or social worker at the hospital helps with discharge coordination. Encourage patients to show their discharge instructions to home care providers.

Other patients, especially older adults, sometimes require discharge to a rehabilitation or skilled nursing center after their hospital recovery. During their recovery, patients work to gain mobility and recovery of their independent living skills. In addition, nurses provide wound care and other specialized services. A case coordinator or social worker works with the patient, family, and nurse to coordinate transfer to the skilled nursing center.

◆ Evaluation

Through the Patient's Eyes. Consult with a patient and family to gather evaluation data, and remember that evaluation is ongoing. During your hourly rounds ask specific questions that evaluate patient expectations and perceptions. For example, you might ask, "Is your pain being managed well?" "How well are you sleeping?" and "Is there anything I can do for you at this time?" Evaluate your patient's level of comfort, and ensure that the patient understands all aspects of nursing care. For example, say, "Tell me if there is anything about your discharge instructions that you do not understand." Resolve any concerns

or issues, and answer the patient's and family caregiver's questions before discharge.

Patient Outcomes. Evaluate the effectiveness of care based on the patient-centered expected outcomes established after surgery for each nursing diagnosis. If a patient fails to progress as expected, revise the patient's care plan based on evaluation findings and the patient's needs.

Make sure to evaluate for pain relief using a pain scale. Determine the efficacy of both pharmacological and nonpharmacological measures. As for other patient problems, use appropriate objective evaluative measures—for example, inspect the condition of a wound, monitor usage of the incentive spirometer, measure the distance or number of times that a patient can ambulate, or monitor the amount of fluid and food intake.

Part of an evaluation is to determine the extent to which the patient and family caregiver learn self-care measures. Use the teach-back method of patient education by having patients restate, in their own words, information that you taught (Bastable, 2019). If a patient must perform any skill at home, such as a dressing change or exercise, evaluate through return demonstration (see Chapter 25). Alper (2020) describes using teach-back frequently and repetitively, starting early on in the hospitalization, to build knowledge, attitudes, and skills more effectively. This strategy showed promise in the reduction of hospital readmissions (Alper, 2020).

Many agencies call patients at home 24 hours after discharge to help evaluate patient outcomes. This allows for monitoring the progress of a patient's recovery and for identifying the development of complications. This also allows the nurse to evaluate and reinforce a patient's understanding of restrictions, wound care, medications, and necessary follow-up.

SAFETY GUIDELINES FOR NURSING SKILLS

Ensuring patient safety is an essential role of the professional nurse. Use sound clinical judgment by communicating clearly with members of the health care team, assessing, analyzing the patient's clinical findings, and incorporating the patient's priorities of care and preferences. Use the best evidence, applying professional standards, when selecting interventions to use in patient care delivery. When performing the skills in this chapter, remember the following points to ensure safe, patient-centered care:

- Coughing and deep breathing are sometimes contraindicated after brain, spinal, head, neck, or eye surgery (prevents intracranial and intraocular pressure increases).

- Patients who are severely obese sometimes have more improved lung function and vital capacity in the reverse Trendelenburg or side-lying position.
- Immediately report to the health care team any signs of VTE, such as pain, tenderness, redness, warmth, or swelling in the upper or lower extremities during postoperative exercises.

SKILL 50.1   TEACHING AND DEMONSTRATING POSTOPERATIVE EXERCISES

Delegation and Collaboration

The skills of preoperative teaching cannot be delegated to assistive personnel (AP). AP can reinforce and help patients perform postoperative exercises. The nurse instructs the AP about:

- Any precautions or safety issues unique to the patient (e.g., fall risks, mobility limitations, bleeding precautions).
- Informing the nurse of any identified concerns (e.g., inability to perform exercise).

Equipment

- Pillow
- Incentive spirometer
- Preoperative education flow sheet
- Positive expiratory pressure (PEP) device
- Stethoscope

STEP	RATIONALE
ASSESSMENT	
1. Identify patient using at least two identifiers (e.g., name and birthday or name and medical record number) according to agency policy.	Ensures correct patient. Complies with The Joint Commission standards and improves patient safety (TJC, 2021).
2. Assess patient's/family caregiver's knowledge, experience, and health literacy.	Ensures that the patient/family caregiver has the capacity to obtain, communicate, process, and understand basic health information (CDC, 2021).

Continued

SKILL 50.1 **TEACHING AND DEMONSTRATING POSTOPERATIVE EXERCISES—cont'd**

STEP	RATIONALE
3. Identify patient's cognitive level and language. If patient does not speak English or is deaf, have a professional interpreter available to assist you.	These factors may alter patient's ability to understand meaning of surgery and can affect postoperative healing if full understanding is not present.
4. Assess patient's knowledge, prior experience with surgery and anesthesia, and feelings about procedure.	Reveals need for patient instruction and/or support.
5. Assess patient's understanding of the intended surgery and anesthesia. Ask patient to offer a description rather than asking a simple yes or no question (e.g., "Tell me what your surgery will involve"). Ask about patient's and family caregiver's expectations of surgery and care. Include questions concerning time frame for surgery and recovery, fears, cultural practices, and religious or spiritual beliefs.	Patients may have misconceptions and incomplete knowledge. Asking about fears, cultural practices, and religious or spiritual beliefs allows you to anticipate priorities of care and adapt teaching and support accordingly.
6. Assess patient's risk factors for postoperative respiratory complications (nursing history and ability to breathe deeply, cough). Check nursing history for patient's height and age.	General anesthesia predisposes patient to respiratory problems (Bittner, 2020; Mills, 2018). Presence of underlying respiratory conditions or patient's inability to perform postoperative respiratory exercises increases the risk for pulmonary complications. Height and age are used to set incentive spirometer parameters.
7. Assess patient's anxiety related to surgery by noting responses and observing nonverbal behavior.	Directs you to provide additional emotional support, which may be needed to facilitate the patient's readiness to learn.
8. Assess who is primary family caregiver and the person's ability and willingness to learn and support patient following surgery.	Family caregiver's presence after surgery is an important factor in patient recovery. Caregiver can coach patient through postoperative exercise, help with medication administration, and observe for postoperative complications.
9. Assess patient's goals or preferences for how skill is to be performed or what patient expects.	Allows care to be individualized to patient.
10. Assess patient's medical record for type of surgery and approach.	The surgical procedure itself may require patients to limit activities postoperatively. Anticipating any limitations that might affect how patient can perform postoperative exercises allows you to adapt your instruction preoperatively.

PLANNING

1. Perform hand hygiene. Prepare equipment and room for instructions and demonstrations.	Reduces transmission of microorganisms. A well-equipped room provides a conducive environment to learning.
2. Provide patient privacy	Maintaining privacy promotes patient dignity and respect.
3. If patient is in health care agency: position the patient in a semi-Fowler's position or upright on the side of the bed as tolerated.	Appropriate positioning allows for increased participation in postoperative exercises and optimal comfort.
4. Plan teaching session for when the patient is not in pain.	Pain distracts patients from focusing on learning. Decreased pain promotes patient participation in the postoperative exercises.
5. Prepare health literacy–appropriate teaching materials. Provide instruction when family caregiver is present (if appropriate).	Promotes patient understanding of instructions. Family caregiver can be important resource for patient's recovery postoperatively.
6. Explain the importance of patient participation in performing postoperative exercises. Discuss surgical procedure and expected postoperative experiences and exercises.	Reduces anxiety and promotes cooperation.

IMPLEMENTATION

1. Inform patient and family caregiver of date, time, and location of surgery; anticipated length of surgery; additional time in postanesthesia recovery area; and where to wait.	Accurate information helps reduce stress of uncertainty associated with surgery.
2. Encourage and answer questions that patient and family caregiver ask.	Responding to patient and family caregiver questions helps to decrease anxiety and demonstrates your concern for them.
3. Instruct patient about preoperative bowel or skin preparations as needed. Check medical orders and agency policy regarding number of preoperative showers and agent to be used for each shower (2% or 4% chlorhexidine gluconate [CHG] is used most often). a. For CHG liquid: • For the liquid, first shower with soap and water. Clean between any skin folds. • Then wash with CHG. Let the liquid stay on the skin for at least 1 minute. • Then use a clean towel to thoroughly dry off. Inform patient that skin may feel sticky after completion. This is normal and will last only a short time. • Use a fresh towel after each bathing. • Have patient don clean clothing. b. For CHG cloths: • Be sure the skin is dry. Use one cloth for each body part (e.g. arms, abdomen, leg and foot, back, groin, and buttocks.	Proper skin preparation is critical element in preventing surgical site infections (SSIs). Showering first with soap and water removes dirt and oil that can prevent CHG from working correctly. Rinsing skin removes residual antiseptic preparation that may cause skin irritation (Mann, 2020). After use, towels contain microorganisms that can grow in presence of moisture. Using a fresh towel after each shower and donning clean clothing minimizes risk of reintroducing microorganisms to clean skin (Berríos-Torres et al., 2017).

CLINICAL JUDGMENT: *Have patient use chlorhexidine only on the skin below the neck, not on the face.*

STEP	**RATIONALE**
4. Instruct patient about extent and purpose of food and fluid restrictions for period specified before surgery (e.g., no clear liquids at least 2 hours before surgery, no light meal [e.g., toast and a clear liquid] 6 hours or more before surgery, no meat or fried foods 8 hours before surgery, unless otherwise specified by surgeon or anesthesiologist) (Crowley, 2020).	During general anesthesia muscles relax, and gastric contents can reflux into esophagus, leading to aspiration. Anesthetic eliminates patient's ability to gag.
5. Describe perioperative routines (e.g., time-out procedure, operative site marking, insertion of IV catheter and therapy, urinary catheterization, hair clipping or removal, laboratory tests, transport to operating room [OR]).	Allows patient to anticipate and recognize routine procedures, reducing anxiety. Empowers patient with information about what the staff does to keep patient safe for operative process.
6. Describe planned effect of preoperative medications.	Provides information about what to expect, decreasing anxiety.
7. Review which routine medications patient needs to discontinue at home before surgery.	Some medications are discontinued before surgery to minimize effects that can cause surgical risks. For example, anticoagulants may increase bleeding and are usually discontinued several days before surgery. Insulin dosages are usually adjusted because of reduced intake of food before surgery.
8. Describe perioperative sensations and sounds to expect in holding area or operating room (e.g., blood pressure cuff tightening, electrocardiogram [ECG] leads, cool room, and beep of monitors).	Misconceptions and concerns about perioperative sensations and sounds have been ranked high among preoperative patients for causing anxiety.
9. Describe pain-control methods to be used after surgery. Discuss what pain is acceptable; explain that patient will not be pain-free, but that pain will be managed. Explain use of PCA (when appropriate).	Patients are fearful of postoperative pain. Explaining pain-management techniques reduces fear. This helps you understand what degree of pain a patient feels is acceptable and allows you to educate patients that although they will not be pain-free, the pain will be managed.
10. Describe what patient will experience after surgery (e.g., where patient will be upon awakening; frequency of vital signs; presence and location of dressing, catheters, drains, tubes; alternating pressure from sequential compression device; postoperative exercises; and the activity level to be expected).	Provides objective description of what patient can expect after surgery so that patient is prepared.
11. Explain any early mobility protocol; purpose and normal progression from sitting on side of bed to ambulation. Demonstrate how to sit on side of bed. Clarify that protocol starts early during recovery.	Full patient participation is essential for early ambulation to be successful.
12. Perform hand hygiene.	Reduces transmission of microorganisms.
13. Teach turning:	
a. Instruct patient on turning and sitting up (especially suited for abdominal and thoracic surgery):	Promotes circulation and ventilation.
(1) Have patient turn onto right side: assume supine position, then move to side of bed (in this case left side) if permitted by surgery. Instruct patient to move by bending knees and pressing heels against mattress to raise and move buttocks (see illustration). Top side rails on both sides of bed should be in upright position.	Positioning begins on side of bed so that turning to other side does not cause patient to roll toward edge of bed. Buttocks lift prevents shearing force against sheets. If patient's bed has a turn-assist feature, use it to help position patient.
(2) Have patient splint incision with right hand or with right hand with pillow over incisional area; keep right leg straight and flex left knee up (see illustration); grab right side rail with left hand, pull toward right, and roll onto right side. Reverse process to turn to left side.	Supports incision and decreases discomfort while turning.
(3) Instruct patient to turn every 2 hours from side to side while awake. Often patient requires assistance with turning after surgery.	Reduces risk of vascular, pulmonary, and pressure injury complications.

CLINICAL JUDGMENT: *Some patients, such as those who have had back surgery or vascular repair, are restricted from flexing their legs after surgery. In addition, some patients are restricted from turning or may need help for positioning.*

STEP 13a(1) Buttocks lift for moving to side of bed. (From Lowdermilk D, Perry SE: *Maternity and women's health care,* ed 9, St Louis, 2007, Mosby.)

STEP 13a(2) Leg position when turning to right. (From Lowdermilk D, Perry SE: *Maternity and women's health care,* ed 9, St Louis, 2007, Mosby.)

Continued

SKILL 50.1   TEACHING AND DEMONSTRATING POSTOPERATIVE EXERCISES—cont'd

STEP	RATIONALE
(4) To sit up on right side of bed, elevate head of bed and have patient turn onto right side. While lying on right side, patient pushes on mattress with left arm and swings feet over edge of bed with nurse's help. To sit up on left side of bed, reverse this process. Assess whether patient feels dizzy while sitting up. Return to bed if dizziness occurs (see Chapter 38).	Sitting position lowers diaphragm to permit fuller lung expansion. Screening for dizziness detects orthostatic hypotension.

> **CLINICAL JUDGMENT:** *Caution patient to always use the nurse call system to ask for assistance when sitting on side of bed to reduce risk of a fall.*

14. Teach coughing and deep breathing:	Patient may hesitate to take deep breaths because of weakness or pain, resulting in secretions remaining in bases of lungs. Collection of secretions increases risk of pulmonary atelectasis and pneumonia. This is especially important for patients with a history of smoking, lung disease, or patients who are confined to bed rest.
a. Assist patient to high-Fowler's position in bed with knees flexed, or have patient sit on side of bed or chair in upright position.	Sitting position facilitates diaphragmatic expansion.
b. Instruct patient to place palms of hands across from one another lightly along lower border of rib cage or upper abdomen (see illustration).	Allows patient to feel rise and fall of abdomen during deep breathing.
c. Have patient take slow, deep breaths, inhaling through nose. Explain that patient will feel normal downward movement of diaphragm during inspiration. Demonstrate as follows:	Helps to prevent hyperventilation or panting. Slow, deep breath allows for more complete lung expansion.
(1) Have patient avoid using chest and shoulder muscles while inhaling.	Increases unnecessary energy expenditure and does not promote full lung expansion.
(2) Have patient take slow, deep breath through the nose, hold for count of 3 seconds, and slowly exhale through mouth as if blowing out candle (pursed lips).	Resistance during exhalation helps to prevent alveolar collapse.
(3) Have patient repeat breathing exercise 3 to 5 times.	Repetition reinforces learning.
(4) Have patient take two slow, deep breaths, inhaling through nose and exhaling through pursed lips.	Deep breaths expand lungs fully to aid gas exchange and remove anesthetic agent so that patient regains consciousness (Harding et al., 2020). Deep breaths also move air behind mucus to facilitate coughing.
(5) Have patient inhale deeply a third time and hold breath to count of 3. Cough fully for two to three consecutive coughs without inhaling between coughs.	Deep breathing moves up secretions in respiratory tract to stimulate cough reflex without voluntary effort on part of patient (Conde and Adams, 2020; Harding et al., 2020).
(6) Caution patient against just clearing throat without deep breathing.	Clearing throat does not remove mucus from deeper airways.
(7) Have patient practice several times. Instruct patient to perform turning, coughing, and deep breathing every 1 to 2 hours while awake (Harding et al., 2020). Have family caregiver coach patient to exercise.	Ensures mastery of technique. Frequent pulmonary exercises and movement decrease risk of postoperative pneumonia (Harding et al., 2020; Smetana, 2020b).
15. Teach use of an incentive spirometer	Provides visual aid of respiratory effort. Encourages deep breathing to loosen secretions in lung bases.
a. Explain purpose of incentive spirometer and how it works. Position patient in sitting position in chair or in reclining position with head of bed elevated at least 45 degrees.	Promotes cooperation. Facilitates diaphragm lowering and lung expansion.

STEP 14b Deep-breathing exercise—placement of hands on upper abdomen during inhalation. (Copyright © Mosby's Clinical Skills: Essentials Collection.)

STEP	RATIONALE
b. Set targeted tidal volume on the incentive spirometer according to manufacturer directions. Explain that this is the volume level to be reached with each breath.	Establishes goal of volume level necessary for adequate lung expansion. Manufacturers determine target on basis of patient height and age.
c. Explain how to place mouthpiece of incentive spirometer so that lips completely cover mouthpiece. Have patient demonstrate until position is correct (see illustration).	Validates patient's understanding of instructions and evaluates psychomotor skills.
d. Instruct patient to exhale completely; then position mouthpiece so that lips completely cover it, and inhale slowly, maintaining constant flow through unit until reaching targeted tidal volume (see illustration).	Promotes complete inflation of lungs and minimizes atelectasis. Aiming toward target volume offers visual feedback of respiratory effort.
e. Once maximum inspiration is reached, have patient hold breath for 2 to 3 seconds and exhale slowly. Compare what patient achieves to set target.	Promotes alveolar inflation. Establishes measure of normal maximum breath by patient. Used to determine outcome postoperatively.
f. Instruct patient to breathe normally for short period between each of the 10 breaths taken on incentive spirometer. Repeat every hour while awake.	Prevents hyperventilation and fatigue.
16. Teach positive expiratory pressure (PEP) therapy and "huff" coughing:	
a. Explain purpose of PEP device and how it works. Set PEP device for setting ordered.	Promotes cooperation. Higher settings require more effort.
b. Instruct patient to assume semi-Fowler's or high-Fowler's position in bed or to sit in a chair. Place nose clip on patient's nose (see illustration).	Promotes optimum lung expansion and expectoration of mucus.
c. Have patient place lips around mouthpiece. Instruct patient to take full breath and exhale 2 or 3 times longer than inhalation. Repeat pattern for 10 to 20 breaths.	Ensures that patient does all breathing through mouth. Ensures that patient uses device properly.
d. Remove device from mouth and have patient take slow, deep breath and hold for 3 seconds.	Promotes lung expansion before coughing.
e. Instruct patient to exhale in quick, short, forced "huffs." Repeat exercise every 2 hours while awake.	"Huff" coughing, or forced expiratory technique, promotes bronchial hygiene by increasing expectoration of secretions.
17. Teach controlled coughing:	Deep breaths expand lungs fully so that air moves behind mucus and facilitates effective coughing.
a. Explain importance of maintaining upright position in bed or chair; have patient lean slightly forward.	Position facilitates diaphragm excursion and enhances thorax and abdominal expansion.
b. Demonstrate coughing. Fold arms across abdomen and take a slow, deep breath, inhaling through the nose.	Expands lungs.

STEP 15d Diagram of use of incentive spirometer.

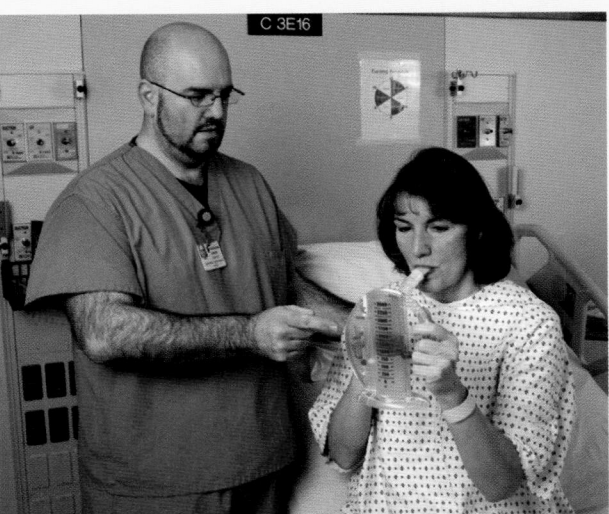

STEP 15c Patient demonstrates incentive spirometry.

STEP 16b Diagram of use of positive expiratory pressure device.

Continued

SKILL 50.1	TEACHING AND DEMONSTRATING POSTOPERATIVE EXERCISES—cont'd

STEP	RATIONALE
c. To exhale, lean forward, pressing arms against abdomen. Cough 2 or 3 times without inhaling between coughs. Cough through a slightly open mouth (see illustration). Coughs should be short and sharp. (Tell patient to push all air out of lungs.)	Clearing throat does not remove mucus from deeper airways. Full, forceful cough is most effective in removing mucus.
d. Breathe in again by "sniffing" slowly and gently through the nose.	Prevents mucus from moving back down airways.
e. Caution patient against just clearing throat instead of coughing deeply. Have patient rest a few minutes and repeat exercise	Clearing throat does not remove mucus from deeper airways.
f. If surgical incision is thoracic or abdominal, teach patient to place either hands or pillow over incisional area and place hands over pillow to splint incision (see illustration). During breathing and coughing exercises, press gently against incisional area for splinting and support.	Surgical incision cuts through muscles, tissues, and nerve endings. Deep-breathing and coughing exercises place additional stress on suture line and cause discomfort. Splinting incision with hands or pillow provides firm support and reduces incisional pulling and pain.
g. Instruct patient to cough 2 to 3 times every 2 hours while awake and to continue to practice coughing exercises, splinting imaginary incision (see illustration).	Deep coughing with splinting effectively expectorates mucus with minimal discomfort.
h. Instruct patient to examine sputum for consistency, odor, amount, and color changes and to notify a nurse if any changes are noted.	Sputum consistency, odor, amount, and color changes may indicate presence of pulmonary complication such as pneumonia.
18. Teach leg exercises:	

CLINICAL JUDGMENT: *Leg exercises are recommended for patients restricted to bed or during times when patients are ambulatory but resting in bed or in a chair. The ideal exercise to promote venous return and improve lung vital capacity is early mobility (see Chapter 38).*

a. Instruct patient to perform leg exercises every 1 to 2 hours while awake: ankle rotation, dorsiflexion and plantar flexion, leg extension and flexion, and straight leg raises.	Leg exercises facilitate venous return from lower extremities and reduce risk of circulatory complications such as venous thromboembolism.
b. Position patient supine.	

STEP 17c Controlled coughing with placement of hands on upper abdomen.

STEP 17f Techniques for splinting incisions.

STEP 17g Patient splinting abdomen with pillow. (From Lewis S, et al: *Medical-surgical nursing: assessment and management of clinical problems*, ed 9, St Louis, 2014, Mosby.)

STEP	**RATIONALE**
c. Instruct patient to rotate each ankle in complete circle and draw imaginary circles with big toe 5 times (see illustration).	Promotes joint mobility.
d. Alternate dorsiflexion and plantar flexion while instructing patient to feel calf muscles tighten and relax (see illustration). Repeat 5 times.	Helps maintain joint mobility and promote venous return to prevent thrombus formation.
e. Perform quadriceps setting by tightening thigh and bringing knee down toward mattress and relaxing (see illustration). Repeat 5 times.	Quadriceps-setting exercises contract muscles of upper legs, maintain knee mobility, and improve venous return to heart.
f. Instruct patient about the hip and leg lift. Have patient alternate raising leg straight up from bed surface. Leg should be kept straight, and then the patient should bend the leg at the knee (see illustration). Instruct patient to do the exercise on the opposite leg. Repeat 5 times.	Causes quadriceps muscle contraction and relaxation, which help promote venous return.
g. Explain to patient the expected progression of activity for early mobility and when it will begin.	Early mobility protocols usually advance from bed rest to sitting on side of bed to sitting in chair and progressive ambulation (see Chapter 38).
19. Have patient continue to practice exercises before surgery at least every 2 hours while awake. Teach patient to coordinate turning and leg exercises with diaphragmatic breathing and use of incentive spirometer.	Leg exercises stimulate circulation, which prevents venous stasis to help prevent formation of deep vein thrombosis (DVT). Coordinating exercises helps patient continuously work toward best outcomes for recovery.
20. Answer questions and verify patient's expectations of surgery. Coach expectations as needed.	Can reduce postoperative anxiety or anger.
21. Reinforce therapeutic coping strategies (e.g., meditation, calming conversation, listening to music).	Therapeutic coping strategies that self-distract patients reduce preoperative anxiety.
22. Help patient to a comfortable position.	Gives patient a sense of well-being.
23. Place nurse call system in an accessible location within patient's reach.	Ensures patient can call for assistance if needed.
24. Raise side rails (as appropriate) and lower bed to lowest position.	Ensures patient safety.
25. Dispose of soiled supplies in appropriate receptacle, remove and dispose of gloves, and perform hand hygiene.	Reduces transmission of microorganisms. Use appropriate disposal receptacle if patient is on hazardous drugs.

EVALUATION

1. If possible, observe patient demonstrating splinting, turning, and sitting, deep breathing, use of incentive spirometer, PEP therapy, and leg exercises.	Validates patient's ability to correctly perform postoperative exercises and use devices.
2. Ask family member(s) to describe postoperative exercises patient is to perform.	Demonstrates learning.
3. Ask family caregivers to describe how they can coach patient with exercises at home before surgery.	Demonstrates understanding of role family members can play to support patient.
4. Use Teach-Back: "I want to be sure I explained what you need to know about the exercises we want you to perform after surgery. Tell me which exercises you will do and how to do them." Revise your instruction now or develop a plan for revised patient/family caregiver teaching if patient/family caregiver is not able to teach back correctly.	Teach-back is an evidence-based health literacy intervention that promotes patient engagement, patient safety, adherence, and quality. The goal of teach-back is to ensure that you have explained medical information clearly so that patients and their families understand what you communicated to them (AHRQ, 2020).

Foot circles

STEP 18c Foot circles. (From Lewis S, et al: *Medical-surgical nursing: assessment and management of clinical problems,* ed 9, St Louis, 2014, Mosby.)

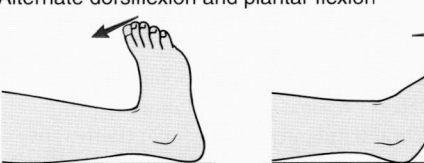

Alternate dorsiflexion and plantar flexion

STEP 18d Alternate dorsiflexion and plantar flexion. (From Lewis S, et al: *Medical-surgical nursing: assessment and management of clinical problems,* ed 9, St Louis, 2014, Mosby.)

Quadriceps (thigh) setting

STEP 18e Quadriceps (thigh) setting. (From Lewis S, et al: *Medical-surgical nursing: assessment and management of clinical problems,* ed 9, St Louis, 2014, Mosby.)

Hip and knee movements

STEP 18f Hip and leg lift. (From Lewis S, et al: *Medical-surgical nursing: assessment and management of clinical problems,* ed 9, St Louis, 2014, Mosby.)

Continued

| **SKILL 50.1** | **TEACHING AND DEMONSTRATING POSTOPERATIVE EXERCISES—cont'd** |

UNEXPECTED OUTCOMES AND RELATED INTERVENTIONS

1. Patient or caregiver identifies incorrect surgical procedure, site, date, or time of surgery.
   - Provide correct information verbally and in writing for patient and family caregiver.
2. Patient incorrectly performs/describes postoperative exercise(s).
   - Explain and demonstrate correct exercise technique.
   - Explain importance of the postoperative exercise as it pertains to patient recovery.
   - Instruct patient to repeat demonstration after clarification.

RECORDING AND REPORTING

- Document preoperative teaching on the appropriate form within the patient's medical record. There is often a preoperative education flow sheet or designated agency form where this information should be documented.
- Document evaluation of patient learning.
- Report patient's inability to identify procedure and site of surgery, as well as understanding of postoperative exercise(s) and teaching, to health care provider.

HOME CARE CONSIDERATIONS

- Incorporate teaching of family members to help patient implement postoperative exercises at home. Be sure family has access to resources (e.g., dressing supplies, dietary food options) at home to support patient appropriately.

KEY POINTS

- Perioperative nursing includes the preoperative, intraoperative, and postoperative phases. Each phase focuses on different aspects of a patient's surgical experience.
- The assessment of risk factors such as history of smoking, obesity, and obstructive sleep apnea allows a nurse to anticipate patient needs and the types of preparation required preoperatively to prevent intraoperative and postoperative complications.
- Malnutrition, diabetes, obesity, smoking, age, obstructive sleep apnea, and cardiac disorders increase patients' risks for perioperative complications.
- A nurse assesses a patient's potential psychological response by identifying the patient's previous experiences with surgery to anticipate needs, providing teaching, addressing fears, and clarifying concerns.
- A standard preoperative teaching plan includes instruction that influences the maintenance of ventilatory function, physical functional capacity, and a sense of well-being, as well as a reduction in patient anxiety and the patient's length of hospital stay.
- Postoperative exercises prevent pulmonary and vascular complications while early ambulation promotes pulmonary and circulatory function as well as prevents deconditioning.
- Using sound clinical judgment during an intraoperative assessment involves a nurse assessing a patient's clinical status, skin integrity, and joint function so that risks for complications can be identified or actual problems recognized to prevent injury if a patient is positioned on the OR table incorrectly.
- The primary differences between intraoperative phases are reflected in the level of monitoring and in the progressive change in focus from acute recovery to preparing patients for convalescence and recovery.
- Hand-off communication ensures that each patient receives the right surgery at the right surgical site by verifying the patient's situation (S) (the patient's problem and type of surgery), background (B) (history), assessment data (A), and recommendations (R) for the interventions that need to be implemented.
- Standardized protocols for hand-off communication between perioperative health care providers minimize surgical risks and promote a seamless transition between each surgical phase.

- Postoperative priorities include maintenance of a patent airway, circulatory and perfusion regulation, temperature control, pain control, fluid and electrolyte balance, and wound care.
- Postoperative patient education should be relevant and specific, culturally appropriate, and accurate to enhance the ability of patients to care for themselves at home.
- When caring for patients who are undergoing ambulatory surgery, prioritize education because of the limited time available, and involve the patient's family or support system.

REFLECTIVE LEARNING

- Think about Mr. Cooper and describe preoperative assessment data that put him at risk for anxiety. (Recognize Cues)
- What priority collaborative problems support or contradict Mr. Cooper's surgical concerns? (Analyze Cues)
- Considering his assessment data and history, what would be the priority clinical issues in caring for Mr. Cooper? (Prioritize Diagnoses)
- Consider Mr. Cooper's clinical situation and describe what postoperative nursing and medical interventions you could use in the management of a patient who has never had surgery and will need a colectomy. (Generate Solutions)
- Which nursing and medical interventions should have priority when implementing Mr. Cooper's care plan? (Take Action)
- Considering the implementation of the orders from Mr. Cooper's health care providers, how would you determine whether they were effective based on current assessment data? (Evaluate Outcomes)

REVIEW QUESTIONS

1. The nurse prepares a patient with type 2 diabetes for a surgical procedure. The patient weighs 112.7 kg (248 lb) and is 157.4 cm (5 feet, 2 inches) in height. Which factors increase this patient's risk for surgical complications? (Select all that apply.)
   1. Obesity
   2. Prolonged bleeding time
   3. Delayed wound healing
   4. Ineffective vital capacity
   5. Immobility secondary to height

2. Which assessment questions should the nurse ask a preoperative patient preparing for surgery? (Select all that apply.)
   1. "Are you experiencing any pain?"
   2. "Do you exercise on a daily basis?"
   3. "When do you regularly take your medications?"
   4. "Do you have any medication allergies?"
   5. "Do you use drugs and/or tobacco products?"

3. Communication between a nurse caring for a patient in the preoperative holding area and the circulating nurse in the operating room (OR) can best be enhanced by which of the following? (Select all that apply.)
   1. Documenting assessment findings in the medical record
   2. Using a standardized SBAR tool
   3. Being responsive in using nonverbal communication techniques
   4. Giving specific information to a transport technician
   5. Listening to the OR nurse's questions

4. Which postoperative intervention best prevents atelectasis?
   1. Use of intermittent compression stockings
   2. Heel-toe flexion
   3. Use of the incentive spirometer
   4. Abdominal splinting when coughing

5. An 85-year-old patient returns to the inpatient surgical unit after leaving the PACU. Which of the following place the patient at risk during surgery? (Select all that apply.)
   1. Stiffened lung tissue
   2. Reduced diaphragmatic excursion
   3. Increased laryngeal reflexes
   4. Reduced blood flow to kidneys
   5. Increased cholinergic transmission

6. A postoperative patient experiences tachypnea during the first hour of recovery. Which nursing intervention is a priority?
   1. Elevate the head of the patient's bed.
   2. Give ordered oxygen through a mask at 4 L/min.
   3. Ask the patient to use an incentive spirometer.
   4. Position the patient on one side with the face down and the neck slightly extended so that the tongue falls forward.

7. Which is the best intervention the nurse should implement to promote bowel function?
   1. Early ambulation
   2. Deep-breathing exercises

3. Repositioning on the left side
4. Lowering the head of the patient's bed

8. Match the nursing interventions on the left with the preventable complication on the right. An intervention may apply to more than one complication.

Nursing Intervention

___ 1. Offering glasses or hearing aid
___ 2. Early ambulation
___ 3. Strict aseptic technique
___ 4. Deep breathing exercise
___ 5. Hydration

Complication

a. Deep vein thrombosis
b. Wound infection
c. Delirium
d. Atelectasis

9. A nurse cares for a postoperative patient in the PACU. Upon assessment, the nurse finds the surgical dressing is saturated with serosanguineous drainage. Which interventions are a priority? (Select all that apply.)
   1. Notify surgeon.
   2. Maintain the intravenous fluid infusion.
   3. Provide 2 L/min of oxygen via nasal cannula.
   4. Monitor the patient's vital signs every 5 to 10 minutes.
   5. Reinforce the dressing.

10. A patient who returned from surgery 3 hours ago following a kidney transplant is reporting pain at a 7 on a scale of 0 to 10. The nurse has tried repositioning with no improvement in the patient's pain report. Unmanaged surgical pain can lead to which of the following problems? (Select all that apply.)
    1. Delayed ambulation
    2. Reduced ventilation
    3. Catheter-associated urinary tract infection
    4. Retained pulmonary secretions
    5. Reduced appetite

Answers: 1. 1, 3; **2.** 1, 4, 5; **3.** 2, 3, 5; **4.** 3; **5.** 1, 2, 4; **6.** 1; **7.** 1; **8.** 1 c, 2 a and c; 3 b, 4 d, 5 a and d; **9.** 1, 5; **10.** 1, 2, 4, 5.

Rationales for Review Questions can be found on the Evolve website.

REFERENCES

Agency for Healthcare Research and Quality (AHRQ): *Patient Safety Network: Never events*, 2019. https://psnet.ahrq.gov/primer/never-events. Accessed July 14, 2020.

Agency for Healthcare Research and Quality (AHRQ): *Health literacy universal precautions toolkit 2nd edition*, Rockville, MD, 2020, Agency for Healthcare Research and Quality.

Alper E, et al: *Hospital discharge and readmission*, 2020, UpToDate. https://www.uptodate.com/contents/hospital-discharge-and-readmission.

American Association of Nurse Anesthetists (AANA): *Malignant hyperthermia crisis preparedness and treatment: position statement, revised*, 2018. https://www.aana.com/docs/default-source/practice-aana-com-web-documents-(all)/malignant-hyperthermia-crisis-preparedness-and-treatment.pdf?sfvrsn=630049b1_8.

American College of Surgeons: *Surgical patient education program: prepare for the best recovery, updated*, 2020. https://www.facs.org/education/patient-education. Accessed July 14, 2020.

American Society of Anesthesiologists (ASA): Practice guidelines for preoperative fasting and the use of pharmacologic agents to reduce the risk of pulmonary aspiration: application to healthy patients undergoing elective procedures, *Anesthesiology* 126(3):376, 2017.

American Society of Anesthesiologists (ASA): *Multimodal approach to pain management reduces opioid use, prescriptions after joint replacement*, 2018. https://www.asahq.org/about-asa/newsroom/news-releases/2018/03/multimodal-approach-to-pain-management-reduces-opioid-use. Accessed July 11, 2020.

American Society of Anesthesiologists: *ASA physical status classification system*, December 13 2020. https://www.asahq.org/standards-and-guidelines/asa-physical-status-classification-system. Accessed September 2021.

American Society of PeriAnesthesia Nurses (ASPAN): *2019-2020 Perianesthesia nursing standards, practice recommendations and interpretive statements*, Cherry Hill, NJ, 2019, ASPAN.

Anderson D, Sexton D: *Overview of control measures for prevention of surgical site infection in adults*, 2020a,

UpToDate. https://www.uptodate.com/contents/overview-of-control-measures-for-prevention-of-surgical-site-infection-in-adults.

Anderson D, Sexton D: *Antimicrobial prophylaxis for prevention of surgical site infection in adults*, 2020b, UpToDate. https://www.uptodate.com/contents/antimicrobial-prophylaxis-for-prevention-of-surgical-site-infection-in-adults.

Association of periOperative Registered Nurses (AORN): *Guidelines for perioperative practice*, Denver, 2020a, AORN.

Association of periOperative Registered Nurses (AORN): *AORN position statement on RN first assistants*, 2020b. RNFA-Standards-of-Practice.pdf. https://www.aorn.org/-/media/aorn/guidelines/position-statements/aorn_position_statement_rnfa.pdf.

Association of periOperative Registered Nurses (AORN): *Prevention of perioperative pressure injury tool kit*, n.d. https://www.aorn.org/guidelines/clinical-resources/tool-kits/prevention-of-perioperative-pressure-injury-tool-kit-nonmembers. Accessed October 2021.

Association of Surgical Technologists (AST): *Guidelines for best practices for the natural rubber latex allergic patient,* 2018. http://www.ast.org/uploadedFiles/Main_Site/Content/About_Us/Guideline_Latex_Allergy.pdf.

Auckley D: *Poor sleep in the hospital: contributing factors and interventions,* 2020, UpToDate. https://www.uptodate.com/contents/poor-sleep-in-the-hospital-contributing-factors-and-interventions/print.

Barnett S: *Anesthesia for the older adult,* 2020, UpToDate. https://www.uptodate.com/contents/anesthesia-for-the-older-adult.

Bastable SB: *Nurse as educator: principles of teaching and learning for nursing practice,* Burlington, MA, 2019, Jones and Bartlett Learning.

Bauer K, Lip GR: *Overview of the treatment of lower extremity deep vein thrombosis (DVT),* 2020, UpToDate. https://www.uptodate.com/contents/overview-of-the-treatment-of-lower-extremity-deep-vein-thrombosis-dvt. Accessed July 11, 2020.

Berríos-Torres SI, et al: Centers for Disease Control and Prevention guidelines for the prevention of surgical site infection, *JAMA Surg* 152(8):784, 2017.

Bittner E: *Respiratory problems in the post-anesthesia care unit (PACU),* 2020, UpToDate. https://www.uptodate.com/contents/respiratory-problems-in-the-post-anesthesia-care-unit-pacu.

Black S, Maxwell L: *General anesthesia in neonates and children: agents and techniques,* 2020, UpToDate. https://www.uptodate.com/contents/general-anesthesia-in-neonates-and-children-agents-and-techniques/print.

Burchum JR, Rosenthal LD: *Lehne's pharmacology for nursing care,* ed 10, St. Louis, 2019, Elsevier.

Butcher HK, et al: *Nursing interventions classification (NIC),* ed 7, St. Louis, 2018, Elsevier.

Centers for Disease Control and Prevention (CDC): *Binge drinking,* 2019, https://www.cdc.gov/alcohol/fact-sheets/binge-drinking.htm.

Centers for Disease Control and Prevention (CDC): *Learn about healthcare-associated venous thromboembolism,* 2020a. https://www.cdc.gov/ncbddd/dvt/ha-vte.html.

Centers for Disease Control and Prevention (CDC): *Target heart rate and estimated maximum heart rate,* 2020b. https://www.cdc.gov/physicalactivity/basics/measuring/heartrate.htm.

Centers for Disease Control and Prevention (CDC): *What is health literacy?* 2021, https://www.cdc.gov/healthliteracy/learn/index.html.

Centers for Medicaid and Medicare Services: *Hospital-acquired condition reduction program (HACRP),* 2020. https://www.cms.gov/medicare/medicare-fee-for-service-payment/acuteinpatientpps/hac-reduction-program.html.

Conde M, Adams S: Overview of the management of postoperative pulmonary complications, *UpToDate,* 2020. https://www.uptodate.com/contents/overview-of-the-management-of-postoperative-pulmonary-complications.

Crowley M: *Preoperative fasting guidelines,* 2020, UpToDate. https://www.uptodate.com/contents/preoperative-fasting-guidelines. Accessed July 14, 2020.

Douketis J, Lip G: *Perioperative management of patients receiving anticoagulants,* 2020, UpToDate. https://www.uptodate.com/contents/perioperative-management-of-patients-receiving-anticoagulants.

European Pressure Ulcer Advisory Panel (EPUAP) and National Pressure Injury Advisory Panel (NPIAP) and Pan Pacific Pressure Injury Alliance: *Treatment of pressure ulcers/injuries: Clinical Practice Guideline. The International Guideline,* Emily Haesler (ED). 2019, EPUAP/NPIAP/PPPIA.

Feinlieb J, et al: *Postoperative nausea and vomiting,* 2020, UpToDate. https://www.uptodate.com/contents/postoperative-nausea-and-vomiting. Accessed July 14, 2020.

Fife C: What really causes pressure ulcers and how can we prevent them? *Today's Wound Clinic,* 13(11):18–21, 2019.

Francis J, Young G: *Diagnosis of delirium and confusional states,* 2020, UpToDate. https://www.uptodate.com/contents/diagnosis-of-delirium-and-confusional-states.

Francone T: *Overview of surgical ostomy for fecal diversion,* 2020, UpToDate. https://www.uptodate.com/contents/overview-of-surgical-ostomy-for-fecal-diversion.

Giger J, Haddad L: *Transcultural nursing: assessment and intervention,* ed 8, St. Louis, 2021, Elsevier.

Hamilton R: *Latex allergy: epidemiology, clinical manifestations, and diagnosis,* 2020, UpToDate. https://www.uptodate.com/contents/latex-allergy-epidemiology-clinical-manifestations-and-diagnosis.

Harding M, et al: *Lewis's medical-surgical nursing: assessment and management of clinical problems,* ed 11, St. Louis, 2020, Elsevier.

Heideman BH: *Helping patients overcome ostomy challenges,* 2017, Wound Care Advisor. https://woundcareadvisor.com/helping-patients-overcome-ostomy-challenges-vol4-no3/.

Inge T: *Surgical management of severe obesity in adolescents,* 2020, UpToDate. https://www.uptodate.com/contents/surgical-management-of-severe-obesity-in-adolescents.

Kawada T: Screening ability of STOP-Bang questionnaire for obstructive sleep apnea, *Anesthesia & Analgesia* 128(3):e48, 2019.

Kline L: *Clinical presentation and diagnosis of obstructive sleep apnea in adults,* 2020, UpToDate. https://www.uptodate.com/contents/clinical-presentation-and-diagnosis-of-obstructive-sleep-apnea-in-adults.

Koutoukidis G, et al: *Tabbner's nursing care: theory and practice,* ed 7, Chatswood, Australia, 2017, Elsevier.

Kozek-Langenecker S: European guideline on perioperative venous thromboembolism prophylaxis: surgery in the elderly, *Eur J Anaesthesiol* 35(2):116, 2018.

Kranz J, et al: Catheter-associated urinary tract infections in adult patients: Preventive strategies and treatment options, *Deutsches Aerzteblatt International,* 117(6):83, 2020.

Lim R: *Bariatric operations for management of obesity: Indications and preoperative preparation,* 2020, UpToDate. https://www.uptodate.com/contents/bariatric-operations-for-management-of-obesity-indications-and-preoperative-preparation.

Litman R: *Malignant hyperthermia: diagnosis and management of acute crisis,* 2020, UpToDate. https://www.uptodate.com/contents/malignant-hyperthermia-diagnosis-and-management-of-acute-crisis.

Ljungqvist O, et al: Enhanced recovery after surgery: a review, *JAMA Surg* 152(3):292, 2017.

Mahanna-Gabrielli E, Eckenhoff R: *Perioperative neurocognitive disorders,* 2020, UpToDate. https://www.uptodate.com/contents/perioperative-neurocognitive-disorders.

Mariano E: *Management of acute perioperative pain,* 2020, UpToDate. https://www.uptodate.com/contents/management-of-acute-perioperative-pain. Accessed July 14, 2020.

Mattison M: *Hospital management of older adults,* 2020, UpToDate. https://www.uptodate.com/contents/hospital-management-of-older-adults/print.

McLendon K, et al: *Deep venous thrombosis risk factors,* 2021, StatPearls, https://www.ncbi.nlm.nih.gov/books/NBK470215/. Accessed October 2021.

Meiner SE, Yeager JJ: *Gerontologic nursing,* ed 6, St. Louis, 2019, Elsevier.

Mills GH: Respiratory complications of anaesthesia, *Anaesthesia* 73(Suppl 1):25, 2018.

Muluk V, et al: *Perioperative medication management,* 2020, UpToDate. https://www.uptodate.com/contents/perioperative-medication-management.

National Council of State Boards of Nursing (NCSBN): *A nurse's guide to the use of social media,* 2018. https://www.ncsbn.org/NCSBN_SocialMedia.pdf. Accessed July 14, 2020.

National Institute on Alcohol Abuse and Alcoholism: *Alcohol Use Disorders Identification Test (AUDIT),* n.d., https://pubs.niaaa.nih.gov/publications/audit.htm. Accessed October 2021.

National Quality Forum (NQF): *Patient Safety, Fall 2018 Cycle: CDP Report TECHNICAL REPORT,* 2019. https://www.qualityforum.org/Publications/2019/08/Patient_Safety_Final_Technical_Report_-_Fall_2018_Cycle.aspx.

Occupational Safety and Health Administration (OSHA): *Healthcare Wide Hazards: latex allergy,* n.d. https://www.osha.gov/SLTC/etools/hospital/hazards/latex/latex.html.

Olson E, et al: *Surgical risk and the preoperative evaluation and management of adults with obstructive sleep apnea,* 2020a, UpToDate. https://www.uptodate.com/contents/surgical-risk-and-the-preoperative-evaluation-and-management-of-adults-with-obstructive-sleep-apnea.

Olson E, et al: *Postoperative management of adults with obstructive sleep apnea,* 2020b, UpToDate. https://www.uptodate.com/contents/postoperative-management-of-adults-with-obstructive-sleep-apnea.

Ricciardi R, et al: *Enhanced recovery after colorectal surgery,* 2020, UpToDate. https://www.uptodate.com/contents/enhanced-recovery-after-colorectal-surgery.

Romanowski KS, Askari R: *Overview of perioperative nutrition support,* 2020, UpToDate. https://www.uptodate.com/contents/overview-of-perioperative-nutritional-support.

Rosenthal L, Association of periOperative Registered Nurses (AORN): *Perioperative assessment of the older adult,* 2019, The Hartford Institute for Geriatric Nursing, NYU Rory Meyers College of Nursing.

Rothrock JC: *Alexander's care of the patient in surgery,* ed 16, St. Louis, 2019, Elsevier.

Ryan M, Sinha M: *Informed procedural consent,* 2020, UpToDate. https://www.uptodate.com/contents/informed-procedural-consent.

Saitz R: *Screening for unhealthy use of alcohol and other drugs in primary care,* 2020, UpToDate. https://www.uptodate.com/contents/screening-for-unhealthy-use-of-alcohol-and-other-drugs-in-primary-care.

Schick L, Windle P: *PeriAnesthesia nursing core curriculum: preprocedure, phase I and phase II PACU nursing,* ed 4, St. Louis, 2020, Elsevier.

Sessler D: *Perioperative temperature management,* 2020, UpToDate. https://www.uptodate.com/contents/perioperative-temperature-management.

Sinha AK, et al: Postoperative malignant hyperthermia- a medical emergency: a case report and review of literature, *J Clin Diagn Res* 11(4):1, 2017.

Smetana G: *Preoperative medical evaluation of the healthy adult patient,* 2020a, UpToDate. https://www.uptodate.com/contents/preoperative-medical-evaluation-of-the-healthy-adult-patient. Accessed July 11, 2020.

Smetana G: *Strategies to reduce postoperative pulmonary complications in adults,* 2020b, UpToDate. https://www.uptodate.com/contents/strategies-to-reduce-postoperative-pulmonary-complications-in-adults. Accessed July 11, 2020.

Sterns R: *Pathophysiology and etiology of edema in adults,* 2020, UpToDate. https://www.uptodate.com/contents/pathophysiology-and-etiology-of-edema-in-adults.

Sviggum H: *Anesthesia for nonobstetric surgery during pregnancy,* 2020, UpToDate. https://www.uptodate.com/contents/anesthesia-for-nonobstetric-surgery-during-pregnancy. Accessed July 13, 2020.

Su X, Wang DX: Improve postoperative sleep: what can we do? *Curr Opin Anaesthesiol* 31(1):83, 2017.

The Joint Commission: *Comprehensive Accreditation and Certification manual, January 1, 2020,* Oakbrook Terrace, IL, 2020, The Commission.

The Joint Commission (TJC): *2021 National Patient Safety Goals,* Oakbrook Terrace, IL, 2021, The Joint Commission. https://www.jointcommission.org/en/standards/national-patient-safety-goals/. Accessed September 27, 2021.

van den Boom W, et al: Effect of A1C and glucose on postoperative mortality in noncardiac and cardiac surgeries, *Diabetes Care* 41(4):782, 2018.

Wahr J: *Safety in the operating room*, 2020, UpToDate. https://www.uptodate.com/contents/safety-in-the-operating-room. Accessed July 15, 2020.

Welch MB: *Patient positioning for surgery and anesthesia in adults*, 2020, UpToDate. https://www.uptodate.com/contents/patient-positioning-for-surgery-and-anesthesia-in-adults.

World Health Organization (WHO): *Surgical safety checklist*, n.d. https://www.who.int/patientsafety/safesurgery/tools_resources/SSSL_Checklist_finalJun08.pdf.

RESEARCH REFERENCES

Arndt K, et al: Vaping: Anesthesia considerations for patients using electronic cigarettes, *AANA J* 88(1):27, 2020.

Becerra A, et al: Prospective observational study of the effectiveness of prewarming on perioperative hypothermia in surgical patients submitted to spinal anesthesia, *Sci Rep* 9:16477, 2019. https://www.nature.com/articles/s41598-019-52960-6. Accessed July 13, 2020.

Bulfone G, et al: Perioperative pressure injuries: a systematic literature review, *Adv Skin Wound Care*, 31(12):556–564, 2018.

Burgess L: The effect of preoperative education on psychological, clinical and economic outcomes in elective spinal surgery: a systematic review, *Healthcare* 21(7):48, 2019.

Cummings KC, et al: Epidural compared with non-epidural analgesia and cardiopulmonary complications after colectomy: a retrospective cohort study of 20,880 patients using a national quality database, *J Clin Anesth* 47(12), 2018.

de Assunção Peixoto C, et al: Risk assessment for perioperative pressure injuries, *Rev Lat Am Enfermagem* 27:e3117, 2019.

Dunwoody D, Jungquist C: Opioid-induced sedation and respiratory depression: are sedation scales enough to prevent adverse drug events postoperatively? *Pain Manag Nurs* 21(1):110–119, 2020

Fracol M, et al: The surgical impact of e-cigarettes: a case report and review of the current literature, *Arch Plast Surg* 44(6):477, 2017.

García-Monasterio E, et al: Post-operative pain management among surgical trauma patients in an acute ward: a best practice implementation project, *JBI Database System Rev Implement Rep* 17(9):1941–1953, 2019.

George J, et al: Use of chlorhexidine preparations in total joint arthroplasty, *J Bone Jt Infect* 2(1):15–22, 2017.

Glick D: *Overview of post-anesthetic care for adult patients*, 2020, UpToDate. https://www.uptodate.com/contents/overview-of-post-anesthetic-care-for-adult-patients.

Grass G, et al: Feasibility of early postoperative mobilisation after colorectal surgery: a retrospective cohort study, *Int J Surg* 56:161, 2018.

Hong-Lin C, et al: The risk factors of postoperative pressure ulcer after liver resection with long surgical duration: a retrospective study, *Wounds* 31(9):242–245, 2019.

Hwang BY, et al: Comparison of patient-controlled epidural analgesia with patient-controlled intravenous analgesia for laparoscopic radical prostatectomy, *Korean J Pain* 31(3):191, 2018.

Iqbal U, et al: Preoperative patient preparation in enhanced recovery pathways, *J Anaesthesiol Clin Pharmacol* 35(Suppl 1):S14–S23, 2019.

Joseph J, et al: Alternating pressure overlay for prevention of intraoperative pressure injury, *J Wound Ostomy Continence Nurs* 46(1):13–17, 2019.

Joshi G: *Anesthetic management for enhanced recovery after major surgery (ERAS) in adults*, 2020, UpToDate. https://www.uptodate.com/contents/anesthetic-management-for-enhanced-recovery-after-major-surgery-eras-in-adults. Accessed July 14, 2020.

Kim JM, et al: Perioperative factors associated with pressure ulcer development after major surgery, *Korean J Anesthesiol* 71(1):48, 2017.

Kim J, et al: Diet modification based on the enhanced recovery after surgery program (ERAS) in patients undergoing laparoscopic colorectal resection, *Clin Nutr Res* 7(4):297–302, 2018.

Koivisto J, et al: Patient education in relation to informational needs and postoperative complications in surgical patients, *Int J Qual Health Care*, 32(1):35–40, 2020.

Mann W: *Overview of preoperative evaluation and preparation for gynecologic surgery*, 2020, UpToDate. https://www.uptodate.com/contents/overview-of-preoperative-evaluation-and-preparation-for-gynecologic-surgery.

Munro CA: *The CMUNRO scale education sheet*, 2019. https://img1.wsimg.com/blobby/go/54e2cb6f-b0b4-4950-9594-41126d75e9fb/downloads/CMUNRO%20SCALE%20Curriculum.pdf?ver=1576268339418

National Institute of Health (NIH): *Sleep apnea*, n.d., National Heart, Lung, and Blood Institute. https://www.nhlbi.nih.gov/health-topics/sleep-apnea.

Pachter C, et al: Smoking is a risk factor for wound complications after direct anterior hip arthroplasty with mesh tape closure, *Adv Skin Wound Care* 33(1):43–46, 2020.

Pai M, Douketis J: *Prevention of venous thromboembolic disease in acutely ill hospitalized medical adults*, 2020, UpToDate. https://www.uptodate.com/contents/prevention-of-venous-thromboembolic-disease-in-adult-nonorthopedic-surgical-patients. Accessed July 14, 2020.

Park S, et al: Development and comparison of predictive models for pressure injuries in surgical patients: a retrospective case-control study, *J Wound Ostomy Continence Nurs*, 46(4):291–297, 2019.

Ramesh C, et al: Effect of preoperative education on postoperative outcomes among patients undergoing cardiac surgery: a systematic review and meta-analysis, *J Perianesth Nurs* 32(6):518, 2019.

Rupich K, et al: The benefits of implementing an early mobility protocol in postoperative neurosurgical spine patients, *Am J Nurs* 118(6):46, 2018.

Saghaleini SH, et al: Pressure ulcer and nutrition, *Indian J Crit Care Med* 22(4):283, 2018.

Skraastad E, et al: Development and validation of the Efficacy Safety Score (ESS), a novel tool for postoperative patient management, *BMC Anesthesiol* 17:50, 2017.

Teleten O, et al: The use of pressure mapping: an educational report. *Wound*, 31(1):e5–e8, 2019.

Weimann A, et al: ESPEN guideline: clinical nutrition in surgery, *Clin Nutr* 36(3):623, 2017.

Wickramasinghe H: *Obstructive sleep apnea, updated (OSA)*, 2019, Medscape. https://emedicine.medscape.com/article/295807-overview#a2. Accessed July 18, 2020.

Zadvinskis I, et al: The impact of nursing work and engagement on patient falls, *J Nurs Adm* 49(11):531–537, 2019.

GLOSSARY

abduction   Movement of a limb away from the body.

abrasion   Scraping or rubbing away of epidermis; may result in localized bleeding and later weeping of serous fluid.

absorption   Passage of drug molecules into the blood. Factors influencing drug absorption include route of administration, ability of the drug to dissolve, and conditions at the site of absorption.

acceptance   Fifth stage of Kübler-Ross's stages of grief and dying. An individual comes to terms with a loss rather than submitting to resignation and hopelessness.

accessory muscles   Muscles in the thoracic cage that assist with respiration.

accommodation   Process of responding to the environment through new activity, thinking, and changing the existing schema or developing a new schema to deal with the new information. For example, a toddler whose parent consistently corrects him when he calls a horse a "doggie" accommodates and forms a new schema for horses.

accountability   State of being answerable for one's actions—a nurse answers to himself or herself, the patient, the profession, the employing institution such as a hospital, and society for the effectiveness of nursing care performed.

accreditation   Process whereby a professional association or nongovernmental agency grants recognition to a school or institution for demonstrated ability to meet predetermined criteria.

acculturation   The process through which an individual or group transitions from one culture to develop the traits of another culture.

acne   Inflammatory, papulopustular skin eruption, usually occurring on the face, neck, shoulders, and upper back.

acromegaly   Chronic metabolic condition caused by overproduction of growth hormone and characterized by gradual, marked enlargement and elongation of bones of the face, jaw, and extremities.

active listening   Listening attentively with the whole person—mind, body, and spirit. It includes listening for main and supportive ideas; acknowledging and responding; giving appropriate feedback; and paying attention to the other person's total communication, including the content, intent, and feelings expressed.

active range-of-motion (ROM) exercise   Exercise to the joint by the patient while doing activities of daily living or during joint assessment.

active strategies of health promotion   Activities that depend on the patient's motivation to adopt a specific health program.

active transport   Movement of materials across the cell membrane by means of chemical activity that allows the cell to admit larger molecules than would otherwise be possible.

activities of daily living (ADLs)   Activities usually performed in the course of a normal day in the patient's life such as eating, dressing, bathing, brushing the teeth, or grooming.

activity tolerance   Type and amount of exercise or work that a person is able to perform without undue exertion or injury.

actual loss   Loss of an object, person, body part or function, or emotion that is overt and easily identifiable.

acuity recording   Mechanism by which entries describing patient care activities are made over a 24-hour period. The activities are then translated into a rating score, or acuity score, that allows for a comparison of patients who vary by severity of illness.

acute care   Pattern of health care in which a patient is treated for an acute episode of illness, for the sequelae of an accident or other trauma, or during recovery from surgery.

acute illness   Illness characterized by symptoms that are of relatively short duration, are usually severe, and affect the functioning of the patient in all dimensions.

adduction   Movement of a limb toward the body.

adolescence   Period in development between the onset of puberty and adulthood. It usually begins between 11 and 13 years of age.

adult day care center   Facility for the supervised care of older adults; provides activities such as meals and socialization during specified day hours.

advanced practice registered nurse (APRN)   Generally the most independently functioning nurse. An APRN has a master's degree in nursing; advanced education in pathophysiology, pharmacology, and physical assessment; and certification and expertise in a specialized area of practice.

advanced sleep phase syndrome   Common in older adults; a disturbance in sleep manifested by early waking in the morning with an inability to get back to sleep. It is thought that this syndrome is caused by advancing of the circadian rhythm of the body.

adventitious sounds   Abnormal lung sounds heard with auscultation.

adverse effect   Harmful or unintended effect of a medication, diagnostic test, or therapeutic intervention.

adverse reaction   Any harmful, unintended effect of a medication, diagnostic test, or therapeutic intervention.

advocacy   Process whereby a nurse objectively provides patients with the information they need to make decisions and supports the patients in whatever decisions they make.

afebrile   Without fever.

affective learning   Acquisition of behaviors involved in expressing feelings about attitudes, appreciation, and values.

afterload   Resistance to left ventricular ejection; the work the heart must overcome to fully eject blood from the left ventricle.

age-related macular degeneration   Progressive disorder in which the macula (the specialized portion of the retina responsible for central vision) degenerates as a result of aging and loses its ability to function efficiently. First signs include blurring of reading matter, distortion or loss of central vision, sensitivity to glare, and distortion of objects.

agnostic   Individual who believes that any ultimate reality is unknown or unknowable.

airborne precautions   Safeguards designed to reduce the risk of transmission of infectious agents through the air that a person breathes.

alarm reaction   Mobilization of the defense mechanisms of the body and mind to cope with a stressor; the initial stage of the general adaptation syndrome.

aldosterone   Mineralocorticoid steroid hormone produced by the adrenal cortex with action in the renal tubule to regulate sodium and potassium balance in the blood.

allergic reaction   Unfavorable physiological response to an allergen to which a person has previously been exposed and has developed antibodies.

alopecia   Partial or complete loss of hair; baldness.

Alzheimer disease   Disease of the brain parenchyma that causes a gradual and progressive decline in cognitive functioning.

AMBULARM   Device used for the patient who climbs out of bed unassisted and is in danger of falling. This device is worn on the leg and signals when the leg is in a dependent position such as over the side rail or on the floor.

amino acid   Organic compound of one or more basic groups and one or more carboxyl groups. Amino acids are the building blocks that construct proteins and the end products of protein digestion.

anabolism   Constructive metabolism characterized by conversion of simple substances into more complex compounds of living matter.

analgesic   Relieving pain; drug that relieves pain.

analogies   Resemblances made between things otherwise unlike.

anaphylactic reaction   Hypersensitive condition induced by contact with certain antigens.

aneurysm   Localized dilations of the wall of a blood vessel; usually caused by atherosclerosis, hypertension, or a congenital weakness in a vessel wall.

anger   Second stage of Kübler-Ross's stages of grief and dying. During this stage an individual resists loss by expressing extreme displeasure, indignation, or hostility.

angiotensin   Polypeptide occurring in the blood, causing vasoconstriction, increased blood pressure, and the release of aldosterone from the adrenal cortex.

anion gap   Difference between the concentrations of serum cations and anions; determined by measuring the concentrations of sodium cations and chloride and bicarbonate anions.

anions   Negatively charged electrolytes.

anthropometric measurements   Body measures of height, weight, and skinfolds to evaluate muscle atrophy.

anthropometry   Measurement of various body parts to determine nutritional and caloric status, muscular development, brain growth, and other parameters.

antibodies   Immunoglobulins essential to the immune system that are produced by lymphoid tissue in response to bacteria, viruses, or other antigens.

anticipatory grief   Grief response in which the person begins the grieving process before an actual loss.

antidiuretic hormone (ADH)   Hormone that decreases the production of urine by increasing the resorption of water by the renal tubules. ADH is secreted by cells of the hypothalamus and stored in the posterior lobe of the pituitary gland.

antiembolic stockings   Elasticized stockings that prevent formation of emboli and thrombi, especially after surgery or during bed rest.

antigen   Substance, usually a protein, that causes the formation of an antibody and reacts specifically with that antibody.

antipyretic   Substance or procedure that reduces fever.

anxiolytics   Drugs used primarily to treat episodes of anxiety.

aphasia   Abnormal neurological condition in which language function is defective or absent; related to injury to speech center in cerebral cortex, causing receptive or expressive aphasia.

apical pulse   Heartbeat as listened to with the bell or diaphragm of a stethoscope placed on the apex of the heart.

apnea   Absence of respirations for a period of time.

apothecary system   System of measurement. The basic unit of weight is a grain. Weights derived from the grain are the gram, ounce, and pound. The basic measure for fluid is the minim. The fluidram, fluid ounce, pint, quart, and gallon are measures derived from the minim.

approximate   To come close together, as in the edges of a wound.

arcus senilis   Opaque ring, gray to white in color, that surrounds the periphery of the cornea. The condition is caused by deposits of fat granules in the cornea. Occurs primarily in older adults.

asepsis   Absence of germs or microorganisms.

aseptic technique   Any health care procedure in which added precautions are used to prevent contamination of a person, object, or area by microorganisms.

assault   Unlawful threat to bring about harmful or offensive contact with another.

assertive communication   Type of communication based on a philosophy of protecting individual rights and responsibilities. It includes the ability to be self-directive in acting to accomplish goals and advocate for others.

assessment   First step of the nursing process. Activities required in the first step are data collection, validation, sorting, and documentation. The purpose is to gather information for health problem identification.

assimilation   The process in which an individual adapts to the host's cultural values and no longer prefers the traditions, values, and beliefs of the culture of origin.

assisted living   Residential living facilities in which each resident has his or her own room and shares dining and social activity areas.

associative play   Form of play in which a group of children participates in similar or identical activities without formal organization, direction, interaction, or goals.

atelectasis   Collapse of alveoli, preventing the normal respiratory exchange of oxygen and carbon dioxide.

atheist   Individual who does not believe in the existence of God.

atherosclerosis   Common arterial disorder characterized by yellowish plaques of cholesterol, lipids, and cellular debris in the inner layers of the walls of the large- and medium-size arteries.

atrioventricular (AV) node   Part of the cardiac conduction system located on the floor of the right atrium; receives electrical impulses from the atrium and transmits them to the bundle of His.

atrophied   Wasted or reduced size or physiological activity of a part of the body caused by disease or other influences.

attachment   Initial psychosocial relationship that develops between parents and the neonate.

attentional set   Mental state that allows the learner to focus on and comprehend a learning activity.

auditory   Related to or experienced through hearing.

auscultation   Method of physical examination; listening to the sounds produced by the body, usually with a stethoscope.

auscultatory gap   Disappearance of sound when obtaining a blood pressure; typically occurs between the first and second Korotkoff sounds.

authority   Right to act in areas in which an individual has been given and accepts responsibility.

autologous transfusion   Procedure in which blood is removed from a donor and stored for a variable period before it is returned to the donor's own circulation.

autonomy   Ability or tendency to function independently.

B

back-channeling   Active listening technique that prompts a respondent to continue telling a story or describing a situation. Involves use of phrases such as "Go on," "Uh-huh," and "Tell me more."

bacteremia   Presence of bacteria in the bloodstream.

bacteriuria   Presence of bacteria in the urine.

balance   Position in which the person's center of gravity is correctly positioned so that falling does not occur.

bandages   Available in rolls of various widths and materials, including gauze, elasticized knit, elastic webbing, flannel, and muslin. Gauze bandages are lightweight and inexpensive, mold easily around contours of the body, and permit air circulation to underlying skin to prevent maceration. Elastic bandages conform well to body parts but can also be used to exert pressure over a body part.

bargaining   Third stage of Kübler-Ross's stages of grief and dying. A person postpones the reality of a loss by attempting to make deals in a subtle or overt manner with others or with a higher being.

baridi   Condition among the Bena people of Tanzania attributed to disrespectful behavior within the family or transgression of cultural taboos. The person experiences physical and psychological symptoms and is usually treated by a traditional healer, who has the person make a public admission or an apology or who treats the person with herbal remedies.

basal cell carcinoma   Malignant epithelial cell tumor that begins as a papule and enlarges peripherally, developing a central crater that erodes, crusts, and bleeds. Metastasis is rare.

basal metabolic rate (BMR)   Amount of energy used in a unit of time by a fasting, resting subject to maintain vital functions.

battery   Legal term for touching another's body without consent.

bed boards   Boards placed under the mattress of a bed that provide extra support to the mattress surface.

bed rest   Placement of the patient in bed for therapeutic reasons for a prescribed period.

benchmarking   Identifying best practices and comparing them with current organizational practices to improve performance. This process helps to support the claims of quality care delivery by the institution.

beneficence   Doing good or actively promoting doing good; one of the four principles of the ethical theory of deontology.

benign breast disease (fibrocystic)   Benign condition characterized by lumpy, painful breasts and sometimes nipple discharge. Symptoms are more apparent before the menstrual period. Known to be a risk factor for breast cancer.

bereavement   Response to loss through death; a subjective experience that a person suffers after losing a person with whom there has been a significant relationship.

biases and prejudices   Beliefs and attitudes associating negative permanent characteristics to people who are perceived as different from oneself.

bi-level positive airway pressure (BiPAP)   Ventilatory support used to treat patients with obstructive sleep apnea, patients with congestive heart failure, and preterm infants with underdeveloped lungs.

bilineally   Kinship that extends to both the mother's and father's sides of the family.

binders   Bandages made of large pieces of material to fit specific body parts.

bioethics   Branch of ethics within the field of health care.

biological clock   Cyclical nature of body function. Functions controlled from within the body are synchronized with environmental factors; same meaning as biorhythm.

biological half-life   Time it takes for the body to lower the amount of unchanged medication by half.

biotransformation   Chemical changes that a substance undergoes in the body such as by the action of enzymes.

blanchable hyperemia   Redness of the skin caused by dilation of the superficial capillaries. When pressure is applied to the skin, the area blanches, or turns a lighter color.

body image   People's subjective concept of their physical appearance.

body mechanics   Coordinated efforts of the musculoskeletal and nervous systems to maintain proper balance, posture, and body alignment.

bone resorption   Destruction of bone cells and release of calcium into the blood.

borborygmi   Audible abdominal sounds produced by hyperactive intestinal peristalsis.

botanica   Place that sells religious and herbal remedies.

bradycardia   Slower-than-normal heart rate; heart contracts fewer than 60 times/min.

bradypnea   Abnormally slow rate of breathing.

bronchospasm   Excessive and prolonged contraction of the smooth muscle of the bronchi and bronchioles, resulting in an acute narrowing and obstruction of the respiratory airway.

bruit   Abnormal sound or murmur heard while auscultating an organ, gland, or artery.

buccal   Of or pertaining to the inside of the cheek or the gum next to the cheek.

buccal cavity   Consists of the lips surrounding the opening of the mouth, the cheeks running along the side walls of the cavity, the tongue and its muscles, and the hard and soft palate.

buffer   Substance or group of substances that can absorb or release hydrogen ions to correct an acid-base imbalance.

bundle of His   Part of the cardiac conduction system that arises from the distal portion of the atrioventricular (AV) node and extends across the AV groove to the top of the intraventricular septum, where it divides into right and left bundle branches.

C

cachexia   Malnutrition marked by weakness and emaciation, usually associated with severe illness.

capitation   Payment mechanism in which a provider (e.g., health care network) receives a fixed amount of payment per enrollee.

capnography   Also known as end-tidal CO_2 monitoring, it provides instant information about how effectively CO_2 is eliminated by the pulmonary system, how effectively it is transported through the vascular system, and how effectively CO_2 is produced by cellular metabolism. Capnography is measured near the end of exhalation.

carbohydrates   Dietary classification of foods comprising sugars, starches, cellulose, and gum.

carbon monoxide   Colorless, odorless, poisonous gas produced by the combustion of carbon or organic fuels.

cardiac index   Adequacy of the cardiac output for an individual. It takes into account the body surface area (BSA) of the patient.

cardiac output (CO)   Volume of blood expelled by the ventricles of the heart, equal to the amount of blood ejected at each beat multiplied by the number of beats in the period of time used for computation (usually 1 minute).

cardiopulmonary rehabilitation   Actively assisting the patient with achieving and maintaining an optimal level of health through controlled physical exercise, nutritional counseling, relaxation and stress management techniques, prescribed medications and oxygen, and compliance.

cardiopulmonary resuscitation (CPR)   Basic emergency procedures for life support consisting of artificial respiration and manual external cardiac massage.

care   To feel concern for or interest in one who has sorrow or difficulties.

care bundle   A group of interventions related to a disease process or condition that, when implemented together, result in better patient outcomes than when the interventions are implemented individually.

caring   Universal phenomenon that influences the way we think, feel, and behave in relation to one another.

carriers   People or animals who harbor and spread an organism that causes disease in others but do not become ill themselves.

case management   Organized system for delivering health care to an individual patient or group of patients across an episode of illness and/or a continuum of care; includes assessment and development of a plan of care, coordination of all services, referral, and follow-up; usually assigned to one professional.

case management plan   Multidisciplinary model for documenting patient care that usually includes plans for problems, key interventions, and expected outcomes for patients with a specific disease or condition.

catabolism   Breakdown of body tissue into simpler substances.

cataplexy   Condition characterized by sudden muscular weakness and loss of muscle tone.

cataracts   Abnormal progressive condition of the lens of the eye characterized by loss of transparency.

cathartics   Drugs that act to promote bowel evacuation.

catheterization   Introduction of a catheter into a body cavity or organ to inject or remove fluid.

cations   Positively charged electrolytes.

center of gravity   Midpoint or center of the weight of a body or object.

centigrade   Denotes temperature scale in which 0° is the freezing point of water and 100° is the boiling point of water at sea level; also called *Celsius*.

cerumen   Yellowish or brownish waxy secretion produced by sweat glands in the external ear.

chancres   Skin lesions or venereal sores (usually primary syphilis) that begin at the site of infection as papules and develop into red, bloodless, painless ulcers with a scooped-out appearance.

change-of-shift report   Report that occurs between two scheduled nursing work shifts. Nurses communicate information about their assigned patients to nurses working on the next shift of duty.

channel   Method used in the teaching-learning process to present content: visual, auditory, taste, smell. In the communication process, a method used to transmit a message: visual, auditory, touch.

charting by exception (CBE)   Charting methodology in which data are entered only when there is an exception from that which is normal or expected; reduces time spent documenting in charting. It is a shorthand method for documenting normal findings and routine care.

chest percussion   Striking the chest wall with a cupped hand to promote mobilization and drainage of pulmonary secretions.

chest physiotherapy (CPT)   Group of therapies used to mobilize pulmonary secretions for expectoration.

chest tube   Catheter inserted through the thorax into the chest cavity for removing air or fluid; used after chest or heart surgery or pneumothorax.

Cheyne-Stokes respiration   Occurs when there is decreased blood flow or injury to the brainstem.

chronic illness   Illness that persists over a long time and affects physical, emotional, intellectual, social, and spiritual functioning.

circadian rhythm   Repetition of certain physiological phenomena within a 24-hour cycle.

circular transactional communication process   Communication model that enhances the linear communication by enabling the sender and receiver to view perceptions, attitudes, and potential reactions of others via a mental picture. This is a continuous and interactive activity.

circulating nurse   Assistant to the scrub nurse and surgeon whose role is to provide necessary supplies; dispose of soiled instruments and supplies; and keep an accurate count of instruments, needles, and sponges used.

civil law   Statutes concerned with protecting a person's rights.

climacteric   Physiological, developmental change that occurs in the female reproductive system between the ages of 45 and 60.

clinical criteria   Objective or subjective signs and symptoms, clusters of signs and symptoms, or risk factors.

clinical decision making   Problem-solving approach that nurses use to define patient problems and select appropriate treatment.

clinical-decision support systems   Computerized programs used within the health care setting to support decision making.

Clinical Information System (CIS)   A computer-based system that collects, stores, and manipulates data to allow health care providers to make informed decisions about patient care.

closed-ended question   Form of question that limits a respondent's answer to one or two words.

clubbing Bulging of the tissues at the nail base caused by insufficient oxygenation at the periphery, resulting from conditions such as chronic emphysema and congenital heart disease.

code of ethics Formal statement that delineates a profession's guidelines for ethical behavior. A code of ethics sets standards or expectations for the professional to achieve.

cognitive learning Acquisition of intellectual skills that encompass behaviors such as thinking, understanding, and evaluating.

collaborative interventions Therapies that require the knowledge, skill, and expertise of multiple health care professionals.

collaborative problem Physiological complication that requires the nurse to use nursing- and health care provider–prescribed interventions to maximize patient outcomes.

colloid osmotic pressure Abnormal condition of the kidney caused by the pressure of concentrations of large particles such as protein molecules that will pass through a membrane.

colon Portion of the large intestine from the cecum to the rectum.

colonization Presence and multiplication of microorganisms without tissue invasion or damage.

comforting Acts toward another individual that display both an emotional and physical calm. The use of touch, the establishment of presence, the therapeutic use of silence, and the skillful and gentle performance of a procedure are examples of comforting nursing measures.

common law One source for law that is created by judicial decisions as opposed to those created by legislative bodies (statutory law).

communicable disease Any disease that can be transmitted from one person or animal to another by direct or indirect contact or by vectors.

communication Ongoing, dynamic series of events that involves the transmission of meaning from sender to receiver.

community-based nursing Acute and chronic care of individuals and families to strengthen their capacity for self-care and promote independence in decision making.

community health nursing Nursing approach that combines knowledge from the public health sciences with professional nursing theories to safeguard and improve the health of populations in the community.

co-morbidity A chronic, long-term condition existing simultaneously with and usually independently of another medical condition.

compassion The feeling that arises when a person is confronted with another's suffering and feels motivated to relieve that suffering. Compassion shows kindness, caring, and a willingness to help others.

competence Specific range of skills necessary to perform a task.

complete bed bath Bath in which the entire body of a patient is washed in bed.

compress Soft pad of gauze or cloth used to apply heat, cold, or medications to the surface of a body part.

computer-based patient record Comprehensive computerized system used by all health care practitioners to permanently store information pertaining to a patient's health status, clinical problems, and functional abilities.

concentration Relative content of a component within a substance or solution.

concentration gradient Gradient that exists across a membrane, separating a high concentration of a particular ion from a low concentration of the same ion.

concept map Care-planning tool that assists in critical thinking and forming associations between a patient's nursing diagnoses and interventions.

confianza Trust.

confidentiality Act of keeping information private or secret; in health care the nurse shares information about a patient only with other nurses or health care providers who need to know private information about a patient to provide care for him or her; information can be shared only with the patient's consent.

conjunctivitis Highly contagious eye infection. The crusty drainage that collects on eyelid margins can easily spread from one eye to the other.

connectedness Having close spiritual relationships with oneself, others, and God or another spiritual being.

connotative meaning Shade or interpretation of the meaning of a word influenced by the thoughts, feelings, or ideas that people have about the word.

conscious sedation Administration of central nervous system–depressant drugs and/or analgesics to provide analgesia, relieve anxiety, and/or provide amnesia during surgical, diagnostic, or interventional procedures.

constipation Condition characterized by difficulty in passing stool or an infrequent passage of hard stool.

consultation Process in which the help of a specialist is sought to identify ways to handle problems in patient management or in planning and implementing programs.

Contact Precautions Safeguards designed to reduce the risk of transmission of epidemiologically important microorganisms by direct or indirect contact.

content The product and information obtained from the system.

continent urinary diversion (CUR) Surgical diversion of the drainage of urine from a diseased or dysfunctional bladder. Patient uses a catheter to drain the pouch.

continuous positive airway pressure (CPAP) Ventilatory support used to treat patients with obstructive sleep apnea, patients with congestive heart failure, and preterm infants with underdeveloped lungs.

convalescence Period of recovery after an illness, injury, or surgery.

coping Making an effort to manage psychological stress.

core temperature Temperature of deep structures of the body.

cough Sudden, audible expulsion of air from the lungs. The person breathes in, the glottis is partially closed, and the accessory muscles of expiration contract to expel the air forcibly.

counseling Problem-solving method used to help patients recognize and manage stress and enhance interpersonal relationships. It helps patients examine alternatives and decide which choices are most helpful and appropriate.

crackles Fine bubbling sounds heard on auscultation of the lung; produced by air entering distal airways and alveoli, which contain serous secretions.

crime Act that violates a law and that may include criminal intent.

criminal law Concerned with acts that threaten society but may involve only an individual.

crisis Transition for better or worse in the course of a disease, usually indicated by a marked change in the intensity of signs and symptoms.

crisis intervention Use of therapeutic techniques directed toward helping a patient resolve a particular and immediate problem.

critical pathways Tools used in managed care that incorporate the treatment interventions of caregivers from all disciplines who normally care for a patient. Designed for a specific care type, a pathway is used to manage the care of a patient throughout a projected length of stay.

critical period of development Specific phase or period when the presence of a function or reasoning has its greatest effect on a specific aspect of development.

critical thinking Active, purposeful, organized, cognitive process used to carefully examine one's thinking and the thinking of other individuals.

crutch gait Gait achieved by a person using crutches.

cue Information that a nurse acquires through hearing, visual observations, touch, and smell.

cultural and linguistic competence Set of congruent behaviors, attitudes, and policies that come together in a system or agency or among professionals that enables effective work in cross-cultural situations.

cultural assessment Systematic and comprehensive examination of the cultural care values, beliefs, and practices of individuals, families, and communities.

cultural awareness Gaining in-depth awareness of one's own background, stereotypes, biases, prejudices, and assumptions about other people.

cultural care accommodation or negotiation Adapting or negotiating with the patient/family to achieve beneficial or satisfying health outcomes.

cultural care preservation or maintenance Retaining and/or preserving relevant care values so that patients are able to maintain their well-being, recover from illness, or face handicaps and/or death.

cultural care repatterning or restructuring Reordering, changing, or greatly modifying a patient's/family's customs for a new, different, and beneficial health care pattern.

cultural competence Process in which the health care professional continually strives to achieve the ability and availability to work effectively with individuals, families, and communities.

cultural encounters   Engaging in cross-cultural interactions; refining intercultural communication skills; gaining in-depth understanding of others and avoiding stereotypes; and managing cultural conflict.

cultural imposition   Using one's own values and customs as an absolute guide in interpreting behaviors.

cultural knowledge   Obtaining knowledge of other cultures; gaining sensitivity to, respect for, and appreciation of differences.

cultural pain   Feeling that a patient has after a health care worker disregards the patient's valued way of life.

cultural respect   Behavior that is respectful and responsive to the needs of the diverse patient.

cultural skills   Communication, cultural assessment, and culturally competent care.

culturally congruent care   Care that fits people's valued life patterns and sets of meanings generated from the people themselves. Sometimes this differs from the professionals' perspective on care.

culturally ignorant or blind   Uneducated about other cultures.

culture   Integrated patterns of human behavior that include the language, thoughts, communications, actions, customs, beliefs, values, and institutions of racial, ethnic, religious, or social groups.

culture-bound syndromes   Illnesses restricted to a particular culture or group because of its psychosocial characteristics.

culture care theory   Leininger's theory that emphasizes culturally congruent care.

culturological nursing assessment   Systematic and comprehensive examination of the cultural care values, beliefs, and practices of individuals, families, and communities.

cutaneous stimulation   Stimulation of a person's skin to prevent or reduce pain perception. A massage, warm bath, hot and cold therapies, and transcutaneous electrical nerve stimulation are some ways to reduce pain perception.

cyanosis   Bluish discoloration of the skin and mucous membranes caused by an excess of deoxygenated hemoglobin in the blood or a structural defect in the hemoglobin molecule.

D

DAR (data, action, patient response)   Format used in focus charting for recording patient information.

data analysis   Logical examination of and professional judgment about patient assessment data; used in the diagnostic process to derive a nursing diagnosis.

database   Store or bank of information, especially in a form that can be processed by computer.

data cluster   Set of signs or symptoms that are grouped together in logical order.

debridement   Removal of dead tissue from a wound.

decentralized management   Organizational philosophy that brings decisions down to the level of the staff. Individuals best informed about a problem or issue participate in the decision-making process.

decision making   Process involving critical appraisal of information that begins with recognizing a problem and ends with generating, testing, and evaluating a conclusion. Comes at the end of critical thinking.

deconditioning   Physiological change following a period of inactivity, bed rest, or sedentary lifestyle. It results in functional losses in such areas as mental status, degree of continence, and ability to accomplish activities of daily living.

defecation   Passage of feces from the digestive tract through the rectum.

defendant   Individual or organization against whom legal charges are brought in a court of law.

defining characteristics   The observable assessment cues that cluster as manifestations of a problem-focused or health promotion nursing diagnosis.

dehiscence   Separation of the edges of a wound, revealing underlying tissues.

dehydration   Excessive loss of water from the body tissues accompanied by a disturbance of body electrolytes.

delegation   Process of assigning another member of the health care team to be responsible for aspects of patient care (e.g., assigning nurse assistants to bathe a patient).

delirium   Acute state of confusion that is potentially reversible and often has a physical cause.

dementia   Generalized impairment of intellectual functioning that interferes with social and occupational functioning.

denial   Unconscious refusal to admit an unacceptable idea.

denotative meaning   Meaning of a word shared by individuals who use a common language. For example, the word *baseball* has the same meaning for all individuals who speak English, but the word *code* primarily denotes cardiac arrest to health care providers.

dental caries   Abnormal destructive condition in a tooth caused by a complex interaction of food, especially starches and sugars, with bacteria that form dental plaque.

deontology   Traditional theory of ethics that proposes to define actions as right or wrong based on the characteristics of fidelity to promises, truthfulness, and justice. The conventional use of ethical terms such as *justice, autonomy, beneficence,* and *nonmaleficence* constitutes the practice of deontology.

depression   (1) Reduction in happiness and well-being that contributes to physical and social limitations and complicates the treatment of concomitant medical conditions. It is usually reversible with treatment. (2) Fourth stage of Kübler-Ross's stages of grief and dying. In this stage the person realizes the full impact and significance of the loss.

dermis   Sensitive vascular layer of the skin directly below the epidermis; composed of collagenous and elastic fibrous connective tissues that give the dermis strength and elasticity.

determinants of health   Many variables that influence the health status of individuals or communities.

detoxify   To remove the toxic quality of a substance. The liver acts to detoxify chemicals in drug compounds.

development   Qualitative or observable aspects of the progressive changes that one makes in adapting to the environment.

developmental crises   Crises associated with normal and expected phases of growth and development (e.g., the response to menopause); same as maturational crises.

diabetic retinopathy   Disorder of retinal blood vessels. Pathological changes secondary to increased pressure in the blood vessels of the retina result in decreased vision or vision loss caused by hemorrhage and macular edema.

diagnosis-related group (DRG)   Classifications based on a hospitalized patient's primary and secondary medical diagnoses that are used as the basis for establishing Medicare reimbursement for patient care.

diagnostic process   Mental steps (data clustering and analysis, problem identification) that follow assessment and lead directly to the formulation of a diagnosis.

diagnostic reasoning   Process that enables an observer to assign meaning to and classify phenomena in clinical situations by integrating observations and critical thinking.

diaphoresis   Secretion of sweat, especially profuse secretion associated with an elevated body temperature, physical exertion, or emotional stress.

diaphragmatic breathing   Respiration in which the abdomen moves out while the diaphragm descends on inspiration.

diarrhea   Increase in the number of stools and the passage of liquid, unformed feces.

diastolic   Pertaining to diastole, or the blood pressure at the instant of maximum cardiac relaxation; the pressure of the blood in the arteries when the heart is filling.

dietary reference intake (DRI)   Information on each vitamin or mineral to reflect a range of minimum-to-maximum amounts that avert deficiency or toxicity.

diffusion   Movement of molecules from an area of high concentration to one of lower concentration.

digestion   Breakdown of nutrients by chewing, churning, mixing with fluid, and chemical reactions.

direct care interventions   Treatments performed through interaction with the patient. For example, a patient may require medication administration, insertion of an intravenous infusion, or counseling during a time of grief.

discharge planning   Activities directed toward identifying future proposed therapy and the need for additional resources before and after returning home.

discrimination   Prejudicial outlook, action, or treatment.

disease   Malfunctioning or maladaptation of biological or psychological processes.

disinfection   Process of destroying all pathogenic organisms except spores.

disorganization and despair   One of Bowlby's four phases of mourning in which an individual endlessly examines how and why the loss occurred.

distress   Damaging stress; one of the two types of stress identified by Selye.

disuse osteoporosis   Reductions in skeletal mass routinely accompanying immobility or paralysis.

diuresis   Increased rate of formation and excretion of urine.

documentation   Written entry into the patient's medical record of all pertinent information about him or her. These entries validate the patient's problems and care and exist as a legal record.

dominant culture   Customs, values, beliefs, traditions, and social and religious views held by a group of people that prevail over another secondary culture.

dorsiflexion   Flexion toward the back.

Droplet Precautions   Safeguards designed to reduce the risk of droplet transmission of infectious agents.

dysmenorrhea   Painful menstruation.

dysphagia   Difficulty swallowing; commonly associated with obstructive or motor disorders of the esophagus.

dyspnea   Sensation of shortness of breath.

dysrhythmia   Deviation from the normal pattern of the heartbeat.

dysuria   Painful urination resulting from bacterial infection of the bladder and obstructive conditions of the urethra.

E

ecchymosis   Discoloration of the skin or bruise caused by leakage of blood into subcutaneous tissues as a result of trauma to underlying tissues.

ectropion   Eversion of the eyelid that exposes the conjunctival membrane and part of the eyeball.

edema   Abnormal accumulation of fluid in interstitial spaces of tissues.

egocentric   Developmental characteristic wherein toddlers are able to assume the view of only their own activities and needs.

electrocardiogram (ECG)   Graphic record of the electrical activity of the myocardium.

electrolyte   Element or compound that, when melted or dissolved in water or other solvent, dissociates into ions and can carry an electrical current.

electronic health record (EHR)   An electronic record of patient health information generated whenever a patient accesses medical care in any health care delivery setting.

electronic infusion device   Piece of medical equipment that delivers intravenous fluids at a prescribed rate through an intravenous catheter.

electronic medical record   Part of the electronic health record that contains patient data gathered in a health care setting at a specific time and place.

embolism   Abnormal condition in which a blood clot (embolus) travels through the bloodstream and becomes lodged in a blood vessel.

emerging adulthood   The time from adolescence to the young adult when responsibilities of a stable job, marriage, and parenthood begin. It includes five features: the age of identity exploration, the age of instability, the age of self-focus, the age of feeling in between, and the age of possibilities.

emic worldview   The inside perspective of a cultural encounter.

emotional intelligence   Assessment and communication technique used to better understand and perceive emotions of oneself. This assists in building a therapeutic relationship.

empathy   Understanding and acceptance of a person's feelings and the ability to sense the person's private world.

empowered   Gave legal authority to or enabled an individual or group; promoted self-actualization of an individual or group.

endogenous infections   Infections produced within a cell or organism.

endorphins   Hormones that act on the mind and produce a sense of well-being and reduction of pain.

endotracheal tube   Short-term artificial airways to administer mechanical ventilation, relieve upper airway obstruction, protect against aspiration, or clear secretions.

enema   Procedure involving introduction of a solution into the rectum for cleansing or therapeutic purposes.

enteral nutrition (EN)   Provision of nutrients through the gastrointestinal tract when the patient cannot ingest, chew, or swallow food but can digest and absorb nutrients.

entropion   Condition in which the eyelid turns inward toward the eye.

environment   All of the many factors (e.g., physical and psychological) that influence or affect the life and survival of a person.

epidermis   Outer layer of the skin that has several thin layers in different stages of maturation; shields and protects the underlying tissues from water loss, mechanical or chemical injury, and penetration by disease-causing microorganisms.

epidural infusion   Type of nerve block anesthesia in which an anesthetic is intermittently or continuously injected into the lumbosacral region of the spinal cord.

erythema   Redness or inflammation of the skin or mucous membranes that is a result of dilation and congestion of superficial capillaries; sunburn is an example.

eschar   Thick layer of dead, dry tissue that covers a pressure injury or thermal burn. It may be allowed to be sloughed off naturally, or it may need to be surgically removed.

ethical dilemma   Dilemma existing when the right thing to do is not clear. Resolution requires the negotiation of differing values among those involved in the dilemma.

ethical principles   Set of guidelines for the expectations of a profession and the standards of behavior for its members.

ethics   Principles or standards that govern proper conduct.

ethics of care   Delivery of health care based on ethical principles and standards of care.

ethnic/cultural identity   Individuals identify consciously or unconsciously with those with whom they feel a common bond because of similar traditions, behaviors, values, and beliefs.

ethnicity   Shared identity related to social and cultural heritage such as values, language, geographical space, and racial characteristics.

ethnocentrism   Tendency to hold one's own way of life as superior to that of others.

ethnohistory   Significant historical experiences of a particular group.

etic world view   The outside perspective of a cultural encounter.

etiology   Study of all factors that may be involved in the development of a disease.

eupnea   Normal respirations that are quiet, effortless, and rhythmical.

eustress   Stress that protects health; one of the two types of stress identified by Selye.

evaluation   Determination of the extent to which established patient goals have been achieved.

evidence-based knowledge   Knowledge that is derived from the integration of best research, clinical expertise, and patient values.

evidence-based practice   Use of current best evidence from nursing research, clinical expertise, practice trends, and patient preferences to guide nursing decisions about care provided to patients.

evisceration   Protrusion of visceral organs through a surgical wound.

exacerbations   Increases in the gravity of a disease or disorder as marked by greater intensity in signs or symptoms.

excessive daytime sleepiness   Extreme fatigue felt during the day. Signs of this include falling asleep at inappropriate times such as while eating, talking, or driving. May indicate a sleep disorder.

excoriation   Injury to the surface of the skin caused by abrasion.

exhaustion stage   Phase that occurs when the body can no longer resist the stress (i.e., when the energy necessary to maintain adaptation is depleted).

exogenous infection   Infection originating outside an organ or part.

exostosis   Abnormal benign growth on the surface of a bone.

expected outcomes   Expected conditions of a patient at the end of therapy or a disease process, including the degree of wellness and the need for continuing care, medications, support, counseling, or education.

extended care facility   Institution devoted to providing medical, nursing, or custodial care for an individual over a prolonged period such as during the course of a chronic disease or the rehabilitation phase after an acute illness.

extension   Movement by certain joints that increases the angle between two adjoining bones.

extracellular fluid (ECF) Portion of body fluids composed of the interstitial fluid and blood plasma.

exudate Fluid, cells, or other substances that have been discharged from cells or blood vessels slowly through small pores or breaks in cell membranes.

F

face-saving Way of speaking or acting that preserves dignity.

Fahrenheit Denotes temperature scale in which 32° is the freezing point of water and 212° is the boiling point of water at sea level.

faith Set of beliefs and a way of relating to self, others, and a Supreme Being.

fajita Cotton binder used on a newborn's abdomen among Hispanics and Filipinos to prevent gas and umbilical hernia.

family Group of interacting individuals composing a basic unit of society.

family as context Nursing perspective in which the family is viewed as a unit of interacting members having attributes, functions, and goals separate from those of the individual family members.

family as patient Nursing approach that takes into consideration the effect of one intervention on all members of a family.

family caregiving A family process that occurs in response to an illness and encompasses multiple cognitive, behavioral, and interpersonal processes.

family diversity The uniqueness of each family unit. For example, some families experience marriage for the first time and then have children in later life.

family durability A system of support and structure within a family that extends beyond the walls of the household.

family dynamics The interactions among family members which is affected by a family's makeup (configuration), structure, function, problem-solving, and coping capacity.

family forms Patterns of people considered by family members to be included in the family.

family function Focuses on the processes used by the family to achieve its goals. Some processes include communication among family members, goal setting, conflict resolution, caregiving, nurturing, and use of internal and external resources.

family hardiness Internal strengths and durability of the family unit; characterized by a sense of control over the outcome of life events and hardships, a view of change as beneficial and growth-producing, and an active rather than passive orientation in responding to stressful life events.

family health Determined by the effectiveness of the family's structure, the processes that the family uses to meet its goals, and internal and external forces.

family resiliency Family's ability to cope with expected and unexpected stressors.

family structure Based on organization (i.e., ongoing membership) of the family and the pattern of relationships.

farmacia Place to obtain prescribed medications.

febrile Pertaining to or characterized by an elevated body temperature.

fecal immunochemical test (FIT) A screening test for colon cancer. It detects occult blood in the stool and is not affected by medication or foods ingested.

fecal impaction Accumulation of hardened fecal material in the rectum or sigmoid colon.

fecal incontinence Inability to control passage of feces and gas from the anus.

fecal occult blood test (FOBT) Measures microscopic amounts of blood in the feces.

feces Waste or excrement from the gastrointestinal tract.

feedback Process in which the output of a given system is returned to the system.

felony Crime of a serious nature that carries a penalty of imprisonment or death.

feminist ethics Ethical approach that focuses on the nature of relationships to guide participants in making difficult decisions, especially relationships in which power is unequal or in which a point of view has become ignored or invisible.

fever Elevation in the hypothalamic set point so that body temperature is regulated at a higher level.

fictive Nonblood kin; considered family in some collective cultures.

fidelity Agreement to keep a promise.

fight-or-flight response Total physiological response to stress that occurs during the alarm reaction stage of the general adaptation syndrome. Massive changes in all body systems prepare a human being to choose to flee or remain and fight the stressor.

filtration Straining of fluid through a membrane.

fistula Abnormal passage from an internal organ to the surface of the body or between two internal organs.

flashback Recollection so strong that the individual thinks that he or she is actually experiencing the trauma again or seeing it unfold before his or her eyes.

flatus Intestinal gas.

flora Microorganisms that live on or within a body to compete with disease-producing microorganisms and provide a natural immunity against certain infections.

flow sheets Documents on which frequent observations or specific measurements are recorded.

fluctuance Soft, boggy feeling when tissue is palpated; usually a sign of tissue infection.

fluid volume deficit (FVD) Fluid and electrolyte disorder caused by failure of bodily homeostatic mechanisms to regulate the retention and excretion of body fluids. The condition is characterized by decreased output of urine, high specific gravity of urine, output of urine that is greater than the intake of fluid in the body, hemoconcentration, and increased serum levels of sodium.

fluid volume excess (FVE) Fluid and electrolyte disorder characterized by an increase in fluid retention and edema, resulting from failure of bodily homeostatic mechanisms to regulate the retention and excretion of body fluids.

focus charting Charting methodology for structuring progress notes according to the focus of the note (e.g., symptoms and nursing diagnosis). Each note includes data, actions, and patient response.

focused cultural assessment Method of evaluating a patient's ethnohistory, biocultural history, social organization, and religious and spiritual beliefs to find issues that are most relevant to the problem at hand.

food poisoning Toxic processes resulting from the ingestion of a food contaminated by toxic substances or bacteria-containing toxins.

food security All members of a household have access to sufficient safe, nutritious food to maintain a healthy lifestyle.

foot boots Soft, foot-shaped devices designed to reduce the risk of footdrop by maintaining the foot in dorsiflexion.

footdrop Abnormal neuromuscular condition of the lower leg and foot characterized by an inability to dorsiflex, or evert, the foot.

friction Effects of rubbing or the resistance that a moving body meets from the surface on which it moves; a force that occurs in a direction to oppose movement.

functional health illiteracy Inability of an individual to obtain, interpret, and understand basic information about health.

functional health patterns Method for organizing assessment data based on the level of patient function in specific areas (e.g., mobility).

functional nursing Method of patient care delivery in which each staff member is assigned a task that is completed for all patients on the unit.

future orientation Time dimension emphasized by dominant American culture. It is characterized by direct communication and is focused on task achievement, whereas past orientation communication is circular and indirect and is focused on group harmony.

G

gait Manner or style of walking, including rhythm, cadence, and speed.

gastrostomy feeding tube Insertion of a feeding tube through a stoma into the stomach to provide enteral nutrition.

general adaptation syndrome (GAS) Generalized defense response of the body to stress; consists of three stages: alarm, resistance, and exhaustion.

general anesthesia Intravenous or inhaled medications that cause the patient to lose all sensation and consciousness.

genomics Describes the study of all the genes in a person and interactions of those genes with one another and with that person's environment.

geriatrics Branch of health care dealing with the physiology and psychology of aging and the diagnosis and treatment of diseases affecting older adults.

gerontology Study of all aspects of the aging process and its consequences.

gingivae Gums of the mouth; mucous membrane with supporting fibrous tissue that overlies the crowns of unerupted teeth and encircles the necks of teeth that have erupted.

glaucoma Abnormal condition of elevated pressure within an eye caused by obstruction of the outflow of aqueous humor. If untreated, it often results in peripheral visual loss, decreased visual acuity with difficulty adapting to darkness, and a halo effect around lights.

globalization Worldwide scope or application.

glomerulus Cluster or collection of capillary vessels within the kidney involved in the initial formation of urine.

gluconeogenesis Formation of glucose or glycogen from substances that are not carbohydrates such as protein or lipid.

glucose Primary fuel for the body; needed to carry out major physiological functions.

glycogen Polysaccharide that is the major carbohydrate stored in animal cells.

glycogenesis Process for storing glucose in the form of glycogen in the liver.

goals Desired results of nursing actions set realistically by the nurse and patient as part of the planning stage of the nursing process.

Good Samaritan laws Legislation enacted in some states to protect health care professionals from liability in rendering emergency aid unless there is proven willful wrong or gross negligence.

graduated measuring container Receptacle for volume measurement.

granny midwives Amateur health practitioners who assist in labor and delivery.

granulation tissue Soft, pink, fleshy projections of tissue that form during the healing process in a wound not healing by primary intention.

graphic record Charting mechanism that allows for the recording of vital signs and weight in such a manner that caregivers can quickly note changes in the patient's status.

grief Form of sorrow involving the person's thoughts, feelings, and behaviors that occurs as a response to an actual or perceived loss.

grieving process Sequence of affective, cognitive, and physiological states through which the person responds to and finally accepts an irretrievable loss.

grounded Connection between the electric circuit and the ground, which becomes part of the circuit.

growth Measurable or quantitative aspect of an individual's increase in physical dimensions as a result of an increase in number of cells. Indicators of growth include changes in height, weight, and sexual characteristics.

guided imagery Method of pain control in which the patient creates a mental image, concentrates on that image, and gradually becomes less aware of pain.

gustatory Pertaining to the sense of taste.

H

halal Foods permissible for Muslims to eat.

hand rolls Rolls of cloth that keep the thumb slightly adducted and in opposition to the fingers.

hand-wrist splints Splints individually molded for the patient to maintain proper alignment of the thumb, slight adduction of the wrist, and slight dorsiflexion.

haram Foods prohibited by Muslim religious standards.

health Dynamic state in which individuals adapt to their internal and external environments so that there is a state of physical, emotional, intellectual, social, and spiritual well-being.

health belief model Conceptual framework that describes a person's health behavior as an expression of his or her health beliefs.

health beliefs Patient's personal beliefs about levels of wellness that can motivate or impede participation in changing risk factors, participating in care, and selecting care options.

health care–acquired infection Infection that was not present or incubating at the time of admission to a health care setting.

health care problems Any conditions or dysfunctions that the patient experiences as a result of illness or treatment of an illness.

health disparities Preventable differences in the burden of disease, injury, violence, or opportunities to achieve optimal health that are experienced by socially and economically disadvantaged populations.

health informatics Application of computer and information science in all basic and applied biomedical sciences to facilitate the acquisition, processing, interpretation, optimal use, and communication of health-related data.

health literacy Patients' reading and mathematics skills, comprehension, ability to make health-related decisions, and successful functioning as a consumer of health care.

health promotion Activities such as routine exercise and good nutrition that help patients maintain or enhance their present level of health and reduce their risk of developing certain diseases.

health promotion model Defines health as a positive, dynamic state, not merely the absence of disease. The health promotion model emphasizes well-being, personal fulfillment, and self-actualization rather than reaction to the threat of illness.

health status Description of health of an individual or community.

heat exhaustion Abnormal condition caused by depletion of body fluid and electrolytes resulting from exposure to intense heat or the inability to acclimatize to heat.

heat stroke Continued exposure to extreme heat that raises the core body temperature to 40.5° C (105° F) or higher.

hematemesis Vomiting of blood, indicating upper gastrointestinal bleeding.

hematoma Collection of blood trapped in the tissues of the skin or an organ.

hematuria Abnormal presence of blood in the urine.

hemolysis Breakdown of red blood cells and release of hemoglobin that may occur after administration of hypotonic intravenous solutions, causing swelling and rupture of erythrocytes.

hemoptysis Coughing up blood from the respiratory tract.

hemorrhoids Permanent dilation and engorgement of veins within the lining of the rectum.

hemostasis Termination of bleeding by mechanical or chemical means or the coagulation process of the body.

hemothorax Accumulation of blood and fluid in the pleural cavity between the parietal and visceral pleurae.

hernia Protrusion of an organ through an abnormal opening in the muscle wall of the cavity that surrounds it.

hilots Amateur health practitioners who assist in labor and delivery among Filipinos.

holistic Of or pertaining to the whole; considering all factors.

holistic health Comprehensive view of the person as a biopsychosocial and spiritual being.

home care Health service provided in the patient's place of residence to promote, maintain, or restore health or minimize the effects of illness and disability.

homeostasis State of relative constancy in the internal environment of the body; maintained naturally by physiological adaptive mechanisms.

hope Confident but uncertain expectation of achieving a future goal.

hospice System of family-centered care designed to help terminally ill people be comfortable and maintain a satisfactory lifestyle throughout the terminal phase of their illness.

Hoyer lift Mechanical device that uses a canvas sling to easily lift dependent patients for transfer.

humidification Process of adding water to gas.

humor Coping strategy based on an individual's cognitive appraisal of a stimulus that results in behavior such as smiling, laughing, or feelings of amusement that lessen emotional distress.

hydrocephalus Abnormal accumulation of cerebrospinal fluid in the ventricles of the brain.

hydrostatic pressure Pressure caused by a liquid.

hyperactive/overactive bladder Common bladder complaint that occurs more frequently with aging and includes the symptoms of urgency, frequency, nocturia, and urge incontinence.

hypercalcemia Greater-than-normal amount of calcium in the blood.

hypercapnia Greater-than-normal amounts of carbon dioxide in the blood; also called *hypercarbia*.

hyperextension Position of maximal extension of a joint.

hyperglycemia Elevated serum glucose levels.

hypertension Disorder characterized by an elevated blood pressure persistently exceeding 120/80 mm Hg.

hyperthermia Situation in which body temperature exceeds the set point.

hypertonic Situation in which one solution has a greater concentration of solute than another; therefore the first solution exerts greater osmotic pressure.

hypertonicity Excessive tension of the arterial walls or muscles.

hyperventilation Respiratory rate in excess of that required to maintain normal carbon dioxide levels in the body tissues.

hypnotics Class of drug that causes insensibility to pain and induces sleep.

hypostatic pneumonia Pneumonia that results from fluid accumulation as a result of inactivity.

hypotension Abnormal lowering of blood pressure that is inadequate for normal perfusion and oxygenation of tissues.

hypothermia Abnormal lowering of body temperature below 35° C, or 95° F, usually caused by prolonged exposure to cold.

hypotonic Situation in which one solution has a smaller concentration of solute than another; therefore the first solution exerts less osmotic pressure.

hypotonicity Reduced tension of the arterial walls or muscles.

hypoventilation Respiratory rate insufficient to prevent carbon dioxide retention.

hypovolemia Abnormally low circulating blood volume.

hypoxemia Arterial blood oxygen level less than 60 mm Hg; low oxygen level in the blood.

hypoxia Inadequate cellular oxygenation that may result from a deficiency in the delivery or use of oxygen at the cellular level.

I

identity Component of self-concept characterized by one's persisting consciousness of being oneself, separate and distinct from others.

idiosyncratic reaction Individual sensitivity to effects of a drug caused by inherited or other bodily constitution factors.

illness (1) Abnormal process in which any aspect of a person's functioning is diminished or impaired compared with his or her previous condition. (2) The personal, interpersonal, and cultural reaction to disease.

illness behavior Ways in which people monitor their bodies, define and interpret their symptoms, take remedial actions, and use the health care system.

illness prevention Health education programs or activities directed toward protecting patients from threats or potential threats to health and minimizing risk factors.

immobility Inability to move about freely; caused by any condition in which movement is impaired or therapeutically restricted.

immunity Quality of being insusceptible to or unaffected by a particular disease or condition.

immunization Process by which resistance to an infectious disease is induced or augmented.

implementation Initiation and completion of the nursing actions necessary to help the patient achieve health care goals.

impression management Ability to interpret others' behavior within their own context of meanings and behave in a culturally congruent way to achieve desired outcomes of communication.

incentive spirometry Method of encouraging voluntary deep breathing by providing visual feedback to patients of the inspiratory volume they have achieved.

incident rates Rate of new cases of a disease in a specified population over a defined period of time.

incident report Confidential document that describes any patient accident while the person is on the premises of a health care agency. (See *occurrence report*.)

independent practice association (IPA) Managed care organization that contracts with physicians or health care providers who usually are members of groups and whose practices include fee-for-service and capitated patients.

indirect care interventions Treatments performed away from the patient but on behalf of the patient or group of patients.

induration Hardening of a tissue, particularly the skin, because of edema or inflammation.

infection Invasion of the body by pathogenic microorganisms that reproduce and multiply.

inference (1) Judgment or interpretation of informational cues. (2) Taking one proposition as a given and guessing that another proposition follows.

infiltration Dislodging an intravenous catheter or needle from a vein into the subcutaneous space.

inflammation Protective response of body tissues to irritation or injury.

informed consent Process of obtaining permission from a patient to perform a specific test or procedure after describing all risks, side effects, and benefits.

infusion pump Device that delivers a measured amount of fluid over a period of time.

infusions Introduction of fluid into the vein, giving intravenous fluid over time.

inhalation Method of medication delivery through the patient's respiratory tract. The respiratory tract provides a large surface area for drug absorption. Inhalation can be through the nasal or oral route.

injections Parenteral administration of medication; four major sites of injection: subcutaneous, intramuscular, intravenous, and intradermal.

inpatient prospective payment system (IPPS) Payment mechanism for reimbursing hospitals for inpatient health care services in which a predetermined rate is set for treatment of specific illnesses.

input For the nursing process, the data or information that comes from a patient's assessment.

insensible water loss Water loss that is continuous and not perceived by the person.

insomnia Condition characterized by chronic inability to sleep or remain asleep through the night.

inspection Method of physical examination by which the patient is visually and systematically examined for appearance, structure, function, and behavior.

instillation To cause to enter drop by drop or very slowly.

institutional ethics committee Interdisciplinary committee that discusses and processes ethical dilemmas that arise within a health care institution.

instrumental activities of daily living (IADLs) Activities necessary for independence in society beyond eating, grooming, transferring, and toileting; include such skills as shopping, preparing meals, banking, and taking medications.

integrated delivery network (IDN) Set of providers and services organized to deliver a coordinated continuum of care to the population of patients served at a capitated cost.

interpersonal communication Exchange of information between two persons or among persons in a small group.

interstitial fluid Fluid that fills the spaces between most of the cells of the body and provides a substantial portion of the liquid environment of the body.

interview Organized, systematic conversation with the patient designed to obtain pertinent health-related subjective information.

intracellular fluid Liquid within the cell membrane.

intradermal (ID) Injection given between layers of the skin into the dermis. Injections are given at a 5- to 15-degree angle.

intramuscular (IM) Injections given into muscle tissue. The intramuscular route provides a fast rate of absorption that is related to the greater vascularity of the muscle. Injections are given at a 90-degree angle.

intraocular Method of medication delivery that involves inserting a medication disk similar to a contact lens into the patient's eye.

intrapersonal communication Communication that occurs within an individual (i.e., people "talk with themselves" silently or form an idea in their own mind).

intravascular fluid Fluid circulating within blood vessels of the body.

intravenous Injection directly into the bloodstream. Action of the drug begins immediately when given intravenously.

intravenous fat emulsions Soybean- or safflower oil–based solutions that are isotonic and may be infused with amino acid and dextrose solution through a central or peripheral line.

intubation Insertion of a breathing tube through the mouth or nose into the trachea to ensure a patent airway.

intuition Inner sensing that something is so.

irrigation Process of washing out a body cavity or wounded area with a stream of fluid.

ischemia Decreased blood supply to a body part such as skin tissue or to an organ such as the heart.

isolation Separation of a seriously ill patient from others to prevent the spread of an infection or protect the patient from irritating environmental factors.

isometric exercises Activities that involve muscle tension without muscle shortening, do not have any beneficial effect on preventing orthostatic hypotension but may improve activity tolerance.

isotonic Situation in which two solutions have the same concentration of solute; therefore both solutions exert the same osmotic pressure.

J

jaundice Yellow discoloration of the skin, mucous membranes, and sclera caused by greater-than-normal amounts of bilirubin in the blood.

jejunostomy tube Hollow tube inserted into the jejunum through the abdominal wall for administration of liquefied foods to patients who have a high risk of aspiration.

joint contracture Abnormality that may result in permanent condition of a joint; is characterized by flexion and fixation; and is caused by disuse, atrophy, and shortening of muscle fibers and surrounding joint tissues.

joints Connections between bones; classified according to structure and degree of mobility.

judgment Ability to form an opinion or draw sound conclusions.

justice Ethical standard of fairness.

K

Kardex Trade name for card-filing system that allows quick reference to the particular need of the patient for certain aspects of nursing care.

karma Asian Indian belief that attributes mental illness to past deeds in one's previous life.

knowing the patient An in-depth knowledge of the patient's patterns of responses; fosters skilled clinical decision making.

Korotkoff sound Sound heard during the taking of blood pressure using a sphygmomanometer and stethoscope.

Kussmaul respiration Increase in both rate and depth of respirations.

kyphosis Exaggeration of the posterior curvature of the thoracic spine.

L

laceration Torn, jagged wound.

la cuarantena Period of rest and restricted physical activity after childbirth that usually lasts 40 days.

language Code that conveys specific meaning as words are combined.

laryngospasm Sudden uncontrolled contraction of the laryngeal muscles, which in turn decreases airway size.

lateral violence Hostile, aggressive, and harmful verbal and nonverbal behavior by a nurse to another nurse via attitudes, actions, words, or behaviors. This behavior includes criticizing, intimidations, blaming, fighting, public humiliation, isolating, withholding assistance, or undermining efforts in completing assignments. This leaves the nurse feeling bullied, inadequate and powerless.

law Rule, standard, or principle that states a fact or relationship between factors.

laxatives Drugs that act to promote bowel evacuation.

learning Acquisition of new knowledge and skills as a result of reinforcement, practice, and experience.

learning objective Written statement that describes the behavior that a teacher expects from an individual after a learning activity.

left-sided heart failure Abnormal condition characterized by impaired functioning of the left ventricle caused by elevated pressures and pulmonary congestion.

leukoplakia Thick, white patches observed on oral mucous membranes.

licensed practical nurse (LPN) Also known as the licensed vocational nurse (LVN) or, in Canada, registered nurse's assistant (RNA); trained in basic nursing skills and the provision of direct patient care.

licensed vocational nurse (LVN) The LVN is the same as a licensed practical nurse (LPN), an individual trained in the United States in basic nursing techniques and direct patient care who practices under the supervision of a registered nurse. The LVN is licensed by a board after completing what is usually a 12-month educational program and passing a licensure examination. In Canada an LVN is called a certified nursing assistant.

lipids Compounds that are insoluble in water but soluble in organic solvents.

lipogenesis Process during which fatty acids are synthesized.

living wills Instruments by which a dying person makes wishes known.

local anesthesia Loss of sensation at the desired site of action.

logroll Maneuver used to turn a reclining patient from one side to the other or completely over without moving the spinal column out of alignment.

lordosis Increased lumbar curvature.

M

maceration Softening and breaking down of skin from prolonged exposure to moisture.

mal de ojo Evil eye.

malignant hyperthermia Autosomal-dominant trait characterized by often fatal hyperthermia in affected people exposed to certain anesthetic agents.

malpractice Injurious or unprofessional actions that harm another.

malpractice insurance Type of insurance to protect the health care professional. In case of a malpractice claim, the insurance pays the award to the plaintiff.

managed care Health care system in which there is administrative control over primary health care services. Redundant facilities and services are eliminated, and costs are reduced. Preventive care and health education are emphasized.

Maslow's hierarchy of needs Model developed by Abraham Maslow that is used to explain human motivation.

matrilineal Kinship that is limited to only the mother's side.

maturation Genetically determined biological plan for growth and development. Physical growth and motor development are a function of maturation.

maturational loss Loss, usually of an aspect of self, resulting from the normal changes of growth and development.

Medicaid State medical assistance to people with low incomes, based on Title XIX of the Social Security Act. States receive matching federal funds to provide medical care and services to people meeting categorical and income requirements.

medical adhesive–related skin injury (MARSI) The presence of erythema and/or other manifestation of cutaneous abnormality that persists 30 minutes or longer after removal of a device or adhesive securing the device.

medical asepsis Procedures used to reduce the number of microorganisms and prevent their spread.

medical device–related pressure injury (MDRPI) Occurs when the skin or underlying tissues are subjected to sustained pressure or shear from medical devices or equipment.

medical diagnosis Formal statement of the disease entity or illness made by the physician or health care provider.

medical record Patient's chart; a legal document.

Medicare Federally funded national health insurance program in the United States for people over 65 years of age. The program is administered in two parts. Part A provides basic protection against costs of medical, surgical, and psychiatric hospital care. Part B is a voluntary medical insurance program financed in part from federal funds and in part from premiums contributed by people enrolled in the program.

medication abuse Maladaptive pattern of recurrent medication use.

medication allergy Adverse reaction such as rash, chills, or gastrointestinal disturbances to a medication. Once a drug allergy occurs, the patient can no longer receive that particular medication.

medication dependence Maladaptive pattern of medication use in the following patterns using excessive amounts of the medication, increased activities directed toward obtaining the medication, or withdrawal from professional or recreational activities.

medication error Any event that could cause or lead to a patient's receiving inappropriate drug therapy or failing to receive appropriate drug therapy.

medication interaction Response that occurs when one drug modifies the action of another drug. The interaction can potentiate or diminish the actions of another drug, or it may alter the way a drug is metabolized, absorbed, or excreted.

melanoma Group of malignant neoplasms, primarily of the skin, that are composed of melanocytes. Common in fair-skinned people having light-colored eyes and in those who have been sunburned.

melena Abnormal black, sticky stool containing digested blood that is indicative of gastrointestinal bleeding.

menarche Onset of a girl's first menstruation.

Ménière's disease Chronic disease of the inner ear characterized by recurrent episodes of vertigo; progressive sensorineural hearing loss, which may be bilateral; and tinnitus.

menopause Physiological cessation of ovulation and menstruation that typically occurs during middle adulthood in women.

message Information sent or expressed by sender in the communication process.

metabolic acidosis Abnormal condition of high hydrogen ion concentration in the extracellular fluid caused by either a primary increase in hydrogen ions or a decrease in bicarbonate.

metabolic alkalosis Abnormal condition characterized by the significant loss of acid from the body or increased levels of bicarbonate.

metabolism Aggregate of all chemical processes that take place in living organisms and result in growth, generation of energy, elimination of wastes, and other functions concerned with the distribution of nutrients in the blood after digestion.

metacommunication Dependent not only on what is said but also on the relationship to the other person involved in the interaction. It is a message that conveys the sender's attitude toward self and the message and the attitudes, feelings, and intentions toward the listener.

metastasize Spread of tumor cells to distant parts of the body from a primary site (e.g., lung, breast, or bowel).

metatheory An area of study that examines the relationships of various components that make up the knowledge of a discipline, including philosophical, theoretical, and empirical components that provide a broad overview of the discipline.

metered-dose inhaler (MDI) Device designed to deliver a measured dose of an inhalation drug.

metric system Logically organized decimal system of measurement; metric units can easily be converted and computed through simple multiplication and division. Each basic unit of measurement is organized into units of 10.

microorganisms Microscopic entities such as bacteria, viruses, and fungi that are capable of carrying on living processes.

micturition Urination; act of passing or expelling urine voluntarily through the urethra.

milliequivalent per liter (mEq/L) Number of grams of a specific electrolyte dissolved in 1 L of plasma.

mindfulness A moment-to-moment present awareness with an attitude of nonjudgment, acceptance, and openness. Mindfulness meditative practices are effective in reducing psychological and physical symptoms or perceptions of stress.

mind mapping Graphic approach to represent the connections between concepts and ideas (e.g., nursing diagnoses) that are related to a central subject (e.g., the patient's health problems).

minerals Inorganic elements essential to the body because of their role as catalysts in biochemical reactions.

minimum data set (MDS) Required by the Omnibus Budget Reconciliation Act of 1987, the MDS is a uniform data set established by the Department of Health and Human Services. It serves as the framework for any state-specified assessment instruments used to develop a written and comprehensive plan of care for newly admitted residents of nursing facilities.

minimum effective concentration (MEC) The plasma level of a medication below which the effect of the medication does not occur.

misdemeanor Lesser crime than a felony; the penalty is usually a fine or imprisonment for less than 1 year.

mobility Person's ability to move about freely.

moderate sedation/analgesia/conscious sedation Administration of central nervous system depressant drugs and/or analgesics to provide analgesia, relieve anxiety, and/or provide amnesia during surgical, diagnostic, or interventional procedures. Routinely used for diagnostic or therapeutic procedures that do not require complete anesthesia but simply a decreased level of consciousness.

monosaturated fatty acid Fatty acid in which some of the carbon atoms in the hydrocarbon chain are joined by double or triple bonds. Monounsaturated fatty acids have only one double or triple bond per molecule and are found as components of fats in such foods as fowls, almonds, pecans, cashew nuts, peanuts, and olive oil.

morals Personal conviction that something is absolutely right or wrong in all situations.

motivation Internal impulse that causes a person to take action.

motivational interviewing Interview technique used to identify patients' thoughts, beliefs, fears, and current health care behavior with the aim of helping them to identify improved self-care behaviors.

mourning Process of grieving.

murmurs Blowing or whooshing sounds created by changes in blood flow through the heart or abnormalities in valve closure.

muscle tone Normal state of balanced muscle tension.

myocardial contractility Measure of stretch of the cardiac muscle fiber. It can also affect stroke volume and cardiac output. Poor contraction decreases the amount of blood ejected by the ventricles during each contraction.

myocardial infarction Necrosis of a portion of cardiac muscle caused by obstruction in a coronary artery.

myocardial ischemia Condition that results when the supply of blood to the myocardium from the coronary arteries is insufficient to meet the oxygen demands of the organ.

N

NANDA International North American Nursing Diagnosis Association, organized in 1973. It formally identifies, develops, and classifies nursing diagnoses.

narcolepsy Syndrome involving sudden sleep attacks that a person cannot inhibit. Uncontrollable desire to sleep may occur several times during a day.

nasogastric (NG) tube Tube passed into the stomach through the nose to empty the stomach of its contents or deliver medication and/or nourishment.

nebulization Process of adding moisture to inspired air by adding water droplets.

necessary losses Losses that every person experiences.

necrotic Of or pertaining to the death of tissue in response to disease or injury.

negative health behaviors Practices actually or potentially harmful to health such as smoking, drug or alcohol abuse, poor diet, and refusal to take necessary medications.

negative nitrogen balance Condition occurring when the body excretes more nitrogen than it takes in.

negligence Careless act of omission or commission that results in injury to another.

neonate Stage of life from birth to 1 month of age.

nephrons Structural and functional units of the kidney containing renal glomeruli and tubules.

neurotransmitter Chemical that transfers the electrical impulse from the nerve fiber to the muscle fiber.

Never Events Serious incidents that are wholly preventable because guidance or safety recommendations that provide strong systemic protective barriers are available at a national level and should have been implemented by all health care providers.

nociceptors Somatic and visceral free nerve endings of thinly myelinated and unmyelinated fibers. They usually react to tissue injury but may also be excited by endogenous chemical substances.

nocturia Urination at night; can be a symptom of renal disease or may occur in persons who drink excessive amounts of fluids before bedtime.

nonblanchable hyperemia Redness of the skin caused by dilation of the superficial capillaries. The redness persists when pressure is applied to the area, indicating tissue damage.

noninvasive positive-pressure ventilation (NPPV) Used to prevent using invasive artificial airways (endotracheal [ET] tube or tracheostomy) in patients with acute respiratory failure, cardiogenic pulmonary edema, or exacerbation of chronic obstructive pulmonary disease. It has also been used following extubation of an ET tube.

nonmaleficence Fundamental ethical agreement to do no harm. Closely related to the ethical standard of beneficence.

nonrapid eye movement (NREM) sleep Sleep that occurs during the first four stages of normal sleep.

nonshivering thermogenesis Occurs primarily in neonates. Because neonates cannot shiver, a limited amount of vascular brown adipose tissue present at birth can be metabolized for heat production.

nonverbal communication Communication using expressions, gestures, body posture, and positioning rather than words.

normal sinus rhythm (NSR) The wave pattern on an electrocardiogram that indicates normal conduction of an electrical impulse through the myocardium.

numbing One of Bowlby's four phases of mourning. It is characterized by a lack of feeling or by feeling stunned by a loss; may last a few days or many weeks.

nurse-initiated interventions Response of the nurse to the patient's health care needs and nursing diagnoses. This type of intervention is an autonomous action based on scientific rationale that is executed to benefit the patient in a predicted way related to the nursing diagnosis and patient-centered goals.

Nurse Practice Acts Statutes enacted by the legislature of any of the states or the appropriate officers of the districts or possessions that describe and define the scope of nursing practice.

Nursing Clinical Information System (NCIS) A system that incorporates the principles of nursing informatics to support the work that nurses do by facilitating documentation of nursing process activities and offering resources for managing nursing care delivery.

nursing diagnosis Formal statement of an actual or potential health problem that nurses can legally and independently treat; the second step of the nursing process, during which the patient's actual and potential unhealthy responses to an illness or condition are identified.

nursing health history Data collected about a patient's present level of wellness, changes in life patterns, sociocultural role, and mental and emotional reactions to illness.

nursing intervention Any treatment based on clinical judgment and knowledge that a nurse performs to enhance patient outcomes.

Nursing Outcomes Classification A systematic organization of nurse-sensitive outcomes into groups or categories based upon similarities, dissimilarities, and relationships among the outcomes.

nursing process Systematic problem-solving method by which nurses individualize care for each patient. The five steps of the nursing process are assessment, diagnosis, planning, implementation, and evaluation.

nursing-sensitive outcomes Outcomes that are within the scope of nursing practice; consequences or effects of nursing interventions that result in changes in the patient's symptoms, functional status, safety, psychological distress, or costs.

nurturant Behavior that involves caring for or fostering the well-being of another individual.

nutrients Foods that contain elements necessary for body function, including water, carbohydrates, proteins, fats, vitamins, and minerals.

O

obesity Abnormal increase in the proportion of fat cells, mainly in the viscera and subcutaneous tissues of the body.

objective data Information that can be observed by others; free of feelings, perceptions, and prejudices.

occurrence report Confidential document that describes any patient accident while the person is on the premises of a health care agency. (See *incident report*.)

olfactory Pertaining to the sense of smell.

oncotic pressure Total influence of the protein on the osmotic activity of plasma fluid.

open-ended question Form of question that prompts a respondent to answer in more than one or two words.

operating bed Table for surgery.

operating room (1) Room in a health care facility in which surgical procedures requiring anesthesia are performed. (2) Informal: a suite of rooms or an area in a health care facility in which patients are prepared for surgery, undergo surgical procedures, and recover from the anesthetic procedures required for the surgery.

ophthalmic Drugs given into the eye in the form of either eye drops or ointments.

ophthalmoscope Instrument used to illuminate the structures of the eye to examine the fundus, which includes the retina, choroid, optic nerve disc, macula, fovea centralis, and retinal vessels.

opioid Drug substance derived from opium or produced synthetically that alters perception of pain and that, with repeated use, may result in physical and psychological dependence (narcotic).

oral hygiene Condition or practice of maintaining the tissues and structures of the mouth.

orthopnea Abnormal condition in which a person must sit or stand to breathe comfortably.

orthostatic hypotension Abnormally low blood pressure occurring when a person stands.

osmolality Concentration or osmotic pressure of a solution expressed in osmoles or milliosmoles per kilogram of water.

osmolarity Osmotic pressure of a solution expressed in osmoles or milliosmoles per kilogram of the solution.

osmoreceptors Neurons in the hypothalamus that are sensitive to the fluid concentration in the blood plasma and regulate the secretion of antidiuretic hormone.

osmosis Movement of a pure solvent through a semipermeable membrane from a solution with a lower solute concentration to one with a higher solute concentration.

osmotic pressure Drawing power for water, which depends on the number of molecules in the solution.

osteoporosis Disorder characterized by abnormal rarefaction of bone, occurring most frequently in postmenopausal women, sedentary or immobilized individuals, and patients on long-term steroid therapy.

ostomy Surgical procedure in which an opening is made into the abdominal wall to allow the passage of intestinal contents from the bowel (colostomy) or urine from the bladder (urostomy).

other provider interventions Therapies that require the combined knowledge, skill, and expertise of multiple health care providers; also called *interdependent interventions*.

otoscope Instrument with a special ear speculum used to examine the deeper structures of the external and middle ear.

ototoxic Having a harmful effect on the eighth cranial (auditory) nerve or the organs of hearing and balance.

outcome Condition of a patient at the end of treatment, including the degree of wellness and the need for continuing care, medication, support, counseling, or education.

outliers Patients with extended lengths of stay beyond allowable inpatient days or costs.

outpatient Patient who has not been admitted to a hospital but receives treatments in a clinic or facility associated with the hospital.

output The product and information obtained from the system.

oxygen desaturation A decrease in oxygen concentration in the blood resulting from any condition that affects the exchange of carbon dioxide and oxygen.

oxygen saturation Amount of hemoglobin fully saturated with oxygen, given as a percent value.

oxygen therapy Procedure in which oxygen is administered to a patient to relieve or prevent hypoxia.

P

pain Subjective, unpleasant sensation caused by noxious stimulation of sensory nerve endings.

palliative care Level of care that is designed to relieve or reduce intensity of uncomfortable symptoms but not to produce a cure. Palliative care relies on comfort measures and use of alternative therapies to help individuals become more at peace during end of life.

pallor Unnatural paleness or absence of color in the skin.

palpation Method of physical examination whereby the fingers or hands of the examiner are applied to the patient's body to feel body parts underlying the skin.

palpitations Bounding or racing of the heart associated with normal emotions or a heart disorder.

Papanicolaou (Pap) smear Painless screening test for cervical cancer. Specimens are taken of squamous and columnar cells of the cervix.

parallel play Form of play among a group of children, primarily toddlers, in which each one engages in an independent activity that is similar to but not influenced by or shared with the others.

paralytic ileus Usually temporary paralysis of intestinal wall that may occur after abdominal surgery or peritoneal injury and that causes cessation of peristalsis; leads to abdominal distention and symptoms of obstruction.

parenteral administration Giving medication by a route other than the gastrointestinal tract.

parenteral nutrition (PN) Administration of a nutritional solution into the vascular system.

parteras Lay midwives.

partial bed bath Bath in which body parts that might cause the patient discomfort if left unbathed (i.e., face, hands, axillary areas, back, and perineum) are washed in bed.

passive range-of-motion (PROM) exercises Range of movement through which a joint is moved with assistance.

passive strategies of health promotion Activities that involve the patient as the recipient of actions by health care professionals.

pathogenicity Ability of a pathogenic agent to produce a disease.

pathogens Microorganisms capable of producing disease.

pathological fractures Fractures resulting from weakened bone tissue; frequently caused by osteoporosis or neoplasms.

patient- and family-centered care Model of nursing care in which mutual partnerships between the patient, family and health care team are formed to plan, implement, and evaluate the nursing and health care delivered.

patient-centered care Concept to improve work efficiency by changing the way that patient care is delivered.

patient-controlled analgesia (PCA) Drug delivery system that allows patients to self-administer analgesic medications on demand.

patrilineal, patrilineally Kinship that is limited to only the father's side.

pay for performance Quality improvement program that rewards excellence through financial incentives to motivate change to achieve measurable improvements and improve patient care quality and safety.

perceived loss Loss that is less obvious to others. Although easily overlooked or misunderstood, a perceived loss results in the same grief process as an actual loss.

perception An individual's mental image or concept of elements in their environment, including information gained through the senses.

percussion Method of physical examination whereby the location, size, and density of a body part is determined by the tone obtained from the striking of short, sharp taps of the fingers.

perfusion (1) Passage of a fluid through a specific organ or an area of the body. (2) Therapeutic measure whereby a drug intended for an isolated part of the body is introduced via the bloodstream. (3) Relates to the ability of the cardiovascular system to pump oxygenated blood to the tissues and return deoxygenated blood to the lungs.

perineal care Procedure prescribed for cleaning the genital and anal areas as part of the daily bath or after various obstetrical and gynecological procedures.

perioperative nursing Refers to the role of the operating room nurse during the preoperative, intraoperative, and postoperative phases of surgery.

peripherally inserted central catheter (PICC) Alternative intravenous access when the patient requires intermediate-length venous access greater than 7 days to 3 months. Intravenous access is achieved by inserting a catheter into a central vein by way of a peripheral vein.

peristalsis Rhythmical contractions of the intestine that propel gastric contents through the length of the gastrointestinal tract.

peritonitis Inflammation of the peritoneum produced by bacteria or irritating substances introduced into the abdominal cavity by a penetrating wound or perforation of an organ in the gastrointestinal or reproductive tract.

PERRLA Acronym for "pupils equal, round, reactive to light, accommodation"; the acronym is recorded in the physical examination if eye and pupil assessments are normal.

personalismo Personalistic.

petechiae Tiny purple or red spots that appear on skin as minute hemorrhages within dermal layers.

pharmacokinetics Study of how drugs enter the body, reach their site of action, are metabolized, and exit from the body.

phlebitis Inflammation of a vein.

physician-initiated interventions Based on the physician's response to a medical diagnosis, the nurse responds to his or her written orders.

PIE note Problem-oriented medical record; the four interdisciplinary sections are the database, problem list, care plan, and progress notes.

pilates A system of exercises based on six basic principles: powerhouse, concentration, control, precision, flow of movement, and breathing.

placebos Dosage form that contains no pharmacologically active ingredients but may relieve pain through psychological effects.

plaintiff Individual who files formal charges against an individual or organization for a legal offense.

planning Process of designing interventions to achieve the goals and outcomes of health care delivery.

plantar flexion Toe-down motion of the foot at the ankle.

pleural friction rub Adventitious lung sound caused by inflamed parietal and visceral pleura rubbing together on inspiration.

pneumothorax Collection of air or gas in the pleural space.

point of maximal impulse (PMI) Point where the heartbeat can most easily be palpated through the chest wall. This is usually the fourth intercostal space at the midclavicular line.

point of view Way of looking at issues that reflects an individual's culture and societal influences.

poison Any substance that impairs health or destroys life when ingested, inhaled, or absorbed by the body in relatively small amounts.

poison control center One of a network of facilities that provides information regarding all aspects of poisoning or intoxication, maintains records of their occurrence, and refers patients to treatment centers.

polypharmacy Use of a number of different drugs by a patient who may have one or several health problems.

polyunsaturated fatty acid Fatty acid that has two or more carbon double bonds.

population Collection of individuals who have in common one or more personal or environmental characteristics.

positive health behaviors Activities related to maintaining, attaining, or regaining good health and preventing illness. Common positive health behaviors include immunizations, proper sleep patterns, adequate exercise, and nutrition.

postanesthesia care unit (PACU) Area adjoining the operating room to which surgical patients are taken while still under anesthesia.

postmortem care Care of a patient's body after death.

postural drainage Use of positioning along with percussion and vibration to drain secretions from specific segments of the lungs and bronchi into the trachea.

postural hypotension Abnormally low blood pressure occurring when an individual assumes the standing posture; also called *orthostatic hypotension*.

posture Position of the body in relation to the surrounding space.

power of attorney for health care Person designated by the patient to make health care decisions for the patient if the patient becomes unable to make his or her own decisions.

preadolescence Transitional developmental stage that occurs between childhood and adolescence.

preanesthesia care unit Area outside the operating room where preoperative preparations are completed.

preload Volume of blood in the ventricles at the end of diastole, immediately before ventricular contraction.

preoperative teaching Instruction regarding a patient's anticipated surgery and recovery that is given before surgery. Instruction includes, but is not limited to, dietary and activity restrictions, anticipated assessment activities, postoperative procedures, and pain-relief measures.

presbycusis Hearing loss associated with aging. It usually involves both a loss of hearing sensitivity and a reduction in the clarity of speech.

presbyopia Gradual decline in ability of the lens to accommodate or focus on close objects; reduces ability to see near objects clearly. This condition commonly develops with advancing age.

prescriptions Written directions for a therapeutic agent (e.g., medication, drugs).

presence Deep physical, psychological, and spiritual connection or engagement between a nurse and patient.

present time orientation Time dimension that focuses on what is happening here and now. Communication patterns are circular, and this time orientation is in conflict with the dominant organizational norm in health care that emphasizes punctuality and adherence to appointments.

pressure injury Inflammation, sore, or ulcer in the skin over a bony prominence.

presurgical care unit (PSCU) Area outside the operating room where preoperative preparations are completed.

preventive nursing actions Nursing actions directed toward preventing illness and promoting health to avoid the need for primary, secondary, or tertiary health care.

primary appraisal Evaluating an event for its personal meaning related to stress.

primary care First contact in a given episode of illness that leads to a decision regarding a course of action to resolve the health problem.

primary health care Combination of primary and public health care that is accessible to individuals and families in a community and provided at an affordable cost.

primary intention Primary union of the edges of a wound, progressing to complete scar formation without granulation.

primary nursing Method of nursing practice in which the patient's care is managed for the duration by one nurse who directs and coordinates other nurses and health care personnel. When on duty, the primary nurse cares for the patient directly.

primary prevention First contact in a given episode of illness that leads to a decision regarding a course of action to prevent worsening of the health problem.

problem-focused diagnosis A clinical judgment concerning an undesirable human response to a health condition/life process that exists in an individual, family, or community.

problem identification One of the steps of the diagnostic process in which the patient's health care problem is recognized as a result of data analysis based on professional knowledge and experience.

problem-oriented medical record (POMR) Method of recording data about the health status of a patient that fosters a collaborative problem-solving approach by all members of the health care team.

problem solving Methodical, systematic approach to explore conditions and develop solutions, including analysis of data, determination of causative factors, and selection of appropriate actions to reverse or eliminate the problem.

productive cough Sudden expulsion of air from the lungs that effectively removes sputum from the respiratory tract and helps clear the airways.

professional standards review organization (PSRO) Focuses on evaluation of nursing care provided in a health care setting. The quality, effectiveness, and appropriateness of nursing care for the patient are the focus of evaluation.

prone Position of the patient lying face down.

proprioception Ability of the body to sense its position and movement in space.

prostaglandins Potent hormonelike substances that act in exceedingly low doses on target organs. They can be used to treat asthma and gastric hyperacidity.

proteins Any of a large group of naturally occurring, complex, organic nitrogenous compounds. Each is composed of large combinations of amino acids containing the elements carbon; hydrogen; nitrogen; oxygen; usually sulfur; and occasionally phosphorus, iron, iodine, or other essential constituents of living cells. Protein is the major source of building material for muscles, blood, skin, hair, nails, and the internal organs.

proteinuria Presence in the urine of abnormally large quantities of protein, usually albumin. Persistent proteinuria is usually a sign of renal disease or renal complications of another disease, hypertension, or heart failure.

protocol Written and approved plan specifying the procedures to be followed during an assessment or in providing treatment.

pruritus Symptom of itching; an uncomfortable sensation leading to the urge to scratch.

psychomotor learning Acquisition of ability to perform motor skills.

ptosis Abnormal condition of one or both upper eyelids in which the eyelid droops; caused by weakness of the levator muscle or paralysis of the third cranial nerve.

puberty Developmental period of emotional and physical changes, including the development of secondary sex characteristics and the onset of menstruation and ejaculation.

public health nursing Nursing specialty that requires the nurse to care for the needs of populations or groups.

public communication Interaction of one individual with large groups of people.

pulmonary hygiene More frequent turning, deep breathing, coughing, use of incentive spirometry, and chest physical therapy (PT) if ordered.

pulse deficit Condition that exists when the radial pulse is less than the ventricular rate as auscultated at the apex or seen on an electrocardiogram. The condition indicates a lack of peripheral perfusion for some of the heart contractions.

pulse pressure Difference between the systolic and diastolic pressures, normally 30 to 40 mm Hg.

Purkinje network Complex network of muscle fibers that spread through the right and left ventricles of the heart and carry the impulses that contract those chambers almost simultaneously.

pursed-lip breathing Deep inspiration followed by prolonged expiration through pursed lips.

pyrexia Abnormal elevation of the temperature of the body above 37° C (98.6° F) because of disease; same as fever.

pyrogens Substances that cause a rise in body temperature, as in the case of bacterial toxins.

Q

QSEN The Quality and Safety in the Education of Nurses (QSEN) initiative is the commitment of nursing to the competencies outlined in the Institute of Medicine report related to nursing education. QSEN encompasses six competencies: patient-centered care, teamwork, collaboration, evidence-based practice, quality improvement, and safety.

quality improvement Monitoring and evaluation of processes and outcomes in health care or any other business to identify opportunities for improvement.

quality indicator Quantitative measure of an important aspect of care that determines whether quality of service conforms to requirements or standards of care.

R

race Common biological characteristics shared by a group of people.

racial identity One's self-identification with one or more social groups in which a common heritage with a racial group is shared.

Ramadan Religious observance held during the ninth month of the Islamic calendar year. It involves fasting from sunrise to sunset.

range of motion (ROM) Range of movement of a joint from maximum extension to maximum flexion as measured in degrees of a circle.

rapid eye movement (REM) sleep Stage of sleep in which dreaming and rapid eye movements are prominent; important for mental restoration.

reaction Component of the pain experience that may include both physiological responses, as in the general adaptation syndrome, and behavioral responses.

reality orientation Therapeutic modality for restoring an individual's sense of the present.

receiver Person to whom message is sent during the communication process.

reception Neurophysiological components of the pain experience in which nervous system receptors receive painful stimuli and transmit them through peripheral nerves to the spinal cord and brain.

record Written form of communication that permanently documents information relevant to health care management.

recovery Period of time immediately following surgery when the patient is closely observed for effects of anesthesia, changes in vital signs, and bleeding. The recovery area is usually in the postanesthesia care unit.

referent Factor that motivates a person to communicate with another individual.

reflection Process of thinking back or recalling an event to discover the meaning and purpose of that event. Useful in critical thinking.

refractive error Defect in the ability of the lens of the eye to focus light such as occurs in nearsightedness and farsightedness.

regional anesthesia Loss of sensation in an area of the body supplied by sensory nerve pathways.

registered nurse (RN) In the United States a nurse who has completed a course of study at a state-approved, accredited school of nursing and has passed the National Council Licensure Examination (NCLEX-RN).

regression Return to an earlier developmental stage or behavior.

regulatory agencies Local, state, provincial, or national agencies that inspect and certify health care agencies as meeting specified standards. These agencies can also determine the amount of reimbursement for health care delivered.

rehabilitation Restoration of an individual to normal or near-normal function after a physical or mental illness, injury, or chemical addiction.

reinforcement Provision of a contingent response to a learner's behavior that increases the probability of recurrence of the behavior.

related factor Any condition or event that accompanies or is linked with the patient's health care problem.

relaxation Act of being relaxed or less tense.

reminiscence Recalling the past to assign new meaning to past experiences.

remissions Partial or complete disappearances of the clinical and subjective characteristics of chronic or malignant disease; remission may be spontaneous or the result of therapy.

renal calculi Calcium stones in the renal pelvis.

renin Proteolytic enzyme produced by and stored in the juxtaglomerular apparatus that surrounds each arteriole as it enters a glomerulus. The enzyme affects the blood pressure by catalyzing the change of angiotensinogen to angiotensin, a strong repressor.

reorganization Last phase of Bowlby's phases of mourning. During this phase, which sometimes requires a year or more, the person begins to accept unaccustomed roles, acquire new skills, and build new relationships.

report Transfer of information from the nurses on one shift to the nurses on the following shift. Report may also be given by one of the members of the nursing team to another health care provider (e.g., a physician or therapist).

reservoir Place where microorganisms survive, multiply, and await transfer to a susceptible host.

residual urine Volume of urine remaining in the bladder after a normal voiding; the bladder normally is almost completely empty after micturition.

resistance stage Third stage of the stress response, when the person attempts to adapt to the stressor. The body stabilizes; hormone levels stabilize; and heart rate, blood pressure, and cardiac output return to normal.

resource utilization group (RUG) Method of classification for health care reimbursement for long-term care facilities.

respeto Respectful.

respiration Exchange of oxygen and carbon dioxide during cellular metabolism.

respiratory acidosis Abnormal condition characterized by increased arterial carbon dioxide concentration, excess carbonic acid, and increased hydrogen ion concentration.

respiratory alkalosis Abnormal condition characterized by decreased arterial carbon dioxide concentration and hydrogen ion concentration.

respite care Short-term health services to dependent older adults either in their homes or in an institutional setting.

responsibility Carrying out duties associated with a particular role.

restorative care Health care settings and services in which patients who are recovering from illness or disability receive rehabilitation and supportive care.

restraint Device to aid in the immobilization of a patient or patient's extremity.

return demonstration Demonstration after the patient has first observed the teacher and then practiced the skill in mock or real situations.

rhonchi Abnormal lung sound auscultated when the patient's airways are obstructed with thick secretions.

right-sided heart failure Abnormal condition that results from impaired functioning of the right ventricle; characterized by venous congestion in the systemic circulation.

risk factor Any internal or external variable that makes a person or group more vulnerable to illness or an unhealthy event.

risk management Function of hospital or other health facility administration that is directed toward identification, evaluation, and correction of potential risks that could lead to injury of patients, staff members, or visitors and result in property loss or damage.

risk nursing diagnosis A clinical judgment concerning the vulnerability of an individual, family, group, or community for developing an undesirable human response to health conditions/life processes.

role performance Way in which a person views his or her ability to carry out significant roles.

root cause analysis Process of data collection and analysis that aids in finding the real cause of the problem and working on dealing with it rather than just dealing with its effects.

S

Sabbath From sundown on Friday to sundown on Saturday, this religious observance is a day of rest and worship for Jews and some Christian sects.

sandbags Sand-filled plastic tubes that can be shaped to body contours. They can immobilize an extremity or maintain body alignment.

saturated fatty acid Fatty acid in which each carbon in the chain has an attached hydrogen atom.

scientific method Codified sequence of steps used in the formulation, testing, evaluation, and reporting of scientific ideas.

scientific rationale Reason why a specific nursing action was chosen based on supporting literature.

scoliosis Lateral spinal curvature.

scope of nursing practice A professional definition of what a nurse is licensed to perform.

scrub nurse Registered nurse or operating room technician who assists surgeons during operations.

secondary appraisal Evaluating one's possible coping strategies when confronted with a stressor.

secondary intention Wound closure in which the edges are separated; granulation tissue develops to fill the gap; and, finally, epithelium grows in over the granulation, producing a larger scar than results with primary intention.

secondary prevention Level of preventive medicine that focuses on early diagnosis, use of referral services, and rapid initiation of treatment to stop the progress of disease processes.

sedatives Medications that produce a calming effect by decreasing functional activity, diminishing irritability, and allaying excitement.

segmentation Alternating contraction and relaxation of gastrointestinal mucosa.

self-concept Complex, dynamic integration of conscious and unconscious feelings, attitudes, and perceptions about one's identity, physical being, worth, and roles; how a person perceives and defines self.

self-esteem Feeling of self-worth characterized by feelings of achievement, adequacy, self-confidence, and usefulness.

self-transcendence Sense of authentically connecting to one's inner self.

sender Person who initiates interpersonal communication by conveying a message.

sensible water loss Loss of fluid from the body through the secretory activity of the sweat glands and the exhalation of humidified air from the lungs.

sensory deficits Defects in the function of one or more of the senses, resulting in visual, auditory, or olfactory impairments.

sensory deprivation State in which stimulation to one or more of the senses is lacking, resulting in impaired sensory perception.

sensory overload State in which stimulation to one or more of the senses is so excessive that the brain disregards or does not meaningfully respond to stimuli.

sequential compression stockings Plastic stockings attached to an air pump that inflates and deflates the stockings, applying intermittent pressure sequentially from the ankle to the knee.

serum half-life Time needed for excretion processes to lower the serum drug concentration by half.

sexual dysfunction Inability or difficulty in sexual functioning caused by physiological or psychological factors or both.

sexual identity How a person thinks about himself or herself sexually; it includes gender identity, gender role, and sexual orientation

sexual orientation Clear, persistent erotic preference for a person of one sex or the other.

sexuality "A function of the total personality … concerned with the biological, psychological, sociological, spiritual and culture variables of life …" (Sex Information and Education Council of the United States, 1980).

sexually transmitted infection Infectious process spread through sexual contact, including oral, genital, or anal sexual activity.

shear Force exerted against the skin while the skin remains stationary and the bony structures move.

side effect Any reaction or consequence that results from medication or therapy.

side rails Bars positioned along the sides of the length of the bed or stretcher to reduce the patient's risk of falling.

simpatia Friendly.

sinoatrial (SA) node Called the *pacemaker of the heart* because the origin of the normal heartbeat begins at the SA node. The SA node is in the right atrium next to the entrance of the superior vena cava.

situational crisis Unexpected crisis that arises suddenly in response to an external event or a conflict concerning a specific circumstance.

situational loss Loss of a person, thing, or quality resulting from a change in a life situation, including changes related to illness, body image, environment, and death.

sitz bath Bath in which only the hips or buttocks are immersed in fluid.

skilled nursing facility Institution or part of an institution that meets criteria for accreditation established by the sections of the Social Security Act that determine the basis for Medicaid and Medicare reimbursement for skilled nursing care, including rehabilitation and various medical and nursing procedures.

sleep State marked by reduced consciousness, diminished activity of the skeletal muscles, and depressed metabolism.

sleep apnea Cessation of breathing for a time during sleep.

sleep deprivation Condition resulting from a decrease in the amount, quality, and consistency of sleep.

SOAP note Progress note that focuses on a single patient problem and includes subjective and objective data, analysis, and planning; most often used in the problem-oriented medical record (POMR).

social determinants of health Factors that contribute to a person's current state of health. These factors may be biological, socioeconomic, psychosocial, behavioral, or social in nature.

socializing Interacting with friends or other people; communicating with others to form relationships and help people feel relaxed.

solute Substance dissolved in a solution.

solution Mixture of one or more substances dissolved in another substance. The molecules of each of the substances disperse homogeneously and do not change chemically. A solution may be a liquid, gas, or solid.

solvent Any liquid in which another substance can be dissolved.

source record Organization of a patient's chart so that each discipline (e.g., nursing, medicine, social work, or respiratory therapy) has a separate section in which to record data. Unlike problem-oriented medical record (POMR), the information is not organized by patient problems. The advantage of a source record is that caregivers can easily locate the proper section of the record in which to make entries.

sphygmomanometer Device for measuring the arterial blood pressure that consists of an arm or leg cuff with an air bladder connected to a tube, a bulb for pumping air into the bladder, and a gauge for indicating the amount of air pressure being exerted against the artery.

spiritual distress State of being out of harmony with a system of beliefs, a Supreme Being, or God.

spiritual well-being Individual's spirituality that enables a person to love, have faith and hope, seek meaning in life, and nurture relationships with others.

spirituality Spiritual dimension of a person, including the relationship with humanity, nature, and a Supreme Being.

standard of care Minimum level of care accepted to ensure high-quality care to patients. Standards of care define the types of therapies typically administered to patients with defined problems or needs.

Standard Precautions Guidelines recommended by the Centers for Disease Control and Prevention (CDC) to reduce risk of transmission of bloodborne and other pathogens in hospitals.

standardized care plans Written care plans used for groups of patients who have similar health care problems.

standing order Written and approved documents containing rules, policies, procedures, regulations, and orders for the conduct of patient care in various stipulated clinical settings.

statutory law Of or related to laws enacted by a legislative branch of the government.

stenosis Abnormal condition characterized by the constriction or narrowing of an opening or passageway in a body structure.

stereotypes Generalizations that are made about individuals without further assessment.

sterilization (1) Rendering a person unable to produce children; accomplished by surgical, chemical, or other means. (2) A technique for destroying microorganisms using heat, water, chemicals, or gases.

stoma Artificially created opening between a body cavity and the surface of the body (e.g., a colostomy formed from a portion of the colon pulled through the abdominal wall).

stress Physiological or psychological tension that threatens homeostasis or a person's psychological equilibrium.

stressor Any event, situation, or other stimulus encountered in a person's external or internal environment that necessitates change or adaptation by the person.

striae Streaks or linear scars that result from rapid development of tension in the skin.

stroke volume (SV) Amount of blood ejected by the ventricles with each contraction. It can be affected by the amount of blood in the left ventricle at the end of diastole (preload), the resistance to left ventricular ejection (afterload), and myocardial contractility.

subacute care Level of medical specialty care provided to patients who need a greater intensity of care than that provided in a skilled nursing facility but who do not require acute care.

subcultures Various ethnic, religious, and other groups with distinct characteristics from the dominant culture.

subcutaneous (sub-Q) Injection given into the connective tissue under the dermis. The subcutaneous tissue absorbs drugs more slowly than those injected into muscle. Injections are usually given at a 45-degree angle.

subjective data Information gathered from patient statements; the patient's feelings and perceptions. Not verifiable by another except by inference.

sublingual Route of medication administration in which the medication is placed underneath the patient's tongue.

Sunrise Model A model developed by Leininger that aids the health care practitioner in designing care decisions and actions in a culturally congruent fashion.

supine Position of the patient in which the patient is resting on his or her back.

suprainfection Secondary infection usually caused by an opportunistic pathogen.

suprapubic catheter Catheter surgically inserted through abdomen into bladder.

surfactant Chemical produced in the lungs to maintain the surface tension of the alveoli and keep them from collapsing.

surgical asepsis Procedures used to eliminate any microorganisms from an area. Also called *sterile technique.*

sympathy Concern, sorrow, or pity felt by the nurse for the patient. Sympathy is a subjective look at another person's world that prevents a clear perspective of all sides of the issues confronting that person.

synapse Region surrounding the point of contact between two neurons or between a neuron and an effector organ.

syncope Brief lapse in consciousness caused by transient cerebral hypoxia.

synergistic effect Effect resulting from two drugs acting synergistically. The effect of the two drugs combined is greater than the effect that would be expected if the individual effects of the two drugs acting alone were added together.

systolic Pertaining to or resulting from ventricular contraction.

T

tachycardia Rapid regular heart rate ranging between 100 and 150 beats/min.

tachypnea Abnormally rapid rate of breathing.

tactile Relating to the sense of touch.

tactile fremitus Tremulous vibration of the chest wall during breathing that is palpable on physical examination.

teaching Implementation method used to present correct principles, procedures, and techniques of health care; to inform patients about their health status; and to refer patients and family to appropriate health or social resources in the community.

team nursing Decentralized system in which the care of a patient is distributed among the members of a team. The charge nurse delegates authority to a team leader, who must be a professional nurse.

teratogens Chemical or physiological agents that may produce adverse effects in the embryo or fetus.

tertiary prevention Activities directed toward rehabilitation rather than diagnosis and treatment.

therapeutic communication Process in which the nurse consciously influences a patient or helps the patient to a better understanding through verbal and/or nonverbal communication.

therapeutic effect Desired benefit of a medication, treatment, or procedure.

therapeutic range The safe therapeutic range is between the minimum effective concentration and the toxic concentration.

thermogenesis The physiological process of heat production in the body.

thermoregulation Internal control of body temperature.

threshold Point at which a person first perceives a painful stimulus as being painful.

thrill Continuous palpable sensation like the purring of a cat.

thrombus   Accumulation of platelets, fibrin, clotting factors, and the cellular elements of the blood attached to the interior wall of a vein or artery, sometimes occluding the lumen of the vessel.

tinnitus   Ringing heard in one or both ears.

tissue ischemia   Point at which tissues receive insufficient oxygen and perfusion.

tolerance   Point at which a person is not willing to accept pain of greater severity or duration.

tort   Act that causes injury for which the injured party can bring civil action.

total patient care   Nursing delivery of care model originally developed during Florence Nightingale's time. In the model a registered nurse (RN) is responsible for all aspects of care for one or more patients. The RN works directly with the patient, family, physician or health care provider, and health care team members. The model typically has a shift-based focus.

touch   To come in contact with another person, often conveying caring, emotional support, encouragement, or tenderness.

toxic effect   Effect of a medication that results in an adverse response.

tracheostomy   Procedure whereby a surgical incision is made into the trachea and a short artificial airway (a tracheostomy tube) is inserted.

transcendence   The belief that there is a force outside of and greater than the person that exists beyond the material world.

transcultural   Concept of care extending across cultures that distinguishes nursing from other health disciplines.

transcultural nursing   Distinct discipline developed by Leininger that focuses on the comparative study of cultures to understand similarities and differences among groups of people.

transcutaneous electrical nerve stimulation (TENS)   Technique in which a battery-powered device blocks pain impulses from reaching the spinal cord by delivering weak electrical impulses directly to the surface of the skin.

transdermal disk   Medication delivery device in which the medication is saturated on a waferlike disk, which is affixed to the patient's skin. This method ensures that the patient receives a continuous level of medication.

transfer report   Verbal exchange of information between caregivers when a patient is moved from one nursing unit or health care setting to another. The report includes information necessary to maintain a consistent level of care from one setting to another.

transformational leadership   A leadership style that focuses on change and innovation through effective communication and team building. Engagement, empowerment, and accountability are critical to team effectiveness.

transfusion reaction   Systemic response by the body to the administration of blood incompatible with that of the recipient.

trapeze bar   Metal triangular-shaped bar that can be suspended over a patient's bed from an overhanging frame; permits patients to move up and down in bed while in traction or some other encumbrance.

trimester   Referring to one of the three phases of pregnancy.

trochanter roll   Rolled towel support placed against the hips and upper leg to prevent external rotation of the legs.

trough   The lowest serum concentration of a medication before the next medication dose is administered.

turgor   Normal resiliency of the skin caused by the outward pressure of the cells and interstitial fluid.

U

unconscious/implicit bias   A bias that an individual is unaware of and that happens outside his or her control; it is influenced by personal background, cultural environment, and personal experiences.

unsaturated fatty acid   Fatty acid in which an unequal number of hydrogen atoms are attached and the carbon atoms attach to one another with a double bond.

ureterostomy   Diversion of urine away from a diseased or defective bladder through an artificial opening in the skin.

urge incontinence   A type of urinary incontinence that results from sudden, involuntary contraction of the muscles of the urinary bladder, resulting in an urge to urinate.

urinal   Receptacle for collecting urine.

urinary diversion   Surgical diversion of the drainage of urine such as a ureterostomy.

urinary incontinence   Inability to control urination.

urinary reflux   Abnormal, backward flow of urine.

urinary retention   Retention of urine in the bladder; condition frequently caused by a temporary loss of muscle function.

urine hat   Receptacle for collecting urine that fits toilet.

urometer   Device for measuring frequent and small amounts of urine from an indwelling urinary catheter system.

urosepsis   Organisms in the bloodstream.

utilitarianism   Ethic that proposes that the value of something is determined by its usefulness. The greatest good for the greatest number of people constitutes the guiding principle for action in a utilitarian model of ethics.

utilization review (UR) committees   Physician-supervised committees to review admissions, diagnostic testing, and treatments provided by physicians or health care providers to patients.

V

validation   Act of confirming, verifying, or corroborating the accuracy of assessment data or the appropriateness of the care plan.

Valsalva maneuver   Any forced expiratory effort against a closed airway such as when an individual holds his or her breath and tightens his or her muscles in a concerted, strenuous effort to move a heavy object or change positions in bed.

value   Personal belief about the worth of a given idea or behavior.

valvular heart disease   Acquired or congenital disorder of a cardiac valve characterized by stenosis and obstructed blood flow or valvular degeneration and regurgitation of blood.

variance   Unexpected event that occurs during patient care and that is different from CareMap predictions. Variances or exceptions are interventions or outcomes that are not achieved as anticipated. Variance may be positive or negative.

variant   Differing from a set standard.

vascular access devices   Catheters, cannulas, or infusion ports designed for long-term, repeated access to the vascular system.

vasoconstriction   Narrowing of the lumen of any blood vessel, especially the arterioles and the veins in the blood reservoirs of the skin and abdominal viscera.

vasodilation   Increase in the diameter of a blood vessel caused by inhibition of its vasoconstrictor nerves or stimulation of dilator nerves.

venipuncture   Technique in which a vein is punctured transcutaneously by a sharp rigid stylet (e.g., a butterfly needle), a cannula (e.g., an angiocatheter that contains a flexible plastic catheter), or a needle attached to a syringe.

ventilation   Respiratory process by which gases are moved into and out of the lungs.

verbal communication   Sending of messages from one individual to another or to a group of individuals through the spoken word.

vertigo   Sensation of dizziness or spinning.

vibration   Fine, shaking pressure applied by hands to the chest wall only during exhalation.

Virchow's triad   The three broad categories of factors that are thought to contribute to formation of a venous thrombosis: hypercoagulability, hemodynamic changes, and endothelial injury or dysfunction.

virulence   Ability of an organism to rapidly produce disease.

visual   Related to or experienced through vision.

vital signs   Temperature, pulse, respirations, and blood pressure.

vitamins   Organic compounds essential in small quantities for normal physiological and metabolic functioning of the body. With few exceptions, vitamins cannot be synthesized by the body and must be obtained from the diet or dietary supplements.

voiding   Process of urinating.

vulnerable populations   Collection of individuals who are more likely to develop health problems as a result of excess risks, limits in access to health care services, or being dependent on others for care.

W

wellness   Dynamic state of health in which an individual progresses toward a higher level of functioning, achieving an optimum balance between internal and external environments.

wellness education   Activities that teach people how to care for themselves in a healthy manner.

wellness nursing diagnosis Clinical judgment about an individual, group, or community in transition from a specific level of wellness to a higher level of wellness.

wheezes, wheezing Adventitious lung sounds caused by a severely narrowed bronchus.

workplace violence The act or threat of violence, ranging from verbal abuse to physical assault, directed toward persons at work or on duty.

work redesign Formal process used to analyze the work of a certain work group and change the actual structure of the jobs performed.

worldview Cognitive stance or perspective about phenomena characteristic of a particular cultural group.

wound culture Specimen collected from a wound to determine the specific organism that is causing an infectious process.

wound drainage evacuators Convenient portable units that connect to tubular drains lying within a wound bed and exert a safe, constant, low-pressure vacuum to remove and collect drainage.

Y

yearning and searching Second phase of Bowlby's phases of mourning. It is characterized by emotional outbursts of tearful sobbing and acute distress.

Z

Z-track injection Technique for injecting irritating preparations into muscle without tracking residual medication through sensitive tissues.

INDEX

NOTE: Page numbers followed by *b* indicate boxes, *f* indicate illustrations, and *t* indicate tables.